Clinical to Digital Medicine

Progress in Medicine 2024

An Official Publication of Indian College of Physicians

Academic Wing of Association of Physicians of India

Clinical to Digital Medicine

Progress in Medicine 2024

Volume 34 | 2024

An Official Publication of Indian College of Physicians

Academic Wing of Association of Physicians of India

Editor-in-Chief

Jyotirmoy Pal MD(General Medicine) FRCP FICP FACP WHO Fellow
Professor (General Medicine)
University College of Medicine and Sagore Dutta Medical College
Kamarhati, West Bengal, India
Dean, Indian College of Physicians (ICP)
President-Elect, Association of Physicians (API)

Editor

Nandini Chatterjee MD FRCP(London, Glasgow) FICP
Professor
Department of Medicine
Institute of Post Graduate Medical Education and Research (IPGMER)
Kolkata, West Bengal, India
Joint Secretary Deans Place
Ex-Editor, Journal of the Indian Medical Association (JIMA)
Editor, Bengal Physician Journal

Forewords

Girish Mathur
Gurpreet Singh Wander

JAYPEE

JAYPEE BROTHERS MEDICAL PUBLISHERS
The Health Sciences Publisher
New Delhi | London

Jaypee Brothers Medical Publishers (P) Ltd

Headquarters
EMCA House
23/23-B, Ansari Road, Daryaganj
New Delhi 110 002, India
Landline: +91-11-23272143, +91-11-23272703
+91-11-23282021, +91-11-23245672
E-mail: jaypee@jaypeebrothers.com

Corporate Office
Jaypee Brothers Medical Publishers (P) Ltd.
4838/24, Ansari Road, Daryaganj
New Delhi 110 002, India
Phone: +91-11-43574357
Fax: +91-11-43574314
E-mail: jaypee@jaypeebrothers.com

Overseas Office
JP Medical Ltd.
83, Victoria Street, London
SW1H 0HW (UK)
Phone: +44-20 3170 8910
Fax: +44(0)20 3008 6180
E-mail: info@jpmedpub.com

Website: www.jaypeebrothers.com
Website: www.jaypeedigital.com

***Progress in Medicine 2024 (Volume 34: 2024)* / Jyotirmoy Pal**

First Edition: **2024**

ISBN: 978-93-5696-623-9

Printed at Sanat Printers

DISCLAIMER

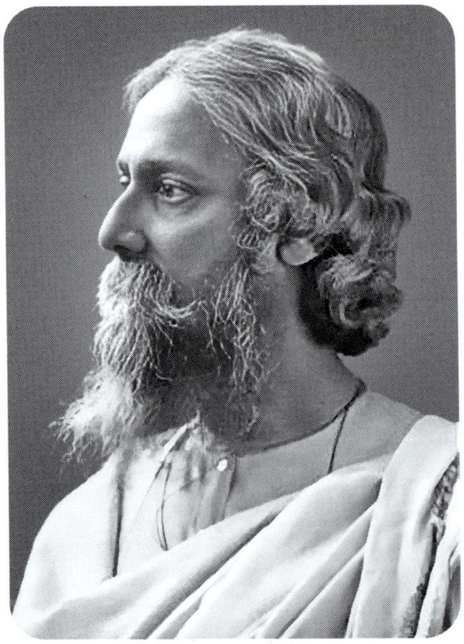

"The highest education is that which does not merely give information but brings our life in harmony with all existence."

—Rabindranath Tagore

Swaroop Kumar Baruah MD(Medicine) MCA FICP
Senior Consultant Physician
Nemcare Super Speciality Hospital
Guwahati, Assam, India

Sweta Amaresh Biradar MD
Consultant Physician
Highborn Poly Clinic
Kalaburagi, Karnataka, India

T Ravikumar MD(General Medicine)
Professor of Medicine
Government Medical College and ESI Hospital
Coimbatore, Tamil Nadu, India

Tahseen Mahmood MD (Endocrinology) SCE Endocrinology (RCP, UK)
Consultant
Classified Specialist in Medicine (Endocrinology)
Combined Military Hospital
Dhaka, Bangladesh

Tapas Kumar MNAMS(Medicine) FICP
Professor
Department of General Medicine
Mata Gujari Memorial Medical College and Lions Seva Kendra Hospital
Kishanganj, Bihar, India

Tarun Kumar Biswas MD(Medicine)
Consultant Physician
Kolkata, West Bengal, India

Tarun Pal MBBS
Junior Resident
Department of Medicine
King George's Medical University (KGMU)
Lucknow, Uttar Pradesh, India

Thamilpavai N MD DM(Neurology)
Professor
Department of Neurology
Madras Medical College
Chennai, Tamil Nadu, India

Tribeni Sharma MD(General Medicine)
Professor of Medicine
Gauhati Medical College and Hospital
Guwahati, Assam, India

TVS P Murthy MD
Medical Superintendent
Professor
Department of Anesthesia
GSL Medical College
Rajahmundry, Andhra Pradesh, India

Uma Sinharoy MD(Medicine) DM(Neurology)
Assistant Professor
Department of Neurology
Bangur Institute of Neurosciences
IPGMER and SSKM Hospital
Kolkata, West Bengal, India

Urza Bhattarai MD
Senior Resident
Department of Internal Medicine
BP Koirala Institute of Health Sciences
Dharan, Nepal

Uttam Kumar Paul MD FICP FIME FAIMER
Professor and Head
Department of Medicine
MGM Medical College
Kishanganj, Bihar, India

Vaibhav Agnihotri MBBS DCH DNB(Pediatrics)
Fellow
Diabetes and Heart Research Centre
Dhanbad, Jharkhand, India

Varun Gupta MD(Thoracic Surgery)
Resident Thoracic Surgery
Lungenklinik Hemer
Hemer, Germany

Veerendra Singh MD(Internal Medicine) FICP FIACM FDI FUPDA
Director
GSSM Cardiorespiratory Centre
Ayodhya, Uttar Pradesh, India

Venkatesh Desai MD(General Medicine)
Associate Professor
Department of General Medicine
Gulbarga Institute of Medical Sciences (GIMS)
Kalaburagi, Karnataka, India

Vijay Garg MD FIAE FICP FCSI FICA(USA) FISE FACC(USA) FACP(USA) FIMSA FISC FESC(Europe)
Professor
Department of Medicine
Ruxmaniben Deepchand Gardi Medical College
Ujjain, Madhya Pradesh, India

Vinay Kumar Meena MD FICP
Assistant Professor
Department of General Medicine
SMS Medical College
Jaipur, Rajasthan, India

Vipasha Garg MBBS
Resident Doctor Final Year (Medicine)
Department of Medicine
Ruxmaniben Deepchand Gardi Medical College
Ujjain, Madhya Pradesh, India

Virendra Verma BSc MBBS MD(Internal Medicine) FUPDA FISCM FISMN
Associate Professor
Department of Medicine
Rajarshi Dashrath Autonomous State Medical College
Ayodhya, Uttar Pradesh, India

Vitull K Gupta MD(Medicine) FICP FCSI FACP FIACM
Health and Human Rights Activist
Consultant, Kishori Ram Hospital and Diabetes Care Centre
Honorary Teaching Faculty, AIIMS
Bathinda, Punjab, India

Y Sathyanarayana Raju MD FICP
Professor
Department of General Medicine
Nizam's Institute of Medical Sciences
Hyderabad, Telangana, India

FOREWORD

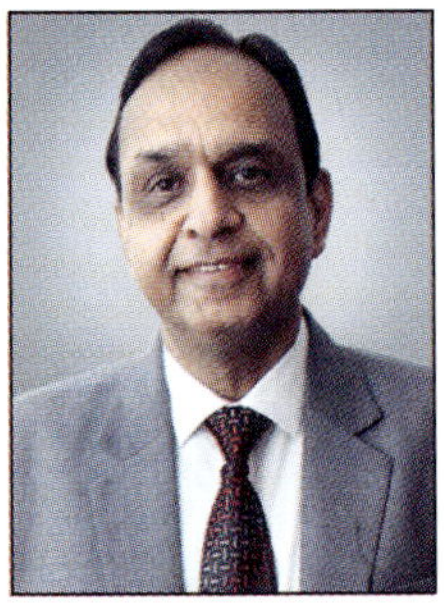

Girish Mathur
MD FICP FACP FRCP(London, Glasgow, Edinburgh) FIACM FRSSDI, Fellow Diabetes India
President, Association of Physicians of India

It is with great pleasure and anticipation that I introduce *"Progress in Medicine 2024,"* a comprehensive compilation poised to make a significant impact on the medical landscape. As we gather at the prestigious annual conference of the Association of Physicians of India (API), APICON 2024, I am honored to be part of this intellectual journey.

Under the expert guidance of our esteemed Chief Editor, Dr Jyotirmoy Pal, Dean of the Indian College of Physicians, this book transcends the boundaries of conventional medical literature. It reflects the collective wisdom and advancements that define the contemporary medical arena.

The pages within encapsulate a symphony of research, innovation, and clinical acumen, showcasing the relentless pursuit of excellence by medical professionals across diverse specialties. From cutting-edge discoveries to nuanced clinical insights, *"Progress in Medicine"* embodies the spirit of evolution that defines the field.

This collaborative effort is a testament to the dedication and expertise of the contributors who have generously shared their knowledge. As we navigate the ever-expanding frontiers of medicine, this compilation serves as a compass, guiding us through the latest breakthroughs and fostering a spirit of continuous learning.

I extend my sincere appreciation to all those who have played a pivotal role in bringing this volume to fruition. May it serve as a source of inspiration, sparking dialogue and fostering a community committed to advancing the science and art of medicine.

In the spirit of shared knowledge and progress, I welcome you to immerse yourself in the insights presented within these pages. May *"Progress in Medicine 2024"* inspire new perspectives, encourage collaboration, and contribute to the collective pursuit of a healthier, more informed future.

Warm regards!

FOREWORD

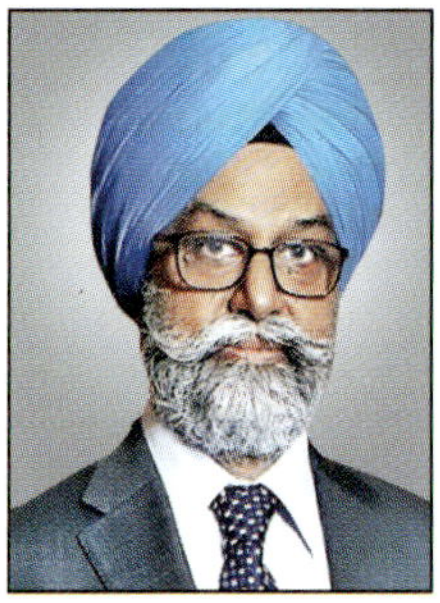

Gurpreet Singh Wander
DM FACC FAMS
Past President, Association of Physicians of India
Director, Physicians Research Foundation, India

The *API Progress in Medicine, 2024* is an excellent compilation of some of the current topics in various subspecialties of medicine by experts in the field. Dr Jyotirmoy Pal has kept the topics that are most relevant for postgraduate students and for young physicians. The experts who have been chosen as authors are some of the best in the field. The special sections on medical education and pharmacotherapeutics will be very useful for the readers. The language of the book is easy to comprehend. The figures, tables, and algorithms will help the readers to understand the topics. Common clinical issues like headache, urine abnormalities, fever with acute kidney injury (AKI), sepsis mimics, and many other topics have been designed and discussed. These clinical problems are generally not addressed in textbooks of medicine. In all these aspects, this is a unique book which I would recommend to physicians across the country. Jaypee Brothers Medical Publishers (P) Ltd has done an excellent work with the setting of the chapters.

PREFACE

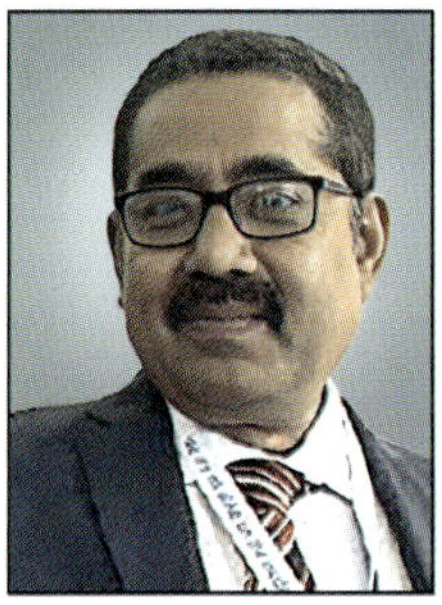

Jyotirmoy Pal
MD(General Medicine) FRCP FICP FACP WHO Fellow
Professor (General Medicine)
University College of Medicine and Sagore Dutta Medical College
Kamarhati, West Bengal, India
Dean, Indian College of Physicians (ICP)
President-Elect, Association of Physicians (API)

It is with pleasure and pride that I write the preface of "*Progress in Medicine 2024*". This voluminous publication of the Association of Physicians of India (API) encompasses the scientific proceedings of the Continuing Medical Education (CME) of APICON 2024. The book has been segregated into sections for various systems and covers a wide range of relevant clinical topics that will assist not only in postgraduate examinations but also in day-to-day decision-making.

There is an ocean of information on the Internet these days, and it is too vast and deep for even the most avid reader to fully encompass. The topics dealt with in Progress in Medicine are chosen to help our students and practitioners update themselves on the latest evidence-based guidelines for management and also emphasize on clinical medicine which is fast becoming a forgotten art.

Medicine is ever changing, and the fields of molecular biology and genetics are expanding day by day. Added to this is the influx of Artificial Intelligence into every aspect of diagnosis and therapeutics. Keeping that in mind, we have kept topics by experts on basic sciences, genetics, and latest technologies. Some writeups are on soft skills that are becoming immensely important these days of the consumer protection act (CPA).

Travel medicine, medical education, medicolegal aspects, and gerontology are oft-neglected areas that have been touched upon.

I thank my entire editorial team for their commendable effort in producing this comprehensive treatise for internists and hope it will be useful in daily practice.

CONTENTS

SECTION 2: DIABETES UPDATE

SECTION 10: NEPHROLOGY

SECTION 11: NEUROLOGY

SECTION 12: PULMONOLOGY

SECTION 13: PHARMACOTHERAPEUTICS

SECTION 14: RHEUMATOLOGY

SECTION 15: MISCELLANEOUS

e-BOOK CONTENTS

Scan the QR Code for above listed e-chapters.

SECTION 1

CARDIOLOGY

1

CHAPTER

Acute Decompensated Heart Failure: Current Guidelines and Management Strategies

Divendu Bhushan, Ajay Bade

ABSTRACT

Heart failure (HF) involves about 64 million people worldwide. In India, it affects almost 4–5 million people with an annual incidence of 0.4–1.8 million. Major causes are coronary artery disease, hypertension, obesity, diabetes, and rheumatic heart disease. It is a critical condition that can be present in various symptoms to a physician. It affects the quality of life and increases morbidity and mortality.

Although the treatment is mainly decongestant like diuretics and vasodilators, management of comorbidity such as anemia, chronic lung disease, hypertension, diabetes, and atrial fibrillation is also important. It becomes complicated if other systems such as the kidney and liver get involved. Nonpharmacological treatment is to be stressed particularly in patients who progressed to a chronic stage. Device therapy gives good results when used in appropriate situations.

INTRODUCTION

Heart failure (HF) is a clinical syndrome caused by inadequate ventricular filling or ventricular output, which is either due to functional or structural abnormality of the heart. Acute decompensated heart failure (ADHF) is a critical condition characterized by the sudden worsening of heart failure symptoms, leading to significant morbidity and mortality. There are divergent trends in incidence, and mortality pertaining to heart failure worldwide. New therapies have promising results.

American College of Cardiology (ACC)/American Heart Association (AHA) classifies stages and types of heart failure which enhances prompt and effective management to improve patient outcomes. These guidelines offer evidence-based recommendations for the diagnosis and management of ADHF, contributing to better patient care and outcomes.

CLASSIFICATIONS AND CAUSES OF HEART FAILURE

American College of Cardiology/AHA defines stages of heart failure—as stage A (at risk), stage B (preheart failure), stage C—symptomatic heart failure, and stage D (advanced) heart failure. This staging identifies the people at risk (diabetic, hypertensive, cardiotoxic medicines, metabolic syndrome, and obesity) and those with preheart failure having structural heart disease, and increased filling pressure.

According to the left ventricular ejection fraction (LVEF), it is divided into—heart failure with reduced ejection fraction (HFrEF) <40%, heart failure with mild reduced ejection fraction (HFmrHF) (41–49%), and heart failure with preserved ejection fraction (HFpEF) >50%. This classification has prognostic and therapeutic implications.

Heart failure is classified in other ways also—high output versus low output and systolic versus diastolic failure.

The most common causes of heart failure are coronary artery disease, hypertension, and valvular heart disease. Other causes include cardiomyopathy, drugs, alcohol, autoimmune, and amyloidosis.

ADHF refers to the acute exacerbation of chronic heart failure or the development of new-onset heart failure, characterized by symptoms, such as dyspnea, fatigue, fluid retention, and congestion. The condition can be classified based on the severity of symptoms, with the AHA/ACC/Heart Failure Society of America (HFSA) guideline categorizing it into stages A–D, while the European Society of Cardiology (ESC) guideline employs NYHA functional classes I–IV.

The main causes of decompensation are new acute coronary syndrome, uncontrolled hypertension, atrial fibrillation (AF) and arrhythmias, acute infection, and anemia, thyroid disorders, and drugs such as verapamil and nonsteroidal anti-inflammatory drugs (NSAIDs).

SYMPTOMS AND SIGNS

Mostly patients present with congestion rather than forward failure and hypoperfusion.

Classical symptoms are shortness of breath, edema, and lethargy. Although mostly the right and left ventricle fails in proportion, at times they have mismatch too. At times in the absence of elevated jugular venous pressure (JVP) and edema, left-sided failure is underestimated. Hypoperfusion is underappreciated in patients with chronic heart failure but can be suspected by narrow pulse pressure and cool extremities. Elevated lactate may indicate hypoperfusion and impending cardiogenic shock.

DIAGNOSTIC EVALUATION

Accurate and timely diagnosis of ADHF is crucial to initiate appropriate management. Key diagnostic tools include:

- *History and physical examination*: Comprehensive assessment of symptoms, medical history, and physical signs of congestion, such as elevated JVP and lung crackles.
- Look for evidence of precipitating factors, such as anemia, fever, infection, and drugs.
- *Biomarkers*: Measurement of B-type natriuretic peptide (BNP) or N-terminal pro-B-type natriuretic peptide (NT-proBNP) levels, which are elevated in heart failure and can aid in diagnosis and prognosis.
- *Electrocardiogram (ECG)*: To identify arrhythmia, ischemic changes, or conduction abnormalities.
- *Echocardiography*: To assess cardiac structure and function, identify valve abnormalities, and estimate ejection fraction.
- Rule out exacerbation of chronic obstructive pulmonary disease (COPD)/asthma, *pneumonia*, and pulmonary embolism.

MANAGEMENT OF ACUTE DECOMPENSATED HEART FAILURE

Treatment of ADHF involves a multidisciplinary approach, with specific therapeutic strategies aimed at relieving symptoms, stabilizing hemodynamics, and improving overall patient outcomes.

Hospital admission is a sentinel event and carries a worse prognosis.

Evaluation of precipitating events, such as acute coronary syndrome (ACS), arrhythmia, anemia, fever, thyroid disorders, and drugs.

Pharmacological Therapy

- *Diuretics*: Loop diuretics like furosemide are first-line agents to reduce fluid overload and alleviate congestion. If the patient is on diuretics—double the dose, and add thiazides or mineralocorticoid receptor antagonist (MRA). The goal is the resolution of symptoms and signs of congestion. At discharge, titration of diuretics is an important issue to reduce mortality and readmission. Diuretics should not be discontinued prematurely because of small changes in serum creatinine (0.3 mg%), as they do not predict a worse outcome but they need a close watch.
- *Vasodilators*: Nitroglycerin and nitroprusside can reduce preload and after-load, easing the workload on the heart. These can be used in acute heart failure to alleviate the symptoms, but there is no benefit in terms of readmission and mortality. Patients with hypertension, coronary ischemia, and mitral regurgitation can be given injection nitroglycerin. For injection of nitroprusside, intensive monitoring is required as it can produce sudden hypotension. Longer infusion can lead to cyanide toxicity, particularly in the setting of renal/liver failure.
- *Inotropes*: It is indicated in cardiogenic shock. Cardiogenic shock in heart failure is caused by acute decompensation of chronic heart failure, acute coronary syndrome, or survivors of cardiac arrest. In case of an acute coronary event, early revascularization is of paramount importance. The choice of inotropic agent depends upon hemodynamic status, arrhythmia, and availability. The first choice of drug is noradrenaline. In severe cases with hypoperfusion with normal blood pressure, inotropes like dobutamine may be considered to improve cardiac contractility. Dopamine use is nowadays decreased due to its arrhythmogenic effects.
- *Beta-blockers*: In stable patients without signs of decompensation, β-blockers play a crucial role in reducing mortality and hospitalizations. According to the OPTIMIZE-HF (Organized Program to Initiate Lifesaving Treatment in Hospitalized Patients with Heart Failure) study, compliance with β-blocker leads to less readmission to hospital and reduces mortality. In a meta-analysis, discontinuation of β-blocker in HFrEF leads to increased mortality, and readmission

to hospital discontinuation or reducing β-blocker should be considered in patients with marked volume overload and marginal low cardiac output.

- *ACEI/ARB*: Angiotensin-converting enzyme inhibitors (ACEI) and angiotensin receptor blockers (ARB) are important drugs for cardiac remodeling in patients with heart failure. Both of these improve outcomes. In the GWTG-HF (Get With The Guidelines-Heart Failure) registry, it was found that discontinuation of ACEI/ARB leads to higher postdischarge mortality and readmission in HFrEF patients.

Treatment of Comorbidities

- *Anemia*: Anemia is associated with poor outcomes of heart failure patients. Iron deficiency is independently associated with poor exercise tolerance and quality of life (QOL). Treatment with IV ferrous carboxymaltose is associated with improved exercise capacity and QOL.
- *Atrial fibrillation*: There is a bilateral cause-and-effect relation between AF and heart failure. Rate control is preferred over rhythm control. Anticoagulation is indicated when heart failure is associated with AF. This can be with direct oral anticoagulant (DOAC) or warfarin. Patients with HF, and difficult-to-control rates, may benefit from atrioventricular node ablation and implantation of a permanent pacemaker if other rate and rhythm control measures fail. If their LVEF is >50%, there is no current evidence that CRT is beneficial compared with RV pacing.
- *Hypertension*: Clinical trials assessing the impact of goal blood pressure reduction on outcomes in patients with HFrEF and concomitant hypertension are lacking. Although adequate antihypertensive treatment in the general population decreases the incidence of heart failure.
- *Diabetes*: ADA recommends sodium-glucose cotransporter-2 (SGLT-2) inhibitors as the first line of treatment in patients with diabetes who are at risk of heart failure. The Food and Drug Administration (FDA) recommends its use in HFrEF patients irrespective of their diabetes status. The SOLOIST-WHF (Effect of Sotagliflozin on Cardiovascular Events in Patients With Type 2 Diabetes Post-WHF) trial extends the benefits of sSGLT-2 inhibitors to patients with diabetes and acute decompensated HF. Patients on SGLT-2 inhibitors should be closely monitored for potential risks, including severe genitourinary infections and, less commonly diabetic ketoacidosis (DKA).
- *Sleep disorders*: Sleep apnea—obstructive or central affects the course of heart failure. These two entities have different lines of management. So, referring a patient for a sleep study is usually a clinical decision.

Central positive airway pressure improves nocturnal hypoxia in patients with central sleep apnea.

Treatment of heart failure needs a close watch on body weight, clinical symptoms, and signs of congestion and hypoperfusion, output, and serum electrolytes.

Nonpharmacological Interventions

- *Fluid and sodium restriction*: To prevent fluid retention and worsening of congestion
- *Oxygen therapy*: In patients with hypoxemia and respiratory distress
- Noninvasive ventilation (NIV)
- *Mechanical ventilation*: In cases of severe respiratory failure
- *Renal replacement therapy*: For patients with refractory fluid overload unresponsive to diuretics

Device Therapy

- *Implantable cardioverter-defibrillator (ICD)*: For primary or secondary prevention of sudden cardiac death in eligible patients.
- *Cardiac resynchronization therapy (CRT)*: In select patients with left bundle branch block and reduced ejection fraction.
- *Mechanical circulatory support*: Temporary devices like intra-aortic balloon pumps may be utilized in critically ill patients awaiting heart transplantation.

Patient Education and Follow-up

- Emphasizing the importance of medication adherence, dietary and lifestyle modifications, and monitoring of symptoms
- Ensuring timely follow-up to assess treatment response and make necessary adjustments

Prognosis and Prevention

The prognosis of ADHF is influenced by various factors, including age, comorbidities, and response to treatment. Regular follow-up, adherence to treatment, and lifestyle modifications are essential to prevent exacerbations and improve outcomes. Efforts should also focus on managing risk factors, such as hypertension, diabetes, and dyslipidemia, which can contribute to the development and progression of heart failure.

HEART FAILURE IN SPECIAL GROUPS

- *Elderly*: Risk of heart failure remains the same at the age of > 80 years in comparison to at 40 years (almost 20%), but two-thirds of elderly patients with heart failure have normal LVEF. Elderly are vulnerable to develop complications due to polypharmacy.

- *Pregnancy*: Heart failure in pregnancy can be due to preexisting illness or peripartum cardiomyopathy (PPCM). PPCM is defined as a systolic failure (LVEF <45%) in the third trimester or just after postpartum. Treatment is multidisciplinary and needs pharmacotherapy modified according to the state of pregnancy and breastfeeding.

CONCLUSION

Acute decompensated heart failure remains a significant clinical challenge, demanding prompt diagnosis and appropriate management. The 2022 AHA/ACC/HFSA and 2021 ESC guidelines provide evidence-based recommendations for the assessment and treatment of ADHF. A comprehensive approach involving pharmacological and nonpharmacological interventions, along with patient education and follow-up, is essential to alleviate symptoms, stabilize hemodynamics, and improve the quality of life for patients with ADHF. With these guidelines as a cornerstone, healthcare providers can optimize patient care and enhance outcomes for individuals living with acute decompensated heart failure.

SUGGESTED READINGS

1. American Heart Association (AHA), American College of Cardiology (ACC), Heart Failure Society of America (HFSA). 2022 AHA/ACC/HFSA Guideline for the Management of Heart Failure.
2. European Society of Cardiology (ESC). 2021 ESC Guidelines for the diagnosis and treatment of acute and chronic heart failure. European Journal of Heart Failure. 2021;23(8):955-1023.

2

CHAPTER

Antiplatelets in High Bleeding Risk Patients

Durga Prasad Chakraborty, Kinkar Lal Paul, Sitaram Pal

ABSTRACT

Use of antiplatelets in high-risk bleeding patients has always been concern regarding their risk of complications that is high risk of bleeding. To manage these complications there has been a parading shift. There are various methods to control bleeding risk using various trials and guidelines by the American College of Cardiology (ACC), American Heart Association (AHA), etc. The total duration of antiplatelet therapy has been cut down from 1 year to 6 months and even 3 months using various modern drug-eluting stents (DESs) and other devices.

The modern DESs and newer devices not only cut down the duration of antiplatelets therapy, but also, reduce the chance of bleeding. Bleeding risk assessment for each individual must be done before starting antiplatelet therapy, so that dosing and duration of antiplatelets can be prescribed easily.

INTRODUCTION

Although, there is a huge advancement in the field of antiplatelet drugs, yet there has always been a concern about the risk arises in using them, especially in the patients having increasing risk of bleeding. Although there are many trials regarding this bleeding issue, which has enlightened us regarding the perfect dosing and duration of antiplatelet drugs, yet many lacunae are there.

We can discuss our whole subject in the following points:

- Assessing the patients who belongs to High Bleeding Risk (HBR) group
- Antiplatelets and there bleeding risk
- Members of antiplatelets agents

ASSESSING THE PATIENTS WHO BELONGS TO HIGH BLEEDING RISK GROUP

Assessing the patients who belong to HBR group is based on various guidelines among which, *Academic Research Consortium-High Bleeding Risk (ARC-HBR)* is more evidence based. The risk was defined based on 14 major and six minor criteria. An individual was considered as HBR if one patient had at least one major or two minor criteria.

Major Criteria

It includes the following:

- Chronic bleeding diathesis
- Active cancer in the past 12 months
- Previous traumatic intracranial hemorrhage (ICH) within the past 12 months
- Nondeferrable major surgery on dual antiplatelet therapy
- Long-term oral anticoagulation
- Spontaneous bleeding requiring hospitalization and transfusion in the past 6 months.
- Liver cirrhosis with portal hypertension
- Previous spontaneous intracerebral hemorrhage (ICH) (at any time)
- Recent major surgery or trauma within 30 days before percutaneous coronary intervention (PCI)
- Presence of known brain arteriovenous malformations
- Sever or end-stage chronic kidney disease (CKD) [estimated glomerular filtration rate (eGFR) <30 mL/min]

- Moderate-to-sever baseline thrombocytopenia (platelet count <100 × 10^9/L)
- Moderate-to-sever ischemic stroke within the past 6 months
- Hemoglobin <11 g/dL for men and 11–11.9 g/dL for women

Minor Criteria

- Age > 75 years
- Moderate CKD (eGFR 30–59 mL/min)
- Hemoglobin 11–12.9 g/dL for men and 11–11.9 g/dL for women
- Spontaneous bleeding requiring hospitalization or transfusion within the past 12 months, not meeting major criterion.
- Long-term use of oral nonsteroidal anti-inflammatory drugs or steroids
- Any ischemic stroke at any time, not meeting major criterion

So this guideline unlike other guidelines divides the patients under two groups. The patient fell into either HBR category or non-HBR category.

ANTIPLATELETS AND THERE BLEEDING RISK

Aspirin

A meta-analysis and prospective and retrospective reviews were conducted by Zheng SL et al. in which 14 different trials containing 164,225 participants were included. There was an increased risk of major bleeding events compare with no aspirin.

Another Scientist De Berardis et al. conducted a population based cohort study at which two things were assessed, viz., major gastrointestinal bleeding and cerebral hemorrhage occurring after the initiation of aspirin therapy.

Result showed the overall incident rate of hemorrhagic events to be 5.58 per 1,000 person-years for aspirin use and 3.60 per 1,000 person-years for those without aspirin use.

Adenosine Diphosphate P2Y12 Inhibitors (For Example, Clopidogrel, Prasugrel, Ticagrelor, and Cangrelor)

Another mega trial CHARISMA (Clopidogrel for High Atherothrombotic Risk and Ischemic Stabilization Management and Avoidance) conducted by Bhatt et al. showed the rate of the primary safety end point [severe bleeding according to Global Use of Strategies to Open Occluded Coronary Arteries (GUSTO) definition] was higher but not statistically significant in the clopidogrel group (1.7%) than in the placebo group (1.3%).

To evaluate a series of ACS patients treated by PCI with newer generation DES using ticagrelor in place of clopidogrel in CHANGE DAPT study. The results were encouraging among the high bleeding risk patients incidence of major bleeding was significantly higher with ticagrelor group compared with copidogrel group.

START-antiplatelet is a prospective observational registry carried out by several Italian cardiologists on patients admitted for ACS management with moto to document the real world therapy for ACS patients with comparison among clopidogrel, ticagrelor, and prasugrel.

GP IIb/IIIa Inhibitors (For Example, Abciximab, Eptifibatide, and Tirofiban)

Once study published among 7,800 patients by Lenderink et al. was published recently which sold that 1,507 patients (19.3%) had bleeding after hospitalization with the diagnosis ACS who were given abciximab infusion major bleeding was seen in 98 patients (1.2%) and ICH in eight patients. Only 2% patients in the study underwent revascularization.

In the *EPIC trial* (with abciximab) in high-risk angioplasty 14% of the patients who receipt bolus dose of abciximab had a thrombolysis in myocardial infarction (TIMI) major bleeding versus 7% in the placebo group.

In the PURSUIT trial (with eptifibatide) there is increased risk of bleeding in patients, in which eptifibatide infusion was given to treat ACS versus placebo. Using TIMI scale there was 10.6% of major in eptifibatide group versus 9.1% of placebo group.

The *PRISM PLUS* study (with tirofiban) infusion in unstable angina a non-Q-wave MI, clearly showed major bleeding in 0.8% in the Heparin group versus 1.4% in the heparin plus tirofiban infusion group.

MEMBERS OF ANTIPLATELETS AGENTS

A brief classification of antiplatelets is as follows:

- *Cyclooxygenase inhibitor*: Acetylsalicylic acid (ASA), aspirin, and triflusal.
- *Adenosine diphosphate (ADP) P2Y12 inhibitor*: Clopidogrel, prasugrel, ticagrelor, and cangrelor.
- *Glycoprotein (GP) IIb/IIIa inhibitor*: Abciximab, eptifibatide, and tirofiban
- *Prostacyclin and analogs*: Prostaglandin I2 (PGI2), ilopros, and treprostinil
- *Phosphodiesterase inhibitors*: Dipyridamole and cilostazol
- *Protease-activated receptor-1 (PAR-1) inhibitor*: Vorapaxar and atopaxar

ASSESSING HIGH BLEEDING RISK

Patients on antiplatelet therapy we should be cautious enough in the following points:

- The risk of bleeding and amount of bleeding in patients on antiplatelet therapy.
- The severity of bleeding.
- Bleeding risk of antiplatelets therapy.

Severity of Bleeding Caused by Antiplatelet Agents

Assessment of severity of bleeding was done by various Scores which were used in different studies.

- *TIMI* bleeding
- *GUSTO*
- *Bleeding Academic Research Consortium* (BARC) definitions.

TIMI Bleeding Definitions

- *Major bleeding*: Intracranial hemorrhage
  - ≥5 g/dL decrease in the hemoglobin concentration
  - ≥15% absolute decrease in hematocrit
- *Minor bleeding*: Observed blood loss

Global Use of Strategies to Open Occluded Arteries Bleeding Definition

- *Severe or life-threatening*: ICH-bleeding that causes hemodynamic compromise and requires intervention
- *Moderate*: Bleeding that requires blood transfusion but does not lead to hemodynamic instability
- *Mild*: Bleeding that does not meet the criteria for severe or moderate bleeding

Bleeding Academic Research Consortium Scoring System

Nowadays we form some sorts of consortium which thoroughly discuss the issue and came up with the BARC scoring system **(Table 1)**.

TABLE 1: BARC scoring system.

Class I	*Bleeding that is not actionable*	• *BARC minor bleeding is class I, II, and IIIA* • *Validation: Diminished quality of life-prolonged hospitalization, and increase costs*
Class II	Any overt, actionable sign of bleeding	
Class IIIA	Overt bleeding with hemoglobin drop of 3–5 g/dL or any transfusion	
Class IIIB	Overt bleeding with hemoglobin drop of ≥5 g/dL bleeding requiring pressors surgical intervention, or due to tamponade	• BARC major bleeding is classes IIIB, IIIC, IV, and V • *Validation*: Bleeding independently associated with a 1-year mortality
Class IIIC	Intraocular or intracranial bleed	
Class IV	CABG-related bleeding: Transfusion of ≥5 units of blood, repeat sternotomy, and chest tube output ≥2 L within 24 hours	
Class V	Fatal bleeding	

(BARC: Bleeding Academic Research Consortium; CABG: coronary artery bypass graft)

Patients on Antiplatelets having Risk of Bleeding

What amount of risk of bleeding the patients have got is determined by following scoring system:

- *DAPT score for ischemic risk*: The range of score is from –2 to 10. The score of ≥2 belongs to high ischemic risk group and <2 indicates low ischemic risk group. This indicates that a score of 2 and >2 favored prolonged DAPT used with DES, while a score of <2 showed poor benefit to risk ratio for using DAPT.
- *Predicting bleeding complications in patients undergoing stent implantation and subsequent dual antiplatelet therapy (PRECISE-DAPT) score*: It include various parameter; Hb%, white blood cell (WBC), age, creatinine clearance test (CCT), and previous bleeding event. Risk group was scored as follows **(Table 2)**:
  - Low bleeding risk (precise-DAPT < 17)
  - Intermediate bleeding risk (17–24)
  - High bleeding risk (≥25)
- *Patterns of non-Adherence to Antiplatelet Regimen in Stented Patients (PARIS) score*: This scoring system predicts OPD group of patients having PCI. It has the

TABLE 2: DAPT score system.

Variable	Points
Age:	
• ≥75 years	–2
• 65–75 years	–1
• ≤64 years	0
DM	1
Current cigarette smoker	1
MI or prior PCI	1
MI at presentation	1
Stent diameter <3 mm	1
Congestive HF or EF <30%	2
Vein-graft PCI	2

(DM: diabetes mellitus; EF: ejection fraction; HF: heart failure; MI: myocardial infarction; PCI: percutaneous coronary intervention) range of score for bleeding from 0 to 14 and patients are grouped at low (0–3), intermediate (4–7) and high (eight or more) bleeding risk.

Various Scenarios Regarding Management of High Bleeding Group of Patients

Are grouped as follows:

Scenario 1

Patient with ACS or non-ACS who undergoes PCI with stenting along with guideline-directed medical therapy (GDMT).

During the time of the first generation DES it was thought that 3–6 months of DAPT therapy was sufficient but unfortunately there is high risk of thrombosis seen; and, that is why duration was prolonged for 12 months. So the newer development of DES decreased duration of DAPT and subsequently decreased risk of bleeding. And it is supported by American College of Cardiology (ACC) and European Society of Cardiology (ESC) guidelines.

There are some recent guidelines have been published which show the noble effect of antiplatelet in HBR patients:

- EVOLVE Short DAPT trial enrolled 2,009 patients at 110 global study sites between February 2016 and March 2018. Among the 1,912 patients with 3-month clinical follow-up, 425 patients were ineligible to discontinue P2Y12 inhibitor at 3 months.

Scenario 2

Patients on anticoagulants for atrial fibrillation (AFib)/venous thromboembolism with antiplated therapy; there are many trials were conducted to compare to safety and efficacy of DAPT with an anticoagulants i.e., triple therapy.

- *WOEST* [What is the Optimal antiplatelet Elet and anticoagulant therapy in patients with oral anticoagulation (OAC) and coronary StenTing]
- *PIONEER AF-PCI* [Rivaroxaban and a dose-adjusted oral vitamin K antagonist (VKA) treatment strategy in subjects with atrial fibrillation who undergo percutaneous coronary intervention]
- *RE-DUAL PCI* (Evaluation Of Dual therapy With Dabigatran vs. Triple Therapy With Warfarin In Patients With AFib that Undergo a PCI With Stenting)
- *AUGUSTUS* (Antithrombotic Therapy After Acute Coronary Syndrome or PCI in Atrial Fibrillation)
- *ENTRUST AF* (Edoxaban-based Antithrombotic Regimen in Patients with AFib)

Based on these trials an updated guidelines from ACC and American Heart Association (AHA) was published in 2020 mentioning pathway for OAC and antiplatelet therapy in patient with AF or venous thromboembolism (VTE).

They have divided patients following groups and recommended the following:

- Patient with AFib on anticoagulation (AC) therapy who now needs PCI
- Patient on antiplatelet therapy with a new diagnosis of AF
- Patient with prior VTE being considered for PCI
- Patient on antiplatelet therapy with new VTE

Scenario 3

Patient with cerebrovascular accidents (CVAs) on antiplatelets; there are several randomized clinical trial regarding this issue.

- *S2TOP-BLEED* [That is male Sex, Smoking, Type of antiplatelet agents, Outcome on modified Rankin Scale (mRS), prior stroke, high blood pressure (BP), lower body mass index (BMI), elderly, Asian ethnicity, and diabetes]

In this trial patients had transient ischemic attack (TIA) or ischemic stroke, data from six randomized clinical trials were used to assess to bleeding risk associated with antiplatelets.

CONCLUSION

There is increased risk of bleeding specially in HBR population during use of antiplatelets. There has been shift of management to cut down the risk of bleeding in HBR population while using antiplatelets. There are various methods to control bleeding risk using various trials and guidelines, (ACC, AHA, etc.) The DAPT has been cut down from, six months to three months or even one month by using various modern DESs. It has also been seen that newer DESs may help to cut down stent-related complication even in short duration of antiplatelet drugs (DAPT, etc.). Bleeding risk assessment for each individual must be done before starting antiplatelets so that proper dosing and duration of antiplatelets can be prescribed.

SUGGESTED READINGS

1. Sabate M, Cequier A, Iñiguez A, Serra A, Hernandez-Antolin R, Mainar V, et al. Everolimus-eluting stent versus bare-metal stent in ST-segment elevation myocardial infarction (EXAMINATION): 1 year results of a randomised controlled trial. Lancet. 2012;380(9852):1482-90.
2. Varenne O, Cook S, Sideris G, Kedev S, Cuisset T, Carrié D, et al. Drug-eluting stents in elderly patients with coronary artery disease (SENIOR): a randomised single-blind trial. Lancet. 2018;391(10115):41-50.
3. Valgimigli M, Bueno H, Byrne RA, Collet JP, Costa F, Jeppsson A, et al. 2017 ESC focused update on dual antiplatelet therapy in coronary artery disease developed in collaboration with EACTS: The Task Force for dual antiplatelet therapy in coronary artery disease of the European Society of Cardiology (ESC) and of the European Association for Cardio-Thoracic Surgery (EACTS). Eur Heart J. 2018;39(3):213-60.
4. Mauri L, Kereiakes DJ, Yeh RW, Driscoll-Shempp P, Cutlip DE, Steg PG, et al. Twelve or 30 months of dual antiplatelet therapy after drug-eluting stents. N Engl J Med. 2014;371(23):2155-66.
5. Mathews R, Peterson ED, Chen AY, Wang TY, Chin CT, Fonarow GC, et al. In-hospital major bleeding during ST-elevation and non-ST-elevation myocardial infarction care: derivation and validation of a model from the ACTION Registry®-GWTG™. Am J Cardiol. 2011;107(8):1136-43.
6. Piccolo R, Gargiulo G, Franzone A, Santucci A, Ariotti S, Baldo A, et al. Use of the Dual-Antiplatelet Therapy Score to Guide Treatment Duration After Percutaneous Coronary Intervention. Ann Intern Med. 2017;167(1):17-25.
7. Subban V. Randomized comparison of six versus twenty-four months clopidogrel therapy after balancing anti-intimal hyperplasia stent potency in all comer patients undergoing percutaneous coronary intervention. Results of the PRODIGY Trial. Indian Heart J. 2012;64(4):428-30.
8. Witberg G, Zusman O, Yahav D, Perl L, Vaknin-Assa H, Kornowski R. Meta-analysis of Studies Examining the External Validity of the DAPT Score. Eur Heart J Cardiovasc Pharmacother. 2019;6(5):285-91.
9. Chichareon P, Modolo R, Kawashima H, Takahashi K, Kogame N, Chang CC, et al. DAPT Score and the Impact of Ticagrelor Monotherapy During the Second Year After PCI. JACC Cardiovasc Interv. 2020;13(5):634-46.
10. Ueda P, Jernberg T, James S, Alfredsson J, Erlinge D, Omerovic E, et al. External Validation of the DAPT Score in a Nationwide Population. J Am Coll Cardiol. 2018;72(10):1069-78.

3

CHAPTER

Happy Heart Syndrome

Rajesh Kumar Jha, Srishti Jha, Surbhi Naik

ABSTRACT

Happy heart syndrome typically explains the role of positive emotional stress in takotsubo syndrome (TTS). It is typically provoked by negative stressors such as grief, anger, and fear leading to the popular term "broken heart syndrome." Broken heart syndrome is a condition which resembles acute coronary syndrome on clinical presentation and thus it becomes very important to differentiate between these two conditions on practical grounds. This chapter explains the details of this condition, its symptoms, evaluation, and management.

INTRODUCTION

Broken heart syndrome is a cardiac condition which is temporary and reversible and clinically mimics acute coronary syndrome. Other words used for it are stress-induced cardiomyopathy or takotsubo cardiomyopathy.

Takotsubo cardiomyopathy was first discovered in Japan in 1991. It is named after the takotsubo, which is a trap used for octopus. Shape of the trap is similar to the appearance of left ventricular (LV) apical ballooning which is seen in these patients.

During systole, the middle part and apex of the left ventricle balloon out, while the base, contracts normally. The shape is similar to a takotsubo **(Figs. 1A and B)**.

A person may think of experiencing a heart attack because symptoms, such as shortness of breath and chest

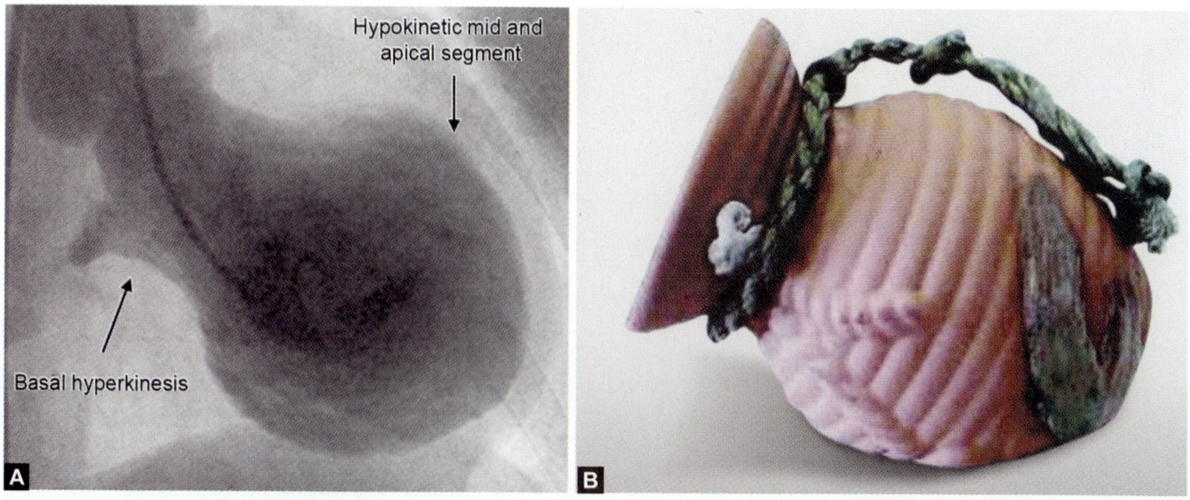

FIGS. 1A AND B: (A) Apical ballooning of left ventricle which looks similar to a (B) takotsubo.
Source: UVA Chemistry.com.

pain, are similar in both conditions. However, in broken heart syndrome, a person does not have blocked coronary arteries or any permanent heart damage, and usually makes a full recovery.

Takotsubo cardiomyopathy is seen more in women, of which 80% cases are seen in postmenopausal women. Thus the mean age for this disease is around 58–75 years. Mortality is at a much lower level with this syndrome (0–8%).

The common triggers for this disease are death of a loved one, some catastrophic event, devastating financial losses, natural disasters, major physical illness/intensive care unit (ICU), etc. Takotsubo cardiomyopathy is also known as apical ballooning syndrome or transient LV apical ballooning syndrome or ampulla cardiomyopathy.

PATHOPHYSIOLOGY

Exact pathophysiology of this syndrome is not known but the postulated physiology behind it states that stressful conditions like death of a loved one, etc., cause excess release of catecholamines causing intense activation of sympathetic system. This induces microvascular spasm or dysfunction causing myocardial stunning or direct myocardial toxicity. Coronary artery spasm or microvascular spasm leads to this acute but reversible condition.

CLINICAL PRESENTATION

Broken heart syndrome presents clinically similar to an acute myocardial infarction (MI) episode. Patient usually comes to the emergency with substernal chest pain and dyspnea and in extreme cases can present in shock or syncope.

Electrocardiogram (ECG) findings are also similar and may include ST elevation (usually anterior precordial leads)—82%; ST-depression, T-wave inversion, QT-prolongation, and abnormal Q-waves **(Fig. 2)**.

The cardiac markers were also found to be elevated in takotsubo cardiomyopathy. There is a rapid but only mild rise of cardiac biomarkers. While in an episode of MI, cardiac biomarkers take longer to rise but peak higher.

EVALUATION

Higher investigations that can help in diagnosing this condition include:

- *Echocardiography*: An echocardiogram shows abnormal movements in the walls of the left ventricle. The main abnormality in takotsubo cardiomyopathy is ballooning of the lower part of the left ventricle (apex). During systole, this bulging ventricle resembles a takotsubo, the octopus trap used mainly by the Japanese fishermen **(Figs. 3A and B)**.

Average LV ejection fraction is 20–49%.

- *Left ventriculography*: Left ventriculography can also be done for evaluation of LV outflow tract obstruction (~16%). It can demonstrate transient dysfunction and ballooning of the LV mid and apical segments.
- *Magnetic resonance imaging (MRI)*: Cardiac MRI may be required in a few cases. Four distinct patterns of dyskinesia and ballooning are recognized—(1) apical (most common), (2) biventricular, (3) midventricular, and (4) basal.

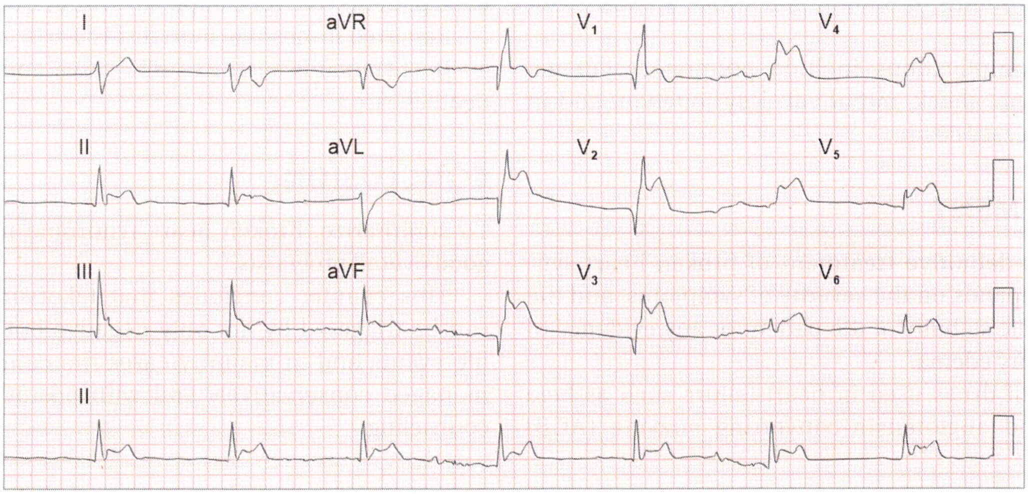

FIG. 2: ECG of a patient of broken heart syndrome mimicking MI.
(ECG: electrocardiogram; MI: myocardial infarction)

CHAPTER 4

Travel Advice in Patients with Congestive Heart Failure

Kamaldeep Chawla, Akashkumar N Singh, Saumitra A Singh, Anil Kulshreshtha

ABSTRACT

Majority of cardiovascular (CV) events are reported in patients with congestive heart failure (CHF), especially during domestic and international air travel compared to general population. The factors that may influence the risk of developing symptoms of heart failure (HF) include choice of destination, travel distance and time, mode of travel, whether condition in the place of arrival, altitude levels, air pollution levels, availability of medical resources, etc. Hence, it is imperative that CHF patients must adhere to specific recommendations such as undergoing pretravel assessments, medication adjustment, adequate fluid intake, access to on-board oxygen supplementation, etc., during travel to minimize the risk of CV events and travel-related illness. This review article focuses on various aspects of travel recommendations for CHF patients planning on national and international air travel to minimize the risk of developing symptoms of HF or CV events.

INTRODUCTION

Patients with congestive heart failure (CHF) most commonly report increased health risks (20–70%) during domestic and international travel. Cardiovascular conditions, such as heart attack, heart failure (HF), and stroke are the most common leading causes of air evacuations, along with injuries and psychiatric emergencies among these patients, especially over the age of 70 years. Cardiovascular disease is reported as the most common cause of death during international travel with a prevalence rate of 1 in 100,000 cases although 1–5% of these patients receive medical help. Majority of the patients with CHF seek medical advice from their healthcare practitioners through specialist consultation prior to planning their travel, especially if they have recently undergone a cardiac surgery or have left ventricular assist devices (LVADs) implanted.

WHO CAN TRAVEL SAFELY?

Patients with below conditions can travel safely by taking appropriate health safety measures as needed.

- Patients with stable health condition
- Patients with controlled blood pressure
- Patients with low risk of developing symptoms of HF as per pretravel risk assessment
- Patients with New York Heart Association (NYHA) class I–II HF after taking appropriate safety measures and undergoing pretravel risk assessment prior to 4–6 weeks of travel date.
- Patients with NYHA class III who are stable and have arrangement for adequate oxygen supplementation during travel especially by air.

WHAT ARE THE CONTRAINDICATIONS FOR TRAVEL?

Patients with below listed health conditions are contraindications for travel:

- Patients who had episode of myocardial infarction (ST-elevation or non-ST-elevation myocardial infarction) within 2 weeks of travel date.
- Unstable angina
- Patients who have undergone complicated percutaneous coronary angioplasty within 2 weeks of travel date. However, short duration travels are recommended in patients who have undergone uncomplicated percutaneous coronary intervention.

- Patients who had cardiac surgery or interventional valve therapy within the previous 3 weeks.
- Patients with NYHA class IV HF or any decompensated HF, unstable angina, untreated arrhythmias (ventricular or supraventricular), Eisenmenger syndrome, uncontrolled pulmonary artery hypertension, and pneumothorax (such as after major cardiac surgery).

WHAT ARE THE GENERAL FACTORS THAT INFLUENCE THE RISK OF HEART FAILURE AMONG PATIENTS WITH CHF?

Several factors that may influence the risk of developing symptoms of HF among these patients include choice of destination, travel distance and time, mode of travel, whether condition in the place of arrival, altitude levels, air pollution levels, availability of medical resources, etc. **(Table 1)**.

PRETRAVEL ASSESSMENT AND EDUCATION FOR CHF PATIENTS

Pretravel risk assessment should be performed by a clinician 4–6 weeks before departure, and patients should receive advice on potential travel-related illness and on strategies to prevent volume depletion. Oxygen supplementation might be useful for patients who are very symptomatic. Special recommendations are needed for patients with cardiac implantable electronic devices or LVADs as well as for those who have undergone major cardiac surgery.

TABLE 1: Factors that influence the risk of heart failure among patients with CHF.

Factor	Explanation
Choice of destination	The choice of destination for travel can have important health implications for patients with HF, particularly when traveling abroad. Considerations include the local climate, air pollution levels, altitude levels, the season upon arrival, the distance and time for traveling, jet lag, and vaccines required
Seasonal changes at destination	Seasonal changes at destination impact rate of hospitalizations due to CHF, especially in elderly patients. The rate of hospitalization is substantially low during warmer periods and high during colder periods as cold climate is known to increase vascular resistance and plasma noradrenaline concentration which may lead to HF decompensation. Temperature had the greatest (inverse) correlation with hospitalizations for HF among other causative environmental factors, such as humidity, precipitation, or irradiation
Time and duration of travel	Time and duration of travel play an important role and have great impact on the health of CHF patients. Appropriate steps should be taken to ensure the patient is not subjected to dehydration or lack of medication. Flight attendants and other personnel need to be informed about the LVAD and the location of the emergency information card. Patients need to maintain fluid intake to avoid low flow alarms from the LVAD pump. For flights longer than 2 hours, support stockings should be considered
Higher altitudes	Patients with HF are more susceptible to the physiological changes induced by high-altitude exposure than the general population. During air travel, cabin pressure is required to be no less than the barometric pressure at an altitude of 2,438 m (8,000 ft), which is classified as an intermediate altitude. Cabin pressures usually remain higher than this altitude, particularly during long distance flights. Travel to high-altitude locations that are >2,500 m above sea level triggers physiological, acclimatization processes within the cardiocirculatory and pulmonary systems. These processes are initiated by a gradual decrease in barometric pressure, which in turn lowers the partial pressure of oxygen in inspired air. Hypobaric hypoxia leads to a fast increase in respiratory rate and tidal volume, which leads to respiratory alkalosis and hypoxic diuresis. Hypoxia induces pulmonary vasoconstriction and eventual pulmonary hypertension, an important trigger for high-altitude pulmonary edema. Therefore, it is safe for CHF patients to travel to destinations at an intermediate altitude (~2,000 m) at sea level
Air pollution	Particulate matter induced pulmonary vasoconstriction results from increases in pulmonary and right ventricular diastolic filling pressures, which affect right ventricular performance. Therefore, given that the effects of air pollutants on cardiovascular performance and outcomes can occur within hours or days of exposure, patients with HF should be advised to avoid traveling to locations with high levels of air pollution
Availability of medical resources	Sufficient medication for the whole journey (consider bringing extra drugs in case of unforeseen delays in returning home). Medication to be kept in carry-on luggage for flights (in case of loss of luggage or emergency). Photocopy of last prescription, insurance card, and patient identification card should be kept handy. List of diagnosed health conditions and prescribed medicines, last discharge letter from hospital, device interrogation printout and list of names and phone numbers of cardiologist, and other relevant clinicians should also be kept readily available

(CHF: congestive heart failure; HF: heart failure; LVAD: left ventricular assist device)

Risk assessment includes examination of full medical history which should include evaluation of current medications, vaccination history, history of any recent surgeries, or device implantation, allergies, pregnancy, or breastfeeding, etc. Prior travel experience or risk tolerance should be analyzed. Any medication or tests suggested by the doctors as part of pretravel assessment such as physical examination, electrocardiogram tracing, biochemistry analysis (plasma levels of creatinine, ferritin, glucose, glycated hemoglobin, N-terminal pro-B-type natriuretic peptide, potassium, sodium, transferrin saturation, thyroid-stimulating hormone, vitamin D and urea, estimated glomerular filtration rate, and lipid profile and liver function tests), full blood count (to identify potential anemia), exercise test, and/or transthoracic echocardiography should be considered. Evaluation of implanted devices should be performed. Administration of any destination-specific vaccines apart from the routine vaccines including measles-mumps-rubella, tetanus-diphtheria-pertussis, coronavirus disease 2019 (COVID-19), pneumococcal disease, and influenza must be administered as needed and as advised by the healthcare provider. Strategies to prevent or treat traveler's diarrhea should be considered.

The patient should be properly educated by the healthcare provider about importance of medical kit (medication and device information) and medical record documents (latest reports, health insurance, etc.) required during travel. Education about medical first aid and basics on how to handle medical emergencies, how to do dose adjustment if needed to avoid dehydration and volume depletion, how to handle any implanted devices such as avoiding strong electromagnetic fields, and factors that lead to volume depletion such as excess alcohol, coffee, salt intake, etc., should be given by the healthcare professional to the patient as part of pretravel risk assessment and education.

VACCINATION OF CONGESTIVE HEART FAILURE PATIENTS

Patients with CHF should be assessed for vaccination status and advised to take all the recommended travel vaccinations during their pretravel assessment. The common vaccines recommended for CHF patients are measles-mumps-rubella, pertussis, tetanus, varicella, influenza, pneumococcal, hepatitis A, hepatitis B, and COVID-19 vaccines. Apart from the commonly recommended travel vaccinations, a few additional vaccinations should also be considered among CHF patients based on the travel destination. **Table 2** summarizes the additional vaccination recommendations in CHF patients based on the travel destination.

TABLE 2: Summary of additional vaccination recommendations in congestive heart failure (CHF) patients based on the travel destination.

Vaccine type	Recommendation
Typhoid: Oral vaccine	To be considered in CHF patients traveling to India and other South Asian countries and South American countries such as Bolivia and Costa Rica
Yellow fever: Single shot vaccine	To be considered in CHF patients traveling to certain African countries such as Cameroon and South American countries such as Bolivia and Costa Rica
Rabies lyssaviruses: Given as series of three vaccines	To be considered in CHF patients traveling to certain African, Asian, and South and Central American countries. This vaccine is mandatory among patients who have high possibility of being in close contact with wild or domestic animals
Poliomyelitis: Given in three shots or as oral vaccine	To be considered in CHF patients traveling to certain African countries such as Benin and Asian countries such as the Philippines
Meningococcal disease: Conjugate vaccine	To be considered in CHF patients traveling to dry places particularly if the travel is in dry season (June to December). These places include Mecca in Saudi Arabia and sub-Saharan African countries, known as the meningitis belt
Japanese encephalitis: Two shot vaccine	To be considered in CHF patients traveling to Japan (Western pacific country) and Southeast Asian countries such as Indonesia

CAPABILITY TO DRIVE

Cardiovascular disease can cause sudden loss of control (also known as sudden cardiac incapacitation) while driving and can lead to accidents. This is due to the pathophysiological mechanisms such as disturbances of brain perfusion (e.g., syncope with or without cardiac arrhythmia, sudden cardiac death due to ventricular fibrillation or asystole, stroke, and aneurysm rupture). General weakness in patients with a recent history of major cardiac surgery or cardiac insufficiency can also lead to sudden loss of control in these patients. Physicians treating patients with CHF should consider the severity of CHF by analyzing the NYHA class and left ventricular ejection fraction (LVEF). Patients with CHF that fall under NYHA class I–III are eligible to drive private vehicles after undergoing health assessment. NYHA class IV patients are not allowed to drive. Patients with a functioning cardiac pacemaker are fit to drive after 1 week while patients with ICDs are not permitted to drive.

Risk stratification can be done using various formulas developed by several health organizations such as "risk of harm" by Canadian Cardiovascular Society to understand the driving capability of the patient with cardiovascular disease. This formula is often considered as the golden standard. The probability of cardiac disease or loss of sudden control in CHF patients mainly depends on the factors such as the time spent by the patient at the wheel, the type of vehicle the patient is driving (private car and truck), and the probability of sudden loss of control. Patients with CHF should ensure that they are permitted to drive in their traveling destination by accessing country-specific driving regulations online.

HEALTH EXPERIENCES DURING TRAVEL

The most common health experiences encountered by the CHF patients during the travel are arrhythmias (atrial fibrillation, ventricular tachyarrhythmia, or premature ventricular contractions) during any sports activities and while flying or staying in higher altitudes, HF decompensation during low adherence to prescribed medication and high sodium food intake, damage to the implanted cardiac lead (fracture or insulation failure) due to exposure to electromagnetic interference, especially while traveling through train or ship, and cardiac device compression with loss of function during diving.

In a questionnaire-based survey performed in a representative cohort of 464 ambulatory patients with stable, well-managed CHF to study the air travel experiences, an expert panel including a cardiologist, an exercise scientist, and a psychologist developed a series of survey questions designed to document travel experiences of CHF patients. The study showed that about 54% of patients have traveled by air since they were diagnosed with CHF. Among these patients about 20% of the patients reported having difficulty in obtaining a travel insurance. Among the 464 patients, about 65% of patients did not have health-related problems whereas 35% of patients had experienced health problems such as cardiovascular problems including fatigue, breathlessness, labored walking, swollen ankles, palpitations, angina, or their defibrillator firing, mainly at the destination, going through security and on the aircraft.

PRECAUTIONS TO FOLLOW

The following precautions should be taken by CHF patients while planning for travel:

- Take frequent breaks after walks, stretching of limbs, sufficient fluid intake and measures to avoid volume depletion, and thromboprophylaxis
- Timely intake of prescribed medication. Keep nitroglycerin spray handy.
- Immediate medical care if acute chest pain or dyspnea occurs
- Implantation of permanent pacemaker before departure if indicated
- Check for blood sugar levels and blood pressure control, especially ambulatory blood pressure measurement for 24 hours before departure
- The physician should always help the patient to prepare a backup plan while traveling to handle unexpected situations during travel such as becoming too ill during the flight or during the vacation. Keep a backup plan for your travel arrangements such as Taxi, hotel accommodation, emergency health service contacts, availability of equipment spare parts, etc.

DISCUSSION

The CHF patients with cardiac symptoms, recent interventions, devices, and surgery are more easily susceptible to have adverse cardiovascular events during travel and need to plan their travel more meticulously. They need to seek medical advice and undergo pretravel risk assessment including physical and medical examination, medication adjustment and dietary, and exercise and lifestyle education if needed by a health-care provider before initiation of the journey. Pretravel risk assessment should also include assessment of travel time, distance, duration, travel insurance, capability to drive private vehicles at destination, vaccination status, destination climate condition, air pollution level, and altitude. Special recommendations and precautions should be taken by patients who have undergone major cardiac surgical treatment or had cardiac rhythm implants or devices such as LVADs. Altitude and cabin pressure may cause hypobaric hypoxia which results in reduced arterial oxygen partial pressure and increased respiratory distress in CHF patients. In-flight oxygen is recommended for these patients traveling with a sea-level partial pressure of oxygen (PaO_2) of 70 mm Hg or lower, or with an expected PaO_2 of 55 mm Hg or lower. The travel induced anxiety-related adverse effects among CHF patients are hemodynamic changes including vasoconstriction, tachycardia, and subsequently decompensated CHF. Thus, it is imperative for these travelers to follow certain relaxation techniques during traveling for long distances. CHF patients are also more prone to experience venous thromboembolism (VTE) following prolonged air travel, especially those with lower LVEF. Thus, it is necessary to identify these patients prior to the commencement of the flight journey and provide proper education about the events that may occur during the flight.

CONCLUSION

Traveling is usually safe in most patients with stable cardiovascular disease. However, it is essential to have a thorough understanding of the physiologic changes that can develop during travel and their potential impact on cardiovascular health of the patients, especially in those with preexisting cardiac conditions or symptoms. It is imperative that the clinicians are aware of the current travel recommendations and precautions to be taken by the CHF patients before and during the travel and advice the patients as needed to avoid any adverse outcomes.

ACKNOWLEDGMENTS

The authors acknowledge the writing support provided by Tatineni Swathi from Arkus Research Pvt Ltd.

Competing interests: The authors declare that they have no competing interests related to this manuscript.

Funding sources: No funding sources were used for the conduct of the study or preparation of this manuscript.

SUGGESTED READINGS

1. Ryan ET, Kain KC. Health advice and immunizations for travelers. N Engl J Med. 2000;342(23):1716-25.
2. von Haehling S, Birner C, Dworatzek E, Frantz S, Hellenkamp K, Israel CW, et al. Travelling with heart failure: risk assessment and practical recommendations. Nat Rev Cardiol. 2022;19(5):302-13.
3. Dharmarajan K, Hsieh AF, Kulkarni VT, Lin Z, Ross JS, Horwitz LI, et al. Trajectories of risk after hospitalization for heart failure, acute myocardial infarction, or pneumonia: retrospective cohort study. BMJ. 2015;350:h411.
4. Alba AC, Bain E, Ng N, Stein M, Brien KO, Ross H. Complications after heart transplantation: hope for the best, but prepare for the worst. Int J Transplant Res Med. 2016;2(2):2
5. Westheim A, Os I, Thaulow E, Kjeldsen SE, Eritsland J, Eide IK. Haemodynamic and neurohumoral effects of cold pressor test in severe heart failure. Clin Physiol. 1992;12(1):95-106.
6. Swenson ER. Carbonic anhydrase inhibitors and high altitude illnesses. Subcell Biochem. 2014;75:361-86.
7. Wold LE, Ying Z, Hutchinson KR, Velten M, Gorr MW, Velten C, et al. Cardiovascular remodeling in response to long-term exposure to fine particulate matter air pollution. Circ Heart Fail. 2012;5(4):452-61.
8. Goodwin T. In-flight medical emergencies: an overview. BMJ. 2000;321(7272):1338-41.
9. Wendt S, Beier D, Paquet D, Trawinski H, Fuchs A, Lübbert C. Medical Advice for Travelers. Dtsch Arztebl Int. 2021;118(21):349-56.
10. Freedman DO, Chen LH, Kozarsky PE. Medical Considerations before International Travel. N Engl J Med. 2016;375(3):247-60.
11. Liew CH, Flaherty GT. Pre-travel health advice for patients with cardiovascular disease. Int J Travel Med Glob Health. 2019;7(3):79-85.
12. Klein HH, Sechtem U, Trappe HJ. Fitness to Drive in Cardiovascular Disease. Dtsch Arztebl Int. 2017;114(41):692-702.
13. Simpson C, Dorian P, Gupta A, Hamilton R, Hart S, Hoffmaster B, et al. Assessment of the cardiac patient for fitness to drive: drive subgroup executive summary. Can J Cardiol. 2004;20(13):1314-20.
14. Izadi M, Alemzadeh-Ansari MJ, Kazemisaleh D, Moshkani-Farahani M. Air travel considerations for the patients with heart failure. Iran Red Crescent Med J. 2014;16(6):e17213.
15. Ingle L, Hobkirk J, Damy T, Nabb S, Clark AL, Cleland JG. Experiences of air travel in patients with chronic heart failure. Int J Cardiol. 2012;158(1):66-70.

5

CHAPTER

The Correlation of Electrocardiography and Echocardiography for Clinicians: A Comprehensive Analysis

Santanu Bhakta, Navaneel Chakraborty, Angik Mukherjee

ABSTRACT

Electrocardiogram (ECG) and echocardiogram (echo) are invaluable tools for cardiovascular evaluation. They differ in terms of principles, methodologies, and the insights they offer. This chapter aims to explore the correlation between ECG and echo, highlight their respective strengths and limitations, and discuss how physicians can effectively utilize the information obtained from these tests. Pertinent research articles, books, and professional guidelines were reviewed, focusing on the clinical correlation between ECG and echo. Additionally, case studies and clinical experiences were analyzed to validate the correlation in different clinical scenarios. The correlation between ECG and echo exhibits varying degrees depending on the underlying cardiac condition. However, in many cases, these two tests are complementary and provide vital information that helps physicians to make accurate diagnoses. Physicians should understand the relationship between these tests, their strengths, and limitations to optimize patient care. Continued research in this field is essential to refine the correlation and ensure more accurate clinical decision-making.

INTRODUCTION

Electrocardiogram (ECG) and echocardiogram (echo) are two important diagnostic tests that are used to assess the heart. An ECG records the electrical activity of the heart, while an echo uses ultrasound waves to create images of the heart's structure and function. Clinical correlation between ECG and echo is the process of interpreting the results of these two tests together in order to make a diagnosis.

In this chapter, we will discuss the basics of ECG and echo, and how they can be used together to assess the heart.

UNDERSTANDING ELECTROCARDIOGRAM AND ITS CLINICAL RELEVANCE

What is an ECG?

A noninvasive diagnostic technology called electrocardiography captures the electrical activity of the heart throughout time. It is frequently used in clinical practice to detect conduction anomalies, ischemic alterations, and cardiac arrhythmias. ECGs are also performed in various clinical scenarios, including regular examinations for asymptomatic people to detect latent or hidden cardiac ailments.

UNDERSTANDING ECHOCARDIOGRAPHY AND ITS CLINICAL RELEVANCE

What is an Echocardiography?

Ultrasound waves are used in the noninvasive imaging procedure known as echocardiography to show the structure and operation of the heart. Clinicians can evaluate irregularities in wall motion, chamber sizes, valve function, and overall cardiac performance using the real-time, dynamic images of the heart it offers.

CORRELATING ECG AND ECHO DATA: KEY CONCEPTS AND EXAMPLES

Evaluating Rhythm and Conduction Abnormalities

The initial signs of rhythm disturbances, such as atrial fibrillation, ventricular tachycardia, or atrioventricular

(AV) block, are frequently provided by ECG data. By exposing the anatomical underpinnings of various rhythm problems, such as atrial or ventricular hypertrophy, the echo can supplement this knowledge.

Identifying Ischemic Changes and Wall Motion Abnormalities

When ST-segment elevations or depressions occur, ischemia alterations are particularly detectable by ECG. Clinicians can pinpoint regions of myocardial ischemia and their effects on regional wall motion by comparing these results with echo.

Assessing Valvular Function

An ECG can reveal problems with the valves, such as left atrial enlargement or atrial fibrillations, brought on by mitral stenosis. By offering a thorough evaluation of valve shape, function, and regurgitation severity, echocardiography assists in the diagnosis and management of valvular diseases.

SPECIFIC CARDIAC CONDITIONS, AND THEIR CORRESPONDING ECG AND ECHO FINDINGS

Case 1

A 43-year-old male comes for routine clinical checkup without specific symptoms. He is obese, hypertensive, and on therapy for about 1 year. His office blood pressure is 142/84 mm Hg and body mass index (BMI) is 29 kg/m^2. Cardiovascular examination reveals nothing except cardiac apex, which is in 5th intercostal space (ICS).

On repeated interrogation, he recognizes a minimal shortness of breath (SOB) nowadays, which he thinks as age- and obesity-related problem.

With normal hematological and biochemical parameters, cardiovascular evaluations are carried out.

This is a prototype example of a clinical scenario where proper history (SOB on exertion), bedside examination (shifting of cardiac apex), ECG [complete right bundle branch block (RBBB) as in **Fig. 1**], and echocardiography [LVH, grade 1 left ventricular diastolic dysfunction (LVDD) as in **Figs. 2 and 3**] can be correlated intelligently for taking a crucial decision to manage the patient.

Left Ventricular Hypertrophy

Left ventricular hypertrophy (LVH) is a condition in which there is either an increase in left ventricular mass or left ventricular cavity enlargement.

ECG Findings

More than 30 criteria are postulated to diagnose LVH. The most commonly used are:

- *The Sokolow–Lyon criteria*: S wave depth in V_1 + tallest R wave height in V_5–V_6 > 35 mm.
- *Non-voltage criteria*:
  - Increased R wave peak time >50 ms in leads V_5 or V_6
  - ST segment depression and T wave inversion in the left-sided leads.

Echo Findings

Total 48% patients with ECG diagnosed LVH have enlarged interventricular septum and posterior walls of the left ventricle (LV) (≥12 mm), 33% without posterior wall thickening have an LV dilated (≥58 mm) according to echocardiography. When the LV mass is calculated using dimensions, it is higher (>200 g) in 78% patients using the Penn approach in all patients. These findings suggest that LV mass estimation by echocardiography is a more accurate predictor of LVH than LV posterior wall and septal thickness.

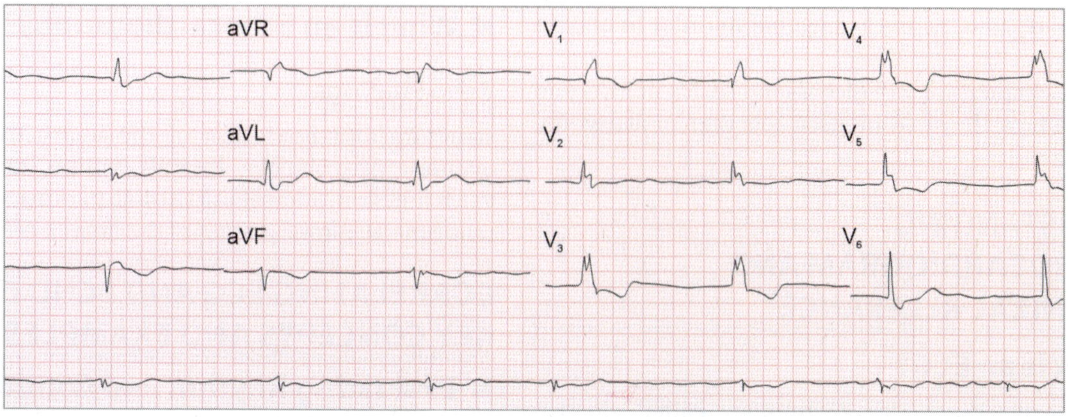

FIG. 1: ECG of case 1 shows complete right bundle branch block (RBBB).

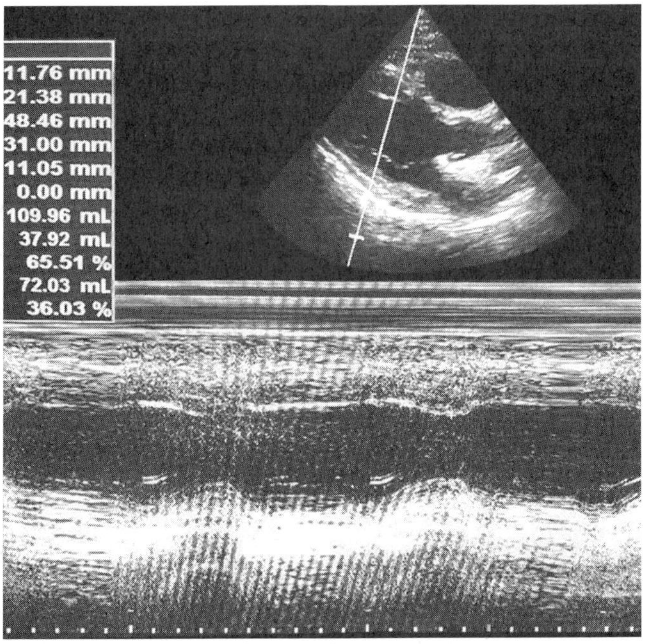

FIG. 2: 2D and M-mode echo with left ventricular hypertrophy (LVH).

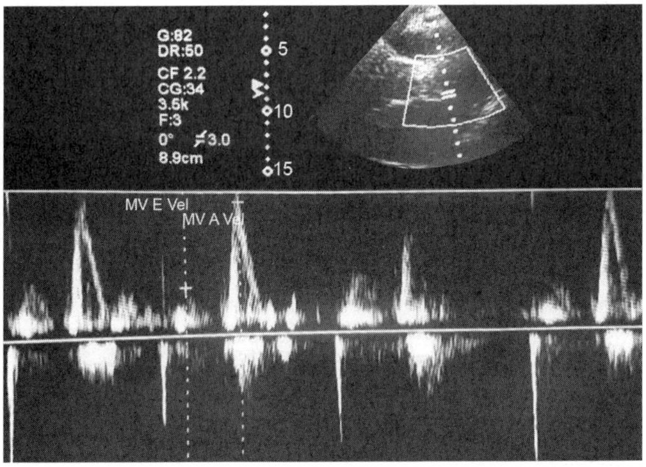

FIG. 3: Echo Doppler study: Grade 1 left ventricular diastolic dysfunction (LVDD).

Chronic Obstructive Pulmonary Disease

The right ventricle, LV, and pulmonary arteries are all significantly impacted by chronic obstructive pulmonary disease (COPD). A linear link exists between the prevalence of pulmonary hypertension and the severity of COPD, and severe pulmonary hypertension is usually accompanied by cor pulmonale.

ECG Findings

- In cases with emphysema, the most frequent ECG abnormalities are:
  - the P-wave axis is shifted to the right, with significant P waves in the inferior leads and flattened or inverted P waves in leads I and aVL.
  - Right-handed rotation of the QRS axis toward +90° (vertical axis)
  - PR and ST segments that "sag" below the TP baseline due to excessive atrial depolarization, especially in the left precordial leads (V_4-V_6)
  - Low voltage QRS complexes
- With the development of cor pulmonale, changes are:
  - Right atrial enlargement
  - Right ventricular hypertrophy
- Distinct P wave morphologies (associated with increased mortality in patients with COPD)

Echo Findings

The most common echocardiographic findings in COPD are right atrial and ventricular enlargement, right ventricular hypertrophy, pulmonary hypertension, and tricuspid regurgitation (TR) (90–100%).

Left ventricular diastolic as well as biventricular systolic dysfunction is also observed in a large amount of COPD patients (30–70%).

Myocardial Infarction

Atherothrombotic occlusion of the coronary artery causes myocardial infarction (MI), also referred to as a heart attack. Chest pain, breathlessness, and perspiration are possible symptoms. It is essential to get medical care right away to save lives, limit damage, and avoid problems.

ECG Findings

Electrocardiogram is the investigation to diagnose acute myocardial infarction (AMI). A series of changes are noted in ST segment, T wave, and QRS complex in MI. A lot of variations of ECG changes are noted in MI, depending on size, site, extent, and duration.

Though various specific changes of ECG are obvious in MI, even in an expert eye, they are frequently confusing and making diagnostic dilemma. Nonconclusive ST-T changes and borderline increased cardiac markers are frequently confusing to make the decision for MI management, especially thrombolysis.

Echo Findings

Echocardiography in AMI is useful for identification of regional wall motion abnormalities (RWMA).

It can be used to ascertain any intracardiac complications, such as systolic dysfunction, acute mitral regurgitation (MR) from chordae tendineae or papillary muscle rupture, ventricular septal defect (VSD), pericardial effusion, tamponade from free wall rupture, mural thrombus, ventricular aneurysm, and pseudoaneurysm.

Over time, infarcted areas will appear thinned and fibrotic, and cardiac remodeling is identified by echo study.

Case 2

After a short course of viral illness, a 40-year-old lady, who was apparently healthy, presented with gradually increasing SOB, cough, and chest discomfort. With moderate anemia and dependent pitting edema, signs of biventricular failure are noted. Left ventricular type of apex with MR murmur is the prominent cardiac finding **(Fig. 4)**.

The utter importance of good history, clinical evaluations, and echo (as in **Figs. 5 and 6**) with support of ECG **(Fig. 4)** is reflected in this example. Some points may favor ischemic heart disease (IHD), whereas some points go in favor of rheumatic heart disease (RHD). But with an integral correlation of all, she is diagnosed as a patient with viral cardiomyopathy.

Keynote: The use of new echocardiographic technologies, such as three-dimensional (3D) echocardiography for more precise evaluation of LV volumes, ejection fraction (EF), and speckle tracking for the study of strain, particularly for early diagnosis, can be beneficial.

Hypertrophic Obstructive Cardiomyopathy

The term hypertrophic cardiomyopathy (HCM) precisely designates a disorder in which the heart muscle thickens (hypertrophies) abnormally. Though it can affect other areas of the heart as well, the LV is most frequently affected. These elements might cause symptoms such as SOB, chest pain (angina), fainting episodes, palpitations, and fatigue. In some cases, individuals with hypertrophic obstructive cardiomyopathy (HOCM) may not experience any symptoms at all.

ECG Findings

- Left ventricular hypertrophy with increased precordial voltages and nonspecific ST segment and T-wave abnormalities
- Deep, narrow ("dagger-like") Q waves in lateral (I, aVL, V_5-V_6) +/- inferior (II, III, aVF) leads
- Giant precordial T-wave inversions in apical HCM
- Left atrial enlargement (P mitrale) and some signs of Wolff–Parkinson–White (WPW) (short PR and delta wave)—ECG features of WPW were seen in 33% of patients with HCM in one study.

Echo Findings

These include asymmetrical septal hypertrophy, systolic anterior motion (SAM) of the mitral valve, a small LV cavity, septal immobility, and premature closure of the aortic valve. LV thickness, evaluated at the septum and free wall level, is considered abnormal when ≥15 mm, and defined as asymmetrical in the presence of a septal to free wall thickness ratio between 1.3 and 1.5.

Left Ventricular Diastolic Dysfunction

Left ventricular diastolic dysfunction [heart failure with preserved ejection fraction (HFpEF)] is a frequently recognized entity of various disease processes. Patient

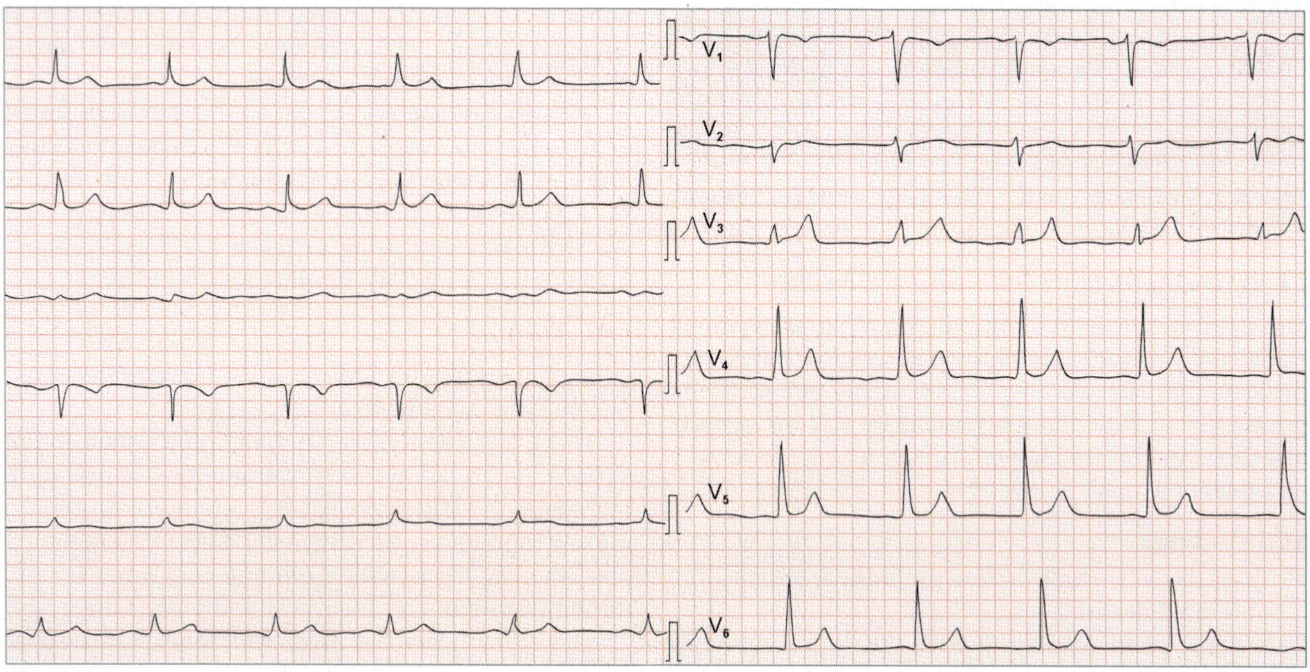

FIG. 4: ECG of case 2 shows a short PR.

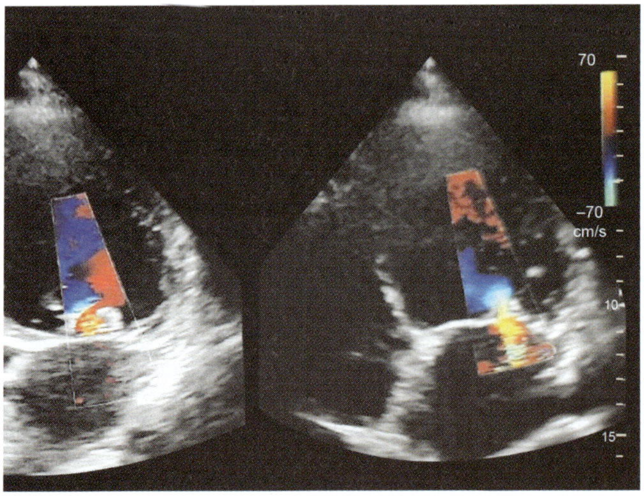

FIG. 5: Echo color Doppler study—moderate mitral regurgitation (MR).

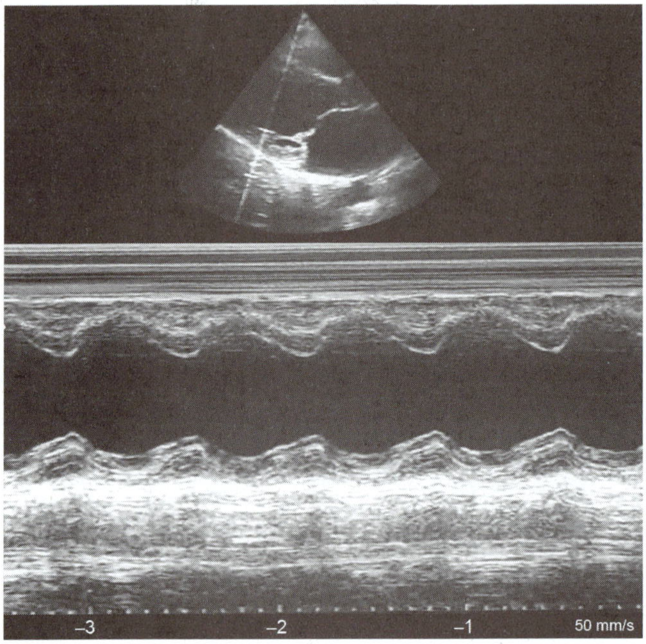

FIG. 6: 2D and M-mode study shows dilated left ventricle (LV).

usually presents with signs of heart failure, and ECG may not be helpful, except in the diagnosis of primary diseases such as LVH, IHD, and cardiomyopathy.

These four parameters are assessed to evaluate LVDD:

1. Medial and lateral mitral annular tissue Doppler velocity (e')
2. Average E/e' ratio. (<8 normal/>14 suggestive of LVDD)
3. Left atrial volume index (LAVI) = LA volume/body surface area
4. TR jet velocity.

ADVANTAGES OF CORRELATING ECG AND ECHO DATA

Improved Diagnostic Accuracy

Electrocardiography and echo can offer complementing information when performed in tandem, improving diagnostic precision and lowering the possibility of misdiagnosis.

Comprehensive Patient Assessment

Clinicians are better able to comprehend a patient's cardiac status when ECG and echo results are correlated. The patient's cardiovascular condition can be evaluated holistically by combining data on electrical activity, rhythm, and anatomical anomalies.

Guidance for Treatment Decisions

Treatment decisions can be guided by integrated ECG and echo data, especially in complex situations.

CHALLENGES AND LIMITATIONS

Technical Considerations

To acquire precise and trustworthy data, trained operators are needed for both ECG and echo. ECG lead placement errors or poor echocardiographic views might produce false results.

Interpretation Variability

As a result of the subjectivity involved in interpreting ECG and echo data, various clinicians may arrive at different diagnoses. This constraint can be lessened by creating standardized processes and enlisting the help of specialists.

CONCLUSION

A more detailed assessment of a patient's cardiovascular health is made possible by correlating ECG and echo data, which is essential in modern clinical practice.

Clinical decision-making, patient care, and diagnostic accuracy can all be enhanced by integrating electrical and structural data. However, difficulties like technical considerations and variations in interpretation underline the necessity of continual education and teamwork among doctors. The correlation of ECG and echo will remain a cornerstone in cardiovascular care as a result of technological and standardization developments, helping to improve patient outcomes and cardiac health in general.

SUGGESTED READINGS

1. Hampton J, Hampton J (Eds). The ECG Made Easy. International Edition, 9th edition. United Kingdom: Elsevier; 2019.
2. Sattar Y, Chhabra L. Electrocardiogram. In: StatPearls [Internet]. Treasure Island (FL): StatPearls Publishing; 2023.
3. Hillis GS, Bloomfield P. Basic transthoracic echocardiography. BMJ. 2005;330(7505):1432-6.
4. Cuspidi C, Sala C, Negri F, Mancia G, Morganti A; Italian Society of Hypertension. Prevalence of left-ventricular hypertrophy in hypertension: an updated review of echocardiographic studies. J Hum Hypertens. 2012;26(6):343-9.
5. Agrawal S, Kumar S, Gabhane V, Acharya S, Wanjari A. Electrocardiography and Echocardiography Correlation in Patients of Left Ventricular Hypertrophy. J Clin Diagnos Res. 2019;13(12):OC01-OC04.
6. Gupta NK, Agrawal RK, Srivastav AB, Ved ML. Echocardiographic evaluation of heart in chronic obstructive pulmonary disease patient and its co-relation with the severity of disease. Lung India. 2011;28(2):105-9.
7. Wilansky S. Echocardiography in the assessment of complications of myocardial infarction. Tex Heart Inst J. 1991;18(4):237-42.
8. Maron BJ, McKenna WJ, Danielson GK, Kappenberger LJ, Kuhn HJ, Seidman CE, et al. ACC/ESC clinical expert consensus document on hypertrophic cardiomyopathy: a report of the American College of Cardiology Task Force on Clinical Expert Consensus Documents and the European Society of Cardiology Committee for Practice Guidelines. J Am Coll Cardiol. 2003;42 (9):1687-713.
9. Nagaonkar VS. Study of correlation between ECG findings and echocardiographically detected left ventricular diastolic dysfunction. 2017;3(3):103-7.
10. Huis In't Veld AE, Man FS, Rossum AC, Handoko ML. How to diagnose heart failure with preserved ejection fraction: the value of invasive stress testing. Neth Heart J. 2016;24(4):244-51.

6

CHAPTER

Cardiomyopathy in Women

Soma Saha

ABSTRACT

Cardiomyopathies are a large group of heterogeneous cardiac muscle disorders characterized by myocardial structural and functional dysfunction in the absence of abnormal loading conditions. There are differences in the prevalence, clinical pattern, management, and outcomes between men and women as some variants of the disease are unique in women. The major impact on gender differences is due to the cellular effect of sex hormones on the renin–angiotensin–aldosterone system (RAAS), endothelial injury, vascular aging, and left ventricular remodeling. The socioeconomic, psychological and cultural factors, reluctance in disease acceptance, and everyday life approach may differ between men and women, leading to differences in approach, prognosis, and disease outcomes. Women are underrepresented in the majority of clinical trials, which may be the reason for the diagnostic bias and underutilization of treatment. The influence of the sex hormones in the pathophysiology of cardiomyopathy in women requires a better understanding of gender-specific cardiomyopathy and may help in early diagnosis and management. Understanding the gender-specific differences in epidemiology, pathophysiology and socioeconomic barriers of the management of heart failure (HF) and cardiomyopathy in women will help in better strategic planning for the better treatment outcomes in women with cardiomyopathy.

INTRODUCTION

Cardiomyopathies are a large group of heterogeneous cardiac muscle disorders characterized by myocardial structural and functional dysfunction in the absence of abnormal loading conditions such as coronary artery disease (CAD), valvular heart disease, congenital heart disease, or hypertension. Cardiomyopathies may be genetically inherited or acquired and exhibit ventricular inappropriate dilation or hypertrophy leading to electrical or mechanical dysfunction and progressive heart failure (HF). There are differences in the prevalence, clinical pattern, management, and outcomes between men and women as some variants of the disease like peripartum cardiomyopathy (PPCM) are specific to women. Some cardiomyopathies such as stress cardiomyopathy, hypertrophy cardiomyopathy (HCM), sarcoidosis, and amyloidosis have sex-specific differences in presentation, treatment, and outcomes. The major impact on gender differences is due to the cellular effect of sex hormones on the renin–angiotensin–aldosterone system (RAAS), endothelial injury, vascular aging, and left ventricular (LV) remodeling. The socioeconomic, psychological and cultural factors, and reluctance in disease acceptance may differ between men and women, leading to differences in the prognosis and disease outcomes. We will discuss the major differences in the epidemiology, genetics, pathophysiology, disease pattern, and treatment outcome of different cardiomyopathies between men and women and the gender-specific cardiomyopathies unique to women.

CLASSIFICATION OF CARDIOMYOPATHY

Cardiomyopathies are classified based on phenotypic information, which includes cardiac morphology, physiology, and cellular-molecular pathology. Various types of cardiomyopathies are as follows:

- Dilated cardiomyopathy (DCM)
- Restrictive cardiomyopathy (RCM)
- Hypertrophic cardiomyopathy
- Arrhythmogenic right ventricular cardiomyopathy (ARVC)
- Inflammatory cardiomyopathy
- Ischemic cardiomyopathy
- Infectious cardiomyopathy

CLINICAL PRESENTATION OF CARDIOMYOPATHY

All types of cardiomyopathies ultimately lead to HF due to either mechanical or electric dysfunction of the myocardium. HF may be classified as HF with preserved ejection fraction (HFpEF) when ejection fraction (EF) $>50\%$ or HF with reduced EF (HFrEF) when EF $<40\%$. HF imposes an economic burden on society due to recurrent hospitalization, and it is the major cause of morbidity and mortality in cardiomyopathy. HF affects 2.6 million women in the United States. There are gender-specific differences in HF regarding epidemiology, pathophysiology, and treatment outcomes.

Heart Failure with Reduced Ejection Fraction

The lifetime risk of HFrEF is lower in women (5.8%) compared to men (10.6%). This may be due to the fact that women have higher levels of natriuretic peptide than men. Women are more likely to have nonischemic cardiomyopathy, whereas men suffer from CAD. According to recent HF trials, PARADIGM-HF [Prospective comparison of Angiotensin Receptor-neprilysin (ARN) inhibitor with Angiotensin-converting enzyme (ACE) inhibitor to Determine Impact on Global Mortality and morbidity in Heart Failure] and ATMOSPHERE (Aliskiren Trial to Minimize Outcomes in Patients with Heart Failure), women have a lower quality of life (QOL) compared to men despite lower mortality due to HF compared to men.

SEX-BASED DIFFERENCE IN MEDICAL THERAPY AND INTERVENTION

Guideline-based medical therapy is the mainstay of treatment in HF. There is limited data from the landmark clinical trials of HF in women due to underrepresentation of women because of sociocultural barriers. Women have better survival benefit from angiotensin II receptor blockers (ARBs) compared to ACE inhibitors as estrogen stimulates increased angiotensin II receptor expression and activation. So, ARB and subsequently ARN inhibitors have better effect on women compared to ACE inhibitor.

SPECIFIC CARDIOMYOPATHIES FOR WOMEN

Some cardiomyopathies are specific and unique to women like PPCM and Takotsubo cardiomyopathy (TC).

Peripartum Cardiomyopathy

Peripartum cardiomyopathy is defined as dilatation of heart in a temporal relationship with pregnancy. It is the major cause of HF and high mortality in pregnancy and postpartum. The incidence of PPCM varies from 1 in 100 in Nigeria to 1 in 2,000 in Japan. The etiology of PPCM is multifactorial and may be associated with risk factors like black race, advanced maternal age, gestational hypertension, gestational diabetes, multifetal pregnancy, and anemia. The genetic predisposition of PPCM is supported by identifying *TTN* truncating variants (TTNtvs) by *DCM* gene sequencing. In a study of 90 families with DCM, 6% were found to have at least one member with PPCM. Hemodynamic stress in pregnancy may be one of the potential factors for PPCM as in vascular-hormonal animal models of pregnancy-associated cardiomyopathy have been studied for the same. The cleavage of nursing hormone prolactin due to oxidative stress to 16-kDa prolactin fragments causes vasculoendothelial toxicity and decreases the expression of vaculo proangiogenic growth factor (VEGF), leading to myocardial injury in the animal model. The cardiomyopathy was partly reversed with bromocriptine in this model and a complete recovery was achieved with the addition of VEGF in this model.

A majority of women present with signs and symptoms of HF in immediate postpartum period of delivery. Though the myocardial dysfunction started in the later phase of pregnancy, but the overt symptoms of HF are masked by the pregnancy. Because the spontaneous resolution of the LV function is known to occur in mild cases in the peripartum or immediate postpartum period, the incidence of PPCM is underreported, and the incidence of PPCM in subsequent pregnancy is underestimated. The usual presentations are breathlessness on exertion, orthopnea, paroxysmal nocturnal dyspnea, palpitation, and pedal edema. Arrhythmia, thromboembolism, and cardiogenic shock are found in a very small number of cases.

An echocardiogram is a diagnostic test to pick up PPCM, which shows LV or biventricular dilatation with systolic dysfunction in the form of reduced EF < 45%. N-terminal pro-B-type natriuretic peptide (NT-proBNP) levels are grossly elevated in HF. Cardiac MRI is a more specific diagnostic tool for the diagnosis of right ventricular (RV) dysfunction. Recovery occurs within 3–6 months of postpartum period but delayed recovery is also reported as late as 2 years.

The management of PPCM is similar to that of other forms of nonischemic DCM, which includes guideline-directed medical therapy (GDMT), considering fetal safety and lactation. Oral anticoagulation therapy in postpartum period and injectables in the third trimester are also suggested, considering the hypercoagulable state of pregnancy. The indication of starting oral anticoagulation is EF between 30 and 35% according to the American College of Cardiology (ACC) and European Society of Cardiology (ESC). The prolactin inhibitor bromocriptine has shown greater improvement in the EF ranging from 27 to 58% when given at the dose of 2.5 mg twice daily for 2 weeks followed by 2.5 mg daily for 6 weeks. The National Institute of Health supported randomized double-blind study for the evaluation of bromocriptine in women with PPCM (the REBIRTH study). It is in the experimental phase and is yet to start in the United State and Canada. The 2018 ESC guidelines included a weak recommendation (class IIb, level of evidence B) for the use of bromocriptine. The 2010 ESC statement advised against breastfeeding based on prolactin hypothesis. However, a small study in the United State showed greater recovery with breastfeeding, and it is not associated with any adverse outcome or persistent myocardial dysfunction.

Hemodynamic instability despite medical therapy should prompt early delivery. Vaginal delivery should be the mode of delivery unless there are obstetric indications for cesarean section. Volume overload in the immediate postpartum period may be treated with diuretics and other GDMT. HF medications should be continued indefinitely with persistent LV dysfunction. After recovery of cardiac function, the duration of continuation of treatment is unknown. There may be subclinical LV dysfunction, which may be a reason for the continuation of HF medications. HF medications should be weaned in a stepwise fashion with frequent clinical assessment and echocardiographic monitoring every 3–6 months.

There is always a subclinical myocardial dysfunction even after recovery from HF. The 2018 ESC guidelines discouraged subsequent pregnancy if left ventricular ejection fraction (LVEF) is not >50–55%. The risk associated with subsequent pregnancy depends upon recovery of LV systolic function and prepregnancy LVEF. Contraception is recommended with progesterone-based oral contraceptives (OCPs) and subcutaneous or intrauterine device avoiding estrogen-containing OCP.

Stress Cardiomyopathy or Takotsubo Cardiomyopathy

Stress cardiomyopathy or TC, also known as apical ballooning syndrome or broken heart syndrome, is a transient and reversible cardiomyopathy in which LV dilatation and acute HF occur following physical or intense emotional stress. It is more common in females than males; the female and male ratio is 9:1. In an International Takotsubo Registry of 1,750 patients, 89.8% were women, the vast majority of them were post-menopausal >55 years of age. Predominant symptoms are chest pain (in 76% patients) followed by dyspnea (in 47%) and syncope (in 7.7%). Preceding physical (in 36%) and emotional (in 28%) triggers with elevated troponin values (in 87%) and ST elevation are found in the ECG in almost half of the patients.

The pathophysiology of TC is uncertain. A different hypothesis suggested that estrogen deficiency and increased autonomic activity lead to sympathetic stimulation, which causes microvasculature disruption and myocardial dysfunction ultimately landing with apical ballooning and pump failure. Echocardiography is one of the standard investigating tools for TC. Typical LV contractile abnormalities involving the apex are found in >80% of the patients. There may be acute LV outflow tract obstruction because of the compensatory hyperdynamic contraction of the basal LV segment with associated apical LV dyskinesia and systolic anterior motion of the mitral valve with associated outflow tract gradient and hypotension. The management of TC is like that of acute HF. The in-hospital mortality rate is 4.1%. Most of the deaths occur due to irreversible cardiogenic shock, LV rupture or malignant ventricular arrhythmia, or rarely complete heart block. TC is a self-limited disorder with complete or nearly complete resolution of LV dysfunction within days to weeks. The use of ACE inhibitors for a long term has been shown to reduce recurrence, though prophylactic beta blockers are not recommended.

Cardiac Amyloidosis

Cardiac amyloidosis is a form of infiltrative myocardial disease caused by the deposition of amyloid fibrils within the myocardium. There are two forms of cardiac amyloidosis, the first is light chain amyloidosis (AL) and the second is transthyretin amyloid cardiomyopathy (ATTR-CM). Male preponderance of ATTR-CM with 80–90% may be due to the protection of female by the female sex hormone against the myocardial involvement in ATTR amyloidosis. Different studies show that females have lesser interventricular and posterior wall thickness, and lower median LV mass compared to males.

Cardiac Sarcoidosis

Cardiac sarcoidosis is an inflammatory granulomatous disease that is more common in black women and residents of Northern Latitude. In a study by Myocardial Inflammatory Disease in Finland (MIDFIN), women have a higher frequency of LV systolic dysfunction and septal wall motion abnormalities. In the United State, a national survey identified female preponderance of cardiac sarcoidosis (n = 200 of 241, 67% women). Women are more susceptible to atrial arrhythmia compared to men who have higher rates of ventricular arrhythmia and require implantable cardioverter-defibrillator (ICD) or cardiac resynchronization therapy (CRT) with defibrillator. LV dysfunction is the strongest predictor of survival in patients with cardiac sarcoidosis. Data on sex differences in cardiac sarcoidosis outcomes are limited and may be due to the under representation of women in the different clinical trials of HF and underutilization of devices (ICD, CRT-D) in women with cardiac sarcoidosis compared to men.

Hypertrophy Cardiomyopathy

Hypertrophy cardiomyopathy is an autosomal dominant inheritance genetic cardiomyopathy with a male preponderance of 55–65%. Women are more likely to have functional disabilities and experience death from HF and stroke than men because of delayed diagnosis and more disabilities in the form of higher outflow gradient, worse diastolic function, and severe HF symptoms at presentation. Compared to male patients, women with HCM and a greater amount of fibrosis at the cellular level contribute to worse outcomes. The sex differences in the mortality and outcome between the cohort despite similar therapy may be attributed to the sex differences in disease phenotype or progression at the time of diagnosis and management.

CONCLUSION

The differences in the epidemiology, etiology, pathophysiology, clinical presentation, and outcomes in different types of cardiomyopathy in women determine the prognosis. Few cardiomyopathies like PPCM and TC are unique in women. Sex hormones play a major role in the etiopathogenesis of cardiomyopathy in women. There is inadequate data on the evaluation and outcome of the cardiovascular disease in women due to under representation of women in the different major clinical trials of cardiovascular diseases. Women should be included in an equal number in the trials. Gender-specific medicine is more personalized for targeted risk stratification and a therapeutic approach for women to reduce inappropriate treatment and optimization of cost effectiveness. The gender-specific approach yields a better understanding and proper utilization of available treatment modalities in women with cardiomyopathies.

SUGGESTED READINGS

1. Pinto YM, Elliott PM, Arbustini E, Adler Y, Anastasakis A, Bohm M, et al. Proposal for a revised definition of dilated cardiomyopathy, hypokinetic non-dilated cardiomyopathy, and its implications for clinical practice: a position statement of the ESC working group on myocardial and pericardial diseases. Eur Heart J. 2016;37:1850-8.
2. Virani SS, Alonso A, Aparicio HJ, Benjamin EJ, Bittencourt MS, Callaway CW, et al.; American Heart Association Council on Epidemiology and Prevention Statistics Committee and Stroke Statistics Subcommittee. Heart disease stroke statistics-2021 update: a report from the American Heart Association. Circulation. 2021;143(8):e254-743.
3. Pandey A, Omar W, Ayers C, LaMonte M, Klein L, Allen NB, et al. Sex and race differences in lifetime risk of heart failure with preserved ejection fraction and heart failure with reduced ejection fraction. Circulation. 2018;137:1814-23.
4. Mentzer G, Hsich EM. Heart failure with reduced ejection fraction in women: epidemiology, outcomes, and treatment. Heart Fail Clin. 2019;15:19-27.
5. Dewan P, Rørth R, Jhund PS, Shen L, Raparelli V, Petrie MC, et al. Differential impact of heart failure with reduced ejection fraction on men and women. J Am Coll Cardiol. 2019;73(1):29-40.
6. Hudson M, Rahme E, Behlouli H, Sheppard R, Pilote L. Sex differences in the effectiveness of angiotensin receptor blockers and angiotensin converting enzyme inhibitors in patients with congestive heart failure-a population study. Eur J Heart Fail. 2007;9:602-9.
7. Kamiya CA, Kitakaze M, Ishibashi-Ueda H, Nakatani S, Murohara T, Tomoike H, et al. Different characteristics of peripartum cardiomyopathy between patients complicated with and without hypertensive disorders. Results from the Japanese Nationwide survey of peripartum cardiomyopathy. Circ J. 2011;75:1975-81.
8. van Spaendonck-Zwarts KY, van Tintelen JP, van Veldhuisen DJ, van der Werf R, Jongbloed JD, Paulus WJ, et al. Peripartum cardiomyopathy as a part of familial dilated cardiomyopathy. Circulation. 2010;121:2169-75.
9. Patten IS, Rana S, Shahul S, Rowe GC, Jang C, Liu L, et al. Cardiac angiogenic imbalance leads to peripartum cardiomyopathy. Nature. 2012;485:333-8.
10. Regitz-Zagrosek V, Roos-Hesselink JW, Bauersachs J, Blomström-Lundqvist C, Cífková R, De Bonis M, et al. 2018 ESC guidelines for the management of cardiovascular diseases during pregnancy. Eur Heart J. 2018;39:3165-241.

11. Templin C, Ghadri JR, Diekmann J, Napp LC, Bataiosu DR, Jaguszewski M, et al. Clinical features and outcomes of takotsubo (stress) Cardiomyopathy. N Engl J Med. 2015;373:929-38.
12. Agdamag AC, Patel H, Chandra S, Rao A, Suboc TM, Marinescu K, et al. Sex differences in takotsubo syndrome: a narrative review. J Womens Health (Larchmt). 2020;29(8):1122-30.
13. Hahn VS, Yanek LR, Vaishnav J, Ying W, Vaidya D, Lee YZJ, et al. Endomyocardial biopsy characterization of heart failure with preserved ejection fraction and prevalence of cardiac amyloidosis. JACC Heart Fail. 2020;8:712-24.
14. Kandolin R, Lehtonen J, Airaksinen J, Vihinen T, Miettinen H, Ylitalo K, et al. Cardiac sarcoidosis: epidemiology, characteristics, and outcome over 25 years in a nationwide study. Circulation. 2015;131(7):624-32.
15. Olivotto I, Maron MS, Adabag AS, Casey SA, Vargiu D, Link MS, et al. Gender-related differences in the clinical presentation and outcome of hypertrophic cardiomyopathy. J Am Coll Cardiol. 2005;46(3):480-7.

7

CHAPTER

Prosthetic Valve Thrombosis

Suresh V Sagarad, Sweta Amaresh Biradar

ABSTRACT

Mechanical heart valve while prolonging the life of patients with severe valvular disease are associated with risk of pannus formation, degeneration, endocarditis, and thrombosis. Though oral anticoagulation is used to prevent thrombosis of mechanical valves, this complication happens in significant proportion of patients despite frequent monitoring. Subtherapeutic international normalized ratio (INR) is the important underlying risk factor in many while hypercoagulable state may contribute in some. Cinefluorography was the gold standard in olden days; however, availability of echocardiography, especially the advent of transesophageal echocardiography (TEE) and three-dimensional (3D) echocardiography has extended diagnostic capabilities. Multidetector computed tomography (CT) is useful wherever available. Optimizing oral anticoagulation is critical in most patients with smaller thrombus and in less symptomatic cases. Thrombolysis is useful in dissolving thrombus, low dose slow thrombolytic infusion is associated with lower complications and higher success rates. Surgery is the preferred choice with larger thrombus with evidence of systemic embolization. Transcatheter manipulation is currently reserved for very high risk for surgery.

INTRODUCTION

Prosthetic heart valves have reduced morbidity and mortality in patients with severe valvular heart disease. Prosthetic heart valves have been used in various clinical situations involving different valves mainly mitral and aortic valves. However, prosthetic heart valves require continued monitoring with lifelong anticoagulation, especially with mechanical prosthesis. Thrombosis, pannus formation, degeneration, and endocarditis are important complications associated with prosthetic heart valves. These can be associated with increased morbidity and mortality. Prosthetic heart valve thrombosis is an important complications which can be asymptomatic or immediately life threatening. All healthcare providers managing these patients with prosthetic heart valves should be aware about this.

INCIDENCE, ETIOLOGY, AND PATHOPHYSIOLOGY

The estimated annual rate of mechanical valve thrombosis (MVT) ranges from 0.1 to 5.7% within 3 months from surgical implantation procedure. High shear stress across prosthetic valve leads to blood cell damage and activation of platelets. Prosthetic valve surface augments clotting through protein adsorption, cellular adhesion, thrombin generation, and activation of complement system.

RISK FACTORS FOR THROMBOSIS

- *Type of valves*: Three major types of valves are commonly used, i.e., (1) caged ball, (2) tilting disk, and (3) bileaflet valves. Caged ball and older tilting disk valves had higher risk of thrombosis. Bileaflet designs are commonly used due to better hemodynamics and low thrombogenicity. However, older tilting disk and caged ball valves can still be encountered in older patients who have undergone surgery long back.

- Subtherapeutic anticoagulation, short interruptions, and poor adherence to medications
- Hypercoagulable state

CLINICAL PRESENTATION

Thrombus formation leads to obstruction and/or regurgitation of the valve. Clinical presentation will depend upon degree of acuity and severity. Clinical presentation can range from incidental with no symptoms to severe cardiogenic shock. Often they present with features of heart failure and cardiogenic shock. Examination may reveal reduced or absent clicking associated with valve opening and closing, new murmur, signs of pulmonary edema, and congestive heart failure. There may be features of pulmonary or systemic embolism. Ischemic stroke may be first presentation of prosthetic valve thrombosis and needs high index of suspicion.

DIAGNOSTIC EVALUATION

Echocardiography, cinefluorography, and multidetector computed tomography (CT) are commonly used imaging modalities to assess prosthetic valve thrombosis. Imaging modality should identify etiology, location, severity, and hemodynamic changes.

Echocardiography

Echocardiography is the initial investigation of choice. Two-dimensional (2D) imaging commonly used and can be supplemented with 3D wherever available. Valve appearance, leaflet mobility, and presence of thrombus can be assessed by 2D imaging.

Depending on the valve position and imaging plane, mechanical valve appears as echogenic structure with varying degrees of shadowing artifact. Characteristic leaflet motion can be appreciated by echocardiography. M mode is useful to improve temporal resolution. Mechanical valves have an expected opening and closing angles depending on the make. Manufacturer does provide that information with observed deviation. Transesophageal echocardiography identifies opening and closing angles better than transthoracic echocardiography (100% vs. 85% in mitral position, 77% vs. 40% in aortic position with single disk valves). Assessment is less accurate for bileaflet prosthesis.

Color Doppler assessment: Obstruction will lead to flow acceleration with increased blood velocity that will be proportional to degree of obstruction generally. Inadequate valve closure will lead to valvular or paravalvular regurgitation that can be detected as regurgitant jet. Valvular and paravalvular regurgitation are due to different etiologies and hence should be clearly identified to initiate specific therapeutic option. Impaired valve disk motion due to vegetation, pannus, or thrombus leading to valve closure will lead to valvular regurgitation. Multiple etiologies may coexist together. Suture line disruption due to technical error, annular disruption, suture failure, or endocarditis will lead to paravalvular leak.

Spectral Doppler

Prosthetic valve obstruction is usually defined as mean transvalvular gradient increase of >50% (or an increase >10 mm Hg across an aortic prosthesis) compared with the postoperative baseline value. Baseline postoperative values should be known for comparison. Delay in peak transvalvular velocity generation. Acceleration time (AT) >100 ms is 86% sensitive and specific for aortic valve obstruction. Indexing the AT to total ejection time (ET) (i.e., the AT/ET ratio) is also more useful to assess for pathologic obstruction; an AT/ET ratio >0.37 provides 96% sensitivity and 82% specificity for stenosis, whereas an AT >128 ms and AT/ET >0.58 is 100% specific for stenosis.

A Doppler velocity index <0.25 is 59% sensitive and 100% specific for stenosis. Comparing the calculated effective orifice area (EOA) with values reported by the manufacturer aids in diagnosis. Normal Doppler echocardiographic parameters that are suggestive of prosthetic valve obstruction for the four valve positions have been provided by the American Society of Echocardiography guidelines. Acoustic shadowing, reverberation artifacts, and poor acoustic windows may lead to erroneous measurement of EOA via miscalculation of the left ventricular outflow tract diameter and velocity-time integral. This problem can be overcome with the use of 3D. EOA derived via three-dimensional-transesophageal echocardiography (3D-TEE) has been shown to yield more accurate results.

Cardiac Computed Tomography and Magnetic Resonance Imaging

Multidetector CT is useful and can accurately measure degree of leaflet restriction. CT can differentiate pannus from thrombus depending on attenuation values. A cutoff of >145 HU more likely pannus while values below this more likely thrombus. Resolution of mass and improvement in leaflet mobility on serial scanning is a sign of therapeutic efficacy. In one of the study, thrombolysis was found to be more beneficial for lesion with <90 HU on CT imaging. Due to significant artifacts during MRI, currently cardiac MRI is not recommended for prosthetic valve evaluation.

MANAGEMENT

Outcome is better if detected early when thrombus size is small. <5 mm thrombus are generally nonobstructive with good response and lesser risk of complications. Obstructive symptoms with higher risk of embolization is more often with >5 mm thrombus. Adequate anticoagulation is critical in the management. For uncomplicated less severe clinical situations optimization of anticoagulation and follow-up imaging to monitor thrombus resolution is recommended. Unfractionated heparin (UFH) or low molecular heparin can be added till adequate anticoagulation with oral anticoagulants is achieved. Larger thrombus >10 mm with evidence of systemic embolization generally requires surgical intervention.

Therapeutic options available for obstructive thrombus include optimizing anticoagulation, thrombolysis, transcatheter manipulation, and surgery.

Anticoagulation

Subtherapeutic anticoagulation is the most common underlying pathogenetic basis for MVT. Heparin with warfarin to achieve optimal international normalized ratio (INR) is the mainstay of treatment. At least partial resolution can be achieved, especially when thrombus is small (<10 mm). Subsequent risk of thrombosis is very high in patients who had MVT. Higher oral anticoagulation dosage is recommended to keep INR in higher range. Strict adherence and monitoring is necessary to prevent further events. Direct oral anticoagulants are attractive agents in nonvalvular anticoagulant indicated situations, however, no recommendations yet to use these agents in MVT.

Thrombolysis

Thrombolytic therapy can be considered in selected patients. Smaller size of the thrombus has the highest prediction for success and low rate of complication. Compared to patients with thrombus size <0.8 cm^2, an incremental increase in thrombus area of 1 cm^2 by TEE measurement was associated with a 2.4-fold increased complication risk, and a history of prior stroke was associated with a 4.5-fold increase in complication rate. Thrombus area of <0.8 cm^2 identified patients with low complication risk (6%), compared to a thrombus area of 0.8–1.6 cm^2 (29%) and >1.6 cm^2 (47%). In the TROIA (Comparison of Different Transesophageal Echocardiography Guided Thrombolytic Regimens for Prosthetic Valve Thrombosis) trial, which included the largest patient cohort with MVT, a low-dose (25 mg) and slow (6 hours) infusion of tissue plasminogen activator (tPA) without bolus the study showed no difference in mortality when compared to higher doses or faster infusions; however, there were fewer nonfatal major complications with a low-dose and slow-infusion regimen. In PROMETE (Prosthetic Mechanical Valve Thrombosis and the Predictors of Outcome) trial, which used a low-dose (25 mg), ultra-slow (25 hours) tPA infusion showed a 90% success rate with low complications (<2% each for mortality, bleeding, and major embolus). In each of these trials, anticoagulation was maintained using UFH and paused during thrombolytic infusion, with interval echocardiographic imaging done to assess need for repeat dosing until resolution was achieved. Important contraindications to thrombolysis included left atrial thrombus, ischemic stroke within 3 weeks of presentation, history of hemorrhagic stroke, or a bleeding diathesis (generally an INR >3). Studies do support use of thrombolysis both in left- and right-sided MVT.

Transcatheter Interventions

Percutaneous transcatheter approach is not part of the guidelines at present; however, the procedure has been proven to be safe and effective in a small number of patients who fail or have a contraindications to thrombolysis, decline redo surgery, and have very high surgical risk. It works as bridge to redo surgery through the acute phase of cardiogenic shock.

Redo Surgery

Clinical outcome of redo surgery is determined by functional class (17.5% mortality in class IV vs. 4.7% mortality in class I–III). Surgery allows replacement of older thrombogenic valves with newer low thrombogenic valves. A definitive diagnosis and treatment is possible if diagnosis is doubtful. Trials comparing redo surgery and thrombolysis have varying results based on inclusion criteria. Redo surgery is required in cases during which thrombolytic therapy does not achieve hemodynamic stability. Thrombolysis and catheter manipulations are more effective if fresh thrombus while organized mature thrombus can be effectively treated with surgery.

CONCLUSION

Patients with prosthetic heart valves presenting with new onset heart failure should be evaluated for prosthetic heart valve thrombosis. Some patients may be asymptomatic or minimally symptomatic which needs high index of suspicion. Multimodality imaging with echocardiography including TEE, cinefluorography, and CT scan are useful to assess these patients. Patients with smaller size thrombus can be managed with optimizing anticoagulation. Low-dose slow thrombolysis has been shown to be effective. Patients with larger thrombus with evidence of systemic embolization are better treated with surgery. Currently transcatheter manipulation is reserved for patients with high risk for surgery and contraindications for thrombolysis.

SUGGESTED READINGS

1. Otto CM, Nishimura RA, Bonow RO, Carabello BA, Erwin JP 3rd, Gentile F, et al. 2020 ACC/AHA Guideline for the Management of Patients With Valvular Heart Disease: Executive Summary: A Report of the American College of Cardiology/American Heart Association Joint Committee on Clinical Practice Guidelines. Circulation. 2021;143(5):e35-e71. Erratum in: Circulation. 2021;143(5):e228. Erratum in: Circulation. 2021;143(10):e784.
2. Yoganathan AP, He Z, Casey Jones S. Fluid mechanics of heart valves. Annu Rev Biomed Eng. 2004;6:331-62.
3. Metzdorff MT, Grunkemeier GL, Pinson CW, Starr A. Thrombosis of mechanical cardiac valves: a qualitative comparison of the silastic ball valve and the tilting disc valve. J Am Coll Cardiol. 1984;4:50-3.
4. Deviri E, Sareli P, Wisenbaugh T, Cronje SL. Obstruction of mechanical heart valve prostheses: clinical aspects and surgical management. J Am Coll Cardiol. 1991;17:646-50.
5. Suh YJ, Kim YJ, Hong YJ, Lee HJ, Hur J, Im DJ, et al. Measurement of Opening and Closing Angles of Aortic Valve Prostheses In Vivo Using Dual-Source Computed Tomography: Comparison with Those of Manufacturers' in 10 Different Types. Korean J Radiol. 2015;16(5):1012-23.
6. Muratori M, Montorsi P, Teruzzi G, Celeste F, Doria E, Alamanni F, et al. Feasibility and diagnostic accuracy of quantitative assessment of mechanical prostheses leaflet motion by transthoracic and transesophageal echocardiography in suspected prosthetic valve dysfunction. Am J Cardiol. 2006;97(1):94-100.
7. Marcoff L, Koulogiannis KP, Aldaia L, Fuschetto DP, Kipperman RM, Laighold S, et al. Color Paucity as a Marker of Transcatheter Valve Thrombosis. JACC Cardiovasc Imaging. 2017;10(1):78-81.
8. Ben Zekry S, Saad RM, Ozkan M, Al Shahid MS, Pepi M, Muratori M, et al. Flow acceleration time and ratio of acceleration time to ejection time for prosthetic aortic valve function. JACC Cardiovasc Imaging. 2011;4(11):1161-70.
9. Zoghbi WA, Chambers JB, Dumesnil JG, Foster E, Gottdiener JS, Grayburn PA, et al. Recommendations for evaluation of prosthetic valves with echocardiography and doppler ultrasound: a report From the American Society of Echocardiography's Guidelines and Standards Committee and the Task Force on Prosthetic Valves, developed in conjunction with the American College of Cardiology Cardiovascular Imaging Committee, Cardiac Imaging Committee of the American Heart Association, the European Association of Echocardiography, a registered branch of the European Society of Cardiology, the Japanese Society of Echocardiography and the Canadian Society of Echocardiography, endorsed by the American College of Cardiology Foundation, American Heart Association, European Association of Echocardiography, a registered branch of the European Society of Cardiology, the Japanese Society of Echocardiography, and Canadian Society of Echocardiography. J Am Soc Echocardiogr. 2009;22(9):975-1014; quiz 1082-4.
10. Ozkaramanli Gur D, Baykiz D, Gur O, Alpsoy S, Akyuz A, Gurkan S. Evaluation of mechanical prosthetic valves: the role of three dimensional echocardiography in calculating effective orifice area in obese vs non-obese individuals. Int J Cardiovasc Imaging. 2021;37(1):215-27.
11. Gündüz S, Özkan M, Kalçik M, Gürsoy OM, Astarcioğlu MA, Karakoyun S, et al. Sixty-Four-Section Cardiac Computed Tomography in Mechanical Prosthetic Heart Valve Dysfunction: Thrombus or Pannus. Circ Cardiovasc Imaging. 2015;8(12): e003246.
12. Vahanian A, Beyersdorf F, Praz F, Milojevic M, Baldus S, Bauersachs J, et al. 2021 ESC/EACTS Guidelines for the management of valvular heart disease. Eur Heart J. 2022; 43(7):561-632.
13. Tong AT, Roudaut R, Ozkan M, Sagie A, Shahid MS, Pontes Júnior SC, et al. Transesophageal echocardiography improves risk assessment of thrombolysis of prosthetic valve thrombosis: results of the international PRO-TEE registry. J Am Coll Cardiol. 2004;43(1):77-84.
14. Özkan M, Gündüz S, Biteker M, Astarcioglu MA, Çevik C, Kaynak E, et al. Comparison of different TEE-guided thrombolytic regimens for prosthetic valve thrombosis: the TROIA trial. JACC Cardiovasc Imaging. 2013;6(2):206-16.
15. Özkan M, Gündüz S, Gürsoy OM, Karakoyun S, Astarcıoğlu MA, Kalçık M, et al. Ultraslow thrombolytic therapy: A novel strategy in the management of PROsthetic MEchanical valve Thrombosis and the prEdictors of outcomE: The Ultra-slow PROMETEE trial. Am Heart J. 2015;170(2):409-18.
16. Hariram V. Percutaneous management of prosthetic valve thrombosis. Indian Heart J. 2014;66(4):427-9.
17. Chen Y, Waksman R, Satler L, Barnett C, Chen A, Rogers T. Percutaneous transcatheter release of stuck mechanical mitral valve leaflet. Eur Heart J. 2020;41(41):4072.
18. Soria Jiménez CE, Papolos AI, Kenigsberg BB, Ben-Dor I, Satler LF, Waksman R, et al. Management of Mechanical Prosthetic Heart Valve Thrombosis: JACC Review Topic of the Week. J Am Coll Cardiol. 2023;81(21):2115-27.

8

CHAPTER

Cardiac Imaging for the Physicians

Mainak Mukhopadhyay

ABSTRACT

Cardiac imaging provides physicians with a comprehensive understanding of the heart's anatomy and function, aiding in the diagnosis of cardiovascular disorders, such as coronary artery disease (CAD), valvular heart disease, congenital heart disease, and diseases of the great arteries. Its accuracy and precision, enhanced by artificial intelligence (AI), make it a valuable tool for heart disease diagnosis and treatment.

INTRODUCTION

In recent years, physicians have relied more and more on cardiac imaging to identify and treat cardiac patients. Both structural and functional advanced imaging of the heart has ushered a new dawn. This kind of imaging is crucial for cardiac care because it enables physicians to make enlightened judgments and provide patients with individualized care. To identify and treat cardiac patients more precisely, this manuscript will look into the quick developments in cardiac imaging technology.

VARIOUS MODALITIES OF CARDIAC IMAGING

Cardiac imaging has developed to the point where a variety of imaging modalities are available to help doctors better diagnose and treat cardiac patients, namely:

- Chest X-ray
- Echocardiography
- Cardiac computed tomography (CT)
- Cardiac magnetic resonance imaging (MRI)
- Nuclear imaging
- Coronary imaging
- Fusion imaging
- Artificial intelligence (AI) in cardiac imaging

Not every patient needs all the imaging modalities. Depending upon the clinical presentation initial diagnostic imaging modality is chosen. Some patients need various modalities for diagnosis, planning of therapy, and for follow-up.

CHEST X-RAY IN CARDIOLOGY

With the advent of various modern cardiac imaging modalities, the reliability of chest X-rays for cardiac evaluation has decreased a lot nowadays. Still, in resource-limited situations, we cannot deny its role. Radiologically the heart size is considered normal if the cardiothoracic ratio (cardiac width/thoracic width) is <50% and cardiac shadow is considered enlarged when the ratio is >50% **(Fig. 1)**. Good quality posteroanterior (PA) chest X-ray with no rotation (the spinous processes are at the midpoint between the medial ends of the clavicles) allows the heart size to be assessed accurately. Taking into consideration both the PA and lateral views, we can have an idea about the chamber of enlargement. Assessment of the vascular congestion is also very important. Normally the upper zone vessels are smaller than the lower zone vessels. The lungs are clear—indicating there is no pulmonary edema. The costophrenic angles are well-defined indicating that there is no pleural effusion. The upper zone vessels' prominence is an indicator of increased pulmonary

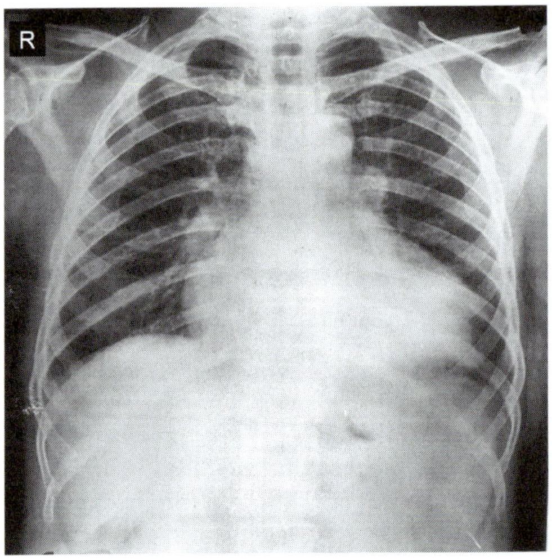

FIG. 1: Chest X-ray showing cardiomegaly with upper lobe venous prominence in a patient of dilated cardiomyopathy (DCM).

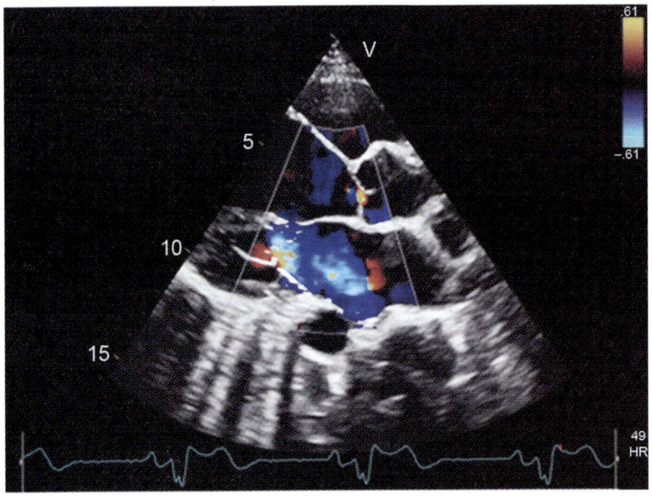

FIG. 2: Parasternal long-axis view in TTE of a DCM patient showing mitral regurgitation jet (blue).
(DCM: dilated cardiomyopathy; TTE: transthoracic echocardiography)

venous pressure. Signs of pulmonary edema are septal lines (Kerley B lines-horizontal lines which contact the edge of the lung) due to interstitial edema, and airspace shadowing due to alveolar edema. The costophrenic angles may be blunt due to bilateral pleural effusions. In the context of acute pulmonary edema, alveolar edema radiates symmetrically from the hilar regions in a "bat's wing" distribution of airspace shadowing.

ECHOCARDIOGRAPHY DOPPLER IMAGING

The application of ultrasound in medical science is ubiquitous. Echocardiography is the second most widely used cardiac diagnostic modality after ECG. The age-old days of only M-mode echocardiography have become the story of the past and at present, we are witnessing the application of AI in the advanced echo modes, viz., three-dimensional (3D) echo, speckled tracking, strain imaging, etc. Echocardiography is performed for structural (anatomical) and hemodynamical assessment of the heart. After the recent application of tissue Doppler and strain imaging, time-specific information (regional time to peak contraction and blood-speckled tracking) is also available. Echocardiography, apart from diagnostic information, also provides us with prognostic information. A good interpretation of the echocardiography study warrants ECG-guided echo and clinical correlation.

There are various types of echocardiography available nowadays, namely:

- *Transthoracic echocardiography (TTE)*: TTE is the most performed echo both for the adult and pediatric group **(Fig. 2)**.
- *Transesophageal echocardiography (TEE)*: TEE is performed through the esophagus. It gives an excellent clear imaging window for the evaluation of prosthetic valves, interatrial septum, aortic root, aorta, left atrial appendage, and pulmonary veins.
- *Intracardiac echocardiography (ICE)*: Nowadays for various cardiac interventional procedures (e.g., septal puncture, ablation, etc.) ICE is being applied.
- *Stress echocardiography*: Dobutamine stress echocardiography is regularly being used for evaluation of hibernating viable myocardium, low-flow low-gradient aortic stenosis, etc. DSE is an alternative to treadmill test (TMT) for patients who cannot perform exercise stress tests. To assess how well the heart pumps under normal and stressful conditions, a stress echocardiogram is performed. Dobutamine or atropine is often used for this procedure, which may be done through transthoracic or transesophageal methods.
- *Contrast echocardiography (CE)*: Commonly used is bubble CE for evaluation of shunts. CE is effective in the evaluation of LV function in TTE if the window is not good enough. CE aids in the assessment of coronary perfusion as well as the imaging of the left ventricle under a better window.
- *3D echocardiography*: Both TTE and TEE 3D echocardiography are available. This advanced instrument gives an excellent structural demonstration of the heart. Due to its full 3D imaging of the heart architecture and thorough examination of left ventricular functional parameters, 3D echocardiography improves the diagnostic accuracy and precision of cardiac structural and functional evaluation **(Fig. 3)**.

- *Fetal echo Doppler*: This is done between 18 and 22 weeks of the antenatal period to exclude any significant cardiac structural anomaly, especially in high-risk individuals.
- *Tissue Doppler echo and strain imaging*: Tissue Doppler imaging is continually gaining popularity since it can be used to evaluate the heart's tissues' and muscles' velocities, allowing for the determination of the regional systolic and diastolic functions of both the left and right ventricles.

Two-dimensional (2D) M-mode echocardiography provides us with an anatomical picture with 2D measurements. Doppler-echo is an integral part of the clinical evaluation of cardiac patients as it provides comprehensive hemodynamic information for accurate assessment of severity. Normal blood flow in circulation is known as laminar flow whereas a disturbed flow (stenotic, regurgitant shunt flows, etc.) is known as turbulent flow. Pulse wave Doppler (PW) records velocity at a particular predetermined site. It is used for diastolic function assessment and is important in continuity equations for valve area calculation. Continuous wave (CW) records high-velocity flow, hence ideal for evaluation of turbulent flow along the whole of the Doppler beam. The gradient is a difference in pressure between two chambers. Peak gradient is related to blood flow and hence tachycardia, exercise, anemia, thyrotoxicosis, or any other high output state can increase the peak gradient. That is why it is advised to record heart rate and blood pressure (BP) at the time of study. Mean gradient means an average of multiple instantaneous gradients in a cardiac cycle. Hence it is more reliable than the peak gradient.

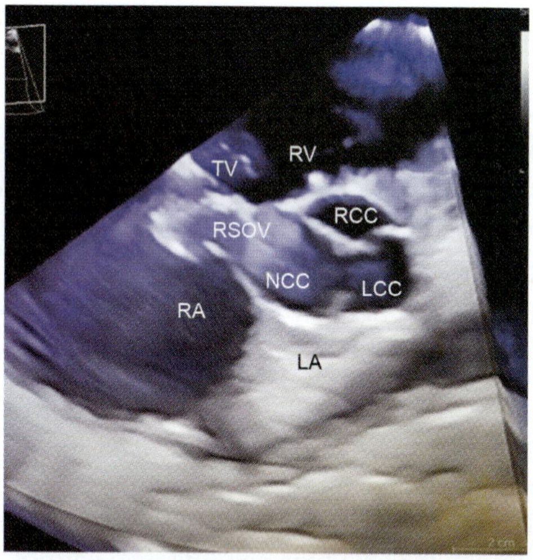

FIG. 3: Basal parasternal short axis 3D view in TTE.
(LA: left atrium; LCC: left coronary cusp; NCC: noncoronary cusp; RA: right atrium; RCC: right coronary cusp; RSOV: ruptured sinus of Valsalva aneurysm; RV: right ventricle; TV: tricuspid valve; 3D: three-dimensional)

CARDIAC COMPUTED TOMOGRAPHY INCLUDING COMPUTED TOMOGRAPHY CORONARY ANGIOGRAPHY AND CORONARY ARTERY CALCIUM SCORE

The detailed cardiac anatomical structure, great vessels, and coronary artery tree may all be accurately seen in three dimensions using cardiac CT **(Fig. 4)**. The most popular noninvasive technique for assessing the risk of coronary artery disease (CAD) is called coronary artery calcium scoring (CACS). In CT the extent of CAD is graded according to the CAC score although this correlation is sometimes controversial.

- *CAC 0*: No evidence of CAD
- *CAC 1–10*: Minimal evidence of CAD
- *CAC 11–100*: Mild evidence of CAD
- *CAC 101–400*: Moderate evidence of CAD
- *CAC > 400*: Extensive evidence of CAD

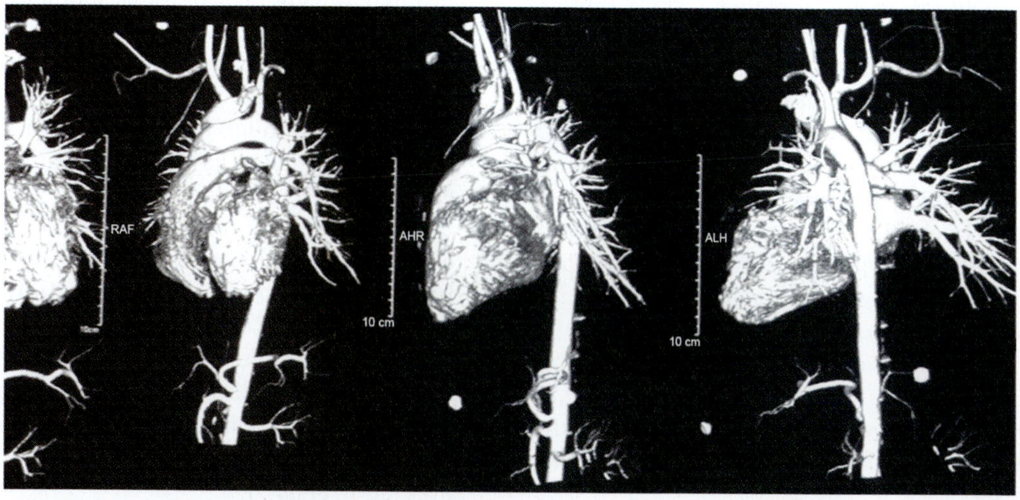

FIG. 4: Cardiac computed tomography (CT) showing normal cardiac and great vessels and coronary artery origin anatomy.

The chance of the next 5 years major adverse clinical events (MACE) remains very low in patients with a CAC score of 0.

Computed tomography coronary angiography (CTCA) may be used to find plaque in asymptomatic people. In the evaluation of suspected individuals with an intermediate risk of CAD, it is a valuable technique for excluding obstructive CAD. With the most recent developments in cardiac CT technology, known as cardiac computed tomography angiography (CTA), it is now possible to create a single picture with great spatial resolution, which incorporates all the data from a single cardiac cycle. The radiation dose has been significantly reduced because of the advent of dual-source CT technology. The CTA is a helpful technique that offers a functional evaluation of CAD and a comprehensive anatomical picture of the coronaries. It offers details on the coronary artery lesions, including their location, degree of stenosis, and plaque distribution. It may also provide information to help with CAD treatment decisions. CTA combines the advantages of anatomical examination for choosing the best revascularization method. CTA can also forecast how cardiac procedures will turn out. It is strongly advised that it be used at facilities with expertise for reliable detection of CAD.

In post bypass surgery patients, CTA has got important role in the follow-up assessment of graft patency in the long run. In the emergency department, when a patient presents with acute chest pain, CTA has an important "Triple Rule Out" protocol to exclude acute coronary syndrome, pulmonary embolism, or aortic dissection.

CARDIAC MAGNETIC RESONANCE IMAGING

Cardiac MRI is a vital tool for the noninvasive observation and evaluation of cardiovascular disease. It is used to diagnose congenital heart disease (CHD), cardiac tumors, and cardiomyopathies [e.g., ARVC **(Figs. 5A and B)**, amyloid, etc.], myocarditis (e.g., sarcoid, TB, etc.), ischemic heart disease, pericardial lesions, and valvular heart disease. Nevertheless, cardiac MRI has the drawback of taking a lot of time to acquire images owing to the requirement of procurement images with different contrasts, high temporal and spatial resolution, and/or whole-heart exposure. Latest technological advancements have put forward the concept of amalgamating AI with cardiac MRI. AI utilizes large data sets to learn the key reconstruction factors and parameters. Particularly, deep learning techniques present a huge potential for using the techniques of deep neural networks (DNN) to study the reconstruction process from prevailing datasets in advance. DNN will then present a faster and more efficient reconstruction which can then be applied to all newly attained data. Compressed sensing for cardiac MRI and learning model techniques, such as cardiac cine imaging, 3D late gadolinium enhancement imaging, and whole-heart coronary magnetic resonance angiography (CMRA) hold the potential.

CORONARY IMAGING

Coronary imaging is commonly done with invasive coronary angiography that gives the detailed anatomy of the luminogram. Invasive coronary angiography is a

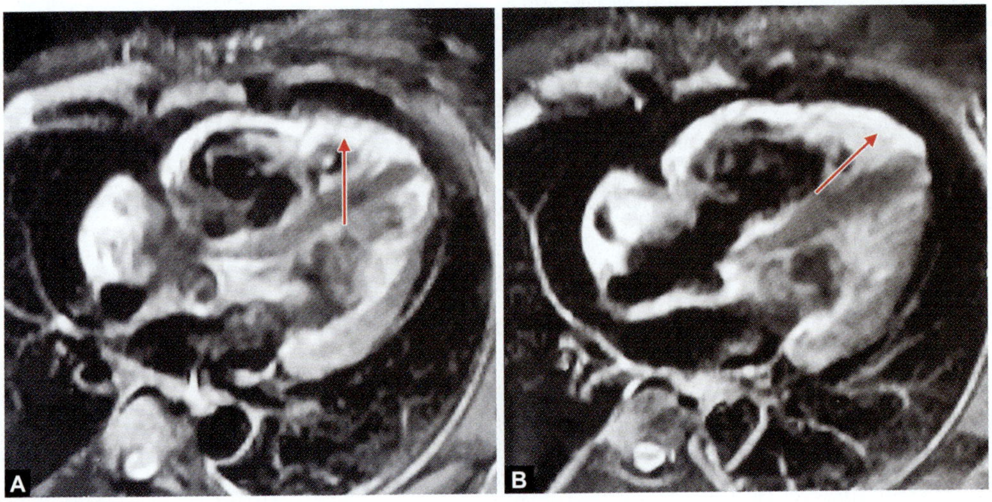

FIGS. 5A AND B: Cardiac MRI showing fibrofatty infiltration (red arrow) of right ventricle-suggestive of ARVC.
(ARVC: arrhythmogenic right ventricular cardiomyopathy; MRI: magnetic resonance imaging)

domain of interventional cardiology and is beyond the scope of this manuscript. The coronary intervention has reached a new height with the advent of intracoronary imaging in the form of intravascular ultrasound (IVUS) and optical coherence topography (OCT). Both these imaging modalities help us to assess the lumen as well as the wall of the coronary artery so that we can identify and quantify the atherosclerotic plaque burden as well as the nature of the plaque (calcified or noncalcified) **(Figs. 6A to F)**. IVUS virtual histology can also give us the entire data of the plaque composition **(Figs. 7A and B)**. Ultramodern functional imaging modality, e.g., fractional flow reserve (FFR) provides us with the functional significance of the atherosclerotic stenosis so that any intervention (stenting

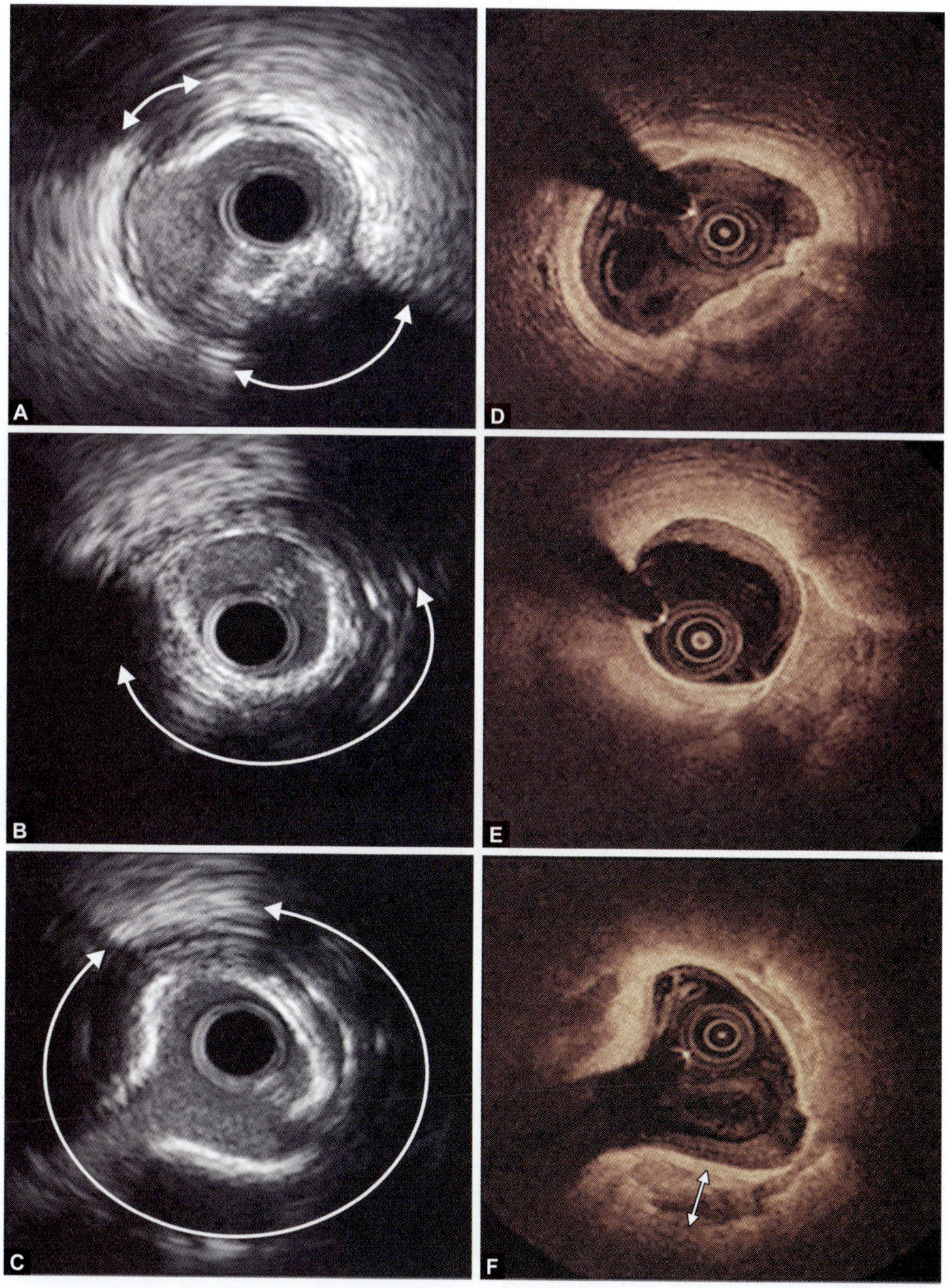

FIGS. 6A TO F: Intravascular ultrasound and OCT images of mild, moderate, and severe calcification. (A to C) Intravascular ultrasound images of mild, moderate, and severe calcification, visualized as superficial hyperechoic tissue with acoustic shadowing, delimited by the arc of calcification relative to the center of the lumen (white arrows). (D to F) Corresponding slices obtained by optimal coherence tomography (OCT). Calcification by OCT is visualized as a signal-poor or heterogeneous region with sharply delineated borders (white arrow in F).

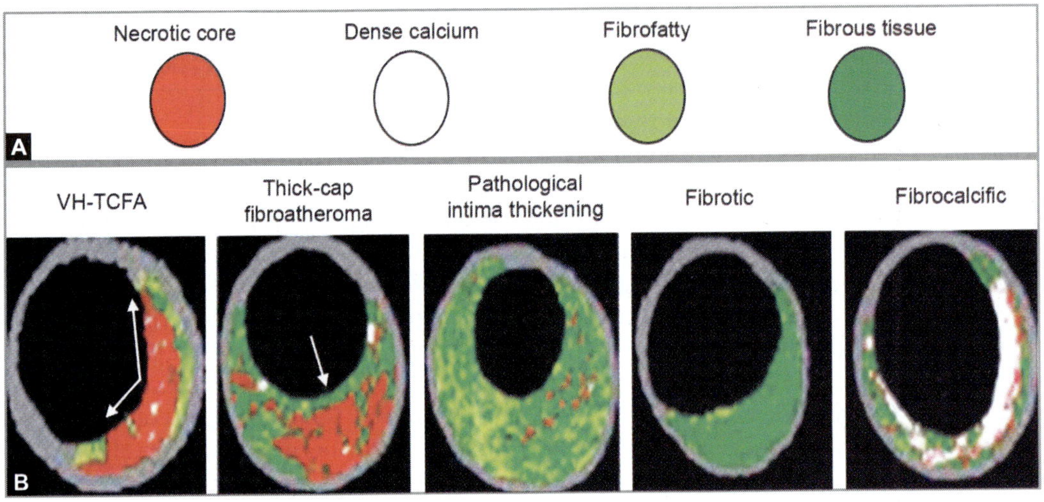

FIGS. 7A AND B: Intravascular ultrasound (IVUS) virtual histology showing various components of atheromatous plaque.

the stenosis) becomes a rational one, rather than just eye assessment (oculostenotic reflex).

NUCLEAR IMAGING

For cardiac imaging, nuclear imaging is a crucial approach. It enables the collection of excellent imaging data together with dynamic functional evaluation. It may be used to infer complicated cardiac architecture as well as myocardial perfusion, wall motion, and viability. To provide noninvasive imaging, radiopharmaceuticals are injected during the process. A small amount of absorbed radiation is given to the patient, and the radiopharmaceutical's gamma rays are used to detect the resulting imaging. The two modalities most often utilized in clinical practice are single photon emission computerized tomography (SPECT) and positron emission tomography (PET). To evaluate the viability and perfusion of the myocardium, SPECT offers a 3D imaging of the myocardium. Due to its superior resolution and accuracy, this method is the nuclear imaging test that is carried out the most often. Unlike SPECT, PET may be utilized to identify myocardial ischemia and transmural microvascular dysfunction. Although it costs more than SPECT, it has far greater sensitivity and resolution. Myocardial tracer activity may also be quantified by PET, which has the potential to be more precise and therapeutically useful. Additionally, it may be utilized for the noninvasive examination of metabolic diseases as well as the measurement of ventricular strain and function.

FUSION IMAGING

Fusion imaging is a method for getting a comprehensive evaluation of the architecture, perfusion, and function of the heart. It is the merging of cardiac images from several imaging modalities, including nuclear, CT, and echocardiography. Using two or more imaging modalities, this approach creates a picture that incorporates the benefits of each modality's best features. To pinpoint the precise location of stenotic arteries and the functional characteristics of the myocardium, fusion imaging combines the benefits of CT and echocardiography.

Transcatheter aortic valve implantation (TAVI) is the main clinical use of fusion imaging. In this treatment, the fusion of the transcatheter aortic valve with the native leaflets is assessed by fusion imaging. It is beneficial to establish the proper valve position and, if required, take remedial action. Percutaneous mitral valve repair, pulmonary valve intervention, and percutaneous coronary intervention (PCI) are a few more treatments that involve fusion imaging. Additionally, it is being utilized more often to address acute strokes and check valves in congenital heart disorders. Combining the benefits of two or more imaging modalities, fusion imaging is a promising imaging technique. It aids in illuminating the functional and anatomical specifics of heart diseases.

ARTIFICIAL INTELLIGENCE IN CARDIAC IMAGING

Due to its many uses, doctors have chosen AI in cardiac imaging as their future preferred technology. The development of automated acquisition and automatic algorithms to help with crucial stages of the diagnostic process has been made possible by AI. AI may be used to analyze CT and echocardiogram pictures for anatomical anomalies and diseases, assisting human professionals in making accurate and timely diagnoses. Deep learning is an AI technology that can analyze complicated, high-dimensional data without the need for manual analysis from human specialists. Additionally, AI may assist in interpreting minute variations in imaging data that would otherwise go unnoticed, resulting in a more precise diagnosis of the illness.

An aberrant cardiac condition may be identified from a single picture using AI, as can more complicated abnormalities. For instance, AI solutions may identify left ventricular and left atrial abnormalities in echocardiograms, as well as coronary artery calcification (CAC). In cardiac CT scans, AI is also utilized to identify CAD. Additionally, an AI tool has been created to identify subendocardial ischemia in PET images. Deep learning, an AI method, is utilized to extract the key elements from the photos, enabling the doctor to make a precise diagnosis. Due to its capacity for analyzing, processing, and interpreting huge amounts of imaging data, AI has shown to be an effective tool in cardiac imaging.

MYOCARDIAL VIABILITY ASSESSMENT BY CARDIAC IMAGING

When evaluating heart disorders, myocardial viability is a crucial factor. The capacity of cardiac imaging to identify myocardial vitality at the cellular level has increased. The existence of normal, stunned, or hibernating myocardium in people with heart problems may be determined by cardiac imaging. The myocardial viability may be evaluated with excellent precision utilizing a range of modalities, including nuclear, CT, and echocardiography.

Stress echocardiography measures myocardial hibernation by revealing regional wall motion abnormalities at rest but contractile during stress (dobutamine or exercise). Nonviable or scarred myocardium remains the same both at rest and during stress.

Cardiac CT imaging may be utilized to detect scar tissues in the left ventricle and to determine if myocardial fibrosis and calcification are present. The injection of radionuclides such as thallium, sestamibi, and rubidium aids in the detection of viable myocardium. PET imaging, which gives a more accurate evaluation than CT imaging, may be used to determine myocardial viability. The metabolic alterations that take place in ischemia and hibernating myocardium may be detected by PET imaging. It helps determine the myocardium's viability and offers useful information about the myocardium's metabolic status. Even cardiac MRI has the potential to pick up nonviable myocardium (>70% of the myocardial thickness is involved).

STRUCTURAL HEART INTERVENTION AND CARDIAC IMAGING

Different interventions are used in the context of valvular, ventricular, atrial, and vascular illnesses in structural heart treatments or therapies. Cardiac imaging is crucial in determining the best course of therapy by assessing the architecture and functioning state of the heart starting from preprocedural planning to intraprocedural execution to postprocedural follow-up. The anatomy of the valve is assessed using TEE and fluoroscopy, and the degree of stenosis or regurgitation is determined. It can assess the left and right heart chamber diameters and identify structural anomalies in natural or artificial valves. Additionally, intraventricular gradient and valve performance may be assessed by echocardiography. Cardiac CT is useful for determining the amount and location of annular calcifications as well as for determining if a patient is a good candidate for percutaneous intervention. Fusion imaging, which combines CT and echocardiography, aids in providing accurate intervention guidance. Fusion imaging technology makes it possible to correctly determine the location of the valve before prosthetic valves are implanted. For placing the device, fluoroscopy can pinpoint the precise position of the catheter's tip.

Cardiac imaging may be used to assess ventricular assist devices. It aids in measuring the atrium's size and determines if a heart transplant is appropriate. Therefore, structural heart interventions need a thorough evaluation of the architecture and operation of the heart, which cardiac imaging offers. It aids in selecting the optimal intervention strategy and achieving the greatest treatment result.

COMPLEX CONGENITAL HEART DISEASE AND CARDIAC IMAGING

Complex CHD may include conditions including tricuspid atresia, coarctation of the aorta, transposition of the major arteries, complete anomalous pulmonary venous return, and single-ventricle physiology. In the identification and treatment of complicated congenital heart disorders, cardiac imaging is crucial. The right-to-left shunt, cardiac anomalies, and the measurement of pulmonary and systemic vascular resistance may all be done with the use of an echocardiogram, which is used to evaluate the structure and function of the heart. Doppler echocardiography may be used to assess the shunt flow between the pulmonary artery and aorta, identify arterial and venous blockage, and more. Better picture quality is provided by TEE, which also aids in the evaluation of atrial and ventricular septal abnormalities. Aortic anomalies are detected by cardiac MRI, which is also used to analyze the anatomy of the heart and quantify shunt flow across different components. Patients with congenital heart disorders may use cardiac CT to assess anomalies in coronary artery architecture and perfusion apart from a complete description of the cardiac anatomy. Due to the higher heart rate in pediatric or neonatal patients, cardiac CT images are a better choice than cardiac MRI. Angiography and cardiac catheter study may be used to quantify the pulmonary and systemic vascular resistances as well as detect abnormal coronary arteries. Cardiovascular imaging is also utilized to evaluate the success of difficult congenital heart operations. It aids in identifying postoperative problems and aids in choosing the appropriate remedial action. Therefore, cardiac imaging is essential for diagnosing and treating complicated congenital heart problems.

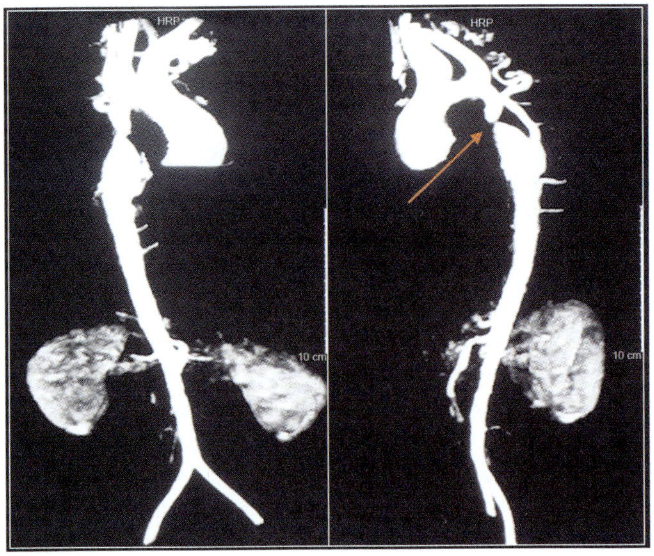

FIG. 8: Magnetic resonance (MR) aortogram showing focal constriction (orange arrow) suggestive of coarctation of the aorta.

IMAGING OF GREAT VESSELS

Cardiovascular imaging is often used to image large blood vessels, such as the thoracic aorta and the pulmonary arteries. It assists in determining the best course of therapy and in determining if any illness is present in the large arteries.

To assess the great vessels' anatomy and function, TEE may be employed. It aids in determining the presence of a thrombus, if any, causing occlusion and preventing the arteries and veins from flowing freely. Additionally, it may be utilized to find aneurysms or great vessel dissections. The major vessels may be precisely mapped anatomically using a CT scan, which can also find diseases including atheromatous plaques, aneurysms, and dissection. For the early identification of vascular disorders, it is more sensitive than echocardiography. Great vessels are imaged using cardiac MRI. It may be utilized to identify various abnormalities of the coronary arteries. It has a very high resolution and is capable of picking up minute details in the thoracic aorta architecture **(Fig. 8)**. To identify and diagnose illnesses of the major arteries, cardiac imaging is crucial. By determining the issues, the best course of action may be chosen.

CONCLUSION

Physicians may get a thorough grasp of the anatomical and functional characteristics of the heart with the use of cardiac imaging. Cardiovascular disorders such as CAD, valvular heart disease, CHD, and diseases of the great arteries may be diagnosed using a variety of cardiac imaging techniques. The development of cardiac imaging has made it possible to image the heart without invasive procedures with greater accuracy and precision. Additionally, it has made it possible to assess cardiac viability and anticipate the results of different therapies. The interpretation of cardiac imaging data has been made easier by AI, which has been shown to be an effective tool. As a result, cardiac imaging has become a useful tool for doctors to diagnose and treat heart disorders.

SUGGESTED READINGS

1. Urzua Fresno C, Sanchez Tijmes F, Shaw KE, Huang F, Thavendiranathan P, Khullar S, et al. Cardiac Imaging in Myocarditis: Current Evidence and Future Directions. Can Assoc Radiol J. 2023;74(1):147-59.
2. Kellman P, Arai AE. Cardiac imaging techniques for physicians: Late enhancement. J Magnetic Reson Imaging. 2012;36(3):529-42.
3. Petersen SE, Abdulkareem M, Leiner T. Artificial Intelligence Will Transform Cardiac Imaging—Opportunities and Challenges. Front Cardiovasc Med. 2019;6:133.
4. Azarine A, Scalbert F, Garçon P. Cardiac functional imaging. Presse Med. 2022;51(2):104119.
5. Saunderson CED, Plein S, Manisty CH. Role of cardiovascular magnetic resonance imaging in cardio-oncology. 2021;22(4): 383-96.
6. Kaminaga T, Takeshita T, Kimura I. Role of magnetic resonance imaging for evaluation of tumors in the cardiac region. Eur Radiol. 2003;13(Suppl 6):L1-10.

7. Douglas PS, Cerqueira MD, Berman DS, Chinnaiyan K, Cohen MS, Lundbye JB, et al. The Future of Cardiac Imaging: Report of a Think Tank Convened by the American College of Cardiology. JACC Cardiovasc Imaging. 2016;9(10):1211-23.
8. Fonseca R, Negishi K, Otahal P, Marwick TH. Temporal changes in appropriateness of cardiac imaging. J Am Coll Cardiol. 2015;65(8):763-73.
9. Jiang B, Guo N, Ge Y, Zhang L, Oudkerk M, Xie X. Development and application of artificial intelligence in cardiac imaging. Br J Radiol. 2020;93(1113):20190812.
10. Baron T, Bergsten J, Albåge A, Lundin L, Sörensen J, Öberg K, et al. Cardiac Imaging in Carcinoid Heart Disease. JACC Cardiovasc Imaging. 2021;14(11):2240-53.
11. Adabifirouzjaei F, Hsiao A, DeMaria AN. Mitral Valve Prolapse—The Role of Cardiac Imaging Modalities. Struct Heart. 2022;6(2):10024.
12. Karamitsos TD, Arvanitaki A, Karvounis H, Neubauer S, Ferreira VM. Myocardial Tissue Characterization and Fibrosis by Imaging. JACC Cardiovasc Imaging. 2020;13(5):1221-34.
13. Marto JP, Kauppila LA, Jorge C, Calado S, Viana-Baptista M, Pinho-E-Melo T, et al. Intravenous thrombolysis for acute ischemic stroke after recent myocardial infarction: case series and systematic review. Stroke. 2019;50(10):2813-8.

9

CHAPTER

Health Hazards of Tobacco Consumption

Tobacco: A Marketed Malady and an Engineered Addiction

Venkatesh Desai, Naveen S Hiremath

ABSTRACT

Tobacco consumption in any form is proven and established to be associated with various health hazards. Tobacco exposure in any form is dangerous, leading to catastrophic complications. The consequences of tobacco exposure range from local oral pathology to systemic diseases. Tobacco affects every system of the body, causing a wide range of diseases, such as coronary heart disease, cerebrovascular disease, cancers of bladder esophagus and lung, chronic obstructive pulmonary disease (COPD), and other respiratory illness, affecting reproductive health in men and women. Hence, reducing tobacco exposure in individuals needs a multidimensional approach. The collective efforts of the individual, society, and the government are required for reducing the tobacco burden in a community. General public awareness, health education, government tax imposition, and a ban on tobacco products can result in the prevention of morbidity and mortality, resulting in the proper use of manpower and resources in the community.

INTRODUCTION

The epidemic of diseases and death due to tobacco and its products' use is increasing very rapidly. India is the second-largest producer and consumer of tobacco in the world. Of the 8 million deaths occurring worldwide each year due to tobacco and tobacco-derived products, 5 million people die prematurely every year. By 2030, the estimated number of premature deaths attributable to tobacco would double to 10 million deaths every year, with about 7 million of them in developing countries.

The prevalence of tobacco use in India among men is >50 % (rural > urban) and among women, it varies between 15 and 60%. Among the adolescents, the prevalence varies from 3.3% in Goa to 62.8% in Nagaland. The cost of tobacco attributable burden was estimated as ₹ 277.611 billion (US$ 6.5 billion) in 1999 **(Table 1)**. This increased to ₹ 308.33 billion (US$ 7.2 billion) in the year 2002–2003.

The National Sample Survey-52nd Round and National Family Health Survey-2 (NFHS-2) found that male tobacco use prevalence was 51.3% in 1995–1996 and 46.5% in 1998–1999 (Rani et al. 2003). The prevalence of smoking is higher among rural women and women in the north and northeast. The prevalence of tobacco use in pregnant women is similar to that in nonpregnant women of the same age. Among children and youth, 2 in every 10 boys and 1 in every 10 girls use a tobacco product (Rani et al. 2003).

Tobacco is the most common substance of abuse in India. 21% of the population uses some form of tobacco according to the National Mental Health Survey, 2015. Smokeless/chewable tobacco use is more prevalent as compared to smoking in India as per Global Adult Tobacco Survey 2 (GATS 2). Both forms are highly addictive. According to the World Health Organization (WHO), there is no safe level of exposure as tobacco kills half of its users.

DIFFERENT FORMS OF TOBACCO

- *Smoking*: *Beedis*, cigarettes, cigars, cheroots, hookah, *hookli*, *chhutta*, *dhumti*, *chillum*, etc.
- *Smokeless*: Betel quid, *pan masala*, tobacco-areca nut and slaked lime, *mishri*, *khaini*, *gutka*, *bajjar*, snuff, and for chewing.
- *E-cigarettes*: Known as electronic nicotine delivery systems (ENDS).

TABLE 1: Prevalence of tobacco use in Indian adults.

Survey	Strata	National Sample Survey-52nd Round, 1995–1996	National Family Health Survey-2, 1998–1999
Age group		15+ years	15+ years
No surveyed	Urban + Rural	396,546	315,597
Regular tobacco users	M (%)	51.3	46.5
	F (%)	10.3	13.8
Regular smokers	M (%)	35.3	29.3
	F (%)	2.6	2.4
	All (%)	19.2	NR
Regular smokeless users	M (%)	24.0	28.1
	F (%)	8.6	12.0
	All (%)	16.4	NR

Note: Confidence intervals were not available for any national survey data.

(NR: not reported; M: male; F: female)

Sources:

1. Rani M, Bonu S, Jha P, Nguyen SN, Jamjoum L. Tobacco use in India: prevalence and predictors of smoking and chewing in a national cross-sectional household survey. Tob Control. 2003;12(4):e4.
2. National data for India on tobacco use, 1995-96 and 1998-99.

SMOKING AND HEALTH RISK

The US Surgeon General's report 2004 states that smoking harms almost every organ of the body. Overall, it causes more than 480,000 deaths annually (including deaths from secondhand smoke). Tobacco use remains the leading preventable cause of death and is responsible for the death of 1 in 10 adults (about 5 million deaths each year) with 2.41 (1.80–3.15) million deaths in developing countries and 2.43 (2.13–2.78) million in developed countries, of which 3.84 million deaths were in men. Even people who smoke fewer than five cigarettes a day can have early signs of cardiovascular disease (CVD). 50% of unnecessary deaths due to tobacco occur in middle age (35–69 years), robbing around 22 years of normal life expectancy. In developed countries, smoking is estimated to cause over 90% of lung cancer in men and about 70% of lung cancer in women. Also, 56–80% of deaths occur due to chronic respiratory disease, and 22% of cardiovascular deaths occur due to tobacco. Attributable mortality is 13.3% in males and 3.8% in females. Globally, smoking-related mortality is about 12% for vascular disease, 66% for cancer of the trachea, bronchus, and lung combined, and 38% for chronic respiratory disease.

Smoking can affect a person's health in many other ways as well, harming nearly every organ in the body **(Box 1)**.

BOX 1: Health consequences related to tobacco exposure.

Heart and blood vessel diseases:
- Atherosclerosis, coronary heart disease
- Cerebrovascular diseases
- Abdominal aortic aneurysm
- Peripheral vascular disease (may cause gangrene in the legs)
- Erectile dysfunction or impotence (atherosclerosis and endothelial dysfunction of the internal pudendal and penile arteries)

Cancer:
- Cancers of the bladder, cervix, esophagus, kidney, larynx, lung, oral cavity and pharynx, pancreas, stomach, and leukemia
- *Precancerous lesions*: Leukoplakia, erythroplakia of the oral cavity

Respiratory diseases:
- *Chronic obstructive pulmonary disease*: Chronic bronchitis
- *Acute respiratory illnesses*: Pneumonia, bronchitis, and other respiratory infections
- *Respiratory effects mediated in utero*: Reduced respiratory function in infants
- *Respiratory effects in childhood and adolescence*: Decreased physical fitness, potential retardation in the rate of lung growth, and the level of maximum lung function among children and adolescents
- *Respiratory effects in adulthood*: Acceleration of age-related decline in lung function among adults
- *Other respiratory effects*: Increased cough, phlegm production, wheezing, respiratory infections, and dyspnea

Reproductive effects:
- *Fetal death and stillbirth*: Sudden infant death syndrome (SIDS)
- *Fertility*: Delayed conception (primary and secondary infertility)
- *Low birth weight*: Fetal growth restriction and preterm delivery
- *Pregnancy complications*: Premature rupture of membranes, abruptio placentae, and placenta previa

Other effects:
- Cataract
- Diminished health status, adverse surgical outcomes related to wound healing, and respiratory complications
- Low bone density among postmenopausal women, and risk of hip fractures
- Peptic ulcer disease, periodontitis

Source: US Department of Health and Human Services, 2004.

TOBACCO AND CANCER

More than 10 million people globally are diagnosed with cancer every year. By 2040, the global burden is expected to grow to 27.5 million new cancer cases and 16.3 million cancer deaths simply due to the growth and aging of the population. Cancer causes 6 million deaths every year, or 12% of deaths worldwide. Smoking causes about 20% of all cancers and about 30% of all cancer deaths in the United States. International Agency for Research on Cancer (IARC) monograph states that tobacco smoking is the major cause of lung cancer (all types), and is associated with oral cancer, cancers of the oropharynx and hypopharynx, esophagus, stomach, liver, pancreas, larynx, nasopharynx, nasal cavity and nasal sinuses, urinary bladder, kidney and cervix, and myeloid leukemia. Secondhand smoke is shown to be carcinogenic to lungs. The US Surgeon General's report, 2004 states that there is sufficient evidence to infer a causal relationship between smoking and cancer of the lung, oral cavity, larynx, esophagus, urinary bladder, kidney, stomach and pancreas, uterine cervix, as well as acute myeloid leukemia.

Lung Cancer

Tobacco contains several toxic and carcinogenic chemicals. The most important group is the tobacco-specific nitrosamines (TSNAs). Nitrosamines are found in tobacco products in abundance and are highly carcinogenic. Tobacco smoke contains highly carcinogenic chemicals called polycyclic aromatic hydrocarbons (PAHs). About 80% of lung cancers, as well as about 80% of all lung cancer deaths, are due to smoking.

Lung cancer is the leading cause of cancer deaths in people in the United States. Lung cancer is the number one cause of cancer deaths among Indian women. Women's death rates due to lung cancer have risen 600% since 1950. About 80% of all lung cancer deaths are attributable to smoking. Chewing tobacco and snuff contain 28 different carcinogens contributing to lung cancer. Smoking *beedis*, hookahs, and cigarettes are associated with similarly elevated risks.

Oral Cavity and Tongue

The risk of oral cancer increases with the use of tobacco in chewing forms. A multicentric study in South Indian cities showed that betel quid (*pan*) chewing women had 25–46 times higher risk, and men had a 3.6–6-fold greater risk of oral cancer. Men chewing dried tobacco (*chadha*) had a nearly fivefold greater risk of oral cancer.

Esophagus

Studies in the Indian subcontinent have shown a 2.6–3-fold greater risk of esophageal cancer in tobacco plus betal quid users and 2–4-fold for *beedi* smokers. Risk of cancer in the lower third of the esophagus for *pan*-tobacco chewers was 6.6-fold greater than for nonchewers. *Beedi* smokers have a significant risk factor for cancers of all the three segments of the esophagus but conferred a sevenfold greater risk for the upper one-third of the esophagus.

Oropharynx and Larynx

Smoking has a sevenfold higher risk, whereas *beedi* has a fivefold higher risk, and tobacco chewing has nearly eightfold risk for cancer of oropharynx. *Beedi* smoking has a 2–7 times greater risk of laryngeal cancer.

Stomach

Smoking has a twofold increased risk of stomach cancer, but chewers have not been found to have the same risk.

Cervix

Pan-tobacco chewing has a direct dose-dependent association with invasive cervical cancer. A study in West Bengal found that 54% of the women with the habit of *pan*-tobacco chewing had cervical dysplasia, while it was only 4.1% among nonchewers. Indian women have cervical cancer rates 3.5 times the national average. One of the behavioral factors considered to elevate the risk of cervical cancer is tobacco.

Gallbladder and Urinary Bladder

Smokers have an 11-fold increased risk of developing gallbladder cancer among patients with gallstones. Smoking is found to be a risk factor for urinary bladder cancer.

Penis

A case–control study in Chennai found a fourfold greater risk of penile cancer in men who used snuff and chewed tobacco, whereas it was 1.7% among smokers.

Women who smoke have increased risks for cancers of the pancreas and kidney. The association of smokeless tobacco has been observed with cancers of oral cavity, pharynx, larynx, and esophagus, and precancerous lesions of the oral cavity. Cigarettes, cigars, and pipes can all cause cancer. There is no safe form of tobacco smoke. There is also an increased risk of acute myeloid leukemia.

TOBACCO AND CARDIOVASCULAR DISEASES

Cardiovascular disease is the largest contributor to deaths globally, accounting for 20.5 million, i.e., almost one-third of all global deaths (from 12.1 million deaths in 1990) (as per World Heart Federation). In India, CVD

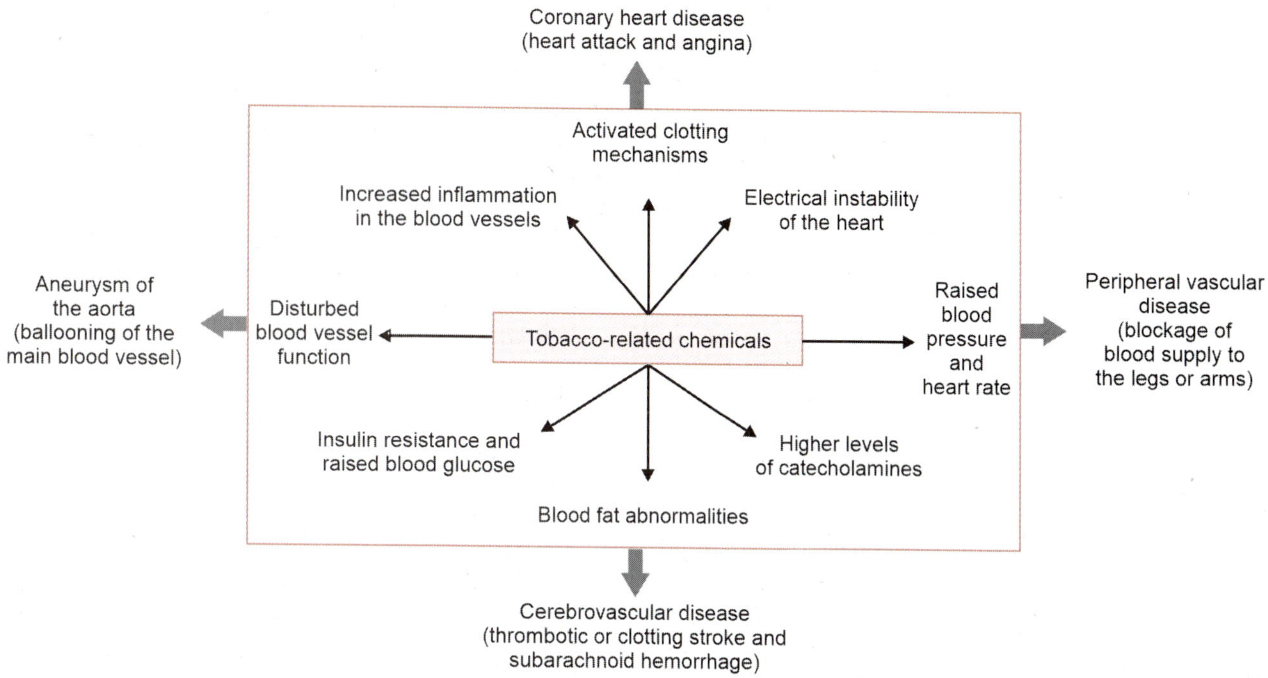

FIG. 1: Effects of tobacco on cardiovascular system.

contributed to 28.1% of total deaths and 14.1% of total disability-adjusted life years (DALYs). By 2020, about 42% of the total deaths in India were projected to be due to cardiovascular causes **(Fig. 1)**.

Tobacco smoke contains nicotine, carbon monoxide, nitrogen oxides, hydrogen cyanide, and tar, with cadmium, zinc, and carbon disulfide being minor constituents; all of which cause vascular injury. Smoking causes endothelial dysfunction, lipid alterations, and platelet activation, leading to a prothrombotic state. Tobacco use also increases the risk and severity of vascular disease by increasing the risk of diabetes, which itself damages the vessels by accelerating atherosclerosis. Smoking is associated with coronary artery disease (CAD), angina, sudden cardiac death (SCD), arrhythmia, stroke, peripheral artery disease, abdominal aortic aneurysms, renal artery stenosis, cor pulmonale, and erectile sexual dysfunction. Thus, smoking affects the entire vascular system.

TOBACCO AND LUNG DISEASE

Tobacco smoke causes inflammation and edema of the respiratory tract. The narrowing of the respiratory tract causes obstruction to the airflow and air trapping in the lungs. Also, there is initiation of several enzymatic reactions causing damage to the lung tissues. These processes are progressive, especially in the presence of continued smoking. The irreversible lung damage results in marked respiratory disability, respiratory failure, and premature death. Smoking is also associated with the increased airway wall remodeling seen in chronic asthma.

In a study, chronic obstructive pulmonary disease (COPD) was observed among 36.4% of *beedi* smokers and 45.4% of cigarette smokers versus 3% among nonsmokers. Tobacco smoking accounts for 80–90% of all COPD cases. Passive smoking is responsible for bronchial hyper-responsiveness, whose risk is maximum in women and children (1.8 times increased risk of asthma). It also increases the risk of lung infections, such as pneumonia and tuberculosis (TB), and it can worsen some existing lung diseases, such as interstitial lung diseases (ILDs). The prevalence and mortality in TB is about 3–4 times higher in smokers than nonsmokers (200,000 deaths per year due to smoking in those with pulmonary TB, out of 700,000 tobacco smoking-related deaths, half of them being men in their third to fourth decade of life).

TOBACCO USE AND REPRODUCTIVE HEALTH

Nicotine leads to decreased blood supply to the uterus and placenta. It also has a significant effect on the functions of the brain and on organ development during the sensitive period of development of the fetus. Carbon monoxide can cause reduced oxygen delivery to the fetal cells. Heavy metals and PAHs induce fetal toxemia, retard fetal growth and development, and disrupt the endocrine system.

Mother and Child

Women who smoke while pregnant have a higher risk of ectopic pregnancy, placenta previa, placental abruption, premature births, and low birth-weight babies. They also have an increased risk of still birth and increased risk of miscarriage. There is also a risk of cleft lip, cleft palate, restricted head growth (length, head circumference, chest circumference, and shoulder circumference all are reduced), and possibly other birth defects. Babies of mothers who smoke during and after pregnancy have a greater risk of sudden infant death syndrome (SIDS). Exposure to secondhand smoke during pregnancy has been associated with lower infant birth weight.

Men

Smoking is associated with a higher risk of erectile dysfunction. This risk increases the more they smoke and the longer they smoke. Men who smoke have a lower sperm count and poorer sperm quality than nonsmokers. There is also an increased risk of birth defects in fetus.

TOBACCO AND ORAL AND DENTAL LESIONS

Tobacco in any form, either smoked or smokeless, can cause a wide spectrum of oral mucosal alterations or lesions. Oral and pharyngeal tissues come into direct contact with carcinogens present in smokeless tobacco products and tobacco smoke. TSNAs are formed in the mouth through the process of nitrosation.

These lesions include:

- *Precancerous or premalignant*: It is a localized tissue alterations, like leukoplakia, erythroplakia, and palatal changes.
- *Premalignant conditions*: These are more generalized and widespread with significant systemic involvement, like oral submucous fibrosis (OSMF), oral lichen planus, and other related lesions. Erythroplakia is the most severe oral premalignant lesion as it carries much greater risk of cancer, while leukoplakia is the most common precancerous lesion associated with tobacco chewing or smoking. OSMF is caused due to areca nut, *pan masala*, and *gutka* chewing practice, and hence is common in youths. 4.5–7.6% of OSMF lesions progress to malignant transformation and oral cancer.

TOBACCO AND DIABETES

Diabetes and smoking both reduce the delivery of oxygen to body tissues, resulting in poor circulation. Smoking alters blood sugar levels, making it harder to control diabetes. Of people with diabetes who need amputations, most of them are smokers as nicotine is a vasoconstrictor. Smoking increases cholesterol levels and leads to atherosclerosis and arteriosclerosis. Diabetes increases low-density lipoprotein (LDL), very low-density lipoprotein (VLDL), and other cholesterol levels. The combined cardiovascular risk of smoking and diabetes is as high as 14 times that of either smoking or diabetes alone **(Table 2)**.

TABLE 2: Relative risk of death from specific causes among people aged >55 years.

	Women				Men			
	Never smoked		Current smoker		Never smoked		Current smoker	
Cause of death	No. of deaths	Relative risk	No. of deaths	Relative risk (95% CI)	No. of deaths	Relative risk	No. of deaths	Relative risk (95% CI)
All causes	31,786	1.0	8,150	2.8 (2.7–2.9)	24,863	1.0	8,325	2.8 (2.8–2.9)
Diseases established as caused by smoking†								
Lip and oral cavity cancer, C00-C14	57	1.0	42	5.6 (3.7–8.6)	82	1.0	64	5.7 (4.1–8.1)
Esophageal cancer, C15	81	1.0	50	5.1 (3.5–7.4)	178	1.0	104	3.9 (3.0–5.0)
Stomach cancer, C16	184	1.0	34	1.7 (1.2–2.5)	154	1.0	45	1.9 (1.4–2.7)
Colorectal cancer, C18–C20	1,016	1.0	174	1.6 (1.4–1.9)	753	1.0	160	1.4 (1.2–1.7)
Liver cancer, C22	228	1.0	40	1.8 (1.3–2.5)	228	1.0	74	2.3 (1.8–3.0)
Pancreatic cancer, C25	948	1.0	184	1.9 (1.6–2.2)	747	1.0	153	1.6 (1.4–1.9)
Laryngeal cancer, C32	2	1.0	27	103.8 (24.2–445.5)	23	1.0	50	13.9 (8.3–23.3)

Continued

Continued

	Women				Men			
	Never smoked		Current smoker		Never smoked		Current smoker	
Cause of death	No. of deaths	Relative risk	No. of deaths	Relative risk (95% CI)	No. of deaths	Relative risk	No. of deaths	Relative risk (95% CI)
Lung cancer, C33–C34	735	1.0	1,872	22.9 (21.0–25.0)	480	1.0	1,754	25.3 (22.8–28.1)
Urinary bladder cancer, C67	123	1.0	48	3.9 (2.8–5.5)	201	1.0	84	3.9 (3.0–5.1)
Kidney and renal pelvis cancer, C64–C66	256	1.0	32	1.2 (0.9–1.8)	237	1.0	62	1.8 (1.4–2.4)
Acute myeloid leukemia, C92.0	180	1.0	22	1.1 (0.7–1.7)	210	1.0	48	1.9 (1.4–2.7)
Diabetes, E10–E14	743	1.0	110	1.5 (1.3–1.9)	729	1.0	142	1.6 (1.3–1.9)
Ischemic heart disease, 120–125	4,119	1.0	1,014	3.0 (2.8–3.2)	4,947	1.0	1,522	2.6 (2.4–2.7)
Other heart disease, 100–109 and 126–151	2,329	1.0	340	1.9 (1.7–2.1)	1,736	1.0	364	2.0 (1.8–2.2)
Total stroke, 160–169	2,435	1.0	385	2.1 (1.8–2.3)	1,399	1.0	279	1.9 (1.7–2.2)
Atherosclerosis, 170	76	1.0	12	2.1 (1.1–4.0)	57	1.0	32	5.0 (3.2–7.9)
Aortic aneurysm, 171	99	1.0	91	10.1 (7.4–13.6)	126	1.0	116	7.5 (5.8–9.7)
Other arterial diseases, 172–178	81	1.0	47	5.6 (3.9–8.2)	57	1.0	36	5.3 (3.4–8.2)
Pneumonia, influenza, and tuberculosis, J10–J18 and A16–A19	723	1.0	100	1.9 (1.6–2.4)	487	1.0	87	2.0 (1.6–2.6)
COPD, J40–J44	410	1.0	941	25.0 (21.2–28.1)	259	1.0	825	27.8 (24.1–32.0)
Additional diseases associated with smoking[‡]								
All infections, A00–B99[§]	598	1.0	137	2.5 (2.1–3.0)	475	1.0	125	2.2 (1.3–2.7)
Breast cancer, C50	1,748	1.0	274	1.3 (1.2–1.5)	—	—	—	—
Prostate cancer, C61	—	—	—	—	1,101	1.0	166	1.4 (1.2–1.7)
Rare cancers[¶]	1,233	1.0	143	1.1 (0.9–1.3)	402	1.0	84	1.6 (1.2–2.0)
Cancers of unknown site	866	1.0	237	2.7 (2.3–3.2)	665	1.0	268	3.2 (2.8–3.7)
Hypertensive heart disease, 111	244	1.0	45	1.9 (1.4–2.7)	193	1.0	75	2.9 (2.2–3.9)
Essential hypertension and hypertensive renal disease, 110 and 115	249	1.0	48	2.4 (1.7–3.4)	175	1.0	49	2.6 (1.9–3.6)
All other respiratory diseases[‖]	442	1.0	69	1.9 (1.5–2.5)	375	1.0	77	2.0 (1.5–2.6)
Ischemic disorders of the intestines, K55	93	1.0	48	6.1 (4.2–8.7)	46	1.0	29	5.6 (3.5–9.0)
Liver cirrhosis, K70 and K74	201	1.0	69	2.6 (2.0–3.5)	174	1.0	109	3.6 (2.3–4.6)
All other digestive diseases[**]	618	1.0	105	2.1 (1.7–2.5)	378	1.0	107	2.6 (2.0–3.2)
Renal failure, N17–N19	504	1.0	77	1.9 (1.5–2.5)	407	1.0	84	2.1 (1.6–2.6)

Continued

Continued

	Women				Men			
	Never smoked		Current smoker		Never smoked		Current smoker	
Cause of death	No. of deaths	Relative risk	No. of deaths	Relative risk (95% CI)	No. of deaths	Relative risk	No. of deaths	Relative risk (95% CI)
Additional rare causes combined††	1,565	1.0	290	2.0 (1.8–2.3)	624	1.0	130	1.9 (1.5–2.2)
Unknown causes	955	1.0	274	2.2 (1.9–2.5)	787	1.0	221	1.9 (1.6–2.2)

†Participants were enrolled in Cancer Prevention Study I (CPS I) in 1959 and in Cancer Prevention Study II (CPS II) in 1982. Analyses of both studies excluded participants younger than 50 years of age.

‡The contemporary cohort consisted of cohorts from five studies. Participants were enrolled in the Nurses' Health Study (NHS) in 1976, the Health Professionals Follow-up Study (HPFS) in 1986, the CPS II Nutrition Cohort in 1992, the National Institutes of Health–American Association of Retired Persons (NIH–AARP) Diet and Health Study in 1995–1996, and the Women's Health Initiative (WHI) in 1993–1998.

§Age at the start of follow-up is shown.

¶For women, the spouse's educational level was used if it was more advanced.

||Race was self-reported.

**Ethnic group was self-reported. The HPFS was not included in this analysis.

††Smoking status was recorded as of 1959 for CPS I, 1982 for CPS II, 1999 for the CPS II Nutrition Cohort, 2000 for the HPFS and the NHS, 1996 for the NIH–AARP cohort, and 1995–2001 for the WHI.

Source: Carter BD, Abnet CC, Feskanich D, Freedman ND, Hartge P, Cora E, et al. Smoking and Mortality—Beyond Established Causes. N Engl J Med. 2015;372:631-40.

CONCLUSION

Health hazards already proven to be associated with tobacco use can be substantially overcome with general public awareness, motivation, government imposition, and a ban on tobacco products. It is possible to prevent morbidity, mortality, and economic expenditure, which leads to proper utilization of manpower and resources.

SUGGESTED READINGS

1. Gupta PC, Ray CS. Epidemic in India. In: Boyle P, Gray N, Henningfield J, Seffrin J, Zatonski W (Eds). Tobacco: Science, Policy and Public Health. Oxford: Oxford University Press; 2004. pp. 253-66.
2. WHO report on the global tobacco epidemic 2023. https://www.who.int/teams/health-promotion/tobacco-control/global-tobacco-report-2023
3. Gupta PC. Health consequences of tobacco use in India. World Smoking and Health. 1988;13:5-10.
4. World Health Organization. (2022). The World Health Report:2002: Reducing risks, Promoting Healthy Life. [online] Available from http://www.who.int/whr/ 2002/chapter4/en/index6.html [Last accessed December, 2023].
5. Office of the Surgeon General (US); Office on Smoking and Health (US). The Health Consequences of Smoking: A Report of the Surgeon General. Atlanta: Centers for Disease Control and Prevention (US); 2004.
6. Gupta PC, Murti PR, Bhonsle RB. Epidemiology of cancer by tobacco products and the significance of TSNA. Crit Rev Toxicol. 1996;26(2):183-98.
7. Benowitz NL. Cigarette smoking and cardiovascular disease: Pathophysiology and implications for treatment. Prog Cardiovasc Dis. 2003;46(1):91-111.
8. Reddy KS, Gupta PC (Eds). Report on Tobacco Control in India. India: Ministry of Health & Family Welfare, Government of India. Centers for Disease Control and Prevention, USA. World Health Organization; 2004.
9. Royal College of Physicians. Smoking and Health: Summary and a report of the Royal College of Physicians of London on smoking in relation to cancer of the lung and other diseases. London: Pitman Medical Publishing Co Ltd; 1962.
10. Krishna K. Tobacco chewing in pregnancy. Br J Gynaecol. 1978;85(10):725-8.
11. Rani M, Bonu S, Jha P, Nguyen SN, Jamjoum L. Tobacco use in India: prevalence and predictors of smoking and chewing in a national cross sectional household survey. Tob Control. 2003;12(4):e4.
12. Ferlay J. GLOBOCAN 2018. Lyon: World Health Organization International Agency for Research on Cancer, 2018.

10

CHAPTER

Peripheral Vascular Disease: A Surrogate of Cardiovascular Disease Risk

Bipul Chandra Kalita, Nitesh Badal

ABSTRACT

Individuals with peripheral vascular disease (PVD) who have coronary artery disease (CAD) are more susceptible to cardiovascular (CV) events than individuals with CAD alone. Globally, cardiovascular disease (CVD) is the primary cause of death. To increase longevity and quality of life, risk factors for CV events must be identified and treated. By identifying the causative factors and giving them more attention during treatment, the excess morbidity linked to PVD in CAD patients may be reduced. A deeper comprehension of the variables contributing to poorer outcomes in PVD patients can be used to pinpoint high-risk patient subgroups and facilitate the creation of focused interventions aimed at lowering morbidity and death rates.

INTRODUCTION

Peripheral vascular disease (PVD) is a chronic, advancing atherosclerotic condition that can result in partial or complete blockage of the peripheral arteries. Usually, PVD affects the iliac arteries, lower limbs, and occasionally, the upper extremities. PVD, which affects about 200 million people globally, is becoming a global health concern. The disease presentation and progression vary, with some remaining asymptomatic and others advancing to arterial ulceration, claudication, resting limb ischemia, and limb amputation. PVD is the cardiovascular disease (CVD) equivalent, with high risk lethal and nonfatal cardiovascular (CV) events such as myocardial infarction and stroke occurring often.

ETIOLOGY

The primary cause of peripheral vascular illness is progressive atherosclerotic disease, which reduces the blood supply to key organs and causes end-organ ischemia. In the development of atherosclerosis, significant modifiable and nonmodifiable risk factors have been discovered.

Risk factors include:

- Tobacco use
- Diabetes mellitus
- Hypertension
- HIV
- Dyslipidemia
- Age > 50 years
- Elevated homocysteine levels
- Body mass index (BMI) > 30
- Family history of CVD

Smoking is associated with the highest risk of PVD development with an odds ratio of 2.7 [(95% confidence interval (CI) 2.4–3.1]. History of CVD and diabetes are also significant risk factors with odds ratios of 2.6 (95% CI 2.2–3) and 1.9 (1.7–2.1), respectively.

EPIDEMIOLOGY

The global prevalence of PVD was 5.6% in 2015.[7] The prevalence of PVD has increased by about 45% globally from 2000 to 2015.

Indian scenario: In people with normal glucose tolerance (NGT), impaired glucose tolerance (IGT), and diabetes, the prevalence rates of PVD were 2.7%, 2.9%, and 6.3%, respectively. 3.2% was the total prevalence rate. When compared to participants who had just been diagnosed with diabetes, known diabetic subjects had a higher prevalence of PVD (7.8%).

PATHOPHYSIOLOGY

The main cause of PVD is the development of atherosclerotic disease, which results in macro- and microvascular dysfunction. A number of vascular cells, thrombotic agents, cholesterol, and inflammatory chemicals are all involved in the pathophysiology of atherosclerosis.

The intimal layer of big arteries accumulates lipoproteins and with the invasion of lymphocytes and macrophages, the presence of lipoprotein in the endothelium causes lipid oxidation and a cytokine response. These oxidized lipids are consumed by macrophages, which create foam cells that result in the formation of "fatty streaks" which progress into plaques with necrotic lipid cores and smooth muscle cells (SMCs). Cytokines and growth factors secreted by SMC and endothelial cells cause SMC to migrate to the luminal side of the plaque, extracellular matrix to be produced, and ultimately the creation of a fibrous plaque.

Over years, atherosclerotic plaque progressively accumulates within the vessel wall. Vascular stenosis and frequent vascular dilatation are caused by plaque build up to maximize end-organ perfusion. Collateral circulatory beds typically form to maintain distal perfusion and tissue viability when constriction advances and blocks the artery.

ARTERY-RELATED DIFFERENCES IN ATHEROSCLEROSIS EXPRESSION

Atherosclerotic plaque onset, progression, and clinical manifestation have been linked with the type and location of the arteries. The carotid arteries frequently have foam cell lesions, which likely explain the dynamics of carotid intima-media thickness. In the femoral arteries, atherosclerosis progresses slowly and fibrous plaques predominate in severe cases. A systemically more susceptible expression of atherosclerosis is indicated by the increased prevalence of lipid core plaques in all arteries in coronary fatalities patients.

Regardless of the level of atherosclerosis, PVD manifests as thrombosis. In two-thirds of individuals with acute limb ischemia, thrombi are associated with little atherosclerosis.

CLINICAL PRESENTATION

The degree of arterial insufficiency and the existence of concomitant diseases, which may change or obfuscate the symptoms of underlying vascular illness, can affect how PVD presents clinically.

Patients with advanced diabetes mellitus, lumbosacral illness, or spinal stenosis often arrive with an unusual presentation. These conditions have the potential to change a patient's sense of pain.

Over 50% of patients with PVD are asymptomatic. The most typical PVD symptom is intermittent claudication. Additionally symptoms include paresthesia, rigidity, and cool extremities in the lower limbs. Pain at rest, nonhealing sores or ulcers, and gangrene in one or both legs are symptoms of critical limb ischemia.

DIAGNOSIS

- The resting ankle-brachial index (ABI) is the primary test for detecting PVD, according to the 2016 American Heart Association (AHA)/American College of Cardiology (ACC) guidelines. ABI should be determined in each limb and is defined as the ratio of the higher reading of the two ankle pressures (dorsalis pedis and posterior tibial) over the higher reading of either the right or left brachial pressure. An ABI of 0.90 or less in each limb indicates PVD. ABI's sensitivity and specificity are typically stated to be >80%.
- A toe-brachial index with a threshold of 0.70 can be utilized to diagnose PVD in the presence of noncompressible and calcific ankle arteries.
- Duplex ultrasonography, computerized tomography angiography, and magnetic resonance angiography.
- The most accurate way is invasive angiography.
- Toe arterial waveform analysis, transcutaneous oxygen pressure, and skin perfusion pressure.
- *Biomarkers*: Numerous biomarkers still in research have been found. Wilson et al. proteomic analysis of plasma samples from individuals with and without PVD revealed that the patients with PVD have higher level of β2-microglobulin. High-sensitivity cardiac troponin T appears to be the most promising circulating biomarker of future PVD risk.

RECOMMENDATIONS FOR THE USE AND INTERPRETATION OF THE ANKLE-BRACHIAL INDEX

- An ABI of <0.90 ought to be taken into account as the threshold for validating the diagnosis of PVD affecting the lower extremities (class I; level of evidence A).

- ABI declines ≥ 0.15 over time may be useful in identifying notable disease progression (class IIa; level of evidence B).
- Regardless of the existence of PVD symptoms and other CV risk factors, subjects with an ABI of ≤ 1.40 are deemed to be at extreme risk of CV morbidity and death (class I; level of evidence A).
- Patients are classified as "borderline" if their ABI falls between 0.91 and 1.00 (level of evidence A; class IIa).

COMPLICATIONS

- Amputation
- Acute limb ischemia
- Higher rate of mortality
- *Other CVDs*: CAD, heart failure (HF) and cerebrovascular accident (CVA)
- Reduced physical function and quality of life

MANAGEMENT

Lifestyle changes are the first step, followed by the addition of medication and interventional therapy.

Cardiovascular risk factor modification:

- Smoking cessation
- Control of hypertension and diabetes
- Statin therapy [to keep low-density lipoprotein cholestrol (LDL-C) < 100 mg%]
- Exercise
- *Pharmacotherapy*:
  - Cilostazol
  - Aspirin
  - Oral anticoagulants
- *Revascularization*: Surgical and percutaneous interventions

LOOKING BEYOND PERIPHERAL VASCULAR DISEASE (LINK BETWEEN PERIPHERAL VASCULAR DISEASE AND CARDIOVASCULAR DISEASE)

Due to the widespread nature of atherosclerosis, PVD frequently coexists with coronary and cerebrovascular illness. According to several epidemiological studies, 40–60% of people with PVD had signs of either cerebrovascular illness, coronary disease, or both. Compared to controls of same age, patients with intermittent claudication had a considerably higher mortality rate. In this patient-population, coronary or cerebrovascular events are primarily to blame for fatalities.

The main cause of death worldwide is CV illness. To increase health and longevity, it is essential to identify and address CV event risk factors. Patients with CAD frequently have PVD, which has a prevalence of 22–42%. Patients with CAD who also have PVD experience worse CV outcomes than those who only have CAD. Whether common risk factors such as hypertension and dyslipidemia can account for the elevated risk of CV events linked to PVD is unknown. Lack of exercise, compromised endothelial function, decreased heart function, and inflammation are among additional causes that have been proposed. Finding these causes and paying more attention to their treatment should reduce the excess morbidity related to PVD in people with CAD.

Acute symptomatic PVD was strongly related with an elevated risk of later CV events, mortality, myocardial infarction (MI), and the requirement for coronary revascularization in a large sample of patients with CAD. Inflammation, glycemic control, the severity of the heart disease, and classic PVD risk variables were all implicated in this connection. Together, they accounted for about half of the increased risk in CV morbidity and mortality conferred by an initial symptomatic PVD event. According to these findings, PVD may still identify a subgroup that is especially at risk for negative CV outcomes and could benefit from more extensive secondary prevention.

Hospitalization for incident PVD also predicts negative CV outcomes, in addition to the poor prognosis brought on by concomitant PVD.

Myocardial infarction is 2.5 times more common in people with clinically severe PVD (ABI < 0.9) than in those without PVD.

Only when the index was ≤0.7 did the risk of a CV event become significant in the Pittsburgh study, because individuals with a lower score had more advanced atheroma, the likelihood ratio of a subsequent event was higher for those with an index ≤ 0.7 than for those with an index ≤ 0.9. An index ≤ 0.9; however, would be more likely to detect individuals with early disease without symptoms for screening purposes, who would not otherwise seek medical attention.

CONCLUSION

An increased risk of lower extremity ulceration, amputation, and death are all connected with PVD as are exertional limb symptoms, functional deterioration, and poor quality of life. Along with the rising burden of atherosclerotic risk factors and an aging population, the prevalence of PVD is rising globally. Although many of the risk factors for PVD are also common to other CV illnesses, other risk variables such as smoking and dyslipidemia, affect PVD risk differently than they do CAD risk. Our understanding of atherosclerotic risk has been advanced by increased attention to PVD, particularly in the context of polyvascular illness, and this paradigm is increasingly utilized in the design of CV treatment trials. Understanding and diagnosing PVD can be useful as it is linked to CVD and other atherosclerotic diseases. In short, PVD can be a guiding light to CVD.

SUGGESTED READINGS

1. European Stroke Organisation; Tendera M, Aboyans V, Bartelink ML, Baumgartner I, Clément D, et al. ESC Guidelines on the diagnosis and treatment of peripheral artery diseases: Document covering atherosclerotic disease of extracranial carotid and vertebral, mesenteric, renal, upper and lower extremity arteries: the Task Force on the Diagnosis and Treatment of Peripheral Artery Diseases of the European Society of Cardiology (ESC). Eur Heart J. 2011;32(22):2851-906.
2. Meijer WT, Grobbee DE, Hunink MG, Hofman A, Hoes AW. Determinants of peripheral arterial disease in the elderly: the Rotterdam study. Arch Intern Med. 2000;160(19):2934-8.
3. Fowkes FG, Rudan D, Rudan I, Aboyans V, Denenberg JO, McDermott MM, et al. Comparison of global estimates of prevalence and risk factors for peripheral artery disease in 2000 and 2010: a systematic review and analysis. Lancet. 2013;382(9901):1329-40.
4. Krishna SM, Moxon JV, Golledge J. A review of the pathophysiology and potential biomarkers for peripheral artery disease. Int J Mol Sci. 2015;16(5):11294-322.
5. Subherwal S, Patel MR, Kober L, Peterson ED, Bhatt DL, Gislason GH, et al. Peripheral artery disease is a coronary heart disease risk equivalent among both men and women: results from a nationwide study. Eur J Prev Cardiol. 2015;22(3):317-25.
6. Sampson UKA, Fowkes FGR, Naidoo NG, Criqui MH. Peripheral Artery Disease. In: Prabhakaran D, Anand S, Gaziano TA, Mbanya JC, Wu Y, Nugent R (Eds). Cardiovascular, Respiratory, and Related Disorders, 3rd edition. Washington (DC): The International Bank for Reconstruction and Development/The World Bank; 2017.
7. Song P, Fang Z, Wang H, Cai Y, Rahimi K, Zhu Y, et al. Global and regional prevalence, burden, and risk factors for carotid atherosclerosis: a systematic review, meta-analysis, and modelling study. Lancet Glob Health. 2020;8(5):e721-9.
8. Premalatha G, Shanthirani S, Deepa R, Markovitz J, Mohan V. Prevalence and risk factors of peripheral vascular disease in a selected South Indian population: the Chennai Urban Population Study. Diabetes Care. 2000;23(9):1295-300.

11

CHAPTER

Surgical Management of Aortic Valvular Disease

Shilpa Basu Roy

ABSTRACT

Patients with diseases of the aortic valve, namely aortic stenosis and aortic regurgitation, are commonly seen in the cardiological department. In this article, we attempt to briefly describe the common clinical manifestations and the line of management of these patients. The various treatment options that are available in the current era have also been discussed in a very concise way.

INTRODUCTION

The aortic valve is involved with the onward blood flow from the left ventricle to the aorta and plays an important role in the maintenance of the systemic circulation. Any lesion of the aortic valve would eventually lead to hemodynamic instability and myocardial dysfunction which may or may not be reversible. The common aortic valve lesions are aortic regurgitation (AR) and aortic stenosis (AS).

AORTIC REGURGITATION

In this condition, there is lack of apposition of the aortic valve leaflets causing insufficiency and leading to back flow of the blood into the left ventricle during diastole.

AORTIC STENOSIS

In this condition, there is obstruction of the blood flow across the aortic valve during left ventricular (LV) systole due to narrowing of the aortic valve orifice.

SIGNS AND SYMPTOMS

Patients presenting with aortic valvular disease (both stenosis and regurgitation) often present with progressive chest pain, palpitation, syncope, and symptoms of heart failure such as dyspnea, orthopnea, and paroxysmal nocturnal dyspnea.

MANAGEMENT

Investigations

- *Transthoracic echocardiography*: This is the investigation of choice and is considered as the gold standard.
- *Transesophageal echocardiography*: This is highly sensitive and often used to describe in details the anatomy of the aortic valve and the lesions there of (e.g., the extent of thickening of leaflets, coaptation, and diameter of the aortic annulus)
- *Carotid artery Doppler of neck vessels*: To see the presence of atherosclerotic plaque and check the patency of the artery
- *Cardiac CT*: Although rarely required, but may be used when any other associated cardiac anomaly is suspected.
- *Coronary angiography*: This is required in most cases as part of preoperative screening, especially in those patients who meet at least one of the following criteria:
  - Are more than 40 years of age
  - Have a history of angina
  - Have a history of previous coronary artery disease
  - Have a family history of coronary artery disease
- *CT aortography*: This is sometimes needed in patients where echocardiography suggests dilated aortic root or ascending aorta. Also to assess the atherosclerotic plaque. This is necessary for planning the surgical repair.

Treatment

Conservative medical management: Most patients with early aortic valvular diseases are managed symptomatically, often with diuretics and digoxin. In patients with regurgitant lesions, the systemic resistance is lowered using vasodilators or angiotensin-converting enzyme (ACE) inhibitors.

Surgery: Patients who meet the criteria for surgical management as per the American Heart Association guidelines are considered for surgery. Grossly the indications are as follows:

For AS, the candidates for aortic valve replacement are:
- Symptomatic patients with severe AS.
- Patients with symptomatic, severe AS undergoing coronary artery bypass surgery.
- Patients with asymptomatic, severe AS undergoing surgery on the aorta or other heart valves.
- Patients with asymptomatic, severe AS and LV systolic dysfunction (ejection fraction < 0.50).

For AR, the candidates for aortic valve replacement are:
- Surgery is recommended for symptomatic patients with severe AR regardless of LV function; for asymptomatic patients with: (A) LV end-systolic diameter (LVESD) >50 mm or >25 mm/m^2 body surface area (if body size is small) or (B) resting LV ejection fraction (LVEF) <50%; and for both symptomatic and asymptomatic patients undergoing coronary artery bypass grafting (CABG) or surgery of the ascending aorta or of another valve.
- Valve-sparing aortic root replacement is recommended for young patients with aortic root dilation. Ascending aortic surgery is indicated for Marfan patients with aortic root disease and maximal ascending aortic diameter >50 mm.

Surgical intervention: There are various surgical interventions available for the patients. All open heart procedures are done by completely arresting the heart using cardioplegia solution while the patient is put on the cardiopulmonary bypass (heart-lung) machine. The various surgical options are as follows:
- Aortic valve repair
- Aortic valve replacement
- *Aortic neocuspidization*: Ozaki procedure

Repair of the aortic valve is always preferred over valve replacement. The most important advantage is—there is no need for postoperative anticoagulation therapy in these patients. However, rheumatic valvular disease is the most common etiology in Indian patients. In these patients, the valvular leaflets are usually thickened and calcified, and are beyond the scope of repair. Valve repair is usually possible in patients where the etiology is connective tissue disorder, such as in patients with Marfan's syndrome.

Types of aortic repair: The following techniques of repair are usually possible in the different aortic valve diseases:

For aortic valve insufficiency:
- Aortic root and annular techniques, e.g., aortic cusp coaptation may be improved in selected patients by subcommissural annuloplasty.
- *Valve-sparing root replacement (VSRR)*: This procedure is usually done in AR caused due to aortic root dilatation. In this procedure, the aortic root is either remodeled by annuloplasty technique, or reimplantation if the aortic root is done after adequate assessment of the aortic cusp.
- *Repair of isolated aortic valve related aortic insufficiency*: This technique is reserved for selected patients, e.g., in those with aortic cusp prolapse.

For AS:
- *Transcatheter balloon aortic valvuloplasty (BAV)*: This is a minimally invasive procedure done by the interventional cardiologists in the cath lab.

For small aortic root:
- Supra-annular valves may be used.
- Aortic root enlargement techniques can be done, which may be either posterior root enlargement techniques (e.g., Nick's or Manouguian's procedure) or anterior root enlargement techniques (e.g., Konno-Rastan procedure)
- *Ross procedure*: In this procedure, the aortic root is replaced by the patient's own pulmonary valve (autograft). The latter is replaced by a pulmonary homograft.

Aortic valve replacement: This is done by completely excising the aortic valve leaflets and replacing them with an artificial valve **(Figs. 1 and 2)**. The artificial valve may be either mechanical (metallic) or bioprosthetic each having specific indications, advantages, and disadvantages.

Mechanical (metallic) valves ***(Fig. 3)***: These are indicated in patients who are younger than 55 years of age because the valves have a longer lifespan of 15–20 years. However, the most important problem with this valve is the lifelong requirement of anticoagulants and its complications. A meticulous monitoring of patients' international normalized ratio (INR) level is also necessary. The target INR level is between 2 and 2.5. Special precautions are needed in pregnant patients with mechanical heart valves.

Bioprosthetic valves ***(Fig. 4)***: These are made using animal tissues (either porcine or bovine) and are indicated in patients above the age of 55 years and also in young females

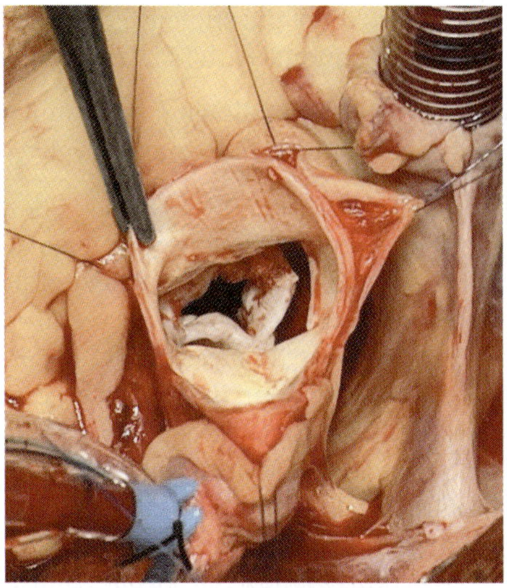

FIG. 1: This is an intraoperative picture of severe aortic stenosis showing grossly thickened and severely calcified aortic cusps.

of reproductive age group where family is not completed. They are also indicated in patients with known bleeding manifestations and coagulopathies. The most important advantage is that lifelong anticoagulation is not necessary. The disadvantage is their shorter lifespan of about 10–20 years. However, the newer generation bioprosthetic valves are being marketed as having comparable lifespan as that of the mechanical valves. These valves are more expensive than mechanical valves. Some intraoperative pictures of implantation of a bioprosthetic aortic valve have been shared here **(Figs. 5 and 6)**.

Sutureless valves ***(Fig. 7)***: These valves have been developed to reduce the operating time of aortic valve replacement surgery and thereby reduce the complications arising due to it. After excising the native aortic cusps, the aortic annulus is sized and the sutureless aortic valve is deployed and implanted using three guiding sutures **(Fig. 8)**. The

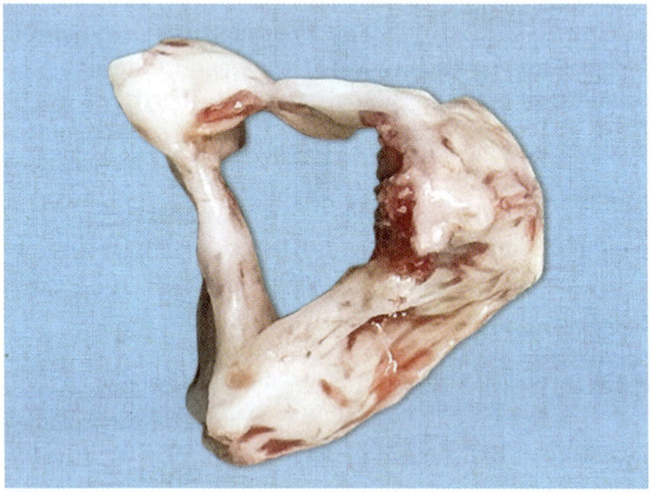

FIG. 2: This shows the excised deceased aortic cusps.

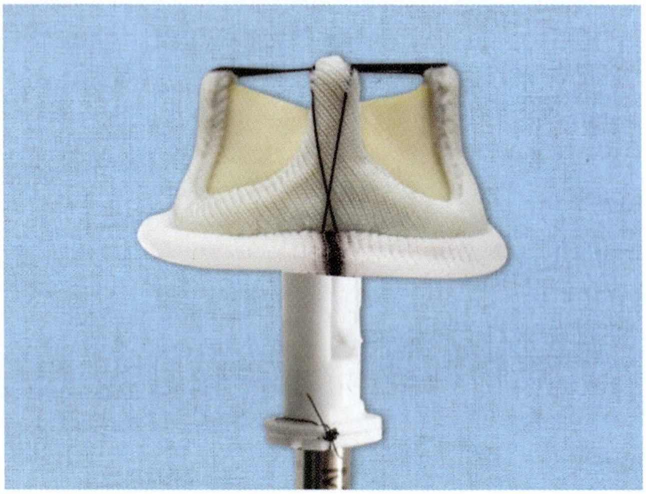

FIG. 4: Biological aortic valve.

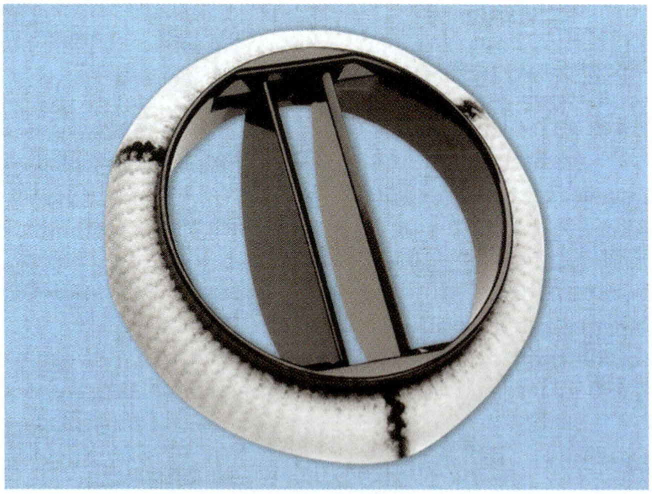

FIG. 3: Mechanical (metallic) aortic valve.

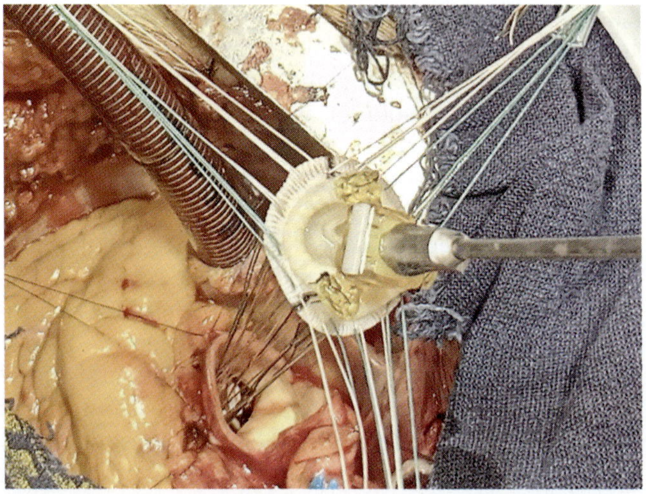

FIG. 5: This is an intraoperative picture showing implantation of a biological aortic valve, using interrupted polyester sutures.

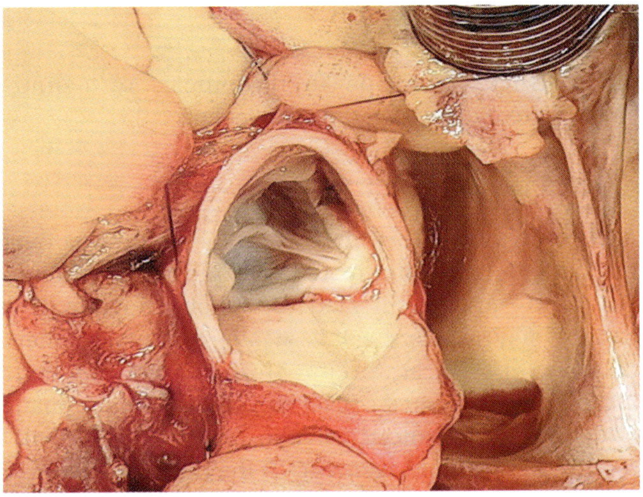

FIG. 6: This is an intraoperative picture showing the biological aortic valve after implantation.

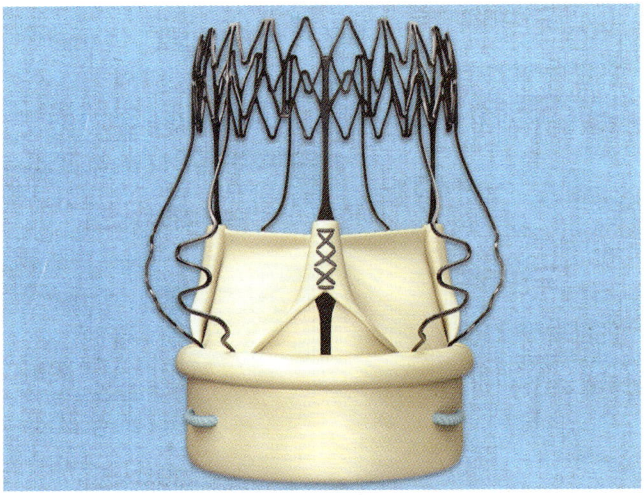

FIG. 7: Sutureless aortic valve.

guiding sutures are removed later on, thus reducing the time for suturing the valve and also the overall time for surgery. This is mostly preferable in patients who are high-risk candidates for prolonged surgery. The reduced operating time helps in preserving the hemodynamic status of these patients.

Transcutaneous aortic valve implantation (TAVI) ***(Fig. 9)***: This is done percutaneously in the cath lab by the interventional cardiologist. These are special valves which are 10 times more costly than the conventional valves used in open surgery. TAVI is indicated either in aged patients who are at high risk for open surgery, or in those patients who want TAVI as per their choice.

Creation of new aortic leaflets (aortic valve neocuspidization or Ozaki procedure): This is a newer

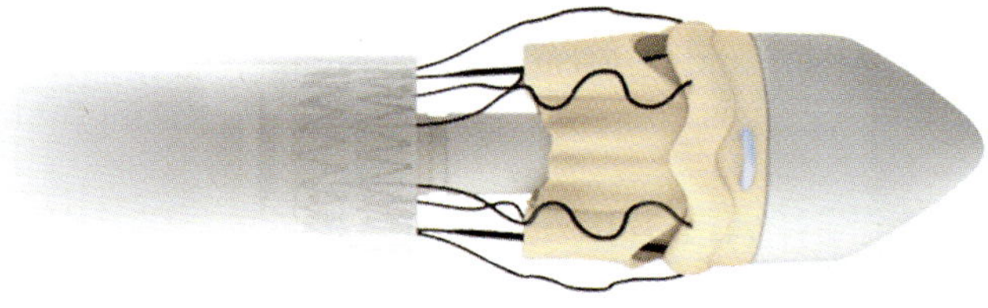

FIG. 8: Deployment device of sutureless valve.

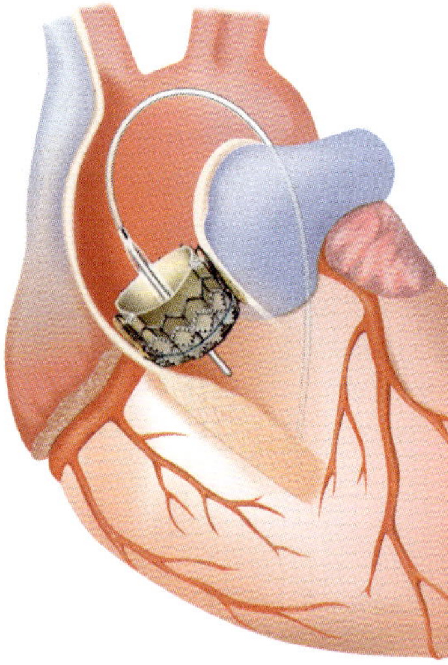

FIG. 9: Deployment of transcutaneous aortic valve implantation (TAVI).

surgical technique developed and pioneered by renowned Japanese cardiac surgeon Dr Ozaki. This technique is applicable for both AR and AS patients. In this procedure, after excising the diseased valve leaflets, new leaflets are created using the patient's own pericardium using standardized tools. As a result, the Ozaki procedure is more cost effective than conventional open surgery and there is no requirement for postoperative anticoagulants. The use of standardized tools has decreased the learning curve for the surgeons.

For dilated aortic root with dilated ascending aorta:

- *Bentall's procedure*: In this procedure, the diseased aortic valve along with the dilated root and ascending aorta is excised, which is then replaced with a valved conduit. The right and left coronary arteries are carefully mobilized and their ostia are preserved in the form of coronary buttons, which are individually anastomosed on holes created on the sides of the conduit.
- *Ozaki procedure with Florida sleeve*: This may be done as an alternative to the Bentall's procedure. In this procedure, the diseased valve leaflets are excised and new aortic cusps are created, i.e., the Ozaki procedure.

The diseased dilated aortic root and ascending aorta is excised and replaced with a conduit, i.e., the Florida sleeve. This is a newer technique with a promising future.

COMPLICATIONS

The most common complications following an aortic valve surgery can be grouped into the following:

- *Immediate postoperative*:
  - Patient prosthesis mismatch
  - Paravalvular leak
  - Bleeding
  - Cardiovascular accident (CVA) which may be either ischemic due to embolism of thrombus, atherosclerotic plaque or air, or due to intracranial hemorrhage
  - Arrhythmias
  - Low cardiac output
  - Infection
  - Death
- *Delayed*:
  - Prosthetic valve endocarditis
  - Struck valve due to thrombosis or pannus formation around the valve leaflets

CONCLUSION

Aortic valvular disease is a common finding among the patients reporting to the cardiology department. Diagnosis can be easily made by echocardiogram. Few patients may need further investigations for management planning or surgical workup. Most patients with early disease can be treated conservatively. The symptomatic patients with advanced valvular diseases will usually require surgical management. In the modern era, there are several options for surgical repair or replacement of the aortic valve depending on the patient's medical profile. Overall, patients with aortic valvular diseases have extremely favorable outcomes if they are treated timely.

SUGGESTED READING

1. Otto CM, Nishimura RA, Bonow RO, Carabello BA, Erwin JP 3rd, Gentile F, et al. 2020 ACC/AHA Guideline for the Management of Patients With Valvular Heart Disease: Executive Summary: A Report of the American College of Cardiology/American Heart Association Joint Committee on Clinical Practice Guidelines. Circulation. 2021;143(5):e35-71.

12

CHAPTER

Dual Antiplatelet Therapy in Coronary Artery Disease

Ankan Pathak, Aparna Tewari, Chandan Sharma

ABSTRACT

Central to the management of coronary artery disease (CAD) includes the usage of dual antiplatelet therapy more commonly known as DAPT. However, despite the rapid strides made in the field of interventional cardiology, there still remains a degree of uncertainty as far as the duration of DAPT in CAD is concerned. As per the latest guidelines, DAPT should be continued for at least 1 year following acute coronary syndrome (ACS) and 6 months following percutaneous coronary intervention (PCI) for stable angina.

INTRODUCTION

Antiplatelet therapy forms the backbone in the treatment of coronary artery disease (CAD) for the treatment of atheroembolic events. Aspirin—often considered the prototype antiplatelet agent, has had multiple studies that have revealed that it reduces the incidence of major adverse cardiovascular events (MACE) by approximately one-fifth. Dual antiplatelet therapy (DAPT) is often defined as the combination of aspirin plus a P2Y12 inhibitor. With the usage of DAPT, it results in greater platelet inhibition and greater reduction in MACE abeilt at the cost of one major side effect—an increased risk of bleeding.

Routine DAPT is currently not a recommendation for patients with stable CAD without a history of acute coronary syndrome (ACS), percutaneous coronary intervention (PCI), or coronary artery bypass graft (CABG) within 12 months.

DURATION OF DUAL ANTIPLATELET THERAPY

Two landmark associations namely the European Society of Cardiology and the American Heart Association have stated that the standard duration of DAPT for patients with ACS is ≥12 months, and ≥6 months for those with CAD undergoing intervention. As far as the choice of P2Y12 inhibitor is concerned, usually in patients with a high risk of ischemic events (patients presenting with ACS, diabetic, smokers, and obese subjects) either prasugrel or ticagrelor is recommended. The standard durations mentioned above may be changed depending upon the clinical scenario. Both the guidelines have also mentioned the DAPT score as a tool to monitor patients.

DUAL ANTIPLATELET THERAPY SCORE

Dual antiplatelet therapy score **(Table 1)** has become a vital cog in the wheel when it comes to assessing the risk-benefit ratio of using DAPT > 12 months after PCI. The score can range from –2 to 10 points, and a score of ≥2 necessitates the use of a longer DAPT and a score of <2 necessitates a standard DAPT.

PRECISE-DAPT SCORE

The PRECISE-DAPT (Predicting Bleeding Complications in Patients Undergoing Stent Implantation and Subsequent Dual Antiplatelet Therapy) score is another

TABLE 1: Components and scoring system of DAPT score.

Variables	Points
Age in years:	
• More than –75	–2
• 65–75	–1
• <65	0
Smoking	1
Diabetes mellitus	1
MI at presentation	1
Prior PCI or MI	1
Paclitaxel eluting stent	1
Stent diameter < 3 mm	1
CHF or LVEF < 30	2
Vein graft stent	2

(CHF: congestive heart failure; DAPT: dual antiplatelet therapy; LVEF: left ventricular ejection fraction; PCI: percutaneous coronary intervention; MI: myocardial infarction)

validated scoring tool vital to making a decision regarding the duration of DAPT in patients who have undergone PCI.

This is calculated using five parameters, namely:

1. Age
2. White blood cell count
3. Hemoglobin level
4. Creatinine clearance
5. History of spontaneous bleeding

A score totaling >25 is deemed to be at higher risk of bleeding. A score >25 also suggests that a standard DAPT duration is more prudent rather than an extended duration of DAPT.

PREVENTING GASTROINTESTINAL BLEEDS

Amongst the leading causes of serious bleeding arising from DAPT therapy is gastrointestinal (GI) bleed. Proton-pump inhibitors (PPIs) are commonly coprescribed along with DAPT to reduce the incidence of GI bleed. However, the ACC/AHA recommends PPI for a specific subset of patients—patients on Warfarin therapy, steroids, or use of nonsteroidal anti-inflammatory drugs (NSAIDs) intake, prior episode of GI bleed, and increased age.

ANTIPLATELET AND ANTITHROMBOTIC THERAPY

With the increasing incidence of CAD and along with it atrial fibrillation (AF), it remains important for clinicians to use both antiplatelets and antithrombotics at the same time. It already complicates the issue of risk-benefit assessment. Dual antiplatelet therapy, i.e., aspirin plus P2Y12 inhibitors, is used for secondary prevention of coronary events and protection against stent thrombosis but does not provide protection against stroke in AF. Also, to complicate matters 10% of the patients who undergo PCI also have AF, hence it is vital to use DAPT and oral anticoagulants (OACs) simultaneously, also called *triple anticoagulation* or *triple therapy*. There is substantial evidence that recommends the use of CHA_2DS_2–VASc and HAS-BLED (Hypertension, Abnormal Renal/Liver Function, Stroke, Bleeding History or Predisposition, Labile INR, Elderly, Drugs/Alcohol Concomitantly) scores when it comes to assessing risk-benefit ratio in patients of AF. There is a general preference in the usage of clopidogrel rather than the more potent prasugrel or ticagrelor in such a group of patients. In patients with a presumable degree of high atherothrombotic risk coupled with a low bleeding risk, triple therapy (aspirin, clopidogrel, and oral anticoagulant) can be prescribed for up to a period of 6 months, with dual therapy (clopidogrel plus oral anticoagulant) continued for up to a period of 12 months after PCI. In individuals with a high bleeding risk, the duration of triple therapy can be shortened to as low as 1-month duration or can be removed altogether. In all cases irrespective of bleeding risk, once 12 months of dual therapy have been completed, individuals can continue oral anticoagulant as monotherapy indefinitely.

CONCLUSION

The decision about DAPT is one that rests with the clinician himself. It is very difficult to balance between preventing an in-stent restenosis but on the flip side, overzealous treatment might increase the risk of major bleeding. The choice of DAPT in addition to the duration is equally important. Validated scoring tools such as the DAPT score and PRECISE-DAPT score do help to individualize treatment schedules. It is important to identify patients who are high thrombotic risk patients and equally important in indentifying patients who are at risk of bleed.

SUGGESTED READINGS

1. Antithrombotic Trialists' (ATT) Collaboration; Baigent C, Blackwell L, Collins R, Emberson J, Godwin J, et al. Aspirin in the primary and secondary prevention of vascular disease: a collaborative meta-analysis of individual participant data from randomised trials. Lancet. 2009;373(9678):1849-60.
2. Yeh RW, Secemsky EA, Kereiakes DJ, Normand SL, Gershlick AH, Cohen DJ, et al. Development and validation of a prediction rule for benefit and harm of dual antiplatelet therapy beyond 1 year after percutaneous coronary intervention. JAMA. 2016;315(16):1735-49.
3. Agewall S, Cattaneo M, Collet JP, Andreotti F, Lip GY, Verheugt FW, et al. Expert position paper on the use of proton pump inhibitors in patients with cardiovascular disease and antithrombotic therapy. Eur Heart J. 2013;34(23):1708-13.
4. Lip GYH, Collet JP, Haude M et al. Management of antithrombotic therapy in AF patients presenting with ACS and/or undergoing PCI: a summary of the joint consensus document of the European Heart Rhythm Association (EHRA), European Society of Cardiology Working Group on Thrombosis, European Association of Percutaneous Cardiovascular Interventions (EAPCI) and European Association of Acute Cardiac Care (ACCA) endorsed by the Heart Rhythm Society (HRS), AsiaPacific Heart Rhythm Society (APHRS), Latin America Heart Rhythm Society (LAHRS), and Cardiac Arrhythmia Society of Southern Africa (CASSA). Eur Heart J. 2018;39:2847-50.

13

CHAPTER

Sudden Cardiac Arrest: Perspectives in Mid-21st Century

Ashish K Thakur, Anshini Thakur

ABSTRACT

Sudden cardiac arrest (SCA)/death continues to be a major global health issue, with wide geographic variations and access to the expected standards of care. Although the mortality with out-of-hospital cardiac arrest (OHCA) has improved over the years in certain population groups, for the general population at large this remains unchanged. The article below covers the current perspectives relating to prediction and prevention, identifying high-risk groups, and offering tailored and advanced therapies. With prehospital care now established as the key prognostic marker of survival in sudden cardiac death (SCD), the relevant aspects are covered, including the just concluded ARREST (Advanced Reperfusion Strategies for Refractory Cardiac Arrest) trial, early and multimodality neuroprognostication, the role of cardiac arrest centers, multidisciplinary (MDT) approach, and specialist clinics. Case selection for invasive tests/treatment and advanced cardiopulmonary resuscitation (CPR) using mechanical circulatory devices have been reviewed, combined with recent aspects of implantable cardioverter-defibrillators (ICDs) and medical therapies. Future perspectives to improve the care of patients and relatives using all available resources and global collaborative approaches are also covered.

INTRODUCTION

Sudden cardiac arrest (SCA), also known as sudden cardiac death (SCD), widely recognized as part of sudden arrhythmic death syndrome (SADS) is a major cause of global mortality and morbidity. SCD is usually defined as sudden death due to a presumed cardiac cause within 1 hour of symptoms, if witnessed, or within the last 24 hours of if unwitnessed. Exact data about its incidence/prevalence varies a lot, due to heterogenous and inconsistent reporting across the world, except in countries having a systematic process of maintaining accurate cardiac arrest data and annual survival rates. Overall, up to 5 million people could have SCD every year globally, with rising age and coronary artery disease (CAD) being the most important variables (average age 60–65 years). An Indian study estimated OHCA incidence at 40–42/100,000 in the general population, mainly in males with CAD. In a postpandemic world with rising trends of cardiovascular risk factors, sedentary lifestyle, and increasing stress, the overall incidence of SCA/SCD seems to be on the rise in developing countries, with numerous other factors contributing to the despicable situation. The survival rates for out-of-hospital cardiac arrest (OHCA) remain a meager low at 10% in the general population, this can be as high as 70% in selected patient populations, based upon circumstances and the rapidity of resuscitation, return of spontaneous circulation (ROSC) and postresuscitation care.

SUDDEN CARDIAC ARREST/SUDDEN CARDIAC DEATH: CHALLENGES IN MANAGEMENT

The OHCA population is quite heterogenous, with successful ROSC in 40–60% with advanced cardiac life support (ACLS), out of which, <15% would be conscious survivors, with the rest being comatose. Initiatives are underway to improve survival rates besides identifying populations at high risk and better prediction and prevention, and refining protocols of resuscitation, mechanical circulatory support, and addressing aspects beyond resuscitation for survivors to maximize their outcomes and have established prognostic processes in place to tailor management and clarify the poor risk and support survivors and families with a multi-disciplinary approach and improving awareness in the general population about bystander cardiopulmonary resuscitation (CPR) and using defibrillators, especially automated external devices (AEDs), which are key to enhancing survival in SCA/SCD. Most sudden deaths occur due to a cardiac cause and up to half of these can be sudden, especially in acute coronary syndromes (ACS). It is also pertinent to remember that the majority of in-hospital arrests are due to nonshockable rhythms/pulseless electrical activity (PEA) due to patient subset/comorbidities. **Figures 1A and B** depict the causes of SCA/SCD across all ages and the young, with the majority due to CAD, followed by a range of arrhythmogenic conditions. It is now being recognized that SCA is an event on a spectrum, invariably leading to death (SCD).

The recently published UK ARREST trial is the first prospective, randomized trial that included patients (≥18 years) with ROSC after OHCA with no ST-elevation on electrocardiogram (ECG). They were randomly assigned at the scene by paramedics (London Ambulance Service) to be transferred to a cardiac catheter laboratory at one of seven dedicated cardiac arrest centers or receive the usual standard of care at the geographically closest emergency department at one of 32 local hospitals. With 411 participants in the cardiac arrest center group and 412 in the standard care group, there was no mortality benefit **(Fig. 2)** between the groups at 30 days, 3 months,

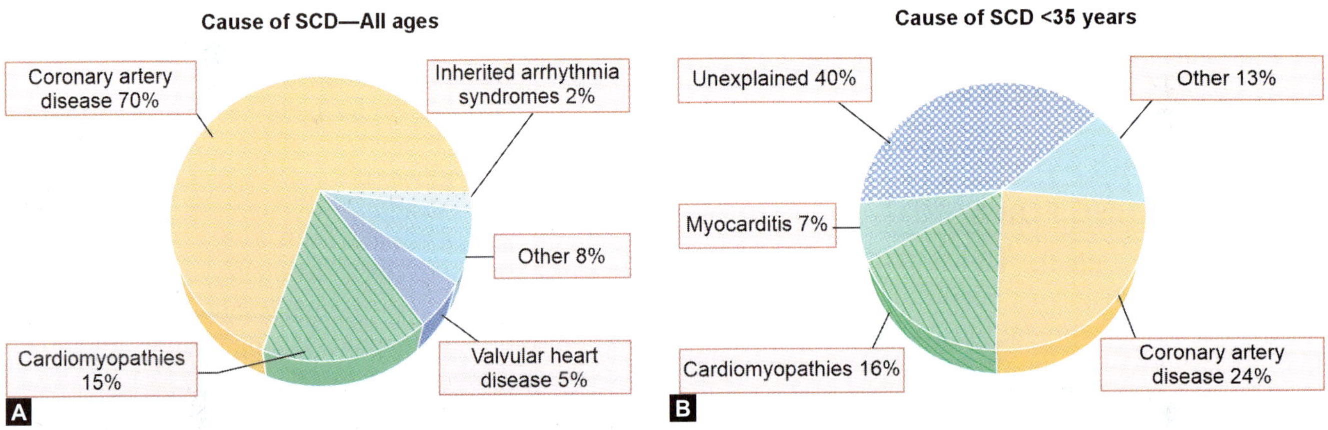

FIGS. 1A AND B: Causes of sudden cardiac death (SCD).
Source: With permission from Isbister J, et al. (2019).

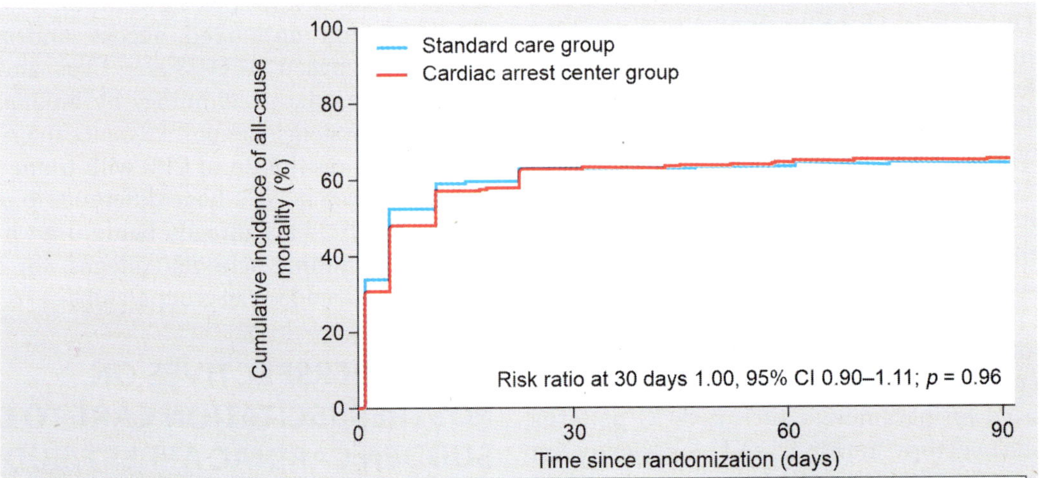

Number at risk				
Standard care group	413	154	153	148
Cardiac arrest center group	414	153	148	148

FIG. 2: The ARREST trial. Kaplan–Meier plot of all-cause mortality up to 3 months (intention-to-treat population).

or any difference in neurological outcomes, further highlighting the relevance of prehospital care.

The challenges to tackling SCA/SCD in current times include:

- Most OHCA events occur indoors, with challenges to recognition and seeking help
- Up to a third to half of events are unwitnessed
- Rising incidence of nonshockable arrests, with poorer prognosis
- Lack of awareness and bystander CPR skills, leading to poor resuscitation and survival rates, especially in low- and middle-income countries
- Universal automated external defibrillator (AED) access and training
- Proper postresuscitation care
- Universal and affordable genetic testing for risk stratification
- Access to screening, diagnostic tests, and medications
- Data/bio-statistical management
- Early and multimodality neuroprognostication
- Access to survivorship support

WHAT CAN HELP PREDICT AND PREVENT SCA/SCD GOING FORWARD?

The strategies to predict and prevent cardiac arrest revolve around identifying people at high risk, both in the general population and those with a family history of SCA/SCD. with specific strategies and varying yields. They comprise population-based initiatives such as screening people into endurance training or competitive sports for abnormal electrocardiography (i.e., hypertrophy), estimating cardiovascular disease (CVD) risk, and enhancing awareness around it, combining these with specific and targeted genetic testing for high-risk features in families (first-degree relatives) of SCA/SCD patients. This is also known as "phenotyping," where one could have Ischemic versus nonischemic heart disease, with further subtyping of both groups as per presence or absence of ischemia or scar, and the pattern of hypertrophy, infiltration, and other markers on advanced imaging [right ventricular dysplasia—arrhythmogenic right ventricular cardiomyopathy (ARVC)], with a heightened risk of potentially fatal ventricular arrhythmias. In the absence of any obvious structural or functional heart disease, this can be difficult, and needs a high index of suspicion based on parameters such as ECG patterns (e.g., Brugada), ectopy burden, and complexity on monitoring, besides a good history of symptoms if any and clinical examination and offering preventive treatments like implantable defibrillators to suitable patients. Patients and their families need ongoing assessments and support via bespoke services (e.g., inherited cardiac conditions clinics) using a multidisciplinary (MDT) approach, including genetic testing was indicated for familial causes. Often very early interventions such as primordial prevention (at the school level) of diabetes and CVD can help reduce the risk of SCA/SCD. The debate on the identification of patients at the highest risk of arrhythmic death continues; however, with pros and cons of offering preventive treatment strategies based upon relatively simple or single versus complex and a set of multiple testing criteria. There is a renewed call for an autopsy of all fatal SCD, especially younger ones to learn about the cause(s) and the practice varies widely on a global basis.

FLOW OF THE SCA/SCD PATIENT: HOW CAN BETTER COMMUNITY CPR AND AEDS CHANGE THE LANDSCAPE?

Good basic life support (BLS) skills, rapid defibrillation, correction of acid–base balance, and ruling out a reversible cause (the Ps and the Ts) are vital to maximizing survival in OHCA. Effective chest compressions have been emphasized over the years, with less evidence for the effectiveness of adjunctive interventions like mouth-to-mouth respiration, especially for bystander CPR, and evidence for drugs such as adrenaline and amiodarone are on the decline, as the focus has shifted on high-quality chest (cardiac) compressions being the most important parameter. AEDs remain the mainstay in treating OHCA, and in the presence of a shockable cause (ventricular fibrillation or pulseless ventricular tachycardia), the prognosis declines with every passing minute, with almost no chance of survival at 10 minutes of lack of cerebral blood flow (no flow time). There is ample evidence that enhanced access and provision of community-based AEDs saves lives and combining them with modern technology by linking to hospital/emergency systems, remote assistance to first responders, and prompt restitution of CPR with trained volunteers/champions can make a huge difference to the outcomes. These initiatives are already being used in a variety of settings, including schools/colleges, for allied health professionals, and social groups/clubs.

NEWER PERSPECTIVES ON POSTRESUSCITATION CARE TO OPTIMIZE SUDDEN CARDIAC ARREST/SUDDEN CARDIAC DEATH OUTCOMES

After successful ROSC, survival and successful discharge from the hospital are entirely dependent upon postresuscitation care. Regardless of etiology, about two-thirds of OHCA patients will die due to hypoxic brain injury, with a cardiac cause for death in only 15% of patients. The key aspects are determined by the initial rhythm, promptness of defibrillation and CPR, no flow time, hemodynamic status, and vital organ function. This led to the development of the MIRACL2 neurologic risk score for neurological prognostication using seven variables at the scene of the arrest. A scoring system (maximum of 10) allows to categorize patients as having good to poor prognosis for neurological outcomes in 6 months, with almost similar (poor) prognosis from score 5–10 and best prognosis from 0 to 3. Younger patients and those with scores up to 4 may benefit from cardiac catheterization to define coronary anatomy, early revascularization, and establish safe/appropriate mechanical circulatory support if necessary. There is also a King's Out of Hospital Cardiac Arrest Registry (KOCAR) culprit lesion probability score for OHCA based on clinical features at presentation, and if combined with the MIRACL2 score, helps rationale decision making about catheter laboratories, mechanical support, escalation of management, and facilitate realistic and objective discussions with survivor's families. The issue of taking all/most OHCA survivors without ST elevation on ECG to catheter laboratory is controversial and there seems to be consensus about appropriate case selection, besides optimizing anticoagulation and antiplatelet therapy due to a high thrombogenic state, "culprit only" intervention and supportive care, besides mechanical circulatory support for carefully selected patients, mainly those in cardiogenic shock. Both KOCAR and MIRACL2 can be assessed before the patient arrives at the hospital and based on hemodynamics and organ function, it is possible to phenotype patients surviving OHCA into four broad categories: (1) Nonshocked, (2) hemodynamically shocked, (3) hypoperfused, and (4) hemometabolic shocked [Society for Cardiovascular Angiography and Interventions (SCAI)-5 classification], with the last group having the worst outcomes and prognosis, with different modes of death across the groups explained by their phenotypes. In highly selected patients (cardiogenic shock), extracorporeal-cardiopulmonary resuscitation (E-CPR) is a resuscitation method combining placing patients on extracorporeal membrane oxygenation (ECMO), which can improve survival rates, compared with standard CPR interventions. The E-CPR is only available at a few centers of excellence and is limited to patients not responding to typical interventions and is another time-critical intervention to improve outcomes in OHCA patients. In patients for whom diagnosis remains unclear after initial evaluation, further tests like advanced ECG, and cardiac imaging can help with diagnostic information in almost half of patients. Eventually, about 5–10% of OHCA events remain unexplained despite extensive workup and could be considered as "idiopathic ventricular fibrillation." This is being studied further, to find an explainable cause, like has been the case for other difficult conditions such as Brugada syndrome, short QT syndrome, and the very recently described widespread ST-segment depression syndrome, and the identification of microstructural epicardial abnormalities.

IMPLANTABLE CARDIOVERTER-DEFIBRILLATOR, MEDICATIONS AND FURTHER: SUMMARY PERSPECTIVES IN SUDDEN CARDIAC ARREST/SUDDEN CARDIAC DEATH

Implantable cardioverter-defibrillator treatment is indicated for survivors with good neurological outcomes and no other treatable cause of arrhythmia, i.e., CAD; however, it should be carefully considered as per further arrhythmic and SCA risk, with an overall benefit for secondary prevention. ICD is now also indicated for myocarditis and coronary vasospasm causing SCA. Although the evidence base is large for primary and secondary prevention, there is a strong need to revisit the primary prevention indications in the modern context of medical management and complex device therapy (CRT), compared with earlier trials comparing medical management with ICD in heart failure. Patients with ischemic left ventricular systolic dysfunction (LVSD) benefit more than nonischemic etiology. Implantable cardioverter-defibrillators need to be affordable and universally available, especially for poor regions. They cannot prevent SCD and there is a need to consider their shock-related aspects, besides device and lead-related complications. ICD benefits reduce with comorbidities, especially in multicomorbid patients, and in women, with reduced risk of SCA, when being considered for primary prevention, with most benefits in younger male patients (<50–60 years) with CAD without significant comorbidities. Besides providing defibrillation and pacing functions, ICDs also provide monitoring benefits. There is a trend toward a rise in the use of subcutaneous ICDs in young and active patients (<40 years), besides the development of strategies for leadless devices, further reducing the morbidity potential, compared with conventional intravascular systems. EP studies and ablation have a role as well, especially for atrial fibrillation with preexcitation [Wolff-Parkinson-White (WPW)] and selected cases of idiopathic ventricular fibrillation (VF). Neuromodulation using sympathetic denervation has a role to play in scenarios with catecholaminergic or idiopathic recurrent ventricular tachycardia (VT)/VF, and long QT syndrome (LQTS) as adjunctive preventive therapies. Further, a great innovation on the horizon is nontraumatic and pain-free optogenetic defibrillation or pacing using epicardial illumination (brief blue light pulses), with modulation of cardiac channel/cells. Some other novel approaches to prevent SCD include a biological pacemaker to treat bradyarrhythmia, and biological substrate modification techniques, injecting exosomes to reduce ventricular scar as highly innovative and futuristic initiatives.

Medical management addresses either the arrhythmogenic substrate or arrhythmia itself, besides guidance-directed medical treatment of CVD and risk factors. Beta-blockers are conventionally used for suppressing arrhythmia and reducing SCD. Statins have a modest beneficial effect on SCD, due to reduced ACS events. Angiotensin converting enzyme (ACE) inhibitors/angiotensin receptor blockers (ARBs) and mineralocorticoid receptor antagonists (MRAs) improve left ventricular reverse remodeling, prevent heart failure deterioration, and improve survival, potentially also with decreased SCD risk via inhibition of myocardial and vascular adverse remodeling, reduced collagen deposition and myocardial stiffness, modulation of nitric oxide synthesis, and prevention of hypokalemia. Entresto (neprilysin inhibition with ARB) might also reduce the risk of SCD with evidence of reduced VT, ICD shocks, and ventricular premature contractions (VPCs). As per recent evidence, sodium-glucose transport protein 2 (SGLT2) inhibitors have pleiotropic effects in heart failure with both reduced and preserved ejection fraction and are associated with lower risk of new-onset atrial and ventricular arrhythmias and SCD in both diabetic and nondiabetic patients with LVSD. Amiodarone is indicated to treat symptomatic ventricular tachycardia and reduce the incidence of ICD shocks, and the risk of hospitalization, with no survival benefits. Quinidine can help patients with Brugada syndrome. There is no specific proven medication for idiopathic VF, a third of whom may receive appropriate ICD therapy within 3 years from the implant. Specific preventive measures play a vital role in reducing SCD risk, including avoidance of competitive/extreme exertional activities for ARVC, hypertrophic obstructive cardiomyopathy (HOCM)/hypertrophic cardiomyopathy (HCM) patients, and using immunosuppressive agents in cardiac sarcoidosis. This also includes using β-blockers and sympathetic denervation for channelopathies, catecholaminergic VT/VF, and LQTS. Targeted medicines like mexiletine for LQTS3 and quinidine and temperature management for Brugada syndrome. Mavacamten, (myocardial myosin inhibitor), is now available for HOCM and acts by reducing myocardial contractility and left ventricular outflow tract (LVOT) obstruction, effectively reducing VT/SCD risk.

NEUROPROGNOSTICATION IN SCA/SCD: THE FUTURE

Neurological prognostication determines the eventual outcomes, survival to discharge, and medium- and long-term prognosis of patients. Although prehospital parameters like the MIRACL2 score are very helpful at the outset, formal prognostication on a day-to-day basis is now being done in centers of excellence in MDT format. The process is complex and involves a dedicated team of specialist health professionals (OHCA specialist team) who besides implementing MIRACL2 on arrival, at 48–72 hours post-ROSC, undertake regular neurological reviews, especially quantitative pupillometry and brainstem reflexes. It also involves neurophysiological testing with electroencephalography (EEG) and somatosensory evoked potentials. This information is combined with other available data such as biomarkers (neuron-specific enolase), computed tomography (CT), and magnetic resonance imaging (MRI) to make treatment decisions and have discussions with relatives. This multimodal prognostication technique allows for as much accuracy as possible and is usually performed after the effect of confounding factors such as sedation and hypothermia is excluded. Decisions like withdrawal of life-sustaining treatment (WLST) can be considered with a confirmed diagnosis of brain death. The neuroprognostication MDT team involves intensive care unit (ICU) consultants, cardiologists, neurologists, specialist nurses, occupational therapists, and physiotherapists as per the established prognostication strategy from the UK Resuscitation Council **(Flowchart 1)** and European Society of Intensive Care Medicine Guidelines 2021. This also avoids inappropriate WLST and continuing with futile treatment, in a fully informed manner with relatives. The Essex Heart Centre in the UK is leading this initiative, besides setting up dedicated care after resuscitation (CARE) clinics for OHCA survivors.

Care after resuscitation clinics are multidisciplinary initiatives for OHCA survivors and their families. With only one in 10 OHCA surviving to hospital discharge and up to half or two-thirds of them having residual brain/organ dysfunction, this one-stop clinic with an MDT approach helps tailor ongoing medical/interventional treatment, device management (ICD), psychosocial aspects, genetic testing of families, occupational and physiotherapy

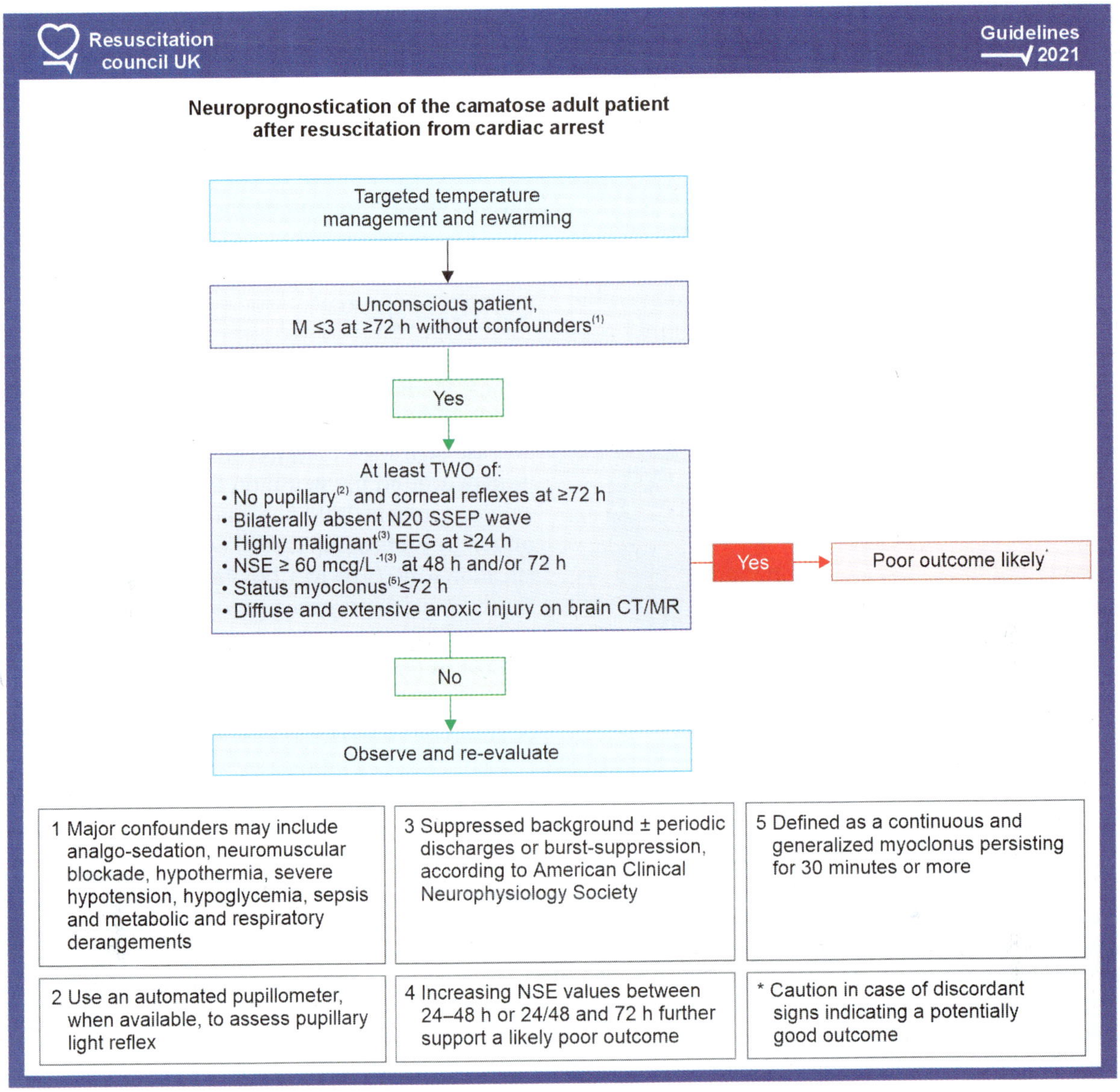

FLOWCHART 1: UK Resuscitation Council Guidelines 2021—neuroprognostication algorithm.
(CT: computed tomography; EEG: electroencephalography; MR: magnetic resonance; NSE: neuron-specific enolase)

and rehabilitation and peer support groups after a life-changing event like OHCA.

The Lancet Commission on SCD **(Fig. 3)** adopts a circle of care concept (pre-, peri-, and post-SCA) is aimed at addressing the global gaps in SCA/SCD management with a unified approach across countries and their governments, hoping to change the shape of cardiac arrest care via major policy and bespoke change in how care is provided currently. This also covers key aspects of prevention and prediction, with a global collaborative approach to enhance awareness, CPR skills, availability of AEDs and their appropriate use, and accurate and valid data management for research purposes.

OUT-OF-HOSPITAL CARDIAC ARREST AND LEARNINGS FROM THE CORONAVIRUS DISEASE 2019 PANDEMIC

There was a trend toward a rise in OHCA during the pandemic and studies done had limitations, varying protocols, and guidelines for resuscitation. The key learnings include the multifactorial impact of the infection, including respiratory distress causing SCD. Other factors include inflammation, increased thrombogenicity, direct myocardial injury, causing myocarditis/infarction, heart failure, pulmonary embolism, stroke, and sepsis-induced SCA. There was no significant rise in ICD-delivered therapies and overall, the number of coronavirus disease 2019 (COVID-19) patients having OHCA was lower than noninfected patients. The trends were lower in the second wave. It was inferred that indirect effects of the pandemic, combined with limitations and often hesitations in timely access to healthcare, contributed to cardiovascular events, often attributed to pandemic/infection induced.

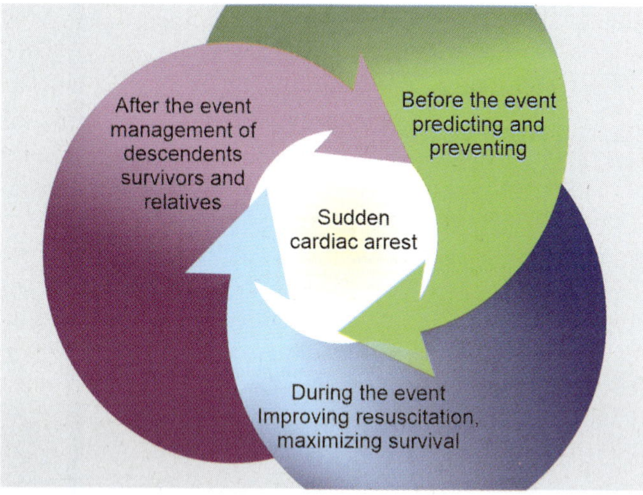

FIG. 3: The circle of sudden cardiac death, from the Lancet Commission on SCD, 2023.

The 2022 European Society of Cardiology (ESC) "10 commandments" for managing ventricular arrhythmias (VA) and preventing SCD factors age, sex, and underlying risk/etiology, linking to the dominant arrhythmia in various groups are enumerated in **Box 1**, giving out the most important takeaways in OHCA management.

CONCLUSION

Global efforts to reduce the burden of SCD call for a radical change in strategies, aimed at better awareness of the condition, wide expansion of bystander CPR skills, and use of AEDs with universal access. The wide variations in data around the world on SCD need an accurate and valid approach. With the majority of prognosis determined by prehospital care of SCD patients, early prognostication with a MIRACL2 score is strongly recommended. Younger patients may benefit by direct transfer to dedicated cardiac arrest centers. Case selection is of the utmost importance for invasive testing and treatments, including PCI, and mechanical circulatory support (e-CPR). Alongside, continued efforts for better and early

BOX 1: About 10 commandments for managing ventricular arrhythmias (VA) and preventing SCD (European Society of Cardiology, 2022).

1. The risk of VA/SCD increases with age. However, the age at presentation, the "age peak" and the subtype of VA potentially leading to SCD, is different for different diseases **(Fig. 4)**
2. Survival rate remains low after out-of-hospital cardiac arrest. Early implementation of resuscitative interventions is pivotal to improving survival. It is important to increase the availability of public access defibrillators at sites where cardiac arrest is more likely to occur and to promote community training in basic life support, especially in schools
3. Sudden cardiac arrest survivors should undergo systematic examination overseen by a multidisciplinary team, to identify the cause of cardiac arrest and those at risk of an inherited cardiac disease needing familiar evaluation
4. Investigation of unexpected SD should be made a public health priority. A comprehensive autopsy is recommended, ideally, in all cases of unexpected SD, and always in those < 50 years of age
5. Genetic testing is increasingly available. Risk stratification, including genetic findings, exists for several diseases and risk calculators have been developed (i.e., LQTS and lamin A/C cardiomyopathies)
6. Risk prediction based on a single parameter does not consider the potential combined effect and interactions between factors. In patients with dilated cardiomyopathy/hypokinetic nondilated cardiomyopathy, indication for primary prevention ICD implantation should not be restricted to a LVEF ≤35% but also clinical presentation, cardiac magnetic resonance imaging, and genetic testing
7. Idiopathic PVCs or VT are a diagnosis per exclusion. CMRI is important if initial evaluation is inconclusive or the presentation is atypical, and in patients with an unexplained reduced LVEF and a PVC burden of ≥10%. For symptomatic idiopathic PVC/VT from right ventricular outflow tract or left ventricular fascicle and for PVC-induced cardiomyopathy catheter ablation is the first-line treatment
8. Catheter ablation is the first-line treatment for recurrent VT in patients after myocardial infarction on amiodarone treatment
9. In patients with a preserved or mildly reduced LVEF after prior myocardial infarction presenting with a hemodynamically tolerated VT, either VT ablation performed in experienced centers or ICD implantation are treatment options requiring shared decision-making
10. Medical treatment like nonselective β-blockers nadolol or propranolol are the preferred β-blockers in LQTS and catecholaminergic polymorphic ventricular tachycardia patients

(CMRI: cardiac magnetic resonance imaging; ICD: implantable cardioverter defibrillator; LVEF: left ventricular ejection fraction; LQTS: long QT syndrome; PVCs: premature ventricular contractions; SD: sudden death; SCD: sudden cardiac death; VA: ventricular arrhythmias; VT: ventricular tachycardia)

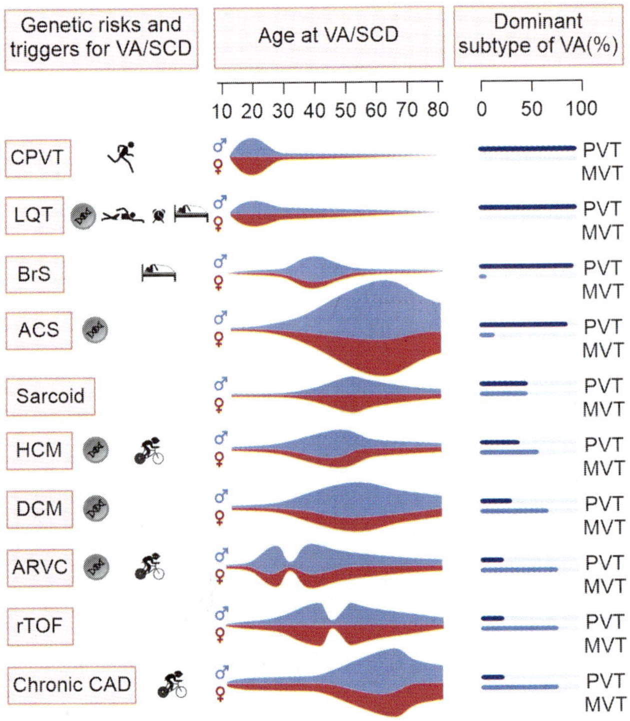

FIG. 4: Central illustration from ESC guidelines for the management of patients with ventricular arrhythmias and the prevention of sudden cardiac death.

(ACS: acute coronary syndrome; ARVC: arrhythmogenic right ventricular cardiomyopathy; BrS: Brugada syndrome; CAD: coronary artery disease; CPVT: catecholaminergic polymorphic ventricular tachycardia; DCM: dilated cardiomyopathy; HCM: hypertrophic cardiomyopathy; ESC: European Society of Cardiology; LQT: long QT syndrome; MVT: monomorphic ventricular tachycardia; PVT: polymorphic ventricular tachycardia; rTOF: repaired tetralogy of Fallot; SCD, sudden cardiac death; VA: ventricular arrhythmia; VF: ventricular fibrillation)

Source: Adapted from Zeppenfeld K, et al. (2023).

risk stratification, optimization of diagnostic imaging, and screening clinics will help identify high-risk individuals, combined with both primordial and primary prevention of cardiovascular disease. The field of genetic testing continues to evolve, and its universal access will be of immense value for screening and offering tailored therapies, including advanced ICDs for secondary and primary prevention. Multimodality neuroprognostication is an invaluable tool in post resuscitation care and the establishment of dedicated MDT-structured cardiac arrest clinics for survivors and families are an extension of how SCD care can be taken to a new level, with bespoke management. A lot more needs to be done in years to come for SCD where the cause is unclear or unknown, with research, autopsy data, and refining genetic testing for inherited causes, especially for deprived regions/countries. Advances in defibrillator technology need to be combined with universal access to cheaper and safer treatments for eligible patients for primary and secondary prevention. Some of the most recent preventive approaches include targeted medical management, advanced defibrillators, neuromodulation, immunotherapeutic strategies to reduce cardiac fibrosis, and genetic testing guided stratification and treatment, including genome editing [clustered regularly interspaced palindromic repeats (CRISPR)–Cas9 system] as targeted gene therapy. Finally, as quoted by the International Commission on SCD, "Understanding the biological, neurological, and psychological foundation of the challenges faced by survivors of SCA must become a priority to facilitate the development of effective rehabilitation programs targeted to survivors and their family and allow the best foundation for returning to a normal life."

SUGGESTED READINGS

1. Zipes DP, Wellens HJJ. Sudden cardiac death. Circulation. 1998;98(21):2334-51.
2. Fishman GI, Chugh SS, DiMarco JP, Albert CM, Anderson ME, Bonow RO, et al. Sudden cardiac death prediction and prevention: report from a National Heart, Lung, and Blood Institute and Heart Rhythm Society Workshop. Circulation. 2010;122(22):2335-48.
3. Isbister J, Semsarian C. Sudden Cardiac Death: an update. Intern Med J. 2019;49(7):826-33.
4. Sasson C, Rogers MAM, Dahl J, Kellermann AL. Predictors of survival from out-of-hospital cardiac arrest: a systematic review and meta-analysis. Circ Cardiovasc Qual Outcomes. 2010;3(1):63-81.
5. Karam N, Pechmajou L, Narayanan K, Bougouin W, Sharifzadehgan A, Anys S, et al. Evolution of incidence, management, and outcomes over time in sports-related sudden cardiac arrest. J Am Coll Cardiol. 2022;79(3):238-46.
6. Lynge TH, Risgaard B, Banner J, Nielsen JL, Jespersen T, Stampe NK, et al. Nationwide burden of sudden cardiac death: a study of 54,028 deaths in Denmark. Heart Rhythm. 2021;18(10):1657-65.
7. Fox CS, Evans JC, Larson MG, Kannel WB, Levy D. Temporal trends in coronary heart disease mortality and sudden cardiac death from 1950 to 1999: the Framingham Heart Study. Circulation. 2004;110(5):522-27.
8. Haukilahti MAE, Holmström L, Vähätalo J, Kenttä T, Tikkanen J, Pakanen L, et al. Sudden cardiac death in women. Circulation. 2019;139:1012-21.
9. Okrainec K, Banerjee DK, Eisenberg MJ. Coronary artery disease in the developing world. Am Heart J. 2004;148(1):7-15.
10. Hinkle LE Jr, Thaler HT. Clinical classification of cardiac deaths. Circulation. 1982;65(3):457-64.
11. Tseng ZH, Olgin JE, Vittinghoff E, Ursell PC, Kim AS, Sporer K, et al. Prospective countywide surveillance and autopsy

characterization of sudden cardiac death: POST SCD study. Circulation. 2018;137(25):2689-700.
12. Ricceri S, Salazar JW, Vu AA, Vittinghoff E, Moffatt E, Tseng ZH. Factors predisposing to survival after resuscitation for sudden cardiac arrest. J Am Coll Cardiol. 2021;77(19):2353-62.
13. Priori SG, Blomström-Lundqvist C, Mazzanti A, Blom N, Borggrefe M, Camm J, et al. 2015 ESC Guidelines for the management of patients with ventricular arrhythmias and the prevention of sudden cardiac death: the Task Force for the Management of Patients with Ventricular Arrhythmias and the Prevention of Sudden Cardiac Death of the European Society of Cardiology (ESC). Endorsed by: Association for European Paediatric and Congenital Cardiology (AEPC). Eur Heart J. 2015;36(41):2793-867.
14. Al-Khatib SM, Stevenson WG, Ackerman MJ, Bryant WJ, Callans DJ, Curtis AB, et al. 2017 AHA/ACC/HRS guideline for management of patients with ventricular arrhythmias and the prevention of sudden cardiac death: executive summary: a report of the American College of Cardiology/American Heart Association Task Force on Clinical Practice Guidelines and the Heart Rhythm Society. Heart Rhythm. 2018;15(10):e190-252.
15. Stiles MK, Wilde AAM, Abrams DJ, Ackerman MJ, Albert CM, Behr ER, et al. 2020 APHRS/HRS expert consensus statement on the investigation of decedents with sudden unexplained death and patients with sudden cardiac arrest, and of their families. Heart Rhythm. 2021;18(1):e1-50.
16. Empana J-P, Lerner I, Valentin E, Folke F, Böttiger B, Gislason G, et al. Incidence of sudden cardiac death in the European Union. J Am Coll Cardiol. 2022;79(18):1818-27.
17. Marijon E, Narayanan K, Smith K, Barra S, Basso C, Blom MT, et al. The Lancet Commission to reduce the global burden of sudden cardiac death: a call for multidisciplinary action. Lancet. 2023;402(10405):883-936.
18. Patterson T, Perkins GD, Perkins A, Clayton T, Evans R, Dodd M, et al. Expedited transfer to a cardiac arrest centre for non-ST-elevation out-of-hospital cardiac arrest (ARREST): a UK prospective, multicentre, parallel, randomised clinical trial. Lancet. 2023;402(10410):1329-37.
19. Remme CA. Sudden Cardiac Death in Diabetes and Obesity: Mechanisms and Therapeutic Strategies. Can J Cardiol. 2022;38(4):418-26.
20. Pareek N, Kordis P, Beckley-Hoelscher N, Pimenta D, Kocjancic ST, Jazbec A, et al. A practical risk score for early prediction of neurological outcome after out-of-hospital cardiac arrest: MIRACLE2. Eur Heart J. 2020;41(47):4508-17.
21. Pareek N, Frohmaier C, Smith M, Kordis P, Cannata A, Nevett J, et al. A machine learning algorithm to predict a culprit lesion after out of hospital cardiac arrest. Catheter Cardiovasc Interv. 2023;102(1):80-90.
22. Sutton RM Friess SH Naim MY, Lampe JW, Bratinov G, Weiland TR 3rd, et al. Patient-centric blood pressure-targeted cardiopulmonary resuscitation improves survival from cardiac arrest. Am J Respir Crit Care Med. 2014;190(11):1255-62.
23. Agerskov M, Hansen MB, Nielsen AM, Møller TP, Wissenberg M, Rasmussen LS. Return of spontaneous circulation and long-term survival according to feedback provided by automated external defibrillators. Acta Anaesthesiol Scand. 2017;61(10): 1345-53.
24. Cheskes S, Verbeek PR, Drennan IR, McLeod SL, Turner L, Pinto R, et al. Defibrillation strategies for refractory ventricular fibrillation. N Engl J Med. 2022;387(21):1947-56.
25. Babini G, Ruggeri L, Ristagno G. Optimizing defibrillation during cardiac arrest. Curr Opin Crit Care. 2021;27(3):246-54.
26. Marijon E. (2023). The circle of sudden cardiac death and new paradigms. The Lancet Commission on sudden cardiac death. [online] Available from https://esc365.escardio.org/presentation/262432 [Last accessed December, 2023].
27. Nolan JP, Deakin CD, Soar J, Perkins GD, Davies R, Rowland M, et al. Post-resuscitation care guidelines. Resuscitation Council UK guidelines 2021. [online] Available from file:///C:/Users/LENOVO/Downloads/Post-resuscitation%20care%20guidelines.pdf [Last accessed December, 2023].
28. Resuscitation Council UK. Neuro-prognostication of the comatose adult patient after resuscitation from cardiac arrest. Resuscitation Council UK guidelines 2021. [online] Available from https://www.resus.org.uk/sites/default/files/2021-04/Neuroprognostication%20Algorithm%202021.pdf [Last accessed December, 2023].
29. Zeppenfeld K, Tfelt-Hansen J, de Riva M, Winkel BG, Behr ER, Blom NA, et al. 2022 ESC Guidelines for the management of patients with ventricular arrhythmias and the prevention of sudden cardiac death. Eur Heart J. 2022;43(40):3997-4126.
30. Suverein MM, Delnoij TS, Lorusso R, Brandon Bravo Bruinsma GJ, Otterspoor L, Elzo Kraemer CV, et al. Early Extracorporeal CPR for Refractory Out-of-Hospital Cardiac Arrest. N Engl J Med. 2023;388(4):299-309.
31. Tfelt-Hansen J, Winkel BG, de Riva M, Zeppenfeld K. The '10 commandments' for the 2022 ESC Guidelines for the management of patients with ventricular arrhythmias and the prevention of sudden cardiac death. European Heart Journal. 2023;44:176-7.
32. Thakur AK. Sudden Cardiac Arrest. In: Kamath S (Ed). API Textbook Medicine, 11th edition. New Delhi: CBS Publishers & Distributors Pvt. Ltd; 2019. pp. 1584-92.
33. Srivatsa UN, Swaminathan K, Sithy AM, Amsterdam E, Shantaraman K, et al. Sudden cardiac death in South India: incidence, risk factors and pathology. Indian Pacing Electrophysiol J. 2016;16(4):121-5.
34. SCAI Shock. (2021). SCAI Previews an Expert Consensus Update to SCAI SHOCK Stage Classification. [online] Available from https://scai.org/scai-previews-expert-consensus-update-scai-shock-stage-classification [Last accessed December, 2023].

14

CHAPTER

Sudden Cardiac Death in Young

Iranna Hirapur

ABSTRACT

In this chapter, we are going to address increasing sudden cardiac death (SCD) and heart attacks in the Indian population. SCD is a major public health problem and these days we are witnessing a high number of young SCDs, and the majority of them are secondary to myocardial ischemia or infarction. Though in India, we do not have proper documentation and research about the same, but there is a general consensus among physicians and cardiologists that a majority of young deaths are because of myocardial ischemia. Smoking or chewing any form of tobacco along with early-onset prediabetes or diabetes is a fatal combination for heart attack and SCD in young people.

INTRODUCTION

Sudden cardiac death (SCD) is a natural death occurring within 1 hour of onset of symptoms due to cardiac causes in a person with or without previously recognized cardiac disease. SCD is increasing more commonly in young Indians.

Around 80% of patients who experience SCD have atherosclerotic coronary artery disease (CAD) as the underlying cause. Other etiologies include coronary artery thrombosis, myocardial infarction (MI), hypertrophic cardiomyopathy (HCM), dilated cardiomyopathy, myocarditis, valvular heart disease, electrophysiological abnormalities, congenital long QT syndrome (LQTS), right ventricular dysplasia, Brugada syndrome (BrS), and catecholaminergic polymorphic ventricular tachycardia (CPVT). Risk factors that predispose to sudden cardiac death are diabetes, hypertension, sedentary life, dyslipidemia, and smoking. Smoking is an important risk factor (causes increase in platelet adhesion and release of catecholamines). One needs to know the differences among cardiovascular collapse, cardiac arrest, and SCD.

Cardiovascular collapse is a sudden loss of effective circulation due to cardiac and/or peripheral vascular factors that may reverse spontaneously (e.g., neurocardiogenic syncope, vasovagal syncope) or require interventions.

Cardiac arrest is an abrupt cessation of cardiac function resulting in loss of effective circulation that may be reversible by prompt emergency medical intervention but will lead to death in its absence.

Sudden cardiac death is sudden unexpected death attributed to cardiac arrest, which if witnessed occurs within 1 hour of the onset of symptoms.

MYOCARDIAL SUBSTRATE, TRIGGERS, AND RISK FACTORS FOR SUDDEN CARDIAC DEATH

Myocardial substrates for SCD are myocardial scar, hypertrophy, fibrosis, myocardial stretch, electrical heterogeneity, ion channel functional modification, and abnormal calcium handling.

Triggers for SCD are heart failure/stretch, ischemia, myocardial inflammation, vigorous exertion, electrolyte abnormality, environmental stress, and psychological stress/depression.

Population-based risk factors are male sex, black race, diabetes mellitus, smoking, hypertension (HTN), chronic kidney disease (CKD), electrocardiogram (ECG) features [QT, QRS prolongation, early repolarization, left ventricular hypertrophy (LVH)], family history of SCD (genetics), diet low in N-3 polyunsaturated fatty acids (PUFA), atrial fibrillation (AF), obstructive sleep apnea (OSA), heavy alcohol intake, low magnesium levels, cardiomyopathies [non-ischemic dilated cardiomyopathy (NIDCM), HCM, arrhythmogenic right ventricular cardiomyopathy (ARVC), etc.], inherited arrhythmia syndrome [LQTS, BrS, CPVT, early repolarization syndrome (ERS), etc.], valvular heart diseases, idiopathic ventricular fibrillation (VF), etc.

CARDIAC RHYTHMS AND SUDDEN DEATH

In the early days of emergency medical services (EMS) systems, over half of the victims were found in VF, giving rise to the hypothesis that ischemic VF or ventricular tachycardia (VT) degenerating to VF was the most common event. The proportion of cardiac arrest found in VF has decreased markedly since 1970s in western world to only 20–25% in recent studies, and pulseless electrical activity (PEA) or asystole is now the most common scenario. Proposed explanations for these changes in PEA versus VF include aging and the increased prevalence of end-stage cardiovascular disease and other severe comorbidities. However, postmyocardial ischemic VT and VF deaths are more common in young Indians (needs more research and data).

There is data about an absolute decrease in VF incidences across the globe. Proposed explanations include decreases in underlying coronary heart disease (CHD) incidence, increased use of beta blockers in CHD, and implantable cardioverter-defibrillator (ICD) in high-risk patients.

DISEASE-SPECIFIC MECHANISMS

Coronary Artery Disease

Coronary artery disease can cause SCD through several mechanisms. Acute MI or transient myocardial ischemia can lead to polymorphic VT and VF, severe bradyarrhythmias such as heart block with a slow escape rhythm, PEA due to a massive MI or associated myocardial rupture. Ventricular scar from prior infarcts increases VT and VF. Post MI, the risk of SCD elevates up to tenfold, with the highest absolute rates in the first 30 days after MI.

Cardiomyopathies and Other Forms of Structural Heart Disease

Scar-mediated reentrant VT can also occur in a host of nonischemic cardiomyopathies in which replacement fibrosis and/or inflammatory ventricular infiltrates occur. Surgical scars due to ventricular septal defect (VSD), tetralogy of Fallot (TOF) repair, etc., can also serve as the substrate for ventricular re-entry. LVH, ventricular stretch due to fluid overload, and cardiomyocyte dysfunction can result in electrical heterogeneity and other electrophysiologic changes that predispose to ventricular arrhythmias, including ion channel alterations that prolong action-potential duration, impair cellular calcium handling, and diminish cellular coupling.

In the Absence of Structural Heart Disease

Ventricular fibrillation can be due to an inherited ion channel abnormality, as in LQTS and BrS, rapid AF associated with Wolff–Parkinson–White (WPW) syndrome, or drug toxicities, such as polymorphic VT due to drugs that prolong the QT interval. PEA can result from pulmonary embolism, exsanguination, i.e., severe loss of blood, or the terminal phase of respiratory arrest.

MANAGEMENT OF CARDIAC ARREST

Community approaches to reduce death focus on the rapid identification of victims and implementation of resuscitation measures by those who first encounter the victim, most likely the lay public. The approach for the "out-of-hospital chain of survival" includes:

- Initial evaluation and recognition of the sudden cardiac arrest (SCA)
- Rapid initiation of cardiopulmonary resuscitation (CPR) with an emphasis on chest compressions
- Defibrillation as quickly as possible usually with an automated external defibrillator (AED) applied by the lay rescuer or emergency medical team.
- Advanced life support (ALS) and postcardiac arrest care

Overall survival for out-of-hospital cardiac arrest in patients receiving CPR in Europe and the United States of America is around 16%, which is far less in India. The initial goal of resuscitation is to achieve the return of spontaneous circulation (ROSC). Success is strongly related to the time between collapse and initiation of resuscitation, decreasing markedly after 5 minutes, and the rhythm at the time of emergency medical technician (EMT) arrival, being best for VT, worse for VF, and poor for PEA and asystole. Outcomes are also determined by the age, clinical state, and comorbidities of the victim prior to the arrest.

Initial Evaluation and Initiation of Cardiopulmonary Resuscitation

The rescuer should check for a response from the victim, shout for help, and call or ask someone else to call ambulance. The rescuer should be present at the patient's side so that the responding dispatcher can provide instructions and queries to the rescuer. Consideration of aspiration or airway obstruction is important, and if suspected a Heimlich maneuver may dislodge the obstructing body. A trained healthcare provider should check for a pulse (taking no longer than 10 seconds so as not to delay the initiation of chest compressions) and assess breathing. Gasping respirations and brief seizure activity are common during SCA and may be misinterpreted as breathing and responsiveness. Chest compressions should be administered at a rate of 100–120/min depressing the sternum by 5 cm (2 inch) allowing full chest recoil between compressions. Chest compressions generate forward cardiac output with sequential filling and emptying of the cardiac chambers. Interruption of chest compressions should be minimized to reduce end-organ ischemia. Ventilation may be administered with two breaths for every 30 compressions if a trained rescuer is present, but for lay rescuers, chest compressions alone ("hands-only CPR") are more likely to have similar benefit. If a second rescuer is present, they should be sent to seek out an ambulance service and AED wherever available.

Rhythm-based Management

The rapidity with which defibrillation/cardioversion is achieved is an important predictor of outcome. A defibrillator, most often a direct current (DC) shock or AED, should be applied as soon as available. AEDs can be easily used by lay rescuers and trained first responders, such as police officers and trained security guards. When the arrest is witnessed, the use of AEDs by lay responders can improve cardiac arrest survival rates. With increasing cardiac arrest in young people, the healthcare system and government should actively make AED available in public places and take the initiative to train one and all. Once AED patches are applied to the chest, a brief pause in chest compressions is required to allow the AED to record the rhythm. An AED will advise delivery of a shock if the recorded rhythm meets the criteria for VF or VT. Chest compressions are continued while the defibrillator is being charged. As soon as a diagnosis of VF or VT is established, a 200-joule biphasic waveform shock should be delivered. Chest compressions are resumed immediately and continued for 2 minutes until the next rhythm check. If VT/VF is still present, a second maximal energy shock is delivered. This sequence is continued until personnel to administer ALS are available, or ROSC is achieved. ECG rhythm strips produced by the AED should be retrieved, for future analysis and management.

When ALS is available, an IV or intraosseous line is inserted for medication, and if possible advanced airway [endotracheal tube (ET) tube or supraglottic airway device] is secured. Epinephrine 1 mg every 3–5 min is administered through IV or intraosseously. If circulation is not restored or the patient is stuporous despite the return of circulation, confirmation that acidosis and hypoxia are adequately addressed should be assessed with arterial blood gas (ABG) test. If metabolic acidosis persists after successful defibrillation and with adequate ventilation, 1 mEq/kg sodium bicarbonate ($NaHCO_3$) may be administered. VT is treated with external shocks synchronized to the QRS when monomorphic, and asynchronous shocks are given for polymorphic VT or VF. If VT/VF recurs after one or more shocks, amiodarone 300 mg is administered as a bolus via IV or intraosseous route in the hope that arrhythmia recurrence will be prevented after the next shock, followed by a 150 mg bolus if the arrhythmia recurs. If amiodarone fails, lidocaine can be administered. Common causes of recurrent VT/VF may be due to ongoing myocardial ischemia or infarction that would benefit from emergent coronary angiography (CAG) and revascularization, or QT prolongation causing the polymorphic VT torsades de pointes that may respond to IV magnesium. Hyperkalemia should respond to calcium, while other measures are implemented to reduce serum potassium. PEA/asystole should be managed with CPR, ventilation, and administration of epinephrine. Causes of PEA/asystole that require specific therapy should be considered including airway obstruction, hypoxia, hypovolemia, acidosis, hyperkalemia, hypothermia, toxins, cardiac tamponade, tension pneumothorax, pulmonary embolism, and MI. Naloxone should be administered if opiate overdose is suspected.

Postcardiac Arrest Acute Management

Following restoration of effective circulation, the possibility of acute MI should be immediately assessed. The majority of patients who have acute ST-elevation myocardial infarction (STEMI) are found to have a culprit coronary stenosis/occlusion and emergent CAG with percutaneous angioplasty, and stenting is recommended. Angiography should also be considered if an acute coronary syndrome (ACS) is suspected, even if ST segment elevation is absent, as approximately half of selected patients undergoing angiography for this concern are found to have a coronary lesion as a potential cause of SCA. However, immediate angiography has not been found to result in better outcomes compared to delayed angiography in patients presenting with out-of-hospital cardiac arrest due to VT/VF with no ECG evidence of ST elevation. Hemodynamic instability is often present

SECTION 2

DIABETES UPDATE

16

CHAPTER

Prevention of Complications of Diabetes Mellitus

Anil Chaturvedi

ABSTRACT

India is currently on the thrown of an epidemic of diabetes mellitus. The economic burden and loss of quality of life experience by diabetic individual are related to the morbidity associated with microvascular and macrovascular complication. Three landmark studies on glycemic control in diabetes mainly DCCT (Diabetes Chronic Complications Trial), UKPDS (United Kingdom Prospective Diabetes Study), and Kumamoto study have documented the beneficial effects of glycemic control in preventive microvascular complications. Early aggressive control is of crucial importance since it influences long term complication. Nearly two-thirds patients are undiagnosed and do not need the glycemic target. Nearly two-thirds of disgylcemic individuals are prediabetic and two-thirds are progressed diabetes. Over two-thirds of diabetes with hypertension and dyslipidemia do not receive insulin as a therapeutic measure. Every 1% decrease in glycated hemoglobin can reduce long term diabetes complications. Glycemic control confers 43% reduction in lower extremity amputations or peripheral vascular disease, 37% decrease in microvascular disease, 19% reduction in incidence of cataracts, 16% reduction in heart failure, 14% reduction in myocardial infarction and 12% reduction in cerebrovascular accidents. Thus early aggressive therapy multidrug therapy approach together with lifestyle modification will prevent the long term complication of diabetes.

INTRODUCTION

There is phenomenal increase in incidence and prevalence diabetes globally, the total number of people with diabetes is projected to grow from 573 million in 2021 to 784 million by 2045. India has second highest number in the world with 74 million people suffering from diabetes. This number is estimated to increase to 92.97 million by 2030 and 124.07 million by 2045.

It is matter of concern that diabetes control and management in India is suboptimal. Patient with self-glucose monitoring have high mean glycated hemoglobin (HbA1c) levels (8.9 ± 2.1%) according to the ICMR-INDIAB (Indian Council of Medical Research-India Diabetes) study. Diabetes is the leading cause of many complications, such as nephropathy 28.5%, retinopathy 10.5–22.6%, peripheral neuropathy 26.1%, peripheral vascular disease 6.3%, diabetes foot 6%, coronary artery disease 40.4%, gastroparesis 56.8%, erectile dysfunction 78%, and periarthritis shoulder 29.6%.

Diabetes complications do not occur in every patient. Those who have longer duration of diabetes, poor blood sugar, and blood pressure control, are inactive, overweight, or obese, and take excess alcohol and tobacco/smoking, are more likely to develop complications. Some people are genetically predisposed to develop complications.

Diabetic complications are the major causes of morbidity and mortality for people with diabetes. They can be grouped into those specific to diabetes (e.g., retinopathy, nephropathy, or neuropathy) and macrovascular diseases which are shared with nondiabetic individuals but occur earlier and in more severe forms in diabetes (e.g., coronary heart disease, cerebrovascular disease, and peripheral vascular disease). Diabetic retinopathy is the most common cause of blindness in young people. Diabetic nephropathy is now the most common cause of end-stage renal disease in the world. Diabetes is the most important condition underlying macrovascular disease such as myocardial infarction and stroke.

CLASSIFICATION OF COMPLICATIONS

Diabetes mellitus is characterized by absolute or relative deficiency, hyperglycemia, and development of diabetic specific microvascular complication in retina, kidney, and nerves. It is also associated with accelerated macrovascular disease affecting arteries in heart, brain, and lower limbs. The macrovascular complication of diabetes are associated with significant mortality and morbidity and cut short the life expectancy of a diabetic by 7–10 years. The main contributing cause of death in 66% of diabetic is macrovascular disease, coronary artery disease in two-thirds, and cerebrovascular disease and peripheral vascular disease in remaining one-third, diabetes is an expensive disease. **Box 1** lists major complications of diabetes.

The screening of microvascular complication is a simple economical and useful method of risk prediction in diabetes. The early initiations of preventive measures not only prevent but also delay this complication. Type 2 diabetes mellitus (T2DM) patients' microvascular complication can many a times manifest at the time of diagnosis, though these complications can typically develop over several years. The duration of diabetes and the combined role of hypertension, dyslipidemia, smoking, and obesity have a greater significance in development and prognosis of these complications. The interplay between genetic and environmental factors do play an important role in microvascular complication of diabetes.

BOX 1: Classification of complications of diabetes mellitus.

Microvascular complications:
- Nephropathy
- Retinopathy
- Neuropathy:
  - Peripheral neuropathy
  - Automatic neuropathy:
    - Cardiovascular autonomic neuropathy:
      - Postural hypotension
      - Loss of circadian rhythm of blood pressure
      - Postprandial hypotension
      - Resting tachycardia and diminished heart rate variability
      - Silent myocardial ischemia
    - Gastrointestinal autonomic neuropathy:
      - Diarrhea
      - Constipation
      - Gastroparesis
    - Genitourinary neuropathy:
      - Sexual dysfunction:
        - Erectile dysfunction
        - Retrograde ejaculation
      - Bladder dysfunction:
        - Sudomotor abnormalities
        - Hypoglycemia unawareness
        - Anemia because of erythropoietin depletion

Macrovascular complications:
- Coronary artery disease
- Cerebrovascular disease
- Peripheral vascular disease

Others:
- Diabetic foot
- Cutaneous complications
- Rheumatic complications
- Ocular complications other than retinopathy
- Infections

PREVENTION OF MICROVASCULAR COMPLICATIONS OF DIABETES

Primary Prevention

The goal of prevention of microvascular complication is intense management of modifiable risk factors and lifestyle modifications. Health promotion and health education is an important aspect of primary prevention. A summary of outpatient department (OPD) evaluation for identification of individuals at high risk of complications is outlined in **Table 1**.

Secondary Prevention

Regular blood pressure and blood sugar monitoring along with intensive management of risk factor helps in preventing and reducing the complications of retinopathy, chronic kidney disease (CKD), foot ulcerations, and peripheral neuropathy.

CLINICAL CONSIDERATIONS

History and Physical Examination

A thorough history of duration of diabetes, smoking, tobacco consumption, alcohol, physical activity, and comorbidities medication should be elaborated. The diabetic retinopathy can be evaluated by enquiring the symptoms of visual impairment and floaters in eye. Assessment of visual activity and retinal examination is

TABLE 1: Outpatient department evaluation for identification of individuals at high risk of complications.

Microvascular complications	*History*: • Burning, numbness, cotton wool sensation, or pain in feet • Swelling of feet • Postural dizziness • Sexual dysfunction including erectile dysfunction or retrograde ejaculation • Constipation, diarrhea, and upper gastrointestinal symptoms • Recurrent urinary tract infection, urinary incontinence, and retention *Physical examination*: • Orthostatic hypotension • Resting tachycardia • Pedal edema and facial puffiness • Comprehensive foot examination (see below)
Macrovascular complications	*History*: • Angina (typical and atypical) • Exercise intolerance • History suggestive of stroke or transient ischemic attack • Intermittent claudication *Examination*: • Palpation of peripheral pulses • Carotid bruit
Other	*Comprehensive foot examination*: • Inspection for any deformities, infection, or ulcer • Palpation of dorsalis pedis pulses • Testing for loss of protective sensation ○ 10 g monofilament ○ Vibration using 128 Hz tuning fork ○ Ankle reflexes

an integral part of the retinopathy evaluation. Diabetic nephropathy can be easily assessed by measuring estimated glomerular filtration rate (eGFR), BP monitoring, and electrolytes in the blood. Foot examination is a very important part of physical examination of any diabetic patient. It includes inspection of the skin, foot ulceration—deformities, neurological examination, and evaluation of arterial pulsation.

Recommendations for Glycemic Control

Glycemic control and patient centric approach and individualization of targets are of paramount importance and sole objective for the prevention of microvascular complication for diabetes. Broad guidelines are given below:

- Maintain HbA1c target of <7% in patients with microvascular complication for diabetes
- Maintain HbA1c target of <6.5% in those patients who are not in risk of hypogylcemia.
- Maintain HbA1c target of <7.5% in older healthy individuals with few coexisting morbidities and good functional and mental status

Recommendations for Blood Pressure Control

In all adults with microvascular complication of diabetes with BP <140/90 mm Hg should be maintained, however, a strict of BP target of <130/80 mm Hg should be achieved in high-risk young people with diabetic kidney disease (DKD). Angiotensin-converting enzyme (ACE) inhibitors or ARBs are preferred first-line drugs for the control of blood pressure as they have added advantage of reducing DKD progression.

Management of Dyslipidemia

Lifestyle modification is the cornerstone of the management of dyslipidemia; weight loss and increase physical activity are most beneficial in adults between 40 and 60 years. Retrospective analysis of the "Scandinavian Simvastatin Survival study" and the CARE (Cholesterol and Recurrent Events) trial have demonstrated that statin therapy reduced the risk of cardiovascular events in diabetic patients with coronary artery disease and elevated or average low-density lipoprotein (LDL) cholesterol by 55 and 24% respectively. Thus, in patients with T2DM above the age of 40 years, statin therapy is clearly beneficial and should be instituted.

Smoking

Smoking cessation is important to halt the progression of to hold diabetes complications retinopathy. Smoking is one of the major avoidable causes of morbidity and mortality and is the most important modifiable cause of premature death. Regular smoking reduces life span by 7.5 years on an average. Smoking cessation results in multiple health benefits. The risk of heart attacks decreases by half in 1 year and becomes similar to nonsmokers in 15 years after quitting smoking. The risk of lung cancers is halved by 10 years after smoking cessation.

Diet

The vegetarian diets consisting of fruits and vegetables, legumes and nuts, whole grains, and monosaturated fats from olive oils not only prevent the complications of diabetes but also help in controlling the diabetes. Dietary

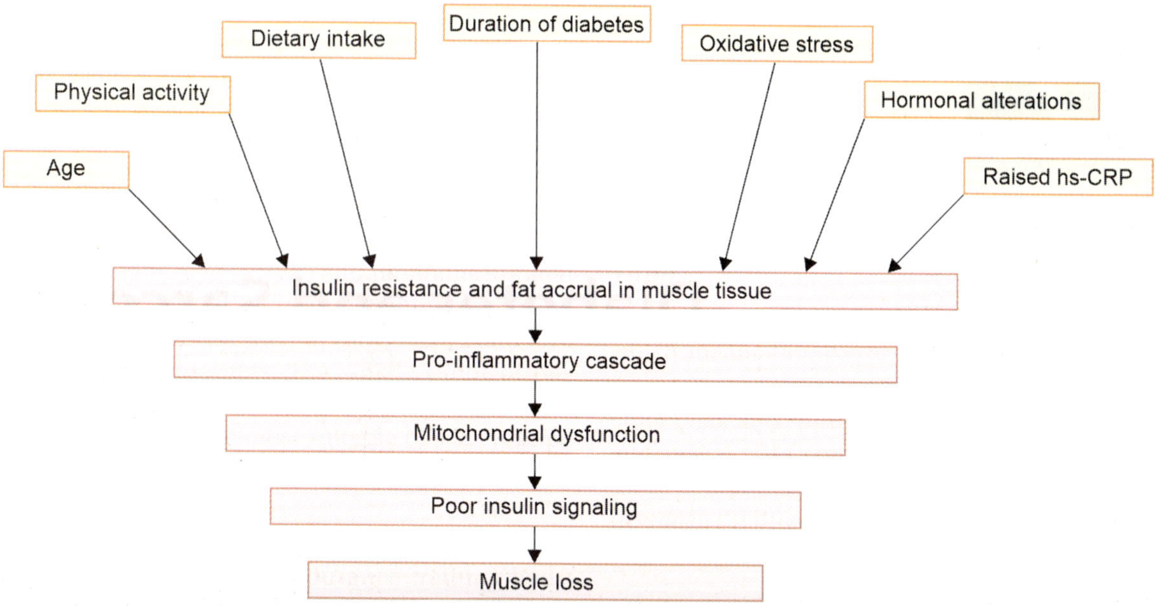

FLOWCHART 1: Etiopathogenesis of sarcopenia in diabetes.
(hs-CRP: high-sensitivity C-reactive protein)

presence of insulin resistance and fat accrual in muscle tissue induce a pro-inflammatory cascade that causes mitochondrial dysfunction, poor insulin signaling, and muscle loss **(Flowchart 1)**. These are primary pathophysiological processes underlying the diabetic association of sarcopenia. The disturbance of glucose storage brought on by the loss of muscle mass further interferes with glucose storage and insulin sensitivity. Reduced oxidative capability in aging skeletal muscle leads to an increase in the formation of reactive oxygen species, which aids in oxidative mitochondrial DNA mutagenesis and pro-inflammatory processes. Insulin resistance is linked to both chronic low-grade inflammation and mitochondrial dysfunction. Additionally, as people age, ectopic fat, such as intramyocellular lipids (IMCL) and adipocytes, found intermuscularly and intramuscularly infiltrates skeletal muscle more frequently. Insulin resistance has been linked to intramuscular and intermuscular adipose tissue (IMAT) and IMCL. Through increased local release of pro-inflammatory adipokines, IMAT-derived adipocytes may adversely affect muscle metabolism and insulin sensitivity, and intermuscular fat may also impede insulin action by decreasing blood supply to muscle.

EPIDEMIOLOGY

In a recent systematic review, diabetic patients had an increased prevalence of sarcopenia compared to controls whilst associated with an increased odds of having DM, suggesting a bidirectional association between diabetes and sarcopenia, particularly when diabetic complications are present. According to recent National Health and Nutrition Examination Survey (NHANES) data, the prevalence of sarcopenia among US elders was 17.8% overall, and it was higher (27.9% vs. 15.7%) among diabetics than without ($p < 0.05$) when gender, age, ethnicity, educational attainment, body mass index (BMI), and muscle-building activity were taken into account as confounders. In another investigation, the diabetic group (DG) had lower calcium and healthy diet intake, a higher BMI, waist circumference, and a lower history of fractures than the control group (CG) ($p < 0.005$). The DG had a greater prevalence of comorbidities (osteopenia—53% and osteoporosis—19%) and aberrant bone mineral density (BMD) ($p < 0.005$). Presarcopenia and sarcopenia were linked to changed BMD ($p < 0.005$) but not to the duration or control of diabetes. In Malaysia, a community-based study of elderly T2DM patients was investigated for a relationship between sarcopenia and diabetic retinopathy. The results showed that the prevalence of diabetic retinopathy was lower in the T2DM group with sarcopenia (28.1%) than T2DM group without sarcopenia (71.2%). In one research, diabetes neuropathy was more common in T2DM patients with sarcopenia (80%) compared to T2DM patients without sarcopenia (70.3%) ($p = 0.07$). In an Indian study, diabetic patients had a significantly higher odds ratio of 1.14 [95% confidence interval (CI) 1.06–1.26, $p < 0.001$] for sarcopenia, establishing diabetes as a risk factor.

DIAGNOSTIC APPROACH

Sarcopenia in diabetic patients must be early identified and treated. As glycemic control and the length of diabetes are highly correlated with sarcopenia, the primary components of a diabetes screening should be a fasting and random plasma glucose test, a 2-hour oral glucose tolerance test, and HbA1c, along with clinical symptoms. Strength, Assistance with walking, Rising from a chair, Climbing stairs, and Falls (SARC-F) questionnaire is one of the screening tools demonstrated to have good specificity.

Additionally, in order to prevent sarcopenia in DM patients, physical assessment of diabetics should be done based on the assessment of BMI and body fat percentage. Handgrip strength and chair stand tests can help in the assessment of sarcopenia. Furthermore, quantification of muscle loss and quality of muscle damage in sarcopenia can be ascertained with various tools that measure body composition such as bioimpedance analysis (BIA), dual-energy X-ray absorption (DXA), computed tomography (CT), and magnetic resonance imaging (MRI). Additionally, air displacement plethysmography (ADP) evaluates total body fat and lean tissue as well as body volume and body density. The importance of early detection and diagnosis of sarcopenia in diabetic patients, even at younger ages, cannot be overstated. To avoid the twin burden of T2DM and sarcopenia, comprehensive care of both conditions, emphasizing exercise and diet, needs to be addressed in all patients.

FUNCTIONAL CONSEQUENCES

Sarcopenia in association with DM has a number of functional consequences linked to higher mortality. Independent of body weight, a decline in muscle strength indicates a higher mortality rate in the elderly. It has been shown that the loss of muscle mass with age is linked to a number of direct and indirect effects, such as a reduction in metabolic rate and maximum oxygen uptake, a reduction in aerobic capacity, and frailty. Diabetes has been found to be 1.5–2 times more common in frail elders than in those without frail. Frailty is also associated with hypertension, peripheral artery disease, and congestive heart failure.

MANAGEMENT

The International Clinical Practice Guidelines for Sarcopenia (ICFSR) 2018 strongly recommend both aerobic and resistance exercise as nonpharmacological primary therapeutic strategy treatment for sarcopenia, to prevent and treat the decline in muscle mass and strength that occurs with aging. Although the exact mechanism is still unclear, getting enough nutritional supplements and proteins can help stop muscle loss and provide adequate energy. Especially, leucine, an essential protein, exhibits strong insulinotropic properties that increase amino acid availability for muscle protein synthesis, reduce muscle protein breakdown, and enhance glucose disposal to help maintain glycemic homeostasis. In addition, omega-3 fatty acids, nicotinamide adenine dinucleotide precursor, and vitamins D and B modify insulin sensitivity, oxidative stress, and inflammation to maintain muscle mass and improve glycemic level. Hormonal treatments such as transdermal testosterone gels and selective androgen receptor modulators are potential therapeutic targets for pharmacotherapy, though lifestyle changes remain the cornerstone of T2DM with sarcopenia management. Antidiabetic medications, such as metformin, are frequently used in T2DM and have been shown to increase muscle mass and strength. Thiazolidinediones work as insulin sensitizers and dipeptidyl peptidase-4 inhibitors increase muscle mass and glycemic control, while sulfonylureas and glinides predispose muscle atrophy. Agonists of glucagon-like peptide 1 are anti-inflammatory and antioxidants. Most importantly, sodium-glucose cotransporter-2 inhibitors are highly effective therapeutic choices for the treatment of elderly T2DM patients by enhancing fatty acid metabolism in muscle and minimizing muscle atrophy.

Beside the physical interventions, nutritional treatments play a significant role in DS. A recent study showed that protein intake is strongly related to skeletal muscle mass in older T2DM patients. The branched-chain amino acids valine, leucine, and isoleucine have been shown to minimize the likelihood of muscle mass loss. Supplementation of essential amino acids (EAAs) has been shown to improve the muscle protein anabolism in sarcopenic individuals. This emphasizes that dietary proteins may play a role in gluco-regulatory function in relation to glucose-insulin metabolism diabetic populations. Few studies have evaluated the role of EAA in sarcopenic individuals. In elderly glucose-intolerant individuals, supplementation of EAA along with arginine two times a day for 16 weeks was shown to improve the lean body mass, lower extremity physical functioning capacity in terms of gait speed, timed 5-step test, and timed floor transfer test. Another study in an Italian cohort of elderly people with a sedentary lifestyle treated with an amino acid mixture 12 g/day orally for 3 months showed a significant increase in 6-minute walk distance along with an increase in the distance, speed, and stairs-walking capacity as assessed by walking impairment questionnaire. There was a substantial increase in muscle strength as well along with improvements in plasma glucose and lipid levels. Similar results were replicated in another study involving elderly individuals with walking impairment. Amino acid supplementation increased muscle strength, walk distance, walk speed, and muscle strength. There was improved myocardial ability in acute overload as indicated by higher peak stress left ventricular ejection fraction. Thus, in individuals who are sarcopenic, supplementation of EAA can help improve muscle strength and walking capacity, thereby increasing the functional gains in these individuals.

CONCLUSION

In patients with diabetes, poor physical performance is a sign of severe sarcopenia and low muscle strength as a key feature of sarcopenia. Low muscle quantity and quality can help ascertain the sarcopenia diagnosis. Healthcare practitioners should adopt practices for early detection and treatment for individuals at risk for sarcopenia. EAA can help improve the muscle strength and walking capacity. Further research in DS is necessary to reduce the negative health outcomes in such individuals.

SUGGESTED READINGS

1. Patterson CC, Harjutsalo V, Rosenbauer J, Neu A, Cinek O, Skrivarhaug T, et al. Trends and cyclical variation in the incidence of childhood type 1 diabetes in 26 European centres in the 25 year period 1989–2013: a multicentre prospective registration study. Diabetologia. 2019;62(3):408-17.
2. Lin X, Xu Y, Pan X, Xu J, Ding Y, Sun X, et al. Global, regional, and national burden and trend of diabetes in 195 countries and territories: an analysis from 1990 to 2025. Sci Rep. 2020; 10(1):14790.
3. Bertoluci MC, Moreira RO, Faludi A, Izar MC, Schaan BD, Valerio CM, et al. Brazilian guidelines on prevention of cardiovascular disease in patients with diabetes: a position statement from the Brazilian Diabetes Society (SBD), the Brazilian Cardiology Society (SBC) and the Brazilian Endocrinology and Metabolism Society (SBEM). Diabetol Metab Syndr. 2017;9(1):1-36.
4. Chung SM, Moon JS, Chang MC. Prevalence of Sarcopenia and Its Association With Diabetes: A Meta-Analysis of Community-Dwelling Asian Population. Front Med. 2021;8:681232.
5. Pacifico J, Geerlings MAJ, Reijnierse EM, Phassouliotis C, Lim WK, Maier AB. Prevalence of sarcopenia as a comorbid disease: A systematic review and meta-analysis. Exp Gerontol. 2020;131:110801.
6. Cruz-Jentoft AJ, Bahat G, Bauer J, Boirie Y, Bruyère O, Cederholm T, et al. Sarcopenia: revised European consensus on definition and diagnosis. Age Ageing. 2019;48(1):16-31.
7. Rubio-Ruiz ME, Guarner-Lans V, Pérez-Torres I, Soto ME. Mechanisms Underlying Metabolic Syndrome-Related Sarcopenia and Possible Therapeutic Measures. Int J Mol Sci. 2019;20(3):647.
8. Feng L, Gao Q, Hu K, Wu M, Wang Z, Chen F, et al. Prevalence and Risk Factors of Sarcopenia in Patients With Diabetes: A Meta-analysis. J Clin Endocrinol Metab. 2022;107:1470-83.
9. Mesinovic J, Zengin A, De Courten B, Ebeling PR, Scott D. Sarcopenia and type 2 diabetes mellitus: a bidirectional relationship. Diabetes, Metab Syndr Obes. 2019;12:1057-72.
10. Kim JA, Wei Y, Sowers JR. Role of mitochondrial dysfunction in insulin resistance. Circ Res. 2008;102(4):401-14.
11. Miljkovic I, Kuipers AL, Cauley JA, Prasad T, Lee CG, Ensrud KE, et al. Greater Skeletal Muscle Fat Infiltration Is Associated With Higher All-Cause and Cardiovascular Mortality in Older Men. J Gerontol A Biol Sci Med Sci. 2015;70(9):1133-40.
12. Veronese N, Pizzol D, Demurtas J, Soysal P, Smith L, Sieber C, et al. Association between sarcopenia and diabetes: a systematic review and meta-analysis of observational studies. Eur Geriatr Med. 2019;10(5):685-96.
13. Dai S, Shu D, Meng F, Chen Y, Wang J, Liu X, et al. Higher Risk of Sarcopenia in Older Adults with Type 2 Diabetes: NHANES 1999–2018. Obes Facts. 2023;16(3):237-48.
14. Trierweiler H, Kisielewicz G, Hoffmann Jonasson T, Rasmussen Petterle R, Aguiar Moreira C, Zeghbi Cochenski Borba V. Sarcopenia: A chronic complication of type 2 diabetes mellitus. Diabetol Metab Syndr. 2018;10:25.
15. Sazlina SG, Lee PY, Chan YM, A Hamid MS, Tan NC. The prevalence and factors associated with sarcopenia among community living elderly with type 2 diabetes mellitus in primary care clinics in Malaysia. PLoS One. 2020;15(5): e0233299.
16. Yang Q, Zhang Y, Zeng Q, Yang C, Shi J, Zhang C, et al. Correlation between diabetic peripheral neuropathy and sarcopenia in patients with type 2 diabetes mellitus and diabetic foot disease: A cross-sectional study. Diabetes Metab Syndr Obes. 2020;13:377-86.
17. Das S. The impact of diabetes on sarcopenia in community-dwelling older adults in India: key findings from the longitudinal ageing study in India (LASI). Diabetes Epidemiol Manag. 2023;12:100158.
18. Xu Z, Zhang P, Chen Y, Jiang J, Zhou Z, Zhu H. Comparing SARC-CalF With SARC-F for Screening Sarcopenia in Adults With Type 2 Diabetes Mellitus. Front Nutr. 2022;9: 803924.
19. Fukuoka Y, Narita T, Fujita H, Morii T, Sato T, Sassa MH, et al. Importance of physical evaluation using skeletal muscle mass index and body fat percentage to prevent sarcopenia in elderly Japanese diabetes patients. J Diabetes Investig. 2019;10(2): 322-30.
20. Kuriyan R. Body composition techniques. Indian J Med Res. 2018;148(5):648-58.
21. Purnamasari D, Tetrasiwi EN, Kartiko GJ, Astrella C, Husam K, Laksmi PW. Sarcopenia and Chronic Complications of Type 2 Diabetes Mellitus. Rev Diabet Stud. 2022;18(3):157-65.
22. Khamseh M, Malek M, Aghili R, Emami Z. Sarcopenia and diabetes: Pathogenesis and consequences. Br J Diabetes Vasc Dis. 2011;11(5):230-4.
23. Dent E, Morley JE, Cruz-Jentoft AJ, Arai H, Kritchevsky SB, Guralnik J, et al. International Clinical Practice Guidelines for Sarcopenia (ICFSR): Screening, Diagnosis and Management. J Nutr Heal Aging. 2018;22(10):1148-61.

24. Dhillon RJ, Hasni S. Pathogenesis and Management of Sarcopenia. Clin Geriatr Med. 2017;33(1):17-26.
25. Chen H, Huang X, Dong M, Wen S, Zhou L, Yuan X. The Association Between Sarcopenia and Diabetes: From Pathophysiology Mechanism to Therapeutic Strategy. Diabetes Metab Syndr Obes. 2023;16:1541-4.
26. Massimino E, Izzo A, Riccardi G, Pepa G Della. The Impact of Glucose-Lowering Drugs on Sarcopenia in Type 2 Diabetes: Current Evidence and Underlying Mechanisms. Cells. 2021;10(8):1958.
27. Miki A, Hashimoto Y, Matsumoto S, Ushigome E, Fukuda T, Sennmaru T, et al. Protein Intake, Especially Vegetable Protein Intake, Is Associated with Higher Skeletal Muscle Mass in Elderly Patients with Type 2 Diabetes. J Diabetes Res. 2017;2017:7985728.
28. Low S, Wang J, Moh A, Ang SF, Ang K, Shao YM, et al. Amino acid profile of skeletal muscle loss in type 2 diabetes: Results from a 7-year longitudinal study in Asians. Diabetes Res Clin Pract. 2022;186:109803.
29. Hamarsland H, Nordengen AL, Nyvik Aas S, Holte K, Garthe I, Paulsen G, et al. Native whey protein with high levels of leucine results in similar post-exercise muscular anabolic responses as regular whey protein: A randomized controlled trial. J Int Soc Sports Nutr. 2017;14:43.
30. Volpi E, Kobayashi H, Sheffield-Moore M, Mittendorfer B, Wolfe RR. Essential amino acids are primarily responsible for the amino acid stimulation of muscle protein anabolism in healthy elderly adults. Am J Clin Nutr. 2003;78(2):250-8.
31. Gulati S, Misra A. Dietary proteins, metabolic syndrome, and sarcopenia: Focus on Asian Indians. Diabetes Metab Syndr Clin Res Rev. 2019;13(6):3091-2.
32. Børsheim E, Bui QU, Tissier S, Kobayashi H, Ferrando AA, Wolfe RR. Effect of amino acid supplementation on muscle mass, strength and physical function in elderly. Clin Nutr. 2008;27(2):189-95.
33. Scognamiglio R, Avogaro A, Negut C, Piccolotto R, de Kreutzenberg SV, Tiengo A. The effects of oral amino acid intake on ambulatory capacity in elderly subjects. Aging Clin Exp Res. 2004;16(6):443-7.

Therapeutic Targets

According to KDIGO study daily dietary sodium intake should be 2 g/day and physical activity >150 minutes of moderate intensity to maintain body mass index between 20 and 25 kg/m^2. Smoking cessation is strongly recommended. Target blood pressure should be <130/80 mm Hg, if albuminuria is present.

Renin-angiotensin-aldosterone system inhibition should be mandatory in all patients with albuminuria. HbA1c <7% for most patients.

Higher target is suggested in patients with risk of hypoglycemia, patients with severe comorbidities and limited life expectancy. In lipid management, statin therapy should be prescribed for all patients with DM and CKD. CKD stage IV and CKD progression were the nephrology referral criteria's.

CONCLUSION

Diabetic nephropathy and end-stage renal disease remain a significant problem despite best efforts to limit the impact of disease on end organ damage. In such a complex milieu of diabetes where no single treatment can halt the disease progression, a multifactorial approach includes glycemic control, ACE normal inhibitor and blood pressure lowering. Disease modifications, such as lipid control, smoking cessation, and weight reduction provide additive renal benefits, particularly in addressing cardiovascular risk.

Effective delivery of these interventions in combination reduces the risk of DKD progression as well as other microvascular complications, cardiovascular events, and mortality.

SUGGESTED READINGS

1. Gross ML, Amann K, Ritz E. Nephron number and renal risk in hypertension and diabetes. J Am Soc Nephrol. 2005;16 Suppl 1: S27-9.
2. Rizvi S, Raza ST, Mahdi F. Association of genetic variants with diabetic nephropathy. World J Diabetes. 2014;5(6):809-16.
3. Anjana RM, Pradeepa R, Unnikrishnan R, Tiwaskar M, Aravind SR, Saboo B, et al. New and Unique Clusters of Type 2 Diabetes Identified in Indians. J Assoc Physicians India. 2021;69(2):58-61.
4. Umanath K, Lewis JB. Update on diabetic nephropathy: core curriculum 2018. Am J Kidney Dis. 2018;71(6):884-95.
5. Mogensen CE, Christensen CK, Vittinghus E. The stages in diabetic renal disease. With emphasis on the stage of incipient diabetic nephropathy. Diabetes. 1983;32 Suppl 2:64-78.
6. Selby NM, Taal MW. An updated overview of diabetic nephropathy: Diagnosis, prognosis, treatment goals and latest guidelines. Diabetes Obes Metab. 2020;22 Suppl 1:3-15.
7. Suneja M. Diabetic Nephropathy and diabetic kidney disease. J Diabetes Mellitus. 2021;11(5):359-77.
8. Giglio RV, Patti AM, Rizvi AA, Stoian AP, Ciaccio M, Papanas N, et al. Advances in the Pharmacological Management of Diabetic Nephropathy: A 2022 International Update. Biomedicines. 2023;11(2):291.
9. Lopez LN, Wang W, Loomba L, Afkarian M, Butani L. Diabetic kidney disease in children and adolescents: an update. Pediatr Nephrol. 2022;37(11):2583-97.

19

CHAPTER

Reversal of Lifestyle-related Disorders: Diabetes Mellitus, Nonalcoholic Steatohepatitis, and Hypertension

Sanjib Kumar Sharma, Urza Bhattarai

ABSTRACT

Unhealthy habits are a major preventable risk factor for the development of any noncommunicable disease (NCD). Unhealthy habits include tobacco use, unhealthy hypercaloric diet or harmful use of alcohol, stressful living, and physical inactivity. Poor lifestyle choices lead to lifestyle-related disorders (LRDs), the impact of which is not only limited to physical health but also associated with mental disorders and a contribution to the global economic burden. In this narrative review, we discuss the reversal of LRDs through nonpharmacological interventions that could significantly improve the quality of life of affected individuals and reduce the increasing NCD threat to the healthcare system. We focus on key nonpharmacological approaches and mechanisms in the reversal of lifestyle disorders such as diabetes mellitus, nonalcoholic steatohepatitis (NASH), and hypertension.

INTRODUCTION

Noncommunicable diseases (NCDs) are a major contributing factor to increasing morbidity and mortality throughout the globe. The underlying risk factors for the development of NCDs include poor self-management, genetics, environmental factors, or socioeconomic concerns. Among these factors, an unhealthy lifestyle is a major preventable risk factor for the development of any NCD. Lifestyle-related disorders (LRDs) occur as a result of unhealthy habits; examples include tobacco use, unhealthy hypercaloric diet or harmful use of alcohol, stressful living, and physical inactivity. Poor lifestyle choices lead to LRDs, the impact of which is not only limited to physical health but also associated with mental disorders and a contribution to the global economic burden.

Lifestyle medicine interventions include comprehensive lifestyle changes through improved healthy food habits, increased physical activity, stress management, and social support. These interventions can undoubtedly prevent and treat lifestyle-related noncommunicable illnesses. Recently, it is increasingly known that these interventions could also possibly reverse LRDs. In this narrative review, we discuss the reversal of these disorders through nonpharmacological interventions that could significantly improve the quality of life of affected individuals and reduce the increasing NCD threat to the healthcare system.

PATHOPHYSIOLOGY OF LIFESTYLE DISORDERS

"New world syndrome" is a term given to a set of NCDs brought on by lifestyle changes, especially common to the indigenous group. Traditional activities included farming and hunting that involved more activity. "New world syndrome" thus occurs as a result of rapid modernization of lifestyle and decreasing healthier traditional habits or cultures. Contributions include change from a previous traditional habit to modern changes, including stressful and sedentary employment.

Today's modern lifestyle consists of increased consumption of processed food, physical inactivity, environmental toxins, and chemicals which are associated

3. Nishimoto S, Sata M, Fukuda D. Expanding role of deoxyribonucleic acid-sensing mechanism in the development of lifestyle-related diseases. Front Cardiovasc Med. 2022;9:881181.
4. Deshpande N, Kapoor N. Reversal of Diabetes and Lifestyle Disorders: The Basis, Effectiveness, and Evidence. Current Trends in Diabetes. 2020;30:68.
5. Wu D, Wang H, Xie L, Hu F. Cross-Talk Between Gut Microbiota and Adipose Tissues in Obesity and Related Metabolic Diseases. Front Endocrinol. 2022 5;13:908868.
6. Kassam Z, Smith M, Alm E. Bariatric surgery versus intensive medical therapy for diabetes. N Engl J Med. 2014;371(7):680.
7. Singla R, Gupta G, Dutta D, Raizada N, Aggarwal S. Diabetes reversal: Update on current knowledge and proposal of prediction score parameters for diabetes remission. Diabetes Metab Syndr. 2022;16(4):102452.
8. Lean ME, Leslie WS, Barnes AC, Brosnahan N, Thom G, McCombie L, et al. Durability of a primary care-led weight-management intervention for remission of type 2 diabetes: 2-year results of the DiRECT open-label, cluster-randomised trial. Lancet Diabetes Endocrinol. 2019;7(5):344-55.
9. Hydes TJ, Ravi S, Loomba R, Gray ME. Evidence-based clinical advice for nutrition and dietary weight loss strategies for the management of NAFLD and NASH. Clin Mol Hepatol. 2020;26(4):383-400.
10. Mikhail N, Golub MS, Tuck ML. Obesity and hypertension. Prog Cardiovascular Dis. 1999;42(1):39-58.
11. Husain K, Ansari RA, Ferder L. Alcohol-induced hypertension: Mechanism and prevention. World J Cardiol. 2014;6(5):245-52.
12. Bäckhed F, Ding H, Wang T, Hooper LV, Koh GY, Nagy A, et al. The gut microbiota as an environmental factor that regulates fat storage. Proc Natl Acad Sci USA. 2004;101(44):15718-23.
13. Cotillard A, Kennedy SP, Kong LC, Prifti E, Pons N, Le Chatelier E, et al. Dietary intervention impact on gut microbial gene richness. Nature. 2013;500(7464):585-8.

20

CHAPTER

Monogenic Diabetes

Srinath KM, Krupa Krishnan

ABSTRACT

Monogenic diabetes is defined as diabetes caused by defects in a single gene, in contrast to type 1 diabetes mellitus and type 2 diabetes mellitus where inheritance is polygenic. The pathophysiological mechanisms of monogenic diabetes are better understood than any other form of diabetes.

Monogenic diabetes is relatively rare and accounts for approximately 1–5% of diabetes but is probably underdiagnosed (80%) owing to insufficient genetic testing. The major monogenic diabetes categories are maturity-onset diabetes of young (MODY), neonatal diabetes mellitus (NDM), and syndromic diabetes.

About >40 subtypes of monogenic diabetes have been identified to date, the most prevalent being deficiencies of glucokinase (GCK) and hepatocyte nuclear factor 1-alpha (HNF1A). Next-generation sequencing has made genetic diagnosis affordable, enabling effective genomic medications in monogenic diabetes. Precision medicine approaches are available for some forms of monogenic diabetes (including GCK and HNF1A diabetes) and raise patients' quality of life.

INTRODUCTION

Monogenic diabetes refers to diabetes mellitus (DM) caused by a mutation in a single gene which includes three major entities namely (1) maturity-onset diabetes of the young (MODY), (2) neonatal diabetes mellitus (NDM), and (3) syndromic diabetes **(Flowchart 1)**.

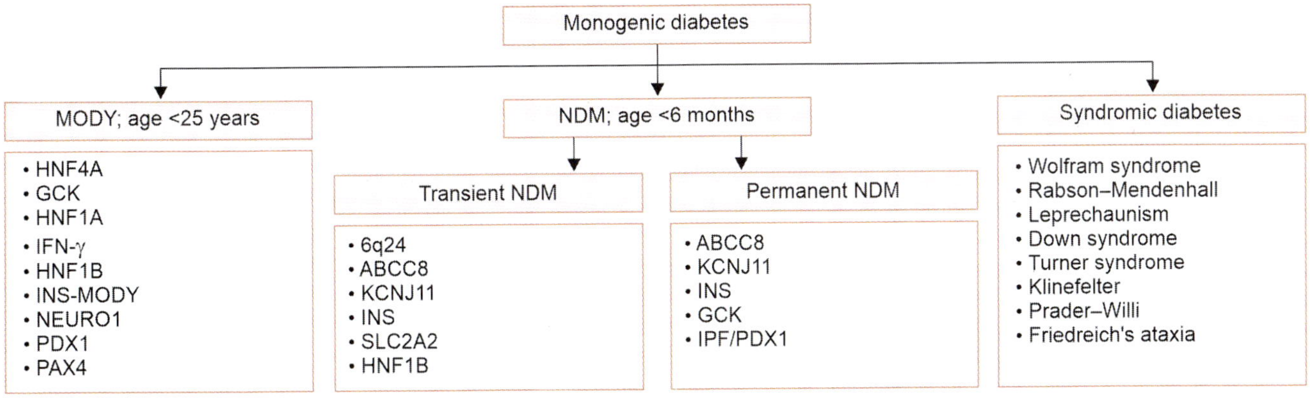

FLOWCHART 1: Classification of monogenic diabetes.

(ABCC8: ATP-binding cassette subfamily C member 8; GCK: glucokinase; HNF4A: hepatocyte nuclear factor 4-alpha; HNF1B: hepatocyte nuclear factor 1-beta; IFN-γ: interferon gamma; INS-MODY: insulin gene maturity-onset diabetes of the young; IPF: insulin promoter factor; PDX1: pancreatic and duodenal homeobox 1; PAX4: paired box 4; SLC2A2: solute carrier family 2 member 2)

MONOGENIC VERSUS POLYGENIC DIABETES

Monogenic diabetes results from variation in highly penetrant variants in a single gene whereas the pathogenesis of polygenic diabetes results from the contribution of multiple genetic variations, including those involving insulin secretion and insulin sensitivity, with smaller yet significant contributions from environmental and lifestyle factors. The lapse in the diagnosis of monogenic diabetes is probably due to several overlapping features such as age of onset, family history, measures of obesity, and markers of insulin resistance with type 1 diabetes mellitus (T1DM) and type 2 diabetes mellitus (T2DM). However, the diagnosis is important to provide an etiology-based treatment.

GENETICS OF MONOGENIC DIABETES

Mutations in one of four genes, including the (1) enzyme glucokinase (*GCK*), (2) transcription factors—hepatocyte nuclear factor 1-alpha (*HNF1A*), (3) hepatocyte nuclear factor 4-alpha (*HNF4A*), and (4) hepatocyte nuclear factor 1-beta (*HNF1B*), account for the bulk of MODY cases while KCNJ11 and ATP-binding cassette subfamily c member 8 (ABCC8) are the ones that are most frequently impacted in neonatal diabetes.

Glucokinase

- *Age*: <30 years
- *Synonym*: MODY 2
- *Gene mutation*: Mutations in the *GCK* gene on chromosome 7p
- *Biochemical abnormality*: Isolated fasting hyperglycemia: 97–150 mg/dL, with relatively normal oral glucose tolerance tests (OGTT) with 75 g anhydrous glucose tolerance test, with glycated hemoglobin (HbA1c) never crossing 7.5%.

Glucokinase-MODY is the most common cause of monogenic diabetes. GCK facilitates the first step in glucose metabolism which is the conversion of glucose to glucose-6-phosphate which further triggers the cascade of events leading to insulin secretion. It is also responsible for the hepatic regulation of glucose release and storage. Impaired GCK activity, resets the threshold glucose level needed for insulin secretion to a higher level, hence patients have isolated fasting hyperglycemia. Individuals remain asymptomatic and are incidentally detected during health checkups. Mild isolated fasting hyperglycemia does not significantly contribute to diabetic complications and hence treatment is not required except in pregnancy due to the risk of fetal macrosomia.

Hepatocyte Nuclear Factor 1-alpha

- *Age*: <30 years
- *Synonym*: MODY 3
- *Gene mutation*: Mutations in the *HNF1A* gene located on chromosome (12q24.2)

Hepatocyte nuclear factor 1-alpha is the most common cause of symptomatic MODY. HNF1A is a transcription factor found in the liver, kidney, intestine, and pancreatic tissue. Thus, mutation in HNF1A causes dysregulation of glucose metabolism, and transport and causes progressive β-cell dysfunction. Most patients at diagnosis are initiated on sulfonylureas, but due to progressive beta cell dysfunction, will eventually require insulin.

Hepatocyte Nuclear Factor 4-alpha

- *Synonym*: MODY 1
- *Gene mutation*: Mutation of the *HNF4* gene on chromosome 20q12-q13.1

This gene is expressed in islets cells, kidneys, liver, and intestines and the clinical profile of individuals with HNF4A is similar to HNF1A. Patients present most commonly occur in the mid-twenties. Individuals with this mutation have been found to have a higher birth weight and increased incidence of macrosomia. Treatment is similar to MODY3.

Hepatocyte Nuclear Factor 1-beta

- *Synonym*: MODY 5 and renal cysts and diabetes (RCAD) syndrome
- *Genetic mutation*: Intragenic and deletion of chromosome 17q12
- *Biochemical abnormality*: RBS is in the range of 200 mg/dL, HbA1c: ~7.5–8.5%

This mutation can affect gene regulation in the liver, kidneys, intestines, lungs, or ovaries. Patients can develop renal abnormalities like renal cysts, which are the most common, detected prenatally as bilateral hyperechogenic kidneys, absent kidney, and renal hypoplasia. Other abnormalities are genital abnormalities, diabetic nephropathy, and early renal failure. Treatment includes insulin initially and switching to orally administered antihyperglycemic agents (OHAs), such as sulfonylureas and meglitinide.

Neonatal Diabetes

- *Age*: <6 months
- *KCNJ11 and ABCC8*: The *KCNJ11* gene encodes the inner part and ABCC8 encodes the outer part of the K^+-ATP channel which is an important channel enabling insulin release and hence mutations in the same lead

to decreased insulin release. Treatment includes insulin and sulfonylureas. Patients with mutations in KCNJ11 may display increased frequency of attention deficit hyperactivity disorder, sleep disturbances, developmental delays, and seizures as the brain contains K^+-ATP channels. In addition to enhancing glycemic management, sulfonylureas may also improve neurological function.

Overexpression of Genes at Chromosome 6Q24

This is the most common cause of transient neonatal diabetes, in which the diabetes spontaneously resolves within the first year of life but typically recurs in adolescence. Insulin is the mainstay treatment.

CLINICAL FEATURES AND DIAGNOSIS

When to Suspect Monogenic Diabetes?

Monogenic diabetes is suspected in individuals with the following features:

- Age of onset of diabetes < 25 years
- Profile not fitting into T1DM with:
  - Negative pancreatic islet autoantibodies
  - Prolonged honeymoon period (i.e., > 3–5 years after the onset of diabetes)
  - Measurable C-peptide in the presence of hyperglycemia
  - Low insulin requirement (i.e., 0.5 U/kg/day) for therapy
  - Absence of ketoacidosis when treating without insulin
- Profile not fitting into T2DM with:
  - Age of onset < 45 years
  - Lack of significant overweight/obesity
  - Lack of markers of insulin resistance (acanthosis nigricans)
  - Normal triglyceride levels and/or normal or elevated high-density lipoprotein (HDL)
- Isolated nonprogressive fasting hyperglycemia
- High sensitivity to sulfonylureas
- Extra pancreatic features (e.g., renal, hepatic, and gastrointestinal)
- Strong family/personal history of neonatal diabetes or neonatal hypoglycemia
- A family history of diabetes consistent with autosomal dominant inheritance that contrasts with T1DM and T2DM in the following ways:
  - T1DM can run in families but is often sporadic—only 2–6% of individuals with T1DM have an affected parent
  - T2DM frequently runs in families; shared environmental factors and risk alleles can result in the development of the disease in several family members. When comparing T2DM with MODY, T2DM has an onset after 45 years and coexists with obesity, whereas MODY has an onset of <35 years and the absence of obesity.

NEED FOR DIAGNOSIS OF MONOGENIC DIABETES

It is important to identify cases of monogenic diabetes for the following reasons **(Flowchart 2)**:

- To provide treatment targeting the specific causative.
- To detect other family members in those with a significant family history.
- Prediction or early identification of other multisystem features that may be associated with the genetic defect.

Barriers in identifying monogenic diabetes cases due to:

- Lack of clinical suspicion or awareness
- Poor access to genetic testing facilities
- Relatively expensive genetic testing

GENETIC TESTING

In the past, clinical phenotypes and the relative occurrence of mutations in a given population have both been used as a guide to genetic testing. But in recent times, with the advancement of technology, sequencing of a single gene that seems specific to a phenotype is possible such as:

- A young nonobese patient with a family history of diabetes presenting with isolated fasting hyperglycemia can undergo GCK testing.
- A child detected with renal cysts and or genitourinary malformations with elevated blood sugar can undergo HNF1B testing.
- A neonate or infant with neurological dysfunction with diabetes diagnosed within the first 6 months can be tested for ABCC8 or KCNJ11.
- Diabetes occurring within the first year of life with recurrence in adolescence should raise the suspicion of overexpression of genes at 6q24.

Genetic Diagnosis: Impact on the Diabetes Treatment

Appropriate diagnosis of the type of diabetes with the help of genetic testing can help direct medical practitioners toward a definitive treatment strategy using either insulin, OHAs, or both. This also helps to prognosticate individuals and foresee complications.

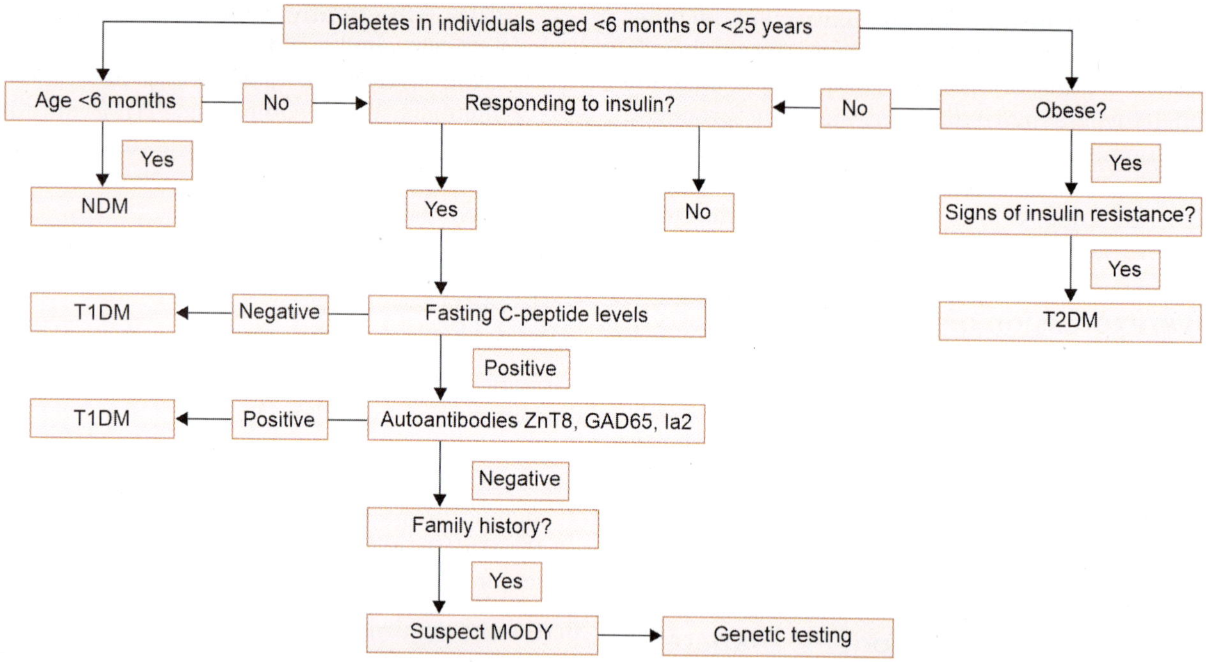

FLOWCHART 2: Algorithm to identify monogenic diabetes.

(GAD65: glutamic acid decarboxylase 65; Ia2: islet antigen 2; MODY: maturity-onset diabetes of the young; NDM: neonatal diabetes mellitus; T1DM: type 1 diabetes mellitus; T2DM: type 2 diabetes mellitus; ZnT8: zinc transporter 8)

TREATMENT (FIG. 1)

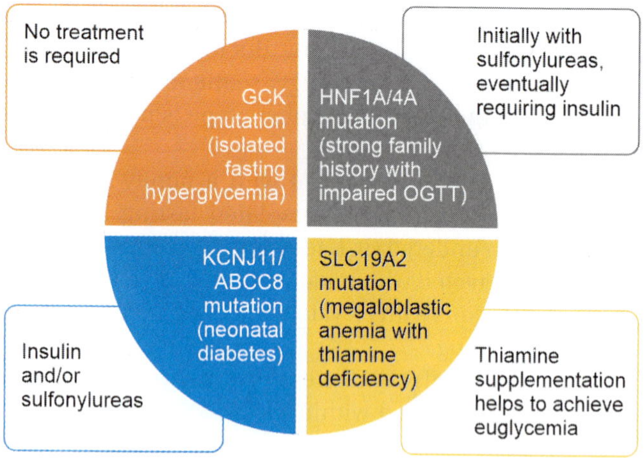

FIG. 1: Treatment of MODY.

(ABCC8: ATP-binding cassette subfamily C member 8; GCK: glucokinase; HNF1A: hepatocyte nuclear factor 1-alpha; MODY: maturity-onset diabetes of the young; OGTT: oral glucose tolerance tests; SLC19A2: solute carrier family 19 member 2)

CONCLUSION

Managing DM in the appropriate manner is essential to reduce the overall morbidity and mortality of individuals. Hence, targeted treatment according to the phenotype and genotype is important. Timely clinical suspicion, with the help of biochemical indicators and genetic testing, can help to personalize the therapeutic options and to achieve glycemic targets set for the individual without causing many side effects. Correct therapy, avoiding the needless use of insulin or other unsuitable medicines, and genetic counseling are all made possible by genetic testing. Increasing the ethnic variety of research participants is crucial to a better understanding of the effects on all communities because most of the present data on monogenic diabetes are based on Caucasian populations.

SUGGESTED READINGS

1. Zhang H, Colclough K, Gloyn AL, Pollin TI. Monogenic diabetes: a gateway to precision medicine in diabetes. J Clin Invest. 2021;131(3):e142244.
2. Misra S, Owen KR. Genetics of monogenic diabetes: present clinical challenges. Curr Diab Rep. 2018;18(12):141.
3. Misra S, Hattersley AT. Monogenic causes of diabetes. In: Holt RIGH, Cockram C, Flyvbjerg A, Goldstein BJ (Eds). Textbook of Diabetes, 5th edition. Malden (MA): Wiley-Blackwell; 2017. pp. 241-61.
4. De Franco E, Flanagan SE, Houghton JA, Allen HL, Mackay DJ, Temple IK, et al. The effect of early, comprehensive genomic

testing on clinical care in neonatal diabetes: an international cohort study. Lancet. 2015;386(9997):957-63.
5. Riddle MC, Philipson LH, Rich SS, Carlsson A, Franks PW, Greeley SA, et al. Monogenic diabetes: from genetic insights to population-based precision in care. Reflections from a *Diabetes Care Editors'* expert forum. Diabetes Care. 2020;43(12):3117-28.
6. Sperling MA, Garg A, Cowie CC, Casagrande SS, Menke AS, Cissell MA, et al. Monogenic forms of diabetes. In: Diabetes in America, 3rd edition. Bethesda (MD): National Institute of Diabetes and Digestive and Kidney Diseases (US); 2018.
7. Naylor RN, Knight Johnson AE, Del Gaudio D, Feldman J, Mirzaa GM, et al. Maturity-onset diabetes of the young overview. In: GeneReviews® [Internet]. Seattle (WA): University of Washington, Seattle; 1993.
8. Delvecchio M, Pastore C, Giordano P. Treatment options for MODY patients: a systematic review of literature. Diabetes Ther. 2020;11(8):1667-85.
9. Lemelman MB, Letourneau L, Greeley SA. Neonatal diabetes mellitus: an update on diagnosis and management. Clin Perinatol. 2018;45(1):41-59.
10. Harris A, Letourneau LR, Greeley SA. Monogenic diabetes: the impact of making the right diagnosis. Curr Opin Pediatr. 2018;30(4):558-67.

21

CHAPTER

Mitochondria as a New Target for Managing Diabetic Complications

Vitull K Gupta, Meghna Gupta, Varun Gupta

ABSTRACT

Diabetes mellitus (DM) is a serious chronic noncommunicable disease (NCD) now being considered as one of the largest global health crises. Management of diabetes and its complications is focused on controlling the blood glucose levels by various nonpharmacological and pharmacological strategies, but still control of blood glucose may not prevent and decrease complications of diabetes, suggesting to search for new strategies and focus on the target to alleviation of root cause of diabetes rather than symptomatic approach. Mitochondria are known as the powerhouses of the cell and have been extensively studied and implicated as an important factor in pathogenesis, development, progression, and complications of type 2 diabetes mellitus (T2DM). Different types of mitochondrial dysfunction have been implicated in pathogenesis of T2DM which has led to research into the role of mitochondrial dysfunction in insulin resistance, diabetes, and its complications. Interventions influencing mitochondria in diabetes include dietary interventions, exercise, pharmacological agents like metformin, thiazolidinediones (TZDs), dipeptidyl peptidase-4 (DPP-4) inhibitors, sodium-glucose cotransporter-2 (SGLT-2) inhibitors, or gliflozins and a few novel therapeutic approaches targeting mitochondria has been explored. This chapter explores new insights into the role of mitochondria in pathogenesis of diabetes and managing complications of diabetes.

INTRODUCTION

Diabetes mellitus (DM) is a serious chronic noncommunicable disease (NCD), presently being considered as one of the largest global health crises with 11.4% Indian prevalence of diabetes and 15.3% prediabetes, more importantly >50% people being unaware of their diabetic status predisposing them to increased incidence of complications of diabetes and mortality.

Interplay of various environmental and genetic factors in DM can result in progressive loss of β-cell function and/or mass or insulin resistance (IR) clinically resulting in hyperglycemia and risk of developing chronic complications of DM for which the progression rates may differ. Type 2 diabetes mellitus (T2DM) comprise about 90% of total diabetic cases.

Triumvirate hypothesis explains the pathogenesis of T2DM involving three organs dysfunction, the pancreas with decreased insulin secretion/sensitivity, liver with increased hepatic glucose production, and muscles with decreased glucose uptake leading to hyperglycemia. Later hypothesis included adipose tissue, gut, kidney, α-cells of pancreas, and nervous system. Chronic complications associated with T2DM have been classified into macrovascular complications including cardiovascular, cerebrovascular, and peripheral vascular diseases whereas microvascular complications include neuropathy, nephropathy, and retinopathy.

MITOCHONDRIA AND TYPE 2 DIABETES MELLITUS

Mitochondria are known as the powerhouses of the cell and have been extensively studied and implicated as an important factor in pathogenesis, development, progression, and complications of T2DM, now being considered as an important target for lifestyle and pharmacological interventions. Mitochondria play a pivotal role in cellular energy metabolism, oxidative phosphorylation (OXPHOS), β-oxidation of fatty acids, and adenosine triphosphate (ATP) production making mitochondria essential for glucose and lipid metabolism including the cellular redox state with production and clearance of reactive oxygen species (ROS), calcium homeostasis, substrate metabolism, and apoptosis.

Different types of mitochondrial dysfunction have been implicated in pathogenesis of T2DM including decreased mitochondrial content, mitochondrial dysbiogenesis, impaired mitochondrial function causing intracellular accumulation of lipids and increased ROS production as a potential cause of IR, β-cell dysfunction, and diabetes complications. A vicious cycle is created with association of T2DM, IR, and mitochondrial dysfunction. Human studies investigating mitochondria in liver, skeletal muscle, and blood cells have shown that in diabetic patients, mitochondrial function is impacted but may be with different tissue-specific mechanisms.

In DM, mitochondrial function has been extensively studied in skeletal muscle, and found an undeniable relationship between mitochondrial dysfunction, T2DM, and IR may be due to intrinsic mitochondrial dysfunction or reduced mitochondrial content, accumulation of intramuscular fat, and lipid products like diacylglycerol and ceramides responsible for inhibition of insulin signaling by activating novel protein kinases C (PKC). Another hypothesis proposed that impaired oxygen supply to the skeletal muscle is responsible for suboptimal muscle mitochondrial function rather than intrinsic impairment of mitochondrial oxidative function. Increased production of ROS because of mitochondrial dysfunction further accentuates muscle dysfunction in DM.

Mitochondrial abnormalities in liver lead to IR and influence glucose homeostasis in liver by affecting various pathways of glucose metabolism including glycogenesis, glycogenolysis, glycolysis, and gluconeogenesis. Cellular subcompartment essential for lipid metabolism, the mitochondrial-associated endoplasmic reticulum membranes (MAMs) is upregulated in hepatic IR and mitochondrial abnormalities are responsible for increased hepatocellular lipid content that is nonalcoholic fatty liver (NAFL), often progresses to nonalcoholic steatohepatitis (NASH) and nonalcoholic fatty liver disease (NAFLD), which play an important role in the development of IR and fatty liver disease in diabetes and more importantly may even precede the manifestation of T2DM.

A research paper that aimed to study mitochondrial parameters like mitochondrial mass, membrane potential, and superoxide production in peripheral blood mononuclear cells (PBMCs) of T2DM patients showed more spherical smaller mitochondria with reduced total mitochondrial mass, increased mitochondrial superoxide production, and mitochondrial membrane potential. Another study done in diabetic patients assessed platelet mitochondria showing reduced oxygen consumption and oxygen-dependent ATP synthesis, induction of mitochondrial antioxidant enzymes, and upregulation of oxidative stress. Evidence showed higher maximal oxygen consumption in PBMCs from patients of DM is consistent with higher ROS production suggesting relationship between mitochondrial and vascular smooth muscle cell dysfunction. Evidence suggests that sirtuin 1 (silent mating-type information regulation 2 homolog 1) (SIRT1) stimulates pancreatic β-cells to secret insulin and decreases oxidative stress. SIRT1 in muscle and liver activates peroxisome proliferator-activated receptor-γ coactivator-1α (PGC-1α) to stimulate mitochondrial biogenesis making sirtuin-activating compounds, novel agents for prevention, and management of DM and its complications.

Mitochondrial dysfunction also affects other tissues implicated in pathogenesis as well as complications of diabetes.

MITOCHONDRIA AND COMPLICATIONS OF TYPE 2 DIABETES MELLITUS

Presently, management of diabetes is focused on controlling the blood glucose levels to prevent and decrease complications of diabetes, but complications develop even with tight control of diabetes suggesting focus on the target to alleviation of root cause of diabetes rather than symptomatic approach. This has led to research into the role of mitochondrial dysfunction in IR and DM and its complications.

In development of diabetic complications, complex relationship between chronic hyperglycemia-induced over production of ROS, diminished antioxidant defense, IR, and mitochondrial dysfunction, where one factor influences the other and vice versa. That is why focus is being shifting to "mitochondrial medicine," that is interventions to stimulate mitochondrial biogenesis, metabolism, and/or reduce mitochondrial dysfunction to ameliorate IR and prevent or reduce complications of DM.

A study reviewed the role of mitochondria in complication of diabetes and indicated that mitochondria dysfunction or damage could be important in development of complications like cardiomyopathy, nephropathy, neuropathy, and retinopathy. Evidence showed dramatic dysfunction in the inner mitochondrial membrane potential, mitochondrial superoxide production, mitochondrial mass leading to endothelial dysfunction. Main reason for coronary arteries dysfunction was suggested to be the increased ROS production resulting

CONCLUSION

Good glycemic control in diabetes is best for prevention, management, and control of complications of diabetes, but despite good glycemic control and meticulous treatment of diabetes, complications may still develop, stimulating research exploring new avenues to treat diabetes and prevent complications leading to investigation into the role of mitochondria in pathogenesis of diabetes, IR, and complications of diabetes. Mitochondria have been extensively studied in diabetes and are increasingly being recognized as an important factor in the causation, progression of diabetes, and its complications, thus considered to be a valuable target for mitochondrial specific interventions and novel drug development. Positive thing is that mitochondrial dysfunction can be improved by interventions, most importantly increasing physical activity and healthy diet along with conventional and mitochondrial targeted pharmacological interventions leading to improvement of metabolic health and prevention of diabetes, its treatment and its complications. Thus, the present chapter stresses on need for opening new avenues for the prevention and treatment of diabetes and its complications with a focus on associated mitochondrial dysfunction.

SUGGESTED READINGS

1. Anjana RM, Unnikrishnan R, Deepa M, Pradeepa R, Tandon N, Das AK, et al. Metabolic non-communicable disease health report of India: the ICMR-INDIAB national cross-sectional study (ICMR-INDIAB-17). Lancet Diabetes Endocrinol. 2023;11(7): 474-89.
2. ElSayed NA, Aleppo G, Aroda VR, Bannuru RR, Brown FM, Bruemmer D, et al. 2. Classification and Diagnosis of Diabetes: Standards of Care in Diabetes-2023. Diabetes Care. 2023;46(Suppl 1):S19-S40.
3. DeFronzo RA. Lilly lecture 1987. The triumvirate: beta-cell, muscle, liver. A collusion responsible for NIDDM. Diabetes. 1988;37(6):667-87.
4. Defronzo RA. Banting Lecture. From the triumvirate to the ominous octet: a new paradigm for the treatment of type 2 diabetes mellitus. Diabetes. 2009;58(4):773-95.
5. Krako Jakovljevic N, Pavlovic K, Jotic A, Lalic K, Stoiljkovic M, Lukic L, et al. Targeting Mitochondria in Diabetes. Int J Mol Sci. 2021;22(12):6642.
6. Townsend LK, Brunetta HS, Mori MAS. Mitochondria-associated ER membranes in glucose homeostasis and insulin resistance. Am J Physiol Endocrinol Metab. 2020;319(6):E1053-E1060.
7. Blake R, Trounce IA. Mitochondrial dysfunction and complications associated with diabetes. Biochim Biophys Acta. 2014;1840(4):1404-12.
8. Ritter O, Jelenik T, Roden M. Lipid-mediated muscle insulin resistance: different fat, different pathways? J Mol Med (Berl). 2015;93(8):831-43.
9. Cree-Green M, Scalzo RL, Harrall K, Newcomer BR, Schauer IE, Huebschmann AG, et al. Supplemental Oxygen Improves In Vivo Mitochondrial Oxidative Phosphorylation Flux in Sedentary Obese Adults With Type 2 Diabetes. Diabetes. 2018;67(7): 1369-79.
10. Widlansky ME, Wang J, Shenouda SM, Hagen TM, Smith AR, Kizhakekuttu TJ, et al. Altered mitochondrial membrane potential, mass, and morphology in the mononuclear cells of humans with type 2 diabetes. Transl Res. 2010;156(1):15-25.
11. Avila C, Huang RJ, Stevens MV, Aponte AM, Tripodi D, Kim KY, et al. Platelet mitochondrial dysfunction is evident in type 2 diabetes in association with modifications of mitochondrial anti-oxidant stress proteins. Exp Clin Endocrinol Diabetes. 2012;120(4):248-51.
12. Hartman ML, Shirihai OS, Holbrook M, Xu G, Kocherla M, Shah A, et al. Relation of mitochondrial oxygen consumption in peripheral blood mononuclear cells to vascular function in type 2 diabetes mellitus. Vasc Med. 2014;19(1):67-74.
13. Kwak SH, Park KS, Lee KU, Lee HK. Mitochondrial metabolism and diabetes. J Diabetes Investig. 2010;1(5):161-9.
14. Hassanpour SH, Dehghani MA, Karami SZ, Dehghani F. Role of mitochondria in diabetes and its complications. IJPSR. 2018;9(6):2185-9.
15. De Felice FG, Ferreira ST. Inflammation, defective insulin signaling, and mitochondrial dysfunction as common molecular denominators connecting type 2 diabetes to Alzheimer disease. Diabetes. 2014;63(7):2262-72.
16. Kizhakekuttu TJ, Wang J, Dharmashankar K, Ying R, Gutterman DD, Vita JA, et al. Adverse alterations in mitochondrial function contribute to type 2 diabetes mellitus–related endothelial dysfunction in humans. Arterioscler Thromb Vasc Biol. 2012;32(10):2531-9.
17. Daniele G, Eldor R, Merovci A, Clarke GD, Xiong J, Tripathy D, et al. Chronic reduction of plasma free fatty acid improves mitochondrial function and whole-body insulin sensitivity in obese and type 2 diabetic individuals. Diabetes. 2014;63(8): 2812-20.
18. Kowluru RA, Kowluru A, Veluthakal R, Mohammad G, Syed I, Santos JM, et al. TIAM1-RAC1 signalling axis-mediated activation of NADPH oxidase-2 initiates mitochondrial damage in the development of diabetic retinopathy. Diabetologia. 2014;57(5):1047-56.
19. Guan Y, Drake JC, Yan Z. Exercise-Induced Mitophagy in Skeletal Muscle and Heart. Exerc Sport Sci Rev. 2019;47(3):151-6.
20. Apostolopoulou M, Pesta D, Karusheva Y, Gancheva S, Jelenik T, Bierwagen A, et al. Effects on Insulin Sensitivity, but Not on Mitochondrial Function Are Dependent on Insulin Resistance Status after High Intensity Interval Training. Diabetes. 2018;67:69.
21. Rena G, Hardie DG, Pearson ER. The mechanisms of action of metformin. Diabetologia. 2017;60(9):1577-85.
22. Alshawi A, Agius L. Low metformin causes a more oxidized mitochondrial NADH/NAD redox state in hepatocytes and inhibits gluconeogenesis by a redox-independent mechanism. J Biol Chem. 2019;294(8):2839-53.

23. Wang Y, An H, Liu T, Qin C, Sesaki H, Guo S, et al. Metformin Improves Mitochondrial Respiratory Activity through Activation of AMPK. Cell Rep. 2019;29(6):1511-1523.e5.
24. Divakaruni AS, Wiley SE, Rogers GW, Andreyev AY, Petrosyan S, Loviscach M, et al. Thiazolidinediones are acute, specific inhibitors of the mitochondrial pyruvate carrier. Proc Natl Acad Sci U S A. 2013;110(14):5422-7.
25. Mima A. Mitochondria-targeted drugs for diabetic kidney disease. Heliyon. 2022;8(2):e08878.
26. Lachaux M, Soulié M, Hamzaoui M, Bailly A, Nicol L, Rémy-Jouet I, et al. Short-and long-term administration of imeglimin counters cardiorenal dysfunction in a rat model of metabolic syndrome. Endocrinol Diabetes Metab. 2020;3(3):e00128.

22

CHAPTER

Importance and Interpretation of Time-in-Range in Clinical Practice

Md Hamid Ali

ABSTRACT

Time-in-range (TIR) is now becoming an important parameter of glucose control in finer tune in comparison to glycated hemoglobin (HbA1c). It is more clearly related to complications of diabetes in a better way. TIR is the amount of time a patient spends within a specific blood glucose (blood sugar) range, which is usually 70–180 mg/dL. Uncontrolled diabetics have a higher incidence of complications. The purpose of this chapter is to find out the answers to two main questions: (i) Can continuous glucose monitoring (CGM) and TIR improve the A1c? and (ii) Can TIR help reduce diabetes complications? Excessive glycemic variability (GV) and sub-optimal TIR can significantly impact the lives of people with diabetes. As per the statements of the American Diabetes Association (ADA) Standards of Medical Care in Diabetes 2022, TIR and GV are key metrics to facilitate effective diabetes management. HbA1c does not provide a measure of GV or hypoglycemia. Patients with abnormal carotid intima-media thickness (CIMT) had significantly lower TIR ($p < 0.0001$). TIR is inversely proportional to diabetic retinopathy (DR) severity. Lower TIR is associated with an increased risk of all-cause and cardiovascular disease (CVD) mortality among patients with diabetes mellitus (DM). Each 10% drop in TIR was associated with a 64% increased risk of retinopathy in people with type 1 diabetes mellitus (T1DM), increased risk of peripheral neuropathy in people with type 2 diabetes mellitus (T2DM) and chronic kidney disease (CKD), increased risk of microalbuminuria in people with T1DM, increased mortality in people with T2DM, 5% increased risk of cardiovascular mortality, and 8% increased risk of all-cause mortality. TIR is an important mental and emotional consideration for people with diabetes, particularly for those taking insulin. The results also serve as a testament to the daily reality of living with diabetes, which is experienced as a physical and psychological battle between hypoglycemia and hyperglycemia. Various guidelines are now recommending TIR as a glucometric measure. The evolution of glucose measurement has been from HbA1c to finger prick test and ultimately to TIR.

INTRODUCTION

Until recently, glycated hemoglobin (HbA1c) was the "gold standard" for the evaluation of glucose control and there is enough supporting evidence of an association between HbA1c and vascular complications in type 1 diabetes mellitus (T1DM) and type 2 diabetes mellitus (T2DM). In spite of that, several limitations of HbA1c exist. Its measurement is jeopardized by factors such as anemia, pregnancy, hemoglobinopathy, and ethnicity. There is discordance between measured HbA1c and the true mean glucose in a substantial number of patients. In addition, HbA1c does not capture hypoglycemia, hyperglycemia, and glycemic variability (GV). In contrast, continuous glucose monitoring (CGM) can track the glucose profile from days to weeks, providing valuable information for the individualization and adjustment of treatment. Importantly, the comprehensive data generated by CGM facilitates the development of new glycemic metrics—TIR is a simple and intuitive metric. In T2DM, TIR is related to the prevalence of diabetic retinopathy (DR), nephropathy, cardiovascular death and all-cause mortality. Beck et al. described association of TIR with the progression of DR and the development of albuminuria in T1D. Moreover, in pregnant women with T1DM, Murphy HR observed that even a small increment (5%) in TIR was associated with improved neonatal outcomes.

EVOLUTION OF GLUCOSE MEASUREMENT: HBA1C TO FINGER PRICK TEST TO CGM/TIR

Baseline data from LANDMARC (LongitudinAl Nationwide stuDy on Management And Real-world outComes of diabetes in India) underscore the extent of suboptimal glycemic control in a vast majority of Indians with T2DM. Only 25.1% of participants had controlled glycemia (HbA1c < 7%). LANDMARC is the first large-scale, longitudinal, prospective, observational real-world study to investigate management and complications in T2DM across India over a period of 3 years. Four out five people with T2DM are uncontrolled in India. Uncontrolled patients have reported a higher incidence of complications.

Could CGM and TIR improve the HbA1c? Can CGM help reduce diabetes complications?

Continuous glucose monitoring, as compared with blood glucose meter monitoring, resulted in significantly lower HbA1c levels (63% vs. 39%) in 8 months. TIR is the amount of time a patient spends within a specific blood glucose (blood sugar) range, which is usually 70–180 mg/dL. TIRs are both appropriate and useful as clinical targets and measurements that complement HbA1c. Every 5% increase in TIR is associated with clinically significant benefits for T1DM or T2DM. Target values should be considered an integral component of CGM data analysis and day-to-day treatment decision-making.

Glycemic Variability

Glycemic variability is a common challenge for people with diabetes. Excessive GV and suboptimal TIR can significantly impact the lives of people with diabetes. International guidelines recommend TIR and GV as key metrics to facilitate effective diabetes management. TIR is associated with the risk of microvascular complications and can be used for assessment of glycemic control.

As per the American Diabetes Association (ADA) Standards of Medical Care in Diabetes 2022, *"A1C does not provide a measure of glycemic variability or hypoglycemia."* Recommendations of the International Consensus on Time-in-Range 2019 state, "The consensus panel identified 'time-in-range' as a metric of glycemic control that provides more actionable information than A1C alone"

Glycemic Variability: Clinical Implications for Diabetes—Comorbidities and Mortality

Patients with abnormal carotid intima-media thickness (CIMT) had significantly lower TIR ($p < 0.0001$). GV is an independent prognostic factor for composite major adverse cardiovascular events (MACE) after 3 months in patients undergoing percutaneous coronary intervention (PCI). Mean glucose, glucose standard deviation (SD), mean amplitude of glucose excursion (MAGE), and night mean amplitude of glycemic excursion (NMAGE) were higher in DM patients with obstructive sleep apnea. The odds of having albuminuria are 0.94 per 10% increase in TIR of 70–180 mg/dL, after adjusting for multiple factors including GV. TIR is inversely proportional to DR severity. Lower TIR is associated with an increased risk of all-cause and CVD mortality among patients with DM. Perioperative TIR (3.9–10.0 mmol/L) and time-below-range (TBR) (<3.9 mmol/L) are significantly associated with major amputation in hospitalized patients with diabetic foot osteomyelitis (DFO). GV is a common challenge in T1DM. 56% of people with T1DM were found to have excess GV (% of CV >36%). 9 h/day are spent outside the target range for an average person with T1DM.

Self-monitoring blood glucose (SMBG) has the following features:

- Provides a single "point-in-time" measurement
- May miss nocturnal and asymptomatic hypoglycemia
- Indicates the direction or rate-of-change of glucose levels
- Reliance on patient-maintained data poses a risk of noncompliance and unreliable results
- Requires finger stick, which is painful and invasive, and the risk of infection is there.

Glycated Hemoglobin: May not Give a Full Picture

- Reflects mean glycemia of an individual in the previous 2–3 months
- Does not provide data as to how to adjust the treatment regimen when the levels are elevated
- Does not reflect inter- and intra-day glycemic excursions
- Does not reflect rapid fluctuations in daily glucose control and hypoglycemia

On the contrary, TIR has the following advantages:

- Compares any time periods
- Captures all glucose levels for the given time frame and identifies time within a safe range
- Immediately detects acute effects of therapy changes
- Good correlation with patient-reported outcomes (PROs)
- Low susceptibility to interference
- Correlation with endpoints unclear, hardly any long-term studies

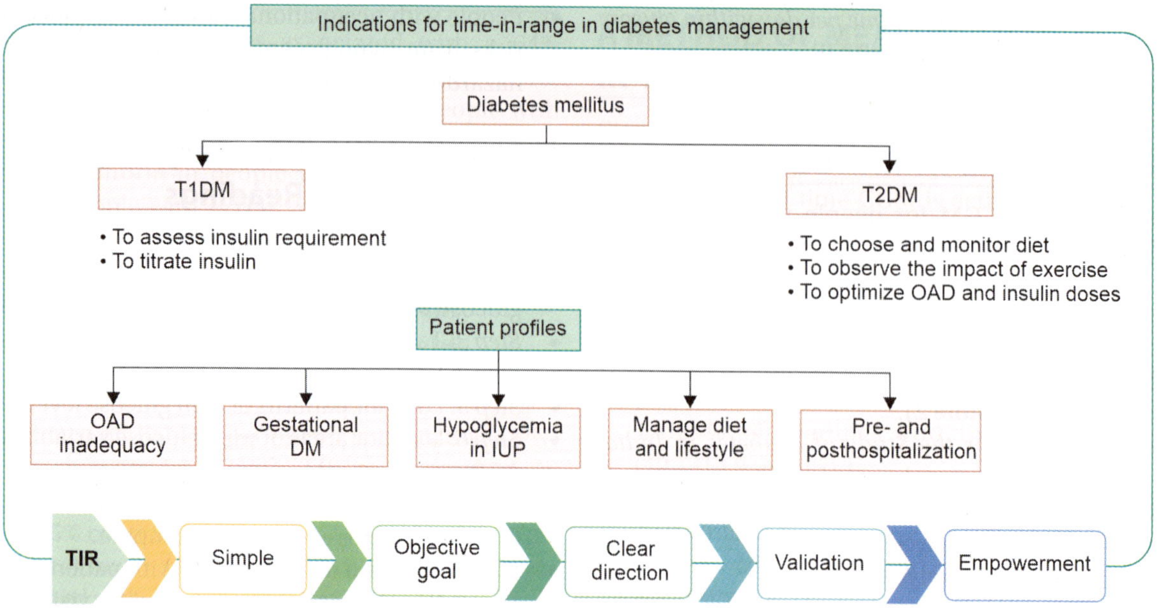

FLOWCHART 1: Indications for time-in-range in diabetes management.

(DM: diabetes mellitus; IUP: intrauterine pregnancy; OAD: oral antidiabetic drug; T1DM: type 1 diabetes mellitus; T2DM: type 2 diabetes mellitus)

TABLE 2: Three main types of CGMS.

Real-time CGMS	Flash glucose monitoring/ intermittently scanned CGM	Professional CGM for doctors
Provides continuous glucose readings in real time and alerts the user when their glucose levels are too high or too low	Provide continuous glucose readings, but they do not transmit data in real time	Patients are implanted with sensor and sent, data is downloaded and reviewed, to guide/plan the treatment
Transmits data wirelessly to a receiver or smartphone app	User scans the sensor with a reader or smartphone app to get a current glucose reading	Sensor glucose readings are recorded every 1–15 minutes
Real-time CGMS include the Dexcom G6, Guardian Connect, and FreeStyle Libre 2	Examples of flash glucose monitoring systems include the FreeStyle Libre	• Retrospective analysis of the sensor data • Patient cannot see the sensor glucose readings

(CGMS: continuous glucose monitoring system)

Recommended Frequency for Repeating CGM/TIR Assessment in Patients with Type 2 Diabetes Mellitus in South Asia

Repeating CGM/TIR assessment in patients with T2DM in South Asia is based on previous AGP report of the patient (nonpregnant).

Practical use of ambulatory glucose profile (AGP) and TIR is given in **Table 3**.

TABLE 3: Practical use of AGP and TIR.

Current AGP	Future recommendation on CGM/TIR
TIR > 90% and TBR < 1%	Once every 6 months
TIR > 70% and TBR > 4%	Once every 3 months
TIR > 50% and TBR > 5%	Once every 2 months
Use clinical judgement/repeat more frequently if vulnerable to hypoglycemia	

(AGP; ambulatory glucose profile; CGM; continuous glucose monitoring; TBR: time-below-range; TIR: time-in-range)

CONCLUSION

Four out of five people with T2DM are uncontrolled in India. TIR impacts the quality of daily life.

TIR correlates better with the patient experience and patient-reported outcomes. To get TIR, CGM is mandatory. Despite their clinical significance, CGM tools are not widely popular. CGM tools help identify high-risk population by providing GV data across different age groups. Real world evidence highlights the benefits of CGM in clinical care. There is some evidence between GV and development of diabetic complications.

If TIR decreases by 10%, retinopathy risk increases by 64%, nephropathy risk increases by 40%, and neuropathy risk increases by 25%. Initial evidences also show increase in the surrogate markers of macrovascular complications like abnormal CIMTs. TIR is an important mental and emotional consideration for people with diabetes and particularly for those taking insulin. The results also serve as a testament to the daily reality of living with diabetes, which is experienced as a physical and psychological battle between hypoglycemia and hyperglycemia. Patients may perceive increased daily TIR as having greater success with their diabetes, whereas HbA1c is not likely to have the same daily relevance or result in the equivalent feelings of personal or therapeutic success.

SUGGESTED READINGS

1. Das AK, Kalra S, Joshi S, Mithal A, Kumar KMP, Unnikrishnan AG, et al. One-year trends from the LANDMARC trial: A 3-year, pan-India, prospective, longitudinal study on the management and real-world outcomes of type 2 diabetes mellitus. Endocrinol Diabetes Metab. 2022;5(1):e00316.
2. Martens T, Beck RW, Bailey R, Ruedy KJ, Calhoun P, Peters AL, et al. Effect of continuous glucose monitoring on glycemic control in patients with type 2 diabetes treated with basal insulin: a randomized clinical trial. JAMA. 2021;325(22):2262-72.
3. Battelino T, Danne T, Bergenstal RM, Amiel SA, Beck R, Biester T, et al. Clinical targets for continuous glucose monitoring data interpretation: Recommendations from the international consensus on time in range. Diabetes Care. 2019;42(8):1593-603.
4. Mayeda L, Katz R, Ahmad I, Bansal N, Batacchi Z, Hirsch IB, et al. Glucose time in range and peripheral neuropathy in type 2 diabetes mellitus and chronic kidney disease. BMJ Open Diab Res Care. 2020;8:e000991.
5. Khaire SS, Gada JV, Utpat KV, Shah N, Varthakavi PK, Bhagwat NM, et al. A study of glycemic variability in patients with type 2 diabetes mellitus with obstructive sleep apnea syndrome using a continuous glucose monitoring system. Clin Diabetes Endocrinol. 2020;6(1):1-9.
6. Yoo JH, Choi MS, Ahn J, Park SW, Kim Y, Hur KY, et al. Association between continuous glucose monitoring-derived time in range, other core metrics, and albuminuria in type 2 diabetes. Diabetes Technol Ther. 2020;22(10):768-76.
7. Wakasugi S, Mita T, Katakami N, Okada Y, Yoshii H, Osonoi T, et al. Associations between continuous glucose monitoring-derived metrics and diabetic retinopathy and albuminuria in patients with type 2 diabetes. BMJ Open Diabetes Res Care. 2021;9(1):e001923.
8. Yin X, Zhu W, Liu C, Yao H, You J, Chen Y, et al. Association of continuous glucose monitoring-derived time in range with major amputation risk in diabetic foot osteomyelitis patients undergoing amputation. Ther Adv Endocrinol Metab. 2022;13:20420188221099337.
9. Monnier L, Colette C, Wojtusciszyn A, Dejager S, Renard E, Molinari N, et al. Toward defining the threshold between low and high glucose variability in diabetes. Diabetes Care. 2017;40:832-8.
10. Agiostratidou G, Anhalt H, Ball D, Blonde L, Gourgari E, Harriman KN, et al. Standardizing clinically meaningful outcome measures beyond HbA_{1c} for type 1 diabetes: A Consensus report of the American Association of Clinical Endocrinologists, the American Association of Diabetes Educators, the American Diabetes Association, the Endocrine Society, JDRF International, the Leona M. and Harry B. Helmsley Charitable Trust, the Pediatric Endocrine Society, and the T1D Exchange. Diabetes Care. 2017;40:1622-30.
11. Sherwani SI, Khan HA, Ekhzaimy A, Masood A, Sakharkar MK. Significance of HbA1c test in diagnosis and prognosis of diabetic patients. Biomark Insights. 2016;11:95-104.
12. Danne T, Nimri R, Battelino T, Bergenstal RM, Close KL, DeVries JH, et al. International consensus on use of continuous glucose monitoring. Diabetes Care. 2017;40(12):1631-40.
13. Beck RW, Bergenstal RM, Riddlesworth TD, Kollman C, Li Z, Brown AS, et al. Validation of time in range as an outcome measure for diabetes clinical trials. Diabetes Care. 2019;42(3):400-5.
14. Lu J, Wang C, Shen Y, Chen L, Zhang L, Cai J, et al. Time in range in relation to all-cause and cardiovascular mortality in patients with type 2 diabetes: a prospective cohort study. Diabetes Care. 2021;44:549-55.
15. Kesavadev J, Misra A, Saboo B, Agarwal S, Sosale A, Joshi SR, et al. Time-in-range and frequency of continuous glucose monitoring: Recommendations for South Asia. Diabetes Metab Syndr. 2022;16(1):102345.
16. Mohan V, Unnikrishnan AG, Kesavadev J, Saboo B. Positioning "time-in-range" in the treatment of diabetes in India. Int J Diabetes Technol. 2022;1(1):32-41.
17. Beck RW, Bergenstal RM, Cheng P, Kollman C, Carlson AL, Johnson ML, et al. The relationships between time in range, hyperglycemia metrics, and HbA1c. J Diabetes Sci Technol. 2019;13(4):614-26.
18. Vigersky RA, McMahon C. The relationship of hemoglobin A1c to time-in-range in patients with diabetes. Diabetes Technol Ther. 2019;21(2):81-5.

23

CHAPTER

Hypoglycemia without Diabetes

Polok Das

ABSTRACT

Hypoglycemia is mostly caused by exposure to insulin or insulin-producing drugs used to treat diabetes, or other drugs, including alcohol. However, many other conditions can cause hypoglycemia, including severe organ failure, sepsis and neonatal death, hormone deficiencies, non-beta cell tumors, insulinoma, and previous gastric surgery.

INTRODUCTION

Hypoglycemia is most commonly caused by insulin or insulin-producing drugs used to treat diabetes mellitus or by exposure to other drugs, including alcohol. However, a number of other disorders, including critical organ failure, sepsis and inanition, hormone deficiencies, non-β-cell tumors, insulinoma, and prior gastric surgery, can cause hypoglycemia.

Hypoglycemia may be documented by *Whipple's triad*:

- Symptoms, signs, or both consistent with hypoglycemia,
- A low reliably measured plasma glucose concentration, and
- Resolution of those symptoms or signs after the plasma glucose concentration is raised.

The lower limit of the fasting plasma glucose concentration is normally ~70 mg/dL (~3.9 mmol/L). The definition of "low" is judgmental, but a plasma glucose concentration of <55 mg/dL (3.0 mmol/L) is unequivocally low.

SYSTEMIC GLUCOSE BALANCE AND GLUCOSE COUNTERREGULATION

Systemic glucose balance is normally maintained, and hypoglycemia and hyperglycemia are prevented, by dynamic, regulation of endogenous glucose production from the liver and kidneys and of glucose utilization by tissues outside the central nervous system (CNS), such as muscle.

Glucose Metabolism

Glucose is derived from three sources—(1) intestinal absorption following digestion of dietary carbohydrates, (2) *glycogenolysis,* and (3) *gluconeogenesis.*

Precursors for gluconeogenesis include lactate and pyruvate, various amino acids such as alanine and glutamine, and also glycerol, to a lesser extent.

The multiple fates of glucose transported into cells can be:

- Glucose can be stored as glycogen or may undergo glycolysis to pyruvate. Pyruvate can be further reduced to lactate, or transaminated to form alanine.
- Or converted to acetyl coenzyme A (CoA). Acetyl CoA, in turn, enters the tricarboxylic acid cycle to form carbon dioxide and the water cycle can be converted to fatty acids which can form triglycerides, oxidized, or utilized for the synthesis of ketone bodies (acetoacetate and β-hydroxybutyrate) or cholesterol.

Glucose-6-phosphatase, the Enzyme Necessary for the Release of Glucose into the Circulation, is Expressed only in the Liver and Kidneys

The liver and kidneys also express the enzymes necessary for gluconeogenesis, including the critical gluconeogenic enzymes pyruvate carboxylase, phosphoenolpyruvate carboxykinase, and fructose-1,6-bisphosphatase. Muscle can store glucose as glycogen, or metabolize glucose (through glycolysis) to form pyruvate, which, can then be reduced to lactate or transaminated to form alanine. Lactate (and pyruvate) released from muscle can be transported to the liver and the kidneys, to enter *the Cori or glucose-lactate cycle.* Alanine, glutamine, and other amino acids can also flow from muscle to liver and kidneys, to enter *the glucose-alanine and glucose-glutamine cycles. Both these cycles contribute to gluconeogenesis.*

Systemic Glucose Balance

- Normally, rates of endogenous glucose production and those of glucose utilization into tissues other than the brain are coordinately regulated—largely by the *plasma glucose-lowering (regulatory) hormone insulin and the plasma glucose-raising (counterregulatory) hormones glucagon and epinephrine.*
- The glucose pool, i.e., free glucose in the extracellular fluids plus in the cells of certain tissues (primarily the liver) is 15–20 g (83–111 mmol). Glycogen contains approximately 70 g (390 mmol) of glucose, with a range of about 25–130 g (135–722 mmol), which can be used as a source of glucose.
- Therefore, the *preformed glucose can provide less than an 8-hour supply of energy*, even at the diminished rate of glucose utilization.
- *If fasting is extended to 24–48 hours*, the plasma glucose concentration declines and then stabilizes; hepatic glycogen content falls to <10 g after which *gluconeogenesis is the sole source of glucose production.*

Systemic glucose balance, maintenance of the normal plasma glucose concentration, is accomplished by a network of hormones, neural signals, and substrate effects **(Fig. 1)**.

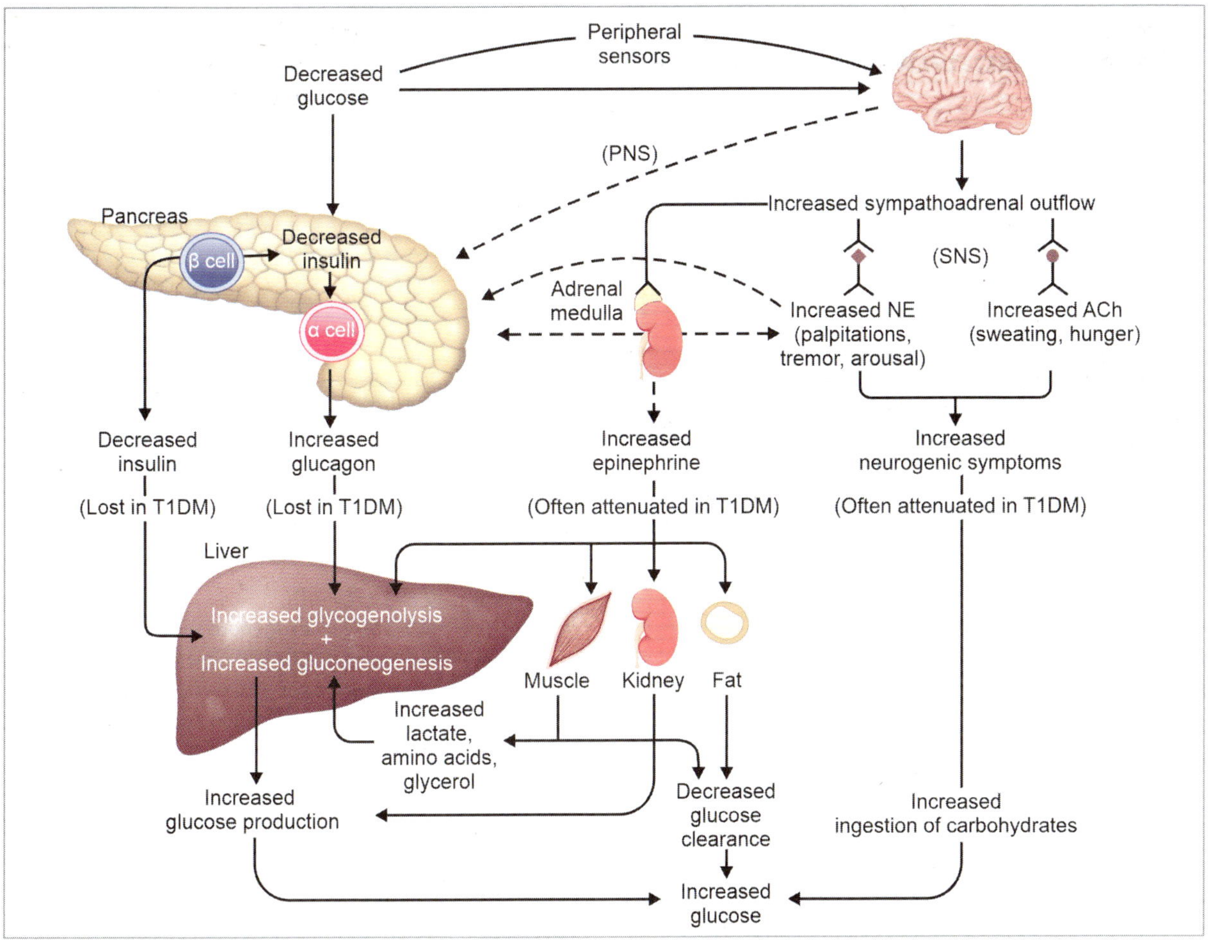

FIG. 1: Physiologic and behavioral defenses against hypoglycemia.

(Ach: acetylcholine; CNS: central nervous system; T1DM: type 1 diabetes mellitus)

Source: Melmed S, Koenig R, Rosen CJ, Auchus RJ, Goldfine AB. Hypoglycemia. In: William's Textbook of Endocrinology, 14th edition. Amsterdam: Elsevier; 2020. p. 1529.

24

CHAPTER

Sleep, Circadian Rhythm, and Diabetes Mellitus

Lekshmi Sudhakaran, Rakesh K Sahay

ABSTRACT

The prevalence of lifestyle diseases in India, including diabetes mellitus (DM), hypertension (HTN), and obesity, has significantly increased over the past few decades. Modern lifestyles, such as increased screen time, shift work, sedentary lifestyles, and irregular eating patterns, have contributed to this rise. The chapter explores the relationship between sleep, circadian rhythm, and diabetes mellitus, emphasizing the importance of quality sleep and stable circadian rhythm in regulating insulin sensitivity and glucose homeostasis. It presents clinical implications, including the potential impact of improving sleep quality and circadian rhythm on diabetes prevention and management, and suggests sleep interventions and lifestyle modifications for diabetic patients.

INTRODUCTION

Recently published data from the Indian Council of Medical Research–India Diabetes (ICMR–INDIAB) study reported the prevalence of lifestyle diseases in India as follows: Diabetes mellitus (DM) at 11.4%, prediabetes at 15.3%, hypertension (HTN) at 35.5%, generalized obesity at 28.6%, abdominal obesity at 39.5%, and dyslipidemia at 81.2%. Over the past six decades, there has been a significant increase in the prevalence of DM. While conventional risk factors for the development of diabetes are well-known, emerging evidence suggests that modern lifestyles, including increased screen time and use of electronic devices, shift work, 24/7 lifestyle, social jet lag, high-stress levels, sedentary lifestyle, caffeine and stimulant use, light pollution, and irregular eating patterns may also contribute to the disease. These lifestyle changes have allowed our behavioral cycles to become independent of natural patterns of sunlight, leading to a disturbance in our circadian rhythms as well as sleep deprivation.

Multiple studies have demonstrated that circadian misalignment leads to dyssynchrony between the functions of different organs and plays a pathological role in the development of systemic metabolic dysfunction. In this article, we aim to explore the relationship between sleep, circadian rhythm, and diabetes mellitus.

SLEEP AND CIRCADIAN RHYTHM

Sleep and Its Stages

In 1834, Robert MacNish described sleep as "the intermediate state between wakefulness and death; wakefulness being regarded as the active state of all the animal and intellectual functions, and death as that of their total suspension." Sleep and wakefulness are endogenous, recurring, behavioral states that reflect coordinated changes in the dynamic functional organization of the brain and that optimize physiology, behavior, and health. Homeostatic and circadian processes regulate the propensity for wakefulness and sleep.

The sleep process is divided into two main phases: Nonrapid eye movement (NREM) sleep and rapid eye movement (REM) sleep. These two types of sleep alternate in cycles throughout the night, with each cycle lasting around 90–120 minutes **(Table 1)**.

TABLE 1: Stages of sleep cycle.

Sleep stage	Description	Characteristics
NREM stage 1	Very light sleep	Transition from wake to sleep, drift in and out of sleep, awaken easily, hypnagogic jerk (sense of falling followed by sudden muscle contractions)
NREM stage 2	Relatively light but maintained sleep	Brain activity is relatively slower, breathing and heart rate slowed and maintained sleep
NREM stage 3	Deep sleep (slow wave sleep)	Lower brain activity, high-awakening threshold, and restoration of body
REM	Rapid eye movement sleep	Very active brain activity, dreams, and paralyzed body

(NREM: nonrapid eye movement; REM: rapid eye movement)

Recently, there has been a lot of focus on sleep research and sleep medicine, aimed at unraveling the intricacies of sleep biology and its effects on human health and disease states. The three key elements of good quality sleep are:

- Depth—sleep is deep enough to be restorative
- Duration—length of the sleep
- Continuity—sleep without fragmentation

Circadian Rhythm and Its Role in Regulating Various Physiological Processes

Our sleep and wake patterns are not just influenced by fatigue, but also by our innate rhythms. These rhythms, known as circadian rhythms, control the 24-hour changes in our physiology and behavior, including body temperature, blood pressure, hormone levels, mood, cognitive ability, and even physical performance. Franz Halberg coined the term "circadian" in 1959 to emphasize the self-sustaining nature of biological clocks. The term "circadian" comes from the Latin words *circa* = "about" and *dies* = "day." In 2017, Michael Rosbash, Jeffrey Hall, and Michael Young were awarded the Nobel Prize in Physiology or Medicine for their discoveries of the molecular mechanisms that control circadian rhythms. Their studies on the fruit fly (*Drosophila melanogaster*) led to these breakthroughs.

The production of melatonin, often referred to as "sleep hormone," is primarily influenced by the light-dark cycle, and it is synthesized and released by the pineal gland. The release of melatonin follows a distinct pattern, with levels rising in the evening as darkness sets in and reaching their peak during the night. This increase in melatonin secretion in response to darkness is a signal to the body that it is night-time, promoting feelings of drowsiness and readiness for sleep. Melatonin production rising in the evening coincides with a decline in core body temperature. During sleep, both melatonin levels and core body temperature remain elevated, reflecting the body's preparation for restorative rest. As morning approaches and external light increases, melatonin production decreases, signaling the body to wake up, while core body temperature rises, contributing to feelings of alertness during the day.

The circadian clock anticipates and adapts our physiology to the different phases of the day. Cortisol levels follow a circadian rhythm that is influenced by sleep. In normal physiology, cortisol levels are lower at the beginning of sleep and increase toward the end of the sleep period, reaching their peak just before waking up. This rhythm is closely associated with the sleep-wake cycle. Cortisol plays a central role in the circadian system and impacts almost every tissue and organ in the body.

Central and Peripheral Clocks in Mammals

In mammals, including humans, the circadian timing system is composed of both central and peripheral clocks. They are organized in a hierarchical manner and they work in synchrony in order to regulate various physiologic processes and behaviors.

- *The central clock*: The master pacemaker of the circadian system is the central clock, which is located in the hypothalamus of the brain and known as the suprachiasmatic nucleus (SCN). The SCN receives direct input from specialized light-sensitive cells in the eyes, enabling it to detect changes in light and darkness. This information helps the SCN synchronize the body's internal rhythms with the external day-night cycle, a process known as entrainment. The SCN generates a rhythmic electrical and hormonal output that impacts other areas of the brain and the body as a whole. It controls a range of bodily functions, such as the sleep-wake cycle, hormone production, body temperature, and metabolism.
- *The peripheral clock*: Peripheral clocks are located in various tissues, producing local rhythms that are mainly reset by feeding. Circadian clocks within the adrenal cortex contribute to diurnal variations in cortisol release by modulating sensitivity to adrenocorticotropic hormone (ACTH). Similarly, the beta cell circadian clock appears to be critical for insulin secretion. Additionally, circadian clocks within target tissues (such as adipose tissue, liver, and skeletal muscle) may modulate sensitivity to endocrine factors in a time-of-day-dependent manner.

HOW DO SLEEP AND CIRCADIAN RHYTHM DISRUPTION CONTRIBUTE TO TYPE 2 DIABETES MELLITUS?

- *Role of sleep deprivation in type 2 diabetes mellitus (T2DM)* **(Box 1)**: Sleep is controlled by the circadian process and the homeostatic S factor, which accumulates during sleep deprivation. The identity of the homeostatic factor is unclear, but adenosine is a well-studied somnogen. Sleep is promoted by adenosine receptors, and wakefulness is promoted by adenosine antagonists, like caffeine. However, adenosine and other somnogens are not the only factors that promote sleep. Recent evidence suggests that the S factor may be encoded by the accumulation of neuronal oxidative stress.

  The consequences of S factor accumulation can be seen by considering the effects of adenosine and reactive oxygen species (ROS) on metabolism. Both disrupt autonomic nervous system balance, resulting in relative sympathetic dominance and lower vagal tone. This imbalance has been shown to affect metabolic function, including increasing the sensitivity of adrenal glands to ACTH before sleep and elevating evening cortisol levels. Cortisol increases neuronal stress by generating more mitochondrial reactive oxygen species. Neural circuits promoting wakefulness may also drive cortisol release and sympathovagal imbalance.

  These shifts in autonomic activity and cortisol release have widespread impacts across the body, affecting immunity, appetite, and metabolism. Roden and Shulman, in their integrative model of T2DM, have described the influence of upregulation of hypothalamic-pituitary-adrenal (HPA) axes and sympathetic dominance on carbohydrate metabolism.

  Sympathetic nervous system (SNS) dominance and cortisol drive lipolysis. Elevated cortisol levels reduce insulin sensitivity, reducing inhibition of lipolysis. Lipolysis releases nonesterified fatty acids (NEFA), which are converted into fatty acyl-CoA to produce triacylglycerol (TAG) in the muscle and liver. The build-up of ectopic fat in the liver and muscle may cause other complications, such as nonalcoholic fatty liver disease, which is also linked to sleep deprivation. When synthesizing TAG, diacylglycerol (DAG) is produced, which activates protein kinase C epsilon (PKCε) in hepatocytes or PKCε/PKCθ in myocytes to inhibit insulin signaling. This effect is compounded by the cortisol-induced reduction in insulin sensitivity at these cells. This reduction in insulin sensitivity in the myocytes reduces glucose transporter type 4 (GLUT4) insertion and, hence, glucose uptake in muscle, and increasing glucose levels. In the liver, the reduced insulin sensitivity and increased levels of acetyl-CoA drive gluconeogenesis. Normally, elevated glucose levels drive insulin release in the pancreas, but the relative increase in SNS activity and cortisol inhibits this response. Therefore, over long periods of time, glucolipotoxicity impairs β-cell function. The autonomic imbalance and cortisol can also directly drive inverse processes to insulin, such as increasing hepatic gluconeogenesis and reducing glucose uptake via GLUT4 at adipose tissue and muscle, also contributing to T2DM. However, the effects of S factor accumulation likely go beyond cortisol and autonomic activity, with observed changes in other metabolic hormones, such as leptin.
- *Role of circadian misalignment in T2DM* **(Box 2)**: Circadian misalignment is a key factor in the development of T2DM. The circadian rhythm is driven

BOX 1: Role of sleep deprivation in T2DM.

Sleep regulation factors:
- Sleep is controlled by circadian rhythm and the homeostatic S factor
- S factor accumulates during sleep deprivation
- Adenosine is a well-studied somnogen
- Adenosine receptors promote sleep, while adenosine antagonists like caffeine promote wakefulness
- Recent evidence suggests S factor may involve neuronal oxidative stress

Autonomic nervous system and cortisol:
- Adenosine disruption and oxidative stress imbalance the autonomic nervous system—sympathetic dominance and lower vagal tone result
- Imbalance affects metabolic function
- Elevated cortisol levels due to stress and disruption

Metabolic impacts:
- Sympathetic dominance and cortisol drive lipolysis
- Elevated cortisol reduces insulin sensitivity
- Lipolysis releases nonesterified fatty acids (NEFA) converted into triacylglycerol (TAG)
- Ectopic fat accumulation in the liver and muscle can lead to complications
- Reduced insulin sensitivity in myocytes reduces glucose uptake
- The liver's reduced insulin sensitivity drives gluconeogenesis
- Glucose regulation is impaired by autonomic imbalance and cortisol
- Long-term effects contribute to β-cell dysfunction and T2DM

Other metabolic hormones:
- S factor accumulation affects other metabolic hormones, such as leptin

BOX 2: Role of circadian misalignment in T2DM.

Circadian rhythm and T2DM:

- Circadian misalignment is linked to the development of T2DM.
- Core clock genes (CLOCK, BMAL1, PER, and CRY) drive the 24-hour circadian rhythm.
- The hypothalamic suprachiasmatic nucleus (SCN) is the master clock, synchronizing peripheral clocks.
- Disruptions to circadian rhythm affect insulin sensitivity, increasing T2DM risk.
- Polymorphisms in clock genes contribute to T2DM risk.

Effects of circadian misalignment:

- Circadian misalignment causes insulin resistance, independent of sleep deprivation.
- Food intake timing influences T2DM risk by affecting metabolic efficiency.
- Desynchrony between central and peripheral clocks contributes to T2DM.

Synchrony and impact on metabolism:

- Alignment of light and other cues maintains synchrony between central and peripheral clocks.
- Central and peripheral clock desynchrony impairs metabolic processes like cortisol release.
- Organ activity follows circadian patterns; misalignment impairs metabolic function.
- Peripheral desynchrony leads to ectopic lipid accumulation, elevated glucose, and TAG.
- Prolonged effects can lead to glucolipotoxicity and β-cell dysfunction.

(CRY: cryptochrome; PER: period; TAG: triacylglycerol; T2DM: type 2 diabetes mellitus)

by 4 core clock genes that cycle every 24 hours—CLOCK, brain and muscle arnt-like protein 1 (BMAL1), period (PER), and cryptochrome (CRY). The master clock is located in the hypothalamic SCN and synchronizes clocks in other areas of the body, including peripheral organs. Disruptions to our circadian rhythm can affect insulin sensitivity, increasing the risk of T2DM. Large-scale studies have shown that polymorphisms in clock genes can increase the risk of T2DM. Additionally, experiments show that circadian misalignment alone can cause insulin resistance, independent of sleep deprivation. The timing of food intake can also contribute to T2DM, with constant exposure to nutrients reducing our ability to metabolize food efficiently.

Desynchrony between peripheral clocks regulating energy metabolism and the central clock regulating behavior and eating can also contribute to T2DM. Alignment of light and other zeitgebers is necessary to maintain synchrony between central and peripheral clocks. When synchrony is maintained, the circadian rhythm of both the central SCN and peripheral clocks are in-phase. However, if our behavioral cycles do not align with external light cycles, the amplitude of SCN circadian oscillations is lower, which impairs the SCN-mediated anticipatory metabolic processes, such as cortisol and growth hormone release. This reduction in central rhythm amplitude, along with the mismatch in behavioral and external light cycles, results in desynchrony not only between the SCN and peripheral clocks but also between the peripheral clocks.

Key metabolic organs undergo constant fluxes in metabolites, with different processes being favored at different times. This means that misalignment across the activity of the organs, due to peripheral desynchrony between the circadian clocks, can impair metabolic function resulting in ectopic lipid accumulation, as well as elevated levels of plasma glucose and TAG. Over longer periods of time, this can lead to glucolipotoxicity, impairing β-cell function. Further research is needed to clarify the mechanisms behind these phenomena.

CLINICAL IMPLICATIONS

The potential impact of improving sleep quality and circadian rhythm on diabetes prevention and management includes:

- *Sleep plays a crucial role in regulating insulin sensitivity*: To maintain overall health and well-being, it is suggested that adults get at least seven hours of sleep each night. Studies show a link between lack of sleep and insulin resistance. This is caused by inflammatory markers like C-reactive protein (CRP) and serum amyloid A (SAA). Other markers such as glucagon-like peptide-1 (GLP-1) and NEFA metabolism may also be involved. Proper sleep is important for metabolic health and preventing T2DM. Sleep loss is a modifiable risk factor that can decrease the prevalence of metabolic complications.
- *Maintaining a stable circadian rhythm helps in regulating glucose homeostasis*: For almost 50 years, it has been known that glucose tolerance follows a daily rhythm in humans. Comparing glucose intake at different times of day leads to higher glucose levels in the evening than in the morning. The causes of this decreased glucose tolerance may include lower insulin sensitivity, excessive glucose production in the liver, and/or reduced beta-cell function. Studies in healthy humans have shown that insulin sensitivity and beta-cell function are lower at dinner than at breakfast. The role of hepatic glucose production in the diurnal regulation of glucose homeostasis in normal humans is

still unclear. Nonetheless, evidence has shown a clear daily rhythm of liver glucose production in patients with T2DM that leads to morning hyperglycemia (dawn phenomenon). Higher glucose production before breakfast could be due to a long overnight fast and the resulting surge of counterregulatory hormones (e.g., cortisol, growth hormones, and norepinephrine) or a circadian modulation of hepatic glucose production, as suggested by studies in rodents.

- *Sleep is crucial for the regulation of various hormones, including cortisol, melatonin, and growth hormones, all of which have an impact on metabolism and glucose regulation*: Growth hormone levels increase during sleep, particularly during slow-wave sleep (SWS). Patients with posttraumatic stress disorder and disturbed sleep exhibit lower night-time growth hormone plasma levels. Melatonin plays an important role in regulating human sleep. Administration of sustained-release or transdermal formulation melatonin reduces sleep latency, increases total sleep time, and improves sleep maintenance. Cortisol levels decrease during SWS, and intravenous infusion of cortisol is known to increase SWS and decrease REM sleep by suppressing corticotropin-releasing hormone (CRH). Leptin levels were increased during the biological night and peaked during the biological morning in one study, but another study reported no fluctuations in leptin levels according to circadian rhythms.
- *Sleep influences hunger and appetite-regulating hormones, such as leptin and ghrelin*: Disruptions in sleep patterns have been found to increase energy intake, particularly from snacking on high-fat and high-carbohydrate foods. There appears to be a reciprocal relationship between sleep and weight loss, and although studies have used different methods and measures, sleep deprivation negatively affects the neuroendocrine appetite control system, leading to alterations in metabolic rate and hindering weight maintenance and loss efforts.
- *Short sleep is associated with diabetes: People with* short sleep duration have a 20–30% higher risk of T2DM, compared to people who get sufficient sleep. Long sleepers are also at risk.
- Rotating night shift work has been linked to obesity, metabolic syndrome, glucose dysregulation, and T2DM.
- Pan and colleagues evaluated the association between rotating night shift work and T2DM in two US women cohorts. They followed 69,269 women aged 42–67 in [Nurses' Health Study-I (NHS I), 1988–2008], and 107,915 women aged 25–42 in NHS-II (1989–2007) without diabetes, cardiovascular disease, and cancer at baseline. In both cohorts, the duration of shift work was associated with an increased risk of T2DM, with the risk increasing as the duration of shift work increased. Further adjustment for body mass index weakened the association. Our results suggest that screening and intervention strategies are necessary to prevent diabetes in rotating night shift workers.
- *Prevention of gestational diabetes mellitus (GDM)*: Studies that look at sleep duration and quality have found that both short and poor sleep are independently associated with an increased risk of GDM. However, this relationship is affected by body mass index (BMI), as both short and long sleep duration are associated with the risk of GDM only in nonobese women.

The sleep interventions and lifestyle modifications for diabetic patients include:

- *Sleep hygiene*: Practices and habits that are necessary to have good night-time sleep quality and full daytime alertness.
- *Maintain a regular sleep schedule*:
  - Go to bed and get up around the same time every day (even on weekends and vacations).
  - Limit naps close to bedtime, early afternoon naps may be better.
- *Sleep environment*:
  - Bedrooms should be quiet, dark, relaxing, and comfortable with cool temperatures.
  - Eliminate light from electronic devices, lamps, etc.
  - Blackout curtains, eye shades, ear plugs, white noise machines, etc., may be used to make the environment relaxing and conducive.
- *Presleep routine*: Relaxing prebedtime routine to help wind down:
  - Warm bath/shower (thermophysiological cascade)
  - Quiet activities (reading and music)
  - Low lights
  - Avoid electronic devices and short-wavelength ("blue") light before bed (change settings, and brightness on devices).
  - Try to avoid emotionally upsetting conversations and activities before attempting to sleep (news and social media).
  - Limit other stimulating activities—caffeine, nicotine, alcohol, fatty or fried meals, spicy dishes, and carbonated drinks.
- *Adequate daytime light exposure*: Together with limited nighttime light exposure, sufficient daytime light helps maintain proper expression and timing of the circadian system and sleep-wake cycle regulation.
- *Exercise*: Even 10 minutes of aerobic exercise (e.g., walking or cycling) can improve nighttime sleep quality.

The possible interventions to correct abnormal circadian rhythms include:

- *Light therapy*: Controlled exposure to natural or artificial light, especially in the morning, can help reset the circadian clock. Studies have shown that light therapy can improve sleep quality, circadian alignment, and insulin sensitivity. For individuals with diabetes, regularly exposing oneself to bright light in the morning may help regulate their circadian rhythms.
- *Behavioral therapy*: Cognitive-behavioral therapy for insomnia (CBT-I) and other behavioral interventions can improve sleep quality and promote better circadian alignment. These therapies address sleep hygiene, relaxation techniques, and cognitive strategies to enhance sleep duration and quality.
- *Melatonin supplementation*: Some studies have suggested that taking melatonin supplements may improve insulin sensitivity and glucose control in diabetics.
- *Meal timing and diet*: Aligning meal timing with the body's natural circadian rhythms may optimize metabolic processes. Strategies such as time-restricted eating (TRE), where food is consumed within a specific window each day, have shown potential benefits for insulin sensitivity and glucose regulation.
- *Medication management*: Some medications used to treat diabetes, such as metformin, may affect circadian rhythms. Researchers are exploring whether adjusting the timing of medication administration can optimize their impact on metabolic processes.
- *Mindfulness and relaxation techniques*: Practicing mindfulness, meditation, and relaxation exercises can help reduce stress and promote better sleep, ultimately contributing to improved circadian rhythms.

FUTURE DIRECTIONS AND RESEARCH GAPS

- Further investigation is needed to understand the biological mechanisms connecting sleep disruption, circadian rhythm disturbances, and diabetes. It is crucial to comprehend the molecular and cellular pathways that regulate glucose metabolism and insulin sensitivity in response to sleep and circadian cues.
- More studies aim to investigate how an individual's chronotype (natural preference for morning or night) affects their susceptibility to diabetes. Researchers should explore how chronotype influences the development and management of the disease.
- Studies aim to create interventions and treatment strategies that are specifically targeted toward improving sleep quality and circadian rhythms, with the ultimate goal of enhancing glucose metabolism and insulin sensitivity in individuals with diabetes, or those who are at risk of developing the condition.
- Further studies can explore the link between sleep deprivation and inflammatory markers to establish a cause-and-effect relationship. This will enable us to stress the significance of sufficient sleep to our patients and enhance their management.
- We need future studies to investigate the effects of sleep and circadian rhythm disruptions on gestational diabetes mellitus and aim to explore interventions that can mitigate these effects.
- Further research should focus on determining the most effective sleep patterns that facilitate and maintain weight loss in overweight and obese individuals while optimizing hormonal and metabolic functions.
- We require studies that aim to evaluate the potential impacts of sleep and circadian rhythm disturbances on public health, particularly in relation to diabetes. The focus is on identifying prevention strategies and relevant healthcare policies that can help mitigate these effects.

CONCLUSION

In conclusion, the intricate relationship between sleep, circadian rhythm, and diabetes mellitus has emerged as a pivotal area of research and clinical consideration. The rising prevalence of lifestyle-related diseases, including diabetes, necessitates a comprehensive understanding of the multifaceted influences of modern living on our biological rhythms. As elucidated in this article, sleep and circadian rhythm disruptions can significantly impact glucose metabolism, insulin sensitivity, and overall metabolic health. The interplay between central and peripheral clocks, the role of key hormones such as melatonin and cortisol, and the effects of sleep deprivation on systemic functions underscore the importance of maintaining a harmonious sleep-wake cycle for diabetes prevention and management.

The integration of sleep and circadian rhythm optimization into diabetes care strategies holds immense potential for improving patient outcomes. Recognizing that sleep is a crucial modulator of insulin sensitivity, and that circadian misalignment can lead to metabolic dysregulation, emphasizes the need for tailored interventions that encompass lifestyle modifications, behavioral therapies, light exposure strategies, and even pharmacological approaches. As we navigate the complexities of modern living, it becomes evident that embracing the natural rhythms of our bodies can empower individuals to take charge of their metabolic health.

Efforts to bridge the research gaps highlighted in this article, such as the mechanisms linking sleep disruption, chronotype, and diabetes risk, and the development of personalized interventions, are imperative. By fostering interdisciplinary collaborations between sleep researchers, endocrinologists, and public health professionals, we can unravel the intricate web of interactions between sleep, circadian rhythms, and diabetes mellitus. Ultimately, a holistic approach that acknowledges the significance of sleep and circadian rhythm alignment has the potential to usher in a new era of diabetes care, enhancing overall well-being and paving the way for healthier, more balanced lives.

SUGGESTED READINGS

1. Anjana RM, Unnikrishnan R, Deepa M, Pradeepa R, Tandon N, Das AK, et al. Metabolic non-communicable disease health report of India: the ICMR-INDIAB national cross-sectional study (ICMR-INDIAB-17). Lancet Diabetes Endocrinol. 2023;11(7):474-89.
2. Rockville MD. (2012). Arousal and Regulatory Systems: Workshop Proceedings. [online]. Available from https://www.nimh.nih.gov/research/research-funded-by-nimh/rdoc/arousal-and-regulatory-systems-workshop-proceedings [Last accessed December, 2023].
3. Chandrashekaran MK. Biological rhythms research: A personal account. J Biosci. 1998;23(5):545-55.
4. Foster RG. Sleep, circadian rhythms and health. Interface Focus. 2020;10(3):20190098.
5. Ferrie JE, Kivimäki M, Akbaraly TN, Tabak A, Abell J, Davey Smith G, et al. Change in Sleep Duration and Type 2 Diabetes: The Whitehall II Study. Diabetes Care. 2015;38(8):1462-72.
6. Cagnacci A, Elliott JA, Yen SS. Melatonin: a major regulator of the circadian rhythm of core temperature in humans. J Clin Endocrinol Metab. 1992;75(2):447-52.
7. Scher A, Hall WA, Zaidman-Zait A, Weinberg J. Sleep quality, cortisol levels, and behavioral regulation in toddlers. Dev Psychobiol. 2010;52(1):44-53.
8. Parameswaran G, Ray DW. Sleep, circadian rhythms, and type 2 diabetes mellitus. Clin Endocrinol (Oxf). 2021;96(1):12-20.
9. Singh T, Ahmed TH, Mohamed N, Elhaj MS, Mohammed Z, Paulsingh CN, et al. Does Insufficient Sleep Increase the Risk of Developing Insulin Resistance: A Systematic Review. Cureus. 2022;14(3):e23501.
10. Qian J, Scheer FAJL. Circadian System and Glucose Metabolism: Implications for Physiology and Disease. Trends Endocrinol Metab. 2016;27(5):282-93.
11. Papatriantafyllou E, Efthymiou D, Zoumbaneas E, Popescu CA, Vassilopoulou E. Sleep Deprivation: Effects on Weight Loss and Weight Loss Maintenance. Nutrients. 2022;14(8):1549.
12. Pan A, Schernhammer ES, Sun Qi, Hu FB. Rotating night shift work and risk of type 2 diabetes: two prospective cohort studies in women. PLoS Med. 2011;8(12):e1001141.
13. Facco FL, Grobman WA, Reid KJ, Parker CB, Hunter SM, Silver RM, et al. Objectively measured short sleep duration and later sleep midpoint in pregnancy are associated with a higher risk of gestational diabetes. Am J Obstet Gynecol. 2017;217(4):447.e1-13.

25

CHAPTER

Diabetic Cheiroarthropathy

Arun Kumar Kedia, Harshpreet Singh Tuteja

ABSTRACT

Diabetic cheiroarthropathy is a well-known and relatively common complication among patients with diabetes mellitus (DM) affecting nearly two-thirds of patients. It is characterized by limited mobility of the hand joints and sometimes manifests in legs, thickening of the skin, and flexion contractures. It has also been reported in over 50% of cases of type 1 DM patients. It is usually a clinical diagnosis and early diagnosis can prevent many major complications. Treatment involves reassurance, physiotherapy, occupational therapy, and medical management.

INTRODUCTION

Diabetic cheiroarthropathy, also known as the limited joint mobility syndrome (LJMS) or stiff hand syndrome, or diabetic sclerosis, occurs in long-standing diabetes. It has been reported in 15–60% of patients with type 1 diabetes mellitus (T1DM) and is also seen equally in type 2 diabetes mellitus (T2DM) patients. The prime pathology includes collagen cross-linking, blood vessel microangiopathy due to hyperglycemia, and the formation of advanced glycation end products (AGEs). It is characterized by a painless noninflammatory reduction in the mobility of feet, hands, and large joints. Early recognition is important because if diagnosed early it can be reversed and secondly it is a useful marker to detect early microvascular complications of diabetes. There is also a strong association between the prevalence of microvascular complications in T1DM and the severity of joint limitation.

PATHOPHYSIOLOGY

This syndrome has a multifactorial genesis with the interplay of various factors. The most important factor includes the proliferation of collagen in the skin, tendons, subcutaneous tissues, and muscles. There is simultaneously an alteration in collagen biochemistry leading to the stiffness of collagen fibers. There is a thickening of the capillary basement membrane leading to ischemia of tissues causing tissue fibrosis ultimately leading to waxy skin. The epidermis and dermis are microscopically deficient in normal skin architecture because of the ischemia. High oxidative stress levels seem to also play an important role. Hyperglycemia causes high levels of oxidative stress and the formation of AGEs. Increased production of reactive oxygen can initiate the inflammatory cascade, producing several cytokines and growth factors causing hyperglycemia-induced cellular damage. AGEs also form cross-links with skin collagen, tendons, and ligaments altering their biological structure and function. Collagen has a long half-life; therefore, the AGE cross links to collagen gradually accumulate in the skin, tendons, and ligaments and are considered to play an important role in the development of LJMS. Abnormalities of matrix metalloproteinases and their tissue inhibitors have also been demonstrated in diabetic fibroblast culture systems ex vivo which explain the pathophysiology.

Recent advances in research on peroxisome proliferator-activated receptor γ (PPAR-γ) better explain the pathogenesis of diabetic tendinopathy. Downregulation of PPAR-γ in diabetes has been found to limit vessel and nerve ingrowth, and can also affect neurogenesis. Hyperglycemia itself may lead to alterations in the redox environment, resulting in increased intracellular water and cellular edema. It also leads to a reduction in proteoglycans levels decreasing the synthesis or sulfation of glycosaminoglycans. Endogenous soluble RAGE (receptor for advanced glycation end products) isoforms found circulating in plasma and tissues are lower in vascular diseases and diabetes, suggesting a significant inverse correlation with vascular damage.

EPIDEMIOLOGY

The reported prevalence in diabetes mellitus (DM) apparently varies between 8 and 58%, depending on the different diabetes patients' cohorts and the applied definitions of LJMS. The prevalence of LJMS in subjects without DM is difficult to estimate and may vary between 4 and 26%. Epidemiological data found no clear gender or racial preferences in the development of LJMS in diabetes.

CLINICAL FEATURES

Patients present with subtle development of skin thickening of fingers which sometimes depicts as scleroderma. Typically, patients present with limitation of extension of the metacarpophalangeal, proximal interphalangeal, and distal interphalangeal joints, starting on the ulnar side and spreading radially.

Some patients develop progressive flexion contractures and stiffness of the hand joints which can be best elicited by prayer sign or table top sign. Incomplete approximation of one or more of the digits when the patient attempts to approximate the palmar surfaces of the proximal and distal interphalangeal joints with palms pressed together and the fingers abducted constitute a positive prayer sign **(Fig. 1)**. In table top sign, the patient is instructed to touch the table with the palmar surfaces of the hands. Failure of the patient to keep his/her palms and digits completely flat on the table is considered as the positive table top sign **(Fig. 2)**.

Another clinical manifestation is flexor tenosynovitis (trigger finger) described as a catching sensation or finger locking with pain in the affected finger occurring in 16–42% of cases. Dupuytren's contracture, resulting from thickening and fibrosis of plantar fascia may be seen in some cases in the early course of the disease.

Carpal tunnel syndrome (CTS) is also one of the complications occurring in 20% of cases resulting from median nerve entrapment resulting from connective tissue alteration. Classical clinical findings of CTS include Tinel's sign (tapping over the median nerve on the volar aspect of the wrist leads to pinpricking sensation over the course of the affected nerve).

Diabetic cheiroarthropathy may also lead to impaired mobility of the toes and foot joints. Charcot joint is a less common manifestation and occurs in <1% of cases. There may be contracture and thickening of the plantar fascia and the skin over the toes. Similar to CTS, tarsal tunnel syndrome may be in long-standing diabetes. The arches of the feet may be exaggerated and the patient may have difficulty in walking along with the risk of frequent falls. Certain parts of the feet may be exposed to high pressure like the plantar surfaces of the great toes and the heels, increasing the risk of ulceration. Deformities can occur with midtarsal collapse ("rocker bottom" feet), predisposing to ulceration and infection of the skin over desensate bony prominences. Diabetic osteolysis is characterized by resorption of the distal metatarsal and proximal phalanges of the feet, giving radiographs a characteristic "licked candy" appearance. Lumbar polyradiculopathy is characterized by pain, dysesthesias, and rapid atrophy of the proximal muscles of one or both thighs.

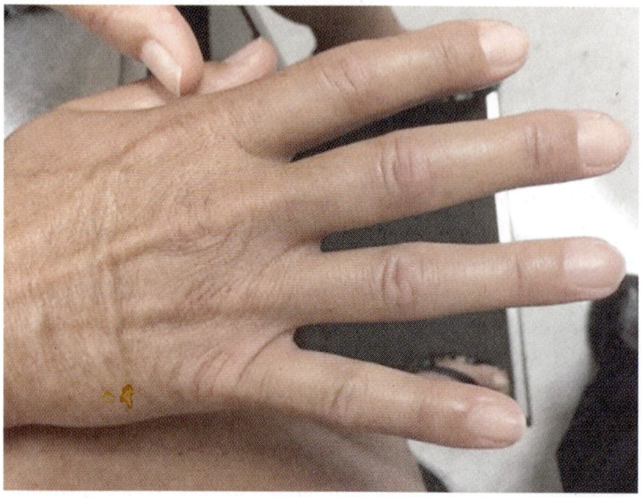

FIG. 1: Diabetic hand with tight, thick waxy skin, and incomplete extension.

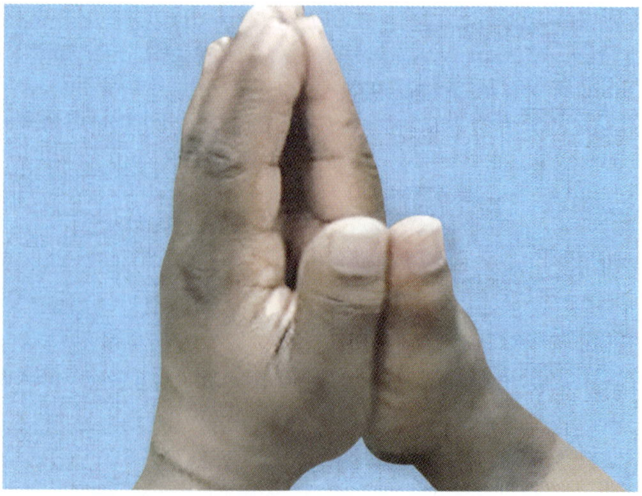

FIG. 2: Positive prayer sign.

CORRELATION WITH MICROVASCULAR COMPLICATIONS

Diabetic cheiroarthropathy has a direct correlation with microvascular complications of diabetes. Diabetic patients with diabetic cherioarthropathy have a higher risk of proliferative retinopathy, neuropathy, and nephropathy. Diabetic retinopathy is most commonly associated with it. Patients with LJMS have shown a greater prevalence of cataracts and retinopathy. Irrespective of glycemic control the presence of diabetic cherioarthropathy has been associated with a higher risk of albuminuria and males have higher rates of protienuria and hypertension. The presence of diabetic cheiroarthropathy warrants better control of the patient's glycemic status to prevent further deterioration of diabetes-related complications.

DIAGNOSIS

The diagnosis of diabetic cheiroarthropathy is essentially clinical. Various clinical signs, like prayer sign, table top sign, and Tinel's sign give a clue to the diagnosis. Role of imaging is increasing nowadays with ultrasound and MRI playing a significant role in the diagnosis of soft tissue disorders and multiple deformities. Sonography findings include thickening of the subcutaneous tissues and flexor tendon sheaths and MRI shows enhancement and thickening of the flexor tendon sheaths. In some cases where carpel tunnel syndrome is present, electromyography/nerve conduction velocity (EMG/NCV) testing can confirm the diagnosis.

TREATMENT

Prevention and strict glycemic control are important because limited joint mobility is directly correlated with the duration of diabetes and hyperglycemia. So, the first and foremost priority is to optimally control blood sugar levels with holistic interventions including dietary modifications, physical activity, and appropriate medication.

Once the patient develops clinical manifestations, physiotherapy plays an important role. Stretching exercises of the hand and foot not only improve joint mobility, they may alleviate pain also. In rare cases of persistent inflammation, use of nonsteroidal anti-inflammatory drugs (NSAIDs) and short course steroid shows some good results.

Many compounds are currently in study and can be divided into inhibitors and breakers of AGE. Inhibitors work as carbonyl-trapping agents and promote excretion or inhibit the uptake of iron and copper ions. Breakers are effective in delaying a range of diabetic complications including nephropathy, neuropathy, retinopathy, and vasculopathy in animal models of diabetes. Breakers include aminoguanidine, pyridoxamine, glucosamine, some angiotensin-converting enzyme inhibitors, aldose reductase inhibitors, genistein, and several natural derivatives (rutin, quercetin, hesperidin, and polyphenols).

New compounds which counteract the negative effects of AGEs may be part of future clinical trials resulting in greater control of AGE-related complications including tendon and ligament damage.

Nonpharmacological treatment modalities include:

- *Physical rehabilitation*: Improves joint motion
- *Manual techniques (soft tissue mobilization and friction massage)*:
  - Decreases spasm and edema
  - Increases range of motion
  - Break adhesions around joint structures
- *Acupuncture*: Target the nervous system inducing biophysical signals to allow for healing responses to occur
- *Heating*: Increases blood flow to the diseased area, increases tissue extensibility, and decreases pain
- *Electrical stimulation (alternating or pulsing, or combined)*: Controls pain and inhibits spasticity
- *Extracorporeal shock wave*: Increases cell proliferation and increases blood flow to joints.

CONCLUSION

Even though the incidence of diabetic cheiroarthropathy is high, it is often neglected. Early diagnosis is important not only to prevent deformities but also to warrant for microvascular complications. Majority of the conditions are treatable through physical rehabilitation and a good collaboration with a sound physiotherapist is essential to take care of the problems. Care of the musculoskeletal system of diabetic patients should be in routine clinical practice.

Bhalla et al. reported that some racial/ethnic minorities with type 2 diabetes mellitus (T2DM) were more prone to having proteinuric DKD rather than nonproteinuric DKD. Unnikrishnan et al. reported that the prevalence of overt nephropathy and microalbuminuria was 2.2 and 26.9%, respectively, among urban Asian Indians with T2DM.

PATHOPHYSIOLOGY OF HYPERGLYCEMIA IN DIABETIC KIDNEY DISEASE

The root problem of hyperglycemia in DKD occurs with following pathophysiology as mentioned in **Figures 1 and 2**:

- Hyperglycemia leads to hyperfiltration, which is followed by metabolic, hormonal, hemodynamic, inflammatory, and epigenetic changes.
- Oxidative stress and hypoxia play a vital role.
- All these precipitate to podocyte injury, mitochondrial distress, tissue death, glomerulosclerosis, and interstitial fibrosis.

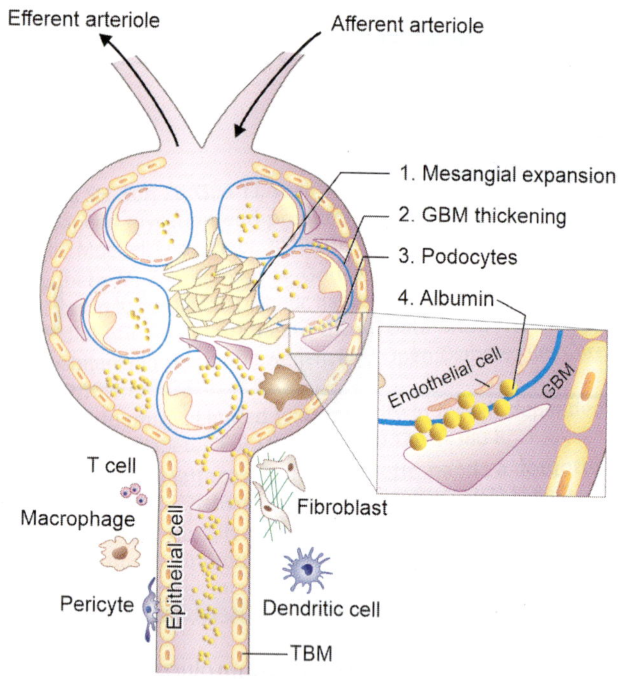

FIG. 2: Pathogenesis of diabetic kidney disease (DKD).
(DKD: diabetic kidney disease; GBM: glomerular basement membrane; TBM: thin basement membrane)

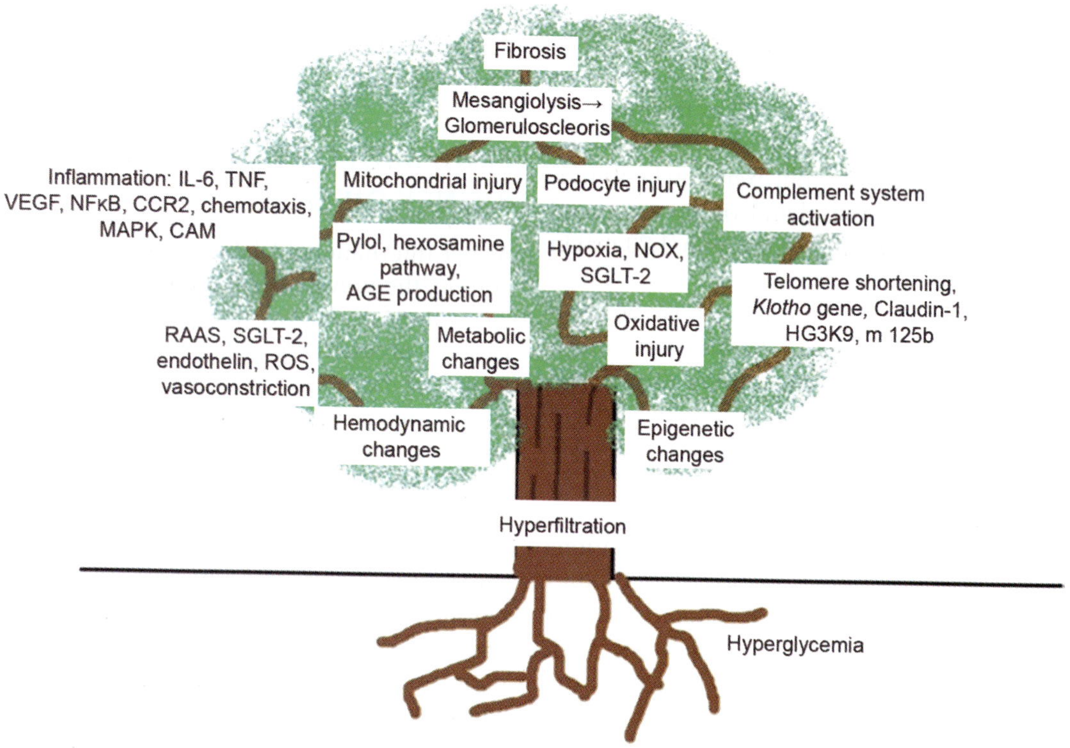

FIG. 1: Hyperglycemia leading to diabetic kidney disease (DKD).
(AGE: advanced glycation end product; CCR2: C chemokine receptor type 2; CAM: CaM kinase II; IL-6: interleukin 6; MAPK: mitogen-activated protein kinase; NFκB: nuclear factor-κB; NOX: NADPH-oxidases; RAAS: renin–angiotensin–aldosterone system; ROS: reactive oxygen species SGLT-2: sodium-glucose cotransporter-2; TNF: tumor necrosis factor; VEGF: vascular endothelial growth factor)

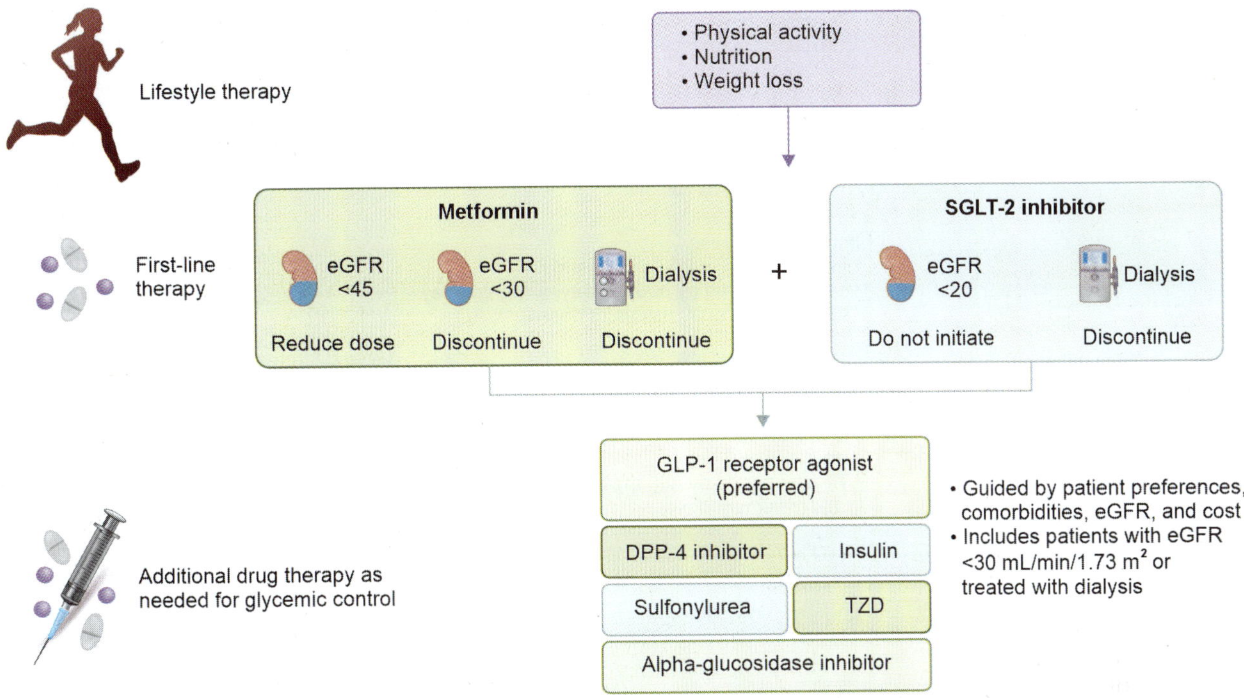

FIG. 3: Treatment algorithm for selecting glucose-lowering drugs for patients with T2DM and CKD.

Note: Kidney icon indicates estimated glomerular filtration rate (eGFR; mL/min/1.73 m^2); dialysis machine icon indicates dialysis.

(CKD: chronic kidney disease; DPP-4: dipeptidyl peptidase-4; GLP-1: glucagon-like peptide 1; SGLT-2: sodium-glucose cotransporter-2; T2DM: type 2 diabetes mellitus; TZD: thiazolidinedione)

Source: Adapted from KDIGO 2022 Clinical Practice Guideline for Diabetes Management in Chronic Kidney Disease. Kidney Int. 2022;102(5S):S1-S127.

Patients on Hemodialysis

The Kidney Disease Improving Global Outcomes (KDIGO) guidelines suggest that insulin, dipeptidyl peptidase 4 (DPP-4) inhibitors, thiazolidinediones, sulfonylureas, or alpha-glucosidase inhibitors may be used for glycemic control in patients on hemodialysis.

The kidneys play an important role in endogenous glucose production mostly during prolonged starvation periods. 80% of exogenous insulin does not go via first-pass metabolism in the liver. It is primarily cleared via renal metabolism. So, impaired renal function in patients with diabetes can result in decreased clearance of insulin and, consequently, prolonged exposure.

Impaired renal function in patients with diabetes can affect the pharmacokinetics of some insulin formulations including regular human insulin and insulin lispro. Insulin aspart and insulin detemir, however, have demonstrated unaffected pharmacokinetics. Published evidence indicates that insulin analogs may maintain their pharmacokinetic profiles in this patient population.

Pharmacokinetic properties of insulin degludec in subjects with varying degrees of renal function—normal, mild, moderate, or severe renal impairment—or ESRD undergoing hemodialysis were evaluated in 30 patients. The ultra-long pharmacokinetic properties of insulin degludec were preserved with no statistically significant differences in absorption or clearance, compared with subjects with normal renal function.

Patients on Peritoneal Dialysis

Choice of Therapy

Patients who were already on an oral agent with good glycemic control prior to starting peritoneal dialysis may continue oral agent, and in patients who develop diabetes after starting peritoneal dialysis, sulfonylurea is preferred. Metformin should not be used for patients on peritoneal dialysis because of an increased risk of lactic acidosis. Over time, many patients will require insulin.

Subcutaneous versus Intraperitoneal Insulin

We and most nephrologists prefer subcutaneous insulin for patients on continuous ambulatory peritoneal dialysis (CAPD) or continuous cycler peritoneal dialysis. Intraperitoneal insulin is not used, as it often does not adequately control blood sugar. Another potential

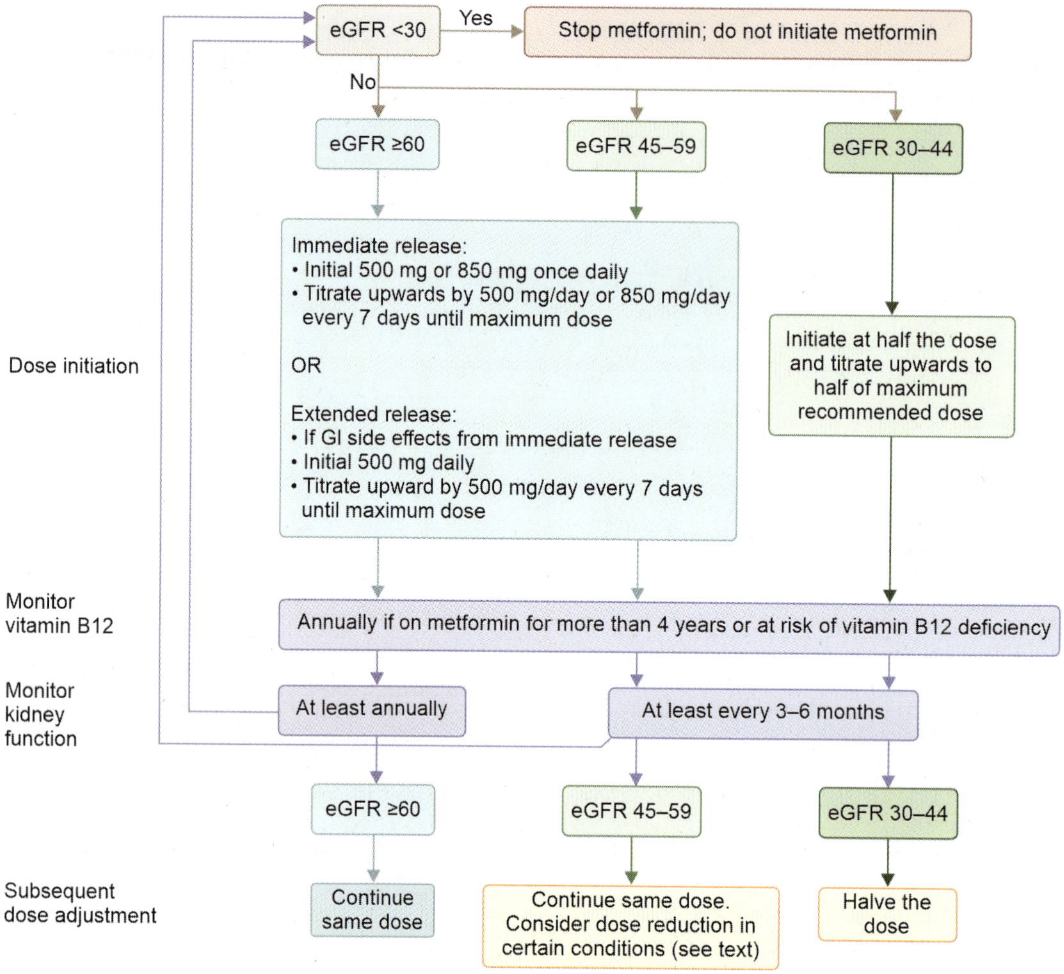

FLOWCHART 1: Suggested approach in dosing metformin based on the level of kidney function.

(eGFR: estimated glomerular filtration rate)

Source: Adapted from KDIGO 2022 Clinical Practice Guideline for Diabetes Management in Chronic Kidney Disease. Kidney Int. 2022;102(5S):S1-S127.

TABLE 3: Patient factors influencing the selection of glucose-lowering drugs other than SGLT-2 inhibitors and metformin in type 2 diabetes mellitus and CKD.

	Practical provider guide to initiating SGLT-2 inhibitors in patients with type 2 diabetes mellitus and CKD		
	Assessment	**Intervention**	**Follow-up**
Patient selection	*Eligible patients*: • eGFR ≥ 20 mL/min/1.73 m^2 *High priority features*: • ACR ≥ 200 mg/g • Heart failure *Potential contraindications*: • Genital infection risk • Diabetic ketoacidosis • Foot ulcers • Immunosuppression	*SGLT-2 inhibitor with proven benefits*: • Canagliflozin 100 mg • Dapagliflozin 10 mg • Empagliflozin 10 mg *Education*: • Sick day protocol* • Perioperative care† • Foot care	• Assess adverse effects • Review knowledge • Anticipate an acute drop in eGFR, which is generally not a reason to stop the SGLT-2 inhibitor

Continued

Continued

Practical provider guide to initiating SGLT-2 inhibitors in patients with type 2 diabetes and CKD				
	Assessment		**Intervention**	**Follow-up**
Glycemia	Hypoglycemia risk: • Insulin or sulfonylurea • History of severe hypoglycemia • HbA1c at or below goal	If high	*Education*: • Hypoglycemia symptoms • Glycemia monitoring • Consider insulin/sulfonylurea dose reduction	• Ask about hypoglycemia • Reduce sulfonylurea or insulin if needed
Volume	Volume depletion risk: • Concurrent diuretic use • Tenuous volume status • History of AKI	If high	*Education*: Volume depletion symptoms consider diuretic dose reduction	• Re-assess volume • Reduce concomitant diuretic if needed

* *Sick day protocol (for illness or excessive exercise or alcohol intake)*: Temporarily withhold SGLT2i, keep drinking and eating (if possible), check blood glucose and blood ketone levels more often, and seek medical help early.

† *Periprocedural/perioperative care*: Inform patients about risk of diabetic ketoacidosis; withhold SGLT-2 inhibitor the day of day-stay procedures and limit fasting to minimum required; withhold SGLT-2 inhibitor at least 2 days in advance and the day of procedures/surgery requiring 1 or more days in hospital and/or bowel preparation (which may require increasing other glucose-lowering drugs during that time), measure both blood glucose and blood ketone levels on hospital admission (proceed with procedure/surgery if the patient is clinically well and ketones are <1.0 mmol/L), and restart SGLT-2 inhibitor after procedure/surgery only when eating and drinking normally.

(ACR: albumin-to-creatine ratio; AKI: acute kidney injury; eGFR: estimated glomerular filtration rate; HbA1c: glycated hemoglobin; SGLT-2: sodium-glucose cotransporter-2)

Source: Adapted from Zoungas S, de Boer IH. SGLT2 inhibitors in diabetic kidney disease. Clin J Am Soc Nephrol. 2021;16:631-33.

TABLE 4: Dosing for available GLP-1 RA and dose modification for CKD.

GLP-1 RA	Dose	CKD adjustment
Dulaglutide	0.75 and 1.5 mg once weekly	• No dosage adjustment • Use with eGFR > 15 mL/min/1.73 m^2
Exenatide	10 μg twice daily	Use with CrCl > 30 mL/min
Exenatide extended-release	2 mg once weekly	Use with CrCl > 30 mL/min
Liraglutide	0.6, 1.2, and 1.8 mg once daily	• No dosage adjustment • Limited data for severe CKD
Lixisenatide	10 and 20 μg once daily	• No dosage adjustment • Limited data for severe CKD
Semaglutide (injection)	0.5 and 1 mg once weekly	• No dosage adjustment • Limited data for severe CKD
Semaglutide (oral)	3, 7, or 14 mg daily	• No dosage adjustment • Limited data for severe CKD

(CKD: chronic kidney disease; CrCl: creatinine clearance; eGFR: estimated glomerular filtration rate; GLP-1 RA: glucagon-like peptide 1 receptor agonists)

Source: Adapted from KDIGO 2022 Clinical Practice Guideline for Diabetes Management in Chronic Kidney Disease. Kidney Int. 2022;102(5S):S1-S127.

concern is that the absorption of insulin may significantly vary among patients or may decline over time in a single individual due to acquired abnormalities in the peritoneal membrane.

Abnormal Variations in Peritoneal Kinetics

The selection of oral agents described above assumes that peritoneal transfer kinetics is relatively normal. Patients treated with CAPD who have uncontrolled hyperglycemia should undergo a peritoneal equilibration test. High transporters, who can have enormous glucose loads from rapid peritoneal glucose absorption, will usually benefit from transfer to nocturnal automated peritoneal dialysis.

CONCLUSION

There is paradigm shift in management of DKD. This chapter focuses on existing evidence including guidelines and recommendations that will assist clinicians to make informed choices while managing diabetic patients with CKD.

SUGGESTED READINGS

1. Levin A, Stevens PE, Bilous RW, Coresh J, De Francisco ALM, De Jong PE, et al. Kidney Disease: Improving Global Outcomes (KDIGO) CKD Work Group. KDIGO 2012 clinical practice guideline for the evaluation and management of chronic kidney disease. Kidney Int. Suppl. 2013;3(1):1-150.
2. de Boer IH, Caramori ML, Chan JCN, Heerspink HJL, Hurst C, Khunti K, et al. Executive summary of the 2020 KDIGO Diabetes Management in CKD Guideline: evidence-based advances in monitoring and treatment. Kidney Int. 2020;98(4):839-48.
3. International Diabetes Federation. (2021). IDF Diabetes Atlas, 10th edition. [online] Available from https://diabetesatlas.org/atlas/tenth-edition/ [Last accessed December 2023].
4. New JP, Middleton RJ, Klebe B, Farmer CKT, de Lusignan S, Stevens PE, et al. Assessing the prevalence, monitoring and management of chronic kidney disease in patients with diabetes compared with those without diabetes in general practice. Diabet Med. 2007;24(4):364-9.
5. Mohan V, Sandeep S, Deepa R, Shah B, Varghese C. Epidemiology of type 2 diabetes: Indian scenario. Indian J Med Res. 2007;125(3):217-30.
6. Liyanage T, Toyama T, Hockham C, Ninomiya T, Perkovic V, Woodward M, Fukagawa M, et al. Prevalence of chronic kidney disease in Asia: a systematic review and analysis. BMJ Glob Health. 2022;7(1):e007525.
7. Bhalla V, Zhao B, Azar KMJ, Wang EJ, Choi S, Wong EC. et al. Racial/ethnic differences in the prevalence of proteinuric and nonproteinuric diabetic kidney disease. Diabetes Care. 2013;36(5):1215-21.
8. Unnikrishnan RI, Rema M, Pradeepa R, Deepa M, Shanthirani CS, Deepa R, et al. Prevalence and risk factors of diabetic nephropathy in an urban South Indian population: the Chennai Urban Rural Epidemiology Study (CURES 45). Diabetes Care. 2007;30(8):2019-24.
9. Fu H, Liu S, Bastacky SI, Wang X, Tian XJ, Zhou D. Diabetic kidney diseases revisited: A new perspective for a new era. Mol Metab. 2019;30:250-63.
10. Ravikumar P, Bhansali A, Walia R, Shanmugasundar G, Ravikiran M. Alterations in HbA(1c) with advancing age in subjects with normal glucose tolerance: Chandigarh Urban Diabetes Study (CUDS). Diabet Med. 2011;28(5):590-4.
11. Fioretto P, Barzon I, Mauer M. Is diabetic nephropathy reversible? Diabetes Res Clin Pract. 2014;104(3):323-8.
12. Bin Rakhis SA Sr, Al Duwayhis NM, Aleid N, AlBarrak AN, Aloraini AA. Glycemic Control for Type 2 Diabetes Mellitus Patients: A Systematic Review. Cureus. 2022;14(6):e26180.
13. Yadav SCB. Glycemic control in diabetic kidney disease patients. Clinical Queries: Nephrology. 2012;1(2):111-4.
14. Kidney Disease: Improving Global Outcomes (KDIGO) Diabetes Work Group. KDIGO 2022 Clinical practice guideline for diabetes management in chronic kidney disease. Kidney Int. 2022;102(5S):S1-27.
15. Dozio E, Corradi V, Proglio M, Vianello E, Menicanti L, Rigolini R, et al. Usefulness of glycated albumin as a biomarker for glucose control and prognostic factor in chronic kidney disease patients on dialysis (CKD-G5D). Diabetes Res Clin Pract. 2018;140:9-17.
16. Konya J, Ng JM, Cox H, Cooke M, Lewis N, Bhandari S, et al. Use of complementary markers in assessing glycaemic control in people with diabetic kidney disease undergoing iron or erythropoietin treatment. Diabet Med. 2013;30(10):1250.
17. Chen CW, Drechsler C, Suntharalingam P, Karumanchi SA, Wanner C, Berg AH. High glycated albumin and mortality in persons with diabetes mellitus on hemodialysis. Clin Chem. 2017;63(2):477.
18. Selvin E, Rawlings AM, Grams M, Klein R, Sharrett AR, Steffes M. et al. Fructosamine and glycated albumin for risk stratification and prediction of incident diabetes and microvascular complications: a prospective cohort analysis of the Atherosclerosis Risk in Communities (ARIC) study. Lancet Diabetes Endocrinol. 2014;2(4):279.
19. Joubert M, Fourmy C, Henri P, Ficheux M, Lobbedez T, Reznik Y. Effectiveness of continuous glucose monitoring in dialysis patients with diabetes: the DIALYDIAB pilot study. Diabetes Res Clin Pract. 2015;107(3):348.
20. MacIsaac RJ, Ekinci EI, Jerums G. Progressive diabetic nephropathy. How useful is microalbuminuria?: contra. Kidney Int. 2014;86(1):50-7.
21. Diabetes Control and Complications Trial/Epidemiology of Diabetes Interventions and Complications Research Group.
22. Adler AI, Stevens RJ, Manley SE, Bilous RW, Cull CA, Holman RR, et al. Development and progression of nephropathy in type 2 diabetes: the United Kingdom Prospective Diabetes Study (UKPDS 64). Kidney Int. 2003;63(1):225-32.
23. Mann JFE, Ørsted DD, Brown-Frandsen K, Marso SP, Poulter NR, Rasmussen, et al. Liraglutide and renal outcomes in type 2 diabetes. N Engl J Med. 2017;377(9):839-48.
24. Marso SP, Bain SC, Consoli A, Eliaschewitz FG, Jódar E, Leiter LA, et al. Semaglutide and cardiovascular outcomes in patients with type 2 diabetes. N Engl J Med. 2016; 375(19):1834.
25. Gerstein HC, Colhoun HM, Dagenais GR, Diaz R, Lakshmanan M, Pais P, et al. Dulaglutide and cardiovascular outcomes in type 2 diabetes (REWIND): a double-blind, randomised placebo-controlled trial. Lancet. 2019;394(10193):121-30.
26. de Boer IH, Khunti K, Sadusky T, Tuttle KR, Neumiller JJ, Rhee CM, et al. Diabetes management in chronic kidney disease: A consensus report by the American Diabetes Association (ADA) and Kidney Disease: Improving Global Outcomes (KDIGO). Diabetes Care. 2022;45(12):3075-90.
27. Del Prato S, Tiengo A. The importance of first-phase insulin secretion: implications for the therapy of type 2 diabetes mellitus. Diabetes Metab Res Rev. 2001;17(3):164-74.
28. National Kidney Foundation. KDOQI clinical practice guidelines for chronic kidney disease: evaluation, classification and stratification. Am J Kidney Dis. 2002;39(2 Suppl 1):S1-266.
29. Snyder RW, Berns JS. Use of insulin and oral hypoglycemic medications in patients with diabetes mellitus and advanced kidney disease. Semin Dial. 2004;17(5):365-70.
30. Holmes G, Galitz L, Hu P, Lyness W. Pharmacokinetics of insulin aspart in obesity, renal impairment, or hepatic impairment. Br J Clin Pharmacol. 2005;60(5):469-76.
31. Jacobsen LV, Popescu G, Plum A. Pharmacokinetics of insulin detemir in subjects with renal or hepatic impairment. Diabetologia. 2002;45(suppl 1):A259.
32. Kiss I, Arold G, Roepstorff C, Bøttcher SG, Klim S, Haahr H, et al. Insulin degludec: pharmacokinetics in patients with renal impairment. Clin Pharmacokinet. 2014;53(2):175-83.
33. Wijewickrama P, Williams J, Bain S, Dasgupta I, Chowdhury TA, Wahba M, et al. Narrative review of glycemic management in people with diabetes on peritoneal dialysis. Kidney Int Rep. 2023;8(4):700.
34. Selgas R, Diez JJ, Muñoz J, Miranda B, de Alvaro F, Rodriguez JC, et al. Comparative study of two different routes for insulin administration in CAPD diabetic patients. A multicenter study. Adv Perit Dial. 1989;5:181.
35. Scavini M, Pincelli A, Petrella G, Galimberti G, Zager PG, Torri M, Pozza G, et al. Intraperitoneal insulin absorption after long-term intraperitoneal insulin therapy. Diabetes Care. 1995;18:56.

27

CHAPTER

Common Mistakes in Insulin Therapy

Nirmalya Roy, Mainak Mandal, Abhishek Chanda

ABSTRACT

Insulin therapy is a fundamental component of diabetes mellitus (DM) management, impacting millions of individuals across the globe. Despite its proven efficacy, the successful implementation of this life-saving treatment is hindered by a myriad of errors and challenges. Addressing insulin therapy errors is essential for patient well-being. Medication errors and preventable mishaps in insulin use can happen at any stage, from prescription to administration, and must be avoided to ensure treatment success.

INTRODUCTION

A substantial number of individuals with diabetes mellitus (DM) rely on insulin therapy to achieve satisfactory glycemic control and reduce the risk of complications. According to the United Kingdom Prospective Diabetes Study (UKPDS) study, approximately 50% of pancreatic beta cells are depleted at the time of type 2 diabetes mellitus (T2DM) diagnosis, resulting in insulin deficiency.

India is home to a staggering 72.9 million people living with diabetes. The Indian Council of Medical Research-India Diabetes (ICMR-INDIAB) study reveals that a significant percentage of these patients require insulin for treatment. Regardless of glycated hemoglobin (HbA1c) levels, insulin remains an unmatched tool for reducing HbA1c, yet a considerable portion of diabetes patients on insulin therapy struggle to attain their desired glycemic targets.

Therefore, addressing errors in insulin therapy remains a crucial and correctable factor for many patients. Medication errors, which encompass any preventable events leading to inappropriate medication use or patient harm while under the care of healthcare professionals, patients, or consumers, must be avoided in individuals on insulin treatment to ensure therapeutic success. These errors can potentially occur at any stage of the insulin administration process, from prescription to actual administration.

PRESCRIPTION ERROR

Challenge

The prevalence of errors stemming from illegible prescriptions and insufficient instructions on storage and administration techniques, both for patients and healthcare personnel, is a significant concern. Additionally, the use of "U" as an abbreviation for "unit" in prescriptions is often misinterpreted as the numeral "4," and the inclusion of "BD" in prescriptions can lead to confusion.

Solution

Addressing this issue necessitates a multifaceted approach. It is imperative to provide comprehensive explanations and counselling to patients and their families. Equally important is the avoidance of improper or potentially misleading abbreviations when drafting prescriptions.

IMPROPER STORAGE

Challenge

Managing the storage of insulin devices such as insulin pens, vials, and unused cartridges can be challenging. Ideally, these items should be stored in a refrigerator

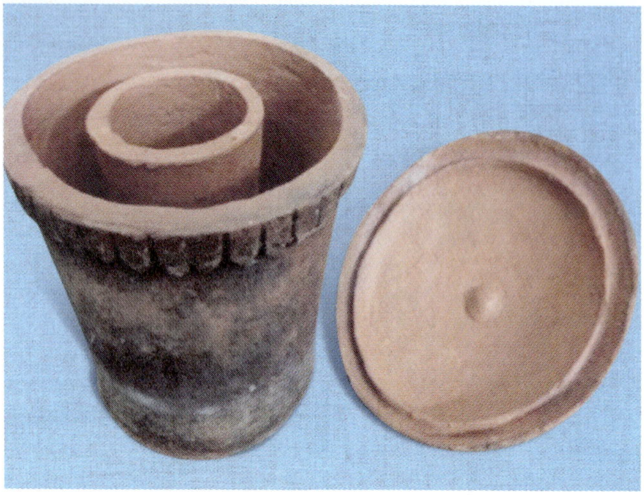

FIG. 1: Zeer pot.

between 2 and 8°C to ensure their effectiveness until their expiration date; however, if insulin is exposed to temperatures below 2°C or above 8°C, it can only be used safely for up to 4 weeks. This poses a significant problem for individuals with diabetes mellitus from low socioeconomic backgrounds who lack access to refrigeration in our country.

Solution

To address this issue, it is crucial to maintain insulin within the recommended temperature range and prevent it from freezing. For those with limited access to refrigeration due to socioeconomic constraints, an effective solution is to use a Zeer pot **(Fig. 1)** for insulin storage. This pot consists of an outer chamber filled with water or wet sand and an inner chamber designed for insulin storage. This simple yet effective method ensures that insulin remains properly stored, even in the absence of a refrigerator.

STORAGE OF INSULIN DURING TRAVEL

Challenge

Managing insulin storage while traveling poses a significant concern, particularly for individuals who require insulin and are frequent travelers.

Solution

When traveling, it is essential to store insulin in insulated containers or bags. If the anticipated temperature exceeds 30°C, consider using ice packs to maintain the appropriate temperature. For air travel, it is advisable to place insulin in cabin baggage to protect it from unfavorable conditions and freezing.

Additionally, for individuals traveling to regions with significant time zone differences, there are dosage adjustments to consider. When traveling eastward, where the day shortens, a reduction in the insulin dose may be necessary. Conversely, when traveling westward, where the day lengthens, an increase in the insulin dose may be warranted to accommodate the changing time zones.

DOSING ERRORS

Challenge

Dosing errors are a concern in India due to the availability of both U40 and U100 insulin, each requiring specific syringes for proper administration. The U40 syringe is designated for U40 insulin, identifiable by its red cap and red scale markings, while the U100 syringe is designed for U100 insulin, distinguished by its orange cap and black scale markings. Many patients mistakenly treat insulin cartridges as vials and incorrectly attempt to pierce the cartridges.

Solution

To mitigate dosing errors, it is crucial to adhere to the appropriate insulin-syringe pairing. U40 insulin should be exclusively used with U40 syringes, and U100 insulin should be administered with U100 syringes. This practice ensures that syringe-vial mismatches are avoided, promoting accurate dosing and patient safety.

COLD INSULIN

Challenge

Storing insulin in the refrigerator can sometimes result in discomfort and irritation at the injection site if administered immediately.

Solution

To minimize the risk of injection site complications, it is advisable to allow the refrigerated insulin to equilibrate at room temperature for at least 30 minutes before injection. This brief period of adjustment helps to alleviate discomfort and ensures a smoother injection experience.

PROBLEMS WITH SPLIT-MIX INSULIN

For patients using split-mix insulin [a combination of regular and neutral protamine Hagedorn (NPH) insulin], it is crucial to maintain the correct sequence when mixing.

Clear insulin should be drawn first, followed by cloudy insulin. Strict adherence to this sequence is essential to prevent alterations in the chemical and pharmacokinetic properties of the insulin components.

PROBLEMS WITH CLEANSING

To prevent local infections and minimize the risk of healthcare-associated infections, it is crucial to follow proper sterilization procedures when preparing for an injection. This involves using alcohol swabs to clean the injection site thoroughly using a circumferential method.

However, it is important to note that while the top portion of the insulin vial should be cleaned, insulin needles should not be cleaned with alcohol. Cleaning the needle with alcohol can strip away the silicone coating on the needle, which may lead to more painful injections.

These measures are essential to safeguard against local infections and soft tissue complications during insulin administration.

FEAR OF NEEDLE

Challenge

The fear of injections, known as trypanophobia or belonephobia, can have a profound impact on an individual's emotional well-being and glycemic control. Similarly, the fear of pricking associated with diabetes management can cause distress and significantly hinder self-care efforts. Needle phobia often stems from a lack of confidence in one's ability to manage insulin therapy, leading to feelings of loss of self-control.

Solution

Addressing these fears and anxieties is essential to ensure effective glycemic control. It is crucial to provide appropriate support and resources to individuals experiencing needle phobia, helping them build confidence in managing their insulin therapy. This holistic approach promotes better emotional well-being and empowers individuals to take control of their diabetes management.

PAIN DURING INJECTION

Challenge

While pain during insulin injection is relatively rare, it can occur when the needle irritates nerve endings. Several factors can contribute to injection pain, including injecting into the tip of hair follicles, using a blunt needle repeatedly in the same site, administering cold insulin, and the formation of abscesses **(Fig. 2)**.

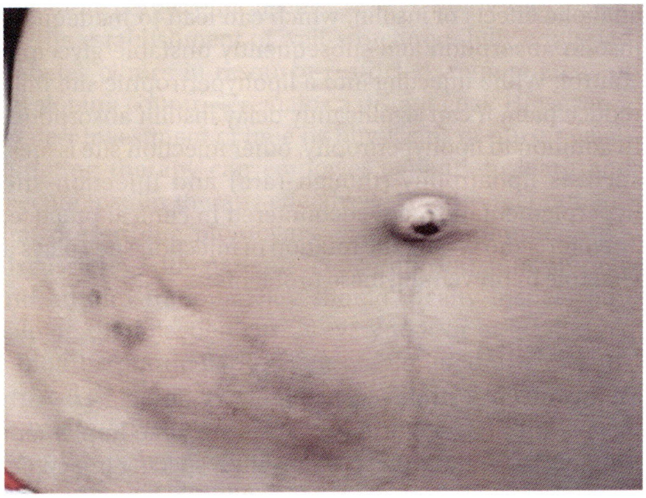

FIG. 2: Injection site abscess.

Solution

To mitigate the risk of pain during insulin injection and related complications, certain steps should be followed:

- *Appropriate site selection*: Choose injection sites carefully, avoiding areas with hair follicles or sites that have been previously traumatized.
- *Use thin gauge needles*: Opt for thin-gauge needles to minimize discomfort during injection.
- *Short needles*: Use shorter needles when possible to reduce the risk of reaching nerve endings.
- *Use new needles*: Always use a new, sharp needle for each injection.
- *Allow insulin to reach room temperature*: Ensure that insulin reaches room temperature before injection to prevent the discomfort caused by cold insulin.
- *Adequate skin fold*: Maintain an adequate skin fold to prevent the needle from reaching deeper tissues.
- *Avoid bruised or traumatized areas*: Avoid injecting into areas that are bruised or have been recently traumatized.
- *Follow a systematic rotation policy*: Implement a systematic rotation policy for injection sites to prevent repeated use of the same area.

By adhering to these guidelines, individuals can reduce the likelihood of pain during insulin injection and enhance their overall injection experience.

INJECTION SITE PROBLEMS

Challenge

Injection site lipohypertrophy, as illustrated in **Figures 3A and B**, resulting from repeated insulin injections in the same location is a common concern among individuals on insulin therapy. This is primarily attributed to the

28

CHAPTER

Hypoglycemia and Cardiovascular Disease: Current Understanding

Apurba Mukherjee, Shilanjan Roy, Tarun Kumar Biswas, SV Ramanamurty, TVS P Murthy

ABSTRACT

There is well-documented association between severe hypoglycemia and adverse clinical outcomes, including increased cardiovascular mortality and all-cause mortality.

Severe hypoglycemia is associated with more than fourfold higher cardiovascular mortality in VADT (Veterans Affairs Diabetes Trial) and a >2.8% mortality rate per year in ACCORD (Action to Control Cardiovascular Risk in Diabetes Study); the hazard ratio for cardiovascular mortality was 3.79 in ADVANCE (Action in Diabetes and Vascular Disease-PreterAx and DiamicroN Controlled Evaluation) trial.

Hypoglycemia is exceedingly common and is mostly attributable to sulfonylurea and insulin therapy. Renal dysfunction and older age are also important risk factors. Severe hypoglycemia may be associated with increased all-cause and cardiovascular mortality in patients with type 2 diabetes mellitus (T2DM). These complications develop from various pro-inflammatory, prothrombotic, proatherosclerotic, and proarrhythmogenic processes. Comparatively metformin, voglibose, and the newer glucose-lowering agents such as the incretin [glucagon-like peptide 1 (GLP-1) receptor agonists and dipeptidyl peptidase 4 (DPP-4) inhibitors] and sodium-glucose cotransporter-2 (SGLT-2) inhibitor classes of agents are associated with much lower rates of hypoglycemia relative to sulfonylureas or insulin and may be accepted as preferred therapies in diabetic patients with a higher risk of hypoglycemia.

INTRODUCTION

Hypoglycemia in diabetic patients has multiple short- and long-term clinical implications. Whether acute or recurrent, hypoglycemia significantly affects the cardiovascular (CV) system.

Several pathophysiological pathways have been postulated linking hypoglycemia to increased CV risk which includes hemodynamic changes, myocardial ischemia, abnormal cardiac repolarization, cardiac arrhythmias, prothrombotic and pro-inflammatory effects, and endothelial dysfunction.

New therapeutic agents for type 2 diabetes mellitus (T2DM) have a very low risk of causing hypoglycemia and have cardioprotective benefits; also, the use of new technologies, such as continuous glucose monitoring (CGM) devices and insulin pumps, has the potential to reduce hypoglycemia and its adverse CV outcomes in patients with diabetes.

CARDIOVASCULAR CONSEQUENCES OF SEVERE HYPOGLYCEMIA

There is a deficiency in understanding the direct/causal association between adverse CV outcomes and severe hypoglycemia.

In patients with diabetes who already have vascular disease, acute hypoglycemia may lead to acute vascular events, including acute myocardial infarction and ischemic stroke.

Among older adults with diabetes, the presence of coronary artery disease (CAD) can lead to acute myocardial ischemia during hypoglycemia.

Hypoglycemia also can induce changes in the electrical system in the heart, such as QT interval prolongation and ST wave changes.

These changes are usually because of hypokalemia, resulting from the catecholamine release triggered by hypoglycemia.

Cardiac arrhythmias may lead to the well-recognized complication of sudden cardiac death during hypoglycemia.

Gill et al. utilized CGM and continuous electrocardiography in type 1 diabetes mellitus (T1DM) patients, 20–50 years old. They documented longer QTc intervals during nocturnal hypoglycemia as well as cardiac rate and rhythm disturbances in 62% of 13 nocturnal hypoglycemia episodes.

A study by Pistrosch et al. found a higher rate of ventricular tachycardia (VT) in patients with a hypoglycemic event, but VT occurred with the same frequency during daytime and sleep, whereas hypoglycemia was recorded twice as often at night than during daytime.

However, Chow et al. observed that bradycardia and ventricular ectopics were strongly associated with nocturnal rather than daytime hypoglycemia.

One study showed that the mortality rate of diabetic patients developing severe hypoglycemia after acute coronary syndromes was twice than that of those who did not experience hypoglycemia. The effect persisted even after adjustments were made for confounding factors.

In patients with ST-elevation myocardial infarction (STEMI), 30-day mortality was greater in patients at the upper and lower extremes of blood glucose during hospitalization, showing a U-shaped curve.

Another study revealed that nondiabetic patients developing spontaneous hypoglycemia in hospitals had a poorer outcome and higher mortality than patients with insulin-treated diabetes exposed to iatrogenic hypoglycemia.

Probably, recurrent antecedent hypoglycemic episodes diminish the cardiac vagal baroreflex sensitivity and the sympathetic response to drug-induced hypotension. This attenuates the autonomic responses to CV stress for up to 16 hours.

This may also be the likely mechanism for inducing arrhythmias making the heart susceptible to recurring hypoglycemia.

EFFECTS OF HYPOGLYCEMIA ON THE BRAIN

The risk of ischemic stroke increases by two- to fourfold in diabetic patients. Also, stroke is more severe with greater cerebral ischemic damage, lower survival rates, higher chances of recurrence, and delayed recovery.

There should be a fine balancing act between hyperglycemia and hypoglycemia in stroke patients because hyperglycemia has detrimental effects on stroke outcomes, but efforts to aggressively control blood sugar can result in hypoglycemia, which can cause further damage to cerebral tissues.

Decreased cognitive function is also an important factor leading to an increased risk of both hypoglycemia and CV events and mortality.

One study examining magnetic resonance imaging (MRI) of the brain in a cohort of T1DM patients showed that brain lesions were more common in patients with T1DM who had a history of repeated (five or more) hypoglycemic episodes.

Whitmer et al. reported a dose-response relationship between the number of episodes of hypoglycemia and the risk for developing dementia.

CLINICAL OUTCOMES IN PATIENTS WITH SEVERE HYPOGLYCEMIA (TABLE 1)

Evidence suggests a clear association between severe hypoglycemia and adverse clinical outcomes, including increased CV mortality and all-cause mortality.

Severe hypoglycemia is associated with more than fourfold higher CV mortality in VADT (Veterans Affairs Diabetes Trial) and a >2.8% mortality rate/year in ACCORD (Action to Control Cardiovascular Risk in Diabetes Study); the hazard ratio for CV mortality was 3.79 in ADVANCE (Action in Diabetes and Vascular Disease-PreterAx and DiamicroN Controlled Evaluation) trial.

Leong et al. followed 285 diabetic patients for the development of incident CADs. Hypoglycemia was associated with a twofold increase in CAD risk [hazard ratio (HR) 2.15]. Among patients with high vascular risk, the risk was threefold (HR 3.01) in the subset aged ≥65 years.

TABLE 1: Hypoglycemia-mediated effects that may contribute to cardiovascular dysfunction.

Risk factor	Hypoglycemia-induced effect
Abnormal cardiac repolarization	QT interval prolongation, increased plasma epinephrine and norepinephrine concentrations, and hypokalemia
Reduced myocardial perfusion	Hemodynamic changes with an increase in cardiac workload and heart rate, fall in central arterial pressure, and large vessel elasticity
Atherosclerosis	Increase in endothelial dysfunction and inflammation
Prothrombotic state	Increased platelet aggregation and increased coagulation

Atrial or ventricular arrythmias were significantly more common at night than during daytime hypoglycemia. Excessive compensatory vagal activation after the counterregulatory phase may explain the bradycardia and associated arrythmias. QT prolongation and alteration of T-wave morphology were also observed during hypoglycemia in some participants.

Beom et al. have shown that QTc interval prolongation can occur in adults with T2DM and severe hypoglycemia even without hypokalemia as well as without any significant differences in the amplitude and morphology of T waves or significant ST-segment changes.

These findings are interesting as several studies have suggested that QTc interval prolongation is due to and an increase in serum catecholamines.

HEART RATE VARIABILITY

The heart rate variability (HRV) is a part of the counterregulatory response to hypoglycemia during mild hypoglycemia in people with and without T2DM.

Soydan et al. demonstrated that attenuated HRV is linked to an increased risk of developing sudden arrhythmia following mild hypoglycemia in adults with T2DM.

Based on these findings, recommendations from the American Diabetes Association (ADA) 2013 suggested that "less stringent glycated hemoglobin (HbA1c) targets" may be appropriate for patients with a history of severe hypoglycemia, advanced microvascular or macrovascular complications, or extensive comorbid conditions.

An analysis of the ADVANCE trial showed that participants with a history of severe hypoglycemia showed an increased risk of not only CV but also nonvascular outcomes [including gastrointestinal (GI), digestive, and skin conditions].

PATHOLOGIC MECHANISM OF CARDIOVASCULAR DISEASE IN HYPOGLYCEMIA (FIG. 1)

Hypoglycemia negatively impacts various pathways that might promote cardiovascular disease (CVD), notably:

- Blood coagulation abnormality
- Inflammation
- Endothelial dysfunction
- Sympathetic system overactivation
- Oxidative stress
- Accelerated atherosclerosis

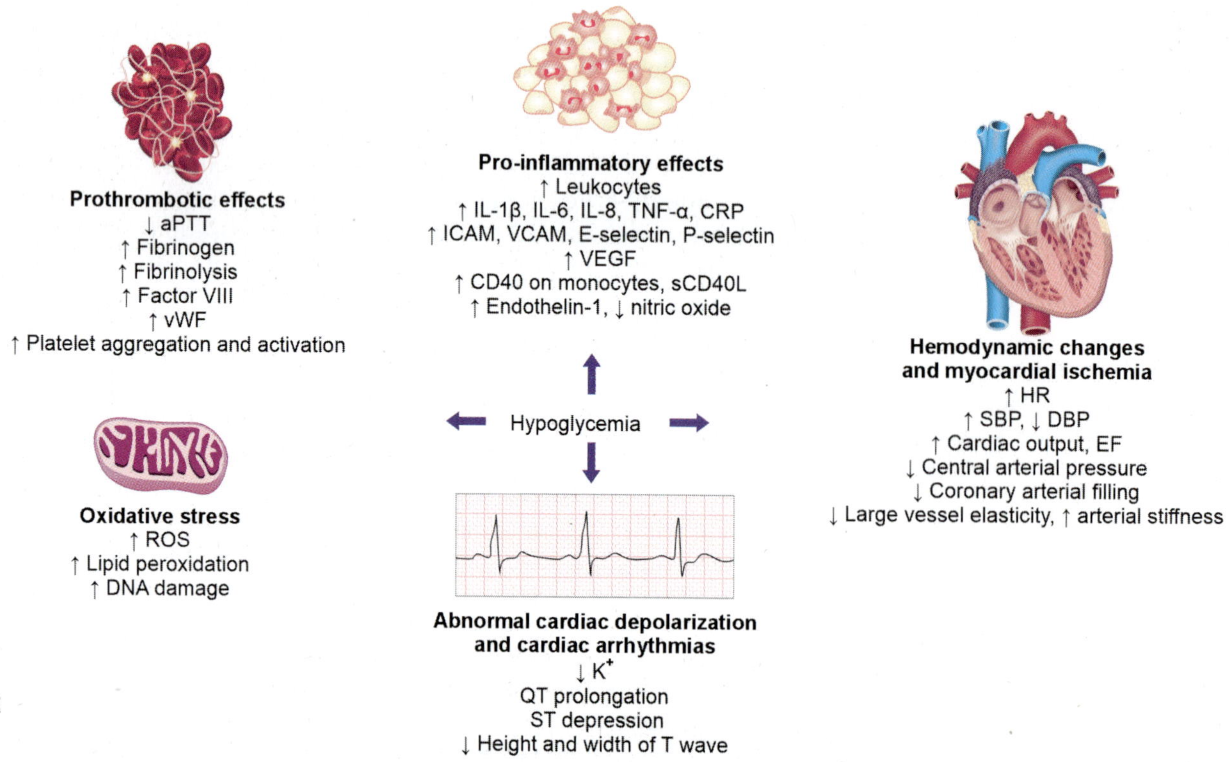

FIG. 1: Pathophysiology linking hypoglycemia to cardiovascular outcomes.

(aPTT: activated partial thromboplastin time; CRP: C-reactive protein; DBP: diastolic blood pressure; EF: ejection fraction; HR: heart rate; ICAM: intercellular adhesion molecule; IL-1β: interleukin 1 beta; ROS: reactive oxygen species; SBP: systolic blood pressure; TNF-α: tumor necrosis factor alpha; VCAM: vascular cell adhesion molecule; VEGF: vascular endothelial growth factor; vWF: von Willebrand factor)

Coagulation Abnormalities

Hypoglycemia can influence platelet aggregation and alter several components of the inflammatory cascade.

This results from an increase in P-selectin expression (a marker of platelet activation), fibrinogen, and factor VIII levels, along with a reduction in plasminogen activator inhibitor 1 (PAI-1) levels. It results in plasminogen generating a denser fibrin clot that is resistant to fibrinolysis as seen in subjects with T1DM. There is also reduced systemic fibrinolytic balance and enhanced platelet-monocyte aggregation providing a pathologic rationale for the increased rates of acute ischemic events seen with diabetes mellitus (DM) and hypoglycemia.

As seen with hyperglycemia, acute insulin-induced hypoglycemia also has a deleterious effect on hemostatic proteins toward creating a prothrombotic, hypofibrinolytic state.

The increased levels of the antifibrinolytic agent PAI-1 following acute and repeated hypoglycemia are associated with increased thrombin generation and increased plasma levels of clotting factor VIII, thereby increasing thrombus formation.

Inflammation

Episodes of hypoglycemia have shown to increase circulating inflammatory markers such as CD40, CD40 ligand, interleukin-6, tumor necrosis factor alpha (TNF-α), adhesion molecules high-sensitivity C-reactive protein, and other pro-inflammatory and atherothrombotic biomarkers.

The common biomarkers involved are vascular cell adhesion molecule-1, intercellular adhesion molecule-1, and E-selectin, vascular endothelial growth factor, along with TNF-α.

An increase in adiponectin levels is reported by Joy et al. with hypoglycemia.

The increases in inflammatory mediators are higher after repeated episodes of hypoglycemia as compared to a single hypoglycemic episode.

Endothelial Dysfunction

Abnormal endothelial function is an early marker of subclinical atherosclerosis.

Sommerfield et al. in a cohort of T1DM found that hypoglycemia resulted in a reduction in arterial wall stiffness and augmentation index, which may be due to the insulin-induced changes in the arterial endothelium.

It is thought that hypoglycemia-induced endothelial dysfunction together with increases in inflammatory biomarkers and blood coagulation abnormalities is likely the pathologic mechanism for accelerated atherosclerosis and CV events.

Sympathoadrenal Response

The sympathetic response to hypoglycemia is a counterregulatory mechanism to combat the impact of abnormally low glucose levels on the system. But the release of catecholamines can profoundly affect the CV system, directly altering cardiac contractility, myocardial work, and cardiac output, and therefore increasing oxygen demand which may precipitate ischemia in the presence of preexisting CAD.

Catecholamine in excess also directly acts on the platelet reactivity and may be proarrhythmic.

Hypokalemia due to catecholamine excess may also induce increased intracellular calcium with prolongation of action potentials. All these can lead to fatal cardiac arrythmias.

Accelerated Atherosclerosis

The VADT trial showed a link between hypoglycemia and progression of atherosclerosis. The study results indicated that serious hypoglycemia in patients on standard therapy, but not intensive therapy, was associated with increased coronary artery calcium (CAC) progression (up to 50%) over a nearly 5-year period.

IS CARDIOVASCULAR DISEASE A RISK FACTOR FOR SEVERE HYPOGLYCEMIA?

In a study done by Jae-Seung Yun et al., compared to patients without CVD, patients with established CVD were older, had a longer duration of diabetes and hypertension, received more insulin, and had more diabetic microvascular complications at baseline. The development of severe hypoglycemia was associated with a history of CVD (HR 1.99; $p = 0.031$) after adjusting for sex, age, diabetic duration, hypertension, HbA1c levels, diabetic complications, CV autonomic neuropathy, and insulin use. *This study documents that a history of CVD is an independent risk factor for the development of severe hypoglycemia in T2DM.*

Thus, in patients with established atherosclerotic cardiovascular disease (ASCVD), modification of glycemic target for the prevention of hypoglycemia should be done.

In another retrospective case-control study, patient groups with CAD and stroke had 1.48 and 2.78 times higher risk of severe hypoglycemia than control groups, respectively.

If myocardial damage or dysfunctional sympathetic innervations preexisted in patients with CVD, hypoglycemia recognition by patients is not easy.

Again, if hypoglycemic episodes are recurrent, hypoglycemia unawareness may occur. Hypoglycemia counter regulation to some extent is triggered by a glucose-sensitive brain region which may be damaged by ischemic events, and thereby response to hypoglycemia may be blunted in patients with diabetes.

Cardiac autonomic neuropathy (CAN) is associated with impaired recognition of hypoglycemia and impaired recovery from hypoglycemia because of defective endocrine counterregulatory mechanisms.

Furthermore, medications such as β-blockers used in CVD, may mask the symptoms of hypoglycemia.

IMPORTANT FACT FOR THE CLINICIANS

Hypoglycemia is exceedingly common and is mostly attributable to sulfonylurea (SU) and insulin therapy. Renal dysfunction and older age are also important risk factors. Severe hypoglycemia may be associated with increased all-cause and CV mortality in patients with T2DM. These complications develop from various pro-inflammatory, prothrombotic, proatherosclerotic, and proarrhythmogenic processes. Comparatively metformin, voglibose, and the newer glucose-lowering agents such as incretin [glucagon-like peptide 1 (GLP-1) receptor agonists and dipeptidyl peptidase 4 (DPP-4) inhibitors] and sodium-glucose cotransporter-2 (SGLT-2) inhibitor classes of agents are associated with much lower rates of hypoglycemia relative to SUs or insulin and may be accepted as preferred therapies in diabetic patients with a higher risk of hypoglycemia.

In 2023, the ADA has endorsed a personalized approach to selecting antidiabetes drugs for individuals with long-standing T2DM taking into consideration five key factors. These factors are as follows:

1. *Comorbidities*: Particularly, patients with a history of ASCVD, heart failure, or chronic kidney disease (CKD)
2. *Hypoglycemia risk*: Emphasizing the importance of avoiding episodes of low blood sugar
3. *Body weight*: Considering the impact of weight management in treatment decisions
4. *Accessibility and cost*: Addressing practical concerns related to medication access and affordability
5. *Efficacy*: Evaluating the effectiveness of antidiabetic drugs in managing blood glucose levels

The avoidance of hypoglycemia has been underscored, especially with the availability of a wider range of incretin-based therapies, such as DPP-4 inhibitors, GLP-1 receptor agonists, in addition to metformin, SGLT-2 inhibitors, pioglitazone, and alpha-glucosidase inhibitors (AGIs), which may be more appropriately utilized. SGLT-2 inhibitors have demonstrated clear benefits in reducing heart failure risk across different categories of systolic function and providing advantages for patients with CKD. Some GLP-1 receptor agonists have shown remarkable benefits in reducing the risk of ASCVD in individuals with T2DM.

CONCLUSION

Anticipated research is expected to reveal more data on dual agonism, involving both GLP-1 and gastric inhibitory polypeptide (GIP), and even triple agonism, encompassing GLP-1, GIP, and glucagon. These innovative therapies hold promise for significant weight reduction, improved glycemic control without the risk of hypoglycemia, potential benefits for CVD regression and kidney health, and the management of fatty liver disease. These findings are likely to emerge within the next 2–4 years. Meanwhile, it is imperative to minimize the risk of hypoglycemia. Complex insulin regimens should be avoided whenever possible, and high doses of SUs and meglitinides should be used sparingly. Recent research indicates that different types of hypoglycemia, such as severe, nonsevere, recurrent, and asymptomatic episodes, can have a substantial impact on CV health and morbidity. Of particular note is the association between hypoglycemia occurring within 3 months of initiating insulin therapy, as observed in both the intensive and standard arms of the ACCORD trial and increased mortality over the subsequent 2–3 years. This association is believed to be linked to heightened inflammation, prothrombotic tendencies, antifibrinolytic properties, increased adhesion molecule expression, and disturbances in electrical conduction. Understanding these intricate mechanisms and counterregulatory responses is crucial for grasping the protective or potentially counterproductive effects of counterregulatory excess in hypoglycemia on CVD in T2DM. Subsequent research in this field is expected to shed further light on these critical issues.

SUGGESTED READINGS

1. Bolognesi R, Tsialtas D, Bolognesi MG, Giumelli C. Marked sinus bradycardia and QT prolongation in a diabetic patient with severe hypoglycemia. J Diabetes Complications. 2011:25(5): 349-51.
2. Gill GV, Woodward A. Casson IF, Weston PJ. Cardiac arrhythmia and nocturnal hypoglycaemia in type 1 diabetes—the 'dead in bed' syndrome revisited. Diabetologia. 2009:52(1):42-5.
3. Pistrosch F, Ganz X, Bornstein SR, Birkenfeld AL, Henkel E, Hanefeld M. Risk of and risk factors for hypoglycemia and associated arrhythmias in patients with type 2 diabetes and cardiovascular disease: a cohort study under real-world conditions. Acta Diabetol. 2015;52(5):889-95.
4. Kosiborod M, Inzucchi SE, Goyal A, Krumholz HM, Masoudi FA, Xiao L, et al. Relationship between spontaneous and iatrogenic

hypoglycemia and mortality in patients hospitalized with acute myocardial infarction. JAMA. 2009;301(15):1556-64.

5. Radermecker RP, Scheen AJ. Management of blood glucose in patients with stroke. Diabetes Metab. 2010:36(Suppl 3): 594-9.
6. Perros P, Deary IJ, Sellar RJ, Best JJ, Frier BM. Brain abnormalities demonstrated by magnetic resonance imaging in adult IDDM patients with and without a history of recurrent severe hypoglycemia. Diabetes Care. 1997;20(6):1013-8.
7. Leong A, Berkowitz SA, Triant VA, Porneala B, He W, Atlas SJ, et al. Hypoglycemia in Diabetes Mellitus as a Coronary Artery Disease Risk Factor in Patients at Elevated Vascular Risk. J Clin Endocrinol Metab. 2016;101(2):659-68.
8. Beom JW, Kim JM, Chung EJ, Kim JY, Ko SY, Na SD, et al. Corrected QT Interval Prolongation During Severe Hypoglycemia without Hypokalemia in Patients with Type 2 Diabetes. Diabetes Metab J. 2013;37(3):190-5.
9. Soydan N, Bretzel RG, Fischer B, Wagenlehner F, Pilatz A, Linn T. Reduced capacity of heart rate regulation in response to mild hypoglycemia induced by glibenclamide and physical exercise in type 2 diabetes. Metabolism. 2013;62(5):717-24.
10. Zoungas S, Chalmers J, Neal B, Billot L, Li Q, Hirakawa Y, et al; ADVANCE-ON Collaborative Group. Follow-up of blood-pressure lowering and glucose control in type 2 diabetes. N Engl J Med. 2014:371(15):1392-406.
11. Ibbotson SH, Catto A, Davies JA, Grant PJ. The effect of insulin-induced hypoglycaemia on factor VIIL: C concentrations and thrombin activity in subjects with type 1 (insulin-dependent) diabetes. Thromb Haemost. 1995;73(2):243-6.
12. Wright RJ, Newby DE, Stirling D, Ludlam CA, Macdonald IA, Frier BM. Effects of acute insulin-induced hypoglycemia on indices of inflammation: putative mechanism for aggravating vascular disease in diabetes. Diabetes Care. 2010;33(7):1591-7.
13. Desouza CV, Bolli GB, Fonseca V. Hypoglycemia, diabetes, and cardiovascular events. Diabetes Care. 2010:33(6):1389-94.
14. Yun JS, Ko SH, Ko SH, Song KH, Yoon KD, Yoon KH, et al. Cardiovascular Disease Predicts Severe Hypoglycaemia in Patients with Type 2 Diabetes. Diabetes Metab J. 2015;39(6):498-506.
15. Lin YY, Hsu CW, Sheu WH, Chu SJ, Wu CP, Tsai SH. Risk factors for recurrent hypoglycemia in hospitalized diabetic patients admitted for severe hypoglycemia. Yonsei Med J. 2010;51(3): 367-74.

29

CHAPTER

A Diabetic Patient with Abdominal Pain and Rectal Bleeding

Ashis K Saha

ABSTRACT

Diabetic patients may experience abdominal pain and rectal bleeding due to lower gastrointestinal tract issues. Diagnosis can be achieved through clinical history, physical examination, hematological or biochemical investigations, endoscopies, and radio imaging. Rectal bleeding can occur in any patient, regardless of prior or current diagnosis, with an incidence of 33–87/100,000 patients.

INTRODUCTION

Rectal bleeding in any patient from any cause starts from any sites of intestine after the attachment of ligament of treitz upto anus. These diseases can be diagnosed from clinical history, physical examination, hematological or biochemical investigations, different methods of endoscopies, and different methods of radio imaging.

Rectal bleeding or hematochezia can be defined as passage of blood per rectum ranging from a streak of blood with stool or on the toilet paper to expulsion of a large volume of blood per rectum. Abdominal pain with rectal bleeding may occur in any patient who may or may not be diagnosed as diabetic prior to the episode of bleeding or diagnosed during investigation of this present episode. The incidence of rectal bleeding is 33–87/100,000 patients.

CAUSES OF ABDOMINAL PAIN ASSOCIATED WITH RECTAL BLEEDING

- *Anus*:
  - Fissure-in-ano
  - Trauma
- *Colon and rectum*:
  - Scarring carcinoma
  - Diverticular disease
  - Inflammatory bowel disease (IBD):
    - Ulcerative colitis
    - Crohn's disease
  - Ischemic colitis
  - Bacillary dysentery
  - Irradiation proctitis
  - Irradiation colitis
- *Small intestine*:
  - Intussusception
  - Mesenteric infarction

HISTORY

Anus

- *Fissure-in-ano*:
  - Occurs in patients under 40 years of age, common in children.
  - Precipitating factor is constipation.
  - There may be associated pain during defecation persisting a few minutes to hours afterward.
  - Patient may be fear of doing defecation because of pain.
  - Bleeding may be seen on the toilet paper or as a streak of blood on the wall of the stool.
- *Trauma*:
  - History of penetrating injury into anal canal
  - May be a history of sexual abuse or homosexuality.

Colorectal Causes

- *Cancer or polyp*:
  - It occurs after middle age, but polyp may occur at a younger age.
  - History of blood mixed with stool
  - History of change in the bowel habit
  - Colicky abdominal pain due to narrowing of a segment of the colon
  - In case of rectal involvement there may be tenesmus along with a streak of blood on the stool.
- *Diverticular disease*:
  - It occurs starting from early adulthood.
  - History of high protein diet or western diet
  - Unexplained abdominal pain with occasional extreme cramping
  - Altered bowel movements
- *IBD*:
  - It occurs in middle age.
  - Sudden onset of passage of blood with mucus during diarrhea, may be passage of fresh blood
  - Associated colicky abdominal pain, fever, and joint pain
  - In case of rectal involvement, there is tenesmus.
- *Ischemic colitis*:
  - Usually occurs in the elderly.
  - Postprandial colicky abdominal pain followed by passage of dark red blood per rectum
  - Diarrhea
- *Bacillary dysentery*:
  - History of intake of outside or hotel food
  - Passage of mucus with blood mixed with scanty stool
  - Associated history includes:
    - Tenesmus
    - Fever with chill
    - Arthralgia
    - Backache
- *Irradiation proctitis or colitis*:
  - Middle aged or elderly are affected.
  - History of cancer in the genital organ
  - History of irradiation
  - History of tenesmus or colicky abdominal pain during and prior to defecation
  - Passage of blood mixed with stool and mucus

Small Intestine

- *Intussusception*:
  - It usually occurs in infants but may occur at any age.
  - History of colicky abdominal pain with drawing of legs up
  - There may be screaming.
  - Passage of blood and mucus mixed with stool—redcurrant jelly stool
- *Mesenteric infarction*:
  - It usually occurs in the elderly.
  - History of metabolic syndrome, diabetes mellitus, or heart disease
  - History of central colicky abdominal pain with bleeding and passage of blood mixed with stool
  - There may be collapse or shock.

PHYSICAL EXAMINATION

General Survey

- *Pallor*: Cancer from any sites in the gastrointestinal tract
- *Jaundice*:
  - In case of extraintestinal involvement in IBD
  - Secondary metastasis in cancer
- *Weight loss*:
  - IBD
  - Cancer
  - Irradiation colitis
- *Lymphadenopathy*: Secondary metastasis in case of cancer
- *Edema*:
  - IBD due to hypoproteinemia
  - Cancer
- *Pulse*: Tachycardia
- *Blood pressure*: Low or there may be a presence of shock. There is finally recumbent hypotension.
- *Dermatological manifestation*:
  - Pyoderma gangrenosum—IBD
  - Erythema nodosum—IBD
- *Eye examination*: This may demonstrate uveitis, scleritis, or episcleritis suggesting extraintestinal manifestation of IBD.

Regional Examination

- *Fissure-in-ano*:
  - It can be examined by separating the buttocks as a sentinel pile is seen in the midline, commonly posteriorly and rarely anteriorly.
  - Digital examination is very painful during the examination.
- *Carcinoma*: Anal ulcer is a central ulcer with a surrounding everted margin, as in early case biopsy should be taken to differentiate it from fissure-in-ano.
- *Trauma*:
  - Presence of bruising
  - Anal skin or mucosa may be split.
  - Digital examination may be painful.

Colon and Rectum

- *Carcinoma*:
    - Left iliac fossa is tender.
    - There may be signs of intestinal obstruction.
    - Digital examination demonstrates hard, irregular, and ulcerating mucosa.
- *Diverticular disease*: There may be tenderness in the left or right side of the colon depending upon the presence of diverticulum.
- *IBD*:
    - Presence of palpable mass in the right iliac fossa—Crohn's disease
    - Abdomen is distended, tender—toxic megacolon
    - Signs of peritonitis—perforation of the colon
- *Ischemic colitis*:
    - Tenderness on the left side of the abdomen
    - There may be a presence of shock
- *Irradiation proctitis or irradiation colitis*:
    - Presence of lower abdominal tenderness
    - In per rectal examination, there may be granular mucosa with the presence of blood at the tip.
- *Rectal prolapse*:
    - Rectum can be seen as decent outside the anus.
    - There may be associated ulceration.

Small Bowel

- *Intussusception*:
    - Presence of mass palpable in the right iliac fossa.
    - In the progression of the disease, right iliac fossa becomes empty.
- *Mesenteric infarction*:
    - Diffuse abdominal tenderness
    - Features of collapse and shock

Risk Assessment

Extremely validated score "Oakland score" should be used for assessing the patient in case of lower gastrointestinal bleeding using seven variables **(Table 1)**.

- If the score is ≤8 and there is no other indication for hospital admission, patient can be safely discharged from the hospital. Safe discharge is characterized by the absence of all of the following:
    - Rebleeding
    - Transfusion of red blood cells
    - Therapeutic intervention to control the bleeding by endoscopic, radiological or surgical hemostasis followed by readmission within 28 days after discharge.
- If the score is >8, it suggests major bleeding.

One has to detect the stability of the patient by assessment of shock index, i.e., the ratio between heart rate and systolic blood pressure. If it is more than 1, the patient is unstable.

TABLE 1: Oakland score.

Predictor	Score
Age	
<40 years	0
40–69 years	1
≥70 years	2
Gender	
Female	0
Male	1
Previous admission for lower gastrointestinal bleeding	
No	0
Yes	2
Digital rectal examination	
No bleeding	0
Bleeding	1
Heart rate	
<70 beats/min	0
70–89 beats/min	1
90–109 beats/min	2
≥110 beats/min	3
Systolic blood pressure	
<90 mm Hg	5
90–119 mm Hg	4
120–129 mm Hg	3
13–159 mm Hg	2
≥160 mm Hg	0
Hemoglobin level	
<7 g/dL	22
7–8.9 g/dL	17
9–10.9 g/dL	13
11–12.9 g/dL	8
13–15.9 g/dL	4
≥16 g/dL	0

GENERAL INVESTIGATIONS

- *Hematological and biochemical investigations*:
    - Hemoglobin: In case of acute lower gastrointestinal bleeding, hemoglobin will be normal or mildly low initially, but in the next 72 hours extravascular fluid will enter into the vessels to restore the blood volume leading to a fall in hemoglobin level.

- There may be leukocytosis in the case of:
  - Associated infection
  - IBD
  - Ischemic colitis
  - Carcinoma
- Erythrocyte sedimentation rate (ESR) is increased in:
  - Carcinoma
  - Associated infection
  - IBD
  - Ischemic colitis
- C-reactive protein (CRP) is increased in:
  - Associated infection
  - IBD
  - Ischemic colitis
- Liver function test will be abnormal in case of liver disease and in case of extraintestinal manifestation in IBD. Raised alkaline phosphatase (ALP) suggests the presence of sclerosing cholangitis.
- International normalized ratio (INR) will be increased in case of liver diseases.
- Blood for sugar and glycosylated hemoglobin (HbA1c)—for diabetes
- Serum insulin and C-peptide to detect the type of diabetes
- Metabolic panel to detect hypokalemia, hypoalbuminemia, and hypomagnesemia
- Serological markers: Antineutrophil cytoplasmic antibodies and anti-*Saccharomyces cerevisiae* antibodies—IBD

- Stool for culture and sensitivity in case of suspected bacillary dysentery
- *Endoscopies*:
  - Upper gastrointestinal endoscopy is performed in case of the following indications:
    - Brisk rectal bleeding with gross hemodynamic compromise
    - Past medical history of peptic ulcer disease
    - Portal hypertension
  - Unless the bleeding is massive or brisk, colonoscopy should be done after oral lavage solution. Patients of >50 years of age with unexplained rectal bleeding should undergo colonoscopy within 2 weeks. But in case of severe or brisk bleeding, colonoscopy should be done within 24 hours of admission.
  - In case of minor bleeding, proctoscopy or proctosigmoidoscopy should be done to detect the lesions in the anal canal or sigmoid colon.
    - Capsule endoscopy: In case of positive findings, treatment should be directed toward the findings. If it is negative and the patient is stable, he/she should be treated for iron deficiency in case of anemia, and second capsule endoscopy should be performed to identify bleeding sources, because it can be diagnosed in 50% cases.
    - Colonoscopy is performed to detect ulcerative colitis, Crohn's disease, and diverticular disease. Colonoscopic finding suggestive of ulcerative colitis with negative stool culture is indicative of ulcerative colitis until proven otherwise. Features of colonoscopy in ulcerative colitis include:
      - Loss of vascular pattern
      - Fragile and granular mucosa
      - Ulceration
      - Pseudopolyposis
    - Double balloon enteroscopy or spiral enteroscopy should be done after capsule endoscopy to detect the lesion and if required, biopsy can be taken from the lesion.
- *Imaging studies*:
  - Radiographic imaging:
    - In case of ischemic colitis:
      - Dilatation of colon is seen early with mucosal edema (thumb printing) and formation of pseudopolyps.
      - After the involvement of small bowel also due to ischemic injury, there is dilatation of small bowel along with thickening of the valvulae conniventes.
      - Later on, haustra become edematous and thickened containing large amount of secretions.
      - With further edema, haustra will disappear completely giving rise to a hose-like appearance of the colon.
      - There may be appearance of localized pneumatosis.
      - Lastly, there is tubular narrowing as well as stricturing of the long segment of the colon.
    - In case of ulcerative colitis:
      - Intraluminal gas pattern to detect pseudopolyps and ulcers
      - Shortening of the colon
      - Loss of colonic haustra
      - Massive dilatation of the colon in case of toxic megacolon which is more pronounced in the transverse colon
      - There may be pneumoperitoneum in case of perforation of the colon
  - Barium enema demonstrates the following features:
    - In case of ischemic colitis:
      - During acute stage, after vascular insult, colonic spasm-associated thickening as well as blunting of the mucosal folds

        - Multiple mucosal scalloping or thumbprinting can be seen along the bowel contour.
        - With further progression of the edema of the mucosa, these folds become ill defined.
        - There is an increase in the intraluminal secretion.
        - During the phase of healing as fibrosis sets in there is flattening along with rigidity of one side of the colon.
        - Finally, there is stricture of the long segment of the colon with dilatation of the proximal bowel leading to the shortening of the bowel ultimately.
    - In case of ulcerative colitis:
        - In case of extensive disease, the whole colon will be involved but in case of segmental involvement, only the left colon will be involved.
        - Colon will be narrowed.
        - Incomplete filling due to colonic spasm.
        - Before the appearance of an ulcer, the mucosa looks granular.
        - With the first appearance of an ulcer, mucosa becomes fine and stippled, when seen on en face.
        - In case of an established ulcer, mucosa becomes coarsely granular due to deposition of the granulation tissue.
- CT scan of the abdomen: It will depict the changes in the blood vessels as well as the bowel wall. Contrast-enhanced CT scan will demonstrate the hemodynamics of the blood flow in the bowel wall. Diagnosis of bowel wall ischemia depends upon:
    - Degree of ischemia
    - Length of the bowel wall involved.
    - Whether both small and large bowels are involved.

Following features are seen in the ischemic colitis:
- Thromboembolization in the mesenteric vessels
- Segmental thickening of the bowel wall
- Intramural or portal venous gas
- Absence of enhancement of the bowel wall with contrast-enhanced CT scan
- Due to mucosal edema there is irregular narrowing of the lumen of the bowel.
- Proximal to the stenotic segment of the bowel, there is a dilatation of the bowel.
- Other nonspecific signs of bowel wall ischemia are:
    - Obstruction of the bowel
    - Mesenteric edema
    - Mesenteric vascular engorgement
    - Ascites

Following features can be found in the case of ulcerative colitis:
- Circumferential and symmetrical wall thickening which is greater in the case of Crohn's colitis
- Enlargement of the folds in the colonic wall
- Proliferation of the perirectal fat
- Inhomogeneous attenuation
- Fistula formation
- Abscess formation
- Target sign in the rectum consisting of:
    - Inner ring consists of attenuation of the soft tissue representing the mucosa, lamina propria, and muscularis mucosae.
    - Middle ring results from widening and fatty infiltration in the submucosa, this suggests the chronicity.
    - Outer ring represents muscularis propria.
- *CT angiography*:
    - It is noninvasive and widely available.
    - It can detect the lesion if the rate of bleeding is more than 0.3–1.0 mL/min.
    - It is performed prior to catheter angiography.
    - It has the highest diagnostic yield in case of hemodynamically unstable patients.
    - After detection of the bleeding site, mesenteric catheter angiography should be performed.
    - It should be the first line of investigation when colonoscopy will not be appropriate.
    - Disadvantages:
        - Low sensitivity
        - It requires radiation exposure.
        - Intravenous contrast is used that may be nephrotoxic.
        - It lacks direct therapeutic capability.
- *Catheter angiography*:
    - Indications:
        - In case of hemodynamically unstable patients, colonoscopy is not appropriate.
        - Persistent or recurrent bleeding
    - This catheterization process should be started in the inferior mesenteric artery before catheterizing the superior mesenteric artery because full contrast in the urinary bladder may obscure the bleeding sites from the branches of the inferior mesenteric artery.
    - If prior CT angiography already detects the bleeding site, then for controlling hemorrhage, gelfoam or coils should be introduced through the catheter or administration of intra-arterial vasopressin.
    - It can detect bleeding if bleeding rate from the lesion is at least 1 mL/min.
- *Radionuclide imaging*:
    - Here, technetium-based tracers are used to tag the red blood cells.

- It can detect bleeding if the bleeding rate is 0.1–0.5 mL/min.
- Repeated imaging is performed up to 24 hours to identify the source of bleeding.

Disadvantage: Though it is more sensitive than CT angiography or catheter angiography, but it can only localize the bleeding site, and therapeutic intervention is not possible.

CONCLUSION

In a diabetic patient with rectal bleeding, proper history, physical examination, and relevant examination should be done to clench the diagnosis, so that proper treatment can be provided to the sufferer to save his/her life.

SUGGESTED READINGS

1. Farrell JJ, Friedman LS. Gastrointestinal bleeding in the elderly. Gastroenterol Clin North Am. 2001;30:377-407.
2. Boley SJ, DiBiase A, Brandt LJ, Sammartano RJ. Lower intestinal bleeding in the elderly. Am J Surg. 1979;137:57-64.
3. The Royal College of Surgeons. (2013). Commissioning Guide: Rectal Bleeding. [online] Available from https://www.rcseng.ac.uk/library-and-publications/rcs-publications/docs/rectal-bleeding-guide/ [Last accessed November, 2023].
4. Khodadoostan M, Shavakhi A, Padidarnia R, Shavakhi A, Ahmadian M. Full colonoscopy in patients under 50 years old with lower gastrointestinal bleeding. J Res Med Sci. 2018;23:45.
5. Counter SF, Froese DP, Hart MJ. Progressive evaluation of formalin therapy for radiation proctitis. Am J Surg. 1999;177:396-8.
6. Rubinstein E, Ibsen T, Rasmussen RB, Reimer E, Sorensen BL. Formalin treatment of radiation-induced hemorrhagic proctitis. Am J Gastroenterol. 1986;81:44-5.
7. Rossini FP, Ferrari A, Spandre M, Cavallero M, Gemme C, Loverci C, et al. Emergency colonoscopy. World J Surg. 1989;13:190-2.
8. Peura DA, Lanza FL, Gostout CJ, Foutch PG. The American College of Gastroenterology Bleeding Registry: preliminary findings. Am J Gastroenterol. 1997;92:928-8.
9. Kochhar R, Sriram PV, Sharma SC, Goel RC, Patel F. Natural history of late radiation proctosigmoiditis treated with topical sucralfate suspension. Dig Dis Sci. 1999;44:973-8.
10. Grigsby PW, Pilepich MV, Parsons CL. Preliminary results of a phase I/II study of sodium pentosanpolysulfate in the treatment of chronic radiation-induced proctitis. Am J Clin Oncol. 1990;13:28-31.
11. Chapuis P, Dent O, Bokey E, Galt E, Zelas P, Nicholls M, et al. The development of a treatment protocol for patients with chronic radiation-induced rectal bleeding. Aust N Z J Surg. 1996;66:680-5.
12. Lipper B, Simon D, Cerrone F. Pulmonary aspiration during emergency endoscopy in patients with upper gastrointestinal hemorrhage. Crit Care Med. 1991;19:330-3.
13. Quine MA, Bell GD, McCloy RF, Charlton JE, Devlin HB, Hopkins A. Prospective audit of upper gastrointestinal endoscopy in two regions of England: safety, staffing and sedation methods. Gut. 1995;36:462-7.
14. Bell GD, Reeve PA, Moshiri M, Morden A, Coady T, Stapleton PJ, et al. Intravenous midazolam: a study of the degree of oxygen desaturation during upper gastrointestinal endoscopy. Br J Clin Pharmacol. 1987;23:703-8.
15. Freeman ML, Hennesy JT, Cass OW, Pheley AM. Carbon dioxide retention and oxygen desaturation during gastrointestinal endoscopy. Gastroenterology. 1993;105:331-9.
16. Griffin SM, Chung SC, Leung JW, Li AK. Effect of intranasal oxygen on hypoxia and tachycardia during endoscopic cholangiopancreatography. BMJ. 1990;300:83-4.
17. Cuellar RE, Gavaler JS, Alexander JA, Brouillette DE, Chien MC, Yoo YK, et al. Gastrointestinal tract hemorrhage. The value of a nasogastric aspirate. Arch Intern Med. 1990;150:1381-4.
18. McArdle K, Leung E, Latif S, Bohra A, Ishaq S. Management of lower gastrointestinal bleeding: endoscopist or radiologist? Gut. 2010;59:1605-79.
19. Khanna A, Ognibene SJ, Koniaris LG. Embolization as first-line of therapy for diverticulosis-related massive lower gastrointestinal bleeding: evidence from meta-analysis. J Gastrointest Surg. 2005;9:343-52.
20. Olds GD, Cooper GS, Chak A, Sivak MV Jr, Chitale AA, Wong RC. The yield of bleeding scan in acute lower gastrointestinal bleeding. J Clin Gastroenterol. 2005;39:273-7.

30 CHAPTER

Dyspepsia in Diabetic Mellitus

Agnibha Maiti, Siladitya Dewasi, Kishen Goel

ABSTRACT

Diabetes mellitus, a global health epidemic, imposes significant medical, social, and economic challenges, affecting various organ systems. Among its complications, gastrointestinal (GI) dysmotility is prevalent, impacting 76% of diabetic patients. This dysfunction, driven by neural, hyperglycemic, and hormonal factors, disrupts the intricate balance of the enteric and extrinsic nervous systems regulating GI functions. Animal studies reveal neural losses, oxidative stress, and apoptosis as underlying mechanisms, yet they are reversible with insulin therapy. In humans, diabetic enteropathy manifests as gastric dysfunctions, dyspepsia, and constipation, leading to delayed gastric emptying (GE), altered sensation, and impaired accommodation. Diagnostic tools such as scintigraphy and the wireless motility capsule aid in accurate assessment, while management strategies focus on nutritional support, glycemic control, and symptom relief. Emerging treatments such as camicinal and relamorelin hold promise, emphasizing the need for continual research in understanding and managing diabetic enteropathy, which significantly impacts patients' quality of life within the complex spectrum of diabetes complications.

INTRODUCTION

Diabetes mellitus, dubbed the epidemic of the 21st century, continues to pose a major medical, social, and economic challenge. Diabetes affects virtually every organ system in the body. The duration and severity of the disease may have a direct impact on organ involvement. Gastrointestinal (GI) dysmotility occurs frequently in diabetes and affects almost 76 percent of diabetic patients. It is caused by extrinsic (i.e., sympathetic and parasympathetic) neural dysfunction, hyperglycemia, and hormonal disturbances. A role of intrinsic (i.e., enteric) neuronal dysfunctions, resulting from loss of excitatory and inhibitory neurons and interstitial cells of Cajal, has also been implicated.

NORMAL GASTROINTESTINAL MOTOR FUNCTIONS AND REGULATION

Gastrointestinal motor function is predominantly regulated by the intrinsic or enteric nervous system, often referred to as the "little brain" within the digestive tract. The extrinsic nervous system modulates these functions. The parasympathetic arm of the extrinsic nervous system stimulates nonsphincteric muscles and inhibits sphincters, while the sympathetic component produces the opposite effects. The enteric nervous system comprises numerous of neurons organized in ganglionated plexus, including the submucous plexus responsible for absorption and secretion, and the myenteric plexus that regulates motility. Pacemaker activity is maintained by the interstitial cells of Cajal. In diabetes, the autonomic and enteric nervous systems within the GI tract can be affected. Disruptions in the extrinsic nerves at any level have the potential to impact GI motility and secretion.

PATHOPHYSIOLOGY IN ANIMAL STUDIES

Extrinsic neural dysfunction in animal models of diabetes is often characterized by a loss of myelinated and unmyelinated fibers, suggesting ischemic injury. Within the enteric nervous system, reduced neuronal staining and loss of nitric oxide synthase (NOS) expressing inhibitory neurons have been observed in diabetic animal models, which may contribute to impaired gastric accommodation and accelerated intestinal transit. Loss of interstitial cells of Cajal, a hallmark of diabetes, is associated with gut dysmotility. Mechanisms underlying neuronal loss and gut dysmotility in diabetes include apoptosis, oxidative stress, advanced glycation end products, and neuroimmune processes. However, these effects are reversible, as insulin treatment and pancreas transplantation have shown improvements in glycemic control and nerve damage in animal models. Insulin also restores NOS expression and gastric emptying, while insulin-like growth factors prevent the loss of interstitial cells of Cajal. Additionally, overexpression of glial cell line-derived neurotrophic factor in transgenic mice reduces enteric neuron apoptosis, improves gastric emptying, and enhances intestinal transit.

PATHOPHYSIOLOGY OF DIABETIC ENTEROPATHY IN HUMANS

Gastric Dysfunctions

Neuropathy and Paresis

Diabetes affects gastric function, leading to alterations in gastric emptying, sensation, and accommodation. Vagal neuropathy can cause antral hypomotility and pylorospasm, delaying gastric emptying. Impaired gastric accommodation due to vagal neuropathy may increase gastric pressure and accelerate the emptying of liquids, but the relationship with rapid gastric emptying is unclear. The impact of vagal neuropathy on postprandial accommodation remains uncertain, as accommodation may be preserved in diabetes, possibly involving nonvagal adaptive mechanisms. Small bowel dysmotility can also contribute to gastric stasis.

Hyperglycemia and Paresis

Acute hyperglycemia delays gastric emptying, but the effects are modest. Hyperglycemia suppresses antral motility and migrating motor activity. Acute modulation of blood glucose within the postprandial range also delays gastric emptying, to a lesser extent. Higher glycated hemoglobin levels are associated with slower gastric emptying and increased GI symptoms in people with diabetes. The impact of strict glycemic control on gastric emptying is unclear. Electrolyte imbalances and iatrogenic factors, such as treatment with amylin analogs such as pramlintide or glucagon-like peptide-1 (GLP-1) receptor agonists such as liraglutide can worsen motor function in diabetes.

Dyspepsia and Paresis

Gastroparesis is a syndrome characterized by symptoms and objective evidence of delayed gastric emptying. Some individuals with gastric retention may be asymptomatic due to afferent dysfunction. Nausea and vomiting can occur in episodes and may lead to hypoglycemia. The term gastroparesis should be used for markedly delayed gastric emptying, while diabetic dyspepsia is appropriate when the delay is not severe. Dyspepsia is characterized by upper GI symptoms, and vomiting is usually not severe. Significant weight loss can occur in people with dyspepsia due to reduced caloric intake. Gastric emptying of <65% at 4 hours is considered a significant delay. Rapid gastric emptying of liquids may be an early manifestation of type 2 diabetes mellitus (T2DM). Symptoms and signs are not reliable predictors of delayed gastric emptying. Measurement of gastric emptying is essential in people with upper GI symptoms. Autonomic tests and upper GI endoscopy are necessary for evaluation **(Table 1)**. Metabolic derangements and certain medications can contribute to dysmotility. Barium X-rays and other tests should be considered based on clinical features. Gastric emptying can be quantified using scintigraphy or stable isotope breath tests, and pressure profiles in the stomach and small bowel can confirm motor disturbances. Enteral feeding may be tailored based on the underlying motility disorder.

Diagnostic Tests

Diagnostic testing for delayed gastric emptying is typically based on symptom pattern and severity. However, gastric emptying assessments should also be considered for individuals with unexplained hypoglycemia, even if they do not have symptoms. Scintigraphy, stable isotope breath tests, or the presence of retained food in the stomach can be used to confirm delayed gastric emptying. Barium studies and scintigraphy with liquid meals have limited value in identifying dysmotility, as they may not accurately reflect the condition. Scintigraphy still now is the gold standard for diagnosis. Intragastric retention of >60% of a standard meal at 2 hours and >10% at 4 hours points toward diabetic gastroparesis. Noninvasive tests for measuring gastric emptying are summarized in **Table 2**.

Solid emptying can be assessed using a radiolabel that tags the solid phase of a meal. This test has a well-defined normal range and a high sensitivity (90%) and specificity (70%) for distinguishing normal function from delayed gastric emptying. It is important to obtain scans for 4 hours after a meal to accurately assess gastric emptying, as it is initially slow. Another useful test involves a standardized meal with a biscuit enriched with

TABLE 1: Commonly performed autonomic test.

Test	Physiological functions tested	Rationale	Comments/Pitfalls
Sympathetic function			
Thermoregulatory sweat test (% surface area of anhidrosis)	Preganglionic and postganglionic cholinergic	Stimulation of hypothalamic temp, control centers	Cumbersome, whole-body test
Quantitative sudomotor axon reflex test (sweat output, latency)	Postganglionic cholinergic	Antidromic stimulation of peripheral fiber by axonal reflex	Needs specialized facilities
• Heart rate and blood pressure responses • Orthostatic tilt test	Adrenergic	Baroreceptor reflex	Impaired responses if intravascular volume is reduced
Postural adjustment ratio	Adrenergic	Baroreceptor reflex	Impaired responses if intravascular volume is reduced
Cold pressor test	Adrenergic	Baroreceptor reflex	Impaired responses if intravascular volume is reduced
Sustained hand grip	Adrenergic	Baroreceptor reflex	Impaired responses if intravascular volume is reduced
Plasma norepinephrine response to postural changes	Postganglionic adrenergic	Baroreceptor stimulation	Moderate sensitivity, impaired response if intravascular volume is reduced
Intravenous edrophonium	Postganglionic adrenergic	Anticholinesterase "stimulates" postganglionic fiber at prevertebral ganglia	False negatives caused by contributions to plasma norepinephrine from many organs
Parasympathetic function			
Heart rate (RR) variation with deep breathing	Parasympathetic	Vagal afferents stimulated by lung stretch	Best cardiovagal test available, but not a test of abdominal vagus
Supine/erect heart rate	Parasympathetic	Vagal stimulation by change in central blood volume	Cardiovagal test
Valsalva ratio (heart rate, maximum/min)	Parasympathetic	Vagal stimulation by change in central blood volume	Cardiovagal test
Gastric acid secretory or plasma pancreatic polypeptide response to modified sham feeding or hypoglycemia	Parasympathetic	Stimulation of vagal nuclei by sham feeding or hypoglycemia	Abdominal vagal test, critically dependent on avoidance of swallowing food during the test
Nocturnal penile tumescence	Pelvic parasympathetic?	Integrity of S2-4	Plethysmographic technique requiring special facilities
Cystometrographic response to bethanechol	Pelvic parasympathetic	Increase in intravesical pressure suggests denervation supersensitivity	Tests parasympathetic supply to bladder, not bowel

Source: Camilleri M, Ford MJ. Functional gastrointestinal disease and the autonomic nervous system: a way ahead? Gastroenterology. 1994;106(4):1114-8.

TABLE 2: Noninvasive tests for measuring gastric emptying.

Feature	Gastric emptying by scintigraphy	Stable isotope breath test	Wireless pressure and pH capsule
Indication/function measured	Gastric emptying	Gastric emptying	Emptying and pressure amplitude
Device, assembly, or special requirements	External gamma camera and isotope-labeled meal	Breath collection vials and stable isotope-labeled meal	Intraluminal capsule with miniaturized strain gauge and pH measurement
Placement of device	–	–	Capsule swallowed
Performance/versatility/ interpretation	Excellent, standardized meals, data acquisition, and interpretation	• Becoming standardized • Performance related to mathematical analysis	Standard acquisition, delayed emptying fairly valid; pressures of unclear significance

Continued

Continued

Feature	Gastric emptying by scintigraphy	Stable isotope breath test	Wireless pressure and pH capsule
Duration of study	Typically, 4 hours, could be added to small bowel and colon transit	3–4 hours	6 hours, could be added to small bowel and colon transit
Availability/potential use	+	+++	+
Costs	++	+	++

Note: The "+" signs signify the lowest (+) to the highest (+++) availability or potential use.

Sources:

1. With permission from Shin AS, Camilleri M. Diagnostic assessment of diabetic gastroparesis. Diabetes. 2013;62(8):2667-73.
2. With permission from American Diabetes Association.

13C, which is metabolized and produces enriched CO_2. Measurement of $^{13}CO_2$ breath content using isotope ratio mass spectrometry allows estimation of gastric emptying half-life.

The wireless motility capsule (SmartPill™) is Food and Drug Administration (FDA)-approved for evaluating gastric emptying, colonic transit time, and measuring pH, temperature, and pressure throughout the GI tract. It is a safe and practical alternative to gastric electrical stimulation. The capsule transmits data to a receiver worn by the patient, recording pH, pressure, and temperature. Gastric emptying time is determined by the rise in pH from the gastric baseline to >4.0, indicating passage from the antrum to the duodenum. Normal emptying should occur within 5 hours, with a maximum of 6 hours assigned if it takes longer. Although not as accurate as scintigraphy with a digestible solid meal, the wireless motility capsule offers point-of-care use, avoids radiation exposure, and has enhanced utility in differentiating individuals with diabetic gastroparesis from healthy individuals based on pressure profile measurements.

In individuals without certain GI conditions, the wireless motility capsule may not detect a specific contraction within 6 hours or may be affected by the presence of a meal, hindering accurate emptying assessment. Challenges with capsule ingestion and the risk of retention or obstruction are additional limitations. The capsule is not recommended for children or those with a history of esophageal stricture. For severe upper GI symptoms, antropyloroduodenal manometry is a specialized technique that evaluates pressure profiles in the stomach and small bowel, guiding management. It can identify hypo motility in the gastric antrum and/or intestinal neuropathy. Some individuals with selective or dominant gastric function abnormalities may tolerate enteral feeding directly into the small bowel, unlike those with more generalized motility disorders. Diabetes can impair gastric accommodation after meal intake, contributing to symptoms, such as nausea, bloating, and early satiety. Imaging the stomach wall with pertechnetate allows measurement of gastric volume postmeal.

For constipation, initial tests include colonic transit, anorectal manometry, and rectal balloon expulsion. These tests can help diagnose or rule out defecation disorders, and additional imaging is only needed in specific cases. Delayed colonic transit is common in people with defecatory disorders. Slow transit constipation can only be diagnosed after excluding defecatory disorders. Intraluminal assessments, such as colonic manometry and barostat, can identify other dysfunctions in individuals with slow transit constipation, such as impaired contractile responses and abnormal tone. Colonic transit can be evaluated with radiopaque markers (5–7 days) or scintigraphy (24–48 hours), and both methods are equally accurate in identifying slow or rapid transit. Small intestinal dysmotility may present with abnormal migrating motor complexes, failure to switch from fasting to postprandial patterns, or features of vagal neuropathy. Stool fat assessment can differentiate diabetic diarrhea caused by malabsorption. Upper endoscopy can help diagnose bacterial overgrowth and exclude celiac disease through duodenal aspirates and small bowel biopsy. Lactose or glucose hydrogen breath tests rely on substrate metabolism by bacteria in the small intestine, but early peaks may be due to rapid delivery to the colon rather than small bowel bacterial overgrowth. To mitigate this, a stricter definition of small intestinal overgrowth may use an early hydrogen peak (20 ppm) caused by small intestinal bacteria, occurring at least 15 minutes before the later prolonged peak. However, even with stricter definitions, the lactulose hydrogen breath test's sensitivity and specificity for detecting small bowel bacterial overgrowth are reported to be only 68 and 44%, respectively, and for the glucose breath test, 62 and 83%, respectively.

MANAGEMENT

The principles of management are to address fluid and nutritional requirements, improve glycemic control, and treat symptoms. Dietary modification is a very important cornerstone of therapy. Fat and fiber intake should be minimized, carbonated liquid be avoided, taking multiple small low-fat meals advised. Severe gastroparesis may require hospitalization for intravenous hydration, correction of metabolic derangements, nasoenteric decompression, and enteral nutrition to manage vomiting and nutritional needs. In cases of malnutrition, parenteral nutrition may be necessary. Endoscopic disruption of bezoars can be done, followed by gastric decompression to remove undigested particles. Erythromycin at a dose of 3 mg/kg body weight intravenously every 8 hours can accelerate gastric emptying. When oral intake is resumed, treatment with oral erythromycin 250 mg TID daily for 1–2 weeks is worthwhile. Thereafter, the prokinetic effects of erythromycin are limited by tachyphylaxis. Anecdotal findings suggest that erythromycin may be effective if courses are separated by a drug-free period, e.g., lasting 2 weeks.

In individuals with severe refractory gastroparesis, a jejunal feeding tube may be needed to bypass the stomach. Prior to this procedure, a trial of nasojejunal feeding with infusion rates of at least 60 mL of iso-osmolar nutrient per hour should be conducted. Liquid or blended food is better tolerated during this phase. It is important to monitor blood glucose frequently, although improved glycemic control does not necessarily improve gastric emptying in people with poorly controlled T2DM.

Jejunal feeding tubes are preferably placed directly into the jejunum using endoscopy, laparoscopy, or minilaparotomy if needed. Gastrectomy does not provide relief from symptoms or improve quality of life, and people with gastroparesis often experience persistent symptoms after gastrectomy due to concomitant small intestinal involvement. Other prokinetic agents may be tried as adjuncts if the patient remains symptomatic. Metoclopramide, is a peripheral cholinergic and antidopaminergic agent. During acute administration, it initially enhances gastric emptying of liquids in diabetic gastroparesis, but its symptomatic efficacy is probably related to its central antiemetic effects. However, its long-term use is restricted by a decline in efficacy and central nervous system (CNS) side effects. Therefore, we prefer to prescribe a dose of 10 mg TID, administered 30 minutes before meals, for a short duration; the higher dose is 20 mg TID. A systematic review of trials concluded that there was limited evidence to support the use of domperidone, which is another dopaminergic antagonist but it is most commonly used because of its lesser side effects. Acotiamide is another prokinetic drug first approved in Japan which acts as a gastric motility modulator and alleviates symptoms of dyspepsia. Endoscopic injection of botulinum toxin into the pylorus was not effective in controlled studies primarily of idiopathic gastroparesis.

Food and Drug Administration recognizes gastric electrical stimulation for refractory gastroparesis, but its use is controversial. Published data suggest the device reduces vomiting frequency only when turned on, but data submitted to FDA indicate a similar reduction with the device on or off, suggesting a placebo response. Additionally, the device is expensive, does not accelerate gastric emptying, and has device-related complications in 10–20% of patients.

NEW MOTILIN AGONIST

Erythromycin, currently used off-label as a gastric prokinetic, has several drawbacks including the potential for antibiotic resistance, tachyphylaxis, and unwanted drug interactions due to its inhibition of cytochrome P-450 CYP3A4. It is extensively metabolized by CYP3A isozymes, and drugs that inhibit CYP3A can increase erythromycin concentrations, raising the risk of ventricular arrhythmias and sudden death. A promising alternative is camicinal, a selective small-molecule motilin receptor agonist that has shown the ability to induce phasic contractions and increase GI motility in conscious dogs. It has also demonstrated preferential activation of the β-arrestin pathway, aiding in faster recovery from receptor desensitization. Studies have shown that GSK962040 (camicinal) has a greater effect on cholinergic activity in the antrum compared to the fundus and small intestine. Results from a phase-II clinical study assessing its effects on gastric emptying, symptoms, safety, tolerability, and pharmacokinetics in individuals with type 1 diabetes mellitus (T1DM) and T2DM with gastroparesis are eagerly awaited.

NEW GHRELIN AGONIST

Relamorelin (RM-131) is a new ghrelin receptor agonist that has shown promising results in animal studies for increasing gastric emptying compared to other ghrelin mimetics. Two crossover studies conducted in individuals with T2DM or T1DM and delayed gastric emptying demonstrated that relamorelin significantly accelerated the gastric half-emptying time of solids compared to placebo. Another phase II study in individuals with T1DM showed that relamorelin reduced upper GI symptoms, particularly in those with high-baseline vomiting symptoms. Additionally, relamorelin has shown potential in accelerating colonic transit in individuals with chronic constipation.

CONCLUSION

Diabetes mellitus, beyond its well-known metabolic implications, significantly impacts the GI system, leading to a spectrum of disorders collectively termed *diabetic enteropathy*. This complication, affecting a substantial portion of diabetic patients, arises from a complex interplay of extrinsic and intrinsic neural dysfunctions, hyperglycemia, and hormonal imbalances. Through a meticulous exploration of the pathophysiology and diagnostic modalities, this review illuminates the challenges faced in diagnosing and managing diabetic enteropathy. Management strategies, rooted in nutritional modification, glycemic control, and symptomatic relief, form the cornerstone of addressing this condition. While traditional prokinetic agents such as erythromycin and metoclopramide have been employed, recent advancements in motilin and by ghrelin agonists, such as camicinal and relamorelin, offer promising avenues for future treatments. However, the intricate nature of diabetic enteropathy necessitates a multifaceted approach, emphasizing the need for ongoing research. In the face of the growing prevalence of diabetes mellitus, understanding and effectively managing its GI complications are paramount. By integrating evolving therapeutic options with a comprehensive understanding of the underlying mechanisms, healthcare providers can enhance the quality of life for patients grappling with diabetic enteropathy. Through continued research and clinical innovation, we strive toward alleviating the burden imposed by this intricate facet of diabetes on global healthcare.

SUGGESTED READINGS

1. Ordog T. Interstitial cells of Cajal in diabetic gastroenteropathy. Neurogastroenterol Motil. 2008;20(1):8-18.
2. Chandrasekharan B, Srinivasan S. Diabetes and the enteric nervous system. Neurogastroenterol Motil. 2007;19(12):951-60.
3. Camilleri M. Integrated upper gastrointestinal response to food intake. Gastroenterology. 2006;131(2):640-58.
4. Schmidt RE. Neuropathology and pathogenesis of diabetic autonomic neuropathy. Int Rev Neurobiol. 2002;50:257-92.
5. Sinnreich M, Taylor BV, Dyck PJ. Diabetic neuropathies. Classification, clinical features, and pathophysiological basis. Neurologist. 2005;11(2):63-79.
6. Vittal H, Farrugia G, Gomez G, Pasricha PJ. Mechanisms of disease: the pathological basis of gastroparesis—a review of experimental and clinical studies. Nat Clin Pract Gastroenterol Hepatol. 2007;4(6):336-46.
7. Watkins CC, Sawa A, Jaffrey S, Blackshaw S, Barrow RK, Snyder SH, et al. Insulin restores neuronal nitric oxide synthase expression and function that is lost in diabetic gastropathy. J Clin Invest. 2000;106:373-84. [Erratum appears in J Clin Invest. 2000;106:803.]
8. Horvath VJ, Vittal H, Lörincz A, Chen H, Almeida-Porada G, Redelman D, et al. Reduced stem cell factor links smooth myopathy and loss of interstitial cells of cajal in murine diabetic gastroparesis. Gastroenterology. 2006;130(3):759-70.
9. Anitha M, Gondha C, Sutliff R, Parsadanian AS, Mwangi S, Sitaraman SV, et al. GDNF rescues hyperglycemia-induced diabetic enteric neuropathy through activation of the PI3K/Akt pathway. J Clin Invest. 2006;116(2):344-56.
10. Samsom M, Szarka LA, Camilleri M, Vella A, Zinsmeister AR, Rizza RA. Pramlintide, an amylin analog, selectively delays gastric emptying: potential role of vagal inhibition. Am J Physiol Gastrointest Liver Physiol. 2000;278(6):G946-51.
11. Cervera A, Wajcberg E, Sriwijitkamol A, Fernandez M, Zuo P, Triplitt C, et al. Mechanism of action of exenatide to reduce postprandial hyperglycemia in type 2 diabetes. Am J Physiol Endocrinol Metab. 2008;294(5):E846-52.
12. van Can J, Sloth B, Jensen CB, Flint A, Blaak EE, Saris WH. Effects of the once-daily GLP-1 analog liraglutide on gastric emptying, glycemic parameters, appetite and energy metabolism in obese, non-diabetic adults. Int J Obese (Lond). 2014;38(6):784-93.
13. Camilleri M. Clinical practice. Diabetic gastroparesis. N Engl J Med. 2007;356(8):820-9. [Erratum appears in N Engl J Med. 2007;357:427].
14. Phillips WT, Schwartz JG, McMahan CA. Rapid gastric emptying of an oral glucose solution in type 2 diabetic patients. J Nucl Med. 1992;33(8):1496-500.
15. Alipour Z, Khatib F, Tabib SM, Javadi H, Jafari E, Aghaghazvini L, et al. Assessment of the Prevalence of Diabetic Gastroparesis and Validation of Gastric Emptying Scintigraphy for Diagnosis. Mol Imaging Radionucl Ther. 2017;26(1):17-23.
16. Camilleri M, Zinsmeister AR, Greydanus MP, Brown ML, Proano M. Towards a less costly but accurate test of gastric emptying and small bowel transit. Dig Dis Sci. 1991;36(5):609-15.
17. Bharucha AE, Camilleri M, Veil E, Burton D, Zinsmeister AR. Comprehensive assessment of gastric emptying with a stable isotope breath test. Neurogastroenterol Motil. 2013;25(1):e60-9.
18. Szarka LA, Camilleri M, Vella A, Burton D, Baxter K, Simonson J, et al. A stable isotope breath test with a standard meal for abnormal gastric emptying of solids in the clinic and in research. Clin Gastroenterol Hepatol. 2008;6(6):635-43.e1.
19. Kuo B, McCallum RW, Koch KL, Sitrin MD, Wo JM, Chey WD, et al. Comparison of gastric emptying of a nondigestible capsule to a radio-labelled meal in healthy and gastroparetic subjects. Aliment Pharmacol Ther. 2008;27(2):186-96.
20. Camilleri M, Bharucha AE, di Lorenzo C, Hasler WL, Prather CM, Rao SS, et al. American Neurogastroenterology and Motility Society consensus statement on intraluminal measurement of gastrointestinal and colonic motility in clinical practice. Neurogastroenterol Motil. 2008;20(12):1269-82.
21. Kloetzer L, Chey WD, McCallum RW, Koch KL, Wo JM, Sitrin M, et al. Motility of the antroduodenum in healthy and gastroparetics characterized by wireless motility capsule. Neurogastroenterol Motil. 2010;22(5):527-33.
22. Simren M, Stotzer PO. Use and abuse of hydrogen breath tests. Gut. 2006;55(3):297-303.

23. Camilleri M, Parkman HP, Shafi MA, Abell TL, Gerson L, et al. Clinical guideline: management of gastroparesis. Am J Gastroenterol. 2013;108(1):18-37;quiz,8.
24. Annese V, Janssens J, Vantrappen G, Tack J, Peeters TL, Willemse P, et al. Erythromycin accelerates gastric emptying by inducing antral contractions and improved gastroduodenal coordination. Gastroenterology. 1992;102(3):823-8.
25. Janssens J, Peeters TL, Vantrappen G, Tack J, Urbain JL, De Roo M, et al. Improvement of gastric emptying in diabetic gastroparesis by erythromycin. Preliminary studies. N Engl J Med. 1990;322(15):1028-31.
26. Bharucha AE, Kudva YC, Basu A, Camilleri M, Low PA, Vella A, et al. Relationship between glycemic control and gastric emptying in poorly controlled type 2 diabetes. Clin Gastroenterol Hepatol. 2015;13(3):466-76.e1.
27. Sugumar A, Singh A, Pasricha PJ. A systematic review of the efficacy of domperidone for the treatment of diabetic gastroparesis. Clin Gastroenterol Hepatol. 2008;6(7):726-33.
28. Friedenberg FK, Palit A, Parkman HP, Hanlon A, Nelson DB. Botulinum toxin A for the treatment of delayed gastric emptying. Am J Gastroenterol. 2008;103(2):416-23.
29. Arts J, Holvoet L, Caenepeel P, Bisschops R, Sifrim D, Verbeke K, et al. Clinical trial: a randomized-controlled crossover study of intrapyloric injection of botulinum toxin in gastroparesis. Aliment Pharmacol Ther. 2007;26(9):1251-8.
30. Thielemans L, Depoortere I, Perret J, Robberecht P, Liu Y, Thijs T, et al. Desensitization of the human motilin receptor by motilides. J Pharmacol Exp Ther. 2005;313(3):1397-405.
31. Murray KT, Meredith S, Narasimhulu SS, Narasimhulu SS, Hall K, Stein CM. Oral erythromycin and the risk of sudden death from cardiac causes. N Engl J Med. 2004;351(11):1089-96.
32. Leming S, Broad J, Cozens SJ, Otterson M, Winchester W, Lee K, et al. GSK962040: a small molecule motilin receptor agonist which increases gastrointestinal motility in conscious dogs. Neurogastroenterol Motil. 2011;23(10):958-e410.
33. Sanger GJ. Ghrelin and motilin receptor agonists: time to introduce bias into drug design. Neurogastroenterol Motil. 2014;26(2):149-55.
34. Van der Ploeg L, Laken H, Sharma S, Datta R, Halem H, Dong J, et al. Preclinical gastrointestinal prokinetic efficacy and endocrine effects of the ghrelin mimetic RM-131. Life Sci. 2014;109(1): 20-9.
35. Shin A, Camilleri M, Busciglio I, Burton D, Smith SA, Vella A, et al. The ghrelin agonist RM-131 accelerates gastric emptying of solids and reduces symptoms in patients with type 1 diabetes mellitus. Clin Gastroenterol Hepatol. 2013;11(11):1453-9.e4.
36. Shin A, Camilleri M, Busciglio I, Burton D, Stoner E, Noonan P, et al. Randomized controlled phase Ib study of ghrelin agonist, RM-131, in type 2 diabetic women with delayed gastric emptying: pharmacokinetics and pharmacodynamics. Diabetes Care. 2013;36(1):41-8.
37. Acosta A, Kolar G, Iturrino J, Szarka L, Boldingh A, Burton D, et al. Sa2051 a phase II, randomized, double-blind, placebo-controlled, multiple-dose, parallel-group study to evaluate the efficacy, safety, and pharmacodynamics of RM-131 in patients with chronic constipation. Gastroenterology. 2014;146(5 Suppl 1):S364.

31

CHAPTER

Diabetes and Vaccination

Anand Shankar

ABSTRACT

The Indian population has grown significantly in recent decades, with infectious diseases accounting for 25% of total mortality. Despite the belief that adults are protected from vaccine-preventable diseases, recent pandemics have highlighted this vulnerability. Immunization is crucial for primary prevention, and adults make up 60% of the population. However, the Universal Immunization Program (UIP) and Expanded Program of Immunization (EPI) have limited coverage for adults above 45 years of age.

INTRODUCTION

Indian population is known to be primarily a young population. However, over the last few decades, there has been a sizable increase in the population of adults and elderly individuals. Infectious diseases are a major health concern as they account for 25% of total mortality in the adult population in India. Overall, 95% of deaths from vaccine-preventable diseases occur in adults. Therefore, the general premise that adults are protected from vaccine-preventable diseases does not hold true.

The recent spate of pandemics and associated morbidity and mortality have only highlighted our susceptibility to infectious diseases. Augmenting the immunity, innate or acquired, is an important mode of primary prevention. Immunization offers an established means of promoting herd immunity against known vaccine-preventable diseases and forms an important part of primary prevention.

Adults constitute 60% of the total population in India. With the Universal Immunization Program (UIP) and Expanded Program of Immunization (EPI) being launched after 1978, the adult Indian population above 45 years of age is unlikely to have received immunization against most vaccine-preventable diseases. With growing age, a decline in immunological function, termed immunosenescence, is noted, which accounts for reduced immunity with increasing age. A summary of the burden and clinical implications of vaccine-preventable diseases is provided in **Table 1**.

IMPORTANCE OF VACCINATIONS

The administration of influenza vaccination has demonstrated a significant reduction in hospitalization associated with respiratory illnesses among individuals diagnosed with diabetes. According to the American Diabetes Association (ADA) 2021, vaccination has been shown to decrease the likelihood of hospitalizations, pneumonia, and mortality associated with influenza. Pneumococcal vaccines, namely PCV13 (13-valent pneumococcal conjugate vaccine) and PPSV23 (23-valent pneumococcal polysaccharide vaccine), provide protection against bacterial infections, such as pneumonia, meningitis, and bloodstream infections, as stated by the Centers for Disease Control and Prevention (CDC) in 2021. The administration of the hepatitis B vaccine is of utmost importance in the prevention of this viral infection and its associated complications, as stated by the ADA in 2021. The administration of the Tdap (tetanus, diphtheria, and pertussis) vaccine is strongly advised for individuals diagnosed with diabetes in order to provide protection against the infectious diseases,

TABLE 1: Disease burden and implications of vaccine-preventable diseases in India.

Diseases	Implications
Rubella	• 40–45% of childbearing women are susceptible • 2 lakh babies are born annually with birth defects • CRS accounts for 10–15% of congenital cataracts
Cervical cancer	• Accounts for 132,000 cases and 74,000 deaths annually • Random screening reveals HPV positivity in 16% of women
Hepatitis B	• 40 million carriers and 2.05 lakh deaths annually • High-risk groups include HCW, frequent blood recipients, IV drug abusers, multiple sex partners, or homosexuals • In Delhi, a mere 50% of HCWs have been administered with a minimum of one dose of the hepatitis B vaccine
Influenza	• Reported 20% of hospital admissions due to influenza during monsoons • Annual mortality of 40,000 • Highest infection rate in children but a higher complication rate in adults over 65 years of age
Hepatitis A	• HAV seroprevalence ranges from 38 to 92% in different age groups • HAV incidence is 3.4–12.3% in adults diagnosed with acute hepatitis
Pneumococcal disease	• *Streptococcus pneumoniae* accounts for 85% of invasive diseases in adults • 70% of the global incidence of pneumonia occurs in Africa and South-East Asia
Meningococcal disease	• Several episodes of meningococcal meningitis have been reported in major cities such as Delhi due to greater overcrowding, climatic conditions, and vulnerable population • Routine immunization of Haj pilgrims and institutional inmates is recommended
Chickenpox	• Primarily known as a disease of childhood • It is noted to affect adolescents and young adults due to low seroconversion rates in tropical countries such as India • Infection during pregnancy increases the risk of congenital varicella syndrome

(CRS: congenital rubella syndrome; HAV: hepatitis A virus; HCW: healthcare workers; HPV: human papillomavirus; IV: intravenous)

such as diphtheria, tetanus, and pertussis (whooping cough). In accordance with individual circumstances, the administration of supplementary vaccinations, such as human papillomavirus (HPV) vaccine, the herpes zoster vaccine (shingles), and other relevant immunizations, may be contemplated.

COVID-19 VACCINE AND DIABETES

Several studies on the effects of immunization of COVID-19 on diabetic individuals have found a link between raised blood glucose and vaccination, or even the production of new-onset diabetes mellitus. These results also suggest that immunization of COVID-19 may cause transitory hyperglycemia in type 1 diabetes mellitus (T1DM) patients. Infection of severe acute respiratory syndrome coronavirus 2 (SARS-CoV-2) has been linked to immunological stress and dysglycemia. The blood glucose levels worsening following immunization is thought to have a pathogenesis with the hyperglycemia associated with infection of SARS-CoV-2. Possible mechanisms for the development of acute insulin reduction and islet cell injury include entry through the islet angiotensin-converting enzyme 2 receptor, induction of a cytokine storm, initiation of oxidative stress, overactivation of the renin–angiotensin–aldosterone system, and dysregulation of stress hormone release, specifically cortisol and catecholamines, resulting in heightened insulin resistance. Although risk and poor prognosis are seen in T1DM and type 2 diabetes mellitus with COVID-19, vaccination must be prioritized in them. Additional investigation is warranted to address outstanding matters pertaining to the administration of COVID-19 vaccines.

VACCINATION CHALLENGES AND IMPACT ON DIABETIC PATIENTS

Adherence to vaccination schedules presents a formidable obstacle for individuals afflicted with diabetes. Various factors, including cognitive impairment, limited knowledge, logistical challenges, and conflicting obligations, may potentially contribute to suboptimal rates of vaccination.

In a recently conducted investigation, it was determined that the administration of influenza vaccination exhibited notable efficacy in mitigating the occurrence of hospitalizations associated with respiratory illnesses within the population of individuals afflicted with diabetes. Influenza vaccination effectively mitigates the occurrence of respiratory infections (severe), thereby aiding individuals with diabetes in maintaining optimal glycemic control, and diminishing the likelihood of complications associated with diabetes.

CURRENT RESEARCH

In a recent investigation, the efficacy of influenza immunization in mitigating hospitalizations associated with respiratory ailments in individuals diagnosed with diabetes was assessed. The results demonstrated a notable decrease in hospitalizations, underscoring the significance of influenza immunization in safeguarding individuals with diabetes against severe respiratory infections. Although the findings demonstrated a noteworthy decrease in such hospitalization study designs, this design choice has the potential to introduce inherent biases that warrant consideration. Furthermore, the investigation primarily centered on hospitalizations as opposed to specific outcomes pertaining to glycemic control, thereby constraining the direct evaluation of the influence on diabetes management.

The current body of research offers valuable insights regarding the effects of vaccinations on the management of diabetes. However, there exist several domains that necessitate additional investigation and inquiry to augment our comprehension and optimize medical practice.

RECOMMENDATIONS

The CDC recommends the administration of pneumococcal vaccination to individuals diagnosed with diabetes, taking into consideration their age and specific risk factors. The administration of the PCV13 is advised for individuals between the ages of 19 and 64 who have been diagnosed with diabetes. Subsequently, it is recommended to administer the PPSV23 vaccine at a later interval.

The following recommendations should be taken into consideration when managing vaccinations in patients diagnosed with diabetes mellitus:

- *Conduct an evaluation of the patient's immunization history*: A comprehensive assessment of the patient's immunization history is warranted in order to ascertain the administered vaccines as well as those that are currently pending. The assessment should encompass the individual's age, presence of comorbidities, and any pertinent risk factors that could potentially impact the recommendations for vaccination.
- *Adhere to the recommendations outlined in the national guidelines*: It is imperative to remain informed about the vaccination recommendations disseminated by national healthcare authorities, including but not limited to the CDC, the World Health Organization (WHO), or pertinent regional guidelines. The present guidelines offer precise recommendations pertaining to vaccinations in individuals diagnosed with diabetes.

Ensuring optimal protection against vaccine-preventable diseases necessitates the attainment of high vaccination rates within the population of individuals diagnosed with diabetes. Effective and compassionate communication has the potential to mitigate vaccine hesitancy and facilitate informed decision-making.

The incorporation of reminder systems is advised for implementation. Reminder systems, including but not limited to phone calls, text messages, or electronic notifications, should be employed to prompt individuals diagnosed with diabetes regarding forthcoming vaccinations or overdue immunizations.

The WHO calls upon all countries to implement strategies for the promotion of healthy aging and align healthcare systems to address the health needs of adults with special emphasis on immunization. **Table 2** describes the vaccinations.

TABLE 2: Vaccinations for adults and adults with diabetes.

Vaccine	Adults	Adults with diabetes	Comments
COVID-19	Yes	Yes	It is strongly advised that all individuals of adult age receive a primary series of the COVID-19 vaccine, followed by subsequent booster doses as per eligibility criteria
Hepatitis A (HepA)	May be	May be	This intervention is highly recommended for individuals presenting with a specific risk factor for HepA.* The administration of the vaccine typically entails a bifurcated approach, involving two separate doses, with a temporal interval ranging from 6 to 18 months
Hepatitis B (HepB)	Yes	Yes	It is recommended that individuals who are under the age of 60 years and those who have been diagnosed with diabetes undergo a series of HepB vaccinations consisting of either two or three doses, depending on the specific brand of vaccine

Continued

Continued

Vaccine	Adults	Adults with diabetes	Comments
Hib (*Haemophilus influenzae* type b)	May be	May be	Certain adults with specific high-risk conditions, such as the absence of a functional spleen, necessitate immunization with Hib vaccine*
Human papillomavirus (HPV)	Yes	Yes	After consulting with their doctor, 27–45yearolds can get HPV vaccines. Depending on the age of the first dosage, the vaccination is administered in 2 or 3 doses over 6 months
Influenza (Flu)	Yes	Yes	Getting vaccinated against influenza every autumn (or even winter or spring) protects you and others
Measles, mumps, rubella (MMR)	May be	May be	A potential requirement for an additional administration of medication may be indicated. Individuals with compromised immune systems are advised against receiving the MMR vaccine*
Meningococcal ACWY (Men ACWY)	May be	May be	The administration of the Men ACWY vaccine is deemed necessary for individuals presenting with various medical conditions*
Meningococcal B (MenB)	May be	May be	The administration of the MenB vaccine is potentially indicated for various medical conditions*
Pneumococcal (PPSV23; PCV15, PCV20)	Yes	Yes	It is imperative for individuals in the adult population diagnosed with diabetes to receive either the 20-valent pneumococcal conjugate vaccine (PCV20) as a stand-alone intervention or the 15-valent pneumococcal conjugate vaccine (PCV15) followed by the 23-valent pneumococcal polysaccharide vaccine (PPSV23) after a period of 1 year
Tetanus, diphtheria, whooping cough (pertussis) (Tdap, Td)	Yes	Yes	It is strongly recommended that individuals who have not previously received a dose of Tdap (tetanus, diphtheria, and pertussis) vaccine should promptly avail themselves of a Tdap immunization at present. Subsequently, it is recommended to administer a Tdap or Td booster dose at intervals of 10 years
Varicella (Chickenpox)	May be	May be	Individuals who have not previously experienced varicella infection, lacked immunization, or received only a single dose of the vaccine are advised to consult a healthcare professional to obtain pertinent information regarding the vaccination*
Zoster (shingles)	Yes	Yes	Individuals who are 19 years of age or older and exhibit a compromised immune system or are within the age range of 50 years or older are advised to undergo a two-dose regimen*

*It is advised to seek consultation from a healthcare provider in order to assess the potential risk of infection and ascertain the necessity of administering this vaccine.

VACCINE POSSIBILITIES IN TYPE 1 DIABETES MELLITUS PREVENTION

While no vaccination for T1DM prevention is presently available, continuing research is investigating potential strategies. Immunomodulatory therapy, aimed at modulating the body's immune response, preservation of insulin-producing beta cells, targeted immunizations to redirect autoimmune responses, and the identification of genetic and environmental risk factors, encompass a range of potential interventions. These initiatives seek to postpone or prevent the onset of T1DM by regulating the immune system or protecting beta cells. It is crucial to emphasize, however, that research is ongoing, and it may be some time before effective preventive vaccines or techniques become available.

CONCLUSION

In conclusion, it is imperative to underscore the indispensability of vaccinations in individuals afflicted with diabetes, as they serve as a crucial measure in averting diseases that can be prevented through immunization, and mitigating the onerous consequences that may ensue. Vaccinations exert a beneficial influence on the management of diabetes through their capacity to enhance glycemic control, mitigate hospitalizations, and optimize overall health outcomes. Continual investigation and cooperative endeavors among healthcare practitioners, researchers, and policymakers are imperative in order to enhance our understanding and optimize vaccination methodologies for individuals afflicted with diabetes.

SUGGESTED READINGS

1. Esposito S, Mariotti Zani E, Torelli L, Scavone S, Petraroli M, et al. Childhood vaccinations and type 1 diabetes. Front. Immunol. 2021;12:667889.
2. Galanos Get, Dimitriou H, Pappas A, Perdikogianni C, Symvoulakis EK, Galanakis E, et al. Vaccination coverage of patients with type 2 diabetes mellitus: challenging issues from an outpatient secondary care setting in Greece. Front Public Health. 2022;10:921243.
3. N Prakash, et al. Adult vaccination: need of the hour. Medicine Update. 2023 (APICON);33:819-22.
4. Chellappan DK, Bhandare RR, Shaik AB, Prasad K, Suhaimi NAA, Yap WS, et al. Vaccine for diabetes—where do we stand? Int J Mol Sci. 2022;23(16):9470.
5. Guidelines for vaccination in normal adults in India. Indian J Nephrol. 2016;26(Suppl 1):S7-S14.
6. Jothydev Kesavadev J, Misra A, Das AK, Saboo B, Basu D, Thomas N, et al. Suggested use of vaccines in diabetes. Indian J Endocrinol Metab. 2012;16(6):886-93.
7. Fradkin J, Rodgers GP. The economic imperative to conquer diabetes. Diabetes Care. 2008;31(3):624-5.
8. Vamos EP, Pape UJ, Curcin V, Harris MJ, Valabhji J, Majeed A, et al. Effectiveness of the influenza vaccine in preventing admission to hospital and death in people with type 2 diabetes. CMAJ. 2016;188(14):E342-E351.
9. Jackson ML, Nelson JC, Weiss NS, Neuzil KM, Barlow W, Jackson LA. Influenza vaccination and risk of community-acquired pneumonia in immunocompetent elderly people: A population-based, nested case-control study. Lancet. 2008; 372(9636):398-405.
10. Martínez-Baz I, Navascués A, Portillo ME, Casado I, Fresán U, Ezpeleta C, et al. Effect of influenza vaccination in preventing laboratory-confirmed influenza hospitalization in patients with diabetes mellitus. Clin Infect Dis. 2021;73(1):107-14.
11. Raviotta JM, Zimmerman RK. Models of health behavior and systems and overcoming barriers to improved immunization rates. In: Rockwell PG (Ed). Vaccine Science and Immunization Guideline. Berlin: Springer; 2017. pp. 235-71.
12. Boey L, Spiessens T, Loix S, Thijssen K, Cools S, Roelants M, et al. Seroprevalence of antibodies against vaccine-preventable diseases in children with chronic diseases. Vaccination in individuals/patients and populations at risk. 2020;27:109.
13. Pal R, Bhadada SK, Anoop Mishre. COVID-19 vaccination in patients with diabetes mellitus: Current concepts, uncertainties and challenges. Diabetes Metab Syndr. 2021;15(2):505-8.

SECTION

3

ENDOCRINOLOGY

32

CHAPTER

Subclinical Cushing Syndrome

Dinesh Kumar Sharma, Sunil Kumar Mahavar, Rohit Ishran

ABSTRACT

Subclinical Cushing's syndrome (SCS) is a milder and often asymptomatic form of Cushing's syndrome (CS), characterized by subtle elevations in cortisol levels without classical clinical manifestations. While the term "subclinical" implies a lack of overt symptoms, accumulating evidence suggests that SCS can have significant clinical implications and may lead to various metabolic and cardiovascular complications. This paper aims to provide a comprehensive review of the current understanding of SCS, including its etiology, pathophysiology, diagnostic challenges, clinical significance, and management approaches.

INTRODUCTION

Cushing's syndrome (CS) is a rare endocrine disorder caused by chronic exposure to excessive glucocorticoids, is characterized by typical signs and symptoms of hypercortisolism such as plethora, moon face, buffalo hump, central obesity, easy bruising, deep purple striae, proximal muscle weakness, menstrual irregularities, acne, hirsutism, osteoporosis, and glucose intolerance. Subclinical Cushing's syndrome (SCS), also known as mild or preclinical CS, is a milder form of the disease with subtle biochemical abnormalities and without the typical clinical features of CS.

Clinically inapparent adrenal masses (incidentalomas) are discovered incidentally in the course of diagnostic testing for other conditions and have no symptoms and signs. First described in case reports, subclinical hypercortisolism was then appreciated as a frequent endocrine disorder, being detected in up to 15–20% of patients with adrenal incidentalomas.

The diagnosis and management of SCS present several challenges, mainly due to the lack of consensus on diagnostic criteria and the varying degrees of cortisol elevation. This paper aims to shed light on the current understanding of SCS, exploring its clinical significance and highlighting the importance of early detection and appropriate management.

ETIOLOGY AND PATHOPHYSIOLOGY

The most common cause of SCS is the incidental discovery of adrenal incidentalomas, asymptomatic adrenal tumors found incidentally during imaging studies performed for unrelated reasons. Other causes include bilateral macronodular adrenal hyperplasia and adrenal microadenomas. In SCS, the excess cortisol production is typically less pronounced than in overt CS, and the pathophysiological mechanisms contributing to this condition are not yet fully understood. Genetic predisposition and alterations in the hypothalamic-pituitary-adrenal axis have been proposed as potential contributing factors, i.e., the degree of 11β-hydroxysteroid dehydrogenase type 1 activity (11βHSD1), also known as cortisone reductase and glucocorticoid receptor genetic variants.

CLINICAL FEATURES AND DIAGNOSTIC CHALLENGES

Patients with SCS are older, more frequently of male gender, and bearing an adrenal instead of pituitary adenoma when compared to patients with mild Cushing's by definition, SCS has no clinical manifestation. However, more detailed questioning and careful second physical examination may reveal subtle evidence for hormone excess, such as recent weight gain, skin atrophy, increased facial fullness central obesity with thin legs and arms, and more pronounced rubeosis (especially of the breasts).

Subclinical Cushing's syndrome often presents with nonspecific and subtle clinical manifestations, making the diagnosis challenging. Commonly observed features include mild hypertension, glucose intolerance, and dyslipidemia.

However, these findings can overlap with those seen in other metabolic disorders, leading to diagnostic difficulties. Additionally, SCS may be masked by concurrent comorbidities or medications that affect cortisol levels. The lack of standardized diagnostic criteria further complicates the identification of SCS cases.

LABORATORY INVESTIGATIONS (BOX 1)

Laboratory assessment of SCS involves measuring cortisol levels in various contexts, such as the 24-hour urinary free cortisol (UFC) test, late-night salivary cortisol (LNSC) test, and low-dose dexamethasone suppression test (LDDST).

The rationale for screening patients with adrenal incidentalomas for early detection and prevention of disease and exclusion of SCS in patients with adrenal incidentaloma scheduled for unilateral adrenalectomy to prevent postoperative adrenal crisis. In these patients, adrenocorticotropic hormone (ACTH) suppression via the negative glucocorticoid feedback resulted in atrophy of the contralateral adrenal with consecutive hypocortisolism after surgery.

The diagnostic criteria and biochemical features of SCS are not defined very well and are used to differ according to different studies.

BOX 1: Stepwise endocrinological investigation of subclinical Cushing's syndrome in patients with adrenal incidentalomas.

- *Step I*:
  - Screening test
  - Serum cortisol after dexamethasone suppression (3 mg dexamethasone at 2300 hours orally)
- *Step II*:
  - Confirmatory test
  - Confirmation by high dose (8 mg) dexamethasone suppression
- *Step III*:
  - Evaluation of the degree of hypercortisolism
  - Plasma ACTH during CRH testing, UFC, diurnal rhythm of cortisol secretion

(ACTH: adrenocorticotropic hormone; CRH: corticotropin-releasing hormone; UFC: urinary-free cortisol)

Higher cortisol concentrations after dexamethasone are correlated with lower plasma ACTH concentrations, lower dehydroepiandrosterone-sulfate (DHEA-S) levels, and higher midnight cortisol concentrations in patients with adrenal incidentalomas.

Missing cortisol suppression after a 1 mg overnight dexamethasone suppression test is the best means to uncover autonomous cortisol secretion.

Missing cortisol suppression (<5 μg/dL or 180 nmol/L) excludes the diagnosis after standard low-dose dexamethasone suppression.

Missing cortisol suppression after high dose dexamethasone suppression and the blunted response of ACTH to stimulation with CRH establish SCS diagnosis.

Blunted diurnal variation of cortisol secretion and blunted ACTH response to CRH are nonspecific findings in SCS.

Elevated UFC is not a useful screening test in SCS and an increased level indicates emerging CS.

However, interpretation of these tests can be challenging due to diurnal variations and assay-specific variations.

IMAGING INVESTIGATIONS

Adrenal magnetic resonance imaging (MRI) is as effective as computed tomography (CT) to play a crucial role in identifying adrenal lesions **(Fig. 1)** and ruling out functional tumors. Positron emission tomography (PET) along with computed tomography (CT) can be used in difficult cases.

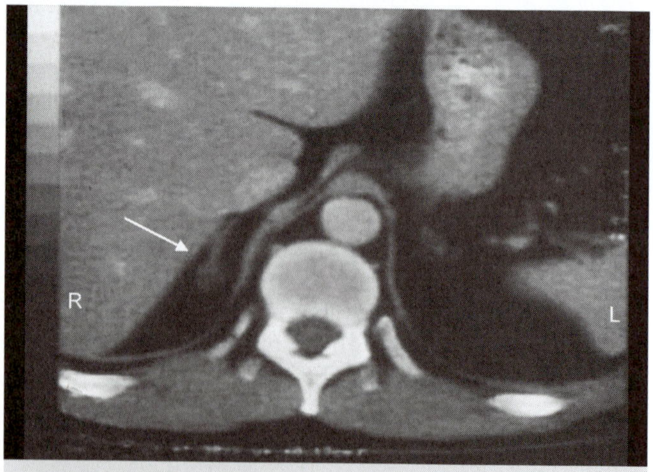

- Small size
- Hypodensity (attenuation value <10 HU)
- Rapid washout of IV contrast
- Round or oval-shaped homogenous mass
- Well-defined margins

FIG. 1: Magnetic resonance imaging (MRI) findings of adrenal incidentaloma.

Adrenal scintigraphy (^{131}I and ^{75}Se norcholesterol) can be used to screen for subclinical and differentiation between benign and malignant lesions to some degree of CS, but usually not done due to high radiation exposure.

CLINICAL SIGNIFICANCE AND ASSOCIATED COMPLICATIONS

Despite the lack of overt clinical symptoms, SCS has been associated with various complications, including cardiovascular disease (mean carotid artery intima-media thickness and atherosclerotic plaques) metabolic abnormalities (i.e., insulin-resistance state), osteoporosis (lower bone mass and increase susceptibility to fractures), and psychological disturbance. However, the causal relationship between hypercortisolism and metabolic, cardiovascular, and bone diseases in SCS is not being established yet.

PROGRESSION OF DISEASE

The natural course of SCS **(Fig. 2)** and the risk of developing overt CS are still unknown. Studies showed that the risk of a nonsecreting adrenal incidentaloma developing subclinical hyperfunction was 3.8% after 1 year and 6.6% after 5 years. For patients with masses with subclinical autonomous glucocorticoid overproduction, the estimated cumulative risk of developing overt CS was 12.5% after 1 year.

These data showed that patients with SCS are at risk of developing overt CS. So, a more vigilant follow-up including biochemical and hormonal profiles is advisable in early nonoperable SCS patients.

MANAGEMENT STRATEGIES

In the treatment of adrenal incidentalomas hormone-producing mass (aldosterone-producing adrenal tumors and pheochromocytoma) should be removed surgically to prevent serious morbidity **(Flowchart 1)**.

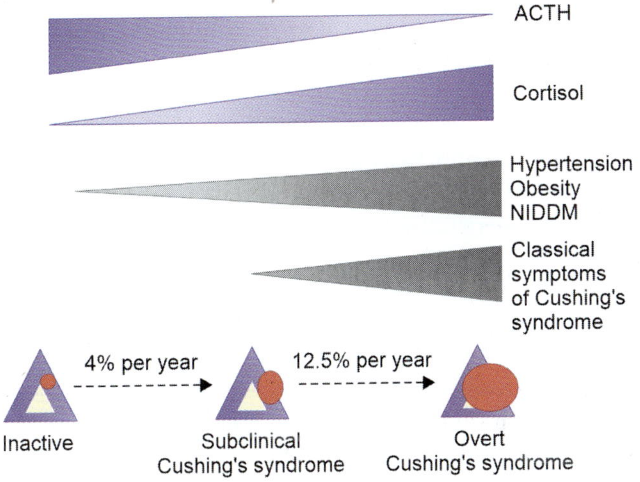

FIG. 2: Spectrum of subclinical Cushing's syndrome.
(ACTH: adrenocorticotropic hormone; NIDDM: noninsulin-dependent diabetes mellitus)

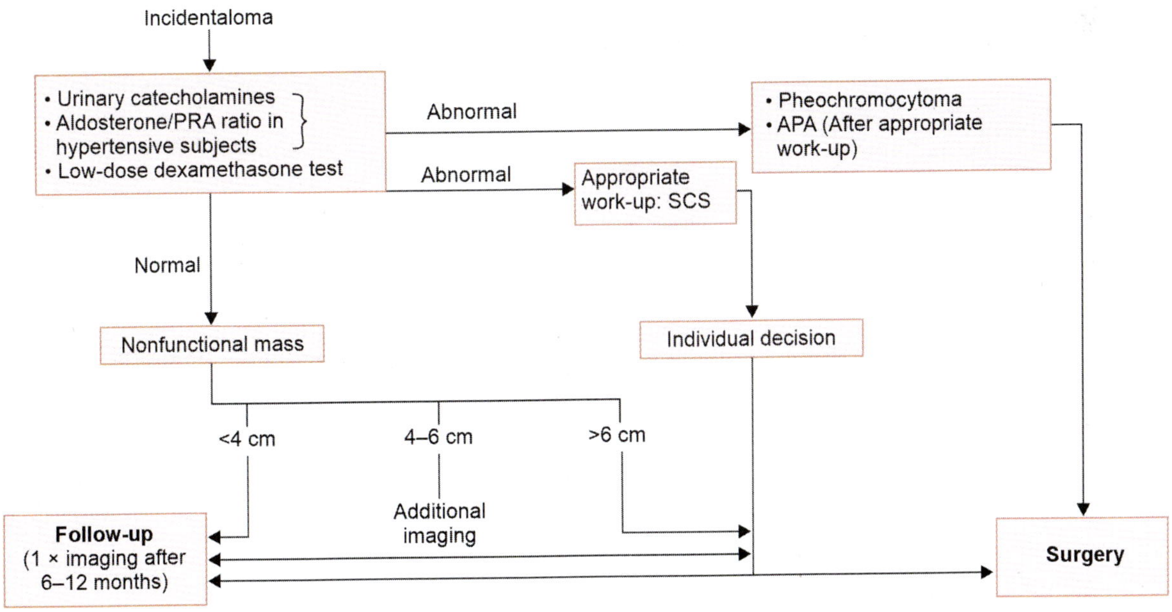

FLOWCHART 1: Workup of adrenal incidentaloma.
(APA: aldosterone-producing adenoma; PRA: plasma renin activity; SCS: subclinical Cushing's syndrome)

The National Institutes of Health (NIH) consensus conference on the management of the clinically inapparent adrenal mass concluded that both adrenalectomy and careful observation can be suggested as treatment options in SCS.

In SCS, surgery should be considered in patients with **(Flowchart 2)**.

- Suppressed plasma ACTH and elevated UFC who have progression to overt CS is imminent
- Normal plasma ACTH and UFC should undergo adrenalectomy if they are young (age <50 years old) or have metabolic disease of recent onset possibly related to CS (hypertension, obesity, and diabetes)
- Nonsecreting adenomas of size >4 cm or size increasing by >1 cm

Studies showed that there was a reduction in blood pressure, insulin resistance, and weight after surgical removal of SCS-producing adrenal masses but these evidences were not sufficient to conclude whether surgery is preferable to nonsurgical medical management of metabolic disease in SCS.

FOLLOW-UP

During and after the operation, glucocorticoid replacement therapy is required in patients with SCS, especially with suppressed plasma ACTH. These patients are likely to develop adrenal insufficiency and should be monitored closely. Glucocorticoid therapy should be continued until the adrenocortical function of the contralateral adrenal is regained.

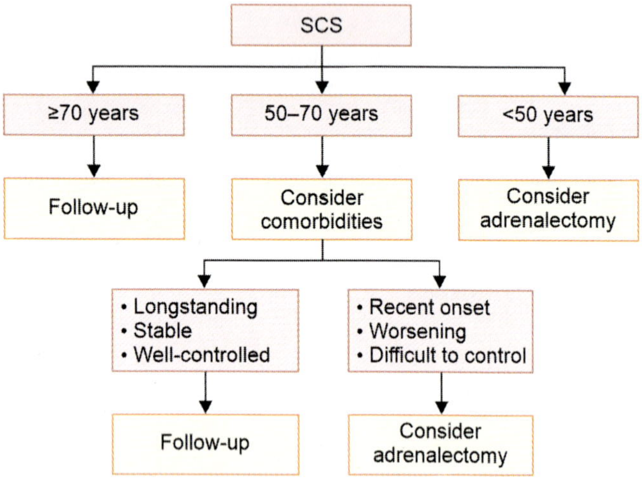

FLOWCHART 2: Management strategy of subclinical Cushing's syndrome (SCS).

CONCLUSION

Subclinical Cushing's syndrome, though lacking classical clinical symptoms, is a condition of clinical significance that warrants attention. Early detection and proper management are crucial to prevent potential complications associated with chronic cortisol excess. Standardization of diagnostic criteria and guidelines for SCS would greatly contribute to improved patient care and outcomes **(Table 1)**.

TABLE 1: Comparison of subclinical Cushing's syndrome and mild Cushing's syndrome.

	Subclinical Cushing	Mild Cushing
Sex	Slight female excess	Clear female excess
Age at diagnosis	Usually, >50 years	Usually, <50 years
Diagnostic modality	• Incidental finding • Radiological tests usually prompt further endocrine work-up	• Finding based on clinical suspect • Endocrine tests usually prompt further radiological work-up
Cause of disease	Usually, adrenal adenoma	Usually, pituitary adenoma
Clinical presentation	• One or more features of the metabolic syndrome • No specific Cushingoid signs (slight facial roundness may be present)	• One or more features of metabolic syndrome • One or more specific Cushingoid signs (usually of minimal to mild intensity)
Biochemical presentation	• Altered response to DST • UFC usually normal • MSC usually normal • ACTH usually low	• Altered response to DST • UFC is usually normal or slightly elevated • MSC usually elevated • Variable ACTH
Disease course	• Usually does not progress to overt Cushing's syndrome • Hypoadrenalism may occur after removal of the adrenal tumor	• Usually progressive to more severe clinical presentation • Hypoadrenalism ensues invariably after removal of the causing tumor

(ACTH: adrenocorticotropic hormone; DST: dexamethasone suppression test; MSC: midnight salivary cortisol; UFC: urinary free cortisol)

SUGGESTED READINGS

1. Reincke M. Subclinical Cushing's syndrome. Endocrinol Metab Clin North Am. 2000;29(1):43-56.
2. Favero V, Cremaschi A, Parazzoli C, Falchetti A, Gaudio A, Gennari L, et al. Pathophysiology of mild hypercortisolism: From the bench to the bedside. Int J Mol Sci. 2022;23(2):673.
3. Terzolo M, Pia A, Reimondo G. Subclinical Cushing's syndrome: definition and management. Clin Endocrinol. 2012;76(1):12-8.
4. Grumbach MM, Biller BM, Braunstein GD, Campbell KK, Carney JA, Godley PA, et al. Management of the clinically inapparent adrenal mass ("incidentaloma"). Ann Intern Med. 2003;138(5):424-9.
5. Tsagarakis S, Roboti C, Kokkoris P, Vasiliou V, Alevizaki C, Thalassinos N. Elevated post-dexamethasone suppression cortisol concentrations correlate with hormonal alterations of the hypothalamo–pituitary axis in patients with adrenal incidentalomas. Clin Endocrinol. 1998;49(2):165-71.
6. Barzon L, Scaroni C, Sonino N, Fallo F, Paoletta A, Boscaro M. Risk factors and long-term follow-up of adrenal incidentalomas. J Clin Endocrinol Metab. 1999;84(2):520-6.

33

CHAPTER

Hyperprolactinemia: Approach

Shriraam Mahadevan, Adlyne Reena Asirvatham

ABSTRACT

Prolactin (PRL) is a vital hormone secreted by the pituitary gland, physiologically responsible for maintaining lactation in the postpartum period. Significantly elevated levels of PRL (>100–150 ng/mL) in nonpregnant settings are associated with suppression of gonadal axis, oligomenorrhea, and galactorrhea in the females. The presentation may be quite late in males due to the absence of the these symptoms. Thus, any male with delayed puberty, halted pubertal progression, gynecomastia, lack of libido, sexual dysfunction, or subfertility should be checked for hyperprolactinemia. Lesser degrees of PRL elevation (<100 ng/mL) are due to drugs many times. Stalk compression-related mild hyperprolactinemia should also be considered and pituitary magnetic resonance imaging (MRI) may be required to rule out the same. Treatment includes dopamine receptor 2 (D2) agonist therapy for tumoral causes of hyperprolactinemia, which is most often curative if managed for adequate time and followed up regularly. Even macroadenoma of pituitary-secreting prolactin is well amenable for medical therapy with cabergoline/bromocriptine. Subfertility due to ovulatory dysfunction as in polycystic ovary syndrome (PCOS) may be an exception to the latter rule and a short-term therapy with D2 agonists to normalize PRL level may be attempted.

INTRODUCTION

Prolactin (PRL) in humans is a polypeptide (198 amino acids) hormone secreted by the lactotrophs, predominantly in the pars distalis of the anterior pituitary gland. The main role of the hormone, especially in females, is milk production during the lactation period. In addition, from animal studies, it is observed that it plays some part in modulating inflammation, immunity, angiogenesis, osmoregulation, reproduction, and other putative functions. With the advent of highly sensitive chemiluminescence assays, elevated serum prolactin level is not uncommonly encountered in clinical practice. This chapter will provide a revision of the basics of PRL secretory physiology and a practical approach to elevated PRL levels.

PROLACTIN ESTIMATION AND NORMAL LEVELS

Normally, the fasting PRL level in nonpregnant, premenopausal females and males is usually <20 ng/mL. Strictly speaking, a few purists may prefer to take three samples at 20-minute interval, pool the plasma together, and get the PRL to average out the pulsatile secretion. The latter is rarely done in practice.

"Hook effect": When PRL levels are very high as observed occasionally in macroprolactinomas, both the binding and capture antibodies may get saturated, resulting in falsely normal to slightly above normal values leading to misdiagnosis. This may be avoided by diluting the sample (preferably 1 in 100) to get the accurate PRL levels. Many

laboratories test PRL in dilution, whenever a pituitary macroadenoma is diagnosed.

It is always worthwhile to know the causes of hyperprolactinemia to approach the problem in clinical practice. This etiology of hyperprolactinemia could be broadly grouped under physiological, pharmacological, pathological, and miscellaneous causes.

PHYSIOLOGICAL CAUSES

As we understand from basic human physiology, pregnancy and lactation are the most important physiological conditions in which PRL is bound to be elevated. In addition, diurnal variations (higher values in sleep), mild PRL elevations after food, exercise, and stress may be useful to remember. Though some reports are contrary, nipple stimulation, breast examination, and sexual activity may also mildly increase PRL.

PHARMACOLOGICAL CAUSES

Prolactin is the only anterior pituitary hormone under predominant inhibitory influence from the hypothalamus, namely dopamine. Any inhibition of dopamine secretion (several drugs as discussed further and given in **Box 1**) or interruption of its transport through the portal system (stalk compression even by a nonfunctioning pituitary macroadenoma or inflammation, as in infundibulo-hypophysitis) may result in disinhibition of lactotrophs and secrete more PRL.

In drug-induced hyperprolactinemia, the PRL levels usually do not rise above 100 ng/mL. Among the commonly encountered drugs in practice are proton pump inhibitors, especially in combination with prokinetics like domperidone and levosulpiride. Among antipsychotics, risperidone is, probably, exceptionally potent to elevate PRL even above 300 ng/mL. Aripiprazole is the only neuroleptic that does not affect PRL levels. Among calcium channel blockers, verapamil for unknown reasons raises PRL levels. In the Indian setting, alternate and complementary forms of therapies may also elevate PRL and need to be considered. In all these situations, if possible, it may be best to avoid the suspected drug for at least a week or two and recheck PRL levels to confirm hyperprolactinemia.

BOX 1: Common drugs that cause hyperprolactinemia.

- Dopamine receptor blockers
- Cimetidine
- Proton pump inhibitors
- Levosulpiride
- Metoclopramide
- Domperidone
- Serotonin reuptake inhibitors
- Tricyclic antidepressants
- Phenothiazines/antipsychotics
- Verapamil
- Methyldopa, reserpine
- Protease inhibitors

PATHOLOGICAL CAUSES

Prolactin is usually secreted only by the pituitary gland even in pathological conditions and here again, in prolactinomas alone, the size of the pituitary tumor correlates with the serum level of prolactin. Thus, in microprolactinomas the prolactin levels are usually between 100 and 300 ng/mL and in macroadenomas, it is usually well above this range. It is again important to remember that prolactin being under the inhibitory influence of the hypothalamus is elevated even in non-PRL-secreting tumors of the pituitary due to stalk compression. On the same note, any inflammatory condition of the pituitary (granulomatous or lymphocytic hypophysitis) that involves the infundibulum (stalk) also raises prolactin levels. The PRL levels in the latter conditions are usually between 50 and 100 ng/mL only.

In significant head injury affecting sellar-suprasellar area, whether pituitary function is intact or not may be assessed to an extent by PRL levels as its elevated level indicates stalk/hypothalamic injury with normal anterior pituitary functions.

Ectopic secretion of PRL, paraneoplastically, by nonpituitary tumors elsewhere is extremely rare. Similarly, PRL receptor's nonfunctioning mutation causing "resistance" to PRL and thus causing hyperprolactinemia is extremely rare with only countable case reports.

Other Endocrinopathies Causing/Associated with Hyperprolactinemia

Primary hypothyroidism causes significant elevation in PRL. The reasons attributed include elevated thyrotropin-releasing hormone (TRH)-stimulating PRL, alteration in dopaminergic tone, and decreased clearance of PRL. It is wise to wait until euthyroid state is achieved before reassessing PRL and addressing it independently if still elevated.

Mildly raised PRL to the tune of around 30–50 ng/mL is observed, though less frequently, in PCOS. The exact reason is unclear but may be related to hypothalamic factors altering the dopaminergic tone and the effect of estrogen.

MISCELLANEOUS CAUSES

Macroprolactin

In contrast to the normal PRL (23 kDa), "macroprolactin" are PRL molecules that are bound to IgG class of immunoglobulins, increasing their molecular weight several fold. The latter drastically reduces the clearance of PRL, and hence assayed in standard immunoassays. If the sample is centrifuged with polyethylene glycol (PEG) and the supernatant reassayed for PRL, the monomeric true value is obtained. Usually, the macroprolactin level is considered significant if <50% of the initial value is obtained after PEG precipitation.

Chronic Kidney Disease

Macroprolactin and chronic kidney disease (CKD) are the main conditions reducing the clearance of PRL. In mild reduction in glomerular filtration rate (GFR), prolactin may be only mildly elevated but in stage 4 and 5 CKD, PRL elevation (if done for some other reasons) may be quite significant. MRI scan to rule out pituitary lesion needs to be carefully decided based on other clinical correlations.

Estrogen Effect on Prolactin

It is observed that macroprolactinoma patients when conceive on dopamine receptor 2 (D2) agonist therapy (cabergoline/bromocriptine) need to be closely monitored with visual fields for possible increase in size of tumor. This is attributed to the estrogen-related effect (in pregnancy) on lactotrophs. It is generally followed in practice that in macro-/microprolactinoma patients, estrogen (in females) or testosterone (in males) is not started till the PRL is normalized. The latter is due to a possible increase in tumor size. However, there are studies to show that in usual dose of estrogens used on combined pills there is little or no effect on the tumor. Another observation is that in normal pregnancy, despite PRL being high there is no galactorrhea. One of the explanations usually suggested is that the high estrogen levels have a PRL-blocking effect at the mammary gland level. In addition, though suckling of the baby causes reflex increase in PRL secretion, the effect of suckling on the pituitary tumor in a patient conceived on treatment for prolactinoma during postpartum period is controversial.

Idiopathic Hyperprolactinemia

In addition to these explainable conditions, a small proportion of patients (may be up to 10%) may have hyperprolactinemia without discernable causes. It is likely that the pituitary tumor is not picked up by the MRI in many of these cases. Most of them may be asymptomatic (in females, without menstrual disturbance or galactorrhea). Unless there are issues like subfertility, one need not treat the mild hyperprolactinemia. However, as mentioned earlier, MRI may be indicated to rule out non-PRL-secreting pituitary tumors with stalk effect.

Chest Wall/Spinal Cord Lesions

Patients with chest wall injury in upper thoracic (D2 to D6) region, spinal cord lesions, even herpes zoster infection in any of the dermatomes may have reflex (neural) stimulation of PRL. In many of these cases, there may be unilateral galactorrhea.

CLINICAL MANIFESTATION

Premenopausal Females

Prolactin > 100 ng/mL as seen in pathological causes alluded to above usually manifests as expected in a postpubertal female with galactorrhea and oligo/amenorrhea. Any one or both symptoms may be present in almost three-fourths of the cases of true hyperprolactinemia. Thus, even microprolactinomas present quite early in females of reproductive age. Other less common presentations include aggravation of hirsutism, subfertility, and declining bone density (osteoporosis). The oligomenorrhea and hirsutism associated with hyperprolactinemia thus overlap with PCOS and listed in the secondary causes of PCOS. Another manifestation of prolactinoma, in pathological cause of macroadenoma, is pressure symptoms—headache and visual field defects. If prolactinomas occur in peripubertal age group [as in multiple endocrine neoplasia type 1 (MEN1)], delayed puberty or failure of progression of puberty (arrested puberty) may be the main presentation and need to be carefully evaluated.

Postmenopausal Females

Since they are already amenorrhoeic, hyperprolactinemia may be suspected only if they complain of galactorrhea. The breasts of a postmenopausal lady though less in glandular density may still be sensitive to circulating PRL levels, especially if previously lactated. Osteoporosis may be severe in perimenopausal ladies. If galactorrhea is lacking, then large adenomas may be present only with pressure symptoms.

Males

In general, males, especially with prolactinomas, present late with more pressure symptoms of pituitary enlargement (headache and visual disturbance). Any male with gynecomastia, rarely expressive galactorrhea, decreased libido, sexual dysfunction, hypogonadism, subfertility, and osteoporosis/fragility fractures should be evaluated for hyperprolactinemia.

HISTORY AND EXAMINATION

History should focus on the chronology of events and mainly details of medications including complementary and alternative medications. Breast discharge in galactorrhea is always bilateral and clear-cut milky in appearance. Direct clinical examination may be required to confirm galactorrhea in cases where spontaneous breast discharge is not forthcoming. A simple microscopic examination may reveal fat globules in typical galactorrhea in doubtful situations as well as positivity for fat staining. Males usually do not complain of breast discharge, but in severe hyperprolactinemic cases even males may have slight expressive galactorrhea. Subtle signs of hypogonadism in males should be actively looked for, viz., gynecomastia, reduced muscle bulk, softer testes, and kyphosis due to asymptomatic severe vertebral osteoporosis. Visual field examination by confrontation is imperative in all cases where macroadenoma is suspected. Features of MEN1 such as collagenomas in skin should be actively looked for, especially in younger patients.

INVESTIGATIONS

Initial testing for a suspected hyperprolactinemia patient is to get fasting PRL, free T4, and thyroid-stimulating hormone (TSH) levels. As discussed earlier, in patients with pituitary macroadenoma, one needs to get PRL in dilution to rule out "hook effect" and get the panel of anterior pituitary hormones as well. In mildly elevated PRL levels with less or no symptoms, macroprolactin estimation may also be done. Visual field objectively by automated perimetry may also be required for follow-up monitoring. MRI imaging of the sellar area with dynamic contrast imaging is required in microadenomas. Contrast-enhanced MRI is very valuable in diagnosing hypophysitis where stalk dimensions and posterior pituitary bright spot need to be carefully examined. MRI imaging is required even in mild hyperprolactinemic cases also to rule out stalk effect by a nonfunctioning adenoma. Since most of the prolactinomas, respond very well to D2 agonist therapy, baseline imaging for accurate assessment of dimensions and extensions is vital in monitoring the case during follow-up.

MANAGEMENT PRINCIPLES

If drug-induced hyperprolactinemia is suspected, all efforts must be taken to try stopping the drug for at least 2 weeks and recheck PRL again. Extra caution is to be taken if antipsychotic drugs are the incriminating agents. Without a detailed discussion with the psychiatrists withholding the antipsychotic agents or switching to another agent should not be attempted as it may worsen the underlying condition. Similarly, in a patient on treatment for psychosis, if pathological (prolactinoma) causes of hyperprolactinemia are diagnosed, cabergoline or bromocriptine should not be started without informing and having a discussion with the psychiatrist to modify the agents accordingly. PRL associated with hypophysitis or stalk compression normalizes once the inciting factor settles. Similarly, chest wall/local conditions causing elevated PRL are likely to regress once the primary condition is treated.

■ Prolactinomas

Regarding prolactinomas, any symptomatic patient with disturbing galactorrhea or amenorrhea, the treatment of choice is D2 agonists. Cabergoline is the mainstay of treatment for more than two decades now and bromocriptine is less commonly used.

■ Macroprolactinomas

Even in a case of sight-threatening macroprolactinoma, a trial of cabergoline (at least 0.5–1 mg twice a week) should be given and the visual field should be examined frequently. A favorable response is obtained in most of the situations and surgery is most often avoided/deferred. With gradually escalating doses of cabergoline based on PRL values monitored once in 6–8 weeks, most of the patients (almost 70–80%) respond very well and the PRL levels normalize in 3- 6 months. The drug is continued for longer periods of time (sometimes in years) for its good antitumor effect. An MRI may be repeated at 6–12 monthly period to document the same. Other hormones, if normal at baseline, do not get affected with cabergoline therapy alone.

■ Microprolactinomas

Microadenomas, PRL secreting, also respond well to cabergoline therapy and the doses required are much less (usually 0.25–0.5 mg/week). The probability of the microadenoma growing into a macroadenoma is less than 20% over 3–5 years. The biochemical response to cabergoline is good and the PRL normalizes in most of the patients, and the symptoms abate in a few months. Subfertility, again if due to hyperprolactinemia, rapidly improves. In contrast, to macroadenoma, the microadenomas require prolonged cabergoline therapy and often do not regress completely in the MRI. Hence, regular MRI scans for monitoring may not be required.

Adverse Effects to Dopamine Receptor 2 Agonists

Giddiness, nasal stuffiness, and headache may be observed in the initial few doses of cabergoline. It is usually preferred to take it at bedtime and gradually up-titrate the dose over a few months to minimize the adverse effects. Prolonged use of cabergoline especially in years, as may be required in macroprolactinomas, is associated with a possible effect on cardiac valvular fibrosis and hemodynamic effect of stenosis. However, the risk is too low and in a clinically higher-risk patient, regular echocardiogram at yearly intervals may be indicated.

Fertility and Pregnancy during Treatment

The ovulatory functions in females rapidly normalize on correcting the high PRL levels, and hence, the possibility of pregnancy should be discussed at the start of cabergoline in a lady anxious to conceive. There have been several occasions in which the amenorrheic lady did not resume menstruation on starting cabergoline but later confirmed that she had conceived. Hence, barrier contraception is advised to avoid pregnancy till PRL normalizes, and conception is attempted in an anticipated manner. Once confirmed to have pregnancy, in microprolactinomas, the general guideline is to stop cabergoline and clinical follow-up during pregnancy and postpartum period. In macroprolactinomas, cabergoline is continued during pregnancy, as there may be an increase in size during pregnancy and vision may be affected. In postpartum period, generally, cabergoline is avoided to continue lactation uninterruptedly. The decision to restart may be taken when breastfeeding is planned to be stopped.

CONCLUSION

Hyperprolactinemia is not an uncommonly encountered clinical problem not only in gynecology or endocrine practice but also in general physician practice. A basic understanding of physiology and the varied presentation, especially in females, would help in managing patients appropriately. A reliable assay showing PRL levels >100–150 ng/mL usually suggest tumor (micro- or rarely macroadenoma of pituitary). Lesser degrees of hyperprolactinemia should be considered for other causes mainly drugs, hypothyroidism, and PCOS among many. D2 agonist therapy like cabergoline is very effective in controlling hyperprolactinemia and is the treatment of choice even for sight-threatening macroadenomas. Other etiologies of elevated PRL should be treated according to the cause (hypothyroidism, drugs to be withdrawn if possible). Regular follow-up with periodic monitoring is mandatory in tumoral causes of hyperprolactinemia and the outcome is very rewarding.

SUGGESTED READINGS

1. Vilar L, Vilar CF, Lyra R, Freitas MDC. Pitfalls in the diagnostic evaluation of hyperprolactinemia. Neuroendocrinology. 2019;109(1):7-19.
2. Chanson P. Treatments of psychiatric disorders, hyperprolactinemia and dopamine agonists. Best Pract Res Clin Endocrinol Metab. 2022;36(6):101711.
3. Samson SL, Hamrahian AH, Ezzat S; AACE Neuroendocrine and Pituitary Scientific Committee; American College of Endocrinology (ACE). American Association of Clinical Endocrinologists, American College of Endocrinology Disease State Clinical Review: Clinical relevance of macroprolactin in the absence or presence of true hyperprolactinemia. Endocr Pract. 2015;21(12):1427-35.
4. Capozzi A, Scambia G, Pontecorvi A, Lello S. Hyperprolactinemia: pathophysiology and therapeutic approach. Gynecol Endocrinol. 2015;31(7):506-10.
5. Kannan S, Mahadevan S, Sathya A, Sriram U. Prolactin and alternative medicines: a word of caution. Trop Doct. 2008;38(3): 195-6.
6. Kaiser U, Ho K. Pituitary physiology and diagnostic evaluation. In: Melmed S, Auchus RJ, Goldfine AB, Koenig RJ, Rosen CJ (Eds). Williams Textbook of Endocrinology, 14th edition. Philadelphia: Elsevier; 2020. pp. 184-235.

34 CHAPTER

Unusual Presentations of Hypothyroidism

Prakash Keswani, Suchitra Garhwal, Ramji Sharma

ABSTRACT

Hypothyroidism is a common endocrine disorder. Sometimes hypothyroidism can present with atypical findings, which leads to delays in diagnosis and treatment. This may alter the prognosis and course of the disease. Hypothyroidism may present with unusual clinical manifestations related to neurological, psychiatric, reproductive, renal, gastrointestinal, or ophthalmic system. Knowledge of these unusual manifestations of hypothyroidism helps in early diagnosis and treatment of disease conditions.

INTRODUCTION

Hypothyroidism is one of the most common endocrine problems in the general population in India with a prevalence rate of around 11%. The most common etiology of hypothyroidism is autoimmune thyroiditis. Typical clinical features of hypothyroidism are tiredness, cold intolerance, hoarse voice, dry coarse skin, constipation, delayed tendon relaxation, puffy face, hands and feet, alopecia, and bradycardia. Patients with these symptoms are easily suspected and diagnosed as hypothyroid. However, some patients may present with atypical clinical features, which can lead to diagnostic dilemmas and mislead our attention to other diseases. These atypical presentations are diagnosed with hormonal analysis and respond well to thyroxine (T4) therapy. So not to miss, we must be aware of such unusual presentations of hypothyroidism and should consider hypothyroidism when we confront such atypical cases in our day-to-day practice. Here we shall be discussing a few such interesting cases of hypothyroidism.

CASE 1

A 7-year-old female child was brought by her mother to outpatient department (OPD), with a complaint of vaginal bleeding for 2 days. The mother also gives a history of enlargement of bilateral breasts for 3 months. On general examination, height was 111 cm, (corresponding to a height age of 5 years 10 months), and weight was 23.1 kg. Thelarche was present up to Tanner stage 3 but without pubic or axillary hair. On vaginal examination, mucosa was estrogenized. Laboratory investigations revealed an estrogen level of 65 pg/mL, follicle-stimulating hormone (FSH) 7 mIU/mL, luteinizing hormone (LH) 1.3 mIU/mL, and prolactin 72 ng/mL. On ultrasonography, multiple ovarian cysts were seen and the uterus was pubertal in size. A wrist X-ray revealed a bone age of 5 ½ years. Primary thyroid hormone deficiency was seen with low T4 (1.2 µg/dL), low triiodothyronine (T3) (30 ng/dL), and high thyroid-stimulating hormone (TSH) (82 µIU/mL) levels. Her magnetic resonance imaging (MRI) cranium showed an enlarged pituitary gland. Based on the clinical presentation of thelarche, vaginal bleeding without adrenarche and pubarche with retarded height and bone age, pubertal estrogen, and low T3, T4, and high TSH a diagnosis of Van Wyk-Grumbach syndrome was considered. She was started with T4 therapy and responded well to it and had no further episodes of bleeding. On follow-up, her clinical condition improved and cysts were absent on ultrasound (USG).

EFFECT OF HYPOTHYROIDISM ON THE PITUITARY AND REPRODUCTIVE SYSTEM

The association in young females of long-standing primary hypothyroidism, isosexual precocious pseudopuberty, and multicystic enlarged ovaries was first described in 1960 by Van Wyk–Grumbach. Because of negative feedback of low T3 and T4 on the hypothalamus and pituitary, increased levels of thyrotropin-releasing hormone (TRH), TSH, and prolactin is secreted. Excess TSH leads to stimulation of gonadal FSH receptors. This is supported by specific FSH/estrogen-dominated clinical pictures and histopathological findings. It is important to recognize this syndrome because initiating simple thyroid hormone replacement completely resolves symptoms and hormone abnormalities, avoiding unnecessary investigations for other serious diseases and surgical intervention. Phenotypically, girls show the classical "hypothyroid" appearance, delayed growth, FSH-mediated secondary sexual characteristics, breast development with or without galactorrhea, and uterine bleeding but the absence of pubic or axillary hair development.[3,4]

CASE 2

A 29-year-old female presented in the emergency room after a suicidal attempt. She has a history of decreased ability to concentrate, anxiety, insomnia, auditory hallucinations, fatigue, and tiredness. There was no drug history. On physical examination, she was avoiding eye contact, having slow speech, dry skin, periorbital puffiness, enlargement of the thyroid, and sluggish deep tendon reflex (DTR). Her pulse rate (PR) was 58/min and her blood pressure (BP) was 100/64 mm Hg. The patient was admitted with a diagnosis of major depressive disorder with psychotic features and treated with Haloperidol and Paroxetine. On further investigation, her complete blood count, electrocardiography (ECG), liver function test (LFT), and kidney function test were within normal limits. The thyroid function test detected overt hypothyroidism (TSH > 150 μIU/mL, T3 41 ng/dl, T4 1.0 μg/dL, and raised antimicrosomal antibody 506 U/L). The treatment was started with levothyroxine 100 μg/day. Clinically condition of the patient improved remarkably. Following this paroxetine therapy was gradually decreased and discontinued. She continued to do well with T4 therapy and was comfortable with up to 1 year of follow-up.

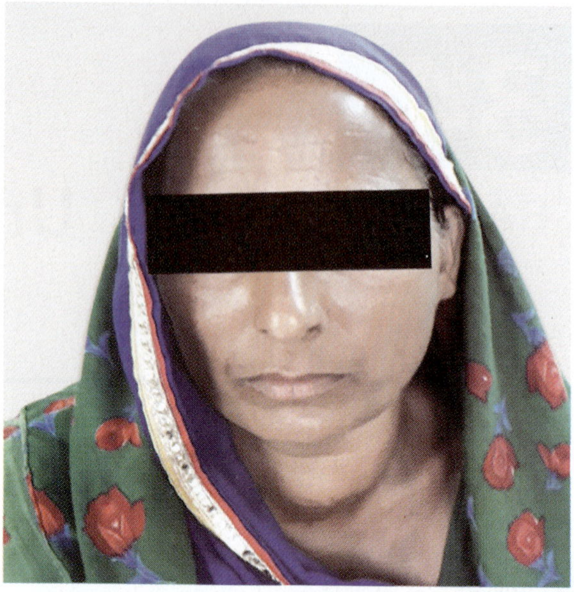

FIG. 1: A case of hypothyroidism with psychiatric manifestation.

CASE 3

A 46-year-old woman presented with altered behavior **(Fig. 1)**. She had a history of irrelevant talks and was anxious, had delusions and hallucinations, and was crying in between. There was no history of psychiatric illness or medical or drug history. On examination, her voice was husky, with slow speech, dry skin, a puffy face, and sluggish DTR. Her PR was 68/min and her BP was 110/80 mm Hg. The rest of the systemic examination was normal. On laboratory examination, overt hypothyroidism was seen (TSH 139 μIU/mL, T3 25 ng/dL, and T4 1.6 μg/dL). Tablet levothyroxine was started at 150 μg/day and her behavioral problems improved. Diagnosis of myxedema madness was considered and haloperidol was discontinued. About 2 months later patient came to the OPD and had no complaints. About 4 months later patient returned back with a recurrence of auditory and visual hallucinations. On evaluation, she gave a history of omission of treatment for 2 months, and repeat TSH was 120 μIU/mL. She was restarted with levothyroxine and 2 weeks later, hallucinations disappeared.

HYPOTHYROIDISM AND PSYCHIATRIC DISORDERS

It is less commonly known that hypothyroidism can induce various psychiatric disorders that include severe depression, frank psychosis, irritability, agoraphobia, dementia, and melancholia, and it has been recognized as early as 1888. Disorganized agitated states also have been described as crying, hyperactivity, insomnia, irritability, anger, and both auditory and visual hallucinations (1947) and have been labeled as "myxedema Madness." Depressive syndrome and manic depression (bipolar) are also described with hypothyroidism. Clinically these patients present with apathy, anergia, depressed mood, disturbed sleep, and fatigue. Patients presenting with such manifestations are often misdiagnosed as having a primary psychiatric illness, which delays treatment.

CASE 4

A 36-year-old female was admitted with a complaint of generalized swelling, generalized weakness, and drowsiness **(Fig. 2)**. On physical examination, the patient was drowsy and had hoarseness of voice, anasarca, and pale conjunctivae. Her PR was 80/min and her BP was 130/100 mm Hg. Investigations done in the emergency laboratory revealed hemoglobin (Hb) 7 g/dL, serum creatinine 2.1 mg/dL, serum protein 4.6 g/dL, serum albumin 2.2 g/dL, random blood sugar (RBS) 76 mg/dL, serum Na 131 mEq/L, serum potassium (sK) 4.1 mEq/L, and serum uric acid 7.3 mg/dL. On the next day morning round provisional diagnosis of renal failure was considered and low dose diuretics were started along with other supportive measures. The next day routine investigations confirmed these reports and her thyroid functions revealed gross hypothyroidism (TSH>150 µIU/mL, T3 30 ng/dL, and T4 1.2 µg/dL). On ultrasonographic examination, kidney size was normal with maintained

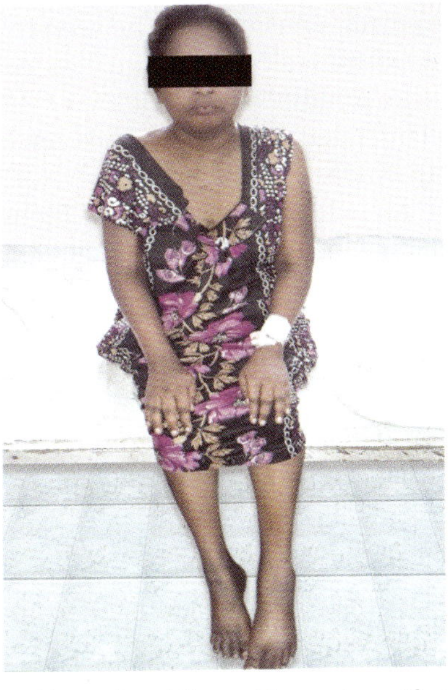

FIG. 2: A case of hypothyroidism with renal manifestation.

corticomedullary differentiation. Diagnosis of primary hypothyroidism was considered and T4 100 µg daily was started and one packed red cell (PRC) transfusion was given. After 5 days of treatment, her swelling reduced, creatinine came down to 1.8 mg/dL and consciousness also improved. On follow-up after 1 month, her creatinine level fell to 1.2 mg/dL and her TSH level was 25 µIU/mL.

EFFECT OF HYPOTHYROIDISM ON RENAL FUNCTION

Hypothyroidism leads to a decrease in renal plasma flow by 25 %, glomerular filtration rate by 20–30%, and also a decrease in renal tubular absorption of secreted solutes. Factors contributing to decreased glomerular filtration rate (GFR) are low serum atrial natriuretic peptide (ANP) levels, afferent renal arteriolar constriction, and thickening of the glomerular basement membrane (GBM). Long-standing hypothyroidism has been found to be associated with decreased creatinine clearance and elevated serum creatinine which are found to revert back with T4 replacement.

In patients with chronic renal failure (CRF), hypothyroidism results in deterioration of renal function, which improves with T4 therapy. Hence, serum TSH should be measured in patients with unexplained deterioration in renal function to rule out hypothyroidism[7].

CASE 5

A 45-year-old female presented with fatigue, lethargy, weakness and breathlessness. On physical examination, periorbital puffiness and pitting edema of feet and hands were present, and jugular venous pulse (JVP) was raised favoring cardiac failure **(Figs. 3A and B)**. Her PR was 90/min, her BP was 90/70 mm Hg, and her apical impulse was absent. On further investigations Hb was 9.8g/dL, RBS was 81 mg/dL, LFT and renal function test were within normal limits. The lipid profile was deranged with serum cholesterol 286 mg/dL, LDL 157 mg/dL, and serum Tg 191 mg/dL. Serum creatine phosphokinase (CPK) was elevated. Her Chest X-ray (CXR) showed typical bottle-shaped cardiomegaly and her echocardiography showed pericardial effusion. On further investigation, a thyroid function test revealed TSH >150 µIU/mL, T3 30 ng/dL, and T4 1.2 µg/dL and was diagnosed as primary hypothyroidism with pericardial effusion. She was started with tab T4 in low doses (50 µg/day) and while keeping a watch on cardiac functions, the dose increased to 125 µg/day in 10 days. She improved symptomatically and her pericardial effusion also decreased significantly.

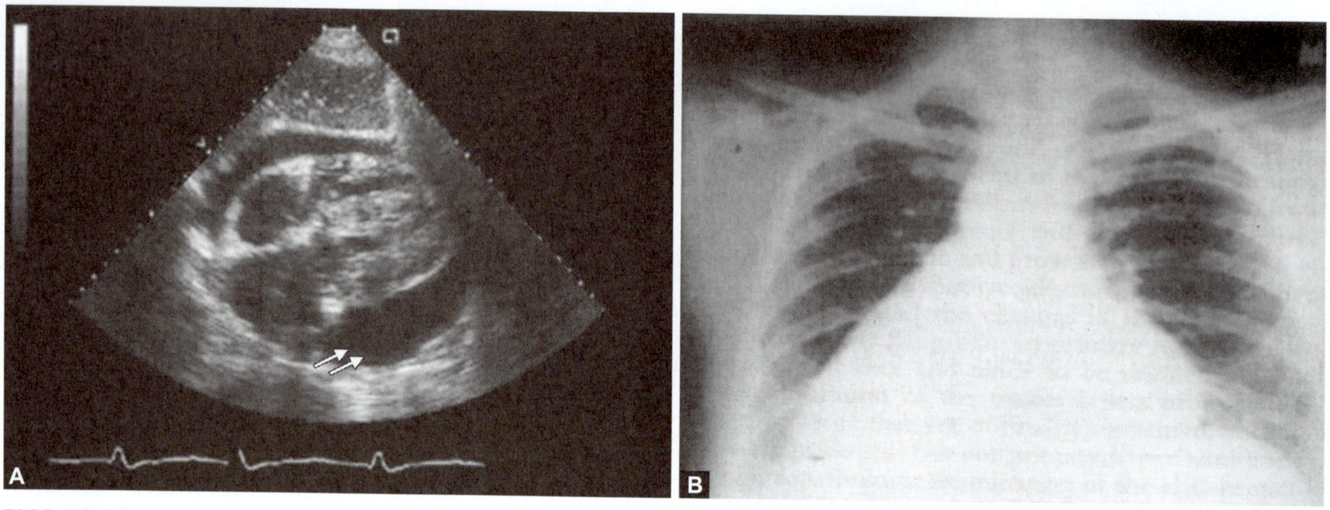

FIGS. 3A AND B: Two-dimensional (2D) echo and chest X-ray showing pericardial effusion.

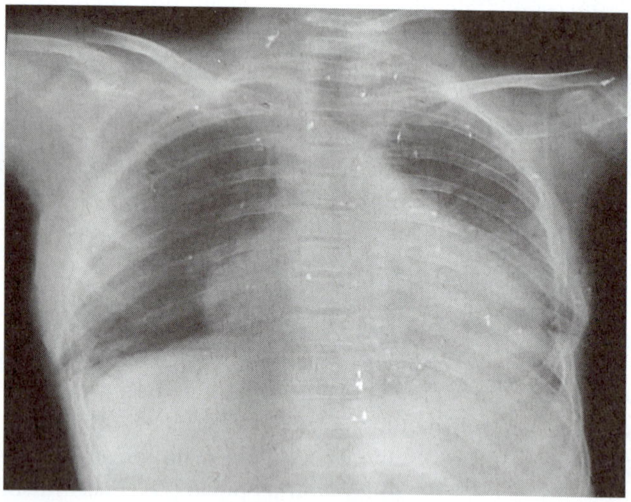

FIG. 4: Chest X-ray showing cardiomegaly.

CASE 6

A 19-year-old female patient presented with a complaint of menorrhagia for 15 days, breathlessness, and severe weakness **(Fig. 4)**. On examination, her pulses were feeble, and severe pallor and edema were present. The patient had oligomenorrhea with menorrhagia for 3 years. The patient received a 2-unit PRC transfusion 1 day ago. As the patient was in shock, inotrope support was started and bleeding was controlled by giving tranexamic acid and ethamsylate. ECG was low voltage and CXR showed cardiomegaly suggestive of pericardial effusion. On investigation, complete blood count (CBC) showed Hb 4.3 g/dL, serum iron was 77, total iron-binding capacity (TIBC) 282, ferritin 113.8, B12 634, and folate 14.73. Advanced hematology report showed reticulocytes at 3% and IPF at 25%. The patient was transfused with multiple PRC and inotrope support was tapered. The thyroid profile of the patient was TSH was 528 μIU/mL, T3 0.01 pg/dL, and T4 0.42 ng/dL. Thyroxine therapy was started with all precautions. The patient's USG showed a follicular cyst of 25 × 21 mm with minimal inter-bowel free fluid. A 2D echo was done which showed moderate pericardial effusion with normal left ventricular (LV) systolic function (EF 55%). After starting treatment, the condition of the patient improved.

EFFECT OF HYPOTHYROIDISM ON FLUID ACCUMULATION

In hypothyroidism, effusions can be seen in pericardial, pleural, and peritoneal spaces and less commonly in joints and the middle ear. Pericardial effusions are usually small but large effusions can be seen in prolonged severe hypothyroidism. Fluid analysis shows high protein and cholesterol with high viscosity. Pleural effusion may be unilateral or bilateral. The exact mechanism of pleural effusion is not clear but changes in permeability is proposed mechanism for effusion. Ascites is a rare and poorly understood complication of severe hypothyroidism. Ascitic fluid is yellow gelatinous peritoneal exudate with a high protein content of the fluid (>2.5 g/dL) and a high serum-ascites fluid albumin gradient.

CASE 7

A 62-year-old hypertensive man came with a complaint of weakness in both lower limbs. He was feeling unsteady on his feet, losing his balance, and was no longer able to walk without assistance. The patient also gave a history of hoarseness of voice and constipation. There was no history of drug or alcohol ingestion. On examination, PR was 74/min, BP was 168/86 mm Hg, along with a hoarse voice and dry skin. On neurological examination, power was normal in all four limbs, but dysarthric speech, finger-nose-finger test, dysdiadokokinesia, heal-shin test, and Romberg test were positive. The gait of the patient was abnormal as the patient had impaired tandem walking. Deep tendon reflexes showed delayed relaxation. A provisional diagnosis of cerebellar ataxia was made, but the etiology was not clear. On laboratory investigations, CBC, renal function test (RFT), and LFT were within normal limits. Serum CPK was 427 U/L and anti-microsomal antibody titer was 1:1,600. The thyroid function test of the patient was abnormal with high TSH (88 mIU/mL), and low T4 (2.1 μg/dL), T3 (50 ng/dL). CT scan of the head was normal. The patient was started with a tablet of levothyroxine 125 μg/day and the patient's condition improved. He was discharged and referred to a rehabilitation center. On follow-up after 3 months, his neurological examination and thyroid function test were normal.

EFFECT OF HYPOTHYROIDISM ON NEUROLOGICAL DISORDERS

Hypothyroidism has been found to affect the central and peripheral nervous system. Mononeuropathy (carpel tunnel syndrome being commonest), polyneuropathy, and cranial nerve (II, V, VII, and VIII) neuropathy are usual presentations, while generalized peripheral neuropathy and cerebellar ataxia are unusual presentations associated with hypothyroidism. Clinical Society of London has described gait unsteadiness in patients of hypothyroidism as early as 1888. Patients may have loss of equilibrium, unsteadiness on their feet, and lack of coordination of their extremities. Other neurologic disorders that may be seen in hypothyroidism are myopathy, pseudomyotonia, muscle hypertrophy, and seizures. Most patients eventually recover by using thyroid hormone treatment.

CASE 8

A 50-year-old male presented with abdominal distension, abdominal pain and not passing stool for the last 3 days. On examination, PR was 74/min, BP was 130/90 mm Hg, abdominal distension was present and bowel sounds were absent. A provisional diagnosis of paralytic ileus and suspicion of intestinal obstruction was considered. On laboratory investigations, CBC, RFT, and LFT were within normal limits, serum Na was 130 mEq/L and sK 3.0 mEq/L. USG abdomen revealed gaseous distension and no other pathology was observed. On further investigations, the thyroid function test detected overt hypothyroidism with TSH 125 μIU/mL, T4 1.6 μg/dL, and T3 35 ng/dL. Hence, a diagnosis of primary hypothyroidism with paralytic ileus was made and the patient was started on levothyroxine 150 μg/day. The patient was given the support of intravenous (IV) fluids constipation was managed conservatively and electrolytes were corrected. After starting treatment, the condition of the patient improved.

EFFECT OF HYPOTHYROIDISM ON GIT

Deficiency of thyroid hormone can cause decreased gut motility and hypotonia throughout the gastrointestinal tract. The pathophysiology may include a decrease in the electric and motor activities of the gut, a decrease in the number and frequency of muscle contractions in the colon and the rectum, and prolonged gastric emptying. Motility disturbance may be severe enough to cause ileus or megacolon and patients may resemble to an intestinal obstruction as in our case. It would be reasonable to rule out hypothyroidism before surgery is undertaken for intestinal obstruction of unclear cause.

CASE 9

An 8-year-old child presented with growth retardation **(Fig. 5)**. His height was 104 cm and weighed 18 kg. His chronological age was 8 years, height age was 4 ¾ years, weight age was 6 years, and bone age was 4 years. This boy was a disproportionate dwarf with retarded bone age.

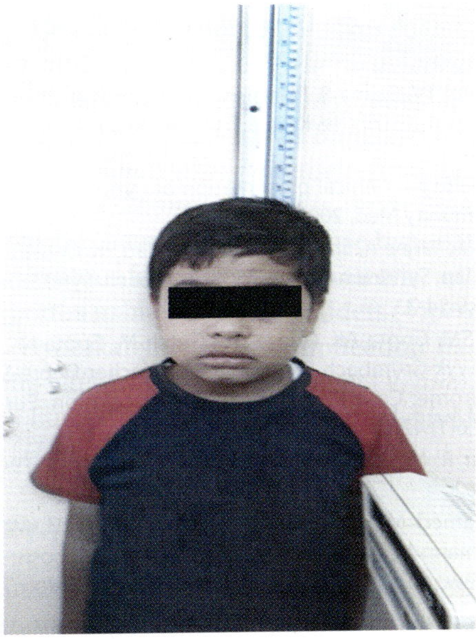

FIG. 5: A case of hypothyroidism with growth failure.

Anterior Pituitary Insufficiency

Anterior pituitary insufficiency is the most well-recognized endocrine manifestation of SBE. This is commonly seen in snakebites due to Russel's viper envenomation (RVE) (*D. russelii* and *D. siamensis*).

Pathophysiology

The pituitary gland which is encased in a bony cavity sella turcica easily gets compressed on getting enlarged or engorged. The anterior pituitary gets its blood supply from the superior hypophyseal artery and is more prone to compression by the enlarged pituitary gland which leads to ischemic damage of the gland it supplies. The following mechanisms have been postulated for the vascular insufficiency of the gland following RVE:

- Engorgement of the gland due to capillary leak syndrome (CLS)
- Microthrombi deposition or hemorrhage due to disseminated intravascular coagulation (DIC) compromising pituitary vascular supply
- Alteration in the pituitary intravascular pressure due to CLS
- Minor alteration in intrasellar pressure compresses the anterior pituitary blood vessels in the compact bony sella turcica.
- Hypotension due to circulatory shock could also result in ischemic damage similar to the pathophysiology seen in postpartum hemorrhage leading to shock and then causing Sheehan's syndrome.
- Direct toxic effects of Russel's viper venom on the pituitary cells as shown in the animal experiments
- Autoantibodies developed against the pituitary antigens which are released due to pituitary tissue necrosis during acute episodes could be contemplated in the pathogenesis of RVE-associated delayed HP.

Clinical Features

Based on the duration at which the clinical features of snake envenomation appear after the bite, hypopituitarism could be categorized as either acute or delayed hypopituitarism.

Acute Hypopituitarism

Acute-onset API has been reported after RVE in many studies starting from the first day to 2 weeks of bite. AI is the cardinal clinical presentation of API but because of the overt systemic presentations of snake envenomation, it is very often missed.

In refractory hypotension which responds only to glucocorticoids, detection of hypoglycemia or hyponatremia could warrant a clinical possibility of this endocrine complication. Along with the secondary AI, central hypothyroidism should also be looked for. Low thyroid-stimulating hormone (TSH) levels along with low or normal thyroxine (T4) levels could help to diagnose central hypothyroidism in the acute phase though several other conditions could mimic it. API may be transient or may continue as a subclinical course into chronic HP.

Chronic or Delayed Hypopituitarism

This is the continuation phase of acute HP, either following an acute presentation or as a result of occult pituitary tissue damage secondary to a venomous snakebite. The mean time to diagnose delayed HP in a South Indian study was around 8 years. Chronic HP could be dormant or may appear slowly many weeks or years after the snake envenomation in the form of vague fatigue, loss of weight, and loss of appetite. Different studies have shown different pituitary axes involvement due to snake envenomation. Cortisol and growth hormone (GH) axes were commonly involved in one study and somatotrophs followed by gonadotroph were involved in another study. Clinical manifestations of the gonadotroph axis depend on whether the pituitary damage occurred before puberty or later. Gonadotroph axis involvement before puberty could lead to primary amenorrhea and loss of secondary sexual characteristics. Pituitary damage occurring later would lead to secondary amenorrhea, erectile dysfunction, infertility, loss of libido, and loss of secondary sexual characteristics.

Precipitating or the Risk Factors for the Development of Anterior Pituitary Insufficiency

Studies have shown that patients with certain complications during the acute phase of RVE could predict the possible development of API as follows:

- Serious manifestations in the form of AKI, mechanical ventilation, CLS, and DIC
- AKI needing hemodialysis, high 20-minute whole blood clotting time at presentation
- Multiorgan dysfunction, thrombocytopenia, and bleeding tendency needing blood transfusions

Diagnosis

Acute Hypopituitarism

Many factors affect the assessment of hormone levels and make the accurate diagnosis of acute HP difficult in acute settings like snake envenomation as levels of cortisol would be otherwise low. We need to prove hypocortisolism to diagnose API, and the criteria are different for the acute phase as given below:

- Fasting serum cortisol <3 μg/dL (83 nmol/L)
- Random serum cortisol <5 μg/dL (138 nmol/L) in suspected pituitary apoplexy

- Random serum cortisol <10 μg/dL (275 nmol/L) in a critically ill patient)
- Postcosyntropin peak cortisol <18 μg/dL (500 nmol/L)
- Postcosyntropin delta cortisol <9 μg/dL (250 nmol/L)
- The diagnosis of involvement of the gonadotropic axis is difficult as the levels of luteinizing hormone (LH), follicle-stimulating hormone (FSH), testosterone, and estradiol are otherwise low in any critical illness.

Thus, the diagnosis of API is done based on the clinical features such as unexplained and refractory hypotension in a patient with AKI, CLS, and DIC with the laboratory evidence of hyponatremia and hypoglycemia with or without imaging modalities showing pituitary hemorrhage or infarction.

Chronic or Delayed Hypopituitarism

Any patient with features of hypogonadism, central hypothyroidism, secondary AI, or GH deficiency with a past history of snake envenomation should alert the clinician regarding the possibility of chronic HP as a complication of venomous snakebite.

Imaging

In the majority of the HP cases, the imaging shows normal sella in the first year following pituitary injury due to RVE but in the later years, it shows partial or total empty sella.

Management

Having suspected API, we need to start intravenous hydrocortisone for the management of AI. But thyroxine supplementation needs to be started only after correcting the AI to avoid an adrenal crisis resulting from the thyroxine-induced accelerated metabolic clearance of cortisol. Maintenance and continuation of hormone replacement depend on the reevaluation of pituitary axes done, 4–6 weeks after the recovery.

Involvement of Posterior Pituitary Following Snake Envenomation

The inferior hypophyseal artery supplies the posterior pituitary gland directly, and hence it would withstand the vascular insult effectively. Thus, it is very rare to find the features of posterior pituitary insufficiency following a venomous snakebite. But there are few reports of central diabetes insipidus following RVE. However, the occurrence is more due to the damage of the hypothalamus rather than the posterior pituitary.

Diabetes insipidus manifests as the passing of large quantities of hypotonic urine which occurs due to absolute deficiency (central) or relative by way of resistance (nephrogenic) to the actions of arginine vasopressin (AVP). The central form of diabetes insipidus due to snake envenomation, though very rare, has been reported in the literature. If there is API in the form of hypocortisolism, the characteristic clinical symptom, the polyurea may not be there but it could promptly appear after the cortisol replacement. The treatment is oral or nasal desmopressin.

ADRENAL INSUFFICIENCY AS A COMPLICATION OF SNAKE ENVENOMATION

Adrenal insufficiency is of two types:

1. Primary AI
2. Secondary AI

Secondary AI occurs as a consequence of API following SBE. However, primary involvement of the adrenal gland due to snake envenomation is very rare. It can occur due to adrenal hemorrhage (AH). Refractory hypotension, hypoglycemia, hyponatremia, and hyperkalemia in a case of snake envenomation should rise suspicion of primary AI.

METABOLIC AND ELECTROLYTE ABNORMALITIES AS COMPLICATIONS OF SNAKE ENVENOMATION

Dysglycemia

Hyperglycemia

Hyperglycemia is a not so common endocrine complication of SBE. The pathophysiology seems to be due to the release of massive amount of catecholamines as seen in scorpion envenomation. Activation of alpha receptors by these catecholamines preventing the release of insulin is thought to be the cause of this. There could be also release of counterregulatory hormones such as glucagon and cortisol which could further increase the blood sugars. This phenomenon is seen in pediatric population as well as adult victims of venomous snakebite.

Hypoglycemia

Intractable hypoglycemia indicates API.

ELECTROLYTE DISTURBANCES

Electrolyte imbalance which is not related to pituitary insufficiency or AI has been observed in snake envenomation.

Hyponatremia

Etiopathogenesis

Studies have confirmed that the decrease in serum sodium is a result of urinary salt loss due to the natriuretic peptides present in the snake venom rather than that of syndrome of inappropriate antidiuretic hormone secretion (SIADH) as thought earlier.

Clinical Features

The clinical features of hyponatremia in snake envenomation could vary in severity from being totally asymptomatic to deep coma depending upon the severity and rapidity with which it occurs.

Management

Since this hyponatremia is not due to SIADH, fluid restriction as a corrective measure is not advised and is promptly corrected by intravenous saline administration. In case of chronic hyponatremia, cautious and slow correction is contemplated in order to prevent osmotic demyelination. When there is a possibility of AI, supplementation of glucocorticoids is mandatory.

Hypokalemia

Life-threatening hypokalemia resulting in muscle weakness which is independent of the neurotoxicity has been described due to snake envenomation. The intracellular redistribution of potassium due to the venom toxins seems to be a more suitable explanation. There could be associated hypomagnesemia due to the venom toxin-induced renal tubular damage resulting in urinary excretion of magnesium, especially following viperine bites.

Hypokalemia could manifest as simple muscle cramps, constipation, abdominal bloating, and polyuria or as serious muscle weakness such as periodic paralysis, cardiac arrhythmias, rhabdomyolysis, and respiratory failure. Management is similar to any other type of hypokalemic periodic paralysis in the form of oral or intravenous potassium replacement. But, since this is a venom-induced redistributive type of hypokalemia, there is always a risk of rebound hyperkalemia which one should look for. Correction of concomitant hypomagnesemia is needed if present.

Hyperkalemia

Hyperkalemia is a complication of snake envenomation which occurs not directly but secondary to the other complications of snake envenomation such as rhabdomyolysis and AKI and could be life-threatening. T4RTA which occurs as a result of venom toxin-induced renal injury can also be a cause of hyperkalemia. The treatment involves potassium-lowering therapy and in severe cases hemodialysis.

Type 4 Renal Tubular Acidosis

Type 4 renal tubular acidosis is characterized by hyperkalemia, normal anion gap metabolic acidosis, and inappropriately low urine transtubular potassium gradient (TTKG). Most of the time, this is a transient phenomenon which occurs due to either direct effect of venom toxins on the renal tubules or renal damage in the early phase of snake envenomation. Most of the time, there has been a good recovery following fludrocortisone therapy. Hyperkalemia needs standard therapy.

CONCLUSION

Clinicians need to be aware and vigilant of endocrine complications of venomous snakebite. Whenever the clinical features do not fit into standard snake envenomation and the response to antisnake venom (ASV) is not satisfactory, endocrine complications should be thought of. Prompt diagnosis and management of endocrine complications could be lifesaving.

SUGGESTED READINGS

1. Waiddyanatha S, Silva A, Siribaddana S, Isbister GK. Long-Term Effects of Snake Envenoming. Toxins (Basel). 2019;11(4):193.
2. Bhattacharya S, Nagendra L, Tyagi P. Snakebite Envenomation and Endocrine Dysfunction. In: Feingold KR, Anawalt B, Blackman MR (Eds). Endotext [Internet]. South Dartmouth (MA): MDText.com, Inc.; 2000. Available from https://www.ncbi.nlm.nih.gov/books/NBK575924/ [Last accessed November, 2023].
3. Bhattacharya S, Krishnamurthy A, Gopalakrishnan M, Kalra S, Kantroo V, Aggarwal S, et al. Endocrine and Metabolic Manifestations of Snakebite Envenoming. Am J Trop Med Hyg. 2020;103(4):1388-96.
4. Roy A, Suryadevara V, Nagarajan K, Sahoo J, Naik D, Perumal NL, et al. Pituitary Dysfunction Following Snakebite Envenomation: A Clinico–Radiological Assessment of 15 Cases and Review of the Literature. Neurol India. 2022;70(5):2093-99.
5. Wolff H. Is it time to denominate hypopituitarism after snake bite? QJM. 2013;106(4):390.
6. Wolff H. Insufici ˆencia hipofis ´aria anterior por picada de of´ıdio. Arq Bras Endocrinol Metab. 1958;7:25-47.
7. Eapen CK, Chandy N, Kochuvarkey KL, Zacharia PK, Thomas PJ, Ipe TI. An Unusual Complication of Snake Bite: Hypopituitarism after Vper Bites. In: Ohsaka A, Hayashi K, Sawai Y, Murata R,

Funatsu M, Tamiya N (Eds). Animal, Plant, and Microbial Toxins. New York: Springer; 1976. pp. 467-73.
8. Tun-Pe, Phillips RE, Warrell DA, Moore RA, Tin-Nu-Swe, Myint-Lwin, et al. Acute and chronic pituitary failure resembling Sheehan's syndrome following bites by Russell's viper in Burma. Lancet. 1987;2(8562):763-7.
9. Burke CW. The anterior pituitary, snakebite and Sheehan's syndrome. Q J Med. 1990;75(276):331-3.
10. Antonypillai CN, Wass JA, Warrell DA, Rajaratnam HN. Hypopituitarism following envenoming by Russell's vipers (Daboia siamensis and D. russelii) resembling Sheehan's syndrome: first case report from Sri Lanka, a review of the literature and recommendations for endocrine management. QJM. 2011;104(2):97-108.
11. Jeevagan V, Katulanda P, Gnanathasan CA, Warrell DA. Acute pituitary insufficiency and hypokalaemia following envenoming by Russell's viper (Daboia russelii) in Sri Lanka: exploring the pathophysiological mechanisms. Toxicon. 2013;63:78-82.
12. Lakhotia M, Pahadiya HR, Singh J, Gandhi R, Bhansali S. Adrenal hematoma and right hemothorax after echis carinatus bite: an unusual manifestation. Toxicol Int. 2014;21(3):325-7.
13. Luksic B, Culic V, Stricevic L, Brizic I, Poljak NK, Tadic Z. Infant death after nose-horned viper (Vipera ammodytes ammodytes) bite in Croatia: A case report. Toxicon. 2010;56(8):1506-9.
14. Mao YC, Liu PY, Chiang LC, Liao SC, Su HY, Hsieh SZ, et al. Bungarus multicinctus multicinctus snakebite in Taiwan. Am J Trop Med Hyg. 2017;96(6):1497-504.
15. Kankananarachchi I, Fernando MP, Denipitiya T, Navabalasooriyar P, Kitulwatte NC. Persistent hyponatraemia following suspected krait envenomation in a 5-year-old Sri Lankan child: a case report. Ceylon Med J. 2018;63(1):24-5.
16. Ho PL, Soares MB, Maack T, Gimenez I, Puorto G, Furtado MF, et al. Cloning of an unusual natriuretic peptide from the South American coral snake Micrurus corallinus. Eur J Biochem. 1997;250(1):144-9.
17. Wium CA, Marks CJ, Du Plessis CE, Muller GJ. Berg adder (Bitis atropos): An unusual case of acute poisoning. South Afr Med J. 2017;107(12):1075-7.
18. de Silva U, Sarathchandra C, Senanayake H, Pilapitiya S, Siribaddana S, Silva A. Hyponatraemia and seizures in Merrem's hump-nosed pit viper (Hypnale hypnale) envenoming: a case report. J Med Case Rep. 2018;12(1):213.
19. Malina T, Krecsak L, Jelic D, Maretic T, Toth T, Sisko M, et al. First clinical experiences about the neurotoxic envenomings inflicted by lowland populations of the Balkan adder, Vipera berus bosniensis. Neurotoxicology. 2011;32(1):68-74.
20. Denis D, Lamireau T, Llanas B, Bedry R, Fayon M. Rhabdomyolysis in European viper bite. Acta Paediatr. 1998;87(9):1013-5.
21. Weerakkody RM, Lokuliyana PN, Lanerolle RD. Transient distal renal tubular acidosis following hump nosed viper bite: Two cases from Sri Lanka. Saudi J Kidney Dis Transpl. 2016;27(5): 1018-20.
22. Gawarammana IB, Mudiyanselage Kularatne SA, Kularatne K, Waduge R, Weerasinghe VS, Bowatta S, et al. Deep coma and hypokalaemia of unknown aetiology following Bungarus caeruleus bites: exploration of pathophysiological mechanisms with two case studies. J Venom Res. 2010;1:715.
23. Struyk AF, Cannon SC. Paradoxical depolarization of BA2+-treated muscle exposed to low extracellular K+: insights into resting potential abnormalities in hypokalemic paralysis. Muscle Nerve. 2008;37(3):326-37.
24. Gopalakrishnan M, Vinod KV, Dutta TK, Shaha KK, Sridhar MG, Saurabh S. Exploring circulatory shock and mortality in viper envenomation: a prospective observational study from India. QJM. 2018;111(11):799-806.
25. Than Than, Francis N, Tin-Nu-Swe, Myint-Lwin, Tun-Pe, Soe Soe, et al. Contribution of focal haemorrhage and microvascular fibrin deposition to fatal envenoming by Russell's viper (Vipera russelli siamensis) in Burma. Acta Trop. 1989;46(1):23-38.
26. Myint-Lwin, Warrell DA, Phillips RE, Tin-Nu-Swe, Tun-Pe, Maung-Maung-Lay. Bites by Russell's viper (Vipera russelli siamensis) in Burma: haemostatic, vascular, and renal disturbances and response to treatment. Lancet. 1985;2(8467):1259-64.
27. Sherif IH, Vanderley CM, Beshyah S, Bosairi S. Sella size and contents in Sheehan's syndrome. Clin Endocrinol (Oxf). 1989;30(6):613-8.
28. Diri H, Karaca Z, Tanriverdi F, Unluhizarci K, Kelestimur F. Sheehan's syndrome: new insights into an old disease. Endocrine. 2016;51(1):22-31.
29. Hart GR, Proby C, Dedhia G, Yeo TH, Joplin GF, Burrin JM. Burmese Russell's viper venom causes hormone release from rat pituitary cells in vitro. J Endocrinol. 1989;122(2):485-94.
30. Goswami R, Kochupillai N, Crock PA, Jaleel A, Gupta N. Pituitary autoimmunity in patients with Sheehan's syndrome. J Clin Endocrinol Metab. 2002;87(9):4137-41.
31. De Bellis A, Kelestimur F, Sinisi AA, Ruocco G, Tirelli G, Battaglia M, et al. Anti-hypothalamus and anti-pituitary antibodies may contribute to perpetuate the hypopituitarism in patients with Sheehan's syndrome. Eur J Endocrinol. 2008;158(2):147-52.
32. Proby, Tha-Aung , Thet-Win, Hla-Mon, Burrin JM, Joplin GF. Immediate and long-term effects on hormone levels following bites by the Burmese Russell's viper. Q J Med. 1990;75(276): 399-411.
33. Rajagopala S, Thabah MM, Ariga KK, Gopalakrishnan M. Acute hypopituitarism complicating Russell's viper envenomation: case series and systematic review. QJM. 2015;108(9):719-28.
34. Golay V, Roychowdhary A, Dasgupta S, Pandey R. Hypopituitarism in patients with vasculotoxic snake bite envenomation related acute kidney injury: a prospective study on the prevalence and outcomes of this complication. Pituitary. 2014;17(2):125-31.
35. Naik BN, Bhalla A, Sharma N, Mokta J, Singh S, Gupta P, et al. Pituitary dysfunction in survivors of Russell's viper snake bite envenomation: A prospective study. Neurol India. 2018;66(5):1351-8.
36. Bhat S, Mukhopadhyay P, Raychaudhury A, Chowdhury S, Ghosh S. Predictors of hypopituitarism due to vasculotoxic snake bite with acute kidney injury. Pituitary. 2019;22(6):594-600.
37. Shivaprasad C, Aiswarya Y, Sridevi A, Anupam B, Amit G, Rakesh B, et al. Delayed hypopituitarism following Russell's viper envenomation: a case series and literature review. Pituitary. 2019;22(1):4-12.
38. Gupta UC, Garg OP, Kataria ML. Cranial diabetes insipidus due to viper bite. J Assoc Physicians India. 1992;40(10):686-7.
39. Christ-Crain M, Bichet DG, Fenske WK, Goldman MB, Rittig S, Verbalis JG, et al. Diabetes insipidus. Nat Rev Dis Primers. 2019;5(1):1-20.
40. Golay V, Roychowdhary A, Pandey R, Pasari A, Praveen M, Arora P, et al. Growth retardation due to panhypopituitarism and central diabetes insipidus following Russell's viper bite. Southeast Asian J Trop Med Public Health. 2013;44(4):697-702.
41. Krishnan MN, Kumar S, Ramamoorthy KP. Severe panhypopituitarism and central diabetes insipidus following

snake bite: unusual presentation as torsades de pointes. J Assoc Physicians India. 2001;49:923-4.
42. Garrahy A, Moran C, Thompson CJ. Diagnosis and management of central diabetes insipidus in adults. Clin Endocrinol (Oxf). 2019;90(1):23-30.
43. Claudet I, Grouteau E, Cordier L, Franchitto N, Bréhin C. Hyperglycemia is a risk factor for high-grade envenomations after European viper bites (Vipera spp.) in children. Clin Toxicol (Phila). 2016;54(1):34-9.
44. Bahloul M, Turki O, Chaari A, Bouaziz M. Incidence, mechanisms and impact outcome of hyperglycaemia in severe scorpion-envenomed patients. Ther Adv Endocrinol Metab. 2018;9(7):199-208.
45. Ronen JA, Gavin M, Ruppert MD, Peiris AN. Glycemic Disturbances in Pheochromocytoma and paraganglioma. Cureus. 2019;11(4):e4551.
46. Audebert F, Sorkine M, Bon C. Envenoming by viper bites in France: clinical gradation and biological quantification by ELISA. Toxicon. 1992;30(5-6):599-609.
47. Trinh KX, Khac QL, Trinh LX, Warrell DA. Hyponatraemia, rhabdomyolysis, alterations in blood pressure and persistent mydriasis in patients envenomed by Malayan kraits (Bungarus candidus) in Southern Vietnam. Toxicon. 2010;56(6):1070-5.
48. Vink S, Jin AH, Poth KJ, Head GA, Alewood PF. Natriuretic peptide drug leads from snake venom. Toxicon. 2012;59(4):434-45.
49. Kumar Keyal N, Shrestha R, Thapa S, Adhikari P. Krait Snake Bite Presenting as a Cerebral Salt Wasting. Indian J Crit Care Med. 2019;23(7):347-8.
50. Höjer J, Tran Hung H, Warrell D. Life-threatening hyponatremia after krait bite envenoming–a new syndrome. Clin Toxicol (Phila). 2010;48(9):956-7.
51. Spasovski G, Vanholder R, Allolio B, Annane D, Ball S, Bichet D, et al. Clinical practice guideline on diagnosis and treatment of hyponatraemia. Eur J Endocrinol. 2014;170(3):G1-47.
52. Kularatne SA. Common krait (Bungarus caeruleus) bite in Anuradhapura, Sri Lanka: a prospective clinical study, 1996-98. Postgrad Med J. 2002;78(919):276-80.
53. Aye KP, Thanachartwet V, Soe C, Desakorn V, Thwin KT, Chamnanchanunt S, et al. Clinical and laboratory parameters associated with acute kidney injury in patients with snakebite envenomation: a prospective observational study from Myanmar. BMC Nephrol. 2017;18(1):92.
54. Weiner ID, Wingo CS. Hypokalemia–consequences, causes, and correction. J Am Soc Nephrol. 1997;8(7):1179-88.
55. Kardalas E, Paschou SA, Anagnostis P, Muscogiuri G, Siasos G, Vryonidou A. Hypokalemia: a clinical update. Endocr Connect. 2018;7(4):R135-46.
56. Batlle D, Arruda J. Hyperkalemic Forms of Renal Tubular Acidosis: Clinical and Pathophysiological Aspects. Adv Chronic Kidney Dis. 2018;25(4):321-33.
57. Karunarathne S, Udayakumara Y, Govindapala D, Fernando H. Type IV renal tubular acidosis following resolution of acute kidney injury and disseminated intravascular coagulation due to hump-nosed viper bite. Indian J Nephrol. 2013;23(4):294-6.

SECTION

4

GASTROENTEROLOGY

36
CHAPTER

Approach to a Case of Refractory Ascites

Meenakshi Bhattacharya, Prashant Gajbhare, Prashant Dhumal, Ashish Gandhi

ABSTRACT

Refractory ascites is recurrence of ascites that cannot be mobilized or prevented from recurring (i.e., after therapeutic paracentesis) by medical therapy. It may be diuretic resistant or diuretic intractable ascites. Approximately 5–10% of patients with cirrhosis and ascites become refractory to standard therapy as indicated by randomized trials. Portal hypertension and renal sodium retention are two important factors for formation of ascites. Prognosis of refractory ascites is poor and it is usually associated with complications, such as hepatorenal syndrome, spontaneous bacterial peritonitis (SBP), and dilutional hyponatremia. Adherence to strict dietary sodium restriction, frequent large volume paracentesis (LVP), albumin infusion, and transjugular intrahepatic portosystemic shunt (TIPS) may help improve patient's quality of life; however, liver transplantation remains the definitive therapeutic intervention for refractory ascites.

INTRODUCTION

Refractory ascites ('intractable ascites', 'resistant ascites', or 'problematic ascites') is defined as ascites that does not recede or that recurs rapidly after therapeutic paracentesis, despite dietary sodium restriction and maximum tolerable doses of diuretics (spironolactone 400 mg/day and furosemide 160 mg/day). Diuretic resistant and diuretic intractable ascites are two subtypes of refractory ascites. Diuretic resistant ascites is ascites not responsive to dietary sodium restriction and intensive diuretic treatment. Diuretic intractable ascites is ascites that is refractory to treatment due to the development of diuretic induced complications. Diuretic induced complications are hepatic encephalopathy (HE) in absence of other precipitating factors, diuretic induced renal failure [increase in serum creatinine by >100% to a value above 2 mg/dL in patients of ascites responding to diuretics, diuretic induced hypokalemia (serum potassium <3 mEq/L) or hyperkalemia (serum potassium >6 mEq/L)].

The modified diagnostic criteria (International Club of Ascites) for refractory ascites are as follows:

- *Treatment duration*: Patients must be on intensive diuretic therapy (spironolactone 400 mg/day and furosemide 160 mg/day) for at least 1 week and on a salt-restricted diet of <90 mmol/day or 5.2 g of salt/day.
- *Lack of response*: Mean weight loss of <0.8 kg over 4 days and urinary sodium output less than the sodium intake.
- *Early ascites recurrence*: Reappearance of grade 2 or 3 ascites within 4 weeks of initial mobilization.
- *Diuretic-induced complications*:
    - Diuretic induced HE: Development of encephalopathy in the absence of any other precipitating factor.
    - Diuretic induced renal impairment: Increase of serum creatinine by >100% to a value >2 mg/dL in patients with ascites responding to treatment.
    - Diuretic-induced hyponatremia: Decrease of serum sodium by >10 mmol/L to a serum sodium of <125 mmol/L.

in ascites formation. TIPS is an effective treatment option for refractory ascites in selected patients. TIPS is superior to LVP in controlling ascites, and recent evidence shows a survival advantage in carefully selected patients with low MELD (Model for End stage Liver Disease) scores. Younger patients with portal hypertension benefit most, while higher age or MELD scores decrease transplant-free survival. TIPS can be a definitive treatment or bridge therapy to liver transplant. TIPS insertion has various complications. Immediate ones include arrhythmia, hemoperitoneum, and liver capsule rupture (rare in experienced hands). Early post-TIPS complications involve shunt migration, shunt kinking, and ischemic hepatitis. Endotipsitis causing continuous bacterial infections can be the troubling complication. Hepatic encephalopathy (HE) is a major clinical complication, affecting 30–50% of patients. Risk factors for HE are age, Child–Pugh/MELD scores, prior spontaneous HE episodes, sarcopenia, and lower portal systemic pressure post TIPS. Under-dilation or smaller diameter stents may reduce post TIPS HE risk. Pre-emptive lactulose and rifaximin improve HE control. Cardiac failure can develop due to increased cardiac output after TIPS, particularly in patients with pre-existing cardiac dysfunction.

Appropriate patient selection is essential for successful TIPS outcomes and reducing complications. Age >70 years, MELD score >18, previous spontaneous HE ≥ grade 2, cardiac failure, pulmonary hypertension, liver cancer, sepsis, or portal vein thrombosis are considered contraindications for TIPS placement.

Automated Low-flow Ascites Pump

It is a rechargeable programmable device which pumps ascites from the peritoneal cavity into the bladder, discharging it as urine. It performs continuous small volume paracentesis for up to 16 hours during awake hours. The device has sensors to stop pumping when there is minimal or no ascites. The discharge rate can be adjusted based on the patient's dietary sodium consumption, allowing individualized management of ascites. Typically, alfapump use does not require concomitant albumin infusions.

Alfapump effectively controls ascites, reducing paracentesis frequency and volume. Initial complications have decreased with improved techniques and prophylactic antibiotics. Some patients may still develop renal dysfunction due to continuous paracentesis. Monitoring and intermittent albumin may be needed. Contraindications to this modality are severe renal dysfunction, previous infections or surgeries, bladder cancer, solid organ transplantation, and high bilirubin levels. Improved quality of life and mortality is observed in patients tolerating alfapump. Survival outcomes are comparable to regular LVP, but formal studies are lacking.

LIVER TRANSPLANTATION

For patients with refractory ascites and advanced liver disease, liver transplantation is the ultimate treatment option. It addresses the underlying liver dysfunction and provides a definitive cure for ascites. Those patients having complications related to portal hypertension, but not having severe liver dysfunction, have lower priority for transplant. After transplantation, ascites may persist temporarily due to hemodynamic adjustments, so a sodium-restricted diet is advised until ascites resolves **(Flowchart 1)**.

PROGNOSIS

Refractory ascites carries poor prognosis, with significantly increased mortality rates. The prognosis depends on the underlying liver disease, the response to treatment, and the availability of liver transplantation. Clearance of ascites with TIPS improves quality of life, nitrogen balance, muscle gain, and survival. Studies suggest improved post TIPS survival with an 8-mm covered stent compared to a 10-mm covered stent.

Refractory ascites poses a significant challenge in the management of patients with advanced liver disease. A multidisciplinary approach involving hepatologists, gastroenterologists, and surgeons is necessary to address the complex nature of this condition. With appropriate diagnostic evaluation and a comprehensive treatment plan, focusing on both medical and procedural interventions, it is possible to improve the quality of life and outcomes for patients with refractory ascites.

CONCLUSION

Refractory ascites is a relatively common condition in patients with decompensated liver cirrhosis. Dietary compliance improves quality of life of RA patients. Various treatment options are available, although definitive treatment is liver transplantation.

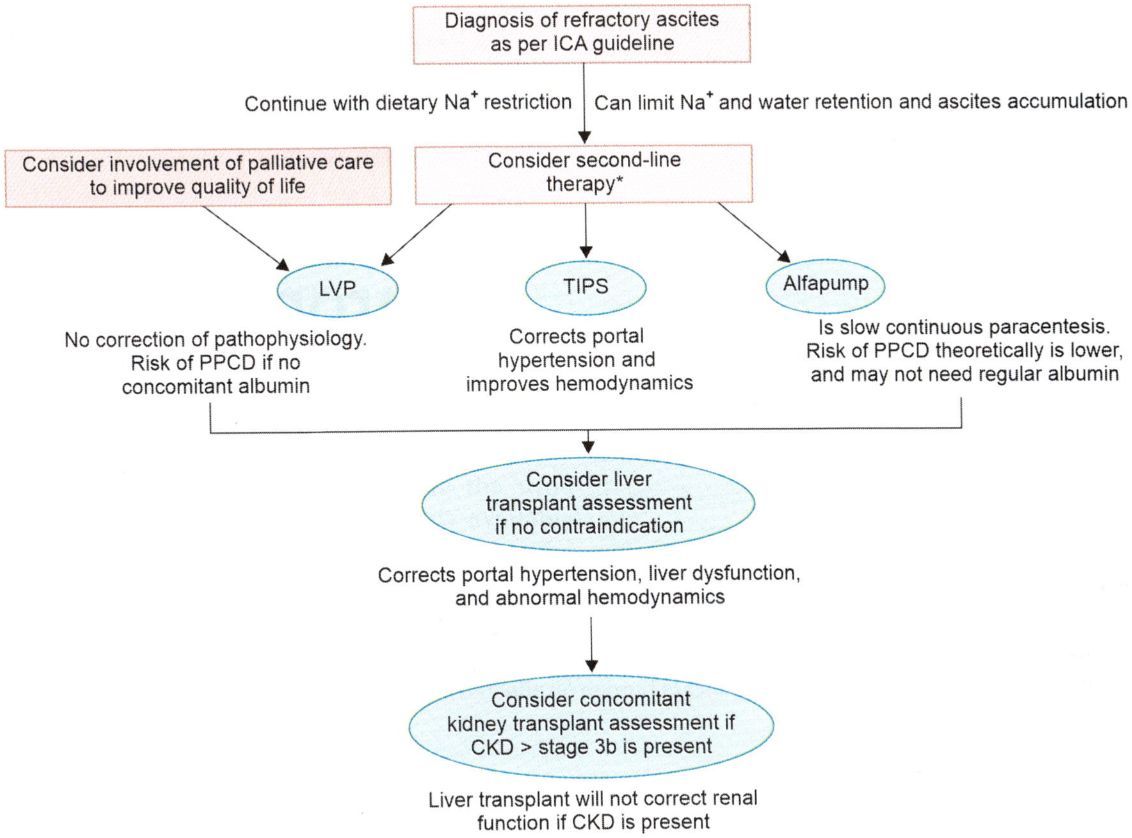

FLOWCHART 1: Algorithm on diagnosis of refractory ascites as per ICA guidelines.

(Alfapump: automated low-flow ascites pump; CKD: chronic kidney disease; ICA: International Club of Ascites; LVP: large volume paracentesis; PPCD: postparacentesis circulatory dysfunction; TIPS: transjugular intrahepatic portosystemic shunt)

SUGGESTED READINGS

1. Siqueira F, Kelly T, Saab S. Refractory Ascites: Pathogenesis, Clinical Impact, and Management. Gastroenterol Hepatol (NY). 2009;5(9):647-56.
2. Salerno F, Guevara M, Bernardi M, Moreau R, Wong F, Angeli P, et al. Refractory ascites: pathogenesis, definition and therapy of a severe complication in patients with cirrhosis. Liver Int. 2010; 30:937-47.
3. Madoff DC, Cornman-Homonoff J, Fortune BE, Gaba RC, Lipnik AJ, Yarmohammadi H, et al. Management of Refractory Ascites Due to Portal Hypertension: Current Status. Radiology. 2021;298(3):493-504.
4. Aithal GP, Palaniyappan N, China L, Härmälä S, Macken L, Ryan JM, et al. Guidelines on the management of ascites in cirrhosis. Gut. 2021;70(1):9-29.
5. Vidal González D, Pérez López KP, Vera Nungaray SA, Moreno Madrigal LG. Treatment of refractory ascites: Current strategies and new landscape of non-selective beta-blockers. Gastroenterol Hepatol. 2022;45(9):715-23.
6. Arroyo V, Ginès P, Gerbes AL, Dudley FJ, Gentilini P, Laffi G, et al. Definition and diagnostic criteria of refractory ascites and hepatorenal syndrome in cirrhosis. International Ascites Club. Hepatology. 1996;23(1):164-76.
7. Wong F. Management of refractory ascites. Clin Mol Hepatol. 2023;29(1):16-32.
8. Runyon BA. Management of adult patients with ascites due to cirrhosis: an update. Hepatology. 2009;49(6):2087-107.
9. Moore KP, Wong F, Gines P, Bernardi M, Ochs A, Salerno F. The management of ascites in cirrhosis: report on the consensus conference of the International Ascites Club. Hepatology. 2003;38(1):258-66.
10. Ginès P, Titó L, Arroyo V, Planas R, Panés J, Viver J, et al. Randomized comparative study of therapeutic paracentesis with and without intravenous albumin in cirrhosis. Gastroenterology. 1988;94(6):1493-502.
11. Salerno F, Cammà C, Enea M, Rössle M, Wong F. Transjugular intrahepatic portosystemic shunt for refractory ascites: a meta-analysis of individual patient data. Gastroenterology. 2007;133(3):825-34.
12. European Association for the Study of the Liver. EASL clinical practice guidelines on the management of ascites, spontaneous bacterial peritonitis, and hepatorenal syndrome in cirrhosis. J Hepatol. 2010;53(3):397-417.
13. European Association for the Study of the Liver. EASL Clinical Practice Guidelines for the management of patients with decompensated cirrhosis. J Hepatol. 2018;69(2):406-60.
14. Martín-Llahí M, Guevara M, Torre A, Fagundes C, Restuccia T, Gilabert R, et al. Prognostic importance of the cause of renal failure in patients with cirrhosis. Gastroenterology. 2011;140(2):488-96.e4.

CAUSES OF CHRONIC DIARRHEA

There is a wide range of possible causes of chronic diarrhea that need to be considered. It may be helpful to attempt to distinguish malabsorptive diarrhea from inflammatory and secretory causes to help focus on investigations. Particularly in malabsorption, steatorrhea or complaints of bulky malodorous stool can be present **(Box 2)**.

INITIAL APPROACH IN PATIENTS WITH CHRONIC DIARRHEA

Patients with persistent diarrhea must undergo a thorough physical examination and medical history taking in order to be evaluated. Clinicians should initially consider the patient's family history of conditions like celiac disease or inflammatory bowel disease when taking the medical history. In the past, the differential diagnosis of diarrhea was focused on the mechanisms that caused it. Therefore, the evaluation of indications, symptoms, and analytical tests that are suggestive of an organic disease constitutes the first step in the diagnostic procedure. Alarming symptoms or unusual blood test results indicate an organic cause as shown in **Flowchart 1**. In these circumstances, diarrhea might be classified as inflammatory, watery, or malabsorption-related (steatorrhea). Alarm signs consist of:

- Development of symptoms after age 50 years
- Rectal bleeding/melena
- Diarrhea or nighttime agony

BOX 2: Possible causes of chronic diarrhea.

Common:
- Functional bowel disorders (including IBS-diarrhea)
- Bile acid diarrhea
- Dietary-related colonic neoplasia
- *Inflammatory bowel disease*: Ulcerative colitis, Crohn's disease, and microscopic colitis
- Celiac disease
- Drug causes
- Overflow diarrhea

Infrequent:
- Small bowel bacterial overgrowth
- Mesenteric ischemia
- Lymphoma
- Chronic pancreatitis
- *Surgical causes*: Small bowel resections, fecal incontinence, internal fistulae, etc.
- Radiation enteropathy
- Pancreatic carcinoma
- *Endocrine causes*: Hyperthyroidism, diabetes, hypoparathyroidism, and Addison's
- Giardiasis (and other chronic infections)

Rare:
- *Other small bowel enteropathies*: Whipple's disease, tropical sprue, amyloid, intestinal lymphangiectasia, etc.
- Autonomic neuropathy
- *Hormone secreting tumors*: VIPoma, gastrinoma, and carcinoid
- Factitious diarrhea

(IBS: irritable bowel syndrome; VIPoma: vasoactive intestinal peptide tumor)

Source: Adapted from British Society of Gastroenterology (BSG) (2018).

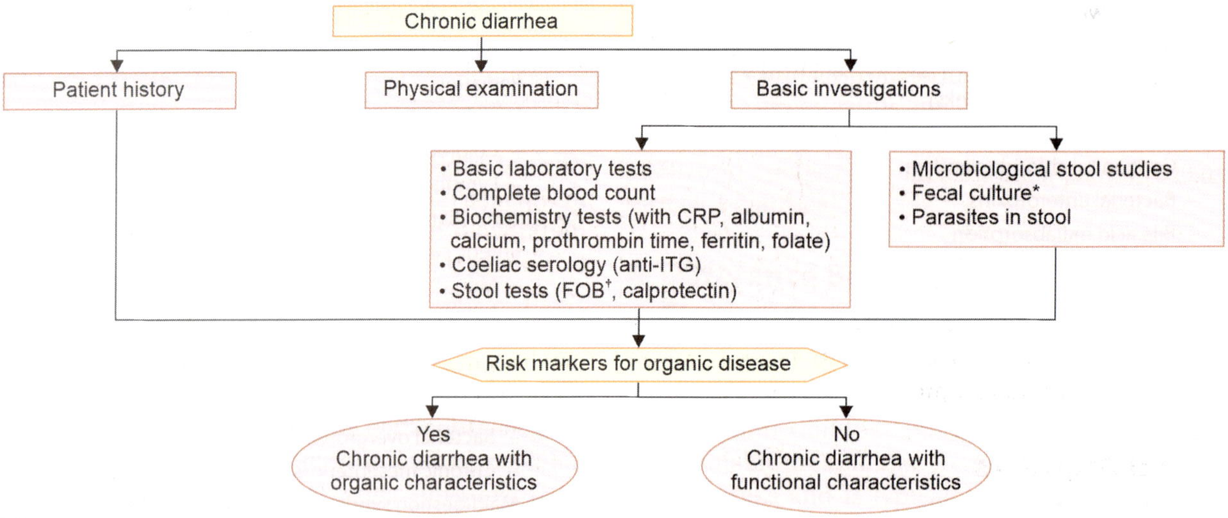

*Fecal culture is only indicated in immunocompromised patients or patients receiving immunosuppressants (in many cases these tests may have been performed during the acute phase of the disease before the duration of symptoms suggests a chronic process).

†The fecal occult blood test has a high sensitivity for intestinal inflammation.

FLOWCHART 1: The initial approach in patients with chronic diarrhea.

(CRP: C-reactive protein; FOB: fecal occult blood; tTG: tissue transglutaminase IgA test)

Source: Adapted from Fernández-Bañares et al.

- Escalating stomach discomfort
- A fever or other unusual systemic symptoms
- Laboratory abnormalities such as high fecal calprotectin or occult blood, raised erythrocyte sedimentation rate (ESR) and C-reactive protein (CRP), iron deficiency anemia
- First-degree relative with colorectal cancer or inflammatory bowel disease

GUIDELINES FOR THE EXAMINATION OF PERSISTENT DIARRHEA IN ADULTS FROM THE BRITISH SOCIETY OF GASTROENTEROLOGY

Clinical Evaluation

- Advocate using a thorough background to organize your inquiries.
- Suggest screening blood tests to rule out conditions, such as anemia and celiac disease, as well as stool testing to check for inflammation.
- Following routine blood and stool tests and recommend a positive diagnosis of irritable bowel syndrome (IBS).

Inflammation or Cancer

- Encourage colonoscopy to rule out colorectal cancer in people with changed bowel habits or rectal bleeding.
- In primary or secondary care, recommend fecal immunochemical testing for fecal blood loss as a rule-out test or to expedite investigations in patients who have lower gastrointestinal symptoms (chronic diarrhea) but no rectal bleeding.
- Fecal calprotectin is advised for IBS suspects under the age of 40 years to rule out colonic inflammation.

Additional Clinical Evaluation

- Referral for additional investigations is advised if symptoms continue despite standard initial tests and therapy.
- Blood and stool testing are advised to rule out malabsorption and recurrent infections (particularly in elderly or immunocompromised patients).

Typical Disorders

- Depending on local availability, either the blood bile acid precursor 7alpha-hydroxy-4-cholesten-3-one (7αHCO or 7αC4) test or the selenium-75-homocholic acid taurine (75SeHCAT) test should be used to confirm a diagnosis of bile acid diarrhea in individuals with functional bowel syndrome or IBS.
- To rule out microscopic colitis, a colonoscopy with nonrectal biopsies of the right and left colon is advised.

Malabsorption

- If lactose maldigestion is thought to be present, suggest having hydrogen breath test (if available) or lactose/carbohydrate avoidance.
- Depending on availability, magnetic resonance imaging (MRI) is advised to evaluate small bowel disorders.
- Depending on local availability, video capsule endoscopy (VCE) is advised for the examination of small intestinal abnormalities.
- Due to their low sensitivity and specificity, barium enteroscopy and barium enteroclysis are not advised for the examination of small bowel disorders.
- Enteroscopy is not advised for the diagnosis of chronic diarrhea; rather, it is only advised for specific lesions found by MRI or VCE.
- If fat malabsorption is thought to be present, a fecal elastase test is advised.
- If chronic pancreatitis is suspected, MRI rather than computed tomography (CT) is advised to evaluate structural abnormalities of the pancreas.
- Since there is little data to support routine hydrogen or methane breath testing, an empirical treatment of antibiotics is advised, if small intestinal bacterial overgrowth is suspected.

Structural and Surgical Issues

- Endoanal ultrasonography and anorectal manometry should only be used when all other conservative therapies have failed, and another local pathology has been ruled out.
- Offer MRI or CT with contrast follow-up as radiologic modalities for the study of fistulae.

Unique Causes

Because hormone-secreting tumors seldom cause diarrhea, testing is only advised after other potential reasons have been ruled out.

TREATMENT/MANAGEMENT

In order to treat chronic diarrhea, one must first identify the underlying reason (if one is known), firm up the bowel motions, and address any difficulties brought on by the diarrhea. When feasible, the underlying cause of chronic

TABLE 1: Treatment options in chronic diarrhea.

Drug class	Mode of action and indication	Agent	Dose
Opiates (mu opiate receptor selective)	Inhibition of motility, proabsorptive, and symptomatic treatment for most cases of chronic diarrhea	Loperamide	2–4 mg, four times daily
		Morphine	2–20 mg, four times daily
		Diphenoxylate	2.5–5 mg, four times daily
		Codeine	15–60 mg, four times daily
		Tincture of opium	2–20 drops, four times daily
Alpha-2 adrenergic agonist	Proabsorptive, diabetic diarrhea, VIPoma, and autonomic neuropathy	Clonidine	0.1–0.3 mg, three times daily
Somatostatin analog	Proabsorptive, hormonal antagonist, neuroendocrine tumors, fistulas, and a small bowel resection	Octreotide	50–250 μg, three times daily (subcutaneously)
NSAID	Inhibition of prostaglandin synthesis, inoperable and villous adenoma, radiation proctitis, and medullary carcinoma	Indomethacin	25 mg, three times daily
Antibiotics	Small bowel bacterial overgrowth (intermittent treatment), *Clostridium difficile*	Metronidazole, rifaximin, quinolones, and vancomycin	
Bile acid-binding resin	Binding of bile acids and bacterial toxins, ileal disease, and postcholecystectomy diarrhea	Cholestyramine	4 g, one to four times daily
		Colesevelam	625 mg, up to six times daily
		Colestipol	4 g, one to four times daily
Fiber supplements	Water binding	Calcium polycarbophil	5–10 g daily
		Psyllium	10–20 g daily

(NSAID: nonsteroidal anti-inflammatory drug; VIPoma: vasoactive intestinal peptide tumor)

diarrhea should be identified and treated. The course of treatment will rely on the precise diagnosis determined by the initial testing. It may be necessary to use empiric treatment if testing reveals no diagnosis or if the disease has no known cure. Opiate receptor agonists with a focus on the gastrointestinal tract are frequently used as first-line empiric therapy. A safe mu-receptor agonist called loperamide is employed to lessen intestinal peristalsis.

Eliminating a meal or medicine may be the only necessary treatment in some circumstances:

- For those who are lactose intolerant, this includes avoiding lactose-containing meals and beverages.
- Some medicines (such as laxatives and antacids) can also cause diarrhea.
- Other components that are known to cause diarrhea include sugar-free products manufactured with sorbitol and foods made with fat substitutes.

Given in **Table 1** is a list of pharmacological treatments for treating chronic diarrhea, many of which are symptomatic. Various additional causative therapy alternatives, such as food in celiac disease or lactose intolerance, or medications targeted against the underlying cause of diarrhea, should not be neglected in favor of symptomatic treatment approaches. There is no simple and logical algorithm to govern the empiric treatment of chronic diarrhea in every patient. Therefore, a thoughtful trial-and-error approach is frequently required to find the most effective therapy or combination of therapies for each patient.

CONCLUSION

Through a comprehensive analysis of published literature, it is concluded that a multidisciplinary approach, including dietary modifications, medication, and lifestyle changes, is essential in effectively managing chronic diarrhea, alleviating symptoms, and improving patients' overall well-being.

SUGGESTED READINGS

1. Nemeth V, Pfleghaar N. Diarrhea. In: StatPearls [Internet]. Treasure Island (FL): StatPearls Publishing; 2023. [online] Available from https://www.ncbi.nlm.nih.gov/books/NBK448082/ [Last accessed December, 2023].
2. Fine KD, Schiller LR. AGA technical review on the evaluation and management of chronic diarrhea. Gastroenterology. 1999;116(6):1464-86.
3. Hammer HF. Management of chronic diarrhea in primary care: The gastroenterologists' advice. Dig Dis. 2021;39(6):615-21.
4. Descoteaux-Friday GJ, Shrimanker I. Chronic Diarrhea. In: StatPearls [Internet]. Treasure Island (FL): StatPearls Publishing; 2023. [online] Available from https://www.ncbi.nlm.nih.gov/books/NBK544337/ [Last accessed December, 2023].
5. Fernández-Bañares F, Accarino A, Balboa A, Domènech E, Esteve M, Garcia-Planella E, et al. Chronic diarrhoea: Definition, classification and diagnosis. Gastroenterol Hepatol. 2016;39(8):535-59.
6. Hiner GE, Walters JR. A practical approach to the patient with chronic diarrhoea. Clin Med (Lond). 2021;21(2):124-6.
7. Arasaradnam RP, Brown S, Forbes A, Fox MR, Hungin P, Kelman L, et al. Guidelines for the investigation of chronic diarrhoea in adults: British Society of Gastroenterology, 3rd edition. Gut. 2018;67(8):1380-99.

38

CHAPTER

Hepatitis in Immunocompromised

BB Rewari, Priyanka Ojha

ABSTRACT

Viral hepatitis, especially B and C, is a major health problem world over and in India. India also has second highest burden of human immunodeficiency virus (HIV) globally (though a low prevalence). HIV response in India has seen significant reduction in new infections and acquired immunodeficiency syndrome (AIDS) related deaths. There has been significant coverage with antiretroviral therapy (ART) over the years after the free ART program was rolled out in 2004. The National Viral Hepatitis Control Program (NVHCP) launched in 2018 is providing free diagnostic and treatment services for persons with chronic hepatitis B and C.

Around 6–8% of people living with HIV also have chronic hepatitis B or C due to common modes of transmission. The natural history of both HIV and hepatitis infections is altered in the presence of other leading to rapid progression. There are some drug–drug interaction among drugs used for their treatment and also decision on which treatment to be initiated may sometime be tricky. The present chapter deals with some of these issues.

INTRODUCTION

Chronic hepatitis B and C infection are major public health problems globally. Approximately 354 million individuals worldwide are chronically infected with hepatitis, 296 with hepatitis B virus (HBV), and 58 million with chronic hepatitis C virus (HCV); among these, approximately 1 million die because of end-stage liver disease (ESLD) or hepatocellular carcinoma (HCC). In 2022, it was reported that 39.0 million (33.1–45.7 million) people globally were living with HIV with 1.3 million new infections and 690,000 acquired immunodeficiency syndrome (AIDS)-related deaths annually. Globally, the estimated prevalence and burden of HCV coinfection among people living with HIV are 6.2% (interquartile range 3.4–11.9%) and HBV coinfection rates are 7.6% (interquartile range 5.6–12.1%).

The guidelines for management of hepatitis B and C have been simplified over the years and availability of direct-acting antivirals (DAAs) for HCV offer a potential for cure in almost 90–95% of those with HCV. HBV can be very well prevented by good vaccination program and managed adequately with simple drugs, though the treatment is lifelong in most of the cases.

However, the management of hepatitis in immunocompromised host needs additional considerations. The most common cause of immune suppression among people is HIV infection with 38 million people living with HIV globally. This chapter will focus mainly on presentation and management of hepatitis among those with HIV but also cover other conditions leading to immune suppression, such as certain autoimmune disorders and those on chemotherapy for malignancy.

HEPATITIS AND HUMAN IMMUNODEFICIENCY VIRUS COINFECTION

Hepatitis B virus, HIV, and HCV share similar transmission routes. In general, concurrent, or sequential infection with these viruses usually results in more severe and progressive liver disease and a higher incidence of cirrhosis, hepatocellular carcinomas (HCC), and mortality. Human immunodeficiency virus and HCV have common routes of transmission, and people living with HIV, especially people who inject drugs and men who have sex with men, have an increased risk of HCV infection.

Liver disease has emerged as a leading cause of death in HIV-infected persons coinfected with either hepatitis B or C, as mortality due to other HIV-related conditions has declined following the introduction of ART. Viral hepatitis is an increasing cause of morbidity and mortality among people living with HIV, including those on ART. In a large study, compared with HIV-only patients, HBV-coinfected patients had 42% higher mortality, HCV-coinfected patients had 65% higher mortality and patients with both HCV and HBV coinfections had 123% higher mortality. A comprehensive approach includes prevention, HBV and HCV testing, hepatitis B vaccination, and treatment and care for people with HIV, who are coinfected with hepatitis B and/or hepatitis C.

Human Immunodeficiency Virus and Hepatitis B Coinfection

Approximately 10% of all the HIV-infected people are also chronically coinfected with HBV, with differences related to the variability in prevalence of HBV in the areas. A factsheet published by National Viral Hepatitis Surveillance Programme in India estimated a national seroprevalence of hepatitis B as 0.95 (0.89–1.01). The risk of developing chronic infection is 90% following perinatal infection (up to 6 months of age) but decreases to 20–60% between the ages of 6 months and 5years. Infection in adulthood leads to chronic hepatitis in <5% of the cases in immunocompetent individuals. However, several studies have documented an increased risk of chronic infection in adults with immunocompromised state including HIV infection.

Natural History among Human Immunodeficiency Virus and Hepatitis B-coinfected Patients

The evidence suggests that HIV infection profoundly influences the course of HBV infection; persons have higher serum HBV-deoxyribonucleic acid (DNA) polymerase activity, lower rates of loss of serum hepatitis B e antigen (HBeAg) leading to rapid progression, increased risk of cirrhosis, liver related mortality, and hepatocellular carcinoma especially at lower CD4 T-cell counts.

The HBV infection also negatively impacts the progression of HIV infection leading to faster immune deterioration and higher mortality. The HIV-hepatitis-coinfected persons show faster CD4 decline, slower CD4 recovery following ART, increased incidence of AIDS and non-AIDS events, increased rate of antiretroviral drug (ARV) toxicity and increased chances of immune reconstitution hepatitis. Hence, all the people newly diagnosed with HIV should therefore be screened for hepatitis B surface antigen (HBsAg).

Evaluation of Human Immunodeficiency Virus and Hepatitis B-coinfected Persons

All persons newly diagnosed with HIV should be screened for HBsAg. Those found positive for HBsAg should be evaluated further following the guidelines for the evaluation of those with hepatitis B infection according to the technical guidelines for management of hepatitis B, National Viral Hepatitis Control Program (NVHCP), MoH&FW. Besides routing clinical evaluation, one should look for sign of cirrhosis and hepatic decompensation, such as jaundice, conjunctival hemorrhages, anemia, spider angioma, palmar erythema, petechiae, clubbing, gynecomastia, testicular atrophy, parotid enlargement, asterixis (liver flaps and flapping tremors), caput medusa, ascites, edema, longitudinal veins alongside of abdomen, hepatomegaly, hepatic bruit, venous hum, and splenomegaly.

The laboratory investigations, besides routine hemogram and chemistry, should specifically include liver function test (LFT), prothrombin time, alpha-fetoprotein (AFP), ultrasound, and upper gastrointestinal (GI) endoscopy wherever indicated. The virological examination should include HBV-DNA quantitative.

One important component in evaluation is the staging of cirrhosis. Earlier invasive techniques like liver biopsy were used and Metavir score (F0–F4) was done. But now, newer techniques like liver elastography (Fibroscan) are used to measure liver stiffness and determine the stage of liver cirrhosis. Noninvasive techniques such as the AST to Platelet Ratio Index (APRI) and fibrosis 4 (FIB-4) score are recommended under the NVHCP.

Treatment of Human Immunodeficiency Virus and Hepatitis B-coinfected Patients

All HIV positive patients with HBV coinfection should start dual anti-HIV and HBV therapy irrespective of CD4 count, HBV viral load or status of liver disease, e.g., ALT level or fibrosis stage.

The recommended nucleotide reverse transcriptase inhibitor (NRTI) regimen presently is tenofovir disoproxil fumarate (TDF) + 3TC + dolutegravir (DTG). Fortunately, TDF, a drug widely included in almost all ART regimens, is also the most effective drug for long-term treatment of HBV, leading to sustained HBV viral suppression, reversal of cirrhosis and fibrosis and reduction in HBV-related mortality. All people coinfected with HIV and HBV should therefore receive a TDF-based ART regimen in combination with 3TC, as the NRTI backbone of an ART regimen, regardless of stage of disease or HBV-DNA level.

This treatment strategy has achieved high rates of HBV-DNA suppression (90%), HBeAg loss (46%), and HBsAg loss (12%) in HBeAg-positive patients after 5 years of the treatment, without evidence of resistance, and has reduced progression to cirrhosis with no significant differences in the response in those with or without HIV coinfection. Till date, no viral resistance to tenofovir in vivo has been described, although resistant strains have been identified in vitro.

If ARVs need to be changed because of HIV drug resistance or some drug toxicity, then tenofovir and lamivudine (LAM) should be continued together with the new ARV drugs unless TDF is specifically contraindicated due to its toxicity.

In situations where tenofovir cannot be used, entecavir (ETV) is the alternative drug. ETV is a guanosine analog given at a daily dose of 0.5 mg and in LAM-resistant.

Hepatitis B virus at 1 mg: It reduces HBV-DNA by 4.20 log copies/mL in HIV/HBV-coinfected patients with HBV resistant to LAM at 48 weeks of therapy. However, ETV is not recommended as monotherapy in HIV/HBV-coinfected patients.

Prevention of Hepatitis B Infection

The risk of HBV infection may be higher in HIV-infected adults, and therefore all persons newly diagnosed with HIV should be screened for HBsAg and immunized if not infected. Those already infected with HBV (HBsAg positive) do not require HBV vaccine. People living with human immunodeficiency virus (PLHIV) who have already suffered from HBV in the past and have developed protective titer of hepatitis B surface antibody (anti-HBs) antibody (>10 μIU/mL) also do not require HBV vaccine.

Those who are surface antigen negative need to be vaccinated against hepatitis B besides following other precautions. Response to HBV vaccine is lower in persons with HIV or with a low CD4 count, and a meta-analysis has shown that a schedule of four double (40 μg) doses of the vaccine provides a higher protective anti-HBs titer than the regular three 20 μg dose schedule.[9]

Besides this, all infants born to hepatitis B positive women need to be immunized within 12 hours of birth (dose: 0) followed by 1, 2, and 6 months of age (dose: 10 μg IM) and HBIG: 0.5 mL IM.

Human Immunodeficiency Virus and Hepatitis C Coinfection

Viral hepatitis C infection is associated with significant morbidity and mortality. Chronic HCV infection can cause a wide spectrum of liver disease, potentially leading to severe liver damage, including cirrhosis, organ failure and hepatocellular carcinoma. It accounts for nearly 12–32% of all cases of liver cancer and 10–20% cases of cirrhosis of liver, both of which have high treatment costs and poor outcomes.

In a recent factsheet released by National Viral Hepatitis Surveillance Programme, it was estimated that national seroprevalence of hepatitis C was 0.32% (0.28–0.36) and it is estimated that a broad range of 5.2–13 million people may be infected with hepatitis C.

Because of shared routes of transmission, certain groups, in particular persons who inject drugs (PWID) have high rates of coinfection with HIV and HCV. Other high-risk groups are those who have a high frequency of injections and a low level of infection control, transmission from HCV infected mothers and people with HCV infected sexual partners.

Spontaneous clearance of acute HCV infection occurs within 6 months of infection in 15–45% of infected individuals in the absence of treatment. Almost all the remaining 55–85% of persons needs to be treated for HCV.

Natural History of Human Immunodeficiency Virus/Hepatitis C Virus Coinfection

Coinfection with HIV adversely affects the course of HCV infection, and coinfected persons, particularly those with advanced immunodeficiency (CD4 count <200 cells/mm^3), have significantly accelerated progression of liver disease to cirrhosis, decompensated liver cirrhosis and HCC than HCV-monoinfected persons. Furthermore, even among patients in whom ART leads to successful control of HIV infection (i.e., undetectable HIV viral load), the risk of hepatic decompensation among coinfected patients is higher than among patients with HCV monoinfection. In persons with HIV infection, HCC tends to occur at a younger age and within a shorter time period. For these reasons, all persons with HIV/HCV coinfection should be considered for HCV treatment.

The natural history of HIV is also affected by coinfection with HCV. Two large European cohorts have shown that after ART initiation, CD4 recovery was impaired in HIV/HCV-coinfected persons when compared to those infected with HIV alone. HIV/HCV-coinfected persons also demonstrated more rapid HIV disease progression compared to those who were HIV-infected alone and had impaired recovery of CD4 cells.

It is recommended to screen all PWID (IDUs), those with history of multiple blood/blood product transfusion, or those with raised liver enzymes (ALT) more than two times the ULN or based on strong clinical suspicion. There are additional risk groups identified under NVHCP that should be prioritized. The test used detects anti-HCV antibodies. In persons who have anti-HCV antibodies, a nucleic acid test (NAT) for HCV RNA, which detects the presence of the virus, is needed to confirm the diagnosis of chronic HCV infection.

Evaluation of Human Immunodeficiency Virus Sand Hepatitis C Virus-coinfected Persons

The assessment of those with HCV/HIV includes clinical evaluation—history, physical examination for jaundice, hepatosplenomegaly, ascites, cirrhosis/decompensation, and laboratory tests including LFT, prothrombin time, complete hemogram, AFP, etc. Other tests required are abdominal ultrasound, endoscopy, assessment of liver fibrosis (APRI/FIB-4/FibroScan), described earlier in the chapter, and HCV RNA quantitative assay.

Treatment of Human Immunodeficiency Virus and Hepatitis C Coinfection

Treating HCV infected persons in the past with interferon and ribavirin combination therapy was very difficult, as many patients had to discontinue treatment due to side-effects. Furthermore, sustained virological response (SVR) rates in patients with coinfection were lower than among HCV monoinfected patients.

The advent of newer drugs, DAA, for HCV treatment has revolutionized the management of HCV. The results of treatment with DAAs in persons with HIV coinfection are comparable to those with HCV monoinfection. Thus, DAA therapy has substantially simplified the treatment of persons with HIV and HCV coinfection. There are a fewer drug-drug interactions between DAAs and ARV medicines. SVR rates with DAA-based therapy among persons with HIV coinfection are comparable to those without HIV infection.

The DAAs available under the NVHCP for management of Hepatitis C include sofosbuvir, daclatasvir, velpatasvir, and ribavirin. Treatment is currently recommended for individuals >18 years of age, and choice of regimen is influenced by stage of disease (cirrhosis or no cirrhosis) and other comorbidities or complications. The recommended regimens under NVHCP are enumerated in **Table 1**.

In general, clinical stabilization of HIV disease with ART is advisable before starting treatment for HCV, especially for people with advanced immunosuppression (CD4 count below 200 cells/mm^3)

While the DAA for treating hepatitis C infection have revolutionized treatment outcomes, it is important to bear in mind that there are some drug interactions between ARV drugs and directly acting antivirals, especially with efavirenz where in dose of daclatasvir has to be modified.

Prevention of Hepatitis C Virus Infection in Human Immunodeficiency Virus—Positive

There is no effective HCV vaccine and Prevention of Parent to Child Transmission (PPTCT) protocol for prevention of hepatitis C. The prevention of HCV infection among IDUs needs to be done by strict maintenance of disposal of needle, syringe, sharps, etc., at the healthcare settings and safe sexual behaviors.

Cytomegalovirus Hepatitis in Immunocompromised Hosts

Human *Cytomegalovirus* (HCMV) is a common pathogen, thought to affect 40–100% of the world population. It is mainly transmitted through close contact by body fluids, such as saliva, blood, urine, breast milk, semen and cervical secretions, and also by organ transplantation. The clinical manifestations are extensive and vary particularly between immunocompetent and immunocompromised hosts. While the vast majority of the immunocompetent hosts have a completely asymptomatic course, the immunocompromised host may experience a wide range of severe complications, including esophagitis, colitis, hepatitis, encephalitis, pneumonitis, bacterial superinfection. In immunocompetent hosts, clinically significant hepatitis is rare and only case reports or small case series are available in the literature. However, hepatitis is a well-known manifestation of HCMV infection

TABLE 1: Recommended regimens of direct-acting antivirals under National Viral Hepatitis Control Program (NVHCP), India.

Regimen type	Category of patients	Regimen recommended	Duration of treatment
I	Patient without cirrhosis (uncomplicated)	Sofosbuvir (400 mg) and daclatasvir (60 mg)*	12 weeks
II	Patient with cirrhosis compensated (Child–Pugh A)	Sofosbuvir (400 mg) + velpatasvir (100 mg)	12 weeks
III	Patient with cirrhosis decompensated (Child–Pugh B and C)	Sofosbuvir (400 mg) + velpatasvir (100 mg) and ribavirin (600–1,200 mg)	12 weeks
		In ribavirin intolerant patients—sofosbuvir (400 mg) + velpatasvir (100 mg)	24 weeks

*Dose adjustments may be required in people living with human immunodeficiency virus (PLHIV), renal inefficiency, etc.

in immunocompromised hosts, particularly in liver transplant patients, in which the incidence is relatively high. Indeed, fulminant hepatitis requiring living-donor liver transplant has been described in this population. Like other herpes viruses, HCMV has the ability to create a lifelong latent infection.

The main approach of management relies on preventing disease occurrence. There are two approaches in prevention, prophylaxis, and preemptive therapy. In prophylaxis, antivirals are started just after transplantation occurs and last for at least 3 months. In preemptive therapy, the recipients are closely monitored for the presence of HCMV replication before any symptoms occur; if HCMV replication is identified, antiviral treatment is promptly initiated.

Hepatitis E in Immunocompromised Individuals

Hepatitis E virus (HEV) is a leading cause of acute icteric hepatitis in developing countries. In majority of cases, HEV infection is a self-limiting hepatitis requiring only symptomatic treatment. However, in immunocompromised individuals, especially those with solid organ or stem cell transplantation, it can be life threatening due to liver cell inflammation and fibrosis with subsequent cirrhosis and death. The need for retransplantation as a result of posttransplant hepatitis is of great concern. In addition, there have been many reported incidents of extrahepatic manifestations, for which the exact mechanisms remain to be elucidated. The cornerstone of the treatment in immunocompromised solid organ transplant recipients is reduction of immunosuppressive therapies, while attempting to minimize the risk of organ rejection. Subsequent treatment options include ribavirin and pegylated interferon alpha in those who have demonstrated ribavirin resistance. Further investigation assessing safety and efficacy of antiviral therapy is imperative given the rising global health burden. Given this concern, vaccination has been approved in China with other investigations underway throughout the world. In this review we introduce the epidemiology, diagnosis, clinical manifestations, and treatment of HEV, with emphasis on immunocompromised individuals in the United States.

Hepatitis B and C Virus Infection in Other Immunocompromised Patients

Hepatitis B virus and HCV reactivation is known to occur is patients receiving chemotherapy for various malignancies due to loss of HBV or HCV immune control. Reactivation of HBV is known to occur in patients with hematologic malignancies, but it can also occur in those with solid tumors. It can lead to liver failure and even death anti-HBV prophylaxis effectively prevents HBV reactivation. The universal HBV testing among patients identified for cancer therapy was found to be both cost-effective and cost-saving and useful to decide candidates for HBV prophylaxis. Hepatitis B virus infection prophylaxis initiated before and continued concomitantly with cancer therapy can effectively prevent HBV reactivation. Prophylaxis should be continued for at least 6–12 months after the end of cancer therapy. Entecavir, TDF, and tenofovir alafenamide (TAF) are found to be quite effective.

The HCV-related cytolysis of liver cells secondary to the attack by cytotoxic T lymphocytes against infected cells leads to an exacerbated response and more rapidly evolutive in immunosuppressed patients. However, HCV infection in situation of immunosuppression may lead to different conditions ranging from enhancement to inhibition of HCV replication/infection and from worsening to improvement of liver damage. For HCV reactivation among immunosuppressed, only prevention is to provide DAAs therapy for all HCV-infected patients and this can provide a potential cure in most cases.

CONCLUSION

In immunocompromised patients the progression of hepatitis is faster and there may be reactivation of latent infection as well. In PLHIV and co infected with hepatitis B or C, the disease progression is faster. People Living with human immunodeficiency virus with advanced immunodeficiency (CD4 count <200 cells/mm^3) shows significantly accelerated progression of liver disease to cirrhosis, decompensated liver cirrhosis, and HCC. HIV/HCV-coinfected persons also demonstrated more rapid HIV disease progression compared to those who were HIV-infected alone and had impaired recovery of CD4 cells and slower CD4 recovery. However, the response to therapy for either disease is same as in monoinfected persons except some change in certain ARV drugs and drug–drug interactions. DAAs offer significant levels of cure in persons with HCV infection while tenofovir used for most PLHIV is drug of choice for the treatment of hepatitis B also. Adequate vaccination for hepatitis B among people with immune suppression is important and must be focused on during management of immune suppression due to any cause.

SUGGESTED READINGS

1. World Health Organization. HO Global progress report on HIV, viral hepatitis and sexually transmitted infections, 2021. Accountability for the global health sector strategies 2016–2021: actions for impact. [online] Available from https://www.globalhep.org/sites/default/files/content/resource/files/2021-05/WHO%20Progress%20Report%202021.pdf [Last accessed November, 2023].
2. Unaids.org. (2023). The Path That Ends AIDS, 2023 UNAIDS GLOBAL AIDS UPDATE. [online] Available from https://thepath.unaids.org/ [Last accessed November, 2023].
3. World Health Organization. Consolidated guidelines on HIV prevention, testing, treatment, service delivery and monitoring: recommendations for a public health approach. [online] Available from https://www.who.int/publications/i/item/9789240031593 [Last accessed November, 2023].
4. Jia J, Zhu Q, Deng L, Lan G, Johnson A, Chen H, et al. Treatment outcomes of HIV patients with hepatitis B and C virus co-infections in Southwest China: an observational cohort study. Infect Dis Poverty. 2022;11(1):7.
5. Sarmati L, Malagnino V. HBV Infection in HIV-Driven Immune Suppression. Viruses. 2019;11(11):1077.
6. National Centre for Disease Control Directorate General of Health Services (Ministry of Health & Family Welfare) National Program for Surveillance of Viral Hepatitis. (2021). Seroprevalence of Hepatitis B and Hepatitis C (Based on National Family Health Survey-4)-Fact sheet 2021. [online] Available from https://nvhcp.mohfw.gov.in/common_libs/Approved%20factsheet_4_10_2021.pdf [Last accessed November, 2023].
7. Ministry of Health & Family Welfare; Department of Health & Family Welfare. (2023). National Guidelines for diagnosis and management of Viral Hepatitis, 2018 NVHCP, MoH & FW, India. [online] Available from https://main.mohfw.gov.in/documents/program-guidelines [Last accessed November, 2023].
8. Ministry of Health and Family Welfare, government of India. (2018). National Laboratory Guidelines for Testing of Viral Hepatitis, 2018 NVHCP, MoH & FW, India. [online] Available from https://nvhcp.mohfw.gov.in/common_libs/national-laboratory-guidelines.pdf [Last accessed November, 2023].
9. National AIDS Control Organization. (2021). National Guidelines on HIV Care and Treatment, 2021. NACO, MoH & FW. [online] Available from https://naco.gov.in/sites/default/files/National_Guidelines_for_HIV_Care_and_Treatment_2021.pdf [Last accessed November, 2023].
10. Sun YH, Sheng WH, Tsai MS, Lee KY, Chang SY, Hung CC. Hepatitis B virus coinfection in human immunodeficiency virus-infected patients: A review. World J Gastroenterol. 2014;20(40):14598-614.
11. Cunha TD, Wu GY. Cytomegalovirus Hepatitis in Immuno-competent and Immunocompromised Hosts. J Clin Transl Hepatol. 2021;9(1):106-15.
12. Damiris K, Meybodi MA, Niazi M, Pyrsopoulos N. Hepatitis E in immunocompromised individuals. World J Hepatol. 2022;14(3):482-94.
13. Hwang JP, Torres HA. Hepatitis B virus and hepatitis C virus infection in immunocompromised patients. Curr Opin Infect Dis. 2018;31(6):535-41.
14. Zignego, Giannini C, Gragnani L, Piluso A, Fognani E. Hepatitis C virus infection in the immunocompromised host: a complex scenario with variable clinical impact. J Transl Med. 2012;10:158.

SECTION

5

GERIATRICS

39

CHAPTER

Medication Reconciliation

Arunima Goswami

ABSTRACT

Medication errors are a common and preventable cause of patient harm in healthcare settings with 40% of errors due to inadequate reconciliation. These errors can cause serious harm and even death. Improper medication reconciliation at discharge can lead to critical conditions in patients and may require readmission. Cursory medication reconciliation at discharge and at transitions of care in and outside the hospital is risk points for medication errors. Physicians should be aware of these common errors which can be rectified by proper medication reconciliation and work toward improving patient safety.

INTRODUCTION

Safety in medication prescription is of utmost importance in the healthcare setup. This is because prescribing medicines is a universal intervention in the treatment of all patients. According to the "Preventing Medication Errors report" of the Institute of Medicine, the average patient has at least one medication error per day. This corroborates with the fact that medication errors represent the most common patient safety error. However, medication errors occur frequently and are considered to be the single most preventable cause of patient harm in hospitals, the community and in residential accommodations. Inadequate reconciliation accounts for >40% of medication errors. Medication errors have the potential to cause serious harm and may even result in death. About 25% of all adverse drug events (ADEs) are due to medication errors. The risk areas are identified as places where a patient is transferred from one level of care to another. For example, when a patient is shifted from the intensive care unit (ICU) to the ward or when a patient is brought into a hospital from a geriatric care center.

Many examples of improper medication reconciliation at discharge abound. A patient may be readmitted 2–3 days after discharge with severe hypoglycemia as he was following a new regimen of oral hypoglycemics in addition to another oral hypoglycemic which he was already taking at home prior to admission. Similarly, duplication of similar drugs, such as pregabalin and gabapentin is seen in the same discharge hand out. A common mistake is not restarting an anticoagulant on a postsurgery discharge, which may lead to the patient ending up with a stroke. Every physician will be able to relate to such medication errors which commonly occur in discharge prescriptions.

DEFINITION

Medication reconciliation is the process of obtaining and documenting a complete and accurate list of current patient medications and comparing this list with new medication orders at each point of transition of care. This helps in rectifying any discrepancies in the new prescription before the patient becomes vulnerable to harmful effects of medications. Medication reconciliation helps eliminate duplication and/or omission of important medications.

DIFFERENT LEVELS OF MEDICATION RECONCILIATION

The *best possible medication history (BPMH)* is the foundation of medication reconciliation. It is not like routine history taking of medications. BPMH involves:

- A structured and systematic interview of the patient and/or family members
- Reliable medication information thus obtained should be cross-checked with at least one other source like government database, information of current medication of patients with pharmacists, previous hospital records, actual inspection of medicines, vials, etc.

Medication reconciliation, as per the National Accreditation Indicator in Canada, has varying levels of intensity from Bronze to Diamond as a continuum. Bronze indicates BPMH with admission reconciliation, silver-bronze level plus reconciliation at discharge, gold-silver level plus interprofessional collaboration, platinum-gold level plus attention to broader medication issues plus medication counseling, and diamond-platinum level plus postdischarge follow-up phone call plus communication with pharmacy and primary care physicians.

Where should medication reconciliation occur?

- *Ambulatory setup*: Literature on medication reconciliation in ambulatory setups are beginning to emerge. As elsewhere BPMH is the foundation of medication reconciliation. Due to the increase in noncommunicable diseases, the patients are seen to consult doctors of multiple specialties leading to generation of multiple prescriptions. This leads to unnecessary duplication of medications.
- *Inpatient setup*: Ideally medication reconciliation should be targeted at both admission and discharge. However in practice, implementation in both the situations is difficult. A good strategy is to target both and also target each point of transition of care in a hospital. It is easy to take a BPMH during an elective admission. However in an emergency setting, a BPMH is not possible and whatever medication history taken is usually cursory. Having said that, the emergency department is a much larger entry point for hospitalized patients and hence, the strategies used for medication reconciliation during an elective admission may not be practically possible in the busy time pressed setting of an emergency department. A good BPMH during admission paves the way for good medication reconciliation at discharge. Even though medication reconciliation is not important for admission orders, it will be easy to outline an accurate discharge if a BPMH already exists and it will be time saving also.

When should medication reconciliation occur?

Medication reconciliation should be started at/or soon after admission, as this will ultimately save time and lead to better implementation. Some studies have pointed out that serious medication errors can occur during internal transfers inside a hospital. Most hospitals target medication reconciliation at admission and/or at discharge. Reconciliation at admission helps in avoiding medication errors at the discharge process. The general discharge process should be integrated with medication reconciliation, though it is already a complex process involving physicians, nurses, pharmacists, etc.

Who should be targeted for medication reconciliation?

Should all patients be targeted for medication reconciliation or only high-risk patients should enjoy this benefit. With limited human resources, some authors have suggested that medication reconciliation can be focused by age (over 65 years) or number of medications (>4). Others have proposed factors such as frequent hospitalization, high alert medication usage and chronic diseases prone to frequent medication change. If we can narrow down the target population requiring medication reconciliation, quality can be assured in the whole process. This is better than an average medication reconciliation drawn out for all patients. But of course if quality can be assured, targeting all patients is the best option.

Who should implement medication reconciliation?

From the qualification and expertise point of view pharmacists seem to be the best persons to lead inpatient medication reconciliation. Alternatives are pharmacy technicians, nurses, resident doctors, and medical students. Nowadays "care coordinators" are also evolving to coordinate the medical care of a patient. These "care coordinators" can take active part in medication reconciliation. It should be remembered that irrespective of whoever carries out medication reconciliation, the patient is an integral partner of the process. A completely perfect reconciliation will serve no purpose, if the patient does not understand his medication orders. However if persons of only one specialty is designated, the responsibility of medication reconciliation, it is only natural that the others will keep themselves away from this tedious responsibility.

How to implement medication reconciliation?

- BPMH should be taken and verified by collecting the list of medications, vitamins, nutritional supplements, herbal medicines, over-the-counter drugs, and vaccines. This should be followed by development of a list of current medications.

- A list of medications to be prescribed should also be prepared.
- The medications of the two lists are to be compared.
- The appropriateness of the dosages of the medications is to be determined.
- Make clinical decisions based on this comparison.
- Any changes in this list are to be documented.
- The definite area of implementation of medication reconciliation should be identified like at admission, at points of transition of care in the same hospital, at discharge, etc.
- Healthcare professionals and team roles and responsibilities for medication reconciliation should be identified
- A dedicated area in the patient chart should be present where exclusively medication history would be written. At the same time, a particular person should be designated to write medication history including the time frame and procedure for documentation. All these should be clearly defined to avoid duplication of history taking of medications.
- Usage of standardized medication forms facilitates an accurate medication reconciliation history.
- Delineate an exact time frame for completion of medication reconciliation. Many organizations review medication reconciliation at every primary care visit and within 24 hours of inpatient admission. High-risk medications, such as antihypertensives, antiseizures, hypoglycemic, antibiotics, may need to be reconciled sooner, e.g., within 4 hours of admission.
- Medication reconciliation is a complex process and hence education programs are necessary from time to time to update the persons who implement medication reconciliation.
- Once the medication reconciliation process is properly integrated into the ambulatory or inpatient setup, monitoring and auditing of the process is necessary with designation of the personnel responsible to do so.
- Patient education and partnership of the patient is the major point of focus. Patients may not be accurate historians, and hence, assistance is needed to make the information as accurate as possible. A process should be established where patients bring their medications, including all over-the-counter preparations, in every healthcare encounter. Additionally, educating patients about their medications allows them to have better track of what medication they are receiving.

BARRIERS

There are many barriers associated with effective and efficient medication reconciliation. Developing and implementing effective programs including standardization of the process is very complex. Garnering leadership and support from physicians and nurses and making them understand the need for medication reconciliation is a big challenge. Implementing the same within a time frame is more so. The main barrier is to make the healthcare personnel understand the importance of medication reconciliation. Next, it is also difficult to convince someone to take up this tedious responsibility. No one wants to go into the details of history taking of different medications including over-the-counter products, herbal medicines, etc. as the procedure is time consuming. Nowadays, in certain settings, specialized "care coordinators" are designated to take up this role.

FUTURE RESEARCH

More research is needed to cover all aspects of medication reconciliation. This will help in building a robust data base, which will impact prevention of adverse drug events. Multisite studies with large sample sizes are required to assess the magnitude and scope of the problem. Various approaches, both paper based and electronic, are needed to determine the accuracy, feasibility, and ease of documenting accurate patient medication lists.

The medication reconciliation process takes time, which may extend up to an additional 30–60 minutes per patient. In a busy inpatient setup, this may translate into a requirement for additional full-time staff. Busy clinicians are bound to resist to a change in their busy schedule. Similarly, nurses will also look into this documentation as an additional burden. A designated person needs to be identified to carry out the medication reconciliation process. This person may be a pharmacist, a care coordinator, a resident doctor, or a nurse. However, the most important point is that patients need to be full partners and self-advocates in the medication reconciliation process.

CONCLUSION

There is ample evidence to demonstrate that medication reconciliation is effective in preventing adverse effects and patient harm. Carrying out a cursory medication reconciliation will do little to prevent catastrophic outcomes and hence is of no use. Therefore, rather than implementing medication reconciliation just for its namesake is a waste of time. Hospitals and healthcare setups should seriously consider investing more time and energy to build up a robust strategy for effective medication reconciliation. Medication reconciliation is a major component of safe patient care in any environment.

SUGGESTED READINGS

1. Cornish PL, Knowles SR, Marchesano R, Tam V, Shadowitz S, Juurlink DN, et al. Unintended medication discrepancies at the time of hospital admission. Arch Int Med. 2005;165:424-9.
2. Coombes R. Death of teenager from a drug error a decade ago has made UK a leader in safety. BMJ. 2012;344:e3826.
3. Nebeker JR, Barach P, Samore MH. Clarifying adverse drug events: a clinician's guide to terminology, documentation and reporting. Ann Int Med. 2004;140:795-801.
4. Coleman EA, Boult C. Improving the quality of transitional care for persons with complex care needs. J Am Geriatr Soc. 2003;51:556-7.
5. Lehnbom EC, Stewart MJ, Manias E, Westbrook JI. Impact of medication reconciliation and review on clinical outcomes. Ann Pharmacother. 2014;48(10):1298-312.
6. Fernandes O. Medication reconciliation in the hospital: what, why, where, when, who and how? Healthc Q. 2012;15:42-9.
7. Bayoumi I, Howard M, Holbrook AM, Schabort I. Interventions to improve medication reconciliation in primary care. Ann Pharmacother. 2009;43(10):1667-75.
8. Coffey M, Cornish P, Koonthanam T, Etchells E, Matlow A. Implementation of admission medication reconciliation at two academic health sciences centres: challenges and success factors. Healthc Q. 2009;12:102-9.
9. Rumball-Smith J, Hider P. The validity of readmission rate as a marker of the quality of hospital care, and a recommendation for its definition. N Z Med J. 2009;122(1289):63-70.
10. Santell JP. Reconciliation failures lead to medication errors. Jt Comm J Qual Patient Saf. 2006;32(4):225-9.
11. Fernandes OA, MacKinnon NJ. Point counterpoint—the "Pro" side—Is the prioritization of medication reconciliation as a critical activity the best use of pharmacist time? Canadian J Hosp Pharmacy. 2008;61:149-50.
12. Barnsteiner JH. Medication reconciliation. Hughes RG (Ed). Patient Safety and Quality; An Evidence-based Handbook for Nurses. Rockville (MD): Agency for Healthcare Research and Quality (US); 2008. pp. 459-72.

40

CHAPTER

Caregiver Communication/ Counseling in Dying Patients

P Krishna Prasanthi

ABSTRACT

Terminally ill patients, due to barriers in communication with family members often manifest uncertainty, negative feelings, diminished self-esteem, negative adaptation, and other psychological problems. Published data suggest that open communication with caregivers of terminally ill patients helps in diminishing psychological distress and maintaining self-protection. A multidisciplinary team of caregivers (clinician, nurse, counsellor, and social workers) is required to engage terminally ill dying patients for open communication. There is a need for generating further evidence regarding the various methods of communication, skills development, and outcomes.

INTRODUCTION

"Effective communication starts with listening"
"Good communication ends lot of bad things, bad communication ends lot of good things"

Caregivers encounter severe difficulties while communicating openly with terminally ill dying patients and their relatives about illness and death. The term "terminal illness" is applied to a disease which cannot be cured and is likely to lead to death. Open communication in this context refers to candid and straightforward conversations about illness and death. These conversations include discussions regarding diagnosis, likely outcomes, prognosis, available treatment options, and treatment goals. Further, these conversations also focus on *end-of-life (EOL)* wishes, goals of care, and plans for the future. Such open communication regarding concerns and feelings has been observed to enhance the abilities of terminally ill patients and their family members. In this chapter, the concerns, methods, challenges while communicating with dying patients and their families will be presented.

EVIDENCE REGARDING BENEFITS OF OPEN COMMUNICATION

Terminally ill patients, due to barriers in communication with family members often manifest uncertainty, negative feelings, diminished self-esteem, negative adaptation, and other psychological problems. Published research data suggest that open communication by caregivers of terminally ill patients helps in diminishing psychological distress and maintaining self-protection.

Terminally ill dying patients by openly expressing their concerns and feelings contribute to enhancing their as well as their family members' abilities to cope with the stressful situation. Open communication also seems to predict higher levels of empathy and intimacy between dying patients and their spouses. It has also been observed to improve physical health not only of the patients but also of their caregivers and reduce feelings of caregiver burden. It has also been shown to alleviate the feelings of powerlessness often encountered by dying patients.

In contrast, some of the recent studies have reported an inverse association between open communication and mental health of patients such as depression, anxiety, and emotional exhaustion and also quality of life of the caregivers, care derived self-esteem, and avoidance of open communication by the caregivers.

SETTINGS OF END-OF-LIFE CARE DELIVERY

Holistic care is provided to terminally ill patients at home, in hospices. There has been an increased use of

9. Buckman R. How to Break Bad News: A Guide for Health Care Professionals. Baltimore, MD: John Hopkins University Press; 1992.
10. Bailey M. (2018). Doctors learn how to talk to patients about dying. [online] Available from https://kffhealthnews.org/news/doctors-learn-how-to-talk-to-patients-about-dying/ [Last accessed November, 2023].
11. Baile WF, Buckman R, Lenzi R, Glober G, Beale EA, Kudelka AP. SPIKES–a six–step protocol for delivering bad news: application to the patient with cancer. Oncologist. 2000;5(4):302-11.
12. Rabow MW, McPhee SJ. Beyond breaking bad news: how to help patients who suffer. West J Med. 1999;171(4):260-3.
13. Everitt R, Wong AK, Wawryk O, Le B, Yoong J, Pisasale M, et al. A multi-centre study on patients dying from COVID-19: communication between clinicians, patients and their families. Intern Med J. 2022;52(12):2068-75.
14. Marcus JD, Mott FE. Difficult conversations: from diagnosis to death. Ochsner J. 2014;14(4):712-7.
15. Crawford GB, Price SD. Team working: palliative care as a model of interdisciplinary practice. Med J Aust. 2003;179(S6):S32-4.
16. Chaturvedi SK, Loiselle CG, Chandra PS. Communication with relatives and collusion in palliative care: a cross-cultural perspective. Indian J Palliat Care. 2009;15(1):2-9.
17. Lakin JR, Koritsanszky LA, Cunningham R, Maloney FL, Neal BJ, Paladino J, et al. A systematic intervention to improve serious illness communication in primary care. Health Aff (Millwood). 2017;36(7):1258-64.
18. Institute for Healthcare Improvement. The Conversation Project. Resources for healthcare professionals. [online] Available from https://theconversationproject.org/ [Last accessed November, 2023].
19. Brighton LJ, Koffman J, Hawkins A, McDonald C, O'Brien S, Robinson V, et al. A Systematic Review of End-of-Life Care Communication Skills Training for Generalist Palliative Care Providers: Research Quality and Reporting Guidance. J Pain Symptom Manage. 2017;54(3):417-25.

41

CHAPTER

Principles of Geriatric Prescribing

Parvati Nandy, Manish Ranwa

ABSTRACT

The geriatric age group presents unique problems for rational prescription of drugs for their multiple comorbidities. Major among the problems are polypharmacy, prescription cascades, use of herbal medications, increased toxicity of drugs used in old age and necessity of adjusting drug doses with liver and kidney function. Principles of proper geriatric prescribing include rational drug use with appropriate doses, de-escalating therapies and stopping medications as and when possible, taking help of adherence aids and preventing over as well as under prescribing.

INTRODUCTION

Increased longevity of humanity today comes with its own charms and challenges. To maintain a steady quality of life of a person as they age and attain geriatric age group requires very careful and long drawn planning as well as monitoring on the part of the individual, as also improvement in health infrastructure which has to be able to cater the increasing population of geriatric individuals in the world today. The number of people > 60 years from year 2000–2050 is expected to double from 11 to 22%.

PROBLEMS ENCOUNTERED IN GERIATRIC AGE GROUP IN PRESCRIBING DRUGS

- Medications need to be used with special caution as there are age related changes in pharmacokinetics (i.e., absorption, distribution, metabolism, and excretion) and pharmacodynamics (physiological effects of drugs).
- Care has to be taken to calculate drug doses in older individuals. There may be increased volume of distribution, due to relative increase in body fat in comparison to skeletal muscles with aging. There may also be a natural decline in renal function with age, both of these lead to increased drug concentration in elderly people.
- Hepatic functions also decline with advancing age, thus there may be significant variability in drug metabolism among older adults. Polypharmacy in decreasing hepatic function may lead to adverse drug reactions.
- Multiple comorbidities in the geriatric age group lead to more and more prescription of drugs. In a survey of medicare beneficiaries discharged after acute hospitalization, patients were prescribed on an average of 14 medications including one-third with the side effects that could exacerbate geriatric syndromes.
- Use of herbal or dietary supplements by older adults has been increasing from 14% in 1998 to 63% in 2010. Herbal medicines may interact with prescribed drug therapies and lead to adverse events, this makes it very important for care givers to routinely note down patient's use of unconventional medications.
- *Prescribing cascades*: Defined as the situation in which a first drug administered to a patient causes adverse event signs and symptoms, that are misinterpreted as a new condition, resulting in a new medication being prescribed. The patient then is at risk of developing additional adverse drug reactions related to new and unnecessary treatment, for example, patients on calcium channel blockers may develop peripheral edema. Thus they may be started on diuretics, if the edema is seen as a new condition.

- *Transition in care settings*: Transition in care between hospitals to institutional care and home care are a common cause in occurrence of medicational error. These may occur due to lapse in handing over of medicine administration duties among care givers and so on. For this improved and full proof communication and documentation between changed team of doctors would be appropriate. Additionally, on discharge, the entire medication chart needs to be revised and unnecessary drugs need to be omitted, which may have been prescribed at different points by different prescribers.
- *Underutilization of appropriate medication*: Stressing on avoiding overprescribing drugs in elderly should go hand in hand with proper clinical judgement and utilization of essential drugs in age appropriate doses, such that the patient receives the adequate drug in acceptable dosage for his most pressing illness. Thus prioritization of health benefits of essential medications should not be overlooked.

PRINCIPLES OF GERIATRIC PRESCRIBING

General Principles

- Match medications with diagnosis
- Consider reducing doses and stopping drugs
- Encourage adherence aids and or consultation with pharmacists to make simple drug schedules, proper labeling, and aids for visually impaired patients. Cognitive impairment patients need to be helped in medications by trained care givers.
- Geriatric patients need to be evaluated thoroughly for identification of all conditions that:
    - Could benefit from drug treatment
    - Be adversely affected by the drug treatment
    - May influence the efficiency of drug treatment
- As such patients have several comorbidities; priority of treatment should be given to the life-threatening issues first and so on, trying to manage certain medical conditions without drugs as often as possible.
- Knowledge of the pharmacology of the drugs being prescribed and awareness about dosage adjustment due to altered liver/kidney functions is essential for rational prescribing in the elderly patients. Renal impairment becomes more common with advancing age, for stable patients, and creatinine clearance can be calculated by standard formulas factoring age in the formula. Because of decreased muscle mass, however, serum creatinine levels may not adequately reflect renal function. Thus, dose reduction of commonly used drugs is necessary in elderly.

Beers Criteria

It was developed by an expert consensus panel in 1991, is the most widely used criteria to assess inappropriate drug prescribing. These criteria constitute a list of medications that are potentially inappropriate for use in older individuals. They are grouped into five categories:

1. Drugs potentially inappropriate in most older patients
2. Drugs to be avoided in older individuals with certain conditions
3. Drugs to use with certain cautions
4. Drug-drug interactions
5. Drug adjusted based on kidney function

These criteria have been updated in 2019, and are available on the American Geriatric Society website.

Some common medication errors that need to be avoided are as follows:

- Avoid the concurrent use of opioids with either benzodiazepines or gabapentinoids as it can cause increased risk of overdose and sedation.
- Hyperkalemia may be precipitated in patients on angiotensin-converting enzyme (ACE)/angiotensin receptor blocker (ARB) medications if given trimethoprim/sulfamethoxazole.
- Aspirin in elderly age group for cardiovascular disease prophylaxis may lead to increased bleeding risk and has to be prescribed with caution.
- Serotonin and norepinephrine reuptake inhibitors (SNRIs) are to be avoided in patients at risk for falls and fractures.
- Avoid sliding scale insulin in elderly without using basal regimens due to risk of hypoglycemia without benefit of improvement in diabetes control.

MEDICATION ALERTS FOR OLDER DRIVERS

Older adults who continue to drive are at highest risk of causing fatal car crashes. Thus they should be routinely assessed for driving skills as well as their ongoing medications should be reviewed periodically.

MEDICATION WITH STRONG POTENTIAL TO AFFECT DRIVING

- Anticholinergics
- Anticonvulsants
- Antidepressants
- Antiemetics
- Antihistamines
- Antihypertensives
- Antiparkinsonian drugs
- Antipsychotic drugs

- Benzodiazepines
- Muscle relaxants
- Narcotic analgesics

PRINCIPALS OF TREATMENT OF SOME COMMON DISEASES IN THE GERIATRIC AGE GROUP

Hypertension

Hypertension has to be controlled in the geriatric age group, but targets of blood pressure (BP) control remains confusing. A delicate balance has to be drawn for optimum BP control, hypotension, and postural hypotension should not be offset. Several research articles HYVET (Hypertension in the Very Elderly Trial) and SPRINT (Systolic Blood Pressure Intervention Trial)—multicentric studies on hypertension done in patients > 80 years old have shown that there is a significant reduction in cardiovascular disease events with optimum control of BP. In the elderly a systolic target < 150 significantly reduced the risk of stroke and heart failure, and also reduced the risk of mortality from significant hypotension, e.g., falls. Thus a person centric approach to hypertension in the heterogeneous geriatric age group is mandatory. For older patients with minimal morbidity, low risk of falls, lower BP targets < 130 may be useful. However, for those with multiple comorbidities and risk, higher systolic targets (<150) is probably safer.

Diabetes

There is a limitation of data on patients above age of 80 years with diabetes and other comorbidities, such patients are prone to increased risk of hypoglycemia, when treated with multiple hypoglycemic agents. The diabetes management in the elderly has to be person centric. These patients tend to have progressive renal decline and cognitive decline and are subject to medication error. In the elderly age group > 80 years, intensive glycemic control does not reduce major macrovascular events for at least 10 years, nor does it result in improved microvascular outcomes for at least 8 years, and at the same time increases the risk of severe hypoglycemia 1.5-3 fold. "Choosing wisely" recommendations of American Geriatric Society states that in most adults > 65 years, the harms associated with glycated hemoglobin (HbA1c) target < 7.5% or 9% are likely to outweigh the benefits. Thus, in the geriatric population treatment of diabetes has to be tailored to patient's medical and functional status, personal goals, and life expectancy. Older diabetic patients have to be regularly screened for neuropathy. While using oral hypoglycemic agent (OHA), personalized treatment based on the individual patients' liver and kidney function, other comorbidities and functional status has to be made. While using insulin therapy, long acting once a day regimens are useful and multiple boluses of short-acting regimens may be complicated for use by the patient. Here, also personalized targets have to be met.

Hyperlipidemia

Usage of statins in patients <75 years of age for primary cardiovascular risk reduction may be feasible, but there are no definite guidelines regarding starting/continuing statin therapy beyond the age of 80 years.

Osteoarthritis

Beyond the age of 65, nonsteroidal anti-inflammatory drugs (NSAIDs) have to be used with caution for joint pain. Concomitant NSAID and proton-pump inhibitor (PPI) use in these situations may have complications such as renal impairment, risk of heart failure, and gastrointestinal (GI) bleed with NSAIDs and increased incidence of pneumonia, C-difficile diarrhea and osteoporosis with PPI.

Paracetamol is the safest in this situation, nonpharmacological therapies such as physiotherapy, local hot and cold compress, and ultrasonic rays may be used for pain relief. Fomentations of NSAIDs also work well in certain cases. *Narcotics* are the last option. Definitive orthopedic procedures like joint replacement surgeries also work well for the selected elderly cases.

Cancer

Half of all the cancers occur after age of 65 years. Such patients may already have multiple comorbidities and functional impairments. Thus a personalized approach yields better results.

CONCLUSION

- Prescribing in elderly is made more complex by the physiological changes associated with aging and increased burden of disease.
- Polypharmacy increases the chance of adverse drug reactions and the prescribing cascade.
- Under prescribing of the essential drugs is also detrimental to the patient care.
- Regular review of the medication charts with omission of nonessential drugs, proper coordination among care givers is very important for geriatric care.
- Recommended dosages for elderly patients are to be adhered to.
- Consider nonpharmacological treatments if appropriate.
- Patients need to be educated about their prescribed drugs and the side effects they may encounter so that they report early and necessary action may be taken.

functional well-being needs to be assessed. A detailed dietary and nutritional assessment and level of physical activity needs to be ascertained. We need to rule out use of off prescription drugs, nonsteroidal anti-inflammatory drugs (NSAIDs), corticosteroids, ephedrine, etc. A detailed physical examination should include routine palpation, auscultation, examination for bruits over the abdominal aorta and bruits over major arteries. Also look for postural hypotension, renal insufficiency and estimated glomerular filtration rate (eGFR), thyroid dysfunction, obstructive sleep apnea, other comorbidities, and drug compliance.

Blood pressure measurement should be done as per the usual guidelines. An average of three different readings in two separate visits must be taken. There should be a standard cuff, obese cuff, and a child cuff for malnourished individuals. BP should be measured in supine and upright positions. An automatic BP machine might give faulty readings; hence, it is advisable to check manual BP.

TRIALS

The Hypertension in the Very Elderly Trial (HYVET) demonstrated a cardiac mortality benefit in octogenarians treated with antihypertensives. The SPRINT (Systolic Blood Pressure Intervention Trial) showed benefits of systolic BP goal <120 mm Hg in elderly aged >75 years. However, these trials were conducted in relatively fit individuals living in the community. Patients with diabetes, cardiovascular diseases, cerebrovascular accidents, multiple comorbidities, cognitive decline, dementia, loss of autonomy, orthostatic hypotension, and metabolic disorders were excluded from the study. Hence, the results of these trials need to be taken with a pinch of salt. The treatment plan needs to be individualized taking into consideration trial data and guidelines of prominent associations.

PRINCIPLES OF TREATMENT

The patient's preferences and needs have to be understood and there should be a shared decision-making between the healthcare provider, patient, and his family to ensure better compliance, follow-up, and long-term adherence. The drug schedule may need to be modified based on the side effects and drug interactions. On every visit, we need to look for drug adverse effects, assess the quality of life and emphasize the need for long-term adherence to the therapy.

Nonpharmacological treatment may not be very effective in very old. Weight loss may be associated with cachexia and loss of muscle mass. Excessive salt reduction may be associated with hyponatremia, postural hypotension, and risk of falls. Physical activity should be adapted to suit the functional capacity in the elderly. Smoking, tobacco, and alcohol should be strongly discouraged.

Different guidelines have defined different cutoff values for initiation of pharmacotherapy and targets to treat hypertension in elderly. The American College of Cardiology/American Heart Association (ACC/AHA) 2017, American Academy of Family Physicians (AAFP) 2017, and European Society of Cardiology 2018 guidelines are summarized in **Table 2**. There is vast heterogeneity among the various guidelines. This could be because of variable demographic, social, cultural, and ethnic factors among the population under study.

Polypharmacotherapy should be strongly discouraged. It is strongly advisable to start with monotherapy and slowly uptitrate/add another class of drug as per individual response and side effect profile. Be very cautious while adding the third class of drug. At every step, the clinician should go very slowly with a close vigil on side effects. The side effects may not be well pronounced as in the young. All international guidelines recommend the five major classes of drugs [calcium channel blockers, angiotensin-converting enzyme (ACE) inhibitors, angiotensin receptor blockers (ARBs), diuretics, and β-blockers] for treatment of hypertension in the elderly and very old.

The treatment should be based on functional status of the patient rather than the chronological age.

- *Older adults with preserved functional status*: These patients have preserved functional status with no comorbidities or relatively well-controlled disease. They are fairly independent. They should be given treatment at par with younger patients to achieve full benefit of treatment.
- *Elderly with moderate functional decline*: These patients have moderate cognitive and functional decline and dependence on activities of daily living.

TABLE 2: Summary of various international guidelines for treatment of hypertension in elderly.

	ACC/AHA 2017	AAFP 2017	ESC/ESH 2018
Elderly	≥65 years	≥60 years	• Elderly 65–79 years • Very old ≥80 years
Rx threshold	≥130/80 mm Hg	SBP ≥150 mm Hg	• Elderly ≥140/90 mm Hg • Very old ≥160/90 mm Hg
BP target	<130/80 mm Hg	SBP <150 mm Hg	130–139/70–79 mm Hg

(AAFP: American Academy of Family Physicians; ACC/AHA: American College of Cardiology/American Heart Association; ESC: European Society of Cardiology; ESH: European Society of Hypertension)

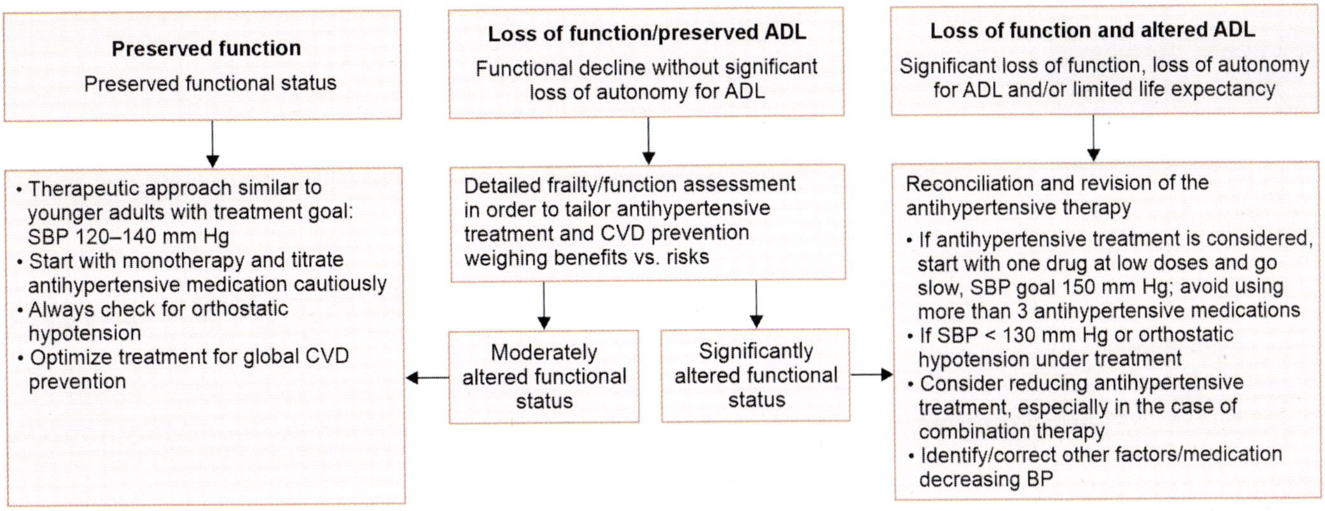

FLOWCHART 1: Treatment plan based on functional status of patients.
(ADL: activities of daily living; CVD: cardiovascular disease; SBP: systolic blood pressure)

They have one or two comorbidities. These patients need a comprehensive geriatric assessment and accordingly therapy should be individually tailored.

- *Elderly with significant loss of function, loss of autonomy for activities of daily living, and limited life expectancy*: These patients are usually >85 years of age and have multiple comorbidities, dementia, and dependency. The aim of treatment should be in alleviating symptoms and achieving a good quality of life. Risk of iatrogenic complications is extremely high in these patients. There should be a focus on de-escalating drug therapy. Antihypertensives should be titrated to achieve a systolic BP between 130 and 150 mm Hg. If there is postural hypotension or BP drops to <130 mm Hg, antihypertensives may even be stopped. There is not enough trial data in this group of patients; hence, clinical judgment with close monitoring is the key to manage these patients **(Flowchart 1)**.

CONCLUSION

The treatment of hypertension in elderly and very old is tricky and different from that in younger patients. Biological age rather than chronological age should be considered. The patients should be assessed based on functional status, frailty levels, activities of daily living, and multiple comorbidities. Comprehensive geriatric assessment should be performed when necessary. We should closely monitor for orthostatic hypotension and other adverse effects. Deprescribing should be done when required. The aim of treatment should be to reduce morbidity, mortality, alleviate symptoms, give good quality of life, and minimize iatrogenic complications.

SUGGESTED READINGS

1. Franklin SS, Larson MG, Khan SA, Wong ND, Leip EP, Kannel WB, et al. Does the relation of blood pressure to coronary heart disease risk change with aging? The Framingham Heart Study. Circulation. 2001;103:1245-9.
2. Lewington S, Clarke R, Qizilbash N, Peto R, Collins R. Prospective Studies Collaboration. Age-specific relevance of usual blood pressure to vascular mortality: a meta-analysis of individual data for one million adults in 61 prospective studies. Lancet. 2002;360:1903-13.
3. Beckett NS, Peters R, Fletcher AE, Staessen JA, Liu L, Dumitrascu D, et al. Treatment of hypertension in patients 80 years of age or older. N Engl J Med. 2008;358(18):1887-98.
4. Williamson JD, Supiano MA, Applegate WB, Berlowitz DR, Campbell RC, Chertow GM, et al. Intensive vs standard blood pressure control and cardiovascular disease outcomes in adults aged ≥75 years: a randomized clinical trial. JAMA. 2016;315:2673-82.
5. Williams B, Mancia G, Spiering W, Agabiti Rosei E, Azizi M, Burnier M, et al. 2018 ESC/ESH Guidelines for the management of arterial hypertension. Eur Heart J. 2018;39:3021-104.
6. Whelton PK, Carey RM, Aronow WS, Casey DE Jr, Collins KJ, Dennison Himmelfarb C, et al. 2017 ACC/AHA/AAPA/ABC/ACPM/AGS/APhA/ASH/ASPC/NMA/PCNA guideline for the prevention, detection, evaluation, and management of high blood pressure in adults: executive summary: a report of the American College of Cardiology/American Heart Association Task Force on Clinical Practice Guidelines. Hypertension. 2018;71:1269-324.

44

CHAPTER

Elderly Thrombocytopenia

Sunita Aggarwal, Sudipta Nandi, Sandeep Garg, Anshul Tomar, Dhananjay Kharche

ABSTRACT

Thrombocytopenia in the elderly is a crucial subject and requires more attention as the risk of bleeding is very high. The elderly are more predisposed to have thrombocytopenia because of the multiple comorbidities, frail clearance of worn-out platelets, and the multiple drugs that the elderly patients are on, which have certain antiplatelet activity.

The other aspect that makes thrombocytopenia in the elderly a special issue, is its association with malignancies, particularly hematological ones. This implies the indication of performing higher investigations in the workup of thrombocytopenia in the elderly.

Immune thrombocytopenia (ITP) in the elderly is an important cause of thrombocytopenia. The ITP here is mainly secondary, associated with malignancy, human immunodeficiency virus (HIV), hepatitis C virus (HCV), or other autoimmune disorders like systemic lupus erythematosus (SLE). History and examination are not very conclusive, as the differentials are very wide for elderly thrombocytopenia. Investigating thrombocytopenia in the elderly is thus very extensive.

INTRODUCTION

The term "elderly" is defined as persons aged 60 years or more considering a national policy for older persons adopted by the Government of India.

Thrombocytopenia is defined as a platelet count below 100,000/μL for adults. Degrees of thrombocytopenia can be further subdivided into mild (platelet count 100,000–150,000/μL), moderate (50,000–99,000/μL), and severe (<50,000/μL).

Age-related changes in the organ and vasculature systems along with the multiple comorbidities increase the risks of thrombocytopenia. Thrombocytopenia in the elderly can be associated with malignancy, autoimmunity, drug intake, bone marrow failure, etc. Thrombocytopenia is a more critical issue for the elderly due to a greater risk of falls secondary to neuromuscular weakness, and loss of subcutaneous fat causing increased bleeding complications.

CAUSES OF ELDERLY THROMBOCYTOPENIA

Pseudothrombocytopenia (Box 1)

BOX 1: Pseudothrombocytopenia (falsely low platelet counts).

- In vitro platelet clumping caused by ethylenediaminetetraacetic acid (EDTA)-dependent agglutinins (naturally occurring antibodies)
- In vitro platelet clumping caused by an insufficiently anticoagulated specimen
- In vitro platelet clumping caused by glycoprotein IIb/IIIa inhibitors (e.g., abciximab) (*Note*: These can also cause true thrombocytopenia)
- Giant platelets counted by the automated counter as white blood cells (WBCs) rather than platelets

TABLE 1: Causes of quantitative platelet dysfunction.

Decreased production	Increased destruction
Bone marrow failure: • Aplastic anemia • Myelofibrosis (postradiation) • Myelodysplasia	*Peripheral consumption*: • Sepsis • Disseminated intravascular coagulation (DIC) • Thrombotic microangiopathy (TMA)—hemolytic uremic syndrome (HUS)/thrombotic thrombocytopenic purpura (TTP)
Nutritional deficiency • B9/B12 deficiency • Copper deficiency	Increased destruction (autoimmune): • Immune thrombocytopenic purpura (ITP)
Malignancies: • Acute leukemia • Chronic lymphocytic lymphoma • Solid malignancies	*Sequestration*: • Hypersplenism (secondary to chronic liver disease)
Drug-induced: • Valproate (direct marrow toxicity) • Oxaliplatin • Gemcitabine • Quinine (megakaryocyte inhibition)	*Drug-induced*: • Abciximab (antibody-mediated platelet destruction) • Penicillin • Rifampicin • Ranitidine • Heparin • Vaccine-induced • Herbal medications
Infections: • Human immunodeficiency virus (HIV) • *Cytomegalovirus* (CMV) • Epstein–Barr virus (EBV)	*Infections*: • Human immunodeficiency virus (HIV) • Hepatitis C virus (HCV)
Persistent comorbidities in the elderly: • Diabetes mellitus • Chronic kidney disease (CKD) • Cerebrovascular accident (CVA)	*Rheumatological diseases*: • Rheumatoid arthritis • Sjögren's syndrome • Systemic sclerosis

Quantitative Platelet Dysfunction

Refer **Table 1** for qualitative platelet dysfunction.

Qualitative Platelet Dysfunction

The change in platelet function is driven by differential messenger ribonucleic acid (mRNA) and microRNA (miRNA) expression, an increase in oxidative stress, and changes in platelet receptors; making the platelets qualitatively weak **(Fig. 1)**.

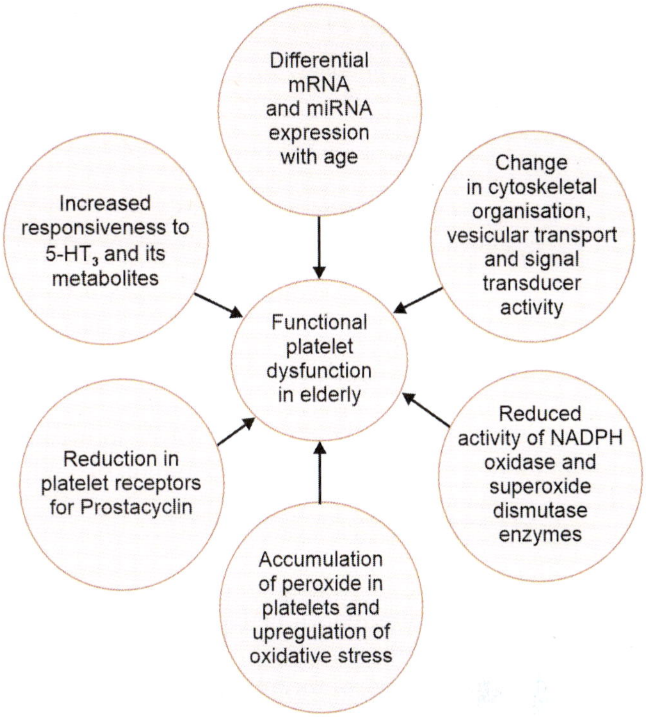

FIG. 1: Molecular level alterations causing qualitative platelet dysfunction.

(mRNA: messenger ribonucleic acid; miRNA: micro-ribonucleic acid; NADPH: nicotinamide-adenine dinucleotide phosphate; 5-HT$_3$: 5-hydroxytryptamine)

MECHANISM AND INCIDENCE OF ELDERLY THROMBOCYTOPENIA

Immune Thrombocytopenia

Immune thrombocytopenia is a common cause of moderate-to-severe thrombocytopenia in otherwise asymptomatic elderly. The incidence of ITP in older males is around 23/100,000 males, a nearly 10-fold increase when compared to men aged between the ages of 30 and 39 years. The mechanism of ITP is antibody-mediated platelet destruction. The ITP occurring in the elderly is mostly secondary to either malignancy or infections like HIV/hepatitis C. It is mandatory to screen these etiologies in the elderly with thrombocytopenia.

Heparin-induced Thrombocytopenia

It is characterized by antibodies against platelet factor 4/heparin complexes causing platelet activation. The elderly age group is an isolated risk factor to develop heparin-induced thrombocytopenia (HIT). Clinical features include new onset thrombocytopenia in a patient exposed to heparin within the prior 5–10 days; a platelet count drop of >50% from baseline, venous or arterial thrombosis, necrotic skin lesions at sites of heparin injection, and acute systemic reactions after intravenous

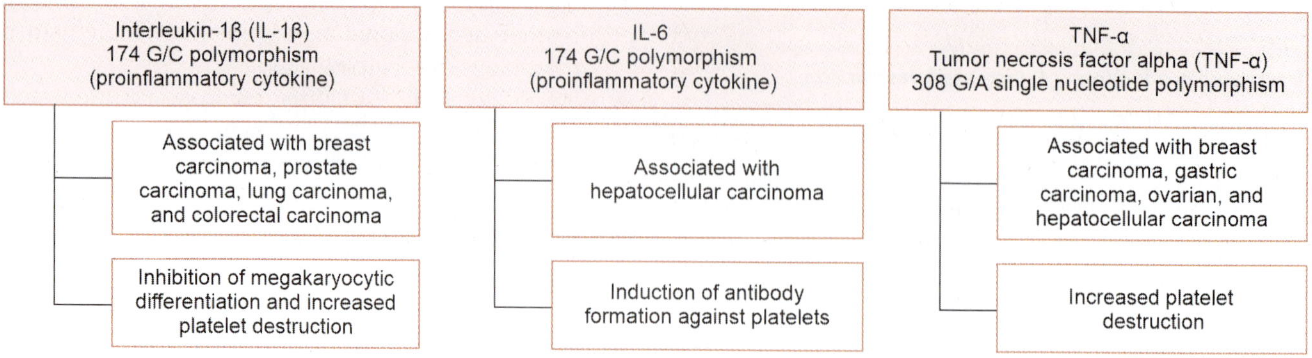

FLOWCHART 1: Mechanisms of various malignancies causing thrombocytopenia.

heparin administration. Treatment involves immediate discontinuation of heparin and administration of a novel oral anticoagulant.

Malignancy

Cancer can cause thrombocytopenia as a component of chronic disseminated intravascular coagulation (DIC), bone marrow infiltration, or thrombotic microangiopathy (TMA). The prevalence of thrombocytopenia in malignancy may be related to many variables, including therapeutic side effects, polymorphism, and mutation in certain transcription factors (TFs) and cytokines, as well as genetic factors. A careful evaluation of these genetic changes and a better understanding of their role in the incidence of thrombocytopenia can be helpful in choosing the most appropriate treatment protocols **(Flowchart 1)**.

Hematological malignancies are more likely to cause thrombocytopenia because of either autoimmune destruction or marrow involvement. Solid organ malignancies tend to cause thrombocytopenia by distant metastasis to bone marrow. Another mechanism of getting thrombocytopenia in malignancy is via chemotherapy. Certain chemotherapeutic agents such as ifosfamide, cyclophosphamide, and rituximab are prone to cause thrombocytopenia due to their cytotoxic effects.

Data on the true prevalence of thrombocytopenia in patients with cancer and concomitant thrombosis are extremely limited. The Flatiron Health Electronic Health Record database discovered a 3-month cumulative incidence of thrombocytopenia of 13% (any grade, platelet count 100,000/L) among patients with solid tumors. Severe thrombocytopenia (platelet count <50,000/μL) occurred in 6% of the patients with solid tumors receiving chemotherapy, and 28% of patients with hematological malignancies receiving chemotherapy.

Nutrient Deficiencies

Deficiency of nutrients required for hematopoiesis (e.g., folate and vitamin B12) typically causes mild pancytopenia, but isolated thrombocytopenia may be seen. Nutrient deficiencies are prevalent in old age due to poor oral intake, certain dietary practices, and indigestion or other gastrointestinal surgeries if supplementation is inadequate.

Bone Marrow Disorders

Particularly important to elderly patients with bone marrow dysplasia is the age-related decline in normal bone marrow function, including the diminished capacity of response to stressors such as infection and myelosuppressive treatments. Autoimmune attack against marrow stem and progenitor cells leads to pancytopenia. These patients can have persistent thrombocytopenia, require regular platelet transfusions, which are expensive and inconvenient and are at risk for further serious bleeding complications. At presentation, virtually all patients with aplastic anemia are thrombocytopenic—platelet counts of <50,000 or 20,000/μL are diagnostic criteria for moderate and severe aplastic anemia, respectively.

Another possibility for thrombocytopenia in older adults is myelodysplastic syndrome (MDS), which affects the megakaryocyte lineage. Although the majority of MDS cases have concomitant thrombocytopenia (65%), isolated thrombocytopenia is less common (12% of the cases). Other cytopenia or macrocytosis on a total blood count, as well as symptoms of dyserythropoiesis and/or dysgranulopoiesis on a peripheral blood smear examination, should induce a bone marrow examination to rule out an MDS.

Thrombotic Microangiopathy

Thrombotic microangiopathies such as thrombotic thrombocytopenic purpura (TTP), and hemolytic uremic syndrome (HUS), are rare in the elderly, but drug-induced thrombotic microangiopathy (DITMA) must be considered in any patient with microangiopathic hemolytic anemia and thrombocytopenia. Mitomycin C, gemcitabine, and oxaliplatin are the most frequently reported chemotherapeutic medications to be related to the development of HUS/TTP. In the limited recent reports of ADAMTS13 (a disintegrin and metalloproteinase with a thrombospondin type 1 motif, member 13) activity, nearly all instances have levels > 10%. Endothelial activation and damage appear to be prevalent in chemotherapeutic agent-related instances.

Comorbidities

Multiple concomitant comorbidities such as diabetes mellitus, hypertension, atherosclerosis, dyslipidemia, and obesity predispose an elderly to subendothelial damage leading to exposure to subendothelial matrix. There is a gradual reduction of vasoprotective factors such as nitric oxide (NO) and prostacyclins (PGI_2) with increasing age. This causes the deposition of platelets at the exposed site leading to a condition of thrombocytopenia along with a greater risk of thrombosis.

Others

- The elderly, who have prosthetic valves can develop thrombocytopenia.
- Post-transfusion purpura is a rare form of immune-mediated platelet destruction following transfusion of platelet-containing blood products.

APPROACH TO THROMBOCYTOPENIA

Our approach to the patient with newly discovered, unexplained thrombocytopenia involves confirmation of the finding by repeating the complete blood count (CBC) to exclude pseudothrombocytopenia, reviewing the peripheral blood smear, obtaining prior platelet counts if available, assessing other hematologic abnormalities.

Evaluation of thrombocytopenia should start with history and physical examination followed by laboratory analysis.

History

- History should be taken for recurrent bleeding, bruising, ecchymosis, and malena to localize the source of bleeding.
- The presence of family history is unlikely in the elderly, but if present should carefully be evaluated for underlying malignancies.

Physical Examination

- Physical examination should focus on finding occult lymphadenopathy and/or hepatosplenomegaly. The liver and spleen should be examined for respective enlargement.
- Splenomegaly can be a sign of liver disease, lymphoma, or other hematologic conditions; hypersplenism of any etiology may cause thrombocytopenia.
- Lymphadenopathy in a patient with thrombocytopenia may suggest infection, lymphoma, or other malignancies including metastasis.

Laboratory Analysis

Hemogram

Thrombocytopenia is initially detected in a hemogram. A combination of thrombocytopenia with leukocytosis favors the diagnosis of infection or hematological malignancy. The presence of pancytopenia is seen more in the elderly than younger population because of the higher incidence of myelodysplasia and malignancy.

Peripheral Blood Smear

It is helpful in the exclusion of pseudothrombocytopenia. Leukoerythroblastic findings and teardrop cells suggest an infiltrative process in the bone marrow. Immature WBC suggests leukemia or myelodysplasia. Multilobed/hypersegmented neutrophils (i.e., >5 lobes) suggest a megaloblastic process (e.g., B12, folate, and copper deficiency).

Mean Platelet Volume

The effective size of the platelet is measured in terms of mean platelet volume (MPV). Antonio et al. quoted that there is a steady rise in MPV with age. A higher MPV means larger platelets, which are seen when peripheral platelet destruction occurs. Lower MPV is suggestive of decreased platelet formation. Smaller platelets tend to be older, so a low MPV could mean the bone marrow is not producing enough new platelets.

Human Immunodeficiency Virus and Hepatitis C Virus Testing

Human immunodeficiency virus and HCV must be ruled out in all cases of thrombocytopenia.

Bone Marrow Assessment

Bone marrow assessment is not required in all patients of thrombocytopenia; however, it is essential for the elderly to rule out malignancy. Normal or increased numbers of megakaryocytes suggest that thrombocytopenia is due to a condition associated with platelet destruction. Decreased megakaryocyte number along with overall hypocellularity may be seen in aplastic anemia. Megaloblastic changes in the red blood cell (RBC) and granulocytic series suggest a nutrient deficiency (e.g., vitamin B12, folate, and copper), while dysplastic changes suggest a myelodysplastic disorder. Granulomata, increased reticulin or collagen fibrosis, or infiltration with malignant cells establishes the diagnosis of bone marrow invasion, especially when a leukoerythroblastic blood picture is also present.

Radiological Evaluation

Radiological investigations are needed to detect the underlying malignancy associated with thrombocytopenia.

Positron Emission Tomography

Positron emission tomography (PET) is a very useful tool to detect occult malignancy. In an elderly with thrombocytopenia, PET does not only help in localizing but also helps in staging the malignancy.

MANAGEMENT OF THROMBOCYTOPENIA

The management of thrombocytopenia depends upon the management of the underlying disorder.

Emergency Management of Bleeding

Urgent management of critical bleeding in the setting of severe thrombocytopenia requires immediate platelet transfusion, regardless of the underlying cause.

Indications for Platelet Transfusion

By convention, most authors use the term "therapeutic transfusion" to refer both to the transfusion of platelets to treat active bleeding and the transfusion of platelets in preparation for an invasive procedure that could cause bleeding. The term "prophylactic transfusion" is used to refer to platelet transfusion given to prevent spontaneous bleeding.

Active Bleeding

Actively bleeding patients with thrombocytopenia should be transfused with platelets immediately to keep platelet counts >50,000/μL in most bleeding situations including DIC, and >100,000/μL if there is intracranial bleed.

Preparation for an Invasive Procedure

If the thrombocytopenia is severe, if there is not enough time to employ other measures to raise the platelet count when necessary, and if the risks of bleeding are considerable, platelets are transfused in advance of an invasive procedure. Certain platelet counts have been set as recommended cutoffs for different surgeries viz **(Table 2)**.

Anticoagulation in Individuals with Thrombocytopenia

Thrombocytopenia may raise the risk of bleeding, but it does not protect against venous thromboembolism (VTE) or stroke.

Decisions about anticoagulation in patients with thrombocytopenia must balance the risks of thrombosis and thrombosis progression with the risks of bleeding due to thrombocytopenia as well as other bleeding risk factors. Cancer-associated VTE is one of the most common scenarios in which VTE and thrombocytopenia coexist.

The management of thrombocytopenia in the elderly should focus on managing the comorbidities along with the management of bleeding, if any.

Immune thrombocytopenia management (Flowchart 2): Treatment of MDS is usually limited to drugs, such as azacitidine and decitabine. If the drugs fail in achieving remission, the patient should be taken up for allogenic or autologous bone marrow transplantation, depending upon the performance status.

Thrombocytopenia which is secondary to nutritional deficiency of should be corrected with adequate supplementation.

Chemotherapy or malignancy-associated thrombocytopenia can be treated with drugs such as roflumilast, eltrombopag, lusutrombopag, and recombinant

TABLE 2: Various invasive procedures and their minimal recommended platelet count.

Procedures/Surgeries	Recommended platelet count
Neurosurgery/Ocular surgery	<100,000/mm^3
Other major surgeries	<50,000/mm^3
Endoscopic procedures	<50,000/mm^3
Bronchoscopy with bronchoalveolar lavage (BAL)	<20,000/mm^3
Central line placement	<20,000/mm^3
Lumbar puncture	<10,000/mm^3
Neuraxial analgesia	<80,000/mm^3
Bone marrow aspiration/biopsy	<20,000/mm^3

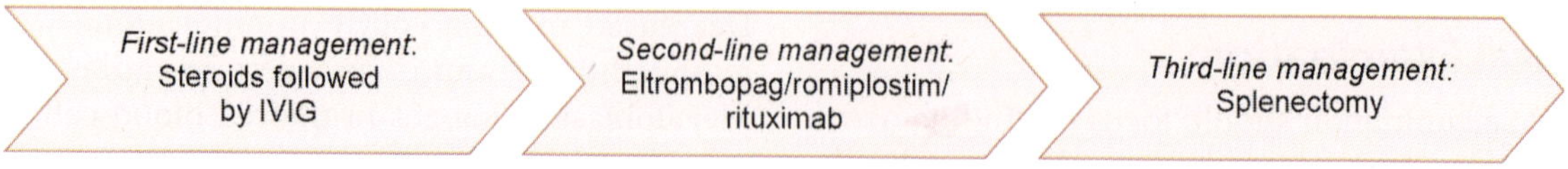

FLOWCHART 2: Step-wise management of ITP.
(ITP: immune thrombocytopenia management; IVIG: intravenous immunoglobulin)

thrombopoietin. Recombinant interleukin 11 (oprelvekin) has been shown to reduce the need for platelet transfusions in individuals who had previously received chemotherapy and platelet transfusions from 96 to 70%. Chemotherapy dose or frequency reductions are the mainstays of treatment in chemotherapy-induced thrombocytopenia.

CONCLUSION

Thrombocytopenia is becoming more common in older people, and the diagnostic workup is largely the same as in younger patients, with a focus on ruling out an underlying malignancy. The mechanisms that cause disease may differ and are likely to be a hot issue for research in the future since it will assist tailor therapy. One of the review's limitations is that evidence-based therapy is scarce among older patients, despite a growing number of retrospective studies concentrating on this demographic. After correcting for other variables, age is associated with the accumulation of chronic diseases but is unlikely to be a prognostic factor in ITP. Thus, rather than age, therapy decisions should be patient-tailored based on the patient's preferences, comorbidities, and fitness.

Thrombocytopenia in the elderly confers a greater risk on their frail physical status. Multiple comorbid conditions in an elderly person confer a greater risk of bleeding. Immune thrombocytopenia occurring in the elderly is by and large associated with HIV-HCV/malignancy. Therapies are tailored according to the disease process and the treatment availability, acceptability, and affordability.

SUGGESTED READINGS

1. Cortelazzo S, Finazzi G, Buelli M, Molteni A, Viero P, Barbui T. High risk of severe bleeding in aged patients with chronic idiopathic thrombocytopenic purpura. Blood. 1991;77(1):31-3.
2. Stasi R, Amadori S, Osborn J, Newland AC, Provan D. Long-term outcome of otherwise healthy individuals with incidentally discovered borderline thrombocytopenia. PLoS Med. 2006;3(3):e24.
3. Rodeghiero F, Stasi R, Gernsheimer T, Michel M, Provan D, Arnold DM, et al. Standardization of terminology, definitions and outcome criteria in immune thrombocytopenic purpura of adults and children: report from an international working group. Blood. 2009;113(11):2386-93.
4. Aster RH. Pooling of platelets in the spleen: role in the pathogenesis of "hypersplenic" thrombocytopenia. J Clin Invest. 1966;45(5):645-57.
5. Waisbren J, Dinner S, Altman J, Frankfurt O, Helenowski I, Gao J, et al. Disease characteristics and prognosis of myelodysplastic syndrome presenting with isolated thrombocytopenia. Int J Hematol. 2017;105(1):44-51.
6. Bloom MB, Johnson J, Volod O, Lee EY, White T, Margulies DR et al. Improved prediction of HIT in the SICU using an improved model of the Warkentin 4-T system: 3-T. Am J Surg. 2020;219(1):54-7.
7. Young NS, Calado RT, Scheinberg P. Current concepts in the pathophysiology and treatment of aplastic anemia. Blood. 2006;108(8):2509-19.
8. Avvisati G, Tirindelli MC, Annibali O. Thrombocytopenia and hemorrhagic risk in cancer patients. Crit Rev Oncol Hematol. 2003;48(Suppl):S13-6.
9. Snoeck HW. Aging of the hematopoietic system. Curr Opin Hematol. 2013;20(4):355-61.
10. Zhang X, Chuai Y, Nie W, Wang A, Dai G. Thrombopoietin receptor agonists for prevention and treatment of chemotherapy-induced thrombocytopenia in patients with solid tumours. Cochrane Database Syst Rev. 2017;11(11): CD012035.
11. Shaw JL, Nielson CM, Park JK. The incidence of thrombocytopenia in adult patients receiving chemotherapy for solid tumors or hematologic malignancies. Eur J Haematol. 2021;106(5):662-72.

45

CHAPTER

Caring for the Elderly in the Intensive Care Unit

Y Sathyanarayana Raju

ABSTRACT

A gradual increase in the elderly population has been observed globally, and it is estimated that this increasing trend is likely to continue in the near future. The disease burden and severity are higher in elderly not only because of physiological alterations that occur with aging but also due to various other factors such as multimorbidity, frailty, polypharmacy, and disability. The number of elderlies requiring intensive care unit (ICU) admission is also increasing. Critical care physicians are adapting and extrapolating the existing evidence obtained from adults in the general population to treat the older adults. In the current critical care delivery model, elderly patients requiring critical care are being admitted according to their presenting condition, under the specialists pertaining to the system involved. Thus, delivery of holistic critical care to the elderly is seldom happening, especially in developing countries like India. The ultimate goal of delivery of critical care to the elderly is to improve the outcome of the elderly individuals admitted to ICUs and optimize their functional status. To tackle this problem, there is a need to develop the specialty of geriatric critical care medicine to deliver the best possible care to critically ill elderly.

INTRODUCTION

In the past two decades, there has been a gradual increase in elderly population. The term elderly has no precise definition. Many studies have used different arbitrary cutoff points, such as over 60, 65, or 70 years old. However, most prospective epidemiological studies define the "elderly population" as the age group ≥ 65 years. According to the World Health Organization (WHO), in 2019, the number of people aged 60 years and older was 1 billion. By 2030, one in six people in the world will be ≥ 60 years. The world population of people aged 60 years and older will be doubled (2.1 billion) by 2050. Almost two-thirds of the world population over 60 years are living in low- and middle-income countries. According to the Census 2011, India has 104 million elderly, constituting 8.6% of the total population.

The disease burden grows with increasing life expectancy. Hence, the diversity, severity, and complexity of illnesses are expected to occur. The disease burden and severity are higher in elderly due to various factors such as multimorbidity, disability, and frailty. Owing to normal physiological alterations that occur with aging, elderly population are more prone to complications due to common chronic diseases when compared to the young. If complications develop, the need for an intensive care unit (ICU) increases and recovery may be prolonged.

Elderly population currently accounts for almost half of the ICU admissions. Critical care physicians adapt the existing evidence to treat older adults admitted in the ICU. However, there is a lack of formal training about principles of geriatric care and management. Hence, a field of "geriatric critical care medicine" is being proposed to give the best care to older adults with critical illnesses. ICU clinicians must be able to manage age-related complexity and vulnerability by integrating geriatrics into clinical practice.

Aging-related common clinical conditions, other than discrete disease processes, which increase the vulnerability to morbidity and lead to poor prognosis are

TABLE 1: Comparison of the causes of ICU admission in elderly.

Variable	Upparakadiyala R	Miniksar ÖH	Fuchs L	Lankoandé M
Place of study	Tirupati	Turkey	Boston	Burkina Faso
Year of study	2022	2021	2012	2018
Age (years)	69.8 ± 7.6*	86–90	>65	71.7 ± 6.1*
Sample size	196	218	7,265	237
Cause for ICU admission				
Central nervous system (CVA, meningitis and seizures)†	83 (42.3)	36 (16.5)	ND	65 (27.4)
Respiratory system (ARDS and pneumonia)†	22 (9.7)	25 (11.5)	822 (11.3)	ND
Cardiovascular system (heart failure/MI)†	14 (7.1)	3 (1.4)	1,635 (22.5)	18 (25)
Gastrointestinal system†	5 (2.5)	9 (4.1)	1,126 (15.5)	13 (5.5)
Genitourinary system†	26 (13.3)	12 (5.5)	216 (0.03)	43 (18.1)
Metabolic†	16 (8.2)	ND	ND	20 (8.4)
Infections (sepsis)†	18 (9.2)	43 (19.7)	814 (11.2)	26 (10.9)
Trauma†	–	5 (2.3)	1,050 (14.4)	25 (10.5)
Miscellaneous†	12 (6)	17 (7.8)	817 (11.2)	27 (11.4)

*Data are expressed as mean ± standard deviation.
†Data are presented as number (%).

(ARDS: acute respiratory distress syndrome; CVA: cerebrovascular accident; ICU: intensive care unit; MI: myocardial infarction; ND: not described)

Sources: Upparakadiyala R, et al. 2022; Miniksar ÖH, et al. 2021; Fuchs L et al. 2012; Lankoandé M, et al. 2018.

collectively termed as "geriatric syndromes". Some of these include delirium, recurrent falls, pressure ulcers, and incontinence. The presence of one or more of these syndromes contributes to increased need for nursing care and reduced quality of life both during and after critical illness. The increasing need for ICU admission in elderly can be attributed to diseases of single or multiple systems. The cause for ICU admission in elderly varies in different geographic regions. A comparison of the causes of ICU admission in elderly is depicted in **Table 1**.

MANAGEMENT OF ELDERLY IN INTENSIVE CARE UNIT

The need for ICU admission should be based on the patient's comorbidities, acuity of illness, and prehospital functional status, which includes quality of life and whether the patient was living independently or was admitted from a subacute/chronic healthcare facility.

The care of elderly patients in the ICU is comparable to care of younger patients. The priorities of management are the same. Because critically ill elderly patients often have impaired physiologic reserves, the clinician must be extra vigilant in searching for early, subtle signs of organ system dysfunction and cautious in weaning physiologic support. Management of various organ systems is detailed further.

Cardiovascular System

In older adults, there is an increased incidence of myocardial infarction (MI) associated with increased in-hospital mortality; presence of comorbidities further increases the risk. Other common cardiac manifestations include heart failure and arrhythmias. It is probably appropriate to set a cardiac index and oxygen delivery goals slightly above resting levels, but every effort must be made to minimize unnecessary stresses that increase metabolic demand such as hypothermia, shivering, exposure to a cool ambient environment, hypovolemia, acidosis, pain, and inappropriate weaning from inadequate mechanical ventilatory support. The oxygen transport system should also be optimized so as to achieve the least demand. Hemodynamic monitoring should be done regularly either physiological or invasive to interpret the abnormalities and intervene as appropriate.

Respiratory System

In elderly patients, there is an impairment of respiratory reserve due to age-related physiological changes which affects respiratory function. There will be a diminished response to hypoxia and hypercarbia, airway protective mechanism also diminishes with age, thus increasing the risk of aspiration. In addition to these, presence of obesity and chronic lung diseases further diminishes the respiratory function. The sedatives and narcotics administered during ICU stay further blunt respiratory function. All these factors increase the need for ventilatory support.

The requirement of mechanical ventilatory support increases as the age advances, and hence, the elderlies are also at risk of developing complications related to ventilatory support. The benefits of ventilator in acute and chronic respiratory function impairment should be measured against the risks associated with prolonged intubation. Intermittent mandatory ventilation with high positive end-expiratory pressure may be required till the sedative effect is weaned off and lung function recovers. A spontaneous breathing trial (SBT) is to be done on a daily basis to assess the respiratory effort and to wean off the ventilator. Timely tracheostomy can be done if there is a prolonged ventilatory requirement.

Neurological

Acute brain dysfunction, or delirium, and long-term cognitive impairment are highly prevalent among ICU patients. Around 60–80% of ICU patients are known to develop delirium during their critical phase of illness. Age is a well-established risk factor for both delirium and cognitive impairment. Routine screening for delirium should be done with validated assessment tools such as Confusion Assessment Method for the ICU (CAM-ICU) or Intensive Care Delirium Screening Checklist (ICDSC). The onset of delirium is an independent predictor of increased duration of mechanical ventilation, duration of ICU and hospital stay, increased healthcare costs, long-term cognitive impairment, and mortality. Serial neurological examination and minimized sleep disturbances should be followed for ICU patients to assess cognitive dysfunction. Analgesics and sedatives should be used cautiously as and when needed.

Nutrition

Malnutrition is associated with functional decline, sarcopenia, anemia, and poor wound healing. Nutritional support should be initiated early following ICU admission. Currently, there is no single best tool for nutritional assessment of elderly in the ICU. The Geriatric Nutritional Risk Index (GNRI) was created to predict nutrition-related risk of morbidity and mortality in hospitalized older patients. Other tools used are Mini Nutritional Assessment (MNA) and Nutrition Risk in the Critically Ill (NUTRIC) score. Enteral nutrition is preferred as it preserves intestinal function. Total parenteral nutrition (TPN) used in enteral nutrition is contraindicated and is associated with increased mortality.

Infection and Immunity

Aging leads to an age-dependent decline in immune system effectiveness, this is known as immunosenescence, these changes include a higher level of proinflammatory cytokine secretion at baseline and a decrease in the ability to stimulate the immune response to antigens. Sepsis may present as hypotension, elevated cardiac index, acidosis, and worsening hypoglycemia or hyperglycemia. In elderly, respiratory infection is the most common source of sepsis followed by urinary source. The decline in immune system function in older patients also increases their risk for secondary infections or hospital-acquired infections. Antibiotics should be used with caution, as the renal clearance diminishes with age and due to usage of multiple concomitant drugs.

Drugs

Multimorbidity in elderly leads to polypharmacy. In a systemic review, polypharmacy has established a strong relationship with negative clinical outcomes. This also leads to increased occurrence of inappropriate doses of medication, adverse drug reactions, and drug–drug interactions, which ultimately results in poor hospital outcome. Excessive usage of sedatives may increase the risk of development of delirium. Aging itself is an independent risk factor for adverse drug reactions. Along with this gradual decrease in renal and hepatic reserve decreases the clearance of drugs, hence, contributing to toxicity.

OUTCOME

Outcome assessment in terms of mortality, functional level, and quality of life is evaluated by various methods and at various times in the course of critical illness and recovery. However, not all individuals of the same age are equally vulnerable to critical illness. Age is not the only predictor of outcomes in a critically ill older adult. Other factors that would determine the outcomes and recovery include pre-existing factors that increase the vulnerability (e.g., frailty), triggering factors that cause acute worsening (e.g., infection and fall), and factors that prolong the recovery period (e.g., delirium).

Immunosenescence (age-associated gradual deterioration of protective immunity) and *inflammaging* (chronic subclinical systemic inflammation) are the two main phenomena that result in systemic deterioration, leading to increased susceptibility to chronic illnesses. Advanced life-support technology that can be provided in the ICU is intended to provide temporary physiologic support to patients with potentially reversible organ failure or dysfunction. With the projected exponential increase in the number of elderly patients and the increasing burden of chronic disease, how can we best select which patients are likely to derive the most benefit from admission to the ICU?

Various scoring systems like acute physiology and chronic health evaluation (APACHE) II and III are used to predict the mortality and morbidity risk. The goal of critical care medicine is to restore patients to a level of functioning, similar to that of their preadmission status and to return the patients back to their routine status. However, despite optimal measures, this is not achieved in many cases and patients are discharged in a suboptimal state.

CONCLUSION

The ultimate goal of delivery of critical care to the elderly is to improve the outcome of the elderly individuals admitted to ICUs and optimize their functional status. To tackle this problem, there is a need for capacity building. Developing the specialty of geriatric critical care medicine to deliver the best possible care to critically ill elderly is the need of the hour.

SUGGESTED READINGS

1. World Health Organization. (2023). Ageing. [online] Available from https://www.who.int/health-topics/ageing. [Last accessed December, 2023].
2. World Health Organization. (2022). Ageing and health. [online] Available from https://www.who.int/india/health-topics/ageing. [Last accessed December, 2023].
3. Fried LP, Ferrucci L, Darer J, Williamson JD, Anderson G. Untangling the concepts of disability, frailty, and comorbidity: implications for improved targeting and care. J Gerontol A Biol Sci Med Sci. 2004;59:255-63.
4. Akinosoglou K, Schinas G, Almyroudi MP, Gogos C, Dimopoulos G. The impact of age on intensive care. Ageing Res Rev. 2023;84:101832.
5. Marik PE. Management of the critically ill geriatric patient. Crit Care Med. 2006;34(9 Suppl):S176-82.
6. Brummel NE, Ferrante LE. Integrating geriatric principles into critical care medicine: the time is now. Ann Am Thorac Soc. 2018;15(5):518-22.
7. Raju YS, Regati M. Critical care in the elderly: Need of the hour. J Clin Sci Res. 2022;11(3):123-4.
8. Upparakadiyala R, Singapati S, Sarkar MK, Swathi U. Clinical profile and factors affecting outcomes in elderly patients admitted to the medical intensive care unit of a tertiary care hospital. Cureus. 2022;14(2):e22136.
9. Miniksar ÖH, Özdemir M. Clinical features and outcomes of very elderly patients admitted to the intensive care unit: a retrospective and observational study. Indian J Crit Care Med. 2021;25(6):629-34.
10. Fuchs L, Chronaki CE, Park S, Novack V, Baumfeld Y, Scott D, et al. ICU admission characteristics and mortality rates among elderly and very elderly patients. Intensive Care Med. 2012;38(10):1654-61.
11. Lankoandé M, Bonkoungou P, Simporé A, Somda G, Kabore RAF. Inhospital outcome of elderly patients in an intensive care unit in a Sub-Saharan hospital. BMC Anesthesiol. 2018;18:118.
12. Brunker LB, Boncyk CS, Rengel KF, Hughes CG. Elderly patients and management in intensive care units (ICU): Clinical challenges. Clin Interv Aging. 2023;18:93-112.
13. Watters JM, Bessey PQ. Critical care for the elderly patient. Surg Clin North Am. 1994;74(1):187-97.
14. Ouimet S, Kavanagh BP, Gottfried SB, Skrobik Y. Incidence, risk factors and consequences of ICU delirium. Intensive Care Med. 2007;33(1):66-73.
15. Ely EW, Inouye SK, Bernard GR, Gordon S, Francis J, May L, et al. Delirium in mechanically ventilated patients: Validity and reliability of the confusion assessment method for the intensive care unit (CAM-ICU). JAMA. 2001;286(21):2703-10.
16. Bouillanne O, Morineau G, Dupont C, Coulombel I, Vincent JP, Nicolis I, et al. Geriatric nutritional risk index: A new index for evaluating at-risk elderly medical patients. Am J Clin Nutr. 2005;82(4):777-83.
17. Vellas B, Guigoz Y, Garry PJ, Nourhashemi F, Bennahum D, Lauque S, et al. The mini nutritional assessment (MNA) and its use in grading the nutritional state of elderly patients. Nutrition. 1999;15(2):116-22.
18. Pawelec G. Age and immunity: what is "immunosenescence"? Exp Gerontol. 2018;105:4-9.
19. Yoshikawa TT. Antimicrobial therapy for the elderly patient. J Am Geriatr Soc. 1990;38(12):1353-72.
20. Maher RL, Hanlon J, Hajjar ER. Clinical consequences of polypharmacy in elderly. Expert Opin Drug Saf. 2014;13(1):57-65.

46

CHAPTER

Anemia in the Elderly: New Therapeutic Concepts

Shyam Chand Chaudhary, Arvind Kumar Verma, Avinash Kumar, Tarun Pal, Kamal Kumar Sawlani

ABSTRACT

The elderly population is growing worldwide day by day. Anemia is a significant concern in the elderly, impacting both physical and cognitive function, and reducing quality of life. It is often linked to chronic diseases and inflammation. The consequences of anemia in the elderly are far-reaching and affect cardiovascular health, cognitive function, and mortality. This chapter explores the multifactorial causes of anemia in the elderly, including nutritional deficiencies, anemia of chronic disease (ACD), and unexplained anemia. Various diagnostic methods, from basic investigations to bone marrow aspiration, are discussed. Managing anemia in the elderly involves a tailored approach, considering underlying causes and comorbidities. Treatment options include supplementation therapy, erythropoiesis-stimulating agents (ESAs), gene therapy, hepcidin inhibitors, and hypoxia-inducible factor (HIF) prolyl-hydroxylase inhibitors.

INTRODUCTION

The world's population is currently experiencing its highest-ever age distribution, marked by a substantial growth in the elderly demographic. Despite not being a disease, advanced age renders individuals susceptible to chronic health issues, resulting in functional limitations. Anticipated projections indicate that by 2050, nearly a quarter of the global population will be elderly, consequently straining healthcare resources and economies.

Anemia is a major public health problem both in developed and developing countries, although the rates are higher in all ages in underdeveloped nations. Anemia per se is not a disease, rather it is a symptom. It is an important health indicator and affects both cognitive and physical functions in the elderly, leading to poor quality of life. Estimates of anemia prevalence reported in the reviewed literature range from 2.9 to 61% in elderly men and from 3.3 to 41% in elderly women. This variability is related to a number of factors, including the setting of the study, the health status of the subject population, and the criteria used to define anemia.

Anemia of chronic disease (ACD), also known as anemia of chronic inflammation, pertains to specific chronic medical conditions, such as chronic renal disease, rheumatoid arthritis, cancer, autoimmune disease, and chronic infection. It is reasonable to anticipate anemia in older individuals grappling with these enduring conditions, similar to their younger counterparts. However, it is not always recognized that older patients with different medical issues, such as cognitive impairment, face a bleaker outlook when they are also anemic. While the connection between anemia and heart failure, myocardial infarction, or mortality is expected, the underlying reasons linking anemia with other health issues are more elusive.

Anemia in the elderly is particularly relevant as it has a number of serious consequences, such as a higher incidence of cardiovascular disease, cognitive impairment, decreased physical performance and quality of life, and increased risk of falls and fractures. Furthermore, the presence of anemia is significantly associated with longer hospital stays and with an increased risk of mortality. Anemia in old age is unique in many aspects. Its diagnosis poses a challenge as there are innumerable presentations of anemia, which are nonspecific and often overlooked. Clinical features of anemia tend to be attributed to advancing age, which may present as worsening of other conditions.

DEFINITION

The World Health Organization defines anemia when (established in 1968) hemoglobin (Hb) is <13 g/dL and hematocrit (HCT) is <0.39 (39%) in males, and Hb is <12 g/dL and HCT is <0.36 (36%) in females.

EPIDEMIOLOGY

The prevalence of anemia in older people presents significant problems for global healthcare systems. Large prospective registry studies have found that anemia affects elderly people on average 10–24% of the time. Low Hb levels increase the risk of heart disease, dementia, sleep disorders, low mood, and a reduced quality of life. Additionally, anemia is linked to diminished physical and mental function. Falls and fractures are more likely to occur in people with low Hb levels.

PRESENTATIONS

Common presentations of anemia are fatigue, loss of appetite, palpitation, breathlessness on exertion, and chest pain. Underlying health conditions like diabetes, hypertension, kidney disease, and cancer can exacerbate the state of anemia.

ETIOLOGY

Anemia in the elderly has a multifactorial origin, resulting from a complex interplay of numerous factors. The various factors causing anemia are illustrated in **Table 1**, and **Table 2** exhibits varying prevalence rates.

TABLE 1: Factors responsible for anemia in the elderly.

Types of anemia	Salient features

Anemia of inflammation (anemia of chronic disease)	• Most common form of anemia in elderly
	• Three mechanisms involved in the development of anemia of chronic disease are:
	  ○ Failure of erythropoiesis
	  ○ Lack of iron for hemoglobin synthesis
	  ○ Decreased RBC survival

Anemia due to blood loss	• By the direct loss of RBCs (posthemorrhagic anemia)
	• Protracted blood loss:
	  ○ Gradually depleting iron stores, eventually resulting in iron deficiency
	  ○ It can result from gastritis, peptic ulcer (due to drugs), varices, hemorrhoids, gastrointestinal tumors, and genitourinary tract.

Anemia due to decreased production of RBC	• Deficiency of raw materials (vitamin B12, folic acids, and iron) • Bone marrow failure (aplastic anemia and myelodysplastic syndrome) • Bone marrow infiltration (leukemia, lymphoma, and secondaries) • Other diseases interfering with normal marrow function (anemia of inflammation)
Unexplained anemia (UA)	Anemia of unknown etiology (AUE)

(RBC: red blood cells)

TABLE 2: Prevalence and subtypes of anemia in the elderly.

Subtypes	Prevalence	Etiology	Prevalence	More frequent in elderly
Anemia of chronic disease	30%	Chronic inflammation	20%	Yes
		Renal disease	8%	Yes
Nutritional anemia	30%	Iron deficiency	15%	No
		Cobalamin deficiency	5–10%	Yes
		Folate deficiency	5–10%	No
Unknown cause	20%	MDS	15%	Yes
		Senescence	Unknown	Unknown
Other	<10%	Various	<10%	No

(MDS: myelodysplastic syndromes)

Anemia in the elderly can be categorized into three broad groups: Nutritional deficiency, ACD, and unexplained anemia (UA). It is important to note that these groups are not mutually exclusive. In a single patient, multiple causes may coexist, and each of them can independently contribute to the development of anemia.

ANEMIA OF INFLAMMATION (ANEMIA OF CHRONIC DISEASE)

Anemia of inflammation (AI), previously recognized as ACD, manifests as moderate normochromic-normocytic anemia arising from systemic inflammation and immune activation. A substantial portion of anemic individuals aged over 65 exhibit a hyperinflammatory condition seen in chronic kidney disease (CKD) or AI-related states such as cancer, autoimmune disorders, and chronic infections. The decline in glomerular filtration rate (GFR), nearly universal among this population, often coincides with reduced erythropoietin (EPO) production. Key underlying mechanisms include inadequate EPO levels and an impaired response of erythroid progenitors to EPO. Notably, various cytokines, such as tumor necrosis factor-alpha (TNF-α), interleukin (IL)-1, and transforming growth factor beta (TGF-β), detrimentally affect erythroid progenitor cell development. Another factor in AI's progression is eryptosis, the phagocytosis of aging erythrocytes prompted by changes in their plasma membrane composition.

Anemia of inflammation is prevalent worldwide and is particularly common among hospitalized patients, emerging as the primary anemia type in intensive care settings. Molecular processes driving AI are intricate and diverse. The overproduction of cytokines, such as IL1-β, TNF-α, and IL-6 by macrophages, along with interferon-gamma (INF-γ) by lymphocytes, leads to reduced EPO production, hindered erythropoiesis response, elevated hepcidin levels, and potential activation of erythrophagocytosis, especially during acute forms of inflammation.

NUTRITIONAL DEFICIENCIES ANEMIA

Nutritional deficiencies constitute a subgroup that can be effectively treated and include deficiencies in iron, vitamin B12, or folate. Among these, the most common type of nutritional anemia arises from iron deficiency, which is typically identified by low levels of serum ferritin and transferrin saturation. It is important to note that even when serum ferritin levels are within the normal or high range, iron deficiency cannot be ruled out entirely. This is because ferritin is an acute phase protein that may become elevated in the presence of inflammation or with advancing age.

Diagnosis of iron deficiency should not be an end in itself but should rather be the initiation of a search for its cause, including looking for a possible site of blood loss and possible underlying malignancy. The pathophysiology of ACD is multifactorial and relates to a reduced efficiency of iron recycling from red blood cells (RBCs), resulting in a functional iron deficiency. Thus, early and correct diagnosis is essential. Therefore, we always include folate and vitamin B12 measurement in our basic laboratory screening in elderly anemic patients.

UNEXPLAINED ANEMIA

Unexplained anemia makes up roughly one-third of all anemia cases in elderly individuals and is primarily a diagnosis reached by eliminating other possible causes since it cannot be classified using current available methods.

The pathophysiology of UA is intricate and not well understood. While undiagnosed malignancies, including myelodysplasia, previously unnoticed CKD, and other unusual factors might account for some cases of UA, their collective impact remains relatively limited. In populations where thalassemia is prevalent, thalassemia trait may account for another proportion of the UAs.

Dissecting the underlying causes of UA is complicated by the prevalence of coexisting health conditions in the elderly. Additionally, age-related elevations in proinflammatory cytokines like IL-6 can reduce the responsiveness of stem cells and progenitors to growth factors while promoting the production of hepcidin in an environment with diminished pluripotent hemopoietic stem cell reserves. Elevated levels of hepcidin have been observed in cases of UA, implying that inflammatory processes may play a role in anemia among the elderly, potentially involving mechanisms akin to those seen in ACD. Hence, a significant portion of UAs still lack a clear cause even after a thorough extended hematologic assessment.

DIAGNOSTIC WORKUP

Diagnostic workup can be tied up starting from basic investigations for determining the cause of anemia to a focused investigation for specific disease **(Table 3)**.

Bone marrow aspiration and biopsy are essential for ruling out hematologic disorders, including myelodysplastic syndromes (MDS), and for establishing an accurate diagnosis, especially when there are additional abnormalities in blood counts or other indications of a clonal hematologic condition.

TABLE 3: Suggested investigations in elderly with anemia.

Primary investigation	Level two investigations	Level three investigations
• Hemoglobin • Differential blood count • RBC indices • Reticulocyte count • Peripheral blood smear • CRP • Creatinine/glomerular filtration rate • Aminotransferase/aspartate • Stool for occult blood	• Serum vitamin B12 • Serum folate • Serum iron • Serum ferritin • Serum copper • Serum lactate dehydrogenase • Serum haptoglobin • Serum EPO level • Serum electrophoresis • Upper GI endoscopy and colonoscopy	• BM aspiration and biopsy • Molecular, cytogenetic, and/or flow cytometry studies

(BM: bone marrow; CRP: C-reactive protein; EPO: erythropoietin; GI: gastrointestinal; RBC: red blood cell)

In individuals with inconclusive results, further molecular, cytogenetic, and/or flow cytometry studies can be valuable in arriving at a definitive diagnosis, especially when there is suspicion of a clonal bone marrow disorder like MDS.

TREATMENT

Managing anemia in older individuals poses a clinical challenge, particularly when the cause is unclear and multiple comorbidities are involved. In many instances, correcting the anemia can be achieved through supplementation therapy or addressing the underlying cause when known. However, in some cases, ongoing treatment with interventional medications, continuous use of EPO, or blood transfusions may be necessary to effectively manage the anemia.

Before devising a treatment strategy, it is crucial to accurately identify the primary diagnosis and any associated conditions, with a focus on disorders that can be treated. Optimal therapy tailored to the patient's age is then introduced, considering potential side effects and impact on their quality of life.

For many individuals dealing with genuine iron deficiency, oral iron supplementation has proven effective. In recent times, novel oral iron variants such as ferric maltose and Sucrosomial iron, boasting heightened effectiveness and fewer adverse effects, have gained approval. If oral iron fails to address anemia, intravenous (IV) iron therapy becomes a valuable option. This is particularly relevant when factors such as reduced gastrointestinal absorption, compliance challenges, or an inflammatory state result in decreased iron utilization.

Various IV iron formulations are accessible, including iron sucrose, ferric gluconate, and ferumoxytol as rapid IV administration. Recently, newer and safer formulations, primarily ferric carboxymaltose and iron isomaltose, have gained approval and are being prescribed more frequently.

New Therapeutic Agents

Erythropoiesis-stimulating Agents

Erythropoiesis-stimulating agents (ESAs) are currently approved for the treatment of anemia in CKD and MDS. An insufficient response to EPO in the presence of anemia may be a central factor in the pathophysiology of anemia of unknown etiology (AUE). ESAs may have a role in the treatment of these patients with AUE. Some examples of newer ESAs include epoetin, darbepoetin, and methoxy polyethylene glycol-epoetin beta. These ESAs are generally prescribed in conditions characterized by impaired RBC production.

Erythropoietin Gene Therapy

Due to potential harm associated with high doses of erythropoietic products, there is an increasing interest in researching the possibility of generating lower yet sustained levels of EPO through gene therapy. The specific cells and sites from which EPO is released into the bloodstream do not seem to be the critical factors, and researchers have explored various delivery systems, including injecting naked DNA, adenovirus transfection, using artificial human chromosomes, and transplanting cells that have been manipulated ex vivo, either from the patient themselves (autologous) or from a donor (allogeneic).

Hepcidin Inhibitors

In individuals with pronounced inflammatory conditions, heightened levels of hepcidin disrupt the absorption of iron and the release of iron from macrophages, leading to anemia.

Lexaptepid pegol is a proprietary RNA oligonucleotide, consisting of a 44-nucleotide L-stereoisomer sequence, linked to a 40 kDa polyethylene glycol (PEG). It has the capacity to counter anemia by targeting hepcidin. When administered via IV or subcutaneous routes, lexaptepid pegol binds to hepcidin, preventing its interaction with ferroportin-a channel for iron, found on the gastrointestinal enterocytes' basolateral surface and macrophage plasma membranes. This action holds the potential to alleviate anemia triggered by inflammation.

Hypoxia-inducible Factor Prolyl-hydroxylase Inhibitors

Hypoxia-inducible factor prolyl-hydroxylase (HIF-PH) inhibitors such as roxadustat, vadadustat, daprodustat, molidustat, enarodustat, and desidustat can be particularly beneficial for elderly patients with naturally low EPO levels. Roxadustat (FG-4592), for instance, operates as an oral inhibitor of HIF-PH, which stimulates the production of RBCs and regulates iron metabolism. This approach provides an alternative to the traditional use of ESAs for the treatment of anemia.

Hypoxia-inducible factor prolyl-hydroxylase inhibitors present a pharmacological solution to overcome the challenges posed by ESA hyporesponsiveness. Unlike ESAs, which act directly on EPO receptors in RBC precursors, erythropoiesis through the HIF-PH pathway depends on cellular oxygen levels. It has been suggested that HIF-PH inhibitors may achieve more consistent and sustained erythropoiesis over time compared to ESAs.

Despite its potential benefits, the use of oral HIF-PH inhibitors has generated discussions regarding their effectiveness in addressing ESA hyporesponsiveness. These inhibitors offer an alternative physiological pathway for anemia treatment. However, uncertainties remain, particularly concerning the suitability and safety of HIF-PH inhibitors usage in elderly patients due to a lack of long-term safety data for this population.

Activin Type II Receptor Agonists

Luspatercept and sotatercept are categorized as EPO-modulating agents aimed at enhancing the effectiveness of EPO. These activin receptor II ligand traps work by inhibiting growth differentiation factor 11 (GDF11), showing promise as therapeutic options for various forms of ineffective erythropoiesis, including MDS and β-thalassemia.

Luspatercept is a fusion protein composed of the extracellular domain of activin receptor type IIB and the Fc portion of human immunoglobulin G1 (IgG1). By obstructing TGF-β superfamily inhibitors, it curtails Smad2 and Smad3 signaling. This action prevents the activation of multiple TGF-β superfamily members responsible for late-stage ineffective erythropoiesis. Luspatercept is also intended for patients who do not respond to ESA and have low-risk MDS with ring sideroblasts.

Similarly, sotatercept functions as another example of this drug category. These agents aim to enhance effective EPO levels, addressing deficiencies present in conditions like lower-risk MDS, β-thalassemia, and primary myelofibrosis. Ongoing research is investigating their use in patients with MDS and CKD.

CONCLUSION

Anemia in the elderly is a complex and widespread problem that has significant consequences for the well-being of older individuals. Diagnosing anemia in this population can be challenging due to the presence of multiple comorbidities and nonspecific symptoms, and its management in the elderly requires a personalized approach. Newer agents such as luspatercept and sotatercept seem promising in its management. Addressing anemia in the elderly is of paramount importance to improve their quality of life and reduce the risk of complications.

SUGGESTED READINGS

1. Beghé C, Wilson A, Ershler WB. Prevalence and outcomes of anemia in geriatrics: a systematic review of the literature. Am J Med. 2004;116(Suppl 7A):3S-10S.
2. Gaskell H, Derry S, Moore RA, McQuay HJ. Prevalence of anaemia in older persons: systematic review. BMC Geriatr. 2008;8:1.
3. Van Puyvelde K, Cytryn E, Mets T, Beyer Ingo. Anaemia in the elderly. Acta Clin Belg. 2009,64(4):292-302.
4. Weiss G, Goodnough LT. Anemia of chronic disease. N Engl J Med. 2005;352(10):1011-23.
5. Nutritional anaemias. Report of a WHO scientific group. World Health Organ Tech Rep Ser. 1968;405:5-37.
6. Ferrucci L, Guralnik JM, Bandinelli S, Semba RD, Lauretani F, Corsi A, et al. Unexplained anaemia in older persons is characterised by low erythropoietin and low levels of pro-inflammatory markers. Br J Haematol. 2007;136(6):849-55.
7. Stauder R, Thein SL. Anemia in the elderly: clinical implications and new therapeutic concepts. Haematologica. 2014;99(7):1127-30.
8. Macdougall IC. Novel erythropoiesis-stimulating agents: A new era in anemia management. Clin J Soc of Nephrol. 2008;3(1): 200-7.
9. Gowanlock Z, Sriram S, Martin A, Xenocostas A, Lazo-Langner A. Erythropoiesis-stimulating agents in elderly patients with

anemia: response and cardiovascular outcomes. Blood Adv. 2017;1(19):1538-45.
10. Van Eijk LT, John ASE, Schwoebel F, Summo L, Vauléon S, Zöllner S, et al. Effect of the antihepcidin Spiegelmer lexaptepid on inflammation-induced decrease in serum iron in humans. Blood. 2014;124(17):2643-6.
11. Kaplan JM, Sharma N, Dikdan S. Hypoxia-inducible factor and its role in the management of anemia in chronic kidney disease. Int J Mol Sci. 2018;19(2):389.
12. Dhillon S. Roxadustat: first global approval. Drugs. 2019;79(5): 563-72.
13. Piga A, Perrotta S, Gamberini MR, Voskaridou E, Melpignano A, Filosa A, et al. Luspatercept improves hemoglobin levels and blood transfusion requirements in a study of patients with β-thalassemia. Blood. 2019;133(12):1279-89.
14. Fenaux P, Platzbecker U, Mufti GJ, Garcia-Manero G, Buckstein R, Santini V, et al. Luspatercept in Patients with Lower-risk Myelodysplastic Syndromes. N Engl J Med. 2020;382(2):140-51.

47

CHAPTER

End-of-life Care: Current Scenario in India

Sudha Sarna, Mukesh K Sarna

ABSTRACT

Advancements in technology and understanding of the disease have led to more patients benefiting from treatment, but the burden on critical care and long-term care for incurable or terminally ill patients in India is increasing. End-of-life care (EOLC) is crucial for managing death painlessly, saving families money, and restoring meaningful life. Physicians have an ethical duty to communicate patients' dismal prognosis with honesty and clarity, and to discuss treatment choices and the acceptability of natural death. However, in India, EOLC decisions have faced challenges due to misunderstandings, societal ignorance, and caregivers' ignorance. To improve EOLC, there is a need for increased awareness among the general population and increased funding for palliative care. Support from the government, community involvement, and integrating palliative EOLC into primary healthcare and medical education is essential. The most underserved area of healthcare in India is palliative and end-of-life care (PEOLC), and integrating palliative EOLC into the nation's healthcare system is urgently needed.

INTRODUCTION

Due to the advancement in technology and understanding of disease, pathophysiology, diagnosis, and management, more and more patients are benefiting and getting cured of disease. On the other side, a greater number of patients with advanced disease are spending longer in intensive care units (ICUs), and the process of dying becomes more prolonged for incurable or terminally ill patients.

India has a population of >140 crores, and there are 13.8 crore elderly or senior citizens. India has a death rate of 9.45 deaths per 1,000 inhabitants. This large number explains the burden on critical care; the availability of beds becomes difficult at times as an increasing number of patients with chronic disease or terminal illness require long-term care. Thus, for many such patients whose treatment trials in intensive care failed, life support will only prolong the dying process.

End-of-life care (EOLC) is about the quality of dying, where death can be managed in such a way that it is painless, has no negative impact on the survivors, and, in the Indian context, can save the family money, rather than a painful, lonely end of life where death seems inevitable or the possibility of restoring meaningful life is less.

The physician has an ethical and constitutional duty to convey the patient's dismal prognosis to the patient or family, with honesty and clarity, as well as reasoning why further active support looks to be useless. The physician is expected to commence open discussions about the patient's impending death or severe impairment, the merits and drawbacks of treatment choices, and the acceptability of letting the patient to die naturally.

In India, EOLC decisions have been viewed as difficult due to a number of hurdles, including misunderstanding of ethical issues, a culture of heroic "fighting till the end,"' societal ignorance, and caregiver's ignorance.

WHAT IS PALLIATIVE CARE AND END-OF-LIFE CARE?

According to the World Health Organization, palliative care (PC) is an approach that enhances the quality of life for patients and their families dealing with the issues brought on by life-threatening illnesses by preventing and relieving suffering through early identification, assessment, and treatment of pain and other distressing physical, psychosocial, and spiritual problems. In India, only 1% of people have access to the pain management and PC. EOLC is a multidisciplinary method of providing "whole person care" to persons with advanced, progressing, incurable, or life-limiting illnesses in order to provide them the best quality of life possible before dying away. Beyond the affected individuals, the care process includes their family members and caregivers **(Figs. 1 and 2)**.

CURRENT STATUS OF END-OF-LIFE CARE AND CHALLENGES IN INDIA

The Economic Intelligence Unit released "The 2015" Quality of Death Index in 2015, with the goal of measuring the availability and quality of PC in 80 countries.

They compared countries based on five criteria: (1) Palliative and healthcare environment, (2) human resources, (3) care affordability, (4) care quality and community engagement, and (5) PC demand and supply.

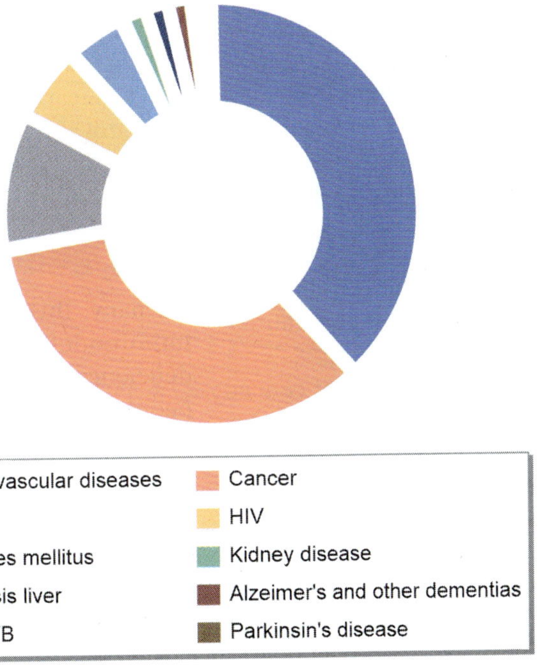

FIG. 1: Distribution of adults in need of end-of-life care (EOLC).
Source: WHO and Worldwide Palliative Care. Global Atlas of Palliative Care, 2nd edition. London, UK: WHO and Worldwide Palliative Care; 2020.

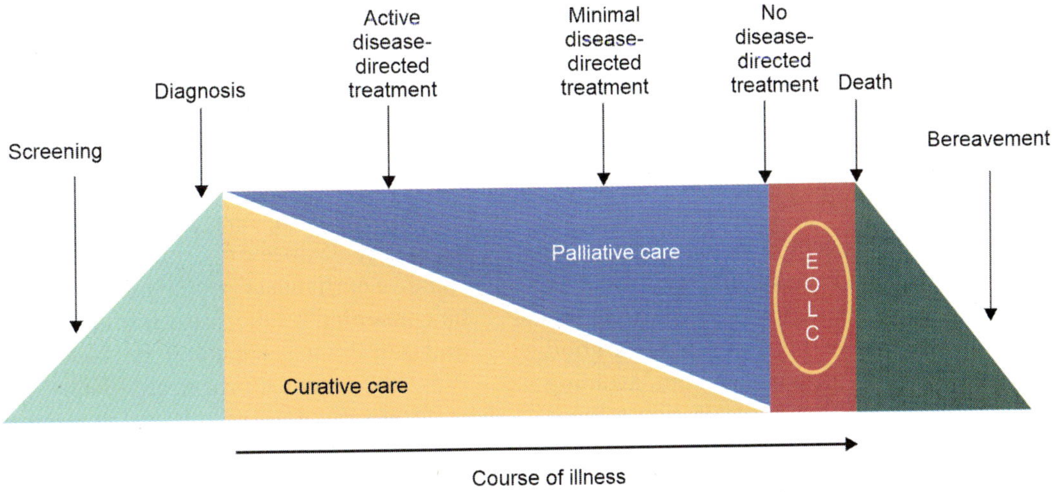

FIG. 2: End-of-life care (EOLC) begins much before the actual death of a patient and continues during the process of death and after death also.

India was placed 67th out of 80 countries and 14th among 21 low-income countries.

Palliative care is estimated to be provided to 5.4 million patients in India each year. While EOLC is fast evolving in the country, the vast gap between supply and demand implies that more work is required to provide proper PC to the majority of the Indian people.

According to a data analysis published on February 6, 2018, in the UK: EOLC profiles, February 2018 update, the number of hospital deaths fell from 57.9% in 2004 to 46.9% in 2016. The percentage of deaths in homes and hospices increased by 5.1 and 0.9%, respectively, in the United Kingdom. However, the scenario is different in our country.

Even though just 1–2% of the population in India has access to it, PC is a crucial part of the country's medical system. Many patients and families who are unable to find comfort throughout their diagnosis phase are ignored due to the medical community's lack of knowledge.

Medical students and practitioners need to take certain factors into account because of the lack of access to pain management and the use of opioids for trauma and terminal diseases.

In India, more than one million new cases of cancer are diagnosed each year, and it is estimated that the cancer burden in India will almost double during the coming twenty years. When the cancer becomes incurable and patient approaches the terminal stage of illness, end-of-life care can avoid unnecessary cost of treatments.

The absence of pain and symptom management in medical syllabuses and higher medical treatment fees contribute to the lack of EOLC. There is a need to include palliative EOLC as primary health education in medical professionals' training **(Box 1)**.

BOX 1: EOLC challenges.

Patient related:
- Patient thinks that he will get cured in the hospital
- Patient could not believe the sudden deterioration of his condition

Related to family members:
- Hope of being cured at the hospital
- Social pressure
- Fear of worsening of patient's condition at home
- Denial in accepting the patient's condition

Physician-related:
- Fear of legal ramifications
- Physician consider disease treatable
- Overestimate the chances of survival
- Verbal agreement with DNR but refuses to sign due to fear of legal implications

(DNR: do not resuscitate; EOLC: end-of-life care)

What Constitutes a Meaningful or Good Death?

In Indian clinical settings, EOLC for quality of life and death is frequently disregarded. Developed countries such as the United Kingdom, the United States, Canada, and Australia are attempting to provide "good death" for terminal illnesses. A meaningful death is one that is free of death anxiety, distress, and suffering and is in accordance with cultural and ethical norms. Physical, psychological, spiritual, and emotional assistance from family, caregivers, and friends is required for a good death. Proper pain and symptom management, avoiding extended dying processes, clear communication, proper preparation, and spiritual or emotional support, are all important aspects of a decent death.

In India, due to difficulty in implementing advance directives in palliative EOLC, making it a place not to die for many. This is particularly true for people with human immunodeficiency virus (HIV)/acquired immunodeficiency syndrome (AIDS), learning disabilities, older people, cancer patients from poverty, dementia, and the third gender community. Modern India requires holistic care, which is an urgent need.

Good EOLC is a human right, and every individual has a right to a good, peaceful, and dignified death.

THE LEGAL POSITION OF END-OF-LIFE CARE IN INDIA

Around 70–90% of deaths of terminally ill in the USA and Europe are mediated through an EOL decision (Prendergast, Ethicus-I and II). Most withdrawal of critical care in India is done via left against medical advice (LAMA) [INDICAPS (Indian Intensive Care Case Mix and Practice Patterns Study)-I and II]. There were a few clinical and court cases, and consensus/guidelines which helped in the development of understanding of EOLC and laws related to EOLC.

- *Aruna Shanbaug versus The Union of India (2011)*: Summary—Supreme Court accepted in principle "passive euthanasia" when burdens are intolerable, to be consented by the "next friend," not by physicians and family to take such decisions without bias. Prescribed a court procedure involving a High Court to decide about the withdrawal of support.
- *Justice Puttaswamy (Retd) versus UOI summary (2017)*: The right to privacy is protected as a fundamental right under Articles 14, 19, and 21 of the Constitution of India. Justice Chelameshwar—it is a right to "privacy of

choice," i.e., "individual autonomy over fundamental personal choices."

- *Common cause versus Union of India (2018)*: Right to autonomy, i.e., sovereignty over one's body and person. Right to refuse treatment, autonomy extends to the incompetent state. The validity of the Advance Medical Directive (AMD) and legally appointed proxy established, permitted withdrawal (WD)/withholding (WH) from persons who neither possess decision-making capacity nor have executed AMD. In such a scenario the "best interest" principle applies. Laid down guidelines for the implementation of AMD and WD/WH of life support.

Developments after Common Cause

- The ISCCM filed an application for clarification and simplification in the Supreme Court.

  End of Life Care in India Taskforce (ELICIT) and the Vidhi Centre for Legal Policy have drafted and published a model legal framework for EOLC
- *Miscellaneous Application No. 1699/2019*: ISCCM versus UOI Supreme Court; January 2023, in which the honorable Supreme Court simplified its order on passive euthanasia, limited the role of officials and hospitals got more say in the cases of EOLC.

THE ETHICAL ISSUES IN END-OF-LIFE CARE

Talking about death is mostly prohibited in many societies, which prevents one from planning for his end time and the survivors after his death.

Palliative EOLC focuses on enhancing the patient's well-being and maximizing their quality of life. Clinicians must maintain medical ethics, policy, and professional treatment standards in all situations. The law advises physicians not to go against patients' wills, even if it causes death. They must provide detailed medical treatment information and leave the individual's decision-making to the individual. Medical ethics govern medical professionals' activities and moral principles, and patients have the right to access their diagnosis information and accept or refuse treatment.

In order to provide care for patients with severe illnesses such as HIV and cancer, medical ethical norms are essential. The principles of beneficence, nonmaleficence, social fairness, and proper care are central to Indian Palliative EOLC. Patient autonomy transcends bothersome difficulties and gives patients complete control over their sickness. For patients to have the highest quality of life and well-being, doctors need to be fully informed about medical treatment policies and the patient's condition. Nonmaleficence entails taking care of the patient's requirements without engaging in harmful behavior and avoiding inefficient treatments that can raise risk factors.

The primary focus is to make dying meaningful, addressing all the needs of the dying individual without fear. Healthcare providers must earn the trust of patients, ensuring quality communication and respecting their wishes. Fair treatment gives patients the right to claim their legitimate rights, emphasizing the importance of ethical principles in EOLC.

CHECKLISTS FOR END-OF-LIFE CARE

In clinical settings we often find ourself in decision dilemmas, and require a decision tree or algorithm, which can help us in reaching a decision. Following are the algorithms which can help us in such situations **(Flowcharts 1 and 2 and Boxes 2 and 3)**.

ADVANCE MEDICAL DIRECTIVE/LIVING WILL

The idea of an AMD supports fundamental human autonomy and dignity in death. When someone loses their ability to make decisions, it enables them to retain autonomy over their medical treatment options. AMDs are formal documents that have sections for updated confirmation of application and revocation in addition to a formal declaration that is signed by qualified witnesses. In the case of Common Cause versus Union of India, where the petitioner contested the constitutionality of Section 306 of the Indian Penal Code (IPC) and the right to pass away with dignity as a fundamental right under Article 21 of the Constitution, the Supreme Court of India addressed the idea of AMD.

The idea of AMD was developed in response to the creation of medications that put families through financial hardship due to the expenditures of long-term medical care. It was created to protect the right to a dignified death and to limit medical intervention in circumstances of incapacitation. An important instrument for preserving fundamental human autonomy and dignity in death is the AMD. The legality, applicability, and alignment of AMDs with the purposes and goals of the author are crucial considerations.

A statement confirming the person's informed decision must be included in advance directives, which must be written with notarized signatures. The only directives deemed legal are those relating to the

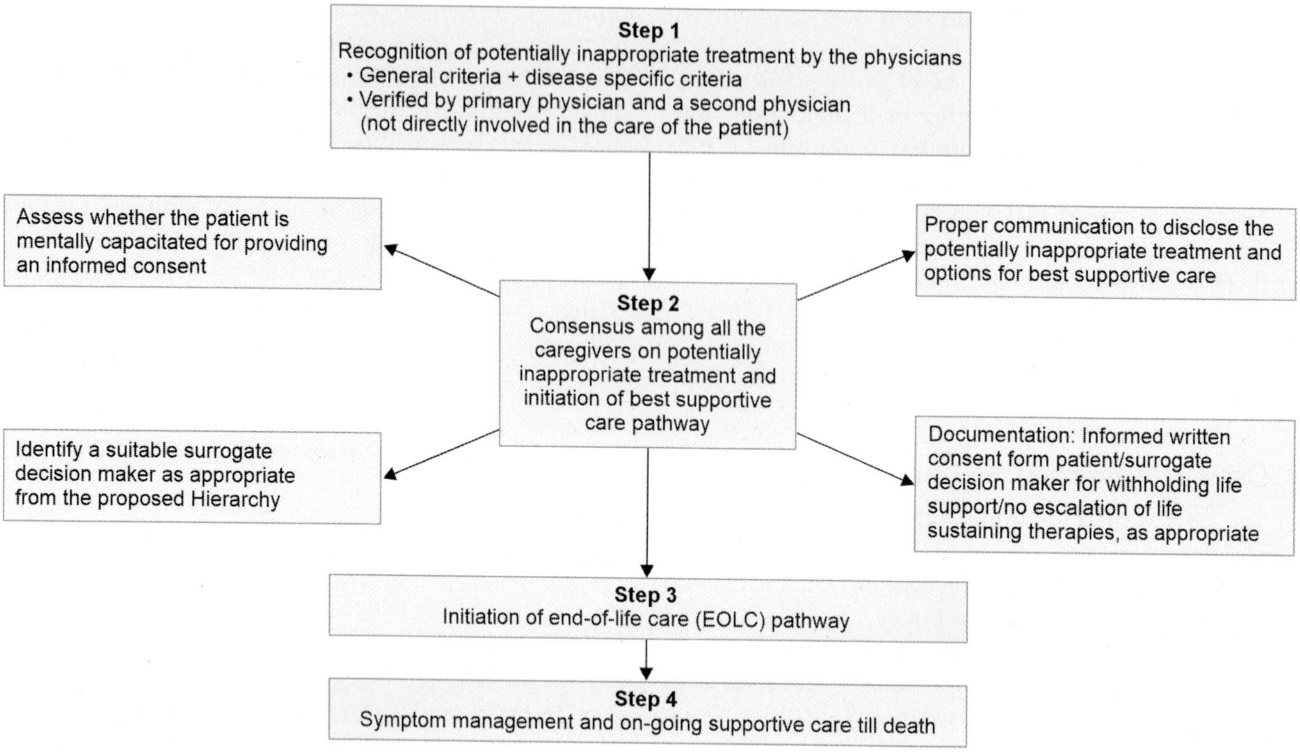

FLOWCHART 1: End-of-life care execution pathway.

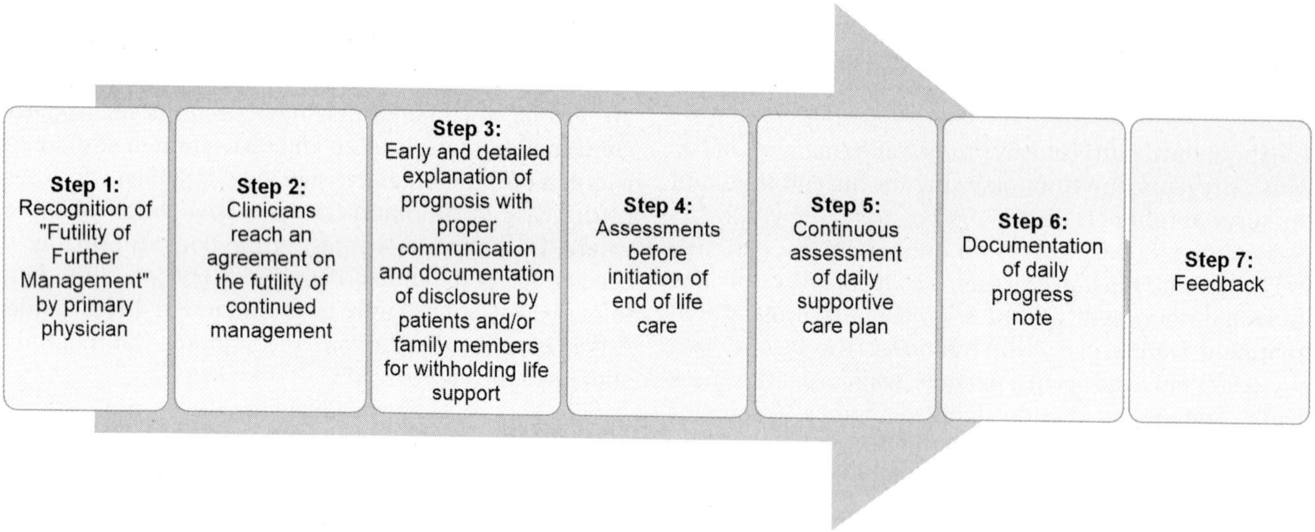

FLOWCHART 2: Guidelines for end-of-life care.

Source: Bhatnagar SM. Guidelines for End of Life Care, AIIMS, New Delhi. [online] Available from https://aiims.edu/images/pdf/notice/irch-9-3-20.pdf [Last accessed December, 2023].

cessation or withholding of life-sustaining care. The High Court may assess the decision's legitimacy and appropriateness if the executor is no longer able to do so. In civil or criminal actions, hospitals and physicians are not held accountable for adhering to a legally executed advance directive. According to their constitutional right under Article 25 of the Constitution, doctors should be permitted to exercise their conscientious objection to the enforcement of advance directives on religious grounds.

WITHDRAWAL OF SUPPORT

The earlier verdict by the honorable Supreme Court advised for a complex procedure, which made it time-consuming and difficult to implement in a terminally ill patient. Supreme Court simplified its order on passive euthanasia in the decision to "Miscellaneous Application No. 1699/2019: ISCCM versus UOI Jan 2023" **(Flowchart 3)**.

BOX 2: Who requires end-of-life care (EOLC)?

- Catastrophic brain injury with coma (other than brain death)
- Critical illness on a background of irreversible severe neurological disability
- Critical illness on a background of chronic irreversible disorders of consciousness
- Postcardiac arrest Glasgow Coma Motor Score less than or equal to 2 for more than 3 days
- Advanced or metastatic malignancy
- Advanced age and frailty with organ failure or comorbidities
- Acute decompensation of chronic end stage organ failure
- Worsening critical illness due to acute conditions refractory to a reasonable trial of organ support
- Any patient who expresses a desire against aggressive care

DO NOT ATTEMPT RESUSCITATION

Cardiopulmonary resuscitation (CPR) may have minima influence on overall illness outcome in some people with specific medical issues and is more likely to aggravate

BOX 3: How to prepare the family for EOLC?

- Meet family regularly. The first meeting should be within 24–48 hours of admission
- All the different departments should be engaged with a senior nurse, in the care of the patient
- Arrange a meeting with colleagues before discussing with attendants and try to reach on a consensus
- Arrange a meeting in a room, not by the bedside
- Arrange a formal meeting using SPIKES protocol
- Debrief the team after a family meeting
- Document everything with signs of family members and members of the team

SPIKES:
S – Setting the context
P – Assessing the patient's Perception
I – Obtaining the patient's Invitation
K – Giving Knowledge and information
E – Addressing the Emotions
S – Strategy and Summary

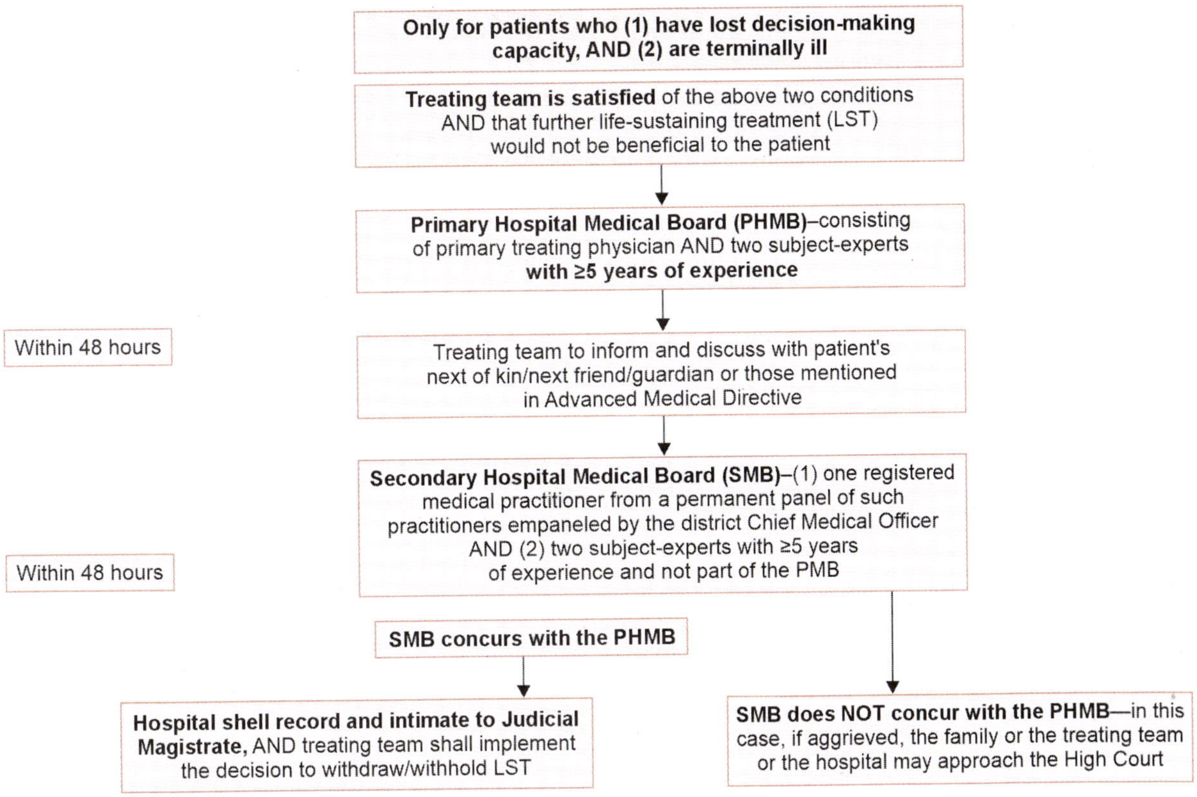

FLOWCHART 3: Algorithm for withdrawal of support.

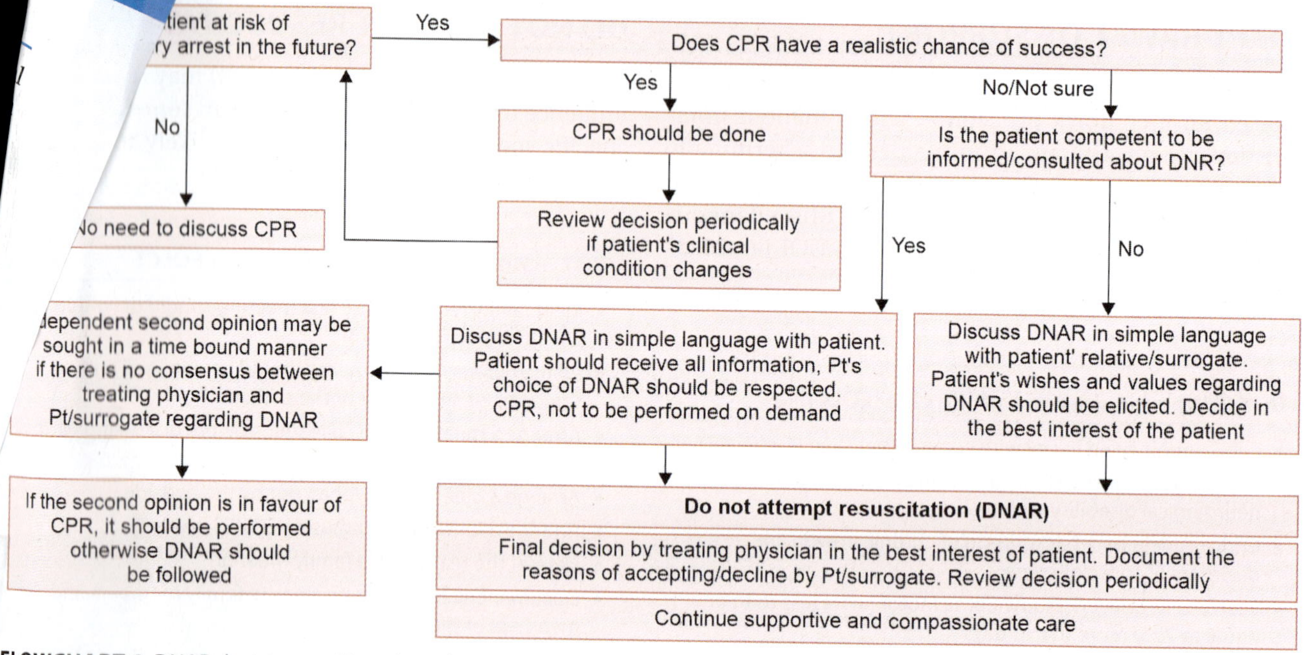

FLOWCHART 4: DNAR decision-making algorithm. The algorithm constantly undergoes evaluation and reflects the current consensus.

suffering and worsen quality of life. In such cases, do not attempt resuscitation (DNAR) has been utilized as an option in several countries to avoid unnecessary CPR and respect the patient's dignity. The DNAR decision should be made by the treating physician who is knowledgeable about the patient's medical condition, and the patient or her/his surrogate should be informed. While DNAR is being ordered on the patient's medical case record, every effort should be made to address the underlying condition and give optimal medical care with compassion. The consent document should be properly signed and stored. This policy document defines the DNAR principles, gives an algorithm and framework for implementation, and addresses frequently asked questions **(Flowchart 4)**.

CONCLUSION

Patients who are terminally ill suffer from machine-related sufferings and are deprived of their autonomy and right to a dignified death. The 2023 ruling, while a step forward, nevertheless has significant flaws. In order for individuals to understand how to make an advance directive, it is essential to increase awareness among the general population. A terminally ill individual on artificial life support systems may experience misery every minute of their lives.

One of the main obstacles to offering EOLC in India is a lack of funding and unequal access to healthcare services. Chronic or life-threatening disease can swiftly plunge an entire family into a cycle of poverty since healthcare costs are so exorbitant and about 75% of them come out of patient's pockets. In India, there is little public awareness of EOLC. A lot of work needs to be done at the local and central level to make PC accessible and inexpensive for the growing number of individuals who require them, despite recent increased attention and hopeful developments. Support from the government, community involvement, and incorporation of PC into primary healthcare and medical education would be beneficial. In most Indian healthcare systems, talking about dying with dignity and having a nice death is uncommon. The most underserved area of healthcare in India is EOLC. Integrating palliative EOLC within the nation's healthcare system is urgently needed. To summarize, current healthcare system is providing inadequate care for dying patients. If the push toward life sustaining treatments is balanced with options of comfort care, more people would have the chance of transition to death with dignity.

MEDICINE is...

"To cure sometimes, to relieve often and to comfort always"

SUGGESTED READINGS

1. Mani RK, Amin P, Chawla RJ, Divatia JV, Kapadia F, Khilnani P, et al. Guidelines for end-of-life and palliative care in Indian intensive care to units: ISCCM consensus Ethical Position Statement. [online] Available from https://www.ijccm.org/doi/IJCCM/pdf/10.5005/ijccm-17-S1-26 [Last accessed December, 2023].
2. Bhatnagar SM. Guidelines for End of Life Care, AIIMS, New Delhi. [online] Available from https://aiims.edu/images/pdf/notice/irch-9-3-20.pdf [Last accessed December, 2023].
3. Mir WAY, Misra S, Sanghavi D. Life before Death in India: A Narrative Review. Indian J Palliative Care. 2023;29(2):207-11.
4. Anjali G, Bimla S, Jayshree S. Legal issues in end-of-life care. Current status in India and the road ahead. Current Med Res Prac. 2023;13(1):32-9.
5. Mani RK, Amin P, Chawla R, Divatia JV, Kapadia F, Khilnani P, et al. Guidelines for end-of-life and palliative care in Indian intensive care units: ISCCM consensus Ethical Position Statement. Indian J Critic Care Med. 2012;16(3):166-81.
6. ICMR Consensus Guidelines on 'Do Not Attempt Resuscitation'. Indian Council of Medical Research Expert Group on DNAR†. Indian J Med Res. 2020;151(4):303-10.
7. Vaiphei SD. Current State of Palliative End-of-Life Care in India. J Palliat Care Med. 2022;12(1):437.

SECTION

6

HEMATOLOGY

48

CHAPTER

B12 Deficiency in India: The Causes and Solutions

PK Sasidharan

ABSTRACT

The major causes of nutritional anemia in India are iron, vitamin B12, and folic acid deficiencies which tend to coexist. More people in India have B12 deficiency than iron deficiency, which is frequently brought on by poor dietary practices, malabsorption, or autoimmune mechanisms. Due to the numerous, frequently subclinical, and concomitant presentations of B12, folic acid and iron deficiency, diagnosis, and treatment are often delayed. Doctors frequently make diagnoses based purely on B12 levels, although this is not always accurate. B12 deficiency is caused by problems with diet, lifestyle, social interactions, and culture. It is possible to make diagnosis with careful study of the dietary practices by being aware of the clinical features and hemogram findings. To make clinical decisions, begin treatment and promote a modified diet plan for patients, doctors must sharpen their clinical capabilities.

INTRODUCTION

Nutritional anemias in India have a very high prevalence which is not declining, and the common causes are iron, B12, and folic deficiencies. B12 deficiency is extremely common, may be more common than iron deficiency in India, seen even among the rich, mostly due to faulty dietary habits, though malabsorption and autoimmunity are other causes. In the Western scenario, B12 deficiency itself is uncommon, and it is often due to malabsorption or autoimmunity. Following the Western guidelines for diagnosis and management is improper in the Indian setting. Despite being a common disorder, affecting all organs and systems, its recognition is delayed due to diverse manifestations which are subclinical most often. In addition, the symptoms of the deficiencies are dominated or masked by comorbidities. To add to the confusion only low B12 levels indicate deficiency, normal values do not rule out deficiency and sometimes laboratory estimations are unreliable even from the best of centers. But diagnosis is easy with proper dietary history predicting the probability and, looking for supportive evidence, which is possible by being familiar with the clinical presentations, the physical signs and red cell indices, but paradoxically doctors tend to rely only on the B12 levels for diagnosis. But the fact is that B12 levels are not always reliable. Since B12 and folic acid work together and since the symptoms and signs of their deficiencies are overlapping, diagnosis and management of them in isolation will lead to unsatisfactory results. The reasons for the deficiency are mostly nutritional and are related to diet, lifestyle, and social and cultural issues. Any of its varied manifestations can occur in isolation and can be coexisting with other deficiencies and comorbidities, giving rise to confusing clinical pictures. These confounding issues leave us with the only option of studying dietary practices, symptoms, and signs, as the most reliable method to identify B12 or any other nutritional deficiencies. In this scenario, doctors must sharpen clinical skill to make a clinical judgment, initiate therapy, and advocate a modified diet plan to give benefit to the patients. The ways and means of picking up those with clinical or subclinical B12 deficiency and the reasons and solutions to the problem are discussed in this chapter.

VITAMIN B12 (COBALAMIN)

In 1855, Thomas Addison described cases of anemia not responding to iron therapy. Addison coined the term "pernicious anemia" to describe the pernicious nature of the problem. The term was used because of the protean manifestations, the severity of anemia, neuropsychiatric problems, lack of response to iron therapy, and the fact that they succumbed to the illness in 1–3 years after the diagnosis. In 1908, Whipple reported the success of a liver diet in experimental dogs which were subjected to repeated phlebotomies. Taking clue from this observation, in 1926, George Richards Minot and William P Murphy subjected 45 patients with pernicious anemia to what they called as liver therapy. The liver therapy included nearly raw liver with mutton/beef and fresh fruits. Now we know that such a diet would provide vitamin B12, iron, and folic acid besides all the essential amino acids needed for hemoglobin synthesis. There was significant improvement in majority and some even recovered completely. For their observations in 1934, Minot, Murphy, and Whipple shared the Nobel Prize. In 1935, William B Castle described the Intrinsic Factor (IF). Castle noticed that all patients with pernicious anemia were not improving with the liver therapy. Some did not respond, and many had only partial recovery. He then hypothesized that the factor which helped in the liver diet needed some kind of IF from the stomach to complete its action, which might be missing in those who failed to respond to the liver diet. He called the factor in liver diet as extrinsic factor, which we now know as B12. To prove his hypothesis, Castle himself consumed mutton and then got his gastric juice aspirated and it was administered to those desperate patients who did not improve. There was a remarkable recovery in all of them. One great thing to note here is that all these innovative discoveries were based on meticulous observation.

Natural sources of B12: Meat is the primary source of it in the diet. The chemical structure of vitamin B12 was identified by Dorothy Crowfoot Hodgkin, and it was isolated in 1948. It is produced industrially by bacterial fermentation synthesis. Leafy vegetables, on regular intake can provide vitamin B12, provided the contaminating harmless bacteria are not removed by thorough washing. Leafy vegetables are the only dietary source of B12 for strict vegetarians. Fish and egg are supposed to provide it, but the observation is that those who do not consume meat regularly have clinical or subclinical B12 deficiency. It may be present only in inadequate amounts in these food items, the bioavailability may be poor, or what is present in them is destroyed by cooking. It could be possible that curry leaves and betel leaves could be providing B12. The problems attributed to betel leaf-chewing appear to be from the unwanted ingredients of the betel quid, especially tobacco and the slaked lime.

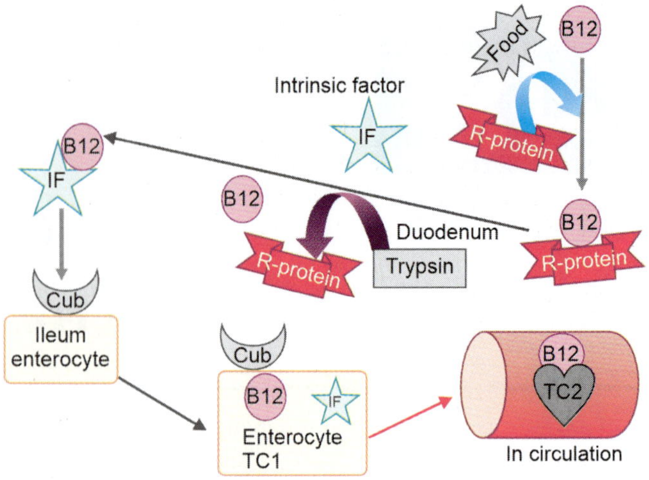

FIG. 1: Absorption of B12.
(R-protein: ribosomal protein; Cub: cubilin receptor; IF: intrinsic factor; TC1: transcobalamin 1; TC2: transcobalamin 2)

Absorption of B12: B12 absorption happens by both passive and active mechanisms. Passive absorption is possible through buccal, duodenal, and ileal mucosa but it is inefficient and only <1% of an oral dose gets absorbed. With 1,000 µg oral or sublingual dose, only <10 µg may get absorbed. Active absorption of B12 occurs in the terminal ileum, it is an efficient mechanism, mediated by IF secreted from the gastric parietal cells **(Fig. 1)**.

Dietary B12 is bound to proteins in the diet. The enzymes present in saliva and stomach digests and frees that B12. It soon combines with cobalamin-binding proteins (haptocorrins or the R-protein) in the salivary and gastric secretions. This travels down to the duodenum where the pancreatic trypsin removes the R-protein and the B12 is now free to combine with the IF secreted from the stomach. The IF–B12 complex is resistant to digestion and it travels down to the ileum, where the IF attaches to the Cubilin receptors on the enterocyte, the complex is then internalized by the process of endocytosis. Inside the enterocyte the IF is catabolized and B12 soon combines with the transport protein, transcobalamin 1 (TC1). The TC1 transports B12 (cobalamin) from IF to enterocytes. Finally, the cobalamin is transferred from the enterocyte into the portal circulation where transcobalamin 2 (TC2) carries B12 in circulation. It is TC2 that delivers B12 to various organs where it is needed.

Enterohepatic circulation of B12: Significant enterohepatic circulation exists for B12. After circulating in the blood, part of B12 is secreted into bile and it binds again with IF, the process is repeated and finally, most of it is reabsorbed. Therefore, deficiency develops rapidly if there is any disease affecting terminal ileum or if this portion is resected or if there is bacterial overgrowth in the terminal ileum due to any cause leading to malabsorption of B12.

Tuberculosis and typhoid fever are two common disorders affecting terminal ileum and their link to the development of B12 deficiency needs to be explored.

Biochemical functions of vitamin B12: There are two active forms, namely (1) methylcobalamin and (2) adenosylcobalamin. Methylcobalamin is involved in the action of methionine synthase which is involved in methylation reactions and DNA synthesis and the defects in this are responsible for homocysteine accumulation, the consequent vascular events, and several cancers. It is much needed in all the rapidly dividing cells of the body including those in the bone marrow and epithelial and mucosal surfaces. The adenosylcobalamin-dependent enzyme, methylmalonyl-coenzyme A (CoA) mutase, is involved in the isomerization of methylmalonyl CoA to succinyl-CoA. This metabolic pathway is important for fatty acid synthesis and is involved in myelin sheath formation. Dysfunction of this pathway causes defective myelin synthesis and could be the metabolic defect behind all the neurological and psychological manifestations of B12 deficiency.

Western scenario of B12 deficiency: Regular consumption of meat gives the daily requirement of 1–3 μg/day of B12 in a typical Western diet. In addition, majority of them consume raw vegetables and fresh fruits as well. Such people would get B12 regularly and if they consume fresh fruits and vegetables, they will get enough folic acid too. On a Western diet, and if dietary B12 is absorbed properly, they would have enough body stores to the tune of 2,000–3,000 μg (but only on a Western diet) which is sufficient for 3–4 years, even if fully cut off from B12 intake or absorption. Due to these reasons, on a proper Western diet, it is impossible to have B12 deficiency unless complicated by malabsorption, autoimmunity, or other reasons.

CAUSES OF B12 DEFICIENCY IN INDIA

B12 deficiency anywhere in the world is due to lack of a balanced diet, more so in the Indian context where most people are vegetarians. Meat consumption is rare even among nonvegetarians and the intake of leafy vegetables is poor in the majority. We seem to forget the fact that hemoglobin synthesis needs a source of complete protein with all essential amino acids, a source of B12, folic acid, and iron taken together in the diet. Indian diet is mostly vegetarian, often there is insufficient or no B12 in the average Indian diet and they have poor body stores of B12. In addition, there are several factors, which could cause malabsorption of B12, like ileocecal tuberculosis, hepatobiliary dysfunction, chronic pancreatitis, and use of proton pump inhibitor (PPI), and/or metformin which interfere with its absorption. To compound the issues further, majority do not take fresh fruits or raw vegetables regularly. Thus, even those who consume meat regularly and getting B12, do not get adequate folic acid and the available folic acid is destroyed by deep cooking. The situation now is that majority do not get both B12 and folic acid together in diet, and if someone gets any one of them, it is only by chance, and the problem is a lack of awareness regarding a balanced diet.

Gastric causes of B12 deficiency: Most important gastric cause described is autoimmune atrophic gastritis with a lack of IF or due to anti-IF antibodies. In clinical practice, atrophic gastritis is often due to B12 deficiency, and leads to a vicious cycle, by decreasing IF secretion, and it cannot be corrected by oral B12, but promptly corrected by parenteral B12 administration with folic acid supplements.

Gastroduodenal causes of B12 deficiency: Most important is gastric bypass surgery, gastrectomy with bypass, with defective production, or utilization of IF. In Zollinger-Ellison syndrome, the excess acid that is secreted enters the duodenum which reduces pH and interferes with trypsin (pancreatic) mediated digestion and removal of B12-binding protein, preventing B12 from getting attached to the IF. For the same reason patients with chronic pancreatitis would have B12 deficiency due to absence of trypsin.

Intestinal causes of B12 malabsorption: Ileocecal tuberculosis, ileal involvement by inflammatory bowel disease, and ileal resections are common causes. It could interfere with the absorption of dietary B12 and could derange enterohepatic circulation. B12 malabsorption could persist even after treatment for ileocecal tuberculosis due to irreparable defects in B12 absorption. Tropical sprue, fish tapeworm infestation, and gluten-induced enteropathy are other rare causes. Human immunodeficiency virus (HIV) infection and radiotherapy are rarely the causes for B12 deficiency due to its malabsorption.

Drugs causing B12 deficiency: Prolonged use of metformin and PPIs is the most important causes. Besides prolonged use of PPIs, it can cause refractory iron deficiency as well. Therefore, PPI may be reserved for emergencies, considering these issues. Patients on metformin need B12 supplements on a regular basis but it should not be given along with metformin. Other drugs known to cause deficiency are anticonvulsants, cytotoxic drugs, alcohol, colchicine, and potassium chloride.

B12-folate-B6 relations: B12 and folic acid always work together, along with B6. **Figure 2** shows the biochemical functions of B12 and the relation between B12 and folic acid to B6. Even if all three are available, unless there is

Supportive findings in hemogram: Hemoglobin can be normal, low normal, or very low, sometimes it could be as low as 4 g/dL. MCV is on the higher side of >90 fl in majority, but when it is >100 fl, in an appropriate clinical setting, it is almost diagnostic. But one needs to exclude other causes of macrocytosis. If clinical indications are very strong, even normal MCV or low MCV does not exclude B12/folic acid deficiency. This is because of the commonly coexisting iron deficiency and sometimes even thalassemia trait. If the dietary history, symptoms, and physical findings are suggestive of B12/folic acid deficiency, a normal red cell distribution width (RDW), or low RDW can favor B12/folic acid deficiency.

White blood count (WBC) in B12 deficiency: Obvious leukopenia, isolated neutropenia, low normal WBC count, or at least an absence of leukocytosis when expected could be due to B12 or folic deficiency. Even in leukopenia, counts are usually >1,500/mm^3.

Platelet counts in B12 deficiency: Some patients are referred for undiagnosed low normal or reduced platelet counts. But in B12 deficiency, the counts are usually >40,000/mm^3. Definite features of iron deficiency with the absence of expected thrombocytosis should also make one suspect coexisting B12 or folic acid deficiency. Finally, it is worth remembering that dietary history is the most useful diagnostic test in predicting all nutritional deficiencies.

Textbook statement that in a nonanemic patient, the presence of a few macrocytes and hypersegmented neutrophils (>5 lobes) in the peripheral blood may be the only indication of B12 deficiency, is not true in clinical practice. In the Indian scenario, when the clinical indications for B12 deficiency are strong, peripheral blood and bone marrow are needed only when there is a need to exclude other causes of cytopenia, that too only if there is no response after B12 and folic acid supplementation. In B12 deficiency, the bone marrow is hypercellular, with the accumulation of primitive cells due to selective death by apoptosis of more mature forms (ineffective hematopoiesis). Because of dyserythropoiesis, besides splenomegaly and unconjugated hyperbilirubinemia, there could be increased urine urobilinogen, and elevated lactate dehydrogenase (LDH) as in hemolysis, due to the death of red cells in the marrow. Reticulocyte count is normal or low, unless B12 and folic acid were already given, and the marrow has started responding to treatment.

Laboratory Diagnosis of B12 Deficiency

B12 levels, even from standard laboratories, are not often reliable due to several reasons. But low B12 levels (160–200 ng/L) confirms its deficiency, but normal or higher than normal values do not rule out the deficiency. It is often falsely normal in 50%, especially if deficiency is due to an autoimmune etiology. Serum methylmalonic acid (MMA) is elevated (950 nmol/L) most often and is said to be more specific. It may be used for early diagnosis, even in the absence of hematological abnormalities. But, it also is not reliable in renal failure and is false positive in 30% of normal individuals and 15% of the elderly. Homocysteine levels are elevated (>28) in both B12 and folic acid deficiencies. But it is elevated in pyridoxine deficiency, chronic kidney disease (CKD), alcoholism, smoking, hypothyroidism, steroid therapy, and cyclosporine and hence not useful for diagnosis. All these clearly indicate that laboratory tests should be used only in research settings, and we should depend on clinical skill alone in routine practice.

Tests for the causes of B12 deficiency: Schilling test has become obsolete and is no longer used in clinical practice. Sometimes a weakly positive direct Coombs test (DCT) is found in those with B12 deficiency, but in that situation, we should suspect collagen vascular disorder with coexisting autoimmune hemolysis. If the erythrocyte sedimentation rate (ESR) is very high, think of underlying systemic lupus erythematosus (SLE) or active tuberculosis with ileocecal involvement. When tuberculosis is suspected by good clinical judgment and reasoning, the presence of a strongly positive Mantoux test (>15 mm induration) would make it almost certain. Antinuclear antibody/anti-double stranded DNA (ANA/anti-dsDNA) is to be done in cases of suspected autoimmune etiology. Bone marrow study is needed only when we clinically suspect other disorders causing cytopenia. Gastric biopsy done to diagnose B12 deficiency, would amount to unnecessary torture. In case if it is done, there could be atrophy of all layers of the body and fundus, with loss of glandular elements, an absence of parietal and chief cells and replacement by mucous cells, a mixed inflammatory cell infiltrate, and perhaps intestinal metaplasia. But all these changes could be the consequences of deficiency rather than the cause of B12 deficiency.

How to Manage B12 Deficiency?

Replenish the body stores with 5–6 intramuscular injections of hydroxocobalamin or cyanocobalamin (1,000 μg/dose) daily or at 3- to 7-day intervals. Maintenance is with 1,000 μg IM every month or at least once in 3 months indefinitely. Always give folic acid and give iron when needed. Prescribe a balanced diet containing appropriate protein, enough vegetables, and fresh fruits. Manage the underlying disorder causing B12 deficiency. Methylcobalamin is not a good choice as it would not provide the other equally important active ingredient, adenosylcobalamin. Oral forms are not ideal during treatment, because there could be malabsorption due to the mucosal atrophy of B12 deficiency, besides other factors like metformin and PPIs interfering with absorption.

CONCLUSION

B12 deficiency is extremely common since majority do not take a balanced diet; many have improper absorption. Strict vegetarians almost always have B12 deficiency and B12 deficiency of autoimmune nature is increasingly seen. Megaloblastic anemia is only a rare manifestation of B12 deficiency. B12 deficiency coexists with folic acid and other nutritional deficiencies. Diagnosis is possible by dietary history, careful physical examination, and supportive evidence in a hemogram. We should not rely on B12 estimations for its diagnosis. Clinical skill and clinical judgment are most important. Look for B12 deficiency in all individuals/undiagnosed issues. Along with B12 always give folic acid ± iron + balanced diet; prompt therapeutic response with B12 is the best proof for diagnosis.

SUGGESTED READINGS

1. Sasidharan PK. B12 deficiency in India. 2017 Arch Med Health Sci. 2017;5(2):261-8.
2. Bunn HF. Vitamin B12 and pernicious anemia—the dawn of molecular medicine. N Engl J Med. 2014;370(8):773-6.
3. Stabler SP, Allen RH. Vitamin B12 deficiency as a worldwide problem. Annu Rev Nutr. 2004;24:299-326.
4. Minot GR, Murphy WP. Treatment of pernicious anemia by a special diet. JAMA 1926;87:470-6.
5. Minot GR, Murphy WP, Stetson RP. The response of the reticulocytes to liver therapy: Particularly in pernicious anemia. Am J Med Sci. 1928;175:581-99.
6. Castle WB. The conquest of pernicious anemia. In: Wintrobe MM (Ed). Blood, Pure and Eloquent. New York: McGraw-Hill; 1980. pp. 284-317.
7. Nielsen MJ, Rasmussen MR, Andersen CB, Nexø E, Moestrup SK. Vitamin B12 transport from food to the body's cells—A sophisticated, multistep pathway. Nat Rev Gastroenterol Hepatol. 2012;9:345-54.
8. Stabler SP. Clinical practice. Vitamin B12 deficiency. N Engl J Med. 2013;368:149-60.
9. Stabler SP. Megaloblastic anemias: Pernicious anemia and folate deficiency. In: Young NS, Gerson SL, High KA (Eds). Clinical Hematology. Philadelphia: Mosby; 2006. pp. 242-51.
10. Sasidharan PK. Malnutrition—our first enemy and the enemy within all nations. HEAL THY WORLD. Chennai: Notion Press India; 2023. pp. 87-94.
11. Sasidharan PK. Nutrition and balanced diet principles and practice. HEAL THY WORLD. Chennai: Notion Press India; 2023. pp. 95-139.
12. de Jager J, Kooy A, Lehert P, Wulffelé MG, van der Kolk J, Bets D, et al. Long term treatment with metformin in patients with type 2 diabetes and risk of vitamin B-12 deficiency: randomised placebo controlled trial. BMJ. 2010;340:c2181.
13. Dipin Kumar PU, Sasidharan PK, Shaan M. Clinicopathological correlation of pancytopenia. Indian J Emerg Med. 2016;2:101-4.
14. Khunger JM, Arulselvi S, Sharma U, Ranga S, Talib VH. Pancytopenia—A clinicohaematological study of 200 cases. Indian J Pathol Microbiol. 2002;45:375-9.
15. Lindenbaum J, Healton EB, Savage DG, Brust JC, Garrett TJ, Podell ER, et al. Neuropsychiatric disorders caused by cobalamin deficiency in the absence of anemia or macrocytosis. N Engl J Med. 1988;318(26):1720-8.
16. Healton EB, Savage DG, Brust JC, Garrett TJ, Lindenbaum J. Neurologic aspects of cobalamin deficiency. Medicine (Baltimore). 1991;70:229-45.
17. Remacha AF, Souto JC, Piñana JL, Sardà MP, Queraltó JM, Martí-Fabregas J, et al. Vitamin B12 deficiency, hyperhomocysteinemia and thrombosis: a case and control study. Int J Hematol. 2011;93(4):458-64.
18. Sasidharan PK, Mohammed A. Cortical vein thrombosis due to acquired hyperhomocysteinemia. Natl Med J India. 2009;22: 300-1.
19. Sasidharan PK. Cerebral vein thrombosis misdiagnosed and mismanaged. Thrombosis. 2012;2012:210676.
20. Agrawala RK, Sahoo SK, Choudhury AK, Mohanty BK, Baliarsinha AK. Pigmentation in vitamin B12 deficiency masquerading Addison's pigmentation: A rare presentation. Indian J Endocrinol Metab. 2013;17(Suppl 1):S254-6.
21. Kannan R, Ng MJ. Cutaneous lesions and Vitamin B12 deficiency: An often-forgotten link. Can Fam Physician. 2008;54:529-32.
22. Baker SJ, Ignatius M, Johnson S, Vaish SK. Pigmentation and vitamin B12 deficiency. Br Med J. 1963;2(5366):1205.
23. Sasidharan PK, Bindya M, Sajeeth Kumar KG. Hematological Manifestations of SLE at Initial Presentation: Is It Underestimated? ISRN Hematol. 2012;2012:961872.
24. Limal N, Scheuermaier K, Tazi Z, Sene D, Piette JC, Cacoub P. Hyperhomocysteinaemia, thrombosis and pernicious anemia. Thromb Haemost 2006;96:233-5.
25. Yang DT, Cook RJ. Spurious elevations of vitamin B12 with pernicious anemia. N Engl J Med. 2012;366:1742-3.
26. Carmel R, Agrawal YP. Failures of cobalamin assays in pernicious anemia. N Engl J Med. 2012;367:385-6.
27. Stabler SP, Marcell PD, Podell ER, Allen RH, Lindenbaum J. Assay of methylmalonic acid in the serum of patients with cobalamin deficiency using capillary gas chromatography-mass spectrometry. J Clin Invest. 1986;77:1606-12.
28. Stabler SP, Allen RH, Savage DG, Lindenbaum J. Clinical spectrum and diagnosis of cobalamin deficiency. Blood. 1990;76:871-81.
29. Bor MV, Cetin M, Aytaç S, Altay C, Ueland PM, Nexo E, et al. Long term biweekly 1 mg oral vitamin B12 ensures normal hematological parameters, but does not correct all other markers of Vitamin B12 deficiency. A study in patients with inherited Vitamin B12 deficiency. Haematologica. 2008;93:1755-8.

49

CHAPTER

Macrophage Activation Syndrome

Rakhi Sanyal

ABSTRACT

Macrophage activation syndrome (MAS) is a subgroup of hemophagocytic lymphohistiocytosis (HLH) with heterogeneous etiology unlike the primary HLH which has a genetic predisposition. It is characterized by a severe cytokine storm seen in the background of various rheumatological conditions, malignancies, and infections. It has a varied presentation from mere subclinical to severe life-threatening condition with a high mortality rate and is often masked by a background of various other clinical conditions making its diagnosis immensely challenging. A high degree of clinical suspicion leading to a prompt diagnosis and timely intervention is very important to reduce the mortality in majority of patients.

INTRODUCTION

Hemophagocytic lymphohistiocytosis (HLH) is a life-threatening condition which includes the great majority of patients with macrophage-related disorders. It is a disease with major diagnostic and therapeutic difficulties and comprises of two different conditions, (1) a primary autosomal recessive form called familial HLH (fHLH) and (2) the other being secondary HLH or secondary macrophage activation syndrome (sMAS). These two are difficult to differentiate from one another. The familial form is a fatal disease if left undiagnosed or untreated. It has its onset during infancy or early childhood. The onset and the recurring bouts of fHLH are triggered by infections. The secondary HLH (sMAS) develops as a result of a strong immunological activation caused by variety of infections, autoimmune disorders and malignancies. The clinical spectrum being nonspecific, various biochemical, radiological, and histopathological features are crucial for diagnosis and strong degree of clinical suspicion is a key to early diagnosis. A timely intervention is necessary to reduce the mortality.

EPIDEMIOLOGY

Due to its under recognition, the actual incidence of MAS is unknown. HLH 2004 criteria is used to diagnose MAS. In systemic juvenile idiopathic arthritis (sJIA), the prevalence of MAS is about 10%, whereas subclinical MAS is reported by 40% as evidenced from bone marrow analysis. MAS in systemic lupus erythematosus (SLE) vary from 0.9 to 4.6%. The mortality rate varies from 8 to 23% in sJIA, 5–35% in SLE, but in adult population it is reported to be around 50%.

HEMOPHAGOCYTIC LYMPHOHISTIOCYTOSIS-2004 CRITERIA

- Molecular diagnosis consistent with HLH (same as in HLH-94 criteria)
- Five out of the following eight criteria: (1) Fever, (2) splenomegaly, (3) cytopenias (affecting at least two of three lineages in the peripheral blood), (4) hypertriglyceridemia and/or hypofibrinogenemia, (5) hemophagocytosis in bone marrow, spleen, or lymph

nodes, or in other tissues, (6) Low or absent NK-cell activity, (7) Ferritin ≥ 500 ng/mL, and (8) soluble CD25 (sIL-2 receptor alfa) ≥ 2,400 U/mL.

TYPES OF MACROPHAGE ACTIVATION SYNDROME

Macrophage activation syndrome (MAS) can be classified into primary and secondary types **(Box 1)**, depending on its association with underlying conditions or triggers.

Secondary MAS typically arises during the course of these underlying conditions and is triggered by factors, such as infections, medication changes, and disease flares.

BOX 1: Types of MAS and their origin.

- *Primary*: Familial HPS or HLH
  - Due to genetic mutations:
    - PRF1 (FHLH2)
    - UNC13D (FHLH3)
    - STX11 (FHLH4)
    - STXBP2 (FHLH5)
- *Secondary*:
  - Viral infections:
    - EBV
    - CMV
    - Parvovirus B-19
    - Herpes simplex virus
    - HIV
    - Novel coronavirus
  - Malignancies:
    - Leukemia
    - Lymphoma
  - Autoimmune/autoinflammatory conditions:
    - Macrophage activation syndrome:
      - sJIA
      - AOSD
      - SLE
      - Systemic sclerosis
  - Others:
    - Tuberculosis
    - Malaria
    - Enteric fever
    - Leishmaniasis

(AOSD: adult-onset Still's disease; CMV: cytomegalovirus; EBV: Epstein–Barr virus; MAS: macrophage activation syndrome; sJIA: systemic juvenile idiopathic arthritis; SLE: systemic lupus erythematosus)

PATHOPHYSIOLOGY OF MACROPHAGE ACTIVATION SYNDROME

The pathophysiology of MAS involves a dysregulated immune response and hyperactivation of macrophages, leading to widespread inflammation and organ dysfunction. Although the exact mechanisms are not fully understood, several key factors contribute to the development of MAS **(Flowchart 1)**.

The interplay between dysregulated T-cell activation, macrophage hyperactivation, cytokine release, and subsequent immune dysregulation resulting in multiorgan dysfunction, and potentially life-threatening complications.

CLINICAL MANIFESTATIONS OF MACROPHAGE ACTIVATION SYNDROME

The clinical manifestations of MAS can vary but generally involve systemic inflammation and multiorgan dysfunction. The signs and symptoms of MAS are as follows **(Table 1)**.

MACROPHAGE ACTIVATION SYNDROME MIMICKERS

The symptoms of MAS can be mimicked by other diseases like severe sepsis, disseminated intravascular coagulation (DIC), SLE and other vasculitis, infective endocarditis, hemolytic uremic syndrome (HUS)/thrombotic thrombocytopenic purpura (TTP), viral infections, complicated malaria, rickettsial infections, coronavirus disease 2019 (COVID-19), and post-COVID syndrome, and drug reactions.

MACROPHAGE ACTIVATION SYNDROME AND CORONAVIRUS DISEASE 2019

In COVID-19 associated MAS, the severe acute respiratory syndrome coronavirus 2 (SARS-CoV-2) virus triggers an aberrant immune response, leading to a cytokine storm and systemic inflammation. This cytokine storm is characterized by elevated levels of proinflammatory cytokines, including interleukin-6 (IL-6), interleukin-1 (IL-1), and tumor necrosis factor alpha (TNF-α), which can contribute to the development of MAS by driving macrophage hyperactivation and amplifying the inflammatory cascade. Here, clinical presentation is same as in other underlying conditions, but with unique features of respiratory symptoms and lung involvement.

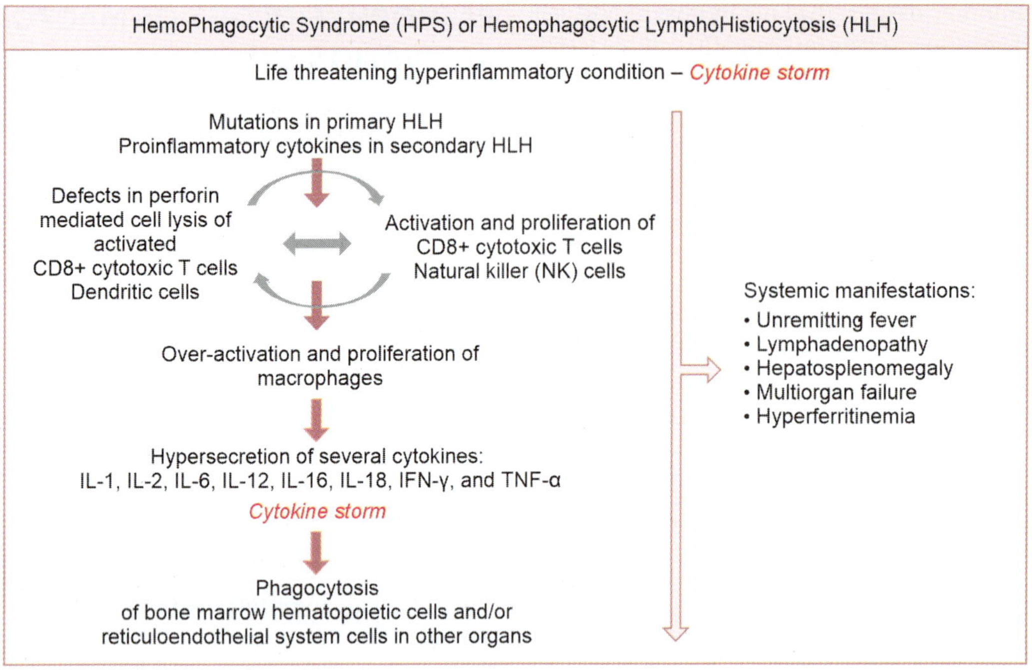

FLOWCHART 1: Schematic representation of pathophysiology of MAS.

(IL: interleukin; IFN-γ: interferon gamma; MAS: macrophage activation syndrome; TNF-α: tumor necrosis factor alpha)

TABLE 1: Clinical presenting features suggestive of MAS.

Clinical presentation	Correlating laboratory findings
Fever of unknown origin	Negative blood cultures, elevated ferritin
Liver failure	Elevated AST
Thrombocytopenia/DIC/ coagulopathy	Prolonged PT, elevated fibrin split products
Encephalitis	Elevated CSF protein, EEG evidence of encephalopathy

(AST: aspartate aminotransferase; CSF: cerebrospinal fluid; DIC: disseminated intravascular coagulation; EEG: electroencephalography; PT: prothrombin time)

DIAGNOSTIC TESTS

No single test can definitively diagnose MAS. A combination of clinical, laboratory, and histopathological findings are considered **(Table 2)**.

- Hematological and biochemical tests for cytopenias, deranged coagulation profile, and elevated transaminases, C-reactive protein (CRP), triglyceride and ferritin, with low fibrinogen.
- *Immunological tests*: Impaired NK cell activity and elevated soluble CD25
- Bone marrow examination for presence of hemophagocytes and to rule out confounding pathologies **(Figs. 1A and B)**
- Imaging studies for hepatosplenomegaly
- *Other tests*: Genetic studies for mutations in familial hemophagocytic lymphohistiocytosis
- Evaluation of underlying diseases

Healthcare providers may thus initiate treatment based on clinical suspicion, even before all diagnostic tests are completed **(Flowchart 2)**.

TREATMENT

Hemophagocytic lymphohistiocytosis has a life-threatening course. Left untreated or undiagnosed or any delay in initiating treatment leads to poor survival chances. Treatments have been developed at pediatric centers targeting mainly FLH. Primary and secondary HLH is difficult to differentiate at presentation; hence specific therapy can be started in severe HLH irrespective of primary or secondary.

The principles of treatment are as follows:

- Stabilization of the patient and organ support
- Active search for the trigger and its aggressive management
- Suppressing the overactive immune response
- Close monitoring of the patient to evaluate the response
- A joint consensus for timely intervention and initiating HLH 2004 protocol

In a vast majority of secondary MAS encountered in acute medical units, mostly in the background of sepsis, treating the primary cause aggressively along

TABLE 2: Diagnostic criteria of MAS based on HScore.

Clinical/Laboratory findings	HLH-2004	HScore
Fever (°C)	≥ 38.5	• *<38.4*: 0 points • *38.4–39.4*: 33 points • *>39.4*: 49 points
Organomegaly	Splenomegaly	• *Absent*: 0 points • *Hepatomegaly or splenomegaly*: 23 points • *Hepatomegaly and splenomegaly*: 38 points
Cytopenia	• Cytopenia of ≥2 series • Hemoglobin < 9 g/dL • Platelet count < 100 × 10^9/L • Absolute neutrophil count < 1 × 10^9/L	• *Single series*: 0 point • *Two series*: 24 points • *Three series*: 34 points
Triglycerides (mmol/L)	Hypertriglyceridemia and/or hypofibrinogenemia triglycerides ≥ 3.0 (65 mg/dL)	• *<1.5*: 0 point • *1.5–4.0*: 44 points • *>4.0*: 64 points
Fibrinogen (mg/dL)[a]	Fibrinogen ≤ 150 mg/dL, (1.5 g/L)	• *>2.5*: 0 points • *≤2.5*: 30 points
Ferritin (ng/L)	≥500 µg/L	• *<2,000*: 0 points • *2,000–6,000*: 35 points • *>6,000*: 50 points
Serum AST (IU/L)	–	• *<30*: 0 points • *≥30*: 19 points
Hemophagocytosis in the bone marrow	Hemophagocytosis in the bone marrow, spleen or the lymph nodes	• *Absent*: 0 points • *Present*: 35 points
Immunosuppression	–	• *Absent*: 0 points • *Present*: 18 points
NK cell activity	Low or absent	–
$_S$CD25 (sIL2Rα)	≥2,400 U/mL	–
Age at onset (years)	–	–

[a]Are used as single parameters for HLH-2004 scoring.

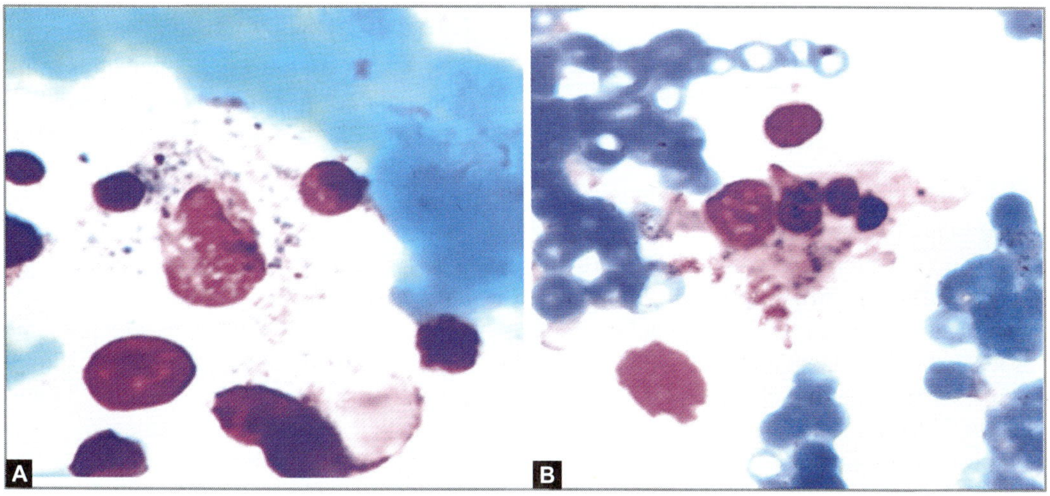

FIGS. 1A AND B: Hemophagocytosis in bone marrow (100×).

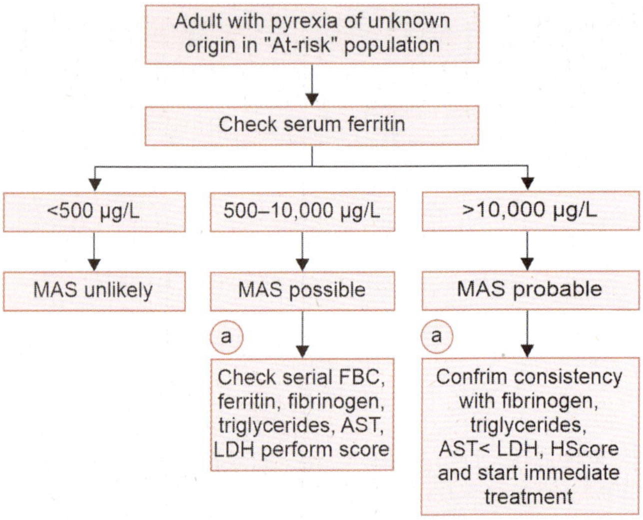

[a] Where underlying cause in not known, investigative approach includes imaging/bone marrow biopsy for malignancy, thorough infectious screen and targeted viral serology dependent on epidemiological risk for exposure to various pathogens (EBV serology and EBV DNA is recommended in all patients).

FLOWCHART 2: Algorithm for diagnosis of MAS in adults.
(AST: aspartate aminotransferase; EBV: Epstein–Barr virus; FBC: full blood count; LDH: lactate dehydrogenase; MAS: macrophage activation syndrome)

with supportive measures results in complete recovery and a continuous monitoring is required whether HLH 2004 protocol to be initiated along with it. This decision is very crucial for secondary MAS especially related to infections where immunosuppressants can be a double-edged sword. Too early initiation can be detrimental while delaying the decision to start HLH protocol can be life threatening too. Hence a MDT with a joint consensus is crucial for decision making.

Earlier the long-term survival was very low. But in 1994, the first international treatment protocol was developed increasing the survival rate. A modified protocol was made in 2004 resulting in decreased early mortality rate.

Initial Therapy (Induction Phase): First 8 Weeks

- Etoposide 150 mg/m^2 twice a week for 2 weeks and then weekly
- Dexamethasone 10 mg/m^2 for 2 weeks followed by 5 mg/m^2 for 2 weeks, 2.5 mg/m^2 for 2 weeks, then 1.25 mg/m^2 for 1 week followed by 1 week of tapering. A close monitoring of clinical and biochemical parameters to be done for the response as well as complications related to the therapy.
- Cyclosporine A can be added as per the severity of the case. Patients who do not respond to the initial therapy within 2–3 weeks or shows recurrence of symptoms and deterioration of laboratory parameters needs salvage therapy.

Patients with nonfamilial disease who undergo resolution are recommended to stop the therapy and a close follow-up is needed. In case of reactivation of the disease, the treatment must have to be restarted.

Supportive measures: Antifungal treatment and continuous cotrimoxazole equivalent to 5 mg/kg of trimethoprim thrice a week as *Pneumocystis jiroveci* prophylaxis.

Continuation Therapy

Is indicated in proven FLH and persistent or relapsing non-fHLH. It consists of dexamethasone pulse therapy (10 mg/m^2/day for 3 days every second week) in combination with daily oral cyclosporine A (aiming at trough levels of 200 μg/L).

The aim of continuation therapy is to keep the patient stable till HSCT can be performed. Intrathecal methotrexate therapy is given in patients with CNS symptoms persisting after 2 weeks. Corticosteroids (prednisolone) can be added in a few subset of patients with above.

Salvage Therapy

In case of nonresponders, partial responders or relapse may be treated with reintensification of standard therapy with various regimens, such as doxorubicin, etoposide, and prednisolone. Others being alemtuzumab, infliximab, daclizumab, anakinra, and vincristine for refractory HLH. Further studies and research needed for strong recommendations.

Secondary Hemophagocytic Lymphohistiocytosis

It is crucial to search for the triggers. In adults most of the patients are diagnosed in intensive care unit (ICU) where initially misdiagnosed as sepsis or multiple organ dysfunction syndrome (MODS). In more severe cases, response to etoposide is good and in less severe cases treatment with steroids and/or intravenous immunoglobulin (IVIG) can be started. Rituximab can be added to the regimen.

Hematopoietic Stem Cell Transplantation

It is the definitive treatment for HLH in the most severe cases which are nonresponders. Therapeutic plasma exchange can be a bridging therapy till other therapies have a chance to work or HSCT.

CONCLUSION

Macrophage activation syndrome is a severe, potentially life-threatening complication associated with varied etiology, involving a dysregulated immune response and hyperactivation of macrophages, leading to widespread inflammation and multiorgan dysfunction. The diagnosis relies on a combination of clinical, laboratory, and histopathological findings. The management of MAS involves a multidisciplinary approach. Treatment aims to control the underlying disorder and suppress the excessive immune response. Early recognition, prompt intervention, and regular follow-up are crucial in reducing the morbidity and mortality. Further research is needed to develop more targeted therapies for this potentially devastating condition.

SUGGESTED READINGS

1. La Rosée P, Horne A, Hines M, von Bahr Greenwood T, Machowicz R, Berliner N, et al; Recommendations for the management of hemophagocytic lymphohistiocytosis in adults. Blood. 2019;133(23):2465-77.
2. Henderson LA, Cron RQ. Macrophage Activation Syndrome and Secondary Hemophagocytic Lymphohistiocytosis in Childhood Inflammatory Disorders: Diagnosis and Management. Paediatr Drugs. 2020;22(1):29-44.
3. Canny SP, Orozco S L, Thulin N K, Hamerman J. Immune Mechanisms in inflammatory anemia. Ann Rev Immunol. 2023;41:405-29.
4. Lerkvaleekul B, Vilaiyuk S. Macrophage activation syndrome: early diagnosis is key. Open Access Rheumatol. 2018;10: 117-28.
5. Henter JI, Horne A, Aricó M, Egeler RM, Filipovich AH, Imashuku S, et al. HLH-2004: diagnostic and therapeutic guidelines for hemophagocytic lymphohistiocytosis. Pediatr Blood Cancer. 2007;48(2):124-31.
6. Parodi A, Davì S, Pringe AB, Pistorio A, Ruperto N, Magni-Manzoni S, et al. Macrophage activation syndrome in juvenile systemic lupus erythematosus: a multinational multicenter study of thirty-eight patients. Arthritis Rheum. 2009;60(11):3388-99.
7. Gavand PE, Serio I, Arnaud L, Costedoat-Chalumeau N, Carvelli J, Dossier A, et al. Clinical spectrum and therapeutic management of systemic lupus erythematosus-associated macrophage activation syndrome: a study of 103 episodes in 89 adult patients. Autoimmun Rev. 2017;16(7):743-9.
8. Soy M, Atagündüz P, Atagündüz I, Sucak GT. Hemophagocytic lymphohistiocytosis: a review inspired by the COVID-19 pandemic. Rheumatol Int. 2021;41(1):7-18.
9. Warmoth T, Ramesh M, Iwuji K, Pixley JS. Macrophage Activation Syndrome in Adults: A Retrospective Case Series. J Investig Med High Impact Case Rep. 2021;9:23247096211026406.
10. Carter SJ, Tattersall RS, Ramanan AV. Macrophage activation syndrome in adults: recent advances in pathophysiology, diagnosis and treatment. Rheumatology (Oxford). 2019;58(1):5-17.

50

CHAPTER

Spectrum of Plasma Cell Dyscrasias

S Usha

ABSTRACT

Plasma cell dyscrasias is also known as plasma cell disorders and plasma cell proliferation disease, in this spectrum of severe progressive monoclonal gammopathies wherein a clone or multiple clones of premalignant or malignant plasma cells secrete a monoclonal antibody called myeloma protein, which is injurious to cause tissue damage in the body and cause a spectrum of disease in dyscrasias.

INTRODUCTION

The spectrum of plasma cell dyscrasias includes at one end, hematological disorders which is a silent disorder monoclonal gammopathy of undetermined significance (MGUS), and the other end of the spectrum, the hematological malignancy is multiple myeloma (MM), Waldenström macroglobulinemia (WM), β-cell-associated neoplasms from MGUS-precursors.

Physicians should understand that this spectrum of diseases can progress to the malignant phase, and complications can arise at any stage of dyscrasias, so monitoring of the patient is necessary to avoid or reduce the clinical impact. Malignancy can be treated at an early stage if monitored at transitions to malignancy.

Dyscrasias of plasma cells are defined as the presence of these genetically unstable clonal plasma cells, lymphoplasmacytoid cells, or β-cells infiltrating bone marrow (BM) or other tissues. Myeloma protein in blood or urine can be detected by various types of gel electrophoresis. The presence of this monoclonal protein is the hallmark of plasma cell dyscrasias including MM, light-chain MM, and plasma cell leukemia.

These plasma cells produce heavy chain antibodies namely, immunoglobulin G-gamma (IgG-γ), immunoglobulin A-alpha (IgA-α), immunoglobulin E-epsilon (IgE-ε), immunoglobulin D delta (IgD-δ), immunoglobulin M mu (IgM-μ) and light-chain antibodies kappa (κ), and lambda (λ), they undergo primary genomic and secondary genomic changes to become malignant.

The plasma cell population has 1900 distinct deoxyribonucleic acid (DNA) alterations in 900 genes in many malignant forms of plasma cell dyscrasias.

MYELOMA PROTEIN TOXICITY

This protein is nonfunctional and formed as a result of gene mutations. In plasma cell dyscrasia, the spectrum toxic effect that occurs in early stages requires treatment irrespective of tissue or mass affected by myeloma protein-producing cells. The toxic effects are proximal tubulopathy, distal tubule affected cause myeloma nephropathy and glomerular nephritis disease.

The κ- and λ-light chains aggregate with each other to cause extracellular amyloid deposits leading to amyloidosis causing injury to the heart, liver, kidney, stomach, and intestine and causing autonomic neuropathies.

In cryoglobulinemia, IgM myeloma protein, rare IgA, free κ- or λ-light-chain proteins increase the viscosity in peripheral vessels leading to gangrene central nervous system (CNS)—involvement causes blurred vision, headache, vertigo, and ataxia, due to IgM monoclonal proteins which may also lead to thrombocytopenia causing bleeding.

In this spectrum of plasma cell dyscrasia, the stages mentioned underneath are to be known by physicians.

Monoclonal Gammopathy of Undetermined Significance Stage

- Monoclonal gammopathy undetermined significance with subtypes of:
  - Non-IgM MGUS
  - IgM MGUS
  - Light-chain MGUS
- Monoclonal gammopathy of renal significance

Smoldering Multiple Myeloma Stage

- Non-IgM MGUS
- S Waldenström myeloma
- Light-chain smoldering multiple myeloma (SMM)

Paraneoplastic Complications

- Amyloidosis of light chain
- Amyloidosis of heavy chain
- Polyneuropathy organomegaly, endocrinopathy, monoclonal gammopathy, and skin changes (POEMS) syndrome
- Nonessential cryoglobulinemia

Malignant Stage

Tumor burden is more and causes life-threatening progression of disease:

- Plasmacytoma
- Plasma cell myeloma with lymphocytic leukemia with B-cell lymphocytosis
- WM
- Plasma cell leukemia
- Light-chain myeloma
- Heavy chain disease like immunoproliferation small intestinal disease (IPSID)

Franklin disease with or without lymphoma and chronic lymphocytic leukemia (CLL).

MONOCLONAL GAMMOPATHY OF UNDERMIND SIGNIFICANCE

This is an incidental finding where protein electrophoresis is done for various reasons where no signs or symptoms in this plasma cell dyscrasia. It has two subtypes which are mentioned underneath.

Nonimmunoglobulin M Monoclonal Gammopathy of Undetermined Significance

It is commonly diagnosed by:

- Bone marrow clonal plasma cells < 10% of total nucleated cells
- Absence of CRAB criteria:
  C: Calcium level > 11 mg/dL
  R: Renal insufficiency serum creatinine > 2 g/dL
  A: Anemia of <10 g/dL
  B: Bone lytic lesion more due to plasmacytoma
- No evidence of plasmacytoma in bone or soft tissue of amyloidosis
- Higher light-chain concentration of >100 mg/dL
- Circulating blood plasma cells < 20% of the total circulating cells

Immunoglobulin M Monoclonal Gammopathy of Undetermined Significance

It forms 20% of MGUS whereas in an increase in B-cell derivative with both plasma cell and lymphocytic cells IgM MGUS protein is <30 g/L. No symptoms of end-organ dysfunction are attributed to WM but can progress to non-Hodgkin lymphoma (NHL), WM, CLL, and systemic amyloidosis.

Light-chain Monoclonal Gammopathy of Undetermined Significance

This can be diagnosed by the immunological method of κ and λ light chain indicating light-chain plasma cell dyscrasia, where in no CRAB criteria and the ratio of κ to λ falls above normal of 0.26–1.65 forms 19% if MGUS can progress to light-chain MM.

Monoclonal Gammopathy of Renal Significance Glomerular Filtration Rate

Monoclonal gammopathy of renal significance glomerular filtration rate (MGRS GFR) reduced to < 40 along with MGUS criteria, biopsy confirmed warrant emergency treatment even if plasma cell dyscrasia suggests nonmalignant disease.

SMOLDERING MULTIPLE MYELOMA STAGE

This is the next stage of MGUS. In this spectrum of plasma cell dyscrasias, though considered premalignant can progress to malignant plasma cell dyscrasia greater than MGUS and has two subtypes, mentioned underneath.

Nonimmunoglobulin M Smoldering Multiple Myeloma

Diagnosed as non-IgM MGUS except intact IgG or IgA myeloma protein > 30 g/L; bone marrow showing bet 10% and < 60% of urine protein—0.5 g or greater levels of Bence Jones lack CRAB criteria.

S Waldenström Macroglobulinemia

They were diagnosed in asymptomatic individuals having S. IgM level 30 g/L or bone marrow lymphoplasmacytoid cells infiltrated. About > 120% of total nucleated cells with no end-organ damage.

Light-chain Smoldering Multiple Myeloma

This is a symptomatic diagnosis by 24 hours of urinary Bence Jones protein.

PARANEOPLASTIC COMPLICATION

Here regardless of tumor burden, myeloma protein levels, the presence of other criteria suggesting dyscrasia enters a life-threatening malignant phase.

- Amyloidosis—AL
- Amyloidosis—AH
- POEMS syndrome
- Nonessential cryoglobulinemia where in type I and type II plasma cells. Dyscrasias in present type-I, WM, MM, or MGUS, and B cell proliferative disorders with type-II cryoglobulinemia with myeloma protein with rheumatoid activity along with hepatitis B and C human immunodeficiency virus (HIV) virus.

MALIGNANT STAGE

- *Plasmacytoma*: This is in between MGUS and MM in the spectrum of plasma cell dyscrasia with pathological bone fracture causing extramedullary plasmacytoma.
- *Nonsecretary MM*: No myeloma protein detected having bone marrow of plasma cells > 10% of nucleated cells with end-organ damage CRAB sign is positive.
- *Plasma cell*: Myeloma with concomitant CLL monoclonal B-cell lymphocytosis. This is a rare form of plasma cell dyscrasia.
- MM-CRAB criteria along with light and heavy chain myeloma protein > 10% bone marrow clonal plasma cell.
- *Plasma cell leukemia*: In this plasma cell dyscrasias which may be primary or secondary plasma cell leukemia lymphoid/spleen/liver enlarged along with thrombocytopenia.

CONCLUSION

Plasma cell dyscrasia is a spectrum of disease from premalignant to the malignant stage of diseases due to genetically unstable plasma cells producing monoclonal antibodies of the heavy chain or light chains or a combination which necessitates to monitor the patient to avoid the clinical impact or to treat at an early stage if transition to malignancy and have a periodic follow up in silent stage.

SUGGESTED READINGS

1. Cestillo JJ. Plasma cell disorders. Prim Care. 2016;43(4):677-91.
2. Willrich AVM, Murray DL, Kyle RA. Laboratory testing for monoclonal gammopathies: Focus on monoclonal gammopathy of undetermined significance and smoldering multiple myeloma. Clin Biochem. 2017;51:38-47.

SECTION

7

HYPERTENSION UPDATE

51

CHAPTER

Ambulatory Blood Pressure Monitoring: Pros and Cons

Anuradha Deuri, Asif Mohammed

ABSTRACT

Hypertension is one of the most widely prevalent diseases globally, and also has emerged to be one of the major causes of global premature morbidity and mortality. Therefore, blood pressure (BP) assessments are crucial for the physicians for the early diagnosis and management of hypertension. But the clinic BP readings only present a snapshot assessment of the patient's BP. Ambulatory blood pressure monitoring (ABPM) assists in decreasing the number of possible fallacious measurements, along with the greater understanding of the dynamic and diurnal variability of BP. This chapter will emphasize on the importance of ambulatory BP, its advantages and limitations compared with the benchmark clinic BP measurement and a quick review on its use and interpretation to detect and treat hypertension.

INTRODUCTION

Hypertension is one of the major causes of global disease burden, and has given rise to a significant number of premature deaths worldwide. Hypertension and associated complications are substantial contributors to death and disability in South Asian countries such as India, Pakistan, Bangladesh, Nepal, Bhutan, and Sri Lanka. A study conducted in India between 2004–2005 and 2011–2012, discovered that the prevalence of hypertension had risen three times, which was more than WHO's (World Health Organization) Southeast Asia's regional level (25%). In India, hypertension causes 5.1% of all mortality and as a major risk factor, which accounts for 15% of all cardiovascular mortality. Hypertension was responsible for 53.8%, 55.7%, and 54.3% deaths due to heart disease, stroke, and chronic kidney disease, respectively in India in 2016.

The 2013 NICE guidelines have emphasized the routine usage of ambulatory blood pressure monitoring (ABPM) to establish the diagnosis of hypertension if the office blood pressure (BP) is ≥140/90 mm Hg. Latest American College of Cardiology (ACC)/American Heart Association (AHA) guidelines have recommended to start antihypertensive medications according to clinic BP readings. However, clinic BP readings present a snapshot estimation of the patient's BP, which might not exhibit patient's true BP. Also, the clinic BP measurement does not give us any information regarding the fluctuations of BP all over the day or the consequence of the anti-hypertensive on the fluctuations. ABPM helps in eliminating the possible fallacious measurements, along with the greater understanding of the dynamic variability of BP. Now we will talk about the importance of ABPM and its pros and cons, in contrast with the conventional clinic BP measurement and its use and interpretation to diagnose and treat hypertension more precisely, so that we can prevent morbidity and mortality.

WHAT IS AMBULATORY BLOOD PRESSURE MONITORING?

Ambulatory blood pressure monitoring is when your BP is measured as you move around, living your normal daily life. It is measured for up to 24 hours. ABPM can find out the diurnal rhythmic changes and BP disparity with different environmental and emotional changes. A small digital BP monitor is attached to a belt around your

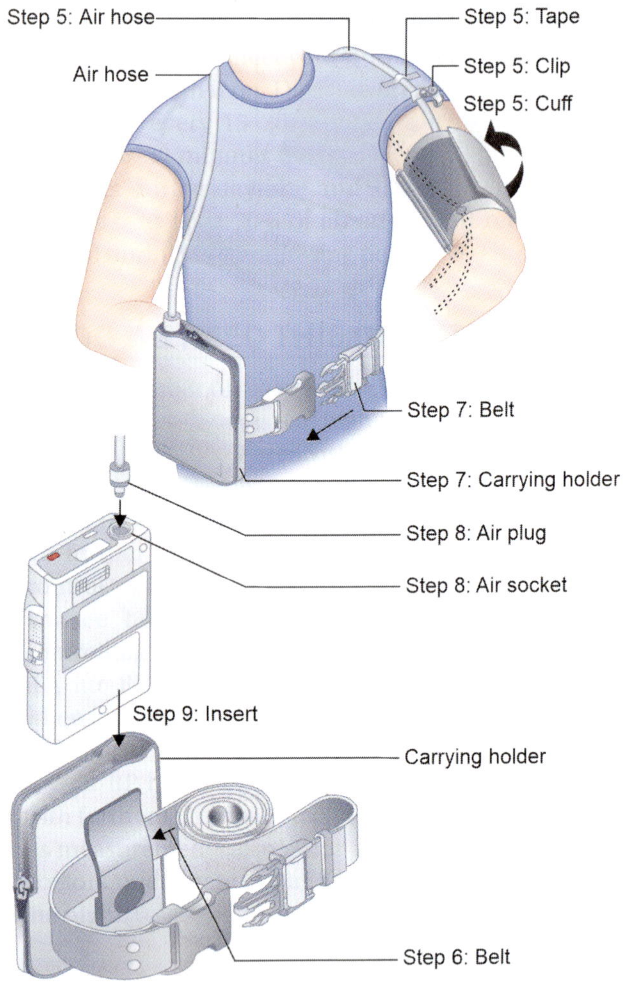

FIG. 4: Steps of application of ambulatory blood pressure monitoring (ABPM) machine (steps 5–9).

ABNORMAL BLOOD PRESSURE VARIABILITY ACCORDING TO AMBULATORY BLOOD PRESSURE MONITORING (FIG. 5)

- *White-coat hypertension:*
  - Untreated individuals with elevated office BP 140/90 mm Hg
  - And, 24 hours ABPM <130/80 mm Hg/awake ABPM <135/85 mm Hg/sleep ABPM <120/70 mm Hg
  - Or, home BP (HBP) <135/85 mm Hg
- *Masked hypertension*
  - Untreated normal office BP <140/90 mm Hg with elevated ABPM measured awake BP of (≥135/85 mm Hg) or
  - HBP ≥135/85 mm Hg
- *Masked uncontrollable hypertension*
  - Treated subjects with office BP <140/90 mm Hg and 24-hour ABPM ≥130/80 mm Hg and/or
  - Awake ABPM ≥135/85 mm Hg and/or
  - Sleep ≥120/70 mm Hg or
  - HBP ≥135/85 mm Hg

PATTERN OF DIURNAL VARIABILITY OF BLOOD PRESSURE ACCORDING TO AMBULATORY BLOOD PRESSURE MONITORING

- *Normal dipping:*
  - Nocturnal systolic and diastolic BP fall >10% of day-time values or
  - Night/day systolic and diastolic BP ratio <0.9 and >0.8
  - Normal diurnal systolic and diastolic BP pattern
- *Reduced dipping:*
  - Nocturnal systolic and/or diastolic BP fall from 1 to 10% of daytime values or
  - Night/day systolic and/or diastolic BP ratio <1 and >0.9
  - Reduced diurnal systolic and/or diastolic BP pattern
  - Associated with increased cardiovascular risk
- *Nondipping and rising:*
  - No reduction or increase in nocturnal systolic and/or diastolic BP or
  - Night/day systolic and/or diastolic BP ratio
  - Associated with increased cardiovascular risk
- *Extreme dipping:*
  - Marked nocturnal systolic and/or diastolic BP fall >20% of daytime systolic and/or diastolic values or
  - Night/day systolic and/or diastolic BP ratio <0.8
  - Debatable association with cardiovascular risk
- *Nocturnal hypertension:*
  - Increased absolute level of night time systolic and/or diastolic BP (120/70 mm Hg)
  - Associated with increased cardiovascular risk—may indicate obstructive sleep apnea
- *Morning surge:*
  - It is defined as a rise in BP >55 mm Hg from the lowest nighttime reading
  - It presents a risk of stroke almost three times greater than that seen in patients without a morning elevation of BP.

PROS OF AMBULATORY BLOOD PRESSURE MONITORING

- Gives a larger number of readings than office BP measurement
- Provides a better profile of BP behavior in the patient's usual daily environment
- Allows identification of white-coat and masked hypertension phenomena **(Table 2)**

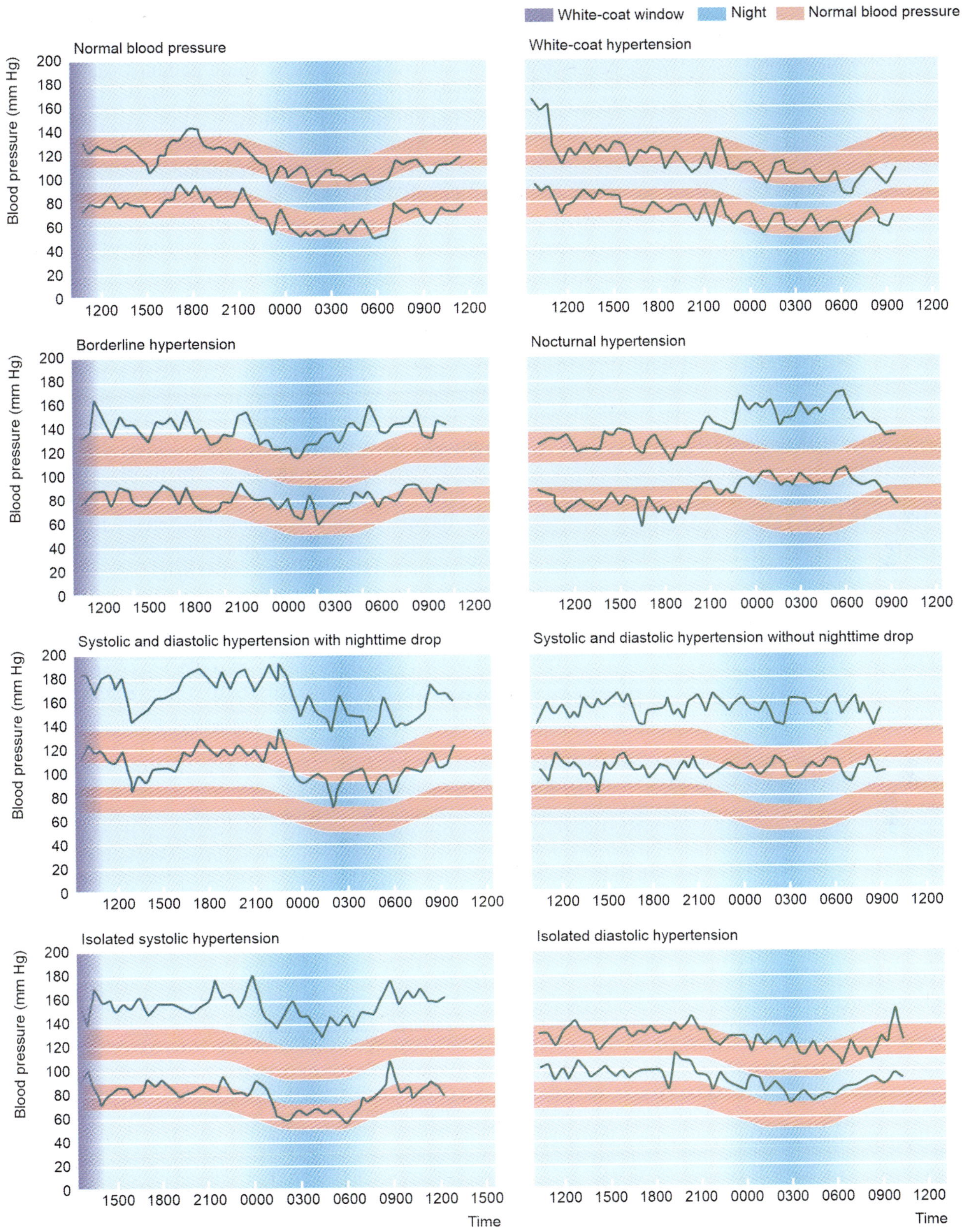

FIG. 5: Variation of blood pressure (BP) in different conditions as identified by ambulatory blood pressure monitoring (ABPM).

TABLE 2: Normal blood pressure variability according to ambulatory blood pressure monitoring (ABPM).

ABPM	Systolic (mm Hg)	Diastolic (mm Hg)
Over 24 hours	≤130	≤80
Awake (daytime)	≤135	≤85
Asleep (nighttime)	≤120	≤70
% allowed above limit	<25%	<25%

Source: Adapted from O'Brien E, et al. (2013).

- Demonstrates nocturnal hypertension
- Assesses BP variability over the 24-hour period
- Assesses the 24-hour efficacy of antihypertensive medication
- Stronger predictor of cardiovascular morbidity and mortality than office measurement
- No placebo effect

CONS OF AMBULATORY BLOOD PRESSURE MONITORING

- Expensive and needs patient training
- Limited availability, lack of knowledge, and awareness
- May cause discomfort, particularly at night and during work
- Reluctance to use by some patients, especially for repeat measurement
- Imperfect reproducibility
- Provision of intermittent measurements in sedentary rather than ambulatory conditions
- Possibility of inaccurate readings during activity
- Inability to detect genuine artifactual measurements
- There is a tendency for electronic devices to overestimate diastolic BP in patients with atrial fibrillation.

CONCLUSION

The superiority of ABPM to office BP in evaluating the diurnal variations, masked hypertension, and the risk for developing cardiovascular and renal events has been studied in a large spectrum of associated diseases and populations. In the modern era of medicine, ABPM must be utilized to diagnose hypertension early and monitor the therapeutic efficacy of antihypertensive treatment to prevent organ damage and premature deaths. Awareness programs and availability of ABPM machine in every setup must be emphasized in hypertension control programs of our country.

SUGGESTED READINGS

1. Lim SS, Vos T, Flaxman AD, Danaei G, Shibuya K, Adair-Rohani H, et al. A comparative risk assessment of burden of disease and injury attributable to 67 risk factors and risk factor clusters in 21 regions, 1990–2010: a systematic analysis for the Global Burden of Disease Study 2010. The Lancet. 2012;380 (9859):2224-60.
2. Krishnan A, Garg R, Kahandaliyanage A. Hypertension in the South-East Asia region: an overview. Reg Health Forum. 2013;17(1):7-14.
3. Patel S, Ram U, Ram F, Patel SK. Socioeconomic and demographic predictors of high blood pressure, diabetes, asthma and heart disease among adults engaged in various occupations: evidence from India. J Biosoc Sci. 2020;52(5):629-49.
4. Registrar General of India. (2017). Report on medical certification of cause of Death. [online] Available from https://censusindia.gov.in/2011-Documents/mccd_Report1/MCCD_Report-2017.pdf [Last accessed November, 2023].
5. IndiaSpend. (2018). High blood pressure killed 1.6 mn Indians in 2016, but most are unaware of its dangers. [online] Available from https://www.ind iaspend.com/high-blood-pressure-killed-1-6-mn-indians-in-201 6-but-most-are-unaware-of-its-dangers-94201/ [Last accessed November, 2023].
6. National Institute for Health and Clinical Excellence (NICE). (2011). Hypertension: the clinical management of primary hypertension in adults. Clinical Guideline 127. [online] Available from www.nice.org.uk/guidance/CG127. [Last accessed November, 2023].
7. Whelton PK, Carey RM, Aronow WS, Casey DE Jr, Collins KJ, Dennison Himmelfarb C, et al. 2017 ACC/AHA/AAPA/ABC/ACPM/AGS/APHA/ASH/ASPC/NMA/PCNA guideline for the prevention, detection, evaluation, and management of high blood pressure in adults: executive summary: a report of the American College of Cardiology/American Heart Association task force on clinical practice guidelines. Hypertension. 2018;71(6):e136-9. Erratum in: Hypertension. 2018;72(3):e33.
8. Grossman E. Ambulatory blood pressure monitoring in the diagnosis and management of hypertension. Diabetes Care. 2013;36(Suppl 2):S307-11.
9. Flynn JT, Urbina EM, Brady TM, Baker-Smith C, Daniels SR, Hayman LL, et al. Ambulatory blood pressure monitoring in children and adolescents: 2022 update: a scientific statement from the American Heart Association. Hypertension. 2022;79:e114-24.
10. Muntner P, Shimbo D, Carey RM, Charleston JB, Gaillard T, Misra S, et al. Measurement of blood pressure in humans: a scientific statement from the American Heart Association. Hypertension. 2019;73:e35-66.

52

CHAPTER

Hypertension in Young

Bharat Agarwal

ABSTRACT

Hypertension alone is a major risk factor for major adverse cardiovascular events as compared to other modifiable risk factors. It affects nearly one-fourth of the world population contributing to significant morbidity and mortality.

Hypertension at a younger age increases the risk of major adverse cardiovascular events, heart failure, ischemic heart disease, strokes, transient ischemic attack (TIA), and chronic kidney disease earlier in life, i.e., in middle age vis-à-vis later in life as life expectancy increases.

As compared to older adults, hypertensive patients below the age of 40 years have lower awareness, slower diagnosis rates, and poorer blood pressure control.

Hypertension may be primary or essential hypertension and secondary hypertension.

- *Primary or essential hypertension*: Nearly 90–95% of all adult hypertension.
- *Secondary hypertension*: 2–10% of adult hypertension secondary to renal, vascular, and endocrine pathologies.

Internationally, all societies for hypertension (American, British, and European) advise to investigate a cause for secondary hypertension in young adults with the following:

- *Young age at onset of hypertension*: <30 years
- *Severe hypertension*: BP >180/110 mm Hg
- Drug-resistant hypertension
- Evidence of end organ damage
- Sudden deterioration in blood pressure control
- Nondipping on ambulatory blood pressure monitoring (ABPM)

INTRODUCTION

Hypertension alone is a major risk factor for major cardiovascular disease events as compared to other modifiable risk factors. It affects nearly one-fourth of the world population contributing to significant morbidity and mortality.

Due to its lack of severe symptoms and potentially fatal effects, hypertension has been known as a silent killer.

People aged 18–31 years had a 33% slower rate of hypertension diagnosis compared with adults aged 60 years or older.

Hypertension at a younger age increases the risk of major adverse cardiovascular events, heart failure, ischemic heart disease, strokes, transient ischemic attack (TIA), and chronic kidney disease earlier in life, i.e., in middle age vis-à-vis later in life as life expectancy increases.

Hypertension at younger age can have adverse health effects in the short-term also.

It has been well documented to have left ventricular hypertrophy (LVH), impact on brain volume, and white matter hyperintensity early in life, thus adversely impacting cardiovascular and neurovascular health in young adults.

A retrospective analysis of the Coronary Artery Risk Development in Young Adults (CARDIA) data demonstrated a significantly higher risk of cardiovascular disease among hypertensives [defined by 2017 American College of Cardiology/American Heart Association (ACC/AHA) guidelines] compared to normotensives (<120/80 mm Hg) in individuals below the age of 40 years at baseline.

Adults, who smoke, chew tobacco, drink alcohol, are obese, engage in sedentary behavior, consume too much salt, and have unhealthy lifestyles are at a higher risk of developing hypertension.

As compared to older adults, hypertensive patients below the age of 40 years have lower awareness, slower diagnosis rates, and poorer blood pressure control.

Blood pressure in adulthood may also be determined by factors occurring many years earlier. Barker et al. proposed the developmental origins of health and disease hypothesis whereby the lifetime trajectory of BP is programmed in the perinatal period. Although fetal growth restriction may play some role, other factors such as genetic and environmental influences are probably more significant. This is supported by studies demonstrating higher BP in adolescents whose mothers had experienced hypertensive disorders of pregnancy and higher rates of antihypertensive prescriptions to young adults born preterm.

Hypertension may be primary or essential hypertension and secondary hypertension.

- *Primary or essential hypertension*: Nearly 90–95% of all adult hypertension which may develop as a result of environmental or genetic causes.
- *Secondary hypertension*: 2–10% of adult hypertension secondary to renal, vascular, and endocrine pathologies.

DIAGNOSIS OF HYPERTENSION

The definition of hypertension has been expanded by the 2017 ACC/AHA Hypertension Clinical Practice Guidelines to include blood pressure above 130/80 mm Hg.

However as per International Society of Hypertension, 2020, hypertension can be diagnosed when systolic blood pressure (SBP) in the office or clinic is ≥140 mm Hg and/or diastolic blood pressure (DBP) is ≥90 mm Hg following repeated examination.

Whenever possible, the diagnosis should not be made on a single office visit. Usually 2–3 office visits at 1–4-week intervals (depending on the BP level) are required to confirm the diagnosis of hypertension.

The diagnosis might be made on a single visit, if BP is ≥180/110 mm Hg and there is evidence of cardiovascular disease.

INVESTIGATE A YOUNG HYPERTENSIVE

Internationally, all societies for hypertension (American, British, and European) advise to investigate a cause for secondary hypertension in young adults with the following:

- *Young age at onset of hypertension*: <30 years
- *Severe hypertension*: BP >180/110 mm Hg
- Drug-resistant hypertension
- Evidence of end organ damage
- Sudden deterioration in blood pressure control
- Nondipping on ambulatory BP monitoring

The most common causes of secondary hypertension in young adults are:

- Hypothyroidism
- Renovascular disease:
  - Fibromuscular dysplasia in 18 to 29-year old
  - Atherosclerosis in 30 to 39-year old
- Renal insufficiency
- Primary hyperaldosteronism
- Cushing's syndrome
- Pheochromocytoma

Investigations recommended to be done for a young hypertensive to evaluate cause and target organ damage:

- *Drugs*: MAO inhibitors, SNRI, TCAs, cyclosporine, cocaine, nicotine
- Complete hemogram
- Fasting blood sugar with a glycated hemoglobin (HbA1c)
- Lipid profile
- *Renal function tests*: Serum creatinine, electrolytes, calcium, and uric acid along with estimated glomerular filtration rate (eGFR)
- Urine for microalbuminuria
- Electrocardiogram (ECG) to look for LVH
- Two-dimensional (2D) echocardiography

Targeted investigations for secondary causes of hypertension:

- *Chronic kidney disease*: Renal function tests with eGFR
- *Coarctation of aorta*: Computed tomography angiography
- *Cushing's syndrome*: Other states of glucocorticoid excess (e.g., chronic steroid therapy)—dexamethasone suppression test
- *Pheochromocytoma*: 24-hour urinary metanephrine and normetanephrine
- *Primary aldosteronism*: Other states of mineralocorticoid excess—plasma aldosterone to renin activity ratio (ARR) and adrenal vein sampling
- *Renovascular hypertension*: Doppler flow ultrasonography, magnetic resonance angiography, and computed tomography angiography

- *Sleep apnea*: Sleep study with oxygen saturation
- *Thyroid/parathyroid disease*: Thyroid-stimulating hormone level and serum parathyroid hormone level

TREATMENT OF HYPERTENSION

The debate is whether a risk-based approach is appropriate in young adults with hypertension?

All three guidelines utilize 10-year cardiovascular models to provide thresholds for the initiation of antihypertensive therapy. Absolute 10-year cardiovascular risk is often low in young adults, irrespective of other risk factors, despite a substantially increased lifetime risk of cardiovascular events.

Nonpharmacological Treatment

The ACC/AHA guidelines advocate treating all stage 2 hypertensives (SBP > 140 mm Hg and DBP > 90 mm Hg) regardless of 10-year cardiovascular risk. When considering stage 1 hypertension (SBP of 130–139 mm Hg or DBP of 80–89 mm Hg), they advise treating those with atherosclerotic cardiovascular disease, estimated 10-year cardiovascular risk ≥10%, or the presence of diabetes mellitus or chronic kidney disease.

The JNC 7 recommendations to lower BP and decrease cardiovascular disease risk include the following, with greater results achieved when two or more lifestyle modifications are combined:

- Weight loss (range of approximate SBP reduction of 5–20 mm Hg/10 kg weight loss)
- Limit alcohol intake to <30 mL of ethanol/day for men or 15 mL of ethanol/day for women and people of lighter weight (range of approximate SBP reduction of 2–4 mm Hg)
- Reduce sodium intake to no >100 mmol/day (2.4 g sodium or 6 g sodium chloride; range of approximate SBP reduction, 2–8 mm Hg)
- Maintain adequate intake of dietary potassium (approximately 90 mmol/day)
- Maintain adequate intake of dietary calcium and magnesium
- Stop smoking
- Reduce intake of dietary saturated fat and cholesterol for overall cardiovascular health
- Engage in aerobic exercise at least 30 minutes daily for most days (range of approximate SBP reduction of 4–9 mm Hg)

The AHA/ASA recommends:

- Diet that is low in sodium and high in potassium
- Consumption of fruits, vegetables, and low-fat dairy products for reducing BP and lowering the risk of stroke.
- Increasing physical activity (30 minutes or more of moderate intensity activity on a daily basis) and losing weight (for overweight and obese persons)

The 2018 European Society of Cardiology (ESC) and the European Society of Hypertension (ESH) guidelines recommend:

- A low-sodium diet—limited to 2 g/day
- Reducing body mass index (BMI) to 20–25 kg/m^2
- Reducing waist circumference to <94 cm in men and <80 cm in women

Higher intensity programs associated with >4 kg weight loss had greater benefits.

Weight loss was found to have a greater impact on blood pressure lowering compared with metoprolol treatment in young overweight patients (age <50 years).

Pharmacological Treatment—When Lifestyle Modifications are not Sufficient

The automatic call dispatcher (ACD) algorithm has been proposed by various guidelines for the treatment of hypertension. The options being:

- Angiotensin-converting enzyme (ACE) inhibitors
- Angiotensin II receptor blockers (ARBs) when ACE inhibitors are not tolerated
- Calcium channel blockers (CCBs)
- Diuretics such as thiazide diuretics
- *Beta-blockers*: The ESC/ESH guidelines and Indian hypertension guidelines recommend that β-blockers be used when there is a specific indication for their use [e.g., angina, postmyocardial infarction, heart failure with reduced ejection fraction (HFrEF), or when heart rate control is required, those with high sympathetic drive]

Hypertension in pregnancy and women of child-bearing age:

- Poor control of chronic hypertension during pregnancy increases the risk of preeclampsia, and good blood pressure control before pregnancy is beneficial.
- ACE inhibitors and ARBs in women of child-bearing age should be avoided during pregnancy because of risk of adverse fetal outcomes.
- Those already taking ACE inhibitors or ARBs should be counseled of the fetal risks in pregnancy and switched to alternative antihypertensives, such as labetalol, nifedipine, or methyldopa if they are planning to conceive.
- It is also important to consider that ≤50% of pregnancies are unplanned, so ACE inhibitors and ARBs should be withdrawn promptly upon awareness of pregnancy and alternative agents offered.

CONCLUSION

Young-onset hypertension is a common condition that increases all-cause mortality and results in subclinical organ damage early in its natural history.

Selected patients need a more detailed assessment, evaluation of subclinical organ damage, and investigation of secondary causes of hypertension.

Due diligence needs to be taken to avoid over-diagnosis and overtreatment. Early intervention with medication in young, mild hypertensives (blood pressure >140/90 mm Hg) free of cardiovascular disease could be considered following a 1-year trial of lifestyle modification.

SUGGESTED READINGS

1. Ezzati M, Lopez AD, Rodgers A, Vander Hoorn S, Murray CJ; Comparative Risk Assessment Collaborating Group. Selected major risk factors and global and regional burden of disease. Lancet. 2002;360:1347-60.
2. Johnson HM, Thorpe CT, Bartels CM, Schumacher JR, Palta M, Pandhi N, et al. Undiagnosed hypertension among young adults with regular primary care use. J Hypertens. 2014;32(1):65-74.
3. Sundström J, Neovius M, Tynelius P, Rasmussen F. Association of blood pressure in late adolescence with subsequent mortality: cohort study of Swedish male conscripts. BMJ. 2011;342: d643.
4. Yano Y, Reis JP, Colangelo LA, Shimbo D, Viera AJ, Allen NB, et al. Association of blood pressure classification in young adults using the 2017 American College of Cardiology/American Heart Association blood pressure guideline with cardiovascular events later in life. JAMA. 2018;320:1774-82.
5. Williamson W, Lewandowski AJ, Forkert ND, Griffanti L, Okell TW, Betts J, et al. Association of Cardiovascular Risk Factors with MRI indices of cerebrovascular structure and function and white matter hyperintensities in young adults. JAMA. 2018;320: 665-73.
6. Meher M, Pradhan S, Pradhan SR. Risk Factors Associated With Hypertension in Young Adults: A Systematic Review. Cureus. 2023 Apr 12;15(4):e37467.
7. Williams B, Mancia G, Spiering W, Agabiti Rosei E, Azizi M, Burnier M, et al. 2018 ESC/ESH Guidelines for the management of arterial hypertension. Eur Heart J. 2018;39(33):3021-104.
8. Rimoldi SF, Scherrer U, Messerli FH. Secondary arterial hypertension: when, who, and how to screen? Eur Heart J. 2014;35:1245-54.
9. Barker DJ, Osmond C, Golding J, Kuh D, Wadsworth ME. Growth in utero, blood pressure in childhood and adult life, and mortality from cardiovascular disease. BMJ. 1989;298:564-7.
10. Whelton PK, Carey RM, Aronow WS, Casey DE Jr, Collins KJ, Dennison Himmelfarb C, et al. 2017 ACC/AHA/AAPA/ABC/ACPM/AGS/AphA/ASH/ASPC/NMA/PCNA guideline for the prevention, detection, evaluation, and management of high blood pressure in adults: a report of the American College of Cardiology/American Heart Association task force on clinical practice guidelines. Hypertension. 2018;71:e13-e115.
11. Unger T, Borghi C, Charchar F, Khan NA, Poulter NR, Prabhakaran D, et al. 2020 International Society of Hypertension Global Hypertension Practice Guidelines. Hypertension. 2020;75: 1334-57
12. Jadhav U, Tiwaskar M, Khan A, Kalmath BC, Ponde CK, Sawhney J, et al. Hypertension in Young Adults in India: Perspectives and Therapeutic Options amongst Clinician's in a Cross Sectional Observational Study. J Assoc Physicians India. 2021;69(11):11-2.
13. James PR, Nelson-Piercy C. Management of hypertension before, during, and after pregnancy. Heart. 2004;90(12): 1499-504.
14. National Institute for Health and Care Excellence. (2019). Hypertension in pregnancy: diagnosis and management NICE guideline [NG133]. [online] Available from https://www.nice.org.uk/guidance/ng133 [Last accessed November, 2023].
15. Hinton TC, Adams ZH, Baker RP, Hope KA, Paton JFR, Hart EC, et al. Investigation and Treatment of High Blood Pressure in Young People: Too Much Medicine or Appropriate Risk Reduction? Hypertension. 2020;75(1):16-22.

53 CHAPTER

Renovascular Hypertension

Bharat Panigrahy, Sambit Das, Mahesh Rath

ABSTRACT

Renovascular hypertension (RVH), a subtype of secondary hypertension, is characterized by elevated blood pressure (BP) resulting from vascular abnormalities within the renal arteries or their branches. This condition arises primarily from two main etiologies: (1) atherosclerosis and (2) fibromuscular dysplasia (FMD). This abstract provides a concise overview of RVH, its pathophysiology, diagnosis, and management. The pathophysiology of RVH involves the narrowing of renal arteries due to atherosclerotic plaques or FMD, leading to decreased renal perfusion and subsequent renin–angiotensin–aldosterone system (RAAS) activation. This cascade ultimately results in elevated BP. Accurate diagnosis is essential for effective management. Imaging modalities, such as Doppler ultrasound, magnetic resonance angiography, and computed tomography angiography play a pivotal role in identifying vascular lesions. Additionally, renal artery angiography remains the gold standard for confirming the diagnosis. Treatment options range from lifestyle modifications and pharmacotherapy to invasive interventions like angioplasty and stent placement. A multidisciplinary approach involving nephrologists, interventional radiologists, and vascular surgeons is often necessary to tailor treatment to the patient's specific needs. In conclusion, RVH is a complex condition that requires a thorough understanding of its pathophysiology and careful consideration of diagnostic and treatment strategies. Early diagnosis and appropriate management can lead to improved outcomes and a better quality of life for affected individuals.

INTRODUCTION

By definition, renovascular hypertension (RVH) is high blood pressure (BP) due to narrowing of the arteries that carry blood to the kidneys, a condition called renal artery stenosis. Early 20th-century research on the relationship between renovascular occlusion and BP regulation is still regarded as one of the key findings in clinical hypertension. They established the kidney's important hemodynamic function and the possibility of finding a treatable cause of elevated systemic BP that directly correlated with clinical cases of RVH. Renovascular disease (RVD), which is brought on by atherosclerosis, has become more common as Western populations have aged over the past few decades. One of the most frequent contributors of secondary and treatment-resistant hypertension is still RVH.

EPIDEMIOLOGY OF RENOVASCULAR DISEASE

There are numerous vascular obstructive lesions that might cause RVH symptoms. The prevalence of these lesions may reach up to 6.8% in the population over 65 years of age and 5.8% in cases of secondary hypertension in young adults, accounting for 1–2% of all cases of hypertension in the general population. The majority of cases are caused by fibromuscular dysplasia (FMD) and atherosclerotic renal artery stenosis (ARAS) while other causes can include iatrogenic renal artery diseases, such as those caused by branch vessel occlusions from renal artery stents put across the mouth of a branch vessel or endovascular aortic stent grafts that migrate to obstruct renal artery segments.

The renal artery's origin is frequently the site of atherosclerotic disease, which is occasionally associated to turbulent flow zones. These lesions frequently appear beyond the age of 50 years and are associated with atherosclerotic risk factors, such as hypertension, diabetes, dyslipidemia, and cigarette use. Imaging studies in "at risk" groups show increasing incidence by decade of age and links to various vascular diseases, such as peripheral, cerebral, and coronary vascular disease. Duplex ultrasonography population-based studies show that >6.8% of people over 65 have RVD with >60% blockage. Doppler studies show that prevalence rates for older patients increase over time, with 25% of people over 70 years old.

PATHOPHYSIOLOGY OF RENOVASCULAR HYPERTENSION

According to investigations by Goldblatt and Loesch from the 1930s, occlusive RVD that results in lower renal perfusion pressures has been proven to increase systemic BP. According to research into this phenomenon, the renin-angiotensin-aldosterone system (RAAS) is responsible for the activation of numerous pressor pathways including inflammation, sodium retention, vascular remodeling, peripheral vasoconstriction, and sympathoadrenergic and endothelin pathways. These effects might be transient and develop across a range of time periods.

CLINICAL MANIFESTATIONS AND DIAGNOSIS OF RENOVASCULAR DISEASE

The foundation for treating RVD is the manifestations and their evolution in specific patients. Mild to severe hypertension, vascular congestion, and kidney failure are only a few possible symptoms. For various reasons, a large number of individuals with atherosclerotic RVD present with incidental disease discovered during vascular imaging. Such individuals are frequently successfully treated with only medical therapy. When renal perfusion is more severely diminished, additional pressor mechanisms may be activated, resulting in severe, occasionally rapid BP rises and hastened target-organ harm on top of preexisting critical hypertension. In individuals with left ventricular dysfunction, sodium and water retention, particularly when both kidneys are afflicted and loss of renal mass is evident, contribute to circulatory obstruction and pulmonary edema. Chronic RAAS activation has been linked to the emergence of aberrant left ventricular remodeling that results in cardiac dysfunction. In the long run, these activities contribute to an accelerated progression of renal and cardiac damage by reinforcing a feedback cycle. In the end, persistently inadequate blood flow combined with tissue hypoxia results in irreversible kidney fibrosis, which is frequently referred to as "ischemic nephropathy".

TREATMENT OF RENOVASCULAR HYPERTENSION

The main objective of treating RVH, like with all types of hypertension, is to lessen the morbidity and death brought on by high BP. The preservation of renal circulation and functionality is a secondary objective. As was already mentioned, numerous pressor pathways, including activation of the RAAS, are activated at poststenotic pressure and blood flow drops that the kidney can tolerate. Antihypertensive medication therapy can therefore frequently be used with little negative effects on the poststenotic kidney(s) and efficient BP lowering.

Choosing a Patient

Controlling BP should be attained by combining medical and revascularization techniques. Attempting renal artery revascularization with percutaneous renal artery angioplasty alone in younger subjects with FMD, many of whom will need lifelong therapy, may limit the need for ongoing medical therapy with low risk. For older subjects with ARAS, the efficacy of revascularization routinely requires stenting, is more limited, and probably would not significantly reduce the need for antihypertensive drug therapy. Many would contend that optimizing medical therapy should be the first step for almost all patients because several prospective and randomized trials have failed to demonstrate significant therapeutic advantages from angioplasty with stenting in atherosclerotic patients, albeit with limited generalizability.

RENOVASCULAR HYPERTENSION MEDICAL MANAGEMENT

Before the development of medications that block the RAAS, pharmacological treatment for RVH was few and frequently poorly tolerated. Patients with RVH were included in reports of accelerated and malignant-phase hypertension, progressive encephalopathy, and/or circulatory congestion, which occasionally necessitated therapeutic nephrectomy as a lifesaving measure. Effective BP control became more feasible in the 1990s with the introduction of angiotensin-converting enzyme (ACE) inhibitors and then angiotensin receptor blockers

(ARBs). For the majority of patients with simple RVH, combining these medications with calcium channel blocking medications, diuretics, and other classes has resulted in effective BP control with pharmacological therapy alone. Numerous people with moderate RVH (often undetected) can obtain good BP control with medication therapy and do not require additional diagnostic testing or treatment.

Should ACE/ARB Therapy be Administered to All RVH Patients?

It makes sense that these drugs should be used as the preferred form of therapy given the crucial role that RAAS activation plays in the emergence of RVH. Many prospective, randomized trials using ACE/ARB therapy for patients with atherosclerotic disease elsewhere suggest a mortality benefit during long-term therapy, particularly for those with reduced estimated glomerular filtration rate (eGFR). ACE inhibitors were not included in the medication regimen in several of the early prospective hypertension trials contrasting medical therapy with revascularization therapy. Preexisting azotemia was associated with reduced use of ACE/ARB medication, but examination of the pretrial use of these drugs in participants in the CORAL study found substantial heterogeneity in their use. Diabetic and proteinuric individuals were more likely to be treated with these drugs.

Renovascular hypertension patients should frequently receive statin medication and lifestyle changes like quitting smoking because atherosclerotic disease is a systemic condition. In experimental studies, statins have been demonstrated to alter the kidney's microvascular environment, reducing fibrosis and inflammatory damage. When totally clogged kidneys are removed via nephrectomy in statin-treated patients, less interstitial fibrosis and transforming growth factor-beta are activated than in statin-untreated individuals. As a result, this procedure should frequently be included in the medical treatment of ARAS patients.

The objectives of treatment for RVH are the same as those for other people at risk for hypertension and cardiovascular disease. Many of these individuals have diabetes, lowered eGFR, and concomitant atherosclerotic disease, such as stage 3 chronic kidney disease (CKD). The relative risks and benefits of lowering BP goals in patients with essential hypertension and diabetes are the subject of recent data from SPRINT and ACCORD. Although there are some disagreements about the relative risks and benefits of lower goals, mortality, and stroke events were decreased in SPRINT and may have been in ACCORD with larger numbers. These trials excluded participants with known RVH, but some were probably included. In the CORAL experiment, participants with diabetes and/or stage 3 chronic renal disease had goal BP values <130/80 mm Hg.

The risk of developing vascular disease throughout the course of long-term treatment is a key component of managing RVH.

Revascularization of the Kidneys in the Treatment of RVH

A significant improvement in the treatment of vascular disease has been the introduction of endovascular interventional techniques. The majority of patients with high-grade ARAS and FMD can now have their vessels' patency restored. Stent insertion is advised for ARAS because it results in longer-lasting vascular patency than angioplasty alone. The complication rates from atheroembolic illness have decreased to low levels, as we have discussed, thanks to low-profile devices and technological advancements to minimize endovascular stress.

CONCLUSION

A significant contributor to secondary and treatment-resistant hypertension is still RVD. Recent studies emphasize both the relative safety of medical therapy to manage BP and the kidney's tolerance to a moderate flow reduction during antihypertensive medication therapy. High-risk and progressive renovascular disorders are considered to be rather resistive to medical therapy solely and react better to combining renal revascularization with continued medical therapy. Clinicians who treat complicated hypertension should be knowledgeable with the pathogenic mechanisms, imaging methods, and contemporary RVH management strategies.

SUGGESTED READINGS

1. Goldblatt H, Lynch J, Hanzal RF, Summerville WW. Studies on experimental hypertension: I. The production of persistent elevation of systolic blood pressure by means of renal ischemia. J Exp Med. 1934;59(3):347-79.
2. Derkx FH, Schalekamp MA. Renal artery stenosis and hypertension. Lancet. 1994;344(8917):237-9.
3. Coen G, Manni M, Giannoni MF, Bianchini G, Calabria S, Mantella D, et al. Ischemic nephropathy in an elderly nephrologic and hypertensive population. Am J Nephrol. 1998;18(3):221-7.
4. de Mast Q, Beutler JJ. The prevalence of atherosclerotic renal artery stenosis in risk groups: a systematic literature review. J Hypertens. 2009;27(7):1333-40.

5. Messerli FH, Bangalore S, Makani H, Rimoldi SF, Allemann Y, White CJ, et al. Flash pulmonary oedema and bilateral renal artery stenosis: the Pickering syndrome. Eur Heart J. 2011;32(18):2231-5.
6. Pettinger WA, Mitchell HC. Minoxidil—an alternative to nephrectomy for refractory hypertension. N Engl J Med. 1973;289(4):167-71.
7. Solomon SD, Rice MM, A Jablonski K, Jose P, Domanski M, Sabatine M, et al. Renal function and effectiveness of angiotensin-converting enzyme inhibitor therapy in patients with chronic stable coronary disease in the Prevention of Events with ACE inhibition (PEACE) trial. Circulation. 2006;114(1):26-31.
8. Onuigbo MA. Reno-prevention vs. reno-protection: a critical reappraisal of the evidence-base from the large RAAS blockade trials after ONTARGET—a call for more circumspection. QJM. 2009;102:155-67.
9. ACCORD Study Group; Cushman WC, Evans GW, Byington RP, Goff DC Jr, Grimm RH Jr, et al. Effects of intensive blood-pressure control in type 2 diabetes mellitus. N Engl J Med. 2010;362(17):1575-85.
10. Cooper CJ, Murphy TP, Cutlip DE, Jamerson K, Henrich W, Reid DM, et al. Stenting and medical therapy for atherosclerotic renal-artery stenosis. N Engl J Med. 2014;370(1):13-22.

54

CHAPTER

Hypertensive Emergency

Kamlesh Tewary

ABSTRACT

Hypertensive crisis is a clinical situation when there is abrupt rise in blood pressure and there is either acute (hypertensive emergency) or impending end-organ damage (hypertensive urgency).

Hypertensive emergency: It is characterized by severe increase in systolic and/or diastolic pressure associated with signs or symptom of acute end-organ damage. No blood pressure threshold for diagnosis but usually:

- Systolic blood pressure (SBP) >180–220 mm Hg
- Diastolic blood pressure (DBP) >120–130 mm Hg
- Mean arterial pressure (MAP) >180 mm Hg

Severe elevation in BP >180/120 mm Hg or more without target organ involvement. Adequate treatment of these conditions, a BP lowering within 24 hours by administration of oral drugs.

Hypertensive emergency:

- Requires an immediate BP reduction in few minutes to hours
- Requires an intensive care unit (ICU) setup
- Requires intravenous (IV) drugs for treatment

Organs involves mostly are brain, heart, kidney, eye, and arteries.

The most common end-organ damage is cerebral infarction, pulmonary edema, ischemic heart disease, eclampsia, and retinopathy.

Inadequate blood pressure control and noncompliance of drugs are the most common cause of this condition.

Common investigations are blood electrolytes, creatinine, urea nitrogen, cell count, electrocardiogram (ECG), chest X-ray (CXR), computed tomography (CT) brain, CT chest/magnetic resonance imaging (MRI).

Management: Normalization of BP is usually not recommended.

The most common IV drugs in use are nitroglycerin, sodium nitroprusside, clevidipine, nicardipine, fenoldopam, labetalol, esmolol, and hydralazine.

INTRODUCTION

Systemic hypertension affects over 1 billion people globally, leading to approximately 7.1 million deaths annually. It is a frequent reason for medical visits and its prevalence continues to rise in both young and older adults. Despite its common occurrence, hypertension is often inadequately treated.

Hypertension is defined as systolic blood pressure (SBP) ≥140 mm Hg and/or DBP ≥90 mm Hg. Prehypertension is SBP 120–139 mm Hg and/or DBP 80–89 mm Hg. As BP increases, cardiovascular risk rises. Levels exceeding 180/120 mm Hg can lead to a hypertensive crisis. Previously termed malignant or accelerated hypertension, it is now referred to as hypertensive crisis, encompassing both hypertensive emergency and hypertensive urgency. Hypertensive crisis involves acute elevation of blood pressure (BP) and requires immediate medical attention.

Among the hypertension population, about 1–2% of the patients will ultimately develop hypertensive crisis. As per 2017 American College of Cardiology (ACC)/American Heart Association (AHA) guideline for management of high BP in adults, *hypertensive emergencies* are defined as severe elevations in BP (>180/120 mm Hg) associated with evidence of new or worsening target organ damage. In contrast, *hypertensive urgencies* are situations associated with severe BP elevation in otherwise stable patients, with no acute or impending change in target organ damage or dysfunction. Hypertensive urgencies typically do not require intensive care unit (ICU) admission. However, prompt treatment with oral BP-lowering medication within 24 hours is necessary.

Hypertensive emergency patients would require prompt hospitalization and BP should be lowered within minutes using parental drugs. The goal of therapy is to reduce the mean arterial pressure (MAP) by 25% over the first hour of therapy (normal MAP: 70–110 mm Hg).

$$\text{MAP} = \frac{2 \times \text{DBP} + \text{SBP}}{3}$$

ALTERED BLOOD PRESSURE REGULATION IN HYPERTENSIVE CRISES

The mechanisms underlying both primary (essential) hypertension and hypertensive crises are not totally understood. There seem to be several mechanisms that are found in both chronic primary hypertension and hypertensive crises **(Box 1)**.

The initial event appears to be an abrupt rise in BP from a known or unknown stimulus followed by compensatory mechanisms arising from the vascular endothelium. Hypertension crisis can develop de novo or can complicate underlying essential or secondary hypertension.

The prime reason for hypertensive emergency may broadly include renovascular disease, pheochromocytoma, nonadherence to antihypertensive medication, hyperaldosteronism, and erythropoietin.

BOX 1: Causes of hypertensive emergency and urgency.

Essential hypertension

Renovascular disease:
- *Renal artery stenosis:* Atheroma or fibromuscular dysplasia
- Polyarteritis nodosa
- Takayasu arteritis

Renal parenchymal disease:
- Glomerulonephritis
- Tubulointerstitial nephritis
- Systemic sclerosis
- Hemolytic uremic syndrome
- Thromboticthrombocytopenic purpura
- Diabetes mellitus
- Systemic lupus erythematosus
- Renal aplasia
- Renal cell carcinoma

Pregnancy related:
- Preeclampsia
- Eclampsia

Endocrine:
- Pheochromocytoma
- Cushing syndrome
- Primary hyperaldosteronism
- Renin-secreting tumor

Autonomic hyperreactivity:
- Guillain–Barré syndrome
- Acute intermittent porphyria

Drugs:
- Cocaine, phencyclidine, sympathomimetics, erythropoietin, cyclosporine
- Antihypertensive medication withdrawal
- Amphetamines
- Lead intoxication
- Interactions with monoamine oxidase inhibitors

Central nervous system disorders:
- Head injury
- Cerebral infarction
- Cerebral hemorrhage
- Brain tumor
- Spinal cord injury

Coarctation of the aorta

Burns

Postoperative pain and/or anesthesia complications

EPIDEMIOLOGY

Approximately 1% of hypertensive patients experience a hypertensive crisis due to inadequate BP control. The annual incidence is 1–2 cases per 100,000 patients. Hypertensive emergencies are reported to be twice as common in men compared to women. If left untreated, the death rate associated with hypertensive emergencies exceeds 79%, and median survival is 10.4 months. Acute pulmonary edema, cardiac ischemia, and neurologic

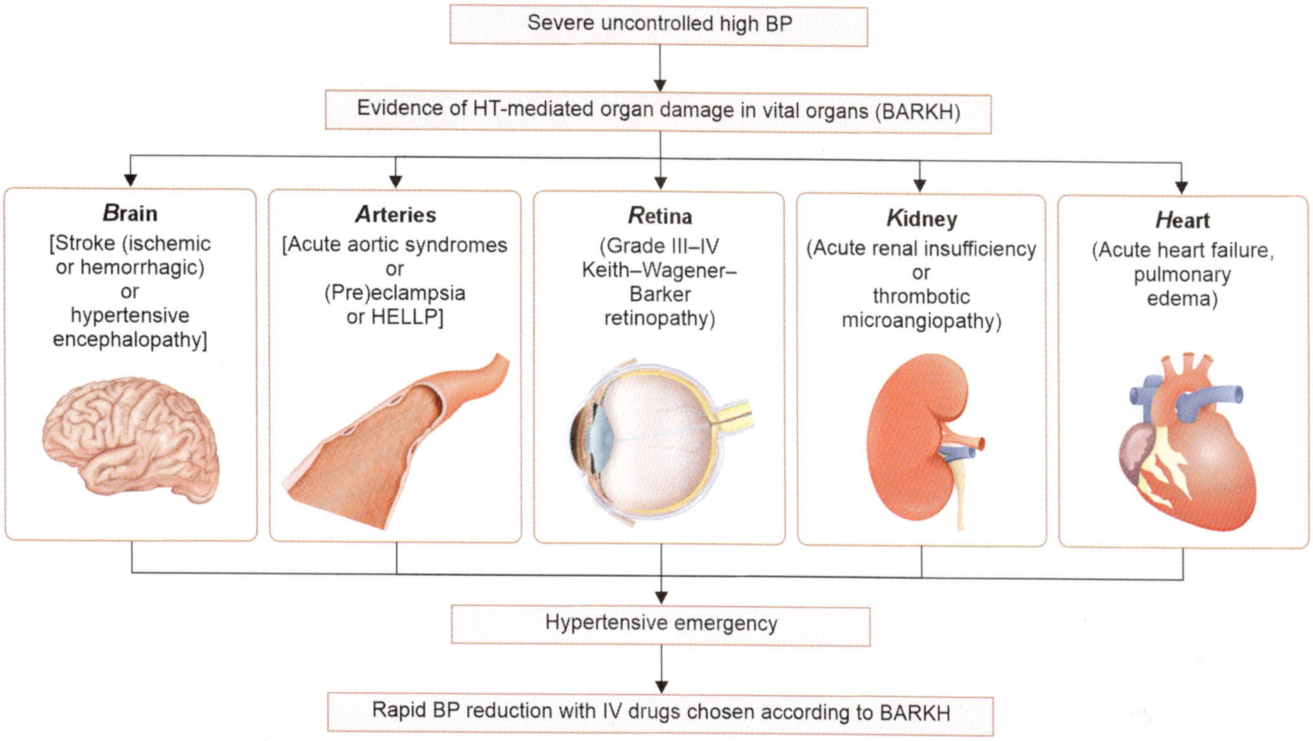

FLOWCHART 1: Severe uncontrolled high BP.

(BP: blood pressure; IV: intravenous)

Source: Rossi GP, Rossitto G, Maifredini C, Barchitta A, Bettella A, Cerruti L, et al. Modern Management of Hypertensive Emergencies. High Blood Press Cardiovasc Prev. 2022;29(1):33-40.

emergencies are the most frequent types of acute target organ dysfunction.

Hypertensive emergencies have a lower prevalence in Asia compared to Western countries, but they remain potentially fatal. Early detection and treatment can prevent morbidity and mortality associated with these emergencies. In-hospital mortality rate is around 2.5%.

COMPLICATION OF HYPERTENSION CRISIS: TARGET ORGAN DAMAGE

Acute increases of BP values are associated with acute life-threatening hypertension-mediated organ damage (HMOD) involving the vital organs. Hence, it becomes crucial for physicians to recognize the patients presenting with hypertensive emergencies.

Brain, arteries, retina, kidney, and/or heart (BARKH)-based algorithm allows a quick identification of the hypertensive emergencies with the associated acute organ damage. BARKH involvement implies the need to reduce BP values with intravenous (IV) treatment with drugs endowed of a titrable BP-lowering effect **(Flowchart 1)**.

Target organ damage may give rise to complications related to target organs. Some of these complications are summarized in **Table 1**.

TABLE 1: The relative frequency of end-organ involvement in hypertensive emergency.

End-organ damage type	Cases (%)
Cerebral infarction	24.5
Intracerebral or subarachnoid bleed	4.5
Hypertensive encephalopathy	16.3
Acute pulmonary edema	22.5
Acute congestive heart failure	14.3
Acute myocardial infarction or unstable angina	12.0
Aortic dissection	2.0
Eclampsia	2.0

Source: Adapted from Zampaglione B, Pascale C, Marchisio M, Cavallo-Perin P. Hypertensive urgencies and emergencies. Prevalence and clinical presentation. Hypertension. 1996;27(1):144-7.

PATHOPHYSIOLOGY

The pathophysiology of hypertensive crisis involves two interrelated mechanisms: (1) failure in autoregulatory mechanisms in the vascular bed and (2) activation of the renin–angiotensin system. Autoregulation is responsible for maintaining stable blood flow regardless of changes in perfusion pressure, but in hypertensive crisis, autoregulation malfunctions, resulting in a sudden

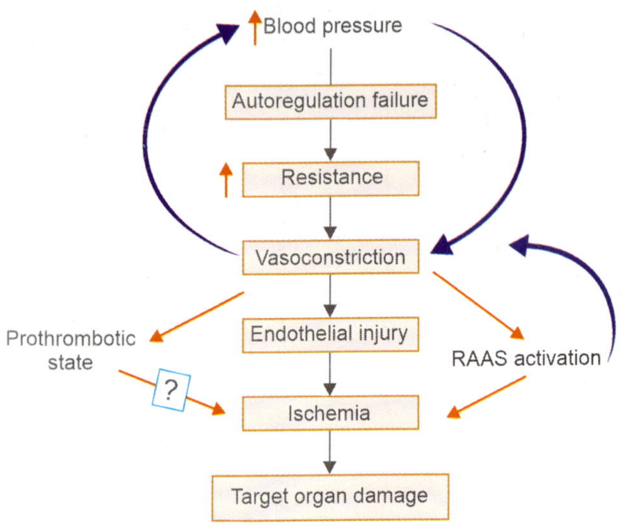

FIG. 1: Pathophysiology of hypertensive crisis.

(RAAS: renin–angiotensin–aldosterone system)

Source: Adapted from Varounis C, Katsi V, Nihoyannopoulos P, Lekakis J, Tousoulis D. Cardiovascular Hypertensive Crisis: Recent Evidence and Review of the Literature. Front Cardiovasc Med. 2017;3:51.

increase in BP and systemic vascular resistance. The renin–angiotensin system activation further contributes to vasoconstriction, perpetuating the cycle of injury, and ischemia.

In addition to these mechanisms, a prothrombotic state and platelet activation may play a role in hypertensive crisis. The abrupt rise in BP promotes acute target end-organ damage, accelerating the rise in BP and causing endothelial damage due to inadequate compensatory mechanisms. The hypertensive emergency BP threshold can vary among individuals, with chronic hypertensive patients having some degree of end-organ protection compared to normotensive individuals.

Hypertensive crisis shares similarities with primary chronic hypertension but is characterized by a more rapid and severe increase in BP, leading to acute target end-organ damage. The precise BP threshold for hypertensive crisis can vary widely among patients, and even small abrupt rises in BP can trigger a hypertensive crisis in normotensive individuals **(Fig. 1)**.

CLINICAL ASSESSMENT: EVALUATION AND DIAGNOSIS

Patients presenting with severe elevated BP are assessed on the following mentioned points:

- Complete history collection (previous history or frequency of the episodes)
- Detailed physical examination
- Duration and degree of preexisting hypertension
- Evidence of target organ damage
- Details of antihypertensive therapy
- Compliance with medications
- Use of the over-the-counter drugs
- Illicit drugs usage

Patients presenting with a history of severely elevated BP should determine any of the following:

- Acute head injury or trauma
- Generalized neurologic symptoms
- Focal neurologic symptoms
- Fundoscopy nausea and vomiting [for raised intracranial pressure (ICP)]
- Chest discomfort or pain
- Acute and severe back pain
- Dyspnea
- Pregnancy
- Use of drugs that can produce a hyperadrenergic state

While examining the patient, following should be checked:

- BP sitting and standing position, if peripheral pulses are markedly reduced
- Respiratory rate (RR) and heart rate (HR)
- O_2 saturation
- Fundoscopic examination.
- Cardiovascular system (CVS)—murmurs S3, gallop, crackles in lung fields, and raised jugular venous pressure (JVP)
- Level of consciousness and focal signs of ischemia
- Renal bruit abdominal mass

INVESTIGATIONS

- ECG
- CXR
- Urinalysis and urine pregnancy test (if appropriate)
- Serum electrolytes and serum creatinine
- Cardiac biomarkers CT or MRI of the brain

Contrast-enhanced CT or MRI of the Chest or Transesophageal Echocardiography

Hypertensive retinopathy, the ocular manifestation of systemic hypertension, can be observed in the eye. The Keith–Wagener–Barker (KWB) classification is a widely used grading system for assessing its severity **(Table 2 and Figs. 2 to 6)**.

Keith–Wagener–Barker Classification

Grades of Hypertensive Retinopathy

Grade 1: Mild hypertensive retinopathy *(in an eye with an unrelated chorioretinal lesion)* with arteriolar narrowing

TABLE 2: Keith–Wagener–Barker classification.

Grade 1	Mild generalized retinal arteriolar narrowing
Grade 2	Definite focal narrowing and arteriovenous nipping
Grade 3	Signs of grade 2 retinopathy plus retinal hemorrhages, exudates, and cotton wool spots
Grade 4	Severe grade 3 retinopathy plus papilledema

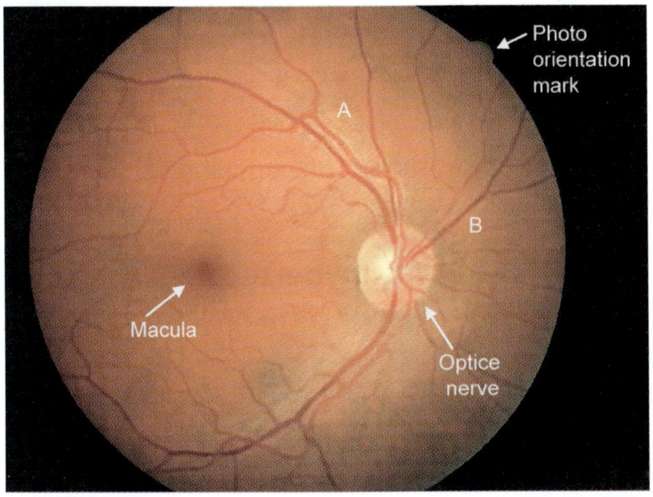

FIG. 2: Normal.

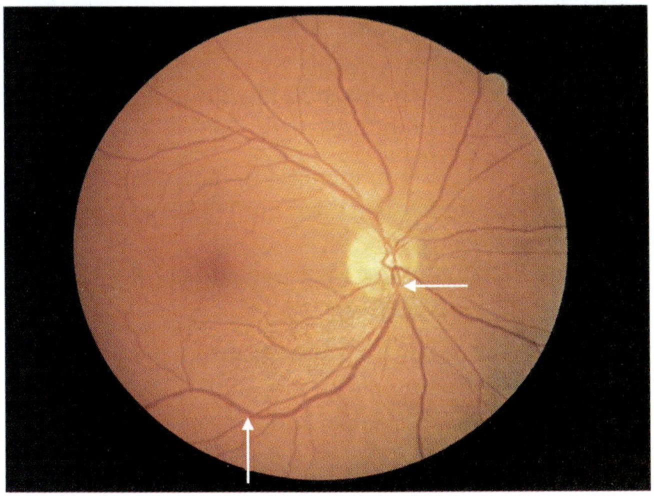

FIG. 3: Grade 1: Mild generalized retinal arteriolar narrowing.

(white arrow), copper wiring (black star), and AV nicking (black arrow).

Grade 2: Moderate hypertensive retinopathy with features of mild hypertensive retinopathy as well as cotton wool spots and intraretinal hemorrhages.

Grade 3: Severe hypertensive retinopathy with features of moderate hypertensive retinopathy and optic disc swelling.

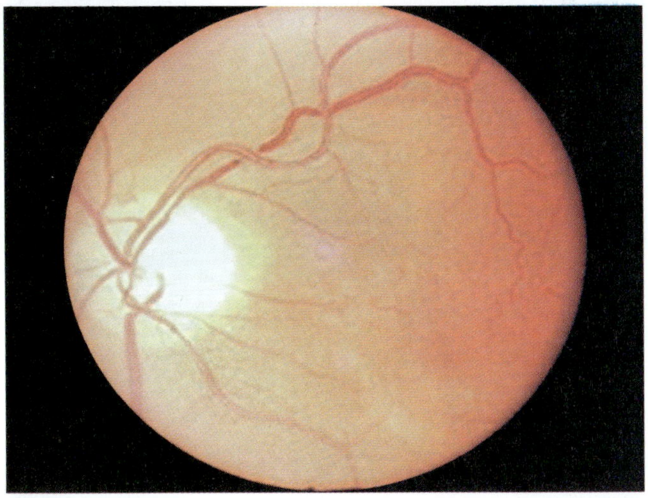

FIG. 4: Grade 2: Definite focal narrowing and arteriovenous nipping.

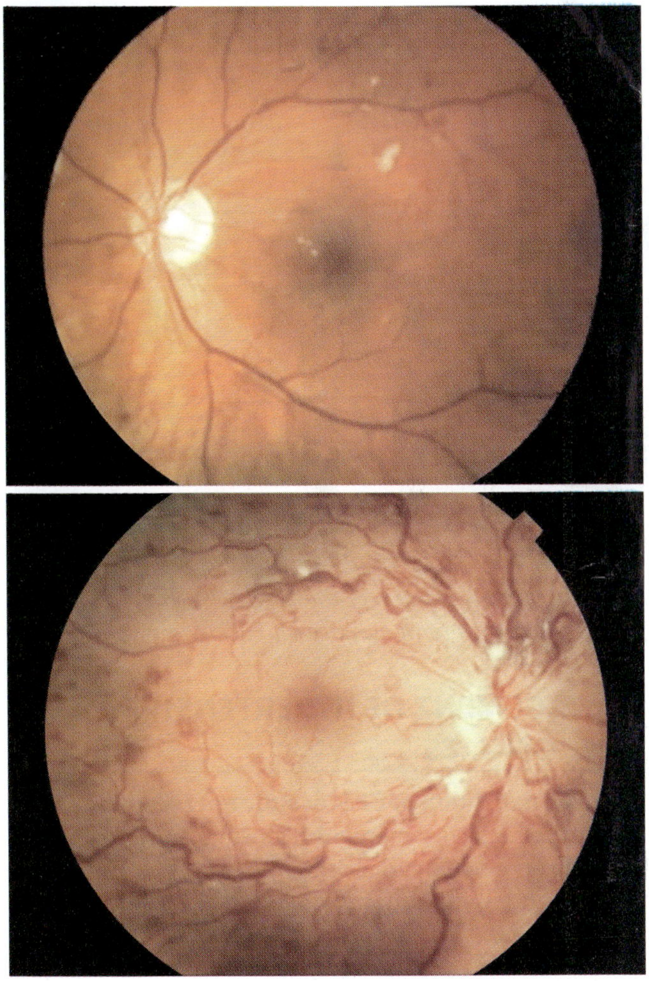

FIG. 5: Grade 3: Signs of grade 2 retinopathy plus retinal hemorrhages, exudates, and cotton wool spots.

Grade 4: Severe hypertensive retinopathy with features of moderate hypertensive retinopathy and optic disc

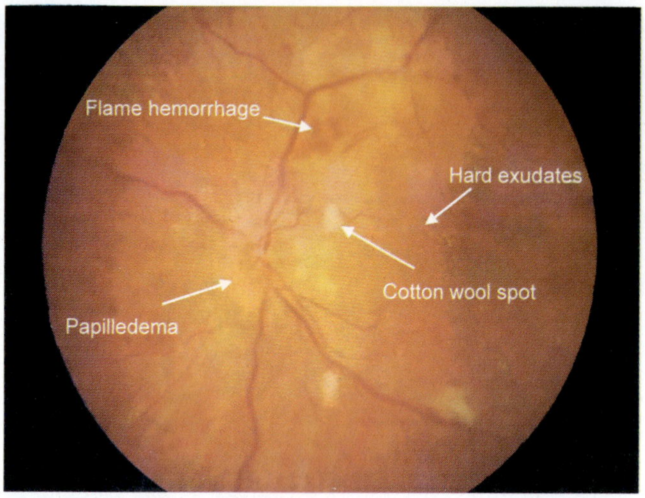

FIG. 6: Grade 4: Severe grade 3 retinopathy plus papilledema.

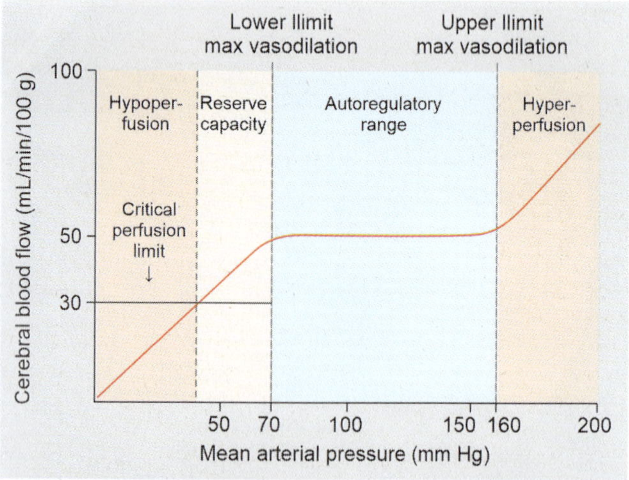

FIG. 7: Management of hypertensive emergencies.

swelling. *Grade 3 and grade 4 highly correlated with progression end-organ damage and decreased survival.*

MANAGEMENT OF HYPERTENSIVE EMERGENCIES

Why normalization of BP is usually not recommended?
In a hypertensive emergency, normalization of BP is usually not recommended as:

- Sudden fall in BP may cause acute hypoperfusion of vital organs and results in myocardial ischemia or infarction, hemiplegia, or acute renal failure.
- Older patients with long lasting hypertension and preclinical organ involvement [left ventricular hypertrophy (LVH), atherosclerosis, and arteriolar remodeling] are at risk of these complications as the lower limit of autoregulation shift to right **(Fig. 7)**.

TABLE 3: BP treatment goals for hypertensive emergency.

Goal time	BP target
First hour	Reduce MAP by 25% (while maintaining goal DBP >100 mm Hg)
2–6 hour	SBP 160 mm Hg and/or DBP 100–110 mm Hg
6–24 hour	Maintain goal for hours 2–6 during first 24 hour
24–48 hours	Outpatient BP goals according to the 2017 guidelines for management of high blood pressure in adults

(BP: blood pressure; DBP: Diastolic blood pressure; MAP: mean arterial pressure; SBP: systolic blood pressure)

In general, use of oral therapy is discouraged for hypertensive emergencies **(Table 3)**.

Intravenous Antihypertensive Drugs for Treatment of Hypertensive Emergencies

Ideal drug for management of hypertensive emergencies should be fast acting, easily titrable, and rapidly reversible and safe. However, finding all the characteristic of an ideal drug in single agent is a challenge.

Nitroglycerin

Intravenous nitroglycerin is a potent vasodilator used for hypertensive emergency, myocardial infarction (MI), and acute heart failure. It causes hypotension and reflex tachycardia but may be used in low doses as adjunctive therapy in certain conditions.

Dosage: Initial 5 μg/min; increase in increments of 5 μg/min every 3–5 minutes to a maximum of 20 μg/min.

Sodium Nitroprusside (Vasodilators—Nitric-oxide Dependent)

Sodium nitroprusside is a potent arterial and venous vasodilator, reducing afterload and preload, but it decreases cerebral blood flow and can increase ICP.

Dosage: Initial 0.3–0.5 μg/kg/min; increase in increments of 0.5 μg/kg/min to achieve BP target; maximum dose 10 μg/kg/min; duration of treatment as short as possible.

Clevidipine

It is a third generation IV dihydropyridine calcium channel blocker (DHP-CCB). It works by relaxing the muscles of heart and blood vessels.

Dosage: An IV infusion at 1–2 mg/h is recommended for initiation and should be titrated by doubling the dose every 90 seconds. The maximum infusion rate for cleviprex is 32 mg/h.

Nicardipine

Nicardipine is a highly selective second-generation CCB with potent cerebral and coronary vasodilatory effects. It can be administered intravenously, with an onset of action between 5 and 15 minutes and a duration of action of 4–6 hours. It improves stroke volume, coronary blood flow, and myocardial oxygen balance.

Dosage: Dose is independent of weight. Infusion rate of 5–2.5 mg/h increments every 5 minutes—maximum being 15 mg/h.

Fenoldopam (Dopamine 1 Receptor Selective Agonist)

Fenoldopam is a short-acting dopamine agonist (DA1 agonist) that increases renal blood flow and sodium excretion. It is highly specific for DA1 receptors and acts as a renal vasodilator. It has a rapid onset of action (within 5 minutes) and duration of 30–60 minutes. Fenoldopam is metabolized in the liver and is often used in hypertensive emergencies with renal dysfunction.

Dosage: Initial 0.1–0.3 μg/kg/min; may be increased in increments of 0.05–0.1 μg/kg/min every 15 minutes until target BP is reached. Maximum infusion rate is 1.6 μg/kg/min.

Labetalol (Adrenergic Blockers Combined α1 and Nonselective β-receptor Antagonist)

Labetalol is a combined α1- and non-selective β-adrenergic receptor blocker. It has a rapid onset of action, lasting for 2–4 hours. It maintains cardiac output and cerebral, renal, and coronary blood flows. Labetalol is commonly used in pregnancy-induced hypertensive crisis due to its limited placental transfer.

Dosage: Initial 0.3–1.0 mg/kg dose (maximum 20 mg) slow IV injection every 10 minutes or 0.4–1.0 mg/kg/h IV infusion up to 3 mg/kg/h. Adjust rate up to total cumulative dose of 300 mg.

Esmolol (Adrenergic Blockers—β1-receptor Selective Antagonist)

Esmolol is an ultra-short-acting, cardioselective β-blocker. It has a rapid onset of action (within 60 seconds) and a short duration (10–20 minutes). Metabolism occurs via ester hydrolysis, independent of renal or hepatic function. Esmolol is considered an ideal β-blocker for critically ill patients and is used intravenously. It is useful in severe postoperative hypertension and situations with increased cardiac output, heart rate, and BP. Esmolol is safe in acute MI, even with relative contraindications to β-blockers.

Dosage: 0.5–1 mg/kg loading dose over 1 minute followed by an infusion—50 μg/kg/min (maximum 300 μg/kg/min). Loading dose 500–1,000 μg/kg/min over 1 minute followed by a 50-μg/kg/min infusion **(Table 4)**.

Additional Drugs

Hydralazine: Initial 10 mg slow IV infusion (maximum 20 mg); repeat every 4–6 hours. BP decreases within 10–30 minutes, lasts 2–4 hours. Not recommended as first-line agent in acute treatment.

Phentolamine: Hydralazine IV bolus—5 mg initially, additional bolus doses every 10 minutes as needed to lower BP in catecholamine-induced hypertensive emergencies.

Enalaprilat: Initial 1.25 mg over 5 minutes, dose increased up to 5 mg every 6 hours as needed for BP control. It is useful in hypertensive emergencies with high renin activity.

TABLE 4: Parenteral medications used for treatment of hypertensive crisis.

	Dosing	Onset of action	Preload	Afterload	Cardiac output
Sodium nitroprusside	0.25–10 μg/kg/min IV infusion	Within seconds to minutes	↓	↓↓	No effect
Nitroglycerin	5–100 μg/min IV infusion	1–5 min	↓↓	↓	No effect
Labetalol	20–80 mg bolus every 10 minutes, or 0.5–2 mg/min IV infusion	5–10 min	No effect	↓	↓
Esmolol	80 mg bolus over 30 seconds then 150 μq/kg/min IV infusion	1–2 min	No effect	No effect	↓
Hydralazine	10–20 mg IV bolus	10–20 min	No effect	↓	↑
Phentolamine	5–15 mg IV bolus	1–2 min	No effect	↓	↑
Nicardipine	2–15 mg/h IV infusion	5–10 min	No effect	↓	↑
Clevidipine	1–2 mg/h then titrate to maximum 16 mg/h IV infusion	1–4 min	No effect	↓	↑
Fenoldopam	0.1–0.6 μq/kg/min IV infusion	5–10 min	No effect	↓	↑
Enalaprilat	1.25–5 mg every 6 hour IV bolus	15–30 min	No effect	↓	↑

Not to Use Sublingual Nifedipine

- Drug is poorly soluble, not absorbed through buccal mucosa.
- Sudden uncontrolled and severe reductions in BP may precipitate cerebral, renal, and myocardial ischemic events.
- Lack of clinical documentation attesting to a benefit from its use
- The Cardio-Renal Advisory Committee of the FDA has concluded that administering sublingual (SL)/oral nifedipine should be abandoned because this agent is neither safe nor efficacious.

CONCLUSION

- Most common cause for hypertension crises is undiagnosed/untreated/inadequately treated hypertension.
- Differentiation of emergency from urgency is absence of target organ damage in the later.
- Clevidipine is the new drug approved for hypertensive emergencies.
- Parenteral nicardipine and labetalol are preferred for most of emergency situations.
- Sublingual or oral nifedipine is not recommended due to lack of safety and efficacy data.

SUGGESTED READINGS

1. Zampaglione B, Pascale C, Marchisio M, Cavallo-Perin P. Hypertensive urgencies and emergencies. Prevalence and clinical presentation. Hypertension. 1996;27(1):144-7.
2. National High Blood Pressure Education Program. The Seventh Report of the Joint National Committee on Prevention, Detection, Evaluation, and Treatment of High Blood Pressure. Bethesda (MD): National Heart, Lung, and Blood Institute (US); 2004.
3. Rossi GP, Rossitto G, Maifredini C, Barchitta A, Bettella A, Cerruti L, et al. Modern Management of Hypertensive Emergencies. High Blood Press Cardiovasc Prev. 2022;29(1):33-40.
4. Varounis C, Katsi V, Nihoyannopoulos P, Lekakis J, Tousoulis D. Cardiovascular Hypertensive Crisis: Recent Evidence and Review of the Literature. Front Cardiovasc Med. 2017;3:51.
5. Papadopoulos DP, Mourouzis I, Thomopoulos C, Makris T, Papademetriou V. Hypertension crisis. Blood Press (2010) 19(6): 328-36.
6. Vidt DG. Hypertensive crises: emergencies and urgencies. J Clin Hypertens (Greenwich). 2004;6(9):520-5.
7. Taylor DA. Hypertensive crisis: a review of pathophysiology and treatment. Crit Care Nurs Clin North Am. 2015;27(4): 439-47.
8. Murphy C. Hypertensive emergencies. Emerg Med Clin North Am. 1995;13(4):973-1007.
9. González Pacheco H, Morales Victorino N, Núñez Urquiza JP, Altamirano Castillo A, Juárez Herrera U, Arias Mendoza A, et al. Patients with hypertensive crises who are admitted to a coronary care unit: clinical characteristics and outcomes. J Clin Hypertens. 2013;15(3):210-4.
10. Marik PE, Varon J. Hypertensive crises: challenges and management. Chest. 2007;131:1949-62.
11. Elliott WJ. Clinical features and management of selected hypertensive emergencies. J Clin Hypertens. 2004;6:587-92.

55

CHAPTER

Hypertension-mediated Organ Damage: Understanding the Impact

Kumudini Jayasinghe

ABSTRACT

Hypertension-mediated organ damage (HMOD) refers to the structural or functional changes that occur in target organs, such as the brain, heart, kidneys, central and peripheral arteries, and eyes, due to hypertension. These changes can manifest in hypertensive emergencies as well as in long-standing hypertension.

A hypertensive emergency is a life-threatening medical condition characterized by significantly elevated blood pressure, leading to progressive or imminent end-organ dysfunction. Timely medical intervention and blood pressure control within minutes to hours are crucial in hypertensive emergencies to prevent progressive or impending end-organ dysfunction.

Hypertension-mediated organ damage can also occur due to long-standing hypertension, and it is more common with severe hypertension. Cardiovascular (CV) risk increases with the presence of HMOD, especially when the damage progresses and affects multiple organs and functions.

Traditionally, CV risk is stratified using charts or calculators that tend to underestimate the real CV risk. However, the diagnosis of HMOD automatically reclassifies patients to the highest level of CV risk.

Subclinical HMOD can be present already at the diagnosis of hypertension. Assessing HMOD is essential, as the progression or regression of HMOD during follow-up visits significantly influences management strategies and the scheduling of further follow-ups.

INTRODUCTION

Hypertension, a pervasive cardiovascular (CV) risk factor for diseases such as stroke, coronary heart disease, and peripheral artery disease, had a global prevalence of 1.13 billion in 2015, with a concerning 235 million in South Asia. Hypertension can harm crucial organs such as the brain, heart, kidneys, blood vessels, and eyes in two instances: (1) Acute or progressive end-organ damage linked to hypertensive emergencies or (2) end-organ damage due to prolonged elevated blood pressure. The damage to organs caused by hypertension is referred to as hypertension-mediated organ damage (HMOD), previously known as target organ damage. HMOD emphasizes the structural and functional alterations occurring in the brain, heart, kidneys, central and peripheral arteries, and eyes due to hypertension.

HYPERTENSION-MEDIATED ORGAN DAMAGE IN HYPERTENSIVE EMERGENCIES

A hypertensive emergency is a life-threatening medical condition characterized by significantly elevated blood pressure, usually with systolic blood pressure (SBP) ≥180 mm Hg or diastolic blood pressure (DBP) ≥120 mm Hg, leading to progressive or imminent end-organ dysfunction. Acute end-organ damage can affect various organs and systems in the body, including the brain, heart, kidneys, blood vessels, and eyes.

Neurological manifestations of hypertensive emergencies encompass hypertensive encephalopathy, ischemic stroke, or hemorrhagic stroke. CV acute end-organ damage may include acute coronary syndrome, acute left-ventricular (LV) failure, and/or aortic dissection. Hypertension caused by conditions such as pheochromocytoma and the usage of sympathomimetic drugs such as methamphetamine and cocaine can trigger acute and severe blood pressure elevation, resulting in acute HMOD. Preeclampsia, eclampsia with hemolysis, elevated liver enzymes, and low platelet count (HELLP) syndrome are also classified as hypertensive emergencies. Malignant hypertension with or without thrombotic microangiopathy or acute kidney failure is a hypertensive emergency characterized by small artery fibrinoid necrosis in the kidney, retina, and brain. A funduscopic examination might reveal flame-shaped hemorrhages and papilledema, alongside microangiopathy, or disseminated intravascular coagulation.

When a patient presents with very high blood pressure values, it is crucial to exclude the presence of a hypertensive emergency through a targeted history, physical examination, and relevant investigations. Timely medical intervention and blood pressure control over minutes to hours are crucial in hypertensive emergencies to prevent progressive or impending end-organ dysfunction. The overall therapeutic goal in patients presenting with hypertensive emergencies is a controlled reduction of blood pressure to safer levels to prevent or limit further hypertensive damage while avoiding hypotension and related complications. The type of acute HMOD is the main determinant of the preferred treatment choice. Labetalol and nicardipine are generally considered safe to use in all hypertensive emergencies and should be readily available wherever hypertensive emergencies are being managed.

HYPERTENSION-MEDIATED ORGAN DAMAGE IN LONG-STANDING HYPERTENSION

Hypertension-mediated organ damage can also occur due to long-standing hypertension, more common with severe hypertension. However, HMOD can also manifest in patients with less severe hypertension due to prolonged elevated blood pressure. CV increases with the presence of HMOD, especially when the damage progresses and affects multiple organs and functions. Overall CV risk is essential for the management of hypertension. CV risk assessment in clinical practice is mostly based on risk estimators, such as the World Health Organization (WHO) risk calculation chart, atherosclerotic cardiovascular disease (ASCVD) risk calculation, Framingham risk score, SCORE (Systemic COronary Risk Evaluation) CV risk calculator, and other risk calculators. CV risk estimators often underestimate the actual CV risk as they do not account for HMOD, which reclassifies low/moderate-risk patients to high risk. Additional detection of HMOD is unlikely to change the management of patients already identified as high-risk [i.e., those with established cardiovascular disease (CVD), stroke, diabetes, chronic kidney disease (CKD), or familial hypercholesterolemia]. However, the presence of HMOD can provide crucial therapeutic guidance for hypertensive patients with low or moderate CV risk, as it automatically reclassifies patients to the highest level of CV risk. This also enables the preferential selection of drug treatment based on the specific impact on HMOD. HMOD, unless treated, gradually progresses from asymptomatic to symptomatic, ultimately leading to overt CVD events. Long-standing hypertension damages vital organs, such as the heart, brain, kidneys, eyes, and blood vessels.

HYPERTENSION-MEDIATED ORGAN DAMAGE IN THE HEART

Hypertensive heart disease (HHD) encompasses LV hypertrophy (LVH), impaired diastolic or systolic function, left atrial enlargement, and arrhythmias. LVH, characterized by increased myocardial mass and ventricular remodeling, significantly contributes to high CV events, such as heart failure, atrial fibrillation, coronary artery disease, and sudden death. In clinical practice, HHD should be evaluated comprehensively, involving an electrocardiogram (ECG) and available imaging techniques.

Left-ventricular hypertrophy detected by transthoracic echocardiogram is a more sensitive marker of LVH than ECG. LV mass index was the single, probably most important predictor of adverse events in patients with hypertension. Furthermore, antihypertensive treatment can be accompanied by a regression of LVH. When LVH is detected, it is recommended to follow patients, preferably by echocardiography for monitoring the evolution or regression of LVH with treatment. The regression may take years, cannot always be achieved, and is less achievable in women, and patients with diabetes and obesity.

Cardiac magnetic resonance is the gold standard for quantification of cardiac structure and function in clinical studies. This allows to detection of interstitial myocardial fibrosis which may precede the development of LVH. However, this modality is expensive and is not available in resource-poor settings.

HYPERTENSION-MEDIATED ORGAN DAMAGE IN THE KIDNEY

Hypertension ranks as the second most significant cause of CKD. Hypertension-induced damage to renal blood vessels impairs glomerular filtration, leading to hypertensive nephropathy and CKD. Renal mechanisms contributing to HMOD include altered tubular sodium handling, glomerular hyperfiltration, and activation of the renin–angiotensin–aldosterone system. The diagnosis of HMOD in the kidney is based on the finding of reduced kidney function or the detection of albuminuria; however, in hypertension-induced kidney disease, albuminuria may not appear until after the reduction in GFR. The albumin:creatinine ratio (ACR) is measured from a spot urine sample (preferably early morning urine) and is the preferred method to quantify urinary albumin excretion. Serum creatinine, estimated glomerular filtration rate (eGFR), and ACR should be documented in all hypertensive patients, and if CKD is diagnosed, these should be repeated at least annually. Early detection and effective blood pressure control are essential in slowing the progression of CKD and reducing the risk of end-stage renal disease.

HYPERTENSION-MEDIATED ORGAN DAMAGE IN THE BRAIN

Hypertension is a major risk factor for cerebrovascular disease, including ischemic or hemorrhagic strokes and cognitive impairment. Long-standing hypertension exerts a cumulative effect on cerebrovascular damage, including atherosclerosis, white matter lesions, silent brain infarcts, microinfarcts, microbleeds, brain atrophy, and dementia. Hypertension management plays a pivotal role in preventing stroke incidence and improving patient outcomes.

ARTERIAL HYPERTENSION-MEDIATED ORGAN DAMAGE

Hypertension induces changes in the small and large arteries characterized by endothelial dysfunction and remodeling. This leads to a reduced dilation capability of the high-resistance vasculature and stiffening of the arteries. Three vascular beds are commonly assessed to detect arterial HMOD: (1) The carotid arteries through carotid ultrasound to detect atherosclerotic plaque burden/stenosis and intima-media thickness (IMT), (2) the aorta by carotid-femoral pulse wave velocity (PWV) assessment to detect large artery stiffening, and (3) the lower extremity arteries by assessment of the ankle-brachial index (ABI). Although, there is evidence to indicate that all three provide added value beyond traditional risk factors, their routine use is currently not recommended.

HYPERTENSION-MEDIATED ORGAN DAMAGE IN THE EYE

Hypertensive retinopathy refers to retinal microvascular signs that are related to raised blood pressure. Fundoscopy is a simple clinical bedside test to screen for hypertensive retinopathy, although interobserver and intraobserver reproducibility are limited. The classification of hypertensive retinopathy based on fundoscopy allows for the detection of retinal lesions, such as hemorrhages, microaneurysms, hard exudates, cotton wool spots (grade 3), papilledema, and/or macular edema (grade 4). These alterations are indicative of severe retinopathy. Retinal damage of grades 1 and 2 such as focal and general arteriolar narrowing and/or arteriovenous nipping, are less specific and reproducible and also have much less predictive value and should ideally be performed by experienced examiners. Damage to the microvasculature may not be apparent on routine funduscopic retinal examination. However, the combined use of adaptive optics (AO) retinal cameras with optical coherence tomography (OCT) has begun to play an important role in detecting the involvement of microvasculature and the development of neovascularization. This presents an early therapeutic target in hypertensive retinopathy.

ASYMPTOMATIC HYPERTENSION-MEDIATED ORGAN DAMAGE

With the wider use of imaging studies, HMOD is increasingly detected in asymptomatic patients. Asymptomatic HMOD includes wide pulse pressure, LVH, microalbuminuria, CKD, and an abnormal ABI, many of which are usually markers of preclinical CVD.

Guidelines support the use of different routine tests and nonroutine tests to assess organ damage in hypertension. Performing a nonroutine test depends on the clinical excellence of the physician. However, the reliance of personal skills in addition to inconsistent availability of services may lead to missing the diagnosis of subclinical HMOD in patients. We can mitigate the problem of under-diagnosing the HMOD to a certain extent, by performing the available laboratory tests and or services in all hypertensive patients.

In the presence of asymptomatic or symptomatic HMOD, patients should be classified and treated as high-risk.

MANAGEMENT OF HYPERTENSION-MEDIATED ORGAN DAMAGE

Some types of HMOD can be reversed by antihypertensive treatment, especially when treatment starts early. However, with long-standing hypertension, HMOD becomes irreversible despite blood pressure control. Nevertheless, blood pressure-lowering treatment is important, as it may delay further progression of HMOD and oppose the trend toward a progressive increase in CV risk. Although poor technical provision and cost may limit the search for HMOD in some countries, it is recommended that basic screening for HMOD be performed in all hypertensive patients, and a more detailed assessment be implemented when the presence of HMOD is important for treatment decisions. Basic tests for HMOD include a 12-lead ECG, urine albumin-to-creatinine ratio, and serum creatinine and eGFR. Extended screening for HMOD includes a two-dimensional (2D) echocardiogram, ultrasound of the kidney/abdomen, special Doppler ultrasonography, brain imaging (CT/MRI), retina microvasculature, CT coronary angiogram, and calcium score. Reassessment of HMOD should be carried out according to the recommendations. HMOD assessment is important, as the progression or regression of HMOD at follow-up visits has a major influence on management strategies and scheduling of further follow-up.

CONCLUSION

Understanding and effectively managing HMOD are pivotal in hypertension management. Comprehensive knowledge of HMOD resulting from hypertensive emergencies and long-standing hypertension, understanding its impact on vital organs, and recognizing its varied manifestations are crucial for providing optimal care to patients. Whether, it is the acute and severe HMOD stemming from hypertensive emergencies or the insidious yet damaging HMOD due to prolonged elevated blood pressure, timely intervention, and tailored treatment plans are paramount. These measures can potentially reverse or halt HMOD progression, ultimately easing the associated CV risks and improving overall patient outcomes. The integration of advanced diagnostic techniques, continuous monitoring, and a multidisciplinary approach in healthcare settings can play a transformative role in addressing HMOD and advancing the field of hypertension management. By prioritizing research, education, and awareness about HMOD, we can work toward a future where its impact is minimized, leading to enhanced CV health and a better quality of life for individuals worldwide.

SUGGESTED READINGS

1. NCD Risk Factor Collaboration (NCD-RisC). Worldwide trends in blood pressure from 1975 to 2015: a pooled analysis of 1479 population-based measurement studies with 19·1 million participants. Lancet. 2017;389(10064):37-55.
2. Unger T, Borghi C, Charchar F, Khan NA, Poulter NR, Prabhakaran D, et al. 2020 International Society of Hypertension Global Hypertension Practice Guidelines. Hypertension. 2020;75(6):1334-57.
3. Mancia G, Kreutz R, Brunström M, Burnier M, Grassi G, Januszewicz A, et al. 2023 ESH Guidelines for the management of arterial hypertension The Task Force for the management of arterial hypertension of the European Society of Hypertension: Endorsed by the International Society of Hypertension (ISH) and the European Renal Association (ERA). J Hypertens. 2023;41(12):1874-2071.
4. Wang X, Hao G, Chen L, Yang Y, Zhou H, Kang Y, et al. Hypertension-mediated organ damage and established cardiovascular disease in patients with hypertension: the China Hypertension Survey, 2012–2015. J Hum Hypertens. 2022;36(12):1092-8.
5. Sehestedt T, Jeppesen J, Hansen TW, Wachtell K, Ibsen H, Torp-Pedersen C, et al. Risk prediction is improved by adding markers of subclinical organ damage to SCORE. Eur Heart J. 2010;31(7):883-91.
6. Kasiakogias A, Rosei EA, Camafort M, Ehret G, Faconti L, Ferreira JP, et al. Hypertension and heart failure with preserved ejection fraction: a position paper by the European Society of Hypertension. J Hypertens. 2021;39(8):1522-45.
7. Wachtell K, Dahlöf B, Rokkedal J, Papademetriou V, Nieminen MS, Smith G, et al. Change of left ventricular geometric pattern after 1 year of antihypertensive treatment: the Losartan Intervention For Endpoint reduction in hypertension (LIFE) study. Am Heart J. 2002;144(6):1057-64.
8. Dziedziak J, Zaleska-Żmijewska A, Szaflik JP, Cudnoch-Jędrzejewska A. Impact of Arterial Hypertension on the Eye: A Review of the Pathogenesis, Diagnostic Methods, and Treatment of Hypertensive Retinopathy. Med Sci Monit. 2022;28:e935135-1-12.
9. Williams B, Mancia G, Spiering W, Rosei EA, Azizi M, Burnier M, et al. 2018 ESC/ESH Guidelines for the management of arterial hypertension. Kardiol Pol. 2019;77(2):71-159.

56

CHAPTER

Resistant Hypertension

BB Thakur

ABSTRACT

Resistant hypertension (RH)-uncontrolled hypertension with three or more antihypertensive agents is common in clinical practice. Clinicians should exclude pseudoresistant hypertension, which results from nonadherence to medications or from elevated blood pressure (BP) related to the white-coat syndrome before the diagnosis of RH.

Resistant hypertension is defined as BP that remains above goal BP of 140/90 mm Hg despite concurrent use of three antihypertensive agents of different classes (one of which is usually a diuretic) at maximum tolerated doses.

The prevalence of RH varies from 10 to 20% in general hypertensive patients. About 5–10% of RH patients have an underlying secondary cause including obstructive sleep apnea (OSA) or primary aldosteronism. Treating these disorders can significantly improve BP beyond medical therapy alone. Patients with RH have almost 50% more chances of adverse cardiovascular events than patients with controlled BP. In patients with true RH, thiazide diuretics, particularly chlorthalidone, should be considered as one of the initial agents. The evidence suggests the use of mineralocorticoid receptor antagonists, such as eplerenone and spironolactone in improving BP control in patients with RH, regardless of circulating aldosterone levels; therefore, this class of drugs should be considered as the preferred fourth drug where serum potassium level is ≤4.5 mmol/L and the BP remains elevated despite treatment with a three-drug regimen to maximal or near-maximal doses. With higher serum potassium levels, increasing the dose of a thiazide-like diuretic should be the preferred choice. New BP-lowering drugs (e.g., nitric oxide donors, vasopressin antagonists, neutral endopeptidase inhibitors, and aldosterone synthase inhibitors) are under trial. The role of device therapy for treating the typical patient with RH remains unclear.

INTRODUCTION

Hypertension is a key determinant of cardiovascular disease morbidity and mortality, directly accounting for approximately 10% of deaths in India. In urban India, the reported prevalence of hypertension ranges between 20 and 33%, and it is of concern that the figure is rising steadily. There is a causal association between the magnitude of blood pressure (BP) elevation and adverse cardiovascular event rate, which provides the rationale for targeting BP reduction in routine clinical practice. However, an estimated 30–50% of the hypertensive population remains uncontrolled with a BP > 140/90 mm Hg, of whom a subgroup fulfills the diagnostic criteria for resistant hypertension (RH). This cohort lies at the extreme end of the cardiovascular risk spectrum, and hence stands to benefit most from BP control.

Most patients with hypertension have other risk factors, such as lipid abnormalities, glucose intolerance and diabetes, family history of early cardiovascular events, obesity, and tobacco use with or without alcohol excess.

Resistant hypertension is defined as BP that remains above the target BP of 140 mm Hg systolic and 90 mm Hg diastolic despite a therapeutic strategy that includes appropriate lifestyle measures plus a diuretic and two other antihypertensive drugs of different classes at maximally tolerated doses. RH also includes patients whose BP is controlled with more than three medications. The suggested target BP in patients with diabetes, chronic kidney disease (CKD), and patients at risk of developing or established cardiovascular disease is 130/80 mm Hg. RH should be diagnosed only after ambulatory blood pressure monitoring (ABPM) when average blood pressure is > 135/85 mm Hg, thereby excluding white-coat hypertension. RH is associated with a high risk of cardiovascular, cerebrovascular, and renovascular events.

PREVALENCE

The aging population, increasing obesity, diabetes, sleep apnea, and CKDs are the main causes leading to the increased prevalence of RH. A number of factors may contribute to the pathogenesis and higher prevalence of RH in CKD, including impaired sodium handling, increased activity of the renin-angiotensin-aldosterone system (RAAS) and sympathetic system, impaired nitric oxide synthesis and endothelium-mediated vasodilation, and increased arterial stiffness. The exact prevalence is unknown due to a lack of proper population studies. More recent observational findings suggest the prevalence to be in the range of 10–20% of hypertensive population, of which only 10% being true prevalence if contributions of poor compliance and white coat effect are excluded. Prevalence has been found to be higher in secondary-care practice.

The status of hypertension awareness, treatment and control status is very low, especially in rural subjects, in India. Prevalence seems to be increasing as suggested by increasing use of multidrug regimens consisting of three or more medications. Whether a genetic factor plays a role in RH is currently being investigated.

CHARACTERISTICS ASSOCIATED WITH RESISTANT HYPERTENSION

- Age > 60 years
- Female gender
- Obesity in 50% of people with RH
- Diabetes
- History of severe hypertension, particularly severe systolic hypertension
- High baseline BP and chronicity of uncontrolled hypertension
- Target organ damage (TOD) [left ventricular hypertrophy (LVH), CKD, atherosclerotic vascular disease]
- Ethnicity (Black people)
- Excessive dietary sodium intake
- Smoking
- Chronic consumption of interfering drugs [nonsteroidal anti-inflammatory drugs (NSAIDs), steroids, etc.]
- Sleep apnea in approximately 74% of people with RH
- High alcohol intake

ETIOLOGY

The etiology of RH is multifactorial and includes both lifestyle and biological factors. RH can be arbitrarily divided into two broad categories: True resistance and apparent, false, or spurious resistance. The prevalence of apparent resistance is higher than true resistance. It is important to distinguish between apparent and true RH.

Apparent Resistance

Causes of apparent RH include poor adherence to recommended lifestyle measures and/or drug treatment, poor BP monitoring technique, and "white-coat effect". Other reasons include the effects of antihypertensive medication, complicated dosing regimens, inadequate patient education, costs of drugs, cuff-related artifacts, psychiatric issues, poor cognition in elderly patients, etc.

Physician-related Factors

- Poor BP measuring technique
- Clinical inertia
- Inadequate doses of antihypertensives
- Inappropriate choice of antihypertensive combinations
- Poor information, education, and communication (IEC)

Cuff-related Artifacts

The cuff should be large enough to encircle at least 80% of the upper arm circumference and extend to at least two-thirds of its length. BP is overestimated when the cuff is too small for the arm. A rare cause of cuff-related artifact is known as pseudohypertension, i.e., marked arterial stiffening (more common in the elderly) due to noncompressibility of severely atherosclerotic or calcified arteries.

White-coat Resistant Hypertension

A significant white-coat effect (clinic BP persistently elevated to 140/90 mm Hg, while out-of-clinic values < 135/85 mm Hg) is observed in 20–30% of resistant hypertensives. About a decade ago, Brown and colleagues reported that 28% of 118 patients with RH, treated with at least three antihypertensive drugs in combination, had normal awake ambulatory BP. A significant white-coat effect is suspected in patients who show signs of overtreatment such as orthostatic hypotension, and in patients with chronically high clinic BP without TOD.

True Resistant Hypertension

Before diagnosing true RH, we should consider and exclude all causes of apparent RH including patient or clinician-related factors, white-coat effect, and pseudohypertension, lifestyle factors (obesity, alcohol, smoking, and dietary sodium), and a thorough search for secondary hypertension should be conducted.

Resistant Hypertension: Secondary Causes

The prevalence of secondary hypertension is greater in people with RH compared to the general hypertensive population. Studies indicate that 5–10% of patients with RH have an underlying secondary cause, with the most common being CKD (may be either the cause or adverse effect of chronic, poorly controlled hypertension), hyperaldosteronism, renal artery stenosis, and obstructive sleep apnea (OSA). It is important to recognize the signs and symptoms that may suggest an underlying disease process **(Table 1)**.

Clinical Evaluation

Medical history, physical examination, and biochemical evaluation should be directed toward confirming true treatment resistance. Assessment of medication adherence is essential to confirm treatment resistance. Home or worksite BP measurements or 24-hour ambulatory monitoring is recommended to exclude a significant "white-coat effect". The possibility of a secondary cause of hypertension should always be considered and excluded. Finally, ABPM should be performed regularly, not only to exclude spurious resistance but also to quantify the degree of BP elevation and subsequent effect of treatment modifications.

Biochemical Evaluation

These help to delineate a potential secondary cause of RH, signals the development of renal dysfunction and helps to monitor response and side effects of antihypertensive agents. These include assessment of the following:
- Urea and electrolytes
- Estimated glomerular filtration rate
- Plasma glucose
- Plasma renin or aldosterone levels
- 24-hour urinary metanephrines or normetanephrines (for pheochromocytoma)
- Urine analysis—microalbuminuria, macroalbuminuria, and hematuria

TARGET ORGAN DAMAGE AND CLINICAL COMPLICATIONS

Left ventricular hypertrophy, hypertensive retinopathy, and renal disease (persistently elevated urinary albumin excretion rate, hematuria, or renal impairment) are the usual TOD in hypertension. Electrocardiography

TABLE 1: Secondary causes in patients with resistant hypertension.

Condition	Clinical features	Initial investigation	Management
Common			
Obstructive sleep apnea (OSA)	Obesity, collar size > 17", daytime somnolence, snoring	Polysomnography	Continuous positive airway pressure
Primary hyperaldosteronism	Fatigue, hypokalemia	Serum aldosterone/plasma–renin ratio (off spironolactone)	Aldosterone receptor antagonists ± surgical resection of secreting adenoma
Renal artery stenosis	Flash pulmonary edema, abdominal bruit	Renal artery imaging: CT, MRI, ultrasound, angiography	Consider renal artery stent
Renal parenchymal disease	Proteinuria, hematuria	Serum creatinine; albumin–creatinine ratio, HbA1c	Correction of underlying etiology
Uncommon			
Hypo- and hyperthyroidism	Eye signs, weight loss or gain, heat or cold intolerance, heart failure	Thyroid-stimulating hormone and free thyroxine	According to underlying process
Coarctation of the aorta	Radioradial or radiofemoral delay, hypertension in a young adult	Chest radiography; imaging of the aorta	Echocardiography, CT, MRI Endovascular or surgical correction
Cushing's syndrome	Abdominal striae, centripetal obesity, hirsutism, interscapular fat deposition	24-hour urine cortisol, low-dose dexamethasone test, evening serum/saliva cortisol	According to underlying etiology

(CT: computed tomography; HbA1c: glycated hemoglobin; MRI: magnetic resonance imaging)

and echocardiography should be performed along with fundoscopy, urine analysis, renal biochemistry, and renal imaging. Evidence of TOD supports the diagnosis of poorly controlled hypertension and may influence decisions about an appropriate treatment target.

In the National Health and Nutrition Examination Survey (NHANES) survey, patients with RH were compared to patients with controlled hypertension taking one to three medications. They were more likely to have reduced renal function and albuminuria. The prevalence of the self-reported medical histories of coronary heart disease, heart failure, and stroke amounted to, respectively, 22, 10, and 10% in RH and 9.4, 4.1, and 3.8% in controlled hypertension ($p < 0.001$ for all comparisons).

REMEDIABLE CAUSES OF RESISTANT HYPERTENSION

Once a diagnosis of true RH has been established, the next step is to evaluate the patient for potentially modifiable contributing factors. We must inquire about the potential use of prescribed and recreational exogenous substances, and wherever possible, the offending agents should be stopped, minimized, or substituted appropriately.

- *Volume overload:*
  - Progressive renal insufficiency
  - High sodium intake, excessive alcohol intake, and obesity
  - Inadequate diuretic therapy
  - Drug-induced hypertension

Agents Contributing to Resistant Hypertension

- Chronic intake of vasopressor or sodium-retaining substances
- NSAIDs
- Cocaine, amphetamines, and other illicit drugs
- Sympathomimetic agents
- Oral contraceptive hormones
- Cyclosporine, tacrolimus
- Erythropoietin
- Glucocorticoids
- Liquorice
- Herbal compounds (ephedra, *mahuang*)

While several drugs may induce preexisting hypertension, NSAIDs are usually the most common due to their frequent use. Oral contraceptives, sympathomimetics (decongestants and anorectics), adrenal steroids, and antineoplastic drugs targeting the vascular endothelial growth factor (VEGF) pathway may also contribute to RH.

MANAGEMENT

A comprehensive management strategy should include the recognition and reversal of contributory factors. Compliance to treatment and lifestyle changes including weight loss, if indicated, aerobic exercise (30 min/day), high-fiber, low-fat, low-salt diet (salt restriction < 6 g/day; a small randomized crossover trial demonstrated that dietary sodium restriction was able to reduce office BP by 20/10 mm Hg in patients with RH), moderation of alcohol (< 21 units/week in men and < 14 units/week in women), and caffeine intake and smoking cessation, as appropriate, are recommended. Potentially interfering substances should be withdrawn or down-titrated as clinically allowable. An effort should be made to increase patient acceptability and compliance and assist them with education, motivation, and self-responsibility in their management program.

DRUG INTERVENTION

Initial Therapy for Resistant Hypertension

Pharmacological treatment of patients with uncontrolled BP despite a triple-drug regimen, usually an angiotensin-converting enzyme (ACE) inhibitor or an angiotensin receptor blocker (ARB) plus a calcium channel blocker (CCB) plus a thiazide-type diuretic (i.e., A + C + D), should begin with optimization of diuretic. A prospective observational study involving 3,550 patients with RH demonstrated that diuretic use is associated with improved BP control after a year of follow-up. Chlorthalidone, a thiazide-like diuretic, is at least twice as potent as hydrochlorothiazide in lowering BP. Chlorthalidone was more effective than lisinopril in reducing the risk of heart failure and stroke in black patients and should be considered as an initial therapy for patients with RH. In the British 2011 National Institute for Health and Clinical Excellence (NICE) consensus statement, indapamide, another thiazide-like diuretic, is recommended over hydrochlorothiazide due to greater antihypertensive efficacy based on a meta-analysis.

Angiotensin-converting Enzyme Inhibitors and Calcium Channel Blockers

After optimizing diuretic therapy, the combination of both ACE inhibitors and CCBs should be prescribed for RH. This combination is superior to the combination of both ACE inhibitors and thiazide diuretics in reducing cardiovascular events in hypertensive patients with a high cardiovascular risk. A recent randomized clinical trial demonstrated that the combination of angiotensin II receptor blockers and CCBs-controlled BP in more than 60% of patients whose previous medication regimens of three drug including a diuretic had failed to achieve their goal BP

Mineralocorticoid Receptor Antagonists, α-blockers, and β-blocker

The aldosterone antagonist spironolactone is an evidence-based fourth-line agent for patients with RH. It should be used cautiously in patients with renal dysfunction and in whom potassium concentrations are >4.5 mmol/L due to the risk of hyperkalemia. If gynecomastia develops in men, due to antiandrogen effects, it can be replaced by eplerenone. Amiloride is another alternative that functions as an indirect aldosterone antagonist. Some thiazides or loop diuretics are available in fixed-dose combination with amiloride. If the baseline potassium is >4.5 mmol/L, doubling the dose of the existing diuretic is recommended. Eplerenone is an alternative aldosterone antagonist that does not cause gynecomastia.

The evidence base for fifth-line therapy is weak. However, in the first instance, the choice would be adrenoreceptor blockade. If the heart rate is <60 beats per minute, an α-blocker would be most appropriate, otherwise an α- and/or β-blocker could be administered. Treatment strategies for treating RH (depending on what agents the patient is already taking) include a vasodilating α-blocker (e.g., labetalol, carvedilol, nebivolol), a direct vasodilator (e.g., hydralazine), or a centrally acting agent such as clonidine (transdermal or oral), guanfacine, or moxonidine. In men with comorbid benign prostatic hyperplasia, an α-blocker (e.g., terazosin) is a reasonable addition. Another strategy that may be particularly useful in patients with comorbid diabetes or CKD is adding a CCB of the alternate class. It is important to note that a nondihydropyridine CCB combined with a β-blocker may promote bradycardia, which can be worsened by clonidine.

It is advisable to use fixed-dose combination therapy to improve treatment adherence and to use at least one drug at night to optimize 24-hour BP control. The combination of ACE inhibitors with ARBs is not recommended due to the increased risk of adverse events (renal dysfunction, hyperkalemia, and syncope) without an increase in benefit as observed in the ONTARGET (ONgoing Telmisartan Alone and in combination with Ramipril Global Endpoint) trial. Similarly, it is not recommended to prescribe aliskiren to patients concurrently on an ACE inhibitor or ARB due to safety concerns (renal dysfunction, hyperkalemia, and stroke).

Newer Drug Therapy

The antagonism of endothelin receptor is a newer approach for the treatment of hypertension using antihypertensive medications which are currently under evaluation. Among the several endothelin receptor antagonists, darusentan, an elective antagonist of endothelin receptors (which causes vasoconstriction and proliferation of vascular smooth muscle), and atrasentan, another highly selective endothelin receptor antagonist, have also shown some favorable reports. However, their future remains unclear as the results in different trials are inconsistent, and they have not been effective in reducing clinic BP in RH and have considerable side effects. Other newer BP-lowering drugs (nitric oxide donors, vasopressin antagonists, neutral endopeptidase inhibitors, aldosterone synthase inhibitors, etc.) are in trial stages. A clinical study conducted on a combination of nitrates with phosphodiesterase-5 inhibitors on six patients resulted in significant BP reduction. A new drug called baxdrostat, a highly selective inhibitor of aldosterone synthase, has been shown to significantly reduce high BP in patients who may not respond to current treatments, according to results from a phase II trial.

Aprocitentan—an oral, once-daily, dual endothelin type A receptor (ETA) and endothelin type B receptor (ETB) endothelin receptor antagonist (ERA)—has a mechanism of action that is ideally suited for the pathophysiology of these difficult-to-treat hypertension, distinct from other and not expected to cause hyperkalemia or renal failure. With its efficacy and promising safety profile particularly in combination with other drugs, including diuretics, may have a promising future in patients at risk of difficult-to-treat hypertension and results of the phase III PRECISION study is awaited.

At times, it might be necessary to stop all current drugs and restart with a simpler treatment regimen under close medical supervision. Hospitalization for hypertension is usually not needed, though a few days in the hospital may be necessary to check the effects of antihypertensive drugs under supervision. Medical therapy is best offered in a "tailored and individualized" fashion, for RH patients under specialist supervision.

Device-based Therapies for Resistant Hypertension

In the past few years, two new procedures have been developed for the treatment of RH: Catheter-based renal denervation (RDN) and electrical stimulation of carotid baroreceptors. These procedures have a strong pathophysiological background, as there is strong evidence that carotid baroreceptors and renal nerves are involved in the pathogenesis of hypertension by potentiating the sympathetic cardiovascular influence, thus promoting the development and progression of elevated BP values. Traditional surgical sympathectomy proposed in the early forties has been discarded due to unacceptable side effects and operative risks.

Renal Denervation

This novel and recently introduced therapeutic approach **(Flowchart 1)** to RH involves bilateral destruction of the renal nerves traveling along the renal artery, using percutaneous catheter-based radiofrequency ablation via the femoral artery. The basis for RDN lies in the importance of sympathetic influences on renal vascular resistance, renin release, sodium reabsorption, and the increased sympathetic tone to the kidney and other organs.

The initial unblinded Symplicity HTN-1 and HTN-2 RDN trials have shown substantial BP reductions in response to RDN, in the order of 30/15 mm Hg, maintained beyond 2 years. RDN resulted in improved BP control, when the patients continued to take antihypertensive drugs at a reduced number or dose.

However, surprisingly, a subsequent randomized sham-controlled trial (Symplicity HTN-3) showed no difference in the office BP or 24-hour ambulatory BP in a denervation group compared with a sham-procedure group treated with medical therapy alone. It remains unclear whether RDN may benefit a subset of patients with RH.

Although there remain many questions to be answered regarding its long-term success, clinical outcomes, and technical issues, further trials are being conducted with new devices. To date, there have not been significant safety concerns except for vascular issues, and no major complications (impairment of renal function, renal artery stenosis/thrombosis) have been reported.

Carotid Baroreceptor Stimulation

The other device option **(Flowchart 2)** allows appropriate physiologic adaptation to elevated sympathetic nervous system (SNS) activation and reduced parasympathetic activation by electrically stimulating the carotid baroreflex, the carotid sinus nerves via implanted devices

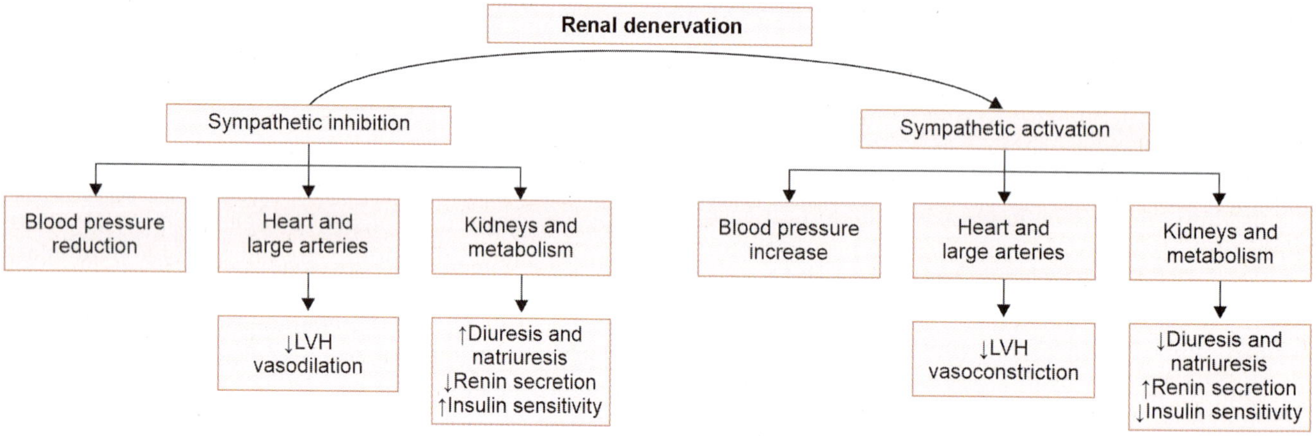

FLOWCHART 1: Scheme illustrating the possible mechanisms through which renal denervation may exert blood pressure-lowering effects: Increase (up arrow) and reduction (down arrow).
(LVH: left ventricular hypertrophy; OSA: obstructive sleep apnea)

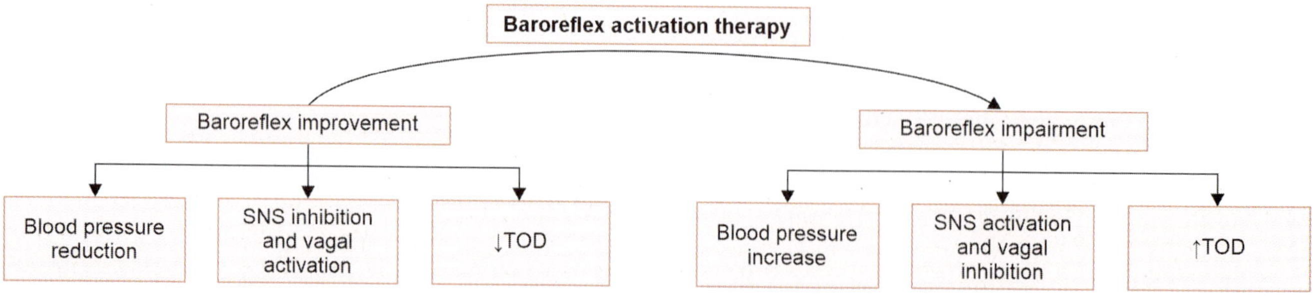

FLOWCHART 2: Possible mechanisms by which electrical stimulation of carotid baroreceptors might help lower blood pressure.
(SNS: sympathetic nervous system; TOD: target organ damage)

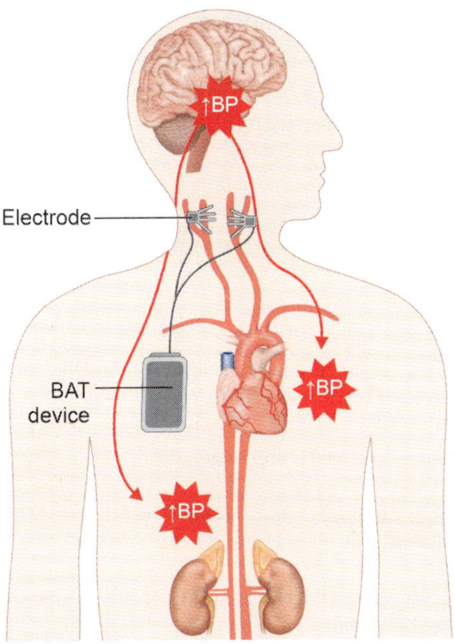

FIG. 1: This device-based treatment consists of an implantable pulse generator and bilateral carotid sinus leads to stimulate the area of greatest response. There is an external programmable device for noninvasive control of the pulse generator. Carotid sinus stimulation acts via a negative loop mechanism through the central nervous system, leading to reflex blood pressure lowering. (BAT: baroreflex activation therapy)

[baroreflex activation therapy (BAT)]. This device-based therapy **(Fig. 1)** has recently been reported to reduce systolic and diastolic BP in RH individuals. The reduction was quite marked when initial BP values were very high, and the effect included ambulatory BP and persisted for up to 53 months.

In several studies, it has been found that unilateral and right-sided BAT has a more profound effect on BP than bilateral or left-sided BAT.

In another study, chronic baroreflex activation markedly and persistently reduced the sympathetic tone of patients with New York Heart Association (NHYA) class III heart failure and reduced left ventricular ejection fraction (LVEF), while increasing baroreflex sensitivity and improving ejection fraction (EF), functional capacity, clinical status, and quality of life, and thereby its scope to be used for patients with severe heart failure. However, a large-scale trial of appropriate design is needed to test this hypothesis.

It seems to be safe with only a few remediable and local side effects (infection, nerve damage, pain of glossopharyngeal nerve origin) reported so far, but a larger database is needed to conclusively establish its safety.

New catheters are being developed to shorten the RDN procedure by other means than radiofrequency, for example, ultrasound.

The experience accumulated in the past few years in the RDN procedure and electrical stimulation of carotid baroreceptors is promising and appears not to be necessarily confined just to RH. Clinical trials are ongoing to determine whether other clinical conditions with a marked sympathetic overdrive, such as congestive heart failure and renal insufficiency might benefit from these interventions by slowing down disease progression and retardation of complications.

PROGNOSIS

The prognosis of patients with RH compared to patients with more easily controlled hypertension has not been specifically evaluated. Prognosis is impaired as such patients typically present with a long-standing history of poorly controlled hypertension and commonly have associated cardiovascular risk factors such as diabetes, OSA, LVH, and/or CKD. The degree to which cardiovascular risk is reduced with the treatment of RH is unknown. The benefits of successful treatment, however, are substantial as suggested by hypertension outcome studies, in general, and the early Veterans Administration cooperative studies, which demonstrated a 96% reduction in cardiovascular events over 18 months with the use of triple antihypertensive regimens compared with placebo in patients with severe hypertension (diastolic BP 115–129 mm Hg).

CONCLUSION

The fundamental approach starts with an accurate diagnosis, excluding pseudoresistance using ambulatory or home BP monitoring, and evaluating treatment compliance. Secondary causes of hypertension are common in the resistant cohort and should be actively searched for. A patient-centered approach, which involves education, lifestyle modification, and a well-tolerated and efficacious treatment regimen, should be followed. Finally, those patients whose BP remains uncontrolled despite multiple pharmacologic agents should be encouraged to enroll into clinical trials investigating novel therapies in RH. Treating RH, particularly in patients who have already been prescribed four or more drugs, is challenging. Selection of additional BP-lowering agents should be based not only on the antihypertensive efficacy but also on the incremental cost, the drugs' adverse effects, and their potential cardiovascular benefits. Until more evidence is available on the long-term efficacy and safety of RDN and baroreceptor stimulation, implementation of these procedures should be restricted to experienced centers/operators with careful case selection.

FUTURE PERSPECTIVES

A prospective epidemiological study is required to know the true prevalence, incidence, and prognostic implications, alongside a global consensus on its definition. Despite the advances made so far, newer therapies need to be explored and are being explored as the disease profile continues to evade physicians with evolving complexities on a continued basis.

SUGGESTED READINGS

1. Beckett NS, Peters R, Fletcher AE, Staessen JA, Liu L, Dumitrascu D, et al. Treatment of hypertension in patients 80 years of age or older. N Engl J Med. 2008;358(18):1887-98.
2. World Health Organization. (2011). Global status report on noncommunicable diseases 2010. [online] Available from https://digitallibrary.un.org/record/706319?ln=en [Last accessed December, 2023]
3. Fagard RH. Resistant hypertension. Heart. 2012;98:254-61.
4. Daugherty SL, Powers JD, Magid DJ, Tavel HM, Masoudi FA, Maragolis KL, et al. Incidence and prognosis of resistant hypertension in hypertensive patients. Circulation. 2012;125(13):1635-42.
5. Gupta AK, Nasothimiou EG, Chang CL, Sever PS, Dahlöf B, Poulter NR, et. al. Baseline predictors of resistant hypertension in the Anglo-Scandinavian Cardiac Outcome Trial (ASCOT): a risk score to identify those at high-risk. J Hypertens. 2011;29(10):2004-13.
6. Pimenta E, Calhoun DA. Resistant hypertension: incidence, prevalence, and prognosis. Circulation 2012;125(13):1594-6.
7. Parati G, Lombardi C, Hedner J, Bonsignore MR, Grote L, Tkacova R, et al. Position paper on the management of patients with obstructive sleep apnea and hypertension: joint recommendations by the European Society of Hypertension, by the European Respiratory Society and by the members of European COST (Cooperation in Scientific and Technological research) ACTION B26 on obstructive sleep apnea. J Hypertens. 2012;30(4):633-46.
8. Vaclavik J, Sedlak R, Plachy M, Navratil K, Plasek J, Jarkovsky J, et al. Addition of spironolactone in patients with resistant arterial hypertension (ASPIRANT): a randomized, double-blind, placebo-controlled trial. Hypertension 2011;57(6):1069-75.
9. Chapman N, Chang CL, Dahlof B, Sever PS, Wedel H, Poulter NR, et al. Effect of doxazosin gastrointestinal therapeutic system as third-line antihypertensive therapy on blood pressure and lipids in the Anglo-Scandinavian Cardiac Outcomes Trial. Circulation. 2008;118(1):42-8.
10. Doumas M, Faselis C, Papademetriou V. Renal sympathetic denervation and systemic hypertension. Am J Cardiol. 2010;105(4):570-6.
11. Symplicity HTN-1 Investigators. Catheter-based renal sympathetic denervation for resistant hypertension: durability of blood pressure reduction out to 24 months. Hypertension 2011;57(5):911-7.
12. Symplicity HTN-Investigators, Esler MD, Krum H, Sobotka PA, Schlaich MP, Schmieder RE, et al. Renal sympathetic denervation in patients with treatment-resistant hypertension (The Symplicity HTN-2 Trial): a randomised controlled trial. Lancet. 2010;376(9756):1903-9.
13. Tsioufis C, Mahfoud F, Mancia G, Redon J, Bruno Damascelli B, Zeller T, et al. What the interventionalist should know about renal denervation in hypertensive patients: a position paper by the ESH WG on the interventional treatment of hypertension. Euro Intervention 2014;9:1027-35.
14. Bakris GL, Nadim MK, Haller H, Lovett EG, Schafer JE, Bisognano JD, et al. Baroreflex activation therapy provides durable benefit in patients with resistant hypertension: results of long term follow-up in the Rheos Pivotal Trial. J Am Soc Hypertens. 2012;6(2):152-8.
15. Zhang Y, Zhang X, Liu L, Wang Y, Tang X, Zanchetti A, et al; FEVER Study Group. Higher cardiovascular risk and impaired benefit of anti-hypertensive treatment in hypertensive patients requiring additional drugs on top of randomized therapy: is adding drugs always beneficial? J Hypertens. 2012;30(11):2202-12.
16. Schmieder RE, Redon J, Grassi G, Kjeldsen SE, Mancia G, Narkiewicz K, et al. ESH position paper: renal denervation-an interventional therapy of resistant hypertension. J Hypertens. 2012;30(5):837-41.
17. Khan NA, Herman RJ, Quinn RR, Rabkin SW, Ravani P, Tobe SW, et al. Canadian Hypertension Education Program. Renal denervation therapy for the treatment of resistant hypertension: a position statement by the canadian hypertension education program. Can J Cardiol. 2014;30(1):16-21.
18. Renal denervation in patients with uncontrolled hypertension (SYMPLICITY HTN-3). Clinicaltrials.gov. 2017.
19. James PA, Oparil S, Carter BL, Cushman WC, Dennison-Himmelfarb C, Handler J, et al. 2014 Evidence-based guideline for the management of high blood pressure in adults: report from the panel members appointed to the eighth joint national committee (JNC 8) JAMA. 2014;311(5):507-20.
20. Mancia G, Fagard R, Narkiewicz K, Redón J, Zanchetti A, Böhm M, et al. ESH/ESC Guidelines for the management of arterial hypertension: The Task Force for the management of arterial hypertension of the European Society of Hypertension (ESH) and of the European Society of Cardiology (ESC). J Hypertens. 2013;31(7):1281-357.
21. Chahal NS, Senior R. Resistant hypertension: evaluation and treatment: Indian Heart J. 2010;62(5):407-9.
22. Sata Y, Xu J, Hering D, Schlaich M. Treating resistant hypertension now and in the future. Medicine Today. 2013;14(1):20-7.
23. Rajeev Gupta, et al. Resistant Hypertension: A Clinical Perspective. Medicine Update. 2011:51-60.
24. Muxfeldt ES, Fiszman R, de Souza F, Viegas B, Oliveira FC, Salles GF. Appropriate Time Interval to Repeat Ambulatory Blood Pressure Monitoring in Patients With White Coat–Resistant Hypertension. Hypertension. 2012;59(2):384-9.
25. Myat A, Redwood SR, Qureshi AC, Spertus JA, Williams B. Resistant hypertension. BMJ. 2012;345:e7473.
26. Boolani H, Sinha A, Randall OS. Resistant Hypertension. 2013;7(5):354-63.
27. Grassi G, Mancia G. New therapeutic approaches for resistant hypertension. J Nephrol. 2012;25(03):276-81.

28. Egan BM, Zhao Y, Li J, Brzezinski WA, Todoran TM, Brook RD, et al. Prevalence of optimal treatment regimens in patients with apparent treatment-resistant hypertension based on office blood pressure in a community-based practice network. Hypertension. 2013;62(4):691-7.
29. Peterzan MA, Hardy R, Chaturvedi N, Hughes AD. Meta-analysis of dose-response relationships for hydrochlorothiazide, chlorthalidone, and bendroflumethiazide on blood pressure, serum potassium, and urate. Hypertension. 2012;59(6):1104-9.
30. ALLHAT Officers and Coordinators for the ALLHAT Collaborative Research Group. The antihypertensive and lipid-lowering treatment to prevent heart attack trial. major outcomes in high-risk hypertensive patients randomized to angiotensin-converting enzyme inhibitor or calcium channel blocker vs diuretic: the antihypertensive and lipid-lowering treatment to prevent heart attack trial (ALLHAT). JAMA. 2002;288(23): 2981-97.
31. Funder JW. Mineralocorticoid receptor antagonists: emerging roles in cardiovascular medicine. Integr Blood Press Control. 2013;6:129-38.
32. Sarwar MS, Islam MS, Al Baker SME, Hasnat A. Resistant hypertension: underlying causes and treatment. Drug Res (Stuttg). 2013;63:217-23.
33. SYMPLICITY HTN-2 Investigators, Esler MD, Krum H, Sobotka PA, Schlaich MP, Schmieder RE, et al. Renal sympathetic denervation in patients with treatment-resistant hypertension (the symplicity HTN-2 Trial): a randomised controlled trial. Lancet. 2010;376(9756):1903-9.
34. Bhatt DL, Kandzari DE, O'Neill WW, D'Agostino R, Flack JM, Katzen BT, et al. A controlled trial of renal denervation for resistant hypertension. N Engl J Med. 2014;370(15):1393-401.
35. De Leeuw, Alnima T, Eric Lovett, Sica D, Bisognano J, Haller H, et al. Bilateral or unilateral stimulation for baroreflex activation therapy. Hypertension. 2015;65:187-92.
36. Ebrahim S, Gopalakrishna G, Mathers C, Patel V, Chatterji S, Chisholm D, et al. Chronic diseases and injuries in India. Lancet. 2011;377(9763):413-28.
37. Kearney PM, Whelton M, Reynolds K, Muntner P, Whelton PK, He J. Global burden of hypertension: analysis of worldwide data. Lancet. 2005;365(9455):217-23.
38. Lewington S, Clarke R, Qizilbash N, Peto R, Collins R; Prospective Studies Collaboration. Age-specific relevance of usual blood pressure to vascular mortality: a meta-analysis of individual data for one million adults in 61 prospective studies. Lancet. 2002;360(9349):1903-13.
39. Patel HC, di Mario C. Renal denervation for hypertension: where are we now? Br J Cardiol. 2013;20:142-7.
40. Pimenta E, Gaddam KK, Oparil S, Aban I, Husain S, Dell'Italia LJ, et al. Effects of dietary sodium reduction on blood pressure in subjects with resistant hypertension: results from a randomized trial. Hypertension 2009;54(3):475-81.
41. Drugs for hypertension. Treat Guidel Med Lett. 2012;10(113): 1-10.
42. Jamerson K, Weber MA, Bakris GL, Dahlöf B, Pitt B, Shi V, et al. ACCOMPLISH Trial Investigators. Benazepril plus amlodipine or hydrochlorothiazide for hypertension in high-risk patients. N Engl J Med. 2008;359(23):2417-28.
43. Ding S, Liu J, Fu Q, Zheng Y. Clinical effects of combined olmesartan medoxomil and amlodipine on clinic and ambulatory blood pressure in elderly patients with resistant hypertension. Arch Gerontol Geriatr. 2013;57(3):423-7.
44. Chapman N, Dobson J, Wilson S, Dahlöf B, Sever PS, Wedel H, et al. Effect of spironolactone on blood pressure in subjects with resistant hypertension. Hypertension. 2007;49(4):839-45.
45. Saha C, Eckert GJ, Ambrosius WT, Chun TY, Wagner MA, Zhao Q, et al. Improvement in blood pressure with inhibition of the epithelial sodium channel in blacks with hypertension. Hypertension. 2005;46:481-7.
46. Saseen JJ, Carter BL, Brown TE, Elliott WJ, Black HR. Comparison of nifedipine alone and with diltiazem or verapamil in hypertension. Hypertension. 1996;28(1):109-14.
47. Bakris GL. A practical approach to achieving recommended blood pressure goals in diabetic patients. Arch Intern Med. 2001;161(22):2661-7.
48. ONTARGET Investigators; Yusuf S, Teo KK, Pogue J, Dyal L, Copland I, Schumacher H, et al. Telmisartan, ramipril, or both in patients at high risk for vascular events. N Engl J Med. 2008;358(15):1547-59.
49. Parving HH, Brenner BM, McMurray JJ, de Zeeuw D, Haffner SM, Solomon SD, et al. Cardiorenal end points in a trial of aliskiren for type 2 diabetes. N Engl J Med.2012;367(23):2204-13.
50. Veterans Administration Cooperative Study Group on Antihypertensive Agents. Effect of treatment on morbidity in hypertension. Results in patients with diastolic blood pressure averaging 115–129 mm Hg. JAMA. 1967;202:1028-34.

57

CHAPTER

Novel Therapies for Resistant Hypertension

Jayanta Datta

ABSTRACT

Despite increase in public awareness about hypertension with its attendant complications and availability and compliance to various therapeutic options, resistant hypertension remains a challenging problem with an estimated prevalence of 13.7%. Therefore, new therapies are still needed to address this problem. Some new drug classes and procedural interventions have shown promising results in the recent clinical trials. Hence, these novel therapeutic approaches are raising our hopes and showing some light at the end of the tunnel in the management of resistant hypertension.

INTRODUCTION

Resistant hypertension describes patients whose blood pressures (BPs) are not controlled despite adherence to at least three antihypertensive agents of different classes, including a (1) diuretic, (2) long-acting calcium channel blocker, and (3) renin–angiotensin–aldosterone system (RAAS) blocker.

Now, if a fourth medicine is added to these patients and the four medicines control BP, then the patient is described as having *controlled resistant hypertension*.

However, if four medicines do not control the BP and a fifth medicine is added, then the patients are labeled as having *refractory hypertension*. More specifically, refractory hypertension describes those patients whose BPs are not controlled despite adherence to at least five antihypertensive drugs of different classes, including a long active thiazide-like diuretic and a mineralocorticoid receptor antagonist (MRA).

Pseudoresistant hypertension refers to poorly controlled hypertension apparently, but the elevated BP is actually attributable to some other factors, such as nonadherence to medications, nonadherence to lifestyle recommendations, white coat effect, suboptimal dosing inaccurate measurements, and poor sleep quality. One must assess for the presence or absence of these factors before labeling a patient as *having true resistant hypertension*.

DIAGNOSIS OF RESISTANT HYPERTENSION

The diagnosis requires ruling out pseudoresistance due to medication nonadherence, improper BP measurement, and white coat effect.

Medication Nonadherence

It is a discrepancy between how a medication is prescribed and how the patient is actually taking it. Studies have shown it ranging from 3 to 86%, with a pooled estimate of 31% in a meta-analysis.

Accurate Measurement

Measuring accurate BP requires proper technique, cuff size, and validated devices. Automated office BP monitoring devices are preferred over conventional auscultatory devices. The results from in-office automated devices are more consistent with ambulatory BP (ABP) monitoring. Two monitoring methods are used: (1) Self-measured and (2) ambulatory. Self-measurement means the patient takes the BP measurement at regular times during the day. Ambulatory monitoring records BP over a 24-hour period. The advantage is its ability to measure nocturnal BP. BP dips typically by 10–20% during sleep, and patients who are "nondippers" are at higher risk of cardiovascular events.

White Coat Hypertension

It is elevated in-office BP readings with normal out-of-office BP in a person not treated with antihypertensive medication. This may be observed in 28–39% of those with resistant hypertension.

LIFESTYLE FACTORS THAT LEAD TO RESISTANT HYPERTENSION

Obesity

The relationship between increased adiposity and elevated BP has been well established. NHANES participants with a body mass index (BMI) of 30 kg/m^2 or higher will be twice as likely to have resistant or apparent treatment-resistant hypertension. Pathogenic mechanisms include increased salt sensitivity, increased sympathetic nervous system (SNS) activity, activation of RAAS system, and aldosterone secretion by adipose tissues.

Dietary Sodium

Dietary sodium raises BP. Certain groups are more salt-sensitive, such as older adults, black people, and patients with chronic kidney disease (CKD). Patients should be counselled to adhere to a diet with <2 g of sodium/day (5 g of table salt) in addition to Dietary Approaches to Stop Hypertension (DASH) diet.

Sedentary Habits

Aerobic exercise has been shown to reduce BP in patients with resistant hypertension. Patients should engage in at least 150 min/week of moderate-intensity aerobic exercises. Both isometric and dynamic resistance exercises have been shown to lower BP.

Alcohol Consumption

Regular alcohol consumption has been shown to increase BP by 1 mm Hg for every 10 g alcohol (1 standard drink), reversible within a few weeks of the cessation.

Smoking/Chewing Tobacco

Nicotine contained in cigarettes and chewing tobacco causes an acute rise in BP. Cessation should be recommended to all patients in general and especially to those with resistant hypertension.

MEDICATIONS THAT RAISE BLOOD PRESSURE

Mediations that can raise BP include the following:
- Nonsteroidal anti-inflammatory drugs (NSAIDs)
- Glucocorticoids
- Serotonin norepinephrine reuptake inhibitors
- Estrogen-containing contraceptives sympathomimetics (pseudoephedrine, ephedrine, cocaine, and amphetamine)
- Vascular endothelial growth factor inhibitors
- Erythropoietin stimulating agents
- Calcineurin inhibitors (cyclosporine and tacrolimus)

EVALUATION FOR SECONDARY HYPERTENSION

Patients with resistant hypertension should be evaluated for secondary hypertension since recognition and directed therapy may improve BP control.

Kidney Parenchymal Disease

Hypertension is both a cause and a consequence of CKD and is common in this patient population. Proposed mechanisms of hypertension in kidney disease include an upregulated RAAS system, increased salt and fluid retention, endothelial dysfunction, and increased SNS activity.

Primary Aldosteronism

Hyperaldosteronism is due to autonomous hypersecretion of aldosterone, leads to salt and water retention and renal potassium wasting. Primary aldosteronism is not uncommon and often goes undiagnosed, with a prevalence ranging from 8 to 30% in various hypertensive population.

Measuring the plasma aldosterone to renin ratio is the test used to screen for primary aldosteronism. The Endocrine Society recommends initial testing with aldosterone-renin ratio followed by a confirmatory test (intravenous and oral salt loading test). Patients at risk include those with resistant hypertension, those with hypertension with spontaneous or diuretic induced hypokalemia, those with adrenal incidentaloma, and hypertensive first-degree relation of patients with primary aldosteronism.

An aldosterone-renin ratio of 20 or higher should undergo investigation if the plasma aldosterone concentration is 15 mg/dL or higher. Patients with very low renin levels, spontaneous hypokalemia, and a plasma aldosterone concentration higher than 20 mg/dL, likely do not require confirmatory testing and should move forward with adrenal imaging.

Obstructive Sleep Apnea

It is commonly associated with resistant hypertension. Proposed mechanisms include endothelial activation, oxidative stress, inflammation, and increased SNS and RAAS activity, which ultimately lead to increased vascular tone and hypertension. Treating obstructive sleep apnea (OSA) with continuous positive airway pressure (CPAP) in patients with resistant hypertension has been shown to decrease 24-hour ABP.

Renovascular Hypertension

It is a syndrome of elevated BP due to diminished renal arterial blood flow resulting in kidney ischemia. It is most commonly caused by atherosclerosis of renal arteries, fibromuscular dysplasia, dissection, and vasculitis.

The diagnosis of renal artery stenosis includes imaging with duplex ultrasonography, computed tomography (CT) angiography or magnetic resonance (MR) angiography. At least 70% of renal artery must be stenosed before the lesion to be considered causing hypertension. Atherosclerotic renal artery stenosis is considered a coronary artery disease (CAD) equivalent, and its treatment consists of medical management focused on BP, lipid and glucose control, and antiplatelet therapy.

Percutaneous revascularization should generally be considered in patients with following high-risk features:

- Recurrent heart failure or unexplained flash pulmonary edema
- Resistant hypertension with failure of optimal medical management
- Unexplained rapid decline in glomerular filtration rate (GFR)
- Bilateral renal artery stenosis or single functioning kidney with stenosis

Other Endocrinopathies

Catecholamine secreting tumors such as pheochromocytoma and paragangliomas are rare cause of hypertension (0.2–0.6%); symptoms that should prompt screening include paroxysmal headaches, diaphoresis, and tachycardia. Endocrine Society 2014 guideline recommended screening by measuring either plasma free metanephrines or 24 hours urine fractionated metanephrines. Normetanephrine and metanephrine levels three or more times higher than the upper limit of normal are highly suggestive.

Cushing's disease or syndrome is a relatively uncommon cause of resistant hypertension. Symptoms include glucose intolerance, acne, osteoporosis, obesity, menstrual changes, hirsutisms, muscle wasting, and moon facies. Patients should be screened by measuring 24 hours urine cortisol level or by low dose dexamethasone suppression test.

Less common endocrine disorders that can contribute to resistant hypertension include disease of thyroid and parathyroid glands.

MANAGEMENT OF RESISTANT HYPERTENSION

All patients diagnosed with resistant hypertension should be screened for causes of secondary hypertension based on history, physical findings, and individual risk factors.

A multifactorial approach to treatment includes a combination of lifestyle modification, pharmacotherapy, and addressing underlying causes.

Patients should be screened for end organ damage, e.g., with serum creatinine and urinalysis for kidney disease, electrocardiography (ECG) and echocardiography to assess for left ventricular hypertrophy, and fundus examination to look for hypertensive retinopathy **(Flowchart 1)**.

PHARMACOLOGIC THERAPY

The initial pharmacologic approach to resistant hypertension consists of three medications at maximally tolerated doses as follows:

1. An angiotensin-converting enzyme (ACE) inhibitor or angiotensin receptor blockers (ARBs) may be better tolerated as they do not carry the same risk of angioedema or cough.
2. A long-acting dihydropyridine calcium channel blocker.
3. A diuretic.

Prescribing antihypertensive therapy begins with identifying comorbidities that require first line agents that have a compelling indication, such as beta blockers for heart failure, a history of myocardial infarction or aortic dissection, or drugs that block RAAS for proteinuria.

If the BP is still not controlled on maximally tolerated therapy with these three agents, an MRA (spironolactone or eplerenone) should be the fourth line agent. The PATHWAY-2 [Prevention And Treatment of Hypertension With Algorithm-Based Therapy Number 2] trial demonstrated that spironolactone was superior

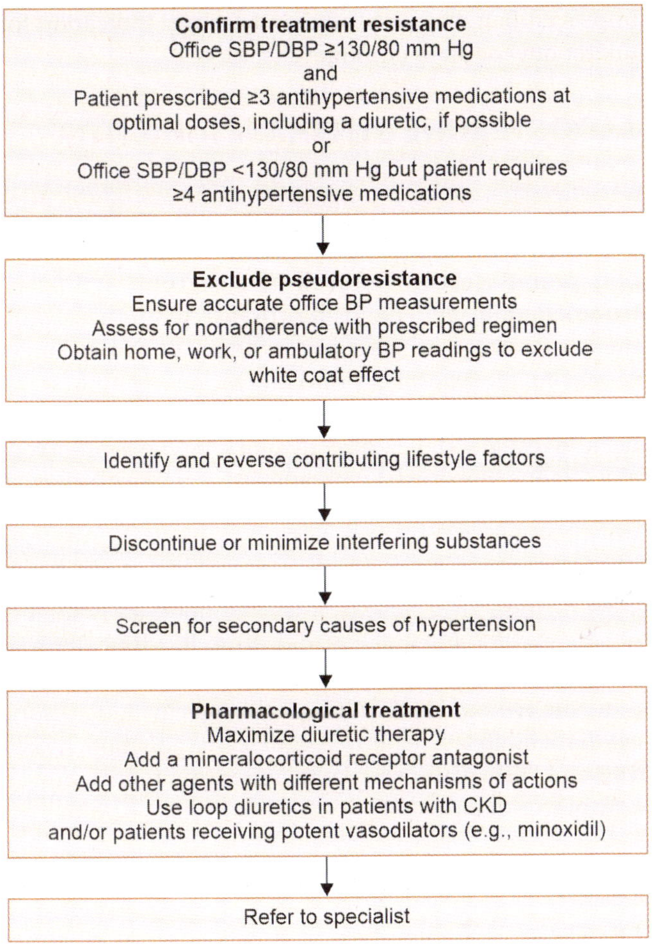

FLOWCHART 1: Algorithm for management of resistant hypertension.

(BP: blood pressure; CKD: chronic kidney disease; DBP: diastolic blood pressure; eGFR: estimated glomerular filtration rate; NSAIDs: nonsteroidal anti-inflammatory drugs; SBP: systolic blood pressure)

Source: American College of Cardiology. (2017). 2017 ACC/AHA guideline for prevention, detection, evaluation and management of high blood pressure in adults). [online] Available from https://www.acc.org/~/media/Non-Clinical/Files-PDFs-Excel-MS-Word-etc/Guidelines/2017/Guidelines_Made_Simple_2017_HBP.pdf [Last accessed November, 2023].

in reducing BP, compared with bisoprolol, doxazosin, or placebo with resistant hypertension.

Vasodilating beta blockers (labetalol, carvedilol, nebivolol, and bisoprolol) may be the preferred fifth-line agents.

Other choices include clonidine, a centrally acting α-2 agonist.

According to American Heart Association (AHA) guidelines, if BP is still not at goal, hydralazine may be initiated at a starting dose of 25 mg three times a day with the addition of a nitrate in presence of heart failure with reduced ejection fraction (EF). Finally, minoxidil may be used if hydralazine is not tolerated. Both are associated with fluid retention and reflex tachycardia.

NOVEL THERAPIES

Six different pharmacologic classes and two procedural interventions were identified as being appropriate for refractory hypertension **(Flowchart 2)**. The pharmacological classes are:

- Nonsteroidal MRA
- Aminopeptidase A inhibitor
- Dual endothelin antagonist
- Aldosterone synthase inhibitor
- Atrial natriuretic peptide inhibitor
- Alternator of hepatic angiotensinogen

Procedural interventions include:

- Renal denervation (RDN)
- Pacemakers improving carotid baroreceptor activity.

ENDOTHELIN SYSTEM AND ITS ROLE IN RESISTANT HYPERTENSION

Endothelin 1 (ET-1) was discovered in 1981 as a potent endothelial derived vasoconstrictor, a complex system

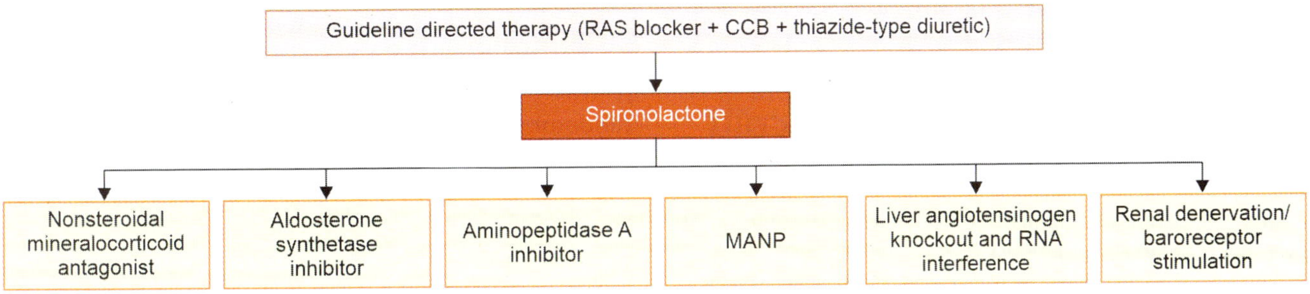

FLOWCHART 2: New antihypertensive treatments for resistant hypertension.

(CCB: calcium channel blocker; MANP: M-atrial natriuretic peptide; RAS: renin–angiotensin system)

Source: Blazek O, Bakris GL. Novel therapies on the horizon of hypertension management. Am J Hypertens. 2023;36(2):73-81.

processing to three peptides (ET-1, 2, and 3) and two receptors [endothelin A receptor (ETA) and endothelin B receptor (ETB)] was discovered. ERAs are the standard of care in PAH. PAH is a disease of alterations of arterioles of the lung with vasoconstrictions and smooth muscle cell proliferation. ERAs improve hemodynamics, 6-minute walk distance, and time to clinical worsening.

PRECISION TRIAL

Aprocitentan—a dual ETA and ETB antagonist was studied in the patients with diastolic blood pressure (DBP) 90–109 mm Hg. Aprocitentan 10, 25, and 50 mg decreased sitting systolic/diastolic automated office BP. Benefit is also seen in ABP. Patients with uncontrolled systolic blood pressure (SBP) ≥ 140 mm Hg despite three or more antihypertensive agents were switched from their current antihypertensive regimen to a triple fixed dose combination if amlodipine, valsartan, and hydrochlorothiazide for 4 weeks, then moved to a blinded placebo run in for four weeks. Those with continuing hypertension were randomized to a placebo or one of the two doses of aprocitentan 12.5 mg or 25 mg daily for 4 weeks. Subsequently, all patients were moved to arocitentan 25 mg for 32 weeks, followed by a 12-week double blind withdrawal period of aprocitentan 25 mg or placebo.

The trial population included 730 patients with resistant hypertension across 22 countries. After 4 weeks of treatment, there was a clinically and statistically significant decline in office SBP from baseline for both the 12.5 and 25 mg dose of aprocitentan versus placebo, $p = 0.0042$ and $p = 0.0046$, respectively. Findings were continued by 24 hours ambulatory SBP measurement. SBP reduction remained consistent during 32 weeks of single-blind use of aprocitentan 25 mg. 12-week double-blind withdrawal phase of aprocitentan versus placebo showed a significant increase in SBP for the placebo arm but not the aprocitentan arm. The most frequent adverse effect was mild to moderate fluid retention.

NONSTEROIDAL MINERALOCORTICOID RECEPTOR ANTAGONIST

Mineralocorticoid receptor antagonists are key agents in guideline-oriented drug therapy for cardiovascular diseases, such as chronic heart failure with reduced EF and resistant hypertension; however, they can be associated with side effects like hyperkalemia. Recently, a new class of nonsteroidal MRAs (esaxerenone, apararenone, and finerenone) has been developed with an improved benefit-risk profile and a novel indication for finerenone for diabetic kidney disease.

ALDOSTERONE SYNTHASE INHIBITOR

Despite the side effects, MRA like spironolactone remains the preferred fourth-line add-on therapy in patients with resistant hypertension. The adverse effects of spironolactone (reduced testosterone synthesis, hyperkalemia, gynecomastia, breast tenderness, and menstrual irregularities) are essentially due to off target blockade of several steroid hormone receptors. To counteract these obstacles, a different approach has been investigated, i.e., directly blocking the synthesis of aldosterone. Baxdrostat embodies an example of selective inhibition of aldosterone synthase without affecting 11β-hydroxylase. *BrigHTN* trial, a randomized double blind placebo-controlled trial was conducted from July 2020 to June 2022. The trial was stopped early for the overwhelming efficiency of the drug. Baxdrostat 1 and 2 mg significantly lowered SBP, meeting the primary outcome of the study. Baxdrostat, the selective aldosterone synthase inhibitor, leads to a significant reduction in both SBP and DBP, with resistant hypertension representing a new powerful tool.

AMINOPEPTIDASE A INHIBITOR

Reducing aminopeptidase A (APA) inhibitor in the brain prevents the conversion of angiotensin II into angiotensin III, regulating vasopressin release and sympathetic nerve activity while increasing baroreflex. The effect is to increase diuresis, lower vascular resistance and control heart rate to reduce BP. However, FRESH (Firibastat in Treatment Resistant Hypertension) trial failed to demonstrate a significant reduction in BP in patients with resistant hypertension.

RENAL DENERVATION

Symplicity HTN-3 Trial

It was a single blind multicentric sham controlled randomized controlled trial (RCT) done in 88 centers in USA. Adults aged 18–80 years with treatment resistant hypertension who had a seated office SBP of 160 mm Hg or more and 24-hour ambulatory SBP of 135 mm Hg or more were randomly assigned (2:1) to receive renal artery denervation or sham control.

The original primary end point was change in office SBP from baseline to 6 months for renal artery denervation group, compared with sham group. Patients were unmasked after 6 months.

535 patients (210 women and 325 men) were randomized, 364 patients received RDN and 171 reduced sham control. At 36 months, change in office SBP was -26.4 mm Hg in RDN group and –5.7 mm Hg in sham control group ($p < 0.0001$). The change in 24 hourly ABP at 36 months was –15.6 mm Hg in RDN group and –0.3 mm Hg in sham control group ($p < 0.0001$).

The final report of the SYMPLICITY HTN-3 trial adds to the evidence supporting the safety of RDN up to 36 months after the procedure. From 12–36 months, patients who were originally assigned to receive RDN had shown a reduction in BP.

The latest trial of RDN to control hypertension SPYRAL HTN-ON MED trial showed reduction in mean ambulatory SBP and DBP in RDN group compared to the sham group at 24 and 36 months. At 36 months mean ambulatory SBP reduction was -10 mm Hg more ($p = 0.0039$), for mean ambulatory DBP treatment difference was –11 mm Hg ($p = 0.016$) and for nighttime SBP the difference was –11.8 mm Hg ($p = 0.0017$). It was concluded that radiofrequency RDN, compared with sham control, showed significant and sustained BP reduction up to 36 months in conjunction with antihypertensive medication.

CONCLUSION

We must diagnose true resistant hypertension first, excluding thereby pseudoresistant hypertension and apparent resistant hypertension. Patient who fails to reach the goal of BP < 130/80 mm Hg despite three antihypertensive drug regimens, including an appropriate diuretic at maximal doses, will be labeled as resistant hypertension. Novel therapies, both in the form of pharmacology and procedures, have demonstrated exciting possibilities for the management of resistant hypertension. Amongst the upcoming drugs, dual endothelial receptor antagonist (ERA) such as aprocitentan and aldosterone synthase inhibitor like Baxdrostat have proven their efficacies in already published trials. Lastly, the SIMPLICITY HTN-3 trial has again ignited our interest in RDN therapy with good results. All these therapies would add to the existing armamentarium in tackling the problem of resistant hypertension.

SUGGESTED READINGS

1. Whelton PK, Carey RM, Aronow WS, Casey DE Jr, Collins KJ, Dennison Himmelfarb C, et al. 2017 ACC/AHA/AAPA/ABC/ACPM/AGS/APhA/ASH/ASPC/NMA/PCNA Guideline for the Prevention, Detection, Evaluation, and Management of High Blood Pressure in Adults: Executive Summary: A Report of the American College of Cardiology/American Heart Association Task Force on Clinical Practice Guidelines. Hypertension. 2018;71(6):1269-1324.
2. Blazek O, Bakris GL. Novel Therapies on the Horizon of Hypertension Management. Am J Hypertens. 2023;36(2):73-81.
3. Schlaich MP, Bellet M, Weber MA, Danaietash P, Bakris GL, Flack JM, et al. Dual endothelin antagonist aprocitentan for resistant hypertension (PRECISION): a multicentre, blinded, randomised, parallel-group, phase 3 trial. Lancet. 2022;400(10367):1927-37.
4. American Heart Association 2022 conference, Nov 5-7, Chicago, IL : 11/5/22 AHA/ESC joint session: BP guidelines.
5. Bhatt DL, Vaduganathan M, Kandzari DE, Leon MB, Rocha-Singh K, Townsend RR, et al. Long-term outcomes after catheter-based renal artery denervation for resistant hypertension: final follow-up of the randomised SYMPLICITY HTN-3 Trial. Lancet. 2022;400(10361):1405-16.
6. Mahfoud F, Kandzari DE, Kario K, Townsend RR, Weber MA, Schmieder RE, et al. Long-term efficacy and safety of renal denervation in the presence of antihypertensive drugs (SPYRAL HTN-ON MED): a randomised, sham-controlled trial. Lancet. 2022;399(10333):1401-10.

58

CHAPTER

Why We Fail to Manage Hypertension?

Hemshanker Sharma, Reeja K Antony

ABSTRACT

Blood pressure simply means the pressure exerted by the blood column to the lateral wall of blood vessels. Any abnormality in this can cause various problems in the body. It can be secondary to some other diseases or can produce complications by itself. Hypertension is a silent epidemic which is increasing morbidity and mortality burden in society. Better management of blood pressure leads to a reduction of complications. In this chapter, we are going to see various barriers to the diagnosis and management of hypertension and how to tackle them.

INTRODUCTION

Hypertension, one of the rising lifestyle diseases, is actually an epidemiological challenge for the treating physicians. It is the third most common cause of death and disability affecting millions of people. It is a major contributor to increased comorbidity and disease burden across the globe. Even though the measurement of blood pressure and treatment is simple, we often fail to manage hypertension effectively. In this chapter, we are going to see the factors behind these failures in hypertension management.

Hypertension is recognized as a silent killer with a significant associated mortality burden. It needs regular screening of blood pressure in people visiting healthcare centers for any diseases and even in people with no symptoms. It will help in the early detection and prevention of complications due to hypertension.

The term hypertension control refers to the percentage of individuals reaching the treatment target, who are aware of their condition and receiving treatment from healthcare providers. Despite a large variety of effective and safe drugs, hypertension control rates have remained at an alarmingly low level for decades. Undiscovered and untreated hypertension significantly increases the risk of developing cardiovascular, brain, and kidney diseases. It accounts for about half of all heart diseases and stroke-related deaths worldwide.

BARRIERS TO DISEASE MANAGEMENT

There are so many barriers to the effective diagnosis and management of hypertensive patients. Factors like poor patient compliance, inadequate dosing, side effects of medications, inability to follow-up regularly, lack of awareness from the patient's part, and lack of surveillance from the physician's part, all contribute to the barriers mentioned above.

According to rule of halves, only 50% of hypertensive patients are diagnosed; of the diagnosed only 50% are put on treatment and of this only 50% have their blood pressure controlled. The management of hypertension focuses on reducing life-threatening complications through appropriate blood pressure control. However, the studies showed unexpected results.

In spite of benefits which are expected through proper blood pressure control like mortality and morbidity reduction, studies have reported a high prevalence (42–89%) of uncontrolled blood pressure among the treated hypertensive patients. So, the thing is that there is a need to explore the burden of uncontrolled hypertension and also determine the factors contributing to failures in achieving the target blood pressure.

So, first of all, we are going to see the enormousness of the problem. Hypertension cases which we are seeing in society are just the tip of iceberg. The hard-hitting fact is that around 60–70% of the total hypertensive people are not even aware that they are suffering from high blood pressure. That means we see only a part of the problem. Even within a visible portion, there are different strata of hypertension with or without controlled blood pressure.

While the primary prevention strategies shall no doubt be most useful, secondary prevention by early diagnosis and treatment also must be equally advocated. This means that we need to explore the unseen part of the spectrum of the hypertensive patients' population.

Lack of Awareness of the Problem

One major factor which hampers the early diagnosis is the lack of awareness in society regarding the seriousness of hypertension as a problem. As mentioned earlier, majority of the people are not aware of the long-term consequences untreated hypertension can lead to. Another misconception about hypertension among people is that once hypertension starts, there is no usefulness of starting medications as it cannot bring blood pressure back to normal, and in such instances, people opt for alternate remedies like changing lifestyle alone. Contrary to this, some other people will start only medications and just ignore the fact that there also should be changes in their lifestyle and diet to bring blood pressure back to a normal level. So, giving proper awareness and different methods of motivational education will be of tremendous help to bring people to the healthcare system.

If we are thinking from another perspective, often treating physicians also lack awareness for properly diagnosing and following up with the patient. Whatever specialties they are in, doctors should be vigilant to diagnose hypertension by proper screening and follow-up of patients when they come to the healthcare setup for the first time. Proper evaluation and starting of treatment at the early stage itself can reduce the burden of the hypertensive population and comorbidities.

Technique of Blood Pressure Measurement

Another important thing that we need to focus on is the technique of measuring blood pressure. The diagnosis, categorization, and treatment of blood pressure depend on its correct way of measurement. Patients are more familiar with having their blood pressure checked in a healthcare provider's office during an appointment. In such cases, a sphygmomanometer is used to measure and record one or two readings during visiting time to the hospital. However, ambulatory blood pressure monitoring (ABPM) is gaining more popularity nowadays as it gives a more accurate picture of fluctuations in the blood pressure of a person over 24 hours, which is most useful in hypertension management. ABPM records your blood pressure over a day, whether you are awake or asleep. This happens outside the healthcare provider's office, as they go about your daily life. Patients wear a cuff on their arm and a small device is attached to a strap or belt. Opting for ABPM over the traditional method will help physicians to properly diagnose hypertension by finding out white coat hypertension, masked hypertension, and nocturnal hypertension.

Diastolic Blood Pressure

Another point where I would like to draw your attention is regarding the "numbers." The thing is that both top and bottom "numbers" matter. When it comes to managing blood pressure, doctors tend to focus on lowering the top, that is, systolic number. It has been well established that aggressively treating high systolic pressure can help lower one's risk for a heart attack or stroke. However, the bottom number, that is, diastolic blood pressure, also plays an essential role in heart health, although it tends to get overlooked. Diastolic pressure plays a critical role in helping coronary vessels supply oxygen to the heart muscle. That means both diastolic and systolic hypertension are related to myocardial infarction (MI)-like diseases. So, it is very important to catch patients with diastolic hypertension also by proper screening.

Management with Drugs

Coming to the drug part, inadequate control of blood pressure may be attributed to both treatment provider-related and patient-related factors. From the physician's side, these factors may include excessive reliance on monotherapy and reluctance to increase drug doses or add additional antihypertensive agents to the treatment regimen. From the patient's side, it is the nonadherence to the prescribed antihypertensive medication that is the villain in the management. Other factors we need to keep in mind are the high cost of therapy and drug side effects occurring to the patients. Steps must be taken to reduce these by the healthcare administration and hospital surveillance system. If we are able to overcome these hurdles, there is a significantly greater likelihood of achieving blood pressure control and consequently lower costs and reduced utilization of healthcare resources. We can adopt strategies such as single pill or fixed-drug combination therapy for improving patient adherence to treatment and thereby better control of blood pressure.

Lack of Follow-up

Often, we lose patients for follow-up after their primary visits. This is also a reason for the increasing burden of ineffectively treated hypertensive patients. Cost of care, long-waiting times, lack of physician continuity, etc., explain the reasons for the lack of follow-up.

TIMELY DIAGNOSIS AND PREVENTION OF COMPLICATIONS

We need to emphasize on the later part of management as well as the initial diagnosis part. Complications of hypertension can develop target organ damage. The primary organs involved are the eye, brain, heart, kidneys, and peripheral blood vessels. It can accelerate atherosclerosis and can lead to cerebrovascular diseases, retinopathy, and heart conditions such as ventricular hypertrophy and hypertensive kidney damage. Failure to diagnose progression to these diseases is failure to manage hypertension itself. So, hospitals should be equipped with facilities such as echocardiography, ophthalmoscope, ultrasonography, and laboratories which can assess hypertension. Treating physicians also should be aware of when to use all these for better management and prevention of complications.

ROLE OF REFERRAL SYSTEM

Last but not the least is the lack of prompt referral. This can cause inadequate management of patients in different strata of society because an effective referral system ensures that there is a close relationship among all levels of healthcare and individuals can receive the best possible care for any diseases. Wherever it is lacking, patients are denied the right to timely diagnosis and prevention of complications of hypertension in this case. Referring to a healthcare facility with much better facilities can ensure patients' adequate treatment and prevention, whether at primary secondary or tertiary levels.

CONCLUSION

In conclusion, we could say that a vast majority of the hypertensive population is not aware of their high blood pressure status; at the same time, a large fraction of the population with increased blood pressure did not have their blood pressure under control. A surveillance system to detect population with high blood pressure, follow-up the detected cases of hypertension, and motivate and counsel the hard-to-treat cases for regular follow-up should be valuable.

SUGGESTED READINGS

1. Lawes CM, Vander Hoorn S, Rodgers A; International Society of Hypertension. Global burden of blood-pressure-related disease, 2001. Lancet. 2008;371(9623):1513-8.
2. Williams B, Mancia G, Spiering W, Agabiti Rosei E, Azizi M, Burnier M, et al. 2018 ESC/ESH guidelines for the management of arterial hypertension. Eur Heart J. 2018;39(33):3021-104.
3. Weiss T. Why do we fail in reaching pressure goals for many hypertensive patients? Eur Soc Cardiol. 2019;17:23-5.
4. Elliott WJ. What factors contribute to the inadequate control of elevated blood pressure?. J Clin Hypertens (Greenwich). 2008;10(1 Suppl 1):20-6.
5. Babiker FA, Moukhyer ME. Awareness of hypertension and factors associated with uncontrolled hypertension in Sudanese adults. Cardiovascular J Afr. 2013;24(6):208-12.

59

CHAPTER

Combination Therapy in Hypertension Do's and Don'ts

Prabhat Pandey

ABSTRACT

More people die each year from cardiovascular (CV) diseases than from any other cause. Over three quarters of the heart disease and stroke-related deaths occur in low-income and middle-income countries. Hypertension or elevated blood pressure (BP) is a serious medical condition that significantly increases the risk of heart, brain, kidney, and other diseases. Hypertension can be defined using specific systolic and diastolic BP levels or reported use of antihypertensive medications. An estimated 1.4 billion people worldwide have high BP, but just 14% have it under the control. However, cost-effective treatment options do exist.

Hypertension is a major preventable risk factor for atherosclerosis and ischemic heart disease. Although modern and effective antihypertensive drugs are available, most patients remain with a suboptimal BP control. Most hypertensive patients will need a combination of antihypertensive agents to achieve the therapeutic goals—recent guidelines recommend initiating treatment with two drugs in those patients with a systolic BP > 20 mm Hg and/or a diastolic BP > 10 mm Hg above the goals, and in those patients with high CV risk. In addition, approximately 25% of the patients will require three antihypertensive agents to achieve the therapeutic targets. In this review, we analyze the latest information available regarding the treatment of hypertension with the combination therapy.

INTRODUCTION

Hypertension is a risk factor for cardiovascular (CV) disease—uncontrolled hypertension increases the relative risk from 2–4 times for coronary disease, stroke, heart failure (HF), peripheral arterial disease, renal insufficiency, atrial fibrillation, and dementia/cognitive impairment. Undoubtedly, poorly controlled hypertensive patients have an increased risk for CV complications.

The goal of antihypertensive therapy is to abolish the risks associated with blood pressure (BP) elevation without adversely affecting the quality of life. Epidemiologic studies and clinical trials have been used to define individual risk and set appropriate BP targets, recognizing that these targets reflect expert consensus based on the available data and are subject to revision as additional evidence is obtained. Drug selection is based on efficacy in lowering BP and in reducing CV endpoints, including stroke, myocardial infarction, and HF. Although, the choice of initial drug therapy exerts some effect on long-term outcomes, it is evident that BP reduction per se is the primary determinant of CV risk reduction. As a result, there has been a progressive lowering of BP targets in large segments of the hypertensive population, including diabetics and patients with established renal or vascular disease. At the same time, increasing emphasis is being placed on the practical tasks involved in consistently achieving and maintaining goal BP in clinical practice.

It is within this context that the American Society of Hypertension presents this Position Paper on Combination Therapy for Hypertension. It will address the scientific basis of combination therapy, present the pharmacologic rationale for choosing specific drug combinations, and review patient selection criteria for initial and secondary use. The advantages and disadvantages of single-pill (fixed) drug combinations (SPCs) and the implications of recent clinical trials involving specific combination strategies will also be discussed.

Achieving recommended goal of BP <140/90 mm Hg in all hypertensives, <130/80 mm Hg in hypertensives with diabetes mellitus (DM) is difficult in majority of patients with hypertension. Various studies have shown that tight control of BP is required to produce the maximum reduction in clinical CV end points. The Framingham Heart Study indicated that a 2 mm Hg reduction in average diastolic blood pressure (DBP) could result in a 14% decrease in the risk of stroke and transient ischemic attacks and a 6% reduction in the risk of coronary artery disease. A meta-analysis of nine major prospective observational studies also showed that prolonged reduction in DBP of 5, 7.5, and 10 mm Hg were associated with 34, 46, and 56% fewer strokes and 21, 29, and 37% lower incidences of coronary heart disease respectively. These data suggest that more aggressive BP lowering might be beneficial. Though, single drug treatment may be effective in some, >50% will require more than one drug for appropriate control of their BP.

RATIONALE FOR USE OF COMBINATION THERAPY

Blood pressure is predominantly determined by three factors namely (1) renal sodium excretion and resultant plasma and total body volume, (2) cardiac performance, and (3) vascular tone, which in turn controls the hemodynamic determinants of BP, such as intravascular volume, cardiac output, and systemic vascular resistance. In real-time, these parameters are regulated by the renin-angiotensin-aldosterone system (RAAS) and sympathetic nervous system (SNS). Other environmental factors that influence BP of an individual patient include the genetic makeup and diet.

In an individual, the elevation of BP is a multifactorial process. In the majority of the cases, the exact etiopathology remains unknown and therefore, treatment for normalization of BP by interfering with only a single pressor mechanism renders futile. Despite the effectiveness of antihypertensive drugs, a vast majority (≈70%) of the patients fail to attain the therapeutic goal of BP < 140/90 mm Hg with monotherapy. Limited BP reduction is seen with monotherapy drug directed at one component of pathophysiologic mechanism along with compensatory (counterregulatory) responses. In such cases, either increased monotherapy dosage or use of drug combination should be considered. While increasing doses of monotherapy are associated with increased risk of adverse effects, patient-specific drug combination with minimal side effects and greater target organ protection should be preferred **(Box 1)**.

BOX 1: Advantages of the combination of antihypertensive drugs.

- *More effective*: Better reductions in blood pressure due to additive effect of complementary drugs as compared to monotherapy
- Fewer dose-dependent side effects
- Fewer metabolic side effects
- *Higher response rate*: Faster control of blood pressure

BOX 2: Advantages of the combination of antihypertensive drugs.

- Greater reductions in blood pressure figures compared with monotherapy
  - *Reduction in adverse effects*:
    - Renin–angiotensin system inhibitors (RASIs) prevent pretibial edema induced by calcium channel blockers
    - RASIs counteract the release of renin caused by natriuretics
    - RASIs block the release of aldosterone induced by natriuretics and the resulting hypokalemia
- Several physiopathological mechanisms of increased blood pressure are blocked
- Greater protection to target organs
- Faster control of blood pressure
- *Combinations may have some effects that are independent of their antihypertensive action*:
  - Anti-inflammatory
  - Metabolic
- *Anticounter regulation*:
  - Diuretics counteract the retention of water produced by vasodilators
  - RASIs compensate for renin release by diuretics

By combining two drugs with different mechanisms of action, an antihypertensive effect of 2–5 times greater than that obtained by monotherapy is possible. Increasing the dose of monotherapy reduces coronary events by 29% and cerebrovascular events by 40%, while combining two antihypertensive agents with a different mechanism of action reduces coronary events by 40%, and cerebrovascular events by 54%. Thus, the use of combination therapy provides greater protection to a target organ than increasing the dose of monotherapy.

In summary, combination therapy looks like a better option than increasing the dose. The advantages of combination therapy are enumerated in **Box 2**.

Fixed-dose combinations (both drugs in the same tablet) offer additional advantages, such as improved adherence by 24%, easier indications, and potentially reduced cost. Their limitation is less possibility of titrating the dose of only one of the drugs.

Both the eighth report of the Joint National Committee for the Prevention, Detection, Evaluation and Treatment of Hypertension (JNC8) and the 2013 guidelines of the European Society of Hypertension and the European Society of Cardiology (ESH/ESC) for the management of hypertension recommend the use of combinations of antihypertensive agents from the beginning for subjects in which the probability of achieving the recommended treatment goals in hypertension with monotherapy is low, as are patients with systolic pressure 20 mm Hg above the target or diastolic pressure 10 mm Hg above the target or more.

COMBINING ANTIHYPERTENSIVE DRUGS

Theoretical Considerations

Careful selection and inclusion of two or more drugs known to long-term incidence of CV endpoints including stroke, myocardial infarction, and HF is highly preferred.

Efficacy

The key objective of any combination of antihypertensive drugs is to efficiently lower BP as compared to its corresponding monotherapies. Selection of combination should be based on drug's ability to act on different pathophysiological mechanisms or to counter-block the regulatory responses that limit the success of monotherapies.

Tolerability

Improving the overall tolerability of the treatment is a key element in designing rational drug combinations. This beneficial effect will occur whenever side effects associated with a particular agent are neutralized by the pharmacologic effects of an added drug. Because most antihypertensive agents produce dose-dependent side effects, high-dose monotherapy may lead to adverse events. In this circumstance, a lower dose of the initial agent in combination with another antihypertensive may be preferable to minimize dose-dependent side effects even if no additional BP reduction is achieved. An example is the use of a low-dose combination of an angiotensin-converting enzyme (ACE) inhibitor and a dihydropyridine calcium-channel blockers (CCBs) in a patient who develops edema at a higher CCB dose. In this instance, reducing the CCB dose and adding an ACE inhibitor will produce comparable BP reduction, but will generally do so without the side effects previously observed.

Adherence

Combination regimens improve long-term adherence to treatment, essential for management of BP. The number of medication and frequency of required dosing both determines the adherence to treatment.

CLINICAL EVIDENCES

Drug Combinations

With seven major classes of antihypertensive drugs and multiple members of each class, the number of possible combinations is quite large. Numerous clinical trials have been conducted to determine the efficacy of rational drug combinations. Some of these commonly used guidelines-recommended drug combinations are mentioned in **Table 1**.

Rational combination therapy lies in the selection of specific drug classes with additive BP reduction, equally or even better tolerated than respective monotherapies, and with evidenced ability to reduce CV events in clinical trials. The clinical trial depicting efficacy of recommended two drug combinations are mentioned in **Table 2**.

TABLE 1: Recommended drug combinations.

American Society of Hypertension	
Preferred	• ACE inhibitors + diuretics • ARBs + diuretics • ACE inhibitors + CCBs • ARBs+ CCBs
Acceptable	• β-blockers + diuretics • CCBs + β-blockers • CCBs + diuretics • DRIs + diuretics • DRIs + ARBs • Thiazide + K^+-sparing diuretics
Less effective	• ACE inhibitors + ARBs • ACE inhibitors + β-blockers • ARBs + β-blockers • Central agents + β-blockers
European Society of Hypertension	
Priority use	• ACE inhibitors + diuretics • ARBs + diuretics • ACE inhibitors + CCBs • ARBs + CCBs • CCBs + diuretics
Avoid	β-blockers + diuretics
Concern	ACE inhibitors + ARBs

(ACE: angiotensin-converting enzyme; ARBs: angiotensin receptor blockers; CCBs: calcium channel blockers; DRI: direct renin inhibitor; K^+: potassium)

TABLE 2: Findings of clinical trials pertaining to two-drug combinations.

Drug combination	Evidence/Clinical trails	Findings
β-blockers + CCBs	Hypertension Optimal Treatment (HOT) study	Intense BP lowering with lower incidence of CV events
Diuretics + RAAS inhibitors	Action in Diabetes and Vascular disease; Preterax and Diamicron-MR Controlled Evaluation (ADVANCE)	*ACE inhibitors + thiazide-like diuretics*: Lower incidence of diabetes-related complications when given to hypertensive type 2 diabetes patients
	Hypertension in the Very Elderly Trial (HYVET)	*ACE inhibitors + thiazide-like diuretics*: Lower incidence of CV events
RAAS inhibitors + CCBs	Avoiding Cardiovascular events through COMbination therapy in Patients Living with Systolic Hypertension (ACCOMPLISH) study	*ACE inhibitors + CCB*: 20% relative risk reduction in CV morbidity and mortality as compared to ACE inhibitors + thiazide-like diuretics
	Anglo-Scandinavian Cardiac Outcomes Trial (ASCOT)	*ACE inhibitors + CCB*: More effective in preventing CV events as compared to β-blocker + diuretic
	OlmeSartan and Calcium Antagonists Randomized (OSCAR) study	*ARB + CCB*: More effective in lowering BP and primary CV endpoints than monotherapies
	Conduit Artery Functional Endpoint (CAFÉ) study	Beneficial effect on central aortic BP, a possible surrogate marker of aortic stiffness
	EXPLOR study	*Amlodipine + valsartan*: In addition to BP-lowering, reduced central systolic BP, central pulse pressure, and augmentation index

(ACE: angiotensin converting enzyme; BP: blood pressure; CCB: calcium channel blockers; CV: cardiovascular)

Diuretics and Renin–angiotensin–aldosterone System Inhibitor

It is most commonly used two-drug antihypertensive treatment where combination of a low dose thiazide such as diuretic and RAAS inhibitor such as ACE inhibitor, angiotensin receptor blocker (ARB) or direct renin inhibitor result in fully additive BP reduction effects. Though, diuretics therapy effectively lower BP, renin activity induced sodium depletion limits its usability. In combined therapy, simultaneous inhibition of RAAS with either an ARB or angiotensin-converting enzyme inhibitor (ACEI), also improves its safety profile by ameliorating diuretic-induced hypokalemia.

RAAS Inhibitors and CCBs

Literature pertaining to benefits of combining a renin-angiotensin blocker, either an ACE inhibitor or an ARB, with a CCB is well-documented. The drug combination has fully additive BP reduction effects and acts at various cardiorenal levels, and limits the deleterious effects of both angiotensin II and increased intracellular calcium. Renin–angiotensin–aldosterone system inhibitors significantly improve the tolerability profile of the CCB via reduction of dose-limiting CCB-induced peripheral edema by postcapillary vasodilation and normalization of hydrostatic pressure.

Calcium Channel Blockers and β-blockers

Calcium channel blockers and β-blockers have complementary pharmacological and additive BP reduction effects. Though the combination of a β-blocker and a dihydropyridine CCB is acceptable; β-blockers should not generally be combined with nondihydropyridine CCBs such as verapamil and diltiazem because their additive effects on heart rate and atrioventricular (AV) conduction may result in severe bradycardia or heart block.

Diuretics and β-blockers

Beta-blockers reduce BP by lowering cardiac output and suppression of renin release. They are relatively less effective than ACE inhibitors, ARBs, and CCBs, β-blockers that attenuate the RAAS activation when given with a thiazide-diuretic since their combination results in full additive BP reduction effect. Various meta-analyses over the years have reported that β-blockers reduce CV endpoints in placebo-controlled trials. Addition of diuretics also been reported to improve the effectiveness of β-blockers in patients of black ethnicity and patients with low renin hypertension. Despite increased risk of associated side effects, such as glucose intolerance, fatigue, and sexual dysfunction, these combinations are classified as acceptable.

Renin–angiotensin–aldosterone System Inhibitors, Calcium Channel Blockers, and Diuretics

In about 15–20% hypertensive patients, often treatment goal reduction in BP cannot be achieved with two-drug combination. In such patients, triple-drug combination

TABLE 3: Antihypertensive efficacy of triple combinations—RAAS inhibitors, thiazide-diuretics, and CCBs.

Year	Study	Combination	Finding
2009	Calhoun et al.	Valsartan 320 mg + amlodipine 10 mg + HCT 25 mg	Better control with triple combination (70.8% vs. 54.1%)
2010	Oparil et al.	Olmesartan 40 mg + amlodipine 10 mg + HCT 25 mg	Better control with triple combination (69.9% vs. 53.4%)
2011	Wright et al.	Valsartan 160 mg + amlodipine 5 mg + HCT 25 mg	Better control with triple combination (57% vs. 46%)
2012	Neutel et al.	Olmesartan up to 40 mg + amlodipine up to 10 mg + HCT up to 25 mg	72.2% within patients on prior CCB and 76.9% within patients with prior ARB
	Lacourciére et al.	Aliskiren 300 mg + amlodipine 10 mg + HCT 25 mg	Better control with triple combination (62.3% vs. 41.3%)

(ARB: angiotensin receptor blockers; CCB: calcium channel blockers; HCT: hydrochlorothiazide)

of renin-angiotensin blocker, a CCB, and a diuretic proves to be beneficial. Most of the associated limitations are significantly reduced by combination therapy as RAAS inhibitors can limit both metabolic alterations induced by diuretics and ankle edema caused by CCBs. Collectively, 70% of the patients have been reported to achieve target BP with complete-dose triple combinations **(Table 3)**.

SPECIAL CONDITIONS AND USE OF COMBINATION THERAPY

Hypertension and Diabetes/Proteinuria

Hypertension act synergistically and increases the risk of macrovascular and microvascular complications of diabetes. While these complications decrease with reduction in BP; target BP is rarely achieved with monotherapy. Antihypertensive drugs such as ACEIs, ARBs, CCBs, diuretics, and β-blockers all have compelling indications in diabetes. Use of RAAS inhibitors (initial therapy) with secondary drug such as CCBs or diuretics, or ACEI plus an ARB combination is recommended. ACEIs and ARBs have renoprotective role in diabetic nephropathy and the combination therapy of an ARB and a CCB has been shown to have antiproteinuric effect in patients with type 2 diabetic nephropathy, with reduced renal function. Although, the treatment with an ARB plus an ACE inhibitor has a greater antiproteinuric effect, it worsens renal anemia and increases serum potassium concentrations in patients with impaired kidney function.

BOX 3: Irrational combinations of hypertensive drugs.

Drug classes without partial or complete additive antihypertensive effects should not be combined:

- CCBs should not be combined with diuretics because both drug classes are natriuretic and cause reflex activation of the RAAS
- ACE inhibitor (or ARB) should not be combined with a β-blocker if the rationale for the combination is to improve BP control
- Drugs directly acting on the RAAS, including ACE inhibitors, ARBs, or renin inhibitors, since it increases the risk of associated side effects, such as hyperkalemia, elevation of creatinine, and hypotension

While some antihypertensive combinations do not have synergistic BP-lowering effects, others may have negative effects:

- *Clonidine and doxazosin (or other α1-receptor blockers)*: Opposite selectivity, elevates BP

Finally, some combinations may even be dangerous:

- *Clonidine and β-blocker*: Both drugs can depress left ventricular function and β-blocker further amplifies the pressor response caused by a sudden clonidine withdrawal
- β-blocker should not be combined with nondihydropyridine calcium antagonists (verapamil or diltiazem) to avoid additive negative chronotropic, dromotropic, and inotropic effects

(ACE: angiotensin-converting enzyme; ARB: angiotensin receptor blockers; BP: blood pressure; CCB: calcium channel blockers; RAAS: renin–angiotensin–aldosterone system)

Irrational combinations of hypertensive drugs are enumerated in **Box 3**.

Hypertension and Dyslipidemia

Dyslipidemia and hypertension coexist frequently, and hypercholesterolemia and hypertension are the two leading risk factors CAD-related events. Telmisartan, apart from its antihypertensive effect through antagonizing AT1 receptors, has a unique property that activates peroxisome proliferator-activated receptor-γ (PPAR-γ) and is suggested to improve insulin sensitivity and reduce triglyceride levels, leading to a reduction of the risk for atherosclerosis. Therefore, use of telmisartan alone or in combination with a diuretic/CCB is recommended in hypertensive patients with dyslipidemia.

Hypertension and Heart Failure

Diuretics, β-blockers, ACEIs, ARBs, and aldosterone antagonists are indicated in the management of HF and have been shown to reduce morbidity and mortality in appropriately selected patients with HF. The severity of HF, left ventricular ejection fraction, history of myocardial infarction and any other associated comorbidities dictates the selection of drug. In such patients, β-blockers and ACEIs treatment has been reported to improve symptoms and reduce the risk of death and hospitalization for worsening HF. β-blocker like carvedilol has now become the most extensively studied class of agents in the treatment of chronic heart failure (CHF). Carvedilol Prospective Randomized Cumulative Survival (COPERNICUS) study, showed improved clinical status and reduced the risk of death with carvedilol as compared to placebo. Addition of angiotensin II type 1 receptor blockers such as candesartan to ACEIs in patients with CHF, have favorable effects on hemodynamic measurements, and leads to reduced CV events and left ventricular ejection fraction. ONTARGET (Ongoing Telmisartan Alone and in Combination With Ramipril Global End Point Trial) reported that both the ARB telmisartan and the ACEI ramipril are equally effective in preventing CV events in high-risk patients and that the combination provides no added benefit and rather causes more side effects than either monotherapy. However, the study does not rule out use of the ACEI plus ARB combination in severe HF, where angiotensin escape mechanisms are expressed and dual blockade may be needed.

Hypertension and Chronic Renal Failure

Both hypertension and chronic kidney disease (CKD) are risk factors for one other; while CKD causes hypertension, hypertension in turn worsens renal failure. The management of hypertension in CKD, primarily focuses on reduction of BP along with reduction of protein excretion. The choice of drug for an individual primarily depends on the presence of degree of proteinuria and its progression to end-stage renal disease.

Angiotensin-converting enzyme inhibitorsor ARBs are first-line drugs of choice and often require an additional CCB or diuretic. Use of thiazide diuretics are recommended if glomerular filtration rate (GFR) is ≥40 mL/min/1.73 m^2 (body surface area), and loop diuretics if GFR ≤ 40–50 mL/min/1.73 m^2.

Hypertension in Elderly Population

While treating hypertension in elderly patients, their altered physiology and concomitant CV and renal disease should be closely monitored before commencement of any drug therapy. HYVET (Hypertension In the Very Elderly Trial) reported reduced incidence of fatal stroke, CV death and HF, and recommends use of monotherapy or combination therapy with thiazide diuretics, ACEIs, and CCBs for hypertension in the elderly.

BOX 4: Drug classes and contraindicated conditions.

- *ACEIs*: Pregnancy, angioneurotic edema, hyperkalemia, and renal artery stenosis
- *ARBs*: Pregnancy, hyperkalemia, and renal artery stenosis
- *β-blockers*: Asthma, marked bradycardia, abnormal glucose tolerance, obstructive pulmonary disease, and peripheral artery disease
- *CCBs*: Heart failure and bradyarrhythmias
- *Diuretics*: Gout, hypokalemia, pregnancy, and impaired glucose tolerance

(ACEIs: angiotensin converting enzyme inhibitors; ARBs: angiotensin receptor blockers; CCBs: calcium channel blockers)

Hypertension in Pregnancy and Breastfeeding

About 5–7% of all pregnancies are complicated by hypertension. New-onset hypertension, proteinuria, and multisystem involvement, the subset of preeclampsia is primarily responsible for majority of maternal and fetal morbidity. Based on the available clinical evidence, the preferred drugs during pregnancy are:

- *First-line*: α-methyldopa, β-blocker (propranolol) and labetalol
- *Second-line*: Metoprolol, atenolol, and CCB (nifedipine)
- *Third-line*: Clonidine and diuretics

For pregnant women with severe hypertension: Hydralazine, labetalol, and nifedipine

Maternal antihypertensive drugs compatible with breastfeeding: Cautious use of captopril, diltiazem, enalapril, hydralazine, hydrochlorothiazide, labetalol, methyldopa, minoxidil, β-blockers, such as propranolol and timolol, spironolactone, and verapamil.

Drug Classes and Contraindicated Conditions

Drugs classes contraindicated in specific conditions are mentioned in **Box 4**.

GUIDELINES AND RECOMMENDATIONS

Combinations as First-step Antihypertensive Therapy

Both guidelines of the European Society of Hypertension and the European Society of Cardiology (ESH/ESC) for the management of hypertension and the eighth report of the Joint National Committee for the Prevention, Detection, Evaluation and Treatment of Hypertension (JNC-8) recommends the antihypertensive combination therapy from the beginning, in patients whom treatment goal in hypertension cannot be achieved with monotherapy. American Society of Hypertension also recommends initiation of combination therapy as first-line treatment in patients with >20/10 mm Hg BP reduction treatment target. International Society of Hypertension 2020 guidelines recommend the use of single-pill combination including a thiazide-like diuretic plus CCB or CCB plus ARB for patients from the African desert.

British Hypertension Society-National Institute for Clinical Excellence (BHS-NICE) guidelines 2019 recommends the use of RAAS inhibitors and CCBs as first-line therapy and that their combination is the preferred two-agent approach if monotherapy fails to achieve target BP.

CONCLUSION

Hypertension, a complex syndrome leads to alternation of both cardiac and vascular structure and function. Since pathogenesis of hypertension is a multifactorial process, often multidrug therapy is essential to attenuate pressor mechanisms. All of the current guidelines recommend the routine initiation of more than one antihypertensive drug in patients with stage 2 hypertension to reach BP goals and effectively reduce the associated CV risk; however, in some patients, a triple combination is often needed, the most rational being those including renin-angiotensin blockers, CCBs and diuretics. Selection of drugs for combination therapy should be tailored according to individual patient based upon the risk factors, presence of comorbidities such as diabetes, renal dysfunction, and the adverse effects. Though strategies for clinical use of combination therapy continue to evolve; available evidence suggests use of ACE inhibitors (but not ARBs) with CCBs for effective protection from clinical events.

SUGGESTED READINGS

1. Drugsincontext.com. Welcome to Drugs in Context. [online] Available from https://www.drugsincontext.com/ [Last accessed December, 2023].
2. Gradman AH, Basile JN, Carter BL, Bakris GL; American Society of Hypertension Writing Group. Combination therapy in hypertension. J Am Soc Hypertens. 2010;4(1):42-50.
3. World Health Organization. Guidelines for the pharmacological treatment of Hypertension in adults. Geneva: World Health Organization; 2021.
4. Ram CVS. Indian Hypertension Guidelines 2023. J Hypertens. 2023;41(12):2072-3.
5. Guerrero-García C, Rubio-Guerra AF. Combination therapy in the treatment of hypertension. Drugs Context. 2018;7:212531.
6. Kalra S, Kalra B, Agrawal, N. Combination therapy in hypertension: An update. Diabetol Metab Syndr. 2010;2:44.

60

CHAPTER

A 74-year-old Diabetes and Hypertensive Male Presents with Dizziness

Boudhayan Das Munshi, Arunima Sarkar, Suman Ghosh, Monidipa Ghosh

ABSTRACT

Dizziness is sensation of disturbed spatial orientation without a distorted sense of motion. It is often referred to as vertigo, lightheadedness, and imbalance. The major causes include general medical conditions, otological, or neurological causes. In a 74-year-old hypertensive with diabetes mellitus, dizziness causes would be evaluated keeping the background comorbidities in mind looking out for complications related to the disease processes or their treatments and also at independent causes of dizziness. An organized clinical approach could provide possible clues to the diagnosis. Definitive treatment would depend on the underlying cause. Acute medical management and supportive treatment would be initiated as necessary.

INTRODUCTION

Dizziness is a nonspecific umbrella term which is used to often describe presyncope, vertigo, disequilibrium, and lightheadedness. It is the sensation of disturbed spatial orientation without a distorted sense of motion.

The synonyms of dizziness and their definitions are as follows:

- *Vertigo:* The sensation of self-motion when no self-motion is occurring or the sensation of distorted self-motion during an otherwise normal head movement.
- *Lightheadedness:* A feeling you are "going to faint".
- *Imbalance:* A state of being out of equilibrium or with loss of balance.
- *Gait disorder:* A problem or difficulty with walking.
- *Acute vestibular syndrome:* Sudden onset of vertigo, nausea, postural instability, and nystagmus lasting for ≥24 hours.
- *Transient vestibular syndrome:* Sudden onset of dizziness, vertigo, or unsteadiness lasting <24 hours.

PRIMER TO CASE ANALYSIS

A 74-old-male with diabetes mellitus and hypertension presenting with dizziness would lead to a case analysis of a middle-old male presenting with the symptom of dizziness in the background of comorbidities. So, causes of dizziness which are dependent and independent of the comorbidities, age, and gender need to be explored with appropriate history taking, clinical examination, investigations, and managed appropriately.

DIFFERENTIAL DIAGNOSIS IN PATIENTS WITH DIZZINESS

- *General medical*:
    - Metabolic: Hypoglycemia and hypercalcemia
    - Cardiovascular: Postural hypotension, dysrhythmia, carotid sinus syndrome, and valvular dysfunction
    - Hematological: Anemia and hyperviscosity syndromes
    - Infectious: Sepsis and meningitis
    - Malignancy: Posterior fossa or brainstem tumors, and paraneoplastic (cerebellar) syndromes
- *Otological*:
    - Benign paroxysmal positional vertigo
    - Ménière's disease
    - Post-traumatic syndrome
    - Perilymphatic fistula

- Vestibular neuritis and labyrinthitis
- Paget's disease
- Tumors
- Autoimmune disorders

- *Neurological*:
  - Stroke
  - Neuroinfectious
  - Multiple sclerosis
  - Neurodegenerative
  - Malignant
  - Psychogenic
  - Migraine
  - Epilepsy
  - Microvascular compression (vestibular paroxysmia)

CLINICAL PRESENTATION AND CLINICAL APPROACH

This presentation could be in the emergency or in the outpatient department. The ultimate diagnosis could range from the common to the uncommon causes. Central causes would require a more urgent diagnosis and management than the peripheral causes.

Each cause presents with its typical symptoms, signs, and needs a different approach to workup and management. So, a detailed history and focused clinical examination is the forerunner of appropriate diagnosis with the relevant investigations **(Table 1)**.

The key elements of history taking include:
- *Timing*: Onset and duration **(Table 2)**
- Has this happened before?
- Associated symptoms
- Triggers

Clinical examination should not miss an elaborate neurological examination including cranial nerves, hearing, and gait assessment.

The others in the list of differential diagnosis will include:
- Acute intoxication with alcohol
- Cholesteatoma

TABLE 1: Differential diagnosis with their respective symptoms, clinical examination, and investigations.

Differential diagnosis	Symptoms	Examination	Investigation
Benign paroxysmal positional vertigo (BPPV)	Vertigo on rolling over in bed and looking up which last for seconds	*Dix–Hallpike test* ***(Fig. 1)***: Diagnostic of BPPV, typically demonstrating nystagmus and symptoms that are delayed by about 15 seconds, peak in 20–30 seconds and then decay with complete resolution of the episode of vertigo; supine lateral head turns: Similar to the Dix–Hallpike maneuver, a positive test is noted when the patient experiences vertigo with nystagmus	• Diagnosis held by Dix–Hallpike test and supine lateral head turns • Pure-tone audiometry and MRI brain normal
Ménière's disease	Spontaneous vertigo attacks (each lasting 20 minutes to 12 hours) with documented low- to midfrequency sensorineural hearing loss in the affected ear before, during, or after one of the episodes of vertigo, with fluctuating aural symptoms (hearing loss, tinnitus, or ear fullness) in the affected ear	Usually normal, Romberg's test may be positive, may have horizontal and/or rotatory nystagmus which is suppressed by fixation	• *Pure-tone audiogram*: Sensorineural hearing loss pattern usually at low frequencies • *Electronystagmography*: Normal or unilateral reduction in function • *Electrocochleography*: Abnormal action potential:summating potential (AP:SP) ratio with abnormal tone burst amplitude measurements • *MRI of internal auditory meatus and brain*: Normal
Diabetes mellitus	Often dizziness may coincide with episodes of hypoglycemia where patient feels ill, clammy, generally weak; may be a preceding peripheral vestibular disorder and prolonged symptoms, particularly with associated peripheral neuropathy (associated numbness in feet and legs and history of painless injuries)	May be signs of peripheral neuropathy including numbness and presence of painless injuries	• *Blood glucose*: Low during attacks • *Serum HbA1c*: Elevated compared with nondiabetic levels, but result may be lower than expected

Continued

Continued

Differential diagnosis	Symptoms	Examination	Investigation
Presyncope	Variable depending on specific cause but may include generalized weakness, giddiness, headache, blurred vision, and diaphoresis; may be paresthesia, nausea, and vomiting; patients have a sensation of an impending loss of consciousness	• *Vasovagal attack*: Hypotension and bradycardia during attack • *Cardiopulmonary disease*: Altered cardiac rhythm, murmurs, evidence of cardiac failure	• *ECG*: May demonstrate arrhythmia, ischemic changes, or signs of structural heart disease • *Echocardiogram*: May be evidence of structural heart disease • *Cardiac or event monitoring*: Arrhythmia may be detected associated with symptomatic episodes • Tilt-table testing may demonstrate evidence of autonomic neuropathy if symptoms are provoked
Orthostatic hypotension	Dizziness on standing from a lying or sitting position, episodes are usually transient, may be a history of hypotension, antihypertensive medication use, dehydration, autonomic dysfunction (e.g., with Parkinson disease, multiple system atrophy, diabetic autonomic neuropathy); if associated with autonomic dysfunction may also have dizziness when standing upright for prolonged periods, swimming, or running and may complain of feeling "spacey" or "foggy" without vertigo during exertion; may be a history of bariatric surgery	Drop in systolic BP by 20 mm Hg or diastolic BP by 10 mm Hg within 3 minutes of standing from a lying position	• Diagnosis usually made clinically without further investigations • Tilt-table testing demonstrates orthostatic fall in BP
Vestibular neuritis	Acute onset of vertigo with nausea and vomiting, lasting days but without hearing loss; single episodes frequently recur; symptoms exacerbated by changes in head position	*Acute episode*: May be nystagmus to the affected side, head impulse test will be abnormal (due to loss of the vestibulo-ocular reflex); loss of balance; between episodes of vertigo exam may be normal	• *Pure-tone audiogram*: Normal pattern • *MRI brain*: Normal
Drugs	History of aminoglycoside antibiotics, cisplatin, or other drugs that may cause dizziness (e.g., antihypertensive or antiarrhythmic medication, diuretics, antipsychotic or antiparkinsonian medication, opioids, phosphodiesterase inhibitors, or anesthetic medication); may be hearing loss and tinnitus with aminoglycosides and cisplatin	May be orthostatic hypotension on examination if taking antihypertensive, antipsychotic, or antiparkinsonian medication, opioids, or phosphodiesterase inhibitors	• *Clinical examination*: The diagnosis is often made clinically from the history and physical findings • *Serum drug levels of aminoglycoside*: May be elevated • *Urine drug-toxicity screen*: Elevated levels of drugs or their metabolites • *Blood drug-toxicity screen*: Elevated levels of drugs or their metabolites • Pure-tone audiogram may be a sensorineural hearing loss pattern or normal • *m.1555A > G mutation screening*: May be present

Continued

Continued

Differential diagnosis	Symptoms	Examination	Investigation
Posterior circulation stroke	Sudden intense vertigo, nausea, and vomiting, dysarthria, unilateral limb weakness, headache, diplopia	Nystagmus present and may be bilateral or vertical (suggesting a central cause), head impulse test is negative, patients usually cannot stand without support; patients may have gait and limb ataxia, facial numbness, Horner syndrome, diplopia	• *Blood glucose*: Normal • *CT head without contrast*: May demonstrate hemorrhage or large infarction • *MRI brain*: Lesions demonstrating cerebellar infarction or hemorrhage
Vertebrobasilar insufficiency	Episodic vertigo lasting between 30 seconds and 15 minutes and typically starting after abruptly standing or turning the head; associated with diplopia, dysarthria, ataxia, drop attack, and clumsiness of the extremities; may have risk factors for stroke such as hypertension, hyperlipidemia, diabetes, smoking, or heart disease	Usually, normal	*MRI brain ± angiogram*: May be lesions demonstrating areas of infarction; vascular occlusion of the cerebellar arteries may be demonstrated on angiography
Psychogenic dizziness	Dizziness on standing and walking; may demonstrate anxiety reactions and avoidance behavior to specific stimuli; may be history of panic disorder with agoraphobia, personality disorders, or generalized anxiety; inappropriate or excessive anxiety or fear	Normal clinical balance tests	*Hospital anxiety and depression scale score*: Abnormally high (>8)
Wallenberg syndrome (lateral medullary infarction)	Double vision, abnormal balance, facial or limb numbness, prolonged vertigo lasting several days	Abnormal eye movements; ipsilateral Horner syndrome; diplopia; ipsilateral limb ataxia; truncal ataxia; dysphagia and hoarseness; loss of pain and temperature sensation of the ipsilateral face and contralateral trunk	• *Blood glucose*: Normal • *CT head without contrast*: May demonstrate hemorrhage or large infarction • *MRI brain ± angiogram*: Occlusion of the ipsilateral vertebral artery may be demonstrated
Vertebral artery dissection	More likely to be a young adult or trauma patient; dizziness, headache, and neck pain; may be history of predisposing factors, such as hypertension, recent infection, connective tissue disorder (e.g., Ehlers–Danlos syndrome, Marfan syndrome, osteogenesis imperfecta, fibromuscular dysplasia	Dysarthria, visual field deficits, ataxia	• *MRI angiogram*: May demonstrate double lumen in artery, evidence of intramural hematoma or pseudoaneurysm • *CT angiogram*: May demonstrate double lumen in artery, evidence of intramural hematoma or pseudoaneurysm • *Carotid ultrasound with color Doppler*: May demonstrate arterial dissection, although operator dependent, and sensitivity varies depending on artery involved

Continued

Continued

Differential diagnosis	Symptoms	Examination	Investigation
Acoustic neuroma	• Progressive unilateral sensorineural hearing loss, often accompanied by tinnitus. Vestibular symptoms—imbalance, unsteadiness • Features of brainstem, cerebellar involvement with raised intracranial tension may be presents	• *Cranial nerves (Vth)*: Reduced corneal sensitivity. Numbness or paresthesia of face • *VIIth*: Hypoesthesia of posterior meatal wall (Hitzelberger's sign), loss of taste and reduced lacrimation on Schirmer's test. Delayed blink reflex may be an early manifestation • *IXth and Xth*: Dysphagia, hoarseness of voice due to palatal, pharyngeal, and laryngeal paralysis • *Other cranial nerves* may be affected if the tumor is large	• *Pure-tone audiometry*: Sensorineural hearing loss especially at higher frequencies • Stapedial reflex decay test • CT scan/MRI with contrast • Vertebral angiography helps to differentiate acoustic neuroma from other CP angle tumors

(CP: cerebellopontine; CT: computed tomography; ECG: electrocardiogram; HbA1c: glycated hemoglobin; MRI: magnetic resonance imaging)

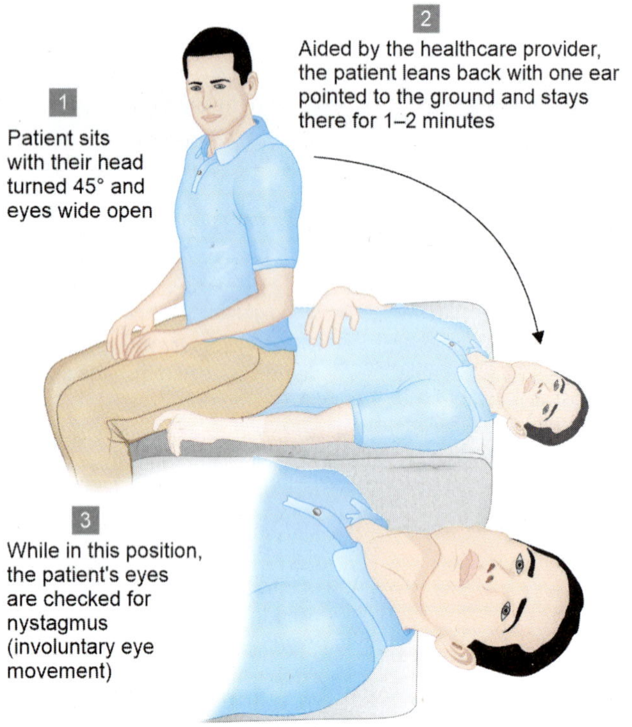

FIG. 1: Dix–Hallpike maneuver.

Source: Cleveland Clinic. Dix-Hallpike Maneuver. [online] Available from https://my.clevelandclinic.org/health/treatments/24859-dix-hallpike-maneuver#:~:text=What%20is%20the%20Dix%2DHallpike [Last accessed November, 2023].

- Superior semicircular canal dehiscence
- Perilymphatic fistula
- Persistent postural perceptual dizziness (PPPD)
- Posterior fossa tumor
- Multiple sclerosis
- Arnold–Chiari malformation type 1
- Normal pressure hydrocephalus
- Idiopathic intracranial hypertension

TABLE 2: Clinical tips—dizziness differentials based on duration.

Time duration	Differential diagnosis
Seconds	BPPV and TIA
Minutes	Migraine, orthostasis, and TIA
Hours	Migraine and Ménière's disease
Days	Migraine, Ménière's disease, and labyrinthitis
Weeks	Labyrinthitis

(BPPV: benign paroxysmal positional vertigo; TIA: transient ischemic attack)

EMERGENCIES

- Posterior circulation stroke
- Vertebral artery dissection
- Acute coronary syndrome
- Arrhythmias
- Pulmonary embolism
- Carbon monoxide poisoning

MULTIFACTORIAL ETIOLOGY OF DIZZINESS IN THE ELDERLY—EVIDENCE

Dizziness in elderly is multifactorial.

- In a population-based study in the elderly 72 years of age and above, about a quarter of the patients had dizziness priorly while seven characteristics were independently found to be associated with dizziness. These include:
  i. Anxiety trait
  ii. Depressive symptoms
  iii. Impaired balance (path deviation and time to turn circle >4 seconds)
  iv. Past myocardial infarction

v. Postural hypotension (mean decrease in blood pressure ≥ 20%)
vi. Five or more medications
vii. Impaired hearing

Only 10% of the study population without the above seven features reported dizziness. Dizziness in the elderly may primarily be due to one problem, a sizeable number of older patients were likely to have multifactorial etiology.

- One study of 417 patients aged 65–95 years found that most, 69%, of patients had presyncope-type dizziness. Underlying cardiovascular disease was the most common contributing factor in 57%, followed by peripheral vestibulopathy (14%) and psychiatric conditions (10%).
- Drug side effects are a contributor to dizziness in 20–25% of older patients.

RED FLAGS IN DIZZINESS

Mandatory Brain Imaging

- Isolated, persistent (>24 hours) vertigo of hyperacute (seconds) onset
- Normal head impulse test
- New-onset headache
- New-onset unilateral deafness
- Cranial nerve weakness or sensory loss (diplopia, dysphagia, dysarthria, and facial weakness) or limb weakness or sensory loss
- Severe (grade 3) ataxia

Acute Brain Imaging not Required

- Subacute onset vertigo (several minutes or hours)
- No other associated neurological symptoms
- No central neurological signs
- An abnormal head impulse test
- Unilateral hearing loss with typical history of Ménière's disease (recurrent episodes of aural fullness, tinnitus, hearing loss, vertigo, and nausea or vomiting lasting >30 min)

TREATMENT

The treatment of dizziness includes management of symptoms and that of the underlying cause.

Acute attacks of dizziness can be treated with vestibular suppressants, antiemetics, antivirals, and steroids. Vestibular suppressants delay the brain's natural compensatory mechanism for peripheral vertigo. So, they should not be used for prolonged periods. Central vestibular compensation is boosted by vestibular rehabilitation.

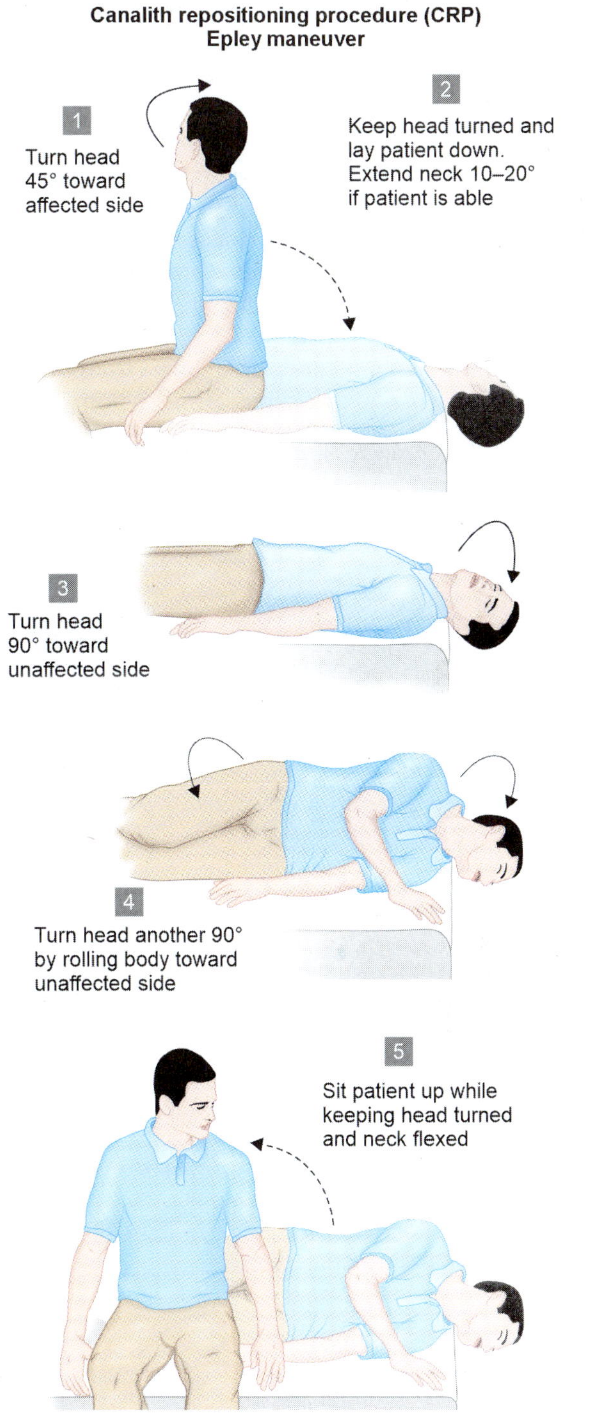

FIG. 2: Epley maneuver.

Source: Cleveland Clinic. (2023). Canalith Repositioning Procedure. [online] Available from https://my.clevelandclinic.org/health/treatments/17930-canalith-repositioning-procedure-crp [Last accessed November, 2023].

Benign paroxysmal positional vertigo is treated by canalith repositioning using the named maneuvers: Epley, Semont, Lempert, and Hamid (horizontal canal cupulolithiasis) **(Fig. 2)**.

Ménière's disease is treated conservatively with diuretics and restricted salt intake. Corticosteroids can be given intratympanically and orally. If used in the early stages of the disease, it is used to stabilize active disease and to recover speech discrimination. Chemical labyrinthectomy using intratympanic gentamicin is minimally invasive procedure in evolution used to treat disabling vertigo of Ménière's disease when hearing loss and speech discrimination have progressed to severe levels. Gentamicin is also useful for treating Tumarkin attacks of Ménière's disease.

Autoimmune inner ear disease differs from Ménière's disease in terms of its rapid progression, bilateral involvement, and response to steroids.

Vestibular migraine is treated with abortive and preventive medications for migraine and prevented by avoidance of triggers.

Hypoglycemia: Dextrose administration (oral or intravenous). Adjust drugs causing hypoglycemia.

Cerebrovascular accident (CVA), multiple sclerosis, and tumors of central nervous system (CNS) are managed as per their respective protocols.

Hypotension: Adjust drugs causing hypotension. Treat the underlying cause like infections with antimicrobial therapy or cardiac conditions with appropriate drugs.

CONCLUSION

An elderly male with diabetes and hypertension would need a multifactorial etiology exploration (common medical, ontological, and neurological) of his dizziness and appropriate management of the causes and comorbidities.

SUGGESTED READINGS

1. Agarwal K, Harnett J, Mehta N, Humphries F, Kaski D. Acute vertigo: getting the diagnosis right. BMJ. 2022;e069850.
2. Bestpractice.bmj.com. BMJ Best Practice. [online] Available from https://bestpractice.bmj.com/topics/en-us/71/urgent-considerations [Last accessed November, 2023].
3. Bisdorff A, Von Brevern M, Lempert T, Newman-Toker DE. Classification of vestibular symptoms: towards an international classification of vestibular disorders. J Vestib Res. 2009;19(1-2):1-13.
4. Bmj.com. BMJ Best Practice. [online] Available from https://bestpractice.bmj.com/topics/en-us/71/diagnosis-approach [Last accessed November, 2023].
5. Cleveland Clinic. Canalith Repositioning Procedure. [online] Available from https://my.clevelandclinic.org/health/treatments/17930-canalith-repositioning-procedure-crp [Last accessed November, 2023].
6. Cleveland Clinic. Dix-Hallpike Maneuver. [online] Available from https://my.clevelandclinic.org/health/treatments/24859-dix-hallpike-maneuver#:~:text=What%20is%20the%20Dix%2DHallpike [Last accessed November, 2023].
7. Lin HW, Bhattacharyya N. Balance disorders in the elderly: epidemiology and functional impact. Laryngoscope. 2012;122:1858-61.
8. Maarsingh OR, Dros J, Schellevis FG, van Weert HC, van der Windt DA, ter Riet G, et al. Causes of persistent dizziness in elderly patients in primary care. Ann Fam Med. 2010;8(3):196-205.
9. Medscape.com. Dizziness, Vertigo, and Imbalance Treatment and Management: Approach Considerations, Management of Peripheral Dizziness, Management of Central Dizziness. [online] Available from https://emedicine.medscape.com/article/2149881-treatment [Last accessed November, 2023].
10. Tinetti ME, Williams CS, Gill TM. Dizziness among older adults: a possible geriatric syndrome. Ann Intern Med. 2000;132:337-44.
11. UpToDate. (2022). Approach to the patient with dizziness. [online] Available from https://www.uptodate.com/contents/approach-to-the-patient-with-dizziness [Last accessed November, 2023].

61

CHAPTER

Isolated Systolic Hypertension

Sangram Biradar

ABSTRACT

Isolated systolic hypertension is a condition characterized by increased aortic stiffness and endothelial dysfunction. It is associated with an increased cardiovascular risk, which is determined by structural components within the vasculature and by functional factors including nitric oxide and endothelin-1.

INTRODUCTION

Isolated systolic hypertension (ISH) is a condition exhibiting a high level of systolic number when the blood pressure is checked. Generally, the systolic blood pressure is >130 mm Hg and diastolic <80 mm Hg.

The systolic blood pressure measures the force of blood pushing against blood vessel walls as heart pumps and diastolic blood pressure measures the arterial resistance to stretch during the time when heart is relaxing.

Isolated systolic hypertension is quite common. Nearly 15% of people aged 60 and above exhibit it. It can be dangerous when it is not treated. Without treatment, it can damage end organs. Further, it is a risk factor for heart attack, cerebrovascular accidents, and damage to the large blood vessels and kidney.

Isolated systolic hypertension is usually not an emergency. However, if systolic blood pressure is >180 mm Hg, it may suddenly without warning may lead to hypertensive crisis. Hence, it should be treated immediately.

PREVALENCE OF ISOLATED SYSTOLIC HYPERTENSION AT NATIONAL AND STATE LEVEL

The overall prevalence of ISH in India is (1.2%). The North-eastern states of Meghalaya (2.3%) and Assam (2.2%) showed highest prevalence of ISH, whereas Andhra Pradesh and Maharashtra had the lowest prevalence of ISH (0.7%).

The highest percentage of males with ISH was seen in Lakshadweep (4.9%), followed by Haryana (4.3%). States with the highest percentage of females with ISH were Meghalaya (2.3%) and Assam (2%).

SYMPTOMS OF ISOLATED SYSTOLIC HYPERTENSION

As with any other types of raised blood pressure, one does not experience any symptoms of ISH initially. But over time, untreated hypertension harms the end organs and causes chest pain, shortness of breath, headaches, and diminished vision.

CAUSES OF ISOLATED SYSTOLIC HYPERTENSION

With advancing age, arteries become stiff and less elastic. They cannot expand and contract like in younger age. When this happens, pulse pressure and systolic blood pressure go up and diastolic pressure goes down due to decreased elasticity of the vessels.

CONDITIONS CAUSING ISOLATED SYSTOLIC HYPERTENSION

Due to deposit of calcium and collagen in the arteries, they become atherosclerotic. The vessels become stiff and less flexible. Loss of elasticity in the arteries leads to the development of ISH **(Fig. 1)**.

RISK FACTORS OF ISOLATED SYSTOLIC HYPERTENSION

The risk factors for development of ISH include high cholesterol, diabetes, sedentary life style, obesity, use of tobacco products, eating processed food containing lot of salt and fat.

ISOLATED SYSTOLIC HYPERTENSION IN YOUNG AND MIDDLE-AGED INDIVIDUALS

The ISH is on rise in young and middle aged, and in those with BMI > 30, and in those using tobacco products.

- Prevalence of ISH among individuals of age between 18–39 years and 40–59 years respectively is estimated to be 1.8% and 6% in US population.

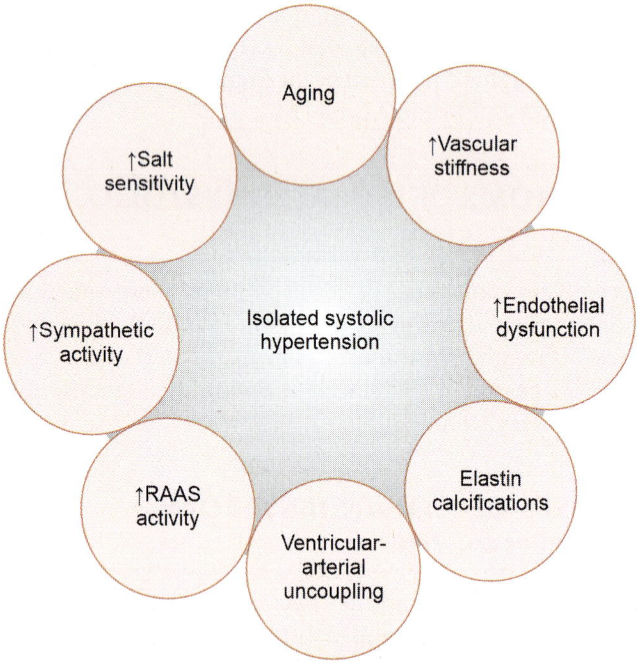

FIG. 1: Pathophysiologic mechanisms associated with isolated systolic hypertension.
(RAAS: renin-angiotensin-aldosterone system)

- In younger individuals, systolic pressure is elevated mainly in peripheral arteries compared to central arteries; this results in higher amplification in upper limb arterial pressure and pulse wave.
- In young patients with ISH and low central blood pressure mainly have lower risk of development of hypertension which needs to be treated.

COMPLICATIONS OF ISOLATED SYSTOLIC HYPERTENSION

If not treated early, ISH can lead to heart failure, heart attack, stroke, chronic kidney disease, and aneurysm.

DIAGNOSIS

Family history of hypertension, diet, activity level and other co-existing medical conditions will help in early diagnosis.

Investigation to Diagnose Isolated Systolic Hypertension

Recording of the blood pressure at two or three different times is required before making a diagnosis. Other tests include EKG, blood tests such as lipid profile, renal function test, and echocardiography.

MANAGEMENT

Nonpharmacological management, such as lifestyle modification, is essential in the treatment of ISH. It includes:

- Less salt in the diet
- DASH diet to following
- Plenty of vegetables and fresh fruits to take
- Decreasing fat intake especially saturated fats
- Weight reduction
- More exercising
- Limiting intake of alcoholic beverages
- Managing stress
- Potassium-rich diet
- Tobacco contents to avoid

There is no outcome data or well-controlled trials to support the use of nonpharmacological treatment measures in ISH. In addition to lifestyle changes, antihypertensive medications are helpful for ISH treatment **(Fig. 2)**.

Medicines to be used are:

- Diuretics
- Calcium channel blockers (CCBs)

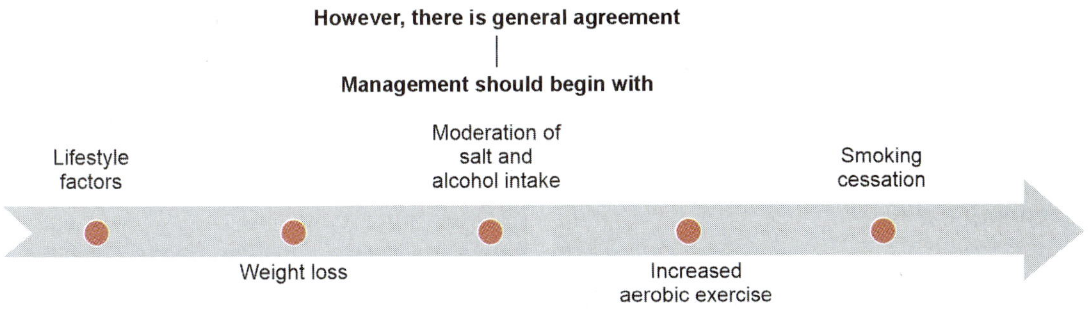

FIG. 2: Use of nonpharmacological treatment measures in ISH.

- Angiotensin-converting enzyme (ACE) inhibitors
- Angiotensin receptor blockers (ARBs)

Selection of drugs depends upon associated conditions and upon body response.

Side effect of drugs includes:
- Headache
- Dizziness
- Loss of appetite
- Dry cough

Antihypertensive agents in ISH:
- ACEi/ARBs can be considered if there are compelling indications such as chronic systolic heart failure, postmyocardial infarction, or chronic kidney disease.
- For patients with diabetes, ACEi/ARBs are better compared to other antihypertensives.
- In elderly patients, recent analysis has shown no significant difference between ACE and other antihypertensive agents on cardiovascular outcomes.
- Choice between different antihypertensive agents should be based on patient's comorbidities, tolerability, and clinical response.

Drug combinations for ISH:
- *Primary*: Calcium channel blocker + Thiazide-like diuretics (Chlorthalidone and Indapamide)
- *Secondary*: Calcium channel blocker + ACE inhibitors or ARBs, Thiazide diuretics (Chlorthalidone and Indapamide) + ARBs or ACEi
- In majority of cases, combination of two or more antihypertensive medications is used to achieve the goal.
- Initial strategy of combining calcium channel blocker and thiazide-like diuretics should be considered as evidence from trials of individual drug therapy has shown not much help.
- The safety and tolerability of this regimen is equivalent to other combinations used in high-risk patients and in patients over age 65 years.
- In the presence of compelling indications for ACEi/ARBs, combination therapy of either ACEi or ARBs with CCBs or thiazide-like diuretics can be considered.
- Thoughtful use of fixed-drug combinations will reduce pill burden and it increases adhere to the therapy.

Management of ISH ***(Flowchart 1)***.

Unmet needs in ISH of the elderly ***(Table 1)***.

PREVENTION

Everyone ages and exhibits some causes of ISH. However, there are things to lower risk of the condition, such as:
- Diabetes management
- High cholesterol content to be reduced
- Regular exercise
- BMI below 30 to maintain
- Tobacco products to avoid
- Avoiding processed food and those food items that contain a lot of salt and fat

PROGNOSIS

Prognosis depends upon how early the diagnosis is made and treatment started to avoid complications of cardiovascular and cerebrovascular systems.

Isolated systolic hypertension is a chronic long-term condition requiring treatment for the rest of life.

Isolated systolic hypertension cannot be cured but can be managed by lifestyle changes and medications. The treatment brings about big difference by decreasing the risk of heart-related events, strokes, and death by 30%.

Living with ISH necessitates regular intake of medicine prescribed, and adherence to dosing schedule. The intake has to be made according to the time fixed. Emergency medical care is required in hypertensive crisis when blood pressure is >180/120 mm Hg, and presence of symptoms like chest pain, shortness of breath, dizziness, and headache.

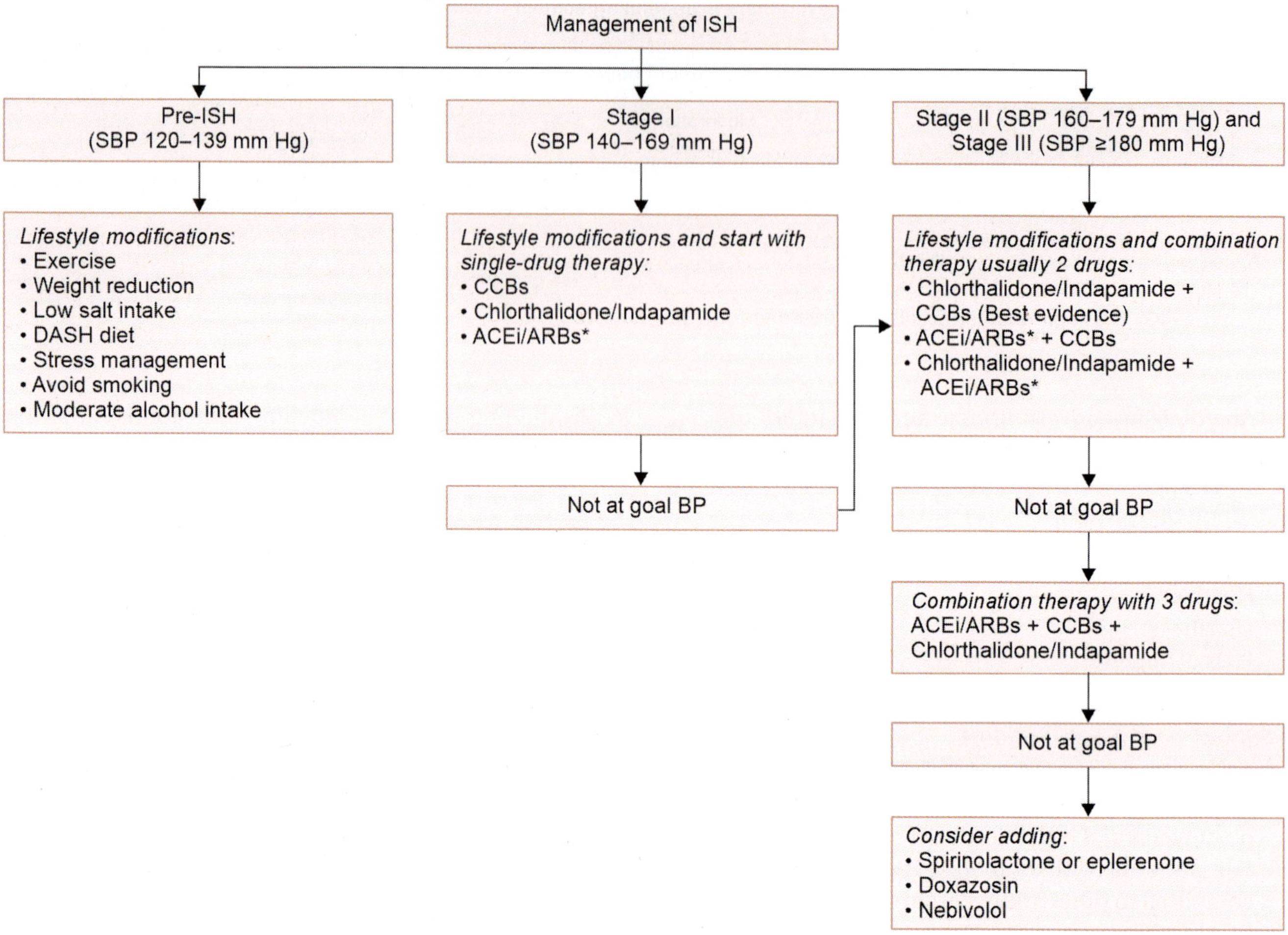

** Compelling indications to prefer ACEi/ARBs*:
- Chronic systolic heart failure
- Postmyocardial infarction
- Chronic kidney disease

FLOWCHART 1: Management of ISH.

(ACE: angiotensin-converting enzyme; ARB: angiotensin receptor blocker; CCB: calcium channel blocker; ISH: isolated systolic hypertension)

TABLE 1: Unmet needs in ISH of the elderly.

Diagnosis	Greater number of diagnostic BP measurements (to cope with increased BP variability)
	Identification of white-coat systolic hypertension
	More common use of central BP measurements
	More common assessment of arterial stiffness
Treatment	Information on protective effect of treatment in patients with comorbidities
	Information on well tolerated on-treatment DBP levels
	Larger use of combination treatment
	New drugs that more effectively counteract age and hypertension-related arterial stiffening
	Greater rate of SBP control

(ISH: isolated systolic hypertension)

SUGGESTED READINGS

1. Saladini F, Palatini P. Isolated Systolic Hypertension in Young Individuals: Pathophysiological Mechanisms, Prognostic Significance, and Clinical Implications. High Blood Press Cardiovasc Prev. 2017;24(2):133-9.
2. Gupta P, Sarkar PG, Verma V, Kumar A, Arora S, Kotwal A, et al. Prevalence and determinants of isolated systolic and isolated diastolic hypertension in India: Insights from the national family health survey (NFHS)-4. J Family Med Prim Care. 2022;11(9):5738-45.
3. Bavishi C, Goel S, Messerli FH. Isolated Systolic Hypertension: An Update after SPRINT. Am J Med. 2016;129(12):1251-8.
4. Angeli F, Verdecchia P, Masnaghetti S, Vaudo G, Reboldi G. Treatment strategies for isolated systolic hypertension in elderly patients. Expert Opin Pharmacother. 2020;21(14):1713-23.
5. Scott H, Barton MJ, Johnston ANB. Isolated systolic hypertension in young males: a scoping review. Clin Hypertens. 2021;27(1):12.
6. Mancia G, Giannattasio C. Diagnostic and therapeutic problems of isolated systolic hypertension. J Hypertens. 2015;33(1):33-43.

62 CHAPTER

The Science of Hypertensive Organ Damage: The Role of Calcium Channel Blockers

Jyotirmoy Pal, Nandini Chatterjee, Piyush Kumar Datta

ABSTRACT

The term 'essential hypertension (HTN)' refers to elevated blood pressure (BP), which can damage vital organs like the heart, brain, and kidneys. Around 1.28 billion adults worldwide suffer from hypertension, with most in low- and middle-income countries. High BP is associated with cardiovascular (CV) complications such as stroke, heart failure (HF), and heart attacks, leading to premature deaths. In India, about 30% of adults have hypertension, with urban areas at 34% and rural areas at 28%. Diabetes and hypertension are traditional risk factors for end organ damage, such as CV disease (CVD), chronic kidney disease (CKD), and stroke. Optimal and comprehensive hypertension management focuses on end-organ protection also and not only on simple BP control.

INTRODUCTION

Over the last few decades, the terminology of 'essential hypertension (HTN)' has defined elevated BP and is an inseparable part of the medical textbooks.

Back in time, when the 'quality' of the pulse of an individual, was an indicator of cardiovascular (CV) health, it was the "hard pulse" that would define hypertension. The Irish-Indian Physician, Frederick Akbar Mahomed (1849–1884) demonstrated that high BP may exist in healthy-looking individuals, was more likely in the elderly, and eventually would end up damaging the crucial organs such as the heart, brain, and kidneys.

Eventually, with the death of President Roosevelt, the revolutionary National Heart Act came into existence which paved the way for many resulting studies, including the Framingham Heart Study, to ponder into and understand this condition, which today is known as *hypertension*.

Globally, around 1.28 billion adults in the age group of 30–79 years suffer from hypertension. Most of them (two-thirds) belong to low- and middle-income countries (LMICs). The Framingham studies over several years showed that hypertension was associated with many CV complications such as stroke, HF, and heart attacks leading to premature deaths and the risk increases with higher BP, both systolic and diastolic.

According to statistics, about 30% of adults in India have hypertension, with urban areas showing a prevalence of 34% and rural areas at 28%. Considering a prevalence of around 7% among young adults aged 20–39 years, it is estimated that there are approximately 27 million young adults in India living with hypertension.

Traditional risk factors for CV disease (CVD), chronic kidney disease (CKD), and stroke are high BP diabetes, and hypertension, the silent epidemic in India, which have been coprevalent in patients as high as 62%. The association of diabetic CKD with hypertension is recorded as high as 78.7% in India.

Over these years, the science of hypertension management has consistently moved toward the significance of end-organ protection over and above the control of BP numbers. While controlling the systolic blood pressure (SBP) and diastolic blood pressure (DBP) numbers is crucial, the major fall-out of hypertension happens on the critical end-organs, such as the heart, kidneys, and brain.

HYPERTENSION-MEDIATED END-ORGAN DAMAGE

Several studies have analyzed the prevalence of hypertension-mediated organ damage (HMOD) in hypertensive patients. These studies suggest that HMOD is common in severe or long-standing hypertension but is also prevalent in less severe hypertension, including asymptomatic people with elevated BP.

About one-third of people with normal levels of BP have some form of HMOD, with the prevalence being higher in older people. The frequency of HMOD in the absence of BP elevation may be attributed to the prevalence of added risk factors for HMOD (diabetes, smoking, advancing age, and obesity).

Also, clinic BP levels misclassify actual hypertension status in some people or the presence of HMOD may be a marker of future hypertension risk. Early detection of hypertensive end organ damage can slow down or prevent damage, or regress the disease with appropriate therapy, where organ damage is yet at a reversible stage. The diagnosis of hypertensive end organ damage is of importance. This is reflected in European, American, and Indian guidelines as well.

HYPERTENSIVE HEART DISEASE

The term hypertensive heart disease encompasses a multitude of functional and structural cardiac changes, important of which is left-ventricular hypertrophy. Hypertensive heart disease is mostly clinically asymptomatic, but at a more advanced stage manifests as angina pectoris, arrhythmia, and dyspnea. These symptoms can be due to reduced coronary reserve, impaired systolic and diastolic left-ventricular function, atrial fibrillation, and ventricular arrhythmia. Hence, coronary heart disease and angina should also raise the possibility of hypertensive heart disease.

HYPERTENSIVE NEPHROPATHY

After 15–20 years, hypertensive nephropathy frequently results in chronic renal failure; mostly unnoticed and without clinical symptoms. It can be detected by means of early symptoms such as the presence of mild albuminuria and a reduced (calculated) glomerular filtration rate (eGFR), both parameters, that can be measured easily.

Microalbuminuria is usually due to structural and functional transformational processes in the glomeruli (endothelium, glomerular basal membrane, and podocytes) that are associated with increased permeability. This permeability disorder is not limited to the renal vessels but is observed in the entire vascular system, which explains why albuminuria is not only a predictor for developing renal dysfunction but is also predictive of CV complications.

Rigorous antihypertensive therapy, mostly in multiple combinations, can prevent the progression of chronic renal failure and proteinuria and thereby improve both the renal and CV prognosis. The LIFE study demonstrated that a reduction in albuminuria in hypertensive patients with LVH was associated with fewer CV complications.

OTHER HYPERTENSION-MEDIATED ORGAN DAMAGE

Cerebrovascular disease, hypertensive retinopathy, and peripheral vascular disease are the other organ damage documented in long-standing hypertension.

INDIAN SCENARIO OF HYPERTENSION-MEDIATED ORGAN DAMAGE

Hypertension is difficult to diagnose since it is asymptomatic, and BP represents a dynamic measure with inherent minute-to-minute variability and the application of incorrect techniques leads to inaccurate measurements. Furthermore, awareness, treatment, and control of hypertension and also techniques available for measurement of BP among healthcare professionals remain suboptimal.

Hence, hypertension acts as a silent killer for many years before overt target organ damage (TOD) is clinically apparent. Most of the patients with hypertension are unaware of their disease, and hence a large number of these subjects have TOD on their first arrival at the hospital.

A study by D Prakash et al. mentioned that 58.6% of patients had stage I HTN and 41.4% had stage II hypertension, according to Joint National Committee-7 (JNC-7). The study population belonged to the urban and semiurban areas, busy in their metro life and as we know hypertension is a silent killer, and most of the patients are unaware of their disease and present to their doctor with relatively high BP values.

This study revealed the presence of hypertensive retinopathy (HR) in 20.67% of patients, having grade 1 or grade 2 HR. Grade 3 HR which was present in stage II hypertensive patients shows association with the severity of hypertension. Indeed, increased BP damages the microvasculature and induces retinal arteriolar narrowing. About 45% of these patients also showed the prevalence of microalbuminuria, which was associated with the severity of hypertension as it was significantly more present in patients of stage II hypertension.

INDIAN GUIDELINES FOR HYPERTENSION

The Indian guidelines propose that angiotensin-converting enzyme (ACE) inhibitors and angiotensin receptor blockers (ARBs) are the preferred agents in young (< 60 years) and calcium channel blockers (CCBs) and diuretics are the preferred agents in those > 60 years.

The choice of an antihypertensive agent is influenced by age, concomitant risk factors, presence of HMOD, other coexisting diseases, socioeconomic considerations, availability of the drug, and past experience of the physician.

> Choice of antihypertensive therapy is to be individualized according to patient characteristics.

Combination therapy in single pills is encouraged for better compliance. It is a known fact that > 70% of patients need a combination of drugs for control of BP. We should start with a two-drug combination, preferably in a single pill for stage 2 hypertension.

Angiotensin-converting enzyme inhibitors/ARBs in combination with CCBs is considered a first-line combination and diuretics may be used as a third agent in combination.

Treatment of hypertension even in octogenarians (> 80 years) has been showing to be beneficial (newer data) and is recommended.

Advanced age, isolated systolic hypertension, angina peripheral vascular disease, carotid atherosclerosis, dementia, and pregnancy are the main conditions favoring use of a dihydropyridine (DHP)-CCB.

MANAGING BLOOD PRESSURE NUMBERS AND END-ORGAN DAMAGE

Calcium channel blockers are safe for senior patients who regularly have large-vessel stiffness and are beneficial in managing hypertension in any age group, CCBs are very effective at reducing BP and decreasing the risk of stroke and CVD. When additional BP lowering is necessary to meet strict targets, CCBs may be added, even in HF or CKD. Dihydropyridines, which were first introduced during the 1960s, have undergone numerous modifications aimed at enhancing their effectiveness and ensuring their safety.

Calcium channel blockers inhibit calcium currents through L-type calcium channels and are potent vasodilators. Some CCBs have the capacity to block additional calcium channels. Dihydropyridines CCBs (e.g., nifedipine, amlodipine, azelnidipine, cilnidipine, and efonidipine) are among the most widely employed drugs managing hypertension, renal, and CVD.

Cilnidipine, a fourth-generation newer dihydropyridine can block both L- and N-type calcium channels. Cilnidipine selectively inhibits the sympathetic nervous system (SNS) because N-type calcium is transported in the brain and along the nerve. Clinical research and animal experiments have shown that cilnidipine has renoprotective, neuroprotective, and cardioprotective properties.

Instrumental Role of Cilnidipine in Hypertension Management and End-organ Protection

The use of long-acting drugs that provide 24-hour efficacy with once-daily administration ensures smooth and sustained control of BP; which in turn is expected to provide greater protection against the risk of major CV events and HMOD.

Cilnidipine has prolonged antihypertensive properties and reduces BP through potent vasodilation and suppression of the sympathetic nervous system at the peripheral sympathetic nerve endings. Thus, it has been shown to not only effectively reduce the BP numbers, but also have beneficial effects on the end organs. A study evaluating the hypertensive effects of cilnidipine found that cilnidipine significantly reduced the 24-hour BP by 6.5 ± 1.7 mm Hg systolic ($p < 0.01$) and 5.0 ± 1.1 mm Hg diastolic ($p < 0.01$).

> Use of long-acting drugs that provide 24-hour efficacy provide greater protection against the risk of major cardiovascular events and hypertension-mediated organ damage (HMOD).

Sympathetic nerve activity is one of the main factors implicated in the development and complications of hypertension, which is a multifactorial and multifaceted disease. Plasma norepinephrine/epinephrine enhances procoagulant platelet activation, increases the risk of coronary thrombosis, and is an important prognostic marker of mortality in congestive heart failure (CHF).

The ACHIEVE-ONE [Ambulatory Blood Pressure Control and Home Blood Pressure (Morning and Evening) Lowering By N-Channel Blocker Cilnidipine], a clinical study on patients (n = 2,319) with essential hypertension, looked at how cilnidipine affected BP and pulse rate in real-world situations. Clinic SBP was significantly lowered after a 12-week treatment of cilnidipine, reduced by 19.6 mm Hg from the baseline value of 155.0 mm Hg. Similarly, morning SBP showed a notable decrease of 17.0 mm Hg from 152.9 mm Hg. The findings of this pivotal study validate the significance of cilnidipine use in hypertension management associated with elevated sympathetic overdrive. It decreases norepinephrine release from sympathetic nerve endings, causing vasodilation, a reduction in heart rate, and an improvement in renal blood flow.

Cilnidipine was also found to significantly lower BP in hypertensive individuals with aberrant nocturnal BP, particularly during sleep when enhanced sympathetic nerve activation takes place. It is helpful in the long-term management of CV issues since it also reduces vascular endothelial dysfunction.

Reduction of Microalbuminuria and Podocyte Protection with Cilnidipine

The N-type calcium channel is inhibited by cilnidipine, which blocks renal sympathetic nerve activity and causes vasodilation of the efferent arterioles. This mechanism can potentially reduce glomerular hypertension, prevent the development of microalbuminuria, and slow the progression of renal disease.

Cilnidipine induces dilation of the efferent arteriole, reducing damage to the glomeruli and suppressing podocyte injury. By reducing oxidative stress, it exerts a renoprotective effect. Cilnidipine exerts higher antioxidant activity than amlodipine and better regulation of proteinuria when compared with L-type CCB.

Due to this, in hypertensive patients with renal disease and significant proteinuria and who are already under a treatment regimen with a renin–angiotensin system (RAS) inhibitor, the addition of cilnidipine can be more effective than amlodipine. The combined treatment approach comprising cilnidipine, and an ARB plays a vital role in not only achieving stringent BP control but also preventing the advancement of kidney disease.

This is validated by the pivotal CARTER (Cilnidipine versus Amlodipine Randomised Trial for Evaluation in Renal Desease) study where the antiproteinuric effects of cilnidipine versus amlodipine were examined in a CARTER. It includes hypertension patients with renal disease (n = 339) who were already under RAS inhibitor treatment.

Regarding the primary endpoint, the cilnidipine group exhibited a significant reduction in the urinary protein/creatinine ratio compared to the amlodipine group. This finding demonstrates that cilnidipine has a more pronounced antiproteinuric effect than amlodipine **(Fig. 1)**.

> Advanced age, isolated systolic hypertension, angina pectoris, peripheral vascular disease, carotid atherosclerosis, dementia, and pregnancy are the main conditions favoring use of a dihydropyridine-calcium channel blocker (DHP-CCB).

Cilnidipine decreases proteinuria by decreasing the intraglomerular pressure, dilates the afferent and efferent arterioles equally, has antioxidative properties, inhibits the renal RAS, and suppresses podocyte injuries, as shown in multiple studies. It leads to minimal pedal edema, <2% versus amlodipine, which causes pedal edema up to 11%.

Due to its high lipophilicity, it has a high volume of distribution and thus ensures 24-hour action, as demonstrated in ambulatory blood pressure monitoring (ABPM)-based studies. It is an effective choice of antihypertensive drug, especially in hypertensive-CKD patients, as a suited early add-on molecule in essential hypertension and younger patients with elevated sympathetic activity.

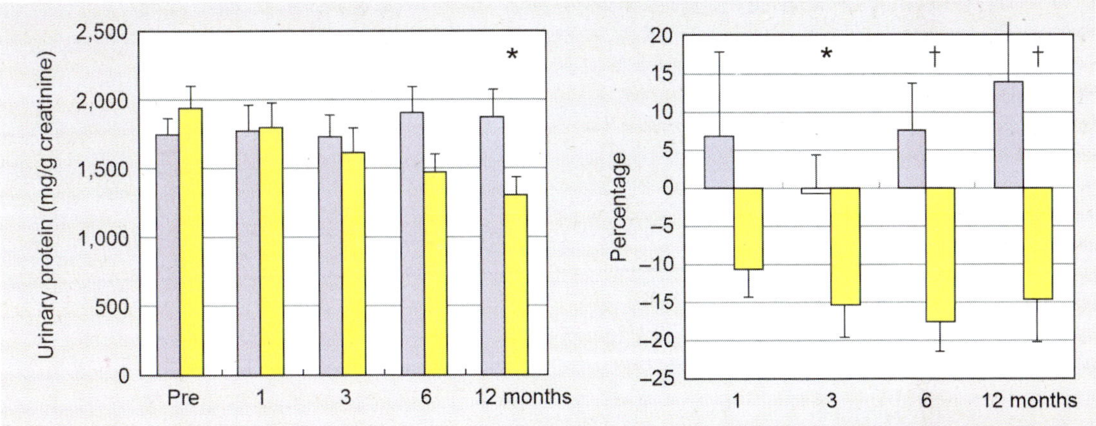

Amlodipine	160	147	142	137	130
Clinidipine	179	168	168	160	146

*$p < 0.05$
†$p < 0.01$, cilnidipine versus amlodipine groups.

FIG. 1: Results are presented as the mean 7 standard error of the mean (SEM). The urinary protein/Cr ratio was reduced in the cilnidipine group but not in the amlodipine group.

CONCLUSION

The majority of the guidelines and studies confirm the significance of treating the resulting end-organ damage due to hypertension. Today, the science of hypertension management encompasses not only the effective control of the BP numbers but use of effective molecules to slow down end-organ damage. Early diagnosis of HMOD is the key to potentially slow down or at times regress organ damage. Renal dysfunction is one of the key outfalls of uncontrolled hypertension and in India, has been seen even in the early stages of hypertension, including in youngsters. It is rather important to include organ-protective molecules early on in the hypertension journey of a patient, to help in slowing down of damage. While ACE inhibitor/ARBs have been the best agents, monotherapy seems ineffective to control the BP numbers, which has led to most guidelines recommending combination therapies to begin with. As the best-suited add-on drug, newer CCBs like cilnidipine have revolutionized hypertension management with their multiple pleiotropic and organ protective features. Adding such organ-protective drugs early on, is beneficial in the management of hypertension.

SUGGESTED READINGS

1. World Health Organization. (2023). Hypertension. [online] Available from https://www.who.int/news-room/fact-sheets/detail/hypertension [Last accessed January, 2024].
2. Saklayen MG, Deshpande NV. Timeline of History of Hypertension Treatment. Front Cardiovasc Med. 2016;3:3
3. Prakash D. Target organ damage in newly detected hypertensive patients. J Family Med Prim Care. 2019;8(6):2042-6.
4. Schmieder RE. End organ damage in hypertension. Dtsch Arztebl Int. 2010;107(49):866-73.
5. Vasan RS, Song RJ, Xanthakis V, Beiser A, DeCarli C, Mitchell GF, et al. Hypertension-Mediated Organ Damage: Prevalence, Correlates, and Prognosis in the Community. Hypertension. 2022;79(3):505-15.
6. Ito T, Fujimoto N, Ishikawa E, Dohi K, Fujimoto M, Murata T, et al. The effect of an L/N-type calcium channel blocker on intradialytic blood pressure in intradialytic hypertensive patients. Clin Exp Hypertens. 2019;41(1):92-9.
7. Kario K, Ando S, Kido H, Nariyama J, Takiuchi S, Yagi T, et al. The effects of the L/N-type calcium channel blocker (cilnidipine) on sympathetic hyperactive morning hypertension: Results from ACHIEVE-ONE. J Clin Hypertens (Greenwich). 2013;15(2):133-42.
8. Aoki S, Hosomi N, Nezu T, Teshima T, Sugii H, Nagahama S, et al. Blood pressure control with cilnidipine treatment in Japanese post-stroke hypertensive patients: The CA-ATTEND study. 1993;39(3):225-34.
9. Kario K, Nariyama J, Kido H, Ando S, Takiuchi S, Eguchi K, et al. Effect of a novel calcium channel blocker on abnormal nocturnal blood pressure in hypertensive patients. J Clin Hypertens (Greenwich). 2013;15(7):465-72. Erratum in: J Clin Hypertens (Greenwich);16(4):316.
10. Nishioka R, Kinoshita S, Shiibashi M, Shimazu T, Nakazato Y, Yamamoto T, et al. Evaluation of the Differences in the Effects of Antihypertensive Drugs on Blood Pressure Variability by 24-Hour Ambulatory Blood Pressure Monitoring in Chronic Cerebrovascular Disease. J Stroke Cerebrovasc Dis. 2015;24(8),1848-54.
11. Nardin C, Rattazi M, Pauletto P. Blood Pressure Variability and Therapeutic Implications in Hypertension and Cardiovascular Diseases. High Blood Press Cardiovasc Prev. 2019;26(5):353-9.

SECTION

8

INFECTIONS

63

CHAPTER

Sepsis Mimics

Ashit Bhagwati

ABSTRACT

Sepsis and sepsis mimics are a common cause of diagnostic dilemmas that occur in critical care units/emergency department proving a challenge to the management of patients due to array of clinical conditions that mimic the condition. Clinical acumen and awareness of this entity can help in diagnosis and required treatment.

INTRODUCTION

Sepsis mimics are a common cause of confusion leading to misdiagnosis in emergency room. Studies have shown around 50% of patients treated as sepsis are in fact cases of sepsis mimics. This confusion occurs because both conditions print with features of systemic inflammatory response syndrome (SIRS) **(Box 1)**. Hence identification is a must to differentiate sepsis from noninfectious diseases which may closely resemble as sepsis, i.e., sepsis mimics. A simple clue to this is unresolving sepsis with appropriate fluid resuscitation and antimicrobials may give clue to this entity.

CAUSES

Common causes of sepsis mimics include:
- Diabetic ketoacidosis
- Kawasaki disease (KD)
- Inborn errors of metabolism (IEM)
- Macrophage activation syndrome (MAS)
- Anaphylaxis
- Adrenal insufficiency
- Acute pancreatitis
- Neuroleptic malignant syndrome (NMS)

BOX 1: Parameters for systemic inflammatory response syndrome (SIRS).

- *Core temperature*: >38°C or <36°C
- *Elevated heart rate*: (>90 beats/min)
- *Respiratory rate*: >20 breaths/min or $PaCO_2$ <32 mm Hg or mechanical ventilation
- *WBC count*: >12,000 cells/mm^3 or <4,000 cells/mm^3, >10% immature cells

(WBC: white blood cell)

Diabetic Ketoacidosis

The hallmark of this disease is uncontrolled high sugars, altered sensorium, hypotension, ketosis and acidosis, and an infective source. Besides base line investigations, fluid administration with insulin drip and electrolyte management especially serum potassium.

Kawasaki Disease

This is an acute febrile multisystem vasculitis with varied presentations. Clinical features are varied, transient, and may not occur at a single time. Diagnosis requires a high degree of suspicion. The presence of thrombocytosis with sterile blood cultures is an important clue. Fluid resuscitation and IV immunoglobulins are standard of care.

Inborn Errors of Metabolism

These are a group of inherited disorders with varied clinical presentations, such as poor feeding, vomiting, and lethargy, leading to confusion with diagnostic challenge.

64 CHAPTER

Update on Scrub Typhus/Scrub Typhus Revisited

Kaushik Kumar Das, Gourav Chakroborty, Asraful Alam

ABSTRACT

Scrub typhus is an under diagnosed re-emerging vector borne disease caused by an intracellular gram-negative bacteria named *Orientia tsutsugamushi*, it is previously known to be endemic in the Asia–Pacific region (in India sub-Himalayan region); however, recent evidence suggested global distribution. The symptom of scrub typhus mimic with other acute febrile illness. That is why diagnosis is challenging, and case of scrub typhus were neglected and underreported. The common symptoms of scrub typhus is fever, headache, dry cough, myalgia, lymphadenopathy and some gastrointestinal disturbances, eschar, may be associated with some severe and life-threatening complications, such as multiorgan failure, disseminated intravascular coagulation (DIC), encephalitis, and myocarditis, that is why early diagnosis and treatment is required to reduce the mortality and complication caused by the disease.

So, any patient presented with fever headache and lymphadenopathy (clinically suspected we should keep in mind about scrub typhus. The diagnosis of scrub typhus mainly based on clinical suspicion confirmed by laboratory and serological testing. Laboratory studies usually reveal leukopenia, thrombocytopenia, deranged hepatic, and renal function. Serological tests consist of polymerase chain reaction (PCR) and indirect fluorescents antibody test to detect scrub immunoglobulin M (IgM).

INTRODUCTION

Scrub typhus, also known as *Rickettsia tsutsugamushi*, is an infectious disease transmitted by the bite of an infected mite. The Chinese were the first to describe this illness in detail in the third century. Antigenically, the gram-negative coccobacillus *Orientia tsutsugamushi* stands apart from the typhus-causing *Rickettsia* family of bacteria. Both shared and unique characteristics set this bacterium apart from other *Rickettsia*.

- It cannot be grown in cell-free media like other *Rickettsia*.
- The laminar outer membrane of *O. tsutsugamushi* is morphologically distinct from that of any other *Rickettsia*.
- Only *O. tsutsugamushi* buds from the plasma membrane of the host cell, allowing it to escape from the infected can. Phospholipase A2 from *Rickettsia* seems to play a mediating role in the intracellular invasion of host cells.

EPIDEMIOLOGY

The Asia–Pacific region is home to the endemic scrub typhus (*O. tsutsugamushi*) virus, which can be found in South Korea, China, Taiwan, Japan, Pakistan, and India. Accurate monitoring data on the prevalence of scrub typhus are lacking since the disease is often misdiagnosed, not recognized, or misidentified as another endemic fever sickness.

- About two-thirds of the cases were found in agricultural
- People between the ages of 40 and 60 years had the highest incidence rates; the summer and fall seasons accounted for around 80% of all the reported cases (June to September)

Vectors

Leptotrombidium are responsible for the transmission and persistence of scrub typhus. The mites can transmit the infection from generation to generation thanks to transovarian transmission. Humans infected by chiggers show symptoms 7–10 days after being bitten (range: 6–19 days).

Incubation Period

Infection commonly presents as an acute febrile illness 7–10 days after the bite of an infected larval from *Trombiculid* mite (chigger).

CLINICAL MANIFESTATIONS

The symptoms of scrub typhus include a rapid onset of fever, chills, and a severe headache. The following symptoms are often experienced by the majority of persons as their illness develops:

- Fever which typically lasts for long period in untreated patients
- Intense generalized headache
- Diffuse myalgia
- *Rash*: Approximately one-half of all patients develop a characteristically nonpruritic macular or maculopapular rash.
- *Eschar*: A painless papule often appears at the site of the infecting chigger bite, subsequent central necrosis occurs, which leads to formation of characteristic eschar with black central necrosis.

NEUROLOGICAL SYMPTOMS

- Scrub typhus causes a wide range of clinical presentations due to the central nervous system (CNS) involvement, including:
  - Meningoencephalitis (more common now days)
  - Cerebral infarction
  - Cyberelites
  - Cranial nerve palsies
  - Plexopathy
  - Transverse myelitis
  - Guillain-Barré syndrome
  - Delirium
  - Coma
  - Transient Parkinsonism
  - Opsoclonus-myoclonus

Scrub typhus causes CNS symptoms such cerebral microinfraction and edema because of vasculitis of the small blood vessels.

Manifestations

Cardiological Manifestations

- Nonspecific ST-T changes
- Premature ventricular complex
- Myocarditis
- New onset atrial fibrillation
- Acute coronary syndrome
- Complete heart block
- Pericardial effusion

Respiratory Manifestations

- Cough
- Acute respiratory distress syndrome (ARDS)
- Diffuse alveolar damage without evidence of vasculitis
- Pathogenesis of ARDS in scrub typhus is not known, thought to be immunological response of the lung to the infection without direct invasion of the organism

Other Signs and Symptoms

Other signs and symptoms may also be seen in scrub typhus

- Localized and subacute generalize lymphadenopathy
- Acute kidney injury
- Patients suffering from scrub typhus often have relative bradycardia. A rise in heart rate of <10 beats/min/°C is considered relative bradycardia.
- Scrub typhus is characterized by hepatic dysfunction, namely elevated aspartate aminotransferases (ASTs) and alanine aminotransferases (ALTs). Low attenuation around the ports and enlarged liver and spleen on abdominal computed tomography (CT); wall thickening in the gall bladder scrub typhus is characterized by hepatic dysfunction, namely elevated AST and ALT. Low attenuation around the ports and enlarged liver and spleen on abdominal CT wall thickening in the gallbladder.

Other Complications

Other complications are as follows:

- Septic shock
- Upper gastrointestinal (GI) bleeding
- Multiorgan dysfunction syndrome

DIAGNOSIS

Scrub typhus, like all *Rickettsia* diseases, lacks an early-stage diagnostic laboratory test. Disease is often diagnosed when epidemiological clues (such as recent exposure to places in which chiggers are known or believed to be present) are correlated with the existence of matching clinical signs and laboratory characteristics.

Patients with scrub typhus may develop the following lab abnormalities:

- Thrombocytopenia
- Elevation of hepatic enzyme, bilirubin, and creatinine

- Leukopenia or leukocytosis enzymes may occur while lab findings are relatively nonspecific. Four methods can be used to confirm the diagnosis.

SEROLOGY

Serological diagnosis continues to rely mostly on the indirect fluorescent antibody (IFA).

For the IFA assay to reliably diagnose an acute case of scrub typhus infection, the titer in paired samples taken at least 14 days apart must have increased by at least a factor of four.

The typical cutoff titer for a single assay is 1:50. Extending from 1:10 to 1:400.

In addition to the passive hemagglutination assay, an enzyme-linked immunosorbent assay (ELISA) has also been developed for the diagnosis of scrub typhus.

BIOPSY

A biopsy taken from a patient with eschar or a broad rash reveals a zone of strong vasculitis surrounding a focal area of cutaneous necrosis and a perivascular collection of lymphocytes and macrophages.

CULTURES

Culture of this organism is available in only a few centers.

POLYMERASE CHAIN REACTION

Scrub typhus can be diagnosed without a doubt using polymerase chain reaction (PCR) technology applied to the patient's blood; PCR has a sensitivity of 82% and a specificity of 100%.

TREATMENT

Antibiotic treatment should be started at the first sign of a *Rickettsia* disease, according to Indian Council of Medical Research (ICMR) recommendations: Do not wait for laboratory confirmation of the *Rickettsia* infection before starting antibiotic treatment.

At Primary Level

Treatment with doxycycline should be initiated before referring the patients.

In Adult

- Tablet doxycycline 200 mg/day in two divided doses for individual above 45 kg for duration of 7 days
- Tablet azithromycin in the single dose orally for 5 days

In Children

- Tablet doxycycline in the dose of 4.5 mg/kg body weight in two divided doses for children below 45 kg for 7 days
- Tablet azithromycin in the single dose of 10 mg/kg body weight for 5 days

In Pregnant Women

- Tablet azithromycin 500 mg in a single dose for 5 days
- Tablet azithromycin is the drug of choice in pregnant women where doxycycline is contraindicated

At Secondary and Tertiary Care

- The treatment as specified above in uncomplicated case
- In complicated cases, the following treatment should be initiated:
    - Doxycycline 100 mg twice daily via intravenous infusion in 100 mL normal saline over half an hour followed by 7–15 days of oral therapy (whenever possible).
    - Infusion of 500 mg of azithromycin in 250 mL of normal saline over 1 hour once day for 1–2 days, then 5 days of oral medication to finish.
    - Chloramphenicol 50–100 mg/kg/day intravenously (IV) as an infusion over 1 hour, then continuing with an oral dose for the remaining 7–15 days of treatment.
    - It is recommended that each issue be treated according to standard procedures.

CONCLUSION

Now the scrub typhus is known to occur in both endemic (sub-Himalayan) area and nonendemic area. The public health importance about the disease is under reported and delayed diagnosed due to lack of specific clinical manifestation and laboratory method, so all the clinicians should be aware of this potentially serious but easily treatable.

SUGGESTED READINGS

1. Walker DH, Feng HM, Popov VL. Rickettsial phospholipase A2 as a pathogenic mechanism in a model of cell injury by typhus and spotted fever group Rickettsiae. Am J Trop Med Hyg. 2001;65(6):936-42.
2. Currie B, O' Conner L, Dwyer B. A new focus of scrub typhus in tropical Australia. Am J Trop Med Hyg. 1993;49(4):425-9.
3. Bonell A, Lubell Y, Newton PN, Crump JA, Paris DH. Estimating the burden of scrub typhus: A systematic review. PLoS Negl Trop Dis. 2017;11(9):e0005838.
4. Sonthayanon P, Chierakul W, Wuthiekanun V, Phimda K, Pukrittayakamee S, Day NP, et al. Association of high Orientia tsutsugamushi DNA loads with disease of greater severity in adults with scrub typhus. J Clin Microbiol. 2009;47(2):430-4.
5. Kim IS, Seong SY, Woo SG, Choi MS, Chang WH. High-level expression of a 56-kilodalton protein gene (bor56) of Rickettsia tsutsugamushi Boryong and its application to enzyme-linked immunosorbent assays. J Clin Microbiol. 1993;31(3):598-605.
6. Kim IS, Seong SY, Woo SG, Choi MS, Kang JS, Chang WS. Rapid diagnosis of scrub typhus by a passive hemagglutination assay using recombinant 56-kilodalton polypeptides. 1993;31(8):2057-60.
7. Kim DM, Yum NR, Yang TY, Lee JH, Yang JT, Shim SK, et al. Usefulness of nested PCR for the diagnosis of scrub typhus in clinical practice: A prospective study. Am J Trop Med Hyg. 2006;75(3):542-5.
8. Ashraf M, Farooq A, Bashir S, Shah S. Renal failure associated with scrub typhus. JK Science. 2010;12(2):81-2.

65

CHAPTER

Metabolic Complications in People Living with HIV

Kaushik Ghosh

ABSTRACT

This article discusses the metabolic complications observed in people living with human immunodeficiency virus (HIV). With the advent of antiretroviral therapy (ART), HIV has become a manageable chronic condition. However, even with effective treatment, HIV infection is associated with a reduced lifespan due to the presence of metabolic complications. The pathophysiology underlying these complications is complex and involves interactions between factors such as viral replication, inflammation, aging, and the effects of ART. Inflammatory markers in the bloodstream have been found to be correlated with insulin resistance and the development of metabolic complications. This phenomenon, known as "inflammaging," is associated with age-related health problems, such as cardiovascular complications, cognitive decline, and low bone mineral density (BMD). Understanding and managing these metabolic complications are essential for improving the long-term health outcomes of people living with HIV (PLWH). Definite guidelines are existed to address various metabolic complications diagnosis and treatment. However, proper management and prevention of future recurrence of these complications are still challenging due to poor understanding of pathophysiology and implementation of available treatment.

INTRODUCTION

After more than four decades since the onset of the human immunodeficiency virus (HIV) pandemic, the once universally fatal infection has undergone a significant transformation. Thanks to the remarkable effectiveness of antiretroviral therapy (ART), HIV is now considered a chronic medical condition that can be managed effectively. This therapy has the ability to suppress active viral replication for extended periods of time, sometimes even spanning several decades. Consequently, people living with HIV (PLWH) who adhere to suppressive ART can expect to have a life expectancy that is nearly equivalent to that of individuals without HIV. However, it is important to note that even with effective treatment, chronic HIV infection is associated with a reduced life span of 6–14 years.[1] This reduction is primarily attributed to the presence of HIV-associated non-acquired immunodeficiency syndrome (non-AIDS) conditions, which are commonly referred to as metabolic complications of HIV.

PATHOPHYSIOLOGY

The pathophysiology underlying the metabolic complications observed in individuals with chronic HIV infection is complex and multifactorial. These complications arise due to intricate interactions between various factors within the host including ongoing low-level viral replication, chronic inflammation, accelerated aging, and long-term adverse effects of ART. Recent research conducted on PLWH has revealed a significant correlation between the presence of inflammatory markers in the bloodstream and the development of insulin resistance and metabolic complications which can be attributed to a process known as "inflammaging."

From a phenotypic perspective, this inflammaging phenomenon in chronic HIV infection is associated with a higher occurrence and increased severity of age-related health problems. These include immunosenescence, cardiovascular complications, age-related malignancies, cognitive decline, frailty, low bone mineral density (BMD), and fragility fractures. Moreover, evidence suggests that inflammaging is also evident at the molecular level. Epigenetic studies examining deoxyribonucleic acid (DNA) methylation in peripheral blood mononuclear cells (PBMCs) from PLWH have revealed an advanced molecular age relative to chronological age. This advancement corresponds to a similar extent (approximately 5–10 years) as the persistent life expectancy deficit observed in these patients.

HIV INFECTION AND ANTIRETROVIRAL THERAPY CAN ALTER GLUCOSE AND FAT METABOLISM

Patients who are infected with HIV face a higher likelihood of developing insulin resistance, impaired glucose tolerance, and subsequent type 2 diabetes mellitus (T2DM) when compared to the general population.

The prevalence of T2DM in patients with HIV infection ranges from 2 to 14%.

The prevalence of obesity, which is defined as having a body mass index of 30 kg/m^2 or higher, is closely linked to the risk of metabolic diseases. Additionally, the accumulation of excess adipose tissue has been found to worsen insulin resistance.

In the context of HIV infection, impaired glucose metabolism has been associated with altered levels of adipokines. These include increased levels of adiponectin and soluble tumor necrosis factor receptor 1 (sTNFR1), as well as decreased levels of leptin. Moreover, HIV-related changes in the functioning of CD4+ and CD8+ T-cells also hinder glycolysis, potentially having a negative impact on glucose metabolism in individuals with HIV.

Chronic HIV infection is characterized by an abnormal activation of the immune system and an increased tendency for blood clotting, as demonstrated by the heightened presence of cardiovascular disease (CVD) biomarkers such as interleukin-6, C-reactive protein, D-dimer, and von Willebrand's factor (vWF). Additionally, there is evidence indicating dysfunction in the endothelium, resulting in impaired relaxation of arteries and elevated levels of monocyte chemoattractant protein 1 (MCP1), P-selectin, vascular cell adhesion molecule 1 (VCAM-1), vWF, and tissue plasminogen activator (t-PA). Lastly, there is a potential for direct damage to endothelial cells and cardiomyocytes caused by viral proteins like gp120 and tat.

Evaluation of Diabetes

The utilization of glycated hemoglobin (HbA1c) as a diagnostic tool for diabetes among individuals receiving ARTs is not advised. It can be falsely low in most instances. However, it can be employed for the purposes of screening and monitoring. Ideally, HbA1c levels should be assessed before initiating ART, if feasible

American Diabetes Association Recommendations

American Diabetes Association (ADA) recommendations are to evaluate the fasting glucose level in order to screen for diabetes or prediabetes in the following instances:

- Prior to initiating ART
- During the process of changing ART
- 3–6 months after initiating or changing ART

If the initial results are within the normal range, it is advised to conduct an annual retesting of fasting glucose. For patients whose fasting glucose test results are close to the diagnostic threshold, it is recommended to retest their fasting glucose every 3–6 months to monitor for any potential progression to diabetes.

HIV Medicine Association and the Infectious Diseases Society of America Recommendations

Prior to initiating ART, it is recommended to acquire fasting or random blood glucose levels as well as HbA1c measurements.

Following the commencement of ART, it is advised to solely rely on plasma glucose criteria for diagnosing diabetes.

It is important to regularly monitor diagnosed diabetes mellitus patients HbA1c levels every 6 months, aiming for a target HbA1c goal of <7%.

Management

Management of diabetes is straightforward according to the guidelines of the country and incorporates a comprehensive approach toward diet, exercise, self-education, and medical nutrition therapy.

It is advisable to engage in proactive management of additional risk factors associated with CVD, such as hyperlipidemia, hypertension, and smoking. Metformin is the recommended initial medication, with caution advised when coadministered with dolutegravir as it can increase metformin concentration.

If patients undergoing ART develop diabetes, it is worth considering a switch to alternative ART agents, especially if they include lopinavir/ritonavir or thymidine analogs such as zidovudine or stavudine.

It is worth noting that there are limited reported interactions between diabetes medications and protease inhibitors, except for saxagliptin, which should be avoided.

CARDIOVASCULAR DISEASE, DYSLIPIDEMIA IN PATIENTS WITH HIV INFECTION

The American College of Cardiology and the American Heart Association have recognized HIV infection as an independent risk factor for dyslipidemia and atherosclerotic cardiovascular disease (ASCVD).

Initially, the identification of HIV infection was primarily associated with a condition known as "slim disease," characterized by severe weight loss. Additionally, the early use of ART resulted in lipodystrophy, which manifested as a loss of subcutaneous fat. This lipodystrophy served as an indicator of underlying dyslipidemia, insulin resistance, and the subsequent development of diabetes.

While contemporary ART treatments have reduced metabolic toxicities, certain agents still carry the risk of causing dyslipidemia. There is a recognized connection between protease inhibitors and dyslipidemia.

The mechanisms behind protease inhibitor-induced dyslipidemia include the inhibition of adipocyte differentiation and lipogenesis, reduced clearance of chylomicrons, and very low-density lipoprotein cholesterol (LDL-C), and increased synthesis of triglycerides in the liver.

Dyslipidemia is more frequently observed with lopinavir/ritonavir, tipranavir, and fosamprenavir, but less often with darunavir and atazanavir. Furthermore, protease inhibitors may interact with lipid-lowering medications.

Evaluations

Human immunodeficiency virus Medicine Association and the Infectious Diseases Society of America (HIVMA-IDSA) recommendations for lipid evaluation in patients with HIV infection.

Prior to commencing ART, it is recommended to evaluate lipid levels.

Additionally, it is crucial to assess all patients for the risk of ASCVD. In cases where patients have elevated levels of LDL-C and/or exhibit a high risk of ASCVD, further evaluation should be conducted in accordance with established guidelines (every 5 years if normal, every 6–12 months if abnormal).

HIV Medicine Association and the Infectious Diseases Society of America

Human immunodeficiency virus Medicine Association and the Infectious Diseases Society of America suggest measurement of lipid levels 1–3 months after initiating ART according to National Lipid Association recommendations.

Management

The primary approach to managing hypercholesterolemia is primarily through the use of statins.

Statins have notable interactions with CYP3A4 enzymes when used alongside protease inhibitors, leading to an increase in statin concentration and subsequently raising the risk of adverse events like rhabdomyolysis. Therefore, the combined administration of protease inhibitors with simvastatin or lovastatin is not recommended.

When considering a statin that undergoes glucuronidation metabolism, one option is pitavastatin, which has been reported to have no interactions with ART. Alternatively, pravastatin may also be considered due to its minimal interactions with ART, except for a potential increase in interactions when combined with the protease inhibitor darunavir.

Non-nucleoside reverse transcriptase inhibitors (NNRTIs) reduce the concentration of statins, thereby diminishing their efficacy. To manage hypertriglyceridemia, fibrates are utilized as they undergo metabolism through CYP4A and do not exhibit significant drug interactions with antiretrovirals.

Occasionally, combination therapy regimens involving niacin, fish oil, and ezetimibe may be necessary but are generally considered safe.

FAT REDISTRIBUTION SYNDROME

Changes in body composition, including alterations in lean body mass and fat distribution, can affect a significant proportion of PLWH, ranging from 10 to 80%. These changes not only pose cosmetic concerns for PLWH but also serve as indicators of increased risk for CVD. The broad prevalence of these changes can be attributed to the absence of universally defined inclusion criteria. Wasting, which refers to the loss of lean body mass, was more commonly observed during the pre-highly active antiretroviral therapy (HAART) era but not uncommon in untreated advanced diseased patients. On the other hand, lipodystrophy syndromes emerged as a consequence of the post-HAART era. These syndromes manifest as either peripheral lipoatrophy (loss of fat in certain areas) or central lipohypertrophy (accumulation of fat in specific regions), or a combination of both.

Factors that increase the likelihood of lipoatrophy consist of older age, a lower initial count of CD4 T cells, a higher viral load, coexistence of hepatitis C, or the usage of NRTI thymidine analogs such as stavudine or zidovudine in treatment, certain mitochondrial haplotypes, and nuclear genetic polymorphisms.

Lipohypertrophy has the potential to manifest in individuals undergoing any ART regimen, as impaired adipogenesis and adipocyte differentiation or function are not limited to older agents alone, but are associated with multiple ART classes. Various risk factors contribute to the development of lipohypertrophy, such as advanced age, female sex, higher baseline body fat, prolonged duration of ART, and inadequate dietary habits. It should be noted that both protease inhibitor-based and NNRTI-based ART regimens have been observed to induce lipohypertrophy.

Evaluation and Treatment

Clinical management of HIV-associated lipodystrophy syndromes often yields unsatisfactory results. Switching ART regimen is recommended. Thiazolidinediones have mixed outcomes and carry risks. Surgical interventions such as gel fillers or autologous fat transplantation are often may not be esthetically pleasing. Lipohypertrophy can be addressed through diet, exercise, and metformin. Suction-assisted lipectomy may be an option for lipohypertrophy.

Tesamorelin, a synthetic form of human growth-hormone-releasing hormone, has demonstrated encouraging outcomes in the reduction of visceral adipose tissue and enhancement of lipid profile, while having no impact on insulin resistance. Nonetheless, discontinuation of tesamorelin has been associated with rapid reaccumulation of adipose tissue, and there is presently a dearth of data on its long-term safety.

THYROID, PITUITARY, ADRENAL, AND GONAD

Hormone replacement therapy (HRT) has decreased pituitary dysfunction and opportunistic infections characterized by pituitary symptoms. The causes of hyperprolactinemia are unknown. Immune dysregulation and macroprolactin may be responsible for this increase. Galactorrhea and elevated prolactin levels can be caused by protease inhibitors, but these side effects are more common in patients taking other prolactin-raising medications. Most affected by hypopituitarism is growth hormone. Patients with HIV should have their anterior pituitary function evaluated. In the United States and Europe, HIV-related growth hormone deficiency cannot be treated with recombinant human growth hormone.

Antiretroviral therapy has substantially decreased the likelihood of thyroid dysfunction in HIV-positive patients. About HIV development, abnormal thyroid function assays include increased thyroxine-binding globulin (TBG), which correlates negatively with a cluster of differentiation (CD4) levels, decreased triiodothyronine (T3), and decreased reverse T3. According to reports, the immune reconstitution inflammatory syndrome (IRIS) may result in thyroid dysfunction. In this situation, Graves' disease is more prevalent than all other forms of thyroid disease. Public health guidelines administer care. Primary adrenal insufficiency is rare in the era of ART. An opportunistic infection causes adrenal insufficiency infrequently. In most cases, exogenous glucocorticoids and ART interact to cause secondary adrenal insufficiency in HIV patients.

BONE DISORDERS

Osteopenia, osteoporosis, and osteonecrosis are more prevalent among HIV-positive patients. Consequently, both acute and nontraumatic fracture rates are up to 7% higher.

Human immunodeficiency virus accelerates bone resorption and loss. T-cell activation and the production of proinflammatory mediators, such as interleukin-6, tumor necrosis factor-alpha, and NF-κB ligand are responsible for its onset. Other soluble immune agents enhance the activity of osteoclasts. According to Veloso et al., the first 2 years of ART therapy result in a 2–6% decrease in BMD. ART does not reverse the decline. IRIS following ART may cause bone loss. When immune function abruptly improves, systemic or local inflammation is accompanied by an increase in cytokine production.

Evaluation and Treatment

Two antiretroviral drugs, (1) protease inhibitors and (2) tenofovir, can cause bone loss. Males older than 49 years and women past menopause should undergo dual-energy X-ray absorptiometry (DEXA) bone density scans. Calcium, vitamin D, and bisphosphonates are safe and effective treatments for osteoporosis in PLWH patients. Using alendronate and zoledronate, researchers have studied osteoporosis in HIV-positive individuals. A single intravenous dosage of zoledronic acid before ART may reduce bone loss. Denosumab, teriparatide, abaloparatide, and selective estrogen receptor modulators alleviate osteoporosis in the general population; however, HIV-infected people have shown little or limited benefit.

CONCLUSION

Antiretroviral therapy has made HIV a chronic and manageable disease. Despite medical improvements, HIV-positive people (PLWH) still have metabolic changes and an increased risk of chronic illnesses. ART now protects metabolism better. The immunological response to the condition and the medications used to treat it have profound metabolic effects on every body part. On a molecular level, the disease accelerates aging. The relationship between HIV infection, ART, and mitochondrial dysfunction is significant. These metabolic abnormalities are associated with increased CVD, T2DM, and nonalcoholic fatty liver disease in HIV-positive individuals (PLWH). Fortunately, medication and lifestyle modifications can assist in regulating these metabolic disorders. The most effective treatments and their underlying mechanisms still require a definitive definition. By remaining informed and embracing the most advanced medical practices, we can ensure that HIV-positive individuals receive the high-quality care they deserve. Together, we can empower PLWH to live healthy, unencumbered lives, free from the obstacles posed by metabolic complications.

SUGGESTED READINGS

1. Marcus JL, Chao CR, Leyden WA, Xu L, Quesenberry CP Jr, Klein DB, et al. Narrowing the Gap in Life Expectancy Between HIV-Infected and HIV-Uninfected Individuals With Access to Care. J Acquir Immune Defic Syndr. 2016;73(1):39-46.
2. Deeks SG. HIV infection, inflammation, immunosenescence, and aging. Annu Rev Med. 2011;62:141-55.
3. Mirza FS, Luthra P, Chirch L. Endocrinological aspects of HIV infection. J Endocrinol Invest. 2018;41(8):881-99.
4. Veloso S, Escote X, Ceperuelo-Mallafre V, Lopez-Dupla M, Peraire J, Vilades C, et al. Leptin and adiponectin, but not IL18, are related with insulin resistance in treated HIV-1-infected patients with lipodystrophy. Cytokine. 2012;58(2):253-60.
5. Tahrir FG, Shanmughapriya S, Ahooyi TM, Knezevic T, Gupta MK, Kontos CD, et al. Dysregulation of mitochondrial bioenergetics and quality control by HIV-1 Tat in cardiomyocytes. J Cell Physiol. 2018;233(2):748-58.
6. Vigouroux C, Maachi M, Nguyen TH, Coussieu C, Gharakhanian S, Funahashi T, et al. Serum adipocytokines are related to lipodystrophy and metabolic disorders in HIV-infected men under antiretroviral therapy. Aids. 2003;17(10):1503-11.
7. Thompson MA, Horberg MA, Agwu AL, Colasanti JA, Jain MK, Short WR, et al. Primary Care Guidance for Persons With Human Immunodeficiency Virus: 2020 Update by the HIV Medicine Association of the Infectious Diseases Society of America. Clin Infect Dis. 2021;73(11):e3572-e3605. Erratum in: Clin Infect Dis. 2021; Erratum in: Clin Infect Dis. 2022;75(11):2052.
8. American Diabetes Association. Standards of Care in Diabetes-2023 Abridged for Primary Care Providers. Clin Diabetes. 2022 Winter;41(1):4-31. Erratum in: Clin Diabetes. 2023;41(2):328.
9. Zaid D, Greenman Y. Human Immunodeficiency Virus Infection and the Endocrine System. Endocrinol Metab (Seoul). 2019;34(2):95-105.
10. Dube MP, Johnson DL, Currier JS, Leedom JM. Protease inhibitor-associated hyperglycaemia. Lancet. 1997;350(9079):713-4.
11. Martinez E, Gatell J. Metabolic abnormalities and use of HIV-1 protease inhibitors. Lancet. 1998;352(9130):821-2.
12. Mhiri C, Belec L, Di Costanzo B, Georges A, Gherardi R. The slim disease in African patients with AIDS. Transactions of the Royal Society of Tropical Medicine and Hygiene. 1992;86(3):303-6.
13. Nduka CU, Uthman OA, Kimani PK, Stranges S. Body Fat Changes in People Living with HIV on Antiretroviral Therapy. AIDS Rev. 2016;18(4):198-211.
14. Cummins NW. Metabolic Complications of Chronic HIV Infection: A Narrative Review. Pathogens. 2022;11(2):197.

66

CHAPTER

Rheumatic Manifestations of Human Immunodeficiency Virus/Acquired Immunodeficiency Syndrome

Gautam Dhar Choudhury

ABSTRACT

Musculoskeletal disorders are common in human immunodeficiency virus (HIV) infection and may result in significant morbidity and impairment of patient's quality of life. An entire spectrum of rheumatic diseases occurs in HIV/acquired immunodeficiency syndrome (AIDS) patient. HIV arthropathy and reactive arthritis are commonly seen in these patients. Rheumatoid arthritis and systemic lupus erythematosus (SLE) found to have a favorable course in these patients. Treatment modalities are almost the same as in non-HIV patient. Aggressive treatment with antiretroviral therapy (ART) and careful monitoring with clusters of differentiation 4 (CD4) count and HIV viral load is vital for disease control.

INTRODUCTION

Musculoskeletal disorders are common in human immunodeficiency virus (HIV) infection and may result significant morbidity and impairment of patient's quality of life. There are three stages where different diseases manifest more commonly. During anytime in course of the disease, advanced HIV disease and with antiretroviral drug therapy (ART). Musculoskeletal syndromes that commonly affects include reactive arthritis, painful articular syndrome, diffuse infiltration lymphocytic syndrome (DILS) and myositis. Incidence and prevalence of rheumatic diseases almost same in HIV and non-HIV patients; however, there is an alteration in clinical presentation and course in preexisting rheumatic disorder.

Common rheumatic conditions encountered in HIV/acquired immunodeficiency disease syndrome (AIDS) patient **(Box 1)**.

BOX 1: Classification of rheumatic disorders in HIV/AIDS patient.

Irrespective CD4 count
- Painful articular syndrome (HIV associated arthropathy)
- Spondyloarthritides, such as reactive arthritis, psoriatic, undifferentiated
- Vasculitis
- Myopathy

Low CD count
- Septic arthritis
- Osteomyelitis
- Pyomyositis

Due to complications associated with HIV treatment
- Osteoporosis
- Myopathy

During immune reconstitution
- SLE
- Sarcoidosis
- RA

(AIDS: acquired immunodeficiency disease syndrome; CD4: clusters of differentiation 4; HIV: human immunodeficiency virus; RA: rheumatoid arthritis; SLE: systemic lupus erythematosus)

HUMAN IMMUNODEFICIENCY VIRUS ASSOCIATED ARTHRALGIA

It is the most common and frequently encountered with incidence around 40% of the patients. Large joints such as knee, shoulder, and elbow are involved. This entity is also mechanisms are HIV-mediated immune activation, cytokine release. Drugs like protease inhibitors also results in osteoporosis.

OSTEONECROSIS

Osteonecrosis occurs mainly in hip joint with prevalence around 4%. Causes are due to chronic inflammation, hypertriglyceridemia as side effect of protease inhibitors and steroid therapy. Patients may require total hip arthroplasty at a younger age.

MANAGEMENT OF HUMAN IMMUNODEFICIENCY VIRUS PATIENTS WITH RHEUMATIC MANIFESTATIONS

Treatment modalities are almost the same as in non-HIV patient. Close monitoring with HIV viral load and CD4 count is necessary during use of immunosuppressive drugs. One can start immunosuppressive drugs when CD4 > 200 copies/μL and viral load < 60,000 copies/μL.

Anti-inflammatory drugs commonly used are indomethacin which has been found to have antiretroviral activity. Same goes for HCQ which has antiretroviral activity.

Biologics are used with cautions and only to those patients who have inadequate response to conventional DMARDs.

CONCLUSION

Almost all the rheumatic conditions are seen in HIV/AIDS patients with special mention of HIV arthropathy and DILS. Standard care for rheumatic diseases in HIV/AIDS patient is the same as in other patients. Antiretroviral agents are vital to contain the disease itself and improve their musculoskeletal symptoms.

SUGGESTED READINGS

1. Berman A, Espinoza LR, Diaz JD, Aguilar JL, Rolando T, Vasey FB, et al. Rheumatic manifestations of Human immunodeficiency virus infection. AmJ Med. 1988;85(1):59-64.
2. Winchester R, Bernstein DH, Fischer HD, Enlow R, Solomon G. The Co-occurence of Reiter's Syndrome and Acquired Immunodeficiency. Ann Intern Med. 1987;106(1):19-26.
3. Wanchu A. Rheumatic manifestations of HIV infection. APLAR J Rheumatol. 2004;7(2):189-91.
4. Ghrenassia E, Martis N, Boyer J, Burel-Vandenbos F, Mekinian A, Coppo P. The diffuse infiltrative lymphocytosis syndrome (DILS). A comprehensive review. J Autoimmun. 2015;59:19-25.
5. Kaye BR. Rheumatologic manifestations of infection with human immunodeficiency virus (HIV). Ann Intern Med. 1989;111(2):158-67.
6. Brown TT, Qaqish RB. Antiretroviral therapy and the prevalence of osteopenia and osteoporosis: a meta-analytic review. AIDS. 2006;20(17):2165-74.
7. Wanchu A, Sud A, Singh S, Bambery P. Human immunodeficiency virus infection in a patient with systemic lupus erythematosus. J Assoc Physicians India. 2003;51:1102-4.
8. Azeroual A, Harmouche H, Benjilali L, Mezalek ZT, Adnaoui M, Aouni M, et al. Rheumatoid arthritis associated to HIV infection. Eur J Intern Med. 2008;19(6):e34-5.
9. Mehsen-Cetre N, Cazanave C. Osteoarticular manifestations associated with HIV infection. Joint Bone Spine. 2016;84(1):29-33.

67

CHAPTER

Re-emerging Zoonosis: A Challenge to Medical Fraternity

Krishna Sen, Sutapa Sen Dutta

ABSTRACT

Day by days zoonotic diseases are becoming significant health problem throughout the world and produce not only a challenge to medical fraternity but also cause huge amount of economic losses especially in the low- and middle-income group countries. Due to various reasons different new pathogens particularly viruses behave in a so unpredictable ways, i.e., epidemic potential, high case fatality ratio, and the absence of specific treatment and vaccines, their control become challenging and a miserable consequences arises.

As the world is now global village, emerging zoonoses of one area easily spread to whole world very rapidly and produce pandemic situation. The important factors responsible for emerging zoonoses are altered human demographics or behavior, the tremendous growth in human population, breakdown in public health measures, changing in climates, changing land use patterns, technological and industrial changes, increase mobility of humans, animals and goods, the increasing virulency of pathogen due to mutation, etc.

So, the prevention of these zoonotic diseases is utmost importance nowadays and "one health approach" is taken by World Health Organization (WHO) on 2007 globally, which should be followed by all countries. Good surveillance system over these zoonoses is also very much required to overcome one of the biggest threat to mankind.

INTRODUCTION

Environment, animals, and humans play important role in the emergence and transmission of different infectious diseases. A major portion of infectious diseases affecting humans is of animal origin. The Asia Pacific Strategy for emerging disease: 2010 report estimated that around 60% of the emerging human infections are zoonotic in nature.

The term zoonosis is derived from the Greek word "Zoon" which means Animal and "Nosos" which means illness. According to World Health Organization (WHO), any disease or infection that is naturally transmissible from vertebrate animals to human or from human to animals is classified as a zoonosis. There are over 200 known types of zoonoses. Some zoonoses, such as rabies are 100% preventable through vaccination and other methods.

Across the Globe, the 13 most common zoonoses were most impactful on poor livestock in the low- and middle-income group countries and an estimated 2.4 billion cases of illness and 2.7 million deaths in humans per year. Worldwide, the direct cost of zoonotic diseases over the last decade has been estimated to be more than $20 billion with over $200 billion indirect losses.

WHY THE EMERGING ZOONOSIS IS SO IMPORTANT?

An interesting finding of these zoonotic diseases is that newer pathogens from animals, especially different viruses emerge and spread across the countries in an unpredictable ways. These emerging zoonoses are also a concern to human health owing to their epidemic potential, high case fatality ratio and the absence of specific treatment and vaccines.

As the world is increasingly interconnected, emerging zoonoses potentially constitute a threat to global health security. However, zoonoses matter not just because they are so common, but because they cause morbidity and mortality, high burden on health systems but more importantly, it causes significant economic loses to the countries by way of losing animal trade, travel as well as loss of economic opportunities for the people through loss of livestock.

If we see an example how zoonosis can adversely impact the economy of a country—severe acute respiratory syndrome (SARS) in 2003 has the cost the world economy over USD$50 billion on account of medical treatment and significantly loss of revenue in tourism industry becoming abruptly half. Another example, the outbreak of Rift Valley Fever (RVF) in Kenya, each household lost on average US$500 as a result of low productivity and cost related to RVF disease control.

CLASSIFICATION OF ZOONOSIS

Classification Based on Etiological Agents

- *Bacterial*: Anthrax, salmonellosis, bovine tuberculosis, campylobacteriosis, listeriosis, plague, brucellosis, Lyme disease, leptospirosis, cat-scratch disease, and psittacosis
- *Viral*: Rabies, human immunodeficiency virus/acquired immunodeficiency syndrome (HIV/AIDS), Ebola, avian influenza, Marburg virus, coronavirus, yellow fever, West Nile, Zika, chikungunya, hantavirus, arenavirus, *Sindbis virus*, Crimean-Congo, sandfly fever, Colorado tick fever, vesicular stomatitis virus, Oropouche virus, Rift valley fever, monkeypox, Kyasanur forest disease, Japanese encephalitis virus, and Chandipura virus.
- *Fungal*: Dermatophytosis, sporotrichosis, Malassezia (pityriasis), cryptococcosis, penicilliosis, lobomycosis, histoplasmosis, coccidioidomycosis, blastomycosis, and pneumocystosis.
- *Parasitic*: Trichinosis, toxoplasmosis, malaria, giardiasis, *Echinococcus*, cryptosporidiosis, leishmaniasis, schistosomiasis, babesiosis, Chagas disease, and intestinal nematodes. *Rickettsia/chlamydial*: Scrub typhus, Rocky Mountain spotted fever (RMSF), and ornithosis
- *Prion*: Spongiform encephalopathy and mad cow disease.

Classification Based on Reservoir Host

- *Anthropozoonoses*: Humans get infected from animal, e.g., rabies
- *Zooanthroponoses*: Animals get infected from human, e.g., tuberculosis in cat and monkey
- *Amphizoonoses*: Infection may pass in any direction, e.g., staphylococcal infection

Classification Based on Transmission Cycle

- *Orthozoonoses*: Transmission is by direct or indirect contact, require single vertebrate species, e.g., anthrax, rabies, tuberculosis, and brucellosis
- *Cyclozoonosis*: Require two or more vertebrate host to complete the transmission cycle:
  i. *Obligatory*: Human is must, e.g., *Taenia solium* and *Taenia saginata*
  ii. *Nonobligatory*: Human is accidentally involved, e.g., hydatid disease and toxoplasmosis
- *Metazoonoses*: Both vertebrate and invertebrate species are involved in transmission, e.g., yellow fever, plague, tick-borne encephalitis, and paragonimiasis
- *Saprozoonoses*: Require a nonanimate substance for completion of life cycle, e.g., histoplasmosis, ancylostomiasis, and cutaneous larva migrans.

EMERGING AND RE-EMERGING ZOONOSES

According to the WHO, emerging zoonosis is defined as a zoonosis that is newly recognized or newly evolved or that has occurred previously but shows an increase of incidence or expansion in geographical, host, or vector range. Re-emerging zoonosis are those which were previously controlled but once again has risen to be a significant health problem. This term also refers to those which were formerly confined to one geographic area, has now spread to other new area. So, emerging and re-emerging, these two terms are used interchangeably. Some of the reemerging diseases are HIV/AIDS, bird flu, Ebola, Marburg disease, mad cow disease, yellow fever, West Nile virus, Zika, corona, dengue, malaria, and chikungunya **(Table 1)**.

FACTORS RESPONSIBLE FOR EMERGENCE OF ZOONOSES

There are numerous factors responsible for emergence of various zoonotic diseases. Among them the important factors are discussed here.

- Altered human demographics or behavior ranging from societal upheaval (e.g., war) that causes humans to leave urban area to simple changes in food habits
- The tremendous growth in human population also exerts pressure resulting in increased contact with wildlife and vectors causing zoonoses

TABLE 1: Emerging viral zoonosis of the last two decades.

Pathogen	Initial outbreak	Geographical distribution	Reservoir	Vector	Lethality
West Nile	1999	Worldwide	Birds	*Culex pipiens*	10–20%
SARS	2004	USA, Canada, Eastern Asia	Bats	None	11%
H1N1 flu	2009	America, Europe, Middle East Asia and Pacific	Birds	None	2–5.4%
MERS-CoV	2012	Middle East and Eastern Asia, Europe and USA	Dromedary Camels	None	35%
Chikungunya	2014	USA and Southern Europe, Sub-Saharan Africa, Eastern Asia, Middle East	Primates, Rodents, birds, and small mammals	*Aedes aegypti* and *Aedes albopictus*	Rare
Zika	2015	America, Africa, and Asia	Primates	*Aedes aegypti* and *Albopictus*	Low
Ebola	2018	West and Central Africa	Bats	None	70%
Crimean–Congo	2018	Sub-Saharan Africa, Eastern Asia and Middle East	Bats	Ticks	10–40%
Yellow fever	2019	South and Central America and Sub Saharan Africa	Primates	*Aedes* and *Haemagogus* species	50%
SARS-CoV-2 (COVID-19)	2020	Worldwide	Bats	None	1–2%

(COVID-19: coronavirus disease 2019; MERS-CoV: Middle East respiratory syndrome coronavirus; SARS: severe acute respiratory syndrome; SARS-CoV-2: severe acute respiratory syndrome coronavirus 2)

Source: Adapted from Marbán-Castro E, Mattar S, González TM. Reemerging zoonoses with "One Health" approach. Rev MVZ Cordoba. 2019;24(3):7280-4.

- Breakdown in public health measures, i.e., sanitation and vaccination directly influence the increased transmission of the zoonotic agents and disease
- Changing in climates may alter the disease pattern, e.g., rickettsia infections are increasing in colder region due to increasing temperature caused by global warming.
- Changing land use patterns may alter the number of reservoir host which encourage the genetic change in pathogen or bring animal hosts or disease vector into close contact with humans.
- Technological and industrial changes in food production can contribute to emergence by increasing the concentration, movements, and mixing of animals.
- Increase mobility of humans, animals, and goods allow disease to spread quickly. Coronavirus disease 2019 (COVID-19) [severe acute respiratory syndrome (SARS)] for instance, spread to nearly 30 countries in six continents within months.
- Occasionally, the pathogen may become more virulent or better adopted to humans or it may undergo changes that affect transmission pattern.
- Increased human susceptibility has also contributed to the emergence of zoonosis.
- Modern medicine also allows more humans, many of them develop chronic disease condition, to survive to an advanced age.
- Finally, some zoonoses are emerging not because they are common but because of the better recognition due to advanced diagnostic technique and better awareness.

IMPORTANT MANIFESTATIONS OF EMERGING ZOONOTIC DISEASES

The majority of emerging zoonotic diseases can be categorized into three different groups (1) disease with no illness, (2) severe illness, and (3) nonspecific syndrome. Several emerging or reemerging zoonosis fall into the second category and these zoonotic diseases are still uncontrolled and far from being eradicated or understood.

Some previous known agents became more infectious due to the alteration in disease patterns, i.e., Oropouche virus or chikungunya. Others such as Nipah or Hendra virus, and coronavirus were not discovered and described until very recently and have a huge pathogenic potential. They are associated with encephalitis (Nipah and tick-borne encephalitis), hemorrhagic fever (hantavirus), flu like signs (avian influenza), and respiratory disease (SARS-coronavirus).

HOW TO CONTROL EMERGENCE OF ZOONOSES?

To prevent the emergence of zoonotic disease various challenging measures should be adopted in individual level and community level. Some of the points are discussed here.

- Reducing domestic-wild animal interaction. For instance, with avian influenza viruses that can be transmitted to domestic poultry population through infected wild birds.
- Sustainable wild life trade, i.e., supporting responsible and proper wildlife use with improving sanitation and animal welfare practices could reduce the risk of zoonosis.
- Safer domestic animal and human interaction, i.e., enhancing hygiene and other biosecurity practices and tracking animals' movements between keepers.
- *Immunization of animals*: Livestock population can be made resistant to diseases by selectively breeding naturally immune animals or through vaccination
- *Good surveillance systems*:
  - Detecting pathogen early in wild or domestic animals before they spread to humans
  - Surveillance for zoonotic disease in humans especially in the farm workers (current infection and previous exposure) and the returning travelers from areas of known emerging disease activity.
- Laboratory services would be more effective in early detection of any zoonoses when there is a common and agreed communication protocol for sharing laboratory surveillance data between animal and human health sectors in real time.
- A mechanism needs to be put in place for sharing of laboratory investigation data within the health sector, principally between the disease surveillance and the clinical services departments. Establishing laboratory networks both within and outside the countries will enhance rapid transfer and shipment of specimens for timely diagnosis of zoonotic disease threats.
- To ensure preparedness of healthcare facilities to the threats of zoonotic infections, an infection prevention and control program should be implemented before the emergence of a disease with the standard precautions as an essential component.
- An integrated vector control management (IVM) approach should be considered for all arthropod-borne viruses as the most rational decision-making process to optimize the use of resources for effective vector control.
- Developing epidemic preparedness and response capacities for emerging zoonoses. The main strategy should begin with developing a national plan involving all important stakeholders. The plan should consider developing a geographic map of the distribution of zoonoses occurring in the countries using geographic information systems and other information technologies, and conducting a detailed risk assessment.

"ONE HEALTH APPROACH" FOR CONTROLLING ZOONOTIC DISEASE

The one health approach concept was launched in 19th century by Rudolf Virchow (1821–1902) after he incorporated veterinary medicine into human health and asserted the absence of dividing line between them. Subsequently, the concept grew worldwide. WHO defines one health "an approach to designing and implementing programs, policies, legislation, and research in which multiple sectors communicate and work together to achieve better health outcomes". In 2007, FAO, WOAH, WHO, UNICEF, WORLD BANK, and UNESCO met in India and developed a joint strategic frame work to respond to the emerging and reemerging infectious diseases. This strategic frame work was entitled "contributing to one world, one health" and built on the lesson of the one health concept.

According to one health concept, the most effective approaches that are commonly used to combat the emerging zoonosis include:

- Joint and/or coordinated disease surveillance between all relevant sectors
- Increase the capacity of laboratories, joint training and laboratory protocol sharing
- Emergency preparedness and response including joint risk assessment and simulation exercise
- Developing work force and technical working group supported by education and legislation
- Effective communication and information sharing between the stakeholders
- Developing local, national, and international strategy's inclusive goal, objectives, and activities for relevant sectors, which describe how collaboration will be accomplished.

CONCLUSION

Emerging zoonoses which are one of the biggest threat to human being, are producing tremendous challenge to medical fraternity in respect of the control and treatment. By the continuous good surveillance and one health approach adopted by WHO, we can prevent these emerging zoonoses significantly.

SUGGESTED READINGS

1. Li A, Kasai T. The Asia Pacific Strategy for Emerging Diseases—a strategy for regional health security. Western Pac Surveill Response J. 2011;2(1):6-9.
2. World Health Organization. (2022). Zoonoses. [online] Available from https://www.who.int/news-room/fact-sheets/detail/zoonoses#:~:text=A%20zoonosis%20is%20an%20infectious,food%2C%20water%20or%20the%20environment [Last accessed November, 2023].
3. Grace D, Mutua F, Ochungo P, Kruska R, Jones K, Brierley L, et al. 2012. Mapping of poverty and likely zoonoses hotspots. Zoonoses Project 4. Report to the UK Department for International Development. Nairobi, Kenya: ILRI; 2012.
4. Chomel BB. Zoonoses. In: Schaechter M (Eds). Encyclopaedia of Microbiology, 3rd edition. University of Carlifonia: Davis CA, USA: Elsevier Inc.; 2009. pp. 820-9.
5. World Health Organization. Emerging Zoonoses. Available online: https://www.who.int/Zoonoses/emerging-zoonoses/en/ [Last accessed on 18th July, 2020].
6. Paweska JT. (2015). Factors affecting the emergence of zoonoses. South Africa: 6th FIDSSA Congress; 2015.
7. Marbán-Castro E, Mattar S, GonzoRLINK http://www.scielo.org.co/scielo.php?pid=S0122-02682019000307280&script=sci_arttext&.
8. Santos R, Monteiro S. Epidemiology, control, and prevention of emerging zoonotic viruses. Viruses Food Water. 2013:442-57.
9. Chomel BB. Control and prevention of emerging zoonoses. J Vet Med Educ. 2003;30(2):145-7.
10. Aggarwal D, Ramachandran A. One Health Approach to Address Zoonotic Diseases. Indian J Community Med. 2020;45(Suppl 1):S6-S8.
11. Erkyihun GA, Bekele M. One Health Approach for the control of Zoonotic Disease. Zoonoses. 2022;2(1).

68 CHAPTER

Infections Causing Nephrotic Syndrome

Krishnendu Roy, Arindam Kargupta, Debapratim Ganguly

ABSTRACT

Nephrotic syndrome, characterized by edema, hypoalbuminemia, dyslipidemia, and proteinuria represents a challenging clinical entity. This review explores the interplay between nephrotic syndrome and various infectious agents. Hepatitis B and C, human immunodeficiency virus (HIV), dengue, malaria, leprosy, syphilis, and schistosomiasis have all been implicated in nephrotic syndrome development. In hepatitis B, viral antigens trigger immune complex deposition within the kidneys, provoking glomerular damage, and proteinuria. Hepatitis C induces glomerular disease through immune complex formation and cryoglobulinemia. HIV-associated nephropathy (HIVAN), primarily presenting as focal segmental glomerulosclerosis (FSGS), poses a significant concern among HIV-infected individuals. Dengue and malaria can lead to acute kidney injury, while leprosy is associated with glomerulonephritis. Nephrotic syndrome in syphilis is characterized by membranous glomerulonephritis. Schistosomiasis manifests as various glomerulonephritis types, with treatment responsiveness varying. Additionally, we explore lesser-known viral culprits, such as cytomegalovirus and Epstein–Barr virus, linked to glomerular lesions. In conclusion, this review underscores the paramount importance of considering infectious etiologies in nephrotic syndrome presentations. Timely diagnosis and targeted treatment of the underlying infection can pave the way for disease remission and improved clinical outcomes. This comprehensive overview offers valuable insights into the intricate relationship between infectious causes and nephrotic syndrome, enhancing clinical awareness, and management strategies.

INTRODUCTION

Nephrotic syndrome (NS) has three defining features, i.e., edema, hypoalbuminemia (3.5 g/dL), and proteinuria (>3.5 g/day). The syndrome is often associated with lipid abnormalities, such as high low density lipoproteins (LDLs) and low high density lipoproteins (HDLs), and lipiduria. Clinically, the patients present with generalized edema with significant facial, eyelid, periorbital edema and frothy urine with normal urinary output. In some :ases penile and scrotal edema can be so severe that it 'n cause urethral obstruction. Despite heavy prote- ria and lipiduria, the urine contains few cells or mainly fatty casts, which is nothing but the tile lipids under low light. NS can lead to serious 'cations, including blood clots that can lead to 'sis, higher risk of infection caused by the loss noglobulins, high-blood pressure, brief or long-lasting kidney problems, including chronic kidney disease, and kidney failure. This is in contrast to nephritic syndrome, which is typically defined as the presence of acute kidney injury (AKI) (renal dysfunction), hypertension, and active urinary sediment (red cells and red cell casts).

CAUSES OF NEPHROTIC SYNDROME

Nephrotic syndrome is not a single disease; it is a constellation of several symptoms that can be caused by many diseases. While the exact causes of NS may vary, here are some common underlying conditions and factors associated with its development. There are some primary causes such as minimal change disease, focal segmental glomerulosclerosis (FSGS), and membranous nephropathy. The secondary causes of NS are enlisted in **Box 1**.

BOX 1: Secondary causes of nephrotic syndrome.

- *Metabolic*
  - Amyloidosis
  - Diabetes mellitus
- *Immunologic:*
  - Cryoglobulinemia
  - Erythema multiforme
  - Henoch-Schönlein purpura
  - Microscopic polyangiitis
  - Polyarteritis nodosa
  - Sjögren syndrome
  - Systemic lupus erythematosus
- Idiopathic/Primary
- *Neoplastic:*
  - Carcinoma (e.g., bronchus, breast, colon, stomach, and kidney)
  - Leukemia and lymphomas
  - Melanoma
  - Multiple myeloma
- *Medication/Drug use:*
  - Heroin
  - Interferon alfa
  - Lithium
  - Nonsteroidal anti-inflammatory drugs
  - Pamidronate
- *Infection:*
  - Bacterial
    - Infective endocarditis
    - Leprosy
    - Syphilis
  - Protozoan
    - Filariasis
    - Helminthiasis
    - Malaria
    - Schistosomiasis
  - Viral
    - Epstein–Barr virus
    - Hepatitis B and C
    - Herpes zoster
    - Human immunodeficiency virus
- *Allergic:*
  - Antitoxins
  - Insect stings and venomous snake bites
  - Poison ivy or oak
- *Genetic syndromes:*
  - Congenital nephrotic syndrome (Finnish type)
  - Familial focal segmental glomerulonephritis
  - Hereditary nephritis (Alport syndrome)
- *Other:*
  - Castleman disease
  - Chronic allograft nephropathy
  - Malignant hypertension
  - Preeclampsia
  - Sarcoidosis

Infectious Causes of Nephrotic Syndrome

Various viral, bacterial, fungal, and protozoal infections are associated with the different type of renal pathology. Common occurring infectious disease which are leading to NS are hepatic B virus, hepatitis C virus, HIV, dengue, malaria, and schistosomiasis, and in certain immunocompromised cases secondary and tertiary syphilitic infection.

VIRAL DISEASE AND NEPHROTIC SYNDROME

Hepatitis B Virus and Nephrotic Syndrome

Nephrotic syndrome is an important extrahepatic manifestation of hepatitis B which is nearly seen in 3–20% of hepatitis B infections. Membranous glomerulonephritis (MGN) is more common in children whereas mesangioproliferative glomerulonephritis (MesPGN) and immunoglobulin A (IgA) deposits are common in adults.

Immune Complex Deposition

In hepatitis B virus (HBV)-associated membranous nephropathy, the immune system produces antibodies against the viral antigens, forming immune complexes. These immune complexes can deposit in the glomeruli, which are the filtering units of the kidneys. The deposition of immune complexes triggers inflammation and damage to the glomerular filtration barrier, leading to protein leakage into the urine.

Podocyte Injury

Podocytes are specialized cells in the glomeruli that play a crucial role in maintaining the integrity of the filtration barrier. In HBV-associated membranous nephropathy, the immune complexes interact with podocytes, causing injury and disruption of their normal function. This disruption further contributes to proteinuria and the development of NS.

and nephrotic) helps distinguish these cases from typical ATN. Treatment strategies remain limited to supportive management in all the categories of dengue.

MALARIA AND NEPHROTIC SYNDROME

Malaria is the one of the most common infectious disease in the tropical countries. Amongst many complication, kidney involvement is relatively frequent and is more common in infections caused by *Plasmodium falciparum* and *P. malariae*, than by *P. vivax*. Kidney complications in malaria mainly occur due to hemodynamic dysfunction and immune response. In *P. falciparum* there is often mild proteinuria associated with subendothelial deposits, mesangial deposits, and MesPGN that usually resolves with treatment. Quartan malaria from infection caused by *P. malariae* is more severe and they can present with resistant NS. They may progress to ESRD as response to steroid is <50%. Patients with NS have thickening of the glomerular capillary walls, with subendothelial deposits of immunoglobulin G (IgG), immunoglobulin M (IgM), and C3 presenting as membranoproliferative glomerulonephropathy. If the patient presents with AKI then early hemodialysis with treatment of complicated malaria can inhibit the progression to end stage renal disease.

NEPHROTIC SYNDROME IN LEPROSY

Different renal lesions have been described in leprosy, including acute and chronic GN, interstitial nephritis, secondary amyloidosis, and pyelonephritis. The exact mechanism that leads to GN in leprosy is not completely understood. The *Mycobacterium leprae* may be directly involved in renal injury and it has already been detected in glomeruli of infected patients. The glomerular lesion is probably caused by immunologic mechanism, with complement decrease and immune complexes deposition in glomerular basement membrane, subendothelial and subepithelial space, detected by electronic microscopy. Sometimes mesangial proliferation and mesangial IgA deposition is also seen. The diversity of histopathological lesions found in leprosy suggests a heterogeneous disease. Immunohistochemical studies with renal tissue have identified the presence of granular deposits of IgG and C3, and less frequently IgA, IgM and fibrin in the mesangium and in the glomerular capillaries, which is characterized by immune complex deposits or in situ formation. Electronic microscopy confirms the presence of dense granular deposits in mesangial-subendothelial and subepithelial regions. Complement consumption in some cases reinforces the hypothesis of an immune complex-mediated disease. Anti-tubercular treatment with immunosuppression with steroids provides the mainstay of treatment.

NEPHROTIC SYNDROME IN SYPHILIS

Syphilis has been called "the great imitator" because it is associated with various clinical presentations. NS is one of the clinical presentations, it usually occurs as a part of secondary syphilis but sometimes it is seen along with the ulcers. The usual histological feature is MGN with subepithelial immune complex deposits. The diagnosis is confirmed with treponemal and nontreponemal tests for *Treponema pallidum*. Penicillin being the mainstay of treatment, alternative drugs can be used if allergic.

NEPHROTIC SYNDROME IN SCHISTOSOMIASIS

Schistosomiasis mainly affects the urinary and gastrointestinal tracts. Immune complex-mediated renal disease occurs with patients *Schistosoma japonicum* and *S. mansoni* but not with *S. haematobium*. It can be of four classes: Class 1—MesPGN, class 2—extracapillary proliferative GN, class 3—MPGN pattern, class 4—FSGS pattern, and class 5—renal amyloidosis. Class 1 and 2 remits with treatment whereas rest three are difficult to treat.

Treatment

The praziquantel is available in the dose of 600 mg, being administered in dose of 50 mg/kg for adults and 60 mg/kg for children. Oxamniquine is presented in pills (250 mg) and solution (50 mg/mL). The recommended dose is 15 mg/kg for adults and 20 mg/kg for children, in unique dose.

Besides the above mentioned causes there are some other unusual and nonsignificant viral causes of glomerular lesions which are not yet established properly. It includes cytomegalovirus causing MPGN and FSGS, influenza causing anti-GBM disease and Epstein-Barr virus producing MPGN.

CONCLUSION

Infections causing NS is a common but underdiagnosed entity. Thus any patient presenting with NS should be thoroughly examined for underlying infections, which if diagnosed and treated properly, can cause complete remission of the disease itself.

SUGGESTED READINGS

1. Loscalzo J, Fauci A, Kasper D, Hauser S, Longo D, Jameson JL. Harrison's Principle of Internal Medicine, 21st edition. New York: McGraw Hill LLC; 2022.
2. Hull RP, Goldsmith DJ. Nephrotic syndrome in adults. BMJ. 2008;336(7654):1185-9.
3. Jaryal A, Kumar V, Sharma V. Renal disease in patients infected with hepatitis B virus. Tropical Gastroenterol. 2016;36:220-8.
4. Cattran DC, Feehally J, Cook HT, Liu ZH, Fervenza FC, Mezzano, SA, et al. Kidney disease: improving global outcomes (KDIGO) glomerulonephritis work group. KDIGO clinical practice guideline for glomerulonephritis. Kidney Int Suppl. 2012;2(2):139-274.
5. Tong X, Spradling PR. Increase in nonhepatic diagnoses among persons with hepatitis C hospitalized for any cause, United States, 2004–2011. J Viral Hepatitis. 2015;22(11):906-13.
6. Prasad N, Patel MR. Infection-induced kidney diseases. Front Med (Lausanne). 2018;5:327.
7. Rosenberg AZ, Naicker S, Winkler CA, Kopp JB. HIV-associated nephropathies: epidemiology, pathology, mechanisms and treatment. Nat Rev Nephrol. 2015;11(3):150-60.
8. Menez S, Hanouneh M, McMahon BA, Fine DM, Atta MG. Pharmacotherapy and treatment options for HIV-associated nephropathy. Expert Opin Pharmacother. 2018;19(1):39-48.
9. Kute VB, Trivedi HL, Vanikar AV, Shah PR, Gumber MR, Kanodia KV. Collapsing glomerulopathy and hemolytic uremic syndrome associated with falciparum malaria: completely reversible acute kidney injury. J Parasit Dis. 2013;37(2)286-90.
10. Singhal PC, Chugh KS, Kaur S, Malik AK. Acute renal failure in Leprosy. Int J Lepr Other Mycobact Dis. 1977;45(2):171-4.

69

CHAPTER

Chemoprophylaxis of Malaria

Parinita Ranjit

ABSTRACT

Malaria is a protozoan infection caused by one of five species of *Plasmodium*, mostly endemic in Africa, East Asia, South America, and parts of Europe and the Middle East. The recommendation regarding malaria prophylaxis depends on individual risk assessment for every traveler and also endemicities of the areas to be visited. The drugs recommended for malaria prophylaxis as per CDC Yellow Book 2024 are mainly atovaquone-proguanil, chloroquine, mefloquine, primaquine, tafenoquine, and doxycycline. Mefloquine is the only drug recommended for pregnant women in all trimesters of pregnancy. Chloroquine and proguanil are considered safe, but their use is restricted because of the emergence of resistance. The drugs used for chemoprophylaxis are generally well tolerated. Gastrointestinal upset, headaches, and transaminitis are the most common side effects. Severe neuropsychiatric manifestations that include seizures and psychosis and cardiac conduction abnormalities may precipitate with mefloquine. Fatal hemolysis may occur in patients with glucose-6-phosphate dehydrogenase (G6PD) deficiency with the use of primaquine and tafenoquine. Hence, G6PD testing is mandatory before using primaquine.

INTRODUCTION

Malaria is a protozoan infection caused by one of five species of *Plasmodium (P. falciparum, P. malariae, P. ovale, P. vivax,* and in Southeast Asia, *P. knowlesi*—the monkey malaria parasite). According to the World Malaria Report 2019 by the World Health Organization (WHO), more than 90 countries reported around 228 million infections and 405,000 deaths in 2018.

IMPORTANCE OF CHEMOPROPHYLAXIS

Malaria is endemic mostly in Africa, East Asia, South America, and parts of Europe and the Middle East. Travelers going to these malaria-endemic countries are at a risk of contracting the disease, and almost 10–30,000 people contract the disease every year. Therefore, all travelers to the endemic areas should be counseled on areas with a malaria risk, mosquito bite avoidance, and chemoprophylaxis.

PRINCIPLES OF CHEMOPROPHYLAXIS

The recommendation regarding malaria prophylaxis involves striking a balance between effectiveness and safety. An individual risk assessment for every traveler should be done by collecting a detailed travel itinerary, including countries and also specific areas to be visited in those countries such as cities, rural areas, or both, types of accommodation, and season of travel. Medicines should be scheduled after assessing traveler's characteristics (e.g., pregnancy and any associated comorbidities) and malarial characteristics at the destination (e.g., rate of transmission and local parasite resistance to drugs).

In humans, the parasite's life cycle occurs in two stages after being transmitted by the bite of a female anopheline mosquito. In the initial liver stage, or pre-erythrocytic schizogony, parasites multiply in the hepatocytes and eventually rupture discharging motile merozoites into the bloodstream. Two species, *P. vivax* and *P. ovale*, have persistent liver stages resulting in relapse months to years later. The second erythrocytic stage occurs when the parasites invade erythrocytes causing clinical illness.

Accordingly, there are two types of malaria chemoprophylaxis, depending on the site of action.

Blood stage prophylaxis refers to drugs that act only on the erythrocytic phase. Chloroquine, mefloquine, doxycycline, etc., are major examples of this. The main disadvantage is that the drugs have to be continued for 4 weeks after travel to eliminate parasites that emerge from the liver as late as 2–4 weeks after exposure. Additionally, they do not have the ability to prevent relapse.

Liver stage prophylaxis refers to the drugs that act on the pre-erythrocytic form of the parasite while invading the hepatocytes. Only two drugs which act on the liver stage—atovaquone-proguanil and primaquine—are recommended, but only primaquine has cidal activity against the hyponozoite. As it kills parasites at an early stage, there is no need to continue drugs after leaving the endemic area.

DRUGS RECOMMENDED FOR CHEMOPROPHYLAXIS

Drugs recommended for malaria prophylaxis as per CDC Yellow Book 2024 are mainly atovaquone-proguanil, chloroquine, mefloquine, primaquine, tafenoquine, and doxycycline **(Table 1)**.

Atovaquone-proguanil

It targets both liver and blood stages and is effective against chloroquine-resistant *P. falciparum*. One adult tablet containing 250 mg of atovaquone and 100 mg of proguanil hydrochloride should be started 1-2 days before the traveler enters the malarial zone until 7 days after exiting the malarial zone. The drug is well-tolerated, but side effects may include gastrointestinal upset, headaches, and transaminitis. It is contraindicated for pregnant women, children under 5 kg, or patients with creatinine clearance < 30 mL/min.

Mefloquine

Mefloquine targets blood schizonts and is effective against chloroquine-resistant *P. falciparum*, though mefloquine resistance has emerged in parts of Southeast Asia. Travelers should begin the medication at least 2 weeks before travel and have to take it weekly until 4 weeks after return. Major adverse effects are neuropsychiatric manifestations that include seizures and psychosis. It should be avoided in people with recent or active depression, schizophrenia, or generalized anxiety disorder. An Food and Drug Administration (FDA) black-box warning exists with rare reports of persistent dizziness following mefloquine use. Also, it is not recommended in people with cardiac conduction abnormalities. Major advantages are that it is a good choice for long trips because it is taken once weekly and it can be used in all trimesters of pregnancy and during breastfeeding.

Chloroquine and Hydroxychloroquine

Chloroquine and hydroxychloroquine both act in the erythrocytic phase. Due to the considerable rise in resistance to these medications, nowadays these drugs are only recommended for travelers visiting areas with chloroquine-sensitive *P. falciparum* (the Caribbean, Central America west of the Panama Canal, and some parts of the Middle East). Travelers have to start the medication 1 week before travel and take it once weekly until 4 weeks after return. The medication is usually well tolerated, but side effects include gastrointestinal upset, headache, dizziness, and flaring of preexisting psoriasis.

TABLE 1: Drugs and recommended doses for chemoprophylaxis of malaria.

Drugs	Dose (adult)	Dose regimen	Beginning of prophylaxis (before exposure)	End of prophylaxis (after exposure)
Atovaquone-proguanil	250 mg/100 mg	Once daily	1–2 days	7 days
Mefloquine	228 mg of base (250 mg of salt)	Once weekly	1–3 weeks	4 weeks
Chloroquine	300 mg of base (500 mg of salt)	Once weekly	1–2 weeks	4 weeks
Doxycycline	100 mg	Once daily	1–2 days	4 weeks
Hydroxychloroquine sulfate	310 mg of base (400 mg of salt)	Once weekly	1–2 weeks	4 weeks
Primaquine (G6PD testing is mandatory before initiation)	30 mg of base (52.6 mg of salt)	Once daily	1–2 days	7 days
Tafenoquine	100 mg	Once daily for 7 days and then once weekly	3 days	1 week

(G6PD: glucose-6-phosphate dehydrogenase)

Primaquine

Primaquine acts against liver hypnozoites and is used as presumptive antirelapse therapy (PART) or terminal prophylaxis, where it is taken once daily for 14 days after returning from a *P. vivax* or *P. ovale* endemic area. It is highly recommended that travelers should be tested for glucose-6-phosphate dehydrogenase (G6PD) deficiency before starting the medication as it can cause fatal hemolytic anemia. Also, it is contraindicated in pregnancy. It can also be used as primary prophylaxis where it should be taken 1–2 days before travel to malaria-endemic areas and daily for 7 days after leaving the area.

Tafenoquine

Tafenoquine is active against both hypnozoites and erythrocytic forms of *Plasmodium* species. It has to be taken daily for 3 days before traveling to an endemic area and then weekly until 7 days after returning. As this drug may also cause fatal hemolytic anemia in patients with G6PD deficiency, testing is mandatory before starting the regimen. Also, it may exacerbate psychotic symptoms. Other side effects are gastrointestinal upset, headache, asymptomatic elevations in methemoglobin levels, and epithelial keratopathy. It is contraindicated in pregnant, breastfeeding mothers, and children below 16 years of age. Inspite of having effects on liver hypnozoites because of its safety profile, from 2020, the Centers for Disease Control and Prevention (CDC) did not recommend tafenoquine for antirelapse therapy but only for primary prophylaxis of *P. ovale* or *P. vivax* malaria.

Doxycycline

Doxycycline targets erythrocytic phase and is effective against chloroquine-resistant *P. falciparum*. The medication needs to be started 1– 2 days before travel and continued daily until 4 weeks after return. Side effects include gastrointestinal upset and photosensitivity. The major advantages are that it is the cheapest medication and can give protection from other infections (e.g., rickettsial infections, leptospirosis). It cannot be used in pregnant, breastfeeding mothers, or children aged < 8 years.

Special Considerations

Pregnant Woman

A pregnant woman should generally be counseled to avoid all nonessential travel as malaria can be more complicated in pregnancy and also there is a potentially increased risk for prematurity, spontaneous abortion, and stillbirth. Mefloquine is the only drug recommended for pregnant women in all trimesters of pregnancy, although data on the first trimester is limited. Chloroquine and proguanil are considered safe, but their use is restricted because of the emergence of resistance. Doxycycline and primaquine are contraindicated in pregnant women. For pregnant women living in malaria-endemic areas, intermittent preventive treatment (IPT) or seasonal malaria chemoprevention (SMC) is preferred. IPT in pregnancy includes giving therapeutic doses of sulfadoxine-pyrimethamine monthly in the second and third trimesters of pregnancy. SMC involves giving monthly treatment doses of amodiaquine and sulfadoxine-pyrimethamine across 3–4 months of the rainy season.

Breastfeeding

Antimalarial drugs are not excreted in enough amount in breastmilk to provide chemoprophylaxis to infants. As mefloquine, chloroquine, and hydroxychloroquine are safe for infants, they may be considered during breastfeeding. Atovaquone-proguanil also has limited safety data and is not recommended for prophylaxis in those breastfeeding infants under 5 kg. Doxycycline and primaquine are also contraindicated. Tafenoquine is also not recommended due to a lack of data.

Children

Atovaquone-proguanil can be given to children over 5 kg. Mefloquine and chloroquine also can be prescribed to children, taking into account the usual contraindications and resistance patterns. Children < 8 years of age should not be administered doxycycline due to concerns of dental discoloration, dysplasia of the teeth, and inhibition of bone growth. Primaquine can be given with prior G6PD testing.

Malaria Prevention in Older Populations

Elderly travelers are more likely to suffer several comorbidities than their younger counterparts. Prescribers should consider creatinine clearance when choosing chemoprophylaxis regimens.

ISSUES OF CONCERN

Concerns Regarding Side-effects of Prophylaxis

The drugs used for chemoprophylaxis are generally well tolerated. Side effects can occur, though minor side effects usually do not require discontinuing the drug. Prophylaxis can be started earlier if a traveler expresses concerns about tolerating a particular medication. For example, mefloquine can be started 3–4 weeks in advance to check for any potential adverse events to occur before travel. If unacceptable side effects develop, the clinician has time to change the medication before the traveler's departure.

Concerns Regarding Missing a Dose of Chemoprophylaxis

A weekly drug, due to having a longer half-life, maintains adequate blood levels for a longer duration compared to drugs that have a daily regimen. If a traveler misses one to two doses, he/she should take the dose as soon as possible and then resume weekly doses on the originally scheduled day. If the traveler is >2 days late, he/she should take a dose as soon as possible and then weekly doses should resume on this new day of the week (the next dose is 1 week later, then weekly thereafter).

For a daily drug, if the traveler is 1–2 days late, protective blood levels are less likely to be maintained. The traveler should take a dose as soon as possible and resume the daily schedule at the new time of day.

Concerns Regarding Change of Prophylaxis

Medications recommended for malaria chemoprophylaxis have different modes of action at different stages of the parasite's life cycle. So, if a patient cannot tolerate the side effects of a drug before completing the full course of an antimalarial drug, another drug needs to be considered having different sites of action; for example, if chloroquine needs to stop, atovaquone-proguanil should be considered. If the switch occurs <3 weeks before departure from a malaria-endemic area, atovaquone-proguanil should be taken once daily for 4 weeks after the switch. If the switch occurs after departure from a malaria-endemic area, atovaquone-proguanil needs to be taken once daily for 4 weeks after leaving the area. Details of switching should be done according to the list provided in the CDC Yellow Book.

CONCLUSION

The interprofessional teams including doctors, primary healthcare clinicians, and nurses need coordinated efforts to execute effective malarial prophylaxis. Due to the emerging resistance, clinicians should consider individual travelers' destination, malarial intensity and pattern of resistance of that area, type of travel, and current medications and health risks while choosing antimalarial chemoprophylaxis.

SUGGESTED READINGS

1. Tan K, Abanyie F. Malaria:CDC Yellow Book 2024: Travel-Associated Infections & Diseases. Georgia: Centers for Disease Control and Prevention; 2024.
2. Andrejko KL, Mayer RC, Kovacs S, Slutsker E, Bartlett E, Tan KR, et al. The safety of atovaquone-proguanil for the prevention and treatment of malaria in pregnancy: a systematic review. Travel Med Infect Dis. 2019;27:20-6.
3. DeVos E, Dunn N. Malaria Prophylaxis. In: StatPearls [Internet]. Treasure Island (FL): StatPearls Publishing; 2023.
4. Angelo KM, Libman M, Caumes E, Hamer DH, Kain KC, Leder K, et al. Malaria after international travel: a GeoSentinel analysis, 2003–2016. Malar J. 2017;16(1):293.

70

CHAPTER

How Benign is Benign Tertian Malaria?

Swaroop Kumar Baruah, Nabanita Barman

ABSTRACT

Malaria is a severe public health problem world over and is responsible for nearly half a million death annually. *Plasmodium falciparum* is well known to cause severe/complicated malaria while *Plasmodium vivax* is usually considered not to lead to severe form and thus neglected in the field of medical research and epidemiological study. Recent evidences however showed vivax to cause nearly all sorts of complications of severe malaria and it needs to be realized to avoid causing delay in proper and timely management with readiness to look for complications and to avoid underestimation of its social and economic burden.

INTRODUCTION

Malaria, an infectious protozoan disease globally present, caused by female *Anopheles* mosquito bite is known since the beginning of human civilization. Out of five species of *Plasmodium* causing malaria, *Plasmodium vivax* and *Plasmodium falciparum* are most widely distributed and pose the greatest threat. While *P. falciparum* is well known to cause severe disease, vivax malaria is supposed to run a benign course. However, there is now robust report with increasing evidence that *P. vivax* infections may also lead to severe clinical complications including variety of hematologic, pulmonary, renal, neurologic, and multiorgan dysfunction.

EPIDEMIOLOGY

Globally, malaria continues to be one of the most important infectious diseases of humankind in terms of morbidity and mortality together with economic burden and loss of human hours. As per malaria report 2022, around 247 million cases of malaria were found to be there worldwide in 2021 with 619,000 deaths. Southeast Asia region accounts for about 2% of global burden of malaria. Although India recorded decrease in malaria prevalence and death, it still accounted for 79% of malaria cases and 83% of malaria deaths in the World Health Organization (WHO) South-East Region in 2021. About 95% of global burden of malaria cases are from African regions with 96% of malarial death.

Out of five species, *P. falciparum* dominates the African region involving 99.7% of the cases while *P. vivax*, the most widespread malarial infection affects majority of tropical and subtropical part of the world. India accounts for the highest burden of *P. vivax* globally with 18% of the total reported 2.14 million confirmed cases in 2014. Mortality from severe malaria remains a significant concern where increasing patients with severe vivax malaria were reported in some endemic countries such as Thailand, Brazil, Indonesia, Papua New Guinea, and India.

CHANGING VIVAX PARADIGM FROM BENIGN TO SEVERE

Contrary to the long-established belief that severe malaria is caused by *P. falciparum* and *P. vivax* runs a benign course; it is now increasingly being acknowledged that *P. vivax* too may lead to severe complications, hospitalization, and death. In 2005, inferred from clinical data of 11 patients from Bikaner that *P. vivax* may lead to both sequestration and nonsequestration-related complications of severe malaria including cerebral malaria, renal failure, severe anemia, circulatory collapse, hemoglobinuria, abnormal bleeding, acute respiratory distress syndrome (ARDS), and jaundice. A systematic review and meta-analysis of Indian literature in 2021 reported that the pooled proportion of severe vivax malaria to be 29.3% with the clinical feature of severe thrombocytopenia, multiorgan dysfunction, and severe anemia, the mortality rate ranged from 0–12.9%. In a trend study from Delhi, it is found that vivax is emerging as the new severe disease in malaria patients.

Recent studies from elsewhere in Asia found that 20–40% of hospitalized malaria patients suffered from *P. vivax* with severe complication with mortality rate of 0.8–1.6%.

In 2012, Brazil reported severe vivax malaria causing anemia, thrombocytopenia, jaundice, acute renal failure, shock, hemoglobinuria, and ARDS in all age groups.

In 2014, in a systematic review of studies from India, USA, Indonesia, and Pakistan found a marked increase in reported case of severe vivax infection like cerebral malaria, generalized seizure, renal dysfunction, respiratory dysfunction, and so on.

All these and many other reports from different corners of the world highlighted the fact that vivax malaria like *P. falciparum* possesses similar risk of severe complicated clinical disease.

CHANGING CONCEPT RELATING TO PATHOPHYSIOLOGY OF VIVAX MALARIA EXPLAINING ITS SEVERE FORM

Continued research with better understanding of pathophysiology of vivax infection revealed the fact that vivax infection causes increased inflammatory response compared to *P. falciparum* and also develops cytoadherence with sequestration and rosette formation similar to *P. falciparum* and so the severe complications. Beside these recent concepts, hypnozoites form of vivax infection persisting in liver cause well-known and many a times debilitating relapses and early gametocyte development challenges prevention of the spread of vivax malaria.

Increased Inflammatory Response

With the rupture of schizont, the parasitized red blood cells (RBCs) get destroyed and release toxic materials with hemozoin which includes glycosylphosphatidylinositol and plasmodial genetic material. *P. vivax* DNA found to have greater genomic content [guanosine-cytosine (GC)] and thus higher concentrations of toll-like receptor 9 stimulating CpG motifs leading to greater monocyte/macrophage activation, endothelial activation, and release of proinflammatory cytokines. This results in imbalance between proinflammatory cytokines like tumor necrosis factor (TNF) and interleukin-γ and anti-inflammatory cytokines like interleukin-10 (IL-10) leading to increased inflammatory response causing severe clinical manifestations of vivax malaria. Low pyrogenic thresholds in *P. vivax* are also attributed to these differences in malarial toxins.

Cytoadherence and Rosetting Phenomenon

The process of cytoadherence and rosetting with sequestration of infected RBCs in endothelial tissue leading to microvascular flow interference with hypoxemic organ damage and inflammatory response is central to the pathogenesis of falciparum malaria. These phenomena of cytoadherence and rosetting, although of moderate level, are now also documented with *P. vivax* infection in organs like lungs. Vivax infected RBCs are shown to bind to endothelial cells via receptors like intercellular adhesion molecule 1 (ICAM-1) however to a lesser degree compared to *P. falciparum*-infected RBCs. Adhesion to chondroitin sulfate A and hyaluronic receptors of endothelial cells in placenta is an important pathogenesis of intrauterine growth retardation and severe anemia in pregnant women.

Relapse

A proportion of intrahepatic forms of *P. vivax* remains inert for a period ranging from 2 weeks and >2 years. These dormant forms known as hypnozoites cause recurrent relapses, resulting in recurrent infection and repeated hemolysis, which sometimes with frequent rapid relapse led to severe hematological complications.

RISK FACTORS PREDISPOSING VIVAX MALARIA TO BECOME SEVERE

Children below 5 years of age are at higher risk of both uncomplicated and severe malaria. Female has more incidences in both young age and adult population with higher incidence of severe malaria.

Genetic polymorphism shows association with severity of clinical course of vivax malaria. Alpha- and beta-thalassemia patients suffer increased risk and Duffy-negative and glucose-6-phosphate dehydrogenase (G6PD)-deficient patients have decreased risk of vivax infection.

Plasmodium vivax now also started to show chloroquine resistance and these cases are more prone to develop severe complications.

COMPLICATIONS OF VIVAX MALARIA

Usually begins with nonspecific symptoms like malaise, headache, fatigue, abdominal discomfort, cough, and muscle aches followed by several days of continued, and irregular fever which then progresses to classical bouts of fever on alternate days (tertian fever). Gradually spleen and liver enlarge, mild jaundice, and anemia develop. Proper and timely treatment including radical cure to prevent relapse helps to recover. Otherwise, *P. vivax* infection may lead to severe complications as reported from all over the world contrary to the previous belief and its reputation of being benign.

Acute Respiratory Distress Syndrome

In a study from Brazil, postmortem characterization of patients with clinical diagnosis of *P. vivax* malaria was done. They demonstrated accumulation of neutrophils in the interalveolar space, heavy infiltrates of intravascular mononuclear cells, diffused endothelial and alveolar damages, and absence of parasite sequestration in the pulmonary vasculature. This suggests that ARDS in *P. vivax* infections might be caused by inflammatory mediators. They have also reported spleen rupture and multiorgan dysfunction syndrome as other complications.

Mild increase in parasite densities in peripheral blood was accompanied by larger increase in circulatory parasite lactate dehydrogenase, suggesting the possibility of parasitized erythrocytes at other sites in the body.

Hematological Complications

Compared to *P. falciparum*-infected RBCs, *P. vivax*-infected RBCs show lower levels of deformability which may contribute to increased fragility of *P. vivax*-infected erythrocytes. Because of less deformability and oxidative stress related to greater inflammatory responses in *P. vivax* infections, lysis of uninfected RBCs is higher in *P. vivax* infections, resulting in greater loss of RBCs and severe anemia.

Most of the *P. vivax* infections result in relapse at 3–4weeks intervals and frequent relapses lead to progressive severe anemia due to hemolysis and dyserythropoiesis before hematological recovery and timely restoration of the erythrocytes population from the preceding infection occurs. Inflammatory cytokine contributing to dyserythropoiesis likely due to direct toxicity of *P. vivax* on erythroblasts or enhanced bone marrow phagocyte activity has been demonstrated in vivax malaria. Moreover, there could have been compounding factors like the impaired immune response of *P. vivax*-infected patients as a result of recrudescence, reinfection, and relapse.

There has been a recent increase in studies in the literature which have assessed the prevalence of thrombocytopenia in *P. vivax* infection. Oxidative stress macrophage colony-stimulating factor immunoglobulin G binding to platelet-bound malaria antigens, spleen pooling, increased plasma cell-free circulating nucleic acid levels in *P. vivax*, and platelet phagocytosis have been postulated as possible mechanisms resulting in thrombocytopenia. The studies suggest that severe anemia and impaired liver and renal functions have been associated with severe thrombocytopenia and in patients with *P. vivax* malaria. This also indicates that multiorgan dysfunction may occur in malaria patients with thrombocytopenia.

Pregnancy-associated Malaria

In endemic regions, young children and pregnant women are particularly vulnerable to the negative health impacts of infection with *P. vivax*. Occurrence of vivax malaria in pregnancy is associated with fetal loss, maternal anemia, low-birth weight, and preterm birth with occasional reports of congenital infection. Production of cytokines, such as IL-1, interferon-γ (IFN-γ), TNF-α, and IL-2 leads to inflammation in the placenta. It has been observed that complement activation plays a pathogenetic role and systemic and placental inflammatory responses along with microvascular dysfunction from vivax malaria may cause deleterious uteroplacental hemodynamic effects and fetal growth restriction. Relapses of vivax malaria in young children result in severe anemia, malnutrition, cognitive impairment, and poor school performance.

Renal Complications

Acute kidney injury manifested by anuria or oliguria is common in patients with severe malaria. It can be multifactorial. Renal cortical necrosis following vivax malaria is increasingly reported from the Indian subcontinent. *P. vivax* has been shown to be associated with atypical hemolytic uremic syndrome. Vivax malaria can cause thrombotic microangiopathy with acute cortical necrosis, acute interstitial nephritis, acute tubular necrosis, and severe endothelial injury. Biomarkers of endothelial activation (angiopoietins 1 and 2) and soluble ang-receptor (Tie 2) are predictors of severe malaria. Endothelial dysfunction, elevated thrombomodulin, von Willebrand factor (vWF), procoagulant activity, and reduction in ADAMTS13 level associated with large vWF polymers are seen in patients with thrombotic microangiopathy caused by *P. vivax* like *P. falciparum*.

Cerebral Malaria

Cerebral malaria due to *P. vivax* is relatively uncommon. Neurological involvement in form of altered consciousness, seizures, and confusion has been reported. Malaria retinopathy is characterized by retinal changes including hemorrhages, cotton wool spots, and papilledema occurring in complicated vivax malaria. Vivax malaria has also been reported to present as cerebral infarct or cerebral venous sinus thrombosis.

Cardiovascular Complications

Plasmodium vivax-infected erythrocytes also may adhere to the endothelium. Likely, accumulation in the capillaries and microcirculation in the myocardium may result in regional dysfunction, leading to pathological alterations in ECG, biomarkers, and echocardiographic parameters and may lead to a greater inflammatory response and endothelial activation.

Hemophagocytic Lymphohistiocytosis

Although uncommon, secondary hemophagocytic lymphohistiocytosis (HLH) might be associated with *P. vivax* infection. It can be fatal if not diagnosed and treated early. HLH is an aggressive inflammatory syndrome that usually presents with fever, cytopenia, hepatitis, lymphadenopathy, and hepatosplenomegaly. The pathogenesis of HLH is thought to be due to impaired function of natural killer cells, cytotoxic T cells, and T regulatory cells that leads to an excessive activation of antigen-presenting cells (macrophages and histiocytes) and CD8+ T cells, which in turn leads to hemophagocytes in the bone marrow and the reticuloendothelial system.

CONCLUSION

Plasmodium vivax infections were thought to be a benign disease. Increasing reports of severe vivax malaria is a matter of concern. The molecular mechanisms for pathophysiology of severe *P. vivax* infection still remain poorly understood. It is possible that drug resistance and evolving alterations in parasites genomic make up and changes in host responses may result in dysregulated immune responses, contributing to severity of infections. Considering that severe malaria and deaths attributable to *P. vivax* is not a rare event, raised clinical awareness of the manifestations of vivax malaria in patients of any age should prompt early detection of malaria.

SUGGESTED READINGS

1. WHO. (2022). World malaria report 2022. [online] Available from https://www.who.int/publications/i/item/9789240064898 [Last accessed December, 2023].
2. WHO. (2023). Malaria: Disease burden. [online] Available from https://www.who.int/news-room/fact-sheets/detail/malaria [Last accessed December, 2023].
3. WHO. (2014). World malaria report 2014. [online] Available from https://www.who.int/publications/i/item/9789241564830 [Last accessed December, 2023].
4. Saini T, Kumhar M, Barjartya HC. Plasmodium vivax malaria—is it benign? J Indian Med Assoc. 2013;111(9):609-11.
5. Kochar DK, Saxena V, Singh N, Kochar SK, Kumar SV, Das A. Plasmodium vivax malaria. Emerg Infect Dis. 2005;11(1):132-4.
6. Kojom Foko LP, Arya A, Sharma A, Singh V. Epidemiology and clinical outcomes of severe Plasmodium vivax malaria in India. J Infect. 2021;82(6):231-46.
7. Matlani M, Kojom LP, Mishra N, Dogra V, Singh V. Severe vivax malaria trends in the last two years: a study from a tertiary care centre, Delhi, India. Ann Clin Microbiol Antimicrob. 2020;19(1):49.
8. Price RN, Douglas NM, Anstey NM. New developments in Plasmodium vivax malaria: severe disease and the rise of chloroquine resistance. Curr Opin Infect Dis. 2009;22(5):430-5.
9. Lacerda MV, Mourão MP, Alexandre MA, Siqueira AM, Magalhães BM, Martinez-Espinosa FE, et al. Understanding the clinical spectrum of complicated Plasmodium vivax malaria: a systematic review on the contributions of the Brazilian literature. Malar J. 2012;11:12.
10. Rahimi BA, Thakkinstian A, White NJ, Sirivichayakul C, Dondorp AM, Chokejindachai W. Severe vivax malaria: a systematic review and meta-analysis of clinical studies since 1900. Malar J. 2014;13:481.
11. Anstey NM, Russell B, Yeo TW, Price RN. The pathophysiology of vivax malaria. Trends Parasitol. 2009;25(5):220-7.
12. Andrade BB, Reis-Filho A, Souza-Neto SM, Clarêncio J, Camargo LM, Barral A, et al. Severe Plasmodium vivax malaria exhibits marked inflammatory imbalance. Malar J. 2010;9:13.
13. Carvalho BO, Lopes SC, Nogueira PA, Orlandi PP, Bargieri DY, Blanco YC, et al. On the cytoadhesion of Plasmodium vivax-infected erythrocytes. J Infect Dis. 2010;202(4):638-47.
14. Udomsanpetch R, Thanikkul K, Pukrittayakamee S, White NJ. Rosette formation by Plasmodium vivax. Trans R Soc Trop Med Hyg. 1995;89(6):635-7.
15. Anstey NM, Handojo T, Pain MC, Kenangalem E, Tjitra E, Price RN, et al. Lung injury in vivax malaria: pathophysiological evidence for pulmonary vascular sequestration and posttreatment alveolar-capillary inflammation. J Infect Dis. 2007;195(4):589-96.
16. Val F, Machado K, Barbosa L, Salinas JL, Siqueira AM, Costa Alecrim MG, et al. Respiratory Complications of Plasmodium vivax Malaria: Systematic Review and Meta-analysis. Am J Trop Med Hyg. 2017;97(3):733-43.
17. Kanodia KV, Shah PR, Vanikar AV, Kasat P, Gumber M, Trivedi HL. Malaria induced acute renal failure: a single center experience. Saudi J Kidney Dis Transpl. 2010;21(6):1088-91.

71

CHAPTER

Fever with Acute Kidney Injury

Chiranjita Phukan, Nitesh Badal

ABSTRACT

Fever with acute kidney injury (AKI) is a common entity encountered in the hospital setup. It can be hospital- or community-acquired AKI. It has a variety of causes attributed to multiple etiological agents—both infectious and noninfectious. The diagnosis can be challenging because of similar clinical presentation. However, prompt diagnosis can make a huge impact in the mortality and morbidity of the patients. Clinical features along with laboratory investigations can help in early identification of the cause as definite treatment can preserve the kidney function.

INTRODUCTION

The Tropics of Cancer and Capricorn serve as the geographic boundaries of the tropical zone, which is characterized by extreme ethnic and socioeconomic diversity. Acute kidney injury (AKI), which has been reported to have incidence rates between 25 and 80%, is characterized by a reversible decline in the glomerular filtration rate, retention of nitrogenous waste products, and an inability to maintain fluid and electrolyte homeostasis, continues to be one of the most puzzling conditions.

EPIDEMIOLOGY

Acute renal failure (ARF) results from 60%, 25%, and 15% of medical, surgical, and obstetrical diseases, respectively, according to two studies from India on patients with AKI conducted over the past three decades.

Acute kidney injury that develops in hospitalized patients [hospital-acquired AKI (HAAKI)] has a different etiology and prognosis than AKI that develops in the community [community-acquired AKI (CAAKI)], particularly in tropical climates. Human health and the emergence of disease in the tropics are significantly influenced by environmental and socioeconomic variables. Most often as a result of the prevalent illness epidemiology and the variable appropriateness of treatment by the local health system, CAAKI makes up the bulk of AKI in the tropics.

Acute kidney injury was seen to occur eight per 1,000 admissions. AKI was acquired in the community in 92.2% of cases and in hospitals in 7.8% of cases. AKI had a medical etiology in 87.4% of patients, a surgical etiology in 9.4%, and an obstetric etiology in 3.2%. Among the medical patients, sepsis was the most frequent (53.1%) cause of AKI. Scrub typhus, urosepsis, and pneumonia were the most prevalent types of sepsis among AKI. Other medical causes of AKI included hypovolemia (9.4%), biological toxins (8.4%), nephrotoxic medications and chemicals (7.4%), cardiac reasons (7.4%), and acute glomerulonephritis (1.9%).

Scrub typhus, falciparum malaria, enteric fever, dengue, and leptospirosis were the most common tropical acute febrile. The incidence of AKI among these patients is 40%.

CAUSES OF FEVER WITH ACUTE KIDNEY INJURY

- *Infections*:
  - Bacterial infection: Sepsis with renal dysfunction
  - Falciparum malaria

- Leptospirosis
- Typhoid
- Hemorrhagic fevers
- Infective diarrhea
- Human immunodeficiency virus (HIV)
- Zygomycosis
- Melioidosis
- Scrub typhus
- Chlamydia
- Legionnaires disease
- Epidemic rift
- Valley fever

- *Plant toxins*:
  - Mushroom
  - Herbal medicine
  - Djenkol beans
  - Propolis
  - *Cleistanthus collinus*
  - *Tripterygium wilfordii*
- *Poisons*:
  - Animal poisons:
    - Snakebites
    - Wasp, hornet, and bee sting
    - Scorpion sting
    - Spider bite
    - Jellyfish sting
    - Carp gallbladder or bile
  - Chemicals:
    - Copper sulfate
    - Ethylene dibromide
    - Chromic acid
    - Paraquat
    - Formic acid
- *Miscellaneous*:
  - Heatstroke
  - Hemolytic uremic syndrome
  - Acute glomerulonephritis
  - Surgical AKI
  - Obstetric AKI
  - Trauma

PATHOPHYSIOLOGY

The main causes of AKI in the tropics continue to be sepsis brought on by bacterial invasion, parasite, and viral infections, poisons, and acute diarrheal illnesses. The incidence of AKI owing to obstetric reasons and acute diarrheal infections has sharply decreased as a result of a significant improvement in maternal and child healthcare in many tropical countries. In-depth discussion is given on the typical tropical diseases that result in AKI as well as how they should be treated under various circumstances.

Malaria Falciparum

One of the primary risks to public health in the tropics continues to be malaria. Less than 1–5% of all occurrences of AKI in endemic areas are caused by malaria, whereas the frequency in nonimmune people is between 25 and 30%. AKI was confirmed in 419 patients in central India, and 22% of those patients had MAKI (malaria-associated kidney infection). AKI alone or as a component of a multiorgan dysfunction may be how MAKI manifests. Predisposing variables include volume depletion, gastrointestinal hemorrhage, sepsis, nephrotoxic medications, and hyperbilirubinemia. Uncertainty surrounds the pathophysiology of MAKI. Several ideas have been put forth including hypovolemia, cytokine- and nitric oxide-mediated arterial vasodilatation, resistance to vasoactive hormones, cytopathic hypoxia resulting in reduced adenosine triphosphate (ATP) synthesis, and mechanical obstruction by infected erythrocytes (cytoadherence). The distal tubules are most affected by acute tubular necrosis (ATN) in the renal histology, which is characterized by a wide range of cell necrosis, edema, and hemosiderin granule deposition. Additionally, glomerulonephritis and interstitial nephritis may be present.

Leptospirosis

Leptospirosis is a zoonotic illness spread by spirochetes of the genus *Leptospira* that affects both visitors and locals in tropical areas. Between 40 and 60% of people with severe leptospirosis develop AKI. Clinical symptoms are typically biphasic, with the immunological phase, which is when nephropathy develops, coming after the initial septicemic phase, which lasts for 3–7 days. Invasion of bacteria, inflammatory processes, changes in hemodynamics, and the direct toxicity of bacterial products are among the pathogenetic pathways proposed. Leptospirosis AKI is primarily nonoliguric, and kaliuresis frequently results in hypokalemia. The initial symptom of leptospirosis is interstitial nephritis. A renal biopsy demonstrates interstitial edema, mononuclear cell infiltration, and a minimal number of eosinophils. It is also possible to have ATN, which mostly affects the proximal tubules. Usually, glomeruli are unharmed. AKI causes the levels of serum creatinine and blood urea nitrogen to rise quickly. In the second phase, serological testing is typically used for diagnosis. Early diagnosis is provided by polymerase chain reaction antigen detection. A screening test that can be utilized is the macroscopic agglutination test. Using dark-field illumination, leptospirae can be found in the urine between 1 and 4 weeks after infection. Doxycycline or crystalline penicillin may speed the improvement of leptospiruria and reduce the length of hospitalization and fever. It has been demonstrated that intravenous ceftriaxone (1 g once day) or cefotaxime (1 g every 6 hours) has penicillin-like effectiveness.

Human Immunodeficiency Virus

Acute kidney injury is a common complication in HIV-positive patients, with a 2.8 odds ratio for developing the condition in those on highly active antiretroviral therapy (HAART) and a sixfold increased risk of in-hospital mortality in HIV patients who have never received HAART. ATN secondary to sepsis, hypotension, dehydration, and nephrotoxins are the known causes of AKI. HIV-related AKI has increased throughout the post-HAART era as a result of the nephrotoxicity of tenofovir and other antibiotics. Other uncommon causes include acute interstitial nephritis (AIN) owing to immunological restoration inflammatory syndrome, extrarenal blockage from retroperitoneal fibrosis, bladder dysfunction, nephrolithiasis, and intrarenal obstruction from medication-induced crystalluria.

Hemorrhagic Viral Fevers

These illnesses are brought on by RNA viruses that are members of the Flaviviridae, Arenaviridae, Bunyaviridae, and Filoviridae families. In around 60% of cases, renal failure has no obvious cause. Rarely dengue fever may result in AKI, which is typically accompanied by hemolysis, rhabdomyolysis, and hypotension. Incidence rates of AKI have been found by Lee et al. to be 4.9% in Chinese patients with severe dengue. The incidence of AKI in dengue fever in India was 14.51%. Tropical Africa has an endemic yellow fever epidemic. Severe cases of anuria and ATN are common. The renal epithelium can be used to demonstrate viral antigens.

Various Other infections

A rare cause of AKI is renal mucormycosis, which manifests as vascular invasion, thrombosis, infarction, and necrosis. These symptoms typically include lumbar pain in a patient with a high fever and hematuria. The kidneys seem enlarged on computed tomography (CT) and ultrasonography, and there is evidence of peri- or intrarenal abscesses. An absence of renal perfusion is visible on a contrast CT scan. Amphotericin B is administered systemically and after severe debridement.

In the tropics, AKI associated with scrub typhus is not uncommon, and it should be suspected in individuals who have been exposed to the environment and have high-grade fever, variable degrees of ARF, and an eschar. In addition to renal biopsy, immunofluorescence methods can be used to make the diagnosis. The processes include *Orientia tsutsugamushi* direct invasion-induced ATN and rhabdomyolysis-induced intravascular hemolysis. Patients respond favorably to doxycycline.

Up to 61% of patients with acute septic melioidosis had AKI. ATN, interstitial nephritis, and very occasionally microabscesses have been observed in renal histology.

Rarely, myoglobinuria or intravascular hemolysis caused by typhoid might result in AKI.

Snakebite

A significant health issue in the tropics is poisonous snakebites, which account for 3% of all AKI cases in India. AKI is caused by snakes from the Elapidae, Viperidae, Colubridae, and Hydrophidae families. Myoglobinuria, proteinuria, hematuria, pigmenturia, rhabdomyolysis, and hematuria are some of the typical clinical manifestations. Within a few hours to 96 hours following the bite, kidney damage can happen and in up to 94% of patients, it is oligoanuric.

The most frequent histologic feature is ATN, which has various degrees of interstitial edema and inflammatory cell infiltration. Additionally discussed are AIN, crescentic glomerulonephritis on occasion, and necrotizing arteritis of the interlobular arteries. The typical pathogenic mechanisms include direct nephrotoxicity, hypovolemia, hemolysis, myoglobinuria, and disseminated intravascular coagulation. Prior to the onset of AKI, early administration of a particular monovalent antivenom is essential. The only antivenom available in most tropical nations is polyvalent. If antivenom is not available, plasmapheresis and blood exchange can be utilized. Early and frequent dialysis procedures are recommended.

Bee sting: Large amounts of venom are released into the bloodstream from several stings following a swarm attack, leading to severe multisystemic consequences, such as hemolysis, rhabdomyolysis, coagulation problems, cardiac, pulmonary, hepatic, and nervous system abnormalities, hypertension, and AKI.

Scorpion: The venom of scorpions induces excessive autonomic activity as well as a significant production of inflammatory cytokines and vasoactive compounds. Renal ischemia brought on by vasoconstriction, hemodynamic instability, rhabdomyolysis, severe systemic inflammation, and direct venom nephrotoxicity are likely the mechanisms of renal injury. ATN, glomerular alterations, interstitial infiltration, thrombotic microangiopathy, and cortical necrosis (CN) are all present in the renal histology.

CLUES TO DIAGNOSIS

Diagnosis of fever with AKI can be very challenging. Investigations do aid us in the diagnosis for the same, however, it takes time. Also, availability of the tests might be limited. For example, serology to diagnose *Leptospira* might not be available in all setups. Hence, it is imperative to have clinical knowledge and clues to diagnose the diseases by following the syndromic approach **(Table 1)**.

DIAGNOSIS

- Diagnosis depends on the clinical presentation. History, clinical examination, and geographical location aid to the diagnosis.
- Complete blood count with liver function test (LFT) and renal function test (RFT) is the basic blood investigations done.
- Chest X-ray along with ultrasound of the abdomen is a must.
- Urinalysis is performed. Blood and urine cultures are sent.
- Further tests are done depending upon presentation. Serologies for *Leptospira*, scrub typhus, typhoid, and dengue are sent.
- Peripheral blood smear helps in the diagnosis of malaria and toxic granules might be seen in sepsis.

MANAGEMENT

Management depends on identification of the offending agents. However, a generalized approach to management is outlined:

- *Input and output monitoring*: This is the most crucial step as it aims to make the patient euvolemic. Fluid bolus with normal saline (NS) is given along with maintenance fluid in dehydrated patients. Periodic monitoring of RFT and electrolytes is mandatory. We can take help of bedside ultrasonography (USG) to assess fluid status by measuring caval index. Pulmonary artery catheterization is an invasive way to assess fluid status.
- *Avoiding nephrotoxic drugs*: It is important to further decrease the damage to nephrons. Also, it is important to modify the drug dosage as per creatinine clearance.
- *Hemodialysis*: It is indicated in patients with uncorrectable acidosis and electrolyte imbalance, dialyzable drug overdose, and uremia. Continuous venovenous hemodialysis (CVVHD) is preferred for patients with hypotension and hemodynamic instability.

TABLE 1: Clues to diagnosis.

Pattern of organ involvement with tropical febrile illness	Differential diagnosis
Fever + jaundice	Leptospirosis, malaria, dengue, hantavirus, rickettsiosis
Biphasic fever + conjunctival suffusion + thrombocytopenia + transaminitis	Leptospirosis
Continuous fever + severe respiratory symptoms leading to acute respiratory distress syndrome (ARDS)	Hantavirus
Fever + severe myalgia + thrombocytopenia + acalculous cholecystitis	Dengue fever
Fever + maculopapular rash + "eschar"	Scrub typhus
Fever + splenomegaly + thrombocytopenia	Malaria
Fever + exposure to unpasteurized milk products	Brucellosis
Fever + diarrhea	Bacterial or viral gastroenteritis

CONCLUSION

A balanced clinical approach to the problem is very important in the tropics due to the changing disease burden, the late presentation of patients to healthcare facilities, and the lack of resources to support patients with established AKI in many regions. The mortality of patients with AKI in the tropics is unacceptably high. In the tropics, a well-rounded clinical approach to the issue is absolutely essential. The treating physician in rural centers should be capable of managing minor causes of AKI and promptly referring patients who need critical care. Treatment of AKI in rural regions is primarily accomplished by transferring the patient to an advanced facility for renal replacement therapy. To accelerate the growth of healthcare in these areas, it is necessary to invest in patient education, fundamental research infrastructure to obtain a true picture of the epidemiology, the use of new clinical biomarkers, and additional resources.

SUGGESTED READINGS

1. Lameire N, Van Biesen W, Vanholder R. Acute renal failure. Lancet. 2005;365(9457):417-30.
2. Jayakumar M, Prabahar MR, Fernando EM, Manorajan R, Venkatraman R, Balaraman V. Epidemiologic trend changes in acute renal failure—a tertiary center experience from South India. Ren Fail. 2006;28(5):405-10.
3. Vikrant S, Gupta D, Singh M. Epidemiology and outcome of acute kidney injury from a tertiary care hospital in India. Saudi J Kidney Dis Transpl. 2018;29(4):956-66.
4. Basu G, Chrispal A, Boorugu H, Gopinath KG, Chandy S, Prakash JA, et al. Acute kidney injury in tropical acute febrile illness in a tertiary care centre—RIFLE criteria validation. Nephrol Dial Transplant. 2011;26(2):524-31.
5. Mishra SK, Das BS. Malaria and acute kidney injury. Semin Nephrol. 2008;28(4):395-408.
6. Andrade L, Daher EF, Seguro AC. Leptospiral nephropathy. Semin Nephrol. 2008;28:383-94.
7. Wyatt CM, Arons RR, Klotman PE, Klotman ME. Acute renal failure in hospitalized patients with HIV: risk factors and impact on in-hospital mortality. AIDS. 2006;20:561-5.
8. Patel ML, Himanshu D, Chaudhary SC, Atam V, Sachan R, Misra R, et al. Clinical Characteristic and Risk Factors of Acute Kidney Injury among Dengue Viral Infections in Adults: A Retrospective Analysis. Indian J Nephrol. 2019;29(1):15-21.
9. Chugh KS, Sakhuja V, Gupta KL, Jha V, Chakravarty A, Malik N, et al. Renal mucormycosis: computerized tomographic findings and their diagnostic significance. Am J Kidney Dis. 1993;22: 393-7.
10. Kim DM, Kang DW, Kim JO, Chung JH, Kim HL, Park CY, et al. Acute renal failure due to acute tubular necrosis caused by direct invasion of Orientia tsutsugamushi. J Clin Microbiol. 2008;46:1548-50.

72

CHAPTER

Kyasanur Forest Disease

Nitin Gupta

ABSTRACT

Kyasanur forest disease is a tick-borne-viral hemorrhagic fever, endemic to five states (Karnataka, Kerala, Tamil Nadu, Maharashtra, and Goa) of India. It is a biphasic disease that occurs usually in the months of December to April in individuals visiting forests or dwelling in nearby areas. It is a biphasic disease with hemorrhagic manifestation in the first phase and neurological manifestations in the second phase. The disease is diagnosed by molecular tests in the early part of the illness and serology in the late part. The treatment is primarily supportive, and a fraction of the patients may need critical care support. Tick protective measures while visiting forests and vaccines play some role in prevention.

INTRODUCTION

Kyasanur forest disease (KFD) is named after the namesake forest area in the district of Shimoga in Karnataka, India. The disease was first reported in the Shimoga district but has now expanded geographically to 16 districts of India. In the year 1957, several cases of deaths were reported in monkeys. This was followed by a large outbreak in humans. A ribonucleic acid (RNA) virus belonging to the Flaviviridae family was identified from samples from monkeys and humans. All the cases presented in the months of December to April and had a definite history of visits to the forest. The outbreaks were heralded by the smell of dead monkeys in forests and most cases reported a history of tick bites. From these clues, it was inferred that KFD is transmitted by the bite of hard ticks that are active in the forests. This chapter summarizes the epidemiology, clinical features, diagnosis, treatment, and prevention of KFD.

EPIDEMIOLOGY

- Kyasanur forest disease has been reported from five states in India. More than 900 cases have been reported so far with an estimated annual number of 160 cases. Karnataka was the first state to report the outbreak in 1957. The disease was initially reported in Shimoga district but has gradually expanded to involve Gulbarga, Chikmagalur, Dakshin Kannada, Udupi, Belgaum, and Chamarajanagara. Since 2012, the states of Tamil Nadu (Mamallapuram), Kerala (Wayanad), Maharashtra (Sindhudurg), and Goa (North) have also reported cases of KFD.
- Kyasanur forest disease is caused by an RNA *Flavivirus* (agent) and is transmitted by the bite of a hard tick, *Haemaphysalis spinigera* (vector). The nymphal forms of the ticks are responsible for transmission and are most active in the dry season. The ticks feed on animals such as rodents, monkeys, and cattle. Agriculturists/woodcutters venture into the forest to retrieve wood in the dry season (December to April). This increases the risk of transmission **(Fig. 1)**. Incidentally, the nymphal forms (responsible for transmission) of the ticks are the most active during this season. In recent times, laborers working in plantations (cashew nut and areca nut) are at the most risk as naturally occurring forests have been replaced by plantations.
- Animals can be reservoirs of the disease and the disease is specifically deadly in monkeys. While the disease is fatal in monkeys (black-faced langur and red-faced bonnet monkey) **(Fig. 2)**, cattle can act as a reservoir. Humans can acquire the infection when they come in

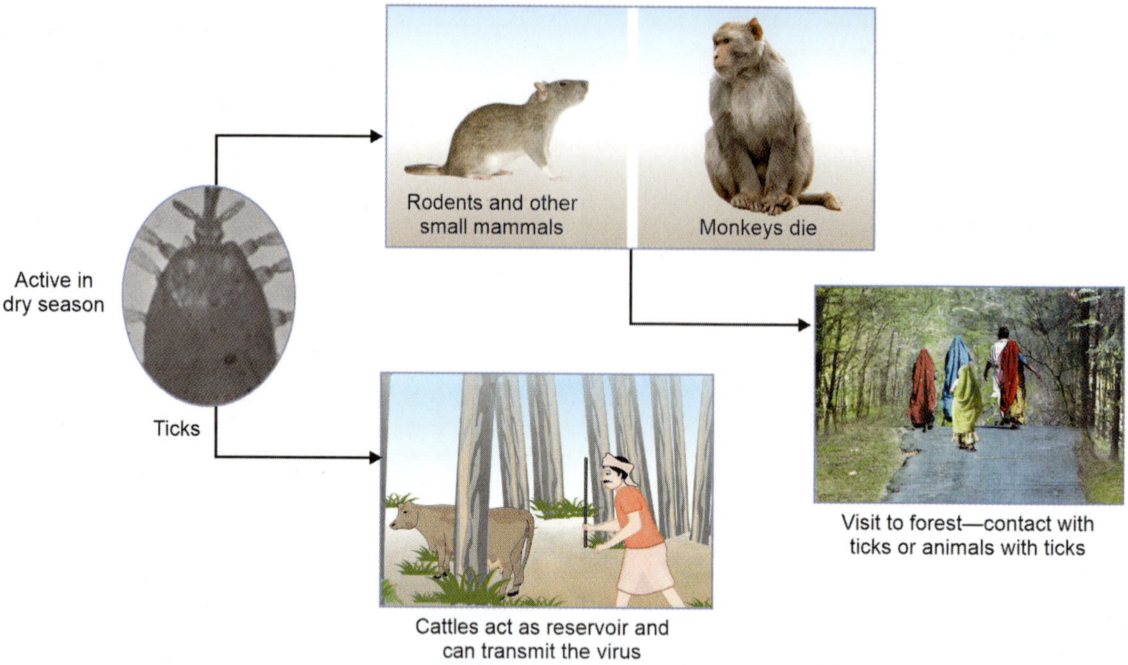

FIG. 1: Schematic diagram showing the transmission cycle of Kyasanur forest disease.

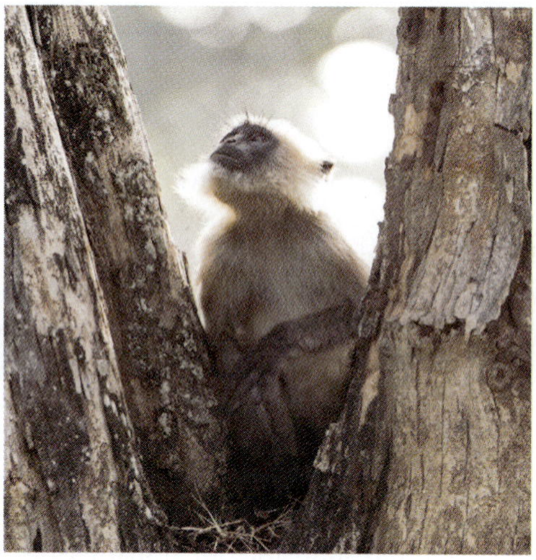

FIG. 2: Black-faced langur photographed in a Kyasanur forest disease endemic area.

contact with the animals harboring these ticks. With increasing deforestation and human activity in the deforestation area, the disease is increasingly being reported in people settled in villages near forests. Cattle grazing in the forest are likely to be responsible for importing the ticks into the villages. Therefore, working with cattle and piled-up dry leaves were risk factors for infection. In some regions of Kerala, tribes hunt monkeys, putting them at risk of acquiring infections.

- One of the first few cases of KFD has been described in **Figure 3** to demonstrate the epidemiology of KFD.

CLINICAL FEATURES

- Most cases are seen in middle-aged male adults (30–45 years). This distribution is primarily due to the acquisition of KFD cases being linked to outdoor work. Since the tick habitats are expanding into the villages with the help of cattle reservoirs and the traditional gender roles are changing, recent reports suggest an increasing number of KFD cases in the female population.
- Kyasanur forest disease is a biphasic disease with two distinct phases **(Table 1)**. The first phase is characterized by fever, severe myalgia, serositis, hemorrhagic manifestations, and encephalopathy. The pathognomonic signs of KFD, conjunctival suffusion, and palatal petechiae are described in the first phase. The second phase has been described to occur in 12–18% of the patients after 1–3 weeks. The manifestations in the second phase are mild and are hypothesized to be immunological in nature. Primarily, aseptic meningitis or cerebellitis has been described in the second phase.

DIAGNOSIS

In the early days of illness, polymerase chain reaction (PCR) in blood to detect the viral RNA is the diagnostic

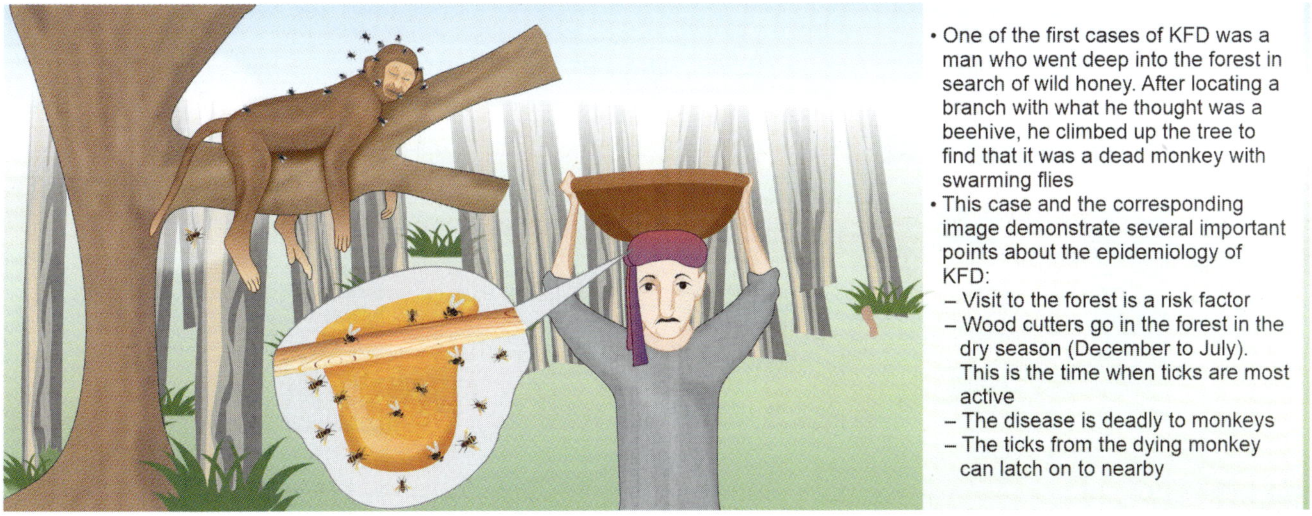

FIG. 3: Clinical case demonstrating epidemiology of Kyasanur forest disease (KFD).

TABLE 1: Comparison of clinical and laboratory features of the first and second phases of Kyasanur forest disease.

Clinical features	First phase	Second phase
Constitutional features	Fever and severe myalgia	Fever and headache
Bleeding manifestations	Present (8–63%)	Absent
Serositis	Present (due to increased vascular permeability)	Absent
Severity	Can be severe	Usually milder
Neurological manifestations	• Altered sensorium, encephalopathy and bleed/infarcts • No CSF pleocytosis	Postinfectious cerebellitis, leptomeningeal enhancement, and CSF pleocytosis
Hematological parameters	High hematocrit, leukopenia, thrombocytopenia and elevated APTT	Leukocytosis
Biochemical parameters	Elevated CPK and AST/ALT	-

(ALT: alanine transaminase; APTT: activated partial thromboplastin time; AST: aspartate transaminase; CSF: cerebrospinal fluid; CPK: creatine phosphokinase)

modality of choice. *NS-5* is the commonly targeted gene for diagnosis. By the second week, enzyme-linked immunosorbent assay (ELISA) to detect antibody response becomes the preferred modality. In the first 3 days of the illness, PCR positivity in KFD is very high. After day 4, it gradually decreases. During this time, the antibody response starts mounting, and the positivity for immunoglobulin M (IgM) increases as the day progresses.

Differential Diagnosis

The following differentials have been identified for KFD:

- Bacterial (scrub typhus, leptospirosis, and enteric fever), viral [coronavirus disease 2019 (COVID-19), dengue, and chikungunya] and parasitic (malaria) infections. The comparative clinical and laboratory manifestations of KFD and its differentials have been summarized in **Table 2**.

TREATMENT

- The treatment of KFD is primarily supportive. In the first phase, due to increased permeability, fluid moves from the intravascular to the extravascular compartment. This leads to hemoconcentration and shock. Prompt management with intravenous fluids is paramount to prevent mortality in such cases. Bleeding manifestations due to severe thrombocytopenia may require management with platelet transfusion and/or fresh frozen plasma.
- In the second phase, the primary challenge is to manage the headache. It must be emphasized here that there is no requirement to treat aseptic meningitis with antibiotics.
- The pooled case fatality rate with KFD in an analysis was found to be 2.4%. Higher age, myocarditis, altered sensorium in the first phase, hypotension at

TABLE 2: Differential diagnosis of patients with Kyasanur forest disease.

Disease	Fever	Palate	Rash	GI	Jaundice	Eyes	LN	HS	Hb↓	TLC↓	TLC↑	Plt↓	LFT↑	Cr↑	CRP↑
COVID-19	Y	N	N	N	N	N	N	N	N	?Y	N	N	N	N	?Y
Dengue	Y	Y	Y	Y	N	N	?Y	N	N	Y	N	Y	Y	N	N
Malaria	Y	N	N	?Y	Y	N	N	?Y	Y	N	N	Y	Y	Y	N
Chikungunya	Y	N	Y	N	N	N	?Y	N	N	Y	N	Y	N	N	N
Scrub typhus	Y	N	?Y	N	?Y	?Y	?Y	Y	?Y	N	Y	Y	Y	?Y	Y
Leptospirosis	Y	N	N	?Y	Y	Y	N	N	?Y	N	Y	Y	Y	Y	Y
Enteric fever	Y	N	?Y	Y	N	N	N	Y	?Y	?Y	Y	Y	?Y		Y
KFD	Y	Y	Y		N	Y	Y	N	N	Y (first)	Y (second)	Y (first)	Y	N	N

Notes:

- Hb↓—anemia, TLC↓—leukopenia, TLC↑—leukocytosis, Plt↓—thrombocytopenia, LFT↑—elevated transaminases (>40 IU/L), Cr↑—acute kidney injury, CRP↑—elevated CRP
- Y: yes; N: no; ?Y: may be seen; First—the first phase of KFD; Second—the second phase of KFD
- Labeling: Red indicates not present, green indicates present, and yellow indicates may be present.

(COVID-19: coronavirus disease 2019; Cr: creatinine; CRP: C-reactive protein; GI: gastrointestinal; Hb: hemoglobin; HS: hepatosplenomegaly; KFD: Kyasanur forest disease; LFT: liver function test; LN: lymphadenitis; Plt: platelet count; TLC: total leukocyte count)

admission, lower platelet count, higher transaminases, higher activated partial thromboplastin time (APTT), and higher creatine phosphokinase (CPK) levels were found to be predictors of mortality in a study from Karnataka. Since more than half of the patients are managed at the primary care level, it is important to identify these predictors and refer these patients early to tertiary care settings.

PREVENTION

- Antitick measures before going to the forest—full-length clothes, use of repellent oils, and washing clothes in warm water after return from the forest
- Avoid cattle grazing in deep forests so that ticks do not latch on to them. Weekly washing and removal of ticks from cattle should be done.
- Indigenously developed formalized virus vaccine has shown to have inadequate efficacy. Two doses one-month apart vaccine followed by boosters are recommended. In a study by Kasabi et al., vaccination did not alter the odds of developing KFD.

CONCLUSION

Kyasanur forest disease should be suspected if a patient presents with febrile illness from endemic areas between December and April and there is a history of forest visits or tick bites. In the first phase, hemorrhage, shock, and altered sensorium are a cause of concern. Eyes and mouth should be examined to look for pathognomonic signs of KFD. The diagnostic investigation of choice in early illness is PCR and IgM ELISA in late illness. The treatment is supportive and early predictors of mortality should be sought for early referral.

SUGGESTED READINGS

1. Work TH, Trapido H, Murthy DPN, Rao RL, Bhatt PN, Kulkarni KG. Kyasanur forest disease. III. A preliminary report on the nature of the infection and clinical manifestations in human beings. Indian J Med Sci. 1957;11(8):619-45.
2. Chakraborty S, Andrade FCD, Ghosh S, Uelmen J, Ruiz MO. Historical Expansion of Kyasanur Forest Disease in India From 1957 to 2017: A Retrospective Analysis. GeoHealth. 2019;3(2):44-55.
3. Kasabi GS, Murhekar MV, Yadav PD, Raghunandan R, Kiran SK, Sandhya VK, et al. Kyasanur Forest Disease, India, 2011–2012. Emerg Infect Dis. 2013;19(2):278-81.
4. Webb HE, Rao RL. Kyasanur forest disease: a general clinical study in which some cases with neurological complications were observed. Trans R Soc Trop Med Hyg. 1961;55:284-98.
5. Gupta N, Chunduru K, Safeer K M, Saravu K. Clinical and laboratory profile of patients with Kyasanur forest disease: A single-centre study of 192 patients from Karnataka, India. J Clin Virol. 2021;135:104735.
6. Gupta N, Nallapati VT, Chunduru K, Vithivattical ARJ, Kadavigere R, Saravu K. Neurological manifestations of Kyasanur Forest disease: a retrospective cohort study from South India. Trans R Soc Trop Med Hyg. 2022;116(10):944-8.
7. Yadav PD, Gurav YK, Shete AM, Jain R, Nyayanit DA, Pardeshi PG, et al. Kinetics of viral RNA, immunoglobulin-M & G antibodies in Kyasanur forest disease. Indian J Med Res. 2019;150(2):186-93.
8. Gupta N, Wilson W, Neumayr A, Saravu K. Kyasanur forest disease: a state-of-the-art review. QJM. 2022;115(6):351-8.

73

CHAPTER

Expanded Dengue Syndrome: The Spectrum

Rantu Barman

ABSTRACT

World Health Organization (WHO) has coined the term expanded dengue syndrome (EDS) for dengue cases that have unusual manifestations with severe organ involvement such as liver, kidneys, brain, and heart reported in dengue hemorrhagic fever (DHF) and also in dengue patients who do not have evidence of plasma leakage. These unusual manifestations may be associated with coinfections, comorbidities, or complications of prolonged shock. There are increasing reports of under-recognized and infrequent manifestations of dengue with severe organ involvement. In this article gives knowledge of the spectrum of EDS which will help to clinch the diagnosis of dengue early, particularly during the ongoing epidemics, and timely interventions which would in turn reduce the mortality and morbidity associated with dengue.

INTRODUCTION

Dengue fever is a mosquito-borne viral infection transmitted to humans via the bite of infected female *Aedes aegypti*, *Aedes albopictus*, *Aedes scutellaris*, and *Aedes polynesiensis*. Dengue virus (DENV) is an arthropod-borne virus of genus *Flavivirus* belonging to the family *Flaviviridae*. It is a single-stranded ribonucleic acid (RNA) virus. There are four genetically related but antigenetically distinct Dengue serotypes (DENV-1, DENV-2, DENV-3 and DENV-4) all of which are prevalent in India.

After dengue virus infection and an average incubation period of 4–7 days, three evolving phases are described, that are (1) febrile phase, (2) critical phase, and (3) recovery phase. In most patients, dengue begins with the typical sudden onset of fever, frontal headache, retro-orbital pain, back pain, severe myalgias, and rash.

Dengue may manifest as asymptomatic, undifferentiated fever, dengue fever, dengue hemorrhagic fever (DHF), and dengue shock syndrome (DSS). Apart from the classical presentation of dengue, there have been many atypical manifestations that have led to diagnostic challenges to the treating physician. Therefore in 2011, WHO incorporated a new terminology known as expanded dengue syndrome (EDS) where patients usually present with atypical manifestations with various systemic involvement.

MANIFESTATIONS OF DENGUE VIRUS INFECTION (FLOWCHART 1)

Dengue may manifest as asymptomatic, undifferentiated fever, dengue fever, DHF and DSS. Apart from the classical presentation of dengue, there have been many atypical manifestations which have led to diagnostic challenges to the treating physician. Therefore in 2011 WHO incorporated a new terminology known as EDS where patient usually presents with atypical manifestations with various systemic involvement.

GLOBAL BURDEN OF DISEASES

The most clinically significant flaviviruses that cause the fever and myalgia syndrome are dengue viruses. Dengue is probably the most prevalent arthropod-borne viral disease worldwide, with 400 million infections occurring per year of which almost 100 million (25%) cause clinical illness. More than half of the world's population is considered to be at risk, although Asia bears 70% of the global burden with an alarming increase over the past decade. Dengue

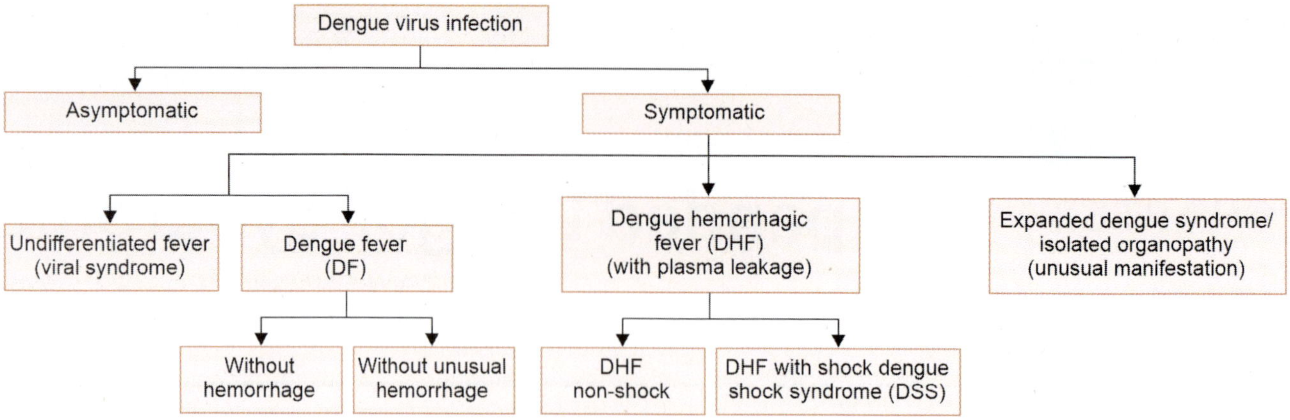

FLOWCHART 1: Manifestations of dengue virus infection (WHO 2011).

cases in India are also on a sharp rise over the past few years to the tune of 28,292 cases in 2010 to 111,880 cases in 2016.

PATHOPHYSIOLOGY

The pathogenesis of dengue virus infection is attributed to the complex interplay between the virus, host factors, and host immune response. Multiple factors including viral load, nonstructural 1 (NS1), anti-NS1 antibodies, infecting serotype and genotype may contribute to the severity of dengue infection. Both innate immunity such as the complement system and NK cells and the adoptive immunity including humoral and cell-mediated immunity are involved in this process.

The hallmark of DHF is the increased vascular permeability resulting in plasma leakage, contracted intravascular volume, and shock in severe cases.

EXPANDED DENGUE SYNDROME-MANIFESTATIONS

Unusual manifestations are uncommon. In recent years with the geographical spread of dengue illness and with more involvement of adults, there have been increasing reports of DF and DHF with unusual manifestations. These include neurological, hepatic, renal, and other isolated organ involvements. These could be explained as complications of severe prolonged shock or associated with underlying host conditions/diseases or coinfections.

High-risk Patients

The following host factors contribute to more severe disease and its complications:
- Infants and elderly
- Obesity
- Pregnant women
- Peptic ulcer disease
- Women who have menstruation or abnormal vaginal bleeding
- Hemolytic diseases, such as glucose-6-phosphate dehydrogenase (G6PD) deficiency and thalassemia
- Congenital heart disease
- Chronic diseases, such as diabetes mellitus, hypertension, asthma, ischemic heart disease, chronic renal failure, and liver cirrhosis
- Patients on steroid or nonsteroidal anti-inflammatory drugs (NSAIDs) treatment

Expanded Dengue Syndrome (Unusual or Atypical Manifestation of Dengue)

See **Table 1**.

Neurological Manifestations

The neurological manifestations of dengue are mainly associated with dengue serotype-2 and dengue serotype-3. Neurological involvement in dengue fever is grouped into three groups:
1. Direct tissue invasion of virus (neurotropicity)—encephalitis, meningitis, meningoencephalitis, and myelitis.
2. Secondary to systemic complications and metabolic alterations—encephalopathy and stroke.
3. Postinfective sequelae including immune-mediated such as acute disseminated encephalomyelitis (ADEM), Guillain-Barré syndrome (GBS), Miller-Fisher syndrome, phrenic neuropathy, oculomotor palsy, Reye's syndrome, maculopathy, and neuropsychiatric manifestations such as amnesia, dementia, and manic psychosis.

   Encephalopathy is the most common neurological manifestation of dengue. The pathophysiology of dengue encephalopathy is multifactorial and is due to

TABLE 1: Expanded dengue syndrome (unusual or atypical manifestation of dengue).

Neurological	• Febrile seizures in young children • Encephalopathy • Encephalitis/Aseptic meningitis • Intracranial hemorrhages/thrombosis • Subdural effusions • Mononeuropathies/Polyneuropathies/ Guillain–Barré syndrome • Transverse myelitis
Gastrointestinal/ Hepatic	• Hepatitis/Fulminant hepatic failure • Acalculous cholecystitis • Acute pancreatitis • Hyperplasia of Peyer's patches • Acute parotitis
Renal	• Acute renal failure • Hemolytic uremic syndrome
Cardiac	• Conduction abnormalities • Myocarditis • Pericarditis
Respiratory	• Acute respiratory distress syndrome • Pulmonary hemorrhage
Musculoskeletal	• Myositis with raised creatinine phosphokinase (CPK) • Rhabdomyolysis
Lymphoreticular/ Bone marrow	• Infection-associated hemophagocytic syndrome • Hemophagocytic lymphohistiocytosis (HLH) and idiopathic thrombocytopenic purpura (ITP) • Spontaneous splenic rupture • Lymph node infarction
Eye	• Macular hemorrhage • Impaired visual acuity • Optic neuritis
Others	• Postinfectious fatigue syndrome, depression, hallucinations, and psychosis • Alopecia

Source: Gulati S, Maheswari A,. Atypical manifestations of dengue. Trop Med Int Health. 2007;12(9):1087-95.

cerebral edema, hypoxia, hemorrhage, and associated systemic dysfunction such as shock, hyponatremia, liver, and kidney failure.

Acute encephalitic syndrome (AES) is an illness where fever is associated with altered sensorium with or without seizures and focal neurological deficits. Initially, it was thought that dengue was an uncommon cause of AES, but due to its increased prevalence dengue has become one of the major causes of AES particularly in dengue-endemic zone after Japanese encephalitis.

Both hemorrhagic and ischemic stroke can occur in DHF. Bleeding manifestations are more common than cerebral infarct due to vasculopathy coupled with thrombocytopenia and platelet dysfunction usually leading to intracranial hemorrhage. Ischemic stroke is caused by disseminated intravascular coagulation (DIC), vasculopathy, and increased level of plasminogen activator inhibitor type 1.

Acute disseminated encephalomyelitis is extremely rare, and usually occurs via molecular mimicry or autoimmune reactions after dengue infection. GBS and mononeuropathies in dengue infection is due to an evoked immune response directed toward the myelin of the axon or peripheral nerve because of the sharing of cross-reactive epitomes (molecular mimicry).

Gastrointestinal/Hepatobiliary Manifestations

Dengue patients with involvement of gastrointestinal and hepatic systems may present with features of asymptomatic elevation of liver enzymes, fulminant hepatic failure, acute pancreatitis, acalculous cholecystitis, peritonitis, subacute intestinal obstruction (SAIO), and rupture of spleen. Transaminitis is observed in 30% of patients. The pathogenesis is a direct viral invasion of hepatocytes and Kupffer's cells, immune mechanism also plays a role. Fulminant hepatic failure is seen in 60–70% of individuals and occurs secondary to shock and DIC in severe dengue fever.

Acalculous cholecystitis has been documented as 27.5%. Direct viral invasion with plasma leakage and serous effusions from increased vascular permeability leads to the thickening of the gall bladder wall and edema in DHF patients.

Acute pancreatitis is an atypical and rare manifestation of dengue. The exact pathogenesis of pancreatic involvement is poorly understood but has been postulated to result either from direct invasion by the virus itself causing inflammation and destruction of pancreatic acinar cells or pancreatic damage due to DSS. Acute pancreatitis in dengue usually is benign and self-limiting.

Cardiovascular Manifestations

A diversity of cardiac manifestations has been reported in dengue infection. Cardiovascular manifestations are caused by serotype 2 and serotype 3 dengue viruses which range from asymptomatic bradycardia to life-threatening myocarditis. Myocarditis is the most common cardiac manifestation. Patients with dengue fever have a variety of rhythm abnormalities which range from sinus tachycardia, heart block, and atrial fibrillation to paroxysmal supraventricular tachycardia (PSVT).

Respiratory Manifestations

Pleural effusion is the most frequent cause of dyspnea in dengue fever, usually bilateral. Lung parenchymal involvement is a less common finding which includes ground glass abnormality, consolidation, interlobular septal thickening, and pulmonary hemorrhage. Extensive lung abnormalities are infrequent even in severe disease and when present should lead physicians to consider other diagnostic possibilities.

Acute lung injury and acute respiratory distress syndrome (ARDS) are the most dreaded complications of DHF/DSS secondary to interstitial and alveolar-capillary membrane permeability leading to interstitial and alveolar edema. Pulmonary hemorrhage is fatal but rare.

Renal Manifestations

The most common renal manifestation is pre-renal acute kidney injury which is related to dehydration and third space fluid loss. Hyponatremia is the most common electrolyte abnormality found in dengue fever. Hyponatremia occurs due to temporary inappropriate antidiuretic hormone secretion and temporary failure of sodium-potassium pump. The incidence of renal manifestations varies from 17 to 62% in dengue fever. Other renal manifestations include proteinuria, glomerulonephritis, IgA nephropathy, hemolytic uremic syndrome, and acute tubular necrosis (ATN).

Hematological Manifestations

Hematological manifestations are thrombocytopenia, atypical lymphocytosis, DIC, hemophagocytic lymphohistiocytosis (HLH), cytopenias, lymphadenopathy, hepatomegaly, and splenomegaly have been reported in dengue fever. Furthermore, idiopathic thrombocytopenic purpura (ITP) and pancytopenia, with bone marrow biopsy revealing aplastic anemia have been described following dengue fever.

Spontaneous and nontraumatic splenic rupture is a rare but potentially lethal manifestation of EDS.

Coinfection

Malaria is the most common coinfection seen with dengue fever. *Plasmodium falciparum* is most commonly associated with malaria with dengue as per Indian studies; however, *Plasmodium vivax* coinfection has also been reported.

Aedes aegypti is common vector for both dengue and chikungunya. Chikungunya fever is often misdiagnosed as dengue infection. However, clinically suspected cases should be listed for both viruses in endemic areas, especially in the monsoon season.

CONCLUSION

Although the atypical presentation of dengue is on the rise, EDS is under-recognized and under-reported. In a clinical scenario, the occurrence of atypical and systemic manifestations should prompt the treating physician to investigate for dengue especially during an epidemic. A thorough and sensible knowledge of EDS and a high degree of clinical suspicion is the key for early diagnosis and treatment. Coinfection and underlying comorbidities should be addressed early and treated accordingly to reduce mortality and morbidity.

SUGGESTED READINGS

1. Pangtey GS, Prakash A, Munjal YP. Role of Carica papaya Leaf Extract for Dengue Associated Thrombocytopenia. J Assoc Physicians India. 2016;64(6):11-3.
2. World Health Organization. Dengue: guidelines for diagnosis, treatment, prevention and control. Geneva: World Health Organization; 2009.
3. Umakanth M, Suganthan N. Unusual manifestations of dengue fever: a review on expanded dengue syndrome. Cureus. 2020;12(9):e10678.
4. Nimagadda SS, Mahabala C, Boloor A, Raghuram PM, Nayak A. Atypical manifestations of dengue fever (DF)-where do we stand today? J Cin Diagn Res. 2014;8(1):71-3.
5. Serufo JC, Nobre V, Rayes A, Marcial TM, Lambertucci JR. Dengue: A reappraisal. Rev Soc Bras Med Trop. 2000;33:465-76.
6. Mohsin N, Mohamed E, Gaber M, Al Obaidani I, Budruddin M, Al Busaidy S. Acute tubular necrosis associated with non-hemorrhagic dengue fever: a case report. Ren Fail. 2009;31(8):736-9.
7. Villamil-Gomez WE, Gonzalez-Camargo O, Rodriguez-Ayubij, Zapata-Serpa D, Rodriguez-Morales AJ. Dengue, chikungunya and Zika co-infection in a patient from Colombia. J Infect Puublic Health. 2016;9(5):684-6.
8. Magalhaes BM, Alexandre MA, Siqueira AM, Melo GC, Gimaque JB, Bastos MS, et al. Clinical profile of concurrent dengue fever and Plasmodium vivax malaria in the Brazilian Amazon: Case series of 11 hospitalized patients. Am J Trop Med Hyg. 2012;87(6):1119-24.

74

CHAPTER

Acute Febrile Illness: Approach and Management

Rajesh M Honnutagi

ABSTRACT

Fever is the most common symptom reported by individuals seeking medical attention, and it may occur either in isolation or in association with other common symptoms. Fever cases that have lasted < 21 days can be undiagnosed in 80% of cases. Acute febrile illness (AFI) is a fever that resolves in 3 weeks without displaying any symptoms or signs specific to a specific organ. The severity of AFIs ranges from mild or self-limiting to life-threatening illness. The most common approach for the management of acute fever depends on the use of antibiotics and supportive therapy with antipyretics. Medical professionals are frequently forced to undertake numerous different analyses in order to conclusively identify an occurrence of AFI due to the vast range of symptoms that fall under the umbrella of AFI. Overlap in the clinical features of AFI and restricted laboratory services make the management of febrile patients in resource-limited settings very challenging. To significantly prevent and reduce the incidence of acute febrile fever, particularly in developing nations, more thorough research is necessary. Several research studies across the nations that clearly describe the causes, symptoms, diagnostic techniques, and therapy approaches to effectively combat AFI will help clinicians in treating these illnesses successfully and more quickly.

INTRODUCTION

Fever is the most common symptom reported by individuals seeking medical attention, and it may occur either in isolation or in association with other common symptoms. Fever that has lasted less than 21 days can be undiagnosed in 80% of cases.

Acute febrile illness (AFI) is a fever that resolves in 3 weeks without displaying any symptoms or signs specific to a specific organ. Patients with infectious diseases often have an AFI. Further, acute febrile illness can be classified based on etiology as nonmalarial AFI, diagnosed AFI, and undiagnosed AFI.

Acute febrile illness signs and symptoms include a high fever lasting > 4 days that fails to subside away after taking the recommended dosage of antibiotics or antivirals, with consistently high body temperatures irritation of the skin, jaundice, typhoid, myalgia, arthralgia, and bleeding problems. The severity of AFIs ranges from mild or self-limiting to life-threatening illness.

ETIOLOGY OF ACUTE FEBRILE ILLNESS

According to the reports, scrub typhus, dengue, malaria, typhoid, and leptospirosis are the major causes of febrile illness in South Asia. Geographical and seasonal diversity, the absence of systematic monitoring, nonspecific syndrome-based fever care guidelines, and a limitation of high-quality diagnostic testing all contribute to the inadequate management of AFIs in India.

The most frequent causes of AFI in hospitalized cases in India include enteric fever, leptospirosis, a form of scrub typhus, dengue fever, and bacterial infections of the circulatory system, particularly those that induce enteric fever. The most common types of fever associated with febrile illnesses in India are dengue and malaria. According to estimates, India accounts for 34% of the global incidence of dengue. According to studies, leptospirosis cases in India range from 3 to 7% **(Flowchart 1)**.

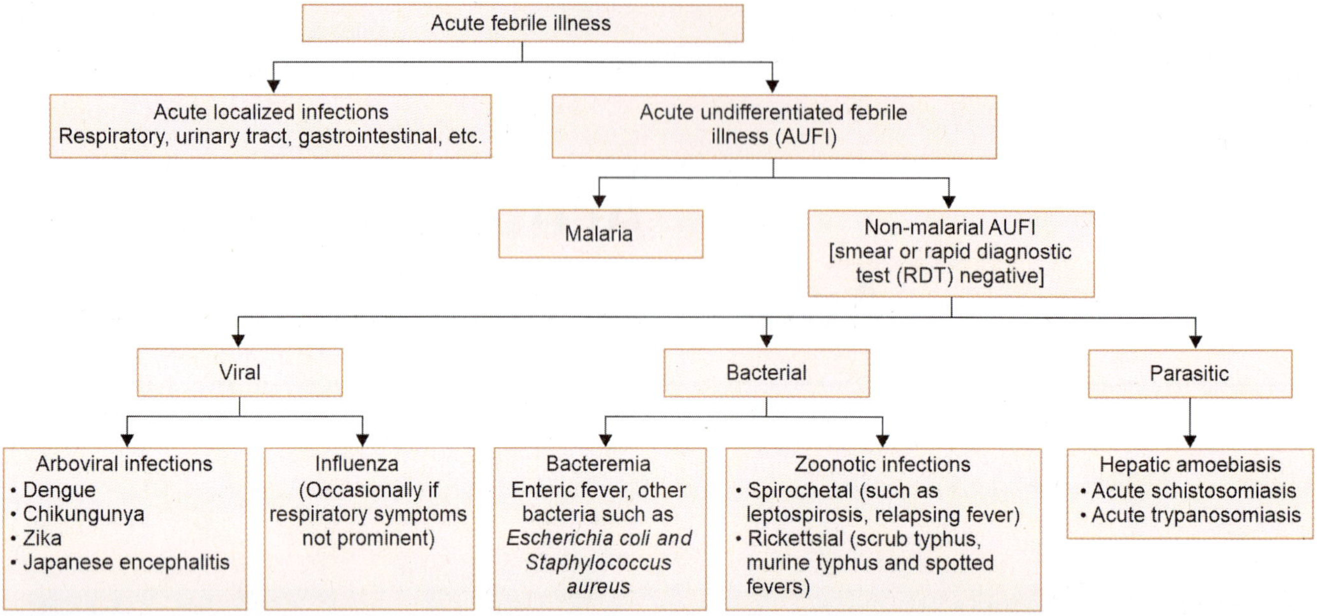

FLOWCHART 1: Etiological factors of acute febrile illness (AFI).

MANAGEMENT OF ACUTE FEBRILE ILLNESS

The care of febrile patients in resource-constrained settings is highly difficult due to an overlap in the clinical manifestations of AFIs and inadequate testing resources. The most common approach for the management of acute fever depends on the use of antibiotics and supportive therapy with antipyretics.

STEPWISE APPROACH FOR EVALUATION OF AFI (TABLES 1 AND 2)

- *Step 1—evaluation of medical history of the patient*: In this step, the patient's previous medical history is evaluated, especially for fevers, infections, or illnesses that are known to predispose to infections. Age, immunosuppression, pregnancy, and comorbidities such as diabetes, chronic kidney disease, cancer, autoimmune illness, rheumatologic fever, and liver impairment that are specific to the patient can help restrict the differential diagnosis and offer valuable information. Assessment of systems must encompass febrile seizures, headache including sinusitis and meningitis, runny nose and congestion, cough or snorting, ear distress or awakening at midnight with symptoms of discomfort (otitis media), abdominal inflammation (pneumonia, strep infections pharyngitis, gastroenteritis, and gastrointestinal abscess), back pain (pyelonephritis) and joint inflammation (osteomyelitis).
- *Step 2—clinical examination of patient*: Preliminary clinical examination should involve the examination of respiratory rate, hydration status, mental status, oropharynx, conjunctiva, skin, chest, heart, and abdomen. Elderly patients need special care if they have underlying medical conditions such as diabetes, problems with swallowing, and cough reflex, ongoing persistent catheters for the urinary tract, prosthetic devices that cause septic arthritis, mental health issues, and chronic immobility.
- *Step 3—evaluation of clinical features and assessment of disease severity*: This involves evaluating the duration of the beginning of the disease, important clinical symptoms to rule in and rule out, and the pattern of organ involvement.
- *Step 4—perform diagnostic tests*: Medical professionals are frequently forced to undertake numerous different analyses in order to conclusively identify an occurrence of AFI due to the vast range of symptoms that fall under the umbrella of AFI. This step involves performing first-line and confirmatory diagnostic tests depending on the day of investigation of the patient and the gravity of the fever. Individuals with fever should undergo a complete blood count, urine analysis, smear microscopy, and/or rapid diagnostic test (RDT), chest X-ray, sputum examination, ultrasound (USG) of the abdomen, etc. In addition to examining the affected person's external signs and symptoms and medical background check is necessary. The main diagnostic procedures include:
    - Peripheral smear examinations
    - RDT

TABLE 1: Evaluation of clinical features of acute undifferentiated febrile illness and assessment of disease severity.

Disease	Onset	Clinical features
Malaria	• *Plasmodium falciparum* (incubation period: 9–14 days) • *Plasmodium vivax* (incubation period: 10–14 days)	• High-intermittent fever with acute onset • Paroxysm of fever, shaking chills, and depending on the type of species, sweating develops every 48 or 72 hours
Dengue	*Incubation period*: 3–14 days with acute onset of high continuous fever (onset of symptom average 4–7 days)	• Headache, retro-orbital pain, myalgia, arthralgia, and rash are all symptoms of dengue fever • Hematocrit increase, mucosal and gastrointestinal bleeding, and thrombocytopenia are all symptoms of dengue hemorrhagic fever • The syndrome of dengue shock low pulse and hypertension • Renal failure, acute respiratory distress syndrome (ARDS), hemophagocytosis, myocarditis, and hepatitis are all symptoms of expanded dengue syndrome
Enteric fever	*Incubation period*: 1–14 days	• *First week*: Comparative bradycardia, a headache, and a fever • *Second week*: Diarrhea, constipation, and abdominal pain • Encephalopathy with hepatosplenomegaly • *Third week*: Multiple organ dysfunction syndrome, perforation, and intestinal hemorrhage
Chikungunya	*Incubation period*: 1–12 days (onset of symptoms: average 3–7 days)	Moderate to high-grade persistent fever, rash, malaise, arthralgia, myalgia, and red eyes that developed suddenly
Leptospirosis	• *Incubation period*: 2–26 days (onset of symptoms: Average 6–10 days) • Moderate-to-high-grade chronic fever with acute onset	• *Anicteric leptospirosis*: ○ Sudden onset of chills, headache, fever, and fatigue ○ An acute skin rash, conjunctival suffusion, and pains in the abdomen • *Icteric leptospirosis*: ○ Jaundice, hematuria, proteinuria, diarrhea, and/or anemia ○ Myocarditis and pulmonary hemorrhages
Scrub typhus	• *Incubation period*: 1–3 weeks	• Myalgia, headache, and fever • Problems with breathing, dizziness, nausea, coughing, and jaundice

TABLE 2: Evaluation of clinical features associated with different types of AFIs due to localized infections.

Fever due to upper respiratory tract infections	• Sore throat, runny or clogged nose, and coughing with or without systemic symptoms such as fever and fatigue, are the main characteristic features of upper respiratory tract infections • *Streptococcal pharyngitis*: Fever and sore throat with swallowing pain develop unexpectedly • *Bacterial sinusitis*: A typical viral upper respiratory tract infection that lasts for 5–6 days. Fever with early onset, headaches, or an increase in discharge from the nose
Fever due to lower respiratory tract infection	Acute lower respiratory tract illness symptoms such as coughing, difficulty in breathing, pleuritic pain in the chest for less than a week, and one systemic feature such as temperature > 37.7°C, cold and rigors, and/or severe fatigue) are a sign of community-acquired pneumonia
Fever due to bone and joint infections	Septic arthritis features include swollen joints along with an aggressively increasing high fever
Fever due to urinary tract infection	Dysuria, along with a fever and chills, is a sign of acute cystitis. Fever coupled with urinary retention and flank pain, and tenderness, are symptoms of acute pyelonephritis
Fever due to server-side template injection	SSTIs involve signs of the inflammatory response, with other manifestations, such as fever and rapid progression of lesions. Cellulitis is characterized by clinically rapidly intensifying pain and redness. Fever and lymphadenopathy may be present
Fever due to intra-abdominal infection	Aggressive bacterial diarrhea is characterized by fever, tenesmus, and grossly bloody feces
Viral fever	Viral pneumonia due to adenovirus, influenza A and B, human metapneumovirus, parainfluenza, rhinovirus, and cytomegalovirus. Characterized by high-grade fever, cough, sore throat, or myalgia

(AFIs: acute febrile illnesses; SSTIs: skin and soft tissue infections)

- Enzyme-linked immunosorbent assay (ELISA)
- Polymerase chain reaction (PCR)
- Treatment options for AFI

CONCLUSION

To significantly prevent and reduce the incidence of AFI, particularly in developing nations, more thorough research is necessary. Several research studies clearly explained the causes, symptoms, diagnostic techniques, and therapy approaches to effectively combat AFIs will help clinicians in treating these illnesses successfully and more quickly. Based on regional or national surveillance information as well as research from hospitals, management guidelines should be evaluated, improved, and locally customized for AFI.

SUGGESTED READINGS

1. Das P, Rahman MZ, Banu S, Rahman M, Chisti MJ, Chowdhury F, et al. Acute febrile illness among outpatients seeking health care in Bangladeshi hospitals prior to the COVID-19 pandemic. PLoS One. 2022;17(9):e0273902.
2. Bhaskaran D, Chadha SS, Sarin S, Sen R, Arafah S, Dittrich S. Diagnostic tools used in the evaluation of acute febrile illness in South India: a scoping review. BMC Infect Dis. 2019;19(1):970.
3. Mørch K, Manoharan A, Chandy S, Singh A, Kuriakose C, Patil S, et al. Clinical features and risk factors for death in acute undifferentiated fever: A prospective observational study in rural community hospitals in six states of India. Trans R Soc Trop Med Hyg. 2023;117(2):91-101.
4. Mørch K, Manoharan A, Chandy S, Chacko N, Alvarez-Uria G, Patil S, et al. Acute undifferentiated fever in India: a multicentre study of aetiology and diagnostic accuracy. BMC Infect Dis. 2017;17(1):665.
5. Bhatt S, Gething PW, Brady OJ, Messina JP, Farlow AW, Moyes CL, et al. The global distribution and burden of dengue. Nature. 2013;496(7446):504-7.
6. Joshi S, Immanuel G, Arulrhaj S, Tiwaskar M, Vora A, Samavedam S. Roadmap for the Management of Acute Undifferentiated Febrile Illness: An Expert Discussion and Review of Available Guidelines. J Assoc Physic India. 2021;69(9):11-2.
7. Bhargava A, Ralph R, Chatterjee B, Bottieau E. Assessment and initial management of acute undifferentiated fever in tropical and subtropical regions. BMJ. 2018;363:k4766.
8. Consolini DM. (2022). Fever in Infants and Children. [online] Available from https://www.msdmanuals.com/en-in/professional/pediatrics/symptoms-in-infants-and-children/fever-in-infants-and-children [Last accessed December, 2023].
9. Indian Medical Association. (2023). Stepwise Guide for Diagnosis and Management of Acute Fever in Primary Care. [online] Available from https://www.ima-india.org/ima/pdfdata/Treatment-Algorithm-Booklet-03122021.pdf [Last accessed December, 2023].
10. Gopalkrishnan R, Ohri VC, Aggarwal S, Walia K. (2019). Treatment guidelines for antimicrobial use in common syndromes. [online] Available from https://main.icmr.nic.in/sites/default/files/guidelines/Treatment_Guidelines_2019_Final.pdf [Last accessed December, 2023].

75

CHAPTER

Changing Clinical Profile of Tropical Infections

Pijush Kanti Mandal, Sandipan Chatterjee

ABSTRACT

Tropical Infections account for a major health problem in those areas. Several factors of the epidemiological triad are responsible for the variation of incidence, prevalence, clinical presentation microbiological resistance, case fatality, and other effects of these infections. Knowledge of these changes is of the utmost importance in better understanding of those diseases and better management.

INTRODUCTION

What are Tropical Infections?

These are infections prevalent in or unique to tropical and subtropical regions and less prevalent in temperate climates. These infections spread via airborne, sexual contact, contaminated food and water, or by insect vectors. Reasons behind the prevalence of these infections in the tropics are the predominant hot climate, a larger volume of rains facilitating the formation of breeding grounds; a larger number of natural reservoirs and a larger number of insects vectors; and poor socioeconomic conditions of tropical countries. Tropical infections may be:

- *Viral*: Dengue, *Rotavirus*, yellow fever, acquired immune deficiency syndrome (AIDS), Ebola, Lassa fever, and rabies
- *Bacterial*: Cholera, *Escherichia coli*, tuberculosis (TB), and leprosy
- *Parasitic*: *Plasmodium*, leishmaniasis, filariasis, schistosomiasis, and trypanosomiasis

NEGLECTED TROPICAL DISEASES

Refers to chronic, debilitating, and often stigmatizing diseases that primarily affect the poorest, particularly in rural areas of tropical and subtropical countries **(Table 1)**.

TABLE 1: Spectrum of neglected tropical diseases (NTD).

Helminth infections	Protozoan infections	Bacterial infections
• Ascariasis • Trichuriasis • Hookworm • Schistosomiasis • Lymphatic filariasis • Onchocerciasis • Dracunculosis	• Leishmaniasis • Chagas disease • African trypanosomiasis	• Trachoma • Leprosy • Buruli ulcer

EPIDEMIOLOGICAL TRIAD

Consists of an external agent, a susceptible host, and an environment that brings the host and agent together. In this model, the disease results from the interaction between the agent and the susceptible host in an environment that supports the transmission of the agent from a source to that host **(Flowchart 1)**.

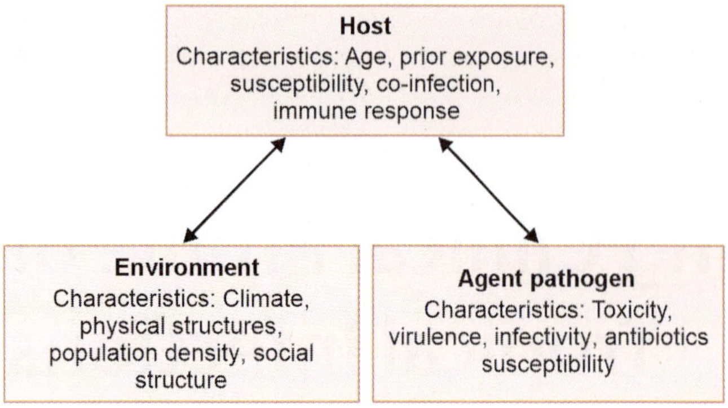

FLOWCHART 1: Epidemiological triad.

FACTORS AFFECTING THE CHANGES IN THE CLINICAL PROFILES OF TROPICAL INFECTIONS

Environment Factors

- Climate changes (such as temperature, precipitation and humidity, wind, and dust).
- Human exploration of tropical rainforest, deforestation, rising immigration, and increased international air travel.
- Changes in hygiene and sanitization status

Agent Factors

Mutation of the agents may lead to different phenotypic changes resulting in variation in the pathogenicity, variable clinical presentation, and changes in antibiotic susceptibility.

Host Factors

- The concerned factors are the level of immunity, genetic factors, and presence of comorbidities over counter antibiotic usage resulting in resistance
- Risk for exposure is affected by behaviors, such as sexual exposure, degrees of hygiene, and protection against mosquito bites.

Alteration in the crucial three elements of the epidemiological triangle leads to variations in the different aspects of the clinical profile of tropical infections. The different elements of the clinical profile of this disease are variously affected.

Disease Transmission

While, personal hygiene, the use of protective devices such as mosquito nets, face masks, and the use of various vaccines prevent disease transmission; on the other hand, poor hygiene, lack of health awareness, and high-risk behavior increase the risk of disease transmission.

Incubation Period

Various climate changes such as temperature changes, rainfall, and humidity as well as antigenic variation in agents result in changes in the incubation period of a disease, e.g., higher temperature facilitates larva development and accelerates the growth of adult *Aedes* and *Anopheles* mosquitos; and also promote higher mosquito-biting rates. Precipitation with a resultant abundance of surface pool waters is strongly correlated with the increased growth of *Anopheles* mosquitoes.

Clinical Presentations

These infections present with a spectrum of clinical features depending upon the virulence, and infectivity of the agent as well as susceptibly, immune response, and presence of comorbidities in the host, e.g., a host who has already been exposed to the dengue virus develops some immunological changes which result in severe manifestations (dengue hemorrhagic fever or dengue shock syndrome) on subsequent exposure by different dengue virus strains.

Sometimes these infections present with uncommon and atypical manifestations, e.g., fever with diarrhea is characteristic of acute gastroenteritis often caused by *E. coli* or cholera; however, diarrhea is present in 38% of malaria (algid malaria) and likewise, a dengue patient may also experience frequent diarrhea with abdominal pain which is considered as intermediate warning symptoms in dengue.

Development of herd immunity results in low virulence of the disease with less incidence of complications.

The predilection for developing severe disease is also changing. While *Falciparum* malaria is known as malignant malaria with several complications and an increased mortality rate over the years, at present we are encountering more and more cases of complicated vivax malaria, which often turns fatal if not treated.

Drug Susceptibility

Variation in the key elements of the epidemiological triad has also resulted in changes in drug susceptibility with a predominance of antibiotic resistance. These may lead to the development of multidrug-resistant and extensively drug-resistant infections with a high case-fatality ratio.

CHANGES IN THE CLINICAL PROFILE OF VARIOUS INFECTIONS

Malaria

Worldwide cases of malaria have reduced in recent years. Malaria case incidence declined by 27% in the period 2000–2015 and mortality rates were reduced by 60%. In India, vivax infection accounts for 60–65% of cases. *Plasmodium vivax* is referred to as benign tertian malaria but presently several cases of severe complicated malaria are due to *P. vivax* infection.

Traditionally vivax malaria is treated with chloroquine and falciparum malaria is treated with quinine or artesunate. However, emerging chloroquine resistance in vivax malaria is another area of concern and accordingly, all cases of complicated vivax malaria are treated with artesunate combination therapy.

The classical features with a paroxysm of fevers are seen in 50–70% of cases. Indiscriminate use of antimalarial drugs, antimalarial drug resistance, and development of immunity has resulted in unusual features as listed here:

- *Atypical central nervous system (CNS) manifestations*: Subarachnoid hemorrhage, dysconjugate gaze, central pontine myelinolysis, cerebellar ataxia, Guillain-Barré (GB) syndrome, personality disturbances and schizophrenia, and postmalaria neurological syndrome
- *Musculoskeletal manifestations*: Myositis, rhabdomyolysis, and periodic paralysis
- *Hematological manifestation*: Hemophagocytic syndrome and cerebral brain thrombosis
- *Renal*: Glomerulonephritis and acute kidney injury (AKI)
- *Pulmonary*: ARDS and interstitial pneumonia
- *Cardiac*: Conduction abnormalities, ventricular hypokinesia, and pericardial effusion
- *GI system*: Hepatic encephalopathy, splenic rupture, acute pancreatitis, and acalculous cholecystitis
- *Endocrine*: Syndrome of inappropriate antidiuretic hormone secretion (SIADH) and diabetes insipidus.
- *Ocular manifestations*: Retinal hemorrhage, subconjunctival hemorrhage, vitreous hemorrhage, keratitis, and uveitis

Dengue

Incidence has grown drastically around the world in recent decades. The majority of cases are asymptomatic or mild and self-managed while others can present with dengue hemorrhagic fever or dengue shock syndrome which are often fatal if not properly treated. Apart from the typical breakbone fever pattern of the disease. Dengue often presents with systemic features.

Dengue hepatitis results from direct viral damage from viral cells or reactive hepatitis. Liver enzymes elevate between the third to the fifth day of fever. A rise in the aspartate transaminase (AST) level is often more than a rise in the alanine transaminase (ALT) level. A negative correlation exists between liver enzyme level and platelet count. Hence dengue hepatitis is considered as poor prognostic marker.

Central nervous system involvement includes dengue encephalitis, stroke, transverse myelitis, and acute disseminated encephalomyelitis (ADEM).

Peripheral nervous system (PNS) involvement: Myositis, facial nerve paralysis, and GB syndrome.

Ophthalmic: Maculopathy, optic neuropathy, and vitreous hemorrhage.

Cardiac manifestations: Majorly asymptomatic but may present with sinus bradycardia, ventricular premature complex (VPC), atrioventricular (AV) dissociation ventricular tachycardia, and even cardiogenic shocks. Accordingly, echocardiography (ECG) should be done in dengue fever with hypotension to rule out cardiogenic shocks from more common vasodilatory shock due to capillary leakage.

Human Immunodeficiency Virus

Better health awareness in common people with the use of protective measures has reduced the transmission of the virus. Globally, the number of new cases has reduced by 59% since the peak in 1995. However, the global prevalence among adults has leveled since 2001 and was 0.7% in 2022. The introduction of more effective drugs with lesser side effects and at low-cost results in increasing drug compliance and consequently increases the number of patients living with human immunodeficiency virus (HIV). The clinical profile of HIV disease is now changing. It may variously present as:

- Acute HIV infection-flu like illness 2–4 weeks after infection
- Cardinal symptoms of AIDS—recurring fever with rapid weight loss, diarrhea, and lymphadenopathy
- Features of various opportunistic infection patterns of which vary from patient to patient and from country to country
- Features of antiretroviral drug toxicity—appetite loss, diarrhea, fatigue, mood changes, dyslipidemia, and lipodystrophy
- Features of immune reconstitution inflammatory syndrome (IRIS)—worsening of features of preexisting opportunistic infections, such as new pulmonary infiltrates and worsening meningeal signs

Influenza

Antigenic variations in the influenza virus result in antigenic drift and antigenic shift. A pandemic like the coronavirus disease 2019 (COVID-19) was a consequence of antigenic shift. Initially, COVID-19 presented with a high case-fatality ratio often complicated with ARDS. With the passage of time after several waves of attack and the use of vaccines, herd immunity developed and there was a significant reduction in fatality. Presently most cases of COVID-19 present as common flu.

Tuberculosis

India's plan of eliminating TB by 2025 is nowhere close to the target. India is way behind the TB reduction goal as well as a target for TB mortality reduction. According to the end-TB strategy, the annual decline in global TB incidence rates must increase to 10% annually by 2025. However, the rate achieved for multidrug-resistant TB (MDR)-TB is 1.36%. The increasing incidence of MDR-TB and extensively drug-resistant TB (XDR-TB) and failure to treat these cases adequately (may be due to delayed diagnosis or poor drug compliance) has emerged as a major health burden. In 2019, there were 25,060 new XDR-TB cases globally which had increased by 22.5% compared with 2010.

The clinical manifestations of TB often differ according to age group. The classical features of fever, cough, hemoptysis, and night sweats are more common in adults. The presentation in elderly patients is more likely nonspecific symptoms and atypical radiological findings, such as breathlessness, loss of appetite, loss of weight, and chest pain. As compared to younger adults, elderly patients have more bilateral involvement and lower zone predominance. Atypical clinicoradiological manifestation in older patients results in delay in diagnosis and treatment, unfortunately, can lead to high mortality and morbidity.

Leprosy

By bringing down the prevalence rate by <1/10,000 at the national level, India officially reached the leprosy elimination goal in 2005. However, leprosy remains endemic in some states and union territories of India, such as Chhattisgarh, Jharkhand, Odisha, Bihar, Maharashtra, Chandigarh, and Dadra and Nagar Haveli. Prevalence has been reduced from 0.69 in 2014–2015 to 0.45 in 2021–2022. The incidence rate per 100,000 population has been reduced from 9.73 in 2014–2015 to 5.52 in 2021–2022.

Apart from cardinal signs of hypopigmented or reddish skin patch with loss of sensation and thickened peripheral nerve, there are some unusual presentations such as psoriatiform plaques, verrucous plaques, hypertrophic scarring, erythema nodosum leprosum and extracutaneous manifestation (fever, neuritis, arthritis, epididymo-orchitis, iridocyclitis, and rarely glomerulonephritis)

Kala-azar

The annual incidence and prevalence of kala-azar worldwide are 0.5 and 2.5 million respectively. About 90% of these cases occur in India, Nepal, Bangladesh, and Sudan. India has made much progress in the past decades with kala-azar. Cases have decreased by 98% in 2021 as compared to 1992, but still cases are getting reported from Bihar, West Bengal, and Uttar Pradesh.

Kala-azar is more prevalent in rural areas and in poor socioeconomic conditions, in people working in fishery, mining, forestry, and farming practices. Visceral leishmaniasis is the most common form of the disease characterized by fever, hepatosplenomegaly, lymphadenopathy, weight loss, anemia, and darkening of skin. Kala-azar can also present as post-kala-azar dermal leishmaniasis (macular, popular, or nodular rash develops as a sequel of visceral leishmaniasis) cutaneous leishmaniasis [several forms—anthroponotic cutaneous. leishmaniasis (ACL), zoonotic cutaneous leishmaniasis (ZCL), diffuse cutaneous leishmaniasis (DCL)] or mucocutaneous leishmaniasis.

Filaria

Despite a substantial decrease in cases of lymphatic filariasis worldwide since 2000, infection rates remain high in endemic areas. India is committed in eliminating lymphatic filariasis by 2027.

Filariasis may be asymptomatic or present with either acute manifestations (fever, dermatolymphangioadenitis tropical pulmonary eosinophilia) chronic manifestations (hydrocele, elephantiasis, and chyluria), or other syndrome (arthritis, thrombophlebitis, and glomerulonephritis).

Scrub Typhus

There has been a sharp increase in the incidence of scrub typhus in recent years. Accordingly, it has become one important differential for undifferentiated fever particularly when associated with rash and eschar.

EMERGING AND RE-EMERGING INFECTIONS

Emerging infections are defined as outbreaks of previously unknown infections or rapid increases in the incidence of known diseases or the persistence of infectious diseases that cannot be controlled.

Including HIV, severe acute respiratory syndrome (SARS), Lyme disease, *E. coli*, hantavirus, dengue, West Nile, and Zika virus.

Re-emerging infections are those that reappear after a significant decrease. It may be due to drug resistance from overuse of antibiotics. Including cholera, influenza, malaria, TB, pertussis, pneumococcal, and gonorrhea.

CONCLUSION

The clinical profile of various tropical infections is changing due to changes in factors. Some common diseases often present with atypical features. Knowledge of such variations is of utmost importance for prompt diagnosis and appropriate treatment of those diseases. prevention and treatment of various complications thereby reducing mortality and morbidity.

SUGGESTED READINGS

1. In: Brent AJ, Seale AC, Blumberg L, Davidson R (Eds). Oxford Handbook of Tropical medicine, 5th edition. United Kingdom: Oxford University Press; 2022.
2. National Centre for Disease Control. National guidelines for Infection prevention and control in healthcare facilities MoHFW 2020 Training Modules. [online] Available from https://ncdc.mohfw.gov.in/index1.php?lang=1&level=2&sublinkid=1019&lid=794 [Last accessed December, 2023].
3. Aschengrau A, Seage GR. Essentials of Epdemiology in Public Health, 3rd edition. Burlington: Jones and Bartlett Publishers, Inc; 2013.
4. Centre for Disease control and Prevention. (2014). Types of healthcare associated infections. [online] Available from https;//www.cdc.gov/hai/infectiontypes.html [Last accessed December, 2023].
5. Sabin NS, Calliope AS, Simpson SV, Arima H, Ito H, Nishimura T, et al. Implications of human activities for (re)emerging infectious diseases, including COVID-19. J Physiol Anthropol. 2020;39(1):29.

76

CHAPTER

Awareness of Tribal Population about Malaria

Uttam Kumar Paul

ABSTRACT

The study aimed to assess the perceptions and practices of a particularly vulnerable tribal group in a rural area of eastern India regarding malaria and its control. An interprofessional intervention was implemented to increase awareness and knowledge of malaria among the tribal population.

A qualitative research intervention was conducted using a partially open-ended questionnaire with 120 participants from a tribal village in West Bengal, India. The questionnaire assessed sociodemographic information and included questions about malaria transmission, prevention, and treatment. Health education workshops were conducted as part of the interprofessional intervention to improve participants' perceptions and practices about malaria.

The study revealed that tribal participants had limited knowledge about malaria, its transmission, and proper prevention and treatment methods before the intervention. However, after the intervention, there were significant improvements in their understanding of malaria breeding places, transmission areas, and treatment options. The study highlights the need for continued efforts to raise awareness among underserved populations with limited access to formal education. Sustainable initiatives, such as environmental cleanups and regular use of mosquito bed nets, can further contribute to reduce mosquito-borne diseases in these areas.

INTRODUCTION

The poor, unschooled, and culturally restricted tribal people are spread out across India. Despite having a precarious health state due to malarial morbidities, people ignore their illnesses and avoid seeing primary care doctors when they are ill for a variety of reasons, including poverty. In many parts of India, malaria, a disease spread by mosquitoes, is on the rise. Both human and animal blood can contain the parasite *Plasmodium*, which causes malaria and is often spread to people by infected mosquitoes.

The community's culture might have an impact on the control approaches since it frequently influences beliefs and practices about malaria. Therefore, understanding local knowledge and practices associated with the condition is necessary to design culturally acceptable, durable, and successful therapies. A thorough assessment of the literature reveals that very little is known about people's overall knowledge, attitudes, and practices about malaria, particularly among the rural and tribal people of the nation. This study was carried out to assess the perceptions and practices and to determine the changes in perceptions and practices after the interprofessional intervention of a particularly vulnerable tribal group in the rural area of eastern India regarding malaria and its control. It also creates the opportunity for the development of control programs that function in different Indian regions.

METHODS

This was a study of qualitative research intervention regarding awareness of a neglected tropical disease namely "Malaria" among the tribal population.

Study area: This study was carried out in a tribal village of Karandighi block, in the district Uttar Dinajpur, West Bengal, India.

Study period: This study was carried out for a period of 18 months from December 21st, 2022 to September 20th, 2023.

Questionnaire preparation: We created a questionnaire with 19 questions with input from the faculty of the medical education department at MGM Medical College and LSK Hospital in Kishanganj, Bihar. The study participants' native language, Bengali, was used to create this schedule. To ensure acceptance, time management, and feasibility, the instrument underwent pretesting on a subsample of 10 individuals in the relevant college's field practice region. Our research team members agreed that an assessment was disregarded if >5% of the data were missing or unanswered. Additionally, to validate the instrument, additional piloting was done if any inquiry went unanswered.

Different parts of the question: In this partially open-ended questionnaire, five questions were from sociodemography, viz., age, gender, educational status, occupation, and family income per month. Of the rest 14 questions, seven questions were prepared to assess the perception regarding malaria transmission; another seven questions were made to assess practice or intended practice or reported practice regarding the treatment of malaria. Out of 14 questions, eight were of multiple choice questions (MCQs) type where multiple responses were allowed, five were of yes or no response type, and the rest one was an open-ended question.

Inclusion criteria: The study included all adult males and females who were willing to participate. A few of the tribal society students who agreed to take part in the study were also included.

Exclusion criteria: The study excluded those who were really unwell and unwilling to participate.

Data collection: Data was gathered by asking them to assemble in a primary school inside the participants' rural neighborhoods. Each participant received a personalized explanation of the study, and their verbal informed permission was collected. The rigorous maintenance of anonymity, confidentiality, and protection of all collected data as well as its usage only for research was guaranteed to the participants. We gave the subjects a well-structured questionnaire. They had already responded. "Interview techniques" were employed for people who could not read or write, and responses were recorded in the questionnaire.

Intervention: The intervention aims to increase tribal people's cognitive, affective, and psychomotor awareness of malaria. During the holidays, the training was delivered in the classrooms of the tribal area's primary school. The intervention consisted of several health education workshops designed as an interprofessional approach including doctors, nurses, other healthcare professionals, and tribal members of the community in response to the shortcomings highlighted in the pre-test assessment's responses.

Post-test: The identical questionnaire that was used for the pretest assessment was given to every participant in the training programs.

Data analysis method: We tabulated and examined all of the responses. The open-ended questions and responses were manually examined using content analysis.

Ethics committee permission: The Institute Ethics Committee (IEC) of the MGM Medical College and LSK Hospital, Kishanganj, Bihar, India, approved this study, and the trial was started after receiving approval from the institute's governing body.

RESULTS

There were 120 total participants, of which 63 (52.5%) were men and 57 (47.5%) were women. Regarding their level of education, 23 participants had no formal education, 59 participants had completed primary school, 30 participants completed secondary school, 7 participants had completed higher secondary education, and one participant had completed graduation. In terms of their employment situation, 39 individuals were unemployed, 52 were nonskilled employees, 19 were skilled workers, and 9 were semi-professional workers. The participants' monthly income varied from below ₹ 2,000 to above ₹10,000. Most of them (69) fell in the lowest income bracket, while only one was in the highest. The rest were distributed among the middle income brackets: 28 earned ₹2,001–4,000, 12 earned ₹4,001–6,000, 7 earned ₹6,001–8,000, and 3 earned ₹8,001–10,000.

The first question about the transmission of malaria was not statistically significant and was not in the 95% range of acceptance in terms of their replies to perception regarding malaria transmission. The second question, which asked where malaria breeds, was statistically significant and had a 95% acceptance rate. The replies to the third question "Where more mosquitoes are found" were statistically significant and in the 95% range of acceptance. Although responses to the fifth question about the primary symptom of malaria were not statistically significant and were not in the 95% range of acceptance, they were statistically significant to the fourth question about the source of information about malaria and were also in the 95% range of acceptance. The sixth question, which asked participants if malaria was curable, had statistically significant responses with a 95% acceptance rate. With a 95% acceptance rate, the responses to the seventh question about the treatment for malaria were statistically significant **(Fig. 1)**.

To assess practice or intended practice or reported practice regarding the treatment of malaria replies to the eighth question, "What you will do if you encounter someone suffering from Malaria," were statistically significant and had a 95% acceptance rate. With a 95% acceptance rate, the ninth question about malaria prevention received statistically significant responses. The tenth question asked respondents how much time they spent on the malaria prevention program, and their replies were statistically significant with a 95% acceptance rate. The eleventh item was a dummy question; hence, the answers on the pre-test and post-test were identical. With a 95% acceptance rate, the responses to the 12th question about malaria detection were statistically significant. The responses on the pre-test and post-test were the same because the thirteenth item was likewise a dummy question. With a 95% acceptance rate, the responses to the fourteenth question addressing the regular usage of bed nets were statistically significant **(Fig. 2)**.

DISCUSSION

Despite the availability of efficient prophylactic measures and antimalarial medications, the burden of malaria disease is rising in many nations. One of the key elements of effective malaria control is an awareness of community perceptions and practices. The study's objective was to determine how well the tribal community members understood how malaria spread and how to prevent it. The primary and most important steps in developing and putting into action a health program are knowledge, attitude, and practice assessment. Additionally, it aids in the creation of community-wide behavioral change strategies for the prevention of malaria that are feasible.

Although the first cognitive domain question on malaria transmission was not statistically significant, the changes regarding malaria breeding places, areas with higher mosquito densities, and the source of information about malaria are statistically significant in the current study. The fifth question on the predominant malaria symptom was not statistically significant, but their understanding of the curability of malaria and the agent used to treat it is statistically significant in the present study. In particular, malaria poses a serious public health threat in India's tribal regions. Malaria is preventable and curable if detected early and given the appropriate care, despite reports of high fatality rates in untreated cases. According to the study's findings, about 40% of respondents knew something about malaria, but even among them, there were muddled about where the disease breeds, how it spreads, how it may be cured, and how to treat it.

The replies to the affective and psychomotor domain questions "What you will do if you see someone suffering from malaria?," "How much time was spent in the malaria control program," "Malaria detection," and "Regular usage

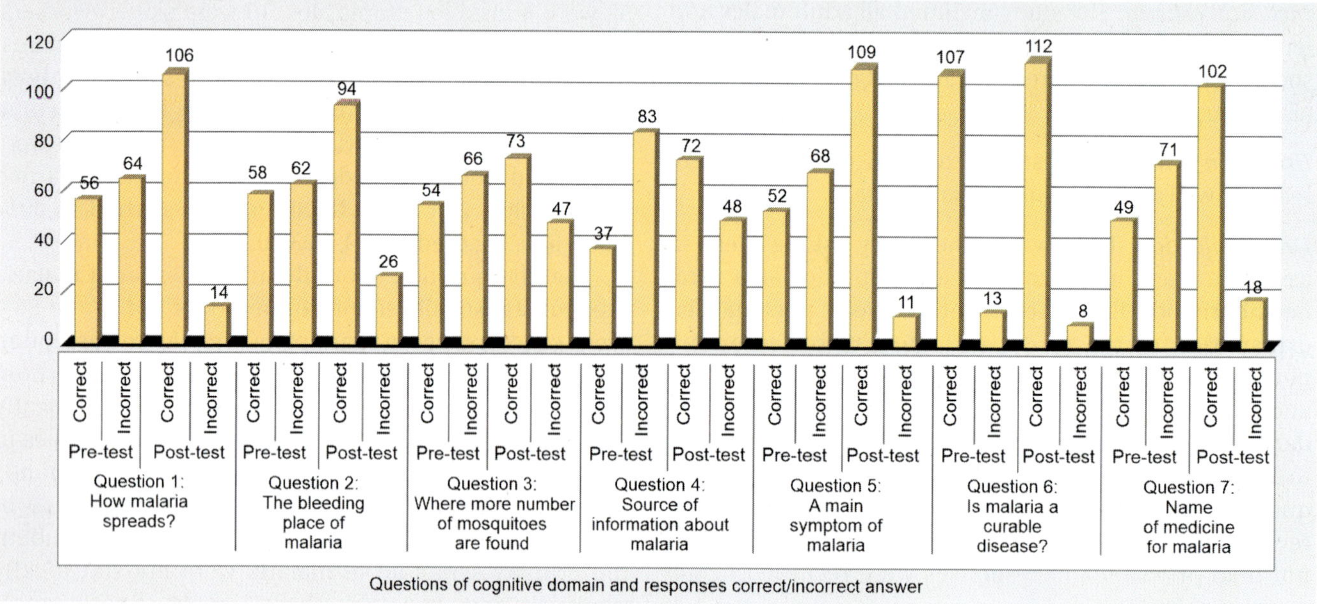

FIG. 1: Analysis of answers to assess the perception regarding malaria transmission.

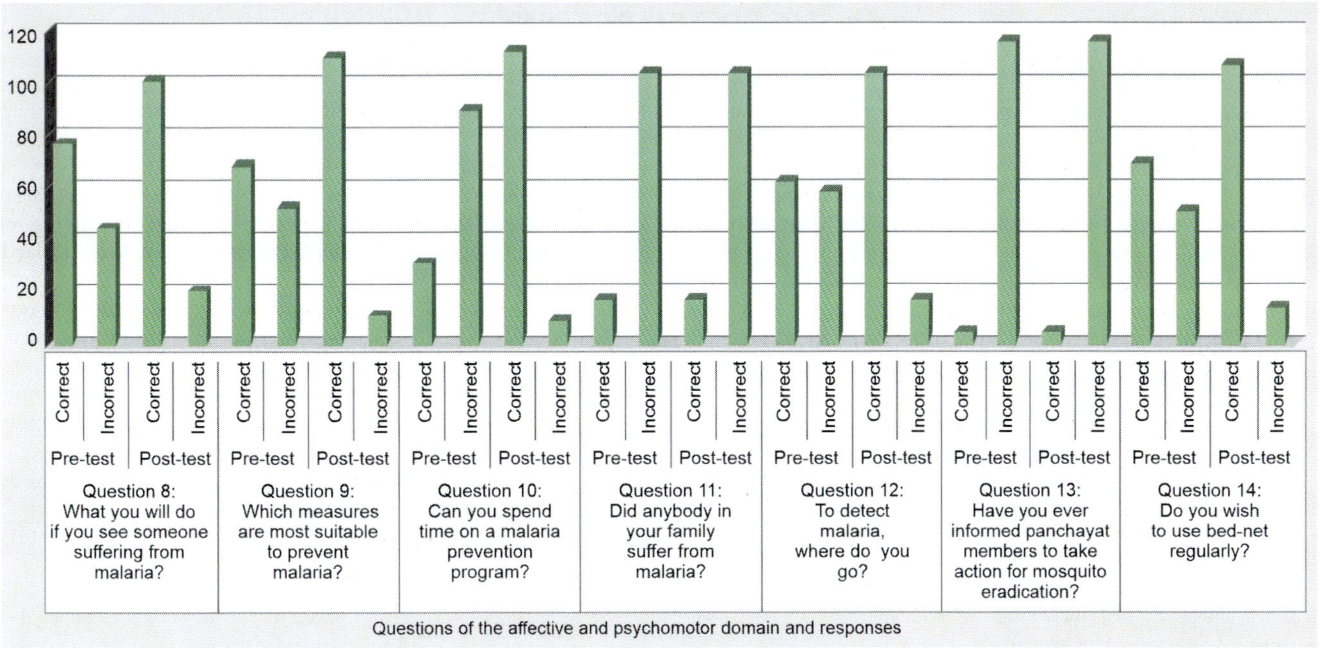

FIG. 2: Analysis of answers to assess practice regarding the treatment of malaria.

of bed-nets?" had statistical significance. As a result, it can be claimed that the intervention program, which took the shape of several health education workshops in their area, significantly altered the affective and psychomotor domain of learning of the tribal community.

Misconceptions about malaria vectors, breeding grounds, and transmission patterns have reportedly been documented as a result of misinformation and the improper application of preventative measures, which are indications of socioeconomic situation, a significant risk factor for malaria.

In the early stages of the study, it was not observed that the tribal people were using any kind of protective method to prevent mosquito bites. However, after the intervention phase, most respondents (86%) supported the use of bed nets and were doing so at night. The earlier research reported somewhat comparable results.

Malaria continues to have a significant negative impact on people's health, well-being, and economy despite several attempts to control it. The main factors influencing the success of mosquito-borne disease control include community knowledge, awareness, and behaviors for prevention as well as an early care-seeking attitude. Concerning mosquito-borne diseases and their control in the community, there is a need to understand and improve current experience and understanding. To improve the cognitive, affective, and psychomotor domain of learning in the tribal society, which will, in turn, have an impact on the burden of disease, novel interventions such as actively incorporating members of the community in the propagation of health education messages must be considered.

FUTURE DIRECTION OF THE RESEARCH

The project's long-term objective is to launch comprehensive activities, such as environmental cleanups, to decrease mosquito breeding grounds by preventing standing water from lingering anywhere in exposed forms for longer than a week. Using mosquito bed nets on a regular basis can also help to reduce cases of other mosquito-borne diseases such as dengue, filaria, and Japanese encephalitis. We want to proceed gradually in order to have a sustainable impact.

CONCLUSION

Our study on malaria awareness intervention in this tribal belt of the northern part of West Bengal in eastern India bordering Bangladesh was reported for the first time to the horizon of our knowledge. It has been observed that a surprisingly high cognitive, psychomotor, and affective learning of malaria in the studied population. In the future, this initiative will receive greater attention and resources in order to raise tribal awareness among people who do not have a formal education.

SUGGESTED READINGS

1. Saha KB, Sharma RK, Mishra R, Verma A, Tiwari BK, Singh N. Establishiing communication mechanism for malaria prevention in Baiga tribal villages in Baiga Chak area of Dindori district, Madhya Pradesh. Indian J Med Res. 2015;141:576-83.
2. Paul UK, Pal R. Intervention on malaria awareness among 'Bedia' tribal community in West Bengal, India. J Family Med Prim Care. 2019;8(9):2820-6.
3. WHO. World Malaria Report 2014. Geneva: WHO; 2014.
4. Paul UK, Bhattacharyya P, Bhattacharyya R, Bandyopadhyay A. Perceptions about malaria among the Bedia tribal people in Uttar-Dinajpur district of West Bengal, India. Int J Res Med Sci. 2017;5:3488-92.
5. Rodríguez AD, Penilla RP, Henry-Rodríguez M, Hemingway J, Francisco Betanzos A, Hernández Avila JE. Knowledge and beliefs about malaria transmission and practices for vector control in Southern Mexico. Salud Publica Mex. 2003;45:110-6.
6. Kumar V, Rathi A, Lal P, Goel SK. Malaria and dengue: Knowledge, attitude, practice, and effect of sensitization workshop among school teachers as health educators. J Family Med Prim Care. 2018;7:1368-74.
7. Ghosh SK, Patil RR, Tiwari S, Dash AP. A community-based health education programme for bio-environmental control of malaria through folk theatre (Kalajatha) in rural India. Malar J. 2006;5:123-8.
8. Regional Medical Research Centre for Tribals, ICMR, Jabalpur. Annual Report 2012-13. [online] Available from http://www.nirth.res.in. [Last accessed December, 2023].
9. Prasad H. Evaluation of malaria control programme in three selected districts of Assam, India. J Vector Borne Dis. 2009;46:280-7.
10. Singh RK, Haq S, Dhiman RC. Studies on Knowledge, Attitude and Practices in Malaria Endemic Tribal Areas of Bihar and Jharkhand, India. J Trop Dis. 2013;1:110.

SECTION

9

METABOLIC DISEASE

77

CHAPTER

Obesity-related Renal Disorders

Arjun Baidya, Puranjoy Chakrabarty, Silima Subhasnigdha Tarenia

ABSTRACT

Obesity is posing to be an incredible healthcare challenge of the modern world. It includes a spectrum rather than a single entity and has its impact on multiple systems. Previously, obesity and its spectrum were well-known for its associations with cardiovascular diseases, surgical complications, diabetes, and hormonal perturbations. However, clinical observations and research work in the last two decades are now indicating for a novel association with renal diseases. As more and more knowledge are being gathered, a distinct pathophysiological correlation is getting established. Expanding from the historical association with focal segmental glomerular sclerosis (FSGS), newer diseases like obesity-related glomerulopathy or the combination of diabetes and obesity effects on renal structure and function is getting unveiled. With the similar increment in chronic kidney disease prevalence worldwide, this newer association needs introduction as well as elucidation for physicians and students to make them aware of the spectrum of involvement as well as pave way for new research ideas which will further enlarge the viewpoint. This chapter aims to present the concept of obesity-related renal diseases and briefly discuss its current understanding and possible impact.

INTRODUCTION

Obesity has become one of the dominant chronic diseases of modern world and it is becoming a worldwide epidemic with a prediction of increase of 40% prevalence in the coming decade. Apart from the well-known associations with risk of type 2 diabetes mellitus (T2DM) and cardiovascular diseases, obesity is also being associated with a myriad of renal diseases extending from focal segmental glomerulosclerosis to chronic kidney disease (CKD). This association is rather new and insights into the pathophysiological mechanisms have been evaluated recently. Having its cohabitancy with other diseases, such as T2DM, hypertension, or cardiovascular diseases, the combined (individual or synergistic) effect on renal physiology and disease is a new concern and challenge for the physicians. This writing is aimed to provide a brief insight into this novel entity and its clinical impact.

EPIDEMIOLOGY OF OBESITY

Prevalence of obesity has increased to enormous proportions in the last 20–30 years with a probable number of 600 million people who were obese worldwide in 2014. Data from the United States suggested around 35% men and 40.4% females were suffering from obesity.

The problem does not spare the young also with an estimate of around 17% prevalence of obesity among 2–19 years age and severe obesity amounting to 5.8%. Although previously considered as a disease of the surplus, obesity is now increasing even in the low- and middle-income countries. The numbers are even more troublesome when we consider India. With the tainted crown of being the "diabetes capital of the world", obesity is not far behind owing to the sedentary lifestyle, urbanization, and unhealthy eating practices prevalent in the country. Over and above, the definition for obesity is different for this part of the world with a lower threshold of body mass index (BMI) and additional concerns of poor waist-hip ratio even with normal BMI. This pattern of central obesity is even more dangerous with greater impact on metabolic and renal diseases. Waist-hip ratio has also been considered as a more appropriate measure of obesity specially in CKD population.

OBESITY: A NEW "NEPHROTOXIC" FACTOR

Higher BMI has long been associated with prevalence and progression of proteinuria. Hyperfiltration and increased glomerular hypertension are among the implicated culprits. Apart from this, a higher BMI is also associated with a low estimated glomerular filtration rate (GFR). Increased visceral adiposity is strongly associated with increased proteinuria among men in some studies. Also, presence of a higher BMI in a CKD patient leads to more rapid loss of GFR and faster progression to end-stage kidney disease (ESKD). When we consider waist-hip ratio or waist circumference as surrogates for obesity, the association remains strong.

The association between obesity and worse renal outcomes is probably independent of the effects of obesity like cardiovascular and metabolic ones; as even on adjustment of the same, the association prevails indicating additional mechanisms of damage.

Another pertinent issue is the poor patient and graft survival following renal transplant in those who had higher BMI compared to lean nonobese individuals which mandates recommendation for weight loss before proceeding for transplant in obese patients to mitigate the immediate perioperative increased mortality and morbidity as well as long term renal outcomes in allograft recipients.

Apart from these, other important associations of obesity and renal diseases include nephrolithiasis and malignancies. Obesity is associated with various types of malignancies, particularly cancers of the kidneys. In a population-based study of 5.24 million individuals from the United Kingdom, a 5 kg/m^2 higher BMI was associated with a 25% higher risk of kidney cancers, with 10% of all kidney cancers attributable to excess weight. The association between obesity and kidney malignancies is quite strong with estimates of around 17–26% of all kidney malignancies attributable to excess weight. Meta-analysis revealed that this association holds for both sexes and across various populations. Among various malignancies, kidney malignancies account for the third highest risk associated with obesity.

PATHOPHYSIOLOGY OF OBESITY-RELATED RENAL DISEASES

Metabolic alterations that are caused by obesity exert variable effects on renal physiology leading to pathological changes in time, although an exact singular pathological construct is still to be elucidated. Many obese individuals do not develop "CKD" which emphasizes that mere increase in weight is not sufficient to cause renal damage. However, direct studies looking into prevalence of CKD in obese or overweight are lacking. Secondly, definition of CKD used is also a concern as GFR-based estimates will be erroneous since obesity leads to glomerulomegaly and subsequent hyperfiltration; so, proteinuria on the other hand can be a reliable early and definite indicator.

Apart from obesity itself, the coexisting comorbidities, such as T2DM, hypertension, hyperuricemia, and metabolic syndrome all by themselves can damage the kidneys. Another novel mechanism is the endocrine aspect of obesity with a disturbance in the various horsmones that puts a metabolic stress which translates to renal damage **(Fig. 1)**. Activation of renin–angiotensin–aldosterone axis, oxidative mechanisms, insulin resistance, and altered lipid metabolism are among the few that contribute. Obesity itself by virtue of increased BMI puts a hyperfiltration stress in the glomeruli which eventually leads to intraglomerular hypertension culminating into proteinuria and ultimately CKD.

The pathological changes that occur have been described from renal biopsies. Excess deposition of renal sinus fat, ectopic lipid accumulation, development of glomerular hypertension, hyperfiltration and increased permeability, and glomerulomegaly are some of the pathological changes; all of which can lead to glomerulosclerosis in the long run **(Fig. 2)**.

Obesity-related glomerulopathy is a pathological term used to describe the changes; although the same is also observed in advanced age and hypertensives.

Obesity is associated with higher prevalence of nephrolithiasis. Increased urinary oxalate and lower urinary pH along with increased urinary uric acid, phosphate, and sodium excretion generate a local milieu for lithogenesis. Concomitant insulin resistance creates important perturbations in ammoniagenesis and tubular Na-H exchange which contributes to urinary acidity necessary for stone formation. Some contribution to nephrolithiasis also stems from therapies for obesity like bariatric surgeries which increase enteral oxalate absorption and increased risk for stone formation.

Pathophysiologic determinants of obesity-related oncogenesis remain unclear. Insulin resistance,

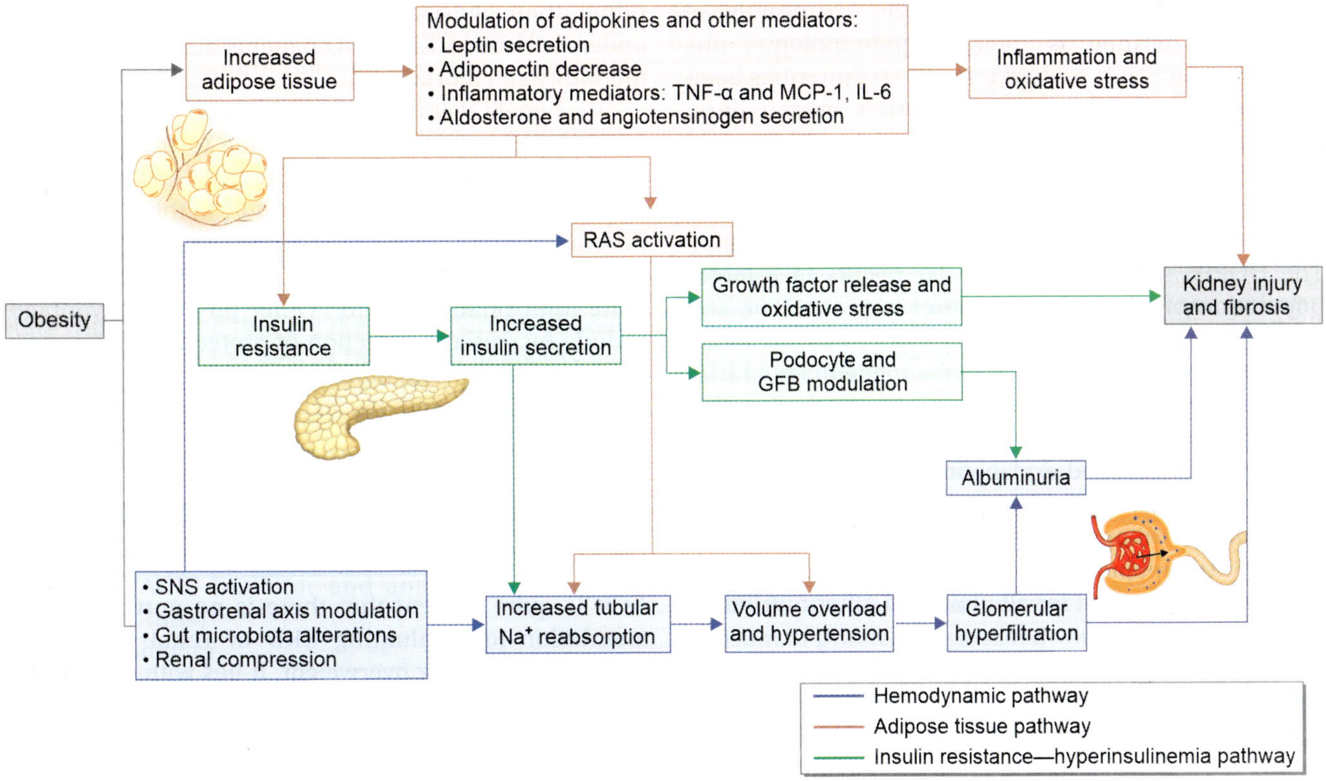

FIG. 1: Pathophysiological mechanisms of obesity-related renal injury.

(GFB: gluten-friendly bread; IL-6: interleukin-6; MCP-1: monocyte chemotactic protein-1; RAS: renin–angiotensin system; SNS: sympathetic nervous system; TNF-α: tumor necrosis factor alpha)

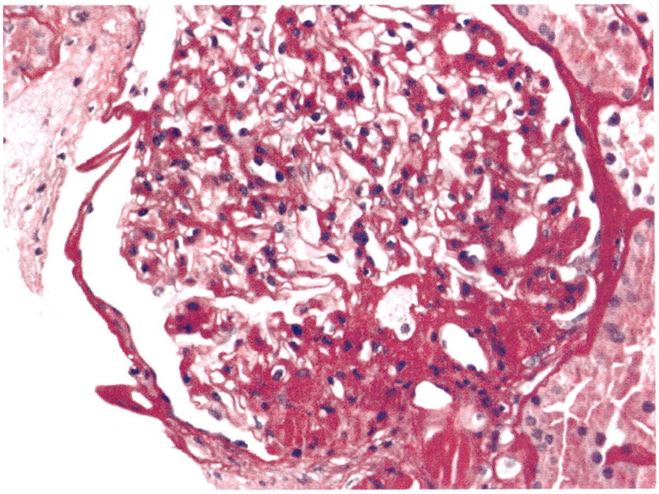

FIG. 2: Obesity-related perihilar focal segmental glomerulosclerosis.

hyperinsulinemia, and increased insulin-like growth factor-1 (IGF-1) were among the usual culprits implicated in oncogenesis. Recently additional contributions from endocrine derangements related to obesity have come into light with its effects on immunity and inflammation that might add to the pathogenesis. Whether these mechanisms are discrete or work in concert need to be elucidated and whether therapeutic advantages can be obtained remain to be seen.

DIABESITY

First described in the 1970s to acknowledge the strong relationship between the two entities and its association with high blood pressure, dyslipidemia, and metabolic syndrome; a toxic cocktail for the kidneys. The synergistic damage that ensues can lead to generation and progression of renal dysfunction faster than that caused by individual components. However, sodium-glucose cotransporter-2 (SGLT-2) inhibitors appears to be a drug tailored to give benefit with its role in controlling diabetes and reducing body weight, blood pressure, and cardioprotective effects.

WHEN OBESITY IS GOOD? OR IS IT?

Although obesity has been implicated in pathogenesis of various renal disorders and CKD, one paradoxical observation is the better outcome of patients with CKD

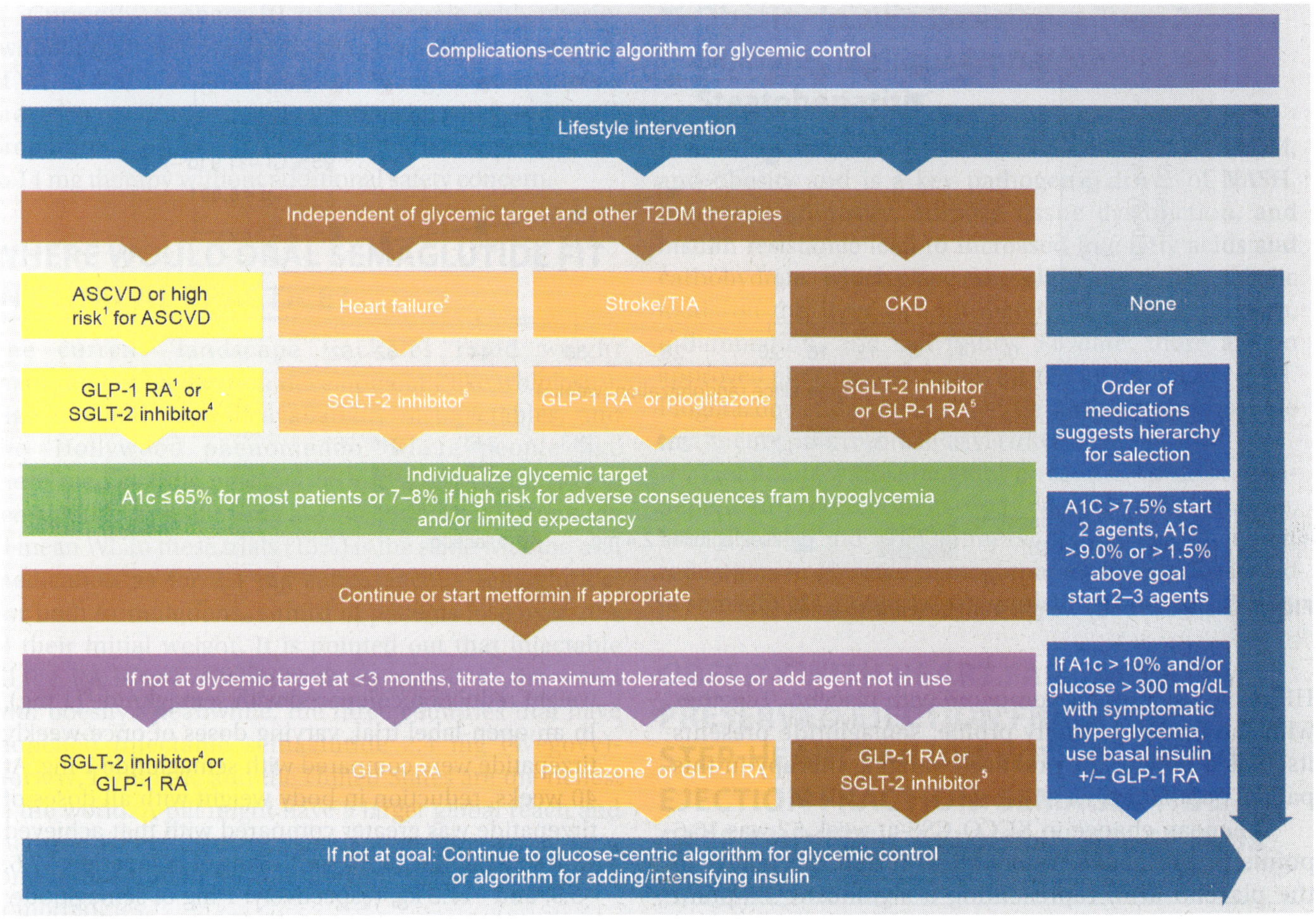

[1]High risk for ASCVD: albuminuria or proteinuria, hypertension, left ventricular hypertrophy, LV systolic or diastolic dysfunction, and ankle-brachial index <0.9.
[2]TZDs are contraindicated in NYHA class IVVHF. ASCVD.
[3]Aglutide/semaglutide/dulaglutide or stroke: semaglutide/dulaglutide.
[4]Canagliflozin/empagliflozin.
[5]Use SGLT-2 or GLP-1 RA with proven benefit.

FLOWCHART 4: Complications-centric glycemic control.

(ASCVD: atherosclerotic cardiovascular disease; CKD: chronic kidney disease; GLP-1 RA: glucagon-like peptide-1 receptor agonist; LV: left ventricular; SGLT-2: sodium-glucose cotransporter-2)

MANAGEMENT OF HYPERGLYCEMIA IN PEOPLE WITH OBESITY

Obesity is the single most modifiable risk factor for the development of hyperglycemia and, although the prevalence of nondiabetic-range hyperglycemia worldwide is not elucidated, it is clear that obesity is the predominant predictor of impaired glucose tolerance (IGT) **(Fig. 9)**.

Why is the Treatment of Hyperglycemia Important in People with Obesity?

People with diabetes and obesity develop more cardiovascular, renal, and neuropathic complications compared with those who are not obese. The effects of obesity on the development of chronic kidney disease (CKD), CVD, obstructive sleep apnea (OSA), nonalcoholic fatty liver disease (NAFLD), and cancer are well recognized. These outcomes might not necessarily be potentiated through insulin resistance or hyperglycemia.

Weight loss appears to lead to improvements in glycemic control. The WL required to significantly improve glycemic control could be as little as 5% of the initial body weight, and significant WL within 6 years of diagnosis from T2DM can lead to its remission **(Flowchart 5)**.

Bariatric Surgery

National Institute for Health and Care Excellence guidelines recommend that patients are referred for a bariatric surgery assessment if they have a BMI of

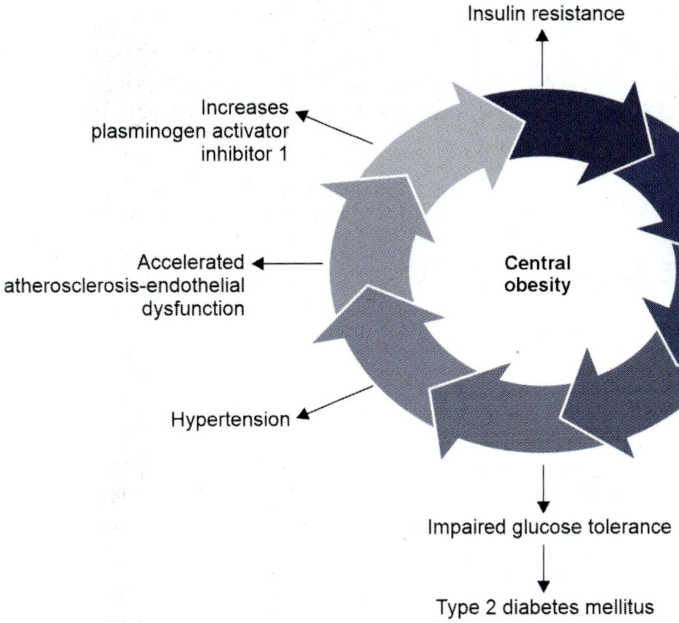

FIG. 9: Central obesity.
(HDL: high-density lipoprotein; LDL: low-density lipoprotein)

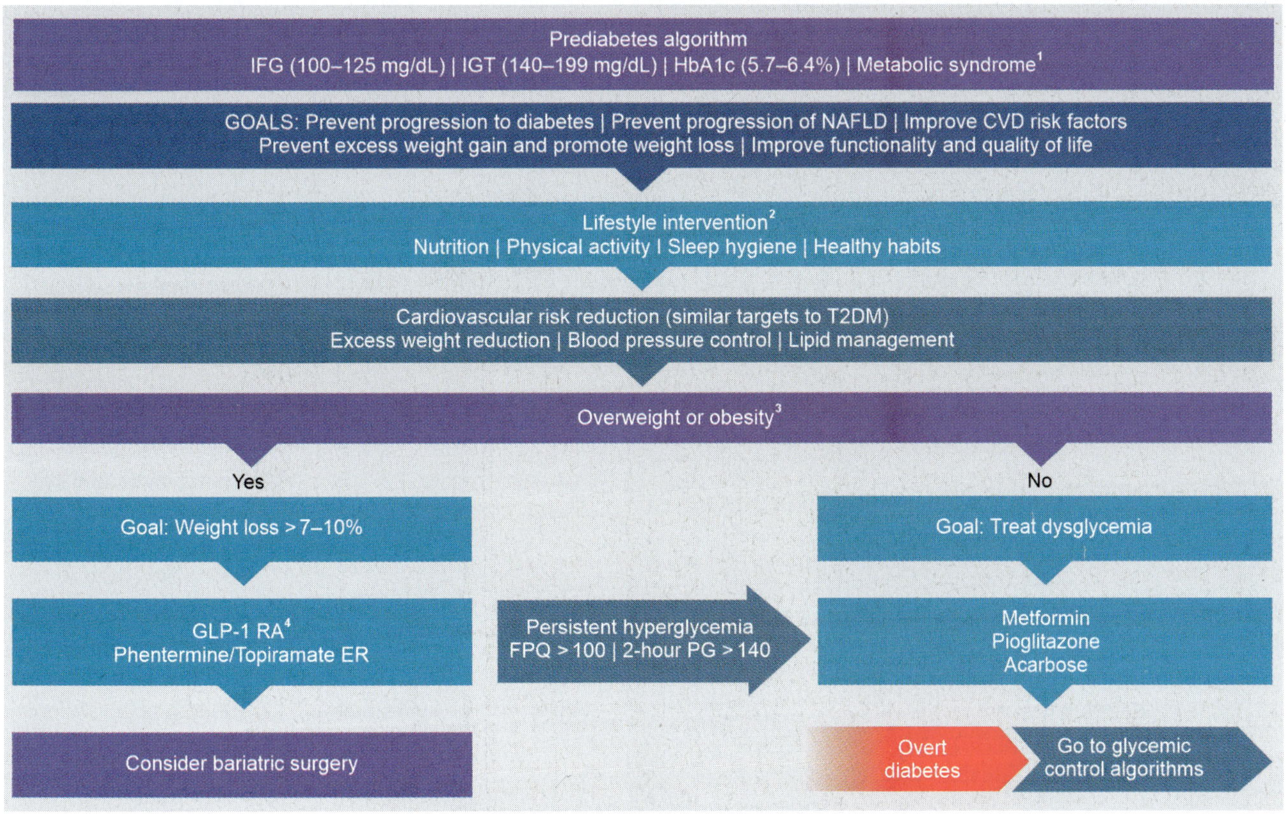

[1]NCEP ATP III Criteria.
[2]See COMPLICATIONS-CENTRIC MODEL FOR THE CARE OF PERSONS WITH OVERWEIGHT/OBESITY.
[3]If no overweight or obesity. Consider T1DM antibody testing for LADA.
[4]Indications for weight-loss medications are obesity or overweight BMI > 27 kg/m^2 with ABCD complication(s) including prediabetes. Choose GLP-1 RA for approved for weight loss. Also consider other approved weight-loss medications [phentermine (short term), orlistat, naltrexone-ER/bupropion-ER].

FLOWCHART 5: Prediabetes.

40 kg/m^2 or above, or 35 kg/m^2 and above with associated multiple health conditions (such as CVDs, diabetes, and OSA) that can be improved with marked WL. Lifestyle modifications and pharmacological interventions are recommended before referral to a Tier 4 bariatric service. Bariatric surgery is the first-line treatment option for individuals with a BMI > 50 kg/m^2. Combined with ongoing lifestyle modifications, bariatric surgery is very effective for long-term WL **(Tables 6 and 7)**.

TABLE 6: Summary of the three most commonly performed bariatric surgery interventions.

Comparison	Roux-en-Y gastric bypass	Gastric banding	Sleeve gastrectomy
Weight loss after 1 year (%)	72%	33%	70%
Diabetes remission (%)	93%	68%	86%
Complications	• Anastomotic leak • Strictures • Internal hernias • Dumping syndrome Nutritional deficiencies • Gallstones	• Band slippage/erosion • Esophageal dilatation • Gastroesophageal reflux Gallstones	• Anastomotic leak • Strictures • Gastroesophageal reflux Gallstones

TABLE 7: Types of bariatric procedures, their respective excess weight loss, and average percentage of resolution of existing obesity-related disease.

Bariatric surgery Type	Average excess weight loss	Resolution of diabetes	Resolution of obstructive sleep apnea	Resolution of hypertension	Resolution of dyslipidemia	Restrictive or malabsorptive	Relative contraindications
RYGB	60–70%	80%	85%	75%	70%	Restrictive and malabsorptive	Severe esophageal reflux, gastroparesis, and IBD
Sleeve gastrectomy	50–60%	60%	70%	60%	55%	Restrictive	Barrett's esophagus, severe esophageal reflux, gastroparesis, and IBD
OAGB	60–70%	80%	85%	75%	70%	Restrictive and malabsorptive	Barrett's esophagus, severe esophageal reflux, gastroparesis, and IBD
Duodenal switch	70–80%	90%	95%	80%	85%	Restrictive and malabsorptive	Barrett's esophagus, severe esophageal reflux, gastroparesis, and IBD
SADI-S	60–70%	85%	90%	75%	70%	Restrictive and malabsorptive	Barrett's esophagus, severe esophageal reflux, gastroparesis, and IBD
Gastric band	40–50%	50%	60%	50%	45%	Restrictive	Previous upper abdominal surgery, high BMI, and eating disorders
Gastric plication	50–60%	60%	70%	60%	55%	Restrictive	Barrett's esophagus, severe esophageal reflux, gastroparesis, and IBD
ESG	25–30%	30%	40%	25%	20%	Restrictive	Previous upper abdominal surgery, active peptic ulcer disease, and large hiatal hernia
Gastric balloon	10–15%	15%	20%	10%	10%	Restrictive	Previous upper abdominal surgery, active peptic ulcer disease, and esophageal stricture

(BMI: body mass index; ESG: endoscopic sleeve gastroplasty; IBD: inflammatory bowel disease; OAGB: one anastomosis gastric bypass-'mini' bypass; Roux en-Y gastric bypass; SADI-S: single anastomosis duodenal-ileal bypass with sleeve)

FUTURE THERAPIES FOR OBESITY

Emerging Obesity Treatments

FORESIGHT-tackling obesities—future choices, danuglipron is another oral GLP-1 RA currently under development (NCT04707313). In early-phase clinical studies, 120 mg twice daily resulted in a placebo-adjusted WL of 5.5% after 28 days in people with T2DM and obesity and it was well tolerated.

Combination of Gut Hormones

The concept of combining gut hormones for obesity management originates from the remarkable results of bariatric surgery on WL, weight maintenance, and obesity-related complications. In the search for the next generation of obesity pharmacotherapies, numerous molecules with diverse metabolic actions are under investigation in combination with GLP-1 RAs (GIP, glucagon, amylin, and peptide YY agonists, and GIP antagonists) aiming to enhance and complement the effect of GLP-1 agonism on weight and metabolism through different mechanisms of actions.

Dual Agonism with Amylin

Amylin is a hormone cosecreted with insulin from pancreatic β-cells in response to food intake. It is implicated in satiety regulation through actions in the brain and improves glycemic control by delaying gastric emptying and inhibiting glucagon secretion. Amylin is being considered as a future treatment for obesity

Cagrilintide

Cagrilintide is a long-acting amylin analog administered once weekly subcutaneously. In a phase II trial, 26 weeks of cagrilintide in doses up to 4.5 mg resulted in greater WL compared with placebo in people with obesity (6.0–10.8% vs. 3.0%) and, at the 4.5 mg dose, cagrilintide was superior to liraglutide 3 mg for WL (10.8% vs. 9.0%).

CagriSema

Weight loss through GLP-1 RAs and amylin analogs is mediated through both distinct and overlapping pathways; thus, combined therapy could yield synergistic effects concerning WL by reducing appetite further. In a phase Ib study, the combination of cagrilintide 2.4 mg plus semaglutide 2.4 mg once weekly (CagriSema) in people with obesity resulted in 17.1% WL after 20 weeks compared with 9.8% WL with placebo plus semaglutide 2.4 mg, without worsening tolerability.

Dual Agonism with Glucagon

Glucagon is secreted from pancreatic α-cells in response to low blood glucose levels. It increases blood glucose through hepatic glucose production, but also reduces food intake, increases energy expenditure, and promotes hepatic fatty acid oxidation.

Combining glucagon with GLP-1 actions could improve WL while protecting against the diabetogenic risk of glucagon agonism—efficacy in early-phase clinical trials with pharmacotherapies based on combinations of gut hormones.

Efinopegdutide

In a phase II trial in people with T2DM and obesity, BI 456906 led to a dose-dependent WL of up to 9.0% at 16 weeks compared with 1.2% with placebo and 5.4% with semaglutide 1 mg.

Cotadutide

About 300 mg was superior for WL (5.02%) compared with placebo (0.68%) and liraglutide 1.8 mg (3.33%) in a 54-week phase IIb trial in people with T2DM and obesity, and reduced glycated hemoglobin (HbA1c) to similar levels to those achieved with liraglutide 1.8 mg.

The most commonly reported adverse effects with dual GLP-1/glucagon agonists were gastrointestinal (nausea and vomiting).

Triple Agonism (Glucagon-like Peptide-1/Glucose-dependent Insulinotropic Polypeptide/Glucagon): Retatrutide

Given the efficacy and benefits of the dual GLP-1/GIP RA tirzepatide and the dual GLP-1/glucagon RAs, a triple agonist targeting all three receptors (GLP-1/GIP/glucagon) could result in superior WL and glycemic control compared with dual agonists. LY3437943 (retatrutide), a new triple agonist, resulted in more WL compared with tirzepatide in preclinical studies and also improved the glucose profile. In a phase Ib trial in people with T2DM, retatrutide once weekly subcutaneously for 12 weeks led to a placebo-adjusted HbA1c reduction of up to 1.6% and dose-dependent placebo-adjusted WL of up to 8.96 kg in the highest dose group.

Other Pharmacotherapies in the Pipeline not Based on Gut Hormones

Bimagrumab, an intravenous 4-weekly human monoclonal antibody against the activin type II receptor,

There is proinflammatory activity and oxidative stress in the bone. This increases muscle fat and adipose tissue inflammation.

Sarcopenic obesity is associated with worse outcomes with knee osteoarthritis, increased risk of falling and fracture, increased risk of depression, and possibly increased cancer risk.

Sarcopenic obesity may increase mortality risk, but the results are conflicting. In a Swedish Cohort study by Berens et al., sarcopenic obesity was found in 4–11% of community-dwelling older adults. 75-year-old women but not men with sarcopenic obesity had an increased risk of dying within 10 years. An 87-year-old man with obesity without sarcopenia was related to a survival benefit over a four-year period.

MANAGEMENT

Individualized management forms the cornerstone of the treatment of obesity in the elderly. Increased physical activity, and dietary management including optimal protein intake are all important.

Exercise reduces oxidative stress, improves muscle oxidative capacity, and promotes mitochondrial synthesis. A combination of aerobic and resistance training exercises promotes muscle synthesis. Exercise-induced minor muscle injury activates the satellite cells to regenerate muscles. The muscle-promoting factors are insulin-like growth factor-1 (IGF-1), fibroblast growth factor, and other mechano growth factor. Aerobic exercise improves cardiorespiratory fitness and has beneficial effects on mortality. Resistance exercise improves muscle and bone mass. At least, 150 minutes of aerobic exercise and two sessions of resistance exercise per week, if necessary, under supervision, improves overall health outcomes. It is important to start low and go slow to minimize injury. This would improve adherence. Aerobic activity should target ~65% of the peak heart rate, aiming to reach 70–85% of the peak heart rate over the duration of the exercise regimen.

If weight loss is intended, a calories restriction of 500–1,000 kcal/day may help. The initial goal for weight loss is 0.5 kg/week. It is important to ensure adequate protein intake of 1 g/kg/day. Higher intake does not improve lean mass and may have adverse effects on kidney function. The mechanisms to improve protein anabolism are subjects of research. It is unclear if protein taken before exercise or spreading out over the day is more helpful. Also, the type of protein, source of protein, and their effects on muscle anabolism need further research. It is also important to limit refined carbohydrates, and saturated fats and to avoid trans fat. A healthy dietary pattern is one rich with complex carbohydrates, pulses, legumes, nuts, fruits and vegetables, mono and polyunsaturated fatty acids, low-fat dairy products, lean meat, and fish.

There are novel treatment modalities in the pipeline that need further evidence. Some of them are whole-body vibration therapy, periodization (systematic variation in physical training specificity, intensity, and volume within a period), selective androgen receptor modulators, ghrelin analog, and myostatin inhibitors.

CONCLUSION

The increasing prevalence of obesity in the elderly is a result of the confluence of the epidemics of obesity and the aging population. Merely diagnosing obesity based on BMI may miss the diagnosis of obesity in the elderly which is often sarcopenic obesity. Increased physical activity in the younger years can help build muscle and bone mass, which may minimize the adverse effects of age-related decline in muscle mass. Sarcopenic obesity has unique challenges that are different from obesity in general. Currently, available treatment modalities are appropriate dietary intake and exercise. There are novel therapies in research, but they need more evidence before they can be applied to the elderly population.

SUGGESTED READINGS

1. NCD Risk Factor Collaboration (NCD-RisC). Trends in adult body-mass index in 200 countries from 1975 to 2014: a pooled analysis of 1698 population-based measurement studies with 19·2 million participants. Lancet. 2016;387(10026):1377-96.
2. Nations United, Department of Economic Population Division. (2017). World Population Prospects: The 2017 Revision, Key Findings and Advance Tables. https://population.un.org/wpp/publications/files/wpp2017_keyfindings.pdf [Last accessed December, 2023].
3. Cruz-Jentoft AJ, Bahat G, Bauer J, Boirie Y, Bruyère O, Cederholm T, et al. Sarcopenia: revised European consensus on definition and diagnosis. Age Ageing. 2019;48(1):16-31.
4. Baumgartner RN, Wayne SJ, Waters DL, Janssen I, Gallagher D, Morley JE. Sarcopenic obesity predicts instrumental activities of daily living disability in the elderly. Obes Res. 2004;12(12):1995-2004.
5. Hirani V, Naganathan V, Blyth F, Le Couteur DG, Seibel MJ, Waite LM, et al. Longitudinal associations between body composition, sarcopenic obesity and outcomes of frailty, disability, institutionalisation and mortality in community-dwelling older men: The Concord Health and Ageing in Men Project. Age Ageing. 2017;46(3):413-20.
6. von Berens Å, Obling SR, Nydahl M, Koochek A, Lissner L, Skoog I, et al. Sarcopenic obesity and associations with mortality in older women and men - a prospective observational study. BMC Geriatr. 2020;20(1):199.

80

CHAPTER

Newer Therapies in Obesity

Smita Thakur, Anshini Thakur

ABSTRACT

Obesity is an epidemic, a global problem, and a public health threat. Obesity affects 60% adults and one in three children. Global Burden of Disease study in 2017 showed that body mass index (BMI) > 25 kg/m^2 is associated with 2.3 and 2.4 million deaths in men and women, respectively. The prevalence of obesity in adults is estimated to be >40% and is increasing globally following coronavirus disease 2019 (COVID-19) pandemic, linked with increased morbidity and mortality from COVID-19.

Leading factors for obesity range from low birth weight (LBW) to aging, diet, sleep patterns, and medications but overall, the burden of lifestyle is the highest contributor. Also, genetics, epigenetics, and environmental factors play a big role.

Obesity is the leading risk factor for disability, causing 7% of years lived with disability. Obesity is the key factor for various noncommunicable diseases (NCDs). It has a strong association with cardiovascular disease (CVD), type 2 diabetes mellitus (T2DM), cancer, musculoskeletal disorders, mental health issues, low self-esteem, underachievement, immune dysfunction, and mortality. Two-thirds of deaths related to high BMI were due to CVD. The prevalence is on the rise due to low-cost food and lack of physical exercise. Obesity affects both developed and underdeveloped countries.

The foremost treatment of obesity is lifestyle change, a healthy diet, and moderate exercise. Randomized controlled trials have shown >8% decrease in weight in the first year; however, cumulative data reveal that most patients cannot sustain the lifestyle changes, and more than half of the lost weight was regained over the next 2 years.

Treatment of obesity is very challenging and evolving. Guidelines agree to a multidisciplinary approach including lifestyle modifications, behavioral therapy, pharmacotherapy, and/or bariatric surgery. Medical and surgical management have revolutionized how we manage obesity currently and in the future. Newer antiobesity medications (AOMs) show very promising results. AOM help patients to lose weight, who have failed to do so with lifestyle modifications. Several drugs have been withdrawn due to cardiovascular (CV) events, and psychiatric, abuse, and dependence risks. There is a need for mandatory placebo-controlled CV safety data for new AOMs and these results show promising results. Future novel AOMs are currently in the pipeline.

Obesity management should focus on managing life courses and tackling an obesogenic environment, including problems with digital marketing to children.

INTRODUCTION

Antiobesity medications (AOMs) are indicated with body mass index (BMI) ≥30 or 27 kg/m^2 in the presence of one or more comorbidities.

Obesity medications including liraglutide, semaglutide, tirzepatide, orlistat, phentermine/topiramate, and bupropion/naltrexone combinations are licensed for nonsyndromic obesity, whereas metreleptin and setmelanotide are indicated for rare obesity syndromes. Tirzepatide is about to be approved by the Food and Drug Administration (FDA).

The majority of AOMs act centrally, reducing appetite, increasing satiety, and slowing gastric emptying. However, current data do not suggest reduction in hard cardiovascular (CV) outcomes, forthcoming data is awaited.

The choice of AOM should take into consideration patient's clinical picture, biochemical profile, comorbidities, expected weight loss, and improvement in CV risk.

MEDICATIONS FOR MONOGENIC SYNDROME OF OBESITY

Monogenic obesity is a rare syndrome constituting <5% of all obesity cases. The medications for monogenic obesity are described here.

Setmelanotide

Setmelanotide is a melanocortin-4 receptor agonist approved in 2020 as a subcutaneous injectable formulation for patients >6 years with obesity due to deficiency of proopiomelanocortin, proprotein convertase subtilisin/kexin type 1 (PCSK9), or leptin receptor deficiency confirmed on genetic testing. The most common adverse effects were injection-site reactions and hyperpigmentation disorders. A total body weight loss of 7.6% was observed in a 1-year trial of patients with Alström and Bardet–Biedl syndrome.

Metreleptin

Metreleptin is a leptin analog, FDA approved in 2014 for leptin deficiency in patients with congenital or acquired lipodystrophy and associated comorbidities. It is administered as subcutaneous daily injections starting at 0.06 mg/kg/day with a maximum dose of 0.13 mg/kg/day. Metreleptin has shown significant improvement in metabolic parameters over 6 months. It has also resulted in a decrease in 24-hour energy expenditure by 5% and 7.9% at 2 weeks and 6 months, respectively. It also resulted in reduction in lean body mass.

MEDICATIONS FOR NONSYNDROMIC OBESITY

Currently approved AOMs target peripheral and central pathways, reducing appetite, and increasing satiety, and hence decreasing energy intake.

Orlistat

Orlistat inhibits gastric and pancreatic lipases, hence decreasing dietary fat absorption. Orlistat causes steatorrhea and causes modest weight loss which depends mainly on diet. It is an oral treatment, 120 mg with meals or within an hour afterward. The XENDOS (XENical in the prevention of diabetes in obese subjects) (n = 3,305) study showed that after 4 years weight loss was higher with orlistat 120 mg TDS as compared to placebo. The ATTEMPT study showed orlistat to be useful in multifactorial treatment of CV risk in patients with metabolic syndrome. If 5% weight loss is not achieved in 3 months, treatment should be discontinued.

Phentermine/Topiramate

Phentermine, a sympathomimetic, stimulates serotonin release at high doses and has a lower risk of substance abuse compared with other amphetamines. As singleton therapy, it is approved for <12 weeks treatment.

Topiramate is a gamma-aminobutyric acid (GABA) agonist, glutamate antagonist, and carbonic anhydrase inhibitor shown to suppress appetite via unclear mechanisms. Phentermine with topiramate is licensed for long-term use.

Patients are started on a low dose and then the dose is increased to mid dose after 2 weeks. If after 12 weeks 3% weight loss is not achieved, the dose can be increased to 11.25/69 mg for 14 days and then to 15/92 mg daily. If 5% weight loss is not achieved after 12 weeks on a high dose, treatment should be gradually tapered and stopped over 1 week. Adverse effects include dry mouth and psychiatric effects such as depression, anxiety, and loss of concentration.

Bupropion/Naltrexone

A combination therapy consisting of bupropion, a dopamine-reuptake inhibitor, and naltrexone, an opioid-receptor antagonist, has a potential for 4–5% reduction in body weight, but its CV safety is questionable. The therapy can cause dizziness, dry mouth, and nausea.

Liraglutide (Saxenda)

Liraglutide is a human glucagon-like peptide-1 (GLP-1) analog with an arginine-for-lysine substitution and a C-16 palmitic acid side chain. The modification prolongs absorption time and decreases deactivation rate of dipeptidyl peptidase. It has a half-life of 13 hours. It acts by increasing insulin secretion, decreasing glucagon production, and delaying gastric emptying and appetite. Its effect relies on oral glucose intake. The SCALE (Satiety and Clinical Adiposity – Liraglutide Evidence in diabetic and non-diabetic individuals) study included four randomized controlled trials (RCTs) on liraglutide 3 mg once daily compared to placebo, extended over 56 weeks. Following 56 weeks of liraglutide with lifestyle intervention, a reduction of 8.4 ± 7.3 kg weight was seen as compared to placebo. 63% patients lost >5% body weight and 33% lost >10% body weight.

Liraglutide reduced prediabetic prevalence, affecting waist circumference, reduction in systolic and diastolic blood pressure, and improvement in dyslipidemia.

Its main side effects were gallbladder-related diseases (cholelithiasis or cholecystitis) and pancreatitis. 78% of these patients underwent surgery and 84% discontinued treatment. Liraglutide is contraindicated in patients with a history or family history of pancreatitis and medullary carcinoma thyroid or multiple endocrine neoplasia.

Semaglutide (Wegovy)

Semaglutide is a GLP-1 analog used in both type 2 diabetes mellitus (T2DM) and obesity. It is available as 2.4 mg once weekly subcutaneous (SC) injection. Oral semaglutide is not approved for obesity treatment. Its starting dose is 0.25 mg, and the dose is titrated every 4 weeks until 2.4 mg is reached (in approximately 16 weeks). Its half-life is 155–184 hours.

The STEP (Semaglutide Treatment Effect in People with obesity) trial evaluated efficacy and safety of semaglutide 2.4 mg weekly dose as compared to placebo for 68 weeks each. The population included men and women with overweight/obesity with at least one treated or untreated weight-related comorbidity. The STEP trial reported a weight reduction of 14.8% in intervention group, compared to 2.4% in placebo group.

The study on the effects of semaglutide on heart disease and stroke in patients with obesity (SELECT study) is ongoing. Gastrointestinal side effects such as nausea, constipation, and diarrhea are common. Contraindications are similar to those of liraglutide.

The STEP 8 study compared semaglutide 2.4 mg once weekly to liraglutide 3 mg daily injections, along with lifestyle intervention. Semaglutide arm showed 15.8% weight reduction as compared to 6.4% weight reduction in liraglutide arm in 68 weeks.

Tirzepatide

Tirzepatide is a new drug with dual coagonist, GLP-1/GIP (glucose-dependent insulinotropic polypeptide).

The SURMOUNT-1 trial evaluated efficacy and safety of tirzepatide once weekly in participants without T2DM who are obese/overweight and have weight-related comorbidities. This randomized controlled, double-blinded trial evaluated 2,539 adults with BMI >30 and >27 kg/m^2 with at least one comorbidity, over 72 weeks. Along with lifestyle intervention, participants were given once weekly tirzepatide injection. Weight loss with tirzepatide 15 mg was 20.9% compared with 3.1% for placebo group.

Tirzepatide has received FDA approval for T2DM but is in the approval process for treatment of obesity.

A meta-analysis compared seven RCTs and reported 9.23 kg more weight loss with tirzepatide 15 mg SC weekly when compared with semaglutide 2.4 mg SC weekly. Tirzepatide is promising in treatment of nonalcoholic fatty liver disease and nonalcoholic steatohepatitis. **Table 1** shows various medications approved by FDA-European Medicines Agency (EMA) per year, their mechanism of action, adverse events, and contraindications.

Figure 1 shows central and peripheral site of actions of various AOMs.

Suggested algorithm for the selection of AOM, taking into consideration the availability of drug safety, contraindications, and preliminary efficacy data for a specific patient profile **(Flowchart 1 and Fig. 2)**.

TABLE 1: Antiobesity medications: approval, mechanism of action, adverse events, and contraindications.

Drug (trade name)	Approval FDA/ EMA (year)	Mechanism of action	Adverse events[a]	Contraindications[b]
Orlistat (Xenical, Alli)	• *FDA*: 1999 • *EMA*: 1998	Gastric and pancreatic lipase inhibitor	Oily rectal leakage, abdominal distress, abdominal pain, flatulence with discharge, fecal urgency, steatorrhea, fecal incontinence, and increased defecation	Patients with chronic malabsorption syndrome or cholestasis, and pregnancy
Phentermine/ Topiramate (Qsymia)	*FDA*: 2012	NE agonist/GABA agonist, glutamate antagonist	Elevation in heart rate, mood and sleep disorders, cognitive impairment, metabolic acidosis, paresthesia, and dry mouth	Glaucoma, hyperthyroidism, during or within 14 days following the administration of monoamine oxidase inhibitors, hypersensitivity to sympathomimetic amines, and pregnancy
Naltrexone/ Bupropion (Contrave/ Mysimba)	• *FDA*: 2014 • *EMA*: 2015	Opioid receptor antagonist/DA- and NE-reuptake inhibitor	Nausea, constipation, headache, vomiting, dizziness, insomnia, dry mouth, diarrhea, and sleep disorder	Chronic opioid use, acute opioid withdrawal, uncontrolled hypertension, seizure disorder, bulimia or anorexia nervosa, abrupt discontinuation of alcohol, benzodiazepines, barbiturates, and antiseizure drugs; concomitant use of MAOIs, patient receiving linezolid or IV methylene blue, and pregnancy

Continued

Continued

Drug (trade name)	Approval FDA/ EMA (year)	Mechanism of action	Adverse events[a]	Contraindications[b]
Liraglutide (Saxenda)	• *FDA*: 2014 • *EMA*: 2015	GLP-1 analog	Increased heart rate, hypoglycemia, constipation, diarrhea, nausea, vomiting, and headache	Personal or family history of medullary thyroid carcinoma or multiple endocrine neoplasia syndrome type 2, and pregnancy
Semaglutide (Wegovy)	• *FDA*: 2021 • *EMA*: 2021	GLP-1 analog	Nausea, vomiting, diarrhea, abdominal pain, constipation, and headache	Personal or family history of medullary thyroid carcinoma or in patients with multiple endocrine neoplasia syndrome type 2, and pregnancy
Setmelanotide (Imcivree)	• *FDA*: 2020 • *EMA*: 2021	MC4R agonist	Injection site reactions, hyperpigmentation, nausea, headache, diarrhea, vomiting, and abdominal pain	None
Tirzepatide[c]	Under consideration by FDA	GIP/GLP-1 dual agonist	Nausea, diarrhea, decreased appetite, vomiting, constipation, dyspepsia, and abdominal pain	Personal or family history of medullary thyroid carcinoma or multiple endocrine neoplasia syndrome type 2, known serious hypersensitivity to tirzepatide or any of the excipients

[a]Adverse events presented here are those that are present in more than 10% of the population, based on the FDA approval leaflet.

[b]Contraindications are based on the FDA approval leaflet.

[c]Under expedited consideration for FDA approval.

(DA: dopamine; EMA: European Medicines Agency; FDA: Food and Drug Administration; GABA: gamma-aminobutyric acid; GI: gastrointestinal; GIP: gastric inhibitory polypeptide; GLP-1: glucagon-like peptide 1; IV: intravenous; MAOIs: monoamine oxidase inhibitors; MC4R: melanocortin-4 receptor; NE: norepinephrine)

Source: Chakhtoura M et al. (2023).

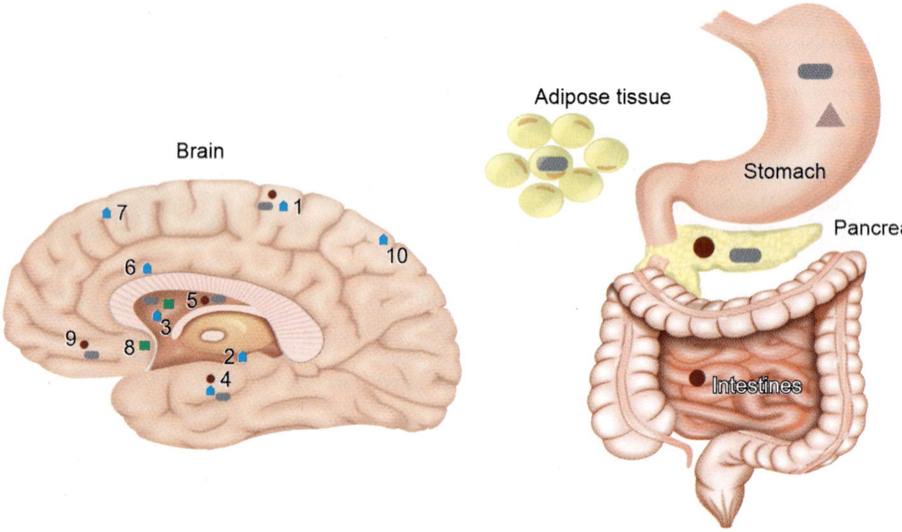

Medication	Central site of action	Peripheral site of action
GLP-1 receptor agonists	1, 3, 4, 5, 9	Gastrointestinal tract
Naltrexone/Bupropion	1, 2, 3, 4, 6, 7, 10	None
Phentermine/Topiramate	2, 3, 8	None
Orlistat	None	Gastrointestinal tract
GIP/GLP-1 dual agonists	1, 3, 4, 5, 9	Adipose tissue, gastrointestinal tract

FIG. 1: Central and peripheral site of actions of various anti-obesity medications.

(GIP: glucose-dependent insulinotropic polypeptide; GLP-1: glucagon-like peptide-1)

Source: Chakhtoura M et al. (2023).

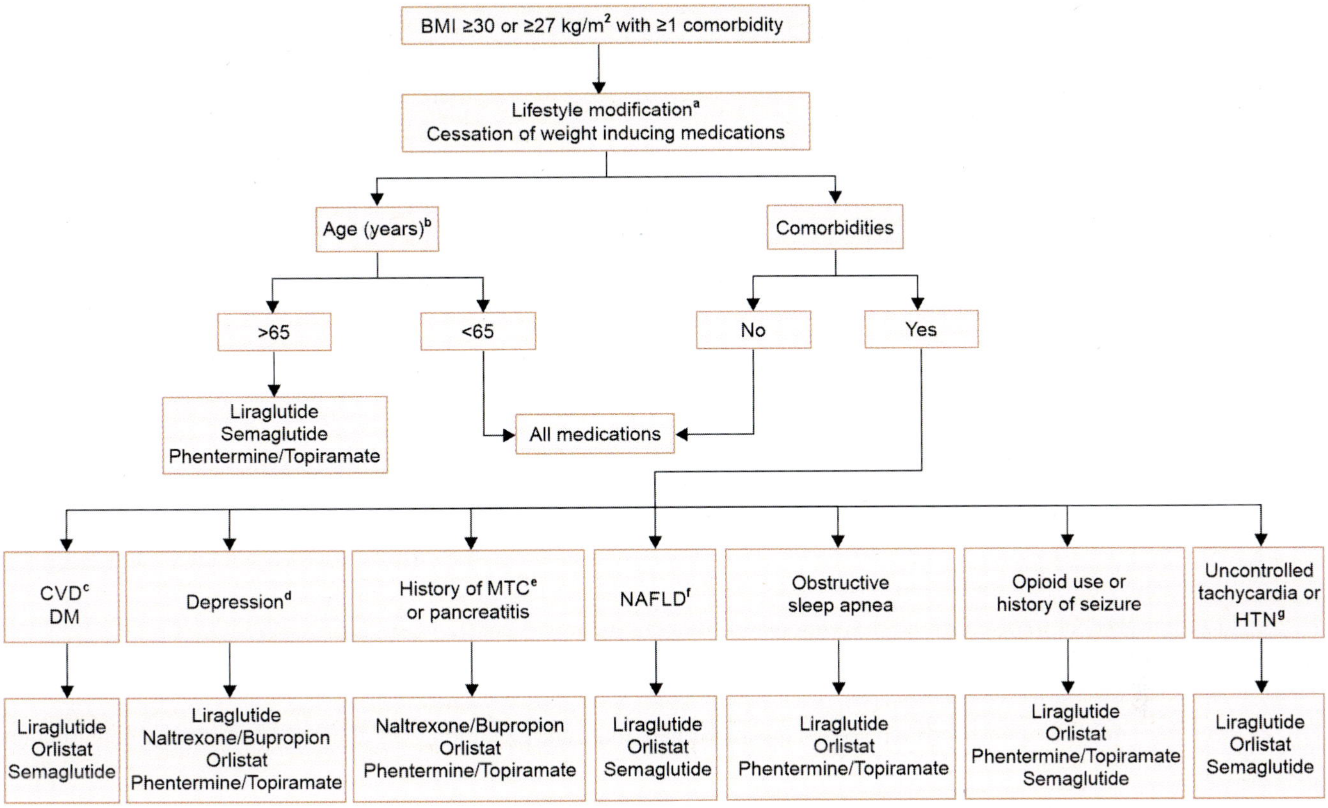

[a] Cardiovascular disease (CVD), diabetes mellitus (DM), hypertension (HTN), medullary thyroid cancer (MTC), nonalcoholic fatty liver disease (NAFLD).
[b] *Age >65 years*: Liraglutide and phentermine/topiramate trials included 7% of participants ≥65 years.
[c] CVD includes patient with previous history of CVD and those at high risk for CVD.
[d] Depression
[e] MTC or family history of MTC, contraindication for liraglutide and semaglutide.
[f] Small trials on orlistat, liraglutide, and semaglutide showed improvement in steatosis, but none of them showed improvement in fibrosis.
[g] The Food and Drug Administration (FDA) leaflet of phentermine states the following under contraindications history of CVD (e.g., coronary artery disease, stroke, arrhythmias, congestive heart failure, uncontrolled HTN).

FLOWCHART 1: Selection of anti-obesity medications.
(BMI: body mass index)
Source: Chakhtoura M et al. (2023).

MEDICATIONS IN THE HORIZON

Several drugs are currently being investigated as potential AOMs, one of those in phase three trials is methylphenidate, a stimulant approved for treatment of attention deficit hyperkinetic disorder. It is a dopamine-reuptake inhibitor and reduces energy intake.

CONCLUSION

Obesity is the biggest public health challenge; all steps must be taken to curb this epidemic. National policies should involve various government sectors and stakeholders.

Evidence indicate that the next few years will revolutionize obesity treatment, improvement in body weight, prevent cardiorenal and metabolic complications of obesity.

Newer AOMs will pave the way for increased weight loss and results may be comparable to bariatric surgery. SC injections may be less tolerated than oral treatments, although their efficacy and safety profile are superior. With wider implementation, the global burden of obesity may decrease.

The OBEsity Diverse Intervention Sharing (OBEDIS) project focuses on dietary and other interventions, streamlines AOM clinical trials, and harmonizes variables and endpoints of AOM clinical trials, to allow data pooling and derivation of prediction models.

Health is influenced by an accumulation of experiences across life course, including the promotion of physical activities.

The World Health Organization recommends that the prevention and management of obesity need coordinated partnerships of various government sectors, communities, mass media, and private sector.

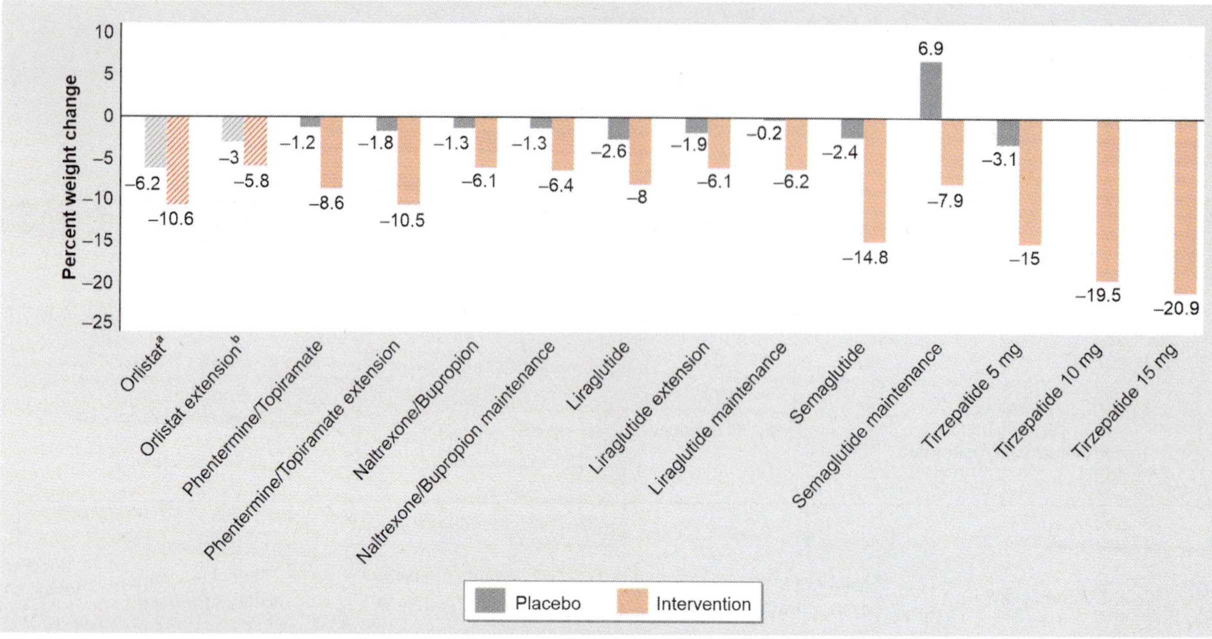

[a] The mean weight change in the orlistat group is in kg not in percent (stripped bar charts).

[b] Under expedited consideration for FDA approval.

FIG. 2: Mean percent (%) weight change reported in the main phase three and extension trials of the Food and Drug Administration (FDA)-approved antiobesity medications.

SUGGESTED READINGS

1. Caklili OT, Cesur M, Mikhailidis DP, Rizzo M. Novel anti-obesity therapies and their different effects and safety profiles: a critical overview. Diabetes Metab Syndr Obes. 2023;16:1767-74.
2. Torgerson JS, Hauptman J, Boldrin MN, Sjöström L. XENical in the prevention of diabetes in obese subjects (XENDOS) study: a randomized study of orlistat as an adjunct to lifestyle changes for the prevention of type 2 diabetes in obese patients. Diabetes Care. 2004;27(1):155-61.
3. West R, Gilsenan A, Coste F, Zhou X, Brouard R, Nonnemaker J, et al. The ATTEMPT cohort: a multi-national longitudinal study of predictors, patterns and consequences of smoking cessation; introduction and evaluation of internet recruitment and data collection methods. Addiction. 2006;101(9):1352-61.
4. Xavier Pi-Sunyer X, Astrup A, Fujioka K, Greenway F, Halpern A, Krempf M. et al. SCALE Obesity and Prediabetes NN8022-1839 Study Group. A randomized controlled trial of 3.0 mg of liraglutide in weight management. NEJM. 2015;373:11-22.
5. Kushner RF, Calanna S, Davies M, Dicker D, Garvey WT, Goldman B, et al. Semaglutide 2.4 mg for the treatment of obesity: key elements of the STEP trials 1 to 5. Obesity (Silver Spring). 2020;28(6):1050-61.
6. Clinicaltrials.gov. (2023). Semaglutide Effects on Heart Disease and Stroke in Patients with Overweight or Obesity (SELECT). [online] Available from https://www.clinicaltrials.gov/study/NCT03574597 [Last accessed December, 2023].
7. Rubino DM, Greenway FL, Khalid U, O'Neil PM, Rosenstock J, Sørrig R, et al. STEP 8 Investigators. Effect of weekly subcutaneous semaglutide vs daily liraglutide on body weight in adults with overweight or obesity without diabetes: The STEP 8 randomized clinical trial. JAMA. 2022;327(2):138-50.
8. Clinicaltrials.gov. (2023). A Study of Tirzepatide (LY3298176) in Participants With Obesity or Overweight (SURMOUNT-1). [online] Available from https://classic.clinicaltrials.gov/ct2/show/NCT04184622 [Last accessed December, 2023].
9. World Health Organization. (2022). WHO European Regional Obesity Report 2022. [online] Available from https://www.who.int/europe/publications/i/item/9789289057738 [Last accessed December, 2023].
10. World Health Organization Europe. (2011). The challenge of obesity. [online] Available from https://www.who.int/europe/news-room/fact-sheets/item/the-challenge-of-obesity [Last accessed December, 2023].
11. Alligier M, Barrès R, Blaak EE, Boirie Y, Bouwman J, Brunault P, et al. OBEDIS Core Variables Project: European Expert Guidelines on a minimal core set of variables to include in randomized, controlled clinical trials of obesity interventions. Obes Facts. 2020;13(1):1-28.
12. National Institute for Health and Care Excellence (NICE). Guidelines on management of Obesity: https://cks.nice.org.uk/topics/obesity/management/management/
13. Dicker D. (2019). European Association for the Study of Obesity. Anti Obesity Medicine. [online] Available from https://cdn.easo.org/wp-content/uploads/2019/08/16195027/Dror-Dicker-Anti-Obesity-Medication.pdf [Last accessed December, 2023].
14. Chakhtoura M, Haber R, Ghezzawi M, Caline Rhayem C, Raya Tcheroyan R, Mantzoros CS. Pharmacotherapy of obesity: an update on the available medications and drugs under investigation. EClinicalMedicine. 2023;58:101882.

81

CHAPTER

Combination Therapy in Lipid Management

Deepak Gupta, Krunal Patel

ABSTRACT

Elevated low-density lipoprotein cholesterol (LDL-C) plays an important role in atherosclerotic cardiovascular disease (ASCVD). Reducing levels of LDL-C lowers the risk for ASCVD. According to scientific studies, the current data suggests very low LDL-C goals in patients at a high/very high cardiovascular (CV) risk because they are associated with fewer CV events and improvements in atherosclerotic plaques. For the past many years, statins have been used for the prevention of numerous atherosclerotic CV events and CV deaths. Certain patients do not show optimal response to statins alone because of several factors. In those patients combination therapy with ezetimibe, bempedoic acid, and proprotein convertase subtilisin/kexin type 9 (PCSK9) inhibitors, is required to control the LDL-C levels and further prevent CV events.

INTRODUCTION

In the past three decades, statins have contributed to the prevention of numerous atherosclerotic cardiovascular (CV) events and CV deaths. Despite its critical role in CV event prevention, heart disease remains one of the leading causes of death. A significant number of studies have shown that lowering circulating low-density lipoprotein cholesterol (LDL-C) is associated with a reduction in the relative and absolute risk of CV diseases (CVDs). Each mmol/L (38.7 mg/dL) reduction in LDL-C is associated with a relative risk (RR) reduction of approximately 22%. This correlation persists even at very low LDL-C levels. The first-line lipid-lowering treatment for atherosclerotic cardiovascular disease (ASCVD) risk reduction continues to be statins. Although many patients achieve lipid-lowering goals with high-intensity statins, certain patients do not have an optimal response because of genetic issues, intolerance, nonadherence, or therapeutic inertia. Strong data from clinical trials supports the effectiveness and safety of nonstatin drugs added to statin therapy in high-risk patients.

SCREENING

Dyslipidemia is an important risk factor for ASCVD, and treatment has been proven to significantly reduce CV risk. According to a study by the American Heart Association, there are approximately 28.5 million people over the age of 20 years old who have high cholesterol, making the prevalence of hypercholesterolemia 11.9%. Therefore, all adults should be screened for plasma lipids. A lipid profile test should be performed, preferably after an overnight fast. In patients with evidence of dyslipidemia, further evaluation, and management are based on evidence of preexisting ASCVD and clinical assessment of CV risk using a risk calculator such as the American Heart Association (AHA) and American College of Cardiology (ACC) risk calculator, such as well as, in some cases, additional approaches to risk assessment, such as apolipoprotein B (ApoB) and lipoprotein (a) [Lp(a)].

Why should lipid-lowering combination therapy be used?

When diet and lifestyle are insufficient to attenuate the risk of atherosclerotic CVD, pharmacotherapy is essential. Statins have long been the first option for LDL-C reduction. However, what matters most is how much, when, and for how long the LDL-C reduction is achieved rather than how it is achieved.

Evidence from a large number of randomized controlled trials (RCTs) strongly supports a dose-dependent association between LDL-C lowering and CV event risk reduction. In the last few years, the IMPROVE-IT (Improved Reduction of Outcomes: Vytorin Efficacy International Trial), FOURIER (Further Cardiovascular Outcomes Research With PCSK9 Inhibition in Subjects With Elevated Risk), and ODYSSEY OUTCOMES trials have demonstrated that achieving an LDL-C below 55 mg/dL is associated with an incremental benefit. Also, the achievement of these very low LDL-C levels is safe and not associated with any increase in side effects, including neurocognitive alterations, cancer, new-onset diabetes, or hemorrhagic stroke, to mention those of major concern.

Combination therapy is necessary to reach these highly challenging low LDL-C values because statins alone will not be able to achieve these objectives. Several drugs, such as cholesterol ester transfer protein (CETP) inhibitors, niacin, and even fibrates failed to show additional benefits to improve CV events. But among the nonstatin therapies, ezetimibe, proprotein convertase subtilisin/kexin type 9 (PCSK9) inhibitors, and bempedoic acid reduce LDL-C by increasing the catabolic rate of the particle through its physiological LDL receptor pathway, so they do not alter the supply of intracellular cholesterol.

The causality of LDL in the process of atherosclerotic lesion development is beyond any doubt. LDL-lowering therapies stop the artery wall damage and progression of atherosclerotic plaques, allowing the action of healing mechanisms, stopping the inflammatory response, cleaning molecular and cell debris, and reducing the atheroma volume, resulting in plaque regression. Thus, the combination of statin and nonstatin therapies **(Table 1)** works synergistically to lower LDL, suppressing the etiology of atherosclerosis.

TABLE 1: Hypolipidemic drugs used in combination therapy.

Drug class	Dose range	Administration	Major side effects	Effect on serum lipid levels (% change)
Statins				
• Atorvastatin • Rosuvastatin • Simvastatin • Pravastatin	• 10–80 mg/day • 5–40 mg/day • 10–40 mg/day • 10–80 mg/day	• Take any time • Take any time • Take in the evening • Take in the evening	• Muscle-related (e.g., myalgia, myopathy, myositis, and rhabdomyolysis), gastrointestinal (e.g., nausea, constipation, dyspepsia, diarrhea), sleep disturbance, elevations in hepatocellular enzymes, and alkaline phosphatase • Statins are dependent on CYP metabolism and/or transmembrane transporters for clearance • Coadministration of drugs that alter CYP metabolism or drug transporters often requires dose limitations or avoidance	• *LDL-C*: ↓ 20–60 • *HDL-C*: ↑ 5–10 • *Triglycerides*: ↓ 10–33
Cholesterol absorption inhibitor				
Ezetimibe	10 mg/day	Take any time	• Generally well tolerated; low risk for potential drug interactions • Increased transaminases may be observed with concurrent statin use; however, coadministration is common	• *LDL-C*: ↓ 17 • *HDL-C*: ↑ 1 • *Triglyceride*: ↓ 7–8

Continued

Continued

Drug class	Dose range	Administration	Major side effects	Effect on serum lipid levels (% change)
PCSK9 inhibitors				
• Alirocumab • Evolocumab	• 75–150 mg every 2 weeks or 300 mg every 4 weeks • 140 mg every 2 weeks or 420 mg every month	• Administer by subcutaneous injection into the thigh, abdomen, or upper arm • Administer by subcutaneous injection into the thigh, abdomen, or upper arm	• Injection site reactions • Low risk for potential drug interactions	• *LDL-C*: ↓ 38–72 • *HDL-C*: ↑ 4–9 • *Triglyceride*: ↓ 2–23
Adenosine triphosphate citrate lyase inhibitor				
Bempedoic acid	180 mg/day	Take any time	• Hyperuricemia, acute gouty arthritis; myalgia, muscle spasms, and arthralgias; and increased aspartate aminotransferase • Potential for significant drug interactions; dose limitations for some statins are recommended during concurrent use	• *LDL-C*: ↓ 15–19 • *HDL-C*: No change to ↓ 4.5 • *Triglyceride*: No change
Fibric acid derivative				
Fenofibrate	• *Nanocrystal*: 145 mg/day • *Micronized*: 90–200 mg/day • *Fenofibric acid*: 105–135 mg/day	• Multiple formulations exist with varying dosing and administration • Some formulations must be administered with food	• Muscle-related (e.g., myalgia, myositis, and rhabdomyolysis), gastrointestinal (e.g., dyspepsia, nausea, bloating, and cramping) • Potential for significant drug interactions; enhances the anticoagulant effect of warfarin, increases the risk of myopathy with statins	• *LDL-C*: ↓ 6–20 • *HDL-C*: ↑ 5–20 • *Triglyceride*: ↓ 41–53

(CYP: cytochrome P450; HDL-C: high-density lipoprotein cholesterol; LDL-C: low-density lipoprotein cholesterol; PCSK9: proprotein convertase subtilisin/kexin type 9)

RISK GROUPS FOR DYSLIPIDEMIA MANAGEMENT

Patients with established atherosclerotic CVD, including those with stable or unstable coronary artery disease, an ischemic stroke of atherosclerotic origin, transient ischemic attack, or peripheral arterial disease, are at high risk of a CVD event.

- *Average-risk* patients are those without any high-risk factors.
- *High-risk* patients are those with a prior CV event or those with other uncontrolled CV risk factors.
- *Very high-risk* patients are those with known CVD and diabetes, recurrent CVD events, or polyvascular disease (atherosclerosis in multiple circulatory beds).

APPROACH TOWARD THE MANAGEMENT OF LOW-DENSITY LIPOPROTEIN CHOLESTEROL

We treat all patients with known CVD with proven lifestyle interventions and high-intensity statin therapy, irrespective of baseline LDL-C. After the successful initiation of high-intensity statin therapy, we remeasure LDL-C within 6–8 weeks. For some patients with CVD in whom the LDL-C remains significantly elevated after high-statin therapy, we consider adding a second drug to further lower the LDL-C. In most cases, we usually choose ezetimibe before a PCSK9 inhibitor for reasons of cost and convenience. After treatment with statins plus ezetimibe, we remeasure LDL-C within 6–8 weeks. For

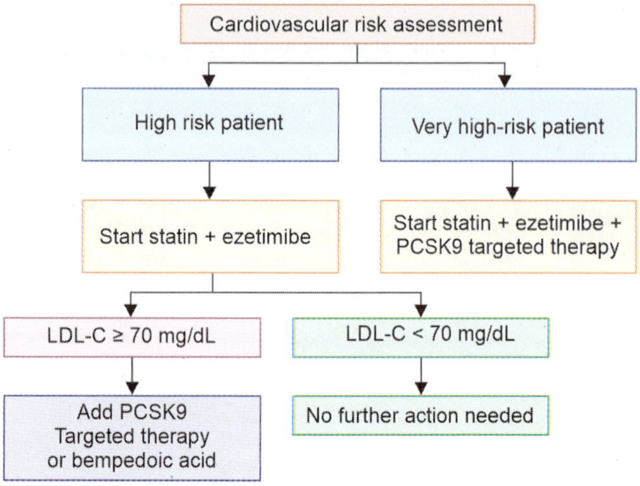

FLOWCHART 1: Approach to manage LDL-C.

(HDL-C: high-density lipoprotein cholesterol; LDL-C: low-density lipoprotein cholesterol; PCSK9: proprotein convertase subtilisin/kexin type 9)

many high-risk patients whose LDL-C remains high, we consider adding a PCSK9 inhibitor.

As outlined in **Flowchart 1**, statin monotherapy, even high-intensity statin monotherapy, will not be sufficient for the majority of patients to achieve the recommended goals.

- For *average-risk* patients whose on-statin treatment LDL-C is ≥ 70 mg/dL, we consider adding ezetimibe. We hardly ever give these individuals PCSK9 inhibitors.
- For *high-risk* patients whose on-statin LDL-C is ≥ 70 mg/dL, we treat them with a second drug and usually start with ezetimibe for cost and convenience. If the LDL-C on statin monotherapy is <70 mg/dL, we usually do not add a second drug.

  If the LDL-C remains above 70 mg/dL on statin plus ezetimibe, we may consider adding a PCSK9 inhibitor.
- For *very high-risk* patients, we consider adding a PCSK9 inhibitor if LDL-C remains above 50 mg/dL even after statin plus ezetimibe therapy.

OTHER POSSIBLE THERAPIES

Although lomitapide may be useful for patients with homozygous familial hypercholesterolemia (HoFH), its price and side-effect profile may discourage doctors from using it.

Bempedoic acid has modest efficacy on LDL-C. It can be used at the same point as ezetimibe, that is when the maximum recommended or tolerated statin dose has failed to achieve the appropriate LDL-C goal and PCSK9 inhibition is not possible. Its efficacy in lowering LDL-C is probably a little less than that of ezetimibe, but the two in combination provide the possibility of substantial LDL-C reduction in the statin-intolerant patient.

Fibrate therapy, which significantly decreases triglyceride levels and increases high-density lipoprotein cholesterol (HDL-C) without significant action on LDL-C, is also associated with a reduction in CV events. The combination of statins and fibrates is emerging as a possible therapeutic approach for many high-risk patients, especially those with atherogenic dyslipidemia. Despite an increase in reports of rhabdomyolysis with statin-fibrate combination therapy, gemfibrozil appears to carry a risk that is roughly 15 times greater than that of fenofibrate when taken with statins. So, this combination is avoided by doctors.

Inclisiran is the first and only small interfering ribonucleic acid (siRNA) therapy to lower low-density lipoprotein cholesterol with two doses a year, one after an initial dose and one at 3 months. The drug was approved in December 2021. The drug is indicated in the United States as a combination with diet and maximally tolerated statin therapy for the treatment of adults with clinical ASCVD or HoFH who require additional lowering of LDL-C (**Table 2**).

Combination Therapy

Combination Therapy in a Special Population

- *Women of childbearing age*: Statin therapy is currently contraindicated during pregnancy. However, recent data suggest that statins may not be uniformly teratogenic. The use of ezetimibe during pregnancy has not been thoroughly explored, so there may be dangers involved.
- *Older patients*: The benefit of LDL-C lowering therapy extends to healthy individuals 75 years of age or older. Statins along with PCSK9 therapy are recommended for these individuals.
- *Familial hypercholesterolemia (FH)*: All FH patients should receive maximally tolerated statin therapy as initial therapy. If, even after three months of compliant statin therapy, the LDL-C target has not been achieved, we add a second drug, ezetimibe a PCSK9 inhibitor, or both, as a second-line therapy. Bempedoic acid might be reasonable to add, if available if LDL-C levels are not achieved even after second-line therapy.

  Investigational and novel therapies such as microsomal triglyceride transfer protein inhibition (lomitapide) and mRNA inhibition of ApoB may be considered.
- *Chronic kidney disease*: When a patient's renal function becomes severely decreased, maximal dose atorvastatin is preferred rather than other statins as it is not dependent on renal function for its metabolism

TABLE 2: Combination therapy regimens and expected LDL-C reduction.

	Expected LDL-C reduction			
	Statin tolerant		**Statin intolerance**	
	>60%	**>80%**	**>35%**	**>60%**
Current options	Rosuvastatin 20–40 + ezetimibe 10	Rosuvastatin 20–40 + alirocumab/evolocumab + (ezetimibe 10)	Ezetimibe 10 + bile acid absorption	
	Atorvastatin 40–80 + ezetimibe 10	Atorvastatin 40–80 + alirocumab/evolocumab (+ ezetimibe 10)		Ezetimibe 10 + alirocumab/evolocumab
	Rosuvastatin 5–10 + alirocumab/evolocumab			
	Atorvastatin10–20 + alirocumab/evolocumab			
Additional emerging options	Rosuvastatin 5–10 + inclisiran	Atorvastatin 40–80 + inclisiran (+ ezetimibe 10)	Bempedoic acid 180 + ezetimibe 10	
	Atorvastatin 10–20 + inclisiran	Rosuvastatin 20–40 + inclisiran (+ ezetimibe 10)		Bempedoic acid 180 + ezetimibe 10 + PCSK9 targeted therapy
	Atorvastatin 20 + ezetimibe 10 + bempedoic acid 180			Ezetimibe 10 + inclisiran

(LDL-C: low-density lipoprotein cholesterol; ; PCSK9: proprotein convertase subtilisin/kexin type 9)

Source: European Society of Cardiology.

and excretion. Concerning second-line therapy, we add ezetimibe for patients who have not met their LDL-C goal.

CONCLUSION

In conclusion, LDL-C lowering is a crucial component of treating plaque lesions and preventing CV events. Greater CV benefits are linked to lowering LDL-C levels. The sooner individuals achieve low LDL-C readings, the better. To tailor the therapy, doctors should take into account all lipid-lowering treatments that are currently accessible. Combination therapy should enable practically all individuals to reach LDL-C targets. Patients at high risk for CV events should get lipid-lowering combo medications as the standard of care.

SUGGESTED READINGS

1. Varughese MG, Deshotels M, Ballantyne CM. (2022). Why Combination Lipid-Lowering Therapy Should be Considered Early in the Treatment of Elevated LDL-C For CV Risk Reduction. [online] Available from https://www.acc.org/Latest-in-Cardiology/Articles/2022/06/01/12/11/Why-Combination-Lipid-Lowering-Therapy-Should-be-Considered [Last accessed November, 2023].
2. Ray KK, Reeskamp LF, Laufs U, Banach M, Mach F, Tokgözoğlu LS, et al. Combination lipid-lowering therapy as first-line strategy in very high-risk patients. Eur Heart J. 2022;43(8):830-3.
3. Rosenson R. (2023). Low-density lipoprotein cholesterol lowering with drugs other than statins and PCSK9 inhibitors. [online] Available from https://www.uptodate.com/contents/low-density-lipoprotein-cholesterol-lowering-with-drugs-other-than-statins-and-pcsk9-inhibitors/print?search=ezetimibe [Last accessed November, 2023].
4. Rosenson RS, Hayward RA, Lopez-Sendon J. Management of low density lipoprotein cholesterol (LDL-C) in the secondary prevention of cardiovascular disease. [online]Available from https://www.uptodate.com/contents/management-of-low-density-lipoprotein-cholesterol-ldl-c-in-the-secondary-prevention-of-cardiovascular-disease [Last accessed November, 2023].

- Identify whether the blood sample is arterial or venous
- Check the validity of blood pH—use the Henderson equation
- Identify the primary disorder
- Identify the causes of the primary disorder.
- Calculate the anion gap (AG) (correct for low albumin, if indicated).
- Calculate the expected compensation (also called *secondary response*)
- Identify the mixed acid-base disorder, if any
- Use $\Delta AG/\Delta HCO_3$—ratio appropriately
- Determine the appropriate treatment

Measure Electrolytes and ABG Simultaneously or Within a Few Minutes Apart (Step 1)

In the evaluation of ABG, if there is a large difference between the measured and calculated HCO_3^-. The ABG and electrolytes should be repeated simultaneously or within a few minutes apart.

The Henderson equation is used to calculate the $[HCO_3^-]$

$$[HCO_3^-] \times (mEq/L) = 24 \times \frac{pCO_2}{[H^+]}$$

Identify whether the Blood Sample is Arterial or Venous (Step 2)

Arterial versus Venous Blood Sample for ABG

Arterial blood is used most of the time to evaluate an acid-base disorder. Venous blood samples can be used because there is an insignificant difference in ABG values between these two samples. There is not much difference between the two samples in normal healthy individuals. Significant differences can be observed in pathological conditions. Large arteriovenous differences can be found in (1) decreased cardiac output and (2) mechanical ventilation.

Check the Validity of Blood pH—Use Henderson Equation (Step 3)

Henderson–Hasselbalch Equation

$$H = pKa + \log\frac{[HCO_3^-]}{[H_2CO_3]}$$

H_2CO_3 cannot be Measured Directly

Its concentration can be estimated from pCO_2 and the solubility coefficient (α) of CO_2 at known temperature and pH. At 37°C and pH of 7.4, the pCO_2 is 40 mm Hg, α is 0.03, and pKa is 6.1. The Henderson-Hasselbalch equation can be appropriately written as:

$$pH = 6.1 + \log\frac{[HCO_3^-]}{[0.03 \times pCO_3]}$$

Henderson Equation

The same information can be obtained by using the Henderson equation, which relates (H^+) to pH. This equation, which calculates (H^+), is expressed as:

$$H^+ (mol/L) = 24 \times \frac{pCO_2}{HCO_3^-}$$

- As an example of how this equation can be used, consider the following ABG values:
  - pH = 7.40
  - pCO_2 = 40 mm Hg
  - HCO_3^- = 24 mEq/L

$$[HCO_3^-] (mEq/L) = 24 \times 40/24 = 40$$

- This $[H^+]$ of 40 corresponds to a pH of 7.40.
- The Henderson equation is thus used clinically to check the validity of pH obtained from the clinical laboratory.
- Please remember the following approximate $[H^+]$ to clinically relevant pH values:
  - pH 7.50 = 30
  - pH 7.40 = 40
  - pH 7.30 = 50
  - pH 7.20 = 60
  - pH 7.10 = 80
  - pH 7.00 = 100
- The Henderson equation can also be used to calculate the $[HCO_3^-]$

$$[HCO_3^-] \times (mEq/L) = 24 \times \frac{pCO_2}{H^+}$$

Primary Acid-base Disturbances (Step 4)

Identify the Causes of the Primary Disorder (Step 5)

Metabolic Acidosis (MAC)

- *Gain of anion*: Hyperchloremic, AG acidosis, and hyperphosphatemic

TABLE 4: Primary acid-base disturbances and their secondary response.

Acid-base disorder	pH	Primary change	Secondary change	Mechanism of secondary change
Metabolic acidosis	<7.40	$\downarrow HCO_3^-$	$\downarrow pCO_2$	Hyperventilation
Metabolic alkalosis	>7.40	$\uparrow HCO_3^-$	$\uparrow pCO_2$	Hypoventilation
Respiratory acidosis	<7.40	$\uparrow pCO_2$	$\uparrow HCO_3^-$	$\uparrow HCO_3^-$ reabsorption
Respiratory alkalosis	>7.40	$\downarrow pCO_2$	$\downarrow HCO_3^-$	$\downarrow HCO_3^-$ reabsorption

- *Loss of cation (Na^+, K^+)*: Renal—renal tubular acidosis (RTA), natriuretic agents, hypoaldosteronism, and excretion of sodium with nonchloride/nonbicarbonate anions (lactate, hippurate, and ketones). Gastrointestinal—diarrhea and vomiting pancreatic secretions.

Metabolic Alkalosis (MAL)

Loss of anion: Gastrointestinal—vomiting, villous adenoma, and chloride secretory diarrheas, renal—chloruretic agents (loop or thiazide diuretics), chloride channelopathies, and hypokalemia. Sweat—cystic fibrosis. Hypoalbuminemic state—malnutrition.

Gain of cation: Sodium bicarbonate, lactate, acetate, and citrate. Hypernatremia (hyperaldosteronism) and hypercalcemia (milk-alkali syndrome and calcium carbonate).

TABLE 5: Respiratory acidosis.

Acute	Chronic
• The central nervous system (CNS) depression • Neuromuscular disorders • Acute airway obstruction • Severe pneumonia or pulmonary edema • Flail chest • Ventilator dysfunction	• Chronic lung disease • Chronic neuromuscular disorders • Chronic respiratory center depression

BOX 1: Respiratory alkalosis.

Etiologies:
- Anxiety hypoxemia lung diseases (e.g., asthma, pneumonia, and PE)
- *CNS diseases*: Drugs—salicylates, catecholamines, and progesterone
- Pregnancy liver disease sepsis hepatic encephalopathy mechanical ventilation

(CNS: central nervous system; PE: pulmonary embolism)

TABLE 6: Unmeasured anions and cations (particularly anions).

Unmeasured cations (mEq/L)	Unmeasured anions (mEq/L)
K^+: 4.5	Albumin: 12
Ca^{2+}: 5.0	Other proteins: 3
Mg^{2+}: 1.5	PO_4^{3-}: 2
	SO_4^{2-}: 1
	Organic acids 5
Total: 11	Total: 23
Anion gap (AG) = 23 – 11 = 12 ± 4	

Calculate Anion Gap (Step 6)

Anion Gap

In plasma, the number of cations must equal the number of anions to maintain electroneutrality. Measurement of all of these cations and anions is not done routinely. Routinely, only Na^+, K^+, Cl^-, and HCO_3^- are measured. From these measurements, the number of unmeasured anions can be calculated.

This sum of unmeasured anions is called the AG:

$$AG\ (mEq/L) = [(Na^+) - (Cl^- + HCO_3^-)]$$

Normal AG Values

The normal reference range for AG is 12 ± 4. It is derived from electrolyte determinations using colorimetry and flame photometry. Newer ion-selective electrode methodology determines the normal AG level is 3–11. These low values are related to high Cl^- determination.

Hyperglycemia and AG

It is always debated whether or not AG should be calculated using measured serum Na^+ or corrected Na^+ in a patient with severe hyperglycemia. Na^+ decreases by 1.6 mEq/dL for each increase in 100 mg/dL glucose above normal glucose levels, but no such number is given for either Cl^- or HCO_3^-. It is, thus, emphasized that only measured Na^+ should be used to calculate the serum AG.

Clinical Use of AG

Traditionally, the AG is classified into *high AG* due to the accumulation of unmeasured anions, normal AG is usually related to a high Cl^- level. *Low AG* implies a substantial decrease in unmeasured anions or an increase in unmeasured cations.

TABLE 7: Most common causes of high AG metabolic acidosis.

Cause	Unmeasured anions causing high AG
• Uremic acidosis (renal failure)	• Sulfate, phosphate, and urate
• Ketoacidosis (diabetes, starvation, and alcohol)	• Acetoacetate and β-hydroxybutyrate
• Lactic acidosis	• L-lactate
• Small bowl resection	• D-lactate
Intoxicants	
• Methanol	• Formate
• Ethylene glycol	• Glycolate and oxalate
• Aspirin	• Salicylate, L-lactate, and ketoacids
• Acetaminophen (Tylenol)	• Pyroglutamate
• Paraldehyde	• Acetaldehyde or acetic acid
• Toluene	• Hippurate and benzoate

Note: Mnemonic to remember AG is GOLD MARK [Glycols (ethylene and propylene), Oxoproline (pyroglutamic acid), L-lactate, D-lactate, Methanol, Aspirin, Renal failure, and Ketoacidosis].

TABLE 8: Nonanion gap metabolic acidosis (NAGMA).

Hardup	Accrued	Panda rush
H: Hyperchloremia	*A*: Ammonium chloride/acetazolamide	*P*: Pancreatic secretion loss
A: Acetazolamide use in Addison's disease	*C*: Chloride intake	*A*: Acetazolamide
R: Renal tubular acidosis	*C*: Cholestyramine	*N*: Normal saline intoxication
D: Diarrhea	*R*: Renal tubular acidosis	*D*: Diarrhea
U: Ureteroenterostomy	*U*: Urine is diverted into the intestine	*A*: Aldosterone antagonists
P: Pancreatoenterostomy	*E*: Endocrine disorders (e.g., Addison's)	*R*: Renal tubular acidosis
	D: Diarrhea	*U*: Ureteric diversion
		S: Small bowel fistula
		H: Hyperalimentation

Note: All involve gain of chloride or loss of bicarbonate (i.e., measured ions).

TABLE 9: Mechanism of common causes of normal AG metabolic acidosis.

Cause	Mechanism
Diarrhea	Loss of HCO_3^- in stool
Ureterosigmoidostomy and ileal conduit	Loss of HCO_3^- in stool
Carbonic anhydrase inhibitors	Loss of HCO_3^- in urine
Recovery phase of ketoacidosis	Less HCO_3^- synthesis from decreased availability of ketones
Chronic kidney diseases (stages 4–5)	Decrease in NH_3 excretion
Proximal renal tubular acidosis (type 2)	Loss of HCO_3^- in urine
Distal renal tubular acidosis (type 1)	Decreased renal acid secretion
Distal renal tubular acidosis (type 4)	Decreased acid secretion and low NH_3 production
Dilutional acidosis	Increased Cl^- due to normal saline administration
Cholestyramine	Release of Cl^- in exchange for HCO_3^-

Low AG MAC and Correction for Low Serum Albumin

- *The most common cause of low AG acidosis in hospitalized patients is hypoalbuminemia.* For each gram decrease in albumin from the normal value, the AG decreases by 2.5.
- *Chronic kidney disease (CKD)* stages 4–5 and low albumin may seem to have a normal AG MAC, but when corrected for normal albumin the acid-base disorder is a high AG MAC. Patient with CKD stages 4–5 has a calculated AG of 12, albumin of 2.0 g/dL, and the laboratory reference AG of 10. This shows that the patient has only 2 excess anions (12 – 10 = 2). However, when AG is adjusted downwards and corrected for hypoalbuminemia, the baseline AG is 5 (10 – 5 = 5), and the excess anions are 7 (12 – 5 = 7) instead of 2. Thus, albumin levels should be obtained whenever an ABG is ordered, particularly in critically ill patients. A decrease in unmeasured anions and an increase in unmeasured cations cause low AG.
- *IgG myeloma* will have low AG because IgG molecules carry a positive charge at a pH of 7.4.
- *Ingestion of bromide or iodine-containing medications or intoxication* of these halides can raise the concentration of unmeasured anions, and lower AG due to measurements of these halides as Cl^-.
- *Severe hypertriglyceridemia* may present with low AG due to a different laboratory measurement.

Calculate the Expected Compensation (Also Called Secondary Response) (Step 7)

Secondary Physiologic Response (or Compensation)

It is a physiologic process that minimizes changes in pH brought about by a primary change. Two types of compensatory responses (secondary physiologic responses) are involved, that are (1) respiratory and (2) renal.

- In a metabolic acid-base disorder, the compensatory response is respiratory. In MAC, the primary change is a decrease in plasma (HCO_3^-), and pH. The compensatory response is a decrease in pCO_2 due to hyperventilation. This decrease in pCO_2 limits the rise in [H^+], and thus the pH is returned to normal. Conversely, hypoventilation is an appropriate physiological response to *MAL*.
- In *a respiratory acid-base disorder, the compensatory response is renal*. In RAC, the primary change is an increase in pCO_2 and a decrease in pH. The renal compensation increases the plasma (HCO_3^-) with a

resultant increase in pH toward normal. It should be pointed out that these compensatory mechanisms return the pH to normal.

Appropriate Compensation

- *MAC*: $\Delta pCO_2/\Delta HCO_3 = 1.2$ ↓
- *MAL*: $\Delta pCO_2/\Delta HCO_3 = 0.7$ ↑
- RAC:
  - *Acute*: $\Delta HCO_3/\Delta pCO_2 = 0.1$ ↑
  - *Chronic*: $\Delta HCO_3/\Delta pCO_2 = 0.4$ ↑
- *RAL*:
  - *Acute*: $\Delta HCO_3/\Delta pCO_2 = 0.2$ ↓
  - *Chronic*: $\Delta HCO_3/\Delta pCO_2 = 0.4$ ↑

Identify the Mixed Acid-base Disorder (Step 8)

How to Evaluate a Mixed Acid-base Disorder?

It is not uncommon for two or three simple or primary acid-base disturbances to coexist in hospitalized patients.

Mixed acid-base disorders should be suspected whenever:

- There is no compensatory response or overcompensation for a primary simple acid-base disorder
- pH and (HCO_3^-) are normal, but the AG is high (mixed MAC and MAL)
- pH is near normal, but (HCO_3^-) is high (mixed MAL and RAC)
- pH is near normal, but (HCO_3^-) is low (mixed MAC and RAL)
- pH is low (<7.4), but (HCO_3^-) is normal (mixed MAC and RAC)
- pH is high (>7.4), but (HCO_3^-) is normal (mixed RAL and MAL)

Use of $\Delta AG/\Delta HCO_3$ (Step 9)

- *Use of $\Delta AG/\Delta HCO_3$—for analyzing mixed acid-base disorders*:

TABLE 10: Common causes of the mixed acid-base disorder.

Metabolic acidosis + respiratory acidosis	Cardiac arrest and respiratory failure + renal failure
Metabolic acidosis + respiratory alkalosis	Salicylate intoxication, sepsis, and advanced liver disease + lactic acidosis
Metabolic alkalosis + respiratory alkalosis	Hepatic cirrhosis + vomit/diuretic overuse, pregnancy + hyperemesis, and overventilation in COPD
Metabolic alkalosis + respiratory acidosis	CDPD with diuretic overuse/vomit
Metabolic acidosis + metabaloic alkalosis	Uremia/ ketoacidosis + vomit
Triple disorders	Ketoacidosis + muntah + liver disease + sepsis

$$\Delta AG = \text{Increase in AG above normal.}$$
$$\Delta HCO_3 = \text{Decrease in } HCO_3 - \text{from normal value.}$$

In a simple or uncomplicated high AG MAC such as ketoacidosis, $\Delta AG/\Delta HCO_3^- = 1$. Any significant deviation from 1 is indicative of a mixed acid-base disorder.

- *Diarrhea:* Typically develops a hyperchloremic or normal AG MAC. A decrease in HCO_3—results in a reciprocal increase in Cl^- so that the AG does not change. It means $\Delta AG = 0$. As a result, the $\Delta AG/\Delta HCO_3^- = 0$.
- *Hypotension and subsequent lactic acidosis when develop* the HCO_3^- decreases even further. The ΔHCO_3^- is greater than ΔAG, and the $\Delta AG/\Delta HCO_3^-$ ratio is < 1 (above 0 but below 1). It indicates a mixed high and normal AG MAC.
- *In pure lactic acidosis, the $\Delta AG/\Delta HCO_3^-$ ratio is usually 1.6* (lactate anions remain in the extracellular compartment because of low urinary excretion. This raises the AG). However, the HCO_3^- concentration does not decrease as non-HCO_3^- buffers participate in buffering lactate anions.
- *In a mixed high AG MAC and MAL*, the HCO_3^- level is inappropriately high relative to the increase in AG. As a result, the $\Delta AG/\Delta HCO_3^-$ ratio is > 2.

DELTA GAP/"DELTA DELTA"

Anion gap metabolic acidosis (AGMA) may overlap with NAGMA or MAL (HCO_3^-) decreases 1 point for every point increase in AG Various methods exist to assess the additional metabolic component (1) corrected bicarbonate, (2) expected bicarbonate, (3) SAG—$aHCO_3$

BOX 2: Delta gap (corrected HCO_3^- method).

- Estimates what [HCO_3^-] would be if the AG process was removed:

$$\Delta AG = AG_{corr} - 12$$
$$[HCO_3^-] + \Delta AG = \text{"corrected"} [HCO_3^-]$$

- "Corrected" [HCO_3^-] elevated, i.e., > 28–30: metabolic alkalosis
- "Corrected" [HCO_3^-] reduced, i.e., < 20: NAGMA

TABLE 11: Corrected HCO_3.

	Cations	Anions	
This is not a real number but estimates what the bicarbonate would be if there was no anion gap process	Na^+	Protein, PO_4, SO_4 (assumed 12) HCO_3^- Cl^-	↑ Anion gap ↑↨ ΔAG — extra AG on the top of normal 12 mEq/L ↓

BOX 3: Delta gap (Na^+-Cl^- effect method).

- Sodium-chloride effect is a derivation of

$\Delta Gap = \Delta AG - \Delta HCO_3^-$

$\Delta Gap = (Na^+) - (Cl^-) - (HCO_3^-) - 12 - (24 - HCO_3^-)$

$\Delta Gap = (Na^+) - (Cl^-) - 36$

< −6 suggests nonanion-gap metabolic acidosis (NAGMA).

> +6 suggests metabolic alkalosis.

BOX 4: Urinary charge gap and urinary anion gap.

$$\text{Urine gap} = (U_{Na^+}) + (U_{K^+}) - (U_{Cl^-})$$

- *Negative urine gap*:
  - Increased excretion of unmeasured cation ammonium
  - Alkalinizing effect via chloride excretion
  - Suggests etiology of NAGMA not intrinsic to kidneys (e.g., diarrhea, diuretics use)
- *Positive urine gap*:
  - Increased excretion of unmeasured anions (bicarbonate, lactate, hippurate, and ketones)
  - Acidifying effect via chloride retention
  - Suggests renal etiology of NAGMA (e.g., RTA)

(NAGMA: nonanion-gap metabolic acidosis; RTA: renal tubular acidosis)

TABLE 12: Urine chloride in metabolic alkalosis.

Urine chloride low (<10–25 mEq/L) (chloride-responsive alkalosis)	Urine chloride high (>20–40 mEq/L) (chloride-nonresponsive alkalosis)
• Vomiting and nasogastric suctioning	• Excess mineralocorticoid activity
• Diuretic use in the past	• Ongoing diuretic use
• Posthypercapnia	• Excess alkali administration
• Contraction alkalosis	• Refeeding alkalosis

(difference), (4) SAG/aHCO_3—(ratio), (5) sodium-chloride effect. No need to conduct if AG is normal.

HOW TO EVALUATE AN ACID-BASE DISORDER CASE-BASED DISCUSSION?

Case 1

A 30-year-old man with a long history of intravenous (IV) drug abuse is admitted for weakness and abdominal pain. His respiratory rate is 24/minute (normal = 12–14/minute). Initial electrolyte and ABG values are:

- Na^+ = 136 mEq/L
- K^+ = 5.1 mEq/L
- Cl^- =100 mEq/L
- HCO_3^- = 14 mEq/L
- H^+ = 120 mg/dL
- Creatinine = 10 mg/dL
- Glucose = 90 mg/dL
- pH = 7.28
- pCO_2 = 30 mm Hg
- pO_2 = 100 mm Hg
- HCO_3^- = 13 mEq/L

Step 1: Electrolytes and ABG were done simultaneously.

Step 2: Check the validity of blood pH. Using the Henderson equation, we obtain:

$$[H^+]\ (nmol/L) = 24 \times 30/14 = 51.4$$

From the section on the Henderson equation, it is evident that the corresponding pH for the $[H^+]$ of 51.4 is approximately 7.28. Therefore, the reported pH for the patient is correct.

Step 3: Identify the primary disorder. The primary disorder is MAC because both pH and HCO_3^- are less than normal.

Step 4: Calculate the AG. 136 – (100 + 14) = 22 (serum albumin not available):

$$[(Na^+) - (Cl^- + HCO_3^-)]$$

Step 5: Identify the cause of the primary disorder. As the AG is 22, this disorder is a high AG MAC. In the laboratory values of the patient, it is evident that the cause is renal failure.

Step 6: Calculate the expected compensation. Since hyperventilation is an appropriate compensatory (secondary response) response, the pCO_2 should be lower than the normal value of 40 mm Hg. This patient's pCO_2 is 30. The following formula is used to determine whether this value is the expected (or predicted) pCO_2:

$$pCO_2 = HCO_3^- \times 1.5 + 8 \pm 2$$

$$= 14 \times 1.5 + 8 + 2 = 29$$

If the patient has an appropriate respiratory response for acidemia of 51.4 (H^+), the expected pCO_2 should be between 27 and 31 mm Hg. Since the patient's pCO_2 is 30, his respiratory response is appropriate.

Step 7: Identify the mixed acid-base disorder, if any. No mixed acid-base disorder is present.

Step 8: Use $\Delta AG/\Delta HCO_3^-$ ratio appropriately.

Step 9: Determine the appropriate treatment. Generally, the treatment for MAC with pH < 7.20 is $NaHCO_3$. In this patient, the pH > 7.20, and thus no treatment is necessary. The patient is symptomatic from his renal failure and needs dialysis to relieve his symptoms. Dialysis will also improve his plasma (HCO_3^-) and blood pH.

Case 2

A 42-year-old man is admitted because of dizziness and weakness. His blood pressure is 120/80 with a pulse rate of 90 beats/min (sitting) and 100/64 with a pulse rate of 110 beats/min (standing). He is not on any medications but admits to vomiting. Admitting laboratory values:

- Na^+ = 129 mEq/L
- K^+ = 2.5 mEq/L
- Cl^- = 58 mEq/L
- HCO_3^- = 58 mEq/L
- Creatinine = 1.9 mg/dL
- BUN = 32 mg/dL
- Glucose = 94 mg/dL
- pH = 7.53
- pCO = 63 mm Hg
- pO_2 = 62 mm Hg
- HCO_3^- = 58 mEq/L

Step 1: Check the validity of pH.
According to the Henderson equation, the (H^+) is 26, which corresponds to the pH of 7.53. Therefore, the reported pH is correct.

Step 2: Identify the primary disorder.
The primary acid-base disturbance is MAL.

Step 3: Calculate the AG.
The AG is 13, which is normal (calculate AG in all primary acid-base disorders so that the hidden MAC is not missed).

Step 4: Identify the cause of the primary disorder.
The cause for MAL is vomiting.

Step 5: Calculate the expected compensation.
The respiratory compensation is appropriate, suggesting that this acid-base disturbance is a simple MAL.

Question 1. How would you treat this acid-base disturbance?

Answer: The treatment is normal saline with KCl supplementation.

Case 3

A 72-year-old woman with a history of type 2 diabetes mellitus, congestive heart failure (CHF), and renal failure is admitted for nausea, vomiting, and shortness of breath. Her medications include insulin and furosemide. Her weight is 60 kg. Admission laboratory values:

- Na^+ = 140 mEq/L
- K^+ = 4.1 mEq/L
- Cl^- = 95 mEq/L
- HCO_3^- = 24 mEq/L
- Creatinine = 4.1 mg/dL
- BUN = 52 mg/dL
- Glucose = 145 mg/dL
- pH = 7.40
- pCO_2 = 40 mm Hg
- pO_2 = 90 mm Hg
- HCO_3^- = 24 mEq/L

Question 1. Characterize the acid-base disturbance in this patient.

Answer: The electrolytes and ABG values reveal no abnormalities. However, a step-by-step approach reveals that a mixed acid-base disturbance is present.

Step 1: Check the validity of pH.
From the Henderson equation, the [H^+] is 40 mmol/L, which is equal to a pH of 7.40.

Step 2: Identify the primary disorder.
From ABG values, no apparent acid-base disturbance is present.

Step 3: Calculate the AG.
The AG is 21, which suggests the presence of a high AG MAC (this case signifies the importance of calculating AG).

Step 4: Identify the cause of the primary disorder.
The cause for this MAC is renal failure.

Step 5: Calculate the expected compensation.
If this were a pure MAC, the pH, serum (HCO_3^-), and pCO_2 levels would be lower than normal. Since the patient has been vomiting and she is also taking furosemide for her CHF, she developed MAL. The coexistence of MAC and MAL normalizes ABG values and gives the impression of no underlying disturbance. The clue for the diagnosis of this mixed MAC and MAL is the presence of a high AG.

Question 2. How would you manage her?

Answer: Since she has shortness of breath due to CHF, IV furosemide can be tried. If the patient fails to respond, nesiritide can be started alone or in combination with dobutamine. If still unresponsive, two to three treatments of hemodialysis can improve her CHF (the patient's symptoms were relieved by two treatments of hemodialysis with low blood flow).

Case 4

A 65-year-old man with a history of chronic obstructive pulmonary disease (COPD) is admitted for management of shortness of breath. On admission, his laboratory values are:

- Na^+ = 134 mEq/L
- K^+ = 3.6 mEq/L
- Cl^- = 90 mEq/L
- HCO_3^- = 34 mEq/L
- Creatinine = 1.1 mg/dL
- BUN = 12 mg/dL
- Glucose = 100 mg/dL
- pH = 7.35
- pCO_2 = 64 mm Hg
- pO_2 = 70 mm Hg
- HCO_3^- = 33 mEq/L

Question 1. Characterize the acid-base disorder.
Answer: As earlier, follow the step-by-step method to analyze this acid-base disorder.

Step 1: Check the validity of pH.
According to the Henderson equation, the (H^+) is 45 nmol/L, which corresponds to a pH of 7.35.

Step 2: Identify the primary disorder.
The primary acid-base disturbance is RAC.

Step 3: Calculate the AG.
The AG is 10, which is normal.

Step 4: Identify the cause of the primary disorder.
The cause for this patient's RAC is COPD.

Step 5: Calculate the expected compensation.
The compensation for RAC is renal reabsorption of HCO_3^-. From, the patient has a primary chronic rather than acute RAC.

Step 6: Determine the appropriate treatment.
The immediate treatment is the administration of oxygen by nasal cannula and subsequent correction of the precipitating factor.

TREATMENT OF ACID-BASE DISORDER

Treatment Metabolic Acidosis

The treatment of MAC consists of the treatment of the primary pathophysiologic process, that is, hypoperfusion, and hypoxia, If pH is severely decreased, administration of $NaHCO_3^-$.

TABLE 13: Classification of metabolic alkalosis.

Chloride-responsive	Chloride-resistant
Urinary chloride < 15 mEq/L	Urinary chloride >25 mEq/L
• Loss of gastric acid • Diuretics • Volume depletion • Posthypercapnia	• Mineralocorticoid excess • Potassium depletion

Hyperventilation, although an important compensatory response to MAC, is not a definitive therapy for MAC. The initial dose of $NaHCO_3$ can be calculated as:

$$NaHCO_3\ (mEq/L) = WT\ (kgs) \times 0.3\ (24\ mEq/L\text{-actual}\ HCO_3)/2$$

Note: 0.3 = the assumed distribution space for bicarbonate and 24 mEq/L is the normal value for (HCO_3^-) on ABG. The calculation markedly underestimates dosage in severe MAC. In infants and children, a customary initial dose is 1.0–2.0 mEq/kg of body weight.

Treatment Metabolic Alkalosis

Etiologic Therapy

Expansion of intravascular volume or the administration of potassium. Infusion of 0.9% saline will dose-dependently increase serum (Cl^-) and decrease serum (HCO_3^-).

Nonetiologic Therapy

Acetazolamide (a carbonic anhydrase inhibitor that causes renal bicarbonate wasting) (5–10 mg/kg IV/PO). Infusion of (H^+) in the form of ammonium chloride, arginine hydrochloride, or 0.1 N hydrochloric acid (100 mmol/L), dialysis against a high-chloride/low bicarbonate dialysate.

0.1 N hydrochloric acid most rapidly corrects life-threatening MAC but must be infused into a central vein; peripheral infusion will cause severe tissue damage.

TREATMENT RESPIRATORY ACIDOSIS

The treatment of RAC depends on whether the process is acute or chronic.

- *Acute RAC*: Require mechanical ventilation unless a simple etiologic factor (i.e., narcotic overdosage or residual muscular blockade) can be treated quickly. Bicarbonate administration rarely is indicated unless severe MAC is also present or unless mechanical ventilation is ineffective in reducing acute hypercarbia.
- Chronic RAC is rarely managed with ventilation but rather with efforts to improve pulmonary function.

TREATMENT RESPIRATORY ALKALOSIS

- Treatment of RAL is often not required.
- The most important steps are recognition and treatment of the underlying cause. For instance, correction of hypoxemia or hypoperfusion-induced lactic acidosis should result in the resolution of the associated increases in respiratory drive. Preoperative recognition of chronic hyperventilation necessitates intraoperative maintenance of a similar $PaCO_2$.

CONCLUSION

Acid-base status is tightly regulated to maintain normal biochemical reactions and organ function. The body uses multiple mechanisms to maintain homeostasis. Abnormalities are extremely common in hospitalized patients with a higher incidence of critically ill with more complex pictures. A standard approach to analysis can help guide diagnosis and treatment.

SUGGESTED READINGS

1. Berend K, de Vries AP, Gans RO. Physiological Approach to Assessment of Acid-base Disturbances. N Engl J Med. 2014;371(15):1434-45.
2. Seifter JL. Integration of Acid-base and electrolyte disorders. N Engl J Med. 2014;371(19):1821-31.
3. Scott MG, LeGrys VA, Hood JL. Blood gases. In: Burtis CA, Ashwood ER, Bruns DE (Eds). Tietz Textbook of Clinical Chemistry and Molecular Diagnostics, 5th edition. St Louis: Elsevier; 2012. pp. 807-35.
4. Quade BN, Parker MD, Occhipinti R. The therapeutic importance of acid-base balance. 2021;183:114278.

83

CHAPTER

Lipoprotein(a): How to Address it?

Vijay Garg, Shivangi Tiwari, Chandrakant Salve, Vipasha Garg

ABSTRACT

Cardiovascular disease (CVD) is the leading cause of death and disability worldwide. High levels of lipoprotein(a) [Lp(a)], an apolipoprotein B100 (ApoB100)-containing lipoprotein, are an independent and causal risk factor for atherosclerotic CVDs through mechanisms associated with increased atherogenesis, inflammation, and thrombosis. Lp(a) is predominantly a monogenic cardiovascular risk determinant, with ≈70% to ≥90% of interindividual heterogeneity in levels being genetically determined. The two major protein components of Lp(a) particles are ApoB100 and apolipoprotein(a). Lp(a) remains a risk factor for CVD development even in the setting of effective reduction of plasma low-density lipoprotein cholesterol and ApoB100. Apart from conventional therapeutic options, various novel therapies are under clinical trial.

INTRODUCTION

Epidemiological, genome-wide association, and Mendelian randomization data provide clear support for a causal role for elevated lipoprotein(a) [Lp(a)] in the development of atherosclerotic cardiovascular disease (ASCVD). The role of apolipoprotein B100 (ApoB100)-containing lipoproteins as the central determinants of atherogenesis and risk for cardiovascular disease (CVD) is well established. Elevated levels of Lp(a) are also found to be associated with stroke, which is more common in men than women, and also target organ damage in patients of essential hypertension. Statin therapy has been the foundation treatment to reduce low-density lipoprotein cholesterol (LDL-C) and to lower the risk of CVD events but it does not seem to reduce Lp(a) significantly.

LIPOPROTEIN(a): STRUCTURE AND FEATURES

Lipoprotein(a) was first described by K Berg in 1963 and is a unique lipoprotein class.

Lipoprotein(a) molecule, structurally similar to the LDL particle, is composed of triglycerides, cholesteryl esters, oxidized phospholipids, and a molecule of ApoB100 covalently bound to apolipoprotein(a) [Apo(a)] **(Fig. 1)**.

Lipoprotein(a) is the preferential lipoprotein carrier for oxidized phospholipids (OxPL), a proatherogenic and proinflammatory biomarker. Lp(a) adversely affects endothelial function, inflammation, oxidative stress, fibrinolysis, and plaque stability, leading to accelerated atherothrombosis and premature coronary artery disease (CAD).

The concentration of Lp(a) is strongly determined by a single gene, the *LPA* gene, which is fully expressed by the age of 2 years. Ethnicity and sex affect the Lp(a) concentrations.

PREVALENCE

Potentially, >1.5 billion individuals worldwide have Lp(a) concentrations associated with increased ASCVD risk.

A global population study [Lp(a) HERITAGE] in 48,135 patients showed that approximately one-fourth of the global population with ASCVD have elevated Lp(a) levels with 10% of the population exhibiting levels >100 mg/dL. The INTERHEART-Lp(a) study showed that elevated Lp(a)

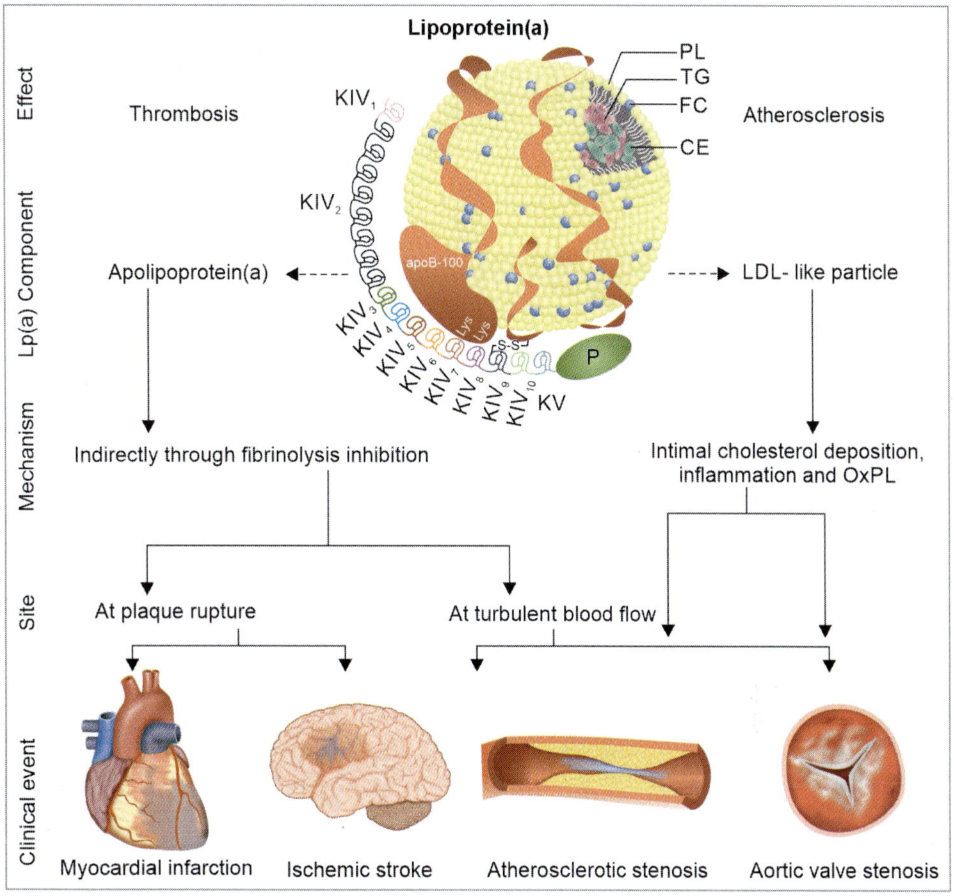

FIG. 1: Structural features of lipoprotein(a) [Lp(a)].

Lp(a) consists of a low-density lipoprotein (LDL)-like particle comprised of a central core of cholesteryl esters (CE) and triacylglycerols (TGs) surrounded by a shell of phospholipids (PL) and free cholesterol (FC) and a single molecule of ApoB100—covalently linked to Apo(a). Apo(a) features 10 different types of plasminogen kringle IV (KIV)-like domains, followed by a kringle V (KV)-like domain and an inactive protease-like domain.

concentration and the risk conferred by elevated Lp(a) vary significantly by ethnicity (seven different ethnic groups were studied).

FACTORS AFFECTING LIPOPROTEIN(a) LEVELS

Primarily, the Lp(a) plasma levels are genetically determined. However, several factors like underlying diseases and therapeutic administration of hormones may increase or decrease the Lp(a) bloodstream levels **(Table 1)**.

TABLE 1: Some factors affecting lipoprotein(a) [Lp(a)] levels.

Increase Lp(a) levels	Decrease Lp(a) levels
Apo(a) gene	Cholestatic liver diseases
Renal disease	Alcohol consumption
Diabetes mellitus	Insulin-like growth factor 1 (IGF-1)
Hypothyroidism	Anabolic steroids and adrenocorticotrophic hormone
Pregnancy	Drugs like tamoxifen, tibolone, and raloxifene
Human growth hormone (HGH)	Obesity
	Diet

Source: Adapted from Jawi MM, Frohlich J, Chan SY. Lipoprotein(a) the Insurgent: A New Insight into the Structure, Function, Metabolism, Pathogenicity, and Medications Affecting Lipoprotein(a) Molecule. J Lipids. 2020;2020:3491764.

LIPOPROTEIN(a) AND CARDIOVASCULAR RISK: WHAT IS THE EVIDENCE?

Multiple epidemiological, Mendelian randomization **(Fig. 2)**, and genome-wide association studies done in the past decade have established Lp(a) as an independent and likely causal risk factor for ASCVD and calcific aortic stenosis.

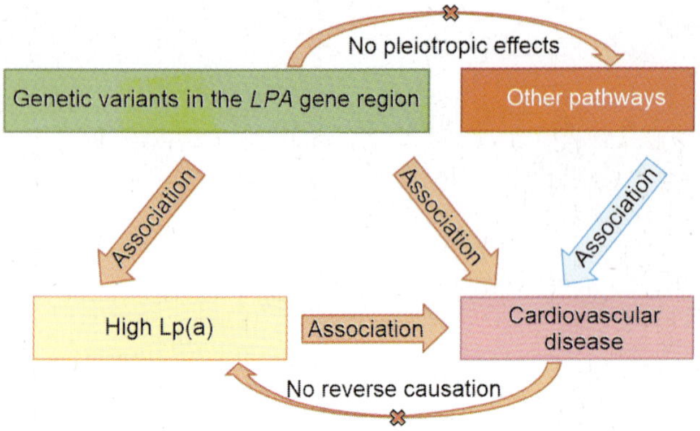

FIG. 2: Schematic illustration of a Mendelian randomization approach using the example of lipoprotein(a) [Lp(a)].

Observational studies showed a significant association of high Lp(a) concentrations with cardiovascular disease. Genetic variants which show a strong association with high Lp(a) concentrations are used as genetic instrument. When these instruments show also an association with cardiovascular disease, a causal association between Lp(a) concentrations and cardiovascular disease is strongly supported and a reverse causation might be excluded. Pleiotropy has to be excluded in the sense that the genetic variant affects the outcome only via the biomarker and not via other independent pathways.

A scientific statement from the American Heart Association (2022) states that Lp(a) is predominantly a monogenic cardiovascular risk determinant, with ≈70% to ≥90% of interindividual heterogeneity in levels being genetically determined.

The results of the FOURIER trial (n = 25,096) demonstrated that higher levels of Lp(a) are associated with an increased risk of cardiovascular events in patients with established CVD irrespective of LDL-C.

ASSOCIATION BETWEEN LIPOPROTEIN(a) AND DIFFERENT CONDITIONS

Evidence from experimental, observational, and genetic studies has demonstrated that increased Lp(a) is associated with increased risk for coronary heart disease (CHD), ischemic stroke (IS), peripheral artery disease, heart failure, calcific aortic valve stenosis (CAVS), mitral valve stenosis, and possibly retinopathy in diabetic patients **(Fig. 3)**.

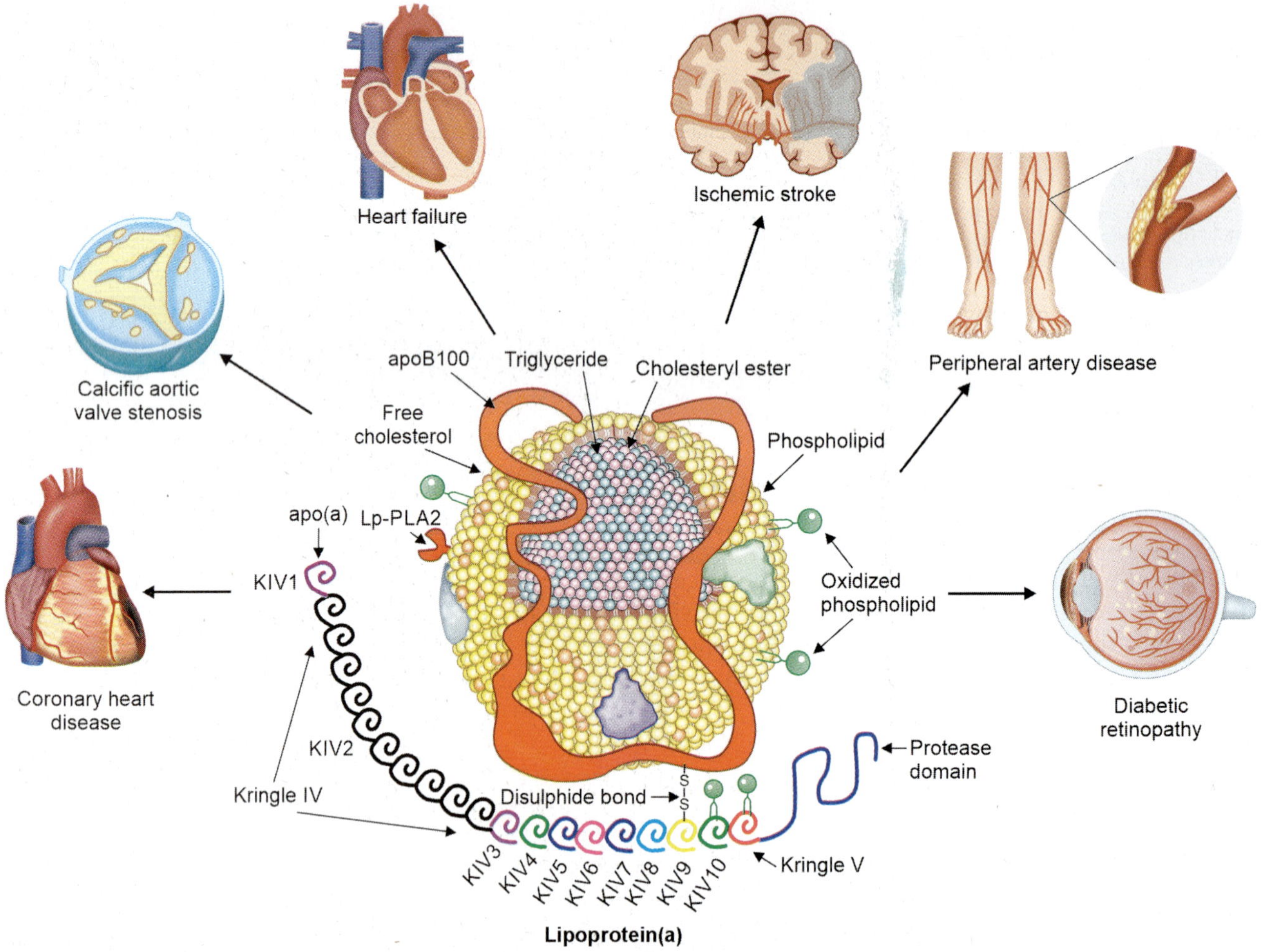

FIG. 3: Pathogenicity of lipoprotein(a) and its association with different conditions.

LIPOPROTEIN(a): ROLE IN ATHEROSCLEROSIS, INFLAMMATION, AND ATHEROTHROMBOSIS

Lipoprotein(a) can be internalized and accumulated in the intima of arteries and the aortic valve leaflets. Furthermore, Lp(a) is more atherogenic than LDL-C as it consists of all of the atherogenic components of both LDL cholesterol and Apo(a).

Inflammation promotes endothelial cell activation, dysfunction and loss of endothelial integrity, failure of endothelial repair, intima lipid deposition, and plaque formation and instability.

Experimental studies have shown that studies have reported that Lp(a) can promote thrombosis, inflammation, and foam cell formation.

Lipoprotein(a) participates in atherothrombosis through several mechanisms. Lp(a) interferes with platelet aggregation, as it can bind to platelet-activating factor (PAF) acetylhydrolase, which degrades and inactivates PAF. This mechanism results in reduced platelet aggregation and activation. **Figure 4** outlines potential impact of Lp(a) on atherosclerotic and thrombotic processes.

LIPOPROTEIN(a) ASSOCIATION WITH OTHER CONDITIONS: CLINICAL EVIDENCES

A meta-analysis of 61 studies demonstrated a significant association between increased levels of Lp(a) and risk of ischemic stroke [IS; standardized mean difference (SMD) 0.76] and its subtypes, large artery atherosclerosis (LAA; SMD-0.68), and intracerebral hemorrhage (ICH; SMD-0.65) compared to control subjects. Increased Lp(a) levels could be considered as a predictive marker for identifying individuals who are at risk of developing IS, LAA, and ICH.

A systematic review and meta-analysis of 13 studies for a total of 1,040 cases and 16,648 controls showed that Lp(a) levels above normal limits were associated with retinal vein occlusion (RVO).

A meta-analysis of 17 studies enrolling 283,328 patients indicated that elevated Lp(a) level was independently associated with an increased risk of cardiac events [relative risk (RR): 1.78] and cardiovascular events (RR: 1.29) in CAD patients.

Clinical studies have indicated that a very low level of Lp(a), approximately below 7 mg/dL, is associated with an increased risk of type 2 diabetes mellitus (T2DM) but the mechanism of this association is unknown.

A meta-analysis of 11 observational studies with 9,304 T2DM patients showed that higher serum Lp(a) in patients with T2DM is independently associated with higher odds of diabetic nephropathy.

A Mendelian randomization analysis suggested a causal relationship between Lp(a) and CHD, aortic aneurysm, and LAA stroke, but *not with* atrial fibrillation, secondary hypertension, heart failure, IS, lacunar stroke, small vessel stroke, and pulmonary embolism (PE).

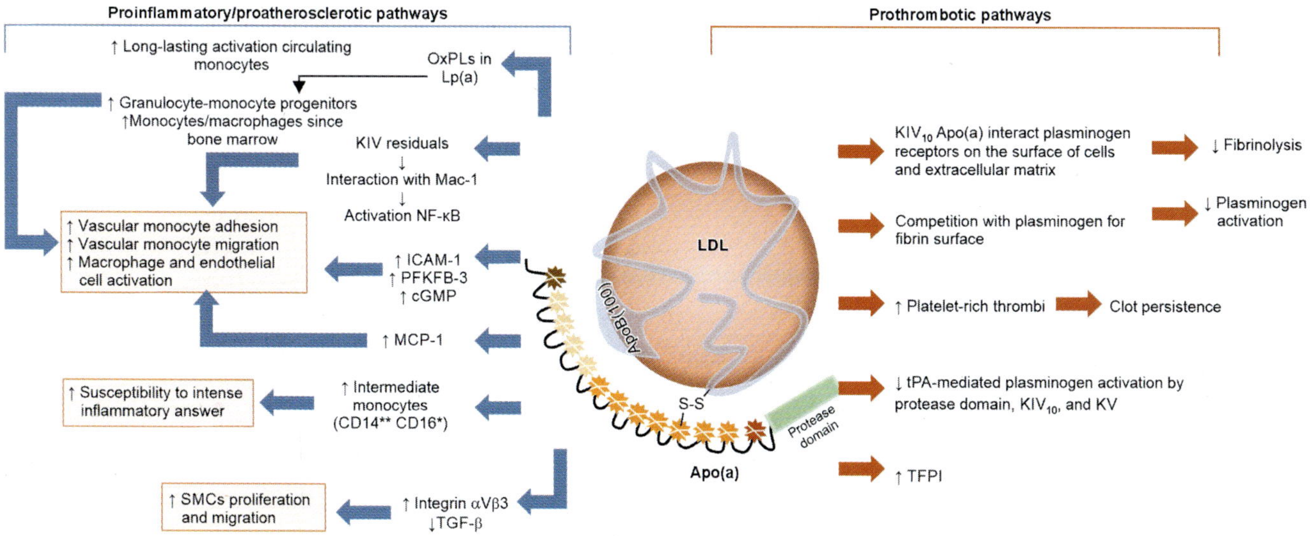

FIG. 4: Main hypothetic mechanisms involved in the pathogenesis of atherosclerosis and thrombosis in patients with higher Lp(a) serum concentrations.

[Apo(a): apolipoprotein(a); CD: cluster of differentiation; cGMP: guanosine 30,50-cyclic monophosphate; ICAM-1: intercellular adhesion molecule-1; KIV: kringle IV; KV: kringle V; LDL: low-density lipoprotein; Lp(a): lipoprotein(a); MCP-1: monocyte chemoattractant protein-1; NF-κB: nuclear factor kappa B; OxPLs: oxidized phospholipids; PFKFB-3: 6-phosphofructo-2-kinase/fructose-2,6-biphosphatase enzyme; SMC: smooth muscle cell; TFPI: tissue factor pathway inhibitor; TGF-β: transforming growth factor-β; tPA: tissue plasminogen activator]

ETHNICITY-BASED LIPOPROTEIN(a) THRESHOLDS

It is known that levels of Lp(a) vary by race and ethnicity. Lp(a) concentrations are lower in Hispanics than in whites; while the European Atherosclerosis Society Consensus Panel recommends a desirable level of <50 mg/dL, the National Heart, Lung, and Blood Institute (NHLBI) recommends that Lp(a) levels in the atherothrombotic range are generally accepted as >30–50 mg/dL. With these differences, there appears to be a need for ethnicity-based Lp(a) thresholds.

LIPOPROTEIN(a) MEASUREMENTS: WHO SHOULD BE SCREENED?

Despite the crucial role of Lp(a), its measurement lacks a globally unified method, and, between different laboratories, results need standardization.

A Scientific Statement from the American Heart Association recommends that Lp(a) should be measured with:

- An isoform-insensitive assay
- Assay that is traceable to the internationally accepted calibrator (World Health Organization/International Federation of Clinical Chemistry Reference Material SRM-2B)
- Assay that is reported in nanomoles per liter (nmol/L).

Lipoprotein(a) should be measured at least once during lifetime, especially in high-risk populations. Screening should be done in the individuals as outlined in **Box 1**.

BOX 1: Screening of lipoprotein(a) [Lp(a)].

Lp(a) should be measured once over a lifespan in individuals with:

- Premature CVD
- Familial hypercholesterolemia or other genetic forms of dyslipidemia
- Recurrent CVD despite optimal lipid-lowering treatment
- ≥5% 10-year risk of fatal CVD according to ESC SCORE guidelines
- Family history of premature CVD and/or elevated Lp(a) (≥50 mg/dL)
- ≥10% 10-year risk of fetal CVD according to US guidelines
- Calcific aortic valve stenosis
- 10–19% Framingham risk according to the 2012 Canadian Cardiovascular Society recommendations

(CVD: cardiovascular disease; ESC: European Society of Cardiology; SCORE: Systematic Coronary Risk Evaluation)

MANAGEMENT STRATEGIES FOR ELEVATED LIPOPROTEIN(a) AND EMERGING NEW TREATMENT STRATEGIES

Lipoprotein(a) levels are refractory to lifestyle interventions.

There are no Food and Drug Administration (FDA)-approved pharmacologic therapies shown to specifically lower Lp(a) and so precise analysis of the contribution of Lp(a) to clinical ASCVD is not yet possible. Among current therapies for lipid modulation, statins are known to increase plasma Lp(a) levels (by ~20%), and PCSK9 (proprotein convertase subtilisin/kexin type 9 antibodies) (alirocumab and evolocumab; ~20–30%) only have a modest effect.

Currently, lipoprotein apheresis (LA) is the only available therapeutic option for patients with elevated Lp(a) and established CVD approved by the FDA.

Hormone replacement therapy: The use of desogestrel-containing oral contraceptives leads to significant reduction in Lp(a).

Ezetimibe—used as adjunct to statins when LDL-C >70 mg/dL and Lp(a) >100 nmol/mL are also some Lp(a) lowering therapies.

Aspirin has been shown to reduce Apo(a) transcriptional activity in hepatocytes.

Cholesteryl ester transfer protein (CETP; e.g., evacetrapib) inhibition can reduce Lp(a) levels in the range of 25–40%. Niacin can also reduce Lp(a) levels in a range between 20 and 30%.

Nucleic acid-based therapies allow for selective gene silencing, thus preventing the production of proteins that may cause or enhance disease. RNA therapies include antisense oligonucleotides (ASOs), small interfering RNAs (siRNAs), microRNAs (miRNAs), RNA aptamers, and mRNAs.

NOVEL THERAPIES

Currently four Lp(a)-reducing RNA interference (RNAi) therapeutics are under clinical trials; three of them, olpasiran, SLN360, and LY3819469, are using the siRNA principle, and one, pelacarsen, is an ASO **(Table 2)**.

CONCLUSION

Lipoprotein(a) is recognized as a risk factor for atherosclerotic and nonatherosclerotic CVDs. The Lp(a) levels are largely genetically determined and mediated by

TABLE 2: RNA-based Lp(a)-lowering therapeutics under clinical development.

Drug	Type	Chemical modification	Delivery system	Targeting gene
Pelacarsen	ASO	2′-O-MOE	GalNAc	*LPA*
Olpasiran	siRNA	2′-O-Me	GalNAc	*LPA*
SLN360	siRNA	2′-O-Me	GalNAc	*LPA*
LY3819469	siRNA	2′-O-Me; 2′-F	GalNAc	*LPA*

(ASO: antisense oligonucleotide; GalNAc: N-acetylgalactosamine; LPA: lipoprotein(a) gene; siRNA: small interfering RNA; 2′-F: 2′-O-fluoro; 2′-O-Me: 2′-O-methoxy; 2′-O-MOE: 2′-O-methoxyethyl)

variations in the *LPA* gene. Despite the recognized role of Lp(a) in atherosclerosis, its measurement lacks a globally unified method. Currently, there is no available therapy dedicated to lowering Lp(a). Novel therapies aimed at clinically significant Lp(a) reduction include RNA interference agents.

SUGGESTED READINGS

1. Genovesi S, Giussani M, Lieti G, Orlando A, Patti I, Parati G. Evidence and Uncertainties on Lipoprotein(a) as a Marker of Cardiovascular Health Risk in Children and Adolescents. Biomedicines. 2023;11(6):1661.
2. Koschinsky ML, Stroes ESG, Kronenberg F. Daring to dream: Targeting lipoprotein(a) as a causal and risk-enhancing factor. Pharmacol Res. 2023;194:106843.
3. Di Fusco SA, Maggioni AP, Scicchitano P, Zuin M, D'Elia E, Colivicchi F. Lipoprotein (a), Inflammation, and Atherosclerosis. J Clin Med. 2023;12(7):2529.
4. Enas EA, Varkey B, Dharmarajan TS, Pare G, Bahl VK. Lipoprotein(a): An independent, genetic, and causal factor for cardiovascular disease and acute myocardial infarction. Indian Heart J. 2019;71(2):99-112.
5. Koutsogianni AD, Liamis G, Liberopoulos E, Adamidis PS, Florentin M. Effects of Lipid-modifying and Other Drugs on Lipoprotein(a) Levels-potent Clinical Implications. Pharmaceuticals (Basel). 2023;16(5):750.
6. Marcovina SM, Shapiro MD. Measurement of Lipoprotein(a): A Once in a Lifetime Opportunity. J Am Coll Cardiol. 2022;79(7): 629-31.
7. Nissen SE, Wolski K, Cho L, Nicholls SJ, Kastelein J, Leitersdorf E, et al. Lipoprotein(a) levels in a global population with established atherosclerotic cardiovascular disease. Open Heart. 2022;9(2):e002060. Erratum in: Open Heart. 2022;9(2).
8. Paré G, Çaku A, McQueen M, Anand SS, Enas E, Clarke R, et al. Lipoprotein(a) Levels and the Risk of Myocardial Infarction among 7 Ethnic Groups. Circulation. 2019;139(12):1472-82.
9. Puri R, Mehta V, Iyengar SS, Narasingan SN, Duell PB, Sattur GB, et al. Lipoprotein(a) and ASCVD risk. J Assoc Physicians India. 2020;68(11[Special]):42-6.
10. Jawi MM, Frohlich J, Chan SY. Lipoprotein(a) the Insurgent: A New Insight into the Structure, Function, Metabolism, Pathogenicity, and Medications Affecting Lipoprotein(a) Molecule. J Lipids. 2020;2020:3491764.
11. Mehta A, Virani SS, Ayers CR, Sun W, Hoogeveen RC, Rohatgi A, et al. Lipoprotein(a) and Family History Predict Cardiovascular Disease Risk. J Am Coll Cardiol. 2020;76(7):781-93.
12. Shah NP, Pajidipati NJ, McGarrah RW, Navar AM, Vemulapalli S, Blazing MA, et al. Lipoprotein (a): An Update on a Marker of Residual Risk and Associated Clinical Manifestations. Am J Cardiol. 2020;126:94-102.
13. Reyes-Soffer G, Ginsberg HN, Berglund L, Duell PB, Heffron SP, Kamstrup PR, et al. Lipoprotein(a): A Genetically Determined, Causal, and Prevalent Risk Factor for Atherosclerotic Cardiovascular Disease: A Scientific Statement from the American Heart Association. Arterioscler Thromb Vasc Biol. 2022;42(1):e48-e60.
14. O'Donoghue ML, Fazio S, Giugliano RP, Stroes ESG, Kanevsky E, Gouni-Berthold I, et al. Lipoprotein(a), PCSK9 Inhibition, and Cardiovascular Risk. Circulation. 2019;139(12):1483-92.
15. Ugovšek S, Šebeštjen M. Lipoprotein(a): The Crossroads of Atherosclerosis, Atherothrombosis and Inflammation. Biomolecules. 2021;12(1):26.
16. Emerging Risk Factors Collaboration; Erqou S, Kaptoge S, Perry PL, Di Angelantonio E, Thompson A, et al. Lipoprotein(a) concentration and the risk of coronary heart disease, stroke, and nonvascular mortality. JAMA. 2009;302(4):412-23.
17. Kumar P, Swarnkar P, Misra S, Nath M. Lipoprotein (a) level as a risk factor for stroke and its subtype: A systematic review and meta-analysis. Sci Rep. 2021;11:15660.
18. Paciullo F, Giannandrea D, Virgili G, Cagini C, Gresele P. Role of Increased Lipoprotein (a) in Retinal Vein Occlusion: A Systematic Review and Meta-analysis. TH Open. 2021;5(3):e295-e302.
19. Wang Z, Zhai X, Xue M, Cheng W, Hu H. Prognostic value of lipoprotein (a) level in patients with coronary artery disease: a meta-analysis. Lipids Health Dis. 2019;18(1):150.
20. Sosnowska B, Surma S, Banach M. Targeted Treatment against Lipoprotein (a): The Coming Breakthrough in Lipid Lowering Therapy. Pharmaceuticals (Basel). 2022;15(12):1573.
21. Ren X, Zhang Z, Yan Z. Association between Lipoprotein (A) and Diabetic Nephropathy in Patients with Type 2 Diabetes Mellitus: A Meta-analysis. Front Endocrinol (Lausanne). 2021;12: 633529.
22. Wang S, Zha L, Chen J, Du D, Liu D, Zhong M, et al. The relationship between lipoprotein(a) and risk of cardiovascular disease: a Mendelian randomization analysis. Eur J Med Res. 2022;27(1):211.
23. Haffner SM, Gruber KK, Morales PA, Hazuda HP, Valdez RA, Mitchell BD, et al. Lipoprotein(a) concentrations in Mexican

Americans and non-Hispanic whites: the San Antonio Heart Study. Am J Epidemiol. 1992;136(9):1060-8.
24. Tsimikas S, Fazio S, Ferdinand KC, Ginsberg HN, Koschinsky ML, Marcovina SM, et al. NHLBI working group recommendations to reduce lipoprotein(a)-mediated risk of cardiovascular disease and aortic stenosis. J Am Coll Cardiol. 2018;71(2):177-92.
25. Nordestgaard BG, Chapman MJ, Ray K, Borén J, Andreotti F, Watts GF, et al. Lipoprotein(a) as a cardiovascular risk factor: current status. Eur Heart J. 2010;31(23):2844-53.
26. Lampsas S, Xenou M, Oikonomou E, Pantelidis P, Lysandrou A, Sarantos S, et al. Lipoprotein(a) in Atherosclerotic Diseases: from Pathophysiology to Diagnosis and Treatment. Molecules. 2023;28(3):969.
27. Kim KA, Park HJ. New Therapeutic Approaches to the Treatment of Dyslipidemia 2: LDL-C and Lp(a). J Lipid Atheroscler. 2023;12(1):37-46.
28. Tsimikas S, Gordts PLSM, Nora C, Yeang C, Witztum JL. Statin therapy increases lipoprotein(a) levels. Eur Heart J. 2020;41(24):2275-84.
29. Nugent AK, Gray JV, Gorby LK, Moriarty PM. Lipoprotein apheresis: first FDA indicated treatment for elevated lipoprotein(a). J Clin Cardiol. 2020;1:16-21.
30. Farina JM, Pereyra M, Mahmoud AK, Chao CJ, Barry T, Halli Demeter SM, et al. Current Management and Future Perspectives in the Treatment of Lp(a) with a Focus on the Prevention of Cardiovascular Diseases. Pharmaceuticals. 2023;16(7):919.

84

CHAPTER

Dyslipidemia: A Clinician's Perspective

Shohael Mahmud Arafat, Tahseen Mahmood, Mehruba Aalm Ananna

ABSTRACT

Atherosclerotic cardiovascular disease (ASCVD) prevention is the main focus for dyslipidemia treatment, with guidelines varying. Risk stratification and achieving lipid goals through lifestyle interventions and pharmacotherapy are key, with new therapies emerging.

INTRODUCTION

The term dyslipidemia refers to abnormal serum levels of cholesterol, triglycerides (TGs), or both, involving abnormal levels of related lipoprotein moieties. Although designated "abnormal," however, it is observed that often there is no precise numeric threshold between normal and abnormal levels as many patients with "normal" cholesterol levels are shown to achieve benefits from further lower levels. As such, rather than merely interpreting the "lipid profile" of the patient per se, it is prudent to judge the patient as a whole based upon the "cardiovascular risk profile" for clinical intervention. This review will try to explore dyslipidemia from a clinician's point of view for which treatment is observed to be beneficial based upon modern updates and evidence.

LIPID BASICS

The major circulating lipids are cholesterol and TGs. Cholesterol, derived from acetyl coenzyme A (acetyl-CoA), serves as a ubiquitous constituent of the cell membrane, and in addition, it can be transformed into hormones and bile salts by specialized cells. TG, derived from gut and liver, are stored or utilized as energy for muscle and adipose tissues. Owing to their poor solubility in organic solvents like blood, lipids require carrier macroparticles called lipoproteins (LPs) to be transported across the aqueous bloodstream. The principal structural proteins of these LP are called apolipoproteins (Apo) that can act as ligands for binding the Lp particles to their cellular receptors and can serve as cofactors for enzymatic reactions. Thus, LPs are large biochemical assemblies of spherical particles that package lipids into a hydrophobic core surrounded by an outer hydrophilic shell of phospholipids (PL), embedded with water-soluble Apo to transport the lipids from one part of the body to other. Based upon the size, lipid composition, function, and Apo content, Lp particles are commonly divided into five classes: Chylomicrons (CM), very-low-density lipoproteins (VLDLs), intermediate-density lipoproteins (IDLs), low-density lipoproteins (LDLs), and high-density lipoproteins (HDLs). Dietary TGs are transported by enterocyte-derived CM and endogenous TGs by hepatocyte-derived VLDLs to muscle and adipose tissues.

CLASSIFICATION OF DYSLIPIDEMIA

The traditional Fredrickson classification based upon observable phenotypes and patterns of elevation in lipids and lipoproteins lack practicality owing to the polygenic basis of most Fredrickson phenotypes and in addition, lipoprotein fractionation methods to delineate them are often inaccessible for most clinicians. Hence, dyslipidemia patterns, observed from the routine laboratory lipid panel, could be classified simply into the following categories:

High cholesterol states (high-LDL-C), high-TG states, combined dyslipidemia (high-non-HDL-C), or others [low-HDL states and high Lp(a) states].

PATHOPHYSIOLOGICAL CONSEQUENCES OF DYSLIPIDEMIA

Oxidation of LDLs followed by uptake by scavenger receptors of arterial wall macrophage generate foam cells that act as a foundation for the development of arterial plaques. These also initiate an inflammatory cascade to further atherogenesis that may lead to plaque rupture causing an occlusive vascular event in the form of stroke, myocardial infarction, or peripheral limb ischemia. As such, a direct relationship between elevated LDL and increased risk of atherosclerotic cardiovascular disease (ASCVD) is well established.

Although epidemiological studies have shown low HDL-C as an independent ASCVD risk factor; however, HDL-C-raising therapies have failed to show any ASCVD benefit. The total cholesterol (TC):HDL ratio reflecting the ApoB:ApoA-I ratio is more predictive of ASCVD risk stratification in this context.

Elevated TG, especially in a nonfasting state is an independent risk factor for ASCVD. Atherosclerotic plaques contain cholesterol esters (CE) that is derived from TG-rich ApoB containing lipoproteins and their remnant particles, such as IDL, CM remnant, and VLDL remnants. In addition, increased levels of VLDL are hypothesized to accumulate small dense low-density lipoprotein (sdLDL) particles with increased infiltrating capabilities to promote atherosclerosis.

SCREENING FOR DYSLIPIDEMIA

The process of atherosclerosis is initiated in childhood and the goal is to reduce the long-term ASCVD risk of a susceptible individual. In order to do so, the primary step is to screen for dyslipidemia by performing a serum lipid profile usually comprising of TC, LDL-C, HDL-C, non-HDL-C, and TG. However, there is no clear consensus on whom and when to screen for **(Table 1)**. Fasting lipid profile is standard whereas non-fasting measurements are also recommended with a repeat fasting lipid profile only if nonfasting TG is >400 mg/dL. A family history of premature ASCVD or familial hypercholesterolemia (FH) should prompt screening in children. Some authorities also recommend measuring ApoB as it integrates all atherogenic LP including VLDL, LDL, IDL, remnants, and Lp(a) for ASCVD risk stratification. Regarding Lp(a), most authorities recommend to measure once in an individual's lifetime.

TABLE 1: Dyslipidemia screening protocol of various authorities.

	ACC/AHA/ ATP-III	EAS/ESC	CCS
Females, age (>years)	20	50 (or post-menopause)	40 (or postmeno-pause)
Males, age (>years)	20	40	40
How to screen	*Standard fasting or nonfasting lipid profile*: TC, LDL-C, HDL-C, non-HDL-C, and TG	*Standard fasting or nonfasting lipid profile*: TC, LDL-C, HDL-C, non-HDL-C, and TG	• *Standard fasting or nonfasting lipid profile*: TC, LDL-C, HDL-C, non-HDL-C, and TG • Lp(a)—once in the patient's lifetime, with initial screening
	Optional: ApoB and Lp(a)	*Lp(a)*: Consider once in the patient's lifetime	*Optional*: ApoB

(ACC: American College of Cardiology; AHA: American Heart Association; ATP: Adult Treatment Panel; CCS: Canadian Cardiovascular Society; EAS: European Atherosclerosis Society; ESC: European Society of Cardiology; HDL-C: high-density lipoprotein cholesterol; LDL: low-density lipoprotein; TC: total cholesterol; TG: triglyceride)

PRACTICAL APPROACH TO EVALUATE DYSLIPIDEMIA

The initial steps are to identify the category of dyslipidemia (elevated LDL-C, elevated TG, elevated non-HDL-C, or low HDL-C) and to rule out possible secondary causes. Correction of secondary causes often improves or normalizes the disturbance. In patients with high LDL-C, serum thyroid stimulating hormone (TSH) is the most important laboratory investigation as other secondary causes are usually obvious from history and clinical examination. In poorly controlled diabetic patients with mild to moderate hypertriglyceridemia (HTG), achievement of glycemic control usually results in marked improvement in serum TG levels. Other common causes of HTG include obesity, chronic kidney disease, inflammatory diseases, and human immunodeficiency virus (HIV). Occasionally, withdrawal of certain drugs significantly improves lipid profile. If secondary causes are not obvious, the next step is to decide whether treatment is required in order to reduce ASCVD risk or prevent other complications. If lipid/lipoprotein abnormality is markedly abnormal or begins at a young age, consideration for monogenetic disorders should be done and a family history of premature cardiovascular disease or pancreatitis should be sought for. In young patients with ASCVD and normal lipid profiles with no obvious risk factors, measurement of Lp(a) should be done where facilities are available. In cases of uncertainty, a cardiac calcium scan is helpful especially in the elderly where a score of 1–99 favors the use of statin and 100 indicates the need for statin therapy.

MANAGEMENT OF PATIENTS WITH DYSLIPIDEMIA

The purpose of treating dyslipidemia is to prevent (primary or secondary) ASCVD and or other complications like pancreatitis through lifestyle interventions and pharmacotherapy.

Lifestyle interventions include dietary management, regular exercise of at least 30 minutes for 5 days a week, attainment of ideal body weight, smoking cessation, and limiting or abstinence from alcohol consumption.

Dietary management is often effective in most patients with HTG. However, as only 15–20% of serum cholesterol is derived from dietary sources, dietary interventions are recommended but often not sufficient enough to substantially lower serum cholesterol.

General dietary measures include reduction of portion sizes, replacing high glycemic index (GI) foods with complex carbohydrates, and opting for lean meat and fish over red meats to replace trans and saturated fats with mono and polyunsaturated fats. Moreover, the inclusion of plant sterols and soluble fibers in the diet has been shown to decrease LDL-C by 6–14%.

For severe HTG and hypercholesterolemia, specialized dietary intervention under the supervision of a registered dietitian is recommended. Usually, low-fat diet comprising $<30\%$ of daily total calorie intake is advised. Individuals with serum TG >10 mmol/L (885 mg/dL) are recommended to take fat $<15\%$ of the daily total calorie intake.

For elevated cholesterol states, available pharmacotherapies are statins, ezetimibe, bempedoic acid, bile acid sequestrants, and proprotein convertase subtilisin/kexin type 9 (PCSK9) inhibitors. The initial drug of choice is a statin categorized as moderate intensity (ability to reduce LDL-C by 30–49%) and high intensity (reduces LDL-C over 50% for high-risk cases) determined by risk stratification. For risk stratification, a number of calculators are available. In the United States, the American College of Cardiology (ACC)/American Heart Association (AHA) risk calculator is the most popular while in Europe, the SCORE calculator is popular. An LDL-C between 70 and 99 mg/dL is a reasonable goal for primary prevention using moderate-intensity statins. Achieving an LDL-C below 55–70 mg/dL (number varies between guidelines) usually by high-intensity statins or combining with ezetimibe or PCSK9 inhibitors, provide the greatest benefit in patients with established ASCVD (secondary prevention).

Hypertriglyceridemia is usually dealt with by fibrates, n-3 fatty acids (e.g., icosapent ethyl), and less commonly niacin (an effective drug limited by side effects). It is to be noted that fibrates lack ASCVD risk reduction benefits and are recommended to be prescribed if TG is >500 mg/dL (885 mg/dL or 10 mmol/L by some authorities) in order to minimize the risk of pancreatitis.

In elevated non-HDL-C states or combined dyslipidemia management goal is that of ASCVD risk reduction by statins and lifestyle modifications. Icosapent ethyl is recommended for accompanied mild to moderate HTG.

Although low HDL-C is an excellent predictor of ASCVD risk, studies have failed to prove any benefit in terms of ASCVD risk reduction by increasing its levels. It is postulated that HDL-C function rather than its quantity would become a potential target in the near future.

MANAGEMENT OF DYSLIPIDEMIA IN SPECIAL SITUATION

Statin-associated Muscle Symptoms

Statin-associated muscle symptoms (SAMS) are the most prevalent among the musculoskeletal, gastrointestinal, and neurocognitive adverse effects of statins that pose a significant barrier to achieve optimum lipid targets. SAMS commonly involves proximal muscle groups including thighs, calves, buttocks, and back muscles in a symmetrical manner typically in the form of myalgia, stiffness, cramps, or tenderness with or without elevations of creatine kinase (CK). If CK is more than five times the upper limit of normal (ULN) and symptoms are tolerable, continuation should be considered after counseling the patients on the benefits of statin therapy. If the patient does not want to continue, reassessment should be done after two to four weeks of discontinuation. If no improvement of symptoms occurs then statin can be reintroduced. If symptoms improve after withdrawing a statin, switching to an alternative statin at the usual starting dose may be considered. Cautious rechallenging with the offending statin is also an option, however, if symptoms recur with this challenge or CK is over more than five times of the ULN at any phase of assessment, the trial of a modified dosing regimen (alternate day, 1/2/3 days interval) with a longer half-life agent (rosuvastatin, atorvastatin, and pitavastatin) or a lower intensity statin (fluvastatin and pravastatin) may be considered. In ultimate statin intolerance, ezetimibe or PCSK-9 inhibitors may be used.

DYSLIPIDEMIA IN PREGNANCY

Statin and fibrates are usually stopped before pregnancy. However, recently in 2021, the United States Food and Drug Administration (FDA) has recommended to continue statin in women with very high ASCVD risk. Although not extensively studied, fibrates are not found to be teratogenic in humans and can be used in patients with severe HTG (>885 mg/dL) beyond the first trimester. Dietary management is the key component to manage dyslipidemia and omega-3 fatty acids may be used in conjunction. In resistant HTG (over 1,770 mg/dL), hospital admission, fluid replacement, diet withholding and plasmapheresis may be considered.

EMERGING THERAPEUTICS IN DYSLIPIDEMIA

In this era of precision medicine, therapies targeting to inhibit molecules that are related to increasing plasma lipids are being introduced. These range from small molecule oral inhibitors, to monoclonal antibodies to ribonucleic acid (RNA) agents that impair translation of the harmful protein product of the targeted genes.

Bempedoic acid (180 mg daily) is an oral small molecule that interferes with adenosine triphosphate (ATP)-citrate lyase to reduce LDL-C by 15–20%. Small interfering RNA inclisiran interferes with intracellular PCSK9 and is notable for its long duration of action for six months following a single subcutaneous injection. Other emerging agents include apolipoprotein C-III (ApoC-III) inhibitor volanesorsen for TG reduction and anti-angiopoietin-like 3 (anti-ANGPTL3) agents such as vupanorsen and evinacumab are worth mentioning with promising results to treat FH.

CONCLUSION

Prevention of ASCVD is the main theme for treating dyslipidemia. A number of guidelines have been published by various authorities that vary significantly between recommendations and treatment strategies. However, the bottom-line task is to stratify risk followed by achieving lipid/lipoprotein goals with a "lower the better" strategy through lifestyle interventions and pharmacotherapy. Newer promising therapies are emerging to fulfill the unmet clinical needs with a ray of hope for the patients.

SUGGESTED READINGS

1. Goff DC Jr, Lloyd-Jones DM, Bennett G, Coady S, D'Agostino RB, Gibbons R, et al. American College of Cardiology/American Heart Association Task Force on Practice Guidelines. 2013 ACC/AHA guideline on the assessment of cardiovascular risk: a report of the American College of Cardiology/American Heart Association Task Force on Practice Guidelines. Circulation. 2014;129(25 Suppl 2):S49-73.
2. Expert Panel on Detection, Evaluation, and Treatment of High Blood Cholesterol in Adults. Executive Summary of The Third Report of The National Cholesterol Education Program (NCEP) Expert Panel on Detection, Evaluation, And Treatment of High Blood Cholesterol In Adults (Adult Treatment Panel III). JAMA. 2001;285(19):2486-97.
3. Pearson GJ, Thanassoulis G, Anderson TJ, Barry AR, Couture P, Dayan N, et al. 2021 Canadian Cardiovascular Society Guidelines for the Management of Dyslipidemia for the Prevention of Cardiovascular Disease in Adults. Can J Cardiol. 2021;37(8):1129-50.
4. Catapano AL, Graham I, De Backer G, Wiklund O, Chapman MJ, Drexel H, et al. 2016 ESC/EAS guidelines for the management of dyslipidaemias. Rev Esp Cardiol (Engl Ed). 2017;70(2):115.

SECTION

10

NEPHROLOGY

85

CHAPTER

Measurement of Immunity in Organ Transplant Recipients

Mukunda Prasad Kafle

ABSTRACT

All organ transplant recipients need immunosuppressive medications for lifetime. These drugs suppress the immunity power of the person so that the "foreign" organ is not destroyed by immunity. At the same time, foreign particles as bacteria, viruses need to be destroyed by the recipient body. So, what is the optimum level to which the immunity should be lowered? We do not have any quantitative tests to answer this question. This is mainly because immunity is a multifactorial entity. The determinants of immunity power may not be the same across individuals. There are some developments in this area. These take indirect factors into account. For example, level of torque teno virus (TTV) viremia may give a rough idea of severity of suppression of immunity.

INTRODUCTION

The intensity of suppression of immunity is the most important element in maintaining the balance between organ survival and adverse effects of immune suppression in people living with transplanted organs. Currently, a state of immune suppression is achieved by the use of multiple drugs which blunt the immune response to foreign antigens (expressed by the donor organ). Each component drug in the current immunosuppressive regimen works at different steps of the body's defense algorithm.

This suppression of immunity brings about long-term graft survival and thus a long-term relief from the complications of end-stage organ failure. Suboptimal immunosuppression can give rise to graft rejection and organ failure whereas oversuppression of immunity can dampen the body's response to serious infections and leads to various opportunistic infections which increase the morbidity and mortality in organ transplant recipients.

An arbitrary measurement of immunosuppression for an optimal outcome on both sides of organ survival and infection avoidance is necessary. There are no available biomarkers to determine optimal degree of immunosuppression thereby helping in predicting ideal outcomes.

RELEVANCE

Let us answer two questions before proceeding further. Why do some people suffer rejection at a certain dose of immunosuppressive drugs while others do not? Why do some people catch infection at a certain dose of immunosuppressive drugs whereas others do not?

These questions can be answered in multiple ways. That means, there is no consensus to one answer to each of these questions and everybody answers these questions according to their comfort. While answering these questions, experts will agree on one common entity that is the "net state of immune suppression (NSI)".

Net State of Immune Suppression

In the immunosuppressed organ transplant recipients, balance between organ survival and risk of infection has been proposed to be a consequence of net state of immune suppression (let's say NSI for simplicity). According to Fishman, NSI is a conceptual measure of the factors contributing to a patient's risk for infection. Currently, NSI is defined as *"a qualitative measure of the risk factors for infection in an individual including both immunosuppressive medications and iatrogenic conditions"*. Clinical tools to quantify this entity are lacking. Therefore, it cannot be measured in individuals to stratify the various levels of immune suppression. If NSI is measurable in some units, then we can examine the impact of various levels of immune suppression in the outcomes of the organ and patient safety. Furthermore, if NSI could be quantified accounting for all the cumulative factors that can modify immune function, then that could be a valuable tool in the management of organ transplant recipients. Apart from that, it could also guide the clinical decision-making in infectious diseases and other areas of medicine, such as allergies, autoimmune diseases, cancer pathogenesis, and cancer chemotherapy.

CURRENT CLINICAL PRACTICE

If such a pivotal tool in immunity is unmeasurable, then how do the clinicians make decisions in current day practice? Current clinical decision-making and immunological monitoring depends largely on therapeutic drug monitoring (TDM) and clinical judgment. Measurements of trough and peak levels of tacrolimus and cyclosporine are widely available. Monitoring the levels of mycophenolate mofetil (MMF) and mammalian target of rapamycin inhibitor (mTORi) are suggested by various authorities but their availability is limited. Moreover, these calcineurin inhibitor (CNI) (or antimetabolite) levels are only one component of the complete state of immunosuppression. There are many other important factors that can contribute to the net state of immunosuppression. Some of these factors are presented in **Box 1**.

Although the clinicians have knowledge of various components that could contribute to NSI, a comprehensive tool to express the total level of immunity is not available. For example, we know that white blood cell (WBC) is the integral part of immunity and we transiently hold antimetabolites during leukopenia but it is not valued while changing the dose of immunosuppressant drugs in the long term. Apart from available information, consideration of innate and adaptive immunity is vital too. Other similar clinical tools, suboptimally utilized in clinical decision-making are presented in **Box 2**.

IMMUNE BACKGROUND

The potential effects of factors that are not direct components of the immune system [e.g., nutrition, duration on dialysis, obesity, disease conditions like diabetes, systemic lupus erythematosus (SLE), polymyalgia rheumatica, giant cell arteritis (GCA)] but still modify NSI in many ways. These factors can potentially contribute to NSI.

BOX 1: Potential factors that contribute to the net state of immunosuppression.

- *Immunosuppressive therapy*: Type, dose, duration, temporal sequence, and intensity
- Underlying immune deficiency (e.g., adrenal insufficiency, systemic lupus erythematosus, and complement deficiencies)
- Post-transplant renal, hepatic, pulmonary or cardiac dysfunction, or diabetes
- Prolonged use of ventilatory support, urinary, vascular access or dialysis catheters, surgical drains, or other breaks in skin or mucosal defenses
- Surgical issues resulting from the transplant procedure, resulting in leaks (blood, lymph, and urine) and fluid collections, devitalized tissue, poor wound healing, and surgical drainage catheters
- White cell counts (e.g., neutropenia, lymphopenia—often drug induced)
- *Metabolic conditions*: Uremia, malnutrition, diabetes mellitus, alcoholism, and cirrhosis
- Prior therapies affecting immunity (chemotherapy or antimicrobials)
- *Viral infections*: CMV, EBV, HSV, VZV, RSV, hepatitis B and C, HIV

(CMV: cytomegalovirus; EBV: Epstein–Barr virus; HIV: human immunodeficiency virus; HSV: herpes simplex virus; RSV: respiratory syncytial virus; VZV: varicella zoster virus)

BOX 2: Clinical tests available for monitoring immunity.

- *Therapeutic drug monitoring*: CNI levels and mTORi levels
- *Immune function assays*:
  - T-lymphocyte counts: (CD4+ and CD8+)
  - T-cell functional assays: sCD30, stimulated intracellular adenosine triphosphate (iATP) levels
  - Lymphocyte transformation test
  - Markers of T-cell exhaustion (e.g., PD-1)
  - Cytokine (e.g., IL-10) levels
  - Gamma globulin levels, C3, and IFN-γ
  - Quantitative molecular viral loads
- *Immunoregulatory genes*:
  - Single-nucleotide polymorphisms in genes for MBL2, ficolin-2, and MBL-associated serine protease 2
  - Polymorphisms of nucleotide-binding oligomerization domain-containing 2 (NOD2)
  - Polymorphisms in pentraxin 3
- *Consideration of comorbid conditions*: Diabetes, lupus, nutrition, and obesity
- *Microbiome dysbiosis*: Reduced amount of gastrointestinal butyrate-producing bacteria
- *Other measurable factors*: White blood cell (WBC) counts, WBC differential count, and NK cells

(CNI: calcineurin inhibitor; IFN-γ: interferon gamma; IL-10: interleukin-10; NK: natural killer; mTORi: mammalian target of rapamycin inhibitor)

TRANSPLANTATION TOLERANCE

Transplantation tolerance is *"a state in which there is a lack of a destructive immune response by the recipient toward the well-functioning donor organ, in the absence maintenance immunosuppression, and with a fully intact immune system"*. Currently, complex chimerism-based algorithms including total lymphoid irradiation followed by bone marrow transplantation and kidney transplantation from the same donor are attempted to induce transplantation tolerance. Some patients themselves skip immunosuppressive drugs for long term after several years of transplantation and still have a functioning allograft. Long-term use of immunosuppressive drugs can theoretically reprogram the immune system in the genetic level. If such reprogramming occurs, allograft recipients could tolerate the organ at lower intensity of immunosuppression.

In simple words, tolerating a foreign organ would mean a negligible degree of immune suppression in the setting of a reprogrammed immune system. Quantification of NSI would potentially help in exploring the development of tolerance after several years of uneventful organ transplantation. Furthermore, if NSI is quantifiable in single unit, the desired value of this entity may be different at various points of time after organ transplantation.

Necessity of a Comprehensive Tool

A comprehensive, routinely applicable, affordable clinical tool is needed for the optimal maintenance immunosuppression in organ transplant recipients. This is because at higher levels of immunosuppression, infection occurs at lower levels of infectious "exposure" or with organisms of lower levels of native virulence. With lower levels of immunosuppression, infection is less common, drug toxicities are less frequent, but graft rejection more prevalent. Researchers have also stressed on the necessity of measurement of NSI. Availability of a comprehensive tool to measure immunity could assist in identifying people who can be withdrawn off immunosuppression and thus reduce the cost and adverse effects of the drugs. For instance, it could be beneficial to reduce overprescribing steroids in children who suffer bone toxicities and growth retardation.

POTENTIAL TOOLS TO MEASURE IMMUNITY

Potential tools to measure the degree of immunosuppression are discussed as follows:

- *TTV viremia*: Torque teno virus, an anellovirus, is ubiquitous but of unknown pathogenic significance. TTV viremia is related to the degree of immunosuppression. According to Roberts and Fishman (2021) *"the only assays that measure all limbs of coordinated immune responses are measurements of circulating viral loads (e.g., intrinsic antiherpesvirus immunity)"*. Epstein–Barr virus (EBV), cytomegalovirus (CMV), varicella zoster virus (VZV), polyomaviruses (BKV and JCV), and herpes simplex virus (HSV) are other potential candidate microorganisms.
- *Immune risk phenotype/immune risk profile (IRP)*: The term "immune risk phenotype" was described as the combination of high CD8 and low CD4 T-cell counts with a poor proliferative response to concanavalin A and low percentages of B-cells. Currently, it is defined as a positive CMV serology plus at least one of the following three criteria:
  i. CD4/CD8 ratio <1
  ii. CD8T-cells >600 cells/μL
  iii. CD28 negative T-cells >300 cells/μL

  Immune risk profile: "Immune risk profile" has been defined as:

  A positive CMV serology with at least one of the following:
  - CD4/CD8 ratio <1
  - CD8 T-cell count >90th percentile

  Positive patients have greater frequency of opportunistic infections and severe bacterial infections but lower acute rejection rates. Mortality rate in individuals with an inverted CD4/CD8 ratio also increased significantly above the age of 60 years. However, it is not routinely utilized in the management of immunosuppressive therapy.
- *Immune function assay*: The ImmuKnow (Cylex Inc, USA) assay was approved as an immune cell function assay to quantify cell-mediated immunity by measuring the concentration of ATP from CD4+ T cells. The assay measures intracellular ATP produced by purified CD4+ T lymphocytes after in vitro whole blood incubation with phytohemagglutinin (PHA). ATP levels have been shown to correlate with T lymphocyte activity and, consequently, cell-mediated immune function. Lower levels of ATP have been associated with a higher risk of infection, whereas increased production of ATP seems to be associated with rejection.
- *Pleximmune™*: This assay assesses the activity of T-cytotoxic memory cells through the expression of CD154 (an inflammatory/activation marker). An increased ratio of expression of CD154 on patient's cells as compared to basal level of expression on third party cells is in favor of an acute rejection.

- *Regulatory T cells (Tregs)*: Low numbers of circulating Tregs before transplantation may help identify recipients at high risk for acute rejection episodes in liver transplant recipients. Similarly, decreased numbers of blood Tregs have been observed in patients who suffered an acute rejection.

CONCLUSION

Quantification of the total intensity of immune suppression in organ transplant recipients could be helpful to optimize the clinical management of organ transplant recipients. Levels of some viruses in the human body might work for the purpose if validated scientifically.

SUGGESTED READINGS

1. Fishman JA. Infection in solid-organ transplant recipients. N Engl J Med. 2007;357(25):2601-14.
2. Lim TY, Heneghan M. Biomarkers of immunosuppression. Clin Liver Dis (Hoboken). 2016;8(2):34-8.
3. Kasiske BL, Zeier MG, Chapman JR, Craig JC, Ekberg H, Garvey CA, et al. KDIGO clinical practice guideline for the care of kidney transplant recipients: a summary. Kidney Int. 2010;77(4):299-311.
4. Fishman JA. Infection in Organ Transplantation. Am J Transplant. 2017;17(4):856-79.
5. Roberts MB, Fishman JA. Immunosuppressive Agents and Infectious Risk in Transplantation: Managing the "Net State of Immunosuppression". Clin Infect Dis. 2021;73(7):e1302-e1317.
6. Albert-Vega C, Tawfik DM, Trouillet-Assant S, Vachot L, Mallet F, Textoris J. Immune Functional Assays, From Custom to Standardized Tests for Precision Medicine. Front Immunol. 2018;9:2367.
7. Salama AD, Womer KL, Sayegh MH. Clinical transplantation tolerance: many rivers to cross. J Immunol. 2007;178(9):5419-23.
8. Fishman JA. Opportunistic infections—coming to the limits of immunosuppression? Cold Spring Harb Perspect Med. 2013;3(10):a015669.
9. Pawelec G, Ferguson FG, Wikby A. The SENIEUR protocol after 16 years. Mech Ageing Dev. 2001;122(2):132-4.
10. Plonquet A, Bastuji-Garin S, Tahmasebi F, Brisacier C, Ledudal K, Farcet J, et al. Immune risk phenotype is associated with nosocomial lung infections in elderly in-patients. Immun Ageing. 2011;8:8.
11. Wikby A, Månsson IA, Johansson B, Strindhall J, Nilsson SE. The immune risk profile is associated with age and gender: findings from three Swedish population studies of individuals 20-100 years of age. Biogerontology. 2008;9(5):299-308.
12. Uemura T, Riley TR, Khan A, Hollenbeak C, Schreibman I, Ghahramani N, et al. Immune functional assay for immunosuppressive management in post-transplant malignancy. Clin Transplant. 2011;25(1):E32-7.
13. He Q, Fan H, Li JQ, Qi HZ. Decreased circulating CD4+CD25 highFoxp3+ T cells during acute rejection in liver transplant patients. Transplant Proc. 2011;43(5):1696-700.

86

CHAPTER

Antidiabetic Agents in Renal Dysfunction

Sandeep Arora, Suchitra Garhwal, Ramji Sharma, Srikant Sharma

ABSTRACT

Patients with diabetes mellitus have high risk of development of diabetic kidney disease (DKD), and good glycemic control can decrease its incidence. Regular screening of diabetic patients for kidney disease can improve outcomes. Management of DKD includes lifestyle modification, management of hyperglycemia with glucose-lowering medication, control of hypertension and hyperlipidemia, and avoidance of tobacco. In the presence of renal dysfunction, because of several metabolic factors, diabetes management becomes difficult. Selection of antidiabetic drugs is important to avoid drug accumulation, hypoglycemia, and drug toxicity in these patients. Some drugs may have hazardous effects while other drugs have been found to improve renal functions. Management of diabetes requires a multidisciplinary approach, and treatment needs individualization for each patient to avoid adverse effects.

INTRODUCTION

Diabetes mellitus is the greatest epidemic in human history and is the leading cause of end-stage renal disease (ESRD). The International Diabetes Federation Diabetes Atlas 2021 states that 10.5% of the adult population (20–79 years) is suffering from diabetes, with unawareness of about 50%. Diabetic kidney disease (DKD) affects approximately 20–40% of adults with diabetes and has come out as the most common cause of chronic kidney disease (CKD) and ESRD, requiring renal replacement therapy. The 2022 American Diabetes Association (ADA) Standards of Medical Care in Diabetes and the Kidney Disease: Improving Global Outcomes (KDIGO) 2022, Clinical Practice Guideline for Diabetes Management in Chronic Kidney Disease each has provided evidence-based recommendations for its management. A joint approach of ADA and KDIGO representatives developed a series of consensus statements to guide clinical care to the patients.

Management of diabetes in CKD is complicated and challenging because of the increased risk of hypoglycemia, renal excretion of most oral antidiabetics, unpredictive appetite of patients with CKD, and the effects of hemodialysis and peritoneal dialysis on glycemic control. These factors need special consideration as far as management of diabetes in CKD patients is concerned.

DIABETIC KIDNEY DISEASE AND HYPOGLYCEMIA

Various factors predispose CKD patients to an increased risk of hypoglycemia. These include:

- As glomerular filtration rate (GFR) decreases (<60 mL/min/1.73m^2), insulin requirement decreases as insulin is cleared by kidneys and can lead to hypoglycemia.
- Depletion of glycogen storage in the patients with CKD and uremia occurs due to suboptimal nutrition and appetite.
- Renal gluconeogenesis is reduced as a result of reduction in renal mass in CKD patients.
- Most of the oral hypoglycemic agents (OHAs) are excreted by kidneys. It results in accumulation of these drugs and their metabolites, which can cause hypoglycemia in CKD patients.

PATHOPHYSIOLOGY OF DIABETIC KIDNEY DISEASE

Chronic hyperglycemia is the main culprit that leads to DKD. DKD has multiple pathophysiologic mechanisms involving the effects of soluble factors (growth factors, endothelin, angiotensin II, and advanced glycosylation end products), structural changes in glomerulus (basement membrane thickening, mesangial expansion, and increased extracellular matrix), and hemodynamic changes in renal microcirculation (glomerular hyperfiltration and hyper perfusion, and increased glomerular capillary pressure). DKD is seen in about 20–40% of patients with diabetes. Additional genetic and environmental factors also contribute to the development of DKD.

SCREENING AND DIAGNOSIS OF DIABETIC KIDNEY DISEASE

Diabetic kidney disease is diagnosed with persistently low GFR (<60 mL/min/1.73m^2), albuminuria [albumin-to-creatinine ratio (ACR) >30 mg/g], or other evidence of kidney damage. As significant fluctuations are seen in above parameters among individuals, a repeat urine sample within 3–6 months is suggested. Annual screening is recommended for patients with diabetes for CKD by ADA-KDIGO. CKD screening should start with diagnosis of type 2 diabetes mellitus (T2DM) and 5 years after the diagnosis of type 1 diabetes mellitus (T1DM).

Albuminuria can be measured by 24-hour collection with creatinine, or by measurement of the ACR in a random spot collection, which is the most convenient method. Alternative etiology of renal involvement other than diabetes should be ruled out, i.e., fever, infection, refractory hypertension, nephrotic syndrome, congestive heart failure (CHF), hematuria, or vigorous exercise.

TARGET GLYCEMIC CONTROL IN DIABETIC KIDNEY DISEASE

The ADA-KDIGO asserts individualization of glycemic targets based on patient characteristics and comorbid conditions. On the basis of randomized controlled trial (RCT) data, KDIGO proposes a glycated hemoglobin (HbA1c) target of <6.5% to <8.0% for DKD, which improves cardiovascular outcomes, microvascular endpoints, survival rates, and slows down CKD progression. The ADA endorses an initial HbA1c target of <7% to curtail microvascular complications in patients with T1DM and T2DM with no hypoglycemia risk; however, higher target (i.e., <8%) are admissible for patients with short life span and with high risk-benefit ratio.

Intensive glycemic control is found to be associated with the advantage of reduced development and slowed progression of nephropathy in several trials. Studies state that by decreasing HbA1c, primary and secondary prevention of nephropathy, retinopathy, and neuropathy can be observed.

ACCURACY OF HbA1c IN DIABETIC KIDNEY DISEASE

The HbA1c measurements sometimes can be erroneous in kidney disease patients. False high values are seen because of anemia due to decreased lifespan of the red blood cells (RBCs), hemolysis, and iron deficiency; falsely high values can also be seen due to carbamylation of hemoglobin and the presence of acidosis. So, in kidney disease, fructosamine (glycation of multiple serum proteins) and glycated albumin (glycation of albumin) can be used, both measure glucose control over last 2 weeks, but there is no clear evidence, which shows their superiority over HbA1c in kidney disease patients.

TREATMENT

In DKD patients, multimorbidity leads to increased risk of CKD progression, cardiovascular events, and premature mortality. Hence, ADA-KDIGO guidelines highlight the significance of comprehensive, holistic, and patient-centered medical treatment to enhance patient outcomes. The aim of a comprehensive approach is to treat the patient as a "whole" and comprise multidisciplinary treatment, patient education for self-management, and primary and secondary prevention of diabetes-related complications such as CKD, atherosclerotic cardiovascular disease (ASCVD), and heart failure. Treatment focuses on optimization of lifestyle, pharmacological therapy for control of glycemia, blood pressure (BP), and lipids.

Education, Self-care, and Patient Empowerment

The ADA-KDIGO guidelines highlight "team-based" integrated approach that involves diabetes care and education specialists such as physicians, nurses, physician assistants, dietitians, exercise specialists, pharmacists, dentists, podiatrists, and/or mental health professionals. Behavioral evaluation should be done for all patients with diabetes and for those who are not able to achieve targets to assess psychosocial barriers to treatment and self-management.

Lifestyle

The ADA–KDIGO guidelines emphasize individualized and balanced diets enriched with vegetables, fruits, and whole grains but low in refined carbohydrates and sugar-sweetened beverages. A low-sodium diet (KDIGO: <2,000 mg/day, ADA: 1,500 to <2,300 mg/day) is endorsed to decrease cardiovascular disease (CVD) risk and to manage BP. A low dietary protein intake is (0.8 g/kg/day) approved but slightly higher quantities of dietary protein (1.0–1.2 g/kg/day) are advised for patients on maintenance dialysis or for those who are malnourished.

The ADA–KDIGO guidelines recommend moderate to intense exercise period of 150 min/week, restraining of sedentary lifestyle, and smoking cessation. In diabetic patients with obesity, ADA–KDIGO recommend achieving healthy weight by diet, physical activity, and behavioral therapy.

Glycemic Control

Metformin

Metformin is the oldest and commonly used oral antihyperglycemic drug. It reduces HbA1c by 1% and does not cause hypoglycemia. Common adverse effects are gastrointestinal (GI) upset, lactic acidosis (overall risk is low), and vitamin B12 deficiency (with use >4 years). Usually, metformin-related lactic acidosis is seen with other comorbid diseases like renal insufficiency.

Because of these factors, metformin can be used safely with estimated GFR (eGFR) <60 mL/min/1.73 m^2. In advanced DKD, it is to be used with caution and dose adjustment to avoid lactic acidosis. It can also be used with precaution up to eGFR > 30 mL/min/1.73 m^2, and with reduction of dose with probability of lactic acidosis. For guarded use in CKD patients, eGFR should be measured every 3–6 months if eGFR falls to <60 mL/min/1.72 m^2.

Sulfonylureas

Sulfonylureas (SUs) act as insulin secretagogues by acting on SU receptors on beta cells. HbA1c reduction of 1.5–2% and risk of hypoglycemia is seen with SU. First generation SUs, especially chlorpropamide and glibenclamide, because of long duration and hypoglycemia, are not used nowadays. Glimepiride, glipizide, and gliclazide are frequently used molecules in management of T2DM. These drugs undergo hepatic metabolism and excretion of metabolites (active metabolites of glimepiride and inactive metabolites of glipizide and gliclazide) by kidney. Glipizide and gliclazide have comparatively low risk of hypoglycemia in CKD patients, and can be used with caution. These drugs should also be avoided if eGFR < 30 mL/min/1.73m^2.

Glinides

Glinides are insulin secretagogues with shorter half-life in comparison to SU. They can cause HbA1c reduction of 0.5–1.5%. Cautious use of nateglinide with eGFR < 60 mL/min/1.73 m^2 is advised because of reduced elimination of active metabolites in CKD. Although repaglinide elimination half-life is slightly more in CKD, it is comparatively safe without dose alteration, but should be used cautiously with eGFR < 30 mL/ min/1.73 m^2.

Thiazolidinediones

Thiazolidinediones (pioglitazone and rosiglitazone) are peroxisome proliferator-activated receptor gamma (PPAR-γ) agonists and improve insulin sensitivity. Presently available drug pioglitazone can cause HbA1c reduction of 0.5–1.4% without risk of hypoglycemia. This drug undergoes hepatic metabolism and has no risk of accumulation in CKD. This drug is better to be avoided in CKD patients because of fluid retention and precipitation of heart failure.

Alpha-glucosidase Inhibitors

Alpha-glucosidase inhibitors act by reducing the lysis of oligo- and disaccharides in the small intestine and retarding glucose absorption. Common adverse effects are bloating, flatulence, and abdominal cramping. HbA1c reduction of 0.5–0.8 % is seen and is weight neutral. Renal excretion of active metabolites prohibits their use in CKD.

Dipeptidyl Peptidase-4 Inhibitors

Dipeptidyl peptidase-4 (DPP-4) inhibitors (sitagliptin, vildagliptin, saxagliptin, and linagliptin) reduce degradation of incretin hormones such as glucagon-like peptide-1 (GLP-1) and gastric inhibitory polypeptide (GIP) by inhibiting DPP-4. HbA1c reduction of 0.5–0.8% is seen and is weight neutral. No evidence of hypoglycemia is there, as their mechanism is glucose dependent. In moderate to severe renal dysfunction, dose adjustment is required except in linagliptin (renal excretion is only 7%).

Sodium-glucose Cotransporter-2 Inhibitors

This newer class (canagliflozin, dapagliflozin, and empagliflozin) inhibits sodium-glucose cotransporter-2 (SGLT-2) in proximal renal tubules and decrease glucose reabsorption from tubular lumen, leading to glycosuria. They also decrease BP by natriuresis and reduce weight. HbA1c reduction of 0.9–1% is seen with this class of drugs. These drugs have similar pharmacokinetics, with quick oral absorption, prolonged elimination, and half-life facilitating once-daily dosing. They are metabolized by the liver to inactivate metabolites via glucuronidation.

This group of drugs have been proved to have multiple benefits. Significant reduction in HbA1c, along with weight reduction and reduced risk of heart failure is observed. Above all these drugs have been found, not only to retard the progression but also reverse the nephropathy and improve renal functions. These benefits make them as drugs of choice in patients of T2DM with nephropathy. The ADA-KDIGO 2022 guidelines state that SGLT-2 inhibitor can be prescribed in DKD patients up to eGFR > 20 mL/min/1.73 m^2, based on results of the Dapagliflozin And Prevention OF Adverse Outcomes in Chronic Kidney Disease (DAPA-CKD) and the Empagliflozin Outcome Trial in Patients with Chronic Heart Failure (EMPEROR) trials.

These drugs may cause hypovolemia, euglycemic ketoacidosis, and urogenital infections, so precautions need to be taken.

Glucagon-like Peptide-1 Agonist

Glucagon-like peptide-1 agonists (GLP-1As) are injectable molecules except for semaglutide, which is now available in oral form also. These drugs act like gut hormones known as incretins, which induce insulin release, retard glucagon secretion, and gastric emptying. They reduce appetite and lead to weight loss. HbA1c reduction of 1% is seen with this class of drugs.

In various cardiovascular outcome trials, it was seen that these molecules decrease albuminuria, retards eGFR decline and also attenuates chance of major adverse cardiovascular events (MACE) in DKD patients. These benefits advocate their use in T2DM with nephropathy.

Common adverse effects are GI upset (nausea, vomiting, and diarrhea) and injection-site reaction (<1%). GLP-1 receptor agonists should not be prescribed to patients at risk for thyroid C-cell tumors (e.g., multiple endocrine neoplasia), pancreatic cancer, or pancreatitis.

Insulin

In CKD, patients are at a higher risk of hypoglycemia. Major excretion route of insulin is renal (30–80%). As eGFR decreases, there is increase in half-life of insulin. Insulin dose and type is modified according to patients' need and comorbidities. Insulins after dose adjustment are safe and effective in all stages of nephropathy.

The rapid-acting insulin analogs (aspart, lispro, and glulisine) have rapid onset within 5–15 minutes. They have peak and short duration of action, which makes them ideal for glycemic control in renal dysfunction. These are used as "basal-bolus therapy" and in insulin pumps.

The short-acting insulin (regular crystalline) has onset within 30–60 minutes, reaches peak levels at 2–3 hours, and their effect remains for 5-8 hours. Their additional benefit is cost effectiveness in contrast to rapid acting analogs.

Intermediate-acting insulin is isophane or neutral protamine Hagedorn (NPH) with onset within 2–4 hours. They reach peak levels at 4–6 hours and their effect remains for 10–14 hours. Their use is restricted because of erratic absorption and longer duration of action.

The long-acting insulin analogs (glargine and detemir) have onset within 2–4 hours, with no prominent peak and effect persisting for 20–24 hours. They should be cautiously used in CKD because of delayed clearance.

Premixed insulins are a combination of fixed percentage of one short- or rapid-acting analog and one intermediate analog. Their main advantage is twice-daily dosing, but this leads to more constraints in titration and dosing at fixed timings.

Blood Pressure Control

Blood pressure management plays a vital role in retarding progression of microvascular complications of diabetes. The importance of BP control in retarding nephropathy is as good as of glycemic control. To decrease the progression of DKD and ASCVD, lower targets (130/80 mm Hg) are recommended.

Management of hypertension includes lifestyle modifications [dietary sodium <2,300 mg/day, dietary approaches to stop hypertension (DASH) diet, avoiding sedentary lifestyle, exercise and reducing alcohol] and pharmacotherapy. Angiotensin-converting enzyme (ACE) inhibitors and angiotensin receptor blockers (ARBs) retard the progression of DKD and are the drugs of choice in T2DM. A 2012 Cochrane review stated that ACE inhibitors decrease the incidence of new-onset albuminuria and mortality.

Aldosterone antagonists should be prescribed cautiously in combination with ACE inhibitors or ARBs, because of hyperkalemia. Calcium channel blockers, thiazides, centrally acting drugs, and beta-blockers are other safely used antihypertensives.

CONCLUSION

Diabetic kidney disease is one of the common causes of CKD. Good glycemic control without additional increase in hypoglycemia can reduce risk of DKD in diabetic patients. Regular screening for development of DKD in diabetic patients can help in treatment optimization and improved outcome. Drug selection for patients with renal dysfunction is important. Recent trials and recommendations advocate for SGLT-2 inhibitors and GLP-1A over the other antidiabetics for clear advantage of avoiding hypoglycemia and renal benefits. Prevention and management of DKD require a comprehensive and multidisciplinary approach for better prognosis.

SUGGESTED READINGS

1. Afkarian M, Zelnick LR, Hall YN, Heagerty PJ, Tuttle K, Weiss NS, et al. Clinical manifestations of kidney disease among US adults with diabetes, 1988-2014. JAMA. 2016;316(6):602-10.
2. de Boer IH, Khunti K, Sadusky T, Tuttle KR, Neumiller JJ, Rhee CM, et al. Diabetes Management in Chronic Kidney Disease: A Consensus Report by the American Diabetes Association (ADA) and Kidney Disease: Improving Global Outcomes (KDIGO). Diabetes Care. 2022;45(12):3075-90.
3. Bansal B, Chauhan J. Management of type 2 Diabetes in patients with chronic kidney disease. Arch Clin Nephrol. 2017;3(1): 053-56.
4. McGrath K, Edi R. Diabetic kidney disease: diagnosis, treatment, and prevention. Am Fam Physician. 2019;99(12):751-9.
5. Kalantar-Zadeh K. A critical evaluation of glycated protein parameters in advanced nephropathy: a matter of life or death: A1C remains the gold standard outcome predictor in diabetic dialysis patients. Counterpoint. Diabetes Care. 2012;35:1625-8.
6. Kidney Disease: Improving Global Outcomes (KDIGO) Diabetes Work Group. KDIGO 2022 Clinical Practice Guideline for Diabetes Management in Chronic Kidney Disease. Kidney Int. 2022;102(5S):S1-23.
7. American Diabetes Association Professional Practice Committee. 4. Comprehensive medical evaluation and assessment of comorbidities: Standards of Medical Care in Diabetes–2022. Diabetes Care. 2022;45(Suppl 1):S46-59.
8. Nathan DM, Buse JB, Davidson MB, Ferrannini E, Holman RR, Sherwin R, et al. Medical management of hyperglycemia in type 2 diabetes: a consensus algorithm for the initiation and adjustment of therapy: a consensus statement of the American Diabetes Association and the European Association for the Study of Diabetes. Diabetes Care. 2009;32(1):193-203.
9. Hahr AJ, Molitch ME. Management of diabetes mellitus in patients with chronic kidney disease. Clinical Diabetes and Endocrinol. 2015;1:2.
10. Lv J, Perkovic V, Foote CV, Craig ME, Craig JC, Strippoli GF. Antihypertensive agents for preventing diabetic kidney disease. Cochrane Database Syst Rev. 2012;(12):CD004136.

Unusual urine colors may indicate potential endogenous (pigmenturia, lipids, etc.) or exogenous (drugs, foods, etc.) processes.

To optimize the yield, 10 mL of urine is centrifuged for a minimum of 5 minutes at a speed of at least 1,500 rpm. After removing 9.5 mL of supernatant urine, using suction or carefully decanting, gentle manual agitation of the test tubes, or using a pipette for gentle suction, expulsion of the sediment is conducted. A single drop of urine sediment is then placed on a standardized glass slide and covered with a slip. The sediment field is examined at both low (original magnification × 10) and high power (original magnification × 40) using either brightfield or phase contrast microscopy. At least 10 fields (ideally 20 fields) should be observed under each power for a thorough examination. During analysis, it is important to take note of urine dipstick findings, especially pH and osmolality, as erythrocyte and leukocyte size and shape may vary depending on osmotic forces **(Table 1)**.

TABLE 1: Urine casts and associated syndromes.

Kidney syndrome	Urine cast/sediment	Urine dipstick
Prerenal azotemia	Hyaline casts, a small number of finely granular casts, and occasional renal tubular epithelial cells	–/+ protein
Acute tubular injury	RTEC casts, RTECs, "muddy brown" casts, course granular casts	–/+ protein
Acute interstitial nephritis	RBCs, occasional RBC casts, WBCs, WBC casts, RTECs, and RTEC casts	–/+ protein, +/++ LE, +/++ blood
Nephritic syndrome	Isomorphic RBCs, dysmorphic RBCs (acanthocytes), RBC casts, WBCs, and WBC casts	+/++ protein, ++/+++ blood
Nephrotic syndrome	Lipid droplets, oval fat bodies, lipid-laden casts, cholesterol crystals, and birefringent Maltese cross	+++/++++ protein
Crystalline nephropathy	RTECs, RBCs, WBCs, some WBCs engulfing crystals, various endogenous or drug-related crystals	–/+ blood, –/+ LE
Osmotic nephropathy	Swollen RTECs with cytoplasmic vacuoles, RTEC/granular casts	–/+ protein

(LE: leukocyte esterase; RBCs: red blood cells; RTEC: renal tubular epithelial cells; WBCs: white blood cells)

ACUTE KIDNEY INJURY

While prerenal AKI is frequently encountered in hospitalized patients, tubular damage due to ischemic, toxic, or combined insults is also a prevalent factor contributing to AKI in this context. Therefore, analyzing the urine sediment for different cell types and casts proves beneficial in determining the underlying cause of AKI in hospitalized individuals. AKI with a purely prerenal origin typically manifests as a urinary sediment that appears unremarkable or contains hyaline casts. A few RTECs might also be observed. In contrast, AKI caused by ischemic and/or toxic damage to the tubules is characterized by the presence of cells and casts indicative of tubular injury and necrosis. A considerable number of RTECs may be visible either alone or accompanied by casts. While leukocytes and RBCs may also be present, they could be attributed to other factors like infection, kidney stones, or concurrent lesions in the glomerulus or interstitium. The presence of RTEC casts, along with RTECs, indicates a relatively recent tubular injury. Additionally, the identification of fine or coarse granular casts, alone or with RTECs, suggests significant tubular injury. The higher the number of casts, the more severe is the AKI.

Renal Tubular Epithelial Cells and Casts

The presence of RTECs and casts in the urine sediment indicates that they have undergone necroptosis due to ischemic and/or toxic injury. Urinary RTECs can exhibit varying shapes such as round, oval, polygonal, or columnar. These cells typically possess a high nucleolar-to-cell diameter ratio, with a mean nuclear diameter of 7.7 ± 1.1 μm and a cell diameter of 13.2 ± 2.2 μm. In comparison, superficial transitional uroepithelial cells have a larger mean nuclear diameter of 10.1 ± 1 μm and a cell diameter of 31.2 ± 9 μm. To visualize the size difference, one can compare RTECs to neighboring erythrocytes, which are typically half the diameter of an RTEC (around 6 μm). Differentiating round RTECs from deep uroepithelial cells can be challenging since they share similar cell diameter and nucleolar size ratios.

Granular Casts

All casts share a common composition, with uromodulin forming their backbone. The initial formation of casts occurs in the loop of Henle and further maturation takes place in the distal tubular lumens. Granular casts, which can be either fine, coarse or a mix of hyaline and granular components (hyaline-granular cast), typically indicate tubular injury. These casts may consist of degraded cell lysosomes (visible as granules under electron microscopy) mixed with ultrafiltered serum proteins or particles from degenerated RTECs along with uromodulin. Casts that appear dense and exhibit a brownish or burnt umber color are referred to as "muddy brown casts". In hospitalized patients experiencing AKI, a significant abundance of these casts is considered a telltale sign of severe ATN. Nevertheless, it is essential to note that the presence of granular casts does not exclusively indicate ATN as they can also be observed in AIN, thrombotic microangiopathy, and other kidney disorders.

Hyaline Casts

Hyaline casts primarily consist of uromodulin, a product of a loop of Henle cells, and are observable when a decrease in renal perfusion leads to sluggish urinary flow. These casts may also appear after exercise, indicating dehydration. In some instances, severe renal hypoperfusion can cause "patchy" tubular injury, coexisting with prerenal physiology, resulting in a hybrid form of AKI. From a clinical perspective, the patient might show a partial response to prerenal treatment, while the urine sediment exhibits hyaline casts, along with a few scattered RTECs and hyaline-granular casts. In such cases, the approach involves correcting the prerenal parameters while simultaneously providing support for the underlying ATN.

ACUTE INTERSTITIAL NEPHRITIS

Making a clinical diagnosis of AIN is notoriously challenging, and it frequently necessitates a kidney biopsy. In cases of AIN, the urine sediment frequently includes RTECs, granular casts, and WBCs (with negative urine culture results). These findings likely indicate tubular injury/tubulitis due to the inflammatory interstitial process. Although WBC casts are uncommon, their presence strongly suggests AIN, especially in the absence of acute/chronic pyelonephritis. However, the presence of dysmorphic RBCs and RBC casts, along with pyuria or WBC casts, shifts the diagnosis toward proliferative glomerulonephritis.

Leukocytes and White Blood Cell Casts

When evaluating hospital-acquired AKI, drug-induced AIN is frequently considered in the list of potential causes due to the extensive exposure of patients to various potential causative medications. Distinguishing leukocyte casts from RTEC casts can pose significant challenges. However, carefully examining their cellular structures (single- vs. multilobed nucleus) and sizes (RTECs larger than WBCs) often enables accurate identification. Typically, neutrophils are the most common type of WBC found in urine, indicating urinary infections, but they can also be observed in the context of inflammatory kidney conditions. Neutrophils have a diameter of approximately 10–15 μm, larger than RBCs (around 6 μm) and smaller than RTECs (approximately 15–30 μm), and they possess a multilobed nucleus. Furthermore, leukocytes have the potential to form blebs, which might be mistaken for dysmorphic RBCs by individuals without adequate training.

NEPHRITIC AND NEPHROTIC SEDIMENT

Nephritic syndrome is characterized by active urine sediment with hematuria, proteinuria, hypertension, and reduced glomerular filtration rate (GFR). Common causes of nephritic syndrome include proliferative glomerulonephritis, small-vessel vasculitis, and antiglomerular basement membrane (anti-GBM) disease, which, when severe, are referred to as rapidly progressive glomerulonephritis. In the nephritic sediment, a significant number of erythrocytes and RBC casts can be observed. The urine sediment in nephritic syndrome is distinguished by an abundance of erythrocytes and RBC casts. One of the key indicators of glomerular bleeding is the presence of "dysmorphic RBCs," which includes acanthocytes or G1 cells. They aid in diagnosis, treatment response as well as recurrence of the disease. Up until now, it has been observed that continuous hematuria is linked to a higher probability of antineutrophil cytoplasmic antibody vasculitis relapse.

Nephrotic syndrome is characterized by edema, hypoalbuminemia, high-grade proteinuria (exceeding 3.5 g/day), and hypercholesterolemia. Generally, patients with nephrotic syndrome exhibit urine sediments that are relatively unremarkable (acellular). Glomerular lesions, as seen on histopathology, are usually nonproliferative and are distinguished by a permeable GBM. Analyzing the urine sediment may reveal indications that corroborate the presence of nephrotic syndrome, such as the identification of lipiduria and lipid casts.

Erythrocytes and Red Blood Cell Casts

Red Blood Cells and RBC casts may appear in urine after vigorous physical activity. Dysmorphic RBCs, including acanthocytes or G1 cells, are more specific for glomerular injury, but their sensitivity is limited. Dysmorphic RBCs can exhibit various shapes, such as a ring shape with single or multiple bullae-like protrusions. These cells are smaller (around 3 μm) than isomorphic RBCs due to membrane loss. The process behind the formation of dysmorphic RBCs is not clearly understood, but it may be because of several injuries faced by RBCs during their passing through the gaps in an injured GBM and then being exposed to an unfavorable tubular environment with osmotic changes and acidic urine. Differentiating acanthocytes from dysmorphic nonG1 cells or pseudoG1 cells (like sickled cells, echinocytes, schistocytes, stomatocytes, poikilocytes, etc.) can be challenging. There are no specific morphologic criteria for G1 cells, but they typically have membranous blebs, a doughnut shape with a target configuration, and fragmented cell contours. Isomorphic erythrocytes can become crenated in concentrated urine, and it is crucial to recognize that these cells are not dysmorphic RBCs. Another type of urinary RBC is the ghost cell, which has low hemoglobin content and exhibits a low refractive index.

Lipiduria and Lipid Casts

Free lipid droplets, oval fat bodies, lipid casts, and cholesterol crystals might be evident in the urine sediment. When circular fat droplets containing cholesterol esters are present, they produce birefringent Maltese crosses under polarized light. Oval fat bodies can represent either macrophages or RTECs that have engulfed fat droplets. These cells endocytose the fat, leading to their engorgement with lipid droplets. In some cases, free lipid droplets, cholesterol crystals, and/or oval fat bodies may become embedded in a cast matrix, giving rise to a lipid or "fatty" cast.

CONCLUSION

In summary, this chapter highlights the vital role of urine analysis, specifically cast examination, in diagnosing and understanding renal disorders. Dr Thomas Addis's quote underscores urine's importance as a real-time source of kidney health information. The chapter explores various casts in urine sediment, detailing their associations with specific renal conditions. It delves into cast formation, emphasizing the role of renal tubular epithelial cells (RTECs) and discusses challenges in interpretation.

The impact of automated urine analysis in centralized labs is acknowledged, but the decline in physicians' cast examination is regrettable. A comparison between automated systems and manual urine microscopy is provided, emphasizing the latter's additional diagnostic value. The chapter concludes by stressing a comprehensive approach to kidney disease diagnosis, combining urine microscopy with medical history, physical exams, and imaging. It underscores manual urine microscopy's importance in predicting outcomes, advocating for a balanced approach that melds automation with healthcare professionals' expertise for a thorough understanding of kidney health.

SUGGESTED READINGS

1. Bakan E, Ozturk N, Baygutalp NK, Polat E, Akpinar K, Dorman E, et al. Comparison of Cobas 6500 and Iris IQ200 fully-automated urine analyzers to manual urine microscopy. Biochem Med (Zagreb). 2016;26(3):365-75.
2. Chawla LS, Dommu A, Berger A, Shih S, Patel SS. Urinary sediment cast scoring index for acute kidney injury: a pilot study. Nephron Clin Pract. 2008;110(3):c145-150.
3. Perazella MA, Coca SG, Hall IE, Iyanam U, Koraishy M, Parikh CR. Urine microscopy is associated with severity and worsening of acute kidney injury in hospitalized patients. Clin J Am Soc Nephrol. 2010;5(3):402-8.
4. Cavanaugh C, Perazella MA. Urine Sediment Examination in the Diagnosis and Management of Kidney Disease: Core Curriculum 2019. Am J Kidney Dis. 2019;73(2):258-72.
5. Zaman Z. The Urinary Sediment: An Integrated View, by Giovanni B. Fogazzi Z. Zaman. Clin Chem. 2011;57:532.
6. Perazella MA. Clinical Approach to Diagnosing Acute and Chronic Tubulointerstitial Disease. Adv Chronic Kidney Dis. 2017;24(2):57-63.

SECTION

11

NEUROLOGY

88

CHAPTER

Newer Insights into Vascular Dementia

Jaydeep Majumdar, Bhaskar Ghosh

ABSTRACT

Vascular dementia is the second leading cause of late-life dementia accounting for almost one-third of dementia cases in India. This vascular brain injury induced disruption of cognitive network has significant impact on quality of life. The term vascular cognitive impairment and dementia (VCID) encompasses the different phenotypic subgroups like subcortical ischemic vascular dementia (SIVD), poststroke dementia, multi-infarct dementia, and mixed dementia. Overlapping clinical profile and cognitive pattern often makes it difficult to differentiate clinically between mixed dementia and pure Alzheimer disease (AD). Apart from well-recognized cardiovascular risk factors, APOE4-related cerebral amyloid angiopathy (CAA) has also been proposed as a risk factor for VCID. Diagnosis of VCID demands careful clinical history, proper general and neurological examination supported by neuroimaging, and sometimes genetic study in appropriate context. Primary prevention that aims to achieve optimal brain health has been emphasized in the management of VCID along with other pharmacological and rehabilitative measures.

INTRODUCTION

Dementia refers to a clinical syndrome characterized by ongoing cognitive decline that interferes with the ability to function independently in everyday activities. Mild cognitive impairment (MCI) is a state intermediate between normal cognition and dementia with preserved day-to-day functional capability. Vascular dementia refers to any dementia that is primarily caused by a cerebrovascular disease or impaired cerebral blood flow or in which these are the chief contributing causative factors. The term vascular cognitive impairment and dementia (VCID) has evolved over time and has been classified into four phenotypic subgroups as per the VICCCS (Vascular Impairment of Cognition Classification Consensus Study) criteria **(Fig. 1)**.

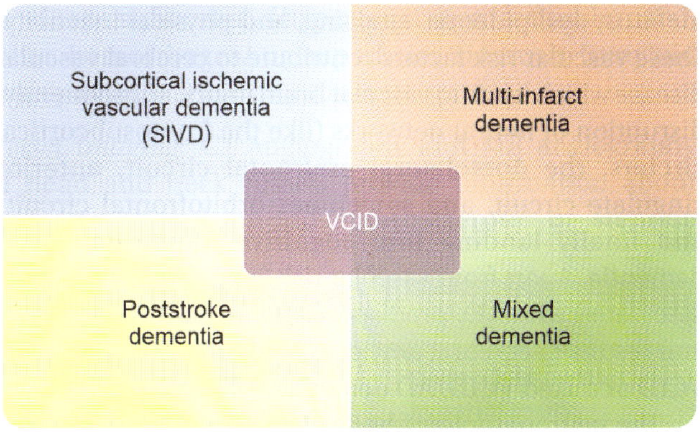

FIG. 1: The VICCCS criteria for classification of VCID.
(VCID: vascular cognitive impairment and dementia; VICCCS: Vascular Impairment of Cognition Classification Consensus Study)

- *Subcortical ischemic vascular dementia (SIVD)*: Slow progression with delayed processing speed, decline in complex attention, and executive dysfunction.
- *Poststroke dementia*: Stepwise progression, presenting either immediately after stroke or within 6 months of stroke. Presenting symptom depend on the location of vascular insult. Infarcts or hemorrhages in specific strategic locations like thalamus, medial temporal cortex, head of caudate nucleus, dominant angular gyrus, or anterior corpus callosum can impair memory, especially episodic memory. Lesions, outside these

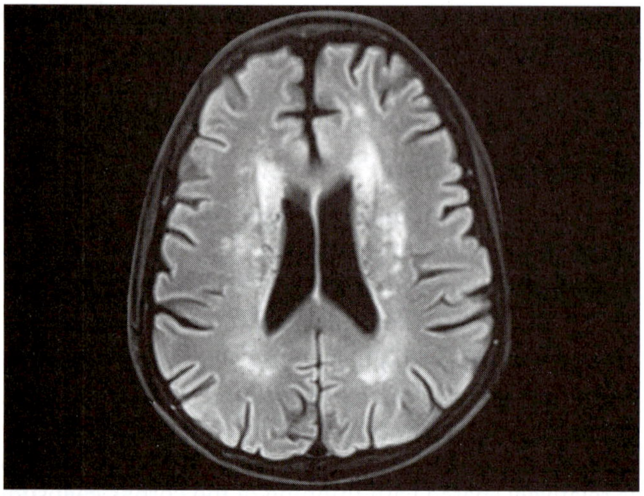

FIG. 2: Magnetic resonance imaging (MRI) brain of a patient of vascular cognitive impairment and dementia (VCID) showing Fazekas grade 3 changes.

pathology. The specificity and sensitivity of CT angiography is better compared to MR angiography but there is additional risk of contrast toxicity and radiation with CT angiography. Carotid Doppler study and transcranial Doppler study can alternatively be ordered for vessel imaging but these modalities are operator dependent.

Fludeoxyglucose-positron emission tomography (FDG-PET): Location-specific hypometabolism may provide additional information differentiating VCID (diffuse subcortical and focal cortical region) from degenerative dementia like AD (temporoparietal area).

Amyloid PET: It helps in assessing AD, mixed dementia, or CAA by detection of fibrillar amyloid-β by specific tracer. In spite of these advanced imaging modalities, due to overlapping clinical profile and cognitive pattern, it is often difficult to differentiate clinically between mixed dementia and pure AD **(Table 2)**.

TABLE 2: Differentiating features between VCID and AD.

Salient pointers	VCID	AD
History:		
• Progression	• Stepwise progression (multi-infarct/ poststroke dementia) or Slow progression (subcortical ischemic vascular disease)	• Slow progression
• Risk factors	• Hypertension, diabetes, dyslipidemia, atrial fibrillation, smoking, physical inactivity, genetic predisposition	• Genetic predisposition
• Past medical/family history	• Stroke, coronary artery disease, or peripheral vascular disease	• AD
General and systemic examination: Clinical evidences of enhanced atherosclerosis and cardiovascular risk factors	Evident	Usually absent in pure AD
Cognitive and neurological assessment	• Depends on the location of involvement. Commonly executive dysfunction, slow processing speed, memory retrieval defect, poor attention • *Focal neurodeficit*: Sensory, motor, autonomic, cranial nerve deficit, or gait abnormality may be associated	• Early memory impairment (amnestic variety) • Other neurological examination usually normal until advanced stage
Laboratory investigations	• Deranged lipid profile (dyslipidemia), altered glycemic index including HbA1c level • *ECG*: It may reveal atrial fibrillation	Usually normal
Structural imaging:		
• CT/MRI	• White matter changes, strategic infarcts, microbleeds, lobar hemorrhages, superficial siderosis	• Medial temporal (particularly, hippocampal) atrophy, parietal and frontal atrophy
• Vessel imaging	• Intracranial/carotid atherosclerotic or stenotic lesion	• None
Metabolic imaging: FDG-PET	Areas of decreased glucose uptake depending on location of vascular insult	Hypometabolism in temporo-parieto-frontal cortex
Biomarkers	None	Cerebrospinal fluid or PET fibrillar amyloid-β or phosphorylated tau

(AD: Alzheimer disease; CT: computed tomography; ECG: electrocardiogram; FDG-PET: fludeoxyglucose-positron emission tomography; MRI: magnetic resonance imaging; VCID: vascular cognitive impairment and dementia)

Genetic Testing

Appropriate clinical settings (young stroke and strong family history of VCID without significant atherosclerotic risk factor) or very suggestive neuroimaging may warrant genetic testing.

MANAGEMENT

Primary Prevention

Primary prevention aims toward effective reduction of cardiovascular risk factors to achieve "optimal brain health", which is defined by seven parameters to preserve cognition. As per American Heart Association/American Stroke Association guidelines, these parameters include hypertension (untreated blood pressure <120/80 mm Hg), fasting blood glucose (<100 mg/dL), total cholesterol (<200 mg/dL), smoking status (non-smoker), moderately intense to vigorous physical activity, body mass index (<25 kg/m^2), diet containing fruits and vegetables, oily fish, fiber-rich whole grains, restricted sodium and restricted sugar-sweetened beverages.

Secondary Prevention

Blood pressure: American Society of Hypertension recommends blood pressure goal of <150/90 mm Hg in 80 years aged or older to reduce stroke risk. Angiotensin-converting enzyme (ACE) inhibitors may protect against VCID.

Lipids: High serum total cholesterol in midlife is associated with VCID in later life. Statins reduce risk of cognitive decline.

Blood sugar: Both hyperglycemia and hypoglycemic spells worsen cognition. A goal of 7–7.9% is adequate enough to retard cognitive decline in VCID.

Antithrombotic medications: These should be avoided for primary prevention. Antiplatelet drugs or anticoagulant (in atrial fibrillation or valvular heart disease) are indicated in secondary prevention of ischemic stroke.

Special consideration in CAA: In patients with CAA, blood pressure needs to be maintained <120/80 mm Hg to prevent additional risk of ICH. Due to effects on coagulation and fibrinolysis, there is increased risk of ICH in CAA patients with the use of statin. Given increased risk of ICH, an estimation of risk-benefit and cautious monitoring is essential with the use of antithrombotic medications.

TREATMENT

Pharmacological Treatment

Cholinesterase inhibitors, though the Food and Drug Administration (FDA) approved for AD, may be reasonable to use in VCID with concomitant AD. Donepezil (5–10 mg/day) or galantamine (8–12 mg/twice a day) can be used in VCID patients not directly attributed to clinical stroke.

Memantine (20 mg/day), an N-methyl-D-aspartate (NMDA) receptor antagonist, the FDA approved for moderate to severe AD, is considered to be of satisfactory cognitive benefit in VCID patients.

Investigational Agents

These include calcium channel blocker (nimodipine and nicardipine), ergot alkaloids (hydergine and nicergoline), cerebrolysin, ginkgo biloba, citicoline, vitamin B_{12}, folic acid, xanthine derivative (propentofylline, pentoxifylline, and denbufylline), and piracetam.

REHABILITATION

Aerobic exercise, nutrition, social interaction, and cognitive rehabilitation program can improve affected cognitive domains by resynchronization of disrupted cognitive networks.

CONCLUSION

Vascular cognitive impairment and dementia is a unique and common cause of dementia that is multifactorial with multimodal pathogenesis. Etiologic entities such as CAA and genetic mutations are needed to be emphasized apart from cardiovascular risk factors. Meticulous history, structured physical and cognitive assessment, and appropriate neuroimaging may point toward VCID. Primary prevention that aims to achieve optimal brain health is the cornerstone of management.

SUGGESTED READINGS

1. Duong S, Patel T, Chang F. Dementia What pharmacists need to know. Can Pharm J (Ott). 2017;150(2):118-29.
2. Smith EE. Clinical presentations and epidemiology of vascular dementia. Clin Sci (Lond). 2017;131:1059-68.
3. Skrobot OA, O'Brien J, Black S, Chen C, DeCarli C, Erkinjuntti T, et al. The Vascular Impairment of Cognition Classification Consensus Study. Alzheimers Dement. 2017;13(6):624-33.

4. Chang Wong E, Chang Chui H. Vascular Cognitive Impairment and Dementia. Continuum (Minneap Minn). 2022;28(3):750-80.
5. Schneider JA, Arvanitakis Z, Bang W, Bennett DA. Mixed brain pathologies account for most dementia cases in community-dwelling older persons. Neurology. 2007;69(24):2197-204.
6. Arshad F, Samim MM, Paplikar A, Rajendran S, Kalkonde Y, Alladi S. Vascular cognitive impairment in India: Challenges and opportunities for prevention and treatment. Cereb Circ Cogn Behav. 2022;3:100034.
7. Alladi S, Mekala S, Chadalawada SK, Jala S, Mridula R, Kaul S. Subtypes of dementia: a study from a memory clinic in India. Dement Geriatr Cogn Disord. 2011;32:32-8.
8. Gorelick PB, Scuteri A, Black SE, Decarli C, Greenberg SM, Iadecola C, et al. Vascular contributions to cognitive impairment and dementia: a statement for healthcare professionals from the American Heart Association/American Stroke Association. Stroke. 2011;42(9):2672-713.
9. Iadecola C. The pathobiology of vascular dementia. Neuron. 2013;80(4):844-899.
10. Wilkinson D, Doody R, Helme R, Taubman K, Mintzer J, Kertesz A, et al. Donepezil in vascular dementia: a randomized, placebo-controlled study. Neurology. 2003;61(4):479-86.

89

CHAPTER

Autoimmune Encephalitis

Kamal Kumar Sawlani, Arzoo Sharma, Ambuj Yadav, Shyam Chand Chaudhary

ABSTRACT

Autoimmune encephalitis (AE) is an immune-mediated inflammatory condition of the brain. Syndromes associated with neuronal cell surface antibodies or synaptic protein antibodies are considered as AE, while paraneoplastic syndromes are often associated with antibodies against intracellular neuronal proteins. The incidence of AE has increased in the previous few years. The most common entity is anti-N-methyl-D-aspartate receptor (NMDAR) encephalitis. AE has a subacute onset with rapid progression of cognitive, psychiatric, and behavioral changes, often with seizures. AE can be diagnosed as possible, probable, and definite AE based on various criteria which include clinical features, neuroimaging, cerebrospinal fluid (CSF) findings, and antibody testing in serum and CSF. CSF may show evidence of inflammation in the form of pleocytosis (cells > 5/mm^3) and mildly elevated protein. Magnetic resonance imaging (MRI) may show signal hyperintensities in the affected brain regions on T2-weighted images or fluid-attenuated inversion recovery (FLAIR) MRI. The differential diagnoses of AE include central nervous system (CNS) infections, metabolic encephalopathy, septic encephalopathy, drug toxicity, vascular disorders, neoplastic disorders, and demyelinating and inflammatory disorders. Early initiation of immunotherapy is crucial in the management of AE and should not be delayed awaiting antibody results. First-line therapy includes intravenous steroids, intravenous immunoglobulin (IVIG), and plasmapheresis. Other treatment modalities include rituximab and cyclophosphamide. Supportive therapy is equally important.

INTRODUCTION

Autoimmune encephalitis (AE) is a rapidly progressive encephalopathy (usually <6 weeks) caused by brain inflammation. Being dwellers of a tropical region, the suspicion of infection is the first reflex that comes to us, but with the refinement of acumen and diagnostic aids, the detection, diagnosis, and treatment of autoimmune pathologies are now becoming increasingly common, the prevalence of which now matches that of infections.

In AE, there are antibodies against certain neuronal antigens. This may or may not be associated with cancers. Those that are come under the purview of paraneoplastic encephalitis. All paraneoplastic encephalitis are autoimmune, but not all AE are paraneoplastic. Autoantibody targets are generally divided into three main categories: (1) Cell surface proteins, (2) Synaptic proteins, and (3) Intraneuronal antigens **(Table 1)**.

Syndromes associated with neuronal cell surface antibodies or synaptic protein antibodies are considered as AE, while paraneoplastic syndromes are often associated with antibodies against intracellular neuronal proteins (onconeuronal proteins).

The AE syndromes encompass a horizon of clinical manifestations which may range from the common limbic encephalitis to complex manifestations such as seizures and coma. The most common of these entities is the anti-N-methyl-D-aspartate receptor (NMDAR) encephalitis. Diagnosing a patient with AE requires a multipronged approach including clinical assessment, neuroimaging, electroencephalogram (EEG), lumbar puncture, and antibody testing [both in the cerebrospinal fluid (CSF) and in serum].

Although the presence of autoantibodies against neuronal antigens clinches the diagnosis of definite AE,

TABLE 1: Antibodies in autoimmune encephalitis.

Antibody	Syndrome
Intracellular antigens	
Anti-Hu ANNA-1 (antineuronal nuclear antibody)	Limbic encephalitis
Anti-Ma2	Limbic encephalitis
Anti-GAD (glutamic acid decarboxylase)	Limbic encephalitis
Cell surface antigens and synaptic protein antigen	
Anti-NMDA receptor (N-methyl-D-aspartate)	Anti-NMDAR encephalitis
Anti-LGI-1 (leucine-rich glioma inactivated protein-1)	Limbic encephalitis
Anti-AMPA receptor (alpha-amino-3-hydroxy-5-methyl-4-isoxazolepropionic acid)	Limbic encephalitis with nystagmus and seizures
Anti-GABAA receptor (gamma-amino butyric acid-A)	Encephalitis with refractory seizures and status epilepticus
Anti-GABAB receptor (gamma-amino butyric acid-B)	Limbic encephalitis, intractable seizures, and orolingual dyskinesias
Anti-GluK2 (glutamate kainate receptor subunit 2)	Encephalitis, cerebellar ataxia, and cerebellitis
Anti-mGluR5 (metabotropic glutamate receptor 5)	Encephalitis
Antidopamine 2 receptors	Basal ganglia encephalitis
Anti-GLY receptor (glycine)	Progressive encephalomyelitis with rigidity and myoclonus, stiff person syndrome
Anti-CASPRA (contactin-associated protein-like 2)	Limbic encephalitis and Morvan syndrome
Antiganglionic AchR (acetylcholine receptor)	Autonomic dysfunction, peripheral somatic neuropathies, and encephalopathies
Anti-MOG (myelin oligodendrocyte glycoprotein)	ADEM, optic neuritis, myelitis, and cortical encephalitis
Anti-IgLON5 (immunoglobulin-like cell adhesion molecule 5)	REM and non-REM sleep parasomnias, abnormal movements, and gait disturbances
Anti-DPPX (dipeptidyl-peptidase-like protein-6)	Hyperreflexia, agitation, myoclonus, tremor, and seizures
Antineurexin-3 alpha	Orofacial dyskinesias and central hypoventilation
Anti-GFAP (glial fibrillary acidic protein)	Headache, optic disc edema and optic papillitis, encephalopathy, autonomic instability, myelopathy, tremor, and psychiatric disturbances
Anti-AK5 (adenylate kinase 5)	Limbic encephalitis refractory to therapy, amnesia, and depression
Anti-AQP 4 (aquaporin 4)	Encephalitis and neuromyelitis optica spectrum disorder
Anti-GQ1b (antiganglioside GQ1b antibody)	Bickerstaff's brainstem encephalitis

(ADEM: acute disseminated encephalomyelitis; REM: rapid eye movement)

the presence of antibodies is not mandatory (possible and probable encephalitis) for the initiation of treatment as these tests are not available in most parts of the world, are costly, and test results are often delayed leading to a delay in management. Furthermore, many patients of AE are seronegative (as many as 50%); therefore, the diagnosis of possible and probable AE relies on clinical assessment (which includes symptomatology of subacute onset of short-term working memory loss, altered mentation, new-onset seizures, and psychiatric manifestations), CSF pleocytosis, and a supportive magnetic resonance imaging (MRI). Detection of the presence of AE-specific immunoglobulin G (IgG) antibody testing in both serum and CSF, CSF IgG index and oligoclonal bands, EEG, and a brain biopsy may aid in the diagnosis of AE.

EPIDEMIOLOGY

The incidence of AE has increased in the previous few years from 0.4 per 10,000 person-years in 1995–2005 to 1.2 per 10,000 person-years in 2006–2015. The most common entity is anti-NMDAR encephalitis. The prevalence of AE, especially anti-NMDAR encephalitis, now matches that of antiviral encephalitis.

PATHOPHYSIOLOGY

Neuronal and glial synaptic membrane proteins are targeted by IgG. It binds to extracellular epitopes of ionotropic, metabotropic receptors, water channels, and neural adhesion proteins. The mechanism implicated is antigen binding, cross-linking, internalization, and degradation. This is particularly specific for anti-NMDAR and aquaporin 4. Antibody-dependent cellular cytotoxicity (ADCC) and complement cascade play a vital role. In case of leucine-rich glioma inactivated-1 (LGI-1) and anticontactin-associated protein (CASPR), there is interference with the protein target's function. Molecular mimicry plays an important role in postviral triggered encephalitis, mostly associated with herpes simplex virus (HSV).

In case of NMDAR encephalitis, the antibodies are directed toward a subunit of NR1 subunit of NMDAR. There is evidence of moderate inflammatory infiltrates consisting of plasma cells, IgG, and microglial activation. In case of myelin oligodendrocyte glycoprotein (MOG) autoimmunity, demyelination is the primary feature.

CLINICAL MANIFESTATIONS

When to suspect autoimmune encephalitis?

Autoimmune encephalitis has a quite classical presentation. It is an entity of subacute onset with rapid progression of cognitive, psychiatric, and behavioral changes, often with seizures. It has a fluctuating clinical course. There may be myoclonus, tremulousness, headache, and blurred vision with a family history of autoimmune diseases. Apart from the detection of neuronal antigens, the presence of non-neuronal antibodies should point in the direction of an autoimmune pathology. Both CSF and MRI show evidence of inflammation in the form of pleocytosis (cells > 5/mm^3), mildly elevated protein in the CSF, and signal abnormalities in the gray white matter on T2-weighted or fluid-attenuated inversion recovery (FLAIR) MRI.

DIAGNOSTIC CRITERIA

Graus et al. in a position paper published in 2016 had provided a practical clinical approach to the diagnosis of AE and defined the criteria for possible, probable, and definite AE.

Diagnostic Criteria for Possible Autoimmune Encephalitis

All three of the following criteria must be met:

1. Subacute onset with rapid progression (within a span of 3 months) of working memory deficit, psychiatric manifestations, and/or altered mentation
2. At least one of the following:
   i. New-onset central nervous system (CNS) findings
   ii. Seizures
   iii. CSF pleocytosis (>5 leukocytes/mm^3)
   iv. MRI, suggestive of encephalitis
3. Exclusion of alternative diagnoses

Magnetic Resonance Imaging

Autoimmune limbic encephalitis is characterized by mesial temporal lobe T2 hyperintensities. Anti-NMDAR encephalitis may have a normal MRI, but a wide variety of T2 signal abnormalities have been reported. In gamma-aminobutyric acid A (GABAA) receptor antibody encephalitis, T2 signal abnormalities are multifocal involving white gray matter. Basal ganglia T1 or T2 hyperintensities may accompany LGI-1 encephalitis.

Magnetic resonance imaging is also helpful in excluding other disorders (cerebrovascular event, or metastatic disease). Patients with AE may present with a normal brain MRI or CSF findings.

Positron Emission Tomography

On positron emission tomography (PET) scan, the most common finding in AE is glucose hypometabolism. In anti-NMDAR encephalitis, hypometabolism is noted in the mesial occipital region whereas in anti-LGI-1 antibody encephalitis, basal ganglia hyper- or hypometabolism is typically seen.

SPECIFIC AUTOIMMUNE ENCEPHALITIS SYNDROMES

Anti-NMDAR Encephalitis

This disease entity is commonly seen in younger age groups, <45 years of age with a high female predominance in the ratio of 4:1. It has been typically linked to the presence of ovarian teratoma so much so that the removal of the same leads to rapid improvement in the clinical status of the patient. The classically described presentation of anti-NMDAR encephalitis is a woman in her 20s presenting with psychiatric disturbances, dyskinesias, seizures, and hypoventilation.

It is subacute in presentation with a prodrome of viral illness with a predominance of neuropsychiatric symptoms including panic, hallucinations, delusions, and incoherence with seizures and memory disturbances. There are oral, buccal, lingual, and facial dyskinesias that are pathognomonic. Hypoventilation is a commonly associated feature and may require mechanical ventilation. It is also associated with autonomic dysregulation such as hypertension, diaphoresis, salivation, pupillary dilatation, and tachycardia followed by episodic bradycardia to the point of asystole due to sinus pauses.

Cerebrospinal fluid shows pleocytosis with cells ranging from 5 to 100/mm^3, a mild increase in protein. MRI shows signal intensity on T2 and FLAIR. EEG shows a classical "extreme delta brush" pattern, which is pathognomonic. The target antigen in the disorder is the NRI antigen, as a subunit of the NMDAR.

Though this form of encephalitis is associated with teratomas, anti-NMDAR encephalitis unrelated to tumors is being increasingly recognized. Also, anti-NMDAR encephalitis is said to have been triggered by HSV infection. Based on a number of studies, approximately 20–30% of the patients who are anti-NMDAR antibody negative in the serum and CSF at the time of herpes simplex virus encephalitis (HSVE) seroconvert to positive NMDAR antibodies with episodes of relapsing symptoms which cannot be associated with HSVE.

Diagnostic Criteria

- *Probable anti-NMDAR encephalitis*:
  - Rapid onset of at least four of the following six symptoms:
    a. Cognitive dysfunction or abnormal psychiatric behavior
    b. Speech dysfunction
    c. Seizures
    d. Movement disorders, dyskinesias, and abnormal posturing
    e. Autonomic dysfunction or cerebral hypoventilation
    f. Impaired consciousness
  - At least one of the following laboratory results:
    a. Abnormal EEG (abnormal slowing or extreme delta brush pattern)
    b. CSF pleocytosis or oligoclonal bands
  - Exclusion of other diagnoses:

  Diagnosis of anti-NMDAR encephalitis can also be made if there is presence of a systemic teratoma and three of the above-mentioned symptoms.
- *Definite anti-NMDAR encephalitis*:
  - IgG anti-GluN1 antibodies
  - One or more of the six major groups of symptoms
  - Exclusion of other disorders

Limbic Encephalitis

Limbic encephalitis is a subacute disease process involving mainly the temporal, deeper medial forebrain region, more specifically the hippocampus, amygdala, and insula. The patient presents with the predominant features of decline in memory, confusion and disorientation, changes in eating habits, disturbed sleep, apathy, and frank psychosis with delusions. Seizures are a common presentation. When the left side of the hippocampus is predominantly involved, the memory dysfunction is more verbal, whereas the dysfunction is more visual if the right side is more involved.

A few patients with anti-LGI-1 encephalitis may present with only seizure and not the entire clinical picture of limbic encephalitis. In such scenarios, in patients presenting with new-onset seizures with an unclear etiology, the possibility of AE must be kept in mind and an autoantibody panel tested for.

Limbic encephalitis, once known to be completely synonymous with paraneoplastic syndromes (intracellular antibodies), is now being increasingly recognized to be seen with neuronal surface antibodies.

The diagnostic criteria for definite autoimmune limbic encephalitis require all four of the below:

1. Subacute onset (rapid progression of <3 months) of memory deficits, seizures, and psychiatric symptoms
2. Bilateral brain abnormalities of T2-weighted FLAIR MRI highly restricted to the medial temporal lobes
3. At least one of the following:
   i CSF pleocytosis [more than five white blood cells (WBCs) per cubic mm]
   ii EEG with slow wave activity involving the temporal lobes.
4. Exclusion of alternative causes

If antibodies specific to neuronal cell surface antigens or synaptic antigens are detected, the diagnosis of limbic encephalitis may be made even if at least two of the first three criteria are met.

The differential diagnoses of limbic encephalitis include HSVE, human herpesvirus 6 (HHV-6) encephalitis, glioma, status epilepticus, neurosyphilis, Whipple's disease, and human immunodeficiency virus (HIV).

Acute Disseminated Encephalomyelitis

Acute disseminated encephalomyelitis (ADEM) is a disease mainly presenting in children and adults aged <40 years. Classically, it follows an acute systemic infection or a vaccination. Clinical manifestations include a variable extent of encephalopathy, ataxia, cranial nerve palsies, hemiparesis, myelopathy, or optic neuritis. CSF analysis shows pleocytosis but finding oligoclonal bands is increasingly uncommon. Brain imaging with MRI shows multiple large (>2 cm) abnormalities on T2-FLAIR. For a diagnosis of definite ADEM, there must be an absence of new clinical and MRI findings 3 months after symptom onset.

Diagnostic Criteria

All five of the below-mentioned criteria must be satisfied:

1. A first multifocal, clinical CNS event of inflammatory demyelinating cause
2. Encephalopathy unexplained by pyrexia
3. Abnormal findings on MRI brain:
   - Diffuse, large (>2 cm) lesions involving the cerebral white matter
   - T1 hypointense lesions
   - Deep gray matter abnormalities

4. No new development after 3 months of symptom onset (clinical or radiological)
5. Exclusion of other causes

Bickerstaff's Brainstem Encephalitis

This disorder is characterized by a subacute onset of gradual impairment of consciousness along with bilateral ataxia and ophthalmoparesis. It is typically preceded by an infection. It has a good prognosis and has antibodies against anti-GQ1b receptor and is related to Miller–Fisher syndrome.

The criteria for diagnosis of probable Bickerstaff's encephalitis are as follows:

- Subacute onset of a decreased level of consciousness, bilateral external ophthalmoplegia, and ataxia
- Exclusion of other diagnoses

Definite diagnoses of Bickerstaff's encephalitis are characterized by the presence of IgG anti-GQ1b antibodies, despite the occurrence of recovery within 12 weeks of onset, and the absence of bilateral external ophthalmoplegia, or ataxia.

DIFFERENTIAL DIAGNOSIS

The few main differential diagnoses of AE include CNS infections, metabolic encephalopathy, septic encephalopathy, drug toxicity, cerebrovascular disease, neoplastic disorders, demyelinating and inflammatory disorders, Creutzfeldt–Jakob disease, epileptic disorders, and rheumatological disorders such as systemic lupus erythematosus and sarcoidosis. It is important to exclude these disorders, especially infectious etiologies before starting immunosuppressive therapy.

TREATMENT

Early initiation of immunotherapy is crucial in the management of AE and may be started on clinical suspicion (possible or probable AE). It should not be delayed awaiting antibody results.

Acute Therapy

The following treatment options may be considered as acute therapy in cases of AE. Other agents used are given in **Table 2**.

- *Intravenous (IV) methylprednisolone*: This is given as 1,000 mg IV daily for 3 days and then once weekly for 5- 11 weeks.
- *Intravenous immunoglobulin (IVIG)*: The recommendation for this is to start with 0.4 g/kg daily for 3 days followed by 0.4 g/kg every week for 5–11 weeks.

TABLE 2: Immunosuppressive agents used in autoimmune encephalitis.

Agent	Dose
Intravenous methylprednisolone	1 g daily for 3 days and then once weekly for 5–11 weeks
Intravenous immunoglobulin	0.4 g/kg daily for 3 days followed by 0.4 g/kg every week for 5–11 weeks
Plasma exchange	3–6 plasma exchanges over consecutive or alternating days
Rituximab	1 g intravenous (IV) initially followed by 1 g after 2 weeks or 4 weekly doses of 375 mg/m^2
Cyclophosphamide	500–1,000 mg/m^2 IV monthly for 3–6 months 1–2 mg/kg/day orally
Tocilizumab	8 mg/kg IV initially, followed by 8 mg/kg after 1 month. The same dose can be given monthly depending on response
Bortezomib	1.3 mg/m^2 per dose IV twice weekly for 2 weeks. A 10-day break is given after every cycle and a maximum of eight cycles can be given
Azathioprine (+prednisone)	2–3 mg/kg/day orally
Mycophenolate mofetil (+prednisone)	1–3 g/day orally
Prednisone	15–30 mg/day orally for 1 year
Cyclosporine	2–5 mg/kg/day orally twice daily
Tacrolimus	0.15–0.30 mg/kg/day orally in two divided doses

- *Plasma exchange*: Three to six plasma exchanges on consecutive or alternative days using a large-bore catheter
- *Rituximab*: This agent is given intravenously in two doses of 1,000 mg each 2 weeks apart or 4 weekly doses of 375 mg/m^2. This can be given every 6 months without the need for monitoring CD20/CD19 counts.
- *Cyclophosphamide*: An IV dose of 500–1,000 mg/m^2 is given monthly for 3–6 months and then an oral dose of 1–2 mg/kg in the morning. A dose reduction by 50% is done when the WBC count is <1,500/mm^3 and absolute neutrophil count (ANC) reduces to <500 cells/mm^3 and a reduction to 25% is to be done when hemoglobin (Hb) is <8.3 g/dL.

Intravenous methylprednisolone is the preferred first-line therapy. IVIG may be given to patients with diabetes or who are not able to tolerate steroids. In case of inadequate response to steroids, plasma exchange can be given. In an acutely ill patient, after the initial therapy is initiated, the patient should be re-evaluated for response to treatment. If there is an evidence of nonresponsiveness, steroid or IVIG therapy should be continued and an immunosuppressant (rituximab or cyclophosphamide) should be added. Patients usually require specialized intensive care and supportive therapies.

Chronic Therapy

If symptoms tend to relapse after short-term acute therapies, maintenance immunotherapies over the long term should be considered. Oral steroids or IVIG may be considered for a duration of approximately 6 months to 1 year with gradual tapering of therapy.

A risk of relapse remains if therapy is tapered fast. When using azathioprine and mycophenolate mofetil, a minimum overlap period of 12 weeks in case of azathioprine and 8 weeks in case of mycophenolate mofetil is advised. If there is no relapse for around 3–5 years, gradual tapering of therapy may be done.

Supportive Therapy

In addition to immunotherapy, a patient may require symptomatic management.

- *Psychosis/agitation/mania*: Benzodiazepines, mood stabilizers, or antipsychotics may be used.
- *Seizures*: Antiepileptics
- *Movement disorders*: Benzodiazepines, anticholinergics, muscle relaxants, dopamine blockers, and dopamine agonists
- *Dysautonomia*: Intensive care unit (ICU) care, beta-blockers and alpha-2 blockers for increased sympathetic drive. Fludrocortisone or midodrine for postural hypotension. Temporary pacemaker placement may be required in severe arrhythmia. Bladder incontinence requires antimuscarinics such as oxybutynin.
- *Sleep disorders*: Good sleep hygiene, benzodiazepines, and melatonin

Patients should be monitored for side effects when using steroids and immunosuppressants with regular monitoring of complete blood count, liver function tests, and renal function tests. As there is a risk of deterioration of bone mineral density when using steroids, patients are advised elemental calcium 1,500 mg/day and vitamin D 1,000 IU/day. When steroids are used for a period of more than 3 months, a baseline bone mineral density scan should be done with treatment with bisphosphonates. Prophylaxis for *Pneumocystis jirovecii* is to be considered (trimethoprim/sulfamethoxazole one double-strength tablet is given thrice a week).

CONCLUSION

Autoimmune encephalitis is a well-known entity. Its incidence is now equal to that of infectious causes. The clinical manifestations include classical disorders such as limbic encephalitis, brainstem encephalitis, and uncommon ones such as autoimmune epilepsy. MRI brain reveals typical findings suggestive of specific disorders but may sometimes be normal. CSF analysis and autoantibody testing provide further clues to the diagnosis, as does PET. Certain patients might be seronegative, requiring reliance on clinical symptoms, MRI, and EEG. Though the definite diagnosis requires the detection of antibodies, the treatment may be initiated based on possible and probable criteria. Early initiation of immunotherapy is crucial in the management of AE.

SUGGESTED READINGS

1. Venkatesan A, Tunkel AR, Bloch KC, Lauring AS, Sejvar J, Bitnun A, et al; International Encephalitis Consortium. Case definitions, diagnostic algorithms, and priorities in encephalitis: consensus statement of the international encephalitis consortium. Clin Infect Dis. 2013;57(8):1114-28.
2. Dalmau J, Rosenfeld MR. Autoimmune (including paraneoplastic) encephalitis: clinical features and diagnosis. In: UpToDate, Wen PY (Ed), UpToDate, Waltham, MA, 2023. [Last assessed December 10, 2023].
3. Dalmau J, Rosenfeld MR, Graus F. Paraneoplastic neurologic syndromes and autoimmune encephalitis. In: Loscalzo J, Kasper DL, Longo DL, Fauci AS, Hauser SL, Jameson JL (Eds). Harrison's Principles of Internal Medicine, 21st edition. New Delhi: McGraw Hill; 2022, pp. 728-36.
4. Orozco E, Valencia-Sanchez C, Britton J, Dubey D, Flanagan EP, Lopez-Chiriboga AS, et al. Autoimmune Encephalitis Criteria in Clinical Practice. Neurol Clin Pract. 2023;13(3):e200151.
5. Lawn ND, Westmoreland BF, Kiely MJ, Lennon VA, Vernino S. Clinical, magnetic resonance imaging, and electroencephalographic findings in paraneoplastic limbic encephalitis. Mayo Clin Proc. 2003;78(11):1363-8.
6. Hacohen Y, Wright S, Waters P, Agrawal S, Carr L, Cross H, et al. Paediatric autoimmune encephalopathies: clinical features, laboratory investigations and outcomes in patients with or without antibodies to known central nervous system autoantigens. J Neurol Neurosurg Psychiatry. 2013;84(7):748-55.

7. McKeon A, Dubey D, Flanagan E, Zekeridou A, Pittock S. Autoimmune encephalitis and meningitis. In: Louis E, Mayer S, Noble J (Eds). Merritt's Neurology, 14th edition. Singapore: Wolters Kluwer; 2022.
8. Graus F, Titulaer MJ, Balu R, Benseler S, Bien CG, Cellucci T, et al. A clinical approach to diagnosis of autoimmune encephalitis. Lancet Neurol. 2016;15(4):391-404.
9. Titulaer MJ, McCracken L, Gabilondo I, Armangué T, Glaser C, Iizuka T, et al. Treatment and prognostic factors for long-term outcome in patients with anti-NMDA receptor encephalitis: an observational cohort study. Lancet Neurol. 2013;12(2):157-65.
10. Wingerchuk DM. The clinical course of acute disseminated encephalomyelitis. Neurol Res. 2006;28(3):341-47.
11. Kesselring J, Miller DH, Robb SA, Kendall BE, Moseley IF, Kingsley D, et al. Acute disseminated encephalomyelitis. MRI findings and the distinction from multiple sclerosis. Brain. 1990;113 (Pt 2):291-302.
12. Koga M, Kusunoki S, Kaida K, Uehara R, Nakamura Y, Kohriyama T, et al. Nationwide survey of patients in Japan with Bickerstaff brainstem encephalitis: epidemiological and clinical characteristics. J Neurol Neurosurg Psychiatry. 2012;83(12): 1210-5.

90

CHAPTER

Neuroimaging in Acute Stroke

K Muralidharan, K Mugundhan

ABSTRACT

Neuroimaging in the diagnosis of acute stroke is mainly used in differentiating hemorrhagic from ischemic stroke, to assess the degree of tissue loss, to identify the vascular lesion that have led to the stroke. Noncontrast computed tomography of (CT) brain is the essential diagnostic modality in acute stroke, as it is cost-effective, easy to acquire, and less time consuming. Multimodal CT along with magnetic resonance imaging (MRI) including perfusion imaging will help to distinguish between the brain tissue which has irreversibly infarcted and those which can be potentially salvageable. This will help in selection of patients for neurointervention like intravenous (IV) thrombolysis and mechanical thrombectomy.

INTRODUCTION

Imaging is an essential component in the workup of patients presenting with symptoms of stroke. Imaging studies in acute stroke have the following aims: Differentiate ischemia from hemorrhage which directs further therapy, assess the extent of brain injury (irreversible infarction or under perfused tissue) and potential complications, such as herniation or midline shift, identify the risk, the possible etiology and identify the type and location of the vascular lesion responsible for the deficit.

The two imaging modalities that are commonly used in acute stroke are MRI and CT. The advantages of CT in acute stroke are the lower price, speed, and ease of getting done, availability round the clock, and not much contraindication. Various modalities in CT are noncontrast CT, computed tomography angiography (CTA), and computed tomography perfusion (CTP).

NONCONTRAST COMPUTED TOMOGRAPHY

Various imaging findings of acute stroke on noncontrast CT is enumerated in **Box 1** and **Figures 1A and B**.

ISCHEMIA

- The early radiologic signs of ischemia in noncontrast CT are:
    - Lentiform nucleus obscuration
    - Loss of differentiation of gray-white matter in the insula, known as insular ribbon sign
    - Loss of differentiation of gray-white matter in cortex, known as cortical ribbon sign

BOX 1: Imaging features on noncontrast CT.

- Any intracerebral, intraventricular, subarachnoid, subdural, or extradural hemorrhage
- Eye deviation
- Hyperdense artery sign
- Early ischemic changes (obscuration of lentiform nucleus, insular ribbon sign, and loss of gray-white differentiation of surface cortex)
- ASPECTS a (good 8–10, intermediate 5–7, and poor 0–4)

(ASPECTS: Alberta stroke program early computed tomography score; CT: computed tomography)

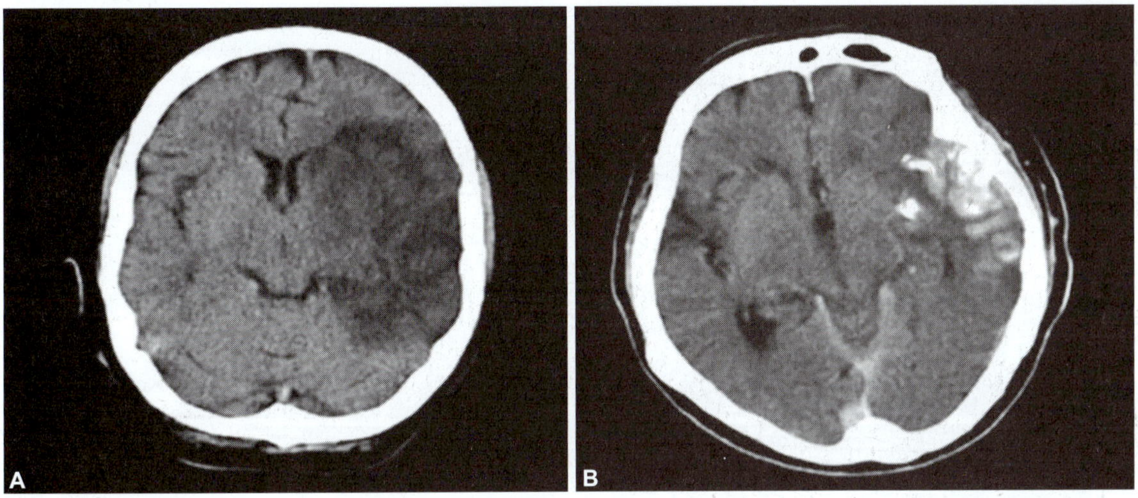

FIGS. 1A AND B: Noncontrast CT in patients with acute stroke. (A) Axial noncontrast CT showing infarction in the left cerebral hemisphere. (B) Axial noncontrast CT showing intracerebral hemisphere in the left temporal region with the extension into the adjacent subarachnoid space.

- Loss of normal gray-white matter differentiation occurs due to blurring as a result of edematous gray matter which happens in severe ischemia. It appears darker on CT
- Alberta stroke program early computed tomography score (ASPECTS) and the one-third of the middle cerebral artery (MCA) rule are the two common methods by which the extent of ischemic changes can be established.
- *One-third MCA rule*: If ischemia involves more than one-third of the MCA territory, then there is limited benefit in thrombolysis and there is higher risk of post-thrombolysis intracerebral hemorrhage.

The ASPECTS is a 10-point score which will measure the areas where there is parenchymal hypoattenuation or loss of gray-white matter differentiation in the MCA territory **(Fig. 2)**.

- It is assessed in axial cuts at the level of:
  - The caudate head (C-caudate head, L-lentiform nucleus, and I-internal capsule)
  - M1–M3 regions (ganglionic level)
  - M4–M6 regions (supraganglionic level)
- On noncontrast CT, brain regions that are darker than the contralateral normal-appearing white matter are a marker of increased risk hemorrhage with thrombolysis.
- The presence of these regions does not mean that thrombolysis is absolutely contraindicated, but they do mean that clinicians should proceed with caution after weighing the risks and benefits of thrombolysis.
- A thrombus inside the artery is seen on the noncontrast CT as the hyperdense artery sign.

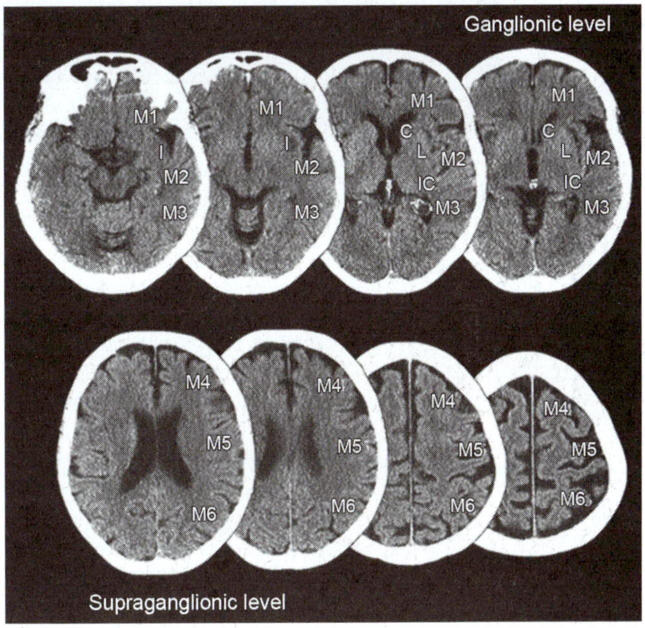

FIG. 2: The Alberta stroke program early CT score (ASPECTS) template applied to noncontrast computed tomography (CT).

DIFFUSION-WEIGHTED MAGNETIC RESONANCE IMAGING FLUID-ATTENUATED INVERSION RECOVERY MISMATCH (FIGS. 3A TO F)

When a mismatch is seen between fluid-attenuated inversion recovery (FLAIR) and diffusion-weighted imaging (DWI), there are only subtle early ischemic changes in NCCT (A, B, and C). When there is no mismatch between DWI and FLAIR, there are subacute changes in NCCT (D, E, and F).

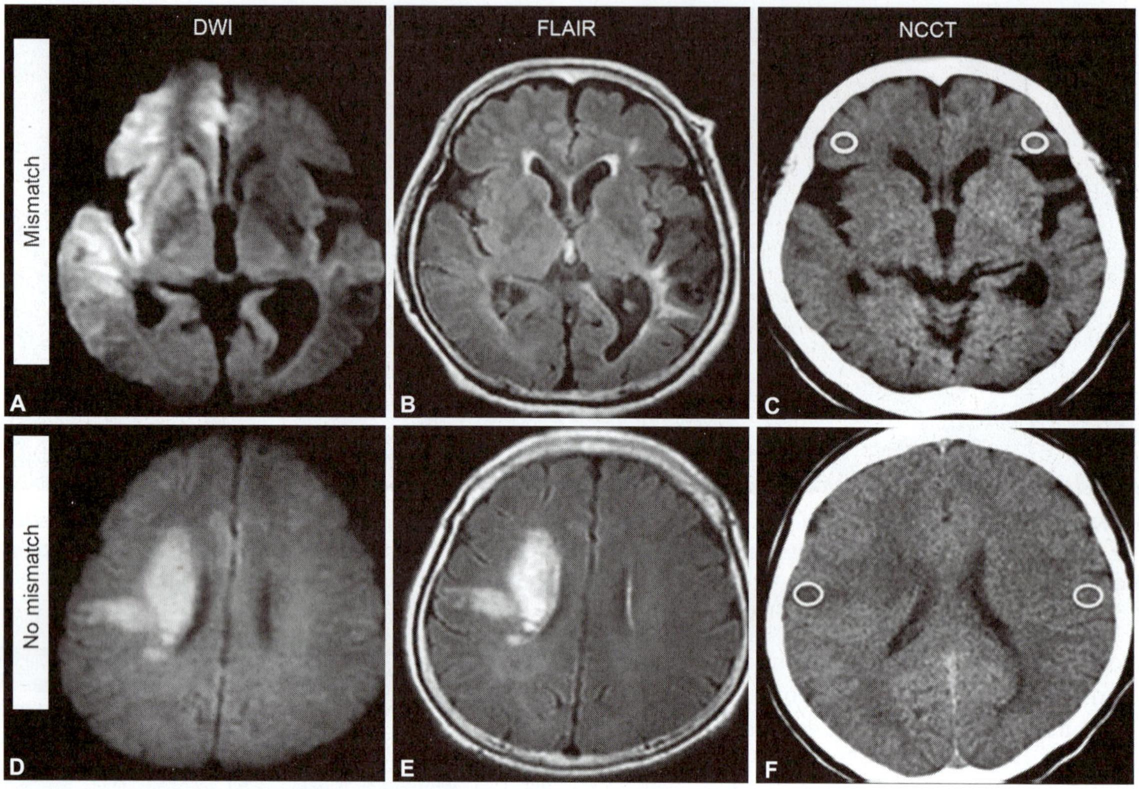

FIGS. 3A TO F: DWI and FLAIR MRI changes with corresponding changes on NCCT.
(DWI: diffusion-weighted imaging; FLAIR: fluid-attenuated inversion recovery; MRI: magnetic resonance imaging; NCCT: noncontrast computed tomography)

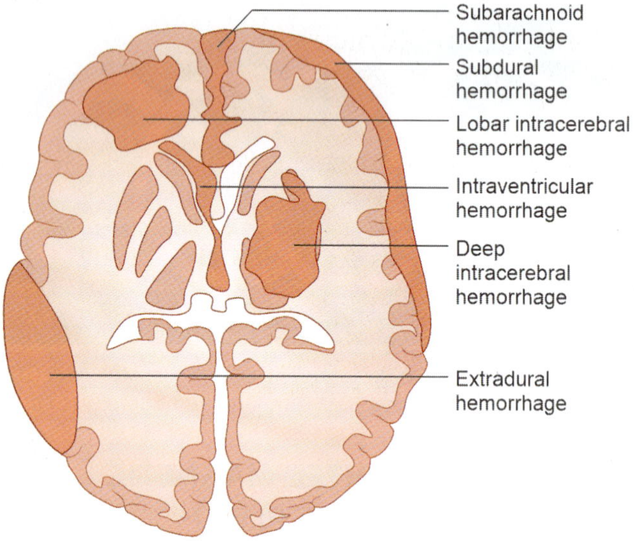

FIG. 4: Location and types of intracranial hemorrhage.

TABLE 1: Etiology of intracerebral hemorrhage (ICH) according to location.

Location	Etiology
Intraparenchymal:	
Lobar	Amyloid angiopathy, bleeding diathesis, hypertension, vascular malformations, tumors, venous thrombosis, and vasculitis
Deep	Hypertension, tumors, and moyamoya syndrome
Intraventricular	Hypertension and tumors
Subarachnoid	Aneurysms, amyloid angiopathy, and trauma
Subdural	Trauma, bleeding diathesis
Extradural	Traumas

HEMORRHAGE

Based on location, hemorrhages are classified into subarachnoid, subdural, extradural, intracerebral, and intraventricular **(Fig. 4)**. This classification aids in finding the likely etiology **(Table 1)**. The CT signs associated with poor prognosis with intracerebral hemorrhage are the black hole sign (hypodense region which is surrounded by a hyperdense region and not connected with the nearby brain tissue), the blend sign (hemorrhage with hyperdense and hypodense foci), and the island sign (minimum of three scattered tiny hemorrhages separate from the main hemorrhagic focus **(Figs. 5A and B)**.

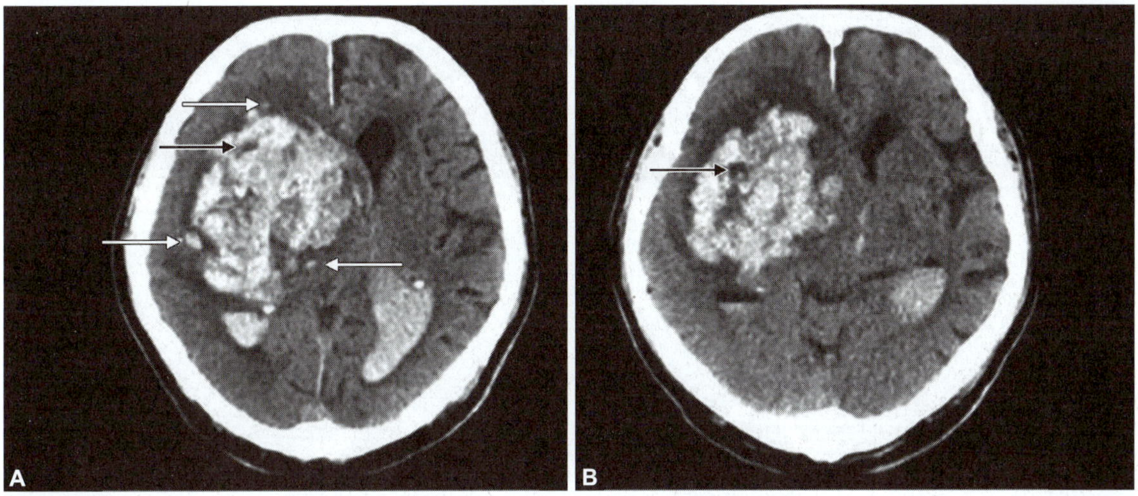

FIGS. 5A AND B: Imaging characteristics of intracerebral hemorrhage associated with poor prognosis. (A) Axial noncontrast CT showing the island sign (i.e., at least three scattered small hemorrhages separate from the main hemorrhage) (white arrows), whereas the hemorrhage has hyperdense and hypodense regions (the blend sign) (black arrow), (B) Axial noncontrast CT showing the black hole sign (a hypodense region surrounded by a hyperdense region not connected with the adjacent brain tissue) (arrow).

COMPUTED TOMOGRAPHY ANGIOGRAPHY

It is the major modality which is used to image blood vessels of the brain. Various imaging features on CTA is enumerated in **Box 2**.

Hemorrhage

- *Spot sign*: The serpiginous or linear contrast density locate within the intraparenchymal hemorrhage **(Fig. 6)**
- The speed of increase in size of the spot sign is a marker of hemorrhage growth.

Ischemia

Computed tomography angiography of head and neck will assist in detection of thrombus within arteries and their severity, collateral status, and other associated pathological findings.

The head and neck CTA, has the following important uses:

- Identifying thrombi in large proximal intracranial arteries [also called large vessel occlusions (LVOs)]. Patients with LVOs can benefit from acute endovascular treatment.
- Determining the location of thrombus within the intracranial arterial tree (e.g., internal carotid artery versus M1 segment of MCA vs. more distal arteries) helps identify the likelihood that a thrombus will respond to IV thrombolysis.

BOX 2: Imaging in computed tomography (CT) angiography.

Imaging features on CT angiography to rapidly assess patients presenting with acute stroke

Intracranial hemorrhage:
- Abnormal-looking vessels
- Spot sign

Ischemia:
- Presence and location of thrombus (intracranial or extracranial)
- Collateral status
- Any extracranial large artery pathology (plaque and dissection)
- Aortic disease
- Other pathologies (carotid web vasculopathy)

Arch and large vessel anatomy

- Assessing thrombus burden will help in determining if endovascular therapy or IV thrombolysis will be successful or not.
- Helps in identifying the patients with minor strokes or transient ischemic attack (TIA), who are at risk of recurrent ischemic events by detecting the thrombus within arteries of the brain.
    - An excellent tool in assessing the collateral status is the multiphase CTA **(Figs. 7A to C)**
    - On multiphase CTA, the arteries which are distal to the blocked artery will be assessed for the extent of arterial contrast, if any delay in filling of contrast, and impaired washout of contrast as compared to arteries on the contralateral side.

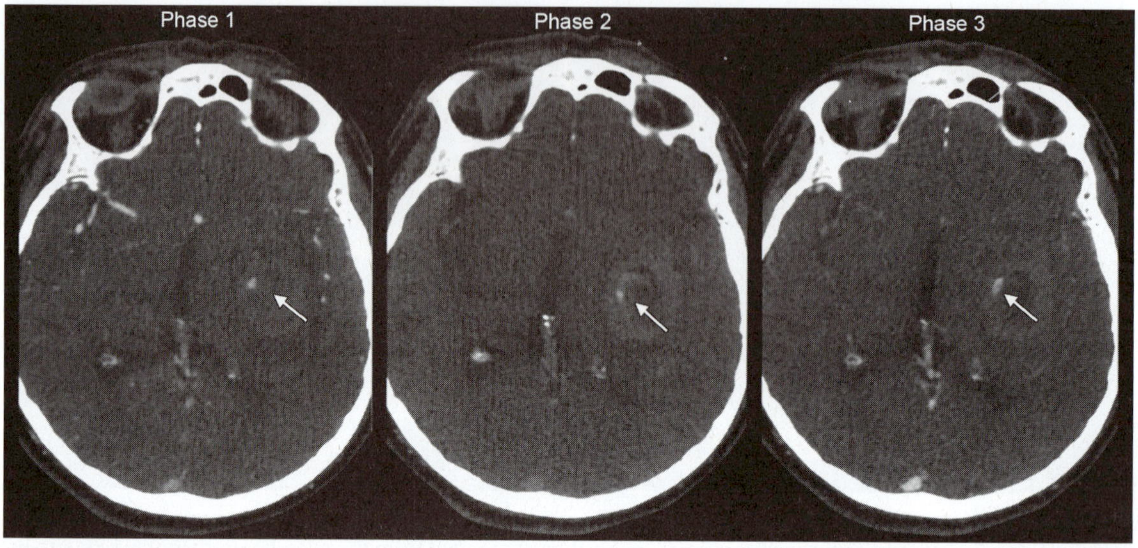

FIG. 6: The spot sign, a marker of intracerebral hemorrhage growth, seen in the three phases (arrows) of a multiphase computed tomography (CT) angiogram.

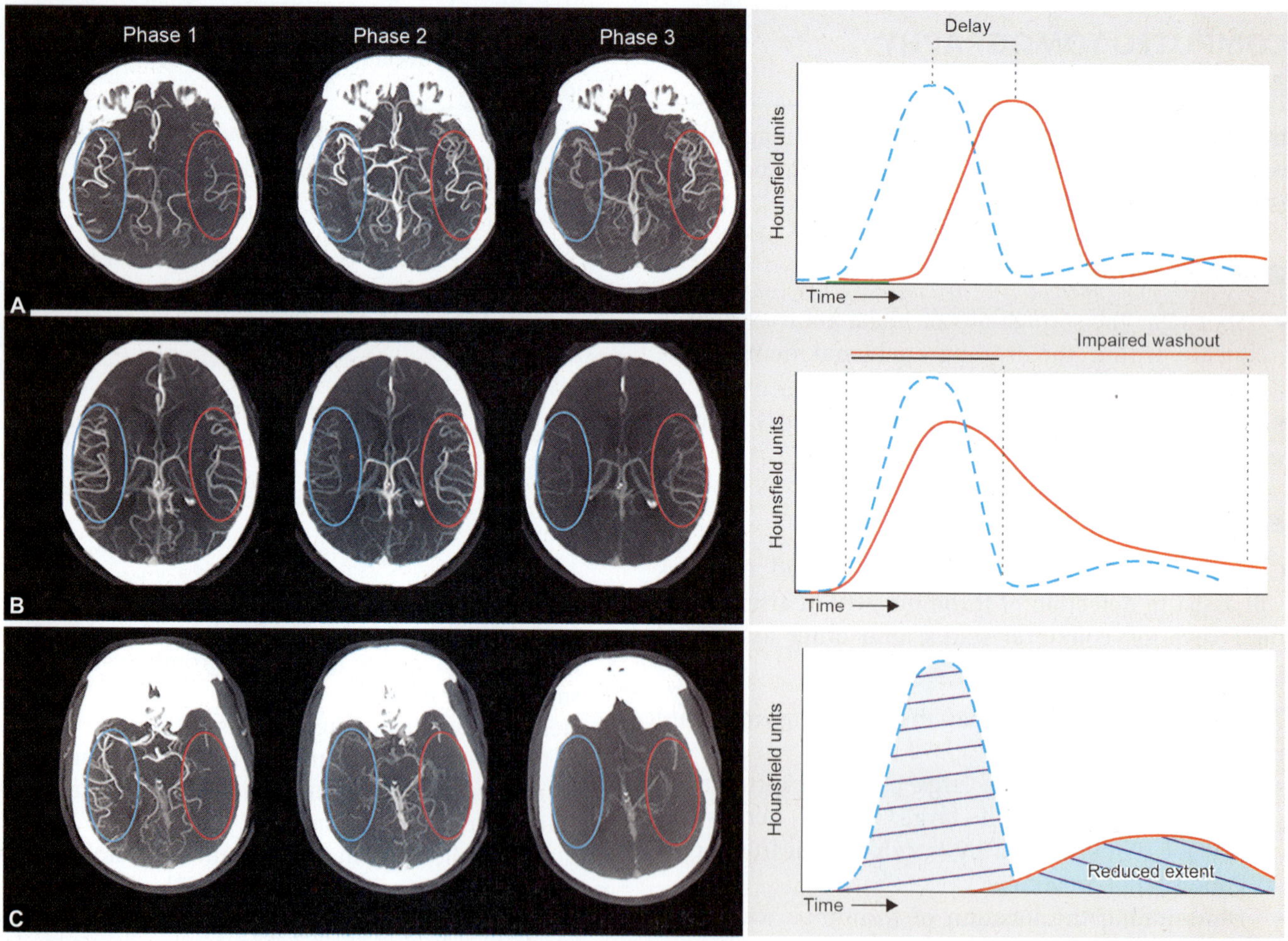

FIGS. 7A TO C: Multiphase computed tomography (CT) angiogram assessment of collateral status in the symptomatic brain in three phases. (A) A one-phase delay is noticed during filling of arterial contrast between the symptomatic left side and the right side, (B) Impairment in the washout of contrast is noticed in the third phase on the symptomatic left side when it is compared to the right side, (C) A decreased number of blood vessels is seen on the symptomatic left side as compared to the right side.

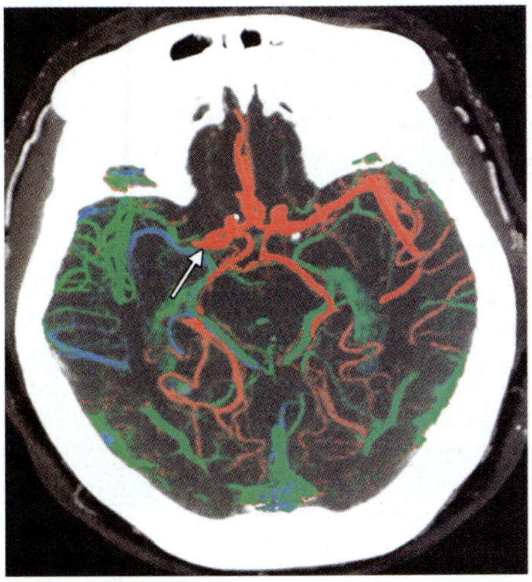

FIG. 8: Composite time-resolved map of collateral filling generated using multiphase computed tomography (CT) angiography.

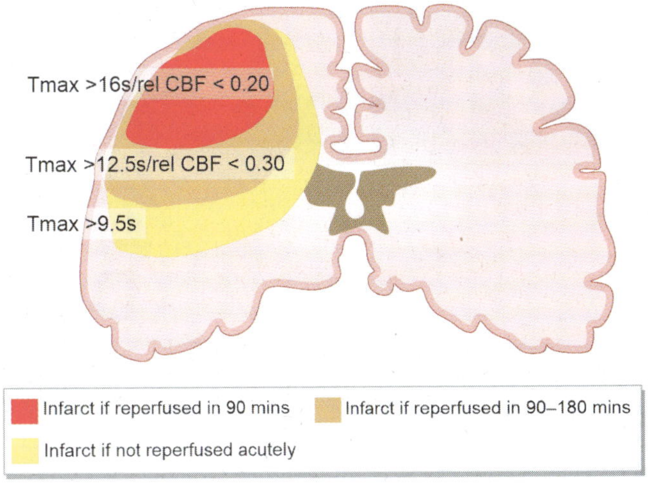

FIG. 9: Time-based CT perfusion thresholds that help predict follow-up infarction.

(CT: computed tomography; rel CBF: relative cerebral blood flow; Tmax: a contrast transit time parameter)

COMPUTED TOMOGRAPHY PERFUSION

Like CTA, CTP is a CT scan obtained after the injection of IV contrast.

The occlusion is noted in the M1 segment of right MCA (arrow). The algorithm classifies all. There are three categories of voxels: (1) red, (2) green, or (3) blue, which is based on whether maximum contrast enhancement happens before or after an identified venous window for that particular patient. Arteries which appear red show peak contrast early, arteries which appears green will show peak contrast at a time almost similar to when the density of contrast goes to peak in the veins on the normal side, and arteries which appear blue will show peak contrast much later than when the density of contrast peaks in veins on the normal side **(Fig. 8)**.

- Brain tissue which has very low blood flow on CTP is likely to get early infarct. By detecting the regions with very low blood flow, CTP can also help in predicting brain regions which are at increased risk of hemorrhage after acute stroke treatment.
- In NCCT, the changes which appear subacute or the regions which has changes seen on DWI and FLAIR images (no DWI-FLAIR mismatch) will also help the clinicians in predicting the risk of hemorrhage after acute treatment.
- Time-based CT perfusion thresholds will help to predict follow-up infarction **(Fig. 9)**

CONCLUSION

Acute stroke diagnosis and treatment is a skillful art which involves rapid assessment of necessary clinical and neuroimaging details and making correct clinical judgment in a timely manner. Physicians should use CT as the first line neuroimaging tool because of its easy availability, ease of use, and the rapidity of acquisition. Noncontrast CT of brain and CTA of the head and neck are the essential modalities in patients who present with acute stroke. They help in the diagnosis of stroke, determining the prognosis, and in identifying the patients who will benefit from the acute stroke treatment. Other techniques such as multiphase CTA and CT perfusion will provide additional help to identify the potentially salvageable brain tissue and assess the risk of treatment.

SUGGESTED READINGS

1. Menon BK. Neuroimaging in acute stroke .Continuum (Minneap Minn). 2020;26(2):287-309.
2. Menon BK, Goyal M. Imaging paradigms in acute ischemic stroke: a pragmatic evidence-based approach. Radiology. 2015;277(1):7-12.
3. Meissner W, Sibon I, Rouanet F, Ménégon P, Orgogozo JM. MRI versus CT in acute stroke. Lancet. 2007;369(9570):1341-2.
4. Menon BK, Puetz V, Kochar P, Demchuk AM. ASPECTS and other neuroimaging scores in the triage and prediction of outcome in acute stroke patients. Neuroimaging Clin N Am. 2011;21(2): 407-23,xii.
5. Menon BK, d'Esterre CD, Qazi EM, Almekhlafi M, Hahn L, Demchuk AM, et al. Multiphase CT angiography: a new tool for the imaging triage of patients with acute ischemic stroke. Radiology. 2015;275(2):510-20.
6. d'Esterre CD, Boesen ME, Ahn SH, Pordeli P, Najm M, Minhas P, et al. Time-dependent computed tomographic perfusion thresholds for patients with acute ischemic stroke. Stroke. 2015;46(12):3390-7.

91

CHAPTER

Approach to Bladder Dysfunction (Neurogenic)

Sathish Kumar M

ABSTRACT

Neurogenic bladder affects a patient's quality of life significantly and makes him/her feel embarrassed. Knowledge about the neural control of micturition is essential for understanding the pathophysiology of bladder dysfunction. Parasympathetic innervation favors emptying, whereas sympathetic outflow maintains storage. Brainstem (pontine) micturition centers ensure coordination between detrusor contraction and sphincter while receiving input from cortical regions. In this chapter, symptoms of storage dysfunction, voiding dysfunction, evaluation, and treatment of neurogenic bladder are discussed.

INTRODUCTION

Bladder dysfunction can be neurogenic or urological in origin. Knowledge about neural control of micturition is essential for understanding bladder symptoms. In this chapter, the neural control of micturition, the pattern of bladder involvement at various neuraxis levels, and the diagnostic approach followed by management are discussed.

NEURAL CONTROL OF MICTURITION

The lower urinary tract (LUT) comprises the bladder, urethra, and internal and external urethral sphincters. LUT dysfunction significantly affects a patient's dignity and quality of life and often makes him/her feel embarrassed or ashamed. The two major functions of LUT include (1) storage and (2) voiding at the appropriate time. The integrated control by the central nervous system and the peripheral nervous system ensures proper periodic evacuation of urine. The internal and external urethral sphincters play a vital role in maintaining continence. The sphincters remain contracted during storage mode. Bladders spend most of the time in storage of urine (98%). A person with 400–600 mL of bladder capacity voids 3–4 hours once. Voiding is a conscious decision and takes 2–3 minutes. Brainstem circuitry is involved in the micturition reflex (coordinated and sustained contraction of detrusor and relaxation of sphincters), modulated by the input from the forebrain. The bladder is innervated by both the somatic and autonomic nervous systems. Parasympathetic preganglionic fibers arise from the second, third, and fourth sacral segments of the intermediolateral gray column (detrusor center of sacral cord) and synapse with parasympathetic ganglia on the bladder wall. The short postganglionic parasympathetic fibers arise from the bladder wall ganglia, innervate the detrusor, and release acetylcholine (ACh) when the detrusor needs to contract. Ach acts on M3 subtype of muscarinic receptor. Sympathetic innervation is from T11 to L2 spinal cord segments and is conveyed to the bladder via inferior mesenteric ganglia and hypogastric nerves (both preganglionic and postganglionic fibers). Norepinephrine (NE) is the primary neurotransmitter from postganglionic sympathetic terminals which act on beta-3 and alpha-1 receptors to relax the detrusor and to contract the smooth muscles of the sphincter, respectively. Onuf's nucleus is a group of motor neurons in the ventral horn of S2 to S4 segments of the cord and they provide somatic efferent to the external urethral sphincter. The striated muscles of the external urethral sphincter respond to the nicotinic effect of ACh. A delta and unmyelinated C fibers convey afferent information from the bladder and sphincter to the sacral center for micturition via pelvic, hypogastric, and pudendal nerves. Pontine micturition center (PMC) receives input from higher centers via periaqueductal gray (PAG) matter of the midbrain and is responsible for switching between storage and emptying modes. Urinary continence is maintained through neural pathways connecting the cerebral cortex to the LUT, which also permits voiding when it is suitable socially. The prefrontal cortex, especially medial frontal cortex, sends a signal to PMC via PAG which activates the parasympathetic system for voiding when it is socially appropriate.

Neurogenic Bladder

Based on the site of lesion in neuraxis, patterns of bladder dysfunction differ **(Fig. 1)**. Suprapontine, infrapontine-suprasacral, and sacral-infrasacral are the three locations of neurogenic LUT dysfunction. Suprapontine and infrapontine-suprasacral lesions result in detrusor overactivity (DO). Sacral-infrasacral lesions predominantly result in voiding dysfunction due to poor detrusor contraction.

Cortical Lesions

Tumors, aneurysms, penetrating wounds, and prefrontal lobotomy that affect the anterior regions of the frontal lobe result in severe urgency and increased frequency of micturition. The patient is socially aware of the urge incontinence and feels embarrassed. Rarely, urinary retention is also reported. There is normal coordination between detrusor and sphincter but DO is noted in cystometry. Urinary incontinence appears early in dementia with Lewy body whereas late in Alzheimer's disease. Small vessel disease or leukoaraiosis can also result in urinary incontinence. In normal pressure hydrocephalus (NPH), urinary incontinence improves after lumbar puncture and cerebrospinal fluid (CSF) drainage.

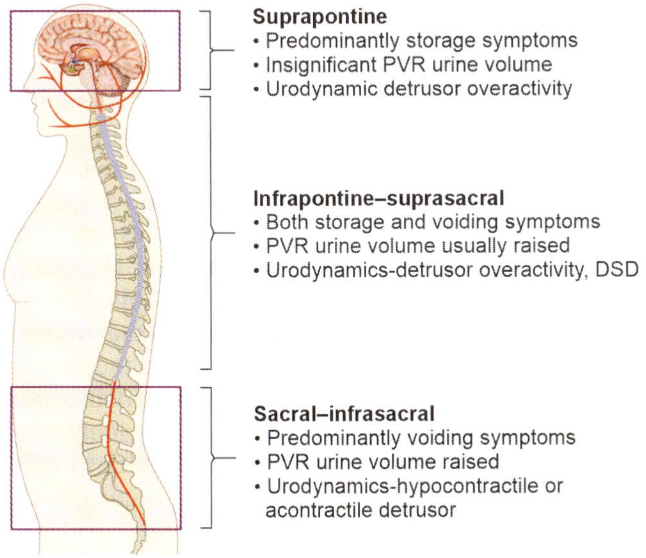

FIG. 1: Three patterns of neurogenic bladder dysfunction.
(DSD: detrusor sphincter dyssynergia; PVR: postvoid residual)

Basal Ganglia Lesions

Bladder dysfunction appears late in Parkinson's disease (PD). About 38–71% of patients report LUT symptoms (LUTS). Nocturia followed by urgency is the most common nonmotor symptom in PD. DO is observed in urodynamics. Loss of circadian rhythm in PD leads to nocturnal polyuria. Prostate enlargement, pelvic floor weakness, and bradykinesia of pelvic floor muscles contribute to LUTS in PD.

Multisystem Atrophy

Lower urinary tract symptoms in the beginning of Parkinsonism signal multisystem atrophy (MSA). Nearly 97% develop LUTS during the course of the disease. Urgency and urge incontinence are the most common symptoms experienced by MSA patients. High postvoid residual (PVR) > 100 mL, detrusor sphincter dyssynergia (DSD), open bladder neck at the start of bladder filling, and neurogenic pattern in electromyogram (EMG) of the anal sphincter are observed in urodynamic evaluation.

Brainstem Lesions

Voiding difficulty is rarely reported in brainstem strokes and posterior fossa tumors. The more the dorsal location of the lesion, the more the possibility of voiding dysfunction.

Spinal Cord Lesions

Spinal cord lesions are the most common cause of neurogenic bladder. The transspinal pathway connecting PMC to the sacral cord gets disrupted and synergic activity is lost leading to DSD. After acute spinal cord injury, there is complete urinary retention during the phase of spinal shock. Later, the detrusor starts to contract in response to low filling volumes. C fibers become major afferent and form a spinal segmental reflex resulting in automatic voiding. Small capacity and overactive bladder leads to urgency and increased frequency. If DO is severe, incontinence occurs. Symptoms of storage dysfunction are more troublesome to the patient than voiding

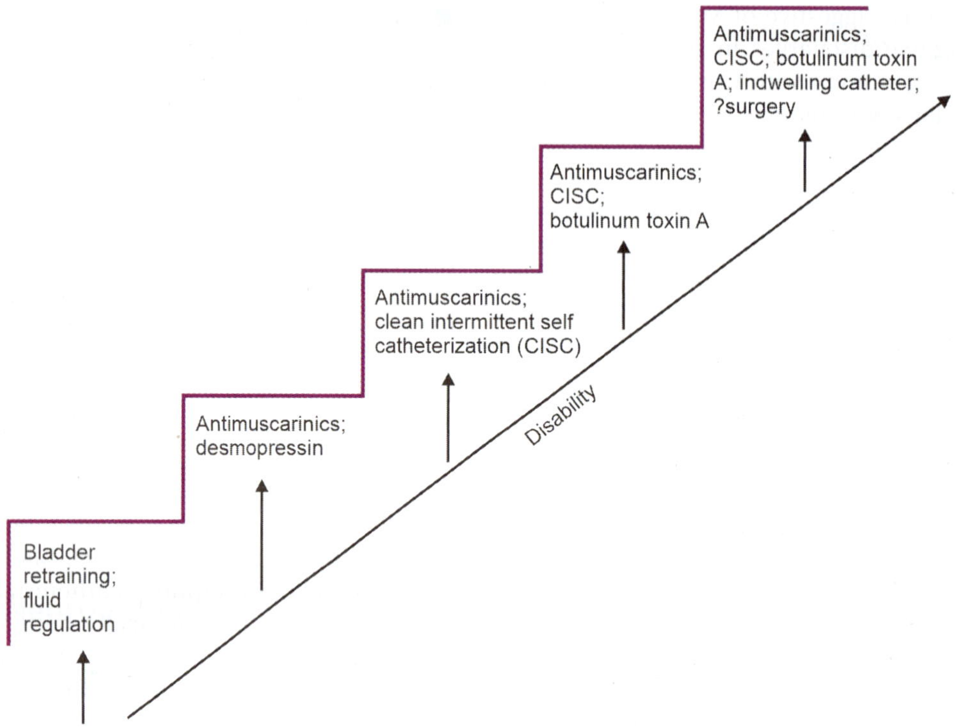

FIG. 2: Stepwise approach to managing neurogenic bladder.

SUGGESTED READINGS

1. Fowler CJ, Griffiths D, de Groat WC. The neural control of micturition. Nat Rev Neurosci. 2008;9(6):453-66.
2. Griffiths DJ. The pontine micturition centres. Scand J Urol Nephrol Suppl. 2002;(210):216.
3. Tish MM. Geerling JC. The Brain and the Bladder: Forebrain Control of Urinary (In)Continence. Front Physiol. 2020;11:658.
4. Ransmayr GN, Holliger S, Schletterer K, Heidler H, Deibl M, Poewe W, et al. Lower urinary tract symptoms in dementia with Lewy bodies, Parkinson disease, and Alzheimer disease. Neurology. 2008;70(4):299-303.
5. Sakakibara R, Kanda T, Sekido T, Uchiyama T, Awa Y, Ito T, et al. Mechanism of bladder dysfunction in idiopathic normal pressure hydrocephalus. Neurourol Urodyn. 2008;27(6):507-10.
6. Sakakibara R, Uchiyama T, Yamanishi T, Kishi M. Genitourinary dysfunction in Parkinson's disease. Mov Disord. 2010;25(1):2-12.
7. Richard C, Amarenco G, Palma JA, Kaufmann H, Drapier S, Gamé X, et al. Early bladder dysfunction in multiple system atrophy: who seek shall find. Clin Auton Res. 2019;29(6):625-6.
8. Panicker JN, Fowler CJ, Kessler TM. "Lower urinary tract dysfunction in the neurological patient: clinical assessment and management." Lancet Neurol. 2015;14(7):720-32.
9. Phé V, Chartier-Kastler E, Panicker JN. Management of neurogenic bladder in patients with multiple sclerosis. Nat Rev Urol. 2016;13(5):275-88.
10. Podnar S, Fowler C. Pelvic organ dysfunction following cauda equina damage. In: Fowler C, Panicker J, Emmanuel A (Eds). Pelvic Organ Dysfunction in Neurological Disease: Clinical Management and Rehabilitation. Cambridge: Cambridge University Press; 2010. pp. 266-77.
11. Osman NI, Chapple CR. Fowler's syndrome—a cause of unexplained urinary retention in young women? Nat Rev Urol. 2014;11(2):87-98.
12. Kessler TM. Diagnosis of urinary incontinence. JAMA. 2008;300(3):283.
13. Rovner E, Dmochowski R, Chapple C, Thompson C, Lam W, Haag-Molkenteller C. OnabotulinumtoxinA improves urodynamic outcomes in patients with neurogenic detrusor overactivity. Neurourol Urodyn. 2013;32(8):1109-15.
14. Bartley J, Gilleran J, Peters K. Neuromodulation for overactive bladder. Nat Rev Urol. 2013;10(9):513-21.
15. Jankovic J, Mazziotta JC, Pomeroy SL. Neurourology. In: Newman NJ (Ed). Bradley and Daroff's Neurology in Clinical Practice, 8th edition. Philadelphia: Elsevier; 2021. pp. 633-49.
16. Przydacz M, Chlosta M, Dudek P, Cudnoch-Jedrzejewska A, Zgliczynski W, Dobruch J, et al. Desmopressin treatment for nocturia caused by nocturnal polyuria: practical guidelines. Cent European J Urol. 2020;73(4):498-505.

92

CHAPTER

Red Flag Sign in Headache

Thamilpavai N, LA Ravi, Arunsaravanan S, Aiswarya G Kumar, Devireddyprasoona

ABSTRACT

Headache patients are commonly encountered in our day-to-day practice. It is important to distinguish between primary and secondary headache disorders. Red flag sign is pertinent to diagnose secondary headache and to determine whether neuroimaging is mandatory to make a diagnosis.

INTRODUCTION

A list of eight categories and 46 subcategories of potential secondary causes are reported in the International Classification of Headache Disorders, 3rd edition (ICHD-3). Detailed history taking and neurological examination is mandatory to make a diagnosis. A change in the pattern warrants immediate attention. Recent or new onset headaches, progressive in nature, atypicality in presentation, and the chances of abnormality are high.

CASE VIGNETTE 1

A 14-year-old girl presented with complaints of headache for the last 10 days which was left-sided associated with recurrent episodes of vomiting followed by altered sensorium for the last 1 day. Headache was intermittent, moderate in intensity, with no postural or diurnal fluctuations, temporarily relieved with medications and not associated with visual disturbances or photophobia. This was followed by altered sensorium in the form of decreased responsiveness, and paucity of speech for the last 1 day before presentation in our hospital. There was no history of fever, seizure, weakness, or sensory disturbances. The patient had a history of one episode of seizure for 3 years and started on antiepileptic medications. She was born to nonconsanguineous parents, previously well and developmentally normal. On examination, the patient was arousable with verbal stimuli, drowsy with confused speech and impaired comprehension. There was no neck rigidity. Bilaterally pupils were equal and reactive. Visual acuity and field of vision were normal and no papilledema on fundoscopy once her general condition improved. Motor system examination revealed equal movement of all four limbs with normal deep tendon reflexes with bilateral flexor plantar response.

Investigations and Management

Her baseline was normal. Cardiac evaluation and vasculitic profile were normal. Carotid vertebral Doppler study was normal. ENT (ear, nose, and throat) and ophthalmology evaluation was normal. Magnetic resonance imaging (MRI) brain showed acute infarct in left inferior medial temporal region and parieto-occipital region and magnetic resonance venography (MRV) showed no significant abnormality **(Figs. 1 to 4)**. The patient was treated with antiedema measures, antiplatelet drugs, and supportive measures and continued on antiepileptic medications. The patient's general condition gradually improved.

Multifocal acute infarcts were noted in left inferior-medial temporal region and parieto-occipital region with diffusion restriction **(Fig. 5)**. MRI and MRV normal study **(Fig. 6)**. Management—antibiotics, antiplatelets, and statins. Genetic analysis for mitochondrial disorders was sent. Reports are awaited.

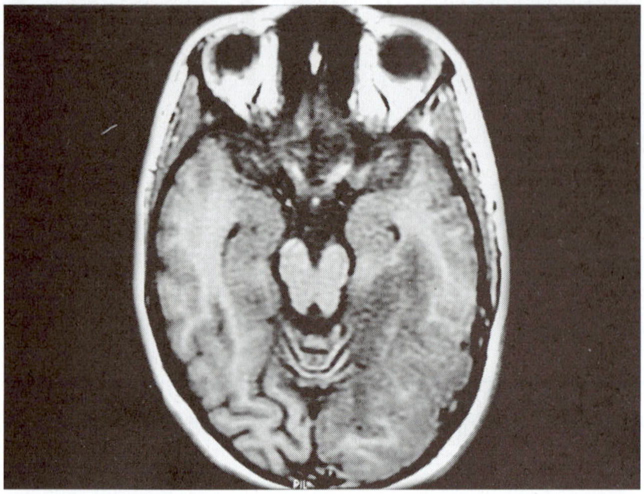

FIG. 1: T1-weighted image axial.

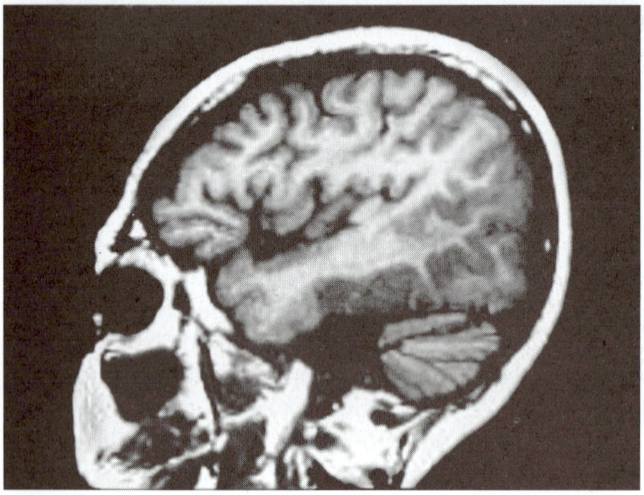

FIG. 2: T1-weighted image sagittal.

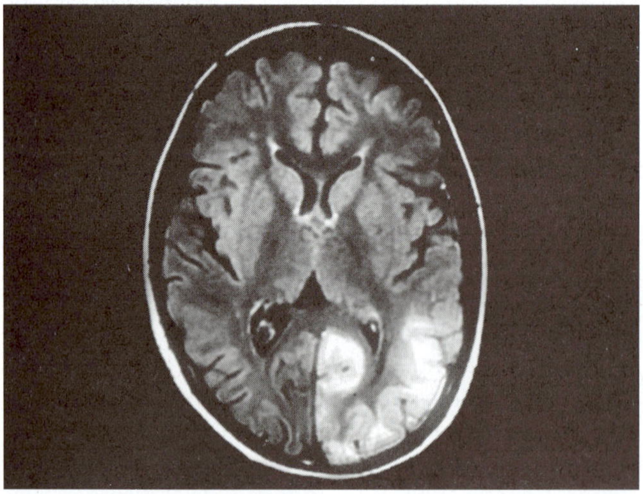

FIG. 3: T2 axial FLAIR image.

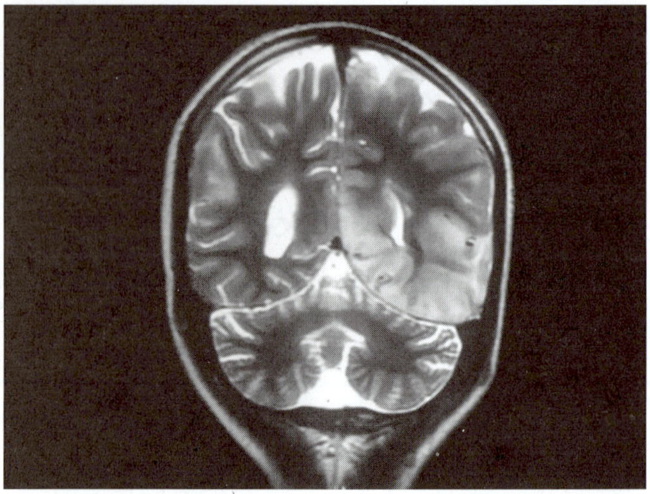

FIG. 4: T2 coronal image.

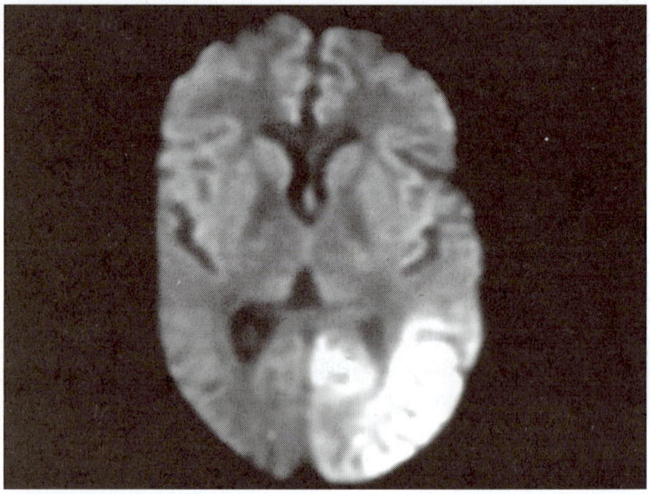

FIG. 5: Diffusion-weighted image—diffusion restriction.

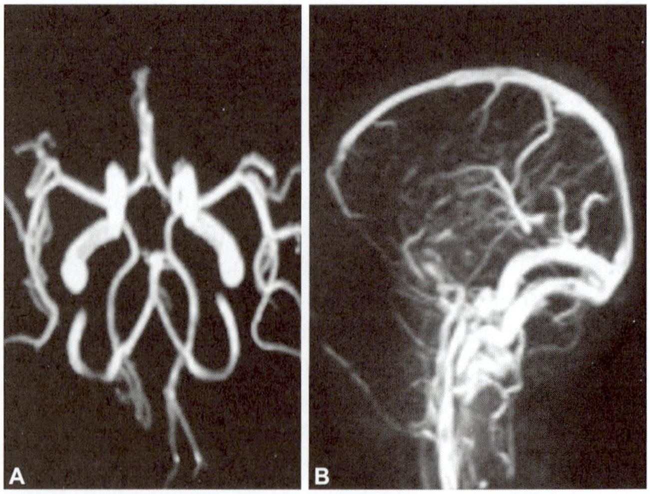

FIGS. 6A AND B: (A) Magnetic resonance arteriogram; (B) Magnetic resonance venogram.

CASE VIGNETTE 2

A 20-year-old female P1L1A1 post-term normal delivery 5 days back with an uneventful first pregnancy presented with complaints of headache and vomiting to our emergency department (ED) of 20 days duration with altered sensorium of 1 day duration. Headache started from the last trimester of pregnancy (36 weeks of gestational age) and was intermittent, mild-moderate intensity, over the occipital area, dull aching with no postural or diurnal fluctuations, temporarily relieved with analgesics, only to return after a few hours. There was no associated photophobia or phonophobia or visual blurring or double vision and no aggravating factors for head pain It was associated with neck pain and recurrent episodes of projectile nonbilious vomiting. She delivered a live male baby by normal vaginal delivery. On day 2 postdelivery, the patient had a worsening headache which became continuous with no relief with analgesics and was severe in intensity. She also developed altered sensorium with decreased responsiveness for the last 1 day before presentation to our hospital. Vitals were stable. There was no history of any febrile illness.

There was history of contact with pulmonary tuberculosis 8 years back. No history of seizures. No history of limb weakness. On examination, the patient was drowsy and irritable with neck rigidity with positive Kernig sign and Brudzinski sign. Bilateral pupils were equal and active with dolls eye movement intact and no papilledema on fundoscopy. Motor system examination revealed power in all four limbs as 3/5 with generalized hyperreflexia with bilateral withdrawal plantars. The patient was initiated on empirical parenteral antibiotics and antiviral with antiedema measures on day 1 of admission.

Investigations

Complete blood count, liver function tests, and renal function tests were normal. MRI brain: T2/FLAIR (fluid-attenuated inversion recovery) hyperintense conglomerate lesions in a left occipitotemporal area with surrounding edema and T2/FLAIR hyperintense lesion in central pons **(Figs. 7 to 10)**. T1 postcontrast shows leptomeningeal and tentorium cerebelli enhancement as well as subpial enhancing nodules with homogenously enhancing lesion in left occipitotemporal as well as cerebellar vermis and left cerebellar hemisphere **(Figs. 10 to 12)**. Possibilities to be considered are central nervous system (CNS) tuberculosis and atypical posterior reversible encephalopathy syndrome (PRES).

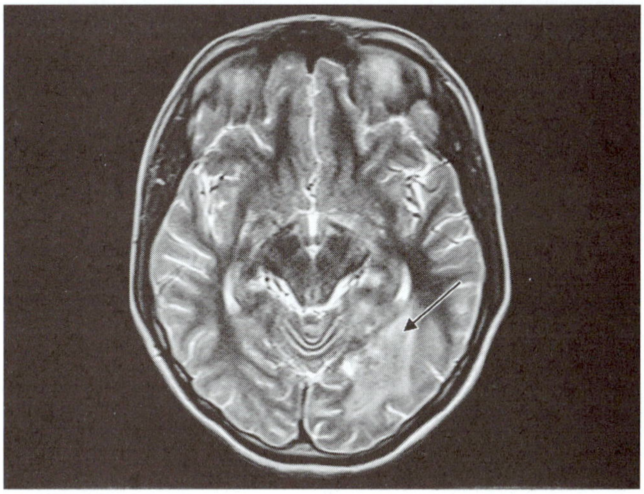

FIG. 7: T2 axial image.

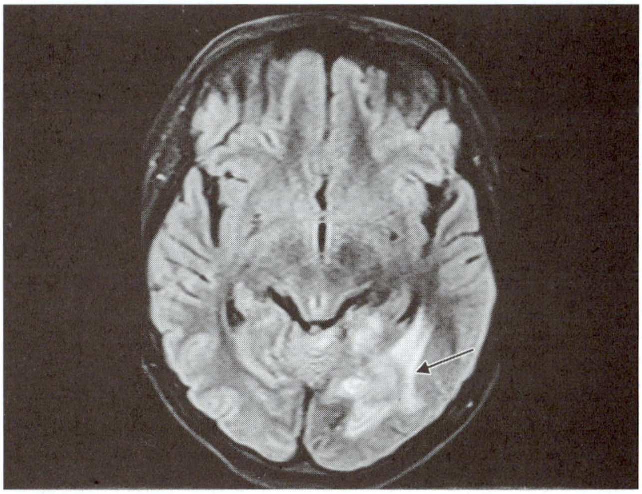

FIG. 8: T2 axial FLAIR image.

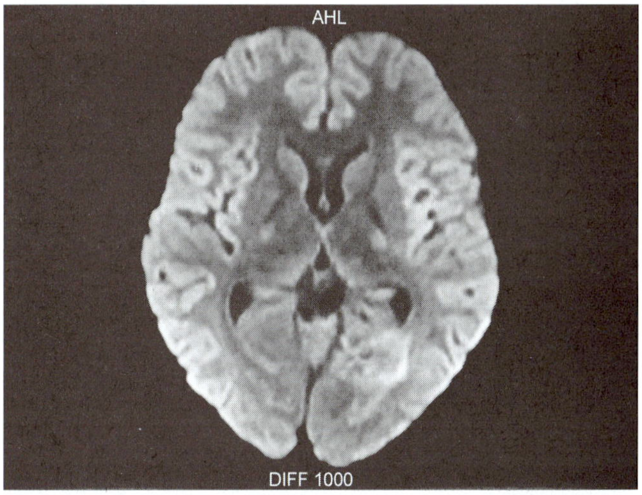

FIG. 9: Diffusion-weighted image.

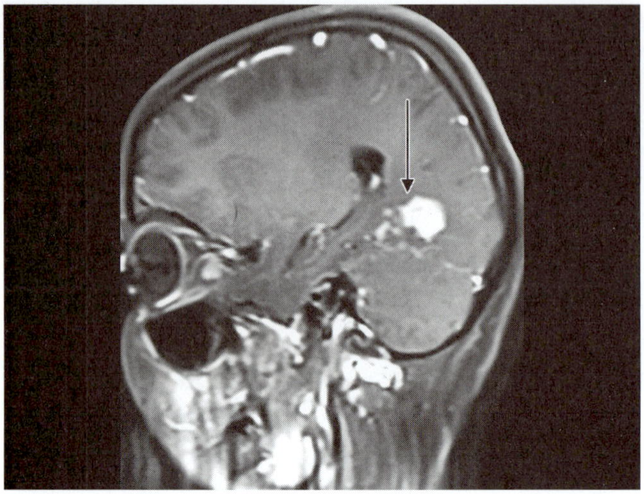

FIG. 10: Postgadolinium T1 sagittal.

Treatment

In view of neuroimaging findings in the background of subacute meningoencephalitis, patient was also initiated on empirical modified antituberculous treatment [tablet INH—300 mg, capsule rifampicin (RIF)—600 mg, tablet levofloxacin—750 mg daily, and tablet pyrazinamide on alternate days with IV steroids]. Patient sensorium and neck stiffness improved and became ambulatory by day 7. Visual acuity, field of vision, and color vision were tested every day and found to be normal. On the 10th day, patient developed sudden onset of blurring of vision. Repeat CT brain revealed acute hydrocephalus. Initial CT and MRI brain was normal **(Fig. 13)**. Neurosurgeons opinion obtained and urgent ventriculoperitoneal (VP) shunt done **(Fig. 14)**.

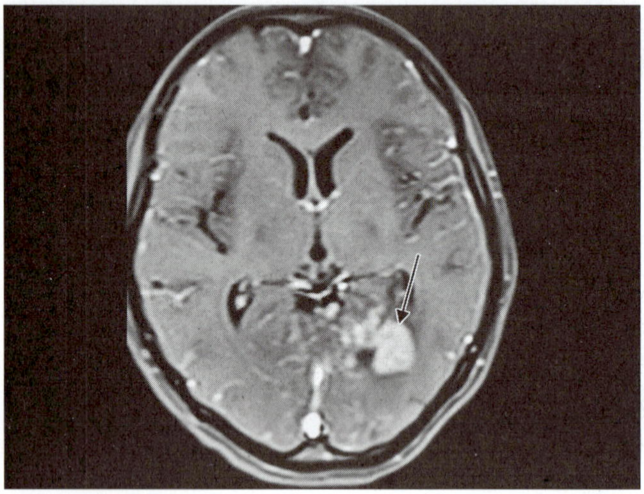

FIG. 11: Postcontrast T1 FS axial.

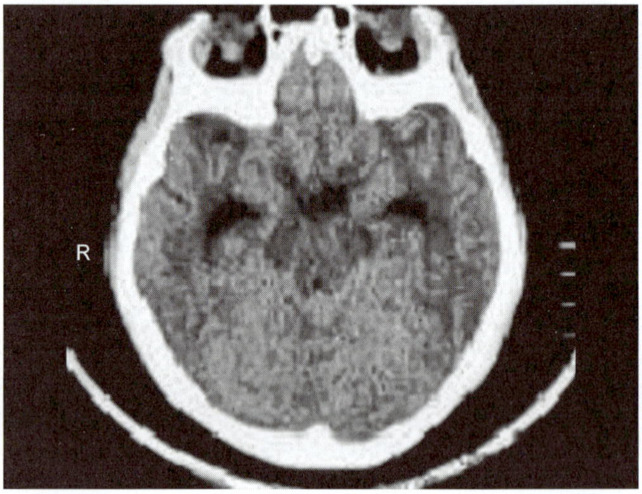

FIG. 13: CT brain—temporal horns of lateral ventricle dilated with periventricular leakage suggestive of hydrocephalus.

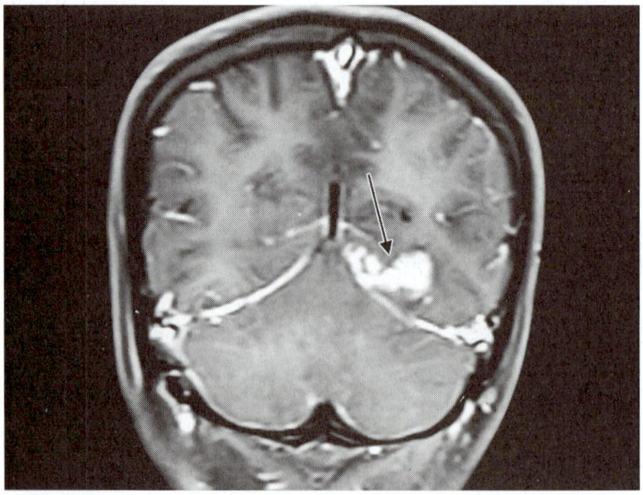

FIG. 12: Postgadolinium FS T1 coronal.

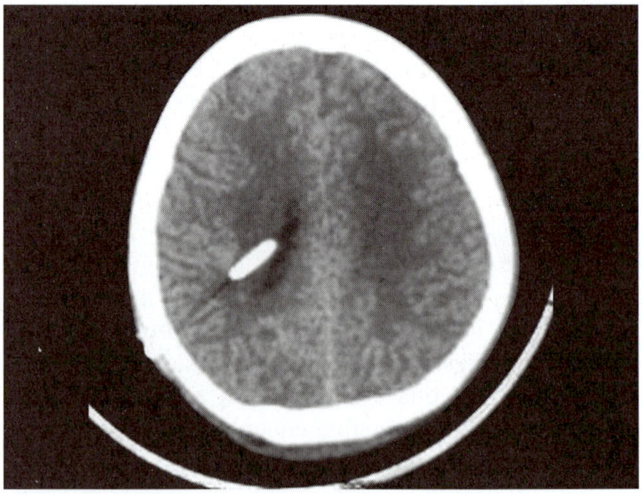

FIG. 14: Post-ventriculoperitoneal (VP) shunt.

Condition at discharge: The patient headache resolved and no focal neurological deficit at present.

CASE VIGNETTE 3

A 45-year-old male with no known comorbidities presented with headache and vomiting of 3 months duration with an altered sensorium of 1 week. Evaluated initially at a private hospital at the onset of headache, imaging at that time was normal. The patient continued to have mild persistent headaches. No history of fever or seizures. On neurological examination, Glasgow coma scale (GCS) was E4, V4, and M5, with pupils equally reacting to light. Fundus with no papillodema was seen. There was no neck stiffness.

Investigation and Management

The routine was normal. The fever workup was negative. CT brain is normal. The patient was treated as a case of meningoencephalitis and started antibiotics and antivirals as per protocol along with steroids. Cerebrospinal fluid (CSF) analysis showed glucose 24 mg/dL, protein 488 mg/dL, and chloride 97 mmol/L. CSF GeneXpert *Mycobacterium tuberculosis* (MTB)/RIF—MTB not detected, RIF resistance not detected. Human immunodeficiency virus (HIV) was reported as reactive. MRI brain with contrast—abnormal meningeal thickening and enhancement in the prepontine, interpeduncular, and bilateral ambient cistern **(Figs. 15 and 16)**. Abnormal enhancement is also seen in the ependymal lining of bilateral lateral ventricles. Diffuse effacement of bilateral cerebral sulci and basal cisterns seen. Diffuse ventricular dilatation of temporal horn of lateral ventricles. Ill-defined patchy enhancement with cytotoxic edema is seen in the left thalamus, bilateral crus cerebri, and over the splenium of corpus callosum. Acute lacunar infarcts is seen in left corona radiata and left posterior parietal parasagittal cortex **(Figs. 17 and 18)**. The patient was treated with antiedema measures and retroviral drugs. The patient developed worsening of the sensorium when a repeat CT brain showed hydrocephalus **(Figs. 19 and 20)**. Attenders are not willing for VP shunt. The patient on conservative measures finally succumbed.

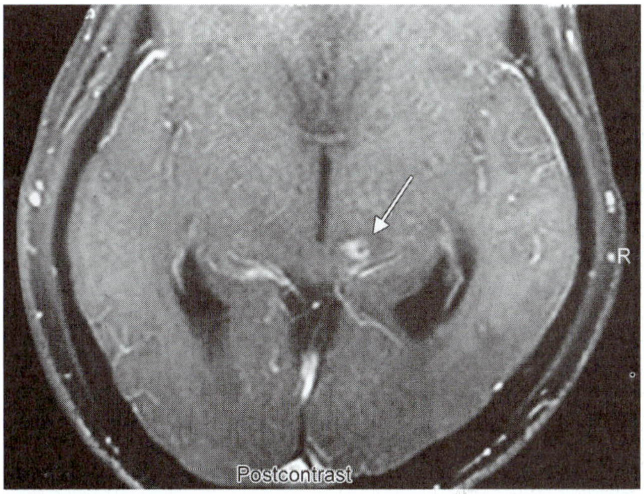

FIG. 16: T1 axial postcontrast.

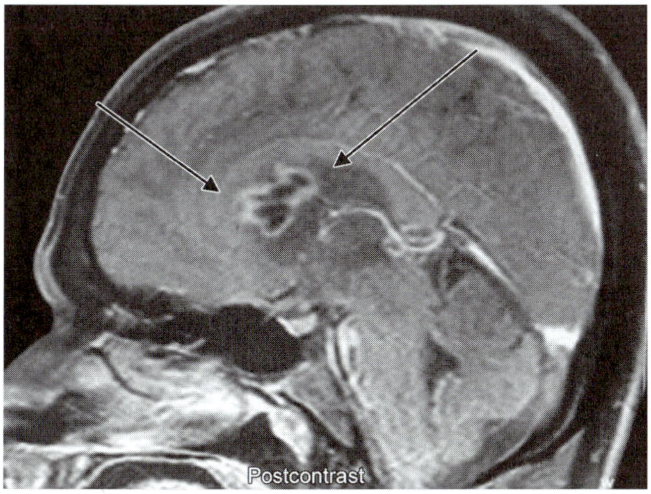

FIG. 15: T1 sagittal.

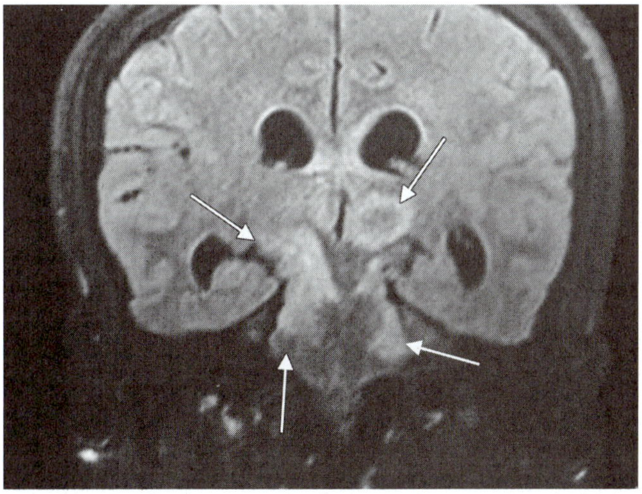

FIG. 17: T2 axial FLAIR.

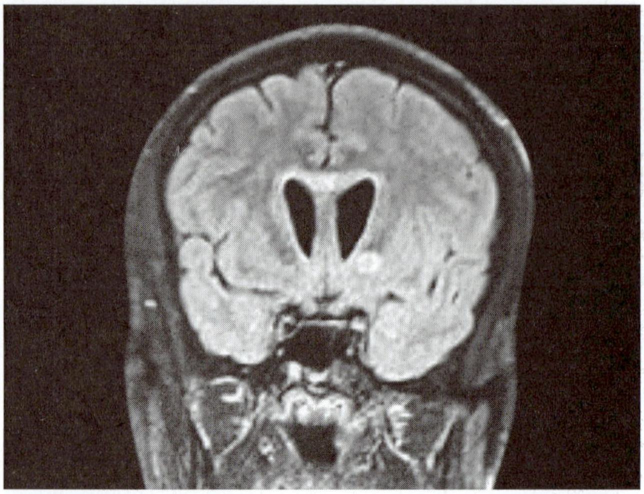

FIG. 18: T2 FLAIR coronal.

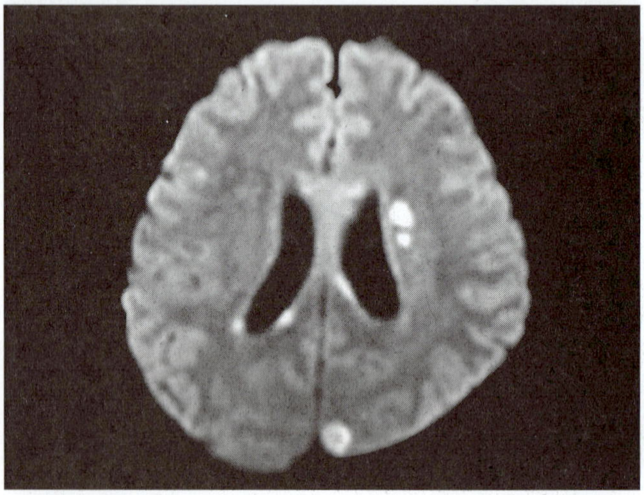

FIG. 19: Diffusion restriction image.

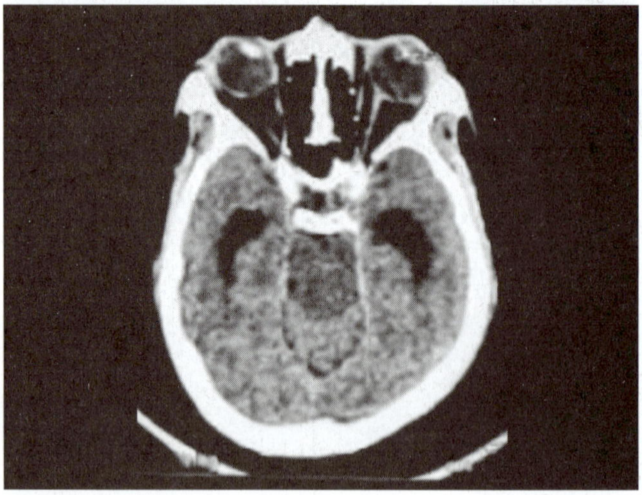

FIG. 20: CT brain—hydrocephalus.

CASE VIGNETTE 4

A 54-year-old female patient with nil comorbidities presented with complaints of acute febrile illness of days duration with associated generalized myalgias, recurrent bouts of nonprojectile, nonbilious vomiting, and headache that was holo-cranial, continuous, moderate-severe intensity of dull aching pain with no postural or diurnal fluctuations, and no aggravating and relieving factors for head pain. No associated visual blurring or double vision. On day 4 of febrile illness, the patient developed altered sensorium in the form of irrelevant self-talk and decreased responsiveness followed by an episode of seizure of generalized tonic-clonic semiology lasting for few minutes followed by sudden onset weakness of left upper and lower limbs that subsequently improved over next few days. No associated facial deviation. On examination, the patient was drowsy, disoriented, and intermittently obeying commands with neck rigidity, bilateral pupils that were symmetrical and reactive to light with preserved oculocephalic reflex, preserved extraocular movements, and normal fundoscopy with mild left hemiparesis.

Investigations

Acute febrile encephalopathy workup revealed thrombocytopenia with dengue NS1 serology positive, typhoid, macroscopic slide agglutination test (MSAT) for leptospirosis, and malarial parasite (MP) was negative. Lumbar puncture—elevated CSF protein (88 mg/dL) with normal glucose and acellular CSF. MRI brain is suggestive of T2/FLAIR hyperintensities showing patchy diffusion restriction and gradient blooming in bilateral frontal parasagittal regions suggestive of bilateral high frontal hemorrhagic infarcts, fluid debris in bilateral occipital horns of lateral ventricles showing diffusion restriction, and decreased flow signal intensity in anterior two-thirds of superior sagittal sinus suggestive of superior sagittal thrombosis which was subsequently ascertained with CT venogram **(Figs. 21 to 24)**. The patient was managed with parenteral fluids and antiepileptics with serial platelet monitoring. Given accompanying thrombocytopenia and no established indication for anticoagulation in postinfectious cerebral venous thrombosis (CVT) in the background of dengue fever, anticoagulation was deferred. Mechanisms for CVT in dengue fever include dehydration secondary to increased capillary permeability, coagulopathy due to endothelial dysfunction, and cytokine storm.

Discussion: The red flags are shown in **Boxes 1 and 2.**

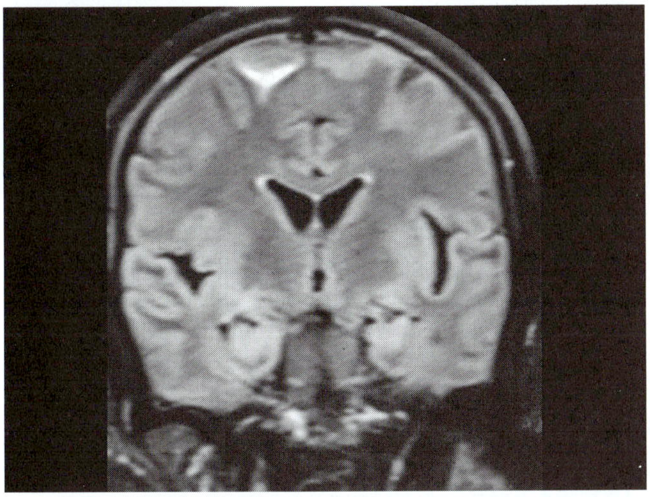

FIG. 21: T2-weighted (T2W) FLAIR image—bifrontal hemorrhagic infarcts.

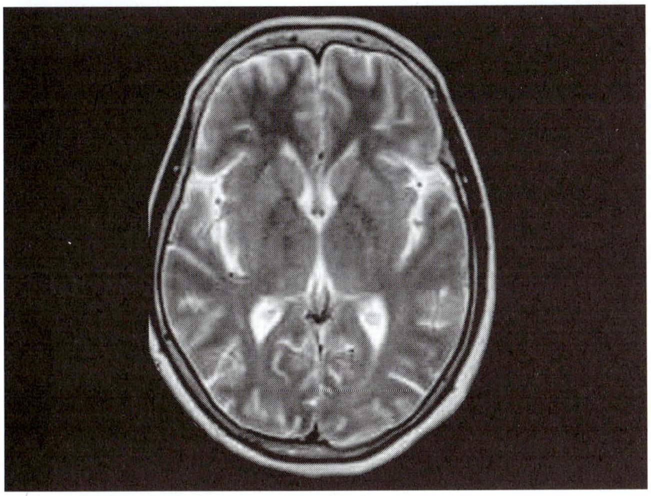

FIG. 22: T2-weighted (T2W) image—fluid-debris levels in occipital horns of bilateral lateral ventricles.

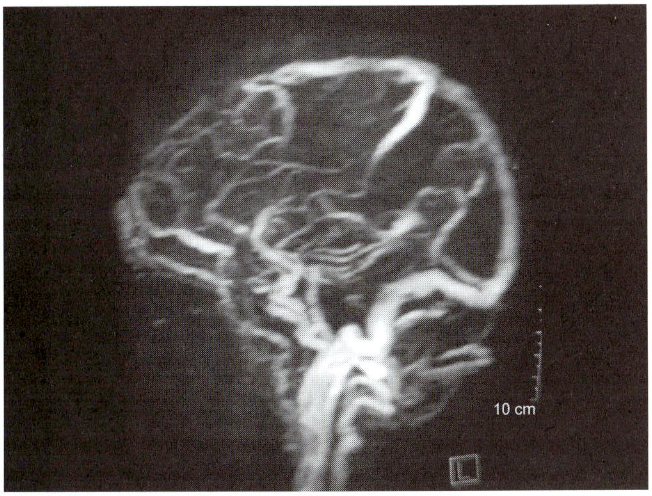

FIG. 23: Magnetic resonance venography (MRV)—thrombosis of the anterior one-third of superior sagittal sinus.

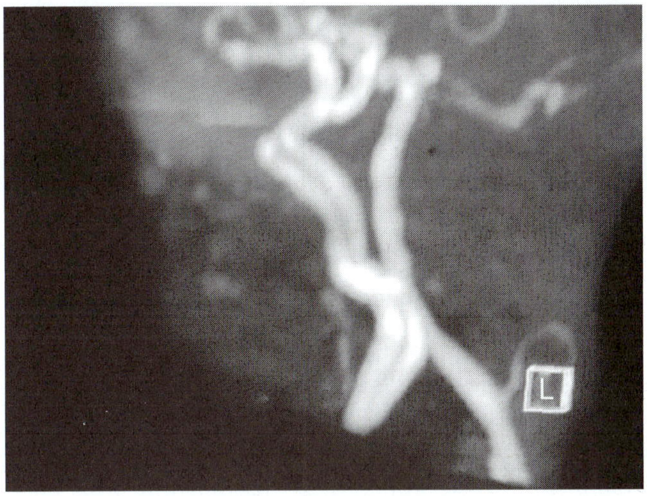

FIG. 24: Magnetic resonance angiography (MRA)—normal.

BOX 1: Red flags.

- Fever with systemic symptoms
- History of neoplasm
- Altered sensorium/neurological deficit
- Abrupt or sudden onset
- Age of onset above 50 years of age
- New onset/changing pattern
- Headache induced by positional changes
- Precipitating factors—coughing, sneezing, and exercise
- Fundus—papilledema
- Atypical presentation, progressive in nature

BOX 2: Red flags.

- Pregnancy or puerperium
- Painful eye with autonomic manifestations
- Headache following trauma
- Human immunodeficiency virus (HIV)
- Medicine overuse

Clues

Systemic symptoms with fever: Rule out systemic or neurologic infection or vasculitis, rheumatic disease, or any other inflammatory disease.

Neoplasm: Intracranial metastasis should be suspected in a patient with new onset headache along with coexistent symptoms like emesis, headache duration ≤10 weeks, atypical headache pattern, pulsating quality, and moderate to severe intensity. Neurological examination might reveal gait instability and extensor plantar response.

Headache in stroke: More common hemorrhagic than in ischemic stroke. Headache after stroke.

Older age (onset after 65 years of age): Increased incidence of secondary causes than primary.

Postural changes: Increased on assumption of upright posture with resolution on lying down—spontaneous intracranial hypotension.

Coughing induced headache: Chiari malformations and posterior fossa lesions.

Fundus examination: Papilledema—most of the patients have increased incidence of abnormal intracranial pathology.

Headache during antepartum, peripartum, and postpartum period: Stringent evaluation is needed to rule out secondary causes. Early identification and aggressive management is needed to prevent mortality. Neurological causes should be evaluated amidst non-neurological causes like postpartum eclampsia and postlumbar puncture headache. Red flags are elevated blood pressure, new onset headache, migraineurs with a longer duration of headache attack, relapsing thunderclap headaches, single thunderclap headache, visual loss, seizures, Horner syndrome, papilledema, and focal neurologic findings.

The differential diagnosis is shown in **Box 3**.

Abrupt onset of headache also known as thunderclap headache: Evaluate for aneurysmal subarachnoid hemorrhage and reversible cerebral vasoconstriction syndrome, which are the most common causes. Other secondary causes are meningoencephalitis, intracerebral hemorrhage, cervical artery dissection, CVT, spontaneous intracranial hypotension (SIH), pituitary apoplexy, and PRES. Early identification and treatment is important for improved outcomes. A lumbar puncture is therefore needed in all cases of thunderclap headache after normal brain imaging. CTA/MRA is done when necessary to exclude other causes and to clinch the diagnosis.

BOX 3: Differential diagnosis of headache in pregnancy.

- Puerperium—pre-eclampsia, eclampsia, reversible cerebral vasoconstriction syndrome, and posterior reversible encephalopathy syndrome
- Complications of anesthesia—postlumbar puncture headache and meningitis
- Hypercoagulable states—arterial stroke and cerebral venous sinus thrombosis
- Valsalva maneuver during labor—rupture of preexisting aneurysm and worsening of preexisting space occupying lesion
- Sheehan syndrome and pituitary apoplexy

Headache with neurological deficit: Hemorrhagic stroke tops the list followed by ischemic stroke. Others disorders implicated are infections, abscesses, and tumors. Hemorrhagic stroke patients with subarachnoid hemorrhage as a presentation almost all of them have headache while only 58% with intracerebral hemorrhage have headache. Headache is more common with posterior circulation, than anterior, cortical, cardioembolic, and large vessel occlusion rather than small vessel or lacunar infarction.

HEADACHE AS THE PRESENTATION OF STROKE (FIG. 25)

Age of onset >65 years (older age): Age itself is a red flag as secondary causes are more common like temporal arteritis, stroke, infections, subdural hematomas, and medication overuse headache.

Management

Early diagnosis and pertinent management are mandatory in all cases of headaches with red flags to avoid catastrophes. Neurological deficits carry a warning even without headache. Postpartum headaches carry a high mortality if not diagnosed early and treated.

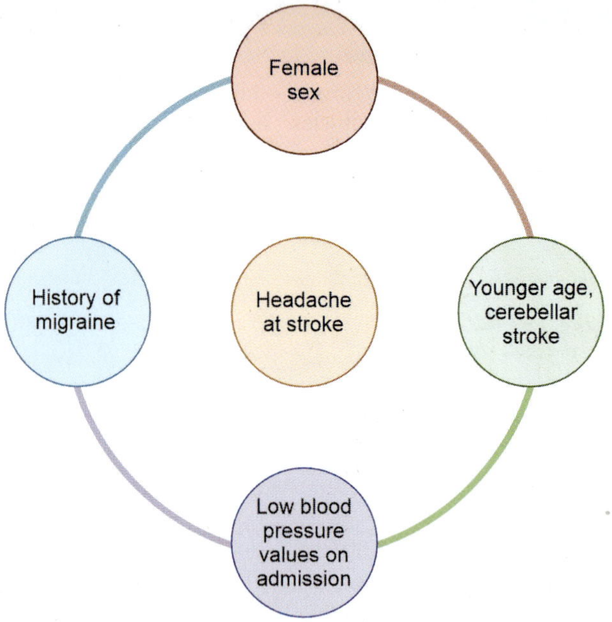

FIG. 25: Headache as a presentation of stroke.

CONCLUSION

Strategic characterization of headache characteristics into red flags (warning signs and symptoms) and green flags (primary headache predictors) is important as the patient steps into the ED department as an outpatient. All patients discharged should have diagnosis as per the ICHD-3 criteria to avoid misdiagnosis.

SUGGESTED READINGS

1. Do TP, Remmers A, Schytz HW, Schankin C, Nelson SE, Obermann M, et al. Red and orange flags for secondary headaches in clinical practice: SNNOOP10 list. Neurology. 2019;92(3):134-44.
2. Rimmele F, Janke J, Kropp P, Kasch R, Walter U, Jürgens TP. Headache in the Neurological Emergency Department-High Degree of Inadequate Documentation Calls for Structured Assessments. Front Neurol. 2022;13:847484.
3. Sharma TL. Common Primary and Secondary Causes of Headache in the Elderly. Headache. 2018;58(3):479-84.
4. Robbins MS. Headache in Pregnancy. Continuum (Minneap Minn). 2018;24(4, Headache):1092-107.
5. Janvier AS, Russell R. Postpartum headache - diagnosis and treatment. BJA Educ. 2022;22(5):176-81.
6. Harriott AM, Karakaya F, Ayata C. Headache after ischemic stroke: A systematic review and meta-analysis. Neurology. 2020;94(1):e75-e86.
7. Ducros A, Bousser MG. Thunderclap headache. BMJ. 2013;346: e8557.

93 CHAPTER

Myelin Oligodendrocyte Glycoprotein Antibody-associated Diseases

K Muralidharan, PR Sowmini

ABSTRACT

Myelin oligodendrocyte glycoprotein antibody-associated disease (MOGAD) is a recently recognized entity with characteristic clinical and paraclinical features, which help in early diagnosis. The median age of onset is within the fourth decade of life. Optic neuritis is the most common presenting phenotype. The disease course is either monophasic or relapsing, with subsequent relapses. Residual disability occurs in 50–80% of patients, with transverse myelitis at onset being the most significant predictor of long-term outcome. Myelin oligodendrocyte glycoprotein (MOG) antibody testing should be done in selected patients who present with clinical and paraclinical features suggestive of MOGAD, using a validated cell-based assay. Magnetic resonance imaging (MRI) features can help in differentiating MOGAD from other neuroinflammatory disorders like neuromyelitis optica spectrum disorder (NMOSD) and multiple sclerosis. High-dose steroids and plasma exchange are used in the treatment of acute attacks, and for immunosuppressive therapies, oral steroids, steroid-sparing agents, and rituximab are used as maintenance treatment.

INTRODUCTION

Myelin oligodendrocyte glycoprotein antibody-associated disease (MOGAD) are a relatively new concept in neurology, which have been recognized only since 2015. Myelin oligodendrocyte glycoprotein (MOG) comprises a minor constituent (0.05%) of the central nervous system (CNS) myelin, which is expressed on the outer lamella of the myelin sheath. MOG autoantibodies were first thought to be a subset of aquaporin 4 (AQP4)-negative cases of neuromyelitis optica (NMO). But now, its clinical spectrum has expanded.

EPIDEMIOLOGY AND CLINICAL COURSE

Unlike multiple sclerosis (MS) and AQP4-positive neuromyelitis optica spectrum disorder (NMOSD), MOG-associated disorders have no clear sex predilection. Males and females appear to be similarly impacted. They are more common in children than in adults. Although the median age of onset is in the early to mid-30s, the disease has a bimodal distribution. They may follow either a monophasic or relapsing course and may emerge in the setting of viral infections and vaccination. They are not strongly linked to other systemic autoimmune disorders which distinguishes them from AQP4-positive NMOSD and, to a lesser extent, MS.

PATHOLOGY

Histopathologic features of MOGAD are cortical demyelination and perivenular, confluent white matter lesions. Lymphocyte infiltrates in MOGAD are predominantly CD4+ cells, whereas it is CD8+ lymphocytes in MS. MOGAD is differentiated from AQP4-positive NMOSD where the AQP4 expression and morphology of astrocyte are preserved. Necrosis and granulocytic cell infiltrates are absent.

CLINICAL PHENOTYPES

Clinical phenotypes include seronegative NMO, MS, acute disseminated encephalomyelitis (ADEM), transverse myelitis, and chronic relapsing inflammatory optic neuritis. The most common clinical manifestations are optic neuritis, ADEM, and myelitis, either alone or in combination. The distribution of different phenotypes in adult and pediatric populations is shown in **Figure 1**.

Optic Neuritis

Optic neuritis is the most common manifestation and occurs in around 41% of pediatric patients and 56% of adult patients. It is usually bilateral and recurrent, and presents simultaneously or sequentially with myelitis or any another clinical phenotype. Optic disc edema and peripapillary hemorrhages are seen on examination. On MRI, we see a longitudinally extensive optic nerve involvement, perineural enhancement, and optic chiasm involvement. Visual loss is severe in both MOGAD and AQP4-positive NMOSD optic neuritis, but the recovery of vision is usually better in MOGAD.

Myelitis

Myelitis frequently arises in the setting of prodromal illness. On MRI, there are multiple spinal lesions, which may be either short-segment or longitudinally extensive and involve the cord anywhere from medulla to conus. Gadolinium enhancement is not common. Spinal cord gray-matter involvement is present disproportionately, which is seen as an 'H pattern' in the axial section and a linear central T2 hyperintensity in the sagittal section. Spinal cord atrophy is rare, and the imaging abnormalities might resolve after clinical recovery.

Neuromyelitis Optica Spectrum Disorder

Around 7–42% of seronegative NMOSD patients have anti-MOG autoantibodies and are classified as MOG-associated disorders. Simultaneous myelitis and optic neuritis or bilateral optic neuritis is found to be more common in MOGAD than AQP4-positive NMO. Area postrema syndrome is rare in MOGAD. The difference between clinic radiological features in NMOSD and MOGAD is shown in **Table 1**, and the site of involvement in various demyelinating disorders is depicted in **Figure 2**.

Acute Demyelinating Encephalomyelitis

Acute demyelinating encephalomyelitis presentation is usually seen in pediatric patients, especially those younger than 10 years of age. MRI shows supratentorial brain lesions bilaterally, involving both subcortical and deep white matter, and involvement of the deep gray matter like the thalamus and basal ganglia. In all pediatric patients presenting with ADEM, MOG autoantibody testing is warranted.

Focal Encephalitis

Very rarely, MOGAD can present with symptoms of focal encephalitis like reduced consciousness, seizures, and focal deficits. MRI shows hyperintense cortical fluid-attenuated inversion recovery (FLAIR) lesions which are usually unilateral, along with corresponding leptomeningeal enhancement.

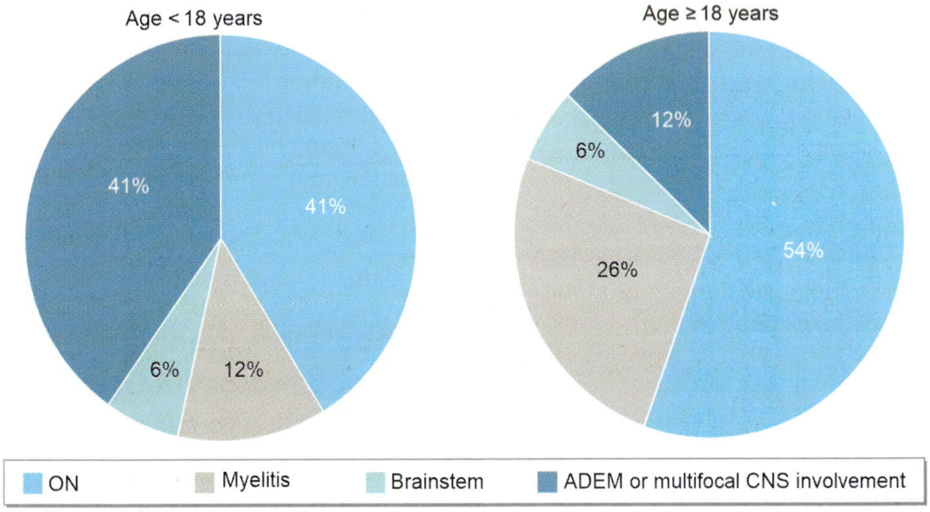

FIG. 1: Age-wise distribution of different phenotypes.
(ADEM: acute disseminated encephalomyelitis; CNS: central nervous system; ON: optic neuritis)

TABLE 1: Clinical and radiological features of NMOSD with AQP4-IgG-positive status versus MOG-IgG-positive status.

Features	AQP4-IgG-positive status	MOG-IgG-positive status
Main target	Astrocytes	Myelin
Evolution	Relapsing	Usually monophasic
Prognosis	Poor	Favorable
Gender	Female predominance	Lower female-to-male ratio or male predominance
Approximate age of onset	More common in adults than in children	Younger age
Phenotypes	Multiple phenotypes, but the most common are the core clinical syndromes of NMOSD	Various phenotypes, but the most common is optic neuritis
Most common magnetic resonance imaging patterns	• *Optic nerve*: Bilateral, long-length, and posterior involvement, usually with chiasmatic extension • *Spinal cord*: LETM, central/gray matter lesions, bright spotty lesions on T2-weighted images, and dark lesions on Tl-weighted images • *Brain lesions*: Periependymal lesions and corticospinal tract involvement • *Gadolinium enhancement*: Cloud-like enhancement; thin periventricular enhancement	• *Optic nerve*: Bilateral, long-length, and anterior involvement; severe optic disk swelling; perineural enhancement; optic chiasm less involved • *Spinal cord*: Involvement of conus or thoracolumbar cord • *Brain lesions*: Deep gray matter lesions, ADEM-like lesions (large cerebral lesions), fluffy lesions in the pons and cerebellar peduncles and adjacent to the fourth ventricle, and periependymal areas rarely involved • *Gadolinium enhancement*: Optic perineural enhancement
Associated disorders	NMOSD, ADEM in children, and autoimmune disorders	AQP4-IgG-negative NMOSD status, multiple sclerosis, ADEM, recurrent optic neuritis, and LETM

(ADEM: acute disseminated encephalomyelitis; AQP4: aquaporin 4; IgG: immunoglobulin G; LETM: longitudinally extensive transverse myelitis; NMOSD: neuromyelitis optica spectrum disorder; MOG: myelin oligodendrocyte glycoprotein)

Chronic Lymphocytic Inflammation with Pontine Perivascular Enhancement Responsive to Steroids

Chronic lymphocytic inflammation with pontine perivascular enhancement responsive to steroids (CLIPPERS) is a rare syndrome characterized by subacute dysfunction of the pontocerebellum, without peripheral nerve involvement. It is steroid responsive. MRI shows small, homogeneous gadolinium-enhancing nodules in the pons and cerebellum.

DIAGNOSTIC WORKUP

Diagnostic workup includes CNS imaging along with cerebrospinal fluid (CSF) and blood testing.

Neuroimaging in Myelin Oligodendrocyte Glycoprotein Antibody-associated Disease

Magnetic resonance imaging shows various distinctive radiologic features corresponding to the clinical phenotype, which are shown in **Figures 3 to 5**.

- *Acute optic neuritis*: Perineural enhancement (50%); long-segment lesions (80%), chiasmal involvement (10–20%)
- *Acute myelitis*: Short-segment lesions and longitudinally extensive lesions; multiple spinal cord lesions; central gray involvement (H sign) and linear sagittal T2 hyperintensity (~30%); involvement of the conus (4–40%); enhancement/edema mild or relatively uncommon (25–70%)
- Acute ADEM-diffuse, poorly demarcated, large (>1–2 cm), bilateral lesions involving subcortical/deep white matter and deep gray matter
- *Non ADEM encephalitis*: Unilateral or bilateral cortical/subcortical lesions (~16%); isolated deep gray matter lesions; meningeal enhancement (<10%)

Laboratory Findings in Myelin Oligodendrocyte Glycoprotein Antibody-associated Disease

Anti-MOG antibodies must be detected in the serum using cell-based assays, and titers > 1:20 are considered positive. Titers of 1:20–1:40 have a positive predictive value of about 51% in diagnosing MOGAD, whereas titers of 1:1,000 or more have a positive predictive value of 100%.

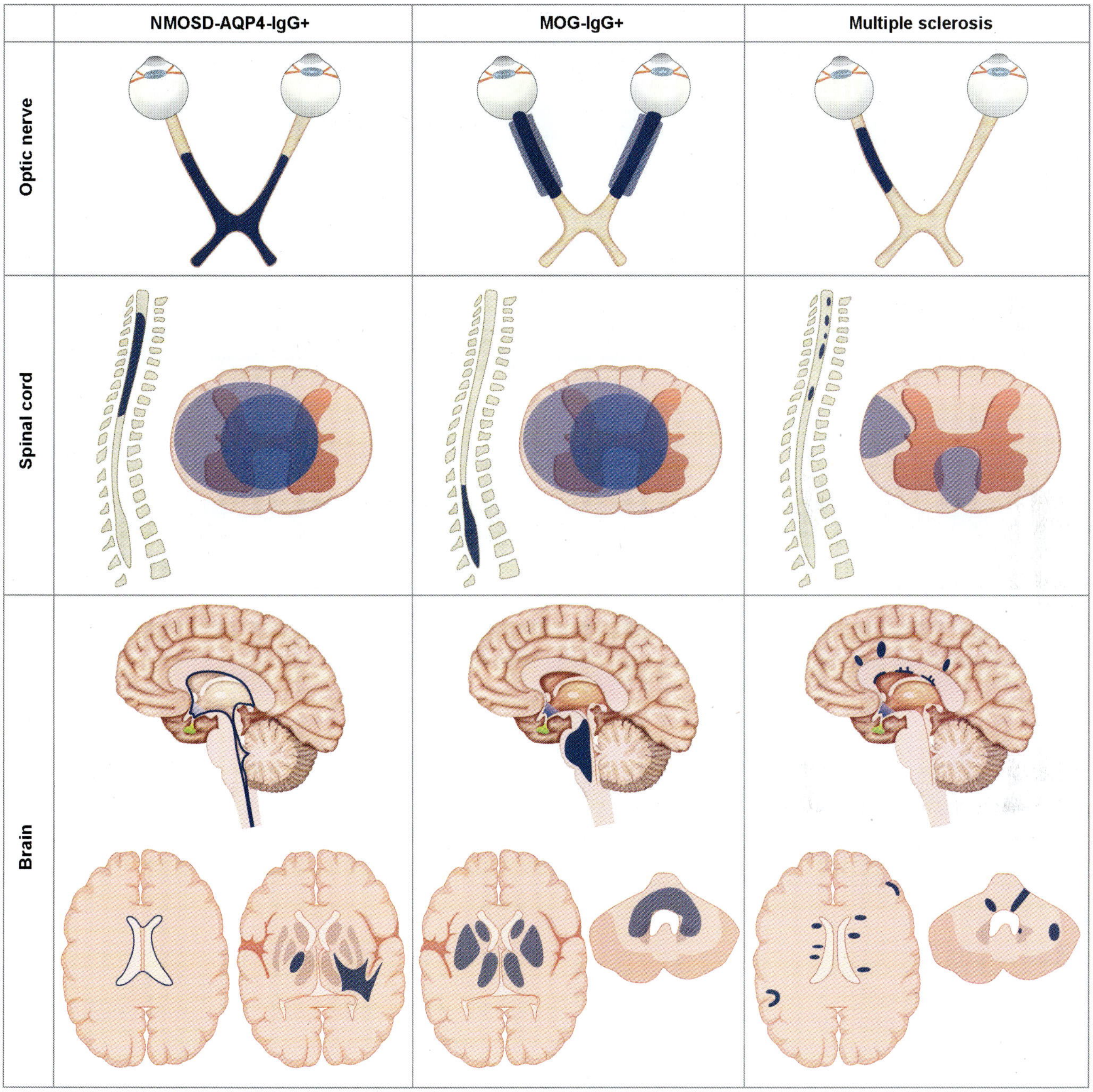

FIG. 2: Site of involvement in NMOSD, MOG and MS.

(AQP4: aquaporin 4; IgG: immunoglobulin G; NMOSD: neuromyelitis optica spectrum disorder; MOG: myelin oligodendrocyte glycoprotein; MS: multiple sclerosis)

Cerebrospinal fluid pleocytosis is common during relapses and is more marked than in MS or AQP4-positive NMOSD. 10–15% of patients show a CSF cell count of 100/ mm^3 or more. Lymphocytes are the predominant cell type, but neutrophils are also found in around half of patients. CSF cell counts are usually higher when patient presents with ADEM or myelitis when compared to isolated optic neuritis. CSF protein may be elevated during relapses, and the oligoclonal band is usually negative.

The summary of demographic, clinic radiological, and laboratory features of various demyelinating disorders is depicted in the **Table 2**.

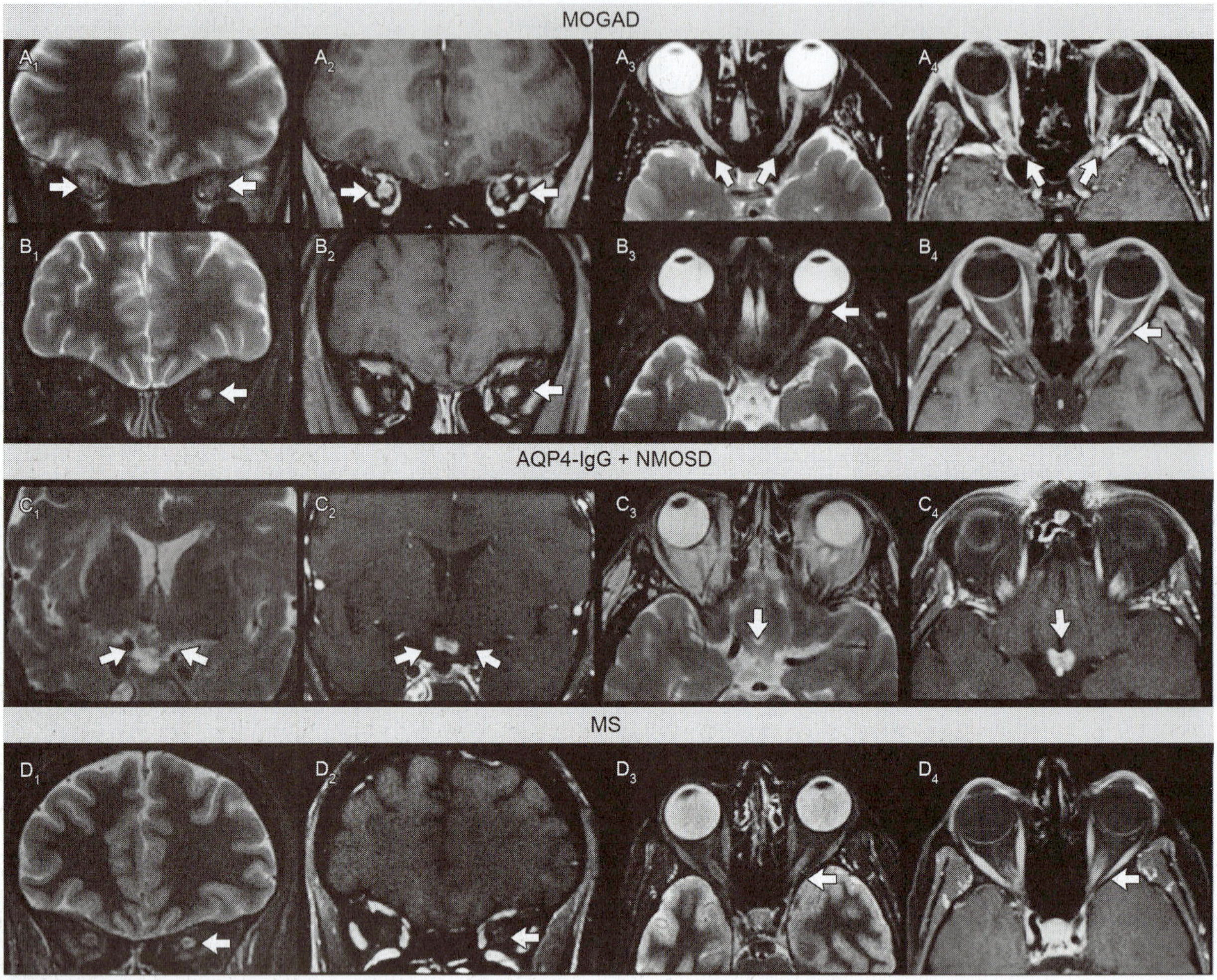

FIG. 3: Orbital fat-saturated MRI in optic neuritis with MOGAD, AQP4-IgG + NMOSD, and MS.

(AQP4: aquaporin 4; IgG: immunoglobulin G; NMOSD: neuromyelitis optica spectrum disorder; MOGAD: myelin oligodendrocyte glycoprotein antibody-associated disease; MRI: magnetic resonance imaging; MS: multiple sclerosis)

TREATMENT

Acute attacks of MOGAD are treated in the same way as other demyelinating disorders. High-dose intravenous (IV) corticosteroids at the dose of 20–30 mg/kg/day methylprednisolone in pediatric patients or 1 g/day methylprednisolone in adults are given for 3–5 days.

There is a higher risk of relapse seen in the months after the acute episode. It is usually seen when the steroid is being withdrawn. Hence, a slow oral steroid tapered up to 3 months is suggested to prevent this relapse. Pediatric guidelines suggest to start oral prednisone at 1–2 mg/kg/day (maximum 60 mg daily) and then tapering it down to 0.5 mg/kg/day over 1–4 weeks. Further tapering should be done very slowly, with the aim to have the patient fully weaned off steroids by around 3 months after relapse. These guidelines can also be extended to adults.

Usually, majority of patients are steroid responsive, and if patients do not respond to steroids, either plasma exchange or intravenous immunoglobulin (IVIg) is used as second-line therapy. Treatment escalation is advised for patients who do not improve after IV methylprednisolone or those who have a severe attack like complete loss of vision, severe weakness, or severe encephalopathy which requires intensive care unit (ICU) admission. Escalation therapies are immunoadsorption, plasma exchange (five exchanges on alternative days), IVIgs (total of 2 g/kg over 2 or 5 days), or plasma exchange followed by IVIgs.

For those presenting with relapsing disease, steroid-sparing agents are used. The most commonly used agents are rituximab, mycophenolate mofetil, azathioprine, tocilizumab, and maintenance IVIg. Patients who are treated with any of these agents generally experience a reduction in the annualized relapse rates, but a high proportion (20–75%) continues to experience relapses. Rituximab, which is usually highly effective in other demyelinating disorders, is found to be relatively less effective for MOGAD.

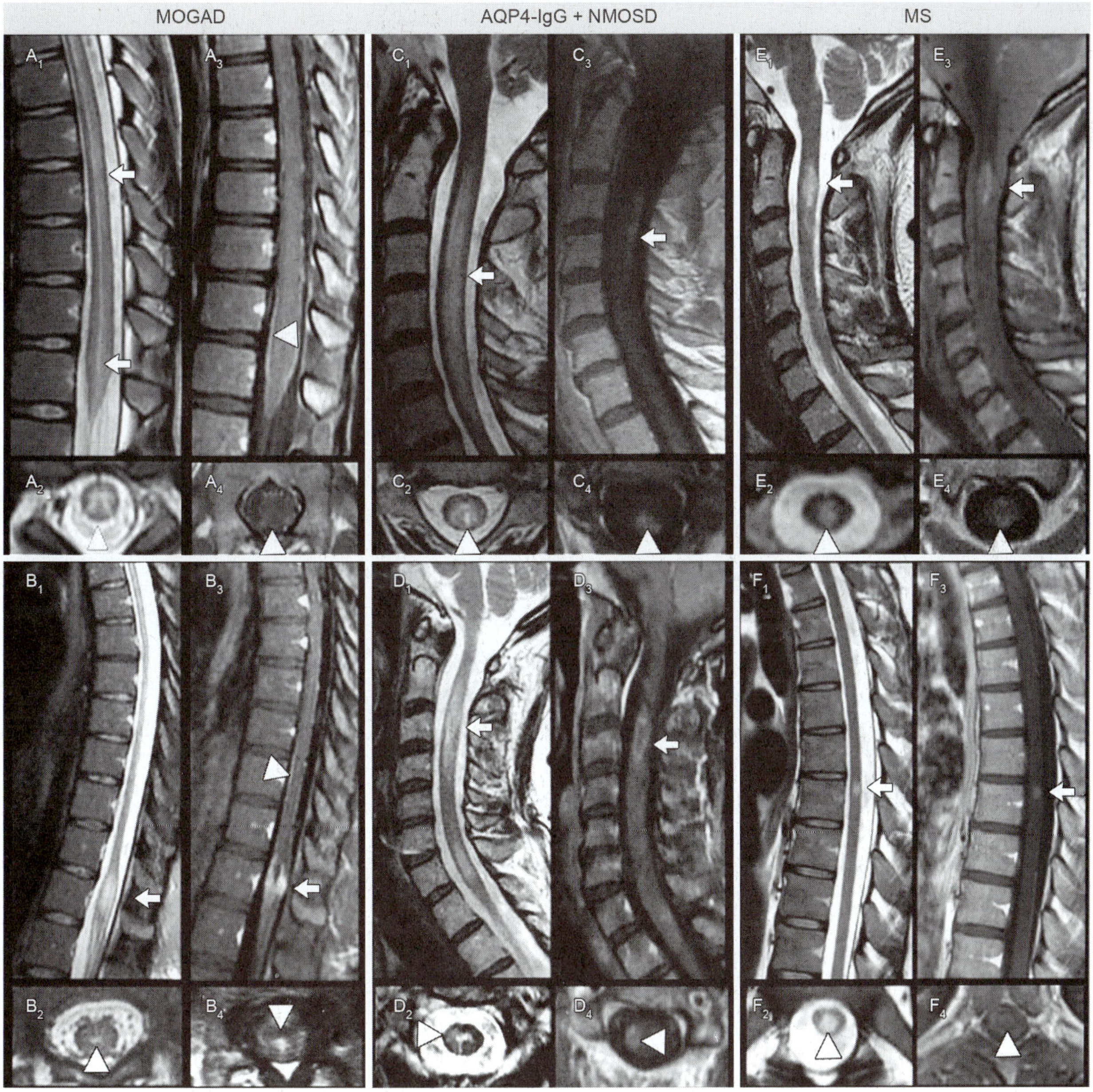

FIG. 4: Spinal cord MRI features in patients with MOGAD, AQP4-IgG + NMOSD, and MS.

(AQP4: aquaporin 4; IgG: immunoglobulin G; NMOSD: neuromyelitis optica spectrum disorder; MOGAD: myelin oligodendrocyte glycoprotein antibody-associated disease; MRI: magnetic resonance imaging; MS: multiple sclerosis)

There is a controversy on when to start patients on long-term immunotherapy. The majority of patients have a monophasic disease, and hence subjecting these patients to lifelong immunosuppression leads to unwanted adverse effects. Hence, it is suggested to initiate the maintenance immunotherapy during the second event (i.e., first relapse). If subsequent relapses occur while the patient is on immunotherapy, then an alternative agent needs to be considered. If relapses continue in spite of adequate treatment with at least two different immunotherapies, then add-on therapy can be used. For example, oral prednisone or pulse IVIg can be added to rituximab.

PROGNOSIS

Good or full recovery is seen in 78% patients. Younger patients have better recovery, and the disability is greater in the patients who have more numbers of attacks and those who did not have full recovery from their initial attack.

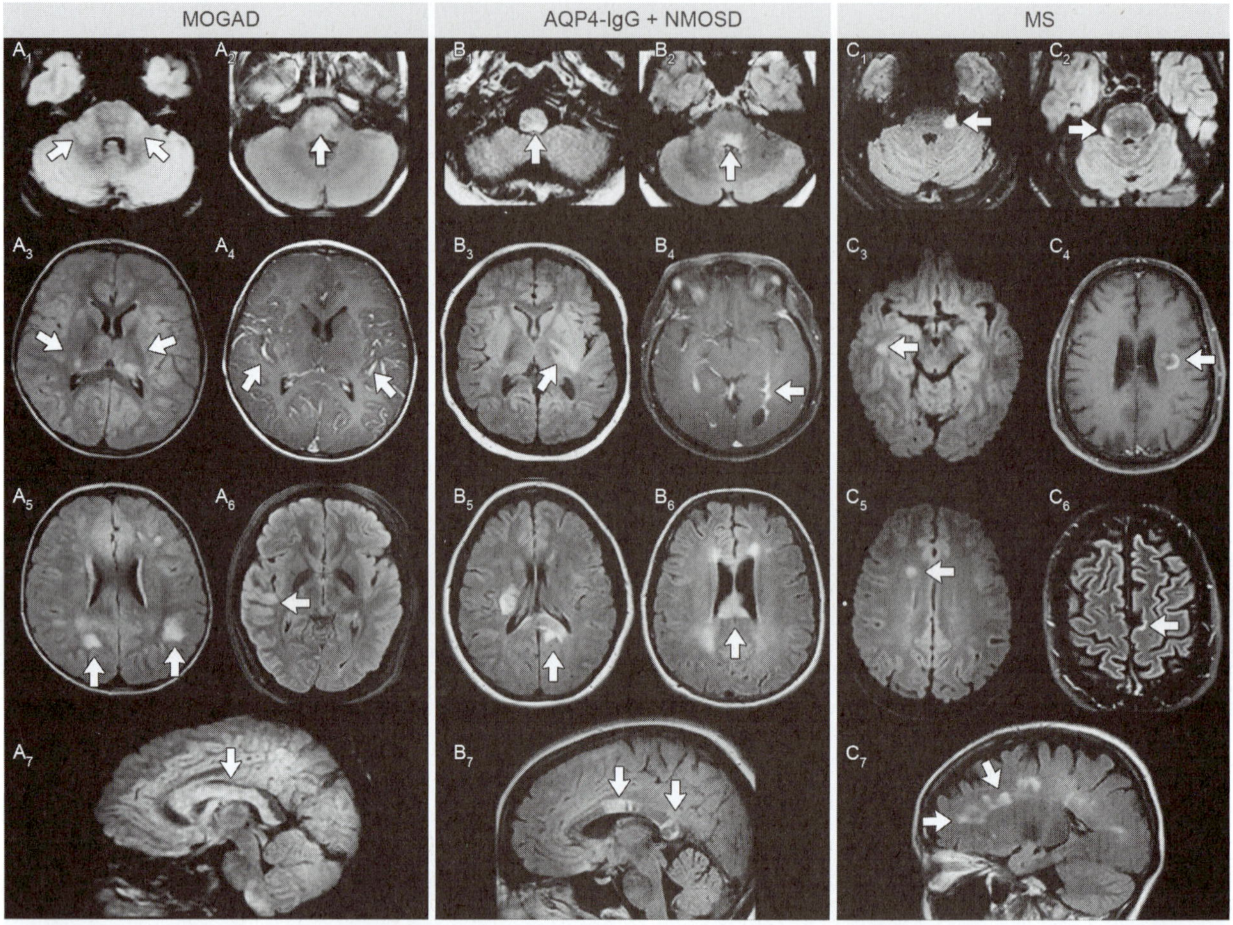

FIG. 5: Brain MRI features in patients with MOGAD, AQP4-IgG + NMOSD, and MS.

(AQP4: aquaporin 4; IgG: immunoglobulin G; NMOSD: neuromyelitis optica spectrum disorder; MOGAD: myelin oligodendrocyte glycoprotein antibody-associated disease; MRI: magnetic resonance imaging; MS: multiple sclerosis)

TABLE 2: Comparison of demographics, clinical, laboratory, and magnetic resonance imaging (MRI) characteristics in MOGAD compared to AQP4-IGG+NMOSD, and MS.

	MOGAD	NMOSD	MS
Demographics			
Age	0–40	30–50	20–40
Sex (F:M)	1:1	9:1	2–3:1
Ethnicity	No racial predominance	African-American, Asian	Caucasian
Clinical features			
Antecedent infection/ immunization	Common	Rare	Rare
Disease course	Relapsing–50%; Monophasic–50%	Generally relapsing	Relapsing–85%; progressive–15%
Optic neuritis	+++	+++	++
Myelitis	++	+++	+++
Area postrema syndrome	Rare	++	Rare
Encephalopathy	++	Rare	Rare
Seizures	+	Rare	Rare

Continued

Continued

	MOGAD	NMOSD	MS
CSF			
Oligoclonal bands	<20% (transient)	<20% (transient)	>85% (persistent)
WBC > 50	35%	13–35%	Rare
MRI			
Optic nerve	Uni-/bilateral, long lesions (>50%), mainly anterior segments, perineural enhancement	Uni-/bilateral, mainly posterior segments including chiasm	Generally unilateral, short lesions, mainly along the intraorbital tract
Spinal cord	Longitudinally extensive (60%), generally more than one lesion, conus involved, H-sign axially, enhancement in 50%	Longitudinally extensive (85%), single lesion. Central/diffuse on axial images. Elongated ring or patchy enhancement	• Multiple short lesions; periphery of cord. • Ring or nodular enhancement
Brain	ADEM-like, 'fluffy' lesions in both white and deep gray matter, extensive involvement of cerebellar peduncles. Cortical hyperintensity may occur	Often nonspecific; area postrema, peri- 3rd/4th ventricle, corticospinal tracts, sometimes extensive white matter lesions	Ovoid periventricular, infratentorial, juxtacortical. Central vein sign. Ring enhancement

(AEDM: acute disseminated encephalomyelitis; AQP4: aquaporin 4; CSF: cerebrospinal fluid; IgG: immunoglobulin G; NMOSD: neuromyelitis optica spectrum disorder; MOGAD: myelin oligodendrocyte glycoprotein antibody-associated disease; MRI: magnetic resonance imaging; MS: multiple sclerosis; WBC: white blood cells)

CONCLUSION

The diagnosis of MOGAD is essential to plan appropriate management. Characteristic clinical and paraclinical features, in association with positive MOG antibody help in the identification of MOGAD from other neuro-inflammatory demyelinating disorders. But, still in many cases, making a definitive diagnosis is difficult. Hence, the definition of MOGAD-specific diagnostic criteria, as well as the identification of markers of disease, is still a matter of research. Once the disease has been diagnosed, uncertainty is there among the best treatment approaches and so, clinical trials for the pharmacological management of MOGAD are still needed.

SUGGESTED READINGS

1. Hor JY, Asgari N, Nakashima I, Broadley SA, Leite MI, Kissani N, et al. Epidemiology of neuromyelitis optica spectrum disorder and its prevalence and incidence worldwide. Front Neurol. 2020;11:501.
2. de Mol CL, Wong Y, van Pelt ED, Wokke B, Siepman T, Neuteboom RF, et al. The clinical spectrum and incidence of anti-MOG-associated acquired demyelinating syndromes in children and adults. Mult Scler. 2020;26(7):806-14.
3. Ciotti JR, Eby NS, Wu GF, Naismith RT, Chahin S, Cross AH. Clinical and laboratory features distinguishing MOG antibody disease from multiple sclerosis and AQP4 antibody-positive neuromyelitis optica. Mult Scler Relat Disord. 2020;45: 102399.
4. Dubey D, Pittock SJ, Krecke KN, Morris PP, Sechi E, Zalewski NL, et al. Clinical, radiologic, and prognostic features of myelitis associated with myelin oligodendrocyte glycoprotein autoantibody. JAMA Neurol. 2019;76(3):301-9.
5. Bruijstens AL, Wendel EM, Lechner C, Bartels F, Finke C, Breu M, et al. E.U. Paediatric MOG consortium consensus: Part 5—treatment of paediatric myelin oligodendrocyte glycoprotein antibody-associated disorders. Eur J Paediatr Neurol. 2020;29: 41-53.

94

CHAPTER

Memory Assessment and Detection of Early Dementia

Tribeni Sharma

ABSTRACT

Dementia is a progressive neurological disorder characterized by a decline in cognitive function, impacting memory thinking and behavior. It is mainly prevalent among older individuals but can also affect young individuals. Alzheimer's disease is the most common form of dementia accounting for 60–70% of cases.

Early detection of dementia plays a crucial role in managing the condition effectively. It allows healthcare professionals to identify the type of dementia and develop appropriate treatment plans and support systems. Early detection can also help make informed decisions about care options and further arrangements. Various tools and assessments have been developed to aid in the early detection of dementia.

In conclusion, early detection of dementia is crucial for effective management and improved outcomes for individuals and their families. By identifying the condition early on, healthcare professionals can tailor treatment plans and support systems to meet the specific needs of individuals. Additionally, early detection offers the opportunity to explore the potential medical interventions and access support services, ensuring the best possible care and quality of life for those affected by dementia.

INTRODUCTION

Dementia is a progressive neurodegenerative disorder characterized by a decline in cognitive functions, including memory, thinking, behavior, and the ability to perform daily activities. Common causes of dementia include Alzheimer's disease, cerebrovascular disease, frontotemporal degeneration, Parkinson's disease, etc. Alzheimer's disease, the most common form of dementia, affects approximately 60–80% of people diagnosed with the condition. It is very crucial though tough to differentiate Alzheimer's disease from typical age-related changes.

SIGNIFICANCE OF EARLY DETECTION

Early detection of dementia is crucial as it allows for timely interventions, access to appropriate care, and better management of the disease.

Early detection of dementia offers numerous advantages for patients, their families, healthcare providers, and society as a whole. Firstly, an early diagnosis allows patients to have more time to plan for their future and make informed decisions regarding their care, treatment options, and legal matters such as advanced care planning, and setting up power of attorney. This knowledge empowers individuals and enables them to maintain control over their lives and financial affairs.

Secondly, early detection provides an opportunity to access appropriate care and support services. It allows patients to engage in therapeutic and supportive interventions that can enhance their quality of life and overall well-being. For example, memory clinics and cognitive rehabilitation programs can aid individuals in developing strategies to cope with memory loss and manage other cognitive impairments effectively.

Furthermore, early detection enables healthcare professionals to educate and support family members, who play a crucial role in caregiving. Informed family members are better prepared to navigate the challenges of dementia caregiving, access support networks, and understand the progression of the disease. This support contributes to the overall well-being of both patients and their families, alleviating emotional distress and promoting a healthier caregiver–patient relationship.

CHALLENGES IN EARLY DETECTION

Despite the significance of early detection, several challenges exist. Firstly, dementia is a complex disorder, and its symptoms can be mistaken for normal aging or other health conditions. The early signs of dementia, such as mild memory loss or occasional forgetfulness, can often be attributed to everyday stressors or fatigue. Consequently, individuals and even healthcare professionals may overlook or underestimate these initial symptoms, leading to delayed diagnosis and intervention.

Secondly, stigma and societal misconceptions about dementia can hinder early detection efforts. Negative stereotypes and fear associated with the diagnosis of dementia may discourage individuals from seeking help or acknowledging their symptoms. Moreover, the lack of awareness in the general population about the early signs and risk factors of dementia can further delay diagnosis, as individuals may not recognize the need for assessment or may be unaware of available resources.

Thirdly, healthcare disparities and limited access to specialized memory clinics or diagnostic services can be significant barriers to early detection. In many regions, there is a shortage of specialists trained in dementia care, leading to long waiting times for appointments and delayed diagnosis. Additionally, financial constraints can restrict access to diagnostic tests, further perpetuating disparities in timely detection.

METHODOLOGIES FOR EARLY DETECTION

Several methodologies are employed to aid the early detection of dementia. These include cognitive assessments, neuroimaging techniques, biomarker analysis, and subjective reports from patients and their families.

Memory assessment plays a central role in the early detection of dementia. Memory impairment is often one of the earliest signs of cognitive decline. It is crucial to conduct a comprehensive memory assessment to identify any subtle changes that may indicate the presence of dementia. Memory tests typically evaluate various aspects of memory, including short-term memory, long-term memory, and working memory. These tests can take the form of questionnaires, interviews, or cognitive assessments specifically designed to measure memory performance. The tools of memory assessment can be divided into patient assessment tools and informant tools.

One commonly used tool for memory assessment is the Mini-Mental State Examination (MMSE). The MMSE assesses various cognitive functions, including memory, orientation, attention, and language. It consists of a series of questions and tasks that evaluate an individual's ability to recall information, follow instructions, and perform simple calculations. However, the MMSE has been criticized for its limited sensitivity in detecting early-stage dementia and its potential for biased scoring.

To address these limitations, more advanced and comprehensive memory assessment tools have been developed. The Montreal Cognitive Assessment (MoCA) is one such tool that is gaining popularity for detecting mild cognitive impairment and early dementia. The MoCA assesses a broader range of cognitive functions, including attention, language, visuospatial abilities, and executive functions, in addition to memory. This comprehensive approach increases the sensitivity of the assessment and improves the accuracy of early detection. Other tools that are gaining popularity to be used in primary healthcare are General Practitioner Assessment of Cognition (GPCOG) and mini-COG.

In addition to standardized assessments, medical professionals should also consider subjective reports from patients and their family members or caregivers. These reports can provide valuable insights into any changes in memory and daily functioning that may indicate cognitive decline. This information, coupled with the results of formal memory assessments, can help build a more comprehensive picture of an individual's cognitive status. Some tools that can be used by informants are Eight-item Informant interview to Differentiate Aging and Dementia (AD8) and short form of the Informant Questionnaire on Cognitive Decline in Elderly (IQCODE).

Early detection of dementia through memory assessment allows individuals to access appropriate care and support. An early diagnosis helps individuals and their families plan for the future and make informed decisions regarding treatment, caregiving, and potential lifestyle changes. It also enables healthcare professionals to provide education and support to family members who may be experiencing emotional distress and uncertainty about the disease.

Neuroimaging techniques, such as magnetic resonance imaging (MRI) and positron emission tomography (PET), provide structural and functional information about the brain. MRI scans can detect brain atrophy (shrinkage) or the presence of abnormalities that contribute to cognitive impairment. PET scans using specific tracers can detect amyloid plaques and tau tangles, which are characteristic hallmarks of Alzheimer's disease. These imaging techniques aid in differential diagnosis and contribute to early detection efforts.

Biomarker analysis involves studying specific substances or molecules in the blood, cerebrospinal fluid, or other body fluids that may indicate the presence of dementia. For instance, beta-amyloid and tau proteins are biomarkers associated with Alzheimer's disease. While biomarker analysis is still predominantly used in research settings, ongoing studies aim to develop reliable and accessible biomarker tests that can aid in early detection and monitoring of dementia.

Moreover, a comprehensive approach employing multiple methodologies may yield the most accurate results in early detection. Combining cognitive assessments, neuroimaging, biomarker analysis, and subjective reports allows for a more robust evaluation of an individual's cognitive status, increasing the sensitivity and specificity of the detection process.

CONCLUSION

Early detection of dementia is vital for timely intervention, access to appropriate care, and improved management of the disease. Despite challenges such as the complexity of dementia symptoms, societal misconceptions, and limited access to specialized diagnostic services, various methodologies, including cognitive assessments, neuroimaging, biomarker analysis, and subjective reports, aid in the early detection of dementia. By addressing these challenges, enhancing awareness, and utilizing a comprehensive approach to detection, healthcare providers can improve patient outcomes, support families, and optimize the quality of life for individuals living with dementia. Ultimately, early detection empowers individuals, enables them to plan for the future, and promotes early access to interventions that can slow disease progression and improve overall well-being.

SUGGESTED READINGS

1. Cordell CB, Borson S, Boustani M, Chodosh J, Reuben D, Verghese J, et al.; Medicare Detection of Cognitive Impairment Workgroup. Alzheimer's Association recommendations for operationalizing the detection of cognitive impairment during the Medicare Annual Wellness Visit in a primary care setting. Alzheimers Dement. 2013;9(2):141-50.
2. Rasmussen J, Langerman H. Alzheimer's Disease-Why We Need Early Diagnosis. Degener Neurol Neuromuscul Dis. 2019;9:123-30.
3. Dubois B, Picard G, Sarazin M. Early detection of Alzheimer's disease: new diagnostic criteria. Dialogues Clin Neurosci. 2009;11(2):135-9.

95

CHAPTER

Approach to a Case of Refractory Seizures

Uma Sinharoy

ABSTRACT

Approach to refractory seizures is complex and multidirectional. Apparent pharmacoresistant to antiseizure medications must be considered as a priority to rule out a misdiagnosis. Epilepsy caused by surgically remediable conditions must be identified by our best possible resources to achieve best possible seizure freedom. For the rest of the nonsurgical patients, there are provinces of alternative treatments, neurostimulations, and ketogenic diet under the supervision of dedicated epilepsy centers.

INTRODUCTION

This is an age-old topic with which medical science is struggling for more than a century but still many questions are unanswered. Patients with refractory seizures are suffering from devastating neurological condition with recurrent unprovoked seizures, focal or generalized. Although criteria for defining "refractory epilepsy" are elusive (number of drugs tried, dose of drugs, duration of treatment, etc.) a hard core of 20–30% of patients continue to have seizures that appear to be resistant to all pharmacological manipulations. Epilepsy is generally considered "refractory," "drug-resistant," or "intractable" when seizures cannot be controlled by at least two or three ASDs (antiseizure drugs) appropriate for the particular epilepsy type. In this regard, the International League against Epilepsy (ILAE) Task Force proposed that "[d]rug-resistant epilepsy (DRE) may be defined as failure of adequate trials of two tolerated and appropriately chosen and used ASD schedules (whether as monotherapies or in combination) to achieve sustained seizure freedom".

BOX 1: Dimensions of refractory epilepsy.

- Intractable seizures
- Excessive drug burden
- Neurobiochemical changes
- Cognitive decline
- Psychosocial dysfunction
- Dependent behavior
- Restricted lifestyle
- Unsatisfactory quality of life
- Increased mortality, increased risk of SUDEP

"Refractory epilepsy", therefore, may come up with constellation of disabilities with recurrent seizures being just one of its manifestations **(Box 1)**.

RESPONSE TO THE FIRST AED IS A POWERFUL PROGNOSTIC INDICATOR

This factor was particularly predictive among patients in whom treatment with the first drug was ineffective.

BOX 2: Predictors of development of refractory seizures.

Patient factors:
- Intellectual or developmental delay at presentation
- Structural malformation evident on imaging
- Seizure onset under 1 year of age

Epilepsy factors:
- Epileptic syndrome associated with intractability
- Multiple seizure types
- Status epilepticus
- Failure to respond to first antiepileptic drug

BOX 3: Contributing factors to the biological basis of refractory epilepsy.

- Syndromic classification, e.g., childhood epileptic encephalopathies
- Causative neuropathology, e.g., mesial temporal sclerosis, cortical dysplasia
- Hyperexcitable and disinhibited neuronal network reorganization, e.g., mossy fiber sprouting
- Altered neurotransmitter receptors, e.g., composition/functioning of GABA/glutamate receptors
- Ion channelopathies, e.g., sodium, calcium, and potassium channels
- Reactive autoimmunity, e.g., autoantibodies against glutamic acid decarboxylase
- Impaired antiepileptic drug penetration, e.g., P-glycoprotein expression at blood–brain barrier; GABA = γ-aminobutyric acid

Therefore, in many patients, refractory epilepsy declares itself early. Predictors of development of refractory seizures are as follows **(Box 2)**.

Refractory epilepsy is a multifactorial condition. Putative factors contributing to the biological basis of refractory epilepsy are summarized in **Box 3**.

MANAGEMENT STRATEGY

Patients with refractory epilepsy carry the greatest burden of treatment. Management strategies of refractory epilepsy fall into three main categories: pharmacotherapy, epilepsy surgery, and alternative treatment strategies including neurostimulation, ketogenic diet, and lifestyle changes **(Box 4)**.

Epilepsy is a clinical diagnosis. Hence, chance of misdiagnosis is as high as 30% even in specialty clinics. Nonepileptic seizures may constitute up to 25% of cases of drug-resistant epilepsy and perhaps cause the greatest diagnostic illusion. The diagnosis is sometimes become more puzzling as in the 10% of those with nonepileptic seizures who also have simultaneous epileptic seizures. **Table 1** summarizes features to differentiate epileptic from nonepileptic seizures.

BOX 4: General principles of managing refractory epilepsy.

- Review the diagnosis and classification
- Review ASDs currently and previously used
- Consider nonpharmacological treatments
- Address comorbidities and lifestyle issues
- Optimize quality of life

(ASD: antiseizure drug)

TABLE 1: Differentiate between epileptic seizures from nonepileptic seizures.

Feature	Epileptic seizures	Nonepileptic/ dissociative seizures
Nature	Predominately stereotypical	Typically lack consistency
Occurrence during sleep	Can occur from sleep	Rarely occur from sleep
Eyes	Rarely closed	Can be closed
Duration	Rarely longer than seconds to minutes several to tens of minutes in duration	
Breathing	Typically apneic in expiration	May have rapid breathing or breath hold in inspiration
Color	May be cyanosed, pale, or flushed	Rarely cyanosed
Amplitude of movements	Tend to reach maximum then decrease	Can "wax and wane"
Seizure frequency	Typically unpredictable and can "cluster"	Frequency can be regular
Injuries	Can sustain injuries and lateral tongue bites	Rarely sustain injuries or lateral tongue bites

PHARMACOLOGICAL THERAPY IN DRUG-RESISTANT EPILEPSY

Therefore, choice of an optimal ASDs regimen for a case of resistant seizure needs to consider many variables like the pharmacodynamics and pharmacokinetics of ASDs, patient-related factors (age, compliance, comorbidities, and concomitant medications) and a systematic diagnosis of epilepsy syndrome and seizure types.

TABLE 2: Causes of pseudoresistance to ASDs in epilepsy.

Reason	Examples
Wrong diagnosis	Syncope, cardiac arrhythmia, or other conditions; psychogenic nonepileptic seizures
Wrong drug (or drugs)	Inappropriate for seizure type; pharmacokinetic or pharmacodynamic interactions
Wrong dose	Too low (overreliance on "therapeutic" blood levels); side effects preventing drug increase
Lifestyle issues	Poor compliance with medication; alcohol or drug abuse

A newly diagnosed patients with epilepsy are commonly initiated with monotherapy since around 50% of patients with untreated epilepsy achieve prolonged seizure control (>12 months) with a first drug regimen. According to expert opinion, polytherapy should be considered only after the failure of at least two or three monotherapies. Furthermore, recent evidences also suggest choosing duotherapy as an alternative to second drug monotherapy after failure of the initial monotherapy, thus achieving seizure remission of 15–20% as around 60% of patients may obtain seizure freedom after the second drug trial.

Patients who failed to respond to the second drug trial, either in monotherapy or duotherapy, fulfill the ILAE criteria for DRE and should be referred to dedicated epilepsy centers. However, they should be re-assessed (i.e., with prolonged video-EEG, neuroimaging) vigorously to exclude pseudo-pharmacoresistance and to make the correct diagnosis of epilepsy as mentioned in **Table 2**.

Patients who may benefit from surgical treatment like those caused by focal epileptogenic lesions have a higher likelihood of seizure remission (about 60–80%) if they are promptly referred to specialized centers rather than continue subsequent drug trials. Otherwise, if the lesion cannot be completely surgically resected without consequent neurologic morbidities, systematic trials of a second duotherapy or a triple therapy may be required, with a lower percentage of remission. If a 5th or 6th drug trial with dual, triple, or quadruple therapy fail, other alternative therapies should be evaluated. Vagus nerve stimulation (VNS) or ketogenic diet may be actively pursued.

Emerging Antiseizure Drugs to Overcome Drug-resistant Epilepsy

Recently approved ASDs as add-on treatment in patients with focal seizures, with or without secondarily generalization, and primary generalized tonic-clonic seizures are perampanel (2012), eslicarbazepine (2013), brivaracetam (2016), everolimus (2016), cannabidiol/Epidiolex (Greenwich Biosciences; 2018), cenobamate (2019), and fenfluramine (2020), and Stiripentol's 2018 approval was based on earlier European data.

Another Interesting Approach at the Age of Genomic is "Precision Medicine"

There is an evergrowing list of genes carrying rare pathogenic variants in epilepsy. These discoveries facilitate a rational treatment approach with a better selection of ASDs. In some situations, it is now possible to correct specific metabolic defects (e.g., the ketogenic diet for GLUT1 deficiency, or pyridoxine for pyridoxine-dependent epilepsies), avoid ASDs that can potentially deteriorate the pathogenic defect (e.g., the administration of sodium channel blocking drugs in SCN1A-related Dravet syndrome). Discovery of the functional defect caused by gene mutation using existing ASDs (e.g., using sodium channel blockers in SCN8A or SCN2A pathogenetic variants with gain-of-function effect) has streamlined our therapy and we are now using medications already available for other indications (e.g., memantine used to treat epileptic encephalopathy caused by GRIN2A mutation of NMDA glutamate receptors).

ALTERNATIVES TO PHARMACOLOGICAL TREATMENT

The best and potentially alternative to ASMs for patients with refractory epilepsy is surgical treatment, whenever it is possible. Presurgical evaluation with functional neuroimaging and comprehensive neuropsychological testing is crucial for precise localization of the epileptogenic zone and identification of eloquent cortical regions **(Boxes 5 and 6)**.

Neurostimulation devices can either provide continuous stimulation (open loop), or can deliver stimulation based upon detected brain activity (closed-loop). The most widely studied and established invasive neurostimulation approach is vagal nerve stimulation (VNS), followed by deep brain stimulation (DBS), and the more recent ones like responsive neurostimulation (RNS), and chronic subthreshold cortical stimulation (CSCS) **(Box 7)**.

Noninvasive alternatives are transcutaneous vagus nerve stimulation (tVNS), trigeminal nerve stimulation (TNS), transcranial magnetic stimulation (TMS), and transcranial direct current stimulation (tDCS). Current evidences support the efficacy and the safety of VNS, DBS, RNS, and tDCS for DRE in adult patients, mainly with focal seizure onset epilepsy. Unfortunately, despite evolution in the field of numerous devices for neurostimulation,

BOX 5: Presurgical evaluation.

- All patients with refractory seizures after treatment with two appropriate AEDs should be referred to a specialist epilepsy center for evaluation
- A comprehensive history, including drug history and physical examination, is performed to guide the investigations
- Baseline metabolic evaluation of blood and urine, karyotype analysis, and fragile X should be considered
- Analysis of cerebrospinal fluid is recommended for all patients with refractory seizures
- Prolonged video-EEG monitoring and appropriate magnetic resonance brain imaging with specific epilepsy protocol sequences should be performed for all
- Magnetoencephalography (MEG) allows further localization of focal epilepsy
- Multidisciplinary input is required to interpret the results and tailor a patient-specific plan
- Invasive monitoring with subdual electrodes allows precise localization of the epileptogenic zone and identification of eloquent cortical regions and their relation to each other
- Timely evaluation and action is important

BOX 6: Common surgical procedures for epilepsy.

- Anterior temporal lobe resection
- Amygdalohippocampectomy
- Neocortical resection
- Lesionectomy
- Hemispherectomy/hemispherotomy
- Multilobar resection
- Corpus callosotomy
- Multiple subpial transection
- Stereotactic ablation

there is relatively poor knowledge about the underlying mechanisms and a lack of guidelines or consensus or awareness across epileptologists on the judicial usage of these techniques.

Among nonpharmacological treatment approach for refractory seizures, there is the scope for ketogenic diet. This strict dietary regimen is characterized by high-fat and low-carbohydrate levels mimicking fasting but has either fasting or nonfasting modified regimen. This has been commonly practiced among specific groups of children with DRE. However, it is not usually continued long term due to its cost, noncompliance, and metabolic and nutritional issues.

BOX 7: Summary: Practical approach to refractory seizures.

- Referral to specialist epilepsy center
- History and physical examination
- Directed diagnostic investigations
- Scalp video EEG monitoring
- Neuroimaging—brain MRI (epilepsy protocol)
- Functional assessment—language lateralization and neuropsychology
- Review results with expert panel
- *Potential surgical candidate*:
  - Curative—lesionectomy/invasive EEG monitoring and resection
  - Palliative—corpus callosotomy and multiple subpial transections
- Nonsurgical candidate—consider vagal nerve stimulation or dietary options like ketogenic diet

CONCLUSION

Drug therapy remains the first and foremost approach to achieve long-term seizure control. After having a systematic diagnostic classification and the selection of patients who are candidates for resective surgery, it is mandatory to have a checklist to monitor the pharmacodynamic and pharmacokinetic profile of drugs, possible adverse effects, in order to choose adequate drug regimens. In the new second, third, and latest generation ASD era, rational polytherapy has acquired more relevance. So, before considering a patient completely unresponsive to drug therapy, it is necessary to re-assess the diagnosis, along with the genetic background and critically consider the rationality of the previous and current therapeutic regimens. Alternative nonpharmacological approaches such as electrical stimulation and diet therapy are also promising, but they are still far away to achieve long-term seizure control.

SUGGESTED READINGS

1. Kwan P, Brodie MJ. Refractory epilepsy: a progressive, intractable but preventable condition? Seizure. 2002;11(2):77-84.
2. Tang F, Hartz AMS, Bauer B. Drug-resistant Epilepsy: Multiple Hypotheses, Few Answers. Front Neurol. 2017;8:301.
3. Fattorusso A, Matricardi S, Mencaroni E, Dell'Isola GB, Di Cara G, Striano P, et al. The Pharmacoresistant Epilepsy: An Overview on Existant and New Emerging Therapies. Front Neurol. 2021;12:674483.
4. Schuele SU, Lüders HO. Intractable epilepsy: management and therapeutic alternatives. Lancet Neurol. 2008;7(6):514-24.

96

CHAPTER

Understanding Sleep: In Health Perspective

Veerendra Singh

ABSTRACT

Sleep constitutes approximately one-third of human life. Two basic types of sleep are non-rapid eye movement (NREM 1, NREM 2, and NREM 3) and rapid eye movement (REM) sleep. Variability in sleep physiology across childhood influences cognitive performance. Sleep enhances adaptive immune response and long-term antigenic memory. Sleep duration and quality are associated with physical, mental, and immunological health. Sleep deprivation has metabolic consequences, such as obesity and diabetes. With decreased sleep, cognitive tasks are impaired disproportionately. Sleep disorders impact the proper functioning of the body. Seizures can interrupt sleep, while sleep disorders can aggravate seizures. Understanding the factors that improve sleep health has the potential to impact physical and mental health.

INTRODUCTION

Sleep is a naturally recurring, rapidly reversible state of reduced responsiveness, motor activity, and metabolism. Three criteria—reversibility, recurrence, and spontaneity—distinguish sleep from hibernation, coma, or anesthesia. Sleep is accompanied by complex changes in spontaneous brain activity, fluctuations in hormone levels, and relaxation of musculature. The purpose of sleep includes restoration, energy conservation, memory consolidation, and removal of toxins in the brain.

STAGES AND PATTERNS OF SLEEP

Two basic types of sleep are non-rapid eye movement (NREM 1, NREM 2, and NREM 3) and rapid eye movement (REM) sleep. NREM 1 is a transition between wakefulness and sleep. Heartbeat, breathing, and eye movements slow down, and muscles relax. In NREM 2, brain wave activity further slows but with brief bursts of electrical activity. NREM 3 is the period of deep sleep. Brain wave activity goes to the lowest levels. Night terrors occur during non-REM sleep.

During REM sleep, eyes move rapidly from side to side behind closed eyelids, breathing becomes faster and irregular, and heart rate increases to near waking levels. Most of dreaming occurs during REM sleep. Virtual paralysis of limbs prevents one from acting out of dreams.

Typically, NREM3 sleep is present more in the first third of the night, whereas REM sleep predominates the last third of the night. Patterns of sleep change across human development. Infant's sleep duration is halved in adolescence. Sleep is consolidated to a single bout by 5–7 years of age.

CIRCADIAN RHYTHMS

Circadian rhythms control the timing of sleep. The suprachiasmatic nucleus in the anterior hypothalamus sets the body clock with light processing in the retina and time cues entraining to a 24.2-hour cycle. Circadian rhythms are disrupted in night shift workers and people traveling across different time zones, called "Jet-lag".

NEUROPHYSIOLOGY OF SLEEP

During sleep, the brain becomes less responsive to visual, auditory, somatosensory, and other environmental stimuli. Ventrolateral preoptic nucleus of the anterior hypothalamus uses gamma-aminobutyric acid (GABA) and galanin to initiate sleep. Hypocretin (orexin) neurons in the lateral hypothalamus help stabilize sleep.

Sleep represents an optimal time window for consolidating encoded labile memory traces. Declarative memories, which can be consciously recalled, have two components: Episodic memory and semantic memory. Napping benefits declarative memory in infants and continues to support it across early childhood. Sleep has an insignificant impact on adolescent memory consolidation. For nondeclarative memories, role of naps in procedural learning in early childhood is ambiguous. Sleep after learning produces long-lasting procedural memory in adolescence. Emotional memories are strengthened through sleep. Studies using magnetic resonance imaging (MRI) found that infants can differentiate emotional content while sleeping.

SLEEP AND IMMUNE RESPONSES

Sleep and immunity are bidirectionally linked. Sleep enhances adaptive immune response and long-term antigenic memory by increasing the proportion of T cells producing proinflammatory and Th1-cytokines like interleukin 2 (IL-2), interferon-γ, tumor necrosis factor-alpha (TNF-α), and enhancing the production of IL-12 by monocytes and myeloid dendritic cells. Human volunteers who slept normally on the first night after vaccination against hepatitis A displayed a twofold increase in antibody titers.

GENES AND NEUROTRANSMITTERS

Genome-wide association studies have identified sites on various chromosomes that increase susceptibility to sleep disorders. Neurotransmitters that shape sleep include GABA, norepinephrine, orexin, acetylcholine, histamine, adrenaline, cortisol, and serotonin.

SLEEP MEASUREMENT

Polysomnography (PSG) is the gold standard for objectively measuring sleep. Actigraphy is a device worn on the wrist to objectively estimate sleep parameters. Sleep diaries and sleep questionnaires allow subjective estimates of various sleep parameters.

THEORIES OF SLEEP

Adaptive or Evolutionary Theory

Inactivity at night is an adaptation to keep organisms out of harm when they would be particularly vulnerable. A simple counterargument to this theory is that it is always safer to remain conscious in order to be able to react to an emergency.

Energy Conservation Theory

According to this theory, sleep evolved as a means of conserving energy as metabolism is significantly reduced during sleep.

Restorative Theories

Sleep provides an opportunity for the body to repair and rejuvenate itself. The build-up of adenosine in the brain during wakefulness leads to the perception of being tired. During sleep, the body clears adenosine from the system.

Information Consolidation Theory

Sleep helps process information acquired during day and consolidate them into long-term memory.

Brain Plasticity Theory

Sleep is correlated to neural restructuring, which involves changes in the structure and organization of the brain, a phenomenon known as brain plasticity.

Although these theories remain unproven, science has made tremendous strides in discovering what happens during sleep. The reasons and meaning of dreams still remain a mystery.

SLEEP AND HEALTH OUTCOMES

Cardiovascular Health

Sleep duration and quality are associated with hypertension, hyperlipidemia, coronary disease, vascular disease, myocardial infarction, and stroke. The mechanisms implicate sympathetic activation, cellular stress, inflammation, and metabolic dysregulation.

Metabolic Health

There is a cross-sectional relationship between habitual sleep duration outside the normative range and obesity-related outcomes. Sleep loss impairs insulin and glucose homeostasis, disrupts metabolic hormones (e.g., leptin and ghrelin), alters adipose tissue function, and contributes to the incidence of type 2 diabetes mellitus.

Immunological Health

Sleep deprivation generates a proinflammatory state, and alters the expression, production, and function of cytokines, antibodies, and leukocytes. Insufficient sleep has been linked to increased infection, reduced recovery capacity, and blunted vaccine responses. Primary sleep disorders, sleep apnea, and insomnia are associated with elevations in circulating immune markers.

Mental Health

Insomnia is a well-established risk factor for depression, anxiety, alcohol abuse and psychosis. In general, sleep disruption produces basic functional impairments in emotion regulation, recognition, reasoning, and memory.

Behavioral Health

Insufficient sleep and poor sleep quality have been associated with suboptimal dietary health, more sedentary behavior, less exercise, more habitual smoking, and greater use of alcohol.

Cognitive Health

In addition to its acute effects on executive function and declarative memory, poor sleep has been linked with the development of Alzheimer's disease. Sleep contributes to the regulation of amyloid beta (Aβ) and tau proteins and discourages their buildup into pathological aggregates.

SLEEP DISORDERS

Sleep disorders are the conditions that affect sleep quality, timing, or duration to impact the ability of the body to properly function during wake period. International Classification of Sleep Disorders (ICSD) is the most widely used classification of sleep disorders **(Box 1)**.

Insomnia Disorders

Insomnia is the inability to initiate or maintain sleep causing daytime distress. Many factors may contribute to insomnia, including stress, medications, and environment. Cognitive and behavioral programs are effective in the long-term management of insomnia.

BOX 1: The International Classification of Sleep Disorders, 3rd edition, text revision (ICSD-3 TR).

- Insomnia disorders
- Sleep-related breathing disorders
- Central disorders of hypersomnolence
- Circadian rhythm sleep-wake disorders
- Parasomnias
- Sleep-related movement disorders

Source: American Academy of Sleep Medicine. International Classification of Sleep Disorders, 3rd edition, text revision. Illinois: American Academy of Sleep Medicine; 2023.

Sleep-related Breathing Disorders

Sleep-disordered breathing is characterized by abnormal respiration during sleep. It includes obstructive sleep apnea (OSA), central sleep apnea (CSA), sleep-related hypoventilation, and sleep-related hypoxemia disorder.

Obstructive Sleep Apnea

Obstructive sleep apnea is characterized by recurrent episodes of partial or complete closure of the upper airway leading to decreased quality of life, daytime sleepiness, obesity, hypertension, coronary artery disease, atrial fibrillation, and stroke.

Central Sleep Apnea

The airway mechanics are healthy, but the brain does not provide the signals needed to breathe during sleep. Established risk factors include cardiovascular problems, narcotics, and high altitude. Treatment of CSA, mainly, is addressing the underlying cause.

Sleep-related Hypoventilation Disorders

Sleep-related hypoventilation disorders involve elevated blood levels of carbon dioxide during sleep. Chronic obstructive pulmonary disease, pulmonary hypertension, obesity, nervous system disease, and certain medications can trigger hypoventilation.

Sleep-related Hypoxemia Disorders

Sleep-related hypoxemia disorder is when oxygen concentrations drop, but carbon dioxide concentration does not rise high enough, as in hypoventilation.

Snoring and Catathrenia

Snoring occurs when air moves around floppy tissue near the back of the throat and causes that tissue to vibrate. Catathrenia is a pattern of abnormal breathing and vocalization that is often referred to as sleep-related groaning. It can be annoying for bed partners.

Central Disorders of Hypersomnolence

The hallmark of central disorders of hypersomnolence is pathologic daytime sleepiness. ICSD, third edition (ICSD-3) classifies eight different types of this disorder: narcolepsy type 1 (with cataplexy), narcolepsy type 2 (without cataplexy), idiopathic hypersomnia, Kleine-Levin syndrome, hypersomnia associated with a psychiatric disorder, hypersomnia due to a medical disorder, hypersomnia due to a medication or substance, and insufficient sleep syndrome.

Core features of narcolepsy type 1 include cataplexy, sleep paralysis, sleep-related hallucinations, and disrupted nocturnal sleep.

Cataplexy is the sudden loss of muscle tone triggered by strong emotions like laughter, fear, surprise, or anger. It can cause slurred speech, head drop, or complete weakness of most muscles. Knees may suddenly lose strength, causing falls.

Circadian Rhythm Disorders

There are two prominent types: Phase-advanced sleep and phase-delayed sleep. In the former, the sleep onset and waking occur earlier and in the latter, delayed than the social norms. Alterations in the sleep-wake cycle occur in shift workers, those who stay up late, take late afternoon naps, or international travelers crossing time zones. Exposure to blue light-emitting devices, such as smartphones and tablets, prior to falling asleep can contribute to sleep problems, presumably because blue light affects levels of melatonin.

Parasomnias: Disruptive Sleep Disorders

Parasomnias are abnormal behaviors during sleep, falling asleep, or waking up. Although more common in children, parasomnias can occur at any age. ICSD classification divides parasomnias into six groups **(Box 2)**. REM sleep behavior disorder is most commonly associated with an underlying neurologic condition. NREM parasomnias are relatively rare, episodic, and often self-limiting events.

BOX 2: Parasomnias: Disruptive sleep disorders.

- *NERM-related*:
  - Sleepwalking
  - Confusional arousal
  - Night terror
- *REM-related*:
  - REM sleep behavior disorder
  - Recurrent isolated sleep paralysis
  - Nightmare disorder
- *Others:* Both NREM and REM related—
  - Enuresis
  - Exploding head syndrome
  - Sleep-related hallucinations
  - Sleep-related eating disorder
  - Sleep-related sexual behavior
- Parasomnia due to drug or substance use
- Parasomnia due to medical condition
- Parasomnia, unspecified

(NREM: non-rapid eye movement; REM: rapid eye movement)

Source: American Academy of Sleep Medicine. International Classification of Sleep Disorders. Illinois: American Academy of Sleep Medicine; 2007.

Sleep-related Movement Disorders

Restless legs syndrome (RLS) and periodic limb movement disorder (PLMD) are two sleep-related movement disorders. In RLS, an uncomfortable sensation in the legs makes movement irresistible. There is a circadian variation in the symptoms and most people experience periodic movements of legs, which can disrupt sleep.

EFFECTS OF SLEEP DEPRIVATION

Total sleep deprivation results in death in animals. Sleep deprivation can interfere with work, school, driving, and social functioning. 13% of work injuries could be attributed to poor sleep. Chronic sleep deprivation increases long-term risk of physical and mental health problems. Under or oversleeping can cause tiredness, headaches, weight gain, low immunity, mood changes, trouble concentrating, and decreased libido. Sleep deprivation has metabolic consequences, such as obesity and diabetes, and impairment of cognitive tasks.

DISORDERS ACCENTUATED DURING SLEEP

Attacks of angina and gastric acid secretions can be augmented by the activation of the autonomic nervous system in REM sleep. NREM sleep can increase epileptic discharge. In general, NREM sleep facilitates interictal epileptiform activity (IEA). REM sleep inhibits IEA and is protective against seizures. Depressed people sleep either too much or not enough.

EFFECT OF SLEEP DISORDERS ON EPILEPSY

Nocturnal seizures can interrupt sleep, while sleep disorders can aggravate seizures. Sleep deprivation is the most potent trigger of epileptic seizures and epileptiform discharges. Patients with epilepsy have reduced NREM (NREM 2 and NREM 3) and REM sleep. Antiepileptic drugs have differential effects on sleep architecture. Gabapentin, tiagabine, pregabalin, clobazam, and carbamazepine reduce sleep latency and improve sleep efficiency. Phenobarbital, carbamazepine, phenytoin, valproic acid, and levetiracetam aggravate daytime sleepiness. Felbamate, zonisamide, and lamotrigine at high doses cause insomnia. Topiramate, vigabatrin, lacosamide, and low-dose zonisamide, lamotrigine, and levetiracetam have minimal effect on sleep architecture.

CONCLUSION

Sleep is accompanied by complex changes in spontaneous brain activity, fluctuations in hormone levels, and relaxation of musculature. Variability in sleep physiology across childhood influences cognitive performance. Sleep deprivation has metabolic consequences, such as obesity and diabetes. Understanding the factors that shape sleep health has the potential to improve intervention strategies and identify therapeutic targets applicable to cardiovascular, neurocognitive, neurodegenerative, and immune-related disorders.

SUGGESTED READINGS

1. Siegel JM. Sleep viewed as a state of adaptive inactivity. Nat Rev Neurosci. 2009;10(10):747-53.
2. Grandner MA, Alfonso-Miller P, Fernandez-Mendoza J, Shetty S, Shenoy S, Combs D. Sleep: important considerations for the prevention of cardiovascular disease. Curr Opin Cardiol. 2016;31(5):551-65.
3. Koren D, Taveras EM. Association of sleep disturbances with obesity, insulin resistance and the metabolic syndrome. Metabolism. 2018;84:67-75.
4. Hertenstein E, Feige B, Gmeiner T, Kienzler C, Spiegelhalder K, Johann A, et al. Insomnia as a predictor of mental disorders: A systematic review and meta-analysis. Sleep Med Rev. 2019;43:96-105.
5. Bazil CW, Short D, Crispin D, Zheng W. Patients with intractable epilepsy have low melatonin, which increases following seizures. Neurology. 2000;55(11):1746-8.

97

CHAPTER

Longitudinally Extensive Transverse Myelitis: Differential Diagnosis

Arunmozhimaran Elavarasi, Kameshwar Prasad

ABSTRACT

Transverse myelitis (TM) is a clinical syndrome characterized by sensory, motor, sphincter, and autonomic involvement due to an inflammatory lesion in the spinal cord. TM is characterized by symmetric bilateral weakness along with sensory loss. When the clinical picture of TM is associated with T2-weighted hyperintensity extending over three or more vertebral segments in sagittal spinal magnetic resonance imaging, the term longitudinally extensive transverse myelitis (LETM) is used. Thus, TM is a clinical syndrome, while LETM is a clinicoradiologic syndrome. Acute TM is a clinical syndrome with onset and progression over hours to days. Some may have weakness as the initial symptom, while others may present with bladder retention, following which weakness occurs after a few hours or days. Though immune-mediated inflammatory myelopathies are the most common cause of LETM, noninflammatory etiologies and other causes of LETM should not be overlooked as they have completely different therapeutics and prognoses. The diagnostic workup of a patient with myelopathy is presented in this chapter.

INTRODUCTION

Transverse myelitis (TM) is a clinical syndrome characterized by sensory, motor, sphincter, and autonomic involvement. TM implies focal spinal cord dysfunction due to an inflammatory lesion. In patients who present with paraparesis or quadriparesis with or without other features, spinal cord localization is always a consideration. TM is characterized by symmetric bilateral weakness along with sensory loss. When the clinical picture of TM is associated with T2-weighted hyperintensity extending over three or more vertebral segments in sagittal spinal magnetic resonance imaging (MRI), the term longitudinally extensive transverse myelitis (LETM) is used. Thus, TM is a clinical syndrome, while LETM is a clinicoradiologic syndrome.

With the availability of high-quality imaging and ease of access to MRI, diagnosing LETM has been made easier. However, the differential diagnosis and diagnostic workup of LETM are expanding with the discovery of newer antibodies. Though immune-mediated inflammatory myelopathies are the most common cause of LETM, noninflammatory etiologies and other causes of LETM should not be overlooked as they have completely different therapeutics and prognoses.

CASE VIGNETTE 1

A 30-year-old male presented with a tingling sensation in both lower limbs, left more than right, starting from the feet and extending up to the knees. The very next day, he felt weakness in both lower limbs such that he could not walk and needed one person's support to walk. This weakness progressed over the next 5 days to a nadir where he could not move his legs at all, and also he felt weakness in his right upper limb with a band-like sensation in the upper chest. He also had retention of urine, for which he was catheterized. He had hyperreflexia of all four limbs and sensory loss for all modalities below the level of T4. History revealed that the patient had refractory hiccoughs lasting a few days a month before presentation, which resolved spontaneously. MRI revealed LETM extending from the lower medulla to the D5 level **(Figs. 1A and B)**. The patient underwent a cerebrospinal fluid (CSF)

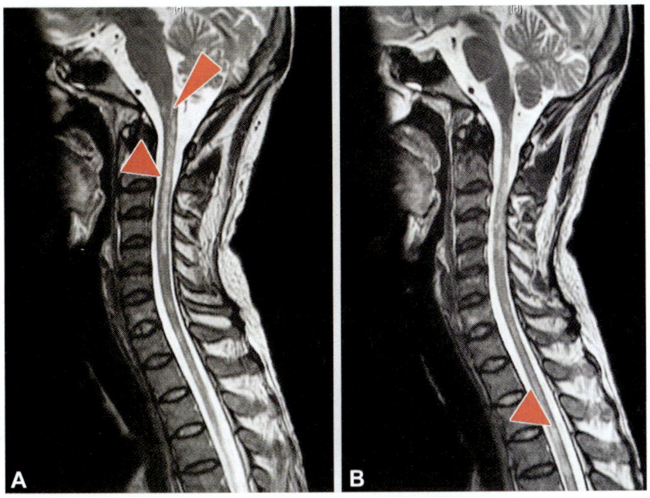

FIGS. 1A AND B: Long segment T2-hyperintense lesion in the spinal cord extending from the lower medulla to C5 cervical cord level (short arrowhead). The lesion extends into the area postrema of the medulla (A: red arrowhead). (B) The lesion extending well below the thoracic spinal cord with skip areas between the cervical and dorsal spine lesions.

examination which revealed lymphocytic pleocytosis with increased protein and normal glucose. Serum aquaporin-4 and myelin oligodendrocyte glycoprotein (MOG) antibodies were negative.

CASE VIGNETTE 2

An 18-year-old man presented with progressive walking difficulty and pain in both lower limbs for 8 months. He was evaluated in another center and started on dexamethasone based on MRI showing LETM. There was a symptomatic improvement for a few weeks, and then he worsened and became bedbound after around 1 month. He developed urinary urgency and urge incontinence, upper limb weakness, and facial and bulbar weakness 2 months later and had three seizures. Based on CSF showing lymphocytic pleocytosis, he was started on antitubercular therapy and corticosteroids. The seizures were thought to be due to sequelae of past head trauma.

On examination, general physical examination was normal, and there was no peripheral lymphadenopathy. He had a right scrotal mass. Neurologic examination revealed bilateral facial, palatal and pharyngeal weakness, and areflexic quadriparesis. MRI revealed LETM. CSF examination showed a T-cell lymphoma restricted to the central nervous system (CNS) as the peripheral smear, bone marrow, and positron emission tomography (PET) scan did not reveal the involvement of other sites.

CLINICAL FEATURES

The spinal cord has several afferent and efferent tracts in a tightly compact structure. The corticospinal tracts, spinothalamic and spinocerebellar tracts, and posterior columns lie in the white matter of the spinal cord. The anterior horn cells lie in the central gray matter of the spinal cord. The spinal cord has both the upper and lower motor neurons and thus can present with weakness with spasticity and hyperreflexia (except in the acute phase when hypotonia and areflexia may be seen due to spinal shock phase) or wasting and fasciculations, depending on the level and extent of involvement. The involvement of specific tracts leads to the clinical features in specific patterns which can be identified based on the deficits.

Transverse myelitis is classically associated with bilateral loss of motor, sensory, and autonomic functions below the level of involvement. It may or may not be symmetrical. The presence of sensory level with reduced or lost sensations below a spinal level is characteristic of a spinal cord lesion.

The acute transverse myelitis (ATM) consortium working group laid down the diagnostic criteria for transverse myelitis (TM) **(Box 1)**.

The initial stages may be associated with flaccid weakness (associated with hypotonia and areflexia) with retention of urine and constipation. This is referred to as the stage of "spinal shock". Later, the patient may develop spasticity with an overactive bladder. Up to one-third of patients with idiopathic TM have a complete to near complete recovery, one-third are left with deficits, and one-third may not recover following treatment.

BOX 1: Acute transverse myelitis consortium working group criteria for diagnosis of transverse myelitis.

- Sensory, motor, or autonomic dysfunction attributable to the spinal cord
- Bilateral symmetric or asymmetric signs and/or symptoms
- Definite sensory level
- Magnetic resonance (MR) spine excluded compressive extra-axial lesion
- Spinal cord inflammation as evidenced by cerebrospinal fluid (CSF) pleocytosis/elevated immunoglobulin G (IgG) index/imaging showing gadolinium enhancement
- If the above criteria are not met, repeat magnetic resonance imaging (MRI) and lumbar puncture evaluation between 2 and 7 days after the onset of symptoms shows the above findings
- Onset to nadir ranges from 4 hours to 21 days, and if the patient woke up with symptoms, some progression should be demonstrated on history

LOCALIZATION AND DIFFERENTIALS

Acute transverse myelitis is a clinical syndrome with onset and progression over hours to days. So, depending on the tempo of progression, the patient may present with forme-fruste of ATM. Some may have weakness as the initial symptom, while others may present with bladder retention, following which weakness occurs after a few hours or days. The onset may be asymmetrical. So, in the initial stages, e.g., if the central part of the cord is involved first, the patient may present with a pure motor syndrome. Weakness and sphincter involvement imply an anterolateral cord syndrome. Loss of proprioception with or without weakness implies a posterior cord syndrome. **Box 2** lists the possible differentials in terms of localization.

OTHER CLINICAL FEATURES

Patients with LETM may have had a history of other deficits such as vision loss, recurrent hiccoughs, and transient weakness, which suggest the involvement of other areas of the CNS such as optic nerves and chiasm or the area postrema, which are characteristic locations of involvement in patients with neuromyelitis optica spectrum disorders (NMOSDs). These symptoms strongly suggest demyelination as the cause of the LETM. However, patients may have vision loss and cerebral involvement in conditions such as systemic lupus erythematosus (SLE), Behçet's disease, leukemia, or lymphoma. Demyelinating disorders have an onset to nadir time of 4 hours to 21 days. Onset to the nadir of <4 hours is usually seen in spinal cord infarction, and longer progression may indicate other etiologies of LETM, as listed in **Box 3**.

BOX 2: Differentials for localization—mimics and chameleons.

Pure motor syndrome:
- Anterior horn cell myelitis
- Acute polyradiculopathy
- Acute polyneuropathy
- Limb-girdle myasthenia
- Acute myositis

Sensory motor syndrome with or without sphincter involvement:
- Acute transverse myelitis
- Acute polyradiculopathy—cauda-conus syndrome
- Parasagittal cerebral lesion

Pure sensory syndrome:
- Posterior cord syndrome
- Ganglionopathy
- Acute inflammatory sensory radiculopathy

DIAGNOSTIC EVALUATION

Magnetic Resonance Imaging Spine

Magnetic resonance imaging spine is the first investigation if myelopathy is a consideration. In patients with myelopathy, MR rapidly differentiates compressive from noncompressive myelopathies. The clinical history and examination lack sensitivity and specificity in ruling out a compressive lesion. ATM, by definition, needs MRI to rule out compressive etiologies.

Longitudinally Extensive Transverse Myelitis

Longitudinally extensive transverse myelitis is a radiologic diagnosis in which the vertical extent of the lesion is more than three contiguous vertebral segments in the T2 sequence of sagittal spinal MRI. The horizontal extent involves at least two-thirds of the spinal cord and involves the central part of the spinal cord. LETM is commonly associated with NMOSD in the setting of acute presentation. This radiologic finding can also occur in other demyelinating conditions such as multiple sclerosis (MS). Though MS lesions are usually characterized by shorter lesions that predominantly involve the periphery of the spinal cord, the presence of confluent lesions in MS may present radiologically with LETM. Spinal cord infarction is characterized by anterior cord lesions with diffusion restriction on MRI and involvement of the vertebral bodies. Sarcoidosis is usually associated with dural lesions. Dural arteriovenous (AV) fistulas have a characteristic appearance with increased flow voids on MRI. Cord contusions, nucleus pulposus embolism, and cord herniation may also be identified on MRI. **Box 3** lists the etiologic differentials for a radiologic case of LETM.

Cerebrospinal Fluid Examination

Cerebrospinal fluid examination can help in the etiologic diagnosis. In LETM, the patient has an inflammatory CSF picture with lymphocytic pleocytosis, raised protein, and low sugar. The cell count is usually <100 cells/mm^3 but may be in several hundreds in case of acute necrotizing myelitis. Nevertheless, a very high CSF cell count should point toward an infectious cause such as viral myelitis. Tuberculosis also can present with a similar picture, but the CSF sugars may be low. CSF hypoglycorrhachia can occur in noninfectious causes, such as sarcoidosis, and neoplastic causes such as leukemias and lymphomas. Noninflammatory CSF picture is seen in other causes of LETM, such as dural AV fistula, spinal cord tumors such as ependymomas and astrocytomas, spinal cord infarction, traumatic concussion, and metabolic myelopathies, which help in the diagnostic pathway.

BOX 3: Radiologic differentials.

Inflammatory:
- Primary demyelination
- Neuromyelitis optica spectrum disorders
- MOG antibody-associated demyelination
- Multiple sclerosis
- Immune-mediated disorders
- Systemic lupus erythematosus
- Behçet's disease
- Sarcoidosis
- Sjögren's myelopathy
- Parainfectious/postvaccinial myelitis

Infectious myelitis:
- Tuberculosis
- Viral myelitis—enteroviruses; herpes viruses—HSV, VZV, CMV, HIV, and HTLV
- Syphilis
- Lyme disease
- Schistosomiasis

Neoplastic myelopathy:
- Lymphoma/leukemia
- Postradiation myelitis
- Paraneoplastic myelitis
- Astrocytomas/ependymomas

Vascular myelopathy:
- Spinal cord infarction
- Dural AV fistula-related myelopathy
- Nucleus pulposus embolism

Toxic/metabolic myelopathies:
- B12 deficiency—subacute combined degeneration
- Nitrous oxide intoxication
- Copper deficiency
- Biotinidase deficiency
- MTHFR mutations and disorders of folate metabolism

Trauma-related causes:
- Hematomyelia
- Traumatic myelopathy—spinal cord contusion

(AV: arteriovenous; CMV: cytomegalovirus; HIV: human immunodeficiency virus; HSV: herpes simplex virus; HTLV: human T-lymphotropic virus; MOG: myelin oligodendrocyte glycoprotein; VZV: varicella zoster virus)

Cerebrospinal fluid polymerase chain reaction (PCR) for viral panels can help clinch the diagnosis in the appropriate setting. With the availability of pan-viral PCR panels and next-generation sequencing, diagnosing infective causes of myelitis has become easier. In the appropriate clinical setting, testing for syphilis, Lyme disease, brucellosis, CSF GeneXpert, and mycobacterial culture may be required.

Antibody Testing

Neuromyelitis optica spectrum disorder may be associated with antibodies to aquaporin-4 in up to 70% of cases. Aquaporin-4-negative patients may show MOG antibody positivity.

Inflammatory diseases such as Behçet's disease, SLE-related myelopathy, and Sjögren's syndrome may lead to LETM. In the appropriate setting, autoantibody profiles, pathergy testing, salivary scintigraphy, Schirmer's test, and lip biopsy for Sjögren's syndrome may help narrow the differentials. Paraneoplastic myelitis may be associated with anti-collapsin response mediator protein 5 (anti-CRMP-5) antibodies. A PET scan may be done in case of a high index of suspicion.

Metabolic Panels

Vitamin B12 deficiency and disorders of folate metabolism may present with LETM. There have been case reports of *MTHFR* mutations and defects of the folate metabolism presenting with vision loss and paraparesis, which is a differential diagnosis for NMOSD. These patients may have a complete response to treatment with L-methyl folate. Reduced serum B12 or folate and raised homocysteine and methylmalonic acid levels suggest these disorders. An exome sequencing can reveal other metabolic disorders, such as biotinidase deficiency, which can have a similar presentation. Copper deficiency may be evaluated with serum ceruloplasmin and copper levels.

CASE VIGNETTE 1 CONTINUED

The patient was treated with corticosteroids and plasma exchange with near-complete recovery. A diagnosis of NMOSD was made since the patient had a history of area postrema syndrome, and imaging confirmed the same. He was treated with rituximab infusions and is now relapse-free.

CONCLUSION

Longitudinally extensive transverse myelopathy is a clinicoradiologic syndrome with several etiologic differentials. Careful clinical history, detailed general examination, and imaging evaluation can guide appropriate investigation panels. Inflammatory demyelination is the most common cause of LETM, with NMOSD topping the list. Early and appropriate management can be rewarding as most diseases on the list have specific therapy, and patients may be restored to their functional baseline.

SUGGESTED READINGS

1. Transverse Myelitis Consortium Working Group. Proposed diagnostic criteria and nosology of acute transverse myelitis. Neurology. 2002;59(4):499-505.
2. Beh SC, Greenberg BM, Frohman T, Frohman EM. Transverse Myelitis. Neurol Clin. 2013;31(1):79-138.
3. Kitley JL, Leite MI, George JS, Palace JA. The differential diagnosis of longitudinally extensive transverse myelitis. Mult Scler. 2012;18(3):271-85.
4. Murphy OC, Barrera P, Villabona-Rueda A, Mealy M, Pardo CA. Identification of specific causes of myelopathy in a large cohort of patients initially diagnosed with transverse myelitis. J Neurol Sci. 2022;442:120425.
5. Nightingale H, Witherick J, Wilkins A. Diagnosis of longitudinally extensive transverse myelitis. BMJ Case Rep. 2011;2011:bcr1020103444.
6. Roman GC. Proposed diagnostic criteria and nosology of acute transverse myelitis. Neurology. 2023;60(4):730-1.
7. Tobin WO, Weinshenker BG, Lucchinetti CF. Longitudinally extensive transverse myelitis. Curr Opin Neurol. 2014;27(3):279-89.
8. Trebst C, Raab P, Voss EV, Rommer P, Abu-Mugheisib M, Zettl UK, et al. Longitudinal extensive transverse myelitis—it's not all neuromyelitis optica. Nat Rev Neurol. 2011;7(12):688-98.
9. Weidauer S, Hattinge E, Arendt CT. Cervical myelitis: a practical approach to its differential diagnosis on MR imaging. Rofo. 2023;195(12):1081-96.
10. ElavarasiA, Dash D, Warrier AR, Bhatia R, Kumar L, Jain D, et al. Spinal cord involvement in primary CNS lymphoma. J Clin Neurosci. 2018;47:145-8.

98

CHAPTER

Approach to Transient Loss of Consciousness

Amit Aggarwal, MPS Chawla

ABSTRACT

Events regarding transient loss of consciousness (TLOC) present diagnostic dilemmas due to diverse etiologies and varied risk factors, and commonly involve multidisciplinary specialties. A systematic classification scheme is required to define the pathophysiology and clinical features of TLOC in a lucid manner in order to aid diagnosis, thus avoiding confusion due to inconsistent terminology. TLOC is defined as short duration, abrupt onset, and apparent loss of consciousness followed by spontaneous and complete recovery. Major forms of TLOC are syncope, generalized epileptic seizures, functional TLOC, and a group of related miscellaneous disorders and mimics. The management of patients experiencing TLOC requires recognition of defining clinical features of each of these major groups, and coordination between different clinical specialties in order to formulate a valid clinical approach.

INTRODUCTION

Brief episodes of unconsciousness are difficult to diagnose because the spells typically terminate by the time the patient consults a physician. The medical description of the episode by the patient is mostly unreliable and often non-contributory towards a specific underlying etiology. The causes of transient loss of consciousness (TLOC) commonly include cardiac arrhythmias, postural hypotension, drugs, epileptic seizures, parasomnias, concussion, functional/psychogenic disorders, and organic encephalopathies. Diagnostic insecurity leads to either a "shotgun" approach targeting all possible causes or conversely, a purely restricted approach to one's own speciality. The latter approach commonly leads to many erroneous diagnoses of epilepsy.

Reflex syncope is one of the most common causes of TLOC affecting up to 40% of individuals in any study cohort. The term "syncope" is used by many clinicians for various causes, whereas some others ascribe it to purely cerebral hypoperfusion. This ambiguity was addressed by the multidisciplinary task force on syncope with the introduction of the term TLOC to describe the wider concept of brief episodes of unconsciousness, rendering syncope as just one form of TLOC under the resulting classification scheme.

DEFINITIONS

The term "unconscious" is commonly used to describe a state ranging from complete alertness, through somnolence or stupor, to coma. "Unconsciousness" is used exclusively in the latter sense in our definition of TLOC, implying an association with loss of postural control and falling. The word "unconscious" may also be used to describe states such as absence and complex partial seizures, where patients seem to be awake but unaware of themselves or their environment, but not included as a form of TLOC, as patients usually remain upright during attacks. The occurrence of loss of consciousness in TLOC is determined by using three key features elicited in the medical history, which are as follows:

1. Loss of normal motor control manifested as either flaccidity or rigidity, and loss of postural control resulting in a fall, which may or may not be accompanied by jerky limb movements.
2. Loss of normal responsiveness.
3. Total amnesia for the event.

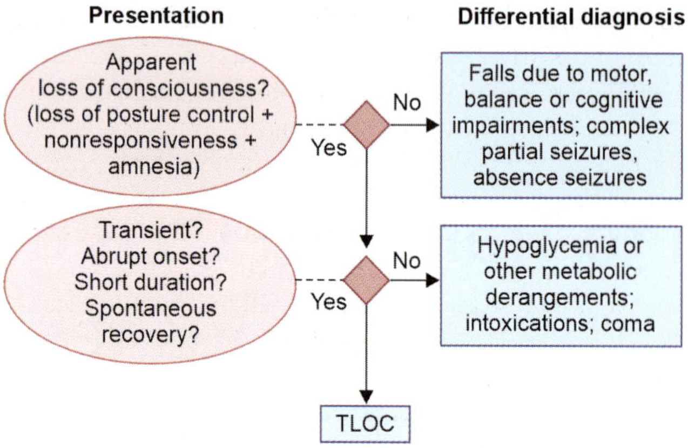

FIG. 1: Main features of transient loss of consciousness (TLOC) and differential diagnosis.

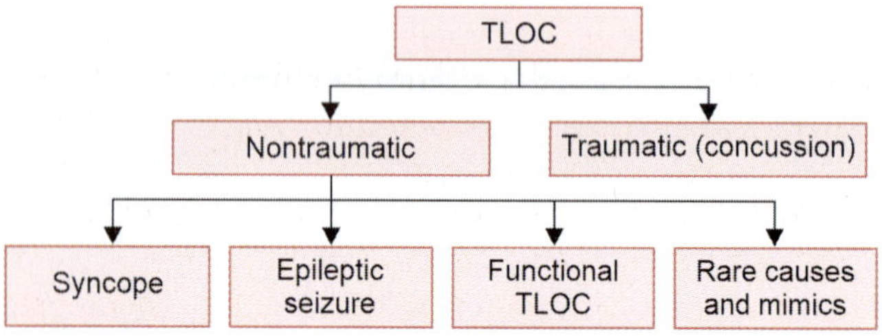

FLOWCHART 1: Main forms of transient loss of consciousness (TLOC).

Transient loss of consciousness is defined as a short duration, rapid onset, and apparent loss of consciousness followed by spontaneous and complete recovery. This description includes disorders where consciousness seems to be lost, such as functional and psychogenic TLOC. The fact that these spells can be mistaken for either epilepsy or syncope warrants their inclusion in the classification. Any deviation from the defining features changes the differential diagnosis; e.g., a longer duration of spell excludes syncope but includes intoxications or metabolic encephalopathies, and lack of unconsciousness would necessitate other causes of falls to be ruled out as outlined in **Figure 1**.

Transient loss of consciousness can be traumatic (concussion), where the underlying cause is obvious, and non-traumatic as described in **Flowchart 1**. The miscellaneous group includes rare disorders that cause TLOC and conditions that can be mistaken for it, and do not share a common underlying pathophysiology or presentation.

A detailed classification scheme of the main forms of TLOC is described in **Box 1**. Transient loss of consciousness due to cerebral concussion is not discussed in detail due to obvious underlying cause.

BOX 1: Classification of transient loss of consciousness (TLOC).

Classification of TLOC

The conditions listed are predominantly those that cause syncope in adults. The group "syncope caused by mechanical and/or hydraulic factors" encompasses forms of syncope in which gravitational stress and increased intrathoracic pressure cause a temporary reduction in cardiac output.

- Syncope:
  - *Reflex (neurally-mediated) syncope*:
    - *Vasovagal syncope*: Triggered by pain, fear, instrumentation (e.g., hypodermic needles) or standing for an extended period
    - *Situational syncope*: Triggered by coughing, sneezing, micturition, or gastrointestinal stimulation (swallowing, defecation, and visceral pain)
    - Carotid sinus syncope
    - *Syncope caused by mechanical and/or hydraulic factors*: Triggers include the "mess trick" (a self-induced form of syncope), playing wind instruments, and straining
  - *Syncope due to orthostatic hypotension*:
    - Primary autonomic failure
    - Secondary autonomic failure
    - Drug-induced autonomic failure
    - Volume depletion
  - *Cardiac syncope*:
    - *Arrhythmias as primary cause*: The causes include bradycardia (due to sinus node dysfunction, atrioventricular node dysfunction, pacemaker or implantable cardioverter-defibrillator malfunction, or drugs) and tachycardia (supraventricular or ventricular)
    - *Structural diseases*: Cardiac disease (valvular disease, infarction and/or ischemia, hypertrophic cardiomyopathy, cardiac masses, pericardial disease or tamponade, and congenital anomalies of coronary arteries), pulmonary embolus, acute aortic dissection, or pulmonary hypertension
- *Epileptic seizures*:
  - *Primary generalized*:
    - Tonic, clonic, and tonic–clonic
    - Atonic
  - Secondary generalized
- *Functional TLOC:*
  - Functional TLOC mimicking epileptic seizures (pseudoseizures)
  - Functional TLOC mimicking syncope (pseudosyncope)
- *Miscellaneous causes and mimics:*
  - Vertebrobasilar transient ischemic attacks and stroke
  - Subclavian steal syndrome
  - Cataplexy
  - Excessive daytime sleepiness
  - Metabolic disorders (hypoglycemia)
  - "Drop attacks"

SYNCOPE

"Syncope" is defined as TLOC due to cerebral hypoperfusion. The clinical features of syncope are related to the consequences of cerebral hypoperfusion and the underlying cause. However, not every clinical feature is manifested in all the episodes, owing to the differences in the rapidity of onset. In cardiac asystole, individuals notice very few features before loss of consciousness culminating in precipitous syncope. Whereas in autonomic failure, more features are observed before the onset of syncope, such as difficulty in thinking and lightheadedness, followed by loss of color vision and blurring of vision. The sounds may seem distant and the individuals lose the ability to act purposefully while still maintaining awareness, just before becoming unconscious. The onset of unconsciousness is accompanied by loss of voluntary motor control and flaccidity during falls, although stiffness may also occur sometimes. Breathing may be shallow and the blood pressure is barely recordable. Usually, the eyes remain open, even if they were closed before the attack began, and is directed upward or straight ahead. Myoclonic jerking of limbs may also occur lasting for a few seconds, are small in amplitude, not cause pronounced bending of knees or elbows, and is not rhythmic or synchronous. But tonic-clonic movements are absent. Tongue biting is very rare in syncope, and even when it occurs it usually involves the tip, rather than the sides as in epilepsy. Unconsciousness usually lasts < 20 seconds in syncope, but can last longer if the patient is kept upright. Falling or lying down results in an increase in venous return and cardiac output, leading to a rise in blood pressure restoring cerebral perfusion and recovery from syncope. After the fainting spell, the patient experiences some residual weakness; but unlike in the postictal phase, confusion, drowsiness, and headaches are not observed.

Causes of Syncope

Reflex or Neurally-mediated Syncope

It is both preceded and followed by autonomic activation, characterized by nausea, a deathly white pallor, and sweating. A key feature is that it is usually triggered, and numerous variants are named as per the inciting trigger.

Vasovagal Syncope

The most common triggers are acute pain, fear, or prolonged standing. It occurs at some point in up to 40% of individuals and has a pronounced familial occurrence. The incidence peaks initially at 13–16 years of age, is relatively rare during most of adult life, but reemerges in old age after the sixth decade. First episodes are uncommon beyond the age of 35 years and alternative causes should be considered. The pathophysiology is poorly understood, particularly in cases of pure emotional syncope, where the mere sight of blood might trigger syncope even in the supine position; however, it is postulated to result from the withdrawal of sympathetic activity, thus releasing vasoconstriction and leading to a fall in systemic vascular resistance. Fall in blood pressure is less steep in the elderly than in younger patients. It is considered that unconsciousness ensues when mean cerebral blood pressure falls to around 40 mm Hg. Arterial hypotension is counteracted by arterial baroreflexes, by increasing systemic vascular resistance and heart rate. In orthostatic vasovagal syncope, the blood pressure and heart rate fall precipitously after a period of instability with oscillations. This later phase is the actual syncopal reflex. Syncope in which bradycardia is a more important contributory factor than hypotension is termed "cardioinhibitory vasovagal syncope." If hypotension occurs without significant bradycardia, the reflex is called "vasodepressive vasovagal syncope." Orthostatic vasovagal syncope consistently occurs when cardiac output decreases by almost 50%, explaining its common occurrence with hypovolemia (blood or fluid losses) or cutaneous vasodilatation (fever, excessive heat, or alcohol use).

Situational Syncope

The term "situational syncope" indicates syncope elicited by various specific triggers, such as micturition, coughing, sneezing, and gastrointestinal stimulation (swallowing, defecation, and visceral pain). The awareness of these specific triggers aids in the diagnosis.

Carotid Sinus Syncope

It encompasses both spontaneous and induced carotid sinus syncope. A spontaneous variant is a rare form (<1% cases) in which external pressure exerted on the carotid sinus (tight-collared clothing or shaving) raises the blood pressure, which is subsequently lowered down by the "baroreflex" through bradycardia and/or vasodilatation. Carotid sinus hypersensitivity is tested in the elderly by carotid sinus massage, usually in the context of a tilt table test. If massage results in a short asystole of at least 3 seconds and/or a blood pressure drop of over 50 mm Hg but no syncope, the response is hypersensitive. Whereas, if massage results in syncope, which requires a longer period of asystole or very low blood pressure, the response is called *induced carotid sinus syncope*.

Syncope Triggered by Mechanical or Hydraulic Factors

The triggers include the "Mess Trick," which is a type of self-induced syncope (fainting lark) precipitated by simultaneous squatting with hyperventilation followed by sudden erect posturing or forced Valsalva maneuver. Other causes may be straining, weightlifting, or playing wind instruments.

Syncope due to Orthostatic Hypotension

Orthostatic hypotension is defined as a fall in systolic blood pressure of 20 mm Hg or more, and/or a drop in diastolic pressure of 10 mm Hg or more, within 3 minutes of standing up. This leads to syncope only if the blood pressure drop is pronounced. The 3-minute period is generally accepted for routine clinical purposes and gives a 50% yield of abnormal results in cases of autonomic dysfunction. **Figures 2A and B** compare the events in orthostatic hypotension with those in vasovagal syncope.

- Standing rarely evokes vasovagal syncope and the timing is not related to the duration of standing. Sweating, nausea, and pallor occur before hypotension or bradycardia, indicating dysfunctional autonomic adjustments to standing. In both vasodepressor and cardioinhibitory vasovagal syncope, a fall in blood pressure signifies the onset of the reflex proper. Syncope causes a fall that rapidly restores blood pressure, except when asystole occurs; when circulation resumes on terminating asystole.
- In syncope due to orthostatic hypotension, blood pressure falls immediately on standing up. Unlike vasovagal syncope while standing, orthostatic hypotension recurs on standing up repeatedly, although to a varied extent. A compensatory increase in the heart rate occurs, depending upon the extent of autonomic dysfunction. Blood pressure declines less rapidly as standing continues and stabilizes at a lower level unless syncope intervenes. The lying down position helps to restore blood pressure.

Orthostatic hypotension occurs usually by drugs that cause vasodilatation or hypovolemia, and less often by autonomic failure, in the context of the inability of the autonomic nervous system to adjust blood pressure on rising to an upright position. "Primary autonomic failure" includes neurodegenerative diseases such as pure autonomic failure, multiple system atrophy, Lewy body dementia, and Parkinson's disease with autonomic failure. "Secondary autonomic failure" denotes diseases that are not primarily neurodegenerative in nature but damage the autonomic system, such as diabetes mellitus and amyloidosis. The clinical features associated with orthostatic hypotension fall under the heading of "orthostatic intolerance," which includes light-headedness and dizziness, and relatively rarely "syncope." The symptoms do not necessarily appear immediately upon standing up. Pain in the neck and shoulders (coat hanger pain) due to ischemia of local muscles, which resolves on lying down, provides a diagnostic clue. Few individuals with orthostatic hypotension due to autonomic failure also get postexercise hypotension, when orthostatic intolerance occurs soon after cessation of physical exercise, such as resting after climbing a flight of stairs and terminating a brisk wall suddenly. Some individuals may suffer from postprandial hypotension after ingestion of heavy meals.

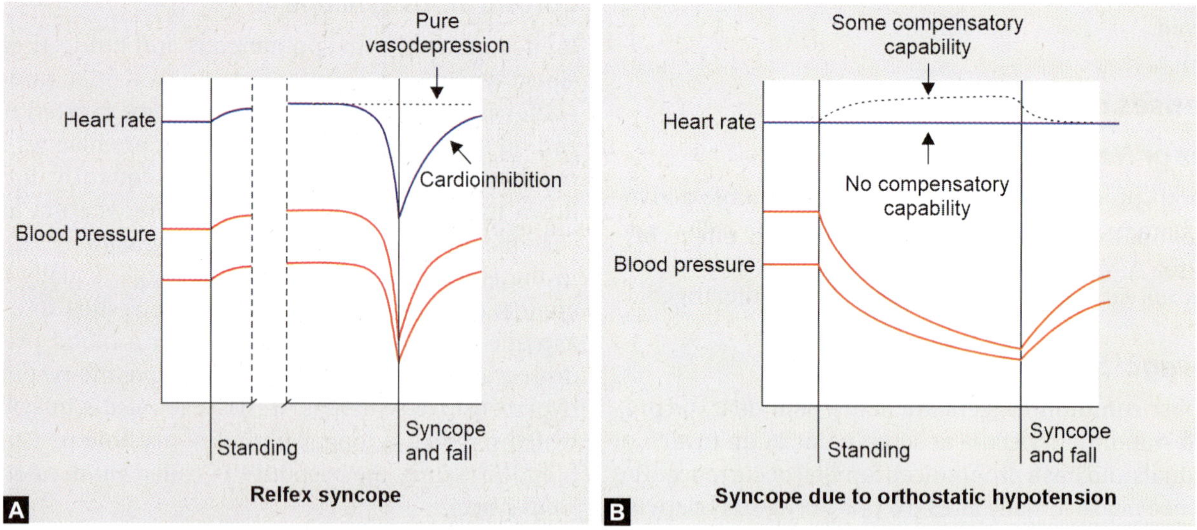

FIGS. 2A AND B: Circulatory patterns in vasovagal syncope evoked by standing and syncope due to orthostatic hypotension.

"Initial orthostatic hypotension" refers to brief lightheadedness and visual blurring on rising suddenly after prolonged rest, or from squatting. This phenomenon may occur in otherwise healthy individuals and sometimes cause syncope. It is attributable to a mismatch between cardiac output and systemic vascular resistance, caused by the failure of an otherwise normal autonomic system to adapt to the hemodynamics promptly to the upright posture. These episodes are so brief that they can only be detected with continuous blood pressure monitoring. "Delayed orthostatic hypotension" appears >3 minutes after standing, the mechanism of which is poorly understood.

Cardiac Syncope

Cardiac syncope primarily occurs due to sudden impairment of cardiac output, but inadequate autonomic vascular responsiveness also plays a contributory factor. During paroxysmal tachyarrhythmia, prompt vasoconstrictor response prevents blood pressure from dropping to symptomatic levels. Although the heart rate in tachycardia is important, the autonomic component determines whether the arrhythmia is hemodynamically tolerated or results in syncope. Similarly, in structural heart diseases (such as aortic stenosis and obstructive cardiomyopathy), an inappropriate reflex response causing vasodilatation instead of vasoconstriction contributes to syncope susceptibility. In elderly individuals, an inadequate increase in cardiac output in response to exertion, due to ventricular dysfunction or chronotropic incompetence, can be aggravated by varying degrees of subclinical autonomic failure, or due to pharmacotherapy associated with hypertension and ischemic heart diseases. Thus, syncope in elderly individuals is frequently multifactorial and far more common than in younger age groups. Cardiac syncope is often associated with a more worrisome prognosis than reflex or orthostatic syncope, and the mortality risk is proportional to the severity of the underlying cardiac condition.

Cardiac arrhythmias are usually associated with structural heart diseases (ischemic diseases or various cardiomyopathies), or as a proarrhythmic effect of drugs used to treat comorbid conditions (e.g., certain antimicrobials, psychotropic agents, and antiarrhythmic drugs). These agents can lead to prolonged ventricular repolarization, predisposing to "torsades de pointes," or increase in the risk of reentrant tachyarrhythmias or various conduction blocks due to already diseased myocardium or the presence of dyselectrolytemia. In structural heart diseases, bradyarrhythmias cause syncope more commonly than tachyarrhythmias due to myocardial fibrosis, ischemic changes, sinus node dysfunction, or atrioventricular conduction block. As a rule, cardiac syncope can be attributable to a sustained low ventricular rate of <35–40 beats/min for 20–30 seconds, or a prolonged sinus pause. The classic example of the latter is Stokes-Adams syncope, which is characteristically sudden in onset, with no premonitory symptoms. Repeated syncope with no recognizable triggering pattern, and reported even when in the supine position, should raise the suspicion of a cardiac cause. The main causes of arrhythmic syncope in the younger age group are hereditary channelopathies, such as long QT syndromes and Brugada syndrome. In Brugada syndrome, the syncope typically occurs during night due to slower heart rates triggering polymorphic ventricular tachycardia. In such cases, there is usually a family history of sudden cardiac death at a young age, necessitating further diagnostic evaluation. The absence of "autonomic activation" is a more consistent marker of cardiac syncope as compared to reflex syncope, where it is present. **Figure 3** summarizes the underlying pathophysiological basis of various types of syncope.

EPILEPTIC SEIZURES

Tonic, tonic-clonic, and atonic epileptic seizures are the only seizure types included as possible causes of TLOC. Epileptic seizures usually last >1 minute, and are longer than most syncopal attacks. Unlike syncope, jerks can begin unilaterally and before the fall, in epilepsy. They are coarse, symmetrical, rhythmic, and involve pronounced bending of knees and elbows. Other important clues to an epileptic etiology are a lateral tongue bite, pronounced head deviation, visual gaze directed to one side, and emission of a cry at the onset of the episode. Convulsive seizures can start as a partial seizure, beginning with mumbling or purposeless acts or focal jerks while still upright. Recovery can be slow, and disorientation may persist for extended periods in epileptic seizures. In rare cases, epileptic fits can precipitate syncope through cardiac arrhythmia or asystole, and conversely, cerebral hypoperfusion in syncope might induce an epileptic attack. **Table 1** compares the differences in the clinical features of syncope and seizures.

FUNCTIONAL TRANSIENT LOSS OF CONSCIOUSNESS

In somatization and conversion disorders, patients exhibit somatic symptoms that have no somatic explanation, but an underlying psychological mechanism is thought to be present. These disorders often occur in the context of prior psychological problems and physical and/or sexual abuse, are more common in females than males, and

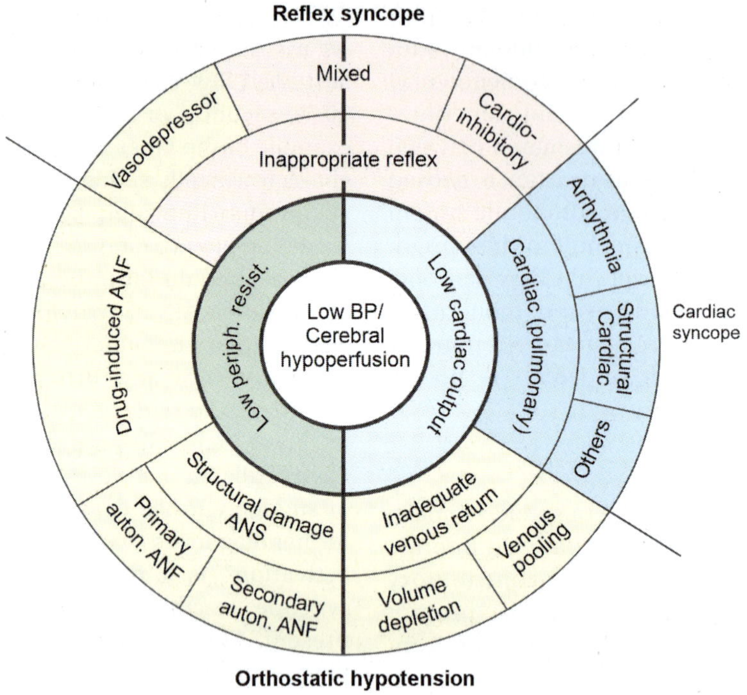

FIG. 3: Pathophysiological basis of the classification of syncope.
(ANF: atrial natriuretic factor; ANS: autonomic nervous system; auton. autonomic; BP: blood pressure; low periph. resist.: low peripheral resistance)

TABLE 1: Comparison of clinical features of syncope and seizures.

Clinical feature	Syncope	Epileptic seizures
Useful features		
Presence of trigger	Very often	Rare
Nature of trigger	*Differs between types*: Pain, standing, emotions for WS—a specific trigger for situational syncope; standing for OH	Flashing lights are best known; also range of rare triggers
Prodromes	Often presyncope (autonomic activation in reflex syncope, light-headedness in OH. Palpitations in cardiac syncope)	*Epileptic aura*: Repetitive, specific for each patient. Includes *déjà vu*. Rising sensation in the abdomen (epigastric aura) and/or an unusual unpleasant smell
Detailed characteristics of myoclonus	• <10, irregular in amplitude, asynchronous, and asymmetrical • Starts after the onset of LOC	• 20–100, synchronous, symmetrical, and hemilateral • The onset mostly coincides with LOC • Clear long-lasting automatisms such as chewing and lip-smacking at the mouth
Tongue bite	Rare, the tip of the tongue	Side of the tongue (rarely bilateral)
Duration of restoration of consciousness	10–30 seconds	Maybe many minutes
Confusion after attack	No understanding of the situation for <10 seconds in most syncope, full alertness, and awareness afterward	Memory deficit, i.e., repeated questions without imprinting for many minutes
Features of limited utility		
Incontinence	Not uncommon	Common
Presence of myoclonus (see below for nature of myoclonus)	Very often	~60%, dependent on accuracy of observation
Eyes open during LOC	Frequent	Nearly always
Fatigue and sleep afterward	Common, particularly in children	Very common
Blue face	Rare	Fairly often

(LOC: loss of consciousness; OH: orthostatic hypotension; VVS: vasovagal syncope) are more prevalent in the younger age group. The term "functional" has replaced "psychogenic," to remove the somewhat offending implication that the condition is "all in the head."

Pseudoepilepsy is a type of functional TLOC resembling epileptic seizures, and has now been termed "psychogenic nonepileptic seizures (PNES)." Tongue bites and incontinence are rare in pseudoseizures. Trauma occurs less often than in true epilepsy but may be observed in over 50% of the cases. Alternating movements of the limbs (arc de cercle) and pelvic thrusting can occur. The movements can change in nature as well as severity, during an attack. In contrast to both syncope and epileptic seizures, the eyes are almost always closed in PNES and are a useful diagnostic feature if observed by trained personnel, but eyewitness accounts are less reliable. **Table 2** compares the differences in clinical traits of functional and epileptic seizures.

The distinguishing features between epilepsy and pseudoseizures are too subtle to allow a definitive diagnosis to be established based on detailed history taking, thus ictal video-EEG recording is the gold standard investigation. In some cases, functional attacks can be induced by verbal suggestions or various provocations for the purpose of video-EEG recording.

"Pseudosyncope" is the second variant of functional TLOC, which is characterized by the absence of jerks. They account for almost 6% of all the presumed syncopal

TABLE 2: Comparison between clinical features of psychogenic and epileptic seizures.

Attack feature	Psychogenic seizure	Epileptic seizure
Stereotypy of attack	Often variable	Stereotypical
Onset or progression	Gradual	More rapid
Duration	May be prolonged	Typically 1–2 minutes
Diurnal variation	Daytime	Nocturnal or daytime
Injury	Rare	Can occur with tonic–clonic seizures
Tongue biting	Rare (typically the tip of the tongue)	Can occur with tonic–clonic seizures (lateral tongue or inside of the cheek)
Ictal eye closure	Common	Rare (eyes typically open)
Urinary incontinence	Rare	Frequent
Vocalization	May occur; variable (often crying, moaning)	Tonic–clonic seizures may have an ictal cry at the onset
Motor activity	Prolonged, uncoordinated; pelvic thrusting, and back arching	Typically unilateral rhythmic jerking, dystonic posturing of a limb, or synchronous tonic–clonic activity
Prolonged loss of muscle tone	Common	Rare
Postictal confusion	Rare	Common (several minutes, often fatigued for hours desiring sleep)
Postictal headache	Rare	Common
Postictal crying	Common	Rare
Relation to medication changes	Unrelated	Usually related
Relation to menses in women	Uncommon	Occasionally increased
Triggers	Emotional disturbances	Sleep deprivation, illness, and medication nonadherence
Frequency of attacks	More frequent, up to daily	Less frequent
Interracial electroencephalogram (EEG) findings	Normal	Frequently abnormal
Reproduction of attack by suggestion	Sometimes	No
Ictal EEG findings	Normal	Abnormal
Presence of secondary gain	Common	Uncommon
Presence of others	Frequently	Variable
Psychiatric disturbances	Very common (though not always apparent)	Variable

99

CHAPTER

Practical Approach to Acute Vestibular Syndrome

G Balaji

ABSTRACT

Acute vestibular syndrome is defined as sudden-onset, continuous vertigo lasting longer than 24 hours with associated nausea and vomiting, all of which are worsened with head movement. It results from a unilateral vestibular lesion that causes a sudden asymmetry of the neuronal nuclei firing rate and is largely associated with severe anxiety and vasovagal responses. The main causes of acute vestibular syndrome (AVS) are vestibular neuritis (VN), which nearly counts for 70% of cases, and posterior circulation stroke (PCS), accounting for 25% of the diagnoses. A methodological clinical approach focusing on comprehensive history and ocular motor findings can improve diagnostic accuracy and is more sensitive and specific than early neuroimaging.

This article provides a comprehensive overview of AVS, including its etiology, clinical presentation, differential diagnosis, diagnostic approach, and treatment modalities. By understanding the intricacies of AVS and following a methodical approach will lead to timely and appropriate intervention in patients with acute vestibular syndrome.

INTRODUCTION

Acute vestibular syndrome (AVS) was originally coined by Hotson and Baloh in 1998, it describes the sudden onset of continuous vertigo lasting longer than 24 hours and associated with nausea, vomiting, unsteadiness, and aggravated by change in head posture. The causes for AVS are myriad ranges from benign to potentially grave. AVS accounts for nearly 20–25% of dizzy patients visiting the emergency department (ED). Among the AVS patients nearly 20–25% will have a cause that is potentially life-threatening, such as posterior circulation stroke. **Table 1** summarizes a list of differential diagnosis causing an AVS.

The most common causes for AVS in patients presenting to the Emergency Room (ER) are inflammatory events of the peripheral labyrinth followed in frequency by ischemic events of the posterior cerebral circulation. It is of prime importance for the primary physician in ER to differentiate between these two conditions as the prognosis and treatment strategies vary greatly. A systematic approach is crucial in evaluating a patient with AVS. By emphasizing the core characteristics of acute vestibular syndrome in history-taking, including quality, timing, triggers, and associated symptoms, it is possible to identify true acute vestibular syndrome. Finally, key examination techniques narrow the causes of true acute vestibular syndrome to central and peripheral etiologies. The following steps are recommended:

APPROACH TO A PATIENT WITH ACUTE VESTIBULAR SYNDROME

The primary vestibular symptoms can be defined as enumerated in **Box 1**.

Step 1: Comprehensive History-taking

Onset and Duration of Symptoms

Determine whether the vertigo appeared suddenly or developed gradually. Establishing the duration of symptoms aid in categorizing the condition as acute or subacute.

TABLE 1: Differential diagnosis of AVS.

Vascular ischemic strokes	• Ischemic strokes • Posterior fossa hemorrhages • Vertebral artery dissection
Inflammatory/ Infectious	• AUVP/vestibular neuritis/labyrinthitis • Brainstem encephalitis • Ramsay Hunt syndrome • Mumps virus • Neuroborreliosis • Neurosyphilis
Neoplastic	• Chronic myeloid leukemia • Primary central nervous system lymphoma • Paraneoplastic • Vestibular schwannoma • Temporal bone metastasis
Degenerative/ Deficiency/Drugs	• Multiple sclerosis Barona • Wernicke encephalopathy
Autoimmune/ Allergic	• Anti-GQ1b antibody syndrome • Behçet's disease • Antiphospholipid syndrome • Cogan syndrome
Traumatic concussion	• Whiplash injuries • Inner ear decompression sickness/barotrauma

(AVS: acute vestibular syndrome; AUVP: acute unilateral vestibulopathy)

BOX 1: Primary vestibular symptoms.

Glossary of primary vestibular symptom definitions in the international classification of vestibular disorders:

- *Dizziness* is the sensation of disturbed or impaired spatial orientation without a false or distorted sense of motion
- *Vertigo* is the sensation of self-motion (of head/body) when no self-motion is occurring or the sensation of distorted self-motion during an otherwise normal head movement
- *Vestibulovisual symptoms* are visual symptoms that usually result from the vestibular pathology or the interplay between visual and vestibular systems. These include false sensations of motion or tilting of the visual surround and visual distortion (blur) linked to vestibular (rather than optical) failure
- *Postural symptoms* are balance symptoms related to maintenance of postural stability, occurring only while upright (seated, standing, or walking)

Characteristics of Vertigo

Ascertain the nature of vertigo. Is it a spinning sensation, a feeling of swaying, or unsteadiness? By highlighting a sensation of false motion or movement, vertigo can be more accurately identified.

Is the Movement Continuous?

An essential differentiation to be made by the examiner is to determine whether vertigo is exquisitely caused by position shift or if it is mostly spontaneous and continuous, merely increased by movement because vertigo worsens with head movement, when a patient's vertigo worsens with position changes, a diagnosis of benign paroxysmal positional vertigo (BPPV) is not certain until distinctive nystagmus generated by canal-plane-specific positioning is evident.

Associated Symptoms

Inquire about accompanying symptoms, such as nausea, vomiting, hearing loss, tinnitus, and visual disturbances. These can provide crucial clues to the underlying etiology.

Previous Episodes

Question the patient about any prior episodes of vertigo or similar symptoms. A history of recurrent episodes may suggest a different set of specific vestibular disorder, such as Ménière's disease, vestibular migraine, and BPPV.

Step 2: Focused Physical Examination

Once the history has confirmed acute onset spontaneous vertigo that is present continuously A thorough physical examination complements the information gleaned and assists in localizing the pathology and narrowing down the differential diagnosis to a peripheral vestibulopathy, i.e., vestibular neuritis (VN) (labyrinthitis if hearing is also involved) and ischemic labyrinthopathy or a central cause that is mainly posterior circulation stroke a lesion along the central vestibular circuit.

Head Impulse-nystagmus-test of Skew Examination

This three-step bedside oculomotor examination [Head Impulse-Nystagmus-Test of Skew (HINTS)] appears more sensitive for stroke than early magnetic resonance imaging (MRI) in AVS. This triad of tests aids in distinguishing between peripheral and central causes **(Table 2)**. The presence of normal horizontal head impulse test, direction-changing nystagmus in eccentric gaze, or skew deviation (vertical ocular misalignment) was 100% sensitive and 96% specific for stroke. Initial MRI diffusion-weighted imaging was falsely negative in 12% (all <48 hours after symptom onset).

Truncal Ataxia Grading

- *Grade 1*: Mild-to-moderate imbalance with walking independently
- *Grade 2*: Severe imbalance with standing, but cannot walk without support
- *Grade 3*: Falling at an upright posture

TABLE 2: Hints findings in central and peripheral acute vestibular syndrome (AVS).

	Head impulse test	Nystagmus	Test of skew
Central	No corrective saccade	• Direction-changing, pure vertical, pure torsional, or vertical-torsional • Nonfatiguing	Abnormal vertical ocular alignment
Peripheral	Corrective saccade with head turn toward side of lesion	Unidirectional, horizontal torsional, and attenuates with fixation point	Absent

Carmona et al. study concluded that ataxia and truncal instability ratings when added to HINTS contributed to an overall sensitivity.

Audiometric Evaluation

Conduct audiometric tests, such as pure-tone audiometry and speech audiometry, to assess for any associated hearing loss. In case of a central pathology hearing loss is present in anterior inferior cerebellar artery stroke, peripheral pathology it is indicative of labyrinthine involvement.

Step 3: Imaging Studies

Magnetic Resonance Imaging

Consider an MRI of the brain if there are concerning neurological signs, atypical features, or if central pathology is suspected.

TREATMENT

The treatment approach to AVS mainly depends on the ability to make a correct etiological diagnosis. The primary clinical objective is to make a quick and accurate distinction between VN and posterior circulation stroke. A delay in the diagnosis of stroke would be detrimental in the form of progression of the disease, worsening of symptoms reduction in therapeutic effects when stroke treatment is administered late. Tissue plasminogen activators and antiplatelet drugs are the two main options for the treatment of cerebral ischemic stroke. Conventional rehabilitation therapy and pharmacotherapy for balance recovery among stroke patients, such as core strength exercises, visual feedback training, and proprioceptive neuromuscular facilitation, yield unsatisfactory results.

The treatment options for VN can be categorized into symptomatic therapy, specific drug therapy, and vestibular rehabilitation. Symptomatic treatment with vestibular suppressants such as antihistamines, benzodiazepines, and anticholinergics, is widely used because they are effective against dizziness, nausea, and vomiting for early treatment of acute VN, they have to be used for short duration as prolonged use can reduce vestibular compensatory mechanism. It has been studied that high doses of glucocorticoids in the acute stage accelerates and improves the recovery of vestibular function. The gold standard and long-term treatment goal would be vestibular rehabilitation. The target is to improve vertigo, gaze stability, postural stability, and daily living activities through vestibular compensation and central neuroplasticity. The prognosis in patients with VN is generally good, but residual dizziness may remain in some patients after the acute phase, similar to persistent disabling imbalance after successful repositioning maneuvers for BPPV.

CONCLUSION

An organized and systematic approach to a patient presenting with acute vestibular syndrome is pivotal in achieving an accurate diagnosis and guiding appropriate treatment. By meticulously gathering a comprehensive history, performing focused physical examinations, employing specialized vestibular tests, and judiciously utilizing imaging studies, one can navigate through the complex landscape of AVS and arrive at an etiological diagnosis of AVS. This methodical approach will lead to timely and appropriate intervention in patients with acute vestibular syndrome.

SUGGESTED READINGS

1. Steenerson KK. Acute Vestibular Syndrome. Continuum (Minneap Minn). 2021;27(2):402-19.
2. Hotson JR, Baloh RW. Acute vestibular syndrome. N Engl J Med. 1998;339(10):680-5.
3. Mantokoudis G, Otero-Millan J, Gold DR. Current concepts in acute vestibular syndrome and video-oculography. Curr Opin Neurol. 2022;35(1):75-83.
4. Bisdorff AR, Staab JP, Newman-Toker DE. Overview of the International Classification of Vestibular Disorders. Neurol Clin. 2015;33(3):541-50.
5. Kattah JC, Talkad AV, Wang DZ, Hsieh YH, Newman-Toker DE. HINTS to diagnose stroke in the acute vestibular syndrome: three-step bedside oculomotor examination more sensitive than early MRI diffusion-weighted imaging. Stroke. 2009;40(11):3504-10.

6. Carmona S, Martínez C, Zalazar G, Moro M, Batuecas-Caletrio A, Luis L, et al. The diagnostic accuracy of truncal ataxia and HINTS as cardinal signs for acute vestibular syndrome. Front Neurol. 2016;7:125.
7. Viola P, Gioacchini FM, Astorina A, Pisani D, Scarpa A, Marcianò G, et al. The pharmacological treatment of acute vestibular syndrome. Front Neurol. 2022;13:999112.
8. Newman-Toker DE, Hsieh YH, Camargo CA Jr, Pelletier AJ, Butchy GT, Edlow JA. Spectrum of dizziness visits to US emergency departments: cross-sectional analysis from a nationally representative sample. Mayo Clin Proc. 2008;83(7):765-75.
9. Machner B, Choi JH, Trillenberg P, HeideW, Helmchen C. Risk of acute brain lesions in dizzy patients presenting to the emergency room: who needs imaging and who does not? J Neurol. 2020;267(Suppl 1):126-35.
10. Sjögren J, Magnusson M, Tjernström F, Karlberg M. Steroids for acute vestibular neuronitis-the earlier the treatment, the better the outcome? Otol Neurotol. 2019;40(3):372-4.

100

CHAPTER

Neuroimaging in Clinical Practice

Aminur Rahman

ABSTRACT

Neuroimaging is a specialization of imaging technique that produce images of the brain or other parts of the central nervous system (CNS) in a noninvasive manner that directly or indirectly assess the structural or functional activity of the nervous system. Computed tomography (CT) and magnetic resonance imaging (MRI) are the most widely used modalities in routine clinical practice. Neuroimaging can be divided into two broad categories, namely, (1) structural, and (2) functional neuroimaging. This article discusses the basics and applications of various traditional, as well as emerging neuroimaging techniques, considering their strengths and limitations with this rapidly expanding field.

INTRODUCTION

Neuroimaging is the use of varied ways to either directly or indirectly image the structure and functional activities of the nervous system. Neuroimaging plays a vital part in the determination of central nervous system (CNS) diseases. Main modalities of neuroimaging approaches are computed tomography (CT) scan and magnetic resonance imaging (MRI). The pioneer method for imaging brain structure was CT. It remains useful because of short imaging times, wide vacuity, ease of access, sensitive spotting of calcification and hemorrhage, and resolution of bony detail. MRI provides excellent detailed structural information and enables the naked eye to distinguish argentine matter (neuronal cell bodies) from white matter (myelinated tracts). MRI offers superior soft-tissue contrast, excellent visualization of vascular structures, minor artifacts, and imaging in any plane. New anatomical methods, similar as diffusion tensor imaging (DTI), have been developed to specifically image myelinated tract. These approaches can be used to trace the normal and anomalous evolution of neural pathways in children. Nowadays, CT and MRI operations that concentrate on functional and physiologic display of the CNS will add greatly to the clinical usefulness of these imaging tools. Neuroimaging techniques are growing increasingly sophisticated and as a result there is a high demand in both clinical and research settings for individuals with neuroimaging skills.

INDICATIONS

- To investigate a patient who has or may have a neurological disorder, such as stroke, headache, syncope, and seizure disorder.
- It is indicated for CT-, MRI- and PET-guided stereotactic surgery or radiosurgery for treatment of intracranial tumors, arteriovenous malformations, and other surgically treatable conditions.
- It is helpful to diagnose metabolic diseases and degenerative diseases (such as Alzheimer's disease, and Parkinson's disease) and also for neurological and cognitive psychology research.

TYPES OF NEUROIMAGING (FIG. 1)

Structural Imaging

- Structural imaging refers to approaches that are specialized for the visualization and analysis of

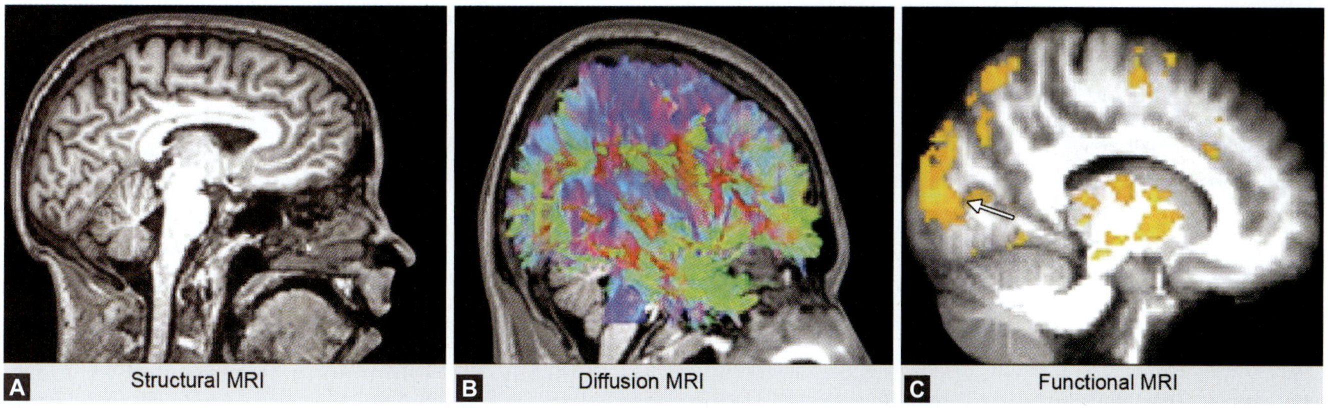

FIGS. 1A TO C: Magnetic resonance imaging (MRI)-based imaging techniques: (A) Structural MRI reveals the gross anatomical structure of the brain with high detail; (B) Diffusion MRI reveals the overall layout of white matter connections and pathways within the brain (known as diffusion tractography); and (C) Functional MRI reveals areas of the brain that are active when individual is asked to perform a particular task. In this case, an individual who is congenitally blind was asked to identify a tactile pattern through touch. Note areas of activation identified throughout the brain (yellow) including within the occipital cortex which is normally associated with visual information processing (arrow).

anatomical properties of the brain. Structural approaches are particularly useful for detecting brain damage and abnormalities.
- It deals with the structure of the nervous system and the diagnosis of gross (large scale) intracranial disease (such as stroke, tumor, infection, and demyelinating disease) and injury.
- It also shares detailed information regarding brain integrity, microstructure, and white matter connections.

Functional Imaging

- Functional imaging has been the dominant force in cognitive neuroscience because it ables to determine when and where neural activity in the brain is associated with the ability to perform a particular cognitive task.
- It localizes the activity of brain associated with performing a cognitive task and/or behavior.
- It is used to diagnose metabolic diseases and lesions on a finer scale (such as Alzheimer's disease) and also for neurological and cognitive psychology research and building brain-computer interfaces.

TECHNIQUE OF NEUROIMAGING

- Computed tomography or computed axial tomography (CAT)
- Magnetic resonance imaging
- Functional magnetic resonance imaging (fMRI)
- Magnetoencephalography
- Positron emission tomography (PET)
- Single-photon emission computed tomography (SPECT)
- Computed tomography angiography
- Magnetic resonance angiography
- Magnetic resonance venography
- MR neurography/MR imaging of peripheral nerve injury (PNI)
- Cerebral digital subtraction angiography

GUIDELINES FOR SELECTING OF NEUROIMAGING TECHNIQUES

- Neuroimaging techniques have advantages and disadvantages that are based on the strengths and limitations of each. The different neuroimaging techniques in terms of the degree of invasiveness, tasks that can be performed, spatial resolution, and temporal resolution.
- Spatial resolution refers to how accurately the measured activity is localized within the brain, and temporal resolution refers to how closely the measured activity corresponds to the timing of the actual neural activity.
- The following guidelines are used for selecting of neuroimaging techniques mentioned in **Table 1**.

COMPUTERIZED TOMOGRAPHY (CT) SCAN OF HEAD

Introduction

- CT scan is an imaging modality that uses X-rays to obtain structural and functional information about the human body. It is also called a CAT scan.
- The word tomography is derived from a Greek word where *tomos* represents "slice" or section and *graphia*

TABLE 1: Guidelines for selecting of neuroimaging techniques.

Conditions	Recommended technique
Hemorrhage:	
Acute parenchymal	CT, MR
Subacute/chronic	MRI
Subarachnoid hemorrhage	CT, CTA, lumbar puncture angiography
Aneurysm	Angiography > CTA, MRA
Ischemic infarction:	
Acute infarction	MRI > CT
Hemorrhagic infarction	CT or MRI
Carotid or vertebral dissection	MRI/MRA
Vertebral basilar insufficiency	CTA, MRI/MRA
Carotid stenosis	CTA > Doppler ultrasound, MRA
Suspected mass lesion:	
Neoplasm, primary, or metastatic	MRI + contrast
Infection/abscess	MRI + contrast
Immunosuppressed with focal findings	MRI + contrast
Vascular malformation	MRI ± angiography
White matter disorders	MRI
Demyelinating disease	MRI ± contrast
Dementia	MRI > CT
Trauma:	
Acute trauma	CT (noncontrast)
Shear injury/chronic hemorrhage	MRI
Headache/migraine	CT (noncontrast)/MRI
Seizure:	
First time, no focal neurologic deficits	CT/MRI as screen ± contrast
Partial complex/refractory	MRI with coronal T2W imaging
Cranial neuropathy	MRI with contrast
Meningeal disease	MRI with contrast
Spine:	
Low back pain	
No neurologic deficits	MRI or CT after 4 weeks
With focal deficits	MRI > CT
Spinal stenosis	MRI or CT
Cervical spondylosis	MRI or CT myelography
Infection	MRI + contrast, CT
Myelopathy	MRI + contrast > myelography
Arteriovenous malformation	MRI, myelography/ angiography

(CT: computed tomography; CTA: computed tomography angiography MRA: magnetic resonance angiography; MRI: magnetic resonance imaging; T2W: T2-weighted)

meaning "description". The term tomography refers to a process for generating two-dimensional (2D) image slices of an examined organ of three-dimensions (3D).

- CT scans can expose patients to levels of radiation 100–500 times higher than traditional X-rays, with higher radiation doses producing better resolution imaging.
- CT scanning uses a computer program that performs a numerical integral calculation (the inverse Radon transform) on the measured X-ray series to estimate how much of an X-ray beam is absorbed in a small volume of the brain.
- Typically the information is presented as cross-sections of the brain. It uses a series of X-rays of the head taken from many different directions. Clinicians of 10 times take multiple scans, with 30% of individuals undergoing at least three scans in one study of CT scan usage.
- While easy to use, increases in CT scan use, especially in asymptomatic patients, is a topic of concern since patients are exposed to significantly high levels of radiation.
- Computed tomography (CT or CAT scan) is a noninvasive diagnostic imaging procedure that uses a combination of X-rays and computer technology to produce horizontal (axial) and vertical (sagittal/coronal) images (often called slices) of the head.
- A CT is a display of the anatomy of thin slide of the body developed from multiple X-ray absorption measurement made around the body's periphery.
- Routine head CT is performed in an axial axis with 15–20° angulations of the gentry to orbitomeatal plane. This angulation provides superior visualization of brainstem and cerebellum. This angulation also decreases radiation to eyes. Routine CT examination of brain involves making (9–10) axial section.
- A CT scan shows detailed images of any part of the brain including the hemorrhage, infarction, calcification, and other pathological conditions. CT scans are more detailed than standard X-rays. Indications of CT scan of brain are given in **Box 1**.

BOX 1: Indications of computed tomography (CT) scan of head.

- Head injury or skull fractures
- Stroke
- Suspected hydrocephalus
- Suspected intracranial hematoma
- Evaluation of headaches
- Diseases or malformations of the skull
- Initial evaluation for space-occupying lesions
- Seizures
- Unexplained change in mental status

BOX 2: Contraindications of CT scan of head.

- Computed tomography (CT) scan has no absolute contraindications
- Caution is indicated in pregnant women, particularly during the first trimester to avoid fetal abnormalities
- Repeated X-ray exposure may increase the patient's risk for cancer

Indications of CT Scan of Head

- A CT brain is considered to look at the structures of the brain and evaluate for the presence of pathology, such as mass/tumor, abscess, and stroke **(Box 1)**.
- It is particularly good for hemorrhage, trauma, or fracture to the skull and for hydrocephalus.
- It will usually exclude nonstroke lesions, including subdural hematomas and brain tumors.
- It will demonstrate intracerebral hemorrhage within minutes of stroke onset.
- CT changes in cerebral infarction may be completely absent or very subtle within the first few hours after symptom onset, though changes usually evolve over time (12–24 hours).
- Contraindications of CT scan of head are given in **Box 2**.

MAGNETIC RESONANCE IMAGING OF BRAIN

Introduction

- Magnetic resonance imaging is an imaging technique used primarily in medical settings to produce high quality images of the soft tissues of the human body.
- Magnetic resonance imaging is based on the magnetic characteristics of the imaged tissue. It involves creation of tissue magnetization (which can then be manipulated in several ways) and detection of tissue magnetization as revealed by signal intensity.
- Imaging is created by the motion of hydrogen protons in response to the applied radiofrequency.
- It is useful in a wide range of clinical situations; e.g., imaging the optic chiasm, small intracanalicular acoustic neuroma, and detection of meningiomas which are sometimes isointense with normal CNS tissue on T2- and T1-weighted unenhanced sequences, intramedullary spinal tumors, leptomeningeal disease, and in demonstrating acute inflammation in multiple sclerosis plaques.
- Indications for brain MRI are given in **Box 3**.
- Contraindications for brain MRI are given in **Box 4**.

BOX 3: Indications for brain MRI.

- Vascular (ischemic and hemorrhagic stroke, AVM, aneurysm, and venous thrombosis)
- Infection (abscess, cerebritis, encephalitis, and meningitis)
- Inflammatory/demyelinating lesions (multiple sclerosis, sarcoidosis, etc.)
- Tumor (primary CNS and metastatic)
- Trauma (epidural hematoma, subdural hematoma, and contusion)
- Hydrocephalus

(AVM: arteriovenous malformation; CNS: central nervous system; MRI: magnetic resonance imaging)

BOX 4: Contraindications for brain MRI.

- Implanted devices and other metallic devices:
  - Pacemakers and other implanted electronic devices
  - Aneurysm clips and other magnetizable materials
  - Cochlear implants
  - Some artificial heart valves
  - Intraocular metallic foreign bodies
  - Screening CT of the orbits if history suggests possible metallic foreign body in the eye
- Unstable patients (most resuscitation equipment cannot be brought into the scanning room)
- Other relative contraindication—severe agitation or claustrophobia (may require anesthesia assistance)

(CT: computed tomography MRI: magnetic resonance imaging)

Magnetic Resonance Imaging Compatible Metals

- *Titanium*: Titanium's nonmagnetic properties make it compatible for use with an MRI as well. Joint replacements, surgical screws, bone plates, and pacemaker cases all use titanium.
- *Cobalt-chromium*: Though cobalt has magnetic properties, implants such as coronary stents made of cobalt-chromium alloy have tested safe during an MRI. The alloy also tests safe for larger items, such as knee and hip replacements.
- *Copper*: Researchers have tested intrauterine contraceptive devices (IUCDs) for MRI safety. Some of these devices have a small copper coil. Copper wiring for pacemakers has also tested safe for an MRI.
- *Stainless steel*: Some stainless steel alloys have a very low reaction, or susceptibility, to magnetic fields. Medical supply companies sell stainless steel tools and accessories that staff can safely use in the MRI room.

Stainless steel items such as dental braces can distort MRI images, however. If the metal interferes too much with the MRI image, the doctor may recommend you have your braces removed.

Limitations of Magnetic Resonance Imaging

- Subject to motion artifact
- Inferior to CT in detecting acute hemorrhage
- Inferior to CT in detection of bony injury
- Requires prolonged acquisition time for many images

MAGNETIC RESONANCE IMAGING OF SPINE

Introduction

- Magnetic resonance imaging of the spine uses radio waves, a magnetic field, and a computer. It creates clear and detailed pictures of the spine and surrounding tissues.
- MRI does not use radiation and may require an injection of gadolinium contrast material.
- MRI scan was developed in the 1980s and has revolutionized our ability to see normal and abnormal spinal structures and helps diagnose those spinal disorders.
- MRI of the spine can be useful in evaluating symptoms such as neck or back pain, leg pain, numbness, tingling or weakness, or problems with bladder, and bowel control.
- It can assess the disks to see whether they are bulging, ruptured, or pressing on the spinal cord or nerves.
- It can also help to diagnose tumors, bleeding, swelling, developmental or structural abnormalities, and infections or inflammatory conditions in the vertebrae or surrounding tissues.
- The indications of MRI spine are given in **Box 5**.

BOX 5: Indications of MRI spine.

- Assess spinal anatomy and alignment
- Detect congenital anomalies of vertebrae or the spinal cord
- Detect bone, disk, ligament, or spinal cord injury after spine trauma
- Assess lower back pain due to intervertebral disk disease (degenerated, bulging, or herniated) and intervertebral joint disease, compression fracture, or bone swelling)
- Assess compression of spinal cord and nerves
- Assess inflammation of the spinal cord or nerves
- Assess infection involving the spine, disks, and spinal contents including spinal cord or its coverings (meninges)
- Assess tumors that arise from or have spread to the vertebrae, spinal cord, nerves, or the surrounding soft tissues

Overview of Spine

- The spine is located in the midline posteriorly, extending from the base of the skull to natal cleft, supporting the head, shoulder girdle, rib cage, and attaching to the pelvis.
- It is composed of 24 vertebrae separated by intervertebral disks, with additional sacral and coccygeal segments which are usually but, variably, fused.
- The vertebrae are grouped together into groups based on similar osteology and regional relations; cervical spine (seven vertebrae), thoracic spine (12 vertebrae), and lumbar spine (five vertebrae).
- The sacrum has five fused vertebral segments and the coccyx has a further 3–5 vertebral segments.

Magnetic Resonance Imaging with or without Contrast

- MRI without contrast cannot generally help in evaluating the given tumor condition. MRI images with contrast are clearer than the images of MRI without contrast. Due to the high clarity of images gathered by MRI with contrast, they are easier for a medical specialist to evaluate and interpret.
- Noncontrast MRI is great option for patients for whom dye is not recommended, pregnant women, and kidney-compromised patients. Noncontrast also provides greater images of blood vessel activity, detecting aneurysms, and blocked blood vessels.

FUNCTIONAL IMAGING

Positron Emission Tomography Imaging

Introduction

- Positron emission tomography is a type of nuclear medicine procedure that measures metabolic activity of the cells of body tissues.
- This imaging technique employs radioactive isotopes and can study a variety of functional or chemical features in normal and pathological brain which are inaccessible to other imaging modalities.
- A positron is a positively charged electron, and in PET imaging, a biological tracer is labeled with a positron-emitting radionuclide.

- PET scans of the brain are used to detect or highlight tumors and diseased tissue, measure cellular and/or tissue metabolism, show blood flow, evaluate patients who have seizure disorders that do not respond to medical therapy and patients with certain memory disorders, and determine brain changes following injury or drug abuse, among other uses.
- The imaging of cerebral metabolism indirectly via perfusion directly with PET using [^{18}F] fluorodeoxyglucose (FDG) is clinically well established.
- Using radioisotopes such as [^{15}O] or [^{18}F] deoxyglucose, it has been possible to quantify cerebral blood flow and metabolism in vivo.
- The tracer is given by intravenous injection or gaseous inhalation, and its distribution in the brain can be demonstrated on tomographic images.
- Radioisotope labels are also used in PET studies to evaluate receptor binding, e.g., the study of dopaminergic receptors in extrapyramidal disease.

Advantages

- PET studies provided considerable insights into aspects of normal brain function and as well disease pathogenesis and pathophysiology.
- Valuable insights have been obtained into the varying anatomical patterns of altered metabolism and flow in a wide range of neurodegenerative diseases, and the patterns of flow and oxygen utilization in infarcts and their surrounding ischemic penumbra.
- Amyloid PET in AD is shown in **Figure 2**.

Disadvantages

- It is an expensive tool and requires immediate access to a cyclotron.
- The opportunity for serial examinations is limited by the constraints of radiation exposure.

Single-photon Emission Computed Tomography

Introduction

- It is a functional nuclear imaging technique performed to evaluate regional cerebral perfusion.
- Because cerebral blood flow is closely linked to neuronal activity, the activity distribution is presumed to reflect neuronal activity levels in different areas of the brain.

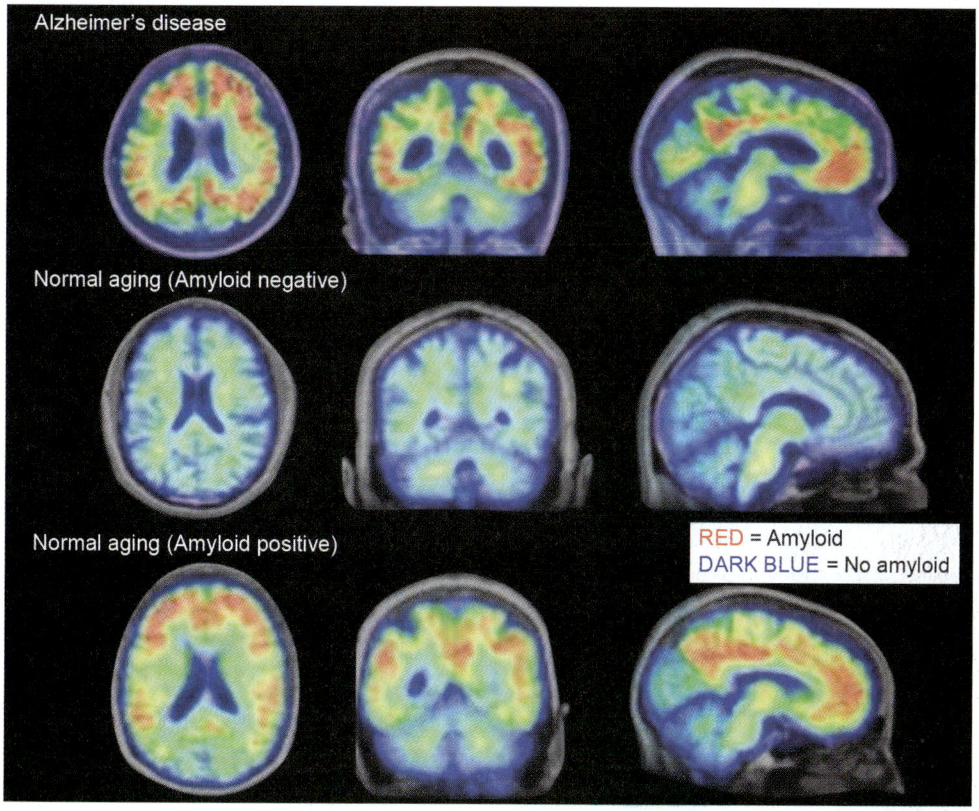

FIG. 2: Positron emission tomography (PET) using fluorodeoxyglucose (FDG), which is taken up by active mitochondria, to measure the metabolic activity of the brain. Patients with Alzheimer's disease show evidence of near-global decreases in metabolic function, particularly in the temporoparietal regions.

- A lipophilic, PH-neutral radiopharmaceutical [most commonly 99mTc-hexamethylpropyleneamine oxime (HMPAO) and 99mTc-ethylene dicysteine diethyl ester (ECD), with a half-life of 6.02 hours] is injected into the patient, which crosses the blood–brain barrier and continues to emit γ-rays.
- A 3D representation of cerebral blood flow can be literated using γ-detectors, allowing for interpretation.
- *Acetazolamide* increases local pCO_2 and causes arteriolar dilation, allowing for assessment of cerebrovascular reserve in transient ischemic attack (TIA), stroke, and vascular anomalies and distinguishing vascular from neuronal causes of dementia. SPECT of stroke is shown in **Figure 3**.
- Indications of SPECT are given in **Box 6**.

Limitations

- SPECT is technically less sophisticated and demanding when compared with PET, but provides lower-resolution images.
- It can be used to evaluate regional variations in blood flow, but its role in everyday clinical practice is, like that of PET, a small one.

Magnetic Resonance Neurography

Introduction

- Magnetic resonance neurography (MRN) or MR neurography, also known as MR imaging of peripheral nerves injury, is an advanced technique that is useful for diagnosing disorders of the peripheral nerves beyond the spinal canal.
- *MRN* is a relatively new noninvasive imaging technique for dedicated assessment of peripheral nerves.
- It is the direct imaging of nerves in the body by optimizing selectivity for unique MRI water properties of nerves. It is a modification of MRI.
- It is used to assess peripheral nerve entrapments and impingements as well as localization and grading of nerve injuries and lesions.
- Nerve trauma, tumor, inflammation, radiation damage, compression related to disk disease, or entrapment are some of the more common nerve diseases that are evaluated with MRN.
- MRN can image nerves anywhere in the body, although it is most commonly used in the diagnosis of abnormalities of the brachial plexus, lumbosacral plexus, thoracic outlet, and sciatic nerves.
- MRN is mostly used to assess major nerve compressions such as those affecting the sciatic nerve (e.g., piriformis syndrome), the brachial plexus nerves (e.g., thoracic outlet syndrome), the pudendal nerve, or virtually any named nerve in the body.
- Many nerves, such as the median and ulnar nerve in the arm or the tibial nerve in the tarsal tunnel, are just below the skin surface and can be tested for pathology with electromyography, but this technique has always been difficult to apply for deep proximal nerves.
- So MRN can characterize nerve morphology, longitudinal variations in signal intensity and caliber, and connections and relations to other nerves or plexuses to help identify pathology in correlation with the patient's clinical history, physical examination, and electrophysiological studies.

Clinical Applications

It is especially beneficial for patients with:

- Persistent nerve-related symptoms despite normal or equivocal routine spine imaging
- Specific nerve abnormalities on electromyelography

Magnetic Resonance Neurography Protocol

- Dedicated high-resolution MR sequences are utilized to optimally increase the conspicuity of nerve tissue

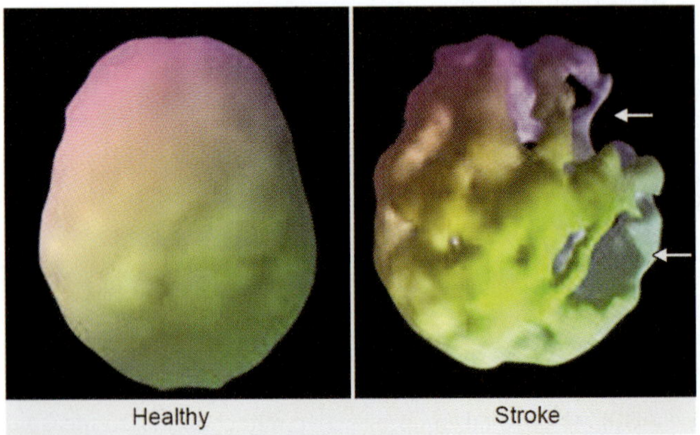

FIG. 3: Single-photon emission computed tomography (SPECT).

BOX 6: Indications of single-photon emission computed tomography (SPECT).

- Detection and evaluation of cerebrovascular disease
- Aid in the diagnosis and differential diagnoses of suspected dementia
- Detection of seizure focus
- Assessment of brain death
- Evaluating suspected brain trauma
- *Neuropsychiatric disorders*: Mood disorders, evaluating and subtyping attention-deficit disorder
- Substance abuse
- Infection/inflammation

BOX 7: Pitfalls and technical limitations of magnetic resonance neurography (MRN).

- Differentiating nerves from adjacent vessels
- Increased perineural T2 signal from adjacent vessels
- Magic angle effect
- Inhomogeneous fat suppression
- Increased specific absorption rate (SAR) at 3 T
- Increased susceptibility artifact at 3 T

signal. Exact parameters, planes, and reconstructions will vary according to anatomical location, scanner constraints, and local preference. Commonly used imaging protocols include:
  - Axial T1-weighted
  - Axial fat-suppressed T2-weighted
  - 3D STIR (short tau inversion recovery)
  - 3D PSIF (reversed fast imaging with steady state precession)
- Diffusion tensor imaging and high-resolution balanced steady state sequences [e.g., 3D constructive interference in steady state (CISS)] may also be useful.
- Use of intravenous gadolinium contrast is usually restricted for assessment of infection, perineural involvement by tumor of further assess mass lesions.
- Pitfalls and technical limitations of MRN are given in **Box 7**.

SUMMARY

- Neuroimaging includes the use of various techniques to either directly or indirectly image the structure, function, or pharmacology of the brain.
- Neuroimaging falls into two broad categories: (1) structural imaging and (2) functional imaging.
- CT scan is used to visualize of gross brain abnormalities, malformations, hemorrhagic stroke, and bone structure.
- Magnetic resonance imaging scans use echo waves to discriminate among gray matter, white matter, and cerebrospinal fluid.
- Electroencephalography (EEG) is used to show brain activity under certain psychological states, such as alertness or drowsiness.
- Positron emission tomography scans show brain processes by using the sugar glucose in the brain to illustrate where neurons are firing.
- Functional magnetic resonance imaging scans are a series of MRIs measuring brain function via a computer's combination of multiple images taken less than a second apart.

CONCLUSION

Neuroimaging is an important crucial approach in clinical neuroscience and modern cognitive of the human brain along with the quantitative examination of the structure, blood flow, blood volume, electrical activity, metabolism, oxygen consumption, and many other physiological activities inside the CNS, it may give a variety of directly or indirectly derived graphical representations. It plays a role in the investigation of structural lesions as well as the physiological underpinnings of mental processes and is crucial to the identification, diagnosis, and treatment of neurological and psychiatric disorders as well as the testing of novel therapeutic interventions.

SUGGESTED READINGS

1. Brammer M. The role of neuroimaging in diagnosis and personalized medicine—current position and likely future directions. Dialogues Clin Neurosci. 2009;11(4):389-96.
2. Eggebrecht AT, White BR, Ferradal SL, Chen C, Zhan Y, Snyder AZ, et al. A quantitative spatial comparison of high-density diffuse optical tomography and fMRI cortical mapping. Neuroimage. 2012;61(4):1120-8.
3. Filler A. The history, development and impact of computed imaging in neurological diagnosis and neurosurgery: CT, MRI, and DTI. Nature Precedings. 2009.
4. Grover VP, Tognarelli JM, Crossey MM, Cox IJ, Taylor-Robinson SD, McPhail MJ. Magnetic Resonance Imaging: Principles and Techniques: Lessons for Clinicians. J Clin Exp Hepatol. 2015 Sep;5(3):246-55.
5. Winegar BA, Kay MD, Taljanovic M. Magnetic resonance imaging of the spine. Pol J Radiol. 2020 Sep 25;85:e550-e574.
6. Lameka K, Farwell MD, Ichise M. Positron Emission Tomography. Handb Clin Neurol. 2016;135:209-227.
7. Yandrapalli S, Puckett Y. SPECT Imaging. [Updated 2022 Oct 3]. Available from: https://www.ncbi.nlm.nih.gov/books/NBK564426/
8. Ku V, Cox C, Mikeska A, MacKay B. Magnetic Resonance Neurography for Evaluation of Peripheral Nerves. J Brachial Plex Peripher Nerve Inj. 2021 May 14;16(1):e17-e23. doi: 10.1055/s-0041-1729176.

SECTION

12

PULMONOLOGY

101

CHAPTER

Noninvasive Ventilatory Support: Another Revolution in Medicine

Roman Jaeschke, Miłosz Jankowski

ABSTRACT

Options of support for critically ill patients, always important, became of particular importance during the recent coronavirus disease 2019 (COVID-19) pandemic. The sheer scale of challenges and the stress on system capacity led to the development and dissemination of newer modes of noninvasive ventilatory support (NIVS) or noninvasive respiratory support (NIRS). Their use, out of necessity, migrated outside their areas of usual use (intensive care units) to lower-level acuity units. This also led to new groups of clinicians being exposed to and responsible for their use. This chapter summarizes basic information on NIVS directed at such nonspecialists.

INTRODUCTION

During the first weeks of the coronavirus disease 2019 (COVID-19) pandemic, intensive care units (ICUs) in my city, Hamilton in Ontario, Canada, have not yet seen their first COVID-19 patient, but we were hearing about such patients from Toronto or Niagara region, both < 100 km from us. We were anxiously discussing management priorities and exchanging late-night emails on hydroxychloroquine, steroids, and azithromycin. However, the most commonly debated topic was how rapidly those patients deteriorate and how to time the initiation of mechanical ventilation.

To start, people used to act very rapidly until two things became clear: first, that we are running out of ventilators or spaces to use them, and second, that we should not do it fast in the first place. The pattern of practice changed from thinking about intubation once we needed more than 40% oxygen to support oxygenation, to observing and following people who were on 100% oxygen.

The major part of our comfort was wider employment of noninvasive ventilatory support (NIVS), in the form of either positive airway pressure (PAP) [continuous (CPAP) or bi-level (Bi-PAP), with the latter representing real noninvasive ventilation (NIV)] or nasal high-flow therapy (NHFT). Practice guidelines in the early stages of the COVID-19 pandemic supported the option of using NIV and NHFT and contributed to their widespread use.

CHANGING PATTERN OF PRACTICE AND CHANGING OPTIONS

In contrast to invasive mechanical ventilation (IMV), which is delivered through either an endotracheal tube (ETT) or a tracheostomy tube, NIV and CPAP can be delivered through many interfaces, such as oral, nasal, oronasal, or full facial masks or a full-head helmet.

Continuous Positive Airway Pressure

Continuous PAP provides constant PAP, which facilitates the recruitment of alveoli, thereby improving gas exchange in the lungs, reduces preload and afterload (of particular importance in pulmonary edema), and reduces the respiratory effort needed in patients with bronchial obstruction by matching airway pressure to the auto-positive end-expiratory pressure (PEEP) distal to the obstruction site. Its primary use in the acute setting is for congestive heart failure.

Noninvasive Ventilation

While many ventilatory modes are theoretically possible during bilevel NIV, the assist/controlled (A/C) mode is quite frequently used. In some ventilators dedicated for NIV, it is called spontaneous/triggered (ST) mode. As with the A/C mode in IMV, the ventilator provides fully supportive breaths at a set rate, but if a patient's inspiratory efforts trigger a breath, these are also supported by the ventilator. A purely spontaneous ventilation mode, such as pressure support ventilation (PSV), which in some NIV-dedicated ventilators is simply called spontaneous (S) mode, may also be used, but it depends on the patient having an adequate respiratory drive.

In addition to the respiratory rate, using NIV the clinician sets the inspiratory positive airway pressure (IPAP) and the expiratory positive airway pressure (EPAP). Due to the lack of a definitive airway and the increasing risk of air leaks, the maximum values of EPAP are ~10–12 cmH_2O and of IPAP are ~20–24 cmH_2O. Beyond these levels (and not infrequently below) many patients do not tolerate NIV, and there is an increasing risk of gastric insufflation, which could lead to vomiting and aspiration.

The greater the difference between these pressures (IPAP - EPAP, i.e., the drive pressure), the greater the tidal volume (Vt) generated. This is important for patients with or at risk of hypercapnia [e.g., in chronic obstructive pulmonary disease (COPD)] or barotrauma. Higher IPAP and/or EPAP levels also result in a higher mean airway pressure compared with CPAP and thus may improve oxygenation. In some ventilators, it is possible to set Vt and IPAP range ($IPAP_{max}$ and $IPAP_{min}$). These ventilators deliver IPAP between $IPAP_{max}$ and $IPAP_{min}$ aiming for set Vt.

In patients who are going to use the device for longer than a few hours, a heated humidifier or heat moisture exchanger may be used to increase the patient's comfort.

Noninvasive ventilation is generally delivered to the patient in a sitting or semirecumbent position. To encourage tolerance of the device, it is important to explain the interface and purpose of the treatment to the patient before initiation and to let them know that the positive pressure may initially feel uncomfortable. The proper size of interface (most commonly the mask) is of crucial importance. Patients should be encouraged to breathe evenly and calmly **(Fig. 1)**.

Ventilation is usually started with an EPAP of 3–4 cmH_2O (in practice, this is the lowest pressure that can be set in individual models) and an IPAP of 10 cmH_2O in order to get the patient accustomed to NIV. The pressure is then gradually increased by 2–3 cmH_2O to the target values every few minutes. In general, the minute ventilation may be further affected by the difference between IPAP and EPAP as well as inspiratory time, and oxygenation may be affected by the fraction of inspired oxygen (FiO_2) and EPAP.

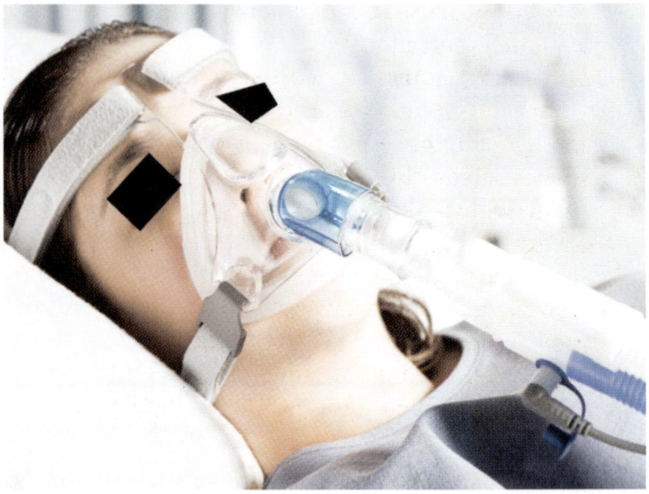

FIG. 1: Noninvasive ventilation (NIV) delivered by a mask covering mouth and nose.

Courtesy: Fisher and Paykel.

The patient's condition should be closely monitored (clinically for respiratory rate and respiratory effort, as well as through oximetry and arterial or venous blood gas analysis) and, in the event of worsening, intubation and mechanical ventilation should not be delayed. The first hour of NIV is crucial, as the NIV failure rate is at its highest during this time, and in common indications for NIV (COPD, congestive heart failure), patients generally rapidly respond to treatment. In significantly agitated patients for whom tolerance is a challenge, administration of a very low dose of a sedative drug (e.g., intravenous midazolam) may be considered, but this requires very close monitoring in an appropriate setting to avoid or at least detect early excessive suppression of respiratory efforts.

Indications for the use of NIV could be acute or chronic. It is most often used in acute hypoxic or hypercapnic respiratory failure in patients who do not have an indication for immediate intubation and who do not respond or are unlikely to fully respond to standard pharmacologic treatment and traditional oxygen therapy (see later on NHFT). One may also try to use it in patients who decline intubation, either as a trial of treatment or as a symptom control. The most common indications for acute NIV include the following:

- Exacerbations of COPD with hypercapnia [consider arterial blood pH < 7.35 and partial pressure of carbon dioxide ($PaCO_2$) >45–49 mm Hg; these values are only approximations and require continuous clinical correlation]—even in patients anticipated to require intubation, NIV should be trialed as intubation is arranged, because some patients may improve and avoid intubation altogether.

- *Cardiogenic pulmonary edema*: Via positive intrathoracic pressure, NIV and CPAP reduce preload and afterload, thus exerting beneficial hemodynamic effects, in addition to improving oxygenation in patients with cardiogenic pulmonary edema.
- Exacerbations of chronic disease-causing hypercapnia, particularly chest deformity (e.g., kyphoscoliosis) and neuromuscular disorders or obesity hypoventilation syndrome
- NIV may be used as an adjunct during withdrawal of mechanical ventilation as a method to reduce extubation failure.

Chronic NIV (including home NIV) may be used in the setting of:

- Neuromuscular diseases, including amyotrophic lateral sclerosis (ALS)
- Chest deformities causing respiratory failure (e.g., advanced kyphoscoliosis)
- Obesity hypoventilation syndrome
- COPD with significant hypercapnia, persisting despite optimization of therapy

Considering the use of NIV (and CPAP), one needs to keep in mind situations that may potentially preclude their use. Those include, among others, lack of cooperation (claustrophobic, anxious, or too uncomfortable), significantly decreased level of consciousness (unless related to rapidly reversible hypercapnia), lack of spontaneous respiratory effort, airway obstruction or the presence of large volume of airway secretions, severe hemodynamic instability, and high risk of aspiration of gastric contents (e.g., ileus obstruction, ongoing vomiting among other causes). CPAP or even NIV following the upper gastrointestinal (GI) or respiratory tract surgery may be used, but this decision should be reviewed with the surgeon as barotrauma or gastric distention may occur, especially with higher applied pressures.

Complications are usually local and caused by a mask (pressure ulcers and abrasions on the nose and other parts of the face, rhinitis, and nasal congestion) or air leakage (conjunctivitis). Hypotension and pulmonary barotrauma (rarely) and gastric distension may also occur. Nutrition may be compromised, as many NIV interfaces prevent reliable enteral access.

Nasal High-flow Therapy

Nasal high-flow therapy provides flow rates up to 60 L/min (in some devices 80 L/min) of inspiratory gas. Oxygen may be added as needed up to ~100% by using an air/oxygen blender or oxygen flow meter. As high flow rates are generated, a heated humidifier is an obligatory element of the system **(Fig. 2)**. The two main parameters that can be set are inspiratory gas (oxygen + air) flow and the FiO_2 or oxygen flow (if oxygen flow is set instead of FiO_2, the device measures FiO_2 and the operator should adjust oxygen flow to desired FiO_2). The temperature of gas is usually set at 37°C, but it can be lowered to a value tolerated by the patient. In general, patients are started with an FiO_2 based on their anticipated requirements and on a flow ranging from a traditionally lower rate (~30 L/min), which is then titrated up to the maximum tolerated flow, to a more recent higher starting rate of 50–60 L/min (in some devices, 60–80 L/min is possible). Higher flows increase dead-space washout (and thus may improve hypercapnia), may produce a higher dynamic PEEP (and thus contribute to improve oxygenation), and reduce the volume of entrained room air during the respiratory cycle, resulting in a more precise titration of FiO_2. Flows are usually maintained at ~50–60 L/min until FiO_2 requirements are lower (<50%), at which point flows are weaned alongside the FiO_2.

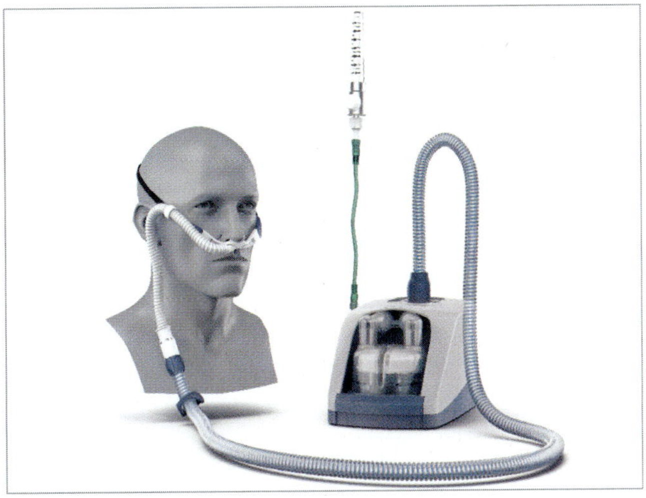

FIG. 2: Schematic setup for nasal high-flow therapy (NHFT).
Courtesy: Fisher and Paykel.

In addition, many patients find NHFT to be more comfortable. NHFT also allows for better communication, oral care, and enteral nutrition. It is suggested for use in acute hypoxemic respiratory failure, as it may reduce the risk of intubation and was routinely used in patients with COVID-19-related hypoxemic respiratory failure in order to avoid intubation, which is a benefit that may be further improved with the use of awake-prone positioning. A recent meta-analysis suggested no major difference in effectiveness between NIV and NHFT in patients with acute hypoxemic respiratory failure.

As noted above, postextubation use of NHFT may increase successful extubation, particularly in patients at some but not too high risk of extubation failure. In patients at higher risk, especially those with hypercapnia, postextubation NIV may be preferred, and NHFT may be used between NIV sessions.

While NHFT may play a role in hypercapnic respiratory failure, there is currently growing but still insufficient evidence for this, especially compared with the robust body of evidence supporting the use of NIV in hypercapnia. The existing evidence is too imprecise to conclude benefit or harm. NHFT can also be used for preoxygenation during endotracheal intubation; however, when used in the peri-intubation period, it may have no effect on peri-intubation hypoxemia compared with conventional oxygen delivery systems.

Lastly, NHFT may be a potential alternative in patients not tolerating NIV (e.g., agitation or secretions) and in patients in whom there is no plan for escalation of interventions, but control of symptoms including dyspnea, excessive work of breathing, or hypoxia is desirable.

CONCLUSION

Technological developments combined with the pandemic and the need for clinical solutions to deal with mounting numbers of patients requiring ventilatory/respiratory support led to the widespread use of newer forms of support. Those new potential modalities of treatment, used with increasing frequency by nonspecialists, have been discussed in this chapter.

ACKNOWLEDGMENTS

This paper used the material included in Oczkowski S, Jaeschke R, Rochwerg B, Jankowski M, Twardowska M. Noninvasive mechanical ventilation and continuous positive Airway Pressure. McMaster Textbook of Internal Medicine. Kraków: Medycyna Praktyczna; 2022. [online] Available from https://empendium.com/mcmtextbook/chapter/B31.IV.24.67.2 [Last accessed December, 2023].

SUGGESTED READINGS

1. Evans L, Rhodes A, Alhazzani W, Antonelli M, Coopersmith CM, French C, et al. Surviving sepsis campaign: International guidelines for management of sepsis and septic shock 2021. Intensive Care Med. 2021;47(11):e1181-247.
2. Rochwerg B, Brochard L, Elliott MW, Hess D, Hill NS, Nava S, et al. Official ERS/ATS clinical practice guidelines: noninvasive ventilation for acute respiratory failure. Eur Respir J. 2017; 50(2):1602426.
3. Osadnik CR, Tee VS, Carson-Chahhoud KV, Picot J, Wedzicha JA, Smith BJ. Non-invasive ventilation for the management of acute hypercapnic respiratory failure due to exacerbation of chronic obstructive pulmonary disease. Cochrane Database Syst Rev. 2017;7(7):CD004104.
4. David-João PG, Guedes MH, Réa-Neto Á, Chaiben VBO, Baena CP. Noninvasive ventilation in acute hypoxemic respiratory failure: A systematic review and meta-analysis. J Crit Care. 2019;49:84-91.
5. Vaschetto R, Pecere A, Perkins GD, Mistry D, Cammarota G, Longhini F, et al. Effects of early extubation followed by noninvasive ventilation versus standard extubation on the duration of invasive mechanical ventilation in hypoxemic non-hypercapnic patients: a systematic review and individual patient data meta-analysis of randomized controlled trials. Crit Care. 2021;25(1):189.
6. Oczkowski S, Ergan B, Bos L, Chatwin M, Ferrer M, Gregoretti C, et al. ERS clinical practice guidelines: High-flow nasal cannula in acute respiratory failure. Eur Respir J. 2022;59(4):2101574.
7. Rochwerg B, Einav S, Chaudhuri D, Mancebo J, Mauri T, Helviz Y, et al. The role for high flow nasal cannula as a respiratory support strategy in adults: a clinical practice guideline. Intensive Care Med. 2020;46(12):2226-37.
8. Chaudhuri D, Trivedi V, Lewis K, Rochwerg B. High-flow nasal cannula compared with noninvasive positive pressure ventilation in acute hypoxic respiratory failure: a systematic review and meta-analysis. Crit Care Explor. 2023;5(4):e0892.
9. Ovtcharenko N, Ho E, Alhazzani W, Cortegiani A, Ergan B, Scala R, et al. High-flow nasal cannula versus non-invasive ventilation for acute hypercapnic respiratory failure in adults: a systematic review and meta-analysis of randomized trials. Crit Care. 2022;26(1):348.

102

CHAPTER

Respiratory Symptoms in Gastroesophageal Reflux Disease

MD Varunn

ABSTRACT

Gastroesophageal reflux disease (GERD) often extends its effects beyond the esophagus, leading to respiratory symptoms in some individuals. These respiratory manifestations, including chronic cough, asthma-like symptoms, and shortness of breath, significantly affect an individual's well-being. The relationship between GERD and respiratory issues is complex, involving direct irritation of the airway and indirect vagal nerve stimulation. Diagnosis requires a comprehensive evaluation, and collaboration between gastroenterologists and respiratory specialists is essential. Management encompasses lifestyle adjustments, medications, and, in severe cases, surgery. Psychological factors can influence treatment outcomes, highlighting the importance of psychological and behavioral interventions. These connections between GERD and respiratory symptoms are not exclusive to adults, as children can also be affected, necessitating tailored approaches. Ongoing research continues to shed light on this intricate relationship.

INTRODUCTION

Gastroesophageal reflux disease (GERD) is a chronic condition characterized by the abnormal reflux of stomach acid into the esophagus. While the hallmark symptoms of GERD include heartburn and regurgitation, respiratory symptoms can also be present in some individuals. These respiratory symptoms, often referred to as "respiratory reflux" or "silent reflux", occur due to the reflux of gastric contents into the upper airway, leading to irritation and inflammation. This chapter aims to explore the relationship between GERD and respiratory symptoms, their underlying mechanisms, and potential treatment approaches.

PREVALENCE AND CLINICAL PRESENTATION

Gastroesophageal reflux-related respiratory symptoms are reported to be prevalent in a significant proportion of individuals with GERD. Various studies have indicated that up to 70% of patients with GERD may experience respiratory manifestations. The respiratory symptoms commonly associated with GERD include chronic cough, asthma-like symptoms, wheezing, shortness of breath, hoarseness, and recurrent respiratory infections. However, it is important to note that the presence of these symptoms does not automatically imply GERD as the cause, as other respiratory conditions must be ruled out **(Box 1)**.

The likelihood of a causal relationship between GERD and respiratory disorders varies across different manifestations and is not uniformly established.

BOX 1: Respiratory disorders associated with gastroesophageal reflux disease.

- Bronchial asthma (reflux asthma syndrome)
- Chronic persistent cough (reflux cough syndrome)
- Pulmonary aspiration complications (bronchiectasis, lung abscess, and aspiration pneumonitis)
- Chronic bronchitis
- Idiopathic pulmonary fibrosis
- Obstructive sleep apnea syndrome
- Chronic obstructive pulmonary disease

MECHANISMS OF RESPIRATORY SYMPTOMS IN GASTROESOPHAGEAL REFLUX DISEASE

The exact mechanisms underlying respiratory symptoms in GERD are not fully understood but are believed to involve both direct and indirect pathways. The direct pathway involves the reflux of gastric acid and other contents into the upper airway, triggering inflammation and irritation of the respiratory mucosa. This can result in bronchospasm, airway hyperreactivity, and increased mucus production.

The indirect pathway involves the stimulation of the vagus nerve, which connects the gastrointestinal and respiratory systems. Vagus nerve stimulation can lead to bronchoconstriction, increased cough reflex sensitivity, and alterations in airway tone. Additionally, microaspiration of small amounts of gastric contents into the lungs may contribute to respiratory symptoms, leading to chronic inflammation and damage **(Fig. 1)**.

DIAGNOSTIC EVALUATION

The diagnosis of GERD-related respiratory symptoms can be challenging due to overlapping symptoms with other respiratory conditions. A thorough clinical history, including symptom assessment and response to empirical treatment, is essential. Diagnostic tools such as esophageal pH monitoring, esophagogastroduodenoscopy (EGD), and imaging studies can help confirm the presence of GERD and evaluate the severity of reflux.

In some cases, specialized tests like multichannel intraluminal impedance (MII) can be utilized to detect nonacidic reflux events that may be missed by pH monitoring alone. Collaboration between gastroenterologists and respiratory specialists is crucial to establish an accurate diagnosis and guide appropriate management **(Box 2)**.

BOX 2: Criteria for determining which individuals with chronic cough should be evaluated for gastroesophageal reflux disease (GERD).

- Chronic cough (> 8 weeks)
- Not on angiotensin-converting enzyme inhibitor
- Not a present smoker or exposed to other environmental irritants
- Chest radiograph is normal (or near normal)
- Symptomatic asthma has been ruled out*
- Postnasal drip syndrome has been ruled out*
- Eosinophilic bronchitis has been ruled out*

*Through relevant tests such as a sinus computed tomography (CT) scan showing normal results, negative histamine provocation, absence of sputum eosinophilia, and no improvement observed with steroid treatment.

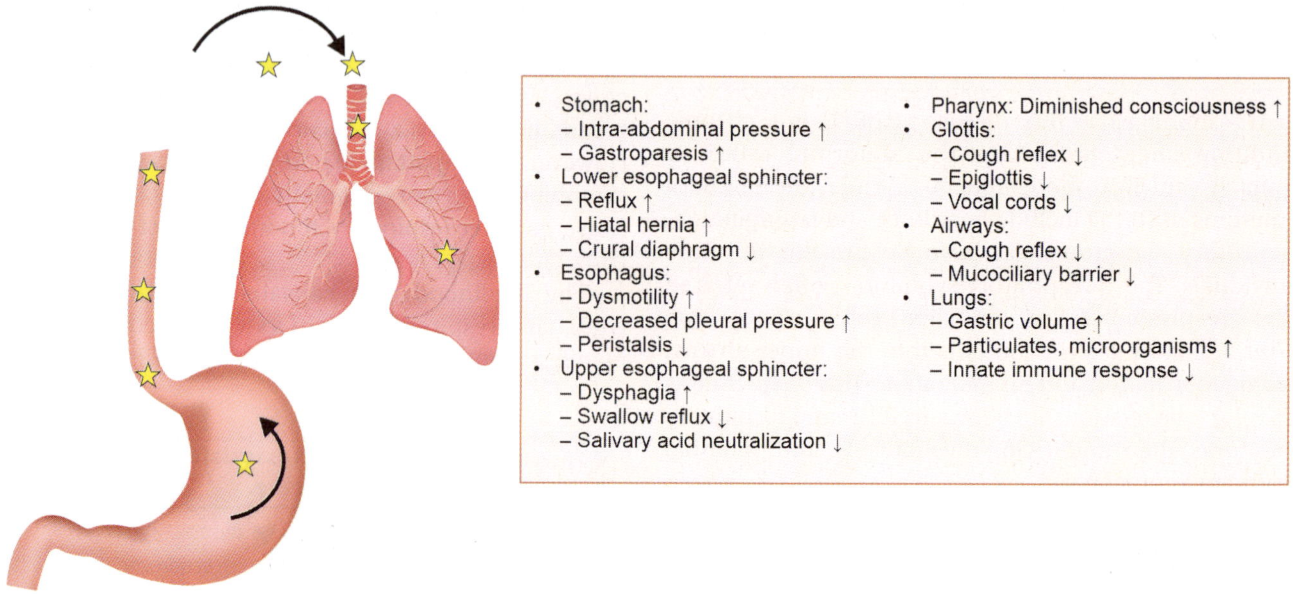

FIG. 1: Gastric-to-pulmonary aspiration: While gastroesophageal reflux is common, the occurrence of refluxate reaching the lower airways necessitates the breakdown of multiple protective mechanisms.

Note: The up arrow (↑) denotes factors that encourage or facilitate aspiration, while the down arrow (↓) represents mechanisms that safeguard against aspiration and its associated consequences.

COMORBIDITIES AND ASSOCIATION WITH ASTHMA

Epidemiological insights underscore the notable overlap between GERD and asthma, revealing a frequent co-existence. However, recent critical literature reviews and meticulously controlled studies have cast a discerning light on the robustness of this association, prompting deliberation about whether it has been somewhat over-emphasized. Proposed mechanisms include micro-aspiration and vagally mediated bronchospasm, although the precise impact of esophageal acid on pulmonary function continues to be a subject of spirited debate within the medical community.

Of paramount importance is the role of nocturnal reflux in the genesis of respiratory complaints. During the nocturnal sleep cycle, the mitigating mechanisms against reflux become less effective, facilitating the potential aspiration of gastric contents into the upper airway. Moreover, asthma itself can be contributory to the prevalence of reflux, with negative pleural pressure during asthma exacerbations increasing the likelihood of reflux events. Notably, the influence of certain bronchodilator medications on reflux has raised intriguing questions that warrant further investigation.

As for interventions, medical therapy has exhibited promise in ameliorating asthma symptoms, particularly in cases of difficult-to-treat asthma. Antireflux therapy, often involving the use of proton pump inhibitors (PPIs), has shown potential in selected patients. However, the decision to pursue surgical intervention, typically in the form of fundoplication, should be carefully weighed, as it may not consistently yield optimal outcomes. The exact patient population that stands to gain the most from surgical antireflux procedures remains a matter of ongoing investigation.

CLINICAL SYNDROMES ASSOCIATED WITH GASTROESOPHAGEAL REFLUX DISEASE

Gastroesophageal reflux disease has been linked to various clinical syndromes affecting the lungs. These include nodular granulomatous bronchiolar disease, bronchiolitis obliterans with organizing pneumonia (BOOP), idiopathic pulmonary fibrosis (IPF), scleroderma, bronchiolitis obliterans post-lung transplantation, and nontubercular mycobacterial (NTM) lung infections. It is important to note that acute lung injury caused by significant aspiration of gastric contents, known as aspiration pneumonitis, represents a distinct clinical syndrome that should be distinguished from the more gradual onset of microaspiration-related diseases.

The nodular granulomatous bronchiolar disease often afflicts patients with neurological disorders and esophageal conditions. Repeated aspiration of gastric contents leads to granulomatous reactions in the bronchioles. Notably, this condition can occur in patients solely with GERD, indicating the complexity of these associations. BOOP is less frequently linked to GERD, yet cases show that GERD treatment can resolve refractory BOOP. Fibrosing lung diseases like IPF and scleroderma share similarities in clinical presentation, characterized by dyspnea, inspiratory rales, and fibrotic radiographic changes. Both conditions involve frequent esophageal dysfunction and recurrent microaspiration, suggesting their connection to GERD. Studies have correlated the severity of esophageal reflux with declining lung function in scleroderma patients.

The prevalence of GERD in IPF patients has given rise to the hypothesis that recurrent microaspiration drives the ongoing inflammation in the disease. However, it is essential to distinguish this from acute exacerbation of IPF, as the pathology may involve organizing pneumonia. Some patients show diffuse fibrosis with bronchiolar damage, implicating a combination of reflux and aspiration.

In the context of lung transplant recipients, bronchiolitis obliterans syndrome (BOS) affects small airways, and GERD is associated with its development and progression. Factors like gastroparesis, vagus nerve dysfunction, oropharyngeal dysphagia, and impaired cough reflex contribute to GERD-related lung disease in this population. Notably, many lung transplant patients with GERD may not exhibit classic symptoms, emphasizing the need for vigilance in diagnosis.

Nontubercular mycobacterial lung infection often presents as nodular bronchiectasis. It has been associated with esophageal disorders, and studies indicate a link between pathological acid reflux and this infection. The exact connection between NTM lung infection and GERD remains speculative. There is some evidence suggesting that acid-suppressing medications may not be the primary factor in its pathogenesis, as *Mycobacterium avium* naturally resists acidic pH.

These associations between GERD and various lung diseases have significant implications for diagnosis and treatment. While some questions remain regarding the causal relationships between GERD and these syndromes, understanding these connections is essential for providing comprehensive care to patients with these conditions.

MANAGEMENT

The management of GERD-related respiratory symptoms involves a combination of lifestyle modifications,

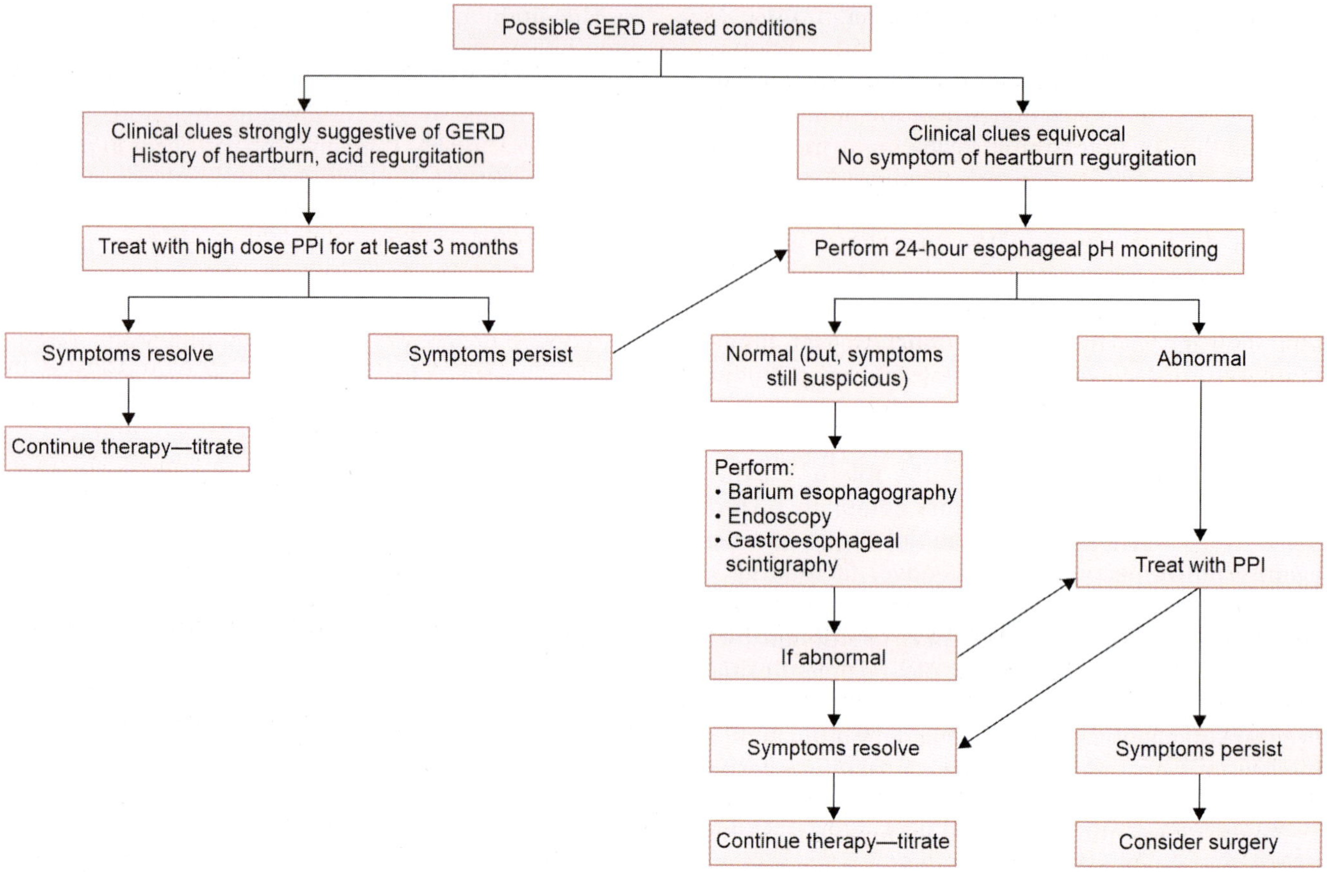

FLOWCHART 1: Approach to diagnosing and managing gastroesophageal reflux disease (GERD)-related extraesophageal symptoms.
(GERD: gastroesophageal reflux disease; PPI: proton pump inhibitor)

pharmacotherapy, and in select cases, surgical interventions. Lifestyle modifications include weight loss (if applicable), avoiding trigger foods, elevating the head of the bed during sleep, and adopting proper dietary habits.

Pharmacotherapy options primarily focus on reducing gastric acid production and improving esophageal motility. PPIs, H2 receptor antagonists, and prokinetic agents are commonly prescribed medications. PPIs, in particular, have shown efficacy in relieving respiratory symptoms associated with GERD.

Surgical interventions such as fundoplication may be considered for patients with severe refractory symptoms, who do not respond to conservative measures or require long-term medication use. However, the decision for surgery should be made on an individual basis after careful evaluation and discussion with a healthcare professional **(Flowchart 1)**.

IMPACT ON QUALITY OF LIFE

Gastroesophageal reflux disease can extend its effects beyond the esophagus, causing a range of respiratory symptoms that significantly influence an individual's quality of life. The persistence of these symptoms, such as chronic cough and shortness of breath, brings physical discomfort, fatigue, and limitations in daily activities. Furthermore, the unpredictable nature of these respiratory symptoms can lead to anxiety and psychological distress. It is imperative for healthcare providers to recognize the comprehensive impact of GERD-related respiratory symptoms on patients' well-being and to implement holistic management approaches.

Patients frequently describe a burning sensation, chest tightness, or the feeling of "something stuck" in the throat. Such chronic discomfort can significantly reduce the overall quality of life, as individuals may find themselves struggling to breathe and sleep properly.

THE ROLE OF DIET AND LIFESTYLE MODIFICATIONS

Effective management of GERD-related respiratory symptoms often begins with lifestyle modifications. Patients are commonly advised to make specific dietary changes, including avoiding trigger foods like spicy foods, caffeine, alcohol, and fatty meals. Weight loss can also be beneficial for those who are overweight or obese, as it can alleviate symptoms by reducing intra-abdominal pressure. Additionally, adopting specific behaviors such as eating smaller, more frequent meals and refraining from lying down immediately after eating can help decrease reflux episodes and ameliorate respiratory symptoms.

Lifestyle changes extend beyond dietary adjustments. Patients are encouraged to elevate the head of their beds and avoid tight clothing. These changes aim to minimize the chances of gastric contents flowing back into the esophagus, reducing the likelihood of aspiration into the airways. Avoiding late-night snacks or meals and refraining from tobacco use and alcohol consumption can further mitigate symptoms.

PSYCHOLOGICAL AND BEHAVIORAL INTERVENTIONS

Psychological factors play a substantial role in GERD symptoms and can significantly affect the outcomes of treatment. Stress, anxiety, and other emotional factors may exacerbate GERD symptoms or hinder the effectiveness of treatment. Consequently, addressing psychological well-being is an important component of comprehensive care. This can be achieved through stress management techniques, relaxation exercises, and cognitive-behavioral therapy.

These interventions aim to reduce stress levels, enhance coping mechanisms, and improve overall treatment responses, ultimately contributing to the relief from GERD-related respiratory symptoms. Stress management can help patients develop healthier ways of responding to the challenges posed by GERD, ultimately reducing the impact of psychological distress on their lives.

PEDIATRIC CONSIDERATIONS

Gastroesophageal reflux disease-related respiratory symptoms are not exclusive to adults, they can also affect children. In pediatric populations, respiratory symptoms such as chronic cough, wheezing, and recurrent respiratory infections may serve as the primary manifestations of GERD. Diagnosing GERD in children requires special attention due to their unique developmental and physiological characteristics.

Children's treatment approaches need to be tailored to their age and specific needs, often with a focus on lifestyle modifications and dietary changes suitable for their developmental stage. Pediatric GERD can often be managed with dietary adjustments and medications to relieve symptoms and reduce the risk of complications.

CONCLUSION

Respiratory symptoms in GERD are a frequently encountered manifestation of the disease. These symptoms can significantly impact an individual's quality of life and require a comprehensive diagnostic approach for accurate identification.

By understanding the underlying mechanisms and employing appropriate diagnostic techniques, healthcare professionals can effectively diagnose GERD-related respiratory symptoms and provide tailored treatment strategies. Collaboration between gastroenterologists and respiratory specialists is crucial for comprehensive management and optimal patient outcomes. The ongoing research in this field will continue to shed light on the complex interactions between GERD and respiratory symptoms, enabling further advancements in diagnosis, treatment, and patient care.

SUGGESTED READINGS

1. Dent J, El-Serag HB, Wallander MA, Johansson S. Epidemiology of gastro-oesophageal reflux disease: a systematic review. Gut. 2005;54(5):710-7.
2. Harding SM. Gastroesophageal reflux, asthma, and mechanisms of interaction. Am J Med. 2001;111(Suppl 8A):8S-12S.
3. Galmiche JP, Zerbib F, Bruley Des Varannes S. Review article: respiratory manifestations of gastro-oesophageal reflux disease. Aliment Pharmacol Ther. 2008;27(6):449-64.
4. Kahrilas PJ, Altman KW, Chang AB, Field SK, Harding SM, Lane AP, et al. Chronic cough due to gastroesophageal reflux in adults: CHEST guideline and expert panel report. Chest. 2016;150(6):1341-60.
5. Irwin RS, Curley FJ, French CL. Chronic cough. The spectrum and frequency of causes, key components of the diagnostic evaluation, and outcome of specific therapy. Am Rev Respir Dis. 1990;141(3):640-7.

103
CHAPTER

Spontaneous Pneumothorax

BL Bhardwaj, RS Bhatia, Rajbir Singh, Prabhpreet Kaur

ABSTRACT

Spontaneous pneumothorax implies air collection in the pleural cavity without any preceding trauma. The presence of preexisting lung disease would differentiate secondary from primary pneumothorax. Apart from a wide range of causative factors, active pulmonary tuberculosis (TB), chronic bronchitis emphysema, bronchogenic carcinoma, suppurative pneumonia, bronchiectasis, etc., are common causes of secondary spontaneous pneumothorax. A common entity in males, spontaneous pneumothorax has smoking as a high-risk factor. Chest X-ray is diagnostic, and high-resolution computed tomography (HRCT) has added new dimensions to diagnostic etiological yield. HRCT suggests a 3–4% yield of spontaneous pneumothorax in coronavirus disease 2019 (COVID-19) pneumonia. The pathological varieties such as closed, open, and valvular types, determine the course of the disease as well as its management. The tension-type spontaneous pneumothorax is a medical emergency and an urgent management action is rewarding. The controversy is still on between physicians' conservative management and surgeon's active measures. In small closed pneumothorax of <20% of hemithorax, no specific treatment is required. Pneumothorax of >20% or with dyspnea requires active management. The ultimate choice is chest tube drainage under a water seal and if not give good results, it has to be assisted by open thoracotomy. With video-assisted thoracoscopic surgery (VATS) National Wilms' Tumor Study (NWTS), recurrence prevention can be targeted, with optimal use of HRCT chest. With underlying lung disease. In case of simultaneous bilateral spontaneous pneumothorax, surgical pleurectomy should be attempted. Chemical pleurodesis using a sclerosing agent such as tetracycline hydrochloride can be of value. The outcome is good in a healthy adult in the absence of preexisting pulmonary disease.

INTRODUCTION

The collection of air in the pleural cavity without any preceding trauma is called spontaneous pneumothorax. It can be primary when there is no demonstrable pulmonary pathology or it can be secondary where associated clinically recognizable pulmonary pathology with structural or functional abnormality. Etiological diagnosis decides the definitive line of treatment. Clinical diagnosis, assisted white matter hyperintensities (WMH) plan X-ray chest is sufficient to sum up the diagnosis of spontaneous pneumothorax. High-resolution computed tomography (HRCT) if available offers investigation. Although a range of simple observations of bilateral thoracostomy has been described management is suggested on having an aggressive approach.

TYPES

Two types of pneumothoraxes have been described: (1) primary spontaneous pneumothorax and (2) secondary spontaneous pneumothorax.

Primary Spontaneous Pneumothorax

It is common in young healthy tall, thin, male adults in the age group of 20–40 years, with male to female ratio being 6:1 and incidence being 7.4 per 100,000/year for males, with a corresponding figure of 1:2 for females in the USA and UK. It affects both tie lungs equally This results from the rupture of small air-spaced measuring 1–2 cm in diameter (subpleural bleb) into the pleural space because of congenital weakness in connective tissue of subpleural alveoli or may arise as an interstitial emphysema. This occurs almost in 90% of cases, often multiple and commonly involving the apices, possibly because of the mechanical stress of regional distending forces which are maximum over the apices. Relative ischemia of lung apices may also contribute. An association between smoking, the high-pulmonary concentration of hydroxyproline (a degradation product of collagen), and specific human leukocyte antigen (HLA) antigen and antitrypsin genotypes (in familial occurrence of spontaneous pneumothorax have been observed).

Secondary Spontaneous Pneumothorax

It occurs as a result of lung disease. Spontaneous pneumothorax occurs because of the rupture of the cavity of the subpleural tuberculous lesion giving way into the pleural cavity. About 1.4% of cases of active pulmonary tuberculosis are complicated by pneumothorax, and 90% of these cases are cavitary. If not treated, these cases get further complicated as empyema or bronchopleural fistula. Rarely pneumothorax may occur in acute miliary tuberculosis possible mechanisms suggested are an initial pneumomediastinum with leakage of air through mediastinal pleura, rupture of caseation or necrosis of subpleural miliary nodule through pleura, rupture of bullous lesion of military tuberculosis or paroxysmal cough causing forceful expiratory effort against a closed glottis causing rupture. Spontaneous pneumothorax in coronavirus disease 2019 (COVID-19) diffuse lung injury is also contributed by barotrauma during oxygen therapy. Chronic bronchitis and emphysema significantly contribute to this type of pneumothorax. Trapped air leaks through weakened walls of dilated and distended alveoli, assisted by high intrabronchial pressure aggravated by cough. Secondary spontaneous pneumothorax can be life-threatening in chronic obstructive pulmonary disease (COPD) patients. In <1% of adults and 2.5% of children, bronchial asthma is the cause of pneumothorax. Staphylococcal pneumonia in children and *Klebsiella pneumonia* in adults are the infections that are commonly associated with pneumothorax. It is the multiple cystic areas (pneumatoceles) that rupture into the pleural space. Iatrogenic pneumothorax may occur during closed/transbronchial/transthoracic biopsy, subclavian/jugular vein catheterization, nasogastric tube placement, tracheostomy, mechanical ventilation, cardiopulmonary (CP) resuscitation or taking a liver biopsy.

A recurrent pneumothorax associated with menstruation, almost always on the right side, and occurring in women over 25–30 years of age has been described by Maurer et al. in 1958 as catamenial pneumothorax. About one-third of the patients have associated pelvic endometriosis. Air leaks occur possibly from the peritoneal cavity into the pleural space through diaphragmatic fenestrations. Acquired immunodeficiency syndrome (AIDS)-related pneumothorax, frequently associated with *Pneumocystis carinii* pneumonia. A virulent form of necrotizing subpleural necrosis results in diffuse air leaks. Due to age >60 years, pulmonary fibrosis, and increased height/weight ratio recurrence are common. Common causes and occurrence of spontaneous pneumothorax with other diseases along with suggested CT scoring are seen in **Boxes 1 to 3** and **Table 1**.

Spontaneous pneumothorax is the main respiratory manifestation of Marian's syndrome also. A basic defect in collagen fiber having fewer side-to-side linkages results in increased tissue friability along with patchy abnormal alveolar elastica, that is more pronounced over the areas of emphysema. Apart from the manifestation of honeycomb lung or cystic fibrosis, it can rarely be seen in bronchogenic carcinoma, sarcoidosis, hydatid cyst of lung, pulmonary alveolar proteinosis, Wegener's granulomatosis, eosinophilic granuloma of lung and aseptic cavitating pulmonary infarction. Three types of pneumothoraxes are recognized pathologically.

Closed

Where the communication with the atmospheric air gets sealed off as the ruptured site closes. Air in the pleural cavity gets absorbed and the lung re-expands to its original

BOX 1: Spontaneous pneumothorax.

Etiology

- *Primary*: Apical blebs
- *Secondary*:
  - Common causes: Pulmonary tuberculosis, chronic bronchitis, and emphysema, bronchial asthma, suppurative pneumonia, lung abscess, bronchiectasis, Birt–Hogg–Dubé syndrome, bronchogenic carcinoma, and cystic fibrosis
  - Rare causes: Cryptogenic fibrosing alveolitis, occupational lung disorders (acute silicosis), Shaver's disease, granulomatous disease (late fibrotic stage of sarcoidosis, histiocytosis X, and Wegener's disease), connective tissue disorders [systemic lupus erythematosus (SLE) and rheumatoid disease], hemosiderosis, pulmonary alveolar proteinosis, hereditary disease (neurofibromatosis and tuberous sclerosis), inherited syndrome (Marfan's syndrome, Ehlers–Danlos syndrome, and Marfanoid hypermobility syndrome), coccidioidomycosis, parasitic disease (hydatid disease), intrathoracic tumors (metastatic sarcomas, germ cell tumors, and metastatic Wilm's tumor), cavitating pulmonary infarction, and catamenial pneumothorax

BOX 2: Occurrence of spontaneous pneumothorax in association with other disease.

Spontaneous pneumothorax may occur:
- *As a complication of:*
  - Bronchial asthma
  - Rupture of staphylococcal
  - Pneumatocele
- *As a manifestation of:*
  - Honeycomb lung
  - Bronchogenic carcinoma
  - Coal worker's pneumoconiosis
  - Sarcoidosis
  - Silicosis
  - Fibrosing alveolitis
- COVID-19 diffuse lung injury
- *Is precipitated during:*
  - Corticosteroid therapy
  - Positive pressure breathing [using positive end-expiratory pressure (PEEP)]
  - Menstruation
- *AIDS-related*: Associated with pneumocystis infection.
- Bilateral spontaneous pneumothorax secondary to osteosarcoma metastasis

BOX 3: Spontaneous pneumothorax.

Equally common among:
- Infectious, e.g., tuberculosis
- Noninfectious, e.g., chronic obstructive airway disease (COAD)

TABLE 1: Signs in etiology of spontaneous pneumothorax.

	Infective	Noninfective
Lesion wall thickness		Present
Solid component		Present
Pleural effusion	Present	
Pleural thickness	Present	
Consolidation	Present	

position over a few weeks. Intrapleural pressure remains lesser than atmospheric pressure.

Open

Where the communication with the atmospheric air remains patent in the form of a bronchopleural fistula as the ruptured site does not close. Intrapleural pressure approximates the atmospheric pressure and does not allow the lung to re-expand. Patent bronchopleural fistula makes the pleural space susceptible to infections resulting in pyopneumothorax.

Tension (Valvular)

Where the communication with the outside air is persistent but is small and valvular, allowing the air to enter only without permitting it to escape. This allows a large amount of air trapping in the pleural cavity. Intrapleural pressure becomes more than atmospheric pressure, resulting in mediastinal displacement toward the opposite side, consequently compressing the opposite lung.

CLINICAL PRESENTATION AND DIAGNOSIS

Small pneumothoraces can be asymptomatic and only detected as accidental radiological findings. Clinical features and functional abnormalities depend on the size of the pneumothorax, the amount of lung collapse, and preexisting lung disease. Its course depends on the type of pneumothorax. Sudden onset of chest pain is the most common clinical symptom, often associated with breathlessness. Pain is continuously invariably exacerbated by deep inspiration or postural change. Severe dyspnea with cardiopulmonary compromise forms the hallmark of tension dyspnea. Restless, anxious, tachypneic patients may have cyanosis as well. Failure in rapid relief of tension may result in a rapid low volume pulse with hypotension and pulsus paradoxus.

Small pneumothoraces are often missed on clinical examination. Otherwise, clinical chest findings include a prominent chest wall, diminished respiratory movements, percussion note is hyperresonant, coin test positive, vocal fremitus, presence of mediastinal shift to the opposite side, and breath sounds are diminished or absent on auscultation. Succession splash may be hard if there is hydropneumothorax. One may find a mediastinal crunch (crepitus) over the precordium that occurs due to close proximity of trapped air and the moving cardiac muscle, (earlier called Hamman's sign). Mediastinal emphysema may cause central chest pain simulating myocardial infarction. Re-expansion pulmonary edema occurring as a rare life-threatening complication in pneumothorax as well as pleural effusion, atelectasis, and postlobectomy is clinically recognized as respiratory failure with circulatory shock. Pinkish sputum, dyspnea, tachycardia, hypothermia, and hypotension are clinical symptoms. X-ray chest reveals pulmonary edema. About 20% mortality may occur. Thoracentesis, thoracotomy with intravenous (IV) fluids, oxygen, and morphine are given. Nasal intermittent positive pressure ventilation (NIPPV) helps. Diuresis should not be attempted.

Diagnosis is often based on clinical findings, confirmed by chest skiagram. Classical radiological features of pneumothorax include a lucent zone devoid of lung marking with a sharply defined lung edge (the lung compressed toward the hilum), with a convexity outward. Small pneumothoraces can be detected in the expiratory film, especially in the lateral view (preferably in children). Exaggerated bronchovascular markings because of increased blood flow to the lung can be seen on the opposite side. In massive compression collapse (complete pneumothorax), the lung is compressed toward the hilum and appears as a dense globular mass. In tension pneumothorax, the mediastinum is shifted to the opposite side. Radiological findings are characteristics of pneumomediastinum. If hydropneumothorax is present, a horizontal at the fluid level is visualized.

A restrictive type of ventilatory impairment is classically seen in pneumothorax, with reduced vital capacity, functional residual capacity, and total lung capacity. Diffusion capacity is reduced; vital capacity is reduced a little. If pneumothorax is >20%, hypoxemia may be present. Initial hypoxemia occurs due to a collapsed lung causing lesser blood flow to the side. It improves gradually because of compensatory hypoxic vasoconstriction that corrects gross ventilation/perfusion imbalance. Cyanosis disappears later due to a reduction in the perfusion of the collapsed lung. The value of HRCT adds meaningfully in diagnosing spontaneous pneumothorax since etiological diagnosis is important for the definitive treatment of any disease. Also, HRCT can detect even lesions, such as eosinophilic granuloma and lymphangioleiomyomatosis. HRCT can also diagnose pulmonary tuberculosis in patients where chest X-ray may be reported normal HRCT findings suggestive of active tuberculosis are:

- Centrilobular nodule with branching linear structures
- Tree-in-bud appearance, having more than one contiguous branching site
- Consolidation of cavitary nodule
- About 5–8 mm diameter poorly defined nodules
- Lobular consolidation with thickening of interlobular septae
- Bronchial wall thickness with or without bronchiectasis

Box 4 shows the differential diagnosis of spontaneous pneumothorax.

BOX 4: Differential diagnosis.

- Myocardial infarction
- Bronchial asthma
- Pulmonary embolism
- Perforated peptic ulcer
- Large emphysematous bulla
- Diaphragmatic hernia

MANAGEMENT

Management of pneumothorax may be conservative or active, depending upon the amount of air in the pleural cavity and the underlying physiological disturbance, e.g., tension pneumothorax is taken as a medical emergency. Conservative therapy is indicated in a healthy non-dyspneic adult, having a pneumothorax of very small volume, occupying <20% of hemothorax. Air will get absorbed at the rate of 1.25%/day, if there is no further leak, thus allowing re-expansion of hemithorax volume at the same rate. Re-expansion pulmonary edema can occasionally complicate decompression procedures in different lung diseases. This would help 20% of pneumothorax re-expanding within 20 days. About 100% supplemental oxygen helps in enhancing the air absorption by several folds, through creating a substantial fall in the total end capillary pressure nearly from 706–146 mm Hg. About 100% oxygen increases 10 times the gradient for movement of gas from capillaries in the parietal and visceral pleura to air in the pleural cavity by replacing nitrogen with oxygen in capillaries. High oxygen concentration may be harmful in cases of COPD with carbon dioxide retention. Since relapse is common in 1/3–1/2 of patients, observation alone should be avoided, except in very small pneumothoraces or apical pneumothoraces. Guidelines have been laid down by a British group for the management of spontaneous pneumothorax.

Pleural cavity air should be removed by simple aspiration or by inserting a chest tube through intercostal space under a water-seal device. Chest X-ray is not as effective as computed tomography (CT) and therefore, for secondary pneumothoraces, intercostal tube drainage offers a better option for those with a distance of >2 cm above which the volume of pneumothorax will be >50%. The tip of the wide bore needle has to be introduced into the pleural cavity above the rib to prevent injury to the intercostal vessels as an emergency measure, followed by replacement with an intercostal catheter (connected to the water seal) to prevent any injury by the needle tip to the expanding lung. Simple aspiration is safe as an initial treatment of choice in patients with normal lungs who present with spontaneous pneumothorax, irrespective of its stay, and may offer a short hospital stay and reduce the rate of pleurectomy with no increase in recurrence rate at one year. Appropriate treatment not just on the size of a pneumothorax on chest X-ray but more importantly, on the clinical status of the patient. Active management is indicated in tension pneumothorax, pneumothorax of >20% of hemithorax, with coexisting pulmonary disease, in a dyspneic patient, in a patient with previous pneumothorax in the opposite lung, in an increasing (progressive) pneumothorax, in bilateral pneumothorax, and also in cases with accompanying pleural effusion or empyema.

The initial simple method includes inserting an intercostal tube connected to an underwater seal that allows re-expansion of the lung. In case of failure of response, suction can be applied. Complications such as hemothorax and thromboembolism can occur. Alternatively, a Heimlich flutter valve can be connected to the tube; although it is cheap and makes the patient mobile, mechanical problems with the value; however, restrict its use. Others have used a urinary bag with a flutter valve. The only drawback is that suction cannot be applied to it, in case it is required for the persistent leak, although the suction application has been found to be unnecessary. Risk of lung laceration and complications such as empyema and chronic pneumothorax are commonly seen with needle aspiration. In open pneumothorax, reexpansion usually does not occur by this method; and persistent air leak following tube drainage for spontaneous pneumothorax is a potentially troublesome complication. Thoracentesis can be of therapeutic value in closed spontaneous pneumothorax only in selected cases since there are more relapses, and more changes of lung laceration and empyema. In case of failure of reexpansion of the lung within 7–10 days despite of good chest tube, parietal pleurotomy is carried out for a posterolateral recurrence, contralateral occurrence, bilateral simultaneous pneumothorax, persistent pleural effusion, and high-risk patients, such as air-crew, divers, and seafarers.

Surgical Management

About 7-9 days would provide a reasonable opportunity for persistent air leaks to resolve with medical treatment with normal lungs. Under thoracoscopic guidance, allowing for both the excision and closure of ruptured blebs in a fashion identical to the traditional approach with open thoracotomy can be done. With video-assisted thoracoscopic surgery (VATS), recurrence prevention can be targeted with optimal use of HRCT chest. The recurrence rate of primary spontaneous pneumothorax after VATS bullectomy combined with surgical pleurodesis is in the range of 1.7–5%. Lesser shoulder dysfunction and pain medication requirements are observed with VATS as compared to postlateral thoracotomy during the postoperative period. Surgical pleurectomy should be attempted early, especially in simultaneous bilateral spontaneous pneumothorax, secondary to underlying lung disease. Tension pneumothorax is treated as a medical emergency, urgently converting the tension pneumothorax into an open variety, by inserting any available wide-bore needle into the pleural space. The needle is then replaced by an intercostal catheter, as early as possible. Minimal invasive management is suggested for first and recurrent pneumothorax. Recurrent pneumothorax, seen in about 20% of cases within a year, treatment with sclerosing agents is more effective in preventing ipsilateral recurrence than chest tube insertion alone. Although thoracotomy remains the current standard treatment, yet chemical pleurodesis can be useful, especially in patients who run the risk of surgery. About 1 g tetracycline hydrochloride solution in 50 mL of normal saline with 10 mL of 1% lignocaine is injected into the chest tube and is allowed to remain there for several hours before drainage. Due to an inflammatory reaction (chemical pleuritis), with visceral and parietal pleurae get adherent, thus leading to pleural symphysis. It is less painful, causes lesser exudation and the patient has a shorter hospital stay. Catamenial hemothorax (and pneumothorax) is also effectively treated with chemical pleurodesis. **Table 2** shows the therapeutic approach to spontaneous pneumothorax.

Autologous blood patch pleurodesis can be used as a simple, painless, and inexpensive alternative treatment

TABLE 2: Spontaneous pneumothorax management.

A. Therapeutic options:
- Observations alone (conservative)
- Thoracentesis
- Chest tube thoracostomy
- Chest tube thoracostomy with chemical pleurodesis
- Surgical interventions
    - Thoracostomy
    - Thoracoscopy with pleurodesis

B. Suggested methods of treatment in spontaneous pneumothorax

Type of pneumothorax	Treatment option
Pneumothorax of < 20% of lung volume • Apical pneumothorax • Closed type pleural leak	Observation alone
Pneumothorax of > 20% • Leak if closed-type • Pneumothorax with clinical symptoms	Thoracentesis
Pneumothorax with open-type chest tube thoracostomy • Pneumothorax with bronchopleural fistula • Pyopneumothorax	
Tension pneumothorax	Urgent chest tube
Thoracostomy	
Ipsilateral recurrent pneumothorax	
Chest tube	Thoracostomy
With chemical	Pleurodesis

in patients with persistent air leaks. Aggressive stepped care management by large bore intercostal chest tube drainage, chemical pleurodesis, and an early video-assisted talc powder age in AIDS-related spontaneous pneumothorax as it carries high mortality. Chronic pneumothorax due to persistent bronchopleural fistula or leak through multiple congenital or emphysematous bullae needs to be treated by decortication, by stripping the parietal pleura, or by suturing the fistulous tract, or segmental resection of a diseased lung. A huge bulla associated with spontaneous pneumothorax should be an indication for VATS, since this giant bulla, can itself be a manifestation of lung carcinoma or a focus for recurrent infection. Analgesics, backrest, oxygen therapy, and prophylactic antimicrobial therapy form important supportive measures. About 3 months follow-up for 1 year, to detect recurrence is recommended. Complications such as hemothorax, infection, and atelectasis can be treated with thoracotomy and clot evacuation, anti-microbials, and physiotherapy respectively. The prognosis is good in healthy adults without any underlying lung diseases. Tension pneumothorax may be rapidly fatal if not urgently treated. Mortality is higher in the elderly with airway obstruction. Complications like hemothorax pose a great hazard. With lowered morbidity and proven safety, VATS can be used in the elderly and pediatric populations.

CONCLUSION

Nontraumatic air collection in the pleural cavity without any cause or secondarily with recognizable abnormal structural or physiological pulmonary pathology is the spontaneous pneumothorax. The definitive course of management is decided by etiology. Although an aggressive approach has been suggested as the choice of management, simple observations to undergoing bilateral thoracostomy have also been employed. High-resolution computed tomography is optimally used and with the help of VATS prevention of recurrence is possible, especially in the absence of preexisting lung disease. Chemical pleurodesis is of great value for good outcomes. The conservative approach stands strong in 20% of cases against the application of surgical management. However, pneumothorax of >20% or with dyspnea requires urgent active surgical management. Chest tube drainage under a water seal stands as the best choice. However, if good results are falling short assistance of open thoracotomy can be taken.

SUGGESTED READINGS

1. Pareek KK, Narsimulu G. Medicine Update. New Delhi: Jaypee Brothers Medical Publishers; 2019. pp. 284-94.
2. Ohata M, Suzuk H. Pathogenesis of spontaneous pneumothorax. With special reference to the ultrastructure of emphysematous bullae. Chest. 1980;77(6):771-6.
3. Sharpe IK, Ahmad M, Braun W. Familial spontaneous pneumothorax and HLA antigens. Chest. 1980;78(2):264-8.
4. Narang PK, Surendra Kumar, Gupta A. Pneumothorax and pneumomediastinum complicating acute miliary tuberculosis. Tubercle. 1997;58(2):79-82.
5. Kedia Y, Awad NT, Nair J, Patil D, Amin P, Vijayan S, et al. Spontaneous Pneumothorax in Patients of COVID 19 Pneumonia. J Assoc Physicians India. 2022;70(2):11-2.
6. RS Bhatia, Suryakant (Eds). COPD. JBS Foundation Lucknow; 2016.
7. Bhatia RS, Bhardwaj BL. Pulmonary changes during perimenstrual period. In: SB Gupta (Ed). Medicine Update. New Delhi: Jaypee Brothers Medical Publishers; 2005. pp. 565-68.
8. Devi BS, et al. Pulmonary disorders in PLWHIV. Med Update. API. 2019;29:296-9.
9. Vidyasagar B, Jayan R, Ranjana SD. Recurrent pneumothorax in Marfan's syndrome. Lung India. 1998;16(1):29-31.
10. Tyagi R, Handa A. Pulmonary sarcoidosis; Med Update; API 2019;29:303-309.
11. Suryakant, RS Bhatia (Eds). Lung Cancer. JBS Foundation Lucknow; 2019.
12. Zbar B, Alvord WG, Glenn G, Turner M, Pavlovich CP, Schmidt L, et al. Risk of renal and colonic neoplasms and spontaneous pneumothorax in the Birt-Hogg-Dubé syndrome. Cancer Epidemiol Biomarkers Prev. 2002;11(4):393-400.
13. Handa AK, Eggleston FC. Pneumothorax caused by hydatid cysts. Indian J Chest Dis Allied Sci. 1982;24(1):47-9.
14. O'Neill S, Sweeney J, Walker F, O'Dwyer WF. Pneumothorax in the Ehlers-Danlos syndrome. Ir J Med Sci. 1981;150(2):43-4.
15. Jaspan T, Davison AM, Walker WC. Spontaneous pneumothorax in Wegener's granulomatosis. Thorax. 1982;37(10):774-5.
16. Bhatia RS, Sibia SS. Management of spontaneous pneumothorax. In: Venkataraman S (Ed). Med Update API; 2004. pp 221-26.
17. Mazarika B, et al. Re-expansion Pulmonary odema. The Pulmonary Face. 2014;14:46-8.
18. MacDuff A, Arnold A, Harvey J; BTS Pleural Disease Guideline Group. Management of spontaneous pneumothorax: British Thoracic Society Pleural Disease Guideline 2010. Thorax. 2010;65 Suppl 2:ii18-31.
19. Khanna A. HRCT. Med Update. API. 2019;29:288-94.
20. Puri H V; VATS in spontaneous pneumothorax; Lung India;2021;38:36-40.
21. Bairwa M, et al. Secondary pneumothorax. JAPI. 2023;71:64-66.
22. Gupta N, Gupta RC. Thoracic endometeriosis syndrome. Lung India. 2000;18(1):32.
23. Sen BK, Basu M, Das S, Chaturvedi AN. Unusual Cause of spontaneous bilateral pneumothorax secondary to osteosarcoma metastasis. J Assoc Physicians India. 2016;64(2):68-9.

104

CHAPTER

Respiratory Complications of Blood Transfusion

Kanchan Bhardwaj, Prabhpreet Kaur, Rajbir Singh, BL Bhardwaj, RS Bhatia

ABSTRACT

Serious lung complications can occur if not recognized in time during a blood transfusion. Therefore, strict vigil on following the guidelines and taking necessary precautions are very vital to prevent unnecessary morbidity and mortality. An informed consent for blood transfusion from the patient or kin, explaining them the infectious and noninfectious complications of the procedure, is necessary. Apart from primary and secondary respiratory complications such as acute lung injury, hypotension, cardiac arrhythmia, transfusion-associated circulatory overload, systemic complications such as sepsis, air embolism, febrile reaction, acute hemolytic reaction, and anaphylaxis need to be urgently looked for.

INTRODUCTION

Blood transfusion is generally a safe procedure, but as with many other medical therapies, adverse effects related to blood transfusion cannot be avoided. The greatest challenge of blood transfusion is the risk of morbidity and mortality from its noninfectious complications. The treating physicians should be aware of such risks when discussing the need for transfusion with the patient. Informed consent for transfusion may include a discussion of the risks of infectious disease as serious complications of blood transfusion.

Many common clinical signs and symptoms are associated with more than one type of adverse reaction. Early recognition, prompt cessation of transfusion, and further evaluation are key to a successful outcome. Signs and symptoms indicators of a transfusion reaction are associated with more than one type of adverse effects. Common signs and symptoms related to respiratory manifestations are:

- Respiratory distress including wheezing, cough, dyspnea, orthopnea, tachypnea, and stridor
- Chest pain
- Hypoxemia, respiratory failure, and bilateral pulmonary edema
- Sudden shortness of breath, acute cyanosis, chest pain, cough, hypotension, and cardiac arrhythmia

The transfusion complications, which primarily present with respiratory symptoms, damage the lungs, leading to respiratory failure, especially in critically ill and postoperative patients are:

- Transfusion-related acute lung injury (TRALI)
- Transfusion-associated circulatory overload (TACO)
- Transfusion-associated sepsis (TAS)
- Air embolism

Other transfusion-related complications presenting with respiratory symptoms are:

- Febrile nonhemolytic transfusion reactions (FNHTRs)
- Anaphylactic transfusion reaction
- Acute hemolytic transfusion reactions (AHTRs)

TRANSFUSION-RELATED ACUTE LUNG INJURY

Transfusion-related acute lung injury is an acute complication of transfusion during or within 6 hours of transfusion presenting with respiratory distress and severe hypoxemia in the absence of other causes of acute lung injury (e.g., aspiration pneumonia, toxic inhalation, lung contusion, near drowning, severe sepsis, shock, multiple traumas, burn injury, acute pancreatitis, cardiopulmonary bypass, and drug overdose). It can be accompanied by fever or hypotension. TRALI is considered

BOX 1: Diagnosis based on clinical and radiological parameters.

- *Onset*: Within 6 hours of transfusion
- *Oxygenation*: $PAO_2/FiO_2 < 300$ mm Hg regardless of positive end-expiratory pressure level

or

Oxygen saturation of <90% on room air

- *Chest X-ray*: Bilateral infiltrates on frontal chest radiography
- *Blood pressure*: Pulmonary artery occlusion pressure < 18 mm Hg when measured

or

No evidence of left atrial hypertension

(FiO_2: fraction of inspired oxygen; PAO_2: partial pressure of arterial oxygen)

the leading cause of transfusion-associated fatalities. Patients with special clinical diagnosis (i.e., infection, surgery, and trauma) have an increased risk of TRALI with a significant impact on morbidity and outcome. **Box 1** shows the clinicoradiological parameters.

Frequency

Transfusion-related acute lung injury is the leading cause of transfusion-related mortality. Recent efforts to decrease the transfusable plasma collected from female donors appear to be decreasing the number of TRALI fatalities in USA.

Pathophysiology

Although the pathogenesis is not fully understood, two hypotheses have been postulated:

1. Immune TRALI
2. Nonimmune TRALI

Immune Transfusion-related Acute Lung Injury

Immune TRALI consists of an antibody-mediated one-hit event. Antibodies against the human leukocyte antigens (HLAs) or human neutrophil antigens (HNAs) in the transfused blood component (up to 89% cases) react with recipient leukocytes, causing aggregates that occlude the pulmonary circulation. Implicated antibodies include HLA I (4–23%), HLA II (34–47%), and HNA (8–28%). Antibodies against class II HLA, anti-HLA-A2 (antibody against class I HLA), and HNA-3a (antibody against human neutrophilic antigens) are frequently associated with severe (ventilator support required) and fatal cases. Blood components implicated are usually donated by multiparous females and are associated with large volumes of plasma; however, blood components with <20 mL of plasma and the presence of anti-HNA-3a have been associated with immune TRALI. In rare instances (6%), the antibodies will be present in the recipient, reacting with the donor leukocytes. Immune TRALI may occur in patients with no underlying lung injury or even in healthy individuals.

Nonimmune Transfusion-related Acute Lung Injury

Nonimmune TRALI consists of a two-hit event. The risk of developing this type of injury depends on the patient's predisposition to this disorder. The first hit (i.e., lung trauma or an infectious inflammatory disease in the patient) may result in priming of the patient's neutrophils. The pro-inflammatory priming event of the patient's endothelium, which primes the patient's neutrophils, is a basic requirement for nonimmune TRALI. The second hit (i.e., transfused biologically active substances accumulated during storage or antileukocyte antibodies) causes the activation of the primed neutrophils. Both the immune and nonimmune TRALI lead to a final common pathway that causes damage to the endothelium, leading to pulmonary capillary permeability and resulting in noncardiogenic pulmonary edema.

Milder forms of respiratory distress (transient dyspnea) may still represent this syndrome. TRALI may be difficult to differentiate from a "possible TRALI" (a transfusion-unrelated acute lung injury that is not only temporarily related to a transfusion but also has at least one other temporally related risk factor for acute lung injury) or TACO. The physician treating the patient of TRALI must communicate promptly with the transfusion services physician.

Differential Diagnosis

Three main conditions that need to be differentiated from TRALI are:

1. Anaphylactic transfusion reactions
2. TACO
3. TAS

In anaphylactic transfusion reaction, bronchospasm, laryngeal edema, severe hypotension, erythema (often confluent), and urticaria are prominent symptoms. Fever and pulmonary edema are not associated with anaphylactic reactions.

Transfusion-associated circulatory overload has a clinical presentation very similar to that of TRALI, with respiratory distress, tachypnea, and cyanosis as the most prominent features. In TACO, the pulmonary edema is cardiogenic, whereas it is noncardiogenic in TRALI.

High-grade fever with hypotension and vascular collapse are prominent features of TAS.

Respiratory distress is infrequently associated with these reactions. With the rapid onset of respiratory distress, in addition to TACO and TRALI, coincident myocardial infarction and pulmonary embolism as well as other causes of acute lung injury should be considered.

■ Treatment

Respiratory and circulatory support with additional oxygen supplementation with or without mechanical ventilation is needed in almost all cases. Typical TRALI cases improve within 48 hours, whereas in some cases it can persist for up to 1 week. Fatality is observed in 6–20% of cases. A TRALI-suspected case should be reported to the blood center for a serological workup of the recipient and the implicated donor for the presence of HLA/HNA antibodies. If such antibodies are present in the donor, he is excluded from further donations. Because TRALI is a clinical diagnosis, the absence of demonstrable immune incompatibility between donor and recipient does not preclude the diagnosis of TRALI.

Blood components that contain large volumes of plasma donated by alloimmunized donors would be at a high risk of causing immune-mediated TRALI, e.g., in multiparous females and multitransfused donors. A preventive policy with a "predominant male policy" resulted in a decrease in TRALI. Removing the plasma from the platelets and resuspending them in platelet additives are helpful in preventing TRALI.

TRANSFUSION-ASSOCIATED CIRCULATORY OVERLOAD

Volume overload can precipitate acute pulmonary edema, especially in the elderly (above 70 years) and infants who are at a greater risk, although all transfusion recipients are susceptible to some degree. Modest volume can also precipitate TACO, and high flow rates are frequently cofactors. There are no diagnostic signs or symptoms of TACO. The patients may develop the following signs and symptoms within 1–2 hours of transfusion: Gallop, jugular vein distension, elevated central venous pressure, elevated pulmonary wedge pressure, dyspnea, orthopnea, new ST-segment and T-wave changes on electrocardiogram (ECG), elevated serum troponin, and elevated brain natriuretic peptide (BNP), a cardiac marker. Increasing blood pressure characterized by a widening of the pulse pressure is a characteristic of TACO. Radiograph shows pulmonary edema, cardiomegaly, and a distended pulmonary artery with a widened cardiothoracic ratio.

■ Frequency

Frequency is not known exactly but is a very common cause of transfusion-related fatalities. Fresh frozen plasma (FFP) was more frequently associated with TACO followed by packed red blood cells (PRBCs).

■ Differential Diagnosis

Transfusion-associated circulatory overload is most commonly confused with TRALI as both these reactions cause pulmonary edema. It is possible for TACO and TRALI to occur concurrently in the same patient. Hypertension is a constant feature of TACO, whereas it is an infrequent and transient manifestation of TRALI. Furthermore, rapid improvement with diuresis or inotropic agents is consistent with TACO.

In congestive heart failure, BNP levels are elevated. Post-transfusion to pretransfusion BNP ratio of 1.5 with a posttransfusion level of at least 100 pg/mL as a cutoff yielded a sensitivity and specificity > 80% in TACO. With rapid onset of respiratory distress, possible causes of acute lung injury, such as coincidental myocardial infarction, pulmonary embolus, and others, should be considered in addition to TACO and TRALI.

■ Treatment

Transfusion should be stopped, and patients should be treated in a seated position, providing supplemental oxygen and reducing intravascular volume with diuretics. If symptoms persist in confirmed TACO, administration of additional diuretics or therapeutic phlebotomy in 250 mL increments may be considered. To prevent complications in situations where rapid loss of blood is occurring, the components should be administered slowly, particularly in patients at risk of TACO (i.e., pediatric patients, severely anemic patients, and patients with congestive cardiac failure). Transfusion rates of 2–4 mL/min and 1 mL/kg of body weight per hour are the most frequently cited infusion rates. Total fluid input and output must be monitored. In patients with volume overload caused by medical reasons existing before transfusion, furosemide can be given prophylactically. The rate of transfusion can be further slowed, if necessary, by dividing a unit of PRBC or another component into smaller aliquots and transfusing a portion at a time over as much as 4 hours, the maximum allowable time a blood component should be kept outside the blood bank-monitored storage. **Table 1** shows a comparison between TACO and TRALI.

TABLE 1: Comparison of features in TRALI and TACO.

Features	TRALI	TACO
Body temperature	Fever can be present	Unchanged
Blood pressure	Hypotension	Hypertension
Respiratory symptoms	Acute dyspnea	Acute dyspnea
Neck veins	Unchanged	Can be distended
Auscultation	Rales	Rales, S3 may be present
Chest radiograph	Diffuse, bilateral infiltrates	Diffuse, bilateral infiltrates
Ejection fraction	Normal, decreased	Decreased
Pulmonary artery occlusion pressure	18 mm Hg or less	>18 mm Hg
Pulmonary edema fluid	Exudate	Transudate
Fluid balance	Positive, even negative	Positive
Response to diuretics	Minimal	Significant
White blood cell count	Transient leukopenia	Unchanged
BNP	<200 pg/mL	>1,200 pg/mL
Leukocyte antibodies	Donor leukocyte antibodies present, cross-match incompatibility between donor and recipient	Donor leukocyte antibodies may or may not be present, positive results can suggest TRALI even with true TACO cases

(BNP: brain natriuretic peptide; TACO: transfusion-associated circulatory overload; TRALI: transfusion-related acute lung injury)

TRANSFUSION-ASSOCIATED SEPSIS

Fever ≥101°F, shaking chills, and hypotension during or shortly after transfusion are the most frequent presenting symptoms of TAS. In severe cases, patients develop shock with accompanying renal failure and disseminated intravascular coagulation (DIC).

Differential Diagnosis

The severity and abruptness of signs and symptoms associated with TAS may be similar to those of AHTRs. Mild cases may be confused with febrile nonhemolytic transfusion reactions. Diagnosis of TAS is done by culturing the same organism from both patient and the remainder of the component. In suspected TAS, the returned component should be visually examined for any color change, especially brown or purple discoloration of red cell components, and bubbles/frothiness in a particular component. A Gram stain should be done on the returned component.

Treatment

In suspected TAS, the transfusion should be stopped immediately, and supportive care of the patient should be initiated. Broad-spectrum antibiotics should be given.

AIR EMBOLISM

Air embolism can occur if blood in an open system is infused under pressure or if an open system is infused under pressure or if air enters the central catheter while blood administration sets are being changed. The minimum volume of air embolism that is potentially fatal for an adult is approximately 100 mL. Symptoms include cough, dyspnea, chest pain, and shock.

If air embolism is suspected, the patient should be placed on the left side with the head down to displace the air bubble from the pulmonic valve. Aspiration of the air is sometimes attempted. Proper inspection of the infusion pumps, instruments for blood recovery or apheresis, and tubing couplers are very essential to prevent this complication.

FEBRILE NONHEMOLYTIC TRANSFUSION REACTIONS

It is the occurrence of ≥1°C rise in temperature above 37°C that is associated with transfusion and for which no other cause is identifiable. Other symptoms may include shaking, chills, tachypnea, change in blood pressure, and anxiety. Symptoms usually occur during transfusion or up to 4 hours after. Most FNHTRs are benign, although they may cause significant discomfort and even hemodynamic or respiratory effects.

Differential Diagnosis

The symptoms associated with an FNHTR may be present in several other types of transfusion reactions, the most serious of which are hemolytic transfusion reactions (HTRs), sepsis, and TRALI. Each of these other reactions has signs and symptoms and associated laboratory results that help to distinguish them from FNHTRs once an investigation is begun; recognition of FNHTRs requires diagnosis by exclusion.

Treatment

In suspected FNHTR, the transfusion is discontinued and transfusion reaction workup is initiated and antipyretics should be given. Prestorage leukocyte reduction, especially if performed at the time of collection, significantly decreases the frequency of FNHTRs.

ANAPHYLACTIC TRANSFUSION REACTIONS

Anaphylactic transfusion reactions vary from mild (urticarial) to life-threatening anaphylaxis. Symptoms occur within seconds to minutes of the start of the transfusion. Extensive cases may be accompanied by angioedema. It can rarely involve the throat, tongue, or lungs, causing respiratory distress. The respiratory system is involved with dyspnea, wheezing, and stridor.

Differential Diagnosis

The respiratory symptoms of anaphylaxis may be suggestive of an acute asthmatic attack or TRALI. However, classic symptoms of allergy, including urticaria, angioedema, and pruritis, do not occur in asthmatic attacks or TRALI.

Treatment

An antihistamine may be administered along with supportive treatment for other symptoms. Premedication with an antihistamine 30 minutes before transfusion may be helpful in patients with a history of multiple allergic reactions. Steroids are of help when antihistamines are not sufficient. Patients with unresponsive recurrent reactions, washed red cells, or platelets can be of help. Plasma reduction or replacement in platelet products may be beneficial. Alternatively, administration of deglycerolized red blood cells (RBCs) has been helpful in cases when washed red cells were not effective. The plasma used for transfusion for patients diagnosed with immunoglobulin A (IgA) deficiency that produces anti-IgA should be from IgA-deficient donors.

ACUTE HEMOLYTIC TRANSFUSION REACTIONS

Rapid hemolysis of as little as 10 mL of incompatible blood can produce symptoms of AHTRs. There is pain in the chest, flank, or back with hypotension, shock, and DIC. Red or dark-/cola-colored urine may be the first sign of intravascular hemolysis.

Differential Diagnosis

Respiratory difficulty is not typically a symptom of AHTR. Fever with hypotension may occur in TRALI and sepsis. Hemolysis may not be detected immediately and does not occur in sepsis and TRALI.

Treatment

Prompt recognition of AHTR and immediate cessation of the transfusion reaction are crucial. Maintain renal flow with normal saline with a goal of the urine flow rate of >1 mL/kg/h. Diuretic furosemide promotes renal cortical flow and promotes urine output. Hyperkalemia and subsequent cardiac arrest may occur. Metabolic acidosis and uremia may necessitate dialysis. DIC may be the first indication of AHTR in an anuric and anesthetized patient. A common cause of AHTR is a clerical error. Institutional policies to reduce such errors should be in place and followed religiously.

CONCLUSION

Respiratory complications are potentially serious ones. Their early recognition is the key to patient safety. Clinicians should have knowledge of these complications so that they can identify them at the earliest and save the patient.

SUGGESTED READINGS

1. Claudia SC, Delaney M, Johnson ST, Katz LM (Eds). Technical Manual: Methods and Appendices, 20th edition. Bethesda, Maryland: AABB; 2020. pp. 627-58.
2. Harmening D (Ed). Modern Blood Banking & Transfusion Practices, 7th edition. Philadelphia: F.A. Davis Company; 2018. pp. 373-95.
3. Simon TL, McCullogh J, Synder EL, Solheim BG, Strauss RG (Eds). Rossi's Principles of Transfusion Medicine, 5th edition. Oxford: Blackwell Publishing Ltd; 2016.

105

CHAPTER

Management of Parapneumonic Effusion and Empyema

Sarvinder Singh

ABSTRACT

Parapneumonic effusions are pleural effusions that occur in the pleural space adjacent to bacterial pneumonia. Empyema is a collection of pus in the pleural cavity. If left untreated, complicated parapneumonic effusion/empyema leads to chronic encasement and pleural thickening. Simple parapneumonic effusions can be managed conservatively with appropriate antibiotics, but complicated parapneumonic effusions often require some kind of drainage along with antibiotics. Clinically, it is diagnosed with persistent fever, stony-dull-tender percussion, and absent breath sounds. Gram-positive as well as gram-negative organisms are also implicated. Majority of cases are due to anaerobic infection. Many cases may have mixed organisms. Tuberculosis should be suspected if no organism is grown in empyema. Chest X-ray, thoracic ultrasound, and CT scan help in the localization of effusion and detection of loculations. Management includes well-selected antibiotics and drainage by tube thoracostomy. Intrapleural fibrinolytics have been used in multiloculated complicated parapneumonic effusions with success. The use of thoracoscopy and video-assisted thoracoscopic surgery (VATS) has left very few cases requiring surgical decortication. Properly treated parapneumonic effusions have a good prognosis.

INTRODUCTION

Parapneumonic effusions are pleural effusions that occur in the pleural space with associated bacterial pneumonia. They are seen in approximately 40% of bacterial pneumonias. The simple parapneumonic effusion is generally small and resolves with antibiotic therapy. A complicated parapneumonic effusion or empyema may result in bacterial invasion of the fluid and may require some intervention.

Empyema has been a matter of concern for centuries. Around 500 BC, Hippocrates recommended treating empyema with open drainage. Tillett et al. used streptokinase and streptodornase for intrapleural debridement in parapneumonic empyema in 1950. Light et al. suggested that a low pleural fluid pH was an indicator of tube drainage. The use of video-assisted thoracoscopic surgery (VATS) has become widespread in the treatment of loculated parapneumonic effusions in the last one decade.

DEFINITION

Any pleural effusion associated with bacterial pneumonia, lung abscess, or bronchiectasis is a parapneumonic effusion. An empyema is defined as pus in the pleural space. Generally, 60% of empyemas are parapneumonic, whereas 20% arise after thoracic surgical procedures, and the remaining 20% arise due to the complications of various conditions such as thoracic trauma, esophageal perforation, thoracentesis, and subdiaphragmatic infection.

PATHOPHYSIOLOGY

The evolution of a parapneumonic pleural effusion can be divided into three stages.

1. *Exudative stage*: The increased pulmonary interstitial fluid crosses the visceral pleura and accumulates in the pleural space. The pleural fluid in this stage is exudative with polymorphonuclear leukocytes

predominance, normal glucose level, and a normal pH.

2. *Fibropurulent stage*: This stage is characterized by infection of pleural fluid with the bacteria. Pleural fluid in this stage contains many polymorphonuclear neutrophils (PMNs), bacteria, and cellular debris. The fibrin is deposited as continuous sheets that cover both the visceral and the parietal pleura. There is a tendency for the fibrin membrane to form multiple locules. The pleural fluid pH and glucose levels decrease, and the lactate dehydrogenase (LDH) level increases progressively in this stage.
3. *Organization stage*: In this stage, the fibroblasts grow into the exudate from both the visceral and the parietal pleural surfaces to produce an inelastic membrane. This membrane/pleural peel can encase the lung and hamper the re-expansion of the underlying lung when the pleural fluid is drained.

CLINICAL PRESENTATION

Common clinical symptoms of bacterial pneumonia with parapneumonic effusion include cough, fever, pleuritic chest pain, dyspnea, and sputum production. Patients with empyema may have a longer course with several days of fever and malaise.

Physical examination may identify the presence of pleural fluid when the typical findings of consolidation, i.e., fine or coarse crackles, bronchophony, and increased fremitus, are replaced by decreased breath sounds and decreased fremitus. Dullness on percussion is a clinical sign of lung consolidation in pneumonia and pleural effusion. These findings may be absent. Hence, an X-ray of chest is a must for a complete evaluation.

BACTERIOLOGY

Before the antibiotic era, the bacteriological species were predominantly gram-positive species comprising pneumococci and beta-hemolytic streptococci. With the wider use of antibiotics, bacteriology has changed to gram-negative species such as *Klebsiella pneumoniae, Pseudomonas aeruginosa, Proteus* species, and *Escherichia coli*, especially if the patient is in the intensive care unit setting. The empyemas are seen in adult patients as a complication of community-acquired pneumonia, predominantly as a result of pneumococcal infection whereas aspiration cases are more likely to contain anaerobes. In most cases of trauma or complicated hemothorax, *S. aureus* is implicated. *S. aureus* is the most common infective organism in infancy, accounting for up to 92% empyemas in childhood, followed by *P. aeruginosa* and *Haemophilus influenzae*. Inoculation of pleural fluid directly into blood culture bottles may improve the microbiologic yield. The putrid smell of empyema fluid is considered to be diagnostic of anaerobic infection.

Patients with diabetes mellitus are at an increased risk of empyema, secondary to *K. pneumoniae*. Methicillin-resistant *S. aureus* (MRSA) often causes a necrotizing pneumonia that is complicated by pleural infection. In patients with influenza, the major causes of bacterial superinfection and empyema have been *S. aureus*, *S. pneumoniae*, and *S. pyogenes*. Gupta in a study on parapneumonic effusions in the rural population of Khammam district, Andhra Pradesh, showed that *S. pneumoniae* was the most frequently isolated organism (26.32%), followed by *S. aureus* (21.05%) and *E. coli* (15.79%).

Tuberculous empyema should be considered in patients with risk factors for tuberculous infection. Tuberculous empyema is a disease in which pus is present in the pleural space and the predominant pleural cell is the PMN. Tuberculous empyema should be differentiated from tuberculous pleurisy, in which a lymphocytic effusion occurs from the immunologic response to tuberculous proteins.

DIAGNOSIS

The possibility of a parapneumonic effusion should be suspected in patients of bacterial pneumonia who do not show satisfactory response to antimicrobial therapy. It is important to diagnose complicated parapneumonic effusion early, as delay in instituting proper pleural drainage in such patients increases morbidity.

Chest X-ray

The blunting of costophrenic (CP) angle on X-ray chest posteroanterior (PA) view is appreciated only when fluid is >500 mL. The presence of pleural fluid is earliest picked up in the lateral chest radiograph. If the posterior CP angle is blunted, pleural effusion should be evaluated with bilateral decubitus chest radiographs, ultrasound of the pleural space, and CT scan of the chest.

Ultrasound

Ultrasound is an excellent tool in the evaluation of pleural effusion. It helps in localizing, looking for septation, and drainage of fluid.

Thoracentesis

Thoracentesis is performed for the further management of the effusion and to provide fluid for culture and sensitivity studies. In general, a parapneumonic effusion should be sampled if it meets any of the following criteria:

- It is free-flowing but has layers > 10 mm on a lateral decubitus film.
- It is loculated.
- It is associated with thickened parietal pleura on a contrast-enhanced CT scan, a finding that is suggestive of empyema.

PLEURAL FLUID ANALYSIS

The pleural fluid is examined grossly for color, turbidity, and odor. Fluid is analyzed for pleural fluid glucose, LDH, protein levels, pH, and adenosine deaminase (ADA). Samples of pleural fluid are also sent for bacterial cultures, Gram stain, cytologic studies, and mycobacterial and fungal smears. Culture yields are higher if the pleural fluid is directly inoculated into blood culture bottles at the time of thoracentesis. The pleural fluid cultures in patients with parapneumonic effusions are frequently negative. To identify the organism responsible for the pneumonia, nuclei acid amplification has been used. Maskell et al. performed this procedure on 404 pleural fluid specimens obtained during the MIST 1 (First Multicentre Intrapleural Sepsis Trial). They reported that the nucleic acid amplification technique identified bacteria in 70 samples that were negative on culture.

The pleural fluid with parapneumonic effusions varies from a clear, yellow exudate to thick, foul-smelling pus. If the odor of the pleural fluid is feculent, the patient is likely to have an anaerobic pleural infection. However, only 60% of anaerobic empyema have a foul odor.

Bad prognostic markers for parapneumonic effusions and empyema are as follows:

- Pus present in pleural space
- Gram stain of pleural fluid positive
- Pleural fluid glucose < 40 mg/dL
- Pleural fluid culture positive
- Pleura fluid pH < 7.0
- Pleural fluid LDH > 3× upper normal limit for serum
- Pleural fluid loculated

As per Light's classification and treatment scheme for parapneumonic effusions and empyema, parapneumonic effusions are classified into seven classes **(Table 1)**.

MANAGEMENT

The management of parapneumonic effusions and empyema involves:

- Appropriate antibiotics
- Management of the pleural fluid

Antibiotic Selection

All patients with parapneumonic effusions or empyema should be treated with antibiotics. The Gram stain of the

TABLE 1: Light's classification and treatment scheme for parapneumonic effusions and empyema.

Class	Nomenclature	Findings	Management
1	• Nonsignificant • Pleural effusion	Small <10 mm thick on decubitus X-ray chest	No thoracentesis is indicated
2	Typical parapneumonic pleural effusion	• >10 mm thick • Glucose >40 mg/dL, pH > 7.2, LDH > 3× upper normal limit • Glucose > 40 mg/dL • Gram stain and culture negative	Antibiotics alone
3	Borderline complicated pleural effusion	• pH <7.0–<7.2, and or LDH > 3× upper normal limit glucose > 40 mg/dL • Gram stain and culture negative	Antibiotics plus serial thoracocentesis
4	Simple complicated pleural effusion	• pH < 7.0 • Glucose < 40 mg/dL • Gram stain or culture positive • Not loculated, no frank pus	Tube thoracostomy plus antibiotics
5	Complex complicated pleural effusion	• pH < 7.0 or glucose > 40 mg/dL or Gram stain/culture positive • Multiloculated	Tube thoracostomy plus fibrinolytics
6	Simple empyema	• Frank pus present • Single locule or free flowing	Tube thoracostomy ± decortication
7	Complex empyema	• Frank pus • Multiple locules	Tube thoracostomy ± fibrinolytics VATS and decortication

(VATS: video-assisted thoracoscopic surgery)

pleural fluid should guide the selection of an antibiotic. The initial antibiotic selection is usually based on whether the pneumonia is community acquired or hospital acquired. Patients hospitalized with community-acquired pneumonias that are not severe are recommended beta-lactam (cefotaxime, ceftriaxone, ampicillin-sulbactam, or ertapenem). Patients with severe community-acquired pneumonia are recommended beta-lactam plus either an advanced macrolide or a respiratory fluoroquinolone. If a *pseudomonas* infection is suspected, an antipseudomonas antibiotic such as piperacillin, piperacillin-tazobactam, imipenem, meropenem, or cefepime should be included. As anaerobic bacteria cause a sizable percentage of parapneumonic effusions, anaerobic coverage is recommended with either clindamycin or metronidazole. In patients with healthcare-associated pneumonia with parapneumonic effusion, coverage should be provided for gram-negative enteric bacteria and methicillin-resistant *Staphylococcus aureus* (MRSA). A reasonable antibiotic selection in such patients is a carbapenem such as meropenem and vancomycin. It is recommended to continue antibiotic therapy till there is radiographic resolution of fluid. This may take 2–4 weeks of therapy.

Intrapleural Antibiotics

Intrapleural antibiotics were first used to treat an infected pneumonectomy space by Clagett and Geraci in 1963. Since that time, there have been several reports regarding the use of intrapleural antibiotics in the treatment of empyema complicating pneumonia. The personal experience of the author has been very rewarding, but some good randomized studies are required to recommend this therapy.

Options for Management of Pleural Fluid

The options available for the management of the pleural fluid in patients with parapneumonic effusion are as follows:

- Conservative
- Therapeutic thoracentesis
- Intercostal chest tube drainage
- Intrapleural fibrinolysis
- VATS
- Thoracotomy with decortication and the breakdown of adhesions, and open drainage

Conservative

Pleural fluid from patients with parapneumonic effusions should be sampled as soon as possible. Evaluation of fluid is necessary to determine if drainage of the fluid is required. Approximately 10% of patients with parapneumonic effusions require drainage.

Therapeutic Thoracentesis

Therapeutic thoracentesis was first practiced as a treatment modality for parapneumonic effusions in the mid-nineteenth century. Some patients with complicated parapneumonic effusion can be treated with repeated thoracocentesis along with appropriate antibiotics.

Intercostal Chest Tube Drainage

The initial management of most patients with complicated parapneumonic effusions has been intercostal chest tube drainage. Large (28–36 F) tubes have been recommended because of the belief that smaller tubes would become obstructed by the thick fluid. The British Thoracic Society (BTS) guidelines state that a small-bore catheter 10–14 F will be adequate for most cases of complicated parapneumonic pleural infection. There is no consensus on the optimal size of the chest tube for drainage. In general, chest tubes should be left in place until the volume of the pleural drainage is < 50 mL for 24 hours and until the draining fluid becomes clear yellow.

Intrapleural Fibrinolytics

Drainage of complicated parapneumonic effusions is difficult due to loculation. Intrapleural fibrinolytics destroy the fibrin membranes and facilitate drainage of the pleural fluid. In a landmark study on the use of intrapleural fibrinolytics for the treatment of complicated parapneumonic effusion, the administration of streptokinase had no effect on the need for surgery or the duration of hospitalization. But this study did not consider the patients who do not have access to surgery like patients in our country and other third-world countries. Indian experience in intrapleural fibrinolysis is encouraging and most of the centers are using it, which are short of surgery that is not easily accessible to our patients.

Video-assisted Thoracoscopic Surgery

Video-assisted thoracoscopic surgery is often used to debride multiloculated empyemas or uniloculated empyemas that fail to resolve with antibiotics and chest tube drainage. VATS can be used as a procedure to assist initial insertion of chest tube under vision. At the time a chest tube is inserted, VATS can be used to irrigate the pleural space and break down all the fibrous strands.

Decortication

Decortication involves removal of all the fibrous tissue from the visceral and parietal pleura along with pus from the pleural space. It eliminates pleural sepsis and thus assists expansion of underlying lung. In the acute stage of infection, decortication helps in control of pleural infection. Decortication should not be performed just to remove thickened pleura, because such thickening usually resolves spontaneously over several months.

Open Drainage Procedures

These procedures are of historical value now. The first is rib resection and inserting short/large bore tubes and irrigating daily with antiseptic solutions. the second is Eloesser flap which is a skin-lined fistula to provide drainage without tube insertion.

CONCLUSION

Parapneumonic effusion and empyema is the collection of fluid and pus in the pleural space adjacent to pneumonias, and presence of this increases morbidity and mortality. Parapneumonic effusions and empyema respond well to appropriate antibiotics and drainage. If untreated in time, it leads to pleural thickening and encasement of lung, and loculated effusions. Intrapleural fibrinolytic therapy is an option in loculated effusion, especially when surgical option is not available or affordable. Most of the complicated effusions and empyema can be treated with VATS. Surgical drainage procedures and decortication are reserved for very few cases. A proposed algorithm for management is shown in **Flowchart 1**.

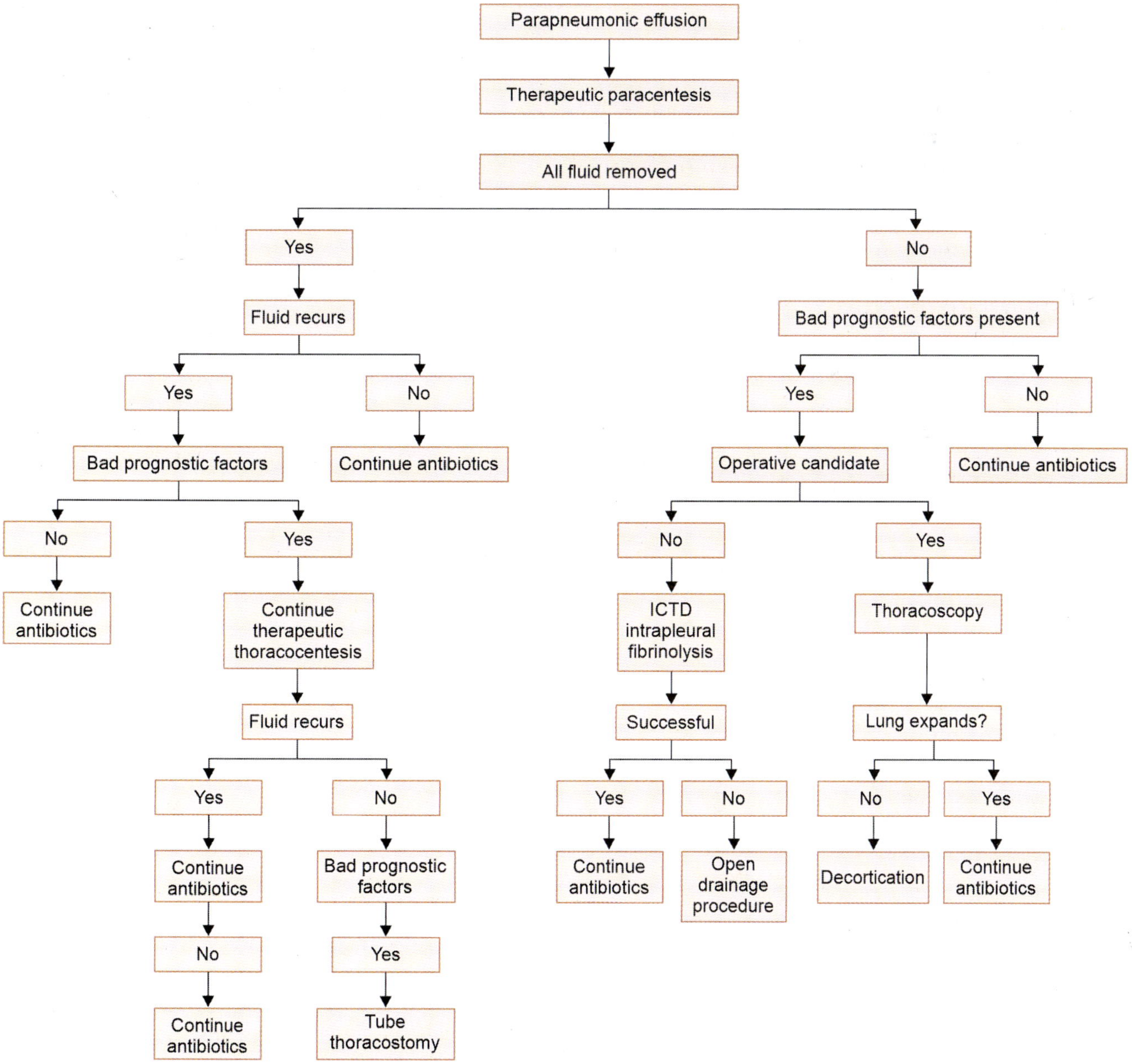

FLOWCHART 1: Algorithm for management of patients with parapneumonic effusions.
(ICTD: intercostal tube drainage)

SUGGESTED READINGS

1. Light RW, Girard WM, Jenkinson SG, George RB. Parapneumonic effusions. Am J Med. 1980;69(4):507-12.
2. Adams F. The Genuine Works of Hippocrates. New York: William Wood and Company; 1886. p. 266.
3. Light RW, Mac Gregor MI, Ball WC Jr, Luchsinger PC. Diagnostic significance of pleural fluid pH and PCO2. Chest. 1973;64(5):591-6.
4. Ferguson MK. Thoracoscopy for empyema, bronchopleural fistula and chylothorax. Ann Thorac Surg. 1993;56(3):644-5.
5. Maede RH. A History of Thoracic Surgery. Springfield: Charles C Thomas; 1961.
6. Maskell NA, Batt S, Hedley EL, Davies CW, Gillespie SH, Davies RJ. The bacteriology of pleural infection by genetic and standard methods and its mortality significance. Am J Respir Crit Care Med. 2006;174(7):817-23.
7. Clagett OT, Geraci JE. A procedure for the management of postpneumonectomy empyema. J Thorac Cardiovasc Surg. 1963;45:141-5.
8. Davies HE, Davies RJ, Davies CWH; BTS Pleural Disease Guideline Group. Management of pleural infection in adults: British Thoracic Society pleural disease guideline 2010. Thorax. 2010;65:ii41-53.
9. Maskell NA, Davies CW, Nunn AJ, Hedley EL, Gleeson FV, Miller R, et al. U.K. controlled trial of intrapleural streptokinase for pleural infection. N Engl J Med. 2005;352(9):865-74.
10. Barthwal MS, Deoskar RB, Rajan KE, Chatterjee RS. Intrapleural streptokinase in complicated parapneumonic effusions and empyema. Ind J Chest Dis Allied Sci. 2004;46(4):257-61.

SECTION

13

PHARMACOTHERAPEUTICS

106

CHAPTER

Prescribing Cascade

Nandini Chatterjee, Prafulla K Nath, Pranab K Datta

ABSTRACT

Prescribing cascades are said to occur when adverse drug events are categorized as new medical conditions and additional medications are prescribed. This may add to potential harm to the health of the patient and also increase financial burden. Elderly patients with multimorbidity and resultant polypharmacy are important predisposing factors. A high degree of clinical suspicion and awareness is necessary to recognize adverse drug reactions (ADRs) to prevent this phenomenon.

INTRODUCTION

Prescribing cascades were first elucidated in 1995 by Rochon and Gurwitz who opened a new vista in the domain of inappropriate prescribing practices.

A prescribing cascade comprises a sequence of events in which an adverse drug event is misinterpreted as a new medical condition, resulting in the addition of another medication **(Table 1)**.

The phenomenon also includes now, unnecessary diagnostic tests, medical devices, and over-the-counter therapies, which may have detrimental effects on the patient.

Prescribing cascades can be:

- Appropriate (potential benefits > risks)
- Inappropriate (risks > potential benefits)

Furthermore, an appropriate prescribing cascade can become inappropriate with the passage of time.

TABLE 1: Examples of prescribing cascades.

Initial treatment	Adverse effect	Subsequent treatment
Nonsteroidal anti-inflammatory drugs	Rise in blood pressure	Antihypertensive treatment
Thiazide diuretics	Hyperuricemia	Treatment for gout
Metoclopramide treatment	Parkinsonian symptoms	Treatment with levodopa

WHO ARE AT RISK?

- Elderly individuals
- Female gender
- Those on multiple medicines
- Patients on drugs with a high risk of adverse events, e.g., cardiovascular drugs, nonsteroidal anti-inflammatory drugs (NSAIDs), anticoagulants, and antibiotics.

FACTORS INFLUENCING PRESCRIBING CASCADES

Multicountry studies have shown variation in prescribing cascade according to the local prescribing trends due to the following:

- Differences in demographics
- Medication availability
- Approved clinical indications
- Help-seeking behavior
- Prescribing culture
- Genetic polymorphisms

HOW TO DETECT PRESCRIBING CASCADES?

- We need to clarify the indication for each drug during the medication review

107

CHAPTER

Transporter-mediated Drug–Drug Interactions: Translation into Clinics

Shambo Samrat Samajdar, Shravan Venkatraman, Saumen Chaudhary

ABSTRACT

Drug–drug interactions are a critical clinical concern, often arising from the modulation of drug transporters responsible for the uptake and efflux of xenobiotics in various organs. Notably, drug transporters in the small intestine, liver, and kidney play pivotal roles in shaping the pharmacokinetic profiles of drugs, significantly impacting their clinical outcomes. This chapter sheds light on the key mechanisms of interactions involving selected intestinal, hepatic, and renal drug transporters, with a particular focus on probe drugs that undergo minimal metabolic alteration. These transporters include organic anion transporting polypeptide (OATP) 1A2, OATP2B1, OATP1B1, OATP1B3, P-glycoprotein (P-gp), organic anion transporter (OAT) 1, OAT3, breast cancer resistance protein (BCRP), organic cation transporter (OCT) 2, and multidrug and toxin extrusion protein (MATE) 1. Furthermore, this chapter delves into genotype-dependent drug-drug interactions, offering valuable insights into the intricate web of factors affecting drug responses.

INTRODUCTION

Drug-drug interactions play a very important and serious role when a patient takes concomitant drugs. The main mechanism is induction or inhibition of drug transporters that are responsible for the cellular uptake and efflux of the drugs. The pharmacokinetic profile of the drug is determined by drug transporters of the small intestine, liver, and kidney. Transporter-mediated drug-drug interactions in these three organs influence the pharmacokinetics and clinical effects of drugs.

CLASSIFICATION OF TRANSPORTERS

There are more than 400 transporters in the entire human genome. They are primarily classified into the uptake and efflux membrane proteins based on the route to which they direct the substances. The transporters are categorized into two major superfamilies, adenosine triphosphate (ATP)-binding cassette (ABC) transporters and the solute carrier (SLC) transporters, based on their underlying mechanism of action.

Based on the direction of the movement of substances, transporters are majorly classified into uptake and efflux transporters. The major uptake transporters are the organic anion transporting polypeptide (OATP), organic anion transporter (OAT), organic cation transporter (OCT), bile acid transporters [Na^+ taurocholate cotransporting polypeptide (NTCP), apical sodium-dependent bile acid transporter (ASBT), and organic solute transporter (OSTα-OSTβ)], peptide transporters (PEPT), concentrative and equilibrative nucleoside transporters, and glucose transporters.

The major efflux transporters are P-glycoprotein (P-gp), bile salt export pump (BSEP), multidrug resistant proteins (MRPs), breast cancer resistance proteins (BCRP), all of which belong to ABC superfamily except the multidrug and toxin extrusion proteins (MATE) which are SLCs.

MECHANISMS OF DRUG–DRUG INTERACTIONS

- If the transporter located in the clearance organs is inhibited by one drug, the systemic exposure of the drug is altered and may result in an alteration in pharmacological or toxicological response.

- If the transporter located at the barrier is inhibited by one drug, the local exposure of the drug is altered without affecting the systemic exposure.
- If the transporter which is involved in the transport of endogenous substrates is inhibited, it leads to the toxicological effect of the inhibitor drug by alteration of the plasma concentration of endogenous substance.

TRANSPORTERS

- Various uptake and efflux transporters belonging to ABC and SLC transporter superfamilies are involved in the drug disposition.
- The SLC transporters are primarily involved in the uptake of drugs.
- Solute carrier class proteins for the transport of substrates across the membrane depend on an electrochemical gradient. They may also rely on the ion gradients generated by ATP-dependent pumps for the movement of the substrates against the concentration gradient.
- Orally administered drugs have to pass through the gut wall mucosa before they may reach the capillaries that lead to the portal vein. There are many drug transporters involved in intestinal drug absorption.
- While transporters of the SLC family facilitate the cellular uptake of their substrates, ABC transporters such as P-gp mediate the ATP-dependent efflux of drugs back into the intestinal lumen.

COMPLEX WORLD OF INTESTINAL UPTAKE TRANSPORTERS

When it comes to orally administered drugs, their journey toward therapeutic action hinges on their ability to navigate the intricate barrier presented by the gut wall mucosa. This mucosal barrier comprises polarized enterocytes firmly interconnected through tight junctions. Inside these enterocytes, a multitude of drug transporters play pivotal roles in the process of intestinal drug absorption. While transporters from the SLC family facilitate the cellular uptake of their substrates, ATP-dependent efflux of drugs back into the intestinal lumen is orchestrated by ABC transporters like P-gp.

Our understanding of drug–drug interactions involving intestinal uptake transporters is currently limited. However, intriguing drug–food interactions, notably with fruit juices, have garnered attention. The concurrent consumption of grapefruit juice, for instance, is known to elevate the plasma concentrations of numerous drugs, largely due to its well-documented inhibition of intestinal CYP3A4. It is noteworthy that the effect of grapefruit juice can be unpredictable, as evidenced by a study by Dresser et al. in 2002, which reported a reduction in plasma concentrations of the antihistaminic drug fexofenadine in the presence of grapefruit, orange, or apple juice. This unexpected outcome is particularly interesting given that fexofenadine is a substrate of P-gp. Furthermore, the study by Glaeser et al. suggests that grapefruit juice affects fexofenadine plasma levels without altering the expression of OATP1A2 or P-gp in the intestine.

Beyond P-glycoprotein: The Role of OATP2B1

One uptake transporter that has been identified at the luminal membrane of enterocytes is OATP2B1.While previous studies did not report statistically significant transport of fexofenadine by OATP2B1 in vitro, recent research reveals that, under acidic extracellular pH conditions, OATP2B1 may mediate the uptake of fexofenadine, and this uptake is inhibited by apple juice in vitro. Coadministration of apple juice also resulted in a reduction in fexofenadine's area under the curve $(AUC)_{0\text{-}\infty}$ and C_{max} in volunteers. This leads to the hypothesis that inhibition of OATP2B1 by fruit juices might contribute to food-fexofenadine interactions within the small intestine.

Broadening the Perspective

Beyond fexofenadine, grapefruit and/or orange juice have shown the potential to decrease the $AUC_{0\text{-}\infty}$ and Cmax of other orally administered substrates of OATP1A2, such as celiprolol, atenolol, and ciprofloxacin. Whether OATP2B1 plays a role in the intestinal uptake of these substances and contributes to these food–drug interactions remains a subject for future investigation.

Aliskiren: A Case Study

The renin inhibitor aliskiren presents another interesting drug–food interaction with grapefruit juice. Aliskiren's pharmacokinetics is characterized by poor oral bioavailability and high interindividual variation in plasma concentrations, primarily due to unchanged biliary elimination. Aliskiren is recognized as a substrate of intestinal CYP3A4, P-gp, and OATP2B1, with OATP2B1 believed to be responsible for its intestinal uptake. Notably, inhibition of intestinal uptake, rather than inhibition of CYP3A4 or P-gp, appears to be the primary mechanism underlying the interaction between grapefruit juice and aliskiren. A similar interaction has been observed with orange and apple juice, likely attributed to the inhibition of OATP2B1 by flavonoids found in these juices

The intricate world of intestinal uptake transporters plays a pivotal role in determining how drugs are absorbed in the body. The complex interplay between drugs and food, particularly fruit juices, adds an extra layer of complexity to drug therapy. Understanding the nuances of these interactions is not only fascinating but also crucial for optimizing drug efficacy and safety. Further research is essential to uncover the full extent of these intricate mechanisms and their implications for drug absorption and drug-food interactions.

INTESTINAL EFFLUX TRANSPORTERS: GATEKEEPERS OF DRUG ABSORPTION

Exploring ATP Binding Cassette Transporter P-glycoprotein

Within the realm of drug transporters, ABC transporter P-gp, encoded by the *ABCB1* gene, stands as one of the most meticulously studied transporters. In the gut mucosa, it takes up residence at the luminal membrane of enterocytes, orchestrating the efflux of its substrates back into the intestinal lumen. As such, P-gp plays a pivotal role in restricting the oral bioavailability of these substrates. Furthermore, intestinal P-gp has implications for the systemic clearance of intravenously administered drugs, contributing to their active secretion into the intestinal lumen. It is noteworthy that the expression of P-gp progressively increases from the proximal to the distal regions of the small intestine. P-gp exhibits its versatility by transporting a wide array of structurally diverse substances.

Partnership between P-glycoprotein and CYP3A4

In addition to P-gp, the enterocytes house the drug-metabolizing enzyme, CYP3A4. Interestingly, numerous substrates of P-gp are also metabolized by CYP3A4, leading to the notion that these two entities work in tandem to diminish the oral bioavailability of drugs. However, it is vital to acknowledge that the overlap of their substrates is not absolute. For instance, midazolam is metabolized by CYP3A4 but is not transported by P-gp, while digoxin, a P-gp substrate, does not succumb to the influence of CYP3A4. Digoxin, with its narrow therapeutic index, has earned its place as a probe drug for scrutinizing P-gp inhibition in clinical investigations

Mechanisms of P-glycoprotein-mediated Drug Interactions

P-gp-mediated drug interactions revolve around two primary mechanisms: Induction and inhibition. Induction of intestinal P-gp elevates the presystemic extraction of its substrates, thereby reducing their oral bioavailability. On the other hand, inhibition increases the oral bioavailability of drugs that rely on P-gp for transport. Let us delve into these mechanisms further, using the P-gp probe drug, digoxin, as an illustrative example.

Induction: The Rifampin Example

A seminal study by Greiner et al. in 1999 explored the effects of the antibiotic rifampin on digoxin's pharmacokinetics. The study involved healthy volunteers who received a single oral dose of 1 mg digoxin, either with or without prior oral treatment of 600 mg rifampin daily for 10 days. Intriguingly, after rifampin pretreatment, digoxin's $AUC_{0\text{-}144h}$ was significantly reduced, and both Cmax and oral bioavailability decreased by 58 and 30%, respectively. Duodenal biopsies revealed a 3.5-fold increase in P-gp expression. The AUC of orally administered digoxin was negatively correlated with P-gp expression in the small intestine. Subsequent studies have corroborated these findings, highlighting the role of rifampin in reducing oral digoxin bioavailability through the induction of intestinal P-gp and, consequently, enhanced presystemic digoxin extraction

Inhibition: The Quinidine Case

Conversely, inhibition of P-gp, a well-documented mechanism underlying drug interactions, leads to an increase in the oral bioavailability of drugs that rely on P-gp for transport. For example, the concomitant administration of quinidine and digoxin results in a substantial increase in digoxin serum concentrations, often accompanied by adverse reactions. Studies, both in vitro and in vivo, confirm that quinidine inhibits P-gp-mediated digoxin transport, supporting the notion that inhibition of P-gp is a significant factor in this interaction.

Beyond P-glycoprotein: Breast Cancer Resistance Protein and Multidrug Resistance Protein 2

In addition to P-gp, the luminal membrane of enterocytes hosts the efflux transporters BCRP and multidrug resistance protein 2 (MRP2). These transporters mirror P-gp in their ability to limit drug absorption, following the same principles that apply to intestinal P-gp-mediated drug interactions. For example, BCRP significantly restricts the oral bioavailability of topotecan in animal models. Clinical trials have affirmed that topotecan's oral bioavailability increases substantially when coadministered with the BCRP and P-gp inhibitor GF120918.

In summary, intestinal efflux transporters, notably P-gp, play a pivotal role in shaping the pharmacokinetics of orally administered drugs, with induction and inhibition as key mechanisms driving drug interactions. These transporters' impact on drug absorption and bioavailability underscores the importance of understanding their functions and their consequences for therapeutic outcomes.

HEPATIC TRANSPORTERS

- The liver is a major contributor to first-pass metabolism of orally administered drugs.
- The amount of blood filtered by the liver per time unit accounts for approximately 1,500 mL/min. The portal vein contributes 70–80% and the remaining percentage comes from the hepatic artery.
- Statins are used to reduce the occurrence of cardiovascular events and death in patients at risk. Statins have a risk of myopathy which increases with a rise in plasma concentration of statins, which is affected by interindividual variability.
- In particular, high-dose therapy with statins and the concomitant use of certain drugs are associated with a significant increase in the incidence of rhabdomyolysis.
- If the hepatocellular uptake of the drug by OATP1B1 is inhibited, it may increase the risk of myotoxic side effects and impair the therapeutic efficacy of statin therapy.

Hepatic Efflux Transporters

- Several ATP-dependent efflux transporters and MATE1, which is driven by the transmembraneous proton gradient, are localized in the canalicular membrane of the hepatocyte.
- These transporters contribute to the biliary excretion of drugs and their metabolites.
- Tubular secretion by kidneys is the main mechanism of elimination for metformin.
- A functional interplay between OCT2-mediated metformin uptake and efflux by MATE1 was important with respect to metformin secretion. Impaired transporter-mediated secretion of metformin increases the risk of metformin accumulation resulting in lactic acidosis.

Hepatic Transporters: Key Players in Drug Metabolism and Interactions

The liver plays a pivotal role in the metabolism and clearance of drugs from the body. Within the liver, a complex network of transporters is responsible for moving drugs and their metabolites into and out of hepatocytes. Understanding the interplay of these hepatic transporters is crucial for predicting and managing drug interactions and optimizing drug therapy.

Hepatic Uptake Transporters

Hepatic uptake transporters, primarily from the SLC family, facilitate the transport of drugs into hepatocytes. These transporters are especially important for drugs like statins, which are used to manage cholesterol levels. Some statins are substrates for these transporters, which means their pharmacokinetics (how the body processes drugs) are significantly influenced by them. In particular, OATP1B1, OATP1B3, and OATP2B1 are key players in the uptake of statins, and genetic variations can affect their transport activity. Inhibitors of these uptake transporters can lead to increased statin concentrations in the bloodstream, potentially causing adverse effects.

Hepatic Efflux Transporters

Hepatic efflux transporters, primarily from the ABC family and MATE1, are located in the canalicular membrane of hepatocytes and are involved in the export of drugs and their metabolites into the bile. One well-known example of interactions at hepatic efflux transporters involves the drug digoxin, which is secreted into the bile. Inhibition of the P-gp transporter by drugs like quinidine and verapamil can reduce the biliary clearance of digoxin, increasing its intracellular concentration within hepatocytes. Understanding these interactions is crucial for predicting and managing drug interactions involving P-gp substrates. Another transporter, MATE1, plays a role in the renal tubular secretion of certain drugs, like metformin. In animal experiments, it has been shown that MATE1 also contributes to metformin export from hepatocytes into the bile, raising questions about potential interactions and their clinical significance in humans.

In summary, hepatic transporters play a vital role in the metabolism, distribution, and elimination of drugs. Interactions at these transporters can lead to significant changes in drug concentrations and therapeutic outcomes, highlighting the importance of understanding these mechanisms to optimize drug therapy and prevent adverse effects.

RENAL UPTAKE TRANSPORTERS

- Inhibition of OATs or OCT2 at the basolateral membrane of renal proximal tubule cells decreases the cellular uptake of their substrates.
- As a result, the renal clearance of drugs which are eliminated to a significant degree by renal tubular secretion may be reduced.

- The uricosuric drug probenecid is the prototypical inhibitor of the OATs, OAT1 and OAT3. Probenecid was originally developed to prolong the plasma half-life of the antibiotic benzylpenicillin. The major route of the elimination of benzylpenicillin, renal tubular secretion, is efficiently inhibited by probenecid.
- A beneficial interaction that reduces the risk of adverse drug reactions is seen with the combination of probenecid and cidofovir. Cidofovir is transported by OAT1 and the tubular secretion of cidofovir is blocked by probenecid (OAT1 inhibitor) leading to less accumulation in renal tubular cells, faster elimination of the drug from the kidney, and overall decreased exposure of the kidney to the drug.

RENAL EFFLUX TRANSPORTERS

- P-glycoprotein is a well-characterized export protein present at the luminal membrane of renal proximal tubule cells.
- Digoxin is mainly excreted through the kidney, and concomitant administration of P-gp inhibitors like quinidine decreases the renal clearance of digoxin. Quinidine also has drug–drug interaction with digoxin by facilitating intestinal absorption and inhibiting the export in bile. There are also other P-gp inhibitors like ritonavir or itraconazole, which inhibit the renal clearance of digoxin.

Renal Transporters: The Significance of Drug Elimination and Interaction

The kidneys play a pivotal role in the elimination of drugs from the body through processes involving glomerular filtration and tubular secretion. Renal tubule cells have an intricate network of uptake and export transporters that play a crucial role in drug elimination. Understanding these renal transporters and their interactions is vital for predicting and managing drug interactions as well as optimizing drug therapy.

Renal Uptake Transporters

Renal uptake transporters, located in the basolateral membrane of renal proximal tubule cells, facilitate the cellular uptake of their substrates. Inhibition of these transporters can decrease the renal clearance of drugs, primarily eliminated through renal tubular secretion. Probenecid is a well-known example of an inhibitor of OATs, affecting OAT1 and OAT3. Probenecid was initially developed to prolong the plasma half-life of antibiotics like benzylpenicillin by efficiently inhibiting renal tubular secretion. Probenecid's inhibition of OAT1 and OAT3 contributes to multiple clinical drug interactions, including reducing the renal clearance of drugs like methotrexate and furosemide. The interaction between gemfibrozil and pravastatin also involves OAT3. Gemfibrozil, primarily known as an inhibitor of hepatic uptake transporters for pravastatin, decreases renal pravastatin clearance, illustrating the importance of both hepatic and renal transporters in this interaction. An example of a beneficial interaction is the combination of probenecid with cidofovir, an antiviral drug known for its renal toxicity. Probenecid inhibits the uptake of cidofovir into renal proximal tubule cells, reducing nephrotoxic effects and increasing cidofovir's therapeutic effectiveness. OCT2 is another transporter involved in drug interactions, facilitating the uptake of various drugs. Inhibitors of OCT2, such as cimetidine, can reduce the renal clearance of OCT2 substrates like metformin and ranitidine. An intriguing interaction involving OCT2 is observed with cisplatin, an anticancer drug with nephrotoxicity as a major limitation. Cimetidine and imatinib can inhibit OCT2-mediated uptake of cisplatin, potentially reducing its nephrotoxic effects. The combination of cimetidine or imatinib with cisplatin has shown partial renoprotective effects in animal studies.

Renal Efflux Transporters

Renal efflux transporters, including MATE1 and P-gp, located in the luminal membrane of renal proximal tubule cells, are involved in the export of drugs into the tubular lumen. MATE1 is an interesting transporter that can act as both an uptake and efflux transporter, driven by an oppositely directed proton gradient. MATE1 is believed to work in coordination with OCT2 to determine the renal tubular secretion of cationic drugs. The interaction between cimetidine and metformin is influenced by MATE1, and further research is needed to clarify the importance of MATE1 in drug interactions. P-gp plays a significant role in the renal clearance of drugs, as inhibition of P-gp can reduce the renal clearance of its substrates. Digoxin, mainly eliminated through renal clearance, is a well-known example of a drug that interacts with P-gp inhibitors like quinidine, leading to increased plasma concentrations. BCRP, an efflux transporter, has also been associated with the renal secretion of certain drugs, such as methotrexate. Polymorphisms in the *ABCG2* gene encoding BCRP may be associated with gout risk, making inhibition of renal BCRP a potential risk factor for this condition. Further studies are needed to elucidate the importance of renal BCRP in transporter-mediated drug interactions.

Understanding the roles and interactions of these renal transporters is essential for optimizing drug therapy, minimizing adverse effects, and preventing potential drug interactions.

ROLE OF PHARMACOGENOMICS

- Genotype-dependent drug–drug interactions are well known for drug-metabolizing enzymes (e.g., CYP2D6 and CYP2C19).
- The extent of these interactions is considerably smaller in poor metabolizers compared with extensive metabolizers.
- Cyclosporine was found to increase plasma concentrations of the oral antidiabetic drug repaglinide by inhibiting both CYP3A4-mediated metabolism and OATP1B1-mediated hepatic uptake of repaglinide.
- In subjects homozygous for the SLC22A2 c.808G>T mutation of OCT2, cimetidine caused only a modest reduction (13%) in renal clearance of metformin while this reduction was more pronounced in individuals with the GT or GG (wild-type) genotypes (26% and 42%, respectively).

Pharmacogenomics of Transporter-mediated Drug–Drug Interactions

It is a well-established fact that drug–drug interactions can lead to significant changes in pharmacokinetic parameters. However, it is important to recognize that these interactions often exhibit considerable interindividual variability. Some of this variability, in the extent of drug–drug interactions, can be attributed to genetic alterations in genes encoding drug-metabolizing enzymes or drug transporters. While genotype-dependent drug interactions are well documented for drug-metabolizing enzymes like CYP2D6 and CYP2C19, there has been limited exploration of genotype-dependent transporter-mediated drug interactions.

EXAMPLES OF GENOTYPE-DEPENDENT TRANSPORTER-MEDIATED DRUG INTERACTIONS

Cyclosporine and Repaglinide Interaction

Cyclosporine is known to increase the plasma concentrations of the oral antidiabetic drug repaglinide. This effect is attributed to the inhibition of both CYP3A4-mediated metabolism and OATP1B1-mediated hepatic uptake of repaglinide. Interestingly, the extent of this interaction was found to be 42% lower in individuals with the SLCO1B1 521TC genotype compared to those with the high-activity 521TT reference genotype.

Metformin and Cimetidine Interaction

The interaction between metformin and cimetidine is another classic example of a transporter-mediated drug interaction. In a study by Wang et al., it was observed that subjects homozygous for the SLC22A2 c.808G>T mutation of OCT2 experienced only a modest reduction (13%) in the renal clearance of metformin when cimetidine was administered. In contrast, individuals with the GT or GG (wild-type) genotypes showed more pronounced reductions (26% and 42%, respectively). This finding is consistent with in vitro data, which indicated that OCT2-mediated metformin uptake was considerably less sensitive to inhibition by cimetidine in cells expressing the variant protein compared to cells expressing wild-type OCT2 (IC50: 45 μM vs. 11 μM).

Apple Juice and Fexofenadine Interaction

In a recent study by Imanaga et al., the impact of apple juice on fexofenadine pharmacokinetics was investigated in relation to SLCO2B1 genotypes (encoding OATP2B1). The study reported a decrease in fexofenadine $AUC_{0-\infty}$ in volunteers with the SLCO2B1 c.1457C>T polymorphism, which has been shown to reduce OATP2B1 transport activity. Intriguingly, the extent of reduction in fexofenadine $AUC_{0-\infty}$ was lower in subjects homozygous for the SLCO2B1 c.1457C>T polymorphism compared to those homozygous for the wild-type allele.

Understanding how genetic variations impact transporter-mediated drug interactions can be crucial for personalized medicine. It allows for the prediction and management of drug interactions based on an individual's genetic makeup, ultimately leading to safer and more effective drug therapies. Further research in this field is expected to uncover more genotype-specific interactions, providing valuable insights into optimizing drug regimens for different patient populations.

CLINICAL IMPLICATIONS

- P-glycoprotein transporter encoded by the *MDR1* gene pumps back certain drugs such as vinblastine and doxorubicin into the maternal circulation, thereby protecting the fetus.
- Protease inhibitors, which are substrates to P-gp, achieve only low fetal concentrations, which have the risk of increase in vertical transmission of HIV infection from the mother to the fetus.
- At birth, the function of drug transporters is low such as in P-gp, which pumps morphine from the blood–brain barrier back to the systemic circulation. Hence, neonates are more sensitive than older children to the

depressant effects of morphine on the central nervous system (CNS).

- OCTs and MATEs share the common inhibitors cimetidine (histamine receptor antagonist), pyrimethamine (antiprotozoal and antimalarial dihydrofolate reductase inhibitor), and the chemotherapeutic tyrosine kinase inhibitors imatinib and erlotinib. Any drug-drug interaction involving these drugs could depend on the dose of the coadministered inhibitors.
- Concurrent administration of statins with gemfibrozil can cause myopathy.
- Losartan can inhibit both URAT1 and OAT4 and may, therefore, lead to the formation of kidney stones.
- The HIV protease inhibitor ritonavir blocks GLUT4, resulting in hyperglycemia in prediabetic patients treated with ritonavir.
- Inhibition of sodium-glucose cotransporters-2 (SGLT-2) results in osmotic diuresis due to the increased glucose load in the urine and has been linked to increased urination and thirst. SGLT-2 inhibitor, dapagliflozin, can cause hypotension and light-headedness due to excessive dehydration.
- The transporters like GAT—GAT-1, GAT-2, GAT-3, and GABA—act as the target for the drug tiagabine used for epilepsy. Other notable transporters used as drug targets include norepinephrine transporter (NET) [for antidepressants like tricyclic antidepressants (TCAs)], serotonin transporter (SERT) [for selective serotonin reuptake inhibitors (SSRIs) (used for depression)], and SGLT-2 (dapagliflozin and canagliflozin for diabetes mellitus).

CONCLUSION

Drug transporters are important determinants of therapeutic response in an individual. They can act as drug targets, and transporter-mediated drug–drug interactions play a vital role in patients, especially the elderly who are at risk of polypharmacy. Understanding about the drug transporters will also help us in targeted drug delivery.

IMPORTANCE OF TRANSPORTER-MEDIATED DRUG–DRUG INTERACTIONS: SUMMARY

- Inhibition or induction of drug transporters in the small intestine, liver, and kidney can significantly impact the pharmacokinetics and pharmacodynamic effects of multiple drugs, potentially influencing drug efficacy and toxicity.
- Transporter-mediated drug–drug interactions are a critical consideration in drug development and regulatory approval processes.
- These interactions may also have beneficial effects, such as reducing the tolerability of cytotoxic drugs through the inhibition of transporter-mediated cellular uptake.
- Genotype-dependent drug interactions play a role and may explain interindividual differences in the extent of drug interactions.

Intestinal Drug Transporters

- Inhibition of intestinal uptake transporters or induction of efflux transporters can decrease the intestinal absorption of drugs.
- Inhibition of intestinal efflux transporters may increase the oral bioavailability of drugs.

Hepatocellular Drug Transporters

- Inhibition of hepatocellular uptake transporters increases the area under the plasma concentration-time curve and maximal plasma concentration.
- Inhibition or induction of drug transporters at the canalicular membrane may decrease or increase, respectively, the secretion of drugs into the bile.

Renal Drug Transporters

- Inhibition of renal drug transporters may decrease the renal clearance of compounds with relevant renal tubular secretion.
- The nephrotoxicity of drugs that need to be taken up by renal tubular cells to cause toxic effects may be decreased by the inhibition of renal uptake transporters.

Conclusion and Future Perspective

- Qualitative prediction of transporter-mediated drug–drug interactions can be made based on cellular localization, substrate specificities, and inhibitors of drug transporters using in vitro data.
- Reliable quantitative predictions of these interactions require further improvements in in vitro methods.

This summary highlights the significance of transporter-mediated drug interactions, their impact on drug efficacy and safety, and the potential for genotype-based variations. It also underscores the importance of understanding these interactions in different organ systems, offering insights into predicting and managing drug–drug interactions for improved patient care.

SUGGESTED READINGS

1. Alexander SP, Kelly E, Marrion NV, Peters JA, Faccenda E, Harding SD, et al. The concise guide to pharmacology 2017/18: Overview. Br J Pharmacol. 2017;174:S1-16.
2. Palleria C, Di Paolo A, Giofrè C, Caglioti C, Leuzzi G, Siniscalchi A, et al. Pharmacokinetic drug-drug interaction and their implication in clinical management. J Res Med Sci. 2013;18(7):601-10.
3. Müller F, Fromm MF. Transporter-mediated drug-drug interactions. Pharmacogenomics. 2011;12(7):1017-37.
4. Kulik A, Brookhart MA, Levin R, Ruel M, Solomon DH, Choudhry NK. Impact of statin use on outcomes after coronary artery bypass graft surgery. Circulation. 2008;118(18): 1785-92.
5. Graham DJ, Staffa JA, Shatin D, Andrade SE, Schech SD, La Grenade L, et al. Incidence of hospitalized rhabdomyolysis in patients treated with lipid-lowering drugs. JAMA. 2004;292(21):2585-90.
6. Wang ZJ, Yin OQ, Tomlinson B, Chow MS. OCT2 polymorphisms and in-vivo renal functional consequence: studies with metformin and cimetidine. Pharmacogenet Genomics. 2008;18(7):637-45.
7. Overbosch D, Van Gulpen C, Hermans J, Mattie H. The effect of probenecid on the renal tubular excretion of benzylpenicillin. Br J Clin Pharmacol. 1988;25(1):51-8.
8. Izzedine H, Launay-Vacher V, Deray G. Antiviral drug-induced nephrotoxicity. Am J Kidney Dis. 2005;45(5):804-17.
9. Leahey EB Jr, Reiffel JA, Drusin RE, Heissenbuttel RH, Lovejoy WP, Bigger JT Jr. Interaction between quinidine and digoxin. JAMA. 1978;240(6):533-4.
10. Kajosaari LI, Niemi M, Neuvonen M, Laitila J, Neuvonen PJ, Backman JT. Cyclosporine markedly raises the plasma concentrations of repaglinide. Clin Pharmacol Ther. 2005;78(4):388-99.
11. Takane H, Shikata E, Otsubo K, Higuchi S, Ieiri I. Polymorphism in human organic cation transporters and metformin action. Pharmacogenomics. 2008;9(4):415-22.
12. Ersoy A, Hoffmaster A. Drug transporters. In: Golan E, Armstrong J, Armstrong W (Eds). Principles of Pharmacology: The Pathophysiologic Basis of Drug Therapy. Philadelphia: Lippincott Williams & Wilkins; 2017. p. 1042.
13. Giacomini KM, Sugiyama Y. Membrane transporters and drug responses. In: Brunton L, Lazo JS, Parker KL (Eds). Goodman & Gilman's: The Pharmacological Basis of Therapeutics, 13th edition. New York: McGraw Hill, 2018. pp. 41-70.
14. Gideon K, Special aspects of perinatal and pediatric pharmacology. In: Katzung G, Trevor J (Eds). Basic and Clinical Pharmacology. New York: McGraw Hill; 2018. pp. 1013-23.
15. König J, Müller F, Fromm MF. Transporters and drug-drug interactions: Important determinants of drug disposition and effects. Pharmacol Rev. 2013;65:944-66.
16. Girennavar B, Jayaprakasha GK, Patil BS. Potent inhibition of human cytochrome P450 3A4, 2D6, and 2C9 isoenzymes by grapefruit juice and its furocoumarins. J Food Sci. 2007;72(8):C417-21.
17. Bressler R. Grapefruit juice and drug interactions: Exploring mechanisms of this interaction and potential toxicity for certain drugs. Geriatrics. 2006;61(11):12-8.
18. Cvetkovic M, Leake B, Fromm MF, Wilkinson GR, Kim RB. OATP and P-glycoprotein transporters mediate the cellular uptake and excretion of fexofenadine. Drug Metab Dispos. 1999;27(8): 866-71.
19. Glaeser H, Bailey DG, Dresser GK, Gregor JC, Schwarz UI, McGrath JS, et al. Intestinal drug transporter expression and the impact of grapefruit juice in humans. Clin Pharmacol Ther. 2007;81(3): 362-70.
20. Kobayashi D, Nozawa T, Imai K, Nezu J, Tsuji A, Tamai I. Involvement of human organic anion transporting polypeptide OATP-B (SLC21A9) in pH-dependent transport across intestinal apical membrane. J Pharmacol Exp Ther. 2003;306(2):703-8.
21. Shimizu M, Fuse K, Okudaira K, Nishigaki R, Maeda K, Kusuhara H, et al. Contribution of OATP (organic anion-transporting polypeptide) family transporters to the hepatic uptake of fexofenadine in humans. Drug Metab Dispos. 2005;33(10):1477-81.
22. Imanaga J, Kotegawa T, Imai H, Tsutsumi K, Yoshizato T, Ohyama T, et al. The effects of the SLCO2B1 c.1457C>T polymorphism and apple juice on the pharmacokinetics of fexofenadine and midazolam in humans. Pharmacogenet Genomics. 2011;21(2):84-93.
23. Vaidyanathan S, Camenisch G, Schuetz H, Reynolds C, Yeh CM, Bizot MN, et al. Pharmacokinetics of the oral direct renin inhibitor aliskiren in combination with digoxin, atorvastatin, and ketoconazole in healthy subjects: the role of P-glycoprotein in the disposition of aliskiren. J Clin Pharmacol. 2008;48(11): 1323-38.
24. Igel S, Drescher S, Mürdter T, Hofmann U, Heinkele G, Tegude H, et al. Increased absorption of digoxin from the human jejunum due to inhibition of intestinal transporter-mediated efflux. Clin Pharmacokinet. 2007;46(9):777-85.
25. Drescher S, Glaeser H, Mürdter T, Hitzl M, Eichelbaum M, Fromm MF. P-glycoprotein-mediated intestinal and biliary digoxin transport in humans. Clin Pharmacol Ther. 2003;73(3):223-31.
26. Mouly S, Paine MF. P-glycoprotein increases from proximal to distal regions of human small intestine. Pharm Res. 2003;20(10):1595-9.
27. Benet LZ. The drug transporter-metabolism alliance: uncovering and defining the interplay. Mol Pharm. 2009;6(6):631-43.
28. Fenner KS, Troutman MD, Kempshall S, Cook JA, Ware JA, Smith DA, et al. Drug–drug interactions mediated through P-glycoprotein: clinical relevance and in vitro–in vivo correlation using digoxin as a probe drug. Clin Pharmacol Ther. 2009;85(2):173-81.
29. Gurley BJ, Swain A, Williams DK, Barone G, Battu SK. Gauging the clinical significance of P-glycoprotein-mediated herb–drug interactions: comparative effects of St. John's wort, Echinacea, clarithromycin, and rifampin on digoxin pharmacokinetics. Mol Nutr Food Res. 2008;52(7):772-9.
30. Kruijtzer CMF, Beijnen JH, Rosing H, ten Bokkel Huinink WW, Schot M, Jewell RC et al. Increased oral bioavailability of topotecan in combination with the breast cancer resistance protein and P-glycoprotein inhibitor GF120918. J Clin Oncol. 2002;20(13):2943-50.
31. Dresser GK, Bailey DG, Leake BF, Schwarz UI, Dawson PA, Freeman DJ, et al. Fruit juices inhibit organic anion transporting polypeptide-mediated drug uptake to decrease the oral availability of fexofenadine. Clin Pharmacol Ther. 2002 ;71(1): 11-20.
32. Greiner B, Eichelbaum M, Fritz P, Kreichgauer HP, von Richter O, Zundler J, et al. The role of intestinal P-glycoprotein in the interaction of digoxin and rifampin. J Clin Invest. 1999;104(2):147-53.

108

CHAPTER

Drug-induced Renal Injury: New Insights and Clinical Implications

Virendra Verma

ABSTRACT

Human kidneys serve to convert >1,700 L of blood per day into about 1 L of a highly concentrated fluid called urine. In so doing, the kidney excretes the waste products of metabolism; precisely regulates the body's concentration of water, salt, calcium, phosphorus and other anions and cations; and maintains the appropriate acid-base balance of plasma. Exposure to certain drugs often results in damage or destruction of normal renal functions. Therefore, early detection of drugs adverse effects in correlation to renal function is important to prevent progression to end-stage renal disease. Clinicians should be familiar with the pathogenesis and clinicopathologic manifestations of these forms of kidney injury and judicious use of these agents in setting where risk of renal injury is high. Several biomarkers have recently proven useful for assessment of nephrotoxicity that can assess kidney damage early and more accurately for effective protection of drug-induced nephrotoxicity. In this chapter, I summarize mechanisms of drug-induced nephrotoxicity and present the list of drugs that cause renal dysfunction, biomarkers that can be used for early assessment of nephrotoxicity, and the management of acute and chronic kidney diseases.

INTRODUCTION

Renal injury refers to damage or impairment to the kidneys, the vital organs that filter waste products and maintain fluid balance. It can manifest in various forms, ranging from mild dysfunction to severe renal failure. Many factors including acute conditions, chronic diseases, medications, toxins, and systemic disorders, can cause it.

A common form of renal injury is acute kidney injury (AKI), also known as acute renal failure. AKI is characterized by a rapid decline in kidney function, resulting in electrolyte imbalances and the accumulation of waste products. Dehydration, sepsis, hypotension, urinary blockage, and nephrotoxic medications can cause it. AKI increases mortality and a study sheds light on its prevalence and outcomes.

Chronic kidney disease (CKD) causes renal function loss and fluid regulation problems and develops over time. It is typically linked to diabetes, hypertension, and glomerulonephritis. The Global Burden of Disease Study 2019 emphasizes the prevalence and burden of CKD globally and the need for efficient management and preventative measures. According to the study, CKD affects approximately 9.1% of the global population, accounting for nearly 700 million individuals worldwide. This prevalence indicates the pressing need for effective prevention and management strategies to address the growing impact of CKD on public health.

In the setting of renal damage, drug-induced renal failure is of paramount concern. Some medications can harm kidney function, despite their essential role in disease management. AKI and worsening CKD are two possible outcomes of drug-induced renal failure. This type of kidney damage has extensive consequences for healthcare systems and places a high cost on individual patients with symptoms and complications. As a result, drug-induced renal failure becomes a major contributor of poor patient outcomes and high healthcare expenditures. However, it can be mitigated by early detection, optimal management measures, and the identification and avoidance of drugs associated with a higher risk of renal injury.

This review aims to comprehensively analyze renal injury including its various forms, such as AKI and CKD. By examining the etiology, epidemiology, diagnostic tools, treatment options, and ongoing research in the field, this review seeks to enhance our understanding of renal injury and its implications. Furthermore, this review aims to identify gaps in current knowledge, highlight active research areas, and emphasize the importance of early detection, effective prevention, and optimal management strategies. By consolidating existing literature and presenting a cohesive overview, this review aims to contribute to advancing renal injury research and clinical practice, ultimately improving patient outcomes and quality of life.

A COMMON MECHANISM OF INJURY IN AKI AND CKD

The common mechanisms of injury in AKI involve several pathophysiological processes. Some of the common injury mechanisms observed in AKI and CKD are mentioned in **Table 1**.

CLASSIFICATION OF DRUGS CAUSING AKI AND CKD

Drug-induced renal injury can occur through various mechanisms including direct toxicity, immune-mediated reactions, and alterations in renal blood flow. Understanding the classification of drugs associated with AKI and CKD is essential for healthcare professionals to make informed decisions regarding medication choices and monitoring strategies. **Table 2** lists the classification of common drugs causing renal injury and their frequency of

GUIDELINES FOR MEDICATION AVOIDANCE IN STAGE III AND BEYOND CKD: PROTECTING RENAL FUNCTION AND IMPROVING PATIENT WELL-BEING

In patients with stage III and beyond CKD, carefully considering medication choices is crucial to protect renal function and promote overall patient well-being. Kidneys play a vital role in drug metabolism and elimination. Hence, impaired kidney function can significantly impact the pharmacokinetics and pharmacodynamics of various medications. Certain drugs can further compromise renal function or lead to adverse effects in patients with advanced CKD. **Table 3** shows the category and drugs to be avoided for patients with caution in renal injury.

STRATEGIES FOR MAINTAINING AWARENESS OF KIDNEY IMPLICATIONS IN CRITICAL CARE SETTINGS

Regular monitoring of serum creatinine, urine output, and estimated glomerular filtration rate (eGFR) is crucial for evaluating kidney function and detecting early signs of AKI and CKD. Risk factors, such as preexisting renal impairment, hypovolemia, sepsis, nephrotoxic medications, and underlying diseases to prevent kidney injury, require optimized medication therapy. This can be achieved by adjusting doses, avoiding concomitant nephrotoxic agents, and considering alternatives with improved renal safety profiles. Maintain fluid balance and engage in collaborative conversations with healthcare professionals to promote optimal patient outcomes. To improve patient outcomes, stay updated on evidence-based guidelines and research.

TABLE 1: Mechanisms of renal injury in acute kidney injury (AKI) and chronic kidney disease (CKD).

Mechanism of injury	Acute kidney injury	Chronic kidney disease
Ischemia and hypoperfusion	Reduced blood flow to the kidneys leads to tissue hypoxia and injury	Gradual decline in renal blood flow over time, often due to underlying conditions like hypertension or diabetes
Inflammation and immune response	Activation of immune cells and release of proinflammatory cytokines contribute to tissue damage	Chronic inflammation, immune-mediated glomerular injury, and interstitial inflammation
Oxidative stress	The imbalance between reactive oxygen species (ROS) production and antioxidant defense mechanisms causes cellular damage	Persistent oxidative stress resulting from multiple factors including inflammation and metabolic abnormalities
Tubular injury	Direct toxic insults (e.g., nephrotoxic drugs or contrast agents) damaging tubular cells	Progressive tubular damage and atrophy, leading to impaired reabsorption and secretion functions
Glomerular injury	Glomerular inflammation, immune complex deposition, or other insults leading to glomerular dysfunction	Glomerulosclerosis, deposition of extracellular matrix, and loss of functional glomeruli
Fibrosis	Not a prominent feature in AKI	Excessive deposition of extracellular matrix proteins, leading to renal fibrosis and loss of functional nephrons

TABLE 2: Classification of drugs causing renal injury.

Category	Most frequently causing AKI/CKD	Infrequently causing AKI/CKD	Moderately causing AKI/CKD
Renal failure/AKI	• NSAIDs (e.g., ibuprofen) • Angiotensin II receptor blockers (ARBs) • Contrast agents (e.g., iodinated) • Antibiotics (e.g., penicillins) • Antivirals (e.g., acyclovir) • Chemotherapy drugs (e.g., cisplatin)	• ACE inhibitors • Diuretics • COX-2 inhibitors • Methotrexate	• Aminoglycosides • Amphotericin B • Cisplatin • Cyclosporine • NSAIDs (e.g., naproxen) • Radiocontrast agents • Tacrolimus • Vancomycin
CKD	• NSAIDs (e.g., ibuprofen) • ARBs • ACE inhibitors • Diuretics	• Lithium • Cyclosporine • Tetracyclines	• Tenofovir • Sulfonamides (e.g., trimethoprim-sulfamethoxazole) • Aminoglycosides • Analgesic mixtures containing phenacetin • Chinese herbal remedies (e.g., aristolochic acid) • Lead • Mercury • Cadmium

(ACE: angiotensin-converting enzyme; AKI: acute kidney injury; CKD: chronic kidney disease; COX-2: cyclooxygenase-2; NSAIDs: nonsteroidal anti-inflammatory drugs)

TABLE 3: Drugs to be avoided or used with caution in renal injury.

Category	Drugs to be avoided or used with caution
Nonsteroidal anti-inflammatory drugs (NSAIDs)	Ibuprofen, naproxen, diclofenac, celecoxib, etc.
Contrast agents	Iodinated contrast agents (e.g., iohexol and iopamidol)
Aminoglycoside antibiotics	Gentamicin, tobramycin, amikacin, neomycin, and streptomycin
Metformin	Requires dose adjustment or discontinuation
Proton pump inhibitors (PPIs)	Omeprazole, pantoprazole, esomeprazole, and lansoprazole

STRATEGIES FOR MAINTAINING AWARENESS OF KIDNEY IMPLICATIONS IN CHRONIC LIFESTYLE DISEASE MANAGEMENT SETTINGS

- Educate patients on medication adherence, blood pressure control, blood sugar management, and lifestyle changes
- Conduct regular assessments of kidney function for early detection of dysfunction
- Foster collaboration among healthcare providers for effective communication, medication review, and lifestyle modifications
- Encourage physical activity, a balanced diet, smoking cessation, and moderation in alcohol consumption
- Stay updated on guidelines and research through continuous professional development

BIOMARKERS FOR RENAL INJURY

Biomarkers play a crucial role in the early detection, diagnosis, and monitoring of renal injury. Common biomarkers include neutrophil gelatinase-associated lipocalin (NGAL), kidney injury molecule-1 (KIM-1), N-acetyl-β-D-glucosaminidase (NAG), cystatin C, cystatin C-based equations, and α1-microglobulin (A1M).

Neutrophil gelatinase-associated lipocalin is a protein produced and released by damaged renal tubular cells in response to injury and has shown promise in the early detection of AKI. KIM-1 is a transmembrane protein upregulated in proximal tubular cells following injury, and elevated levels in urine or blood samples may indicate ongoing kidney injury and help monitor disease progression.

N-acetyl-β-D-glucosaminidase is an enzyme in the brush border of renal tubular cells. Increased urinary NAG levels indicate a tubular injury and can be used as a biomarker for nephrotoxicity. Urinary NAG levels can help identify and monitor renal tubular damage caused by various factors including exposure to nephrotoxic drugs or other insults.

Cystatin C is an endogenous protein freely filtered by the glomerulus and reabsorbed by renal tubules, making it a valuable biomarker for estimating kidney function. Cystatin C-based equations have been developed to estimate glomerular filtration rate (GFR), providing an alternative to serum creatinine-based estimates.

Alpha-1-microglobulin is a low molecular weight protein filtered by the glomerulus and reabsorbed by the proximal tubules. Elevated urinary levels of A1M can be used as a biomarker for tubular injury, assisting in renal damage identification and monitoring disease progression. These biomarkers have potential applications in diagnosing and monitoring various renal conditions.

MANAGEMENT OF DRUG-INDUCED ACUTE KIDNEY INJURY

Managing drug-induced AKI involves several key strategies. Firstly, it is crucial to identify and immediately discontinue using drugs or chemicals that may be causing kidney injury. Prompt action in stopping the offending agents is essential to prevent further kidney damage. Supportive care also plays a vital role in AKI management. This includes maintaining hydration, optimizing oxygenation, and ensuring hemodynamic stability. Adequate fluid resuscitation and careful blood pressure management can improve renal perfusion and promote kidney recovery.

Close monitoring of serum creatinine, urine output, and electrolytes is critical to pharmacovigilance in AKI management. Regular monitoring allows healthcare professionals to assess kidney function, track changes over time, and make informed decisions regarding treatment adjustments. In addition to discontinuing nephrotoxic medications, efforts should be made to avoid prescribing such medications to patients at risk of AKI, as this can further prevent harm to the kidneys. In severe cases where conservative management fails to improve kidney function, renal replacement therapy (RRT) may be initiated. RRT, such as hemodialysis or continuous RRT, provides temporary support to the kidneys and aids in kidney recovery.

MANAGEMENT OF DRUG-INDUCED CHRONIC KIDNEY DISEASE

Managing drug-induced CKD involves a comprehensive approach to slow the progression of renal damage. A crucial step is discontinuing medications that can worsen renal function or contribute to CKD progression. Medication dosing should be adjusted based on eGFR or other renal function tests to minimize further renal damage.

Controlling blood pressure and reducing proteinuria are key therapeutic targets in managing drug-induced CKD. Medications such as angiotensin-converting enzyme (ACE) inhibitors and angiotensin receptor blockers (ARBs) are commonly prescribed to regulate blood pressure and reduce proteinuria, which can help slow down the progression of CKD. Maintaining fluid and electrolyte balance by effective management of sodium, potassium, and phosphate levels contributes to preserving optimal kidney function.

The management of drug-induced CKD also involves addressing and managing cardiovascular risk factors. This includes managing conditions, such as hypertension, diabetes, and dyslipidemia, commonly associated with CKD. By effectively managing these risk factors, healthcare practitioners can prevent or slow down the progression of CKD.

For patients with advanced CKD and end-stage renal disease (ESRD), RRT options should be considered. Depending on the patient's specific needs and clinical situation, these options may include hemodialysis, peritoneal dialysis, or kidney transplantation.

PHARMACOGENOMICS AND PERSONALIZED MEDICINE

Understanding how genetic variations influence an individual's response to medications in pharmacogenomics can significantly optimize treatment outcomes. By incorporating pharmacogenomic testing, healthcare professionals can personalize medicine selection and dose based on a patient's genetic profile. This approach helps minimize the risk of adverse drug reactions and enhances the efficacy of pharmacotherapy.

CONCLUSION

Drug-induced kidney damage poses a significant concern in clinical practice, emphasizing the importance of early recognition, appropriate management, and collaborative efforts among healthcare professionals. Awareness of drugs and substances that can potentially cause renal injury, understanding the underlying mechanisms, and prompt withdrawal of offending agents are crucial for preventing and managing drug-induced renal injury. Close monitoring of renal function parameters, maintaining hydration and electrolyte balance, and leveraging pharmacogenomics for personalized treatment approaches are essential strategies for minimizing the risk of kidney damage. By implementing these measures, healthcare providers can enhance patient safety, improve outcomes, and optimize the overall management of drug-induced renal injury.

SUGGESTED READINGS

1. GBD Chronic Kidney Disease Collaboration. Global, regional, and national burden of chronic kidney disease, 1990-2017: a systematic analysis for the Global Burden of Disease Study 2017. Lancet. 2020;395(10225):709-33.
2. Kellum JA, Lameire N, Aspelin P, MacLeod AM, Barsoum RS, Mehta RL, et al. Kidney disease: Improving global outcomes (KDIGO) acute kidney injury work group. KDIGO clinical practice guideline for acute kidney injury. Kidney Int Suppl. 2012;2(1):1-138.
3. Perazella MA, Butler AM. Drug-induced acute kidney injury: A focus on recent medications and injurious mechanisms. Am J Kidney Dis. 2016;68(5):804-17.
4. Matzke GR, Aronoff GR, Atkinson AJ Jr, et al. Drug dosing consideration in patients with acute and chronic kidney disease—a clinical update from kidney disease: Improving Global Outcomes (KDIGO). Kidney Int. 2011;80(11):1122-37.
5. Parikh CR, Devarajan P, Zappitelli M, Sint K, Thiessen-Philbrook H, Li S, et al. Postoperative biomarkers predict acute kidney injury and poor outcomes after pediatric cardiac surgery. J Am Soc Nephrol. 2011;22(9):1737-47.
6. Vaidya VS, Ferguson MA, Bonventre JV. Biomarkers of acute kidney injury. Annu Rev Pharmacol Toxicol. 2008;48:463-93.
7. Mulay SR, Linkermann A, Anders HJ. Necroinflammation in kidney disease. J Am Soc Nephrol. 2016;27(1):27-39.
8. Dharnidharka VR, Kwon C, Stevens G. Serum cystatin C is superior to serum creatinine as a marker of kidney function: a meta-analysis. Am J Kidney Dis. 2002;40(2):221-6.
9. Grubb A, Simonsen O, Sturfelt G, Truedsson L, Thysell H. Serum concentration of cystatin C, factor D, and beta 2-microglobulin as a measure of glomerular filtration rate. Acta Med Scand. 1985;218(5):499-503.
10. Tantisattamo E, Tantisattamo N. Pharmacogenomics and personalized medicine in chronic kidney disease. Pharmacogenomics. 2020;21(2):93-110.

109

CHAPTER

Drug-induced Cholestasis

Manuj Kumar Sarkar, Subhra Dey, Boudhayan Das Munshi

ABSTRACT

The liver is the first defense organ after drugs get absorbed from the gastrointestinal system; therefore, it is predisposed to many types of injuries by external agents, including drugs. Drug-induced liver injury (DILI) can mainly present with either hepatitis or cholestatic or mixed type of presentation. Cholestatic liver injury accounts for 20–40% of DILI. Prompt identification and withdrawal of offending drugs is essential to stop the progression of chronic liver disease, which may rarely progress to the requirement of liver transplantation.

INTRODUCTION

The liver is the body's primary organ that deals with detoxifying endogenous and exogenous toxins in the body. The clinical presentation of drug-induced cholestasis includes vanishing bile duct syndrome (VBDS), secondary sclerosing cholangitis, bland cholestasis, and cholestatic hepatitis. Mortality of cholestatic drug-induced liver injury (DILI) can be as high as 10%. Risk factors for drug-induced cholestasis include older age, genetic determinants, and chemical and physical properties of drugs. Among these three patterns, cholestatic injury occurs in 20–40% of cases.

TYPES OF DRUG-INDUCED LIVER INJURY BASED ON ETIOLOGY

Drug-induced liver injury can present similar to acute or chronic liver disease, complicating the diagnosis and treatment of primary liver disease. DILI can be classified into two forms: (1) Intrinsic DILI and (2) idiosyncratic DILI. When DILI is dose-dependent and predictable, it is called intrinsic DILI. More than 50% of cases of acute liver failure are due to intrinsic DILI, which occurs usually due to a high dosage of drug administration and typically resolves by reducing the dose or stopping the drug.

While idiosyncratic, the DILI course is unpredictable, found less commonly, presents slowly and late, and is often asymptomatic to mild liver enzyme elevation and sometimes in advanced liver failure. Prompt recognition of idiosyncratic DILI is pivotal, and complete withdrawal of the offending drug is essential for response to treatment. This form of DILI is a diagnosis of exclusion, which is very difficult. Idiosyncratic DILI usually presents with chronic DILI, the definition of which has constantly changed over the last 30 years since the introduction of the term in 1990 by CIOMS; presently, EASL defines liver inflammation of > 12 months since the initiation of DILI as chronic DILI, whereas USA and Chinese guidelines recommend 6 months as cut-off criteria.

RISK FACTORS FOR DRUG-INDUCED LIVER INJURY

- *Chemical properties of drug*: Lipophilic drugs have more chances of cholestatic liver injury, for example, trovafloxacin has a fluorinated side chain, making it more lipophilic, leading to more DILI cases. Similarly, drugs excreted in bile have more chances of developing cholestatic DILI, 70%, compared with 40% with drugs of minimal biliary excretion.

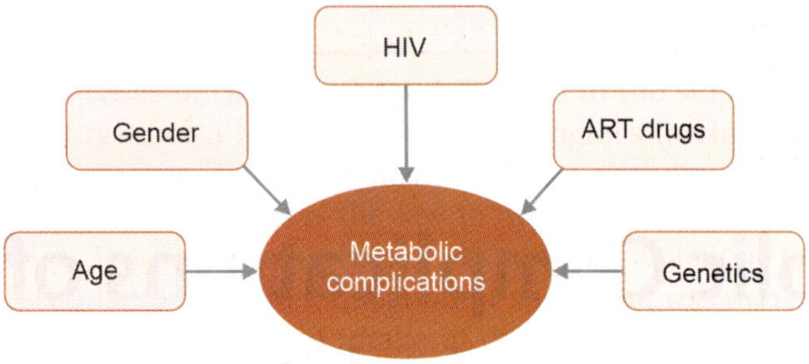

FIG. 1: Factors associated with metabolic complications in HIV patients.
(ART: antiretroviral therapy; HIV: human immunodeficiency virus)

the specific drugs, but earlier studies reported a prevalence of 10–80%. PLHIV either presents lipohypertrophy and lipoatrophy alone or its combination. From the published studies, it is evident that certain classes of antiretroviral drugs are the primary risk factors for lipodystrophy in HIV-infected patients. Apart from the ART duration, age, gender, and genetic predisposition are a few other risk factors for the development of lipodystrophy. Lipodystrophy syndrome manifestation is different from person to person. In lipoatrophy, loss of subcutaneous fat occurs in the face, arms, legs, and buttocks, resulting in a sunken appearance. Whereas, lipohypertrophy results in fat accumulation in the abdomen, neck, and breasts. Lipodystrophy is found to be associated with metabolic abnormalities, such as hyperlipidemia, insulin resistance (IR), and diabetes mellitus. Prior use of NRTI-class drugs like stavudine or ZDV has been linked with lipoatrophy of which stavudine has a strong association with lipoatrophy. Whereas, abacavir and tenofovir alafenamide (TAF) were not linked with lipoatrophy. Lipohypertrophy, especially trunk fat increase, has been reported with efavirenz, PIs, and raltegravir.

METABOLIC SYNDROME

As per the Adult Treatment Panel III (ATP III) report, metabolic syndrome is a cluster of metabolic abnormalities including abdominal obesity, high blood pressure, elevated triglycerides (TGs), elevated fasting glucose levels, and reduced high-density lipoproteins (HDLs). If three or more of these criteria are satisfied, then the condition is referred to as metabolic syndrome. These metabolic abnormalities increase the risk of heart disease, stroke, and type 2 diabetes mellitus (T2DM). The pathogenesis of ART-related metabolic syndrome is not yet fully understood. Some unproven hypotheses on this topic are chronic inflammation of HIV or alterations in gut flora. IR, dyslipidemia, lipodystrophy, and consequently cardiovascular risk are associated with the use of PI or NRTI.

DYSLIPIDEMIA

Dyslipidemia due to the HIV treatment is associated with a range of values of serum concentrations of total cholesterol (TC) and TG, depending on the class of ART being used. Few drugs of the first-generation combinations in ART are associated with changes/abnormalities in lipid metabolism.

From the NRTI class, ZDV is more significantly associated with dyslipidemia as compared to abacavir, causing increased low-density lipoprotein (LDL) levels and TG. Elevated TG, LDL, and HDL levels have been reported with TAF. Tenofovir disoproxil fumarate (TDF) has been associated with lower lipid levels than abacavir or TAF. Efavirenz which is an NNRTI drug is associated with elevated levels of TG, LDL, and HDL. All ritonavir or cobicistat-boosted PIs showed an increase in TG, LDL, and HDL levels. A higher increase in TG levels was noted with ritonavir-boosted lopinavir (LPV/r) than boosted darunavir (DRV/r), or boosted atazanavir (ATV/r). Elvitegravir/cobicistat results in higher levels of TG, LDL, and HDL.

INSULIN RESISTANCE AND DIABETES

Though antiretroviral drugs in combination have improved the ART and prognosis of HIV infection, these drugs are associated with long-term complications such as IR, especially associated with older age. Published studies reported the approximate incidence of glucose metabolism disorders in PLHIV is around 2–25%, which leads to a two times higher risk of type 2 diabetes in this population. Adipose tissue has a major role in the pathogenesis of systemic IR. IR further contributes to other diseases including T2DM and a cluster of cardiovascular risk factors.

Diabetes mellitus and IR have been associated with the use of ZDV and ritonavir-boosted lopinavir (LPV/r), while no such associations have been reported with boosted atazanavir (ATV/r) or darunavir (DRV/r).

BONE DENSITY LOSS

Osteoporosis is one of the serious adverse effects caused by long-term ART. It is a multifactorial systemic skeletal disease followed by low bone mineral density, deterioration of bone architecture, bone fragility, and consequently increased fracture risk. Loss of bone mineral density is commonly observed in patients with HIV infection receiving ART. HIV patients on PI-containing regimens demonstrate bone loss in the spine, while those on NRTI-containing regimens show bone loss in the hip. Some studies state that combining NRTI drugs with PI-containing regimens also leads to bone loss among patients with HIV infection. Also, the correlation between ART usage, timing, dosages, and adherence with osteoporosis risk among patients with HIV infection remains unclear. ZDV is associated with anemia and neutropenia.

METABOLIC COMPLICATIONS ASSOCIATED WITH ANTIRETROVIRAL DRUGS CLASSWISE

A review by Thet and Siritientong (2020) summarized various metabolic complications associated with each antiretroviral drug. **Table 1** is the concise summary of the review representing metabolic complications associated with each antiretroviral drug reported in the published studies. From this table, individual drugs and types of ART associated with different metabolic complications can be differentiated. These incidences are not specific to drugs; however, the prevalence and severity change as per the drug class.

SWITCHING ANTIRETROVIRAL DRUGS DUE TO ADVERSE EVENTS

Nearly all antiretroviral drugs are associated with adverse effects that cause treatment discontinuation, nonadherence to medication, or switching to alternate ART. Newer regimens are associated with fewer adverse effects. Below 10% of treatment-limiting adverse events are reported in randomized trials involving treatment-naive patients. Most clinical trials involve specific inclusion criteria and are conducted for a short duration; hence, they cannot be directly related to real-world scenarios. But in reality, ART is recommended in all patients and therapy must be continued indefinitely. While selecting the ARV regimen, healthcare practitioners must consider the following points:

- Potential adverse effects
- Individual's comorbidities
- Concomitant medications
- Prior history of drug intolerances

MANAGEMENT OF METABOLIC COMPLICATIONS ASSOCIATED WITH ANTIRETROVIRAL THERAPY: SUBSTITUTION WITH ALTERNATE ANTIRETROVIRAL AGENTS

Metabolic complications by the current antiretroviral drugs can be reduced or reversed by switching to alternate drugs. Published studies reported various switching strategies. Few metabolic complications by ongoing antiretroviral drugs and the appropriate switching options reported are discussed here.

Peripheral lipoatrophy which is characterized by loss of subcutaneous fat of the limbs, face, and buttocks is associated with the use of prior NRTI class drugs, especially stavudine and ZDV. Switching from nucleoside analogs such as ZDV or stavudine to abacavir showed improvement in lipoatrophy, but the study recommended a larger study population and longer follow-up to clinically conclude improvement in lipoatrophy. As per the US, Department of Health and Human Services (DHHS) reports, switching from NRTI class drugs, especially stavudine and ZDV, a slow (several years) and incomplete fat recovery noted.

Antiretroviral therapy is associated with lipohypertrophy, i.e., accumulation of visceral, truncal, dorsocervical, and breast fat. Lipohypertrophy is more common with older PIs like indinavir. However, there are no clinical pieces of evidence that support switching to another first-line regimen that could reverse lipohypertrophy.

Among different ritonavir-boosted PIs, boosted lopinavir (LPV/r) and boosted fosamprenavir (FPV/r) more commonly elevate TG and LDL levels than other ritonavir-boosted PIs. Switching from a saquinavir/ritonavir (PI-based) regimen to an abacavir-based regimen showed significant improvements in lipid abnormalities. Many studies reported switching from ritonavir or cobicistat boosted efavirenz to INSTI—doravirine, or rilpivirine for hypertriglyceridemia (with or without elevated LDL level). Switching from boosted lopinavir (LPV/r) to atazanavir or boosted atazanavir (ATV/r) also improved TG and LDL levels. Atazanavir coadministration with TDF should be avoided as TDF reduces the ATV levels.

Switching from boosted lopinavir (LPV/r) to INSTI and NNRTI gave conflicting results for IR. The studies from the HIV-negative subjects yielded a causal relationship between boosted lopinavir and IR. A switch from a stable PI regimen to ritonavir-boosted atazanavir (ATV/r) was found to improve IR and dyslipidemia in HIV-infected men. According to the reports, traditional risk factors of IR exacerbate more influence than any of the PIs.

Switching from TDF to TAF or abacavir (abacavir should be used only in HLA-B*5701 negative patients), or NRTI sparing regimens, or NRTI regimens using only lamivudine or emtricitabine also reported for the bone density effects. Switching from TDF to other antiretroviral drugs improved bone density with unknown clinical significance. A smaller decrease in bone mineral density is reported in TAF as compared to TDF, and hence patients

TABLE 1: Common metabolic effects of antiretroviral drugs.

	Nucleoside reverse transcriptase inhibitors								Non-nucleoside reverse transcriptase inhibitors				Protease inhibitors							Integrase inhibitors	
Effects	ABC	ZDV	3TC	D4t	TDF	TAF	ddI	FTC	NVP	EFV	ETR	RPV	LPV	RTV	ATV	DRV	IDV	NFV	SQV	DTG	RAL
Lipodystrophy	✓	✓	✓																✓		✓
Limb fat loss							✓											✓			
Lipoatrophy				✓	✓		✓	✓		✓			✓								
Facial atrophy		✓	✓	✓													✓				
Lower limb atrophy		✓	✓	✓													✓				
Buttock atrophy		✓	✓	✓													✓				
Lipid abnormalities													✓	✓		✓				✓	
Hypertriglyceridemia	✓	✓	✓	✓	✓			✓	✓	✓	✓		✓	✓	✓	✓		✓	✓		
Hypercholesterolemia	✓	✓	✓	✓	✓			✓	✓	✓	✓	✓	✓	✓	✓	✓		✓			✓
Hyperbilirubinemia			✓										✓	✓	✓	✓					
Increased AST										✓	✓	✓	✓		✓	✓		✓			
Increased ALT										✓		✓	✓		✓	✓		✓			
Hyperlactatemia				✓																	
Lactic acidosis	✓	✓		✓																	
Leukopenia		✓																			
Anemia		✓	✓	✓	✓			✓	✓	✓											
Metabolic and nutritional disorder													✓	✓		✓					
Gastrointestinal disorders													✓		✓					✓	✓
Hyperglycemia													✓	✓		✓					
Peripheral neuropathy		✓	✓	✓					✓	✓											
Osteopenia					✓	✓															
Decreased BMD at lumbar spine			✓	✓	✓	✓		✓	✓	✓			✓	✓	✓		✓				
Decreased BMD at hip			✓	✓	✓	✓		✓	✓	✓			✓	✓			✓				

(3TC: lamivudine; ABC: abacavir; ATV: atazanavir; BMD: bone mineral density; D4T: stavudine; ddI: didanosine; DRV: darunavir; DTG: dolutegravir; EFV: efavirenz; ETR: etravirine; FTC: emtricitabine; IDV: indinavir; LPV: lopinavir; NFV: nelfinavir; NVP: nevirapine; RAL: raltegravir; RPV: rilpivirine; RTV: ritonavir; SQV: saquinavir; TAF: tenofovir alafenamide; TDF: tenofovir disoproxil fumarate; ZDV: zidovudine) show improvement in bone mineral density when they are switched from TDF to TAF. However, studies on the long-term effects of TAF in osteopenia or osteoporosis patients are essential.

Zidovudine from the NRTI class has been associated with neutropenia and macrocytic anemia. Hence, switching from ZDV to a regimen without ZDV has been suggested.

MANAGEMENT STRATEGIES FOR THE METABOLIC COMPLICATION IN PEOPLE LIVING WITH HUMAN IMMUNODEFICIENCY VIRUS

Antiretroviral drugs must be studied for their long-term as well as short-term metabolic abnormalities associated with them. HIV infection and ART develop metabolic complications which affects nutritional status in PLHIV. Hence, long-term monitoring and management of metabolic complications are essential to avoid aggravation by poor nutritional status in PLHIV. Also, dietary management is needed for the treatment of related complications such as dyslipidemia, glucose abnormalities, and limb fat loss. Nutritional counseling and intervention, lifestyle management, and pharmaceutical interventions as per the individual patient's requirement are some of the management strategies to overcome metabolic complications in PLHIV.

CONCLUSION

Important goals for ART are to achieve and sustain viral suppression for a prolonged period; and to anticipate and manage both long- and short-term ART-related adverse effects. The information regarding metabolic complications associated with each antiretroviral drug and drug class can be useful for finding new regimens with fewer side effects or switching to some simplified regimen with improved tolerability. Several other factors that are also involved in metabolic complications in PLHIV need to be addressed. Genetic analysis, nutritional counseling, and management may also help to reduce the metabolic complications in PLHIV on ART.

SUGGESTED READINGS

1. Ergin HE, Inga EE, Maung TZ, Javed M, Khan S. HIV, Antiretroviral therapy and metabolic alterations: A review. Cureus. 2020;12(5):e8059.
2. Anuurad E, Semrad A, Berglund L. Human immunodeficiency virus and highly active antiretroviral therapy-associated metabolic disorders and risk factors for cardiovascular disease. Metab Syndr Relat Disord. 2009;7(5):401-10.
3. World Health Organization. (2021). Consolidated Guidelines On HIV prevention, testing, treatment, service delivery and monitoring: recommendations for a public health approach. [online] Available from https://www.who.int/publications/i/item/9789240031593 [Last accessed December, 2023].
4. Chow DC, Day LJ, Souza SA, Shikuma CM. Metabolic complications of HIV therapy. IAPAC Mon. 2006;12(9):302-17.
5. Guzman N, Vijayan V. HIV-Associated Lipodystrophy. In: StatPearls [Internet]. Treasure Island (FL): StatPearls Publishing; 2023. [online] Available from https://www.ncbi.nlm.nih.gov/books/NBK493183/ [Last accessed December, 2023].
6. Department of Health and Human Services. (2023). Panel on Antiretroviral Guidelines for Adults and Adolescents. Guidelines for the Use of Antiretroviral Agents in Adults and Adolescents with HIV. Available from https://clinicalinfo.hiv.gov/en/guidelines/adult-and-adolescent-arv. [Last accessed December, 2023].
7. Samaras K, Wand H, Law M, Emery S, Cooper D, Carr A. Prevalence of metabolic syndrome in HIV-infected patients receiving highly active antiretroviral therapy using International Diabetes Foundation and Adult Treatment Panel III criteria: associations with insulin resistance, disturbed body fat compartmentalization, elevated C-reactive protein, and [corrected] hypoadiponectinemia. Diabetes Care. 2007;30(1):113-9. Erratum in: Diabetes Care. 2007;30(2):455.
8. Pedro MN, Rocha GZ, Guadagnini D, Santos A, Magro DO, Assalin HB, et al. Insulin Resistance in HIV-Patients: Causes and Consequences. Front Endocrinol (Lausanne). 2018;9:514.
9. Kelesidis T, Currier JS. Dyslipidemia and cardiovascular risk in human immunodeficiency virus infection. Endocrinol Metab Clin North Am. 2014;43(3):665-84.
10. Honnapurmath VK, Patil VW. Antiretroviral Therapy-induced Insulin Resistance and Oxidative Deoxy Nucleic Acid Damage in Human Immunodeficiency Virus-1 Patients. Indian J Endocrinol Metab. 2017;21(2):316-21.
11. Chiu ML, Liang WM, Li JP, Cheng CF, Chiou JS, Ho MW, et al. Timing, Dosage, and Adherence of Antiretroviral Therapy and Risk of Osteoporosis in Patients With Human Immunodeficiency Virus Infection in Taiwan: A Nested Case-Control Study. Front Pharmacol. 2021;12:631480.
12. Thet D, Siritientong T. Antiretroviral Therapy-Associated Metabolic Complications: Review of the Recent Studies. HIV AIDS (Auckl). 2020;12:507-524.
13. O'Brien ME, Clark RA, Besch CL, Myers L, Kissinger P. Patterns and correlates of discontinuation of the initial HAART regimen in an urban outpatient cohort. J Acquir Immune Defic Syndr. 2003;34(4):407-14.
14. Carr A, Workman C, Smith DE, Hoy J, Hudson J, Doong N, et al. Abacavir substitution for nucleoside analogs in patients with HIV lipoatrophy: a randomized trial. JAMA. 2002;288(2):207–15.
15. Clumeck N, Goebel F, Rozenbaum W, Gerstoft J, Staszewski S, Montaner J, et al. Simplification with abacavir-based triple

111 CHAPTER

Disease-modifying Antirheumatic Drugs in Pregnancy and Lactation

H Basavanagowdappa, R Subramanian, Praveen Kulkarni

ABSTRACT

Prevalence of rheumatic diseases is more in women when compared to men, barring ankylosing spondylitis and gout. Course of autoimmune rheumatic disease (AIRD) is often fluctuating with frequent remissions and exacerbations, the causes of which are multifactorial. Pregnancy in patients with AIRD is complicated by physiological, immunological, and hormonal imbalances which may have a direct impact on AIRD activity. Managing AIRDs in pregnancy and lactation is just not limited to prescription of compatible drugs; we need to precisely plan to minimize adverse effects in the conceptus and neonates. The timing of pregnancy depends on the disease activity and the half-life of immunomodulatory agents which may either required to be discontinued or switched to drugs which are safe and compatible with pregnancy. In this chapter, authors have described the uses of various disease-modifying antirheumatic drugs (DMARDs) during pregnancy and lactation.

INTRODUCTION

Prevalence of rheumatic diseases is more in women when compared to men, barring ankylosing spondylitis and gout. Managing autoimmune rheumatic diseases (AIRDs) in pregnancy and lactation is just not limited to prescription of compatible drugs; we need to precisely plan to minimize adverse effects in the conceptus and neonates. The process and therapeutic plan must concentrate on maintaining a low disease activity for a successful pregnancy outcome. In the era of biologicals and small molecules, in addition to optimal use of conventional synthetic disease-modifying antirheumatic drugs (csDMARDs), it is possible to achieve and maintain an adequate disease control. However, it is not uncommon to encounter flares of AIRD during pregnancy and lactation, in the event of which, it is prudent to strike a balance between the change of drugs and the potential benefits and risks to the mother and fetus. Utilization of csDMARDs effectively in pregnancy and lactation is a shared decision making between the caregiver and the patient with AIRD.

The level of evidence of safety of csDMRADs', biologicals, and small molecules in pregnancy and lactation is based on large registries and postmarketing surveillance rather than randomized controlled trials wherein pregnancy and lactation is excluded. Furthermore, most AIRD require combination of DMARDs' which makes it difficult to attribute adverse maternal and fetal outcomes to one particular drug.

BACKGROUND

Course of AIRD is often fluctuating with frequent remissions and exacerbations, the causes of which are multifactorial. Pregnancy in patients with AIRD is complicated by physiological, immunological, and hormonal imbalances which may have a direct impact on AIRD disease activity **(Fig. 1)**.

It is generally known that rheumatoid arthritis (RA) improves during pregnancy and flare ups are more likely during postpartum period. Other conditions like systemic lupus erythematosus (SLE) and Sjögren's syndrome have an unpredictable course during pregnancy. Spondyloarthritis (SpA) and systemic sclerosis (SSc) remain fairly stable throughout pregnancy. Most AIRDs do not affect fertility significantly, however SLE can cause a concerning issue of pregnancy loss, and in other

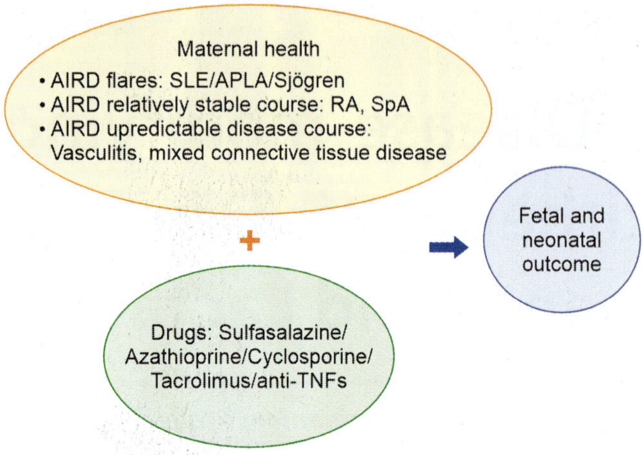

FIG. 1: AIRD course in pregnancy and drug usage.

(AIRD: autoimmune rheumatic disease; anti-TNFs: anti-tumor necrosis factors; APLA: antiphospholipid antibody; SLE: systemic lupus erythematosus; RA: rheumatoid arthritis; SpA: spondyloarthritis; TNFs: tumor necrosis factors)

disorders, the fecundity may be affected. The usage of csDMARDs' and biological in AIRDs may however have an effect on fertility, fecundity, and teratogenicity depending on the drug used.

PRINCIPLES IN PRESCRIBING DMARDS' IN AIRD AND PREGNANCY

- Maternal health status is prioritized over potential fetal outcomes in severe/life-threatening AIRD, in case alternative agents which are compatible with pregnancy are not available.
- Stable disease prior to conception will ensure a favorable pregnancy outcome.
- All patients with AIRD who are planning a family should undergo preconception counseling, documentation of potential risks/benefits, and contraceptive advice.
- Avoid drugs that are incompatible during pregnancy and switch to immunomodulatory drugs that are compatible with pregnancy to ensure adequate disease control.
- Usage of steroids should be at a minimum effective dose and whenever possible it should be stopped.
- Biologic DMARDs may be continued throughout pregnancy if required to control disease activity/bring down severe maternal disease.
- There can be unpredictable efficacy and bioavailability of live vaccine in neonate, if the mother is exposed to biologic DMARDs and hence there will be need of modification in immunization schedules
- There is no convincing data about adverse fetal development or pregnancy outcome with paternal exposure of DMARDs. However, some drugs may affect fertility and men who take these medicines should be reassured about the safety of conception and pregnancy outcome in spouse.

Antimalarials

Hydroxychloroquine (HCQ) is one of the commonly used DMARDs. This drug has pleiotropic effects and helps in controlling inflammation, vascular, and thrombotic effects. There are evidences of its safety in pregnancy. In addition, it is known to reduce the incidence of congenital heart block in neonates of mothers with Ro/La positivity. At a dose of 200–400 mg/day, the benefits of treatment with HCQs far outweigh the risks of disease flares and pregnancy outcomes and it is recommended to be continued throughout pregnancy and lactation.

Corticosteroids

Corticosteroids are frequently used in rheumatic diseases (prednisolone, prednisone, and methylprednisolone). They are metabolized in the placenta; hence, 10% or less of the active drug reaches the fetus. The fluorinated steroids are used to prevent or treat preterm labor and improvement of fetal lung maturity. The adverse effects of concern with the use of steroids in pregnancy are:

- Low birth weight
- Hypertension and hyperglycemia
- Premature rupture of membranes
- *Congenital malformations*: This is often confounded by the use of concomitant drugs rather than steroid alone.

In pregnancy and lactation, prednisolone is found to be safe. The dose of prednisone should be as low as possible and should be tapered to minimum required for disease control. Steroid sparing drugs which are compatible with pregnancy can be used.

CONVENTIONAL SYNTHETIC DMARDS

Methotrexate

Methotrexate (MTX) is contraindicated in pregnancy and was previously recommended to be stopped at least 3 months in advance of conception. Risk of severe teratogenicity is known with MTX, craniofacial defects, defects in spine, and ribs and malformations of the digits in the fetus are reported **(Table 1)**.

Methotrexate should be avoided in pregnancy and stopped, and conception planning can be done only after 1 month of stopping. "*In unintended pregnancy on low-dose (25 mg/week) MTX, where there is minimal risk to the fetus; the drug should be stopped immediately, folic acid supplementation (5 mg/day) continued*", it is always

TABLE 1: DMARDs' safety in pregnancy and lactation.

DMARDs to be avoided in preganancy and lactation	DMARDs to be used only in severe life-/organ-threatening maternal disease	DMARDs considered safe in pregnancy and lactation
• Methotrexate • Leflunomide • Cyclophosphamide* • Mycophenolate mofetil • Janus kinase (JAK) inhibitors	• Cyclophos-phamide • Rituximab† • Belimumab† • IL-1/IL-6/IL-17/IL-23† • Abatacept†	• Hydroxychlo-roquine • Sulfasalazine • Azathioprine • Cyclosporine/Tacrolimus • Intravenous immuno-globulins • Anti-TNFs‡

*Cyclophoshamide may be used only in severe organ or life-threatening maternal disease and is to be avoided paternal exposure.

†Avoid live vaccinations in the neonate if used in the third trimester

‡All anti-TNF except certolizumab will affect live vaccine immunization schedule in the neonate.

(TNFs: tumor necrosis factors; DMARDs: disease-modifying antirheumatic drugs; IL-1: interleukin-1)

TABLE 2: DMARDs' associated effects on paternal exposure.

DMARDs to be avoided for paternal exposure	DMARDs considered to be safe in paternal exposure
Cyclophosphamide	• Methotrexate • Leflunomide • Hydroxychloroquine • Sulfasalazine* • Azathioprine • Cyclosporine/Tacrolimus • Intravenous immunoglobulins • Anti-TNFs • Mycophenolate mofetil • Rituximab • Belimumab • IL-1/IL-6/IL-17/IL-23 • Abatacept • Janus kinase (JAK) inhibitors

*Consider stopping sulfasalazine if pregnancy is delayed by >12 months and work up for other causes of infertility in paternal exposure.

(TNFs: tumor necrosis factors; DMARDs: disease-modifying antirheumatic drugs; IL-1: interleukin-1)

advisable to seek help from fetal medicine specialist. It is not advisable to give MTX during breastfeeding as the risk benefit data is insufficient.

Sulfasalazine

Sulfasalazine (SSZ) should be used with caution in ill or preterm infants, hyperbilirubinemia or infants with glucose-6-phosphate dehydrogenase (G6PD) deficiency. SSZ along with folic acid is considered safe in pregnancy and lactation and doses do not confer any additional risk. In males **(Table 2)**, it is known to cause oligozoospermia and may need to be withdrawn in case the baseline low sperm counts. This adverse effect is however reversible.

Leflunomide

Leflunomide is a category X drug in women who are pregnant. It is a dihydroorotase inhibitor and due to extensive enterohepatic circulation, it can be detected in plasma years after discontinuation. Hence, cholestyramine washout is recommended for clearance of the drug and to keep the plasma drug levels to a minimum. Recommended dosing is 8 g thrice a day for 11 days.

Azathioprine

It is a purine analog and is a Food and Drug Administration (FDA) category D drug in pregnancy and is a precursor of 6 mercaptopurine. There is no increase in major birth defects or preterm births in patients on azathioprine. It is considered safe in pregnancy and lactation and has no effect on paternal exposure.

Mycophenolate Mofetil

Mycophenolate mofetil (MMF) interferes with guanine synthesis and results in decreased lymphocyte generation. It is FDA category D in pregnancy and birth defects, such as microtibia, cleft palate, ocular defects, and agenesis of corpus callosum has been reported with MMF used in pregnancy. It is recommended to be stopped 6 weeks prior to conception.

Cyclosporine and Tacrolimus

Both are calcineurin inhibitors which prevent T-cell activation by inhibiting interleukin-2 (IL-2). They fall into FDA category C and are considered safe in pregnancy, paternal exposure, and lactation.

Cyclophosphamide

This is an alkylating agent which is cytotoxic. It is both teratogenic and gonadotoxic. It is associated with increased risk of infertility and its use is contraindicated in maternal or paternal exposure except in severe life or organ-threatening disease with limited treatment options.

Intravenous Immunoglobulin

Intravenous immunoglobulin (IVIG) is often considered as a rescue therapy in diseases, such as SLE and antiphospholipid antibody syndrome and is considered to be safe in pregnancy, lactation, and paternal exposure.

Biologicals

Biologicals are increasingly used in AIRD; biologicals are composed of varying degrees of immunoglobulins which neutralize the effects of target molecules. These molecules actively cross the placental barrier which accelerates after the 16th week of pregnancy. Half-life, bioavailability, and rates of placental transfer of biologic DMARDs' vary and hence can affect the vaccination schedule in a neonate of a mother who has been prescribed these drugs during pregnancy. Anti-tumor necrosis factors (anti-TNFs) except certolizumab if given beyond the midsecond trimester is a contraindication for live vaccine immunization in the neonate. Studies of maternal exposure did not report an increased risk of preterm birth, miscarriage, low birth weight, or congenital malformations.

Certolizumab is compatible with all three trimesters of pregnancy, has negligible placental transfer compared with other TNF inhibitors, and does not require any alteration to the infant vaccination schedule. For normal vaccination schedule, anti-TNF withdrawal is listed in **Table 3**. Anti-TNFs are recommended for use in lactation.

Limited evidence has not shown rituximab, belimumab, IL-1/IL-6/IL-17/IL-23 antagonists, and abatacept to be teratogenic. However, there remains insufficient evidence that these are compatible with pregnancy. Their use is limited to life-threatening or organ-threatening AIRD if no other alternative is available. Live vaccination is contraindicated for up to 6 months with the use of these agents.

TABLE 3: Anti-TNFs stoppage at gestation for live vaccine safety in neonate.

Anti-TNF	Gestational age at which anti-TNFs are recommended to be discontinued for vaccine safety in neonates
Infliximab	20 weeks
Adalimumab	28 weeks
Golimumab	28 weeks
Etanercept	32 weeks
Certolizumab	May be continued throughout pregnancy

Janus Kinase Inhibitors

These are small molecule inhibitors (tofacitinib, baricitinib, and upadacitinib) which could theoretically cross the placenta. There is insufficient data of the use of these agents in pregnancy and lactation and are hence avoided.

CONCLUSION

The management of AIRDs in pregnancy and lactation requires a multidisciplinary approach with a team of physicians, obstetrician, and fetal medicine specialists. The timing of pregnancy depends on the disease activity and the half-life of immunomodulatory agents which may either required to be discontinued or switched to drugs which are considered to be safe and compatible with pregnancy. Preconception counseling and tailored treatment strategies for different AIRDs' are prudent to ensure successful pregnancy. It is pertinent to address issues related to vaccinations in the newborn, especially in mothers on biological disease response modifiers. Paternal exposure to DMARDs' other than cyclophosphamide (contraindicated) and SSZ (known to cause reversible oligozoospermia) and biologics/small molecules is relatively safe.

SUGGESTED READINGS

1. Oliver JE, Silman AJ. Why are women predisposed to autoimmune rheumatic diseases? Arthritis Res Ther. 2009;11(5):252.
2. Russell MD, Dey M, Flint J, Davie P, Allen A, Crossley A, et al. British Society for Rheumatology guideline on prescribing drugs in pregnancy and breastfeeding: immunomodulatory anti-rheumatic drugs and corticosteroids. Rheumatology (Oxford). 2023;62(4):e48-e88.
3. Georgiou PE, Politi EN, Katsimbri P, Sakka V, Drosos AA. Outcome of lupus pregnancy: a controlled study. Rheumatology (Oxford). 2000;39:1014-9.
4. Flint J, Panchal S, Hurrell A, van de Venne M, Gayed M, Schreiber K, et al. BSR and BHPR guideline on prescribing drugs in pregnancy and breastfeeding-Part I: standard and biologic disease modifying anti-rheumatic drugs and corticosteroids. Rheumatology (Oxford). 2016;55(9):1693-7.
5. Østensen M, Khamashta M, Lockshin M, Parke A, Brucato A, Carp H, et al. Anti-inflammatory and immunosuppressive drugs and reproduction. Arthritis Res Ther. 2006;8(3):209.
6. Cooper WO, Cheetham TC, Li DK, Stein CM, Callahan ST, Morgan TM, et al. Brief report: Risk of adverse fetal outcomes

associated with immunosuppressive medications for chronic immune-mediated diseases in pregnancy. Arthritis Rheumatol. 2014;66(2):444-50.

7. Chambers CD, Johnson DL, Robinson LK, Braddock SR, Xu R, Lopez-Jimenez J, et al. Birth outcomes in women who have taken leflunomide during pregnancy. Arthritis Rheum. 2010;62(5):1494-503.
8. Moretti ME, Verjee Z, Ito S, Koren G. Breast-feeding during maternal use of azathioprine. Ann Pharmacother. 2006; 40(12):2269-72.
9. Tsao NW, Sayre EC, Hanley G, Sadatsafavi M, Lynd LD, Marra CA, et al. Risk of preterm delivery and small-for-gestational-age births in women with autoimmune disease using biologics before or during pregnancy: a population-based cohort study. Ann Rheum Dis. 2018;77(6):869-74.
10. Berkhout A, Clark JE, Wen SC. In utero exposure to biologic disease-modifying anti-rheumatic drugs and effects to the infant: infectious complications, vaccine response, and safety of live vaccine administration. Expert Rev Vaccines. 2019;18: 495-504.

112 CHAPTER

Metabolic Complications in Autoimmune Diseases

Rajdip Sen

ABSTRACT

Metabolic syndrome (MetS) encompasses multiple risk factors that result from insulin resistance resulting in abnormal adipose deposition and function. Complex interactions occur between the metabolic and immune systems and they are regulated through genetics, nutritional status, and the intestinal microbiome. Changes in the immune-metabolic interface contribute to the development of autoimmune diseases. Adipokines are involved in the regulation of both inflammatory processes and autoimmunity which have participation in rheumatic diseases. The incidence of coronary vascular disease remains high in acute rheumatic diseases in spite of recent advances in the treatment of rheumatic diseases. Altered secretion patterns of proinflammatory adipokines and MetS could be the link between cardiovascular disease (CVD) and rheumatological disorders. Also, in acute rheumatic disease, there occurs activation of proinflammatory signaling pathways resulting in the induction of chronic inflammation contributing to the coronary vascular disease.

INTRODUCTION

Link between Metabolic Syndrome and Autoimmune Diseases

Inflammatory markers such as tumor necrosis factor-alpha (TNF-α), interleukin-6 (IL-6), and other adipokines produced by visceral adipose tissue, and hypoadiponectinemia contribute to the development of metabolic syndrome (MetS)-associated cardiovascular disease (CVD). Proinflammatory molecules, such as complement C3 and TNF are also produced more by abdominal adipose tissue than subcutaneous adipose tissue and it also induces increased lipolysis and free-fatty acids, which also cause insulin resistance. There is a close interrelation between the inflammatory immune response and metabolic pathways in adipose tissue. In this way, cells of the adaptive immune system, including T and B cells, contribute significantly to adipose tissue inflammation. Lymphocytes regulate recruitment of innate immune cells into adipose tissue and produce cytokines that influence the inflammatory balance. Obesity-induced alterations in the balance of T helper cell type 1 (Th1)- and T helper cell type 2 (Th2)-type signals influence macrophage recruitment and phenotype in adipose tissue, generating a pathogenic environment. The proinflammatory cytokines implicated in metabolic syndrome, consist of different families of cytokines: IL-1 family which are involved in the regulation of immune responses that participate in atherosclerosis, myocardial infarction, stroke, and other CVDs. In systemic autoimmune/inflammatory diseases, such as rheumatoid arthritis (RA), systemic lupus erythematosus (SLE), ankylosing spondylitis (AS), psoriatic arthritis (PsA), antiphospholipid syndrome (APS) and systemic sclerosis (SSc), IL-23/IL-17 family are increased. These cytokines have a proatherogenic role, participating from early stage to advanced stage of the disease. Moreover, the proinflammatory state of MetS interrelated with insulin resistance and endothelial dysfunction, provides a connection between inflammation and metabolic processes.

Microbial dysbiosis, described as the decrease of useful bacteria and the increase of harmful bacteria, occur in metabolic disorders and contribute to the pathogenesis of several diseases such as obesity, MetS and type 2 diabetes mellitus (T2DM). This imbalance in gut microbiota may also contribute to the occurrence of autoimmune rheumatic disease (ARD), such as RA and SLE.

METABOLIC SYNDROME AND RHEUMATIC DISEASES

In rheumatic diseases, especially SLE or RA, insulin resistance may be important in increasing the risk of cardiovascular complications.

METABOLIC SYNDROME AND GOUT

Comorbidities such as obesity, arterial hypertension, and abnormal lipid and glucose homeostasis included in MetS, have been traditionally associated with gout. The prevalence of MetS in gout varies between 37 and 51%. Hyperuricemia may lead to insulin resistance and cause endothelial dysfunction and also inhibition of nitric oxide bioavailability leading to subsequent hyperinsulinemia, so that the relationship between MetS and gout may be linked to insulin resistance. Monosodium urate gout inflammation is induced by IL-1 which is produced by innate immunity and inflammasome. Adipose tissue plays an important role in gout, obesity being an independent risk factor for it. The accumulation of visceral fat is harmful, even in patients without generalized obesity. The possible explanations about fat accumulation in the development of gout are the correlation between fat accumulation and hyperuricemia, and that fat affects uric acid metabolism resulting in increase in serum uric acid levels. Hyperuricemia induces vascular dysfunction and CVD. Endothelium damage and consequent dysfunction is the first step in the development of coronary vascular disease. It has been demonstrated that hyperuricemia is capable of beginning endothelial injury by increasing platelet aggregation, proinflammatory activity, inhibition of nitric oxide production and increase of expression of inflammatory cytokines, IL-6, interleukin-8 (IL-8), and TNF. In relation with adipokines, a positive correlation between serum uric acid and leptin levels has been reported and a negative correlation with adiponectin. In gout a significant increase of adiponectin in patients who received benzbromarone, a potent uricosuric drug was found. This increase is created by an agonist effect on peroxisome proliferator activated receptors gamma with anti-inflammatory consequences.

METABOLIC SYNDROME AND RHEUMATOID ARTHRITIS

Rheumatoid arthritis and MetS share common features, such as increase in free radicals, deficiency of antioxidant systems, increase in proinflammatory cytokines, endothelial damage, and the formation and destabilization of atherosclerotic plaques. A large proportion of patients with RA have only alterations in body fat composition without obesity, such as high cholesterol levels, low high-density lipoprotein (HDL) cholesterol and high-triglyceride levels, observed even in preclinical RA. High caloric intake and lack of physical activity are other important factors. In fact, there is a relation between sarcopenia and obesity in RA, with improvement of the former after IL-6 blocking. Patients with RA have a higher frequency of glucose metabolism disorders compared to general population, including T2DM. Insulin resistance is probably due to obesity, the cascade of proinflammatory cytokines (including TNF, IL-1, and IL-6) and B-cell dysfunction. Therapeutic blockade of TNF improves insulin sensitivity and reduces insulin resistance (IR) in RA patients. Various adipokines may also play a pathogenic role in RA. Leptin (a proinflammatory adipokine) levels are elevated in patients with RA, especially in those with high-disease activity. In preobese and obese patients with RA, elevated levels of leptin and its soluble receptor have been found associated to anticyclic citrullinated peptide antibodies compared to controls. Elevated circulating levels of adiponectin have been found in RA patients compared to controls, but no association with disease activity has been demonstrated. Circulating levels of resistin, leptin, IL-6, and IL-17 correlated with disease activity regardless of the subject's body mass index (BMI). Visfatin, a growth factor for B-cell precursors, is an adipokine with proinflammatory properties implicated in joint damage in RA patients. Even a decrease in serum levels of visfatin has been associated with a reduction in the activity in early RA, suggesting that such a decrease may be a predictor of response to treatment. Vitamin D deficiency is also associated with MetS and dyslipidemia suggesting a potential role in CVD risk; however, further studies are necessary to determine if vitamin D supplementation contributes to diminish cardiovascular (CV) risk in these patients. Patients with RA also have significant modification of the intestinal flora and decreased gut microbiome variety in comparison to healthy controls.

METABOLIC SYNDROME AND SYSTEMIC LUPUS ERYTHEMATOSUS

Systemic lupus erythematosus is characterized by autoantibodies against cellular and extracellular components with deposition of immune complexes in several tissues leading to systemic manifestations. Patients with SLE develop premature atherosclerosis and vascular stiffening, leading to higher risk for CVD. The risk of CV events in patients with SLE is 7–17 times higher than that in the general population. This increased risk cannot be fully explained by traditional Framingham risk factors alone. The pathogenesis of CVD in SLE is not completely understood; however, it is related to the greater activity of the disease leading to increase of inflammation, steroid therapy, and IR. Therefore, MetS may be a bridge between chronic inflammation and accelerated atherosclerosis in patients with SLE.

Pathogenesis of Metabolic Syndrome in Systemic Lupus Erythematosus

The overproduction of proinflammatory factors such as IL-6, leptin, resistin, plasminogen activator inhibitor-1, TNF-α results in a state of chronic inflammation in SLE. SLE patients with MetS have a significantly higher serum level of uric acid, inflammatory biomarkers such as homocysteine, IL-8, or complement molecules. The presence of MetS has been linked to an increased organ damage score, a decreased percentage of circulating endothelial progenitor cells and increased arterial stiffness. A high prevalence of 25-hydroxyvitamin D [25(OH)D] deficiency and insufficiency in patients with SLE has been reported in several studies. Deficiency of 25(OH)D was associated with increased MetS prevalence, a decreased level of high-density lipoprotein and fasting glucose in premenopausal SLE patients. As in other ARD a strong connection between SLE and the composition of gut microbiota has been described. Therefore, dietary interventions, like administration of probiotics, may contribute to correct dysbiosis observed in SLE and other ARD's.

METABOLIC SYNDROME AND PRIMARY ANTIPHOSPHOLIPID SYNDROME

The coexistence of primary APS and MetS may detect a subgroup of patients with higher risk of arterial events, suggesting that MetS may aggravate existing endothelial abnormalities of primary antiphospholipid syndrome (PAPS). Adipocytokines, plasminogen activator inhibitor (PAI-1), glucose, acute phase reactants and lipid profiles were measured in PAPS patients in order to evaluate the association between adipocytokines and MetS, inflammation and other CV risk factors as well as the presence of MetS and insulin resistance using the homeostasis model assessment (HOMA) index. The authors concluded that adipocytokines may be involved in low-grade inflammation, insulin resistance and MetS in these patients. Increased IL-17 and Th17-inducing cytokines, IL-23 and transforming growth factor (TGF) in blood of PAPS patients were found indicating an amplified Th17 response possibly associated with vascular manifestations of the disease.

METABOLIC SYNDROME AND SPONDYLOARTHROPATHIES

Tumor necrosis factor-alpha blockade in ankylosing spondylosis patients improves insulin sensitivity in nondiabetic patients and may slow atherosclerosis progression, with beneficial effects on adipokines, biomarkers of atherosclerosis, and MetS-related biomarkers. In nondiabetic patients with AS on treatment with infliximab, leptin and visfatin serum levels did not correlate with disease activity or systemic inflammation. An increased oxidative stress, impaired endothelial function, and IMT have been reported in AS patients as compared with controls. Papadakis et al. found that men with AS have a higher prevalence of CV risk factors and MetS in comparison with controls and it was associated with increased 10-year CVD risk.

TREATMENT FOR METABOLIC SYNDROME IN AUTOIMMUNE RHEUMATIC DISEASE

The most important and first line treatment for MetS lies on the lifestyle changes including diet and exercise. However, the use of medication is required, due to the fact that combination of comorbidities makes diet and exercise insufficient to pursue this goal. Metformin, a biguanide having insulin-sensitizing effect, reduces low-density lipoprotein and cholesterol levels, and has pleiotropic vascular effects as statins, thus they can be used for treatment of MetS. Hydroxychloroquine has various immunomodulatory and anti-inflammatory properties. Furthermore, chloroquine induces an increase in insulin activity and serum glucagon levels, decreases calcium and potassium levels and total protein content improving glucose tolerance with a decrease of glucose levels in normal subjects. Statin therapy reduces CV risk through reducing oxidative stress, thereby improving endothelial function. They also have anti-inflammatory properties. As weight loss is desirable in patients with MetS, antiobesity drugs such as phentermine, extended release phentermine/topiramate, lorcaserin, orlistat may be considered. Cilostazol, an antiplatelet agent, also improves atherogenic dyslipidemia, increases nitric oxide levels and decreases proinflammatory state. Another target would be the reduction of oxidative stress with acetylcysteine. Vitamin D, a new immunomodulator, is considered to play a protective role against CVD, IR, and obesity with anti-inflammatory effects and protective role against MetS in RA patients; hence, it could be used in other ARD.

CONCLUSION

Metabolic syndrome has a great impact on the quality of life of patients with rheumatological disorders. In SLE patients, MetS is associated with new organ damage, new vascular events, and increased mortality. MetS and acute rheumatological disease share immunological mechanisms inherent to metabolic control, ARD development, and coexistence of both conditions. Our aim should be to control MetS and ARD to restore immunological balance.

SUGGESTED READINGS

1. Zmora N, Bashiardes S, Levy M, Elinav E. The role of the immune system in metabolic health and disease. Cell Metab. 2017;25(3);506-21.
2. Popovic-Kuzmanovic D, Novakovic I, Stojanovich L, Aksentijevich I, Zogovic N, Tovilovic G, et al. Increased activity ofinterleukin-23/interleukin-17 cytokine axis in primary antiphospholipid syndrome. Immunobiology. 2013;218(2):186-91.
3. Li C, Hsieh MC, Chang SJ. Metabolic syndrome, diabetes, and hyperuricemia. Curr Opin Rheumatol. 2013;25(2):210-6.
4. Cao H, Lin J, Chen W, Xu G, Sun C. Baseline adiponectin and leptin levels in predicting an increased risk of disease activity in rheumatoid arthritis: a meta-analysis and systematic review. Autoimmunity. 2016;49(8):547-53.
5. Ruiz-Irastorza G, Egurbide MV, Olivares N, Martinez-Berriotxoa A, Aguirre C. Vitamin D deficiency in systemic lupus erythematosus: prevalence, predictors and clinical consequences. Rheumatology (Oxford). 2008;47(6):920-3.
6. Rodrigues CE, Bonfá E, Caleiro MT, Vendramini MB, Bueno C, Lopes JB, et al. Association of arterial events with the coexistence of metabolic syndrome and primary antiphospholipid syndrome. Arthritis Care Res (Hoboken). 2012;64(10): 1576-83.
7. Han C, Robinson Jr DW, Hackett MW, Paramore LC, Fraeman KH, Bala MV. Cardiovascular disease and risk factors in patients with rheumatoid arthritis, psoriatic arthritis, and ankylosing spondylitis. J Rheumatol. 2006;33(11):2167-72.
8. Ladeiras-Lopes R, Fontes-Carvalho R, Bettencourt N, Sampaio F, Gama V, Leite-Moreira A. Novel therapeutic targets of metformin: metabolic syndrome and cardiovascular disease. Expert Opin Ther Targets. 2015;19(7):869-77.
9. Curr Hu C, Lu L, Wan JP, Wen C, The pharmacological mechanisms and therapeutic activities of hydroxychloroquine in rheumatic and related diseases. Med Chem. 2017;24(20):2241-9.

113

CHAPTER

Paraneoplastic Arthropathy

Sarbani Sengupta

ABSTRACT

Paraneoplastic arthropathy (PA) is a distinct group of joint disorders that should be considered in any patient presenting with features mimicking inflammatory arthropathy but clinical, radiological, blood parameters, and treatment outcomes do not match properly with the particular inflammatory arthritis thought of. The primary cause of PA is the effect of humoral factors or cytokines released from the tumor itself or due to cellular or humoral immunity directed against the tumor cells or antigenic cross-reactivity between the tumor and synovium. That is why the symptoms of arthritis may develop at a site distant from the site of actual malignancy. Usually, there is a temporal relationship between the development of arthropathy and malignancy. PA may present before, concurrent with, or after the diagnosis of malignancy. In suspected PA, age-appropriate investigation to diagnose malignancy should be contemplated. Early diagnosis helps in early treatment of cancer. Treatment of underlying malignancy alleviates the arthritis symptoms in most cases, but symptoms may recur if the malignancy relapses.

INTRODUCTION

Paraneoplastic arthropathy, though rare, may present with joint pain or musculoskeletal problems to a clinician. It is a usual practice to focus primarily on confirming the occurrence of primary rheumatological diseases (RDs), but a variety of musculoskeletal symptoms (MSKs) may be associated with malignant diseases.

There can be several types of association between malignancy and MSKs, which are as follows:

- A direct triggering of a new-onset rheumatological condition by a tumor or its metastases
- Development of cancer within a temporal interval of up to 20 years in individuals with established RD, e.g., development of non-Hodgkin lymphoma (NHL) among patients with systemic lupus erythematosus (SLE)
- Risk of malignancy with immunosuppressive and disease modifying antirheumatic drugs (e.g., cyclophosphamide, azathioprine, mycophenolate, and methotrexate) as well as certain antirheumatic biologic agents increase the risk of hematologic and other malignancies.
- Rheumatic disorders associated with treatments for malignant diseases like secondary gout
- Paraneoplastic syndromes where the rheumatological manifestations have a temporal relationship with malignancy. To consider a syndrome truly paraneoplastic, a causal relationship needs to be established.

In this chapter, we shall focus on paraneoplastic rheumatic disorder (PRD) and more specifically on PA.

Paraneoplastic rheumatic disorder is a disorder that may present before, concurrent with, or after the diagnosis of malignancy. PRDs are a clinical expression of occult cancer that is not directly related to a tumor or metastasis and manifests as MSKs. In PRD, MSKs may occur in bones, joints, fasciae, vessels, muscles, cutaneous structures, and a mixture of these generally no longer than 2 years (although maybe more) before the diagnosis of an associated neoplasm. Hence, it is of utmost clinical importance to think of PRD during clinical evaluation and laboratory investigation so that the underlying malignancy is detected and treated early. The primary cause of PA is the effect of humoral factors or cytokines released from the tumor itself or due to cellular or humoral immunity directed against the malignant tumor cells.

As paraneoplastic syndrome can affect other systems also, it is heterogeneous in nature. That is why it is a mimicker of so many conditions. Clinicians should be very alert in picking up such PA early during consultation. Approximately 7–10% of patients with paraneoplastic syndrome have rheumatological symptoms.

PARANEOPLASTIC ARTHROPATHY

The main types of PA are mentioned in **Box 1**. Some of the more common and classical diseases are discussed in the following text.

Hypertrophic Osteoarthropathy

Hypertrophic osteoarthropathy (HOA) is a syndrome characterized by abnormal proliferation of the skin and osseous tissues at the distal parts of the extremities. It is called secondary HOA associated with malignancy and is different from primary or idiopathic HOA. Clinical features of secondary HOA include digital clubbing, increased periosteal activity of the tubular bones (clinically characterized by tenderness over the involved area), arthralgias, and joint effusion which are noticed predominantly around large joints. Some patients may present even before the appearance of clubbing with a painful arthropathy resembling inflammatory arthritis.

A typical patient of HOA presents with tibial and femoral bone pain, arthralgia, and synovitis of the adjacent joints. The radiographic feature of HOA is a smooth, symmetric, and continuous periosteal reaction of the tubular bones (tibia, fibula, radius, and ulna are most common). Isotopic bone scan shows increased tracer uptake due to the formation of new osseous tissue. Positron emission tomography (PET) also detects increased metabolic activity of the involved long bones.

Malignancy associated with the secondary form of HOA is usually lung cancer (most are adenocarcinoma and least are small-cell carcinoma). It is less often associated with other conditions (e.g., Hodgkin lymphoma).

Pathogenesis of secondary HOA suggested the roles of platelet-derived and other growth factors. Circulatory bypass of the lung by megakaryocytes could release growth factors in the distal extremities leading to this condition.

Treatment with nonsteroidal anti-inflammatory drugs (NSAIDs) or other analgesics may provide significant symptomatic relief. Removal of lung cancer or treatment of the other causes results in regression in the clinical manifestations in many patients but is not always effective. In patients with refractory disease, bisphosphonates, like pamidronate and zoledronic acid, may be tried.

BOX 1: Paraneoplastic arthropathy.

- Hypertrophic osteoarthropathy (HOA)
- Carcinoma polyarthritis
- Amyloid arthritis
- Palmar fasciitis and polyarthritis syndrome
- Remitting seronegative symmetrical synovitis with pitting edema (RS3PE)
- Relapsing polychondritis
- Polyarthritis with panniculitis
- Multicentric reticulohistiocytosis

Paraneoplastic Polyarthritis

Paraneoplastic polyarthritis is probably the classical form of paraneoplastic arthritis which is seen by the clinicians. Joint symptoms may be the initial presentation of an underlying malignancy or may precede malignancy by months. Arthritis may present like rheumatoid arthritis involving small and large joints in a symmetrical fashion or may present as an asymmetric polyarthritis involving predominantly the lower extremities. Most patients are male (usually >50 years of age) and have an explosive onset of the disease. Family history of rheumatoid arthritis, high titer of rheumatoid factor positivity, rheumatoid nodules, and radiographic findings like erosive joint disease are characteristically absent. However, some cases may show low titer rheumatoid factor and anti-cyclic citrullinated peptide (anti-CCP) antibody positivity. Synovial fluid analysis data is sparse. As paraneoplastic polyarthritis is a great mimicker of other inflammatory arthritis, sometimes steroids and other immunosuppressive agents are used to treat this condition. As the improvement of symptoms are not encouraging, with treatment which actually delays the diagnosis of underlying malignancy.

Paraneoplastic polyarthritis may be associated with solid tumors (lung, breast, colon, stomach, and kidney) and hematological malignancies (leukemia, lymphoma, and myeloma). The articular symptoms may be the initial presentation of the disease and may precede the diagnosis of the underlying malignancy by months.

There is no definite treatment for this condition. However, treatment of the underlying malignancy usually results in a resolution of arthritic symptoms. But symptoms can again recur if the malignancy relapses.

Patients with myelodysplastic syndromes (MDSs) sometimes also develop polyarthritis that may be confused with seronegative rheumatoid arthritis. So, an appropriate hematological investigation is warranted if clinical and routine blood tests indicate such conditions.

Amyloid Arthritis

Primary or AL [immunoglobulin (Ig) light chain] amyloidosis is a plasma cell disorder characterized by overproduction and tissue deposition of monoclonal Ig light chains or fragments. Amyloid arthropathy may occur in 0.1–6% of patients with multiple myeloma, with an onset either coincident with or subsequent to the diagnosis of myeloma. Amyloid deposits in AL amyloidosis can involve the synovium, leading to rheumatic symptoms. Classical presentations of arthropathy in AL amyloid are subacute, low grade, progressive, and symmetric. Arthropathy has a predilection for the shoulders, knees, wrists, metacarpophalangeal and proximal interphalangeal joints, and, to a lesser degree, the elbows and hips. There is usually a little morning stiffness. Joints are usually nontender or mildly tender. Patients may have subcutaneous nodules which can be confused with rheumatoid nodules, but biopsy shows amyloid deposition. Macroglossia, submandibular gland involvement, and carpal tunnel syndrome are other common manifestations. Congo red staining of synovial spun sediment can show amyloid deposits from synovial fragments. Arthropathy as well as tendinopathy may improve with appropriate chemotherapy.

Palmar Fasciitis and Polyarthritis Syndrome

This condition is sometimes also referred to as palmar fibromatosis. Patients present with hand pain and stiffness; firm, painful nodules with thickening and erythema of the palmar fascia; and digital swelling with flexion contractures. Sometimes, other joints like shoulders and knees are also involved. Polyarthritis may accompany the fibrosis. It is a rare disorder associated with a variety of malignant neoplasms. The most frequently reported tumor is ovarian cancer, but other solid tumors of stomach, pancreas, lung, colon, and prostate have also been described in association with this disorder. There is no known effective treatment although some improvement may be seen with treatment of the underlying malignancy.

Remitting Seronegative Symmetrical Synovitis with Pitting Edema

Remitting seronegative symmetrical synovitis with pitting edema (RS3PE) usually develops acutely in elderly people. Generally, there is symmetric arthritis involving predominantly the small joints associated with marked pitting edema of the dorsum of hands and feet. Rheumatoid factor is negative in these patients. Concurrent malignancy has been found to be from 16 to 30% with RS3PE. The list of malignancies associated with RS3PE includes hematologic (leukemia, MDS, and lymphoma) as well as solid tumors (prostate, breast, gastrointestinal, lung, ovary, bladder, and endometrium). Initial evaluation of a patient with RS3PE should include a careful history for any symptoms that suggest an underlying malignancy as well as age-appropriate cancer screening.

Relapsing Polychondritis

Relapsing polychondritis (RPC) is a rare immune-mediated condition associated with inflammation in cartilaginous structures and other tissues throughout the body, particularly the ears, nose, eyes, joints, and respiratory tract. Other organs that can be involved include the vasculature, inner ear, central nervous system, and skin. Some of the patients with RPC present with a malignant or premalignant condition. Historically, MDS has been described in association with RPC. MDS can occur before, simultaneously with, or after RPC. The etiology of this conglomeration of symptoms and bone marrow involvement is likely the genetically described disease called VEXAS (vacuoles, E1 enzyme, X-linked, autoinflammatory, somatic) syndrome. Isolated instances of Hodgkin lymphoma, NHL, and carcinoma of a variety of types have been described.

Polyarthritis with Panniculitis

Lobular panniculitis with extensive fat necrosis on skin biopsy along with arthritis and/or bone necrosis have been described in association with pancreatic disease [i.e., pancreatitis, panniculitis, and polyarthritis (PPP) syndrome] and pancreatic tumors. The ankles, knees, wrists, and metacarpophalangeal joints are most commonly affected. Characteristic radiographic findings include loss of joint space, osteolytic lesions, pathologic fractures, and progression to osteonecrosis. Joint disease does not respond well to NSAIDs and glucocorticoids. No other proven beneficial treatment has been described.

Multicentric Reticulohistiocytosis

This rare non-Langerhans cell proliferative histiocytosis of an unknown cause presents with rapidly destructive polyarthritis. It may progress to arthritis mutilans. The disease may be associated with papules and nodules. Multicentric reticulohistiocytosis (MRH) is associated with an underlying malignancy in 25% of cases and tends to be relatively resistant to glucocorticoids and disease-modifying antirheumatic drugs.

CONCLUSION

Paraneoplastic arthropathy is a clinically challenging condition. Any arthropathy patient presenting with atypical features requires a thorough clinical examination and detailed evaluation of the systems for the search of an underlying malignancy. Diagnostic evaluation should include hematological parameters, biochemical parameters, inflammatory markers, autoimmune markers, and age-specific neoplasm-related search. As PA is relatively rare, case reports and reviews are necessary to raise awareness. Management of PA and cancer requires oncologists and rheumatologists to work collaboratively. As early diagnosis helps to manage the cancer early, proper management of suspected PA is of utmost importance.

TAKE HOME MESSAGE

- Paraneoplastic arthropathy, though rare, can be the first sign of an occult malignancy or its recurrence.
- In a paraneoplastic situation, the strongest argument is usually based on a close temporal relationship between the advent of MSKs and the diagnosis of a tumor although tumor may be manifested/detected later on.
- Lung cancer and hematological malignancies are the most frequent type of tumors associated with an inflammatory articular disease but paraneoplastic syndromes also occur with other solid tumors too.
- The main kinds of hematological diseases held responsible for this paraneoplastic manifestation are NHL, AML, and multiple myeloma.
- Underlying malignancy should be suspected in patients with rheumatologic diseases who do not respond as expected to therapy.
- Classical PA presents in male patients of age >50 years. Polyarticular arthritis with symmetric involvement of the limbs mimics rheumatoid arthritis. Family history of rheumatoid arthritis, high titer of rheumatoid factor, rheumatoid nodules, and radiographic findings like erosive joint disease are characteristically absent. Response to treatment is also poor.
- In suspected PA, age-appropriate investigation to diagnose malignancy should be contemplated.
- Early diagnosis helps in early treatment of cancer.
- Treatment of underlying malignancy alleviates the arthritis symptoms in most of the cases.

SUGGESTED READINGS

1. Manger B, Schett G. Paraneoplastic syndromes in rheumatology. Nat Rev Rheumatol. 2014;10(11):662-70.
2. Fam AG. Paraneoplas rheumatic syndromes. Baillieres Best Pract Res Clin Rheumatol. 2000;14(3):515-33.
3. Martinez-Lavin M, Pineda C. Hypertrophic osteoarthropathy. In: Rheumatology, Hochberg MC, Silman AJ, Smolen JS, Weinblatt ME, Weisman MH (Eds). London: Mosby; 2003. p. 1763.
4. Mody GM, Cassim B. Rheumatologic features of hematologic disorders. Curr Opin Rheumatol. 1996;8(1):57-61.
5. Morel J, Deschamps V, Toussirot E, Pertuiset E, Sordet C, Kieffer P, et al. Characteristics and survival of 26 patients with paraneoplastic arthritis. Ann Rheum Dis. 2008;67(2):244-7.
6. Prokaeva T, Spencer B, Kaut M, Ozonoff A, Doros G, Connors LH, et al. Soft tissue, joint, and bone manifestations of AL amyloidosis: clinical presentation, molecular features, and survival. Arthritis Rheum 2007;56(11):3858-68.
7. Li H, Altman RD, Yao Q. RS3PE: Clinical and Research Development. Curr Rheumatol Rep. 2015;17(8):49.
8. Yanagi T, Matsumura T, Kamekura R, Sasaki N, Hashino S. Relapsing polychondritis and malignant lymphoma: is polychondritis paraneoplastic? Arch Dermatol. 2007;143(1):89.
9. Tannenbaum H, Anderson LG, Schur PH. Association of polyarthritis, subcutaneous nodules, and pancreatic disease. J Rheumatol. 1975; 2(1):15-20.
10. El-Haddad B, Hammoud D, Shaver T, Shahouri S. Malignancy-associated multicentric reticulohistiocytosis. Rheumatol Int. 2011;31(9):1235-8.

114
CHAPTER

Leprosy Rheumatology Interface

Tapas Kumar, Animesh Paul

ABSTRACT

Leprosy, though predominantly a dermatological problem, has many extracutaneous features among which articular and vascular manifestations are protean. Leprosy has a worldwide distribution varying in prevalence in different countries. India is among the top five countries where the incidence is quite high.

Apart from the typical cutaneous manifestations leading to different classes of diseases like tuberculoid and lepromatous, there is a mixture of different types leading to myriad presentations. Taking into account the rheumatological aspects, such as articular, vascular, and musculoskeletal features, makes it a dilemma in reaching a diagnosis.

Many a times conditions labeled as rheumatoid arthritis (RA), vasculitis, or other musculoskeletal diseases turn out to be leprosy-related. Leprosy type I and type II reactions are the most common components.

Treatment of the underlying leprosy leads to amelioration of the articular and vascular symptoms. Treatment is not always rewarding specifically in long-standing cases.

INTRODUCTION

Leprosy (also known as Hansen's disease) is a chronic granulomatous infection caused by *Mycobacterium leprae*. Leprosy was well recognized in the oldest civilizations of Egypt, China, and India. Its causative agent was first described by GH Armour Hansen. Even after five centuries, the disease is largely associated with social stigma.

Human is the only natural reservoir of leprosy. Active cases, especially multibacillary (MB) cases, are the main source of infection. The incubation period varies from a few months to years (2–10 years) and may be longer in MB cases.

The differing immune responses to *M. leprae* result in a spectrum of diseases ranging from tuberculoid to lepromatous leprosy. Its clinical manifestations are primarily confined to skin and peripheral nerves. The musculoskeletal system is the third most commonly involved.

Rheumatologists should be aware of this since some form of joint involvement occurs in about 75% of cases of leprosy, and at times, it may be the only obvious manifestation.

EPIDEMIOLOGY

In 2019, 202,256 new cases were reported by 118 countries. The top five countries reporting new cases were India, Brazil, Indonesia, Nepal, and Bangladesh. The epidemiological data regarding the prevalence of arthritis in leprosy vary, depending upon the geographical area and the reporting center.

CLINICAL MANIFESTATION

Leprosy classically affects the skin and peripheral nervous system. Musculoskeletal system involvement in leprosy is very important because it leads to the most dreaded facet of leprosy, i.e., deformities and disabilities.

Bone Changes

The bone changes may be specific or nonspecific:

- *Specific*: From direct invasion by *M. leprae*
- *Nonspecific*: When affected indirectly

The nonspecific involvement is much more common and includes osteomyelitis, osteoporosis, atrophy, and absorption of the bones.

Joint Involvement

Joint involvement is seen across the whole spectrum of leprosy. It is most severe and common in lepra reactions. *Four types of joint involvement have been noted*:

1. Chronic insidious onset arthritis
2. Acute arthritis seen during reactionary episodes
3. Neuropathic or Charcot's arthropathy
4. Septic arthritis

The insidious arthritis occurs without any reactionary episode and tends to involve multiple peripheral joints, especially the small joints of hands and feet in a symmetrical manner.

The polyarthritic symmetrical small joint arthritis of leprosy can easily be confused with that of rheumatoid arthritis (RA).

The juxta-articular erosions seen in RA at times can be seen in leprosy radiologically. The often positive immunological markers, i.e., rheumatoid factor (RF) and antinuclear antibodies (ANA), in lepromatous leprosy further complicate the diagnosis. Anticyclic citrullinated peptide (anti-CCP) is usually absent.

The Charcot's arthropathy develops insidiously and painlessly. It is related to impaired sensations in joints and the surrounding tissues. The arthropathy usually involves the weight-bearing joints though other joints, like wrist, have been reported to be affected.

The leprae reactions, both type I and type II, may be associated with the development of acute arthritis. The arthritis appears to have an immunological basis and is usually associated with constitutional symptoms or other features of reactionary episodes. Clinically, the arthritis may be polyarticular and symmetrical, mimicking RA.

Skeletal Muscle Involvement

Skeletal muscles are rarely involved. Myositis may present with pain in the affected muscle. The histopathological specimens may reveal lepromatous granulomas between muscle fibers and connective tissue coverings of the muscle. The fibers surrounding the granuloma are degenerated. Acid-fast bacillus (AFB) can be seen in the macrophages, leprae cells, and even lying freely between the muscle fibers.

Rare Musculoskeletal Manifestation

Tenosynovitis in leprosy has been reported. Agarwal et al. described five cases of pure neuritic leprosy confirmed by nerve biopsy, presenting with tenosynovitis and arthritis.

Cryoglobulinemic vasculitis and enthesitis isolated tenosynovitis are some of the other uncommon manifestations of leprosy.

Sacroiliitis was also reported in only one study with a very high incidence of 64% in their cohort of leprosy.

Dactylitis presenting as a fusiform swelling is confined to the finger only, often of the right hand, and is a rare manifestation.

Specific changes due to bacillary deposits in the bones and their feeding vessels are less common and are seen as osteitis, periostitis, lytic lesions, erosions, and bone cysts in phalangeal bones **(Table 1)**.

TABLE 1: Various rheumatological and autoimmune manifestations observed in leprosy.

Rheumatological and autoimmune manifestations	*n* (%)
Arthralgias	3 (10.3)
Acute symmetric polyarthritis	5 (17.2)
Chronic symmetric polyarthritis (RA-like)	7 (24.1)
Charcot's arthropathy (neuropathic joint)	1 (3.4)
Spondyloarthritis-like:	
• Symmetric lower limb oligoarthritis/ReA-like	2 (6.8)
• With back pain and sacroiliitis	3 (10.3)
Leprosy arthritis with subsequent RA	3 (10.3)
Tenosynovitis only	5 (17.2)
Arthritis, foot edema with tenosynovitis (gout-like)	2 (6.8)
SHFS	6 (20.6)
Ankle arthritis with erythema nodosum (sarcoid/Poncet's-like)	2 (6.8)
Relapsing polychondritis (ear/saddle nose/tracheal cartilage)	1 (3.4)
Lucio leprosy	1 (3.4)
Lepra reaction/ENL	15/13 (51.7/44.8)
Autoantibody positivity	
• RF	7 (24.1)
• Anti-CCP	3 (10.3)
• ANA	3 (10.3)
• ANCA	1 (3.4)

(ANA: antinuclear antibodies; ANCA: antineutrophil cytoplasmic antibodies; Anti-CCP: anticyclic citrullinated peptide; ENL: erythema nodosum leprosum; RA: rheumatoid arthritis; ReA: reactive arthritis; RF: rheumatoid factor; SHFS: swollen hand and feet syndrome)

Source: Wakhlu A, Sawlani KK, Himanshu D. Rheumatological manifestations of Hansen's disease. Indian J Rheumatol. 2018;13:14-9.

PATHOGENESIS

Mycobacterium leprae enters the body and starts pathogenesis in the peripheral nerves. The bacilli are engulfed by Schwann cells and histopathological changes begin in nerve and skin. The type of leprosy developed depends on predominantly cell-mediated immune response of the person. The pathogenesis of articular involvement in leprosy is still not fully understood. There could be several mechanisms which include immune reactional states (types I and II lepra reaction), direct infiltration of the synovium, and peripheral sensory neuropathy (Charcot's or neuropathic joints) leading to joint destruction.

LEPRA REACTION

There are two types of reaction: Type I and II. These affect 30–50% of all leprosy patients **(Table 2)**.

LUCIO'S PHENOMENON

Lucio's phenomenon is observed in diffuse leprosy of Lucio and Latapí and may be a variant of erythema nodosum necroticans. Marked vasculitis and thrombosis of the superficial and deep vessels result in hemorrhage and infarction of the skin.

Clinically, the skin reaction begins as slightly indurated, bluish-red, ill-defined, painful, and rarely palpable plaques with an erythematous halo, usually developing on one limb but sometimes on other areas of the body. It is not commonly observed in India.

CASE 1

A 22-year-old student was suffering from arthritis and a burning sensation in hands for 6 months. His RF and antinuclear antibodies (ANA) were positive, and erythrocyte sedimentation rate (ESR) was high (60 mm).

He was being treated with disease-modifying antirheumatic drugs (DMARDs) and prednisolone. There was a marginal improvement, but he was still having the pain. When he turned to a rheumatology center, on careful inspection, it was found that there was tell-tale evidence of white patches on the palmar aspect of both the hands **(Fig. 1)**. Skin smear showed *M. leprae*.

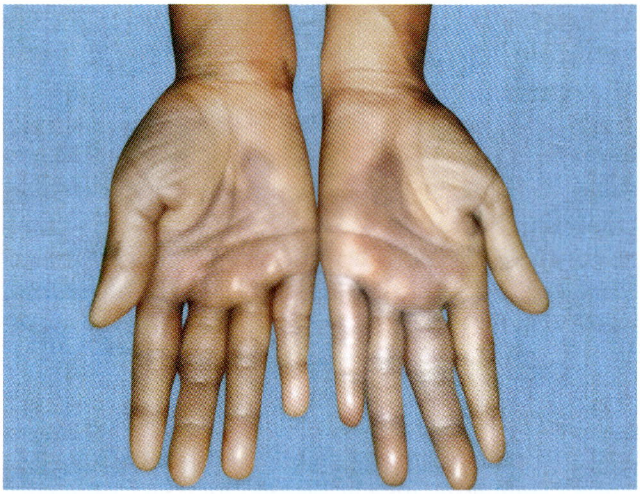

FIG. 1: White patches on the palms of both the hands.

Courtesy: Dr PS Mahapatra, Professor, Institute of Postgraduate Medical Education and Research (IPGMER), Kolkata, India.

TABLE 2: Lepra reaction.

Leprosy stage	Type 1 reaction: Reversal reaction (RR)	Type 2 reaction: Erythema nodosum leprosum (ENL)
Occurrence	Occurs in borderline disease (BT, BB, and BL)	Occurs in BL and LL
Skin	Acute onset of redness and swelling in leprosy skin lesions, and sometimes may ulcerate. Marked edema of the hands, feet, and face may occur. No new lesions appear	New painful and tender red papules or nodules occur in crops in limbs or trunk and face. Ulceration of nodules may occur. Edema of the hands, feet, or face may occur. Original leprosy skin patches remain as they were
Nerve	New nerve damage manifesting as numbness, or muscle weakness in the hands, feet, or face. Pain or tenderness in one or more nerves, with or without loss of nerve function	New nerve damage manifesting as numbness, or muscle weakness in the hands, feet, or face. Pain or tenderness in one or more nerves, with or without loss of nerve function
Systemic	Unusual	Common, including fever, malaise, lymphadenitis, uveitis, neuritis, arthritis, dactylitis, and orchitis
Immunological profile	Increased TNF-α, IFN-γ, IL-2 and IL-4 are suggestive of Th1 type reaction	ENL is thought to be the consequence of immune complex deposition, given its Th2 cytokine profile, and high levels of IL-6. IL-8, and IL-10
Diagnosis	Clinical	Clinical
Treatment	Steroids	Steroids

(BB: borderline borderline; BL: borderline lepromatous; BT: borderline tuberculoid; IFN: interferon; IL: interleukin; LL: lepromatous leprosy; TNF: tumor necrosis factor; Th: T helper)

Later on, by treatment with multidrug therapy (MDT) (rifampicin, 600 mg/clofazimine, 300 mg once a month, and 100 mg of dapsone daily), the patient improved after 6 months.

This was lepra I reaction of leprosy.

CASE 2

A lady aged 35 years was suffering from swollen hands with arthritis in all the joints of hand with swelling and arthritis of both the ankle joints. She was treated with steroids and nonsteroidal anti-inflammatory drugs (NSAIDs). There was marginal improvement, but the deformities were persisting. She also had positive RF and atrial natriuretic factor (ANF), and her ESR was raised.

On presentation to a rheumatologist, it was found that she had classic infiltrative skin lesions on face, and scaly lesions over abdomen and both hands and feet **(Figs. 2A to C)**:

A split skin smear was taken, and it was positive for *M. leprae*

It was of MB type.

On treatment with antileprotic therapy, the arthritis and skin lesions resolved.

This was type II lepra reaction, classically known as erythema nodosum leprosum (ENL) reaction.

CASE 3

A 32-year-old nonsmoker male with biopsy-proven Hansen's disease [borderline lepromatous (BL)] on long-term treatment with prednisolone and clofazimine for last 4 years was referred to the rheumatology clinic with acute onset of feeling cold in index, middle and ring fingers of left hand. The patient did not have any history of diabetes.

Two days later, he developed painful gangrene on the digital pulps of the affected fingers **(Fig. 3)**. On examination, thickening of ulnar and peroneal nerves and hypopigmented, hypoesthetic patches were found.

His RF, ANA, anti-CCP, anti-double-stranded DNA were positive in low titer. The Doppler studies of digital arteries in right hand are suggestive of reduced blood flow.

A right subclavian angiography was consistent with the focal distal arteritic lesion. Other causes like cervical rib and proximal subclavian arterial lesions were ruled out.

A diagnosis of vasculitis was made and considered a likely complication of leprosy.

A short course of prednisolone, 30 mg daily for 6 weeks, and later 5 mg daily, and hydroxychloroquine, antiplatelet drugs, along with antileprosy drugs were started. The patient slowly improved. His digital pulp lesions were healed with some residual disease.

This was a case of vasculitis due to leprosy.

CASE 4

Figure 4 shows the presence of arthritis with thickening of the ulnar nerve bilaterally and characteristic wasting.

The patient was suffering from chronic arthritis with typical claw hand deformity. So, it is a case of chronic arthritis of leprosy with a claw hand deformity.

CASE 5

A 58-year-old-male laborer presented to his general practitioner with an acute onset of episodic pain and swelling in feet and ankles along with progressive swelling of the hands for the last 4 months. He was treated

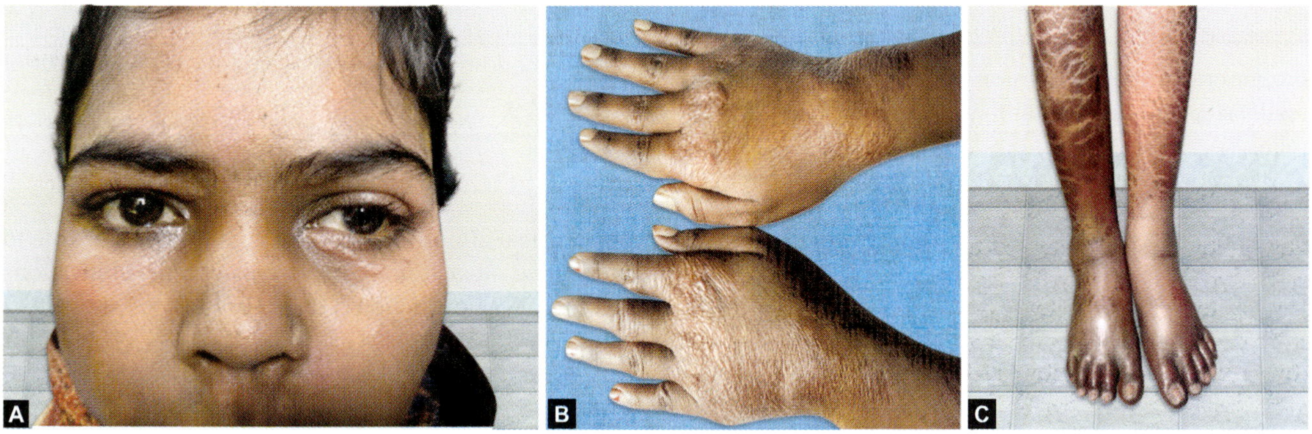

FIGS. 2A TO C: (A) Classic infiltrative skin lesions on face; (B and C) Scaly lesion over hands and feet.

Courtesy: Dr Shyamashis Das, Professor, Institute of Neurosciences, Kolkata, India.

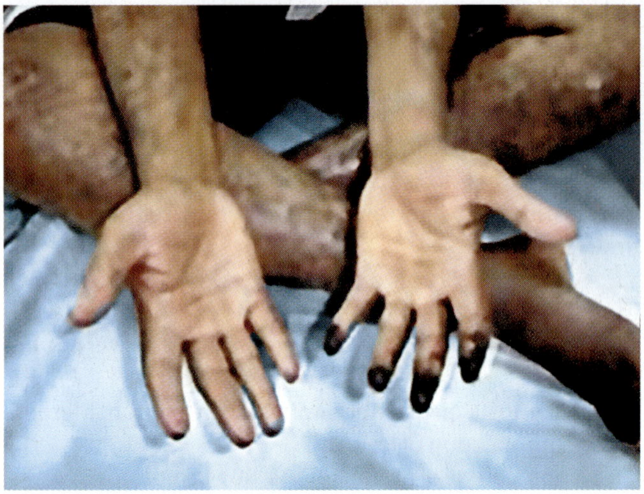

FIG. 3: Gangrene on digital pulps of the index, middle, and ring fingers of left hand.

Courtesy: Dr Arvind Chopra and Dr Sheetal Salvi, Center for Rheumatic Disease, Pune, India.

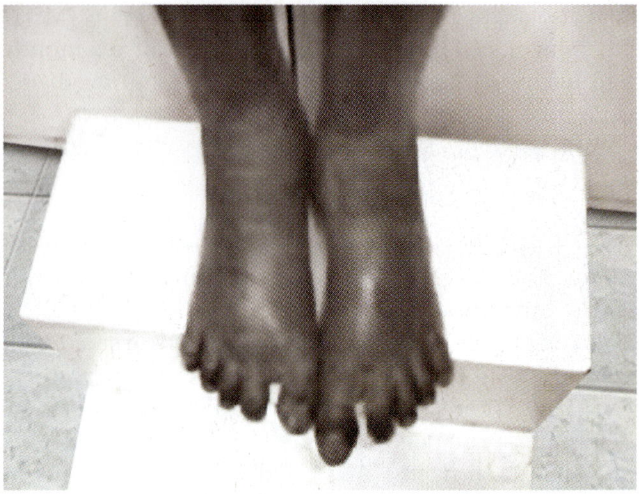

FIG. 5: Dactylitis in case of borderline lepromatous in lepra reaction type I.

Courtesy: Dr Arvind Chopra and Dr Sheetal Salvi, Center for Rheumatic Disease, Pune, India.

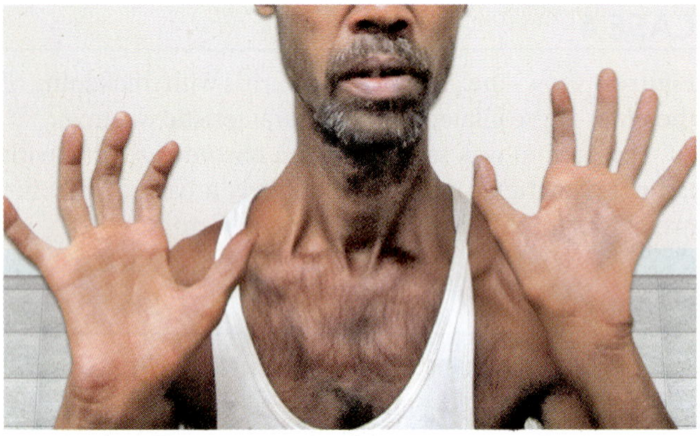

FIG. 4: Chronic arthritis of leprosy causing typical claw hand deformity.

Courtesy: Dr PS Mahapatra, Professor, Institute of Postgraduate Medical Education and Research (IPGMER), Kolkata, India.

by general practitioners for possible RA with several analgesics and anti-inflammatory drugs but found little relief.

He was then referred for a rheumatology opinion. On careful examination, it was found that the fingers of the feet had a darkened sausage-like appearance to suggest dactylitis **(Fig. 5)**. The palms appeared red and flushed. However, he had bilateral painful, tender knee synovitis. Both the ankles were tender and painful on movement. The skin on hands and feet appeared shiny and taut (sclerodactyly appearance) and felt thickened over the ankles, distal legs, forearms, and upper face. Although his skin complexion was fairly brown, a few large faintly hypopigmented patches with reduced touch sensation could be discerned on upper arms and the back. His ulnar nerves and peroneal nerves felt thickened but nontender. The sensations of touch and sharp pain were reduced on distal extremities, and the small muscles of hands and feet appeared wasted.

He was seronegative for RF, C-reactive protein (CRP), and antistreptolysin-O (ASO) titer, but strongly sero-positive for ANA. X-ray of hands and wrists showed degenerative distal interphalangeal joint disease and juxta-articular osteoporosis, but bone resorption was absent.

The skin clip from the lumbar region tested positive for lepra bacilli (+ +). He was confirmed with a case of Hansen's disease—BL in lepra reaction type I. He was begun on a standard regimen, including steroids. The patient made dramatic improvement over 12 weeks of follow-up.

RADIOLOGICAL MANIFESTATION

Radiological abnormalities in patients of arthritis due to leprosy can range from normal joints to joint subluxations and complete destruction **(Figs. 6A and B)**. Juxta-articular erosions were also seen.

Periostitis, bone resorption, sacroiliitis, and deformed joints have all been described in arthritis associated with leprosy.

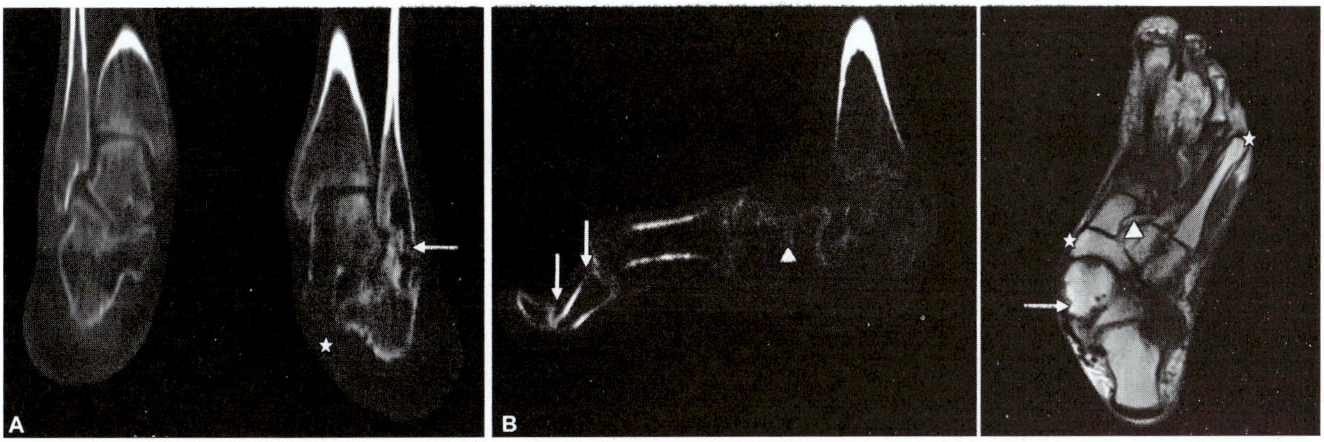

FIGS. 6A AND B: (A) Computed tomography (CT); (B) Magnetic resonance imaging (MRI) images of ankle joints show radiological features of neuropathic arthritis. Debris/loose bodies in joint (white triangle), subarticular erosions (horizontal arrow), dislocations (vertical arrow) and deformities (star).

Courtesy: Dr Rituparna Das, Mata Gujri Memorial Medical College, Bihar, India.

DIAGNOSIS AND DIAGNOSTIC DILEMMA

In rheumatic conditions, we should always see for skin manifestation and nerve involvement. The presence of autoantibodies like RF, ANF, and infrequently anti-CCP often creates confusion. Multisystemic involvement of leprosy, specifically during lepra reactions, often misleads toward alternate diagnoses like septicemia.

Deformed joints appear to be like flexion contracture. So, a more thorough examination may reveal the underlying etiology. Leprosy may often mimic lupus and scleroderma due to predominant skin affection.

TREATMENT

Only one multidrug regimen is recommended by the World Health Organization (WHO) for the treatment of leprosy.

Multibacillary Leprosy

- Monthly dose of rifampin 600 mg + dapsone 100 mg + clofazimine 300 mg
- Daily doses of dapsone 100 mg + clofazimine 50 mg
- *Duration*: 12 months

Paucibacillary Leprosy

- Monthly doses of rifampin 600 mg
- Daily doses of dapsone 100 mg
- *Duration*: 6 months

Type 1 Reactions

Oral, short-acting glucocorticoids (prednisolone 1 mg/kg of body weight once a day, usually with a maximum of 60–80 mg)

Type 2 Reactions (or ENL)

Steroids, pentoxifylline, and thalidomide (a dose of 100–200 mg is given either once or twice daily).

CONCLUSION

Rheumatological conditions in leprosy may present either as part of disease process or as the presenting manifestation. A high degree of suspicion is the first requirement to diagnose arthritis.

Leprosy is a great mimicker of various rheumatological conditions as has been illustrated in the cases depicted earlier. Leprosy should be diligently searched in patients with unexplained articular manifestations. Even in endemic areas, arthritis due to leprosy is overlooked. However, antileprosy treatment is usually rewarding in long run.

SUGGESTED READINGS

1. Chauhan S, Wakhlu A, Agarwal V. Arthritis in leprosy. Rheumatology. 2010;49(12):2237-42.
2. World Health Organization. (2023). Leprosy (Hansen's disease). [online] Available from. vbs://www.who.int/news-room/fact-sheets/detail/leprosy [Last accessed December, 2023].
3. World Health Organization. (2021). Leprosy: Number of new leprosy cases 2021. [online] Available from vbs://apps.who.int/neglected_diseases/ntddata/leprosy/leprosy.html [Last accessed December, 2023].
4. Haroon N, Agarwal V, Aggarwal A, Kumari N, Krishnani N, Misra R. Arthritis as presenting manifestation of pure neuritic leprosy—a rheumatologist's dilemma. Rheumatology (Oxford). 2007;46:653-6.
5. Thappa DM, Karthikeyan K, Vijaikumar M, Koner BC, Jayanthi S. Leg ulcers in active lepromatous leprosy associated with cryoglobulinaemia. Clin Exp Dermatol. 2002;27(6):451-3.
6. Carpintero-Benitez P, Logrono C, Collantes-Estevez E. Enthesopathy in leprosy. J Rheumatol. 1996;23(6):1020-1.
7. Cossermelli-Messina W, Festa Neto C, Cossermelli W. Articular inflammatory manifestations in patients with different forms of leprosy. J Rheumatol. 1998;25(1):111-9.
8. Messner RP. Arthritis due to mycobacteria and fungi. In: Hollander JL, McCarty DJ (Eds). Arthritis and Allied Conditions: A Textbook of Rheumatology. Philadelphia: Lippincott Williams & Wilkins; 1979. pp. 1380-4.

115 CHAPTER

Biomarkers in Rheumatology: How to Interpret?

Arup Kumar Kundu, Abhra Chandra Chowdhury

ABSTRACT

Laboratory tests are useful in the diagnosis of autoimmune diseases but practitioners should be aware of the limitations of these tests. Usually, a thorough history and meticulous physical examination can help in making diagnosis of autoimmune diseases. Tests should be ordered in the appropriate clinical context, otherwise interpretation of these tests becomes difficult. Some of the common tests are rheumatoid factor (RF), anti-cyclic citrullinated peptide (anti-CCP) antibodies, antinuclear antibodies (ANAs), HLA-B27, anti-neutrophil cytoplasmic antibody (ANCA), antiphospholipid (aPL) antibodies, serum uric acid (SUA), antistreptolysin O (ASO) titer, C-reactive protein (CRP), and erythrocyte sedimentation rate (ESR).

INTRODUCTION

The biological markers are extensively used in rheumatology; these are totally different from clinical markers, which depend entirely on physical variables like assessment of pain, tender, swollen joint count, etc. The biomarkers, serological or proteomic, help to detect and diagnose rheumatic diseases earlier, and assess the disease activity more precisely. The biomarkers have been included in the recent classification criteria of many diseases to enable an early diagnosis and in time commencement of treatment. They help in more accurate subclassification of various diseases and more focused monitoring of certain organ involvement like lung or kidney. With the assistance of biomarkers, the assessment of disease activity as well as response to treatment becomes more reliable.

RHEUMATOID FACTOR

Rheumatoid factor (RF) is a frequently ordered test during evaluation of a patient with joint symptoms **(Table 1)**. RF is immunoglobulin M (IgM) autoantibody targeting the Fc portion of human IgG. It is called so as it was first described in the sera of patients with rheumatoid arthritis (RA). RF is present in up to 70% of patients with

TABLE 1: Conditions associated with rheumatoid factor (RF) positivity.

Conditions	Frequency (%)
Rheumatoid arthritis	70–75
Other rheumatic conditions	
Primary Sjögren's syndrome	75–95
Systemic lupus erythematosus (SLE)	20–35
Progressive systemic sclerosis (PSS)	20–30
Systemic vasculitis	5–20
Juvenile idiopathic arthritis (JIA)	5
Mixed connective tissue disease (MCTD)	50–60
Dermatomyositis	20
Infections (RF is transient and harmless)	
Infective endocarditis	40
Malaria	15–18
Hepatitis B	25
Hepatitis C	40–75
Human immunodeficiency virus (HIV)	20
Tuberculosis	15
Syphilis	10–35

Continued

116 CHAPTER

Pregnancy and Autoimmune Rheumatic Diseases

Prashasti Gupta, Preeti Kumari, Ghan Shyam Pangtey

ABSTRACT

Autoimmune rheumatic diseases (ARDs) include diseases such as rheumatoid arthritis, systemic lupus erythematosus, spondyloarthritides, psoriatic arthritis, systemic sclerosis, Sjögren's disease, antiphospholipid antibody (APLA) syndrome, etc. The burden of autoimmune disorders is several times higher in women compared to male. In various studies, it has been found that ARDs are more severe in women and also associated with poorer outcome. The peak incidence often occurs during the reproductive years and usually affects both fertility and pregnancy outcomes. Impacts on pregnancy can lead to early miscarriages, low birth weight infants, as well as adverse maternal outcomes with increased morbidity and mortality. The management of the disease becomes more complicated with many of the antirheumatic drugs can itself lead to teratogenicity, infertility, and fetal loss. Managing women with autoimmune disease is complex in our Indian patriarchal society, as there is almost no social or family support for their illness. Many females are abandoned or divorced by their in-laws after learning about their autoimmune illness. Most females suffering from ARDs can have pregnancies that turn out successful when these are carefully planned with a team-based approach involving multiple specialists like rheumatologist/treating clinician, obstetrician-gynecologist, and infertility expert. For obtaining best fetomaternal outcomes, conception should be planned at a time of disease quiescence and with the mother on medications that would be compatible throughout gestation and lactation. Prepregnancy assessment includes estimation of activity and severity of disease, ensuring safe medication, and testing certain antibodies. Use of appropriate contraception is a must at all other times, especially for those taking medications with potential teratogenicity or when sufficient drug safety data is lacking.

INTRODUCTION

Autoimmune rheumatic diseases (ARDs) are chronic systemic illnesses that commonly affect the joints, but can have a variety of extra-articular manifestations. Although greater than 200 ARD are known to affect children and adults, relatively more common ones include systemic lupus erythematosus (SLE), rheumatoid arthritis (RA), systemic sclerosis (SSc), Sjögren's disease, antiphospholipid syndrome (APS), and spondyloarthritides such as ankylosing spondylitis (AS) and reactive and psoriatic arthritis. These bring with them considerable morbidity and also premature mortality due to either infections, organ, or life-threatening complications as well as accelerated adverse cardiovascular outcomes. In addition, these assume particular importance when they afflict young adults because of the impact on their productive years of life as well as negative implications on reproductive health issues.

The management of reproductive health issues in patients with ARD is a little different from that in the healthy population. Thus, rheumatologists and other clinicians attending to these patients should always discuss with them about aspects, such as contraception, conception timing, medication safety in pregnancy and lactation, assisted reproductive technology (ART), fertility preservation when indicated, and hormone replacement therapy (HRT), provide appropriate counseling and also collaborate with specialists from obstetrics-gynecology, reproductive endocrinology, and infertility.

The latest update (2020) on the recommendations by the American College of Rheumatology (ACR) for the management of reproductive health in patients suffering from ARD serves as a useful guide for managing them, however, the ultimate decision regarding their application rests with the treating clinician in light of patient's individual circumstances including patient's values, preferences, and comorbidities reflecting and promoting a shared decision-making process.

Pregnancy and these diseases are reciprocally related; a flare in disease activity can occur in pregnancy and disease activity also negatively affects pregnancy course and outcome. Nevertheless, the impact pregnancy has on ARD varies by condition. It is of particular importance to realize that all patients with ARD are especially prone to develop a disease flare postpartum. Certain general principles that apply to management of ARD and pregnancy are outlined below with specifics of different diseases and medication use dealt with under separate sections.

GENERAL CONSIDERATION: PREGNANCY AND RHEUMATIC DISEASES

Women with ARD should be counseled during pregnancy planning and preconception counseling should include assessment of disease activity, review and modification of antirheumatic drugs to nonteratogenic and pregnancy compatible one, stabilization of disease, assessing the antibody status, and determination of end-organ damage.

- Contraception and pregnancy planning should be discussed at initial or early visit with women of childbearing age. Highly effective contraceptives like intrauterine devices (IUDs) or hormonal contraceptives like subdermal implants are advisable. Women taking mycophenolate mofetil (MMF) for maintenance or induction of disease should use an IUD alone or two other methods of contraception together because MMF may reduce serum estrogen and progesterone levels reducing the efficacy of oral contraceptives.
- Proper conception timing is crucial. Disease activity should be low, obtained with medications that may be continued safely throughout pregnancy. So, if the patient is on a pregnancy incompatible medication, a switch should be made to a compatible one and appropriate time should be given to assess disease response to it as well as side effects if any. The recommended duration of remission before the patient can safely conceive differs among the ARDs, in general 3–6 months of remission is deemed sufficient.
- If there is a presence of any end-organ damage secondary to the disease like pulmonary hypertension, interstitial lung disease, and heart or renal failure, the decision regarding pregnancy should be jointly taken by a multidisciplinary group of experts with the couple apprised of the elevated risk of pregnancy-related adverse outcomes.
- All patients with SLE as well as any ARD patient with an adverse obstetric history or history of thrombosis should be evaluated for the presence of antiphospholipid (aPL) antibodies. Also in view of the risk of fetal complete heart block (CHB), prepregnancy screen should include anti-Ro and anti-La antibodies for all patients with ARD.
- While fertility is not affected in women suffering from ARDs (unless treated with gonadotoxic medication), it does decrease with age and ART may be needed by few. This may include techniques like ovarian stimulation (which elevates estrogen levels) in vitro fertilization and embryo transfer. So, caution should be taken to preferably proceed with it only when disease is in the quiescent phase. Also, it should be noted that cyclophosphamide (CYC) can affect maturing follicles, so should be discontinued before these procedures.
- Disease-modifying antirheumatic drugs (DMARDs), such as CYC, MMF, and methotrexate (MTX) should be ideally stopped 3 months prior to attempting conception, but folic acid continued through preconception till end of pregnancy. CYC however may be used for life-threatening conditions in the second/third trimester.
- Women with ARD receiving monthly intravenous CYC who are yet to complete their family should be given monthly gonadotropin-releasing hormone agonists, preferably about 2 weeks before scheduled CYC administration. Also, for men with ARD treated with CYC, sperm cryopreservation is suggested.
- Since women with ARD may experience disease flare postpartum and require treatment, it is important to strike a balance between the benefits of disease control and risk of drug exposure to the nursing baby through breast milk. The lactation-compatible medications may further have to be customized based on a review of individualized risks and benefits.
- In pregnant patients with RA as well as SLE, certain complications, such as pregnancy-induced hypertension, preeclampsia, intrauterine growth retardation, and premature delivery (often requiring cesarean section) occur significantly more commonly than in the healthy pregnant women. Thus all pregnant patients with ARD, especially SLE and aPL+ should receive preventive treatment with low dose aspirin (75–100 mg/day), beginning in the first trimester.

Systemic Lupus Erythematosus

The lupus activity during pregnancy in patients with SLE is complicated and difficult to predict. The various studies on lupus activity during pregnancy are very heterogeneous with definition of flare, study population, and with multiple confounders. During pregnancy differentiating between preeclampsia and SLE activity becomes very difficult as renal flares are more common than arthritis or other manifestations. Certain studies indicate that 35–70% of women with SLE may experience a flare during pregnancy or postpartum, especially in patients with preexisting kidney disease and high disease activity around the time of conception.

Prolonged remission of disease activity before pregnancy reduces the likelihood of lupus flare. Decreased flare rate in third trimester has been reported in a recent study presumably because of blunted interleukin-6 (IL-6) response due to lower levels of estrogen. Up to 33% of patients may develop disease flares during postpartum period. The following factors may be associated with better prediction of lupus disease flare in pregnancy:

- Active disease during the 6 months prior to conception
- Nephritis in past
- Discontinuation of hydroxychloroquine (HCQ)
- Primigravida

As far as contraception in SLE is concerned, it is advisable to avoid use of the transdermal estrogen-progestin patch. In SLE, patients with moderate or severe disease activity including nephritis, progestin-only, or IUD contraceptives over combined estrogen-progestin contraception are recommended, because of the potential increased risk of worsening disease due to hormonal influence (estrogen). Same is recommended in women with SLE with aPL positivity because estrogen increases risk of thromboembolism. For those requiring ART, an acute lupus flare might result because of the attendant hormonal surge from ovarian induction.

Neonatal SLE is a clinical syndrome which can develop in the fetus of mothers with ARD and who are positive for anti-Ro and anti-La autoantibodies and characterized by cardiac and cutaneous manifestations. They need to be closely followed up after 16-week of pregnancy with cardiologist and fetal echocardiography (management discussed in Sjögren's syndrome section).

Rheumatoid Arthritis

As per World Health Organization (WHO) 2019 data, world over, 18 million people were found to be living with RA, out of which approximately 70% were women. In RA, some women improve, some have increased disease activity, while others remain the same. A systematic review conducted in 2019 by Jethwa H et al. reported that RA improved in 60% of patients through pregnancy and flared in approximately 47% of cases after delivery.

Systemic Sclerosis

About systemic sclerosis, studies have shown that the disease seems to remain largely stable. In a comprehensive review done by Betelli M et al., almost 61% of patients remained stable and approximately 20% got better or worse during pregnancy. Regarding specific SSc symptoms, a temporary improvement of Raynaud's phenomenon and digital ulcers may be found during the second trimester as opposed to a worsening of esophageal reflux. This could be partly related to physiological changes in pregnancy. Diffuse cutaneous SSc patients should generally avoid pregnancy in early disease due to an elevated risk of scleroderma renal crisis.

Sjögren's Disease

As far as Sjögren's syndrome is concerned, no large-scale studies document a pregnancy-associated increase in disease activity.

Anti-Sjögren's-syndrome-related antigen A (Anti-SSA) and anti-SSB antibodies may be present not only in Sjögren's syndrome, but also in other ARD. These antibodies are capable of passing across the placenta from the 16th week of gestation, which may cause atrioventricular blockage in the fetal heart (mostly between 18 and 24 weeks of gestation), or even neonatal lupus. The risk of CHB in the fetus of a mother with presence of these antibodies is 2%; however, it increases to 18% if it happened in a past pregnancy. Detection by screening with serial fetal echocardiograms will help with supervising atrioventricular conductivity in the fetal heart. Following the recommendations of the American Heart Association, monitoring of such a fetus should start at 16 weeks of gestation with measurements performed weekly, until 26 weeks of gestation. HCQ has a protective role in this regard for both the ongoing as well as future pregnancies. Also, for such women with fetal first- or second-degree heart block shown on echocardiography, treatment with dexamethasone 4 mg/day could help to prevent CHB.

Antiphospholipid Syndrome

Antiphospholipid syndrome is also known as antiphospholipid antibody (APLA) syndrome is a systemic autoimmune disease resulting in arterial and venous thrombosis and pregnancy morbidity affecting both mother and fetus. In early pregnancy it may present as recurrent fetal loss and abortion, while in late pregnancy it may be associated with vascular thrombosis or preeclampsia. In obstetric APS, the aim of management is ensuring adequate anticoagulation and maternal and fetal well-being through regular monitoring. Perinatal counseling is important to reassure the couple that a good outcome is possible through proper monitoring and regular follow up with both the rheumatology and obstetric teams.

Being a hypercoagulable state in itself, pregnancy confers an additional risk factor for thrombotic events in APS patients. It is crucial to note that pregnancy can be a trigger for the catastrophic antiphospholipid syndrome (CAPS), a rare but life-threatening emergency. For patients with aPL antibody positive [lupus anticoagulant (LAC), anticardiolipin antibodies (aCL), and beta-2-glycoprotein I (β2GPI)], primary or secondary APS undergoing ovarian induction, there could be a risk of potentially life-threatening thrombosis.

Low-dose aspirin and prophylactic-dose low molecular weight heparin (LMWH) are recommended for patients with obstetric APS. In addition, prophylactic-dose LMWH should be continued for 6–12 weeks postpartum. For patients with thrombotic APS, low-dose aspirin and therapeutic dose LMWH should be given throughout pregnancy. In the postpartum period, heparin is continued till 6 weeks and then discontinued in obstetric APS. In contrast, in vascular APS, reinitiation of vitamin K oral antagonist should be done as this is safe in lactation.

MEDICATION USE DURING PREGNANCY

Anti-inflammatory Medication and Conventional DMARDs

- *Nonsteroidal anti-inflammatory drugs (NSAIDs)* used in a wide variety of ARD are often required during pregnancy, but because of the potential risk of premature closure of the ductus as well as bleeding and oligohydramnios, their use in the third trimester is not recommended.
- *Glucocorticoids* can be used during pregnancy for treating flares, when indicated. Prednisone and prednisolone are rapid acting with negligible transplacental transfer, so are preferred. However, betamethasone and dexamethasone can cross the placenta easily and therefore are of use in preventing fetal CHB (in case of maternal Ro/La positivity) as well as preventing neonatal respiratory distress syndrome in preterm labor cases by accelerating lung maturation.
- *Methotrexate* is contraindicated during pregnancy [Food and Drug Administration (FDA) category X drug—causes abortions, fetal congenital anomalies involving heart, nervous system, and skeleton].
- *Mycophenolate* use is also associated with an increased first trimester loss and development of various congenital malformations, hence is contraindicated.
- *Sulfasalazine, colchicine, and azathioprine* are considered safe for use in pregnancy.
- *Hydroxychloroquine* use in pregnant patients with SLE is associated with reduced disease activity and also brings down the risk of flares. So, it is recommended to continue this drug in patients with SLE and other ARD like RA and Sjögren's syndrome throughout pregnancy.
- *Leflunomide* (FDA category X drug) can take up to 2 years to get fully eliminated from the body due to its long half-life. An accelerated drug elimination procedure (cholestyramine washout 8 g TDS for 11 days) should be provided to a patient on therapy who wishes to conceive with the aim of achieving plasma concentration of the active metabolite (teriflunomide <0.02 mg/L). Additionally, it is advisable to wait out three menstrual cycles after achieving this before attempting to conceive.
- *Intravenous immunoglobulin (IVIG), cyclosporine, and tacrolimus* are also considered compatible with pregnancy.

Biological DMARDs and Small Synthetic DMARDs

The management of ARDs has changed drastically with the advent of biological disease-modifying antirheumatic drugs (bDMARDs). Common ARDs treated with bDMARDs include SLE, RA, spondyloarthritides, and juvenile idiopathic arthritis (JIA).

However, the experience with the use of biologics in pregnancy is limited because of the observational nature of the available studies and restricted capability to conduct experimental trials in pregnancy.

- *Tumor necrosis factor (TNF) inhibitor* therapy with infliximab, etanercept, adalimumab, or golimumab can be given preconception as well as during pregnancy. Certolizumab is considered especially safe with negligible placental transfer owing to absence of Fc chain in its structure.

  The recommended duration for discontinuing medication prior to the scheduled delivery may rely on the half-life of the specific drug. This measure ensures the absence of the medication in the baby's bloodstream during delivery, as it may pose a risk of infections if the baby receives live vaccines. As per established protocols, only infants exposed to biologics before 22 weeks are eligible to receive live vaccines. While babies exposed to biologics during the second and third trimesters can adhere to the vaccination program, they should refrain from receiving live vaccines in the initial 6 months of their life.
- Anakinra (IL-1 receptor antagonist), belimumab (monoclonal antibody against B-cell activating factor),

TABLE 2: Conditions where autoantibodies may be positive.

Autoantibody	Rheumatoid factor (RF)	Anti-CCP	ANA	ANCA
Rheumatic conditions with positivity	• Rheumatoid arthritis • Sjögren's syndrome • Cryoglobulinemia • MCTD • SLE • Interstitial lung disease (ILD)	• Rheumatoid arthritis • Overlap syndrome • SLE • ANCA-vasculitis	• SLE • Systemic sclerosis • MCTD • Sjögren's syndrome • Drug-induced lupus • Myositis • JIA	• ANCA-associated vasculitis (GPA, MPA, and EGPA) • SLE • Crohn's disease • Ulcerative colitis • PSC • IgA nephropathy
Nonrheumatic conditions with positivity	• Myeloma • Subacute bacterial endocarditis • TB • Viral and bacterial infections	• Malignancy • TB	• TB • Autoimmune thyroiditis • Pulmonary HTN • Malignancy • Drugs (sulfa drugs, penicillamine, and minocycline)	• TB • Syphilis • HIV • Lymphoma • Drugs (propylthiouracil, cocaine, and methimazole)

(ANA: antinuclear antibodies; ANCA: antineutrophil cytoplasmic antibody; CCP: cyclic citrullinated peptide; GPA: granulomatosis with polyangiitis; HIV: human immunodeficiency virus; HTN: hypertension; IgA: immunoglobulin A; ILD: interstitial lung disease; JIA: juvenile idiopathic arthritis; MCTD: mixed connective tissue disease; PSC: primary sclerosing cholangitis; SLE: systemic lupus erythematosus; TB: tuberculosis)

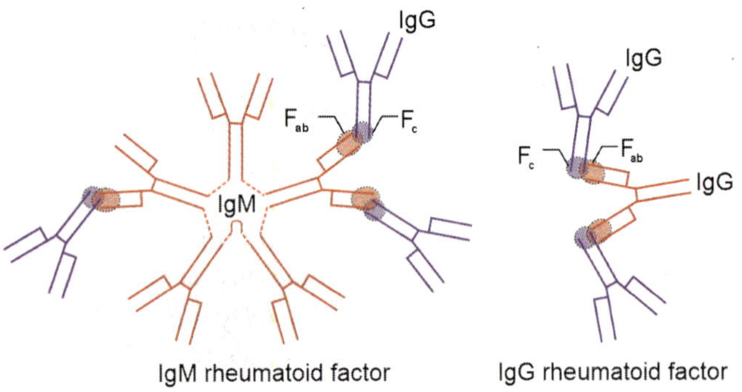

FIG. 1: Rheumatoid factor IgM and IgG subtypes.
(IgG: immunoglobulin G; IgM: immunoglobulin M)

Anti-cyclic Citrullinated Peptide

- *Antibodies against citrullinated proteins*: Citrunillation of proteins is carried out by Peptidylarginine deiminases (PAD enzymes).
- Anti-cyclic citrullinated peptide (anti-CCP) antibodies are more specific for RA, but they can also be seen in certain other conditions.
- Anti-CCP-positive patients can develop RA later, and these seropositive patients also usually have a higher disease burden and a chance of extraarticular manifestations
- Newer generation assays (CCP2 or CCP3 assays) have a higher sensitivity (65–70%) and specificity (95%) for RA

Antinuclear Antibodies

- Antinuclear antibodies refer to a host of autoantibodies directed against various cellular components.
- Some of the antigenic targets may not be nuclear components (e.g., anti-Ro and antisynthetase), so the term "anticellular antibody" may be more correct.
- Historically, the presence of ANA was established through the discovery of the "LE cell," a macrophage that had ingested the nuclear matter of a lymphocyte, in the bone marrow of a patient with SLE.
- The usual test for ANA positivity is through indirect immunofluorescence microscopy (IIF) using HEp-2 cells to test for patient sera containing these antibodies.
- An ANA report using HEp-2 cells is expressed under the following headings: Titer, pattern, and intensity. Some common causes for ANA positivity are mentioned in **Table 3**.
  - *Titer*: The dilution ratio of patient serum at which ANA is positive. Titers up to 1:80 may be seen in 20% of normal individuals, especially in older females. Higher titers like 1:160 and above are more sensitive for ANA positivity.
  - *Pattern*: Depending on the type of antigen targeted by the patient antibodies, a pattern of immunofluorescence is seen.
  - *Intensity*: Scored from 1+ to 4+ depending on the reader's opinion of the intensity of fluorescence.
- The specific antibodies responsible for ANA positivity are mentioned in **Table 3**, and testing for them

TABLE 3: Common autoantibodies responsible for antinuclear antibodies (ANA) positivity.

Antibody targets	Pattern (IIF)	Disease association	Importance
dsDNA	Nuclear homogenous	SLE	Predicts renal involvement, flares
Histone	Nuclear homogenous	Drug-induced lupus	Not specific but sensitive
Sm	Nuclear coarse speckled	SLE	Relatively specific
U1RNP	Nuclear coarse speckled	MCTD	Required for labeling MCTD
Ro(SSA) and La(SSB)	Nuclear fine speckled	Sjögren's syndrome and SLE	Neonatal lupus, subacute cutaneous lupus, and risk of lymphoma
CENP (A to F)	Centromeric	Systemic sclerosis	Raynaud's phenomenon, pulmonary HTN, and less ILD
Scl-70 (topoisomerase 1)	Nucleolar	Systemic sclerosis	Diffuse cutaneous disease, and risk of ILD
Antisynthetase (Jo-1, PL-7, PL-12, EJ, OJ, etc.)	Cytoplasmic or sometimes "negative"	Antisynthetase syndrome/ myositis	Arthritis, mechanic's hands, ILD, cutaneous rash, and myositis

(CENP: centromere protein; dsDNA: double-stranded deoxyribonucleic acid; HTN: hypertension; ILD: interstitial lung disease; MCTD: mixed connective tissue disease; SLE: Systemic lupus erythematosus; U1RNP: U1 ribonucleoprotein particle)

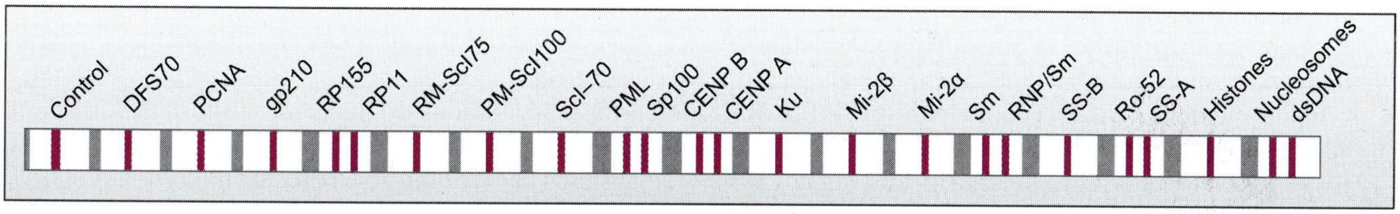

FIG. 2: Line immunoassay for antinuclear antibody (ANA) profile test.

requires an enzyme-linked immunosorbent assay (ELISA) or immunoblot (line immunoassay). These tests determine which of the several antibodies is present **(Fig. 2)**. This is called the ANA Profile or "extractable nuclear antigen (ENA)" test, as the antigens are extracted on a nitrocellulose membrane and antibodies against them are tested.

- The ANA profile test can reveal antibodies pathogenic for certain diseases, or even help in prognostication.
- ANA may be negative on IIF, in cases such as Ro and antisynthetase antibody positivity, where the antigens are cytoplasmic and therefore fluorescence may not be reported. In cases with a high suspicion of Sjögren's or inflammatory myositis, it is therefore necessary to test for the specific antibodies using an ENA test, even in the absence of ANA positivity.

Antineutrophil Cytoplasmic Antibodies

- Directed against the granular components of the neutrophilic cytoplasm
- Often associated with some of the small vessel vasculitides
- Commonly directed against two major antigens: (1) Myeloperoxidase (MPO) or (2) proteinase-3 (PR3) in neutrophils
- Similar to ANA, can be reported using IIF microscopy as p-ANCA or c-ANCA (perinuclear staining or cytoplasmic staining)
- p-ANCA or c-ANCA reports only refer to the immunofluorescence pattern. This positivity may be due to antibodies against any neutrophil protein [(e.g., MPO, PR3, elastase, bactericidal increasing protein (BPI), lactoferrin, and catalase]
- Antibodies against MPO or PR3 have been associated with pathologic conditions. p-ANCA with MPO positivity, or c-ANCA with PR3 positivity, will give a clearer picture of truly pathogenic antibodies.
- Recent guidelines state that testing for anti-MPO or anti-PR3 using ELISA or LIA methods is preferable to simply reporting p/c-ANCA.
- *Patients with high suspicion of small vessel vasculitis are those with any of the following features*: Alveolar hemorrhage, subglottic stenosis, vasculitic ulcers with arthritis, chronic suppurative otitis media, or rapidly progressive glomerulonephritis.

GENETIC TESTS

The immune pathways in our body are regulated by several genes, but the MHC-associated genes [human leukocyte antigen (HLA) complex] have been most widely studied. None of the genetic tests need to be repeated if once performed using a good laboratory setup, especially if the polymerase chain reaction (PCR) method is used.

Human Leukocyte Antigen B27

- Occurs in 6–8% of the normal Indian population, even without diseases.
- Has been associated with axial spondyloarthritis or ankylosing spondylitis with variable prevalence.
- Several hypotheses exist on the pathogenicity of HLA-B27 in arthritis, but none have been proven without fault.
- HLA-B27 is not an absolute requirement to diagnose spondyloarthritis, and it is quite possible to have HLA-B27 positivity without any inflammatory disease in an individual.
- With the clinical picture of spondyloarthritis, HLA-B27 can add to the evidence for diagnosis. However, the diagnosis is based on clinical features and imaging.

Human Leukocyte Antigen B51

- Associated with a proportion of patients with Behçet's disease, but may also occur in the normal population.
- Behçet's disease is unusual in the Indian population, so testing for HLA-B51 without a relevant clinical scenario can only lead to confusion.

CONCLUSION

- Laboratory tests help in the diagnosis of rheumatologic diseases only 10% of the time.
- They are a useful adjunct to proper history taking and clinical examination.
- The presence of autoantibodies or elevated inflammatory markers is usually just a sign of immune activity, rather than always being a pointer to a specific diagnosis.
- Interpreting a laboratory result requires an understanding of the pretest probability of a positive test, as well as the chances of false positives or false negatives.
- Only a few laboratory tests have a prognostic value, but they can help to detect disease activity early in the absence of very objective clinical findings.

SUGGESTED READINGS

1. Abernethy TJ, Avery OT. The occurrence during acute infections of a protein not normally present in the blood: I. Distribution of the reactive protein in patients' sera and the effect of calcium on the flocculation reaction with C polysaccharide of Pneumococcus. J Exp Med. 1941;73(2):173-82.
2. Fautrel B, Le Moël GI, Saint-Marcoux BE, Taupin PI, Vignes ST, Rozenberg SY, et al. Diagnostic value of ferritin and glycosylated ferritin in adult onset Still's disease. J Rheumatol. 2001;28(2):322-9.
3. Correia ML, Carvalho S, Fortuna J, Pereira MH. Comparison of three anti-CCP antibody tests and rheumatoid factor in RA and control patients. Clin Rev Allergy Immunol. 2008;34(1):21-5.
4. Agmon-Levin N, Damoiseaux J, Kallenberg C, Sack U, Witte T, Herold M, et al. International recommendations for the assessment of autoantibodies to cellular antigens referred to as anti-nuclear antibodies. Ann Rheum Dis. 2014;73(1):17-23.
5. Bossuyt X, Cohen Tervaert JW, Arimura Y, Blockmans D, Flores-Suárez LF, Guillevin L, et al. Position paper: Revised 2017 international consensus on testing of ANCAs in granulomatosis with polyangiitis and microscopic polyangiitis. Nature Reviews Rheumatology. 2017;13(11):683-92.

118

CHAPTER

Environmental Influences on Rheumatology

Partha Sarkar, Anustup Mukherjee

ABSTRACT

The environment has its share of influence on human health apart from genes and behavioral activity of humans. Environmental influence on rheumatic diseases is being increasingly recognized recently like in other diseases. Air pollution, through the agents such as particulate matters, gases emitted mainly from automobiles and industries, and organic and inorganic dusts and fumes, has the greatest impact on rheumatic diseases. Domestic and industrial sewage, heavy metals, and pesticides are the waterborne mediators of health effects on autoimmunity. Ultraviolet (UV) rays and ambient temperature also have their share of impact on human health. Knowledge regarding environmental factors is critical to undertaking preventive efforts against the development and/or exacerbation of rheumatic diseases.

INTRODUCTION

Our environment plays a central role in the development and exacerbation of rheumatic and musculoskeletal diseases (RMDs). Environmental pollution is a major cause of mortality and morbidity. Environmental pollutants originate from a source and are transported by air, water, or soil before affecting humans. With time, our environment is getting more polluted mostly because of human activities. Air pollution has the greatest impact on human health among others. Its effect on cardiovascular and respiratory systems is well established. But its impact on RMDs is also substantial as suggested by recent studies. Besides air pollution, other sources of pollution have also been found to exert an effect on the course of RMDs.

AIR POLLUTION

The major conduit of environmental influence on human health is air quality. Automobiles, industries, and domestic usage account for the major sources of air pollution. Particulate matters, organic dusts, gases like NO_2, SO_2, CO, and O_3, and other industrial pollutants are the chief mediators of health effects. Smoking, active as well as passive, is a behavioral as well as an environmental factor which is one of the most hazardous health habits having deleterious effects on autoimmune diseases but is beyond the scope of discussion in this chapter. The major mechanism of damage by air pollutants is oxidative stress. Chronic exposure to air pollutants generates oxidative stress which further generates reactive oxygen species (ROS) to modify the immune system (**Fig. 1**).

Effect of Air Pollution on Rheumatic and Musculoskeletal Diseases

Rheumatoid Arthritis

There is an increased association between air pollution and rheumatoid arthritis (RA) disease severity. Exposure to high levels of pollutants has been found to be associated with higher C-reactive protein (CRP) levels and a higher risk of flares. Air pollution also diminishes the response to certain biological disease-modifying antirheumatic drugs (bDMARDs), as per few studies.

Systemic Lupus Erythematosus

Increased particulate matters ($PM_{2.5}$) and O_3 in the air increased hospital admissions in systemic lupus

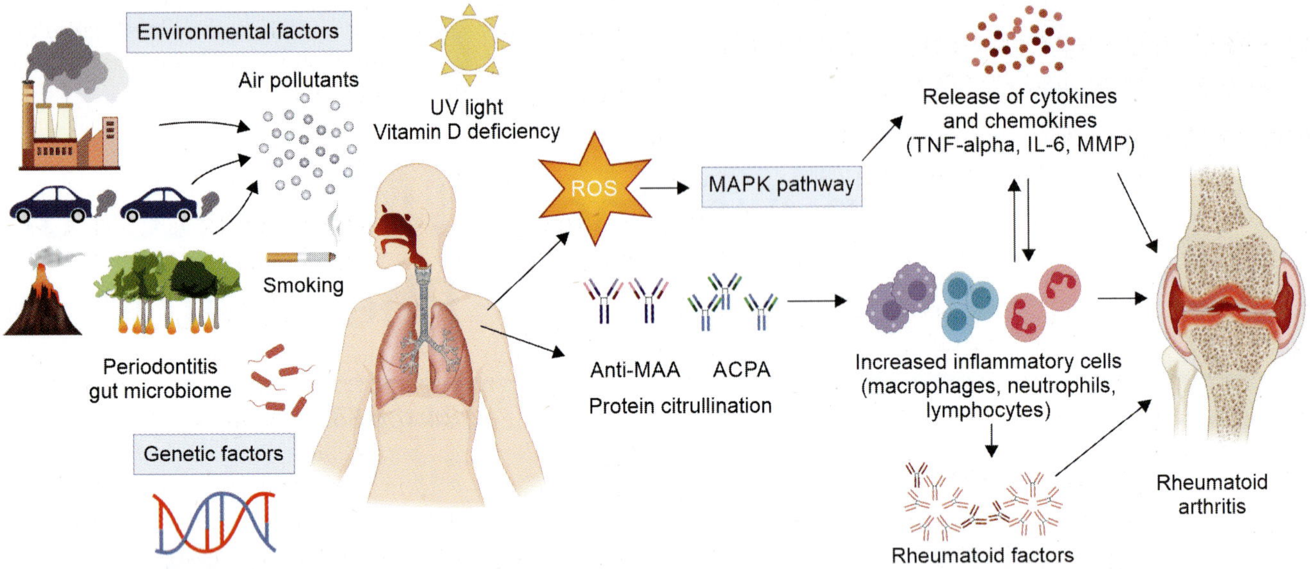

FIG. 1: Mechanism of development of rheumatoid arthritis due to air pollutants.

(ACPA: anticitrullinated peptide antibody; IL-6: interleukin 6; MAA: malondialdehyde-acetaldehyde adduct; MAPK: mitogen-activated protein kinase; MMP: matrix metalloproteinase; ROS: reactive oxygen species; TNF: tumor necrosis factor; UV: ultraviolet)

erythematosus (SLE) patients. In a few studies, NO_2 and CO were found to be independent risk factors for SLE nephritis. Exposure to poor air quality is associated with the development of pleuropulmonary manifestations in SLE patients.

Sjögren's Syndrome

Increased dry organic air pollutants increase the risk for sicca symptoms in Sjögren's syndrome (SS) patients. As in SLE, $PM_{2.5}$ and NO_2 exposure increases the number of outpatient department (OPD) visits in SS, whereas in a few studies, O_3 exposure appeared to be associated with decreased risk.

Systemic Sclerosis

Benzene concentration in air is positively correlated with the extent of skin involvement and also the reduction of diffusing capacity of the lungs for carbon monoxide (DLCO) in systemic sclerosis (SSc) patients. Like in other connective tissue diseases, NO_2, SO_2, and $PM_{2.5}$ negatively impact health by increasing the likelihood of interstitial lung diseases (ILDs).

Spondyloarthritis

Like in RA, air pollution diminishes the response to bDMARDs in spondyloarthritis (SpA) patients. Long-term exposure to poor-quality air has a negative correlation with BASMI (Bath Ankylosing Spondylitis Metrology Index)/BASFI (Bath Ankylosing Spondylitis Functional Index)/BASDAI (Bath Ankylosing Spondylitis Disease Activity Index) scores of patients.

TABLE 1: Inflammatory myositis.

Factors	Association	Myositis phenotype
Ultraviolet (UV) rays	Risk	Dermatomyositis
Silica dust	Risk	Dermatomyositis
Inorganic dust	Risk	All
Automobile gas/fumes	Risk	Antisynthetase syndrome

Vasculitis

Exposure to inhaled particulate matters and silicon tetroxide has been found to increase the incidence of antineutrophil cytoplasmic antibody (ANCA)-associated vasculitis.

Gout

Environmental factors such as particulate matters, SO_2, and CO increase hospitalization risk for gout. Also, the changes in temperature and humidity induced by air pollution impact the crystallization of uric acid in joints.

Inflammatory Myositis

Factors that contribute to inflammatory myositis are given in **Table 1**.

WATER POLLUTION

Effect of Water Pollution on Rheumatic and Musculoskeletal Diseases

Rheumatoid Arthritis

Polycyclic aromatic hydrocarbons (PAHs) are environmental pollutants found in barbecued foods, urban traffic pollution, burning of garbage, etc. Excessive amounts of PAHs are found in waste incinerators and decomposition products of oil burning. PAHs act via aryl hydrocarbon receptors (AHRs) which, via ligand-dependent signal transduction pathways, increase the activity of TH1 and TH17 cells, thereby precipitating RA **(Fig. 2)**.

Systemic Lupus Erythematosus

Ingestion of nitrates, heavy metals, pesticide residues, industrial wastewater, domestic sewage, and other pollutants entering drinking water increases the risk of SLE. Exposure to trichloroethylene, trichloroethane, inorganic chromium, and other chemicals obtained from wells in industrial areas hastens SLE progression.

Spondyloarthritis

Increased burden of heavy metals such as lead, cadmium, and mercury in drinking water is associated with faster progression of deformities in SpA patients.

RADIATION AND THERMAL HAZARDS

Environmental radiation such as ultraviolet (UV) rays and other radioactive substances has an enormous impact on health.

In several studies, it was seen that working in a cold environment is associated with an increased risk of developing both anticyclic citrullinated peptide (anti-CCP) positive and -negative RA patients.

It is now an established fact that UV radiation exposure is associated with photosensitivity, rashes, and flares in SLE patients. SLE patients are hence advised to avoid direct sunlight between 10 AM and 4 PM and use sunscreen with a sun protection factor of at least 30.

Sunlight is the source of vitamin D for humans. Vitamin D has an enormous role in immune regulation. Vitamin D deficiency/insufficiency due to lack of sunlight

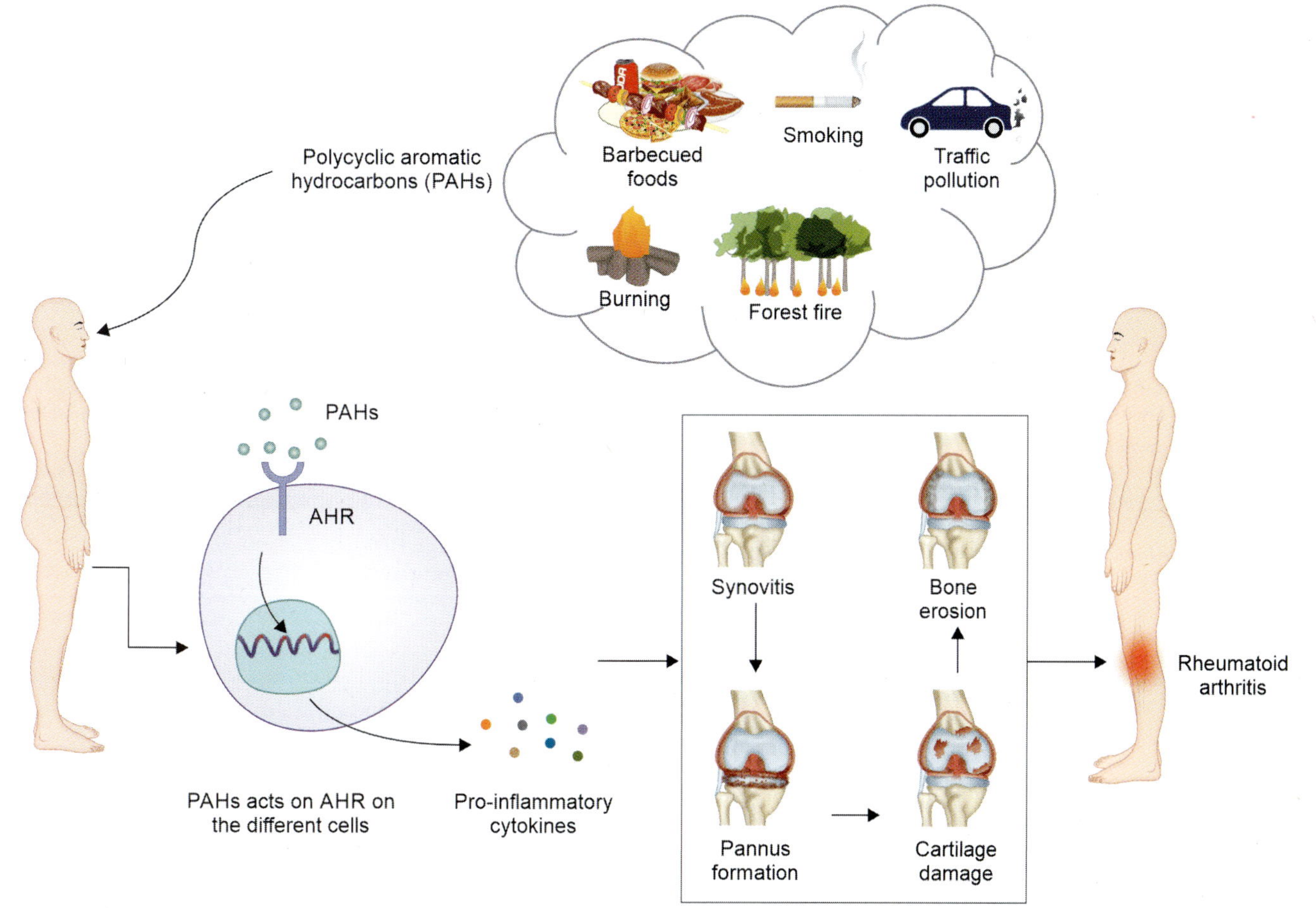

FIG. 2: Mechanism of development of rheumatoid arthritis due to polycyclic aromatic hydrocarbons.
(AHR: aryl hydrocarbon receptor)

exposure has been attributable to the onset of many autoimmune diseases.

OTHER SOURCES OF POLLUTION

The usage of organic pesticides is an independent modifier in the pathogenesis of SLE. Nonbiodegradable plastic materials, which are converted to microplastics, aggravate RA by affecting the proliferation, migration, and inflammation of fibroblast-like synovial cells by regulating mitochondrial homeostasis.

CONCLUSION

For long, autoimmune RMDs were considered to be mainly a genetic disorder with human leukocyte antigens (HLA) and non-HLA genes involved. With progress in research, RMDs were found to have a strong environmental influence. The complex interplay of environment and genes brings about the clinicopathological features of these diseases. Research on environmental influence has paramount importance because in many cases, they are avoidable and are hence effective preventive options.

SUGGESTED READINGS

1. Adami G, Viapiana O, Rossini M, Orsolini G, Bertoldo E, Giollo A, et al. Association between environmental air pollution and rheumatoid arthritis flares. Rheumatology (Oxford). 2021;60(10):4591-7.
2. Shin J, Lee J, Lee J, Ha EH. Association Between Exposure to Ambient Air Pollution and Rheumatoid Arthritis in Adults. Int J Environ Res Public Health. 2019;16(7):1227.
3. Rezayat AA, Niloufar Jafari, Mir Nourbakhsh SH, Hasheminezhad Hoseini FS, Hooshmand N, Ghasemi Nour M, et al. The effect of air pollution on systemic lupus erythematosus: A systematic review and meta-analysis. Lupus. 2022;31(13):1606-18.
4. Bai H, Jiang L, Li T, Liu C, Zuo X, Liu Y, et al. Acute effects of air pollution on lupus nephritis in patients with systemic lupus erythematosus: A multicenter panel study in China. Environ Res. 2021;195:110875.
5. Chen Y, He YS, Feng YT, Wu ZD, Wang J, Yin KJ, et al. The effect of air pollution exposure on risk of outpatient visits for Sjogren's syndrome: A time-series study. Environ Res. 2022; 214(Pt 3):114017.
6. Galperín G, Berra M, Marquez MI, Mandaradoni M, Tau J, Berra A. Impact of environmental pollution on the ocular surface of Sjögren's syndrome patients. Arq Bras Oftalmol. 2018;81(6): 481-9.
7. Borghini A, Poscia A, Bosello S, Teleman AA, Bocci M, Iodice L, et al. Int J Environ Res Public Health. 2017;14(11):1297.
8. Roeser A, Sese L, Chassagnon G, Chaigne B, Dunogue B, Tran Ba S, et al. The association between air pollution and the severity at diagnosis and progression of systemic sclerosis-associated interstitial lung disease: results from the retrospective ScleroPol study. Respir Res. 2022;60:1513.
9. Adami G, Rossini M, Viapiana O, Orsolini G, Bertoldo E, Pontalti M, et al. Environmental Air Pollution Is a Predictor of Poor Response to Biological Drugs in Chronic Inflammatory Arthritides. ACR Open Rheumatol. 2021;3(7):451-6.
10. Soleimanifar N, Nicknam NH, Bidad K, Jamshidi AR, Mahmoudi M, Mostafaei S. Effect of food intake and ambient air pollution exposure on ankylosing spondylitis disease activity. Adv Rheumatol. 2019;59(1):9.
11. Zhao WM, Wang ZJ, Shi R, Zhu YY, Zhang S, Wang RF, et al. Environmental factors influencing the risk of ANCA-associated vasculitis. Front Immunol. 2022;13:991256.
12. Wu ZD, Yang XK, He YS, Ni J, Wang J, Yin KG, et al. Environmental factors and risk of gout. Environ Res. 2022;212(Pt C):113377.
13. Xi X, Ye Q, Fan D, Cao X, Wang Q, Wang X, et al. Polycyclic Aromatic Hydrocarbons Affect Rheumatoid Arthritis Pathogenesis via Aryl Hydrocarbon Receptor. Front Immunol. 2022;13:797815.
14. Kilburn KH, Warshaw RH. Prevalence of symptoms of systemic lupus erythematosus (SLE) and of fluorescent antinuclear antibodies associated with chronic exposure to trichloroethylene and other chemicals in well water. Environ Res. 1992;57(1):1-9
15. Hashmi GMM, Shah MH. Comparative Assessment of Essential and Toxic Metals in the Blood of Spondyloarthropathy Patients and Healthy Subjects. Biointerface Res Appl Chem. 2022;12(2):1935-50.
16. Zeng P, Bengtsson C, Klareskog I, Alfredsson L. Working in cold environment and risk of developing rheumatoid arthritis: results from the Swedish EIRA case–control study. RMD Open. 2017;3(2):e000488.

SECTION

15

MISCELLANEOUS

119

CHAPTER

Improving Communication Skills in the Practice of Medicine

RK Singal, Atul Bhasin

ABSTRACT

Good communication skills are extremely important for medical professionals in the present era. Effective communication between healthcare provider and patients and their family members results in improved healthcare outcomes. Effective communication requires the physician to be an active listener and spend time with patients. The importance of listening extends far beyond the academic and professional settings and is extremely important in creating a trustworthy doctor-patient relationship. Disclosure of errors in medical practice involves a frank conversation with plain language, referring to the incident as an error, providing necessary details, and an honest apology. Healthcare providers must communicate clearly and effectively when working with patients and teams in our complex healthcare system. Communication skills can be learned, practiced, and mastered. Good communication skills among doctors are crucial in building a trustworthy doctor-patient relationship.

INTRODUCTION

Good communication skills have been extremely important for medical professionals in the Western world for decades. Its significance is now well acknowledged in our country too and it is the "need of the hour" in the present era.

Communication skills are a backbone, over which a lot of areas of patient care rest such as first contact patient interviews, probing for associated and additional problems, counseling the patient, explaining treatment options, its complications, and advising follow-up. It is also necessary for explaining risks to the patient, counseling in case of bereavement or mishap, providing information about a surgical procedure and its complications, taking informed consent, and a lot more other areas of patient care. Effective communication between healthcare providers and patients (and their family) results in improved healthcare outcomes and is positively correlated with patient adherence to therapeutic interventions.

Despite increasing awareness of the importance of communication skills in modern medical practice, Indian Medical Colleges have not incorporated the training in their curricula. Best teaching practices and evaluation methods to improve the skills of medical students, and to communicate optimally with patients, families, and health team members can be incorporated in undergraduate years.

COMPONENTS OF COMMUNICATION

Effective communication requires the physician to be an active listener and spend time with patients. Physicians need to listen to their patients stories and how the illness affected their patients life. Active listening takes time but can yield essential clues about the patient's health.

There are three basic components of communication verbal, nonverbal, and paraverbal. The verbal component deals with the content of the message including a selection of the words. The nonverbal component includes body language such as posture, gesture, facial expression, and spatial distance. Paraverbal components include tone, pitch, pacing, and volume of the voice. While communicating, most of us focus on the verbal component that constitutes only ten percent of the message delivered, whereas nonverbal and paraverbal components contribute ninety percent of the total message delivered.

The verbal component is quite important and it includes information about the nature, course, and prognosis of the disease; various treatment options available; nature, cost, and yield of the investigations, and risks/benefits of invasive procedures. Although the nonverbal component of communication is frequently considered less important, literature suggests that it significantly influences important outcomes, such as patients satisfaction, adherence to advice, and clinical outcomes.

BARRIERS TO GOOD COMMUNICATIONS

There are several barriers to effective communication between patients and doctors. The most important one is a lack of insight due to inadequate knowledge and training in communication skills. Many a times, doctors do not give enough heed to the importance of keeping patients adequately informed. Nonverbal components of the communication are frequently neglected. The language barrier is also important. It is not unusual for patients speaking in their local languages and giving tough time to doctors. Another important barrier is the lack of adequate knowledge about the disease or treatment options. Finally, human failings such as stress, tiredness, and lack of time are major contributing factors in an overburdened setting.

LEARN TO LISTEN TO PATIENTS PATIENTLY

The importance of listening extends far beyond the academic and professional settings and is extremely important in creating a trustworthy doctor-patient relationship, which is a prerequisite for therapeutic success. Studies exploring the reasons for filing litigations against doctors found that a significant proportion of the patients were dissatisfied, because the doctor had not listened, or understood their problem fully.

COMMUNICATING WITH ATTENDANTS

This scenario usually comes when a doctor is treating an indoor patient. Attendants are apprehensive and at times full of doubts and queries. Communicating with the attendants assumes great importance, especially when the patient is critically ill or admitted in the intensive care unit (ICU).

Certain tips to improve one's ability to communicate are summarized below:

- Never be informal with them. Conduct conferences once and if possible, twice daily.
- Talk about and appreciate the efforts made by them.
- Most of the attendants surf the internet and gather lots of information. Try to satisfy their queries by giving better references.
- Always explain the dynamic nature of the disease. This is especially important for critically ill patients.
- Second opinion should be sought proactively. This is important not only in patient management when one is in doubt, but also helpful in building the attendant's confidence.
- Never express shock. Try to convince that all efforts are being made to bring the situation under control or will be controlled.
- Consent taking is a very important part of counseling. Never neglect this and give it to paramedical staff or interns, who may fail to explain convincingly.

COMMUNICATING WITH COLLEAGUES

Junior doctors including postgraduate students, fellows, and interns along with nursing and supportive staff are part of the team. It is important to keep them united and motivated. The following principles should be followed:

- Never talk low about your colleagues or scold residents, fellows, or other students in front of patients or attendants. One should be extremely cautious while asking questions from Junior Residents on rounds. Patients may feel insecure in the absence of senior consultants, who may not be present at all the time.
- Greatest courtesy should be displayed for all staff including nurses, paramedical, and other supporting staff. Make them realize that they are a part of the team and their role and responsibility is also important. A system with effective teamwork can improve the quality of patient care and reduce workload among healthcare professionals.

MANAGING DIFFICULT ENCOUNTERS

Difficult encounters are not uncommon in medical practice. It is worth noting that difficult encounters may be consequent to a combination of factors related to the doctor, patient, and even the circumstances. It is precipitated by an imbalance between the expectations, perceptions, and conduct of the doctor and the patient involved.

At times, a patient may present with misleading information from the internet and pose a challenging situation leading to professional burnout of the physician. Furthermore, lack of adequate knowledge or time or even negative bias toward the patient's ailment maybe attributed to difficult encounters. Besides, poor communication skills and psychosocial attitudes along with lesser job satisfaction among the doctors may also be contributory.

HEALTH COMMUNICATION AND SEXUAL ORIENTATION

Medical professionals need to recognize the unique obstacles often encountered by lesbian, gay, bisexual, transgender, queer, intersex, and asexual (LGBTQIA) persons and communities. We need to create and foster the patient-clinician relationship with a population that has and continues to face discrimination from healthcare systems. One should use language that does not assume patient orientation, gender, or relationship to other persons and allows an open dialogue with patients to address a variety of issues unique to LGBTQIA persons and communities.

ROLE OF INFORMED CONSENT IN CLINICAL SETTINGS

Informed consent plays an integral role in the patient-physician relationship. The informed consent is an integral component of any clinical or research interaction with patients. The process of informed consent has evolved over the past century through numerous lessons learned from malpractice and unethical conduct of human research. The need for informed consent has been codified to highlight fundamental human rights including autonomy and integrity. The modern process of informed consent is thus regarded as a legal obligation rather than an ethical duty toward patients.

Informed consent is grounded in the principles of autonomy and respect involving a mutual understanding of the diagnosis, available treatment options, and consequences of opting for these different options. Informed consent should be provided by a capacitated patient or their proxy except for life-threatening emergencies where seeking consent would delay necessary treatment. For informed consent to be legally and ethically valid, patients must receive the necessary disclosures for decision-making, voluntarily give consent, and comprehend the information being communicated.

ESTABLISHING GOALS OF CARE

Modern patient-centered care should be respectful of and responsive to individual patient preferences, needs, and values and we should try to ensure that patient values guide all clinical decisions. However, extensive gaps exist between the patient and the care team, when establishing a patient's goals of care (GOC).

The role of the physician during GOC discussion is to provide accurate medical information about the patient's prognosis and answer any clinical questions. Challenges occur when prognosis is unclear, whether from lack of information, multiple comorbidities, or disagreement among medical providers. With evermore treatment options and new diagnoses, it is difficult to expect patients to be fully informed without the guidance of a physician. During recent years, misinformation has become a growing challenge. Most of the misinformation that patients bring to GOC discussions come from online sources, such as social media, blogs, and unreliable internet sites. As a result, physicians must not only provide accurate medical information, but also identify and correct misinformation.

BREAKING BAD NEWS

Bad news means any information that has a potential to have a devastating influence on one's life. However, its impact is highly dependent on the recipient's expectations and understanding. Disclosing bad news is a complex communication art, that not only involves the verbal component of actual news breaking, but also includes the empathetic response of the doctor to tackle the reaction. Poor communication skills of an inexperienced clinician can ruin the goal of providing support to the patient and eliciting the patient's collaboration for future treatment.

The bad news exists, regardless of whether and how we give it. Giving it well, cannot make the bad news better, but it can allow the patient to experience a caring and human connection at a difficult time, to feel that their experience is valued. It is useful to follow a strategic approach as described below, while breaking bad news and provide information according to the patient's own knowledge or expectations as well as to condense the emotional turmoil into an effective future management plan in the same setting.

Be Primed-up for the Interview

Breaking bad news is a daunting task and one should mentally rehearse the act of disclosure and the manner of reacting to the patient's emotions. Following the key communication skills such as maintaining privacy, sitting relaxed with the patient, maintaining constant eye-to-eye contact, and avoiding any time pressure, and interruptions allows an undistracted and focused discussion. If the patient wishes someone else to be with them, allow the patient to choose among relatives or friends.

Assess the Patient's Knowledge and Attitude

By asking open-ended questions, the doctor not only gains insight into the patient's perception of his medical problem, but also gets the opportunity to assess the patient's preparedness for the bad news.

Assess the Patient's Desire to Get the Level of Details of Information

Some patients may express the desire for full information about their diagnosis, prognosis, and details of their illness, while others only want to have a broad idea. Such information makes it easy for the doctor to reveal the information according to the desire of the patient.

ACTUAL BREAKING OF BAD NEWS

It is better to plan an agenda with the patients including diagnosis, treatment, prognosis, and support or coping. An initial warning may decrease the shock that can follow the disclosure of bad news. The use of simple and nontechnical words, giving information in small portions, and periodic assessment of the impact are some of the communication tools that can be extremely useful.

Addressing Patient's Emotions

The patient's emotional reaction may vary from silence to disbelief, crying, denial, or anger. It is the physician's duty to support the patient by making an empathic response. Moving closer to the patient, holding hands, and using empathic statements help the physician to not only support the patient, but also to acknowledge their own sadness and emotion. Sometimes when the patient becomes silent or tearful, allow them time to recover. Exploratory questions may be helpful, when the patient's reaction is ambiguous.

Treatment Plan and Summarize

It is important to formulate and discuss future plans of treatment with patients and/or attendants by involving them in the decision-making. Those who are having a definite plan of action are less likely to get anxious or panic. Summarizing the whole discussion in the last is extremely useful and helps in assessing if the patient has understood the facts correctly or not.

CLASSIFYING AND DISCLOSING MEDICAL ERRORS

Medical errors are common in medical practice and include adverse events, delays in care, near misses, delays in diagnosis, and unanticipated outcomes. Harm from medical error is classified as potential or actual harm, and graded in severity from no harm to death. Medical errors cause significant harm to patients and their families, including physical and emotional harm. Disclosing medical errors minimizes perceived harm of error by patients, decreases litigation, and rebuilds trust between provider and patient. Error disclosure should contain facts and an apology.

Guidelines for disclosure of errors involve a frank conversation with plain language, referring to the incident as an error, providing necessary details, and an honest apology. These conversations begin by clearly stating there was an error. They then describe the course of events, using nontechnical language. Importantly, the disclosure must contain an apology. The discussion should not be defensive, nor a statement of regret, but should provide objective facts along with a clear apology as a means of empathic human connection. Then, elicit questions or concerns and address them. Finally, plan the next steps and next contact with the patient in very clear, discrete terms. After the initial conversation, it is important to follow words with action. This includes minimizing further harm to the patient, and making institutional changes to prevent future similar events.

HANDLING HOSTILE PATIENTS

Difficult patient encounters are common, and many involve patient hostility. Patient hostility generally occurs from broken communication and/or a mismatch in goals in the patient-physician dyad. Healing the breach in the healthcare alliance requires inquiry into the cause of the patient's anger, active listening, collaboration on the next steps, and patient empowerment in creating a common goal.

Interactions between physicians and patients, like any interpersonal experience, have the potential to be challenging. Physicians have a unique opportunity to use their medical knowledge and communication skills to collaborate with even the most challenging of patient circumstances, with the understanding that it is natural to have fraught encounters from time to time.

IMPROVING COMMUNICATION SKILLS OF PHYSICIANS

Healthcare providers must communicate clearly and effectively when working with patients and teams in our complex healthcare system. Communication skills can be learned, practiced, and mastered. Foundational skills improve with deliberate practice and feedback. Many communication skills can be developed and honed, including creating rapport, setting an agenda, eliciting the patient's perspective, naming and managing emotion, providing information, checking for understanding, and collaborating on treatment plans. Studies show that effective use of communication skills leads to improved patient outcomes, patient and clinician satisfaction, and institutional metrics.

Communication skills can improve at individual, group, or systems level. Ultimately, the goal is not merely to make skills better, but also for the development and enhancement of the community, ongoing peer reinforcement of effective communication skills, and support of healthcare staff in the context of arduous work with high burnout risk. Through enhancing communication skills and thereby these individual and community connections, we can make the work of healthcare more sustainable, higher quality, and increasingly humanistic.

CONCLUSION

To conclude, good communication skills among doctors are crucial in building a trustworthy doctor-patient relationship that not only helps in therapeutic success by providing holistic care to the patient, but also leads to job satisfaction among the doctors. By actively listening, practicing empathy, and employing clear and culturally sensitive communication, internists can provide the highest level of care to their patients, while fostering positive healthcare experiences. Not many doctors are naturally blessed to have good communication skills and there is the necessity of formal training in this. Inculcating habits of good communication skills during formative years will help the medical students and future practitioners. Regular components for improving effective communication should be included in the medical school curriculum.

SUGGESTED READINGS

1. Stewart MA. Effective physician-patient communication and health outcomes: a review. CMAJ. 1995;152(9):1423-33.
2. Main CJ, Buchbinder R, Porcheret M, Foster N. Addressing patient beliefs and expectations in the consultation. Best Pract Res Clin Rheumatol. 2010;24(2):219-25.
3. Roter DL, Frankel RM, Hall JA, Sluyter D. The expression of emotion through nonverbal behavior in medical visits. Mechanisms and outcomes. J Gen Intern Med. 2006;21(Suppl 1):S28-34.
4. Lester GW, Smith SG. Listening and talking to patients. A remedy for malpractice suits? West J Med. 1993;158(3):268-72.
5. Kurtz SM. Doctor-patient communication: principles and practices. Can J Neurol Sci. 2002;29(Suppl 2):S23-9.
6. Teutsch C. Patient-doctor communication. Med Clin North Am. 2003;87(5):1115-45.
7. Lerner S, Magrane D, Friedman E. Teaching teamwork in medical education. Mt Sinai J Med. 2009;76(4):318-29.
8. Hull SK, Broquet K. How to manage difficult patient encounters. Fam Pract Manag. 2007;14(6):30-4.
9. The SUPPORT Principal Investigators. A controlled trial to improve care for seriously ill hospitalized patients. The study to understand prognoses and preferences for outcomes and risks of treatments (SUPPORT). The SUPPORT Principal Investigators. JAMA. 1995;274(20):1591-8 [Erratum: Pejic RN. The symbol of medicine: Aesculapius or cadeuceus. JAMA. 1996;24;275(16):1232].
10. Committee on Approaching Death: Addressing Key End of Life Issues; Institute of Medicine. Dying in America: Improving quality and honoring individual preferences near the end of life. Washington (DC): The National Academies Press; 2015.
11. Baile WF, Buckman R, Lenzi R, Glober G, Beale EA, Kudelka AP. SPIKES-A six-step protocol for delivering bad news: Application to the patient with cancer. Oncologist. 2000;5(4):302-11.
12. Gallagher TH, Studdert D, Levinson W. Disclosing harmful medical errors to patients. N Engl J Med. 2007;356(26):2713-9.
13. Stewart M, Brown JB, Donner A, McWhinney IR, Oates J, Weston WW, et al. The impact of patient-centered care on outcomes. J Fam Pract. 2000;49(9):796-804.

120

CHAPTER

An Approach to a Patient with Unknown Poisoning: A Toxicological Dilemma

N Madhuwanthi Hettiarachchi, Suranga Ravinda Manilgama

ABSTRACT

Self-poisoning with salicylate is potentially fatal. Salicylates are commonly used and easily accessible as over-the-counter medications, making them susceptible to abuse. While acute toxicity can be identified with an ingestion history, both acute and chronic salicylate toxicity often go unnoticed, and delayed diagnosis can result in higher morbidity and mortality rates, particularly among the elderly. When adults present with uncertain acid–base abnormalities and accompanying neurological symptoms, salicylate toxicity should be considered as a potential cause. Treatment for salicylate toxicity involves alkaline diuresis and occasionally dialysis, and the prognosis greatly depends on early recognition and prompt intervention.

INTRODUCTION

A poisoning is defined as any illness which is caused by exposure to a toxic substance. Poisoning can occur as a result of deliberate self-harm occupational, warfare hazards, or accidental exposures and due to overuse of recreational drugs and alcohol.

EPIDEMIOLOGY

Deliberate self-harm results in about 800,000 deaths each year intentional self-poisoning has become a major health burden in Sri Lanka. Impulsive poisoning is common in the young and many deaths occur due to late presentations and inability to identify the poisons. Overdoses with pharmacological substances are becoming more and more common even in Sri Lanka when compared with poisoning due to agrochemicals. The pattern of self-poisoning in Sri Lanka represents that of industrialized countries but has a higher fatality ratio.

According to a police report in Sri Lanka (in 2019) suicide mortality rate was 14.1/100,000/population.

Managing patients with suspected poisoning can be challenging due to the unknown nature of the poison and its potential consequences. In the emergency department, clinicians must adopt a systematic approach to assess and manage these cases. This approach increases the chances of identifying the cause of poisoning and providing effective treatment.

Efficiently gathering information from the patient and collateral sources is crucial. This includes prehospital care, vital signs, physical examination findings, and key clinical data. The goal is to identify potential toxicological causes while considering nontoxicological causes as well. In this context, applying the knowledge about toxidromes will be beneficial to the clinician.

Toxidrome refers to the combination of signs and symptoms that occur as a result of exposure to specific toxic agents **(Table 1)**. These toxidromes are characterized by changes in vital signs and noticeable effects on the body. The toxidromes are defined according to the size of the pupil texture of the skin secretions and vital signs and the mental status of the patient and it is a clinical diagnosis. Most poisonings do not exhibit specific toxidromes, and there can be a combination of signs and symptoms or nonspecific findings. Additionally, individuals may have varying physiological responses, leading to different outcomes. The investigations may not show a distinct pattern either. However, certain expanded toxidromes or patterns of illness related to specific organ systems can provide clues about potential causes or help rule out others.

TABLE 1: Summary of toxidromes.

Toxin	HR/BP	Respiration	Temperature	Eyes	Skin/Secretion	Mental status
Sympathomimetic	↑↑	↑	↑	●	Diaphoretic	Agitated
Anticholinergic	↑↑	↑	↑↑	●	Dry	Agitated
Cholinergic	↓↓	↓	↓	•	Copiously wet	Somnolent
Sedative Hypnotics	–	– or ↓	–	●	Normal	Somnolent/Coma
Opioids	–	↓↓	–	•	–	Somnolent-coma

(BP: blood pressure; HR: heart rate)

The complexity increases due to drugs that mimic specific classes of drugs, exposures to multiple substances, and the emergence of new synthetic illicit drugs with nonspecific clinical presentations. As only a handful of antidotes are available, management is mostly centered around administering symptomatic care, enhancing the existing physiological clearance mechanisms, and supporting the systems.

Managing complex toxicology patients with multiple coingestion is a dilemma due to the lack of consensus guidelines. In these cases, clinical expertise and a multidisciplinary approach are crucial to develop individualized patient management plans.

HISTORY AND VITAL SIGNS

When a patient with an unknown poisoning is admitted to a toxicological emergency where a patient is unable to provide a medical history, it is necessary to gather information from various other sources. Collateral history should be obtained from bystanders relatives or friends. Further information should be gathered from the scene of the incident, including details about the substances involved, any available materials such as empty pill bottles, blister packs, sachets, or chemical containers, and the possible route of exposure. It is also important to consider the number of victims and the specific situation, such as the location (indoor/outdoor and residential/nonresidential) or if it occurred in a correctional facility. Emergency medical services may have conducted environmental testing, such as measuring carbon monoxide and hydrogen sulfide levels. If the exposure happened in an occupational setting, contacting the facility to gather information on potential chemical exposures is vital. Involving family and friends can provide insights into the patient's past medical history, medication history, and social background. In cases where medication history is unreliable, reaching out to the patient's pharmacy or reviewing the state Prescription Drug Monitoring Program can reveal recent prescriptions. Electronic medical records and integrated systems across multiple institutions can also be valuable sources of information in these situations.

DIFFERENTIAL DIAGNOSIS

After assessing the vital signs look for differential diagnoses and evaluate the patient for a possible toxidrome.

Case History

A 53-year-old healthcare worker, a diagnosed patient with hypertension, dyslipidemia, and epilepsy was transferred from the peripheral hospital where he used to work early morning in a drowsy and confused state, under the influence of alcohol. The incident was suspected to have happened during his night shift. On admission his airway was patent and his respiratory rate (RR) was 14, without any features of respiratory distress. Bilateral breath sounds were equal without any added sounds and saturation of peripheral oxygen (SpO_2) was 99% on room air. His heart rate (HR) was 88 beats/min, blood pressure was 100/85 mm Hg, with normal cardiac rhythm. His Glasgow Coma Scale (GCS) was 12/15, (E4, V4, and M4) but he was drowsy and confused, bilateral pupils were 3 mm in size and were equally reacting to light. There were no neurological abnormalities. Random blood sugar was 85 mg/dL. The alcohol smell was there and there were no external injuries. His temperature was 36°C, and the clinic records were not available.

According to the information available the possible differential diagnoses were antiepileptic overdose or antihypertensive overdose or any other recreational drug abuse, methanol or ethylene glycol poisoning, alcohol overdose or alcohol withdrawal were possible toxicological etiologies.

The possibility of any other diagnosis apart from a toxicological diagnosis had to be considered as well. When the toxidrome approach is applied in this patient a sedative hypnotic syndrome is the most possible diagnosis with the available findings.

Sedative-hypnotic intoxication typically manifests as central nervous system (CNS) depression while vital signs remain within the normal range **(Table 1)**. However, in cases of severe toxicity or when combined with certain substances, vital signs may be affected. Additionally, when multiple substances are involved, changes in vital signs over time can occur, reflecting the different mechanisms of action and pharmacokinetics of each agent.

The possibility of an antihypertensive overdose as the blood pressure was slightly toward the lower side. Investigations are necessary to further narrow down the possibilities computer tomography of the brain was done at the emergency treatment unit to exclude any intracranial pathology.

When assessing and managing a patient with poisoning Resus-RSI-DEAD pathway mnemonic will be adhered to.

ASSESSMENT AND MANAGEMENT OF A POISON PATIENT

- *Resus*: Resuscitation
- *R*: Risk assessment
- *S*: Supportive care
- *I*: Investigations
- *D*: Decontamination
- *E*: Enhanced elimination
- *A*: Antidotes
- *D*: Disposition

The following investigations are usually done to arrive at a diagnosis and assess and manage the patient:

- Arterial blood gas (ABG)
- Electrocardiography (ECG)
- Random blood sugar (RBS) serum creatinine
- Full blood count (FBC)
- Creatine phosphokinase (CPK)
- Serum glutamic oxaloacetic transaminase (SGOT)/serum glutamate pyruvate transaminase (SGPT)
- International normalized ratio (INR)/activated partial thromboplastin time (aPTT)
- Serum potassium/sodium
- Ionized calcium and magnesium
- Grouping and cross matching

After the initial assessment and stabilization, conducting specific laboratory tests can provide valuable information about the cause of the illness. It is crucial to measure blood glucose immediately, followed by blood gas, electrolytes, and cooximetry. Liver function tests and renal functions are also considered as first-line investigations. Calculating the anion gap will give important clues to the diagnosis. Anion gap metabolic acidosis is a frequently observed toxicological condition with a defined set of possible causes, which can be further narrowed down based on whether blood lactate levels are elevated or within the normal range.

If facilities are available looking at ethanol level and paracetamol level will exclude the possibilities of any coingestion also.

Our patient showed evidence of a normal pH in the initial ABG.

INVESTIGATIONS

Arterial Blood Gas Results (Table 2)

The patient was managed as per the Resus–RSI–DEAD pathway. Our patient showed evidence of a normal pH (toward the alkalosis side) with normal CO_2 and normal HCO^-_3. There was a high-lactate level. The anion gap was not measured due to the unavailability of chloride. The elevated lactate level would have been due to tissue ischemia and hypoxia, evidence of dehydration, alcoholic ketoacidosis, sepsis, or may be due to metformin overdose. Gastric lavage was not done and activated was not given due to late presentation and low GCS. The patient was hydrated well with a 120 mL/h. The urine pH was 7.5. ECG was normal. He was closely monitored in the ICU. After 6 hours of admission, ABG is done. His serum calcium was corrected second ABG showed an alkaline pH with low CO_2 and low HCO^-_3.

Serum electrolytes showed persistent hypokalemia with increased lactate. RBS level was increasing.

At this juncture, the patient was having deep Kussmaul-type breathing and he was hyperventilating washing out CO_2. The patient was becoming drowsy.

After 10 hours of admission, the patient was in a deeply sedated state. RR and work of breathing increased. He was electively intubated, sedated, and ventilated. He was found to have persistently high blood pressure with early evidence of pulmonary edema He was managed with high positive end-expiratory pressure (PEEP), intravenous (IV) glyceryl trinitrate (GTN) infusion, and IV frusemide.

TABLE 2: Arterial blood gas (ABG) results.

	Day 1(1)	Day1(2)	Day1(3)	Day 2	Day 3
pH	7.417	7.47	7.37	7.6	7.2
pO_2 mm Hg		70	238	336	
pCO_2 mm Hg	39	20	27.9	12.3	42.9
Na^+ mmol/L	150	147	149	149	172
K^+ mmol/L	3.7	3.8	3.98	3.1	2.5
Ca^{2+} mmol/L	0.83	0.74	0.84	0.79	
Glucose (mg/dL)	176	168	126	118	
Lactate mmol/L	5.9	7.5	8.3	4.5	8.3
HCO_3 (mmol/L)	25.8	14.3	16.2	12.4	17.4
Cl^-	Slope	Slope	Slope		

He developed metabolic acidosis later. The possibility of salicylate poisoning was considered. Later a small note he had written on a prescription pack that he had overdosed, which contained aspirin, was found.

SALICYLATE POISONING

Salicylate is used as an analgesic, antipyretic, and antiplatelet agent. Salicylates irreversible block the cyclooxygenase-1 (COX-1) pathway and modify the COX-2 pathway.

Salicylates are found in a variety of medications, such as:

- Analgesics
- Antipyretics
- Antidiarrheal medications
- Acne treatments
- Chinese herbal preparations
- Oral antiseptic rinses

Topical ointments (e.g., oil of wintergreen): Oil of wintergreen contains 98–100% methyl salicylate, and 1 tablespoon (5 mL) contains approximately 7,000 mg of salicylate, which is equivalent to nearly 22 adult's strength aspirin tablets.

Salicylate poisoning can be categorized as either acute or chronic. Acute poisoning typically occurs in young adults with a history of psychiatric issues or previous overdose. Acute toxicity is more common in younger patients and commonly occurs due to intentional poisoning.

They often consume salicylate alone or in combination with other drugs in suicide attempts.

Chronic toxicity or therapeutic salicylate poisoning is most common in elderly patients taking aspirin for chronic inflammatory conditions. These patients may not offer a history of salicylate overdose. Chronic toxicity in the elderly is more common due to age-related decrements in renal function, hypoalbuminemia, altered end-organ sensitivity to medications, and the nonrecognition of the presence of salicylates in off-the-counter medicinal products account for an increased risk of toxicity. Chronic toxicity can result in nonspecific, delirium, confusion, dehydration, fever, and unexplained metabolic acidosis.

Cerebral edema and pulmonary edema are more common than with acute toxicity; therefore the salicylate levels should be a part of your delirium screen.

There are several differential diagnoses of salicylate poisoning.

Differential Diagnosis of Salicylate Poisoning

- Sepsis
- Acute delirium
- Organic psychosis
- Alcohol withdrawal/alcoholic ketoacidosis/acute alcohol intoxication
- Encephalopathy
- Adult respiratory distress syndrome
- Lactic acidosis or ketoacidosis, or any other cause of high anion-gap
- Metabolic acidosis
- Pulmonary embolism
- Congestive heart failure

INVESTIGATIONS

Screening should be done with ABG, 12 lead ECG, blood sugar levels, and paracetamol levels. The therapeutic range of salicylate is 1.1–2.2 mmol/L (15–30 mg/dL and 150–300 mg/L). Levels correlate poorly with the severity of toxicity but can be done every 4 hours to identify ongoing or delayed absorption from a bezoar or modified-release preparation.

Investigations will show evidence of hyper/hypoglycemia and hypokalemia acid-base disturbance—initial respiratory alkalosis, followed by elevated anion gap metabolic acidosis. If acidosis is present this is a late sign and indicates imminent demise without intervention.

Electrocardiography will show widened QRS, AV block, and ventricular arrhythmias. Full blood count and C-reactive protein (CRP) are needed to exclude any infections and sepsis, evidence of aspiration or pulmonary edema is shown by chest X-ray (CXR). Renal functions need to be checked with serum electrolytes including serum calcium and magnesium levels.

Initial respiratory alkalosis is due to stimulation of the medullary respiratory center in the brain. Over time, the uncoupling of oxidative phosphorylation (it halts the electron transport chain in the mitochondria) leads to hyperthermia, and elevated anion gap metabolic acidosis develops. However, many bedside gas machines record a normal or low anion gap by mistaking salicylate ions for chloride ions.

CLINICAL SYMPTOMS AND SIGNS

Clinical symptoms and signs may take up to 6–12 hours to manifest. There will be a rapid clinical deterioration.

Salicylate affects hydrogenase and transaminase enzymes, disrupting carbohydrate metabolism and resulting in increased production of ketone bodies as well as the buildup of lactic and pyruvic acids. Salicylate intoxication. These patients commonly present with dehydration due to volume depletion. At high doses, salicylates interfere with oxidative phosphorylation, leading to elevated body core temperature and consequent

122 CHAPTER

Implementation of New Trends in the Field of Medicine in the Consumer Protection Act Era

RM Chhabra, Sunil Kumar Bakshi, Manoj Vimal

ABSTRACT

As science is advancing, the treatment of diseases with new trends, either with drugs or technology, is on changing with the emergence of drugs or technologies. With lots of research, trials, studies, clinical experiences, and clinical trials various treatment options are available. They are approved by authorities, such as Central Drugs Standard Control Organization (CDSCO), and Food and Drug Administration (FDA), and then implemented in clinical practice.

Research, trials, studies, clinical experiences, and clinical trials with various trends require a lot of finances, manpower, government approvals, healthcare providers, laboratories, etc. After clinical trials, these new trends are used for treatment purposes.

INTRODUCTION

Implementation of new drugs, trends, and technology, a clinician requires proper guidelines laid down by authorities after proper research and clinical trials approved by the government of respective departments, especially in this era.

IMPLEMENTATION OF NEW TRENDS

Incorporating new trends in medicine in the Consumer Protection Act (CPA) era is a complex process that requires collaboration between government agencies, healthcare providers, industry stakeholders, and patients' advocates. The overarching goal should be to balance innovation and patient protection, ensuring that consumers have access to cutting-edge medical care while also safeguarding their rights and well-being.

Change in Scenario after Consumer Protection Act

The CPA, 1986 has had a significant impact on the health-care delivery system in India. It has brought about several changes in the healthcare landscape, benefiting patients and improving the quality of healthcare services. Here are some of the key changes and their effects:

- *Informed consent*: The Act ensures that patients are fully informed about the risks and benefits of new medical treatments or procedures.
- *Regulatory oversight*: The Act strengthens regulatory agencies responsible for overseeing medical practices, drugs, and devices. These agencies should have the capacity to assess the safety and efficacy of emerging medical technologies and treatments.
- *Clinical trials and evidence-based medicine*: The Act encourages healthcare providers to participate in clinical trials and adopt evidence-based practices. It supports research institutions and collaborations that generate high-quality data on new medical interventions.
- *Transparency*: The Act promotes transparency in medical pricing and outcomes.
- *Personalized medicine*: The Act emphasizes the development and implementation of personalized medicine approaches. These treatments are tailored to individual patients' genetic, environmental, and lifestyle factors, potentially improving outcomes and reducing side effects.

- *Artificial intelligence (AI) and data security*: The Act embraces AI and data analytics in healthcare for improved diagnostics, treatment planning, and patient management. However, it establishes robust data security and privacy regulations to protect patients' information.
- *Alternative therapies*: The Act acknowledges and regulates alternative and complementary therapies. It ensures that practitioners of these therapies meet appropriate standards of education and training.
- *Patient advocacy*: The Act encourages the formation of patient advocacy groups and empowers them to participate in healthcare decision-making processes. These groups can help ensure that patient perspectives are considered in the development and implementation of new medical trends.
- *Conflict of interest disclosure*: The Act requires healthcare providers to disclose any financial interests they have in pharmaceutical companies or medical device manufacturers. This transparency can help mitigate conflicts of interest that may compromise patient care.
- *Continuing education*: The Act promotes continuing education and training for healthcare professionals to keep them updated on the latest medical trends and technologies.
- *Insurance coverage*: The Act ensures that insurance providers cover new and innovative treatments that have been proven effective and safe, thus making these options accessible to a wider range of patients.
- *Ethical considerations*: The Act maintains a strong focus on ethical considerations, including equitable access to healthcare, especially in the context of emerging trends that may be expensive or inaccessible to certain populations.
- *Enhanced patient rights*: The Act has reinforced the rights of healthcare consumers, ensuring that patients are informed about their rights, including the right to information, choice, and redressal. This has empowered patients to actively participate in their healthcare decisions and demand quality services.

Implementation of New Trends in the Field of Medicine

The implementation of new trends in the field of medicine can be challenging due to several limitations and barriers. These limitations can hinder the adoption of innovative medical practices and technologies. Some of the key limitations include:

- *Regulatory hurdles*: The stringent regulatory requirements for new medical treatments and technologies can slow down their adoption. Clinical trials, approvals, and compliance with regulatory agencies can be time-consuming and expensive.
- *Cost*: Many innovative medical treatments and technologies are expensive to develop and implement. The high costs can limit their accessibility to a broader population, especially in resource-constrained healthcare systems.
- *Lack of evidence*: New medical trends often lack a robust body of evidence supporting their efficacy and safety. Healthcare providers may be hesitant to adopt these trends without clear data on their benefits.
- *Resistance to change*: Healthcare professionals and institutions may resist adopting new trends due to the inertia of established practices. There can be a reluctance to change clinical routines and procedures.
- *Limited access*: Inequality in access to healthcare can hinder the implementation of new trends. Patients in rural or underserved areas may have limited access to innovative treatments and technologies.
- *Insurance coverage*: Limited or lack of insurance coverage for new treatments can discourage patients from pursuing them. Insurers may be slow to adapt their coverage policies to include emerging trends.
- *Healthcare infrastructure*: Inadequate healthcare infrastructure, such as a lack of advanced diagnostic equipment or trained personnel, can limit the implementation of new medical technologies.
- *Ethical and legal issues*: New trends may raise ethical and legal questions, such as those related to patient privacy, consent, and liability. Addressing these issues can delay implementation.
- *Patient education*: Patients may lack awareness and understanding of new trends in medicine, making it difficult for them to make informed choices or request specific treatments.
- *Data privacy and security*: The collection and use of patient data in innovative healthcare technologies can raise concerns about privacy and security. Ensuring data protection can be a significant challenge.
- *Health disparities*: New trends may exacerbate health disparities, as certain populations may not have equal access or resources to benefit from these innovations.
- *Resource allocation*: Deciding where to allocate limited healthcare resources can be a complex issue. Choices must be made about which new trends to be prioritized for implementation.
- *Cultural and societal factors*: Cultural beliefs, societal attitudes, and patients' preferences can affect the acceptance and implementation of new medical trends.

- *Healthcare workforce training*: Preparing healthcare professionals to use new technologies and treatments effectively often requires specialized training, which can be time-consuming and costly.
- *Market dynamics*: Market forces and competition among healthcare providers and pharmaceutical companies can influence the adoption of new trends. Profit motives may not always align with patients' needs.

Overcoming these limitations often requires a coordinated effort among healthcare stakeholders, including governments, healthcare providers, insurers, researchers, and patient advocacy groups. It involves not only addressing the technical and scientific aspects of new trends, but also addressing the socioeconomic and ethical considerations associated with their implementation. Policymakers play a crucial role in creating an environment that supports the responsible adoption of new trends while ensuring patient safety and equitable access to healthcare innovations.

FIVE MAJOR RIGHTS

In India, consumers of healthcare services have certain rights that are protected by law. These rights are essential to ensure that patients receive quality care and are treated fairly within the healthcare system. Here are five major consumer rights in healthcare in India.

Right to Information

Patients have the right to be informed about their medical condition, diagnosis, treatment options, and potential risks and benefits. Healthcare providers are obligated to provide clear and accurate information in a language that the patient understands. Additionally, patients have the right to access their medical records and reports.

Right to Quality Care

Patients have the right to receive healthcare services that meet a certain standard of quality. This includes the right to treatment by qualified and competent healthcare professionals, the use of up-to-date medical practices, and access to safe and effective medications and medical devices.

Right to Privacy and Confidentiality

Patients have the right to privacy and confidentiality regarding their medical information. Healthcare providers must ensure that patient records and personal health information are kept confidential, and are only disclosed to authorized individuals or entities with the patient's consent or as required by law.

Right to Choose

Patients have the right to choose their healthcare provider and treatment options, and they have the right to refuse medical treatment or interventions. This includes the right to seek a second opinion, and the right to be informed about the cost of treatment.

Right to Redressal

Patients have the right to seek redressal and compensation for any harm or negligence experienced during healthcare treatment. There are various mechanisms in place, such as consumer forums and healthcare Ombudsman, which patients can utilize to file complaints and seek resolution.

It is important to note that these rights are protected under various laws and regulations in India, including the CPA, 2019 and the Clinical Establishments (Registration and Regulation) Act, 2010. Patients should be aware of their rights and should not hesitate to assert them when seeking healthcare services. Additionally, healthcare providers are expected to respect and uphold these rights to ensure that patients receive ethical and quality care.

CONCLUSION

In the era of the CPA, the implementation of new trends in the field of medicine represents a complex and delicate balancing act. While innovation in healthcare holds the promise of improved patient outcomes and expanded treatment options, it must occur within a framework that prioritizes patient safety, rights, and equitable access to care.

Key considerations include navigating stringent regulatory requirements, ensuring affordability and access to new treatments, relying on robust scientific evidence, addressing ethical concerns, promoting healthcare equity, and maintaining patient privacy and data security.

Moreover, healthcare providers and policymakers must uphold the principles of transparency, informed consent, and quality care while fostering an environment that encourages patient education and empowerment.

Ultimately, the successful implementation of new medical trends under the CPA requires a multidisciplinary approach involving healthcare stakeholders, regulators, patients, and advocates. It is a dynamic process that seeks to harmonize innovation and consumer protection to ensure the highest standards of healthcare for all.

SUGGESTED READINGS

1. Balarajan Y, Selvaraj S, Subramanian SV. Health care and equity in India. Lancet. 2011;377:505-15.
2. Ministry of Health and Family Welfare, Government of India. (2017). National Health Accounts: Estimates for India 2014-15. [online] Available from https://nhsrcindia.org/sites/default/files/2021-06/NHA%20Estimates%20Report%20-14-15.pdf [Last accessed December, 2023].
3. Rao M, Rao KD, Shiva Kumar AK, Chatterjee M, Sundararaman T. Human resources for health in India. Lancet. 2011;377:587-98.
4. Rao KD. (2012). Situation Analysis of the Health Workforce in India. Human Resources Technical Paper I. Public Health Foundation of India. [online] Available from https://api.semanticscholar.org/CorpusID:3938944 [Last accessed January, 2024].
5. Tamanna MZ, Eram U, Al Harbi TM, Alrashdi SA, Khateeb SU, Aladhrai SA, et al. Clinical value of leukocyte counts in evaluation of patients with suspected appendicitis in emergency department. Ulus Travma Acil Cerrahi Derg. 2012;18:474-8.
6. He Y, Aliyu A, Evans M, Luo C. Health care cybersecurity challenges and solutions under the climate of COVID-19: Scoping review. J. Med. Internet Res. 2021;23(4):e21747.
7. Ekblaw A, Azaria A, Halamka JD, Lippman A; MIT Media Lab, Beth Israel Deaconess Medical Center. (2016). A case study for blockchain in healthcare: "MedRec" prototype for electronic health records and medical research data. [online] Available from https://www.healthit.gov/sites/default/files/5-56-onc_blockchainchallenge_mitwhitepaper.pdf [Last accessed January, 2024].
8. Gulliford M, Figueroa-Munoz J, Morgan M, Hughes D, Gibson B, Beech R, et al. What does 'access to health care' mean? J Health Serv Res Policy. 2002;7:186-8.
9. World Health Organization. (2023). Maternal mortality. [online] Available from http://www.who.int/mediacentre/factsheets/fs348/en/ [Last accessed December, 2023].
10. Ministry of Health and Family Welfare. (2018). Charter of Patients' Rights for adoption by NHRC. [online] Available from https://main.mohfw.gov.in/sites/default/files/PatientCharterforcomments.pdf [Last accessed December, 2023].

diagnostic electrocardiogram (ECG) findings. Approximately 30% of such patients have a completely blocked coronary artery without the characteristic ECG ST-segment elevation. Additionally, around 25% of patients diagnosed with acute myocardial infarction (MI) initially exhibit a negative troponin blood test for myocardial injury. Addressing this concern, Al-Zaiti et al. conducted a study developing a risk score and tested it for prospective assessment and external validation across independent health systems.

Remarkably, the "SMART" AI-derived risk score accurately reclassified 1 in 3 patients. The study focused on elucidating the 25 most critical features contributing to the model's accuracy. This AI model outperformed both clinical experts and commercial ECG interpretation systems. The study marked a pioneering effort, leveraging machine learning and novel ECG features for optimizing the detection of occlusive heart attacks (MI) in patients presenting with negative ST elevation MI patterns on their initial ECGs.

- *Newer versions of large language models are answering medical questions increasingly correctly*: A recent report by Google AI researchers, led by Karan Singhal, tracked the progression of their language models from Flan-PaLM to Med-PaLM. In addition to surpassing the passing threshold for the United States Medical Licensing Examination (USMLE), Med-PaLM exhibited substantial advancements in accurate comprehension, retrieval, and reasoning for 140 medical questions, compared to Flan-PaLM.

  The clinician panel evaluation demonstrated that while 61.9% of Flan-PaLM's long-form answers aligned with scientific consensus, Med-PaLM's score surged to 92.6%, approaching parity with clinician-generated answers (92.9%). However, the AI models performed unfavorably in terms of incorrectness. Although increased bias was not observed, the AI models demonstrated weaker performance in inappropriate/incorrect content and potential harm likelihood. The authors acknowledged these limitations and emphasized the need for robust evaluation frameworks and method development in crafting safe and effective clinical large language models (LLMs).

  Notably, the Med-PaLM2 model showcased superior performance compared to the published "Nature" paper on Med-PaLM. This acceleration in fine-tuning LLMs surpasses the pace of peer-reviewed publications, suggesting a promising trajectory for future improvements. The competitive landscape includes Google, Microsoft, and other tech giants alongside startups with impressive LLMs, with a notable emphasis on healthcare applications, as highlighted in a recent Wall Street Journal (WSJ) article.
- *AI outshines in health care at paperwork*: New York Times front-page article highlighted the use of AI-generated conversations during clinic visits to streamline note-taking, treatment planning, and billing. This AI application aims to alleviate the documentation burden on doctors and combat burnout, with the synthetic note cross-checked against spoken words for accuracy. The software simplifies medical terms and provides a color-coded recording of the visit, allowing patients to review medical moments. While the potential to reduce documentation is promising, robust data and prospective peer-reviewed studies are currently lacking. This application does not require regulatory oversight, distinguishing it from other AI uses. The discussed advantages and challenges of AI emphasize responsible implementation and ethical considerations.

CONCLUSION

Our actual intelligence lies in our ability to make the best use of AI, considering its constraints and deploying it to maximize its benefits while mitigating its pitfalls. By continuously advancing AI research, implementing robust regulations, and fostering a harmonious collaboration between humans and AI systems, we need to endeavor to shape a future where AI stands as a formidable instrument of advancement without infringing upon human welfare.

SUGGESTED READINGS

1. Flanagin A, Bibbins-Domingo K, Berkwits M, Christiansen SL. Nonhuman "Authors" and Implications for the Integrity of Scientific Publication and Medical Knowledge. JAMA. 2023;329(8):637-39.
2. Else H. Abstracts Written by ChatGPT Fool Scientists. Nature. 2023;613(7944):423.
3. Beutel G, Geerits E, Kielstein JT. Artificial hallucination: GPT on LSD? Crit Care. 2023;27:148.
4. HIMSS. (2020). AI in Healthcare: How It's Changing the Industry. [online] Available from https://www.himss.org/resources/ai-healthcare-how-its-changing-industry [Last accessed December, 2023].

5. Houssami N, Kirkpatrick-Jones G, Noguchi N, Lee CI. Artificial Intelligence (AI) for the early detection of breast cancer: a scoping review to assess AI's potential in breast screening practice. Expert Rev Med Devices. 2019;16(5): 351-62.
6. National Cancer Institute. (2022). Can Artificial Intelligence Help See Cancer in New, and Better, Ways? [online] Available from https://www.cancer.gov/news-events/cancer-currents-blog/2022/artificial-intelligence-cancer-imaging [Last accessed December, 2023].
7. Paul D, Sanap G, Shenoy S, Kalyane D, Kalia K, Tekade RK. Artificial intelligence in drug discovery and development. Drug Discov Today. 2021;26(1):80-93.
8. Johnson KB, Wei WQ, Weeraratne D, Frisse ME, Misulis K, Rhee K, et al. Precision Medicine, AI, and the Future of Personalized Health Care. Clin Transl Sci. 2021;14(1):86-93.
9. Pyrros A, Borstelmann SM, Mantravadi R. Zaiman Z, Thomas K, Price B, et al. Opportunistic detection of type 2 diabetes using deep learning from frontal chest radiographs. Nat Commun. 2023;14(1):4039.
10. Ueda D, Matsumoto T, Ehara S, Yamamoto A, Walston SL, Ito A, et al. Artificial Intelligence-Based Model to Classify Cardiac Functions from Chest Radiographs: A Multi-Institutional, Retrospective Model Development and Validation Study. Lancet Digital Health. 2023;5(8):e525-33.
11. Al-Zaiti S, Martin-Gill C, Zègre-Hemsey JK, Bouzid Z, Faramand Z, Alrawashdeh MO, et al. Machine Learning for ECG Diagnosis and Risk Stratification of Occlusion Myocardial Infarction. Nat Med. 2023;29(7):1804-13.
12. Singhal K, Azizi S, Tu T, Mahdavi SS, Wei J, Chung HW, et al. Large Language Models Encode Clinical Knowledge. Nature. 2023;620(7972):172-80.
13. Lohr S. (2023). A.I. May Someday Work Medical Miracles. For Now, It Helps Do Paperwork. [online] Available from https://www.nytimes.com/2023/06/26/technology/ai-health-care-documentation.html?searchResultPosition=1 [Last accessed December, 2023].

124

CHAPTER

Sodium-glucose Cotransporter-2 Inhibitor and Genital Tract Infection: How to Tackle in Clinical Practice

NK Singh, Vaibhav Agnihotri, Leena Singh, Richa Manaswita

ABSTRACT

Sodium-glucose cotransporter-2 (SGLT-2) inhibitor medications have shown a significantly increased risk of genital tract infections (GTIs), although there is inconsistent reporting regarding the incidence of urinary tract infections (UTIs) compared to other antidiabetic drugs.

The glycosuria induced by SGLT-2 inhibitor predisposes individuals to the development of GTIs, including balanitis and balanoposthitis in men and vulvovaginitis in women. Moreover, GTIs occur more frequently in uncircumcised men. *Candida albicans* has been identified as the most common pathogen causing these infections.

Various factors contribute to the predisposition of individuals with type 2 diabetes mellitus to genital infections and UTIs, including glucosuria, bacterial adherence to the uroepithelium, and immune dysfunction. However, the precise role of glucosuria as a causative factor for these infections is not yet fully understood.

Some recent trials and pharmacovigilance databases support the notion that combination therapy with a dipeptidyl peptidase 4 (DPP-4) inhibitor may reduce the frequency of GTIs associated with SGLT-2 inhibitors.

In the era of SGLT-2 inhibitors, physicians need more awareness about when to suspect and how to tackle GTIs.

INTRODUCTION

Patients with type 2 diabetes mellitus are more likely to have genital tract colonization with *Candida* species, and the risk of genital mycotic infections (GMIs) is higher in patients with diabetes. In a population-based study conducted in the United Kingdom, it was found that diabetic women had a risk ratio of 1.81 [95% confidence interval (CI) 1.64–2.0] for vaginitis and diabetic men had a risk ratio of 2.85 (95% CI 2.84–4) for balanitis compared to individuals without diabetes. These findings suggest an increased susceptibility to fungal infections in individuals with diabetes.

Furthermore, several systematic reviews and meta-analyses have shown a four- to eightfold increased risk of GMIs in patients taking sodium-glucose cotransporter-2 (SGLT-2) inhibitors compared to those taking a placebo or other hypoglycemic agents.

MECHANISTIC CONSIDERATIONS

The urinary glucose excretion in patients taking SGLT-2 inhibitors can indeed reach high levels, with reported values of up to 90 g/day. This high concentration of glucose in the urine provides an ideal environment for the growth of microorganisms, including *Candida* species.

The average daily volume of urine excreted in individuals corresponds to a urinary glucose concentration of approximately 30 g/L. This concentration is similar to that of Sabouraud agar, which is a culture medium commonly used to promote the growth of yeast, including *Candida* species. The similarity in glucose concentrations between urine and Sabouraud agar provides a biologically plausible explanation for the increased risk of GMIs observed in patients taking SGLT-2 inhibitors **(Boxes 1 and 2)**.

BOX 1: Factors contributing to an increased risk of genital mycotic infections.

- High glucose concentration in the urine
- Altered immune response often associated with diabetes
- Impaired mucosal defense mechanisms
- Changes in vaginal pH
- Increased adherence of *Candida* species to the genital tract
- Anatomical abnormalities

BOX 2: Predisposing factors contributing to genital infections.

- Poor hygiene
- Topical corticosteroid use
- Pharmacologically induced glucosuria
- Pregnancy, estrogen, and oral contraceptive use
- Moist and warm environment of the genital area
- Genital infections in diabetes are often not transmitted sexually
- Circumcision in men—indirectly related to lower incidence of genital infection

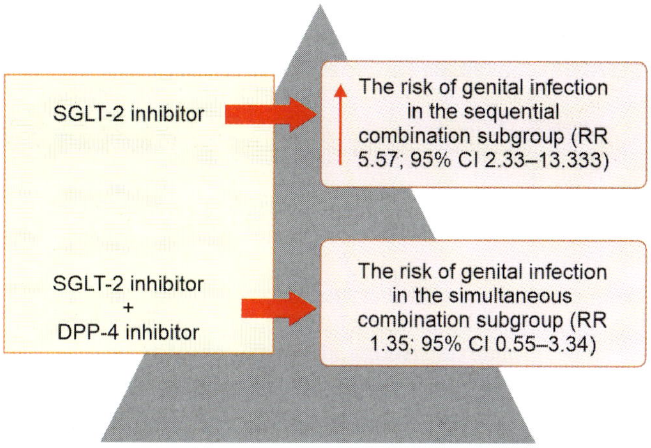

FIG. 1: Simultaneous combination versus the sequential combination.

(CI: confidence interval; DPP-4: dipeptidyl peptidase 4; RR: relative risk; SGLT-2: sodium-glucose cotransporter-2)

Source: Min SH, Yoon JH, Moon SJ, Hahn S, Cho YM. Combination of sodium-glucose cotransporter 2 inhibitor and dipeptidyl peptidase-4 inhibitor in type 2 diabetes: a systematic review with meta-analysis. Sci Rep. 2028;8(1):4466.

URINARY TRACT INFECTION-RELATED ISSUES

Based on early reports and concerns raised by a limited number of cases, there were initial concerns regarding an increased risk of urinary tract infections (UTIs) associated with SGLT-2 inhibitors. However, subsequent data from large randomized clinical trials and real-world population-based studies have not demonstrated a significant elevation in the risk of UTIs among patients using SGLT-2 inhibitors.

ADDING DIPEPTIDYL PEPTIDASE 4 INHIBITOR WITH SODIUM-GLUCOSE COTRANSPORTER-2 INHIBITOR: REALITY VERSUS HYPE

The exact nature of the interaction between dipeptidyl peptidase 4 (DPP-4) and SGLT-2 proteins and its impact on GTIs require further investigation. Some studies have suggested that DPP-4 inhibitors may have antimicrobial properties by inhibiting the DPP-4 enzyme in these microbes, rendering them inactive or less virulent.

It is important to note that these are hypothetical explanations, and the precise mechanisms underlying the observed moderation of GTIs with fixed-dose combinations (FDCs) compared to SGLT-2 inhibitor monotherapy are not yet fully understood.

The analysis of the Food and Drug Administration (FDA) Adverse Event Reporting System revealed that the frequency of genitourinary tract infections (GUTIs) among reports listing both SGLT-2 and DPP-4 inhibitors as suspect or concomitant drugs was significantly lower compared to reports listing SGLT-2 inhibitors without DPP-4 inhibitors.

SIMULTANEOUS COMBINATION VERSUS SEQUENTIAL COMBINATION

Taken together, the data from randomized controlled trials (RCTs) and pharmacovigilance databases provide consistent evidence that combination therapy involving a DPP-4 inhibitor can effectively reduce the frequency of GUTIs associated with SGLT-2 inhibitors. These findings have important implications for clinical practice, as GUTIs are a common adverse effect of SGLT-2 inhibitors and can significantly impact the patient's well-being.

Incorporating a DPP-4 inhibitor as part of combination therapy may therefore be considered as a strategy to mitigate this particular side effect and enhance the overall safety profile of SGLT-2 inhibitors **(Fig. 1)**.

RESTARTING SODIUM-GLUCOSE COTRANSPORTER-2 INHIBITOR AFTER URINARY TRACT INFECTION/GENITAL TRACT INFECTION (BOX 3)

It is worth noting that while the recommendations by South Asian Federation of Endocrine Societies (SAFES) are specific to the South Asian region, they may provide

BOX 3: South Asian Federation of Endocrine Societies (SAFES) consensus statement advocates.

- *Perineal hygiene*: The consensus statement emphasizes the importance of maintaining perineal hygiene to prevent GTIs
- *Prophylactic antifungal coverage*: In patients with a history of GTIs, the consensus statement suggests considering prophylactic antifungal coverage when initiating SGLT-2 inhibitor therapy
- *Avoidance in specific cases*: The consensus statement recommends avoiding SGLT-2 inhibitors in certain situations. These include cases with a previous history of upper UTIs, complicated GTIs, or refractory/resistant GTIs

(GTIs: genital tract infections; SGLT-2: sodium-glucose cotransporter-2; UTIs: urinary tract infections)

TABLE 1: Keep watch on possible GTIs with SGLT-2 inhibitor.

Men	
Balanitis	Skin cuts at glans, soreness, and redness
Balanoposthitis	Watch for thick curdy discharge under the foreskin
Urethritis	Burning sensation and itching
Epididymo-orchitis	Scrotal area pain
Women	
Vaginitis	Itching, burning, and red skin of the vulva
Vulvovaginitis	• Thrush patches–usually found loosely adherent to the vulva • Thick, white, and curd-like vaginal discharge • Foul smell
Pelvic inflammatory disease	Pelvic pain

(GTIs: genital tract infections; SGLT-2: sodium-glucose cotransporter-2)

valuable insights and considerations for healthcare professionals globally.

TREATMENT PEARLS (TABLE 1)

Education to Patient is Essential

It is important to provide patient education regarding perineal hygiene as a proactive measure for all diabetic patients, regardless of the type of antidiabetic therapy they are receiving **(Box 4)**.

Treatment of *Candida* Balanitis

Balanitis refers to inflammation of the head of the penis, and when caused by the *Candida* species, it is referred to as *Candida* balanitis **(Box 5)**.

BOX 4: Some key recommendations for perineal hygiene that must be followed.

- Washing the genital organs after urination or defecation using clean water or mild soap if necessary
- Using routine hygienic wipes or sprays for additional cleanliness
- Advising women to wash from front to back to prevent the spread of bacteria from the anal area to the urinary tract
- Uncircumcised males should retract the prepuce before washing and use clean water or mild soap if needed
- It is advisable not to use alcohol-based disinfectants for washing the genital area

BOX 5: Key points regarding the treatment of *Candida* balanitis.

- *Frequent normal saline washes*: Maintaining good hygiene is essential in the management of balanitis. Frequent washing of the affected area with normal saline (a saltwater solution) can help in reducing inflammation and preventing infection spread
- *Antifungal cream*: Topical antifungal therapy is the mainstay of treatment for *Candida* balanitis. Clotrimazole cream 1% is commonly recommended and should be applied twice a day for a duration of 10 days. Miconazole cream 2% can be used as an alternative to clotrimazole
- *Treatment duration*: While relief from symptoms is often immediate, it is crucial to continue the treatment for the full recommended duration of 10 days. This ensures complete eradication of the *Candida* infection and reduces the risk of recurrence
- *Addition of topical steroids*: In mild cases, the use of topical steroids is generally not recommended. However, in cases with marked inflammation, 1% hydrocortisone (a mild topical steroid) can be used in combination with topical antifungal agents such as imidazole. The addition of steroids helps to reduce inflammation and alleviate symptoms
- *Topical therapy sufficiency*: In most cases of *Candida* balanitis, topical therapy alone is sufficient for effective treatment. Systemic (oral) antifungal medications are typically reserved for more severe or recurrent cases

Vulvovaginitis

The diagnosis of a suspected *Candida* infection can be achieved by performing a wet-mount preparation using saline and 10% potassium hydroxide. This method helps identify the presence of yeast or hyphae, in addition to assessing the vaginal pH, which should fall within the normal range of 4.0–4.5. If the findings from the wet-mount preparation are negative, vaginal cultures for *Candida* should be obtained to ensure an accurate diagnosis.

Early initiation of antifungal therapy, guided by appropriate culture results, is crucial for effectively managing severe systemic *Candida* infections. Azoles, particularly fluconazole, have become the primary choice of treatment in recent years. A single dose of fluconazole or a short course of fluconazole for 3 days has shown response rates exceeding 90%.

In complicated cases of vulvovaginal candidiasis, intravaginal therapy with topical agents or oral fluconazole may be required. While most *Candida* species respond well to treatment, *C. krusei* and *C. glabrata* infections pose challenges. Managing *C. glabrata* infections may involve alternative approaches, as azole therapy may be ineffective. Additionally, although rare, resistance to fluconazole and azole-class drugs has been observed in *C. albicans* infections, particularly in individuals with prolonged exposure to these medications.

Recurrent vulvovaginal candidiasis is typically caused by azole-susceptible *C. albicans*, and contributing factors such as diabetes are uncommon. Treatment involves induction therapy followed by maintenance therapy, with a weekly dose of 150 mg of fluconazole being the most convenient option. After discontinuing maintenance therapy, a recurrence rate of 40–50% can be expected. Alternative options include topical clotrimazole cream, clotrimazole vaginal suppositories, or intermittent use of other oral or topical antifungal treatments.

In addition to the currently available treatments, there are several newer investigational agents that are currently undergoing clinical trials for the management of candidiasis. One such agent is ibrexafungerp, which is a glucan-synthase inhibitor. It has received approval in 2021 for oral formulation and is used for the treatment of vulvovaginal candidiasis. However, the parenteral formulation of ibrexafungerp is still under investigation for its efficacy in treating candidemia and invasive candidiasis.

Another promising investigational agent is rezafungin, which belongs to the echinocandin class of antifungal drugs. Rezafungin is unique in that it is a long-acting formulation administered once a week.

ONGOING GENIUS STUDY 2023

At present, no clear real-world data exists in India about the prevalence of GTI and UTI and its association with various factors such as ethnicity, regionality, hygiene, circumcision, and climate. Wide variation in the prevalence of GTI and UTI with the use of SGLT-2 inhibitors exists from single-center studies from India. A study to estimate the prevalence of GTI/UTI in patients receiving SGLT-2 inhibitors and the impact of gliptins on the prevalence is going on at pan Indian in 44 centers by author's initiated research.

CONCLUSION

It is important for individuals with diabetes who are taking SGLT-2 inhibitors to be aware of this potential risk and to promptly seek medical attention if they experience symptoms of genital fungal infections such as itching, burning, discharge, or discomfort in the genital area.

Considering the cultural background in South Asia, it is important to recognize that women may feel hesitant to disclose information regarding GTIs.

Therefore, it is crucial to prioritize privacy and approach the collection of this information with empathy.

SUGGESTED READINGS

1. Bartolo C, Hall V, Friedman ND, Lanyon C, Fuller A, Morrissey CO, et al. Bittersweet: infective complications of drug-induced glycosuria in patients with diabetes mellitus on SGLT2-inhibitors: two case reports. BMC Infect Dis. 2021;21(1):284.
2. Perkovic V, Jardine MJ, Neal B, Bompoint S, Heerspink HJL, Charytan DM, et al. Canagliflozin and Renal Outcomes in Type 2 Diabetes and Nephropathy. N Engl J Med. 2019;380(24):2295-306.
3. Heise T, Seewaldt-Becker E, Macha S, Hantel S, Pinnetti S, Seman L, et al. Safety, tolerability, pharmacokinetics and pharmacodynamics following 4 weeks' treatment with empagliflozin once daily in patients with type 2 diabetes. Diabetes Obes Metab. 2013;15(7):613-21.
4. Nyirjesy P, Zhao Y, Ways K, Usiskin K. Evaluation of vulvovaginal symptoms and Candida colonization in women with type 2 diabetes mellitus treated with canagliflozin, a sodium glucose co-transporter 2 inhibitor. Curr Med Res Opin. 2012;28(7):1173-8.
5. Wiegley N, So PN. Sodium-Glucose Cotransporter 2 Inhibitors and Urinary Tract Infection: Is There Room for Real Concern? Kidney360. 2022;3(11):1991-3.
6. Min SH, Yoon JH, Moon SJ, Hahn S, Cho YM. Combination of sodium-glucose cotransporter 2 inhibitor and dipeptidyl peptidase-4 inhibitor in type 2 diabetes: a systematic review with meta-analysis. Sci Rep.2028;8(1):4466.
7. Fadini GP, Bonora BM, Mayur S, Rigato M, Avogaro A. Dipeptidyl peptidase-4 inhibitors moderate the risk of genitourinary tract infections associated with sodium-glucose co-transporter-2 inhibitors. Diabetes Obes Metab. 2018;20(3):740-4.
8. Kalra S, Ghosh S, Aamir AH, Ahmed MT, Amin MF, Bajaj S, et al. Safe and pragmatic use of sodium-glucose co-transporter 2 inhibitors in type 2 diabetes mellitus: South Asian Federation of Endocrine Societies consensus statement. Indian J Endocrinol Metab. 2017;21(1):210-30.
9. Pappas PG, Kauffman CA, Andes DR, Clancy CJ, Marr KA, Ostrosky-Zeichner L, et al. Clinical Practice Guideline for the Management of Candidiasis: 2016 Update by the Infectious Diseases Society of America. Clinical Infectious Diseases. 2016;62(4):1-50.
10. Colombo RE, Vazquez JA. An evaluation of ibrexafungerp for the treatment of invasive candidiasis: the evidence to date. Expert Opin Pharmacother. 2021;22(7):797-807.

125

CHAPTER

Artificial Intelligence and Electrocardiogram

SB Gupta

ABSTRACT

Artificial intelligence (AI) is the latest technology to train the computer systems. Using AI techniques, with deep-learning processes, making use of sophisticated networks like convolution neural network (CNN), will be boon to health industry. AI has been used to detect various parameters and cardiovascular conditions, which is beyond the imagination.

INTRODUCTION

Artificial intelligence (AI) has revolutionized the science by predictions using computer-based algorithms that no one expected. Machine learning is the basis of AI where computers are allowed to learn, directly from the vast data. In medicine, the principle is utilized to differentiate between healthy and disease. In healthcare system, AI is being used for screening, disease detection and classification, risk-stratification, and proper therapy selection.

Computers are made to work like human brain with interconnected nodes called as neurons, arranged in a network layout. This process is called deep learning and the network is called convolutional neural network.

Basically, there are three steps of deep learning:

1. Training
2. Internal validation
3. Testing

For example, lakhs of electrocardiograms (ECGs) of males are fed to a machine, so that it learns to identify the ECG of males. Similarly, lakhs of ECGs of females are fed to the machine to learn the ECG of females. Then, a set of ECGs, again in lakhs, are fed and machine identifies whether the ECG is of male or female, and the accuracy is estimated. This process is known as internal validation. If accuracy is acceptable, then the machine is subjected to test the data given.

AGE AND SEX ESTIMATION USING ARTIFICIAL INTELLIGENCE FROM STANDARD 12-LEAD ECGS

Convolutional neural networks were trained to predict age and sex using 10-second, 12-lead ECG from 499,727 patients by Attia et al. 399,750 patients were in the training set and 99,977 patients were in the internal validation set. Mean age of the patients was 58.6 ± 16.2 years and 52% were males. Then, 275,056 ECGs were the testing set. Apart from the above data set, 100 patients were selected randomly and their multiple ECGs over two decades were also tested for their chronological age against convolution neural network (CNN)-predicted age at that year of life.

For all patients, clinical history was extracted for previous history of diabetes, hypertension, coronary artery disease (CAD), myocardial infarction (MI), low ejection fraction (EF), arrhythmias, and any cardiac surgery. For the set of 100 patients, in the follow-up period, history for any incident events was recorded like history of hospitalizations for any hemodynamic shock, new diagnosis of CAD, heart failure (HF), any thromboembolic events, and cardiac transplantation.

For each ECG, the algorithm output gave a probability number for sex determination. Number closer to zero had high probability of being female, while a number closer to 1 means high probability of being male. The overall accuracy was 90.4%–90.6% for females and 90.3% for males. When 10% of the ECGs with intermediate probability (0.31<P<0.69) were rejected, the accuracy improved to 94.3% and if 20% ECGs with p values between 0.17 and 0.83 were excluded, the accuracy for sex determination further improved to 96.8%. Sex differentiation was more accurate in younger patients (<45 years of age) as compared to patients older than 55 years, 93% versus 89%, respectively. Lower accuracy of sex determination in older individuals can be due to changes in the hormonal status and its effect on the ECGs. Another limitation was the comparison of the data with the self-reported sex.

The output of the age-estimation network was a continuous variable. The mean absolute error was 6.9 ± 5.6 years ($p < 0.0001$). The area under the curve (AUC) was 0.94 for detection of age ≥ 40 years, with 87.8% sensitivity, 86.8% specificity, and accuracy of 87%. It was noted that where CNN-predicted age was >7 years from the chronological age, the patients had a higher incidence of pre-existing comorbidities, such as previous MI, low EF, CAD, hypertension, and atrial fibrillation (AF). It appears that CNN-predicted age is more of physiological age of a person than just the chronological age and is a better marker. In the cohort of 100 patients where multiple ECGs were taken over decades, a sicker cohort of patients with a need of serial ECGs were selected. There were no significant morbidities and patients were otherwise healthy where the CNN-predicted age was <7 years or ±7 years of the chronological age. However, where the CNN-predicted age was >7 years of the chronological age, new-onset low EF, incident MI, new-onset hypertension and diabetes mellitus, cardiac transplantation, and major events like hemodynamic shock occurred during follow-up period. In one patient, CNN-predicted age decreased after the cardiac transplant.

Attia et al. concluded that using CNN, trained computer can identify from 12-lead standard ECG "whether the individual is male or female and can determine age within 7 years of the actual age." And if CNN-predicted age is >7 years of the chronological age, likely to have higher chance of cardiovascular morbidities.

DETECTION OF ASYMPTOMATIC LEFT VENTRICULAR DYSFUNCTION USING AN AI-ENABLED ECG

Asymptomatic left ventricular dysfunction (ALVD) is common in elderly population (~ 9%) and 3–6% in general population, and lead to increased morbidity, mortality, and reduced life expectancy. Identification of ALVD can lead to proper medical treatment with angiotensin-converting enzyme (ACE) inhibitors, angiotensin receptor blockers (ARBs) and/or beta-blockers, and device therapies like implantable cardioverter-defibrillators (ICDs) and cardiac resynchronization therapy (CRT) to retard the progression of the disease to symptomatic HF, thereby reducing mortality. Currently, we do not have a noninvasive, inexpensive tool to determine ALVD and either echocardiography or estimation of B-type natriuretic peptide (BNP) levels are the basic investigations to identify it. Using AI-enabled ECG with paired 12-lead ECG and echocardiogram (echo) data, Attia et al. hypothesized to identify ALVD.

A cohort of 625,326 patients with paired ECG and transthoracic echo (TTE) were screened for analysis. Finally, 97,829 patients where ECG and echocardiography were performed within 2 weeks constituted the analysis data set, with 89% within 1 day—35,970 patients in training set, 8,989 patients in internal validation set, and 52,870 patients in testing set. The mean age of the patient population was 61.8 ± 16.5 years. In the testing data set, EF ≤ 35% was present in 4,131 patients (7.8%), 6,740 (12.7%) patients had EF between 35 and <50%, and 41,999 (79.5%) patients had EF ≥ 50%.

Higher degree of discrimination between EF ≤ 35% and EF = 35% was seen in the test data with the overall accuracy of 85.7%, sensitivity of 86.3%, and specificity of 85.7%. When patients with no known comorbidities were analyzed separately, the accuracy improved to 92.5%, with 95.6% sensitivity and 92.4% specificity. Across all age and sex groups, the network performance was strong.

1,335 patients, having normal EF on echo, were labeled as having low EF on CNN-ECG (false positive), when followed up, 147 patients developed left ventricular dysfunction (LVD) over a median follow-up of 3.4 years, suggesting network identified the ECG abnormalities of LVD earlier before the overt LVD. Such "false positive" patients who had normal EF, but network reported low EF, had a fourfold increased risk of developing ventricular dysfunction over next 5 years. AUC of CNN-predicted low EF was 0.93 as compared to AUC for BNP and N-terminal prohormone of BNP (NTproBNP) to screen for systolic and diastolic function was 0.60 and 0.70, respectively.

To conclude, AI-enabled ECG screening for ALVD is low cost, powerful tool, and can identify the individuals who are at increased risk for developing LVD in future.

DETECTION OF HYPERTROPHIC CARDIOMYOPATHY USING AI-ENABLED ECG

Ko et al. published a study for detection of hypertrophic cardiomyopathy (HCM) using AI-enabled ECG. Digital

12-lead ECGs, obtained from 2,448 verified patients of HCM and 51,153 non-HCM, were age- and sex-matched, control trained, and validated by the CNN. A separate dataset from 612 HCM patients and 12,788 control subjects were used as the testing set.

The mean age for HCM group was 54.8 ± 15.9 years, and 57.5 ± 15.5 years for the control group. The AUC of CNN was 0.96 with 87% sensitivity and 90% specificity. In younger patients, the performance of CNN was better with 95% sensitivity and 92% specificity.

To conclude, AI based algorithm can detect HCM on ECG by trained and validated CNN with high diagnostic accuracy.

NONINVASIVE DETECTION OF HYPERKALEMIA FROM AI-ENABLED ECG

Hyperkalemia is a medical emergency, if not detected early and treated appropriately. Seen commonly in patients with HF, chronic kidney disease (CKD) and with the medications to treat these conditions like ACE inhibitor/ARBs. Hyperkalemia carries high arrhythmia risk and mortality. ECG changes have been described in hyperkalemia, but they are not consistent and appear late. As patients are mostly asymptomatic, diagnosis of hyperkalemia is challenging.

Electrocardiogram and serum potassium levels within 12 hours of ECG were extracted from Mayo Clinic Data between 1994 and 2017. 709,000 patients, 2.1 million ECGs, and 4.0 million serum potassium values made the data for the study. 5.0 mmol/L was taken as the threshold, and repeated positive results were taken to avoid false positive tests. Finally, 20,196 positive and 2.0 million negative tests were the dataset. Using ECG leads I and II, deep neural network was trained with AI algorithm to detect hyperkalemia. Tests were performed on 698,939 ECGs from 224,690 patients and the AUC was 0.87, with 85% sensitivity and 72% specificity.

The study concluded that AI algorithm is a viable tool for detecting even mild hyperkalemia from a two-lead ECG.

DETECTION OF AORTIC STENOSIS USING AN AI-ENABLED ECG

263,570 patients with ECG and echo performed within 180 days were the study dataset. CNN was trained to detect at least moderate aortic stenosis (AS) (aortic valve velocity ≥ 3 m/sec and/or area ≤ 1.5 cm^2) using 12-lead ECG. 50% of the patients were used for the training, 10% for internal validation, and 40% for the testing. Out of 105,461 testing patients, 5,088 (4.8%) patients were of at least moderate AS category and were labeled as "positive". CNN could identify at least moderate AS with 75% accuracy, 78% sensitivity, and 75% specificity.

To conclude, AI-enabled ECG can be used to detect AS early, and can become a powerful tool for screening of asymptomatic AS in community using 12-lead ECG.

ARTIFICIAL INTELLIGENCE-ENABLED ECG ALGORITHM FOR ATRIAL FIBRILLATION

Atrial fibrillation is the most common type of cardiac arrhythmia and affects 1–4% of the general population and is an important risk factor for stroke, HF, and mortality. Prevalence of AF is predicted to double over the next 30 years and is associated with a fivefold increased risk of ischemic stroke. Screening for AF remains a challenge, as the present common screening methods like single ECG or 24-hour ambulatory ECG recording (Holter) have very low yield.

Identifying AF from a sinus rhythm ECG using AI seems to be a good proposition. From the Mayo Clinic dataset between 31st December 1993 and 21st July 2017, digital standard 12-lead ECG having sinus rhythm of patients 18 years or older was the study material. If the patients had at least one ECG of AF or atrial flutter, they were taken as positive for AF. 180,922 patients were included with 649,931 sinus rhythm ECGs. 454,789 ECGs from 126,526 patients were used for the training set. 6,430 ECGS from 18,116 patients used for internal validation and 130,802 ECGs from 36,280 patients comprised the testing dataset. 3,051 (8.4%) patients out of testing dataset had verified AF or atrial flutter. Patients were categorized into two categories: First, having AF within 31 days of the index ECG (window of interest) and second, AF later than 31 days.

Overall AUC was 0.87, accuracy of 79.4% with 79.0% sensitivity and 79.5% specificity. If taken for ECGs within window of interest, AUC improved to 0.90 with overall accuracy of 83.3%, sensitivity of 82.3% and 83.4% specificity. For the second group of patients where the AF occurred beyond 31 days of index ECG, the AUC remained 0.90.

Study concluded that AI-enabled ECG in sinus rhythm can identify patients with history of AF or impending AF quiet accurately.

Super-human diagnostic abilities have been provided to the clinicians by the application of AI to the ECG interpretation.

CONCLUSION

Artificial intelligence-enabled ECG can identify age and sex from the ECG and may reflect physiological age more than the biological age. It can identify whether the patient had AF or likely to have AF from sinus rhythm ECG. AI-enabled ECG can detect asymptomatic AS, hyperkalemia, HCM, and individuals with low EF. It is an universally available and inexpensive technology to screen population and identify the individuals who are at risk, and necessary medical attention can prevent the progression of the disease.

SUGGESTED READINGS

1. Attia ZI, Friedman PA, Noseworthy PA, Lopez-Jimenez F, Ladewig DJ, Satam G, et al. Age and sex estimation using artificial intelligence from standard 12-lead ECGs. Circ Arrhythm Electrophysiol. 2019;12(9):12e007284.
2. Attia ZI, Kapa S, Lopez-Jimenez F, McKie PM, Ladewig DJ, Satam G, et al. Screening for cardiac contractile dysfunction using an artificial-enabled electrocardiogram. Nat Med. 2019;25(1):70-4.
3. Ko WY, Siontis KC, Attia ZI, Carter RE, Kapa S, Ommen SR, et al. Detection of Hypertrophic Cardiomyopathy Using a Convolutional Neural Network-Enable Electrocardiogram. J Am Coll Cardiol. 2020;75(7):722-33.
4. Galloway CD, Valys AV, Petterson FL, Gundotra VP, Treiman DL, Albert DE, et al. Non-invasive detection of Hyperkalemia with a Smartphone Electrocardiogram and Artificial Intelligence. J Am Coll Cardiol. 2018;71(11):A272.
5. Shelly M, Attia ZI, Ko WY, Ito Saki, Essayagh B, Michelena HI, et al. Detection of aortic stenosis using an artificial intelligence-enabled electrocardiogram. J Am Coll Cardiol. 2020; 75(11):2115.
6. Godin R, Yeung C, Baranchuk A, Guerra P, Healey JS. Screening for atrial fibrillation using a mobile, single-lead electrocardiogram in Canadian primary care clinics. Canadian J Cardiol. 2019;35(7):840-5.
7. Jones NR, Taylor CJ, Hobbs FDR, Bowman L, Casadei B. Screening for atrial fibrillation: a call for evidence. Eur Heart J. 2020;41(10):1075-85.
8. Attia ZI, Noseworthy PA, Lopez-Jiminez F, Asirvatham SJ, Deshmukh AJ, Gersh BJ, et al. Artificial Intelligence-Enabled ECG Algorithm for the identification of patients with atrial fibrillation during sinus rhythm: a retrospective analysis of outcome prediction. Lancet. 2019;394:861-7.
9. Attia ZI, Harmon DM, Behr ER, Friedman PA. Application of artificial intelligence to the electrocardiogram. Eur Heart J. 2021;42(46):4717-30.

126

CHAPTER

Organs-on-Chips: Past, Current, and Future

Alladi Mohan, G Bindhu Madhavi, B Venkata Rami Reddy

ABSTRACT

Organs-on-a-chip, also called microphysiological systems or "tissue chips" are microengineered biomimetic systems which represent the structural and functional characteristics of human tissue. These bioengineered microdevices recapitulate key functional aspects of organs and tissues and have been observed to bridge the gap between extensively studied animal models and human-based clinical trials. Organs-on-a-chip have been found to be useful in significantly reducing the failure rate in current drug development with better safety and efficacy compared to the existing models. Over the past decade tremendous advances have occurred in developing several models of organs-on-a-chip for different organs. Further advances are focussed on the development of human-on-a-chip, which helps in holistic approach toward individual care. This chapter details the structure, applications, limitations, and future advances of organs-on-a-chip.

INTRODUCTION

Drug development is an extremely slow and expensive process. To produce drugs which treat chronic and complex diseases, trials involving large number of patients studied for long duration and complex analyses are required. Thus, the cost of drug development and the time duration required for this is huge. In addition, only a miniscule few drugs will eventually reach the market after clinical testing; hence, drug development requires new approaches and tools that can reverse these trends and deliver the appropriate science for patient. Preclinical drug development uses animal models, which contribute enormously for understanding the physiology of disease and development of new medicines. Despite the significant contributions, the lack of human-relevant preclinical models results in high failure rates and has led to a rise in healthcare costs as well as a smaller number of effective drugs that are reaching the patients. This chapter summarizes the principles, techniques of fabrication, and recent progress of organs-on-a-chip research and the role of this innovative approach in drug development.

To overcome these, drug development inefficiencies newer approaches that include molecular pathways are emerging which include the development of cell culture analogs, two-dimensional (2D) culture, microfluidics, and microfabrication. Cell culture refers to growth and maintenance of cells in a controlled environment. The 2D cell culture systems were used to study functions of various cells or cell products; later it became evident that the 2D cultures fail to accurately simulate the physiology of living tissues/organs, and microenvironmental factors. These limitations have led to other more complex three-dimensional (3D) models, which better represent the spatial and chemical complexity of living tissues. The 3D models have been in vogue for >50 years to study the molecular basis of tissue function and drug responsiveness in some diseases. Gradually, it became evident that even 3D models also have many limitations due to lack of multiscale architecture, absence of fluid flow and tissue-tissue interfaces.

To overcome all these limitations, using microfluidics and microfabrication have emerged as the most relevant and direct methods to study human physiology. Microtechnology has enabled to mimic the physiological environment of tissues and organs, which led to the development of novel *in vitro* organ systems which are termed *"organs-on-a-chip" systems*. These devices (also called microphysiological systems or "tissue chips") combine bioengineered 3D culture with microfluidic systems to simulate human tissue responses and diseases. The organs-on-a-chip are microdevices that represent the key functional aspects of organs and tissues.

ORGANS-ON-A-CHIP: PAST—WHAT DO WE KNOW?

Structure of Organs-on-a-Chip

The development of the organs-on-a-chip was initiated three decades ago, beginning with the application of microfluidic devices for cell culture and biological analysis. Microfluidics includes study and manipulation of fluids in a measure of microliter (μL) confined within channels with dimensions of few tens to hundreds of micrometers. The first-generation microfluidic biological devices referred as "cells on a chip." The combination of microfluidics 3D cell cultures leads to better representation of in vivo cell environment and allows study of biological organs with minute volumes of fluids. Organs-on-a-chip approach aims at mimicking the cellular architecture and biochemical factors which serves the purpose for disease modeling and drug screening.

Organs-on-a-chip comprise advanced *in vitro* technology which enables the experimentation with biological cells and tissues outside the body. For any given target organ, the process of creating its on-chip representation starts by reducing the organ to its most basic anatomical and functional unit responsible for organ-specific physiological function. The functional units of the organ are then examined to identify their key cellular constituents, structural organization of different cell and tissue types, and biochemical and/or mechanical cues that are present in their local microenvironment. These features are individually assessed for inclusion into the organ-chip model. Organs-on-a-chip are more superior to the existing drug development methods in many ways. The advantages of organs-on-a-chip are mentioned in **Box 1** and different functions of organs-on-a-chip are mentioned in **Box 2**.

BOX 1: Advantages of organs-on-a-chip.

- Replicate the physiological and pathological environment
- High throughput and smart analysis
- Continuous flow of nutrients can be maintained
- Human-derived cells are used, therefore physiologically more relevant results are obtained
- Multiple cell types can be layered which may mimic various organs and organ systems

BOX 2: Functions of organs-on-a-chip.

- Single cell analysis
- Cell–cell interactions
- Fluid gradient involving bacterial chemotaxis
- Axon growth
- Neuronal modules
- Cancer cell migration
- Drug development
- Precision medicine

Source: Ma C, Peng Y, Li H, Chen W. Organ-on-a-chip: a new paradigm for drug development. Trends Pharmacol Sci. 2021;42(2):119-33.

While designing the chip structure, some key issues need to be addressed. First, the design must address the properties to emulate and measure. Second, different cells must be incubated into the device. Third, cellular growth, differentiation and function are established in order for the chip to operate like an organ. Fourth, data are obtained through chemical and physical testing.

ORGANS-ON-A-CHIP: CURRENT

Applications of Organs-on-a-Chip

In recent years different models of organs-on-a-chip were developed for different organs. This includes lung on a chip, heart on a chip, kidney on a chip, skin on a chip, pancreas on a chip, brain on a chip and blood brain barrier on a chip. Various application of all these organs-on-a-chip are mentioned in **Table 1**.

ORGANS-ON-A-CHIP: THE FUTURE

Single organ chips fail to fully reflect the complexity and integrity of organ function. This leads to the development of multiorgans-on-a-chip or human-on-a-chip in which cells of different organs and tissues simultaneously connected by channels to depict multi-organ interaction. Designs including 2–10 organs-on-a-chip are being developed. As the number of organs-on-a-chip increases, the complexity of system also enhances.

This system enables in vitro insight into organ–organ interactions. It helps in simultaneous operation of multiple multiorgan culture units., for example, implementation of human-on-chip for cancer model helps to study metastasis, tumor growth and pathophysiology of tumor cells. Similarly lab-on-chip is used to study cell biology, proteomics, and molecular biology. Novel microfluidic designs are being developed where the tissues are able to perform the function required to support other tissues. Other future prospects include the advances in design, modeling, and usability of organs-on-a-chip.

K

L

M

Q

R

T

U

V

W

X

Y

Z

CONTRIBUTORS

Aaliya Jabbar MBBS
Junior Resident
Department of Medicine
Era's Lucknow Medical College
Lucknow, Uttar Pradesh, India

Aarathy Kannan MD (Dip Diab) MBA
Consultant Physician and Diabetologist
Sundaram Arulrhaj Hospitals
Tuticorin, Tamil Nadu, India

Aayushi Rathi DNB
Resident (Final Year)
Department of Respiratory Medicine
Apollo Gleneagles Hospital
Kolkata, West Bengal, India

Abdul Haroon Shah MBBS
PG Student (3rd Year)
Sardar Patel Medical College
Bikaner, Rajasthan, India

Abha Gupta MD
Professor and Head
Department of Medicine
Lala Lajpat Rai Memorial Medical College
Meerut, Uttar Pradesh, India

A Bhagwati MD(Medicine) FICP FICCM ADHA(Hospital Administration)
Honorary Physician and Intensivist
Department of Internal Medicine and Critical Care
Bhatia Hospital
Honorary Physician
Saifee Hospital
Wockhardt Hospital
Smt Motiben Dalvi Hospital
Mumbai, Maharashtra, India

Abhishek Borkotoky MBBS
Junior Resident
Department of General Medicine
Institute of Medical Sciences
Banaras Hindu University
Varanasi, Uttar Pradesh, India

Abhishek Kumar MD(General Medicine) FICP FIACM
Consultant Medicine, Avni Care
Patna, Bihar, India

Abhishek Kumar Tiwari MD
DM Resident Cardiology
Coimbatore Medical College and Hospital
Coimbatore, Tamil Nadu, India

Abhishek Singhai MD(Medicine)
Associate Professor
Department of Medicine
All India Institute of Medical Sciences
Bhopal, Madhya Pradesh, India

Aditi Aggarwal MBBS
Junior Resident (DNB)
Nemcare Hospital
Guwahati, Assam, India

Aditya Chakravorty MBBS
Post Graduate Student
Department of General Medicine
School of Medical Sciences and Research
Sharda University
Greater Noida, Uttar Pradesh, India

Aditya Prakash Misra MD FICP
Senior Consultant
Department of Internal Medicine
Fortis Flt Lt Rajan Dhall Hospital
Medeor (Rockland) Qutab Hospital
New Delhi, India

AG Unnikrishnan MD DM(Endocrinology) DNB MNAMS
CEO and Chief Endocrinologist
Chellaram Diabetes Institute
Pune, Maharashtra, India

Aishwarya N Udupa MBBS
Resident of General Medicine
Jawaharlal Nehru Medical College
KLE Academy of Higher Education and Research
Belagavi, Karnataka, India

Ajay K Pandey MD(Medicine) DM(Cardiology) FACC FESC FSCAI(USA)
Consultant Interventional Cardiologist and Head (Cardiology)
Galaxy Hospital
Varanasi, Uttar Pradesh, India

Ajaypal Singh MBBS
PG Student (3rd Year)
Sardar Patel Medical College
Bikaner, Rajasthan, India

Ajeet Singh Chahar MD(General Medicine)
Associate Professor in Medicine
PG Department of Medicine
SN Medical College and Hospital
Agra, Uttar Pradesh, India

Ajoy Tewari MD FRCP FACP FICP
Director Consultant Diabetologist
Jai Clinic and Diabetes Care Centre
Lucknow, Uttar Pradesh, India

A Kader Sahib MD MRCP DNB
Consultant Cardiologist
Apollo and Ayesha Hospital
Trichy, Tamil Nadu, India

Akanksha Gautam MS(Obstetrics and Gynecology)
Senior Resident
Department of Gynaecology
Eternal Hospital
Jaipur, Rajasthan, India

Akashkumar Navinprakash Singh MD(Internal Medicine) MSc(Diabetes) FACP FICP FIACM FRSSDI Fellow Diabetes India
Consultant Physician
Spandan Multispeciality Hospital
Vadodara, Gujarat, India

Akash Panigrahi DM(Endocrinology)
Consultant Endocrinologist
Tata Main Hospital
Jamshedpur, Jharkhand, India

Anupama YJ MD(Medicine) DNB(Nephrology)
Consultant Nephrologist
Nanjappa Hospital
Shivamogga, Karnataka, India

Anupam Dey MD FICP FACP
Professor and Head
Department of General Medicine
All India Institute of Medical Sciences
Bhubaneswar, Odisha, India

Anupam Prakash MD(General Medicine)
Director Professor
Department of Medicine
Lady Hardinge Medical College
New Delhi, India

Anup Kumar Das MD FICP
Professor of Medicine
Assam Medical College
Dibrugarh, Assam, India

Anurag DM(Gastroenterology)
Resident Doctor
JLN Medical College and Hospital
Ajmer, Rajasthan, India

Anurag Varma MD(Psychology) FIPS FIACAM
Consultant Psychiatrist
MLN Medical College
Prayagraj, Uttar Pradesh, India

Anusha Yadav MBBS
PG Student (3rd Year)
Sardar Patel Medical College
Bikaner, Rajasthan, India

Anushka Deogaonkar MBBS
Intern, Bharti Vidyapeeth
Pune, Maharashtra, India

Anyam Borpuzari MBBS
Medical Officer
Government of Assam
Sivasagar, Assam, India

Aparna Agrawal MD
Director Professor of Medicine
Lady Hardinge Medical College
New Delhi, India

Aparna Tewari MD(Anesthesiology and Critical Care Medicine)
Postgraduate Trainee
Kolkata Medical College
Kolkata, West Bengal, India

Appandraj Jain MD(General Medicine)
Professor and Head
Department of Internal Medicine
Melmaruvathur Adhiparasakthi Institute of Medical Sciences and Research (MAPIMS)
Melmaruvathur, Tamil Nadu, India

Aqsa Jafri MD(General Medicine Student)
Junior Resident
PG Department of Medicine
SN Medical College and Hospital
Agra, Uttar Pradesh, India

Aradhana Singh MD(Medicine)
Professor and Founder Head
Department of Clinical Immunology and Rheumatology
SMS Medical College and Hospital
Jaipur, Rajasthan, India

Aradhya Sekhar Bagchi MD(Medicine)
Consultant Physician
Nil Ratan Sircar Medical College
Kolkata, West Bengal, India

Arathi Darshan MD FICP
Professor of Medicine
KLE Academy of Higher Education and Research
Jawaharlal Nehru Medical College
Belagavi, Karnataka, India

Arghya Chattopadhyay MD(Medicine) DM(Clinical Immunology and Rheumatology)
Assistant Professor
Department of Rheumatology
North Bengal Medical College and Hospital
Siliguri, West Bengal, India

Arijit Sinha MD DNB(General Medicine) FICP
Professor, Department of General Medicine, NRS Medical College
Kolkata, West Bengal, India

Arjun Tandon MD(Medicine)
Senior Resident
Department of Cardiology
Banaras Hindu University
Varanasi, Uttar Pradesh, India

Arkadip Choudhury MD(Medicine)
Assistant Professor
Department of General Medicine
Tripura Medical College and Dr BRAM Teaching Hospital, Hapania
Agartala, Tripura, India

Arpit Jain MD(Radiation Oncology) DrNB(Medical Oncology)
Consultant
Department of Medical Oncology
Rajiv Gandhi Cancer Institute and Research Centre
New Delhi, India

Arun Kumar Kedia MD(Medicine)
Consultant Physician
Lifeworth Hospital
Raipur Chhattisgarh, India

Arup Kumar Kundu MD FRCP FICP MNAS
Ex-Professor of Medicine and In-Charge, Division of Rheumatology
Department of Medicine
RG Kar Medical College
Kolkata, West Bengal, India

Ashee Verma MBBS
Locum Resident
Government Medical College
Kota, Rajasthan, India

Ashima Katyal MD
Assistant Professor
Kalpana Chawla Government Medical College
Karnal, Haryana, India

Ashish Goel MD
Professor and Head
Department of Medicine
Dr BR Ambedkar State Institute of Medical Sciences (AIMS)
Mohali, Punjab, India

Ashok K Taneja MD DipCARD FRCP FACP FICP FIAE FDI
Director
Taneja Heart Diabetes Centre
Gurugram, Haryana, India

Ashok Kumar MD
Professor and Head
Department of Medicine
Santosh Medical College and Hospital
Ghaziabad, Uttar Pradesh, India

Ashutosh Kumar Karn MD DM(Neurology)
Chief Medical Officer
Department of Medicine
ABVIMS and Dr Ram Manohar Lohia Hospital
New Delhi, India

Ashwini Nigam MD(Medicine)
Professor of Medicine
PG Department of Medicine
SN Medical College
Agra, Uttar Pradesh, India

Asish Mondal MD(Internal Medicine)
Assistant Professor
Kolkata Medical College
Kolkata, West Bengal, India

AS Mohan MD FICP
Retired Professor and Head (Medicine)
Tirunelveli Medical College
Tirunelveli, Tamil Nadu, India

AS Senthilvelu MD
Managing Trustee
Erode Diabetes Foundation
Physician, Diabetologist and Medical Superintendent
Maaruthi Medical Centre and Hospitals
Erode, Tamil Nadu, India

Aswin Sasikumar MBBS
Resident of General Medicine
Jawaharlal Nehru Medical College
KLE Academy of Higher Education and Research
Belagavi, Karnataka, India

Atanu Chandra MD(Internal Medicine) DNB(Internal Medicine) MRCP (UK)
Assistant Professor
Department of Internal Medicine
Bankura Sammilani Medical College
Bankura, West Bengal, India

Atanu Thakur MD(Medicine)
Associate Professor
Department of Medicine
Veer Surendra Sai Institute of Medical Science and Research (VIMSAR)
Burla, Odisha, India

Atul Bhasin DNB(Internal Medicine, Army Hospital R&R) MNAMS FIACM FICP FACP(USA) FRCP(London)
Senior Director
Department of Internal Medicine
BLK-MAX Super Speciality Hospital
New Delhi, India

Atul Gupta MBBS
Junior Resident 3rd Year
Department of Medicine
GSVM Medical College
Kanpur, Uttar Pradesh, India

Atul Kumar MD
Consultant, Dr Prasad Diabetes and Hypertension Care Clinic
Patna, Bihar, India

Atul Mehrotra DTCD MD(Medicine) FICP FISC FACP PGDDM
Consultant Physician
Mehrotra Family Clinic
Lucknow, Uttar Pradesh, India

Ashutosh Chaturvedi MD(Medicine) Certified in Diabetes(Chennai)
Assistant Professor
Department of Medicine
Mahatma Gandhi Medical College
Jaipur, Rajasthan, India

Avik Chakraborty MD(Medicine) FICP FIACM
Professor
Department of General Medicine,
Tripura Medical College and Dr BRAM Teaching Hospital, Hapania
Agartala, Tripura, India

Avina Jain MD(Dermatology, Venereology and Leprosy)
Chief Dermatologist
Auro Skin Clinic
Mumbai, Maharashtra, India

Balakrishnan Kannan MD DM(Neurology)
Consultant Neurologist
Sundaram Arulrhaj Hospitals
Tuticorin, Tamil Nadu, India

Balbir Singh Kohli MD DNB(Medicine) AFIH FAIMS
Head
Department of Critical Care and Emergency
Hira Mongi Navneet Hospital
Consultant Physician
Fortis and Jupiter hospital
Mumbai, Maharashtra, India

Basabbijay Sarkar MD
Consultant Physician and Head
Department of Internal Medicine
Fortis Hospitals
Kolkata, West Bengal, India

BD Goswami MD(Medicine) PhD(Gastroenterology, Russia) FISG FACG(USA) AGAF(USA) FSGEI FRCP(Edinburgh, Glasgow)
Senior Consultant Gastroenterologist
Dispur Hospital
Former Professor and Head
Department of Gastroenterology
Gauhati Medical College and Hospital
Guwahati, Assam, India

Bharat Bhushan Sharma MD(Internal Medicine)
Senior Professor and In-Charge
Respiratory Allergy Clinic
Department of Medicine
SMS Medical College
Jaipur, Rajasthan, India

Bharath HR MD
Senior Resident
Department of Gastroenterology
Dr SN Medical College,
Jodhpur, Rajasthan, India

Gaurav Singh MD(Medicine)
Senior Resident
Department of Medicine
Narayan Medical College and Hospital
Sasaram, Bihar, India

Gautam Bhandari MD
Senior Consultant
Manidhari Hospital
Jodhpur, Rajasthan, India

GC Khilnani MD FCCP(USA) FAMS FICCM FICP FNCCP FISDA
Chairman
PSRI Institute of Pulmonary
Critical Care and Sleep Medicine
PSRI Hospital
New Delhi, India

GD Ramchandani MD FICP FRCP(London, Ireland, Glasgow, Edinburg) FACE FACP FRSSDI FIACM FDI FGSI
Professor
Department of Internal Medicine
Daswani Dental College
Senior Physician and Consultant Diabetologist
Ramchandani Diabetes Care and Research Center
Kota, Rajasthan, India

Geeta Kampani MD(General Medicine) FICP
Professor and Consultant
Department of Medicine
ABVIMS and Dr RML Hospital
New Delhi, India

Girish Mathur MD(Medicine) FICP FIACM FACP(USA) FRCP(Glasgow, London, Edinburgh)
Senior Consultant Physician
Alka Diagnostic Centre
Kota, Rajasthan, India
President- API

Girish Verma MD(Medicine) FRCP(Edinburgh) FICP FIACM FIAE F.Diab. India FRSSDI
Professor of Medicine
Geetanjali Medical College and Hospital
Udaipur, Rajasthan, India

Gopika Dineshan MBBS
Postgraduate in Geriatric Medicine
Bangalore Medical College and Research Institute
Bengaluru, Karnataka, India

(Maj) Gowri Shanker R MB DA PG(DipDiab) FCD
Physician, IIT Madras
Chennai, Tamil Nadu, India

G Prakash MD DDiab FICP
Professor and Head
Department of Diabetology
Government Mohan Kumaramangalam Medical College Hospital
Salem, Tamil Nadu, India

Gurinder Mohan MD(Medicine)
Professor and Head
Department of Medicine
Sri Guru Ramdas University of Medical Sciences and Research
Amritsar, Punjab, India

G Usha MD(General Medicine)
Consultant Physician
Fernandez Hospital
Hyderabad, Telengana, India

Harbir Kaur Rao MD FICP FGSI FIMSA
Professor and Head (Retired)
Medicine and Cardiology
Government Medical College
Patiala, Punjab, India
Professor and Head (Retired)
Medicine
MM Institute of Medical Sciences and Research
Mullana, Haryana, India

Hardik Rughwani MD DM
Consultant Gastroenterologist
AIG Hospitals
Hyderabad, Telangana, India

Harikishan Boorugu MD
Consultant Physician
Fernandez Hospital
Hyderabad, Telangana, India

Harpreet Singh MD
Associate Professor Medicine
Unit In-Charge
Government Medical College
Amritsar, Punjab, India

Harshita Lachhwani MBBS
Intern
Shri Ram Murti Institute of Medical Sciences
Bareilly, Uttar Pradesh, India

Hemshanker Sharma MD FICP FIAMS MACP FICCD
Professor of Medicine
Department of Postgraduate Medicine
JLN Medical College
Bhagalpur, Bihar, India

HK Aggarwal MD FIACM FICP FRCP(Edinburgh, London)
Senior Professor and Head
Department of Medicine
Pandit Bhagwat Dayal Sharma Post Graduate Institute of Medical Sciences
Rohtak, Haryana, India

HS Pathak MD(Medicine) DBMS FICP FIACM
Retired Professor and Head
Department of Medicine
College of Medicine and JNM Hospital
Kalyani, West Bengal, India

Iman Kalyan Sarkar DNB(Medicine)
Senior Resident
Department of Medicine
College of Medicine and JNM Hospital, WBUHS
Kalyani, West Bengal, India

Ishan Mishra MBBS
Area Medical Advisor
Pfizer Oncology
Bhopal, Madhya Pradesh, India

ISM Giridhar MD
Senior Resident
Department of Neurology
MS Ramaiah Medical College
Bengaluru, Karnataka, India

Jacquiline D Shira MD
Assistant Professor of Medicine
Nagaon Medical College Hospital
Nagaon, Assam, India

Jagdeep Chugh MD(Medicine) FICP
Senior Consultant
Department of Internal Medicine and Diabetes, Satyam Medical Centre, Gujranwala Town
Fortis Hospital, Shalimar Bagh
New Delhi, India

Jaisuresh K DM(Nephrology)
Consultant Nephrologist and Transplant Physician
Assured Best Care Hospital
Tiruchirappalli, Tamil Nadu, India

Jalees Fatima MD(Medicine) FACP FICP FRSSDI FIMSA
Professor and Head
Department of Medicine
Era's Lucknow Medical College
Lucknow, Uttar Pradesh, India

Jananee Muralidharan MD MRCP(UK)
Assistant Professor
Department of Medicine
Faculty
Department of Medical Education
St John's Medical College and Hospital
Bengaluru, Karnataka, India

Javal Bhatt DNB(Medicine)
Consultant Physician, Jupiter Hospital
Thane, Maharashtra, India

Jaya Bhanu Kanwar MD(General Medicine) DM(Endocrinology)
Professor and Head
Department of Endocrinology
Institute of Medical Sciences and SUM Hospital
Bhubaneswar, Odisha, India

Jayanta K Panda MD(Internal Medicine) FACP(USA) FICP FRSSDI FIMAMS
Consultant in Diabetes, Metabolic and Critical Care Medicine
Professor, Department of General Medicine, SCB Medical College
Cuttack, Odisha, India

Jayanta Sharma MD FICP FIACM FIAMS FCCS FCSI FGSI FACP FRCP(Glasgow) FRCP(Edinburgh)
Senior Consultant
Department of Internal Medicine
Apollo Multispeciality Hospitals
Kolkata, West Bengal, India

Jay Tewari MBBS
Final Year Student
King George's Medical University
Lucknow, Uttar Pradesh, India

Jeevan Prakash MD(Medicine)
Head (Critical Care Medicine)
Era's Lucknow Medical College
Lucknow, Uttar Pradesh, India

Jitendra Singh MD(General Medicine) CCCKD(Kidney Disease) PGDC(Cardiology) PGDRM(Diabetes and Renal Management) Postgraduate Diploma in Advanced Diabetes Care & Clinical Endocrinology FICN FIACM FICP
Co-Incharge of Emergency and Assistant Professor
Department of General Medicine
Institute of Medical Sciences, Banaras Hindu University
Varanasi, Uttar Pradesh, India

Jothydev Kesavadev MD FACE(USA) FRCP(London, Glasgow, Edinburgh) FACP(USA)
Chairman and Managing Director
Jothydev's Diabetes Research Centers
Kerala, India

Joydeep Samanta MD(Medicine) DM(Clinical Immunology and Rheumatology)
Assistant Professor
Rheumatology Unit
Department of Internal Medicine
All India Institute of Medical Sciences
Raipur, Chhattisgarh, India

Jugal Kishor Sharma MD(Medicine) FICP FRCP(London, Ireland, Glasgow and Edinburgh) FACP FACE FICN FRSSDI FGSI FISH FIACM FIMSA FDiab(India)
Medical Director
Central Delhi Diabetes Centre
New Delhi, India

Jyoti Chugh MD DNB
Senior Consultant (Obstetrics and Gynecology)
Satyam Medical Centre, Gujranwala Town
Fortis Hospital, Shalimar Bagh
New Delhi, India

Jyoti Kiran DM PDT(Neurology)
Neurologist
Calcutta National Medical College and Hospital
Kolkata, West Bengal, India

Kamal Garg MD
Postgraduate
Maulana Azad Medical College
New Delhi, India

Kanupriya Goel DM(Cardiac Anesthesia)
2nd Year
Dr Ram Manohar Lohia Hospital
New Delhi, India

Karandeep Kaur MBBS
Junior Resident
Department of Medicine
Sri Guru Ramdas University of Medical Sciences and Research
Amritsar, Punjab, India

Karnati Prudhveer Reddy MBBS
Postgraduate
Department of General Medicine
JSS Hospital
Mysuru, Karnataka, India

Kashish Gupta MD(Medicine)
Senior Resident
SMS Medical College and Hospital
Jaipur, Rajasthan, India

Kauser Usman MD FIMSA FIACM FICP FACP(USA) FRCP(Edinburgh)
Professor
Department of Medicine
Officiating Head
Department of Geriatric Medicine
King George's Medical University
Lucknow, Uttar Pradesh, India

Kaushik Basu MD DM(Rheumatology and Clinical Immunology)
Associate Professor
Department of Rheumatology
Medical College
Kolkata, West Bengal, India

Kaushik Hazra DTCD MD(General Medicine)
Associate Professor of Medicine
Jagannath Gupta Institute of Medical Sciences and Hospital (JIMSH)
Budge Budge, West Bengal, India

Kaushik Sen MD DM(Endocrinology)
Associate Professor
Department of General Medicine
Barasat Government Medical College
Kolkata, West Bengal, India

Kaustubh Dilip Salagre MD(Medicine)
Associate Professor
Department of Medicine
Seth GS Medical College and KEM Hospital
Mumbai, Maharashtra, India

Ketan K Mehta MD FCPS FICP FISE FGSI
Consulting Physician
Asian Heart Institute
Mumbai, Maharashtra, India

K Nagesh MD FICP FCCP
Consultant Physician and Director
Nagesh Hospital
Hassan, Karnataka, India

Krishna Pawan Jaldu MBBS
Resident
Department of Medicine
Santosh Medical College and Hospital
Ghaziabad, Uttar Pradesh, India

Krunal Patel MD(General Medicine)
2nd Year PG Resident
Mahatma Gandhi Hospital
Jaipur, Rajasthan, India

Kshitija Gadekar MD DM
Professor and Head
Department of Nephrology
MGM Medical College
Aurangabad, Maharashtra, India

Kuldeep Gurjar MBBS
3rd Year Post graduate Student
Department of Medicine
Maulana Azad Medical College
New Delhi, India

Kunal Ahuja DNB
Associate Consultant
PSRI Institute of Pulmonary Critical Care and Sleep Medicine
PSRI Hospital
New Delhi, India

Kushal Markanday MD(Medicine)
Assistant Professor
Department of Medicine
Maharishi Markandeshwar Institute of Medical Sciences and Research
Mullana, Haryana, India

Lalatendu Mohanty MD
Professor and Head
PG Department of Medicine
Kalinga Institute of Medical Sciences
Bhubaneswar, Odisha, India

Lalita Verma MD(Microbiology)
Senior Demonstrator
Department of Microbiology
SMS Medical College
Jaipur, Rajasthan, India

LH Ghotekar MD MNAMS FIACM FIMSA
Director-Professor and Head
Department of Medicine
Head, Department of Neurology
Lady Hardinge Medical College and SSKH
New Delhi, India

Liyakat Ali Gauri MD(General Medicine)
Senior Professor
Department of General Medicine
Sarder Patel Medical College
Bikaner, Rajasthan, India

LP Meena MD
Professor
Department of General Medicine
Institute of Medical Sciences
Banaras Hindu University
Varanasi, Uttar Pradesh, India

Madhulata Agarwal MD(Internal Medicine)
Assistant Professor
Department of Medicine
SMS Medical College
Jaipur, Rajasthan, India

Madhuri Matta MD(Medicine)
Head
Department of Medicine
INHS Kalyani
Visakhapatnam, Andhra Pradesh, India

Madhur Rai MD(Physiology)
Associate Professor
Postgraduate Department of Physiology
MGM Institute of Health Sciences
Navi Mumbai, Maharashtra, India

Mahabir Thakur MD(General Medicine) DTM&H
Consultant
Department of Internal Medicine
Cardiac Care and Research Centre
Sitamarhi, Bihar, India

Mahesh Choudhary DNB(Medicine)
Trainee, Jupiter Hospital
Thane, Maharashtra, India

Manabendra Nayak MD PhD FICP MRCP FRCP(Edinburgh, Glasgow, London) FACP(USA) FCCP(USA)
Head, Department of Medicine
Down Town Hospital
Guwahati, Assam, India
Postgraduate Teacher of Medicine
NBEMS

Manab Narayan Baruah MD(Pediatrics)
Associate Professor
Department of Paediatrics
Jorhat Medical College and Hospital
Jorhat, Assam, India

Manas Das MD(General Medicine)
Senior Resident
Department of Medicine
Lady Hardinge Medical College
New Delhi, India

Manas Thakur MD(Internal Medicine)
Resident (DM Cardiology)
Mahatma Gandhi Medical College
Jaipur, Rajasthan, India

Manikandan DNB(General Medicine)
DNB Post Graduate
Sundaram Arulrhaj Hospitals
Tuticorin, Tamil Nadu, India

Manisha MBBS
PG Student (3rd Year)
Sardar Patel Medical College
Bikaner, Rajasthan, India

Manish Kumar MD DTM&H(UK) FICP FIACM FIAMS Certified Echocardiologist (IAE) Fellow Royal Society of Tropical Medicine(UK)
Consultant Physician and Chief
Noninvasive Cardiac Lab
Department of Medicine
Arc Hospital
Bhagalpur, Bihar, India

Manish Pahariya MD
Professor of Medicine
Mahatma Gandhi Medical College and Hospital
Jaipur, Rajasthan, India

Manish Sharma MBBS
Third Year Postgraduate Student
Department of Medicine
ABVIMS and Dr RML Hospital
New Delhi, India

Manjari Saha MD(General Medicine)
Associate Professor
Department of Internal Medicine
Kolkata Medical College
Kolkata, West Bengal, India

Manoj Khanal MD DM(Neurology)
Associate Director and Head
Department of Neurology
Max Super Speciality, Shalimar Bagh
New Delhi, India

Manoj K Srivastav MD(Medicine)
Professor
Department of Medicine
Narayan Medical College and Hospital
Sasaram, Bihar, India

Manoranjan Behera MD FICP
Professor and Head
Department of Medicine
Bhima Bhoi Medical College
Balangir, Odisha, India

Masum Talesara MD(Medicine)
Junior Resident
Department of Medicine
RD Gardi Medical College
Ujjain, Madhya Pradesh, India

Mathew Thomas MD FRCP(London) FRCP(Edinburgh) FICP FISHTM
Professor of Internal Medicine and Hematology and Senior Consultant
KIMS Hospital
Thiruvananthapuram, Kerala, India

Mayank Gupta MD(Internal Medicine)
Assistant Professor, Department of Medicine, NIMS Medical College
Jaipur, Rajasthan, India

Meenakshi MS(Obstetrics and Gynaecology)
Professor
JLN Medical College and Hospital
Ajmer, Rajasthan, India

Meenaxi Sharda MD(Medicine) DCH FIAE FICP
Senior Professor of Medicine
Head Geriatric Medicine
Government Medical College
Kota, Rajasthan, India

Meghna Aggarwal MD(Medicine)
Senior Resident
Department of Nephrology
Government Medical College
Kota, Rajasthan, India

Meghna Dutta DNB(Family Medicine)
Junior Consultant
Department of Internal Medicine
Apollo Multispeciality Hospitals
Kolkata, West Bengal, India

Mehdi Ali Mirza MD DM
Assistant Professor
Department of Pharmacology
ESIC Medical College and Hospital
Hyderabad, Telangana, India

ME Yeolekar MD(General Medicine and Therapeutics) MNAMS(Medicine) FICP
Senior Consultant Physician (Internal Medicine)
Ex-Professor and Head (Medicine)
Sion Hospital
Past Dean LTMG/KEM Hospital
Former DMER (MCGM)
Mumbai, Maharashtra, India

M Gunasekaran MD FICP
Senior Consultant Physician
Dravidian Speciality Hospital
Pattukkottai, Tamil Nadu, India

Minal Harde MD DNB(Anesthesia)
Associate Professor
Department of Anaesthesia
Topiwala National Medical College and BYL Nair Charitable Hospital
Mumbai, Maharashtra, India

M Jawahar Farook DNB(Medicine) DNB(Cardiology) MNAMS FNB(Interventional Cardiology) FESC FCSI FSCAI
Senior Interventional Cardiologist
Meenakshi Mission Hospital and Research Centre (MMHRC)
Madurai, Tamil Nadu, India

ML Patel MD MNAMS FIACM FICP FACP
Professor
Department of Medicine
King George Medical University
Lucknow, Uttar Pradesh, India

Molly Mary Thabah MD FRCP(Edinburgh)
Professor
Department of Clinical Immunology
Jawaharlal Institute of Postgraduate Medical Education and Research
Puducherry, India

Monica Gupta MD(Medicine) DNB(Medicine) FICP
Professor
Department of General Medicine
Government Medical College and Hospital
Chandigarh, India

Monika Maheshwari DNB MD PhD DM(Cardiology) FACC FRCP(Glasgow, Edinburgh) FESC FAPSC FEAC FCSI FISE FIAE FICP FIACM MAMS FICA
Former Professor of Medicine and Assistant Professor
Department of Cardiology
Jawahar Lal Nehru Medical College
Ajmer, Rajasthan, India

MPS Chawla MD FACP FRCP FICP FIACM FISC FIMSA
Professor and Head
Department of Medicine
ABVIMS and Dr Ram Manohar Lohia Hospital
New Delhi, India

MP Sharma DM(Gastroenterology)
Head
JLN Medical College and Hospital
Ajmer, Rajasthan, India

M Raveendran MD(General Medicine)
Professor of Medicine and Dean
Government Medical College and ESI Hospital
Coimbatore, Tamil Nadu, India

Mrinal Kanti Roy MD DM(Neurology) FIACM FICP FRCP(Glasgow) FACP(USA)
Retired Professor, Calcutta National Medical College and Hospital
Kolkata, West Bengal, India

Mritunjay Kumar MBBS
Junior Resident
Department of General Medicine
Institute of Medical Sciences
Banaras Hindu University
Varanasi, Uttar Pradesh, India

M Sabir MD(General Medicine)
Senior Consultant Physician and Pulmonologist, Kothari Medical and Research Institute
Retired Professor and Head
Respiratory Division
Department of Medicine
SP Medical College
Bikaner, Rajasthan, India
Former President: Indian Chest Society

MS Prasad MS
Consultant Surgeon
MedIndia Hospitals
Chennai, Tamil Nadu, India

Mukesh K Sarna MD FACP FRCP(London, Edinburgh, Glasgow) FICP FISH FRSSDI FIACM FDI
Professor and Unit Head
Department of General Medicine
Mahatma Gandhi Medical College and Hospital
Jaipur, Rajasthan, India

Mukulesh Gupta MD(General Medicine) PG Diploma in Diabetes (Cardiff, UK) FICP FRSSDI FUPDA FInSH FISCM FIACM FISMN Fellow Diabetes, India FACP(USA)
Director
Udyan Health Care Pvt Ltd
Lucknow, Uttar Pradesh, India

Murugesh Pastapur MD
Consultant Physician
Ex-Professor of Medicine
MR Medical College
Kalaburagi, Karnataka, India

Nadeem Liyakat MD(Radiodiagnosis)
Senior Resident
Department of Radiodiagnosis
SP Medical College
Bikaner, Rajasthan, India

Nalini Humaney MD(General Medicine) FICP
Professor in Medicine
NKPSIMS & RC and LMH
Nagpur, Maharashtra, India

Narayan Deogaonkar MD FRCP(London) FICP
Director
Deogaonkar Hospital
Nashik, Maharashtra, India

Narayan Prasad MD DM FRCP
Professor and Head
Department of Nephrology
Sanjay Gandhi Postgraduate Institute of Medical Sciences
Lucknow, Uttar Pradesh, India

Naresh Kumar Midha MD(Medicine)
Associate Professor
Department of Medicine
All India Institute of Medical Sciences
Jodhpur, Rajasthan, India

Narinder Pal Singh MD MBA
Dean Research
Eternal University
Baru Sahib, Himachal Pradesh, India
Consultant
Academic Program in Nephrology
Max Super Speciality Hospital
Saket, New Delhi, India

Nasir Hussain MBBS
Medical Officer
Jain Chest Care Center
Jaipur, Rajasthan, India

Naween Kumar MD
Assistant Professor
Department of Medicine
Darbhanga Medical College
Darbhanga, Bihar, India

Neeti Agrawal MD DM
Senior Resident
Department of Endocrinology and Metabolism
Medical College Superspeciality Block (SSB)
Kolkata, West Bengal, India

Niharika Sinha MBBS PG Diploma in Rheumatology EULAR
Consultant Rheumatologist
Joint Pain and Arthritis Clinic
Patna, Bihar, India

Nikita Srivastava MD
Ex-Senior Resident
Department of Medicine
Lady Hardinge Medical College and SSKH
New Delhi, India

Nilanjan Mal MBBS
PGT-3
Department of General Medicine
Rajendra Institute of Medical Sciences
Ranchi Jharkhand, India

Nilesh Kumar MD(General Medicine)
Associate Professor and
Co-Nodal Officer
COE for Hemoglobinopathies and
Bleeding Disorder
Department of General Medicine
Institute of Medical Sciences
Banaras Hindu University
Varanasi, Uttar Pradesh, India

Nipun Goel MBBS
PG Resident
Department of General Medicine
Mahatma Gandhi Medical College
and Hospital
Jaipur, Rajasthan, India

Niraj Lodha MD FICP PGD in Clinical Endocrinology and Diabetes
Senior Consultant Physicians and
Diabetologist, Lodha Hospital and
Test Tube Baby Center
Pali, Rajasthan, India

Nirmal Das Vaishnav MD
DrNB Resident (Medical Oncology)
Bhagwan Mahaveer Cancer Hospital
and Research Center
Jaipur, Rajasthan, India

Nirupam Prakash MD(Medicine) FICP PGCC(Diabetes) PGCC(Cardiology)
Consultant Physician, CGHS
Lucknow, Uttar Pradesh, India

Niteesh Singh MD
Junior Resident III
PG Department of Medicine
SN Medical College
Agra, Uttar Pradesh, India

Nitin Jain MD(Respiratory Medicine)
Consultant and Director Intervention
Jain Chest Care Center
Jaipur, Rajasthan, India

Nitin Sinha MD(Medicine) PGDHHM(IGNOU)
Professor, Department of Medicine
ABVIMS and Dr RML Hospital
New Delhi, India

Nitu Chauhan MD(Pathology)
Associate Professor and Head
Department of Transfusion Medicine
SN Medical College and Hospital
Agra, Uttar Pradesh, India

N Subramanian MD MRCP(UK) MRCP CCT(Rheumatology) FRCP FICP
Consultant Rheumatologist
Rosemary Mission Hospitals,
Tirunelveli
Assistant Professor of Rheumatology
and Medicine
Velammal Medical College Hospital
and Research Institute
Madurai, Tamil Nadu, India

Om Prakash Sharma MD FICN FICP FIAMS FCGP FGSI FACM FIMSA FRCP(Edinburgh) FGAPIO
Senior Consultant Geriatric Medicine
Indraprastha Apollo Hospitals
Sarita Vihar, New Delhi, India
Emeritus Clinical Tutor
Apollo Hospitals Educational and
Research Foundation

Paila Deepika MBBS
Resident
Department of Medicine
Lady Hardinge Medical College
New Delhi, India

Pankaj Manoria MD DM FACC FESC
Director
Manoria Heart and Critical Care
Hospital
Bhopal, Madhya Pradesh, India

Pankaj Nand Choudhry MD(Medicine) FICP FIACM
Senior Consultant and Academic
Head
Department of Internal Medicine
Max Super Speciality Hospital
Ghaziabad, Uttar Pradesh, India

Pankaj R Jawandhiya MD DM DNB
Nephrologist
NewEra Hospital
Nagpur, Maharashtra, India

Pankaj Verma MD(Medicine)
Assistant Professor
Department of Medicine
Dr Ram Manohar Lohia Institute of
Medical Sciences
Lucknow, Uttar Pradesh, India

Paramita Bhattacharya DNB(Medicine)
Assistant Professor
Department of Medicine
College of Medicine and JNM
Hospital, WBUHS
Kalyani, West Bengal, India

Partha Karmakar MD(Medicine) DNB(Medicine) Dip Cardiology FICP FACP
Professor
Department of Medicine
College of Medicine and Sagore Dutta
Hospital
Kolkata, West Bengal, India

Partha Pratim Chakraborty MD DM DNB MNAMS FRCP FACE FICP
Assistant Professor
Department of Endocrinology and
Metabolism
Medical College Superspeciality
Block (SSB)
Kolkata, West Bengal, India

Parth Deogaonkar MD(Medicine) DNB(Nephrology)
Consultant
Deogaonkar Hospital
Nashik, Maharashtra, India

Pawan Suri MD DM FRCP FESC FSCAI FCSI
Director and Chief Cardiologist
Global Super Speciality Hospital
Jalandhar, Punjab, India

Payal Jain MD(General Medicine) FIACM FICP FIMSA
Professor
Department of General Medicine
Government Institute of Medical
Sciences
Greater Noida, Uttar Pradesh, India

PC Manoria MD DM FACC FESC FCAPSC
Director
Manoria Heart and Critical Care Hospital
Bhopal, Madhya Pradesh, India

Pearl Samaria MBBS(Student)
Mahatma Gandhi University of Medical Sciences and Technology (MGUMST)
Jaipur, Rajasthan, India

Pinaki Mukhopadhyay DM FICP FASN FRCP(London)
Head, Department of Nephrology
Nil Ratan Sircar Medical College
Kolkata, West Bengal, India

Piyush Manoria DTCD MD(Medicine) DM(Gastroenterology)
Chief Gastroenterologist and Hepatologist
Manoria Hospital
Bhopal, Madhya Pradesh, India

PK Maheshwari MD DM(Neurology) MAMS FFIACM FRCP(Edinburgh) FIAN FICP
Professor and Head
Department of Neurology
Superspeciality Block
SN Medical College
Agra, Uttar Pradesh, India
President, Agra Academy of Neurology

P Paranthaman MD DTCD FICP FRCP(Glasgow) FACP FIMSA MHSc(Diabetology)
Professor of Medicine and Head
Department of General Medicine
Government Kilpauk Medical College
Chennai, Tamil Nadu, India

Prabhakar K MD(General Medicine) FICP MNAMS
Principal and Dean
Sri Devaraj Urs Medical College
Kolar, Karnataka, India

Prabhat Pandey MD(Medicine) MIP FCCP FICA FICP FCSI FCGP FIAMS PG Dip(Diabetology) FDiab India
Professor and Head
Department of Medicine
DNB Faculty
Chandulal Chandrakar Memorial Superspeciality Hospital
Bhilai, Chhattisgarh, India

Prakhar Gupta MBBS
Practitioner
Osmo Kidney Care Centre
Varanasi, Uttar Pradesh, India

Pramod Kumar Agrawal MD(Medicine) FICP FRCP(Glasgow)
Professor and Head
Department of Medicine
Katihar Medical College
Katihar, Bihar, India

Pramod Kumar Sinha MD(Medicine) FICP FCSI Dip(Echocardiography)
Associate Professor and Head
Department of Medicine
Anugrah Narayan Magadh Medical College and Hospital
Gaya, Bihar, India

Prasanta Kumar Bhattacharya MD PhD FACP FICP
Senior Professor (HAG) and Head
Department of General Medicine
Member Secretary, Institutional Ethics Committee
North Eastern Indira Gandhi Regional Institute of Health and Medical Sciences
Shillong, Meghalaya, India

Prashant Prakash MD(Medicine) MD(Chest) MAMS FICP FIACM
Professor and Head
Super Specialty Department of Pulmonary Medicine
SN Medical College
Agra, Uttar Pradesh, India

Prashasti Gupta MD
Assistant Professor of Medicine
Lady Hardinge Medical College
New Delhi, India

Preeti Sarma MD
Registrar
Department of Gastroenterology
Gauhati Medical College and Hospital
Guwahati, Assam, India

Pritam Gupta MD(Medicine) FRCP FICP FIMS
Senior Consultant
Fortis Hospital, Shalimar Bagh
New Delhi, India

Priyank Rastogi MD
Associate Professor
Department of Medicine
ESI Post Graduate Institute of Medical Sciences and Research
Basaidarapur, New Delhi, India

Priyanshu Shah MD
Assistant Professor
Medical ICU
Department of Medicine
LTM Medical College and General Hospital, Sion
Mumbai, Maharashtra, India

Puneet Rijhwani MD FICP FRCP(Edinburgh) FACP FIACM FDI
Professor and Head
Department of Medicine
Mahatma Gandhi University of Medical Sciences and Technology
Jaipur, Rajasthan, India

Radha TR MD(General Medicine) MD(Pediatrics) DNB(Pediatrics)
Professor and Head
Department of Medicine
Government Medical College
Kottayam, Kerala, India

Rahul Ramchandani MBBS
Final Year Resident
Department of Internal Medicine
Institute of Medical Sciences and SUM Hospital
Bhubaneswar, Odisha, India

Rahul T Chakor MD(Medicine) DM(Neurology)
Professor and Head
Department of Neurology
TN Medical College
BYL Nair Hospital
Mumbai, Maharashtra, India

Rajat Chaudhary MD(Medicine)
Senior Resident
Department of Cardiology
GIPMER
New Delhi, India

Rajinder Singh Gupta MD FICP FGSI FIMSA
Professor and Head (Retired)
Medicine
Government Medical College
Patiala, Punjab, India
Professor (Retired)
Medicine
MM Institute of Medical Sciences and Research
Mullana, Haryana, India

Rajiv Kumar Bandaru MD(General Medicine)
Associate Professor
Department of General Medicine
ESIC Medical College and Hospital
Hyderabad, Telangana, India

Raj Kamal Choudhary MD(Medicine) FICP
Associate Professor
Department of Post Graduate Medicine
Jawaharlal Nehru Medical College
Bhagalpur, Bihar, India
Former SRTL, WHO
Former Consultant, CDC

Rajneesh Sachan MD
Resident
Department of General Medicine
Institute of Medical Sciences
Banaras Hindu University (IMS-BHU)
Varanasi, Uttar Pradesh, India

Rakesh Bhadade MD(Internal Medicine) FICP FRCP(London)
Associate Professor
Department of Medicine and In-Charge EMS
Topiwala National Medical College and BYL Nair Charitable Hospital
Mumbai, Maharashtra, India

Rakesh Kumar Goel MD(Medicine) PG Dip(Public Health) PG Dip(Hospital Administration)
Senior Professor and Head
Department of Medicine
Maharaja Agrasen Medical College (MAMC), Agroha
Hisar, Haryana, India

Rakesh M Parikh FCPS(Medicine) Dip. Diabetology
Consultant Diabetologist
CKS Hospital Jaipur and Diabecity
Jaipur, Rajasthan, India

Raman Sharma MD
Professor of Medicine
Mahatma Gandhi Medical College and Hospital
Jaipur, Rajasthan, India

Ramesh Aggarwal MD FRCP(Edinburgh) FICP
Professor
Department of Medicine
Lady Hardinge Medical College
New Delhi, India

Ramesh Duraisamy MD
Assistant Professor of Medicine
Coimbatore Medical College and Hospital
Coimbatore, Tamil Nadu, India

Ramesh Mundle MD
Professor
Department of Medicine
NKP Salve Institute of Medical Sciences
Nagpur, Maharashtra, India

Ranjan Kumar MD
Chief Consultant
Ranjan Heart Clinic
Patna, Bihar, India

Ranjit Mohan Anjana MD DipDiab(UK) PhD FACP FICP FRCP(Glasgow Edinburgh, London) FACE
Managing Director
Dr Mohan's Diabetes Specialities Centre
President
Madras Diabetes Research Foundation
Chennai, Tamil Nadu, India

Rashi Maheshwari MD DM(Rheumatology and Clinical Immunology)
Assistant Professor
Department of Clinical Immunology and Rheumatology
SMS Medical College and Hospital
Jaipur, Rajasthan, India

Raveendran AV MD FRCP(Edinburgh)
Assistant Professor of Medicine (Former)
Government Medical College
Kottayam, Kerala, India

Ravikeerthy M MD(Medicine) FRCP(Glasgow) FICP PGDM(London)
Professor of Medicine
Meenakshi Medical College and Research Centre
Kanchipuram, Tamilnadu, India

Ravindra Kumar Modi MD FICP
Senior Consultant
Modi's Diabetes Research Centre
Purnea, Bihar, India

R Dharini DNB(General Medicine)
Consultant Physician
Chellaram Diabetes Institute
Pune, Maharashtra, India

Renu Saigal MD FICP MAMS FRCP FACP
Consultant Rheumatologist
Former Senior Professor and Head
Department of Medicine
SMS Medical College
Jaipur, Rajasthan, India

Ripun Borpuzari MD(Medicine) FICP
Retired Joint Director
Health and Family Welfare
Government of Assam
Senior Physician
Sivasagar, Assam, India
Chairperson, RSSDI Assam 2022–2023

Rishabh Kochar MD(General Medicine)
Senior Resident (DM fellow)
Department of Pulmonary Medicine
All India Institute of Medical Sciences
Jodhpur, Rajasthan, India

Ritu Karoli MD(Medicine) FICP MAMS
Additional Professor
Department of Medicine
Dr Ram Manohar Lohia Institute of Medical Sciences
Lucknow, Uttar Pradesh, India

RK Singal MD FACP(USA) FRCP(Glasgow) FICP FIAMS
Principal Consultant and Head
Department of Internal Medicine
BLK-MAX Super Speciality Hospital
New Delhi, India

R Lakshmi Narasimhan
DM(Neurology) DNB(Neurology) PhD FAAN FRCP(London, Glasgow) FIAN FEBN
Director and Professor of Neurology
Institute of Neurology
Madras Medical College
Chennai, Tamil Nadu, India

RM Chhabra MD(Medicine) FIMSA FICP FDI FRCP(Edinburgh)
Senior Consultant Physician
Department of Medicine
Max Super Speciality Hospital, Shalimar Bagh
Saroj Super Speciality Hospital
New Delhi, India

Rohini Handa MD DNB FAMS FICP FACR FRCP(Glasgow)
Professor and Senior Consultant Rheumatologist
Apollo Indraprastha Hospitals
New Delhi, India

Rohith Velusamy DNB
Postgraduate of Internal Medicine
Sundaram Arulrhaj Hospitals
Tuticorin, Tamil Nadu, India

Rohit Ihran MD
Assistant Professor
Department of General Medicine
SMS Medical College and Hospital
Jaipur, Rajasthan, India

Rohit Ram Kumar MD(General Medicine)
Senior Resident (DM Neurology)
Government Medical College
Kottayam, Kerala, India

Rosemarie de Souza MD(Internal Medicine)
Professor and Head,
Department of Medicine
Topiwala National Medical College and BYL Nair Charitable Hospital
Mumbai, Maharashtra, India

RS Chejara MD
Associate Professor of Medicine
Department of Medicine
SMS Medical College
Jaipur, Rajasthan, India

Ruchi Kapoor MD
National Head – Lab Clinical Excellence and Quality Assurance
TATA 1mg Labs
Gurugram, Haryana, India

Rupa Kasaraneni MBBS
Junior Resident
Sri Devaraj Urs Medical College
Kolar, Karnataka, India

Sahil Langde MD
Postgraduate Student (Medicine)
Seth GS Medical College and KEM Hospital
Mumbai, Maharashtra, India

Sahubar Sadiq MD DM
Consultant Physician and Neurologist
Ramnad Neuro Care Center
Ramanathapuram, Tamil Nadu, India

Saibal Chakravorty MD(Medicine) FRCP FICP FIACM Diploma in Diabetes(UK)
Senior Consultant Physician and Unit Head
Department of Internal Medicine
Diabetology and Critical Care
Metro Multispeciality Hospital
Noida, Uttar Pradesh, India

Sajid Ansari MD(Medicine) FACP(USA) FICP FISC FISH FEAC FIAE FCSI
Director
SS Heart Care Centre
Lucknow, Uttar Pradesh, India

Sambit Das MD(Medicine) DM(Endocrinology)
Professor
Department of Endocrinology
Kalinga Institute of Medical Sciences
Bhubaneswar, Odisha, India

Sameer Gulati MD FICP FIACM FIMSA
Professor
Department of Medicine
Lady Hardinge Medical College and Associated Hospitals
New Delhi, India

Samir Sahu MD(Medicine) FICP
Professor and Head
PG Department of Medicine
Institute of Medical Sciences and SUM Hospital
Bhubaneswar, Odisha, India

Sandeep Garg MD(Medicine)
Director Professor
Department of Medicine
Maulana Azad Medical College
New Delhi, India

Sandeep Rai DNB(Medicine) PG DipDiab MNAMS FACP(USA) FRCP(UK)
Senior Professor and Unit Head
Postgraduate Department of Medicine
MGM Institute of Health Sciences
Navi Mumbai, Maharashtra, India

Sandeep Suri MD(Medicine)
Consultant Physician and Diabetologist
Holy Help Hospital
Hisar, Haryana, India

Sanjay Bandyopadhyay MD DNB DM(Gastrology) MNAMS FRCP
Head
Department of Gastroenterology
ILS Hospitals Dumdum
Kolkata, West Bengal, India

Sanjay Gupta MD(Medicine) DNB FRCP(Edinburgh)
Senior Consultant
SG Diabetes Centre
New Delhi, India

Sanjay Kumar MD
Chief Consultant, Chest Clinic
Patna, Bihar, India

Sanjay Mehndiratta MD(Medicine)
Consultant Physician
MRG Hospital
Jaipur, Rajasthan, India

Sanjay Tandon MD(Medicine) FICP FISC FACP FACC FRCP
Director
Tandon Clinic
Lucknow, Uttar Pradesh, India

Sanjay V Patane MD AFIH PGDMT
Professor and Head
Department of Emergency Medicine
Indian Institute of Medical Science (IIMSR)
Jalna, Maharashtra, India

Santosh Salagre MD MBA FAIMER Fellow
Professor of Medicine
Seth GS Medical College and KEM Hospital
Mumbai, Maharashtra, India

Sarabmeet Singh Lehl MD(Medicine) FIACM FAIMER Fellow
Professor
Department of General Medicine
Government Medical College and Hospital
Chandigarh, India

S Arulrhaj MD PhD FRCP(Glasgow and London) MBA
Chairman, Chief Physician and Intensivist
Sundaram Arulrhaj Hospitals
Tuticorin, Tamil Nadu, India

Satyabrata Ganguly MD(General Medicine)
Emeritus Professor
Apollo Multispeciality Hospital
Kolkata, West Bengal, India

Saumik Datta MD DM(Endocrinology) FICP FISH
Professor and Head
Department of General Medicine
Burdwan Medical College and Hospital
Bardhaman, West Bengal, India

Saumitra Ray MD FRCP FCSI FICP FESC FACC FSCAI
Ex-Professor
Vivekananda Institute of Medical Sciences
Director, Invasive Cardiology
Advanced Medical Research Institute
Kolkata, West Bengal, India

Saumitra Singh MBBS
Medical Officer
Spandan Multispeciality Hospital
Vadodara, Gujarat, India

Saurabh Puri DNB(General Medicine) DNB SS(Nephrology)
ILBS Hospital
New Delhi, India

Saurabh Srivastava MD(General Medicine) FRCP(Edinburgh, Glasgow) FACP FICP FIMSA FIACM FIAMS FGSI FISH FUDA FDI MAMS
Professor and Head
Department of Medicine
Government Institute of Medical Sciences
Greater Noida, Uttar Pradesh, India

Sayan Kar DNB(General Medicine)
Junior Resident
Department of General Medicine
Medica Superspecialty Hospital
Kolkata, West Bengal, India

Sayantani Bhattacharya MBBS
Associate Physician
Urban Healthcare Hospital
Kolkata, West Bengal, India

Sayonee Das MD(General Medicine, Gold Medal)
Resident (DrNB Nephrology)
Apollo Multispeciality Hospital
Kolkata, West Bengal, India

SB Gupta MD FACC FISE FCSI FICP FICC
Ex-Head, Medicine and Cardiology
Central Railway HQ Hospital
Ex-Consultant Physician Cardiologist
Asian Heart Institute
Mumbai, Maharashtra, India

S Chiranth MBBS
Postgraduate 3rd Year
Department of Medicine
VMMC and Safdarjung Hospital
New Delhi, India

Shaibal Guha MD
Director
Positive Health Center
Patna, Bihar, India

Shailendra Kumar MD
Associate Professor and Head
Department of TB and Chest
SK Medical College
Muzaffarpur, Bihar, India

Sharad N Deshmukh MD MNAMS
Former Associate Professor of Medicine
IGMC Nagpur, NKPSIMS
Nagpur, Maharashtra, India

Shashidhara KC MD
Professor
Department of General Medicine
JSS Medical College
Mysuru, Karnataka, India

Sheila Nainan Myatra MD FCCM FICCM
Department of Anaesthesiology, Critical Care and Pain
Tata Memorial Hospital
Parel, Mumbai, India

Shikhar Bansal MD(General Medicine)
Resident (DM Cardiology)
IPGMER and SSKM Hospital
Kolkata, West Bengal, India

Shikhar Garg MD
Senior Resident (1st Year DM)
Department of Cardiology
Dr Ram Manohar Lohia Institute of Medical Sciences
Lucknow, Uttar Pradesh, India

Shilpa Gupta MD(General Medicine)
Senior Physician
Punjab Cancer Care and Multispeciality Hospital
Bhathinda, Punjab, India

Shivangi Maheshwari MBBS
Clinician
Sri Hari Kamal Diabetes and Heart Clinic
Lucknow, Uttar Pradesh, India

Shiv Ghodasara MD(Medicine)
Resident (DM Oncology)
Geetanjali Medical College and Hospital
Udaipur, Rajasthan, India

Shouvik Datta MBBS
Post Graduate (JR-3)
Department of General Medicine
SRMS Institute of Medical Sciences
Bareilly, Uttar Pradesh, India

Shrivarthan Radhakrishnan MD(Medicine) DM(Neurology) DrNB(Neurology)
Associate Consultant
Department of Neurology
MGM Healthcare
Chennai, Tamil Nadu, India

Shubha Laxmi Margekar MD
Professor
Department of Medicine
Lady Hardinge Medical College and SSK Hospital
New Delhi, India

Shubham MD(Medicine)
Resident Doctor
JLN Medical College and Hospital
Ajmer, Rajasthan, India

Shubhransu Patro MD(General Medicine) FICP
Professor
Postgraduate Department of General Medicine
Kalinga Institute of Medical Sciences
KIIT Deemed to be University
Bhubaneswar, Odisha, India

Shuchita Mundle MD
Professor
Department of Obstetrics and Gynecology
All India Institute of Medical Sciences
Nagpur, Maharashtra, India

Shweta Saxena MD(Obstetrics and Gynecology)
Consultant Gynecologist
Lucknow, Uttar Pradesh, India

Sidhartha Gautam Senapati MBBS
Research Fellow
Mayo Clinic College of Medicine and Sciences
Rochester, Minnesota, USA

Simi Patoa MD(Medicine)
Registrar
Silchar Medical College and Hospital
Silchar, Assam, India

Sirshendu Pal MD(Medicine) FRCP(Glasgow, Edinburgh)
Senior Consultant Physician and Diabetologist
Mitra's Multi Speciality Hospital
Siliguri, West Bengal, India

Siwalik Banerjee MD
Consultant Rheumatologist
Department of Rheumatology
University Hospitals Coventry and Warwickshire NHS Trust
Coventry, UK

SK Gautam MD(Medicine) FACP(USA) FICP FIACM FInSH
Professor of Medicine
GSVM Medical College
Kanpur, Uttar Pradesh, India

S Meenakshi-Sundaram MD(General Medicine) DM(Neurology)
Associate Professor of Neurology
Department of Neurosciences
Apollo Speciality Hospitals
Madurai, Tamil Nadu, India

Smita Gupta DNB(General Medicine) MNAMS
Professor and Head
Department of General Medicine
SRMS Institute of Medical Sciences
Bareilly, Uttar Pradesh, India

Smit Shrivastava MD PGDHHM DM (Cardiology) FACC FSCAI FESC FICP FIMSA FICN FISE
Professor and Head
Advance Cardiac Institute
PT JNM Medical College and Dr BRAM Hospital
Raipur, Chhattisgarh, India

SM Mishra MD FICP
Head
Department of Respiratory Medicine
Bhagwan Mahavir Institute of Medical Sciences, Pawapuri
Nalanda, Bihar, India

Sneha Modi MBBS
DNB Trainee Medicine
Sri Balaji Action Medical Institute
New Delhi, India

Somnath SM MD DNB(Medicine) FICP FRCP
Consultant Physician
Sanjana Diabetes and Eye Care
Ballari, Karnataka, India

Sonam Spalgais DNB(Pulmonary Medicine) MNAMS
Assistant Professor
Department of Pulmonary Medicine
Vallabh Bhai Patel Chest Institute
New Delhi, India

Sourav Paul MBBS
Junior Resident
Department of Internal Medicine
Kolkata Medical College
Kolkata, West Bengal, India

SP Sondhi MD
Guest Faculty
Department of Medicine
Subharti Medical College
Director
Omnibus Healthcare India Pvt Ltd
Meerut, Uttar Pradesh, India

Sreelakshmi R PhD
Research Scientist
Jothydev's Diabetes Research Center
Thiruvananthapuram, Kerala, India

Srina Ray MBBS(Cal)
Clinical Assistant
Heart Clinic
Kolkata, West Bengal, India

SS Dariya MD(Medicine) FACP FGSI FDI FIPA
Senior Consultant Physician
SMS Hospital
Jaipur, Rajasthan, India

S Sreenivas MD DM(Neurology)
Consultant Neurologist and Professor
Department of Medicine/Neurology
GSL Medical College
Chairman
Sri Padma Madhav Super Speciality Hospital
Rajahmundry, Andhra Pradesh, India

Subhita Choudhary MD(General Medicine)
Assistant Professor
Department of General Medicine
Shri Kalyan Government Medical College
Sikar, Rajasthan, India

Sudhanshu Pandey BPT MPT
Consultant Physical Therapist
Department of Physiotherapy and Rehabilitation
CISF Hospital
New Delhi, India

Sudha Sarna MD(Anesthesia)
Professor and Head
Department of Palliative Medicine
Mahatma Gandhi Medical College and Hospital
Jaipur, Rajasthan, India

Sudhir Bhandari MD DNB MNAMS FRCP (London, Edinburgh) DSc
Vice-Chancellor
Rajasthan University of Health Science (RUHS)
Professor Emeritus
SMS Medical College and Attached Group of Hospitals
Jaipur, Rajasthan, India

Sudhir Chandra Jha MD(Medicine) DNB(Medicine)
Associate Professor
Department of Medicine
Darbhanga Medical College
Darbhanga, Bihar, India

Sudhir Kulkarni MD DM
Emeritus Professor
Department of Nephrology
MGM Medical College
Aurangabad, Maharashtra, India

Sudhir Mehta MD(Internal Medicine)
Senior Professor and Head
Department of Medicine
SMS Medical College
Jaipur, Rajasthan, India

Sudipta Modak MD
Retired Associate Professor
Department of Chemistry
Calcutta University
Kolkata, West Bengal, India
Chairman BMC, CMC

Sugandha Sharma MS(Obstetrics and Gynecology)
Consultant Gynecologist
Global Heart and General Hospital
Jaipur, Rajasthan, India

Sujoy Ghosh DM FRCP FACE
Professor
Department of Endocrinology
Institute of Post Graduate Medical Education and Research
Kolkata, West Bengal, India

Sumbul Mazhar MD
Resident
Department of General Medicine
Institute of Medical Sciences
Banaras Hindu University (IMS-BHU)
Varanasi, Uttar Pradesh, India

Sumita Chaudhry MD
Consultant and Clinical Incharge, BMT
Department of Hematology
Safdarjung Hospital & VMMC
New Delhi, India

Sunil K Dadhich MD DM
Senior Professor and Head
Department of Gastroenterology
Dr SN Medical College
Jodhpur, Rajasthan, India

Sunil Kumar Bakshi MD(Medicine) FIAMS FGSI
Senior Consultant Physician
Department of Medicine
Metro Multispeciality Hospital
Noida, Uttar Pradesh, India

Sunil Kumar Mahavar MD
Professor
Department of General Medicine
SMS Medical College and Hospital
Jaipur, Rajasthan, India

Sunita Aggarwal MD(Medicine) FACP FRCP FICP FIACM FIMSA
Director Professor
Maulana Azad Medical College
New Delhi, India

Supriya Sarkar MD(Respiratory Medicine) FICP FCCP
Professor and Head
Department of Respiratory Medicine
College of Medicine and Sagore Dutta Hospital
Kolkata, West Bengal, India

Surabhi Talwar MD
Consultant Nephrologist
Department of Nephrology, University Hospitals Coventry and Warwickshire NHS Trust
Coventry, UK

Suraj S Yadav PhD
Assistant Professor
School of Pharmacy
National Forensic Sciences University
Gandhinagar, Gujarat, India

Surendra Kumar MD(General Medicine) Fellowship in Clinical Endocrinology PG Dip(Diabetology) AMU FACP FRCP FIACM FICP
Senior Professor and Unit Head
Department of Medicine
Sardar Patel Medical College
Bikaner, Rajasthan, India

Suryasnata Rath MS FRCS
Network Director—Operations
Ophthalmic Plastic Surgery Services
LV Prasad Eye Institute
Bhubaneswar, Odisha, India

Suvarthi Ray MBBS
Postgraduate Trainee
Department of General Medicine
All India Institute of Medical Sciences
Patna, Bihar, India

SV Ramanamurty MD FICP FIACM FACP
Professor
Academic Director—PG Education
Department of General Medicine
GSL Medical College
Rajahmundry, Andhra Pradesh, India

Swaroop Kumar Baruah MD(Medicine) MCA FICP
Senior Consultant Physician
Nemcare Hospital, Guwahati
Former Professor and Head
Department of Medicine
Gauhati Medical College
Guwahati, Assam, India

Swati Srivastava MD FACE FACP FICP
Senior Professor and Unit Head
SMS Medical College and Hospital
Jaipur, Rajasthan, India

Tanuja Manohar MD(Internal Medicine)
Professor and Head
Department of Medicine
NKPSIMS & RC and LMH
Nagpur, Maharashtra, India

Tanushree Debgupta MD(Medicine)
Assistant Professor
Silchar Medical College and Hospital
Silchar, Assam, India

Tapas Bandyopadhyay MD(Medicine) FICP FDI
Senior Consultant
Department of General Medicine
Medica Superspecialty Hospital
Kolkata, West Bengal, India

Tapas Kannu Vyas MBBS
Resident, Mahatma Gandhi Medical College and Hospital
Jaipur, Rajasthan, India

T Geetha MD
Professor of Medicine
Coimbatore Medical College and Hospital
Coimbatore, Tamil Nadu, India

Thair Al Jumaily Arab Board of Medicine Arab Board of Cardiology
Consultant, Interventional Cardiologist
Fujairah Hospital, Emirates Health Services (EHS)
Fujairah, UAE

Tribhuwan Gupta DM(Nephrology)
Director, Osmo Kidney Care Centre
Varanasi, Uttar Pradesh, India

Triven Sagar Sandepogu MD(General Medicine) FGID(CMC Vellore)
Professor
Department of General Medicine
Malla Reddy Institute of Medical Sciences and Hospital
Hyderabad, Telangana, India

TR Sirohi MD
Professor of Medicine
Subharti Medical College
Meerut, Uttar Pradesh, India

Trupti Trivedi MD
Professor of Medicine, Medical ICU
Department of Medicine
LTM Medical College and General Hospital, Sion
Mumbai, Maharashtra, India

TS Chandrasekar MD DM DSc FRCP(Edinburg, Glasgow, Ireland and London) FASGE FACG AGAF MWGO
Founder, Chairman and Chief Interventional Gastroenterologist
MedIndia Hospitals
Chennai, Tamil Nadu, India

Tuhina Gupta MS(Obstetrics and Gynecology) FMAS DMAS
Assistant Professor
SGT Medical College and Hospital
Gurugram, Haryana, India

Udas Chandra Ghosh MD(General Medicine) DNB(General Medicine) DNB(Respiratory Diseases) DTCD FICP FRCP(Glasgow)
Professor
Department of Medicine and In-Charge of Rheumatology Division
Medical College Kolkata
Kolkata, West Bengal, India

Umar Faruque MD
Registrar
Department of Medicine
Dhubri Medical College and Hospital
Dhubri, Assam, India

Ummed Singh MD(General Medicine)
Associate Professor
Department of General Medicine
Shri Kalyan Government Medical College
Sikar, Rajasthan, India

Upal Sengupta MD(General Medicine) DM(Nephrology)
Associate Professor
Department of Nephrology
KPC Medical College and Hospital
Kolkata, West Bengal, India

Upendra Sharma MD(General Medicine) DM(Clinical Hematology)
Senior Consultant Hematologist and Hemato-oncologist
Bhagwan Mahaveer Cancer Hospital and Research Center
Jaipur, Rajasthan, India

Utkarash Mishra MD DM(Nephrology)
Assistant Professor
Department of Nephrology
Christian Medical College
Vellore, Tamil Nadu, India

Uttam Kr Nath MD(Medicine) DFID(Diabetology)
Associate Professor
Department of Medicine
Jorhat Medical College and Hospital
Jorhat, Assam, India

Vaibhav Shukla MD(Medicine) FRCP(Edinburgh) FICP
Professor
Department of Medicine
Era's Medical College
Lucknow, Uttar Pradesh, India

VA Kothiwale MD PhD
Professor of General Medicine
Jawaharlal Nehru Medical College
KLE Academy of Higher Education and Research
Belagavi, Karnataka, India

Vamsi Krishna Annamdevula MD(Medicine)
Senior Resident
PG Department of Medicine
Institute of Medical Sciences and SUM Hospital
Bhubaneswar, Odisha, India

Vanita Arora MD DNB(Cardiology) MNAMS FRCP(Edinburgh) FESC FHRS
Senior Consultant
Apollo Hospital
New Delhi, India

Varun Vinayak Prakash Rao MD
MS Ramaiah Medical College
Bengaluru, Karnataka, India

Vasantha Kamath MD(Medicine) FICP
Professor Emeritus
Department of Medicine
MVJ Medical College and Research Hospital
Bengaluru, Karnataka, India

(Lt Gen) Ved Chaturvedi MD DM
Senior Consultant Rheumatologist
Sir Ganga Ram Hospital
New Delhi, India

Veerendra Singh MD(Internal Medicine) FICP FIACM FDI FUPDA
Director
GSSM Cardiorespiratory Centre
Ayodhya, Uttar Pradesh, India

Vibha Sharma MBBS MD
Postgraduate Resident (Medicine)
Department of General Medicine
Kalinga Institute of Medical Sciences
KIIT Deemed to be University
Bhubaneswar, Odisha, India

Vidita Kalra MD(Medicine)
Final Year Postgraduate Student
Mahatma Gandhi University of Medical Sciences and Technology
Jaipur, Rajasthan, India

Vijaya Prasanna Parimi MD DM(Rheumatology)
Consultant Rheumatologist
Department of Clinical Immunology and Rheumatology
ESIC Medical College and Hospital
Hyderabad, Telangana, India

Vijay Budhwar DM(Endocrinology) PDT
Department of Endocrinology
Institute of Post Graduate Medical Education and Research
Kolkata, West Bengal, India

Vijay Garg MD FIAE FICP FCSI FICA(USA) FISE FACC(USA) FACP(USA) FIMSA FISC FESC(EUROPE)
Professor
Department of Medicine
RD Gardi Medical College
Ujjain, Madhya Pradesh, India

Vijaykumar G Warad MD(General Medicine)
Professor, Department of Medicine
BLDE Deemed to be University
Shri BM Patil Medical College Hospital and Research Centre
Vijayapura, Karnataka, India

Vijay Kumar MD(General Medicine) FICP FDI FIACM PGDHM
Additional Professor
Department of General Medicine
All India Institute of Medical Sciences
Patna, Bihar, India

Vikash Khandelia DM(Nephrology)
Professor and Head
Department of Nephrology
Government Medical College
Kota, Rajasthan, India

Vineet Behera MD DM FACP FASN FICP
Professor of Medicine and Nephrologist
INHS Kalyani
Visakhapatnam, Andhra Pradesh, India

Vineet Talwar MD(Medical Oncology) FRCP(UK) DNB FICP FIMSA MNAMS
Director
Department of Medical Oncology
Rajiv Gandhi Cancer Institute and Research Centre
New Delhi, India

Vinod Ravindran MD MRCP(UK) CCT(Rheumatology, UK) FRCP(Edinburgh)
Consultant Rheumatologist
Centre for Rheumatology
Kozhikode, Kerala, India
Adjunct Professor
Department of Medicine
Kasturba Medical College
Manipal, Karnataka, India

Vipul Chavda MD FRCP FACP
Chairman and Endocrine Physician
Rudraksha Institute of Medical Sciences
Ahmedabad, Gujarat, India

Virendra Kumar Goyal MD FICP FACP FIACM FDI FRCP(Edinburgh, Glasgow, London)
Professor and Head
Department of Medicine
American International Institute of Medical Sciences
Udaipur, Rajasthan, India

Vishwanath Krishnamurthy MD FICP
Professor of Medicine
MS Ramaiah Medical College
Bengaluru, Karnataka, India
Honorary Secretary API Karnataka Chapter

Vishwas Galav MD(Medicine)
Second Year DM(Cardiology)
Resident
Department of Cardiology
Jawahar Lal Nehru Medical College
Ajmer, Rajasthan, India

Viswanathan Mohan MD PhD DSc FRCP(London, Edinburgh, Glasgow and Ireland) DSc(Honoris Causa) FAMS FNASc FASc FNA FAMS FACE FTWAS MACP FRS (Edinburgh)
Chairman
Dr Mohan's Diabetes Specialities Centre and Madras Diabetes Research Foundation
Chennai, Tamil Nadu, India

VK Katyal MD FACC(USA)
Head
Department of Medicine
Positron Multispeciality and Cancer Hospital
Rohtak, Haryana, India

VN Mishra MD(Medicine) FACP FICP FIACM FIAOG
Professor, Department of Medicine
All India Institute of Medical Sciences
Bhopal, Madhya Pradesh, India

V Palaniappan MD FICP FRCP(London)
Managing Director
Sri Sakthi Vinayaga Multispeciality Hospital and Dr V Palaniappan's Diabetes Specialities Center
Guziliamparai, Tamil Nadu, India

V Palanikumaran MD DDiab(MMC)
Senior Assistant Professor
Madurai Medical College
Madurai, Tamil Nadu, India

Wesley Hannah BDS MPH PhD
Research Associate
Dr Mohan's Diabetes Specialities Centre (IDF Centre of Excellence in Diabetes Care) and
Madras Diabetes Research Foundation (ICMR Centre for Advanced Research on Diabetes)
Chennai, Tamil Nadu, India

Yashasvi Gautam MD FICP FIACM
Honorary Senior Consultant Physician
Sudha Hospital and Jaiswal Hospital
Kota, Rajasthan, India

Yogesh Kumar Govil MD FACP FACG AGAF MRCP(E)
Senior Consultant
Department of Gastroenterology
Einstein Jefferson Medical Centre
Philadelphia, Pennsylvania, USA

Yogita Pendurkar DNB(Medicine)
Consultant Physician
Department of Medicine
Jupiter Hospital
Thane, Maharashtra, India

Yojana Gokhale MD
Professor of Medicine and In-Charge of Rheumatology
Lokmanya Tilak Municipal Medical College
Mumbai, Maharashtra, India

Zairemliana Chenkual MBBS
Post Graduate Trainee
Department of Emergency Medicine
All India Institute of Medical Sciences,
Patna, Bihar, India

FOREWORD

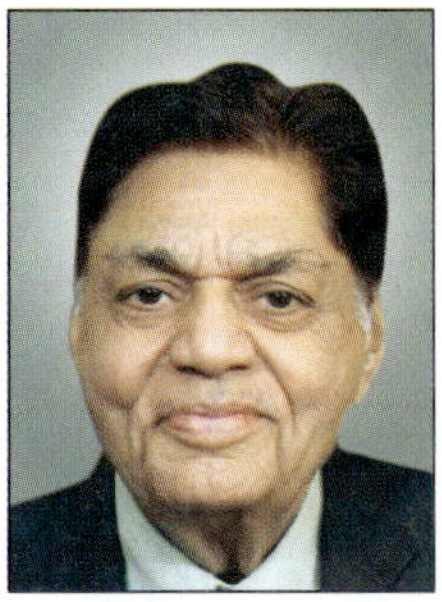

KK Pareek MD FICP FRCP
Past President API
Past Dean API
Immediate Past President IACM
Chairman API House Committee

It is both a privilege and an honor to contribute the foreword for "*Medicine Update 2024*", the annual publication of the *Association of Physicians of India (API)*. As we come together to celebrate the wealth of knowledge encapsulated within these pages, we pay tribute to the visionary physicians who, in 1944, laid the foundation for API with the noble aim of fostering collaboration, sharing experiences, and advancing medical science in our diverse and dynamic nation on one platform.

In the ever-evolving landscape of healthcare, where learning is a perpetual journey, the Medicine Update plays a pivotal role. In a country like India, with its vast expanse and varied healthcare challenges, disseminating knowledge becomes a necessity to stay updated with the cutting-edge developments in medicine. API has been at the forefront of this mission, providing a common platform for physicians across the nation to converge, exchange ideas, and stay abreast of the latest advancements.

Dr Milind Nadkar, the Scientific Chairman for APICON 2024 and the President-Elect of the API, stands as a beacon of leadership in the physician community. His wealth of experience, dedication to academic pursuits, and dynamic approach to healthcare have been instrumental in shaping its annual scientific program. Dr Nadkar's expertise has been evident through his tenure as the Chief Editor of the Journal of API and as the Honorary Secretary of API.

Medicine, as a field, is undergoing a transformative journey, and the theme of APICON 2024, "Clinical to Digital Medicine," reflects this paradigm shift. We are witnessing the integration of traditional clinical practices with cutting-edge digital technologies, promising to revolutionize patient care, diagnostics, and medical research. This forward-looking theme demonstrates a commitment to not only addressing current clinical challenges but also embracing the potential of digital interventions to shape the future of medicine in India.

The substantial undertaking of crafting the extensive scientific program for APICON 2024 spanning over 3½ days and featuring >500 lectures is a testament to the unwavering dedication of Dr Nadkar and his editorial team. Medicine Update 2024 serves as a tangible manifestation of their commitment to delivering a comprehensive and enlightening experience for conference delegates and readers alike, with each chapter authored by experts in their respective fields.

Dr Nadkar's meticulous curation ensures that the content is tailored to meet the diverse needs of practicing physicians, adeptly translating theoretical concepts into practical applications for the benefit of our patients.

I extend my heartfelt appreciation and congratulations to Dr Milind Nadkar and his editorial team for their exceptional work in creating this invaluable resource.

May *Medicine Update 2024* persist as a guiding beacon of knowledge, supporting physicians on their journey of lifelong learning.

Wishing all the delegates of APICON 2024 an enriching and enlightening experience.

PREFACE

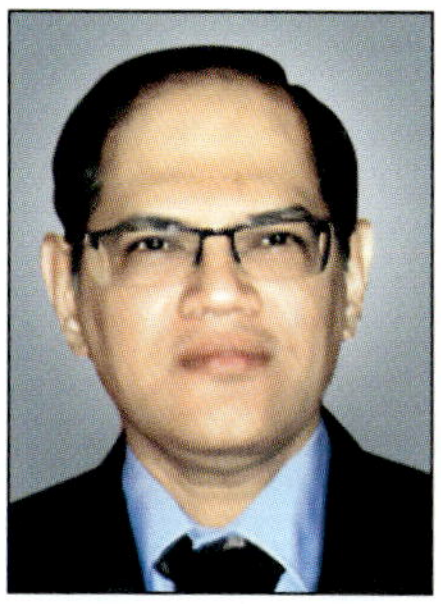

Milind Y Nadkar MD FICP FACP
President-Elect
Association of Physicians of India
Professor and Head
Department of Medicine and
Chief of Rheumatology Services
Seth GS Medical College and KEM Hospital
Mumbai, Maharashtra, India

With immense pleasure, I present before you the two volumes of "*Medicine Update 2024*" on the occasion of the 80th Annual Conference of the Association of Physicians of India—APICON 2024—being held at New Delhi from February 22 to 25, 2024.

I first go down to the memories of my mentor, Late Dr Siddhrath N Shah, who has guided me throughout my API career. His teachings and insights have greatly helped me in formulating the Scientific Program for APICON 2024 and also in editing of this book "Medicine Update 2024". Without his hand-holding over the years, I could not have moved a step further.

Truly, it was a herculean task to put up such a huge Scientific Program and to publish Medicine Update 2024. I thank my entire Scientific Committee and the Editorial Board for their relentless support in this venture.

Internal medicine and all its subspecialties are undergoing a tremendous transformation with new research every day. A lot of research is published every day. It is extremely difficult for a physician to update his knowledge by reading the literature in their busy schedule. The Scientific Program of APICON 2024 attempts to breach the gap in the knowledge of physicians. During the scientific program, we have planned interactive lectures, scientific celebrations, orations, panel discussions, and workshops.

The theme of this year's scientific program is "*clinical to digital*". On these lines, the Scientific Committee has tried to strike a balance between clinical medicine, laboratory medicine, and therapeutic advances. The scientific content of the program is published in this book with over 281 Chapters that will be a ready reference for future use.

There will be 12 workshops with hands-on training in the subjects of Ventilator Management, Biological and Nuclear Warfare, Communication Skills, Sleep, Intraarticular Injections, etc. A quiz has been organized for the interest of PG students.

There are over 1,500 research papers that will be presented on the platform or as e-posters which will give an opportunity to young physicians and postgraduate students to showcase their research.

I hope that the readers will find "Medicine Update 2024" worth our efforts and help in enhancing their knowledge and clinical skills.

ACKNOWLEDGMENTS

It was an enormous responsibility to compile and publish a book of the magnitude of "*Medicine Update 2024*" and I find myself absolutely short of words to thank enough all who have helped and guided me in executing this mammoth task.

I would express my deep appreciation and indebtedness to all the authors from across the country for their outstanding contribution and sharing their learnings and knowledge through the chapters of this book.

I extend a very special gratitude to Dr Yash Pal Munjal, stalwart of the Association of Physicians of India (API), for being on my side ever guiding me. Dr KK Pareek needs a special mention and gratitude for the support I received from him and for his kind words for me in the "Foreword" of the book.

It was not possible to successfully complete the task of publishing this book without the support and help of the members of the Scientific Committee and the members of the Editorial Board. I am grateful to them for providing timely inputs which were crucial in bringing everything together.

I express my very sincere thanks to my friend and close associate Dr Rakesh Bhadade for his constant support and standing shoulder to shoulder with me. I extend my special thanks to Dr Anupam Prakash for his tireless help in formulating this book.

I express my sincere gratitude and appreciation to the efforts of Shri Jitender P Vij (Group Chairman), Mr MS Mani (Group President), and Mr Ankit Vij (Managing Director), Jaypee Brothers Medical Publishers (P) Ltd, New Delhi, India, for their sincere efforts in publishing this book. Furthermore, I am thankful to Ms Chetna Malhotra (Senior Director—Professional Publishing, Marketing and Business Development), Ms Pooja Bhandari (Director—Production), Ms Nedup Bhutia Pillai (Team Leader—Print Publishing), Ms Tamali Deb (Manager—Copyediting), Mr Ajay Kumar Sharma (DGM—Production), Mr Sunil Dogra [Assistant Manager Production (Designing Department)], Mr Keshav Kumar (Assistant Manager—Production), Mr Manoj Kumar (Team Leader—Production), Ms Seema Dogra (Cover Visualizer), and Mr Varun Rajoria (Senior Graphic Designer) and the entire team of M/s Jaypee Brothers Medical Publishers (P) Ltd, New Delhi, India, who have been instrumental in giving the final shape to this book. Their sincere efforts are truly praiseworthy.

I extend my very sincere thanks and deep sense of appreciation to the members of the editorial office Mr Aniruddha Sapatnekar, Director, OneMD, for all his help. He has worked tirelessly and diligently at every step of giving final shape to this book.

I also express my very sincere thanks to the members of the Governing Body, API; Faculty Council, Indian College of Physicians (ICP); and Members of Board of Directors, Physicians Research Foundation (PRF), for helping me with their valuable suggestions, inputs, and guidance.

I appreciate the help and cooperation of API office members, especially Mrs Sunita Shukla and Mr Rajanikant Parmar.

I am grateful to all the honorable members of API who gave me the opportunity to publish this book as Chairman Scientific Committee APICON 2023 and President-Elect of the elite organization, API.

The compilation of this book would not have been possible without the participation and assistance of so many people whose names may not all be enumerated, but their contribution is sincerely appreciated and gratefully acknowledged.

In the end, I would like to thank the Almighty God for his blessings without which I would not have been able to do any of this.

Milind Y Nadkar

CONTENTS

VOLUME 1

SECTION 1: CARDIOLOGY

SECTION 2: CRITICAL CARE

SECTION 3: DIABETES

SECTION 8: HEPATOLOGY

SECTION 9: HYPERTENSION

SECTION 10: IMMUNOLOGY

VOLUME 2

SECTION 11: INFECTIONS

SECTION 14: NEUROLOGY

SECTION 18: PULMONOLOGY

SECTION 20: MISCELLANEOUS

SECTION

11

INFECTIONS

144

CHAPTER

Emerging Infectious Disease

Anchin Kalia, Krunal Patel

ABSTRACT

Emerging infectious diseases are the ones that either have appeared and affected the population for the first time or have existed previously but are now rapidly spreading, with either increase in the number of people getting infected or via spreading to new geographical areas, and thus pose a constant threat, especially in healthcare settings. Pandemics tend to occur when there is disruption to the ecosystem such as introducing a strain of virus into humans or animals against which they are not immune. There is an ongoing risk of the emergence of infectious diseases with the growth of the human population and the increase in urbanization. The emergence and re-emergence of infectious diseases are influenced by multiple factors such as climate, demographic changes, and ecological factors. As humans may have little or no immunity to emerging infectious diseases, their impact on the health system, economy, and society is difficult to predict. Novel human coronavirus [severe acute respiratory syndrome-coronavirus (SARS-CoV)], Crimean Congo hemorrhagic fever (CCHF), Avian influenza [H5N1], and others discussed here in this chapter are examples of diseases that have recently emerged and have affected the World Health Organization (WHO) South East Asia region. This chapter contains key information regarding the emergence and re-emergence of major infectious diseases.

INTRODUCTION

An emerging infectious disease is defined as one that has appeared and affected a population for the first time or has existed previously, declined, or was controlled, but is rapidly increasing, in terms of either the number of new cases within a population or its spread to new geographical areas.

Sometimes, an old disease appears in a new clinical form that may be severe or fatal. These are known as re-emerging infectious diseases. Human behavior affects re-emergence. For example, overuse of antibiotics has led to the growth of disease-causing organisms that are resistant to medicines. It has allowed a re-emergence of diseases that once were treatable and controllable.

Emerging infectious diseases are categorized into two types:

1. *Zoonotic diseases*: These are the which are transmitted from animals to humans through direct contact or via food, water, and environment. For example, Hantavirus pulmonary syndrome, brucellosis, Q fever.
2. *Vector-borne diseases*: These are the ones which are caused by bacteria, parasites, and viruses that are transmitted by vectors (mosquitoes, ticks, flies) such as malaria, zika virus disease, chikungunya, dengue fever.

HOW INFECTIONS EMERGE?

Infectious disease emergence involves two main steps:

1. An agent is introduced into a new host population.
2. The agent is established and transmitted within the new host population.

Between 60 and 80% of emerging infectious diseases are derived from animal sources. From HIV-1 and HIV-2, to the 1918 influenza virus to Middle East respiratory syndrome coronavirus, to severe acute respiratory syndrome-coronavirus 2 (SARS-CoV-2), all have emerged

TABLE 1: Emerging diseases in India.

Disease	Agent	Vector	Mode of transmission	Clinical signs and symptoms	Treatment
Avian Influenza [H5N1]	–	–	• Infection of humans from poultry is rare • Most likely occurs through direct or indirect contact with sick or dead birds or contaminated products • Human to human rare and is by direct respiratory route	• Rapid onset of flu-like symptoms (fever, chills, body ache, headache, sore throat, dry cough) • Frequent watery diarrhea, and progression to severe pneumonia and multiorgan failure	• *Early stage*: Antiviral medicines • Family member, if any, develops a fever after body aches or running nose-like symptoms should contact the nearest health center or doctor
Chikungunya (Incubation period: Usually 3–7 days)	Alphavirus *Togaviridae* family of arboviruses	*Mosquitoes*: *Aedes aegypti* and *Aedes albopictus*	Bite of infected female mosquito	• Sudden onset of fever, severe headache, chills, nausea and vomiting, severe joint pains • Serious complications are not common but can cause death in older people	• Symptomatic treatment with anti-inflammatory drugs • People with persistent joint pain may require analgesics and long-term anti-inflammatory therapy
Crimean–Congo hemorrhagic fever (CCHF) (Incubation period: 1–3 days following tickbite)	Nairovirus *Bunyaviridae* family	*Ticks*: *Hyalomma* genus commonly	Direct contact with blood or tissues of livestock, tick bites, affected people	• With sudden onset of high fever and chills, headache, dizziness, muscle pain • Also, gastrointestinal (GI) symptoms, flushing of face and neck, bleeding manifestations, and congested conjunctiva	• Antiviral agents have shown some benefit • But the mainstay of management is general supportive therapy
Dengue (breakbone fever) (Incubation period: 4–6 days after mosquito bite)	Dengue virus *Flaviviridae* family	*Mosquitoes*: *Aedes* genus recognized by black and white strips/spot markings on their bodies and legs	Bite of infected female mosquito	• Fever with rash, severe headache, pain behind the eyes, muscle and joint pains • Some may develop severe dengue or dengue shock syndrome (high-grade fever with facial flushing, bleeding manifestations, low BP, circulatory failure, critical state of shock)	• No specific drug or vaccine available for dengue treatment • Paracetamol is a drug of choice for fever and joint pain • Avoid aspirin as it increases the risk of bleeding • Use IV fluids judiciously
Novel human coronavirus (SARS-CoV) (Incubation period: 2–14 days)	SARS coronavirus (SARS-CoV)	–	Close person-to-person contact, i.e., by inhaling droplets when the infected person coughs or sneezes, and can be transmitted during air travel	• *Sudden onset of flu-like symptoms*: Fever, muscle pain, lethargy, cough, and sore throat • Severe cases progress to respiratory disease and pneumonia that can be fatal	• *Recently approved by FDA*: Nirmatrelvir/ Ritonavir (Paxlovid) (dosing depends on renal function) • Symptomatic and supportive therapy is required

Continued

Continued

Disease	Agent	Vector	Mode of transmission	Clinical signs and symptoms	Treatment
Scrub typhus (Incubation period: 5–20 days after the initial bite)	*Orientia tsutsugamushi*	–	Species of Chigger mites (*Leptotrombidium deliense* and others)	• Chigger bite is painless, maybe noticed as transient localized itch, scab at the bite site • Sudden shaking chills, fever, severe headache, infection of mucous of the conjunctiva, and swollen lymph nodes • Spotted rash on the trunk may be present and sometimes muscle or GI pain • Complications may include pneumonia and myocarditis	Treatable with antibiotics, mainly doxycycline
Japanese encephalitis (Incubation period: 5–15 days)	*Flavivirus* genus *Flaviviridae* family	*Mosquitoes*: *Culex vishnui* and *Culex tritaenio-rhynchus*	Bite of infected Culex mosquitoes, usually during the rainy season	• Rapid onset of high fever, stiff neck, coma, tremors, and convulsions • Can be clinically confused with cerebral malaria, meningitis, Chandipura virus, and West Nile virus	• No specific treatment • Supportive treatment and good nursing care can significantly reduce the number of deaths

information about vaccines. It is interesting to note that the debate over vaccines and vaccination coverage received extra focus during the novel coronavirus pandemic.

Testing and Diagnosis

The interplay of five components is what influences how testing affects the outcome of an infectious disease outbreak:

- *First*: Diagnosing the disease
- *Second*: Preventing it from spreading
- *Third*: Identifying the communities or populations most impacted
- *Fourth*: Mapping the most severe hotspots and making preventive strategies
- *Fifth*: Identification of viral strains and controlling of outbreaks and epidemics

Treatment

Infections must be treated to control certain diseases at the population level. Treating infectious disease can significantly improve the quality of life for those who are infected by minimizing the disease's negative effects on social and economic spheres as well as preventing potential co-infection-related complications for the patient. An example of this is HIV-infected individuals under antiretroviral therapy and with undetectable viral load do not transmit the virus through sexual contact.

CONCLUSION

The dynamic landscape of emerging infectious diseases demands a unified global effort. As we have explored various pathogens and their unpredictable patterns, it becomes evident that vigilance and preparedness are crucial. Prevention through robust surveillance, timely intervention, and vaccination strategies, emerges as a linchpin in our defence against these dynamic threats. The narrative of emerging infectious diseases is ever-evolving, and our commitment to understanding, addressing, and preventing these threats must evolve with it.

SUGGESTED READINGS

1. GOV.UK. (2023). Emerging infections: how and why they arise. [online] Available from https://www.gov.uk/government/publications/emerging-infections-characteristics-epidemiology-and-global-distribution/emerging-infections-how-and-why-they-arise#:~:text=Between%2060%25%20and%2080%25%20of,within%20the%20new%20host%20population. [Last accessed December, 2023].
2. Baker RE, Mahmud AS, Miller IF, Rajeev M, Rasambainarivo F, Rice BL, Takahashi S, et al. Infectious disease in an era of global change. J Microbiol. 2022;20:193-205.
3. Ellwanger JH, da Veiga ABG, de Lima Kaminski V, Valverde-Villegas JM, de Freitas AWQ, Chies JAB. Control and prevention of infectious diseases from a One Health perspective. Genet Mol Biol. 2021;44(1 Suppl 1):e20200256.

145

CHAPTER

Biomarkers in Sepsis: Present and Future

A Bhagwati

ABSTRACT

Biomarkers serve an important value for diagnosis, prognosis and early detection of disease, and risk stratification theragnostic in patients with sepsis or presumed sepsis. Significant advances have occurred in the use of biomarkers and their predictive values.

INTRODUCTION

Sepsis is characterized by a dysregulated immune response which leads to organ dysfunction. This process generates host-response biomarkers, which play an important role in diagnosis, early detection of organ dysfunction, risk stratification, prognosis, patient management, and antimicrobial stewardship. There are many biomarkers, but only a few are commonly used in clinical procedures. They also may assist in stratifying septic patients into phenotypes, i.e., hyperinflammatory versus immunosuppressive.

BIOMARKERS (FLOWCHART 1)

- *Review of sepsis biomarkers*:
  - 178 different biomarkers
  - Most of them had been tested clinically:
    - Primarily as prognostic markers
    - Relatively few have been used for diagnosis
- *Large numbers of markers:*
  - Cytokines
  - Receptor biomarkers
  - Coagulation biomarkers
  - Biomarkers related to vascular endothelial damage
  - Markers related to organ dysfunction
  - Acute-phase protein biomarkers
  - Others

The biomarkers in use are:

Commonly in use—

- Procalcitonin (PCT)
- Mid-regional proadrenomedullin (MR-proADM)

Biomarkers under investigation with encouraging results:

- Pancreatic stone protein (PSP)
- Soluble triggering receptor expressed on myeloid cells-1 (sTREM-1)
- Presepsis

Older but still in use biomarkers include:

- Lactate
- C reactive protein (CRP)

Procalcitonin

Procalcitonin is a 116-amino acid peptide precursor of calcitonin and has been extensively investigated as an aid in critically ill patients with sepsis. It is produced by parafollicular cells of the thyroid and neuroendocrine cells of the lung and the intestine (extrathyroidal). It is raised in a response to a proinflammatory stimulus, especially of bacterial origin (mainly from the cells of lung and the intestine).

Characteristic of Procalcitonin

- Fast response (2–4 hours)
- Peak values (8–24 hours)

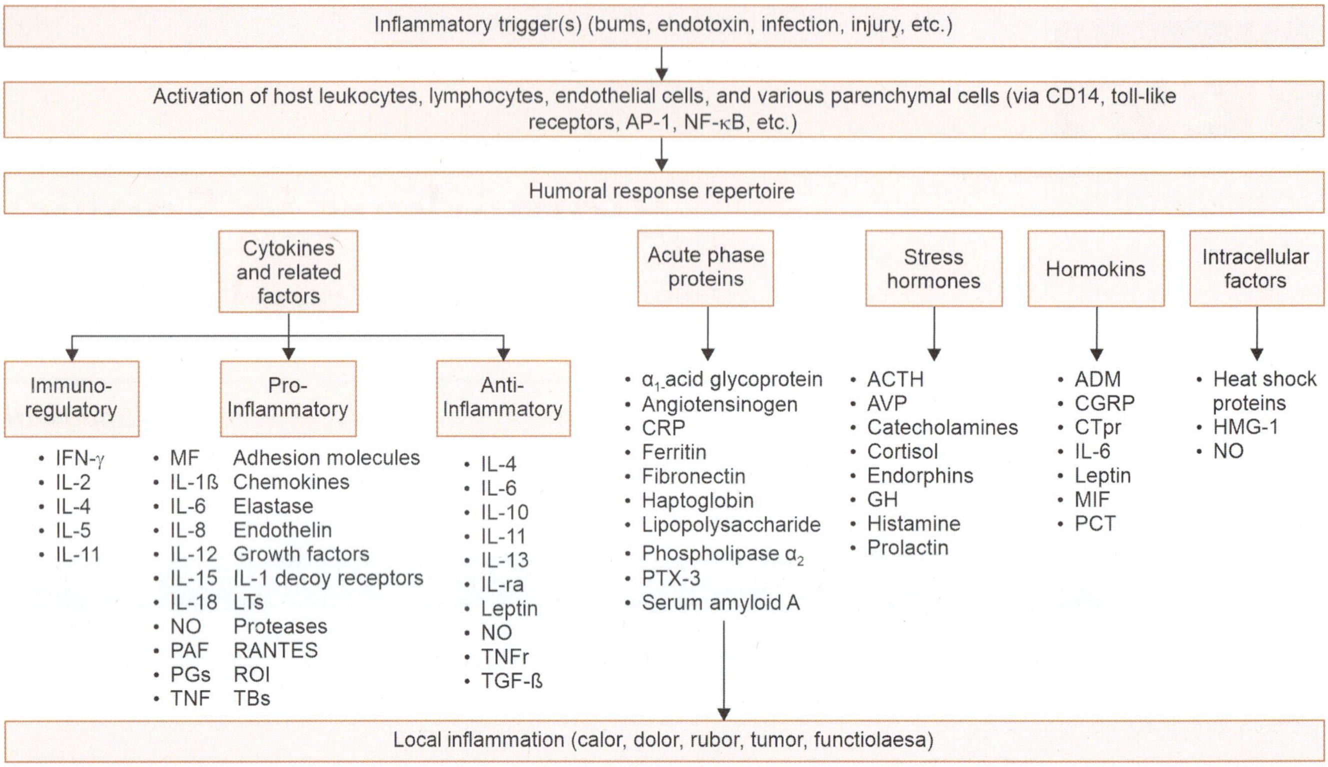

FLOWCHART 1: Biomarkers.

- Short half-life (~24 hours) independent of renal function
- Easy to measure in serum and plasma (stable in vivo and in vitro)
- Plasma concentration approximately <0.05–1,000 ng/mL

Reference Values of Procalcitonin (Except Children) (Table 1)

Above ten important systemic inflammatory response syndrome (SIRS), exclusively due to severe bacterial sepsis or septic shock. Suggest daily PCT measurement.

Uses of Procalcitonin

- Diagnosis of sepsis
- Antibiotic guidance **(Flowchart 2)**
- Prognostication

Nonbacterial Infections: Viruses, Fungi, and Parasites

Procalcitonin tends to be low in infection in girls. However, in systemic viral infection, the PCT value can be as high as 16 mg/mL.

TABLE 1: Procalcitonin (PCT) reference values.

<0.05 ng/mL	Healthy individuals
<5 ng/mL	Probability of sepsis is low, local infection possible
0.5–2 ng/mL	Moderate SIRS, in case of proven infection-diagnosis of sepsis PCT repeated after 6–24 hours
>2 ng/mL	Probability of sepsis is high

(SIRS: systemic inflammatory response syndrome)

A low serum PCT cannot be used to exclude bacterial from viral infections, but a combination of PCT, CRP, white blood cell (WBC), and clinical illness scoring system might be more useful.

Presepsin (Soluble CD14 Subtype)

The molecule is released into circulation after activation of a proinflammatory signal cascade on contact with infectious agents.

It is used in initial diagnosis and sepsis risk stratification. The diagnostic accuracy of PCT and presepsin in a meta-analysis of 19 studies that had enrolled 3,012 patients showed that the diagnostic accuracy of PCT and presepsin in identifying infection was similar, and both were useful in diagnosis of bacterial infections.

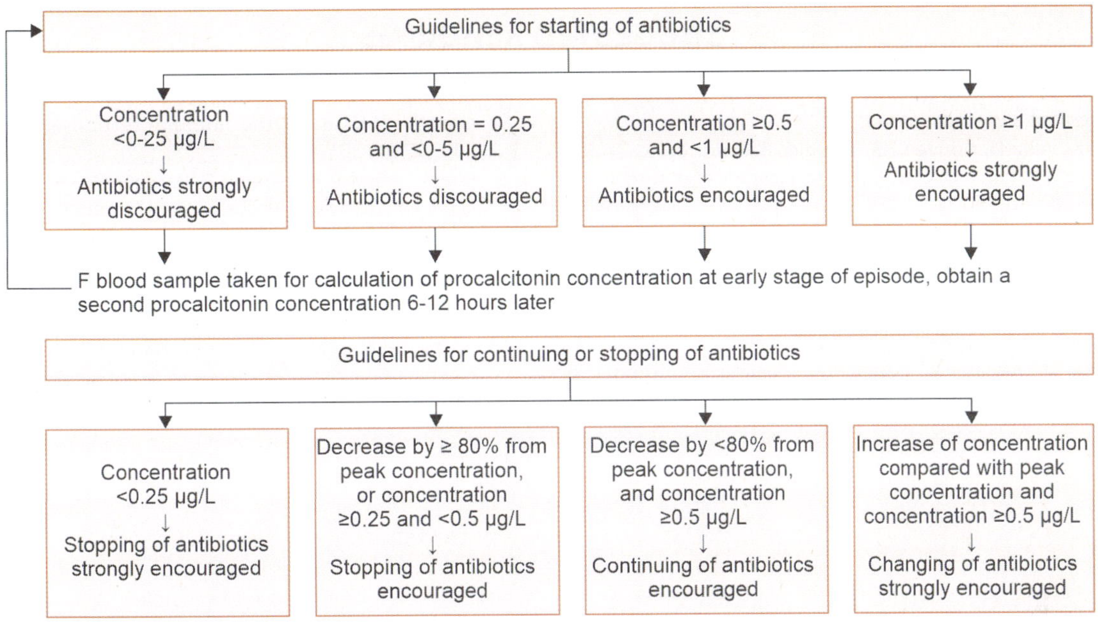

FLOWCHART 2: Guidelines for starting, continuing, or stopping of antibiotics according to procalcitonin concentrations.

Pancreatic Stone Protein

Pancreatic stone protein is a 14 kDa insoluble polypeptide encoded by a single transcript of the *reg* gene, resulting in a 144-amino acid length glycoprotein. PSP plays an important role in the immune and inflammatory response to infection, as a result of which it is identified to have potential. A biomarker of infection and sepsis was made. Various studies and analysis showed that PSP started to increase 5 days before the clinical diagnosis of sepsis. Hence, serial measurement demonstrated that there is an increase of this marker approximately 5 days prior to clinical diagnosis of sepsis, which plays a major role in the clinical diagnosis of sepsis. Hence, it is also shown to be a good prognostic marker of sepsis.

Mid-regional Proadrenomedullin

Mid-regional proadrenomedullin is a potent vasodilator agent with immune-modulating metabolic properties which rise in sepsis.

It is synthesized in different tissues, including the adrenal cortex, kidney, lung, blood vessels, and heart. MR-proADM is a good application in the prompt identification of sepsis patients with a moderate illness severity. It has the highest predictive value for mortality and is a reliable marker of mortality and disease severity along time in sepsis. Hence, it is a good organ dysfunction marker, which helps in discrimination of survivors and nonsurvivors. The higher clearance of MR-proADM levels during an intensive care unit (ICU) stay indicates a favorable outcome.

Soluble Triggering Receptor Expressed on Myeloid Cells-1

The Triggering Receptor Expressed on Myeloid Cells (TREM) family has several isoforms which share low sequence homology with each other and have only one immunoglobulin-like domain. Activation of toll-like receptors (TLRs) upregulates and amplifies the expression of TREM-1. Its expression is significantly enhanced in skin, biological fluids, and tissues infected by gram-positive and gram-negative bacteria, including fungi.

This molecule plays a role in nearly distinction between sepsis and SIRS. It also serves as a prognostic marker of infection and plays some role as a diagnostic marker of sepsis. However, further data is awaited.

CONCLUSION

Clinical management in critical illness, particularly in sepsis, becomes an interplay between the application of clinical parameters and the use of sepsis biomarkers. An important consideration that much prevents routine serial use of these biomarkers in the ICU is the high cost of the test. Also, recent progress in several areas of biomarker research can transform the application of biomarkers for diagnosis, prognosis, risk stratification, molecular phenotypic, and monitoring of therapeutic response in treatment.

SUGGESTED READINGS

1. Jaun Carlos Ruiz-Rodriguez JC, Chiscano-Canon L, et al. ICU Management and Practice. 2023.
2. Andaluz-Ojeda D, Nguyen HB, Meunier-Beillard N, Cicuéndez R, Quenot J-P, Calvo D, et al. Superior accuracy of mid-regional proadrenomedullin for mortality prediction in sepsis with varying levels of illness severity. Ann Intensive Care. 2017; 7(1):15.
3. Becker KL, Snider R, Nylen ES. Procalcitonin assay in systemic inflammation, infection, and sepsis, clinical utility and limitations. Criti Care Med. 2008;36(3):941-52.
4. Bleharski JR, Kiessler V, Buonsanti C, Sieling PA, Stenger S, Colonna M, et al. A role for triggering receptor expressed on myeloid cells-1 in host defence during the early-induced and adaptive phases of the immune response. J Immunology. 2003;170(7):3812-8.
5. Boeck L, Graf R, Eggimann P, Pargger H, Raptis DA, Smyrnios N, et al. Pancreatic stone protein; a marker of organ failure and outcome in ventilator associated pneumonia. Chest. 2011;140(4):925-32.
6. Enguix-Armada A, Escobar-Conesa R, García-De La Torre A, De La Torre-Prados MV. Usefulness of several biomarkers in the management of septic patients: C-reactive protein, procalcitonin, presepsin and mid-regional pro-adrenomedullin. Clin Chem Lab Med. 2016;54(1):163-8.

146

CHAPTER

Malaria: Are We on the Path to Eradication?

Bhaskar Kanti Nath, Umar Faruque

ABSTRACT

Malaria eradication has been a global health priority for many years. While progress has been made in reducing malaria-related deaths, there are still significant challenges to overcome. These challenges include limited healthcare accessibility, diagnostic difficulties, drug resistance, and social and cultural barriers. However, innovative strategies and tools such as vector-control methods, chemoprevention and newer methods like gene drive mosquito technology, sterile insect technology (SIT), and newer drugs are being explored to intensify the fight against malaria. With continued dedication, collaboration, and innovation, there is hope for a world free from the burden of malaria.

INTRODUCTION

Malaria has been a long-standing global health challenge. Whereas previously the idea of eliminating malaria at the regional level appeared out of reach, the international conversation has now shifted to an even loftier goal—total eradication of malaria. Finding agreement on the viability and the way to eradicating malaria has proven challenging, despite greater funding, technological advancements, and a significant decline in annual mortality. While the road ahead is still fraught with challenges, there is hope that with continued efforts and innovations, we may eventually rid the world of this deadly disease.

GLOBAL FIGHT AGAINST MALARIA

The global fight against malaria is a determined and ongoing effort to combat one of humanity's oldest and deadliest foes. Malaria, caused by the *Plasmodium* parasite and transmitted by bite of a female anopheles mosquito, is a scientifically complex and life-threatening disease. Its prevalence is highest in the tropical and subtropical regions of the world. Approximately 247 million cases and 6,19,000 deaths due to malaria have been reported in 2021 worldwide with *Plasmodium falciparum* being the most common cause.

Over the years, significant progress has been made, resulting in a substantial reduction in malaria-related mortality rates. This progress is attributed to a combination of factors including the widespread distribution of insecticide-treated bed nets, indoor residual spraying (IRS), the development of more effective antimalarial medications, and the pursuit of innovative solutions such as malaria vaccines.

However, considerable challenges remain including drug resistance, insecticide resistance, and limited healthcare access in vulnerable regions. Despite these obstacles, international partnerships, research advancements, and political commitment offer hope for a future where malaria is no longer a global health threat (**Fig. 1**).

PROGRESS TOWARD MALARIA ERADICATION

Progress toward malaria eradication has been both promising and challenging. Significant strides have been made in reducing malaria-related deaths and improving access to prevention and treatment in many parts of the world. A few facts include the following.

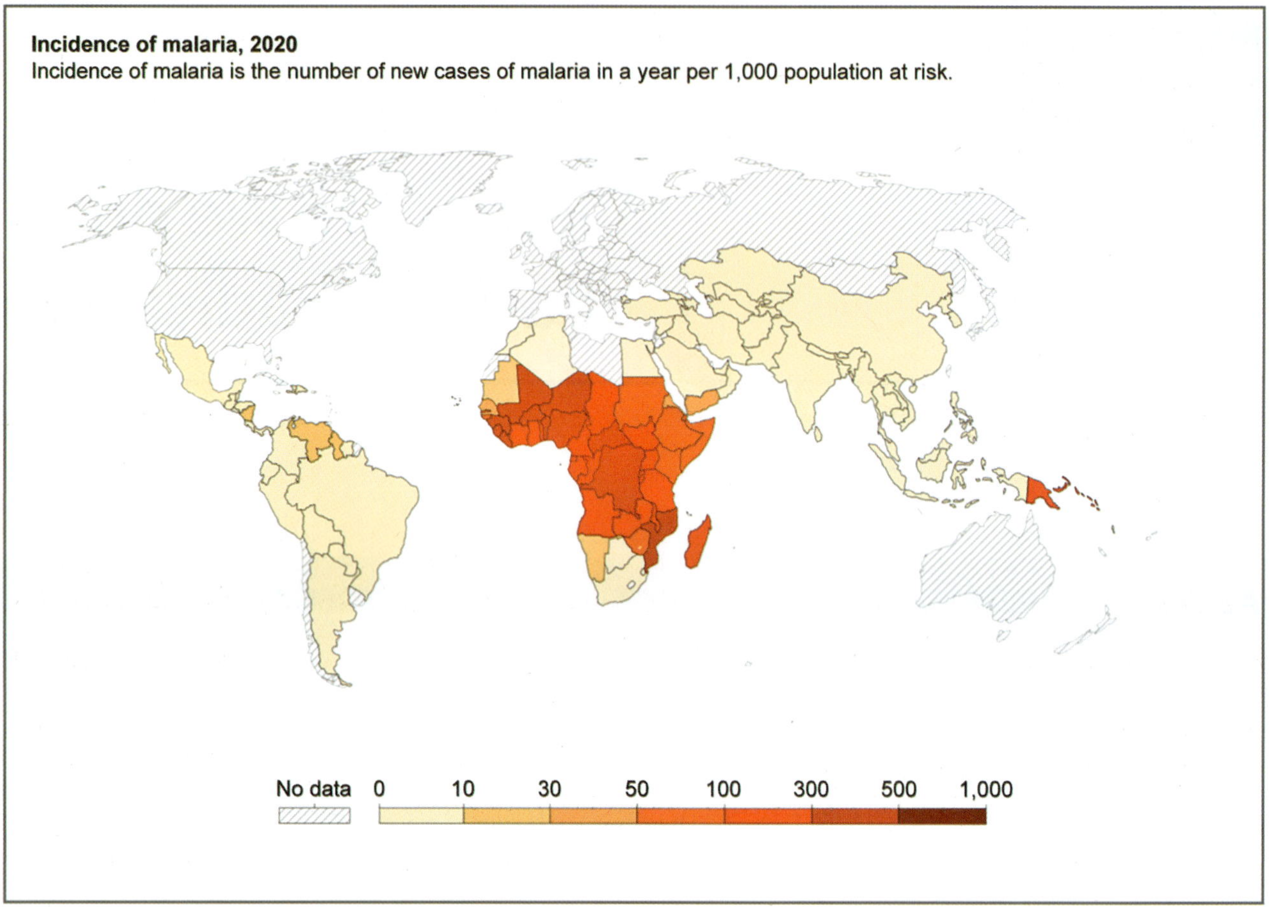

FIG. 1: Incidence of malaria.

Source: World Health Organization (via World Bank).

The latest data shows that malaria-endemic countries have reduced from 108 in year 2000 to 84 in 2021.

The number of nations that were malaria endemic in 2000 and reported fewer than 100 malaria cases climbed from 6 in 2000 to 27 in 2021, maintaining steady in 2021 when compared to 2020.

However, there has been a noticeable increase in the number of *Plasmodium knowlesi* infections in humans in some countries in the South-East Asia (SEA) region, particularly in Malaysia with 13 deaths from 3,575 *Plasmodium knowlesi* cases that were documented in 2021 alone.

Despite the setbacks, several countries continue to make significant progress; between 2011 and 2021, the classification rates among the E-2025 countries (WHO launched the E-2025 initiative to halt the transmission of malaria in 25 identified countries by 2025) climbed from 7.6 to 90.8%, suggesting sustained efforts by governments in pursuit of their elimination targets. On the other hand, no country that was declared to be free of malaria between 2000 and 2021 has been discovered to have malaria transmission re-established.

CHALLENGES IN ELIMINATING MALARIA

The history of malaria dates back to 2700 BCE when scriptures like the Chinese Nei Ching (the Canon of Medicine) described recurrent fevers with signs and symptoms similar to malaria. The prevalence and distribution of many hemoglobinopathies, including sickle cell anemia, and the selection for specific features that gave carriers a minor survival advantage have all been directly influenced by malaria.

It is hardly surprising that malaria eradication has been a top priority of global public health, for almost a century, given the burden and history of the disease. However, there are several obstacles to overcome, which are as follows:

- *Healthcare accessibility:* Access to healthcare services continues to be a serious issue in many nations. In Africa, just one in five pregnant women who live in areas with moderate to high malaria transmission can get the medication they need to prevent malaria.
- *Diagnostic challenges:* Rapid diagnostic tests (RTDs) used to diagnose *P. falciparum* primarily

detect the histidine-rich protein 2 (HRP2). Studies regarding Pfhrp2 along with Pfhrp3 deletions have been conducted in 47 countries and the presence of deletions has been confirmed in 40 countries. Such false-negative RDT results due to such deletion pose a threat to malaria eradication.

- *Insecticide resistance:* All of the major anopheline vectors around the world have been documented to have insecticide resistance. More than 78 nations have reported verified resistance to at least one type of insecticide in the most recent decade, and 29 nations confirmed resistance to four insecticide classes—pyrethroids, organophosphates, carbamates, and organochlorines—in at least one malaria vector species across different sites in the country.
- *Antimalarial drug resistance:* In SEA nations, artemisinin-based combination therapy has replaced the long-used chloroquine and the recently discontinued sulfadoxine-pyrimethamine as the first-line treatments for *Plasmodium falciparum* malaria. However, *Plasmodium falciparum* artemisinin resistance was first reported in 2008 in Cambodia. Later, it was discovered that the mutation in the kelch 13 propeller gene, which was linked to this resistance, had spread to several nations, including India. Even though substantial resources have been invested in creating more effective antimalarial drugs over the past few decades, the emergence and rapid spread of resistance is a hefty challenge for malaria eradication.
- *Social and cultural barriers to eliminating malaria:* Understanding how communities perceive and respond to malaria is crucial for designing effective control programs. Communities may have diverse beliefs and behaviors related to malaria, and these can influence the success of intervention measures. Studies have found that the disease was more prevalent among those who have low income, poor knowledge of basic malaria facts, inhabit remote areas, and hesitate to use bed nets. These factors need to be tackled to successfully curb the disease.

INNOVATIVE STRATEGIES AND TOOLS

To control and ultimately eradicate malaria, it is necessary to develop new tools and technologies as well as improved mechanisms for maintaining detailed surveillance and spatial decision support systems (SDSS), which enhance improved reporting and timeliness of interventions.

Strategies that are currently in use to control malaria include the following:

- Vector-control methods (i.e., diminishing the vectors' capacity to bite people and spread the parasite, hence lowering the risk of infection)
- Chemoprophylaxis methods (i.e., giving patients antimalarial medications to halt disease progression as prophylaxis during visit to endemic regions)
- Environmental management and chemical control (such as IRS)
- Biological control (such as genetically modified mosquitos)
- Personal protective behavior [such as sleeping under long-lasting insecticidal bed nets, (LLINs) and applying insect repellents—though they have a limited impact on elimination]

Strategies and tools under trials that hold the potential to further intensify the fight against the eradication of malaria include the following:

- *Gene drive mosquito technology:* This involves CRISPR-Cas9-based technology to create genetic alternation in mosquitoes that targets inhibiting mosquito reproduction or viability, thereby aiming to eradicate or decrease the population to levels incapable of supporting disease transmission. However, the effect of transmission of modified genes to mosquito species that do not transmit diseases and the effect of total eradication of the mosquitoes on the ecosystem are some issues that researchers are trying to find out.
- *Sterile insect technology (SIT):* The SIT method relies on the idea that releasing sterile males with native females will reduce the females' capacity for reproduction and, if enough males are released over a long enough period, result in the local eradication or suppression of the mosquito population. Unlike "gene drive" systems, which might reduce disease vectors permanently by transferring desirable genetic modifications from one generation to the next, SIT is self-limiting and is not expected to persist or spread in the environment. Although the strong record of success against a range of agricultural pest insects has been documented, the same is under research to control malaria.
- *Malaria vaccine:* RTS,S/AS01 (RTS,S) is a vaccine developed for the prevention of *Plasmodium falciparum* infection. Although the effectiveness is moderate, the RTS,S/AS01 vaccination nonetheless has a major positive impact on public health. According to the phase 3 results for this vaccine, for every 1,000 children who received four doses of the vaccine, 1,744 clinical cases of malaria were averted. Children in sub-Saharan Africa and other areas with moderate to high *Plasmodium falciparum* malaria transmission are advised to receive the RTS,S/AS01 (RTS,S) malaria vaccine, as recommended by the World Health Organization (WHO). The recommendation is supported by findings from a running pilot program in Ghana, Kenya, and Malawi.

- *Ivermectin for malaria control:* Ivermectin, a common and inexpensive anti-helminthic medicine used to treat onchocerciasis (river blindness) and other parasitic infections, has been discovered by Senegal and Colorado State University researchers to have the potential to significantly reduce malaria transmission. The study discovered that over 2 weeks after participants in different Senegalese villages took the medicine ivermectin as part of a campaign to battle onchocerciasis, collaterally reduced transmission of malaria parasites by mosquitoes. The medication seems to kill mosquitoes that transmit malaria. However, further studies are needed regarding this before mass drug administration of ivermectin can be used as a strategy to control malaria transmission.
- *Next-generation antimalarial medications:* There is an unmet need for newer drugs for malaria treatment, provided that artemisinin-based therapy is developing resistance. Some drugs under trial include ganaplacide-lumefantrine, M5717-pyronaridine, ZY19489-ferroquine, and cipargamin.
- *Piperonyl butoxide (PBO) nets:* Bed nets sprayed with pyrethroid insecticides have been widely used to cut down on the spread of malaria. The malaria-carrying mosquitoes are now becoming resistant to this class of insecticide, though. The addition of PBO, a different molecule, to the bed nets is one strategy for overcoming this resistance. Although PBO is not an insecticide, it does operate by blocking an enzyme that the mosquito contains and which prevents the action of pyrethroids.
- *Attractive toxic sugar baits (ATSBs):* ATSBs are regarded as a new paradigm for vector control. Due to their ease of production and low cost, they are technologically acceptable. ATSBs can be used both indoors and outdoors to kill mosquitoes that are attracted to sugar and feed on a sugary solution containing a mosquitocidal chemical like malathion, Pirimiphos-methyl, etc.
- *Drone-mediated larvae control:* Some researchers effectively used drones to control vectors of malaria by aerial application of Aquatain Mosquito Formulation (AMF), a monomolecular surface film with larvicidal activity at targeted zones. However, this strategy merits further development in terms of cost and application due to the urgent demand for outdoor malaria mosquito-control techniques.

FUTURE PROSPECTS FOR MALARIA ERADICATION

While complete eradication of malaria remains a formidable challenge, the progress made in recent years is encouraging. With continued dedication, collaboration, and innovation, we have a real chance of seeing a world free from the burden of malaria. It is a goal that, while difficult, is worth pursuing for the health and well-being of millions around the globe.

In conclusion, the path to malaria eradication is a challenging one, but it is not insurmountable. By building on the progress made and embracing innovative approaches, we can move closer to a world where malaria is a thing of the past. It is a path that requires commitment, resources, and a global effort, but the potential rewards in terms of lives saved and communities thriving make it a journey well worth taking.

SUGGESTED READINGS

1. Hemingway J, Shretta R, Wells TN, Bell D, Djimdé AA, Achee N, et al. Tools and strategies for malaria control and elimination: What do we need to achieve a grand convergence in malaria? PLoS Biol. 2016;14(3):e1002380.
2. Dhiman S. Are malaria elimination efforts on right track? An analysis of gains achieved and challenges ahead. Infect Dis Poverty. 2019;8(1):14.
3. Laurens MB. RTS,S/AS01 vaccine (MosquirixTM): An overview. Hum Vaccin Immunother. 2019;16(3):480-9.
4. Kobylinski KC, Sarr MD, Sylla M, Foy BD, Chapman PL. Ivermectin mass drug administration to humans disrupts malaria parasite transmission in Senegalese villages. Am J Trop Med Hyg. 2011;85(1):3-5.
5. Alphey L, Benedict M, Bellini R, Clark GG, Dame DA, Service MW, et al. Sterile-insect methods for control of mosquito-borne diseases: An analysis. Vector-Borne Zoonotic Dis. 2010;10(3): 295-311.
6. Fiorenzano JM, Koehler PG, Xue R-D. Attractive toxic sugar bait (ATSB) for control of mosquitoes and its impact on non-target organisms: A review. Int J Environ Res Public Health. 2017;14(4):398.
7. World Health Organization. (2022). World malaria report 2022 [online] Available from https://www.who.int/teams/global-malaria-programme/reports/world-malaria-report-2022 [Last accessed December, 2023].

147

CHAPTER

Dengue: Pathophysiology and Clinical Aspects of Dengue Fever

Raman Sharma, Tapas Kannu Vyas, Anil Mahla, Manish Pahariya

ABSTRACT

Dengue is an arthropod vector-borne disease affecting millions and causing significant mortality globally. The four serotypes (DENV 1–4) of this Flavivirus are transmitted to humans by Aedes aegypti and Aedes albopictus mosquitoes. Transmission in humans through the vector is highly efficient with secondary attack rates, sometimes reaching up to 50–70%.

Antibody dependent enhancement is the current accepted pathogenesis for clinical manifestations of severe dengue resulting from an enhanced cytokine storm.

Diagnosis is primarily established in two stages—in stage I (stage of fever and viremia) by nonstructural protein 1 antigen (NS1 Ag) testing (sensitivity 90% in febrile phase) and in stage 2 (early post febrile period) by immunoglobulin M (IgM) capture enzyme-linked immunosorbent assay (ELISA) (sensitivity of 90–97%). Management is relatively simple, cost efficient, and highly effective in saving lives if instituted timely and precisely. Untreated mortality of dengue shock syndrome may reach up to 40% but with treatment it may be < 1%.

Cornerstone of management is appropriately instituted volume replacement.

Early identification of pre-shock stage through warning signs can be the game changer.

For an infection which has been present since centuries together no efficacious antiviral has been found to work. Prevention is limited to personal protection, and difficult to achieve vector control measures.

INTRODUCTION

Dengue virus (DENV) is responsible for an estimated 100 million symptomatic cases of infection out of 390 million infections and 10,000 deaths annually.

Dengue fever (DF) is the most prevalent arthropod-borne disease caused by Flavivirus documented since 1779-1780 and has shown no decline with frequent resurgences. Tropics and subtropical areas host to the vector and the agent **(Figs. 1 to 3)**.

The four serotypes of DENV (DENV 1-4) are transmitted to humans primarily by the bite of *Aedes aegypti* mosquito and *Aedes albopictus* **(Fig. 1)** without any crisscross immunity.

Dengue (DEN) 2 is the most prevalent serotype over the past 50 years in India with serotypes 3 and 4 frequenting in some outbreaks.

Risk of disease is presumed to be higher with areas having multiple circulating endemic serotypes. "Asian genotype" DEN 2 and 3 are associated with severe disease

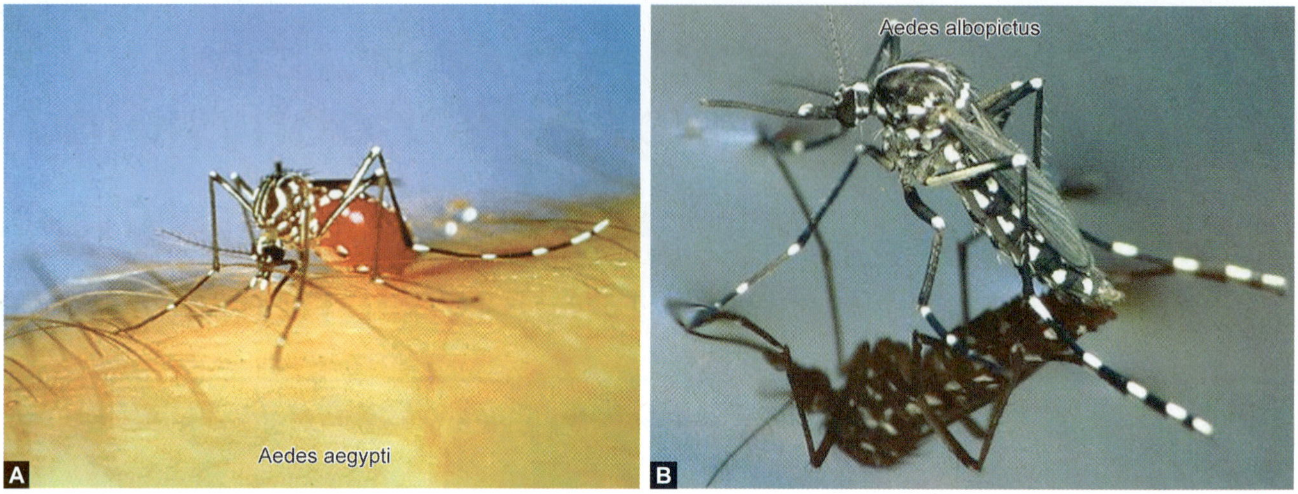

FIGS. 1A AND B: Asian tiger mosquito with tiger-like stripes. (A) *Aedes aegypti*; (B) *Aedes albopictus*.

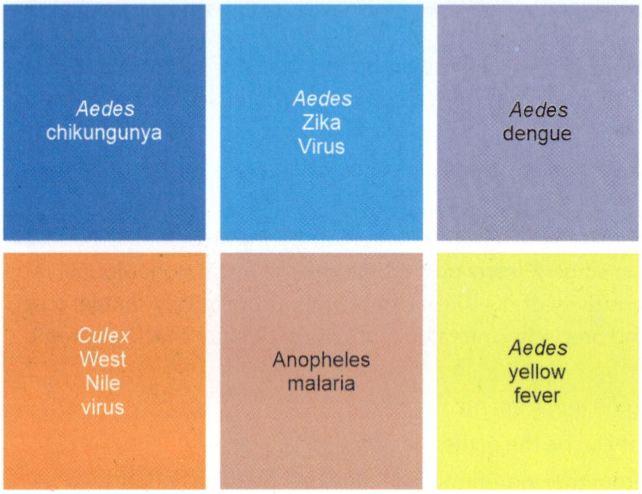

FIG. 2: Deadly mosquito-borne diseases.

and epidemic outbreaks. The secondary attack rate in dengue may reach up to 50–70%.

THE VECTOR

Mosquitoes, a "Spanish word for little fly", are the deadliest predators, responsible for devastating illnesses, there are >3,000 species, they are found in every part of the world except Antarctica **(Figs. 3 and 4)**.

It is an efficient vector because it is highly susceptible to DENV, feeding preferentially on human blood, causing an almost imperceptible bite, is a daytime feeder, is capable of biting several people in a short period for one blood meal and covers 50 or more households in a closed community. The mosquito is well adapted to life in urban settings and typically breeds in clean, stagnant water in containers that collect rainwater, such as coolers, tires, tin cans, pots, and buckets.

GLOBAL AGE-STANDARDIZED MORTALITY, INCIDENCE, AND DALY RATE OF DENGUE FEVER IN 2017

The precise burden of the disease in different populations cannot be assessed accurately. Disability-adjusted life year (DALY) is thus, used to assess the overall burden of the disease, a time-based measure that combines years of life lost due to premature mortality (YLLs) and years of life lost due to time lived in states of less than full health, or years of healthy life lost due to disability (YLDs).

One DALY represents the loss of the equivalent of one year of full health.

Two identifiable syndromes (primary/secondary):
1. Dengue fever (mostly primary)
2. Dengue hemorrhagic fever (DHF)/dengue shock syndrome (DSS) (mostly secondary) resulting from two sequential infections

Rest: Unclassified/intermediate/subclinical infection as shown in **Figure 5**.

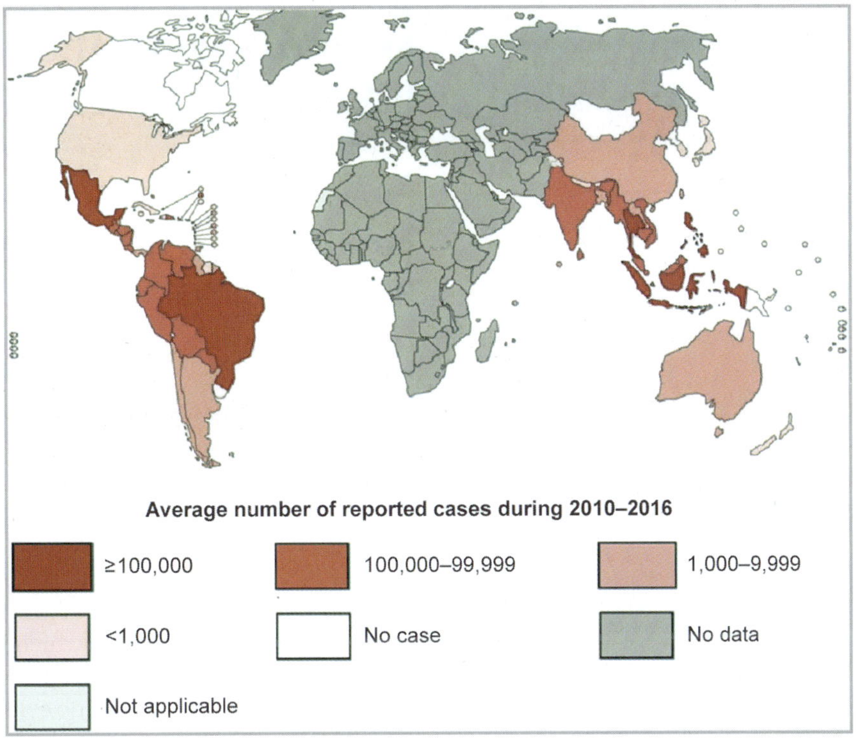

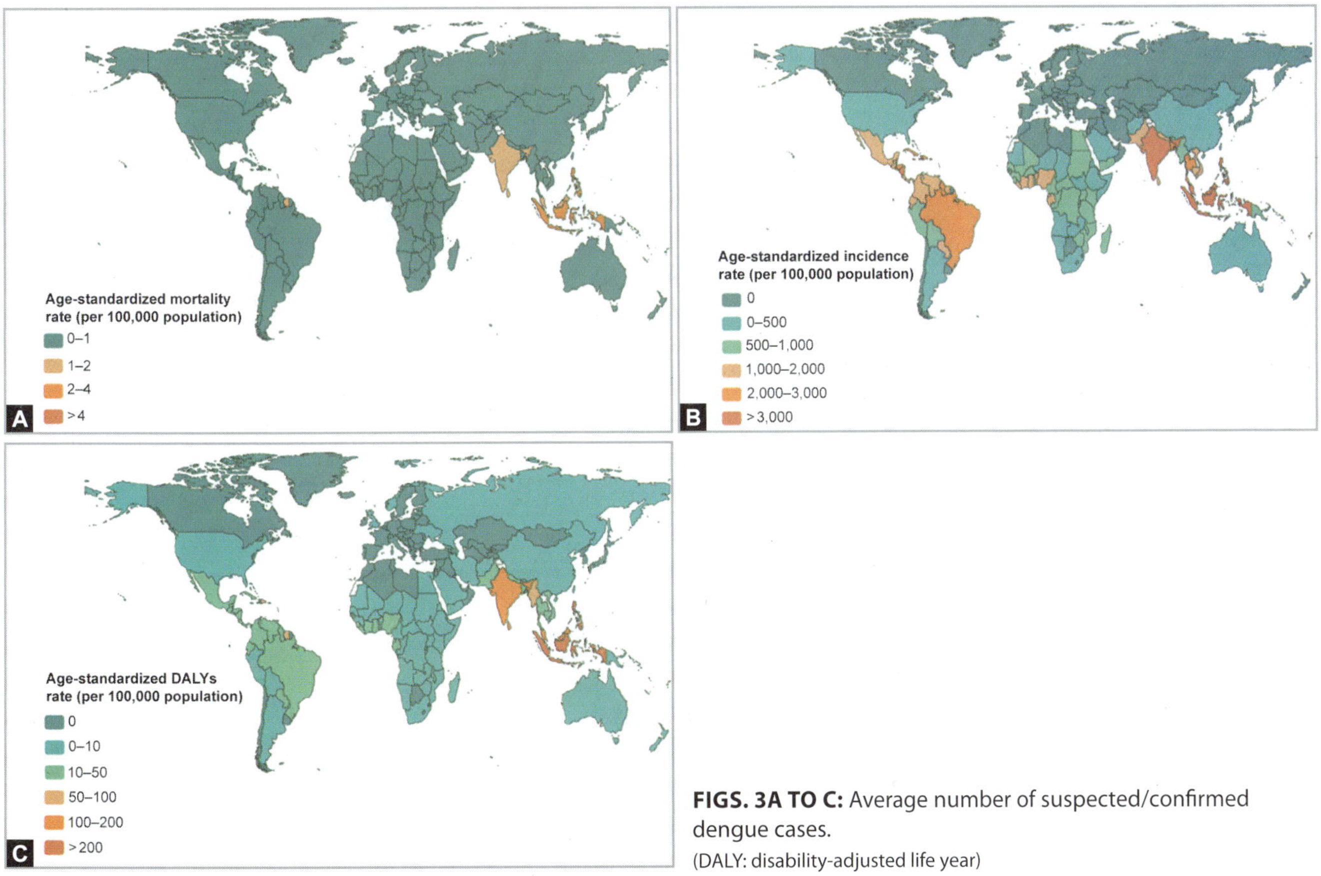

FIGS. 3A TO C: Average number of suspected/confirmed dengue cases.
(DALY: disability-adjusted life year)

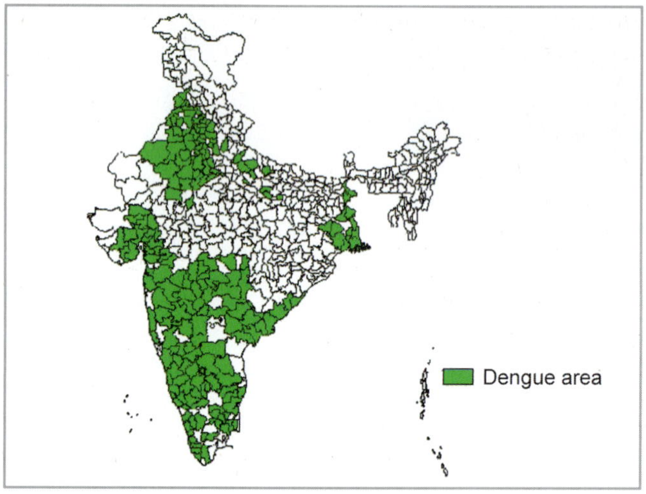

FIG. 4: Dengue areas of India by viral research and diagnostic laboratories (VRDL).

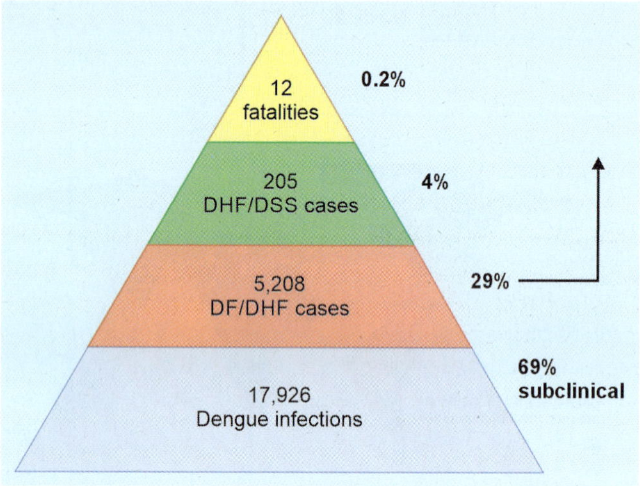

FIG. 5: ICEBERG characteristics of dengue (proportionate district of dengue cases during 1997 Cuban epidemic).

WORLD HEALTH ORGANIZATION 2012 REVISED CLASSIFICATION OF DENGUE (FIG. 6)

- Dengue fever
- Severe dengue

RISK FACTORS (FIG. 7) AND PATHOGENESIS

Current concept centers on the phenomenon of "antibody dependent enhancement" (ADE) which means infection by a new serotype virus leads to partnering with immunoglobulin G (IgG) due to a previous dengue infection and consequently infecting the macrophages and dendritic cells leading to liberation of inflammatory mediators causing the cytokine storm. Nonstructural protein 1 (NS1) modulates the glycocalyx with release of heparan sulfate.

The typical coagulopathy, which is usually manifested as an increase in activated partial thromboplastin time with low fibrinogen levels and no evidence of procoagulant activity is caused primarily due to loss of essential

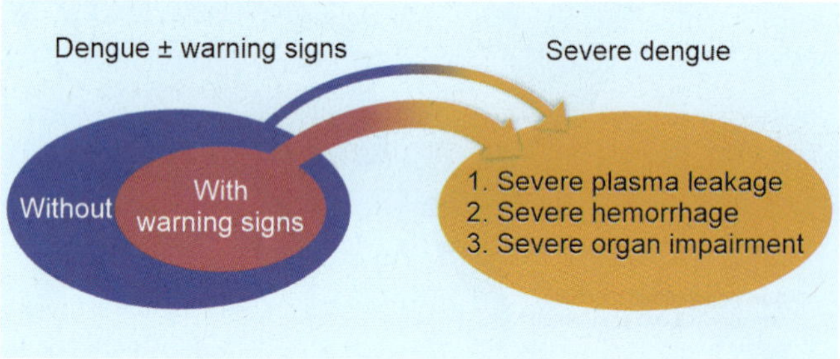

FIG. 6: Dengue case classification by severity.

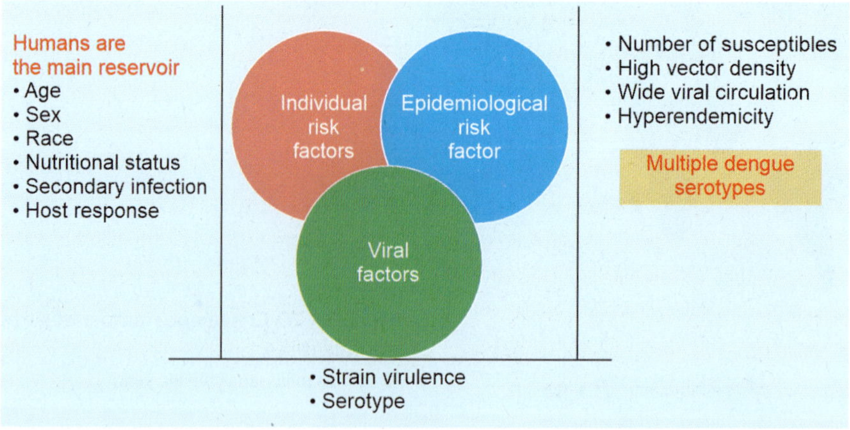

FIG. 7: Risk factors for dengue hemorrhagic fever/dengue shock syndrome (DHF/DSS).

coagulation proteins. Heparan sulfate may also contribute to the coagulopathy by acting as an anticoagulant.

Capillary leak syndrome: Plasma leakage, due to an increase in capillary permeability, is a cardinal feature of DHF but is absent in DF. Electron microscopy demonstrates widening of endothelial tight junction hence, establishing the fact that augmented capillary permeability is due to endothelial dysfunction rather than injury.

Blood and bone marrow: Leukopenia, thrombocytopenia, and a hemorrhagic diathesis are the typical hematologic findings in DENV infections. Leukopenia is apparent early in illness and is of similar degree in DHF and DF it is thought to represent a direct effect of DENV on the bone marrow.

CLINICAL FEATURES

- Febrile phase
- Critical phase
- Recovery phase

Dengue Fever (Febrile Phase)

Incubation: 7–10 days

Fever: 5–7 days associated with retro-orbital pain, myalgias, back pain, and polyarthralgias (break bone fever)

Rash **(Fig. 8)**:
- Centrifugal distribution
- Erythematous/urticarial/scarlatiniform
- Palmoplantar edema and pruritus

Dengue Hemorrhagic Fever (Critical Phase) WHO Classification 1997

(If untreated then leads to mortality of 10–20%)

Fever/H/O Fever

+

Thrombocytopenia < 100 k

Hemorrhagic manifestations

Evidence of plasma leakage

(The plasma leakage is more specific than hemorrhage)

↑ HCT > 20%

Hypoproteinemia

Effusions

Laboratory tests confirmed dengue infection in as many as 90% of these cases.

DSS/Severe Dengue (Critical Phase)

(Predicted mortality around 20–40%)

- SBP < 90 mm
- Narrow pulse pressure < 20 mm
- Fluid accumulation
- Severe bleeding
- SGOT/SGPT elevation > 1,000
- Neurological involvement
- Acute kidney injury (AKI) or
- Multiorgan dysfunction syndrome (MODS)

In 2011, the WHO South-East Asia Regional Office published new guidelines for the prevention and control of dengue and introduced the concept of the *expanded dengue syndrome*. The syndrome includes patients with severe organ involvement (liver, kidney, brain, or heart) but without evidence of plasma leakage **(Fig. 9)**.

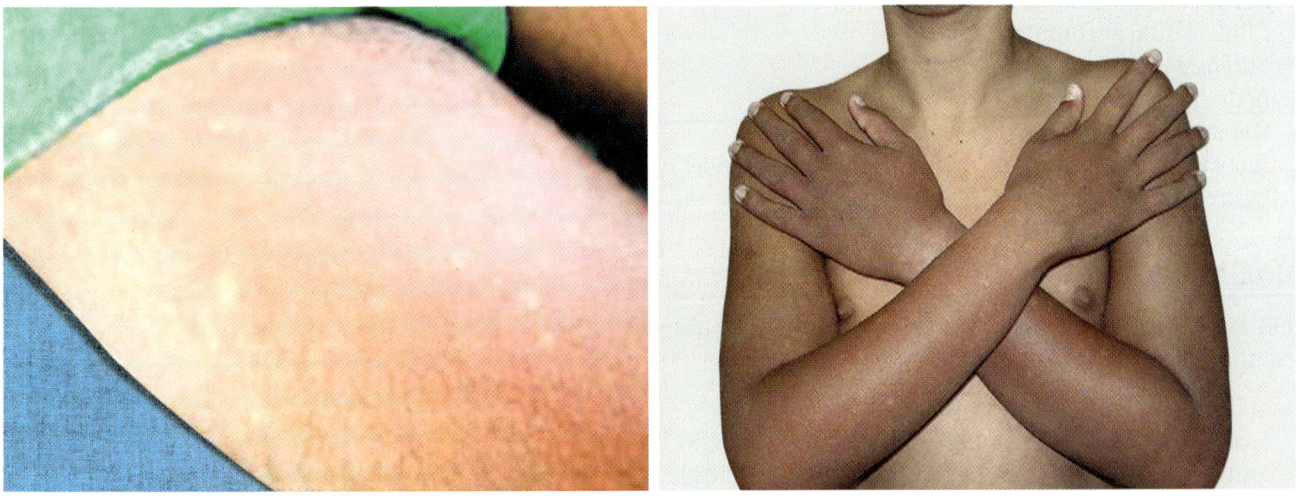

Rash with sparing of skin islands of Whites

Measly rash

FIG. 8: Rash—centrifugal distribution.

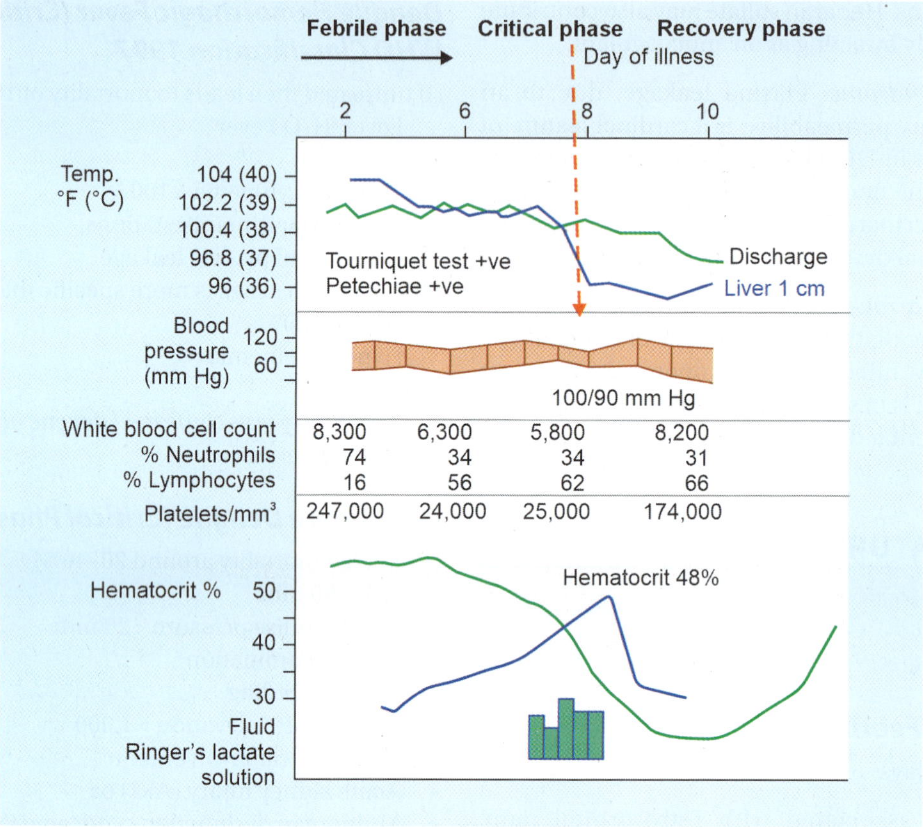

FIG. 9: Typical clinical course of dengue hemorrhage fever.

IDENTIFY PRESHOCK STAGE BY WARNING SIGNS (TABLE 1)

- Abdominal pain and tenderness
- Persistent vomiting
- Abrupt change from fever to hypothermia
- Clinical fluid accumulation
- Mucosal bleeding
- Lethargy/restlessness
- Hepatomegaly > 2 cm
- Increasing hematocrit (HCT) and decreasing platelet
- Decreased urine output

DIAGNOSIS (FIG. 10)

Real-time reverse transcriptase-polymerase chain reaction (RT-PCR) is most confirmative.

Diagnosis of dengue falls in two stages:

- *Stage I:* Fever and viremia accompanied by NS1 antigens in blood (rapid, sensitive, and specific). Diagnostic sensitivity of NS1 during febrile phase can

TABLE 1: Main signs and symptoms observed in DHF fatal cases studied in Cuba.

Clinical manifestation	1981	1997
Fever	88	100
Vomiting	81	100
Hepatomegaly	35	66.6
Abdominal pain	58	83.3
Ascites	8	91.6
Pleural effusion	8	58.3
Shock	100	100
Hemorrhagic manifestations	65	100
Petechiae	38	41.6
Hematemesis	35	58.3
Melena	4	25
Vaginal bleeding	44	42.8
Hemoconcentration	92	91.6
Thrombocytopenia	71.8	83.3

Note: Numbers given as %.

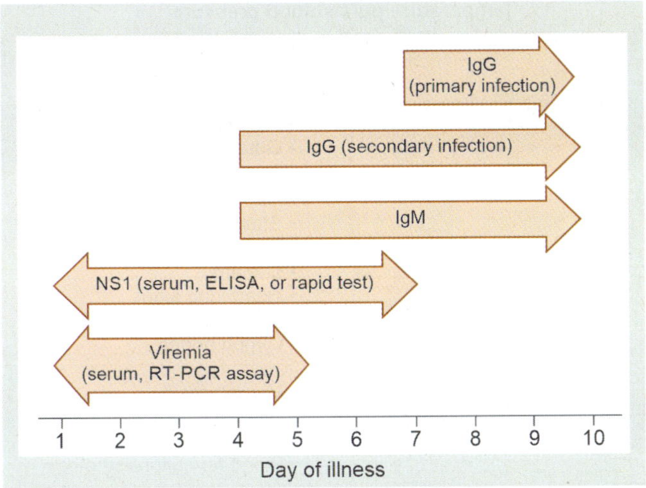

FIG. 10: Laboratory diagnostic options in a patient with suspected dengue infection. Detection of viral nucleic acid, nonstructural protein 1 (NS1), or IgM seroconversion is a confirmatory finding in patients in whom dengue is a possible diagnosis. Day 0 is the first day when the patient noted any symptom during this illness. (Diagnosis according to duration of fever)

exceed 90%, lower (70%) in secondary dengue because of presence of cross reactive NS1 antibodies that impede detection of free NS1.

- *Stage II:* Early post-febrile period lasting a few weeks when immunoglobulin M (IgM) and IgG antibodies are in excess. IgM enzyme-linked immunosorbent assay (ELISA) (capture). Sensitivity is 90–97%, detectable after 5–6 days and lasts 2–3 months. False positive after yellow fever/Japanese encephalitis (JE) vaccination. IgG lasts lifelong.

MANAGEMENT

Management of dengue is relatively simple, inexpensive, and highly effective in saving lives and reducing mortality and morbidity as long as it is correct and instituted timely, albeit it is highly complex and involute manifestations.

AIMS OF TREATMENT

- Assess the severity of dengue infection
- Assurance - usual clinical outcome good
- Intercept the progression early by prompt fluid replacement
- Use of blood/plasma substitute/platelets in patient with falling HCT or continuous bleeding

CLINICAL MANAGEMENT

Identify Preshock Stage by Warning Signs

- *Need of IV fluids*:
  - Plasma volume is reduced
  - Volume loss may be up to 20% because of plasma leakage

Antipyretics

- Paracetamol 500 mg; use in minimum dosage required (not exceeding 6 doses per 24 hours). No intramuscular injections in such patients.
- Oral fluids—fruit juices/ORS (40–50 mL/kg/day) is preferable to plain water.

Fluid Chart

- *Total fluid requirement/day*: 1,500 mL + 20 mL/kg for each kg > 20 kg
- Maintenance fluid should *not* exceed—3 L/day

Signs of over hydration: Rapidly falling HCT/wide pulse pressure.

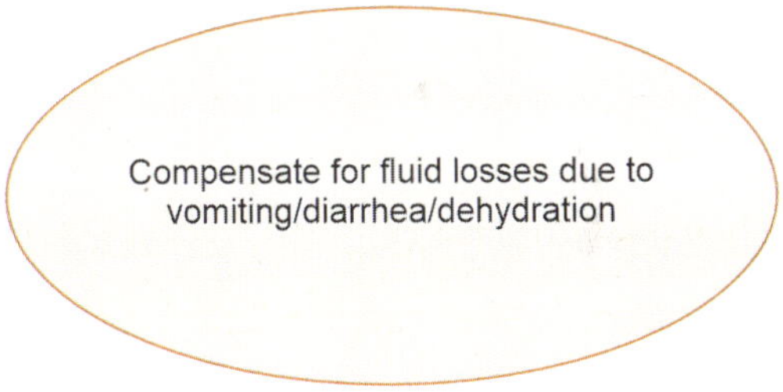

Type of Fluid

Crystalloids—normal saline (NS)/Ringer's lactate (initially NS preferred but if hyperchloremic acidosis occurs use ringer lactate); use ringer acetate, if patient has lactic acidosis and glucose saline if sugar < 80 mg.

- Initial rate of infusion at rate of 6 mL/kg/h.
- Watch for recovery by monitoring PR, BP - 1–2 hours, urine output HCT 8 hourly.
  If no improvement sequentially increase infusion rate: Infuse at the rate of 10 mL, 12 mL upto 20 mL/kg/h.

If still no improvement, consider colloids.

Fresh frozen plasma (FFP): Prepared from single units of whole blood or from plasma collected by apheresis techniques. Appropriately stored—usable for 1 year. Use

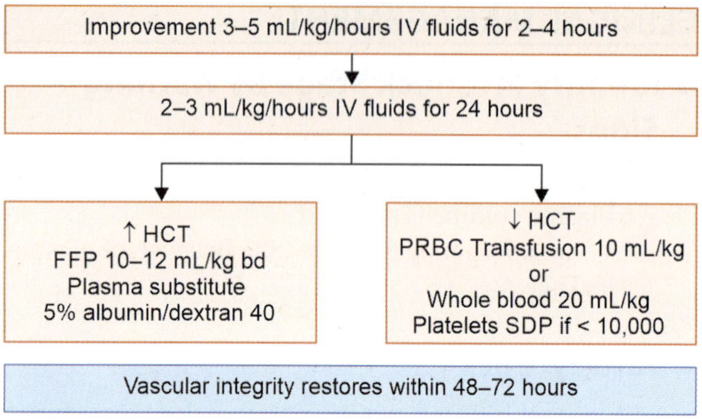

FLOWCHART 1: Fluid resuscitation in dengue.

as soon as it is thawed. One unit of FFP—250 mL FFP contains all of the coagulation factors and other proteins present in the original unit of blood **(Flowchart 1)**.

D/D: Acute febrile illnesses such as measles, enterovirus, adenovirus or influenza virus infections and others namely malaria, typhoid, Scrub typhus, leptospirosis, viral hepatitis or sepsis.

Antivirals: None

Steroids: Increase incidence of gastrointestinal (GI) bleed, hence, not recommended

Artesunates: Avoid injudicious use (post-artesunate delayed hemolysis/resistance)

Correction of electrolyte imbalance:

- Antiemetics
- Antihistaminics
- *Antibiotics:* AVOID: (i) Cefoperazone C/I (ii) Gram-negative sepsis only in 0.5%

ADDITIONAL COMPLICATIONS

- Liver failure possibly due to prolonged shock/hypoxia
- Disseminated intravascular coagulation (DIC)
- Acute respiratory distress syndrome (ARDS)
- *Neurological manifestations:* Encephalopathy, seizures, meningitis, stroke, mononeuropathies, polyneuropathies, Guillain-Barré syndrome, transverse myelitis, myositis with rhabdomyolysis
- Myocardial dysfunction, arrhythmias, myocarditis
- AKI in 3%
- Gram-negative sepsis 0.5%
- Retinal vasculitis
- Hemophagocytic lymphohistiocytosis (HLH)

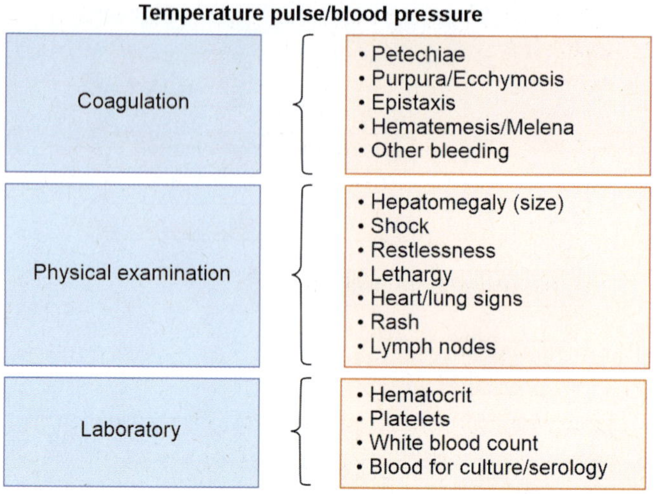

FIG. 11: Daily record of parameters.

DAILY RECORD OF PARAMETERS (FIG. 11)

It is impertinent to note that physician should record vital parameters such as vitals (blood pressure, temperature, pulse), coagulation profile (petechiae, melena, epistaxis), physical examination (hepatosplenomegaly, rash, shock) and lab values (hematocrit, platelet counts) daily and compare with previous day values to infer about the progress of patient's condition.

SIGNS OF RECOVERY

Stable pulse, blood pressure, breathing rate, normal temperature, no evidence of external or internal bleeding, return of appetite, no vomiting, good urinary output, stable HCT, and convalescent confluent petechiae rash.

WHEN TO DISCHARGE?

- Absence of fever for at least 24 hours without the use of antipyretics
- Return of appetite
- Visible clinical improvement
- Good urine output
- Stable HCT
- Passing of at least 2 days after recovery from shock
- No respiratory distress
- Platelet count of > 50,000/mm^3

PROPHYLAXIS: VACCINE

- *CYD-TDV (Dengvaxia):* Live attenuated tetravalent vaccine; licensed in over 20 countries in Latin America and Southeast Asia *first licensed in 2015* (indicated

in individuals having laboratory confirmed previous dengue infection and residing in endemic zones).
- *Vaccine efficacy:* 30.2%.
- *Vaccines in advanced clinical development:*
  - *TAK-003:* Live attenuated tetravalent vaccine, efficacious in both seropositive and negative individuals.
  - Tetravalent, live-virus vaccine attenuated through directed mutagenesis with a DENV-2/-4 chimeric strain

Vaccine response: 4 weeks to13 months after the last vaccine

Approved for use in dengue-endemic territories for those aged 9–45 years preferably seropositive individuals and not for travelers to endemic areas.

PRACTICE POINTS

- Identify preshock stage by warning signs
- Decreasing platelet and increasing HCT is unique to dengue
- Leucopenia and anicteric hepatitis (SGOT/SGPT 2–5 times elevation) are good predictor of clinical dengue
- Prophylactic platelet transfusion does not improve outcome in nonbleeding patient
- Over hydration is sometimes associated with ARDS (stop fluids when HCT normalizes)
- Drop in HCT with stable vitals denotes recovery whereas drop in HCT with ongoing bleeding and unstable signs is worrisome
- Overall mortality in severe dengue is < 1%

VECTOR CONTROL MEASURES

- *Personal prophylactic measure*:
  - Use of mosquito repellent creams, liquids, coils, mats, etc.
  - Wearing of full sleeve shirts and full pants with socks
  - Use of bed nets for sleeping infants and young children during day time to prevent mosquito bite.
- *Biological control*:
  - Use of larvivorous fishes in ornamental tanks, fountains, etc.
  - Use of biocides
- *Chemical control*:
  - Use of chemical larvicides like abate in big breeding containers
  - Aerosol space spray during day time.
- *Environmental management and source reduction methods*:
  - Detection and eliminating of mosquito breeding sources
  - Management of roof tops, porticos, and sunshades
  - Proper covering of stored water
  - Reliable water supply
  - Observation of weekly dry day
- *Health education*: Impact knowledge to common people regarding the disease and vector through various media sources such as TV, radio, cinema slides, etc.
- *Community participation*: Sensitizing and involving the community for detection of *Aedes* breeding places and their elimination.

SUGGESTED READINGS

1. Zeng Z, Zhan J, Chen L, Chen H, Cheng S. Global, regional, and national dengue burden from 1990 to 2017: A systematic analysis based on the global burden of disease study 2017. eClin Med. 2021;32:100712.
2. https://hmis.mohfw.gov.in: National Vector Borne Disease Control Programme Dengue and Dengue Hemorrhagic fever https://hmis.mohfw.gov.in/downloadfile?filepath=publications/Other/HMIS%20Annual%202019-20%20Report.pdf
3. Murthy S, Keystone J, Kissoon N. Infections of the developing world. Crit Care Clin. 2013;29(3):485-507.

148

CHAPTER

Vaccination of Healthcare Workers

Triven Sagar Sandepogu

ABSTRACT

Healthcare workers (HCWs) are at a greater risk of exposure as well as the spread of vaccine-preventable diseases as they are in constant touch with patients and infectious materials. Knowledge regarding vaccinations is better among healthcare workers than the public. Education and academic leadership play a role when comes to vaccination in HCWs. Strategies that can be adopted for increasing the coverage include free vaccination, education to break the myths about vaccination, vaccination sessions on nights as well as weekends, and adequate staff and mobile units. Various vaccine administration schedules are mentioned underneath.

INTRODUCTION

Vaccine-preventable diseases are a significant cause of morbidity and mortality. Patients harboring vaccine-preventable diseases are treated regularly by healthcare workers (HCWs), who may or may not have received corresponding vaccinations.

Healthcare workers are at a greater risk of exposure as well as the spread of vaccine-preventable diseases as they are in constant touch with patients and infectious materials. To control these risks, public health authorities have introduced vaccine recommendations for HCWs, aside from personal protection, vaccination of HCWs is recommended in many countries to fulfill legal requirements minimizing potential exposure of patients to infectious agents.

Vaccination programs among HCWs form an integral part of infection prevention.

Here, is the list of vaccines recommended for HCW by the World Health Organization (WHO) **(Table 1)**.

TABLE 1: Vaccines recommended by WHO.

Vaccine	Recommendation
Hepatitis B	HCWs who have chances of exposure to blood and blood products at work
Influenza	Annual immunization with a single dose is recommended
Tetanus, diphtheria, and pertussis (Tdap)	A one-time dose of Tdap as soon as possible if not received previously
Measles, mumps, and rubella (MMR)	All HCWs to be immune to measles and rubella
Meningococcal	One booster every 3–5 years may be considered for HCW
Varicella	Two doses for susceptible HCWs
COVID-19	Two doses for all HCWs
Hepatitis A	
HCWs infected with HIV	MMR vaccine, enhanced inactivated poliovirus vaccine (IPV), influenza, and pneumococcal vaccines
Typhoid	
Meningococcal disease	

(COVID-19: coronavirus disease 2019; HCWs: healthcare workers; HIV: human immunodeficiency virus)

The risk of hepatitis B infection from occupational exposure depends on the degree of contact with blood or other body fluids. As part of standard precautions vaccination is the major tool for preventing hepatitis B virus (HBV) infections, The risk is higher if the infected person is hepatitis B e antigen (HBeAg) positive. They are given at dose series of 0, 1, and 6 months. Prevaccination serologic screening for prior infection is not indicated for persons being vaccinated because of occupational risk. Postvaccination testing for antibody to hepatitis B surface antigen (anti-HBs) response is indicated for HCWs who have blood or patient contact and are at ongoing risk for injuries with sharp instruments or needlesticks (e.g., physicians, nurses, dentists, phlebotomists, medical technicians, and students of these professions). Knowledge of antibody response aids in determining appropriate postexposure prophylaxis.

Vaccine-induced antibodies to HBV decline gradually over time, and less than or equal to 60% of persons who initially respond to vaccination will lose detectable antibodies over 12 years. Studies among adults have demonstrated that, despite declining serum levels of antibodies, vaccine-induced immunity continues to prevent clinical disease or detectable viremic HBV infection. Therefore, booster doses are not considered necessary. Periodic serologic testing to monitor antibody concentrations after completion of the three-dose series is not recommended.

Influenza is a viral respiratory disease that affects humans and animals. The virus mutates quickly, and its seasonal strains cause outbreaks yearly, mostly during winter. However, they mostly cause absenteeism among medical staff rather than life-threatening complications. In the case of the influenza vaccine annual vaccinations are recommended due to constant changes in the virus. In a recent study of long-term care facilities with uniformly high patient influenza vaccination levels, patients in facilities where >60% of the staff had been vaccinated against influenza experienced less influenza-related mortality and illness than patients in facilities with no influenza-vaccinated staff.

Guillain–Barré syndrome is the most severe and well-established side effect of the influenza vaccine. Despite the universal recommendation of annual influenza vaccination, the vaccination rates remain low.

Primary vaccination of previously unvaccinated adults for tetanus, diphtheria consists of three doses of adult tetanus-diphtheria (Td) toxoid: 4–6 weeks should separate the first and second doses; the third dose should be administered 6–12 months after the second. After primary vaccination, a Td booster is recommended for all persons every 10 years. HCWs should be encouraged to receive recommended Td booster doses.

Measles, mumps, and rubella (MMR) are highly contagious viral infections that can result in severe complications, sequelae, and congenital anomalies. Nosocomial measles transmission is facilitated by its highly contagious nature and its ability to persist in aerosol suspension for at least 1 hour. Transmission from patients to unprotected HCWs can occur via infected individuals who seek medical care before developing clinically recognizable disease, i.e., before rash onset. Thus, measles represents an occupational risk for HCWs.

Mumps is no longer a common disease in most high-income countries. Nosocomial mumps outbreaks have been infrequent. The WHO has not provided any specific recommendations or evidence of measles immunity in HCWs.

Pertussis causing whooping cough is a highly-transmissible respiratory disease caused by *Bordetella pertussis*, is life-threatening for unvaccinated infants and remains a public health concern, pertussis outbreaks in nosocomial settings are well-described in many countries with more than 30 reported nosocomial outbreaks The index cases were often found among healthcare staff, and *B. pertussis* transmission occurred more frequently among colleagues than between HCWs and their patients. Healthcare workers and patients may serve as pertussis sources in nosocomial outbreaks, resulting in substantial morbidity and constraining infection control measures.

Varicella-zoster virus (VZV) is one of the herpes viruses. It is responsible for chickenpox in primary infections (mostly in children, teenagers, and young adults) and for herpes zoster (mostly in older people) when it reactivates, after a latent period in sensory nerve ganglia. Epidemiology varies between temperate/climate areas, where transmission is seasonal (winter-spring) and affects young children, and tropical areas, where infections occur later, resulting in higher rates of susceptible adults in tropical regions. Varicella transmission in healthcare settings from HCWs to susceptible patients has been reported, mostly in tropical countries or in HCWs who received only one vaccine dose. The vaccination recommendations are not routinely recommended to all healthcare professionals.

The coronavirus disease 2019 (COVID-19) is a highly transmittable and pathogenic viral infection caused by severe acute respiratory syndrome coronavirus 2 (SARS-CoV-2), which emerged in Wuhan, China, and spread around the world. All HCWs are recommended to take two doses of COVID-19 vaccines followed by a single booster dose.

Routine pre-exposure hepatitis A vaccination of HCWs and routine immunoglobulin (IG) prophylaxis for hospital personnel providing care to patients with hepatitis A are not indicated. Rather, sound hygienic practices should be emphasized. Staff education should emphasize precautions regarding direct contact with potentially infective materials (e.g., hand washing). In documented outbreaks of hepatitis A, administration of IG to persons who have close contact with infected patients (e.g., HCWs and other patients) is recommended. A single intramuscular dose (0.02 mL/kg) of IG is recommended as soon as possible and less than or equal to 2 weeks after exposure.

For HCWs infected with human immunodeficiency virus (HIV), the MMR vaccine is recommended for all asymptomatic HIV-infected HCWs who do not have evidence of severe immunosuppression. Administration of MMR to HIV-infected HCWs who are symptomatic, but who do not have evidence of severe immunosuppression, should be considered. Measles vaccine is not recommended for HIV-infected persons with evidence of severe immunosuppression. Enhanced inactivated poliovirus vaccine (IPV) is the only poliovirus vaccine recommended for HIV-infected persons. Live oral poliovirus vaccine (OPV) should not be administered to immunocompromised persons. Influenza and pneumococcal vaccines are indicated for all HIV-infected persons (influenza vaccination for persons aged greater than or equal to 6 months and pneumococcal vaccination for persons aged ≥ 2 years).

Workers in microbiology laboratories who frequently work with *Salmonella typhi* should be vaccinated with any one of the three typhoid vaccines: oral live-attenuated Typhoid Vaccine Live Oral Ty21a vaccine (one enteric-coated capsule taken on alternate days to a total of four capsules), the parenteral heat-phenol inactivated vaccine (two 0.5 mL subcutaneous doses, separated by greater than or equal to 4 weeks), or the capsular polysaccharide parenteral vaccine (one 0.5 mL intramuscular dose). Under conditions of continued or repeated exposure to *S. typhi*, booster doses are required to maintain immunity, every 5 years if the oral vaccine is used, every 3 years if the heat-phenol inactivated parenteral vaccine is used, and every 2 years if the capsular polysaccharide vaccine is used. Live-attenuated Ty21a vaccine should not be used among immunocompromised persons, including those infected with HIV.

Routine vaccination of civilians, including HCWs, is not recommended for meningococcal vaccine. HCWs who have intensive contact with oropharyngeal secretions of infected patients, and who do not use proper precautions should receive antimicrobial prophylaxis with rifampin (or sulfonamides, if the organisms isolated are sulfonamide-sensitive). Ciprofloxacin and ceftriaxone are reasonable alternative drugs; ceftriaxone can be administered to pregnant women. Vaccination with quadrivalent polysaccharide vaccine should be used to control outbreaks of serogroup C meningococcal disease. Surveillance for serogroup C disease and calculation of attack rates can be used to identify outbreaks and determine whether the use of meningococcal vaccine is warranted.

CONCLUSION

In conclusion, even though the levels of knowledge regarding the vaccinations are better among HCWs than the public the immunization rates never attain 100% they may be due to various factors, such as doubts over its safety and efficacy, fear of adverse effects, and difficulties in getting vaccines. To reach good immunization rates, we must acknowledge that vaccines have benefits and risks, about which misunderstanding or misinformation can occur among healthcare communities, as in the rest of the population.

Education and academic leadership play a role here, but other interventions can be useful and must continue to be tried and implemented. Public education on vaccines may take a more operational approach in the future, perhaps translating to the general public some of the strategies that have proved successful in HCWs.

Strategies that can be adopted for increasing the coverage include (1) free vaccination (2) education to break the myths about vaccination, (3) vaccination sessions on nights and weekends, and (4) adequate staff and mobile units.

Further multicentered studies can be done to assess the factors that play a decisive role in vaccination among HCWs and amidst the COVID pandemic, it is an ideal time to frame a national policy on immunization of HCWs.

SUGGESTED READINGS

1. Hadler SC, Margolis HS. Hepatitis B immunization: vaccine types, efficacy, and indications for immunization. Curr Clin Top Infect Dis. 1992;12:282-308.
2. Centers for Disease Control and Prevention. Hepatitis B virus: a comprehensive strategy for eliminating transmission in the United States through universal childhood vaccination. Recommendations of the Immunization Practices Advisory Committee (ACIP). MMWR Recomm Rep. 1991;40(RR-13):1-25.
3. Potter J, Stott DJ, Roberts MA, Elder AG, O'Donnell B, Knight PV, et al. Influenza vaccination of health care workers in long-term-care hospitals reduces the mortality of elderly patients. J Infect Dis. 1997;175(1):1-6.
4. Centers for Disease Control and Prevention. Diphtheria, tetanus, and pertussis: recommendations for vaccine use and other preventive measures. Recommendations of the Immunization Practices Advisory committee (ACIP). MMWR Recomm Rep. 1991;40(RR-10):1-28.

5. Centers for Disease Control and Prevention. Prevention of hepatitis A through active or passive immunization: recommendations of the Advisory Committee on Immunization Practices (ACIP). MMWR Recomm Rep. 1996;45(RR-15): 1-30.
6. Centers for Disease Control and Prevention. Poliomyelitis prevention in the United States: introduction of a sequential vaccination schedule of inactivated poliovirus vaccine followed by oral poliovirus vaccine. recommendations of the Advisory Committee on Immunization Practices (ACIP). MMWR Recomm Rep. 1997;46(RR-3):1-25.
7. Centers for Disease Control and Prevention. Typhoid immunization: recommendations of the Advisory Committee on Immunization Practices (ACIP). MMWR Recomm Rep. 1994;43(RR-14):1-7.
8. Haviari S, Bénet T, Saadatian-Elahi M, André P, Loulergue P, Vanhems P. Vaccination of healthcare workers: A review. Hum Vaccin Immunother. 2015;11(11):2522-37.
9. Hajure M, Tariku M, Bekele F, Abdu Z, Dule A, Mohammedhussein M, et al. Attitude Towards COVID-19 Vaccination Among Healthcare Workers: A Systematic Review. Infect Drug Resist. 2021;14:3883-97.

149

CHAPTER

Neglected Tropical Diseases

Swaroop Kumar Baruah, Aditi Aggarwal

ABSTRACT

Neglected tropical diseases (NTDs) are group of diseases of diverse etiology, a subset of infectious diseases consisting of bacterial, viral, parasitic, and fungal origin. Predominantly, they involve poor people, these diseases are mainly found in tropics and their affinity for hot places results in more prevalence in remote rural areas, urban slums, and displaced people around the Equator. It can be considered as disease of the poorest one-sixth population of the world. It can cause massive suffering in the form of acute illness, long-term morbidity and death. Currently, World Health Organization (WHO) has listed 20 diseases to be categorized under NTD. As part of a general disregard for the developing world, and more recently due to focus on human immunodeficiency virus (HIV)/acquired immunodeficiency syndrome (AIDS), tuberculosis and malaria, they have been neglected for decades. Some of these infections are in part attributable to inadequate access to safe water, sanitation, and appropriate housing. Many NTDs are therefore preventable. India, being a tropical country is home to several NTDs. India accounts for most of dengue, visceral leishmaniasis, trachoma, leprosy, cysticercosis, lymphatic filariasis, rabies, ascariasis, and hookworm infestation. There have been recent notable successes in NTD control. Dracunculiasis is approaching eradication. Leprosy and onchocerciasis are in decline.

INTRODUCTION

Neglected tropical diseases (NTDs) are a group of diverse infections that predominantly affect populations in tropical and subtropical regions, particularly in low-income countries. Despite their widespread prevalence and significant impact on public health, they are termed as "neglected" because these diseases often affect marginalized and impoverished communities, receiving scant attention from governments, pharmaceutical companies and global health organizations. NTDs are mostly disabling and chronic in nature. India is the domicile of millions of people who are poor and live in impoverished environments, and hence, are at risk of these diseases.

CLASSIFICATION (WORLD HEALTH ORGANIZATION)

- Buruli ulcer (*Mycobacterium ulcerans*)
- Chikungunya
- Chagas disease
- Cysticercosis
- Dengue fever
- Dracunculiasis (Guinea worm disease)
- Echinococcosis
- Fascioliasis
- Food-borne trematodiasis
- Human African trypanosomiasis (sleeping sickness)
- Leishmaniasis (Kala-azar)
- Leprosy

- Lymphatic Filariasis
- Mycetoma
- Onchocerciasis (river blindness)
- Rabies
- Schistosomiasis
- Soil-transmitted helminthiasis
- Trachoma
- Yaws

RISK FACTORS

These NTDs are often fuelled by a complex interplay of environmental, socioeconomic, and behavioral factors. Poverty and limited access to basic services such as lack of access to clean water, proper sanitation, and adequate healthcare are fundamental drivers of NTDs. Limited education and awareness about disease prevention and transmission play a significant role in persistence of NTDs. Unsanitary living conditions and poor waste management provide breeding grounds for disease vectors and pathogens. Limited access to healthcare facilities and treatment options, especially for people living in remote and underserved areas prevent timely intervention and management of NTDs. Population movement whether due to conflict, displacement or migration can contribute to the spread of NTDs. Cultural practices such as walking barefoot in areas with soil-transmitted helminths or using traditional healing practices instead of modern medicine can perpetuate the spread of NTDs. Also, the neglect of NTDs by pharma industry due to limited profit incentives has led to a dearth of research and development for new drugs and treatment.

All of these risk factors contribute to the prevalence, transmission and persistence of NTDs in the affected communities and require a multifaceted approach that involves collaboration among governments, international organizations, nongovernmental organizations, and local communities.

PREVALENCE

Neglected tropical diseases affect over a billion people worldwide, predominantly in low- and middle-income countries. But the highest burden of NTDs is borne by India, along with other countries of South Asia. These countries account for approximately one-quarter of the world's soil-transmitted helminths infections, one-half or more of the global burden of lymphatic filariasis, visceral leishmaniasis, and leprosy and one-third or more of the global deaths from rabies. These countries are also facing an emerging problem with major arbovirus infections, i.e., dengue, Japanese encephalitis.

India, being a tropical country with diverse ecological and socioeconomic conditions and factors like poverty etc., is home to several NTDs. They are often concentrated in specific regions of India, with higher prevalence in rural and economically disadvantaged areas.

India accounts for half of the total cases of dengue, visceral Leishmaniasis, and trachoma. India also accounts for one-third of the cases of leprosy, cysticercosis, lymphatic filariasis and rabies, approximately one quarter of ascariasis and hookworm infestation. The prevalence of amebiasis and giardiasis is not clear.

PREVENTIVE STRATEGIES

Over the last decade, NTDs have started receiving the increased recognition that they deserve. This was made possible by recognizing what these diseases had in common and grouping them all under the "NTD brand" in global health.

For the sake of program, the WHO classified NTDs into two groups, which are: (1) Preventive chemotherapy and transmission control (PCT) NTDs, and (2) Innovative and intensified disease management (IDM) NTDs. The most prominent examples of NTDs that are included in the PCT group are lymphatic filariasis, onchocerciasis, schistosomiasis, and soil-transmitted helminthiasis; the main approach for their control is regular administration of efficacious, safe, and inexpensive (usually donated) drugs to entire at-risk populations. IDM-NTDs include Buruli ulcer, Chagas disease, human African trypanosomiasis, and leishmaniasis. Currently they lack appropriate tools for large-scale use.

Various preventive strategies have been undertaken by WHO to combat these diseases globally.

- *Preventive chemotherapy:* Coordinated use of antimicrobial and antihelminthic medicines along with complimentary public health interventions is a mainstay of WHO's recommended strategy. The drus that are needed to treat the NTDs are now on the WHO "essential medicines" list and are being provided free of cost by pharma companies through their donation campaigns. These mass drug administration programs through community-directed interventions and school health programs have made it possible to tackle some of the NTDs (trachoma, filiariasis, soil trasmitted helminths, onchocerciasis) on a massive scale.
- *Vector control:* WHO advocates for vector control measures such as insecticide-treated bed nets, indoor residual spraying, and source reduction to control diseases spread by vectors such as mosquitoes and flies (e.g., malaria, dengue and chagas disease). It basically focusses on developing guidelines that are based on

the principles of integrated vector management which also includes judicious use of pesticides.

- *Imroved sanitation and hygiene:* Providing safe water, sanitation, and hygiene also known as WASH Strategy is an important component of the global NTD strategy. Since many of the pathogens that cause these diseases thrive in the unsanitary water and environment, WASH strategy plays an important role in controlling the transmission of such diseases especially those spread via soil-trasmitted helminths.
- *Vaccination programs:* Vaccines do play a critical role in preventing some NTDs. For example, ensuring widespread coverage of vaccines for diseases like polio has led to significant reductions in its cases. WHO is making efforts to develop vaccines for diseases such as dengue and Chagas disease are still ongoing.
- *Veterinary public health services:* This strategy is particularly revelant in cases of neglected zoonotic diseases, a subset of NTDs that are naturally transmitted from vertebrate animals to humans and vice versa. Examples of which include rabies, echinococcosis, taeniasis and cysticercosis, and foodborne trematodiases. Mutifactoral approach is needed to combat this particular subset of diseases.
- *Health education and awareness:* Raising awareness about NTDs, their causes, and preventive measures through global campaigns and partnerships is an essential strategy undertaken by WHO. Educating communities about disease transmission, symptoms and the importance of seeking medical care can lead to early detection and treatment.
- *Community engagement and integrated disease management:* WHO involves local communities in the planning and implementation of preventive measures, leveraging their knowledge and recognizing the importance of community participation. Combining different strategies such as medication distribution with vector control measures can have a synergistic effect on disease reduction.
- *Surveillance, data collection, and research:* WHO assists countries in establishing surveillance systems to track NTDs, identify outbreaks, and monitor progress in disease control. Not only that, but WHO also supports research efforts to develop new diagnostics, drugs and vaccines for NTDs, fostering innovation to improve prevention and control.
- *Targeted interventions:* WHO tailors interventions based on the specific diseases and local texts in different regions, ensuring strategies are appropriate and effective.
- *Global partnerships:* WHO collaborates with International organisations such as center for disease control (CDC), governments, nongovernment organisations, and academic institutions to coordinate efforts and pool resources for NTD control.
- *Monitoring and evaluation:* CDC conducts evaluations to assess the impact of interventions and programs, helping WHO to refine strategies and improve the effectiveness of NTD control efforts. CDC also contributes to the development of policies, guidelines, and recommendations related to NTD prevention, control and elimination.
- *Capacity building:* WHO and CDC both recognizes that strengthening the healthcare systems in endemic areas is crucial. Training healthcare workers, improving laboratory facilities, and enhancing the overall healthcare infrastructure can contribute to better disease management.

Most of these strategies revolves around the principle that engaging communities in the design and implementation of interventions empowers them to take ownership of their health and ultimately leads to a significant progress in tackling these NTDs globally.

RECENT ADVANCES

In the past two decades, we have been increasingly become aware that existing therapies for NTDs suffer from some hard to ignore loopholes such as high degree of side-effects, low bioavailability, toxicity, improper targeting, and problematic application for affected group. Progress in the field of nanotechnology in last decades came up with this intervention of nanocarriers to take over and drive the research and development to the next level. This is by incorporating previous drugs into the nanocarriers rather than discovering newer one which become an expensive affair. These nanocarriers are believed to be a sure shot technique to fight infections at root level by virtue of its nano size and ability to reach at cellular level. Different ways by which nanotechnology is being utilized in today's era include:

- *Drug delivery systems:* Like mentioned above nanoparticles can be engineered to deliver drugs directly to specific cells or tissues, enhancing the effectiveness of treatments while reducing side effects.
- *Improved drug formulations:* Nanotechnology has also allowed for the development of improved drug formulations, such as nanoscale formulations of existing drugs. This enhances drug solubility, stability, and bioavailability, which is particularly important for drugs used in NTD treatment.
- *Diagnostic tools:* Nanoparticles can also be designed to detect specific biomarkers or pathogens associated with NTDs. Microfluidic devices can manipulate small volumes of fluid and samples and enable rapid testing. These cutting-edge diagnostic tools offer increased

sensitivity, rapid results, and the potential for point-of-care testing, especially in resource limited settings.

- *Vector control and vaccine development:* Nanoparticles can also be incorporated into insecticides and insect repellents which can enhance their efficacy. They can also serve as carriers for vaccine antigens, improving the immune response, and potentially leading to more effective vaccines for NTD. This approach holds promise for diseases such as Leishmaniasis and Schistosomiasis.
- *Theranostics:* Combining diagnostics and therapy, nanotechnology-enabled theranostics can simultaneously diagnose and treat NTDs allowing for personalized and targeted interventions. It also provides tools for studying the molecular and cellular mechanisms of NTDs helping in research.

PROGRESS MADE TILL NOW

Much progress has been made over the past decade in the field of tackling NTDs. By 2022, around 47 countries have eliminated at least one NTD. Over 1 billion people were treated for at least one NTD each year from 2015 to 2019. The population requiring NTD interventions decreased by 25% between 2010 and 2021, from 2.19 to 1.65 billion. Countries such as Ghana, Sudan, and Burkina Faso have successfully eradicated Guinea worm disease. Multiple countries have achieved elimination of lymphatic filariasis through MDA programs. Papua New Guinea and India have made significant strides in controlling yaws, a bacterial infection affecting skin, bones, and joints. Many countries such as Oman, Morocco, Cambodia, and Ghana have also made progress in eliminating trachoma, a leading cause of preventable blindness. Onchocerciasis (river blindness) have also been eliminated as a public health problem in countries such as Columbia, Ecuador, Mexico, and most recently Senegal.

CONCLUSION

Neglected tropical diseases represent a complex and multifaceted challenge that affects some of the world's most vulnerable populations. These diseases, often thriving in areas with limited access to healthcare, sanitation, and education, have long been overlooked on the global health agenda. However, concerned efforts by governments, international organizations, nongovernment entities, and dedicated individuals are reshaping the landscape of NTD prevention, control, and eradication.

The fight against NTD is not only a matter of health but also a testament to social justice and human dignity. The progress made in recent years, from elimination of Guinea worm disease in multiple countries to the reduction of trachoma- related blindness, highlights the potential of collaborative and innovative strategies.

Innovations in technology, such as nanotechnology and advanced diagnostics, offer promising tools for early detection, treatment and prevention of NTDs. Equally important are the holistic approaches that encompass community engagement, education, and improved access to clean water and sanitation.

SUGGESTED READINGS

1. Hotez PJ, Damania A. India's neglected tropical diseases. PLoS Negl Trop Dis. 2018;12(3):e0006038.
2. Mitra AK, Mawson AR. Neglected tropical diseases: epidemiology and global burden. Trop Med Infect Dis. 2017;2(3):36.
3. Acharya AS, Kaur R, Goel AD. Neglected tropical diseases-challenges and opportunities in India. Ind J Med Special. 2017;8(3):102-8.

150

CHAPTER

Management of Multidrug Resistant Gram-negative Sepsis in Today's Practice

Basabbijay Sarkar, Sayantani Bhattacharya

ABSTRACT

Multidrug resistant (MDR) gram-negative sepsis is a formidable challenge in modern healthcare. Prompt diagnosis, broad-spectrum empirical antibiotic therapy, and source control are cornerstones of effective management. Antimicrobial stewardship, tailored therapies based on resistance mechanisms, and rapid diagnostics are crucial for optimizing treatment. Individualized care, infection-control measures, and immunomodulatory therapy enhance outcomes, particularly in critically ill patients.

Collaborative interdisciplinary care, including infectious disease specialists and microbiologists, is essential. Continuous monitoring permits therapy adjustments, including de-escalation, while adjunctive treatments address septic shock. Ethical considerations in treatment decisions underscore patient autonomy and quality of life.

Investment in research and development of novel antibiotics remains pivotal in combating MDR gram-negative infections. Patient education about sepsis, antibiotic resistance, and responsible antibiotic use is paramount.

INTRODUCTION

Multidrug resistant (MDR) gram-negative sepsis poses a significant challenge in modern healthcare. Gram-negative bacteria, including strains like *Escherichia coli*, *Klebsiella pneumoniae*, and *Pseudomonas aeruginosa*, have developed resistance to multiple antibiotics, making infections caused by them difficult to treat. This chapter discusses the current approaches to managing MDR gram-negative sepsis in contemporary clinical practice.

DIAGNOSIS AND EARLY IDENTIFICATION

Early diagnosis is crucial for the effective management of MDR gram-negative sepsis. Clinical suspicion should arise in patients with compatible symptoms, such as fever, hypotension, altered mental status, and organ dysfunction. Diagnostic tools include blood cultures, which should be obtained promptly, as well as imaging studies to identify the source of infection **(Flowchart 1)**.

EMPIRICAL ANTIBIOTIC THERAPY

Empirical antibiotic therapy should be initiated as soon as possible after obtaining blood cultures. Due to the risk of MDR pathogens, broad-spectrum antibiotics are often warranted. A common initial regimen includes a combination of antibiotics such as carbapenems (e.g., meropenem or imipenem-cilastatin) or cephalosporins (e.g., cefepime) with agents that cover resistant gram-positives (e.g., vancomycin or linezolid) **(Table 1)**.

ANTIMICROBIAL STEWARDSHIP

Antimicrobial stewardship programs are essential to combat the emergence of antibiotic resistance. Hospitals should establish guidelines for antibiotic use, monitor prescribing practices, and provide education to healthcare providers. De-escalation of antibiotic therapy is recommended once culture results and susceptibility data become available.

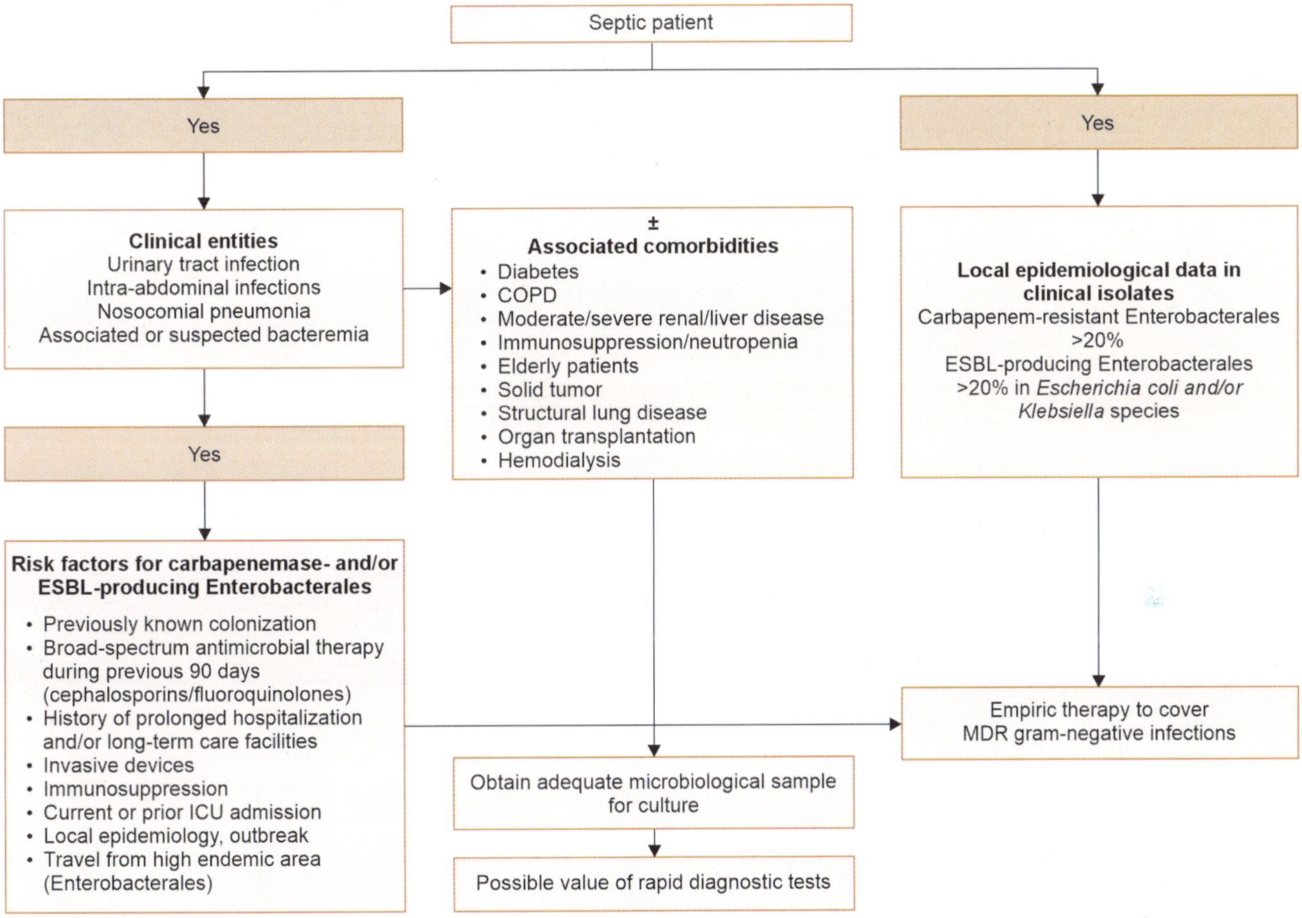

FLOWCHART 1: Algorithm of a septic patient.

(COPD: chronic obstructive pulmonary disease; ESBL: extended spectrum beta-lactamase; ICU: intensive care unit)

TABLE 1: Suggested dosing of antibiotics for the treatment of antimicrobial-resistant infections in adults, assuming normal renal and hepatic function.*,†

Amikacin	• *Uncomplicated cystitis*: 15 mg/kg IV as a single dose • *Pyelonephritis or complicated urinary tract infections*: 15 mg/kg IV once; subsequent doses and dosing interval based on pharmacokinetic evaluation
Ampicillin/Sulbactam	• Total daily dose of 6–9 g of sulbactam • *Potential infusion strategies include the following*: ○ 9 g of ampicillin-sulbactam (6 g ampicillin, 3 g sulbactam) IV every 8 hours, infused over 4 hours ○ 27 g of ampicillin-sulbactam (18 g ampicillin, 9 g sulbactam) IV as a continuous infusion ○ 3 g of ampicillin–sulbactam (2 g ampicillin, 1 g sulbactam) IV every 4 hours, infused over 30 minutes
Cefepime	• *Uncomplicated cystitis*: 1 g IV every 8 hours, infused over 30 minutes • *All other infections*: 2 g IV every 8 hours, infused over 3 hours (if possible)
Cefiderocol	2 g IV every 8 hours, infused over 3 hours
Ceftazidime/Avibactam	2.5 g IV every 8 hours, infused over 3 hours
Ceftazidime/Avibactam PLUS aztreonam	• *Ceftazidime–avibactam*: 2.5 g IV every 8 hours, infused over 3 hours PLUS • *Aztreonam*: 2 g IV every 6–8 hours (every 6-hour dosing preferred if possible), infused over 3 hours
Ceftolozane/Tazobactam	• *Cystitis*: 1.5 g IV every 8 hours, infused over 1 hour • *All other infections*: 3 g IV every 8 hours, infused over 3 hours

Continued

Continued

Ciprofloxacin	• *Cystitis*: 400 mg IV every 12 hours or 500 mg PO every 12 hours • *All other infections*: 400 mg IV every 8 hours OR 750 mg PO every 12 hours
Colistin	Refer to international consensus guidelines on polymyxins (Tsuji et al.)
Eravacycline	1 mg/kg per dose IV every 12 hours
Ertapenem	1 g IV every 24 hours, infused over 30 minutes
Fosfomycin	*Uncomplicated cystitis*: 3 g PO as a single dose
Gentamicin	• *Uncomplicated cystitis*: 5 mg/kg/dose IV as a single dose • *Pyelonephritis or complicated urinary tract infections*: 7 mg/kg IV once; subsequent doses and dosing interval based on pharmacokinetic evaluation
Imipenem–cilastatin	• *Uncomplicated cystitis*: 500 mg IV every 6 hours, infused over 30 minutes • *All other infections*: 500 mg IV every 6 hours, infused over 3 hours (if possible)
Imipenem–cilastatin/ Relebactam	1.25 g IV every 6 hours, infused over 30 minutes
Levofloxacin	750 mg IV/PO every 24 hours
Meropenem	• *Uncomplicated cystitis*: 1 g IV every 8 hours, infused over 30 minutes • *All other infections*: 2 g IV every 8 hours, infused over 3 hours (if possible)
Meropenem/Vaborbactam	4 g IV every 8 hours, infused over 3 hours
Minocycline	200 mg IV/PO every 12 hours
Nitrofurantoin	• *Macrocrystal/monohydrate (Macrobid®)*: 100 mg PO every 12 hours • *Oral suspension*: 50 mg PO every 6 hours
Polymyxin B	Refer to international consensus guidelines on polymyxins (Tsuji et al.)
Tigecycline	200 mg IV as a single dose, then 100 mg IV every 12 hours
Tobramycin	• *Cystitis*: 5 mg/kg/dose IV as a single dose • *Pyelonephritis or complicated urinary tract infections*: 7 mg/kg IV once; subsequent doses and dosing interval based on pharmacokinetic evaluation
Trimethoprim–sulfamethoxazole	• *Cystitis*: 160 mg (trimethoprim component) IV/PO every 12 hours • *Other infections*: 8–12 mg/kg/day (trimethoprim component) IV/PO divided every 8–12 hours (consider maximum dose of 960 mg trimethoprim component per day)

*Dosing suggestions limited to organisms and infectious syndromes discussed in the Infectious Diseases Society of America (IDSA) AMR treatment Guidance document.

†Dosing suggested for several agents in the table may differ from that recommended by the United States Food and Drug Administration.

(IV: intravenous; mg/kg: milligrams per kilogram; PO: enterally)

SOURCE CONTROL

Identifying and controlling the source of infection is paramount. This often involves surgical or interventional procedures, such as drainage of abscesses, debridement of infected tissue, or removal of infected devices (e.g., central venous catheters or prosthetic joints).

COMBINATION THERAPY

In severe cases of MDR gram-negative sepsis, combination antibiotic therapy may be necessary. This approach helps reduce the risk of resistance development and improve treatment outcomes. Synergistic combinations, such as a beta-lactam with an aminoglycoside or colistin, can be considered based on susceptibility testing **(Table 2)**.

RESISTANCE MECHANISMS

Understanding the mechanisms of resistance is crucial in managing MDR infections. Common resistance mechanisms include extended-spectrum beta-lactamases (ESBLs), carbapenemases, and efflux pumps. Tailoring antibiotic therapy to target the specific resistance mechanism is important for successful treatment.

ANTIBIOTIC RESISTANCE SURVEILLANCE

Hospitals should regularly monitor antibiotic resistance patterns within their facilities. Surveillance data can guide empirical therapy choices and help identify emerging resistance trends, allowing for timely interventions.

TABLE 2: Potential in vitro activity of antibiotics against target carbapenem-resistant gram-negative bacteria and approved indications.

	CRAB	ESBLs	CRPA non-MBL	CRE non-CP	CRE-KPC	CRE-OXA-48	CRE-MBL	Current clinical indications/approval
Newer antibiotics								
Ceftolozane–Tazobactam	No	Yes	Yes	No	No	No	No	FDA and EMA approved for cUTI, cIAI, HAP, and VAP
Ceftazidime–Avibactam	No	Yes	Yes	p/e	Yes	Yes	No	FDA and EMA approved for cIAI and cUTI, HAP and VAP, and (in EMA only) for the treatment of gram-negative infections in patients with limited treatment options
Meropenem–Vaborbactam	No	Yes	No	p/e	Yes	No	No	FDA approved for cUTI, EMA approved for cUTI, HAP and VAP, and for the treatment of gram-negative infections in patients with limited treatment options
Imipenem–cilastatin/ Relebactam	No	Yes	Yes	p/e	Yes	No	No	• FDA approved for cUTI and cIAI • EMA approved for HAP and VAP and for BSI with a suspected respiratory source, and for the treatment of gram-negative infections in patients with limited treatment options
Plazomicin	No	Yes	p/e	Yes	Yes	Yes	p/e	• FDA approval cUTI, EMA application withdrawn
Eravacycline	Yes	Yes	No	Yes	Yes	Yes	Yes	• FDA and EMA approved for cIAI
Cefiderocol	Yes	Yes	Yes	Yes	Yes	Yes	Yes	FDA cUTI, HAP and VAP; EMA for the treatment of infections due to aerobic gram-negative organisms in adults with limited treatment options
Older antibiotics								
Polymyxins	Yes	Yes	Yes	Yes	Yes	Yes	Yes	• *FDA*: Serious infections caused by susceptible strains, when less potentially toxic drugs are ineffective or contraindicated • *EMA*: Treatment of serious infections due to aerobic gram-negative pathogens in patients with limited treatment options
Aminoglycosides	p/e	p/e	p/e	p/e	p/e	p/e	p/e	*EMA and FDA*: For the treatment of a variety of bacterial infections
Fosfomycin IV	No	Yes	p/e	p/e	p/e	p/e	p/e	• *EMA*: To treat serious infections when other antibiotic treatments are not suitable • *FDA*: Under review
Aztreonam	No	No	p/e	No	No	No	p/e	*EMA and FDA*: For the treatment of infections caused by susceptible gram-negative microorganisms
Tigecycline	Yes	Yes	No	Yes	Yes	Yes	Yes	*EMA and FDA*: Complicated SSTI and IAI (FDA also CAP)
Temocillin	No	Yes	No	No	p/e	No	No	*EMA and FDA*: Orphan drug status for the treatment of infections caused by Burkholderia cepacia in patients with cystic fibrosis

Note: The table presents the spectrum of potential in vitro activity of the listed antibiotics; resistance can develop and treatment should be directed by susceptibility testing.

(BSI: bloodstream infection; CAP: community-acquired pneumonia; cIAI: complicated intra-abdominal infections; CRAB: carbapenem-resistant *Acinetobacter baumannii*; CRE non-CP: non-carbapenemase-producing carbapenem-resistant Enterobacterales; CRPA non-MBL: carbapenem-resistant *Pseudomonas aeruginosa* non-metallo-b-lactamase-producing; cUTI: complicated urinary tract infections; EMA: European Medicines Agency; ESBLs: extended-spectrum b-lactmases; FDA: US Food and Drug Administration; HAP: hospital-acquired pneumonia; MBL: metallo-b-lactamase; SSTI: skin and soft-tissue infections; VAP: ventilator-associated pneumonia; p/e: partially effective)

Source: Paul M, Carrara E, Retamar P, Tängdén T, Bitterman R, Bonomo RA. European Society of Clinical Microbiology and Infectious Diseases (ESCMID) guidelines for the treatment of infections caused by multidrug-resistant Gram-negative bacilli (endorsed by European society of intensive care medicine). Clin Microbiol Infect. 2022;28(4):521-47.

RAPID DIAGNOSTIC TESTS

Advancements in molecular diagnostics and biomarkers enable the rapid identification of pathogens and their resistance profiles. Technologies like polymerase chain reaction (PCR) and MALDI-TOF (matrix-assisted laser desorption ionization–time of flight) can provide results within hours, allowing for more precise and timely antibiotic selection.

INDIVIDUALIZED THERAPY

Consideration of patient-specific factors, such as comorbidities, immunosuppression, and previous antibiotic exposure, is essential for tailoring therapy. Individualized treatment plans can optimize outcomes and minimize adverse effects.

Infection-control Measures

Preventing the spread of MDR pathogens within healthcare facilities is crucial. Stringent infection-control measures, including hand hygiene, isolation precautions, and environmental cleaning, help reduce transmission.

IMMUNOMODULATORY THERAPY

In some cases, adjunctive therapies targeting the host's immune response may be beneficial. This includes the use of agents like granulocyte colony-stimulating factor (G-CSF) or monoclonal antibodies to enhance immune function.

COLLABORATIVE CARE

Interdisciplinary collaboration among healthcare professionals, including infectious disease specialists, microbiologists, surgeons, and pharmacists, is essential for optimizing patient care. Regular case discussions and antimicrobial stewardship meetings facilitate shared decision-making.

MONITORING AND DE-ESCALATION

Continuous monitoring of clinical and laboratory parameters is necessary to assess treatment response. Once the patient stabilizes and culture results are available, de-escalation of antibiotic therapy should be considered to minimize the risk of antibiotic-related adverse events and resistance.

Adjunctive Therapies

In patients with septic shock, aggressive fluid resuscitation, vasopressor support, and close hemodynamic monitoring are crucial. Additionally, consideration of adjunctive therapies such as corticosteroids or activated protein C may be warranted in specific cases.

ETHICAL CONSIDERATIONS

Managing MDR gram-negative sepsis may involve complex ethical decisions, such as balancing the potential benefits of aggressive therapy with the patient's quality of life and wishes. In some cases, discussions about goals of care, palliative care, or end-of-life care may be necessary.

RESEARCH AND DEVELOPMENT

Investment in research and development of new antibiotics and alternative treatment modalities is essential to combat MDR gram-negative infections. Encouraging pharmaceutical companies and researchers to develop novel therapies is critical in addressing this global healthcare challenge.

PATIENT EDUCATION

Patients and their families should be educated about sepsis, its risks, and the importance of adhering to prescribed treatments. Communication about the potential consequences of antibiotic resistance and the need for responsible antibiotic use is vital.

CONCLUSION

Managing MDR gram-negative sepsis in contemporary clinical practice demands a multifaceted approach. Early diagnosis, appropriate antimicrobial therapy, infection control, and individualized patient care are essential components of effective management. With the continued emergence of antibiotic resistance, ongoing research, antimicrobial stewardship, and interdisciplinary collaboration are crucial in ensuring successful outcomes for patients with MDR gram-negative sepsis.

SUGGESTED READINGS

1. Cassini A, Hogberg LD, Plachouras D, Quattrocchi A, Hoxha A, Simonsen GS, et al. Attributable deaths and disability-adjusted life-years caused by infections with antibiotic-resistant bacteria in the EU and the European Economic Area in 2015: a population-level modelling analysis. Lancet Infect Dis. 2019;19:56-66.
2. Tacconelli E, Carrara E, Savoldi A, Harbarth S, Mendelson M, Monnet DL, et al. Discovery, research, and development of new antibiotics: the WHO priority list of antibiotic-resistant bacteria and tuberculosis. Lancet Infect Dis. 2018;18:318e27.
3. World Health Organization. (2022). 2020 Antibacterial agents in clinical and preclinical development: an overview and analysis. [online] Available from https://www.who.int/publications/i/item/9789240021303 [Last accessed December, 2023].
4. Clancy CJ, Nguyen MH. Estimating the size of the United States market for new antibiotics with activity against carbapenem-resistant Enterobacteriaceae. Antimicrob Agents Chemother. 2019;63:e01733e819.
5. Scudeller L, Righi E, Chiamenti M, Bragantini D, Menchinelli G, Cattaneo P, et al. Systematic review and meta-analysis of in vitro efficacy of antibiotic combination therapy against carbapenem-resistant Gram-negative bacilli. Int J Antimicrob Agents. 2021;57:106344.
6. Zusman O, Avni T, Leibovici L, Adler A, Friberg L, Stergiopoulou T, et al. Systematic review and meta-analysis of in vitro synergy of polymyxins and carbapenems. Antimicrob Agents Chemother. 2013;57:5104e11.
7. Liberati A, Altman DG, Tetzlaff J, Mulrow C, Gotzsche PC, Ioannidis JP, et al. The PRISMA statement for reporting systematic reviews and meta-analyses of studies that evaluate healthcare interventions: explanation and elaboration. BMJ. 2009;339:b2700.
8. Singer M, Deutschman CS, Seymour CW, Shankar-Hari M, Annane D, Bauer M, et al. The third international consensus definitions for sepsis and septic shock (Sepsis-3). JAMA. 2016;315:801e10.
9. Gutierrez-Gutierrez B, Salamanca E, de Cueto M, Hsueh PR, Viale P, PanoPardo JR, et al. A predictive model of mortality in patients with bloodstream infections due to carbapenemase-producing Enterobacteriaceae. Mayo Clinic Proc. 2016;91:1362e71.
10. Palacios-Baena ZR, Gutierrez-Gutierrez B, De Cueto M, Viale P, Venditti M, Hernandez-Torres A, et al. Development and validation of the INCREMENTESBL predictive score for mortality in patients with bloodstream infections due to extended-spectrum-beta-lactamase-producing Enterobacteriaceae. J Antimicrob Chemother. 2017;72:906e13.
11. Tsuji BT, Pogue JM, Zavascki AP, Paul M, Daikos GL, Forrest A. International Consensus Guidelines for the Optimal Use of the Polymyxins: Endorsed by the American College of Clinical Pharmacy (ACCP), European Society of Clinical Microbiology and Infectious Diseases (ESCMID), Infectious Diseases Society of America (IDSA), International Society for Anti-infective Pharmacology (ISAP), Society of Critical Care Medicine (SCCM), and Society of Infectious Diseases Pharmacists (SIDP). Pharmacotherapy. 2019;39:10-39.

151

CHAPTER

Restricted Antibiotics in the Era of Antimicrobial Resistance

Amitav Mohanty

ABSTRACT

Multidrug resistant (MDR) bacteria pose a serious threat to public health, as they can cause infections that are challenging to manage and have higher mortality rates. Common examples include methicillin-resistant *Staphylococcus aureus* (MRSA), carbapenem-resistant Enterobacteriaceae (CRE), etc. These bacteria have acquired genetic mutations or acquired resistance genes, allowing them to survive exposure to various antibiotics. Reserve antibiotics, also known as last-resort antibiotics or antibiotic "drugs of last resort," are a subset of antimicrobial agents that are preserved for the treatment of severe infections caused by MDR bacteria. These antibiotics are reserved as a last line of defense when other treatment options have failed or are ineffective. The purpose of reserving these antibiotics is to minimize the development and spread of further antibiotic resistance. The development of new antibiotics is crucial to replenish the arsenal of reserve antibiotics. Research and development efforts are ongoing to discover novel antimicrobial agents and alternative treatment strategies. In addition to discovering new antibiotics, it is essential to implement comprehensive infection prevention and control measures to reduce the incidence of drug-resistant infections and safeguard the effectiveness of reserve antibiotics in the long-term.

INTRODUCTION

In the sphere of medicine, the growth of multidrug resistance (MDR) has turned into a potentially fatal problem. The prognosis of people with bacterial illnesses was significantly changed by the development of antibiotics. However, their excessive and careless use has resulted in the development of "superbugs" that jeopardize their effectiveness. Global public health is seriously threatened by antimicrobial resistance (AMR). Due to the stress on healthcare, it raises morbidity and mortality and is linked to substantial economic expenses. MDR bacterial infections also significantly affect clinical and financial consequences. Currently, AMR causes 700,000 patient deaths annually around the globe. According to projections, this number of fatalities will rise to 10 million by 2050, which will cause the gross domestic product (GDP) to fall by at least 2.5%.

INCIDENCE OF RESISTANCE AGAINST DIFFERENT ANTIMICROBIALS

The World Health Organization's (WHO) recent report [Global Antimicrobial Resistance and Use Surveillance System (GLASS) Report: Early implementation 2020] published some key facts about the increasing AMR rates from 78 countries. The major findings of the reports were as follows: (1) A significantly higher rate of AMR against common bacterial infections; (2) median frequency of resistance in pathogens isolated from patients with bloodstream infections: (i) Methicillin-resistant *Staphylococcus aureus* (MRSA): 12.11%, (ii) *Escherichia coli* resistant to third-generation cephalosporins: 36.0%, (iii) *Klebsiella pneumoniae* resistant to third-generation cephalosporins: 57.6%, with 12 countries reporting 80–100% resistance, (iv) *Acinetobacter* species: aminoglycosides 41.2% and carbapenems 63.2%; (3)

median resistance to ciprofloxacin in urinary tract infections: (i) 43.29% for *Escherichia coli* in 33 reporting countries, territories, and areas and (ii) 38.1% for *Klebsiella pneumoniae* in 34 reporting countries, territories, and areas. India has been reported to have one of the highest rates of antibiotic resistance worldwide. According to the authors' calculations using data from the Global Burden of Disease 2019 for India, the mortality rate from infectious diseases in the country is 216.4 per 100,000 people, with an estimated 56,524 newborn fatalities each year due to sepsis brought on by antibiotic resistance. With a 47% growth from 5,411 to 7,976 million defined daily doses between 2010 and 2020, India has the second-highest global consumption of antibiotics. The over-the-counter (OTC) availability of affordable antibiotics in the context of lax compliance and enforcement of prescription-only restrictions has led to increased usage.

WHO PATHOGENS PRIORITY LIST

In the WHO's list, bacteria are divided into three priority categories: (i) Critical, (ii) high, and (iii) medium, depending on how urgently new antibiotics must be developed to tackle these pathogens. The pathogens in the most dangerous category are MDR bacteria, which are a hazard to people requiring medical devices such as ventilators and blood catheters as well as to people residing in nursing homes and hospitals. *Acinetobacter*, *Pseudomonas*, and certain Enterobacteriaceae, including *Klebsiella pneumoniae*, *Escherichia coli*, and *Enterobacter* species, are among the microorganisms with a critical priority. These pathogens can cause serious and frequently fatal infectious illnesses such as bloodstream infections and pneumonia and are resistant to numerous medications. Bacteria such as *Enterococcus faecium* and *Staphylococcus aureus* that are resistant to a variety of antibacterials, including vancomycin and fluoroquinolones, fall under the high priority group. *Shigella* and *Streptococcus pneumoniae* are examples of bacteria in the medium priority category that, despite some resistance, are still treatable with the available effective medicines.

ACCESS, WATCH, RESERVE (AWARE) CLASSIFICATION FOR ANTIBIOTICS USE

The WHO Expert Committee on Selection and Use of Essential Medicines developed the AWaRe classification of antibiotics in 2017 as a tool to support antibiotic stewardship efforts at local, national, and international levels. It stands for Access (to be widely available and affordable), Watch (to be used only for specific indications because their use increases the potential for the emergence of AMR), and Reserve (for situations when all other alternatives have failed). To emphasize the significance of their proper usage, antibiotics are divided into three categories: Access, Watch, and Reserve. These categories take into account the effects of various antibiotics and antibiotic classes on AMR. A total of 258 antibiotics are included in the 2021 update of the AWaRe classification. Countries can use this classification as a tool to support monitoring and stewardship initiatives for antibiotics. However, this classification model does not propose its use in determining the inclusion of antibiotics in national essential medication lists **(Table 1)**.

TABLE 1: Reserve group antibiotics and antibiotic classes (WHO Aware 2021).

Antibiotic	Class	Category	Listed on EML 2021
Aztreonam	Monobactams	Reserve	No
Carumonam	Monobactams	Reserve	No
Cefiderocol	Other-cephalosporins	Reserve	Yes
Ceftaroline fosamil	Fifth-generation cephalosporins	Reserve	No
Ceftazidime/avibactam	Third-generation cephalosporins	Reserve	Yes
Ceftobiprole medocaril	Fifth-generation cephalosporins	Reserve	No
Ceftolozane/tazobactam	Fifth-generation cephalosporins	Reserve	No
Colistin IV	Polymyxins	Reserve	Yes
Colistin oral	Polymyxins	Reserve	No
Dalbavancin	Glycopeptides	Reserve	No
Dalfopristin/quinupristin	Streptogramins	Reserve	No
Daptomycin	Lipopeptides	Reserve	No
Eravacycline	Tetracyclines	Reserve	No
Faropenem	Penems	Reserve	No
Fosfomycin IV	Phosphonics	Reserve	Yes
Iclaprim	Trimethoprim derivatives	Reserve	No
Imipenem/cilastatin/relebactam	Carbapenems	Reserve	No
Lefamulin	Pleuromutilin	Reserve	No
Linezolid	Oxazolidinones	Reserve	Yes
Meropenem/vaborbactam	Carbapenems	Reserve	Yes
Minocycline IV	Tetracyclines	Reserve	No
Omadacycline	Tetracyclines	Reserve	No
Oritavancin	Glycopeptides	Reserve	No

Continued

Continued

Antibiotic	Class	Category	Listed on EML 2021
Plazomicin	Aminoglycosides	Reserve	Yes
Polymyxin-B IV	Polymyxins	Reserve	Yes
Polymyxin-B oral	Polymyxins	Reserve	No
Tedizolid	Oxazolidinones	Reserve	No
Telavancin	Glycopeptides	Reserve	No
Tigecycline	Glycylcyclines	Reserve	No

(EML: essential medicines list)

Antibiotics and antibiotic classes included in the reserve group should only be used to treat infections caused by known or suspected MDR organisms. Antibiotics from the reserve group should only be used as a "last resort". Some of the antibiotics from the reserve group are also included in the WHO Model Lists of Essential Medicines when they have a favorable risk–benefit profile and clinical activity against "critical priority" or "high priority" bacterial pathogens according to the WHO Priority Pathogens List 1, notably carbapenem-resistant Enterobacteriaceae. These antibiotics should be used in the patients only when all other options have been exhausted or are inappropriate for the patient and the situation demanding a highly specific intervention. To maintain their effectiveness, these antimicrobials could be protected and prioritized as essential priorities of national and international stewardship programs that involve monitoring and utilization reporting of them in specific settings.

ANTIMICROBIAL STEWARDSHIP

Antimicrobial stewardship (AMS) is defined as "an organizational or healthcare-system-wide approach for fostering and monitoring judicious use of antimicrobials to preserve their effectiveness." In order to improve patient treatment outcomes and safety by reducing AMR development, AMS brings together healthcare leaders, microbiologists, infectious disease experts, doctors, nurses, farmers, veterinarians, IT experts, and clinical chemists. The major core principles of antibiotic stewardship program mainly consist of (1) leadership commitment to the required human, financial, and information technology; (2) accountability for program management and results through a single doctor/pharmacist leader; (3) utilizing a single pharmacy leader's drug expertise that will aid in directing implementation efforts to increase antibiotic use; (4) taking steps to put interventions into effect, such as preauthorization, prospective audit, and feedback; (5) monitoring prescription usage, the effects of therapies, patterns of resistance, and other significant outcomes; (6) directly informing hospital administration, chemists, nurses, and prescribers of prescription and resistance information; and (7) educating patients and healthcare workers (prescribers, chemists, and nurses) on adverse antibiotic reactions, antibiotic resistance, and appropriate prescribing.

Antimicrobial Stewardship Implementation to Curb Antimicrobial Resistance

Implementing a proper AMS policy and its benefits was justified by a prospective real-world Indian study conducted to evaluate the prudent use of high-end antibiotics among inpatients for a period of 3 months. Department-specific educational interventions were used, and feedbacks revealed that meropenem was the most frequently used high-end antibiotic. After the feedback and intervention, there was a 51.2% decrease in the unjustified antibiotic usage. From the preintervention observation of 77% to the postintervention observation of 88%, the appropriateness of the usage rose. The study came to the conclusion that it is necessary to maintain the rising compliance of prudent use of expensive antibiotics. Therefore, it is essential to continually develop AMS practices. Antimicrobial usage must be drastically reduced if AMR is to be eradicated. Long-term AMR containment treatments would place a focus on laws and policies that support a more rational and appropriate use of antibiotics. There are numerous instances where modifications to antibiotic-prescribing practices have significantly reduced the occurrence of resistant disease outbreaks. A key tactic for maintaining antibiotic efficacy in the treatment of infectious illnesses is their prudent use. 90% of all antibiotics are used in the community for nonhospitalized patients. But it was discovered that more than half of these were either superfluous or improper. Drug use evaluation (DUE) for the more expensive antibiotics would not only increase the effectiveness of the treatment but also aid in cost conservation and AMR prevention.

The main reason why doctors employ broad-spectrum antibiotics is that it is difficult to quickly and accurately identify the microorganisms that cause infectious diseases and their susceptibility profiles. Poor outcomes, including increased morbidity and mortality rates and longer stays in healthcare institutions, are linked to ineffective treatment of infections. Narrowing the spectrum of antibiotics and combining chemotherapeutic principles can improve efficacy, reduce toxicity and the overall cost of care, and prevent AMR in the population. An alternative approach to decreasing the cost is the repurposing of withdrawn and underused antimicrobial drugs which can provide an alternative or additional approach to de-novo drug discovery and the impact of latency with new drug discovery and clinical trials. This is evident with the return of colistin and fosfomycin use for MDR gram-negative infections.

CONCLUSION

In conclusion, the MDR pathogens can lead to drastic fatality and outcomes. Although these bacteria differ genetically, they share a number of resistance mechanisms, including reduced drug uptake, altered drug targets, drug inactivation, and activation of drug efflux pumps, which underlie the existence and persistence of these pathogens. This makes it crucial to be more vigilant in the surveillance and application of AMS in order to restrict the spread of the resistant infections and antibiotic resistance. The reserve antibiotics as classified by the WHO AWaRe classification should be only used against specific targeted organisms which have a proven susceptibility against them. The nationwide implementation of these programs, along with the creation of novel antibiotics or treatment modalities, will probably be the only means of limiting the global spread of MDR bacteria.

SUGGESTED READINGS

1. Jayalakshmi J, Priyadharshini MS. Restricting high-end antibiotics usage-challenge accepted. J Family Med Prim Care. 2019;8(10):3292.
2. Ghosh C, Sarkar P, Issa R, Haldar J. Alternatives to conventional antibiotics in the era of antimicrobial resistance. Trends Microbiol. 2019;27(4):323-38.
3. World Health Organization. Global Antimicrobial Resistance Surveillance System (GLASS) Report: Early Implementation. Geneva: World Health Organization; 2020.
4. Mehta A, Brhlikova P, McGettigan P, Pollock AM, Roderick P, Farooqui HH. Systemic antibiotic sales and WHO recommendations, India. Bull World Health Organ. 2022;100(10):610-9.
5. Mancuso G, Midiri A, Gerace E, Biondo C. Bacterial antibiotic resistance: The most critical pathogens. Pathogens. 2021;10(10):1310.
6. World Health Organization. (2021). 2021 AWaRe classification. [online] Available from https://www.who.int/publications/i/item/2021-aware-classification [Last accessed December, 2023].
7. Majumder MA, Rahman S, Cohall D, Bharatha A, Singh K, Haque M, et al. Antimicrobial stewardship: Fighting antimicrobial resistance and protecting global public health. Infect Drug Resist. 2020:4713-38.
8. Leekha S, Terrell CL, Edson RS. General principles of antimicrobial therapy. Mayo Clin Proc. 2011;86(2):156-67.

152 CHAPTER

Growing Threat of Carbapenem-resistant Enterobacteriaceae: How to Tackle?

Aditya Prakash Misra

ABSTRACT

Carbapenem-resistant Enterobacteriaceae (CRE) have become a serious threat to modern medicine all over the world. The World Health Organization (WHO) in 2017 mentioned in a policy statement that it is critically important to develop newer antibiotics against CRE. Most of the carbapenemases, *Klebsiella pneumoniae* carbapenemase (KPC), metallo-β-lactamases (MBLs), and OXA-48 are plasmid-mediated and have horizontal spread from one species to another. Various newer tests have been developed to quickly diagnose the CRE. Treatment of various infections caused by CRE is difficult and there are limited treatment options. There is an urgent need to develop newer antibiotics and evolve new strategies to effectively control and treat various infections caused by CRE.

INTRODUCTION

Enterobacteriaceae family comprises gram-negative bacteria living in intestines of humans and animals. The important pathogens of this family are *Escherichia coli, Klebsiella, Enterobacter, Salmonella, Shigella, Serratia, Yersinia, Proteus*, etc. In 2017, the World Health Organization (WHO) said that carbapenem-resistant Enterobacteriaceae (CRE) constitute a serious threat against which newer antibiotics should be developed. These bacteria cause pneumonitis, bloodstream infections, complicated urinary tract infections (UTIs), and intra-abdominal infections.

Carbapenems were introduced in the 1980s to tackle extended-spectrum β-lactamase (ESBL) producers and were highly efficacious. However in 1990, *Serratia* resistant to carbapenem-producing imipenem (IMP) was discovered in Japan. This was followed by discovery of VIM-1 (Verona integron-encoded metallo-β-lactamase) in Italy first in *Pseudomonas* and later in Enterobacteriaceae. In the Unites States of America (USA), *Klebsiella pneumoniae* (*K. pneumoniae*) with resistance to carbapenems was discovered in 1996. CRE refers to bacteria of Enterobacteriaceae family that survive and grow in presence of therapeutic concentrations of carbapenems. Centers for Disease Control and Prevention (CDC) defines CRE as enterobacteria not susceptible to any carbapenem or documented to produce carbapenemase.

Highest rates of carbapenem resistance are seen in *K. pneumoniae* over other species of Enterobacteriaceae and this is seen across the globe. CRE cause mainly hospital-associated infections which are difficult to treat and cause significant morbidity and mortality. In Indian subcontinent, community-acquired CRE infections, producing New Delhi metallo-β-lactamase (NDM) type of enzymes are also reported.

Carbapenem-resistant Enterobacteriaceae are divided into two main groups—carbapenamase-producing CRE (CP-CRE) and non carbapenemase-producing CRE. CP-CRE can be divided into three subgroups according to Ambler classification.

Within class A carbapenemases is *K. pneumoniae* carbapenemase (KPC), which is plasmid-encoded. It is most prevalent in the world. Initially, KPC was found only in *K. pneumoniae*; however now, KPC producing *E. coli, Proteus mirabilis, Serratia marcescens, Enterobacter, Salmonella*, and *Citrobacter* have been identified. A total of 12 bla_{KPC} gene variants exist globally.

Class B carbapenemases are metallo-β-lactamases (MBLs). These enzymes are most problematic and possess broad hydrolytic properties. The most common MBLs are NDM-1, which are most frequently found in Indian subcontinent.

The third group of carbapenemases are OXA-48 and like it, belonging to Ambler class D. these have low activity against carbapenems.

Noncarbapenemases-producing CRE have alternative mechanisms, namely AmpC type of β-lactamase, porin loss, and efflux pumps overexpression.

Currently, MBLs are most prevalent in Indian subcontinent, KPCs though found all over the globe, are most common in Northern and Southern Americas. OXA-48-like carbapenemases are endemic in Turkey, Middle east, and North Africa. Among all gram-negative bacteria, KPCs-producing organisms are most successful in causing pandemics in the world.

DETECTION OF CARBAPENEMASES

Detection of carbapenemases includes phenotypic and genotypic tests.

Phenotypic: Following are the various tests:

- *Modified Hodge test*: Sensitivity and specificity are good and do not require special equipment; however, it is operator dependent.
- *Carbapenem inactivation method*: It has a sensitivity of 99% for detecting various types of CRE. As per Clinical and Laboratory Standards Institute (CLSI), this should be the first-line confirmation test for CRE. It has low cost and does not need special equipment.
- Ethylenediaminetetraacetic acid (EDTA) inhibition test is used to detect MBLs. Boronic acid inhibition is used to detect KPC producers.
- *Carba NP test*: A rapid colorimetric test, highly sensitive in detecting KPC and most MBL-producing strains. It may not identify OXA-48 and GES-5. This test has been endorsed by CLSI.
- *MALDI-TOF (Matrix-assisted laser desorption ionization—time of flight mass) spectrometry assay*: Sensitivity and specificity are 100% with turnaround time of 30 minutes; however, it may show false-negative in OXA-48 and slime-producing organisms.
- *Genotypic tests*: These are conventional polymer chain reaction (PCR)/real-time PCR, Verigene and BioFire FilmArray. Sensitivity and specificity of BioFire is 100% in detecting KPCs and results are available in about 1 hour.
- *Xpert Carba R*: Uses rectal swab and detects carbapenemase. It does not tell species carrying them.
- Genome and metagenome sequencing are also being done as a research tool.

TREATMENT

The worldwide spread of multidrug-resistant CRE strains are causing a serious threat. In our country, resistance to various antibiotics is steadily increasing. Problem is further aggravated by absence of a central collating body, ineffective antibiotic stewardship program, and rampant misuse of available antibiotics. Major pharmacological companies are not doing enough research for discovering newer antibiotics. There is no gold standard treatment for KPC-producing *Klebsiella*. The choice of treatment depends upon site and severity of infection, local antibiogram, and host factors. Various strategies to effectively treat these infections are discussed further.

Combination Therapy

Most of the retrospective studies have found that combination therapy is associated with lower mortality. Choice of the combination should be guided by local antibiogram. For KPC-producing CRE, it will be prudent to use polymyxins with carbapenems. However, this combination may not show good results if minimal inhibitory concentration (MIC) levels are >16 μg/mL. A study from intensive care unit (ICU) patients in North India showed polymyxin resistance in *Klebsiella* isolates in blood, urine, and sputum samples as 8.75%, 4.26%, and 4.4%, respectively.

Dual Carbapenem Therapy

Dual carbapenem therapy refers to the use of ertapenem with either meropenem or doripenem. Ertapenem has highest affinity for carbapenemase and may consume most of it and allowing larger part of the other carbapenem to exert its bactericidal effect.

Triple Combination Therapy

Triple combination of polymyxins, carbapenem, and tigecycline has been found to significantly reduce the mortality in infections due to KPC-producing CRE. The emergence of polymyxin-resistant strains during the treatment is a serious concern.

NEWER AGENTS

Avibactam is a *non-β-lactam β-lactamase* inhibitor that has activity against class A and C β-lactamases, including KPC and AmpC. Its combination with ceftazidime has been approved by Food and Drug Administration (FDA) in 2015 for complicated UTI, including pyelonephritis. It may not be effective if MIC levels are >8 μg/mL. Meropenem with another β-lactamase inhibitor vaborbactam is also being tried. IMP-cilastatin along with relebactam, another new β-lactamase inhibitor, is also being used. Plazomicin a new aminoglycoside with efficacy against multidrug-resistant Enterobacteriaceae bacteria is also available now. Eravacycline, a semi-synthetic tetracycline with efficacy against KPC and NDM carbapenemase, is showing promise.

INFECTIOUS DISEASE SOCIETY GUIDANCE

For pyelonephritis and complicated UTI (cUTI), ciprofloxacin, levofloxacin, and trimethoprim-sulfamethoxazole may be preferred if sensitive. For ertapenem-resistant KP, meropenem in prolonged infusion should be given. Extended infusion of meropenem is preferred for infections outside urinary tract, caused by ertapenem-resistant but meropenem-susceptible Enterobacteriaceae. For infections outside of urinary tract resistant to both ertapenem and meropenem ceftazidime-avibactam, meropenem-vaborbactam and IMP–cilastatin–relebactam are the preferred drugs. For our country, where metallo-β enzymes are encountered often, combination of ceftazidime-avibactam and aztreonam should be preferred in case of meropenem resistance or if susceptibility results are not available. Cefiderocol may be used as an alternative in CP-CRE, where carbapenemase is other than MBL (VIM and IMP).

To emphasize again, for KPC type CP-CRE, ceftazidime-avibactam, meropenem-vaborbactam, IMP–cilastatin–relebactam are the preferred drugs. Cefiderocol may be used as an alternate agent. For NDM producers, ceftazidime-avibactam and aztreonam combination or cefiderocol as a monotherapy are the recommended antibiotics. For OXA-48 producers, ceftazidime-avibactam or cefiderocol are the preferred agents.

The emergence of resistance when using these novel β-lactam antibiotics is a concern. The likelihood of developing resistance is highest in ceftazidime-avibactam. Although β-lactam antibiotics are preferred for CP-CRE, tigecycline and eravacycline may be used as alternate in certain situations. Tetracycline derivatives should not be used as monotherapy for UTI and bloodstream infections. Higher doses of tigecycline are to be used for better results. Polymyxin B and colistin are not recommended for CP-CRE. Colistin may be used for carbapenem-resistant *K. pneumoniae* (CPKP) cystitis.

SUGGESTED READINGS

1. Suay-Garcia B, Perez-Gracia T. Present and future of Carbapenem-resistant Enterobacteriaceae (CRE) Infections. Antibiotics. 2019;8:122.
2. Lovleva A, Doi Y. Carbapenem-resistant Enterobacteriaceae. Clin Lab Med. 2017;37(2):303-15.

153
CHAPTER

Bacterial Diversity and Antibiotics Resistance Pattern in Diabetic Patients

Pankaj Nand Choudhry, Saurabh Puri

ABSTRACT

Sepsis and septic shock are the leading cause of morbidity and mortality in both diabetic and nondiabetic patients with a wide diversity of bacteria prevalent in the community. Local data about antimicrobial resistance in both diabetic and nondiabetic patients should be available for the proper initiation of empirical therapy. Our aim is to evaluate the spectrum of pathogens causing sepsis and septic shock and their profiles of antimicrobial resistance in a series of diabetic and nondiabetic patients.

A prospective observational study with 495 participants was conducted targeting the diabetic and nondiabetic patients admitted with sepsis or septic shock in the intensive care unit (ICU). An antibiotic sensitivity test was done on each of the isolates and the results of the antibiogram were compared between diabetic and nondiabetic patients. The statistical analysis was done by Chi-square test, Fisher's exact test using statistical product and service solutions known as statistical package for the social sciences (SPSS), 17.0 version (Chicago, IL, USA).

The most common isolated organism was *Klebsiella* followed by *Escherichia coli*, *Staphylococcus*, *Acinetobacter*, and *Enterococcus* in both diabetic and nondiabetic patients. The highest sensitivity was seen for tigecycline and colistin whereas highest resistance was seen for cephalosporin, fluoroquinolones, and carbapenems in both diabetic and nondiabetic patients. Statistically significant results were seen for sensitivity of trimethoprim-sulfamethoxazole for *Acinetobacter* and *E. coli*. Statistically significant results for carbapenem, beta-lactam + beta-lactamase inhibitor, and cefepime were observed for *Klebsiella* and for teicoplanin and vancomycin were observed for *Enterococcus*.

This study helps to understand the diversity of bacteria prevalent in community and formulate a better empirical antibiotic usage policy with proper implementation of antibiotic stewardship in a better way. Empirical antibiotic therapy should be prescribed only after performing antimicrobial susceptibility testing in order to obtain a better outcome.

INTRODUCTION

Sepsis and septic shock, with subsequent multiorgan failure, are the leading causes of mortality in intensive care units (ICU). Sepsis accounts for >10% of inhospital mortality. The risk of developing infections and sepsis is high in patients with type 2 diabetes mellitus (T2DM). Also, the prognosis of infection can be worsened by the presence of T2DM. Sepsis leads to an increased rate of mortality and morbidity in T2DM.

Sepsis that is complicated by acute organ dysfunction accounts for around half of the ICU resource utilization. Its associated morbidity and mortality are higher when compared to sepsis without acute organ dysfunction. The mortality rate caused due to severe sepsis varies from 28.6 to 49.6%. Advanced age, chronic alcoholism, and an immunosuppressed state are the various factors that can negatively impact the treatment outcome of severe sepsis.

Different types of organisms can cause sepsis. The most common organism isolated in septic patients is the gram-negative bacteria. Recently, the proportion of patients with severe infections due to gram-positive bacteria has increased. It accounts for half of the incidents of septicemia and severe systemic infections.

The hospital mortality rate identified in the bacteremic diabetic and nondiabetic patients is 24.1 and 44.0%, respectively. Diabetic patients with bacteremia are less likely to develop septic shock and acute renal failure with a 4 and 7% risk compared to nondiabetic patients with 13 and 19% risk, respectively. The mortality rate for diabetic and nondiabetic patients with bacteremia is identified to be 21.6 and 37.2%, respectively.

The appropriate selection of empirical antibiotics based on the pattern of local antibiotic resistance can reduce the mortality rate and increase the rational use of antibiotics. Pradipta et al. conducted a retrospective observational study in which levofloxacin, ceftazidime, ciprofloxacin, cefotaxime, ceftriaxone, and erythromycin were the most frequently used antibiotics in patients with sepsis showing an average resistance of above 50%. In a cross-sectional study conducted by Anvarinejad et al., multidrug resistance was identified in 91% of the isolates and methicillin resistance in 78% of *Staphylococcus aureus* isolates. Whereas 53% of the gram-negative species were identified as positive for extended-spectrum β-lactamase.

The mortality ascribed to sepsis is decreasing because of improvements in treatment and nursing, but still, sepsis remains a critical problem, especially in diabetic patients. The influence of diabetes mellitus on the outcomes of sepsis remains controversial. The antimicrobial resistance of bacterial pathogens in the diabetic population with infection is less investigated. Routine bacteriological profiling along with antibiotic resistance patterns should be considered as a necessary component in the management of sepsis. A knowledge of these patterns is essential when local policies on the use of antibiotics are being devised. The present study was conducted to compare the bacterial diversity in sepsis patients under ICU care and their antibiotic resistance pattern in diabetic and nondiabetic patients.

PATIENTS AND METHODS

The prospective study included bacterial isolates identified from various samples collected at the inpatient department (IPD) of Max Super Specialty Hospital, Vaishali, a tertiary care facility of Delhi-NCR between March 2018 and March 2019.

The study was approved by the Ethical Committee of Max Super Specialty Hospital, Vaishali, Ghaziabad, Uttar Pradesh, India.

Bacterial Identification Method and Antibiotic Susceptibility Testing

Bacterial isolates were recovered from different clinical samples including blood, urine, respiratory secretions, and others. The isolates were identified by standard microbiological methods and the automated VITEK 2 system. All repeat isolates and the isolates recovered from the regions of most likely colonization such as throat swab and perianal swab were excluded from the study. Six major classes of antibiotics, namely beta-lactams, fluoroquinolones, carbapenems, macrolides, aminoglycosides, and sulfamethoxazole-trimethoprim, in addition to colistin and tigecycline, were used to determine the antibiotic susceptibility pattern of isolates.

Statistical Analysis

Statistical analysis was performed by the statistical package for the social sciences (SPSS) program for Windows, version 17.0 (SPSS, Chicago, IL, USA). Continuous variables are presented as mean ± standard deviation (SD), and categorical variables are presented as absolute numbers and percentages. Data were checked for normality before statistical analysis. Normally distributed continuous variables were compared using the unpaired *t*-test, whereas the Mann–Whitney U test was used for those variables that were not normally distributed. Categorical variables were analyzed using either the Chi-square test or Fisher's exact test. $p < 0.05$ was considered statistically significant.

RESULTS

A total of 495 participants were included in the final analysis, with 240 participants in the diabetic group and 255 participants in the nondiabetic group. The mean age of participants in the diabetic group was 65.43 ± 10.36 and 60.75 ± 15.15 in the nondiabetic group. The difference in mean age between the study groups was statistically significant (p value < 0.05). Out of 240 diabetic patients, 133 (55.42%) were male, and 107 (44.58%) were female. Out of 255 nondiabetic patients, 171 (67.06%) were male, and 84 (32.94%) were female. Lower respiratory tract infection (LRTI) was observed in 101 (42.26%) diabetic patients, whereas in nondiabetic patients, it was found in 133 (52.16%) patients. Other sources of sepsis were bloodstream infection (BSI), which was present in 58 (24.27%) diabetic patients and 55 (21.57%) nondiabetic patients, urinary tract infection (UTI) was observed in 57 (23.85%) and 47 (18.43%) diabetic and nondiabetic patients, respectively along with skin and subcutaneous tissue infection (SSTI) in 23 (9.62%) and 20 (7.84%) diabetic and nondiabetic patients, respectively. The most common isolated organism was *Klebsiella* in both diabetic [70 (31.25%)] and nondiabetic patients [82 (33.33%)]. Other organisms isolated were *E. coli* [52 (23.21%) in diabetic and 42 (17.07%) in nondiabetic patients], *Staphylococcus* [25 (11.16%) in diabetic, 30 (12.2%) in nondiabetic patients], *Acinetobacter* [22 (9.82%) in diabetic, 29 (11.79%) in nondiabetic patients], *Enterococcus* [19 (8.48%) in diabetic, 13 (5.28%) in nondiabetic patients], and other organisms such as *Citrobacter, Providencia, Morganella, Stenotrophomonas, Proteus, Myroides*, and *Elizabethkingia* [21 (9.38%) in diabetic and 18 (7.32%) nondiabetic patients] **(Table 1)**.

Out of the total isolates, culture revealed growth of *Candida* in 16 (6.67%) diabetic patients and 9 (3.53%) nondiabetic patients. Diabetic patients had growth of *Candida albicans* [10 (62.5%)], and nondiabetic patients had growth of *Candida tropicalis* [6 (66.67%)].

Among 223 diabetic patients, *Acinetobacter* was primarily isolated in patients with LRTI [15 (68.18%)] whereas prevalence in BSI, SSTI, and UTI was in 4 (18.18%), 2 (9.09%), and 1 (4.55%) patients, respectively. A major source of *Enterococcus* was patients with UTI [10 (52.63%)], whereas prevalence in BSI, LRTI, and SSTI was in 5 (26.32%), 3 (15.79%), 1 (5.26%) patients, respectively. *E. coli* was isolated in 22 (43.14%) patients with UTI, the rest of the other sources revealed 11 (21.57%) patients from LRTI, 9 (17.65%) from BSI, and 9 (17.65%) from SSTI. *Klebsiella* was isolated in 43 (61.43%) LRTI patients, the rest of the other sources revealed 12 (17.14%) patients in UTI, 12 (17.14%) in BSI, and 3 (4.29%) in SSTI. A major source of *Pseudomonas* was LRTI [7 (46.67%)], other sources revealed 4 (26.67%) in SSTI, 2 (13.33%) in BSI, and 2 (13.33%) in UTI. *Staphylococcus* was isolated in patients with BSI [17(68%)], rest of other sources were UTI [4 (16%)], LRTI [3(12%)], and SSTI [1(4%)], respectively. For others, the major source was LRTI for 13 (61.9%) patients. The difference in culture reports among the sources was statistically significant ($p < 0.05$) **(Table 2)**.

TABLE: 1 Comparison of culture report between study groups ($n = 470$).

Culture report	Diabetes mellitus	
	Yes ($n = 224$)	No ($n = 246$)
Acinetobacter	22 (9.82%)	29 (11.79%)
Enterococcus	19 (8.48%)	13 (5.28%)
Escherichia coli	52 (23.21%)	42 (17.07%)
Klebsiella	70 (31.25%)	82 (33.33%)
Others	21 (9.38%)	18 (7.32%)
Pseudomonas	15 (6.7%)	32 (13.01%)
Staphylococcus	25 (11.16%)	30 (12.2%)

Among the nondiabetic patients, the major source of *Acinetobacter* was in LRTI patients 19 (65.52%), the rest of the other sources revealed 8 (27.59%) in BSI, and 2 (6.9%) in SSTI patients. *Enterococcus* was isolated in BSI and UTI patients 4 (30.77%) respectively, while 2 (15.38%) was isolated in SSTI patients. For *E. coli*, the major source was UTI patients 17 (40.48%), and prevalence in other sources were LRTI patients 13 (30.95%), BSI patients 8 (19.05%), SSTI patients 4 (9.52%). For *Klebsiella*, the major source was LRTI for 54 (65.85%) patients, and the rest of the other sources revealed BSI patients 12 (14.63%), UTI patients 10 (12.2%), and SSTI patients 6 (7.32%). For *Pseudomonas*, the major source was LRTI for 19 (59.38%) patients, the rest of the other sources revealed UTI, BSI, and SSTI patients 7 (21.88%), 3 (9.38%), 3 (9.38%). For *Staphylococcus*, the major source was BSI for 16 (53.33%) patients and LRTI for 11 (36.67%) patients. For others, the major source was LRTI for 9 (50%) participants **(Table 3)**.

Among the study population with culture report for *E. coli*, there was not a statistically significant difference in drugs belonging to nitrofurantoin, cefepime, cefuroxime, ceftriaxone, ciprofloxacin, imipenem, ertapenem, meropenem, amoxicillin, ampicillin, and piperacillin/tazobactam, cefoperazone/sulbactam, amoxicillin/clavulanic acid between the study groups ($p > 0.05$) while for trimethoprim-sulfamethoxazole there was a statistically significant difference between study groups ($p < 0.05$). Among the study population with culture report for *Klebsiella*, there was not a statistically significant difference in the following drugs, nitrofurantoin, cefuroxime, ceftriaxone, amoxicillin, ampicillin, and

TABLE 2: Comparison of culture report across sources in diabetic patients ($n = 223$).

Culture report	Source				Chi-square	p value
	BSI	LRTI	SSTI	UTI		
Acinetobacter ($n = 22$)	4 (18.18%)	15 (68.18%)	2 (9.09%)	1 (4.55%)		
Enterococcus ($n = 19$)	5 (26.32%)	3 (15.79%)	1 (5.26%)	10 (52.63%)		
Escherichia coli ($n = 51$)	9 (17.65%)	11 (21.57%)	9 (17.65%)	22 (43.14%)		
Klebsiella ($n = 70$)	12 (17.14%)	43 (61.43%)	3 (4.29%)	12 (17.14%)	82.463	<0.001
Others ($n = 21$)	4 (19.05%)	13 (61.9%)	2 (9.52%)	2 (9.52%)		
Pseudomonas ($n = 15$)	2 (13.33%)	7 (46.67%)	4 (26.67%)	2 (13.33%)		
Staphylococcus (n=25)	17 (68%)	3 (12%)	1 (4%)	4 (16%)		

(BSI: bloodstream infection; LRTI: lower respiratory tract infection; SSTI: skin and subcutaneous tissue infection; UTI: urinary tract infection)

TABLE 3: Comparison of culture across sources in nondiabetic patients ($n = 246$).

	Source			
Culture report	**BSI**	**LRTI**	**SSTI**	**UTI**
Acinetobacter ($n = 29$)	8 (27.59%)	19 (65.52%)	2 (6.9%)	0 (0%)
Enterococcus ($n = 13$)	4 (30.77%)	3 (23.08%)	2 (15.38%)	4 (30.77%)
Escherichia coli ($n = 42$)	8 (19.05%)	13 (30.95%)	4 (9.52%)	17 (40.48%)
Klebsiella ($n = 82$)	12 (14.63%)	54 (65.85%)	6 (7.32%)	10 (12.2%)
Others ($n = 18$)	2 (11.11%)	9 (50%)	3 (16.67%)	4 (22.22%)
Pseudomonas ($n = 32$)	3 (9.38%)	19 (59.38%)	3 (9.38%)	7 (21.88%)
Staphylococcus ($n = 30$)	16 (53.33%)	11 (36.67%)	0 (0%)	3 (10%)

(BSI: bloodstream infection; LRTI: lower respiratory tract infection; SSTI: skin and subcutaneous tissue infection; UTI: urinary tract infection)

tigecycline between the study groups ($p > 0.05$) while for imipenem, ertapenem, meropenem, cefoperazone/sulbactam, piperacillin/tazobactam, amoxicillin/clavulanic acid and cefepime, there was a statistically significant difference between study group ($p < 0.05$). Among the study population with culture report for *Staphylococcus*, there was not a statistically significant difference in any of the drugs belonging to oxacillin, ampicillin, benzylpenicillin, clindamycin, gentamicin, linezolid, teicoplanin, vancomycin, nitrofurantoin, cefoxitin, ciprofloxacin, levofloxacin, and erythromycin between the study groups ($p > 0.05$). Among the study population with culture report for *Pseudomonas*, there was not a statistically significant difference in drugs belonging to ceftazidime, cefepime, piperacillin/tazobactam, ticarcillin/clavulanic acid, cefoperazone/sulbactam, netilmicin, amikacin, gentamicin, tobramycin, benzylpenicillin, lincomycin, nitrofurantoin, ciprofloxacin, levofloxacin, imipenem, meropenem, doripenem between the study groups ($p > 0.05$). Among the study population with culture reports as *Enterococcus*, there was not a statistically significant difference in drugs belonging to linezolid, gentamicin, nitrofurantoin, and tetracycline between the diabetes mellitus ($p > 0.05$), while for teicoplanin, vancomycin there was a statistically significant difference between the study groups ($p < 0.05$).

Out of 240 participants in the diabetic group, 110 (46.03%) participants had outcomes as death, and 130 (53.97%) participants had outcomes as discharged. Out of 255 participants in the nondiabetic group, 103 (40.39%) participants had the outcome as death, and 152 (59.38%) participants had the outcome as discharged. The difference in outcome between the study group was not statistically significant ($p > 0.05$).

DISCUSSION

The risk of developing infections and sepsis is high in patients with T2DM. Also, the prognosis of infection can be worsened by the presence of T2DM. Sepsis leads to an increased rate of mortality and morbidity in T2DM patients with sepsis. Antimicrobial stewardship is defined as the optimal selection, dosage, and duration of antimicrobial treatment that can result in the best clinical outcome for the management or prevention of infection, with minimal toxicity to the patient and minimal impact on subsequent resistance. Working with healthcare practitioners in order to help each patient receive the most appropriate antimicrobial with the correct dose and duration; prevention of antimicrobial overuse, misuse, and abuse; and minimizing the development of resistance are the goals associated with antimicrobial stewardship. Antimicrobial resistance of bacterial pathogens in the diabetic population with infection is less investigated. Routine bacteriological profiling along with antibiotic resistance patterns should be considered as a necessary component in the management of sepsis. A knowledge of these patterns is essential when local policies on the use of antibiotics are being devised. The present study was conducted to compare the bacteriological diversity in patients with sepsis under ICU care and compare their antibiotic resistance patterns in diabetic and nondiabetic patients.

A total of 495 participants were included in the final analysis, with 240 participants in the diabetic group and 255 participants in the nondiabetic group.

In the present study, the mean age of participants in the diabetic group was higher compared to the nondiabetic group. Similarly, in the retrospective study by Trivedi et al., in 115 participants, the mean age of the participants was greater in the diabetic group compared to the nondiabetic group. The present study was conducted in a tertiary care hospital that caters to both urban and rural populations and has a huge burden of critical referral cases with aging population. In the current study, the majority of the participants were males in the diabetic and nondiabetic groups. In the study by Trivedi et al., the majority of the participants were females in the diabetic group, whereas in the nondiabetic group majority were males. The diabetic group showed contradictory results, whereas the nondiabetic group showed resembles our study results.

In the present study, the source was identified as LRTI in the majority of cases, followed by BSI, UTI, and SSTI in both the diabetic and nondiabetic groups. In a prospective cohort study performed by Muller et al., URTI was identified as the major source followed by UTI, MSMI, and LRTI in the diabetic and nondiabetic group, which is contradictory to our study results. In the study of Esper et al., the source of infection of most participants was found in the respiratory tract in both the diabetic and nondiabetic population followed by genitourinary, gastrointestinal, skin and soft tissue, and bone.

In the diabetic population, the culture report showed *Acinetobacter, Enterococcus, E. coli, Klebsiella, Staphylococcus*, and *Pseudomonas* species, whereas in nondiabetic patients, *Acinetobacter, Enterococcus, E. coli, Klebsiella, Staphylococcus*, and *Pseudomonas* species were identified in the culture report. Acharya et al. conducted a prospective cross-sectional study in 180 patients in which *E. coli, Klebsiella, Enterococcus, Enterobacter, Citrobacter*, and *Proteus* species were identified in diabetic and nondiabetic patients. In a population of 200 participants, Akhand et al. performed a study in which the culture report showed *E. coli* 64.5% and 66.7%, *Klebsiella* 22.6% and 12.5%, *Enterococcus* 6.5% and 4.2%, *Enterobacter* 0% and 4.2%, *Citrobacter* 3.2% and 0%, and *Proteus* 0 and 8.4% in diabetic and nondiabetic population, respectively.

Among the diabetic people, BSI and UTI were identified as the major source of *Enterococcus* and *Staphylococcus*. Whereas the major source was LRTI and UTI for *E. coli* and *Klebsiella*. For *Pseudomonas*, the major sources were LRTI and SSTI, while BSI and LRTI were the sources of infection in *Acinetobacter* growing isolates.

Among the nondiabetic people, BSI, LRTI, and UTI were identified as the major sources of *Acinetobacter, Enterococcus, E. Coli, Klebsiella, Staphylococcus*, and *Pseudomonas* species, respectively.

In the present study, the *Acinetobacter* was most sensitive to colistin, trimethoprim-sulfamethoxazole, and tigecycline, whereas resistant to cefepime, ceftriaxone, ciprofloxacin in diabetic patients. Similarly, in nondiabetic patients, *Acinetobacter* was most sensitive to colistin and tigecycline and resistant to cefepime, ciprofloxacin, and imipenem. Ahmadishooli et al. conducted a study in 84 diabetic patients in which the *Acinetobacter* was sensitive to ampicillin-sulbactam, cefepime, ceftriaxone, gentamycin, ciprofloxacin, cotrimoxazole, amikacin, meropenem, imipenem, ceftazidime, and piperacillin/tazobactam, whereas resistant to amikacin.

In the current study, the *E. coli* was sensitive to tigecycline, colistin, and amikacin, while it was resistant to amoxicillin, ampicillin, and ciprofloxacin in diabetic patients. Similarly, in nondiabetic patients, *E. coli* was sensitive to tigecycline, colistin, and amikacin and resistant to amoxicillin, ampicillin, and ciprofloxacin. In Thapa et al., *E. coli* isolates were sensitive to amikacin, nitrofurantoin, cotrimoxazole and resistant to nalidixic acid, norfloxacin, ciprofloxacin in diabetic patients. Whereas in nondiabetics, all *E. coli* isolates were sensitive to cotrimoxazole, amikacin, nitrofurantoin, and resistant to nalidixic acid, norfloxacin, and cotrimoxazole.

In the current study, *Klebsiella* was most sensitive to colistin and tigecycline and resistant to amoxicillin, ceftriaxone, and cefuroxime in diabetic patients. Whereas in nondiabetic patients, *Klebsiella* was most sensitive to colistin and tigecycline and resistant to amoxicillin, ceftriaxone, and cefuroxime. In Thapa et al., all the *Klebsiella* isolates were sensitive to almost all antibiotics and did not show any resistant pattern in diabetic patients. In nondiabetic patients, all isolates were sensitive to cotrimoxazole, amikacin, and nitrofurantoin and resistant to nalidixic acid.

In the present study, the *Staphylococcus* was most sensitive to daptomycin, teicoplanin, and vancomycin and resistant to ampicillin and benzylpenicillin in diabetic patients, whereas in nondiabetic patients, *Staphylococcus* was most sensitive to daptomycin, teicoplanin, and vancomycin and resistant to ampicillin and benzylpenicillin. Thapa et al. performed an cross-sectional descriptive study in 601 subjects in which the *S. aureus* isolates were sensitive to gentamicin, cefotaxime, cotrimoxazole, and ciprofloxacin and resistant to amikacin, oxacillin, and azithromycin in diabetic patients, whereas in nondiabetic all isolates were sensitive to azithromycin, gentamicin, cefotaxime, cotrimoxazole, vancomycin, and levofloxacin and resistant to oxacillin, which was contradictory to our study results.

In the present study, *Pseudomonas* was most sensitive to amikacin, imipenem, and meropenem and resistant to ticarcillin/clavulanic acid, netilmicin, and tobramycin in diabetic patients, whereas in nondiabetic patients, the *Pseudomonas* was sensitive to amikacin, imipenem, and doripenem and resistant to ticarcillin/clavulanic acid, netilmicin, and tobramycin. In Jain et al., the *Pseudomonas* culture isolates were sensitive to amikacin, imipenem, meropenem, piperacillin-tazobactam combination, tigecycline, ciprofloxacin, and levofloxacin in diabetic patients.

In the present study, *Enterococcus* was most sensitive to tigecycline and linezolid and resistant to ciprofloxacin and levofloxacin in diabetic patients. Whereas in nondiabetic patients, *Enterococcus* was most sensitive to

TABLE 4: Comparison of outcome between study groups (*n* = 494).

Outcome	Diabetes mellitus		Chi-square	*p* value
	Yes (*n* = 240)	No (*n* = 255)		
Death	110 (46.03%)	103 (40.39%)	1.469	0.226
Discharge	130 (53.97%)	152 (59.38%)		

tigecycline and linezolid and resistant to ciprofloxacin and levofloxacin in diabetic patients. Jain et al. performed a study on 185 subjects in which *Enterococcus* culture isolates were sensitive to linezolid, daptomycin, teicoplanin, tigecycline, benzylpenicillin, vancomycin, ciprofloxacin, levofloxacin, erythromycin, and tetracycline in diabetic patients.

In the present study, the mortality rate was identified as high in the diabetic group compared to the nondiabetic group. Whereas the discharge rate was high in the nondiabetic patients compared to diabetic patients. Similarly, in the study by Moutzouri et al., the mortality in diabetic septic patients was higher compared to the mortality in the nondiabetic population **(Table 4)**.

CONCLUSION

Antimicrobial resistance has been increasing at an alarming rate worldwide. One of the few major factors that lead to an increase in resistance is the indiscriminate, injudicious use, and underdosing of antibiotics. Uncontrolled blood sugar in the sea of an existing pandemic of diabetes mellitus adds to the increasing resistance, leading to a high mortality.

The isolates in the present study revealed *Klebsiella* to be the most prevalent organism in both diabetic and nondiabetic patients, whereas the lowest prevalence in diabetic patients was that of *Pseudomonas. Enterococcus* was the lowest in prevalence among nondiabetic patients. Colistin was found to be highly sensitive in *Klebsiella, Acinetobacter,* and *E. coli* in both diabetic and nondiabetic patients. *Acinetobacter* showed high resistance to cephalosporin, fluoroquinolones, and carbapenems in both diabetic and nondiabetic patients; however, sensitivity was lower for tigecycline in diabetic patients when compared to nondiabetic patients.

Escherichia coli was highly resistant to beta-lactam, beta-lactam/beta-lactamase inhibitors, cephalosporins, and fluoroquinolones in both diabetic and nondiabetic patients, whereas tigecycline sensitivity was much lower in diabetic patients when compared to nondiabetic patients. Isolates showing the growth of *Klebsiella* revealed significant resistance to cefepime, beta-lactam, beta-lactam/beta-lactamase inhibitor, carbapenems, aminoglycosides, nitrofurantoin among diabetic patients in comparison to nondiabetic patients. *Pseudomonas* was highly sensitive to polymyxin B in both groups, whereas diabetic patients showed increased resistance to carbapenems, beta-lactam/beta-lactamase inhibitors, aminoglycosides, cephalosporins, and fluoroquinolones. *Enterococcus* and *Staphylococcus* were gram-positive bacteria that were seen in a significant number of isolates. *Enterococcus* showed high resistance to beta-lactams, aminoglycosides, fluoroquinolones, and macrolides in both diabetic and nondiabetic patients. However, in the group of diabetic patients, there was a significant increase in resistance to linezolid, glycopeptides, nitrofurantoin, and tetracycline, when compared with nondiabetics. Tigecycline showed resistance in half isolates among both diabetic and nondiabetic patients. Another gram-positive bacterium, *Staphylococcus,* revealed high resistance to beta-lactams, linezolid, fluoroquinolones, and macrolides in both groups. This study conducted in a tertiary care hospital will help in understanding the diversity of bacteria prevalent in our community, which would help in formulating a better empirical antibiotic usage policy with proper implementation of antibiotic stewardship. Empirical antibiotic therapy should be prescribed only after taking a sample for performing antimicrobial susceptibility testing and targeted therapy is to be done according to the results of the culture and susceptibility testing in order to obtain a better outcome.

SUGGESTED READINGS

1. Berg D, Gerlach H. Recent advances in understanding and managing sepsis. F1000Res. 2018;7:F1000 Faculty Rev-1570.
2. Frydrych LM, Fattahi F, He K, Ward PA, Delano MJ. Diabetes and Sepsis: Risk, recurrence, and ruination. Front Endocrinol (Lausanne). 2017;8:271.
3. Angus DC, Linde-Zwirble WT, Lidicker J, Clermont G, Carcillo J, Pinsky MR. Epidemiology of severe sepsis in the United States: analysis of incidence, outcome, and associated costs of care. Crit Care Med. 2001;29(7):1303-10.
4. Yang Y, Yang KS, Hsann YM, Lim V, Ong BC. The effect of comorbidity and age on hospital mortality and length of stay in patients with sepsis. J Crit Care. 2010;25(3):398-405.
5. Beale R, Reinhart K, Brunkhorst FM, Dobb G, Levy M, Martin G, et al.; PROGRESS Advisory Board. Promoting Global Research Excellence in Severe Sepsis (PROGRESS): lessons from an international sepsis registry. Infection. 2009;37(3):222-32.
6. O'Brien JM Jr, Lu B, Ali NA, Martin GS, Aberegg SK, Marsh CB, et al. Alcohol dependence is independently associated with

sepsis, septic shock, and hospital mortality among adult intensive care unit patients. Crit Care Med. 2007;35(2):345-50.

7. Pradipta IS, Sodik DC, Lestari K, Parwati I, Halimah E, Diantini A, et al. Antibiotic resistance in sepsis patients: evaluation and recommendation of antibiotic use. N Am J Med Sci. 2013;5: 344-52.
8. Anvarinejad M, Pouladfar G, Japoni A, Bolandparvaz S, Satiary Z, Abbasi P, et al. Isolation and antibiotic susceptibility of the microorganisms isolated from diabetic foot infections in Nemazee Hospital, Southern Iran. J Pathog. 2015;2015:328796.
9. Doron S, Davidson LE. Antimicrobial stewardship. Mayo Clin Proc. 2011;86(11):1113-23.
10. Trivedi U, Parameswaran S, Armstrong A, Burgueno-Vega D, Griswold J, Dissanaike S, et al. Prevalence of multiple antibiotic resistant infections in diabetic versus nondiabetic wounds. J Pathog. 2014;2014:173053.
11. Muller LM, Gorter KJ, Hak E, Goudzwaard WL, Schellevis FG, Hoepelman AI, et al. Increased risk of common infections in patients with type 1 and type 2 diabetes mellitus. Clin Infect Dis. 2005;41(3):281-8.
12. Esper AM, Moss M, Martin GS. The effect of diabetes mellitus on organ dysfunction with sepsis: an epidemiological study. Crit Care. 2009;13(1):R18.
13. Acharya D, Bogati B, Shrestha G, Gyawali P. Diabetes mellitus and Urinary Tract Infection: Spectrum of Uropathogens and their Antibiotic Sensitivity. JMMIHS. 2015;1(4):24-8.
14. Akhand A, Biswas D, Tilkar M, Tenguriya M, Tilkar Y. Comparative study of urinary tract infection in patients with or without diabetes: A prospective study from central India. International Journal of Medicine Research. 2018;3(1):75-8.
15. Ahmadishooli A, Davoodian P, Shoja S, Ahmadishooli B, Dadvand H, Hamadiyan H, et al. Frequency and antimicrobial susceptibility patterns of diabetic foot infection of patients from Bandar Abbas District, Southern Iran. J Pathog. 2020;2020:1057167.
16. Thapa P, Sunar A, Lamichanne D, Dhungana A, Paudel R, Jaiswal S, et al. Antimicrobial sensitivity pattern of bacteria causing urinary tract infection among diabetic patients. Research Square. 2020.
17. Jain SK, Barman R. Bacteriological profile of diabetic foot ulcer with special reference to drug-resistant strains in a tertiary care center in North-East India. Indian J Endocrinol Metab. 2017;21(5):688-94.
18. Moutzouri AG, Athanassiou GA, Dimitropoulou D, Skoutelis AT, Gogos CA. Severe sepsis and diabetes mellitus have additive effects on red blood cell deformability. J Infect. 2008;57(2):147-51.

154

CHAPTER

Outpatient Antimicrobial Therapy

Yashasvi Gautam, Akanksha Gautam

ABSTRACT

Outpatient parenteral antimicrobial therapy (OPAT) has rapidly grown since its inception due to factors such as cost containment, daily antimicrobial agents, technological advancements, increased patient acceptance, and skilled community services. However, more information is needed on its benefits, safety, and limitations.

INTRODUCTION

The practice of administering intravenous antimicrobial therapy in the home and in alternate care settings has grown rapidly since it was first described in 1974 by Rucker and Harrison. The growth of outpatient parenteral antimicrobial therapy (OPAT) has been fueled by a variety of factors including the push for cost containment, the development of antimicrobial agents that can be administered once daily, technological advances in vascular access and infusion devices, increased acceptance of such therapy by both patients and health care personnel, and the availability of reliable and skilled services for OPAT in the community. Although OPAT has become widely accepted as a form of medical therapy, more information is needed regarding its benefits, safety, and limitations.

DEFINITION OF OUTPATIENT PARENTERAL ANTIMICROBIAL THERAPY

Outpatient parenteral antimicrobial therapy is defined as the administration of parenteral antimicrobial therapy in at least two doses on different days without intervening hospitalization.

- A method for delivering intravenous antibiotics without requirement for inpatient stay
- In the community or outpatient setting
- Infections whose requirement for IV antibiotics are the only reason for admission to or barrier to discharge from hospital

TYPES OF OUTPATIENT PARENTERAL ANTIMICROBIAL THERAPY (DELIVERY MODELS)

- Home based
- Infusion center based
- Skilled nursing facility (SNF) based

Home Based

All medications are administered in the home by the patient, patient's family member, or a home health nurse. Critical to the success of home-based OPAT is the presence of a competent and adherent patient and/or caregiver. Minimal features required for safe home infusion include adequate refrigeration and storage and the presence of at least one adult who can reliably learn and perform sterile infusion technique and communicate with the treatment team.

Patient convenience; regular skilled clinical assessments; opportunity for home inspection; availability of a registered nurse on 24-hour basis.

Requires patient/caregiver competence and compliance; requires reliable home infusion nursing;

increased cost to patient in the absence of home infusion insurance benefit; may entail substantial co-pays.

Infusion Centers Based

This model is resource intensive, requiring reliable transportation, availability of a skilled nurse to infuse antimicrobial agents, and all the accompanying office resources but offers additional oversight with daily in-person visits.

- High degree of clinical oversight; usually covered by medicare; minimizes out-of-pocket costs to patient.
- Cost effective
- Can be based in community hospitals, clinics, or acute hospitals
- Can be used to teach patients and staff, deliver therapy, check bloods, and monitor patients
- Patient has to travel but less delay in waiting for staff
- Drop in for problems

Skilled Nursing Facility Based

Skilled nursing facility is a healthcare facility, patients are more likely to encounter resistant organisms, including *Clostridium difficile*. Overall, this option is significantly more expensive to the healthcare system compared to any of the other OPAT models but may minimize the patient's out-of-pocket expense.

Usually covered by payers/medicare; other skilled nursing needs (e.g., physical therapy, wound care) can be met; may be less labor intensive for supervising physicians when treating patients with multiple comorbid conditions; minimizes out-of pocket expanses.

Variable levels of clinical oversight; patients may dislike staying in SNF; may exhaust patient's SNF benefits; most expensive for overall healthcare system costs to patient.

EMERGING TRENDS IN OUTPATIENT PARENTERAL ANTIMICROBIAL THERAPY

The role of remote-access delivery of OPAT oversight is currently under investigation. The use of telemedicine to support OPAT in geographically isolated locations is appealing but challenged in the United States by reimbursement models and interstate regulatory requirements. Also unknown, but promising, are the roles of the long-acting semisynthetic lipoglycopeptides dalbavancin and oritavancin, currently approved narrowly, but offering potential promise because of their very long half-lives and infrequent dosing requirements. The role of these expensive agents, particularly in persons who inject drugs (PWID), remains to be defined. Additionally, one source of complications during OPAT is the ventricular assist device (VAD). Delivery of antimicrobials by subcutaneous administration has the potential to avoid the need for a VAD.

TEAM MEMBERS IN OUTPATIENT PARENTERAL ANTIMICROBIAL THERAPY

The typical OPAT team consists:

- Physician—treating physician addresses the indication of OPAT selection of antimicrobial requirement, duration of therapy, and subsequent medical evaluation.
- OPAT nurse specialist with IV access expertise
- Pharmacist
- The patient and the caregiver

PATIENT EVALUATION AND SELECTION FOR OUTPATIENT PARENTERAL ANTIMICROBIAL THERAPY

Initiation of OPAT requires that a physician determine that such therapy is needed to treat a defined infection that hospitalization is not needed to control the infection, and that alternate routes of drug delivery are not feasible or appropriate.

General guidelines and recommendations for patient selection have been published. The patient must be compliant and have the physical ability to complete therapy. Either the patient, a family member, or a designated friend must have the cognitive ability and manual dexterity to infuse antibiotics. Patients must also be able to keep their clinic appointments. The patient's home must have a telephone, running water and, if necessary, a refrigerator for medications.

The patient and care givers should understand the benefit, risk, economic consideration involved in OPAT.

Outpatient parenteral antimicrobial therapy has been used for a wide variety of infections. Any discussion of safety and efficacy needs to focus on the specific infection being treated.

- *Osteomyelitis:* Long course needed for care, most patient are stable, fulminant infection.
- *Endocarditis:* Stringent patient selection criteria. Contraindicated in prosthetic valve, persistently positive blood culture, congestive heart failure (CHF), recurrent embolism, and conduction defects.
- *Central nervous system (CNS) infections:* Good success rate, need close monitoring, higher risk for complication, and rehospitalization.
- *Skin and soft tissue infection:* Complicated and drug-resistant skin and soft tissue infection (SSTI) can also be treated by novel bovine serum albumin (BSA).
- Surgical site infection

- Febrile neutropenia
- *Other infections:* Lyme borreliosis, cellulitis, septic arthritis, sinusitis, abdominal abscesses, pyelonephritis, and cytomegalovirus retinitis are some of the other infections for which OPAT is used. The safety and success of OPAT for each of these diagnoses rest on good clinical judgment during patient selection. OPAT should not be started until the patient is medically stable and the risk of complications has decreased to a minimal level.

COMPLICATIONS OF OUTPATIENT PARENTERAL ANTIMICROBIAL THERAPY

Intravenous (IV) line infection, thrombosis, mechanical and chemical phlebitis, HAL (health care-associated infections).

Antimicrobial Selection and Administration

When selecting an antimicrobial for OPAT, multiple factors must be taken into account, including the probable infecting organism, the pharmacodynamic and pharmacokinetic properties of candidate drugs, and drug stability. Although almost any antimicrobial can be used, drugs with long half-lives continue to be extensively prescribed, although specific choices will vary with the patient population, the likely diagnosis, the anticipated duration of therapy, and physician preference. Use of agents that can be administered once daily reduces disruption of daily activities and limits the potential for complications. The choice of antimicrobials for OPAT needs to be continually evaluated as new oral agents may replace some parenterally administered choices, and antimicrobial resistance is an ongoing issue.

The initial dose of an intravenous agent should be administered in a supervised setting, such as a physician's office, ambulatory care department, or the hospital, before a patient's discharge to home care. Personnel trained in resuscitation and appropriate equipment should be readily available.

For OPAT it is easiest to divide antibiotics into three categories, outlined in **Box 1**.

BOX 1: Categories of antibiotics for use in outpatient parenteral antibiotic therapy.

- *Category 1:* Can typically be dosed daily
  - Aminoglycosides
  - Amphotericin B
  - Caspofungin
  - Ceftriaxone
  - Daptomycin
  - Ertapenem
  - Vancomycin
- *Category 2:* Are stable for >24 hours either at room temperature or if refrigerated. These medications can be given via a syringe pump or an electronic infusion pump
  - Aztreonam
  - Cefazolin
  - Cefepime
  - Ceftazidime
  - Clindamycin
  - Nafcillin
  - Oxacillin
  - Penicillin
  - Piperacillin ± tazobactam
  - Ticarcillin ± clavulanate
- *Category 3:* Have limited stability and are difficult to use in the outpatient setting. These medications should be used for OPAT only under very unusual circumstance
  - Ampicillin
  - Imipenem
  - Meropenem

Clinical monitoring: The frequency of patient follow-up visits with the supervising physician needs to be determined when a patient begins a course of OPAT. In most circumstances, patients see the managing physician once or twice each week. Some patients need to be seen daily by a physician, especially at the beginning of OPAT. Patients with endocarditis, meningitis, or other life-threatening infections may also require more frequent visits. Less frequent visits may be appropriate for patients with stable chronic infections, few comorbid conditions, and appropriate caregiver support.

Laboratory monitoring: The guidelines displayed in **Table 1** address the minimum frequency of monitoring for adverse reactions and toxicity. Additional studies may be needed for determination of the response to therapy.

Adverse effects in patients receiving antimicrobial therapy are not unusual. If laboratory parameters show an adverse trend, the frequency of laboratory monitoring should be increased; in some cases, the medication may need to be changed or its use discontinued. Data suggest that some adverse reactions, such as renal or vestibular toxicity and leukopenia, become more frequent as the length of therapy increases. Even though an infection is responding, the need for regular laboratory monitoring remains.

TABLE 1: Monitoring for adverse reactions and toxicity.

Antimicrobial agent(s), by class	Frequency of testing Number of times per week				Other
	Complete blood count[a]	Renal function tests[b]	Potassium level	Liver enzyme levels	
Aminoglycosides (gentamicin, tobramycin, amikacin)	Once	Twice	……	……	Clinical monitoring for vestibular and hearing dysfunction at each visit; serum concentrations as clinically indicated
β-Lactams (penicillins, cephalosporins, aztreonam, carbapenems)	Once	Once	…….	….[c]	
Antipseudomonal penicillins	Once	Once	Once		
Fluoroquinolones	……	…..	…..	Once	
Miscellaneous:					
• Clindamycin	Once	Once	…	Once	
• Daptomycin	Once	Once	….	Once	Creatine phosphokinase (CPK) at least weekly
• Linezolid	Once	……	….	…..	….
• Pentamidine	Twice	Twice	Twice	…..	Blood glucose level daily; chemistry profile[d] twice per week
• Quinupristin-dalfopristin	…..	……	……	Once	Monitor for arthralgias
• Trimethoprim-sulfamethoxazole	Once	Once	Once	……	
• Vancomycin	Once	Once	……	…….	Serum levels as clinically indicated
Antifungals:					
• Amphotericin B, including lipid formulations	Once	Twice	Twice	Once	Magnesium level once per week
• Azole antifungal agents	Once	Once		Once	
• Caspofungin				Once	
Antivirals:					
• Ganciclovir	Twice	Once			
• Acyclovir	Once	Once			Magnesium level once per week
• Foscarnet	Once	Twice	Twice	Once	Chemistry profile[d] with calcium and magnesium level once per week
• Cidofovir	Once	Once	Once		Urinalysis and chemistry profile[d] once per week

[a]Should include a differential count of leukocytes and platelet count.

[b]Renal function tests may include serum creatinine and blood urea nitrogen levels and urinalysis. Trough levels appear to be the earliest indication of aminoglycoside toxicity.

[c]Weekly liver enzyme tests with oxacillin, nafcillin, and carbapenems.

[d]A chemistry profile should include liver enzyme levels as well as electrolyte levels.

Note: Frequencies are minimal criteria for patients with normal or stable renal function. Different criteria may apply for children.

TYPES OF INTRAVENOUS ACCESS USED FOR OUTPATIENT PARENTERAL ANTIMICROBIAL THERAPY

There are three basic types of IV access used for OPAT:

- Peripherally inserted central catheter (PICC) lines
  A PICC line should be considered for any treatment course lasting >2 weeks
- Midline catheters
- Peripheral lines

Risk of Outpatient Parenteral Antimicrobial Therapy

The administration of intravenous antimicrobial therapy is potentially hazardous. These are:

- Misdiagnosis and inappropriate treatment
- Inappropriate OPAT therapy when oral would be effective
- Inappropriate duration of therapy
- Inappropriate place of care
- Increased antimicrobial resistance

Advantages of Outpatient Parenteral Antimicrobial Therapy

- Prevents social/psychological problems
- Allows choices of therapy to suit individual needs
- Preferred by patients
- Allows for earlier discharge or prevent hospitalization
- Eases pressure on hospital beds
- Improved efficiency of resource use
- Reduces hospital medical/nursing staff workloads
- Avoids hospital acquired infection
- Allows for effective antibiotic stewardship and auditing of prescribing

ANTIMICROBIAL STEWARDSHIP AND OUTPATIENT PARENTERAL ANTIMICROBIAL THERAPY

- Antimicrobial stewardship is a locally based program to ensure safe, effective, and prudent use of antimicrobials in order to optimize outcome and minimize unintended consequences such as clostridioides difficile-associated disease (CDAD), methicillin-resistant *Staphylococcus aureus* (MRSA) infection, and drug-related toxicity.
- Minimizing unnecessarily prolonged IV therapy,
- Promoting early switching from IV to oral treatment and, whenever possible,
- Simplification of antimicrobials to the narrowest spectrum possible.
- Outpatient parenteral antibiotic therapy should have antibiotic plan and that is reviewed regularly and adapted as circumstances evolve.

OUTPATIENT PARENTERAL ANTIBIOTIC THERAPY IN ASIA

With help of colleagues and their personal networks, Fisher D et al. surveyed healthcare facilities across 17 countries in Asia to ascertain the current means (if any) of providing OPAT. In that survey they also sought to explore the capacity and interest of these facilities in developing systematized OPAT services.

Australia, New Zealand, and Singapore remain the only countries in the Asia Pacific to have implemented such comprehensive OPAT services nationally. The literature identifies Japan as the only other country to undertake OPAT in a healthcare institution in a systematic way.

After exclusions the survey contained responses from 171 different institutions in 17 Asian countries: Bangladesh (4), Brunei (4), Cambodia (3), China (13), Hong Kong (2), India (29), Indonesia (21), Japan (36), Malaysia (9), Mongolia (1), Myanmar (7), Philippines (6), Singapore (9), Sri Lanka (5), Taiwan (5), Thailand (16), and Vietnam (1). Most were university or tertiary referral centers (124) with 62% government funded and the remainder private. Most respondents were doctors (89%) and nurses (8%).

This survey supported the hypothesis that parenteral antibiotics are commonly provided in an outpatient setting, but the delivery is likely to be performed with suboptimal oversight.

The lack of a systematic approach to OPAT in most countries prevents stakeholders from understanding the appropriateness of antibiotic usage. This is contrary to worldwide efforts targeting antibiotic use in the struggle against emerging multiple drug resistance (MDR) organisms. Furthermore, individual patient care risks a lack of oversight, coordination, and outcomes monitoring in such infusion services.

Outpatient parenteral antibiotic therapy has well-documented strength in its potential to address bed shortages and therefore best utilize hospital inpatient resources; in fact this is a feature of publications reporting outcomes. In the only matched-comparison cost analysis of OPAT in Asia, OPAT was found to cost 40% less than inpatient-only care in terms of cost per day, although length of treatment in OPAT was prolonged.

The risk of infection related to home care appears to be much less than the risk of nosocomial infections, and the chances of acquiring an antimicrobial-resistant organism from the home environment are likewise lower.

CONCLUSION

- Outpatient parenteral antibiotic therapy allows patient requiring IV antibiotics to be treated outside hospital.
- Outpatient parenteral antibiotic therapy is suitable for many infections, especially cellulitis, bone and joint infections, and infective endocarditis.
- Antibiotic can be administered in an outpatient unit, at home by nurse, or at home by patient or a carer.
- Patient should be assessed by a doctor and specialist nurse to determine medical and social suitability.
- Evidence suggests that OPAT is safe as long as it is administered through a formal service structure to minimize risk.
- Largely underutilized in Asia including India.

SUGGESTED READINGS

1. Rucher RW, Harrison GM. Outpatient intravenous medications in the management of cystic fibrosis. Pediatrics. 1974;54:358-60.
2. Chapman ALN, Seaton RA, Cooper MA, Hedderwick S, Goodall V, Reed C, et al. Good practice recommendations on out-patient parenteral antimicrobial therapy (OPAT) in adults in the UK: a consensus statement. J Antimicrob Chemother. 2012;67:1053-62.
3. Matthews PC, Conlon CP, Berendt AR, Kayley J, Jefferies L, Atkins BL, et al. Outpatient parenteral antimicrobial therapy (OPAT): is it safe for selected patients to self-administer at home? A retrospective analysis of a large cohort over 13 years. J Antimicrob Chemother. 2008;61:226-7.
4. Chapman ALN, Dixon S, Andrews D, Lillie PJ, Bazaz R, Patchett JD. Clinical efficacy and cost-effectiveness of outpatient parenteral antibiotic therapy (OPAT): a UK perspective. J Antimicrob Chemother. 2009;64(6):1316-24.
5. Török ME, Chapman AL, Lessing MP, Sanderson F, Seaton RA. Outpatient antimicrobial therapy: recent developments and future prospects. Curr Opin Investig Drugs. 2010;11(8):929-39.
6. Poretz DM, Woolard D, Eron LJ, Goldenberg RI, Rising J, Sparks S. Outpatient use of ceftriaxone: a cost-benefit analysis. Am J Med. 1984;77:77-83.
7. Eisenberg JM, Kitz DS. Savings from outpatient antibiotic therapy for osteomyelitis: economic analysis of a therapeutic strategy. JAMA. 1986;255:1584-8.
8. Yong C, Fisher DA, Sklar GE, Li SC. A cost analysis of outpatient parenteral antibiotic therapy (OPAT): an Asian perspective. Int J Antimicrob Agents. 2009;33(1):46-51.
9. Nathwani D. The management of skin and soft tissue infections: Outpatient parenteral antibiotic therapy in the United Kingdom. Chemotherapy. 2001;47(Suppl 1):17-23.
10. Chambers S, Gallagher K, Metcalf S, Pithie A. Home intravenous antimicrobial service—twelve months experience in Christchurch. NZ Med J. 2002;115:216-8.
11. Barr DA, Semple L, Seaton RA. Outpatient parenteral antimicrobial therapy (OPAT) in a teaching hospital-based practice: A retrospective cohort study describing experience and evolution over 10 years. Int J Antimicrob Agents. 2012;39:407-13.
12. Bazaz R, Chapman AL, Winstanley TG. Ertapenem administered as outpatient parenteral antibiotic therapy for urinary tract infections caused by extended-spectrum-beta-lactamase-producing Gram-negative organisms. J Antimicrob Chemother. 2010;65:1510-3.
13. Bernard L, El-Hajj, Pron B, Lotthé A, Gleizes V, Signoret F, et al. Outpatient parenteral antimicrobial therapy (OPAT) for the treatment of osteomyelitis: Evaluation of efficacy, tolerance and cost. J Clin Pharm Ther. 2001;26:445-51.
14. Esposito S, Noviello S, Leone S, Tice A, Seibold G, Nathwani D, et al. Outpatient parenteral antibiotic therapy (OPAT) in different countries: A comparison. Int J Antimicrob Agents. 2004;24:473-8.
15. Fisher DA, Kurup A, Lye D, Tambyah PA, Sulaiman Z, Poon EY, et al. Outpatient parenteral antibiotic therapy in Singapore. Int J Antimicrob Agents. 2006;28:545-50.
16. Gray A, Dryden M, Charos A. Antibiotic management and early discharge from hospital: An economic analysis. J Antimicrob Chemother. 2012;67:2297-302.
17. Kieran J, O'Reilly A, Parker J, Clarke S, Bergin C. Self-administered outpatient parenteral antimicrobial therapy: A report of three years' experience in the Irish healthcare setting. Eur J Clin Microbiol Infect Dis. 2009;28:1369-74.
18. Wai AO, Frighetto L, Marra CA, Chan E, Jewesson PJ. Cost analysis of an adult outpatient parenteral antibiotic therapy (OPAT) programme. A Canadian teaching hospital and Ministry of Health perspective. Pharmacoeconomics. 2000;18:451-7.
19. Theocharis G, Rafailidis PI, Rodis D, Kontopidis I, Barbas SG, Falagas ME. Outpatient parenteral antibiotic therapy (OPAT) at home in Attica, Greece. Eur J Clin Microbiol Infect Dis. 2012;31:2957-61.
20. Ingram PR, Lye DC, Fisher DA, Goh WP, Tam VH. Nephrotoxicity of continuous versus intermittent infusion of vancomycin in outpatient parenteral antimicrobial therapy. Int J Antimicrob Agents. 2009;34:570-4.
21. Fisher D, Michaels J, Hase R, Zhang J, Kataria S, Sim B, et al Outpatient parenteral antibiotic therapy (OPAT) in Asia: missing an opportunity. J Antimicrob Chemother. 2017;72(4):1221-6.
22. DeMaio J. Outpatient parenteral antibiotic therapy. Infect Med. 2004;21(10).
23. Norris AH, Shrestha NK, Allison GM, Keller SC, Bhavan KP, Zurlo JJ, et al. 2018 Infectious Diseases Society of America Clinical Practice Guideline for the management of outpatient parenteral antimicrobial therapy. Clin Infect Dis. 2019;68(1):e1-e35.

155

CHAPTER

Challenging Fungal Lung Infections in Diabetes

P Paranthaman

ABSTRACT

Infections in diabetes occur frequently, spread more widely, and heal less rapidly, due to impaired innate and adaptive immunity. The increased morbidity and mortality in fungal lung infections are attributed to delayed diagnosis coupled with rapidly progressive angioinvasive nature of the pulmonary mucormycosis and invasive aspergillosis which pose great challenges in management of pulmonary fungal infections in diabetes. It is estimated that the prevalence of mucormycosis is 70 times higher in India than the global data. Diabetes is the most common risk factor followed by hematological malignancies and organ transplantation. We had come across more number of cases of invasive aspergillosis and pulmonary mucormycosis during the coronavirus disease 2019 (COVID-19) pandemic due to dysfunctional innate and adaptive immunity coupled with new onset of diabetes following COVID-19 infection, as well as immunosuppression following glucocorticoid use in the treatment of COVID pneumonia. Early diagnosis is primarily with high index of suspicion because most of the time, invasive aspergillosis and pulmonary mucormycosis present with mild symptoms such as cough, breathlessness, chest discomfort, and mild hemoptysis with minimal or no clinical signs which may be missed; hence, with the high index of clinical suspicion and imaging, we can arrive at the reasonably correct diagnosis and start empirical antifungal therapy till we get the confirmation by sample culture due to highly invasive and relentlessly progressive nature of invasive aspergillosis and primary mucormycosis.

INTRODUCTION

Fungal infections in diabetes are more common in poorly controlled diabetes. When glycated hemoglobin (HbA1C) > 12.3%, it impairs the neutrophil function which is the initial defense against fungal invasion. There are several limitations in diagnosis due to nonspecific symptoms and signs in early disease and often diagnosis is missed and we also face a lot of challenges in management of angioinvasive fungi, owing to rapid progression and inadequate penetration of drugs at the site of infection secondary to vascular thrombosis. More than half of pulmonary mucormycosis is diagnosed during autopsy.

RISK FACTORS

- *Host factor*: Impairment of immune response—hyperglycemia impairs neutrophil chemotaxis and adherence to vascular endothelium, resulting in impaired opsonophagocytosis because more nicotinamide adenine dinucleotide phosphate hydrogen (NADPH) is derived from superoxide production in polyol pathway and also intracellular bactericidal activity and cell-mediated immunity are depressed in diabetic patients. Vascular insufficiency results in tissue ischemia and also impairs oxygen-dependent bactericidal function of leukocytes.
- *Organism-specific factors*: *Rhizopus* species have ketone reductase which allows them to thrive in high glucose and acidotic conditions, typically in diabetic ketoacidosis (DKA).

ASPERGILLUS LUNG DISEASE

Aspergillus species is ubiquitous spores in outdoor and indoor; it rarely causes disease in healthy individuals but causes significant disease in patients with diabetes. *Aspergillus fumigatus* is responsible for >90% of human *Aspergillus* infection, but in diabetes, *Aspergillus niger* is more common. Depending on the susceptibility of the host, aspergillosis can cause aspergilloma, allergic bronchopulmonary aspergillosis, invasive pulmonary aspergillosis, and chronic cavitary pulmonary aspergillosis.

Aspergilloma (Fungal Ball)

Aspergilloma usually occurs in preexisting lung cavities without invasion into cavity wall. Majority of patients will be asymptomatic and blood-mixed sputum in 45–85% of cases may be recurrent but rarely life-threatening. It can occasionally present with constitutional symptoms such as fever, weight loss, and fatigue; physical findings may be nonspecific. In the chest radiography, we may see partially filled cavity with crescent air shadow usually seen in upper lobe changes with posture Monod sign **(Fig. 1)**, eosinophilia is common and serum precipitin is positive in 93–100% of cases; its absence makes the diagnosis unlikely.

Treatment

For life-threatening hemoptysis, surgical resection is the treatment of choice; we may have unpredictable results for intracavitary and systemic antifungals. Steroids may be useful when constitutional symptoms are present.

Allergic Bronchopulmonary Aspergillosis

Allergic bronchopulmonary aspergillosis is a hypersensitive lung disease due to *Aspergillus* antigen and it is more common during the winter season when ambient air contains the greatest quantities of *Aspergillus* spores; patients with bronchial asthma and atopic individuals are commonly affected; pathological changes predominantly occur in the proximal airway as ectasia and mucus impaction; but it usually spares distal airways. The histological hallmark of the disease is eosinophil infiltration in the bronchial wall and granulomas. Present usually with cough and expectoration of mucus plugs and episodic wheeze, sputum may be brownish color with abundant mycetoma elements and eosinophils. Sputum culture may be positive in 60–80% cases, screening for total immunoglobulin E (IgE) is useful. Pulmonary function test will show restrictive pattern in 87–100% of cases.

Clinical presentation alone may not be contributory in making diagnosis but useful when coupled with serial X-ray which shows patchy infiltrates (fleeting opacities), which is more common in the upper lobe, and mucoid impaction seen as tram-like and ring shadow and thickened bronchial wall. Bronchography with high-resolution computed tomography (HRCT) can identify central bronchiectasis.

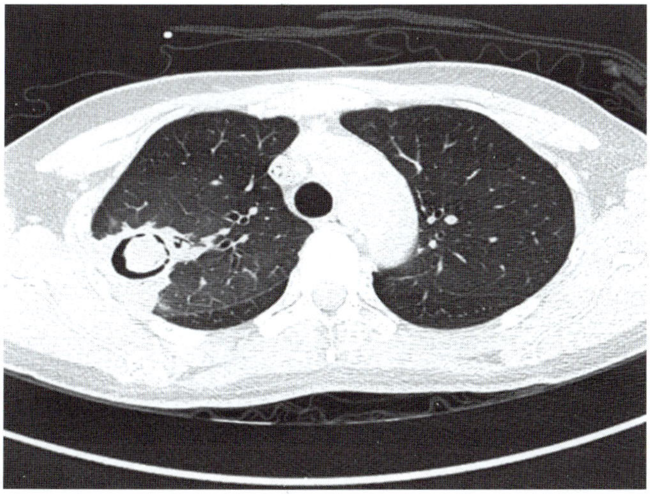

FIG. 1: Monod sign.

Invasive Aspergillosis

Invasive aspergillosis occurs commonly in immune-compromised patients. The major risk factors are diabetes mellitus, high-dose glucocorticoids, and patients with prolonged neutropenia. They usually arise from endogenous commensals with high *Aspergillus* spore count in the winter season. Diabetic patients are more prone to microbial infections particularly fungal infections. Invasive aspergillosis can involve lungs in >90% patients, can present as focal or multifocal-necrotizing bronchopneumonia, and pathological studies reveal that invading *Aspergillus* hyphae growing in pulmonary vessels often results in infarction of lung tissue and aggressive spread is the hallmark of this disease. A significant mortality rate is associated with invasive fungal infection—a form of fatal fungal infection. Aspergillosis may cause lung hemorrhage owing to angioinvasion and extend to heart, kidney, and brain.

Clinical Features

Majority of patients are asymptomatic or it may present with fever, dry cough, atypical chest pain, trivial hemorrhage, shortness of breath, and weight loss. Key to early diagnosis are high index of clinical suspicion and screening for circulating antigens (leukemic patients) in the serum. The classical feature of chronic cavitary pulmonary aspergillosis is the presence of one or more pulmonary cavities expanding over a period of months and years in association with pulmonary symptoms; multiple cavities are more common than single cavity and most cavities occur in the upper lobe. Pleural thickening and pericavitary thickening are typical.

Chronic Cavitary Pulmonary Aspergillosis

Chronic cavitary pulmonary aspergillosis is caused by *Aspergillus fumigatus*, but *Aspergillus niger* is common in diabetic patients. *Aspergillus* IgG antibodies are detected in >90% cases. The most common, life-threatening complication is massive hemoptysis.

Diagnosis

In acute invasive pulmonary aspergillosis, because of the presence heavy load of fungus in affected organs, antigen detection by polymerase chain reaction (PCR), microscopy, and histopathology confirm the diagnosis. Histopathology reveals infarction with invasion of pulmonary vessels by many fungal hyphae or acute necrosis **(Fig. 2)**. Hyphae are narrow and septate, branching at 45° (unlike mucormycosis in which hyphae branch at 90°) **(Fig. 3)** and no yeast forms are present in the infected tissue. The raised galactomannan levels in the sputum are more sensitive than in the serum. Positive antigen test usually precedes radiological and clinical evidence by several days.

Diagnostic Criteria for Invasive Aspergillosis

- Culture positivity—sample taken directly from the sight
- Positive histology specific to *Aspergillus* and molecular confirmation of *Aspergillus* species
- Radiological—presence of halo sign and localized ground-glass opacification (GGO) represent hemorrhagic infarct surrounding nodule or consolidation. Halo sign is present for 7 days early in course of illness in neutropenic patients. Elevated total IgE and *Aspergillus*-specific IgE are seen in chronic aspergillosis.

Treatment

Effective treatment includes modifying underlying immunocompromised state of the host—empirical antifungal drug even before the culture report to arrest the progression of angioinvasion of invasive aspergillosis.

Antifungal drugs that are effective against aspergillosis are voriconazole, itraconazole, posaconazole, isavuconazole, caspofungin, micafungin, and amphotericin B.

Intravenous Preparations in Invasive Aspergillosis

Voriconazole, isavuconazole, posaconazole, and amphotericin B are not active against *Aspergillus nidulans* and terreus. *Aspergillus niger* is resistant to itraconazole and isavuconazole.

Duration of therapy in invasive aspergillosis varies from 3 months to several years. Voriconazole is currently preferred drug for chronic aspergillosis because chronic pulmonary aspergillosis responds slowly, so therapy is given for more than 6 months. Glucocorticoids should be used in chronic cavitary pulmonary aspergillosis only if covered with adequate antifungal therapy.

Acute exacerbation of aspergillosis will respond to voriconazole, itraconazole, and short course of steroids. Antifungal response to *Aspergillus* is gratifying, but relapse after 4 months of therapy is common. Surgical treatment of chronic pulmonary aspergillosis poses a lot of challenges; hence, bronchial artery embolization is preferred.

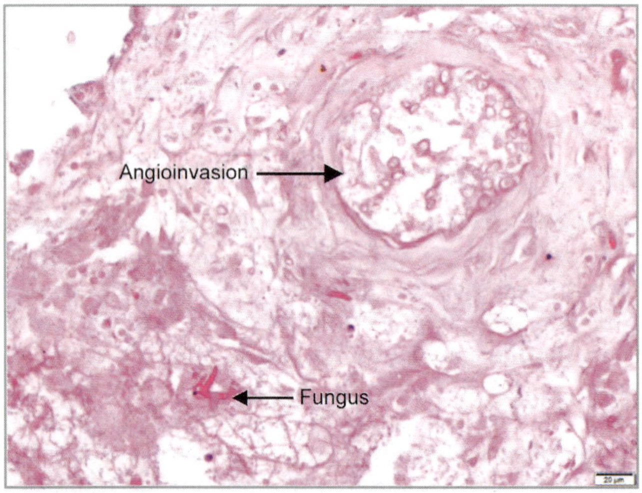

FIG. 2: Angioinvasion by aspergillosis.

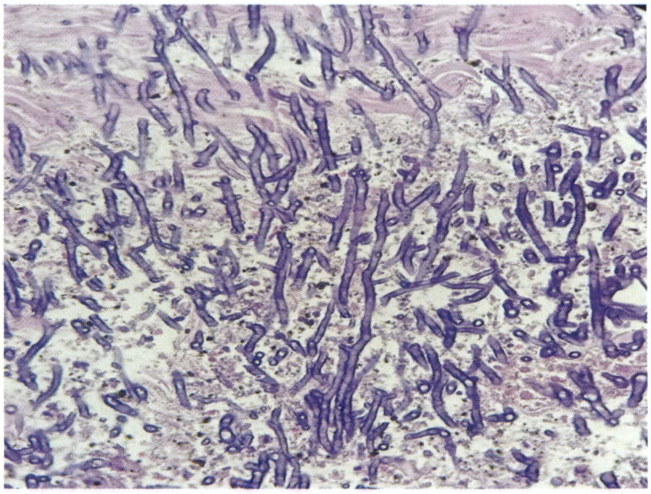

FIG. 3: Aspergillosis.

MUCORMYCOSIS

Mucorales are ubiquitous environmental fungi to which humans are constantly exposed. They are particularly common in uncontrolled diabetes mellitus and neutropenic patients due to defective phagocytosis. DKA and other conditions which cause acidosis result in dissociation of iron for sequestering protein; the elevated levels of free iron support fungal growth in serum and tissues. Mucormycosis is highly invasive and relentlessly progressive and mortality depends on underlying predisposing conditions. Mucormycosis has also emerged as important superinfection in COVID-19 patients; but even before COVID-19, India was hyperendemic for mucormycosis. Increase in the number of cases of mucormycosis during the COVID-19 pandemic has been likely attributed to combination of prevalence and new onset of diabetes and also increased use of corticosteroids in treatment of COVID pneumonia.

Clinical Manifestations

Mucormycosis presents as one of the five well-defined clinical syndromes:

1. Rhino-orbito-cerebral mucormycosis
2. Pulmonary mucormycosis
3. Cutaneous mucormycosis
4. Gastrointestinal mucormycosis
5. Disseminated mucormycosis

Patients with diabetes or DKA typically develop rhino-orbito-cerebral form but rarely develop pulmonary mucormycosis. However, pulmonary mucormycosis occurs more commonly in patients with leukemia on chemotherapy and in patients undergoing hematopoietic stem cell transplantation.

Pulmonary Mucormycosis

Pulmonary mucormycosis is the second most common manifestation of mucormycosis. Symptoms may be dyspnea, cough, chest pain, and fever (not invariably present). Angioinvasion results in necrosis, cavitation, and/or hemoptysis; chest X-ray shows wedge-shaped infarction, nodules, cavities, and masses of lobar consolidation. HRCT chest is sensitive in detecting pulmonary changes earlier than chest X-ray.

- Presence of >10 nodules
- Pleural effusion
- Concomitant sinusitis makes diagnosis of mucor mycosis more likely.

Voriconazole is the first-line drug in the management of aspergillosis, which may exacerbate mucormycosis; hence, if we have doubt that the infection is aspergillosis or mucormycosis, treatment with itraconazole/posaconazole is a reasonable option.

Diagnosis

Despite high index of suspicion in making early diagnosis, unfortunately, half of cases of mucormycosis are diagnosed only at postmortem.

- Culture positive from sterile site (tissue biopsy, needle aspirate, or pleural fluid)
- Histopathological evidence of invasive mucormycosis

Probable Diagnosis

- Positive culture from nonsterile samples
- Sputum or bronchoalveolar lavage
- Detecting Mucorales in histopathological samples
- Patients with appropriate risk factors with clinical and radiological evidence of the disease

In such cases, empirical antifungal therapy may be started till you get the confirmed diagnosis. Biopsy with histopathological examination remains the most sensitive and specific modality for definitive diagnosis. Biopsy reveals characteristic wide, thick-walled, ribbon-like aseptate hyphal elements that branch at 90° **(Fig. 4)**. Mucorales are most effectively visualized with periodic acid–Schiff (PAS) staining.

Polymer chain reaction of Mucorales are useful in diagnosis of mucormycosis.

Culture is positive only in 50% cases.

Treatment

General principles:

- Early initiation of therapy
- Surgical debridement when possible
- Rapid reversal of underlying predisposing risk factor
- Proceeding to treat underlying malignancy

Because disease presents subtly at first, therapy must be started empirically before definitive diagnosis is established.

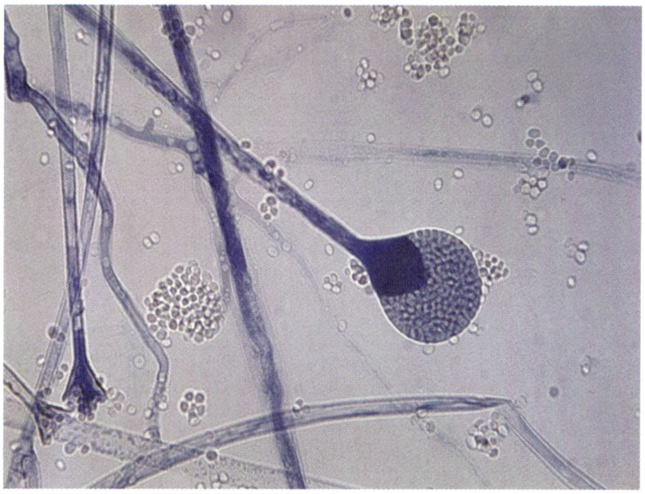

FIG. 4: Mucormycosis with aseptate hyphae.

Blood vessel thrombosis resulting in tissue necrosis in mucormycosis can result in poor penetration of antifungal agents to the site of infection. Debridement of all necrotic tissue can help to eradicate the infection.

Rapidly reversing hyperglycemia, avoidance of iron overload, and withholding corticosteroids are important to improve recovery.

Eradicate mucormycosis before underlying malignancy is treated.

Antifungal Therapy

- Lipid formulation of amphotericin B is less nephrotoxic than amphotericin B deoxycholate.
- Liposomal amphotericin B is preferred over lipid formulation for brain infection. Liposomal amphotericin B is less nephrotoxic.
  - Amphotericin B deoxycholate—1 mg/kg/day
  - Liposomal amphotericin B—5 mg /kg/day
- Multiple studies revealed combination of LAmB and echinocandins (capsofungin, micafungin, and anidulafungin) improves survival rate.
- Deferasirox is contraindicated in patients with active malignancy.
- Posaconazole and isavuconazole are Food and Drug Administration (FDA) approved for mucormycosis.
- Usually, amphotericin B is the first-line therapy followed by oral stepdown therapy with isavuconazole and posaconazole.
- In resistant cases, amphotericin B and echinocandins and posaconazole are rationale of choice.

Adjuvant Therapy

- Hyperbaric oxygen therapy
- Sodium bicarbonate in DKA

In general, antifungal therapy for mucormycosis should be continued until resolution of signs and symptoms.

After several weeks of daily therapy, substitute to thrice a week and twice week.

Stepdown in azoles for chronic supportive therapy is continued.

SUGGESTED READINGS

1. Prakash H, Chakrabarti A. Epidemiology of Mucormycosis in India. Microorganisms. 2021;9(3):523.
2. Pickup JC, Crook MA. Is type II diabetes mellitus a disease of the innate immune system? Diabetologia. 1998;41(10):1241-8.
3. Gong Y, Li C, Wang C, Li J, Ding M, Chen D, et al. Epidemiology and Mortality-Associated Factors of Invasive Fungal Disease in Elderly Patients: A 20-Year Retrospective Study from Southern China. Infect Drug Resist. 2020;13:711-723.
4. Lewis RE, Chamilos G, Prince RA, Kontoyiannis DP. Pretreatment with empty liposomes attenuates the immunopathology of invasive pulmonary aspergillosis in corticosteroid-immunosuppressed mice. Antimicrob Agents Chemother. 2007;51(3): 1078-81.

156

CHAPTER

Rabies Prevention: What is New?

Uttam Kr Nath, Manab Narayan Baruah

ABSTRACT

Rabies is endemic in both humans and animals in most countries in Asia, which causes acute encephalomyelitis. As no treatment has emerged in curing this 100% fatal disease, the postexposure prophylaxis (PEP) is the key to prevent and should be started immediately after reporting to health facility irrespective of time lapse from exposure. An important aspect of PEP is rabies vaccination, but traditionally it consists of long and costly regimens of intramuscular (IM) injections. Most human deaths from rabies are caused by delayed access to the healthcare, unaffordability, or ineffective delivery of PEP. To reduce these barriers, in 2022, the World Health Organization (WHO) published new guidance for PEP with a shortened 1-week intradermal (ID) regimen which is as efficacious as other established regimens. The WHO/Drugs Controller General of India (DCGI) approved the Updated Thai Red Cross regimen for ID PEP in India. This ideal ID route offers economic benefits, safety, and efficacy and reduces the cost of vaccination by about 68%, which is surely an acceptable option for resource-poor countries such as India. Monoclonal antibodies (mAbs) could be better option in PEP in terms of supply, cost, and efficacy rather than equine or human rabies immunoglobulin in the near future.

INTRODUCTION

Rabies is a zoonotic disease caused by ribonucleic acid (RNA) Lyssavirus, belonging to members of the Rhabdoviridae family. It causes acute encephalomyelitis in almost all the warm-blooded animals including man. The causative agent is found in domestic and wild animals and is transmitted to humans and other animals by close contacts with their saliva through bites, scratches, licks on broken skin, and mucous membranes. Dogs are the principal reservoirs of rabies in most of the developing countries as 99% of human rabies is from dog bite. An estimated 59,000 human deaths per year are due to rabies mainly in continents such as Asia (59.6%) and Africa (36.4%) and around 40% of the victims are children below 15 years of age. The World Health Organization (WHO) estimated that one death every 15 minutes is due to rabies and 4 out of 10 deaths are in children. In India, rabies is an endemic disease with a yearly burden of 6–7 million animal bites with 20,000 deaths and 36% of global rabies mortality, with majority of the patients being children and adult males. The WHO, the Food and Agriculture Organization of the United Nations, the World Organization for Animal Health, and the Global Alliance for Rabies Control in 2018 set the global target of achieving zero human deaths from dog-transmitted rabies by 2030 ('zero by 30'). As rabies is 100% fatal, its prevention, both in humans and dogs is the key to reaching this goal.

ANIMALS THAT TRANSMIT RABIES IN INDIA

- *Domestic animals*: Dogs and cats
- *Peridomestic animals*: Cows, buffaloes, sheep, goats, pigs, donkeys, horses, camels, etc.
- *Wild animals*: Foxes and jackals, mongoose, leopards, bears, monkeys, etc.
- *Not reported*: Birds, squirrels, bats, and rodents

In India, dogs are responsible for about 95% of human rabies followed by cats (2%). Jackals, mongoose, and others account for only ~1% of cases.

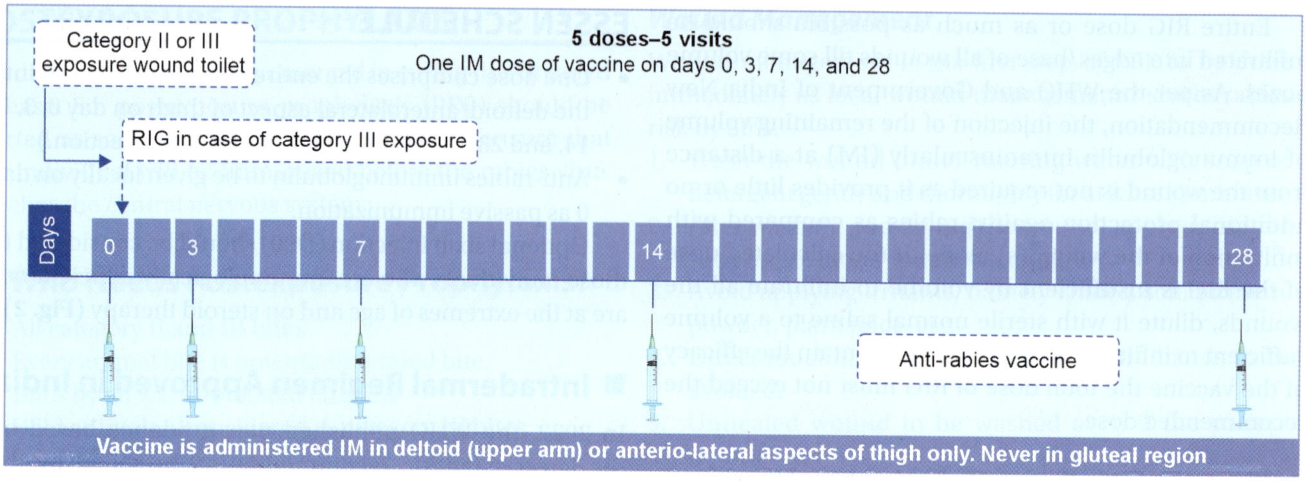

FIG. 2: Five-dose intramuscular regimen: 1-1-1-1-1.
(IM: intramuscular; RIG: rabies immunoglobulin)

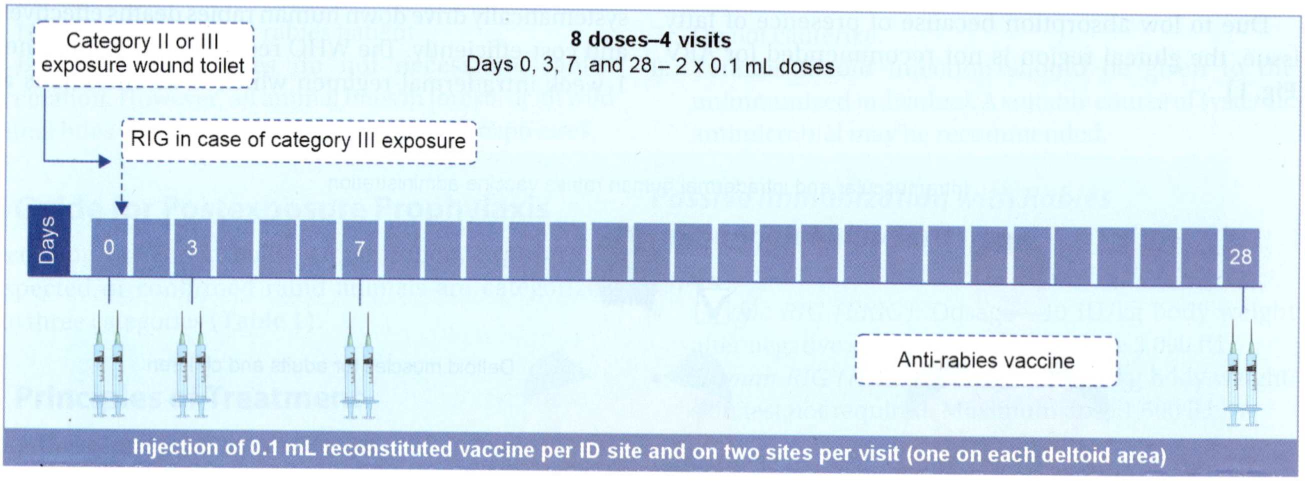

FIG. 3: Updated Thai Red Cross regimen.
(ID: intradermal; RIG: rabies immunoglobulin)

other established regimens. ID vaccination saves up to 85% of the available vaccine, thereby preventing shortages due to supply issues or financial constraints in the healthcare system. The WHO/DCGI approved the ID Updated Thai Red Cross (UTRC) regimen in the National Rabies Control Program for PEP **(Fig. 3)**.

Updated Thai Red Cross 2 Site Regimen

Dose: 0.1 mL (two doses per visit)

Site: Upper arm over each deltoid/anterolateral aspect of thigh

Schedule: 2-2-2-0-2

- *Day 0*: Two sites
- *Day 3*: Two sites
- *Day 7*: Two sites
- *Day 14*: No dose
- *Day 28*: Two sites

Vaccines Approved for Updated Thai Red Cross Schedule

- Purified Vero cell rabies vaccine (PVRV)
- Purified chick embryo cell rabies vaccine (PCECV)

POINTS TO BE REMEMBERED DURING POSTEXPOSURE PROPHYLAXIS

- Intradermal rabies vaccination (IDRV) when given should raise a visible and palpable "bleb" in the skin.
- If ID dose is inadvertently given subcutaneously or IM, a new dose should be given at a nearby site.
- Animal bite victims who are on chloroquine therapy and immune-suppressed persons, ARV should be given by IM route.
- While using ID route, complete course of vaccination should be given irrespective of the status of the animal.

- Reconstituted vaccine to be used immediately, preferably within 6 hours of reconstitution in unforeseen delay with proper storage at 2–8° C.
- For all age groups and sexes, including pregnancy and infancy dose remains same.
- Switching the route of administration from IM to ID or vice versa and switch over from one type of rabies vaccine to the other is not recommended.
- In case of IM regimen if the animal is alive and healthy till 10 days after bite, the PEP may be discontinued after 10 days or PEP can be converted to pre-exposure prophylaxis (PrEP) by skipping the vaccine dose on day 14, with administering the dose of day 28. However, this provision is applicable for dogs or cats only.

POSTEXPOSURE PROPHYLAXIS IN PREVIOUSLY VACCINATED INDIVIDUALS

- *Upon exposure/re-exposure with documented vaccination*:
  - Wound toileting
  - No RIG
- *If full course of PEP/PrEP taken within last 3 months*: No ARV required
- *If >3 months*: Give ID/IM 0 and 3
- *Incomplete/undocumented vaccination*: Treat as a fresh unvaccinated

PRE-EXPOSURE PROPHYLAXIS

Pre-exposure vaccination facilitates PEP by eliminating the need for RIG and may provide protection following an unrecognized exposure.

Who Needs Pre-exposure Prophylaxis?

High-risk groups as follows:

- Laboratory staff handling virus and infected material
- Veterinarians, animal handlers, and dog catchers
- Wildlife wardens and quarantine officers
- Clinicians and paramedicals attending to hydrophobia cases
- Travelers from rabies-free areas to rabies endemic areas

Doses

Three-dose series IM (entire vial × one site) or intradermal regimen (0.1 mL × two sites) at day 0, 7, and either day 21 or 28. Persons at high risk of exposure should be monitored by measuring serum antibody level every 6 months and a booster dose will be required if the level drops below 0.5 IU/mL.

Newer Advances in Postexposure Prophylaxis: Monoclonal Antibodies

Monoclonal antibodies which neutralize the rabies virus could be better option in PEP than ERIG or HRIG in terms of supply, cost, and efficacy. The WHO (2018) recommends that if available, the use of monoclonal antibodies (mAbs) instead of RIG to be encouraged. Currently, two human rabies mAb (single mAb—Rabishield™ and Cocktail of RmAbs (Docaravimab and Miromavimab-Twinrab™) are recommended in India. Further multicentric studies in Indian setting are required prior to incorporation in National Guidelines.

SUGGESTED READINGS

1. Bote K, Nadal D, Abela B. WHO's Latest Rabies Recommendations And Guidance Save Lives And Reduce The Cost Of Treatment. One Health Implement Res. 2023;3:11-5.
2. Ministry of Health and Family Welfare Government of India. (2022). Rabies: General Aspects & Laboratory Diagnostic Techniques 2022. [online] Available from https://ncdc.mohfw.gov.in/WriteReadData/linkimages/RabiesGeneralAspectsLaboratoryDiagnosticTechniques2022.pdf [Last accessed January, 2024].
3. Epidemic Branch Commissionerate of Health, Medical Services And Medical Education, Gandhinagar. National Rabies Control Program: Management of Animal Bites. Guidelines for use of Intra-dermal inoculation of Tissue Culture Vaccines. [online] Available from https://gujhealth.gujarat.gov.in/images/pdf/rabies-control-guideline.pdf [Last accessed January, 2024].
4. National Rabies Control Programme. Guideline For Animal Bite Management & Frequently Asked Questions. Government of West Bengal: PH & CD Branch Directorate Of Health Services; 2021.
5. Fan L, Zhang L, Li J, Zhu F. Advances in the progress of monoclonal antibodies for rabies. Hum Vaccin Immunother. 2022;18(1):2026713.

157

CHAPTER

Pitfalls in the Diagnosis and Management of Central Nervous System Tuberculosis

Jalees Fatima, Aaliya Jabbar

ABSTRACT

Central nervous system (CNS) tuberculosis (TB) is among the least common yet most devastating forms of human mycobacterial infection. The incidence and prevalence of the CNS–TB are unknown but roughly account for 1–10% of all TB cases. CNS–TB conceptually comprises three clinical manifestations and stages. The neurological manifestations of tuberculous meningitis (TBM) are numerous and varied. The diagnosis remains a challenge due to inconsistent clinical presentation. The chapter highlights pitfalls in neurological burden of CNS–TB with various molecular-based methods, including immunoassays and polymerase chain reaction (PCR)-based assays emerged as alternative diagnostic tools due to their sensitivity, and specificity and also throws light upon challenges in its management.

INTRODUCTION

Central nervous system (CNS) tuberculosis (TB) is one of the most severe forms of TB, as its exact incidence and prevalence rates are unknown.

However, its incidence is expected to be relatively high, especially in children, human immunodeficiency viruses-(HIV) infected individuals, and people living in countries with a high burden of pulmonary TB like India.

Central nervous system TB can be broadly grouped into:

- Subacute or chronic meningitis
- Intracranial TB
- Spinal tuberculous arachnoiditis

All the three forms mentioned above occur with equal frequencies in endemic regions like India. CNS–TB occurs in 1–2% of all patients with active TB and accounts for about 8% of all extrapulmonary TB in immunocompetent individuals. Tuberculous meningitis (TBM) is the most devastating of all CNS-TB cases. The case fatality rate of TBM is 15–40% despite effective therapy. Uncertainty and doubt dominate all aspects of TBM. The variable natural history and accompanying clinical features of TBM hinder the diagnosis and the lack of accurate diagnostic tests poses difficulties in treatment **(Box 1)**.

BOX 1: Clinical syndromes of central nervous system (CNS) tuberculosis (TB).

- Tuberculous meningitis (TBM)
- Optochiasmatic arachnoiditis cerebral infarcts due to TBM hydrocephalus
- Tuberculoma/tubercular abscess
- Tuberculosis of the spine (Pott's spine)
- Human immunodeficiency virus (HIV)

In this chapter, we will focus on the challenges and pitfalls faced in the diagnosis and treatment of TBM.

ETIOPATHOGENESIS

Bacillemia (*Mycobacterium tuberculosis*) due to hematogenous spread from the lung (primary site of infection), reactivation, or other organ results in seeding of the brain and meninges is the most common mechanism of infection.

These granulomatous foci in the meninges (tubercles) may caseate (Rich focus) and rupture into the subarachnoid space causing meningitis, or they remain dormant depending on host immunity and other local factors.

Rupture of rich focus leads to release of bacilli into the subarachnoid space, dense gelatinous exudates develop at the base of the brain, which is most florid in the interpeduncular fossa encasing optic chiasma and extend throughout the prepontine cistern up to and around the spinal cord. Three general processes produce the subsequent neurological pathology, i.e., *obliterative vasculitis, adhesion formation, and encephalitis or myelitis*. A characteristic inflammation affects the blood vessels which traverse the exudates. Small- and medium-sized arteries are most frequently involved. The adventitial layer of vessels develops caseation necrosis and tubercles, occluding blood vessels and causing infraction. These are most commonly seen in the distribution of middle cerebral and lateral striate arteries. Infarction through vasculitis accounts for an appreciable part of irreversible neurological sequelae. The adhesion formation of the basal subarachnoid cistern characterized by granulomatous inflammatory exudate can result in obstruction of cerebrospinal fluid (CSF) and lead to hydrocephalus, which can be communicating type or obstructive, depending on the site of the blockage. Adhesions around the interpeduncular fossa can compromise cranial nerves, most commonly involving II, III, IV, and VI.

CLINICAL FEATURES

The disease course runs in three phases:

1. Prodromal phase
2. Meningitis phase
3. Paralytic phase

The usual clinical picture consists of a prodrome of insidious onset of fever, malaise, and headache, followed by prominent neurologic findings, including cranial nerve palsies and long tract signs. Continuous low-grade fever is typically present in about 20–70% of patients. Cranial nerve palsies occur in 20–30% of patients. The sixth cranial nerve is most frequently and commonly affected. Vision loss is due to multiple processes like papilledema due to increased intracranial pressure, optochiasmatic arachnoiditis, third ventricular dilation causing compression of optic chiasma (in hydrocephalus), optic nerve granuloma, or drug-induced (ethambutol) toxicity. Hemiplegia or quadriplegia can occur secondary to infarction or tuberculoma. At times, abnormal movements may dominate the clinical picture in the form of chorea or hemiballismus, athetosis, myoclonic jerks, or ataxia. Seizures, focal or generalized, may occur during acute illness or months after treatment in 10–15% of patients. Examination reveals evidence of meningeal signs in 35–90% of patients in addition to cranial nerve palsies and other focal deficits. Fundoscopy may reveal optic atrophy, papilledema, retinal nerve fiber layer and choroid tubercles in about 10% of patients with TBM. A staging system was introduced in 1947, which has since been widely adopted in the initial assessments of such patients and can be used to estimate prognosis **(Table 1)**.

TABLE 1: Clinical staging of tuberculous meningitis (TBM).

Stage I (early)	• Nonspecific symptoms and signs • No clouding of consciousness • No neurologic deficits
Stage II (intermediate)	• Lethargy or behavioral changes • Meningeal irritation • Minor neurologic deficits, such as cranial nerves
Stage III (late)	• Stupor or coma • Abnormal movements • Seizures severe neurologic deficits, such as paresis

DIAGNOSIS AND ITS PITFALLS

Inconsistent Clinical Presentation

Diagnosis of TBM is difficult for clinicians as it can clinically present similarly to other forms of meningitis. The difficulty in diagnosis often leads to a delay in treatment and subsequent mortality. Classically, TBM presents as a subacute meningitic illness. However, the classical symptoms of subacute meningitis are absent in many cases. The difficulty in diagnosing TBM by clinical assessment alone leads to a delay in early diagnosis and treatment initiation. Symptoms are diverse and inconsistent. In adults, the most predictive symptom of TBM is a duration of illness >5 days.

Pitfalls in the Laboratory Diagnosis of TBM

Cerebrospinal fluid: The traditional way of cytochemical analysis of CSF to differentiate between various forms of meningitis has a low sensitivity and specificity. There is always an element of doubt with the CSF report. Pitfalls lie in the observer-dependent assessment of the type of cells (lymphocyte versus neutrophil) and amount of proteins. Total CSF leukocyte count in TBM can vary from 5 to 1,000 10^3/mL with a predominance of lymphocytes (30–90%) compared to neutrophils (10–70%). Neutrophils can predominate early in the disease process, and their presence is associated with improved survival. Protein is usually elevated but can range from 45 to 360 mg/dL. The above parameters are nonspecific and there is a considerable overlap with other types of meningitis viral and septic meningitis.

Microscopy: Direct microscopy of acid-fast bacilli (AFB) smears is quick and relatively inexpensive. CSF is stained for AFB with the use of the Ziehl-Neelsen staining technique. However, traditional visualization of CSF to evaluate AFB by microscopy has been demonstrated to have a poor sensitivity of 10–20%. This limitation is likely due to the small number of bacilli in CSF, as TBM is a paucibacillary infection. Because of the low sensitivity of microscopy, further diagnostic tests are usually needed.

Mycobacterial diagnosis: Lack of sensitivity of the gold standard test.

The definitive diagnosis of TBM is made by isolation of *M. tuberculosis* from the CSF, by direct staining, or by culture. However, Ziehl–Neelsen smear sensitivity can vary between 10 and 60% and culture positivity rates are between 25 and 75%, but results are only available after 2–6 weeks of incubation.

Increasing the CSF sample volume (minimum 6 mL) and duration of slide examination increases the sensitivity of smear microscopy (to 60%).

Newer Methods of Diagnosis

Many newer tests have been developed for the early diagnosis of TBM, such as polymerase chain reaction (PCR), interferon-gamma release assays (IGRAs), and tuberculostearic acid and adenosine deaminase (ADA) in CSF.

CSF GeneXpert MTB/RIF (Cartridge-based Nucleic Acid Amplification Test)

Xpert MTB/RIF is a cartridge-based fully automated PCR test that has allowed for rapid (within 2 hours) TB diagnostics in resource-limited settings and the detection of rifampin resistance. A 2014 World Health Organization (WHO) review of 18 Xpert MTB/RIF studies for the diagnosis of extrapulmonary TB found a pooled sensitivity of 80.5% [95% confidence interval (CI), 59.0–92.2%] compared to traditional culture and 62.8% (95% CI 47.7–75.8%) against a combined reference standard (CRS). For TBM specifically, Xpert MTB/RIF had a sensitivity of 80.5% (95% CI 59.0–92.2%) and specificity of 97.8% (95% CI 95.2–99.0%).

Based on these results, the WHO at that time recommended the use of Xpert MTB/RIF as the preferred initial test for the diagnosis of TBM. A new version of the Xpert MTB/RIF test called Xpert MTB/RIF Ultra (Xpert Ultra) has been recently developed to improve sensitivity for *M. tuberculosis* detection and to improve rifampin resistance detection. However, these tests have not been assessed completely and are not available in the developing world where most cases of the disease are seen. Xpert Ultra had a higher sensitivity than Xpert MTB/RIF, but the specificity of Xpert Ultra was lower than Xpert MTB/RIF compared to culture results. These results led to the updated current WHO recommendation that Xpert Ultra be used as first-line for the diagnosis of TBM **(Table 2)**.

TABLE 2: Limits of detection of diagnostic tests for tuberculous meningitis (TBM).

Diagnostic test	Limit of detection (CFU/mL)	Sensitivity (%)	Specificity (%)
GeneXpert	116	71	98
Xpert Ultra	15.6	90	90
Culture	1–10	50–70	*

*Gold standard

Adenosine Deaminase

Adenosine deaminase is an enzyme that is found primarily in T-lymphocytes. A recent review and meta-analysis including data from 20 studies found the pooled sensitivity of CSF ADA measurement for the diagnosis of TBM to be 89% with a specificity of 91%. Given the high sensitivities and specificities, ADA CSF testing may be a reasonable test in the evaluation of TBM. However, past studies have noted a high number of false positives in patients with HIV.

CSF Interferon-gamma Release Assays

Typically, IGRAs are used in the diagnosis of latent TB. However, recently CSF testing via IGRA has been studied in the evaluation of TBM. These tests generally require high volumes of CSF, around 5–10 mL. The sensitivity of CSF IGRA is 50–70% with a specificity of 70–90%, making these tests good for ruling in the diagnosis of TBM but not adequate for ruling out TBM.

The role of IGRA is still not clear in the diagnosis of TBM.

Lipoarabinomannan Testing

Patients with advanced HIV/AIDS (acquired immunodeficiency syndrome) may be evaluated with the use of lipoarabinomannan (LAM) testing. LAM is a glycolipid-forming component of the *M. tuberculosis* cell wall and can be found in multiple body fluids of patients with TB especially in urine as it is filtered by kidney resulting in LAM-antigenuria, including CSF. Investigators have found higher sensitivities and specificities in HIV patients.

IMAGING FINDINGS

Brain computed tomography (CT) findings of patients with TBM may exhibit basal meningeal enhancement, infarcts, hydrocephalus, and tuberculomas. These features are highly suggestive of TBM in adults. Magnetic resonance imaging (MRI) can better define the neuroradiological features of TBM, particularly when evaluating brainstem disease. It is characterized by focal or diffuse dural thickening and fluid-attenuated inversion recovery (FLAIR) sequence is specially useful for visualization of thickened dura. Granulomas can be differentiated with the use of MRI. For example, noncaseating granulomas appear hypointense on T1 and hyperintense on T2. In contrast, caseating granulomas appear hypointense or isointense on T1 and isointense with rim-enhancement on T2. Tuberculous abscesses tend to be much larger, faster growing than tuberculomas (usually >3 cm in diameter), solitary, thin-walled, and often multi-loculated. MRI is the modality of choice for evaluating TBM-related vascular disease.

Single photon emission computed tomography (SPECT) can be useful to evaluate vasculitis due to TBM. Patients with TBM can have increased uptake in focal brain lesions, specifically in the meninges and cerebellum on FDG PET (fluorodeoxyglucose positron emission tomography). On the contrary to one study from India found that FDG PET did not detect granulomas which were visible on brain MRI.

Given the fatal consequences of delayed treatment, clinicians frequently initiate empirical therapy in the setting of compatible clinical, epidemiological, and laboratory findings.

CLINICAL SCORING SCALES

Several scales can be used to grade the severity of TBM. The modified British Medical Research Council (BMRC), the Lancet consensus scoring system, the Thwaites diagnostic scoring index, and the Marais diagnostic scoring system with the Thwaites criteria were found to have a sensitivity of 86% and specificity of 79%, and Lancet consensus scoring system from 2010 was based on 20 clinical parameters including clinical features, CSF findings, imaging findings, and evidence of TB elsewhere. With a maximum score of 20. Classifications in this system include definite TBM, probable TBM, possible TBM, and not TBM.

BOX 2: Estimated ratio of cerebrospinal fluid (CSF): Plasma concentration of first-line and second-line drugs.

First-line drugs:
- *Rifampicin*: 20–30%; essential drug despite poor penetration, higher doses may be required
- *Isoniazid*: 80–90%; essential drug good CSF penetration throughout treatment
- *Pyrazinamide*: 90–100%; excellent CSF penetration throughout treatment
- *Ethambutol*: 20–30%; poor CSF penetration once meningeal inflammation is resolved

Second-line drugs:
- Streptomycin, kanamycin, amikacin—10–20%; poor CSF penetration once meningeal inflammation is resolved
- *Moxifloxacin, levofloxacin*: 70–80%; good CSF penetration
- *PAS*: No data
- *Ethionamide, prothionamide, cycloserine*: 80–90%; good CSF penetration

PITFALLS IN MANAGEMENT

- Difficult to diagnose correctly due to atypical presentations
- Limited number of drugs having good CSF penetration **(Box 2)**
- High prevalence of hepatotoxicity as patients are often having disseminated TB and multiple organs may be involved at the same time.
- Lack of clear guidelines on duration of treatment especially those cases who develop toxic hepatitis and remain on modified antituberculosis therapy (ATT) for a substantial time.
- Difficult to diagnose drug resistance in cases presenting only with tuberculoma without meningitis
- Patients often are quite debilitated and are having poor tolerance to therapy and a big subset is left with substantial neurological sequelae.

SUGGESTED READINGS

1. Gupta M, Munakomi S. CNS Tuberculosis. In: StatPearls [Internet]. Treasure Island (FL): StatPearls Publishing; 2023. Gupta M, Munakomi S. CNS Tuberculosis. In: StatPearls [Internet]. Treasure Island (FL): StatPearls Publishing; 2023.
2. Thwaites G, Chau TT, Mai NT, Drobniewski F, McAdam K, Farrar J. Neurological aspects of tropical disease: Tuberculous meningitis. J Neurol Neurosurg Psychiatry. 2000;68(3):289-99
3. Manyelo CM, Solomons RS, Walzl G, Chegou NN. Tuberculous meningitis: Pathogenesis, immune responses, diagnostic challenges, and the potential of biomarker-based approaches. J Clin Microbiol. 2021;59(3):e01771-20.
4. Shah H, Joshi A, Dobish E, Thomas AK. Lessons learned from a fatal case of tuberculous meningitis with a rapid decline in an infant. J Clin Imaging Sci. 2022;12:1.
5. Litjens CHC, Aarnoutse RE, Te Brake LHM. Preclinical models to optimize treatment of tuberculous meningitis—A systematic review. Tuberculosis (Edinb). 2020;122(101924):101924.

158
CHAPTER

Injectable Antiretrovirals: Game Changer Shots

Murugesh Pastapur

ABSTRACT

Treatment of HIV/AIDS (human immunodeficiency virus/acquired immunodeficiency syndrome) is simplified by once-a-day antiretroviral (ART) combination pill in most of the cases. In view of multidrug resistance, pill stigma, toxicity and adherence, we need more new ART in novel formulation, route and mode of administration. Many such investigational ARTs are in pipeline. Instead of daily pills, the infectious disease (ID) consultant prescribing six intramuscular (IM) injections in a year may revolutionize the HIV treatment. Prescribing long-acting antiretroviral therapy (LA-ART)—two injections of ART in a year is not too far in the armamentarium of HIV treatment. Basically these new methods should be noninferior in effectiveness compared to current ART and also match the safety. Already few LA-ART are approved by US FDA (US Food and Drug Administration), EMA (European Medicines Agency), and Health Canada.

INTRODUCTION (TABLE 1)

Enfuvirtide: First injectable antiretroviral (ART) search started at Duke University in 1996, it was called T-20. It was approved by US Food and Drug Administration (US FDA) on March 2003, as a new class of *human immunodeficiency virus (HIV) fusion inhibitor*. Enfuvirtide (Fuzeon) is indicated in treatment of HIV-1 in combination of other ART. It needs to be given daily twice subcutaneously (90 mg bd SC). It has local injection site reactions in almost 100% of patients. It costs around $3,785 per month (60 vials). Landmark studies which showed effectives of T-20 are TORO 1 and 2.

Ibalizumab (IBA)—uiyk: IBA is a humanized monoclonal immunoglobulin G (IgG) antibody which is classified under *HIV* entry inhibitor and it is a CD4-directed post-attachment HIV-1 inhibitor. It is used in combination with

TABLE 1: Timeline of US FDA (US Food and Drug Administration) approved injectable antiretrovirals (ARTs).

Injectable ART	Acronym	US FDA approval details	Class	Dosage frequency	Route
Enfuvirtide	T-20	March, 2003	Fusion inhibitor	Daily injection	SC
Ibalizumab	IBA uiyk	March, 2018	Monoclonal antibody	Every 2 weeks	IV
Rilpivirine	RPV	May, 2021	Second-generation NNRTI	Every 4 weeks or 8 weeks	IM
Cabotegravir	CAB	December, 2021	INSTI	Every 4 weeks or 8 weeks	IM
Cabenuva	–	• January, 2021 monthly dose • February, 2022 every 2 months • March, 2022 oral lead-in phase made optional	Combination of CAB and RPV	Every 4 weeks or 8 weeks	IM
Lenacapavir	LEN	December, 2022	Capsid inhibitor	Every 6 months	SC

(IM: intramuscular; IV: intravenous; INSTI: integrase strand transfer inhibitor; NNRTI: non-nucleoside reverse transcriptase inhibitor; SC: subcutaneous)

other ART in heavily treatment experienced multidrug resistant HIV-1 positive adults. It is available in the brand name of Trogarzo by THERAtechnologies Inc and is administered intravenous 2,000 mg loading dose followed by 800 mg every 2 weeks. Common side effect is diarrhea. It can be used regardless of trophism. Routine HIV drug resistance testing does not give information of IBA. It is rarely used in clinical practice as a salvage therapy. It is approved by US FDA in March 2018. TMB 301 and TMB 311 are the therapeutic studies which supported the use of IBA.

Rilpivirine (RPV): This was approved in May 2021 under the brand name of Edurant and Rekambys. It is a *second-generation NNRTI* (non-nucleoside reverse transcriptase inhibitor) with higher potency, longer half-life, and less side effects. It can be administered once a month (Edurant) intramuscular (IM) or once in 2 months IM (Rekambys) 900 mg/3 mL. Oral form is used 25 mg/day for a month before starting injection to assess the tolerability (costs $1,431 for 30 tablets). This lead-in dose is made optional in new guidelines.

Cabotegravir (CAB): In December 2021 US FDA approved CAB for PrEP (pre-exposure prophylaxis). Long-acting CAB (CAB-LA) was approved by World Health Organization (WHO) as a part of comprehensive HIV prevention in July 2022. Two landmark randomized control studies, HPTN 083 and HPTN 084, showed that use of CAB-LA resulted in 79% relative reduction in HIV risk compared to oral PrEP. Oral PrEP often faced adherence issues. Both oral and long-acting CAB are available. It is given as 600 mg IM injection (Apretude) in buttocks initially two injections 1 month apart and every 2 months one injection for PrEP. It is usually preceded by oral CAB 30 mg once a day for a month. Cost of CAB is $3,964 for a single vial (600 mg/3 mL).

Cabenuva: This is the first and only complete LA injectable ART *regimen.*

It is available as 3 mL kit (600/900) or 2 mL kit (400/600).

- 3 mL injection for every 2 monthly—CAB 200 mg/mL (600 mg total)
  PLUS
- 3 mL injection for every 2 monthly—RPV 300 mg/mL (900 mg total)
  OR
  2 mL injection for every month—CAB 200 mg/mL (400 mg total)
  PLUS
- 2 mL injection for every month—RPV 300 mg/mL (600 mg total)

It needs to be refrigerated. To be used within 6 hours at room temperature. It should be used within 2 hours after loading in the syringe. To be given in each buttock. Patient has to be observed for 10 minutes to see for any reactions.

TABLE 2: Dose schedule.

Day 1	300 mg	2 OD	Oral
Day 2	300 mg	2 OD	Oral
Day 8	300 mg	1 OD	Oral
Day 15	463.5 mg vial	2 SC shots	SC
Every 6 months	463.5 mg vial	2 SC shots	SC

(OD: once a day; SC: subcutaneous)

The policy of 'white bagging' is preferred—injection transferred from directly pharmacy to healthcare provider (who is in charge of giving injection) to maintain cold chain (cannot be directly sent to patient). Cost of 4 mL kit (monthly use) 200–300 mg/mL use is $4,456. Cabenuva was approved based on ATLAS and FLAIR studies. According to SOLAR (Switch Onto Long-Acting Regimen) study by Ramgopal et al. [Conference on Retroviruses and Opportunistic Infections (CROI) 2023, OA #191], 90% of participants who switched from oral BIC/FTC/TAF (bictegravir/emtricitabine/tenofovir alafenamide) to CAB + RPV long-acting injection, preferred complete long-acting regimen to daily medication. This study showed that every 2 months injection of CAB + RPV was noninferior to efficacy compared to continuation of daily oral BIC/FTC/TAF.

Indications of Cabenuva:

- HIV-1-positive patients with virologically suppressed [viral load (VL) < 50 copies/mL]
- Age > 12 years
- Weight >35 kgs
- No resistance to CAB and RPV

Lenacapavir (LEN): This is a capsid inhibitor. It is developed by Gilead Sciences. It is approved for medical use in the European Union in August 2022 and in USA in December 2022. The US FDA granted the application of LEN (SUNLENCA) to Gilead Sciences. Proposed indication for use of LEN—heavily treated persons with multidrug resistance; it is available in oral and injection form (long-acting SC). 1-year therapy costs around $42,250 (oral lead-in and two injections). CAPELLA study showed LEN in combination with other ART demonstrated sustained virologic suppress ion and CD4 recovery in patients with multidrug resistance HIV.

Lenacapvir dosing schedule is shown in **Table 2**.

FUTURE OF LONG-ACTING ANTIRETROVIRAL

Other LA-ART which are tried are islatravir implants. subdermal implant of TAF every 6 months. Even dolutegravir is been used in research as ultra-long-acting removable drug delivery system, which may act up to

9 months. Another monoclonal antibody in pipeline is leronlimab, which is humanized IgG4 monoclonal antibody, directed toward CCR5 and can be used in CCR5-tropic HIV. It is effective against maraviroc-resistant virus. The advantage is that it can be given SC injection every week (unlike IBA which needs to given intravenous). RPV has been tried as microarray patch (MAP) or microneedle technology. This method uses intradermal method. Dapivirine (NNRTI) monthly vaginal ring has already been approved by European Medicines Agency (EMA) for HIV prevention in women. Refillable implants using nanochannels has been tried with TAF and emtricitabine which act >2 months. Another promising regimen in phase I trial is LEN plus dual bNAbs (broadly neutralizing antibodies) every 6 months.

LIMITATIONS

Injection Cabenuva is temperature-sensitive and requires a cold chain at 2–8°C. This is one of the hurdle in LMIC (low- and middle-income countries). Possibility of development of drug resistance during the tail end of LA-ART has to be considered pharmacokinetic (PK) tail. Most of these drugs have local injection site side effects, of which few may persist for weeks. We should know that the LA injectable ART once administered cannot be removed and if any major side effects occur then it becomes difficult to handle. Almost all the LA-ARTs are costly. Even though LA injectable ART regimen are potent and effective, cost of these regimens remains major limitation in both LMIC and developed countries.

CONCLUSION

The present one-size-fit-for-all" LA-ART, irrespective of sex, weight, and race, can be fine-tuned in future by different weight band, gender, and race. It needs more future studies and research. The paradigm shift of daily ART to six injections' regimen in a year is a ground-breaking innovation.

SUGGESTED READINGS

1. Thoueille P, Choong E, Cavassini M, Buclin T, Decosterd LA. Long-acting antiretrovirals: a new era for the management and prevention of HIV infection. J Antimicrob Chemother. 2022;77(2):290-302.
2. World Health Organization. (2022). WHO recommends long-acting cabotegravir for HIV prevention. [online] Available from https://www.who.int/news/item/28-07-2022-who-recommends-long-acting-cabotegravir-for-hiv-prevention [Last accessed December, 2023].
3. Venkatesan P. Long-acting injectable ART for HIV: a (cautious) step forward. Lancet Microbe. 2022;3(2):e94.
4. GSK. (2023). ViiV Healthcare announces positive data demonstrating long-acting injectable Cabenuva (cabotegravir, rilpivirine) is as effective as daily oral Biktarvy (BIC/FTC/TAF) for the treatment of HIV-1. [online] Available from https://www.gsk.com/en-gb/media/press-releases/viiv-healthcare-announces-positive-12-month-findings-from-the-solar-study/ [Last accessed December, 2023].

159

CHAPTER

Sepsis: Diagnose Early and Act Fast

Pramod Kumar Sinha

ABSTRACT

Sepsis is a life-threatening situation occurring due to dysregulated immune response to infection and continues to be a significant global healthcare challenge.

Delay in initiating effective sepsis management increases mortality. Healthcare providers are required to keep vigilance in relevant clinical scenario and utilize appropriate screening tool like systemic inflammatory response syndrome (SIRS), SOFA (Sequential Organ Failure Assessment), qSOFA (Quick Sequential Organ Failure Assessment), or NEWS (National Early Warning Score) for early recognition and risk stratification of sepsis.

Upon suspicion or confirmation of sepsis, time-sensitive interventions including fluid resuscitation, administration of broad-spectrum antibiotics matching with the clinical scenario, and source control measures should be implemented without delay followed by other needed measures.

Thus, sepsis represents a critical medical emergency and requires early diagnosis with timely intervention.

INTRODUCTION

Sepsis is a major public health problem all over the world with case fatality rate as high as >40%. Sepsis is a complex syndrome that can rapidly progress to multiple organ dysfunction with or without septic shock. The consequences of delayed diagnosis and treatment are dire. Every 1 hour of delay in initiating appropriate antibiotics increases the mortality rate. The timely diagnosis and prompt initiation of appropriate treatment are of paramount importance in improving patients' outcome and reducing the burden of sepsis.

Immediate intervention requires the updated understanding of protocols developed by Surviving Sepsis Campaign (SSC)—the International Guidelines for Management of Sepsis and Septic Shock 2021.

With the current understanding of pathophysiology, Society of Critical Care Medicine (SCCM) and the European Society of Intensive Care Medicine (ESICM) in 2016 came with the Third International Consensus definition (Sepsis-3) describing sepsis as a dysregulated host response to infection that leads to acute organ dysfunction and septic shock as a subset of sepsis cases in which underlying circulatory and cellular/metabolic abnormalities are profound enough to substantially increase mortality risk. Acute organ dysfunction is defined as an increase of ≥2 points in the SOFA (Sequential Organ Failure Assessment) score **(Table 1)**. Septic shock recognition criteria includes sepsis with persistent hypotension requiring vasopressors to maintain mean arterial pressure (MAP) ≥65 mm Hg and have serum lactate level >2 mmol/L (18 mg/dL) despite adequate fluid resuscitation. These criteria helps in identifying patients with increased risk of both mortality and prolonged intensive care unit (ICU) stay. qSOFA (Quick Sequential Organ Failure Assessment) score has also been proposed for identifying septic patients outside of ICU **(Table 2)**.

DIAGNOSING EARLY

Early diagnosis requires high index of suspicion in the relevant clinical scenario especially in those with known

TABLE 1: SOFA (Sequential Organ Failure Assessment) score.

	SOFA score				
Organ system	**0**	**1**	**2**	**3**	**4**
Respiratory pO_2/FiO_2 mm Hg (kPa)	≥ 400 (53.3)	< 400 (53.3)	< 300 (40)	< 200 (26.7) With respiratory support	< 100 (13.3) With respiratory support
Coagulation Platelets × $10^3/mm^3$	≥ 150	< 150	< 100	< 50	< 20
Liver Bilirubin mg/dL	< 1.2	1.2–1.9	2.0–5.9	6.0–11.9	> 12.0
Cardiovascular	MAP ≥ 70 mm Hg	MAP < 70 mm Hg	Dopamine < 5 or dobutamine (any dose)	Norepinephrine ≤ 0.1, or epinephrine ≤ 0.1, or dopamine 5.1–1.5 (μg/kg/min)	Norepinephrine > 0.1, or epinephrine > 0.1, or dopamine > 1.5 (μg/kg/min)
CNS Glasgow Coma Scale	15	13–14	10–12	6–9	< 6
Renal, creatinine mg/dL Urine output mL/day	< 1.2	1.2–1.9	2.0–3.4	3.5–4.9 < 500	> 5.0 < 200
The SOFA score ranges from 0 to 24 points, with up to 4 points accrued across six organ systems. With ≥ 2 new SOFA points, the infected person is considered septic and may be at ≥ 10% risk of inhospital death.					

(CNS: central nervous system; FiO_2: fraction of inspired oxygen; MAP: mean arterial pressure; pO_2: partial pressure of oxygen)

TABLE 2: The qSOFA (Quick Sequential Organ Failure Assessment) score.

qSOFA Criteria	**Points**
Respiratory rate ≥ 22/breaths/min	1
Change in mental status	1
Systolic blood pressure ≤ 100 mm Hg	1
2 or more qSOFA points with infection: Greater risk of death or prolonged intensive care unit stay.	

TABLE 3: Systemic inflammatory response syndrome (SIRS) criteria.

Tachycardia	Heart rate > 90 beats/min
Tachypnea	Respiratory rate > 20 breaths/min
Fever or hypothermia	Temperature > 38° or < 36°C
Leukocytosis, leukopenia, or bandemia	WBC ≥ 12,000/mm³, ≤ 4,000/mm³ or bandemia ≥ 10%
Patients who met two or more of these criteria in addition to a known or suspected infection.	

risk factors such as advanced age, immunosuppression, chronic illness, or recent invasive procedures. Common presenting features are nonspecific and include fever, hypotension, altered mental status, and signs of organ dysfunction. qSOFA and systemic inflammatory response syndrome (SIRS) **(Table 3)** have been proposed as a screening tool but none is sufficient alone. NEWS (National Early Warning Score) and MEWS (Modified Early Warning Score) has been found to be a sensitive screening tool for predicting sepsis-related outcomes. However, qSOFA/SIRS can be rapidly scored at the bedside without the need for blood tests, and it is hoped that it will facilitate prompt identification of an infection that poses a greater threat to life. Serum lactate measurement is recommended for identifying sepsis. Rapid diagnostic tools including biomarkers such as procalcitonin and C-reactive protein aid in the early identification of infection and monitoring treatment response. Culture of blood, urine, and other relevant sites along with radiological imaging are required to identify the causative organism and the source of infection.

ACT FAST

Bundle concept: SSC presented a well-defined bundle therapy to facilitate implementation at the bedside to improve outcome. In 2018 SSC revised the task completion time frame and suggested to start resuscitation bundle treatment within 1 hour of arrival or earlier if presenting from another center. Named as 1-hour bundle, this aims to achieve five elements: (1)measuring the lactate level, (2) obtaining blood culture prior to administration of antibiotics, (3) administering broad-spectrum antibiotics, (4) beginning rapid administration of 30 mL/kg crystalloid fluid for hypotension or lactate ≥ 4 mmol/L, and (5) administering vasopressors if the patient remains hypotensive during or after fluid resuscitation to maintain MAP at ≥ 65 mm Hg within 1 hour from sepsis recognition. However, completing the task within 3 hours (3-hour bundle) is found equally good as suggested by SSC in 2015.

INITIAL RESUSCITATION

Sepsis and septic shock are medical emergencies so treatment and resuscitation must begin immediately. Sepsis guideline 2021 suggests to give at least 30 mL/kg of intravenous (IV) crystalloid within the first 3 hours to manage sepsis-induced hypoperfusion which is manifested by acute organ damage +/– hypotension and increased serum lactate level. The PROCESS, ARISE, and PROMISE trials have supported this measure. Further IV fluid therapy should be guided by careful assessment of intravascular volume status and organ perfusion. Systolic blood pressure (BP), heart rate, and central venous pressure (CVP) are poor guides, so dynamic measurements like passive leg raising combined with cardiac output (CO) measurement, fluid challenges with measurement of stroke volume variation (SVV), systolic pressure or pulse pressure variation (PPV), and increases of stroke volume (SV) in response to changes in intrathoracic pressure are recommended. For fluid therapy beyond the initial 30 mL/kg if required, repeated small boluses can be given guided by objective measures of SV and/or CO. However, in resource-limited places, a >15% increase in pulse pressure on a passive leg raise test for 60–90 seconds could be utilized as an indicator of patient fluid responsiveness. In patients with persistent hypotension despite adequate fluid resuscitation, it is recommended to use vasopressor to achieve initial target MAP of 65 mm Hg and also suggested for guiding resuscitation to normalize lactate in patients with elevated lactate levels.

Where advanced hemodynamic measurement system is not available, temperature of extremities, skin mottling, and capillary refill time (CRT) could be used as they very are useful and validated indicators for tissue perfusion. The ANDROMEDA-SHOCK STUDY supported their utility.

For adults with sepsis or septic shock who require ICU admission, SSC 2021 suggests admitting the patients to the ICU within 6 hours.

ANTIMICROBIAL THERAPY

Antimicrobial therapy is one of the most important pillars of sepsis/septic shock management. However, it is recommended that appropriate routine microbiologic cultures (including blood) should be obtained before starting antimicrobial therapy in patients with suspected sepsis and septic shock, if it results in no substantial delay in the start of antimicrobials (i.e., <45 minutes).

Timing of Antimicrobial Drug Administration

A study of 49,331 patients treated at 149 New York hospitals, 35,000 patients treated at Kaiser Permanente Northern California 10,811 patients treated in four Utah hospitals, each additional hour of time from emergency department arrival to administration of antimicrobials was associated with increased inhospital mortality. So antimicrobials must be given as early as possible; however, they must be balanced against the potential harm of unnecessary antimicrobial administration.

International clinical practice guideline 2021 recommended administration of antimicrobials immediately, and within 1 hour, in all patients with potential septic shock and also for patients with confirmed/very likely sepsis.

For patients with possible sepsis without shock, a rapid assessment of infectious and noninfectious etiologies of illness be undertaken to determine, within 3 hours, whether antibiotics should be administered or whether antibiotics should be deferred while continuing to monitor the patient closely.

Selecting an Antimicrobial Regimen

Early antimicrobial treatment for sepsis/septic shock requires empiric broad-spectrum parenteral antibiotic coverage. The appropriate choice depends on the suspected site of infection, the location of infection site (i.e., a community, nursing home, or hospital), the patient's medical history, and local microbial susceptibility pattern.

Initially empiric antimicrobial regimens with a wide spectrum of activity like piperacillin/tazobactam or carbapenems or cefepime covering all the pathogens suspected should be used.

Two antimicrobials with gram-negative coverage for empiric treatment over one gram-negative drug is suggested in cases of high suspicion for multidrug-resistant organisms (like *Pseudomonas aeruginosa*, *Acinetobacter baumannii* or Enterobacteriaceae).

Also combination therapy with double gram-negative coverage is suggested for definitive therapy once causative organism and its sensitivity is identified. Aminoglycosides or levofloxacin or colistin can be used as one of the drugs with others for definitive therapy for gram-negative bacteria.

Dual coverage for gram-positive organisms and methicillin-resistant *Staphylococcus aureus* (MRSA) is recommended that is addition of vancomycin or linezolid or daptomycin against MRSA for patients with a high risk of infection due to these pathogens.

The SSC guideline also recommends against the use of antimicrobials with MRSA coverage and dual gram-negative agent in patients with low risk of MRSA and low risk of multidrug-resistant (MDR) organisms respectively.

Antifungal Therapy

Empirical antifungal therapy is suggested for high-risk but not for low-risk patient of fungal infection. Patients with high risk for fungal infection include immunocompromised patients and patients with febrile neutropenia who fail to defervesce after 4–7 days of broad-spectrum antibacterial therapy. The choice of antifungal agent for empiric therapy depends on multiple issues including host factors, prior colonization and infection, prior exposure to prophylactic or therapeutic antifungal therapy, comorbidities, and the toxicities and drug interactions of the therapeutic options.

Delivery of Antimicrobials

An initial loading dose is suggested to achieve therapeutic blood level rapidly followed by extended or continuous IV infusion of antimicrobials. As opposed to conventional intermittent infusion (infusion ≤ 30 minutes), giving prolonged IV infusion, either as an extended infusion (antibiotic infused over at least half of the dosing interval) or as a continuous infusion leads to sustained concentrations above the minimum inhibitory concentration (MIC), provided the pharmacokinetics and pharmacodynamics of the selected antimicrobials justifies this protocol.

Source control: It is recommended to rapidly identify and remove the source of infection.

This may need drainage of an abscess, debriding infected necrotic tissue, removal of a potentially infected device, or definitive control of a source of ongoing microbial contamination

De-escalation of Antimicrobials

Daily reassessment for antimicrobial de-escalation is suggested. De-escalation requires stopping an antimicrobial that is no longer necessary (in case of combination therapy) or stopping all antimicrobials if infection is ruled out or changing an antimicrobial to narrow the spectrum once the causative pathogen(s) and susceptibilities are identified. A meta-analysis of 13 studies including one randomized controlled trial (RCT) observed improved short-term mortality in patients de-escalated timely.

Duration of Antimicrobials

Shorter duration of antimicrobials is suggested in a patient with adequate source control and clinical improvement; biomarker—procalcitonin is helpful in unclear clinical situation and is suggested.

HEMODYNAMIC SUPPORT

Managing Fluid

Crystalloids are recommended as the first choice for fluid management with a suggestion that balanced crystalloid is better than normal saline. A meta-analysis of 14 RCTs showed decreased mortality with balanced crystalloids compared with normal saline, however, further RCTS like SPLIT trial, SALT pilot trial, and SMART failed to confirm the findings.

Additional use of albumin infusion is suggested in face of need of large volume of crystalloid infusion. Use of starch is not recommended. Gelatin is also not suggested.

Using Vasopressor and Inotropes

Norepinephrine (NE) (at a dose of 0.1–1.2 μg/kg/min) is recommended as the first-choice vasopressor agent for managing septic shock; dopamine and epinephrine are suggested only if NE is not available especially in patients at risk of arrhythmia.

Addition of vasopressin suggested instead of increasing the dose of NE if target MAP level (65 mm Hg) is not achieved with 0.25–0.5 μg/kg/min of NE. If still target MAP is not reached, adding epinephrine suggested. Terlipressin is avoided.

Adding dobutamine to NE is suggested for patients with *septic shock and cardiac dysfunction* with persistent hypoperfusion despite adequate volume status and arterial BP.

RESPIRATORY SUPPORT

High-flow Nasal Oxygen Therapy and Noninvasive Ventilation

Patients with hypoxia without hypercapnia are given high concentrations of inhaled oxygen delivered conventionally with interfaces including nasal prongs, facemask with reservoir, or Venturi mask. When escalation of support required, high-flow oxygen is suggested over noninvasive ventilation as it provides high flow rates to better match patient demand, washout of nasopharyngeal dead space with modest positive airway pressure effect, and keeps secretions warm and humidified.

Mechanical Ventilation

Mechanical ventilation is a critical intervention in patients with hypoxemic hypoxia or ventilatory failure to maintain adequate oxygenation and ventilation in sepsis-induced acute respiratory distress syndrome (ARDS). Important principles are as follows:

- *Tidal volume and plateau pressure*: In accordance with the observation from several meta-analysis, protective ventilation using a low tidal volume strategy (≤6 mL/kg) over a high tidal volume strategy (>10 mL/kg) and using an upper limit goal for plateau pressures of 30 cm H_2O over higher plateau pressures is recommended for managing ARDS due to sepsis/septic shock. This strategy has shown reduced mortality compared with the higher tidal volume and higher plateau pressure in ARDS.

  In non-ARDS respiratory failure, although there is no strong evidence favoring a low tidal volume strategy, still it is suggested.
- *Positive end-expiratory pressure (PEEP)*: In line with a systemic review and meta-analysis by Briel et al., higher PEEP over lower PEEP is suggested in patients of sepsis-induced moderate-to-severe ARDS [PaO_2/FiO_2 (partial pressure of arterial oxygen/fraction of inspired oxygen) ≤200 mm Hg]. The use of higher PEEP (>5 cm H_2O) in ventilation found to decrease mortality.
- *Recruitment maneuvers*: In face of the need to increase ventilatory effort in sepsis-induced moderate/severe ARDS traditional recruitment methods are suggested with close monitoring so as to stop it soon possible. Nontraditional recruitment method with incremental PEEP titration strategy is not recommended.
- *Prone ventilation*: A meta-analysis by Sud et al. in 2010 and another by Minshi et al. in 2017 observed improved survival with prone ventilation of >12 hours daily and is recommended by the SSC guideline.
- *Neuro muscular blocking agents (NMBAs)*: It is used to facilitate mechanical ventilation. SSC 2021 guideline has suggested NMBA to be used in intermittent bolus fashion over continuous infusion strategy in sepsis-induced moderate-severe ARDS. Adequate sedation and analgesia need to be ensured if NMBA is in use. Several trials including ROSE study led to this conclusion.
- *Extracorporeal membrane oxygenation (ECMO)*: Venovenous ECMO suggested in severe ARDS where conventional mechanical ventilation fails if needed infrastructure is available.

ADDITIONAL THERAPY

Corticosteroids

Intravenous corticosteroids suggested in patients of septic shock with ongoing requirement of vasopressor, i.e., requirement of NE or epinephrine at a dose of ≥0.25 µg/kg/min for at least 4 hours after initiation to maintain the target MAP. IV hydrocortisone 200 mg/day given as 50 mg/6 hours or as continuous infusion is the choice.

Blood Product Use

Red blood cell (RBC) transfusion suggested: In accordance with the observation of TRISS trial, TRICC trial, and recent TRICOP trial, SSC 2021 recommended using a restrictive over liberal transfusion strategy which proposes 7 g/dL of hemoglobin as cutoff value for initiating transfusion.

Platelet transfusion suggested when:

- Platelet <10,000/dL
- ≤20,000/dL with bleeding risk
- ≤50,000/dL if invasive procedure/surgery required

STRESS ULCER PROPHYLAXIS

Surviving Sepsis Campaign guideline 2021 issued a weak recommendation for the use of stress ulcer prophylaxis in at-risk patients.

Venous Thromboembolism Prophylaxis

For patients of sepsis/septic shock, venous thromboembolism (VTE) prophylaxis is recommended for critically ill patients. Low-molecular-weight heparin (LMWH) is the choice over unfractionated heparin (UFH). Mechanical VTE prophylaxis in addition to pharmacological therapy is not suggested.

Glucose Control

Initiating insulin therapy at a glucose level of ≥180 mg/dL (10 mmol/L is recommended with aim to achieve target blood glucose range of 144–180 mg/dL, so as to save the patient from deleterious effect of hyperglycemia without inducing harm of hypoglycemia.

Renal Replacement Therapy

Renal replacement therapy (RRT), continuous or intermittent, is suggested in patients of sepsis/septic shock with acute kidney injury (AKI) with definite indication like uremic complications, refractory academia, refractory fluid overload, or hyperkalemia and not only for increase in serum creatinine or oliguria. The IDEAL-ICU trial favors delayed than early initiation of RRT.

Bicarbonate Therapy

This is suggested for adults with septic shock suffering from severe metabolic acidemia (pH ≤7.2) and AKI [AKIN

(Acute Kidney Injury Network) score 2 or 3] but not suggested for hypoperfusion-induced lactic academia.

The SSC 2016/SSC 2021 guideline suggested against the use of:

- Immunoglobulins
- IV vitamin C
- Blood purification strategy

Nutrition

Early (within 72 hours) enteral nutrition is suggested by SSC 2021 in patients who can be fed enterally.

Shared decision-making with patient during treatment and for planning discharge: Recommended

Proper information to patient on discharge: Suggested

CONCLUSION

The "Diagnosis Early and Act Fast for Sepsis" approach represents a crucial step in the battle against this life-threatening condition. By improving recognition, enhancing communication, and implementing evidence-based guidelines such as SSC, healthcare systems can make significant strides in reducing sepsis-related morbidity and mortality.

SUGGESTED READINGS

1. Rhodes A, Evans LE, Alhazzani W, Levy MM, Antonelli M, Ferrer R, et al. Surviving sepsis campaign: International guidelines for management of sepsis and septic shock: 2016. Intensive Care Med. 2017;43:304-77.
2. Levy MM, Evans LE, Rhodes A. The surviving sepsis campaign bundle:2018 update. Intensive Care Med. 2018;44:925-8.
3. Dugar S, Choudhary C, Duggal A. Sepsis and septic shock: Guideline-based management. Cleve Clin J Med. 2020;87:53-64.

160

CHAPTER

What Happens When You do not Recover from COVID-19?

Raj Kamal Choudhary

ABSTRACT

During the early coronavirus disease-2019 (COVID-19) pandemic, public health systems focused on avoiding hospitalization and death. However, the lingering effects of severe acute respiratory syndrome coronavirus 2 (SARS-CoV-2) infections are a concern for everyone, even if initial symptoms are mild. Long COVID symptoms can vary and have different causes, and while certain groups are at greater risk, anyone can develop lasting symptoms. Vaccination may reduce the risk of long COVID, but not reliably prevent it.

INTRODUCTION

During the early months of the coronavirus disease-2019 (COVID-19) pandemic, the main focus of public health systems was on avoiding hospitalization and death. Yet the lingering effects of severe acute respiratory syndrome coronavirus 2 (SARS-CoV-2) infections are something we should all be worried about, even if our initial symptoms are mild. Now, most people will have experienced at least one COVID-19 infection, and in some cases three or more. If you are lucky, you will have escaped relatively unscathed, but for hundreds of millions of people around the world, COVID-19 is proving to have a very long tail. Symptoms of long COVID, or postacute sequelae of COVID-19 (PASC)/post-COVID-19 condition, as it is officially known, can vary, and may have different underlying causes—the mechanics of which still are not fully understood. But although certain groups are at greater risk, it is increasingly clear that anyone can develop lasting symptoms, and that they can be debilitating. Mounting evidence also suggests that vaccination reduces the risk of long COVID, even if it does not reliably prevent it.

PREVALENCE AND RISK FACTORS

Estimating the true prevalence of long COVID has been challenging because people's experiences are so varied. Some have multiple ongoing symptoms, which change over time, while others just have one persistent problem. The severity and duration of people's symptoms can also be very mixed. Gradually though, experts have settled on a clearer working definition of what long COVID is, which makes it easier to estimate how common it is. According to the World Health Organization (WHO), it is "the continuation or development of new symptoms 3 months after the initial SARS-CoV-2 infection, with these symptoms lasting for at least 2 months with no other explanation". The author's experiences with COVID-19 patients based on these criteria, it estimates that around 10–20% of people may go on to develop symptoms that can be diagnosed as long COVID. In the WHO European Region alone, >17 million people are estimated to have experienced it during the first 2 years of the pandemic, with some still living with ongoing symptoms today.

LONG CORONAVIRUS DISEASE SUBTYPES

The most frequently reported symptoms are fatigue, shortness of breath, and brain fog, although people have reported around 200 different symptoms in total. Interestingly though, some of these symptoms appear to cluster together, prompting some researchers to suggest there may be different subtypes of long COVID—

potentially with different underlying causes. According to the Zoe Health Study, which has collected self-reported daily data on people's symptoms, infection and vaccination status over the past 3 years, the largest group of long COVID sufferers report clusters of neurological symptoms such as fatigue, brain fog, headache, and an altered or absent sense of smell. However, these types of symptoms tended to be more common among people infected during the Alpha and Delta waves of the pandemic. Another group experienced predominantly respiratory symptoms, including shortness of breath and chest pain, which could be associated with lingering lung damage caused by the infection. Such symptoms were more common during the early days of the pandemic, before anyone was vaccinated. The final group they identified were people with a diverse range of symptoms including heart palpitations, muscle aches and pains, and skin or hair changes. However, this study only focused on symptoms logged during 2020 and 2021. The team is still analyzing data collected during the Omicron era to see if other clusters have emerged since then. US researchers have also identified distinct clusters of long COVID symptoms, based on health records from nearly 35,000 US patients, with some similarities to those identified by the Zoe team. The first group, accounting for around 34% of patients, was marked by heart and kidney problems, and included a relatively high proportion of patients infected during the first few months of the pandemic. The second, accounting for roughly 33% of people, included ongoing breathing difficulties, together with anxiety, sleep problems, chest pain, and headaches. Nearly two-thirds of those experiencing these kinds of symptoms were women. Musculoskeletal and nervous system problems dominated the third group, including joint and muscle pain, headaches, and sleep problems. This accounted for roughly 23% of patients. The final subtype was characterized by a mixture of respiratory and digestive problems, and accounted for around 10% of patients.

POSSIBLE CAUSES

Investigations into the underlying cause of such symptoms continue, but currently four main theories predominate. The first is residual organ or tissue damage. For instance, body scans have identified tiny blood clots and lung scarring in some patients who have recovered from COVID-19, which might underpin some of the ongoing breathing, heart, or circulatory problems that people experience. An overactive immune system is another possibility. Several research teams have identified autoantibodies—antibodies directed against the body's own tissues—in some groups of long COVID patients. Another theory is that small pockets of active SARS-CoV-2 virus can linger in the body, and continue to trigger immune responses, even though the individual no longer tests positive on standard polymerase chain reaction (PCR) tests. Various studies have identified abnormal immune activity in patients with ongoing COVID-19 symptoms up to 8 months after they initially tested positive for the infection. Others have detected viral spike proteins in the blood of long COVID patients many months after they recovered. Viral reservoirs in the gut are one potential candidate, as genetic material from SARS-CoV-2 has been detected there, sometimes months after the initial infection. It is quite possible that more than one of these factors are involved to some degree in some individuals. For instance, damage from scarring of the lungs and blood vessels from COVID-19 may be compounded by ongoing immune system activity. Finally, some studies have found that long COVID symptoms may not always be due to previous COVID-19 infection. For example, one study in France found that an individual's belief that they had COVID-19 "was associated with most persistent physical symptoms, whereas laboratory-confirmed COVID-19 infection was associated with only (decreased sense of smell)." The different clusters of long COVID symptoms all resemble the symptoms of other diseases, so some long COVID patients' symptoms may be the result of medical problems not dependent on previous COVID-19 infection. This does not mean that their symptoms should be dismissed or that long COVID is not real, but it underscores the importance of careful examination and diagnostic testing for long COVID patients to ensure they receive the most appropriate care. Research into long COVID continues, but this much is clear, even after the pandemic is declared over, COVID-19 will cast a long shadow over the lives of many.

SUGGESTED READINGS

1. Adhikari SP, Meng S, Wu YJ, Mao YP, Ye RX, Wang QZ, et al. Epidemiology, causes, clinical manifestation and diagnosis, prevention and control of coronavirus disease (COVID-19) during the early outbreak period: a scoping review. Infect Dis Poverty. 2020;9(1):29.
2. Gorbalenya AE, Baker SC, Baric RS, de Groot RJ, Drosten C, Gulyaeva AA, et al. (2020). Severe acute respiratory syndrome-related coronavirus: The species and its viruses—a statement of the Coronavirus Study Group. [online] Available from https://www.biorxiv.org/content/10.1101/2020.02.07.937862v1. [Last accessed December, 2023].
3. Lam Ung CO. Community pharmacist in public health emergencies: Quick to action against the coronavirus 2019-nCoV outbreak. Res Social Adm Pharm. 2020;16(4):583-6.

4. Cao M, Zhang D, Wang Y, Lu Y, Zhu X, Li Y, et al. (2020). Clinical features of patients infected with the 2019 novel coronavirus (COVID-19) in Shanghai, China. [online] available from https://www.medrxiv.org/content/10.1101/2020.03.04.20030395v1. [Last accessed December, 2023].
5. Huang C, Wang Y, Li X, Ren L, Zhao J, Hu Y, et al. Clinical features of patients infected with 2019 novel coronavirus in Wuhan, China. Lancet. 2020;395(10223):497-506.
6. Yang X, Yu Y, Xu J, Shu H, Xia J, Liu H, et al. Clinical course and outcomes of critically ill patients with SARS-cov-2 pneumonia in Wuhan, China: a single-centered, retrospective, observational study. Lancet Respir Med. 2020;8(5):475-81.
7. Li T, Wei C, Li W, Hongwei F, Shi J. Beijing Union Medical College Hospital on "pneumonia of novel coronavirus infection" diagnosis and treatment proposal (V2. 0). Med J Peking Union Med Coll Hosp. 2020;6:672-5.
8. Disilvio B, Young M, Gordon A, Malik K, Singh A, Cheema T, et al. Complications and outcomes of acute respiratory distress syndrome. Crit Care Nurs Q. 2019;42(4):349-61.
9. Moldofsky H, Patcai J. Chronic widespread musculoskeletal pain, fatigue, depression and disordered sleep in chronic post-SARS syndrome; a case-controlled study. BMC Neurol. 2011; 11(1):37.
10. Zhou F, Yu T, Du R, Fan G, Liu Y, Liu Z, et al. Clinical course and risk factors for mortality of adult inpatients with COVID-19 in Wuhan, China: a retrospective cohort study. Lancet. 2020;395(10229):1054-62.

161

CHAPTER

Coronavirus Disease Vaccines in 2024

Vasantha Kamath, Kushal Markanday

ABSTRACT

With the World Health Organization (WHO) declaring an end to coronavirus disease 2019 (COVID-19) as a global health emergency, the management of the recently concluded COVID-19 pandemic reflects the technological evolution of humans in fighting such infections. Vaccines proved to be a potent weapon in limiting the repercussions secondary to this global tragedy. Due to the short development time and the novelty of the technologies adopted, several types of vaccines were deployed while we were still in the middle of the pandemic which would have been a sinking boat to sail otherwise. With varying efficacy and resultant side effects; messenger ribonucleic acid (mRNA), inactivated virion, virion vector, viral protein, and deoxyribonucleic acid (DNA)-based vaccines proved beneficial. However, there is a vast scope for improvement with numerous challenges still left to address. With the advent of newer COVID variants, there will be an unending demand for an ideal vaccine that is easier to produce and provides lifelong immunity to all COVID variants, which indeed is a tedious task.

INTRODUCTION

A virus-based pandemic overwhelming the entire healthcare infrastructure in this 21st century raised several questions about our evolution over the last 100 years. However, with the help of the effective mobilization of resources toward disease management and its globalization, we were able to control it within the initial three years.

Rapid development and distribution of safe and effective vaccines proved an important milestone in the control of the pandemic as it boosted the host immunity and ensured the speedy recovery of those affected by limiting coronavirus disease 2019 (COVID-19)-associated complications. The vaccine development began soon after delineating the etiopathogenesis of the disease. The vaccines targeted the viral nuclear and cytoplasmic components thereby limiting the viral multiplication and limiting its transmission.

This chapter highlights the road traveled so far in COVID vaccination along with the challenges including the emergence of newer variants and vaccine-related side effects.

VACCINE DEVELOPMENT

The development of vaccines is considered a tedious and time-consuming task requiring years altogether to define the efficacy, safety, risk rate, dosing, failure rate, and adverse effects of a particular agent. This research and development curve was significantly constricted this time with the first batch of mRNA-based vaccine being released within two months of the genomics reveal of the severe acute respiratory syndrome coronavirus 2 (SARS-CoV-2) virus because of the urgency of producing the vaccine. Gradually the global players came out with several options for COVID-19 vaccines.

World Health Organization (WHO)-United Nations Children's Fund (UNICEF) along with Coalition for Epidemic Preparedness Innovations (CEPI) and GAVI-the vaccine alliance established a vaccine subunit of the access to COVID-19 tools (ACT) accelerator by the name of COVID-19 Vaccines Global Access (COVAX) to augment and facilitate the global development, production, and distribution of vaccines equitably thereby targeting to benefit each country of the world. The Immunization Strategic Advisory Group of Experts (SAGEs) at WHO spearheaded building a network for rapid evidence-based policies for immunization and thereby harmonizing emergency use listings (EUL)/prequalification of several vaccine entrants. **Table 1** highlights the four major categories of vaccines currently in circulation globally.

DEOXYRIBONUCLEIC ACID VACCINES

Deoxyribonucleic acid vaccines are based on plasmid DNA containing mammalian expression promoters and viral protein-encoding genes thereby resulting in in-situ production of the target antigen. Escherichia coli is nowadays being used for large-scale production of such vaccines. Despite being significantly less potent than other vaccines, these intradermal needle-less vaccines rely on needle-free applicators instead of traditional syringes to attain efficiency. Also, these vaccines are stable at 25°C and are hence easily stored and transportable.

Several COVID-19 DNA vaccines are being developed across the globe and are in different phases of clinical trials.

ZyCov-D, a much-anticipated COVID-19 DNA vaccine being manufactured by Zydus Cadila is currently in phase III trials and has shown an efficacy of 67% against severe COVID-19 manifestations.

MUCOSAL VACCINES

Unlike others, these are not injectable vaccines but rather enter our bodies along the path traversed by coronavirus, i.e., via the mucosal tissues. With the USA allocating five billion dollars for its project NextGEN aimed at enhancing the production of mucosal vaccines, several global players have forayed into this field too. Including Bharat Biotech's nasal vaccine intranasal COVID-19 vaccine candidate (iNCOVACC) which is claimed to be more potent than Covaxin and is available in India, several other nations have developed these novel vaccines such as China's Pneucolin (viral vector nasal spray) and Convidecia Air (nebulizer inhaled viral vector Ad5-nCoV), Razi Cov Pars from Iran (intranasal protein unit), America's USSF/VaxForm (oral protein subunit) and Canada's Symvivo (oral live

TABLE 1: Types of vaccines available globally.

Types of vaccines	Whole virus (inactivated vaccines)	Protein subunit (subunit/acellular vaccines)	Viral vector (delivers spike protein genetic code)	Nucleic acid (RNA and DNA)
Examples	Bharat Biotech-ICMR-NIV-*COVAXIN* BBV152, BIBP COVID-19 vaccine, WIBP COVID-19 vaccine	• *Novavax* NVX-CoV2373 (spike protein nanoparticle) • *Corbevax*-RBD protein subunit	*Sputnik*, Oxford-AstraZeneca Covishield (ChAdOx1), and Johnson and Johnson vaccine	• Pfizer–BioNTech Bnt162 mRNA and Moderna mRNA 1273 (RNA) • ZyCoVD (DNA)
Efficacy	70–80%	80–90%	70–90%	95% for mRNA vaccines
Dosage	Two doses for 28 days apart	• Novovax: Two doses 8 weeks apart • Two boosters at 4–6 months interval each, Corbevax-2 doses 28 days apart	Two doses for 3–12 weeks apart	• Two doses for 4–8 weeks apart • Dosage to be adjusted as per age, two boosters at 4–6 months of interval each
Special points	COVAXIN® is included along with immune-potentiators	Works well for α, β, and δ strains. Insufficient data for omicron	• Covishield: Chimpanzee adenovirus vector • Sputnik: Ad5 and Ad26 vectors	DNA vaccines have 60–67% efficacy, when given intradermally via a needle-free applicator
Age group	>18 years of age, can be given to pregnant and breastfeeding females	• All above 12 years of age including pregnant females • Corbevax is in trials for the 5–18 years age group	• >18 years of age • Not well-researched for use in pregnancy	>6 months of age including pregnant females
Advantage	Ready to use, stable at 2–C, heterologous	Proven effective in children and adolescents	Fridge-stable and easily transportable	Moderate efficacy for omicron
Disadvantage	No data available for immunogenicity against the omicron variant	Myocarditis and pericarditis-associated morbidity and mortality are seen in a few cases who used Novavax	Cases of thrombosis with thrombocytopenia has to be reconstituted before use	Needs ultracold storage, vaccine-induced myocarditis has been reported by use of mRNA vaccines

(BIBP: Beijing Institute of Biological Products; DNA: deoxyribonucleic acid; ICMR: Indian Council of Medical Research; NIV: National Institute of Virology Pune; RBD: receptor binding domain; WIBP: Wuhan Institute of Biological Products)

attenuated). Similar to these vaccines mentioned here, there have been a total of 24 mucosal vaccines currently registered in various phases of clinical trials worldwide with five such vaccines currently in use in four countries, that are (1) China, (2) India, (3) Iran, and (4) Russia. Serum Institute of India is currently manufacturing a live attenuated nasal spray from Codagenix (US) which is currently in Phase III trials. The efficacy of these vaccines varies greatly and also report several side effects including nasal irritation and anaphylaxis. It is hypothesized that mucosal vaccines help in preventing asymptomatic COVID, as they potentiate local immunoglobulin A (IgA) response thereby blocking the transmission chain.

GLOBAL AND INDIAN CORONAVIRUS DISEASE 2019 VACCINATION PROGRAM

Globally, as of June 2023, there have been 768,187,096 confirmed cases of COVID-19, including 6,945,714 deaths, reported to WHO and a total of 13,461,344,203 vaccine doses have been administered across 131 nations globally. **Figure 1** gives a pictorial representation of the same as per the WHO COVAX Dashboard.

India initiated its vaccination drive on January 16, 2021, and as of June 2023; 1,025,823,086 persons were vaccinated with at least one dose per 100 population achieving a score of average of 74 persons per 100 population.

CORONAVIRUS DISEASE 2019 VACCINE MYTH-BUSTERS

Coronavirus disease 2019 vaccines do not lead to a positive reverse transcription polymerase chain reaction (RT-PCR) or rapid antigen test result because these tests detect active disease rather than checking a person's immune status. However, immunological serology assays may test positive. People with known atopy to food, drugs, or latex are safe to be administered with COVID-19 vaccines.

Similar to those who got COVID-19 disease after receiving the first dose of the vaccine, the vaccination is also delayed in people with a previous history of COVID-19 and plasma therapy or monoclonal antibody recipients by at least 3 months.

People with all comorbidities including those with immunocompromised states secondary to any cause can be safely vaccinated. However, vaccines have been demonstrated to be less immunogenic among people on high-dose steroids hence lowering the dose for at least 6 weeks is advisable in such cases.

Vaccination is safe for people on anticoagulants and thrombolytics. However, the international normalized ratio (INR) should be tested in such patients to prevent injection site hematoma. The preferable INR in such cases is <3. Also, there is no known cross-reactivity with alcohol intake in the pre/postvaccination period.

Several studies based on serial monitoring of disease-protective immunoglobulins have noted that neither the natural COVID-19 infection nor COVID-19 vaccines provide lifelong immunity. The serum immunoglobulin G (IgG) levels decline over a due period despite the initial peak in such cases. Hence, most of the vaccines are nowadays administered with booster doses for prolonged immunity, especially among high-risk individuals, such as those with age > 65 years, comorbidities, immunocompromised states, and front-line workers.

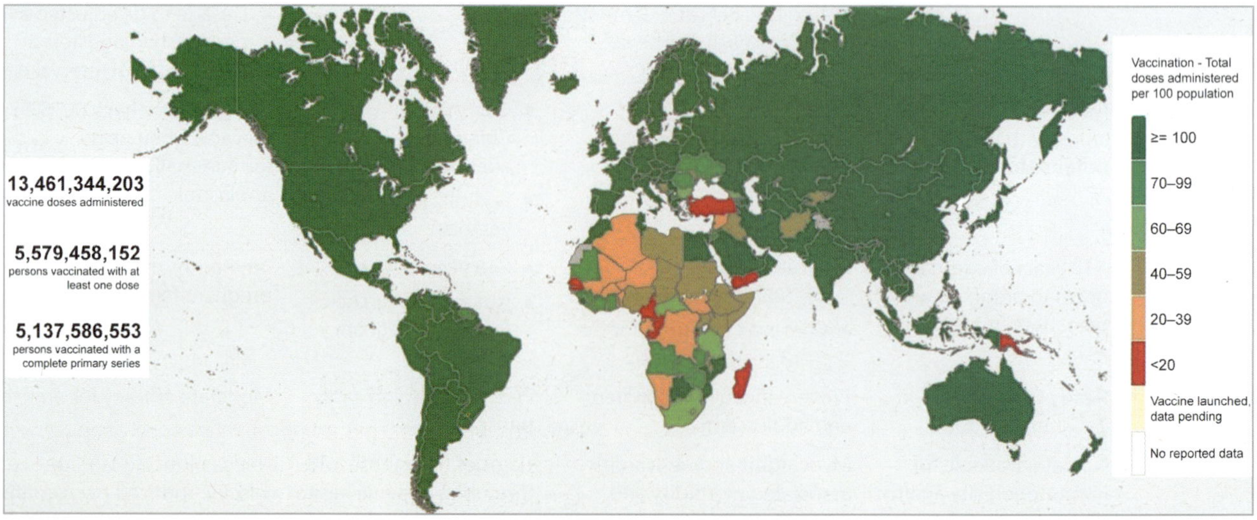

FIG. 1: The global coronavirus disease (COVID) vaccine program—categorizing nations as per total vaccine doses administered per 100 population (June 2023).

Source: United Nations International Children's Emergency Fund. COVID-19 Market Dashboard. [online] Available from https://www.unicef.org/supply/covid-19-market-dashboard [Last accessed January, 2024].

VACCINE-RELATED ADVERSE EVENTS

The common adverse effects related to COVID-19 vaccines include injection site pain, pyrexia, transient blurred vision, abdominal discomfort, nausea, backache, dyspnea, calf swelling or tenderness, pain in head or body, and confusion/irritability to name a few.

Apart from those mentioned in **Table 1**, few specific side effects are seen with particular vaccines, for example, incidences of thrombotic events alongside thrombocytopenia have been reported with the Janssen/Johnson and Johnson (Ad26.COV2.S) and Oxford-AstraZeneca (AZD-1222) vaccines with some cases of cerebral venous sinus or splanchnic vein thrombosis also being reported. However, judging on the grounds of the risk-to-benefit ratio, the vaccine is still being used although it is now labeled with a word of caution for this exclusive but rare adverse event.

Thrombocytopenia in these cases has been implicated to be due to autoantibodies against platelet factor IV (PF-IV). This can however be treated by the use of intravenous immunoglobulins and anticoagulants. This event is now termed as, vaccine-induced immune thrombotic thrombocytopenia.

A few cases of vaccine-induced myocarditis leading to arrhythmia and sudden cardiac deaths have also been seen in patients who received Novavax and Pfizer/Moderna vaccines.

Even though direct vaccine-related type 1 hypersensitivity responses are rare, delayed hypersensitivity reactions like "The COVID Arm" hallmarked by large cutaneous erythematous reactions at the injection site are often documented following the mRNA vaccines. These are often self-limiting but can also be treated using topical corticosteroid ointments.

Local side effects also include more debilitating conditions like Parsonage-Turner syndrome (PTS)/brachial plexopathy which is characterized by the onset of shoulder pain on the injected side. This progresses to patchy sensory impairment in the affected limb and further progresses to weakness in the entire upper limb. PTS is usually self-limiting with complete resolution documented within 2–3 years. Although a majority of PTS cases had been vaccinated by mRNA vaccines, few cases were also seen with the AstraZeneca vaccine.

EFFECT OF CORONAVIRUS DISEASE 2019 ON EMERGING VARIANTS

With 12 variants being monitored (VBM) and newer variants emerging rapidly, the latest being the EU11 strain as of June 2023, Omicron (B.1.1.529) and its descendant lineages (XBB.1.5-23A and XBB.1.16-23B, i.e., recombinants of BA.2.10.1 and BA.2.75 sublineages, i.e., BJ1 and BM.1.1.1) remain two major variants of concern (VOC). Despite several mutations in the structure of SARS-CoV-2 and growing vaccine resistance, the current vaccines are expected to render some protection because of their broader immune response therefore, ruling out the possibility of these vaccines being completely ineffective soon. Several studies have reported the effectiveness of BNT162b2 (Pfizer-BioNTech), ChAdOx1 nCoV-19 (AstraZeneca), mRNA-1273 (Moderna), and CoronaVac vaccines against the Omicron and Delta variants. However, the global focus is now shifting toward monovalent Omicron-specific vaccines latest addition to the arsenal is India's Gennova Biopharmaceuticals' GEMCOVAC-OM which is an Omicron-specific mRNA-based Booster vaccine which is stable at 2–8°C and can be easily stored in a normal refrigerator.

Changing Trends in COVID-19 Vaccination

WHO now recommends routine revaccination every 6–12 months for HCWs, elderly, immunocompromised, and those with comorbidities. Updated Mono/bi/tri-valent vaccines for specific strains are replacing ancestral COVID-19 vaccines. Yearly variant-specific booster shots for COVID-19 are becoming routine, similar to the influenza virus. Newer variants like JN.1 (BA2.86) are escaping immune barriers, so complacency and stasis are not an option.

CHALLENGES AHEAD AND FUTURE PERSPECTIVES

Breakthrough Infections

No vaccine provides 100% immunity against COVID-19, hence many cases of COVID-19 infection even after complete vaccination are being seen worldwide; however, these infections are of lesser severity as compared to those in unvaccinated populations. Hence, a vaccine providing absolute immunity against COVID-19 needs to be developed.

Peltzman Effect

Effective vaccination had resulted in a reduced perception of risk due to COVID-19 hence, the COVID preventive behavior became much relaxed leading to increased propagation of harmful COVID-19 variants hence, resulting in still looming threat of a possible outbreak in the future. Hence, learning from the past and devising appropriate tools to prevent such pandemics in future is both a challenge and a future perspective.

Herd Immunity

With the entry of newer variants and declining immune status with the passage of time herd immunity appears to be a myth. However, the concepts of hybrid immunity (combined immunity secondary to vaccine and infection) alongside the emergence of immune imprinting potentiates the prospects of achieving herd immunity.

CONCLUSION

With the rapid advent of vaccines in the arena of the COVID-19 pandemic, humanity found a silver line over the dark clouds. This helped in controlling the spread of infection and reducing morbidity and mortality secondary to COVID-associated complications. However, there is a long list of pending challenges yet to be addressed necessitating a need for persistent efforts to develop an ideal vaccine.

SUGGESTED READINGS

1. Kamath V, Nivea B. COVID-19 Vaccines: A weapon for global security. APIK J Intern Med. 2021;9(4):200-5.
2. Focosi D. From Co-Administration to Co-Formulation: The Race for New Vaccines against COVID-19 and Other Respiratory Viruses. Vaccines (Basel). 2023; 11(1):109.
3. Srivatsav S, Kamath V, Anand R, Sunil S. Study of adverse events and breakthrough infection following covid-19 vaccination. Eur J Pharm Med Res. 2023;10(1):401-6.

162

CHAPTER

Atypical Manifestations of Dengue

Shashidhara KC, Karnati Prudhveer Reddy

ABSTRACT

Aedes aegypti mosquitoes are the primary vectors of dengue fever (DF). Rapid population growth and urbanization, a lack of sanitary practices, a rise in mosquito populations, and subsequent dengue infections have all been attributed to an estimated 30-fold increase in incidence. As disease burden increases, atypical manifestations have increased as well, although most of them go unnoticed because of ignorance. Our goal was to seek DF's atypical manifestations.

Some of the atypical DF manifestations are no longer uncommon. Since several of these manifestations have the potential to be lethal, clinical vigilance for them is essential for prompt detection and treatment.

INTRODUCTION

Aedes aegypti mosquitoes are the primary vectors of dengue fever (DF). There are four different serotypes of the flavivirus family that causes dengue: DEN-1, DEN-2, DEN-3, and DEN-4. One's infection serotype provides identical serotypes with permanent immunity. An estimated 30-fold increase in prevalence of dengue infections over the previous five decades has been attributed to the multiplication of mosquitoes, rapid urbanization, and inadequate sanitary measures.

Undifferentiated fever and DF are two less serious manifestations of DF, but dengue hemorrhagic fever (DHF) and dengue shock syndrome (DSS) are significantly more serious conditions. Atypical signs have developed with rising illness load but are frequently overlooked due to ignorance. The study's objective was to check for unusual DF manifestations.

ATYPICAL MANIFESTATIONS OF DENGUE

In dengue and DHF, the endothelium is the target of the immunopathological processes. Vascular permeability and coagulation problems are the defining features. These processes can account for different types of systemic involvement. According to the World Health Organization's (WHO) guidelines for addressing DF, a range of unusual or atypical manifestations known as "*expanded dengue syndrome*" is included.

Atypical Neurological Manifestations of Dengue

Neurological involvement was first mentioned in 1976. The neurological manifestations can be grouped into three categories.

1. Mild nonspecific symptoms of headache, giddiness, inattention, slight alteration in sensorium, reduced sleep, and restlessness; postinfectious fatigue syndrome, hair loss
2. Severe syndromes of altered sensorium, lethargy, confusion, seizures, meningismus, myelitis, encephalitis, or encephalopathy
3. Delayed syndromes of paralysis of extremities, Guillain–Barré syndrome (GBS), bulbar palsy, seizures, memory impairment, sensory loss, and various psychiatric manifestations

Encephalopathy: The most common neurological manifestation is encephalopathy. It includes a clinical picture of diminished awareness that can be caused on by encephalitis and complications such liver failure, renal impairment, electrolyte imbalance, hypoxia, and shock due to coagulation disorders in DHF and DSS. Reduced sensitivity, cognitive impairment, seizures as well as personality and behavioral disorders such acute mania, sadness, emotional lability, anxiety, psychosis, and agoraphobia are also seen.

Encephalitis: Inflammation of the brain's parenchyma is usually due to infection. Fever, headache, seizures, altered sensorium, focal neurological impairments on clinical examination, focal abnormalities in neuroimaging are seen. Clinically, it might not be distinguished from encephalopathy. The virus, an antibody, or pleocytosis may be seen in the cerebrospinal fluid (CSF). Dengue encephalitis cannot be ruled out by normal CSF cellularity. In patients with viral meningitis and encephalitis in dengue-endemic areas, dengue is a key contributing factor to encephalitis with normal CSF cellularity. The most often reported serotypes to cause encephalitis are DEN-2 and DEN-3. Immunohistochemistry has been used to isolate the DEN-4 virus from the medulla and cerebellum.

Myelitis: Peripheral nerve system involvement by the dengue virus (DENV) is rarely reported. DENV has been linked to mononeuropathies like phrenic neuropathy, long thoracic neuropathy, isolated Bell's palsy, abducens nerve palsy, and oculomotor palsy as well as acute polyradiculopathy, lumbosacral plexopathy, GBS, Miller Fisher syndrome, and others. Acute disseminated encephalomyelitis (ADEM), postinfectious myelopathy, or transverse myelitis are possible symptoms. In the acute stage of the illness, it may manifest as flaccidity, and in the delayed stage as spasticity. Intrathecal production of dengue immunoglobulin G (IgG) antibodies provides evidence that the pathogenesis is due to immune-mediated processes and direct virus invasion.

Guillain-Barré syndrome: GBS is seen during recover stage of illness due to an abnormal immune response that damages the nerves. According to reports, GBS is the most typical form of dengue in the peripheral nerve system. The cause of this is molecular mimicry. Tumor necrosis factor (TNF), interleukins (ILs), and complement proteins are examples of proinflammatory cytokines that are important in the destruction of peripheral nerve components like myelin or axons.

Atypical Renal Manifestations of Dengue

In cases of DF, acute renal failure typically manifests as shock-induced acute tubular necrosis. If these people are not identified in the earliest possible stage, there is a likelihood that they might develop renal failure.

Proteinuria, hematuria, rhabdomyolysis, and acute kidney injury (AKI) are common renal manifestations. AKI may have a considerable impact on mortality and morbidity. Raised serum creatinine, proteinuria, glomerulonephritis, and hemolytic uremic syndrome (HUS) are some of the manifestations of AKI. Clinically severe AKI is less frequent in DHF, despite the fact that a slight increase in serum creatinine is typical. Other risk factors include concomitant bacteremia. rhabdomyolysis, HUS, and acute glomerulonephritis are potential etiopathogenesis contributors.

Atypical Cardiovascular Manifestations of Dengue Fever

During episodes of DHF, cardiac rhythm abnormalities like atrioventricular blocks, atrial fibrillation, sinus node dysfunction, and ectopic ventricular beats have been described. Clinical cardiac symptoms can range from mild, potentially lethal myocarditis, to severe, life-threatening signs. Direct viral invasion, immune system damage due to cytokines, or both may cause myocardial involvement. The severity of the disease may be correlated with myopericarditis and myocarditis. According to studies, the arrhythmia and reduced left ventricular function cause raised resting diastolic myocardial calcium ion levels and elevated CPK-MB (creatine phosphokinase-myocardial band) levels.

Investigations show alterations in the electrocardiogram (ECG), including sinus tachycardia, sinus bradycardia, T wave inversions, and heart block, as well as changes in the two-dimensional echocardiogram (ECHO), including systolic and diastolic dysfunction, and increased cardiac enzymes (such as troponin T and CPK-MB). Due to the high rate of cardiac involvement in dengue patients, cardiac screening with ECG, ECHO, and CPK-MB levels should be performed on all dengue patients.

Atypical Respiratory Manifestations of Dengue

Acute lung injury (ALI) and acute respiratory distress syndrome (ARDS) are one of the dreaded complications of DHF, secondary to increased alveolar and interstitial edema caused by permeability of the alveolar–capillary membrane. To stop DSS from progressing to ARDS, it is essential to restore adequate tissue perfusion as soon as possible. Equal caution must be taken to prevent excessive fluid infusion after adequate volume replacement, as fluid overload can trigger ARDS.

Pulmonary hemorrhage is another deadly complication to be on the lookout for in these patients. Pleural effusion, pneumonitis, noncardiogenic pulmonary edema (ARDS), and hemorrhage/hemoptysis are possible manifestations. In endemic locations, DSS is listed as the third most common cause of ARDS. Increased levels of von Willebrand factor, tissue factor, tissue plasminogen activator, plasminogen activator inhibitor-1, and fractional catabolic rate of fibrinogen can cause thromboembolic events, which can result in pulmonary embolism. Bilateral pleural effusions and areas of ground-glass opacity or consolidation are the most frequent imaging findings.

Ocular Manifestations

Ocular involvement is now being reported increasingly, with most conditions resolving spontaneously. Ocular findings encompass a spectrum from subconjunctival hemorrhage to complications such as optic neuropathy and panophthalmitis leading to permanent impairment of vision in certain cases. Ocular complications comprise dengue maculopathy, retinal edema, retinal hemorrhages, optic disc swelling, and vitritis **(Fig. 1)**.

It usually occurs bilaterally with macular involvement. When patients with severe episodes of hypotension or encephalopathy are present with ocular symptoms, anterior ischemic optic neuropathy should be suspected. Other rare lesions include superficial punctate erosions, keratitis, scleritis, cotton wool spots, oculomotor palsies, optic neuropathies, neuromyelitis optica, neurogenic ptosis, and significant permanent visual deficits.

Atypical Gastrointestinal Manifestations of Dengue

The most important DF symptoms are those involving the abdomen. They were observed in two-thirds of patients. Dyspepsia, abdominal pain, nausea, and vomiting made up most symptoms. As a physician, one must be extremely alert for symptoms like abdominal pain and vomiting since they are early warning signs to severe dengue. Dengue's gastrointestinal manifestations, includes hepatitis, fulminant hepatic failure, acalculous cholecystitis, acute pancreatitis, and febrile diarrhea. DENV antigen is found in Kupffer cells and sinusoidal lining cells in the liver. Hepatocytes harboring dengue antigen virus may facilitate viral replication. Acute hepatitis symptoms, such as pain in the hypochondrium, hepatomegaly, jaundice, and elevated aminotransferase levels, may serve as indicators to identify hepatic abnormalities.

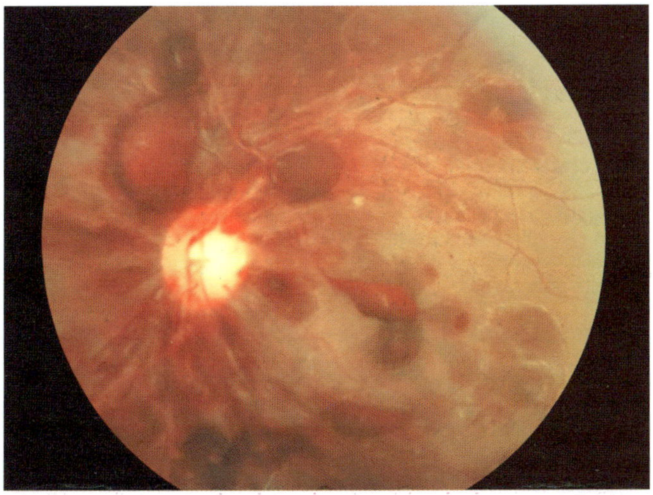

FIG. 1: Fundus photograph showing extensive retinal and preretinal hemorrhages.

Acute liver failure predisposes to encephalopathy, disseminated intravascular coagulation, and fatal hemorrhage. An early sign of dengue infection is a rise in aminotransferases, which has been linked to an increase in disease severity. An unusual DF consequence is acute pancreatitis. Other manifestations include subacute intestinal obstruction, bilateral enlargement of the parotid gland, acalculous cholecystitis, and "febrile diarrhea".

Atypical Musculoskeletal Complications of Dengue Fever

Dengue fever has been described classically as break bone fever as it causes severe muscle, joint, and bone pain. Muscle biopsy samples have been studied, and a variety of results have been found, ranging from mild lymphocytic infiltrate to foci of severe myonecrosis. If left untreated, rhabdomyolysis can result in acute renal failure and electrolyte imbalances.

Pure motor weakness may be found in dengue patients. In cases where electromyography and muscle biopsy results are compatible with myositis and creatinine phosphokinase is high, the differential diagnosis of acute flaccid paralysis should take myositis-related acute pure motor quadriplegia into consideration.

Myositis: This is characterized by widespread skeletal muscle inflammation occurs due to viremia-induced cytokines like TNF leading to severe inflammation and eventual damage to muscle fibers. Its severity can range from mild, self-limiting muscle weakness to severe dengue myositis, which can cause quadriplegia and in rare cases, respiratory failure. Common features include an increased CPK, normal deep tendon reflexes, and soreness while stretching the calf and thigh muscles.

Lymphoreticular Complications of Dengue

Dengue virus antigen is found predominantly in cells of the spleen, thymus, and lymph nodes. There are few reported cases of splenic rupture and infarction of lymph node. There may be subcapsular hematomas in a congestive spleen. In endemic areas, one to be on the lookout for is splenic rupture, **(Fig. 2)** a rare but lethal consequence.

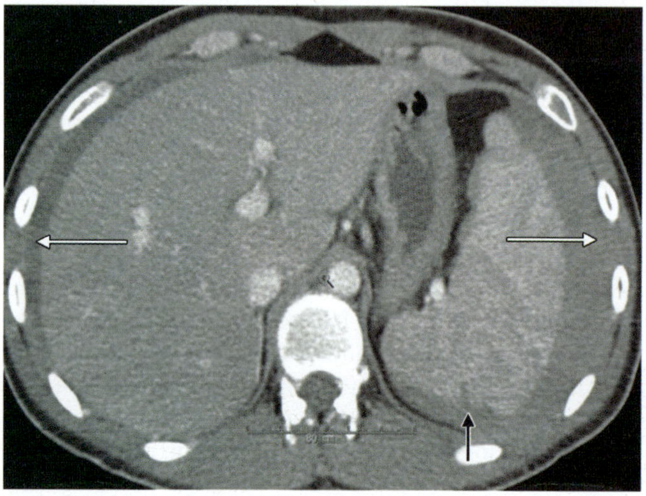

FIG. 2: Computed tomography of the patient's abdomen demonstrating splenic laceration (black arrow) and free fluid in abdomen (white arrows).

A rare consequence known as hemophagocytic lymphohistiocytosis (HLH) is characterized by the activation and unregulated nonmalignant proliferation of T cells and macrophages, which causes a cytokine storm. Fever, hepatosplenomegaly, multiorgan failure, and fulminant pancytopenia approaching severe sepsis are all features of the presentation. A suspicion of HLH is aroused in dengue patients by the persistence of fever for longer than 7 days, chronic progressive cytopenias, elevated ferritin, and organomegaly.

CONCLUSION

Since atypical manifestations of DF are no longer a rare condition and will continue to increase, clinicians should have a high index of suspicion to identify and promptly manage **(Fig. 3)**. It is possible that the atypical manifestations mentioned here go unreported and unrecognized. However, considering the global health issue that dengue poses, it is essential to be aware of all these manifestations for clinical diagnosis and effective care. As a result, they ought to be covered under the case definition for severe dengue. Even in the absence of shock, they require immediate detection and active treatment.

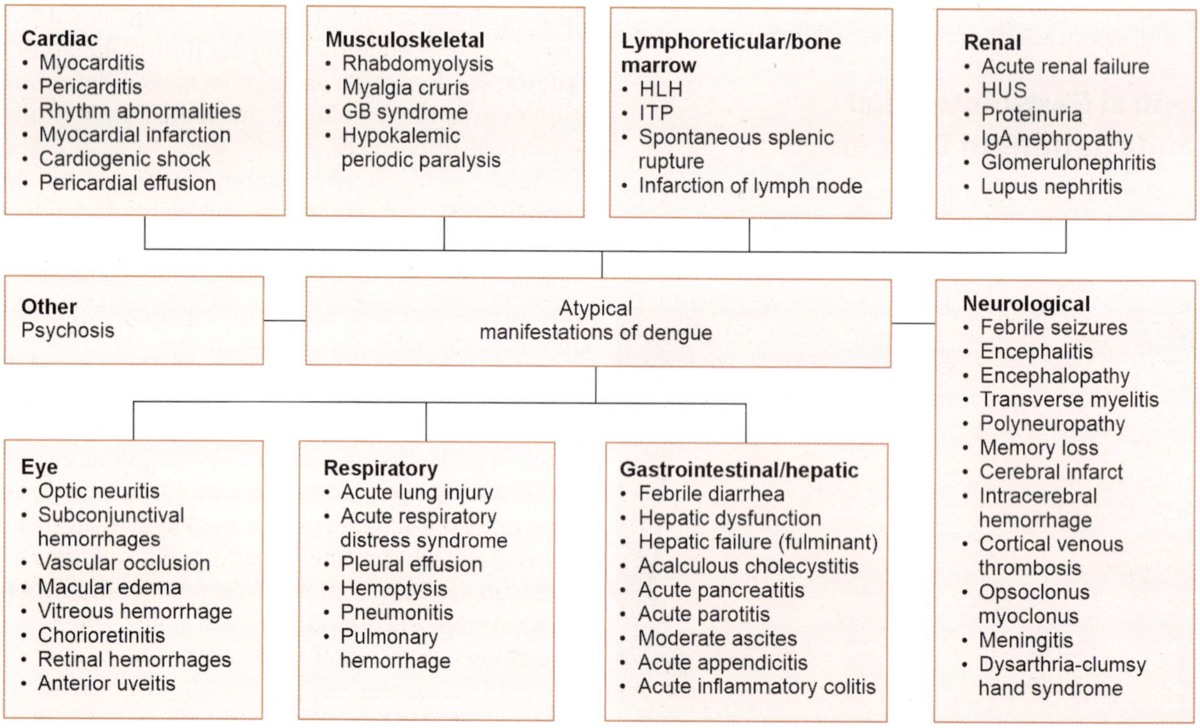

FIG. 3: Atypical manifestations of dengue.

(GB: Guillain–Barré; HLH: hemophagocytic lymphohistiocytosis; HUS: hemolytic uremic syndrome; IgA: immunoglobulin A; ITP: immune thrombocytopenic purpura)

SUGGESTED READINGS

1. World Health Organization. Comprehensive guideline for prevention and control of dengue and dengue haemorrhagic fever.
2. Prabhat N, Ray S, Chakravarty K, Kathuria H, Saravana S, Singh D, et al. Atypical neurological manifestations of dengue fever: A case series and mini review. Postgrad Med J. 2020;96(1142):759-65.
3. Garg RK, Malhotra HS, Jain A, Malhotra KP. Dengue-associated neuromuscular complications. Neurol India. 2015;63(4):497.
4. Malheiros SM, Oliveira AS, Schmidt B, Lima JG, Gabbai AA. Dengue. Muscle biopsy findings in 15 patients. Arq Neuropsiquiatr. 1993;51(2):159-64.
5. Gulati S, Maheshwari A. Atypical manifestations of dengue. Trop Med Int Health. 2007;12(9):1087-95.
6. Biswas S, Kumar P, Tansir G, Biswas A. Case report: Cardiac tamponade in dengue hemorrhagic fever: An unusual manifestation of a common disease. Am J Trop Med Hyg. 2019;101:448-50.
7. Abhinayaa J, James S, Jebaraj R, Vinoth PN. Incidence of cardiac manifestations in children with dengue fever: A cross-sectional study. Rambam Maimonides Med J. 2021;12:e0014.
8. Gupta S, Singh L, Tandon R. Study of pulmonary manifestations among dengue patients in tertiary care hospital of North India. Int J Contemp Med Res. 2020;7:1-5.
9. de Almeida RR, Paim B, de Oliveira SA, Souza AS Jr, Gomes AC, Escuissato DL, et al. Dengue hemorrhagic fever: A state-of-the-art review focused in pulmonary involvement. Lung. 2017;195:389-95.
10. Poletto F, Cerruti L, Spiezia L. Dengue fever as a rare cause of pulmonary embolism. J Thromb Thrombolysis. 2020;49(4):690-3.
11. Karoli R, Fatima J, Siddiqi Z, Kazmi KI, Sultania AR. Clinical profile of dengue infection at a teaching hospital in North India. J Infect Dev Ctries. 2012;6(7):551-4.
12. World Health Organization. (2009). Dengue: Guidelines for Diagnosis, Treatment, Prevention and Control. [online] Available from https://iris.who.int/bitstream/handle/10665/44188/9789241547871_eng.pdf?sequence=1 [Last accessed December, 2023].
13. Nimmagadda SS, Mahabala C, Boloor A, Raghuram PM, Nayak A. Atypical manifestations of dengue fever (DF)—where do we stand today? J Clin Diagn Res. 2014;8(1):71.
14. Sharma N, Mahi S, Bhalla A, Singh V, Varma S, Ratho RK. Dengue fever related acalculous cholecystitis in a North Indian Tertiary Care Hospital. J Gastroenterol Hepatol. 2006;21(4):664-7.
15. Gulati S, Maheshwari A. Atypical manifestations of dengue. Trop Med Int Health. 2007;12:1087-95.
16. Mohanty B, Sunder A, Pathak S. Clinicolaboratory profile of expanded dengue syndrome—our experience in a teaching hospital. Fam Med Prim Care. 2019;8:1022-7.
17. Verma R, Sahu R, Holla V. Neurological manifestations of dengue infection: A review. J Neurol Sci. 2014;346:26-34.

163

CHAPTER

Treatment and Target of Dengue Infection

Surendra Kumar, Ajaypal Singh, Abdul Haroon Shah, Anusha Yadav, Manisha

ABSTRACT

Dengue viruses (DENV) are flaviviruses, transmitted by mosquitos. DENV infection causes dengue fever, dengue hemorrhagic fever, and dengue shock syndrome. It is estimated that a third of the world's population is at risk for infection, with an estimated 390 million infections annually. With increasing geographic spread, frequency, and magnitude of outbreaks, dengue continues to pose a major public health threat worldwide. Dengue fever is one of the major health problems in India. Infection with any of the four dengue virus serotypes results in a diverse range of symptoms, from mild undifferentiated fever to life-threatening hemorrhagic fever and shock. Interaction with specific receptor(s) at the cell surface is one of the first events in the pathogenesis of DENV. However, relatively little is known about these receptors. Cellular receptors in human monocytes and mouse neural cells are main target for the viral infection. The envelope protein of the virus (E-protein) plays an important role in attachment of virus to target cells and their interaction with cellular receptors. The modulation of receptor gene(s) and/or protein(s) can be used as a method for interfering with virus entry and can thus become a new method for disease prevention. DENV infection elicits such a broad range of clinical symptoms, early and accurate laboratory diagnosis is essential for appropriate patient management.

INTRODUCTION

Dengue, an acute febrile illness, is caused by infection with any of four related single-stranded RNA viruses of the genus *Flavivirus*, dengue virus 1, 2, 3, or 4 (DENV-1 to 4). Infection with one DENV confers long-term immunity to that virus but conveys only short-lived protection against the other DENVs. The risk for severe dengue is greater during a second DENV infection; although severe dengue also can occur during the first, third, or fourth infection.

TRANSMISSION

Almost all DENV transmission occurs through the bite of infected *Aedes* species mosquitoes, primarily *Aedes aegypti* and *Aedes albopictus.*

EPIDEMIOLOGY

Dengue is endemic throughout the tropics and subtropics and occurs in >100 countries and destinations worldwide.

PHASES OF SYMPTOMATIC DENGUE

1. *Febrile phase:* Fever typically lasts 2–7 days and can be biphasic. Other signs and symptoms include severe headache; retro-orbital pain; bone, joint, and muscle pain; macular or maculopapular rash; and minor hemorrhagic manifestations, including ecchymosis, epistaxis, bleeding gums, hematuria, petechiae, purpura, or a positive tourniquet test result.
2. *Critical phase:* The critical phase of dengue begins at defervescence and typically lasts 24–48 hours. Most patients improve clinically during this phase, but those with substantial plasma leak (resulting from marked increase in vascular permeability) progress to severe dengue.
3. *Convalescent phase:* As plasma leakage subsides, patients enter the convalescent phase and well-being improves; extravasated intravenous fluids and abdominal and pleural effusions are reabsorbed, hemodynamic status stabilizes.

LABORATORY DIAGNOSIS

Antigen Detection

- ELISA and ICT methods are available for detection of NS1 antigen.
- NS1 is highly specific and becomes detectable from day 1 of fever and remains positive up to 9 days.

Antibody Detection

- IgM antibody appears after 5 days of fever and disappear within 90 days.
- IgG antibody is detectable in 14–21 days and slowly increases.
- In secondary infections IgG titers increases rapidly.
- *MAC-ELISA (IgM antibody capture ELISA)*: It's the recommended serological test in India, all positive RDT of dengue must be confirmed by ELISA.

Other methods are virus isolation, molecular methods like RT-PCR and genotype detection **(Fig. 1)**.

TARGET IN DENGUE TREATMENT

- Manage hematological manifestation.
- Manage cardiac complication.
- Manage renal complication.
- Manage hepatitis and liver failure.
- Manage respiratory complication.
- Manage neurological complication.

ASSESSMENT

Dengue fever is assessed by considering warning signs, the presence of comorbidities, and subsequently categorizing the findings into specific groups **(Flowchart 1)**.

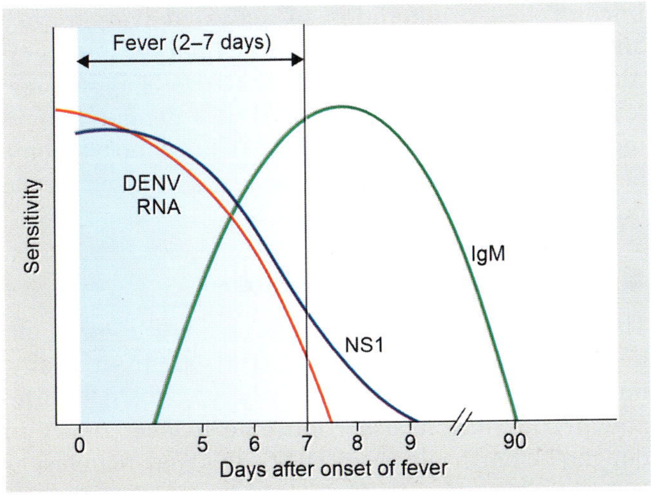

FIG. 1: Dengue viruses RNA nonstructural protein 1 (NS1) antigen, immunoglobulin M (IgM)-antibody enzyme-linked immunosorbent assay (ELISA).

Management of Group A

Outpatient management is provided to patients devoid of warning signs and maintaining vital stability, while attentively monitoring for any potential progression into the critical phase **(Flowchart 2)**.

Management of Group B

Patients exhibiting warning signs, assigned to Group B, undergo inpatient management primarily focusing on the administration of intravenous fluids. This approach includes continuous monitoring of vital signs, vigilant observation for early signs of shock, and periodic reassessment of hematocrit levels **(Flowchart 3)**.

Management of Group C

Patients experiencing dengue shock are classified under Group C, necessitating admission to the ICU. In this setting, their hemodynamic status is closely monitored every 1–2 hours, and aggressive fluid administration is implemented (**Flowcharts 4 and 5**).

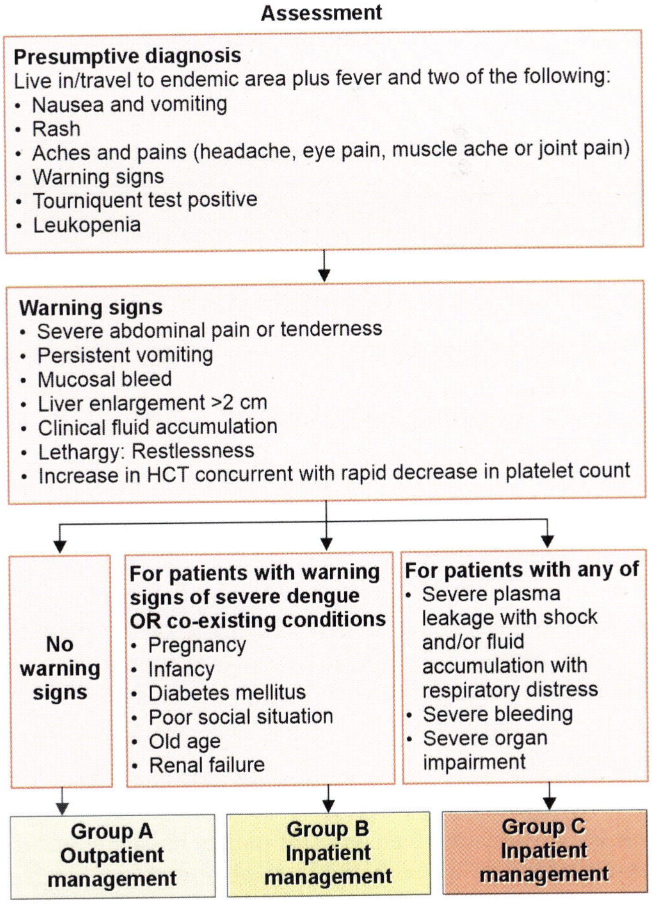

FLOWCHART 1: Dengue case management.
(HCT: hematocrit)

During the febrile phase (may last 2–7 days) and subsequent critical phase (1–2 days), your clinic should

- Follow CBCs
- Watch for dehydration
- Watch for warning signs, including decreasing platelet count and increasing hematocrit
- Watch for defervescence (indicating beginning of critical phase)

Advise patient or their family to do the following:

Control the fever

- Give acetaminophen every 6 hours (maximum 4 doses per day). Do not give ibuprofen, aspirin, or aspirin-containing drugs.
- Sponge patient's skin with tepid water when temperature is high.

Prevent dehydration which occurs when a person loses too much fluid (from high fever, vomiting, or poor oral intake). Give plenty of fluids (not only water) and watch for signs of dehydration. Bring patient to clinic or emergency room if any of the following signs develop:

- Decrease in urination (check number of wet diapers or trips to the bathroom)
- Few or no tears when child cries
- Dry mouth, tongue or lips
- Sunken eyes
- Listlessness, agitation, or confusion
- Fast heartbeat (>100/minute)
- Cold or clammy fingers and toes
- Sunken fontanel in an infant

Prevent spread of dengue within your house

- Place patient under bed net or have patient use insect repellent while febrile to avoid infecting mosquitoes that can infect others within 2 weeks.
- KILL all mosquitoes in house
- Empty containers that carry water on patio
- Put screens on windows and doors to prevent mosquitoes from coming into house

Watch for warning signs as temperature declines 3–8 days after symptoms began. Return IMMEDIATELY to clinic or emergency department if any of the following warning signs appear:

- Severe abdominal pain or persistent vomiting
- Red spots/patches on skin
- Bleeding from nose or gums
- Vomiting blood
- Black, tarry stools
- Drowsiness or irritability
- Pale, cold, or clammy skin
- Difficulty breathing

FLOWCHART 2: Group A: Outpatient management.

Hematological Complication

Thrombocytopenia: Several causes have been implicated in causing thrombocytopenia in dengue.

- Bone marrow suppression with attenuation of megakaryocyte maturation.
- Peripheral destruction of platelets through activation of complement cascade, antibody-mediated destruction, and phagocytosis.

Prophylactic platelet transfusion: Several studies in adult dengue patients have shown that prophylactic platelet transfusion had no significant benefit over supportive care alone, and it did not prevent bleeding or hasten platelet recovery. Consider transfusing platelets once the count is $<10,000/mm^3$.

Platelet transfusion in patients with minor and major bleeds: Do transfuse platelets if the patient has acute severe mucosal bleed, which is not controlled with supportive care. A cut-off immature platelet fraction (IPF) level of ≥10% predicts platelet recovery within the next 72 hours.

Hemophagocytic lymphohistiocytosis (HLH): Secondary HLH is a potentially fatal complication of dengue characterized by a hyperinflammatory state due to the uncontrolled proliferation of activated lymphocytes and the production of proinflammatory cytokines. Although the clinical features may be overlapping, some features that could suggest HLH in a dengue patient include persistent fever, persistent thrombocytopenia beyond 10 days, hyperferritinemia, and elevated lactate dehydrogenase (LDH) levels.

Hepatitis and Liver Failure

The dengue virus has a direct cytopathic effect on hepatocytes causing their apoptosis. Additionally, immune-mediated hepatocyte injury, cytokine storm, and hypoperfusion also contribute to liver injury in dengue hemorrhagic fever (DHF). This may manifest as hepatomegaly, jaundice, elevated transaminases, and acute liver failure (ALF). Management is similar to that of ALF due to other causes.

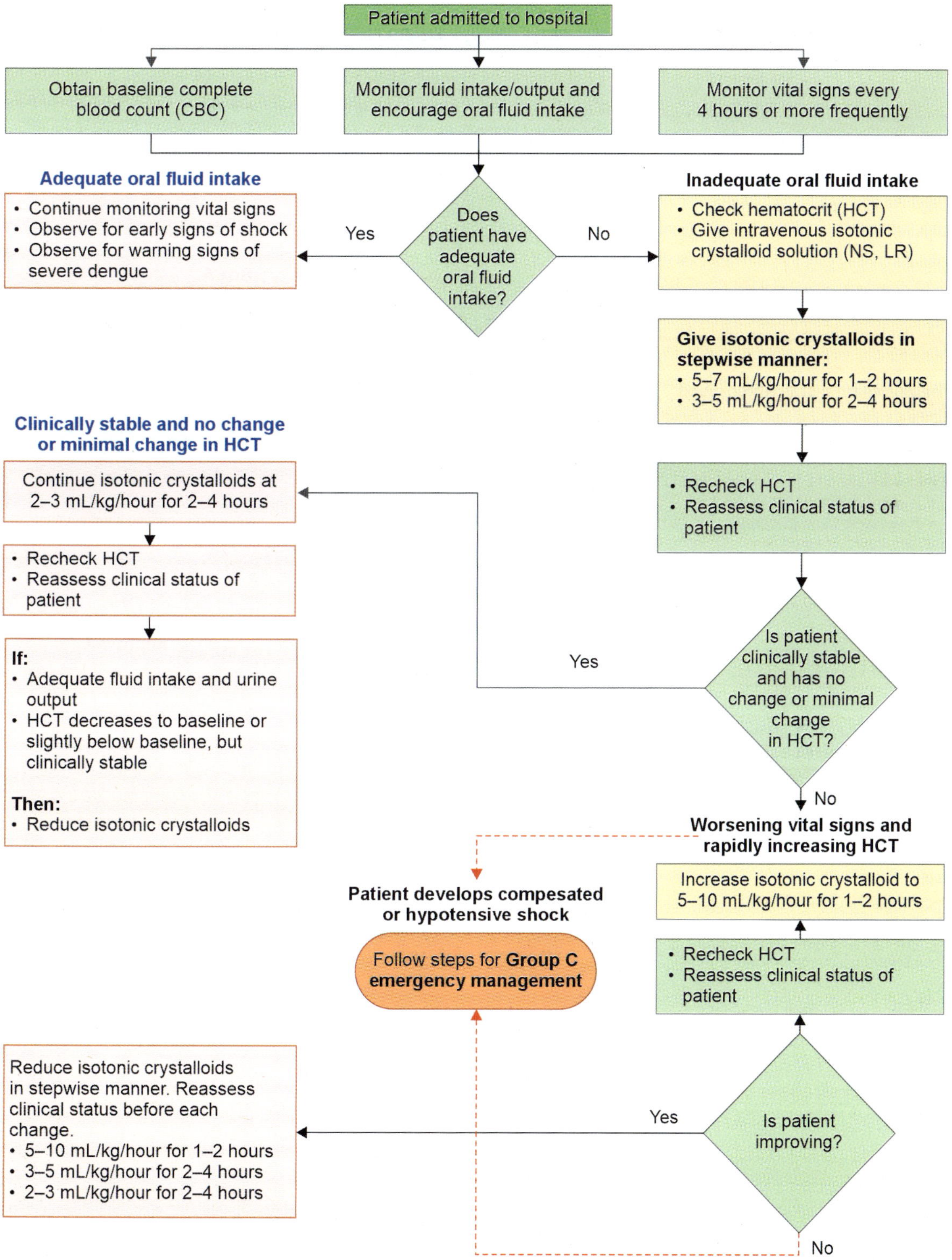

FLOWCHART 3: Group B: Inpatient management for dengue patients with warning signs.
(NS: normal saline; RL: Ringer's lactate)

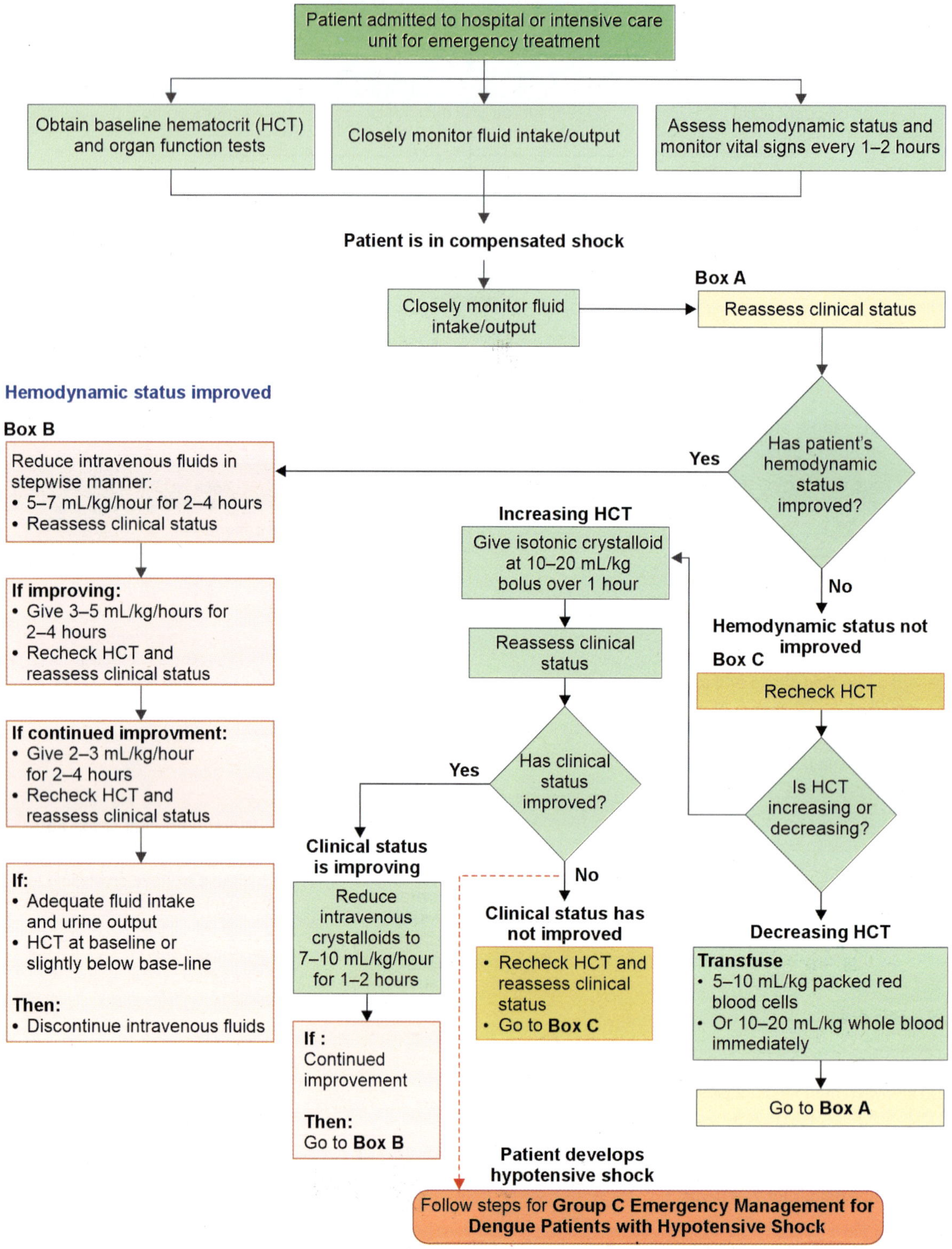

FLOWCHART 4: Group: Emergency management for dengue patients with compensated shock.

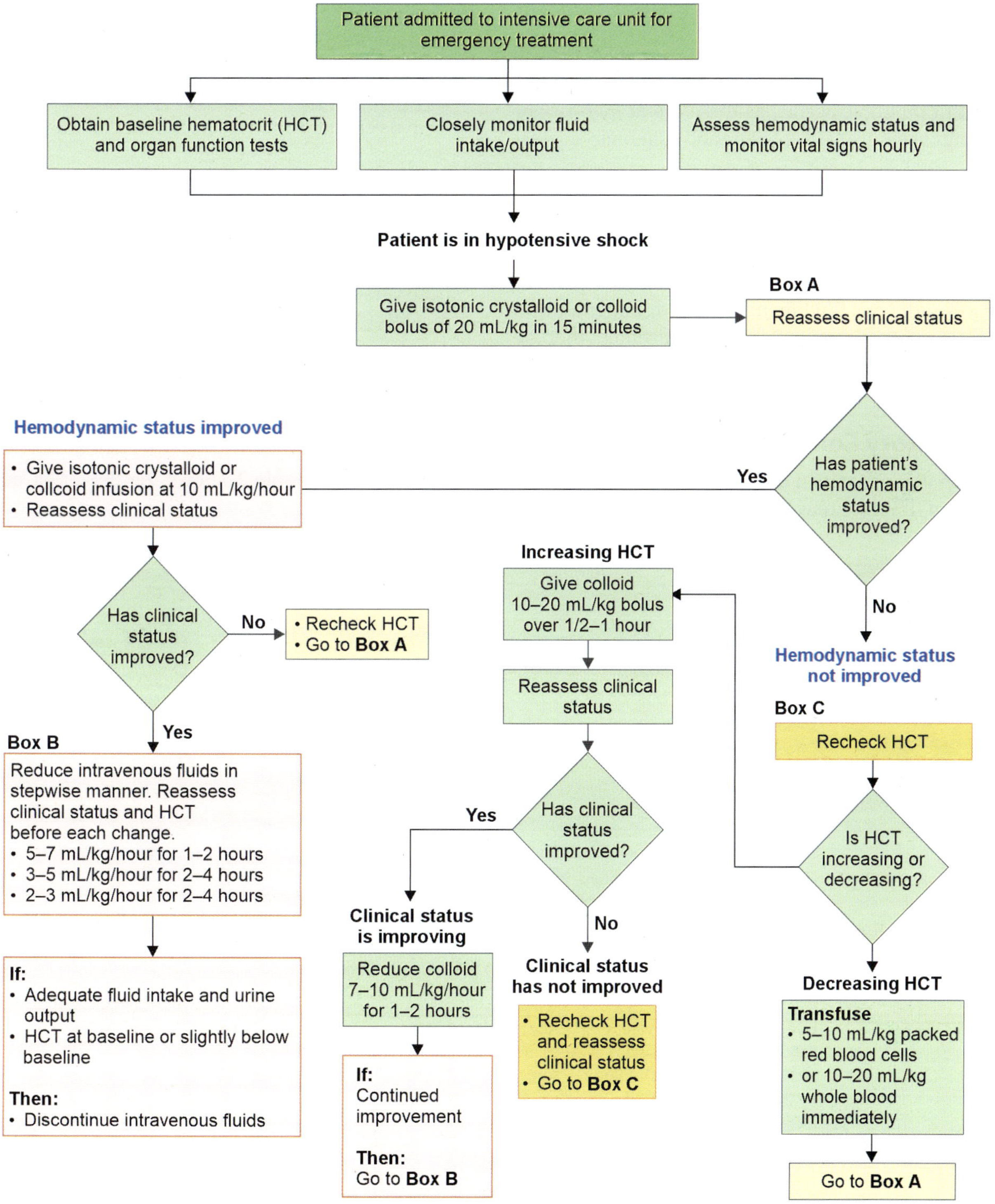

FLOWCHART 5: Group C: Emergency management for dengue patients with hypotensive shock.

Cardiac Complications

Dengue patients with myocarditis and cardiogenic shock need extremely careful fluid resuscitation followed by early initiation of inotropic agents, as these are at high risk of developing congestive cardiac failure and pulmonary edema.

Acute Kidney Injury

Hypoperfusion, rhabdomyolysis, and hemolysis, apart from the direct effects of DENV and immune-mediated injury may lead to renal impairment in dengue. Management comprises judicious fluid management to target a urine output > 0.5 mL/kg/h and early renal replacement therapy when indicated. Continuous venovenous hemofiltration (CVVH) is the preferred modality.

Respiratory Complications

Pleural tap is best avoided in dengue; rarely, therapeutic pleural fluid drainage may be needed in situations where massive pleural effusion leads to an inability to ventilate the patient. Patients with refractory shock have to be intubated and mechanically ventilated. Few patients may develop acute respiratory distress syndrome (ARDS); lung protective ventilation should be initiated in this setting.

Neurological Complication

- *Dengue encephalopathy, encephalitis, Intracranial hemorrhage, immune-mediated syndromes:* Acute transverse myelitis, acute disseminated encephalomyelitis (ADEM), neuromyelitis optica;
- *Neuromuscular:* Guillain-Barré syndrome (GBS), transient muscle dysfunctions, rhabdomyolysis, and neuro-ophthalmic complications. They are managed accordingly.

Dengue vaccine: Table 1 shows the details of dengue vaccines.

TABLE 1: Details of dengue vaccine.

Vaccine/Candidate vaccine	Description	Efficacy/Immune response	Current status
1. Dengvaxia (CYD-TDV)	Live-attenuated, chimeric, tetravalent vaccine built on a yellow fever 17D backbone Developed by Sanofi Pasteur	• Vaccine efficacy against confirmed dengue pooled across two trials was 59.2% in the year following the primary series (per protocol analysis) • During this initial time period, pooled vaccine efficacy against severe dengue was 79.1%	• Phase 3 trials completed • Marketed in some countries
2. TAK-003	Tetravalent dengue vaccine candidate, based on a live-attenuated dengue serotype-2 virus, which provides the genetic "backbone" for all four vaccine viruses Developed by Takeda	Primary efficacy data from part 1 of the TIDES trial showed an overall efficacy to be over 80%. Cumulative efficacy after 3 years of vaccination is 62% (95% CI 56.6–66.7) against virologically confirmed dengue (VCD) and 83.6% (76.8–88.4) against hospitalized VCD	Currently undergoing phase 3 trials; demonstrated efficacy regardless of serostatus before immunization
3. TVOO3/TV005	Live-attenuated tetravalent vaccine developed using recombinant DNA technology by the US NIH's National Institute of Allergy and Infectious Diseases (NIAID)	A single dose of the vaccine has been shown to induce immune response against all four serotypes in 70–90% of flavivirus-naive recipients	Currently undergoing phase 2 trials

SUGGESTED READINGS

1. Sánchez-González L, Adams L, Paz-Bailey G. (2024). Center for Disease Control and Prevention. Dengue: CDC Yellow Book 2024. [online] Available from https://wwwnc.cdc.gov/travel/yellowbook/2024/infections-diseases/dengue [Last accessed January, 2024].
2. Centers for Disease Control and Prevention Guideline. https://www.cdc.gov/dengue/resources/dengue-clinician-guide_508.pdf.
3. Tayal A, Kabra SK, Lodha R. Management of Dengue: An Updated Review. Indian J Pediatr. 2023;90(2):168-77.

164
CHAPTER

The Challenge of Diagnosing and Treating Melioidosis

Avik Chakraborty, Arkadip Choudhury

ABSTRACT

Melioidosis is caused by *Burkholderia pseudomallei*, a facultative intracellular gram-negative bacterium. Southeast Asia forms the heartland of the disease with an increasing number of cases reported from India in recent years. With a wide variety of clinical presentations and radiological features and hardly any specific for itself, melioidosis more often than not mimics an equally large gamut of other diseases. Diagnosis of melioidosis therefore requires a high index of clinical suspicion with a robust laboratory infrastructure for microbiological confirmation which also ensures the initiation and an appropriate treatment regimen at the earliest to minimize both morbidity and mortality associated with the disease.

INTRODUCTION

First reported by pathologist Alfred Whitmore and his assistant Krishnaswami in 1912 during autopsy of beggars and morphine addicts at erstwhile *Rangoon*, presently Myanmar, melioidosis has now broken its usual boundaries of endemicity once limited to Southeast Asia (approximately 44% of disease burden) including India, Northern Australia, and China to almost all the continents.

Melioidosis is caused by *Burkholderia pseudomallei*, a facultative intracellular gram-negative bacterium. It is a widely distributed environmental saprophyte found to be present in soil and fresh surface water in endemic regions. Transmission to humans occurs mainly by contact with infested soil or water through wounds (inoculation), inhalation, or ingestion with person-to-person or animal-to-human transmission being extremely rare. Cases of mother-to-infant transmission in the setting of *B. pseudomallei* mastitis have however been reported as have been laboratory-acquired infections and iatrogenic infections from contaminated hospital or surgical instruments although all of these contribute to a rather small fraction of reported cases.

EPIDEMIOLOGY

Based on a mathematical model published in 2016, about 1,65,000 people are infected by melioidosis every year, of which approximately 89,000 die. Within South Asia, Bangladesh and Sri Lanka are considered endemic for melioidosis; a few cases have been reported each from Nepal and Pakistan. India has experienced an increase in numbers of melioidosis cases in the recent years.

Most infections with *B. pseudomallei* are either asymptomatic or subclinical. Of the symptomatic cases, most (more than 80%) present with acute infection (within 2 months of diagnosis) with overall mortality ranging from 10 to 40%.

The incubation period for acute melioidosis ranges from 4 to 12 days with a mean incubation period of 9 days. Persons experiencing near-drowning in contaminated water can develop symptoms as early as within 24 hours.

Once symptoms persist beyond 2 months, it is referred to as chronic melioidosis and accounts for around 10% cases of symptomatic disease. Chronic infections tend to be more indolent and are associated with significantly lower mortality of about 2%.

Uncommonly (<5%), however, *B. pseudomallei* infections can remain latent for variable periods of time only to activate subsequently, quite analogous to tuberculosis.

CLINICAL FEATURES

Melioidosis is characterized by a wide variety of highly nonspecific clinical features earning it the nickname of "the great mimicker." A brief description of the varied clinical features of melioidosis is furnished in **Box 1**.

DIAGNOSIS

In endemic regions, melioidosis should be routinely considered as a differential diagnosis in any case with of any of the above clinical features. Outside endemic regions, melioidosis should be suspected in those with similar clinical features and having a history of travel to either an endemic zone or a place with an increasing number of reported cases. The possibility of chronic melioidosis or rarely activation of a latent infection should also be considered in those individuals who have an

BOX 1: Clinical features of melioidosis.

Pneumonia

In acute setting:

Very similar to community-acquired pneumonia, characterized by fever with rigors, productive cough, and respiratory distress with or without shock

Chest X-rays may show anything from discrete, patchy, or even diffuse consolidations involving single or multiple lobes to necrotizing lesions, pleural effusions, and even cavitary lesions with abscesses showing fluid levels. Mediastinal lymphadenopathy related to inhalational melioidosis has also been reported, although unlike tuberculosis, calcification of the nodes is rather uncommon

In chronic setting:

Presents similar to tuberculosis with chronic cough, purulent sputum, hemoptysis, and night sweats

Chest X-rays show cavitating, nodular, or streaky infiltrates with fibrotic changes, all of which can be found in those with pulmonary TB with upper lobe consolidation being specially common

Skin infections

Nonspecific features such as skin ulcers, abscesses, pustules, furuncles, crusted erythematous lesions, macular lesions, and rarely diffuse cellulitis.

Failure to respond to conventional antibiotic therapies targeting the usual skin pathogens raises suspicion

Genitourinary infections

Prostatic infections or abscesses, renal abscesses, and urinary tract infections with nonspecific symptoms such as fever with suprapubic pain, dysuria, and difficulty in passing urine or frank retention requiring catheterization

Presence of associated diarrhea can hint toward genitourinary melioidosis although it is not a hallmark

Neurological involvement

Meningitis, meningoencephalitis, encephalomyelitis, isolated myelitis, cerebral and epidural abscesses primarily effecting the brainstem resulting in UMN type of limb weakness, cerebellar signs, cranial nerve (particularly VIth, VIIth) palsies, bulbar palsy, and even flaccid paraparesis with an almost intact level of consciousness during early parts of presentation.

CSF examination reveals leukocytosis in ranges of 30–775 cells/cumm with monocytic pleocytosis and elevated protein with normal or slightly decreased sugar levels while cultures often grow nothing.

MRI shows a notable increase in T2-weighted signal intensities in the region of the brainstem in cases of encephalomyelitis and in the spinal cord in patients with flaccid paraparesis. CT scan reveals no significant finding

Other presentations

Solid organ or parenchymal abscesses in the liver and spleen (often multifocal) associated with fever with chills and rigor. *Symptoms are seldom localizing*

Suppurative parotitis characterized by parotid pain, swelling and tenderness seen especially in children of South Asian origin, partly explained by the ingestion of contaminated water

Septic arthritis of lower limb (most common), upper limbs, vertebra, and pelvis with or without associated osteomyelitis

Mycotic aneurysms

Primary bacteremia in the absence of any localized sign of infection

(CSF: cerebrospinal fluid; TB: tuberculosis; UMN: upper motor neuron)

association with endemic areas and are being evaluated for suspected pulmonary TB.

Sample Collection

Once melioidosis is suspected, specimens from the following sites need to be collected:

- Blood
- Sputum or deep respiratory secretions
- Urine
- Throat swab
- Rectal swab
- Swab from any ulcer or skin lesion
- Pus or fluid from drainable collection or abscess
- Cerebrospinal fluid (CSF) from individuals with features of encephalitis or meningitis

Any and all samples thus collected need to be subjected to both microscopy and culture with culture being the primary method of diagnosis.

Microscopy

Gram staining of sputum samples or purulent drainage form abscesses reveals gram-negative bacilli, while those from culture isolates often show a characteristic bipolar staining giving it a safety pin-like appearance. However, Gram stain alone is not diagnostic.

Culture

A positive culture for *B. pseudomallei* from any site is diagnostic. Blood cultures give positive results in up to 70% cases. *B. pseudomallei* tend to grow readily in standard blood cultures. But the use of selective media such as MacConkey agar, blood agar, and chocolate agar ensures a better growth of the organism. If a sample is collected from a nonsterile site in which case the commensal flora may outgrow *B. pseudomallei*, use of Ashdown agar containing gentamicin or Ashdown liquid transport broth containing colistin enhances the recovery of *B. pseudomallei*. Automated blood culture systems can detect *B. pseudomallei* as early as within 24 hours; however, such systems possess lower sensitivity (~74%) as compared to conventional broth cultures (~90%).

A timely transport of the specimen and maintaining cultures at close to body temperatures (~37°C) is of utmost importance here, as low temperatures during transport and desiccation decrease the viability of *B. pseudomallei*. In fact, samples collected from throat, rectum, or skin lesion are preferably inoculated or plated directly if possible and clinical laboratories are made aware of the same in cases where melioidosis is suspected.

Postculture Identification

Identification of *B. pseudomallei* from culture isolates is made by combining a series of screening tests with commercially available API 20 NE (99% sensitivity in identifying *B. pseudomallei*) or 20 E biochemical kits. The screening system includes Gram stain (already discussed), oxidase reaction (*B. pseudomallei* being oxidase positive), and growth character (*B. pseudomallei* being nonlactose fermenting) and resistance to certain antibiotics. Molecular methods such as 16s rDNA sequencing, multiplex polymerase chain reaction (PCR), and real-time PCR are also being increasingly used for the identification of *B. pseudomallei*.

Serology

Since different groups of people have different levels of circulating antibodies, no standard cutoff can be ascertained for quantitative antibody-based diagnosis of melioidosis. Therefore, tests such as the indirect hemagglutination test (IHAT) have a limited role in endemic areas.

TREATMENT

The treatment of melioidosis is divided into two stages, an intensive phase of intravenous therapy to prevent mortality from severe illness associated with melioidosis and an eradication phase to prevent recurrence.

Initial Intensive Phase

This phase is carried out for 10–14 days with longer durations of up to 4–8 weeks warranted in prolonged critical illness, extensive pulmonary disease, deep-seated collections, organ abscesses, osteomyelitis, septic arthritis, or neurological melioidosis.

An overview of preferred treatment regimens for the intensive phase is given in **Table 1**.

Subsequent Eradication Phase

The preferred drug is trimethoprim-sulfamethoxazole (TMP-SMX) with folic acid given at the same dosage as mentioned earlier.

When TMP-SMX cannot be used due to intolerance or toxicity, doxycycline 100 mg BD or 200 mg BD is considered as an alternative as is Co-amoxiclav at a dose of 20/5 mg/kg orally thrice daily in certain settings for pregnancy and in younger children.

The suggested duration of the eradication phase is a minimum of 3 months but extended to 6 months in

TABLE 1: Preferred regimens for initial intensive phase.

Clinical scenario	Suspected or confirmed melioidosis not requiring ICU or not having features of CNS involvement	Critically ill patients requiring ICU admission but without CNS involvement	Patients with CNS melioidosis	Patients with nonpulmonary focal infections such as prostatic, bones, joints, cutaneous, or soft-tissue melioidosis
Preferred antibiotic	*Recommended dosage and route*			
Ceftazidime	50 mg/kg IV up to 2 g every 6 hours or 1 g IV every 3 hours* or continuous infusion*			As per clinical scenario
Meropenem		25 mg/kg IV every 8 hours†	40/kg IV up to 2 g every 8 hours	Do
Imipenem		25 mg/kg IV every 6 hours‡		Do
Cotrimoxazole add-on				*Children*: 6 mg/kg of TMX component PO BD *Adults: 40–60 kg*—240 mg of TMX component PO BD *Adults > 60 kg*: 320 mg of TMX component PO BD *plus folic acid* 0.1 mg/kg up to 5 mg PO OD (to reduce the potential toxicity due to the antifolate activity of TMP–SMX)
Switchovers and alternatives				
Ceftazidime		Once a patient gets past the severe illness and ceases to require ICU care†		
Meropenem–imipenem	Potential alternatives as well as for switchover therapy if patients continue to be persistently blood culture positive or clinically worsening after 7 days of ceftazidime therapy			

(CNS: central nervous system; MIC: minimum inhibitory concentration; TMP–SMX: trimethoprim/sulfamethoxazole)

*More frequent or continuous dosing tends to maintain plasma drug concentration at levels beyond MIC for extended periods of time.

†Of the above three drugs, only meropenem confers mortality benefits in critically ill patients but has the potential for development of resistance during ongoing treatment.

‡Associated with higher CNS side effects.

Patients with sepsis and septic shock require similar supportive measures to patients with shock due to any other cause. Other additional measures include drainage of prostatic abscesses under CT or transrectal US guidance (other internal collections usually resolve with medical therapy) and surgical removal of mycotic aneurysms.

patients with osteomyelitis and neurologic melioidosis. Patients undergoing vascular surgery with grafts for mycotic aneurysm may even need a lifelong therapy.

Postexposure Prophylaxis

TMP-SMX (Trimethoprim-sulphamethoxazole), double dose of intensive phase (as in **Table 1**), i.e., 640 mg Trimethoprim component PO BD used for intensive phase or eradication phase in adults weighing > 60 kg or amoxicillin–clavulanate (1,500 mg/375 mg every 8 hours in adults weighing > 60 kg) for 21 days and should be started as soon as possible.

Despite emerging data regarding the global disease burden of melioidosis, a large majority of cases go unreported, especially from counties where it is endemic. The major reason for this remains lack of awareness among clinicians regarding the manifestations. This coupled with the fact that most cases of melioidosis occur in the lower socioeconomic group and in villages where health care is approached only in terminal stages and the fact that human-to-human transmission is unlikely create a general barrier toward urging for a diagnostic compulsion. It is true that cultures do yield well, but postculture identification still requires setups not within the reaches of most of the endemic zones from where cases are supposed to be reported. Besides the presence of broad-based clinical features, radiological and laboratory findings together with the intrinsic resistance of *B. pseudomallei* to penicillin, ampicillin, second-generation cephalosporins and aminoglycosides such as streptomycin or tobramycin make both diagnosing and treating melioidosis a challenge. Constant efforts to improve its diagnostic methods and simplify treatment regimens as well as increasing the general awareness about the disease in both general population and treating clinicians, specially those residing in endemic areas, therefore lay at the heart of an effective management of what Sir Aurthur Conan Doyle in his *"Adventures of the Dying Detective"* referred to as the dreaded tropical disease *"Tapanuli fever"* effecting his beloved friend, Sherlock Holmes.

RECENT ADVANCES

Bacterial genes such as fliC encoding for flagellin, rpsU gene encoding for ribosomal protein, and TTS gene encoding for type III secretion system are being employed. Matrix-assisted laser desorption/ionization time-of-flight mass spectrometry (MALDI-TOF MS) is employed for bacterial identification from culture isolates although mis-identification with *Burkholderia thailandensis* has been reported.

Enzyme-linked immunosorbent assays (ELISAs) targeting specific antigens such as the hemolysin co-regulator protein 1 (Hcp 1) and O-polysaccharide (OPS) are new to the market and under evaluation.

Cefiderocol, a novel siderophore cephalosporin, and ceftazidime-avibactam (CZA), a new β-lactam β-lactamase inhibitor combination, have shown promising in vitro results for the treatment of *B. pseudomallei.*

Adding recombinant granulocyte colony-stimulating factor (G-CSF) at a dose of 300 μg IV daily for at least 10 days may be considered in cases of septic shock although data regarding the same is still inadequate.

SUGGESTED READINGS

1. Mohapatra PR, Mishra B. Burden of melioidosis in India and South Asia: challenges and ways forward. The Lancet Regional Health-Southeast Asia. 2022;2:100004.
2. Mukhopadhyay C, Shaw T, Varghese GM, Dance DA. Melioidosis in South Asia (India, Nepal, Pakistan, Bhutan and Afghanistan). Trop Med Infect Dis. 2018;3(2):51.
3. Cheng AC, Currie BJ. Melioidosis: epidemiology, pathophysiology, and management. Clin Microbiol Rev. 2005;18(2):383-416.
4. Wiersinga WJ, Currie BJ, Peacock SJ. Melioidosis. New England J Med. 2012;367(11):1035-44.

165

CHAPTER

PUO—Simplified to Reveal the Unrevealed

Partha Karmakar, Aayushi Rathi, Devendra Gupta

ABSTRACT

Pyrexia of unknown origin (PUO) or fever of unknown origin (FUO) (as called in US) has been the most challenging diagnostic dilemma not only for the internists, but also the infectious disease specialist or the rheumatologist. Since antiquity, fever has been the cardinal manifestation of infectious disease, but throughout the ages different patterns of fever, their associations with infectious and noninfectious causes have been recognized. Even with a standardized protocol, the cause for FUO cannot be identified in a large proportion of patients.

Despite recent advances and imaging techniques such as ^{18}FDG-PET (fluorodeoxyglucose-positron emission tomography), clinical judgment still remains an essential component of care.

INTRODUCTION

Although the original definition by Petersdorf and Beeson included >3 weeks of fever of ≥38.3°C on two occasions and an uncertain etiology despite 1 week of inpatient evaluation. With improving outdoor services, the terms "*inpatient evaluation" has been dropped from the definition*. Also the patients with known immunocompromised state were left out from the classical definition because the workup is different.

So, pyrexia of unknown origin (PUO) is now defined as:

- Fever ≥ 38.3°C/101°F on at least two occasions
- Illness duration of ≥3 weeks
- No known immunocompromised state
- Diagnosis that remains uncertain after thorough history-taking, physical examination, and following obligatory investigations:
  - Complete blood count (CBC), erythrocyte sedimentation rate (ESR), C-reactive protein (CRP)
  - Kidney function test (KFT), liver function test (LFT)
  - Lactate dehydrogenase (LDH), creatine kinase (CK)
  - Ferritin
  - Antinuclear antibody (ANA), rheumatoid factor (RF)
  - SPEP (serum protein electrophoresis)
  - Blood culture ($n = 3$), urine culture (once)
  - Chest X-ray (CXR), ultrasonography (USG) abdomen
  - Tuberculin skin test or interferon-γ release assay (IGRA)

TYPES OF PUO

In 1991, Durack and Street, proposed a classification into four distinct subclasses:

1. Classical FUO (fever of unknown origin)
2. Nosocomial FUO (healthcare-associated)
3. Neutropenic FUO (immune-deficient)
4. Human immunodeficiency virus (HIV)-related PUO

Causes of HIV-related FUO include:

- Disseminated *Mycobacterium avium* complex
- Pneumocystis
- Cytomegalovirus (CMV)
- Histoplasmosis
- Viral/parasitic/tubercular
- Lymphoma/Kaposi sarcoma
- Drug fever/Castleman

PUO vis-à-vis inflammation of unknown origin (IUO):
- IUO is analogous to PUO except for the fever (<38.3°C/101°F)

EVOLVING ETIOLOGIES OVER DECADES

Long fever in early 20th century, was the proposed name for PUO of Dr Richard Cabot of Massachusetts General Hospital observed common causes for PUO were tuberculosis (TB), abscessed, and endocarditis.

In 1930s, Alt and Barker added tumors as an important cause to the list.

In 1961, Petersdorf and Beeson found in a prospective study, "Fever of Unexplained Origin", collagen vascular disease to be responsible for 20% of their 100 cases of PUO.

With the dawn of the millennium special focus has been laid on autoinflammatory diseases [like familial Mediterranean fever (FMF), cryopyrin-associated periodic illness, mevalonate kinase deficiency, etc.] and the better understanding of the connective tissue diseases.

A study in Netherlands conducted between 2003 and 2005 yielded the following distribution as causes of PUO:
- Systemic rheumatic disease [e.g., vasculitis, systemic lupus erythematosus, polymyalgia rheumatica (PMR)]—22%
- Infection—16%
- Malignancy—7%
- Miscellaneous—4%
- No diagnosis—51%

In Asian countries including India infectious causes are the foremost one for PUO as opposed to Western Europe **(Table 1)**.

In Middle East countries pooled data from three studies showed infection caused almost 62% of total cases of PUO.

MISCELLANEOUS CAUSES OF PUO

Drugs

- Virtually all drugs can cause fever, even after long-term use.
- *DRESS* (drug reaction with eosinophilia and systemic symptoms including fever) with or without lymphadenopathy (can be extensive).
- All nonprescription drugs and nutritional supplements to discontinue.
- Fever persists beyond 72 hours after withdrawal is unlikely for drug fever.

Exercise-induced Hyperthermia

- Lasting from half an hour up to several hours
- Moderate to strenuous exercise
- No increase in CRP level or ESR

Factitious Fever (Artificially Induced by the Patient)

- Should be considered in all patients if initial protocol-based evaluation is not fruitful. *It is more common among young women in healthcare professions.*
- For example, by intravenous (IV) injection of contaminated water.

Fraudulent Fever

- The patient is *normothermic but manipulates the thermometer.*
- Simultaneous measurements at different body sites (rectum, ear, mouth) should rapidly identify this diagnosis.
- Important clue—dissociation between pulse rate and temperature.

WHEN TO SUSPECT FACTITIOUS AND FRAUDULENT FEVER

- *Clinical clue*: Not sick in appearance; clinical examination and tests are within normal limits.
- *Biochemical clue*: One of the first steps should be to rule out factitious or fraudulent fever, particularly in patients without signs of inflammation in laboratory tests.

SIMPLIFIED STEPS TO REVEAL THE UNREVEALED CAUSE

Importance of clinical history and examination: History-taking is an art and PUO is a scenario where the artist is put to the test.

TABLE 1: Causes of pyrexia of unknown origin (PUO) (regionwise)—pooled data from last three decades (approximately).

Region	Number of patients (pooled data—number of cohorts)	Infection % in median (range)	Noninfectious inflammatory % in median (range)	Malignancy in median % (range)	Miscellaneous in median % (range)	No diagnosis in median % (range)
Asia	3,802 (20)	42	20	13	9	18
Western Europe	1,820 (10)	17 (11–32)	25 (12–32)	10 (3–20)	10 (0–15)	37 (26–51)

Thorough clinical history and examination is a must to search for potentially diagnostic clues (PDCs). Special attention needs to be laid upon the lymph nodes, temporal arteries, eyes, liver, spleen, entire skin surface, sites of previous surgery, and mucous membranes.

Information about previous illnesses, localizing symptoms like ear or dental symptoms, recreational habits including alcohol intake, medications like over-the-counter (OTC), immunization history, occupational exposures, animal contact or pets, travel to any endemic area, blood transfusion, tattooing or sexual exposure, and familial disorders should not be overlooked.

While hallmark features when present easily suggest particular FUO categories, simultaneously some findings essentially eliminate a pyrexia-of-unknown-origin category, for example, *rigors eliminate the rheumatic/inflammatory category of fever*.

Significant weight loss of >2 lbs/week, specially if accompanied by early anorexia, is a hallmark of neoplastic PUO.

Post-hot bath pruritus suggests a malignant/neoplastic disorder.

Special emphasis has to be laid to specific points attributable to specific disorders, for example:

- Oral ulcers for Behçet's disease or lupus
- Raynaud's phenomena for lupus or scleroderma
- Unpasteurized milk for Q fever
- Contact with birds for *Chlamydia psittaci*
- Joint pain and swelling for most rheumatological diseases

Examination also needs undivided attention for a rapid diagnosis. Not-to-miss checklist includes:

- Sternal tenderness for hematological malignancies
- Unequal pulses for Takayasu arteritis
- Skin lesions like Apple jelly nodule for cutaneous TB
- Panniculitis like erythema nodosum for sarcoidosis
- Fundoscopy for uveitis, Purtscher-like retinopathy
- Splenomegaly for adult onset still disease, Felty syndrome
- Tophi for gout
- Lymphadenopathy for Castleman, Kikuchi, etc.
- Prostatic tenderness for prostatic abscess

INVESTIGATIONS

Stepwise Approach

1. Detailed history and examination
↓
2. Obligatory investigations (as per definition)
↓
3. Ruling out miscellaneous causes:
   a. Factitious and fraudulent fever (thermometer manipulation)
   b. Stopping/replacing suspected drug/s (drug fever)
↓
4. Clinical feature guided-related tests
↓
5. ^{18}FDG-PET/CT (fluorodeoxyglucose-positron emission tomography with computed tomography) or labeled leukocyte scintigraphy or gallium scan
↓
6. Histopathological examination (HPE) of tissue obtained by excisional/incisional biopsy or laparotomy (CT-guided has higher yield)
↓
7. *Other specialized tests*: Sometimes may be of help depending on clinical scenario:
   a. Cryoglobulins
   b. Temporal artery biopsy (if ≥55 years old even in the absence of localizing sign)
   c. Chest and abdominal CT
   d. Bone marrow biopsy
   e. Fungal cultures
   f. CSF study, if CNS symptoms/signs demand
   g. Molecular genetic testing (e.g., next-generation sequencing) for FMF

Therapeutic trials are often helpful as they can help solve some selected cases. It is exemplified in autoinflammatory diseases of unknown origin, where anti-interleukin 1 (IL-1) therapy like *anakinra* have shown success. Other examples are aspirin, corticosteroids, and antimicrobial agents in carefully selected subjects. Like rifampicin, a component of antitubercular regimen is highly active against other species like meningococci. Conversely, fluoroquinolone given for other reasons have activity against TB and Q fever.

Naproxen test: Although not thoroughly validated, this test is used to differentiate between malignant and infectious causes, based on the belief that malignant fevers respond better to nonsteroidal anti-inflammatory drugs (NSAIDs) than paracetamol.

An *ESR > 100 mm/h* narrows down differential for PUO to mostly six entities, namely, *endocarditis, osteomyelitis, drug fever, abscesses, collagen vascular disease, and malignancies.*

Serum ferritin when raised slightly in an acutely ill patient can be attributed to acute phase reaction but like a PUO patient who is *subacutely or chronically ill, persistent hyperferritinemia should hint toward a diagnosis of rheumatic or neoplastic disease.*

Lymph nodes biopsy is among the most common invasive test for PUO. More likely to be diagnostic are *posterior cervical, supra/infraclavicular, or epitrochlear node biopsies.*

IF INITIAL STAGE FAILS, WHAT NEXT?

When the first-stage thorough clinical and diagnostic tests do not lead to a diagnosis:

- *^{18}F-FDG (PET/CT)*: An established imaging procedure in FUO, it accumulates in those tissues with a *high rate of glycolysis* (i.e., malignant cells and activated leukocytes), *thereby enabling imaging of acute and chronic inflammatory processes.* Total diagnostic yield for FDG-PET in PUO is of ~50%.

Or, if not available:

- Radiolabeled leukocyte scintigraphy should be performed, especially when the ESR or the CRP level is elevated.

It is important to note that up to 51% of cases remain undiagnosed (a study in Netherlands). However, the prognosis for these patients is usually good, and it is highly probable that FUO will spontaneously resolve in weeks to months.

PUO IN ELDERLY

Following points are important in elderly suffering from PUO:

- Cause is more likely Atypical manifestation of a common disease
- *Most common diseases*:
  - Noninfectious inflammatory disease (NIID)—giant cell arteritis (GCA) and PMR
  - Infectious disease—TB

As many of these diseases are treatable, it is well worth pursuing the cause of fever in elderly patients.

CONCLUSION

In summary, PUO poses diagnostic puzzles, necessitating a comprehensive approach to uncover the elusive cause behind these clinical manifestations. The prognosis of PUO is determined by the cause of the fever and the nature of the underlying disease with most fever recovering even before reaching diagnosis. The frequency with which infections and neoplasms have been identified as the causes of classical FUO has decreased steadily, whereas the proportion of miscellaneous causes and undiagnosed conditions has risen in recent years. The role of FDG-PET can never be overemphasized as now it has become the investigation of choice for PUO and IUO cases. Thus, it cannot be overemphasized that in medicine, PUO remains one of the most challenging diagnoses. Future advances in microbial studies through gene amplification methods and better understanding of the pathogenesis of systemic rheumatic diseases will continue to alter the distribution of FUO.

The frequent use of empiric antimicrobials can delay the detection of some occult abscesses and infections and simultaneously increase the number of drug fevers. Aggressive use of immunosuppressive regimens, frequent exposure to potentially allergenic medications, lengthy critical care unit admissions, and the rise in multiresistant organisms as resident hospital flora have all changed the types of PUOs encountered.

SUGGESTED READINGS

1. Larson EB, Featherstone HJ, Petersdorf RG. Fever of undetermined origin: diagnosis and follow-up of 105 cases, 1970-1980. Medicine (Baltimore). 1982;61(5):269-92.
2. Durack DT, Street AC. Fever of unknown origin—reexamined and redefined. Curr Clin Top Infect Dis. 1991;11:35-51.
3. Armstrong WS, Katz JT, Kazanjian PH. Human immunodeficiency virus–associated fever of unknown origin: a study of 70 patients in the United States and review. Clin Infect Dis. 1999;28:341-5
4. Vanderschueren S, Del Biondo E, Ruttens D, Van Boxelaer I, Wauters E, Knockaert DD. Inflammation of unknown origin versus fever of unknown origin: two of a kind. Eur J Intern Med. 2009;20(4):415-8.
5. Petersdorf RG, Beeson PB. Fever of unexplained origin: report on 100 cases. Medicine (Baltimore). 1961;40:1-30.
6. De Kleijn EM, Vandenbroucke JP, van der Meer JW. Fever of unknown origin (FUO). I. A prospective multicenter study of 167 patients with FUO, using fixed epidemiologic entry criteria. The Netherlands FUO Study Group. Medicine (Baltimore). 1997;76:392-400.
7. Loscalzo J, Fauci A, Kasper D, Hauser S, Longo D, Jameson JL. Harrison's principles of internal medicine, 21st edition. New York: The McGraw-Hill Companies, Inc.; 2022.
8. Manfredi R, Calza L, Chiodo F. Primary cytomegalovirus infection in otherwise healthy adults with Fever of unknown origin: a 3-year prospective survey. Infection. 2006;34(2):87-90.
9. Brusch JL, Weinstein L. Fever of unknown origin. Med Clin North Am. 1988;72(5):1247-61.
10. Zenone T. Fever of unknown origin in rheumatic diseases. Infect Dis Clin North Am. 2007;21(4):1115-35, x-xi.
11. Zhang J, Chen B, Xu X, Lin Z, Huang B, Song J, et al. Clinical features of 66 lymphoma patients presenting with a fever of unknown origin. Intern Med. 2012;51(18):2529-36.

12. Cunha BA. Fever of unknown origin: focused diagnostic approach based on clinical clues from the history, physical examination, and laboratory tests. Infect Dis Clin North Am. 2007;21(4):1137-87, xi.
13. Carsons SE. Fever in rheumatic and autoimmune disease. Infect Dis Clin North Am. 1996;10(1):67-84.
14. Epperly TD, Moore KE, Harrover JD. Polymyalgia rheumatica and temporal arteritis. Am Fam Physician. 2000;62:789-96.
15. Garg S, Wynne K, Omoyinmi E, Eleftheriou D, Brogan P. Efficacy and safety of anakinra for undifferentiated autoinflammatory diseases in children: a retrospective case review. Rheumatol Adv Pract. 2019;3(1):rkz004.
16. Chang JC, Gross HM. Utility of naproxen in the differential diagnosis of fever of undetermined origin in patients with cancer. Am J Med. 1984;76(4):597-603.
17. Cunha BA. Fever of unknown origin: focused diagnostic approach based on clinical clues from the history, physical examination, and laboratory tests. Infect Dis Clin North Am. 2007;21(4):1137-87, xi.
18. Brown I, Finnigan NA. Fever of Unknown Origin. In: StatPearls [Internet]. Treasure Island (FL): StatPearls Publishing; 2023.
19. Lorenzen J, Buchert R, Bohuslavizki KH. Value of FDG PET in patients with fever of unknown origin. Nucl Med Commun. 2001;22:779-83.

SECTION 12

METABOLISM

166

CHAPTER

Fetal Origin of Adult Metabolic Disorders

Saurabh Srivastava, Amit Gupta, Deepak Sharma

ABSTRACT

There is considerable evidence now to suggest that most of the later health outcomes and noncommunicable diseases such as metabolic syndrome, diabetes mellitus, cardiovascular disease, and stroke are programmed during fetal stage and manifest during adulthood. Maternal nutrition plays a major role in this programming. Both maternal undernutrition and overnutrition carry risk for future disorders, but nutritional deprivation leading to low birth weight has great impact, more so when faced with overnutrition in later life, forming the basis for the 'thrifty phenotype' hypothesis. The evidence in support of these associations comes largely from retrospective cohort studies in which adult outcomes were correlated with birth weight records. The greatest risk from the mismatch of early nutritional deprivation and later nutritional affluence is seen in developing countries and children in these countries are at major risk of future diseases. This manuscript explores the importance of the fetal origin of health and disease.

INTRODUCTION

It is a widely accepted fact both by epidemiological and clinical studies that fetal status during pregnancy is related to future diseases in adulthood. Current studies have shown that intrauterine fetal programming has a substantial impact on the future health of an individual after birth. The 'developmental origin of adult disease' hypothesis was first described by David Barker and his colleagues in 1989. This hypothesis proposed that the intrauterine adaptation due a transient phenomenon induces structural and functional changes in cells and tissues which then become permanent or 'programmed' because they occurred during the critical period of early fetal development. These early life insults due to this 'programming' can lead to a plethora of metabolic disorders in adulthood such as noninsulin-dependent diabetes mellitus (DM), insulin resistance, hypertension, cardiovascular disorders, stroke, and osteoporosis.

FETAL PROGRAMMING

Fetal programming describes the activity in which the transient stimulus or insult has lifelong or permanent effects occurring at critical development period of organogenesis. The adult outcomes are affected by nature, timing, and duration of insult and adversely affect those organs that undergo rapid growth. The adverse events or insults that primarily affect the gestational milieu as well as fetus occur prior to or during pregnancy, such as obesity, overnutrition, undernutrition, preeclampsia, smoking, and uteroplacental insufficiency. The 'thrifty phenotype' hypothesis has been further developed to suggest that developmental programming is only one of a series of adaptations that occur in an external environment predicted during development. The other phenomenon that contributes to fetal programming is 'predictive adaptive response', which signifies that fetus adapts itself based on the predicted postnatal environment. This is also known as developmental (phenotypic) plasticity and allows the organism to thrive in the anticipated environment of adulthood. Diseases occur when there is mismatch between the prenatal and postnatal environment **(Flowchart 1)**.

EPIGENETICS

Epigenetic modifications are the structural changes in the deoxyribonucleic acid (DNA) without changing the DNA sequence and invariably resulting in altered gene expression. It includes DNA methylation, histone modification with acetylation and methylation (of lysine residues), and micro-ribonucleic acid (RNA) regulation of gene expression. Intrauterine environment affects the epigenetic mechanism establishing fetal developmental genotype and programming which affects large number of metabolic and physiological genes, influencing health and adult chronic metabolic disorders **(Flowchart 2)**.

DNA Methylation

The candidate undergoing epigenetic regulation and implicated in type 2 diabetes mellitus (T2DM) is peroxisome proliferator-activated receptor gamma (PPAR-γ) coactivator-1 alpha (PGC-1α). Its regulation is shown in pancreatic islets and skeletal muscle of T2DM subjects. This hypermethylation alone has no functional impact, but when exposed to high-fat diet, it leads to reduced gene expression of PGC-1α. This shows that a second insult is required to unmask epigenetic modification.

Histone Modification

Histone modification in the form of deacetylation and di-methylation at sites in glucose transporter type 4 (*GLUT4*) genes causes corepressor complex formation, resulting in decreased *GLUT4* gene transcription at birth which persists even in adulthood and importantly, these changes are in absence of any DNA methylation.

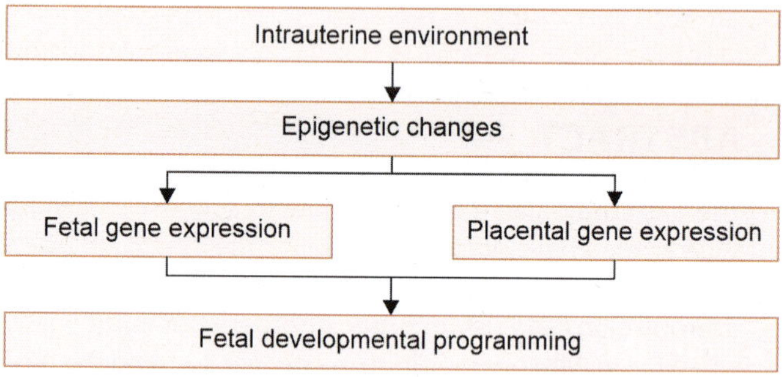

FLOWCHART 2: Epigenetics in fetal programming.

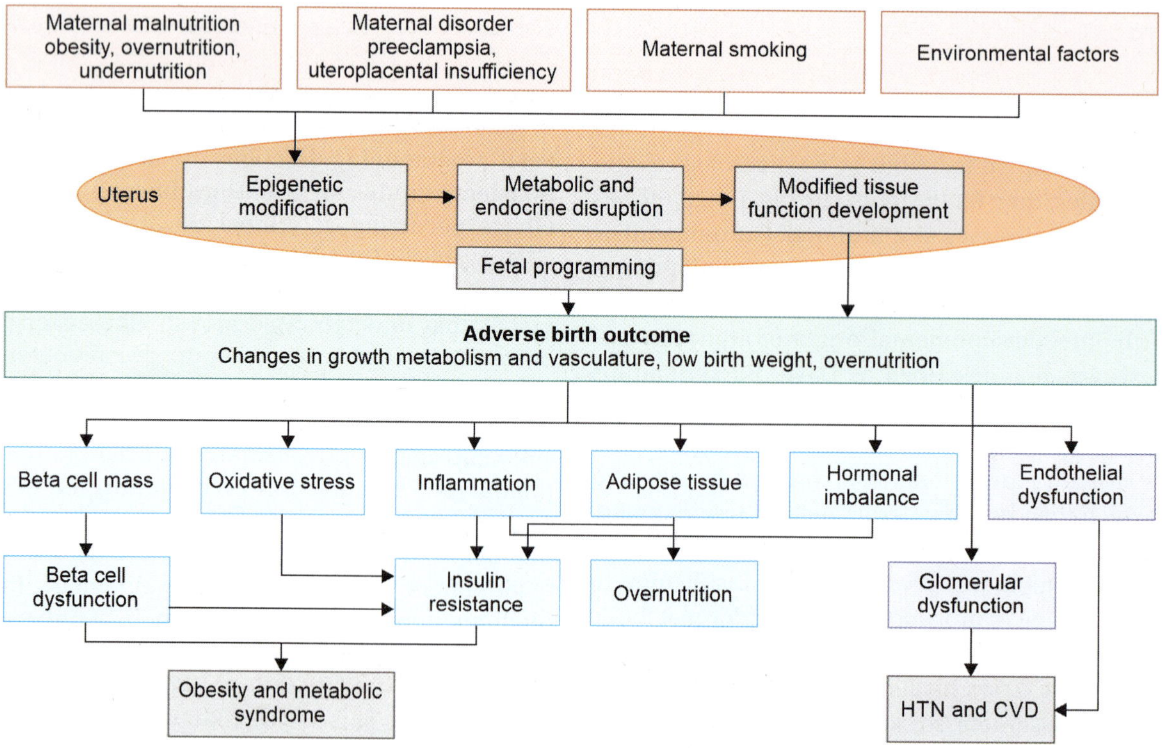

FLOWCHART 1: Summary of fetal programming effects on adult diseases.
(CVD: cardiovascular disease; HTN: hypertension)

Micro-RNAs are small noncoding RNA affecting transcription of genes. Epigenetic regulation is affected by micro-RNA and few studies have shown its role in offspring development.

Maternal Nutrition

The nutrition of expecting mothers is a fundamental public health issue because it influences not only the health of women but also the health of future generations. It is an important factor responsible for fetal origin of adult disease. Both overnutrition as well as undernutrition are responsible for such change.

Nutrition can affect DNA methylation through the action of the one-carbon pathway and its associated metabolites, including folate, riboflavin, choline, etc. Nutritional deprivation of mother during gestational period causes impaired nutrition to fetus, leading to intrauterine growth restriction (IUGR) or low-birth-weight babies. Such nutritional deprivation leads to fetal programming to be thrifty, i.e., efficient in storing the surplus nutrients. These changes help in survival benefit if the postnatal environment is deprived of nutrients, but when the postnatal environment is having adequate or overnutrition, these changes become detrimental, leading to insulin resistance and T2DM in adult life. It has also been seen that nutrient restriction impairs the development of beta-cells in pancreas and causes hyperphagia due to leptin resistance. This hyperphagia along with surplus nutrient postnatally leads to increased adipose tissue and obesity results from multiple cohort studies suggest that an energy-dense diet, independent of maternal obesity, resulting in a hostile intrauterine metabolic environment that poses a risk for insulin resistance DM.

The epidemiological studies supporting this concept are Dutch Hunger Winter study and Chinese Famine study; however, the Leningrad Siege study did not support this concept, probably due to fewer number of subjects and extension of famine into childhood. Various animal studies have shown that maternal global nutrient restriction and low-protein diet during gestation impairs placental amino acid transfer, leading to IUGR and obesity in adulthood.

It has been seen that offspring of obese high-fat fed mothers had a potential to develop metabolic disorders in adulthood, namely nonalcoholic fatty liver disease, insulin resistance, obesity, hypertension, and cardiovascular disorders. High-fat diet and obesity during pregnancy lead to increased transport of lipids into the fetal circulation and increased levels of free-fatty acids, triglycerides, and cholesterol are observed in placenta and fetus. This increased circulating lipids induces widespread inflammation and activation of inflammatory signaling pathways, leading to altered gene expression and may play a role in future disease development.

Vitamin and Microelements

Intrauterine programming is triggered by shortage or excess of vitamins and macro- and micronutrients. Low zinc levels are associated with development of obesity, high leptin levels, insulin resistance, and diabetes in adulthood. Low iron levels in maternal blood predispose to low birth weight and hypertension in later life. Diet deficient in vitamin B12 leads to low birth weight, high visceral fat, and dyslipidemia. Low calcium intake might adversely affect fetal development and is important to recommend calcium supplementation during pregnancy. Reduced concentration of vitamin D in mothers during late pregnancy was associated with reduced whole-body and lumbar-spine bone-mineral content in children **(Fig. 1)**.

CONTRIBUTION OF DIFFERENT ORGANS AND TISSUES TO FETAL PROGRAMMING

To understand the fetal programming key tissues that regulate or respond to changes are to be observed **(Fig. 2)**.

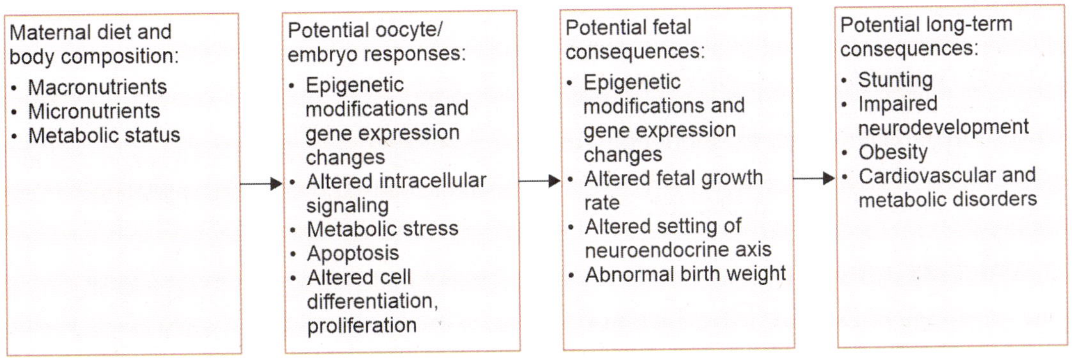

FIG. 1: Effect of maternal nutrition on fetal programming.

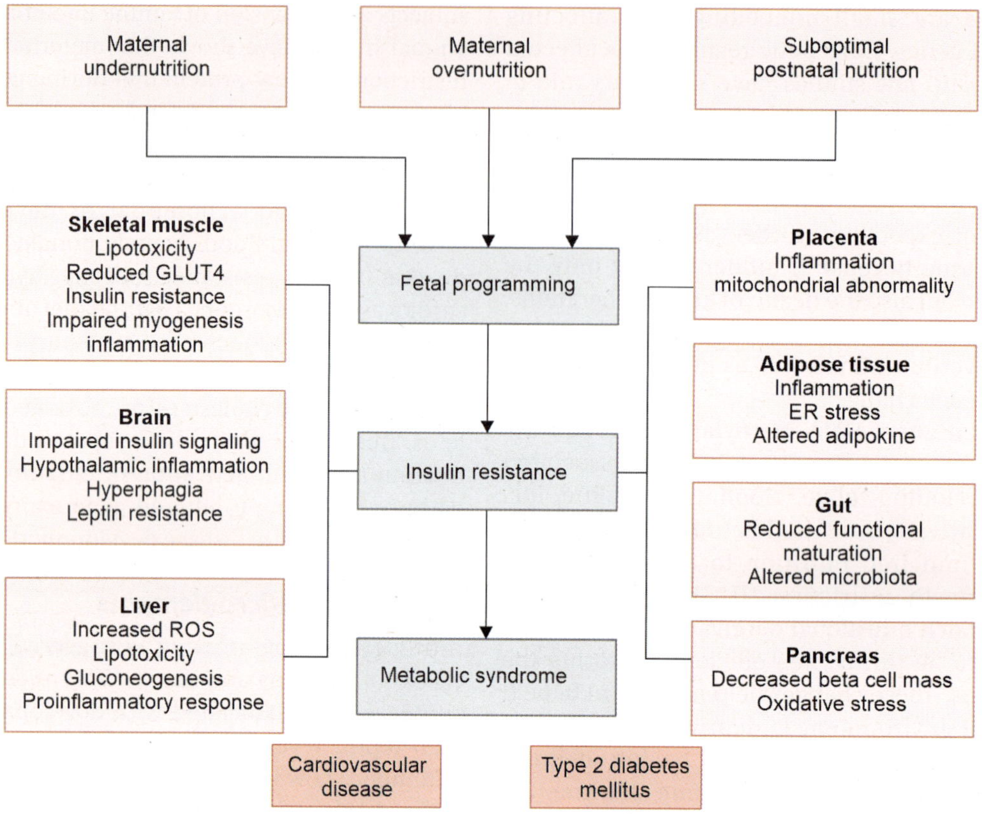

FIG. 2: Contribution of different organs and tissues in fetal programming.
(GLUT4: glucose transporter type 4; ER: endoplasmic reticulum; ROS: reactive oxygen species)

Placenta

The communication between mother and fetus is through placenta. Maternal overnutrition leads to inflammation in placenta which affects the nutrient supply to fetus. Similarly, maternal undernutrition induces placental mitochondrial abnormality and reduces adenosine triphosphate (ATP) production in animal model.

Brain and Hypothalamus

The development of hypothalamus starts from embryonic life and continues into early postnatal life and is very sensitive to perinatal nutrition. High-fat diet causes hypothalamic inflammation, leading to leptin resistance and hyperphagia; however, undernutrition causes impairment of hypothalamic insulin signaling. The progressive loss of hypothalamic neurons to leptin and insulin leads to development of central insulin and leptin resistance and risk of future obesity and diabetes.

Skeletal Muscles

The skeletal muscle development starts in fetal period and at the time of birth, muscle fiber number is established. It has been observed in animal studies that maternal high-fat diet leads to impaired myogenesis and reduced number of GLUT4 in skeletal muscle, causing insulin resistance. It has been observed in low-birth-weight individuals that protein kinase 3, GLUT4, and subunits of phosphoinositide 3-kinase (PI3K) are reduced, leading to insulin resistance.

Adipose Tissue

The suboptimal nutrition in fetal life results in adipocyte dysfunction and thus results in inflammation, increased adiposity, and alteration in adipokine secretion. The role of sympathetic nervous system, which has influence on lipolysis and adipocyte proliferation has been suggested in such programming.

LIVER

Liver is the main source of glycogen and glucose during fasting. High-fat diet during gestation leads to decreased insulin sensitivity and increased risk of nonalcoholic fatty liver disease. Similarly, fatty liver appears to be an early consequence of IUGR. The mechanisms involved appear to be increased reactive oxygen species with decrease in antioxidant defenses, lipotoxicity, increased expression of gluconeogenic enzymes, decreased insulin signaling, and activation of inflammatory pathways.

Pancreas

The pancreatic beta-cells are the only cells that produce insulin. It has been observed in various animal studies that suboptimal maternal nutrition such as overnutrition or undernutrition can compromise pancreatic development in offspring, decreasing beta-cell mass and function and ultimately leading to DM in adulthood.

Gut

The colonization of microbiota in gut starts in utero and this process is affected by maternal microbiota, vaginal microbiota, and nutrition. It has been observed in human studies also that maternal body mass index (BMI), weight, and weight gain during pregnancy influence the composition of microbiota in fetus and there is emerging evidence that gut microbiota are implicated in metabolic disorders.

There are possible mechanisms that explain the fetal programming in adult diseases. The various factors can integrate in any individual, leading to various diseases in adult life **(Fig. 3)**.

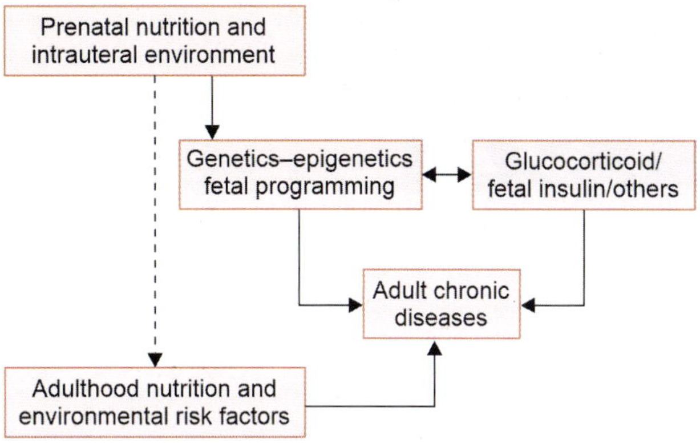

FIG. 3: Various integrating mechanisms in fetal programming.

CONCLUSION AND FUTURE RESEARCH

There is an upsurge of metabolic diseases and intense research on causes and mechanism implicated in current increasing obesity epidemic has addressed role of environment, prenatal, natal, and postnatal conditions responsible for development of disease. The expectant mothers should be informed about fetal programming factors and the pregnancies should be planned accordingly. With education provided to expectant mothers, the health of the next generation could be preserved; this would lead to a decrease in the health system's expenditure on chronic diseases and reduce their negative impact on the economy of the country.

The future research is based on three pillars—the understanding of these processes, availability of biomarkers for diagnosis, and assessment of preventive and curative measures.

SUGGESTED READINGS

1. Stevenson K, Lillycrop KA, Silver MJ. Fetal programming and epigenetics. Curr Opin Endocr Metab Res. 2020;13:1-6.
2. Barker DJP. Foetal origins of coronary heart disease. BMJ. 1995;311:171-4.
3. Barker DJ, Osmond C, Golding J, Kuh D, Wadsworth ME. Growth in utero, blood pressure in childhood and adult life, and mortality from cardiovascular disease. BMJ. 1989;298:564-7.
4. Hocher B. More than genes: the advanced fetal programming hypothesis. J Reprod Immunol. 2014;104-105:8-11.
5. Elsakr JM, Dunn JC, Tennant K, Zhao SK, Kroeten K, Pasek RC, et al. Maternal Western-style diet affects offspring islet composition and function in a non-human primate model of maternal over-nutrition. Mol Metab. 2019;25:73-82.
6. Marciniak A, Patro-Małysza J, Kimber-Trojnar Ż, Marciniak B, Oleszczuk J, Leszczyńska-Gorzelak B. Fetal programming of metabolic syndrome. Taiwan J Obstet Gynecol. 2017;56:133-8.

167

CHAPTER

Adiposity, Obesity Phenotypes, and Cardiovascular Diseases

Ashok Kumar, Shubha Laxmi Margekar, Krishna Pawan Jaldu

ABSTRACT

The prevalence of obesity has become a worldwide epidemic affecting individuals of all ages, and it is linked to various coexisting medical conditions such as hypertension (HTN), type 2 diabetes mellitus (T2DM), dyslipidemia, obstructive sleep apnea and sleep-disordered breathing, specific types of cancer, and significant cardiovascular (CV) disorders. Obesity exerts significant influence on cardiovascular diseases (CVDs), including heart failure (HF), coronary heart disease (CHD), sudden cardiac death, and atrial fibrillation, due to its maladaptive effects on various CV risk factors and its adverse impact on CV structure and function. Furthermore, obesity is linked to diminished overall survival. The identification of obesity is determined by anthropometric parameters that have been linked to both adiposity and its distribution. The indices, either individually or in various combinations, adhere to a comprehensive framework that assigns distinct values to ascertain the level of risk. Anthropometric indices possess the capacity to serve as valuable tools for the identification of risks, implementation of interventions, and evaluation of impacts on nutritional status or health. Consequently, it is appropriate to refer to them as anthropometric health indicators. This chapter focuses on various obesity phenotypes and discusses the impact of obesity on CVDs, so that the proper tools for assessing it and practical management techniques may be conceived to enhance CV consequences.

INTRODUCTION

The prevalence of obesity is reaching epidemic proportions among both adults and children. Both the World Heart Federation (WHF) and the World Obesity Federation (WOF) categorize it as a chronic ailment. Individuals who exhibit excessive body weight or obesity are at a heightened risk of experiencing adverse health outcomes associated with cardiovascular disease (CVD), including both morbidity and mortality. Increased adiposity, particularly in the visceral or abdominal region, has been associated with numerous pathophysiological pathways that directly and indirectly impact cardiovascular (CV) risk and the development of CVD. The development of CVD is influenced by many changes in metabolism, endocrine function, immune response, tissue structure, humoral factors, hemodynamics, and physiological function that are associated with obesity.

According to the Asia-Pacific regional guidelines set by the World Health Organization (WHO), individuals with a body mass index (BMI) falling between the range of 18.5 and 25.0 kg/m^2 are categorized as nonobese, while those with a BMI exceeding 25.0 kg/m^2 are categorized as obese. According to recent studies, there is a stronger association between obesity and morbidity compared to smoking, drinking, and poverty. If current patterns persist, obesity is projected to exceed cigarette misuse as the primary contributor to avoidable mortality in the United States. Additional anthropometric indices, such as body fatness, waist circumference (WC), waist-to-hip ratio (WHR), and weight-to-height ratio (WHtR), have been employed in certain studies, albeit with less frequency, and may possess enhanced predictive capabilities. Ectopic fat accumulation, a result of excessive calorie consumption, is linked to various health conditions, including insulin resistance, dyslipidemia, hypertension (HTN), systemic inflammatory response, type 2 diabetes mellitus (T2DM), CVD, and cancer.

The National Family Health Survey (NFHS) in India has used WC for the first time in the fifth round of the NFHS (2019–2021) to assess abdominal obesity prevalence, with a high rate observed among women. The survey found that 40% of women and 12% of men in India have abdominal obesity. However, 49.3% of women aged 30–39 years and 56.7% of men aged 40–49 years surpass the established threshold for obesity. Only 23% of the female population exceeds the BMI threshold, suggesting that some women with normal BMI also exhibit obesity. The prevalence rates vary across states, with Kerala and Tamil Nadu having high rates of 65.4 and 57.9%, respectively. Abdominal obesity is associated with demographic factors such as older age groups, urban residency, higher socioeconomic status, nonvegetarian dietary patterns, and the religious minority group of Sikhs.

ADIPOSITY

Adiposity refers to the excessive accumulation of bodily fat, with a particular emphasis on central or abdominal fat, which has been well recognized as a significant risk to health. Visceral obesity gives rise to a cascade of cellular and molecular processes that are modulated by both lifestyle variables and genetic susceptibility. The obesogenic environment, distinguished by the consumption of high-calorie foods and the adoption of sedentary lifestyles, interacts with genetic predisposition to contribute to the occurrence of weight gain. Hormonal imbalance, specifically involving insulin and leptin, is among the supplementary variables that contribute to the onset of obesity. These outcomes include the development of insulin resistance, the enlargement of visceral adipocytes, and the secretion of inflammatory mediators. Abdominal visceral fat has been identified as a prominent contributing factor associated with an increased susceptibility to the metabolic syndrome. The utilization of BMI as a common method for evaluating obesity is limited due to its inability to differentiate between muscle mass and body fat mass. Consequently, an individual with a higher muscle mass may erroneously be categorized as overweight or obese. Consequently, a greater number of anthropometric measurements are necessary in order to assess visceral obesity in the abdominal region.

PHENOTYPES

Obesity was defined as BMI ≥30 kg/m^2 for Western or ≥25 kg/m^2 for Asia-Pacific region and metabolically unhealthy was considered at least two metabolic disorders based on the International Diabetes Federation (IDF) criteria **(Table 1)**. As per IDF criteria, four obesity has been classified in four phenotypes: Metabolically unhealthy obesity (MUO), metabolically healthy obesity (MHO), metabolically unhealthy nonobesity (MUNO), and metabolically healthy nonobesity (MHNO) **(Table 2)**.

As per IDF, five cardiometabolic risk factors (NCEP-ATP III) have been taken into consideration for classification of obesity.

TABLE 1: Metabolic derangement parameters for phenotypic classification of obesity.

Parameter	Value
Blood glucose	≥ 100 mg/dL or taking antidiabetic medication
Blood pressure	≥ 130 mm Hg systolic BP and ≥ 80 mm Hg diastolic BP or taking antihypertensive medication
Waist circumference	≥ 90 cm in men or ≥ 80 cm in women
High-density lipoprotein	< 50 mg/dL in men or < 40 mg/dL in women
Triglyceride	≥ 150 mg/dL

TABLE 2: Obesity phenotype as per International Diabetes Federation (IDF) criteria.

	Nonobese (BMI < 30 kg/m^2 for Western or < 25 kg/m^2 for Asia–Pacific region)		Obese (BMI ≥ 30 kg/m^2 for Western or ≥ 25 kg/m^2 for Asia–Pacific region)	
Risk factors/ Class	**MHNO**	**MUNO**	**MHO**	**MUO**
	Presence of at most one metabolic risk factor	Presence of at least two metabolic risk factors	Presence of at most one metabolic risk factor	Presence of at least two metabolic risk factors

(BMI: body mass index; MHNO: metabolically healthy nonobese; MHO: metabolically healthy obese; MUNO: metabolically unhealthy nonobesity; MUO: metabolically unhealthy obesity)

MEASURES OF OBESITY

Obesity is characterized by the excessive accumulation of adipose tissue within the body, with the distribution of this fat playing a pivotal role in influencing metabolic risk. Obese individuals typically display two distinct body forms based on the distribution of fat accumulation: (1) Gynecoid or pear-shape, characterized by fat accumulation in the lower body, specifically the hips and thighs, and (2) android or apple-shape, characterized by fat accumulation in the upper body, particularly the visceral or abdominal region. Abdominal or visceral obesity, sometimes referred to as central obesity, is regarded as the more severe manifestation of fat distribution due to its association with a higher susceptibility to a range of metabolic problems and diseases. Asian Indians exhibit a heightened susceptibility to abdominal obesity and the deposition of visceral fat, rendering them more prone to the concomitant health hazards.

There are several methods that can be utilized for evaluating obesity, one of which is the BMI. The BMI, which is calculated by dividing weight (in kilograms) by the square of height (in meters), is commonly employed as a measure of excessive weight. WC, WHR, and WHtR have stronger predictive capabilities for fat distribution and central obesity and demonstrate a more significant correlation with morbidity. The visceral adiposity index (VAI) is a measurement used to assess the amount of visceral fat in an individual's body. The VAI serves as a reliable measure for assessing body fat distribution and the buildup of visceral fat. Its calculation involves the utilization of anthropometric indices such as BMI and WC, as well as a lipid index comprising triglyceride and high-density lipoprotein (HDL)-cholesterol. The lipid accumulation product (LAP) is composed of WC and triglyceride levels and has been associated with both CVD and all-cause mortality. In addition, CT scans, MRI scans, 3D scans, and dual energy X-ray absorptiometry (DEXA) are employed.

Pathogenesis

The role of the adipocyte as an endocrine organ considerably influences the pathophysiology and problems associated with obesity. Leptin, an endocrine hormone synthesized by adipocytes, plays a crucial role in the regulation of energy metabolism and the control of food intake. Elevated levels of leptin may have a distinct association with the occurrence of CVD. The findings of this study indicate a positive correlation between elevated levels of both C-reactive protein (CRP) and leptin, and an augmented likelihood of experiencing major CV events. This observation has particular significance due to the fact that endogenous hyperleptinemia does not exhibit the expected effects of suppressing appetite or enhancing energy expenditure. CRP has the potential to play a role in the pathogenesis of leptin resistance. Obesity has been found to have detrimental effects on hemodynamic and CV structure and function across various dimensions. Obesity is associated with an elevation in both total blood volume and cardiac output, resulting in an augmented stress on the heart.

Obesity is linked to HTN and dyslipidemia, with high-risk patients exhibiting a combination of metabolic and CV risk factors. Studies show a progressive increase in CVD risk with higher BMI values. The obesity paradox, which suggests improved survival in established CVDs, has been a topic of controversy. Factors contributing to this paradox include misclassification bias, unmeasured confounding factors, and potential bias due to illness-related weight loss. Obese individuals often develop CVD at a younger age, despite being generally healthier with fewer comorbid conditions.

Obesities and Cardiovascular Risk

Many large cardiometabolic imaging studies (CT and MRI) have confirmed that excess visceral adiposity is strongly associated with metabolic disorders. Excess visceral adiposity can be found not only in patients who are obese but also in those who are overweight or even have normal weight, and because excess visceral adiposity and ectopic fat accumulation are the main drivers of the insulin resistance syndrome, even after control for BMI or the amount of total body fat, individuals with high levels of visceral adipose tissue (VAT) show insulin resistance, hyperinsulinemia, glucose intolerance, a typical atherogenic dyslipidemia [high triglyceride and apolipoprotein B levels, increased proportion of small, dense low-density lipoprotein (LDL) particles, low HDL cholesterol levels, and small HDL particles], inflammation, and increased blood pressure levels.

ADIPOSITY AND CORONARY ARTERY DISEASE

The Jackson Heart Study and Framingham Heart Study have highlighted the significant role of obesity and metabolic disorders in the CV system, leading to an increased susceptibility to CVD and its associated symptoms. The presence of excessive adiposity, particularly visceral and ectopic adiposity, plays a significant role in determining the risk of CVDs, particularly in those who acquire coronary artery disease. The Health, Aging and Body Composition Study found that the presence of excess VAT was a significant predictor of myocardial infarction among women aged 70–79 years. The presence of excessive adiposity hastens the advancement of atherosclerosis years before the appearance of clinical symptoms of CVD, particularly in individuals with abdominal adiposity. Cardiac adipose tissue deposits, such as pericardial and epicardial fat, have been linked to coronary events in the general population, regardless of conventional CV risk factors.

ADIPOSITY AND HEART FAILURE

The Framingham Heart Study and TOPCAT studies have shown that obesity is a significant risk factor for HF, with individuals with a two-fold higher risk of HF compared to those with normal body weight. Each rise in BMI by 1 unit is linked to a 5% higher risk of HF in males and a 7% higher risk in women. Around half of the population with obesity experience HF with preserved ejection fraction (HFpEF), presenting a significant obstacle in clinical practice. The prevalence of abnormal subclinical cardiac function in individuals with obesity varies between 37 and 54%. Surgical management of obesity serves as a preventive measure against the onset of HF and demonstrates efficacy in ameliorating existing HF, particularly HFpEF. Emerging research indicates that visceral adipose tissue (VAT) significantly contributes to the progression, pathogenesis, and detrimental consequences observed in obese patients with HFpEF.

ADIPOSITY AND ARRHYTHMIAS

The Framingham Heart Study found a significant positive association between obesity and the occurrence of atrial fibrillation, with a relative rise of almost 50%. The study also found a positive correlation between a one-unit increase in BMI and a 4% heightened likelihood of developing new-onset atrial fibrillation. The mechanistic significance of left atrial enlargement in individuals with obesity is noteworthy, as the relationship between BMI and atrial fibrillation becomes considerably attenuated after accounting for variations in left atrial dimensions. The presence of excess weight and obesity elevates the likelihood of atrial fibrillation by various pathways, including alterations in the structure and electrical properties of the atria. The study also revealed that pericardial fat, as evaluated by CT scans, emerged as a significant predictor of prevalent atrial fibrillation, even after accounting for established risk factors and other indicators of adiposity, such as BMI.

ADIPOSITY SUDDEN DEATH

The Framingham Heart Study and MADIT (Multicenter Automatic Defibrillator Implantation Trial) have found a significant correlation between obesity and cardiac dysrhythmias, indicating an increased risk of sudden cardiac mortality. Both mild and severe obesity are linked to an increased risk of ventricular tachycardia/fibrillation, resulting in a higher occurrence of intricate ventricular dysrhythmias. Obesity is also correlated with a delay in ventricular repolarization, which is independently indicative of CV death. The MADIT II study identified obesity as a distinct risk factor for ventricular tachyarrhythmias in individuals with ischemic cardiomyopathy who had treatment with an implanted cardioverter-defibrillator. Abdominal adiposity may have a significant influence on body fat distribution, with central adiposity independently linked to sudden cardiac death.

Cardiovascular Risks from Severe Obesity

Severe obesity, defined by a BMI of 40 kg/m^2, is a significant determinant of CVD and cardiac dysfunction. Around 33% of patients with severe obesity have HF, and the likelihood of developing HF increases as obesity duration persists. Severe obesity impacts cardiac structure and function, leading to left ventricular remodeling, reduced systolic performance, and impaired diastolic function. Metabolic, inflammatory, and neurohormonal abnormalities are common in individuals with severe obesity. Bariatric surgery can potentially improve heart structure and function, reducing the risk of CV complications. However, contemporary guidelines acknowledge the substantial risk linked to severe obesity, with a 49% increase in the lifetime probability of developing atrial fibrillation.

Changes in Myocardium Structure and Function

The Dallas Heart Study highlights the negative impacts of obesity on heart function and hemodynamics. Obesity-associated comorbidities, neurohormonal and metabolic changes, and visceral adiposity increase the susceptibility to cardiac dysfunction and HF. The study found that individuals with obesity exhibit left ventricular diastolic performance abnormalities, with incidence rates ranging from 23 to 75%. Abnormal subclinical cardiac function in patients with obesity is also documented, with rates ranging from 37 to 54%. The study suggests that abnormal distribution of body fat can result in unfavorable cardiac responses, leading to remodeling of the left ventricle, concentric left ventricular hypertrophy, and, ultimately, HF. Identifying individuals with high-risk obesity and detecting subclinical cardiac structural and functional abnormalities are crucial to preventing HF progression and improve patient outcomes.

High-risk Obesities, Type 2 Diabetes Mellitus, and Cardiovascular Outcomes

Heart failure is a significant risk associated with high-risk obesity, particularly when accompanied by an increased WC, WHR, or elevated levels of VAT. The metabolic syndrome and insulin resistance are associated with CV morbidity and mortality. The MESA (Multi-Ethnic Study of Atherosclerosis) investigation found that the presence of metabolic syndrome can predict the development of HF in a population without preexisting CVD. The coexistence of metabolic syndrome characteristics in individuals with T2DM exacerbates the CVD risk observed in those with persistently high blood sugar levels and impaired regulation of plasma glucose levels. Both conditions are expected to significantly elevate the risk of CV events.

CONCLUSION

The problem of obesity is multifaceted, with a multitude of risk factors that interact with one another. The escalating incidence of abdominal obesity, specifically among middle-aged women, highlights the imperative necessity for additional research aimed at discerning the causative components of obesity and the associated risk factors. Abdominal obesity exhibits a higher prevalence within demographic groups characterized by middle to older age ranges, urban residency, higher socioeconomic status, and nonvegetarian dietary patterns. Considering the substantial amount of the nation's populace residing in rural areas of India, the potential escalation of abdominal obesity and its concomitant health hazards could prove to be a formidable challenge. Hence, it can be argued that the effectiveness of a singular strategy may be limited due to the socioeconomic heterogeneity prevalent inside the nation. Additional investigation is required in order to comprehensively comprehend the potential health hazards linked to abdominal obesity. Indian individuals, specifically women, exhibit a heightened susceptibility to this form of obesity, hence exposing them to considerable risks associated with noncommunicable ailments.

SUGGESTED READINGS

1. Poirier P, Giles TD, Bray GA, Hong Y, Stern JS, Pi-Sunyer FX, et al. Obesity and cardiovascular disease: pathophysiology, evaluation, and effect of weight loss: an update of the 1997 American Heart Association scientific statement on obesity and heart disease from the obesity committee of the council on nutrition, physical activity, and metabolism. Circulation. 2006;113:898-918.
2. Klein S, Burke LE, Bray GA, Bray GA, Blair S, Allison DB, et al. Clinical implications of obesity with specific focus on cardiovascular disease: a statement for professionals from the American Heart Association Council on Nutrition, Physical Activity, and Metabolism: endorsed by the American College of Cardiology Foundation. Circulation. 2004;110:2952-67.
3. Litwin SE. Which measures of obesity best predict cardiovascular risk? J Am Coll Cardiol. 2008;52:616–9
4. Stefan N, Kantartzis K, Machann J, Schick F, Thamer C, Rittig K, et al. Identification and characterization of metabolically benign obesity in humans. Arch Intern Med. 2008;168:1609-16.
5. Kahn SE, Hull RL, Utzschneider KM. Mechanisms linking obesity to insulin resistance and type 2 diabetes. Nature. 2006;444:840-6.
6. Van Gaal LF, Mertens IL, De Block CE. Mechanisms linking obesity with cardiovascular disease. Nature. 2006;444:875-80.
7. Chaudhary M, Sharma P. Abdominal obesity in India: analysis of the National Family Health Survey-5 (2019–2021) data. The Lancet Regional Health-Southeast Asia. 2023;14.
8. Hwang Y-C, Hayashi T, Fujimoto WY, Kahn SE, Leonetti DL, McNeely MJ, et al. Visceral abdominal fat accumulation predicts the conversion of metabolically healthy obese subjects to an unhealthy phenotype. Int J Obes. 2015;39:1365-70.
9. Yu SR, Shin KA. Visceral Adiposity Index and Lipid Accumulation Product as Effective Markers of Different Obesity Phenotypes in Korean Adults: A Cross-Sectional Analysis. Diabetes Metab Syndr Obes. 2023;16:495-504.
10. Gesta S, Tseng YH, Kahn CR. Developmental origin of fat: tracking obesity to its source. Cell. 2007;131(2):242-56.
11. Piqueras P, Ballester A, Durá-Gil JV, Martinez-Hervas S, Redón J, Real JT. Anthropometric indicators as a tool for diagnosis of obesity and other health risk factors: a literature review. Front Psychol. 2021;12:631179.
12. Alpert MA. Obesity cardiomyopathy: pathophysiology and evolution of the clinical syndrome. Am J Med Sci. 2001;321:225-36.
13. Neeland IJ, Ross R, Després JP, Matsuzawa Y, Yamashita S, Shai I, et al. Visceral and ectopic fat, atherosclerosis, and cardio-metabolic disease: a position statement. Lancet Diabetes Endocrinol. 2019;7(9):715-25.
14. Abraham TM, Pedley A, Massaro JM, Hoffmann U, Fox CS. Association between visceral and subcutaneous adipose depots and incident cardiovascular disease risk factors. Circulation. 2015;132(17):1639-47.
15. Hubert HB, Feinleib M, McNamara PM, Castelli WP. Obesity as an independent risk factor for cardiovascular disease: a 26-year follow-up of participants in the Framingham Heart Study. Circulation. 1983;67(5):968-77.
16. Tsujimoto T, Kajio H. Abdominal obesity is associated with an increased risk of all-cause mortality in patients with HFpEF. J Am Coll Cardiol. 2017;70(22):2739-49.
17. Pietrasik G, Goldenberg I, McNITT S, Moss AJ, Zareba W. Obesity as a risk factor for sustained ventricular tachyarrhythmias in MADIT II patients. J Cardiovasc Electrophysiol. 2007;18(2):181-4.
18. Wanahita N, Messerli FH, Bangalore S, Gami AS, Somers VK, Steinberg JS. Atrial fibrillation and obesity—results of a meta-analysis. Am Heart J. 2008;155(2):310-5.
19. Wilner B, Garg S, Ayers CR, Maroules CD, McColl R, Matulevicius SA, et al. Dynamic relation of changes in weight and indices of fat distribution with cardiac structure and function: the Dallas Heart Study. J Am Heart Assoc. 2017;6(7):e005897.
20. Bahrami H, Bluemke DA, Kronmal R, Bertoni AG, Lloyd-Jones DM, Shahar E, et al. Novel metabolic risk factors for incident heart failure and their relationship with obesity: the MESA (Multi-Ethnic Study of Atherosclerosis) study. J Am Coll Cardiol. 2008;51(18):1775-83.

168 CHAPTER

Metabolic (Dysfunction)-associated Fatty Liver Disease: A Silent Epidemic

Tanuja Manohar

ABSTRACT

Metabolic (dysfunction)-associated fatty liver disease (MAFLD) is a serious health condition that affects billions of people worldwide. It is now considered as most important cause of chronic liver disease. In spite of its alarming and rapidly increasing prevalence, it is largely not known to the general population. Even due importance is not given to this entity by the medical fraternity. It is considered a silent killer, as it can go unnoticed until the development of complications. While heavy drinking is often associated with fatty liver disease (FLD), metabolic dysfunction, secondary to dysglycemia, a sedentary lifestyle, and obesity, have emerged as equally important causes of fatty liver disease. Because of the recognition of the role of metabolic dysfunction in causation of fatty liver, nomenclature is changed from nonalcoholic fatty liver disease (NAFLD) to MAFLD. Globally, owing to the pandemic of obesity and type 2 diabetes mellitus (T2DM), MAFLD has become the leading cause of end-stage liver disease in all age groups. Considering its impact on health, it is now included in National Program for Prevention and Control of Cancer, Diabetes, Cardiovascular disease and Stroke (NPCDCS). Its pathogenesis is multifactorial, and treatment is aimed toward management of risk factors like T2DM and obesity.

INTRODUCTION

Metabolic (dysfunction)-associated fatty liver disease (MAFLD) is defined as a condition characterized by liver fat accumulation (>5%) in the presence of at least one of the following three metabolic conditions, overweight/obesity, type 2 diabetes mellitus (T2DM), or at least two of following seven metabolic risk abnormalities in lean nondiabetic patients.

1. Waist circumference ≥90 in men and ≥80 cm in women
2. Blood pressure ≥130/85 mm Hg or on antihypertensive treatment
3. Plasma triglycerides ≥150 mg/dL or specific drug treatment
4. Plasma high-density lipoprotein (HDL)-cholesterol <40 mg/dL for men and <50 mg/dL for women or on treatment
5. Prediabetes
6. Homeostasis model assessment (HOMA) of insulin resistance (IR) score ≥2.5
7. Plasma high-sensitivity C-reactive protein (hs-CRP) level>2 mg/L.

Metabolic (dysfunction)-associated fatty liver disease is inclusive of alcoholic fatty liver disease, nonalcoholic fatty liver disease (NAFLD), and also fatty liver disease (FLD) caused by infection and toxins.

SPECTRUM OF METABOLIC (DYSFUNCTION)-ASSOCIATED FATTY LIVER DISEASE

Metabolic (dysfunction)-associated fatty liver disease is an umbrella term. It describes a histological spectrum ranging from excess fat deposits in the liver (steatosis) to inflammation in the liver, i.e., metabolic dysfunction-associated steatohepatitis (MASH), progressive fibrosis in the liver, ultimately leading to cirrhosis of liver and hepatocellular carcinoma. MAFLD always starts with simple steatosis, and then 5–20% progress to hepatic inflammation or MASH. Almost 20% patients with MASH develop significant fibrosis and 5% end up with cirrhosis and hepatocellular carcinoma.

EPIDEMIOLOGY AND NATURAL HISTORY OF METABOLIC (DYSFUNCTION)-ASSOCIATED FATTY LIVER DISEASE

The prevalence of MAFLD is rising globally parallelly with prevalence of obesity and T2DM. The global prevalence of MAFLD ranges from 13 to 32% with about 27% in Asian population. In India, prevalence ranges from 9 to 32%. Obesity is associated with a 3.5-fold increased risk of developing MAFLD. The relationship between MAFLD and T2DM is bidirectional with a higher prevalence of FLD is seen in patients with T2DM and an increased incidence of T2DM in patients with MAFLD. Majority of patients are diagnosed during the fourth to sixth decade of their life. With the increasing prevalence of childhood obesity and growing awareness about this important entity, statistics are going to change drastically. Gender wise it is more commonly seen in men.

RISK FACTORS FOR METABOLIC (DYSFUNCTION)-ASSOCIATED FATTY LIVER DISEASE

- Any component of metabolic syndrome
- Dietary habits, such as high-calorie and high-carbohydrate diet
- Sedentary lifestyle
- Gut dysbiosis
- Genetic and epigenetic factors

PATHOGENESIS OF METABOLIC (DYSFUNCTION)-ASSOCIATED FATTY LIVER DISEASE

Metabolic (dysfunction)-associated fatty liver disease is a heterogeneous and multifactorial disease. Pathogenetic mechanism can very well be explained by multiple hit hypotheses. MAFLD is thought to be the result of synergistic effects of pathological factors such as IR, disordered lipid metabolism, oxidative stress, endoplasmic reticulum stress, and mitochondrial dysfunction. All these factors exacerbate inflammation and fibrogenesis.

- *Insulin resistance*: IR plays a central role in the development of MAFLD. IR acts on adipose tissue and causes its dysfunction. It stimulates lipolysis and releases adipokines and proinflammatory cytokines. It also increases lipogenesis in the liver, resulting in elevated free fatty acids and lipid accumulation within hepatocytes, predisposing to liver injury and inflammation.
- *Deranged lipid metabolism*: An imbalance between uptake, synthesis, and export of free fatty acids in the liver can result in excessive fat accumulation in hepatocytes leading to simple steatosis. Abnormal lipid metabolism, including high levels of triglycerides and low levels of HDL cholesterol, can contribute to MAFLD.
- *Inflammation:* Low-grade inflammation is a critical factor in the progression of simple steatosis to progressive fibrosis.
- *Oxidative stress*: The fat accumulation in hepatocytes leads to the generation of free oxygen radicals inducing oxidative stress, which further damages hepatocytes and exacerbates inflammation.
- *Genetic factors*: Genetic factors can influence individual's susceptibility to MAFLD. Some genetic variations are associated with an increased risk of developing MAFLD.
- *Gut microbiota*: Changes in the gut microbiota can affect the absorption of nutrients and contribute to inflammation. Functional cross talk between the liver and the complex microbial composition has been identified to play crucial role in pathogenesis of MAFLD.
- *Diet*: A diet high in added sugars, saturated fats, and processed foods can promote the development and progression of MAFLD.
- *Lifestyle factors*: Sedentary lifestyle and obesity are associated with an increased risk of MAFLD.
- *Environmental factors*: Environmental toxins and pollutants may also play a role in the pathogenesis of MAFLD.

CLINICAL FEATURES OF METABOLIC (DYSFUNCTION)-ASSOCIATED FATTY LIVER DISEASE

- In the majority of cases, MAFLD entity remains asymptomatic for years together and gets detected accidentally.
- Patients may have nonspecific symptoms such as extreme tiredness, weakness or fatigue, or discomfort in right upper abdomen.
- Patients can present with complications like cirrhosis and hepatocellular carcinoma.
- Extrahepatic complications of MAFLD include cardiovascular disease associated with increased risk of fatal and/or nonfatal cardiovascular events, cancers,

obstructive sleep apnea (OSA), chronic kidney disease (CKD), polycystic ovarian syndrome (PCOS), and osteoporosis.

DIAGNOSIS OF METABOLIC (DYSFUNCTION)-ASSOCIATED FATTY LIVER DISEASE

- *Ultrasonography (USG) abdomen*: USG abdomen is the most preferred imaging modality for detection of MAFLD due to its low cost and widespread availability. USG can accurately detect steatosis when >30% liver parenchyma has fatty infiltration.
- *FibroScan*: A FibroScan is an important noninvasive test vital for the diagnosis of MAFLD. It measures the amount of fibrosis in the liver. FibroScan provides two parameters, the liver stiffness measurement (LSM) that assesses degree of fibrosis, and controlled attenuation parameter (CAP) that assesses degree of steatosis.
- *Magnetic resonance imaging (MRI)*: MRI-based techniques such as MRI-proton density fat fraction (PDFF) and proton magnetic resonance spectroscopy (MRS) are useful in quantifying fat percentage in liver.
- *Simple biomarker scores*: Biomarker scores such as fibrosis-4 (FIB-4), NAFLD fibrosis score (NFS) score, and aspartate aminotransferase to platelet ratio index (APRI) are based on routine laboratory tests, hence are inexpensive and have good negative predictive value.
- *Liver biopsy*: This is a gold standard for assessing degree of steatosis and fibrosis. It is important for prognostication and response to treatment. However, it is an expensive and invasive procedure. Liver biopsy is not mandatory for the diagnosis of MAFLD.

All high-risk patients should be screened for FLD. Initially, by USG and routine biochemical liver parameters and then by noninvasive biomarkers scores like FIB-4. As depicted in **Flowchart 1**, risk stratification is done as per result of FIB-4 score. Patients with intermediate risk are further subjected to FibroScan to decide plan of management.

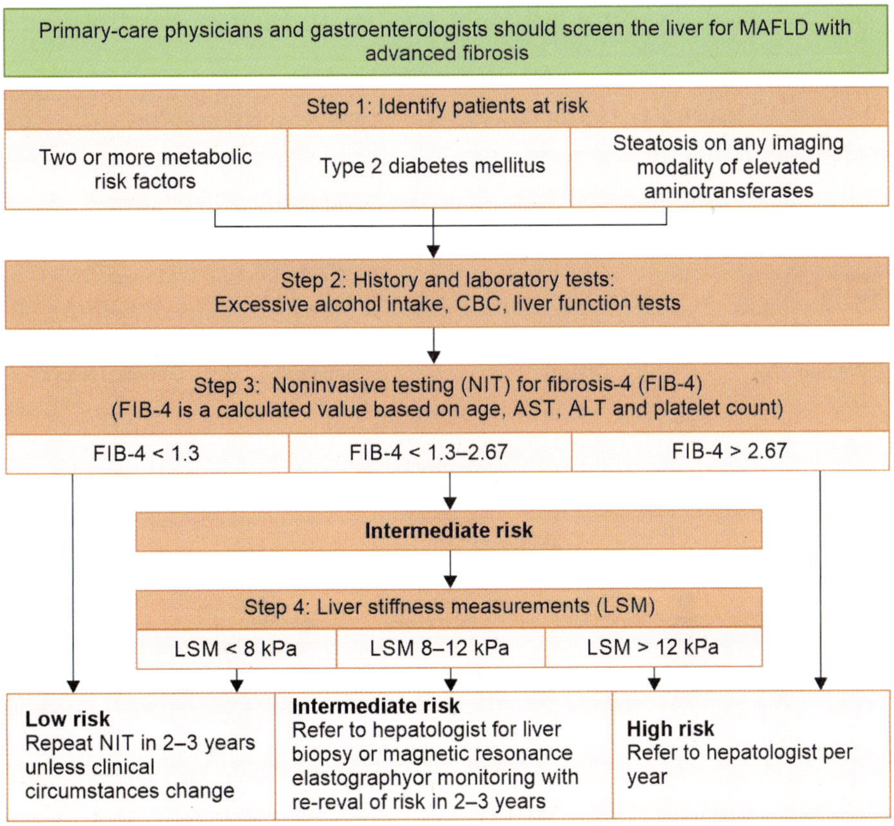

FLOWCHART 1: Algorithm for patients suspected to have MAFLD. Step-by-step approach in triaging patients with MAFLD.
[ALT: alanine transaminase; AST: aspartate transaminase; CBC: complete blood count; MAFLD: metabolic (dysfunction)-associated fatty liver disease]

MANAGEMENT OF METABOLIC (DYSFUNCTION)-ASSOCIATED FATTY LIVER DISEASE

Metabolic (dysfunction)-associated fatty liver disease patients should be evaluated for cardiovascular disease and cardiovascular risk. All patients should be screened for dyslipidemia, hypertension, and diabetes mellitus, and treated aggressively to reduce the risk of cardiovascular and kidney disease. They should be assessed for severity of fibrosis by noninvasive methods and simple noninvasive scores like FIB-4 or NFS score.

Nonpharmacological Treatment

The current approach comprises lifestyle modifications to promote 7–10% weight loss, improve insulin sensitivity by dietary changes and increase physical activity. Sustained weight loss has proved to cause improvement in histological as well as biochemical parameters of MAFLD. A healthy diet, increased physical exercise, and weight reduction are the cornerstones in the management of MAFLD **(Fig. 1)**.

A calorie-restricted diet with a regular calorie deficit can cause sustained benefits. Calorie-restricted diet can promote effective expenditure of body energy stores and also decrease oxidative damage to cells.

Indian diet is comprised of high-carbohydrate content and is one of the contributory factors to MAFLD. Hence, regular consumption of a low-carbohydrate diet has beneficial effect on weight loss as well as MAFLD. A diet high in fructose is associated with rapid progression of MAFLD, and hence should be avoided. A high-fat diet should also be avoided and adequate protein and high-fibre intake has positive impact in halting the progression of disease. Vegetarian diet comprising of fruits and vegetables and also omega-3 supplementation have protective effects on liver.

Aerobic exercises along with resistance exercises has desired effect on patients with MAFLD. It causes improvement in deranged hepatic parameters and also reduces cardiovascular risk. It improves all risk factors associated with MAFLD.

Pharmacological Treatment

Till date, no specific pharmacological therapy for MAFLD has been approved. However, several therapeutic options have shown promising results. The following approaches are suggested as it is proved, beyond doubt, that IR is the

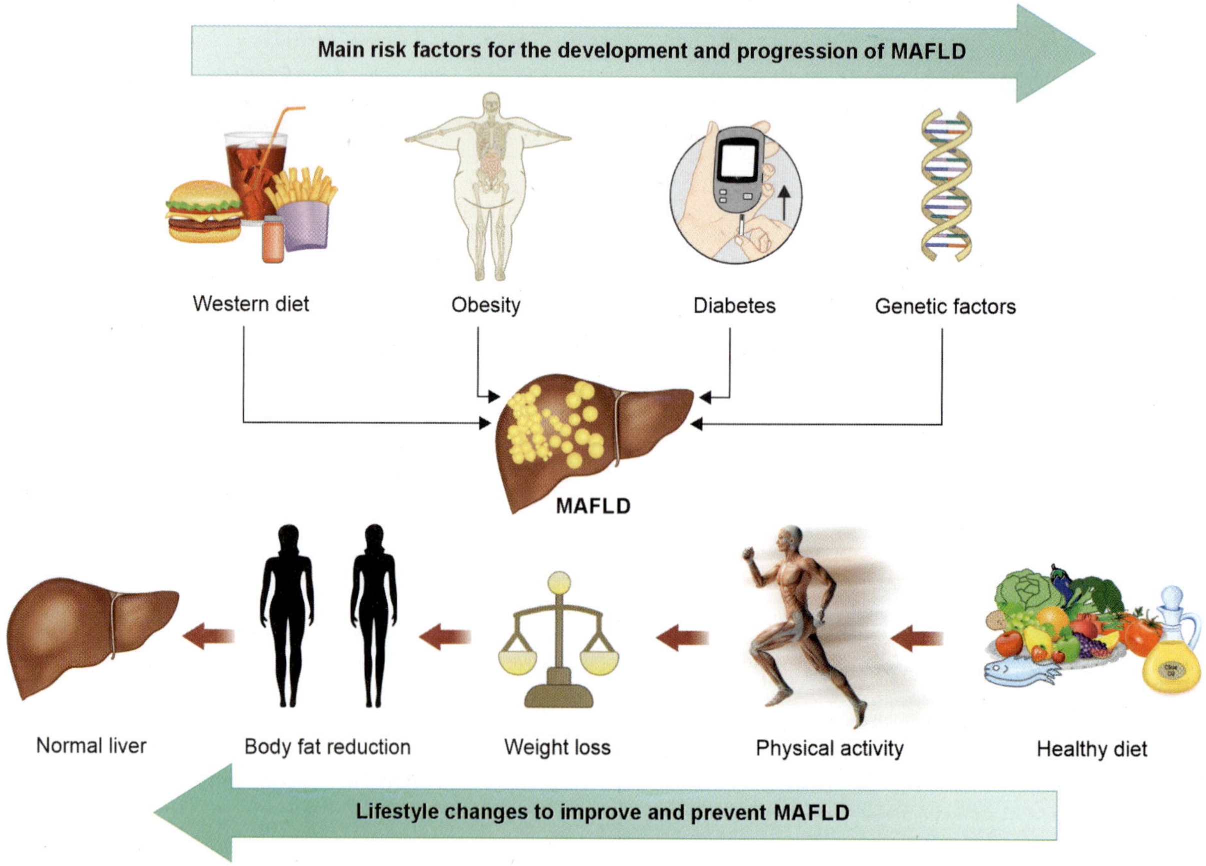

FIG. 1: Risk factors and nonpharmacological treatment of metabolic (dysfunction)-associated fatty liver disease (MAFLD).

most important pathogenetic mechanism responsible for MAFLD. Antihyperglycemic agents, especially insulin sensitizers, have emerged as the potential therapeutic options.

- *Pioglitazone*: It causes significant improvement in liver histology and liver enzymes, in addition to its primary effect as an insulin sensitizer causing control of blood sugar.
- *Glucagon-like polypeptide 1-receptor agonist (GLP-1 RA)*: GLP-1RAs have proved to exhibit many beneficial effects in MAFLD patients. They stimulate glucose-dependent insulin secretion, inhibit glucagon secretion, stimulate β-cell proliferation, increase satiety, and delay gastric emptying. These drugs not only cause decrease in glucose levels but also significantly cause weight reduction and have cardioprotective and renoprotective actions. GLP-1 RA like semaglutide and liraglutide have shown to improve or reverse MAFLD.
- *Dual peroxisome proliferator-activated receptors (PPAR) agonist, saroglitazar*: It acts on many pathogenetic factors responsible for MAFLD. It activates fatty acid oxidation, decreases triglyceride synthesis, and increases insulin sensitivity. It is approved in India for the management of MAFLD.
- *High-dose vitamin E*: 800 mg/day of vitamin E is found to be useful in patients with MAFLD. Vitamin E acts as an antioxidant. It is a potential treatment option for suppressing oxidative stress and metabolism-related liver diseases.
- *Antiobesity drugs*: Drugs like obeticholic acid also cause improvement by reducing weight.

SURGICAL THERAPY

In morbidly obese patients, bariatric surgery has proved to be a boon for reducing the severity of MAFLD along with significant weight loss. Bariatric surgery is known to achieve improvement in steatosis, steatohepatitis, fibrosis, and biochemical parameters in a significant proportion of MAFLD patients. In present scenario, comparatively bariatric surgery outperforms pharmacological therapy in the management of morbid obesity and its consequences like MAFLD.

CONCLUSION

Metabolic (dysfunction)-associated fatty liver disease has evolved as an important cause of chronic liver disease. It is extremely important to recognize this entity as it is associated with long-term hepatic as well as extrahepatic complications having significant morbidity and mortality. It is the need of the hour to create awareness about MAFLD among medical fraternity as well as general public. Educating people about the importance of a healthy diet and exercise remains the main method of prevention and management of this condition. Pharmacological treatment is still in evolving phase although many drugs have shown promising results.

SUGGESTED READINGS

1. Ramírez-Mejía MM, Qi X, Abenavoli L, Romero-Gómez M, Eslam M, Méndez-Sánchez N. Metabolic dysfunction: The silenced connection with fatty liver disease. Ann of Hepatol. 2023;28(6):101138.
2. Pipitone RM, Ciccioli C, Infantino G, Mantia CL, Parisi S, Tulone A, et al. MAFLD: a multisystem disease. Ther Adv Endocrinol Metab. 2023;14:1-23.
3. Persons PA, Bersoux S, Whited MH. Is your patient at risk for NAFLD? Cleve Clin J Med. 2022;89(12):719-27.
4. Stefano JT, Duarte SMB, Ribeiro Leite Altikes RG, Oliveira CP. Non-pharmacological management options for MAFLD: a practical guide. Ther Adv Endocrinol Metab. 2023;14:20420188231160394.
5. Sangro P, de la Torre Aláez M, Sangro B, D'Avola D. Metabolic dysfunction–associated fatty liver disease (MAFLD): an update of the recent advances in pharmacological treatment. J Physiol Biochem. 2023;79:869-79.
6. Kaya E, Yilmaz Y. Metabolic-associated Fatty Liver Disease (MAFLD): A multi-systemic disease beyond the liver. J Clin Transl Hepatol. 2022;10(2):329-38.
7. Kulkarni AV, Sarin SK. The bidirectional impacts of alcohol consumption and MAFLD for progressive fatty liver disease. Ther Advin Endocrinol Metab. 2023;14:20420188231178370.
8. Muangpaisarn P. Metabolic associated fatty liver disease (MAFLD). J Prapokklao Hosp Clin Med Educ Cent. 2022:39(1).
9. Eslam M, Sarin SK, Wong VW, Fan JG, Kawaguchi T, Ahn SH, et al. The Asian Pacific Association for the Study of the Liver clinical practice guidelines for the diagnosis and management of metabolic associated fatty liver disease. Hepatol Int. 2020;14(6):889-919.
10. Clark JM, Cryer DRH, Morton M, Shubrook JH. Nonalcoholic fatty liver disease from a primary care perspective. Diabetes Obes Metab. 2023;25:1421-33.
11. Stefano JT, Duarte SMB, Ribeiro Leite A, Itikes RG, Oliveira CP. Non-pharmacological management options for MAFLD: a practical guide. Ther Adv Endocrinol Metab. 2023;14:20420188231160394.

169

CHAPTER

Metabolic Syndrome and Cardiovascular Disease: An Enigmatic Association

Girish Mathur, Rahul Ramchandani, Divyansh Mathur, Ashutosh Chaturvedi

ABSTRACT

Cardiovascular disease (CVD) has attracted worldwide attention and accounts for a significant number of deaths from noncommunicable diseases. The clustering of obesity-associated cardiovascular risk factors, such as lower high-density lipoprotein (HDL) cholesterol, impaired glucose tolerance (IGT), hypertriglyceridemia, and/or hypertension, are known as the metabolic syndrome (MetS). A variety of cardiovascular disorders, such as microvascular dysfunction, coronary atherosclerosis and calcification, cardiac dysfunction, myocardial infarction, and heart failure, are more common and severe when these risk factors are combined. Each MetS component is a separate risk factor for CVD. The MetS also includes a number of additional, unique risk factors. They include biomarkers for thrombophilia [such as plasminogen activator inhibitor-1 (PAI-1)], endothelial dysfunction (such as E-selectin), increased oxidative stress [such as oxidized low-density lipoprotein (LDL)], and chronic mild inflammation [such as C-reactive protein (CRP)]. As a result, individuals with the MetS may be at an increased risk of atherosclerosis and clinical cardiovascular events.

INTRODUCTION

Ever from the beginning of the metabolic syndrome (MetS) narrative, there has been speculation that one possible consequence for those impacted could be cardiovascular disease (CVD). Subsequently, it became evident from a large body of epidemiological data and a paucity of clinical findings that the metabolic abnormalities associated with the syndrome were major risk factors for CVD **(Fig. 1)**. It was therefore proposed that there is

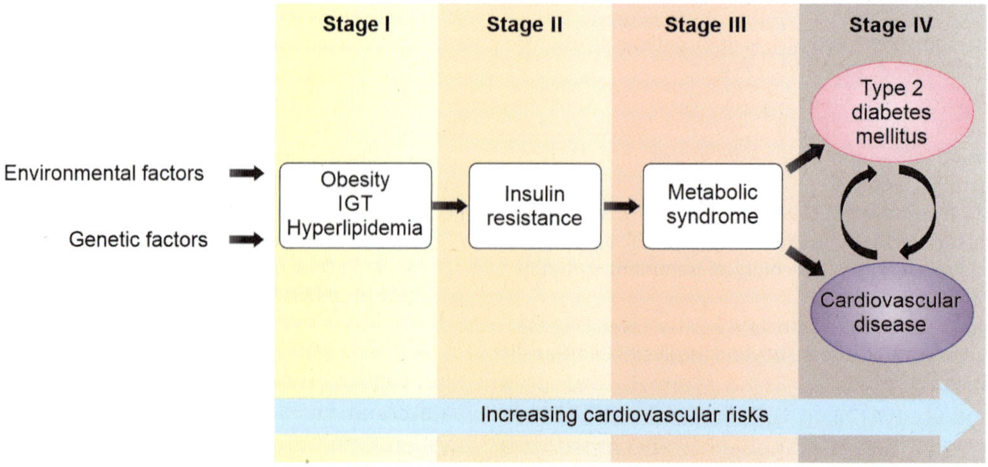

FIG. 1: Progression of metabolic syndrome to cardiovascular diseases.
(IGT: impaired glucose tolerance)

a considerable cardiovascular risk associated with the illness in its subjects. Independent of how MetS is defined, numerous investigations have shown a link between CVD and MetS. These studies have typically shown that people with MetS are more likely to experience CVD events. The largest systematic review and meta-analysis ($n = 951{,}083$) found a 1.5-fold increase in the risk of all-cause death and a twofold increase in the risk of stroke, CVD, and CVD mortality. However, more recent research has found either no or very little correlation between MetS and CVD outcomes. Furthermore, the question whether MetS is a cardiovascular risk factor beyond the individual sum of all its single components remains controversial, and the risk of CVD has been reported to differ by the number of its traits.

CLASSIC FEATURES AND PATHOPHYSIOLOGY OF METABOLIC SYNDROME

There are various criteria used to define MetS, but according to the most widely used criteria given by the National Cholesterol Education Program (NCEP) Adult Treatment Panel III (ATP III) report there are six main components of MetS that affect the risk of developing CVD, i.e., abdominal obesity, atherogenic dyslipidemia, high blood pressure, insulin resistance (with or without glucose intolerance), a proinflammatory state, and a prothrombotic condition. Obesity and insulin resistance are the main underlying risk factors for the development of CVD **(Tables 1 and 2)**.

It is still unclear what pathophysiological mechanism the MetS uses to raise cardiovascular risk. The World Health Organization and the European Group for the Study of Insulin Resistance have already defined the MetS with an emphasis on insulin resistance's autonomous role as the fundamental element. Insulin resistance causes hyperglycemia and hyperinsulinemia, which in turn cause salt retention and peripheral vasoconstriction. Very-low-density lipoprotein (VLDL) is also produced more frequently by the liver, which raises the risk of hypertriglyceridemia, low high-density lipoprotein (HDL) cholesterol, raised apolipoprotein B, elevated tiny low-density lipoprotein (LDL) cholesterol, and atherosclerosis. People with the MetS often have prothrombotic and proinflammatory states as a result of these lipid abnormalities. The International Diabetes Federation, revised NCEP (rNCEP), and NCEP have all released more recent definitions that place a stronger emphasis on central adiposity as the fundamental factor. Tumor necrosis factor (TNF), leptin, adiponectin, and resistin are some of the mediators secreted by adipocytes that cause

TABLE 1: NCEP ATP III proposed diagnostic criteria of metabolic syndrome.

Diagnostic criteria (any three below)	Defining points
Elevated waist circumference*	• *Men*: > 102 cm (> 40 inches) • *Women*: > 88 cm (> 35 inches)
Elevated TG	≥ 150 mg/dL Or Drug treatment for elevated TG
Reduced HDL-C	• *Men*: < 40 mg/dL • *Women*: < 50 mg/dL Or Drug treatment for reduced HDL-C
Elevated blood pressure	≥ 130 mm Hg systolic blood pressure Or ≥ 85 mm Hg diastolic blood pressure Or Drug treatment for hypertension
Elevated fasting glucose	≥ 100 mg/dL Or Drug treatment for elevated glucose

*In non-Asian men and women with a marginally increased waist circumference (37–39 inches in men and 31–34 inches in women), there may be a strong genetic contribution to insulin resistance, and they should benefit from changes in lifestyle. In Asian Americans, there appears to be a lower cutoff point in waist circumference of 35 inches in men and 31 inches in women.

(HDL-C: high-density lipoprotein cholesterol; NCEPATP III: National Cholesterol Education Program Adult Treatment Panel III; TG: triglycerides)

insulin resistance. In these definitions, it is postulated that central obesity causes systemic hypertension and dyslipidemia independently and through the induction of insulin resistance.

IMPAIRED GLUCOSE REGULATION AND CARDIOVASCULAR DISEASE

The MRFIT (Multiple Risk Factors Intervention Trial), the Framingham study, and numerous other longitudinal studies have all amply demonstrated the link between diabetes and higher rates of cardiovascular morbidity and death. Moreover, diabetes worsens the outcome of any acute cardiovascular incident. It has also been studied that the prediabetic states of impaired fasting glucose (IFG) and impaired glucose tolerance (IGT) are already featured by an increased cardiovascular risk and this is why the incidence of CVD did not significantly decline as a result of improvement of glucose control in type 2 diabetes mellitus (T2DM). In fact, glycemic management in diabetic patients should be lowered to normoglycemia

TABLE 2: Proposed definitions and criteria of metabolic syndrome.

Clinical measure	NHLBI/AHA (2005)	WHO (1998)	EGIR	IDF (2005)
Insulin resistance	None Any three of the following:	IGT, IFG, T2DM, or lowered insulin sensitivity plus any two of the following:	Plasma insulin >75th percentile plus any two of the following:	None
Body weight	Waist circumference: • *Men*: ≥102 cm • *Women*: ≥88 cm	Waist-to-hip ratio: • *Men*: >0.9 • *Women*: >0.85; and/or BMI >30 kg/m^2	Waist circumference: • *Men*: ≥94 cm • *Women*: ≥80 cm	Increased waist circumference plus any two of the following:
Triglycerides	TG ≥150 mg/dL or Rx for TG	TG ≥150 mg/dL	TG ≥150 mg/dL	TG ≥150 mg/dL or Rx for TG
HDL-C	• *Men*: HDL-C <40 mg/dL • *Women*: <50 mg/dL; or Rx for reduced HDL-C	• *Men*: HDL-C <35 mg/dL • *Women*: <39 mg/dL	Men or women: HDL-C <39 mg/dL	• *Men*: HDL-C <40 mg/dL • *Women*: <50 mg/dL; or Rx for reduced HDL-C
Blood pressure	≥130 mm Hg systolic or >85 mm Hg diastolic; or Rx for HTN	≥140/90 mm Hg	≥140/90 mm Hg or Rx for HTN	≥130 mm Hg systolic or ≥85 mm Hg diastolic; or Rx for HTN
Glucose	≥100 mg/dL or Rx for glucose (includes diabetes)	IGT, IFG, or T2DM necessary	IGT or IFG (not diabetes)	>100 mg/dL fasting glucose (includes diabetes)
Other	None	Microalbuminuria	None	None

(BMI: body mass index; EGIR: European Group for the Study of Insulin Resistance; HDL-C: high-density lipoprotein cholesterol; HTN: hypertension; IDF: International Diabetes Federation; IFG: impaired fasting glucose; IGT: impaired glucose tolerance; NHLBI/AHA: National Heart, Lung, and Blood Institute/American Heart Association; Rx: prescription; T2DM: type 2 diabetes mellitus; TG: triglycerides; WHO: World Health Organization)

in order to significantly lower the risk of CVD in these persons. In fact, to achieve a substantial reduction of CVD in diabetic individuals their glycemic control should be brought down to the condition of normoglycemia.

VISCERAL ADIPOSITY, LIVER FAT, AND CARDIOVASCULAR RISK

Abdominal obesity is linked to increased CVDs. Evidence support that waist circumference (WC) measurements with body mass index (BMI) applied in the clinical practice may add vital information and successful prediction of cardiovascular risk and mortality focusing on visceral adiposity. Obesity is associated with overt atherosclerotic lesions. Fat streaks that thicken the intima artery layer are the first sign of atherosclerosis. Obesity is considered to accelerate this process by several mechanisms such as insulin resistance through adipocytokines, endothelial dysfunction, hypercoagulability, and inflammation. Several prospective epidemiological studies demonstrate that obesity and higher risk of incident coronary artery disease (CAD) are strongly linked. Instead of body weight, a higher risk of cardiovascular events has been related to excess visceral fat.

HYPERTRIGLYCERIDEMIA AND CARDIOVASCULAR DISEASE

Recently, it has been reported that even mild hypertriglyceridemia can significantly increase the risk of myocardial infarction and stroke. Although the danger of hypertriglyceridemia is smaller than that of hypercholesterolemia, vascular injury appears to be directly influenced by triglyceride-rich lipoproteins, or VLDL.

LOW HIGH-DENSITY LIPOPROTEIN CHOLESTEROL AND CARDIOVASCULAR RISK

Low levels of HDL cholesterol have long been associated with increased risk for CVD and have been documented as a critical risk factor for estimating 10-year risk of CVD. This is biologically plausible since HDL particles drive reverse cholesterol transport and may exert a variety of antiatherogenic effects. High HDL levels are associated with longevity and are protective against the development of atherosclerotic disease. The Framingham study found that as HDL levels steadily decline below 40 mg/dL, the risk for CAD substantially rises. In the Québec Cardiovascular Study, for every 10% reduction in HDL, risk for CAD increased 13%.

HYPERTENSION AND CARDIOVASCULAR RISK

The risk of myocardial infarction and stroke increases steadily with blood pressure, as shown by the Framingham study and the MRFIT. The new observation that even a slight rise in blood pressure can predispose to clinical outcomes led to a reduction in the cutoff levels for diagnosing hypertension. One of the conditions that damages the vascular wall more severely and results in endothelial dysfunction is hypertension which leads to the atherosclerotic process and subsequent clinical vascular events. Meanwhile, elevated blood pressure in turn inhibits the blood flow to pancreas and leads to decrease of insulin secretion, which further exacerbates insulin resistance and MetS.

CONCLUSION

Because the majority of the MetS's clinical and biochemical characteristics, both classic and nonclassic, are cardiovascular risk factors, the majority of individuals with the syndrome are believed to be at risk for CVD. Individuals with the MetS have a twofold to fourfold increased risk of CVD compared to those without the syndrome. Compared to men, women have a roughly fourfold higher risk of developing the syndrome (approximately twofold). When affected individuals already have diabetes, CVD, chronic mild inflammation [high C-reactive protein (CRP)], or both, the risk is increased. Despite the lack of defined diagnostic criteria for MetS, it is crucial to recognize the known risk factors. Patients can be carefully evaluated and followed up on for the emergence of this syndrome and the eventual risk of CVD by identifying the various components. Before asserting that the risk of CVD in persons with the MetS is not more than the total of the risk associated to its individual components, it is critical to establish an acceptable reference category. In this sense, a more accurate estimate of genuine individual risk can be obtained by evaluating the number of risk variables that cluster in the particular subject and comparing them to people who do not have any disorders. The idea that altering one's lifestyle can treat underlying illnesses like obesity and/or insulin resistance. Emphasis should be placed on the MetS and CVD modifications or medicine that improves various classic and auxiliary components of the MetS and, thus, significantly lowers the risk of CVD.

SUGGESTED READINGS

1. National Cholesterol Education Program (NCEP) Expert Panel on Detection, Evaluation, and Treatment of High Blood Cholesterol in Adults (Adult Treatment Panel III). Third report of the National Cholesterol Education Program (NCEP) Expert Panel on Detection, Evaluation, and Treatment of High Blood Cholesterol in Adults (Adult Treatment Panel III) final report. Circulation. 2002;106:3143-421.
2. Grundy SM, Cleeman JI, Daniels SR, Donato KA, Eckel RH, Franklin BA, et al. Diagnosis and management of the metabolic syndrome: an American Heart Association/National Heart, Lung, and Blood Institute Scientific Statement. Circulation. 2005;112:2735-52.
3. Kannel WB, McGee DL. Diabetes and cardiovascular disease. The Framingham Study. JAMA. 1979;241:2035-8.
4. Stamler J, Vaccaro O, Neaton JD, Wentworth D. Diabetes, other risk factors, and 12-yr cardiovascular mortality for men screened in the Multiple Risk Factor Intervention Trial. Diabetes Care. 1993;16:434-44.
5. Mottillo S, Filion KB, Genest J, Joseph L, Pilote L, Poirier P, et al. The metabolic syndrome and cardiovascular risk: A systematic review and meta-analysis. J Am Coll Cardiol. 2010;56:1113-32.
6. van Herpt TTW, Dehghan A, Hoek M, Ikram MA, Hofman A, Sijbrands EJGG, et al. The clinical value of metabolic syndrome and risks of cardiometabolic events and mortality in the elderly: the Rotterdam study. Cardiovasc Diabetol. 2016;15:69.
7. Ju SY, Lee JY, Kim DH. Association of metabolic syndrome and its components with all-cause and cardiovascular mortality in the elderly. Medicine (Baltimore). 2017;96:e8491.
8. Miller M, Seidler A, Moalemi A, Pearson TA. Normal triglyceride levels and coronary artery disease events: the Baltimore Coronary Observational Long-Term Study. J Am Coll Cardiol. 1998;31:1252-7.
9. Tanne D, Koren-Morag N, Graff E, Goldbourt U. Blood lipids and first-ever ischemic stroke/transient ischemic attack in the Bezafibrate Infarction prevention (BIP) Registry: high triglycerides constitute an independent risk factor. Circulation. 2001;104:2892-7.
10. Vasan RS, Larson MG, Leip EP, Evans JC, O'Donnell CJ, Kannel WB, et al. Impact of high-normal blood pressure on the risk of cardiovascular disease. N Engl J Med. 2001;345:1291-7.

170

CHAPTER

War Against Lipids: The New Weapons in the Armory

PC Manoria, Pankaj Manoria

ABSTRACT

Lipids play a very important role in the pathogenesis of atherosclerotic cardiovascular disease (CVD). Low-density lipoprotein cholesterol (LDL-C) is the primary target and non-high-density cholesterol (HDL-C) cholesterol is the coprimary target. HDL cholesterol is a fallen angel because all trials of pharmacological alleviation of HDL-C on top of statins have been flop trials. Triglycerides (TG) are still in search of a positive cardiovascular outcome trial, which is nonexistent at the present time. The Reduction of Cardiovascular Events with Icosapent Ethyl-Intervention Trial (REDUCE-IT) was positive, but the benefit was not related to the lowering of TG. There is no evidence-based target for lipoprotein(a) [LP(a)] at the present time, but the trial assessing the impact of lipoprotein(a) lowering with pelacarsen on major cardiovascular events in patients with CVD (HORIZON) is ongoing and in the future, we may have an evidence-based target for it. So at the present time, the focus is on targeting LDL-C and non-HDL-C. We have a panoply of drugs to lower LDL-C, such as statins, ezetimibe, bempedoic acid, proprotein convertase subtilisin/kexin type 9 (PCSK9) monoclonal antibodies, and inclisiran. These agents have declared war on lipids and currently LDL-C can be cut to any size.

INTRODUCTION

Dyslipidemia is the most common major, modifiable risk factor for atherosclerotic cardiovascular disease (ASCVD) and lipids play a crucial role in the development of atherosclerosis.

Dyslipidemia results in the formation of plaques in the arteries, which are the major culprit for cardiovascular disease (CVD). They put us at risk of heart attacks and strokes. Heart attack is the leading cause of death, and stroke is the most common cause of disability. The lipid management of ASCVD has made great strides during the last couple of years. When we look at the issue of plaque stabilization, the answer is yes and there is overwhelming data on statins to support this. Plaque stabilization results in a decrease in the incidence of acute coronary events. Lipid management with high-intensity statins such as atorvastatin has shown arrest of the progression of atherosclerosis in the effect of intensive lipid lowering on progression of coronary atherosclerosis—evidence for an early benefit from the REVERSAL (Reversal of Atherosclerosis with Aggressive Lipid Lowering) trial. The arrest of the progression of atherosclerosis occurs when the low-density lipoprotein cholesterol (LDL-C) is lowered below 65 mg/dL. Interestingly, the GLAGOV (Global Assessment of Plaque Regression with a PCSK9 Antibody as Measured by Intravascular Ultrasound) trial has shown that with evolocumab, regression of atherosclerosis can also be achieved and this is indeed a big advance in the ongoing war against lipids. Regression of atherosclerosis occurs when the LDL-C is below 50 mg/dL. Due to these developments, the targets for LDL-C are progressively declining. The European Society of Cardiology/European Atherosclerosis Society (ESC/EAS) 2019 guideline recommended a target of 55 mg/dL for the very high-risk group. However, the target recommended for this group by the 2018 American College of Cardiology/America Heart Association (ACC/AHA) guidelines was 70. The Lipid Association of India guideline recommended a target of 50 mg/dL in 2016, and in 2021, it created a new extreme risk group with category A with an LDL-C target < 50 mg/dL (optional goal < 30 mg/dL) and for group B < 30 mg/dL. The FOURIER (Further Cardiovascular Outcomes Research with PCSK9 Inhibition Subjects with Elevated Risk) trial has shown that there is incremental benefit to lowering LDL-C up to 10 mg/dL without any side effects, which clearly implies that lowering LDL-C is very safe. In fact, the side effects that are encountered while lowering LDL-C are related to the drug and not to the lowering of LDL-C. For example, diabetes due to statins is caused by statins and not by lowering LDL-C.

STATINS

Statins are the foundational drugs for lipid management, both for primary prevention and secondary prevention, but in about 50% of patients, they failed to reach the LDL goal. When statins failed to achieve the LDL-C goals, ezetimibe was added.

EZETIMIBE

Ezetimibe was evaluated in the IMPROVE-IT (Improved Reduction of Outcomes: Vytorin Efficacy International Trial). The trial compared simvastatin 40 mg with a combination of simvastatin 40 mg plus ezetimibe 10 mg and showed that there was a statistically significant reduction of 10%, hazard ratio (HR) 0.90; confidence interval (CI) (0.84, 0.97); $p = 0.003$ in the primary ischemic endpoint, which was a composite of cardiovascular (CV) death, myocardial infarction (MI), hospital admission for unstable angina, coronary revascularization (≥ 30 days after randomization), or stroke. The LDL-C level achieved in the simvastatin arm was 69.5 mg/dL, while in the simvastatin plus ezetimibe arm, it was 53.7 mg/dL. The benefit was seen particularly in diabetic patients. There was a decrease in nonfatal MI, nonfatal stroke, and revascularization, but unstable angina and CV death were not affected. Unlike statins, it does not have pleiotropic effects. Ezetimibe is approved as a Class IB indication by guidelines to be used on top of statins if LDL-C goals are not achieved. But if LDL targets are still not achieved with statins and ezetimibe, bempedoic acid (BA) (180 mg/day) is added.

BEMPEDOIC ACID

Bempedoic acid is a useful addition to the therapeutic armamentarium for statin intolerance. It is a prodrug that is converted into its active form, bempedoyl-coenzyme-A, by the enzyme very long-chain acyl-CoA synthetase-1 (ASCVL1). This enzyme is not present in the skeletal muscles and therefore, this drug does not produce muscle symptoms, unlike statins. It inhibits the synthesis of cholesterol by inhibiting the enzyme adenosine triphosphate-citrate lyase (ACL), which is an enzyme upstream of hydroxymethylglutaryl-coenzyme A (HMG-CoA) reductase in the cholesterol biosynthesis pathway. The inhibition of cholesterol synthesis in the liver increases the expression of LDL-C receptors in the liver, resulting in greater clearance of LDL-C, and thereby decreasing its levels in the blood. It is administered at a dose of 180 mg once daily.

Patients with mild-to-moderate renal impairment do not require dose adjustment, but it has not been studied in patients with severe end-stage kidney disease [estimated glomerular filtration rate (eGFR) < 30 mL/min/1.73 m^2] or in patients on dialysis. No dosage adjustment is necessary in patients with mild-to-moderate hepatic impairment, but it has not been studied in patients with severe hepatic impairment (Child–Pugh Class C). The drug is excreted to the kidneys through the channel organic anion transporter 2 (OAT2), which is the same transporter that excretes uric acid and creatinine. So BA has the potential to produce a mild increase in uric acid and creatinine levels. Unlike statins, it has no tendency to produce new-onset diabetes and has favorable effects on glycemic control.

Clinical Studies

BA was evaluated in four phase III trials with about 3,600 participants **(Table 1)**. The effect of BA in patients with ASCVD or high-risk ASCVD or heterozygous familial hypercholesterolemia (HeFH) on maximally tolerated statin background therapy was evaluated in the Cholesterol Lowering via BA, an ACL-inhibiting Regimen (CLEAR Harmony) and CLEAR Wisdom trials **(Table 1)**. Patients with hypercholesterolemia and statin intolerance were evaluated in the CLEAR Tranquility and CLEAR Serenity trials.

In BA trials on maximally tolerated statins, i.e., CLEAR Harmony and CLEAR Wisdom trials, the reduction

TABLE 1: Four phase III trials of bempedoic acid.

Trial	Subset	Duration
Statin-tolerant patients		
CLEAR Harmony	Maximally tolerated statin background therapy	52 weeks
CLEAR Wisdom	Maximally tolerated statin background therapy	52 weeks
Statin-intolerant patients		
CLEAR Serenity	Low, very low, or no statin background therapy	24 weeks
CLEAR Tranquility	Low, very low, or no statin background therapy	12 weeks

in LDL-C was -18.1 ($p \leq 0.001$) and -17.4 ($p \leq 0.001$), respectively, while in statin-intolerant patients in CLEAR Tranquility and CLEAR Serenity trials, the reduction in LDL-C was greater, i.e., -28.5 ($p \leq 0.001$) and -21.4 ($p \leq 0.001$), respectively. The reduction in high-sensitivity C-reactive protein (HsCRP) in the CLEAR Harmony and CLEAR Wisdom trials was -21.5 ($p = 0.001$) and -8.7 in ($p \leq 0.039$), respectively. The reduction in HsCRP in the CLEAR Tranquility trial was -31.1 ($p \leq 0.001$) and -24.3 in the CLEAR Serenity trial ($p \leq 0.001$).

Adverse Effects

Hyperuricemia is an important side effect but is seen only in a minority of patients on BA. It reversibly increases uric acid levels. This occurs within the first 4 weeks of treatment and the levels stabilize thereafter. It has the potential to precipitate gout or increase the risk of gout in patients who do not have the disease, but the incidence of gout during treatment with BA was low in all the trials. Uric acid must be tested in patients who experience symptoms. The pooled analysis of all four phase III randomized control trial showed a minor increase in hepatic enzymes, blood urea, and serum creatinine. A minor decrease in hemoglobin was also reported. In studies, a combination of BA plus ezetimibe in patients who are unable to take statins has shown a reduction of LDL-C by 39.2% and 36.2%, respectively.

CLEAR Outcomes Trial

The CLEAR Outcomes trial carried out in patients with statin intolerance who had or were at high risk for CVD has shown positive results. The trial enrolled 13,970 patients of statin intolerance, out of which 6,992 were randomized in the BA group and the remaining 6,978 in the placebo group. The patients were randomized to receive oral BA 180 mg daily or placebo. The primary endpoint was a composite of death from CV causes, nonfatal infarction, nonfatal stroke, or coronary revascularization. The primary endpoint was significantly lower in the BA compared to placebo, HR 0.87; 97% CI 0.79–0.96; $p = 0.004$. There was also a statistically significant benefit in deaths from CV causes, fatal or nonfatal MI, and coronary revascularization. The mortality rate was not affected. Gout and cholelithiasis were more commonly seen with BA compare to placebo group (3.1% vs. 2.1% and 2.2% vs. 1.2%, respectively).

If the LDL-C goals are not achieved with the triple combo of high-intensity statins plus ezetimibe plus BA because the LDL-C is very high or if there is statin intolerance, then the choice is proprotein convertase subtilisin/kexin type 9 (PCSK9) monoclonal antibodies, evolocumab, and alirocumab.

PROPROTEIN CONVERTASE SUBTILISIN/KEXIN TYPE 9 INHIBITORS

Proprotein convertase subtilisin/kexin type 9 monoclonal antibodies are the molecule of the decade for the management of dyslipidemia and for minimizing ASCVD. All guidelines have approved the use of evolocumab and alirocumab. They are used in very high-risk and extreme-risk groups if LDL-C goals are not achieved by statins plus ezetimibe plus BA. Both monoclonal antibodies have been categorized as class IB recommendation. They decrease LDL-C by about 60%, LP(a) by 20–25%, and have a favorable effect on all other lipoproteins. They also have pleiotropic effects.

Evolocumab

Evolocumab was evaluated in chronic stable angina in the FOURIER trial. The study showed a statistically significant 15% benefit [HR 0.85 (95% CI 0.79–0.92; $p = 0.001$)] in the primary endpoints of CV death, MI, stroke, hospitalization for unstable angina, uric acid, and revascularization. The FOURIER trial result had a reduction in MI by 27% ($p \leq 0.001$), stroke by 21% ($p = 0.01$), and coronary revascularization by 22% ($p \leq 0.001$). All-cause mortality or CV mortality did not show any significant benefit.

The risk reduction at 2 years had a number needed to treat (NNT) of 74 to prevent CVD, MI, and stroke, but at 3 years, it fell to 50. It seems that long-term follow-up could have produced more fruitful results.

Evolocumab is available on the market as a 1 mL pen containing 140 mg. It is given in doses of 140 mg biweekly/420 mg monthly subcutaneously (SQ).

Alirocumab

The ODYSSEY trial was conducted in acute coronary syndrome (ACS) patients after 1–12 months of the acute episode. In this trial, alirocumab was randomized against placebo for all lipid-lowering therapies. The LDL-C dropped from 101.4 to 53.3 mg/dL after a 4-year follow-up. The primary endpoint, a composite of coronary heart death, nonfatal MI, ischemic stroke, or unstable angina requiring hospitalization, occurred in 9.5% versus 11.1%, a relative risk reduction (RRR) of 15%, $p = 0.0003$. Nonfatal MI, Ischemic stroke, and unstable angina requiring hospitalization showed a statistically significant reduction. All-cause mortality showed a nonsignificant reduction and coronary heart disease deaths were not decreased. Patients with LDL > 100 mg/dL benefitted the most. The trial showed incredible safety for alirocumab.

Alirocumab is available as a 1 mL pen containing 75 mg or 150 mg and is given in doses of 75 mg biweekly

BOX 1: Use of PCSK9 MoAbs.

- ASCVD who have not achieved LDL-C goals despite maximally tolerated statins + ezetimibe + bempedoic acid
- Intolerance to statin
- HoFH and HeFH

(ASCVD: atherosclerotic cardiovascular disease; HeFH: heterozygous familial hypercholesterolemia; HoFH: homozygous familial hypercholesterolemia; LDL-C: low-density lipoprotein cholesterol; PCSK9: proprotein convertase subtilisin/kexin type 9)

TABLE 2: Effect of various drugs and combinations on LDL-C.

Drugs	Average LDL-C reduction
Ezetimibe mono	20%
Low/moderate-intensity statin	30%
Low-dose statin plus ezetimibe	30–40%
Bempedoic acid + ezetimibe in statin-naive	45%
High-intensity statin	50%
High-intensity statin plus ezetimibe	65%
High-intensity statin plus ezetimibe plus bempedoic acid	70%
PCSK9 inhibitor	50–50%
PCSK9 inhibitor + high-intensity statin	75%
PCSK9 inhibitor + high-intensity statin + ezetimibe	85%

(LDL-C: low-density lipoprotein cholesterol; PCSK9: proprotein convertase subtilisin/kexin type 9)

or 150 mg monthly SQ. The current use of PCSK9 MoAbs is mentioned in **Box 1**.

The LDL-C cholesterol can be reduced to any level by current drug therapy in various combination **(Table 2)**.

INCLISIRAN

Despite the exciting results of PCSK9 monoclonal antibody trials, two problems were noted with them, i.e., the drug needs multiple injections per year and adherence data is like statins. To circumvent this, a new drug called inclisiran has been developed. It inhibits the synthesis of PCSK9 in the liver.

The beauty of inclisiran is that a single injection decreases LDL-C cholesterol by 50%, which is maintained for the next 6 months.

The drug is being evaluated in the ORION program. ORION phase III pooled analysis of ORION-9, ORION-10, and ORION-11 has been published and has shown exciting results.

PROPROTEIN CONVERTASE SUBTILISIN/KEXIN TYPE 9 VACCINE

Proprotein convertase subtilisin/kexin type 9 is a new therapeutic innovation. A single dose of vaccine decreases LDL-C by 50%, which is maintained for 12 months. If the results of the ongoing future trials come out positive, then a booster dose every year will be a new way of targeting ASCVD.

LIPOPROTEIN(A)

Lipoprotein(a) is a deadly lipoprotein and has a prevalence of about 10% in Asia. Initial screening should be done at 18 years and at 2 years if there is a family history of familial hypercholesterolemia (FH) and premature coronary artery disease (CAD). According to the Lipid Association of India, LP(a) levels > 20 mg/dL are considered to be at increased risk of ASCVD, 20–49 is a moderate risk factor, and >50 mg/dL is at high risk. Lp(a)-driven CVD is considered a slow death sentence with a gloomy prognosis because of the malignant progression of ASCVD and aortic stenosis. The horizon trial with pelacarsen is ongoing and it is likely to emerge as a new potential blockbuster for reducing Lp(a)-driven CVD and becoming a salvageable disease in the future.

GENE EDITING

Gene editing is a new, upcoming technology based on clustered regularly interspaced short palindromic repeats (the CRISPR-Cas9 system). It has two components—guided ribonucleic acid (gRNA) and casein-9 protein. The *gRNA* locates the specific gene and the *Cas9* protein deactivates gene. With this technology, the *PCSK9* gene has been successfully targeted. The beauty of this technology is that after a single sitting, the *PCSK9* gene is deactivated and the LDL-C drops to 20–25 mg/dL for the rest of your life. The first successful patient has already been treated in New Zealand and a trial with VERVE-101 is ongoing in 40 patients with FH.

CONCLUSION

With the availability of many lipid-lowering drugs, we are amidst a golden era of lipid management. In the current scenario, LDL-C can be targeted at any level with great safety. If the horizon trial comes out positive, pelacarsen will improve the outcome of deadly LP(a)-induced CVD. Gene editing is going to be the future of cardiology in terms of lipid management.

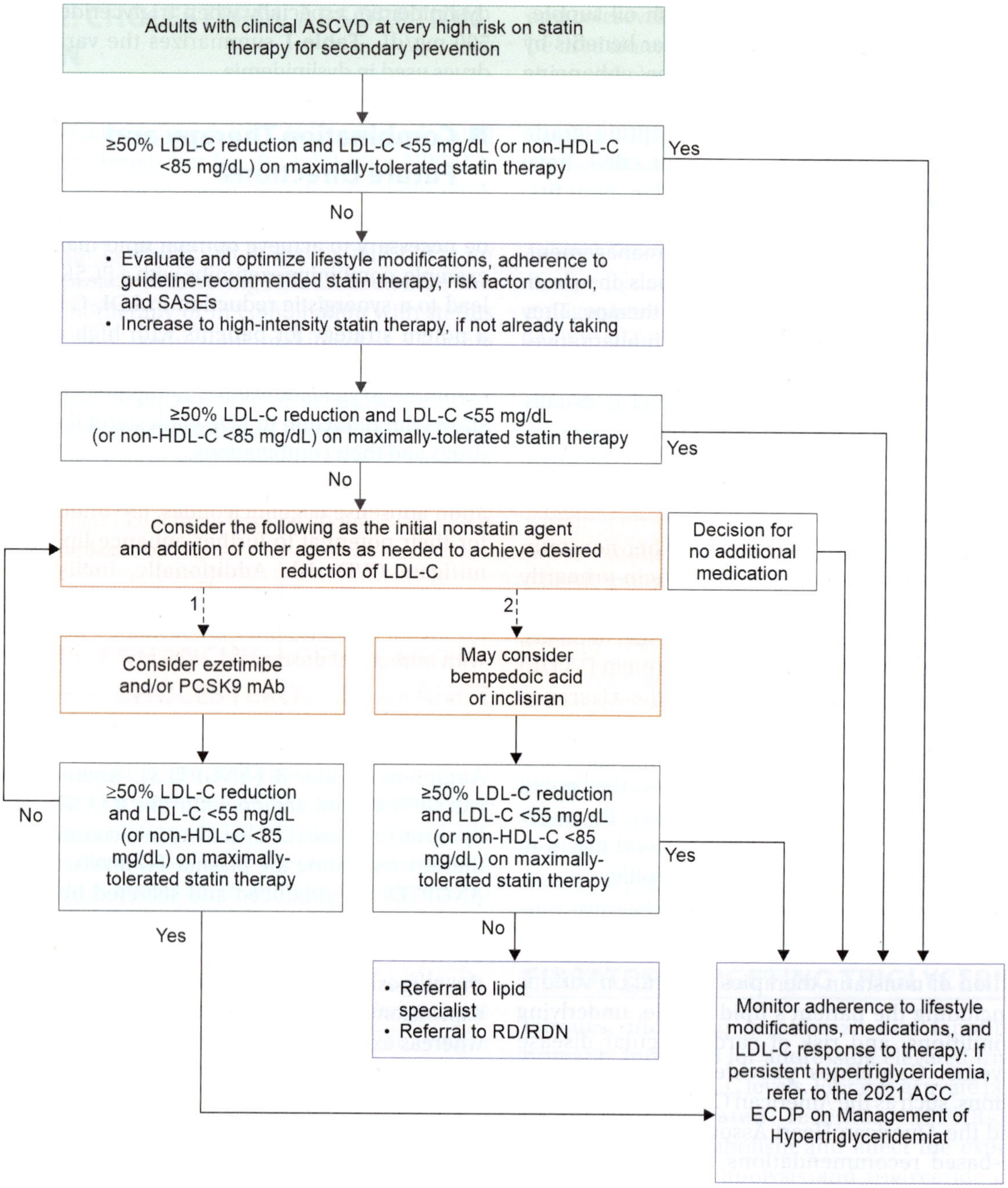

FLOWCHART 1: The algorithm for ASCVD with very high risk.

(ACC: American College of Cardiology; ASCVD: atherosclerotic cardiovascular disease; ECDP: Early Childhood Development Program; LDL-C: low-density lipoprotein cholesterol; non-HDL-C: non-high density lipoprotein cholesterol; PCSK9: proprotein convertase subtilisin/kexin type 9; RD: registered dietitians; RDN: registered dietitian nutritionists; SASEs: statin associated side-effects)

INCLISIRAN

Inclisiran is a synthetic small interfering RNA (siRNA), which works by targeting the PCSK9 and is conjugated to triantennary N-acetylgalactosamine carbohydrates (GalNAc), which targets the siRNA to the liver. There is upregulation of LDL receptors thereby increasing the clearance of LDL-C. In the trial to evaluate the effect of inclisiran treatment on LDL-C in subjects with heterozygous familial hypercholesterolemia (HeFH) (ORION)-10, inclisiran reduced plasma LDL-C levels by 51.3%. The plasma half-life is 5–10 hours. It is given as a subcutaneous injection at days 0, 90 and 6 monthly thereafter. Presently it is not approved by the Food and Drug Administration (FDA).

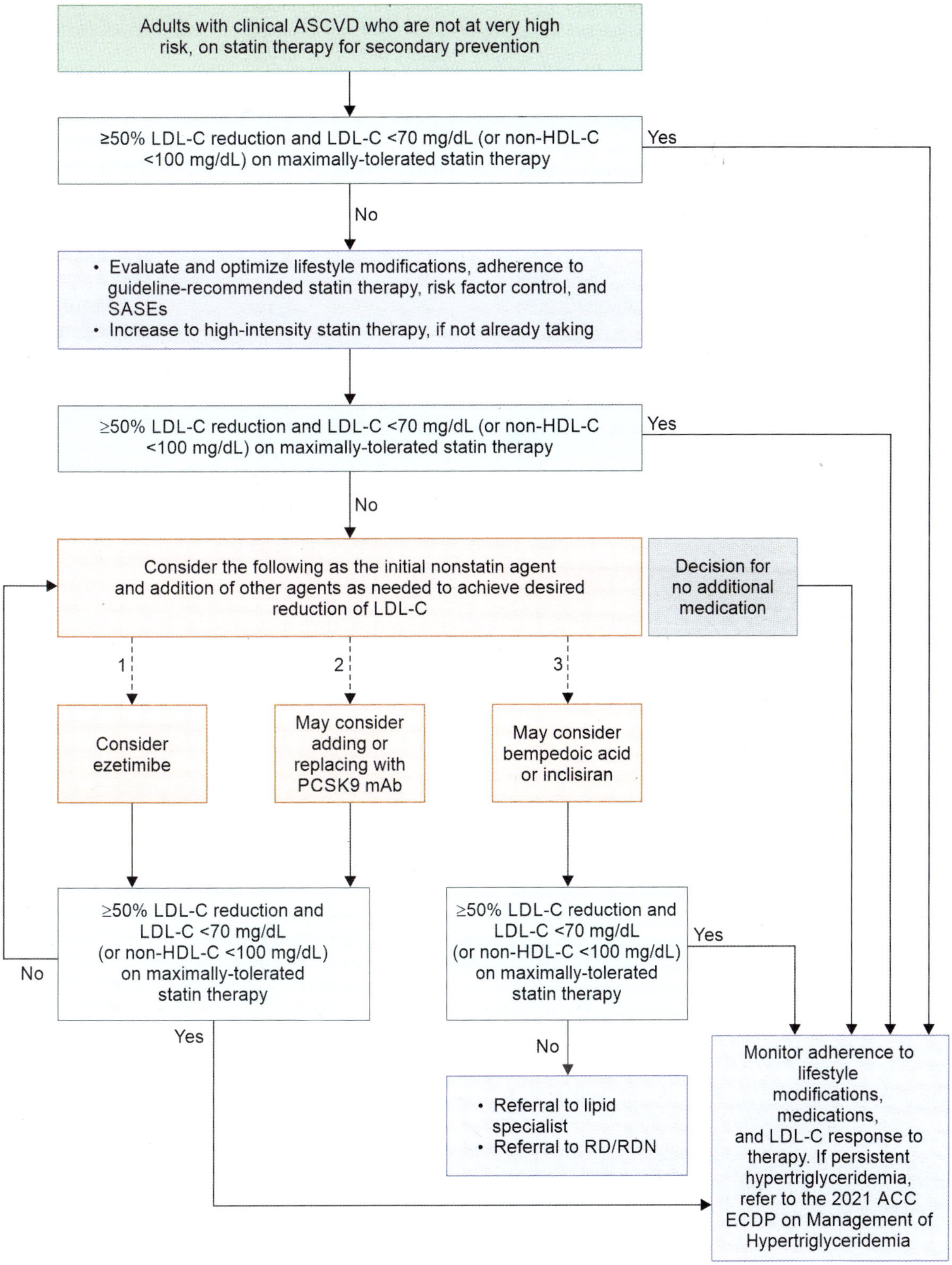

FLOWCHART 2: The algorithm to be adopted for ASCVD who are not at a very high risk.

(ACC: American College of Cardiology; ASCVD: atherosclerotic cardiovascular disease; ECDP: Early Childhood Development Program; LDL-C: low-density lipoprotein cholesterol; non-HDL-C: non-high density lipoprotein cholesterol; PCSK9: proprotein convertase subtilisin/kexin type 9; RD: registered dietitians; RDN: registered dietitian nutritionists; SASEs: statin associated side-effects)

TABLE 1: Various nonstatin drugs used in dyslipidemia.

Drug name	Mechanism of action	Dosage	Frequency	Route of administration	LDL-C lowering (%)	Adverse drug effects
Ezetimibe	Inhibit sterol transporter and NPC1L1	10 mg	Daily	Oral	−18.0	Diarrhea, arthralgia, upper respiratory tract symptoms
Alirocumab	Inhibit PCSK9 from binding to the LDL-C receptors	75 mg/mL 150 mg/mL	Q2W Q4W	Subcutaneous	−47.0 to −57.0	Injection site reactions, nasopharyngitis, and flu-like symptoms
Evolocumab		140 mg/mL 420 mg/mL	Q2W Q4W	Subcutaneous	−53.0	
Bempedoic acid	Inhibits ATP citrate lyase	180 mg	Daily	Oral	−21.4	Gout, thrombocythemia, leukopenia, upper respiratory tract, and symptoms
Inclisiran	Inhibits the production of PCSK9 and blocks PCSK9 from binding to LDL-C receptors	300 mg/mL	Twice yearly	Subcutaneous	−29.9 to −46.4	Injection site reactions

TABLE 2: Intensity of lipid-lowering treatment.

Treatment	Average LDL-C reduction
Moderate intensity statin	≈30%
High-intensity statin	≈50%
High-intensity statin plus ezetimibe	≈65%
PCSK9 inhibitor	≈60%
PCSK9 inhibitor plus high-intensity statin	≈75%
PCSK9 inhibitor plus high-intensity statin plus ezetimibe	≈85%

CONCLUSION

Nonstatin drugs have transformed the management of dyslipidemia, providing clinicians with an array of options to tailor treatment based on individual patient needs and preferences. Ezetimibe, PCSK9 inhibitors, bile acid sequestrants, bempedoic acid fibrates, omega-3 fatty acids, and niacin have each contributed to a more nuanced and comprehensive approach to lipid control. As our understanding of dyslipidemia deepens and new therapeutic avenues emerge, the role of nonstatin drugs will further be enhanced.

SUGGESTED READINGS

1. Joshi SR, Anjana RM, Deepa M, Pradeepa R, Bhansali A, Dhandhania VK, et al. ICMR-INDIAB collaborative study group. Prevalence of dyslipidemia in urban and rural India: the ICMR-INDIAB study. PLoS One. 2014;9(5):e96808.
2. Sullivan D, Olsson AG, Scott R, Kim JB, Xue A, Gebski V, et al. Effect of a monoclonal antibody to PCSK9 on low-density lipoprotein cholesterol levels in statin-intolerant patients: the GAUSS randomized trial. JAMA. 2012;308(23):2497-506.
3. Ballantyne CM, Banach M, Mancini GBJ, Lepor NE, Hanselman JC, Zhao X, et al. Efficacy and safety of bempedoic acid added to ezetimibe in statin-intolerant patients with hypercholesterolemia: a randomized, placebo-controlled study. Atherosclerosis. 2018;277:195-203.
4. Raal FJ, Rosenson RS, Reeskamp LF, Hovingh GK, Kastelein JJP, Rubba P, et al. Evinacumab for homozygous familial hypercholesterolemia. N Engl J Med. 2020;383(8):711-20.
5. Ray KK, Wright RS, Kallend D, Koenig W, Leiter LA, Raal FJ, et al. Two phase 3 trials of inclisiran in patients with elevated LDL cholesterol. N Engl J Med. 2020;382(16):1507-19.

172
CHAPTER

Role of Dual Glucagon-like Peptide Analogs in the Management of Obesity

Sandeep Garg, Kuldeep Gurjar, Sunita Aggarwal

ABSTRACT

Obesity is a chronic disease affecting millions worldwide and often associated with comorbidities like type 2 diabetes mellitus, liver disease, cardiovascular disease, and hypertension. As obesity prevalence increases, new strategies are needed to prevent this condition at both population and individual levels. Energy balance is maintained through various feedback mechanisms, and hormones from peripheral tissues regulate appetite. Initial interventions include diet and exercise, but often fail or show short-term efficacy. Adjunctive pharmacologic therapy and bariatric surgery are considered for those unable to achieve or sustain weight loss.

INTRODUCTION

Obesity is a chronic disease affecting millions of people worldwide, and is often associated with numerous comorbidities, including type 2 diabetes mellitus (T2DM), liver disease, cardiovascular disease, hypertension, and other diseases. As the prevalence of obesity continues to sharply increase at global level, it is crucial to develop newer strategies to prevent this chronic condition at a population level and individual level.

Energy balance is maintained by an intricate network of interacting feedback mechanisms involving the hypothalamus, brain stem, higher brain centers and in the periphery, the stomach, gut, liver, thyroid, endocrine pancreas, and adipose tissue. Hormones from peripheral tissues such as leptin, ghrelin, cholecystokinin, pancreatic polypeptide, peptide YY (PYY) 3–36, glucagon-like peptide-1 (GLP-1), and oxyntomodulin have been shown to regulate appetite. Resistance to the actions of some of these hormones appears to be associated with common obesity.

Initial interventions against obesity are diet and exercise. But unfortunately, these often fail or show only short-term efficacy. After that we have surgical modalities or drug therapy as alternatives. Adults who are unable to achieve or sustain bodyweight loss with comprehensive lifestyle modifications, who have either a body mass index (BMI) ≥ 30 or ≥ 27 kg/m^2 with one or more comorbidities, can be considered for adjunct pharmacologic therapy. Bariatric surgery is an option for individuals with a BMI ≥ 40 or ≥ 35 kg/m^2 and with comorbidities for which appropriate nonsurgical methods have failed.

In this chapter, we briefly overview currently Food and Drug Administration (FDA)-approved drugs and upcoming drugs which are in clinical trials (phases II and III).

OVERVIEW OF CURRENTLY AVAILABLE DRUGS FOR OBESITY (FDA-APPROVED)

An integrated approach for the treatment of obesity should have targets for multiple mechanisms such as feeding circuits, glucose metabolism, and energy expenditure. Agents which have multiple mechanisms for weight loss are likely to be more efficacious than single-target agents. Currently available agents include centrally acting appetite suppressants and peripherally acting compounds.

TABLE 1: Various types of antiobesity drugs and their mechanism of actions.

Drug	Mechanism of action	Dose	Weight change relative to placebo	Side effects
Semaglutide	GLP-1r agonists, decreases appetite, and delays gastric emptying and gut motility	2.4 mg once per week subcu-taneous injection	2.4–14.9%	Abdominal pain, constipation, diarrhea, nausea, vomiting, and pancreatitis (rare)
Liraglutide	GLP-1r agonists, decreases appetite and delays gastric emptying and gut motility	3.0 mg/day subcutaneous injection	2.6–8%	Diarrhea, nausea, vomiting, constipation, dyspepsia, abdominal pain, pancreatitis, and gallstones
Naltrexone SR/ bupropion SR	Opioid receptor antagonist/dopamine and noradrenaline reuptake inhibitor causing appetite suppression	32/360 mg oral twice daily	Dose-dependent (1.3–6.1%)	Headaches, hypertension, sleep disorders, nausea, constipation, vomiting, diarrhea, palpitation, dizziness, tremor, and others
Orlistat	Pancreatic lipase inhibitor causing excretion of 30% of ingested triglycerides in stool	120 mg three times daily	6.1–10.2%	Nausea, diarrhea, steatorrhea, abdominal bloating, and hepatitis
Phentermine/ Topiramate	Sympathomimetics/anticonvulsant causing appetite suppression	15/92 mg once daily oral	Dose-depending (1.2–7.8%)	Tachycardia, xerostomia, constipation, headache, sleep disorder, anxiety, depression, suicidal ideation, and cardiovascular event
Phendimetra-zine	Sympathomimetics causing appetite suppression	Short-term (< 12 weeks) 17.5–35 mg two or three times daily	Not available	Hypertension, ischemic events, palpitations, tachycardia, headache, insomnia, overstimulation, psychosis, and others

(GLP-1r: glucagon-like peptide-1 receptor; SR: sustained release)

- *Centrally acting appetite suppressing drugs*:
  - Phentermine/topiramate
  - Naltrexone/bupropion/setmelanotide
- *Peripherally acting anti-obesity drugs*:
  - Orlistat
- *Anti-obesity agents with mixed central and peripheral action*:
  - Liraglutide
  - Semaglutide

The doses, mechanism of action, percentage weight loss, and side effects of the above are shown in **Table 1**.

ROLE OF INCRETINS IN DIABETES AND OBESITY

Incretin hormones are secreted in the intestine when nutrients are present in its lumen. The term 'incretin effect' was coined based on the discovery that the impact on insulin secretion differs between oral and parenteral glucose administration, reinforcing the notion that presence of certain substances in the gut promote insulin release postingestion. This phenomenon is a component of the enteroinsular axis in glucose homeostasis and is believed to account for a minimum of 50% of insulin secretion.

The primary incretin hormones include GLP-1 and glucose-dependent insulinotropic polypeptide (GIP). GLP-1, a 30-amino acid peptide, is produced by the L cells in the distal ileum and colon's enteroendocrine cells, while GIP, a 4-amino acid peptide, is produced by the K cells in the duodenum and jejunum. Both hormones are rapidly released postingestion, apparently regulated by neural signals, and they stimulate insulin production in pancreatic beta cells in a glucose-dependent manner. During the fasting state, plasma concentrations of GLP-1 and GIP are minimal, and rise occur 15–30 minutes after ingestion. The incretin effect is transient, and remains active for 1–2 minutes postsecretion before being deactivated by dipeptidyl peptidase-4 (DPP-4) enzyme. While GIP predominantly affects pancreatic beta cells, receptors for GLP-1 (R-GLP1) are widely distributed in the endocrine pancreas (alpha and beta cells), heart, stomach, adipose tissue, vagus nerve, and various regions of the central nervous system (CNS).

ROLE OF GLUCOSE-DEPENDENT INSULINOTROPIC POLYPEPTIDE

After released by K cell in duodenum and jejunum, GIP travels to the pancreas's beta cells to reduce glucose levels. It activates GIP receptors (GIPr) through class-II G-protein-coupled receptors, cause increase in intracellular cyclic adenosine monophosphate (cAMP) and calcium, which leads to the release of insulin. GIP has additional roles, including promoting fat metabolism and the proliferation of beta cells. Additionally, the hormone reduces the secretion of gastrin and stomach acid by parietal cells inhibition, promotes the growth of osteoblasts in bones while inhibiting osteoclasts, and potentially participates in neurosignaling, which is evident by the widespread expression of GIPr in the brain. Although their precise function is uncertain, GIPr are also found in other organs such as the heart, kidneys, and skin.

ROLE OF GLUCAGON-LIKE PEPTIDE-1

Glucagon-like peptide-1 binds to GLP-1 receptors (GLP-1r) and induces glycemic effect similar to GIP on the pancreas. Agonists attach to G-protein-coupled receptors, initiating an increase in intracellular cAMP and calcium, which results in the release of insulin. Additionally, GLP-1 inhibits gastric emptying, reduces food intake, and lowers glucagon secretion, leading to a decrease in endogenous glucose production. Furthermore, GLP-1 has also been shown to protect beta cells from apoptosis and stimulate the proliferation of beta cells.

Glucagon-like peptide-1 induces an increase in satiety and a reduction in hunger, resulting in decreased food intake. Additionally, incretins seem to affect the vagus nerve in the CNS, cause a decrease in gastrointestinal motility and a slowdown in gastric emptying. This, in turn, prolongs the sensation of fullness and reduces acid production. It is suggested that GIP works similarly, potentially impacting lipid metabolism and enhancing weight loss effects. GIP influences the body's capacity to expand its white adipose tissue storage in a healthful manner, facilitating increased lipid breakdown and decreasing the overflow of lipids and ectopic fat accumulation in various organs. The reduction in ectopic lipid accumulation may also contribute to improved insulin sensitivity.

ROLE OF GLUCAGON

Glucagon released from alpha cells of pancreas following amino acid stimulation as part of the liver–alpha cell axis. Glucagon regulates glucose homeostasis, counteracting the actions of insulin by stimulating hepatic glucose production (glycogenolysis and gluconeogenesis). Glucagon stimulates beta oxidation of fatty acids and inhibits the formation of malonyl-coenzyme A, the first intermediate of fatty acid synthesis and thus suppressing the hepatic fat synthesis. Along with lipolytic action at pharmacological dose glucagon increases total body energy expenditure.

The role of various important hormones in producing the weight loss is shown in **Figure 1**.

DUAL ANALOGS

Due to peptide nature of incretins and presence of degrading enzyme DPP-4, these analogs lack of oral bioavailability and have short half-lives. Subcutaneous injections resolved the issue of bioavailability of incretins and short half-lives by manufacturing incretins those are resistant to DPP-4 enzyme by altering binding site for DPP-4. At present GLP-1r agonists are approved for diabetes and obesity.

Rationale for Using Dual Analogs

Although GIP was first incretin to be discovered but studies show GIP and its analogs are ineffective in decreasing blood glucose and weight loss when used alone. But when stimulated simultaneously with GLP-1r, GIP appears to enhance not only the weight loss mechanism of the incretin but also its glucose-lowering effects. Activation of GIP may further amplify the insulin secretion induced by GLP-1 activation in the pancreas and the weight loss effects caused by GLP-1 activation in the CNS. Additionally, GIP activation may offer complementary mechanisms by enhancing the expansion of white adipose tissue and improving lipid handling. Ultimately, GIP-r agonism might alleviate the nauseating effects associated with GLP-1 agonism through inhibitory neurons in the area postrema, potentially enabling higher therapeutic doses of GLP-1 analogs with reduced adverse effects; GLP-1r agonist and glucagon (oxyntomodulin analog) also being under trials to know safety and efficacy in obesity and other metabolic disorder **(Table 2)**.

TIRZEPATIDE: DUAL GLP-1/GIP ANALOG

Glucose-lowering Effects

Tirzepatide, a subcutaneous injection administered once weekly, received FDA approval in May, 2022 as an additional treatment, in combination with diet and exercise, to enhance glycemic control in adults diagnosed with T2DM. Its approval followed the completion of five clinical phase III trials known as the SURPASS trials, which involved comparing tirzepatide doses of 5, 10,

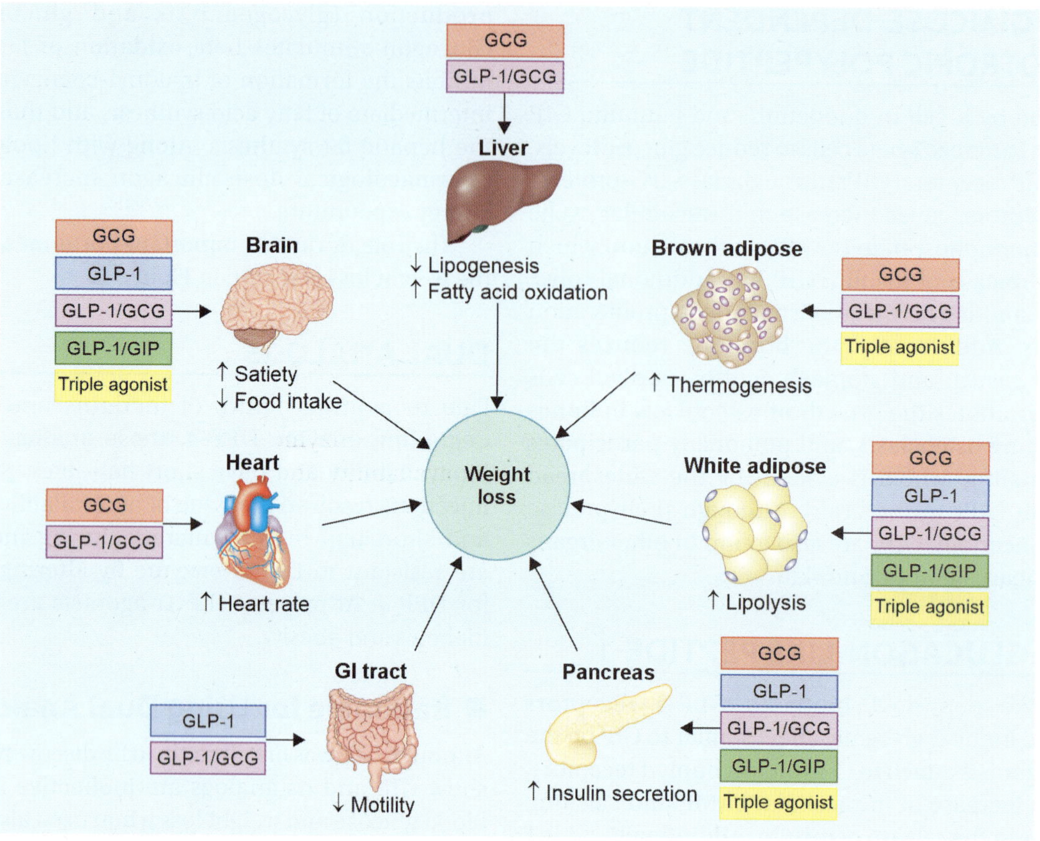

FIG. 1: Incretin/glucagon-targeting agents achieve their weight loss effect through a variety of mechanisms in several organs.

(GCG: glucagon; GLP-1: glucagon-like peptide-1; GI: gastrointestinal; GIP: glucose-dependent insulinotropic polypeptide)

TABLE 2: Dual glucagon-like peptide-1 (GLP-1) analog with either glucose-dependent insulinotropic polypeptide (GIP) agonism or glucagon agonism.

Drug	Mechanism	Company	Clinical trial phase	Disease under trial
Tirzepatide	GLP-1/GIP agonist	Lilly	Phase III	Obesity
Survodutide	GLP-1/Glucagon	Boehringer	Phase II	Obesity
Cotadutide	GLP-1/Glucagon	AstraZeneca	Phase III	Obesity
Mazdutide	GLP-1/Glucagon	Lilly	Phase III	Obesity
Pemvidutide	GLP-1/Glucagon	Altimmune	Phase II	Obesity and nonalcoholic fatty liver disease (NAFLD)
Efinopegdutide	GLP-1/Glucagon	Merck/Hanmi	Phase II	NAFLD

and 15 mg with other antidiabetic medications. Over a 40-week period, the estimated difference between the 15-mg tirzepatide group and the semaglutide group was –0.45 percentage points. Tirzepatide exhibited enhanced efficacy in reducing A1c levels, surpassing placebo outcomes across all doses, and demonstrating superiority over dulaglutide 1.5 mg a once-weekly GLP-1r injectable by 1.1% in another Phase II randomized-controlled trial.

Effects on Weight Loss

Tirzepatide was studied for weight loss and obesity in SURMOUNT trials. SURMOUNT-2 completed recently in April 2023. SURMOUNT-3, 4 are still going on. SURMOUNT-1 assessed The efficacy and safety of tirzepatide were compared to placebo in individuals with a BMI of 30 or higher, or a BMI of 27 with at least

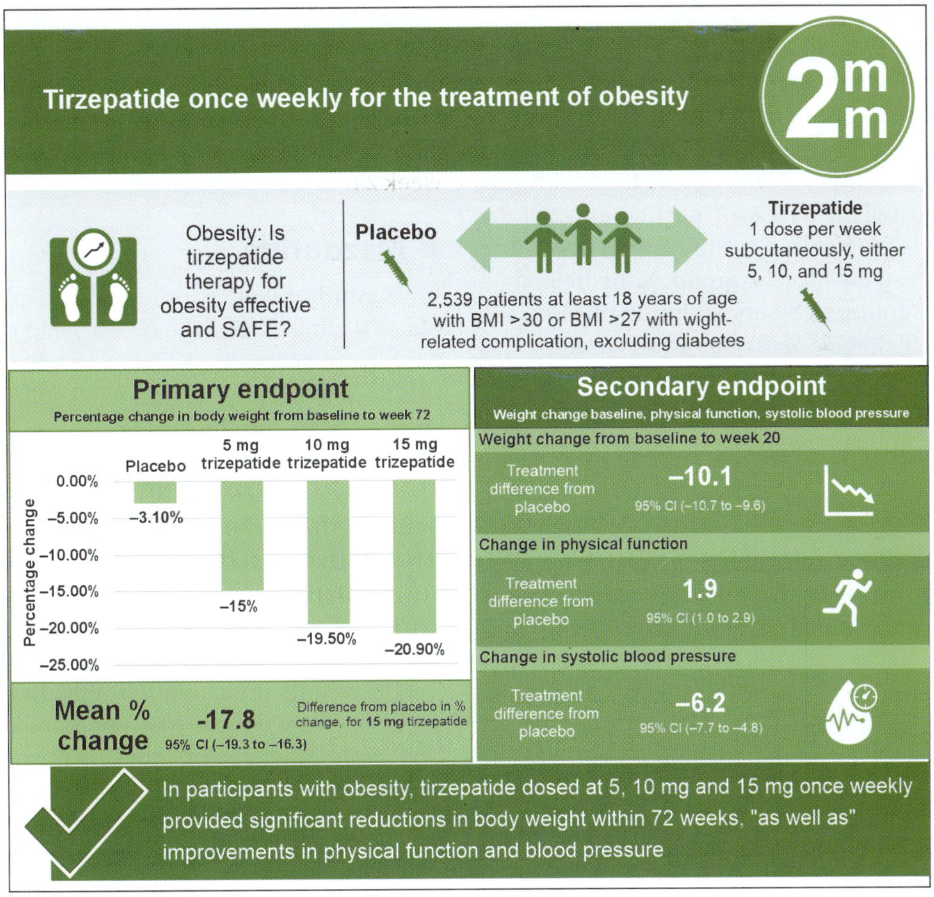

FIG. 2: Effect of tirzepatide in SURMOUNT-1 trial.
(BMI: body mass index; CI: confidence interval)

one weight-related complication, excluding diabetes. The dosages of tirzepatide administered were 5, 10, and 15 mg in a total of 2,539 patients over a 72-week period. The average percentage change in weight from the baseline was 15.9%, 19.5%, and 20.9%, respectively ($p < 0.001$), when compared to the placebo at the 72-week. The study indicated that tirzepatide not only results in a dose-dependent reduction in blood glucose, but also a dose-dependent decrease in weight.

The SURMOUNT-2 trial assessed the use of 10- and 15-mg tirzepatide in 938 adult participants, demonstrating that tirzepatide led to a substantial weight loss of up to 17.8% compared to the placebo over a 72-week period. Although direct comparisons are not available, tirzepatide appears to be more effective in reducing weight than any other currently available weight loss medication. In the SURPASS-2 trial, the 15-mg tirzepatide dosage resulted in an 11.2 kg reduction in body weight, surpassing the 5.7 kg reduction observed with 1-mg semaglutide. Prior to tirzepatide trials, semaglutide had exhibited the most significant placebo-subtracted weight loss when compared to other medications. The summary of the Tirzepatide Trial is shown in **Figure 2**.

American Diabetes Association (ADA) 2023 emphasizes the importance of losing weight stating that >10% weight loss can be disease-modifying and may even lead to disease remission. The SURPASS and SURMOUNT trials have impelled ADA to consider tirzepatide, along with semaglutide, to be 'very highly efficacious for weight loss'.

GLUCAGON-LIKE PEPTIDE-1/GLUCAGON AGONISTS

Survodutide

In a randomized, double-blind, placebo-controlled, dose-finding trial, 387 participants with a BMI of 27 kg/m^2 or higher were enrolled. They were randomly assigned to receive weekly subcutaneous injections of survodutide at various doses (0.6, 2.4, 3.6, or 4.8 mg) or a placebo over a 46-week period. The study incorporated a 20-week rapid, biweekly dose escalation phase, followed by a 26-week maintenance phase. The primary endpoint was the percentage change in body weight from baseline at week 46, with secondary endpoints including the proportion of participants achieving at least 5%, 10%, or 15% weight loss from baseline at week 46. Although the phase II clinical trial results of survodutide indicated up to 18.7% weight loss in overweight or obese individuals within the 46-week timeframe and there were numerous patient discontinuations due to adverse drug reactions. Adverse events were reported in 90.9% of participants in the survodutide group, primarily gastrointestinal in nature, compared to 75.3% in the placebo group. Nonetheless, no unexpected safety concerns emerged during the 46-week study period. The incidence of serious adverse events was comparable between the survodutide group (4.2%) and the placebo group (6.5%). The completion of phase III for this clinical trial is anticipated in 2024.

Cotadutide

Cotadutide, a dual GLP-1 and glucagon receptor agonist, is under development for nonalcoholic steatohepatitis (NASH) and chronic kidney disease with T2DM and obesity.

In phase IIb study by Rajaa Nahra et al., 834 adults with a BMI ≥ 25 kg/m^2 and inadequately controlled T2DM on metformin [with glycated hemoglobin (HbA1c) levels between 7.0 and 10.5%], participants were randomized to receive double-blind cotadutide at doses of 100 μg ($n = 100$), 200 μg ($n = 256$), or 300 μg ($n = 256$), placebo ($n = 110$), or open-label liraglutide 1.8 mg ($n = 110$). All treatments were administered subcutaneously. The primary endpoints were changes in HbA1c and body weight at week 14, and the initially assigned interventions were continued until week 54. Liver damage biomarkers and liver fibrosis algorithms were also evaluated.

Cotadutide demonstrated a significant reduction in HbA1c and body weight at both weeks 14 and 54 compared to the placebo (all $p < 0.001$). Moreover, cotadutide at the 300 μg dose showed improvements in lipid profile, aspartate aminotransferase (AST) and alanine aminotransferase (ALT) levels, propeptide of type III collagen level, fibrosis-4 index, and nonalcoholic fatty liver disease (NAFLD) fibrosis score compared to the placebo, whereas liraglutide did not produce these improvements. Over the course of 54 weeks, cotadutide treatment enhanced glycemic control and facilitated weight loss in participants with overweight/obesity and T2DM. Ad hoc analyses revealed positive changes in hepatic parameters, supporting the need for further evaluation of cotadutide in NASH.

Pemvidutide

The MOMENTUM Obesity phase II trial's results were announced in recently in March, 2023 (week 24 interim analysis of 160 subjects). Mean weight loss of 10.7% (placebo-adjusted 9.7%) at 2.4-mg dose at week 24. Mean weight loss of 11.9% (placebo-adjusted 11.1%) in subjects weighing 115 kg or less at baseline at 2.4-mg dose at week 24. Approximately 50% of subjects achieved 10% or more weight loss and approximately 20% of subjects achieved 15% or more weight loss at the 1.8- and 2.4-mg doses at week 24.

Mazdutide

In a randomized, double-blind, placebo-controlled phase II clinical trial, the efficacy and safety of mazdutide 9 mg were assessed in Chinese individuals with obesity (BMI ≥ 30.0 kg/m^2). A total of 80 subjects were enrolled, with a mean baseline weight of 96.9 kg, mean height of 168.0 cm, and mean BMI of 34.3 kg/m^2. They were randomly assigned in a 3:1 ratio to either the mazdutide 9-mg group or the placebo group, receiving treatment once a week for 24 weeks. The primary endpoint was the percentage change in body weight from baseline compared to placebo after 24 weeks of treatment, and the study extended the treatment period to 48 weeks.

The results indicated that mazdutide 9 mg exhibited superior body weight loss compared to the placebo in Chinese individuals with obesity. The treatment difference in the mean change in body weight from baseline versus placebo was –14.7 kg [95% confidence interval (CI) –17.9 kg, –11.5 kg, $p < 0.0001$]. Additionally, 81.7%, 65.0%, 31.7%, and 21.7% of subjects in the mazdutide 9-mg group achieved 5% or more, 10% or more, 15% or more, and 20% or more weight loss from baseline, respectively, while no subjects in the placebo group achieved a 5% or more reduction in body weight from baseline.

FUTURE PERSPECTIVES

In the search for newer anti-obesity pharmacotherapeutic agents which can lead to significant weight loss without much of safety concerns research and development on gut hormone coagonists is gaining momentum. GLP-1/GIP analog like tirzepatide and GLP-1/glucagon coagonists such as cotadutide and efinopegdutide offer the promise of increased efficacy while minimizing side effects. Furthermore, with enhanced glucagon action the GLP-1/glucagon coagonist has the advantage of being tailored to treat NAFLD directly. Recently published data from the high-dose semaglutide STEP phase III trials and the SURPASS phase III trials on GLP-1/GIP coagonist tirzepatide have set the efficacy bar high in terms of weight loss and glycemic improvement. Triple agonist also being tested for weight loss and antiglycemic effects and showing promising results in phase II trials like retatrutide. With increasing beneficial effects, it is likely that with in next 1–2 years first dual anti-obesity drug will be available in market. There is great hope and bright future for the obese patient.

SUGGESTED READINGS

1. Kang JG, Park CY. Anti-obesity drugs: a review about their effects and safety. Diabetes Metab J. 2012;36(1):13-25.
2. Del Prato S, Gallwitz B, Holst JJ, Meier JJ. The incretin/glucagon system as a target for pharmacotherapy of obesity. Obes Rev. 2022;23(2):e13372.
3. Andraos J, Muhar H, Smith SR. Beyond glycemia: Comparing tirzepatide to GLP-1 analogues. Rev Endocr Metab Disord. 2023;24(6):1089-101.
4. Syed YY. Tirzepatide: First approval. Drugs. 2022;82(11):1213-20.
5. Frías JP, Davies MJ, Rosenstock J, Pérez Manghi FC, Fernández Landó L, Bergman BK, et al. Tirzepatide versus semaglutide once weekly in patients with type 2 diabetes. New Engl J Med. 2021;385(6):503-15.
6. ElSayed NA, Aleppo G, Aroda VR, Bannuru RR, Brown FM, Bruemmer D, Collins BS, Hilliard ME, Isaacs D, Johnson EL, Kahan S. 7. Diabetes technology: standards of care in diabetes—2023. Diabetes Care. 2023;46(Suppl 1):S111-27.
7. Jastreboff AM, Aronne LJ, Ahmad NN, Wharton S, Connery L, Alves B, et al; SURMOUNT-1 Investigators. Tirzepatide once weekly for the treatment of obesity. New Engl J Med. 2022;387(3): 205-16.
8. Nahra R, Wang T, Gadde KM, Oscarsson J, Stumvoll M, Jermutus L, et al. Effects of cotadutide on metabolic and hepatic parameters in adults with overweight or obesity and type 2 diabetes: a 54-week randomized phase 2b study. Diabetes Care. 2021;44(6):1433-42.
9. Ji L, Gao L, Jiang H, Yang J, Yu L, Wen J, et al. Safety and efficacy of a GLP-1 and glucagon receptor dual agonist mazdutide (IBI362) 9 mg and 10 mg in Chinese adults with overweight or obesity: a randomised, placebo-controlled, multiple-ascending-dose phase 1b trial. eClinicalMedicine. 2022;54:101691.
10. Klein S, Nestor JJ, Harris MS, Suyundikov A, Casper R, Steele SM, Payne JD, Krishnan V, ROBERTS M, Browne SK. 334-OR: pemvidutide (ALT-801), a balanced (1: 1) GLP-1/glucagon dual receptor agonist, induces rapid and marked weight loss without the need for dose titration in people with overweight/obesity. Diabetes. 20221;71(Suppl 1).

173

CHAPTER

Proprotein Convertase Subtilisin/Kexin Type 9 Inhibitors Physician's Perspective

VA Kothiwale, Aishwarya N Udupa, Aswin Sasikumar

ABSTRACT

Proprotein convertase subtilisin/kexin type 9 (PCSK9) inhibitors are the most promising among all the newer dyslipidemic drugs, with the potential to be the next wonder drug. Landmark trials have shown additional significant clinical outcomes in patients with high-intensity statin treatment. PCSK9 inhibitors affect all the lipid molecules low-density lipoprotein (LDL), triglycerides, lipoprotein(a) [LP(a)], and high-density lipoprotein (HDL). PCSK 9 Inhibitors are safe and well tolerated. PCSK9 inhibitors have already been approved for use in familial hypercholesterolemia (FH), statin intolerance, and failure to achieve low-density lipoprotein cholesterol (LDL-C) goals despite optimal doses of statins in high-risk individuals.

INTRODUCTION

Proprotein convertase subtilisin/kexin type 9 (PCSK9) are proprotein convertase (PPC) subtilisin kexin 9 inhibitors are potent medications that lower low-density lipoprotein cholesterol (LDL-C) and have been developed very recently for the treatment of atherosclerotic cardiovascular disease. PPC is a family of proteins that activate other proteins. PPCs are involved in processing cellular proproteins, which causes activation, inactivation, or functional changes of hormones, neuropeptides, growth factors, and receptors. Until today, there are nine PCSK9 with varying functions and tissue distribution, and the discovery of these molecules has come from different groups simultaneously. To eliminate the confusion, all these molecules have been named 1–9.

HISTORY

The group headed by Nabil Seidah from Montreal, working on the chemistry and function of a family of PPCs, identified PCSK9 encoded by a gene on chromosome 1. They later worked with a French group and found that among a French family, hypercholesterolemia was associated with a gain of function mutation of a gene on chromosome 1.

Further in the OSLO study, 51 Norwegian subjects with familial hypercholesterolemia (FH) underwent gene sequencing, where it was found that mutations in the *PCSK9* gene were the cause of their autosomal dominant hypercholesterolemia. Dallas heart study, a multidisciplinary study initiated in the 2000s, has provided essential insight into the field of cardiovascular research and showed that loss of function mutation of the *PCSK9* gene was associated with very low cholesterol levels and marked reduction in cardiovascular diseases.

EXPERIMENTAL STUDIES

Maxwell and Breslow conducted preclinical trials on mice to study the function of PCSK9 and their effect on low-density lipoprotein (LDL) receptors and atherosclerosis. Mice with loss of the *PCSK9* gene showed decreased aortic atherosclerosis in contrast to mice with overexpression of PCSK9, which showed marked aortic atherosclerosis. Further, mice with LDL receptors deficient and overexpression of PCSK9 showed no effect on atherosclerosis. This showed that the *PCSK9* gene is responsible for atherosclerosis and acts through LDL receptors.

MECHANISM OF ACTION

Proprotein convertase subtilisin/kexin type 9 is a PPC that is involved in the degradation of LDL receptors in the liver. When there is an increase in PCSK9 there occurs an increase in the degradation of LDL receptors in the liver, which further decreases in LDL receptors in turn leading to an increase in LDL levels in plasma.

Inhibition of PCSK9 convertase leads to decreased degradation of LDL receptors which increases the LDL receptors in the liver. This further results in an increase in the uptake of LDL by the liver which further decreases the plasma LDL levels.

Mutations in the *PCSK9* gene cause FH in a subset of patients by reducing the number of LDL receptors on the surface of hepatocytes. This decreases their ability to clear LDL-C from plasma.

Conversely, other PCSK9 mutations result in unusually low concentrations of plasma LDL-C and a reduced risk of atherosclerotic disease. Blocking the activity of PCSK9 with PCSK9 inhibitors reduces the degradation of LDL receptors and increases the clearance of LDL-C.

CLINICAL APPROACH

Considering the experimental studies and specific mechanisms much research has been implemented to develop a drug that blocks the *PCSK9* gene. Many leading pharmaceutical companies started developing drugs to inhibit PCSK9 and are in many phases of clinical trials.

From laboratory modules, PCSK9 inhibitors can be developed by monoclonal antibodies (mAbs), antisense oligonucleotides (ASOs), small interfering ribonucleic acids (siRNAs), and small molecule inhibitors.

Proprotein convertase subtilisin/kexin type 9 inhibitors as monoclonal antibodies evolocumab (Repatha-Amgen), alirocumab (Praluent-Sanfori Regeneron), and bococizumab (Pfizer) have been developed and completed phase III clinical trials. The first two molecules have been approved by the United States Food and Drug Administration (US FDA) and are available for the treatment of dyslipidemia in cardiovascular disease.

ATHEROSCLEROTIC BURDEN AND CARDIOVASCULAR DISEASE

Atherosclerosis is a chronic progressive inflammatory condition involving the medium and large-sized blood vessels resulting in various vascular events. Lipids play an important role in the development of atherosclerosis. Among lipids, LDL has a very crucial and important role in the initiation and progression of atherosclerosis. With the advent of statins which are β-hydroxy β-methylglutaryl-CoA (HMG-CoA) reductase enzyme inhibitors, which reduces LDL-C levels significantly thereby achieving a reduction of atherosclerosis and associated cardiovascular events. Today statins have become the mainstay in the treatment of primary and secondary cardiovascular events.

There are a number of clinical trials available that support as well as confirm the role of statins in cardiovascular diseases. However, statins also have some limitations.

Limitations of Statins

Statins typically reduce LDL-C levels by 30–40% at best even on optimum dose therapy. Side effects of statins such as muscle weakness, gastrointestinal (GI) intolerance, risk of type 2 diabetes mellitus, and liver failure have resulted in poor compliance with statins therapy. Despite their widespread use, discontinuation and non-adherence remain a major gap in both the primary and secondary prevention of atherosclerotic cardiovascular disease. At its maximum dose target level for LDL-C is not met consistently. Many patients have shown poor adherence to long-term regimens.

Many clinical trials and Adult Treatment Panel (ATP) guidelines suggest that lowering the LDL better the cardiovascular outcome. However, statins at their maximum dose are not able to meet the required reduction in LDL levels to prevent further cardiovascular events. So, there is a need for newer molecules that can decrease LDL-C to prevent cardiovascular mortality and morbidity.

LANDMARK TRIALS OF PROPROTEIN CONVERTASE SUBTILISIN/KEXIN TYPE 9

FOURIER Trial

Further cardiovascular outcomes research with PCSK9 inhibition in subjects with elevated risk (FOURIER) is a randomized, double-blind trial that took into consideration 27,564 stable subjects aged 40–85 years with cardiovascular disease and LDL levels > 70 mg/dL despite high-intensity statin or maximum tolerated statin dose.

The primary endpoints composed of cardiovascular death, myocardial infarction, stroke, hospitalization for unstable angina, and coronary revascularization were found to be lesser in patients on evolocumab (12.6%) compared with the placebo group (14.6%). The secondary end point of cardiovascular death, myocardial infarction, and stroke was also found to be lesser in the evolocumab group (5.9%) compared to the placebo group (7.4%).

ODYSSEY Trial

The ODYSSEY trial is a randomized multicenter double-blinded placebo-controlled trial with a sample size of 18,924 with a median duration of follow-up of 2.8 years, provided evidence that alirocumab, when added to standard therapy, effectively reduced LDL-C levels and, in some cases, reduced the risk of cardiovascular events in high-risk patient populations.

Primary endpoints such as coronary heart disease death, nonfatal myocardial infarction, ischemic stroke, and unstable angina requiring hospitalization occurred in 903 patients (9.5%) in the alirocumab group and 1,052 patients (11.1%) in the placebo group.

FOURIER (evolocumab) and ODYSSEY trial (alirocumab) showed that there is reduction of LDL-C 36–62%, apolipoprotein B (Apo B) to 54%, non-high-density lipoprotein cholesterol (non-HDL-C) to 52%, triglycerides to 17%, lipoprotein A [LP(a)] 20–36%, and increase in high-density lipoprotein (HDL) to 4.6%.

GLAGOV

Global Assessment of Plaque Regression with a PCSK9 Antibody as Measured by Intravascular Ultrasound (GLAGOV) is a randomized, double-blind, placebo-controlled study that enrolled 968 patients with symptomatic coronary artery disease and other high features from 197 centers around the world. The study found that after 18 months of treatment, patients receiving statin monotherapy had a mean LDL-C of 93 mg/dL, which was essentially unchanged from the start of the study. Patients receiving statin therapy with the addition of the PCSK9 inhibitor evolocumab had a mean LDL-C of 36.6 mg/dL and a trough level of 29 mg/dL two weeks after dosing. The study also studied the regression of coronary atheroma and further concluded that patients on statin monotherapy had neither progression nor regression, and the percent change from the baseline was not statistically significant. However, patients receiving the addition of the PCSK9 inhibitor had a statistically significant change in percent atheroma volume.

Meta-analysis of 16 randomized controlled trials (RCTs) of PCSK9 inhibitors (39,104 patients) showed a significantly lower risk of stroke, peripheral artery disease, and decreased LDL levels in FH. A comparative meta-analysis of statins and PCSK9 inhibitors was done, which showed that statins magnify the risk of hemorrhagic stroke and brain injury, whereas PCSK9 inhibitors do not increase hemorrhagic stroke risk. So, PCSK9 inhibitors may be preferred to statins as a lipid-lowering agent class in patients with elevated hemorrhagic stroke risk.

Effects of PCSK9 inhibitor on favorable limb outcomes in patients with chronic limb-threatening ischemia—evolocumab was administered in a patient with critical limb ischemia, and the results were favorable, showing a decrease in the incidence of amputation and better survival. Also, long-term administration of evolocumab over 12 months contributed to improving the proportion of wound-free limb salvage.

NEWER ADVANCES

The growing research in the field of PCKS9 receptors and the promising results from those studies have motivated the scientific and medical community to further explore and experiment on various new aspects of the gene. These have led to newer modalities, such as siRNA (inclisiran), *PCSK9* gene therapy, PCSK9 vaccination, and oral PCSK9 inhibitors.

Inclisiran

It is an alternative approach, inhibiting PCSK9 in plasma with antibodies to inhibit the translation of the protein in the cytoplasm by interfering with the messenger ribonucleic acid (RNA). Two approaches exist to inhibit messenger ribonucleic acid (mRNA) via the use of antisense oligonucleotides and the use of siRNA; siRNA blocks the translation of PCSK9 in RNA and promotes RNA degradation through RNA-induced silencing complex (RISC).

Proprotein Convertase Subtilisin/Kexin Type 9 Gene Therapy

Individuals homozygous for PCSK9 deficiency have been identified and have phenotypes of being healthy though profoundly hypercholesterolemia. Clinical interventions to knock out PCSK9 using gene therapy technology, such as clustered regularly interspaced short palindromic repeats (CRISPR) associated protein 9 (CRISPR-CAS 9), may be feasible to deliver a cure for FH.

Proprotein Convertase Subtilisin/Kexin Type 9 Vaccines

Proprotein convertase subtilisin/kexin type 9 is antigenic and can be used to produce antibodies. Experimental results in animals vaccinated with bacteriophage-like particles (BLP) conjugated with PCSK9 epitopes adjacent to the LDL receptor-binding domain have been encouraging. In various mouse models, vaccination has been shown to decrease LDL-C, decrease cardiovascular disease (CVD), and decrease systemic and vascular inflammation.

Oral PCSK9 inhibitor—MK-0616. Orally, bioavailable cyclic peptide is in Phase 2b RCT. Dosing of once daily.

The studies have shown a reduction in LDL-C at week 8 up to 60.9%.

PROPROTEIN CONVERTASE SUBTILISIN/ KEXIN TYPE 9 BENEFICENCE

Patients whose LDL-C cannot be controlled with intensive statin with other current therapies. Most patients with heterozygous FH. Almost all patients with homozygous FH. Statin intolerance or statins are not clinically appropriate (e.g., drug-drug interactions).

SAFETY AND EFFICACY

In all the clinical trials associated with PCKS9 inhibitors, it was found to be a very safe and effective medication along with statins for LDL reduction. A possible side effect of the therapeutical dose of (cholesterol-lowering) monoclonal antibody might be irritation at the injection site.

Few patients in clinical trials reported the side effects of myalgia, muscle cramps, nausea, vomiting, and epigastric distress. There was no specific organ damage or toxicity reported.

SUGGESTED READINGS

1. Zhang L, Song K, Zhu M, Shi J, Zhang H, Xu L, et al. Proprotein convertase subtilisin/kexin type 9 (PCSK9) in lipid metabolism, atherosclerosis, and ischemic stroke. Int J Neurosci. 2016;126(8): 675-80.
2. Seidah NG, Garçon D. Expanding Biology of PCSK9: Roles in Atherosclerosis and Beyond. Curr Atheroscler Rep. 2022; 24(10):821-30.
3. Hajar R. PCSK 9 Inhibitors: A Short History and a New Era of Lipid-lowering Therapy. Heart Views. 2019;20(2):74-5.
4. Maxwell KN, Breslow JL. Adenoviral-mediated expression of PCSK9 in mice results in a low-density lipoprotein receptor knockout phenotype. Proc Natl Acad Sci USA. 2004;101(18): 7100-5.
5. Page MM, Watts GF. PCSK9 inhibitors—mechanisms of action. Aust Prescr. 2016;39(5):164-7.
6. Barlas S. Health Plans and Drug Companies Dip Their Toes into Value-based Pricing: The Pressure is on P&T Committees to Monitor Utilization. PT. 2016;41(1):39,40,41,53.
7. Mortensen MB, Tybjærg-Hansen A, Nordestgaard BG. Statin Eligibility for Primary Prevention of Cardiovascular Disease According to 2021 European Prevention Guidelines Compared with Other International Guidelines. JAMA Cardiol. 2022;7(8):836-43.
8. Pinal-Fernandez I, Casal-Dominguez M, Mammen AL. Statins: pros and cons. Med Clin (Barc). 2018;150(10):398-402.
9. Talwalkar PG, Sreenivas CG, Gulati A, Baxi H. Journey in guidelines for lipid management: From adult treatment panel (ATP)-I to ATP-III and what to expect in ATP-IV. Indian J Endocrinol Metab. 2013;17(4):628-35.
10. Schwartz GG, Steg PG, Szarek M, Bhatt DL, Bittner VA, Diaz R, et al. Alirocumab and Cardiovascular Outcomes after Acute Coronary Syndrome. N Engl J Med. 2018;379(22): 2097-107.
11. Sinnaeve PR, Schwartz GG, Wojdyla DM, Alings M, Bhatt DL, Bittner VA, et al. Effect of alirocumab on cardiovascular outcomes after acute coronary syndromes according to age: an ODYSSEY OUTCOMES trial analysis. Eur Heart J. 2020;41(24): 2248-58.
12. Nissen SE, Nicholls SJ. Results of the GLAGOV trial. Cleve Clin J Med. 2017;84(12 Suppl 4):e1-5.
13. Sanz-Cuesta BE, Saver JL. Lipid-Lowering Therapy and Hemorrhagic Stroke Risk: Comparative Meta-analysis of Statins and PCSK9 Inhibitors. Stroke. 2021;52(10):3142-50.
14. Sato Y, Uzui H, Morishita T, Fukuoka Y, Hasegawa K, Ikeda H, et al. Effects of PCSK9 Inhibitor on Favorable Limb Outcomes in Patients with Chronic Limb-threatening Ischemia. J Atheroscler Thromb. 2021;28(7):754-65.
15. Voevoda MI, Gurevich VS, Ezhov MV, Sergienko IV. Inclisiran - a new era in lipid-lowering therapy. Kardiologiia. 2022;62(6): 57-62.
16. Katzmann JL, Cupido AJ, Laufs U. Gene Therapy Targeting *PCSK9*. Metabolites. 2022;12(1):70.
17. Toth S, Pella D, Fedacko J. Vaccines Targeting PSCK9 for the Treatment of Hyperlipidemia. Cardiol Ther. 2020;9(2):323-32.
18. Burnett JR, Hooper AJ. MK-0616: an oral PCSK9 inhibitor for hypercholesterolemia treatment. Expert Opin Investig Drugs. 2023;32(10):873-8.

174

CHAPTER

Statin Intolerance: How to Manage?

Kaushik Sen, Arijit Sinha

ABSTRACT

Statin intolerance (SI) is an important problem in clinical medicine. Patients with high dose of statin in prevention of atherosclerotic cardiovascular disease (ASCVD) are more vulnerable. Commonly faced adverse effects—dizziness, abdominal discomfort, muscle pain, and elevated liver enzymes—can be managed without much difficulties. The most important concern is statin-associated muscle symptoms (SAMS). If myopathy or rhabdomyolysis occurs, statins should be stopped immediately. Overall prevalence of SI, as shown in well-conducted meta-analysis, is 9.1%. Intolerance should be judged meticulously to avoid unnecessary discontinuation of statins. Common adverse effects are managed by counseling, dose adjustment, de-challenge and re-challenge, or switching to another statin. At the same time lifestyle modification and correction of modifiable risk factors are to be stressed. Alternative lipid-lowering drugs, either as monotherapy or combination therapy should be used to reach low-density lipoprotein cholesterol (LDL-C) goal. Ezetimibe, bile acid sequestrants, adenosine triphosphate lyase (ACL) inhibitors, proprotein convertase subtilisin/kexin type 9 (PCSK9) inhibitors, long-acting synthetic small interfering RNA (siRNA), lomitapide, and mipomersen may help in selective cases of SI.

INTRODUCTION

Statins are clinically used for treatment in different types of dyslipidemias, for primary and secondary prevention of atherosclerotic cardiovascular disease (ASCVD). Apart from that, its anti-inflammatory, antioxidant, and pleiotropic actions may benefit as adjuvant therapy of various neuropsychiatric disorders and noninfectious uveitis. ASCVD is the leading cause of death globally. Cholesterol plays a key role in the development of atherosclerosis and low-density lipoprotein cholesterol (LDL-C) lowering therapy, especially statins, which lower the risk of ASCVD events. Statins reduce cardiovascular disease (CVD) events by multiple mechanisms such as plaque stabilization, reduction of inflammation, and regression of atherosclerosis. In spite of these unequivocal benefits, the use of statins can be undermined in practice due to the perceived or actual intolerance to statins. Statins are in general well tolerated. However, one of the causes of nonadherence to statin is the so-called statin intolerance (SI). Any adverse event considered intolerable by the patient and/or some laboratory abnormalities attributable to statin treatment may lead to its discontinuation. The most common cause of discontinuation of statins is the muscle-related complaints.

DEFINITION OF STATIN INTOLERANCE

Statin intolerance is defined by different organizations such as International Lipid Expert Panel (ILEP), European Atherosclerotic Society (EAS), and National Institute for Health and Care Excellence (NICE). According to the 2022 new National Lipid Association (NLA) definition, SI is defined as one or more adverse effects associated with statin therapy which resolve or improve with dose reduction or discontinuation and can be classified as complete inability to tolerate any dose of a statin or partial intolerance with inability to tolerate the dose necessary to achieve the patient specific therapeutic objective. To classify a patient as having SI, a minimum of two statins should have been attempted, including at least one at the lowest approved daily dosage.

TYPES OF STATIN INTOLERANCE

One of the major differences of definition of SI between the 2014 and 2022 in NLA scientific statement on SI is that in 2022, NLA classified intolerance as either partial or complete taking into consideration the ability to achieve therapeutic targets on maximally tolerated statins. Partial intolerance means that the patient can tolerate a lower statin dose, a different statin, or alternative regimen, but to an extent that is insufficient for the desired goal of low-density lipoprotein (LDL) reduction. SI exists as a spectrum of muscle-related symptoms which may or may not be related to statin therapy directly and has got a significant "nocebo effect" that is perceived symptoms.

Nocebo Effect

Whether the association between statin therapy and adverse experiences that produce intolerance is due to causality is debated. Well-conducted studies suggest that the incidence of muscle-related symptoms with statin therapy may at least be partly attributable to nocebo effect, which means that the expectation of harm actually results in perceived side effects that may be unrelated to the pharmacological effects of the drug.

Is statin intolerance common?

Among several statin-related adverse effects, new onset diabetes mellitus, elevated liver enzymes, intracerebral hemorrhage, myopathy and rhabdomyolysis need special attention.

Statin treatment is very well tolerated in general. As a whole some form of SI noticed in 5–30% cases which are higher in observational studies and lower in clinical trial group. A systematic review of 26 trials have shown that muscle symptoms are described by 12.7% of patients treated with statins and 12.4% patients treated with placebo. So, it is important to identify patients who are truly statin intolerant because no other currently available treatment option reduces the cardiovascular morbidity and mortality to such an extent like statins do.

A recent meta-analysis of more than 4 million patients including 176 studies, of them 112 randomized control trials (RCTs) and 64 cohort studies, found that the overall prevalence of SI was 9.1%. Interestingly, the prevalence of SI in that particular meta-analysis in RCTs was significantly lower compared to the cohort studies that were included. Furthermore, the prevalence of SI in studies that included both primary and secondary prevention were much higher than when primary or secondary prevention patients were analyzed separately. The prevalence was similar when defined using NLA, ILEP, and EAS criteria 7.0%, 6.7%, and 5.9%, respectively. So, it could be concluded that the prevalence of SI is low when properly diagnosed according to the recent international definitions. It is important to note that the prevalence of complete SI might be overestimated and hence it's very important on the part of physicians to make careful assessment of patients when attributing potential symptoms to SI. The factors associated with more chances of SI are given in **Table 1**.

TABLE 1: Factors associated with more chances of statin intolerance.

Endogenous	Exogenous
• *Age*: >80 years • Female sex • Asian ethnicity • Pre-existing neuromuscular dysfunctions • Pre-existing serious liver or kidney dysfunction • Untreated hypothyroidism	• High-dose statin therapy • *Co-administration of certain drugs*: Fibrates (especially gemfibrozil), antipsychotics, verapamil, macrolides, azole antifungals, amiodarone, cyclosporine, protease inhibitors, etc. • Vitamin D deficiency • Excessive alcohol intake • Heavy exercise

STATIN-ASSOCIATED MUSCLE SYMPTOMS AND CLINICAL PRESENTATION

The most common form of statin-associated muscle symptoms (SAMS) is myalgia, which is symmetrical and usually affects larger muscle groups such as shoulder and pelvic girdle arms and legs, usually without creatine kinase (CK) elevation. Onset time is usually 4–6 weeks after initiation of therapy, after increasing dose. Patients may also complain of cramps, muscle weakness, or tenderness during exercise. The prevalence of myalgia with statins varies from 1 to 5% in RCTs to 29% in observational studies. True myopathy or rhabdomyolysis with statins is very rare, with an incidence of about 1 in 10,000 patients per year and 1 in 100,000 patients per year, respectively, simvastatin being the most commonly implicated agent. SAMS-CI is a clinical index scoring system to assess muscle symptoms. Myopathy to be suspected if CK elevation > 4 × upper limit of normal (ULN) to < 10 × ULN with complete resolution on de-challenge. In severe myopathy CK elevation > 10 × ULN to < 50 × ULN. Rhabdomyolysis to be suspected if CK is > 50 × ULN or > 10 × ULN with renal impairment and muscle symptoms. If there is progressive increase of CK and muscle weakness, statin-induced necrotizing autoimmune myositis (SINAM) to be kept in mind.

Which statins are safer?

There are differences in the incidence of SAMS between statins. More lipophilic statins, such as simvastatin, atorvastatin, lovastatin are more likely to be associated with SAMS because of their ability to nonselectively diffuse into the extrahepatic tissues such as skeletal muscle. In contrast, more hydrophilic statins such as pravastatin and fluvastatin are less likely to penetrate into the muscle and therefore, carry lower risk of development of SAMS.

MANAGEMENT

Management of complete SI, which fortunately is rare, is difficult. Clinicians should understand that most of the patients can tolerate some form of statin, may be an alternative agent, or a reduced dose, or an altered dosing schedule.

Lifestyle modification is important in the form of smoking cessation, maintenance of healthy diet, regular exercise, reduced intake of saturated fat and trans-fat (cakes, cookies, fried foods, pizza, etc.), consumption of red rice yeast, consumption of plant sterols and viscous fiber (vegetables, olive oil, beans, asparagus, etc.)

Correction of modifiable factors, e.g., untreated overt hypothyroidism or vitamin D deficiency, so that after the corrections, an attempt can be made of restarting statins. Coadministered drugs to be reviewed.

De-challenge and re-challenge drugs to identify SI is necessary. Stop statins for 4–6 weeks and observe. If the patient is asymptomatic for 2 weeks, restart with lower dose or alternate statin. If symptoms recur, consider alternatives. An alternative statin, e.g., fluvastatin or pravastatin may be tried. An occasional patient may also tolerate a reduced dose, an alternate-day or twice-weekly dose regimen. In simple words, every attempt should be made to accommodate a statin in patients who require lowering of LDL-C for reduction of ASCVD risk.

In rare patients, who cannot be managed with the above-mentioned protocol, nonstatin pharmacologic therapies may be tried. Among the currently available antihyperlipidemic drugs, only ezetimibe has been shown to reduce the CVD risk significantly as monotherapy without a background therapy with statins. Studies with bempedoic acid are underway. All the other agents, which have been shown to have benefits in reducing the ASCVD risk, have been tried on a background of statin therapy. So, they are difficult to recommend in this clinical scenario as sole agent. Bile acid sequestrants (cholestyramine and colestipol) may be used as an alternative.

A recent double-blind, randomized, placebo-controlled trial with 13,970 patients, where bempedoic acid was used at a dose of 180 mg daily among 6,992 patients showed a lower risk of major adverse cardiovascular events, reduces LDL-C and associated with low muscle-related adverse reactions at the end of 40.6 months (mean duration) follow-up. Fixed-dose combination (FDC) of bempedoic acid and ezetimibe may be tried.

Proprotein convertase subtilisin/kexin type 9 (PCSK9) inhibitor (alirocumab–75 mg SC every 2 weeks, evolocumab–140 mg SC every 2 weeks) lowers LDL-C with lesser muscle symptoms. ORION-3 study reveals that sustained and effective reduction of LDL-C and PCSK9 concentration over 4 years with twice yearly subcutaneous dosing of Inclisiran, a long-acting synthetic siRNA. Lomitapide—a inhibitor of microsomal triglyceride transfer protein (MTP)—reduces LDL-C by 50% and mipomersen (an antisense oligonucleotide inhibitor) by 25%. Evinacumab (an antibody inhibitor of angiopoietin-like 3) is approved for 4-weekly intravenous infusion in homozygous familial hypercholesterolemia to reduce LDL-C level. LDL apheresis is indicated in severe hypercholesterolemia, where drug therapy fails or there is intolerance.

Statins to be stopped immediately if evidences of severe myopathy, rhabdomyolysis, or statin-induced severe necrotizing autoimmune myositis occur. Adequate hydration, renal function and restoration are essential. Immunosuppressive treatment may be required in specific situations.

The management algorithm of SI is given in **Flowchart 1**.

CONCLUSION

Statins has a key role in prevention of coronary artery disease and may have to be used in higher dose. Though statin has low prevalence of intolerance, careful judgment and clinical monitoring are necessary. Early recognition of alarming symptoms is important. Physicians must understand that even low-dose statin is better than no statin.

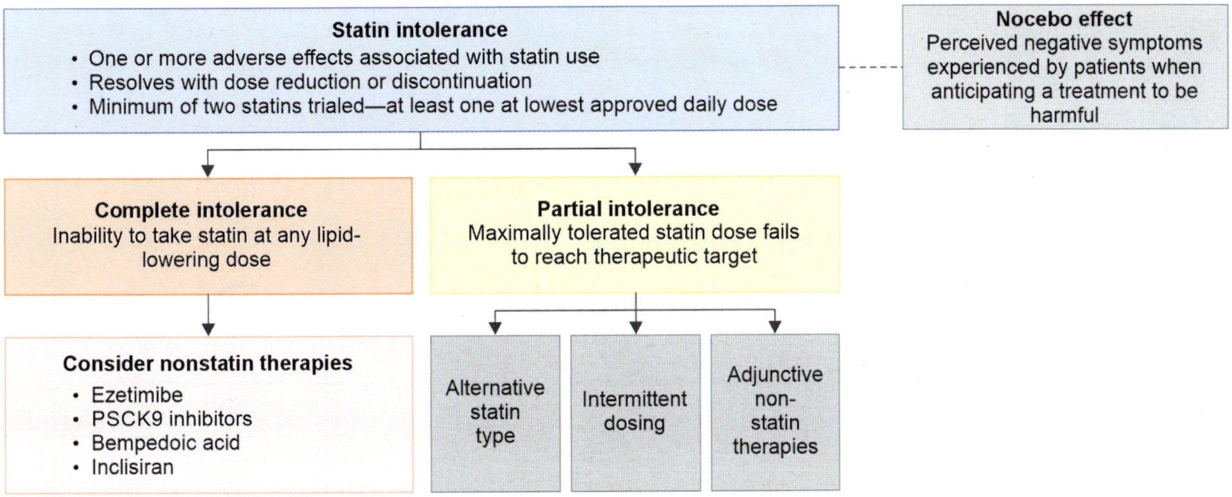

FLOWCHART 1: Algorithm showing management of statin intolerance.

(PCSK9: proprotein convertase subtilisin/kexin type 9)

Source: Gaine SP, Agarwala A, Dixon DL, Patel J. NLA 2022 definition of statin intolerance and approaches to management. [online] Available from https://www.acc.org/Latest-in-Cardiology/Articles/2022/08/08/12/27/NLA-2022-Definition-of-Statin-Intolerance. [Last accessed December, 2023].

SUGGESTED READINGS

1. Cheeley MK, Saseen JJ, Ararwala A, Ravilla S, Ciffone N, Jacobson TA, et al. NLA scientific statement on statin intolerance: a key considerations for ASCVD risk reduction in the statin intolerant patient. J Clin Lipidol. 2022;16(4):361-75.
2. Alonso R, Cuevas A, Cafferata A. Diagnosis and management of statin intolerance. J Atheroscler Thromb. 2019;26:207-2015.
3. Nissen SE, Lincoff AM, Brennan D, Ray KK, Mason D, Kastelein JJP, et al, Bempedoic acid and cardiovascular outcome in statin intolerant patients. N Engl J Med. 2023;388(15):1353-64.

175

CHAPTER

Obesity and Venous Disorders

Sirshendu Pal

ABSTRACT

Obesity predisposes individuals to venous stasis which may trigger deep vein thrombosis and chronic venous insufficiency. Too much weight puts additional load on the circulatory system because the excess body mass implies that our body must work harder to distribute, deliver, and return blood to the cardiac pump. Impaired return of the blood increases the pressure in the lower extremity veins. Venous hypertension due to higher reflux or obstruction is a vital cause of chronic venous insufficiency. The increased pressure in the veins may lead to leaky valves causing varicose veins. Increased body weight is also related to changes in the coagulation system including fibrinolytic activity and increased plasma concentration of coagulation factors.

INTRODUCTION

India is the third most obese country in the world after US and China according to a study published in the Lancet in 2013. The study titled "Global, regional and national prevalence of overweight and obesity in children and adults during 1980–2013: A systematic analysis for the Global burden of disease study 2013" was based on data from international organizations and bodies in different countries like India over three decades. Obesity is also more common in females than males. Venous disorders constitute an important public health problem. According to estimates from different countries, management of venous disorders constitutes 1–3% of the total healthcare expenditure. The actual financial burden is perhaps even greater as the price of cosmetic products and societal costs are not included in healthcare expenditure. Societal costs include hired help for homemaking activities, work absenteeism causing loss of productivity, and intangible costs. Obesity is an important cause of venous disorders and so this review is undertaken to create awareness and focus on the various venous disorders in obesity.

Pathophysiology

The complication of chronic venous insufficiency hinders the person's ability to involve in routine occupation or social activities and also puts a financial burden on the patient and family due to loss of duty hours. Factors contributing to deep vein thrombosis formation as per Virchow's triad of hypercoagulability, stasis, and injury to veins lead to chronic venous insufficiency. Chronic venous insufficiency can lead to difficult-to-heal and recurrent venous ulcers. Danielsson et al. found that there was a significant association between body mass index (BMI) of 28.9 kg/m^2 or more and higher clinical scores of chronic venous disease. The study of Kruger K et al. showed a strong relationship between the cross-sectional areas of veins of lower extremity and increasing BMI. Pathological changes due to hyperglycemia may be etiologically linked to vascular dysfunction in diabetes patients. Local angiogenesis and reduced peripheral blood flow are some of the known vascular complications.

A number of epidemiological studies give strong credence to the hypothesis that obesity is a risk factor for chronic venous insufficiency. Obesity is also related to changes in the coagulation parameters including altered fibrinolytic activity and increased concentration of clotting factors. These changes in endothelial function and coagulation are thought to be important not only for arterial but also for venous thrombosis. Besides obesity is considered to cause venous stasis which may trigger both chronic venous insufficiency and deep vein thrombosis.

Arfvidsson B et al. demonstrated that in morbidly obese patients, the pressure in the iliofemoral vein was significantly more than in nonobese individuals. The increased intra-abdominal pressure is thought to be transmitted to the extremities by the femoral veins causing venous stasis and distension of the veins in the lower extremities favoring venous valve dysfunction and thrombosis.

A waist circumference of > 100 cm may increase the risk of venous thromboembolism by 4 times. Similarly, post-thrombotic syndrome occurs more in obese patients after venous thromboembolism. Increased body weight is a risk factor for not only a first venous thromboembolism event as recently reported but also for recurrent venous thromboembolism events. The prevalence of iliac vein compression is more in women than in men.

TYPES OF VENOUS DISORDERS

Blood Clots

Blood clots can occur on legs, arms, kidneys (renal vein thrombosis), brain (cerebral vein thrombosis), lungs (pulmonary embolism), or other internal organs like liver or pelvic organs.

Deep Vein Thrombosis

The blood clots in the deep veins of legs and arms may cause inflammation. It may be initially asymptomatic but may lead to the dangerous pulmonary embolism.

Superficial Thrombophlebitis

The blood clots in a vein close to the surface of the skin cause inflammation. This causes pain, but the clots usually do not lead to pulmonary embolism unless they move first to the deep venous system.

Chronic Venous Insufficiency

The condition causes stagnation of blood, chronic leg swelling, increased pressure, increased pigmentation or discoloration of skin, or even leg ulcers called venous stasis ulcers.

Venous Ulcers

Ulcers are wounds or open sores that do not heal or keep coming again and again. Venous stasis ulcers occur usually below the knee, on the inner aspect of leg or just above the ankle. Venous leg ulcers are present in 1% of adults.

Arteriovenous Fistulas

Arteriovenous fistulas are arteries and veins that connect with each other directly with nothing in between.

Varicose Veins

Varicose veins are twisted, swollen veins near the surface of the skin and are formed when weak or defective valves allow blood to flow backward or blood stagnates in the vein. Chronic venous obstruction can also cause varicose veins. Women are affected twice as men. Almost 33% of adults have varicose veins.

TESTS TO DIAGNOSE VENOUS DISORDERS

- Ankle brachial index
- Ultrasound
- Intravascular ultrasound
- Computed tomography
- Magnetic resonance imaging
- Angiogram

MANAGEMENT

Lifestyle

It is most important to adopt a healthy lifestyle on a regular basis. Caloric intake should be limited and diet should be low in simple carbohydrates and high in fiber. We should choose foods that are full of antioxidants and essential fatty acids, especially omega-3, to protect the wall of the veins. We should quit tobacco. Weight loss decreases venous pressure and regular exercise increases the tone of the calf muscles to support the vein wall. Exercise also ensures energy expenditure and promotes weight loss. Walking, swimming, and cycling increase venous tone. Sports such as tennis and squash exert pressure by jerks and compress the calf. Heat dilates the veins, and we should avoid sunbathing, saunas, and hot baths. On the contrary, cold water may help if given in a precise direction from the bottom to the top, i.e., from ankles to thigh.

Prolonged standing should be avoided and legs to be elevated at the end of the day. Compression stockings or bandages may be used. Massage may improve lymphatic drainage which relieves the pain.

Medication

Antibiotics may be given to clear skin infections or ulcers. Pentoxifylline may improve blood flow. Anticoagulants or blood thinners may be used to treat blood clots or prevent development of clots. Injection heparin may be used for 3–6 months. Occasionally, thrombolytics such as urokinase or tissue plasminogen activators may be used.

Endovenous Laser Ablation

Endovenous laser ablation is a minimally invasive procedure. A catheter placed in the vein provides heat and obliterates the vein. Thus, less blood pools in the leg and overall blood flow improves.

Sclerotherapy

In serious cases, a sclerosant is injected into the affected veins and the veins become sclerosed. Blood then returns to the heart through other veins. The scarred vein is resorbed.

Vein Surgery

- *Ligation and stripping*: Here, the vein may be tied off (ligation) or if vein or its valves are heavily damaged, the vein may be removed (stripping).
- *Microincision/ambulatory phlebectomy*: This is a minimally invasive procedure in which the superficial varicose veins near skin surfaces are targeted. Needle punctures or small incisions are made over the veins. A phlebectomy hook is then used to remove the involved veins.
- *Subfascial endoscopic perforation surgery (SEPS)*: It is a minimally invasive procedure in which perforating veins above the ankle are targeted. A clip is used to block the veins, thus preventing blood flow. It helps to heal ulcers and prevent their recurrence.

Vein Bypass

In vein bypass, healthy veins from another part of the body are used to create a bypass to re-route the blood from a damaged vein. This is only used in severe cases when no other treatment is effective.

CONCLUSION

Obesity is a well-established risk factor for the development and progression of chronic venous disorders. It has a relevant influence on venous hemodynamic parameters of lower extremities. There is a mechanical role of abdominal adipose tissue in the elevated risk of venous disorders.

SUGGESTED READINGS

1. Eberhardt RT, Raffetto JD. Chronic venous insufficiency. Circulation. 2014;130:333-46.
2. Jawien A. The influence of environmental factors in chronic venous insufficiency. Angiology. 2003;54(Suppl 1):S19-31.
3. Danielsson G, Eklof B, Grandinetti A, Kistner RL. The influence of obesity on chronic venous disease. Vasc Endovascular Surg. 2002;36:271-6.
4. Kruger K, Ose C, Rudofsky G, Roesener J, Weiland D, Hirche H, et al. Peripheral veins: Influence of gender, body mass index, age and varicose veins on cross-sectional area. Vasc Med. 2003;8:249-55.
5. Das Evcimen N, King GL. The role of protein kinase C activation and the vascular complications of Diabetes. Pharmacol Res. 2007;55:498-510.
6. Agemo W, Piantanida E, Dentali f, Steidl L, Mera V, Squizzato et al. Body mass index is associated with the development of the post thrombotic syndrome. Thromb Haemost. 2003;89;305-9.
7. Darvall KA, Sam RC, Silverman SH, Bradbury AW, Adam DJ. Obesity and thrombosis. Eur J Vasc Endovasc Surg. 2007;33:223-33.
8. Tsai KA, Cushman M, Rosamond WD, Heckbert SR, Polak JF, Folsom AR. Cardiovascular risk factors and venous thromboembolism incidence: the longitudinal investigation of thromboembolism etiology. Arch Intern Med. 2002;162: 1182-9.
9. Arfvidsson B, Eklof B, Balfour j. Ilio-femoral venous pressure correlates with intraabdominal pressure in morbidly obese patients. Vasc Endovascular Surg. 2005;39:505-9.
10. Stein PD, Beemoth A, Olson RE. Obesity as a risk factor in venous thromboembolism. Am J Med. 2005;118:978-80.
11. Ageno W, Piantanida E, Dentali F, Steidl L, Mera V, Squizzato A et al. Body mass index is associated with development of post thrombotic syndrome. Thromb Haemost. 2003;89(2):305-9.
12. Eichinger S, Hron G. Bialonczyk C, Hirschi M, Minar E, Wagner O, et al. Overweight, obesity, and the risk of recurrent venous thromboembolism. Arch Intern Med. 2008;168:1678-83.
13. O'Sullivan GH, Semba CP, Bittner CA, Kee ST, Razavi MK, Sze DY et al. Endovascular management of iliac vein compression (May Thurner) syndrome. J Vasc Interv Radiol. 2000;11:823-36.

SECTION

13

NEPHROLOGY

176

CHAPTER

Molecular Mechanisms of Kidney Crosstalk with Distant Organs

Biva Bhakat

ABSTRACT

Interorgan communication is a key factor in maintaining homeostasis of body. Due to this communication, dysfunction in one organ led to dysfunction in multiple organs. Clinical evidence suggests that acute kidney injury (AKI) is a common complication following other organ dysfunction. Similarly, injury in kidney leads to multiorgan dysfunction. The mechanism by which kidney communicates with distant organs is not clearly understood. So, this is an area of active research/interest to identify the underlying mechanism and the important mediators of kidney crosstalk with distant organ. Adequate knowledge about this interaction is very crucial to develop new diagnostic approaches and therapeutic strategies for better outcome in patients with kidney injury.

INTRODUCTION

Organ crosstalk in case of kidney injury is a process by which acute kidney injury (AKI) executes different changes in functions of other organs such as liver, heart, and brain by using different modes of communication—signal transduction pathway, endocrine or paracrine way, or using the neural pathway. Interorgan crosstalk is mainly mediated by soluble mediators, target receptor of the mediators, cellular mediators such as immune cells (organ resident, circulating). Injury to any organ leads to activation of stress response at cellular level, resulting in release of cytokines that leads to activation of innate immune system. Cell death occurs as a result of cell stress followed by release of cell debris and deoxyribonucleic acid (DNA) and ribonucleic acid (RNA) material. These molecules are increased at the site of injury as well in the circulation and in the distant organ also. It has been seen that similar sequence of events is also evident in the remote organs. So, this is an area of active interest in how the inflammatory response of one organ is spreading to distant site and causing multiorgan dysfunction. Various underlying mechanisms have been postulated for this. In the event of kidney injury, the mortality increases significantly because of the involvement of remote organs, i.e., multiorgan dysfunction. For example, AKI alone is associated with 15–30% mortality which rises to 60–80% when associated with multiorgan failure. AKI-induced complications mainly include acute lung injury (ALI) and injury to the heart, brain, gut, and liver. There is also increased susceptibility to infection, resulting in sepsis because of the associated immune dysfunction. In this chapter, the various molecular mechanisms of kidney crosstalk with distant organs will be discussed.

KIDNEY–LUNG CROSSTALK

Acute kidney injury has several adverse effects on lungs as manifested by increased susceptibility of respiratory failure, requirement of invasive mechanical ventilation, prolonged duration of ventilation, and difficulty in weaning from the ventilation. The molecular mechanism of kidney–lung crosstalk involves mainly the following mediators:

- *Increased inflammatory mediators and imbalanced immune response*: Patient with kidney injury usually develops systemic inflammatory response syndrome (SIRS), characterized by elevated levels of various cytokines—interleukin 1 (IL-1), IL-6, IL-8, monocyte chemoattractant protein-1 (MCP1), and tumor necrosis factor-alpha (TNF-α). These cytokines cause inflammation in the lungs and cell apoptosis, oxidative stress, and increased endothelial barrier permeability, resulting in pulmonary edema. Most critical mediator of kidney-lung crosstalk is IL-6 as evidenced by the fact that IL-6 deficiency protects against AKI-induced lung injury by reducing the level of IL-8.

- *Uremic toxin accumulation*: Uremic toxin retention adversely affects lung function as evidenced by reduction in vital capacity. Besides fluid accumulation, the fluid-clearing capacity of lung also reduced because of downregulation of epithelial sodium channels (ENaC), pulmonary sodium-potassium adenosine triphosphatase (Na^+/K^+-ATPase), and aquaporin-5 expression. Indoxyl sulfate and protein-bound uremic toxin is mainly involved in this downregulation. It also induces IL-6 expression.
- *Novel molecules*: mt-DAMPs (mitochondrial damage-associated molecular patterns) is an example of high-mobility group protein 1/alarmins. Their levels are elevated in patients with kidney injury and they promote inflammation in the lung by activating the innate immune system. Osteopontin, an example of immunoregulatory molecule, is the most recently discovered biomarker of kidney injury-induced lung inflammation and endothelial leakage. Alpha-Klotho, coreceptor of fibroblast growth factor 23, upregulates autophagy, inhibit cell senescence, fibrosis, and apoptosis, thereby reducing inflammation. In AKI patients, there is reduction in the circulating alpha-Klotho level that promotes lung inflammation.

KIDNEY–HEART CROSSTALK

In homeostasis, cardiovascular system is regulated by various substances released by kidney such as erythropoietin, renin, prostaglandins, and endothelins. Myocardium also influences kidney function by releasing vasopressin, brain natriuretic peptide, and atrial natriuretic peptide. Thus, kidney and heart regulate blood volume and pressure through interorgan communications. AKI leading to heart failure is considered as cardiorenal syndrome type 3; chronic kidney disease (CKD) causing heart failure is known as cardiorenal syndrome type 4 and systemic disease, affecting both heart and kidney is called cardiorenal syndrome type 5. Important molecular mediators are as follows:

- *Neurohormonal hyperactivity*: Abnormal activation of sympathetic nervous system results in high level of angiotensin-II that causes cardiac remodeling.
- *Inflammatory stress*: In renal dysfunction patients, elevated level of IL-1, IL-6, TNF-α, and interferon alpha (IFN-α) are observed. These cytokines cause endothelial dysfunction and recruit neutrophils in the cardiac tissue, resulting in cardiotoxicity. The hyperactive inflammatory state negatively affect the hematopoietic function, resulting in anemia which exacerbates the heart failure further.
- *Novel mediators*: Stem cell growth factor-β, INF-γ, and calcium/calmodulin-dependent protein kinases (CaMKs) play important role in cardiorenal syndrome by regulating the inflammation and oxidative stress in the body. Various levels of stem cell growth factor-β and INF-γ are seen according to the severity of AKI; CaMKs mainly play role in patients with CKD.

KIDNEY–VASCULAR SYSTEM CROSSTALK

In physiology, kidney receives around 20% of cardiac output which is necessary for providing nutrients and oxygen to renal tubules to maintain their physiological function. One such example is tubule-glomerular feedback. Thus, any pathology in vascular system aggravates the kidney injury. Plasma endothelial injury molecules such as angiopoietin 2 and thrombomodulin are elevated in AKI. Endothelial cells mount rapid response to renal injury by the following mechanisms:

- *Increased permeability*: Increased expression of vascular endothelial growth factor (VEGF) and VEGF receptor (VEGF-R) occurs in patient with kidney injury as a stress response. These lead to angiogenesis and increase vascular permeability, causing vascular leakage.
- *Thrombosis*: Imbalance in the blood coagulation system seen in patients with AKI. The mechanism differs in in arterioles and capillaries, leading to failure of single anticoagulant agents in improving thrombosis. There is loss of endothelial protein C receptor in the arterioles and thrombomodulin in capillaries.
- *Inflammatory cell recruitment*: Upregulation of various adhesion molecules such as E-selectin, P-selectin, intercellular adhesion molecule 1, and vascular cell adhesion molecular 1 occur in endothelial cells. This led to recruitment of neutrophils, macrophages, and lymphocytes, which causes inflammatory reaction locally at the injury site and in the systemic circulation.

KIDNEY–LIVER CROSSTALK

Acute kidney injury exerts several effects on liver, resulting in abnormal hepatic function which contribute to excess mortality in AKI. Though we do not have enough evidence on this like the hepatorenal syndrome, few clinical reports are available in this regard. The following mechanisms have been postulated:

- *Increased metabolic load*: Different drugs or toxic substances are inactivated or their solubility got increased in liver to be excreted by kidney. In case of AKI, the renal excretion is diminished. So, the substances don not get excreted immediately and the liver must function more to inactivate them, leading to hepatic damage.
- *Metabolic acidosis*: It causes resistance to various hormones. It increases insulin resistance, resulting in impaired glucose metabolism. It also causes growth hormone (GH) resistance by decreasing the production of insulin-like growth factor 1 (IGF-1) and diminished hepatic expression of receptor for GH and IGF-1. Hepatic ornithine cycle is also hampered.
- *Altered metabolomics*: Hyperuricemia or hyperphosphatemia in AKI causes altered metabolism in liver. There is disbalance in hepatic ornithine cycle. In AKI, hepatic production of arginine may be hampered because of accumulation of toxins such as asymmetric dimethylarginine (ADMA). Hepatocellular regeneration is also hampered as there is failure of high consumption of ATP. Activation of hydroxymethylglutaryl-CoA (HMG-CoA) reductase may occur.
- *Altered drug metabolism*: Hepatic metabolism of drugs are altered because of altered hepatic clearance or intrinsic clearance. This occurs because of altered expression of drug transporter and metabolic enzymes.
- *Increased acute phase response*: Elevated IL-6 level in AKI-downregulated CYP3A4, thereby inhibiting metabolism of CYP substrates. IL-6 increased production of acute phase response by acting on IL-6 receptor-gp130 glycoprotein complex.

KIDNEY–GUT CROSSTALK

The gastrointestinal tract contains around 70–80% immune cells and about 100 trillion microbial cells. Thus, it is the largest reservoir of immune cells. As AKI is associated with activation of immune and inflammatory cells, the gut is altered by renal injury and any alteration in the gut microbiota or intestinal permeability affect the course of AKI, demonstrating a bidirectional relationship. The mechanisms are as follows:

- *Reduced short-chain fatty acids (SCFAs)*: Renal injury-induced dysbiosis is associated with reduced SCFA production. SCFA have a prominent barrier-strengthening and anti-inflammatory activities. SCFAs exert their protective effect by activating G protein-coupled receptors (GPCRs)—GPR43, GPR41, Olfr78, and GPR109 and by inhibiting histone deacetylase. It decreases the production of cytokines—IL-1, IL-6, TNF-α, MCP-1, and reactive oxygen species (ROS). It also inhibits nuclear factor κB (NF-κB) signaling and toll-like receptor 4 (TLR-4) expression. It stimulates mitochondrial biogenesis. Thus, decreased SCFAs have a deleterious effect on AKI.
- *Altered inflammatory cell pattern*: There is accumulation of neutrophils, pro-inflammatory macrophages, and Th17 cells in the lamina propria. Paneth cell degranulation produce IL-17A which contribute further to intestinal inflammation. Accumulated macrophages show change in phenotype. The mature resident macrophage (Ly6clowCX3CR1high) in state of inflammation undergoes differentiation into Ly6clowCX3CR1int macrophages which is highly proinflammatory. It induces Th17 cells that leads to potentiation of systemic inflammation.
- *Uremic toxin*: Microbiota produces different toxin which undergoes renal excretion. In the setting of renal injury, the excretion is hampered and the uremic toxin gets accumulated in kidney. Few such toxins are indoxyl sulfate, para-cresyl sulfate, indole 3 acetic acid, and trimethylamine-N-oxide. Their accumulation causes endothelial dysfunction, proinflammatory factor expression, ROS production, and leukocyte extravasation. These factors cause further renal injury. Increased urea level increases intestinal permeability. The urea diffuses from blood into gut lumen and converted into ammonia by urease and subsequently into ammonium hydroxide. This damages the tight junction protein, resulting in increased gut permeability.

KIDNEY–BRAIN CROSSTALK

During renal injury, brain is also affected that further increases compatibility. The brain–kidney crosstalk mainly involves cytokines, oxidative stress, and ion transporter disturbances. The central nervous system disturbances occur mainly by the following mechanisms:

- *Disruption of blood–brain barrier*: Normally, transport across the blood–brain barrier is highly regulated. In AKI, the integrity is disrupted. There is infiltration of the various cytokines such as TNF-α, IL-6, MCP-1, and chemokine ligand 1 (CXCL-1), leading to cerebral injury.
- *Acid–base imbalance*: The metabolic acidosis disrupts the neuronal function. Intracellular acidosis increases affinity toward ammonia. This increases the oxidative deamination of glutamate. The excess ammonia cycling between neurons and astrocytes results in altered neurotransmitter balance. Metabolic acidosis also changes the free and bound fraction of calcium

and magnesium. This affects the neurotransmission, electrical gradient, and ion flux, resulting in neurotoxicity.

- *Dysfunction of ion transporter*: Interference with the function of different ion channel changes the concentration of various amino acids and neurotransmitters. Few examples are dysfunction in the Na^+-independent cationic amino acid transporter 1 (CAT1/SLC7A1), associated with influx of L-arginine alters level of taurine, glycine, alanine, etc., excitatory amino acid transporter responsible for efflux of aspartic acid, glutamate and glycine, and gamma aminobutyric acid is also dysfunctional. Organic anion transporter 3 (OAT3) and organic cation transporter 3 (OCT3) also show dysregulation, causing reduced efflux of drugs or organic solutes. These cause neurotoxicity.
- *Increased risk of cerebrovascular accident*: Renal injury-induced dysfunction of endothelial cells, platelets, and altered coagulation cascade leads to increased occurrence of cerebral thrombosis and hemorrhage.

CONCLUSION

Renal injury leads to dysfunction in the multiple organs via complex interaction. In the chapter, we have tried to simplify this to understand the proper pathophysiological mechanism of multiorgan dysfunction in patients with AKI. This is of utmost importance to develop new diagnostic approaches and therapeutic strategy in patients with renal dysfunction. If we can identify and target the molecular mediators involved, kidney injury-related morbidity and mortality will be reduced significantly.

SUGGESTED READINGS

1. Hasegawa S, Inagi R. Molecular mechanisms of kidney crosstalk with distant organs. Nat Rev Nephrol. 2023;19(2):75-6.
2. Feltes CM, Van Eyk J, Rabb H. Distant-organ changes after acute kidney injury. Nephron Physiol. 2008;109(4):80-4.
3. Lee SA, Cozzi M, Bush EL, Rabb H. Distant Organ Dysfunction in Acute Kidney Injury: A Review. Am J Kidney Dis. 2018;72(6): 846-56.

177

CHAPTER

Urinary Biomarkers for Kidney Disease

Pinaki Mukhopadhyay

ABSTRACT

Despite of having serum creatinine as an important biomarker to evaluate kidney dysfunction, search of novel biomarkers is ongoing to circumvent the limitations of creatinine adapting early intervention. There are both serum and urine biomarkers which are often raised in nephron injury in site specific manner. Numerous biomarkers addressing acute kidney injury and chronic kidney disease have been investigated namely cystatin C, kidney injury molecule-1 (KIM-1), neutrophil gelatinase-associated lipocalin (NGAL), liver-type fatty acid-binding protein (L-FABP) have been detected. A combination of biomarkers in detecting kidney dysfunction may predict the outcomes better. There are also insights regarding posttransplant graft dysfunction. However further investigations are needed to find out the potentiality of new biomarkers.

INTRODUCTION

A good biomarker is defined as an easily available organ-specific marker that can be easily interpreted in a cost-effective way. For acute kidney injury (AKI), the biomarkers should be able to identify the insult to kidney as earliest so that intervention can be done with ability to differentiate among prerenal, renal, and postrenal factors.

In chronic kidney disease, the biomarkers that can identify its onset are hard to find but the site of injury whether glomerular, tubular or interstitial and mechanism, progression and prognosis of disease may be estimated from biomarkers.

There are both serum and urine biomarkers available with own advantages and disadvantages. Though creatinine is widely used in kidney injury in cost-effective manner, there are many disadvantages, e.g., creatinine is influenced by age, muscle mass, diet, and its rise is not site specific and also influenced by drugs. Serum biomarkers are often unstable with interference with plasma proteins. Urinary biomarkers though stable are often influenced by volume status and hydration. To circumvent this, urinary biomarkers are often normalized by urinary creatinine concentrations.

DIAGNOSTIC BIOMARKERS IN ACUTE KIDNEY INJURY

Urinary Kidney Injury Molecule-1

Kidney injury molecule-1 (KIM-1), being a transmembrane glycoprotein with ectodomain, is a marker of proximal tubular injury. Other than AKI, it is also showing promising result in chronic renal tubular damage following vesicoureteral reflux, posttransplantation delayed graft function (DGF), human immunodeficiency virus (HIV), and diabetic nephropathy. The ectodomain of KIM-1 is a soluble fragment that can be measured in urine by immunoassay. Biomarker dipstick for KIM-1 is available for rapid detection. A case control study was done among children with cardiopulmonary bypass comparing urinary KIM-1 level with or without AKI. It was observed that urinary KIM-1 levels were increased 6–12 hours following surgery and remained elevated up to 48 hours in patients who sustained a >50% increase in serum creatinine within the first 48 hours but not in children who had normal kidney function.

Urinary Tubular Enzymes

Proximal renal tubular antigens such as alpha-glutathione S-transferase (α-GST), pi-glutathione S-transferase (pi-GST), gamma-glutamyl transpeptidase (GGT), and alanine aminopeptidase (AAP) are released within 12 hours of insult and detectable for 4 days, even before rise of serum creatinine.

Urinary Low-molecular-weight Proteins

Alpha-1-microglobulin, beta-2-microglobulin, retinol-binding protein, adenosine deaminase-binding protein, and urinary cystatin C are urinary low-molecular-weight proteins which are filtered at glomerulus with tubular absorption.

Urine Cystatin C

Its level detected AKI 1–2 days before changes in serum creatinine level and its level was also associated with severity of AKI according to a study by Herget-Rosenthal and associates. Urinary cystatin C is having disadvantages of high-cost burden and lack of standardization. It may be influenced also by inflammatory conditions, glucocorticoid therapy, and hyperthyroidism. Immuno-nephelometric assay for cystatin C measurement provides rapid measurement in minutes.

Neutrophil Gelatinase-associated Lipocalin

Neutrophil gelatinase-associated lipocalin (NGAL) is a promising biomarker in identifying early acute tubular necrosis, differentiating it from prerenal AKI. Urine NGAL is proposed to help AKI up to 48 hours and testing later may not provide promising results.

In contrast-induced nephropathy, rise of both urine NGAL (4 hours) and plasma NGAL (2 hours) levels were documented, even before rise of cystatin C. However many systemic inflammatory conditions and infections may influence this biomarker.

Urinary Interleukin-18

Though urinary interleukin-18 (IL-18) level is elevated in acute tubular necrosis, its role as biomarker needs to be studied further.

Urinary Liver-type Fatty Acid-binding Protein

Urinary level of liver-type fatty acid-binding protein (L-FABP) is associated with proximal tubular injury. Portilla and associates had described the rise of L-FABP within 4 hours of cardiac surgery in children, predicting development of AKI.

Urinary L-FABP levels are also investigated in contrast-induced nephropathy and the results showed its significant rise after 4 hours of cardiac catheterization with persistence of its high level up to 48 hours.

Furosemide Stress Test

In euvolemic patients, furosemide administration at a dose of 1 mg/kg in furosemide naïve and 1.5 mg/kg in non-naïve patient intravenously in stage 1 and stage 2 AKI can produce urine output > 200 mL within 2 hours indicating furosemide responsiveness that can predict progression to stage 3 AKI and mortality.

DIAGNOSTIC BIOMARKERS IN CHRONIC KIDNEY DISEASE

Fibroblast Growth Factor-23

Fibroblast growth factor-23 (FGF-23) level is raised from chronic kidney disease (CKD) stage 4, even in absence of rise of serum phosphorus or parathyroid hormone (PTH). Its rise is prognostically associated with cardiovascular disease in CKD and there is documentation of decline in FGF-23 level in post-kidney transplantation.

Soluble Urokinase Plasminogen Activator Receptor

Soluble urokinase plasminogen activator receptor (suPAR) is thought to be used as a biomarker in AKI within first 7 days of ICU admission but its level is confounded by infection, diabetes, and cardiovascular disease.

Its level is also documented regarding connection between CKD and focal segmental glomerulosclerosis (FSGS) and diabetic nephropathy. Higher baseline suPAR levels were associated with a greater decline in estimated glomerular filtration rate (eGFR)/year.

PROGNOSTIC BIOMARKER

A prognostic biomarker predicts risk of disease progression.

Urinary Renin and Angiotensinogen

Ratio of urinary angiotensinogen to urinary creatinine predicts longer hospital stay. Urinary renin to creatinine ratio is another prognostic biomarker.

Urinary Insulin-like Growth Factor Binding Protein 7 and Tissue Inhibitor of Metalloproteinase 2

Urinary insulin-like growth factor binding protein 7 (IGFBP7) and tissue inhibitor of metalloproteinase 2 (TIMP2) act to arrest cell cycle in AKI. In response to cellular stress in tubular cells, IGFBP7 and TIMP2 are released which cause cell cycle arrest at G1-S phase to provide opportunity for deoxyribonucleic acid (DNA) repair. However, sustained cell cycle arrest can result in fibrosis. Sapphire validation study was performed among 744 patients with critical illness and the primary endpoint of this study was Kidney Disease: Improving Global Outcomes (KDIGO) stage 2 and 3 after 12 hours of enrolment. These two biomarkers were found to be superior among existing biomarkers providing additional information over clinical variables and adding mechanistic insight into AKI.

URINARY RENAL FIBROSIS MARKER

Excessive production of profibrotic molecules such as connective tissue growth factor (CTGF) and transforming growth factor beta 1 (TGF-β1) are associated with renal fibrosis. CTGF expression is upregulated in immunoglobulin A (IgA) nephropathy, FSGS, and diabetic nephropathy. Urinary CTGF is associated with interstitial fibrosis. Elevated urinary TGF-β1 levels were found in patients with glomerulonephritis and diabetic nephropathy, as well as in renal allograft recipients **(Table 1)**.

COMBINATION OF BIOMARKERS

Although the conventional biomarkers (urea, creatinine, and albuminuria) are aiding in diagnosis and staging of kidney injury, the concept of newer biomarkers may be helping early diagnosis, staging, prognostication, and guiding early interventions in kidney injury.

Utilizing the characteristics of biomarkers, it is possible to stratify kidney disease into acute or chronic, prerenal or renal, and glomerular or tubular origin. Kidney disease, being a complex pathophysiological process, may be defined by the change of different biomarkers levels rather single one.

There are many multicenter, prospective studies that support the role of combination biomarkers. One prospective multicenter cohort study with 1,635 emergency patients underwent investigations for five biomarkers (urinary NGAL, KIM-1, urinary L-FABP, urinary IL-18, and cystatin C). Though all biomarkers were elevated in acute intrinsic kidney injury, urinary NGAL level was found to be most useful.

Another prospective study was conducted on AKI patients with cirrhosis investigating the role of biomarkers to differentiate prerenal cause, acute tubular necrosis and hepatorenal syndrome which would be the possible etiologies and understanding the cause to plan the treatment. Urinary biomarkers were found to elevate in cirrhosis with AKI.

The combined urine biomarkers product of [TIMP-2]*[IGFBP7] can improve risk stratification of kidney injury.

RECENT ADVANCES ON BIOMARKERS OF EARLY AND LATE KIDNEY GRAFT DYSFUNCTION

To detect DGF, especially in the setting of expanded criteria donor, kidney biomarkers can be used before

TABLE 1: Important markers defining site-specificity of injury of nephron.

Glomerular injury markers	Proximal tubular injury markers	Loop of Henle injury markers	Distal tubular injury markers	Interstitial fibrosis markers	Markers not site-specific
Albumin	Urine cystatin C	Furosemide stress test	Urine NGAL	Urine TGF-beta	TIMP-2/IGFBP7-G1 cell cycle arrest
Serum cystatin C	Urine KIM-1			Tumor necrosis factor receptor	
Creatinine	Urine IL-18				
	Urine L-FABP				
	Alpha-1-microglobulin				
	Beta-2-microglobulin				

(**IGFBP7: insulin-like growth factor binding protein 7; IL-18: interleukin-18; KIM-1: kidney injury molecule-1; L-FABP: liver-type fatty acid-binding protein; NGAL:** neutrophil gelatinase-associated lipocalin; TGF: transforming growth factor; TIMP-2: tissue inhibitor of metalloproteinase 2)

transplant in the donor or in the recipient immediately after transplant. Urinary extracellular vesicles which are shed from parent cells are used to correlate with DGF. Urinary CD133 + EV are used to predict DGF and found to decrease in graft dysfunction and vascular damage.

- Donor urine derived complement C5a is also a potential marker of DGF, providing a potential rationale for complement blocking therapies to prevent DGF.
- Exosomal messenger ribonucleic acid (mRNA) for NGAL and NGAL concentration in the perfusate of machine-perfused kidneys were associated with DGF also in another study.
- Urinary microRNAs were also studied in a cohort study and found to elevate in DGF.
- Many trials had analyzed mRNA transcripts in urinary sediment cells and identified a 3 gene signature (CD3ε mRNA, CXCL10 mRNA, and 18S rRNA) predicting T cell-mediated rejection (TCMR) even before biopsy proven diagnosis.
- Urinary CXCL9 and CXCL10 are promising biomarkers in TCMR and antibody-mediated rejection (ABMR). Additionally urinary CXCL3 is associated with subclinical inflammation and predict chronic damage.
- Metabolomic profiling led to identification of a panel of five potential biomarkers (guanidinoacetic acid, methylimidazoleacetic acid, dopamine, 4-guanidobutyric acid, and L-tryptophan) can predict the graft dysfunction.
- Elevated expression of FOXP3 in blood and urine samples of kidney transplant recipients is associated with graft dysfunction.

AREAS OF RESEARCH

Metabolomics, proteomics, extracellular vesicles, microRNA, inflammatory markers (IL-6 and IL-10), and monocyte chemoattractant factor 1 are areas of further investigation to find out the potentiality to be used as novel biomarkers.

SUGGESTED READINGS

1. Han WK, Waikar SS, Johnson A, Betensky RA, Dent CL, Devarajan P, et al. Urinary biomarkers in the early diagnosis of acute kidney injury. Kidney Int. 2008;73:863-9.
2. Herget-Rosenthal S, Marggraf G, Hüsing J, Göring F, Pietruck F, Janssen O, et al. Early detection of acute renal failure by serum cystatin C. Kidney Int. 2004;66(15327406):1115-22.
3. Ling W, Zhaohui N, Ben H, Leyi G, Jianping L, Huili D, et al. Urinary IL-18 and NGAL as early predictive biomarkers in contrast-induced nephropathy after coronary angiography. Nephron Clin Pract. 2008;108(18287807):176-81.
4. Portilla D, Dent C, Sugaya T, Nagothu KK, Kundi I, Moore P, et al. Liver fatty acid-binding protein as a bio marker of acute kidney injury after cardiac surgery. Kidney Int. 2008;73(18094680): 465-72.
5. Nakamura T, Sugaya T, Node K, Ueda Y, Koide H. Urinary excretion of liver-type fatty acid-binding protein in contrast medium-induced nephropathy. Am J Kidney Dis. 2006;47(16490622): 439-44.
6. Kashani K, Al-Khafaji A, Ardiles T, Artigas A, Bagshaw SM, Bell M, et al. Discovery and validation of cell cycle arrest biomarkers in human acute kidney injury. Crit Care. 2013;17(1):R25.
7. Honkanen E, Teppo AM, Törnroth T, Groop PH, Grönhagen-Riska C. Urinary transforming growth factor-beta 1 in membranous glomerulonephritis. Nephrol Dial Transplant. 1997;12(9430852):2562-8.
8. Cha DR, Kim IS, Kang YS, Han SY, Han KH, Shin C, et al. Urinary concentration of transforming growth factor-beta-inducible gene-h3(beta ig-h3) in patients with type 2 diabetes mellitus. Diabet Med. 2005;22(15606685):14-20.
9. Nickolas TL, Schmidt-Ott KM, Canetta P, Forster C, Singer E, Sise M, et al. Diagnostic and prognostic stratification in the emergency department using urinary biomarkers of nephron damage: a multicenter prospective cohort study. J Am Coll Cardiol. 2012;59(3):246-55.
10. Belcher JM, Sanyal AJ, Peixoto AJ, Perazella MA, Lim J, Thiessen-Philbrook H, et al. Kidney biomarkers and differential diagnosis of patients with cirrhosis and acute kidney injury. Hepatology. 2014;60(2):622-32.
11. Cappuccilli M, Capelli I, Comai G, Cianciolo G, La Manna G. Neutrophil Gelatinase-Associated Lipocalin as a Biomarker of Allograft Function after Renal Transplantation: Evaluation of the Current Status and Future Insights. Artif Organs. 2018;42: 8-14.
12. Khalid U, Newbury LJ, Simpson K, Jenkins RH, Bowen T, Bates L, et al. A urinary microRNA panel that is an early predictive biomarker of delayed graft function following kidney transplantation. Sci Rep. 2019;9:3584.
13. Suthanthiran M, Schwartz JE, Ding R, Abecassis M, Dadhania D, Samstein B, et al. Urinary-cell mRNA profile and acute cellular rejection in kidney allografts. N Engl J Med. 2013;369:20-31.

178

CHAPTER

Climate Change and Kidney Disease: Threats and Opportunities

Anupama YJ

ABSTRACT

Climate change and global warming are new threats to kidney health. Heat stress impacts kidney functioning and is associated with acute kidney injury and electrolyte imbalances. It is also associated with a new form of chronic kidney disease (CKD) that is seen in laborers of Central America and may be one of the important causes for CKD in Sri Lanka and parts of India. In addition, there are indirect effects on kidney diseases due to an increase in infections and vector-borne diseases. Extreme weather events are on the rise and can have deleterious consequences on health and may impact access to hospitals and dialysis facilities. On the other hand, dialysis services are also important contributors to carbon footprint and add to the ecological burden due to the tremendous demand on resources and the generation of large quantities of biomedical waste. There is an increasing need for health professionals to understand the consequences of climate change on health. This chapter provides an outline of the possible effects on kidney health and also the methods that may be undertaken to mitigate the challenges.

INTRODUCTION

Climate change is a newly recognized threat to life on earth and has far-reaching consequences on human health status. The environmental changes that have accelerated after the Industrial Revolution since the late 19th century have affected the prevalence of many diseases and caused newer diseases to originate. Global efforts are focusing on effective ways to control global warming and contain many diseases, and this requires a multidisciplinary approach. It is now well documented that worldwide, ambient temperature is showing an increasing trend. The global mean temperature has increased by nearly 1.1°C since 1880 (~ 2°F). In addition, there is a marked increase in extreme heat events, called heat waves, which cause increased mortality. The extra heat is driving regional and seasonal temperature extremes, reduces snow cover and sea ice, intensifies heavy rainfall causing sea water levels to rise, and has a cascading effect on habitats of plants and animals, with expansion in some and shrinkage of others. The increase in surface temperature of oceans results in increased rains and untimely snowfall. It also means more precipitation and chaotic weather patterns.

Kidneys are affected by climate change in more ways than one. While there is much attention to global warming and heat stress-related kidney disease, the other changes such as excessive rainfall, snowfall, and flooding can also disturb the lives of patients with kidney disease either directly or indirectly. It is the objective of this chapter to summarize the important effects of changing climate in kidney diseases and give an outline of global efforts to alleviate the damage.

EFFECT OF HEAT STRESS ON KIDNEYS IN HEALTH AND DISEASE

Kidneys are important organs that regulate fluid, electrolyte, and acid-base balance in the body. In addition, they have a large share of the cardiac output flowing through them each minute and are metabolically very active organs. They have an important role in excretion of toxins and are exposed to the concentrated toxic material during their elimination. They also play a role in dissipation of heat along with skin and lungs and regulate body temperature.

In healthy humans, the resting core temperature fluctuates between 36.5 and 37.5°C. Heat stress is the net heat load to which a person is exposed and is a function of environmental factors, physical exertion, and clothing. With exercise, there is active heat production due to metabolism. Thermoregulation aims to balance heat gain with heat loss. When heat gain exceeds heat loss, positive heat balance occurs, and core body temperature rises. Under normal mechanisms, heat loss is mostly through the kidneys and to a lesser extent, water loss occurring through sweat loss, evaporation from the skin, respiration, and the gut. The kidneys respond to heat stress by decreasing urine output and/or increasing the urinary concentration to mitigate water and electrolyte losses.

EFFECTS OF ENVIRONMENTAL CHANGES ON KIDNEY HEALTH

The environmental changes can affect kidney health in four broad areas as outlined in **Box 1**.

Heat Stress Nephropathy

The most studied kidney disease that is associated with heat stress is the Mesoamerican nephropathy, also known as heat stress nephropathy, in the Central American countries. It was first reported in 2002 when an unusually high incidence of chronic kidney disease (CKD) not attributable to the usual causes was recognized in El Salvador. It was later described from other neighboring countries like Nicaragua, Costa Rica, and Guatemala. An overall CKD prevalence of 15–21% has been described in this population. It affected predominantly men, in the age group of 20–40 years, who were actively engaged in agriculture. These patients usually had no known cause of CKD, and it was called chronic kidney disease of uncertain etiology (CKDu). Multiple evaluation and epidemiological surveys later, the cause is still obscure. However, there are pointers toward heat stress as the dominant cause **(Flowchart 1)**. Epidemiologic studies have suggested that the workers in sugarcane fields, and especially sugarcane cutters, are more affected compared to those involved in less strenuous fieldwork. It is also seen in construction workers, miners, and corn field and rice field laborers, while women are less commonly affected. Workers at high altitudes such as coffee workers were usually spared, which explains that heat and humidity play an important role. The pathophysiologic mechanisms involved are multiple as seen in **Flowchart 1**.

Chronic kidney disease of uncertain etiology has been described in agricultural laborers of Sri Lanka and farmers along the east coast of India too, although there are subtle differences between presentations among the different geographic areas. Studies in the Sri Lankan patients implicate the toxins such as agrochemicals and heavy metals such as cadmium, arsenic, and glyphosate. This form of CKDu is seen more in the northern province of Sri Lanka, again documenting increased ambient temperatures compared to other provinces. Many scientists believe that the drying surface water and relying on ground water in the hot temperatures lead to higher concentration of these toxins in drinking water and chronic exposures to such toxins may be the cause of CKDu.

BOX 1: Effects on kidney diseases due to environmental change.

- *Heat stress-related kidney disease*:
  - Acute kidney injury
  - Chronic kidney disease
  - Kidney stones
  - Electrolyte disturbances
  - Increased risk of urinary infections
- *Changing patterns of vector-borne infections*: Infection-related kidney disease
- *Compromised water quality and quantity*:
  - Contamination with nephrotoxic heavy metals and agrochemical residues
  - Lack of access of water to hemodialysis
- *Rising metabolic diseases*:
  - Diabetic kidney disease
  - Obesity-related glomerulopathy

Source: Adapted from Bharati J, et al. (2022).

Heat Stress and Acute Kidney Injury

Heat stress is also associated with acute kidney injury (AKI) and electrolyte disturbances. The California heat wave in 2006 resulted in increased hospitalization from AKI. Studies in sugarcane workers in Nicaragua revealed increased serum creatinine at the end of work shifts, the creatinine levels being more in people who were actively engaged in farming such as sugarcane cutters, which is associated with the most strain. Elevated levels of urinary markers of AKI such as neutrophil gelatinase associated lipocalin (NGAL) and kidney injury molecule-1 (KIM-1) have also been demonstrated in those workers.

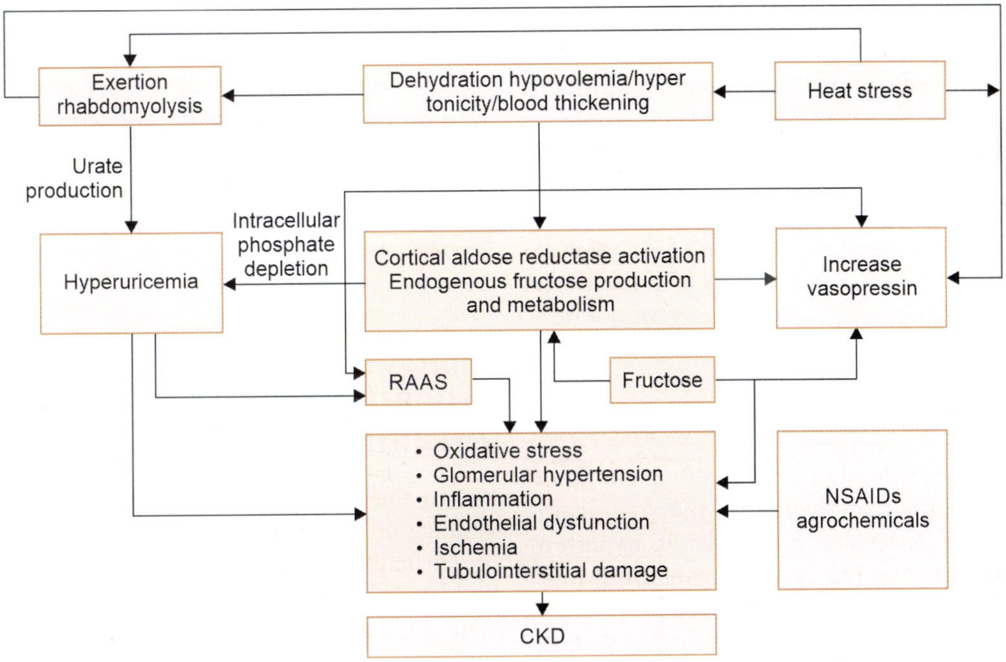

FLOWCHART 1: Pathophysiology of heat stress nephropathy.

(CKD: chronic kidney disease; NSAIDs: nonsteroidal anti-inflammatory drugs; RAAS: renin–angiotensin–aldosterone system)

Source: Singh NP, Gupta AK, Kaur G, Khanna T. Chronic kidney disease of unknown origin: What do we know? J Assoc Physicians India. 2020;68(2):76-9.

Heat Stroke and Acute Kidney Injury

Heat stroke is defined as hyperthermia with body temperature exceeding 106°F and anhidrosis associated with altered sensorium. It can be either of exertional or of epidemic type. Exertional heat stroke follows exertion in hot climate, such as in military personnel or marathon runners. Epidemic or classic heat stroke occurs during heat waves and affects the vulnerable population in the extremes of age, diabetics, and malnourished. Heat stroke is associated with AKI which may be of two types. Exertional heat stroke usually causes acute tubular necrosis, due to rhabdomyolysis, hyperuricemia, and dehydration. AKI in epidemic heat stroke appears to be acute interstitial nephritis and may be due to temperature-induced oxidative stress. Varying combinations of electrolyte disturbances such as hyponatremia, hypokalemia, hypophosphatemia, hypocalcemia, and hypomagnesemia are seen in 30–50% patients. These are due to tubular dysfunction. Dialysis may also be required in 10–30% of patients. Some may progress to CKD with features of chronic interstitial nephritis on kidney biopsy.

Kidney stones are precipitated in the presence of dehydration due to low urine pH as well as urinary concentration. There is also an increased incidence of urinary tract infection.

Increase in Tropical Infections and their Effect on Kidney Disease

Infections are an important cause of AKI in tropical regions. Flooding and heavy rainfalls have been associated with outbreaks of leptospirosis in parts of Southeast Asia. Diarrheal diseases are still one of the leading causes of AKI in the tropics, especially during summer months. Shift of infectious agents and vectors to cooler climates can cause infections in different areas. Westward movement of migratory birds due to environmental change has been linked to emergence of West Nile Virus encephalitis in North America. Natural disasters can also affect access to dialysis facilities. Evacuation causing disaster-induced stress resulted in hypertension, and incident CKD rate following the 2011 Japan earthquake was higher in evacuees compared to nonevacuees.

EXTREME WEATHER EVENTS

Global warming results in increased frequency and duration of extreme weather events. Rainfall can be excessive and unpredictable. Floods, droughts, storms, and wildfire are known to occur with increasing frequency. Rising levels of sea water can make inroads to coastal areas and increase salination of fresh water sources and soil. It has been shown that drinking such water is associated with hypertension and worsening proteinuria. Damage to crops, livestock, fisheries, and poultry affects food security, with resultant malnutrition. Maternal malnutrition directly impacts nephron numbers in the fetus, resulting in the birth of low-birth-weight babies, who are at risk of CKD in later life. Water scarcity can affect dialysis delivery because at least 200–300 L of treated water is required per hemodialysis sitting per person. Disruption of dialysis can also occur to displacement of population due to extreme weather events.

RISK OF NONCOMMUNICABLE DISEASES

Environmental changes such as increased air pollution are incriminated in the pathogenesis of many noncommunicable diseases (NCDs) such as diabetes, hypertension, asthma, and cancer. Rising saline content in fresh water due to rising sea water levels has been proposed to cause increased hypertension in a study from Bangladesh. Global dietary transition to high salt and processed foods leads to obesity. Depletion of fisheries, decreased agricultural productivity, and poor quality of crops may cause undernutrition, with a resultant increase in NCD in the long run.

CONTRIBUTION OF DIALYSIS SERVICES TO ENVIRONMENTAL CHANGE

Hemodialysis services contribute significantly to environmental change. The water requirements of one dialysis sitting are considerable, as already stated. In addition, there is nearly double that water consumption indirectly as the reject water rate of a reverse osmosis unit that is required in processed water supply for dialysis is nearly 50–60%. The considerable use of consumables and electricity contributes to a large carbon footprint. Peritoneal dialysis (PD) contributes to nearly 2.5 kg waste per day, which is nonrecyclable, and its disposal carries a carbon cost.

MEASURES TO MITIGATE ENVIRONMENTAL EFFECTS ON KIDNEY DISEASE

Given the widespread ramifications of environmental change on the biosphere in general and human health in particular, it is quite clear that efforts require a multipronged approach and require efforts at multiple levels. The governments and society must come together to enforce and enact various measures at the legislative level and implementation level. Educating the public regarding the harmful health hazards of climate change and their contribution toward mitigating the adverse effects is an important aspect of the strategy, which requires coordination of all stakeholders **(Fig. 1)**.

Kidney-specific Measures

The adverse effects of heat stress on kidney health can be mitigated by educating people at risk to adopt adequate hydration measures. It is important to avoid sugary drinks

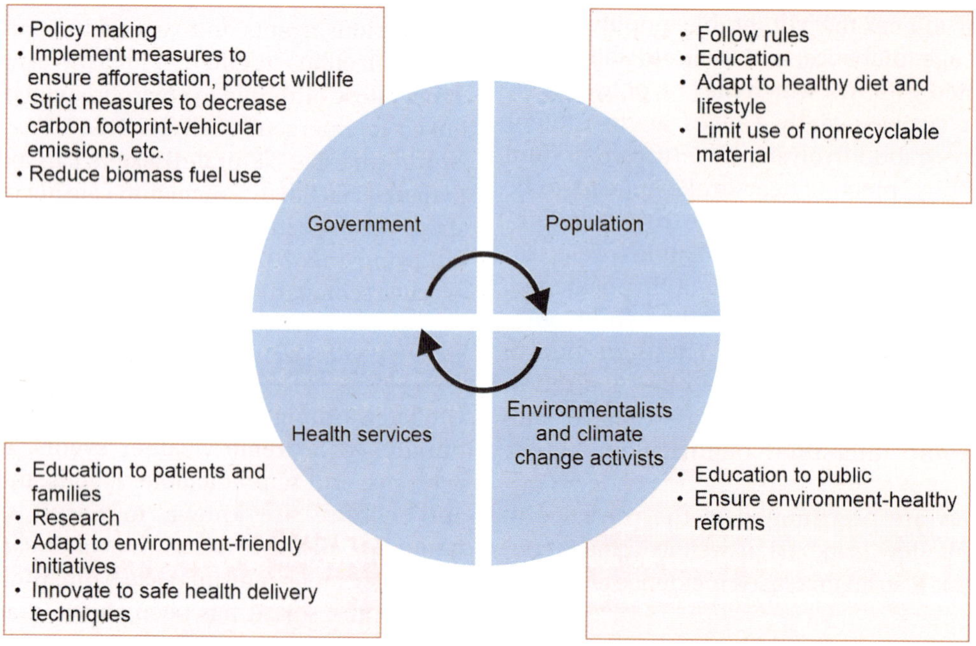

FIG. 1: Interplay between stakeholders to mitigate effects of climate change on kidney health.

TABLE 1: Environmental impact of dialysis: Opportunities for improvement.

Strategies that can be adopted	Pros and cons
Recycle reverse osmosis (RO) reject water	Water can be utilized for housekeeping/laundry
Efficient RO with lower reject water rates can be installed	Decreases water wastage; expensive
Incremental dialysis where appropriate	May be suitable in some patients
Solar energy can be tapped as source of electricity	Capital investment required.
Central dialysis delivery system can be commissioned	• Reduces plastic wastage • *Con*: Microbial contamination with use of long dialysis piping
Waste segregation	Minimizes need for incineration and/or disinfection prior to waste disposal
Paperless clinical documentation	Difficult in resource-poor settings
Tele-health for clinician's review	Can be done
Use of energy-efficient lighting system like motion detector lighting in dialysis units	High cost

Source: Adapted from Yeo SC, Ooi XY, Tan TSM. Sustainable kidney care delivery and climate change: a call to action. Global Health. 2022;18:75.

and sweetened beverages for hydration as they increase fructose levels which can increase oxidant damage. Ensuring that the workers exposed to occupational heat stress take adequate rest between the work hours has gone a long way in mitigating some of the adverse effect of heat stress in Central American countries. The kidney professionals must engage in research in climate change-related kidney disease. Acceptable and reliable biomarkers are required for early diagnosis of kidney disease. They must adapt strategies to implement sustainable methods to minimize carbon footprint in dialysis units **(Table 1)**.

CONCLUSION

Climate change is a new threat to human health. Kidneys bear the brunt of environmental changes as they are responsible for both heat dissipation and toxin removal. Heat stress can cause AKI as well as CKD, including a distinct type of tubulointerstitial disease called heat stress nephropathy. Dialysis delivery also contributes hugely to carbon footprint. Employing environment-friendly ways to provide safe dialysis and "green dialysis" is the need of the hour.

SUGGESTED READINGS

1. Johnson RJ, Sánchez-Lozada LG, Newman LS, Lanaspa MA, Diaz HF, Lemery J, et al. Climate Change and the Kidney. Ann Nutr Metab. 2019;74(Suppl 3):38-44.
2. Barraclough KA, Blashki GA, Holt SG, Agar JWM. Climate change and kidney disease-threats and opportunities. Kidney Int. 2017;92(3):526-30.
3. Bharati J, Nayak S, Jha V. Environmental change and kidney health. Wits J Clin Med. 2022;4(3):141-50.

179
CHAPTER

Management of Complications of Chronic Kidney Disease

Chilaka Rajesh, Utkarash Mishra

ABSTRACT

Chronic kidney disease (CKD) is a progressive condition that effects >10% general population worldwide. It is the one of the leading causes of morbidity and mortality. The complications like anemia, mineral bone disorder (MBD), metabolic acidosis, and cardiovascular complications contribute to higher morbidity, mortality, and poor quality of life in CKD. These complications require specific management approach to improve disease outcome. This chapter illustrates guideline-based evaluation and management of these complications.

INTRODUCTION

Chronic kidney disease (CKD) is defined as abnormalities of kidney structure or function, present for 3 months, with implications for health. CKD is classified based on Cause, glomerular filtration rate (GFR) category, and Albuminuria category (CGA) **(Fig. 1)**.

MEASURES TO PREVENT THE PROGRESSION OF CHRONIC KIDNEY DISEASE

Flowchart 1 shows steps to prevent the progression of CKD.

COMPLICATIONS ASSOCIATED WITH LOSS OF KIDNEY FUNCTION

The complications of CKD are given in **Flowchart 2**.

ANEMIA IN CHRONIC KIDNEY DISEASE

Anemia in CKD is defined as adults and children >15 years with hemoglobin (Hb) concentration < 13.0 g/dL in males and <12.0 g/dL in females.

Investigation of Anemia in CKD

In patients with CKD and anemia (regardless of age and CKD stage), the following tests should be included in initial evaluation:

- Complete blood count
- Absolute reticulocyte count
- Serum ferritin level
- Serum transferrin saturation (TSAT)
- Serum vitamin B12 and folate levels

Frequency of Testing for Anemia

For CKD patients *without anemia*, measure Hb concentration when clinically indicated and:

- At least annually in patients with CKD 3
- At least twice per year in patients with CKD 4–5 nondialysis (5ND)
- At least every 3 months in patients with CKD 5 on hemodialysis (5HD) and CKD 5 on peritoneal dialysis (5PD)

For CKD patients *with anemia* not being treated with an erythropoietin-stimulating agent (ESA), measure Hb concentration when clinically indicated and:

- At least every 3 months in patients with CKD 3–5ND and CKD 5PD
- At least monthly in patients with CKD 5HD

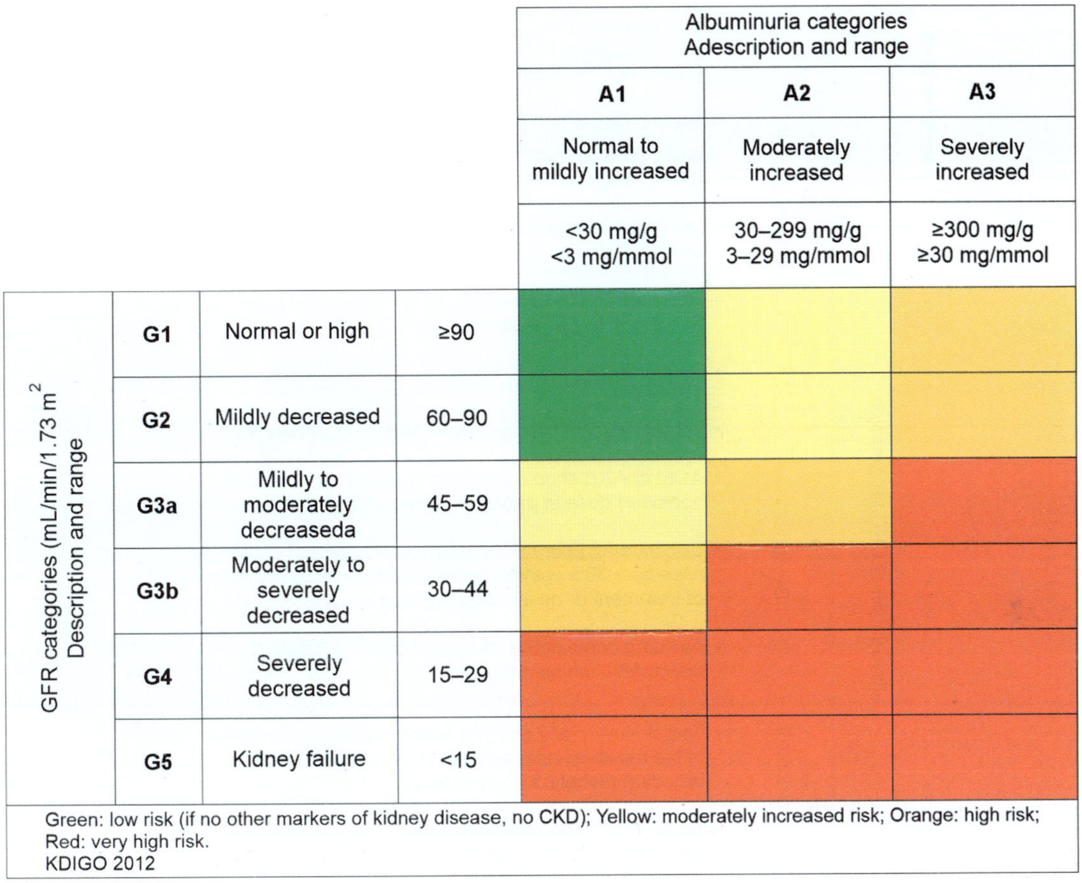

FIG. 1: Prognosis of chronic kidney disease (CKD) by glomerular filtration rate (GFR) and albuminuria categories.

(KDIGO: Kidney Disease: Improving Global Outcomes)

Use of Iron to Treat Anemia in CKD

For adult CKD patients with anemia not on iron therapy (irrespective of ESA therapy status) a trial of intravenous (IV) iron (or in CKD ND patients alternatively a 1–3 month trial of oral iron therapy) can be given if an increase in Hb concentration is desired and *TSAT is <30% and ferritin is <500 ng/mL*.

Use of Erythropoietin-stimulating Agents to Treat Anemia in CKD

All correctable causes of anemia (including iron deficiency, vitamin B12 and folic acid deficiency, hyperparathyroidism, and inflammatory states) should be addressed prior to initiation of ESA therapy.

For adult CKD ND (nondialysis) patients with Hb concentration <10.0 g/dL, ESA therapy should not be initiated.

For adult CKD 5D (dialysis) patients, ESA therapy should be initiated when Hb concentration is between 9.0 and 10.0 g/dL.

Erythropoietin-stimulating agents should not be used to maintain Hb concentration above 11.5 g/dL in adult patients with CKD.

Initial dosing of ESA:

- *Epoetin alfa*: 50–100 units/kg administered three times per week
- *Methoxy polyethylene glycol-epoetin (pegylated epoetin beta)*: 0.6 µg/kg administered every 2 weeks
- *Darbepoetin*: 0.45 µg/kg every week or 0.75 µg/kg every 2 weeks

Newer Agents

Hypoxia-inducible factor–prolyl hydroxylase domain inhibitors (HIF-PHIs) are a class of orally administered drugs for the treatment of anemia of CKD. HIF-PHIs activate the HIF oxygen-sensing pathway and are efficacious in correcting and maintaining hemoglobin levels in patients with nondialysis- and dialysis-dependent CKD **(Flowchart 3 and Table 1)**.

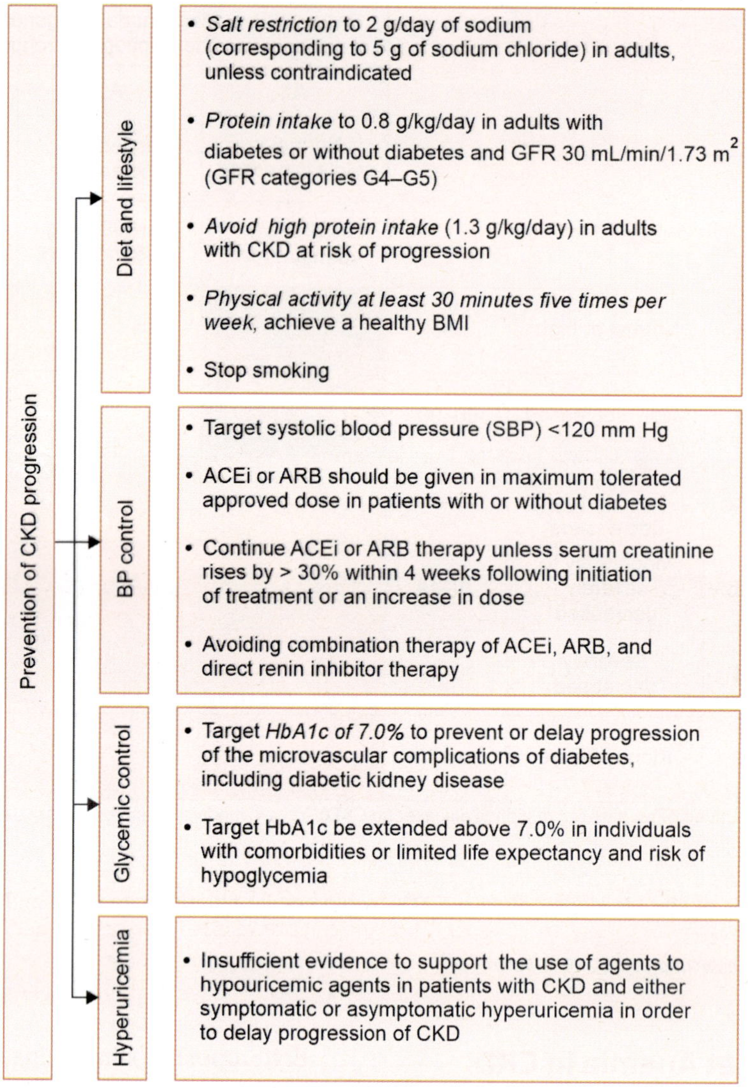

FLOWCHART 1: Prevention of progression of chronic kidney disease (CKD).

(ACEi: angiotensin-converting enzyme inhibitor; ARB: angiotensin receptor blocker; BMI: body mass index; BP: blood pressure; GFR: glomerular filtration rate; HbA1c: glycated hemoglobin)

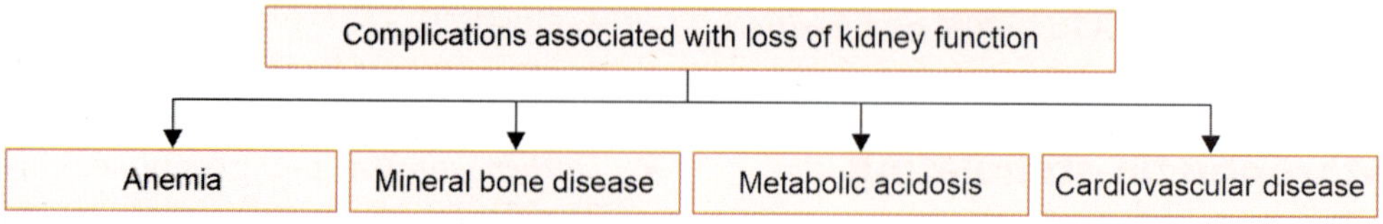

FLOWCHART 2: Complications due to loss of kidney function.

CHRONIC KIDNEY DISEASE—MINERAL BONE DISEASE

Mineral bone disease (MBD) is defined as a systemic disorder of mineral and bone metabolism manifested by one or a combination of:

- Abnormalities of calcium, phosphorus, parathyroid hormone (PTH), or vitamin D metabolism
- Abnormalities in bone turnover, mineralization, volume, linear growth, or strength.
- Vascular or other soft-tissue calcification **(Fig. 2)**

High Turnover Disease

Abnormalities of calcium, phosphate, and vitamin-D metabolism, fibroblast growth factor-23 (FGF-23), and

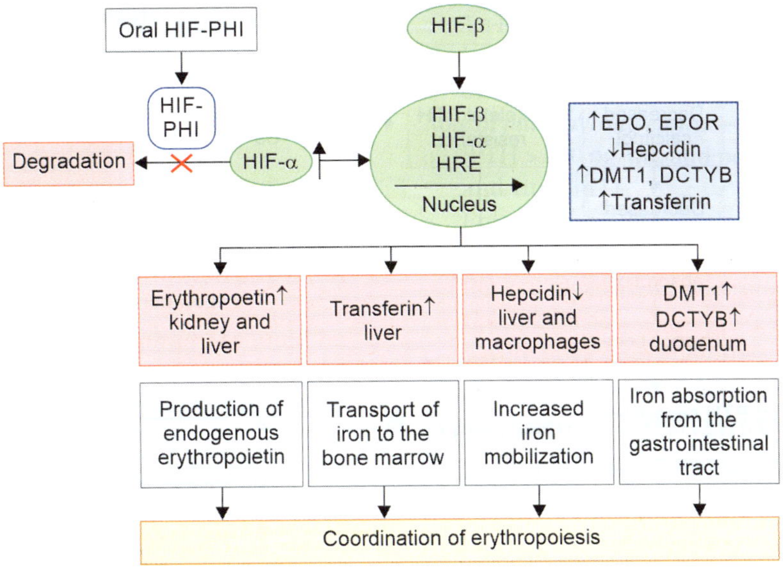

FLOWCHART 3: Mode of action of HIF-PHI (hypoxia-inducible factor–prolyl hydroxylase domain inhibitor).
(DCYTB: duodenal cytochrome B; DMT1: divalent metal transporter; EPO: erythropoietin; EPOR: erythropoietin receptor; HRE: hypoxia responsive element)
Source: Borawski B, Malyszko JS, Kwiatkowska M, Malyszko J. Current Status of Renal Anemia Pharmacotherapy—What Can We Offer Today. J Clin Med. 2021;10(18):4149.

TABLE 1: HIF–PH (hypoxia-inducible factor–prolyl hydroxylase domain) inhibitor.

HIF–PH inhibitor	Dosage
Vadadustat	300 mg once daily (OD) → Can increase up to 600 mg OD
Desidustat	100 mg thrice a week
Daprodustat	2 mg OD → can increase to 4 mg OD
Roxadustat	100 mg thrice a week

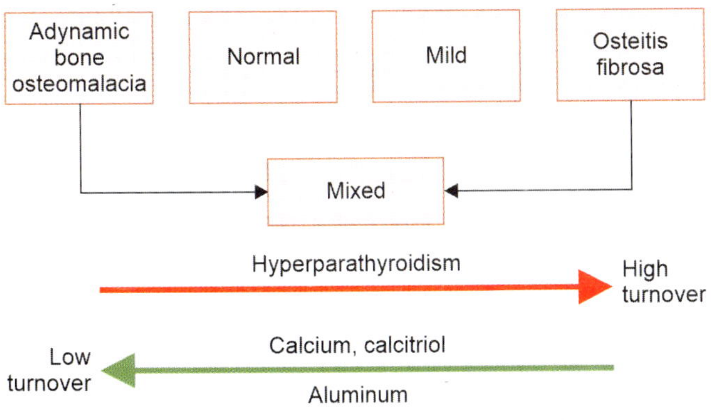

FIG. 2: Skeletal abnormalities in renal osteodystrophy.
Source: Freehally J, Floege J, Tonelli M, Johnson RJ. Text book of Comprehensive Clinical Nephrology, 6th edition. Netherlands: Elsevier; 2018.

abnormal skeletal response to PTH play important role in the pathogenesis of high turnover disease.

Abnormalities in Calcium Metabolism

- Persistent hypocalcemia is a powerful stimulus for hyperparathyroidism
- Total serum calcium decreases in CKD due to:
  - Phosphate retention
  - Decreased production of 1,25-dihydroxyvitamin D
  - Decreased intestinal calcium absorption
  - Skeletal resistance to the calcemic action of PTH

Abnormalities of Phosphate and Vitamin D Metabolism

With progressive CKD, phosphate is retained **(Flowchart 4)**.

Abnormalities of Fibroblast Growth Factor-23

- FGF-23 is secreted by osteocytes and osteoblasts. In CKD patients, increased FGF-23 occurs due to decreased clearance. Primary function of FGF-23 is to maintain normal serum phosphate by reducing renal phosphate reabsorption, reducing intestinal phosphate absorption through decreased calcitriol production.

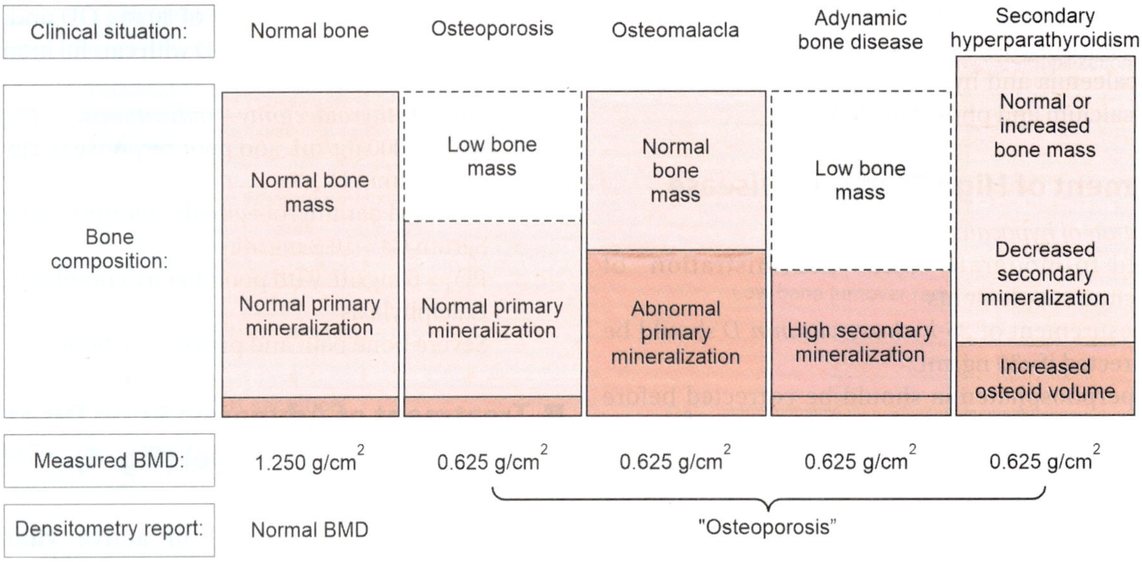

FIG. 4: The value of bone density measurements in the assessment of chronic kidney disease (CKD)-related bone disease.
(BMD: bone mineral density)
Source: Freehally J, Floege J, Tonelli M, Johnson RJ. Text book of Comprehensive Clinical Nephrology, 6th edition. Netherlands: Elsevier; 2018.

TABLE 2: KDIGO (Kidney Disease: Improving Global Outcome) guidelines—monitoring mineral bone disease (MBD) parameters and hemoglobin.

CKD stage	Calcium and phosphate	PTH	Hemoglobin
G3a–3b	Every 6–12 months	Based on baseline	Every 3 months
G4	Every 3–6 months	6–12 months	Every 3 months
G5	Every 1–3 months	3–6 months	Every 3 months
G5D	Every 1–3 months	3–6 months	Every 3 months
CKD G4–G5D—alkaline phosphatase—every 12 months			
G3a–G5D—25-hydroxy vitamin D levels			

(CKD: chronic kidney disease; PTH: parathyroid hormone)

 - ○ Diabetes mellitus
 - ○ Prior ischemic stroke
 - ○ Estimated 10-year incidence of coronary death or nonfatal myocardial infarction >10%
- In adults with dialysis-dependent CKD, statins or statin/ezetimibe combination not be initiated.
- In dialysis patients, already receiving statins or statin/ezetimibe combination at the time of dialysis initiation, these agents be continued

CHRONIC KIDNEY DISEASE AND RISK OF INFECTIONS—VACCINATION

All adults with CKD should be offered annual vaccination with influenza vaccine, and those at high risk of pneumococcal infection should receive vaccination with polyvalent pneumococcal vaccine unless contraindicated.

All adults who are at high risk of progression of CKD and have GFR < 30 mL/min/1.73 m^2 should be immunized against hepatitis B **(Table 2)**.

WHEN TO REFER CKD PATIENTS TO SPECIALIST SERVICES?

- Acute kidney injury (AKI) or abrupt sustained fall in GFR
- GFR < 30 mL/min/1.73 m^2 (GFR categories G4–G5)
- A consistent finding of significant albuminuria
- Progression of CKD
- CKD and hypertension refractory to treatment with four or more antihypertensive agents
- Persistent abnormalities of serum potassium
- The progressive CKD should be managed in a multidisciplinary care setting. The multidisciplinary

team should include or have access to dietary counseling, education and counseling about different renal replacement therapy (RRT) modalities, transplant options, vascular access surgery, and ethical, psychological, and social care.

- Dialysis to be initiated when one or more of the following are present:
  - Symptoms or signs attributable to kidney failure (serositis, acid-base or electrolyte abnormalities, pruritus)
  - Inability to control volume status or blood pressure
  - A progressive deterioration in nutritional status refractory to dietary intervention or cognitive impairment
- Living donor preemptive renal transplantation in adults should be considered when the GFR is <20 mL/min/1.73 m^2, and there is evidence of progressive and irreversible CKD over the preceding 6–12 months.

SUGGESTED READINGS

1. Kidney Disease Improving Global Outcomes (KDIGO) guidelines for the management of evaluation of CKD and managment of CKD complications, Anaemia, Aug 2012, MBD, Jul 2017.
2. Freehally J, Floege J, Tonelli M, Johnson RJ. Text book of Comprehensive Clinical Nephrology, 6th edition. Netherlands: Elsevier; 2018.
3. Reddi AS. Absolute Nephrology Review An Essential Q & A Study Guide. Switzerland: Springer International Publishing; 2022.

180

CHAPTER

Nephrotic Syndrome

Ashwini Nigam, Niteesh Singh

ABSTRACT

Nephrotic syndrome is a clinicopathological entity characterized by heavy protienuria, hypoalbuminemia, generalized edema, and hyperlipidemia. Nephrotic syndrome can be primary or due to secondary causes. In adults, membranous glomerulonephritis and focal segmental glomerulonephritis are the common primary causes and diabetes mellitus is the most common secondary cause of nephrotic syndrome. Most patients present with early mornings' periorbital edema. There are no definite guidelines on diagnostic workup or management of nephrotic syndrome. Renal biopsy is generally not required but used in selective cases to diagnose specific disorder to guide treatment and to describe prognosis. Treatment should include fluid and sodium restriction, oral or intravenous diuretics, angiotensin-converting enzyme (ACE) inhibitors, and some adults with nephrotic syndrome may benefit from corticosteroid treatment, although research data is limited.

INTRODUCTION

Nephrotic syndrome is one of the pathognomonic presentations of glomerular diseases. This clinical syndrome is characterized by pentad of proteinuria: (adult > 3.5 g/day; child > 40 mg/h/m^2), hypoalbuminemia < 3.5 g/dL, edema, hypercholesterolemia, lipiduria. While most of patients may have nephrotic syndrome with preserved renal function, but in a subset of patients with progressive nephrotic syndrome, the progressive loss of renal function eventually results. Although, the disease is self-limiting in a few patients, it requires the specific therapy in few others [e.g., corticosteroids in minimal change disease (MCD)] and often major subset of patients either have a relapsing-remitting or chronic course.

ETIOLOGY

The relative frequency of the different glomerular diseases varies with age. Although predominantly a disease of childhood, individuals in all ages may develop MCD. The prevalence of focal segmental glomerulosclerosis (FSGS) is more in African Americans, which may explain why FSGS is becoming more common in US adults but not in European adults. The most common cause in children is MCD.

Primary causes:

- Minimal change disease
- Membranous glomerulonephritis
- Focal segmental glomerulonephritis
- Membranoproliferative glomerulonephritis
- Immunoglobulin A (IgA) nephropathy

Secondary causes:

- Diabetes mellitus
- Autoimmune disease:
  - Systemic lupus erythematosus (SLE)
  - Rheumatoid arthritis (RA)
- Amyloidosis
- *Cancer*: Multiple myeloma, lymphoma
- *Drugs*:
  - Gold
  - Penicillamine
  - Captopril
  - Nonsteroidal anti-inflammatory drug (NSAID)
  - Lithium
  - Interferon alpha

- *Infection*:
  - Human immunodeficiency virus (HIV)
  - Hepatitis B and C
  - Cytomegalovirus
  - Syphilis
  - Malaria
- *Congenital*:
  - Alport's syndrome
  - Congenital nephrotic syndrome finnish type
  - Pierson's syndrome

PATHOPHYSIOLOGY

Hypoalbuminemia

Increased urinary albumin loss is the chief reason of hypoalbuminemia along with a blunted response from liver to increase albumin synthesis. The compensatory increase in protein synthesis is not selective for albumin and therefore, other protein with higher molecular weight that are not lost in urine increases in plasma, which are further linked with pathogenesis of hyperlipidemia and hypercoagulability.

Edema

Underfill and overfill are the two important mechanisms responsible for edema in patients with nephrotic syndrome. The underfill mechanism is based on decrease in the oncotic pressure due to loss of serum albumin leads to seepage of intravascular fluids to extravascular spaces. The resultant decrease in circulating intravascular volume causes secondary activation of renin-angiotensin-aldosterone system (RAAS), which leads to retention of sodium and water mediated by action of aldosterone in distal tubules in an attempt to counteract hypovolemia but to only end in causing more hydrostatic pressure and consequent edema in a low oncotic pressure condition. Another more common mechanism seen in some patients is proteolytic enzymes mediated damage to epithelial sodium channels (ENaC) in distal part of nephrons resulting in more sodium retention and volume overload. This suppresses renin, angiotensin, and vasopressin and results in hypertension rather than hypotension. These proteolytic enzymes enter the tubular lumen due to heavy proteinuria. The relative resistance of atrial natriuretic peptide in kidney also results in rise of plasma volume.

CLINICAL PRESENTATION

Edema is a common feature of nephrotic syndrome and in beginning it develops around eyes and leg. Overtime, edema becomes generalized and is responsible for weight gain and development of ascites and pleural effusion.

Tiredness and lack of appetite are common.

Metabolic Consequences of Nephrotic Syndrome

Negative Nitrogen Balance

Low serum albumin level is the biochemical marker of heavy proteinuria. Although 10–20% loss of lean body mass occurs but it remains covert unless the edema subsides. Altered proteins in tubular lumen undergo catabolism and this increased catabolism which further adds to negative nitrogen balance.

Hypercoagulability

Various proteins and factors of coagulation cascade have altered levels which along with enhanced platelet aggregation are responsible for hypercoagulability seen in these patients. This is further enhanced by contraction of intravascular volume. Not only the risk of venous thrombosis is increased, but also arterial thrombosis is a major risk. A clinical episode of thromboembolism is seen in about 10% of adults and 2% of children with nephrotic syndrome, with a particularly high risk in patients with membranous nephropathy. The serum albumin levels serves as a surrogate marker for this risk of thromboembolism with a greatly increased risk at serum albumin levels of < 2 g/dL.

Hyperlipidemia and Lipiduria

A frequent association of hyperlipidemia with heavy proteinuria makes it an integral part of nephrotic syndrome. Xanthelasma frequently seen in these patients and may have a rapid onset. Nephrotic syndrome for 5–10 years may lead to development of additional cardiovascular risk factors such as hypertension and uremia. Patients with nephrotic syndrome have five-fold increased risk for coronary death (except for those with MCD). The mechanism behind hyperlipidemia include increased synthesis of very low-density lipoproteins (VLDL), lipoprotein(a) and low-density lipoproteins (LDL) accompanied by increased urinary loss of high-density lipoproteins.

Other Metabolic Effects of Nephrotic Syndrome

Loss of vitamin D-binding protein in urine causes low levels of plasma 25-hydroxyvitamin D levels but with a normal free vitamin D levels and therefore, clinically obvious osteomalacia or uncontrolled hyperparathyroidism is not usual unless there is associated impairment of renal function. Similarly, thyroid-binding globulin is lost in the urine, although total circulating thyroxine reduced, but due to normal free thyroxine and thyroid-stimulating hormone levels patients maintain euthyroid status. Occasionally, copper, iron, or zinc deficiency can occur due to loss of binding proteins in the urine.

INFECTION

Infections remains the major concern in patients with nephrotic syndrome, even before the use of corticosteroids started for patients with childhood MCD, infection-related deaths was the major reported event. Primary peritonitis, characteristic of nephrotic children, which is caused by pneumococci. β-hemolytic streptococci are responsible for cellulitis. The various factors that contribute to this immunocompromised state are fragile skin, large collection of fluids, loss of complement factor -B and IgG.

ACUTE AND CHRONIC CHANGES IN KIDNEY FUNCTION

Acute Kidney Injury

Various mechanisms are involved that leads to increased risk of AKI in patients with nephrotic syndrome. Prerenal AKI resulting from depletion of intravascular volume and septicemia or direct acute tubular necrosis may be the cause; apart from this progression of underlying renal disease, bilateral renal vein thrombosis, drugs such as angiotensin-converting enzyme (ACE) inhibitors or, diuretics. Intrarenal edema with compression of tubules may be rarely associated with prerenal AKI and may be benefitted from albumin transfusion along with a loop diuretic.

Chronic Kidney Disease

Except for MCD, most other causes of nephrotic syndrome invariably lead to progressive kidney failure, with degree of proteinuria being the major risk factor. At daily protein excretion of >5 g/day, the risk of progression to chronic kidney disease (CKD) is marked. Direct toxic effect of proteinuria on tubulointerstitium is also a major cause of chronic injury.

DIAGNOSTIC EVALUATION OF NEPHROTIC SYNDROME

Typical clinical history and laboratory features of nephrotic syndrome are sufficient to establish the diagnosis of nephrotic syndrome.

Sequence of investigations for a person presenting with nephrotic syndrome:
- Confirm proteinuria present by urine dipstik positive 3+/4+.
- Check for concomitant invisible microscopic hematuria
- Urinary protein to creatinine ratio > 3 mg/dL
- Serum albumin < 2.5 g/dL
- Serum lipid profile fasting
- Renal function tests
- Blood glucose and HbA1c
- Autoimmune screening
- Ultrasonography to assess presence of both kidneys, their size and echotexture
- Serum complement level (C3 and C4)
- Serum protein electrophoresis
- HBsAg, anti HCV antibody, HIV screening

RENAL BIOPSY

Renal biopsy is indicated for the following congenital nephrotic syndrome, children older than 8 years at the onset, steroid resistance, frequent relapses, steroid dependency, and significant nephritis manifestations.

DEFINITIONS

Complete remission: Reduction of proteinuria to <3.5 g/dL (or 35 g/L) or urine polymerase chain reaction (PCR) <3.5 g/dL (or 35 g/L) , stable serum creatinine, and serum albumin >3.5 g/dL (or 35 g/L).

Partial remission: Reduction of proteinuria to 0.3–3.5 g/day or urine PCR 300–3500 mg/g (or 30–350 mg/mmol) and a decrease >50% from baseline.

Relapse: Proteinuria >3.5 g/day or urine PCR >3500 mg/g (or 350 mg/mmol) after complete remission has been achieved or an increase in proteinuria by >50% during partial remission.

Frequent relapse: Patients with ≥2 relapses within 6 months after initial therapy or > 3 relapses in any 12-month period.

Infrequent relapser: 1 relapse occurring in 6 months of initial response or 1–3 relapses in any 12-month period.

Steroid-resistant: Persistence of proteinuria >3.5 g/day or urine PCR >3,500 mg/g (or 350 mg/mmol) with 3.5 g/day or urine PCR >3,500 mg/g (or 350 mg/ mmol) with <50% reduction from baseline despite prednisone 1 mg/kg/day or 2 mg/kg every other day for at least 16 weeks.

Steroid-dependent: Relapse occurring during or within 2 weeks of completing glucocorticoid therapy. Persistence of proteinuria >3.5 g/day or urine PCR >3500 mg/g (or

350 mg/mmol) with <50% reduction from baseline despite cyclosporine treatment at trough levels of 100–175 ng/mL or tacrolimus treatment at trough levels of 5–10 ng/mL for >6 months.

Calcineurin inhibitor (CNI)-dependent: Relapse occurring during or within 2 weeks of completing cyclosporine or tacrolimus therapy for >12 months.

TREATMENT OF GLOMERULAR DISEASE

General Principles

Before the starting of treatment, all secondary causes of glomerular disease should be ruled out as with them the treatment is mainly the treatment of underlying disease. In the primary glomerular diseases, both general and specific therapies are to be given. Supportive treatment includes treatment of hypertension, proteinuria, edema, and other metabolic consequences of nephrotic syndrome.

Treatment of Proteinuria

Reduction of proteinuria to levels below 0.5 g/day can minimize progressive loss of kidney functions. ACE inhibitors and angiotensin II receptor blockers (ARBs) used for treatment of proteinuria can reduce proteinuria by average 40–50%, especially when patient is on dietary sodium restrictions, act by reducing intraglomerular hypertension, and reducing increased glomerular capillary wall permeability . The combination is not used due to increased risk of AKI and hyperkalemia. Action of ACE inhibitors and ARBs is independent of reduction of systolic blood pressure and therefore, can be used in normotensive proteinuric patients. Hyperkalemia is a common side effect and in those cases, a loop diuretic can be added. For proteinuria persisting even after maximum tolerable dose of ACE inhibitors or ARB, the low-dose aldosterone antagonist can be added with safety for hyperkalemia to be monitored closely.

Treatment of Hyperlipidemia

Guideline-directed medical therapy for treatment of hyperlipidemia in cardiovascular diseases must be here also to address the hyperlipidemia in nephrotic syndrome along with dietary restrictions. Statins are recommended alone in younger patients with significant comorbidities; a statin/ezetimibe combination is recommended in adults older than 50 years with CKD stage 3–5. Statins alone are also recommended in adults over 50 years with earlier-stage CKD.

Special Therapeutic Issues in Patients with Nephrotic Syndrome

Treatment of Nephrotic Edema

Diuretic therapy accompanied by moderate dietary sodium restriction (60–80 mmol/24 h) remains the mainstay of treatment of nephrotic edema. Hypoalbuminemia reduces protein binding of diuretics and subsequent transport from peritubular capillaries and results in diuretic resistance. Alternatively, loop diuretic with a thiazide diuretic or with metolazone combination may be used to overcome diuretic resistance. Because nephrotic syndrome is associated with activation of ENaC channel, amiloride may be combined with diuretics. Hypovolemic shock is more common in children than in adults. Daily weight should decrease by no >1–2 kg/day in a stepwise manner .

Correction of Hypoproteinemia

High carbohydrate diet along with daily protein intake of (0.8–1 g/kg/day) is recommended along with addition of daily urinary protein losses in patients with heavy proteinuria.

Treatment of Hypercoagulability

Prophylactic low-dose anticoagulation (e.g., heparin 5,000 U subcutaneously twice daily) is recommended in high-risk patients, such as those with relative immobilization in the hospital and albumin levels between 2 and 2.5 g/dL. Full-dose anticoagulation with low molecular weight heparin or warfarin is mandatory if a thrombosis or pulmonary embolism is documented and should be considered if serum albumin decreases to <2 g/dL. Warfarin [target international normalized ratio (INR) 2 to 3] is the long-term treatment of choice but should be used with close monitoring due to altered protein binding.

Disease-specific Therapies

Immunosuppressive therapy is the cornerstone of most pathologies presenting as nephrotic syndrome due to immunogenic damage. In patients developing RPGN, more cytotoxic intensive regimen are used for shorter duration. Most of the immunosuppressants are nonspecific with multiple targets. The mainstays of treatment include corticosteroids, cyclosporine, tacrolimus, cyclophosphamide, mycophenolate mofetil, and/or rituximab.

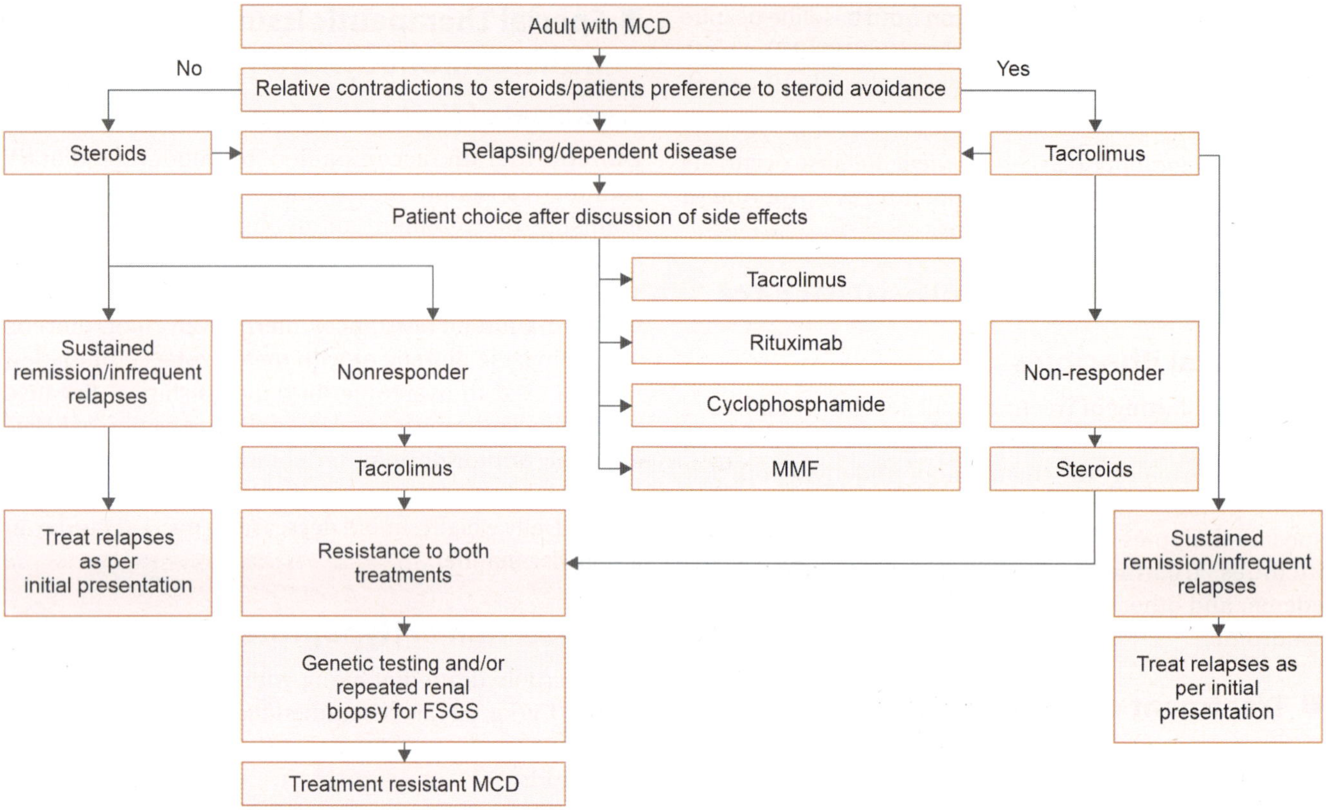

FLOWCHART 1: Algorithm for treatment of adult-onset nephrotic syndrome.

In MCD, steroids are widely used as the initial therapy with slightly lower doses of oral prednisolone (1 mg/kg/day, up to maximum 80 mg/day). Response is often delayed in comparison with that in children, with a median time to remission of 10 weeks, and 25% fail to remit after 3–4 months. The initial high dose of steroids, if tolerated, should be maintained for a minimum of 2 weeks after complete remission is achieved and for a maximum of 16 weeks if complete remission is not achieved. After this, steroids should be tapered over 24 weeks. In case of steroid resistance other immunosuppressive drugs such as CNI (tacrolimus and cyclosporine), mycofenolate mofetil, cyclophosphamide, or rituximab may be used.

Treatment algorithm for adult-onset nephrotic syndrome (MCD) is given in **Flowchart 1**.

In FSGS, mainstay of treatment is high-dose corticosteroids (1 mg/kg/day) for a period of 16 weeks or when there is resolution of proteinuria after which steroids are tapered at a rate of 5 mg every 1–2 weeks with a total duration of 6-month therapy. In case of steroid resistance other immunosuppressive agents such as CNI (cyclosporine and tacrolimus), mycophenolate mofetil can be used for a period of 12 months.

In membranous nephropathy, specific immunosuppressive drug therapy should not be considered unless the patient has had persistent nephrotic-range proteinuria (>4 g/day) and the proteinuria has not declined by >50% from baseline, over a minimum observation period of 6 months, despite maximum antihypertensive and antiproteinuric therapy. In case of risk of progression, a significant benefit has been described with a regimen beginning with methylprednisolone pulses 1 g intravenously for 3 days at the start of months 1, 3, and 5 followed by oral prednisone 0.5 mg/kg/day for 27 days, and each cycle followed by 1 month of treatment with an oral cytotoxic agent (cyclophosphamide or chlorambucil). Nonresponders are treated with either cyclosporine (3.5 mg/kg) for 12 months or mycophenolate mofetil (2–3 g/day) for a period of 12–36 months or rituximab to achieve remision.

SUGGESTED READINGS

1. Orth SR, Ritz E. The nephrotic syndrome. N Engl J Med. 1998;338(17):1202-11.
2. Cameron JS. Nephrotic syndrome in the elderly. Semin Nephrol. 1996;16(4):319-29.
3. Hanko JB, Mullan RN, O'Rourke DM, McNamee PT, Maxwell AP, Courtney AE. The changing pattern of adult primary glomerular disease. Nephrol Dial Transplant. 2009;24(10):3050-4.
4. Kaysen GA, Gambertoglio J, Felts J, Hutchison FN. Albumin synthesis, albuminuria and hyperlipemia in nephrotic patients. Kidney Int. 1987;31(6):1368-76.
5. Humphreys MH. Mechanisms and management of nephrotic edema. Kidney Int. 1994;45(1):266-81.
6. Svenningsen P, Friis UG, Versland JB, Buhl KB, Frederiksen BM, Andersen H, et al. Mechanisms of renal NaCl retention in proteinuric disease. Acta Physiol. 2013;207(3):536-45.
7. Barbour SJ, Greenwald A, Djurdjev O, Levin A, Hladunewich MA, et al. Disease-specific risk of venous thromboembolic events is increased in idiopathic glomerulonephritis. Kidney Int. 2012;81(2):190-5.
8. Wheeler DC, Bernard DB. Lipid abnormalities in the nephrotic syndrome:causes, consequences, and treatment. Am J Kidney Dis. 1994;23(3):331-46.
9. Smith JD, Hayslett JP. Reversible renal failure in the nephrotic syndrome. Am J Kidney Dis. 1992;19(3):201-13.
10. Jennette JC, Falk RJ. Adult minimal change glomerulopathy with acute renal failure. Am J Kidney Dis. 1990;16(5):432-7.
11. Lennartz DP, Seikrit C, Wied S, Fitzner C, Eitner F, Hilgers RD, et al. Single versus dual blockade of the renin-angiotensin system in patients with IgA nephropathy. J Nephrol. 2020;33(6):1231-9.
12. Parving HH, Brenner BM, McMurray JJ, de Zeeuw D, Haffner SM, Solomon SD, et al. Cardiorenal end points in a trial of aliskiren for type 2 diabetes. N Engl J Med. 2012;367(23):2204-13.
13. Lee T, Biddle AK, Lionaki S, Derebail VK, Barbour SJ, Tannous S, et al. Personalized prophylactic anticoagulation decision analysis in patients with membranous nephropathy. Kidney Int. 2014;85(6):1412-20.
14. Talar-Williams C, Hijazi YM, Walther MM, Linehan WM, Hallahan CW, Lubensky I, et al. Cyclophosphamide induced cystitis and bladder cancer in patients with Wegener granulomatosis. Ann Intern Med. 1996;124(5):477-84.

181
CHAPTER

Retarding the Progression of Chronic Kidney Disease with Newer Therapies

Narayan Prasad

ABSTRACT

Chronic kidney disease (CKD) is a progressive and irreversible loss of renal function. Conventionally, dietary salt and protein restriction, lifestyle modification with smoking cessation, reducing obesity, regular exercise, dyslipidemia management, glycemic control, blood pressure control, and use of renin–angiotensin system (RAS) blockers are advocated for retarding the progression of CKD. Newer therapies have emerged with the discovery of sodium-glucose cotransporter-2 (SGLT-2) inhibitors, glucagon-like peptide-1 receptor agonists (GLP-1 RAs), and finerenone. SGLT-2 inhibitors have been increasingly used in nondiabetic kidney diseases, as well. Endothelin receptor antagonists and Bardoxolone methyl are other promising agents of the future.

INTRODUCTION

Chronic kidney disease (CKD) is defined as a progressive and irreversible loss of renal function evidenced by an estimated glomerular filtration rate (eGFR) of < 60 mL/min/1.73 m^2, and persisting kidney damage (proteinuria, active urine sediments, histological damages, structural abnormalities, or a history of kidney transplantation), or both for more than 3 months. Any reversible factor is considered an acute factor, or acute kidney injury, on top of CKD.

There are four major steps in the management of CKD:
1. Identification of risk factors
2. Slowing down the progression
3. Management of complications and smooth transition from CKD to renal replacement therapies
4. Renal replacement therapy

The foremost step in managing CKD is identifying factors responsible for susceptibility, initiation, and progression of CKD, shown in **Table 1**, and curtailing it. Beyond many well-established factors such as salt and protein restriction, lifestyle modification with cessation of smoking, reducing obesity, regular exercise, and dyslipidemia management.

In this chapter, we will discuss the newer ways of slowing the progression of CKD.

TABLE 1: Management of chronic kidney disease.

Susceptibility factors	Initiation factors	Progression factors
Increased susceptibility of individuals to kidney damage	Initiate kidney damage	Cause progressive decline in renal function after initiation of kidney damage
• Age • Family history of kidney disease • Renal transplantation	• Diabetes mellitus • Hypertension • Autoimmune diseases • Systemic infections • Nephrotoxic agents	Persistent activity of the underlying disease, persistent proteinuria, elevated blood pressure, poor glycemic control, high dietary intake of high protein, salt, phosphate diet, hyperphosphatemia, hyperlipidemia, metabolic acidosis, anemia, cardiovascular disease, smoking

DELAYING PROGRESSION OF CHRONIC KIDNEY DISEASE

Measures indicated to delay or halt the progression of CKD are as follows:

- *Treatment of the underlying active diseases, if possible*: Any acute factors such as dehydration, contrast agents, use of nonsteroidal anti-inflammatory drugs (NSAIDs), infections, and nephrotoxic antibiotics should be avoided in a patient with CKD. The underlying active ongoing glomerular diseases, progressive interstitial diseases, systemic infection, obstruction of the urinary tract, and cyst infection in autosomal polycystic kidney diseases should be identified and treated.
- *Blood pressure (BP) control to target values*: Target BP should be preferably 130/80 mm Hg, maximum of 140/90 mm Hg. Lower BP may be preferred in proteinuric CKD patients. The preferred antihypertensives are renin–angiotensin blockers [angiotensin-converting enzyme inhibitor/angiotensin II receptor blockers (ACE inhibitors/ARBs)]. Other antihypertensives such as calcium channel blockers (CCBs), diuretics, centrally acting drugs, and alpha-blockers can be added to achieve the target BP.

  Angiotensin-converting enzyme inhibitor/ARB slows the progression by decreasing intraglomerular hypertension, thus hyperfiltration injuries and proteinuria besides systemic hypertension. It delays the dialysis requirement and reduces the composite endpoint of dialysis and death by 6% lower than those who do not use these drugs. However, a nonsignificant rise in hyperkalemia may be noticed. Other antihypertensives can also reduce proteinuria by controlling BP, and some newer CCBs may have an effect on podocytopathy.
- *Glycemic control to target value [target glycated hemoglobin (HbA1c) < 7%]*: The American Diabetes Association (ADA) recommends HbA1c to 7% or less. DCCT (Diabetes Control and Complications Trial) in type 1 diabetes mellitus (T1DM) and The United Kingdom Prospective Diabetic Study (UKPDS) trials in type 2 diabetes mellitus (T2DM) have established the role of tight glycemic control in reducing albuminuria and slowing down in decline in renal function in diabetic kidney disease.
- *Newer interventions*:
  - Sodium-glucose cotransporter-2 (SGLT-2) inhibitors act through multiple actions to slow the progression of CKD in both diabetic and nondiabetic CKD, which were evidenced through multiple clinical trials.
  - Sugar control: SGLT-2 inhibitors reduce HbA1c by 0.6–1% and preserve renal function, primarily by glucosuria resulting from the blockade of the SGLT-2 channel in the S1 segment of the proximal convoluted tubule. The glucose-lowering effect of SGLT-2 inhibitors is attenuated in patients with eGFR < 60 mL/min/1.73 m^2 and minimal when eGFR is < 30 mL/min/1.73 m^2.
  - Weight loss: SGLT-2 inhibitor also results in caloric loss from glucosuria typically results in 1–3 kg of weight loss mainly because of fat.
  - Blood pressure control: It also reduces systolic BP by approximately 3–6 mm Hg and diastolic BP by about 1–2 mm Hg. BP lowering is mediated through natriuresis and associated plasma volume contraction, reductions in arterial stiffness, and improvement in endothelial function. Reduction in BP is generally observed, irrespective of hypertension status and is also achieved in patients with lower eGFR levels.
  - Reduction in intraglomerular pressure: In patients with diabetes, decreased sodium delivery to the macula densa results in increased proximal tubular sodium reabsorption and afferent arteriolar vasodilatation by tubuloglomerular feedback leading to glomerular hypertension and hyperfiltration. SGLT-2 inhibitors increase distal sodium delivery and inhibit tubuloglomerular feedback resulting in afferent vasoconstriction and reduction in intraglomerular pressure resulting in reduced hyperfiltration injuries.
  - Other pleiotropic effects: Other putative mechanisms through which SGLT-2 inhibitors may be beneficial include reduction in inflammatory mediators, including interleukin-6, nuclear factor-kB, and profibrotic factors, such as transforming growth factor-β. In addition, by conserving the energy required to reabsorb the filtered load of glucose and associated sodium, SGLT-2 inhibition may attenuate renal hypoxia and is simultaneously associated with a rise in hematocrit level.
  - Clinical trial evidences: There are three kidney outcome-directed randomized controlled trials published in the last 5 years, and all showed beneficial effects in reducing proteinuria, slowing down the decline in eGFR, and death of patients, as shown in **Figure 1**.

In the CREDENCE (Canagliflozin and Renal Events in Diabetes with Established Nephropathy Clinical Evaluation) trial, the addition of canagliflozin to renin-angiotensin system (RAS) blockers showed a lower relative risk of end-stage kidney disease (ESKD), a doubling of the creatinine level, or death from renal causes, by 34% [hazard ratio (HR) 0.66; 95% CI 0.53–0.81; $p < 0.001$] at 2.6 years of follow-up. It is also effective in lowering cardiovascular (CV) death and hospitalization for heart failure (HF) in adults with T2DM and diabetic nephropathy with albuminuria >300 mg/day.

In the DAPA-CKD (Dapagliflozin and Prevention of Adverse Outcomes in Chronic Kidney Disease) trial, Dapagliflozin also showed a similar outcome over a median of 2.4 years, a primary outcome event sustained decline in eGFR by 50%, ESKD, and death from renal causes by 9.2% in the dapagliflozin group and 14.5% in the placebo group (HR 0.61; 95% CI 0.51–0.72; $p < 0.001$). In addition, a subanalysis of data also showed a beneficial effect in nondiabetic CKD, particularly IgA nephropathy.

In the most recent EMPA-KIDNEY (The Study of Heart and Kidney Protection With Empagliflozin) trial, Empagliflozin also showed reduced progression of kidney disease or death from CV causes occurred in 432 of 3,304 patients (13.1%) who received empagliflozin, compared with 558 of 3,305 patients (16.9%) who received placebo (HR: 0.72; 95% CI 0.64–0.82; $p < 0.001$). Results were consistent among patients with or without diabetes and across eGFR ranges.

These flozins are the most promising agents to retard the progression of CKD if used with a maximum tolerated dose of RAS blockers. It can be used up to eGFR of 20 mL/min, it may be continued in ESRD patients already on flozins before the ESRD.

A few notable side effects are increased incidence of urinary tract infection and euglycemic ketoacidosis. Very rarely, gangrenous foot and amputations are not observed in larger trials.

- *Glucagon-like peptide-1 receptor agonists' (GLP-1 RAs') renoprotective action:* The impact of GLP-1 RAs) on reducing CV risk with an excellent safety profile is well established. The clinical trials also revealed a renoprotective action through both indirect (improvement of BP and glycemic control, weight loss) and direct (restoration of normal intrarenal hemodynamics, prevention of ischemic and oxidative damage) effects. This results in a reduced incidence of albuminuria and a slower decline of renal function.

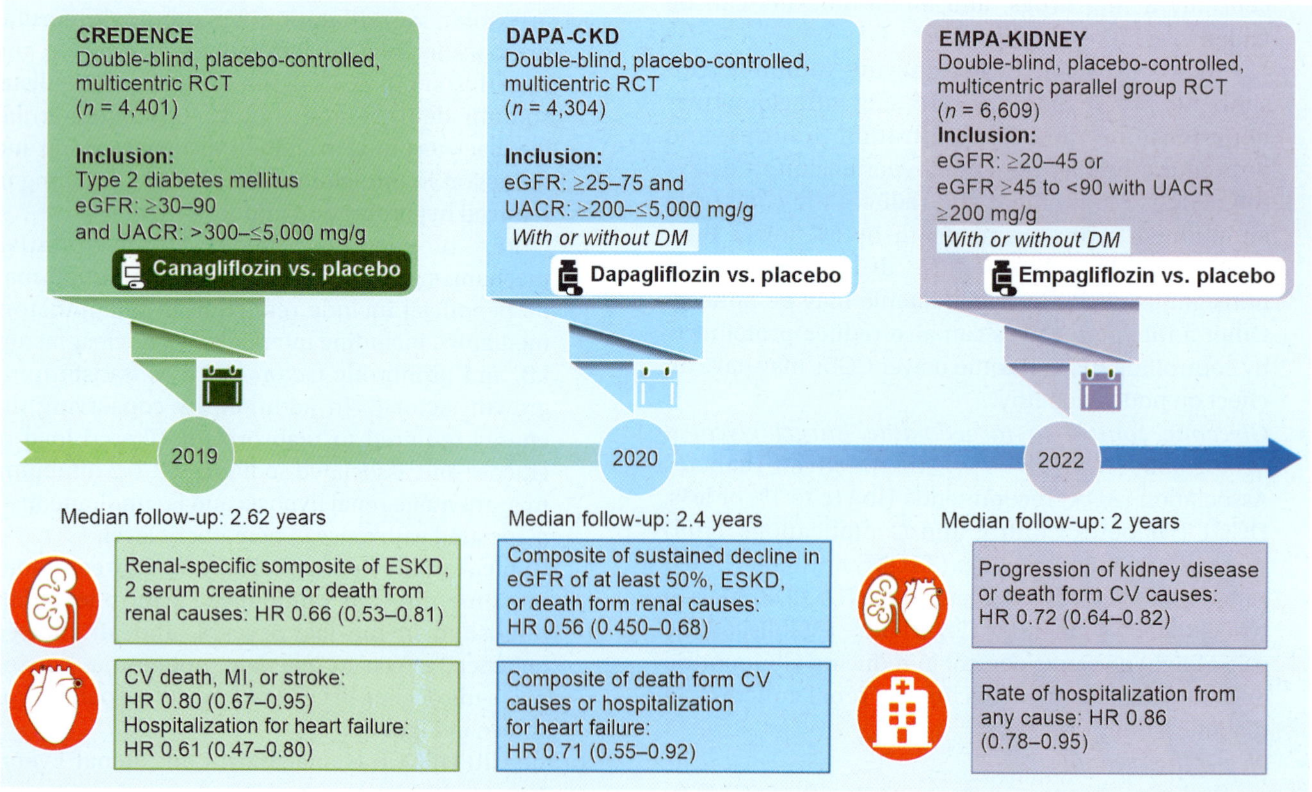

FIG. 1: Randomized controlled trials showing kidney and cardiovascular outcomes with SGLT-2 inhibitors.

(CREDENCE: Canagliflozin and Renal Events in Diabetes with Established Nephropathy Clinical Evaluation; CV: cardiovascular; DAPA-CKD: Dapagliflozin and Prevention of Adverse Outcomes in Chronic Kidney Disease; DM: diabetes mellitus; eGFR: estimated glomerular filtration rate; EMPA-KIDNEY: The Study of Heart and Kidney Protection With Empagliflozin; ESKD: end-stage kidney disease; HR: hazard ratio; RCT: randomized controlled trial; T2DM: type 2 diabetes mellitus; UACR: urine albumin-creatinine ratio)

Presently, the cost is a barrier to common use, these drugs could be advantageous compared with insulin treatment with lower side effects, better therapeutic adherence, and positive effects on body weight.

- *Mineralocorticoid receptor antagonists (MRAs)*: MRAs, such as spironolactone and eplerenone, have traditionally been used to treat conditions such as refractory and resistant hypertension and HF. MRAs also benefit in CKD progression by blocking the effects of aldosterone, a hormone involved in sodium and fluid balance, and by reducing proteinuria, BP, and inflammation in the kidneys. The use remains limited in CKD patients because of side effects, particularly hyperkalemia.

A recent advancement has been furnished with the invention of non-steroidal MRAs and finerenone. Finerenone, a dihydropyridine-based nonsteroidal MRA antagonist, binds to the MR receptor is mineralocorticoid receptor, reduces inflammation, fibrosis, and albuminuria in patients with diabetes and lowers the risk of first onset of kidney failure. Finerenone also reduces mortality and morbidity in patients with chronic severe congestive HF with a reduced ejection fraction. MRA receptor, through which finerenone work, is distributed relatively equally between the heart and the kidney. In comparison, spironolactone and eplerenone receptors have higher concentrations in renal tissue than in cardiac tissue. Finerenone has no significant affinity or activity at androgen, progesterone, estrogen, and glucocorticoid receptors. The drug binds selectively to the mineralocorticoid receptor, and it is at least as potent as spironolactone, with a lower incidence of hyperkalemia and other adverse effects compared with both spironolactone and eplerenone.

The FIDELIO-DKD (Finerenone in Reducing Kidney Failure and Disease Progression in Diabetic Kidney Disease) trial, after a median follow-up of 2.6 years, finerenone was associated with a 3.4% absolute reduction in the rate of kidney failure, renal death, and a drop in eGFR of at least 40% from baseline. In a pooled analysis of FIDELIO-DKD and FIGARO-DKD (Finerenone in Reducing Kidney Failure and Disease Progression in Diabetic Kidney Disease), the FIDELITY (Combined FIDELIO-DKD and FIGARO-DKD Trial Program Analysis) analysis in 13,171 patients, with CKD and T2DM, from 48 countries randomized 1:1 to receive finerenone (10 mg or 20 mg daily) versus placebo and a median duration of 3 years follow-up. It was demonstrated that on top of an optimized RAS blockade, finerenone significantly reduced the risk of the composite CV outcome, time to cardiovascular death, nonfatal myocardial infarction, nonfatal stroke, or hospitalization for HF by 14%. Finerenone also reduced the risk of the composite kidney outcome, time to kidney failure, sustained ≥57% decrease in eGFR from baseline, or kidney death by 23%. In July 2021, the United States Food and Drug Administration (US-FDA) approved finerenone to reduce the risk of sustained eGFR decline, ESKD, CV death, nonfatal myocardial infarction, and hospitalization for HF in individuals with CKD associated with T2DM, based on results from the FIDELIO-DKD study.

- *Anti-inflammatory agents (bardoxolone methyl)*: Bardoxolone methyl is an oral anti-inflammatory and antioxidant agent that activate a cellular pathway known as Nrf2, which regulates the body's defense against oxidative stress. Clinical trials have demonstrated that bardoxolone methyl can improve kidney function and reduce the progression of CKD in patients with T2DM.
- *Endothelin receptor antagonists (ERAs)*: Endothelin (ET) are a family of peptides that act as potent vasoconstrictors and profibrotic growth factors. ET-1 is integral to renal and cardiovascular pathophysiology and exerts effects via autocrine, paracrine, and endocrine signaling pathways tied to the regulation of aldosterone, catecholamines, and angiotensin. It promotes inflammation and fibrosis in the kidneys. In the kidney, ET-1 is critical to maintaining renal perfusion and controls glomerular arteriole tone and hemodynamics. The use of ERAs in hypertensive nephropathy has the potential to decrease proteinuria, and in diabetic nephropathy, has the potential to restore glycocalyx thickness and decrease proteinuria. ERAs show promise in decreasing proteinuria and slowing tissue damage in focal segmental glomerular sclerosis. ET-1 is a potential biomarker for autosomal dominant polycystic kidney disease progression, so it is thought that ERAs may be of some therapeutic benefit.
- *Antifibrotic agents (pirfenidone)*: Pirfenidone is an antifibrotic drug that has been used in the treatment of idiopathic pulmonary fibrosis. It has also shown promise in reducing kidney fibrosis and slowing the progression of CKD in preclinical studies. Clinical trials are currently underway to evaluate its efficacy and safety in CKD patients.
- *Bicarbonate supplementation (target serum bicarbonate 22 mEq/L)*: Growing evidence suggests that correction of metabolic acidosis in patients with CKD may have beneficial effects on protein and bone metabolism. Patients with CKD who receive bicarbonate supplementation show a slower decline in renal function. It also impacts nutritional parameters and reduces protein catabolism.
- *Hypoxia-inducible factor (HIF)-prolyl hydroxylase inhibitors*: HIF stabilizers, such as daprodustat and roxadustat, are novel drugs that aim to stimulate the

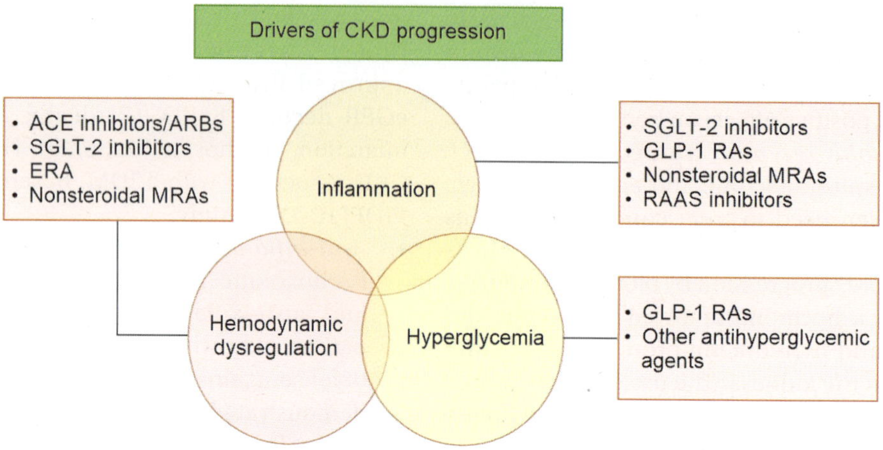

FIG. 2: Pharmacological interventions retarding the progression of CKD.

(ACE: angiotensin-converting enzyme; ARBs: angiotensin II receptor blockers; CKD: chronic kidney disease; ERA: endothelin receptor antagonists; GLP-1 RAs: glucagon-like peptide-1 receptor agonists; MRA: mineralocorticoid receptor antagonists; RAAS: renin–angiotensin–aldosterone system; SGLT-2: sodium-glucose cotransporter-2)

production of erythropoietin, a hormone that regulates red blood cell production. These drugs can potentially improve anemia in CKD patients while also protecting against hypoxia-related kidney damage.

- *Other interventions*: Reduction in protein intake (0.6–0.8 g/kg/day) and salt intake (< 100 mEq/day), reduces hyperfiltration, and had an additive effect with RAS blocker. Smoking cessation, anemia correction, and corrections of CKD-bone-mineral disorder (hyperphosphatemia, hypocalcemia, and hyperparathyroidism) all positively impact CKD-related complications and their progression.

In summary, the pharmacological intervention in retarding the progression of CKD is expanding. A summary of pharmacological intervention in retarding progression is shown in **Figure 2**. SGLT-2 inhibitors, finerenone, and GLP-1 RA, may be used on top of RAS blockers to retard the progression of CKD.

SUGGESTED READINGS

1. Perkovic V, Jardine MJ, Neal B, Bompoint S, Heerspink HJL, Charytan DM, et al; CREDENCE Trial Investigators. Canagliflozin and Renal Outcomes in Type 2 Diabetes and Nephropathy. N Engl J Med. 2019;380(24):2295-306.
2. Heerspink HJL, Stefánsson BV, Correa-Rotter R, Chertow GM, Greene T, Hou FF, et al; DAPA-CKD Trial Committees and Investigators. Dapagliflozin in Patients with Chronic Kidney Disease. N Engl J Med. 2020;383(15):1436-46.
3. The EMPA-KIDNEY Collaborative Group; Herrington WG, Staplin N, Wanner C, Green JB, Hauske SJ, Emberson JR, et al. Empagliflozin in patients with chronic kidney disease. N Engl J Med. 2023;388(2):117-127.
4. Zelniker TA, Wiviott SD, Raz I, Im KA, Goodrich EL, Furtado RHM, et al. Comparison of the effects of glucagon-like peptide receptor agonists and sodium-glucose cotransporter 2 inhibitors for prevention of major adverse cardiovascular and renal outcomes in type 2 diabetes mellitus. Circulation 2019;139:2022-31.
5. Pitt B, Filippatos G, Agarwal R, Anker SD, Bakris GL, Rossing P, et al; FIGARO-DKD Investigators. Cardiovascular Events with Finerenone in Kidney Disease and Type 2 Diabetes. N Engl J Med. 2021;385(24):2252-63.
6. Bakris GL, Agarwal R, Anker SD, Pitt B, Ruilope LM, Rossing P, et al; FIDELIO-DKD Investigators. Effect of finerenone on chronic kidney disease outcomes in type 2 diabetes. N Engl J Med. 2020;383(23):2219-29.
7. Agarwal R, Filippatos G, Pitt B, Anker SD, Rossing P, Joseph A, et al; FIDELIO-DKD and FIGARO-DKD investigators. Cardiovascular and kidney outcomes with finerenone in patients with type 2 diabetes and chronic kidney disease: the FIDELITY pooled analysis. Eur Heart J. 2022;43(6):474-84.
8. Wang YY, Yang YX, Zhe H, He ZX, Zhou SF. Bardoxolone methyl (CDDO-Me) as a therapeutic agent: an update on its pharmacokinetic and pharmacodynamic properties. Drug Des Devel Ther. 2014;8:2075-88.
9. Kohan DE, Barton M. Endothelin and endothelin antagonists in chronic kidney disease. Kidney Int. 2014;86(5):896-904.
10. Cho ME, Kopp JB. Pirfenidone: An anti-fibrotic therapy for progressive kidney disease. Expert Opin Investig Drugs. 2010;19(2):275-83.

182

CHAPTER

Metabolic Bone Disease in Chronic Kidney Disease: Newer Insights

Tribhuwan Gupta, Prakhar Gupta

ABSTRACT

Metabolic bone disease in chronic kidney disease (CKD) is a well-defined entity and has various impacts on mortality and morbidity in kidney patients. There has been lots of changes in classification and diagnosis of this in past 30 years. Current classification and management is based on Kidney Disease: Improving Global Outcomes (KDIGO) guidelines published in 2009 and updated in 2017. Various studies showed conflicting outcomes measures in management of chronic kidney disease—mineral and bone disorder (CKD-MBD) (new term). Calcium-based phosphate binder should be avoided in adults and older populations and parathyroid hormone (PTH) lowering agents should be used cautiously.

INTRODUCTION

Mortality and morbidity in chronic kidney disease (CKD) patient depends on various factors including cardiovascular disease, anemia, chronic inflammation, malnutrition, immune-compromised state, infections, dialysis, etc. Metabolic bone disease which is now termed as chronic kidney disease—mineral and bone disorder (CKD-MBD) since 2006, also contribute toward mortality and morbidity including increased fracture risk and growth retardation in children. CKD-MBD includes biochemical abnormalities, skeletal abnormalities, and vascular calcification in CKD population. The parameters which are altered in CKD-MBD are: (1) serum calcium, phosphorus, parathyroid hormone (PTH), and fibroblast growth factor 23 (FGF23), (2) bone remodeling and mineralization or impaired linear growth in children, and (3) extra skeletal calcification in soft tissue and arteries. A detailed guideline for management of CKD-MBD was published by Kidney Disease: Improving Global Outcomes (KDIGO) in 2009 and updated in 2017. This review chapter will emphasize on newer pathophysiology and management of the same.

PATHOPHYSIOLOGY OF CHRONIC KIDNEY DISEASE—MINERAL AND BONE DISORDER

In CKD, there are altered mineral and endocrine functions that are very important in regulating initial bone formation during growth (bone modeling) and bone structure and function during adulthood (bone remodeling). This leads to bone abnormalities in all patients on dialysis and most patients with CKD-stage 3-5.

Phosphorus (Inorganic Phosphate)

With the decline in glomerular filtration rate (GFR) to 50–60 mL/minute, the kidney ability to control inorganic phosphate (Pi) becomes impaired. Most patients will have increased Pi level once GFR reaches <20–25 mL/minute. This increase in Pi level leads to increase level of PTH and FGF23, which in turn increases renal excretion of phosphorus. This rise in serum PTH at the expense of maintaining normal serum Pi, is a measure mechanism by which secondary hyperparathyroidism develops and is often called "trade-off-hypothesis" **(Flowchart 1)**.

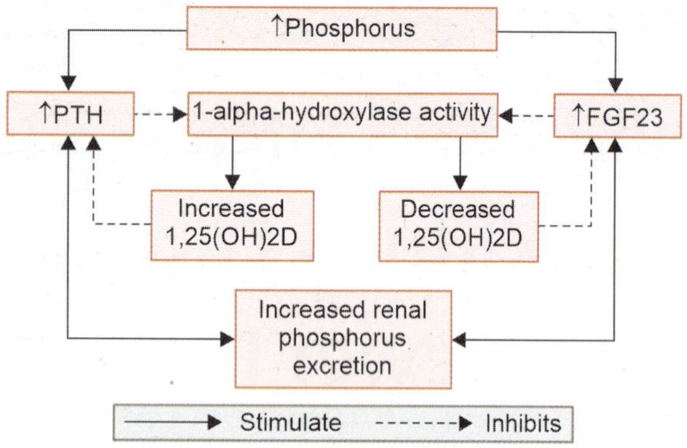

FLOWCHART 1: Regulations of serum phosphorus in CKD.
(CKD: chronic kidney disease; FGF23: fibroblast growth factor 23; PTH: parathyroid hormone)

Calcium

Ionized serum calcium levels are maintained in a range of 8.5–10 mg/dL by inducing increase in secretion of PTH. PTH in turn increases bone resorption, enhanced absorption of calcium in kidneys and increase conversion of 25(OH)D to 1,25(OH)2D in kidney, thereby increasing intestinal calcium absorption. In patients with advancing CKD, there is reduced conversion of 25(OH) D to 1,25(OH)2D due to decreased activity of 1-alpha-hydroxylase activity, reduced renal calcium absorption, and reduced phosphorus excretion. Calcium sensing receptors have been found in parathyroid, kidneys, bone, and vasculature.

Vitamin D

In presence of ultraviolet B sunlight, cholesterol is converted to vitamin D3. Further there are dietary sources of vitamin D2 (ergocalciferol) and vitamin D3 (cholecalciferol) from plant and animal, respectively. Vitamin D-binding protein (DBP) in blood carries these two to liver where they are hydroxylated by CYP27A1 (25-hydroxylate) to yield 25(OH)D, often known as calcidiol. Calcidiol is then converted to 1,25(OH)2D in kidneys by 1-alpha-hydroxylase. This lost step is disturbed in patients with CKD.

Parathyroid Hormone

The main action of PTH is to maintain calcium level by increasing bone mineral dissolution thus releasing calcium and Pi; increasing renal absorption of calcium and excretion of Pi; increasing intestinal absorption of calcium; and increasing production of active D3. CKD leads to hyperparathyroidism and exact interrelationship of calcium, Pi, and vitamin D3 for initiating causation of this is complex because changes in one lead to rapid changes in others. However as per current data, it appears that decline in calcium is more important in stimulating PTH release and calcitriol in inhibiting PTH release.

CLINICAL IMPACT OF CHRONIC KIDNEY DISEASE-MINERAL AND BONE DISORDER

Various randomized controlled trials and epidemiological data suggest that increased levels of phosphorus is associated with increased mortality and morbidity by enhancing cardiovascular disease in patients with CKD. For serum calcium level, no data suggest an increased risk of fracture or mortality in CKD population. Similarly there is no data which suggest any specific level of PTH which has improved outcome in CKD population **(Table 1)**.

METABOLIC BONE DISEASE IN CHRONIC KIDNEY DISEASE

The earlier classification of metabolic bone disease, used parameters of osteoid (unmineralized bone) area as a percentage of total bone area and fibrosis. These two static parameters, i.e., osteoid and fibrosis, along with dynamic bone turnover assessed by bone formation rate (BFR) have been used to classify various forms of renal osteodystrophy over last 30 years, but now it have been replaced by a new KDIGO, *bone turnover, mineralization, and volume (TMV)* system. In *osteitis fibrosis*, a high turnover disease, there is increased rate of bone formation, increased resorption, extensive osteoclastic, and osteoblastic activities. The alignment of strands of collagen in the bone matrix has an irregular woven pattern in contrast to normal lamellar (parallel) in normal bone. These kinds of bone have less strength and fractures easily. *Adynamic (low turnover) bone diseases* are characterized histologically by absence of osteoclastic and osteoblastic activity, osteoid formation, and endosteal fibrosis. Most common cause was aluminum bone disease, which is very uncommon these days. *Mixed uremic osteodystrophy*, where there was features of both secondary hyperparathyroidism and evidence of poor mineralization, is not a well-defined entity.

In the new classification of bone disease by KDIGO, renal osteodystrophy is only one dimension of CKD-MBD that is measured by histomorphometry of bone. The newer TMV classification can have any combination and more accurately defines, the disease process, prognosis, and management aspects **(Table 2)**.

Vascular calcification is another new aspect of CKD where there is arterial calcification, mainly medial which along with intimal calcification (atherosclerosis) and can

TABLE 1: Few studies on clinical outcome of CKD-MBD.

Study (year)	Type	Sample size	Population	Outcome	Observation
Lopes et al. (2020)	Prospective cohort study	17,414 patients	HD	CV mortality	Patients with poor control of serum phosphorus levels (expressed as AUC) during a 6-month period have a higher risk of CV mortality (for AUC > 2 = HR 2.03; 95% CI 1.53–2.69)
Hou Y et al. (2017)	Meta-analysis of 9 cohort studies	1,992,869 patients	HD or PD	All-cause mortality	Compared to reference phosphorus category, both very high (HR 1.39; 95% CI 1.31–1.47) and very low (HR 1.16; 95% CI 1.06–1.28) phosphorus levels are associated with a greater risk for all-cause mortality
Bellasi et al. (2011)	Observational retrospective study	1,716 patients	CKD 3–5, not requiring dialysis	Composite end point of progression to ESKD or death	A worse control of phosphorus levels (4.3 mg/dL) exposes to an increased risk of progression to ESKD or death (HR 2.04; 95% CI 1.44–2.90)
Borrelli et al. (2018)	Observational prospective study	543 patients	CKD 1–5, not requiring dialysis	Renal death (composite of ESKD or all-causes death before ESKD)	In the same subject, higher PTH variation over time (DPTH) with respect to baseline value is associated with an augmented risk of renal death (for the highest DPTH quartile = HR 1.91; 95% CI:1.08–3.38; $p = 0.026$)
Floege J et al. (2011)	Observational prospective study	7,970 patients	HD	All-cause mortality	Compared to reference PTH range (150–300 pg/mL), both elevated (>600 pg/mL) and low (<75 pg/mL) PTH levels are, respectively, associated with a twofold (HR 2.10; 95% CI 1.62–2.73, $p < 0.001$) and 1.5-fold (HR 1.46; 95% CI 1.17–1.83, $p = 0.001$) risk of death

(AUC: area under the curve; CI: confidence interval; CKD-MBD: chronic kidney disease—mineral and bone disorder; CV: cardiovascular; ESKD: end-stage kidney disease; HD: hemodialysis; HR: heart rate; PD: peritoneal dialysis; PTH: parathyroid hormone)

TABLE 2: KDIGO, TMV classification.

Turnover	Mineralization	Volume
Low	Normal	Low
Normal	Abnormal	Normal
High		High

(KDIGO: Kidney Disease: Improving Global Outcomes; TMV: turnover, mineralization, and volume)

increase risk of myocardial infarction, arterial stiffening, and arrhythmias.

MANAGEMENT OF CHRONIC KIDNEY DISEASE-MINERAL AND BONE DISORDER

Chronic kidney disease is defined as abnormalities of kidney structure and function, present for >3 months, with implications for health. CKD is classified based on cause, GFR category (G1–G5) and albuminuria category (A1–A3), CGA **(Table 3)**. There has been few changes in management guidelines from KDIGO-2006 and KDIGO-2017. The new updated guideline is discussed here.

TABLE 3: Classification and prognosis of chronic kidney disease (CKD).

		Albuminuria category		
		A1	A2	A3
Glomerular filtration rate (GFR) category		<30 mg/g/day	30–300 mg/g/day	>300 mg/g/day
G1	>90 mL/minute	G1A1	G1A2	G1A3
G2	60–89 mL/minute	G2A1	G2A2	G2A3
G3a	45–59 mL/minute	G3aA1	G3aA2	G3aA3
G3b	30–44 mL/minute	G3bA1	G3bA2	G3bA3
G4	15–29 mL/minute	G4A1	G4A2	G4A3
G5	<15 mL/minute	G5A1	G5A2	G5A3

(Green—low risk; yellow—moderate risk; orange—high risk; red—very high risk)

Monitoring

- Monitor serum level of calcium, Pi, PTH, and alkaline phosphatase in the beginning of CKD G3a in adults and in children at the beginning of CKDG2. Follow-up measurement at interval of 6–12 months. Those in CKDG4, monitor at interval of 3–6 months for calcium and phosphorus and PTH at 6–12 months and in CKDG5 and on dialysis calcium and phosphorus every 1–3 months and PTH at 3–6 months.

- Vitamin D level (calcidiol) to be measured, corrected and monitored depending on baseline value.
- Those patients with CKDG3a to CKDG5D with evidence of CKD-MBD and or having risk factor for osteoporosis, *bone mineral density (BMD)* to be done.
- It is reasonable to perform a *bone biopsy* in CKDG3a-G5D, if one thinks knowing the type of renal osteodystrophy may impact treatment decision.
- It is recommended that infants with CKDG2-G5D should have their length measured at least quarterly while children annually.
- For diagnosing vascular calcification, it is suggested that, a lateral abdominal radiograph and echocardiogram done at CKDG3a-G5D.

Treatment

- Treatment is targeted taking all parameters altogether; Pi, calcium, and PTH level.
- Elevated phosphate level should be lowered to normal range.
- In adult populations, avoid hypocalcaemia and using calcium-based phosphate binders.
- In children, maintain calcium in age appropriate normal range.
- Use a dialysate calcium concentration between 2.5 and 3.0 mEq/L
- Decision for phosphate lowering treatment should be based on progressively or persistently elevated serum phosphate levels.
- Avoid long term use of aluminum containing phosphate binders and avoid dialysate aluminum contaminations.
- Dietary intake of phosphate to be lowered.
- In patients with CKDG3-G5 not on dialysis, the optimal PTH level is not known. It is suggested that patients with level of PTH rising or persistently above normal limit, should be evaluated and treated for modifiable factors such as calcium, Pi, and vitamin D deficiency.
- Calcitriol and vitamin D analogs not to be routinely used and reserved for CKD patients with severe and progressive hyperparathyroidism.
- In patients on dialysis maintain PTH level to two to nine times the upper normal level of reference. PTH lowering agents used are calcimimetics, calcitriol, or vitamin D, alone or in combination.
- In patients with CKD G3a–G5D with severe hyperparathyroidism, who fail to respond to medical or pharmacological therapy, they suggested parathyroidectomy.
- In patients with CKD G1–G2 with osteoporosis and/or high risk of fracture, as identified by the World Health Organization criteria, they recommended management as for the general population.
- In patients with CKD G3a–G5D with biochemical abnormalities of CKD-MBD and low BMD and/or fragility fractures, they suggest that treatment choices take into account the magnitude and reversibility of the biochemical abnormalities and the progression of CKD, with consideration of a bone biopsy.
- In children and adolescents with CKDG2–G5D and related height deficits, they recommended treatment with recombinant human growth hormone when additional growth is desired, after first addressing malnutrition and biochemical abnormalities of CKD-MBD.

CONCLUSION

Chronic kidney disease is a diverse disease and it has its own risk factors for mortality and morbidity. Furthermore, the outcome of management of CKD-MBD is not well-defined till now, however, it is recommended that optimal treatment must be instituted as per latest guidelines available.

SUGGESTED READINGS

1. Kidney Disease: Improving Global Outcomes (KDIGO) CKD–MBD Work Group. KDIGO clinical practice guideline for the diagnosis, evaluation, prevention, and treatment of chronic kidney disease–mineral and bone disorder (CKD–MBD). Kidney International. 2009;76 (Suppl 113):S1-S130.
2. Kidney Disease: Improving Global Outcomes (KDIGO) CKD-MBD Update Work Group. KDIGO 2017 Clinical Practice Guideline Update for the Diagnosis, Evaluation, Prevention, and Treatment of Chronic Kidney Disease–Mineral and Bone Disorder (CKD–MBD). Kidney Int Suppl. 2017;7:1-59.
3. Taal MW. Brenner and Rector's the Kinney, 9th edition. Amsterdam: Elsevier Health Sciences; 2011.

183

CHAPTER

Kidney–Heart Connection

Vikash Khandelia, Meghna Aggarwal

ABSTRACT

Cardiorenal syndrome (CRS) involves a collection of various pathophysiological pathways that comes into play when there is dysfunction of either of the organs. Sometimes, systemic disease affects the normal functioning of these organs which is classified under CRS type V. A lot of mechanisms have been explained to understand CRS. Diagnosis requires a careful history to know the inciting event to decide target of therapy, laboratory parameters to know the creatinine and glomerular filtration rate (GFR) trend over time, urine routine examination for albuminuria and active urine sediments, and cardiac and renal imaging. Management includes decongestion with diuretics (loop diuretics are preferred, mineralocorticoid receptor antagonists, and thiazides), renin–angiotensin–aldosterone system (RAAS) inhibitors, and beta-blockers. Dose modification of these drugs is required according to stages of renal disease (stages 1–3). Therapy is individualized in renal failure stages 4 and 5, weighing risk–benefit ratio. Newer therapies with sodium-glucose cotransporter-2 (SGLT-2) inhibitors, vasopressin receptor antagonists, neprilysin inhibitors, and ultrafiltration have been studied in various trials. None of these therapies has any proven role in modifying mortality outcome. Prognosis is poor in patients with worsening renal function, with every 10 mL/min reduction in GFR, mortality increased by approximately 15%.

INTRODUCTION

Human kidneys get 25% blood supply of total cardiac output and are highly prone to being affected by acute or chronic cardiac disorders. Cardiorenal syndromes (CRSs) are broadly defined as "disorders of the heart and kidneys whereby acute or chronic dysfunction in one organ may induce acute or chronic dysfunction of the other" **(Table 1)**.

TABLE 1: Classification.

Type	Terminology	Definition
CRS I	Acute cardiorenal syndrome	When acute heart failure leads to AKI or worsening of renal function
CRS II	Chronic cardiorenal syndrome	Chronic heart failure leading to renal injury or progressive renal failure
CRS III	Acute renocardiac syndrome	AKI causing acute cardiac event (inclusive of heart failure)
CRS IV	Chronic renocardiac syndrome	Chronic kidney disease leading to cardiac injury or progression of underlying cardiac disease
CRS V	Systemic cardiorenal syndrome	Any systemic disease, causing acute heart and kidney injury

(AKI: acute kidney injury; CRS: cardiorenal syndrome)

EPIDEMIOLOGY

There are 64.3 million adults living with heart failure (HF) worldwide. It is estimated that the risk of heart failure in patients suffering from chronic kidney disease (CKD) with glomerular filtration rate (GFR) < 60 mL/min/1.73 m^2 is 2–20 times more compared to those patients with preserved GFR. Mortality increases by approximately 15% for every 10 mL/min reduction in GFR. The prevalence of moderate-to-severe kidney impairment (defined as a GFR < 60 mL/min per 1.73 m^2; normal being >90 mL/min per 1.73 m^2) is approximately 30–60% in patients with HF. About 30% patients undergoing treatment for acute or chronic HF frequently develop an increase in serum creatinine, which fulfills criteria for type 1 or type 2 CRS.

Inhospital mortality rate of around 50% is observed in patients with cardiogenic shock and declining renal function. Mortality increased by approximately 15% for every 10 mL/min reduction in GFR. Patients with CKD have an increased risk of both atherosclerotic cardiovascular disease and HF **(Box 1)**.

BOX 1: Risk factors for cardiorenal syndrome (CRS).

- Preexisting chronic kidney disease
- Diabetes
- High-dose diuretics
- Iodinated contrast use
- Old age
- Anemia
- Prior history of heart failure
- Uncontrolled hypertension

PATHOPHYSIOLOGY (FIG. 1)

- *Neurohumoral adaptations*: Renin-angiotensin-aldosterone system (RAAS) activation—nonosmotic release of antidiuretic hormone (arginine vasopressin) and endothelin 1, which leads to free-water retention, hyponatremia, and systemic vasoconstriction, which in turn decrease renal perfusion. Reduced cardiac index is not the primary driver for renal dysfunction in patients hospitalized for HF (ESCAPE trial); in fact, higher cardiac index was paradoxically associated with worsening of GFR.
- *Reduced renal perfusion*: Blunting of tubuloglomerular feedback (TGF) signaling in CRS leads to reduction in renal perfusion due to alteration in levels of angiotensin, renin, nitric oxide, and prostaglandin levels.
- *Venous congestion*: As central venous pressure (CVP) increases, renal venous pressure also increases, which leads to a rise in renal interstitial pressure. Kidney is an encapsulated organ and this rise in interstitial pressure causes a compression of Bowman's capsule and tubules leading to salt and water retention.
- *Right ventricular (RV) dysfunction*: RV dilatation impairs left ventricular (LV) filling and thereby reducing forward output via a ventricular

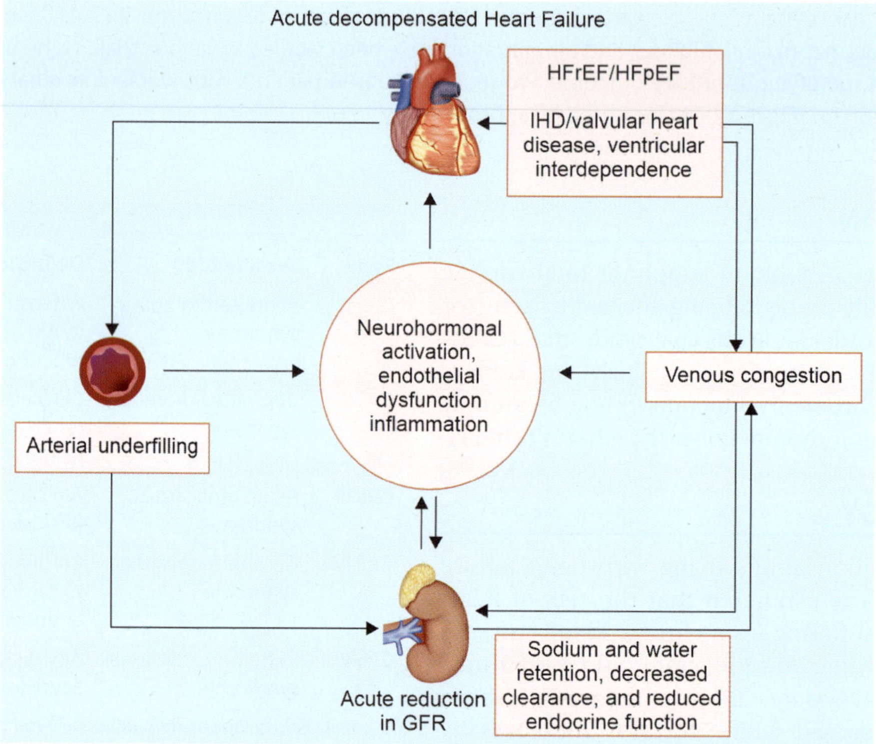

FIG. 1: Pathophysiology of cardiorenal syndrome.
(GFR: glomerular filtration rate; HFrEF/HFpEF: heart failure with reduced ejection fraction/heart failure with preserved ejection fraction; IHD: ischemic heart disease)

interdependent effect (also known as the reverse Bernheim phenomenon) where increased pressure within a distended RV reduces LV transmural pressure for any given intracavitary LV pressure and inducing leftward interventricular septal bowing.

- *Chloride handling*: In patients with HF, chloride plays an important role as chloride is a primary modulator of TGF. In patients with HF who are receiving diuresis, hypochloremia is frequently accompanied by a metabolic alkalosis due to chloride depletion. Despite clinical evidence of persistent volume overload, alkalosis in this setting is frequently and inappropriately attributed to intravascular volume depletion (i.e., "contraction alkalosis"), which may lead to premature de-escalation of decongestive therapies. If the patient has evidence of hypervolemia, metabolic alkalosis in this setting is more likely attributable to abnormal electrolyte homeostasis that results in chloride depletion alkalosis, which is characterized by elevated urine chloride levels.

The trigger for activation of this pathway leading to CRS is acute decompensation of heart leading to arterial under filling and venous congestion. This causes activation of neurohormonal system along with systemic inflammation and dysfunction of endothelium. Due to activation of RAAS due to the abovementioned processes, there is sodium and water retention, decreased clearance of solutes, and disturbed endocrine function of the kidney. Venous congestion and RAAS activation complement each other, leading to a vicious circle of reduced ejection fraction due to further cardiac decompensation. HF with reduced ejection fraction (HFrEF < 40%), HF with preserved ejection fraction (HFpEF > 50%).

DIAGNOSIS

In patients with HF with elevated serum creatinine, it is important to distinguish underlying CKD/primary kidney disease and renal dysfunction associated with CRS. Some patients may have both disorders simultaneously.

Findings in favor of underlying kidney disease include significant proteinuria (>1 g/day), active urinary sediments with hematuria or cellular casts, and/or small-sized kidneys. However, bland urine sediments with insignificant proteinuria, which is typically present in CRS without underlying kidney disease, can also be seen in variety of renal diseases including nephrosclerosis and obstructive nephropathy.

Measurement of the urine sodium concentration (UNa) below 25 mEq/L would be expected with HF since renal perfusion is reduced. Urine sample taken 1–2 hours after a dose of loop diuretic may be a guide to intervene if natriuretic response is low, prompting aggressive diuretic titration. A position statement on use of diuretics in HF from the European Society of Cardiology (ESC) proposes a spot UNa of <50–70 mEq/L after 2 hours or an hourly urine output < 100–150 mL during the first 6 hours to identify a patient with insufficient diuretic response.

In patients with HF, diuretic therapies should be used if there is evidence of clinical congestion even if an elevated blood urea nitrogen/creatinine ratio (BUN/Cr) is present, which suggests prerenal condition **(Table 2)**.

One of the challenges that clinicians face is to assess fluid status of the patient, which is important for calculating input/output and deciding diuretic dose. There are various clinical findings and laboratory and ultrasonography parameters to assess the fluid status of the patient.

TABLE 2: Volume assessment.

Assessment	Volume overload	Volume depleted
History	Increased dietary salt intake and dyspnea	Decreased appetite, diarrhea, and vomiting
Clinical examination	Increasing weight, distended neck veins, peripheral edema	Postural hypotension, low BP in previously hypertensive patient, reduced skin turgor, decreased capillary refill, sunken eyes
Laboratory parameters	Increased levels of ANP and BNP, dilutional hyponatremia, low albumin levels	Increased albumin, decreased ANP and BNP
Chest X-ray	Increased cardiothoracic ratio, bilateral pleural effusion, or costophrenic angle blunting	Normal cardiothoracic ratio
Ultrasound: • Lung • Abdomen	>10 B lines	<5 B lines
IVC collapsibility index	<50% collapse	>50% IVC collapse
Bioimpedance analysis	↑ ECW/ICW	↓ ECW/ICW

(ANP: atrial natriuretic peptide; BNP: B-type natriuretic peptide; ECW: extracellular water; ICW: intracellular water; IVC: inferior vena cava)

BIOMARKERS

Biomarkers are helpful to differentiate between true kidney injury and pseudo-worsening of renal function in the setting of HF. Cystatin C represents a valid surrogate to test renal function, recognized as more predictive of long-term mortality and rehospitalization for acute decompensated HF (ADHF) than serum creatinine or serum B-type natriuretic peptide (BNP). Cystatin C production is less dependent upon muscle mass and therefore less influenced by nutritional status.

Other biomarkers:

- Kidney injury molecule-1 (KIM-1)
- Liver type fatty acid-binding protein (L-FABP)
- Interleukin-18 (IL-18)
- Neutrophil gelatinase-associated lipocalin (NGAL)

Neutrophil gelatinase-associated lipocalin correlates with renal function markers and adverse outcomes or death in ADHF patients.

MANAGEMENT

- *Tackle congestion*: A transient deterioration of estimated GFR or its surrogate increase in serum creatinine is not a marker for worse prognosis provided that relief of congestion is achieved. By contrast, deterioration of GFR with persistence of congestion indicates a worse prognosis and an increased mortality. Hence, decongestion is a major target in acute HF (AHF).
- *Disease-modifying therapies*: Angiotensin-converting enzyme (ACE) inhibitors and angiotensin II receptor blockers (ARBs) are the most prescribed drugs that are established to improve cardiovascular health. These drugs are given safely in patients with CKD stages 1–3 with dose modification. Major side effect is hyperkalemia as many CKD patients are oliguric or anuric and the risk of precipitating hyperkalemia is increased compared to their counterparts who have HFrEF but normal renal function.
- *Removing fluid from third space*: Paracentesis of ascites reduces intra-abdominal pressure and improves GFR. Compression therapy of lower extremities improves lymphatic drainage of interstitial fluid and improves systemic circulation and improves GFR.
- *Inotropes*: Intravenous administration of drugs such as dobutamine, dopamine, and milrinone has a role in treatment of cardiogenic shock and ADHF; now these drugs, especially dopamine, are being reevaluated for improving renal function. It increases renal blood flow, and thereby increasing GFR. In a dose of 2–10 µg/kg/min, dopamine increases renal blood flow which is due to dilation of large conductance vessels and small resistance renal vessels. Dopamine in similar dose (5–10 µg/kg/h) also increases cardiac output. The trials conducted showed variable results in improving renal function when dopamine was combined with diuretic therapy. The role is still controversial.
- *Intravenous vasodilators*: These drugs have essential role in patients with HFrEF, but in patients with CRS, it was seen that kidney function worsened with combined use of diuretics and vasodilators compared to diuretics alone. However, a causal relationship could not be established, so therapy is individualized according to clinical status of the patient.
- *Targeted therapies*: In patients presenting with CRS type V, e.g., Fabry's disease which is an X-linked lysosomal storage disorder involving both heart and kidney, Agalsidase beta-enzyme replacement therapy (Fabrazyme) is prescribed. Similarly, patients suffering from sarcoidosis with heart and kidney involvement are managed with corticosteroid therapy.
- *Newer therapies*: Sodium-glucose cotransporter-2 (SGLT-2) inhibitors—proven to improve cardiovascular and renal outcome in patients presenting with HFrEF in various trials but not effective in reducing mortality in patient with HFpEF.
- *Ultrafiltration*: Removal of fluid from vascular compartment through filtration across a semipermeable membrane. Dialysis is not indicated in all patients but those who present with diuretic resistance, renal injury or failure, or acute cardiac decompensation. The therapy does not alter the outcome and does not offer a better response compared to medical management.

  In the CARESS-HF trial, a comparison of ultrafiltration and pharmacological therapy (diuretics, vasodilators, and inotropic agents) was done. Decongestion and volume loss were similar in both groups, but ultrafiltration was associated with increased rate of adverse events and a rise in serum creatinine levels.
- *Vasopressin receptor antagonists*: Due to neurohormonal activation, there is nonosmotic release of antidiuretic hormone which causes water retention, leading to dilutional hyponatremia. Tolvaptan is a selective vasopressin receptor 2 antagonist which is used in HF patients with hyponatremia. In contrast to other diuretic agents which cause salt diuresis, tolvaptan causes water diuresis only. In various studies, tolvaptan was found to give early symptomatic relief and clinical improvement, but there was no effect on mortality outcome and led to a greater increase in serum creatinine levels compared to placebo.

PROGNOSIS

A baseline reduction in GFR was associated with increased mortality and morbidity. However, an acute reduction in GFR or rise in serum creatinine levels from the baseline failed to show any prognostic significance in the long term.

A systematic review of various studies showed mortality rate at 1 year follow-up which was 51% in patients with moderate-to-severe reduction in GFR, 38% mortality rate in mild increase in GFR, and 24% in patients with normal GFR. With every 10 mL/min reduction in GFR, mortality increased by approximately 15%.

SUGGESTED READINGS

1. McCallum W, Sarnak MJ. Cardiorenal Syndrome in the Hospital. Clin J Am Soc Nephrol. 2023;18(7):933-45.
2. Damman K, McMurray John JV. Cardiorenal syndromes. In: Yu ASL, Chertow GM, Luyckx V, Marsden PA, Skorecki K, Taal MW (Eds). Brenner and Rector's The Kidney, 2-Volume Set, 11th edition. Philadelphia: Elsevier; 2019. pp. 1380-90.
3. Ahmad T, Jackson K, Rao VS, Tang WHW, Brisco-Bacik MA, Chen HH, et al. Worsening renal function in patients with acute heart failure undergoing aggressive diuresis is not associated with tubular injury. Circulation. 2018;137(19):2016-28.

184

CHAPTER

Peritoneal Dialysis: A Physician's Perspective

Vineet Behera, Madhuri Matta

ABSTRACT

Peritoneal dialysis (PD) is a form of renal replacement therapy (RRT) in acute kidney injury (acute PD) or end-stage kidney disease (chronic PD) where the peritoneum membrane acts as a dialyzer. The dialysis is done by multiple exchanges (instillation of PD fluid into peritoneum, dwell time of a few hours, and draining out) of PD fluid (available in different concentrations and different solutes like dextrose) into the peritoneal cavity. This is done through a PD catheter (straight, coiled, or swan-neck type), which may be inserted by an open surgery, laparoscopically, or by percutaneous technique. PD may be of two types, continuous ambulatory peritoneal dialysis (which involves manual exchanges) and automated peritoneal dialysis/continuous cyclic PD in which the exchanges are done by a cycler. Peritonitis is a dreaded complication, which is managed by intraperitoneal antibiotics. The other complications include exit-site infections, mechanical problems like catheter migration or omental wrap, and other metabolic complications. PD is 'home-based' dialysis and is equally effective as hemodialysis and may be preferable in infants and young children, patients with cardiac comorbidities, patients with lack of arteriovenous (AV) fistula/vascular access, or in those having inadequate access to hemodialysis facilities.

INTRODUCTION

Peritoneal dialysis (PD) and hemodialysis are the modalities for renal replacement therapy (RRT). PD may be done in acute settings in patients of acute kidney injury (AKI) by acute PD or for maintenance therapy of patients with end-stage renal disease, as chronic PD. In PD, the peritoneal membrane acts as the dialyzer. Even though both PD and hemodialysis are equally effective, PD has its own advantages being more physiologic (as it is a slow continuous process), and being a home-based dialysis, it does not require a vascular access.

PRINCIPLES OF PERITONEAL DIALYSIS

The peritoneal barrier of capillary blood vessels, intercellular matrix, and peritoneal membrane act as dialyzer in PD. This endogenous dialyzing membrane has multiple pores of different sizes, namely specialized water channels (Aquaporin-1), small pores of 40–50 Å, and large pores of 150 Å, through which the exchange of solutes, electrolytes, and water occurs.

The major principles of dialysis through the peritoneal membrane are diffusion (which is driven by concentration gradients) and convection (which is driven by osmotic or hydrostatic pressure gradients). During the diffusion process, the solute concentration gradient between capillary blood and PD solution permits the solute to move from higher to lower concentration compartment.

PERITONEAL DIALYSIS PROCEDURE

The key component of PD is the PD catheter, which has one end in the peritoneum (open end with multiple pores), while another end exits out of the skin to lie outside, as shown in **Figures 1A and B**. In continuous ambulatory peritoneal dialysis (CAPD), 3–4 exchanges are done in a day. In a typical exchange, 2–2.5 L of dialysis fluid is instilled into the peritoneal cavity and kept inside

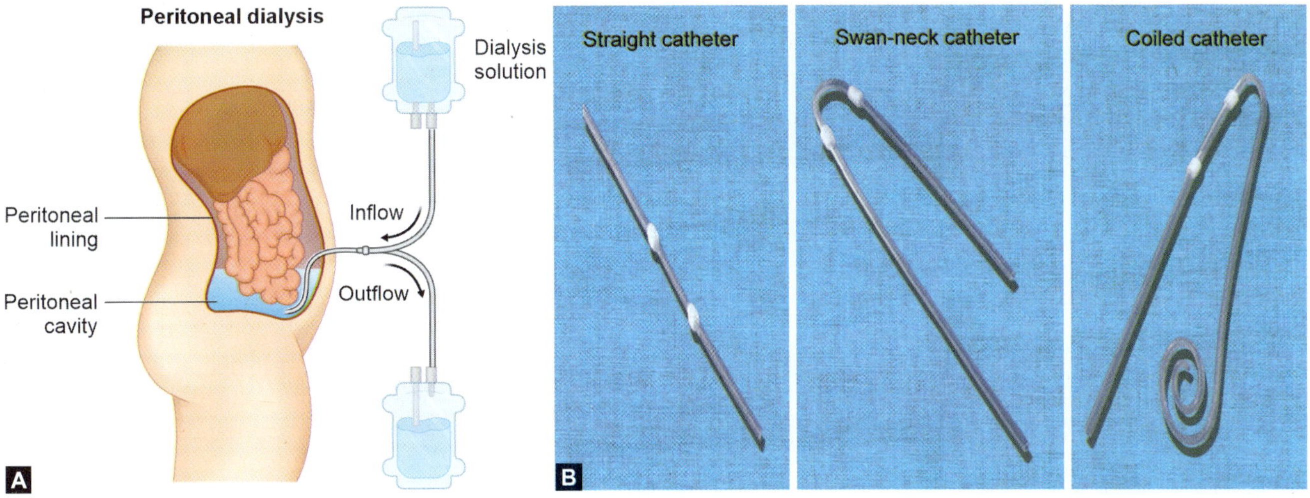

FIGS. 1A AND B: (A) The basic functioning of peritoneal dialysis with the catheter in situ and the double-bag system with Y-set tubing. (B) Common types of peritoneal dialysis catheters.

for few hours. This is done using a double bag system with a Y-set tubing system, as shown in **Figure 1A**.

Peritoneal Dialysis Catheter and Insertion

The commonly used PD catheter is a silastic or polyurethane tube that has side pores present along its intraperitoneal part. It has one or two Dacron cuffs, which allow tissue ingrowth and fibrosis in the connective tissue. This helps to fix the catheter, prevent leakage of fluid around the catheter, and prevent infection. The most commonly used types are straight catheters, swan-neck catheters, and coiled catheters as shown in **Figure 1B**.

Catheters were traditionally inserted by an open surgical technique that involved open surgical laparotomy to expose the peritoneum and then inserting the catheter into the peritoneal cavity under vision. Laparoscopy/peritoneoscopy is a less invasive technique, which is done using laparoscopic ports or peritoneoscope, as shown in **Figures 2A to D**. The percutaneous technique has become very popular and is commonly adopted by nephrologists. This is a minimally invasive method that involves a percutaneous puncture to enter the peritoneum after which the insertion is done by modified Seldinger technique. All techniques have been found to have similar outcomes, with no method superior to the others.

TYPES OF PERITONEAL DIALYSIS AND PRESCRIPTION

There are two broad types of PD, which are described here.

Continuous Ambulatory Peritoneal Dialysis

The peritoneal exchanges are performed manually 3–4 times a day by the patient or his attendant, using 2–2.5 L bags as shown in **Figure 3A**. These bags contain PD fluid, which is a lactate-buffered, balanced salt solution containing glucose (1.5%, 2.5%, or 4.5%) as the osmotic agent. Other alternative osmotic agents include icodextrin (available as 7.5% solution) or amino acid-based fluids. The standard prescription consists of 3–4 exchanges of various concentrations of PD fluids (e.g., 2 cycles × 2 L of 1.5% dextrose × 4 hours each, 01 cycle × 2 L of 2.5% dextrose × 6 hours, and 1 cycle × 2 L of 7.5% icodextrin × 10 hours).

Automated Peritoneal Dialysis or Continuous Cyclic Peritoneal Dialysis

The manual fluid exchanges as done in CAPD are replaced by the use of a cycler or an automated peritoneal dialysis (APD) machine, with fluid bags of generally 5 L size of different concentrations. The exchanges by the cycler can be done at night while the patient is asleep. It is used for patients who cannot do manual exchanges like those with busy daytime routine, patients who are old and debilitated, patients with neurological conditions like stroke, or children. After the nighttime continuous cyclic peritoneal dialysis (CCPD), daytime can be left dry or a long-acting 7.5% icodextrin fluid exchange may be done as shown in **Figure 3B** (like six cycles of 1.5% APD with a dwell time of 1 hour per cycle, with a day dwell of 2 L of 7.5% icodextrin).

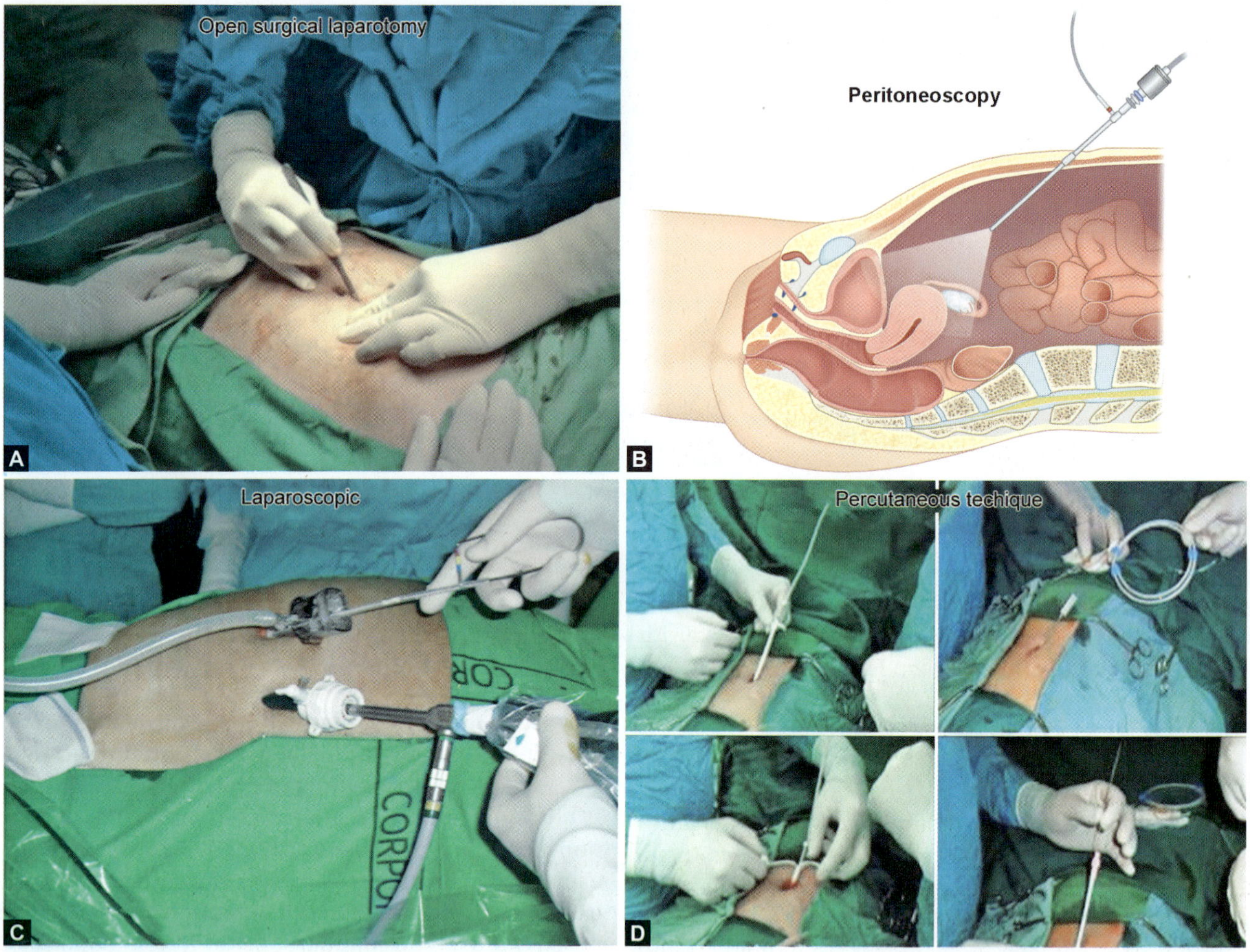

FIGS. 2A TO D: Various types of peritoneal dialysis catheter insertion.

The choice between APD and CAPD should be guided by patient and physician preference, membrane transport status, urine output, and resource availability.

Acute Peritoneal Dialysis

Peritoneal dialysis may be done in the acute setup in AKI or chronic kidney disease (CKD), without any vascular access. It is done using a stiff, rigid polyurethane catheter (without cuff) that is inserted into the peritoneum at the midline infraumbilical area. The previously mentioned soft-cuffed PD catheter may also be used. 1 L PD fluid bottles (1.5% or 2.5% dextrose) or CAPD fluid bags may be used. Acute PD catheters may be used for 3–5 days, after which they pose a risk of infection or pericatheter leaks. The use of this technique has steadily declined over the years, in view of better availability of hemodialysis. However, it is still a commonly used modality in resource-limited settings without hemodialysis and in infants or neonates.

Peritoneal Equilibration Test

A peritoneal equilibration test (PET) can be performed to assess peritoneal membrane characteristics. It is done using the serum and PD-effluent creatinine and glucose values checked in a sequential manner with respect to a PD cycle. The transporter status of peritoneum may vary from high transporter, high-average to low-average, low transporter.

COMPLICATIONS OF PERITONEAL DIALYSIS

Peritonitis

Peritoneal dialysis peritonitis presents with abdominal pain with turbid PD effluent as shown in **Figure 4A**. It is diagnosed by the presence of at least two of the three features, typical clinical features of peritonitis like fever, abdominal pain, and turbid PD fluid; PD

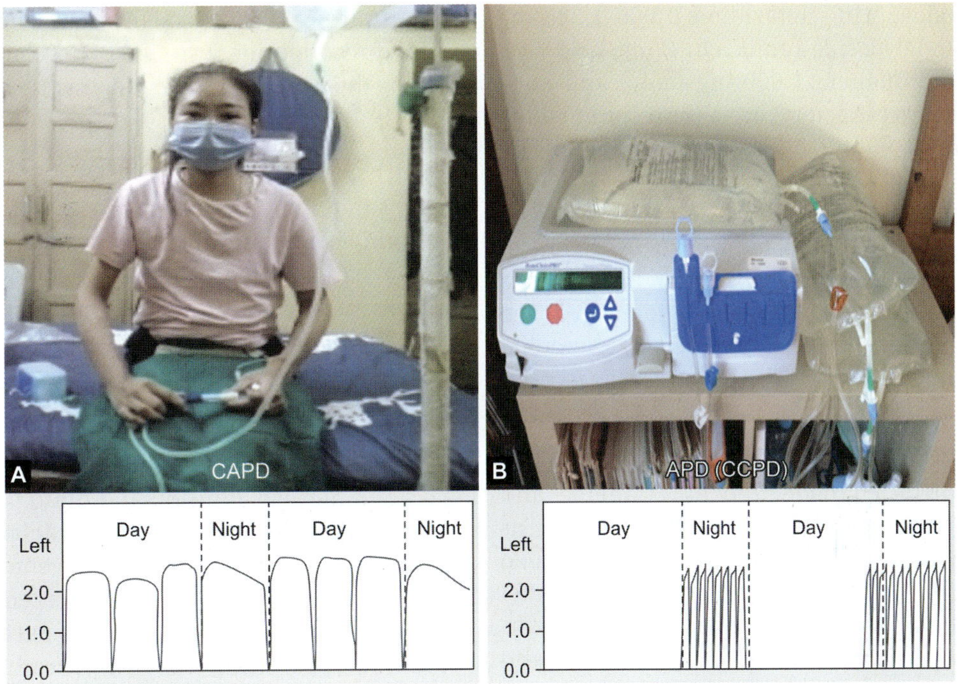

FIGS. 3A AND B: (A) A patient doing manual continuous ambulatory peritoneal dialysis (CAPD) exchanges. (B) Automated peritoneal dialysis (APD) machine with fluid bags.
(CCPD: continuous cyclic peritoneal dialysis)

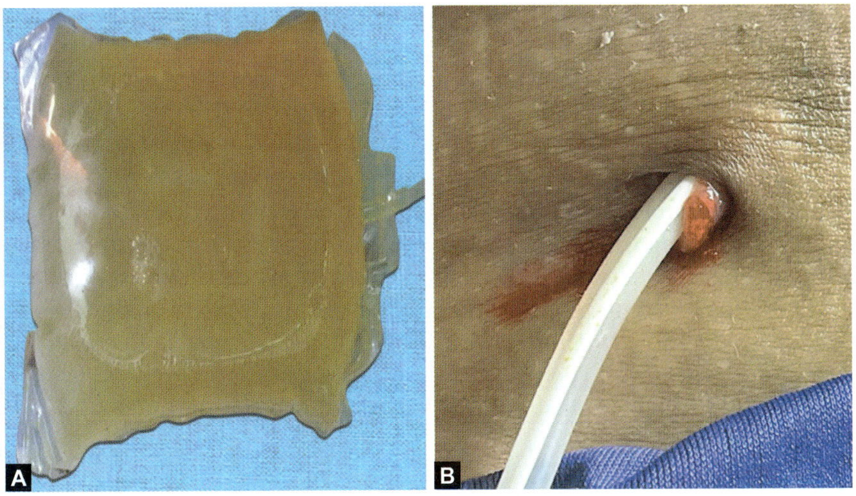

FIGS. 4A AND B: (A) Cloudy peritoneal dialysis fluid in peritonitis. (B) Exit-site infection of peritoneal dialysis catheter.

fluid effluent white blood cell (WBC) count > 100/μL [with > 50% polymorphonuclear (PMN) leukocytes]; and a positive culture from PD effluent. The common organisms causing PD peritonitis are gram-positive organisms like *Staphylococcus aureus*, coagulase-negative *Staphylococcus*; gram-negative organisms like *Pseudomonas*, *Escherichia coli*; and other rarer organisms like fungi or mycobacteria.

The treatment of peritonitis involves early administration of antibiotics. Intraperitoneal (IP) is the preferred route of administration, except in cases of severe sepsis or shock, where intravenous antibiotics are preferred. Empirical antibiotic therapy [generally consisting of a third-generation cephalosporin (like ceftazidime) with an antistaphylococcal agent like vancomycin] may be initiated as soon as possible, which can further be modified after the culture reports.

Gram-positive organisms are treated by a first-generation cephalosporin or vancomycin (15–30 mg/kg every 5–7 days) and gram-negative organisms by a third-generation cephalosporin (ceftazidime 1,000–1,500 mg daily) or an aminoglycoside (amikacin 2 mg/kg daily). Carbapenems (meropenem 1,000 mg daily) and antifungals may be used in refractory cases. The recommended duration of therapy is for 2–4 weeks depending on the type of organism.

Peritoneal dialysis catheter should be removed for refractory (defined by the failure of resolution of peritonitis after 5 days of appropriate antibiotics), relapsing (infection caused by the same organism as the original infection occurring within 4 weeks), tubercular, and fungal peritonitis.

Exit-site Infection

Exit-site infection is characterized by erythema and swelling with discharge coming from the exit site, as shown in **Figure 4B**. It may or may not be accompanied by an infection of the tunnel space, known as tunnel infection. *S. aureus* is the most prevalent infection-causing agent. A minimum of 2 weeks of treatment with gram-positive covering antibiotics is advised, with 3 weeks being advised in case of *Pseudomonas* infections.

Ultrafiltration Failure

Ultrafiltration failure (UFF) is characterized by reduced functioning of PD leading to ultrafiltration volume <400 mL after a dwell time of 4 hours with 2.5% dextrose fluid. It presents with a reduced ultrafiltrate leading to fluid overload. This condition may be of different types.

Type 1 UFF occurs due to a hyperpermeable peritoneum causing a high solute transport leading to a more rapid diffusion of solute across the membrane, while type 2 UFF occurs due to aquaporin dysfunction leading to high average transport. In patients on long-term PD, the peritoneum undergoes both structural and functional changes with time, owing to exposure to hyperosmolar glucose solution. This leads to type 3 UFF, causing a low solute transport. Management of UFF consists of alteration of PD prescriptions, use of APD cyclers or, ultimately, shifting the patients to hemodialysis.

Encapsulating Peritoneal Sclerosis

Encapsulating peritoneal sclerosis is a rare but serious PD complication, in which the bowel and intraperitoneal contents are covered by a thick cocoon of fibrous tissue, causing intestinal obstruction. This requires stopping PD and surgical modalities like adhesiolysis.

Mechanical Problems

Mechanical complications of PD include pericatheter leaks and hernias, infusion and drain pain, flow failure, catheter tip migration, and superficial cuff extrusion. Catheter tip migration leads to movement of tip to right or left upper quadrants of the abdomen leading to poor inflow or outflow. In rare cases, especially in children, omentum may wrap the CAPD catheter leading to mechanical obstruction and floor CAPD flow. These mechanical problems often require surgical management by open or laparoscopic repair, and repositioning of PD catheter.

CONCLUSION

Peritoneal dialysis offers a 'home-based' RRT. There is no requirement for a permanent vascular access. It avoids any chances of blood-borne or cross infections. It is particularly useful in infants and young children, patients with cardiac comorbidities, hypotension, or those having inadequate access to hemodialysis facilities. Even though the overall mortality of patients on PD compared with hemodialysis is not significantly different, but the quality of life and patient satisfaction are better with PD compared to hemodialysis.

SUGGESTED READINGS

1. Blake PG, Daugirdas JT, Ing TS (Eds). Physiology of Peritoneal Dialysis. Handbook of Dialysis, 5th edition. Philadelphia: Lippincott Williams & Wilkins; 2015. pp. 392-407.
2. Peritoneal Dialysis Adequacy Work Group. Clinical practice guidelines for peritoneal dialysis adequacy. Am J Kidney Dis. 2006;48(Suppl 1):S98-129.
3. Li PK, Chow KM, Cho Y, Fan S, Figueiredo AE, Harris T, et al. ISPD peritonitis guideline recommendations: 2022 update on prevention and treatment. Perit Dial Int. 2022;42(2):110-53.

SECTION

14

NEUROLOGY

185

CHAPTER

Approach to a Case of Coma

S Chiranth, Geeta Kampani

ABSTRACT

Coma is a medical emergency commonly encountered in the emergency room. It represents a severe derangement in cerebral function due to structural or nonstructural causes. Most of the underlying processes leading to coma can be life-threatening. Some of these are reversible following timely institution of medical or surgical therapy. It mandates a structured evaluation for the potential reversible etiology of coma.

INTRODUCTION

Coma is a neurologic emergency characterized by alteration of sensorium. There is a continuum of states of decreased responsiveness with multiple terminologies as follows:

- *Stupor*: It is a state of altered consciousness in which a patient can be aroused by vigorous repeated stimulation.
- *Catatonia*: It is a severe psychomotor syndrome associated with pathognomonic features such as verbigeration and waxy flexibility.
- *Vegetative state*: It is a chronic state of lack of cognitive function which occurs after brain injury or on recovery from coma. When this state persists for several months, the prognosis becomes poor and after 1 year is almost nil. This state is termed as persistent vegetative state.
- *Akinetic mutism*: It refers to partially or fully awake patient able to think but akinetic and occurs due to lesions in medial thalamic nuclei, frontal lobes, or massive hydrocephalus.
- *Locked in syndrome*: It is characterized by awake, mute, and immobile patient due to transection of corticospinal and corticobulbar fibers seen in hemorrhage in the bilateral ventral pons and in basilar artery thrombosis. Vertical eye movements and lid elevation remain intact.

ETIOLOGY OF COMA (BOX 1)

Consciousness is a function of the ascending reticular activating system (ARAS) and its connections. Any injury involving the ARAS or its cortical connections can alter the level of consciousness. These may be:

- Lesions involving the upper pons and midbrain
- Diffuse bilateral or large unilateral cerebral lesions
- Toxic, infectious, or metabolic etiologies that impair oxygen or substrate delivery that leads to alteration in cerebral metabolism

HISTORY

- *Time course of loss of consciousness*:
  - Abrupt—seizure/subarachnoid hemorrhage (SAH)
  - Gradual—intracranial space occupying lesion
  - Fluctuating—subdural hemorrhage (SDH) and metabolic encephalopathy
- *Associated clinical features*:
  - Headache and vomiting—intracranial hemorrhage (ICH) and infection
  - Visual symptoms—posterior reversible encephalopathy syndrome
  - Motor deficits—structural lesions
  - Fever—infection and ICH

BOX 1: Causes of coma.

Causes with normal imaging studies and no focal neurological deficit:
- Intoxications: Alcohol and sedatives
- Metabolic disturbances: Uremia, hepatic coma, dyselectrolytemia, diabetic ketoacidosis, and hypoglycemia,
- Shock
- Posterior reversible encephalopathy syndrome and eclampsia
- Severe hypothermia and hyperthermia
- Postseizure states and status epilepticus
- Severe systemic infections

Causes with meningeal irritation and CSF abnormality: Imaging shows no mass lesion:
- Meningitis and encephalitis
- Subarachnoid hemorrhage
- Cholesterol and fat embolism

Causes with abnormal imaging, with or without CSF abnormality:
- Cerebrovascular accident
- Brain abscess
- Massive bilateral cerebral injury
- Intracranial space occupying lesion
- Metabolic causes with coexisting focal brain damage
- Sagittal sinus thrombosis
- CNS vasculitis
- Miscellaneous: Viral encephalitis

(CNS: central nervous system; CSF: cerebrospinal fluid)

- History of preceding fall—SDH
- Recent confusion or delirium—metabolic or toxic cause
- Comorbid illness—diabetes mellitus and hypertension

PHYSICAL EXAMINATION

Hyperthermia

- Infections—cerebral malaria and meningoencephalitis
- Vascular—pontine hemorrhage
- Metabolic—thyrotoxicosis
- Toxic—salicylate and belladonna poisoning
- Heat stroke
- Neuroleptic malignant syndrome

Hypothermia

- Toxic—barbiturate and phenothiazine poisoning
- Metabolic—myxedema coma
- Circulatory failure
- Hypothermia per se can cause coma

Respiratory Patterns

- *Cheyne-Stokes respiration*: Characterized by apneic spells followed by hyperpnea and it is seen in bilateral cerebral hemisphere lesion or bilateral thalamic lesion.
- *Kussmaul breathing*: Seen in metabolic or pontomesencephalic lesion.
- *Apneustic breathing*: Characterized by long inspiratory pause following which air is retained for several seconds and then released it is seen in lower pontine lesions.
- *Agonal gasps*: It indicates a terminal state seen in brainstem lesions.

Bradycardia

- Heart block
- Raised intracranial pressure
- Inferior wall myocardial infarction
- Myxedema coma

Hypertension

- Hypertensive encephalopathy
- Intracranial bleed
- Head injury

Hypotension

- Acute coronary syndrome
- Myxedema coma
- Addisonian crisis
- Sepsis

Skin Discoloration

- *Petechiae—bleeding diathesis associated with*:
  - Intracerebral bleed
  - Meningococcemia
  - Staphylococcal endocarditis
  - Rickettsial infections
- Jaundice—seen in liver disease
- Reddish discoloration—seen in carbon monoxide poisoning
- Cyanosis—seen in circulatory failure and CO_2 narcosis

Odor of Breath

- Burnt almond odor—cyanide poisoning
- Musky/fecal odor—hepatic coma
- Ammoniacal odor—uremia
- Acetone breath—diabetic ketoacidosis
- Alcohol intoxication

FUNDUS EXAMINATION

- Papilledema
- Hypertensive changes
- Retinal hemorrhages

NEUROLOGIC EXAMINATION

The neurologic examination in a comatose patient is done to determine whether the etiology is structural or due to a metabolic dysfunction. It is done under the following headings:

- Level of consciousness
- Motor responses
- Brainstem reflexes

Level of Consciousness

Level of consciousness is assessed by:

- *Glasgow coma scale (GCS)*:
  - It is a useful index to assess the severity of coma and for prognosis but is not useful in ascertaining the etiology of coma and in assessment of mild impairment of consciousness.
- *Full Outline of UnResponsiveness (FOUR)*:
  - It is more recent scoring system which has advantages in intubated patients wherein scoring is done under categories such as eye response, motor response, brainstem reflexes, and intubation.

Motor Examination

Motor examination involves assessment of posturing, muscle tone, power, and reflexes.

Posturing

- *Decorticate posturing*: Suggestive of lesion rostral to midbrain
- *Decerebrate posturing*: Suggestive of lesion below the red nucleus

Muscle tone is usually not affected by most metabolic conditions. Bilateral rigidity can be seen in neuroleptic malignant syndrome, malignant hyperthermia, and hepatic coma. Multifocal myoclonus is suggestive of metabolic/toxic etiology. Asterixis and tremors are suggestive of metabolic/toxic encephalopathy.

Pupils

Disruption of the pupillary light reflex in patients with coma occurs because of either:

- Primary midbrain involvement
- Oculomotor nerve compression due to herniation

Pinpoint pupils can be seen in opioid poisoning and pontine tegmentum lesions. Anticholinergic and sympathomimetic poisoning produce dilated pupils. Pupils are usually spared in metabolic conditions.

Ocular Movements

Central structures involved in extraocular movements lie in the brainstem and are controlled by the frontal eye fields. According to the dictum *"the eyes look toward a cortical lesion and away from a brainstem lesion"*, large cerebral lesions produce a persistent conjugate deviation of eyes toward the side of lesion whereas pontine lesions result in deviation of the opposite side. Irritative lesions usually results in deviation of the eye to the opposite side of the lesion. Downward and medial deviation of the eyeballs is typical of a thalamic bleed.

Ocular Bobbing

Rapid vertical downward movement with slow upward return that are seen in bilateral brainstem lesion. No horizontal eye movements are seen.

Ocular Dipping

Slow downward movement of eyeballs with fast upward return with normal horizontal movements that occur due to diffuse cortical hypoxic damage.

In patients with coma, complete bilateral conjugate roving eye movements usually indicate an intact brainstem. In their absence, horizontal eye movements can be tested with vestibulo-ocular reflexes (VOR).

Brainstem Reflexes

Oculocephalic Reflexes (Doll's Eyes)

Cervical spine fractures should be ruled out before performing oculocephalic maneuver. In the oculocephalic maneuver, the head is rotated abruptly from one side to the other in the horizontal plane. When the oculocephalic reflex is present, the eyes do not turn with the head but in the opposite direction as if the patient is maintaining fixation on a single point. This reflex is usually absent in conscious patients. Absence of doll's eye reflex indicates brain stem involvement.

Oculovestibular Reflex (Caloric Testing)

The test is performed by irrigating the external auditory canal with cold water. After a brief latency, it causes a tonic deviation of both eyes to the side of cold water irrigation and nystagmus toward the opposite side. In comatose patients with brainstem lesions, nystagmus may not occur. This can be remembered by the acronym "COWS" for the direction of nystagmus, cold water opposite and warm water same side. However, this does not always hold true as nystagmus may also be seen toward the opposite direction in frontal lobe lesions with no brainstem involvement.

Corneal Reflex

The corneal reflex's afferent limb is comprised by the trigeminal nerve and nucleus with the interneurons then activating bilateral facial nuclei in the pons resulting in contraction of both orbicularis oculi. Connections with the oculomotor nucleus cause the eyelids to move upward along with closure of eyelids.

Pontine function can be assessed by examining for spontaneous and reflex eye movements and corneal reflex. Medullary function can be assessed by respiratory and pharyngeal responses. Conjugate reflex horizontal movements are dependent on the medial longitudinal fasciculus (MLF) interconnecting the sixth and contralateral third nerve nuclei.

INVESTIGATIONS

- Complete hemogram
- Metabolic profile
- Microbiological profile
- Radiological investigations
- Electroencephalogram (EEG)
- Cerebrospinal fluid (CSF)
- Toxicological analysis

Metabolic Profile

- Blood profile
- Renal function
- Serum electrolytes
- Liver function tests
- Serum ammonia
- Arterial blood gas (ABG)
- Thyroid function tests
- Serum cortisol

Microbiological Investigations

- Malarial antigen and peripheral smear (PS) for malarial parasite
- Blood culture and sensitivity
- Urine culture and sensitivity
- CSF Gram-stain and culture sensitivity
- CSF Ziehl–Neelsen (ZN) staining and tuberculosis (TB) polymerase chain reaction (PCR)
- CSF viral studies

Electroencephalogram Testing

- Diagnostic in herpes encephalitis
- Creutzfeldt–Jakob disease

Radiological Investigations

- CT useful in detecting hemorrhage, tumor, or hydrocephalus
- MRI is highly sensitive in acute ischemic stroke, cerebral venous sinus thrombosis, cerebral edema, and diffuse axonal injury

MANAGEMENT

- GCS ≤ 8, hypoxemia, vomiting, or poor cough/gag reflex requires endotracheal intubation to protect airway.
- In any case of unknown poisoning, a trial of dextrose 25 g is warranted. In case of any malnourished patient, thiamine should be given with or before dextrose infusion.
- In cases of suspected toxin ingestion/drug poisoning presented early to the emergency, gastric lavage can be done.
- In patients with a strong suspicion of raised intracranial tension or herniation, mannitol (1 g/kg IV) can be administered.
- In cases of hyperthermia, temperatures should be reduced with antipyretics and immediate cooling.
- Empirical antibiotic and antiviral therapy in suspected infective meningoencephalitis.

Definitive therapy depends on establishment of the diagnosis.

PROGNOSIS

This depends on the etiology and the severity of coma. Coma due to structural causes, the nature of the lesions and the rapidity with which it is corrected are important determinants of prognosis. Coma due to metabolic causes are usually reversible unless associated with hypoxic brain damage.

SUGGESTED READINGS

1. Cooksley T, Rose S, Holland M. A systematic approach to the unconscious patient. Clin Med (Lond). 2018;18(1):88-92.
2. Zakaria Z, Abdullah MM, Halim SA, Ghani ARI, Idris Z, Abdullah JM. The Neurological Exam of a Comatose Patient. An Essential Pratical Guide. Malays J Med Sci. 2020;27(5):108-23.
3. Loscalzo J, Fauci A, Kasper D, Hauser S, Longo D, Jameson J. Harrison's Principles of Internal Medicine, 21st edition. New York: McGraw Hill; 2022.
4. Schmidt WU, Ploner CJ, Lutz M, Mockel M, Lindner T, Braun M. Causes of brain dysfunction in acute coma: a cohort study of 1027 patients in the emergency department. Scand J Trauma Resusc Emerg Med. 2019;27(1)101.

186

CHAPTER

Acute Encephalitis Syndrome: An Update

Anupam Dey

ABSTRACT

Acute encephalitis syndrome (AES) is characterized by acute onset of fever with alteration in consciousness. In India, AES is primarily caused by the Japanese encephalitis (JE) virus. It can have various infectious and noninfectious etiologies. The first AES case in India case was reported in the state of Tamil Nadu in 1955. India launched a JE vaccination program in 2006, which was integrated with the national immunization program in 2014. Approach to the patient should include a thorough general and neurological examination and relevant investigations including infectious screen as well as neuroimaging. Early suspicion and diagnosis are very important. Management aims at providing general support for various systemic complications as well as specific therapies wherever available.

INTRODUCTION

Acute encephalitis syndrome (AES) has been defined by the World Health Organization (WHO) as an illness in a person of any age at any time of year characterized by acute onset of fever with alteration in consciousness ranging from stupor to coma and/or new-onset convulsion excluding simple febrile seizure. In India, AES is primarily caused by the Japanese encephalitis (JE) virus, mostly among children. It can cause case fatality and lifelong sequelae among survivors.

DEFINITION OF ACUTE ENCEPHALITIS SYNDROME

The International Encephalitis Consortium (IEC) in 2013 provided a consensus definition for presumed acute encephalitis which includes major and minor criteria as given in **Table 1**.

EPIDEMIOLOGY OF ACUTE ENCEPHALITIS SYNDROME IN INDIA

The first AES case in India case was reported in the state of Tamil Nadu in 1955. It has now become endemic in 171 districts of 19 states of India. The first major JE virus epidemic was reported in West Bengal in 1973 (700 cases and 300 deaths). In 1978, Uttar Pradesh reported an epidemic during October and November with 1,100

TABLE 1: Major and minor criteria according to the International Encephalitis Consortium (IEC) in 2013.

Major criteria: Altered mental status for >24 hours without an alternative cause	*Possible AES:* Presence of major and two minor criteria
Minor criteria: • Fever > 38°C • New-onset focal neurological findings. • CSF pleocytosis > 5 cells/mm³ • Brain imaging showing parenchymal changes • Electroencephalography findings consistent with encephalitis	*Probable AES:* Presence of major criteria with three or more minor criteria
	Definite AES: If there is microbiological evidence of organism, or CSF evidence of autoimmune encephalitis, or pathological changes on biopsy

(AES: acute encephalitis syndrome; CSF: cerebrospinal fluid) deaths. A significant outbreak was recorded in Gorakhpur district of UP in 2005 affecting 6,061 cases with 1,500 deaths. State of Bihar, particularly the Muzaffarpur district, has been reporting cases of acute encephalitis among children since 1995. Malkangiri in Odisha state had an outbreak in early September 2016 accounting for 325 AES cases including 91 deaths. India launched a JE vaccination program in 2006, which was integrated with the National immunization program in 2014.

SURVEILLANCE OF ACUTE ENCEPHALITIS SYNDROME

Japanese encephalitis mass immunization campaign was launched in 2006 in 11 districts (endemic regions) of India. In the same year, a national-level AES surveillance guideline was developed by National Vector Borne Disease Control Programme (NVBDCP) for reporting of AES cases and suspected or confirmed JE cases. This led to a finding of other non-JE AES etiologies such as enterovirus, dengue virus, scrub typhus, and other viral, bacterial, and rickettsial etiologies **(Table 2)**.

TABLE 2: Etiology of AES.

Infectious	Noninfectious
Viral: • **Arbovirus:** Japanese encephalitis, Dengue, West Nile encephalitis, Equine encephalitis • **Herpes:** Herpes simplex virus I and II, Varicella zoster, Epstein-Barr, Cytomegalovirus, Human herpes virus 6 • **Myxo and paramyxovirus:** Influenza, measles, mumps, parainfluenza, Nipah virus • **Adeno, parvovirus**	**Inflammatory diseases:** • Acute disseminated encephalomyelitis • Autoimmune encephalitis • Vasculitis • Behcet's disease
Bacterial: • Pyogenic meningitis • Tuberculous meningitis • Leptospira • *Salmonella* • Lyme, Borrelia • *Listeria, Mycoplasma*	**Metabolic toxic encephalopathy:** • Electrolyte imbalance • Hepatic coma, uremic coma • Diabetic ketoacidosis • Hyperosmolar coma • Septic encephalopathy • Toxins induced (lead, mercury)
Rickettsial: • Scrub typhus, Endemic and epidemic typhus, Rocky Mountain spotted fever	**Drug induced**
Fungal: • *Candida*, Cryptococcal, Coccidioidomycosis	**Mitochondrial encephalopathy**
Protozoal: • *Acanthamoeba, Naegleria, Toxoplasma*	
Parasitic: • Malaria, cysticercosis, *Toxoplasma*	

(AES: acute encephalitis syndrome)

DESCRIPTION OF MAJOR AES-CAUSING INFECTIOUS AGENTS

Herpes Simplex Encephalitis

Herpes simplex encephalitis (HSE) occurs due to two viruses: HSV-1 an HSV-2. HSE is a complication of HSV-1 infection and is the most common sporadic focal encephalitis worldwide. Primarily a disease of adults, it has no seasonal variation or gender preference. HSE typically localizes to medial temporal and orbitofrontal cortex.

Clinical Features

Disease course ranges from insidious to a fulminant. Fever and headache are common early symptoms. Seizures can occur in up to 70% of patients. Focal neurological symptoms such as hemiparesis, aphasia, ocular and sensory disturbances can be found. Personality changes and behavioral alterations such as fear and hallucination can be seen.

Diagnosis

Cerebrospinal fluid (CSF) analysis reveals mononuclear pleocytosis (100–200/mm^3), elevated CSF protein (up to 500 mg/dL) and low or normal glucose level. HSV nucleic acid can be detected in CSF using polymerase chain reaction (PCR) in the first week, and IgM enzyme-linked immunosorbent assay (ELISA) in the second week and beyond. Electroencephalography (EEG) may show focal or generalized slowing, and sharp waves in temporal lobe distribution. Magnetic resonance imaging (MRI) shows T2 hyperintensity in medial temporal and basifrontal regions.

Treatment

Acyclovir in a dose of 10 mg/kg IV 8 hourly for 2–3 weeks: Treatment of seizure, status epilepticus, and raised intracranial pressure is vital. Corticosteroids have no proven benefit.

Japanese Encephalitis

It was first reported from Tokyo (Japan) in 1933 and since being primarily reported from the Asian countries. Epidemics occur mainly during the post-monsoon period related to rainfall, flooding, paddy cultivation, pig farming, and mosquito breeding. It is transmitted by infected female *Culex* mosquitoes with humans being dead-end host. Pigs are the amplifying host. *Culex tritaeniorhynchus* is the most efficient vector. The incubation period of JEV is 6–16 days. Children are commonly affected while adults are usually spared due to herd immunity. Subclinical infection is common.

Clinical Features

There are three stages: Prodromal, encephalitis, and convalescent phases. The prodromal stage is characterized by fever (up to 40°C), headache, anorexia, nausea, and vomiting. The encephalitic stage is characterized by features ranging from headache, behavioral abnormalities, seizures, and focal deficits to altered sensorium and deep coma. Seizures commonly occur in children and may be focal or secondary generalized types. Focal deficits such as hemiplegia, quadriplegia, wasting, and cerebellar involvement can be found. In the convalescent stage movement disorders can be seen such as tremor, choreoathetosis, and dystonias.

Diagnosis

Cerebrospinal fluid reveals pleocytosis (10–200/mm^3), elevated proteins, and normal glucose. Diagnosis can be confirmed by reverse transcriptase PCR in CSF or IgM ELISA. MRI imaging reveals thalamic involvement commonly, followed by mid-brain, basal ganglia, and brainstem involvement.

Dengue

Dengue virus is an RNA virus transmitted by bite of infected *Aedes aegypti* mosquito. The disease manifests with fever, headache, myalgia, arthralgia, retro-orbital pain, conjunctival congestion, nausea, and vomiting. Rash may be seen. Severe dengue fever can manifest with thrombocytopenia, mucosal bleeding, hemorrhagic manifestations, and evidence of plasma leakage (ascites, pleural effusion, pericardial effusion, interstitial edema, and pulmonary edema). Thrombocytopenia, coagulopathy, increased vascular permeability, and complement activation are pathophysiological mechanisms of complications.

Clinical Features

Neurological involvement in dengue can be seen in the form of dengue encephalopathy, dengue encephalitis, and immune-mediated syndromes. Dengue encephalopathy presents with altered sensorium, behavioral abnormality, and seizures. Laboratory investigations usually reveal normal CSF study and general slowing in EEG. Dengue encephalitis presents similarly to dengue encephalopathy with higher incidence of seizures. Brain imaging in dengue is usually normal. Immune-mediated syndromes such as Guillain–Barré syndrome, transverse myelitis, and acute disseminated encephalomyelitis (ADEM) can be found in dengue.

Diagnosis

It is based on detection of NS1 antigen in early stage and IgM ELISA after 5–7 days. The management of severe dengue infection requires tertiary level care, proper fluid management, management of raised intracranial pressure (ICP), seizures, dyselectrolytemia, blood sugars, and other vital support.

Chikungunya

It is an arboviral disease which spreads by *Aedes* mosquitoes. Neurological manifestations are rare but encephalitis has been reported. Immune-mediated syndromes including Guillain–Barré syndrome, transverse myelitis, and myoclonus have been reported. CSF in CHIK infection is usually normal. MRI is either normal or reveals nonspecific changes. The diagnosis of CHIK is done by detection of viral RNA by RT-PCR and IgM antibodies by ELISA.

West Nile Virus Encephalitis

West Nile virus is prevalent in Africa, America, Middle-East, and Asia. It spreads by the bite of *Culex* mosquitoes. Neurological illness is rare and manifests with meningitis, encephalitis, and acute flaccid paralysis. Patients may have fever, neck rigidity, myoclonus, Parkinsonian features, seizures, and altered sensorium. Cranial nerve palsies, optic neuritis, and polyradiculopathy are other possible manifestations.

Diagnosis

Cerebrospinal fluid shows lymphocytic pleocytosis (<150 cells/mm^3), elevated protein (<500 mg/dL), and normal glucose. Detection of IgM antibody in serum or in CSF using IgM antibody capture ELISA are diagnostic tests.

PCR is useful in the diagnosis. MRI brain may reveal FLAIR hyperintensity in brainstem, thalamus, basal ganglia, or spinal cord. There is no specific antiviral treatment. Patients are treated symptomatically.

Scrub Typhus

A rickettsial disease is transmitted by the bite of trombiculid mite. It affects various organs such as liver, kidney, lungs, and brain. Neurological manifestations include meningitis, encephalitis, intracranial hemorrhage, demyelination syndromes such as transverse myelitis and cranial nerve palsy.

Diagnosis

Demonstration of IgM antibodies and a four-fold rise in paired sera provide definite evidence. Weil–Felix agglutination test, immunofluorescence assay (IFA), and ELISA can be used.

EXAMINATION OF THE PATIENT WITH ACUTE ENCEPHALITIS SYNDROME

- Assessment of airway, breathing, circulation, neurologic disability including Glasgow Coma Scale (GCS)
- General physical examination—pallor, icterus, skin rashes, parotid swelling, herpes labialis, orchitis, bite marks, and lymphadenopathy
- Systemic examination—Hepatosplenomegaly, lymphadenopathy
- Neurological examination—level of consciousness, pupils, signs of raised intracranial tension, signs of meningeal irritation, focal neurologic deficit, flaccid paralysis, evidence of seizures, and movement disorders

GENERAL INVESTIGATIONS FOR ACUTE ENCEPHALITIS SYNDROME

Following investigations are generally required:
- Complete blood count, electrolytes/blood glucose, liver and kidney function tests, blood culture, and chest X-ray, ABG, and plasma lactate
- CSF analysis (if no contraindications)
- Neuroimaging studies
- EEG in event of seizure or suspicion of nonconvulsive status epilepticus (NCSE) or autoimmune encephalitis (AE)
- Workup for specific infectious etiologies
- Autoimmune workup (if infectious etiologies are negative)—antinuclear antibody (ANA), erythrocyte sedimentation rate (ESR), neuromyelitis optica (NMO) and myelin oligodendrocyte glycoprotein (MOG IgG), and antineuronal antibodies [N-methyl-D-aspartate (NMDA) receptor, voltage-gated potassium channel (VGKC)]

NEUROIMAGING IN ACUTE ENCEPHALITIS SYNDROME

Magnetic resonance imaging is preferred over computed tomography (CT) as it is more sensitive.

Specific areas involved:
- *Medial temporal, orbito-frontal, insular*: HSV
- *Basal ganglia/thalamus*: Japanese encephalitis, West Nile
- *Brainstem and spinal cord (anterior horn cells)*: Enterovirus

GENERAL MANAGEMENT PRINCIPLES

Goals of management are initial stabilization, reaching a specific diagnosis and preventing significant brain injury and sequelae. Red flag features of raised intracranial pressure, status epilepticus, and shock will need critical care support. Supportive care includes maintaining proper hydration, normal sugars, and preventing dyselectrolytemia. Hyperthermia should be avoided. Secondary infections should be treated promptly. Rehabilitation for neurological sequelae should also be given due importance.

Immunotherapy: Steroids are used in ADEM, Hashimoto encephalopathy, and autoimmune encephalitis. Pulse steroids can be given initially followed with low dose oral prednisolone (1–2 mg/kg/day) to taper over 4–6 weeks. Intravenous immunoglobulin (IVIG) is used in ADEM. Plasmapheresis is another first-line treatment option for immune-mediated encephalitis with 5–7 exchanges every other day showing favorable outcome. Other immunosuppressants such as rituximab or cyclophosphamide should be considered in immune-mediated encephalitis, which is refractory to steroid, intravenous immunoglobulin (IVIG) and plasmapheresis.

CONCLUSION

Acute encephalitis syndrome is a potentially serious condition. It has varied etiologies. Neurological deficits and sequelae are causes of concern. Early suspicion and diagnosis are very important. Management aims at providing general support for various systemic complications as well as specific therapies wherever available. With expansion of laboratory investigations and neuroimaging facilities, management of AES should be early and proper.

SUGGESTED READINGS

1. Venkatesan A, Tunkel AR, Bloch KC, Lauring AS, Sejvar J, Bitnun A, et al. Case definitions, diagnostic algorithms, and priorities in encephalitis: Consensus statement of the international encephalitis consortium Clin Infect Dis. 2013;57:1114-2.
2. Misra UK, Kalita J. Changing spectrum of acute encephalitis syndrome in India and a syndromic approach. Ann Indian Acad Neurol. 2022;25(3):354-66.
3. Narain JP, Dhariwal AC, MacIntyre CR. Acute encephalitis in India: An unfolding tragedy. Indian J Med Res. 2017;145(5): 584-7.
4. Banerjee B, Hafis M, Acharya U. Acute encephalitis syndrome: Approach to a changing paradigm. Pediatr Inf Dis. 2019;1(3): 86-94.

187

CHAPTER

Evolving Spectrum of Autoimmune Encephalitis

Nalini Humaney

ABSTRACT

Autoimmune encephalitis (AE) represents an array of diseases occurring when the healthy brain cells are being attacked erroneously by the body's immune system resulting in inflammation. It is at least as common as infectious encephalitis. It includes two major categories: (1) Paraneoplastic (always cancer-related) refers to a condition associated exclusively with cancer, where antibodies target antigens located within cells, and (2) autoimmune (may or may not be cancer-related) refers to a condition that can be either cancer-related or unrelated, where antibodies specifically target antigens present on the surface of cells, and distinction is important between these two entities because antibodies against cell surface cause reversible neuronal dysfunction and show good response to treatment. This condition is marked by noticeable neuropsychiatric symptoms, cognitive decline, movement disorders, and seizures. It is attributed to the presence of antibodies that target neuronal cell surface proteins, ion channels, or receptors. Owing to the inadequacy of diagnostic anomalies on investigations [such as magnetic resonance imaging (MRI) brain, electroencephalogram (EEG), and cerebrospinal fluid (CSF) study] in subgroups of patients and varied clinical presentations including psychiatric manifestation, it can be challenging to diagnose AE. An early diagnosis and timely treatment with short- or long-term immunotherapy can improve the outcome and help the patient to recover from a debilitating and sometimes life-threatening condition.

INTRODUCTION

Historical Perspective

In 2004, young women presented with acute behavioral disturbances and were labeled as encephalitis of unknown etiology. In 2005, such similar states of agitation and psychosis were observed in four young women with ovarian teratomas. In 2007, synaptic protein N-methyl-D aspartate receptor (NMDAR) antibodies and in 2010 autoantibodies against extracellular proteins LGI1 and CASPR2 were detected. The most prevalent noninfectious form of encephalitis, autoimmune encephalitis (AE) is brought on by autoantibodies that target intracellular antigens, such as onconeural antigen, or synaptic surface components, such as surface protein, receptors, and ionic channels. Due to the ongoing discovery of several neuronal autoantibodies that target the extracellular domain of neurological proteins during the past 15 years, the spectrum of AE has grown, and its prevalence is predicted to be similar to that of infectious encephalitis.

EPIDEMIOLOGY

Due to variable presentation and numerous diagnostic antibodies, data on AE is under-reported. An incidence of between 0.7 and 12.6% has been reported in adults, with studies showing that anti-NMDAR encephalitis is the most common form of AE to date. About 80% of those with AE were female, with onset at a median age of 21 years and 30% had underlying malignancies, primarily ovarian teratomas.

PATHOPHYSIOLOGY

In AE, the exact mechanism to immune tolerance collapse is unknown till date. There are two types of antibodies: (1) extracellular against synaptic surface protein (e.g.,

NMDAR, LGI1, AMPAR) and (2) intracellular cytoplasmic (YO, CV2/CRMP5) or nuclear Hubris onconeural antigen. By facilitating the crosstalk between peripheral adaptive immunity and central nervous system (CNS) innate immunity, these circulating neuronal autoantibodies damage the CNS via the inflamed blood–brain barrier and in turn lead to breakdown of immune tolerance. Immune triggers to pathogenesis are tumors, infections (herpes simplex, varicella zoster, mycoplasma), human leukocyte antigen (HLA) class II antigens, or unknown.

CLINICAL SPECTRUM

A variety of clinical features can be observed, depending on the specific neuronal antigen and brain area targeted during the autoimmune reaction. It is of subacute onset with rapid progression, behavioral changes, intractable seizures, decline in memory and cognitive defect, abnormal movements, dysautonomia, and decreased level of consciousness. In NMDA encephalitis, 80% of patients have psychiatric presentation. Strange behaviors, symptoms of mania or depression, agitation, anxiety, and hallucinations are common. These often respond poorly to antipsychotic medications with higher incidence of adverse effects. If the presenting feature is seizure, they are usually intractable and resistant to antiepileptic medications. In late stages of disease, movement disorders like orofacial dyskinesia, dystonia, chorea, tremor, myoclonic jerks, and cerebellar ataxia are seen. The presence of motor-facial dystonic seizures affecting both the face and the limbs at the same time strongly suggests an anti-LGI1 encephalitis. Anti-GLyR encephalitis manifests as progressive encephalomyelitis which is usually accompanied by rigidity and myoclonus. Myokymia and neuromyotonia are seen in anti-CASPR2 encephalitis and opsoclonus myoclonus in anti-GABA-B encephalitis. Cognitive impairment (memory deficit, executive function, apraxia, rapid deterioration of long-term and short-term memory) is seen with inadequate or delayed treatment. Sleep disorder is not a common feature. However, sleep-related problems/sleep disorder can be a presenting feature in immunoglobulin-like cell adhesion molecule 5 (IgLON5) encephalitis. **Flowchart 1** shows clinical features in different types of autoimmune encephalitis.

WHEN TO SUSPECT AUTOIMMUNE ENCEPHALITIS?

Adapted Criteria for Possible Diagnosis of AE

1. Subacute onset within 3 months with psychiatric symptoms or change in the level of consciousness or memory impairment and

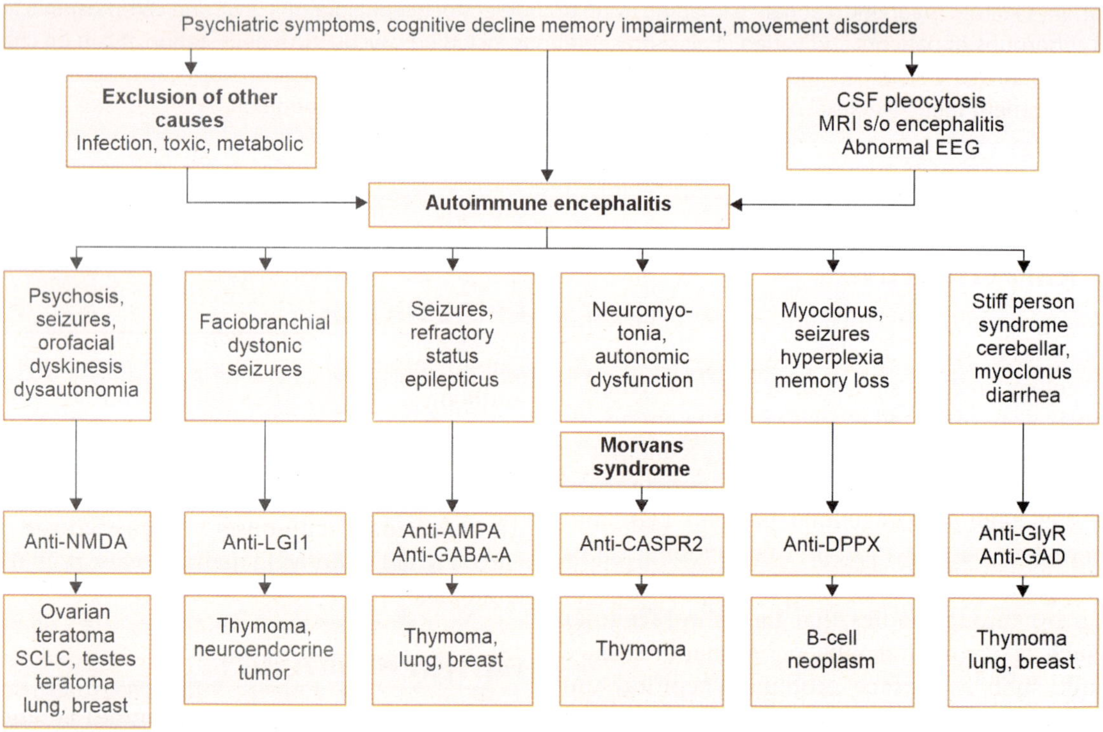

FLOWCHART 1: Different types of autoimmune encephalitis.
(CSF: cerebrospinal fluid)

2. *At least one of the following*:
Seizures not explained by a previously diagnosed seizure disorder:
   - New focal clinical CNS findings
   - Magnetic resonance imaging (MRI) brain findings suggestive of encephalitis
   - Cerebrospinal fluid (CSF) pleocytosis [>5 white blood cells (WBC)/mm^3]
3. With exclusion of other causes

All the above three criteria must be met.

To *definitively diagnose autoimmune limbic encephalitis*, the following criteria should be met:

1. Symptoms with a subacute onset (occurring within a period of <3 months), involving the limbic system and characterized by memory deficits, neuropsychiatric symptoms, or seizures.
2. T2 weighted FLAIR brain imaging should reveal a specific abnormality confined to both the medial temporal lobes.
3. Presence of either of the following findings:
   - Electroencephalogram (EEG) showing patterns consistent with slow-wave or epileptic activity in the temporal lobes
   - CSF analysis demonstrating pleocytosis, with a white blood cell count >5 WBC/mm^3
4. Reasonable exclusion of alternative causes: Infectious meningoencephalitis, septic encephalopathy, metabolic encephalopathy

The above four criteria are required for definitive diagnosis of limbic encephalitis.

If one of the above four criteria is not matched, then a definitive diagnosis can be made if there is presence of antibodies against cell surface protein in both serum and CSF.

DIAGNOSIS

A wide spectrum of clinical presentations makes it challenging to diagnose this condition as symptoms usually begin between a few weeks and 3 months after onset; also, MRI brain rarely shows diagnostic abnormalities, EEG changes are nonspecific, and immunoglobulin G (IgG) neuronal autoantibodies cannot be identified in blood or CSF.

- *Paired CSF and serum antibody assay*: In order to diagnose encephalitis associated with neuronal surface antibodies, CSF IgG antineuronal antibodies must be detected and can provide important insight into the course of the disease, management, and prognosis. In the anti-LGI1 subtype, antibodies are more positive in serum than in CSF. Among all the NMDAR encephalitis patients with antibodies found in CSF, 14% had no detectable antibodies in serum. Therefore, to detect antibodies, it is recommended to collect both CSF and serum.
- The antibody titers of CSF as compared to serum may correlate with clinical severity but to a lesser extent, thus making it difficult to determine clinical recovery based on titers.
- Furthermore, assessing the clinical course, therapeutic response, and overall prognosis is relatively reliable based on accompanying comorbidities and clinical picture.

It is fundamentally vital to screen for the presence of neoplasm since a clinical subtype of antibody detection is often seen to be associated with a coexisting neoplasm (**Flowchart 1**). In females, gynecological examinations including breast examination and ovarian ultrasound/MRI should be performed according to clinical judgment and sensitivity. Additionally, a testicular ultrasound should be performed as part of a urological examination for males. It is advisable to perform a whole-body ^{18}F-fluorodeoxyglucose (FDG)-positron emission tomography (PET) if the above imaging appears to be inconclusive.

- *Serum* testing for thyroid-stimulating hormone and vitamin deficiency (B1, B12, folic acid) should be done.
- *Brain neuroimaging study* T2 weighted (FLAIR) sequence of MRI brain revealed increased signals in one or both medial temporal lobes (limbic encephalitis) or in multifocal gray and white matter areas.
- *EEG*: Nonspecific changes, periodic lateralized discharges, or delta brush in NMDAR encephalitis.
- *CSF study* shows mild to moderate lymphocytosis, high protein, elevated IgG index and positive autoantibodies in CSF.

TREATMENT

Autoimmune encephalitis of synaptic type is life threatening and debilitating and reversible with early timely treatment with effective immunotherapy.

Treatment is shown in **Flowchart 2**.

■ Acute Treatment

When first-line immune therapies are unsuccessful or relapse occurs, second-line treatments such as rituximab or cyclophosphamide are considered.

In order to prevent a relapse, maintenance therapy with immunosuppressants is recommended for 1–2 years for patients who are responding to treatment. It takes approximately 2 years for complete recovery. Details of pharmacotherapy are shown in **Table 1**.

DIFFERENTIAL DIAGNOSIS

- *Toxic encephalopathy*: Ethanol, opiates, benzodiazepines, tricyclic antidepressants, neuroleptics, carbon monoxide usually present with focal neurological deficit
- *Metabolic*: Wernicke's encephalopathy, uremic or hepatic encephalopathy, Hashimoto's encephalopathy
- *Infectious encephalitis*: Herpes simplex virus (HSV) 1, Japanese B encephalitis, Creutzfeldt-Jakob disease (CJD), etc.
- *Encephalopathy as a part of multiorgan dysfunction syndrome (MODS)*: For example, dengue, scrub typhus, cerebral malaria, leptospirosis, and sepsis.

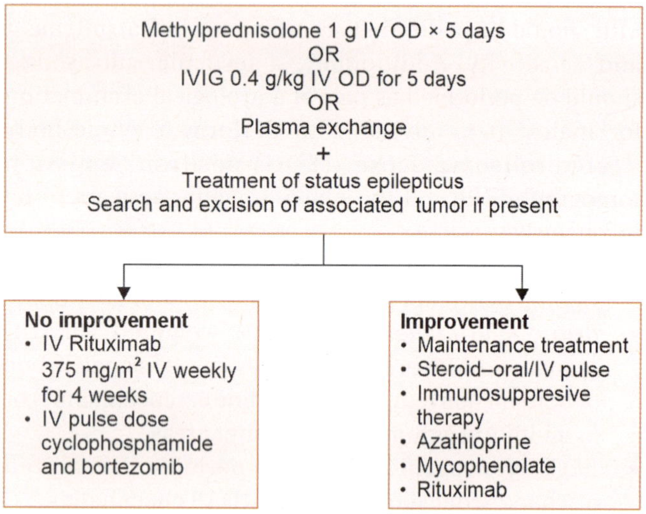

FLOWCHART 2: Treatment of autoimmune encephalitis.

Table 2 shows differences between infectious and noninfectious encephalitis.

PROGNOSIS

There is a better prognosis for autoimmune encephalitis caused by cell surface antibodies than those caused by intracellular antibodies.

Within 4 weeks of treatment with first-line immunosuppressive agents or tumor removal, there was a good outcome.

TABLE 2: Infectious and noninfectious encephalitis.

	Autoimmune encephalitis	Infectious encephalitis
Clinical presentation	Psychosis, language dysfunction, autonomic instability, movement disorder. Rash not seen	Fever, altered sensorium, seizures; rash may appear in HSV/VZV encephalitis
MRI findings	May be normal in anti-NMDAR encephalitis. The lateral temporal lobes and insula are less commonly involved; basal ganglia is often involved	Mesial temporal lobe involvement; lateral temporal lobe and insula may also be involved, basal ganglia spared
CSF findings	Lymphocytic pleocytosis milder	More severe lymphocytic pleocytosis
Treatment	Immunotherapy (+/– tumor removal)	Antiviral agents (Acyclovir)

(CSF: cerebrospinal fluid; HSV: herpes simplex virus; NMDAR: N-methyl-D-aspartate receptor; VZV: varicella zoster virus)

TABLE 1: Pharmacotherapy.

Drug	Route	Dose	Frequency	Side effects
• Glucocorticoids • Methylprednisolone/ oral prednisone	IV/PO	1,000 mg (up to 1 mg/kg prednisone)	Daily for 3–5 days and then weekly for 4–8 weeks	Psychiatric disturbance—psychosis, diabetes, cataract, osteoporosis, hip avascular necrosis
IVIG	IV	0.4 g/kg	(3–5 days) and then weekly	Aseptic meningitis, deep venous thrombosis, renal failure, pulmonary edema
Rituximab	IV	1,000 mg repeat in 2 weeks or 375 mg/m^2 4 doses	Every 6-month based on CD19	Infusion reaction, edema, rash, cytopenias, neutropenic fever, liver toxicity, hepatitis B reactivation
Azathioprine	PO	1 to 2–3 mg/kg/day	BID	Leukopenia, thrombocytopenia, myelotoxicity, liver toxicity, lymphoma, hypersensitivity
Cyclophosphamide	IV or PO	• 500–1,000 mg/m^2/ monthly (IV) • 1–2 mg/kg/day (PO)	• Monthly (IV) • Daily (PO)	Alopecia, infertility, hemorrhagic cystitis, myelotoxicity
MMF	PO	500–3,000 mg/day	BID	Hypertension, creatinine elevation, edema, lymphoma, myelotoxicity, teratogenicity

(IVIG: intravenous immunoglobulin; MMF: mycophenolate mofetil)

CONCLUSION

The discovery of various neuronal autoantibodies has led to an increase in research into the pathophysiology of AE over the past decade, rapidly expanding our understanding of its spectrum and treatment. Due to the broad spectrum of clinical manifestations, low threshold for serum/CSF assays, and nonspecific changes in EEG and MRI brain, the diagnosis can be challenging. AE can masquerade as many common neurological illnesses as enumerated in the differential diagnosis. Most of the patients with behavioral abnormalities often are initially treated as purely psychiatric patients, so diagnosis and treatment of AE get delayed. However, early recognition and prompt immunotherapy can significantly improve the outcome and ensure complete recovery. Emerging therapies offer new hope for patients. The recognition of environmental triggers and initiation of increased awareness among clinicians will be crucial for improving patient outcome in the future.

SUGGESTED READINGS

1. Dalmau J, Graus F. Antibody mediated encephalitis. NEJM. 2018;378;9:840-51.
2. Titulaer MJ, Balu R. Clinical approach to diagnosis of autoimmune encephalitis. Lancet Neurol. 2016;15(4):391-404.
3. Shin Y-W, Lee S-T, Park KI, Jung KH, Jung KY, Lee SK. Treatment Strategies for Autoimmune Encephalitis. Ther Adv Neurol Disord. 2017;11:175628561772234.

188

CHAPTER

Encephalitis and its Mimics in the Critical Care Unit

Chennakesavulu Dara

ABSTRACT

Encephalitis is a frequent cause of neurological consultations for hospitalized patients. However, understanding this syndrome is just one piece of the puzzle. The clinical presentation of encephalitis often shares similarities with infections, parainfections, postinfections, and various immune-mediated diseases. Our primary objective is to distinguish encephalitis from other conditions such as encephalopathy, which can result from factors such as toxins, inherited metabolic disorders, hypoxia, trauma, and vasculopathies. Therefore, we comprehensively explore both common and less common causes of acute encephalitis syndrome (AES) while delving into their clinical, laboratory, and radiological features. This in-depth understanding aids in specific diagnosis, guides treatment, and ultimately enhances patient outcomes.

INTRODUCTION

Acute encephalitis syndrome (AES) is a frequently encountered issue in clinical settings, posing unique challenges due to its abrupt onset necessitating intensive care. AES can stem from various etiologies, encompassing infections and noninfectious central nervous system (CNS) inflammatory conditions, frequently with limited microbial identification. Encephalitis-like symptoms can arise from toxic, metabolic, neoplastic, autoimmune, and cardiovascular etiologies. It is imperative to differentiate these from infectious encephalitis to ensure appropriate treatment. Infectious encephalitis and its noninfectious counterparts exhibit distinctive imaging and clinical characteristics. Consequently, a combined evaluation of imaging and clinical findings often facilitates accurate diagnosis even before laboratory results become available.

In this clinical context, we differentiate among three conditions: Encephalopathy, meningitis, and encephalitis, which share initial symptoms, including systemic issues and cognitive changes. Encephalopathy, the most common and less severe, describes consciousness and cognition changes from systemic disorders without structural brain damage. Triggers for toxic metabolic encephalopathy" include abnormal blood sugar, sodium imbalances, oxygen deprivation, high body temperature, sepsis, and organ dysfunction, all altering the brain's environment and function.

Meningitis involves inflammation in the subarachnoid space surrounding the brain and spinal cord. Bacterial meningitis is particularly destructive as it begins there but progresses to harm the nearby arteries, veins, and the brain itself. Encephalitis, on the other hand, signifies inflammation within the brain's tissue, potentially causing profound CNS damage, leading to permanent neurological impairment or death. While infections are the common cause, some rare conditions trigger this inflammation primarily due to immunological factors.

CAUSES

The cause varies based on the season and geographical location. Viruses have been mainly attributed to be the cause of AES in India though other microbes and toxins have been reported over the past few decades. Noninfective causes of acute encephalitic presentation are increasingly being recognized worldwide **(Box 1)**.

BOX 1: Causes of acute encephalitis.

Infective:
- Viral: Herpes simplex virus, Japanese encephalitis virus, Enteroviruses, parechovirus in neonates
- Bacterial: Acute bacterial meningitis
- Tubercular meningitis
- Dengue
- Neurobrucellosis
- Enteric
- Rickettsial
- Malaria

Noninfective:
- Immune-mediated
- Acute disseminated encephalomyelitis
- Neuromyelitis optica spectrum disorder
- Autoimmune encephalitis- Anti-N-methyl-D-aspartate receptor, limbic encephalitis
- Hashimoto's encephalopathy
- Bickerstaff brainstem encephalitis
- Probable inflammatory
- Acute necrotizing encephalopathy
- Febrile infection-related epilepsy syndrome
- Others
- Inborn errors of metabolism
- Nonconvulsive status epilepticus

INFECTIOUS

Most cases of infectious encephalitis are viral in origin, although bacteria (especially intracellular organisms such as Rickettsiae), fungi, and parasites can also be culprits. When evaluating a patient with suspected CNS infection, it is crucial to consider factors such as age, location, season, immune status, and psychosocial factors, which help identify potential pathogens. Human immunodeficiency virus (HIV) testing is essential since it can predispose to CNS infection and cause meningoencephalitis during primary infection.

The pattern of neurological involvement offers important clues **(Table 1)**. For instance, herpes simplex virus type 1 often affects the mesial temporal lobes, while some flavivirus infections such as Japanese encephalitis and West Nile virus, more commonly target deep gray matter. Brainstem encephalitis, characterized by cranial neuropathies, dysautonomia, and myoclonus, can result from various infections, including certain arthropod-borne viruses, enteroviruses, listeriosis, brucellosis, and tuberculosis. Encephalomyelitis presenting with acute flaccid paralysis can occur with enteroviruses such as poliovirus and EV-71 as well as flaviviruses.

Patients suspected of CNS infection should undergo a lumbar puncture, unless contraindicated. The cerebrospinal fluid (CSF) profile can confirm inflammation and help differentiate between various infectious causes. Viral encephalitis typically presents with lymphocytic pleocytosis, though polymorphonuclear cells may predominate early in the disease. Certain bacterial infections, such as listeriosis, brucellosis, and tuberculosis, may also exhibit lymphocytic predominance but are often associated with higher protein, a low CSF/plasma glucose ratio, and elevated CSF lactate levels. The CSF profile of immune-mediated and inflammatory encephalitis can resemble that of viral encephalitis. Acellular CSF is rare in infectious encephalitis but can occur early and is more common in immunosuppressed patients. CSF eosinophilia is observed in coccidioidomycosis and specific parasitic CNS infections.

Herpes simplex virus encephalitis is the most common form of sporadic encephalitis, primarily caused by herpes simplex virus type 1 (and occasionally type 2). Typical presentations include fever, disorientation, aphasia, behavioral disturbances, and convulsive seizures in some cases. Neuroimaging may initially be negative but usually shows abnormalities within 48 hours, especially on T2-weighted and fluid-attenuated inversion recovery (FLAIR) images, indicating involvement of the limbic system, medial temporal lobes, insular cortices, and inferolateral frontal lobes and clinicians should be aware of important imaging mimics **(Box 2)**.

Cerebrospinal fluid herpes simplex virus polymerase chain reaction (PCR) is highly sensitive and specific, typically confirming the diagnosis, although it may be negative during the acute phase. Repeated CSF examination 24–72 hours later is often diagnostic.

Acute Disseminated Encephalomyelitis

It is typically a single-phase inflammatory demyelinating disorder of the CNS, with a higher incidence in children but affecting all age groups. It manifests suddenly with neurological symptoms emerging days to weeks after infections or vaccinations. In cases lacking a clear history of prior infection or immunization, distinguishing acute disseminated encephalomyelitis (ADEM) from infectious encephalitis based solely on symptoms can be challenging. ADEM exhibits a diverse range of symptoms that evolve over hours to days, including encephalopathy, optic neuritis, and long tract signs. CSF findings in ADEM are similar to those in viral encephalitis. Neuroimaging typically reveals asymmetrical, bilateral areas of heightened signal intensity in regions such as the subcortical white matter, brainstem, cerebellum, periventricular white matter, and deep gray matter.

TABLE 1: Clues to specific diagnosis in acute encephalitis.

Diagnostic entity	Clues on history/Examination	Laboratory investigations
Viral meningoencephalitis	Geographic trends	MRI
	Rapid progression often with seizures/raised ICP	CSF-multiplex PCR
Complicated pyogenic meningitis	Evolving neurologic signs, toxic look with meningeal signs	CSF CT/MRI
Rickettsial	Typical vasculitic rash involving palms/soles, eschar	• PCR on blood samples • Serology • Response to doxycycline
Cerebral malaria	Endemic area/travel, seizure often status, anemia	Smear for MP
Dengue	Seasonal, facial blanching rash, narrow pulse pressure	NS1 antigen, antibody after 5 days, thrombocytopenia
Enteric	Rash, splenomegaly, mild encephalopathy, >1 week fever	Blood culture
Tubercular	Fever >5 days, meningeal signs, cranial nerve palsies, history of contact, evidence of TB elsewhere	• CSF-NAAT for TB, AFB culture • CT/MRI • GA for AFB, CXR
ADEM	Encephalopathy with multifocal neurologic deficits of acute/subacute onset often with recent febrile illness/vaccination	• Neuroimaging • Biomarkers-MOG, NMO IgG in serum
ANE	Abrupt onset of encephalopathy, raised ICP tone abnormalities with/without autonomic dysfunction	• Typical findings on MRI • Liver transaminases
Autoimmune encephalitis	Acute/subacute-onset neuropsychiatric illness with movement disorder, sleep disturbance	• MRI • CSF-antibodies • Serum antibodies
Neurometabolic disorders	Recurrent encephalopathy/family history	• High anion gap metabolic acidosis, ketosis, hyperammonemia, persistent hypoglycemia, TMS/GCMS • Neuroimaging

(ADEM: acute disseminated encephalomyelitis; AFB: acid-fast bacilli; ANE: acute necrotizing encephalopathy; CSF: cerebrospinal fluid; CT: computed tomography; CXR: chest X-ray; GA: gastric aspirates; ICP: intracranial pressure; IEM: inborn errors of metabolism; MP: malarial parasite; MOG: myelin-oligodendrocyte-glycoprotein; MRI: magnetic resonance imaging; NAAT: nucleic acid amplification test; NMO: neuromyelitis optica; PCR: polymerase chain reaction; TB: tuberculosis; TMS-GCMS: trimethylsilyl gas chromatography-mass spectrometry)

BOX 2: Herpes simplex encephalitis mimics.

Infectious:
- Varicella zoster virus
- Human herpes virus 6 (in the immunocompromised)
- Enterovirus
- West Nile virus
- Neurosyphilis
- Tuberculosis

Noninfectious:
- Glioma/lymphoma/metastatic malignancy
- Vasculitis
- Autoimmune limbic encephalitis
- Unilateral posterior reversible encephalopathy syndrome

Acute hemorrhagic encephalomyelitis represents a more rapid and severe variant of ADEM, often triggered by infections or vaccinations. Brain imaging usually indicates hemorrhagic lesions in the white matter. CSF analysis often reveals polymorphonuclear cells and a significant presence of red blood cells.

Hemophagocytic Lymphohistiocytosis

It is characterized by excessive inflammation resulting from abnormal immune activation, likely due to a failure in the regular suppression of activated macrophages and lymphocytes. Histopathological examination of bone marrow, liver, spleen, or lymph nodes can reveal evidence of hemophagocytosis. Elevated levels of soluble CD25 (soluble interleukin-2 receptor alpha) and impaired natural killer cell function are typically observed in conjunction with standard diagnostic investigations.

Influenza-related encephalitis/encephalopathy is a rapidly progressing condition that occurs shortly after the initial flu symptoms. Its exact underlying mechanisms remain unclear. An identifiable imaging pattern involves temporary focal swelling and restricted diffusion in the corpus callosum, which can also be seen in other infections and specific metabolic disorders. Typically, this pattern follows a benign course and is referred to as mild encephalitis/encephalopathy with reversible splenial lesion. Another pattern associated with influenza and other infections leads to bilateral necrosis in regions such as the thalami, brainstem, cerebellum, and cerebral white matter. This condition is termed "acute necrotizing encephalopathy" and carries a more severe clinical course with a poorer prognosis.

Cerebral Malaria

Cerebral malaria is primarily associated with *Plasmodium falciparum* infection and is more likely in certain risk groups such as young individuals, pregnant women, those with HIV infection, and individuals who have had their spleens removed. In adults, this condition is more prevalent among nonimmune individuals compared to those residing in endemic regions. Clinically, it typically starts with a prodrome marked by irregular fevers, malaise, abdominal pain, headache, anorexia, and vomiting, followed by the onset of encephalopathy, seizures, and ultimately, coma. In adults, neurological symptoms emerge approximately 7 days after the initial symptoms and rapidly progress to a comatose state. In children, retinal changes are common and include macular and extramacular whitening, along with orange or white discoloration of blood vessels, representing areas where the parasites accumulate. Diagnosis is confirmed through the examination of thick and thin blood films, which may initially yield negative results, especially in individuals who have been using antimalarial prophylaxis.

NONINFECTIOUS ENCEPHALITIS

Autoimmune Encephalitis Associated with Paraneoplastic or Neuronal Surface Antibodies

Autoimmune encephalitis encompasses a diverse range of neurological disorders linked to antineuronal autoantibodies. These disorders can be categorized into two main groups based on the location of the targeted antigen. The first group involves classic paraneoplastic disorders, associated with antibodies that target intracellular antigens. While these antibodies strongly correlate with underlying malignancies, they are not themselves pathogenic. The second group involves antibodies directed at neuronal surface antigens, which are likely to be pathogenic. Importantly, patients in this category typically respond positively to immunotherapy. Cancer associations vary but remain significant, such as the link between ovarian teratomas and anti-N-methyl-D-aspartate receptor (NMDAR) encephalitis.

Clinicians should consider autoimmune encephalitis in patients who exhibit subacute progressive encephalopathy with new-onset prominent psychiatric symptoms, as well as those with new-onset seizures and cryptogenic status epilepticus. Abnormal movements including orolingual and limb dyskinesias, dystonia, myoclonus, and hyperekplexia are more frequent in autoimmune encephalitis compared to infectious encephalitis. Detecting a known autoantibody aids in diagnosing the condition and determines the necessity to screen for an underlying malignancy.

Bickerstaff's Brainstem Encephalitis

It is characterized by a subacute onset of progressively impaired consciousness, ataxia, and bilateral, relatively symmetrical ophthalmoparesis. Typically, it follows an infectious prodrome, presents as a single-phase illness, and generally carries a favorable prognosis. Additional clinical features may include bilateral facial palsies, bulbar palsy, hyperreflexia, and pupillary abnormalities. Brain magnetic resonance (MR) scans often appear normal. The presence of anti-GQ1b antibodies in the serum can support the diagnosis, but it may be negative in up to 32% of patients. The absence of fever at the onset of neurological symptoms and the relatively symmetrical nature of findings are typically helpful in distinguishing Bickerstaff's encephalitis from infectious rhombencephalitis.

Vasculitis

Central nervous system vasculitis typically manifests with headache and subacute progressive encephalopathy. It can be classified as primary, limited to the CNS, or secondary, associated with an infection or systemic inflammatory disease. Primary CNS vasculitis lacks the systemic symptoms and signs often seen in secondary vasculitis, such as fever, weight loss, joint issues, eye inflammation, or rash. Diagnostic tools include magnetic resonance imaging (MRI), angiography, fludeoxyglucose-18 (FDG), positron emission tomography (PET) scans, with histopathology serving as the definitive method.

Neuromyelitis Optica Brain

Brain lesions observed in neuromyelitis optica brain (NMO) spectrum disorder typically appear in regions rich in aquaporin-4 (AQP-4), such as the area postrema, hypothalamus, or periaqueductal brainstem. Confirming the diagnosis involves the detection of autoantibodies to AQP-4, although 20–30% of patients may test seronegative. Some patients with seronegative NMO spectrum disorder have antibodies to myelin oligodendrocyte glycoprotein (MOG). MOG-IgG associated encephalomyelitis is now recognized as a distinct disease entity, characterized by recurrent (though occasionally monophasic) optic neuritis, myelitis, rhombencephalitis, and ADEM-like presentations.

Neurosarcoidosis

Nervous system manifestations of sarcoidosis encompass cranial neuropathies, myeloradiculopathies (including cauda equina syndrome), peripheral neuropathy, and myopathy. In some cases, patients may present with symptoms such as headache, encephalopathy, psychosis, and seizures. Serum angiotensin-converting enzyme (ACE) levels exhibit poor sensitivity and specificity in diagnosis while CSF ACE concentration is also relatively insensitive and moderately specific. A CSF CD4/CD8 T cell ratio exceeding 5 can support the diagnosis. A definitive diagnosis of sarcoidosis requires the histopathological identification of non-necrotizing granulomas in affected tissue, which may pose challenges in obtaining suitable samples. FDG-PET scans may detect systemic sarcoidosis and aid in identifying potential biopsy sites.

Transient headache and neurological deficits with cerebrospinal fluid lymphocytosis (HaNDL) is a self-limiting condition that can mimic encephalitis. As the name implies, patients typically experience episodes of severe migraine-like headaches along with transient neurological deficits and lymphocytic pleocytosis in the CSF. Common neurological deficits include hemiparesis, hemisensory disturbances, aphasia, and occasionally visual disturbances and encephalopathy.

Toxic and Metabolic Syndromes Encompass a Range of Conditions

Septic Encephalopathy

This is the most common form of infection-related encephalopathy, occurring in up to 70% of sepsis patients. Clinically, individuals with septic encephalopathy initially display confusion and inattention, which can progress to delirium, stupor, and coma.

Toxic Syndromes

In cases of ingestion or overdose, patients often exhibit clinical features that may resemble encephalitis such as alterations in mental status and fever. Identifying the specific toxic syndrome can be crucial for making a diagnosis, especially when there is no immediate history of exposure.

Posterior Reversible Encephalopathy Syndrome

This is a diverse clinical syndrome marked by acute neurological symptoms linked to blood pressure fluctuations, autoimmune and metabolic disorders, infections, eclampsia, transplantation, or exposure to immunosuppressive or cytotoxic drugs. Its sudden onset, which includes seizures, encephalopathy, and, less commonly, focal deficits, can mimic encephalitis. Typically, brain imaging reveals relatively symmetrical signal abnormalities in the cerebral white matter of both hemispheres, with a preference for the parieto-occipital regions. Other brain regions often affected include the frontotemporal lobes, basal ganglia, brainstem, and cerebellum.

Mitochondrial Encephalomyopathies

Among mitochondrial disorders, mitochondrial encephalomyopathy with lactic acidosis and stroke-like symptoms (MELAS) is the one most likely to resemble infectious encephalitis. Clinically, MELAS presents with nonischemic stroke-like episodes leading to symptoms such as hemiparesis, hemianopia, aphasia, encephalopathy, and cortical blindness. Focal and generalized seizures are also common. Patients often have a prior history of migraine headaches, vomiting, muscle weakness, psychiatric issues, growth problems, and hearing loss, although these may be overshadowed by the more dramatic stroke-like manifestations. Neuroimaging reveals hyperintense T2 lesions primarily in the gray and subcortical white matter, with a predilection for the temporal, parietal, and occipital regions. MR spectroscopy demonstrates a significant lactate peak and a low ratio of N-acetyl aspartate to creatine, providing supportive evidence. The definitive diagnosis relies on mitochondrial DNA studies.

Neoplasia

Temporal-lobe tumors can sometimes resemble herpes simplex virus encephalitis. However, MRI signal changes in tumors typically differ from viral encephalitis as they tend to be unilateral and contiguous. It is worth noting that bilateral involvement can occur in conditions such as gliomatosis or lymphomatosis cerebri.

Intravascular Large Cell Lymphoma

Neurologically, this condition manifests as a swiftly advancing encephalopathy. Constitutional B symptoms and skin manifestations are prevalent. Serum lactate dehydrogenase and beta-2-microglobulin levels are often elevated but lack specificity. Brain imaging may reveal related gyriform, perivascular, or homogeneous gadolinium enhancement, along with restricted diffusion.

Subacute Radiation-induced Meningoencephalitis

Subacute radiation-induced meningoencephalitis (SMART) is a rare syndrome that typically arises years after successful treatment of CNS neoplasia with therapeutic cranial irradiation. Clinically, it manifests as recurrent episodes of headache along with seizures, confusion, and focal deficits. Neuroimaging reveals elevated T2 signal and swelling in cortical gyri within the prior radiation area, accompanied by gadolinium enhancement. Generally, both the neurological deficits and imaging abnormalities are reversible, but there is a possibility of permanent sequelae.

DIAGNOSTIC APPROACH

Acute encephalitis syndrome is a medical emergency with diverse potential causes, making initial presentation similar. It is crucial to maintain a high index of suspicion, be aware of conditions that mimic encephalitis, and conduct a swift, focused clinical evaluation, emphasizing history-taking and initial stabilization **(Flowchart 1)**.

When there is evident neurological involvement such as seizures and persistent focal deficits, it is vital to concurrently assess potential neurological diseases along with the overall medical condition. The initial general examination should prioritize vital signs and search for indications of pulmonary, hepatic, or renal issues. Subsequently, a brief neurological assessment focusing on language, orientation, and cranial nerve function is necessary. Essential biochemical markers such as glucose, sodium, liver and renal function, and blood gases if applicable, should be evaluated promptly. If these do not reveal significant non-neurological disease, attention should turn to the nervous system.

Obtaining a history and conducting an examination that suggests a primary CNS process is critical. Brain

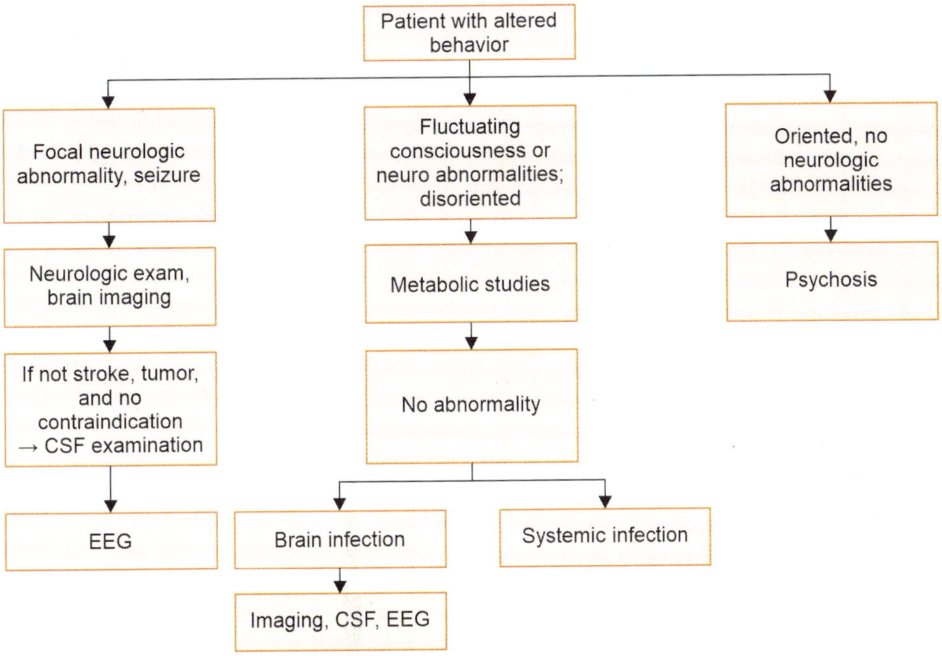

FLOWCHART 1: Clinical approach to the patient with altered brain function.
(CSF: cerebrospinal fluid; EEG: electroencephalography)

imaging can help exclude conditions that mimic encephalitis, determine the presence and extent of inflammation, identify radiological signs of increased intracranial pressure, and provide clues about the etiology through pattern recognition. Additional studies involve CSF analysis, immunological tests, multiplexed PCR testing, along with routine investigations. Early initiation of management is crucial for a better and favorable outcome.

CONCLUSION

While various disorders can cause changes in nervous system function, a systematic clinical approach can often lead to a swift diagnosis. Thankfully, CNS infection is statistically uncommon. However, when encephalitis does occur, the consequences can be severe. In general, initiating treatment as early as possible improves the chances of a favorable outcome.

SUGGESTED READINGS

1. Newton PJ, Newsholme W, Brink NS, Williams IG. Acute meningoencephalitis and meningitis due to primary HIV infection. BMJ. 2002;325:1225-7.
2. Toledano M, Davies NWS. Infectious encephalitis: mimics and chameleons. Pract Neurol. 2019;19:225-37.
3. Wingerchuk DM, Weinshenker BG. Transverse myelitis, and neuromyelitis optica. Continuum. 2013;19:944-67.
4. Kitley J, Woodhall M, Waters P, Leite MI, Devenney E, Craig J, et al. Myelin-oligodendrocyte glycoprotein antibodies in adults with a neuromyelitis optica phenotype. Neurology. 2012;79:1273-7.

189

CHAPTER

Neuromyelitis Optica and Myelin Oligodendrocyte Glycoprotein Autoimmune Disorders and Recent Management

Manoj Khanal

ABSTRACT

Neuromyelitis optica (NMO) is a devastating demyelinating syndrome characterized by optic neuritis (ON) and myelitis, either simultaneously or in sequential relapses. Classical symptoms of NMO are ON, myelitis, or area postrema syndrome. The key diagnostic test is the NMO antibody [anti-aquaporin-4 (AQP4) antibody] with sensitivity 70–80% and specificity close to 100%. There may be overlap syndrome with Sjögren and lupus and vasculitic antibody being positive. Cerebrospinal fluid (CSF) analysis shows oligoclonal bands in only 10% patients with mild elevation in white blood cell (WBC) counts and protein commonly. There is no cure for NMO but it is treatable. Some patients recover but many are left with impairment of vision and limbs weakness which can be severe in some cases. High dosage of intravenous (IV) methylprednisolone pulse is given for 5 days followed by a prednisolone taper. Depending on treatment response, plasmapheresis or IV immunoglobulin (IVIg) may be used for relapses with incomplete recovery after steroids. Azathioprine, mycophenolate mofetil, rituximab, cyclophosphamide, and mitoxantrone, all have been used for preventive treatments. Some improvement appears in few weeks, but disability may persists. Unlike multiple sclerosis (MS), NMO rarely has a secondary progressive phase. 20% with monophasic NMO have permanent visual loss, 30% permanent paralysis in one or both legs.

INTRODUCTION

Neuromyelitis optica (NMO) is a devastating demyelinating syndrome characterized by optic neuritis (ON) and myelitis, either simultaneously or in sequential relapses. It was coined by Eugène Devic in the late 1800s. Until 2004, NMO was considered as a severe variant of multiple sclerosis (MS). in 2004, anti-aquaporin-4 (AQP4) antibody was identified in a majority of patients with the clinical syndrome of NMO with high specificity. Thus it was separated and considered as a separate entity from MS.

PATHOPHYSIOLOGY

NMO Antibody (Anti-aquaporin-4 Antibody)

Aquaporin-4 is a transmembrane protein which facilitates water transport in the central nervous system (CNS). It is expressed at the astrocytic foot processes at the blood-brain barrier (BBB). There is compliment activation leading to 'rim and rosette' pattern of immune complexes in the NMO lesion causing astrocyte death and tissue necrosis in both gray and white matter with accumulation of T cells, B cells, and macrophages similar to MS with additional neutrophils and eosinophils also contribute to tissue damage.

EPIDEMIOLOGY

Neuromyelitis optica is a rare condition. The prevalence is 2–4/100000 in most populations. The female to male ratio is 9:1. The age of onset is older (median age of 40 years). Non-Caucasian (Hispanic and African descent) being commonly affected. The course of NMO is more devastating. The disability accumulated through relapses is more severe with total blindness and paralysis more commonly which is uncommon in MS patients. The majority of NMO patients have no affected relatives and it is regarded as a nonfamilial condition.

CLINICAL FEATURES

The classical symptoms of NMO are ON, myelitis, or area postrema syndrome.

Optic Neuritis

Optic neuritis is severe, bilateral more commonly, and recovery may not be complete. Total blindness can also occur.

Longitudinally Extensive Transverse Myelitis

The hallmark of NMO is spinal cord relapses.

Longitudinally extensive transverse myelitis (LETM) is defined as spinal cord lesion that is contiguous and greater than three vertebral segments, often extending from the cervical junction to the cervical and thoracic cord with motor, sensory, and/or bladder and bowel functions involvement.

Area Postrema Syndrome

Neuromyelitis optica spares the brain but involvement is seen in 10% patients. Brainstem symptoms includes intractable nausea, vomiting, hiccups (area postrema syndrome), double vision, dysphagia, and respiratory compromise. Cerebral symptoms include motor and sensory deficits and encephalopathies.

DIAGNOSIS

The key diagnostic test is the NMO antibody (anti-AQP4 antibody) with sensitivity 70–80% and specificity close to 100%. There may be overlap syndrome with Sjögren and lupus and vasculitic antibody being positive. Cerebrospinal fluid (CSF) analysis shows oligoclonal bands in only 10% patients with mild elevation in white blood cell (WBC) counts and protein commonly.

Wingerchuk Diagnostic Criteria (2015)

A patient with AQP4-IgG (immunoglobulin G) with history of core clinical syndrome (ON, myelitis, area postrema syndrome, brain stem syndrome, narcolepsy, acute diencephalic syndrome, symptomatic cerebral syndrome) along with a positive antiaquaporin-IgG test and exclusion of other causes **(Box 1)**.

BOX 1: Diagnostic criteria for NMOSD (neuromyelitis optica spectrum disorder) with AQP4-IgG (aquaporin-4–immunoglobulin G).

Diagnostic criteria for NMOSD with AQP4-IgG:
- At least one core clinical characteristic
- Positive AQP4-IgG test
- Exclusion of other alternative diagnosis

Diagnostic criteria for NMO without AQP4-IgG or NMOSD with unknown AQP4-IgG status:
- At least two core clinical characteristics occurring as a result of one or more clinical attacks and meets all requirements:
  - At least one core clinical characteristics must be ON, acute LETM or area postrema syndrome.
  - Dissemination in space (two or more different clinical characteristics)
  - Fulfillment of additional MRI requirements
- Negative test for AQP4-IgG or unavailable
- Exclusion of alternate diagnosis

Core clinical characteristics:
- Optic neuritis (ON)
- Acute myelitis (LETM)
- *Acute postrema syndrome*: Episodes of unexplained hiccups or nausea and vomiting
- Acute brainstem syndrome
- Symptomatic narcolepsy or acute diencephalic syndrome with NMOSD typical diencephalic MRI lesions
- Symptomatic cerebral syndrome with NMOSD typical brain lesions

Additional MRI requirements for NMOSD without AQP4-IgG and NMOSD with unknown AQP4-IgG status:
- *Acute ON*: Brain MRI showing (1) normal findings or only nonspecific white matter lesions or (2) optic nerve MRI with T2 hyperintense lesion or T1-weighted Gad-enhancing lesion extending over more than half optic nerve length or involving optic chiasma
- *Acute myelitis*: Associated intramedullary MRI lesions over >3 contagious segments of focal spinal cord atrophy in patients with history of acute myelitis.
- *Acute postrema syndrome*: Associated dorsal medulla/area postrema lesions
- *Acute brainstem syndrome*: Associated periependymal brain stem lesions

(Gad: gadolinium; LETM: longitudinally extensive transverse myelitis; MRI: magnetic resonance imaging; NMO: neuromyelitis optica)

Source: Wingerchuk DM, Banwell B, Bennett JL, Cabre P, Carroll W, Chitnis T, et al. International consensus diagnostic criteria for neuromyelitis optica spectrum disorders. Neurology. 2015;85(2):177-89.

MOG-ASSOCIATED AUTOIMMUNE DISORDERS

- Myelin oligodendrocyte glycoprotein (MOG) antibody is seen in a subset of AQP4 seronegative neuromyelitis optica spectrum disorder (NMOSD) patients.

- Transient seropositivity of MOG antibody is associated with monophasic disease/course.
- Persistently high titer is associated with high risk for relapsing disease.
- MOG-associated disorders also include ON, myelitis, and brainstem syndrome; subtle differences between NMO and MOG disorders
- More common in males
- Acute disseminated encephalomyelitis (ADEM) is the common presenting feature.
- *ON*: presents with disc edema, long section of the optic nerve, and is bilateral.
- *Myelitis*: Lower in the spinal cord (LETM or involve only a small segment)
- *Area postrema syndrome*: Less common
- *Prognosis*: It is better than AQP4-IgG disorders.
- *Relapses*: It is less likely to have severe neurological deficits after a relapse. More likely to maintain motor function; bladder/bowel/erectile dysfunction may be permanent **(Table 1)**.

MANAGEMENT

Approach to treatment in both disorders is identical and comprises three parts:

1. Treatment of relapse
2. Prevention of relapse
3. Treatment of chronic symptoms

Treatment of Relapse

- Prompt and aggressive
- There is no cure for NMO but it is treatable. Some patients recover but many are left with impairment of vision and limbs which can be severe in some cases.
- High dosage of intravenous (IV) methylprednisolone pulse is given for 5 days followed by a prednisolone taper.
- Depending on treatment response, plasmapheresis or IV immunoglobulin (IVIg) may be used for relapses with incomplete recovery after steroid.
- Early plasmapheresis is encouraged for patients with serious deficits or those who do not respond to steroids and treatment of subsequent attacks with plasmapheresis has shown better outcome. This treatment involves the patient's own blood being pumped out, blood cells being removed from the plasma and mixed with a solution, then the new blood mixture being pumped back in.

Prevention of Relapse

Low-dose Prednisolone/Prednisone

Low-dose oral corticosteroids used in many neurological diseases. Tapering dosage of oral steroids are given for few months.

The data on long-term use of steroids are limited. A few studies show a decrease in annual relapse rate by low-dose steroid therapy. It is known from treatment with azathioprine that additional oral prednisone is effective to reduce disease activity during the first 3–6 months until azathioprine reaches full efficacy.

In MOG disease, low-treatment failure rates were achieved with oral prednisone. There can be occurrence of relapses post-tapering and stopping of IV methylprednisolone, but a long-term therapy should be carefully used in view of known side effects.

- Azathioprine, mycophenolate mofetil, rituximab, cyclophosphamide, mitoxantrone all have used for preventive treatments.
- *Azathioprine*: It is a purine analog.

TABLE 1: Differences between NMOSD (neuromyelitis optica spectrum disorder) and MOG (myelin oligodendrocyte glycoprotein) disease.

	NMOSD	MOG disease
Mean age at onset	40–46 years	27–37 years
Female to male ratio	7.2:1–10:1	1:1.6–1.3:1
Median EDSS at last follow-up	4.0–5.8	0–1.5
Coexisting autoimmune disease	16–45%	6–11%
Localization of optic nerve lesions	Orbital, chiasma	Orbital, canalicular, intracranial
Features of optic neuritis	• *OCT*: Prominent • *RNFL*: Thinning	Severe optic nerve swelling at onset; frequently simultaneous or rapidly sequential optic neuritis and LETM
Localization of spinal cord lesions	Cervical, thoracic	Thoracic, lumbar, conus
MRI brain lesions	Frequently lesions in medulla oblongata, area postrema	ADEM like brain lesions, deep gray matter lesions, lesions in pons, thalamus

(ADEM: acute disseminated encephalomyelitis; EDSS: Expanded Disability Status Scale; LETM: longitudinally extensive transverse myelitis; MRI: magnetic resonance imaging; OCT: optical coherence tomography; RNFL: retinal nerve fiber layer)

TABLE 2: Different drugs and their mechanism of action.

Drug	Mechanism of action	Note
Azathioprine	Inhibits purine metabolism	Reported effective in 1998 and mainstay of treatment combined with steroids due to months long onset of action
Mycophenolate mofetil	Inhibits purine metabolism	Better efficacy and tolerability; combined with steroids due to months long onset of action
Methotrexate	Inhibits folate metabolism	–
Cyclophosphamide	DNA crosslinker	–
Rituximab	Antibody against CD20 B cells depletion	Most commonly used treatment for NMOSD
Intravenous immunoglobulins	–	–
Mitoxantrone	DNA synthesis/repair inhibitor	–
Hematopoietic stem cell transplantation	–	It is used in severe case of NMO. Short-term benefit by reduction of inflammation but majority of them relapse within 5 years

(NMO: neuromyelitis optica; NMOSD: NMO spectrum disorder)

- *Eculizumab*: Complement inhibitor is now United States Food and Drug Administration (USFDA) approved for the treatment of NMOSD. It showed a 94% reduction risk for new relapses when it was added on to patients who were given placebo and continued their previous disease-modifying treatment (DMT).
- *Satralizumab and inebilizumab*: Both showed marked reduction in new NMOSD relapses versus the comparison group.
- Multiple DMTs used in MS like interferons and natalizumab can worsen the disease course of NMO. So early and accurate diagnosis is critical for NMO management **(Table 2)**.

It is important to note that interferon beta, fingolimod, natalizumab, and alemtuzumab worsen NMO disease progression and should not be used to treat NMO.

PROGNOSIS

Some improvement appears in few weeks, but disability may persist. It has a monophasic phase also but usually 85% have a relapsing course with repeated episodes of transverse myelitis and/or ON. In the monophasic form, the transverse myelitis and ON occur simultaneously, but relapsing form have weeks or months between initial attacks and have better motor recovery after the initial transverse myelitis event. 55% have a relapse in first year and 90% in the first 5 years. Unlike MS, NMO rarely has a secondary progressive phase. 20% with monophasic NMO have permanent visual loss; 30% permanent paralysis in one or both legs.

SUGGESTED READINGS

1. Wingerchuk DM, Banwell B, Bennett JL, Cabre P, Carroll W, Chitnis T, et al. International consensus diagnostic criteria for neuromyelitis optica spectrum disorders. Neurology. 2015;85(2):177-89.
2. Jankovic J, Mazziotta JC, Pomeroy SL, Newman NJ. Bradley and Daroff's Neurology in Clinical Practice, 8th edition, volumes 1 and 2. Netherlands: Elsevier; 2021. pp. 1252-3.

190

CHAPTER

Acute Stroke Management in the Emergency Department

Divendu Bhushan, Zairemliana Chenkual

ABSTRACT

Cerebrovascular accidents are one of the most common causes of mortality worldwide. It is prudent to recognize it fast as treatment is time dependent and delay can lead to extreme morbidity. In India, it causes 3.5% disability adjusted life year (DALY). As availability of computed tomography (CT) scan and MRI increasing day by day, the facility of treatment is also available in semiurban and rural areas. It needs a teamwork of physician, neurologists, neurosurgeons, and neuroradiologists. With the advancement of technologies, there are facilities of mobile stroke units at various regions of India. As awareness is increasing day by day, patients are benefiting with advanced treatments available such as thrombolysis, mechanical thrombectomy, and aneurysm clipping/coiling. Even early aspiration of brain hemorrhage improves the outcome.

The diagnosis of stroke in the emergency room rests on the bedrock of a focused, accurate history, and physical examination. To enhance clinical outcomes, it is critical in the emergency department (ED) to quickly diagnose and treat it.

INTRODUCTION

The initial few hours after the onset of an acute stroke are very crucial. When a patient exhibits signs and symptoms of an acute stroke, it is critical to act quickly to minimize brain damage. The goal of acute stroke management in the emergency department is to quickly identify, exclude stroke mimics, and treat the underlying cause of the stroke while also ensuring the patient's safety.

The first step is *to notify a stroke team* and initiate a stroke protocol to ensure that treatment can be given as soon as possible. Early care including thrombolysis within 3–4.5 hours has been proven in studies to greatly improve a stroke victim's prognosis. As a result, the initial assessment should be quick and thorough, including an airway assessment, vital sign evaluation, blood tests, electrocardiogram (ECG), and a focused neurological examination.

The *National Institutes of Health Stroke Scale (NIHSS)* is an 11-category (15 items) neurologic assessment tool with a score range of 0 to 42 that is quick (5–10 minutes) and has a high inter-rater reliability and generates a baseline score that can be used to predict patient outcomes; it is the standard tool for stroke evaluation, assessing the severity of the stroke, and the amount of ne urological damage.

A *noncontrast head computed tomography (CT)* scan is also required to determine whether the stroke is ischemic or hemorrhagic. However, a noncontrast brain CT does not show most acute ischemic strokes in the early hours of the stroke. As a result, the first brain CT is primarily useful for ruling out intracranial bleeding, abscess, tumor, and other stroke mimics, as well as detecting current thrombolytic contraindications (e.g., extensive regions of clear hypoattenuation).

ACUTE ISCHEMIC STROKE THROMBOLYSIS: CANDIDATE SELECTION AND TREATMENT

With the advent of endovascular therapies, it is critical to identify the presence of intracranial large-vessel stenosis or occlusion for therapeutic decisions. These lesions can be detected using CT angiography or magnetic resonance angiography **(Flowchart 1)**. If a patient is a candidate for endovascular therapy, vascular imaging

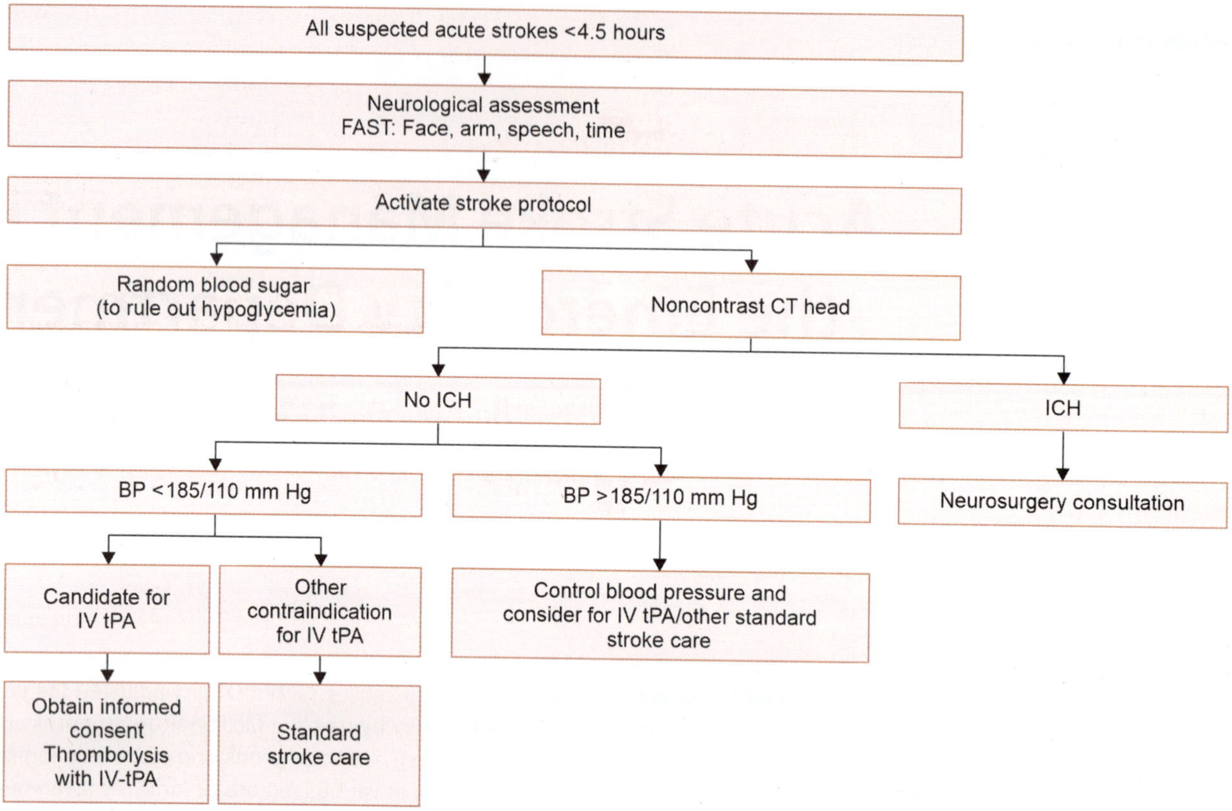

FLOWCHART 1: Acute stroke management in patient presenting with <4.5 hours of symptoms onset.

(CT: computed tomography; ICH: intracranial hemorrhage; IV-tPA: intravenous tissue plasminogen activator)

Note: Stroke patients receiving thrombolytics should not be given antiplatelet for 24 hours after initiation ofthrombolytics. Antiplatelets should be started after 24 hours after initiation of thrombolytics

typical CT angiography of the head and neck should be performed concurrently with the initial head CT; however, these additional studies should not delay thrombolytic administration.

After an ischemic stroke is detected, the attention changes to finding the best candidate for thrombolysis, a treatment that can break down clots and restore cerebral blood flow.

Tissue plasminogen activator (tPA) is the only Food and Drug Administration (FDA)-approved approach medicine, and studies have indicated that if provided within the first hours after onset and within the permitted time range, it can be highly successful.

Tenecteplase (0.25 mg/kg, total dose: 25 mg) can be an alternative to tPA. Contraindications of thrombolysis are mentioned in **Box 1**.

After thrombolysis, serial blood pressure, neurological, and imaging evaluations should be performed accurately to track the patient's recovery and detect and manage symptoms such as intracerebral hemorrhage (ICH) and angioedema.

BOX 1: Absolute contraindications of thrombolytic therapy in stroke patients.

- Hemorrhagic CVA in past
- Nonhemorrhagic CVA in past 3 months
- Blood pressure >180/120 mm Hg
- Structural cerebral vascular lesion
- Malignant intracranial neoplasm
- Suspected aortic dissection
- Active bleeding/bleeding diathesis (except menses)
- Significant closed head trauma/facial trauma within 3 months

(CVA: cerebrovascular accident)

ENDOVASCULAR THERAPY: TIME IS BRAIN

Thrombectomy is an endovascular therapy for ischemic stroke that physically removes clots to restore brain circulation. Its indications include—prestroke mRS 0–1, NIHSS >6, ASPECT of >6, occlusion of ICA or

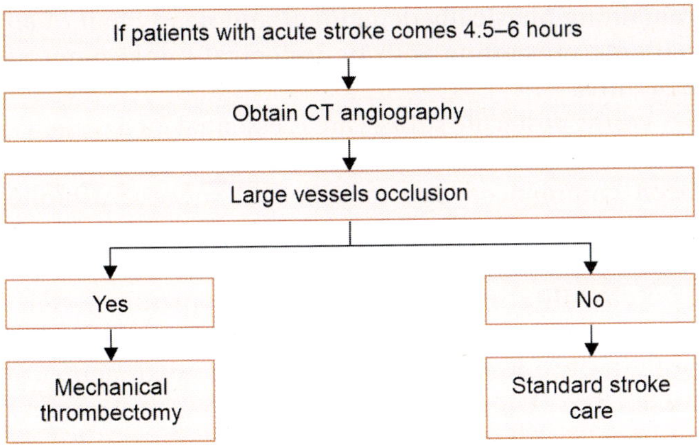

FLOWCHART 2: Acute stroke management in patient presenting within 6 hours of symptoms onset.
(CT: computed tomography)

MCA (M1), age >18 years, and onset of symptoms <6 hours. Endovascular therapy, which swiftly accesses and dislodges clots and can aid when tPA is not a viable therapeutic option, has been shown in studies to enhance patient outcomes. Mechanical thrombectomy can be considered in selected patients after thrombolysis and we should not wait for response of thrombolysis **(Flowchart 2)**.

According to a recent meta-analysis, endovascular management outperforms best medical management alone in early patients with moderate-to-low symptom burden, preexisting collateral driver skills, and larger vessel occlusions, resulting in slow but straightforward depopulation in efforts to beat time of onset. Three randomized controlled trials found that endovascular therapy was more effective in mild-to-severe large anterior circulation strokes.

Also, patients who have a better grasp of the function of endovascular management may benefit from being informed, examined, and swiftly moved to a complete stroke care facility if necessary.

ANTIPLATELETS AND ANTICOAGULATION

- Antiplatelets, aspirin 150 mg and clopidogrel 300 mg, loading to be given followed by aspirin 150 mg daily and clopidogrel 75 mg daily for 3 weeks. This will be followed by single antiplatelet lifelong. In patients who underwent thrombolysis, antiplatelet can be delayed for 24 hours.
- Anticoagulation is not found to be beneficial in ischemic stroke.

ACUTE SPONTANEOUS INTRACEREBRAL HEMORRHAGE

Acute ICH is a medical emergency that ruled out easily by doing noncontract CT brain in suspected cases. Early minimal invasive procedures to evacuate it in supratentorial and intraventricular bleed shows better outcome. Improvement in functional outcome is although not observed and its neutral in clinical trials. In cases of cerebellar bleed indications for evacuation with or without drain extended from neurological deterioration, brainstem compression and hydrocephalus to include large volume (>15 mL bleed) too.

Anticoagulant-induced ICH carries poor prognosis.

There is no benefit of corticosteroids, prophylactic antiepileptic, and neuroprotective agents.

GENERAL MANAGEMENT OF ACUTE STROKE

For all patients, it is critical to adhere to general treatment guidelines because not all patients will be qualified for thrombolytics.

- *Head position*: No beneficial role of keeping patient propped up.
- *Maintain hydration*: Dehydration can worsen outcomes in patients with ischemic stroke due to increased blood viscosity, hypotension, renal impairment, and venous thromboembolism. Routine volume expansion and hemodilution, however, do not enhance stroke patients' outcomes. Therefore, dehydration, if present, should be corrected with intravenous (IV) crystalloids, but not overcorrect.
- *Oxygen*: Routine oxygen supplementation is not recommended in stroke and should be administered only if necessary to maintain oxygen saturation above 94%.
- *Temperature*: Fever is associated with increased morbidity and mortality in stroke, which could be attributed to fever-related inflammatory responses, increased metabolic demands, and free radical production. Determine the source of the fever and address the underlying cause. While it is common practice to treat a fever with paracetamol, strong evidence of positive outcomes remains elusive. Induced hypothermia is not shown benefit in outcome of ischemic stroke patients.

BLOOD PRESSURE CONTROL

The optimal blood pressure for acute ischemic stroke victims is unknown; however, the current American Heart Association/American Stroke Association (AHA/ASA) acute stroke guidelines recommend that hypotension and hypovolemia be corrected with colloids or crystalloids to maintain organ perfusion; however, there is no specific target blood pressure for patients who are not candidates for reperfusion therapy.

BLOOD SUGAR CONTROL

The current AHA/ASA guidelines recommend keeping the blood glucose levels between 140 and 180 mg/dL. Avoid and treat hypoglycemia (< 60 mg/dL).

Hyperglycemia is common in acute stroke and glycemic control has been recommended based on data linking hyperglycemia to poorer outcomes. However, there is a lack of data to support improved outcomes with tight glycemic control.

We have to keep in mind that both hypoglycemia as well as hyperglycemia are important stroke mimics.

LIPID MANAGEMENT

Statins are recommended in acute stroke patients. High-intensity statins should be recommended with target to reduce > 50% low-density lipoprotein (LDL) cholesterol.

ANTIEPILEPTIC DRUGS

No use of prophylactic antiepileptic medicines. If patient developed seizures, appropriate antiepileptic drug (AED) can be used.

POSTSTROKE INTERVENTIONAL MANAGEMENT AND REHABILITATION

Stroke survivors have a high rate of long-term disabilities and complications, with up to one-third remaining physically dependent and nearly half of all patients presenting with neurological impairment at 6 months.

Lastly, postacute stroke care is essential for a patient's full recovery. This phase begins after thrombolysis has been commenced due to safe and successful blood pressure and glucose control, which aids in recovery beyond the initial intervention.

Rehabilitation is critical in supporting patient recovery after a stroke (including spasticity control), potentially improving activity. Such advancements lessen the strain on patients, families, and society while also resulting in significant long-term cost savings.

The care team should establish goals to aid mobility, speech therapy evaluation, and dysphagia evaluation, and should be swiftly examined to optimize strengths and resilience in mild-to- moderate stroke patients.

CONCLUSION

Stroke is a major, widespread health issue that necessitates early care to enhance clinical outcomes. Identifying it early, seeking treatment to a center equipped with stroke unit is need of hour. Timely intervention can save brain and decrease mortality and morbidity. Poststroke rehabilitation is a challenge which can be done with a multidisciplinary team approach.

SUGGESTED READINGS

1. Greenberg SM, Ziai WC, Cordonnier C, Dowlatshahi D, Francis B, Goldstein JN, Hemphill JC 3rd, et al. 2022 Guideline for the management of patients with spontaneous intracerebral hemorrhage: A Guideline from the American Heart Association/ American Stroke Association. Stroke. 2022;53(7):e282 361.
2. Guidelines for the Early Management of Patients with Acute Ischemic Stroke: 2019 Update to the 2018 Guidelines for the Early Management of Acute Ischemic Stroke: A Guideline for Healthcare Professionals From the American Heart Association/ American Stroke Association

191

CHAPTER

Management of Hypertension in Acute Stroke

Jacquiline D Shira, Dwijen Das

ABSTRACT

Stroke is one of the most common causes of mortality and morbidity worldwide and management of hypertension is an essential part of its treatment as well as prevention but despite considerable research effort, the optimal post-stroke blood pressure (BP) management remains controversial and unresolved. A wealth of hemodynamic data provides insights into the pathophysiologic relationship between BP and cerebral blood flow. Different guidelines have been set to guide us to manage the patients with stroke. In this chapter, the authors provided an updated review on the management of arterial hypertension in acute stroke.

INTRODUCTION

Stroke stands as the second most common cause of mortality and third most common cause of disability. Management of hypertension for stroke prevention as well as acute treatment is a cornerstone but even after vigorous research effort, the optimal post-stroke blood pressure (BP) management remains controversial and unresolved. According to the latest guidelines of the American College of Cardiology/American Heart Association (ACC/AHA), BP is considered high if it is 130/80 mm Hg or more. The European Society of Cardiology (ESC) considers 140/90 mm Hg or more as hypertension. Systolic blood pressure (SBP) is considered to be a better predictor than diastolic blood pressure (DBP) as a risk factor for stroke.

ISCHEMIC STROKE

In hospitalized patients with acute ischemic stroke (AIS) not treated with reperfusion therapies (intravenous thrombolysis (IVT) or mechanical thrombectomy (MT)):

- In such patients, hypotension and hypovolemia should be avoided to facilitate systemic perfusion.
- Early treatment of hypertension may be considered in certain comorbid conditions such as heart failure, aortic dissection and myocardial infarction, and coexistent chronic kidney disease (CKD).
- If BP is ≥220/120 mm Hg and there are no associated comorbid conditions, then BP can be reduced acutely initially by 15%, although the benefit of the same in the first 48–72 hours is uncertain. Optimal BP lowering reduces the risk of hemorrhagic transformation and edema, whereas high BP may protect the brain by maintaining cerebral perfusion pressure.
- It is reasonable to lower BP with medications who have a BP of >140/90 mm Hg once the patient is neurologically stable.

There are few studies such as SCAST (The Scandinavian Candesartan Acute Stroke Trial) where patients with AIS and SBP >140 mm Hg were treated with Candesartan within 30 hours of onset and the ENOS (Efficacy of nitric oxide in stroke) trial where patients with SBP > 140 mm Hg were treated with transdermal patches of glyceryl trinitrate (GTN) and compared with placebo. No significant differences and benefit on the final outcome was found between the test and placebo group in both the studies.

In hospitalized patients with AIS and undergoing IVT:

- Before the initiation of intravenous fibrinolytic treatment, BP should be < 185/110 mm Hg and to be maintained < 180/105 mm Hg during the first 24 hours but not < 130–140 mm Hg post-treatment.
- It has been seen that elevated BP levels before and during IVT leads to adverse clinical outcomes such as

symptomatic intracranial hemorrhage (sICH), a lower likelihood of complete recanalization and 3-month good functional outcome.
- It has been seen that with each 10 mm Hg rise in baseline SBP after adjustment for baseline stroke severity, the odds of sICH increased by 10%.

In hospitalized patients with large vessel occlusion and undergoing MT:
- According to the AHA patient's BP undergoing MT should be ≤185/110 mm Hg before and ≤180/105 mm Hg in the first 24 hours after the procedure.
- From the European Stroke Organization (ESO) and ESMINT (European Society for Minimally Invasive Neurological Therapy) recommend BP < 180/105 mm Hg during and the first 24 hours after the procedure and specify the importance of avoiding drops in SBP during the procedure.
- The ESCAPE (Endovascular Treatment for Small Core and Proximal Occlusion Ischemic Stroke) trial stated that SBP ≥ 150 mm Hg is probably useful in keeping the collateral flow adequate, while the artery remain occluded and that controlling BP once reperfusion has been achieved and aiming for a normal BP for that individual.
- Labetalol or an intravenous beta-blocker in low doses is recommended for postprocedural management of BP.

In patients with AIS not treated with reperfusion therapies and with clinical deterioration, does induced hypertension by any vasopressor drug has any role?

The rationale for pharmacologically inducing hypertension is to maintain adequate cerebral perfusion and low BP where reperfusion therapy is not indicated.

In the SETIN-HYPERTENSION (Safety and Efficacy of Therapeutic Induced Hypertension) trial where intervention group received treatment with intravenous phenylephrine with a target of 20% increase in SBP from baseline and compared with control group. Patients with SBP > 170 mm Hg were excluded. The mortality at 90 days in intervention group (1.3%) did not differ much from control group (0%; $p = 0.313$).

Hence, it is suggested that:
- It is reasonable to stop existing BP-lowering medications, where hemodynamic mechanism is suspected for the deterioration.
- Administer IV fluids.
- Introduce nonpharmacological measures to raise BP.
- If necessary, consider use of vasopressor agents.

In patients with AIS, does oral BP-lowering therapy should be continued or temporarily stopped?

There is uncertainty over the benefits and risks, although it is suggested by the ESO to stop oral antihypertensives in patients with dysphagia until swallowing is stored or a nasogastric tube is in place.

HEMORRHAGIC STROKE

In patients with acute intracerebral hemorrhage (ICH):

According to the AHA guidelines:
- When SBP is 150–220 mm Hg, lowering of BP acutely may be effective in relation to functional outcome and is safe.
- When SBP is > 220 mm Hg, it is reasonable to lower BP with intravenous infusion medications and monitoring BP frequently.
- It is reasonable to aim for a target of SBP 140–160 mm Hg early, after the onset of ICH.

According to the ESO:
- In patients with hyperacute (< 6 hours) ICH, lowering BP to < 140 but above 110 mm Hg to reduce hematoma expansion is reasonable
- Initiate antihypertensive treatment as early as possible (ideally < 2 hours of symptom onset). The decrease should not exceed 90 mm Hg from the baseline (risk of acute renal injury increases with > 90 mm Hg reduction from baseline).

The INTERACT2 (Intensive Blood Pressure Reduction in Acute Cerebral Hemorrhage Trial2) was a randomized trial, where BP was reduced within 6 hours of acute sICH in two groups (< 140 and < 180 mm Hg), where there was significant shift to better outcome in group with lower BP arm in comparison to higher arm but mortality was similar in both arms.

Most hematoma expansion occurred within the first 3 hours after the onset of ICH and the probability of hematoma expansion increased with the initial lesion volume of 75 mL.

In order to achieve rapid BP control, drugs need to be fast-acting with short half-life to reduce the risk of excessive reduction of BP but most of the currently used drugs such as labetalol, esmolol, and nicardipine only partially fulfill these criteria. Clevidipine is a calcium-channel blocker with a half-life 1.5 minutes. Graffagnino and his coworkers published a small prospective case-series of 35 patients with acute ICH who were treated with clevidipine. Mean time to target pressure between 140 and 160 mm Hg was only 5.5 minutes and mean volume of ICH was negligible (0.01 mL).

In patients with acute ICH, does oral BP-lowering therapy should be continued or temporarily stopped?

In patients who need BP-lowering medications to maintain BP within the recommended range and who do not have dysphagia or a nasogastric tube is in place, continuation of previous oral antihypertensive has been suggested.

SUBARACHNOID HEMORRHAGE

Increased BP variability is seen to be associated with worse outcomes and excessive BP lowering may compromise cerebral perfusion pressure and induce ischemia in patients with acute subarachnoid hemorrhage (aSAH).

The AHA recommends lowering BP acutely in patients presenting with a SBP of >180–200 mm Hg in aSAH ensuring strict avoidance of hypotension (Mean arterial pressure, i.e., MAP <65 mm Hg).

According to the ESO, until coiling or clipping, SBP should be maintained <180 mm Hg, which may be achieved by nimodipine. If SBP remains high despite these measures, BP-lowering medications should be considered keeping in mind to keep MAP >90 mm Hg.

CONCLUSION

Blood pressure is a powerful determinant of risk for ischemic stroke as well as ICH and there are evidences that suggest that controlling BP reduces the risk of stroke. The management, however, is complex in adults due to its heterogeneous cause. Hence, future studies should focus on the optimal timing and targets for BP reduction as well as the ideal hypertensive medication for the different categories of stroke patients.

SUGGESTED READINGS

1. Lozano R, Naghavi M, Foreman K, Lim S, Shibuya K, Aboyans V, et al. Global and regional mortality from 235 causes of death for 20 age groups in 1990 and 2010: a systematic analysis for the Global Burden of Disease Study 2010. Lancet. 2012;380:2095-128.
2. Whelton PK, Carey RM. The 2017 American College of Cardiology/American Heart Association Clinical Practice guideline for high blood pressure in adults. JAMA Cardiol. 2018;3(4):352.
3. Williams B, Mancia G, Spiering W, Agabiti Rosei E, Azizi M, Burnier M, et al. 2018 ESC/ESH Guidelines for the management of arterial hypertension. Eur Heart J. 2018;39(33):3021-104.
4. Stamler J, Stamler R, Neaton JD. Blood pressure, systolic and diastolic, and cardiovascular risks. US Population Data. Arch Intern Med. 1993;153(5):598-615.
5. Gorelick PB, Whelton PK, Sorond F, Carey RM. Blood pressure management in stroke. Hypertension. 2020;76(6):1688-95.
6. Sandset EC, Anderson CS, Bath PM, Christensen H, Fischer U, Gąsecki D, et al. European Stroke Organisation (ESO) guidelines on blood pressure management in acute ischaemic stroke and intracerebral haemorrhage. Eur Stroke J. 2021;6(2).
7. Sandset EC, Bath PM, Boysen G, Jatuzis D, Kõrv J, Lüders S, et al. The angiotensin-receptor blocker candesartan for treatment of acute stroke (SCAST): A randomised, placebo-controlled, double-blind trial. The Lancet. 2011;377(9767):741-50.
8. ENOS Trial Investigators. Efficacy of nitric oxide, with or without continuing antihypertensive treatment, for management of high blood pressure in acute stroke (ENOS): A partial-factorial randomised controlled trial. Lancet. 2015;385(9968):617-28.
9. Tsivgoulis G, Saqqur M, Sharma VK, Lao AY, Hill MD, Alexandrov AV. Association of Pretreatment Blood Pressure with tissue plasminogen activator-induced arterial recanalization in acute ischemic stroke. Stroke. 2007;38(3):961-6.
10. Berge E, Cohen G, Lindley RI, Sandercock P, Wardlaw JM, Sandset EC, et al. Effects of blood pressure and blood pressure–lowering treatment during the first 24 hours among patients in the Third international stroke trial of thrombolytic treatment for acute ischemic stroke. Stroke. 2015;46(12):3362-9.
11. Turc G, Bhogal P, Fischer U, Khatri P, Lobotesis K, Mazighi M, et al. European Stroke Organisation (ESO) – EUROPEAN society for Minimally Invasive Neurological Therapy (ESMINT) guidelines on mechanical thrombectomy in acute ischaemic stroke endorsed by Stroke Alliance for Europe (SAFE). Eur Stroke J. 2019;4(1):6-12.
12. Goyal M, Demchuk AM, Menon BK, Eesa M, Rempel JL, Thornton J, et al. Randomized assessment of rapid endovascular treatment of ischemic stroke. N Engl J Med. 2015;372:1019-30.
13. Bang OY, Chung J-W, Kim S-K, Kim SJ, Lee MJ, Hwang J, et al. Therapeutic-induced hypertension in patients with noncardioembolic acute stroke. Neurology. 2019;93(21).
14. Al-Shahi Salman R, Frantzias J, Lee RJ, Lyden PD, Battey TWK, Ayres AM, et al. Absolute risk and predictors of the growth of acute spontaneous intracerebral haemorrhage: a systematic review and meta-analysis of individual patient data. Lancet Neurol. 2018;17:885-94.
15. Graffagnino C, Bergese S, Love J, Schneider D, Lazaridis C, LaPointe M, et al. Clevidipine rapidly and safely reduces blood pressure in acute intracerebral hemorrhage: The accelerate trial. Cerebrovascular Diseases. 2013;36(3):173-80.
16. Hoh BL, Ko NU, Amin-Hanjani S, Hsiang-Yi Chou S, Cruz-Flores S, Dangayach NS, et al. 2023 guideline for the management of patients with aneurysmal subarachnoid hemorrhage: A guideline from the American Heart Association/American Stroke Association. Stroke. 2023;54(7).
17. Steiner T, Juvela S, Unterberg A, Jung C, Forsting M, Rinkel G. European stroke organization guidelines for the management of intracranial aneurysms and subarachnoid haemorrhage. Cerebrovasc Dis. 2013;35(2):93-112.

192

CHAPTER

Neuroimmunological Disorders: An Overview

Rahul T Chakor

ABSTRACT

Neuroimmunology is a specialty that focuses on interactions between the nervous system and immune system. Antibody-associated neurological diseases are characterized by a wide range of clinical symptoms, such as memory impairment, behavioral abnormalities, dementia, seizures, movement disorders, weakness, etc. Neuroimmune disorders may affect any part of the nervous system, the brain, and spinal cord [central nervous system (CNS)] or the peripheral nerves, neuromuscular junction and skeletal muscle [peripheral nervous system, (PNS)]. Systemic rheumatologic disorders also frequently affect the nervous system. Paraneoplastic syndromes are a result of exaggerated immune response against a neuronal protein expressed by the tumor. Several drugs such as immune checkpoint inhibitors cause neuroimmunological disorders. We discuss classification and few common neuroimmunological disorders in this chapter.

INTRODUCTION

Neuroimmunology is one of the most rapidly advancing subspecialties in neurology. A field where nervous system and immunology intersect. Neuroimmunological disorders may affect any part of the nervous system **(Box 1)**. Several autoantibodies targeting the central and peripheral nervous system (PNS) have been discovered in the last decade **(Tables 1 to 5)**. Disorders earlier thought as infectious, idiopathic or psychogenic are now reclassified as immune mediated (e.g., NMDA encephalitis). More than 30 new types of pathogenic autoantibodies have been described recently in patients with neurological disease. Thus, representing new clinical entities. Paraneoplastic syndromes are immune-mediated disorders against a neuronal protein expressed by the tumors. There are several classical and non-classical paraneoplastic syndromes **(Box 2 and Table 6)** due to antibodies against intracellular antigens or cell surface antigens **(Tables 1 and 2)**. Systemic and non-systemic vasculitis, autoimmune neurology diseases due to systemic rheumatologic diseases are also neuroimmunological diseases **(Boxes 3 and 4)**. Discovery of antibody mediated neurological disease has diagnostic, therapeutic implications. Technological advances in antigen, antibody detection has hastened detection of new diseases. Antibodies are detected by cell-based assay and novel antigens are discovered by immunoprecipitation and mass spectrometry. Treatment of relapses with high dose steroids, immunoglobulins, and plasmapheresis followed by maintenance therapy with chronic immunosuppression is the usual protocol for most of neuroimmunological disorders **(Box 5)**. We will discuss some common neuroimmunological disorders in this chapter.

AUTOIMMUNE DEMENTIA, ENCEPHALITIS, AND EPILEPSY

These can be due to antibodies to neuronal surface antigen or intracellular/onconeural antigen. Intracellular autoimmune dementia responds poorly to immunotherapy as compared to cell surface autoimmune dementia.

BOX 1: Neuroimmune disorders.

CNS

- Autoimmune encephalitis (NMDA, LGI-1, CASPR 2, GAD-65, amphiphysin, glycine, GABA-A, GABA-B, AMPA, mGluR5, D2R, Neurexin 3α, DPPX, IgLON5, synapsin)
- Autoimmune cerebellitis (Hu/ANNA-1, Ri/ANNA-2, ANNA-3, Yo, PCA-2, GAD-65, Zic-4, Sox1 (glial nuclear antibody), Tr, Protein kinase C gamma, NB (beta-NAP), Carp VIII, mGluR1, septin 5)
- Multiple sclerosis
- Neuromyelitis optica spectrum disorder (NMOSD, AQP4)
- Acute disseminated encephalomyelitis
- GFAP astrocytopathy
- Acute transverse myelitis
- Optic neuritis
- Tropical spastic paraparesis-HTLV1-associated myelopathy
- Post infectious encephalomyelitis
- Rasmussen encephalitis
- Stiff person syndrome (CRMP5, GAD-65, amphiphysin, glycine)
- Poststreptococcal movement disorders
- Pediatric autoimmune neuropsychiatric disorders
- Post infectious cerebellitis
- Hashimoto's encephalopathy/encephalitis
- Paraneoplastic syndromes of the CNS (refer **Box 2**)
- CNS vasculitis
- CLIPPERS (Chronic lymphocytic inflammation with pontine perivascular enhancement responsive to steroids)
- Susac syndrome
- IgGLON-related diseases

PNS

Peripheral nerve

- Guillain–Barré syndrome
- Chronic relapsing/inflammatory demyelinating polyneuropathy
- Multifocal motor neuropathy with conduction block
- Other immune polyneuropathies (MAG, sulfatide, GALOP, CANOMAD, POEMS, etc.)
- Paraneoplastic syndromes of the PNS *(see **Box 2**)*
- Peripheral neuropathy associated with monoclonal proteins (Waldenström macroglobulinemia, MGUS, Multiple myeloma, POEMS etc.)

*Neuromuscular junction (see **Box 2**)*

- Myasthenia gravis
- Lambert–Eaton myasthenic syndrome
- Arthrogryposis multiplex congenital

*Muscle (see **Box 2**)*

- Inflammatory muscle diseases
- Inclusion body myositis (degenerative plus inflammation components)

(CANOMAD: chronic ataxic neuropathy, ophthalmoplegia, IgM paraprotein, cold agglutinins, disialosyl antibodies; GALOP: gait ataxia, late-onset polyneuropathy; POEMS: Polyneuropathy, organomegaly, endocrinopathy, monoclonal protein, skin changes)

TABLE 1: Antibodies against intracellular/cytoplasmic or nuclear antigens.

Onconeuronal antibodies	
Antibody	**Symptoms and disorders**
Anti-Hu/ANNA-1	Sensory neuronopathy, cerebellar degeneration, limbic encephalitis chronic gastrointestinal pseudo-obstruction Lambert–Eaton myasthenic syndrome (uncommon), brainstem encephalitis neuropathies, multifocal nervous system involvement
Anti-Ri/ANNA-2	Opsoclonus/myoclonus, Lambert–Eaton myasthenic syndrome (uncommon), cerebellar ataxia, Jaw dystonia, laryngospasm, cranial neuropathies, myelopathy
ANNA-3	Limbic encephalitis, cerebellar ataxia sensorimotor neuropathy, myelopathy
Anti-Yo	Cerebellar degeneration
Anti-PCA-2	Cerebellar degeneration, limbic encephalitis brainstem encephalitis
Anti-Ma	Limbic encephalitis, brainstem encephalitis
Anti-Ma2	Limbic encephalitis, cranial neuropathies brainstem encephalitis
Anti-CRMP5	Lambert–Eaton myasthenic syndrome, limbic encephalitis, opsoclonus myoclonus stiff person syndrome, optic neuropathy movement disorders (chorea), ataxia myelopathy
Anti-GAD-65	Stiff person syndrome, limbic encephalopathy, cerebellar degeneration, epilepsy, cerebellar ataxia, dyskinesia
Anti-amphiphysin	Stiff person syndrome, limbic encephalitis
Zic-4	Cerebellar degeneration
Sox1 (anti-glial nuclear antibody)	Cerebellar degeneration, Lambert–Eaton myasthenic syndrome, limbic encephalitis sensorimotor neuropathy
Anti-Tr	Cerebellar degeneration
Anti-protein kinase C gamma	Cerebellar degeneration
Anti-ubiquitin conjugating enzyme	Encephalomyelitis
Anti-NB (beta-NAP)	Cerebellar degeneration
Anti-Carp VIII	Cerebellar degeneration

TABLE 2: Antibodies against neuronal surface antigens.

Antibody target	Clinical syndromes/symptoms
AQP4	NMOSD
NMDAR	Encephalitis, psychosis, movement disorder, orofacial lingual dyskinesias, amnesia, behavioral abnormalities, seizures, dysautonomia
LGI-1	Limbic encephalitis (seizures, cognitive impairment), faciobrachial dystonic seizures (FBDS), neuromyotonia
CASPR2	LGI-1-like, neuromyotonia and Morvan's syndrome, neuropathic pain
Glycine receptor	Encephalomyelitis, rigidity, myoclonus, seizures, stiff person syndrome
$GABA_A$ receptor	Seizures, status epilepticus, psychosis
$GABA_B$ receptor	Limbic encephalitis, seizures, memory loss
AMPA receptor	Limbic encephalitis, seizures, memory loss
mGluR5	Limbic encephalitis, confusion, psychosis, memory loss, seizures, movement disorder
DPPX	Confusion, hallucinations, memory loss, hyperexcitability, prodromal diarrhea
D2R	Parkinsonism, chorea, psychosis, dystonia
IgLON5	Sleep disorder, gait abnormalities, bulbar symptoms, cognitive impairment, gaze palsy, hypo-hyperkinetic movement disorder
Neurexin 3α	Clinical overlap with NMDAR encephalitis
mGluR1	Cerebellar ataxia
MOG	Optic neuritis, myelitis, ADEM
Potential transient exposure to surface (during synaptic vesicle exocytosis)	
Amphiphysin	Stiff person syndrome, encephalomyelitis
Septin 5	Cerebellar syndrome, oscillopsia
Synapsin	Limbic encephalitis, in multiple neuropsychiatric disorders

Neuronal Surface Antigen

- *Leucine-rich glioma-inactivated-1 (LGI-1) receptor antibody encephalitis:* This presents with limbic encephalitis in elderly. Faciobrachial dystonic seizures (FBDS) are pathognomonic. Focal motor, generalized tonic clonic seizures, cognitive dysfunction leading to dementia, behavioral symptoms, and insomnia are frequently present. Some patients may have hyponatremia. MRI brain reveals temporal lobe T2/FLAIR hyperintensity. LGI-1 syndrome is usually autoimmune, but rarely is associated with malignancies

TABLE 3: Antibodies seen in inflammatory myopathies.

Autoantibody	Clinical presentation
Anti-Jo 1	Anti-synthetase syndrome
Anti-PL-7, 12	Polyarthritis
Anti-EJ	ILD
Anti-KS	Mechanic hands
Anti-OJ	Myositis
Anti-SRP	Anti-SRP syndrome (muscle, cardiac involvement, steroid resistant)
Anti-Mi2	DM ± ILD
Anti-Scl-PM	Scleroderma, myositis, scleroderma/PM or DM
Anti-Ku	Scleroderma/PM or DM overlap syndromes, SLE, scleroderma, MCTD, Sjögren's, thyroiditis, pulmonary hypertension
Anti-PMS	PM and DM
Anti-56 kDa	PM and DM of childhood onset

TABLE 4: Antiganglioside antibodies associated with different subtypes of Guillain–Barré syndrome (GBS).

GBS subtype	Antibodies
Acute inflammatory demyelinating polyradiculoneuropathy (AIDP)	Unknown
Acute motor and sensory axonal neuropathy (AMSAN)	GM1, GM1b, GD1a
Acute motor axonal neuropathy (AMAN)	GM1, GM1b, GD1a, GalNac-GD1a
Miller Fisher syndrome	GQ1b, GD1b, GT1a
Oculopharyngeal variant	GT1a

TABLE 5: Antibodies seen in myasthenia gravis subtypes.

MG subtype	Auto antibody
Ocular	AchR
Early onset (generalized)	AchR
Late onset (generalized)	AchR, titin, ryanodine
Thymoma	AchR, titin, ryanodine
Musk (facial, bulbar, neck, respiratory weakness, wasting)	MuSK
LRP4	LRP4
Seronegative (generalized)	Antibody against clustered AchR, agrin or cortactin, ColQ
Striated muscle (striational) antibodies	Titin, myosin, actin, ryanodine receptors

- *Contactin-associated protein-like 2 (CASPR2)* receptor antibody presents with cognitive decline, dysautonomia, and sleep disturbances. Involvement of PNS resulting in Morvan's syndrome (peripheral nerve

BOX 2: Paraneoplastic disorders.

Paraneoplastic neurological syndromes

Syndromes affecting the central nervous system

- Cerebellar degeneration
- Encephalomyelitis
- Limbic and brainstem encephalitis
- Opsoclonus-myoclonus
- Stiff person spectrum disorders
- Necrotizing myelopathy
- Motor neuron syndromes (ALS; Subacute motor neuropathy, upper motor neuron dysfunction)

Syndromes affecting the peripheral nervous system

- Sensory neuronopathy/ganglionopathy
- Vasculitis of the nerve and muscle
- Subacute and chronic sensorimotor peripheral neuropathy
- Sensorimotor neuropathies associated with plasma cell dyscrasias and B cell lymphoma
- Autonomic neuropathy
- Brachial neuritis
- Acute polyradiculoneuropathy (Guillain–Barré syndrome)
- Peripheral nerve hyperexcitability

Syndromes Affecting the neuromuscular junction and muscle

- Lambert–Eaton myasthenic syndrome
- Myasthenia gravis
- Dermatomyositis
- Necrotizing autoimmune myopathy

Syndromes affecting the visual system

- Retinopathy
- Optic neuritis
- Uveitis (usually in association with encephalomyelitis)
- Bilateral diffuse uveal melanocytic proliferation

BOX 3: Vasculitis.

Large vessel vasculitis

- Giant cell arteritis
- Takayasu arteritis
- Idiopathic aortitis (IgG4)

Medium vessel vasculitis

- Polyarteritis nodosa
- Kawasaki disease

Small vessel vasculitis

ANCA-associated vasculitis

- Microscopic polyangiitis, granulomatosis with polyangiitis (Wegener), eosinophilic granulomatosis with polyangiitis (Churg–Strauss)

Immune-complex vasculitis

- Cryoglobulinemic vasculitis, IgA vasculitis (Henoch–Schönlein), hypocomplementemic urticarial vasculitis (IgA Vasculitis)

Variable vessel vasculitis

- Behçet disease, Cogan syndrome

Vasculitis associated with collagen vascular disease

- Systemic lupus erythematosus, rheumatoid arthritis

Vasculitis due to substance abuse

- Amphetamines, cocaine, opioids

Vasculitis and infection

- Bacteria, viruses, neurosyphilis, mycoses, parasites, HIV/AIDS

Vasculitis due to drugs

- Penicillamine, minocycline, propylthiouracil, methimazole, carbimazole, hydralazine, minocycline, immune checkpoint inhibitors, levamisole, isoniazid, ethambutol, infliximab, etanercept etc.

Primary CNS vasculitis

TABLE 6: Classical and non-classical paraneoplastic syndromes.

Classical and non-classical paraneoplastic syndromes classified by location		
Neuraxis	**Classical**	**Non-classical**
Supratentorial brain	• Encephalomyelitis • Limbic encephalitis	• Demyelinating encephalopathy, chorea • Parkinsonism
Brainstem and cerebellum	• Cerebellar degeneration • Opsoclonus/myoclonus	• Brainstem encephalitis
Cranial nerves	Cancer-associated retinopathy, melanoma-associated retinopathy	• Optic neuropathy • Bilateral diffuse uveal melanocytic proliferation (BDUMP)
Spinal cord	Subacute motor neuronopathy	• Necrotizing myelopathy • Neuromyelitis optica Inflammatory myelitis • Motor neuron disease, stiff person syndrome
Dorsal root ganglia and peripheral nerve	• Sensory neuronopathy • Chronic gastrointestinal pseudo-obstruction, • POEMS	• Autonomic neuropathy • Acute sensorimotor neuropathy • Polyradiculopathy • Brachial neuropathy • Chronic sensorimotor neuropathy • Neuromyotonia
Neuromuscular junction and muscles	Lambert–Eaton myasthenic syndrome, dermatomyositis	• Myasthenia gravis • Polymyositis • Necrotizing myopathy Myotonia

BOX 4: Neurologic manifestations of systemic rheumatologic diseases.

Neurosarcoidosis

- Cranial neuropathies, meningeal sarcoidosis, pachymeningitis, hypophysitis, granulomas, stroke, encephalopathy, myelopathy, neuropathy (sensorimotor, pure motor or sensory, Guillain–Barré-like syndromes, mononeuritis multiplex, plexopathies)

IgG4 diseases

- Infiltration (pachymeningitis), Tolosa–Hunt syndrome, pituitary gland and/or stalk (IgG4-related hypophysitis), peripheral nerves and rarely brain parenchyma or leptomeninges)

Behçet disease

- Parenchymal (brainstem encephalitis, meninges, cranial nerves, thalamus, basal ganglia, white matter, cerebral cortex, spinal cord. Non-parenchymal (CVST, arterial thrombosis). Peripheral neuropathy (sensorimotor polyneuropathy, mononeuritis multiplex, autonomic neuropathy, Guillain–Barré) necrotizing myositis

Sjögren syndrome

- Peripheral neuropathy-sensory ganglionopathy, sensorimotor, mononeuritis, multiplex, cranial, neuropathies trigeminal neuralgia), radiculoneuropathy, and autonomic dysfunction, myelitis

SLE

- Central nervous system—stroke, vasculopathy, embolism (Libman–Sacks) antiphospholipid antibodies, vasculitis (rare), seizures, migraine (association, likely not causation)
- Demyelinating disease, optic neuritis, brain and brainstem encephalitis, myelitis, meningitis, organic brain syndrome, cognitive dysfunction, dementia, psychosis, peripheral neuropathies

Rheumatoid arthritis

- Atlantoaxial subluxation (myelopathy), neuropathy (pure sensory, sensorimotor, entrapment neuropathies, mononeuritis multiplex

BOX 5: Acute therapy and maintenance therapy for neuroimmunology disorders.

Immunotherapeutic drugs in neurology

Acute/maintenance therapy

Glucocorticoids, intravenous immunoglobulins, therapeutic plasma exchange

Maintenance therapy

Antimetabolites or antiproliferative agents

Azathioprine, mycophenolate mofetil, methotrexate, cyclophosphamide, mitoxantrone, teriflunomide, cyclosporine, tacrolimus

Monoclonal antibodies (Multiple sclerosis)

B cell depletors

- Rituximab, alemtuzumab, ocrelizumab, ofatumumab, ublituximab, natalizumab

Monoclonal antibodies (Myasthenia gravis)

Compliment C5 inhibitor

- Eculizumab, ravulizumab

Neonatal Fc receptor blocker (Myasthenia gravis)

- Efgartigimod,

Recombinant cytokines (Multiple sclerosis)

- Interferon-1a, interferon beta-1b

Synthetic polypeptide

- Glatiramer acetate

Sphingosine 1-phosphate modulator (Multiple sclerosis)

- Fingolimod, siponimod, ozanimod, ponesimod

Nrf2 (nuclear factor erythroid-derived 2-like 2) activators (Multiple sclerosis)

- Dimethyl fumarate, monomethyl fumarate, diroximel fumarate

Miscellaneous

- Isoprinosine, levamisole, thalidomide

Autologous hematopoietic stem cell transplantation

hyperexcitability, neuromyotonia, and continuous muscle fiber activity). Muscle cramps and twitching are typical. EMG shows myokymia. Serum assay for antibodies is sensitive (100%) sensitivity than CSF (88%). These antibodies can be rarely paraneoplastic [breast, small cell lung cancer (SCLC), thymoma, and prostate].

- *NMDA receptor* antibody encephalitis was the first autoimmune encephalitis characterized molecularly. It is commonly seen in young females. Patients present with behavioral and psychiatric disturbances such as paranoia, hallucinations, and psychosis with seizures. Orofacial dyskinesia is diagnostic of NMDA encephalitis. Other movement disorders such as chorea, stereotypies, and repetitive motor behaviors, rigidity are common. Cognitive decline with speech and language disturbances, autonomic disturbances, hypoventilation, and coma is seen in severe cases. Anti-NMDAR antibodies are seen in both serum and CSF. MRI brain reveals abnormality in around 50% patients (hippocampal and basal ganglia T2/FLAIR hyperintensity). EEG reveals a characteristic delta brush pattern. Ovarian teratoma is seen in 60% of women in 18 years and older. Other triggers are infections, HSV encephalitis. Removal of teratoma results in significant recovery.
- *AMPA receptor* antibody encephalitis is a limbic encephalitis (cognitive decline, behavioral symptoms, hallucinations, confusion, and seizures) with cerebellar symptoms and hypersomnia.
- *DPPX receptor* antibody encephalitis presents with cognitive decline, seizures, agitation, tremors, hallucinations, and confusion. Progressive encephalomyelitis with rigidity and myoclonus (PERM) is seen in some patients. Prodromal diarrhea due to dysmotility is frequent.

- *Gamma amino butyric acid B receptor antibody associated encephalitis:*
  Only few cases are reported in the literature. Almost all presented with limbic encephalitis and prominent seizures or status epilepticus. Most common neoplasm associated is small cell lung carcinoma.
- *Gamma amino butyric acid A receptor* antibody encephalitis is rare. Patients present with limbic encephalitis in some patients. Refractory status epilepticus with multifocal cortical MRI abnormalities is seen.
- *Glycine receptor* antibody encephalitis presents as stiff person syndrome and PERM. Rarely limbic encephalitis is reported. These are autoimmune in etiology and rarely associated with thymoma or cancer.

Intracellular Antigen

- *Anti-Hu or antineuronal nuclear antibody 1 (ANNA1)*-associated dementia is commonly associated with small cell lung carcinoma (SCLC). They present with cognitive and behavioral manifestations, neuropathy, cerebellar ataxia, and dysautonomia.
- *Anti-collapsin response mediator protein 5 (CRMP5)*-associated dementia has different manifestations such as cerebellar syndrome, movement disorders like chorea, seizures, cranial and peripheral neuropathy, and cognitive behavioral disturbances. All cases are associated with malignancy hence periodic screening is essential as in other intracellular antibody associated dementia.
- *Glutamic acid decarboxylase (GAD)* antibody-associated dementia. These present with stiff person syndrome and type 1 diabetes mellitus. GAD antibodies are also seen incidentally in asymptomatic individuals. They are rarely paraneoplastic.
- *Purkinje cell cytoplasmic antibody (PCA)* type 2 has a strong association with SCLC. The common manifestations are dementia, involvement of brainstem, neuromuscular junction, peripheral nerves, cerebellum, and autonomic nervous system.
- *Antineuronal nuclear antibody 3 (ANNA3)*-associated dementia. These present with brain stem encephalitis, sensory neuropathy, motor neuropathy, cerebellar ataxia, and myelopathy. There is association with SCLC.

AUTOIMMUNE CNS DEMYELINATING DISORDERS

- *Multiple sclerosis (MS)* is an autoimmune demyelinating disease of the CNS with both inflammatory and neurodegenerative components. It has a relapsing remitting and progressive course. The first clinical event of MS is a clinically isolated syndrome which presents as an episode of optic neuritis, hemiparesis, ataxia, diplopia, vertigo or spinal cord syndromes such as partial transvers myelitis, and Brown–Séquard syndrome. The typical duration of clinical symptomatology is a minimum of 24 hours. Definite neurological signs are required to meet clinical criteria. Two clinical episodes disseminated in space and time, at least 1 month apart with objective clinical evidence and no better explanation fulfil the criteria for clinical diagnosis of MS (Schumacher, Posner criteria). McDonald 2017 criteria are based on MRI evidence of dissemination in space and time. Dissemination in space criteria can be met by demonstrating T2-hyperintense MRI lesions in two of the four typical anatomic locations of MS (periventricular, juxtacortical/cortical, infratentorial, and spinal cord). Dissemination in time criteria can be fulfilled by demonstrating the simultaneous presence of gadolinium-enhancing and non-enhancing lesions. 2017 McDonald criteria state that dissemination in time can be demonstrated by the presence of CSF-specific oligoclonal bands, in a typical clinical syndrome. These criteria facilitate rapid diagnosis of MS with improved sensitivity for a diagnosis of MS in people presenting with typical clinical syndromes. Acute attacks of MS are treated with pulse methylprednisolone. Several disease modifying drugs (DMD) are available **(Box 5)**. Early use of DMD prevents relapses, reduces brain lesions, decreases disability, and conversion to secondary progressive stage.
- *Neuromyelitis optica spectrum disorders (NMOSD)* are inflammatory demyelinating diseases of the CNS associated with episodes of optic neuritis, transverse myelitis, postrema syndrome, acute brainstem syndrome, symptomatic narcolepsy, or acute clinical syndrome. These manifestations that can mimic MS. AQP4-IgG diencephalic antibody is the biomarker of NMO, seen in 80% of cases. Devic disease, opticospinal MS, or Asian MS are all NMOSD. A relapsing course, with severe attacks resulting in permanent deficits is typical of NMOSD. In contrast to MS myelitis attacks are often quite disabling. Optic neuritis episodes in NMOSD tend to be more severe, are associated with less recovery, and are more frequently bilateral than in MS. Systemic autoimmunity-like systemic lupus erythematosus, Sjögren syndrome, and antiphospholipid antibody syndrome frequently coexists with NMOSD. The presence of optic neuritis, transverse myelitis, or intractable vomiting in a patient with one of these disorders suggests NMOSD. The MRI lesions in the optic nerve, brain, and spinal cord

accompanying NMOSD are different than MS. Optic nerve involvement is often bilateral, typically involves the optic chiasm and posterior optic pathway, lesions are adjacent to the third and fourth ventricles (dorsal medulla/area postrema), longitudinally extensive transverse myelitis (LETM), with a T2-hyperintense lesion spanning three or more contiguous. AQP4-IgG antibody testing is available commercially and is best tested in blood as CSF testing is less sensitive. Cell-based assays are more sensitive. Diagnosis of criteria NMOSD needs AQP4 IgG and at least one core clinical characteristic with exclusion of alternative diagnoses. During acute attack high-dose corticosteroids (1,000 mg IV methylprednisolone daily for 5 days) is used initially followed by the use of plasma exchange for five to seven exchanges for severe, corticosteroid-refractory. The goals maintenance therapy is to prevent relapses while limiting side effects. The three most commonly used medications are azathioprine, mycophenolate mofetil, and rituximab. Long-term immunosuppression is currently recommended in all patients with NMOSD.

- *Myelin oligodendrocyte antibody disorder (MOGAD)* presents as a subset of aquaporin-4 (AQP4) negative neuromyelitis optica (NMO) cases. MOG antibodies are detected in patients with ADEM, recurrent optic neuritis, and autoimmune encephalitis. The clinical spectrum of MOGAD has continued to expand. MOGAD are more common in children than in adults, have a monophasic or relapsing course. Seroconversion to MOG-autoantibody negative, decreases the risk of relapse. MOGAD optic neuritis frequently has a relapsing course. MOGADs may emerge as post viral immune-mediated disorder. MOGAD overlaps phenotypically with seronegative NMO, MS, ADEM, transverse myelitis, and chronic relapsing inflammatory optic neuritis. Multifocal relapses with the combination of optic neuritis and myelitis are most common. Optic neuritis in MOGAD is associated with optic disc edema and peripapillary hemorrhages. Long anterior segment optic nerve distinguishes MOGAD from AQP4-positive NMOSD and MS. Vision loss is frequently severe for both MOG-associated and AQP4-positive NMOSD optic neuritis, but recovery of visual acuity is usually better for MOGAD.
- Myelin oligodendrocyte antibody disorder myelitis frequently arises in the setting of prodromal viral illness. It is often multi-segmental, may be either short-segment or longitudinally extensive (three or more spinal segments) and can involve the cord anywhere from the medulla to the conus. There is involvement of spinal gray matter and sometimes asymptomatic lesions are present. There is overlap in clinical features of optic neuritis and myelitis and a subset of patients with MOGADs meet clinical criteria for NMOSD. Between 7 and 42% of seronegative patients with NMOSD have anti MOG autoantibodies and are thus accurately classified as having MOGAD.
- *Chronic lymphocytic inflammation with pontine perivascular enhancement responsive to steroids (CLIPPERS)* is a clinical syndrome of subacute pontocerebellar dysfunction, without peripheral nerve involvement, that is responsive to steroids. MRI shows homogeneous gadolinium-enhancing nodules in the pons and cerebellum. Gadolinium enhancement improves with steroids. Anti-MOG autoantibodies have been detected in several cases of CLIPPERS.

Myelin oligodendrocyte antibody disorders are defined by the presence of anti-MOG antibodies in the serum by using cell-based assays. Acute attacks of MOG-associated disorders are treated similarly to acute events in other demyelinating syndromes with pulse methylprednisolone for 3–5 days. Plasma exchange or IVIg can be used as second-line therapy. Steroid sparing agents such as azathioprine, mycophenolate mofetil, rituximab, tocilizumab, and maintenance IVIg are used for those with relapsing disease.

IMMUNE-MEDIATED NEUROPATHIES

Immune-mediated neuropathies may be acute and self-limited, relapsing-remitting, or chronically progressive. The various immune-mediated neuropathies are, Guillain–Barré syndrome (GBS), CIDP, vasculitic neuropathies **(Box 3)**, autoimmune nodopathies, CANOMAD, paraneoplastic neuropathies, and neuropathy with other systemic rheumatologic conditions **(Box 4)**.

- *Guillain–Barré syndrome* is as an acute ascending neuropathic weakness with strength decreasing to a nadir within 4 weeks along with generalized areflexia. Majority of GBS cases show facial or bulbar weakness. Respiratory muscle weakness is common. Autonomic dysfunction complicates nearly two-thirds of GBS cases. Sensory deficits are mild and reflect preferential involvement of large sensory fibers. About 90% of GBS cases reveal CSF albumino-cytological dissociation. Electrodiagnostic studies typically reveal a picture of AIDP with evidence of a demyelinating polyneuropathy affecting motor more than sensory fibers. Later, more classic features evolve, showing conduction block, temporal dispersion, and prolonged distal and F-wave latencies with sural sparing. GBS variants are AIDP, acute primary axonopathies, such as AMAN, AMSAN, Miller Fisher variant or other regional variants. These axonal subtypes show no evidence of demyelination on nerve conduction studies and typically present as quadriparesis with low amplitude or absent motor potentials and marked evidence of denervation on EMG. Other less common variants of GBS include pure sensory, pure autonomic presentations, as well as regional weakness (oropharyngeal variant). Treatment choice includes PE or IVIg depending on availability and cost.

- *Chronic inflammatory demyelinating neuropathy (CIDP)* presents as progressive symmetric weakness of proximal and distal muscles beyond 8 weeks with sensory disturbance and generalized hypo/areflexia. Temporal evolution may be chronically progressive, stepwise progressive, or relapsing-remitting. Involvement of cranial nerves occurs less frequently in CIDP than in AIDP. Respiratory decompensation and dysautonomia are less prevalent in CIDP. Lymphoproliferative disorders including lymphomas, lupus and other collagen vascular diseases, diabetes, and monoclonal gammopathies are commonly associated with CIDP. The CIDP variant includes multifocal acquired demyelinating sensory and motor neuropathy (MADSAM), distal acquired demyelinating symmetric (DADS) neuropathy, pure sensory CIDP, and multifocal motor neuropathy. Electrodiagnostic studies typically reveal motor and sensory conduction abnormality suggesting demyelination satisfying EAN/PNS criteria. CSF albumino-cytological dissociation is supportive. Treatment with corticosteroids, PE, and IVIg shows roughly equal efficacy. The choice of initial treatment for CIDP should weigh speed of response and side effect profile against convenience and cost. For those refractory, alternative immunosuppressants such as cyclophosphamide cyclosporine or periodic IVIg, PE may be beneficial. Rituximab is beneficial to the subset of treatment-resistant patients with antibodies against nodal and paranodal of proteins such as CNTN1 and NF155.
- *Neuropathies associated with monoclonal gammopathy* Several immune-mediated neuropathies are associated with hematological disorder such as monoclonal gammopathy of undetermined significance (MGUS), Waldenstrom's macroglobulinemia (WM), multiple myeloma (MM), polyneuropathy, organomegaly, endocrinopathy, M protein, skin changes (POEMS), primary amyloidosis, and mixed cryoglobulinemia. MGUS is marked by painless, gradual, distal loss of large fiber sensory modalities. This along with distal weakness leads to a slowly progressive gait disorder. In WM sensory deficits predominate, involving both large and small fiber modalities with distal weakness. In MM typically, the neuropathy is sensory motor distal symmetric with features of primary axonal degeneration. Less frequently, both MGUS and MM can cause mononeuropathy multiplex due to infiltration or deposition of amyloid. In osteosclerotic myeloma, as part of POEMS syndrome, subacute, painful, distal, symmetrical, sensorimotor neuropathy is seen. Many patients fulfil criteria for CIDP. Neuropathies associated with hematological disorders often improve after treating the underlying disorder.

INFLAMMATORY MYOPATHIES

These are characterized by the subacute (over weeks to months) limb girdle weakness, neck flexors, pharyngeal muscles, diaphragmatic weakness, elevated muscle enzymes, and signs of immune dysfunction on muscle biopsies. Dermatomyositis, antisynthetase syndrome, immune-mediated necrotizing myopathy, and overlap myositis are the different types of inflammatory myopathies. Immune-mediated necrotizing myopathy, associated with anti-signal recognition particle (SRP) antibodies have rapid progression over days to weeks. Skin findings of dermatomyositis include the heliotrope sign (periorbital and upper eyelid violaceous discoloration), Gottron sign (erythematous, scaly plaques over the metacarpophalangeal and interphalangeal joints), erythematous rash in sun-exposed areas in the anterior chest (V sign), the posterior neck and shoulders (shawl sign), or the lateral thigh (holster sign). Calcinosis cutis occurs in juvenile dermatomyositis with anti-NXP-2 antibodies. Mechanic's hands are hyperkeratotic eruption over the thumb and the radial aspect of other fingers. It is seen in antisynthetase syndrome and overlap myositis with systemic sclerosis. Interstitial lung disease is a prominent feature of dermatomyositis with anti-MDA-5 antibodies, antisynthetase syndrome, and myositis with systemic sclerosis. Creatine phosphokinase (CPK), lactate dehydrogenase, SGPT, are SGOT are elevated in inflammatory myopathies. CPK can be normal in dermatomyositis and antisynthetase syndrome, especially when the inflammatory muscle fiber pathology is minimal or absent. CPK >20 times normal is seen in necrotizing myopathy. The typical electrophysiologic pattern is the combination of spontaneous activity (fibrillations, positive waves, complex repetitive discharges, and true myotonic discharges) and early recruitment with small, short-duration, polyphasic motor unit potentials. Muscle MRI shows T2 bright signal due to muscle edema. Lung, breast, ovarian, gastrointestinal cancers, lymphoma, and melanoma can occur in inflammatory myopathies, hence screening should be performed in all adults over age of 40 years with dermatomyositis. Patients positive for anti-TIF1-γ16, NXP-2, HMG-CoA reductase IgG antibodies should be screened regularly. First-line treatment is oral or injectable corticosteroids depending on severity of weakness. Second-line treatment is with azathioprine, methotrexate, and mycophenolate mofetil. For refractory cases IVIg, rituximab, and cyclosporine are options.

SUGGESTED READINGS

1. Rizvi SA, Cahill JF, Coyle PK. Clinical Neuroimmunology Multiple Sclerosis and Related Disorders, Current Clinical Neurology. Humana Press; 2020.
2. Dalmau J, Graus F. Autoimmune Encephalitis and Related Disorders of the Nervous System. Cambridge University Press; 2022.

193

CHAPTER

Headache: The Best Clinical Approach

S Sreenivas

ABSTRACT

Headache is a symptom of pain anywhere in the region of the head or neck. There are more than 200 types of headaches. Some are harmless and some are life-threatening. Headache is among the most common reasons patients seek medical attention, on a global basis being responsible for more disability than any other neurologic problem. History (his-story) is the corner stone for the diagnosis of headache type. About 90% of headache is due to primary headache. Migraine at its most basic level is headache with associated features and tension type headache is headache that is featureless. Most patients with disabling headaches probably have migraine. Although 90% of headache patients have underlying primary headache, it is always necessary to rule out secondary headaches that may be dangerous. In an emergency, CT scan is preferred. However when there is a suspicion of an underlying serious disorder MRI is preferred. Fear of missing an underlying secondary cause for the headache is the single most important reason why we investigate headache patients.

INTRODUCTION

The international classification of headache disorders characterizes headache as primary or secondary.

- Primary headaches are those in which headache and its associated features are the disorder itself. They are benign, recurrent headaches not caused by underlying disease or structural problems, e.g., tension-type headache and migraine.
- Secondary headaches are those caused by exogenous disorders. They are caused by an underlying disease such as an infection, brain bleed, or tumors. Secondary headaches may be dangerous.
- Painful cranial neuropathies, other facial pains, and other headaches.

CLASSIFICATION OF HEADACHE DISORDERS

From Headache Classification Committee of the International Headache Society 2018 classification of headache disorders are given in **Box 1**.

BOX 1: Headache classification.

Part one: The primary headaches—
- Migraine
- Tension-type headache
- Trigeminal autonomic cephalalgias
- Other primary headache disorders

Part two: The secondary headaches—
- Headache attributed to trauma or injury to the head and/or neck
- Headache attributed to cranial and/or cervical vascular disorder
- Headache attributed to nonvascular intracranial disorder
- Headache attributed to a substance or its withdrawal
- Headache attributed to infection
- Headache attributed to disorder of homeostasis
- Headache or facial pain attributed to disorder of the cranium, neck, eyes, ears, nose, sinuses, teeth, mouth, or other facial or cervical structure
- Headache attributed to psychiatric disorder

Part three: Painful cranial neuropathies, other facial pain, and other headaches—
- Painful lesions of the cranial nerves and other facial pain
- Other headache disorders

Part four: Appendix

TABLE 1: Mnemonic for headache.

SNOOP red flags	Stands for....	Example...	Think of....
2S	• Systemic symptoms • Secondary risk factors	Fever, weight loss, and fatigue	Infections, inflammation, and metastatic cancer carcinomatous meningitis
N	Neurologic symptoms/signs	Altered consciousness and focal deficits	Encephalitis, mass lesion, and stroke
O	Onset	Thunderclap and abrupt	SAH, ICH, and RCVS
O	Older	New after age 50 years	Temporal arteries
P	• Positional • Prior headache • Papilledema	• Change upright versus lying down • Different in quality • Visual obscurations	• Intracranial hypotension • Intracranial hypertension • Posterior fossa pathology

(ICH: intracerebral hemorrhage; RCVS: reversible cerebral vasoconstriction syndrome; SAH: subarachnoid hemorrhage)

HEADACHE CLINICAL APPROACH—RED FLAGS

The American Headache Society recommends using "SNOOP" a mnemonic to remember the red flags for identifying a secondary headache **(Table 1)**.

PAIN SENSITIVE STRUCTURES

- The brain itself is not sensitive to pain, because it lacks pain receptors.
- However, several areas of the head and neck do have pain receptors and can thus sense pain.
- These include meninges, vessels, cranial and spinal nerves, and head and neck muscles.
- Headaches often result from traction to or irritation of the meninges and blood vessels.

PRIMARY HEADACHE

- About 90% of all headaches are primary headaches.
- Primary headache usually start when people are between 20 and 40 years old.
- *The primary headaches are*:
  - Migraine—unilateral and pulsating accompanied by nausea or vomiting
  - Tension-type headache—bilateral, band-like pressure on both sides of the head usually without nausea or vomiting
  - Trigeminal autonomic cephalalgias
  - Other primary headaches

Migraine

They are recurrent headache attacks of moderate to severe pain intensity with the duration of 4–7 hours with normal physical examination and no other reasonable cause for the headache.

Diagnosis (4, 3, 2, 1 Rule)

- *Duration*: 4 hours to 3 days (72 hours).
- *At least two of the following features*: Unilateral pain, throbbing pain, aggravation by movement, and moderate or severe intensity.
- *Plus at least one of the following features*: Nausea/vomiting, photophobia, and phonophobia.

Migraine versus Tension-type Headache

- Migraine at its most basic level is headache with associated features, and tension-type headache is headache that is featureless.
- Most patients with disabling headache probably have migraine.

Management of Migraine (Flowchart 1)

- Nonpharmacological management
- *Pharmacological management*:
  - Acute attack therapies for migraine
  - Preventive treatments for migraine (in general, a preventive medication to be considered in patients with four or more attacks a month)

Clinical Features of the Trigeminal Autonomic Cephalalgias

Clinical features of the trigeminal autonomic cephalalgias are given in **Table 2**.

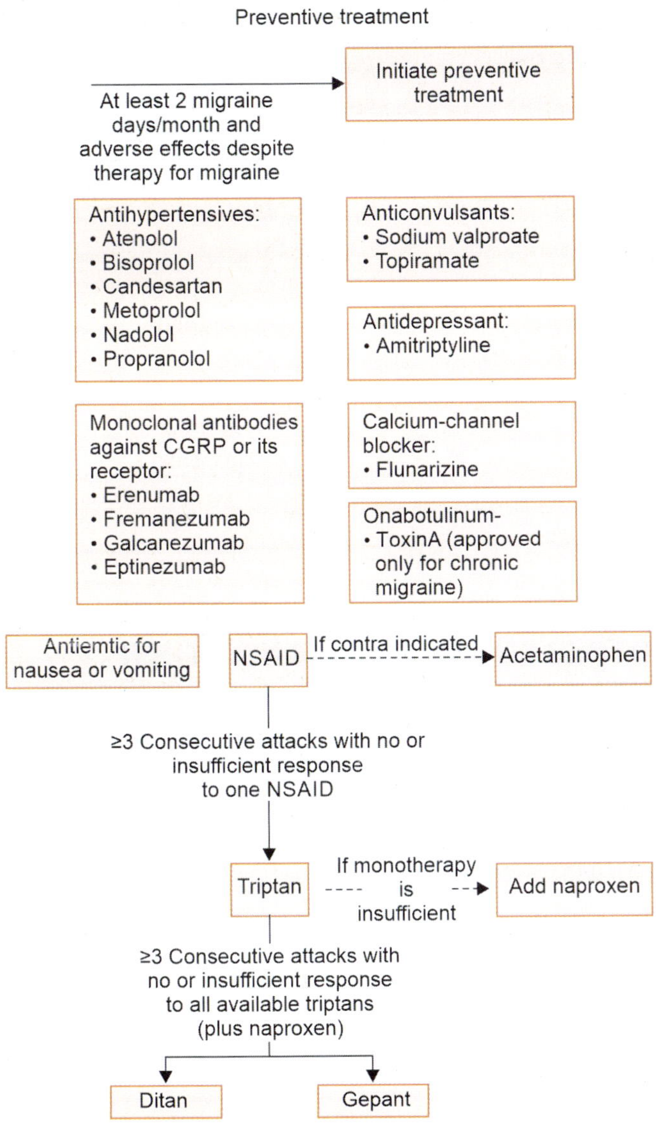

FLOWCHART 1: Management of migraine.

(CGRP: calcitonin gene-related peptide; NSAID: nonsteroidal anti-inflammatory drug)

Other Primary Headaches

- Primary cough headache
- Primary exercise headache
- Primary headache associated with sexual activity
- Primary thunder clap headache
- Cold stimulus headache
- External pressure headache
- Primary stabbing headache
- Nummular headache
- Hypnic headache
- New daily persistent headache

Note:

- These headaches as the name suggests are self-explanatory
- Most of these headache types are responsive to indomethacin

SECONDARY HEADACHES

- *Headache attributed to trauma or injury to the head and or the neck*: The diagnosis depends largely on the close temporal relation between a trauma and headache onset usually within 7 days of trauma.
- *Headache attributed to cranial or cervical vascular disorders*: Vascular disorders cause headache and the new subtype of this category is reversible cerebral vasoconstriction syndrome (RCVS).
- *Headache attributed to nonvascular intra cranial disorder*: Both increased and decreased cerebrospinal fluid (CSF) pressure can lead to headache.
- Headache attributed to a substance or its withdrawal
- Headache attributed to infection
- Headache attributed to a disorder of homeostasis: Hypoxia/hypercapnia and postural hypotension are present in this category

TABLE 2: Clinical features of the trigeminal autonomic cephalalgias.

	Cluster headache	Paroxysmal hemicrania	SUNCT/SUNA
Gender	Male > female	Female = Male	Female ~ Male
Pain			
Type	Stabbing and boring	Throbbing, boring, stabbing	Burning, stabbing, sharp
Severity	Excruciating	Excruciating	Severe to excruciating
Site	Orbit and temple	Orbit, temple	Periorbital
Attack frequency	1/alternate day-8/day	1–20/day (>5/day for more than half the time)	3–200/day
Duration of attack	15–180 min	2–30 min	5–240 seconds

Continued

Continued

	Cluster headache	Paroxysmal hemicrania	SUNCT/SUNA
Autonomic features	Yes	Yes	Yes (prominent conjunctival injection and lacrimation)
Migrainous features	Yes	Yes	Yes
Alcohol trigger	Yes	No	No
Cutaneous triggers	No	No	Yes
Indomethacin effect	—	Yes	—
Abortive treatment	Sumatriptan injection or nasal spray Oxygen	No effective treatment	Lidocaine (IV)
Prophylactic treatment	• Verapamil • Methysergide • Lithium	Indomethacin	• Lamotrigine • Topiramate • Gabapentin

(IV: intravenous; SUNA: short-lasting unilateral neuralgiform headache attacks with cranial autonomic symptoms; SUNCT: short-lasting unilateral neuralgiform headache with conjunctival injection and tearing)

- Headache or facial pain attributed to disorders of the cranium, neck, eyes, ears, nose, sinuses, teeth, mouth, or other facial or cervical structures
- *Headache attributed to psychiatric disorder*: Headache and psychiatric disorder occur together at frequencies higher than expected by chance.

PAINFUL CRANIAL NEUROPATHIES, OTHER FACIAL PAINS, AND OTHER HEADACHES

- Painful cranial neuropathies and other facial pains.
- Other headache disorders.

SUGGESTED READINGS

1. Ashina M. Migraine. N Engl J Med. 2020;383:1866-76.
2. Hoffmann J, May A. Diagnosis, pathophysiology, and management of cluster headache. Lancet Neurol. 2018;17:75-83.

194

CHAPTER

Peripheral Neuropathy: A Clinical Approach

SV Ramanamurty, ISM Giridhar

ABSTRACT

Peripheral neuropathies are the most common neurological conditions encountered by physicians in outpatient department. Peripheral nervous system consists of neural structures present outside the brain and spinal cord, i.e., outside the pia mater. The term peripheral neuropathy is used for involvement of any of the structures, which may be roots, plexus, individual nerves or in combination. Peripheral nerves consist of motor, sensory, and autonomic elements in different proportions. Tingling and numbness or weakness and thinning of limbs or autonomic symptoms like postural hypotension, or loss of hairs or excess sweating, are suggestive of peripheral neuropathy. A stepwise clinical approach is required for correct diagnosis and management, whenever a patient is seen presenting with such symptomatology.

Guillain–Barré syndrome (GBS), chronic inflammatory demyelinating polyneuropathy (CIDP), polyneuropathy due to diabetes mellitus (DM), and nutritional deficiency are some important conditions.

INTRODUCTION

Physicians often come across patients presenting with sensory complaints like pain, tingling, numbness, and sometimes coupled with motor symptoms like weakness or thinning of limbs, suggestive of peripheral neuropathy. A thorough knowledge of organization of peripheral nervous system is required to understand and manage these problems.

The estimated prevalence of peripheral neuropathy ranges from 2.4% in general population to 8% in the elderly above 55 years.

The term "peripheral neuropathy" is used in general for involvement of any structure of peripheral nervous system.

BACKGROUND

- It is believed that John Fothergill (1712–1780) provided the first description of neuropathy in 1773.
- The first description of neuralgia was made by John Fothergill in a medical article, titled "Clinical Lecture on Lead Neuropathy" which was later published in 1924.
- The first known use of the term peripheral neuropathy was in 1936.

ANATOMICAL ASPECTS

- Peripheral nervous system consists of the neural structures outside the brain and spinal cord, i.e., outside the pia mater.
- It consists of anterior root, posterior root, plexus, spinal nerves neuromuscular junction, motor end plate and sensory receptors and cranial nerves excepting first and second cranial nerves, after leaving the cranium, subserving sensory, motor, or autonomic or a combination of the functions.
- *Organization*: Root-trunk-cord-division (for spinal nerves)
- *Peripheral sensory receptors*:
  - Krause bulb—cutaneous sensitivity to cold
  - Merkel's disk—vibration
  - Meissner's corpuscle—light touch

- Ruffini's nerve endings touch—skin stretch
- Pacinian corpuscle—pressure in skin/vibration

TERMINOLOGY

- *Plexopathy*: One side brachial or sacral plexus involved; signs and symptoms are asymmetric.
- *Radiculopathy*: Weakness of distal or proximal muscular weakness or both
- *Mononeuropathy*: Single spinal or cranial nerve affected, e.g., single nerve injury, nerve thickening
- *Mononeuropathy multiplex*: Simultaneous or sequential involvement of multiple noncontiguous spinal nerves, usually bilaterally symmetrical, e.g., diabetes mellitus (DM), vasculitis, sarcoidosis
- *Polyneuropathy*: Symmetrical involvement of multiple nerves, length dependent with weakness along glove and stocking type of distribution, e.g., vitamin B6 deficiency

The classification and causes of peripheral neuropathy are mentioned in **Tables 1 and 2**.

PATHOLOGY

Note: Pathology varies from condition to condition.

- *Demyelinating*:
  - Myelin sheath disruption, acute Guillain-Barré syndrome (GBS), chronic inflammatory demyelinating polyneuropathy (CIDP)
  - Conduction block, recovery occurs in weeks to months

TABLE 1: Classification of peripheral neuropathy.

Pattern of involvement	• Mononeuropathy • Mononeuropathy multiplex • Symmetrical polyneuropathy • Plexopathy • Radiculopathy
Time course	• Acute • Subacute • Insidious
Type of deficit	• Predominantly motor • Predominantly sensory • Mixed sensory–motor • With autonomic involvement
Underlying pathology	• Demyelinating • Axonal
Fiber size	• Large fiber • Small fiber

- *Axonopathy*:
  - Disruption of axis cylinder dying back, from periphery
  - Recovery takes months to years

  Note: It is essential to differentiate axonal and demyelinating neuropathies in view of prognosis **(Table 3)**.
- *Wallerian degeneration*:
  - There is disruption of axon, myelin, and surrounding connective tissues.
  - Recovery will be incomplete or never complete.

TABLE 2: Causes of peripheral neuropathy.

Medical disorders	Renal failure, vitamin B12 deficiency, chronic liver disease, etc.
Vasculitis	• SLE, polyarteritis nodosa • Rheumatoid arthritis, scleroderma, etc.
Hematologic	Lymphomas, chronic leukemias, monoclonal gammopathies, etc.
Endocrine	• Diabetes mellitus, acromegaly • Hypothyroidism, hyperthyroidism, etc.
Toxins	Arsenic, alcohol, hexacarbons, mercury, etc.
Infectious	Lyme disease, HIV, etc.
Inherited	Hereditary motor sensory neuropathy, etc.

(HIV: human immunodeficiency virus; SLE: systemic lupus erythematosus)

TABLE 3: Comparison between axonal and demyelinating neuropathies.

Features	Axonal neuropathies	Demyelinating neuropathies
Motor nerve conduction studies		
Distal latency	Normal	Prolonged
Compound to muscle action potential (CMAP) amplitude	Decreased	Normal
Conduction velocity	Normal	Slow
Temporal dispersion	Absent	Present
F wave	Normal or absent	Prolonged or absent
H reflex	Normal or absent	Prolonged or absent
Sensory nerve conduction studies		
Sensory nerve action potential	Decreased	Normal
Distal latency	Normal	Prolonged
Conduction velocity	[illegible]	Slow

- *Compression*:
  - Carpal tunnel syndrome (median nerve compression) leads to focal and local demyelination, e.g., myxedema
- *Infarction*:
  - Involvement of vaso nervosum leads to multiple infarcts
  - For example, polyarteritis nodosa
- *Infiltration*:
  - Infiltration of the nerves can occur due to leprosy

EXTENT OF INVOLVEMENT OF PERIPHERAL NERVES

- *Neurapraxis*:
  - Here there is no structural damage.
  - Recovery occurs completely in days to weeks.
- *Axonotmesis*:
  - Only axon cylinder is disrupted, recovery takes some months to years
- *Neurotmesis*:
  - There is complete disruption of the nerve.
  - Incomplete recovery

APPROACH

- Analyze the symptoms in chronological order
- Decide the nature of onset whether acute, subacute, or chronic
- Consider the pattern of distribution of weakness
- Workup with relevant investigations
- Manage accordingly

CLINICAL ASPECTS

History

Depending on the etiology and fibers involved, patient may present with varied symptoms and signs.

Symptoms

Motor:
- *Positive symptoms*: Twitching, cramps, myokymia
- *Negative symptoms*: Weakness, fatigue, or wasting (thinning of the limbs)

Sensory:
- *Positive symptoms*: Burning or lancinating pain, tingling paresthesias or hyperalgesia
- *Negative symptoms*: Hyperesthesia, gait abnormalities, loss of balance, especially in dark, difficulty to differentiate between cold and hot

Autonomic:
- Bloating, constipation, diarrhea, impotence, early satiety, light headedness with change in posture
- Examination of limbs may show dryness, scaling, edema, excess sweating, trophic changes, or skin discoloration.
- Some neuropathies may be predominantly with autonomic involvement **(Box 1)**.

General day-to-day activities impairment:
- Patients may feel difficulty to perform their everyday tasks, like writing work, wearing the clothes especially buttoning or unbuttoning, inserting and turning the keys, raising from low-level chair or toilet seat, and moving from side to side on the bed.
- Evolution of the complaints, i.e., onset, duration, and progression
- *Acute*: Inflammatory, e.g., GBS **(Box 2)**
- *Insidious onset*: With slow progression degenerative, e.g., hypothyroidism
- Presence since birth denotes hereditary neuropathy, e.g., Charcot–Marie–Tooth disease

Personal/Social History

- Dietary habits, vegetarian or mixed, smoking, alcohol, drug abuse for pleasure
- Sexual history, lack of libido

BOX 1: Important causes of acute neuropathy.

- Guillain–Barré syndrome
- Vasculitis
- Botulism
- Tick paralysis
- Acute porphyric neuropathy
- Infectious neuropathy
- Critical illness neuropathy

BOX 2: Neuropathies with predominant autonomic features.

- Diabetic autonomic neuropathy
- Guillain–Barré syndrome
- Toxic neuropathies heavy metals, organic solvents, vincristine, cisplatin
- Paraneoplastic and immune mediated neuropathies
- Hereditary sensory and autonomic neuropathies (HSAN), porphyrias, Fabry's disease
- Neuropathy related to amyloidosis
- Human immunodeficiency syndrome (HIV), botulism, Chagas disease

Medical History

- Associated diseases like DM, hypothyroidism, renal failure, connective tissue disorders, cancer or liver disease
- *Drug use*: History of use of chemotherapeutic drugs, steroids, pyridoxine, antibiotics, etc.
- History of orthopedic surgeries, or bariatric surgeries with likely gross reduction of nutrients

Family History

Suggestive of hereditary neuropathies.

PHYSICAL EXAMINATION

General Examination

- Blood pressure (BP) for orthostatic hypotension, resting tachycardia indicating autonomic involvement
- Fragile nails, Koilonychia, Mees' lines
- Pallor, jaundice, oral aphthous ulcers
- Hair loss, malar rash, hyperpigmentation, erythematous photosensitive rash, leonine facies, hypopigmented patches, poorly healing ulcers, linear hyperpigmentation
- Examine for pes cavus, hammer toes or kyphoscoliosis in suspected cases of hereditary neuropathies, clumsiness in walking since childhood without sensory complaints (Charcot-Marie-Tooth disease)
- Thickening of nerves should be examined if leprosy, CIDP suspected
- *Most commonly palpated nerves*: Ulnar nerve at the elbow, peroneal nerve at the fibular head, superficial radial at dorsum of the wrist, greater occipital nerve, great auricular nerve over the neck
- Paraneoplastic syndrome with neuropathy, sensory motor neuropathy, autonomic neuropathy, sensory ganglionopathy (small cell carcinoma of lung)

Cranial Nerve Assessment

- *Anosmia*: Vitamin B12 deficiency
- Optic atrophy in cases of inherited mitochondrial diseases with inherited neuropathy
- Ophthalmoplegia in GBS
- Facial weakness in some neuropathies

Motor Examination

- Neuropathies usually result in distal weakness with involvement of flexors and extensors of lesser toes and extensors of greater toes in legs.
- Weakness of abductors of second and fifth fingers in hands
- Ankle dorsiflexors are more involved compared to plantar flexors.
- Absent ankle jerk

Sensory Examination

Pain, temperature, and touch sensations, joint sense, vibration sense, and position sense are blunted over glove and stocking distribution of varying degrees depending on the duration

GAIT

- Foot drop results in high steppage gait.
- Difficulty in walking on heels than on toes is the typical feature.

Diagnosis

Medical History

- Relevant history suggestive of weakness (loss of motor, sensory, and autonomic function) in glove and stocking distribution
- Gradual onset of abnormal gait (high steppage)
- History of associated diseases like DM, chronic kidney disease (CKD)
- Use of chemotherapeutic drugs, alcohol, etc.
- History of preceding viral infection GBS

Investigations

- Physiologic tests of nerve function
- *Cerebrospinal fluid (CSF) analysis*: Albuminocytological dissociation; usually protein is raised whenever there is infection with raised cell count in CSF. But in GBS protein only raised without rise in cells.
- *Nerve conduction velocity (NCV)*: NCV tests measure signal strength and speed along specific large motor and sensory nerves.
- They can reveal nerves and nerve types affected and whether symptoms are caused by degeneration of the myelin sheath or the axon **(Table 3)**.
- The parameters assessed on NCS include latency, amplitude, sensory nerve action potential, compound to muscle action potential (CMAP).
- F-wave studies reflect conduction over entire length of a motor nerve.
- Erb's point, axillary, and cervical or lumbosacral root stimulation help in assessing conduction block and slowing in proximal nerve segments.
- *Electromyography (EMG) tests*: Detect abnormal muscular electrical activity in motor neuropathy and can help to differentiate between muscle and nerve disorders.

- Nerve biopsy—especially sural nerve
- Neurodiagnostic skin biopsy to examine nerve fiber endings by specialists
- Tests for autonomic function one of which is a the "Quantitative Sudomotor Axon Reflex Test" (QSART) that measures the ability to sweat in several sites in the arm and leg. Abnormalities in QSART are associated with small-fiber polyneuropathies.
- Magnetic resonance imaging/computed tomography/ultrasound (MRI/CT/US) of the offending nerve in selective cases

Ancillary Investigations

Investigations relevant to the clinical setting are as follows:

- Urine analysis
- Complete blood counts
- Antinuclear antibodies, antineutrophil cytoplasmic antibody (ANCA)
- *Serum*: Antiganglioside antibodies
- Blood sugar, serum B12 levels, proteins
- Fasting serum levels of thyroid-stimulating hormone
- Para proteins in patients with chronic demyelinating neuropathy
- Serum heavy metal analysis in suspected cases of exposure
- Testing for vitamin E and copper levels in cases of malabsorption syndrome
- Genetic analysis, e.g., peripheral myelin protein 22 (PMP22)

Note: Gene mutation is responsible in 70% cases of hereditary demyelinating neuropathies.

Management

Principles

- Avoid the offending agent
- Treat the cause
- Treat the symptoms

Symptomatic Medical Therapy

- Tricyclic antidepressants
- Anticonvulsants like gabapentine, carbamazepine, vitamin supplementation (B1, B12, and B6), selenium, zinc, and others

Physiotherapy (Both for Cases of Acute and Chronic Onset)

- Neurodynamic mobilization that moves and glides the nerves to relieve symptoms of peripheral neuropathy
- Anodyne therapy is monochromatic infrared energy; it increases microcirculation and collagen synthesis.
- Balance training such as one leg stance and tandem walking or sit to stand—all will go a long way.
- Faradic current is an interrupted direct current with pulse duration from 0.1 to 1 ms. This frequency and duration cause contraction and relaxation in muscles with intact nerve supply.
- Galvanic current used for stimulation for denervated muscles due to injury
- Cryotherapy with frozen gloves is useful in reducing both the sensory and motor symptoms of the chemotherapy-induced peripheral neuropathy.
- Electric stimulation of individual nerve may provide a novel treatment option for large- and small-fiber neuropathy.
- Interferential therapy (IFT) to alleviate from pain

Surgery

- For entrapment neuropathy, e.g., surgical decompression for carpal tunnel syndrome
- Relevant surgical methods like nerve repair in partial nerve injury

Treatment of the Cause

Early recognition of conditions like GBS will save the patient

Addressing the medical conditions like DM, hypothyroidism, CKD or other specific conditions

Prevention

- Avoid exposure to drugs, toxins, infections
- Treat comorbid conditions
- Control of DM, leprosy, human immunodeficiency virus (HIV)
- Corticosteroids
- Thyroxin

IMPORTANT CONDITION

Guillain–Barré Syndrome/Acute Inflammatory Demyelinating Polyneuropathy (Fig. 1)

- GBS is the most common acute demyelinating anterior polyneuritis.
- It is an autoimmune disorder, which affects people at any age.
- It usually follows viral infection; antiganglioside antibodies are seen in at least one-third of patients.
- Multifocal demyelination with inflammation results in conduction block.
- Severe forms show secondary axonal degeneration.

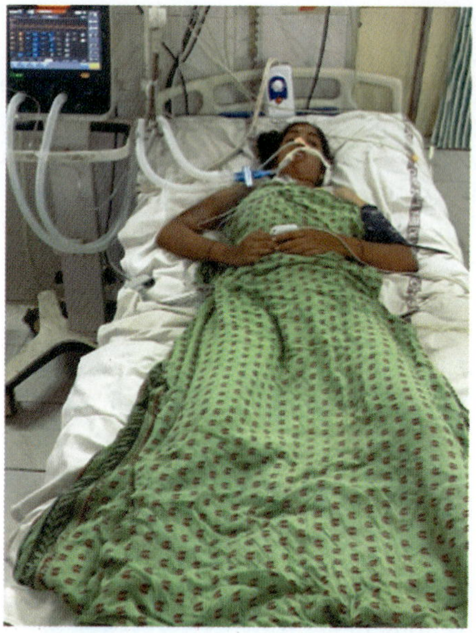

FIG. 1: A 38-year-old female with GBS/AIDP (Guillain–Barré syndrome/acute inflammatory demyelinating polyneuropathy).

Notes:
- Patient complains of difficulty in swallowing since 3 days to solids and liquids aggravated since 1 day
- Weakness of both lower limbs since 1 day notice, while she was unable to stand from squatting position followed by weakness of upper limbs from afternoon
- Vitals stable at admission
- Lumbar puncture was done, cerebrospinal fluid (CSF) revealed raised protein 1.05 g/dL and 5 cells, sugar 85 mg/dL, chloride 112 mg/dL
- With a provisional diagnosis of GBS, intravenous immunoglobulin (0.4 g/kg/day) and other supportive measures were started.
- After 1 day of admission complaining of shortness of breath around 5.30 PM, hence, intubated on the same day at 6.30 PM

Clinical Features

- It is an acute disorder, predominantly a motor neuropathy usually progresses for a few days but rarely up to 1 month. Sensory findings are minimum and consist of distal paresthesias with mildly disturbed joint/position sense.
- Motor paralysis is more striking, and symmetrical, involving mostly proximal muscles. It begins in legs progressing over several days to involve arms, face, and eyes (ascending type of paralysis)
- Deep tendon reflexes (DTR) are blunted, 50% of patients show bilateral facial palsy. Some show bulbar muscle weakness. Respiratory paralysis occurs in a few.
- Autonomic disturbances occur in a few and sudden fluctuations in BP and heart rate may occur.
- Bladder is usually spared.

Variants:
- Acute motor and sensory axonal neuropathy (AMSAN)
- Miller Fisher syndrome

Investigations

- CSF becomes abnormal after 1 week of illness, and shows raised protein >45 mg/dL, normal sugar and cell count
- Nerve conduction studies show slowing of velocities and conduction block (demyelinating pattern)

Treatment

- Maintenance of circulation, airway, breathing, ventilatory support if there is respiratory paralysis
- Monitor pulse, BP, and cardiac activity using a cardiac monitor when the patient develops autonomic instability
- Intravenous immunoglobulin (2 g/kg in divided doses over 5–7 days) have been shown to accelerate recovery.
- Plasma exchange 50 mL/kg on five separate occasions over 1–2 weeks
- Daily plasma exchange in severe GBS helps in early weaning from ventilator
- Physiotherapy for at least 3–4 months

Note: Glucocorticoids have no role.

CONCLUSION

The problem of peripheral neuropathy is often easy to diagnose but difficult to get satisfactory results. Sometimes exhaustive workup is required. It is highly essential to diagnose GBS at earliest and start intravenous immunoglobulin immediately to save the patient. A systematic approach is required to deal with cases of peripheral neuropathy.

SUGGESTED READINGS

1. Remiche G, Kadhim H, Maris C, Mavroudakis N. Peripheral neuropathies, from diagnosis to treatment, review of the literature and lessons from the local experience. Rev Med Brux. 2013;34(4):211-20.
2. Seneviratne U. Guillain-Barré syndrome. Postgrad Med J. 2000;76(902):774-82.

195

CHAPTER

Clinical Approach to Ataxia

MPS Chawla, Ashutosh Kumar Karn, Amit Aggarwal

ABSTRACT

The correct diagnosis of "ataxia" remains a clinical challenge owing to the heterogeneity of the underlying causes. In patients with an early onset of disease before the age of 25 years with healthy parents, an autosomal recessive inheritance is most likely. A familial disorder affecting successive generations is suggestive of autosomal dominant spinocerebellar ataxia. However, in adult neurology, a more frequent and challenging diagnostic situation is that of an ataxic patient with adult-onset sporadic disease, usually after 40 years of age. In such a case, almost the entire spectrum of non-genetic and genetic causes needs to be considered before reaching a diagnosis. Magnetic resonance (MR) brain imaging provides diagnostic clues identifying structural causes, such as tumors and multiple sclerosis. Advances in molecular genetics including the availability of 'next-generation sequencing' have enabled the clinicians to identify many more genetic causes. Autoimmunity is perhaps an under-recognized cause of progressive ataxia, like subjects with antigliadin antibodies and those associated with paraneoplastic syndromes. In this chapter, we provide a step-by-step approach to diagnose and investigate the possible causes of ataxia.

INTRODUCTION

The word "ataxia" originates from the Greek language meaning "incoordination". Neurologically, it is a state of disorder characterized by lack of coordination and balance in different regions of the body including gait, limbs, eye, and speech. Balance and coordination are products of complex circuitry involving the basal ganglia, cerebellum, cerebral cortex, peripheral motor, and sensory pathways. Dysfunction of any part of this intricate circuitry leads to ataxia. It results in errors in the rate, range, force, and direction of movements. Identifying the underlying cause can be challenging, but it indicates cerebellar dysfunction, impaired vestibular function, or a lack of proprioceptive afferent input to the cerebellum.

CLASSIFICATION OF ATAXIA

There are three main types of ataxia, each determined by where it occurs in the body. *Vestibular ataxia* is caused by problems with the semicircular canals, otolith organs, or their connections. *Sensory ataxia* is caused by damage to small or large nerve fibers, the dorsal column, or neuronopathy. *Cerebellar ataxia* is a result of changes in the cerebellar pathways. Additionally, diseases that affect the fronto-ponto-cerebellar fibers can cause gait abnormalities, also known as frontal ataxia or gait apraxia. A patient may experience symptoms of multiple types of ataxia, but the diagnosis is based on the primary type. **Table 1** describes their characteristic traits of various types of ataxia and **Box 1** depicts the various etiological causes of ataxia.

ANATOMIC BASIS OF CLINICAL SIGNS

The cerebellum has different functional regions corresponding to their connections—motor, sensory, visual, and auditory.

- Middle zone lesions affect axial functions and produce nystagmus, disorders of ocular motility, dysarthria, oscillation of head and trunk, instability of stance, and gait ataxia

TABLE 1: Differentiating features of ataxia.

	Vestibular	Cerebellar	Sensory
Vertigo	Present	May be present	Absent
Nystagmus	Present	Often present	Absent
Dysarthria	Absent	May be present	Absent
Limb ataxia	Absent	Usually present (one limb, unilateral, legs only, or all limbs)	Present (typically legs)
Stance	May be able to stand with feet together; typically worse with eyes closed	Unable to stand with feet together and eyes either open or closed	Often able to stand with feet together and eyes open but not with eyes closed (Romberg sign)
Vibration and position sense	Normal	Normal	Impaired
Ankle reflexes	Normal	Normal	Depressed or absent

BOX 1: Etiology of ataxia.

- *Acute causes (minutes to a few days)*:
  - Ischemic or hemorrhagic cerebellar strokes
  - Medications (phenytoin, carbamazepine, phenobarbital, and lithium)
  - Toxins (mercury, thallium, toluene, and solvents)
  - Ethanol intoxication
  - Meningitis (particularly basilar meningitis)
  - Viral cerebellitis
  - Cerebellar abscess
  - Wernicke's encephalopathy/thiamine deficiency
  - Multiple sclerosis
- *Subacute causes (weeks to months)*:
  - Paraneoplastic cerebellar degeneration
  - Superficial siderosis
  - Antiglutamic acid decarboxylase ataxia
  - Creutzfeldt–Jakob disease
  - Brain tumors
- *Chronic causes (months to years)*:
  - Ataxia associated with gluten sensitivity
  - Multiple system atrophy
  - Idiopathic late-onset cerebellar ataxia
  - Genetic ataxia [autosomal dominant spinocerebellar ataxia (SCA) 1–48, autosomal recessive cerebellar ataxia (ARCA), episodic ataxia, mitochondrial ataxia, and X-linked ataxia]
- *Episodic causes (hours to days)*:
  - Genetic episodic ataxia
  - Mitochondrial disease
  - Psychogenic ataxia

- Lateral cerebellum lesions affect limb coordination, tone, and ipsilateral gaze. They cause ipsilateral hemiataxia, limb hypotonia, transient ipsilateral gaze paresis, and nystagmus.

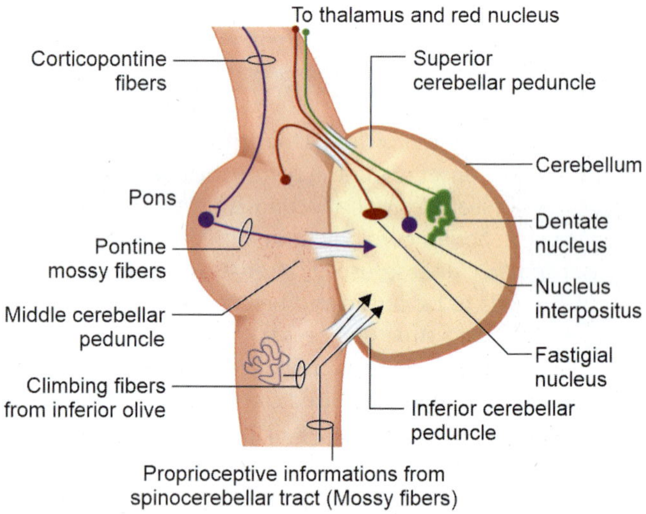

FIG. 1: Afferent and efferent connections of cerebellum.

- Diffuse cerebellar disorders affect the cerebellum, combining midline, and bilateral hemisphere disease features.

Figure 1 shows the various intricate afferent and efferent connections of the cerebellum, which is important for the understanding of anatomical basis of the clinical signs. **Table 2** describes the exact anatomical localization for the associated clinical signs.

Box 2 enumerates all the clinical features associated with ataxia in detail, like gait imbalance, dysarthria, dysphagia, vision disturbances, and loss of fine movements.

NEUROLOGIC EXAMINATION FOR ATAXIA

The neurologic examination of ataxia can be divided into several domains: eyes, speech, hands, legs, and gait. **Box 3** explains the abnormalities of eye movement associated with ataxia syndromes.

TABLE 2: Anatomical localization of clinical signs.

Pattern of involvement	Signs	Causes
Midline	Nystagmus, dysarthria, head and trunk titubation, gait ataxia	Tumor, multiple sclerosis
Superior vermis	Gait ataxia	Wernicke encephalopathy, alcoholic cerebellar degeneration, tumor, multiple sclerosis
Cerebellar hemisphere	Nystagmus, ipsilateral gaze paresis, dysarthria, ipsilateral hypotonia, ipsilateral limb ataxia, gait ataxia, falling to side of lesion	Infarction, hemorrhage, tumor, multiple sclerosis
Pancerebellar	Nystagmus, bilateral gaze paresis, dysarthria, bilateral hypotonia, bilateral limb ataxia, gait ataxia	Sedative drug intoxication, hypothyroidism, autosomal dominant spinocerebellar ataxias, paraneoplastic cerebellar degeneration, Wilson disease, infectious and parainfectious encephalomyelitis, Creutzfeldt–Jakob disease, multiple sclerosis

BOX 2: Clinical features of ataxia.

- Gait imbalance (difficulty walking, running, turning, trouble walking in high heels or barefoot on the beach, and veering toward one side, walking like a drunkards, and frequent falls)
- Loss of hand dexterity with bad handwriting and difficulty performing delicate hand tasks
- Slurred speech
- Swallowing difficulty
- Dizziness
- Associated symptoms of peripheral neuropathy, parkinsonism, sleep dysfunction, autonomic symptoms, seizures, and hearing loss
- Blurry vision, resulting from transient and mild double vision, is also common especially during quick head turn

BOX 3: Eye movement abnormalities associated with ataxia.

- Saccadic intrusion in fixed gaze (i.e., square-wave jerks), which can be seen especially in Friedreich's ataxia
- Horizontal or vertical end-gaze nystagmus, which occurs in many types of ataxia, among which downbeat nystagmus can often been seen in [spinocerebellar ataxia type 6 (SCA6)]
- Ophthalmoplegia/ophthalmoparesis, which can be observed in sensory ataxic neuropathy, dysarthria, and ophthalmoparesis (SANDO)
- Ptosis, which can occur in SANDO and ataxia associated with mitochondrial genome mutations
- Hypometric or hypermetric saccades, which can be observed in many types of ataxia
- Breakdown of smooth pursuit, often encountered in SCA3 and 5
- Slow saccades, typical for SCA2 and 5
- Among these signs, nystagmus, and hypometric or hypermetric saccades are commonly shared by ataxic disorders; these signs are helpful in differentiating cerebellar ataxia from sensory ataxia, especially in the early stages of the disease when no cerebellar atrophy is found on neuroimaging

Speech

Patients with ataxia typically exhibit scanning speech, characterized by syllable-separation and disrupted speech patterns. Speech may be slow and variable in volume.

Limb Ataxia

The ataxic hand examination includes three tasks: (1) finger-nose-finger test, (2) finger chase, and (3) fast alternating movements. Patients with ataxia will have difficulty performing these tasks. In heel-to-shin tests, patients will have difficulty keeping the heel on the shin. Patients are also tested for balance abnormalities using maneuvers, such as standing with feet together, standing on either foot, or hopping on either foot.

Gait

Observing the patient's gait is crucial when diagnosing ataxia. Characteristics of the gait may vary depending on the stage of the disease. A narrow-based gait with frequent missteps and veering may indicate mild cases, while a wide-based gait may develop in moderate cases. Shortened stride length and compensation may occur in advanced stages. Observing stair and running ability can also aid in diagnosis. Once examination establishes the presence of ataxia, other associated extracerebellar signs **(Table 3)** help in the specific diagnoses.

DIAGNOSTIC WORKFLOW FOR CEREBELLAR ATAXIA

A systematic approach to evaluate ataxia involves step-by-step algorithm given in **Flowchart 1**.

Determining the underlying causes of ataxia, various tests are done in a step-by-step approach **(Table 4)**.

TABLE 3: Extracerebellar signs for genetic ataxia.

Signs	Ataxias
Motor neuronopathy	Spinocerebellar ataxias (SCAs) 2, 3, and 36
Severe neuropathy or areflexia	Primarily autosomal recessive ataxias
Pyramidal signs (spasticity and hyperreflexia)	Common in autosomal dominant ataxias, uncommon in autosomal recessive ataxia [e.g., autosomal recessive spastic ataxia of Charlevoix–Saguenay (ARSACS), hereditary spastic paraplegia (HSP), ataxia telangiectasia (AT), Friedreich's ataxia (FA), and cerebellar ataxia with neuropathy and vestibular areflexia syndrome (CANVAS)]
Myopathy, strokes, visual impairment, cardiac disease, seizures, cognitive impairment, liver disease	Mitochondria associated (MELAS, MERRF, NARP, POLG-associated)
Parkinsonism, dystonia, tremor, myoclonus	Common in multiple system atrophy (MSA), variable in inherited ataxias
Chorea	Huntington disease (HD), HD-like, SCA17, Dentato-rubro-pallidoluysian atrophy (DRPLA)
Autonomic dysfunction, rapid eye movement (REM) sleep behavior disorder (RBD)	Most common in MSA; also seen in SCAs 1, 2, 3, and CANVAS
Seizures	Most common in SCA10
Neuropathy and retinitis pigmentosa	NARP (neuropathy, ataxia, and retinitis pigmentosa), a mitochondrial ataxia
Visual impairment or blindness	Most common in SCA7; also in FA, spastic paraplegia (SPG) 7, ataxia with vitamin E deficiency (AVED), POLG-related ataxia
Downbeat nystagmus	SCAs 5, 6, Arnold–Chiari malformation, basilar invagination
Oculomotor apraxia	Ataxia with oculomotor apraxia (AOA) 1, 2, 4 and AT
Tendon xanthoma, early cataracts, seizures, cognitive impairment	Cerebrotendinous xanthomatosis (CTX)
Intellectual disability	SCAs 13, 27
Hyperkeratotic skin lesions, retinitis pigmentosa	SCA34
Chronic cough	CANVAS
Psychiatric features	SCAs 12, 17, 27
Palatal myoclonus	Alexander disease, SCA20
Tremor	SCA12, SCA15/16, FXTAS

NEUROIMAGING FOR ATAXIA

Patients with ataxia should have a brain magnetic resonance imaging (MRI) to check for issues like tumors, strokes, or multiple sclerosis. Cerebellar atrophy is the most common finding. Neurologists examine the degree of atrophy in different areas of the cerebellum to determine the cause of ataxia. Other MRI findings may indicate specific diagnoses, and special attention should be paid to the spinal cord in patients with certain types of ataxia as described in **Table 5**. If multiple system atrophy (MSA) is suspected, dopamine transporter scan (DAT scan) can determine presynaptic dopamine terminal loss.

Genetics of Ataxia

Patient with family history of ataxia, the diagnosis process involves categorizing it into four types based on inheritance patterns: (1) autosomal dominant ataxia, (2) autosomal recessive ataxia, (3) X-linked ataxia, and (4) mitochondrial disorders. Ataxia is caused by various genetic factors, but there are reliable methods for diagnosis and categorization. The Online Mendelian Inheritance in Man (OMIM) is a trusted source of current information on ataxia genetics. Autosomal dominant cerebellar ataxia is classified under the spinocerebellar ataxia (SCA) nomenclature, ranging from type 1 to 48. Each SCA type has distinct but overlapping clinical

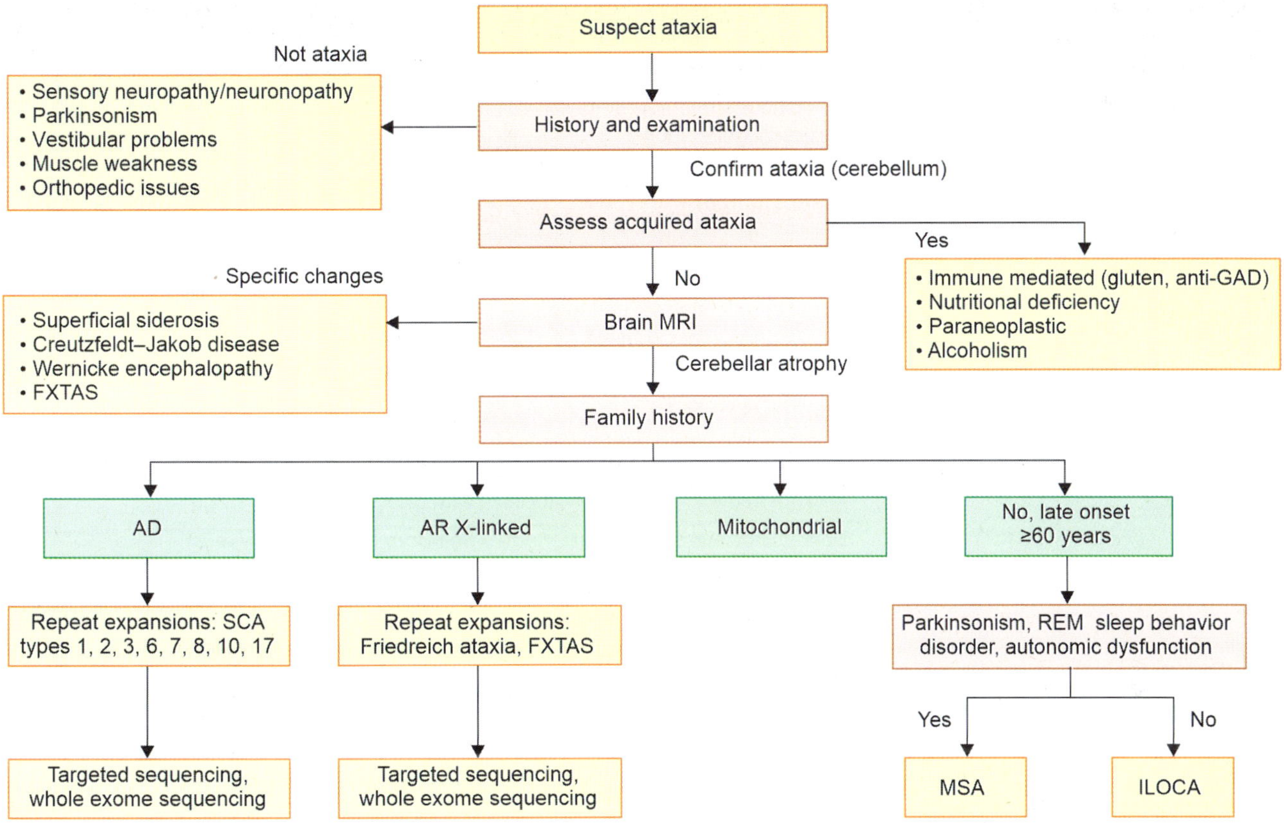

FLOWCHART 1: Diagnostic workflow for ataxia.

(anti-GAD: anti-glutamic acid decarboxylase; AR: autosomal recessive; ILOCA: idiopathic late-onset cerebellar ataxia; MRI: magnetic resonance imaging; MSA: multiple system atrophy; REM: rapid eye movement; SCA: spinocerebellar ataxia)

TABLE 4: Diagnostic investigations in ataxia.

Primary care	Serum urea and electrolytes, serum creatinine, full blood count ESR/C-reactive protein	Liver enzymes, serum GGT, thyroid function tests, vitamin B12	Serum folate, plasma glucose, chest X-ray
Secondary care (first line)	• α-FP • Blood film • Ceruloplasmin/Copper • Celiac disease screen, serum creatine kinase • Genetic tests for Friedreich's ataxia, SCA1, 2, 3, 6, 7 (12, 17) and fragile X tremor-ataxia syndrome	• Lactate • Lipid-adjusted vitamin E and lipoproteins • Lumbar puncture (cells, protein, glucose, cytology, oligoclonal bands, lactate, ferritin) • MR scan of brain and cervical spine	• Anti-Hu/Yo and other paraneoplastic antibodies • Anti-GAD antibody • Anti-voltage-gated calcium channel antibody • CT scan of chest, abdomen, pelvis 14-3-3 and other proteins in CSF (prion diseases)
Secondary care (second line)	• Cholestanol • Plasma oxysterols • Bile acids • Coenzyme Q10 (ubiquinone) • Electroencephalography • Very-long-chain fatty acids	• Muscle biopsy • Ophthalmology/Optical coherence tomography • Peripheral nerve conduction studies • Phytanic acid	• Remaining genetic tests (next-generation sequencing) • Total body PET scan • White cell enzymes

(CSF: cerebrospinal fluid; CT: computed tomography; ESR: erythrocyte sedimentation rate; FP: fetoprotein; anti-GAD: anti-glutamic acid decarboxylase; GGT: gamma-glutamyl transferase; MR: magnetic resonance; SCA: spinocerebellar ataxia; PET: positron emission tomography)

TABLE 5: Brain MRI findings associated with specific forms of ataxia.

Brain MRI findings	Associated findings and pathology	Associated ataxia
No cerebellar atrophy	No obvious structural cerebellar cortical degeneration	Friedreich's ataxia, ataxia with vitamin E deficiency, abetalipoproteinemia, immune-mediated ataxia
Hot cross bun sign	Pontine atrophy	Multiple system atrophy, spinocerebellar ataxia type 2
Cervical spinal cord atrophy	Cervical spinal cord atrophy	Friedreich's ataxia
T2 hyperintensity in the middle cerebellar peduncles	Degeneration/Demyelination of middle cerebellar peduncles	Multiple system atrophy, fragile X tremor-ataxia syndrome
T2 hyperintensity in the mammillary bodies, periaqueductal gray, and paraventricular thalamus	Possibly petechial hemorrhages in these brain regions	Wernicke's encephalopathy
T2 hyperintensity in the bilateral inferior olivary nuclei	Hypertrophic degeneration of the neurons in the inferior olivary nuclei	POLG ataxia, adult-onset Alexander disease, ataxia with gluten sensitivity
Dentate nucleus calcification (CT)	Dentate nucleus calcification	Spinocerebellar ataxia type 20
T2 hyperintensity in the white matter	Leukoencephalopathy	Cerebrotendinous xanthomatosis, adult-onset Alexander disease
Medullary atrophy	Medullary atrophy	Adult-onset Alexander disease
T2 gradient recalled echo showing linear hypointensity around the cerebellum and brainstem	Iron deposition on the surface of the brain parenchyma	Superficial siderosis
Diffusion-weighted imaging hyperintensity in the cerebral cortex, basal ganglia, or thalamus	Spongiform degeneration	Creutzfeldt–Jakob disease
Hypointense pontine stripes, atrophy of superior cerebellar vermis, thinning of posterior mid-body of corpus callosum		Autosomal recessive spastic ataxia of Charlevoix-Saguenay (ARSACS)

(CT: computed tomography; MRI: magnetic resonance imaging)

features **(Table 6)**. Different cytosine adenine guanine (CAG)-repeat SCAs have varying rates of progression. SCA1 progresses the fastest, followed by SCA3 and SCA2, while SCA6 has the slowest progression rate among these subtypes. The common CAG-repeat SCAs are believed to be caused by polyglutamine, and the associated repeats exert toxic effects on neurons or cause the loss of normal function in respective proteins.

Autosomal recessive ataxia can be classified into three categories depending on the presence of associated neuropathy. The first category is characterized by cerebellar ataxia with predominant sensory neuronopathy and includes Friedreich's ataxia. The second category is ataxia with sensorimotor axonal neuropathy, and the third category is ataxia without sensory neuropathy. Identifying the type of ataxia in patients can be helpful in providing appropriate management and treatment. Mitochondrial DNA mutations have been known to cause ataxia, and fragile-X tremor-ataxia syndrome is a prevalent form of X-linked ataxia. Various phenotype-genotype correlations for ataxia are given in **Table 7** that help in arriving at the clinical diagnosis.

TABLE 6: Spinocerebellar ataxia (SCA) subtypes and distinguishing features.

SCA subtypes	Clinical features
SCA1	Pyramidal involvement, ophthalmoplegia
SCA2	Slow saccades, peripheral neuropathy
SCA3	Also known as Machado–Joseph. Pyramidal involvement, ophthalmoplegia, peripheral neuropathy, in a subgroup parkinsonian phenotype
SCA6	Allelic with EA2/familial hemiplegic migraine, mild ataxic syndrome
SCA7	Macular degeneration
SCA8	No specific test
SCA10	Seizures, Mexican origin
SCA11	
SCA12	Tremors, common in India
SCA13	Mental retardation
SCA15	
SCA17	Psychiatric features, dementia, chorea
SCA28	Slow saccades, ophthalmoplegia

TABLE 7: Phenotype diagnostic test-genotype correlations for ataxia.

Clinical features of (in addition to ataxia) phenotype	Neuroimaging and other diagnostic biomarkers	Gene: Disease
Pyramidal signs, amyotrophy, hypermetric saccades	Global cerebellar and brainstem atrophy, "hot cross bun" sign	*ATXN1*: SCA1
Hyporeflexia, hypometric saccades, amyotrophy, autonomic dysfunction, parkinsonism, dystonia; may mimic MSA or ALS	Global cerebellar and brainstem atrophy olivopontocerebellar pattern; "hot cross bun" sign	*ATXN2*: SCA2
Pyramidal signs, "bulging eyes", amyotrophy, neuropathy, parkin sonism, RBD symptoms, autonomic dysfunction; may mimic atypical parkinsonism, MSA, ALS	Global cerebellar atrophy	*ATXN*: SCA3
Neuropathy, areflexia, Babinski signs, scoliosis, pes cavus, cardiomyopathy, diabetes	Spinal cord atrophy, mild or no cerebellar atrophy, elevated cholesterol, serum glucose, and HbA1c	*FXN*: FA
Neuropathy, areflexia, vestibulopathy, chronic cough, autonomic dysfunction	Cerebellar vermian atrophy, abnormal vestibular tests, diminished VOR, gain on HIT on vestibular testing	*RFC1*: CANVAS
XY heterozygote with tremor, ataxia, neuropathy, parkinsonism	T2 hyperintensities in the MCP, mild cerebellar atrophy	*FMR1*: FXTAS
Spasticity, peripheral neuropathy, hearing loss, autonomic dysfunction, seizures; predominantly French-Canadian ancestry	Superior vermian and spinal cord atrophy T2 linear hypointensities in mid pons near pyramidal tracts, thinning of corpus callosum	*SACS*: ARSACS
Sensory myeloneuropathy, visual impairment, areflexia: FA-like picture without musculoskeletal abnormalities	Cerebellar and/or spinal cord atrophy, low serum vitamin E	*TTP*: AVED
	Cerebellar and/or spinal cord atrophy, low serum vitamin E, abnormal lipoprotein profile, PBS shows acanthocytes	*MTTP*: ABL
Oculomotor apraxia, ± telangiectasias, polyneuropathy, chorea, dystonia, sensitivity to ionizing radiation, chorea, infections, immune deficiency	Cerebellar atrophy, hemosiderin deposits and telangiectasias seen in GRE sequences; elevated AFP, low IgA levels	*ATM*: AT
Oculomotor apraxia, polyneuropathy	• Cerebellar atrophy, elevated AFP • Cerebellar atrophy, low albumin, elevated cholesterol	• *SETX*: AOA2 • *APTX*: AOA1
Sensory neuropathy, ophthalmoplegia, myopathy, myoclonus, seizures, visual impairment, liver dysfunction	Cerebellar vermian atrophy, T2 hyperintensities of inferior olivary nucleus (ION); abnormal liver function tests, elevated lactate and pyruvate, abnormal muscle biopsy	*POLG1*: POLG-ataxia
Diverse central and peripheral nervous system involvement, visual, cardiac, hepatic symptoms, including acute stroke-like symptoms, neuropathy, myoclonus, and myopathy	T2 hyperintensities resembling strokes; elevated lactate, pyruvate, abnormal muscle biopsy, EEG may show epileptiform activity	MELAS, MERRF, other mitochondrial disorders
Ataxia, early cataracts, cognitive impairment, seizures	T2 peridentate hyperintensities and gliotic lesions; elevated cholestanol	P450 *CYP27A1*: CTX
XY heterozygote with pyramidal signs, neuropathy, adrenal insufficiency, visual impairment, impotence, cognitive impairment	Abnormal T2 MRI signal in posterior cerebral hemispheres, cerebellum, and spinal cord; elevated fasting very long-chain fatty acids (VLCFAs)	*ABCD1*: ALD

(ABCD1: ATP-binding cassette, subfamily D member 1; AFP: α-fetoprotein; ALD: adrenoleukodystrophy; ALS: amyotrophic lateral sclerosis; AOA: ataxia with oculomotor apraxia; APTX: apraxin; ARSACS: autosomal recessive spastic ataxia of Charlevoix-Saguenay; AT: ataxia-telangiectasia; ATM: AT mutated; ATXN: ataxin; AVED: ataxia with vitamin E deficiency; CANVAS: cerebellar ataxia with neuropathy and vestibular areflexia syndrome; CTX: cerebrotendinous xanthomatosis; FA: Friedreich ataxia; FMR1: fragile X messenger ribonucleoprotein 1; FXN: frataxin; FXTAS: fragile X-associated tremor/ataxia syndrome; HIT: head-impulse test; MCP: middle cerebellar peduncle; MELAS: mitochondrial encephalopathy, lactic acidosis, and stroke-like episodes; MERRF: myoclonic epilepsy with ragged red fibers; MSA: multiple system atrophy; MTTP: microsomal triglyceride transfer protein; PBS: peripheral blood smear; POLG: DNA polymerase; RBD: rapid eye movement sleep behavior disorder; RFC1: replication factor C subunit 1; SACS: sacsin; SCA: spinocerebellar ataxia; SETX: senataxin; TTP: tocopherol transfer protein; VOR: vestibular-ocular reflex)

Episodic Ataxia

Episodic ataxia is a group of genetic conditions that can cause intermittent ataxia attacks ranging from a few minutes to several days as explained in detail in **Table 8**. These conditions are often triggered by exertion and may have a progressive ataxia underlying the episodic attacks. When diagnosing episodic ataxia, it is important

TABLE 8: Episodic ataxia syndromes.

Disease	Phenotype	Onset	Mutation
EA1	Very brief episodes of ataxia; interictal skeletal myokymia	Early childhood	KCNA1
EA2	Ataxic episodes lasting hours; interictal nystagmus	Childhood to young adult	CACNA1A
EA3	Episodic vertigo and tinnitus	–	Linked to 1q
EA4	Episodic vertigo; interictal nystagmus	Late onset	–
EA6	Associated with hemiplegic migraine	–	–
EA7	Attacks of vertigo, weakness, slurred speech	<20 years	Linked to 19q

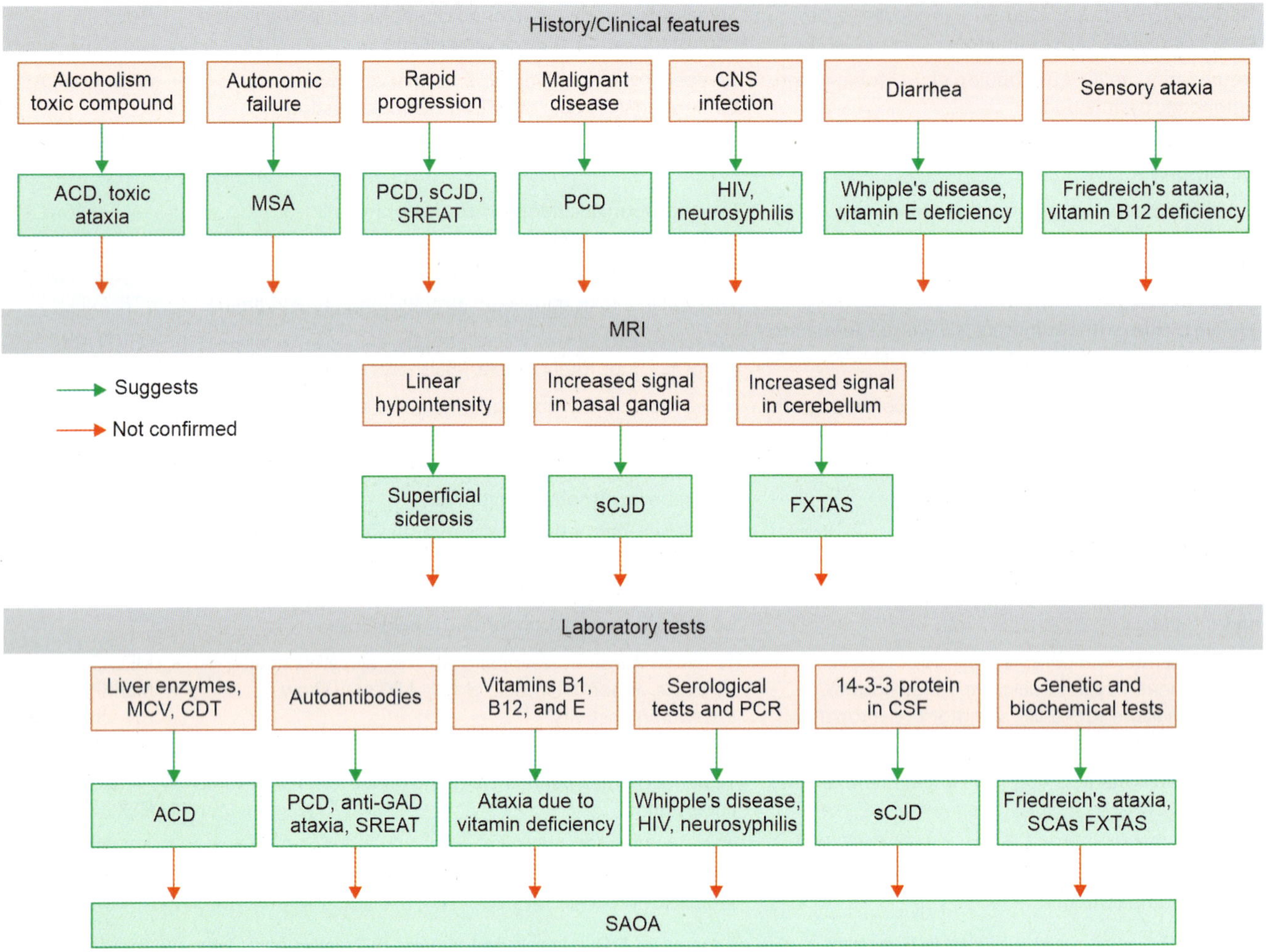

FLOWCHART 2: Summary of diagnostic approach to sporadic adult-onset ataxia.

Note: History and clinical features are often highly suggestive of a specific diagnosis. Similarly, typical MRI features might suggest a particular diagnosis. If the suspected diagnosis is not confirmed by appropriate laboratory tests, wider laboratory screening is required, which will eventually lead to the final specific diagnosis. If all tests are negative, then a diagnosis of SAOA is made by exclusion.

(ACD: alcoholic cerebellar degeneration; CDT: carbohydrate-deficient transferrin; CNS: central nervous system; FXTAS: fragile X-associated tremor/ataxia syndrome; GAD: glutamic acid decarboxylase; MCV: mean corpuscular volume; MSA: multiple system atrophy; PCD: paraneoplastic cerebellar degeneration; SAOA: sporadic adult-onset ataxia of unknown etiology; SCA: spinocerebellar ataxia; sCJD: sporadic Creutzfeldt–Jakob disease; SREAT: steroid-responsive encephalopathy associated with autoimmune thyroiditis)

to consider other possibilities such as multiple sclerosis or psychogenic ataxia, but with thorough evaluation and proper diagnosis, the condition can be identified with confidence. Genetic mutations linked to episodic ataxia are frequently found in ion channels or membrane proteins that have a crucial role in neuronal excitability.

Degenerative Ataxia

Degenerative ataxia typically affects patients over 60 years old with no family history of the condition. MSA and idiopathic late-onset cerebellar ataxia (ILOCA) are the most common diseases in this category. MSA is characterized by cerebellar ataxia, parkinsonism, autonomic instability, and pyramidal signs. It is divided into MSA—parkinsonism or MSA—cerebellar types. Patients with the cerebellar type have a slower disease progression than those with the parkinsonism type. MSA has a poor prognosis, whereas, ILOCA progresses slowly, and present as cerebellar ataxia only and does not affect the patient's lifespan. Patients with ataxia onset later in life should undergo autonomic tests and sleep studies to support the diagnosis of MSA when clinical symptoms are not yet evident.

Flowchart 2 summarizes the clinical approach to diagnose sporadic adult-onset ataxia.

TREATMENT OF ATAXIA

Ataxia treatment can be categorized as symptomatic or disease-modifying. For acquired cases, thiamine, gluten-free diet, and IV immunoglobulin can be used. Genetic ataxias require vitamin E replacement, miglustat, and ketogenic diet. Riluzole, varenicline, and 4-aminopyridine have been proven effective. Exercise, dietary supplementation, and medication regulation are being explored as potential treatments. Antisense oligonucleotides have shown promise in mouse models of SCA2 and SCA3.

Treatment options for various different ataxia types are described in **Table 9**.

CONCLUSION

The causes of cerebellar ataxia are many and can present as diagnostic challenges. The acquired causes of ataxia should first be considered, followed by genetic and degenerative forms of ataxia. If genetic ataxia is suspected, pathologic repeat expansions in the ataxic genes should be determined first, followed by assessing for sequence alterations. Among late-onset cerebellar ataxias, MSA is most common and should be considered. Although the treatment for cerebellar ataxia remains only modestly effective, several novel therapies are currently being tested including pharmacologic therapy, brain stimulation, and antisense oligonucleotides.

TABLE 9: Treatment of hereditary ataxia.

Disorder	Therapy	Dose
SCAs and other HAs	Riluzole	100 mg/day
SCA3	Varenicline	1 mg twice daily
SCAs	Buspirone	30 mg twice daily
SCA3	Zinc	50 mg twice daily
SCA3	Insulin-like growth factor 1	50 μg subcutaneously twice daily
EA2	Acetazolamide	250–1,000 mg/day
EA2	4-amino pyridine	5 mg thrice daily
SCA3	Mexiletine and carbamazepine	For cramps
SCA3	Botulinum toxin type A	For dystonia and spasticity
Friedreich ataxia	Idebenone CoQ10	5–20 mg/kg/day, 30 mg/kg/day
Ataxia with vitamin E deficiency	Vitamin E	800–1,200 mg/day
Abetalipoproteinemia	Vitamin E, vitamin A low-fat diet, medium-chain triglyceride	150 mg/kg
Refsum's disease	• Low phytanic acid diet • Plasma exchange	Below 10 mg/day
Niemann–Pick type C	Miglustat	200 mg thrice daily
Cerebrotendinous xanthomatosis	Chenodeoxycholic acid	750 mg/day
Ataxia with coenzyme Q10 (CoQ10) deficiency	CoQ10 supplementation	30 mg/kg/day
Ataxia with GLUT1 deficiency	Ketogenic diet, modified Atkins diet	–

(GLUT1: glucose transporter 1; HAs: hereditary ataxias; SCA: spinocerebellar ataxia)

SUGGESTED READINGS

1. Aggarwal A, Garg D, Mohd F. Treating Hereditary Ataxias-Where Can We Help? Ann Natl Acad Med Sci (India). 2019;55:182-8.
2. de Silva RN, Vallortigara J, Greenfield J, Hunt B, Giunti P, Hadjivassiliou M. Diagnosis and management of progressive ataxia in adults. Pract Neurol. 2019;19(3):196-207.
3. Khemani P. Adult-onset cerebellar ataxias. Pract Neurol, 2022;21(7):49-58.
4. Kuo SH. Ataxia. Continuum (Minneap Minn). 2019;25(4):1036-54.
5. Kuo SH, Lin CC, Ashizawa T. Cerebellar Ataxia. In: Jankovic J, Mazziotta JC, Pomeroy SL, Newman NJ (Ed). Bradley and Daroff's Neurology in Clinical Practice, 8th edition. Philadelphia: Elsevier; 2021. pp. 208-308.

196

CHAPTER

Approach to Bladder Disorders

Gurinder Mohan, Karandeep Kaur

ABSTRACT

The bladder and urethra have two functions storage and voiding. Voiding is mediated by parasympathetic innervation to the meshwork of smooth muscle in the bladder wall, the detrusor. The brain and the lumbosacral spinal cord together with other complicated neural control systems mediate the coordination between these components, disturbance of which leads to various disorders of bladder function collectively known as *neurological bladder*. Lapides classified bladder dysfunction into five major types: Uninhibited, autonomic (spinal bladder), autonomous, and sensory atonic and motor atonic bladder. Level of lesion determines the presenting features with varying degrees of bladder dysfunction. Evaluation of bladder dysfunction involves history-taking, addressing the symptoms suggesting the various types of bladder dysfunction, and physical examination to localize the lesion in neurological bladder, supplemented by investigations. Management of neurogenic bladder ranges from anticholinergics to catheterization to neuromodulation.

INTRODUCTION

The familiar functions of bladder and lower urinary tract (LUT)—storage and intermittent evacuation of urine are served by the coordinated contraction of the smooth and striated muscles in the two functional units of the LUT, the bladder with the bladder neck, the urethra and the urethral sphincter. The brain and the lumbosacral spinal cord together with other complicated neural control systems mediate the coordination between these components, disturbance of which leads to various disorders of bladder function collectively known as neurological bladder.

STRUCTURE AND INNERVATION OF HUMAN BLADDER

The detrusor, which is compressed as the deep trigone behind the bladder neck, is a network of smooth muscle that makes up the bladder. The smooth muscle that surrounds the bladder neck in males is known as the internal sphincter. It functions as the proximal portion of the urethral sphincter mechanism and is continuous with the prostate capsule. The external sphincter is made up of the intramural striated muscle, which is compressed around the prostatic urethra to create the striated portion of the distal of the sphincter.

Sympathetic fibers to the bladder arise from T12 to L2. Sympathetic stimulation (through beta-adrenergic receptors predominantly on bladder wall and alpha receptors in the bladder neck) and pudendally mediated constriction of the internal and external urethral sphincters, respectively, maintain continence throughout the storage period. Detrusor contractions are avoided by inhibiting the parasympathetic outflow (S2–S4) **(Fig. 1)**.

Effective bladder emptying is achieved by relaxing the detrusor muscles and the external and internal urethral sphincters while simultaneously contracting the parasympathetically mediated detrusors **(Flowchart 1)**.

NEUROLOGICAL BLADDER DYSFUNCTION

The phrase "neurogenic bladder" is an oversimplification of LUT dysfunction that follows neurological disease; lesions of the nervous system can cause distinctive

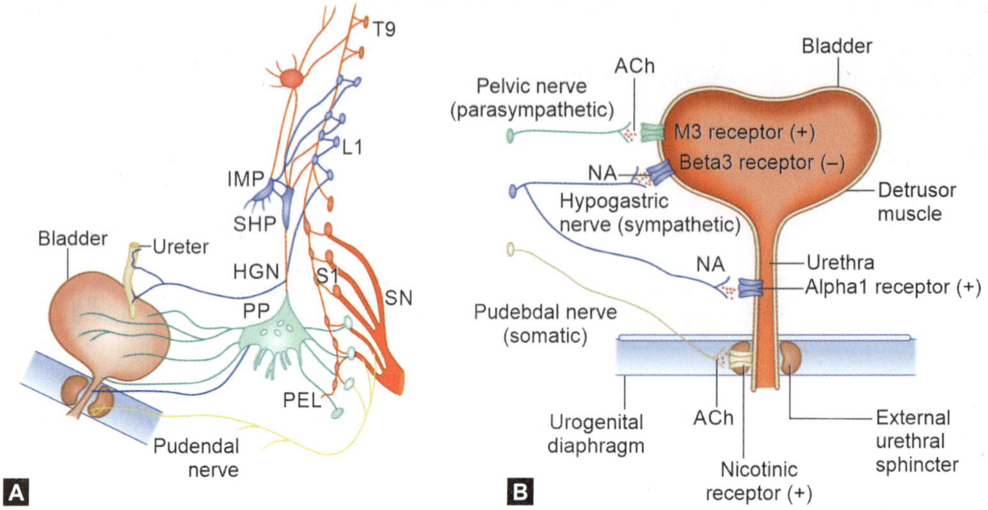

FIGS. 1A AND B: (A) Sympathetic fibers running through the inferior mesenteric ganglia IMP and HGN or through the paravertebral chain to enter pelvic nerves at the base of the bladder and urethra; parasympathetic preganglionic fibers (shown in green) travel in sacral roots and pelvic nerves (PEL) to ganglia in the PP and bladder wall. Somatic motor nerves (shown in brown) that supply the striated muscles of the external urethral sphincter arise from S2 to S4 motor neurons and pass through pudendal nerves. (B) Efferent pathways and neurotransmitter mechanisms that regulate lower urinary tract; parasympathetic postganglionic axons in pelvic nerve release ACh, which produces bladder contraction by stimulating M3 muscarinic receptors in bladder smooth muscle. Sympathetic postganglionic neurons release NA, which activates beta-3 receptors to relax bladder smooth muscle and activates beta-1 adrenergic receptors to contract urethral smooth muscle. Somatic axons in pudendal nerve also release ACh, which produces contraction of external sphincter striated muscle.

(SHP: superior hypogastric plexus; SN: sciatic nerve; IMP: inferior mesenteric plexus; HGN: hypogastric nerve; PP: pelvic plexus; AChL: acetylcholine; NA: noradrenaline)

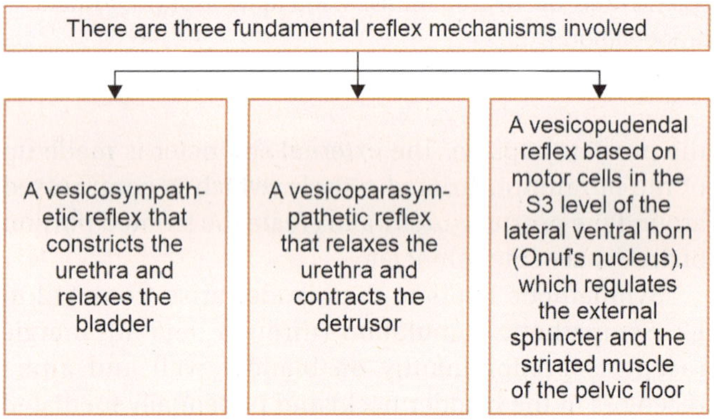

FLOWCHART 1: Fundamental reflex mechanisms.

alterations in LUT functions depending on the site of the lesions in the neurological axis **(Table 1)**.

Uninhibited Bladder

Pathology: Cortical lesions affecting the second frontal gyrus and the corticopontine pathways cause uninhibited bladder.

The typical clinical picture:

- Frontal lobe incontinence as severe urgency and frequency of micturition and urge incontinence but without dementia; the patient is socially aware and embarrassed by the incontinence.

TABLE 1: Lapides classification.

Level of lesion	Bladder
Loss of supraspinal control	Uninhibited
Spinal cord lesion above sacral level	Automatic
Spinal cord lesion involving sacral level	Autonomous
Lesion involving afferent neurons	Sensory neurogenic
Lesions involving efferent neurons	Motor paralytic

- Normal coordination of micturition
- Detrusor overactivity
- *Various lesions*:
  - Stroke
  - Urgency incontinence is linked to small vessel disease of the white matter (leukoaraiosis), more in elderly.
  - Incontinence in patients with increasing cognitive decline in advanced stages of Alzheimer's disease, but it may develop earlier in dementia with Lewy bodies.
  - Patients with normal pressure hydrocephalus (NPH) have shown improvement in urodynamic function within hours following lumbar puncture.
  - *Parkinson's disease (PD)*: Nocturia followed by urinary urgency are the most common nonmotor

symptoms in PD. It is thought that neuronal loss in the substantia nigra may disinhibit the normal effect of basal ganglia on the micturition reflex, resulting in detrusor overactivity.

Spinal (Automatic) Bladder

The most typical cause of neurogenic bladder dysfunction is spinal cord disease.

Pathology: Pontine micturition centers are linked to the sacral cord by transspinal routes. The detrusor and sphincter's reciprocal activity, which is required to switch between storage and voiding, can only be carried out by intact connections, when disturbed leads to detrusor-sphincter dyssynergia.

The typical clinical picture:
- Bladder fullness is not recognized, and increase in intravesical pressure
- Reflex emptying of the bladder may occur without warning.
- Small contracted bladder
- *Various lesions*:
  - Multiple sclerosis
  - Spinal cord injury

Autonomous Bladder

Pathology:
- *Subsacral lesions*: Damage occurs to the motor and sensory components in the cauda equina or pelvis.
- Since the postganglionic parasympathetic innervation is preserved, damage to the cauda equina causes the detrusor to become decentralized rather than denervated.

The typical clinical picture:
- Sensation of full bladder is lost leading to a large atonic bladder.
- Dribbling or overflow incontinence
- Significant residual urine with high infection risk
- It may be associated with loss of perineal sensations and sexual function.
- *Various lesions*:
  - Cauda equina
  - Pelvic surgery
  - Pelvic malignant disease
  - Spina bifida

Sensory Bladder

Pathology: It appears likely sensory deafferentation of the bladder and loss of the spinal reflex result in diminished bladder filling awareness and impaired bladder contractility.

The typical clinical picture:
- Gradual loss of bladder sensation
- Chronic low-pressure urine retention
- Dribbling incontinence
- It is possible to void but with sense of incomplete evacuation
- Urodynamic studies show decreased bladder feeling, increased post-void residual (PVR) volume, decreased urine flow, and impaired detrusor contractility
- *Various lesions*:
  - Diabetes mellitus: Other generalized neuropathy symptoms and signs must be present in affected patients since bladder dysfunction does not happen in isolation.
  - Tabes dorsalis
  - Subacute combined degeneration of the cord (SACD)
- *Others*: Amyloid neuropathy, autoimmune autonomic ganglionopathies

Motor Atonic Bladder

Pathology: Lesion involving efferent motor neurons.

The typical clinical picture:
- Bladder sensation is intact.
- Painful retention
- Initiation of micturition is not possible
- Bulbocavernosus and anal reflexes are absent.
- Opiates, drugs with anticholinergic effects (antipsychotics, antidepressants, and antimuscarinic agents for the bladder), and alpha-adrenergic agonists may all be linked to voiding dysfunction, ranging from mild to severe.

DIAGNOSIS AND EVALUATION

Evaluation of bladder dysfunction involves history-taking, addressing the symptoms suggesting the various types of bladder dysfunction, physical examination to localize the lesion in neurological bladder, supplemented by investigations **(Table 2)**.

URODYNAMIC STUDIES

Uroflowmetry

A spinning disc is located at the bottom of the collection system; urine flowing onto this disc tends to lower its rotation speed, which is maintained constant by a

TABLE 2: Evaluation of bladder dysfunction.

History		
Storage dysfunction (Overactive bladder)	**Voiding dysfunction**	**Urine retention**
• Frequent micturition • Nocturia • Urgency • Urgency incontinenc	• Difficult micturition • An interrupted urinary stream • The need to strain to pass	Complete urinary retention
Physical examination		
Central causes	**Bladder dysfunction with additional findings of**	
Stroke	Motor deficit and personality changes (frontal lobe lesions)	
Parkinson's disease	Rigidity, tremors, and postural instability	
Multisystem atrophy	Akinetic rigidity, cerebellar ataxia, and postural hypotension, characterized by early urinary incontinence and ED	
Cord lesions	**Bladder dysfunction with**	
Spinal cord injury (supra sacral lesions)	Lower limb deficits	
Conus medullaris and cauda equina (infrasacral lesions)	Saddle anesthesia and absence of anal or bulbocavernosus reflex	
Congenital malformations of the spine	Dimpling, a tuft of hair, a nevus, or a sinus in the sacral region	
Peripheral neuropathy	Signs and symptoms of sensorimotor neuropathy	
Investigations		
Screening for UTI	Urine microscopic examination and culture	
Bladder scan	To assess the PVR urine because the degree of incomplete bladder emptying cannot be predicted from history or examination 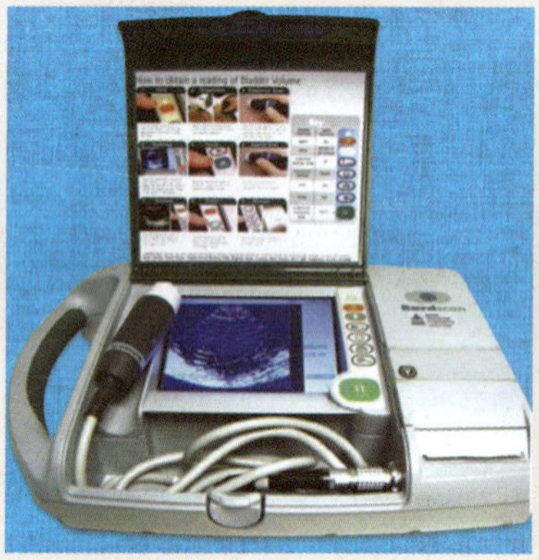 (A) Bladder scan 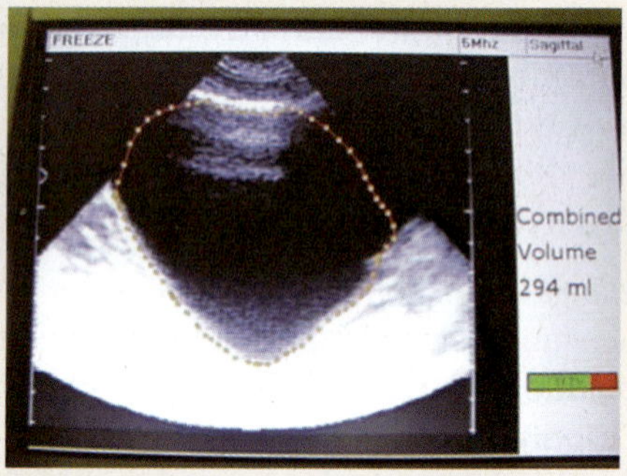 (B) Measured PVR urine	
Ultrasound scan	Surveillance ultrasonography to screen for upper tract disease to check for signs of damage like renal scarring or dilatation of the upper urinary tract. Additionally, consequences of neurogenic bladder dysfunction may be identified with ultrasound, such as bladder stones	
Urodynamic studies	• Uroflowmetry • Cystometry	
Neurophysiological studies	Patients presenting with unexplained pelvic organ or perineal problems, neurophysiology testing assessing the pelvic somatic motor and sensory innervation may be helpful in the evaluation	
Assessing motor and sensory innervation	• Sphincter EMG • Pudendal somatosensory evoked potentials • Assessing the sacral reflex arc	

(ED: erectile dysfunction; EMG: electromyography; PVR: post-void residual; UTI: urinary tract infection)

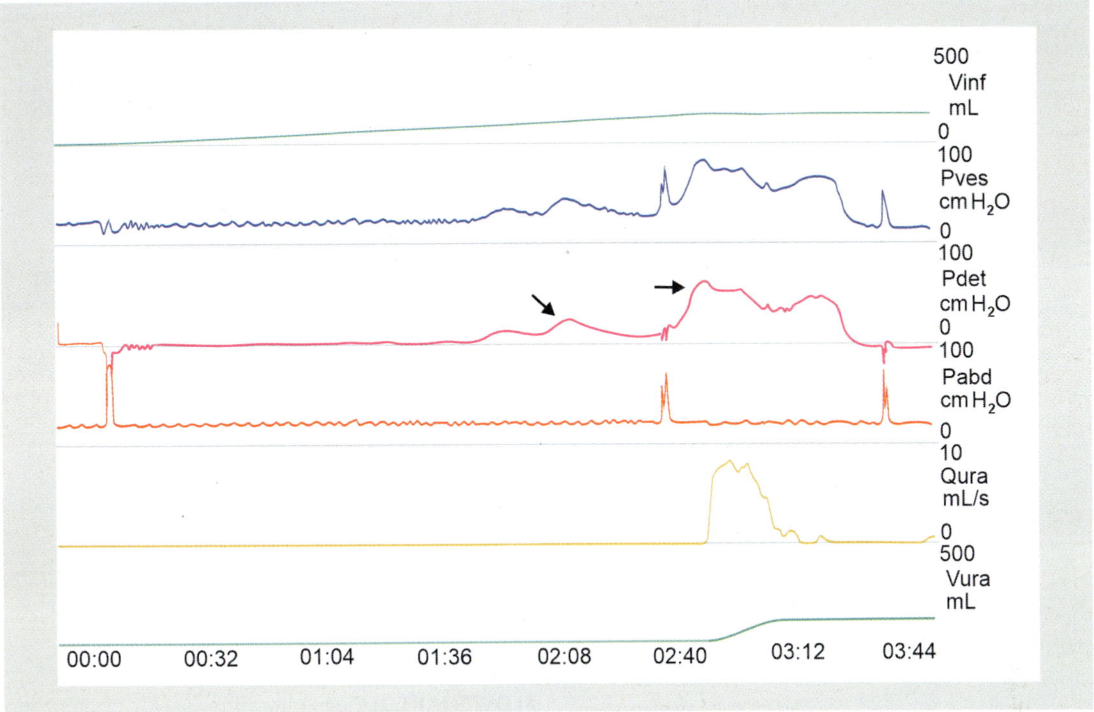

FIG. 2: Filling cystometry demonstrating detrusor overactivity.

servomotor. Based on rotational speed and the amount of time needed to reach maximum flow, the urine flow is computed. The patient must complete the test with a comfortably full bladder that contains, if possible, a volume of at least 150 mL **(Fig. 2)**.

The red trace (Pabd) is the intra-abdominal pressure recorded by the rectal catheter; the dark blue trace (Pves) is the intravesical pressure recorded by the bladder catheter. The pink trace (Pdet) is the subtracted detrusor pressure (Pves–Pabd). Green traces represent volume infused (Vinf) during the test and the volume voided (Vura); the orange trace represents urinary flow (Qura). The black arrow demonstrates detrusor overactivity, and the black arrowhead indicates associated incontinence.

■ Cystometry

Cystometry assesses the pressure–volume relationship during voiding and nonphysiological bladder filling. The intravesical pressure, determined using a catheter in the rectum, is subtracted from the detrusor pressure, which is determined using a catheter in the bladder. First sensation of bladder filling may be reported at 100 mL and 400–600 mL is when it reaches its maximum capacity. In healthy individuals, the bladder enlarges to accommodate this volume of fluid without causing the pressure to rise above 15 cm H_2O. When a bladder acts in this manner, it is termed to be "stable". Detrusor overactivity is the primary aberration detected during filling cystometry.

MANAGEMENT OF NEUROGENIC BLADDER DYSFUNCTION (FIG. 3)

- *General measures*: Bladder retraining to reestablish the regular pattern of micturition by having patients voluntarily "hold on" for longer and longer amounts of time as the clock strikes voiding time
  - Reduced caffeine intake, may lessen urgency and frequency
  - If voiding dysfunction has been ruled out, pelvic floor exercises and neuromuscular stimulation may be effective in reducing overactive bladder (OAB) symptoms.
- *Pharmacologic therapy*:
  - Antimuscarinic agents: The majority of treatment for detrusor overactivity is by antimuscarinic agents, oxybutynin, tolterodine, etc.
  - Beta-3 agonists: Recently, the beta-3 receptor agonist mirabegron has received approval for OAB symptoms.

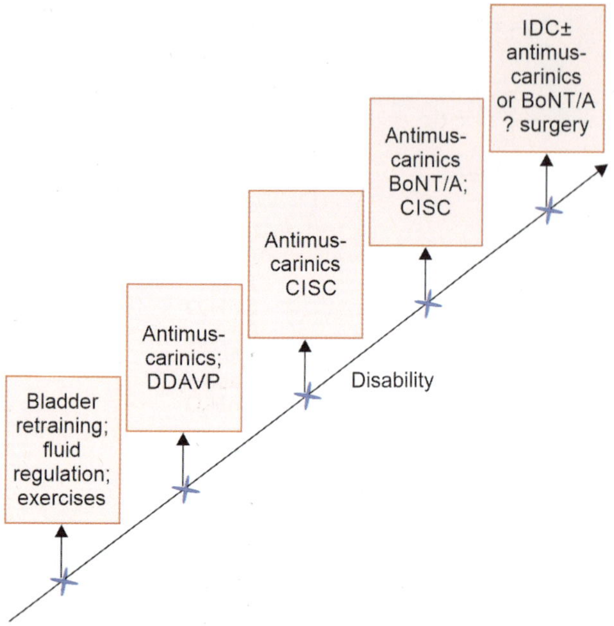

FIG. 3: Stepwise approach toward management of bladder dysfunction.

(BoNT/A: botulinum toxin A; CISC, clean intermittent self-catheterization; DDAVP: desmopressin; IDC: indwelling catheter)

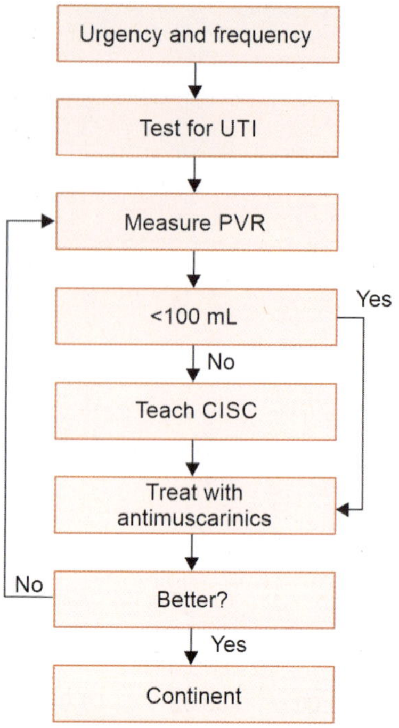

FLOWCHART 2: Clean intermittent self-catheterization (CISC).

(PVR: post void residual; UTI: urinary tract infection)

TABLE 3: Treatment of bladder dysfunction.

Types of bladder	**Uninhibited**	**Automatic**	**Autonomous**	**Sensory atonic**	**Motor atonic**
Site of lesion	Suprapontine	Infrapontine but suprasacral	Subsacral	Peripheral nerve	Peripheral nerve
Pathology	Detrusor hyperreflexia	Detrusor sphincter dyssynergia	• Cauda equina syndrome • Conus medullaris • Spinal shock	Atonicity	Atonicity
Bladder sensation	Intact	Lost	Lost	Lost	Intact
Size of the bladder	Normal	Small	Large	Large	Large
Initiation of micturition	Intact	Lost	Lost	Intact	Lost
Type of incontinence	Urge	Urge	Overflow	Overflow	Overflow
Post-void residual	Nil	Less	Significant	Significant	Significant
Perianal sensation	Intact	Intact	Lost	Lost	Lost
Bulbocavernosus reflex	Intact	Intact	Absent	Absent	Intact
Treatment	Anticholinergics	Clean intermittent self-catheterization	Continuous catheterization	Continuous catheterization	Continuous catheterization

- Botulinum toxin-detrusor overactivity can be improved with intramuscular botulinum toxin type A injections under cystoscopic guidance effective for 8–11 months **(Flowchart 2)**.
- *Others*:
  - Peripheral nerve stimulation (dorsal penile or clitoral nerves, tibial, pudendal, and sacral nerve roots)
  - Sacral neuromodulation

CONCLUSION

Bladder dysfunction is a multifaceted pathology.

Extensive investigation and a precise diagnosis are required before the clinician can initiate individualized therapy.

Treatment must take into account the patient's medical and physical condition and expectations with regard to his or her future social, physical, and medical situation **(Table 3)**.

SUGGESTED READINGS

1. Jankovic J, Mazziotta JC, Pomeroy SL, Newman NJ. Bradley and Darroff's Neurology in Clinical Practice, 8th edition volumes 1 and 2. 2021. pp. 633-4.
2. Fowler CJ, Griffiths D, de Groat WC. The neural control of micturition. Nat Rev Neurosci. 2008;9(6):453-66.
3. Paten JP. The Neurological Differential Diagnosis. United States: Springer; 1995. pp. 268-71.

197

CHAPTER

Multiple Sclerosis: An Update

Shrivarthan Radhakrishnan, R Lakshmi Narasimhan, S Meenakshi-Sundaram

ABSTRACT

Knowledge about multiple sclerosis (MS) continues to evolve and expand. This chapter provides a practical update on the disease and reviews the pathophysiology, clinical features, investigations, diagnostic approach, therapeutic guidelines, and the prognosis. Major advances in the recent times include the advent of newer diagnostic modalities and highly effective disease-modifying therapies. Physicians must have an updated knowledge regarding the benefits and adverse effects of the various treatments while making therapeutic decisions.

INTRODUCTION

Multiple sclerosis (MS) is a presumed autoimmune demyelinating central nervous system (CNS) disease that results in a chronic, debilitating neurological illness resulting from the disruption of normal myelin (demyelination). It leads to a myriad of CNS manifestations affecting the brain, spinal cord, and optic nerves.

EPIDEMIOLOGY

Multiple sclerosis is the most frequent among the various demyelinating diseases described. The disease is more common among white people compared to other races. It is estimated that 2.8 million people across the globe suffer from MS. In India, the prevalence of MS is estimated to be 11/100,000 with an incidence of 0.5/100,000. The disease inherently has a gender predisposition with women being commonly affected than men (3-4:1).

Age group: Most individuals are aged 20–40 years during the first attack of MS (adult-onset MS). However, any age group can be affected, and entities like pediatric MS (onset < 18 years) and late-onset MS onset > 50 years are well described.

Mortality: No significant difference in the mortality rates is observed between patients with MS and the general population in the first 20 years of the illness. However, studies demonstrate a 6.5–7 years reduction in life expectancy with a mortality rate increase of threefold in patients with MS compared to matched general population.

The various risk factors associated with MS are listed in **Table 1**.

GENETICS

A strong genetic susceptibility to MS has been increasingly identified and two human leukocyte antigen (HLA) alleles (*HLA-DQB1* and *HLA-DRB1*) are believed to be associated with a threefold increased risk of MS susceptibility. In addition, close to 100 other genetic factors are believed to contribute to the etiopathogenesis of MS.

PATHOPHYSIOLOGY

The pathological hallmark of MS is an autoimmune-mediated inflammation (by T-cells, B-cells, and plasma cells), resulting in demyelination of central axons with eventual loss of axons and gliotic scarring. This lesion is

TABLE 1: Risk factors for the development of multiple sclerosis.	
Age	**Between 20 and 40 years**
Gender	Female sex
Race	White race
Family history	Monozygotic twins have a higher concordance
Genetic factors	Strong association with HLA-DQB1 and HLA-DRB1 alleles
Climate	More common in temperate countries compared to tropical countries ('latitude gradient')
Vitamin deficiency	Low serum vitamin D levels and lesser sunlight exposure
Infections	Especially Epstein–Barr virus (EBV); sometimes cytomegalovirus (CMV) and varicella zoster virus (VZV)
Associated autoimmune disorders	Hashimoto's thyroiditis, pernicious anemia, psoriasis, type 1 diabetes mellitus, and inflammatory bowel disease
Miscellaneous	Smoking, childhood obesity

referred to as a 'plaque', and it consists of demyelinated axon, decreased number of oligodendrocytes, and astrocyte proliferation with lymphocyte and macrophage infiltrates. The contribution of B-cells to MS pathology is crucial and pathological immortalized B-cells are found in clusters within the brain with a morphology resembling a germinal center. The inflammation is initially perivenular before progressing further radially. Remyelination, which begins after the acute inflammation subsides, is often partial.

CLINICAL FEATURES

The characteristic feature (sine qua non) of MS is the distribution of symptoms and signs over time (relapses) and space (different areas of the CNS affected at different times). The clinical symptoms of MS can broadly be classified into three major groups: (1) relapse, (2) pseudo-relapse, and (3) paroxysmal symptoms **(Table 2)**. Some patients present with a predominant physical disability, while others develop primary cognitive dysfunction.

The various clinical symptoms of MS are summarized in **Table 3**.

TABLE 2: Relapse, pseudorelapse, and paroxysmal symptoms in multiple sclerosis (MS).

Relapse	• A relapse is a patient-reported symptom or objective sign consistent with MS that lasts at least 24 hours in the absence of a fever or infection • For a second relapse to be considered a distinct event, the symptoms/signs must develop at least 30 days after the most recent event
Pseudorelapse/ Pseudoexacerbation	A pseudorelapse is an event similar to relapse occurring in the absence of new central nervous system (CNS) inflammation due to trigger like infection, stress, or increase in body temperature
Paroxysmal symptoms	Paroxysmal symptoms are sudden onset, brief, transient, MS-specific stereotypical symptoms lasting < 24 hours (e.g., trigeminal neuralgia, Lhermitte's sign, paroxysmal dyskinesia, and pruritus)

TABLE 3: Signs and symptoms of multiple sclerosis (MS).

Structure affected	Clinical manifestations
Optic nerve (ON)	• ON is the presenting manifestation in 15–20% of patients in MS and 40–50% of patients develop ON at some point • Clinical features include subacute vision loss (mainly central), color vision impairment, pain with eye movements, and presence of relative afferent pupillary defect (RAPD) • Fundus examination is mostly normal and rarely demonstrates papillitis-related changes
Other cranial nerves	• Bilateral trigeminal neuralgia and glossopharyngeal neuralgia are some of paroxysmal manifestations of MS • Facial myokymia, hemifacial spasm, and unilateral facial paresis can be seen • Rare involvement of III, IV, and VI cranial nerves can be seen
Brainstem	• Supranuclear gaze abnormalities in the form internuclear ophthalmoplegia (INO) and one-and-a-half-eye syndrome are common • Vertigo is seen in up to 50% of the cases and is due to combination of central as well as peripheral causes • Pseudobulbar palsy due to involvement multiple lower cranial nerve nuclei is a late manifestation

Continued

Continued

Structure affected	Clinical manifestations
Cerebellum and connections	• Dysarthria and ataxia due to involvement of cerebellum and its connections is quite common in patients with MS • Several kinds of nystagmus including gaze-evoked, acquired pendular and central positional nystagmus can be seen
Spinal cord	• Can lead to numbness, band like sensation, positive Romberg's sign, Brown–Séquard syndrome, paraplegia, and spastic paraparesis • Bladder involvement in the form of detrusor overactivity and detrusor sphincter dyssynergia can be seen when the cord is involved above the sacral segments. When the sacral segments are affected bladder hypoactivity develops • Sexual dysfunction in the form of decreased libido, erectile dysfunction (in men), and inability to achieve orgasm (in women) can develop • Patients with chronic MS can develop significant gait impairment
Miscellaneous	• Uhthoff phenomenon (abnormal heat sensitivity that usually manifests as visual blurring during a hot shower) • Lhermitte's sign (paroxysmal electric shock-like sensation radiating to back and then to lower limbs on attempted neck flexion) • Cognitive impairment and fatigue

DIAGNOSIS

The four diagnostic tools commonly used to diagnose or exclude MS include:

1. Clinical assessment and neurological evaluation
2. Radiological assessment of the neuraxis
3. Multimodality evoked potentials (MMEPs) study
4. Cerebrospinal fluid (CSF) analysis

Clinical Assessment

Clinical assessment plays a key role in MS management, and there are a few scenarios that raise the likelihood of MS (bilateral trigeminal neuralgia, internuclear ophthalmoplegia, etc.). Also, periodic assessment helps identify new symptoms consistent with relapse and for measuring disease progression.

Radiology

Magnetic resonance imaging (MRI) is the most common and widely used modality that has revolutionized the diagnosis of MS. It is used to confirm the diagnosis, assess response to treatment, and help determine the disease pattern. The use of gadolinium (Gd) contrast [best when used with T1-weighted (T1W) imaging] can help differentiate between inflammatory and noninflammatory etiologies, as well as between active and inactive MS lesions.

The typical MRI finding in MS is referred to as a plaque and can be seen anywhere in the CNS white matter, with the most typical locations being the periventricular white matter, subcortical/juxtacortical white matter, brainstem, cerebellum, and spinal cord. The most specific lesions involve the callososeptal interface. In the posterior fossa, the cerebellum, middle cerebellar peduncles, and the area adjacent to the fourth ventricle are commonly affected. In the spinal cord, the cervical cord is the most commonly involved, followed by the dorsal cord and the conus. The sequences commonly used in MS and MRI findings are summarized in **Table 4**. The typical brain and spinal MRI features of MS are shown in **Figures 1 and 2**.

Multimodality Evoked Potentials Study

Since MS is primarily a demyelinating disorder, the densely myelinated tracts (optic nerve, vestibulocochlear nerve, medial longitudinal fasciculus, medial lemniscus, corticospinal tract, cerebellar pathways, and the posterior column in the spinal cord) are affected early in the disease. Evoked potential (EP) is an electrophysiological measure of the electrical activity of the cerebral cortex following stimulation of a neural tract by an appropriate sensory stimulus. Demyelination of the densely myelinated tracts (which are most susceptible) leads to a prolongation of these latencies. Severe demyelination can also result in a decrease in the amplitude or absence of the potential. EP study was used to diagnose silent and clinically significant lesions before the advent of MRI. In order to increase the sensitivity and specificity of the test, MMEP combining several different forms of EP studies are used and are listed in **Box 1**.

Cerebrospinal Fluid

Cerebrospinal fluid analysis provides useful information mainly to exclude alternate etiologies and to establish the diagnosis in patients with atypical clinical or MRI features. Routine CSF features like color, clarity, and opening pressure are normal in MS. A mild lymphocytic

TABLE 4: MRI sequences commonly used in multiple sclerosis and their significance.	
FLAIR (axial and sagittal)	• Lesions are uniformly hyperintense • Discrete focal lesions which are ovoid and oriented perpendicular to the lateral ventricle (called Dawson's bars or fingers) are seen along the course of the deep medullary veins • Involvement of the callososeptal interface, in the early stages, produces an interrupted appearance, called the 'Dot-Dash sign'
T2 axial	• Lesions appear hyperintense and acute lesions may have surrounding edema • In patients with optic neuritis, the affected optic nerve appears hyperintense (usually the intraocular portion)
T1 (3D inversion recovery-prepared gradient Echo) + Gd	• Lesions appear iso- to hypointense • Profound and persistent hypointensity reflect irreversible tissue damage and permanent demyelination, referred to as T1 black holes • Active lesions show enhancement which are often incomplete around the periphery—open ring sign
DWI axial	High DWI signal with corresponding low ADC indicates restricted diffusion seen in the active stage
Proton density imaging	• Specifically useful for detecting spinal cord lesions • Spinal cord lesions are typically short segment lesions (< 2), eccentric in location, smooth, involving < 50% of the cross section of the cord
MR spectroscopy	Reduced NAA peak and elevated lactate and choline peaks are seen in the sites of demyelination
Double inversion recovery (DIR)	Helps identifying early lesions that preferentially involve the gray matter

(3D: three-dimensional; ADC: apparent diffusion coefficient; DWI: diffusion-weighted imaging; FLAIR: fluid-attenuated inversion recovery; Gd: gadolinium; MRI: magnetic resonance imaging; NAA: N-acetylaspartate)

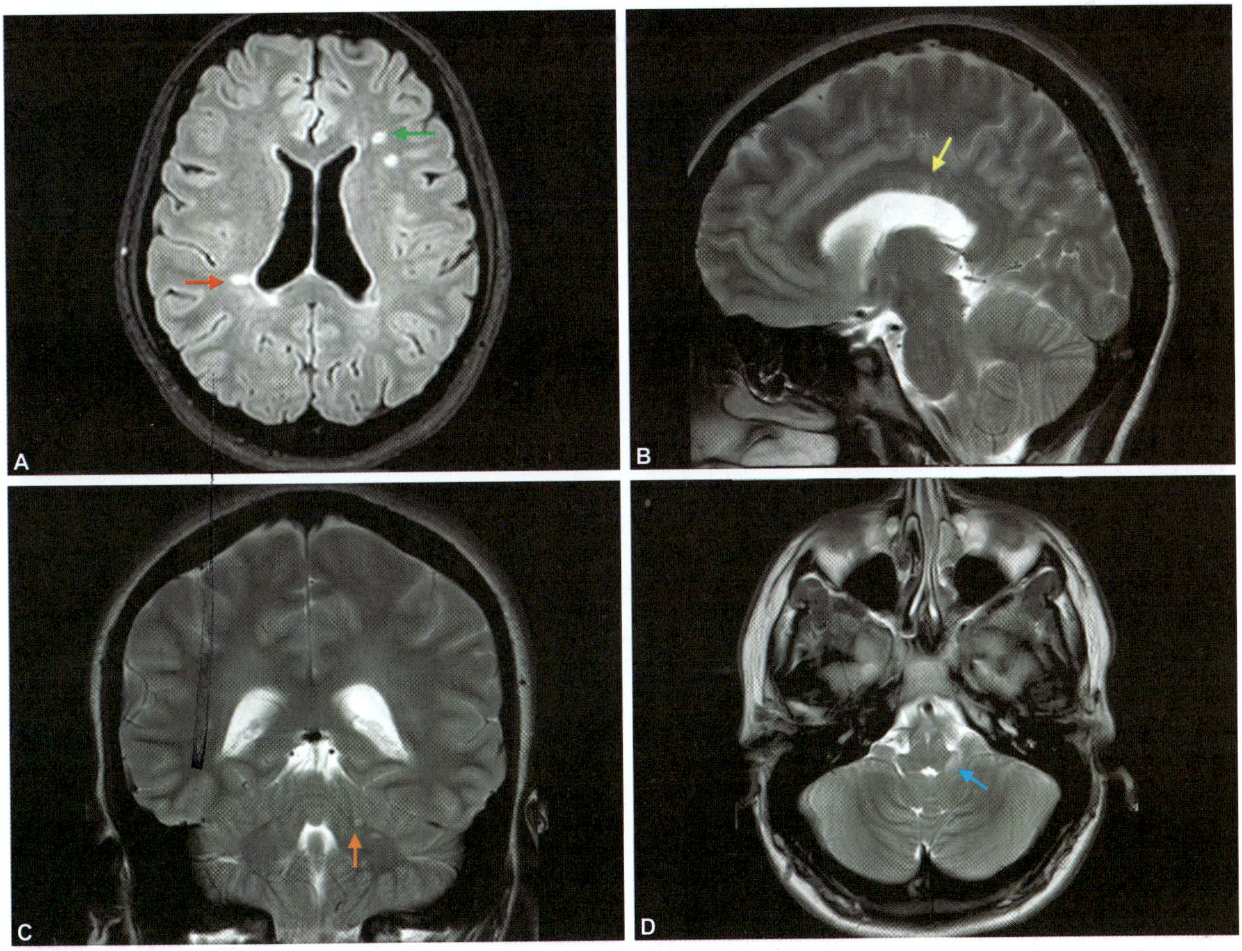

FIGS. 1A TO D: Typical brain imaging findings in multiple sclerosis. (A) Fluid-attenuated inversion recovery (FLAIR) axial showing multiple subcortical (green arrow) and periventricular ovoid lesions (red arrow) typical of MS. (B) T2 sagittal sequence showing lesions in the callososeptal interface (yellow arrow). (C) T2 coronal sequence showing hyperintense lesions in the left superior cerebellum (brown arrow). (D) T2 axial sequence showing demyelinating lesion in left dorsolateral medulla (blue arrow).

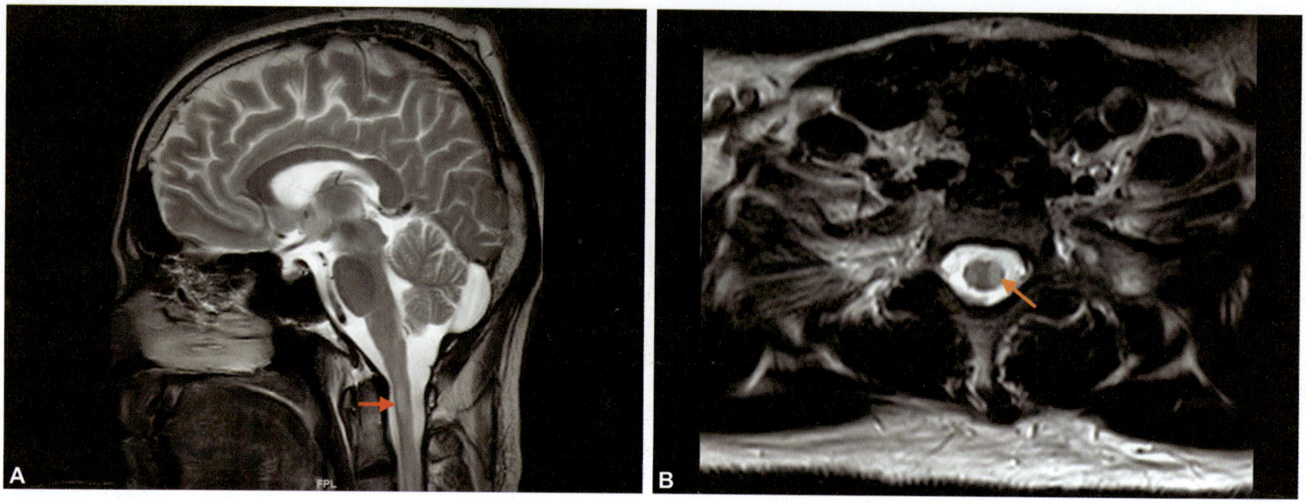

FIGS. 2A AND B: Typical spinal imaging findings in multiple sclerosis (MS). (A) T2 sagittal sequence showing demyelinating short segment MS plaque in the cervical cord (red arrow). (B) T2 axial sequence showing a MS plaque in the spinal cord which is eccentrically located (brown arrow).

BOX 1: Components and clinical application of multimodality evoked potential studies in multiple sclerosis (MS).

Components:

- *Visual evoked potentials (VEPs)*: Optic nerves are stimulated using light and the response picked up over the occipital cortex
- *Brainstem auditory evoked responses (BAERs)*: Auditory nerves are stimulated using sound and response picked up over temporal cortex
- *Somatosensory evoked potentials (SSEPs)*: Median or ulnar nerves in upper limbs and tibial nerves in lower limbs are stimulated and responses picked up over the parietal cortex

Clinical applications:

- Can serve as a measure of the functional impairment in MS
- Can detect subclinical disease
- Can predict the course of the disease in that it can be used to demonstrate worsening of the impulse conduction (disease progression), as well as improvement in the impulse propagation (treatment response)

pleocytosis is seen in 15–20% of the patients, while the rest have normal cell count. The total protein level in CSF in MS is usually normal or shows mild elevation (because of a transient breach in the blood–brain barrier). The diagnostic hallmark is the detection of oligoclonal bands (OCBs) that represent excess antibodies (of IgG class) produced intrathecally by one or more clones of plasma cells that have sequestrated into CSF. They are present in >95% of patients with MS. OCBs are detected by isoelectric focusing in both the serum and the CSF samples, and the presence of two or more bands in the CSF sample coupled with their absence in the paired serum sample is significant. The presence of OCBs provides crucial information in the form of:

- An association with increased disease activity and disability
- Prediction for a greater risk of relapse
- Utility as surrogate 'dissemination in time' marker
- Conferring a higher risk of conversion from a clinically isolated syndrome (CIS) to relapsing-remitting multiple sclerosis (RRMS)
- Risk of greater brain atrophy
- Helping differentiate MS from other demyelinating diseases like neuromyelitis optica spectrum disorders, myelin oligodendrocyte glycoprotein immunoglobulin G (MOG-IgG) antibody-associated syndromes, and acute disseminated encephalomyelitis.

DIAGNOSTIC CRITERIA AND CLINICAL PHENOTYPES

The updated 2017 McDonald criteria are used for the diagnosis of MS and they require unequivocal demonstration of dissemination in space and time. In patients with two or more characteristic attacks affecting different parts of the neuraxis with radiological changes, the diagnosis is straightforward. However, in patients with a single attack (CIS) or those who have two or more attacks, in whom clinical data are insufficient to demonstrate dissemination, additional radiological findings can be used as mentioned in **Table 5**.

There are two major phenotypes of MS which include the RRMS characterized by complete or partial recovery of the relapse, and progressive variants of MS (primary

TABLE 5: 2017 McDonald criteria for demonstration of dissemination in space and time by MRI.

Dissemination in space	Presence of one or more T2-hyperintense lesions characteristic of multiple sclerosis in two or more of the following four areas of the CNS—(1) periventricular, (2) cortical or juxtacortical, (3) infratentorial brain regions, and (4) spinal cord
Dissemination in time	Simultaneous presence of gadolinium-enhancing and nonenhancing lesions at any time or a new T2-hyperintense or gadolinium-enhancing lesion on follow-up MRI, with reference to a baseline scan

(CNS: central nervous system; MRI: magnetic resonance imaging)

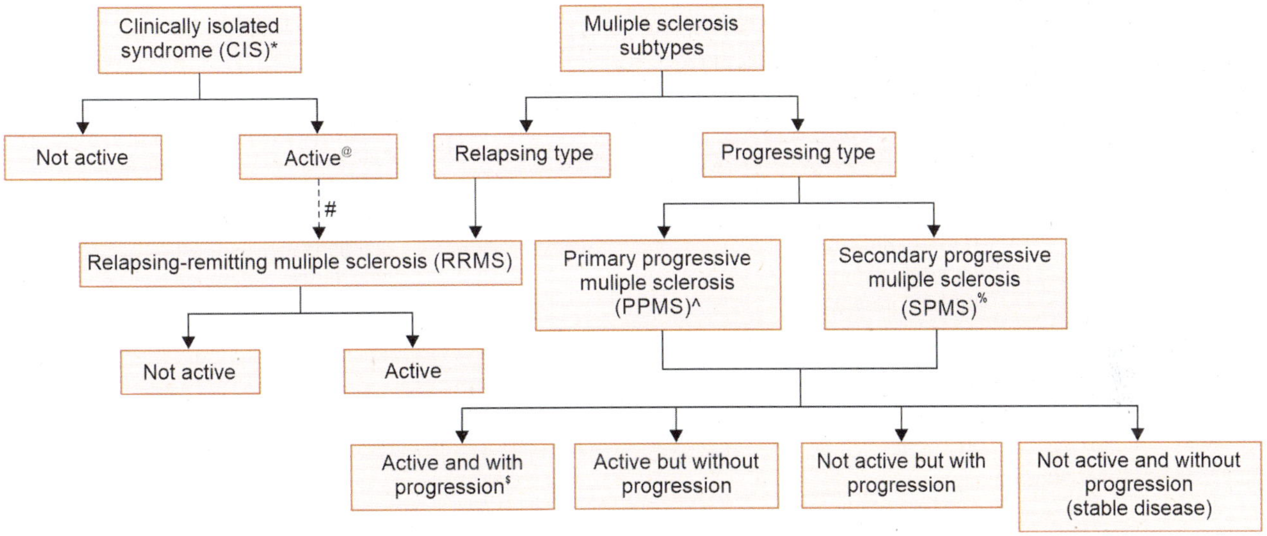

* CIS—first presentation of characteristic inflammatory demyelination seen in MS that does not fulfil the 'dissemination in space and time'.

@ Disease activity refers to development of new clinical relapse and/or new MRI changes (new contrast enhancing lesions and/or development of new T2 lesions and/or unequivocally enlarging lesions in T2).

CIS with a new disease activity qualifies to be called an RRMS.

^ PPMS—progressive accumulation of disability from the onset of disease

% SPMS—progressive accumulation of disability after an initial relapsing course

$ Disease progression is an objective measure of clinical evaluation (e.g., EDSS score).

FLOWCHART 1: The 2013 classification of the subtypes of multiple sclerosis (MS).
(EDSS: Expanded Disability Status Scale)

or secondary) which show a progressive disease course with or without an acute relapse. CIS is a monophasic episode similar to an acute relapse happening for the first time in a patient who is not diagnosed to have MS. CIS is not a subtype of MS, however, if a patient with CIS fulfills the additional criteria for dissemination in space and dissemination in time it qualifies to be called RRMS **(Flowchart 1)**.

TREATMENT

The goal of treatment in acute MS is to restore neurological functions at the earliest, and this is usually achieved with a pulse intravenous methylprednisolone 1 g daily for 5 days. An oral taper is subsequently administered, although this recommendation is not universal. In patients who are refractory to pulse steroids, therapeutic plasma exchange (TPE) can be considered.

Disease-modifying therapies (DMTs) are used to reduce the subsequent risk of relapses in patients with RRMS and CIS. They are broadly divided into three categories as listed in **Table 6**. There is no single 'perfect' drug for MS, and several factors, such as safety, efficacy, tolerability, patient compliance, and disease severity need to be considered before initiating therapy. Oral agents are moderately effective (except cladribine which is a highly efficacious agent) but have the convenience of administration. Monoclonal antibodies are usually intravenously administered (except ofatumumab) and are highly efficacious. Stem cell therapy, especially autologous hematopoietic stem cell transplantation, is an emerging treatment for MS and has niche indications. Other immunomodulators, such as azathioprine, cyclophosphamide, mitoxantrone, and intravenous immunoglobulin are of uncertain/unproven/limited value in MS treatment.

TABLE 6: Disease-modifying therapies (DMTs) in multiple sclerosis.

Drug		Mechanism of action	Route of administration	Dose	Common adverse effects	Pregnancy category
Injectables						
Recombinant human interferon-β	1b	Increases expression of anti-inflammatory cytokines and downregulation of expression of proinflammatory cytokines, alteration of T-cell subsets	Intramuscular	0.25 mg every other day	Flu-like symptoms, mild asymptomatic transaminitis, rarely neuropathy	Category C
	1a—intramuscular form		Intramuscular	30 μg once a week		Category C
	1a—subcutaneous form		Subcutaneous	22 or 44 μg thrice a week		Category C
	1a—pegylated form		Intramuscular or subcutaneous	125 μg every 2 weeks		Category C
Glatiramer acetate (copolymer 1)		Antigenically similar to myelin basic protein, competes with myelin antigens for their presentation to T cells, induces specific T helper 2 type suppressor cells that migrate to the brain	Subcutaneous	20 mg daily or 40 mg thrice a week	Lipoatrophy, transient systemic postinjection reactions such as chest pain, flushing, dyspnea, palpitations, rarely liver dysfunction	Category B
Oral therapies						
Fumarates	Dimethyl fumarate	Activation of nuclear factor-like 2 (Nrf2) pathway	Oral	120 mg increased after 7 days to 240 mg twice daily	Flushing, gastrointestinal side effects, lymphopenia, liver function test derangement	Category C
	Diroximel fumarate			231 mg increased after 7 days to 462 mg twice daily		–
	Monomethyl fumarate			95 mg increased after 7 days to 190 mg twice daily		–
Fingolimod		Sphingosine 1-phosphate (S1P) receptor modulator	Oral	0.5 mg once daily	Macular edema, bradycardia (especially during first dose administration with fingolimod) hypertension, zoster reactivation	Category C
Siponimod				0.25 mg uptitrated to 2 mg once daily		–
Ozanimod				0.23 mg uptitrated over 7 days to 0.92 mg once daily		–
Ponesimod				2 mg uptitrated over 15 days to 20 mg once daily		–
Teriflunomide		Pyrimidine synthesis inhibition	Oral	7 mg or 14 mg once daily	Nausea, diarrhea, hair thinning, headache, asymptomatic transaminitis, teratogenicity	Category X

Continued

Continued

Drug	Mechanism of action	Route of administration	Dose	Common adverse effects	Pregnancy category
Cladribine	Purine synthesis inhibition, promotes lymphocytic apoptosis	Oral	• 3.5 mg/kg divided into 2 yearly treatment courses • Each course: 1.75 mg/kg • Each course divided into two cycles, 4 weeks apart • Each cycle given over 4–5 days	Lymphopenia and bone marrow suppression	Category X
Infusion therapies					
Natalizumab	Antiadhesion molecule α-4 integrin	IV infusion	300 mg over 1 hour, every 4 weeks	Progressive multifocal leukoencephalopathy (PML)	Category C
Ocrelizumab	Anti-CD20		300 mg first dose and repeated after 2 weeks, followed by 600 mg every 6 months	Infusion reaction, reactivation of hepatitis B, hypogammaglobulinemia and neutropenia	Category C
Rituximab			1,000 mg first dose and repeated after 2 weeks, followed by 1,000 mg every 6 months		Category C
Alemtuzumab	Anti-CD52		12 mg daily for 5 days, repeat after 1 year and then 3-day course after 1 more year	Autoimmune disorders, bone marrow suppression, stroke	Category C
Ofatumumab	Anti-CD20	Subcutaneous	20 mg at weeks 0, 1, and 2 followed by 20 mg every month	Injection site reactions, infections	Category C

Unlike RRMS, progressive variants of MS [especially primary progressive multiple sclerosis (PPMS)] have minimal inflammatory activity. Hence, the available DMTs are not very effective. In secondary progressive multiple sclerosis (SPMS) with evidence of disease activity, all the currently available DMTs may be used. In PPMS, ocrelizumab is the only agent that has shown benefit.

Approach to Therapy

There are two major treatment approaches in MS—(1) escalation therapy and (2) early intensive therapy.

Escalation therapy is a 'safety-first' approach where low-efficacy DMT is instituted first and subsequently escalated to a highly effective DMT based on disease response and progression.

result from various intrinsic factors, such as arachnoid granulations, septations, or organized thrombus. It has been debated for a long whether this stenosis is a cause or consequence of raised ICP. In literature, there are studies showing the utility of performing catheter venography with manometry showing a pressure gradient across the stenosis. Lumbar puncture has a crucial role. Firstly, it confirms the presence of increased CSF opening pressure; secondly, CSF content study is done to rule out other infective, inflammatory, or neoplastic causes of raised ICP. Ideally, lumbar puncture should be performed in left lateral decubitus, legs extended, head in a neutral position, and patient breathing normally. An opening pressure of >25 cmH_2O is taken positive for IIH. However, >20 cmH_2O is borderline elevated and should be interpreted with caution in patients with high suspicion of IIH. Return of CSF to normal pressure temporarily relieves headache and other visual symptoms like transient obscuration of vision. The cut-off for pediatric patients is >28 cmH_2O as normal ICP is a little higher in this group of patients. In IIH patients, CSF constituents (sugar, protein, and cell count) remain normal. One of the mandatory ophthalmological investigations done to evaluate and monitor patients of IIH is a formal perimetry examination which can reveal enlarged blind spot initially and later peripheral visual field constriction with sparing of central vision until late. Occasionally, arcuate visual field defects especially in the inferonasal quadrant of the field can also develop. Other ocular investigations such as fundus fluorescence angiography and ultrasound examination are helpful in suspected pseudopapilledema. Optical coherence tomography (OCT) plays a role in quantifying papilledema. Although OCT measures nerve fiber layer thickness and it should be interpreted with caution as there is coexistent edema.

TREATMENT

Apart from alleviating symptoms related to IIH, the goal of therapy also includes prevention of permanent visual field loss. The various modalities to treat this condition include lifestyle intervention (weight reduction), medical management, and surgical intervention. Studies have shown positive results with respect to reduction in CSF opening pressure, papilledema, and headache disability with significant weight reduction but other treatments must be initiated in parallel to get benefits in the short term. Bariatric surgery has been tried in some centers in patients who are morbidly obese. Carbonic anhydrase inhibitors such as acetazolamide remain the mainstay of medical therapy. The mechanism of action is through the reduction in CSF production rate and a mild diuretic effect. It is started with small doses (250 mg twice a day) and gradually increased if required and tolerated. The maximum dose is 2 g twice a day. Most of the patients tolerate this medication very well but the common side effects include paresthesia, dysgeusia, nausea, vomiting, and diarrhea. Topiramate, often used for primary headache disorders, has shown comparable efficacy as acetazolamide in patients of proven IIH. In addition to weak carbonic anhydrase inhibitor, it also causes weight reduction which can have added benefits in these patients. Important side effects include paresthesia, renal stone, and angle closure glaucoma. The dose ranges from 25 mg twice a day up to 100 mg twice a day. Corticosteroids have been used in the past but due to various long-term complications, weight gain and most importantly rebound increase in ICP on withdrawal have warranted its use further in this condition. Still in patients of fulminant presentation, IV steroid is sometimes used for short-term treatment as a bridge therapy before surgical intervention is done. Patients who fail with conservative management or worsen despite maximum tolerated medical therapy are candidates for surgical intervention. This includes optic nerve sheath fenestration, CSF shunting, and transverse venous sinus stenting. Optic nerve sheath fenestration has opted when vision is threatened. A fistula is created between the subarachnoid space and the orbital cavity which releases pressure in the intracranial cavity. In most patients, unilateral optic nerve sheath fenestration suffices and there is improvement in papilledema and visual function on the contralateral side also. But few patients require bilateral sequential optic nerve sheath fenestration. CSF shunting using stereotactic ventriculoperitoneal shunts or lumboperitoneal shunt is effective for rapidly reducing ICP. Unfortunately, this procedure has significant complication rates, such as infection, obstruction, and migration of stents. Recent surgical intervention which has shown promising results includes transverse venous sinus stenting. Patients with imaging evidence of transverse venous sinus stenosis with a pressure gradient of >8 mm Hg across the stenosis are suitable candidates for this procedure. The potential complications are stent thrombosis, subdural hemorrhage, and the development of recurrent stenosis just proximal to the stent. A few trials are going on regarding clear indications of surgery in IIH patients, their timing, and choice of surgical intervention but to date, it remains unclear.

SUGGESTED READINGS

1. Smith JL. Whence pseudotumor cerebri? J Clin Neuroophthalmol. 1985;5(1):55-6.
2. Markey KA, Mollan SP, Jensen RH, Sinclair AJ. Understanding idiopathic intracranial hypertension: mechanisms, management, and future directions. Lancet Neurol. 2016;15(1):78-91.
3. Wall M, Kupersmith MJ, Kieburtz KD, Corbett JJ, Feldon SE, Friedman DI, et al. The idiopathic intracranial hypertension treatment trial: clinical profile at baseline. JAMA Neurol. 2014;71(6):693-701.
4. Capobianco DJ, Brazis PW, Cheshire WP. Idiopathic intracranial hypertension and seventh nerve palsy. Headache. 1997;37(5):286-8.
5. Avery RA, Shah SS, Licht DJ, Seiden JA, Huh JW, Boswinkel J, et al. Reference range for cerebrospinal fluid opening pressure in children. N Engl J Med. 2010;363(9):891-3.
6. Dinkin MJ, Patsalides A. Venous sinus stenting in idiopathic intracranial hypertension: results of a prospective trial. J Neuroophthalmol. 2017;37(2):113-21.

199
CHAPTER

Management of Medical Comorbidities in Dementia: A Comprehensive Approach

Radha TR, Rohit Ram Kumar

ABSTRACT

The global demographic shift toward an aging population has highlighted the increasing prevalence of dementia, particularly in countries like India where approximately 7% of the population is aged above 65. This brings forth the challenge of managing medical comorbidities in individuals with dementia. The coexistence of lifestyle diseases, infections, inflammatory conditions, nutritional disorders, malignancies, and hematologic diseases complicates dementia care and necessitates a multidisciplinary approach.

INTRODUCTION

Dementia, characterized by cognitive decline, memory loss, and impaired daily functioning, poses significant challenges to the healthcare system. The aging population, particularly in India, faces a substantial burden of dementia, with 7% of individuals aged 65 and above affected. The association of dementia with various medical comorbidities underscores the need for a comprehensive management strategy.

CHALLENGES OF DIABETES MANAGEMENT IN INDIVIDUALS WITH DEMENTIA

Diabetes, a disease heavily reliant on self-monitoring, presents unique challenges when coupled with dementia. The intricacies of diagnosis and management have become particularly cumbersome in this vulnerable population.

Diagnosis and Self-monitoring of Glucose

The cognitive decline, forgetfulness, and behavioral issues prevalent in individuals with dementia significantly impede glycemic control. The fear of pricking for blood glucose monitoring becomes a substantial barrier, leading to a reluctance to engage in this crucial aspect of diabetes management. Moreover, the dementia group often faces difficulties in recognizing and documenting their glucose records, introducing complexities in the assessment of their diabetes status. Noncompliance with prescribed medications or inadvertent overdosing becomes a pervasive issue, further exacerbating the challenges associated with diabetes self-management.

Exercise Regimen

Sticking to an exercise regimen poses additional hurdles for individuals with dementia. The cognitive limitations make it challenging to adhere to structured exercise plans, contributing to a sedentary lifestyle. Microvascular complications that accompany diabetes, and the struggle to maintain a consistent exercise routine further amplifies the magnitude of the problem. Balancing the need for physical activity with the cognitive limitations of dementia patients becomes a delicate task in controlling diabetes.

Nutritional Management

Nutritional management in dementia-related diabetes introduces a multifaceted set of challenges. Forgetfulness in relation to eating patterns, development of food fads, and drug-induced nutritional problems (metformin-induced vitamin B12 deficiency) complicate the nutritional aspect of diabetes care. Patients may forget to eat or develop preferences for certain foods, leading to irregular dietary habits. The impact of these challenges on glycemic control necessitates a tailored and vigilant approach to nutritional management.

Basic Principles of Treatment

- Tailored to individuals, depending on the type of diabetes, severity of dementia, comorbidities, and type of dementia care
- Simple regimen, easy to follow
- Avoid hypoglycemia
- Avoid wide fluctuations in blood sugar
- Minimize the number of injections
- Drugs that are best avoided, long-acting sulfonylurea, glitazones
- Short-acting drugs which are easy to titrate with meals are best.
- Metformin, glipizide, sodium-glucose cotransporter-2 (SGLT-2) inhibitors, gliptins, and meglitinide can be used.
- Long-acting peakless insulins are better in dementia patients.

Various devices to assist in choosing insulin/drugs are available:

- Recording and alarm devices
- Insulin pen with memory of time and last injection (novoPen ECHO, or Timesulin memory cap pen device)
- GPS (global positioning system) trackers and alarm devices like wristbands
- Picture phones
- Electrical use monitors
- Continuous glucose monitoring (CGM) devices.

The American Diabetes Association (ADA) 2016 guidelines recommend an HbA1c goal of <7.5% for older adults with intact cognition, <8.0% for those with mild-to-moderate cognitive impairment, and <8.5% for those with moderate-to-severe cognitive impairment. Unfortunately, although raising HbA1c targets may be helpful in reducing hypoglycemia, it is insufficient in preventing hypoglycemia, especially in the elderly. Therefore, raising HbA1c targets cannot be the sole means of preventing hypoglycemia in patients.

HYPERTENSION AND DEMENTIA

Prevalence and Impact of Hypertension in Dementia

The prevalence of hypertension in individuals with dementia is notably high, ranging from 35 to 84%. Among the elderly above 80 years old, approximately 80% are hypertensive, significantly increasing their vulnerability to end-organ damage affecting the heart, brain, kidneys, and eyes. About 73% of these individuals are on at least one antihypertensive medication, with diuretics being the most commonly prescribed.

Complex Link between Cognitive Decline and Hypertension

Hypertension is a risk marker for Alzheimer's disease, associated both with the pathological features of the condition (including plaques, tangles, and hippocampal atrophy) and other vascular risk factors (including obesity and diabetes). The neuropathology of dementia is complex, due to the mixed pathology commonly found in older adults. Small vessel cerebrovascular disease combined with Alzheimer's pathology appears to be a particularly potent cause of dementia. The treatment of hypertension should reduce the progression of the pathological processes and the risk of dementia. Hypertension causes microvascular disease, which not only predisposes to stroke but also affects "neurovascular coupling", the regulation of cerebral blood flow to match the blood supply with the demands of different brain regions.

The hypotension/hypoperfusion damage hypothesis posits that episodes of poor cerebral perfusion due to hypotension worsen deep white matter ischemia and increase the progression of dementia.

Blood pressure (BP) management in patients with dementia requires an individualized approach due to the variability in responses and potential side effects of antihypertensive medications.

Antihypertensive Treatment and Considerations

No single drug has consistently shown superior benefits over others in managing hypertension in individuals with dementia. However, studies suggest that treating hypertension in this population does not cause harm. Balancing the benefits of BP control against potential adverse effects is crucial in the absence of a clear standout medication.

The Systolic Blood Pressure Intervention Trial (SPRINT) included a preplanned subgroup analysis of the population 75 years or older. SPRINT found lower rates of events (including acute coronary syndrome, myocardial infarction, decompensated heart failure, and stroke) in those who had intensive BP lowering targeted to <120 mm Hg compared with those targeted to <140 mm Hg [hazard ratio (HR) 0.66; 95% confidence interval (CI) 0.51–0.85]. However, a subanalysis of the meta-analysis of 15 trials of people older than 60 years showed that treatment was not associated with reduced mortality in those older than 85 years.

Lifestyle Modifications and Exercise Protocols

Lifestyle changes, including exercise, play a pivotal role in managing hypertension. However, implementing exercise protocols in individuals with dementia requires careful consideration to avoid exacerbating sarcopenia. Group exercises, engaging activities like dancing, and varying exercise patterns can improve performance while minimizing adverse effects.

Salt Restriction and Medication Approach

Prescribing salt restriction should be cautious, especially if salt intake is not exceptionally high (>10 g/day), as it might affect food palatability and lead to nutritional deficiencies.

In elderly patients with dementia, a "start low and go slow" approach with medications is prudent, emphasizing lower drug doses with gradual adjustments. The choice of drugs should consider coexisting medical conditions. Multiple drugs in lower doses together are preferable.

CARDIOVASCULAR CONDITIONS

Persons with dementia have a high risk of atherosclerotic vascular disease and they are eligible for treatment for hypertension and hyperlipidemia.

Considerations should include the age, longevity, benefit of aggressive therapy, and hypertension treatment as per guidelines.

Hyperlipidemia should be less rigorously controlled than those without dementia. Hypotension should be avoided, particularly orthostatic. Patient preferences should be given importance. Deprescription of drugs as and when needed should be done.

Surgical treatment of cardiovascular diseases requires individual decision.

MOOD DISORDERS AND MENTAL HEALTH CONDITIONS

Depression, anxiety, and behavioral changes are frequently observed alongside dementia. These mental health conditions often coexist, exacerbating the cognitive decline and diminishing the individual's quality of life. Depression, in particular, can sometimes manifest as an early symptom or as a consequence of coping with the challenges of dementia.

INFECTIONS AND DEMENTIA

Cognitive decline, a hallmark of dementia, also renders individuals more susceptible to various infections. The intricate relationship between infections and dementia poses unique challenges in their diagnosis, management, and impact on the progression of the condition.

Vulnerability to Infections

Individuals experiencing cognitive decline are at an increased risk of infections affecting the skin, genitourinary tract, and respiratory system due to a combination of impaired immune function, difficulties in self-care, and challenges in expressing symptoms, leading to delays in seeking medical attention.

Silent Infections and Atypical Presentations

One of the complexities in diagnosing infections in individuals with dementia is the lack of typical clinical signs. Fever, a common indicator of infection, may not always be present, especially in frail elderly individuals with cognitive decline.

Infections can exacerbate cognitive decline in individuals with dementia. Changes related to infection, such as sepsis or a cytokine storm, can worsen the symptoms of dementia and lead to increased confusion, agitation, and delirium.

Antibiotic Guidelines for Infections in Dementia Patients

Given the complexity of diagnosing infections in individuals with dementia, the following guidelines aim to assist healthcare providers in recognizing potential infections and starting timely antibiotic therapy.

Indications for Antibiotic Treatment in Different Infections

- *Genitourinary tract infections*: In the absence of an indwelling catheter, signs like acute dysuria or fever alongside frequency, urgency, costovertebral angle tenderness, hematuria, suprapubic pain, changes in mentation, or rigor warrant antibiotic treatment.
- *Respiratory tract infections*: Suspected respiratory infections presenting with fever, tachypnea, productive sputum, new productive cough with accompanying symptoms like tachycardia, rigors, or changes in

mental status require consideration for antibiotic therapy, especially in chronic conditions like chronic obstructive pulmonary disease (COPD).
- *Skin infections*: Evidence of purulent discharge with signs of inflammation signifies the need for antibiotic treatment.
- *Unexplained symptoms*: In the absence of a clear focus on infection, alterations in mental status, unstable vital signs, or rigors may necessitate antibiotic therapy.

MUSCULOSKELETAL PROBLEMS AND DEMENTIA

Understanding the interplay between muscular activity, bone health, and dementia reveals profound implications for both prevention and management strategies in dementia.

Muscular Activity and Brain Function

Experimental studies in mice have demonstrated a correlation between muscular activity and brain function. Neurotrophic factors such as brain-derived neurotrophic factor (BDNF), myokines like irisin, and osteokinesis such as osteocalcin have been identified as key elements that not only increase synaptic connections but also enhance neural activity. This connection underscores the importance of maintaining muscular health to potentially slow down cognitive decline in conditions like dementia.

Sarcopenia, Exercise, and Dementia

Sarcopenia, characterized by the loss of muscle mass and strength, is a concern for individuals with dementia. Regular physical activity not only helps prevent sarcopenia but also contributes to increasing synaptic connections and improving brain health.

Osteopenia, Fracture Risk, and Dementia

Osteopenia, the precursor to osteoporosis, often coexists with dementia due to a lack of exercise and nutritional deficits. This leads to an increased risk of fractures, further complicating the health management of individuals with dementia. Interventions like exercise, supplemental calcium, and vitamin D have demonstrated some efficacy in mitigating osteopenia-related risks and improving bone health.

Frailty and Degenerative Joint Diseases

Frailty, often associated with dementia, necessitates specialized attention. However, degenerative joint diseases pose a significant hurdle, limiting exercise and physical activity. Pain stemming from these degenerative conditions requires careful management with minimal medication use.

INFLAMMATORY DISEASES AND COGNITIVE FUNCTION

Inflammatory diseases like rheumatoid arthritis (RA) have been extensively studied in relation to dementia. Active inflammation is known to detrimentally impact cognitive function. Proper management of RA with appropriate medications has been shown to slow the progressive decline in cognitive function, emphasizing the importance of addressing inflammatory diseases in dementia care.

SUGGESTED READINGS

1. Jinkook L, Meijer E, Langa KM, Ganguli M, Varghese M, Banerjee J, et al. Prevalence of dementia in India: National and state estimates from a nationwide study. Alzheimer's Dement. 2023;19(7):2898-12.
2. Hopkins R, Shaver K, Weinstock RS. Management of adults with diabetes and cognitive problems. Diabetes Spectr. 2016;29(4):224-37.
3. Mancia G, Kreutz R, Brunström M, Burnier M, Grassi G, Januszewicz A, et al. 2023 ESH Guidelines for the management of arterial hypertension the Task Force for the management of arterial hypertension of the European Society of Hypertension: Endorsed by the International Society of Hypertension (ISH) and the European Renal Association (ERA). J Hypertens. 2023;41(12):1874-2071.

200

CHAPTER

Neuropsychiatric Aspects of Epilepsy

PK Maheshwari, Akhilesh Kumar Singh, Eish Kumar Dalla

ABSTRACT

Individuals diagnosed with epilepsy encounter a significantly heightened risk, ranging from two to five times, of developing various psychiatric conditions. Around one-third of epilepsy patients eventually receive a psychiatric diagnosis during their lifetime. The coexistence of psychiatric issues alongside epilepsy is often considered an adverse sign, as it can lead to less effective responses to treatment—be it medication or surgery—along with increased health complications and elevated mortality rates. To tackle these associated psychiatric concerns, there exist reliable screening tools specifically tailored to assess mood disorders, anxiety disorders in adults diagnosed with epilepsy. Timely detection and proper management of psychiatric conditions in epilepsy patients play a pivotal role in enhancing treatment outcomes and enhancing the overall quality of life for these individuals.

INTRODUCTION

Psychiatric conditions impact one-third of people with epilepsy, stemming from a complex interconnection of psychosocial and biological elements. The stigma surrounding epilepsy exacerbates discrimination and social seclusion among those affected. From a neurobiological perspective, research has unveiled irregularities within brain networks common to primary psychiatric ailments like depression or schizophrenia, reflecting similar patterns found in conditions such as temporal lobe epilepsy (TLE).

Effectively handling individuals contending with both epilepsy and psychiatric disorders poses significant challenges, regardless of their origins. Hence, it is crucial for healthcare providers to actively identify concurrent psychiatric conditions and incorporate them into personalized and comprehensive management strategies.

EPIDEMIOLOGY

In a comprehensive analysis combining data from 14 population-based studies involving over 1,000,000 participants, active depression in epilepsy was found to have an overall prevalence of 23.1% among adults, indicating a 2.7 times higher risk compared to the general population. Additionally, an examination encompassing 27 studies and over 3,000 individuals with epilepsy highlighted a collective prevalence of 20.2% for anxiety disorders, with generalized anxiety disorder emerging as the most prevalent form. Looking at psychosis and related conditions, an analysis of 57 studies involving >40,000 subjects revealed a combined prevalence of 5.6%, which rose to 7% specifically in individuals with mesial TLE. Moreover, a focused meta-analysis exploring psychogenic nonepileptic seizure (PNES) among people with epilepsy unveiled a prevalence of 12%. Conversely, the prevalence of epilepsy in individuals with PNES was observed to be 22%.

IMPLICATIONS FOR CLINICAL PRACTICE

Psychiatric comorbidities, especially depression, are significant contributors to cognitive complaints in individuals with epilepsy. These comorbidities are linked to a fourfold increased risk of drug resistance in both focal and generalized epilepsies. Additionally, psychiatric comorbidities are associated with premature mortality in epilepsy. Addressing psychiatric comorbidities is crucial for enhancing overall well-being and reducing associated risks in individuals with epilepsy.

SCREENING FOR PSYCHIATRIC COMORBIDITIES

Barriers to the diagnosis and management of psychiatric comorbidities in individuals with epilepsy are intricate and multifaceted. These barriers encompass various factors, including cultural impediments to addressing mental health issues, insufficient training of neurologists and psychiatrists in recognizing and managing these comorbidities, and a lack of allocated resources for implementing a comprehensive multidisciplinary approach. Addressing these barriers is crucial for improving the overall care and outcomes of individuals dealing with both epilepsy and psychiatric conditions. Efforts to enhance awareness, education, and resource allocation can contribute to a more effective and integrated approach to managing these complex health issues **(Table 1)**.

In a systematic review of 16 depression screening tools for adults with epilepsy, the Neurological Disorders Depression Inventory for Epilepsy (NDDI-E) stands out as the most efficient and practical tool, validated in 13 languages. It is effective for detecting major depressive episodes and suicidality, enabling clear suicide prevention pathways. Additionally, the Beck Depression Inventory II (BDI-II), Patient Health Questionnaire 9 (PHQ-9), and Hamilton Depression Rating Scale (HDRS) are validated for depression in epilepsy. For anxiety symptoms, the Hospital Anxiety and Depression Scale (HADS) and Generalized Anxiety Disorder 7 (GAD-7) are validated in adults with epilepsy. Data on pediatric instruments are limited, with the NDDI-E-Youth for ages 12–17 needing further study.

DIAGNOSTIC ISSUES

Following a positive screening for psychiatric symptoms in individuals with epilepsy, it is crucial to confirm the diagnosis. Psychiatric symptoms can manifest in various clinical scenarios, including peri-ictal symptoms (around the time of seizures), side effects of medications, or comorbid psychiatric disorders. Historically, psychiatric symptoms in epilepsy have been categorized based on their temporal relationship with seizures. This categorization is practical as it helps define different clinical scenarios and aids in the accurate diagnosis and management of psychiatric comorbidities in individuals with epilepsy.

Psychiatric symptoms in epilepsy can be classified based on their temporal relationship with seizures.

- *Peri-ictal*: The symptoms that precede a seizure, known as preictal symptoms or auras, often manifest in the context of TLE. These symptoms can include irritability, insomnia, and dysphoria. The prevalence of these symptoms is not precisely known, and they are commonly associated with bilateral tonic-clonic seizures. The duration of preictal symptoms can vary,

TABLE 1: Barriers to access to mental healthcare in people with epilepsy.

Healthcare provider related		Potential solutions
Neurologist related	• Lack of training about the psychiatric aspects of neurological disorders • Lack of knowledge about the management of psychiatric disorders and the use of psychotropic drugs • Lack of time in the outpatient setting misconceptions about seizure risk with psychotropic medications • Failure to educate people with epilepsy and their family members about psychiatric comorbidities • Lack of communication with psychiatrists	• Neurology and psychiatry residency programs with expanded curricula covering psychiatric aspects of neurological disorders and vice versa • To implement routine use of screening instruments in clinical practice • Well-defined clinical pathway to access mental healthcare for people with epilepsy. Tertiary epilepsy centers should have a psychiatrist as part of the team. Information leaflets about psychiatric disorders available for individuals and to be given in clinic routinely
Psychiatrist related	• Lack of training about the psychiatric aspects of neurological disorders • Failure to recognize all the aspects of the clinical manifestations of psychiatric comorbidities in epilepsy • Misconception about the association between psychiatric comorbidities and the underlying epilepsy leading to refusal to treat people with epilepsy • Misconceptions about seizure risk with psychotropic medications. Lack of communication with neurologists	• Neurology and psychiatry residency programs with expanded curricula covering psychiatric aspects of neurological disorders and vice versa • Well-defined clinical pathway to access mental healthcare for people with epilepsy • Tertiary epilepsy centre should have a psychiatrist as part of the team

ranging from a few hours to up to 2 days before the onset of the seizure. Understanding and recognizing these preictal symptoms can be valuable for individuals with epilepsy and their healthcare providers, as they may serve as warning signs of an impending seizure.

- *Ictal*: This include main manifestation of seizure and their presentation is as:
  - Focal aware seizures, which can be nonmotor or emotional (e.g., ictal fear or ictal depression)
  - Nonconvulsive status epilepticus (e.g., ictal psychosis)
- *Postictal*: These are the symptoms following a seizure, mostly bilateral tonic-clonic seizures. Postictal psychoses have a prevalence of around 2%. They are characterized by florid brief psychotic episodes that can last from hours to weeks. These symptoms have a subtle onset after a 48-hour lucid interval from the seizure. There is a high mortality risk due to high suicidal ideation and violent behavior associated with postictal psychoses. Postictal mood and anxiety symptoms have an unknown prevalence, although case series suggest it can be up to 40% in people with drug-resistant TLE.

TREATMENT ISSUES

Striving for complete remission remains the ultimate objective in treating psychiatric comorbidities alongside epilepsy. It is prudent to adhere to established psychiatric treatment norms, considering the distinctive characteristics of individuals with epilepsy, such as potential drug interactions and seizure risks. Ultimately, the goal is to optimize well-being while minimizing adverse effects and the potential for increased seizures.

Psychological Interventions

Psychological interventions take precedence as the primary treatment for anxiety disorders and mild to moderate depression in the general population. A recent International League Against Epilepsy (ILAE) report endorses the use of psychological interventions, particularly cognitive behavioral therapy, for individuals with epilepsy experiencing mild to moderate depressive symptoms, despite the evidence level being moderate. In the case of PNES, psychoeducation and psychological interventions remain the forefront of treatment strategies. This underscores the significance of psychological approaches in addressing mental health aspects across various conditions, including epilepsy and PNES.

Pharmacological Treatments

Placebo-controlled trials, along with open studies, examining sertraline, citalopram, fluoxetine, reboxetine, and mirtazapine, indicate the safety and efficacy of selective serotonin reuptake inhibitors (SSRIs) and newer antidepressants in the context of epilepsy. However, these studies are limited by small sample sizes. For depression in chronic health conditions, citalopram and sertraline are first-line options. No studies on drug treatments for anxiety disorders in epilepsy exist, but SSRIs are typically the first-line treatment. Risperidone, olanzapine, and quetiapine are commonly first-line treatments for first-episode psychosis **(Table 2)**.

TABLE 2: Management of psychiatric comorbidities in epilepsy.

	Management	Comments
Major depression	• *Mild to moderate*: Psychological treatment • *Severe*: Selective serotonin reuptake inhibitors (SSRIs) (either sertraline 50 mg or citalopram 20 mg) ± psychological treatment • If suicidal ideation or psychotic symptoms urgent referral to psychiatry	• Consider interaction with inducers • Consider side effects of SSRIs (i.e., hyponatremia, sexual dysfunction, osteoporosis, bleeding, and weight gain)
Anxiety disorders	• *Mild-to-moderate*: Psychological treatment • *Severe*: SSRIs (either sertraline 50 mg or citalopram 20 mg) ± psychological treatment • If fails two interventions refer to psychiatry	• Consider interaction with inducers • Consider side effects of SSRIs (i.e., hyponatremia, sexual dysfunction, osteoporosis, bleeding, and weight gain)
First episode psychosis	• Urgent referral to psychiatry • *First choice*: Risperidone • *Second choice*: Olanzapine or quetiapine	• Consider interaction between quetiapine and inducers (i.e., undetectable levels of quetiapine up to 700 mg when in combination with carbamazepine) • Consider side effects of antipsychotics (i.e., sedation and weight gain with olanzapine)

Seizure Risk

Traditionally, there was a belief that psychotropic drugs might elevate the risk of seizures, although this assumption lacked substantial clinical evidence. In the case of antipsychotic drugs, clozapine presents the highest seizure risk compared to a placebo. Olanzapine and quetiapine also pose some risk, albeit to a lesser degree, while all other antipsychotics demonstrate no discernible difference from a placebo in terms of seizure risk. This underscores the importance of considering the seizure profile of specific psychotropic medications, with a nuanced understanding of the associated risks.

CONCLUSION

Psychiatric comorbidity in epilepsy is common. Epilepsy clinics require access to mental healthcare. In the absence of specific guidelines, adopt internationally recognized psychiatric disorder guidelines. High-quality studies are needed for evidence-based treatment of mood, anxiety disorders, and psychoses in epilepsy.

SUGGESTED READINGS

1. Mula M, Kanner AM, Jetté N, Sander JW. Psychiatric Comorbidities in People with Epilepsy. Neurol Clin Pract. 2021;11(2):e112-20.
2. Fiest KM, Dykeman J, Patten SB, Wiebe S, Kaplan GG, Maxwell CJ, et al. Depression in epilepsy: a systematic review and analysis. Neurology. 2013;80:590-9.
3. Scott AJ, Sharpe L, Hunt C, Gandy M. Anxiety and depressive disorders in people with epilepsy: A meta-analysis. Epilepsia. 2017;58:973-82.
4. Clancy MJ, Clarke MC, Connor DJ, Cannon M, Cotter DR. The prevalence of psychosis in epilepsy; a systematic review and meta-analysis. BMC Psychiatry. 2014;14:75.
5. Kutlubaev MA, Xu Y, Hackett ML, Stone J. Dual diagnosis of epilepsy and psychogenic nonepileptic seizures: Systematic review and meta-analysis of frequency, correlates, and outcomes. Epilepsy Behav. 2018;89:70-8.
6. Nogueira MH, Yasuda CL, Coan AC, Kanner AM, Cendes F. Concurrent mood and anxiety disorders are associated with pharmacoresistant seizures in patients with MTLE. Epilepsia. 2017;58:1268-76.
7. Stevelink R, Koeleman BPC, Sander JW, Jansen FE, Braun KPJ. Refractory juvenile myoclonic epilepsy: a meta-analysis of prevalence and risk factors. Eur J Neurol. 2019;26:856-64.
8. Fazel S, Wolf A, Långström N, Newton CR, Lichtenstein P. Premature mortality in epilepsy and the role of psychiatric comorbidity: a total population study. Lancet. 2013;382:1646-54.
9. Gill SJ, Lukmanji S, Fiest KM, Patten SB, Wiebe S, Jetté N. Depression screening tools in persons with epilepsy: A systematic review of validated tools. Epilepsia. 2017;58:695-705.
10. Mula M, McGonigal A, Micoulaud-Franchi J-A, May TW, Labudda K, Brandt C. Validation of rapid suicidality screening in epilepsy using the NDDIE. Epilepsia. 2016;57:949-55.
11. Mula M, Iudice A, La Neve A, Mazza M, Mazza S, Cantello R, et al. Validation of the Hamilton Rating Scale for Depression in adults with epilepsy. Epilepsy Behav. 2014;41:122-5.
12. Fiest KM, Patten SB, Jetté N. Screening for Depression and Anxiety in Epilepsy. Neurol Clin. 2016;34:351-61.
13. Wagner JL, Kellermann T, Mueller M, Smith G, Brooks B, Arnett A, et al. Development and validation of the NDDI-E-Y: a screening tool for depressive symptoms in pediatric epilepsy. Epilepsia. 2016;57:1265-70.
14. Michaelis R, Tang V, Goldstein LH, Reuber M, LaFrance WC Jr, Lundgren T, et al. Psychological treatments for adults and children with epilepsy: Evidence-based recommendations by the International League Against Epilepsy Psychology Task Force. Epilepsia. 2018;59:1282-302.
15. Gasparini S, Beghi E, Ferlazzo E, Beghi M, Belcastro V, Biermann KP, et al. Management of psychogenic non-epileptic seizures: a multidisciplinary approach. Eur J Neurol. 2019;26:205-e15.
16. Mula M, Sander JW. Current and emerging drug therapies for the treatment of depression in adults with epilepsy. Expert Opin Pharmacother. 2019;20:41-5.
17. Agrawal N, Mula M. Treatment of psychoses in patients with epilepsy: an update. Ther Adv Psychopharmacol. 2019;9:2045125319862968.
18. Alper K, Schwartz KA, Kolts RL, Khan A. Seizure incidence in psychopharmacological clinical trials: an analysis of Food and Drug Administration (FDA) summary basis of approval reports. Biol Psychiatry. 2007;62:345-54.

201

CHAPTER

Clinical Bedside Test for Autonomic Neuropathy

Balakrishnan Kannan, Rohith Velusamy

ABSTRACT

Autonomic disorders provide a fascinating insight into the complexity of the nervous system, and their effects on human health can range from benign to severe. Understanding the symptoms and signs of autonomic disorders draws on the cognitive skills and the personal interest in the condition of patients that first drew many physicians to neurology. This chapter provides tools to enhance those skills. Recent advances in autonomic neuroscience and accumulated clinical knowledge have led to the classification of autonomic disorders as specific syndromes based on clinical phenotypes and physiological responses to standardized stimuli in the autonomic laboratory. One of the most significant advances has been the capacity to distinguish neurogenic orthostasis from other causes of hypotension. Quantifying sudomotor responses is useful in diagnosing thermoregulatory and small fiber neuropathies, such as those associated with diabetes mellitus. More attention is being paid to autonomic failure as the defining characteristic of neurodegenerative and multiple system atrophy. The once obscure term of dysautonomia is now widely used.

INTRODUCTION

The autonomic nervous system, which innervates every organ system in the body, uses a complex network of autonomously functioning central and peripheral neurons to maintain biological homeostasis both at rest and in reaction to stress. Clinical practice frequently involves autonomic disorders. Their symptoms might be mild or severe, localized or generalized, episodic or continuous, temporary or progressive, common or rare, and benign or severe. They may show themselves in different ways. The amplitude or timing of peripheral autonomic effectors can be affected by the deafferentation of central autonomic centers.

An organized approach is required for the clinical evaluation of a patient with autonomic symptoms. The importance of a detailed medical history in the autonomic evaluation should be emphasized. The autonomic component of the neurological examination comes in next, followed by a laboratory evaluation tailored to each patient's unique presentation. Evaluation is to determine the presence of an autonomic disorder, characterize and localize its spread, and assess the severity of the disorder. Diagnosing significant, curable illnesses is very important.

AUTONOMIC PHYSICAL EXAMINATION

General Evaluation

It is important to note the patient's posture, facial expression, capacity to comprehend, and how old they appear to be in comparison to their actual age. Signs of hypothalamus involvement, such as dwarfism, sexual immaturity, hypothermia, and pallor, must be looked for.

Vital Orthostatic Signs

After the patient has been standing for at least 3 minutes, blood pressure and heart rate (HR) should be monitored. It is a sign of generalized baroreflex-sympathoneural and baroreflex-cardiovagal failure, when orthostatic hypotension (OH) is present without reflex tachycardia. Hypothermic patients could have a cold injury or have hypothalamic issues. Quantitative documentation of OH is crucial. Because patients with chronic neurogenic OH frequently may tolerate surprisingly low blood pressure without symptoms, relying just on orthostatic intolerance symptoms will understate the existence of OH. OH is defined as a fall in systolic blood pressure (SBP) ≥20 mm Hg or of diastolic blood pressure (DBP) ≥10 mm Hg between supine rest and standing for at least 3 minutes.

Blood Pressure in Response to Stress

The sustained hand grip, mental stress, and cold pressor tests all look for increases in DBP of at least 15 mm Hg or an increase in HR of >10 beats/minute in response to peripheral vasoconstriction **(Fig. 1)**.

Heart Rate Variability

The HR should not increase by >30 beats/min above baseline on standing.

Inference

Orthostatic hypotension with reflex tachycardia can denote hypovolemia. OH with absence of reflex tachycardia suggests autonomic failure. Only reflex tachycardia without OH signifies postural tachycardia syndrome (POTS). Resting tachycardia indicates sign of parasympathetic dysfunction.

Head-up Tilting

Baroreflex-cardiovagal gain (baroreflex sensitivity) measurement of beat-to-beat blood pressure, now noninvasive, allows quantification of baroreflex-cardiovascular gain (also called baroreflex sensitivity). Normally, HR increases, so the interbeat interval decreases as blood pressure falls during the fall in Valsalva maneuver. After release of Valsalva maneuver, the interbeat interval reflexively increases as blood pressure exceeds the baseline value. In patients with baroreflex-sympathoneural failure, there is usually a loss of the pressure overshoot as well as a loss of reflexive bradycardia.

Signs of syncope include a gradual decrease in blood pressure, especially diastolic, in total peripheral and/or forearm vascular resistance, and in pulse pressure. Patients with baroreflex-sympathoneural failure have a gradual decrease in pressure. The HR response is usually attenuated. When tilting head-up, blood pressure decreases in the first minute and recovers in 1 minute. Tilt >10 minutes may be needed if later changes are sought (e.g., neurocardiogenic syncope or delayed OH).

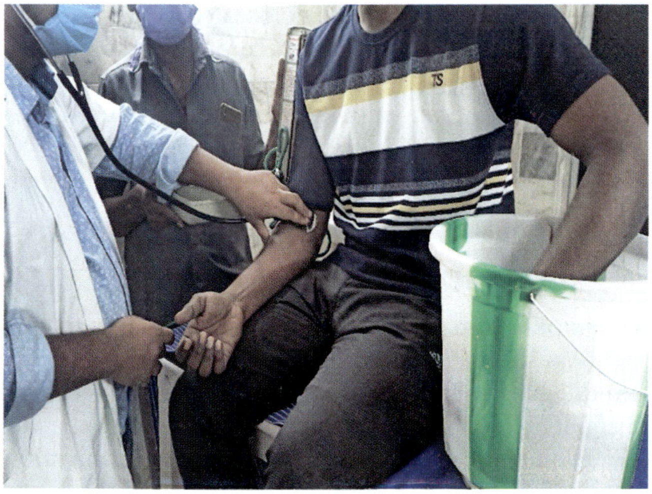

FIG. 1: Blood pressure measurement.

Isometric Handgrip Test

Isometric pressing of a handgrip dynamometer at approximately one-third of maximum contraction strength for 3–5 minutes and BP measured in the other arm at 1 -minute interval is isometric handgrip test. A rise of DBP >15 mm Hg is normal.

Other tests for cardiovascular and vascular autonomic regulation include cardiovascular response to standing and the 30–15th R-R ratio, head-up tilt table testing, HR variation with respiration (sinus arrhythmia; R-R interval analysis), and Valsalva test.

TESTS OF THERMOREGULATORY FUNCTION

Tests of thermoregulatory function include sympathetic skin response (SSR), quantitative sudomotor axon reflex test (QSART), thermoregulatory sweat test, and sweat imprint test.

Thermoregulatory Sweat Test

It focuses on visualizing skin humidity responses to increasing environmental temperature. The patient's body is covered with a powder that turns color when wetted; for example, alizarin red mixed with cornstarch and sodium carbonate is brushed onto the patient's skin. The orange-red mixture turns dark purple when humidified.

Sympathetic Skin Response

This test focuses on measuring skin electrical conductance responses to standard stimuli (e.g., electricity or startle). The skin sympathetic test is sensitive to lesions at either station (e.g., brain, central regulation) or at any station (sensory receptors). Sensory receptors at both stations

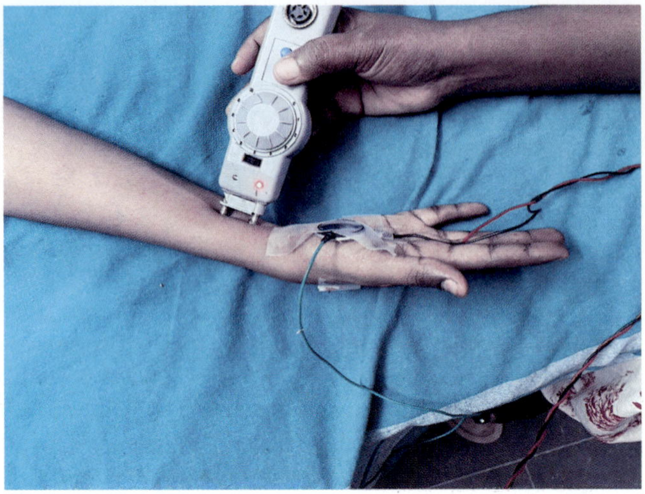

FIG. 2: Measurement of the electrical conductivity of the skin.

include sympathetic parenteral outflow, sympathetic postganglionic neurotransmission, muscarinic cholinergic. SSR requires integrity of hypothalamus, brainstem, spinal circuits, and postganglionic sympathetic neurons. It is performed by applying a strong electrical stimulus to median nerve for a long time course (2 seconds). The active electrode is placed in the palm or sole and the reference electrode in the dorsum of the respective body part. A potential change linked to the median nerve stimulus is generated in the skin by the activation of sweat glands. Following a latency period, a typical response includes a negative response (upward deflection) followed by a positive (downward) correction (can be triphasic also), symmetric in homologous body regions. Hands have larger amplitudes and short latencies than feet. SSR is usually recorded as present/absent in hand and in foot. It elicits an axon reflex mediated by postganglionic sympathetic sudomotor axon **(Fig. 2)**.

Quantitative Sudomotor Axon Reflex Test

The QSART assesses postganglionic and postsudomotor cholinergic and sudomotor functions in a quantifiably and reproducibly way. However, the QSART does involve the administration of an active drug (i.e., acetylcholine). The neural pathway is mediated by an axon "reflex" mediated by a postsugarized sudomotor (sugary) axon (sugary nerve node). Acetylcholine activates the axon terminal of the nerve. It is performed by giving a stimulus to one compartment of a multicompartmental sweat cell. Sweat response is recorded from a second compartment with a sudorometer. Multicompartmental sweat cells are attached to sites on upper and lower limbs. Distribution permits the detection of dysfunction localizable to one specific peripheral nerve territory or of a length-dependent autonomic neuropathy. An absent response indicates a lesion of the postganglionic axon.

Skin and Mucous Membranes

Examination of skin and mucous membranes should be done to look for any changes in acral vasomotor movements, including changes in foot color with standing. Signs of acrocyanosis or pallor, such as mottling or redness, should be looked for. The skin must be checked for any signs of allodynia, which is pain caused by nonpainful stimuli, and for signs of hyperalgesia, which is indicated by increased sensitivity to a painful stimulus.

Sudomotor changes, such as dryness and resistance to a gentle touch, must be checked for. Alopecia and hypertrichosis are signs of skin changes and thickening and distortion are the nail signs. Lipodystrophy and wasting, as well as atrophic skin changes, can also be observed.

Spoon Test

A simple bedside test to demonstrate the distribution of abnormal skin dryness related to loss of sweating is spoon test. When a spoon is drawn over the skin, it glides smoothly over dry (sympathectomized) skin but irregularly and unevenly over moist skin.

Visualization of Sweat Droplets

Sweat droplets may be seen using the +20D ophthalmoscope.

Cold Pressor Test

It is a sensitive semiquantitative test of sweating. It is done by submerging the hand in ice-cold water. A color indicator (alizarin red with cornstarch and sodium carbonate) is applied to the skin. The environmental temperature is increased until an adequate core temperature rise is attained (usually 2°C rise in core temperature/38.5°C, whichever is less) and noting an increase in SBP by 20 mm Hg and DBP by 10 mm Hg.

Pupillary Dysfunction

The pupil shape, pupil size, light, and accommodation response should be noted. If pupils are not responsive to direct light, we should observe the response to 1 minute of sustained light to show the presence of tonic pupils. Redilatation after constriction, if Delayed or slow, is a major symptom of Horner syndrome.

AUTONOMIC FUNCTION TESTS: MISCELLANEOUS TESTS

Tests for Exocrine and Pupillary Regulation

Usage of pharmacological drugs like pilocarpine.

Schirmer's Test for Lacrimation

The patient is instructed to look upward, and the patient's eyelid is pulled down. The bent end of the test strip is placed in the eye such that it rests between the palpebral conjunctiva of the lower eyelid and the bulbar conjunctiva of the eye. Schirmer's test uses paper strips inserted into the eye for several minutes to measure the production of tears. Both eyes are tested at the same time. Most often, this test consists of placing a small strip of filter paper inside the lower eyelid (inferior fornix). The eyes are closed for 5 minutes The paper is then removed and the amount of moisture is measured. After a 5 minutes, the patient is asked to open both eyes and look upward so the test strips may be removed. The Schirmer test score is determined by the length of the moistened area of the strips (using the scale packaged with the strips). The use of the anesthetic ensures that only basal tear secretion is being measured.

Joints

Loss of sympathetic vascular innervation results in high peripheral blood flow through arteriovenous (AV) shunts and abnormal local reflex vascular control, leading to increased osteoclastic activity resulting in reduced bone density, making the bones more prone to fractures. In case of neuropathic joints, the joint may have too much movement. Pain is common in Charcot joint but is less in neuropathic joints due to the disorganization of the joint and the lack of range of motion. Patients with postural tachycardia syndrome may have hypermobility in the joint.

Tests of gastrointestinal autonomic regulation are done by video fluoroscopy and pharyngoesophageal studies, barium enema, and anorectal manometry.

Genitourinary Function

Clinical assessment of bladder function is done by looking for evidence of distension by palpation and percussion, and post void residual urine volume is determined by catheterization after voiding. It can also be tested clinically, by checking the anal wink and bulbocavernosus reflexes. Other tests include urodynamic study, cystometrogram, papaverine injection, and bulbocavernosus reflex.

CONCLUSION

A number of autonomic function tests are considered reliable, reproducible, simple, and quick to carry out. Autonomic function testing should be undertaken after a thorough clinical evaluation. Wider implementation of these techniques, especially those that are the most objective, together with their competent interpretation, may contribute to a better understanding of the role of the autonomic nervous system in the pathogenesis of diabetes and translate into improved patient care. There is still an educational gap that needs to be closed in order to increase the number of healthcare professionals in identifying the signs and symptoms of autonomic disorders. There is also a long way to go in terms of developing more effective treatment options for patients with an autonomic disorder.

SUGGESTED READINGS

1. Goldstein DS, Holmes C, Cannon RO 3rd, Eisenhofer G, Kopin IJ. Sympathetic cardioneuropathy in dysautonomias. N Engl J Med. 1997;336(10):696-702.
2. Low PA. Autonomic nervous system function. J Clin Neurophysiol. 1993;10(1):14-27.
3. Vogel ER, Sandroni P, Low PA. Blood pressure recovery from Valsalva maneuver in patients with autonomic failure. Neurology. 2005;65(10):1533-7.

SECTION

15

NUTRITION

202

CHAPTER

Vegan Diets: Benefits and Dangers

Mayank Gupta, Madhulata Agarwal

ABSTRACT

Vegan diet or plant-based diet is the new health choice of the modern era. Global urbanization and industrialization have created a necessity for transition toward healthy and environmentally sustainable food sources. Replacing animal products with plant-based products has also caused a reduction in greenhouse gas emission apart from all its other health benefits. Thus, vegan diet has gained immense popularity and is the present health mantra. According to the vegan society, 2021 survey; globally the number of vegans is on a rise with 6% of population being strict vegans in US, 4% in Europe, and 13% in Asia. An umbrella review of systematic reviews and meta-analysis by Selinger E et al. (2022); it was found that vegan diet in a general healthy population reduced body weight [95% confidence interval (CI)]: 2.52 kg (−3.06 and −1.98) from eight randomized controlled trials (RCTs); and was also beneficial in reducing incidence of cancer (95% CI): 0.84 (0.75 and 0.95) from two RCTs; and also lowered risk for all-cause mortality (95% CI); 0.87 (0.75 and 1.01) from two RCTs. Vegan diets are rich in nutrients and low in saturated fats and hence vegans have lower body mass index (BMI) and lower risk of cardiovascular diseases. Although vegans have enormous health benefits they do lack in certain nutrients such as calcium, zinc, vitamin D3 and B12, and omega-3 fatty acids and need fortification or supplementation to reduce improve bone health and reduce adverse effects. The reasons to choose veganism as way of life might be several but the crux is optimizing nutrient intake by making healthy choices is essential no matter what diet choice is adopted.

INTRODUCTION

Albert Einstein quoted aptly, "*Nothing will benefit human health and increase chances of survival on earth as much as the evolution to a vegetarian diet.*" Contemporary few decades have seen a massive transformation to vegetarian diets all over the world with growing popularity among teenagers and young adults, especially females. India, the land of diversities, harbors the largest number of vegetarians at ~35% and has done so for generations. The nutritional choice of vegetarians for decades has pivoted around health benefits of plant-based diet, preservation of earth's resources and environment, ethical issues about animals, animal borne diseases and use of antibiotics and growth stimulants to increase meat production.

A well planned and adequately balanced vegan diet is adequate for all stages of lifecycle including infancy, childhood, and adolescence as concluded after several reviews by experts from American Dietetic Association and Dieticians of Canada. Vegetarian diet is further subclassified into vegan (exclude all animal source food and their byproducts), lacto-ovo-vegetarian (no meat, only eggs and dairy products), lacto-vegetarian (no meat, eggs or fish and only dairy products included), ovo-vegetarian (no meat, fish, or dairy products included only eggs), and pescatarian (no meat except fish and shellfish). Vegan diet albeit rich in fiber, folic acid, vitamin C and E, potassium, magnesium, many phytochemicals, and unsaturated fats resulting in low cholesterol, low blood pressure, and reduced cardiovascular disease (CVD) risk, elimination of all animal products leads to certain micro- and macronutrient deficiencies resulting in adverse effects on bone health, immune system as well as mental health. Hence, it is prudent to see both sides of the picture before we make appropriate food and nutrient choices for a holistic healthy life.

DIETARY CHARACTERISTICS OF VEGETARIAN DIETS

Nutritional Status of Vegetarians

Vegetarian diets largely comprise of intake of large amounts of cereals, pulses, nuts, fruits, and vegetables and hence are rich in carbohydrates, dietary fiber, carotenoids, folic acid, n-6 fatty acids, vitamin C, vitamin E, and magnesium. However, they are deficient in proteins, saturated fats, long-chain n-3 fatty acids, retinol, calcium, vitamin B12, vitamin D, and zinc. Vegan diets in particular are more severely deficient in vitamin B12 and calcium. Vegans as compared to nonvegans are more likely to attain the recommended targets for fruit intake, dietary reference values for saturated fatty acids of 10% of total energy, and non-starch polysaccharide intake of 18 g/day as recommended by UK department of health (1991).

Potential Nutritional Short Falls and Advantages

Vegan diets are nutritionally deficient in n-3 fatty acids, vitamin D and B12, iron, calcium, and zinc due to complete elimination of animal source foods and their byproducts resulting in adverse health impacts **(Table 1)**.

TABLE 1: Potential nutritional short falls and advantages.

Nutritional components of diet	Vegan diet: Short falls and advantage
Long-chain n-3 polyunsaturated fatty acids	• Vegan diets are deficient in eicosapentaenoic acid (EPA) and docosahexaenoic acid (DHA) which are essential for brain and eye functions and cardiovascular health • Although, plant n-3 fatty acid alpha-linoleic acid (ALA) can be converted to EPA and DHA, conversion efficiency is very low in females and very low in males. Thus, vegans can obtain DHA from microalgae supplements or foods fortified with DHA and EPA from oil of brown algae (kelp) • DHA supplements elevate total and low-density lipoprotein (LDL) cholesterol, impair immune responses, and prolong the bleeding time • The potential adverse health effects of low circulating levels of EPA and DHA are yet unknown
Vitamin B12	• It is significantly low in vegans in comparison to ovo-, lacto-ovo, lacto-vegetarians • The major sources for vegetarians are eggs, dairy products, and fortified foods • The daily recommended intake is 1.5 μg/day in adults (UK Health Department, 1991). Even though daily intake of 0.3 g/day adequately prevent anemia and macrocytosis, they lead to elevated levels of homocysteine that are detrimental to health
Vitamin D	• Vegans depend on sunlight and vitamin D fortified foods meeting recommended targets as they have lowest mean intake (0.88 μg/day) of vitamin D, which is almost one-fourth that of nonvegans • People living at high altitudes, elderly, those who extensively cover their bodies for cultural reasons or those who use sunscreens are deficient in vitamin D • Low vitamin D levels result in high parathyroid hormone levels and reduced lumbar spine bone mineral density (BMD) by almost 12% in vegans versus nonvegans
Iron, zinc, and calcium	• Vegetarian diet has iron content similar to nonvegetarian diet, but it is less bioavailable than heme iron. Females need to consume iron with vitamin C to increase absorption • Phytates in grains, seeds, and legumes binds zinc and causes its deficiency in vegans • Vegans have calcium deficiency and high risk of fracture due to reduced mean intake of as compared to vegetarians or ovo-lacto vegetarians
Potassium and magnesium	Vegan diet is enriched in potassium and magnesium which helps maintain bone health by providing alkaline environment and reducing bone resorption
Vitamin K and isoflavones	• Vitamin K from green leafy vegetables also reduce risk of fractures in elderly and postmenopausal females • Isoflavones in soy protein also promote bone health and reduce risk of hip fracture

BENEFITS VERSUS HARMS OF VEGAN DIET

The Academy of Nutrition and Dietetics states that appropriately balanced vegan diet is nutritionally apt and healthful for all stages of lifecycle including infancy, childhood, adolescence, older adulthood, pregnancy, lactation, and athletes and has advantage in prevention of certain conditions like diabetes, hypertension, ischemic heart disease (IHD), obesity, and cancer.

Cardiovascular Diseases

In a study by Toohey et al., it was notable that the African American vegans had low body mass index (BMI) versus ovo-lacto vegetarians and Latin American vegetarians had lower BMI as compared to omnivores and it was the lowest among vegans. EPIC-Oxford follow-up study among 21,966 individuals revealed a mean increase in body weight of ~400 g/year with remarkably less weight gain among vegans versus vegetarians and meat-eaters. This difference has not been well understood but might have been due to difference in composition of diet and high fiber content as noted by Spencer et al. (2003). The total plasma cholesterol levels are lower in vegetarians and vegans by 0.61 mmol/L in Health Food Shoppers study and by 0.39 mmol/L and 0.35 mmol/L in men and women respectively in EPIC-Oxford study by Key et al. The effect on cholesterol levels depends on the dietary composition and in particular on the ratio of the saturated and unsaturated fats consumed. Diets rich in soy proteins and nuts lowers serum low-density lipoprotein (LDL) and is cardioprotective. Beilin et al. (1988) noted lower systolic and diastolic blood pressures with difference of almost 2–10 mm Hg among vegans when compared to omnivores. However, EPIC -Oxford study among 11,004 men and women showed a significantly low difference of ≤1 mm Hg in vegans versus meat-eaters, emphasizing that several other factors play a crucial role in determining blood pressure among individuals such as salt intake and alcohol consumption. Albeit low BMI in vegans did result in lower blood pressures of 2–3 mm Hg in comparison to meat-eaters (Appleby et al. 2002).

A collaborative reanalysis of five major prospective studies revealed mortality from IHD was 24% lower in vegans versus nonvegans (Key et al. 1999) and this difference was due to the notifiable difference of almost 0.40 mmol/L in levels of serum cholesterol among vegans as compared to nonvegetarians (Law et al. 1994) and was not attributable to low BMI. Meta-analysis of five prospective studies revealed stroke related death rate ratio of 0.93 among vegetarians as compared to nonvegetarians with major determinant being hypertension. Overall, it was noted that vegan diet being rich in whole grains, soy, nuts, fruits, and vegetables was rich in cardioprotective elements due to increased amounts of fiber, folic acid, potassium, magnesium, isoflavones, phytochemicals, and antioxidants resulting in low BMI, low cholesterol, and low blood pressures and thus, reduced the risk of cardiovascular events such as stroke and IHD.

Cancer

Vegan diet is substantially rich in fiber, vitamin C, carotenoids, flavonoids, other phytochemicals, lycopene, and several other antioxidants and hence are protective for several cancers including colorectal, stomach, mouth, esophagus, prostate, and lungs. Tomatoes that are rich in lycopene are protective for prostate cancer, allium vegetables are protective for stomach cancer, garlic for colorectal cancer, legumes for stomach and prostate cancer, and fruits and vegetables for cancers of lungs, mouth, stomach, esophagus, and colon. Phytochemicals in vegan diet inhibit cell proliferation, deoxyribonucleic (DNA) adduction, phase 1 enzymes, activation of nuclear factor-κB, angiogenesis, and oncogene expression as well as induce phase 2 enzymes and cell cycle arrest.

Vegans also consume more of isoflavone rich soy products that protect them against breast cancer in females and prostate cancer in males. Vegans have reduced risk of breast cancer, although inconclusive due to decreased circulating levels of insulin-like growth factor-1 (IGF-1) attributable to soy products rich in phytoestrogens (Allen et al. 2002; Peeters et al. 2003). Increased consumption of red meat has been associated with moderately increased incidence of liver, esophagus, and colorectal cancers (Key et al. 2004; Norat et al. 2005). Dairy products have been linked to increased risk of colorectal and prostate cancer. Despite this the reduction in incidence of cancer among vegans is not statistically significant as compared to nonvegans attributable to vitamin D deficiency and decreased bioavailability of phytochemicals that is subjected to the methods of food preparation. Apparently, more epidemiological studies are essential to extemporize the understanding and gather convincing evidence regarding beneficial effects of vegan diet on cancer.

Bone Health

Recent studies in postmenopausal women and elderly adults have shown reduced bone mineral density (BMD) leading to increased risk of fracture among vegans as compared to lacto-vegetarians and ovo-lacto vegetarians attributable to reduced protein and inadequate calcium intake, however, no difference was seen in fracture risk among vegans taking >525 mg of calcium/day versus omnivores (EPIC-Oxford study). Bone health also depends on vitamin D, vitamin K, potassium, magnesium, and maintenance of acid base balance. High fruits and vegetable contents of vegan diet provide adequate vitamin K, potassium, and magnesium that provide an alkaline ash for maintenance of bone health by preventing calcium resorption from bones. Framingham heart study showed a 65% decreased risk of hip fracture in elderly men and women with increased vitamin K intake (≥1 serving of green leafy vegetables/day). Randomized clinical trials have shown decreased bone resorption and increased BMD in postmenopausal females with increased soy isoflavone intake.

Mental Health

Vegans have increased prevalence of mental health problems leading to poor quality of life. A systematic review of 18 studies including 160,257 individuals from various geographical areas aged 11–96 years with 149,559 meat-eaters and 8584 meat-abstainers; 11 out of the 18 studies showed adverse mental health among meat-abstainers in terms of increased life-term prevalence of depression (35.2% vs. 19.1%) and anxiety (31.5% vs. 18.4%) as compared to meat-eaters. Women were more adversely affected with mental disorders such as stress.

Overall Mortality

Pooled analysis of five prospective studies and EPIC-Oxford study shows a death rate ratio of 0.95 (95% CI 0.82, 1.11; Key et al. 1999) and 1.05 (95% CI 0.86, 1.27; Key et al. 2003) respectively among vegetarians versus nonvegetarians which is almost similar and comparable. However, standardized mortality ratios observed in three UK cohorts was lower in vegetarians earmarking their overall good health.

SPECIAL CONDITIONS

Children and Adolescents

Childhood and adolescence are the age groups of maximum growth spurt requiring an adequately balanced nutritious diet rendering recommendation of vegan diet intriguing in this age groups. Vegans and vegetarians were found to be shorter than omnivores (–0.32 and –0.57 height Z-scores, respectively), albeit the difference among vegetarians was insignificant (Desmond et al.). Vegan children were found to have significantly low vitamin D levels and reduction in BMD versus omnivores. It is thus recommended to provide apt supplements of Vitamin D and calcium in these age groups in order to maximize childhood BMD to attain peak BMD in order to avoid risk of fractures in adulthood and promote good bone health. Further, prospective longitudinal studies are obligatory to have a better understanding of effects of vegan diet in children and adolescents.

Pregnancy and Lactation

Pregnancy requires balanced diet to ensure optimal fetal growth. Mothers on strict vegan diet are nutritionally deficient in vitamins like B12 associated with adverse fetal outcomes in terms of small for gestational age (SGA) babies, preterm term delivery, and neural tube defects. A study of 273 pregnant women including, 112 omnivores and 60 vegans, observed substantial risk of SGA babies among vegans [relative risk (RR) = 5.9, 95% CI, 1.2–21.8]; also, it was observed that mean gestational weight gain was significantly low in vegans as compared to omnivores (11.6 ± 4.2 kg vs. 14.3 ± 4.6 kg, $p = 0.001$). Also, studies have found vegan mothers to have low nutritional reserves resulting in low fat reserves for breast feeding. Hence, women on strict vegan diets need heightened awareness regarding consumption of diets fortified with essential nutrients and vitamins as recommended by international guidelines during pregnancy and lactation to improve maternal and fetal outcomes.

CONCLUSION

Vegans have good average health comparable to nonvegetarians with the same demographic profile and background, this might partly be due to their health choices and awareness like avoiding drinking or smoking, also they have healthy eating patterns in terms of fat consumption. In most studies, vegans have low BMI compared to nonvegetarians and hence have low cholesterol and decreased risk of hypertension and CVD. However, no difference has been observed in mortality related to malignancies such as colorectal cancer and stroke. Vegans have relatively low circulating levels of IGF-1 and thus, might have reduced incidence of breast and prostrate cancer. Albeit myriad benefits vegan diets are poor sources of calcium, vitamin D, vitamin B12 and omega-3 fatty acids [alpha-linoleic acid (ALA) and docosahexaenoic acid (DHA)] and need fortification to improve bone health and avoid deficiencies. Large studies are needed to strongly establish the benefits of vegan diet and to study its relation to cancer, diabetes, and osteoporosis. The bottom line hence remains, eat healthy to live healthy.

SUGGESTED READINGS

1. Selinger E, Neuenschwander M, Koller A, Gojda J, Kühn T, Schwingshackl L, et al. Evidence of a vegan diet for health benefits and risks—an umbrella review of meta-analyses of observational and clinical studies. Crit Rev Food Sci Nutr. 2023;63(29):9926-36.
2. Key T, Appleby P, Rosell M. Health effects of vegetarian and vegan diets. Proc Nutr Soc. 2006;65(1):35-41.
3. Craig WJ. Health effects of vegan diets. Am J Clin Nutr. 2009;89(5):1627S-33S.
4. Bali A, Naik R. The Impact of a Vegan Diet on Many Aspects of Health: The Overlooked Side of Veganism. Cureus. 2023;15(2):e35148.
5. Selinger E, Neuenschwander M, Koller A, Gojda J, Kühn T, Schwingshackl L, et al. Evidence of a vegan diet for health benefits and risks – an umbrella review of meta-analyses of observational and clinical studies. Crit Rev Food Sci Nutr. 2023;63(29):9926-36.
6. Toohey ML, Harris MA, DeWitt W, Foster G, Schmidt WD, Melby CL. Cardiovascular Disease Risk Factors are Lower in African-American Vegans Compared to Lacto-Ovo-vegetarians.J Am Coll Nutr. 1998;17(5):425-34.
7. Spencer EA, Appleby PN, Davey GK, Key TJ. Diet and body mass index in 38,000 EPIC–Oxford meat-eaters, fish-eaters, vegetarians and vegans. Int J Obes Relat Metab Disord. 2003; 27(6):728-34.
8. Davey GK, Spencer EA, Appleby PN, Allen NE, Knox KH, Key TJ. EPIC–Oxford: lifestyle characteristics and nutrient intakes in a cohort of 33 883 meat-eaters and 31 546 non meat-eaters in the UK. Public Health Nutr. 2003;6(3):259-69.
9. Allen NE, Appleby PN, Davey GK, Kaaks R, Rinaldi S, Key TJ. The Associations of Diet with Serum Insulin-like Growth Factor I and Its Main Binding Proteins in 292 Women Meat-Eaters, Vegetarians, and Vegans. Cancer Epidemiol Biomarkers Prev. 2002;11(11):1441-8.
10. Peeters A, Barendregt JJ, Willekens F, Mackenbach JP, Al Mamun A, Bonneux L, et al. Obesity in adulthood and its consequences for life expectancy: a life-table analysis. Ann Intern Med. 2003 Jan 7;138(1):24-32.
11. Beilin LJ, Rouse IL, Armstrong BK, Margetts BM, Vandongen R. Vegetarian diet and blood pressure levels: incidental or causal association? Am J Clin Nutr. 1988;48(3);Suppl:806-10, ISSN 0002-9165.
12. Key TJ, Schatzkin A, Willett WC, Allen NE, Spencer EA, Travis RC. Diet, nutrition and the prevention of cancer. Public Health Nutr. 2004;7(1A):187-200.
13. Norat T, Bingham S, Ferrari P, Slimani N, Jenab M, Mazuir M et al. Meat, fish, and colorectal cancer risk: the European Prospective Investigation into cancer and nutrition. J Natl Cancer Inst. 200515;97(12):906-16.
14. Appleby PN, Davey GK, Key TJ. Hypertension and blood pressure among meat eaters, fish eaters, vegetarians and vegans in EPIC–Oxford. Public Health Nutr. 2002;5(5):645-54.
15. Key TJ, Fraser GE, Thorogood M, Appleby PN, Beral V, Reeves G, McPherson K. Mortality in vegetarians and nonvegetarians: detailed findings from a collaborative analysis of 5 prospective studies. Am J Clin Nutr. 1999;70:516S-524S.
16. Law MR, Wald NJ, Wu T, Hackshaw A, Bailey A. Systematic underestimation of association between serum cholesterol concentration and ischaemic heart disease in observational studies: data from the BUPA study. BMJ. 1994;308(6925):363-6.
17. Key TJ, Appleby PN, Davey GK, Allen NE, Spencer EA, Travis RC. Mortality in British vegetarians: review and preliminary results from EPIC–Oxford. Am J Clin Nutr. 2003;78(3);Suppl:533S-8S, ISSN 0002-9165.
18. Desmond MA, Sobiecki JG, Jaworski M, Płudowski P, Antoniewicz J, Shirley MK et al. Growth, body composition, and cardiovascular and nutritional risk of 5- to 10-y-old children consuming vegetarian, vegan, or omnivore diets. Am J Clin Nutr. 2021;113(6):1565-77.

203

CHAPTER

Embracing Complexity: Making Sense of Diet

Sandeep Suri

ABSTRACT

Diabetes is a metabolic disorder in which blood glucose levels get elevated, causing free movement of glucose in cells and organs. It was observed that most of the population has obesity-related diabetes, especially the youth. This condition is known as diabesity. It was observed that diet and adequate nutrition play a crucial role in diabetes prevention. However, debate of unhealthy, healthy, and optimal has made people with diabetes, medical practitioners, and other population confused. Some recent progressions have been made in order to conclude some diet-related data. This chapter determines some risk factors by mainly focusing on the types of diet and their impact on weight loss and management along with prevention of diabetes and its management. Discussions have been made to examine interrelationship between nutrients, dietary habits, and types of food they consume together with some future developments and challenges. It is also a hotly debatable topic that which type of diet is best suited for weight loss and diabetes prevention and management. Confusion over low-fat, low-carb, and other therapeutic diets hovers from here to there, but no specific data was seen or observed in this regard.

INTRODUCTION

Diet is a Complex Risk Exposure

Diet is nonbinary, unlike, for example, tobacco, for which zero is best. Foods belong within food groups and may be consumed unprocessed (e.g., beef or pork) or processed (e.g., ham or bacon). Foods contain nutrients (e.g., meat fat or protein as macronutrients; heme iron as a micronutrient) or additives and preservatives if processed and are part of overall dietary patterns (e.g., the Mediterranean diet with relatively low intakes of red meat or a low-carbohydrate diet regimen with relatively high intakes of meat). The continuum of dietary exposures should be considered, as well as 'food substitution effects' because when more or less of one food type is consumed, it impacts the consumption of other foods as part of the overall energy intake.

Diet is Hard to Measure

Hierarchy of diet is variable, hence making it difficult to provide a firm conclusion about what to include and what to exclude from the diet. Dietary tools such as 24-hour recall method and food frequency questionnaire are some commonly used tools to observe the lifestyle and dietary pattern of individuals. It also provides a vision about what type of food groups were generally consumed by that particular population. In the scarcity of suitable alternatives for food measurements, digital media comes to the rescue by introducing many diet-related platforms and diet apps, but they are also not of 'research grade'. No single method is perfect, but with the use of consistent and continuous use of dietary methods and mixture of that can lead to planning a better diet for the individuals with type-2 diabetes mellitus (T2DM).

Study Design of Nutritional Research is Challenging

The randomized controlled trial (RCT) design is considered the gold standard in the hierarchy of evidence-based medicine framework, but for complex behavioral exposures such as diet, unlike for pharmaceuticals, RCTs are more challenging. The bulk of the evidence base for nutrition and health has come from long-term observational prospective cohort studies. Dietary RCTs have several challenges. They have a specific set of limitations including a lack of blinding, lack of an appropriate control group, issues with feasibility and cost, and challenges of adherence and attrition. The inability to pinpoint the specific nutritional component(s) is another challenge, such as in some of the abovementioned RCTs, which could not separate the effects of macronutrient type and energy intake.

New concepts are emerging, such as "n-of-1" trials and adaptive trial design, which need robust testing in the nutrition field. There is strong concordance in findings from prospective observational studies and RCTs and the two study designs should complement each other **(Fig. 1)**.

Reality and Relevance of Different Nutrients and Food Types

A cross-sectional trial between ketogenic and Mediterranean style diet was done to observe the optimal weight loss and significant improvement in the T2DM. Food restrictions along with carbohydrates was done in people with T2DM over a period of 12 weeks. Carbohydrate composition < 20% of the total energy in ketogenic diet and < 40% in low-carb Mediterranean style diet were compared. Both types of diet comprises nonstarchy vegetables and no added sugars or refined grains; legumes, most fruits, and whole grains were avoided in keto diet and incorporated into Mediterranean-style diet. Both diets have shown improvements, but these were not statistically significant. It was observed that 9%

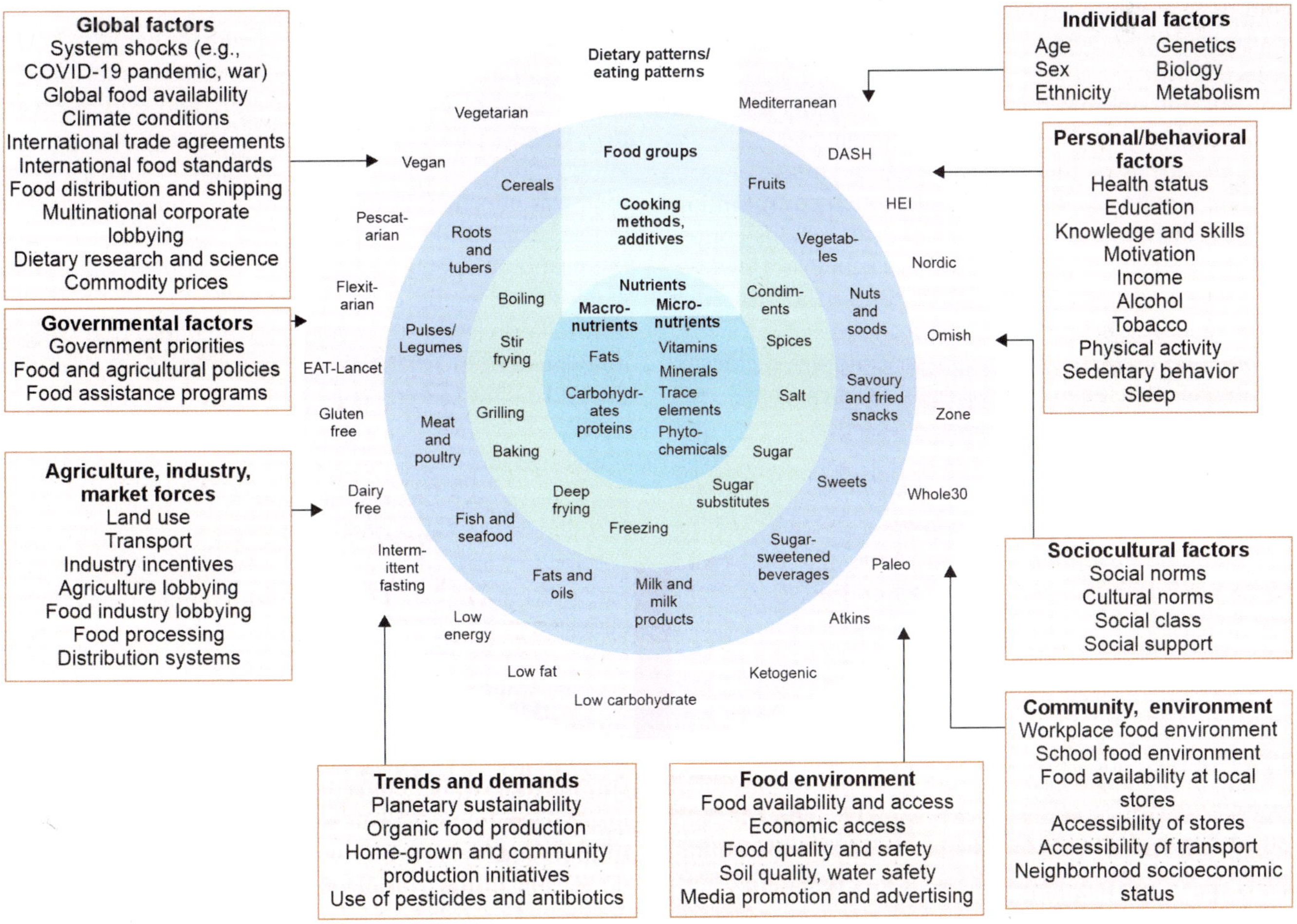

FIG. 1: The complexities of the diet and multiple influences affecting food intake.

(COVID-19: coronavirus disease 2019; DASH: dietary approaches to stop hypertension; HEI: healthy eating index) and 7% decrease in glycated hemoglobin (HbA1c) levels in keto and Mediterranean diets, respectively, whereas only 8% and 7% weight loss is observed in keto diet and Mediterranean diet, respectively. This study was done for a very short duration; hence, more research is needed to build a firm observation in this regard.

NAVIGATING GRAY AREAS IN DIET AND NUTRITION FOR THE TREATMENT OF OBESITY AND TYPE 2 DIABETES MELLITUS

The role of diet and nutrition in managing these conditions has been a subject of ongoing research, clinical practice, and public discussion. Yet, this landscape is characterized by numerous gray areas where the right path is not always clear.

Dietary Patterns

One of the fundamental gray areas in addressing obesity and T2DM through nutrition is the choice of dietary patterns. While there is consensus that reducing calorie intake is crucial for weight management and blood sugar control, the optimal dietary pattern remains a topic of debate. Some popular dietary patterns include:

- *Low-carb diet*: These diets restrict the intake of carbs and emphasize higher fat and protein consumption. Proponents argue that reducing carbs helps control blood sugar levels and promote weight loss. However, long-term adherence and potential nutrient deficiencies are concerns.
- *Low-fat diet*: These diets aim to minimize dietary fat intake, focusing on lean proteins and carbohydrates. They are designed to lower calorie intake and reduce saturated fats. Yet, some critics argue that low-fat diets may not be as effective in managing blood sugar.
- *Mediterranean diet*: This diet emphasizes whole grains, healthy fats, lean proteins, and a variety of fruits and vegetables. It is praised for its heart-healthy components and potential in managing T2DM and obesity.
- *Plant-based diet*: These diets are gaining popularity for their potential in improving metabolic health. They focus on fruits, vegetables, legumes, and whole grains while minimizing or excluding animal products.

The gray area here lies in the fact that no one-size-fits-all approach is universally effective. Individual factors, including metabolic rate, insulin sensitivity, and personal preferences, can greatly influence the success of a particular dietary pattern. Hence, it is essential to tailor the approach to the specific needs and responses of the individual.

Low-fat or Low-carbohydrate Diets for Weight Management?

The Look-AHEAD: The Action for Health in Diabetes (Look-AHEAD) trial compared an intensive lifestyle intervention with a control condition of support and education in people with T2DM. The weight loss strategy, comprising energy reduction (1,200–1,800 kcal/day) through a low-fat diet, was effective. In contrast, in the energy-deficit diet in the T2DM DiRECT (Diabetes Remission Clinical Trial), the proportions of macronutrients were inconsequential, with >50% of energy coming from carbohydrates. A recent umbrella review of the evidence concluded that weight management in T2DM using hypocaloric diets does not depend on any macronutrient profile **(Figs. 2A and B)**.

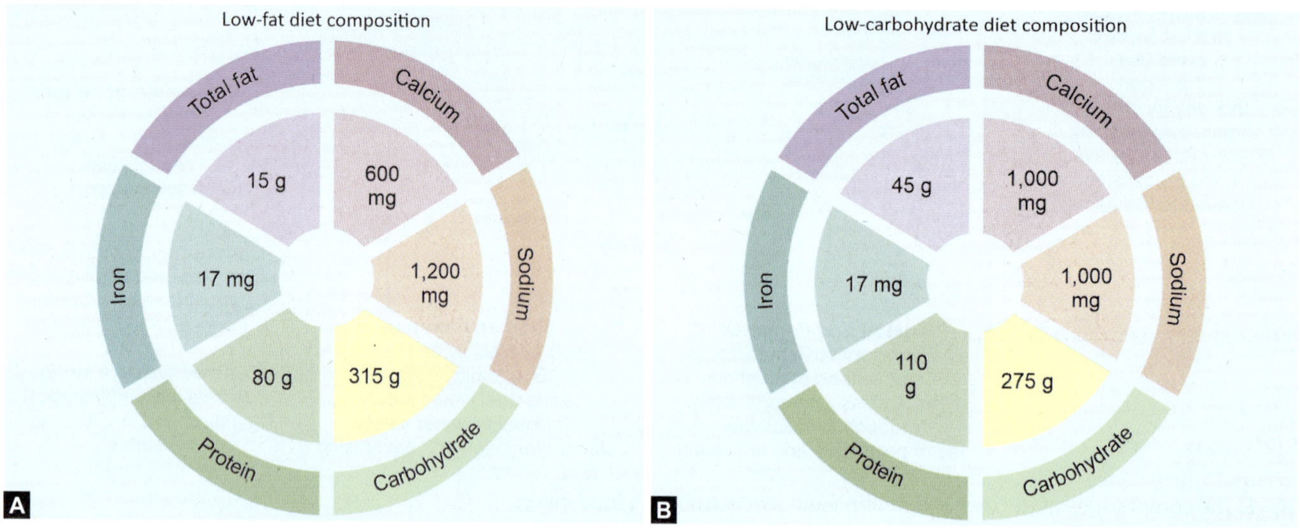

FIGS. 2A AND B: Detailed composition of low-fat and low-carbohydrate diets.

Macronutrient Composition

Another contentious issue in diet and nutrition for obesity and T2DM treatment is the macronutrient composition of the diet. The balance of carbohydrates, fats, and proteins plays a pivotal role in metabolic outcomes.

- *Carbohydrates*: Carbohydrates are often under scrutiny due to their direct impact on blood sugar levels. While reducing refined carbohydrates is widely recommended, the ideal amount and type of carbohydrates remain unclear. Complex carbohydrates found in whole grains, vegetables, and legumes are generally considered healthier choices than simple sugars.
- *Fats*: The type of fats consumed is crucial. Healthy fats such as those from avocados, nuts, and olive oil are recommended, while saturated and trans fats found in many processed foods should be limited. The debate around the amount of fat in the diet continues.
- *Proteins*: Adequate protein intake is essential for satiety and muscle maintenance. However, excessive protein intake, particularly from animal sources, may have implications for kidney health and cardiovascular risk.

Balancing these macronutrients depends on the specific dietary pattern chosen and the individual's health goals, making it another gray area in nutrition therapy for obesity and T2DM.

Calorie Counting versus Food Quality

While managing calorie intake is central to weight management, focusing solely on calorie counting can sometimes undermine the importance of food quality. In this gray area, the idea that a calorie is not just a calorie comes into play. Whole foods that are rich in essential nutrients can be more satiating and support better metabolic health compared to processed, calorie-dense foods.

Emphasizing food quality, such as consuming whole grains, lean proteins, and a variety of fruits and vegetables, is often encouraged. In practice, this approach can lead to better overall health, making it more sustainable for long-term weight management and T2DM control. However, finding a balance between calorie control and food quality remains an ongoing challenge.

Role of Sugar and Artificial Sweeteners

The impact of sugar and artificial sweeteners on obesity and T2DM is a topic of ongoing debate. Reducing added sugars is a widely accepted recommendation as they provide empty calories and can lead to insulin resistance and weight gain. However, the role of sugar substitutes such as artificial sweeteners remains a gray area.

While artificial sweeteners may help reduce calorie intake, concerns about their long-term health effects persist. Some studies suggest that artificial sweeteners may alter taste preferences, disrupt the gut microbiome, and even contribute to weight gain. Therefore, it is essential to approach artificial sweeteners with caution and monitor individual responses.

Meal Timing and Frequency

Meal timing and frequency have gained attention in recent years, with concepts like intermittent fasting becoming popular. This approach involves cycling between periods of eating and fasting. Proponents argue that intermittent fasting can help improve insulin sensitivity and promote weight loss.

However, the gray area here is that individual responses to meal timing and frequency can vary significantly. While some people may benefit from intermittent fasting, others may experience adverse effects, such as increased hunger and irritability. Personalization is key in determining the most suitable meal timing and frequency for individuals.

Individual Variability

The notion of individual variability in response to dietary approaches cannot be overstated. Genetics, metabolism, and personal preferences all contribute to how individuals respond to different diets. What works effectively for one person may not yield the same results for another.

This individual variability underscores the importance of personalized nutrition plans. Healthcare professionals often conduct thorough assessments, considering factors such as genetics, medical history, and current health status to tailor dietary recommendations. Navigating these gray areas requires a holistic approach to healthcare that accounts for the uniqueness of each patient.

Sustainability

Sustainability is a crucial but often overlooked aspect of dietary approaches for obesity and T2DM management. While rapid weight loss methods and extreme diets may yield short-term results, their long-term sustainability is questionable. This is a critical gray area in the treatment of these conditions.

Crash diets or highly restrictive eating plans may not be sustainable for many individuals. The key to success often lies in finding a dietary approach that a person can adhere to over the long term. Long-lasting results come from gradual and sustainable changes in eating habits, rather than extreme and short-lived measures.

Emotional and Behavioral Factors

Emotional eating, stress, and other behavioral aspects can significantly impact the success of dietary interventions for obesity and T2DM. Stress, for instance, can trigger unhealthy eating habits and contribute to weight gain. Emotional eating may lead to overconsumption of comfort foods that are often calorie-dense and low in nutrients. Addressing these emotional and behavioral factors is critical for achieving long-term success.

SUGGESTED READINGS

1. Forouhi NG. Embracing Complexity: Making Sense Of Diet, Nutrition, Obesity And Type-2 Diabetes. Diabetologia. 2023;66:786-99.
2. Evert AB, Dennison M, Gardner CD, Garvey WT, Lau KHK, MacLeod J, et al. Nutrition therapy for adults with diabetes or prediabetes: a consensus report. Diabetes Care. 2019;42:731-54.
3. Ryan DH, Espeland MA, Foster GD, Haffner SM, Hubbard VS, Johnson KC, et al. Look AHEAD (Action for Health in Diabetes): design and methods for a clinical trial of weight loss for the prevention of cardiovascular disease in type 2 diabetes. Control Clin Trials. 2003;24(5):610-28.

204

CHAPTER

Keto Diet: Where do We Stand Today

Virendra Kumar Goyal, Akhani S Krupa

ABSTRACT

Ketogenic diet (KD) is a normocaloric diet composed of high fat and low carbohydrates. It induces a state of nutritional ketosis in which, under shortage of glucose, there is overproduction of ketone bodies which are used as a source of energy, especially in the central nervous system (CNS), as it cannot use fat as an alternative source of energy. KD has been of interest since a century back (early 1920s), when they were first tried for resistant epilepsy. Since then, the benefits of KD have been explored in various other conditions. Many active researches are underway, since then, to prove KD role in other areas as well. As of our current knowledge, KD has proven to be beneficial in—diabetes, cardiovascular diseases, obesity, and epilepsy. Improving neurocognitive and motor functions in many CNS disorders, certain cancers, acne, etc., have shown promising results as well. However, the benefits of KD come with certain risks such as hypoglycemia, worsening renal functions, renal stones, and gut dysbiosis, hence both sides of coin are to be watched and weighed in starting KD. Keto-medicine has ongoing research and innovation continue to shape the field of medicine.

INTRODUCTION

Ketogenic diet (KD) is composed of high fat, adequate protein and low carbohydrates (usually <50 g/day). Despite the change in proportion of its contents, it has normal caloric value. The carbohydrate content provides <10% of total daily calorie requirement. It induces a state of nutritional ketosis in body which has a fasting-like effect in the blood with increased levels of ketone bodies.

Ketogenic diet has been of interest since 1920s when it was used as a therapy for epilepsy by Russel Wilde who also coined the term "ketogenic diet". The novel study by Cahill and colleagues in 1960s showed the metabolic benefits of KD and subsequently the benefits of KD in other areas were explored. KD now has shown to be of proven benefits in obesity and weight loss, diabetes, epilepsy, and cardiovascular disease while there is emerging evidence of benefits in metabolic syndrome, neuromotor and neurocognitive functions, cancers, etc.

WHAT MAKES A KETOGENIC DIET?

Ketogenic diet is a very low carbohydrate diet, rich in fat and provides normal caloric requirement. The carbohydrate component provides <10% of the daily caloric requirement of 2,000-kcal diet. This is equivalent to 20–50 g of carbohydrate/day.

The high content of fat in KD is kept at a ratio of 4:1 (4 g of fat for every 1 g of protein and carbohydrate combined).

There are a variety of options KD, mostly ones with high fat content. The examples of various food items are:

- *Nuts and seeds*: Almonds, walnuts, cashews, sunflower seeds, chia seeds, pumpkin seeds, and flax seeds.
- *Nonstarchy vegetables*: Green cauliflower, broccoli, tomatoes, mushrooms, and peppers.
- *Full-fat dairy*: Yogurt, butter, and cream.
- *Healthy fats*: Coconut oil, olive oil, avocado oil, coconut butter, and sesame oil.

TYPES OF KETO DIET

- *Standard keto diet (SKD):* This type of diet includes low intake of carbohydrate, high intake of proteins, and fat. The typical daily food intake of from these groups is 5% carbs, 20% proteins, and 75% fats.
- *Targeted keto diet (TKD):* This type of keto diet includes low intake of carbs, high intake of protein, and fats. It also includes small amount of carbs consumption before and after workouts to boost metabolism.
- *Cyclic ketogenic diet (CKD):* This type of keto diet cycles between low intake of carbs and high intake of carbs. Throughout a week, 5 or 6 days will include low intake of carb, high intake of proteins and fats. For the remaining 1 or 2 days, the nutrient intake is switched to high carb diet. This method is to trick the body to keep the metabolism up and avoid plateauing in the weight loss process.
- *High protein keto diet (HPK):* This regime is very similar to standard KD. The only difference is the higher amount of protein and lower amount of fat are consumed the recommended ratio is around 5% carbs, 35% proteins, and 60% fats.

METABOLIC CHANGES IN KETOSIS

After being on KD, there is a drastically reduced carbohydrate consumption, hence the glucose reserves in body becomes insufficient for utilization by CNS.

Fat oxidation: This occurs by supply of oxaloacetate from Krebs cycle, which is dependent on glucose supply. After 3–4 days without carbohydrate consumption, the CNS derives energy from alternative sources by production of acetyl coenzyme A (CoA).

During ketosis and relative hypoglycemia, there are low levels of insulin, which diverts pathway toward production of ketone bodies (acetoacetate, β-hydroxybutyric acid, and acetone). This condition leads to ketonemia and ketonuria. When serum ketone levels reach a concentration of about 4 mmol/L, ketone bodies are then used by tissues as a source of energy. This state of ketosis can be seen in:

1. *Pathological ketosis:* Prolonged fasting, also in type 1 diabetes mellitus.
2. *Physiological ketosis:* While consuming KD.

In physiological ketosis, serum ketone levels reach a maximum of 7–8 mmol/L with no change in pH, whereas in uncontrolled diabetic ketoacidosis (i.e., pathological ketosis) it can exceed to >20 mmol/L.

Some unique features to note about this metabolic change are:

- Ketone bodies are able to produce more energy than glucose.
- Although there is a reduction in serum glucose, there is never hypoglycemia, as glucose is formed from two sources during this time—from glucogenic amino acids and from glycerol liberated via lysis of triglycerides.

BENEFITS OF KETOGENIC DIET

- *Proven benefits:* Epilepsy, diabetes, weight reduction, and cardiovascular risks.
- *Emerging evidences:* Neurological diseases, cancers, acne, polycystic ovaries (PCOS), CKD, Crohn's disease, and respiratory diseases.
- *Weight loss:* There is very strong evidence of the role of KD in weight loss. However, the exact mechanism of weight loss is still not completely understood. There are several proposed mechanisms (in order of their supportive evidence):
  - Appetite reduction due to satiety effect and also a direct suppressant action on diet.
  - Reduction in lipogenesis and increased lipolysis.
  - Fat consumption has greater metabolic efficiency by reducing respiratory quotient.
  - Increased metabolic costs of gluconeogenesis and the thermic effect of proteins.
- *Cardiovascular benefits:* Recent studies have shown clear cardiovascular benefits from KD. The benefit seems to be due to reduction of levels of atherogenic molecules in body. The metabolic changes that reduce cardiovascular risks are:
  - *Reduced cholesterol synthesis:* Nutritional ketosis decreases the blood insulin levels, which otherwise on a carbohydrate-rich fed diet, causes cholesterol synthesis.
  - Ketogenic diet increases the levels of high-density lipids.
  - Ketogenic diet increases the volume of very low-density lipid molecules, which reduces the cardiovascular risk, as smaller low-density lipoprotein (LDL) particles are considered to have more atherogenic potential.
  - Ketogenic diet also decreases the triglyceride level (LOE: 3).
- *Insulin resistance:* Due to insulin resistance, the skeletal muscles are not able to utilize glucose for their energy needs. High insulin level leads to diversion of this unutilized glucose to liver where it is converted to fatty acids (de novo lipogenesis).
  Ketogenic diet, by reducing the carbohydrate load of the body, has shown beneficial effects both in improving biomarkers of risk of disease [i.e., fasting plasma glucose (FPG), glyclated hemoglobin (HbA1c)] and also improving insulin sensitivity.

- *Neurological diseases:* KD has shown to be useful in many neurodegenerative and neurocognitive conditions. This is an area of ongoing research and many potential benefits have been proposed from KD. Some of the conditions where KD have shown benefits are:
  - *Epilepsy:* KD has been used historically for refractory epilepsies. Based upon the available evidence, a 2018 expert consensus panel recommended that KD therapy should be offered to children with drug-resistant epilepsy after unsuccessful treatment trials of two antiseizure drugs. Several hypotheses have been put forward to explain the mechanism of action of KD:
    - Anticonvulsant effect of ketone bodies;
    - A reduced excitability of neurons by ketone bodies;
    - An effect on the mammalian target of rapamycin pathway (mTOR).

    The efficacy of KD was reported in a recent review where studies showed marked reduction (30–40%) in seizures, and was also reported that the effects were comparable to modern antiepileptic drugs, at least in children.
  - *Alzheimer's disease:* Recent studies have shown that KD has resulted in gain in daily motor activity and also improved cognitive function. It is proposed that KD causes reduction in deposition of amyloid proteins in neurons and improved the neuronal energy utilization.
  - *Amyotrophic lateral sclerosis (ALS):* Mitochondrial dysfunction in energy production is the key pathologic mechanism in this disease. KD have shown improvements in energy utilization and have resulted in longer maintenance of motor function.
  - *Parkinson's disease:* Although not many studies have been done and benefits remain uncertain early results have shown improvement in motor functions by protection of dopaminergic neurons from degeneration.
- *Others:* Apart from the above, KD has also shown benefit in various other conditions.

  The following diseases where KD have shown potential benefit:
  - Angelman syndrome
  - Mitochondrial myopathy
  - Rett syndrome
  - Spinal cord injury and traumatic brain injury
- *Chronic kidney disease:* Traditionally, a hypoproteinemia diet is proposed for CKD. However, recent trials have proved KD are effective in ameliorating metabolic disturbances in CKD, delaying the initiation of dialysis by almost 1 year and slowing down the rate of decline in renal function by 57%.
- *Crohn's disease:* Crohn's disease is known to be characterized by a progressive worsening of symptoms. In one of the studies, an advanced state of Crohn's disease was treated with KD. It was able to reverse the cluster of symptoms and abnormalities associated with the disease by normalizing the intestinal permeability.
- *Cancers:* Preliminary data points toward potential benefits in certain cancers.

  Ketogenic diet also results in "glucose starvation" of cancer cells.
- *Acne:* KD reduces acne by decreasing Insulin-like growth factor-1 (IGF-1) levels. (IGF-1) levels. This results in reduction in:
  - Androgen-mediated production of sebum
  - Excessive desquamation of the follicular epithelium
  - Proliferation of basal keratinocytes and
  - *Propionibacterium acnes (P. acnes)* colonization and hence inflammation.
- *Respiratory functions:* KD results in fatter oxidation to meet energy requirements, which leads in turn to reduced respiratory exchange ratio and of metabolic carbon dioxide output, and a decrease in arterial carbon dioxide partial pressure. These effects might be useful in respiratory failure; however, this aspect of KD remains to be investigated.

RISKS OF KETOGENIC DIET

Much of the risks proposed to be associated with KD have come from the trials on pediatric patients treated for epilepsy. Some of the common problems associated with KD are:

- *Ketone flu:* The most common short-term side-effects include nausea, vomiting, dizziness, headache, insomnia, fatigue, referred to as keto flu which resolve in a few days to weeks.
- *False-positive breath alcohol test:* Due to ketonemia, acetone in the body can sometimes be reduced by dehydrogenase which can give a false positive alcohol breath test result.
- *Hypoglycemia:* KD can also cause hypoglycemia in certain patients who have risk factors for the same [older age, previous history, on administered oral hypoglycemic agents (OHAs)].
- *Gastrointestinal system:* KD have shown to cause diarrhea, vomiting, and abdominal discomfort in some patients. KD causes gut dysbiosis by reducing the supply of carbohydrate to gut biota, which in turn results in reduced fermentation in the gut leading to decreased butane levels which is thought to decrease inflammation. This may cause many guts inflammatory diseases.

- *Bone and calcium metabolism:* KD has shown to decrease bone mass and cause frequent fractures. In addition, KD has also shown to increase the incidence of renal stones.
- *Cardiovascular:* There have been case reports of patients developing cardiomyopathies secondary to nutritional deficiencies (e.g., selenium and others). Some reports have even shown development of arrhythmias.
- *Hematological:* KD has shown to cause bone marrow suppression and anemia.

CONCLUSION

Ketogenic diet is a normocaloric diet composed of high fat, low carbohydrate and provides adequate calories. It includes a state of nutritional ketosis in which, under shortage of glucose, there is overproduction of ketone bodies which are used as a source of energy, especially in the CNS as it cannot use fat as an alternate source of energy. KD has been explored in various other conditions. Many active research is underway to prove their role in other area as well. As of current knowledge KD has been proven to be beneficial in—diabetes, cardiovascular disease, obesity, and epilepsy. Many other areas have shown promising result as well—improving neurocognitive and motor functions in many CNS disorders, certain cancers, acne, etc.

However, the benefit of KD comes with certain risks such as hypoglycemia, worsening renal functions, and gut dysbiosis. KD has certain side-effects and should be avoided in at-risk patients.

SUGGESTED READINGS

1. Masood W, Annamaraju P, Uppaluri KR. Ketogenic Diet. In: StatPearls. Treasure Island (FL): StatPearls Publishing; 2020.
2. Westman EC, Tondt J, Maguire E, Yancy WS Jr. Implementing a low-carbohydrate, ketogenic diet to manage type 2 diabetes mellitus. Expert Rev Endocrinol Metab. 2018;13(5):263-72.
3. Bando H, Ebe K, Manabe T, Bando M, Yonei Y. Less carbohydrate intake increases serum ketone bodies in low carbohydrate diet. Endocrinol Metab. 2018;2(1):109.
4. Rusek M, Pluta R, Ułamek-Kozioł M, Czuczwar S. Ketogenic Diet in Alzheimer's Disease. Int J Mol Sci. 2019;20(16):3892.
5. Bostock ECS, Kirkby KC, Taylor BV, Hawrelak JA. Consumer Reports of "Keto Flu" Associated with the ketogenic diet. Front Nutr. 2020;7:20.
6. Masood W, Annamaraju P, Uppaluri KR. Ketogenic Diet. In: StatPearls. Treasure Island (FL): StatPearls Publishing; 2020.

SECTION

16

POISONING AND TOXICOLOGY

205

CHAPTER

Slow Poisoning in Modern Era

Appandraj Jain

ABSTRACT

Slow poisoning, a persistent, long-lasting poison, has evolved over time, impacting diagnosis and treatment. Historically used in lead, thallium, and arsenic, it is now considered an adverse event after drug use, causing significant morbidity and mortality. This chapter focuses on common slow poisoning based on clinical experience.

INTRODUCTION

Slow poisoning has always been a part of human life. The causes and understanding of the biological sciences have changed over time, as have their implications for diagnosis and treatment. Chronic poison is a poison that persists for many years. It can kill without patients' knowledge. "You don't even realize you're affected". In the past, lead, thallium, and arsenic were commonly used as slow poison, but in the modern era, slow poisoning is referred to as adverse events that occur after the use of drugs and is one of the important causes of morbidity and mortality. Since there is no trial or studies conducted in the modern era for slow poison, this chapter will deal with common slow poisoning based on my clinical experience.

BETA-BLOCKER POISON

Beta-blocker drugs carry a high risk of potentially causing fatal poisonings because of their strong therapeutic effect and rapid onset of action. The mortality rate of beta-blocker exposures is 1.4% among 280 patients. Among this group, propranolol was common as shown in **Figure 1**.

The first clue for presentation of propranolol poisoning will be bradycardia associated with hypotension to diagnose. Also, some patients have hypoglycemia and altered mental status.

ECG changes will be like wide QRS and a tall R wave in aVR. This is due to sodium channel blocking **(Fig. 2)**.

Calcium Channel Blocker

Calcium channel blocker is the next common poison which mimics beta blockers in symptoms. There are two important findings that may help in differentiating a calcium channel blocker poisoning from a beta blocker poisoning. They are blood glucose and level of consciousness. Calcium channel blocker poison tends to cause hyperglycemia compared to a beta blocker poison in which normal-to-low blood. Also, beta blockers tend to cause a depressed level of consciousness due to

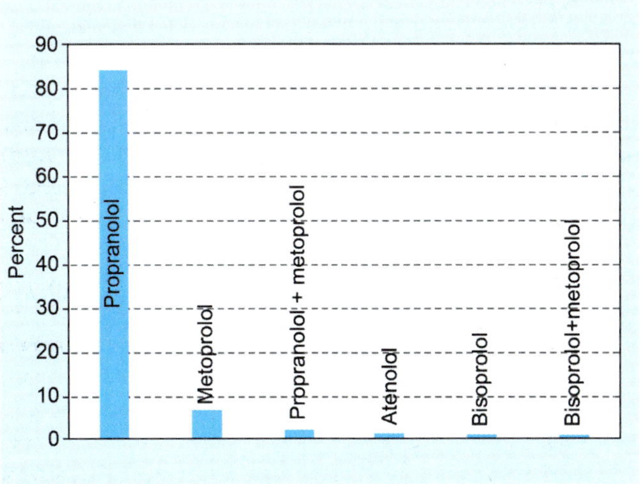

FIG. 1: Frequency of beta-blocker poisoning.

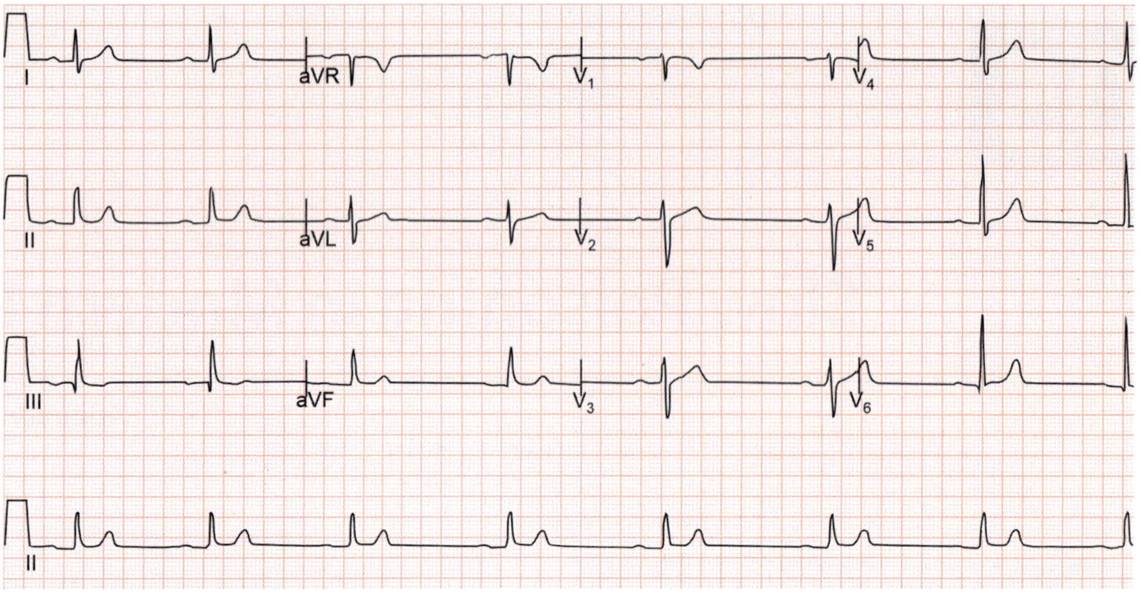

FIG. 2: ECG changes in beta blockers' slow poison.

lipophilicity, and calcium channel blockers have a normal consciousness.

MANAGEMENT

Management of Seizure in Poisoning

- Avoid sodium channel-blocking drugs because many poisons cause sodium channel block which results in cardiac instability.
- Benzodiazepine is the preferred group. If not controlled, give barbiturates.

Bradycardia is managed initially by 0.5 mg IV atropine in patients.

Glucose level should be monitored every 30 minutes initially for up to 4 hours to maintain normal glycemic control (100–200 mg/dL) by starting D10% infusion and D50% IV boluses if needed.

Supportive treatment with vasopressor may be needed since the inotropic effect of high-dose insulin euglycemia may be delayed by up to 15–60 minutes. Inamrinone and milrinone increase inotrophy by increasing the cyclic adenosine monophosphate (cAMP).

Even though there is no randomized controlled trial (RCT) to support glucagon as an antidote, glucagon is considered a useful treatment of choice. But premedication with antiemetic ondansetron 8 mg can be considered because glucagon may induce vomiting **(Flowchart 1)**.

Digoxin Toxicity

Digoxin toxicity is the most common slow poison among geriatric patients with cardiac disorder. Slow digoxin poisoning has a higher fatality. The symptoms will be vaguer like being weak and dizzy followed by emesis and low and slow vitals. This is the reason why it is more difficult to diagnose since it mimics many diseases. It is confirmed by history taking of medication and ECG.

ECG changes seen in patients who are taking normal therapeutic dosage is scotted ST segment, like in **Figure 3**, otherwise known as "The Salvador Dali Moustache."

Digoxin toxicity can cause any dysrhythmia except rapid atrial fibrillation, and death is due to ventricular dysrhythmia.

Management of slow digoxin toxicity **(Box 1)**.

Approach to the patient with a beta blocker or calcium channel blocker overdose

Apply monitors, obtain IV access, check blood glucose and obtain an EKG. Consider co-ingestions. Involve your local poison center early

↓ Observe for signs of toxicity

Decontamination
- Activated charcoal if patient protecting airway and based on timing of ingestion and formulation of drug (i.e., < 1 hour post-ingestion or longer if slow-release/enteric coated)
- Dose charcoal based on a ratio of 1:10 of drug ingested to charcoal

↓ Hypotension and bradycardia

- **Fluids** for hypotension
- **Atropine/transcutaneous pacing** if bradycardia present
- **Calcium**
  - Calcium gluconate (peripheral IV), or calcium chloride (central line)
- **Pressors** (in patients with hemodynamic instability, until insulin infusion takes effect)
  - Epinepherine if poor cardiac contractility on bedside ultrasound
  - Norepinepherine if normal cardiac contractility on beside ultrasound

↓

High dose insulin therapy:
- Bolus 1 U/kg of regular insulin by IV push with 2 amps of D50W
- Infusion of 1 U/kg/h of regular insulin with dextrose infusion if blood glucose < 11 Titrate insulin infusion up every 15 minutes by 0.25–0.50 U/kg/h until adequate cardiac contractility
- Monitor blood glucose every 15 minutes until stable, then monitor hourly. Check potassium frequently

↓ Refractory shock or peri-arrest

Lipid emulsion therapy
- 1.5 mL/kg of 20% lipid emulsion as a bolus, repeated up to two times as needed until clinically stable. Then an infusion of 0.25 mL/kg/min for 30–60 minutes is given
- Extracorporeal membrane oxygenation

FLOWCHART 1: Management of beta blocker and calcium channel blocker poisoning.

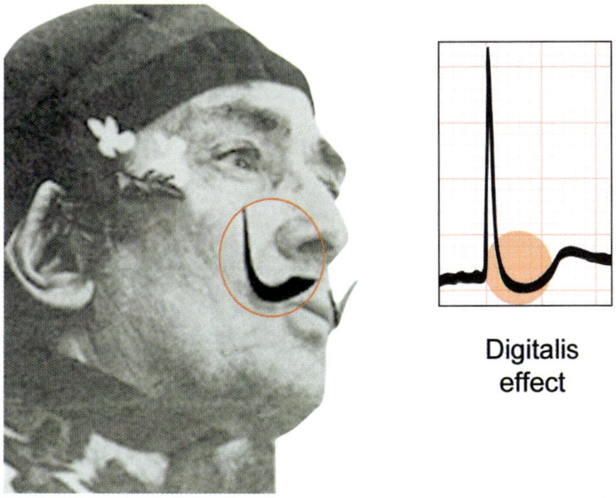

FIG. 3: For the digitalis "effect," remember Salvador Dali.

BOX 1: Management of slow digoxin toxicity.

- *First line*:
  - Depends on blood pressure
  - 0.5 mg IV trial of atropine
  - If the patient has severe hypokalemia and digoxin toxicity, it is important to correct the serum potassium
- *Arrhythmia Mx*:
  - Lignocaine can be used for ventricular tachyarrhythmias
  - Atropine for bradyarrhythmias
- *DigiFab*:
  - In cardiac arrest due to digoxin poisoning, give 10 vials of DigiFab and repeat in 15 mins prn × 1 for a total of 20 vials
  - In chronic digoxin poisoning, give 1 vial and repeat prn based on clinical condition, ECG, and serum potassium (usually requires approximately 5 vials total)
  - In acute digoxin poisoning, give 2 vials and repeat prn based on clinical condition, ECG, and serum potassium (usually requires approximately 10 vials in total)

CONCLUSION

As we progress in scientific development, poisoning becomes more common which mimics other diseases and is also commonly available. Therefore, poisoning circumstances must be thoroughly investigated to screen for coexposure to combined drugs. Follow-up of patient and psychiatrist counseling are must after treatment.

SUGGESTED READINGS

1. Nepovimova E, Kuca K. The history of poisoning: from ancient times until modern ERA. Arch Toxicol. 2019;93(1):11-24.
2. Love JN, Love J, Howell JM, Litovitz TL, Klein-Schwartz W. Acute beta blocker overdose: factors associated with the development of cardiovascular morbidity. J Toxicol . 2000;38(3):275-81.
3. Eizadi-Mood N, Adib M. A clinical-epidemiological study on beta-blocker poisonings based on the type of drug overdose. J Toxicol.2023;2023:1064955
4. Helman A, Thompson M, Austin E. (2017). Low and slow poisoning. emergency medicine cases. [online] Available from https://emergencymedicinecases.com/aortic-dissection-em-cases-course/. [Last accessed December, 2023].
5. Wetherell H. Digoxin and the heart. Br J Cardiol. 2015;22:96-7.
6. Ip D, Syed H, Cohen M. Digoxin specific antibody fragments (Digibind) in digoxin toxicity. BMJ. 2009;339:b2884.
7. Mégarbane B, Karyo S, Baud FJ. The role of insulin and glucose (hyperinsulinemia/euglycemia therapy in acute calcium channel antagonist and beta blocker poisoning. Toxicol Rev. 2004;23(4):215-22.

206

CHAPTER

Snakebite: The First Few Hours

K Nagesh

ABSTRACT

Snakebite is a life-threatening rural medical emergency. Majority of the victims are farmers, they reach the rural small hospitals for treatment. Antisnake venom (ASV) is the important treatment for envenomated bites, as ASV neutralizes only the circulating venom and ASV administration is not useful once the venom is fixed to tissue receptors, ASV need to be administered as early as possible to prevent the complications and there by deaths due to snakebites. The small rural hospitals can play a game changer role in this regard. In this chapter, the author has shared his huge experience in rural and suburban hospitals for the last three decades, blending it with the recent WHO guidelines for the management of snakebite in Southeast Asia.

INTRODUCTION

Snakebite is one of the common medical emergency we come across in rural India. In view of the varied geographical distribution of snakes, the complexity of the snake venom, its variation from species to species, and wide range in the amount of venom injected makes snakebite a challenging clinical situation. There are about 3,000 species of snakes identified all over the world, out of which India harbors about 236 species including 56 species of venomous snakes.

PROLONGED NEGLECT

Snakes are not taken seriously as agents of human diseases. There are very few proper clinical studies. Also, the funding bodies are not encouraging studies on snakebite. There is no emphasis in medical education on snakebite in both undergraduate and postgraduate studies. Current medical textbooks have failed to impart proper knowledge to doctors on snakebite. There is failure of mass education to public.

THE INVISIBLE BURDEN IN INDIA

The path breaking "million death studies" reveals a heartbreaking news that around 46,000 people are dying in India due to snakebite annually. On the other hand, the Government of India statistics shows about two lakh bites and around 1,400 deaths due to snakebite in India yearly. Whereas the WHO data shows 11,000–20,000 deaths annually. So, snakebite in India is vastly underreported and underestimated.

THE FIRST FEW HOURS

Snakebite is predominantly a rural phenomenon, affecting the poor farmers, agricultural laborers, and their children. Majority of the victims reach the rural hospitals like primary health centers (PHCs). Antisnake venom (ASV) neutralizes only the circulating venom and not the venom which is already fixed to tissue receptors. Hence, to be effective ASV should be administered as early as possible to all envenomated patients. The *"bite to needle time"* should be preferably <4 hours. Therefore, the first few hours are the golden hours in the management of snakebite. The small hospitals can play a game changer role in reducing the mortality due to snakebite.

CLINICAL PRESENTATION

Nonpoisonous Snakebite

- Patient walks into the hospital with history of snakebite
- Bite mark present
- No pain, no burning, and no local swelling
- No signs of systemic envenomation
- Anxiety features such as over breathing, cold extremities, and tetany of the hands may be present.
- Vomiting due to herbal medicine may be present
- Laboratory parameters are normal
- 70% of the bites are by nonpoisonous snakes
- 50% of the bites by poisonous snakes are "dry bites"
- Totally 85% of bites are nonpoisonous
- Observe for 24 hours and discharge with injection TT

> ☛ *No role for prophylactic ASV administration*

Viper Envenomation (Fig. 1)

- Prominent bite mark
- Swelling and local pain
- Tenderness along the lymphatic and regional lymph node.
- Bleeding as evidence by the epistaxis, hematemesis, gum bleeding **(Figs. 2A and B)**, petechiae, purpura, ecchymoses, etc.
- Acute abdominal pain
- Hypotension and shock
- Passing reddish or dark brown urine
- Muscle pain, conjunctival edema, and hemorrhage

Triad of Russell's Viper Envenomation

- Swelling
- Bleeding
- Renal involvement

Cobra Envenomation (Figs. 3A and B)

- Prominent bite mark
- Local swelling and blistering
- Descending paralysis as evidenced by ptosis, ophthalmoparesis, and paralysis of the jaw, tongue, and limbs
- Broken neck sign

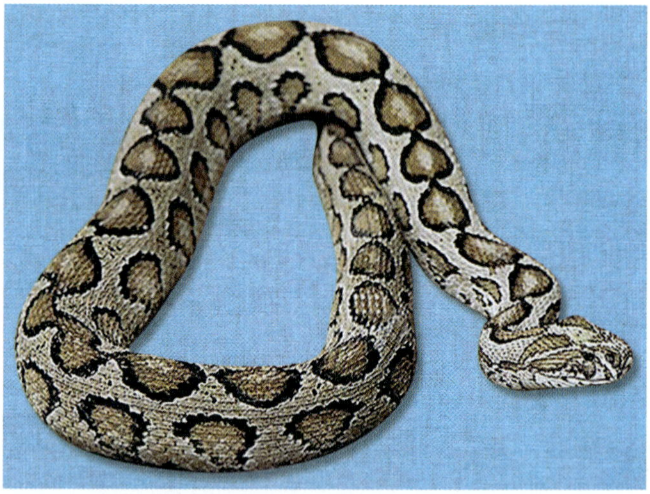

FIG. 1: Russell's viper.

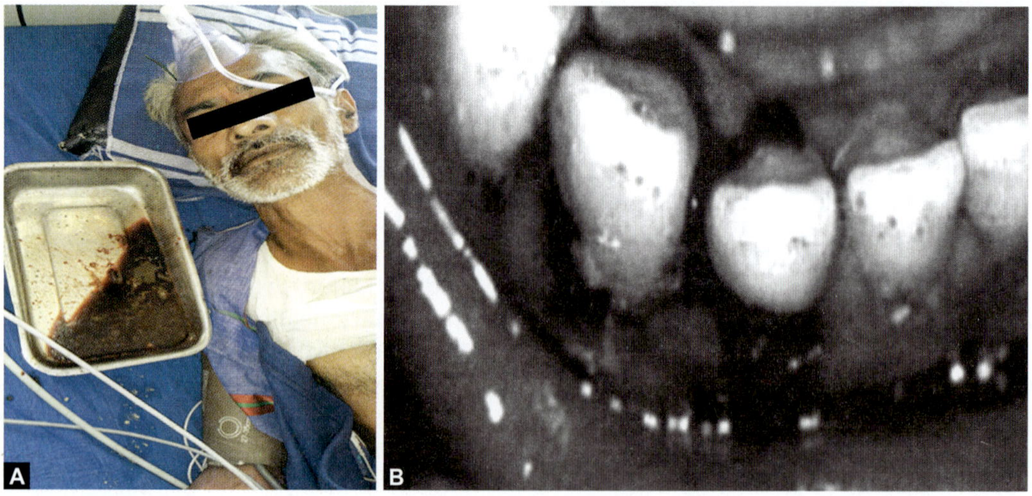

FIGS. 2A AND B: Bleeding from gums and upper gastrointestinal (GI) in a viper bite patient.

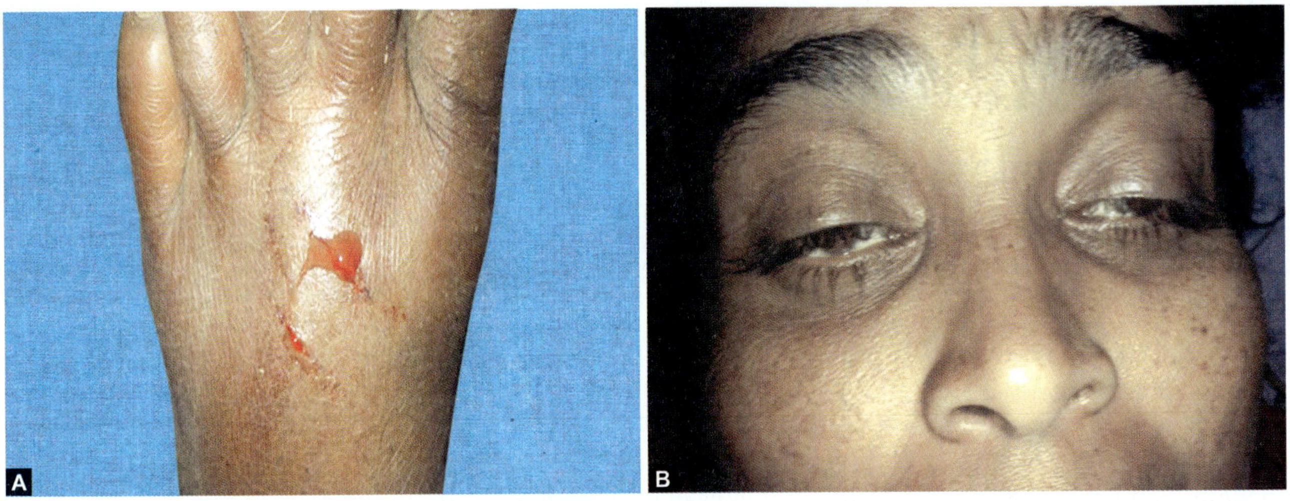

FIGS. 3A AND B: A prominent bite mark and ptosis in a cobra bite patient.

- Hypoxia and altered sensorium/coma
- No bleeding, no renal involvement

Triad of Cobra Envenomation

- Prominent bite mark
- Swelling
- Descending paralysis

Triad of Krait Envenomation

- Faint/no bite mark
- Descending paralysis
- Early morning presentation

SPEECHLESS FARMERS!

Many times, farmers working in the field may not notice the bite particularly bite by a krait, hours later they are brought speechless to the health centers. They are speechless, have ptosis, external ophthalmoplegia, dilated pupils, and generalized paralysis. There are incidences where farmers are buried alive thinking that they are dead by the villagers.

> ☛ *Just paralyzed, not brain dead, they need neostigmine, atropine, ASV, and oxygen to be back into life.*

FIRST AID TREATMENT PROTOCOL

Most of the traditional first aid methods have now proved to be ineffective and even more dangerous.

Tourniquets: They do not Work!

Ineffectiveness of the technique in retarding the venom flow has been proved in many experimental and field studies.

- Increase the risk of ischemia and loss of limb
- Increases the risk of embolism if used in viper bite
- Increased risk of massive neurotoxic blockage when released
- Gives false sense of security, which may delay their journey to hospital

Cutting and Suction: No More Recommended

- Increases the risk of severe bleeding in incoagulable blood in viper bite
- Increase the risk of infection
- No venom is removed by this technique
- This may inhibit the natural oozing out of the venom from wound
- Washing the wound, electrotherapy, and cryotherapy are abandoned as the methods of first aid.
- Pressure immobilization technique (PIM) is not recommended in India for technical reasons **(Box 1)**.

INVESTIGATIONS

20-minute Whole Blood Clotting Test

A simple bedside test, does not require any laboratory or skilled technician. 2 mL of patient's fresh blood is added to a clean, dry, glass test tube and kept vertically aside undisturbed for 20 minutes, tilt the test tube after

BOX 1: Recommended methods of first aid in India.

CARRY, NO, "R.I.G.H.T"*

Carry the victim, should not walk

No tourniquet, no cutting, no electrotherapy

R: Reassure the patients

I: Immobilize in the same way as the fractured limb

G.H: Get to hospital immediately (traditional remedies such as herbal medicine and snake stone have no role)

T: Tell the doctor of any symptoms such as ptosis and blackish vomiting that happened on the way to hospital

*Indian National Snakebite Protocol, 2016.

20 minutes, if blood is still in the liquid state indicates "incoagulable blood", which is diagnostic of viper bite.

Other Useful Tests

Complete blood count (CBC), prothrombin time (PT), activated partial thromboplastin time (APTT), fibrin degradation product (FDP), D-dimer, urine routine, blood urea, serum creatinine, serum potassium, oxygen saturation, electrocardiogram (ECG), etc., will help in managing the victims accurately.

ANTISNAKE VENOM ADMINISTRATION

A polyvalent ASV effective against the four common venomous snakes; cobra, krait, Russell's viper, and saw-scaled viper (big 4) is used in India. As ASV is a scarce and costly element, which can cause severe life-threatening anaphylaxis, should be used only when it is indicated and only when the benefits overweigh the risk.

- *Mere presence of bite mark even by a venomous snake is not indication to administer ASV.*
- *70% of the bites are by nonpoisonous snakes and 50% of the bites by poisonous snakes are dry bites (poisonous snake not envenoming the victims).*

Indications for Antisnake Venom

- *Evidence of neurotoxicity*: Ptosis, external ophthalmoplegia, muscle paralysis, and inability to lift the head.
- *Evidence of coagulopathy*: Visible spontaneous bleeding, prolonged 20-minute whole blood clotting test (WBCT), thrombocytopenia, abnormal PT, APTT, etc.
- *Cardiovascular abnormalities*: Hypotension, shock, and cardiac arrhythmias.
- Severe local swelling involving more than half of the limb or crossing the major joint (in the absence of tourniquet).
- Rapid extension of the swelling within few hours of bite.
- Persistent and severe vomiting or abnormal pain.
- *Evidence of renal involvement*: Passing of dark brown urine, raised blood urea, and serum creatinine.

- *Small local swelling alone, even if accompanied by bite mark from an apparently venomous snake is not the grounds for administration of ASV.*
- *Static swelling of hours old is not an indication to give ASV.*
- *Tourniquet-induced swelling will grossly decrease or disappear by 1 hour after removing it.*

Antisnake Venom Dosage

Antisnake venom administration is the single most important treatment. The dose and dosage of which was highly controversial till recently. Majority of the Western books being followed, does not include the Indian protocols, also the articles published in various journals does not have a consensus opinion.

Initial Doses of Antisnake Venom

The prognosis of the envenomed victims depends on how early and completely the circulating venom is inactivated before the venom gets bound to various tissue receptors, hence the administration of sufficient neutralizing initial dose is the key point in saving the lives and limiting the complications.

The drawbacks in calculating the initial dose:

- Nonavailability of enzyme-linked immunosorbent assay (ELISA) testing to assess the severity of poisoning.
- Symptomatology is not a useful guide to the level of envenomation.

Current Recommendations for Initial Dose

- 100 mL (10 vials) of ASV dissolved in 5–10 mL/kg body weight of normal saline (NS) dextrose, administered over 1 hour at a constant speed as an intravenous (IV) infusion.
- Patient should be closely monitored for 2 hours for any evidence of allergy or anaphylaxis.

- *Children should receive the same dose of ASV as adults*

Response to Antisnake Venom

Is indicated by following improvements in the patient:
- Spontaneous bleeding stops within 15–30 minutes.
- Blood coagulability is restored in 6 hours.
- Neurological symptoms will improve.
- Active hemolysis and rhabdomyolysis may cease.
- Urine returns to normal color.
- In shocked patients, blood pressure (BP) returns to normal.

Repeat Dose of Antisnake Venom

In majority of the patients, the initial dose of 100 mL is sufficient to neutralize the circulating venom, in a subset of patients additional dose is needed as judged by clinical or laboratory evidence. In antihemostatic group if the patient continues to bleed after 1–2 hours after initial dose, a repeat dose of 100 mL should be given; 20-minute WBCT should not be repeated within 6 hours, as liver takes 6 hours to replenish the coagulating factors. If incoagulability persists after 6 hours as evidenced by the 20-minute WBCT, half the initial dose (5 vials) should be administered. In neurotoxic group, if persistence or deterioration of the neurological symptoms occurs after 1–2 hours of the initial dose, a repeat dose of 100 mL should be given.

Maximum Dose of Antisnake Venom

As ASV is costly, scarce, and becomes unavailable in the peak seasons, it should be judiciously used. There are instances where ASV is loaded on neuroparalytic patients who are on ventilators, for no use. The argument that, there need not necessarily be an upper limit for ASV is baseless, as herpetological evidences say that the maximum amount of venom injected by a snake is 147 mg (Russell's viper) and each mL of ASV neutralizes 0.6 mg of venom, that means the maximum dose, one can use in antihemostatic bites is 30 vials, whereas in neuroparalytic bites, once the patient receives 20 vials (10 + 10) the ASV administration is completed.

> ☛ *No justification for massive dose of ASV in India.*

ANAPHYLAXIS

It can occur in 3–50% of the cases receiving ASV; many of the clinicians in remote areas are afraid to take up snakebite cases for the fear of life-threatening anaphylaxis. It can manifest as urticaria, itching, fever, shaking chills, nausea, vomiting, abdominal cramps, tachycardia, hypotension, bronchospasm, angioedema, shock, and death.

Treatment of Anaphylaxis

A syringe loaded with adrenaline should be always kept ready before starting ASV. Infusion of ASV should be stopped temporarily, 0.5 mg of 1:1,000 adrenaline should be given intramuscularly at the first sign of reaction. A second dose can be given if no improvement is seen after 10 minutes. In addition, 100 mg of hydrocortisone + 22.5 mg of pheniramine or 10 mg of chlorpheniramine maleate can be given intravenously. Once the patient has recovered ASV can be restarted slowly for 10–15 minutes keeping the patient under close observation and then normal drip rate should be resumed.

No Antisnake Venom Test Dose must be Administered

Test dose has no predictive value for anaphylaxis or late serum sickness reactions, as these reactions are complement activated, not immunoglobulin E (IgE) mediated; in fact, they may sensitize the patient and create greater risk and may delay the treatment also.

Anticholinesterase Usage

In neuroparalytic victims, ASV alone cannot be relied upon to save the lives, particularly in postsynaptic neuromuscular blockage induced by cobra bite, anticholinesterase can be lifesaving and they may abort the need for artificial respiration **(Figs. 4A and B)**. As the krait envenomation induces presynaptic blockage, the response to these drugs are not predictable in krait bites.

Neostigmine Dosage Intravenously

Injection neostigmine 1.5 mg intramuscularly preceded by injection atropine 0.6 mg IV, if improvement in neuroparalysis, continue with injection neostigmine 0.5 mg IV/intramuscular (IM) every half an hour till complete reversal of neuromuscular blockade. IV atropine has to be given SOS to combat the muscarinic symptoms of neostigmine.

> ☛ *Timely administration of neostigmine maybe lifesaving and can alleviate the need for mechanical ventilation.*

Handling the Tourniquet

If the patient has come with the tourniquet and swollen limb distal to it, should not be removed immediately. If there is evidence of systemic envenomation, initial dose of ASV should be administered before removing the tourniquet. If there are no signs of systemic envenomation, it can be removed with slow decompression using a

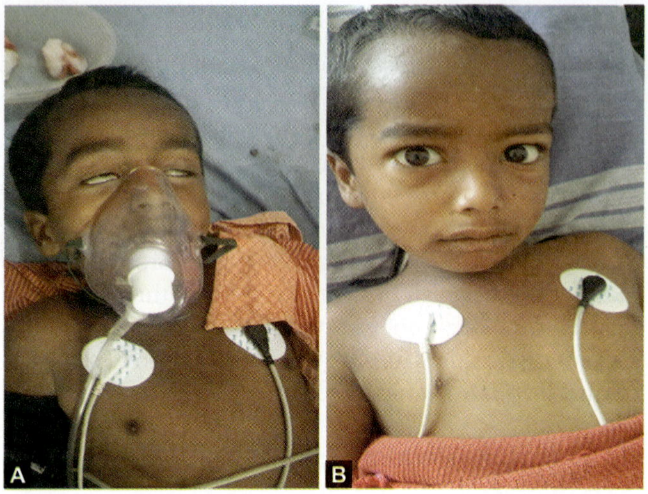

FIGS. 4A AND B: A child who completely recovered from neuroparalysis after neostigmine administration.

sphygmomanometer cuff; however, an IV saline should be on the line.

SUPPORTIVE TREATMENT

- Correction of shock
- Mechanical ventilation
- Hemodialysis
- Administration of blood/blood products
- Antibiotics
- Acute compartmental syndrome

Correction of Shock

Shock could be due to hypovolemia as a result of vomiting, bleeding, increased capillary permeability (venom induced), or anaphylaxis induced by venom itself. Should be managed with adequate administration of crystalloid IV fluids, ionotropic drugs, and adrenaline, if needed.

Mechanical Ventilation

Antivenom treatment alone cannot be relied upon to save the life of the patient with respiratory paralysis due to neurotoxic envenomation. Although artificial ventilation was first suggested for neurotoxic envenoming 140 years ago, patients continued to die of asphyxiation because some doctors believe that antivenom alone is sufficient.

Ambu Bag Ventilation

As majority of the patient of snakebite, present to primary care hospitals, respiratory support using a simple Ambu bag and mouth gag/laryngeal mask airway (LMA) plays an important role in the management of neurotoxic bites. Thousands of patients around the developing world have been kept alive for days using airways and an Ambu bag.

Indications for Intubation

- Absent neck lift
- Pooling of saliva
- Grade 3 power
- Blood gas measurements (if available) showing respiratory acidosis

Unlike in organophosphorus poisoning patients, the need for mechanical ventilation in elapid envenoming, particularly in cobra is only for few hours to 1 or 2 days. A study revealed the mean duration of mechanical ventilation is 26.5 hours.

Hemodialysis

Acute renal failure (ARF) can occur in few patients of Russell's viper and hump nosed pit viper.

Contributing Factors for Acute Renal Failure

- Intravascular hemolysis
- Disseminated intravascular coagulation (DIC)
- Direct nephrotoxicity
- Hypotension

> ☛ *Recovery from ARF is excellent with conservative treatment, few cases need dialysis.*
>
> ☛ *A cautious fluid challenge and furosemide challenge should be given before considering for dialysis.*

Indications for Dialysis

- Clinical uremia (encephalopathy, pericarditis, etc.)
- Fluid overload, not responding to diuretics
- Plasma potassium concentration >7 mmol/L (or hyperkalemic ECG changes)
- Symptomatic acidosis
- *Blood biochemistry*: Serum creatinine >5 mg%, blood urea >140 mg%

> ☛ *Biochemical criteria alone is not sufficient to start dialysis*

Administration of Blood/Blood Products

These can be considered when clinical bleeding continues even after completion of 30 vials of ASV, in antihemostatic envenoming.

Antibiotics

Since many organisms can enter through the bitten wound from the mouth of the snake, a coverage of broad-spectrum antibiotics such as third-generation cephalosporins and metronidazole is needed in majority of the patients.

Acute Compartmental Syndrome

- The role of fasciotomy is highly questionable **(Fig. 5)**.
- Should be considered if intracompartmental pressure is >40 mm Hg measured by striker manometer or by any indigenous method.
- Clinically, pulselessness, pallor, paresthesia, paralysis, pain on passive movements (5 P's) of the affected limb can be an indication for fasciotomy.

To conclude, snakebite is predominantly an occupational hazard of farmers, who mostly present to the rural small hospitals. As in acute myocardial infarction the first few hours are very important in saving the lives.

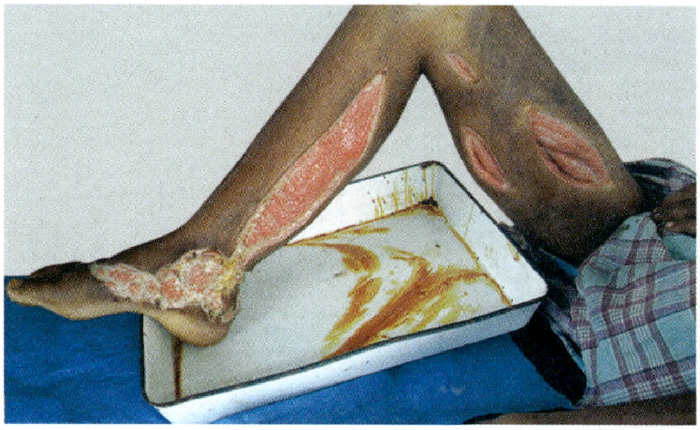

FIG. 5: Indiscriminate, devastating fasciotomy should be discouraged.

Hence, the healthcare facilities in the rural area should be geared up. The primary care physicians should be trained adequately with the local protocols, so that the treatment is timely and effectively carried out. The first few hours of bite, which can be called as the *golden hours*, is very crucial in the management of snakebite.

SUGGESTED READINGS

1. World Health Organization. Guidelines for Clinical Management of Snake Bite in South-East Asia Region. Geneva: World Health Organization; 2010.
2. Management of snake bite, January 2016 by Ministry of health & family welfare, Govt. of India.
3. Warrell DA. Snake bite. Lancet. 2010;375:77-88.
4. Ralph R, Faiz MA, Sharma SK, Ribeiro I, Chappuis F. Managing snakebite. BMJ. 2022;376:e057926.

207
CHAPTER

Long-term Complication of Snakebite

Biranchi Narayan Mohapatra, CBK Mohanty

ABSTRACT

Snakebite mortality is highest in India affecting rural and young people. More than three times of them survive with life changing disabilities. Compared to assumption, more people suffer from long-term complications such as amputation of digit/limb, chronic ulcer, local deformity, functional disability, chronic pain, chronic kidney disease, neurological deficit, hypopituitarism, psychiatric manifestation like depression, and post-traumatic stress disorder causing great health-related economic burden on person and society. There is a gap in actual knowledge and community-based study to ascertain its effect and application of intervention to reduce long-term complication which needs urgent attention.

INTRODUCTION

Worldwide snakebite cases are estimated to be around 1.8–2.7 million with 80,000 to 138,000 deaths annually and nearly three times of death (400,000) survive with life-changing disability. India is the country with highest snakebite mortality (50,000) per year mostly involving rural people (94%), 25% cases are young (<15 years). Most of the snakebite death occur outside hospital (77%) suggesting most of the snakebite victims do not come to healthcare system. Even, those cases admitted are discharged early and no followed up. As a result, long-term complications are not dictated or treated. No attempts have been made to study preventive interventions to reduce long-term complications.

Among the common poisonous snakebite viper and cobra bite produce local manifestations such as swelling and tissue necrosis. Cobra and krait bite produces neuroparalysis leading respiratory paralysis and cardiovascular collapse due to neurotoxin and cardiotoxin. Viper bite produce consumption coagulopathy, bleeding manifestations, and acute kidney injury which are effectively managed by administration of antisnake venom (ASV) early which will prevent death but cannot prevent long-term complications effectively.

In the absence of adequate community-based prospective study, the knowledge on extent and mechanism of long-term complications are largely unknown. This chapter is meant to describe the reported long-term complications for early detection and interventions which will improve the morbidity and economical burden on snakebite victims and on society.

LONG-TERM COMPLICATIONS

Signs and symptoms presenting or persisting beyond 6 weeks following snakebite is considered as long-term complications in this chapter.

Musculoskeletal Disabilities

In a study from Sri Lanka, musculoskeletal disabilities were present in 3.2% of survivors even after several years. Among the survivors with disabilities 15.4% have *amputation* of digit/limb. In viper and cobra bite cases, toxin-mediated tissue necrosis spreading edema, compartmental syndrome leading to limb ischemia compounded by secondary infections which leads to amputation of digit/limb to stop further tissue injury.

Among the snakebite survivors 19.2% have fixed deformities. Joint stiffness and reduced range of movement are common. Necrosis of the muscles, heals with fibrosis and contractures resulted in limb deformity. This can be prevented by proper interventions.

Chronic ulcers at site of bite, local swelling, local pain discoloration, and abnormal skin peeling have been observed in bitten limbs in many cases long after the bite.

African and Asian spitting cobra can produce blindness, but fortunately has not been present in India.

Chronic Kidney Disease

Acute kidney injury occurs in viper bite due to consumption coagulopathy, microangiopathy, and direct toxin effect resulting in acute tubular necrosis in 10–20% cases during acute presentations. Some of them require renal replacement therapy for recovery. Among the survivors 37% in Sri Lanka and 28.7% in India had persisted renal dysfunctions long after the snakebite. 5% of cases who required hemodialysis during acute stage progress to end-stage renal disease requiring lifelong renal replacement therapy. Interventions have to be studied to prevent this progression of kidney functions.

Neurological Deficit

Neurotoxic snakebite such as cobra and krait bite produces post- and presynaptic block at myoneural junctions producing neuroparalysis which usually recovers completely in several days, but subclinical neurotransmission abnormality has been observed in 6 weeks following krait bite in India, which returned to normal by 6 months. In a study from Sri Lanka, subclinical demyelinating type polyneuropathy has been reported 1 year after neurotoxic snakebite.

Brain ischemia due to thrombosis and intracranial hemorrhage have been observed in viper bite with residual neurological deficit even after recovery.

Snakebite cases survived from hypoxic encephalopathy due to respiratory paralysis or cardiac arrest have also been reported with neurological deficit. Blindness, abnormal taste and smell sensation, and decreased parasympathetic activity have been reported long after snakebite.

Endocrine Abnormality

15% of Russell's viper bite has developed *hypopituitarism* at 6 months following the bite. The diagnosis of hypopituitarism is difficult and costly. Hence, remain undictated for long affecting the quality of life and death. Anterior pituitary hormones are mostly reduced. It manifests in patients with secondary amenorrhea, asthenia, loss of libido, weight loss, hypoglycemia, infertility, and hypothyroidism. MRI of brain reveals empty sella in many cases. Early detection and treatment will save the patients.

Mental Health

About 8–43% developed post-traumatic stress disorder and 25–54% snakebite survivors developed depressions. Its detection and interventions can be taken up.

Economic Burden

Chronic disabilities, cost of prolonged healthcare, unable to work due to long-term complications, and social stigma push the snakebite survivors into poverty.

CONCLUSION

There is a lack of community-based study on burden of long-term complication following snake envenomation. Considering India having large number of snakebite affecting mostly rural population and 25% is nearly pediatric population. The burden of snake envenomation needs proper evaluation and development of strategy to reduce the long-term complications and its management **(Box 1)**.

BOX 1: Long-term complication of snake envenomation.

- *Musculoskeletal disabilities:*
  - Amputation digit/limb
  - Contracture of muscle and deformity
  - Chronic ulcer at snakebite site
  - Chronic local pain and swelling
- Chronic kidney disease
- *Neurological deficit:*
  - Following intracerebral hemorrhage (ICH)
  - Posthypoxia or ischemic events
  - Neuromuscular paralysis
  - Blindness, changes in taste, and smell sensation
  - Reduced parasympathetic activity
- *Endocrine dysfunction:* Hypopituitarism
- *Mental health:*
  - Post-traumatic stress disorder
  - Somatization symptoms
  - Depression

SUGGESTED READINGS

1. Waiddyanatha S, Silva A, Siribaddana S, Isbister GK. Long-term Effects of Snake Envenoming. Toxins (Basel). 2019;11:193.
2. Bhaumik S, Gopalakrishnan M, Meena P. Mitigating the chronic burden of snakebite: turning the tide for survivors. Lancet. 2021;398(10309):1389-90.
3. Suraweera W, Warrell D, Whitaker R, Menon G, Rodrigues R, Fu Sh, et al. Trends in snakebite deaths in India from 2000 to 2019 in a nationally representative mortality study. eLife. 2020; 9:e54076.

208

CHAPTER

Blue-green Algae

Sanjay V Patane

ABSTRACT

Blue-green algae (BGA) poisoning occurs after blooms which tend to grow in warm weather and favorable nutrients increasing algal concentration, and breakup in blooms releases toxins which are hepatotoxins and neurotoxins. Animal deaths are common, while human exposures are limited to allergic reactions and mild liver enzyme elevation, and human mortality cannot be ruled out in extremes of cases.

INTRODUCTION

Many cases presenting in emergency department (ED) may have signs and symptoms, like organophosphorus (OP) poisoning, but the treating physician should be alert in not being mislead, but follow the guidelines for treating critical cases, and attempt to diagnose the cause of poisoning. This will prevent overmedication. Cholinergic crisis can be seen with overdose of the substances such as arecoline, pilocarpine, Urecholine (bethanechol), carbachol, choline, and methacholine.

Some types of mushrooms (*Boletus* species, *Clitocybe* species, and *Inocybe* species) can present with symptoms with cholinergic crisis which may suggest OP poisoning.

CASE PRESENTATION

A 24-year-old male patient, farmer by profession was brought to casualty from a rural center. He was semi-conscious and was already intubated and he was on Ambu bag support. He was reported to have impending respiratory failure.

His brother gave history that he had gone to the jungles, and after he consumed water from an old, neglected, and unused pond, he had vomitings, loose motions and tremors, and abdominal pain. This was 2 hours later. Considering some occult poisoning; patient was taken to local civil hospital, where he was intubated with endotracheal tube due to seizures and impending respiratory failure. He also had excessive salivation and mild hypoxia. He was later shifted to our hospital for further management.

On admission, patient was drowsy, but arousable and had excessive sweating and salivation. He had bilateral extensive crepitations. He had passed motions in his clothes. He was restless and his oxygen saturation was ~86 on pulse oximetry, suggesting mild hypoxia. His pupils were small size and were sluggishly responding to light. He responded to injection atropine and his secretions dried-up. He was managed with assisted ventilation support, intravenous (IV) antibiotics, injection atropine, and oximes (PAM) on a presumptive diagnosis of insecticide poisoning. However, his gastric lavage aspirate was not smelling like any OP compound. His serum cholinesterase levels were reported to be normal.

On subsequent day, patient was fully conscious, obeying oral commands and attempting spontaneous breaths but neck holding was unsatisfactory. Weaning trial was attempted, but the patient was having tachypnea and saturation was dropping, hence continued on assisted ventilation with injection atropine to maintain mild atropinization, i.e., drying of secretions. His electrolytes and other metabolic parameters were monitored.

All cyanobacteria are not poisonous, and while the cyanobacteria that generate poisonous toxins may not always do so.

Toxins from these bacteria, called as cyanotoxins, are poisonous to humans, nearly all livestock and wildlife, including cattle, horses, sheep, pigs, chickens, ducks, pigeons, geese, herons, songbirds, dogs, rabbits, small wild and domestic animals, and even frogs, fish, and snakes. These toxins are primarily neurotoxic and hepatotoxic. Drinking stagnant water containing high concentration of these toxins, exposes to toxicity by BGA.

Exposure can cause conjunctivitis, rhinitis, earache, sore throat, and swollen lips. Respiratory symptoms include atypical pneumonia and a hay fever-like syndrome. Exposure can also cause electrolyte imbalances, headache, malaise, and muscle weakness/pain in joints, and limbs. Hepatic failure has been reported in dialysis patients treated with dialysis water contaminated with microcystins. Glycosuria, proteinuria, and occasionally hematuria also have been reported.

Increase in the symptoms of autoimmune diseases such as multiple sclerosis (MS), lupus [systemic lupus erythematosus (SLE)], rheumatoid arthritis (RA), pemphigus vulgaris (a skin condition), etc., as the BGA is known to stimulate the immune system.

Types of toxins commonly produced by cyanobacterial harmful algal blooms (cHAB) are as follows:

• Microcystin	Hepatotoxin
• Nodularin	Hepatotoxin
• Cylindrospermopsin	Cytotoxin
• Anatoxin-a	Neurotoxin, potent rapidly acting
• Anatoin-a(s)	Neurotoxin
• Lyngbyatoxin	Dermatitis
• Saxitoxins	Neurotoxin

There is very limited toxicological data relating to different cyanotoxin concentrations in water and effects on livestock. In a study with lactating dairy cattle, cows were provided drinking water with 1×10^5 cells of *Microcystis aeruginosa* per milliliter (mL), or a microcystin-LR concentration in water of about 9.8 µg/L for 21 days, which is an ingestion rate of microcystin-LR of 1.21 µg/kg of bodyweight per day.

Toxicological data exits for microcystin-LR which is a potent cyanotoxin. No effects were reported in animal health, and no detectable amounts of microcystin were found in the milk.

Yearling beef cattle were given a similar dose of 1×10^5 cells of *Microcystis aeruginosa* in drinking water for 28 days, at an average ingestion rate of microcystin-LR of 1.42 µg/kg of bodyweight per day. There were no significant health effects and no detectable microcystins in liver tissue or blood plasma.

The World Health Organization (WHO) has issued a guideline value for microcystin-LR of 1 µg/L for human drinking water. Many countries have developed human drinking water guidelines for microcystins between 1 and 1.5 µg/L based on lifetime exposures. For recreational water with possible exposure through contact, ingestion and inhalation (from <10 to >2,000 µg/L), and associated with a relative probability of acute health effects, the WHO guidance values for microcystin-LR are higher.

Boiling water will not destroy algae toxins and could actually increase toxin levels. There is no antidote available and the toxin acts very fast. Multiple treatment steps are typically needed to remove algae toxins.

Toxins from algae can accumulate in the entrails (guts) of fish and occasionally in the muscle (fillet). Levels in fish depend upon the severity of the bloom in the area where the fish are caught.

SYMPTOMS OF CYANOBACTERIAL POISONING

Blue-green algae can produce two types of toxins:

1. Microcystins
2. Anatoxins

Microcystins are hepatotoxic while the anatoxins target the nervous system. The clinical signs depend on which toxin is involved.

Microcystins

- Microcystins are hepatotoxic and hence can cause organ failure.
- As liver is an important organ in metabolism and many body systems depend on a functioning liver, a broad list of symptoms arises due to hepatic dysfunction. The gastrointestinal tract affection results in vomiting, diarrhea, and tarry stools. Later deepening icterus, hypoglycemia, hypoproteinemia, bleeding disorders, etc., occur with organ failure.
- Detoxification and metabolism of by-products from the body is an important function of liver. Hepatic encephalopathy may develop with disorientation and seizures due to a buildup of toxins. Shock may eventually follow and the animal becomes comatose. With terminal hepatic failure and rising liver enzymes, death is imminent within days; however, some fatalities occur within 12–24 hours of algae ingestion.

Symptoms of Microcystins Toxicity

- Weakness
- Lethargy
- Lack of appetite
- Vomiting

- Diarrhea (dark and tarry stool)
- Bleeding
- Pale gums
- Icterus (yellow tint to gums and skin)
- Shock
- Seizures
- Collapse and coma
- Death

Anatoxins

- The prognosis is worse with anatoxins.
- Signs of poisoning occur within 30–60 minutes of exposure and nervous system symptoms predominate.
- Drooling of saliva and tears is due to overactive secretions.
- Muscle tremors occur and while some muscles become very rigid others are paralyzed.
- Cyanotic tinge is due to decreased oxygen delivery to mucus membranes and skin.
- Respiratory failure is due to paralysis of the diaphragm (also a muscle) results in death.
- Postexposure with anatoxin, death is quick, often within minutes to hours. In fact, livestock that drink from contaminated ponds are often found dead right by the water's edge.

Symptoms of Anatoxin Toxicity

- Weakness or inability to walk
- Excessive salivation
- Difficulty in breathing
- Blue discoloration of skin and mucous membranes, and tremors
- Seizures
- Muscle rigidity
- Paralysis
- Disorientation
- Coma
- Death

Weight loss, in livestock that do survive cyanobacterial poisoning, is seen and, in some cases, they also develop photosensitivity.

Livestock that develop photosensitivity are prone to sunburns affecting lighter areas of skin, including the muzzle, udder, vulva/anus, and areas with white hide. Affected skin will dry out, turn black and peel, exposing fresh, new skin.

DIAGNOSIS

You can determine the presence of cyanobacteria in a number of ways, which are as follows:

- When you suspect concentrations of cyanobacteria in a water body, walk around to the downward side of the water body. Presence of any dead animals such as mice, muskrats, birds, snakes, or fish is a sign that poisonous condition exists.
- A veterinarian should conduct a necropsy on deceased livestock to rule out other causes of death. If you suspect cyanobacteria, contact your veterinarian to determine which samples would be appropriate for your situation.
- Microscopic examination is one way to determine the presence of potentially poisonous cyanobacteria, but the presence of the bacteria does not mean the water is toxic. Laboratory analysis and testing the water is the most accurate method of determining whether poisonous toxins are present. A water sample of at least 500 mL should be collected from the suspected water source after the discovery of death. Water testing only will determine if the water source contains cyanobacteria.

TREATMENT

- Prompt intervention is needed in all cases of poisoning, but since BGA attacks so fast, speedy intervention is critical. Seek immediate medical care.
- If symptoms detected early and you suspect algae poisoning, measures for toxin elimination from the body should be initiated.
- Induced vomiting was practiced earlier to remove the algae from the stomach but it is relatively contraindicated in unprotected airways. Ryles tube stomach wash removes the toxin from the stomach if the patient is brought early.
- Oral activated charcoal may be given to adsorb some of the toxin and if the patient is brought early.
- The toxins enter the system so fast that regardless of species, he is quite bad before reaching medical care. It is often too late to remove the toxin. Worse still, there is no specific antidote for BGA poisoning. Treatment is limited to supportive care focused on affected organ systems.
- Aggressive therapy including IV fluids and plasma may replenish electrolytes, regulate blood glucose, support organ function, and prevent shock.
- Muscle relaxants to patients with muscle tremors are not advocated but in patients on assisted controlled ventilation, injection lorazepam does help.
- Antiseizure drugs are administered if convulsions occur. Atropine may reduce excess salivation and bronchorrhea.
- Treatment for hepatic failure should be on standard lines, with serial monitoring of enzymes, sugars, electrolytes, and bleeding diathesis.

- Nutraceuticals may be needed to support waning liver function.

No known antidotes are available for poisoning resulting from cyanobacteria. The best solution is to be aware of conditions that spawn cyanobacterial blooms. Avoid exposure to such water and keep cattle from drinking in areas having accumulated bacterial concentrations.

SUGGESTED READINGS

1. Kratz WA, Myers J. Nutrition and Growth of Several Blue-Green Algae. Am J Bot. 1955;42(3):282-7.
2. Spoerke DG, Rumack BH. Blue-green algae poisoning. J Emerg Med. 1985;2(5):353-5.
3. Fogg GE. The comparative physiology and biochemistry of the blue-green algae. Bacteriol Rev. 1956;20(3):148-65.

SECTION

17

PREGNANCY MEDICINE

209

CHAPTER

Antibiotic Use in Pregnancy

G Usha, Harikishan Boorugu

ABSTRACT

Antibiotics are frequently used in pregnancy. About 25% of women would have received at least one antibiotic prescription during the antenatal period. The physiological and immunological changes which occur in pregnancy make the antenatal women prone for infections, some of which could be severe. This necessitates the use of appropriate antibiotics. Like all other classes of drugs used in pregnancy, caution should be exercised while prescribing these drugs in view of the adverse effects they might have on the fetus. Beta-lactams and macrolides can be safely prescribed whereas fluoroquinolones and tetracyclines should be avoided if possible. Since untreated or inappropriately treated infections have adverse consequences on maternal and fetal health, judicious use of antibiotics results in good pregnancy outcome.

INTRODUCTION

Antibiotics are among the most common class of drugs pregnant women receive. They constitute nearly 80% of prescription medications during antenatal period. Women during pregnancy are predisposed to urinary tract infections, severe respiratory tract infections, and maternal sepsis because of physiological and immunological changes. In 2017, globally 11.9 million cases of maternal infections were reported. While antibiotics are useful in reducing morbidity and mortality in these infections, irrational use of it could result in short-term and long-term effects in the fetus. Hence, careful use is warranted while prescribing them in order to maximize maternal benefits and minimize fetal risk.

SAFETY PROFILE OF COMMONLY USED ANTIBIOTICS DURING PREGNANCY

Despite the understanding that antibiotic exposure during fetal development is associated with multiple risks, only 10% of medications have sufficient safety data. Due to ethical and logistical issues, the information on drug safety is limited in pregnancy due to paucity of trials. It is also difficult to establish a causal relationship to a single factor such as drug as a cause for major malformation. Historically, earlier the FDA established 5-letter risk categories as A, B, C, D, and X, which was followed to indicate the potential of a drug to cause teratogenicity. This was replaced with the more descriptive Pregnancy and Lactation Labeling Rule (PLLR) with a summary of the risks during pregnancy and lactation, and a discussion of the data supporting that summary in 2015. But in this article, we will be referring to the safety profile with the earlier system because of familiarity. Apart from risk of teratogenicity, there are other adverse effects such as hypoxia in fetus if there is maternal anaphylaxis, altered gut microbiome, atopy, and described with the maternal use of antibiotics. This article aims at safety and risk profile of groups of antibiotics and their clinical use.

As far as the safety profile of antibiotics in lactation is concerned, guidelines from American Academy of Pediatrics (AAP), UK Drugs in Lactation Advisory Service (UKDILAS), LactMed (Drugs and Lactation Database), and Hale's Risk definition are to be followed.

■ Beta-lactams

This bactericidal group comprising of Penicillin and cephalosporins are the most used antibiotics and have been in use for long period. These can be safely prescribed in pregnancy. They are the first drug of choice in group B Streptococcal and methicillin-sensitive *Staphylococcus aureus* (MSSA) infections.

Cephalosporins are indicated in various gram-positive and gram-negative infections and depending on the generation they are effective against methicillin-resistant *Staphylococcus aureus* (MRSA) and vancomycin-resistant *Enterococcus*. They are safe in lactation.

Beta-lactamase Inhibitor with or without Beta-lactams

This broadens the spectrum and can be used in pregnancy. In those women with a risk of preterm delivery. Amoxyclav should be avoided because of reported risk of necrotizing enterocolitis in the newborn. In lactation, it can be used after benefit/risk assessment.

Piperacillin and tazobactam can be used during pregnancy and lactation.

Macrolides

Macrolide are bacteriostatic drugs primarily. Erythromycin and azithromycin can be safely used in pregnancy and lactation. Azithromycin is used for infections such as community-acquired and *Mycoplasma* pneumonia. Pneumonia is the most common nonobstetric cause of infection, which results in hospitalization and is associated with increased fetal and maternal risk.

Clarithromycin should be avoided unless there is compelling maternal indication.

Tetracyclines

Tetracyclines, which are broad-spectrum bacteriostatic drugs, are teratogenic. Exposure of the fetus after 15th week of gestation is associated with staining of teeth and it also affects bone growth.

Doxycycline, a commonly used drug in this group has not been reported to carry any risk for the fetus in the first trimester. Use of it for prolonged period can cause fulminant hepatitis in the mother. It could be used in life-threatening tick-borne infections, where it might be absolutely indicated. During lactation, it must be used with caution.

Sulfonamides with or without Trimethoprim

These are folate antagonists and were reported to cause two-to-three-fold increase in congenital anomalies including neural tube defects when used in the first trimester. But a recent systematic review did not reveal major teratogenicity and the rate of congenital deformities was comparable to that in general population. Sulfamethoxazole should be avoided after 32 weeks due to risk of kernicterus. Trimethoprim-sulfamethoxazole (TMP-SMX) is indicated for chemoprophylaxis of pneumocystis pneumonia and reactivation toxoplasmosis in those who are HIV-positive in view of the benefit which outweighs the theoretical risk. It is compatible with lactation.

Fluoroquinolones

These rapidly bactericidal drugs are contraindicated in pregnancy though there are some reports of their safe use. They can cause fetal arthropathy and urinary system malformations. The Food and Drug Administration (FDA) has approved ciprofloxacin for postexposure prophylaxis in Anthrax. They are to be avoided in lactation.

Nitrofurantoin

This has a narrow spectrum and is indicated in uncomplicated lower UTI and for long-term suppression in those women with chronic bacteriuria. It is contraindicated in women at term during labor and delivery or when onset of labor is imminent because of the risk of hemolytic anemia in the newborn. It can be used in lactation.

Aminoglycosides

These bactericidal drugs are effective against gram-negative organisms. Streptomycin is contraindicated due to its association with hearing loss in newborns. Short-term use is acceptable with other drugs in this class with monitoring. It can be used in lactation with caution.

Metronidazole

This antiprotozoal drug is bactericidal against anaerobic bacteria. There is no teratogenicity associated with it. There were reports of preterm births which were subsequently not confirmed. It can be used in lactation.

Carbapenems

Data on safety is limited. Ertapenem, meropenem, and dorepenem are Category B and Imipenem-Cilastatin is Category C. Infections resistant to penicillin and cephalosporin can be treated with these drugs Lactation data is limited but can be used with caution.

Monobactams

Aztreonam use should be limited to those patients who have Penicillin allergy though safety data in pregnancy is limited.

Clindamycin

Clindamycin is a lincosamide. Oral preparations are considered safe but vaginal route administration is contraindicated in view of adverse fetal effects in later half of pregnancy. It can be used during lactation.

Linezolid

Linezolid, which is an oxazolidinone, can be used in pregnancy where there are potential benefits. Lactation data is limited but can be used with caution.

Vancomycin

Limited available data suggests that vancomycin can be safely used in pregnancy and lactation.

Fosfomycin

This drug is not known to be associated with any adverse effects on fetus. The oral preparation is considered safe in pregnancy. It is useful in urinary tract infection (UTI) with multidrug-resistant organisms. The data in lactation is limited and must be used with caution **(Tables 1 to 3)**.

INDICATIONS FOR ANTIBIOTICS DURING PREGNANCY

The indications for antibiotics in pregnancy are for infections that are related to pregnancy, for those which are unrelated but may have consequences for maternal and fetal health and prophylactic use of antibiotics for surgery. When initiating antibiotic therapy, it should be remembered that there could be noninfectious conditions which mimic sepsis and efforts should be made to exclude such conditions.

TABLE 1: The FDA risk category.

Pregnancy category rating	Risk
A	Safe in pregnancy
B	Can be used if indicated
C	Can be used if benefits more
D	To be avoided
X	Contraindicated

(FDA: Food and Drug Administration)

PREGNANCY-SPECIFIC INFECTIONS

Maternal Sepsis

Sepsis is the third most common cause of obstetric mortality. The threshold to start antibiotics empirically should be low when there is clinical suspicion. The common organisms are beta-hemolytic *Streptococcus* and

TABLE 2: Safety profile of commonly used antibiotics.

Drug	Category in pregnancy	Lactation
Penicillins	B	Can be used
Cephalosporins	B	Can be used
Macrolides	B/C	Can be used
Aminoglycosides	D	Can be used with caution
Fluoroquinolones	C	Use with caution if needed
Sulfonamides/ Trimethoprim	C	Can be used
Carbapenems	B/C	Can be used with caution
Metronidazole	B	Can be used
Nitrofurantoin	B	Can be used
Fosfomycin	B	Can be used
Doxycycline	D	Can be used, short courses
Linezolid	C	Use with caution
Vancomycin	B	Use with caution

TABLE 3: Hale's classification of lactation risk.

Risk definition	Compatible	Probably compatible	Possibly hazardous	Hazardous	Comments
L1	Yes				• No risk on controlled studies • Risk of harm remote
L2		Yes			Limited studies show no adverse effects, risk remote
L3		Yes			• Risk possible • Risk, benefit analysis
L4			Yes		Positive evidence of risk, avoid unless benefit outweigh risk
L5				Yes	• Significant risk • Contraindicated

Escherichia coli. Amoxyclav, metronidazole, clindamycin, piperacillin-tazobactam, and aminoglycosides are the antibiotics of choice. Antibiotics prophylaxis, when indicated, and appropriate treatment of infection reduce the risk of sepsis.

Chorioamnionitis

This refers to infection of placenta, membranes, and amniotic fluid. It is polymicrobial and may cause maternal complications and labor abnormalities. Aminoglycosides, ampicillin, and metronidazole are the drugs of choice.

Preterm Premature Rupture of Membrane

Prophylactic antibiotic is indicated in stable women who can be managed expectantly to prevent preterm labor. The antibiotic of choice is erythromycin.

Urinary Tract Infections and Asymptomatic Bacteriuria

Untreated, 30–40% of pregnant women with asymptomatic bacteriuria develop symptomatic UTIs. The risk for pyelonephritis is more in pregnancy and there could be fetal complications such as preterm birth, low birth weight, and perinatal mortality. *E. coli* is the commonest organism. Screening for asymptomatic bacteriuria is suggested at least once at 12–16 weeks of gestation with urine culture. Antibiotics therapy is indicated based on culture report.

Prophylactic Antibiotic for C-section

Prophylactic antibiotics are recommended by the World Health Organization (WHO) for women undergoing elective or emergency C-section and a single dose of antibiotic 60 minutes before skin incision is suggested. C-section increases the risk ok postpartum infection by 5- to 20-folds. The drug of choice is first- or second-generation cephalosporin. Continuing postoperatively for longer period depends on other risk factors.

Other Maternal Bacterial Infections

Other maternal infections which are not related to pregnancy should be treated as they would be treated in the nonpregnant patients. If there is an indication for a specific drug with an adverse safety profile, it should be used according to individual case scenario with maternal health being the prime concern.

Antibiotic Resistance and Antimicrobial Stewardship

With the emergence and spread of resistant pathogens, there is a threat in treating even common infections. There is a spread of pan-resistant bacteria and there has to be caution while prescribing antibiotics in pregnancy also. Antimicrobial stewardship is a tool for optimizing the use of these drugs and this along with infection prevention and control is important to address infections in obstetric care setting.

CONCLUSION

The use of antibiotics in pregnancy requires a careful assessment of risk versus benefit to mother and fetus. Though some of the commonly used antibiotics can be used safely in pregnancy, the data for many other in this class of drugs are not available. Emerging resistance is a problem and prescriptions should be for definite indications. The selection, dosing, duration, and monitoring for adverse reactions of the antibiotic would all play a major role in achieving the objective.

SUGGESTED READINGS

1. Bookstaver PB, Bland CM, Griffin B, Stover KR, Eiland LS, McLaughlin M. A review of antibiotic use in pregnancy. Pharmacotherapy. 2015;35(11):1052-62.
2. Latisha M, McGovern PG. Antibiotic use in pregnancy. Topics Obstet Gynecol. 2018;38(7):1-8.
3. World Health Organization. (2021). WHO recommendation on Prophylactic antibiotics for women undergoing caesarean section. [online] Available from https://www.who.int/publications/i/item/9789240028012. [Last accessed December, 2023].

210

CHAPTER

Acute Kidney Injury in Pregnancy

ML Patel

ABSTRACT

Acute kidney injury (AKI) is a clinical syndrome with progressive deterioration of kidney function leading to accumulation of nephrotoxic waste products in circulating blood. It is a major issue in hospitalized patients, with incidence ranging from 1 to 7% of all hospitalized patients and from 30 to 50% of intensive care unit (ICU) patients. Morbidity and mortality associated with AKI remain high, ranging from 20 to 60%, despite improvements in management strategies. AKI can also lead to the development or progression of chronic kidney disease (CKD), proteinuria, and cardiovascular diseases. The best treatment of AKI is prevention with avoidance of nephrotoxic agents and hemodynamic optimization. Renal replacement therapy (RRT) remains the mainstay of treatment for severe AKI in ICU. There are at present multiple disparities in uniform definition, diagnosis, and other areas of AKI and RRT that need to be addressed.

INTRODUCTION

Acute kidney injury (AKI) in pregnancy is a hazard for public health and a major factor in the morbidity and death of both mothers and fetuses. 15–20% of AKI in poor nations is caused by pregnancy-related acute kidney disease, which significantly put up to the total burden of the disease. Up to 20% of all AKI cases in India involve pregnancy-related acute kidney injury (PRAKI), which affects 1 in 50 births. AKI is linked to a high death rate (>30% in most studies). However, in affluent countries, the prevalence of AKI has significantly decreased from 1 per 2,000 to 1 in 20,000 births. Despite the fact that the prevalence of pregnancy-related acute kidney disease is low in developed nations due to better prenatal care, the rates have nearly tripled in the past 10 years in the Western countries. This may be because of increasing maternal age with more comorbidities, higher AKI disclosure rates, increasing incidence of hypertensive disorders of pregnancy, and obesity.

PHYSIOLOGIC AND ANATOMIC CHANGES IN KIDNEY DURING PREGNANCY (TABLE 1)

Anatomical Changes

Size: During pregnancy, both kidneys lengthen by 1–1.5 cm. Up to 30% more volume can be seen in the kidneys, mostly because of an increase in renal vascular and interstitial volume.

Over 90% of women have physiological hydronephrosis of pregnancy, which is characterized by calyces, renal pelvis, and ureter dilatation.

Physiological Changes

Hemodynamic changes: Higher blood volume, decreased systemic vascular resistance, and higher cardiac output are the main modifications. Nitric oxide and relaxin levels are up throughout the body, and angiotensin II is relatively

TABLE 1: Renal changes in pregnancy.

Variable	Change in pregnancy
Kidney size	The kidney size increases by 1–1.5 cm and volume of kidney increases by up to 30%
Hydronephrosis	Physiological dilation of urinary collecting system with hydronephrosis in up to 80% of women (right > left)
Renal blood flow	May increased up to 80% from baseline
GFR	Increased than normal (150–200 mL/min)
Serum creatinine	Falls to 0.4–0.5 mg/dL (*n* = 0.8)*
Uric acid	Falls to 2.0–3.0 mg/dL (*n* = 4–5)
BUN	Falls to 8–10 mg/dL (*n* = 13)*
Sodium	Mild hyponatremia (fall of 4–5 mol/L)
Osmolality	Decreased up to 270 mOsm/kg

*Considered normal in a nonpregnant individual, reflects renal impairment in pregnant women.

(BUN: blood urea nitrogen; GFR: glomerular filtration rate)

less effective at constricting blood vessels. Systemic blood pressure typically drops, typically nadir by 20 weeks' gestation.

Glomerular filtration rate (GFR): In the presence of hyperfiltration, increases by roughly 50%, resulting in a physiological drop in serum creatinine.

Renal plasma flow: During second trimester of pregnancy plasma flow may increase up to 85%.

Serum creatinine: Serum creatinine >0.87 mg/dL should be considered outside the normal range for pregnancy.

Urine protein excretion increases over the course of normal pregnancy, from 60–90 to 180–250 mg/day, as measured by a 24-hour urine collection. As a consequence of this physiologic increase in proteinuria, the threshold for elevated proteinuria in pregnancy has been set at a higher level of 300 mg/day.

ETIOLOGY OF ACUTE KIDNEY INJURY IN PREGNANCY

Development of AKI during pregnancy follows a dual mode distribution with two peaks: initial peak in the first trimester caused by septic abortion and the other peak in the third trimester and/or postpartum due to late obstetrical complications. AKI is a diverse syndrome in pregnant women and is having multiple etiologies. Healthy women developed obstetrical complications or pregnancy-related hypertension and hemolysis, elevated liver enzymes, and low platelet count (HELLP) syndrome. Etiology not related to pregnancy like (acute gastroenteritis, malaria, pyelonephritis, lupus nephritis, and acute interstitial nephritis) is reported to cause renal dysfunction. The causes of AKI in pregnant women are divided into three main groups:

1. *Obstetrical complications*: Septic abortion, abruptio placentae, placenta previa, uterine hemorrhage [antepartum hemorrhage (APH) and postpartum hemorrhage (PPH)], intrauterine fetal demise, puerperal sepsis
2. *Pregnancy-specific disorders*: Preeclampsia, eclampsia, HELLP syndrome, acute fatty liver of pregnancy (AFLP), hyperemesis gravidarum
3. *Miscellaneous causes*: Acute postinfectious glomerulonephritis, lupus nephritis, acute pyelonephritis, dehydration, and calculus of urinary tract

Acute kidney injury in pregnant women can be divided into three groups: prerenal, intrarenal, and postrenal causes. Gestational age and clinical presentation are important determinants of AKI in a pregnancy. Some of the important causes of AKI during pregnancy are mentioned in **Table 2**.

DIAGNOSIS OF AKI IN PREGNANCY

There is no established standard for diagnosing AKI during pregnancy. Due to hyperfiltration, serum creatinine is often lower during pregnancy. However, it is likely that modest increases in serum creatinine (<0.3 mg/dL) may be more sensitive for detecting early injury. There are currently no specific criteria for the diagnosis of AKI in pregnancy.

The Kidney Disease: Improving Global Outcomes (KDIGO) definition and staging system is the most recent and preferred definition.

According to *KDIGO 2012 guidelines*, AKI is defined as any one of the following:

- Increase in serum creatinine by ≥0.3 mg/dL within 48 hours
- Increase in serum creatinine to ≥1.5 times baseline, which is known or presumed to have occurred within the prior 7 days
- Urine volume <0.5 mL/kg/h for 6 hours

ACUTE KIDNEY INJURY NETWORK

The Acute Kidney Injury Network (AKIN) is shown in **Table 3**.

TABLE 2: Causes of acute kidney injury during pregnancy.

Prerenal	Intrinsic renal	Postrenal
Early pregnancy:		
Bleeding—miscarriage	Anticardiolipin antibody syndrome	Renal stones
Hyperemesis gravidarum	Sepsis (i.e., septic abortion)	Ureteral obstruction
Ovarian hyperstimulation syndrome	Autoimmune disease	
Ectopic pregnancy	CKD progression	
Late pregnancy:		
Second trimester bleeding/miscarriage, placenta previa, placental abruption	• Severe preeclampsia, HELLP • Acute fatty liver of pregnancy • HUS/TTP • Pyelonephritis • Glomerulonephritis, interstitial nephritis, lupus nephritis	• Polyhydramnios • Multifetal gestation • Large uterine fibroids • Ureteral obstruction • Renal stones
Postpartum:		
Bleeding—atonic uterus, rupture of uterus, obstetrical (vulvovaginal and perineal tears and lacerations)	• Severe preeclampsia, HELLP • HUS • Puerperal sepsis • Glomerulonephritis, interstitial nephritis, lupus nephritis • Nephrotoxic drugs (NSAIDS) antibiotics, proton-pump inhibitors, CKD progression	Renal stones

Causes of AKI in pregnancy	Timing in pregnancy	Signs and symptoms	Cause of AKI	Treatment options
Hyperemesis gravidarum	First trimester	Intractable nausea, vomiting	Volume depletion, possible acute tubular necrosis	Oral hydration, intravenous hydration if necessary
Septic abortion	First trimester	Fever, abdominal pain	Septic acute tubular necrosis	Broad-spectrum antibiotics, surgical removal of products of conception
Preeclampsia/ Eclampsia	After 20 weeks	New-onset hypertension (SBP ≥ 140 mm Hg and DBP ≥ 90 mm Hg) and proteinuria	Endothelial damage, coagulopathy/ thrombotic micro-angiopathy, possible acute tubular necrosis	Supportive care, delivery when able, expectant management for preterm pregnancies
Urinary tract infection/ acute pyelonephritis	More common after 20 weeks	Flank pain, dysuria, fever, chills	Prerenal AKI secondary to infection, possible acute tubular necrosis	Directed antibiotic therapy
HELLP syndrome	Late second or third trimester	Hemolysis, elevated liver enzymes, low platelets; can be seen concomitantly with preeclampsia	Endothelial damage, coagulopathy/ thrombotic micro-angiopathy, possible acute tubular necrosis	Delivery when able, imaging for right upper quadrant to rule out hepatic bleeding, hypertension control if severe
TTP/HUS	Usually late second trimester or third trimester for TTP, commonly postpartum for HUS	Hemolytic anemia, thrombocytopenia, neurologic abnormalities	Thrombotic microangiopathy	Plasma exchange +/– rituximab
Acute fatty liver disease of pregnancy	Third trimester	Nonspecific-nausea, vomiting, abdominal pain, hypoglycemia, elevated liver enzymes	Prerenal AKI, possible hepatorenal syndrome appearing picture	Delivery when able, liver transplant if warranted

Continued

Continued

Causes of AKI in pregnancy	Timing in pregnancy	Signs and symptoms	Cause of AKI	Treatment options
Lupus nephritis	Delay in pregnancy recommended after 6 months of disease quiescence, kidney manifestations more common postpartum, extrarenal manifestations are more common in second and third trimester	Lupus flare diagnosed with markers of disease activity such as low complement levels, presence of double-stranded DNA, and proteinuria	Increased disease activity worsening kidney function	Immunosuppression, continue hydroxychloroquine during pregnancy
Obstructive uropathy	Second and third trimester	Worsening abdominal pain, oliguria	Reflux and obstruction can cause hydronephrosis	Analgesics, increase in fluid intake, stent or percutaneous nephrostomy tube if conservative management unsuccessful
Placental abruption and placental hemorrhage	Third trimester	Increased vaginal bleeding, abdominal pain	Can cause renal cortical necrosis (rare), prerenal AKI from acute blood loss anemia	Control bleeding, supportive care, delivery of infant
Postpartum NSAIDs use	Postpartum	No specific symptoms, elevated creatinine and bland urine analysis	Worsening prerenal AKI in setting of hypovolemia and NSAIDs-induced vasoconstriction	Stop NSAIDs, increase hydration, supportive care

(CKD: chronic kidney disease; DBP: diastolic blood pressure; HELLP: hemolysis, elevated liver enzymes, and low platelet count; HUS: hemolytic uremic syndrome; NSAIDs: nonsteroidal anti-inflammatory drugs; SBP: systolic blood pressure; TTP: thrombotic thrombocytopenic purpura)

TABLE 3: Acute Kidney Injury Network.

Stage	Serum creatinine	Urine output
1	1.5–1.9 times from baseline OR ≥ 0.3 mg/dL (≥ 26.5 μmol/L) increase	< 0.5 mL/kg/h for 6–12 hours
2	2.0–2.9 times from baseline	< 0.5 mL/kg/h for ≥ 12 hours
3	3.0 times from baseline OR Increase in serum creatinine to ≥ 4.0 mg/dL (≥ 353.6 μmol/L) OR Initiation of renal replacement therapy OR in patients < 18 years, decrease in estimated glomerular filtration rate (eGFR) to < 35 mL/min/1.73 m^2	< 0.3 mL/kg/h for ≥ 24 hours OR Anuria for ≥ 12 hours

TREATMENT OF ACUTE KIDNEY INJURY IN PREGNANCY

Three factors are taken into account in the management of acute kidney injury in pregnancy (P-AKI): dialysis, supportive treatments to maintain renal function, and therapy of the underlying pregnancy-specific illness are all options.

Strategies to Support Renal Function

Beginning as soon as feasible should be the main general action to reduce renal injury (such as treating the etiology, avoiding nephrotoxic medicines, or treating an infectious disease).

The next step is giving intravenous fluids to maintain or restore renal perfusion. Additionally, this treatment guards against hypovolemia, guarantees appropriate uteroplacental perfusion, and promotes fetal health.

Acute kidney injury's known consequences, including hypertension, hyperkalemia, metabolic acidosis, and anemia, are treated with medication. Due to the increased risk of volume depletion, angiotensin-converting enzyme inhibitors and angiotensin II receptor antagonists should not be used during pregnancy. Methyldopa and labetalol are the first-line treatments for pregnant women with hypertension. For the treatment of hyperkalemia, the administration of insulin, glucose, and ion exchange resin is advised.

Although the erythropoiesis-stimulating drug is safe during pregnancy, greater doses are frequently necessary to give pregnant women the desired therapeutic effect.

Dialysis

In PRAKI, uremic symptoms (such as nausea, vomiting, pericarditis, or encephalopathy), volume overload, hyperkalemia, and/or metabolic acidosis that is refractory to early medical treatment are among the reasons for dialysis. However, when GFR drops to below 20 mL/min/1.73 m^2, an early commencement of dialysis is advised. The majority of patients select intermittent hemodialysis as their preferred kind of dialysis. When dialysis is recommended for pregnant women with AKI, it is important to keep a few things in mind. They consist of (1) increased dialysis dosage (daily dialysis lasting longer than 20 h/week). This would lessen hemodialysis's hemodynamic fluctuations and enhance the uremic milieu, which is a high-risk factor for preterm and polyhydramnios.

Treatment of the Underlying Condition Unique to Pregnancy

The underlying source of the injury determines the specific treatment for AKI. The delivery of the fetus must happen quickly in order to treat severe preeclampsia, HELLP syndrome, and AFLP. If birth occurs before 34 weeks' gestation, glucocorticoids are given to reduce the risk of neonatal respiratory distress syndrome. Plasmapheresis and eculizumab [for atypical hemolytic uremic syndrome (aHUS)] are two treatments for thrombotic microangiopathies, such as thrombotic thrombocytopenic purpura (TTP) and aHUS. The aim of plasma exchange in ADAMTS13-deficient TMA (thrombotic microangiopathy) is to restore enzyme activity, and rituximab therapy is a possibility if plasma exchange is ineffective. When starting steroid and immunosuppressive therapy in a pregnant patient with glomerulonephritis, the risks and benefits should be balanced.

SUGGESTED READINGS

1. Selcuk NY, Onbul HZ, San A, Odabas AR. Changes in frequency and etiology of acute renal failure in pregnancy (1980-1997). Ren Fail. 1998;20(3):513-7.
2. Prakash J, Niwas SS, Parekh A, Pandey LK, Sharatchandra L, Arora P, et al. Acute kidney injury in late pregnancy in developing countries. Ren Fail. 2010;32:309-13.
3. Ympa YP, Sakr Y, Reinhart K, Vincent JL. Has mortality from acute renal failure decreased? A systematic review of the literature. Am J Med. 2005;118(8):827-32
4. Gonzalez Suarez ML, Kattah A, Grande JP, Garovic V. Renal Disorders in Pregnancy: Core Curriculum 2019. Am J Kidney Dis. 2019;73(1):119-30.
5. Roy C, Saussine C, Jahn C, Le Bras Y, Steichen G, Delepaul B, et al. Fast imaging MR assessment of ureterohydronephrosis during pregnancy. Magn Reson Imaging. 1995;13:767.
6. Stratta P, Besso L, Canavese C, Grill A, Todros T, Benedetto C, et al. Is Pregnancy-Related Acute Renal Failure a Disappearing Clinical Entity? Ren Fail. 1996;18(4):575-84.
7. Wiles K, Bramham K, Seed PT, Nelson-Piercy C, Lightstone L, Chappell LC. Serum Creatinine in Pregnancy: A Systematic Review. Kidney Int Rep. 2019;4(3):408-19.
8. Gonzalez Suarez ML, Kattah A, Grande JP, Garovic V. Renal Disorders in Pregnancy: Core Curriculum 2019. Am J Kidney Dis. 2019;73(1):119-30.
9. Jeong JY, Kim SH, Lee HJ, Sim JS. Atypical low-signal-intensity renal parenchyma: Causes and patterns. Radiographics. 2002;22:833-46.
10. Anantharaman P, Schmidt R, Holley J. Pregnancy and renal diseases. In: Nissenson A, Berns J, Lerma E (Eds). Current Diagnosis and Treatment: Nephrology and Hypertension. United States: McGraw-Hill International Edition; 2009. pp. 497-8.
11. Krane NK, Hamrahian M. Pregnancy: Kidney diseases and hypertension. Am J Kidney Dis. 2007;49:336-45.

211

CHAPTER

Urinary Tract Infection in Pregnancy

Ramesh Mundle, Shuchita Mundle

ABSTRACT

Asymptomatic and symptomatic urinary infections are a common problem in pregnancy. Due to potential risk to mother and fetus, early detection and prompt treatment of urinary tract infections (UTIs) remains the gold standard. It is advisable to assess the risk factors for UTI in pregnancy. Asymptomatic bacteriuria (ASB) should be diagnosed by routine screening during pregnancy. Untreated asymptomatic infections can progress to lower and upper urinary tract, with persistent and recurrent symptoms and signs. Pyelonephritis is associated with adverse pregnancy outcomes such as intrauterine growth restriction, preeclampsia, and premature delivery.

Acute pyelonephritis is a serious complication and needs hospitalization and parenteral antibiotics.

INTRODUCTION

Urinary tract infections (UTIs) are the common during pregnancy. UTIs can present as asymptomatic bacteriuria (ASB), symptomatic cystitis, or pyelonephritis. ASB is associated with preeclampsia, preterm births, and low birth weight babies.

EPIDEMIOLOGY

The prevalence of ASB varies between 2 and 10%, acute cystitis is seen in about 1 to 4% of pregnant women, and the prevalence of acute pyelonephritis ranges between 0.5 and 2% of pregnancies. The prevalence of UTI in women attending antenatal clinic was reported as 15% in rural Bangalore and 12.2% in a study in New Delhi.

SIGNIFICANCE OF UTI IN PREGNANCY

Risk of UTI begins in the 6th week and has its peak during the 22nd to 24th weeks.

About 25% of women with untreated ASB will progress to symptomatic infection during pregnancy. Untreated UTI or ASB during pregnancy increases the risk of pyelonephritis, sepsis, and transient renal failure. All women should be screened for ASB at the first antenatal visit.

A meta-analysis of 19 cohort studies, among women with ASB showed that untreated ASB during pregnancy significantly increased rates of low birth weight babies and preterm delivery.

There is an increased risk of preeclampsia in women with either ASB or symptomatic UTI as was seen in a case control study of over 15,000 pregnant women.

Pyelonephritis is associated with adverse pregnancy outcomes such as intrauterine growth restriction, preeclampsia, and premature delivery.

PHYSIOLOGICAL CHANGES DURING PREGNANCY

Pregnancy leads to both structural and functional changes in urinary tract. There is an increase in size of kidney with dilatation of renal calyces and ureters, starting before 14 weeks due to the relaxation effect of progesterone, increasing in mid pregnancy due to ureteral compression by the gravid uterus. Stasis of urine, vesicoureteral reflux, and gestational diabetes predisposes to symptomatic upper urinary infections.

Puerperal urinary tract infections are common due to decreased sensitivity of the bladder to intravesical fluid tension in women who have labor trauma or conduction analgesia and anesthesia. Episiotomy, periurethral lacerations, and vaginal wall hematoma may add to bladder insensitivity and urinary retention with the need for catheterization, contributing to infection.

Risk factors that predispose a woman to urinary tract infections, especially during pregnancy are low socioeconomic status, sexual activity, older age, multiparity, anatomical urinary tract abnormalities, sickle cell disease, and diabetes. Bacteriuria is acquired by many women before pregnancy. Bacteriuria and urinary tract infection before pregnancy are two strongest predictors for urinary tract infection and pyelonephritis after 20 weeks' gestation.

Organisms Leading to Urinary Tract Infection in Pregnancy

The organisms that cause UTI in pregnancy are those from normal perineal flora, *Escherichia coli* strains cause approximately 90% of the infections. *E. coli* has adhesins such as P and S fimbriae; these are cell surface proteins that enhance bacterial adherence to uroepithelial cells, through expression of *papG* gene. This gene encodes F fimbriae tip by production of toxins and other virulence factors. Other bacteria that can cause infection are *Klebsiella*, coagulase-negative staphylococci, staphylococci aureus, and Group B streptococci.

Asymptomatic bacteriuria is defined as presence of positive urine culture in a given woman without any clinical manifestations. Cystitis during pregnancy is more likely in women who have ASB before pregnancy. Screening for bacteriuria at first antenatal visit and a positive urine culture (>100,000 organisms/mL) is diagnostic. Unlike nonpregnant females, ASB during pregnancy needs treatment to reduce the maternal and fetal risks. A low colony count of 20,000–50,000 should also be treated to prevent pyelonephritis which may be occur in about 30% women who have ASB.

Asymptomatic bacteriuria responds to empirical treatment with any of the several antimicrobial agents listed in **Table 1**. Longer duration is preferred over single-dose therapy to prevent covert upper urinary tract infection. In persistent or frequent bacteriuria, suppression therapy with nitrofurantoin 100 mg orally can be given throughout pregnancy.

Lower urinary tract infection (LUTI) includes urethritis and cystitis. The symptoms are dysuria, urinary frequency, urgency, painful urination, lower abdominal discomfort, and sometimes hematuria. ASB may progress to acute cystitis/urethritis three to four times more frequently in

TABLE 1: Treatment of asymptomatic bacteriuria (ASB) and lower urinary tract infection (LUTI).

Antibiotic	Dose	Duration
Nitrofurantoin	100 mg, twice a day	5–7 days
Amoxicillin	• 500 mg, thrice a day • 875 mg orally twice a day	5–7 days
Amoxicillin–clavulanate	• 500 mg, thrice a day • 875 mg orally twice a day	5–7 days
Cephalexin	250–500 mg orally every 6 hours	5–7 days
Cefpodoxime	100 mg orally every 12 hours	5–7 days
Fosfomycin	3 g orally as single dose	–
Trimethoprim–sulfamethoxazole	800/160 mg (1 double-strength tablet) every 12 hours	3 days

pregnant women due to the anatomical and physiological changes of pregnancy.

Management in most cases of lower UTI should be guided by culture and sensitivity testing. The optimum duration of treatment should be about 5–7 days. A follow-up urine culture should be done after 1–2 weeks of treatment. Women who have recurrent cystitis, antimicrobial urinary suppression may be given in small doses on a daily basis.

Acute pyelonephritis is the most common medical problem affecting 2% of all pregnancies mostly in the second and third trimester. It is usually as a consequence of undiagnosed and inappropriately treated LUTI or ASB. Other risk factors for acute pyelonephritis are age, nulliparity, sickle cell anemia, diabetes, nephrolithiasis, past history of pyelonephritis, and maternal urinary tract defects.

Women with acute pyelonephritis present with of high-grade fever (>38°C), chills, nausea, vomiting and lumbar pain. Septicemia may complicate acute pyelonephritis in about 20% of the cases. Pyelonephritis is unilateral and right-sided in more than half the cases. Tenderness can be elucidated on one or both costovertebral angels. The differential diagnosis includes preterm labor, chorioamnionitis, appendicitis, placental abruption, or red degeneration in a leiomyoma. Complications of acute pyelonephritis include anemia, septicemia, transient renal dysfunction, and pulmonary insufficiency. Endotoxin-induced alveolar injury may result into pulmonary edema and may occur and in severe cases with acute respiratory distress syndrome (ARDS).

According to 2005 Infectious Disease Society of America guidelines, all suspected cases of pyelonephritis should be hospitalized for initial 48 hours of treatment. Basic laboratory tests like complete blood count (CBC), renal function test, liver function test, coagulation profile, urine and blood culture should be done. An ultrasound scan is mandatory to exclude other causes with similar clinical profile such as liver abscess, ureteric obstruction and other abdominal infections.

Appropriate hydration and parenteral antibiotics should be given to all patients empirically for and laboratory tests like CBC, renal function test, liver function test, coagulation profile, and urine and blood culture should be done. An ultrasound scan will exclude other causes with similar clinical profile such as liver abscess, ureteric obstruction, and other abdominal infections.

Appropriate hydration and parenteral antibiotics should be given to all patients empirically for at least first 48 hours until resolution of fever. A change of antibiotics is required after obtaining microbial sensitivity test results. Oral administration of drugs can is possible after 48 hours of resolution of symptoms if the intravenous (IV) antibiotic has a suitable oral substitute. If fever persists for >48 hours, possible causes like perirenal abscess, urolithiasis, and congenital and acquired changes of the urinary tract should be considered.

Usual duration of antibiotic therapy is 10–14 days, although there are no guidelines for its optimum duration. Beta lactam antibiotics are the most commonly prescribed drugs as they are relatively safe for the fetus. Fluoroquinolones and aminoglycosides, which are often used for pyelonephritis in nonpregnant individuals, should be avoided during pregnancy.

Higher antibiotics are reserved for treatment of more severe cases or those caused by multi-drug-resistant bacteria. Recurrences of episodes of pyelonephritis can be troublesome. In such cases, during the asymptomatic period, prophylactic treatment is recommended with nitrofurantoin or cephalexin at bedtime.

The problem of rapid antibiotic resistance, specially gram-negative bacilli is emerging rapidly. Currently more than half of the *E. coli* strains and one-third of *Klebsiella* are extended-spectrum beta-lactamases (ESBL)-positive, causing resistance to third-generation cephalosporins. Enterobacteriaceae strains are resistant to all beta lactam and carbapenem antibiotics. Methicillin-resistant gram-positive cocci also pose a grave problem **(Table 2)**.

TABLE 2: Diagnosis and treatment of acute pyelonephritis.

Diagnosis	*Symptoms + urine culture*: Fever > 38°C, lumbar pain, skeletal and joint pains, nausea/vomiting with or without accompanying dysuria, polyuria ≥ 10^5 CFU/mL in mid-stream urine specimen
Mild or moderate acute pyelonephritis	• Ceftriaxone 1 g every 24 hours • Cefepime 1 g every 24 hours • Amoxicillin with clavulanic acid 1.2 g every 12 hours • Aztreonam 1 g every 8–12 hours
Severe acute pyelonephritis immunosuppression/ urinary stasis	• Ticarcillin with clavulanic acid 3.1 g every 6 hours • Piperacillin with tazobactam 3.375 g every 6 hours • Meropenem 0.5 g every 8 hours • Ertapenem 1 g every 24 hours • Doripenem 500 mg every 8 hours

KEY POINTS

- The changes in pregnancy and childbirth increases the risk of urinary tract infections.
- All women should have a routine screening for ASB during their first antenatal visit.
- Urinary tract infections during pregnancy increases the risk for preeclampsia, intrauterine growth restriction, and preterm birth.
- Due to potential risk to mother and fetus, early detection and prompt treatment of UTIs remains the gold standard. It is advisable to assess the risk factors for UTI in pregnancy.
- Acute pyelonephritis, is a serious maternal infection, needs hospitalization and parenteral antibiotics to avoid complications of septicemia and ARDS.
- Most of the antibiotics are safe during the second and third trimester, but should be used judiciously to avoid emergence of bacterial resistance.

SUGGESTED READINGS

1. Corrales M, Corrales-Acosta E, Corrales-Riveros JG. Which Antibiotic for Urinary Tract Infections in Pregnancy? A Literature Review of International Guidelines. J Clin Med. 2022;11:7226.
2. Gupta K, Calderwood SB, Lockwood CJ, Bloom A. (2023). Urinary tract infections and asymptomatic bacteriuria in pregnancy. [online] Available from https://medilib.ir/uptodate/show/8065 [Last accessed December, 2023].
3. Cunningham F, Leveno KJ, Bloom SL, Dashe JS, Hoffman BL, Casey BM, Spong CY. Renal and urinary tract disorders. Williams Obstetrics, 25th edition. Italy: McGraw Hill; 2018.

212

CHAPTER

Management of Thyrotoxicosis in Pregnancy

Saumik Datta

ABSTRACT

The management of thyroid disorders in pregnancy, particularly thyrotoxicosis, always starts with a concern whether it is a physiological change related to pregnancy or Graves' disease. Gestational transient thyrotoxicosis (GTT) does not need antithyroid drug. In case of preexisting Graves' disease, management policy should be planned before pregnancy. Thyroid stimulating hormone (TSH) receptor antibody (TRAb) should be evaluated. The scope of definitive therapy before conception, either surgery or radioactive iodine (RAI) ablation, must be discussed. In case of antithyroid drug use, the risk-benefit ratio of both propylthiouracil (PTU) and methimazole should be explained to the patient with emphasis on teratogenicity. PTU is recommended in the first trimester and methimazole for the remaining part of pregnancy. Thyrotoxicosis and its management during pregnancy always involve a concern for the fetus. This concern is not confined only within teratogenicity, but also involves the chance of fetal hypothyroid as well as thyrotoxicosis. This remains an issue even after the birth of the baby.

INTRODUCTION

Proper functioning of thyroid axis is very much needed for growth and reproduction. Thyrotoxicosis is always a difficult condition to detect, diagnose, and manage. In the background of pregnancy, the situation becomes more difficult not only because one has to take care of the fetus but also because one may fail to detect features of thyrotoxicosis, as clinical features of pregnancy may overlap with thyrotoxicosis.

Heat intolerance, exertional dyspnea, palpitations, etc., are common in both conditions. But the threshold of suspicion should always be low, particularly if the lady had a prior history of thyroid disorder, family history of the same, goiter, eye signs, or other features of an autoimmune disorder. One should consider the possibility of thyroid-related disorder with priority. However, routine thyroid function testing in pregnancy has now become easier with the wide availability of thyroid function tests. This has reduced the chance of missing the case.

GESTATIONAL TRANSIENT THYROTOXICOSIS

Once a report comes that is suggestive of thyrotoxicosis, clinicians must be very much judicious about the possibility of gestational transient thyrotoxicosis (GTT). It is not rare in pregnancy. This high human chorionic gonadotropin (hCG) dependent condition is prevalent in the first trimester. hCG can cause thyroid stimulation due to its structural similarity to thyroid-stimulating hormone (TSH). GTT is more common in multiple pregnancies and hydatidiform mole for obvious reasons. Hyperemesis gravidarum is another condition which may lead to GTT. In the preconception euthyroid clinical state, the absence of goiter or eye features favors the possibility of GTT. Serum free thyroxine (FT4) is elevated and TSH is suppressed. In contrast to Graves' disease, triiodothyronine (T3) is not much elevated. Labetalol is enough to control thyrotoxic features. Atenolol should be avoided because of the low-birth-weight (LBW) potential associated with it. Antithyroid drugs are not required in most cases.

GRAVES' DISEASE

The severity of Graves' disease is highly influenced in different trimesters of pregnancy. The first trimester of pregnancy shows exacerbation, whereas the second half of pregnancy is associated with some attenuation of symptoms. The postpartum period may come again come up with exaggerated symptoms.

Thyroid hormones from mothers can cross the placenta and the fetus can present with features of hyperthyroidism and 1–5% of the neonates can develop hyperthyroidism or Graves' disease. Untreated hyperthyroidism in pregnancy may be associated with LBW and prematurity. Eclampsia is also a known complication. However, the outcome is usually good when the hyperthyroid state is managed well by a skilled person throughout the pregnancy.

Preconception Management

Management of hyperthyroidism during pregnancy in a prospective mother with Graves' disease should be planned beforehand with preconception counseling. It is better to avoid pregnancy while in a hyperthyroid state.

Patients may be counseled for ablative therapy. In the case of radioactive iodine (RAI) ablation, one should defer pregnancy for 6 months. This window will help to stabilize the dose of levothyroxine. Following RAI ablation, the TSH receptor antibody (TRAb) value is initially increased and remains elevated for more or less than 12 months, followed by a gradual lowering. If the initial TRAb is on the higher side, then the patient may be planned for surgical intervention. The TRAb value comes down relatively fast following thyroidectomy.

Role of Antithyroid Drugs

In demanding situations, the patient may need to continue antithyroid drugs. Both drugs are associated with teratogenic effects and enjoy similar placental transfer kinetics. However, malformations due to propylthiouracil (PTU) are less frequent and less severe. Methimazole can produce aplasia cutis, a localized punched-out lesion on the parietal part of the scalp. Choanal atresia and esophageal atresia have also been reported in infants born to mothers on methimazole. If the lady is on methimazole therapy at the time of planning pregnancy or conception, she should be switched to PTU. The initial dose is 50 mg twice or thrice daily. However, it should not be continued beyond the first trimester because of apprehension of fatal hepatotoxicity. After the first trimester, a mother should be put on methimazole again within a dose range of 10–20 mg/day. The target of treatment is to make the mother euthyroid as fast as possible with the application of a minimum amount of drug. The thyroid axis should be tested every 4 weeks. The biochemical goal is to keep FT4 at or just above the normal range. However, TSH may remain suppressed for a long time. Normalization of TSH indicates lowering of dose. Otherwise, the fetus may develop hypothyroidism. Most mothers improve within 4–6 weeks. The dose should be adjusted accordingly; it may be halved. Because the TRAb level is reduced in the second part of pregnancy, thyrotoxic features also improve with progression of pregnancy. Sometimes, it has led to a drug-free period.

Often, hyperdynamic features are prominent. We can tackle it with either propranolol or labetalol. Tablet labetalol may be used twice daily within a dose range of 100–400 mg/day. Once the hyperdynamic features are under control, beta-blockers can be withdrawn after the initial few weeks.

Surgery

Thyroidectomy may be indicated in certain conditions. Sometimes, patients do not tolerate antithyroid drugs. Often, they are noncompliant. Rarely, if the goiter is large, the patient may not respond well. Surgery should be planned in the second trimester with adequate preparation. Beta-blocker will reduce hyperdynamic features. A short-term potassium iodide solution will reduce the vascularity of the thyroid gland.

Radioactive Iodine

Radioactive iodine ablation with iodine-131 therapy in pregnancy is contraindicated. It can produce fetal hypothyroidism.

Fetal and Neonatal Thyroid Dysfunction

Fetal and neonatal thyroid dysfunction is always a matter of concern while treating a mother with active Graves' disease or dealing with a mother with a past history of Graves' disease.

A high maternal serum TRAb value may produce fetal hyperthyroidism. Therefore, the maternal serum TRAb value should be assessed on initial evaluation, whenever possible. If the value is high, it should be repeated around 18–20 weeks. This is the time when fetal TSH receptors start responding to TRAb. A TRAb value more than 2–3 times indicates the possibility of fetal thyrotoxicosis. Fetal goiter appears first followed by fetal tachycardia. Fetal tachycardia means fetal heart rate is > 160 beats/min. Fetal heart monitor tracing can show a unique pattern. It can pick up a sustained baseline value of around 170 beats/min along with moderate variability that exhibits acceleration more than deceleration. Intrauterine growth retardation and oligohydramnios are other common features of fetal thyrotoxicosis. Accelerated bone maturation is an important point to note. It is defined by distal femoral ossification before 31 weeks' gestation. Cordocentesis can be applied for the direct assessment of fetal thyroid function. However, it is always a risky procedure and may lead to fetal loss

On the other hand, antithyroid drugs may insult the fetal thyroid gland. The fetal thyroid gland is more sensitive to antithyroid drugs than a mother's gland. Hence, dose reduction must be done once the maternal thyroid function report comes within the normal range.

From the above discussion, it is clear that dose adjustment of antithyroid drugs should also be guided by fetal growth and fetal heart rate.

Lactation

Lactation is another issue. Both drugs are secreted in breast milk. However, breastfeeding is not harmful to the baby if the daily dose of PTU is <450 mg or that of methimazole is <20 mg.

TOXIC NODULAR GOITER

Toxic nodular goiter is another common cause of hyperthyroidism. However, it is not so common in childbearing age. If detected, it is better to go for definitive treatment. Antithyroid drugs should be used very carefully. They can lead to fetal hypothyroidism more frequently than Graves' disease, as there is no TRAb to counteract the effect of antithyroid drugs.

CONCLUSION

Management of thyrotoxicosis in pregnancy needs passion and patience. It is a highly skilled job and treatment must be optimized. Both undertreatment and overtreatment of a mother may lead to fetal hyperthyroid and hypothyroid states, respectively. Judicious selection of treatment option and dose monitoring with fine-tuning guided not only by maternal thyroid function test report but also by fetal condition will help in smooth sailing through this phase.

SUGGESTED READINGS

1. Glinoer D, Spencer CA. Serum TSH determinations in pregnancy: How, when and why? Nat Rev Endocrinol. 2010;6:526-9.
2. Tamaki H, Itoh E, Kaneda T, Asahi K, Mitsuda N, Tanizawa O, et al. Crucial role of serum human chorionic gonadotropin for the aggravation of thyrotoxicosis in early pregnancy in Graves' disease. Thyroid. 1993;3(3):189-93.
3. Weetman AP: Graves' disease. N Engl J Med. 2000;343:1236-48.
4. Azizi F, Amouzegar A. Management of hyperthyroidism during pregnancy and lactation. Eur J Endocrinol. 2011;164:871-6.
5. Moore LE. Thyroid disease in pregnancy: A review of diagnosis, complications and management. World J Obstet Gynecol. 2016;5:66-72.

SECTION 18

PULMONOLOGY

213

CHAPTER

Health Effects of Air Pollution

AS Mohan

ABSTRACT

Air is crucial for all living organisms, and air pollution is a hazardous environmental issue. It causes vital damage, including respiratory issues, and cancer, and harms plants, animals, and ecosystems. Air pollution has been present since ancient times and is linked to global warming, caused by high levels of fumes and chemicals from oil and coal, leading to temperature rise and potential human death.

INTRODUCTION

Air is part and parcel of living organisms both for plants and animals. We cannot live without air for more than a few minutes. But we can live without food and water for a few days. What is air pollution? It is the presence of gas, liquid, and solid matters in excess than required for the survival of the cells. Oxygen (O_2) present in the air is essential for the cells to survive. Air pollution is the most dangerous environmental pollution. Air pollution has been there since the Stone Age when people learned to cook food with fire. Air pollution occurs inside houses, schools, cities, across continents, and globally. Air pollution makes people sick. It causes breathing problems and promotes cancer. It harms plants, animals, and the ecosystem. Air pollution directly leads to global warming. It is due to the presence of high levels of fumes and poisonous chemicals present in the atmosphere. These are mainly produced by the burning of oil and coal by the heavy industries. This in turn causes a rise in atmospheric temperature. This causes morbidity and mortality in many organisms including humans.

CAUSES OF AIR POLLUTION

We will discuss about the major causes of air pollution.

Burning Fossil Fuels

Natural gas, coal, and oil in industries and motor vehicles. These emit harmful chemical components into the atmosphere. They are carbon dioxide, carbon monoxide, sulfur dioxide, nitrogen oxides, and tiny solid particles like lead-called particulates.

Motor Vehicles

When fuels are incompletely burned various volatile organic chemicals (VOCs) enter into the atmosphere.

Decomposed Garbage

In landfills and solid waste disposal sites emits methane gas.

Pollutants from Natural Sources

Forest Fires

Emit VOCs and particulates into the atmosphere.

Volcanos

Spew out sulfur dioxide (SO_2) and large amounts of pulverized lava rock known as 'volcanic ash'.

Unlike pollutants from human activity, naturally occurring pollutants tend to remain in the atmosphere for a short time and do not lead to permanent atmospheric change or damage. Once in the atmosphere, pollutants often undergo chemical reactions that produce additional harmful compounds. Air pollution is subject to weather patterns that can trap it in valleys or blow it across the globe to damage a pristine environment far from the original sources.

EFFECTS OF AIR POLLUTION

- Greenhouse effects
- Particulate contamination
- Increased ultraviolet (UV) radiation
- Acid rain
- Increased ground-level ozone concentration
- Increased levels of nitrogen oxides

MAJOR POLLUTANTS PRODUCED BY HUMAN ACTIVITIES

Sulfur Oxides

Sulfur oxides, particularly SO_2. SO_2 is produced by volcanoes and various industrial processes. Coal and petroleum often contain sulfur compounds and their combustion generates SO_2. Industrial processes such as extracting metal from ore will produce SO_2. Oxidation of SO_2 usually in the presence of a catalyst such as nitrogen dioxide (NO_2) forms H_2SO_4 (sulfuric acid) and thus produces acid rain.

Nitrogen Oxides

Nitrogen dioxide is produced from high-temperature combustion. It is also produced during thunderstorms. This reddish-brown toxic gas has a pungent smell.

Carbon Monoxide

Carbon monoxide (CO) is produced by the incomplete combustion of natural gas, coal, wood, etc. It is a colorless, odorless, and nonirritant toxic gas. Exhaust from vehicles using fuels is the major source of CO. Naturally CO is formed from photochemical reactions in volcanoes and forest fires.

Volatile Organic Compounds

Volatile organic compounds are well-known outdoor air pollutants such as methane and nonmethane gases. Methane causes global warming. The aromatic nonmethane VOCs such as benzene, toluene, and xylene are suspected carcinogens and may lead to leukemia with prolonged exposure.

Particulates

They are known as particulate matter (PM), atmospheric particulate matter or fine particles are tiny particles of solid or liquid suspended in a gas. 'Inhalable coarse particles found near roadways and industries, are larger than 2.5 μm and smaller than 10 μm in diameter'. Fine particles, are found in smoke and haze and are 2.5 μm in diameter. These particles are emitted from forest fires, power plants, industries, and automobiles. Particulate matter contains microscopic solids or liquid droplets when inhaled cause serious health problems.

Aerosol

Some particulates occur naturally, originating from volcanoes, dust, storms, forest and grassland fires, living vegetation, and sea spray, human activities, such as the burning of fossil fuels in vehicles, power plants, and various industrial processes also generate significant amounts of aerosols. Worldwide anthropogenic aerosols, those made by human activities currently account for 10% of our atmosphere. Increased levels of fine particles in the air are linked to health hazards such as heart disease, altered lung functions, and lung cancer.

Chlorofluorocarbons

Harmful to the ozone layer. Currently banned from use.

Ammonia

Ammonia (NH_3) is emitted from agricultural processes. Normally encountered as a gas-characteristic pungent odor. Contributes significantly to the nutritional needs of terrestrial organisms by serving as a precursor to foodstuffs and fertilizers. Ammonia either directly or indirectly is also a building block for the synthesis of many pharmaceuticals. Ammonia is both caustic and hazardous.

Lead

Major sources of lead in the air are ore and metals processing, aircraft operating on leaded aviation fuel, waste incinerators, utilities, and lead-acid battery manufacturers. The highest air concentrations of lead are found near lead smelters. Volcanic activity is the primary natural source of atmospheric lead. As a result of the government's regulatory efforts, the removal of lead from motor vehicle gasoline, levels of lead in the air decreased by 98% between 1980 and 2014.

Radioactive Pollutants

Nuclear reactors do not produce air pollution or carbon dioxide while operating. Radioactive pollutants are produced by nuclear explosions, nuclear accidents, war explosives, and natural processes such as the radioactive decay of Radon.

Pollution occurs when:

- The process of mining uranium releases high amounts of carbon dioxide into the environment.
- Carbon dioxide is also released into the environment when new nuclear plants are built.
- Transport of radioactive waste also causes carbon dioxide emissions.
- Nuclear disasters, e.g., atomic bomb during World War II (1945), Chernobyl disaster (1986), and Fukushima Nuclear Disaster (2011).

Persistent Organic Pollutants

These are organic matter that are resistant to environmental degradation through chemical, biological, and photolytic processes. It is observed that they persist in the environment to be capable of long-range transport, bioaccumulate in human and animal tissue, and biomagnify in food chains. They have significant impacts on humans and the environment.

Ground Level Ozone

Ozone is formed when energetic UV radiation dissociates molecules of O_2 into separate O_2 atoms.

If a free oxygen atom (O-2) collides with an O_2 molecule, it joins up, forming ozone (O_3).

Odors

From garbage, sewage, and industrial processes.

EFFECTS OF AIR POLLUTION

Air pollution causes many diseases without awareness. Air pollution will cause short and long-term effects on the human body.

Short-term Effects

Air pollution will cause the following short-term effects. Constant itching of the nose, and sore throat, which may cause difficulty in breathing. Causes itching and watering in the eyes. It causes headaches and dizziness by its bad smell which is made by smoke or car emissions. A large number of microorganisms can be transmitted through air in an area.

Long-term Effects

It will last for an entire lifetime. They cause increased morbidity and mortality. One-third of deaths from stroke, carcinoma, and heart conditions are because of air pollution.

CARBON MONOXIDE(CO)

Breathing air with a high concentration of CO reduces the amount of O_2 that can be transported to vital organs like the heart and brain. At very high levels, in enclosed environments, CO can cause dizziness, confusion, unconsciousness, and even death.

LEAD

Lead is distributed throughout the body via blood and is accumulated in the bones. High levels of exposure, to lead affect the nervous system, kidney, immune system, reproductive, and cardiovascular systems. Lead exposure also affects the O_2-carrying capacity of the blood.

OZONE

Breathing ozone can cause a variety of health problems, particularly for children, the elderly, and people with lung diseases. Ground-level ozone can also have harmful effects on sensitive vegetation and ecosystems.

PARTICULATE MATTERS (FIG. 1)

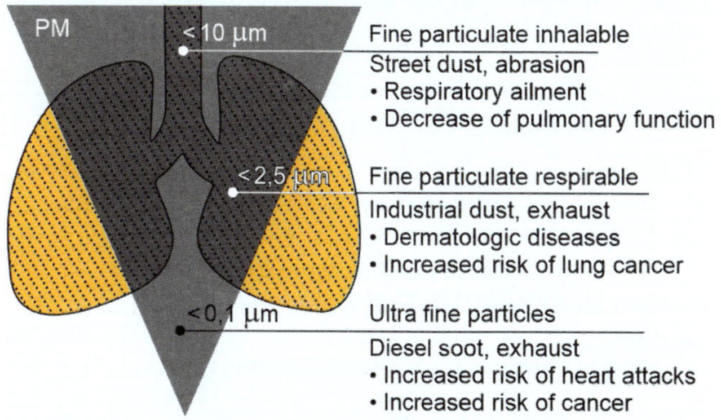

FIG. 1: Types and effects of particulate matter (PM).

NITROUS OXIDE

High concentrations of NO_2 will irritate the airway. Even after short exposure will cause damage to the respiratory system leading to respiratory illnesses. Longer exposures to elevated concentrations of NO_2 may contribute to the development of asthma and potentially increase susceptibility to respiratory infections. People with asthma, especially children and the elderly are generally at greater risk for the health effects of NO_2. NO_2 along with other NO_x reacts with other chemicals in the air to form both particulate matter and ozone. Both of these are also harmful when inhaled due to their effects on the respiratory system.

SULFUR OXIDES

Sulfur dioxide in high concentrations will damage the plants by decreasing their growth. It will cause acid rain and damage the ecosystem. Even brief exposure will affect the lungs leading to dyspnea.

NUCLEAR AIR POLLUTION

Nuclear pollution consists of radiation emitted from atomic nuclei. These radiations are highly injurious to living beings.

Nuclear waste contains highly poisonous chemicals, such as plutonium and uranium pellets. These extremely toxic materials remain highly radioactive for thousands of years posing a threat to agricultural land, fishing waters, freshwater sources, and humans.

Exposure to very high levels of radiation such as being close to an atomic blast can cause acute health effects such as skin burns and acute radiation syndrome (vomiting, diarrhea, fatigue, and reduction in immunity). It can also result in long-term health effects, such as cancer, anemia, birth defects, genetic damage, and cardiovascular disease.

METHODS TO REDUCE AIR POLLUTION

- Drive your car less
- Keep your car in good repair
- Switch to electric motors and equipment
- Do not burn your garbage
- Control of dust particles by improving sanitary conditions within the houses and in public.
- Stop deforestation. Any kind of plant helps the environment's air to be clean. Plants inhale CO_2, which is one of the most common causes of air pollution, and exhale O_2 which makes the air go back to its original composition.
- Produce clean energies, such as solar and wind energies. It does not lead to long-term health damage, because it does not need to burn fossil fuels to produce energy.
- Publish the idea of air pollution and its effects on magazines and social media to educate people.

School children to be taught about environmental pollution.

CONCLUSION

Air pollution plays a significant role in the environment. Air pollution has many effects on every organism living on this earth. Humans are most prone to pollution-related diseases which can lead to death. Air pollution directly results in global warming. We can reduce the effects of air pollution. The first is to produce solar and wind energy which does not affect the natural environment. Stop cutting down the trees since they are very helpful in producing fresh air. Finally, raising people's awareness about air pollution. We should do our best to reduce air pollution to make our globe clean and our bodies healthy.

SUGGESTED READINGS

1. Dawson K, Allan J, Fergusson D. Asthma, air pollution, and climate: a Christchurch study. NZ Med J. 1983;96(727):165-7.
2. Scoggins A, Kjellstrom T, Fisher G, Connor J, Gimson N. Spatial analysis of annual air pollution exposure and mortality. Sci Total Environ. 2004;321(1-3):71-85.
3. Clelland P, Lyne M, Salmond JA, Chelimo C, Dirks KA. Nitrogen dioxide exposure at early childhood centres next to high and low-traffic roads in Auckland, New Zealand. Air Quality and Climate Change. 2015;49(1):28-31.
4. Loscalzo J, Fauci F, Kasper D, Hauser S, Longo D, Jameson JL. Harrisson's Text Book of Internal Medicine, 21st edition. New York: McGraw Hill; 2022.

214

CHAPTER

Changing Trends in Etiopathogenesis of Asthma

M Sabir, Rishabh Kochar

ABSTRACT

Asthma is amongst the most common chronic respiratory diseases. It is characterized by variability in symptoms and airflow obstruction which is usually worsened by environmental triggers acting in concordance with presensitization to environmental antigens, airway inflammation, and airway hyperresponsiveness. Global warming, pollution, climate change and its effects on the weather pattern, and obesity epidemic are some of the newly identified and modifiable risk factors for asthma. With these emerging threats, we are also better understanding the pathogenesis of asthma and how the environmental factors act in synchrony with genetic and host factors leading to eventual development of asthma. Asthma involves both the conducting airways—large and the small, and is characterized by varying combination of inflammation and structural remodeling that might begin in utero. In many patients asthma can spontaneously remit or begin de novo in adulthood, and the factors that lead to the emergence and regression of asthma, irrespective of age, are poorly understood. Better understanding of the pathogenesis has allowed us to provide targeted and highly effective therapies for controlling asthma and reducing the morbidity. Despite significant advances, much work needs to be done for primary prevention of asthma and reducing the asthma-related mortality. Following section deals with newly identified risk factors, pathogenic mechanisms, and therapeutic targets for asthma.

INTRODUCTION

Asthma is common chronic inflammatory disease of the airways characterized by variable symptoms with variable airflow obstruction. It affects >300 million children and adults worldwide. Common symptoms associated with asthma are wheezing, cough with or without sputum, chest tightness, and breathlessness. The hallmark of the disease lies in the variable nature of both symptoms and airflow obstruction which is frequently reversible on treatment with inhaled beta agonists. The variability varies from patient to patient and may have specific patterns like diurnal, seasonal, work-related or exercise- and effort-related to note a few. Pathogenesis of asthma involves a complex interplay of multiple genetic, environmental, and host factors which influence the course and outcome of the disease. With newer threats such as global warming, environmental pollution, changing weather patterns, and newer infectious agents, we are unraveling newer mechanisms into the pathogenesis of asthma. While these are causing increased incidence of asthma and worsening control among preexisting asthmatics, their identification as a problem also offers an opportunity to target these issues before they grow out of control. The following sections will discuss established and emerging risk factors for asthma and newer insights into the pathophysiology.

Few risk factors have been strongly associated with asthma and are supported by data from large number of patients.

- *Allergy*: Personal and family history of allergy and atopic symptoms are one of the strongest risk factors of asthma-increasing the risk by three- to fourfold.
- *Viral and bacterial infections*: Respiratory viral infections by respiratory syncytial virus (RSV) in childhood increases risk of subsequent wheezing illness and asthma by up to four times. Similarly, *Chlamydia pneumoniae* and *Mycoplasma pneumoniae* have been implicated in asthma exacerbations.
- *Hygiene hypothesis*: This hypothesis implies that rise in allergic diseases in childhood and adulthood is a

consequence of reduced rate of exposure to infections and bacterial and environmental antigens such as house dust mite and pollen.

- *Air pollution*: Air pollution is associated with both development of new asthma and exacerbation of preexisting asthma. Exposure to air pollution in children leads to nearly 4 million more new cases per year.
- *Early life factors*: Maternal obesity and excess weight gain during pregnancy, maternal vitamin D and E deficiency, acute viral respiratory infections (RSV, rhinovirus), antibiotic use, birth by cesarean section, nutritional disorders (overweight, obesity), food sensitization (not very common), inadequate physical activity, second hand smoke exposure (parental smoking) while breast feeding are other factors known to increase the risk of asthma specially among children.
- *Occupational exposures*: These include organic dusts derived from plant and animal matter, synthetic compounds such as aniline dyes, acrolein, and inorganic compounds such as metal fumes and smokes.

NEWER INSIGHTS AND NOVEL RISK FACTORS ASSOCIATED WITH ASTHMA

Many new factors are emerging as risk for asthma and its exacerbation. Meanwhile we are also increasing our knowledge on previously poorly understood factors such as thunderstorms and how they affect asthma. One important point to understand is that unlike other organs of the body, human lung is incompletely developed at birth and continues to grow by up to 20 years of age. Thus, any insult to lungs in childhood, be it from infections, pollution, malnutrition and many other agents, predisposes to arrested development of the lung leading to desynapsis and alveolar underdevelopment.

- *Microbiome*: The environmental, airway, and gut microbiome influence each other and in turn the development and outcome of asthma. The influence of microbes on asthma development has been discussed time and again in hygiene hypothesis and childhood infections, but the mechanism by which they lead to asthma was not known. With newer isolation methods such as whole genome sequencing light is being shed on the microbial composition of lung and its impact on diseases.

Studies have shown that lungs are not sterile as previously believed but have a microbiome derived from oropharynx and upper airways. The lung microbiome is responsible for development of immune tolerance, immune activation, and maturation of lymphocytes, and host defense. Infection with pathogenic organisms, change in environmental microbial composition and alteration in gut biome all disrupts this balance and lead to dysbiosis. This results in replacement of normal lung flora with pathogenic organisms like *Mycoplasma*, pneumococcus, *Pseudomonas*, and others **(Fig. 1)**.

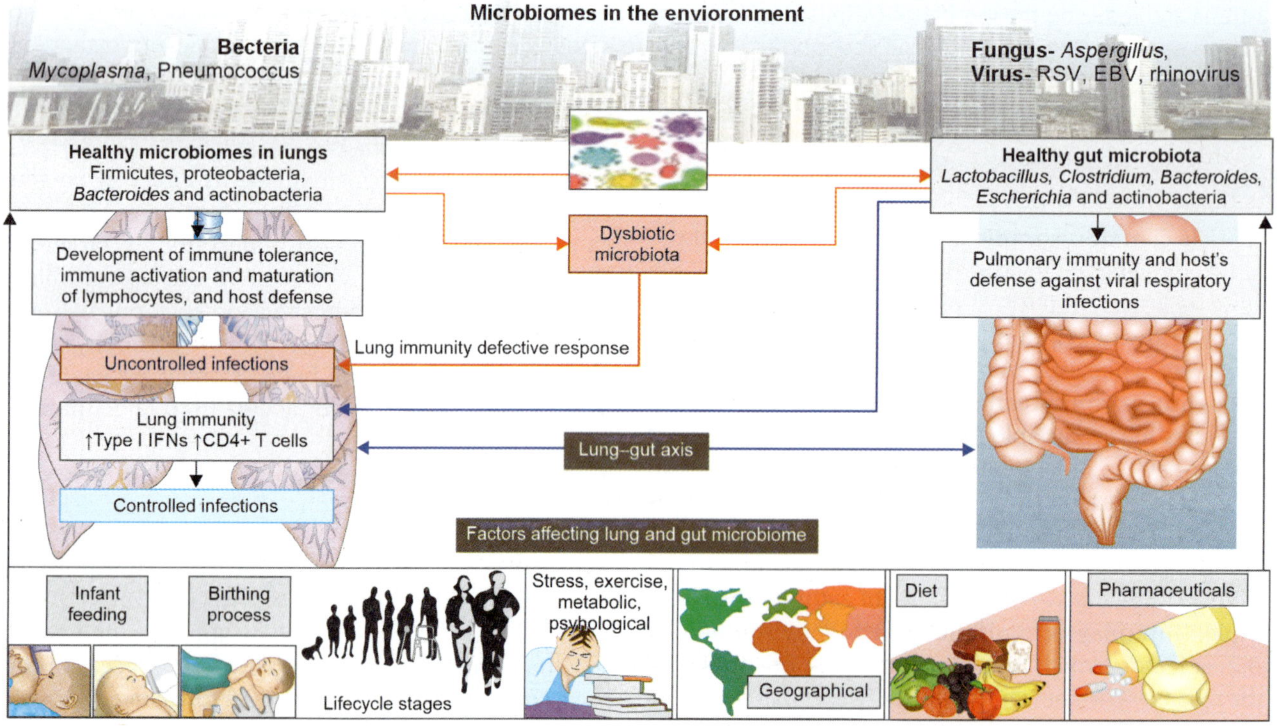

FIG. 1: Interactions between environmental, gut, and lung microbiome.
(EBV: Epstein–Barr virus; IFNs: interferons; RSV: respiratory syncytial virus)

- *Environment-gut-lung axis*: Environmental microbiome affects both gut and lung flora which in turn is responsible for development of immune tolerance. Also, studies are showing evidence that gut and lung are not isolated organ systems but a cross-communication and cross-influence exists between two. The gut represents most distinct and numerous collections of microbes within the body and has a tolerogenic effect on host immune response **(Fig. 1)**.
- *Dysbiotic drift*: Dysbiosis in simple terms means a shift or imbalance in the normal microbiome. Dysbiotic drift is a concept where environmental forces lead to dysbiosis which disproportionately impacts disadvantaged populations and can be a unifying concept on development of asthma by including socioeconomic, environmental, microbiological, and ecological aspects altogether **(Fig. 1)**.

- *Environmental factors*: Global warming has caused chaotic changes in the weather and the weather patterns around the globe with change in the usual climate cycles and increasing frequency of natural disasters. Some of these natural and manmade phenomena are strongly linked to changes in asthma prevalence and control. A few factors are discussed in **Table 1**.
- *Obesity*: Although obesity is long known to be associated with asthma, it has been discussed here in view of rising incidence of obesity and related asthma and recent newer insights into the pathophysiology of obesity-related asthma. Obesity is associated with a state of low level of systemic inflammation (meta-inflammation) which exhibits a non-T helper 2 (Th2) phenotype and is difficult to treat. This is due to cytotoxic T-cell dysfunction and macrophage activation within the fat tissues. Obesity decreases the effectiveness of asthma therapy and increases the rate of hospitalizations due to asthma exacerbations to levels nearly five times greater than those of asthmatic subjects without obesity.
- *Psychosocial factors*: Studies are showing increasingly frequent linkages of childhood asthma with maternal stress during pregnancy and stress during early childhood. The exact pathogenesis is yet to be delineated but it can be a focus of studies in future.

New research on asthma should focus on these emerging risk factors and their control while at the same time taking strong steps to mitigate the pollution and global warming. With all the above factors in consideration, we may still be looking only at the tip of the iceberg of new threats that may emerge if global warming continues unchecked.

UNDERSTANDING ASTHMA PHENOTYPE AND BIOMARKERS

We are moving into an era of precision medicine where treatment is getting increasingly individualized. The same applies to asthma and now we have an armamentarium of investigations to identify, classify, and treat asthma with precision. There are two major phenotypic classifications of asthma.

1. *Cellular phenotypes*: These include Th2 or type-2 asthma and non-Th2 or Th1 asthma. This classification is based on the predominant inflammatory cell subtypes and cytokines involved in asthma pathogenesis:
   a. *Th2 asthma*: Usually associated with childhood onset of symptoms, atopy, eosinophilia, and shows good response to inhaled corticosteroids (ICS). The inflammation is initiated and sustained by Th2 cells that secrete interleukin 4 (IL-4), IL-5, IL-9, and IL-13. Patients have high levels of fraction of exhaled nitric oxide (FeNO) and sputum eosinophilia and exhibit good asthma control.
   b. *Th1 asthma*: It is characterized by onset of symptoms later in life, predominantly neutrophilic inflammation of the airways with poor control of symptoms, need for higher ICS dose, and frequent exacerbation. The inflammation in this subtype is mediated predominantly by IL-17, IL-2, interferon-gamma (IFN-γ). Patients with non-type 2 asthma usually show poor response to treatment; also, the newer therapies and biologicals for asthma control are ineffective in this subgroup.

   There is emerging evidence to demonstrate that inflammation-independent processes also contribute to asthma pathogenesis. Protein kinases, adapter protein, microRNAs, ORMDL3, and gasdermin B are newly identified molecules that drive asthma progression, independent of inflammation.
2. *Clinical phenotypes*: These are based on disease development and behavior. There are multiple classifications of clinical phenotypes of asthma with no uniform agreement. The Global Initiative for Asthma (GINA) guidelines classify asthma into five clinical phenotypes: (1) allergic asthma which is Th2 type, (2) nonallergic asthma, (3) adult-onset asthma, (4) asthma with persistent airflow limitation, and (5) asthma with obesity, all four of which frequently exhibit Th1 type of inflammation **(Fig. 2)**.

TABLE 1: Various environmental factors and their impact of asthma pathogenesis.

Environmental factor	Impact on asthma	Mechanism of action
Air pollution	Increased incidence and exacerbation	• Air pollution constitutes particulate matter, hydrocarbons, dust, and gases such as oxides of nitrogen and sulfur, ozone, and free radicals • Free radicals and particulate matter hamper lung development in children, act as irritant increasing airway inflammation and mucus secretion
Thunderstorm	Increased incidence and exacerbation	• Thunderstorms are associated with dry updraft from ground and increased water in atmosphere • Dry updraft lifts the pollen and subsequent exposure to water causes osmotic shock—pollen grains ruptures and release carbohydrate coated, highly antigenic microparticles which trigger asthma
Sandstorm	Increased exacerbation	• Sandstorms carry fine dust particles coated with minerals like magnesium, iron, aluminum, manganese, and others. Also, bacteria and fungi in the air increase by 40–100% • Metal and minerals are irritants, cause oxidative damage, and activate inflammatory cascade whereas microorganisms present antigenic challenge
Climate change	Increased incidence and exacerbation	• Hot temperatures lead to hot urban islands with increased formation of ozone and other secondary pollutants—act as airway irritants • Due to hot weather pollen seasons are longer and plants produce more pollen—patients are exposed to higher antigen burden
Rain, humidity, dampness, and mold	Increased incidence and exacerbation	• Humidity is conducive to proliferation of bacteria and fungi—increased environmental antigen and microbial burden • Environmental fungi act as sensitizer and antigenic triggers for asthma—known association such as allergic bronchopulmonary aspergillosis and asthma with fungal sensitization • Abnormal environmental microbiome alters host lung microbiome
Wildfires	Increased exacerbation	Wildfires produce smoke and particulate matter (PM)—inhaled products of combustion, PM10 and PM2.5 increases airway inflammation
Migration	Change in epidemiology, increased incidence	• Human migration from rural to urban areas is associated with increased incidence of asthma in urbanized population • Introduction (migration) of non-native plant and animal species by humans into new areas increases exposure to new antigens and potential triggers
Medications	Increase in incidence	Antibiotic and acetaminophen use during pregnancy and early infancy is associated with greater incidence of asthma

Molecular Pathogenesis

In one of the first genome-wide association study of asthma, *ORMDL3 GSDMB* gene was found to be strongly associated with childhood onset asthma. Evaluation revealed that this gene is associated with regulation of unfolded protein response, Th2 cytokine expression, and regulation of pro-inflammatory genes and increased expression of *ORMDL3* is associated with increased risk of asthma. Th2 cells are a distinct lineage of CD4+ T cells which produce IL-4, IL-5, IL-13, and IL-9. On first exposure to antigen or sensitization antigen-presenting cells process and present the allergens to Th2 cells which in turn produce IL-5, IL-4, and IL-13. IL-4 and IL-13 activate B cells to produce immunoglobulin E (IgE) which binds to mast cells, and IL-5 is responsible for differentiation and maturation of eosinophils. On repeat exposure, the antigen binds to IgE causing mast cell degranulation and eosinophil recruitment. There is also release of histamine, leukotrienes, and other mediators causing airway constriction, mucus secretion, airway inflammation, and features of asthma.

The pathogenesis of Th1 asthma is less clearly understood. IL-17 is proposed to play a major role in Th2 low asthma with higher than normal levels being found in serum, sputum and bronchoalveolar lavage (BAL) fluid of patients. It is hypothesized that IL-17 cytokines may stimulate epithelial cells and fibroblasts to release chemoattractants CXCL1/5/8 and granulocyte-macrophage colony-stimulating factor (GM-CSF) recruiting neutrophils to lungs and airway smooth muscle contraction.

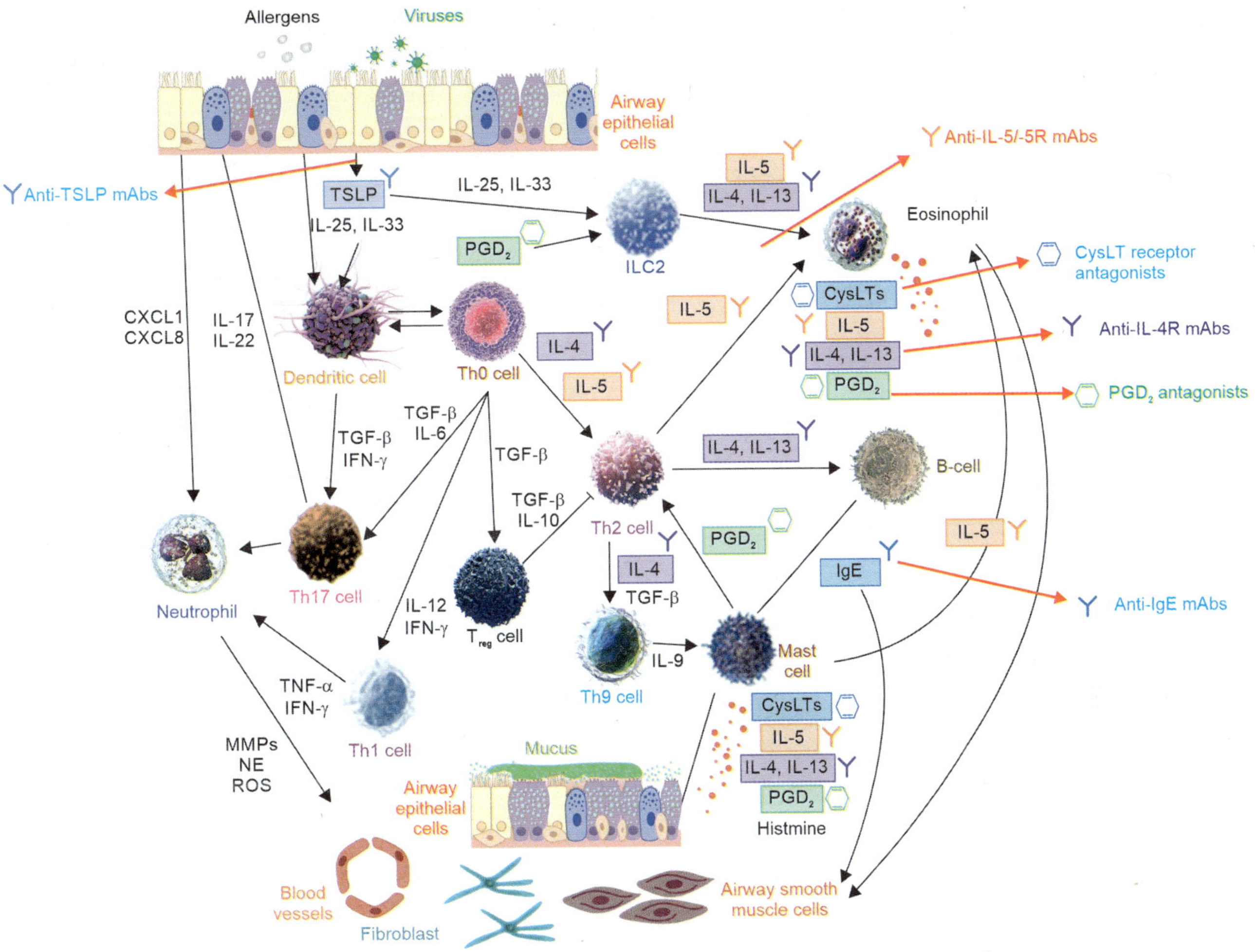

FIG. 2: Inflammatory cascade in asthma and target cytokines.

(CysLTs: cysteinyl leukotrienes; IFN-γ: interferon-gamma; IgE: immunoglobulin E; IL: interleukin; ILC2: group 2 innate lymphoid cell; MMPs: matrix metalloproteinases; NE: neutrophil elastase; PGD_2: prostaglandin D2; ROS: reactive oxygen species; TGF: transforming growth factor; Th: T helper; TSLP: thymic stromal lymphopoietin)

Other cytokines also involved in asthma pathogenesis include interferon-γ (IFN-γ), tumor necrosis factor alpha (TNF-α), transforming growth factor beta (TGF-β) and numerous others which are responsible for sustaining inflammation, increase in mucus secretion, airway smooth muscle contraction and hypertrophy, fibrosis, and airway remodeling.

Micro-RNA and Protein Kinases

Micro-RNAs are noncoding molecules responsible for controlling gene expressions and protein kinases play a role in post-translation modification of proteins. These are intricately linked to each other as micro-RNA can alter the expression of protein kinases. One such kinase identified in asthma is c-Abl (Abelson tyrosine kinase, Abl, ABL1). It regulates smooth muscle contraction, migration, and proliferation and is upregulated in asthmatic smooth muscle cells. Moreover, miR-203 which inhibits c-Abl expression is downregulated in asthmatics. We are only beginning to understand these complex genetic and molecular interactions that shape asthma and hopefully future research will shed more light on these mechanisms.

Biomarkers for asthma and targeted therapy: Scientific advances over last 10 years have revolutionized diagnosis and management of asthma and have enabled precise and personalized treatment. A few biomarkers for asthma are as follows:

- *Sputum and serum eosinophil*: A marker for Th2 inflammation, sputum and serum eosinophils serve both as a diagnostic clue in asthma and as a marker of treatment response. Especially when using biologicals like mepolizumab and dupilumab, serum absolute eosinophil count (AEC) are both predictors and markers of response.

- *Serum IgE level*: IgE levels are nonspecific markers of atopy and type-2 inflammation. High levels of IgE are usually associated with eosinophilia and are suggestive of a response to anti-IgE monoclonal antibody therapy with omalizumab. Levels are also used to monitor treatment response with biological and in allergic bronchopulmonary aspergillosis (ABPA).
- *FeNO*: FeNO is a noninvasive, cheap and reproducible marker of type 2 airway inflammation and treatment response. High FeNO (>50 ppb) levels are representative of active airway inflammation and need for escalation of therapy and low levels (<20 ppb) are usually suggestive of controlled disease activity. The only disadvantage of FeNO is that it is not a good marker for Th1 asthma.
- *Serum periostin*: It is also considered as a surrogate marker of Th2 inflammation and serum periostin levels are higher in patients with eosinophilic asthma. Further researches on the clinical utility of periostin are ongoing.

Unlike Th2 asthma, we have no reliable markers or prognostic indicators for Th1 asthma. Its diagnosis is usually made by excluding Th2 phenotype. Research is needed for finding reliable diagnostic and prognostic markers for Th1 phenotype.

Newer Treatment Modalities

Last 10 years have shown significant advances in therapeutics of asthma and biologicals are becoming the forefront of the management of severe asthma where only corticosteroids were the only reliable option. Detailed discussion on biological is beyond the scope of this text but following **Table 2** shows a summary of currently available modalities.

TABLE 2: Biologicals for asthma, their targets and patient selection.

Agent	Mechanism of action	Patient selection
Omalizumab	Anti-IgE antibody binds to circulating IgE	Age ≥ 6 years, IgE ≥ 30–700 IU/mL allergic sensitization on skin prick or serology
Mepolizumab	Anti-IL-5 antibody	Age ≥ 12 years, AEC ≥ 150 cells/µL at time of testing or ≥ 300 cells/µL in previous year
Benralizumab	Anti-IL-5 receptor antibody	Age ≥ 12 years and AEC ≥ 300 in previous year
Reslizumab	Anti-IL-5 antibody	Age ≥ 18 years, AEC ≥ 400 in previous year
Dupilumab	Anti-IL-4 receptor antibody	Age ≥ 12 years, AEC ≥ 300 and FeNO > 25 ppb

(AEC: absolute eosinophil count; FeNO: fraction of exhaled nitric oxide; IgE: immunoglobulin E; IL: interleukin)

TREATABLE TRAITS IN ASTHMA

Treatable traits are phenotypic or endotypic characters which can be assessed and targeted with treatment. The pivot of management is shifting toward personalized approach with focus on patient's individual problems and needs rather than blanket treatment. This approach focuses on finding treatable traits in individual patients in order to achieve overall disease control. These treatable traits may include airway obstruction, mucus hypersecretion, depression, effort limitation, and many others.

Emerging threats like global warming, changing weather patterns, migration, and pollution also brings an opportunity for us to gain insight into disease pathogenesis and remediate these issues in a timely manner. With expanding risks our knowledge of the disease behavior is also increasing with better diagnostic and treatment modalities and shift in focus toward individualized treatment. Despite all this, we should not ignore the environmental damage and its long-term impact. Though we cannot hope to counteract the harm already done, we can still halt its progression and use measures to protect ourselves from the threats associated with it.

SUGGESTED READINGS

1. Global Initiative for Asthma. (2023). 2023 GINA Main Report. [online] Available from https://ginasthma.org/2023-gina-main-report/ [Last accessed December, 2023].
2. D'Amato G, Holgate ST, Pawankar R, Ledford DK, Cecchi L, Al-Ahmad M, et al. Meteorological conditions, climate change, new emerging factors, and asthma and related allergic disorders. A statement of the World Allergy Organization. World Allergy Organ J. 2015;8(1):1-52.
3. Pelaia C, Crimi C, Vatrella A, Tinello C, Terracciano R, Pelaia G. Molecular targets for biological therapies of severe asthma. Front Immunol. 2020;11:603312.

215
CHAPTER

Phenotypic Management of Bronchial Asthma

Prashant Prakash, Sonam Spalgais

ABSTRACT

Asthma is a heterogenous disease, usually characterized by chronic airway inflammation. It is defined by a history of respiratory symptoms such as wheezing, shortness of breath, chest tightness, and cough that vary over time and in intensity, together with variable expiratory airflow limitation. The word heterogenous in the definition of asthma itself is an indicator of the fact that there are different types of asthma. Recognizable clusters of demographic features, clinical characteristics, lung function, and inflammation are called "asthma phenotypes". Asthma endotypes, on the other hand, are the subtypes defined by a distinct biological mechanism that links clinical characteristics with molecular pathway. Asthma endotypes are broadly categorized as type 2 (T2)-high or T2-low. About half of asthma patients have T2-high asthma. This is even more common in severe asthma patients. The biomarkers used to denote T2-high asthma include sputum and blood eosinophil count, blood periostin level, fractional exhaled nitric oxide (FeNO), allergen-specific immunoglobulin E (IgE). T2-low asthma constitutes neutrophilic, mixed, or paucigranulocytic asthma and there is an absence of markers of T2-high disease such as eosinophilia. This variant has lack a of response to corticosteroids. Phenotypic management of asthma is especially crucial when it comes to managing severe asthma.

INTRODUCTION

Asthma is a heterogenous disease, usually characterized by chronic airway inflammation. It is defined by a history of respiratory symptoms such as wheezing, shortness of breath, chest tightness and cough that vary over time and in intensity, together with variable expiratory airflow limitation. The word heterogeneous in the definition of asthma itself is an indicator of the fact that there are different types of asthma. In the past two decades, a greater insight into the disease has shown that atopic/allergic does not explain all asthma trends and patterns, and thus, the concept of asthma endotypes and phenotypes was proposed.

Phenotypes are defined as observable characteristics that result from a combination of hereditary and environmental influences. Recognizable clusters of demographic features, clinical characteristics, lung function, and inflammation are called "asthma phenotypes". Asthma endotypes, on the other hand, are the subtypes defined by a distinct biological mechanism that links clinical characteristics with molecular pathway. Asthma endotypes are broadly categorized as type 2 (T2)-high or T2-low. Traditionally, asthma is thought of as excessive T helper type 2 (Th2) cell responses and specific immunoglobulin E (IgE) hyper-responsiveness, which only conveys mechanisms of allergic asthma, while asthma now is an umbrella term for the collection of certain endotypes and varying phenotypes.

Type 2-high is defined as the asthma type having cytokines released by Th2 cells such as interleukin (IL-4), IL-5, and IL-13. Biologics target the inflammatory markers that are specifically present in the T2-high subset of asthma patients.

Type 2-high asthma: About half of asthma patients have T2-high asthma. It is even more common in the severe asthma patients. The biomarkers used to denote T2-high

TABLE 1: Endotypes and phenotypes of asthma.

Endotype	Phenotype	Clinical characteristics	Biomarkers	Natural history
T2-high asthma	Atopic	Well-defined, early onset, steroid sensitive	Blood/sputum eosinophil count, serum-specific allergen IgE, high FeNO, high total IgE	Identifiable and treatable, preserved lung function
	Late-onset	Steroid refractory	Blood/sputum eosinophil count, high FeNO	Severe from onset, more frequent exacerbation
	AERD	Adult-onset	Blood/sputum eosinophil count, urinary LTE-4	Severe from onset, more frequent exacerbation
Non-T2 asthma	Nonatopic	Adult onset: Paucigranulocytic or neutrophilic	Induced sputum neutrophil count, MMP-9 in BAL	Variable course and lung function
	Smokers	Older adults	Induced sputum neutrophil count	More frequent exacerbation, lower lung function
	Obesity-related	Gender: Female	Serum IL-6	Severe symptoms, preserved lung function
	Elderly	>50 to >65 years at onset	Induced sputum neutrophil count	Steroid resistant

(AERD: aspirin-exacerbated respiratory disease; BAL: bronchoalveolar lavage; FeNO: fractional exhaled nitric oxide; IL: interleukin; LTE-4: leukotriene E-4; MMP-9: matrix metalloproteinase-9)

asthma include sputum and blood eosinophil count, blood periostin level, fractional exhaled nitric oxide (FeNO), and allergen-specific IgE.

Type 2-low asthma: About 37% of patients with severe asthma belong to this group. This constitutes neutrophilic, mixed, or paucigranulocytic asthma and there is an absence of markers of T2-high disease such as eosinophilia. This subset of asthma phenotype is not very well understood and occurs most likely due to corticosteroid-suppressing underlying eosinophilia. These patients have fewer allergic symptoms and have older age at the time of disease presentation. This neutrophilic asthma has been associated with chronic infection with atypical bacteria, obesity, smoking, and smooth muscle abnormalities. T2-low asthma is probably mediated with IL-25 and IL-33. IL-17, CXCR2, and c-KIT influence the pathogenesis. Presently, the treatment of this subset of patients includes controller medicines and probably bronchial thermoplasty as this variant has lack of response to corticosteroids. The various endotypes and phenotypes of asthma along with their clinical characteristics and biomarkers are shown in **Table 1**.

TYPE 2-HIGH ENDOTYPE/ATOPIC/ ALLERGIC ASTHMA

In cases of allergic asthma, environmental allergens trigger the asthma. This is a common asthma phenotype and is found to occur in about 40–50% of patients with asthma. There is presence of allergic sensitization defined by the presence of serum IgE antibodies and/or a positive skin-prick test to common inhaled or ingested allergens such as house dust mites, animal dander, fungal spores, plant or tree pollen, or peanuts. In up to 80% of cases, patients with allergic asthma have concurrent allergic rhinitis. T2-high asthma has been classified into three groups: Early-onset allergic asthma, late-onset eosinophilic asthma, and aspirin-exacerbated asthma.

Early-onset Allergic Asthma

The clinical presentation of early-onset allergic asthma can range from mild to severe. This phenotype can be distinguished from T2-high nonatopic asthma by positive allergy skin tests and increased serum-specific IgE. The treatment plan for these patients includes decreasing allergen exposure, antihistamines, and corticosteroids. Allergen immunotherapy may also be recommended. Biological therapies that target the allergic response pathway (including the medications omalizumab, mepolizumab, dupilumab, and reslizumab) may also be considered.

Late-onset Eosinophilic Asthma

This is an adult-onset phenotype and shows steroid-resistant eosinophilia. The molecular mechanism remains unknown. Airway T2 inflammation is not reversed by inhalational steroids in these patients. These individuals are of advanced age and exhibit more severe asthma symptoms characterized by a persistent limitation in airflow. The vast majority of these individuals have concurrent chronic rhinosinusitis with nasal polyps, which typically occurs before the onset of asthma. This phenotype is typically distinguished by a noticeable elevation of eosinophils in the blood and sputum, which does not respond to therapy with inhaled or oral corticosteroids. There is typically no indication of atopy. These individuals typically exhibit elevated levels of FeNO and have either normal or increased levels of blood total IgE.

Aspirin-exacerbated Asthma

Aspirin-exacerbated asthma is also a late-onset phenotype. Patients with aspirin-exacerbated asthma have a flare-up of their asthma when they take aspirin or a nonsteroidal anti-inflammatory drug (NSAID). Patients with this asthma phenotype may also have chronic rhinitis or nasal polyps.

TYPE 2-LOW ENDOTYPE/NONATOPIC ASTHMA

Patients with the nonallergic asthma phenotype do not demonstrate evidence of allergic sensitivity. Although asthma is classically associated with eosinophilia and Th2 cytokines, these patients show a neutrophil-predominant disease with an absence of Th2 cytokines. These patients have an asthma diagnosis, but they do not show sensitization to indoor or outdoor allergens, and they do not have elevated eosinophil counts and/or total IgE levels. Nonallergic asthma often develops late in life and this form of the disease is more common in women. It is often associated with chronic rhinosinusitis and nasal polyps, as well as obesity, and is difficult to treat, often requiring long-term treatment with systemic steroids. It is typically identified by the presence of neutrophils in the sputum (>40–60%) or by normal levels of both eosinophils and neutrophils in the sputum. Additionally, it does not show any improvement with corticosteroid treatment. The processes responsible for the recruitment and persistence of neutrophilic airway inflammation are still not understood. Chronic infection with atypical microorganisms, obesity, smoking, and underlying smooth muscle abnormalities are known to be related to severe neutrophilic asthma. These patients have T2-low phenotypes and have been categorized based on clinical attributes, such as obesity, smoking, and age.

Obesity-related Asthma

Obesity is a significant contributing factor to the morbidity of asthma. The typical patient with obesity-related asthma is a middle-aged lady who is not allergic and experiences significant symptoms despite having modestly preserved lung function. The relationship between obesity and asthma is intricate and has multiple aspects. However, the majority of evidence suggests that noneosinophilic inflammatory processes play a significant role at the molecular level. Obesity has the interesting effect of causing CD4 cells to favor Th1 differentiation, which is linked to steroid-refractory asthma.

Smoking-associated Asthma

The mechanisms responsible for smoking-associated asthma remain unknown; however, it is commonly characterized as a T2-low neutrophilic, steroid-resistant phenotype. Possible pathways involve oxidative stress, which triggers epigenetic alterations leading to the activation of neutrophils and macrophages. Nevertheless, smoking also heightens the likelihood of becoming sensitized to allergens and raises the overall levels of IgE, thereby establishing a connection between asthma and chronic obstructive pulmonary disease (COPD).

Very Late-onset Asthma

The diagnosis of very late-onset asthma is not consistently defined, but it is generally considered to occur in individuals over the age of 50 years in some studies and over the age of 65 years in others. Decreased lung function in the aging lungs is caused by the lack of elastic recoil, resulting in mechanical disadvantages.

Broadly, the clinical features and course of T2-high and T2-low asthma are summarized in **Figure 1**.

DEFINITIONS: UNCONTROLLED, DIFFICULT-TO-TREAT, AND SEVERE ASTHMA

Understanding the definitions of difficult-to-treat and severe asthma starts with the concept of uncontrolled asthma.

Uncontrolled Asthma

Uncontrolled asthma includes one or both of the following:

1. Poor symptom control (frequent symptoms or reliever use, activities limited by asthma, and night waking due to asthma).
2. Frequent exacerbations (>2/year) requiring oral corticosteroids (OCS), or serious exacerbations (>1/year) requiring hospitalization.

Difficult-to-treat Asthma

Difficult-to-treat asthma is uncontrolled despite prescribing medium- or high-dose inhaled corticosteroids

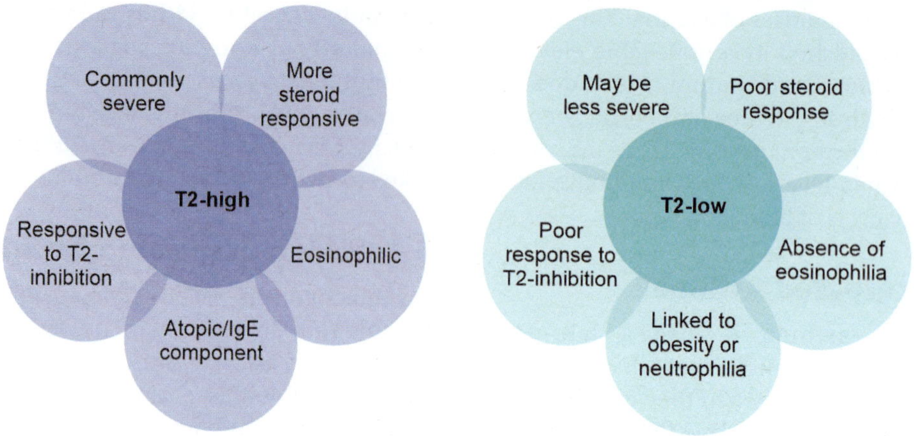

FIG. 1: Phenotypes of type 2-high and type 2-low asthma.
(IgE: immunoglobulin E; T2: Type 2)
Source: Woodruff PG, et al. 2009.

(ICS) with a second controller [usually a long-acting beta-agonists (LABA)] or with maintenance OCS, or that requires high-dose treatment to maintain good symptom control and reduce the risk of exacerbations. It does not mean a "difficult patient". In many cases, asthma may appear to be difficult to treat because of modifiable factors such as incorrect inhaler technique, poor adherence, smoking, or comorbidities, or because the diagnosis is incorrect.

Severe Asthma

Severe asthma is a subset of difficult-to-treat asthma. It means asthma that is uncontrolled despite adherence to maximal optimized high-dose ICS-LABA treatment and management of contributory factors, or that worsens when high-dose treatment is decreased. Therefore, at present, "severe asthma" is a retrospective label. It is sometimes called "severe refractory asthma" since it is defined by being relatively refractory to high-dose inhaled therapy. However, with the advent of biologic therapies, the word "refractory" is no longer appropriate.

Asthma is not classified as severe if it markedly improves when contributory factors such as inhaler technique and adherence are addressed.

Phenotypic management of asthma is especially crucial when it comes to managing severe asthma.

ASSESSMENT OF SEVERE ASTHMA PHENOTYPE

The next step is to assess the patient's inflammatory phenotype, whether is it T2-high or T2-low. Phenotyping a patient with severe asthma for the purpose of management is summarized in **Flowchart 1**.

What is Type 2 Inflammation?

Type 2 inflammation is found in the majority of people with severe asthma. It is characterized by cytokines such as IL-4, IL-5, and IL-13, which are often produced by the adaptive immune system on recognition of allergens. It may also be activated by viruses, bacteria, and irritants that stimulate the innate immune system via the production of IL-33, IL-25, and thymic stromal lymphopoietin (TSLP) by epithelial cells. T2 inflammation is often characterized by elevated eosinophils or increased FeNO, and it may be accompanied by atopy and elevated IgE, whereas non-T2 inflammation is often characterized by increased neutrophils.

In many patients with asthma, T2 inflammation rapidly improves when ICS are taken regularly and correctly; this is classified as mild or moderate asthma. In severe asthma, T2 inflammation may be relatively refractory to high-dose ICS. It may respond to OCS, but their serious adverse effects mean that alternative treatments should be sought.

In adult patients with uncontrolled asthma, despite medium- or high-dose ICS plus LABA or other controllers, a history of exacerbations in the previous year, higher blood eosinophil counts, and higher FeNO levels are associated with a greater risk of severe exacerbations.

Could the Patient have Refractory or Underlying Type 2 Inflammation?

The possibility of refractory T2 inflammation should be considered if any of the following are found while the patient is taking high-dose ICS or daily OCS:

- Blood eosinophils ≥ 150/μL
- FeNO ≥ 20 ppb

- Sputum eosinophils ≥ 2%
- Asthma is clinically allergen driven.

Patients requiring maintenance OCS may also have underlying T2 inflammation. However, biomarkers of T2 inflammation (blood eosinophils, sputum eosinophils, and FeNO) are often suppressed by OCS. Therefore, if possible, these tests should be performed before starting OCS (a short course, or maintenance treatment), or at least 1–2 weeks after a course of OCS, or on the lowest possible OCS dose.

Consider repeating blood eosinophils and FeNO up to three times (e.g., when asthma worsens, before giving OCS, or at least 1–2 weeks after a course of OCS, or on the lowest possible OCS dose), before assuming asthma is non-T2.

ROLE OF BIOLOGICALS IN TYPE-2 TARGETED TREATMENTS

The eligibility criteria for biologicals in T2-high asthma (both severe allergic and severe eosinophilic asthma) are summarized in **Tables 2 and 3**.

Add-on Anti-IgE for Severe Allergic Asthma

- *Regulatory approvals:* These may include omalizumab for ages ≥ 6 years, given by subcutaneous (SC) injection every 2–4 weeks, with dose based on weight and serum IgE. These may also be indicated for nasal polyps and chronic spontaneous (idiopathic) urticaria. Self-administration may be an option.

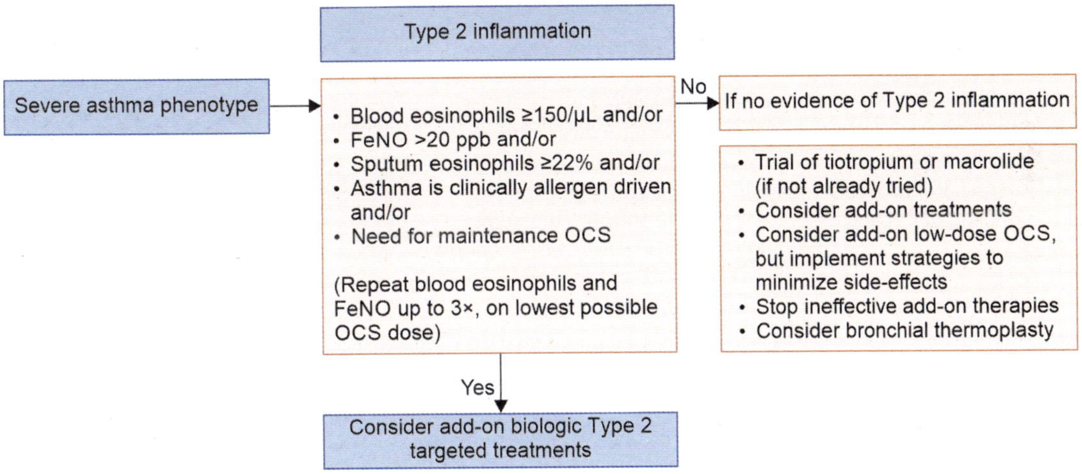

FLOWCHART 1: Phenotyping a patient with severe asthma.

(FeNO: fractional exhaled nitric oxide; OCS: oral corticosteroids)

Source: Global Initiative for Asthma. 2019.

TABLE 2: Eligibility criteria for biologics.

Anti-IgE	Anti-IL-5/Anti-IL-5R	Anti-IL-4R
• Sensitization on skin-prick testing or specific IgE • Total serum IgE and weight within dosage range • Exacerbation in last year	Is the patient eligible for **anti-IL-5/ anti-IL-5R** for severe eosinophilic asthma? • Exacerbation in last year • Blood eosinophils ≥ 300 /μL	Is the patient eligible for **anti-IL-4R** for severe eosinophilic/Type 2 asthma? • Exacerbation in last year • Blood eosinophils ≥ 150 /μL or FeNO ≥ 25 ppb or because of need for maintenance OCS?
What factors may predict good response to anti-IgE? • Blood eosinophils ≥ 260 /μL ++ • FeNO ≥ 20 ppb + • Allergen-driven symptoms + • Childhood-onset asthma +	*What factors may predict good response to anti-IL-5/IL-5R?* • Higher blood eosinophils +++ • More exacerbation in previous year +++ • Adult-onset of asthma ++ • Nasal polyposis ++	*What factors may predicts good response to anti-IL-4R?* • Higher blood eosinophils +++ • Higher FeNO +++

(IgE: immunoglobulin E; FeNO: fractional exhaled nitric oxide; IL: interleukin; OCS: oral corticosteroids)

Source: Global Initiative for Asthma. 2019.

TABLE 3: Summary of the biologics currently approved for the treatment of moderate-to-severe persistent asthma with type 2-high phenotype.

Therapy	Mechanism of action	Indication	Dosing and route	Adverse effects
Omalizumab	Anti-IgE; prevents IgE from binding to its receptor on mast cells and basophils	≥ 6 year old with moderate-to-severe persistent asthma, positive allergy testing, incomplete control with an ICS, and IgE: 30–1,300 IU/mL (United States, age 6–11 years), 30–700 IU/mL (United States, age ≥ 12 years), or 30–1,500 IU/mL (European Union)	0.016 mg/kg per IU of IgE (in a 4-weeks period) administered every 2–4 weeks SC (150–375 mg in the United States; 150–600 mg in European Union)*	Black box warning: ~0.1–0.2% risk of anaphylaxis in clinical trials
Mepolizumab	Anti-IL-5; binds to IL-5 ligand; prevents IL-5 from binding to its receptor	≥ 12 year old with severe eosinophilic asthma unresponsive to other GINA step 4–5 therapies. Suggested AEC ≥ 150–300 cells/μL	100 mg SC every 4 week	Rarely causes hypersensitivity reactions; can cause activation of zoster
Reslizumab	Anti-IL-5; binds to IL-5 ligand; prevents IL-5 from binding to its receptor	≥ 18 year old with severe eosinophilic asthma unresponsive to other GINA step 4–5 therapies. Suggested AEC ≥ 400 cells/μL	Weight-based dosing of 3 mg/kg IV every 4 week	Black box warning: ~ 0.3% risk of anaphylaxis in clinical trials
Benralizumab	Anti-IL-5; binds to IL-5 receptor α; causes apoptosis of eosinophils and basophils	≥ 12 year old with severe eosinophilic asthma unresponsive to other GINA step 4–5 therapies. Suggested AEC ≥ 300 cells/μL	30 mg SC every 4 weeks for three doses; followed by every 8 weeks subsequently	Rarely causes hypersensitivity reactions
Dupilumab	Anti-IL-4R; binds to IL-4 receptor α; blocks signaling of IL-4 and IL-13	≥ 12 year old with severe eosinophilic asthma unresponsive to other GINA step 4–5 therapies. Suggested AEC ≥ 150 cells/μL and/or FENO level ≥ 25 ppb	200 or 300 mg SC every 2 weeks	Rarely causes hypersensitivity reactions; higher incidence of injection site reactions (up to 18%) and hypereosinophilia (4–14%)

*Upper limits exist for the dosing of omalizumab in patients with high IgE levels and increased weight.

(AEC: absolute blood eosinophil count; FENO: fractional exhaled nitric oxide; GINA: Global Initiative for Asthma; ICS: inhaled corticosteroids; IgE: immunoglobulin E; IV: intravenous; SC: subcutaneous)

Source: McGregor MC, et al. 2019.

- *Mechanism*: Omalizumab binds to Fc part of free IgE, preventing the binding of IgE to FcεR1 receptors, reducing free IgE, and downregulating receptor expression.
- *Eligibility criteria (in addition to criteria for severe asthma):* These may vary between payers, but usually include:
  - Sensitization to inhaled allergen(s) on skin-prick testing or specific IgE
  - Total serum IgE and body weight within local dosing range
  - More than a specified number of exacerbations within the last year
- *Outcomes*: Summarized in **Table 4**.
- *Potential predictors of good asthma response to omalizumab:*
  - Baseline IgE level does not predict the likelihood of response.
  - In a post-hoc analysis of one clinical trial, a greater decrease in exacerbations was observed (cf. placebo) with blood eosinophils ≥ 260/μL or FeNO ≥ 19.5 ppb (these criteria represent their median value in that study), but in two large observational studies, exacerbations were reduced with both low or high blood eosinophils or FeNO.
  - Childhood-onset asthma
  - Clinical history suggesting allergen-driven symptoms.
- *Adverse effects*: Summarized in **Table 3**.
- *Suggested initial trial*: At least 4 months.

Add-on Anti-IL-5 or Anti-IL-5R for Severe Eosinophilic Asthma

- *Regulatory approvals:* These may include: For ages ≥ 12 years: Mepolizumab (anti-IL-5), 100 mg by SC injection every 4 weeks, or benralizumab (anti-IL-5 receptor alpha), 30 mg by SC injection every 4 weeks for 3 doses then every 8 weeks. For ages ≥ 18 years: Reslizumab (anti-IL-5), 3 mg/kg by IV infusion every 4 weeks is recommended. For ages 6–11 years, mepolizumab (anti-IL-5), 40 mg by SC injection every 4 weeks is advised. Mepolizumab may also be indicated for eosinophilic granulomatosis with

TABLE 4: Efficacy of the biologics that are US Food and Drug Administration approved for the treatment of moderate-to-severe persistent asthma with type 2-high phenotype.

Therapy	Asthma exacerbation	Lung function	Corticosteroid weaning	Special considerations
Omalizumab	Reduces by 25%	Minimal or equivocal improvement	Decreases use of ICS, but no data that it helps with OCS weaning	Only SC biologic approved for children 6–11 years old
Mepolizumab	Reduces by ~50%	Inconsistent effect	Decreases total use of OCS and has been shown to facilitate complete weaning from chronic OCS (14%)	Standard SC dosing has not been shown to decrease sputum eosinophilia; approved at higher dosing for EGPA
Reslizumab	Reduces by ~50–60%	Improved	Has not been specifically evaluated for this indication	Only weight-based dosing IV biologics approved for asthma
Benralizumab	Reduces by ~25–60%	Improved	Decreases total use of OCS and has been shown to facilitate complete weaning from chronic OCS (50%)	Only SC biologic that offers every 8-week dosing
Dupilumab	Reduces by ~50–70%	Improved	Decreases total use of OCS and has been shown to facilitate complete weaning from chronic OCS (50%)	Only biologic that can be self-administered SC; showed benefit with FENO >25 ppb regardless of eosinophil count

(EGPA: eosinophilic granulomatosis with polyangiitis; FENO: fractional exhaled nitric oxide; ICS: inhaled corticosteroid; IV: intravenous; OCS: oral corticosteroids; SC: subcutaneous)

Source: McGregor MC, et al. 2019.

polyangiitis (EGPA), hypereosinophilic syndrome, and chronic rhinosinusitis with nasal polyps. Self-administration may be an option.

- *Mechanism*: Mepolizumab and reslizumab bind to circulating IL-5; benralizumab binds to IL-5 receptor alpha subunit leading to apoptosis (cell death) of eosinophils.
- *Eligibility criteria (in addition to criteria for severe asthma)*: These vary by product and between payers, but usually include:
  - More than a specified number of severe exacerbations in the last year
  - Blood eosinophils above locally specified level (e.g., ≥150 or ≥300/μL). There is sometimes a different eosinophil cut point for patients taking OCS.
- *Outcomes*: Summarized in **Table 4**.
- *Potential predictors of good asthma response to anti-IL-5 or anti-IL-5R:*
  - Higher blood eosinophils (strongly predictive)
  - Higher number of severe exacerbations in previous year (strongly predictive)
  - Adult-onset asthma
  - Nasal polyps
  - Maintenance OCS at baseline
  - Low lung function [forced expiratory volume in 1 second (FEV_1) < 65% predicted in one study].
- *Adverse effects*: Summarized in **Table 3**.
- *Suggested initial trial*: At least 4 months.

Add-on Anti-IL-4Rα for Severe Eosinophilic/Type 2 Asthma or Patients Requiring Maintenance Oral Corticosteroids

- *Regulatory approvals*: These may include: For ages ≥ 12 years: Dupilumab (anti-IL-4 receptor alpha), 200 mg or 300 mg by SC injection every 2 weeks for severe eosinophilic/T2 asthma; 300 mg by SC injection every 2 weeks for OCS-dependent severe asthma or if there is concomitant moderate/severe atopic dermatitis. For children of age 6–11 years with severe eosinophilic/T2 asthma by SC injection with dose and frequency depending on weight. Dupilumab also be indicated for treatment of skin conditions including moderate to severe atopic dermatitis, chronic rhinosinusitis with nasal polyps, and eosinophilic esophagitis. Self-administration may be an option.

- *Mechanism*: Dupilumab binds to IL-4 receptor alpha, blocking both IL-4 and IL-13 signaling.
- *Eligibility criteria (in addition to criteria for severe asthma):* These vary between payers, but usually include:
  - More than a specified number of severe exacerbations in the last year
  - T2 biomarkers above a specified level (e.g., blood eosinophils ≥ 150/μL and ≤ 1500/μL; or FeNO ≥25 ppb); or requirement for maintenance OCS
- *Outcomes*: Summarized in **Table 4**.
- *Potential predictors of good asthma response to dupilumab*:
  - Higher blood eosinophils (strongly predictive)
  - Higher FeNO (strongly predictive)
- *Adverse effects*: Summarized in **Table 3**.
- *Suggested initial trial*: At least 4 months.

SUGGESTED READINGS

1. Global initiative for asthma. (2023). GINA Main Report. Global strategy for Asthma Management and Prevention. [online] Available from https://ginasthma.org/2023-gina-main-report/ [Last accessed January, 2024].
2. American Academy of Allergy, Asthma and Immunology. (2019). Asthma is a disease of different phenotypes. [online] Available from https://www.aaaai.org/Tools-for-the-Public/Conditions-Library/Asthma/Asthma-is-a-disease-of-different-phenotypes [Last accessed January 2024].
3. Woodruff PG, Modrek B, Choy DF, Jia G, Abbas AR, Ellwanger A, et al. T-helper type 2-driven inflammation Defines Major Subphenotypes of Asthma. Am J Respir Crit Care Med. 2009;180:388-95.
4. Global initiative for asthma. (2019). GINA Difficult-to-treat and severe asthma in adolescent and adult patients: Diagnosis and Management. [online] Available from https://ginasthma.org/wp-content/uploads/2019/04/GINA-Severe-asthma-Pocket-Guide-v2.0-wms-1.pdf [Last accessed January, 2024].
5. McGregor MC, Krings JG, Nair P, Castro M. Role of Biologics in Asthma. Am J Respir Crit Care Med. 2019;199(4):433-45.

216

CHAPTER

Recent Developments in Asthma Education

Bharat Bhushan Sharma, Sudhir Mehta

ABSTRACT

Asthma is a chronic respiratory disease with episodic course and variable frequency of exacerbations. Effective inhaled therapy has revolutionized treatment, with bronchoconstriction being the main pathophysiological mechanism. Inhaled corticosteroids (ICS) provide ideal disease control by controlling inflammation. Asthma is manageable under normal circumstances but not curable. Continuous efforts are needed to educate patients about their disease and make adjustments to medications. Understanding the role of allergenic triggers and the right timing, delivery methods, and medication adjustments is crucial for effective asthma management.

INTRODUCTION

Asthma is a chronic respiratory disease characterized by episodic course with diurnal and seasonal fluctuations along with variable frequency of exacerbations ranging from mild, moderate and at times of life-threatening severity. This episodic course and reversibility of symptoms make it a special entity among all chronic respiratory diseases. Availability of effective inhaled therapy has revolutionized the treatment landscape for this disease.

Until a few decades ago, bronchoconstriction was considered as the main pathophysiological mechanism of asthma and inhaled bronchodilator were the mainstay of treatment. The advent of inhaled corticosteroids (ICS) provided ideal disease control measure by controlling underlying inflammation. Use of both of the above medications now is standard of care for most of the cases of bronchial asthma; however, some additional medications may be required to be added depending on severity of disease and occurrence of exacerbations.

The presence of a specific type of chronic underlying inflammation substantiates the concept that asthma is manageable most of the time under usual circumstances but is not curable. There is, therefore, a need for continuous efforts for educating patients about their own disease and making then useful partners in day-to-day and longer-term adjustments required in controlling asthma with currently available medications.

Right time, delivery methods, and adjustment of medications are crucial aspects of asthma management. Patient needs to understand all these factors and the role of allergenic or other triggers for effective asthma management. However, despite enormous advancements in the understanding of pathophysiology, diagnosis, and management of this disease, it still remains a disease of major public health importance across the globe.

BURDEN OF ASTHMA IN INDIA

The Indian Study on Epidemiology of Asthma, Respiratory Symptoms and Chronic Bronchitis (INSEARCH) using a validated International Union Against Tuberculosis and Lung Diseases (IUALTD) questionnaire, estimated burden of asthma in India was 17.23 million in 2011.

Using data from the National Family Health Survey-3, Agrawal et al. estimated the prevalence of self-reported asthma to be around 2% in India.

The Global Burden of Disease (GBD, 1990–2019) estimated the total burden of asthma in India to be about 13% of the global burden while it has three times higher proportionate mortality as compared to the global data. This disparity from global trends in mortality may be attributed to poor disease management in our country.

NEED OF ASTHMA EDUCATION

The western world recognized the importance of asthma education in management of asthma many centuries ago. Hippocrates was probably the first to educate about associated environmental asthma triggers but the concept of modern asthma education started taking shape only a few decades ago.

Clinical practice guidelines developed by the National Heart, Lung and Blood Institute (NHLBI) stressed on the need of formal and comprehensive asthma self-management education as a key component of optimal asthma care.

The much-awaited focused updates to the NHLBI asthma management guidelines were published in 2020. These guidelines help the clinician integrate the new recommendation on clinical and individually tailored management of asthma. In this update of the US guidelines, patient education factors such as assessment tools for asthma control, adherence, and other factors including inhaler technique were not covered due to availability of sufficient high-quality evidence in these areas in the standard medical literature.

The Centers for Disease Control and Prevention (CDC) has introduced a technical package for improvement of asthma control, the *EXHALE* which highlights the role of asthma education as a vital strategy in management of asthma.

Asthma education is virtually nonexistent in India despite having a high burden of disease and even more importantly having high mortality burden as mentioned above. In a study conducted by *Kotwani et al.*, the formal asthma education was missing in a carefully selected group of people with asthma from an urban community from India. Patients did not have any knowledge of causative factors, mechanism of disease, or treatment of asthma. They also did not know how to assess the severity of their asthma.

In a similar cross-sectional interview-based study on children with asthma and their parents attending outpatient clinics in two major tertiary care institutes of the same city, it was found that no asthma education sessions were offered to patients or parents, beyond a usual clinical consultation with the physician.

While, the same group of researchers conducted an interventional study with a comparison group of usual care using practical and child-friendly educational programs based on locally prevalent asthma medication use. They reported a clear advantage of intervention by simple measures including written asthma action plan in their patients.

STRUCTURE OF ASTHMA EDUCATION

Asthma education can be imparted in a variety of settings and a number of packages are available for this purpose. Some packages focus on adults with asthma while others talk about adolescent or younger children. Most of the packages are designed to be used directly by end users, i.e., patients or children or their parents. Others are intended to include clinicians, social workers, or peers as educators.

These packages incorporate symptom trackers and written asthma action plans and can be compatible with websites or apps, or use more traditional tools printed on paper. Asthma education can be given face-to-face to individual or small groups, or a telephone or a computer can be utilized.

A systematic review encompassing 270 randomized controlled trials (RCTs) about asthma education packages found that it improves asthma control and reduces healthcare utilization by the patients. Other reviews have also suggested the utility of asthma education for improving asthma outcomes and quality of life.

The asthma education is mainly based on the aspects like what is asthma; when to use medications; and how to identify triggers. Knowing about asthma paves the way to defeat asthma. Knowledge of controller and rescue medications and when to use these medications empower patient in the self-management of asthma. Knowledge of triggers strengthens the effectiveness of management strategies.

GUIDELINE-BASED ASTHMA EDUCATION AND WRITTEN ACTION PLANS

The existing asthma self-management plans are mainly of two types **(Flowchart 1)**. In patient-centered plans, patient decides about changing the medications according to the written action plan. While in doctor-centered plans, the major planned decisions are taken by doctors. These plans include self-monitoring by symptoms/peak flow, a written action plan to guide change of medications as per the requirement and regular review of asthma treatment and control by doctors.

Short-term as well as long-term monitoring by symptoms or by peak flow help in identifying exacerbations, change in medications and noting the triggers such as occupational or domestic triggers. Internet- or mobile-based monitoring may be more useful in severe asthma.

Written asthma action plans may be in the form of printed, digital, or picture-based material. According to National Asthma Education and Prevention Program,

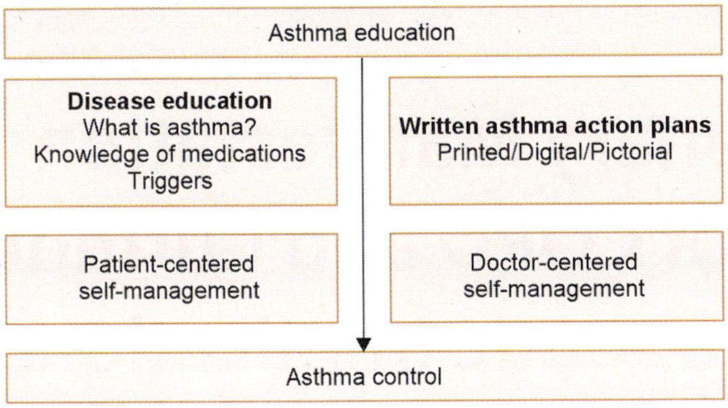

FLOWCHART 1: Core components of asthma education.

USA, green coding means the lungs are functioning well. The symptoms are not present or are well controlled. The patient can typically continue regular medicines and activities. Yellow means the asthma symptoms are more frequent or more severe. This is treated with a short-term increase in medication as per the written action plan provided by doctor. Red means the symptoms are severe and require immediate treatment adjustment, often with several medications or a visit to the doctor as per the written action plan.

Action-based plan that include step-up ICS or oral steroids are more effective. Similarly, peak flow-based plans incorporating personal best are more effective than predicted value-based plans.

Western countries have their own Asthma Management Programs and protocols. The CDC USA, the national public health agency made a self-management education program "*Breathe well, live well*" that helps people with asthma. The program helps people develop skills and confidence in tackling asthma efficiently. The main components of this program are: Understanding of asthma, building asthma support, and using tools for daily self-management and healthy habits. The American Lung Association provides in-person and virtual structured training and materials on asthma education for adults as well as organizations. Breathe well, live well program also provides technical assistance call with the American Lung Association staff for registered participants.

Indian asthma guidelines strongly recommend self-management of asthma involving a combination of patient education, self-monitoring, regular review by physician, and optimal self-management using a written asthma action plan.

Importantly, these guidelines recognize the fact that patient education when used alone is unlikely to improve health outcomes in asthma. However, when asthma education is used as a part of an optimal self-management plan which includes self-monitoring of symptoms or a peak expiratory flow measurement, along with regular physician review and self-management using a written asthma action plan significantly leads to reduction in hospitalizations and other adverse health outcomes related to asthma.

CONCLUSION

The evidence-based asthma education and self-management plans need to be implemented more effectively in India. The education plans are required to tailored according to need of individual patient and should be based on locally prevalent best evidence practices for management of asthma. Structured and competency-based asthma education should be included in undergraduate curriculum and recognized courses for asthma educator are to be developed in order to cater to the healthcare requirements of people suffering from asthma.

SUGGESTED READINGS

1. National Asthma Education and Prevention Program, Third Expert Panel on the Diagnosis and Management of Asthma. Expert Panel Report 3: Guidelines for the diagnosis and management of asthma. Summary report 2007. Bethesda (MD): National Heart, Lung, and Blood Institute (US); 2007. p. 74.
2. Global Strategy for Asthma Management and Prevention. 2023 GINA Report. Available from https://ginasthma.org/wp-content/uploads/2023/05/GINA-2023-Full-Report-2023-WMS.pdf. [Last accessed December, 2023].
3. Agarwal R, Dhooria S, Aggarwal AN, Maturu VN, Sehgal IS, Muthu V, et al. Guidelines for diagnosis and management of bronchial asthma: Joint ICS/NCCP (I) recommendations. Lung India. 2015;32:3-42.
4. Kotwani A, Chhabra SK, Tayal V, Vijayan VK. Quality of asthma management in an urban community in Delhi, India. Indian J Med Res. 2012;135(2):184-92.

217

CHAPTER

Extrapulmonary Manifestations of COPD and Current Therapeutic Implications

Debaprasad Chakrabarti, Birata Debbarma

ABSTRACT

Chronic obstructive pulmonary disease (COPD), a chronic inflammatory lung disease (chronic bronchitis and emphysema) which leads to extrapulmonary complications in the long run, results mainly from smoking and it is accounted as the third leading cause of mortality globally according to recent World Health Organization (WHO) data. In spite of its tremendous burden on global healthcare, effective treatment options remain very limited except symptomatic control by inhaled corticosteroids and beta-adrenergic agonists, leading to some long-term side effects. Several biologic agents are currently developed for the treatment of COPD and have shown promising results. This chapter will focus on extrapulmonary manifestations of COPD, complications, currently available treatment implications, and future therapeutic options.

INTRODUCTION

The joint American Thoracic Society and European Respiratory Society guidelines for chronic obstructive pulmonary disease (COPD) define it as *"a preventable and treatable disease characterized by airflow limitation that is not fully reversible. The airflow limitation is usually progressive and is associated with an abnormal inflammatory response of the lungs to noxious particles or gases, primarily caused by cigarette smoking."*

This particular disease entity mainly involves respiratory system but also may have systemic manifestations. COPD is an umbrella term consisting chronic bronchitis (cough and sputum production for at least 3 months in each of two consecutive years) or emphysema (abnormal distention of airspaces beyond the terminal bronchioles and destruction of the walls of the alveoli) or both **(Fig. 1)**.

As per the World Health Organization (WHO) data, around 3.23 million deaths occurred in 2019 due to COPD, making it the third leading cause of death globally. COPD deaths occur mainly (~90%) in low- and middle-income countries (LMIC) under the age of 70 years. In high-income countries, >70% of COPD cases are caused by tobacco smoking, whereas in LMIC, tobacco smoking is responsible for 30–40% of COPD cases and household air pollution also contributes as a major risk factor. The other important risk factors are exposure to occupational and environmental chemical fumes, dust, and other lung irritants accounting for 10–20% of cases. People who had a history of severe lung infections in childhood are more prone to suffer from COPD. Those who develop emphysema before the age of 40 years or lack any significant risk factors, alpha-1 antitrypsin deficiency should be suspected, although it is a rare cause of COPD.

Extrapulmonary manifestation and complications of COPD have significant effects among COPD patients which often contribute to exacerbations, recurrent hospital admissions, and increased mortality. Cardiovascular [heart failure, ischemic heart disease (IHD), etc.], musculoskeletal, and psychological complications are common among the extrapulmonary complications. IHD is counted as the leading cause of mortality among COPD patients. In addition, the clinical manifestations, pathophysiology, and management strategies of extrapulmonary complications of COPD are different from the COPD patients.

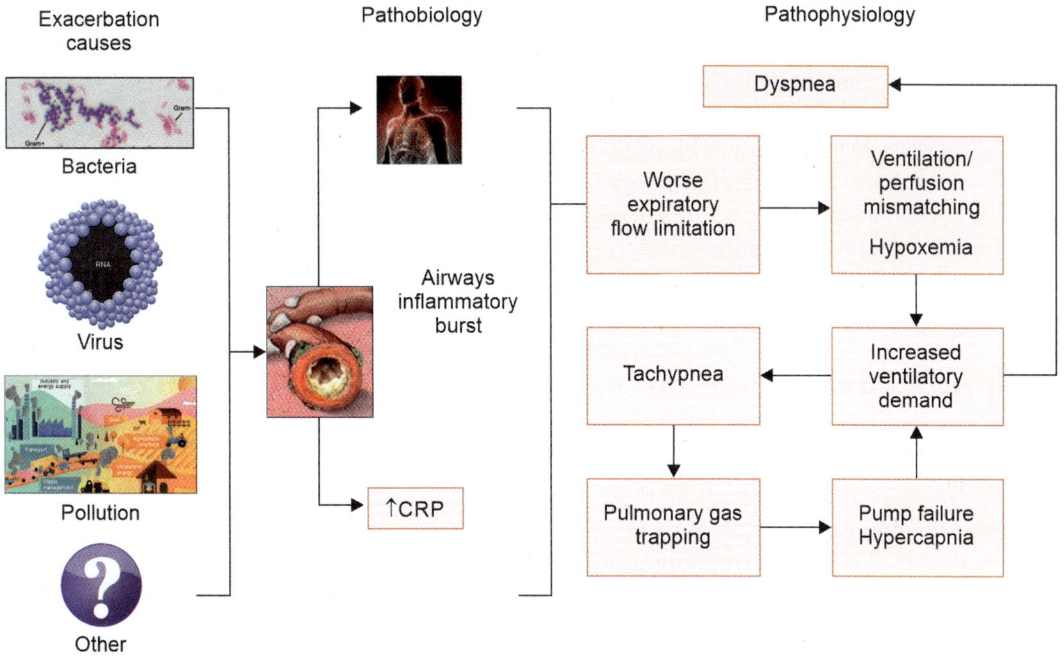

FIG. 1: Pathophysiology of extrapulmonary manifestation of chronic obstructive pulmonary disease (COPD).
(CRP: C-reactive protein)

MUSCLE DYSFUNCTION AND MALNUTRITION IN COPD

Studies on skeletal muscle have shown alteration of muscle function and its structure in COPD patients manifested as atrophy of skeletal specific to muscle fiber type IIA/IIX. These abnormalities lead to impairment of respiratory muscle function, exercise intolerance, increased healthcare utilization, ventilator support, and mortality **(Table 1)**.

TABLE 1: Extrapulmonary manifestations of COPD.

Metabolic disorder	T2DM, metabolic syndrome, dyslipidemia, cachexia, obesity
Neurologic	Stroke, depression, anxiety
CVS	Cor pulmonale, IHD, PHTN, arrhythmia
Muscles	Muscle wasting and dysfunction
Bones	Osteoporosis, osteopenia
Hematological	Anemia of chronic disease, polycythemia
Respiratory system	Obstructive sleep apnea, hyperinflation, lung cancer (small and non-small)
Renal	CKD

(CKD: chronic kidney disease; COPD: chronic obstructive pulmonary disease; CVS: cardiovascular system; IHD: ischemic heart disease; PHTN: pulmonary hypertension; T2DM: type 2 diabetes mellitus)

CARDIOVASCULAR DISEASE

The cardiovascular disease and COPD share common risk factors such as cigarette smoking, increased age, etc., as well as pathophysiology such as vascular dysfunction (smoking), neurohumoral activation, systemic inflammation, and hyperinflation leading to atherosclerosis. The other mechanism is dysfunction of the primary lung disease from secondary pulmonary hypertension (HTN) and ventricular dysfunction due to increased intrathoracic mechanical loads.

Coronary Artery Disease and Atherosclerosis

In the Lung Health trial, which was followed-up for 14 years in 6,000 study subjects, forced expiratory volume in 1 second (FEV_1) was an independent risk factor for mortality for developing myocardial infarction. A large-scale study (sample size of 5,201) by Mannino DM et al. showed that patients with severe and very severe COPD had more than twofold higher risk of developing cardiovascular disease and 1.6-fold more chances of having HTN and hospitalization.

Left Ventricular Failure

An elevated plasma N-terminal prohormone of brain natriuretic peptide (NT-proBNP) is correlated with poor physical activity in COPD patients, suggesting that defective left ventricular function may contribute to reduced performance. There is some evidence that, if anything, the cardiac size is decreased at least in patients with emphysema and that the actual volume of intrathoracic blood is also decreased in patients with hyperinflation. The increase in intrathoracic blood volume after lung volume reduction surgery and the suggested improvement in left ventricular function improvement appear more related to changes in intrathoracic pressures than to a parallel pathological deterioration of lung and cardiac function with inflammation at its center.

Pulmonary Arterial Hypertension

Around 1–3% of COPD patients have severe pulmonary arterial hypertension (PAH), usually disproportionate to airway impairment resembling primary PAH. Recent evidence shows that the natural history of PAH in COPD might be due to endothelial injury by smoking products leading to downregulation of endothelial nitric oxide (NO) synthase and prostacyclin synthase expression, causing dysfunction of endothelium. Selective vasodilators are not recommended in these subsets of patients as decrease in pulmonary arterial pressure with or without improvement of cardiac output is related to worsening of gas exchange and also there is no evidence of long-term clinical benefits. Only oxygen therapy has been found to delay progression of PAH.

NORMOCYTIC ANEMIA

In COPD patients, there is high prevalence of anemia (normochromic normocytic type) which accounts for 15–30%, characteristic for diseases of chronic inflammation in comparison to polycythemia (6%). Therapeutic erythropoietin in not helpful in these patients as end-organ erythropoietin resistance exists.

Anemia plays a significant role in functional capacity as well as poor quality of life.

OSTEOPOROSIS

Even in early stages of COPD, studies have showed that there is increased prevalence of osteoporosis and low bone mineral density (BMD). In the TORCH (Toward a Revolution in COPD Health) trial which included 6,000 cases, it was found that >50% had osteoporosis or osteopenia screened by dual-energy radiograph absorptiometry dual-energy X-ray absorptiometry (DEXA)]. It is observed that the prevalence of osteoporosis is more in males than in females, whereas the incidence of traumatic and nontraumatic fracture is similar in both genders. In COPD patients, vertebral compression fractures are common leading to kyphosis which worsen pulmonary capacity further.

DEPRESSION

The prevalence of major depression requiring medical intervention ranges from 19 to 42%. Due to their reduced physical capacity, COPD patients are unable to participate in social activities and frequently remain isolated. Very often, depression and anxiety symptoms may be masked with COPD symptoms, leading to difficulty in diagnosis in clinical practice. Some simple tools are available to screen depression for clinicians, but if in doubt, referring the patients to a psychiatrist may benefit the individual patients.

LUNG CANCER

Patients with severe COPD cases are at increased risk of developing lung cancer (mainly small and squamous cell carcinomas) by three- to fourfold and is one of the common causes of death. It is also evident from a large-scale prospective trial that lung cancer is also common in COPD patients among almost half a million nonsmokers. Females have higher risk of developing COPD and lung cancer and they might be attributed by hormone-stimulated metabolism of carcinogens in tobacco smoke **(Fig. 2)**.

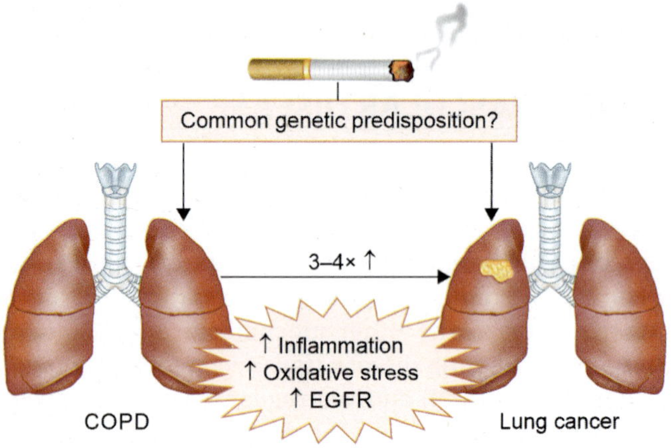

FIG. 2: Pathogenesis of lung cancer.

(COPD: chronic obstructive pulmonary disease; EGFR: estimated glomerular filtration rate)

DIABETES

Chronic obstructive pulmonary disease patients, regardless to severity, have greater risk of developing diabetes by 1.5–1.8 times. The risk factor of diabetes cannot be contributed by corticosteroid alone as it is observed that steroid-naïve COPD patients also have increased prevalence of diabetes. On the contrary, asthmatic patients do not have tendency to suffer from diabetes which might indicate that there may exist separate types of inflammation in COPD and other risk factors such as sedentary lifestyle, age factor, etc.

OBSTRUCTIVE SLEEP APNEA

Around 20% of obstructive sleep apnea (OSA) cases coexist with COPD patients, whereas 10% of OSA patients are associated with COPD independent to severity of the disease.

Recent studies have shown that there is upper airway inflammation among OSA patients, as well as systemic inflammation and oxidative stress other than being associated with many comorbidities such as heart failure, diabetes, and metabolic syndrome.

MISCELLANEOUS

Peripheral neuropathy (including increased phrenic nerve conduction time) and increased excitability of diaphragm has frequent associations with COPD. In the ECLIPSE study, among COPD patients, gastroesophageal reflux disease (GERD) was common, which might be attributed to the flattening of the diaphragm impairing gastroesophageal (GE) sphincter.

IMPLICATIONS FOR THERAPY

In management of extrapulmonary manifestations and complications of COPD, the initial important step is to suppress inflammation adequately to prevent extrapulmonary comorbidities by spillover of inflammatory mediators from the lung to other organs, then the treatment of associated systemic disease or complication, and to observe whether it minimize the COPD severity or not. Emerging evidence has shown that appropriate treatment of certain comorbidities may benefit COPD and such outcome may give new direction for future therapeutic options.

Statins

Statin has several pharmacological actions (pleotropic effects) such as antioxidant, anti-inflammatory, and immunomodulatory effects, which might have beneficial effect in COPD.

Angiotensin-converting Enzyme Inhibitors

Angiotensin-converting enzyme (ACE) inhibitors used in comorbidities such as in HTN and heart failure have been associated with decrease exacerbations and mortality of COPD patients. ACE inhibitors were also found to reduce pulmonary HTN to some extent and other beneficial anti-inflammatory effects might reduce the disease severity of COPD.

Peroxisome Proliferator-activated Receptor Agonists

Peroxisome proliferator-activated receptors (PPARs) have some beneficial effects in several extrapulmonary manifestations of COPD such as cachexia, skeletal muscle dysfunction, and systemic inflammation. PPAR agonists have immunomodulatory effects on interleukin 17 (IL-17) and interferon c (IFN-c) secretion is of particular relevance to COPD **(Fig. 3)**.

Lung Volume Reduction Surgery

Those COPD patients with extrapulmonary comorbidities on medical therapy, Lung volume reduction surgery (LVRS) on them have found to improve body mass index (BMI), metabolic syndrome, osteoporosis, intrathoracic lung volume, and cardiac function, leading to better mortality outcome. But there is no large pharmacological trial to address its long-time survival benefits to evaluate this hypothesis.

Pulmonary Rehabilitation

Meta-analyses have shown that pulmonary rehabilitation has some beneficial effects on functional capacity, quality of life, dyspnea, and low BODE (BMI, obstruction, dyspnea, exercise capacity) index among the COPD patients.

New Therapies

Usage of corticosteroids alone in COPD cannot adequately suppress inflammation such as in patients with asthma; therefore, many alternative anti-inflammatory agents are being evaluated. Broad spectrum anti-inflammatory agents such as phosphodiesterase 4 (PDE4), p38 mitogen-activated protein kinase (MAPK), and nuclear factor kappa B (NF-κB) inhibitors are to be administered orally, thereby having properties of reducing systemic inflammation as well as associated extrapulmonary diseases. Currently, most of the alternative broad-spectrum anti-inflammatory drugs in trials do have certain systemic side effects as they are widely distributed **(Table 2)**.

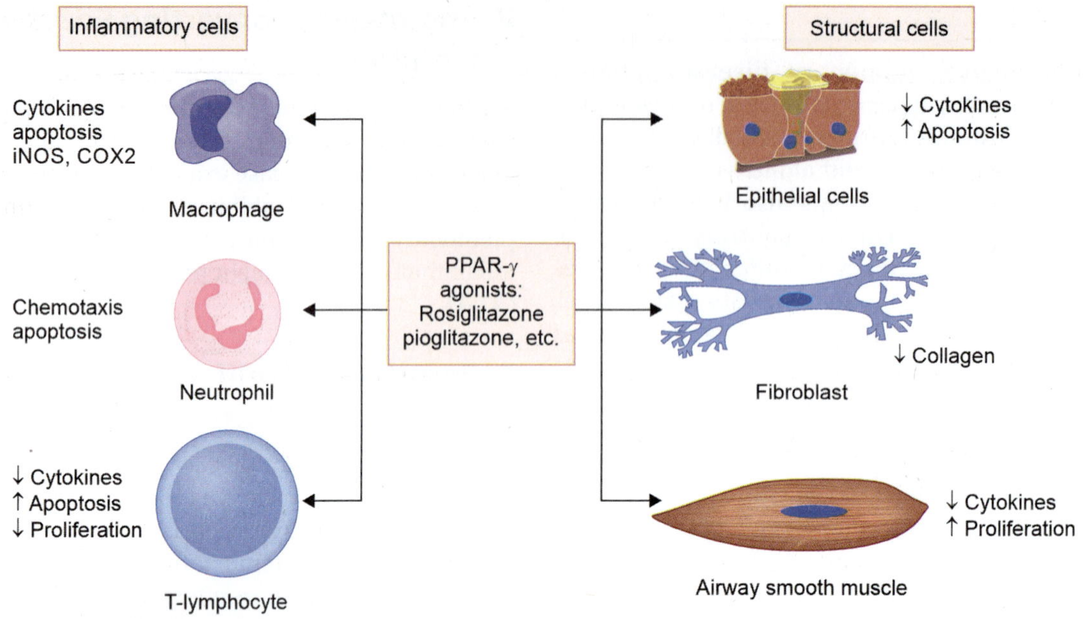

FIG. 3: Peroxisome proliferator-activated agonist (PPAR)-c effects on inflammatory and structural cells.

Note: Small arrows indicate an increase or decrease.

(COX: cyclooxygenase; iNOS: inducible nitric oxide synthase)

TABLE 2: Management of extrapulmonary manifestation of chronic obstructive pulmonary disease (COPD).

Complication	Mechanism	Management
Skeletal muscle dysfunction	• Reduced physical activity • Inflammation • Smoking • Hypoxia • Genetic susceptibility	• Pulmonary rehabilitation • Maintain/improve nutrition • Promote physical activity • Smoking cessation
Osteoporosis	• Reduced physical activity • Inflammation • Smoking • Hypoxia • Steroids	• Pulmonary rehabilitation • Maintain/improve nutrition • Promote physical activity • Smoking cessation • Investigate and treat
Cardiovascular disease	• Smoking • Vascular dysfunction • Neurohumoral activation	• Promote physical activity • Treat hypoxia • Smoking cessation • Optimize bronchodilation • Investigate for and treat cardiovascular risk factors and disease
Cognitive dysfunction	• Hypoxia • Systemic inflammation • Smoking • Depression	• Antidepressant therapy • Correct hypoxia • Promote physical activity • Smoking cessation

FUTURE DEVELOPMENTS

As broad-spectrum oral administration has significant side effects; inhaled form also has some spillover effects from lung. Another concern is to overcome corticosteroid resistance and to understand its molecular mechanisms which may lead to new therapeutic avenues in future.

The future drugs need to be considered in COPD and its comorbidities such as heart failure, osteoporosis, and diabetes which are more common in elderly population. In these conditions, drugs having antiaging properties such as sirtuin 1 and peroxisome proliferator-activated-c coactivator 1a might be tried.

TABLE 3: Summary of biologics currently undergoing clinical trials in the treatment of COPD.

Drug	Target	Clinical effects	Other indications (FDA approved)
Mepolizumab	IL-5	Significant reduction in annual disease exacerbation rates in phase III trials	Severe eosinophilic syndrome, Churg–Strauss syndrome, hypereosinophilic syndrome
Benralzumab	IL-5-Rα	Did not significantly reduce exacerbation and adverse event rates in previous COPD studies	Severe eosinophilic syndrome
Astegolimab	ST2	Significant improvements in QOL questionnaire scores, FEV_1, and reductions in blood eosinophils in phase IIa trial	None
Tozorakimab	IL-33	Favorable safety and pharmacokinetics profiles shown in phase I clinical trial	None

(FDA: Food and Drug Administration; FEV_1: forced expiratory volume in 1 second; IL: interleukin; QOL: quality of life)

Benralizumab is under investigations in phase III RESOLUTE trial for COPD to assess the efficacy and safety in patients with moderate-to-very severe COPD with a history of frequent COPD exacerbations and elevated peripheral blood eosinophils. The results of the RESOLUTE trial are to be published in 2025.

Astegolimab is an anti-ST2 monoclonal antibody (mAb), which has been tested in a randomized phase IIa clinical trial named COPD-ST2OP, which did not reduce exacerbation rates as compared to placebo but did improve patient health status as estimated by eosinophil counts, FEV_1, and St George's Respiratory Questionnaire for COPD scores. These results encouraged for further phase IIb) and phase III randomized controlled trials (RCTs) at a much larger scale, with 1,290 patients each which is slated to complete in 2025.

The TITANIA and OBERON are a pair of parallel phase III randomized clinical trials on the efficacy and safety of tozorakimab with symptomatic COPD and a history of COPD exacerbations in the previous 12 months. In earlier studies, tozorakimab (anti-IL-33 mAb) has been found to be safe with favorable pharmacokinetics profile. The results of these clinical trials are to be published in late 2025.

Of late, several studies on COPD have shown very significant and promising discoveries such as efficacy of targeting neutrophilic inflammation and cytokines with biologic treatments and information on its adverse effects. Therapies targeting eosinophilic infiltration have given commendable results, although not as effective as in asthma. This difference might be due to separate mechanisms, leading to eosinophilic inflammation in COPD and asthma.

Inferences can be drawn from the abovementioned studies that if subset of COPD patients is identified, the greater will be the direct benefits to these subgroups of COPD.

Targeting thymic stromal lymphopoietin (TSLP) and IL-33, which are upstream signaling molecules, make further biologics for treating chronic infections improve extrapulmonary manifestations of COPD patients **(Table 3)**.

CONCLUSION

A systematic approach to evaluate extrapulmonary manifestations and complications needs to be considered, incorporating updated clinical data on new drugs technology to be adopted in screening, investigations, and treatment. There are ongoing new efforts for newer molecules to be added in COPD therapeutic armamentarium with minimized adverse effects.

SUGGESTED READINGS

1. Singh D, Agusti A, Anzueto A, Barnes PJ, Bourbeau J, Celli BR, et al. Global Strategy for the Diagnosis, Management, and Prevention of Chronic Obstructive Lung Disease: the GOLD science committee report 2019. Eur Respir J. 2019;53(5): 1900164.
2. Minnix JA, Karam-Hage M, Blalock JA, Cinciripini PM. The importance of incorporating smoking cessation into lung cancer screening. Transl Lung Cancer Res. 2018;7(3):272-80.
3. Alisamir M, Ebrahimi M, Rahim F. Anemia in chronic obstructive pulmonary disease: A systematic review. Respir Investig. 2022;60(4):510-21.
4. Bitar AN, Sulaiman SAS, Ali IABH, Khan AH. Prevalence, risk assessment, and predictors of osteoporosis among chronic obstructive pulmonary disease patients. J Adv Pharm Technol Res. 2021;12(4):395-401.
5. Rahi MS, Thilagar B, Balaji S, Prabhakaran SY, Mudgal M, Rajoo S, et al. The Impact of Anxiety and Depression in Chronic Obstructive Pulmonary Disease. Adv Respir Med. 2023;91: 123-34.
6. Kim DH, Kim B, Han K, Kim SW. The relationship between metabolic syndrome and obstructive sleep apnea syndrome: a nationwide population-based study. Sci Rep. 2021;11:8751.

7. A multicenter, randomized, double-blind, chronic-dosing, parallel-group, placebo-controlled phase 3 study to evaluate the efficacy and safety of benralizumab 100 mg in patients with moderate to very severe chronic obstructive pulmonary disease (COPD) with a history of frequent COPD exacerbations and elevated peripheral blood eosinophils (RESOLUTE) (2023).
8. A randomized placebo-controlled trial of anti-ST2 in COP Genentech, Inc. A phase IIb, randomized, double-blind, placebo-controlled, multicenter study to evaluate the efficacy and safety of astegolimab in patients with chronic obstructive pulmonary disease (2023).
9. A phase III, multicenter, randomized, double-blind, chronic-dosing, parallel-group, placebo-controlled study to evaluate the efficacy and safety of two dose regimens of tozorakimab in participants with symptomatic chronic obstructive pulmonary disease (COPD) with a history of COPD exacerbations (TITANIA) (2023).

218

CHAPTER

Update in GOLD in the Management of COPD

Kaushik Hazra

ABSTRACT

Chronic obstructive pulmonary disease (COPD) is a prevalent and preventable disease that can be effectively treated. However, the widespread underdiagnosis of COPD often result in inappropriate treatment to patients. Understanding that factors beyond tobacco smoking can contribute to COPD and it can manifest early in life and affect younger individuals, and the existence of conditions ["Pre-COPD", "PRISm" (preserved ratio impaired spirometry)] present new opportunities for its prevention, early detection, and timely therapeutic intervention. There are various pharmacological and non-pharmacological treatments available that have demonstrated efficacy in reducing the mortality of COPD patients. However, for these treatments to be effectively implemented, accurate diagnosis of COPD is crucial. Therefore, there is a need to strengthen any strategy aimed at addressing and improving the significant underdiagnosis of COPD within the community. Recently GOLD (The Global Initiative for Chronic Obstructive Lung Disease) 2023 guidelines have brought noteworthy updates on definition, pathogenesis, risk factors, and management of COPD.

INTRODUCTION

The Global Initiative for Chronic Obstructive Lung Disease (GOLD) has recently unveiled the highly anticipated GOLD report for the year 2023 which is available on the official website at www.goldcopd.org.

This latest edition of the report brings about significant changes compared to its predecessors.

DEFINITION OF CHRONIC OBSTRUCTIVE PULMONARY DISEASE

The GOLD 2023 report introduces a fresh perspective by proposing a novel definition for chronic obstructive pulmonary disease (COPD).

The GOLD 2023 defines COPD as "a heterogeneous lung condition characterized by chronic respiratory symptoms (dyspnea, cough, expectoration, and/or exacerbations) due to abnormalities of the airways (bronchitis, bronchiolitis) and/or alveoli (emphysema) that cause persistent, often progressive, airflow obstruction".

PATHOGENESIS AND RISK FACTORS

The development of COPD is due to different complex factors. These are genetic factors (COPD-G), environmental factors (COPD-P due to pollution and COPD-C due to smoking), due to abnormal lung development (COPD-D), due to infections (COPD-I) or may be due to unknown cause (COPD-U).

ENVIRONMENTAL RISK FACTORS

Cigarette smoking is a significant risk factor for COPD. Individuals who smoke are more likely to experience respiratory symptoms, faster decline in forced expiratory volume in 1 second (FEV_1), and a higher mortality rate due to COPD compared to nonsmokers. However, it is important to note that not all heavy smokers (< 50%) develop COPD. In addition to active smoking, passive exposure to smoke as well as other forms of tobacco smoke like pipe, cigar, water pipe, and even marijuana, are also considered risk factors for COPD.

Chronic obstructive pulmonary disease in nonsmokers are more common in younger age and female patients. Indoor air pollution and occupational exposures are important risk factors.

The burning of biomass, including wood, animal dung, crop residues, and coal, often in inefficient stoves, can result in significant levels of indoor air pollution within households.

GENETIC FACTORS AND DEVELOPMENTAL ABNORMALITIES

The primary genetic risk factor associated with COPD is the presence of mutations in the *SERPINA1* gene, which causes a *deficiency of alpha-1 antitrypsin.*

Numerous studies have shown that *asthma* and atopy during infancy could potentially increase the risk of developing COPD in adulthood.

Abnormal lung development during childhood can result in symptoms resembling asthma, but individuals who were diagnosed as "asthma" during infancy and adolescence may have actually been experiencing symptoms related to COPD.

CHRONIC OBSTRUCTIVE PULMONARY DISEASE ASSOCIATED WITH INFECTIONS

The presence of respiratory tract infection, especially with *Pseudomonas aeruginosa*, is associated with an accelerated decline in FEV_1. Additionally, tuberculosis and human immunodeficiency virus (HIV) infection are significant risk factors for the development of COPD.

Clinical Presentation

Patients with COPD present with various symptoms such as *dyspnea, wheezing, chest tightness, fatigue, limited physical activity, and coughing, with or without sputum production.* They may experience acute respiratory events known as *exacerbations*, characterized by a sudden worsening of respiratory symptoms.

Diagnosis and Grading of Severity

In patients with symptoms of dyspnea, chronic cough, increased sputum production, history of recurrent lower respiratory tract infections, and exposure to known risk factors for COPD, the possibility of a COPD diagnosis should be considered.

However, to confirm the diagnosis, a post-bronchodilator FEV_1/FVC (forced vital capacity) ratio below 0.7 in spirometry is required.

Forced expiratory volume in 1 second is also used to assess the degree of airflow obstruction and classify its severity according to the GOLD grading system. The grades range from *1 (mild) to 4 (very severe), categorizing the airflow obstruction as mild, moderate, severe, or very severe.*

PRE-CHRONIC OBSTRUCTIVE PULMONARY DISEASE

A term "pre-COPD" has been proposed to describe individuals, regardless of age, who exhibit respiratory symptoms, and/or show detectable structural abnormalities (such as emphysema) and/or functional abnormalities (like hyperinflation, rapid FEV_1 decline) *but do not demonstrate airflow obstruction in post-bronchodilator spirometry (i.e., FEV_1/FVC ≥ 0.7).* These patients may or may not develop persistent airflow obstruction as time progresses.

PRESERVED RATIO IMPAIRED SPIROMETRY

The term PRISm (preserved ratio impaired spirometry) is used to identify individuals with FEV_1/FVC >0.7 and FEV_1 <80% of the reference value after bronchodilation. Its prevalence ranges from 7.1 to 20.3%, with a higher occurrence among current and former smokers. PRISm can evolve into normal, obstructive, or restrictive patterns in future.

ASSESSMENT OF SEVERITY

After confirming the diagnosis, primary objectives of the initial assessment are to guide therapy by determining the following:

- Severity of airflow limitation, classified according to GOLD spirometric grades
- Nature and intensity of current symptoms
- History of moderate and severe exacerbations, which are risk for future exacerbations
- Presence and specific type of comorbidity

From ABCD to ABE

In the GOLD 2023 update, there are modifications to the ABCD assessment tool from previous editions to acknowledge the clinical impact of exacerbations regardless of the patient's symptom level. A and B groups remain unchanged, while the *former C and D groups have been merged into a single group now referred to as "E"* (for "exacerbations") **(Fig. 1)**.

CHEST X-RAY AND COMPUTED TOMOGRAPHY THORAX

Radiographic findings associated with COPD may reveal features of lung hyperinflation. Chest X-ray can also be useful in ruling out other potential diagnoses and confirming the presence of significant comorbidities such as *fibrosis, bronchiectasis, pleural diseases,* and *cardiomegaly.*

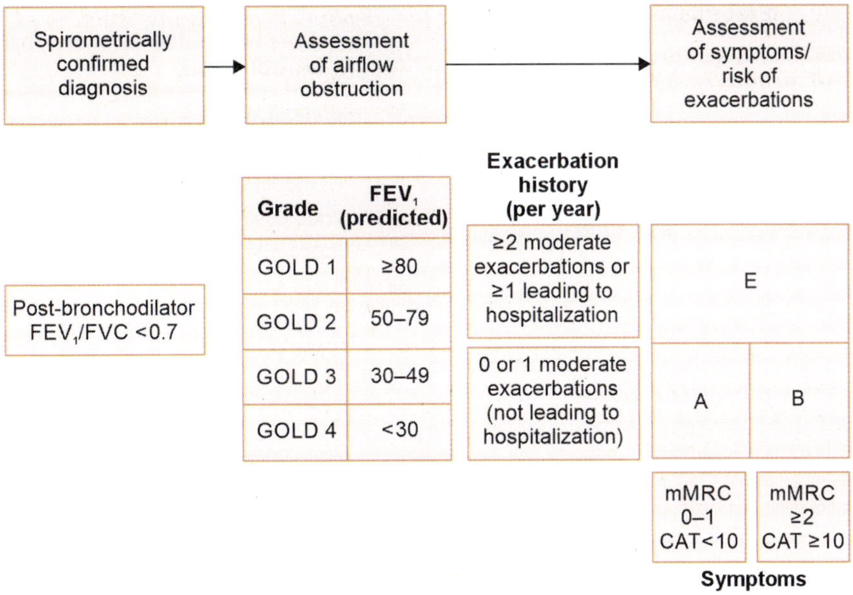

FIG. 1: Severity of chronic obstructive pulmonary disease (COPD) and ABE assessment tool.

(CAT: COPD assessment test; FEV_1: forced expiratory volume in 1 second; FVC: forced vital capacity; mMRC: modified Medical Research Council)

Chest computed tomography (CT) scans are recommended in persistent exacerbations, *lung cancer screening.*

TREATMENT

Pharmacological Therapy

Appropriate Use of Inhaler Devices

In COPD treatment, inhaled therapy plays a fundamental role, and it is vital to ensure the proper use of these devices **(Fig. 2)**.

In the 2023 GOLD recommendation for initiating pharmacological therapy, there are some changes.

- Patients classified in Group A continue to receive the same treatment.
- For patients in Group B, the recommendation now includes initiating a combination of *dual long-acting bronchodilators [a combination of long-acting beta-2 agonist (LABA) and Long-acting muscarinic antagonist (LAMA) bronchodilators].*
- Dual therapy has shown to be more effective than monotherapy.
- In Group E, the initial therapy recommendation is also a LAMA-LABA combination, except for those with *blood eosinophils exceeding 300 cells/μL.* In such cases, *triple therapy* [LABA-LAMA-inhaled corticosteroid (ICS)] is recommended.
- *Using a single inhaler* can offer both convenience and improved effectiveness compared to managing multiple inhalers.

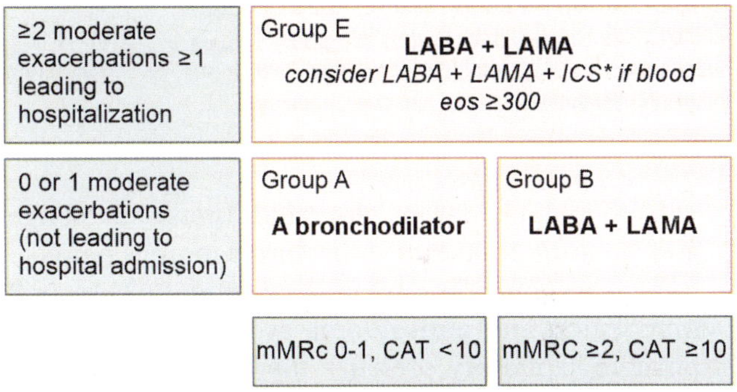

FIG. 2: Appropriate choice of inhalers in different group as per GOLD (The Global Initiative for Chronic Obstructive Lung Disease) 2023 update.

(CAT: chronic obstructive pulmonary disease assessment test; eos: eosinophil count; ICS: inhaled corticosteroid; LABA: long-acting beta-2 agonist; LAMA: long-acting muscarinic antagonist; mMRC: modified Medical Research Council)

- The use of LABA-ICS combination therapy in COPD *is not recommended.*
- If patients on LABA-LAMA treatment with persistent exacerbations and have blood eosinophils *levels above 100 cells/μL,* escalation to LABA-LAMA-ICS therapy is recommended.
- In cases where patients continue to experience exacerbations despite therapy with LABA-LAMA-ICS or have an eosinophil count below 100 cells/μL, the addition of *roflumilast* (particularly for those with chronic bronchitis and an FEV_1 below 50% predicted) or a *macrolide* (especially for nonsmokers) may be considered **(Flowchart 1)**.

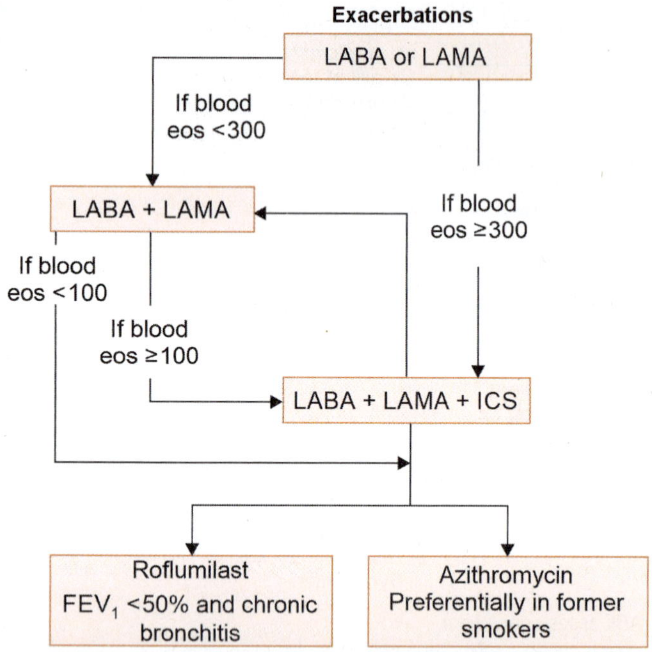

FLOWCHART 1: Role of inhaled corticosteroid (ICS), roflumilast, and azithromycin according to GOLD (The Global Initiative for Chronic Obstructive Lung Disease) 2023 update.

(eos: eosinophil count; FEV_1: forced expiratory volume in 1 second; ICS: inhaled corticosteroid; LABA: long-acting beta-2 agonist; LAMA: long-acting muscarinic antagonist)

- The treatment of chronic bronchitis (persistent cough and sputum production for at least 3 months per year for 2 years) include smoking cessation, LAMAs, oral mucolytics, and antioxidants as well as oscillating positive expiratory pressure therapy. Furthermore, novel treatments such as liquid nitrogen metered cryospray, rheoplasty, and targeted lung denervation are currently being evaluated.

INDICATIONS FOR USING INHALED CORTICOSTEROID IN CHRONIC OBSTRUCTIVE PULMONARY DISEASE

Box 1 shows the indications for using ICS in COPD.

BOX 1: Role of inhaled corticosteroid (ICS) according to eosinophil count.

- *Strongly indicated*:
  - History of hospitalization
  - >2 moderate exacerbations per year
  - Blood eosinophil ≥ 300/μL
  - Concomitant asthma
- *Indicated/can be used*:
  - 1 moderate exacerbation per year
  - Blood eosinophils 10–300 cells/μL
- *Contraindicated*:
  - History of repeated pneumonia
  - Blood eosinophils < 100 cells/μL
  - Associated mycobacterial infection

NONPHARMACOLOGICAL INTERVENTIONS

In COPD management, there is a significant role of nonpharmacological interventions.

Education

It is essential to provide all patients with fundamental knowledge concerning COPD and its treatment, including respiratory medications, *inhalational devices and techniques* to alleviate dyspnea, and guidance on when to seek medical assistance.

Smoking Cessation

Despite being aware of their COPD diagnosis, nearly 40% of individuals continue to smoke, adversely affecting their disease prognosis and progression. Hence, it is important to offer assistance and treatment to all patients who continue to smoke and aiding them in their journey toward quitting.

Vaccination

As per local guidelines, patients should be provided with the option of getting vaccinated against influenza, pneumococcus, coronavirus disease 2019 (COVID-19), pertussis, and herpes zoster, if they have not already received these vaccinations.

Physical Activity and Pulmonary Rehabilitation

All COPD patients should be encouraged to keep active. Technology-based interventions have the potential to provide convenient and accessible means to enhance exercise self-efficacy, and to educate and motivate patients to make healthy lifestyle changes.

Participating in structured pulmonary rehabilitation (PR) programs, be it community-based or home-based, brings significant benefits. It is recommended that patients of GOLD groups B and E, with higher symptom burden and exacerbation risk, should be encouraged to attend PR programs.

Tele-rehabilitation has emerged as a proposed alternative to traditional approaches. It has gained even more significance for delivering rehabilitation services remotely.

Oxygen Therapy

Long-term oxygen therapy (LTOT) is prescribed for patients who meet the following criteria:

- Partial pressure of arterial oxygen (PaO_2) at or below 55 mm Hg (7.3 kPa) or arterial oxygen saturation (SaO_2) at or below 88%, with or without hypercapnia, confirmed twice over a 3-week period.
- PaO_2 is between 55 mm Hg (7.3 kPa) and 60 mm Hg (8.0 kPa), or SaO_2 is 88%, with evidence of pulmonary hypertension, peripheral edema suggesting congestive cardiac failure, or polycythemia (hematocrit > 55%).

Patients should be re-evaluated within 60–90 days with repeat arterial blood gas (ABG) analysis.

Noninvasive Ventilation

Noninvasive ventilation (NIV) may be considered for a selected group of patients having significant daytime hypercapnia [partial pressure of arterial carbon dioxide ($PaCO_2$) is > 53 mm Hg] and recent hospitalization, in patients with coexisting COPD and obstructive sleep apnea.

Surgical Treatment

For certain patients with symptomatic emphysema and significant hyperinflation unresponsive to optimized medical treatment, there is a possibility of considering surgical or bronchoscopic lung volume reduction methods like *surgical bullectomy* and *lung transplantation*.

TREATMENT OF COMORBIDITIES

Chronic obstructive pulmonary disease is almost always accompanied by other coexisting medical conditions which can significantly impact the patient's overall clinical state and prognosis and COPD can also influence the outcomes of comorbidities.

Cardiovascular diseases, ranging from congestive heart failure to ischemic heart disease, arrhythmias, peripheral vascular disease, and hypertension, are commonly found in individuals with COPD. For *lung cancer screening* due to smoking, *an annual low-dose CT scan is recommended.*

Other prevalent comorbidities include sleep apnea, osteoporosis, diabetes, metabolic syndrome, gastroesophageal reflux, anemia, and secondary polycythemia, which may be associated with pulmonary hypertension, venous thromboembolism, and mortality. Anxiety and depression are significant comorbidities in COPD patients.

To prevent severe acute respiratory syndrome coronavirus 2 (*SARS-CoV-2*) *infection*, individuals with COPD should adhere to basic infection control measures.

EXACERBATIONS

Previously the definition of exacerbations of COPD (ECOPD) by GOLD was nonspecific. In GOLD 2023 ECOPD is now defined as an *event characterized by worsening dyspnea and/or cough and sputum over a period of less than 14 days*. This deterioration is often linked to increased local and systemic inflammation, triggered by factors like airway infection, pollution, or other airway insults **(Flowchart 2)**.

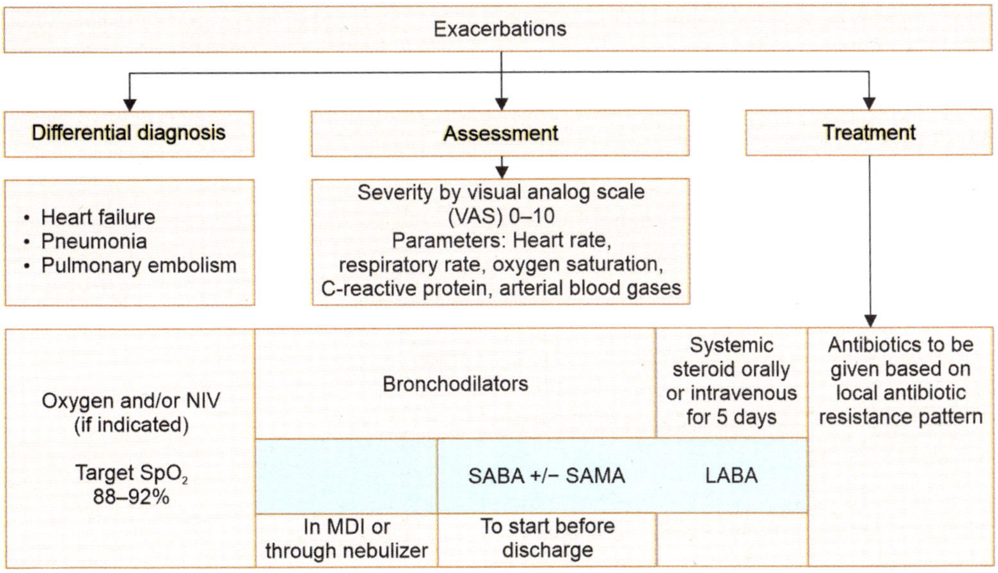

FLOWCHART 2: Diagnosis assessment and treatment of exacerbations of chronic obstructive pulmonary disease (ECOPD).

(LABA: long-acting beta-2 agonist; MDI: metered dose inhaler; NIV: noninvasive ventilation; SABA: short-acting beta-2 agonist SAMA: short-acting muscarinic antagonist; SpO_2: peripheral oxygen saturation)

KEY MESSAGE

Based on the above discussion, the latest GOLD 2023 guidelines have brought about noteworthy updates that include the following:

- A *new definition* of COPD is now proposed.
- They have proposed *taxonomy (etiotypes)* for COPD.
- The use of *CT in COPD* was discussed.
- It covers current and proposed *surgical and bronchoscopic interventions* in COPD.
- The evidence supporting a reduction in mortality with *pharmacotherapy and nonpharmacotherapy* in COPD has been updated.
- There was a detailed discussion on basic principles for *appropriate inhalation device choice.*
- A *new definition and classification of the severity of ECOPD* were updated.
- The *vaccination recommendations* for people with COPD have been updated.
- A section on *tele-rehabilitation* has been added.
- The *ABCD assessment tool has been revised to the ABE* assessment tool.
- *COPD and comorbidities* have been thoroughly updated.
- A section on *COVID-19 and COPD* is updated.

SUGGESTED READINGS

1. Global Initiative for Chronic Obstructive Lung Disease. (2023). Global strategy for prevention, diagnosis and management of COPD: 2023 report. [online] Available from https://goldcopd.org/2023-gold-report-2/ [Last accessed December, 2023].
2. Agustí A, Celli BR, Criner GJ, Halpin D, Anzueto A, Barnes P, et al. Global Initiative for Chronic Obstructive Lung Disease 2023 Report: GOLD Executive Summary. Eur Respir J. 2023;61:2300239.
3. Agustí A, Melén E, DeMeo DL, Breyer-Kohansal R, Faner R. Pathogenesis of chronic obstructive pulmonary disease: understanding the contributions of gene-environment interactions across the lifespan.Lancet Respir Med. 2022;10: 512-24.
4. Kohansal R, Martinez-Camblor P, Agustí A, Buist AS, Mannino DM, Soriano JB. The natural history of chronic airflow obstruction revisited: an analysis of the Framingham offspring cohort. Am J Respir Crit Care Med. 2009;180:3-10.
5. de Marco R, Accordini S, Marcon A, Cerveri I, Antó JM, Gislason T, et al; European Community Respiratory Health Survey (ECRHS). Risk factors for chronic obstructive pulmonary disease in a European cohort of young adults. Am J Respir Crit Care Med. 2011;183:891-7.
6. Wan ES. The clinical spectrum of PRISm. Am J Respir Crit Care Med. 2022;206:524-25.
7. Rodriguez-Roisin R, Rabe KF, Vestbo J, Vogelmeier C, Agustí A; all previous and current members of the Science Committee and the Board of Directors of GOLD (goldcopd.org/committees/). Global Initiative for Chronic Obstructive Lung Disease (GOLD) 20th Anniversary: a brief history of time. Eur Respir J 2017;50:1700671.
8. National Lung Screening Trial Research Team; Aberle DR, Adams AM, Berg CD, Black WC, Clapp JD, Fagerstrom RM, et al. Reduced lung cancer mortality with low-dose computed tomographic screening. N Engl J Med. 2011;365:395-409.
9. Lipson DA, Barnhart F, Brealey N, Brooks J, Criner GJ, Day NC, et al; IMPACT Investigators. Once-daily single-inhaler triple versus dual therapy in patients with COPD. N Engl J Med. 2018;378:1671-80.
10. Agusti A, Fabbri LM, Singh D, Vestbo J, Celli B, Franssen FME, et al. Inhaled corticosteroids in COPD: friend or foe? Eur Respir J. 2018;52:1801219.
11. Montes de Oca M. Smoking cessation/vaccinations. Clin Chest Med. 2020;41:495-512.
12. Spruit MA, Singh SJ, Garvey C, ZuWallack R, Nici L, Rochester C, et al; ATS/ERS Task Force on Pulmonary Rehabilitation. An official American Thoracic Society/European Respiratory Society statement: key concepts and advances in pulmonary rehabilitation. Am J Respir Crit Care Med. 2013;188:e13-e64.
13. Celli BR, Fabbri LM, Aaron SD, Agusti A, Brook R, Criner GJ, et al. An updated definition and severity classification of COPD exacerbations: the Rome proposal. Am J Respir Crit Care Med. 2021;204:1251-8.
14. Mannino DM, Thorn D, Swensen A, Holguin F. Prevalence and outcomes of diabetes, hypertension and cardiovascular disease in COPD. Eur Respir J. 2008;32:962-9.
15. Talic S, Shah S, Wild H, Gasevic D, Maharaj A, Ademi Z, et al. Effectiveness of public health measures in reducing the incidence of COVID-19, SARS-CoV-2 transmission, and COVID-19 mortality: systematic review and meta-analysis. BMJ. 2021;375:e068302.

219

CHAPTER

Asthma Chronic Obstructive Pulmonary Disease Overlap Syndrome: What is New?

Rakesh Kumar Goel, Kanupriya Goel

ABSTRACT

The Global Initiative for Chronic Obstructive Lung Disease (GOLD) in its 2023 report lists asthma as a risk factor for the development of chronic airflow obstruction and chronic obstructive pulmonary disease (COPD) stating that separating asthma from COPD in adults may be clinically difficult at times. The GOLD 2023 report classifies COPD and asthma, particularly childhood asthma as COPD-A. Gibson et al. was the one who coined the term asthma COPD overlap syndrome (ACOS) in 2009 later named as asthma COPD overlap (ACO) to describe patients having features of both COPD and asthma. The 2021 GOLD strategy states that the term "ACO" will no longer be used to refer to patients having both COPD and asthma and instead COPD and asthma are two different disorders that may coexist in the same individual. Despite ample literature on the subject, the diagnosis and treatment of this condition become challenging for clinicians in the current scenario. Triple therapy with inhalational corticosteroids (ICS), long-acting bronchodilating agents (LABA) and long-acting muscarinic antagonists (LAMA) seems to be an appropriate therapy. We aim to review the latest literature and guidelines to elicit relevant information in order to facilitate diagnosis and management of an individual presenting with features of asthma and COPD.

INTRODUCTION

Asthma-COPD overlap (ACO) is a heterogeneous condition describing patients with persistent airflow limitation and clinical and inflammatory features of both asthma and chronic obstructive pulmonary disease (COPD). Asthma and COPD have unique clinical features. Nevertheless, these clinical features can coexist, making it difficult to distinguish between the two conditions in a clinical setting. As a result, the term "ACO" was introduced. However, despite the increased research interest in ACO, there is still much controversy about its existence as a distinct entity, and from 2020 the Global Initiative for Chronic Obstructive Lung Disease (GOLD) stopped referring to ACO, emphasizing the absence of a universally accepted definition due to the lack of substantial evidence.

In 2017, the American Thoracic Society (ATS) and the National Heart, Lung, and Blood Institute (NHLBI) collaborated on an ACO workshop report. The panel concluded that ACO, such as asthma and COPD, does not represent a singular unique disease entity. Instead, ACO should be utilized to describe patients with a prolonged history of asthma, a modest smoking history, and fixed-airflow obstruction. Concurrently, those who exhibit asthma-like symptoms, such as peripheral eosinophilia and bronchodilator responsiveness, may have ACO. While both patient groups are clinically and likely pathologically unique, they are both within the purview of ACO. However, in the 2021 GOLD report the term ACO no longer exists and the authors state that COPD and asthma are two distinct entities which can coexist in a single individual. Despite the removal of ACO from the most important reports on the management of asthma and COPD, i.e., the Global Initiative for Asthma (GINA) and the GOLD, this entity still continues to be important and receive attention in both clinical research and clinical practice.

Our review covers clinical presentation, diagnosis, followed by nonpharmacological and pharmacological treatment options and further directions.

DEFINITION

A number of authors and different consensus guidelines have proposed various definitions of ACO during the last decades, usually using several major and minor criteria. Most of them emphasize the heterogeneity of clinical features and functional and laboratory findings that should be considered as diagnostic criteria that could apply for the identification of individuals with a possible diagnosis of ACO. According to "Dutch hypothesis", obstructive airway diseases share a common genetic pathway, with bronchial hyperresponsiveness being important in both asthma and COPD, while environmental factors determine whether one would have asthma or COPD. This could be differentiated from the "British hypothesis" provided in 1965 by Charles Fletcher, who proposed that an individual with certain genetic predisposition may present the clinical phenotypes of COPD and asthma after exposure to smoking and antigen sensitization, respectively.

The most widely accepted ACO definition is the one of the 2015 GINA/GOLD documents. In this report, the patient should have a chronic airway disease (medical history of cough, sputum production, wheezing, or repeated lower respiratory tract infections) in combination with features of both asthma and COPD.

EPIDEMIOLOGY

The prevalence of ACO in the overall population ranges from 2 to 3%, whereas the prevalence of asthma and COPD ranges from 5 to 17% and 2 to 12%, respectively. However, in COPD patients, the prevalence of ACO may be as high as 25%, and in asthma patients, the estimated prevalence of ACO ranges from 10 to 31%.

In 2023, [Asthma-COPD Overlap in Clinical Practice (ACO_CP 2023): Toward Precision Medicine] study published which characterized ACO patients' bacterial respiratory microbiome in both stable and exacerbation states. In this study, the lower airways of clinically stable ACO patients were found to have bacterial colonization, which makes it challenging to establish the role of bacteria in exacerbation. In the exacerbation condition, the taxonomic richness of bacteria decreased, and the evenness of microbiota increased compared to stable states in ACO patients. The *Prevotella* genus was found to be substantially more abundant in exacerbation samples than in stable samples, suggesting that some species of Prevotella may contribute to ACO pathogenicity. Similar to earlier COPD investigations utilizing culture techniques, this study found substantial abundances of the bacterial aerobic genera *Streptococcus, Haemophilus, Pseudomonas,* and *Moraxella*. The investigation also detected high frequencies of *Prevotella, Veillonella*, and *Actinomyces anaerobes*, suggesting a rich spectrum of taxa.

CLINICAL PRESENTATION AND DIAGNOSIS

Refer to **Table 1**.

TABLE 1: Clinical presentation and diagnosis.

Field	Criteria	Comments
Demographic data	Age ≥ 40 years	
Medical history	• A documented asthmatic history before the age of 40 years • Prior symptoms of asthma or allergic rhinitis • History of atopy and/or allergies. ≥10-pack-year of tobacco smoking or equivalent air pollution	
Symptoms	• The frequency, intensity, and duration of respiratory symptoms • Exercise limitation	Respiratory symptoms (e.g., dyspnea including exertional dyspnea, cough, sputum) are persistent, but variability in symptoms may be prominent
Spirometry	• Post-BD FEV_1/FVC <70% or LLN and BD increase in FEV_1 >12% and 400 mL • FEV_1 < 80%	• The assessment of ACO must involve spirometry before and after BD. These tests confirm airflow limitation (obstruction) and evaluate its reversibility • The airflow limitation is not completely reversible, however there has been historical variance • ACO patients usually have a BD response, defined as a post-BD rise in FEV_1 or FVC of < 10% of the predicted value; however, asthma patients usually have an increase in FEV_1 or FVC of more than 15% of their predicted value. Post-BD FEV_1 and FEV_1/FVC are poor in ACO patients. Normal post-BD values suggest asthma

Continued

Continued

Field	Criteria	Comments
	Persistent partially reversible airflow obstruction (without normalization of obstruction)	While airflow limitation is required for ACO diagnosis, it does not assist distinguish ACO from asthma or COPD
Laboratory tests	• A high level of total serum IgE (>100 international units/mL) • Elevated peripheral blood eosinophil count (>300 cells/μL) • Evidence of allergic disease • Elevated sputum eosinophil counts • Alpha-1 antitrypsin deficiency	• Not routinely obtained. May point a practitioner to asthma or ACO • May point a practitioner to asthma or ACO • Not routinely obtained. May point a practitioner to asthma or ACO • Not routinely obtained. More common in asthma or ACO than COPD • Recommended for all patients with fixed-airflow limitation
Imaging	• A chest radiograph is often used to diagnose chronic symptoms or an exacerbation. The chest radiograph may indicate hyperinflation in ACO patients, but it does not distinguish between asthma, COPD, and ACO • If there is diagnostic uncertainty, high-resolution computed tomography may be helpful. Small airway disease without emphysema may be ACO, although asthma (without COPD) and bronchiolitis obliterans should be evaluated. Severe emphysema is more common in COPD than ACO	

(BD: bronchodilator; LLN: lower limit of normal; ACO: asthma–COPD overlap; COPD: chronic obstructive pulmonary disease; FEV1: forced expiratory volume in 1 second)

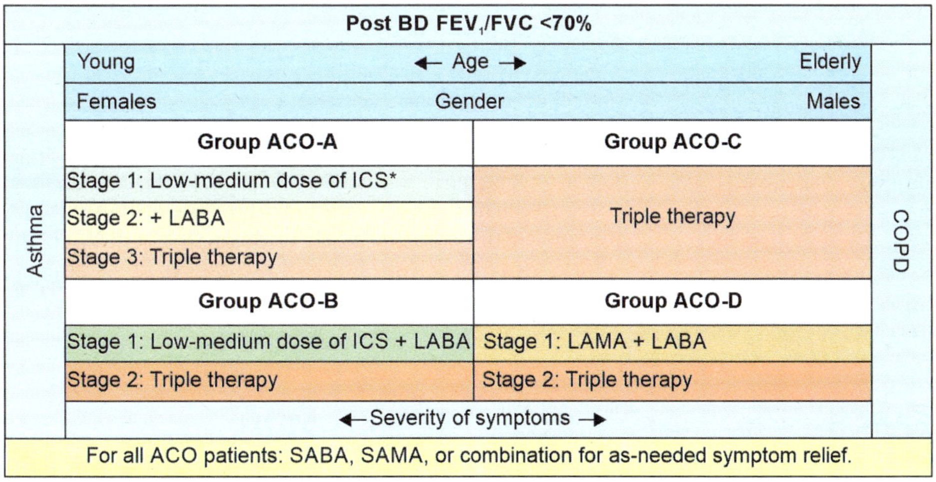

*This stage can be skipped for patients with frequent exacerbations.

FIG. 1: The treatment scheme for ACO patients based on the four phenotypes.

NON-PHARMACOLOGIC TREATMENT

- Smoking cessation
- Vaccination
  - Annual influenza vaccine
  - Pneumococcal vaccine
- Allergen avoidance
- Inhaler technique
- Pulmonary rehabilitation

PHARMACOLOGIC TREATMENT (FIG. 1, TABLES 2 AND 3)

Agreement over the effective management of ACO is in its infancy, and there is limited consensus among medical professionals on the most effective approach. The initial pharmacological options indicated in the joint GINA and GOLD statement on ACO depend on the expert opinion of medical professionals.

TABLE 2: The treatment scheme for asthma–COPD overlap (ACO) patients based on the four phenotypes.

Group ACO-A	• Asthmatics, non-smokers, most probably females. These patients may exhibit eosinophilic inflammation signs • Inhaled corticosteroids (ICS) are appropriate in this group of ACO, as ICS are a mainstay of asthma treatment • Adding a long-acting beta-agonist (LABA), long-acting muscarinic antagonist (LAMA), or both may be essential for symptom control. Nevertheless, as in asthma, LABA monotherapy should be avoided. Leukotriene receptor antagonists can be considered add-on treatments
Group ACO-B	• Asthmatics, smokers, patients having a fixed airway obstruction. These patients are typically younger females with a higher prevalence of atopic characteristics • Given the limited data, starting with ICS plus LABA, then moving to the triple therapy for patients non-responsive to the first stage
Group ACO-C	• Chronic obstructive pulmonary disease (COPD) accompanied by eosinophilia. Patients in this group tend to be older men with a higher eosinophil count than smokers (>300 cells/μL) and T helper cell type 2–related indicators • However, the 2023 GOLD recommends starting LABA and LAMA combination for group B COPD patients and triple therapy for group E (previously known as group C and D). Taking these into consideration, ACO_CP 2023 guide recommends starting with the triple therapy for this ACO phenotype
Group ACO-D	• COPD with a substantial BD response (FEV_1 ≥15% and ≥400 mL), as defined by previous publications. These patients have numerous characteristics of COPD with eosinophilia phenotype, as they are usually older males with comparable baseline lung function. Their blood eosinophil level is typically <300 cells/μL • ICS are not used as monotherapy for COPD. However, in the 2023 GOLD, they recommend starting LABA and LAMA combination for group B COPD; considering that, ACO_CP 2023 guide recommends starting with LAMA plus LABA as initial therapy for this ACO phenotype. Adding ICS (triple therapy) can be considered for unresponsive cases

TABLE 3: The use of biologic agents in patients with asthma–COPD overlap (ACO) features.

Class	Biologic agents	Evidence
Anti-IgE therapy	Omalizumab	Reduces exacerbations and improves symptoms moderately in allergic asthma patients with elevated serum IgE levels and sensitivity to perennial allergens; may be advantageous in ACO
Anti-IL-5/IL-5 receptor alpha (IL-5Ra) therapies	• Benralizumab • Mepolizumab • Reslizumab	Minimizes asthma exacerbations, improves asthma symptoms and quality of life, and reduces systemic corticosteroid use
IL-4 receptor alpha (IL-4Ra) and IL-13 therapies	Dupilumab	Enhances lung function and decreases exacerbations in severe asthma, with patients with higher blood eosinophil levels benefiting the most. However, efficacy in chronic obstructive pulmonary disease (COPD) and ACO is not established
Anti-thymic stromal lymphopoietin-IgG2λ	Tezepelumab	Add-on controller treatment of severe asthma in adults and children ≥ 12 years of age

FUTURE RESEARCH

To better understand ACO and its treatment, further investigation is needed to identify the types of biomarkers and phenotypes that can identify patients who are most sensitive to particular therapies.

Current research on ACO traits has not utilized all possible classification methods. Longitudinal studies are required to enable a deeper understanding of these phenotypes and how they influence management decisions. In addition, performing detailed omics research, including the respiratory microbiome, could considerably improve phenotyping.

CONCLUSION

Asthma and COPD have characteristic symptoms, yet patients with both are prevalent. However, there is no globally accepted definition of ACO, and it may not be considered a distinct disease or clinical entity.

Besides the age and smoking history of the patient, recurrent pulmonary infections and inflammation have been considered as provoking factors contributing to the worsening of pulmonary function in elders.

No single biomarker can be used to identify and classify ACO phenotypes.

Non-pharmacologic treatment options for ACO patients include smoking cessation, annual influenza, and pneumococcus vaccinations, inhaler technique education, avoidance of provoking allergy factors for people susceptible to known allergens, and pulmonary rehabilitation. The treatment of ACO tends to be escalated to counteract clinical manifestations and prevent further worsening. This may involve increasing ICS doses or adding LAMA, ICS, and LABA (triple therapy). However, despite triple inhaled treatment in patients with persistent symptoms or exacerbations, they should be assessed for manifestations that indicate a potential advantages from monoclonal based pharmacotherapy. It is essential to conduct large-scale trials to evaluate clinically relevant outcomes in patients with well-defined ACO.

SUGGESTED READINGS

1. Boulet LP, Boulay M, Dérival JL, Milot J, Lepage J, Bilodeau L, et al. Asthma-COPD Overlap Phenotypes and Smoking: comparative features of asthma in smoking or non-smoking patients with an incomplete reversibility of airway obstruction. COPD J Chron Obstruct Pulm Dis. 2018;15:130-8.
2. Soler-Cataluña JJ, Novella L, Soler C, Nieto ML, Esteban V, Sánchez-Toril F, et al. Clinical characteristics and risk of exacerbations associated with different diagnostic criteria of asthma-COPD Overlap. Arch Bronconeumol (Engl Ed). 2020;56:282-90.
3. Tommola M, Ilmarinen P, Tuomisto LE, Lehtimäki L, Haanpää J, Niemelä O, et al. Differences between asthma-COPD overlap syndrome and adult-onset asthma. Eur Respir J. 2017;49(5):1602383.
4. Woodruff PG, van den Berge M, Boucher RC, Brightling C, Burchard EG, Christenson SA, et al. American Thoracic Society/National Heart, Lung, and Blood Institute Asthma-Chronic Obstructive Pulmonary Disease Overlap Workshop Report. Am J Respir Crit Care Med. 2017;196(3):375-81.
5. Reddel HK, Bacharier LB, Bateman ED, Brightling CE, Brusselle GG, Buhl R, et al. Global Initiative for Asthma Strategy 2021: Executive summary and rationale for key changes. Eur Respirat J. 2022;59:17-35.
6. Global Initiative for Chronic Obstructive Lung Disease – GOLD. (2020). Global Strategy for the Diagnosis, Management and Prevention of COPD. [online] Available from: http://www.goldcopd.org. [Last accessed January, 2024].
7. Gibson PG, Simpson JL. The overlap syndrome of asthma and COPD: What are its features and how important is it? Thorax. 2009;64:728-35.
8. Global Initiative for Chronic Obstructive Lung Disease (GOLD). (2014). Global Strategy for the Diagnosis, Management and Prevention of COPD. [online] Available from: http://www.goldcopd.org. [Last accessed January, 2024].
9. Soler-Cataluña JJ, Cosío B, Izquierdo JL, López-Campos JL, Marín JM, Agüero R, et al. Consensus document on the overlap phenotype COPD-asthma in COPD. Arch Bronconeumol. 2012;48:331-7.
10. Koblizek V, Chlumsky J, Zindr V, Neumannova K, Zatloukal J, Zak J, et al. Chronic Obstructive Pulmonary Disease: Official diagnosis and treatment guidelines of the Czech Pneumological and Phthisiological Society; a novel phenotypic approach to COPD with patient-oriented care. Biomed Pap Med Fac Univ. 2013;157:189-201.
11. Cosio BG, Soriano JB, López-Campos JL, Calle-Rubio M, Soler-Cataluna JJ, de-Torres JP, et al. Defining the Asthma-COPD Overlap Syndrome in a COPD Cohort. Chest. 2016;149:45-52.
12. Sin DD, Miravitlles M, Mannino DM, Soriano JB, Price D, Celli BR, et al. What is asthma-COPD overlap syndrome? Towards a consensus definition from a round table discussion. Eur Respir J. 2016;48:664-73.
13. Cataldo D, Corhay JL, Derom E, Louis R, Marchand E, Michils A, et al. A Belgian survey on the diagnosis of asthma-COPD overlap syndrome. Int J Chron Obstr Pulmon Dis. 2017;12:601-13.
14. Miravitlles M, Alvarez-Gutierrez FJ, Calle M, Casanova C, Cosio BG, López-Viña A, et al. Algorithm for identification of asthma-COPD overlap: Consensus between the Spanish COPD and asthma guidelines. Eur Respir J. 2017;49:1700068.
15. Fletcher CM. Chronic bronchitis. Its prevalence, nature, and pathogenesis. Am Rev Respir Dis. 1959;80:483-94.
16. GINASTHMA.ORG. (2015). Diagnosis of Diseases of Chronic Airflow Limitation. Asthma, COPD and Asthma-COPD Overlap Syndrome (ACOS). A Joint Project of GINA and GOLD. [online] Available from: www.ginasthma.org. [Last accessed January, 2024].
17. Leung JM, Sin DD. Asthma-COPD overlap syndrome: pathogenesis, clinical features, and therapeutic targets. BMJ. 2017;358:j3772.
18. Alshabanat A, Zafari Z, Albanyan O, Dairi M, FitzGerald JM. Asthma and COPD Overlap Syndrome (ACOS): a systematic review and meta analysis. PLoS ONE. 2015;10:e0136065.
19. Alsayed AR, Abu-Samak MS, Alkhatib M. Asthma-COPD Overlap in Clinical Practice (ACO_CP 2023): Toward Precision Medicine. J Pers Med. 2023;13:677.
20. Alsayed AR, Abed A, Jarrar YB, Alshammari F, Alshammari B, Basheti IA, et al. Alteration of the respiratory microbiome in hospitalized patients with asthma–COPD overlap during and after an exacerbation. J Clin Med. 2023;12:2118.
21. Sethi S, Evans N, Grant BJB, Murphy TF. New strains of bacteria and exacerbations of chronic obstructive pulmonary disease. N Engl J Med. 2002;347:465-71.
22. Murphy TF, Brauer AL, Eschberger K, Lobbins P, Grove L, Cai X, et al. Pseudomonas aeruginosa in chronic obstructive pulmonary disease. Am J Respir Crit Care Med. 2008;177:853-60.
23. Global Initiative for Chronic Obstructive Lung Disease (GOLD). (2022). Global Strategy for the Diagnosis, Management, and Prevention of Chronic Obstructive Pulmonary Disease. [online] Available from: https://goldcopd.org/wp-content/uploads/2021/12/GOLD-REPORT-2022-v1.1-22Nov2021_WMV.pdf. [Last accessed January, 2024].
24. Rhee CK. Phenotype of asthma-chronic obstructive pulmonary disease overlap syndrome. Korean J Int Med. 2015;30:443-49.
25. Adrish M, Anand MP, Hanania NA. Phenotypes of asthma-chronic obstructive pulmonary disease overlap. Immunol Allerg Clin N Am. 2022;42:645-55.

PATHOGENESIS OF ALLERGIC BRONCHOPULMONARY ASPERGILLOSIS

Aspergillus, a ubiquitous mold found in soil, water, and air, releases conidia that can easily enter the airways. *Aspergillus* spores are released and inhaled routinely but are normally cleared from airways without any harmful effects. Approximately 8,000–10,000 mL of air is inhaled by an average adult along with 100 *A. fumigatus* conidia on a daily basis. While exposure to a large number of *A. fumigatus* conidia can cause ABPA, not all asthmatics develop the disorder despite living in the same environment. The exact pathogenesis of ABPA remains unclear.

However, it is believed to involve an immune response triggered by *Aspergillus* antigens, resulting in a complex interplay between genetic and environmental factors. Upon inhalation of *Aspergillus* spores, susceptible individuals mount an exaggerated Th2-mediated immune response, leading to the production of immunoglobulin E (IgE) antibodies against *Aspergillus* antigens. This immune response triggers a cascade of inflammatory processes, resulting in bronchial hyperresponsiveness, eosinophilic infiltration, and airway remodeling.

DIAGNOSTIC CHALLENGES

The diagnosis of ABPA can be challenging and often requires a multidimensional approach. Clinical presentation, radiological findings, serological markers, and immunological assessments are all important components in establishing a diagnosis. However, the lack of standardized diagnostic criteria and the overlap of symptoms with other respiratory conditions contribute to diagnostic difficulties.

The International Society for Human and Animal Mycology (ISHAM) has formed an ABPA Working Group to streamline the recognition and diagnosis of this disorder. The working group has proposed recommendations for the diagnosis and classification of ABPA complicating asthma, aiming to improve diagnostic accuracy and reduce misdiagnosis which are discussed in the later section.

CLINICAL PRESENTATION AND RISK FACTORS OF ALLERGIC BRONCHOPULMONARY ASPERGILLOSIS

Allergic bronchopulmonary aspergillosis is more commonly diagnosed in the third decade of life and with no gender predilection. It presents with a wide range of symptoms, often mimicking other respiratory conditions. In a known case of asthma, it can be diagnosed on regular screening as it can be with mild symptoms. In other instances, patients may experience worsening asthma symptoms, including cough, expectoration of brownish mucus plugs (called 'currant jelly' sputum), wheezing, and shortness of breath. Recurrent episodes of bronchial obstruction can lead to irreversible lung damage, resulting in chronic respiratory symptoms and reduced lung function.

In addition to respiratory symptoms, patients with ABPA may also present with systemic manifestations such as fever, weight loss, and malaise. These systemic symptoms are more commonly observed in advanced stages of the disease. In CF patients, ABPA can lead to deteriorating lung function and exacerbate existing respiratory symptoms.

Several risk factors have been associated with the development of ABPA. These include a history of atopy, prolonged exposure to *Aspergillus* spores, poorly controlled asthma, and genetic predisposition. Understanding these risk factors can aid in the early identification and management of patients at a higher risk for ABPA.

DIAGNOSIS OF ALLERGIC BRONCHOPULMONARY ASPERGILLOSIS

The diagnosis of ABPA is based on a combination of clinical, radiological, immunological, and microbiological criteria. The ISHAM has proposed recommendations for the diagnosis and classification of ABPA complicating asthma **(Box 1)**. It was modified in 2021 after Saxena et al. analysis (Modified ISHAM ABPA Working Group criteria, 2021) and was validated in a large cohort of asthmatics attending a tertiary referral center **(Box 2)**. These recommendations aim to simplify the recognition of the disorder and facilitate early intervention.

BOX 1: International Society for Human and Animal Mycology (ISHAM) criteria for diagnosis of ABPA.

- *Predisposing conditions (one must be present)*:
  - Asthma
  - Cystic fibrosis
- *Obligatory criteria (both must be present)*:
  - Serum IgE > 1,000 IU/mL
  - Positive immediate skin test or increased IgE antibody to *Aspergillus*
- *Supportive criteria (≥2 should be present)*:
  - Precipitating serum antibodies to *A. fumigatus* or elevated serum *Aspergillus* IgG
  - Radiographic opacities consistent with ABPA
  - Total eosinophil count > 500 in glucocorticoid naïve patient

(ABPA: allergic bronchopulmonary aspergillosis; CT: computed tomography; IgE: immunoglobulin E; IgG: immunoglobulin G)

The diagnostic criteria for ABPA include a history of asthma, immediate cutaneous hyper-reactivity to *A. fumigatus* antigen, elevated total serum IgE levels, and specific IgE against *A. fumigatus*. Radiological findings such as fleeting pulmonary opacities, central bronchiectasis, **(Figs. 1A and B)** and mucus plugging **(Fig. 2)** are also indicative of ABPA. Microbiological testing, including sputum culture and serological tests, can provide further evidence.

BOX 2: Modified ISHAM ABPA Working Group criteria 2021 (Saxena et al. analysis).

- *Presence of all the following*:
  - Asthma
  - Aspergillus specific IgE > 0.35 kUA/L
  - Serum total IgE > 500 IU/mL
- *And at least two of the following*:
  - *Aspergillus fumigatus* IgG > 27 mgA/L
  - Bronchiectasis on CT chest
  - Peripheral blood eosinophilia > 500 cells/mL

Lung Function Testing

Pulmonary function tests (PFTs) are essential for evaluating the lung function and monitoring disease progression in ABPA. Spirometry, measurement of lung volumes, and diffusion capacity assessments help assess the severity of airflow obstruction, bronchial hyperresponsiveness, and gas exchange abnormalities. Serial monitoring of lung function parameters is valuable for guiding treatment and assessing response to therapy.

Immunological Tests

Immunological tests play a significant role in the diagnosis and management of ABPA. Measurement of total serum IgE levels is a key component of the diagnostic criteria for ABPA. Elevated IgE levels are commonly observed in ABPA patients and can help differentiate ABPA from other respiratory conditions. Additionally, *Aspergillus*-specific IgE and IgG antibodies can be measured to support the diagnosis of ABPA and monitor treatment response.

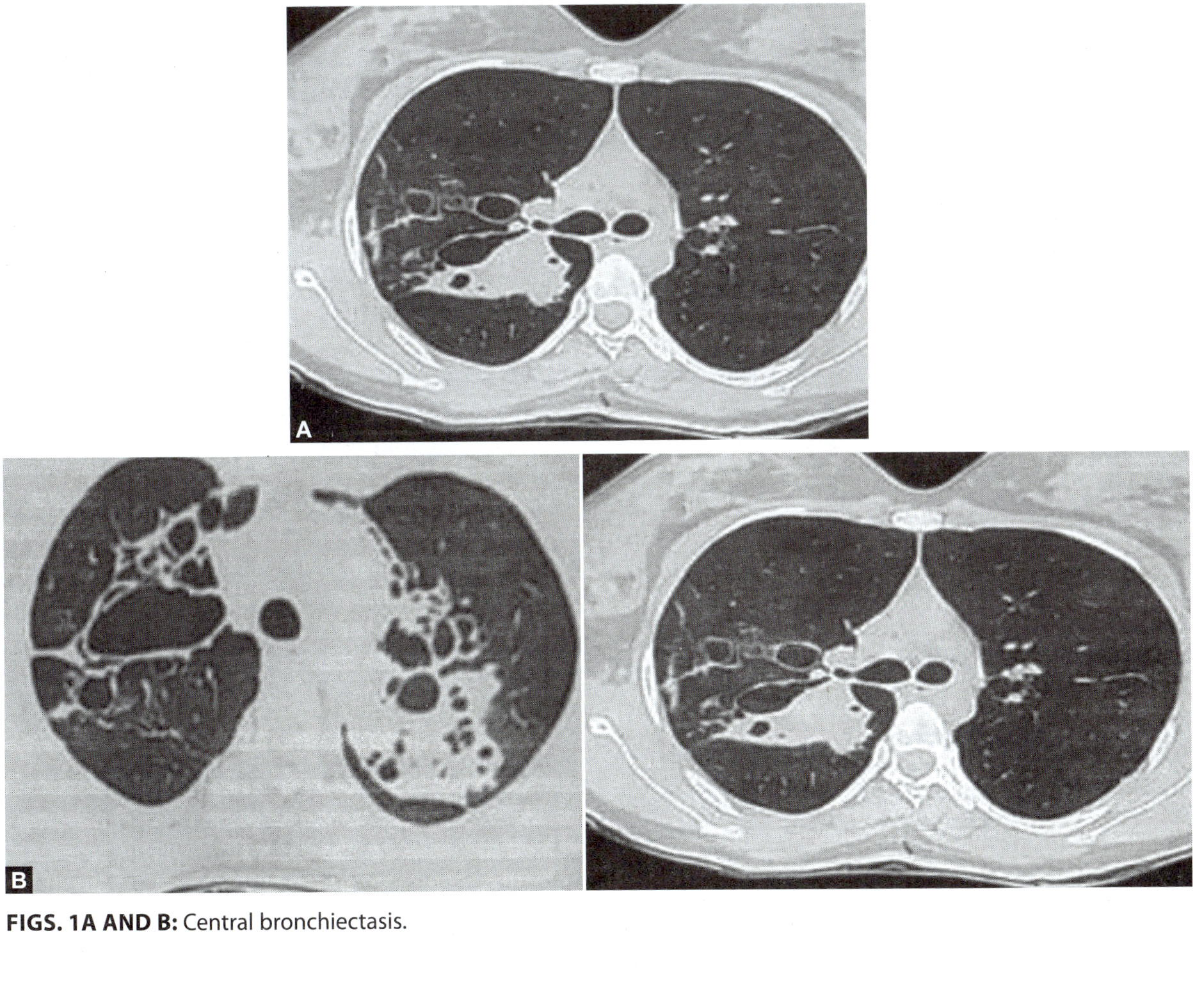

FIGS. 1A AND B: Central bronchiectasis.

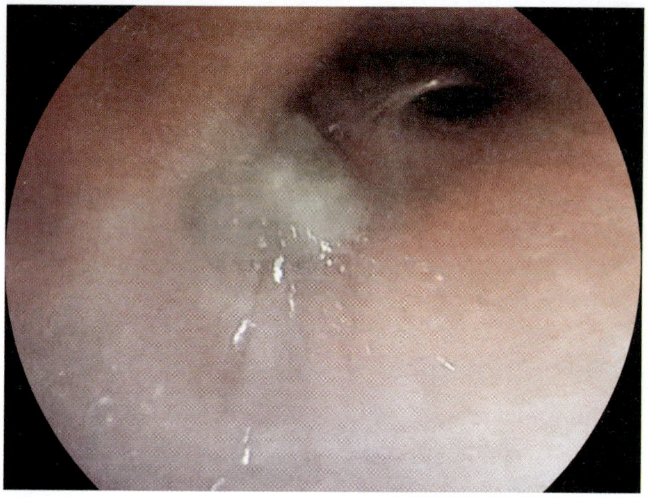

FIG. 2: Mucus plugging of the left upper lobe.

Fungal Biomarkers

The measurement of fungal biomarkers, such as serum galactomannan or β-D-glucan, can provide additional diagnostic and monitoring information in ABPA. These biomarkers reflect the presence and activity of *Aspergillus* species and can be used in conjunction with other clinical and radiological findings. However, their utility in ABPA is not yet well established and requires further research.

Bronchoscopy

Bronchoscopy may be indicated in select cases of ABPA, particularly when there is diagnostic uncertainty or to evaluate complications such as fungal colonization or bronchial obstruction. At times, collapse of a segment and blockade with ploughing can be visualized during bronchoscopy **(Fig. 2)**. Bronchoalveolar lavage (BAL) can be performed during bronchoscopy to collect samples for microbiological and cytological analysis, including identification of *Aspergillus* species, eosinophil count, and fungal culture. BAL galactomannan can also be performed in selected cases where there is suspicion of invasive aspergillosis of the lung.

Molecular Diagnostics

Advances in molecular diagnostic techniques, such as polymerase chain reaction (PCR), have shown promise in the diagnosis of ABPA. PCR-based assays can detect *Aspergillus* DNA in respiratory samples, providing rapid and sensitive identification of the fungal pathogen. These molecular methods hold potential for early detection and improved diagnostic accuracy in ABPA.

Therapeutic Drug Monitoring

Therapeutic drug monitoring (TDM) involves measuring drug levels in the blood to optimize dosage regimens and ensure therapeutic efficacy. TDM is particularly relevant in ABPA patients receiving antifungal agents, such as azoles. Monitoring drug levels helps to maintain adequate systemic exposure, optimize dosing intervals, and prevent suboptimal antifungal therapy.

NEWER ADVANCED MODALITIES

Recombinant *Aspergillus* Antigens

Historically, crude antigens have been employed to monitor immune responses to *A. fumigatus*. There are currently commercially available recombinant *A. fumigatus* antigens, including rAsp f1, rAsp f2, rAsp f3, rAsp f4, and rAsp f6. While the rAsp f3 and f6 cross-react with other fungi, the rAsp f1, f2, and f4 are thought to be highly specific.

Serum Galactomannan

The cell wall of *A. fumigatus* releases galactomannan, a polysaccharide. However, because serum galactomannan has limited sensitivity and specificity, it is not useful for diagnosing ABPA.

Serum Carcinoembryonic Antigen and Periostin

Carcinoembryonic antigen (CEA) levels in the blood and periostin may serve as indicators of eosinophilic inflammation in ABPA. These are still not used as a routine method as they require further studies to establish their role.

RADIOLOGICAL FINDINGS IN ALLERGIC BRONCHOPULMONARY ASPERGILLOSIS

Radiological imaging, particularly high-resolution computed tomography (HRCT), plays a crucial role in the diagnosis and monitoring of ABPA. The characteristic radiological findings seen in ABPA help differentiate it from other respiratory conditions and aid in treatment decisions. The key radiological features observed in ABPA are described in the following text.

Central Bronchiectasis (Figs. 1A and B)

Central bronchiectasis is the hallmark radiological finding in ABPA. It refers to the dilation and thickening of the bronchial walls in the central airways, predominantly involving the larger bronchi. The dilated bronchi are usually cylindrical or varicose in shape. Central bronchiectasis is typically present in a middle lobe or upper lobe distribution.

Mucoid Impaction

Mucoid impaction refers to the accumulation of thick, tenacious mucus within the dilated bronchi seen in ABPA. These mucus plugs can obstruct the bronchial lumens and lead to distal atelectasis or areas of consolidation. Mucoid impaction can be visualized as branching opacities or 'finger-in-glove' opacities on radiological imaging. A classical finding is high attenuating mucus (HAM) **(Figs. 3A and B)**.

Peribronchial Infiltrates

Peribronchial infiltrates are commonly observed in ABPA and reflect the inflammatory response in the bronchial walls. These infiltrates appear as patchy or nodular opacities surrounding the bronchi on HRCT. The infiltrates are often associated with areas of bronchial wall thickening and can extend into adjacent lung parenchyma.

Ground-glass Opacities

Ground-glass opacities (GGOs) can be seen in ABPA and represent areas of increased lung attenuation without obscuration of underlying bronchial or vascular structures. GGOs are indicative of airway inflammation and edema and may be present in areas of bronchial wall thickening or adjacent to mucoid impaction.

Fibrosis and Scarring

In advanced or chronic cases of ABPA, fibrosis and scarring can develop. These findings manifest as linear opacities, traction bronchiectasis, and architectural distortion on HRCT. Fibrotic changes typically occur in areas of resolved or persistent mucoid impaction and represent irreversible lung damage.

Radiological imaging, particularly HRCT, provides valuable information regarding the extent and severity of lung involvement in ABPA. It helps in establishing the diagnosis, assessing disease activity, and monitoring treatment response.

The presence of central bronchiectasis, mucoid impaction, peribronchial infiltrates, and other characteristic findings supports the diagnosis of ABPA and aids in distinguishing it from other respiratory diseases. Radiological findings, combined with clinical and immunological criteria, contribute to the accurate diagnosis and optimal management of ABPA.

DIFFERENTIAL DIAGNOSIS (TABLE 1)

When evaluating a patient with suspected ABPA, it is important to consider and rule out other respiratory conditions that can present with similar clinical features. Some of the key differential diagnoses of ABPA are given in **Table 1**.

CLINICAL STAGING OF ALLERGIC BRONCHOPULMONARY ASPERGILLOSIS PATIENTS

Currently, ABPA is divided into seven stages; however, all the patients do not always move through them in order. About 40–50% of patients experience an exacerbation, most commonly in the first year after stopping treatment. Patients with ABPA frequently see a brief rise in blood total IgE, although this is not important until there is clinical or radiological worsening. **Table 2** shows clinical stages of ABPA.

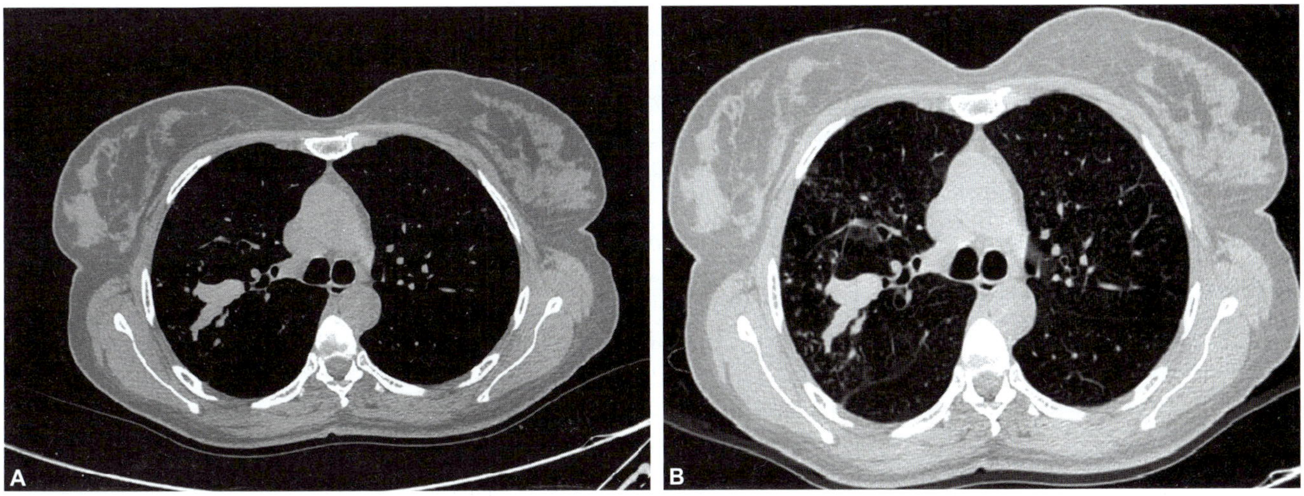

FIGS. 3A AND B: High attenuated mucus.

TABLE 1: Differential diagnosis of ABPA.

Differential diagnosis	Key clinical features	Immunological findings	Radiological findings
Asthma	Chronic airway inflammation, bronchial hyperresponsiveness, reversible airflow obstruction	Elevated total serum IgE levels, *Aspergillus*-specific IgE	Central bronchiectasis may be present
COPD	Chronic airflow limitation, chronic bronchitis/emphysema	Total serum IgE levels may be elevated in exacerbations	Central bronchiectasis may be present
CF	Recurrent pulmonary exacerbations, chronic lung disease in CF patients	Elevated total serum IgE levels, *Aspergillus*-specific IgE	Central bronchiectasis, mucoid impaction
BAFS	Asthma symptoms, positive fungal skin prick test/IgE to fungi	Elevated total serum IgE levels, *Aspergillus*-specific IgE	Central bronchiectasis may be present
Other fungal infections	Vary based on the type of fungal infection (CPA, IPA, aspergilloma)	Variable depending on the specific fungal infection	Radiological findings may differ based on the specific fungal infection
Eosinophilic pneumonia	Cough, dyspnea, peripheral blood eosinophilia	Variable depending on the specific eosinophilic pneumonia	Radiological findings may show peripheral infiltrates, ground-glass opacities
Other allergic pulmonary diseases	Allergic symptoms, exposure history (e.g., allergens, occupational)	Variable depending on the specific allergic pulmonary conditions	Radiological findings may show patchy or nodular opacities, consolidation

(ABPA: allergic bronchopulmonary aspergillosis; BAFS: bronchial asthma with fungal sensitization; CF: cystic fibrosis; COPD: chronic obstructive pulmonary disease CPA: chronic pulmonary aspergillosis; IPA: invasive pulmonary aspergillosis)

TABLE 2: Clinical staging of allergic bronchopulmonary aspergillosis (ABPA) in patients of asthma.

Stage	Definition	Features
0	Asymptomatic	• No previous diagnosis of ABPA • Controlled asthma • Fulfilling diagnostic criteria of ABPA
1	Acute	• No previous diagnosis of ABPA • Clinical presentation consistent with ABPA • Conforming the diagnostic criteria of ABPA
1a	With mucoid impaction	Mucoid impaction present on chest imaging
1b	Without mucoid impaction	Absence of mucoid impaction on chest imaging
2	Response	• Either clinical or radiological improvement, and • Decline in IgE ≥ 25% of baseline (at 8 weeks)
3	Exacerbation	• Either clinical or radiological worsening, and • Increase in IgE by >50% from the 'new baseline' established during response/remission
4	Remission	• Sustained clinicoradiological improvement, and • IgE levels persisting at or below the 'new baseline' (or increase by <50%) for >6 months off treatment
5a	Treatment-dependent ABPA	• >2 exacerbations within 6 months of discontinuing treatment, or • Clinical or radiological worsening and rise in serum total IgE levels, on tapering oral steroids/ azoles
5b	Glucocorticoid-dependent asthma	Systemic glucocorticoids required for asthma control, while ABPA is inactive (as indicated by stable IgE levels and thoracic imaging)
6	Advanced ABPA	• Extensive bronchiectasis due to ABPA on CT chest, and • Cor pulmonale or chronic type II respiratory failure

(CT: computed tomography; IgE: immunoglobulin E)

MANAGEMENT OF ALLERGIC BRONCHOPULMONARY ASPERGILLOSIS

The management of ABPA involves a combination of pharmacological and nonpharmacological interventions. The primary goals of treatment are to control asthma symptoms, prevent exacerbations, and reduce the inflammatory response caused by *Aspergillus* antigens.

Pharmacological Management

Oral Corticosteroids

Prednisone or prednisolone is the mainstay of treatment for ABPA. It helps reduce airway inflammation and control symptoms. The dose and duration of corticosteroid therapy depend on the disease severity and response to treatment.

There have been two dose regimens for oral glucocorticoid therapy studied in the literature:

Medium and high dose: The medium-dose regimen consisted of prednisolone *0.5 mg/kg/day for 1–2 weeks*, then alternate-day therapy for 6–8 weeks, and finally tapering by 5–10 mg every 2 weeks until ceasing after 3–5 months.

The high-dose regimen consisted of prednisolone *0.75 mg/kg/day for 6 weeks* followed by 0.5 mg/kg/day for 6 weeks.

The dose is then reduced by 5 mg every 6 weeks to complete a treatment duration of 6–12 months. Gradual tapering of corticosteroids is necessary to minimize side effects.

Inhaled Corticosteroids

Inhaled corticosteroids (ICS), such as fluticasone or budesonide, can be used as maintenance therapy to reduce airway inflammation and control symptoms in milder stages of ABPA. ICS are often combined with long-acting beta-agonists (LABAs) for better control of symptoms.

Antifungal Therapy

Antifungal agents like itraconazole may be considered in selected cases, especially in patients with moderate-to-severe ABPA or those who fail to respond adequately to corticosteroids alone. Antifungal therapy helps in reducing fungal burden and preventing disease progression. The duration and choice of antifungal agent should be determined by a specialist.

Bronchodilators

Short-acting bronchodilators, such as salbutamol, can be used to relieve bronchospasm and improve airflow in patients with ABPA who have underlying asthma or bronchial hyperreactivity.

Immunomodulatory Agents

In some cases, immunomodulatory agents like omalizumab (anti-IgE monoclonal antibody) or mepolizumab (anti-IL-5 monoclonal antibody) may be considered as an adjunctive therapy, particularly in patients with severe or steroid-dependent ABPA. These agents help reduce allergic inflammation and can lead to improved disease control.

Nonpharmacological Management

Allergen Avoidance

Patients with ABPA should try to minimize exposure to *Aspergillus* antigens by avoiding environments with high mold spore concentrations, such as damp or moldy environments. Proper ventilation and regular cleaning of living spaces can help reduce *Aspergillus* exposure.

Patient Education

Providing education to patients regarding ABPA, its management, and the importance of medication adherence is crucial. Patients should be aware of triggers, signs of exacerbations, and when to seek medical attention.

Pulmonary Rehabilitation

Pulmonary rehabilitation programs can be beneficial for patients with ABPA, particularly those with persistent respiratory symptoms or impaired lung function. These programs involve exercise training, breathing techniques, and education to improve overall lung function and quality of life.

Psychological Support

Allergic bronchopulmonary aspergillosis can have a significant impact on a patient's emotional well-being. Psychological support and counseling can help patients cope with the challenges of living with a chronic respiratory condition.

It is important to note that the management of ABPA should be individualized based on the patient's specific characteristics, disease severity, and response to treatment.

Regular monitoring of symptoms, lung function, and medication side effects is essential for optimizing treatment outcomes. A guided management plan should be made for every patient for better outcomes.

PROGNOSIS AND COMPLICATIONS

The prognosis of ABPA can vary depending on the stage of the disease and the individual patient's response to treatment. Early recognition and appropriate management can significantly improve outcomes and prevent long-term complications.

With appropriate management, many patients with ABPA can achieve good control of symptoms and prevent disease progression. However, it is important to note that ABPA is a chronic condition that requires ongoing monitoring and treatment. The potential complications and long-term outcomes associated with ABPA are as follows:

Bronchiectasis: Bronchiectasis, which is the permanent dilation of the bronchioles, can develop in patients with ABPA, particularly in the advanced stages. This can lead to chronic respiratory symptoms, recurrent infections, and further decline in lung function.

Recurrent exacerbations: Despite treatment, some patients with ABPA may experience recurrent acute exacerbations characterized by worsening respiratory symptoms, increased cough, sputum production, and decreased lung function. These exacerbations require prompt medical intervention to manage the inflammation and prevent complications.

Lung fibrosis: In severe or inadequately controlled cases of ABPA, progressive lung fibrosis can develop over time. Lung fibrosis refers to the formation of scar tissue in the lungs, which can lead to irreversible damage, impaired lung function, and respiratory impairment.

Aspergilloma: In rare cases, ABPA can lead to the formation of aspergillomas, which are ball-like masses consisting of *Aspergillus* fungi in the lung cavities. Aspergillomas may cause symptoms such as hemoptysis and require specific management, including antifungal therapy and sometimes surgical intervention.

Complications from treatment: Prolonged use of systemic corticosteroids, which are often necessary for managing ABPA, can lead to various side effects, such as osteoporosis, adrenal suppression, weight gain, increased susceptibility to infections, and mood disturbances. Close monitoring and appropriate management of these complications are essential.

Early diagnosis, prompt initiation of treatment, and regular follow-up are crucial in minimizing complications and improving the long-term outcomes for patients with ABPA. Adherence to medication, avoidance of triggers, and proactive management of comorbidities such as asthma or CF (if present) are important in optimizing the prognosis.

Each patient's prognosis can vary, and individual factors should be taken into account when assessing the long-term outlook.

FUTURE DIRECTIONS AND RESEARCH NEEDS

While significant progress has been made in understanding and managing ABPA, several areas of research need further exploration. These include the development of standardized diagnostic criteria, the identification of novel biomarkers, and the evaluation of new treatment options. Large-scale epidemiological studies are needed to accurately determine the prevalence and burden of ABPA in different populations. Further research is also required to optimize treatment strategies and assess the long-term outcomes of patients with ABPA.

CONCLUSION

Allergic bronchopulmonary aspergillosis is a complex respiratory disorder that requires early recognition and appropriate management. It is often overlooked or misdiagnosed due to overlapping symptoms with other respiratory disorders. The prevalence of ABPA complicating asthma remains uncertain, highlighting the need for increased awareness and diagnostic accuracy. A multidisciplinary approach involving clinicians, radiologists, and microbiologists is crucial for timely diagnosis and optimal treatment.

SUGGESTED READINGS

1. Salo PM, Arbes SJ Jr, Jaramillo R, Calatroni A, Weir CH, Sever ML, et al. Prevalence of allergic sensitization in the United States: results from the National Health and Nutrition Examination Survey (NHANES) 2005-2006. J Allergy Clin Immunol. 2014;134(2):350-9.
2. Agarwal R, Denning DW, Chakrabarti A. Estimation of the burden of chronic and allergic pulmonary aspergillosis in India. PLoS One. 2014;9(12):e114745.
3. Agarwal R, Chakrabarti A, Shah A, Gupta D, Meis JF, Guleria R, Moss R, Denning DW; ABPA complicating asthma ISHAM working group. Allergic bronchopulmonary aspergillosis: review of literature and proposal of new diagnostic and classification criteria. Clin Exp Allergy. 2013;43(8):850-73.
4. Saxena P, Choudhary H, Muthu V, Sehgal IP, Dhooria S, Prasad KT, et al. Which are the optimal criteria for the diagnosis of allergic bronchopulmonary aspergillosis? A latent class Analysis. J Allergy Clin Immunol Pract. 2021;9(1):328035.e1.
5. Agarwal R, Muthu V, Sehgal IS, Dhooria S, Prasad KT, Aggarwal AN. Allergic Bronchopulmonary Aspergillosis. Clin Chest Med. 2022;43(1):99-125.

221

CHAPTER

Eosinophilia: A Pragmatic Approach for Diagnosis and Treatment

Abha Gupta, Priyank Rastogi

ABSTRACT

Eosinophilia is frequently encountered in clinical practice and is associated with a wide variety of conditions ranging from allergic, rheumatologic, infective, and neoplastic to some rare idiopathic conditions. Arriving at an etiological diagnosis can be challenging and time consuming at times. Although advances in molecular diagnostic techniques have enabled the identification of uncommon causes, but still a large number of cases remain undiagnosed with respect to the cause of eosinophilia. This article presents a pragmatic and simplistic approach for the diagnosis and treatment of eosinophilia.

INTRODUCTION

Eosinophilia is a condition which is commonly seen yet there remains an element of ambiguity regarding its management for many clinicians. Advancements in molecular diagnostic techniques and targeted therapies make it imperative to keep updating with the management principles as they have to be continually revised to cater to such advancements.

BIOLOGY OF EOSINOPHILS

These are mostly bilobed cells, larger than red blood cells (RBCs); lymphocytes and basophils and have affinity for eosin dye. They are produced in bone marrow in response to presence of eosinophil promoting cytokines, like interleukin-5 (IL-5) and granulocyte macrophage colony-stimulating factor (GM-CSF), stromal cells, and mast cells. While these cytokines are the main drivers in reactive eosinophilia, in case of clonal eosinophilia, the triggers include tyrosine kinase gene fusion.

FUNCTIONS OF EOSINOPHILS

Eosinophils have been traditionally thought to be effector cells in the body's defense against parasitic infections and their proposed mechanism of action includes release of toxic eosinophil granule proteins and antibody-dependent cytotoxic cell death. Similar mechanisms may also come into play in causing tissue damage and inflammation during other conditions associated with eosinophilia.

DEFINITIONS

Eosinophilia, defined as an absolute eosinophil count (AEC) >500/μL in blood, is quite common, occurring in 1–2% of the general population. The severity of eosinophilia can be divided into mild (500–1,500 cells/μL), moderate (AEC 1,500–5,000 cells/μL), and severe (AEC >5,000 cells/μL). Hypereosinophilia is defined as moderate to severe eosinophilia ≥1,500 cells/μL. To meet the definition for hypereosinophilic syndrome (HES) requires AEC ≥1,500/μL (on two occasions ≥1 month apart) plus organ dysfunction attributable to hypereosinophilia without any alternate cause.

DIFFERENTIAL DIAGNOSIS

Eosinophilia is associated with several medical conditions and disease states. These conditions are summarized in **Table 1**. The broad category of these conditions includes:

TABLE 1: Differential diagnosis of eosinophilic disorders.

Category	Diseases
Infections	• Helminthic infection (especially those with a tissue invasive phase) • Ascariasis, hookworm infection, strongyloidiasis, and filariases • Fungal infections • Viral infection (HIV and COVID-19) • Protozoal infection (limited to *Sarcocystis* and *Cystoisospora*) • Tuberculosis (rare)
Drugs	• *Antibiotics*: Penicillins, cephalosporins, dapsone, and sulfa-based antibiotics • *Xanthine oxidase inhibitor*: Allopurinol • *Antiepileptics*: Phenytoin, phenobarbitone, lamotrigine, and valproic acid • *Antiretrovirals*: Nevirapine and efavirenz • Nonsteroidal anti-inflammatory drugs • DRESS
Atopy and hypersensitivity	Allergic rhinitis, asthma, atopic dermatitis, eczema, and urticaria
Connective tissue, rheumatologic, and autoimmune disorders	Eosinophilic granulomatosis with polyangiitis (Churg–Strauss vasculitis), bullous pemphigus, inflammatory bowel disease, celiac disease, dermatomyositis/polymyositis, rheumatoid arthritis, progressive systemic sclerosis, Sjögren syndrome, systemic lupus erythematosus, and sarcoidosis
Neoplastic	*Blood-related neoplasms*: • Acute and chronic eosinophilic leukemia • Lymphoma (T cell) and Hodgkins *Solid tumors*: Adenocarcinoma of GI tract- gastric colorectal
Rare conditions	*HES clinical variants*: • Myeloproliferative HE/HES (M-HE/M-HES) • Lymphocytic variant HE/HES (L-HE/L-HES) • Overlap HES • Associated HE/HES • Familial HE/HES • Idiopathic HES Hypereosinophilia of unknown significance (HEUS)

(COVID-19: Coronavirus disease 2019; DRESS: drug reaction with eosinophilia and systemic symptoms; GI: gastrointestinal; HES: hypereosinophilic syndrome; HIV: human immunodeficiency virus)

Infections

The major infections associated with eosinophilia are listed in **Table 1**. Of these, the common ones include helminthic infections like of ascaris and hookworms.

Medications

Numerous drugs have been known to be associated with eosinophilia and such reactions range from mild transient eosinophilia to a life-threatening condition known as "drug reaction with eosinophilia and systemic symptoms (DRESS)". The common drugs reported to have been associated with DRESS include anticonvulsants (valproic acid, lamotrigine, carbamazepine, and levetiracetam), antibiotics, antiretroviral drugs, sulfasalazine, and allopurinol.

Atopy and Hypersensitivity

The conditions associated with mild degree of eosinophilia include allergic rhinitis, asthma, atopic dermatitis, eczema, and urticaria whereas moderate to severe degree of eosinophilia is seen in conditions, such as chronic sinusitis, allergic bronchopulmonary aspergillosis, and chronic eosinophilic pneumonia.

Immune/Connective Tissue Disorders

A number of autoimmune disorders are associated with mild to moderate blood eosinophilia. In some cases, apart from blood, eosinophils are also found at the site of disease such as in eosinophilic granulomatosis with polyangiitis (EGPA, formerly known as Churg-Strauss syndrome).

Neoplastic Conditions

Eosinophilia can be found in association with certain neoplasma like adenocarcinoma of gastrointestinal (GI) tract and ovary as a paraneoplastic condition. However, many blood-based neoplasms are also associated with clonal proliferation of eosinophils and usually lead to condition known as HES.

Hypereosinophilic Syndrome

The definition of HES has been a subject of controversy and has undergone multiple revisions ever since the first comprehensive description of HES was made by Chusid et al. in 1984.

For the sake of simplicity and ease of understanding, HES is defined as: (1) hypereosinophilia (a peripheral eosinophil count of >1,500 cells/μL documented on at least two occasions 1 month apart) or marked tissue eosinophilia and (2) clinical manifestations directly attributable to the eosinophilia. The following six classification categories of HES have been proposed:

1. *Myeloproliferative HE/HES (M-HE or M-HES):* These include HES with documented or presumed clonal eosinophilic involvement. Most of these patients have a deletion in chromosome 4q12 causing the constitutively active fusion tyrosine kinase, FIP1L1-PDGFRA, which can be detected by fluorescence in situ hybridization (FISH) or reverse transcriptase-polymerase chain reaction (RT-PCR) in peripheral blood or bone marrow. Clonal eosinophilia is also present in chronic eosinophilic leukemia-not otherwise specified (CEL-NOS) and can also occur in systemic mastocytosis and lymphoid/myeloid neoplasms.
2. *Lymphocytic variant HES (L-HES)*: This includes HES with either a clonal proliferation or aberrant lymphocytes producing cytokines that lead to eosinophilia. It is associated with skin and soft tissue manifestations and elevated serum immunoglobulin E (IgE). In a special subtype of L-HES known as episodic angioedema with eosinophilia (EAE; Gleich's syndrome), the patients have cyclical episodes of angioedema with urticaria every month accompanied by rise in serum IL-5 levels and eosinophilia.
3. *Overlap HES*: This includes eosinophilic disease restricted to a single organ system accompanied by peripheral hypereosinophilia. Eosinophilic granulomatosis with polyangiitis, also known as Churg–Strauss syndrome, is a special category of overlap HES.
4. *Associated HES:* It includes HES occurring secondary to a defined diagnosis like parasitic helminthic infections, drug hypersensitivity, or primary immunodeficiency.
5. *Familial HES:* A rare autosomal dominant disorder occurring in multiple members of a single family.
6. *Idiopathic HES:* HES of unknown cause that does not satisfy criteria for any of the other categories after comprehensive evaluation.

Experts also consider another category in differential of HES known as hypereosinophilia of undetermined significance (HEUS). This condition refers to long lasting hypereosinophilia in the absence of clinical symptoms.

APPROACH TO DIAGNOSIS

The evaluation of eosinophilia is centered primarily on achieving two goals:

1. Investigating for a possible underlying cause
2. Assessing possible eosinophilia associated end-organ damage or dysfunction

The investigations for achieving these two goals are usually performed in parallel.

Step 1: Initial Evaluation—History, Examination, and Basic Investigations

The diagnostic process begins with a detailed medical history including history of allergic disorders, such as asthma, eczema, and urticaria. A history of skin rashes or lymphadenopathy should also be elicited. Cardiorespiratory symptoms, GI symptoms, and constitutional symptoms, such as fever, night sweats, weight loss, and pruritus should be noted. A detailed travel and food history should be taken. A detailed drug history should be taken and finally, a thorough physical examination should be performed.

Initially, all patients should have a full blood count performed and a blood film examined. Routine testing for kidney and liver function, lactate dehydrogenase, erythrocyte sedimentation rate (ESR), and C-reactive protein should be performed. The latter tests may be helpful in excluding an inflammatory or reactive process associated with eosinophilia. Vitamin B_{12} levels should also be assayed since they may be elevated in myeloid disorders.

Step 2: Testing for End-organ Damage

Eosinophils have potential to migrate into varied tissues to cause organ damage and dysfunction, most common sites being lungs, GI tract, heart, and central nervous system (CNS). Investigations are focused on the particular organ, such as chest radiography and/or computed tomography (CT) of the chest, echocardiography, serum troponin T, and pulmonary function testing. An unprovoked thromboembolic event is also recognized as a consequence of hypereosinophilia.

Step 3: Further Testing Dependent on the Suspected Cause

At this point, further investigations are directed toward confirming the eosinophilia-related condition suspected in step 1. In those with a suspected allergic etiology, further investigations include serum total IgE, allergen-specific IgE tests, and skin prick testing for specific allergies.

In case of suspected infectious cause, stool microscopy for ova, cysts and parasites, and serological tests for suspected parasitic infections, such as strongyloidiasis, schistosomiasis, filariasis, and toxocariasis may be carried out wherever appropriate. In patients with probable opportunistic infections, testing for human immunodeficiency virus (HIV) or human T-lymphotropic virus 1 (HTLV-1) may be carried out.

In patients with a suspected connective tissue disorder, tests include antinuclear antibody (ANA) activity, anti-double-stranded DNA (anti-dsDNA) antibodies, antibodies to cyclic citrullinated peptide (CCP), antineutrophil cytoplasmic antibodies (ANCAs), and serology for hepatitis B and hepatitis C virus.

In patients with a suspected neoplastic condition, such as lymphoma or nonhematological malignancy or T-cell driven eosinophilia, appropriate imaging and tissue biopsy needs to be performed.

Step 4: Investigations to Diagnose Subtypes of Hypereosinophilic Syndromes

These are usually carried out in those cases where there is persisting hyperosinophilia despite treatment for >1 month along with end-organ damage. The important investigations here include peripheral blood analysis for FIP1L1-PDGFRA by FISH or RT-PCR, serum mast cell tryptase levels, peripheral blood T-cell immunophenotyping, T-cell receptor gene rearrangement studies, bone marrow aspirate, trephine biopsy, and cytogenetic analysis.

TREATMENT

Infections

Treatment is targeted at the underlying infection. Although resolution of infection is associated with decrease or resolution of eosinophilia, however, this might not occur immediately.

Drug-induced Eosinophilia

Treatment for drug-related eosinophilia involves withdrawal of the offending drug. In case of DRESS, skin manifestations can be treated with topical corticosteroids whereas in patients with visceral organ involvement, high-dose corticosteroids are used. Complete recovery after drug withdrawal can take weeks to months.

Atopic Disorders

Treatment of most of these diseases consists of corticosteroids (topical or systemic) which target the inciting cells including both eosinophils and other immune cells such as lymphocytes. Recently, eosinophilic asthma patients have been treated with eosinophil-targeted therapies including anti-IL-5 drugs like mepolizumab, which led to improvement of pulmonary function and decrease in diseases flare, and have been approved by the United States Food and Drug Administration (US-FDA) for use as add-on therapy in severe asthma with eosinophilic phenotype.

Autoimmune Disorders

Generally, treatments of autoimmune disease with or without blood eosinophilia are the same and the mainstay of treatment revolves around steroid administration. However, recent studies have employed anti-IL-5 therapy to treat eosinophilic granulomatosis with polyangiitis successfully.

Treatment of Hypereosinophilic Syndromes

The treatment approach in HES is summarized in **Flowchart 1**. As depicted in the **Flowchart 1**, in case of eosinophil-mediated end-organ damage as evidenced by cardiac, neurologic, or thromboembolic complications and/or the presence of extremely high or rapidly increasing eosinophil counts, immediate therapy becomes necessary. In such cases, corticosteroids (1 mg/kg up to 1 g methylprednisolone) are the initial treatment of choice. However, ivermectin (0.2 mg/kg/day for 2 days) should be administered concomitantly to all patients with a history of potential exposure to the helminth, *Strongyloides stercoralis*, so as to prevent the potentially fatal corticosteroid-induced *hyperinfection syndrome*.

In HES, corticosteroids are the mainstay of treatment. The dose of corticosteroids should be tapered slowly once the eosinophil counts normalize and symptoms show improvement. However, in case of patients who do not show the desired response or experience significant side effects, a second agent should be considered.

Here, it is also important to identify subgroups of patients for whom therapies other than corticosteroids are preferable as initial therapy. These include patients with secondary causes which require specific therapy to treat

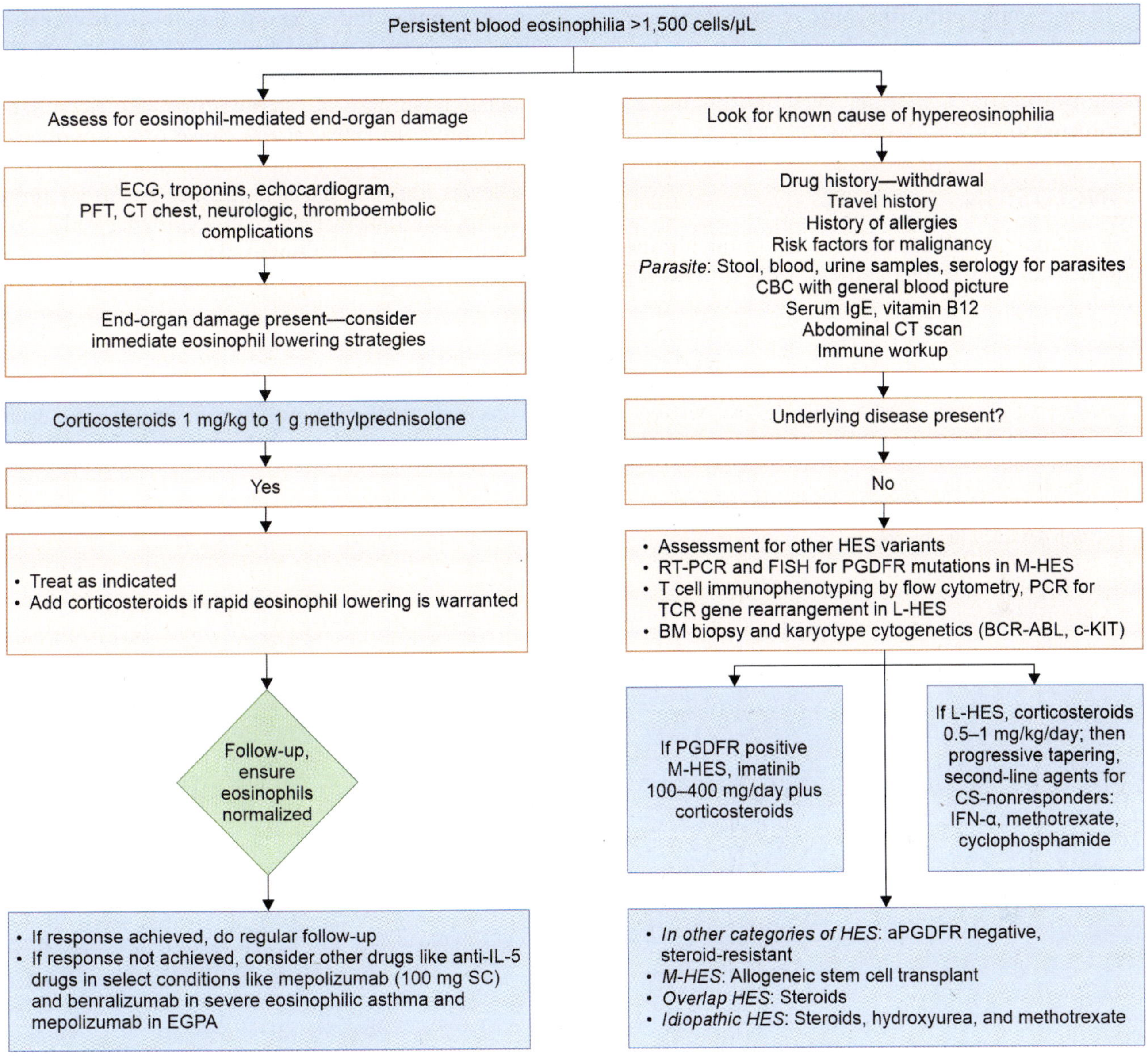

FLOWCHART 1: Approach to hypereosinophilia.

(BM: bone marrow; CBC: complete blood count; CT: computed tomography; EGPA: eosinophilic granulomatosis with polyangiitis; FISH: fluorescence in situ hybridization; HES: hypereosinophilic syndrome; IFN-α: interferon-α; IgE: immunoglobulin E; M-HES: myeloproliferative HES; PFT: pulmonary function test; RT-PCR: reverse transcriptase-polymerase chain reaction; SC: subcutaneous)

the underlying cause (as in case of associated HE/HES), patients with known imatinib sensitive mutations [such as PDGFRA-associated myeloproliferative neoplasms (MPNs) with eosinophilia M-HES], overlap HES, and patients with familial eosinophilia or HEUS.

The majority of M-HES patients (approximately 80%) have a PDGFRA-associated MPN. These patients respond very well to imatinib mesylate and should be treated with this agent as first-line therapy. In cases of resistance to imatinib, newer second- and third-generation tyrosine kinase inhibitors (TKIs) including sorafenib, midostaurin, and ponatinib should be considered. Finally, in steroid-resistant, PDGFRA-negative subjects with HES, allogeneic stem cell transplantation may be considered.

In case of lymphocytic variant HES (L-HES), most patients respond to corticosteroid therapy. Interferon-α is often used as the preferred second-line therapy by virtue of its dual effect on eosinophils and T lymphocytes. Other agents including methotrexate, cyclophosphamide, cyclosporine, and alemtuzumab have also been used as steroid-sparing agents in L-HES.

In case of idiopathic HES, beyond steroid therapy, the commonly used second-line agents for the treatment of idiopathic HES are hydroxyurea, chlorambucil, cytarabine, methotrexate, cyclosporine, cyclophosphamide and alemtuzumab.

CONCLUSION

Eosinophilia is an elevation in the total number of bloodstream eosinophils and can exist in mild to very severe forms. Mild eosinophilia is usually seen in allergic diseases, parasitic disease and drug allergy while severe forms can occur in conditions like DRESS and in association with MPNs. Careful history and examination is imperative to arrive at the cause of eosinophilia. If no apparent cause of the eosinophilia is discernible and levels above 1,500 cells/μL persist for >1 month duration, an exhaustive search in accordance with clinical presentation should be undertaken so as to prevent the risk of eosinophils-induced organ damage.

SUGGESTED READINGS

1. Valent P, Klion AD, Horny HP, Roufosse F, Gotlib J, Weller PF, et al. Contemporary consensus proposal on criteria and classification of eosinophilic disorders and related syndromes. J Allergy Clin Immunol. 2012;130(3):607-12.e9.
2. Kuang FL. Approach to Patients with Eosinophilia. Med Clin North Am. 2020;104(1):1-14.
3. Shomali W, Gotlib J. World Health Organization-defined eosinophilic disorders: 2022 update on diagnosis, risk stratification, and management. Am J Hematol. 2022;97(1): 129-48.

222
CHAPTER

Interstitial Pneumonia with Autoimmune Features: Clinical Clues and Role of Physicians

Udas Chandra Ghosh, Antarleena Ray

ABSTRACT

Interstitial lung diseases (ILD) are a heterogeneous group of disorders affecting the lung parenchyma. The concept of interstitial pneumonia with autoimmune features (IPAF) was introduced in 2015 by the European Respiratory Society (ERS) and American Thoracic Society (ATS) as an initial step to uniformly define, identify, and study the patients with ILD who have features of autoimmunity, yet fall short of a characterizable connective tissue disease.

The task force offers classification criteria organized around three domains: A clinical domain consisting of specific extrathoracic features, a serologic domain consisting of specific autoantibodies, and a morphologic domain consisting of specific chest imaging or histopathologic features.

Treatment must be based on careful evaluation of benefit:risk ratio and should ideally be discussed in multidisciplinary approach.

Majority of patients are treated with glucocorticoids and/or immunosuppressive therapy and occasionally rituximab, illustrating that clinicians would treat subjects with IPAF just like connective tissue disease-associated ILD (CTD-ILD).

Interstitial pneumonia with autoimmune features is a complex clinical entity that lies at the interface of idiopathic interstitial pneumonias (IIP) and CTD-ILD. Its diagnosis and management require a multidisciplinary approach and collaboration between different specialties offer hope for improved outcomes and a better understanding of IPAF in the future.

INTRODUCTION

Interstitial lung disease (ILD) refers to a heterogeneous group of lung disorders associated with varying degrees of inflammation and/or fibrosis of the pulmonary interstitium, resulting in parenchymal damage. ILDs are assessed by clinical, radiologic, and histopathological features and classified according to possible etiology, such as exposure-related (environmental, occupational, and drug reactions), systemic or autoimmune associated [rheumatic disease (RD) and sarcoid], and idiopathic pulmonary fibrosis (IPF). Patients usually present with dry cough and dyspnea on exertion. The disease can be progressive and leads to the need for supplemental oxygen, reduced quality of life, causing significant morbidity and mortality.

Such patients undergo a thorough work-up including a history focused on potential exposures and extra-pulmonary symptoms, physical examination, serology, high-resolution computed tomography (HRCT) thorax, and histopathology of the lung tissue, if indicated. ILD is a major contributor to disease burden in multiple RD such as rheumatoid arthritis (RA), systemic sclerosis (SSc), Sjögren's syndrome (SS), and idiopathic inflammatory myopathies (IIM). However, some patients fail to meet the American College of Rheumatology (ACR) or European League Against Rheumatism (EULAR) classification criteria for various RD and yet their clinical features, serology, and radiographic or histopathological findings indicate an underlying autoimmune pathogenesis of their ILD. Such patients were previously labeled with terms such as "lung-dominant connective tissue disease

(CTD)," "undifferentiated CTD- (UCTD)-associated ILD," and "autoimmune-featured ILD."

In 2015, the European Respiratory Society (ERS) and American Thoracic Society (ATS) coined the term "interstitial pneumonia with autoimmune features" (IPAF). The concept of IPAF was introduced as an initial step to uniformly define, identify, and study patients with ILD who have features of autoimmunity, yet fall short of a characterizable CTD.

Interstitial pneumonia with autoimmune features is a relatively new and evolving clinical entity that lies at the intersection of idiopathic interstitial pneumonias (IIPs) and CTD-associated ILDs (CTD-ILDs). It represents a challenging diagnostic dilemma for clinicians and researchers alike.

DIAGNOSTIC CRITERIA

The ILDs are classified on the basis of specific patterns of clinical, radiographic, and histopathologic parameters **(Flowchart 1)**.

As per guidelines, newly diagnosed patients with ILD should undergo a thorough evaluation, including history and clinical examination, pulmonary function testing (PFT), HRCT scan of thorax, surgical lung biopsy if indicated, and multidisciplinary discussion between clinicians, pulmonologists, rheumatologists, radiologists, and pathologists to provide the most accurate diagnosis **(Fig. 1)**.

The diagnosis of an IIP, of which IPF is most common, is made only after thorough evaluation and careful exclusion of other causes.

Though reliable determinants of prevalence are lacking, it is quite common to encounter patients with IIP who have features suggestive of an autoimmune etiology and yet do not meet the criteria of any particular connective tissue disorder **(Fig. 2)**.

The criteria for diagnosis of IPAF are ***(Table 1)***:
- Presence of an interstitial pneumonia by HRCT or lung biopsy
- Exclusion of alternative etiologies
- Does not meet the criteria for a definite CTD

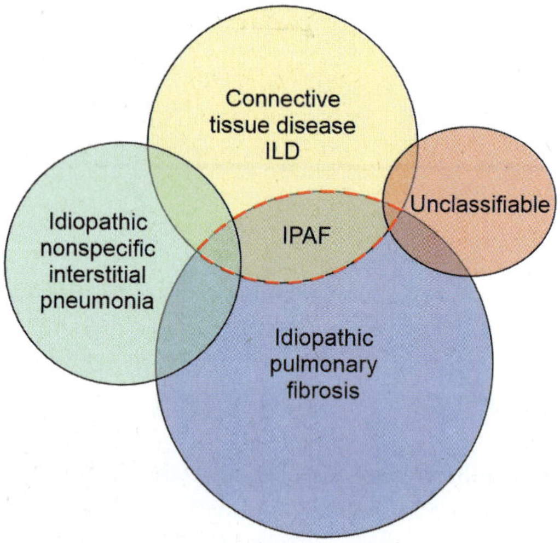

FIG. 1: Interstitial pneumonia with autoimmune features (IPAF) in the scheme of clinical interstitial lung disease (ILD).

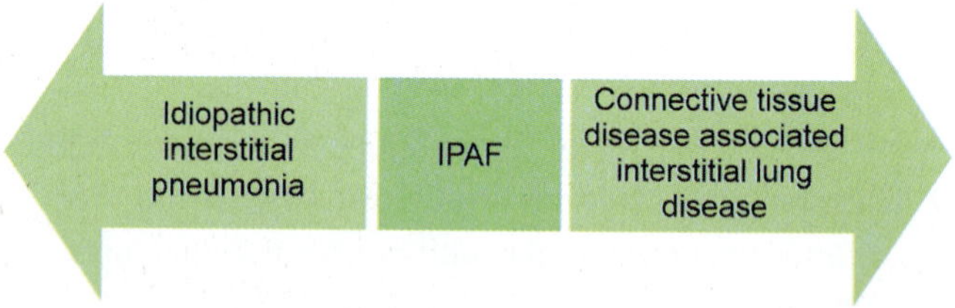

FIG. 2: Interstitial pneumonia with autoimmune features (IPAF) is a relatively newer and evolving clinical entity that lies at the intersection of idiopathic interstitial pneumonias and connective tissue disease-associated interstitial lung diseases.

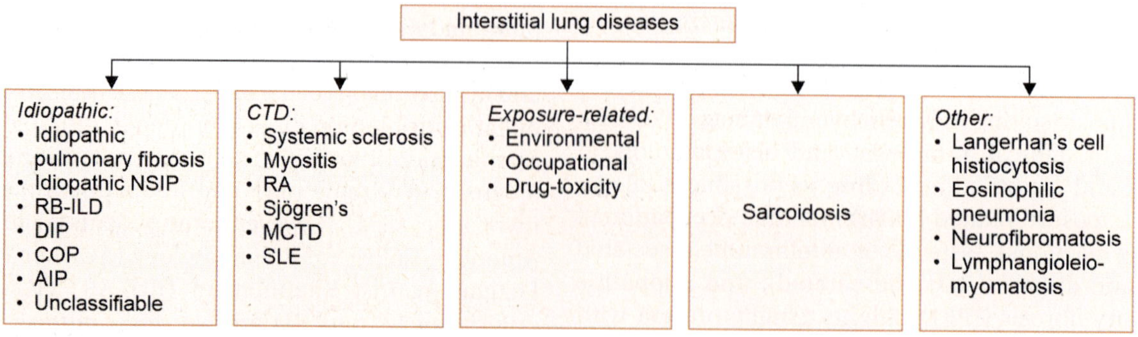

FLOWCHART 1: Classification of interstitial lung diseases.

(AIP: acute interstitial pneumonia; COP: cryptogenic organizing pneumonia; CTD: connective tissue disease; DIP: desquamative interstitial pneumonia; MCTD: mixed connective tissue disease; NSIP: nonspecific interstitial pneumonia; RA: rheumatoid arthritis; RB-ILD: respiratory bronchiolitis-associated interstitial lung disease; SLE: systemic lupus erythematosus)

TABLE 1: Classification criteria for interstitial pneumonia with autoimmune features.

1. Presence of an interstitial pneumonia by HRCT or SLB and
2. Exclusion of alternative etiologies and
3. Does not meet criteria for a defined CTD and
4. At least one feature from at least two of the following domains:

A. Clinical domain	B. Serologic domain	C. Morphologic domain

• Distal digital fissuring (i.e., "mechanic hands")
• Distal digital tip ulceration
• Inflammatory arthritis or polyarticular morning joint stiffness ≥ 60 min
• Palmar telangiectasia
• Raynaud phenomenon
• Unexplained digital edema
• Unexplained fixed rash on the digital extensor surfaces (Gottron sign)
	• ANA ≥ 1 :320 titer, diffuse, speckled, homogeneous patterns or
	  ○ ANA nucleolar pattern (any titer) or
	  ○ ANA centromere pattern (any titer)
	• Rheumatoid factor ≥ 2 × upper limit of normal
	• Anti-CCP
	• Anti-dsDNA
	• Anti-Ro (SS-A)
	• Anti-La (SS-B)
	• Anti-ribonucleoprotein
	• Anti-Smith
	• Anti-topoisomerase (Scl-70)
	• Anti-tRNA synthetase (e.g., Jo-1, PL-7, PL-12; others are: EJ, OJ, KS, Zo, tRS)
	• Anti-PM-Scl
	• Anti-MDA-5
		• Suggestive radiology patterns by HRCT:
		  ○ NSIP
		  ○ OP
		  ○ NSIP with OP overlap
		  ○ LIP
		• Histopathology patterns or features by surgical lung biopsy:
		  ○ NSIP
		  ○ OP
		  ○ NSIP with OP overlap
		  ○ LIP
		  ○ Interstitial lymphoid aggregates with germinal centers
		  ○ Diffuse lymphoplasmacytic infiltration (with or without lymphoid follicles)
		• Multicompartment involvement (in addition to interstitial pneumonia):
		  ○ Unexplained pleural effusion or thickening
		  ○ Unexplained pericardial effusion or thickening
		  ○ Unexplained intrinsic airways disease (by PFT, imaging or pathology)
		  ○ Unexplained pulmonary vasculopathy

Source: Adapted from Fischer A, et al. (2015).

- At least one feature from two of the three domains as follows:
  1. *Clinical domain*:
     a. Distal digital fissuring (i.e., mechanic hands)
     b. Distal digital tip ulceration
     c. Inflammatory arthritis or morning stiffness ≥ 60 minutes
     d. Palmar telangiectasia
     e. Raynaud phenomenon
     f. Unexplained digital edema
     g. Unexplained fixed rash on the digital extensor surfaces (Gottron sign)
  2. *Serologic domain:*
     a. Antinuclear antibody (ANA) ≥ 1:320 titer, diffuse, speckled, homogeneous patterns or ANA nucleolar pattern (any titer) or ANA centromere pattern (any titer)
     b. Rheumatoid factor ≥ 2 × upper limit of normal
     c. Anti-cyclic citrullinated peptide (CCP)
     d. Anti-double-stranded deoxyribonucleic acid (dsDNA)
     e. Anti-Ro (SS-A)
     f. Anti-La (SS-B)
     g. Anti-ribonucleoprotein (RNP)
     h. Anti-Smith
     i. Anti-topoisomerase (Scl-70)
     j. Anti-transfer ribonucleic acid (tRNA) synthetase (e.g., Jo-1, PL-7, and PL-12)
     k. Anti-PM/Scl
     l. Anti-melanoma differentiation-associated gene 5 (anti-MDA5)
  3. *Morphologic domain **(Fig. 3)**:*
     a. *Suggestive radiology patterns by HRCT*: Nonspecific interstitial pneumonia (NSIP)/organizing pneumonia (OP)/NSIP with OP overlap/lymphocytic interstitial pneumonia (LIP)
     b. *Histopathology patterns or features by surgical lung biopsy*: NSIP/OP/NSIP with OP overlap/LIP/interstitial lymphoid aggregates with germinal centers/diffuse lymphoplasmacytic infiltration (with or without lymphoid follicles)

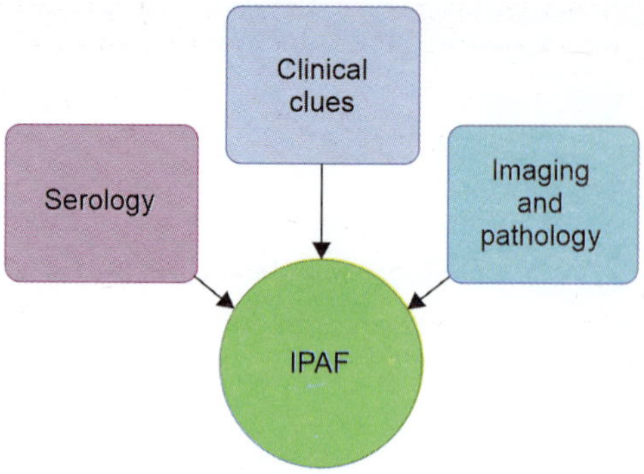

FIG. 3: Three domains contributing to the diagnosis of interstitial pneumonia with autoimmune features (IPAF).

c. *Multicompartment involvement*:
   i. Unexplained pleural effusion or thickening
   ii. Unexplained pericardial effusion or thickening
   iii. Unexplained intrinsic airway disease (by pulmonary function test, imaging, or histopathology)
   iv. Unexplained pulmonary vasculopathy

CLINICAL CLUES

With respect to demographic characteristics, the mean age varies from 60 to 65 years with no gender predisposition, although some studies reported a younger mean age and a predominance of white nonsmoking women. IPAF is mostly associated with smokers or ex-smokers.

According to three published cohorts, there was a significantly high prevalence of patients meeting clinical criteria, around 47–63% of IPAF patients had at least one clinical sign. The most common clinical signs were Raynaud phenomenon, followed by mechanics' hands, arthritis or morning stiffness, and Gottron sign.

SEROLOGY

More than 90% of patients with IPAF have at least one of the serological criteria. The main autoantibody found was positive, high-titer ANA (48–82%). Anti-SS-A, antisynthetase antibodies, as well as rheumatoid factor were also frequently positive.

IMAGING AND PATHOLOGY

The radiological subdomain of the morphological domain describes patterns from HRCT such as NSIP, OP, NSIP with OP overlap, and LIP. The NSIP pattern at HRCT and histopathology (41% and 25%, respectively) was the most frequent finding. It was noted that the histological usual interstitial pneumonia (UIP) pattern observed in IPAF patients has been reported as nontypical, with diffuse lymphoplasmacytic infiltrates, interstitial lymphoid aggregates, or involvement of the airways.

The last subdomain of the morphologic domain is the multicompartment designation, which includes pleural or pericardial effusions or thickening, pulmonary vasculopathy, or intrinsic airway disease. Thus, patients with CTD often demonstrate involvement of pulmonary structures other than the parenchyma, including airways, pleura, and the pulmonary vasculature.

TREATMENT

A significant challenge in treating ILD patients, and especially IPAF, is deciding when to initiate treatment. A significant proportion of IPAF patients demonstrates long-term stability without the need for immunosuppressive therapy. The decision to start treatment should be weighed against the potential risks. Therapy is usually initiated if the patient experiences progressive fibrosis of the lungs (significant symptoms or by PFT parameters or HRCT), is at high risk of progressive disease (such as cases of MDA-5 antibody positive), or if there are extrapulmonary manifestations that warrant therapy (such as debilitating arthritis). Treatment should be individualized.

In the series of IPAF data published to date where treatment is reported, a majority of patients have received glucocorticoids and/or immunosuppressive therapy, including azathioprine, cyclophosphamide, mycophenolate mofetil, calcineurin inhibitors (cyclosporine and tacrolimus), and occasionally rituximab, illustrating that many clinicians would treat subjects with IPAF just like CTD-ILD. Mycophenolate seemed to improve the slope of forced vital capacity (FVC) and of diffusing capacity of the lung for carbon monoxide (DLCO) in a small cohort of IPAF. Cyclophosphamide is considered as the mainstay of therapy for severe or life-threatening forms of CTD-ILD, while rituximab (anti-B-cell CD20 monoclonal antibody) is used in patients with refractory CTD-ILD.

A small minority of patients in published series have received antifibrotic agents (nintedanib); however, efficacy of management is virtually impossible to assess as in most studies, there is absence of a control group and high clinical heterogeneity.

Similar to other ILDs, pulmonary rehabilitation, long-term oxygen therapy, and treatment of gastroesophageal reflux if present are indicated. Prevention of secondary infection including vaccination and bone health assessment are also important. In advanced disease, lung transplantation may be considered.

Treatment decisions in patients classified as IPAF must be based on careful evaluation of benefit:risk ratio in the individual subject and should ideally be discussed in multidisciplinary approach. While a histological NSIP pattern would support an immunosuppressive approach, histological identification of a UIP pattern would warrant a more cautious approach to immunosuppression and early consideration of antifibrotic therapy. Finally, the finding of associated morphological features of IPAF on a biopsy, otherwise characterized by a UIP pattern, would lead to further evaluation and monitoring over time to detect additional features suggestive of an underlying CTD.

The demographic, clinical, and autoimmune features, as well as the imaging phenotype should be taken into consideration and management should be individualized.

PROGNOSIS

The GAP index, a score developed for IPF and based on *G*ender, *A*ge, and lung *P*hysiology (FVC and DLCO) has been used for baseline mortality prediction.

The presence of a UIP pattern at HRCT and/or histopathology is associated with a poor outcome as compared to a non-UIP pattern. Although in general, the diagnosis of IPAF was associated with a better outcome than IPF (a progressive ILD with an estimated survival of only 3–5 years from diagnosis) but worse than in RD-ILD.

Factors associated with a longer transplant-free survival include presence of the clinical domain, higher partial pressure of oxygen (PaO_2) and myositis-specific antibodies, particularly Jo-1 antibody.

Factors associated with worse prognosis include increasing age, history of smoking, lower baseline pulmonary function (FVC and/or DLCO), presence of pulmonary hypertension, RNP antibody, and multi-compartment feature.

Interstitial lung disease may be the initial manifestation of a CTD and it is possible for patients with ILD, including IPAF, to manifest a defined CTD at a later time. Sebastiani et al. observed IPAF evolution to a definite CTD in 13.5% of cases.

MONITORING AND ROLE OF PHYSICIANS

Interstitial pneumonia with autoimmune features is a heterogeneous disorder with undefined pathogenesis, prognosis, and management. The revision of the classification criteria is possibly looming in the future with further refining of our understanding of this complex disease. The management of the IPAF patient is multidisciplinary with pulmonology, rheumatology, pathology, radiology, rehabilitation medicine, and pulmonary transplant providers, all serving major vital roles. The physician/rheumatologist has a significant role in reaching the diagnosis by confirming the autoimmune features and excluding a defined RD and in selection of appropriate therapeutic agents with monitoring for toxicity. All patients with an ILD should be routinely evaluated for the presence of CTD symptoms and signs, monitoring for emergence of a distinct RD, with reevaluation occurring at each visit and for a prolonged duration of follow-up.

SUGGESTED READINGS

1. Raghu G. Interstitial lung disease: a diagnostic approach. Am J Respir Crit Care Med. 1995;151:909-14.
2. Mackintosh JA, Wells AU, Cottin V, Nicholson AG, Renzoni EA. Interstitial pneumonia with autoimmune features: challenges and controversies. Eur Respir Rev. 2021;30(162):210177.
3. Fischer A, Antoniou KM, Brown KK, Cadranel J, Corte TJ, Du Bois RM, et al. An official European Respiratory Society/American Thoracic Society research statement: interstitial pneumonia with autoimmune features. Eur Respir J. 2015;46(4):976-87.
4. Vergara K, Saavedra S, Reyes F, Goecke A, Chesta C, Chavez S. AB1109 Characterization of patients with interstitial pneumonia with autoimmune features (IPAF) and its comparison with patients with scleroderma-related interstitial lung disease and with idiopathic fibrosis. Ann Rheum Dis. 2018;78(Suppl 2).
5. Mathai SC, Danoff SK. Management of interstitial lung disease associated with connective tissue disease. BMJ. 2016;352:h6819.

223

CHAPTER

Smoking-related Interstitial Lung Disease

Devendra Prasad Singh, Manish Kumar

ABSTRACT

A group of diseases which show strong an etiological link with smoking are said to constitute smoking-related interstitial lung diseases (ILDs). They are respiratory bronchiolitis-associated ILD, desquamative interstitial pneumonia, and pulmonary Langerhans cell histiocytosis (PLCH). There is an increased risk of interstitial pulmonary fibrosis and combined pulmonary fibrosis and emphysema in current and ex-smokers as suggested by various epidemiological studies. The most sensitive tool to diagnose different smoking-related interstitial lung diseases (SR-ILDs) is high-resolution computed tomography (HRCT). The distinctive CT features include centrilobular ground glass opacity in respiratory bronchiolitis interstitial lung disease, diffuse ground glass opacity in desquamative interstitial pneumonia, and nodules and cysts in upper lobe in PLCH. The final diagnosis requires the combined efforts of pulmonologist, radiologist and pathologist as there is an overlap of features of different SR-ILDs.

INTRODUCTION

Tobacco smoking is one of the most common addictions afflicting people all over the globe. The devastating impact on our pulmonary as well as nonpulmonary systems caused by smoke is due to its >6,000 harmful substances. Lung cancer and chronic obstructive pulmonary disease (COPD) are well-known smoking-related lung diseases, and this spectrum also includes some less-known lung diseases such as respiratory bronchiolitis-associated interstitial lung disease (RB-ILD), desquamative interstitial pneumonia (DIP), and pulmonary Langerhans cells histiocytosis (PLCH). The causative link and/or epidemiological association between smoking and some of these interstitial lung diseases (ILDs), which are called smoking-related interstitial lung diseases (SR-ILDs), have been shown by some of the recent studies.

CLASSIFICATION

Smoking-related ILDs may be classified into four groups based on the magnitude of the association between smoking and ILDs:

- There is strong association between smoking and ILDs as shown by epidemiological data in the first group, and they are as follows:
  - RB-ILD
  - DIP
  - PLCH
- The etiological association is less strong in the second group. The two ILDs in this group are acute eosinophilic pneumonia and pulmonary hemorrhage syndrome.
- Smoking is more prevalent in the third group of important diseases. Studies show that smoking influences the mortality and morbidity in these diseases. Idiopathic pulmonary fibrosis (IPF), combined pulmonary fibrosis and emphysema (CPFE), and rheumatoid arthritis related ILD (RA-ILD) can be classified in this group.
- Sarcoidosis and hypersensitivity pneumonitis constitute the fourth group of diseases. They seem to be protected from the damaging impact of smoke by virtue of suppressed T helper cell (Th1) immunity. In spite of the above fact, ILDs in smokers are associated with a worse outcome as compared to nonsmokers.

PATHOGENESIS

Tobacco smoking induces chronic inflammation in bronchioles and pulmonary interstitium in a genetically predisposed host, resulting in injury to the endothelium and alveolar epithelium. Lung cells are stimulated by tobacco smoking to produce a large number of reactive oxygen species (ROS), which lead to oxidative stress. Virus-induced parenchymal inflammation is also enhanced. Emphysema and fibrosis are caused by different mediators of smoking-generated oxidative stress, resulting in chronic inflammation and apoptosis **(Flowchart 1)**.

CLINICAL FEATURES

Smoking-related ILDs comprise a heterogeneous group of lung diseases characterized by nonproductive cough and breathlessness.

Respiratory illnesses such as RB-ILD, DIP, PLCH, CPFE, and IPF have a strong association with smoking. Patients presenting with dyspnea and dry cough should be considered for the above differential diagnosis. A thorough clinical evaluation is imperative for a case of ILD.

- *RB-ILD*: It is most common among heavy smokers in the age group of 20–50 years. The exact incidence is unknown, but few studies have shown that it varies from 2 to 13%.

  The clinical presentation is usually asymptomatic, but it may present with cough and dyspnea rarely.
- *DIP*: Smokers or ex-smokers constitute 90% of cases of DIP. Systemic diseases or infections and exposure to occupational agents and drugs may also be associated with DIP occasionally. There is an accumulation of a large number of smoker's macrophages in the alveolar spaces with inflammation and/or fibrosis of pulmonary interstitium. The most common age group of presentation is 20–50 years.

  It is usually insidious in onset with progressive dyspnea and dry cough. The physical examination reveals digital clubbing in around 50% of cases and inspiratory crackles in approximately 60% of cases.
- *PLCH*: Tobacco smoking triggers this polyclonal disorder. It most commonly affects persons of the age group of 20–40 years. Nonproductive cough and dyspnea are common clinical features. It may be associated with weight loss, fever, and night sweats simulating tuberculosis in 33% of cases as per some studies.
- *CPFE*: It is a distinct syndrome in which there is combination of emphysema in upper lobes and fibrosis in lower lobes amongst smokers. The common age of onset is between fifth and seventh decades.
- *IPF*: There is limited evidence to suggest that smoking per se directly causes IPF. However, smokers have an increased incidence of IPF. It is the most common idiopathic interstitial lung disease. Usually, the age of onset is over 50 years, and there is strong history of smoking. There is a strong epidemiological association. IPF presents with progressive dyspnea which is gradual in onset, chronic cough, digital clubbing (60%), and bibasilar inspiratory crackles.

Differential diagnoses of all these SR-ILDs are shown in **Table 1**.

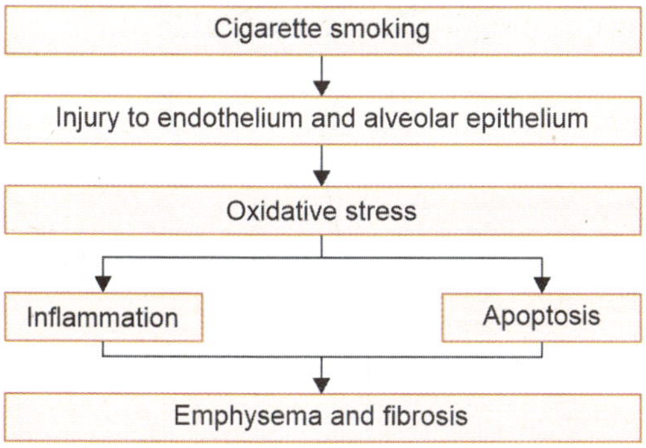

FLOWCHART 1: Pathogenesis of smoking-related-interstitial lung diseases.

TABLE 1: Diagnostic features of smoking-related interstitial lung diseases.

	DIP	RB-ILD	PLCH	CPFE	IPF
Smoking	90%	100%	>90%	Strong	41–83%
Age	20–50 years	20–50 years	20–40 years	50–70 years	Over 50 years
Sex M:F	Nearly 2:1	Slight male dominance	1:1	9:1	1:1 to 2:1
Onset	Insidious	Insidious	Insidious	Insidious	Insidious
Presenting symptoms	• Exertional dyspnea • Dry cough	• Frequently asymptomatic • Dyspnea • Cough	• Exertional dyspnea • Dry cough	Exertional dyspnea	• Exertional dyspnea • Dry cough
Crackles	60%	~50%	Usually absent	87%	Nearly all
Clubbing	Nearly 50%	Occasional	Occasional	43%	50–70%

(CPFE: combined pulmonary fibrosis and emphysema; DIP: desquamative interstitial pneumonia; IPF: idiopathic pulmonary fibrosis; PLCH: pulmonary Langerhans cells histiocytosis; RB-ILD: respiratory bronchiolitis interstitial lung disease)

INVESTIGATIONS

Diagnostic clues of different ILDs have been enumerated in **Table 2**.

In RB-ILD, DIPLD and PLCH, pulmonary function test (PFT) shows an obstructive, restrictive, or mixed pattern. The hallmark of IPF, including CPFE, is a severe restrictive pattern. Honeycombing with bi-basilar predominance in chest radiograph is seen with IPF. The characteristic in CPFE includes emphysema in upper lobe and fibrosis in lower lobe. DIP and RB-ILD have normal or interstitial patchy ground opacity. In PLCH, a cystic or nodular lesion with basilar sparing is noted commonly.

High-resolution computed tomography (HRCT)-radiologist has a very vital role in diagnosis as the characteristic patterns of different ILDs eliminate the need of lung biopsy. In RB-ILD **(Fig. 1A)** and DIP **(Fig. 1B)**, patchy ground glass opacity in upper lobe and ground glass opacity predominantly in the lower lobe are distinctive patterns respectively. In PLCH **(Fig. 1C)**, nodules and cysts with basilar sparing are diagnostic. In CPFE **(Fig. 1D)**, bullous, paraseptal, or centrilobular emphysema in the upper part and fibrosis in the lower part of lung are seen. In IPF **(Fig. 1E)**, subpleural honeycombing with basilar predominance, traction bronchiectasis with an interface sign is diagnostic.

High-resolution CT Chest in Smoking-related Interstitial Lung Disease (Figs. 1A to E)

High-resolution CT chest in SR-ILDs are shown in **Figures 1A to E**.

TREATMENT

General Treatment

- The principal advice in all cases of SR-ILD is cessation of smoking. A number of studies have shown improvement in patients of SR-ILD if they quit smoking. However, there is no robust data to prove that there is a favorable prognosis upon stopping smoking.
- *Oxygen treatment*: Long-term oxygen therapy is indicated if there is significant hypoxia. This treatment may prolong life.
- *Rehabilitation*: It is a very useful modality of conservative treatment which may improve functional capacity in progressive SR-ILD and preserve the quality of life (QoL).
- *Transplantation*: Patient under the age of 65 years may be considered for lung transplantation provided there are no contraindications and they are suffering from refractory progressive disease **(Table 3)**.

TABLE 2: Differential diagnosis of smoking-related interstitial lung diseases based on investigations.

Investigations	RB-ILD	DIP	PLCH	CPFE	IPF
PFT	Mixed defect or normal	Restrictive	Obstructive or restrictive	Severe restriction of diffusion capacity	Restrictive
Chest radiograph	Interstitial or normal	Interstitial, patchy ground glass	Interstitial/cystic or nodular, with basilar sparing	Emphysema in upper part and fibrosis in lower part of lung	Interstitial, honeycombing with basilar predominance
HRCT	• Patchy ground glass • No honeycombing	• Ground glass with lower lung predominance • No honeycombing	Nodules and cysts; basilar sparing	Bullous, paraseptal, or centrilobular emphysema in the upper part and fibrosis in the lower part of lung	Subpleural honeycombing basilar predominance
Bronchoalveolar lavage	Increased total cell count and high number of smoker's macrophages	High total cell count, sometimes pronounced eosinophilia and neutrophilia. Smoker's macrophages regularly seen	Increase in Langerhans cells to >4% is highly specific for the presence of histiocytosis smoker's macrophages regularly seen	Frequently nonspecific, mild neutrophilia. Smoker's macrophages regularly seen	Mild neutrophilia and eosinophilia pronounced lymphocytosis rules out IPF

(CPFE: combined pulmonary fibrosis and emphysema; DIP: desquamative interstitial pneumonia; HRCT: high-resolution computed tomography; IPF: idiopathic pulmonary fibrosis; PFT: pulmonary function test; PLCH: pulmonary Langerhans cells histiocytosis; RB-ILD: respiratory bronchiolitis interstitial lung disease)

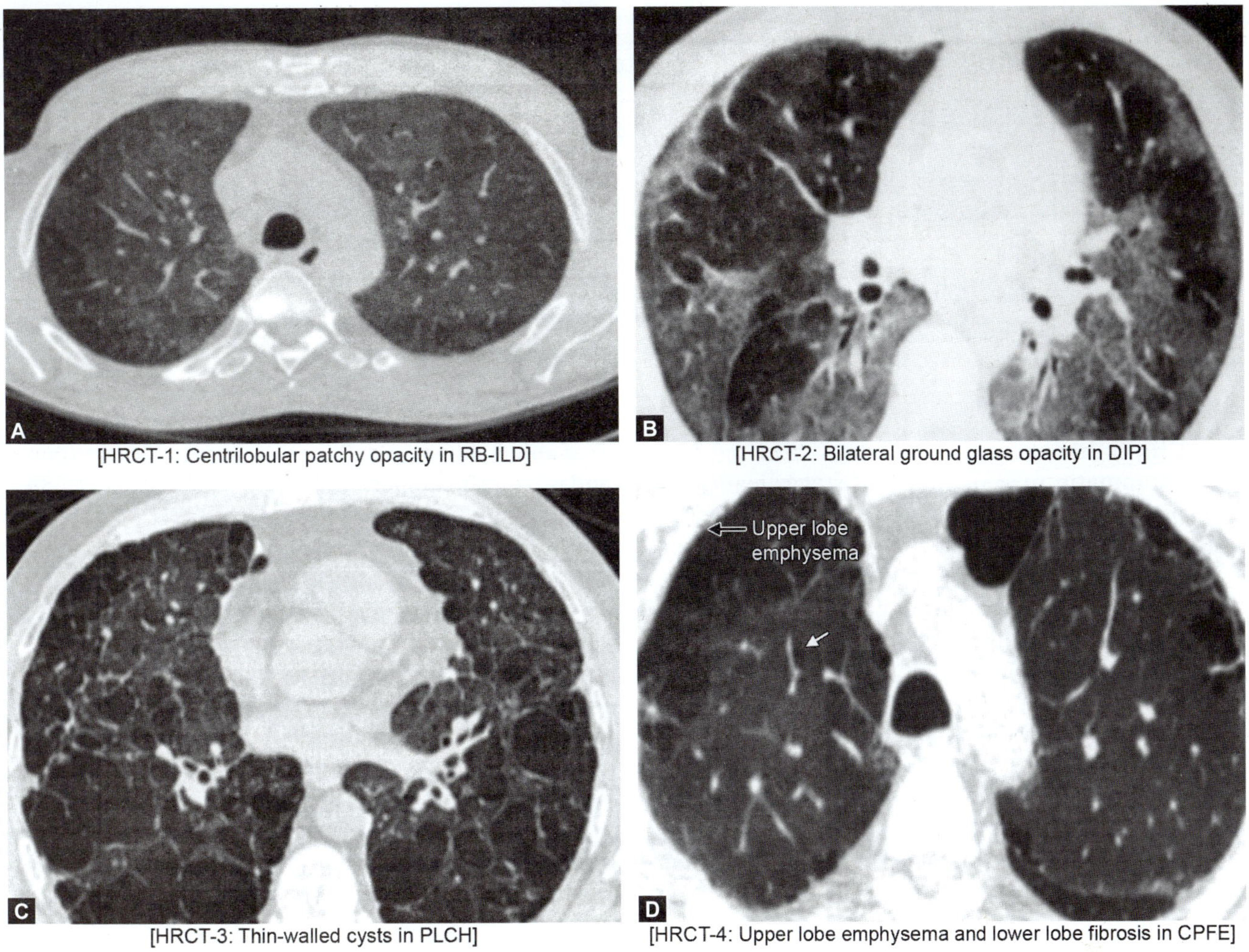

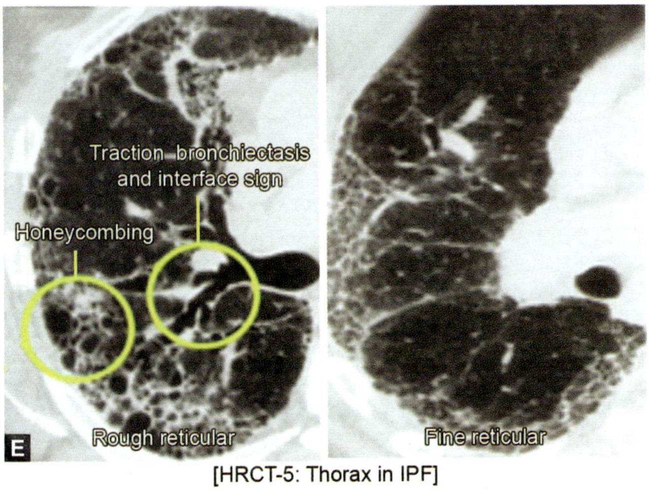

FIGS. 1A TO E: Image showing the diagnostic of CT chest finding of smoking-related interstitial lung diseases.

(CPFE: combined pulmonary fibrosis and emphysema; DIP: desquamative interstitial pneumonia; HRCT: high-resolution computed tomography; IPF: idiopathic pulmonary fibrosis; PLCH: pulmonary Langerhans cells histiocytosis; RB-ILD: respiratory bronchiolitis interstitial lung disease)

Specific Treatment

- *RB-ILD*: The cessation of smoking is the most important factor in the management of RB-ILD. There is a good response to steroid and complete recovery may be possible.
- *DIP*: Regression of disease is seen by cessation of smoking. It is the primary treatment. Oral steroids are indicated in progressive disease; however, the response to steroid therapy is not uniform. Different studies have shown the survival to be 5–10 years.

TABLE 3: Modalities of treatment and prognosis of smoking-related interstitial lung diseases.

Treatment	RB-ILD	DIP	PLCH	CPFE	IPF
• Preventive treatment • Drug treatment • Lung transplant	Smoking cessation	Smoking cessation, steroids	Smoking cessation, steroids?	• Smoking cessation • Long-term oxygen treatment • Lung transplant last option	• Smoking • Steroids? Cytotoxic drug Antifibrotic drugs? • Lung transplant
Response to steroid	Good	Good	Fair	Poor	Poor
Prognosis	Good	Good	Good	Poor	Poor

(CPFE: combined pulmonary fibrosis and emphysema; DIP: desquamative interstitial pneumonia; IPF: idiopathic pulmonary fibrosis; PLCH: pulmonary Langerhans cells histiocytosis; RB-ILD: respiratory bronchiolitis interstitial lung disease)

- *PLCH*: It has a variable course ranging from asymptomatic to a debilitating stage, leading to respiratory failure and even death. The cornerstone of treatment is smoking cessation and steroid therapy.
- *IPF*: It is a progressive disease with a median survival of around 2.5–3.5 years. Treatment is mostly supportive, but capacity and ascend trials have shown a mortality benefit with the use of pirfenidone. Similarly, TOMORROW trial with nintedanib shows preservation of health-related QoL in IPF. The only option in the treatment of IPF is lung transplantation.
- *CPFE*: The prognosis of CPFE is determined by the high prevalence of pulmonary hypertension. Studies have shown the median survival to be better than IPF (around 6.1 years)

Table 3 shows modalities of treatment, drug response, and prognosis of different SR-ILDs.

CONCLUSION

Patients with a positive history of smoking suffering from a nonproductive cough and dyspnea should be considered in the differential diagnosis of SR-ILD. A multidisciplinary approach among pulmonologist, radiologist, and pathologist is essential to confirm the diagnosis of any ILD, including SR-ILDs. HRCT is the most important tool to guide in the diagnosis of ILD. An early diagnosis is imperative for initiating early treatment. The key to treatment is cessation of smoking, as it may improve prognosis. Lung transplant must be considered in refractory SR-ILD.

SUGGESTED READINGS

1. Vassallo R, Ryu JH. Smoking-related interstitial lung diseases. Clin Chest Med. 2012;33:165-78.
2. George AM, Vasarmidi E, Jacob J, Athol UW, Katerina MA. Smoking and interstitial lung diseases. Eur Respir Rev. 2015;24:428-35.
3. Vassallo R. Eyu JH, Schroeder DR, Decker PA, Limper AH. Clinical outcomes of pulmonary Langerhans-cell histiocytosis in adults. N Engl J Med. 2002;346(7):484-90.
4. HagmeverL, Randerrath W. Smoking-related Interstitial Lung Disease. Dtsch Arztebi Int. 2015;112(4):43-50.
5. Bjoraker JA Ryu JH, Edwin MK, Myers JL, Tazelaar HD, Schroeder DR et al. Prognostic significance of histopathologic subsets in idiopathic pulmonary fibrosis. Am J Respir Crit Care Med.1998;157:199-203.
6. Nicholson AG, Colby TV, du Bois RM, Hansell DM, Wells AU The prognostic significance of the histologic pattern of interstitial pneumonia in patients presenting with the clinical entity of cryptogenic fibrosing alveolitis. Am J respire Crit Care Med. 2000;162:2213-7.
7. Park JS, Brown KK, Tuder RM, Valerie A E Hale VA E, Talmadge E, Lynch DA Respiratory bronchiolitis-associated interstitial lung disease: radiologic features with clinical and pathologic correlation. J Comput Assist Tomogr. 2002;26:13-20.
8. Hartman TE, Primack SL, Swensen SI, Hansell D, McGuinness G, Müller NL. Desquamative interstitial pneumonia: thin-section CT findings in 22 patterns. Radiology. 1993;187:787-90.
9. Attrill AK, Kazerooni EA, Gross BH, Flaherty KR, Myers JL, Martinez FJ Smoking-related interstitial Lung Disease: Radiologic-Clinical-Pathologic Correlation. Radiograhics. 2008:28:1383-98.
10. Heyneman LE, S Ward, D A Lynch, M Remy-Jardin, T Johkoh, N L Müller.RB. RB-ILD, DIP different entities or part of the spectrum of the same disease process. Am J Roentgenol. 1999;173:1617-22.
11. Ryu JH, Myers JL, Capizzi SA, Douglas WW, Vassallo R, Decker PA. Desquamative Interstitial Pneumonia and Respiratory Bronchiolitis-Associated Interstitial Lung Disease. Chest. 2005:127:178-84.
12. Suri HS, Eunhee S Yi, Nowakowski GS, Vassallo R. Pulmonary Langerhans cell histocytosis. Orphanet Journal of Rare Disease. 2012;7:16.
13. Protnoy J, Veraldi K, Schwarz MI, Cool CD, Curran-Everett D, Cherniack RM, . Respiratory Bronchiolitis-interstitial lung disease: long-term outcome. Chest. 2007;131:664-71.

224

CHAPTER

Connective Tissue Disease-associated Interstitial Lung Disease: Diagnostic and Therapeutic Dilemmas

Aradhana Singh, Rashi Maheshwari

ABSTRACT

Interstitial lung diseases (ILD) are an important extra-articular feature of autoimmune rheumatic diseases and a major cause of mortality. Systemic sclerosis (SSc) is most frequently associated with ILD and manifests as a nonspecific interstitial pneumonia (NSIP) pattern whereas, in rheumatoid arthritis, the usual interstitial pneumonia (UIP) pattern is more commonly seen. High-resolution computed tomography (HRCT) chest is the investigation of choice and pulmonary function test (PFT) for assessing the functional progression. Identifying patients who need treatment and choosing the appropriate therapy are important to minimize the risk of therapy-related toxicity. Immunosuppressive and/or antifibrotic agents for symptomatic and fibrosing connective tissue disease-associated interstitial lung diseases (CTD-ILDs) can be used in patients who require treatment.

INTRODUCTION

Interstitial lung diseases (ILD) encompass a heterogenous group of lung diseases characterized by diffuse involvement of the pulmonary parenchyma by varying degrees of inflammation and/or fibrosis. ILD exists in approximately 40–50% of patients with connective tissue diseases (CTDs) and is the main cause of morbidity and mortality. Approximately 15% of ILDs will have a background CTD.

Prevalence of ILDs in various CTDs is as follows: Systemic sclerosis (SSc)—30%, rheumatoid arthritis (RA)—2–8%, mixed connective tissue disease (MCTD)—50%, and idiopathic inflammatory myositis (IIM)—20–78%.

Interstitial pneumonia with autoimmune features (IPAF) is a concept widely being used in the literature classifying patients of ILD with some features of CTDs like Raynaud's phenomenon or antinuclear antibody (ANA) positivity but do not meet the criteria for CTD. It predicts response to treatment and hence has favorable prognosis.

Post-COVID, ILD has also been reported in a large number of observational studies; however, a substantial number of patients either will have a static form or may have a progressive type leading to rapid deterioration of lung function.

CLASSIFICATION

The currently used classification of CTD-ILD is the histological classification of idiopathic interstitial pneumonia (IIP), and its relative prevalence in CTDs is given in **Table 1**.

Differential diagnosis for CTD-ILD includes the following:

- *Acute (hours to days)*: Infection, diffuse alveolar damage, acute eosinophilia pneumonia, vasculitis, diffuse alveolar hemorrhage
- *Subacute (weeks to months)*: Hypersensitivity pneumonitis, sarcoidosis, chronic eosinophilia pneumonia
- *Chronic (months to years)*: Pneumoconiosis, amyloidosis, idiopathic interstitial fibrosis

PATHOGENESIS

Genetic factors associated with SSc-ILD are HLA DRB1 alleles, DQB1*05, IRF5, STAT4, CD226, NLRP1, and IRAK1.

TABLE 1: Prevalence of histological patterns of IIP in CTD.

Pattern of ILD	IIP	Rheumatoid arthritis	Systemic sclerosis	SLE	Polymyositis/ dermatomyositis	Sjögren's syndrome
Usual interstitial pneumonia	+++	++	+	+	+	+/-
Nonspecific interstitial pneumonia	++	++	+++	++	++	++
Organizing pneumonia	++	+	+/–	+/–	++	+/–
Lymphocytic interstitial pneumonia	+/–	+/–	+/–	+/–	+/–	++

(CTD: connective tissue disease; IIP: idiopathic interstitial pneumonia; ILD: interstitial lung disease; SLE: systemic lupus erythematosus)

The MUC5B promoter region polymorphisms have been associated with ILD at large and also with RA-ILD.

Fibrosis develops in response to lung injury, and many cell types are implicated in pathogenesis.

The stages are as follows:
1. *Initiation*: Epithelial damage, endothelial activation, immune cell infiltration, inflammation
2. *Progression*: Fibroblast proliferation, fibrocyte recruitment, epithelial–mesenchymal transition, ongoing epithelial damage
3. *Failed resolution*: Myofibroblast persistence, altered matricellular interaction, perturbed epithelial repair

Generation of profibrotic myofibroblasts after lung injury is the key inducer of fibrotic response.

It arises from resident fibroblasts, transdifferentiation of epithelial cells, and circulating progenitor cells including fibrocytes.

DIAGNOSTIC EVALUATION (FIGS. 1A AND B)

Diagnosis of CTD-ILDs is clinicoradiological supported by the demonstration of autoantibodies.

- *Clinical evaluation*: A thorough systemic clinical history and examination should be performed in order to identify subtle features of CTD: Raynaud's phenomenon, arthritis, skin lesions, gangrene, ulcers, dryness of eyes and mouth, alopecia, and muscle weakness. Proper past history of infections, exposure to pets, and smoking and environmental triggers is to be taken in order to rule out the mimics of ILD. Occupational history of patients (mining, textile workers, coal workers) is to be considered before stamping the diagnosis of CTD-ILD in such patients.
- *Role of computed tomography (CT)*: The gold standard for ILD detection is high-resolution CT (HRCT), and very early diseases may be better picked up on prone imaging. HRCT is employed for diagnosis and follow-up. Quantitative CTs have the advantage of being able to quantify the progression. Concerns regarding radiation exposure have led to the development and validation of low-dose CT for CTD-ILD. It has been suggested to perform biannual CT scans to document disease progression. Use of ultra-low-dose CT and artificial intelligence-based quantitative CTs may make this possible in recent future.

  High-resolution CT might be too sensitive as a screening tool for CTD-ILD in unselected patients with CTD. Hence, it should be used to confirm CTD-ILD in the higher risk group (SSc positive for anti-topoisomerase or anti-RNA polymerase III antibodies) or according to symptoms, clinical examination, chest radiography, or pulmonary function abnormalities.
- *Ultrasound screening*: It is used for prognosis. In SSc, the presence of more than five B-lines is associated with worsening ILD. Subpleural disease has a higher risk of progression. Moreover, it is inexpensive, less time-consuming, and widely available.
- *Serum biomarkers*: The strongest evidence is for SP-D (surfactant protein), KL-6 (Krebs von den Lungen-6), and chemokine ligand 19 (CCL19) in SSc-ILD. In RA-ILD, Cancer Antigen 125(CA-125), CA 19-9, carcinoembryonic antigen (CEA), and KL-6 have been validated as biomarkers, including genetic polymorphisms of *MUC5B* gene and serum interleukin 13 (IL-13) levels.
- *Lung biopsy*: It is rarely required in the diagnosis or management of CTD-ILD. Biopsy may be required to rule out airway-centric complications.
- *Evaluation of disease severity*: Pulmonary function test (PFT) provides the most precise measurement of disease severity. In isolated ILD typically, a restrictive ventilatory defect exists, with reduced forced vital capacity (FVC) and total lung capacity (TLC), increased forced expiratory volume 1 to FVC ratio of >0.8, and reduced carbon monoxide diffusing capacity (DLCO) and lung compliance.

  Severity should be assessed by a combination of PFT, HRCT fibrosis score, and exercise-induced changes in blood oxygen saturation (6-minute walk test).

  Early/stable/mild disease should be monitored every 3–6 months.

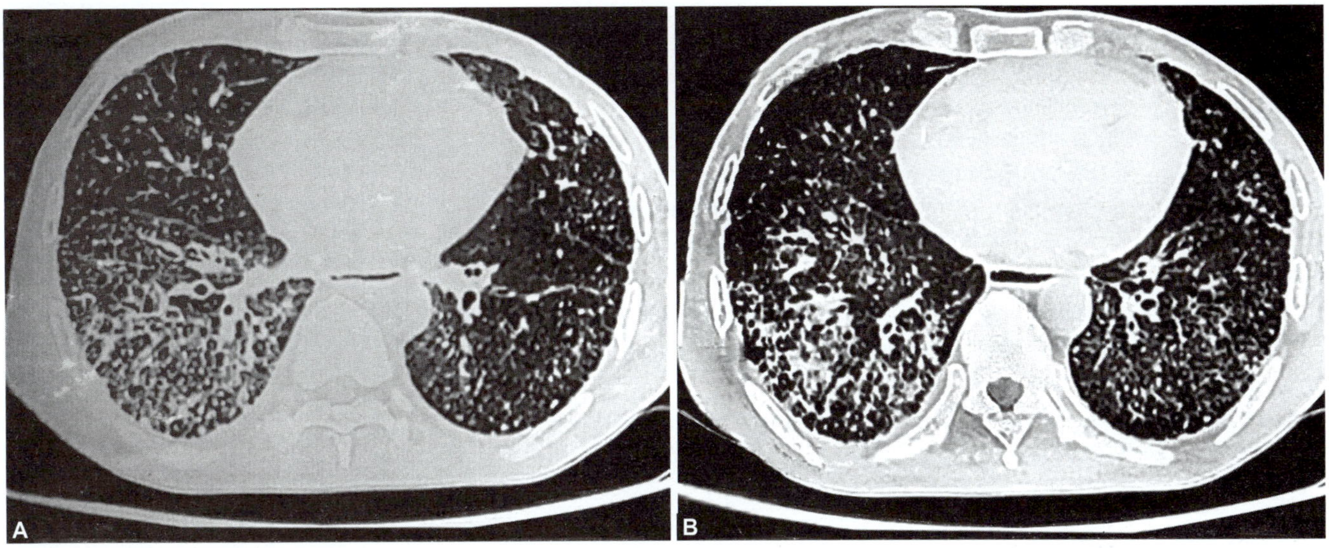

FIGS. 1A AND B: Diagnostic dilemma: High-resolution computed tomography (HRCT) chest showing basal predominance of reticular opacities and ground glass haziness with subpleural sparing suggestive of interstitial lung disease-nonspecific interstitial pneumonia (ILD-NSIP). Along with that, bilateral fields show nodular opacities, suggestive of chronic silicosis in a 42-year-old male patient, stone worker by profession, presenting with diffuse systemic sclerosis.

Source: Picture taken form personal picture gallery.

- *Evaluation of pulmonary comorbidities*: Reduction of DLCO that are disproportionate to lung volumes may be due to coexistent pulmonary vascular limitation. Hence, 2D echocardiography is to be done to rule out pulmonary hypertension.

  Preservation of lung volumes with severe restriction in DLCO may represent coexistent ILD and smoking-related emphysema.
- *Autoantibodies*: In SSc, following antibodies are associated with risk of developing ILD: Anti-Scl70, anti-RNA polymerase III, anti-Th/To, anti-U11/12, anti-Pm/Scl, and anti-U1RNP.

  In myositis, the following antibodies are associated with ILD: Ant-Jo1, anti-Pl-7, anti-PL-12, anti-EJ, anti-OJ, anti-Zo, anti-Ku, anti-KS, anti-MDA5, Pm-Scl, anti-Ro52/60, and anti-U1RNP.

TREATMENT

- *Identification of patients who require treatment*: Patients with dyspnea with Medical Research Council (MRC) classes III and IV require treatment. Patients with clinically meaningful progression of CTD-ILD with >10% relative decline in FVC or >5% to <10% relative decline in FVC with >15% relative decline in DLCO require treatment. A decision to treat could be made if visually estimated volume of interstitial abnormalities is >20% of the total lung volume on CT imaging or the absolute FVC is <70%. The PaO_2/FiO_2 ratio is one of the strongest individual parameters to predict survival in CTD-ILD. In RA-ILD, the presence of honeycombing, regardless of the underlying pattern, is strongly associated with poor prognosis.
- *Role of corticosteroids*: In SSc, corticosteroids are avoided as the possible harms outweigh the benefit. In MCTD-ILD and RA-ILD, prednisolone 0.5 mg/kg/day is used as the usual starting dose with gradual taper over weeks to months. In IIM-ILD, higher doses of corticosteroids (1 mg/kg/day prednisolone) maybe required at the time of the initiation. Lymphocytic interstitial pneumonia and nonspecific interstitial pneumonia (NSIP) show better response to corticosteroids than usual interstitial pneumonia (UIP).
- *Standard immunosuppression used in different CTD-ILD* **(Table 2)**: There are limited trials on CTD-ILD; most of the evidence is derived from the trials conducted in SSc-ILD. The Scleroderma Lung Study I showed favorable outcome in the cyclophosphamide (CYC) arm compared to placebo. The Scleroderma Lung Study II showed comparable results in both the arms (CYC vs. mycophenolate mofetil). FaSScinate trial comparing tocilizumab versus placebo did not meet its primary endpoint but did demonstrate a difference in FVC between the two arms. FocuSSed trial showed a favorable response for subcutaneous tocilizumab.
- *Antifibrotics*: In phase III SENSCIS trial, nintedanib (tyrosine kinase inhibitor) proved to be efficacious in reducing annual decline in FVC versus placebo in patients with SSc-ILD. Nintedanib was subsequently approved by the United States Food and Drug

TABLE 2: Immunosuppressive agents used in CTD-ILD.

CTD	Drugs	Remarks

SSc-ILD	• Mycophenolate 2–3 g daily
	• Cyclophosphamide
	  ○ Oral: 2–3 mg/kg body weight/day
	  ○ Intravenous: 600 mg/m^2 IV every month for a maximum of 6 months
	• Nintedanib may be added to either of the above: 150 mg 12 hourly orally
		Second-line agents:
		• Rituximab (2 g induction as given below)
		• Tocilizumab (162 mg subcutaneously weekly)

RA-ILD	• Rituximab 1 g IV infusion 2 weeks apart • Azathioprine 2–3 mg/kg body weight/day orally • Cyclophosphamide as mentioned above • Mycophenolate 2–3 g daily orally	Methotrexate and leflunomide may be continued in early minimally symptomatic disease
Myositis-ILD	*High-dose steroid (prednisolone 1 mg/kg body weight) with either of the following*: • Rituximab • Mycophenolate • Azathioprine • Cyclophosphamide	Rapidly progressive disease

(CTD: connective tissue disease; ILD: interstitial lung disease; RA: rheumatic arthritis; SSc: systemic sclerosis)

Administration (US FDA) and European Medicines Agency (EMA) for the treatment of SSc-ILD in September 2019 and April 2020, respectively.

The phase III INBUILD study has shown that nintedanib is also efficacious in treating a pooled group of patients with fibrosing ILD with progressive phenotype.

The Scleroderma Lung Study III evaluated the combination of antifibrotic effects of pirfenidone with mycophenolate mofetil and showed more rapid improvement in the FVC% (0–6 months) but overall similar results at the end of 18 months.

- *Role of stem cell transplantation*: Rapidly progressing patients with SSc-ILD without pulmonary hypertension can be managed by autologous hematopoietic stem cell transplant. The SCOT (Scleroderma: Cyclophosphamide or Transplantation) study showed clear benefit in the transplant arm. In ASSIST (American Scleroderma Stem Cell versus Immune Suppression Trial), no patients showed disease progression in the transplant arm, whereas the ASTIS (Autologous Stem Cell Transplantation International Scleroderma) trial demonstrated survival benefit.
- *Nonpharmacological therapies*:
    - *Vaccination*: Influenza and pneumococcal vaccines are recommended for patients having CTD-ILD.
    - *Pulmonary rehabilitation*: Physical activity and exercise training can improve the functional status and quality of life of the patient. The patient should be advised to stop smoking.
- *Management of comorbidities*: Dyspnea in ILD maybe due to underlying pulmonary hypertension, associated myositis, or cardiac disease. Hence, care should be taken for these conditions.
- *Palliative care and oxygen therapy*: Long-term oxygen therapy is a standard care for resting hypoxemia and ambulatory oxygen may help in hypoxemia on exertion. Guidelines exist for effective home oxygen therapy that may be utilized for CTD-ILD.
- *Lung transplantation*: Lung transplantation maybe considered for end-stage CTD-ILD. Combined heart–lung transplant maybe needed in patients with associated pulmonary hypertension. Patients with myositis-associated CTD-ILD have worse postoperative period and poorer outcomes.

CONCLUSION

The heterogeneity of ILD and its underlying CTD often leads to confusion among clinicians. Moreover, clinical progression and treatment response vary among patients. Hence, a clear distinction should be made between patients who need aggressive immunosuppression versus meticulous observation in order to balance out infections in these patients. The future lies in personalized precision medicine which will combine various -nomics (genetic, transcriptomics, and proteomics) and classify patients into rapid and slow progressors further guiding the management of such patients.

SUGGESTED READINGS

1. Wells AU, Denton CP. Interstitial lung disease in connective tissue disease-mechanisms and management. Nat Rev Rheumatol. 2014;10:728-39.
2. Ahmed S, Handa R. Management of connective tissue disease-related interstitial lung disease. Curr Pulmonol Rep. 2022;11: 86-98.
3. Spagnolo P, Distler O, Ryerson CJ, Tzouvelekis A, Lee JS, Bonella F, et al. Ann Rheum Dis 2021;80:143-50.
4. Shao T, Shi X, Yang S, Zhang W, Li X, Shu J, et al. Interstitial Lund disease in connective tissue disease: A common lesion with Heterogenous Mechanisms and treatment considerations. Front Immunol. 2021;12:684699.

225

CHAPTER

Oxygen Therapy

Sanjay Kumar, Ranjan Kumar

ABSTRACT

All of us know that oxygen is essential for life. We receive the required amount of oxygen from atmosphere through breathing. But sometimes additional amount of oxygen is required either due to disease or some physiological condition, so oxygen may be needed for medical uses. Oxygen use for medical purposes needs utmost caution and care. The knowledge of oxygen source, indications to use, delivery system, precautions, and adverse effect is necessary for proper patient care.

INTRODUCTION

A simple audit of drugs and support system used at all levels of healthcare will show that oxygen is one such thing that is used most widely everywhere in healthcare either in wards, operation theaters, intensive care unit (ICU), and even in long-term domiciliary treatment for certain diseases, particularly chronic lung conditions. We must consider oxygen as a pharmacological agent; hence, it is prudent to know its indications, possible side effect, and prescribing information.

DEFINITION

First, we must understand what oxygen therapy means. The ambient air at normal atmospheric pressure has 21% of oxygen. So, we breathe 21% of oxygen from normal air, i.e., fraction of inspired oxygen (FiO_2) 0.21. Supplemental oxygen given to a person increases the FiO_2 over and above 0.21. So, oxygen therapy is basically enhancing the percentage of oxygen in breath over the atmospheric oxygen, i.e., 21%.

INDICATIONS

The basic indication of oxygen therapy is to correct hypoxia. The gold standard to measure hypoxia is arterial blood gas (ABG) measurement and look for partial pressure of arterial oxygen, i.e., PaO_2. But obtaining ABG and seeing PaO_2 is not possible at all times due to time constraints or logistic issues. So, clinical assessment of hypoxia is of utmost importance. Clinically hypoxemic patient may have varied symptoms and signs involving multiple organ system. The hypoxemic patient's skin may be cool and clammy to cyanosed depending upon the degree of hypoxia, and the respiration may be shallow, labored, or in severe case, agonal. The patient may have dyspnea with tachypnea. Similarly cardiac disturbances may also manifest as rate and rhythm disturbances. There may be bradycardia to tachycardia, ectopic beats, and different arrhythmias. Coming to the central nervous system (CNS) manifestations, mild-to-moderate hypoxia may give rise to confusional or agitated state to lethargy and mental obtundation in severe cases.

In ABG the level of PaO_2 denotes the level of hypoxemia. PaO_2 between 60 and 80 mm Hg denotes mild-to-moderate hypoxemia, while PaO_2 <60 mm Hg is indicative of severe hypoxemia.

OXYGEN DELIVERY

In health system, the basic source of oxygen delivery is either through conventional oxygen cylinders or centralized oxygen distribution system which provides bedside source of oxygen through adequately laid down manifold gas pipeline. Cylinders are cheap and easy to use and do not need any power supply while centralized pipeline supply needs more logistic support, but it has distinct advantage of continuous supply and is more cost-effective in the long term. The common cylinder types used in healthcare facilities are shown in **Table 1**.

Conventionally, oxygen is delivered to the patient by interfaces which are classified into low-flow system and high-flow system.

Low-flow System

The low-flow system does not meet the total demand of oxygen required to fulfill total minute ventilation (MV). It also does not deliver a fixed FiO_2. The FiO_2 varies from breath to breath and it depends on the inspiratory flow rate of the patient. The rate of flow of oxygen through different types of low-flow delivery system is limited up to 6 L/min.

The low-flow delivery systems are described in the following text.

Nasal Cannula/Prongs

This is most commonly used device to deliver oxygen. It consists of lightweight tube which splits into two forks or prongs at the terminal end. The prongs deliver the oxygen through nose and it is directed toward nasopharynx, where the work of humidification and heat exchange takes place to some extent. The maximum flow rate is up to 4 L/min. The flow rate of >4 L/min is discomfortable to the patient, as it dries and irritates the nasal mucosa. The estimated FiO_2 through this system is 0.24–0.44, i.e., 24–44%. The advantage of this device is that it is cheap, easy to use, and the patient can eat and drink while using this system.

Simple Face Mask

It is also known as Hudson mask. It is the next common interface in low-flow system. Like nasal prongs, it is also very simple, lightweight, cheap, and easy to use. The caveat in using this device is the proper flow rate, as low-flow rate <4 L/min may not fill the mask space fully and there remains some empty space, where expired carbon dioxide (CO_2) may accumulate and inspired in subsequent breaths. So, the minimal flow rate through mask should be >4 L/min and the maximum flow rate is 8 L/min, providing maximum FiO_2 0.6, i.e., 60%. In comparison to nasal prongs, it is slightly disadvantageous in the form that it keeps patient face and mouth accesses limited, so it is difficult to eat and drink while using this device.

TABLE 1: Types of cylinders.

Type	Normal oxygen capacity (L)	Normal service pressure (psi)	Approximate weight (kg)
D	2.3	1,987	3.9
E	4.7	1,987	6.5
F	9.4	1,987	17
G	23.6	1,987	39
J	47.2	1,987	78

Partial Rebreathing and Nonrebreathing Mask

The partial rebreathing and nonrebreathing masks have a reservoir attached to the face mask, in which oxygen is first collected and then delivered to patient with breath. The main difference between these two is the one-way valve present in nonrebreathing mask that prevents accumulation of expired gases in reservoir bag. The nonrebreathing mask does not entrain the atmospheric air, and if filled with oxygen properly and applied properly, it can provide 100% FiO_2. In order to fill the reservoir properly the flow rate of oxygen should be high enough to the tune of 10–15 L/min. The disadvantage of these devices is same as face mask.

High-flow System

It is another set of devices which may be termed as fixed performance system as it is sans patient factors in oxygen delivery. It delivers consistent FiO_2, independent of patient ventilatory pattern and also meets the full MV requirement of the patient.

There are many devices in high-flow system like Venturi mask and other high-flow aerosol system. The Venturi mask is the most common device in this category. In this system the face mask is fitted with a jet device. The size of jet varies the FiO_2. The oxygen passes through this jet and entrains the atmospheric air to a predictable dilution. The FiO_2 can be adjusted to 24–60% through the different sizes of jet in Venturi system.

High-flow Nasal Cannula

This specialized system to giving oxygen at very high flow rate renewed our attention during coronavirus disease 2019 (COVID-19) pandemic. This highly specialized system uses oxygen from a large-volume source controlled through a flow meter and is admixed with ambient air in a blender to a desired FiO_2. This blended mixture of air and supplemental oxygen is further warmed and humidified in special system and finally delivered to the patient through a specially designed nasal cannula.

It has multiple beneficial physiological effects like decreasing anatomical dead space by washing out CO_2 from upper airways that further helps work of breathing and decreases the respiratory rate. Humidification and warming also improves the work of breathing and spares the body energy cost of normal humidification and warming by body. The very high flow rate in high-flow nasal cannula (HFNC) also generates low level of positive end-expiratory pressure (PEEP) which increases the lung volume and improves gas exchange. The HFNC system may deliver oxygen from 21 to 100%.

MONITORING

The oxygen therapy needs proper monitoring also.

The idea is not only to provide proper oxygen saturation in blood for physiological needs but high doses may produce deleterious effect on body also.

The ideal way of monitoring is to measure PaO_2 and or peripheral oxygen saturation (SpO_2) through ABG measurement and bedside pulse oximetry.

The goal is to maintain PaO_2 level above 80 mm Hg.

SIDE EFFECTS

High oxygen may cause tracheobronchitis, mucociliary dysfunction, and lung parenchymal damage. In neonates, it may also cause retrolental fibroplasia. So, there must be every caution in using oxygen, as is taken in using drugs.

SUGGESTED READINGS

1. Jindal SK, Agarwal R. A Practical Guide to Oxygen Therapy, 3rd edition. New Delhi: Jaypee Brothers Medical Publishers; 2022.
2. Campbell EJM. Oxygen and hypoxia. Seminar Respir Med. 1981;3:59.
3. Cornet AD, Kooter AJ, Peters MJL, Smulders YM. The potential harm of oxygen therapy in medical emergencies. Crit Care. 2013;17:313.

226
CHAPTER

Noninvasive Ventilation for Acute Respiratory Failure in Clinical Practice

Atul Bhasin, RK Singal, Sunil Kumar Bakshi

ABSTRACT

Noninvasive ventilation (NIV) is a ventilatory support that assists breathing without bypassing the upper airway. It plays a crucial role in respiratory failure, reducing both morbidity and mortality. Both continuous positive airway pressure (CPAP) and noninvasive positive pressure ventilation (NPPV) modes help deliver oxygen and clear carbon dioxide, relieving dyspnea, reducing breathing work, respiratory muscle fatigue, and ventilator-associated pneumonia (VAP) incidence. Early detection of NIV failure encourages intubation and ventilation.

INTRODUCTION

Noninvasive ventilation (NIV) is a ventilatory support to assist breathing with an interface without bypassing the upper airway. Respiratory failure could be hypoxemic (failure to maintain adequate oxygenation) or hypercarbia (retention of carbon dioxide) due to any cause leading to impaired arterial blood gases. The role of NIV in respiratory failure has been proven beyond doubt.

Both continuous positive airway pressure (CPAP) and noninvasive positive pressure ventilation (NPPV) modes of NIV help in delivering adequate oxygen and clearing carbon dioxide. The additional benefits of relieving dyspnea, reducing the work of breathing, reducing respiratory muscle fatigue, reducing the incidence of VAP, and being noninvasive have significantly reduced both morbidity and mortality. Early detection of failure of NIV should encourage the physicians to intubate and ventilate patients to reduce both morbidity and mortality.

A continuous positive pressure throughout its cycle prevents atelectasis and collapse of alveoli while NPPV supports the flow during inspiration by creating pressure support. Both the modes provide relief in all types of respiratory failure whether acute, acute-on-chronic, or chronic failure in a conscious patient.

RESPIRATORY FAILURE

Hypoxemic respiratory failure or type 1: PaO_2 <8 kPa and $PaCO_2$ which is normal or low.

Hypercapnic respiratory failure or type 2: PaO_2 <8 kPa and $PaCO_2$ of 6 kPa.

An arterial blood gas analysis will help in differentiating various types of failure in an ideal clinical setting. Patients with acute hypercapnic failure on arterial blood gas (ABG) will reveal a high $PaCO_2$ with low pH and normal bicarbonate values while a chronic hypercapnic failure will have an evidence of chronic respiratory disease and an ABG will have high $PaCO_2$, normal pH and high bicarbonate values. Compensated chronic hypercapnic failure generally does not require NIV support until unless already on oxygen support and NIV for maintenance therapy. These patients when once decompensate due to any precipitating event, e.g., infection especially lung, cardiac failure, or any other illness will immediately require supportive therapy for oxygenation or hypercarbia thus fulfilling the definition of *acute-on-chronic* hypercapnic respiratory failure where an ABG shows sudden increase in $PaCO_2$ from previous chronic levels with low pH and high bicarbonate.

MODES OF NONINVASIVE VENTILATION

Most Commonly Used Modes

- Continuous positive airway pressure
- Bilevel pressure support

Special Modes Available for Invasive Ventilators in ICU

- Controlled mechanical ventilation
- Assist/control ventilation
- Assisted spontaneous breathing (pressure support)
- Proportional assist ventilation

Special Modes of Noninvasive Ventilation

High-flow nasal cannulae (HFNC).

Initiating NIV and it's Prerequisite

All NIV are equipped with triggering mechanisms, oxygen support system, humidifiers, and alarms for their efficient functioning and safety measures. An interface is part of the circuit which needs to create a channel of interaction between the ventilator and patient for the efficient delivery of pressures or volumes with no leakages. As these masks have a very small dead space they are efficient in delivering the inspiratory pressure support generated by the machine. It can vary as per personal choice of physician and facial anatomy of the patient. Varying sizes of nasal masks and full-face masks are available and all very effective for initial treatment of acute respiratory failure. Ideally, initiation of NIV should be done with a full-face mask and subsequently switched over to a nasal mask once patient stabilizes or as an initial step toward weaning. Interactive education and demonstration of the use of face mask can allay the apprehension of patients toward initial discomfort and claustrophobia. Adequate nasal guard support can reduce the incidence of pressure necrosis to skin and surrounding soft tissues. Strict monitoring of the patient can detect early risk of airway compromise in patients with emesis.

High-flow nasal cannulae are new devices with very high-flow rates of humidified oxygen. They deliver high-flow rate of up to 60 L/min without the use of any interface directly through special nasal cannulas. The additional advantages are better compliance, no claustrophobia, and low-level positive end-expiratory pressure (PEEP) and these lead to reduced failure rates and improved parameters. Oral feeding, verbal communication with patients, and no postural discomfort during sleep add to better patient compliance.

INDICATIONS FOR NONINVASIVE VENTILATION

Chronic Obstructive Pulmonary Disease

Chronic obstructive pulmonary disease (COPD) exacerbations most commonly present with hypercapnic respiratory failure usually as acute or acute-on-chronic respiratory acidosis. Reduced oxygenation due to any exacerbating cause or precipitating event leads to hypoxemia along with hypercarbia. These catastrophic changes are primarily due to reduced alveolar ventilation, intra-alveolar gaseous exchange defect, and reduced vital capacity due to respiratory muscle fatigue. Reduced central respiratory drive due to CO_2 narcosis further leads to hypoventilation and increased shallow respiratory rate along with loss of tidal volume. Thus for the correction of both hypercapnia and hypoxemia, ventilatory support is necessary. NIV plays a major role in reversing the above pathophysiological process in a conscious patient. Drowsy or unconscious patients need to be ventilated invasively till the time the precipitating event is controlled.

Cardiogenic Pulmonary Edema

Cardiogenic pulmonary edema leads to hypoxemic respiratory failure in patients with left ventricular failure. Pathophysiologically, the pulmonary edema leads to reduced alveolar compliance. NIV along with pharmacological management improves respiratory mechanics, reduces respiratory muscle distress thus in turn improving work of breathing, and improving compliance. All these in turn cause reduction in left ventricular afterload thus facilitating recovery.

Pneumonia

Acute pneumonias usually, when severe, lead to acute hypoxemic respiratory failure even if there is no evidence of previous lung compromise or evidence of any underlying chronic disease.

The aim is to reduce the work of breathing, improving oxygenation, and avoid intubation till the recovery of underlying pneumonia occurs. The pressures required to treat acute respiratory failure in pneumonias is very high which is disadvantageous as it leads to increased air leaks from the mask, reduced compliance, insufficient recruitment, gastric inflation, and relapse to hypoxemia on intermittent NIV support. In patients intolerant to NIV, alternative HFNC have shown equally good results. It also has advantages of reducing the dead space during ventilation.

Asthma

Asthma being a reversible of bronchoconstricting disease and pathophysiologically it leads to both hypoxemic and hypercapnic failure by various mechanisms. CPAP substantially decreases the pressure-time product of the respiratory muscles which is an index of energy utilization.

Chest Trauma

There is a growing body of evidence that NIV may alleviate acute respiratory failure secondary to blunt chest injuries. NIV improves oxygenation and reduces the incidence of invasive ventilation.

Other Conditions

Noninvasive ventilation has been documented to improve acute respiratory failure in the following conditions with direct impact on mortality of patients.

- Cystic fibrosis/bronchiectasis
- Neuromuscular disease
- Decompensated obstructive sleep apnea
- Postsurgery

CONTRAINDICATIONS

Absolute

- Unconscious patients
- Confusion or agitation
- Poor respiratory drive
- Patients requiring sedation
- Fixed upper airway obstruction

Relative

- Recent facial or upper airway surgery, facial burns, or trauma
- Vomiting
- Inability to protect the airway
- Copious respiratory secretions
- Life-threatening hypoxemia
- Pneumothorax (intercostal drain insertion prior to NIV should be done)

Urgent intubation and ventilation facilities should be available in case there is failure in improvement to NIV. Early detection by trained staff and ABG will improve the detection of failure of NIV.

MONITORING

Clinical Evaluation

- Patient compliance, comfort, and coordination
- Conscious status
- Respiratory movements and chest wall paradox
- Accessory muscle activity and excursions
- Respiratory and heart rate

Laboratory Parameters

- Arterial blood gas analysis should be done as early as two hours after initiation of NIV. The patient should be monitored for clinical improvement and ABG should be performed. In case there is improvement, a decision to intubate should be deferred. If ABG deteriorates the patient should be intubated and ventilated.
- Oxygen saturation (target saturations between 85 and 90%)

Once the patient improves, optimizing of settings can be planned and weaning procedure started as per clinical guidelines. Regular intermittent breaks from NIV for verbal communication (medical staff and relatives), oral meals, fluids, and physiotherapy under supervised care, help in better compliance of patient, and confidence building in therapy.

Treatment Failure

Noninvasive ventilation failure is associated with higher rates of intubation and prolonged hospital stay.

High severity score, elderly, acute respiratory distress syndrome (ARDS) or pneumonia with copious secretions, failure of clinical condition or respiratory distress, and persistently impaired ABG are suggestive of NIV failure.

Plant et al. found that pH of below 7.30 had higher failure rates of NIV and they require invasive ventilatory support.

Limitation's of Noninvasive Ventilation

Apprehension of patient, leakage from circuit, ill-fitting masks, unconscious, or uncooperative patient are limiting the use of NIV. Absence of intensive care unit to provide back in case of failure of NIV is another limiting factor in few centers. Inadequate training of healthcare workers is another reason for poor initiation, maintenance of NIV, and subsequent failures in therapy for acute respiratory failure. Better resource utilization especially of trained respiratory care paramedics can go a long way in better outcome of NIV therapy.

SUGGESTED READINGS

1. Frat JP, Ragot S, Coudroy R, Constantin JM, Girault C, Prat G, et al. Predictors of Intubation in Patients With Acute Hypoxemic Respiratory Failure Treated With a Noninvasive Oxygenation Strategy. Crit Care Med. 2018;46(2):208-215.
2. Messika J, Ben Ahmed K, Gaudry S, Miguel-Montanes R, Rafat C, Sztrymf B, et al. Use of High-Flow Nasal Cannula Oxygen Therapy in Subjects With ARDS: A 1-Year Observational Study. Respir Care. 2015;60(2):162-9.
3. Plant PK, Owen JL, Elliott MW. Early use of non-invasive ventilation for acute exacerbations of chronic obstructive pulmonary disease on general respiratory wards: a multicentre randomised controlled trial. Lancet. 2000;355(9219):1931-5.

227

CHAPTER

Obstructive Sleep Apnea

BK Sundar

ABSTRACT

Obstructive sleep apnea (OSA) is a condition characterized by apnea, hypopnea, and respiratory arousals due to the collapse of the upper airway during sleep. This results in fragmented, nonrestorative sleep, with symptoms including loud snoring, witnessed apnea, and excessive daytime somnolence. OSA is associated with excessive daytime sleepiness and is often referred to as OSA-hypopnea syndrome.

INTRODUCTION

Obstructive sleep apnea (OSA) is an illness that is characterized by apnea, hypopnea, and/or respiratory-related arousals caused by repetitive collapse of the upper airway during sleep, associated with a decrease in oxygen saturation. This results in fragmented, nonrestorative sleep. Loud and disruptive snoring, witnessed apnea during sleep, and excessive daytime somnolence are some of the symptoms associated with OSA. Sleep is a normal body process that allows your body and brain to rest. As quite simple as it seems, sleep is one of the most complex and mysterious body processes. Without enough quality sleep, our body and brain cannot work as it should. OSA that is associated with excessive daytime sleepiness is commonly called obstructive sleep apnea syndrome and obstructive sleep apnea-hypopnea syndrome.

Figure 1 illustrates sleep-related breathing disorder continuum ranging from simple snoring to OSA. Upper airway resistance syndrome (UARS) is sandwiched between snorers and OSA.

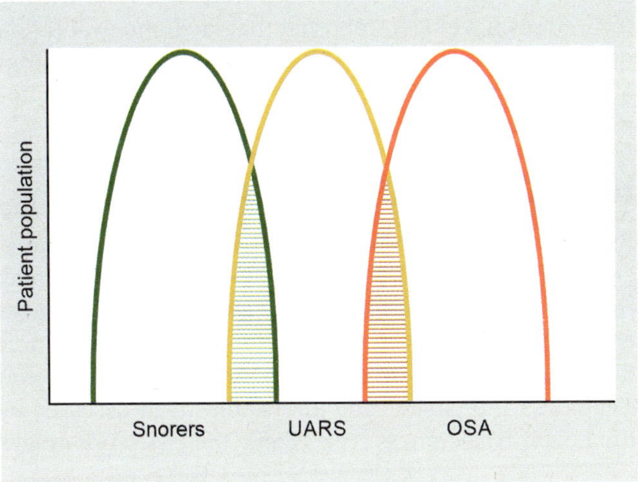

FIG. 1: Breathing disorder continuum ranging from simple snoring to OSA.
(OSA: obstructive sleep apnea; UARS: upper airway resistance syndrome)

Obstructive sleep apnea is an important condition to recognize by physicians as it has a strong association with medical conditions, which include hypertension, cardiovascular disease, coronary artery disease, insulin-resistant diabetes, depression, and sleep-related accidents. It is helpful if spouses can inform about the sleep habits as usually, these patients regard themselves as 'good sleepers' as they can sleep anywhere and anytime (e.g., in office, physician's waiting room, traffic, while reading paper, etc.).

EPIDEMIOLOGY

Obstructive sleep apnea affects almost 1 billion people globally, with 425 million adults aged 30–69 years having moderate to severe OSA. With increasing age, prevalence also increases, and above 50 years of age, there are as many women as men who develop the disorder. An increase in obesity contributes to increasing prevalence of OSA. A combination of obesity, dyslipidemia, insulin resistance, and hypertension is seen in people with OSA.

PATHOPHYSIOLOGY

Negative collapsing pressure during inspiration leads to upper airway obstruction during sleep. Anatomical and neuromuscular factors contributing to airway obstruction are evidenced by airway narrowing during sleep and its relation to body mass index (BMI). Recently, the relevance of physiological, nonanatomical factors has been investigated and several additional factors have been identified, such as:

- Inadequate responsiveness of the genioglossus dilating muscle
- Decreased arousal threshold
- Instability of the respiratory control system

These factors have clinical relevance as they may be amenable to specific treatment approaches. Several novel techniques have been reported that facilitate evaluation of these nonanatomical factors. Whether these findings are reproducible over time and between research groups is yet unknown.

HISTORY AND PHYSICAL FINDINGS

Excessive daytime somnolence is one of the most common symptoms, albeit a majority of patients may remain asymptomatic. **Table 1** gives the list of most common symptoms of OSA. Many patients only report daytime fatigue. There should be a distinction between sleepiness and fatigue, and this is objectively assessed by the Epworth sleepiness scale (ESS). The ESS score ranges from 0 and 24, and a score >9 indicates the presence of excessive daytime sleepiness and requires additional assessment. A fatigue severity scale (FSS) can also be used to assess fatigue severity symptoms. Using both ESS and FSS is helpful as both can be present concomitantly. Other symptoms are morning headache and self-reported insomnia to nocturia. Sleep-onset insomnia and sleep-maintenance insomnia were reported by women.

TABLE 1: Common symptoms associated with obstructive sleep apnea (OSA).

Nocturnal	Diurnal
Snoring	Excessive sleepiness
Witnessed apnea	Morning headaches
Choking at night	Depression/Irritability
Nocturia	Memory loss
Decreased libido	

STOP-BANG questionnaire is a widely accepted screening tool for OSA.

- *S*noring: Do you snore loudly?
- *T*ired: Do you often feel tired, fatigued, or sleepy during the daytime?
- *O*bserved: Has your bed partner observed you stop breathing during your sleep?
- Blood *P*ressure: Are you having/being treated for high blood pressure?
- *B*MI: >35 kg/m^2
- *A*ge: >50 years
- *N*eck circumference: Men > 43 cm, women > 37 cm
- *G*ender: Male

High risk, if 'yes' to >3 items and low risk, if 'yes' to <3 items.

Other physical findings are crowded oropharynx (Mallampati score 3–4), retrognathia, micrognathia, tonsillar hypertrophy (kissing tonsils), low-lying palate/high-arched palate, large tongue, congestive heart failure, pulmonary hypertension, and stroke.

EVALUATION

Any unexplained daytime sleep-related symptoms such as excessive sleepiness, fatigue or not getting up fresh from sleep (nonrestorative sleep) in an adult should be evaluated for OSA. Important symptoms of sleep apnea include '*3S*'—*s*noring, *s*leepiness, and *s*ignificant-other's report of sleep apnea episodes. Regardless of symptoms, patients with comorbidities such as refractory atrial fibrillation, resistant hypertension, and a history of stroke can be screened for sleep apnea.

Nighttime in-laboratory level I polysomnography (PSG) is the gold standard test for the diagnosis of OSA. The test procedure includes monitoring with electroencephalogram (EEG) leads, pulse oximetry, temperature, and pressure sensors to detect nasal and oral airflow; respiratory impedance plethysmography belts around the chest and abdomen to detect motion; an electrocardiogram (ECG) lead; and an electromyogram (EMG) sensor to detect muscle contraction in the chin, chest, and legs.

TABLE 2: Obstructive sleep apnea (OSA) severity based on the apnea-hypopnea index (AHI).

AHI	OSA severity
<5	Normal or primary snoring
5–20	Mild
20–40	Moderate
> 40	Severe

American Academy of Sleep Medicine defines hypopnea based on one of the two criteria:

1. At least 30% airflow reduction for >10 seconds associated with at least 4% oxygen desaturation (medicare criteria)
2. Airflow reduction of at least 30% for >10 seconds associated with at least 3% oxygen desaturation or an EEG showing arousal from sleep

Two criteria for apnea are:

1. Peak signal excursion drop by >90% of baseline, pre-event flow
2. More than 10 seconds duration of drop-in flow

Table 2 shows a list of OSA severity based on the apnea-hypopnea index (AHI).

Routine blood tests are not helpful in diagnosis of OSA. However, thyroid function test, blood sugar, and hemoglobin are done. Pulmonary function testing is not indicated either to make a diagnosis of, or treatment plan for OSA.

Polygraphy, more suitable for ambulatory studies over PSG, lacks the recording of neurophysiological signals. As such, it is not a sleep study as sleep stages and EEG arousals are not documented. Assessment of AHI can be imprecise.

One sleep test is a home sleep testing device that uses NightOwl sensor backed by a NightOwl app and is a simple, safe, and almost accurate way to diagnose your sleep quality. It measures heart rate, oxygen saturation, and movement. NightOwl sensor is strapped to your finger and once you activate it, you can measure your quality and duration of sleep for three consecutive nights. Based on the findings, physicians decide on further analysis.

TREATMENT/MANAGEMENT

A multipronged approach should be individualized for each patient in treating OSA. Treating moderate to severe OSA improves clinical outcomes. Available evidence is lacking or inconsistent on the impact of treating mild OSA on mood, vehicle accidents, neurocognition, cardiovascular events, stroke, and arrhythmias.

Lifestyle modification and treatment of underlying medical conditions are important. Overweight and obese patients should be encouraged to lose weight to decrease the severity of OSA, although it may not be curative. At least 7–8 hours of sleep is recommended. Patients should be counseled to avoid alcohol, smoking, benzodiazepines, opiates, and antidepressants. Optimizing treatment of heart failure and asthma, if any, is recommended. Concomitant nasal obstruction is treated with nasal steroid spray for allergic rhinitis or surgery for nasal valve collapse.

Obstructive sleep apnea is more pronounced in a supine position and can be treated by positioning device to keep patients on their sides.

Pharmacotherapy, which is generally not a preferred primary treatment option, can be considered as an adjunctive for excessive daytime somnolence. Drugs used are central nervous system stimulants (such as modafinil and armodafinil), and dopamine/norepinephrine reuptake inhibitors, such as solriamfetol.

Mechanical measures in the treatment include nasal continuous positive airway pressure (CPAP), bilevel positive airway pressure (BiPAP), and oral appliance therapy. CPAP is considered as gold standard for the treatment of OSA, although it is a challenge to initiate it and convince patients to adhere to the treatment. It was first described by Sullivan et al. in 1981. Flow generator delivers air via a tube, and an oral mask or nasal mask is used to produce a fixed positive pressure in the upper airway. This positive airway pressure (PAP) splints the upper airway, thereby preventing closure and repeated collapse, oxygen saturation is stabilized and sleep fragmentation is reduced. Both fixed CPAP and auto PAP devices are available. No particular clinical advantage is conferred by auto-PAP over fixed CPAP for long-term treatment. A systematic meta-analysis of 36 randomized controlled trials (RCTs) showed effectiveness of CPAP in reducing AHI, sleepiness symptoms, and also improving quality of life in people with moderate to severe OSA. Long-term compliance with CPAP is poor, and in one study only 68% patients were using it at the end of 5 years. Few studies have shown 50% patients discontinue use of CPAP within first year, most of them within 1 month. Acceptable compliance is if one has used CPAP for at least 4 hours and on 70% nights **(Fig. 2)**.

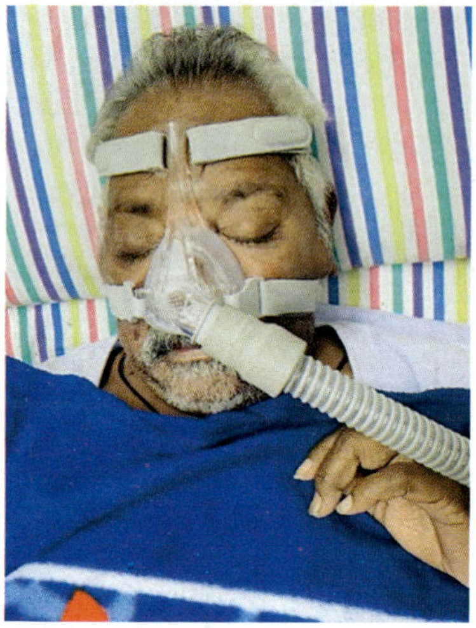

FIG. 2: Nasal continuous positive airway pressure (CPAP) use.

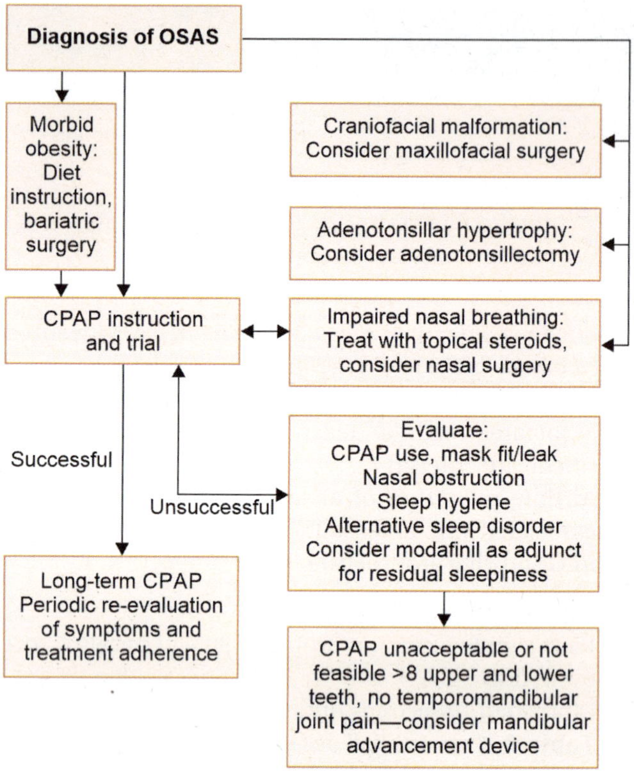

FLOWCHART 1: Treatment options for OSA.

(OSA: obstructive sleep apnea; OSAS: obstructive sleep apnea syndrome; CPAP: continuous positive airway pressure)

Source: Reproduced from Bloch KE et al. 2006.

CONCLUSION

Adult OSA is a chronic condition, with increasing prevalence associated with increasing obesity and aging. Various other physiological and anatomical factors also play a role in the pathogenesis of OSA, like craniofacial features, respiratory control system stability (loop gain), arousal threshold, and upper airway dilator muscle activity. Laboratory-based PSG is the gold standard for the diagnosis; however, home-based testing is also useful, coupled with specialist follow-up. Various home-based sleep studies are under trial (like NightOwl). CPAP is the first-line treatment for severe OSA and moderate OSA with symptoms. Second-line management options include surgical intervention and oral appliances. Involving patients and their relatives and taking note of comorbidities make approach to treatment more holistic. **Flowchart 1** outlines OSA treatment options.

SUGGESTED READINGS

1. Randerath W, Bassetti CL, Bonsignore MR, Farre R, Ferini-Strambi L, Grote L, et al. Challenges and perspectives in obstructive sleep apnoea: Report by an ad hoc working group of the Sleep Disordered Breathing Group of the European Respiratory Society and the European Sleep Research Society. Eur Respir J. 2018;52(3):1702616.
2. Smith IE, Quinnell TG. Obstructive Sleep Apnea: relevance to non-sleep clinicians. Clin Med. 2011;11(3):286-9.
3. Usmani ZA, Chai-Coetzer CL, Antic NA, McEvoy RD. Obstructive Sleep apnoea in adults. Postgrad Med J. 2013;89(1049):148-56.
4. Himanshu Wickramasinghe W, Rowley JA. (2020). Obstructive Sleep Apnea (OSA) Treatment and Management. Medscape. [online] Available from https://emedicine.medscape.com/article/295807-treatment [Last accessed January, 2024].
5. Slowik JM, Sankari A, Collen JF. Obstructive sleep apnea. In: StatPearls [Internet]. Treasure Island (FL): StatPearls Publishing; 2023. [online] Available from https://www.ncbi.nlm.nih.gov/books/NBK459252/ [Last accessed January, 2024].
6. Spicuzza Lucia, Caruso D, Maria GD. Obstructive sleep apnoea syndrome and its management. Ther Adv Chronic Dis. 2015;6(5):27385.
7. Bloch KE. Alternatives to CPAP in the treatment of the obstructive sleep apnea syndrome. Swiss Med Wkly. 2006;136(17-18):261-7.

228

CHAPTER

Extrapulmonary Tuberculosis: Standard Treatment Guidelines

Shailendra Kumar

ABSTRACT

Pulmonary tuberculosis (PTB) remains a global problem despite well-documented and widely disseminated methods of prevention and treatment. Human immunodeficiency virus (HIV) infection and poverty are significant factors in its persistence. Extrapulmonary tuberculosis (EPTB) can affect the tongue, brain, cervical lymph nodes, spinal column, skeletal structures, muscular tissues, integumentary system, eye, pleural cavity, oral cavity, pericardium, peritoneum, genitourinary tract, and gastrointestinal tract. This chapter explicates recent developments in the clinical diagnosis, treatment modalities, and drug resistance patterns of pulmonary and EPTB.

INTRODUCTION

Extrapulmonary tuberculosis (EPTB) cases constituted approximately 16% of the total 7.5 million incident cases reported globally in the year 2019. The diagnosis and management of EPTB pose significant challenges. The majority of cases exhibit constitutive symptoms, including malaise, night sweats, fever, and weight loss, accompanied by organ-specific systemic symptoms. Typically, individuals presenting with symptoms undergo radiologic imaging of the affected organs to assess and strategize a more precise and targeted diagnostic examination. Typically, the extrapulmonary specimen acquired through the process of fine-needle aspiration or biopsy is utilized for the purposes of microscopy, histopathology, culture, biochemical/immunological, and molecular testing. These diagnostic procedures, including drug susceptibility testing, are essential in initiating an efficacious therapeutic intervention.

Pulmonary tuberculosis (PTB) is the most prevalent manifestation; however, EPTB is also a significant clinical concern. Tuberculosis (TB) is a global public health priority, with 10.4 million individuals acquiring the disease in 2016 (10% of whom were coinfected with HIV), resulting in 1.67 million fatalities and six lack cases of multidrug-resistant (MDR) TB. Among HIV-positive patients, EPTB accounts for over 50% of all TB cases. In previous times, prior to the HIV pandemic, and in studies involving individuals with a competent immune system, it has been observed that EPTB constituted approximately 15–20% of all TB cases.

The presentation of tuberculous meningitis (TBM) is characterized by the emergence of neurological sequelae, including cephalalgia, pyrexia of mild intensity, general discomfort, emesis, and cognitive impairment. Untreated TBM may give rise to a constellation of neurological manifestations, including but not limited to coma, seizures, and stupor. The observed clinical manifestations are indicative of the following stages—stage I (characterized by complete consciousness and absence of focal deficits); stage II (marked by consciousness accompanied by fatigue, confusion, and moderate focal neurological manifestations, such as cerebral nerve paralysis or hemiparesis); and stage III (characterized by drowsiness seizures, cerebral palsies, or hemiplegia).

The emergence and proliferation of MDR strains of *Mycobacterium tuberculosis* (MTB), characterized by resistance to isoniazid (INH) and rifampicin (RIF), pose a grave threat to the management and control of TBM. At present, there exists no established or validated treatment protocol, with the exception of the regimen endorsed by the World Health Organization (WHO) for PTB. According to available literature, the utilization of fluoroquinolones, specifically levofloxacin and moxifloxacin, has been proposed as an adjunct to the conventional treatment regimen for MDR-TBM. This recommendation stems from the favorable characteristics exhibited by these medications, including their notable cerebrospinal fluid (CSF) penetration capabilities and efficacy against MDR strains.

The initial indicators for the diagnosis of ocular toxoplasmosis [ocular tuberculosis (OTB)] involve conducting an ophthalmic examination along with a blood test to assess the inflammation markers and white blood cell (WBC) counts. The diagnosis of TB poses a significant challenge due to the absence of accompanying classical symptoms typically observed in patients. Given the rarity of OTB, there is currently no specific molecular diagnostic test recommended for OTB diagnosis. Diagnostic dilemmas in EPTB, bacteriological and molecular diagnosis is not possible in every case because many lesions are paucibacillary. Numerous imaging modalities, such as fundus autofluorescence imaging, fluorescein and indocyanine angiography, fundus fluorescein angiography, optical coherence tomography, microperimetry, and ultrasonography, are now commonly used to assess the severity of ocular impairment and the efficacy of therapeutic interventions.

EXTRAPULMONARY TUBERCULOSIS RISK FACTORS

Tuberculosis exhibits a strong correlation with both overcrowding and malnutrition, rendering it a prominent affliction associated with impoverished conditions. TB can affect any part of the body except hair and nail. Individuals at an elevated risk encompass those who engage in the injection of illicit substances, individuals residing or working in environments where vulnerable populations congregate (such as correctional facilities and homeless shelters), communities lacking adequate medical resources and privileges, ethnic minorities with a heightened susceptibility to adverse outcomes, children who have close proximity to individuals classified as high-risk, and healthcare professionals who provide care to these aforementioned patients.

DIAGNOSIS

- *EPTB*: The choice of diagnostic tests should be guided by the selection of specimen and availability of suitable facilities. Priority is given to the use of cartridge-based nucleic acid amplification test (CB-NAAT) over alternative diagnostic tests. In the evaluation of EPTB, chest radiography, ultrasonography, computed tomography (CT), and magnetic resonance imaging (MRI) are additional diagnostic modalities that may be utilized.
- *Pleural TB*: Imaging can aid in the diagnosis and quantification of an effusion, as well as the differentiation of its cause. All patients with a suspected pleural effusion should have a chest radiograph taken. Other tuberculous manifestations, such as pulmonary consolidation, can aid in the diagnosis. Radiographs are also useful for monitoring the treatment response and are recommended 2 months after therapy initiation and 6 months after therapy initiation. A bedside ultrasonographic examination is beneficial for diagnosing pleural effusion **(Table 1)**.
- *Lymph node TB*: Tuberculous lymphadenitis must be distinguished from lymphadenopathy resulting from specific causes. Differential diagnosis should be considered when diagnosing lymph node TB, particularly when multiple lymph nodes from the same region are affected. The diagnostic modalities for lymph node TB can be categorized as (1) primary diagnostic studies and (2) supplementary diagnostic studies. Primary diagnostic tests consist of fine needle aspiration cytology (FNAC), lymph node biopsy,

TABLE 1: Treatment for extrapulmonary tuberculosis.

For cases that have been treated previously	For cases that have been reported as new
The inpatient (IP) duration will be 12 weeks. Injection streptomycin will be discontinued after 8 weeks, and the remaining four drugs will be administered daily according to the weight band for an additional 4 weeks	The treatment regimen implemented during inpatient care will entail an 8-week course of isoniazid (INH), rifampicin, pyrazinamide, and ethambutol. These medications will be administered on a daily basis, with the dosage adjusted according to the patient's weight, categorized into four distinct bands
There is no requirement for extending the inpatient duration	There will be no indication of the extension of the intravenous infusion pump
Pyrazinamide will be discontinued at the initiation of the treatment for CP, while the remaining medications will be maintained at their current dosages for an additional duration of 20 weeks, administered on a daily basis	Pyrazinamide will be discontinued in the context of continuation phase (CP) treatment, while the remaining three medications will be maintained at their current daily dosages for an additional 16-week period

culture, and molecular assays. The tuberculin skin test and interferon-gamma release assays (IGRAs) are, however, supplementary diagnostic tests.

- *Abdominal TBP*: Serum markers/IGRAs have emerged as a crucial diagnostic instrument for TB of the abdomen. Imaging modalities such as abdominal ultrasound (USG) and CT can assist in the evaluation of peritoneal or omental thickening, ascites, mesenteric alterations, and thickening of the bowel wall. Adenosine deaminase (ADA) and laparoscopy in peritoneal fluid provide a practical, sensitive, and highly specific test for abdominal TB.
- *Genitourinary TB*: Urine routine microscopy and culture, urine NAAT, urine culture for MTB, and Ziehl-Neelsen Staining are preferred tests for genitourinary TB. Ultrasonography of the urinary tract, kidneys, ureters, and bladder, intravenous urography, contrast-enhanced CT (CECT) with CT urography, and cystourethroscopy with or without biopsy are also recommended.

EXTRAPULMONARY TUBERCULOSIS TREATMENT PROCEDURE

The treatment approach for TB has undergone a shift toward a daily regimen, wherein patients are prescribed a fixed dose combination of first-line anti-TB drugs on a daily basis, in accordance with their appropriate weight bands.

EXTRAPULMONARY TUBERCULOSIS MANAGEMENT

The duration of the continuation phase may be prolonged for a period of 3–6 months in specific cases of TB, including those involving the central nervous system, skeletal system, disseminated TB, and other similar presentations. This decision is made by the attending physicians based on clinical judgement and evaluation. Extension beyond a duration of 3 months shall only be granted upon the recommendation of experts specializing in the relevant field.

Timely and precise identification of a medical condition, along with the conduction of drug susceptibility testing, is imperative in order to promptly commence the appropriate therapeutic course of action. **Flowchart 1** provides a concise overview of frequently employed diagnostic tests for diverse EPTB conditions.

In general, a comparatively modest percentage 5–15% of individuals who contract MTB will manifest TB pathology over the course of their lifespan. The likelihood of developing TB disease is significantly elevated in individuals who are infected with the HIV. Additionally, the probability of TB disease is heightened in individuals

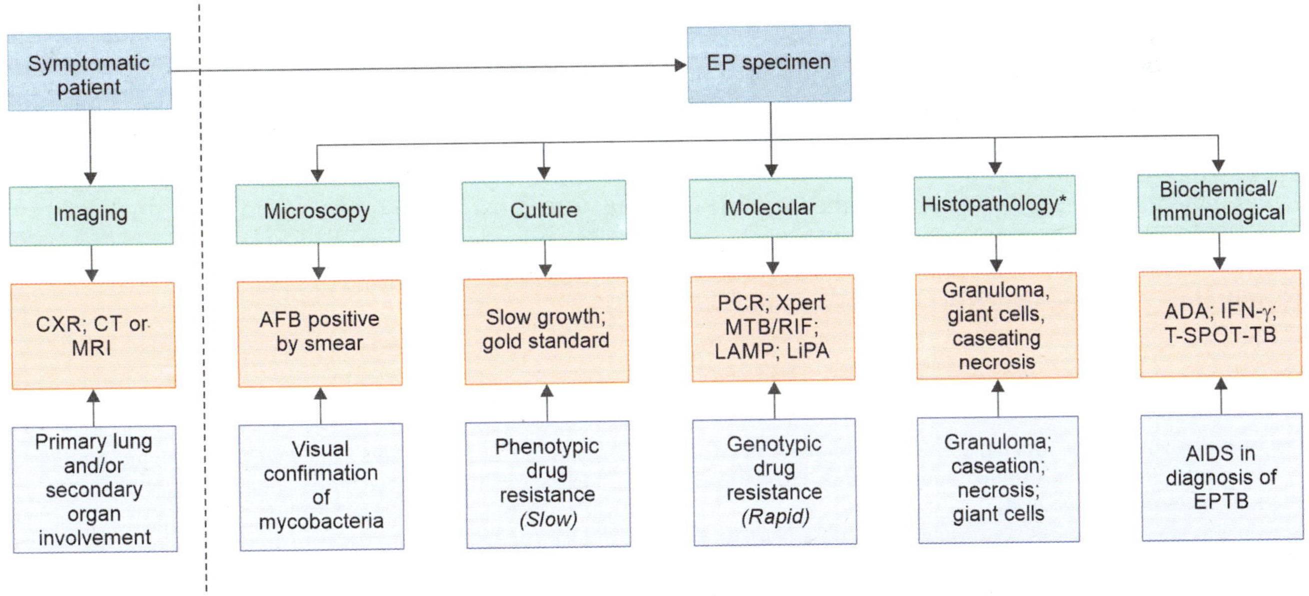

* Modified from Extrapulmonary Tuberculosis, Evangel Publications, Indian College of Physician, Page 3.

FLOWCHART 1: *Mycobacterium tuberculosis* complex EPTB diagnostic panel.

(ADA: adenosine deaminase; CT: computed tomography; CXR: chest X-ray; EPTB: extrapulmonary tuberculosis; IFN-γ: Interferon gamma; LAMP: loop-mediated isothermal amplification; LiPA: line probe assay; MRI: Magnetic resonance imaging; MTB: mycobacterium tuberculosis; PCR: polymerase chain reaction; RIF: rifampin) who are affected by various risk factors, including undernutrition, smoking, type 2 diabetes mellitus, and alcohol consumption.

Close monitoring of patients is imperative to assess treatment progress and evaluate the response of the disease. Follow-up consists of two essential components:

1. Clinical follow-up, which involves the assessment and monitoring of the patient's condition.
2. Laboratory follow-up, which entails the analysis and evaluation of laboratory test results.

The recommended frequency for clinical follow-up is a minimum of once per month. The patient may seek consultations at the clinical facility for periodic assessments, or alternatively, the medical officer may perform the assessment during home visits. Enhancement of thoracic condition, manifestation of augmented body mass, among other indications, may suggest a favorable prognosis. The management of concurrent medical conditions such as HIV and diabetes through appropriate therapeutic interventions is imperative in order to optimize the prognosis of TB treatment. It is imperative to inquire about the precise manifestation and indication of untoward responses to pharmacological agents.

Laboratory investigations may encompass a range of diagnostic procedures aimed at evaluating the prognostic implications of the disease or addressing concurrent medical conditions and potential adverse reactions. In the event of PTB, it is recommended to perform sputum smear microscopy at the conclusion of the intensive phase (IP) as well as at the conclusion of the treatment regimen. A negative sputum smear microscopy outcome observed upon completion of the IP may be indicative of a favorable prognosis.

Long-term follow-up following the conclusion of therapeutic intervention, it is imperative to conduct regular patient follow-up assessments at the intervals of 6, 12, 18, and 24 months. In the presence of any clinical symptoms and/or cough, it is recommended to consider the utilization of sputum microscopy and/or culture for diagnostic purposes. Early detection of TB recurrence is of paramount significance in clinical practice.

The utilization of chest radiography serves as a valuable modality for evaluating the advancement of drug-sensitive PTB in patients, to be administered as deemed necessary and accessible. Clinical assessment is considered the most optimal method for evaluating the efficacy of treatment in cases of EPTB. Assistance from radiological and other pertinent investigations may be sought.

Nevertheless, when faced with clinical deterioration, the attending physician may opt to perform a repeat analysis of sputum smear microscopy, even in the midst of continuous positive airway pressure (CPAP) treatment. This will afford the patient an early opportunity to undergo drug susceptibility testing in the event that they are determined to be sputum smear positive. Upon the conclusion of the therapeutic intervention, it is imperative to conduct a comprehensive evaluation of each patient by means of a sputum smear and/or culture. The significance of this matter lies in the fact that culture, in comparison to smear microscopy, is a more delicate and precise diagnostic method for identifying the presence of MTB in biological samples.

CONCLUSION

The “End Tuberculosis Strategy”, as formulated by the WHO, endeavors to achieve a 95% reduction in TB mortality and a 90% decrease in new TB cases by the year 2035. The attainment of this objective necessitates the implementation of enhanced diagnostic techniques, therapeutic interventions, and more efficacious immunizations in the battle against TB. In order to effectively manage these conditions on a global scale, it is of the uttermost importance to address the effects of EPTB and its escalating drug resistance on the global health landscape and economy, in conjunction with PTB.

SUGGESTED READINGS

1. WHO. (2020). Global Tuberculosis Report. [online] Available from https://www.who.int/publications/i/item/9789240013131 [Last accessed January, 2024].
2. Golden MP, Vikram HR. Extrapulmonary tuberculosis: An overview. Am Fam Phys. 2005;72:1761-8.
3. Ministry of Health and Family welfare. Training Module on Extrapulmonary Tuberculosis. India: Ministry of Health and Family welfare, Govt. of India; 2023.

229

CHAPTER

Pleural Tuberculosis: Diagnosis and Management

SM Mishra

ABSTRACT

Tuberculosis is very important disease, which involves pulmonary and extrapulmonary systems. Pleura is the second most common extrapulmonary site involved, leading to pleural effusion. Etiological diagnosis of pleural tuberculosis is essential for proper management, since apart from tuberculosis there are other important causes also. Chest X-ray, ultrasonography (USG), computed tomography (CT) of chest, pleurocentesis and biochemical examination, cytology, and microbiological investigations generally provide sufficient clue for confirmation of diagnosis. Pleura biopsy, histological examination or culture for *Mycobacterium tuberculosis* sometimes required. Standard treatment regimen for tuberculosis, along with clinical and radiological monitoring is required.

INTRODUCTION

Tuberculosis (TB) is an important infectious disease worldwide, as far as morbidity and mortality is concerned. TB is considered to be a disease of respiratory system as it affects lungs in >80% of cases. But in about 20–30% cases, it involves extrapulmonary sites also, either with or without concomitant involvement of lungs. Pleura is the second most common extrapulmonary site involved (first being the peripheral lymph nodes).

Pleural involvement leads to pleural effusion. Untreated pleural effusion usually resolves spontaneously but it can manifest again. As per different studies in about 65% of untreated patients with pleural effusion, pulmonary TB develops in the next 5 years. There are a number of causes of pleural effusion, other than TB, so as soon as pleural effusion is suspected confirmation of cause of pleural effusion diagnosis is necessary.

CAUSES OF PLEURAL EFFUSION (TABLE 1)

TABLE 1: Common and uncommon causes of pleural effusion.

Common causes	Uncommon causes
• Tuberculosis • Parapneumonic effusion • Malignancy • Pulmonary infarction • Cardiac failure • Subdiagphragmatic disorders (subphrenic abscess, pancreatitis)	• Hypoproteinemia (nephrotic syndrome, liver failure, and malnutrition) • Connective tissue diseases (SLE, rheumatoid arthritis) • Uremia • Meigs syndrome

(SLE: systemic lupus erythematosus)

CLINICAL FEATURES

Cough is the most common presenting complaint in about 94% of cases. Other common symptoms are chest pain (78%), fever (66%), shortness of breath, other constitutional symptom such as night sweats, and weight loss are also seen.

DIAGNOSIS OF PLEURAL EFFUSION

Careful history and clinical examination is the first step in the diagnosis. The systemic examination of chest is inspection, palpation, percussion, and auscultation gives clue about the presence of free fluid in the pleural cavity, whether it is unilateral or bilateral.

INVESTIGATIONS

After clinical confirmation of pleural effusion, for etiological diagnosis following investigations may be undertaken.

Imaging

Investigations generally give clue of the cause of effusion and amount of pleural effusion. In pleural effusion due to TB, generally only one hemithorax (90–95%) is involved and occupies one-third to two-thirds of the hemithorax.

Chest X-ray

This is generally the first investigation and is very useful. X-ray chest posteroanterior (PA) view may help in the quantification of fluid and parenchymal involvement (cavitations, infiltrations, fibrosis, consolidation, etc.). Sometimes, lateral decubitus view is required to detect small effusion. A chest X-ray must be done in all patients with suspected pleural effusion. PA view of chest X-ray requires about 200 mL of fluid for the effusion to be detectable. Chest X-ray is commonly available in most of the health centers and is economical also. This is helpful in monitoring the treatment response and advised 8 weeks (2 months) after the commencement of therapy and at 6 months of therapy.

Ultrasonography

Ultrasonography of chest is more sensitive than X-ray and help in detection of minimal effusion (as little as 50 mL of fluid can be detected), it can be done bedside also. It helps in detection of pleural thickening and loculations, and in guiding interventions.

Computed Tomography Scan

This is a better tool to detect parenchymal involvement, loculations, and pleural thickening. Although not necessary in all cases, but sometimes required in excluding malignancy or causes of recurrent pleural effusion.

Comparison of Different Methods of Imaging (Table 2)

Role of CT Scan in the Diagnosis of Pleural Tuberculosis (Table 3)

TABLE 2: Imaging method comparison.

Findings	Use	Advantage	Disadvantage	Sensitivity	Specificity
• Chest radiograph • Costophrenic angle blunting, with homogenous opacity in lung field	All patients	• Detected when there is >200 mL fluid in posteroanterior (PA) film • Pulmonary involvement can be seen and progress can be monitored	• Small amount of fluid may be missed • Radiation exposure	• *Supine anteroposterior (AP)*: 33–92% • *PA lateral decubitus*: 94% • *Upright*: 82% • *Upright lateral*: 86%	• 70–89% • 100% • 81% • 88%
• Ultrasound • Anechoic region (black) • Below pleural line (white)	Selected patients	• Bedside investigation • Detects as little as 50 mL of pleural fluid • Septations visualized • No radiation	Lung involvement cannot be ruled out in all cases	92–94%	93–100%

TABLE 3: Diagnosis of pleural tuberculosis by computed tomography (CT) scan.

Findings	Use	Advantage	Disadvantage
Hypodense effusion with pleural enhancement with/without pleural thickening	Selected patients—when diagnosis not clear, suspected malignancy, HIV-positive patients	Reference standard in most studies sensitive than X-ray to check for primary lung involvement	• Difficult to distinguish small effusion and pleural thickening • Low sensitivity for septations • High radiation exposure • High cost

Pleurocentesis

This is very important investigation for the diagnosis and confirmation of etiology of pleural effusion. About 50 mL of fluid is required for essential tests recommended for diagnosis of cause of pleural effusion. If clinically indicated to reduce respiratory problem more, fluid must be aspirated.

During procedure, clinical condition of patient must be observed to avoid complications of thoracocentesis.

Postprocedure chest X-ray must be done to detect any complications such as pneumothorax or hydropneumothorax.

Collected pleural fluid is transferred to sterile container before transportation to laboratory. The maximum accepted time delay for pleural fluid sample is 2 hours, but it can be stored for up to 48 hours at 4°C for most tests, except for microbiological culture.

For different tests, pleural fluid must be divided as follows:

- *Cell count*: About 3–4 mL pleural fluid collected in an anticoagulant-coated tube [ethylenediamine-tetraacetic acid (EDTA)/heparin].
- *Biochemical analysis*: 5 mL of pleural fluid is collected in sterile container, without any additive.
- *Microbiological analysis*:
  - 5 mL for Gram-stain and nucleic acid amplification technique (NAAT) in sterile container
  - 5 mL into aerobic and anaerobic culture media
  - 5 mL inoculated into liquid culture media for *Mycobacterium tuberculosis*

The first-line investigations done for diagnosis of cause of pleural effusion are:

- *Cell count*: Total count/differential count
- Glucose
- Protein
- Lactate dehydrogenase (LDH)
- Adenosine deaminase (ADA)

Light's Criteria (Box 1 and Table 4)

Adenosine Deaminase

Adenosine deaminase level in pleural fluid is a semispecific biochemical marker for diagnosis of tuberculous pleural effusion, with cut-off level >40 IU/L. As per different studies, tuberculous pleural fluid contains higher levels of ADA than do most other exudates. The sensitivity and specificity of ADA are approximately 92% and 90%, respectively as per different studies. ADA has high negative predictive value, low ADA (<40 IU/L) values almost rules out possibility of tuberculous pleural effusion. Still, controversies exist over the definitive diagnostic value of pleural fluid ADA. Generally, ADA level >40 IU/L with appropriate clinical situations is diagnostic of tuberculous pleural effusion **(Tables 5 and 6)**.

Two different isoforms of ADA exists—ADA1 and ADA2. ADA1 is found in all cells and ADA2 reflects monocyte/macrophage activation. In patients with tuberculous pleural effusion ADA2 is predominant, while in those with empyema and parainfective effusions, ADA1 is predominant form. Measurement of ADA2 in pleural fluid increases the specificity, ADA1:ADA2 ratio <0.45 in raised ADA levels is highly specific for tuberculous pleural effusion.

BOX 1: Light's criteria for distinguishing pleural transudate from exudate.

Exudate is likely if one or more of the following criteria is met:

- *Pleural fluid protein*: Serum protein ratio >0.5
- *Pleural fluid LDH*: Serum LDH ratio >0.6
- Pleural fluid LDH > two-thirds of upper limit of normal serum LDH

(LDH: lactate dehydrogenase)

Nucleic Acid Amplification Tests

Nucleic acid amplification test for MTB/RIF test of pleural fluid has a sensitivity of about 49.5% and specificity of about 98.9%.

TABLE 4: Pleural fluid analysis in tuberculous pleural effusion.

Pleural fluid	Frequency
Exudative with protein >3 g /dL	Almost all
Pleural fluid > 60 mg /dL	80–85%
>50% lymphocyte	93.3%
Pleural fluid ADA > 40 IU/L	81–100%

TABLE 5: Interpretation of pleural fluid adenosine deaminase (ADA) level in diagnosis of tuberculous pleural effusion.

Level	Interpretation
>70 IU/L	Highly likely to be pleural tuberculosis (TB)
40–70 IU/L	Intermediate level, other risk factors to be considered
<40 IU/L	Low likelihood of TB, investigate for other causes

TABLE 6: Cause of false-negative and false-positive adenosine deaminase (ADA) levels.

False positive	False negative
• Very early stage • Elderly • Current smoker	• Lymphoma • Q fever • Late parapneumonic effusion • Rheumatoid effusion • Mesothelioma

Pleural Biopsy

Sometimes, the results of mentioned tests are inconclusive or not suggestive of TB but clinical suspicion is high. In such cases, pleural biopsy is required, the diagnostic test of choice is thoracoscopy with pleural biopsy. Depending upon the available facility and opinion of specialist either, percutaneous pleural biopsy or thoracoscopic pleural biopsy is done. Better result is seen in thoracoscpic pleural biopsy than percutaneous pleural biopsy (93.2% vs. 84%).

About four to six samples from parietal pleura is collected to maximize the yield. These are used for culture for mycobacteria. Sample should be sent for NAAT also, this test also helps in diagnosis.

Sputum Microscopy

Sputum microscopy should not be ignored in cases of suspected pleural TB, many patients of pleural TB have associated parenchymal involvement. Sputum microscopy and culture confirm the diagnosis.

Tuberculin Skin Testing

In TB pleural effusion, it can positive or negative. Negative test does not rule out its presence. The positive response rate shown in various studies ranges between 40.9 and 66.5%. Immunocompromised and immunosuppressed patients may not show a response.

Screening for Comorbidities

All patients must be screened for HIV and diabetes mellitus. Depending upon history and clinical examination, screening for chronic liver disease and chronic renal disease must be done.

Management of Pleural Tuberculosis

Goal of management are:

- Treatment of active disease
- Symptomatic relief secondary to pleural effusion
- Prevention of complications

Antitubercular therapy is the mainstay of treatment. As per the guidelines, 6 months of treatment is recommended as follows:

2HRZE + 4HRE (total 6 months), 4 drugs rifampicin, isoniazid, pyrazinamide, and ethambutol are given daily for 2 months. Followed by rifampicin, isoniazid, and ethambutol on daily basis as per weight band, as per the National Tuberculosis Elimination Programme (NTEP) guidelines.

In most cases, clinical improvement is observed in 2 weeks following initiation of antitubercular therapy, significant reduction in pleural effusion is noted in 6–8 weeks. Clinical improvement in appetite and defervescence, weight gain, and reduction in shortness of breath is observed.

Follow-up chest X-ray is recommended 8 weeks after initiation of treatment, radiologically amount of pleural effusion decreases. The increasing size of effusion or lack of response indicates paradoxical reaction or alternate diagnosis.

ROLE OF CORTICOSTEROID

As per different studies conducted to evaluate the role of corticosteroid in pleural TB, it is indicated that use of corticosteroid may reduce the time to resolution of effusion and decrease the risk of chronic pleural changes (thickening/adhesion), but no improvement in long-term improvement was observed. But due to lack of sufficient data to support major improvements in respiratory function or clinically relevant outcomes, corticosteroids are not recommended for the treatment of pleural TB.

Pleural fluid drainage: If the effusion causing respiratory distress (shortness of breath, increase in respiratory rate) pleural fluid drainage can be done.

COMPLICATIONS

Lack of Response

In some patients, clinical and radiological improvement is not seen even after 2 months of initiation of proper treatment. In such cases, causes may be:

- Immune reconstitution inflammatory syndrome (IRIS)
- Drug resistance
- Alternate diagnosis
- Superadded infection

Pleural Thickening

It may occur in up to 50% cases of pleural TB. In most of the cases, it remains asymptomatic and causes no major limitation of lung function, but in some of the cases, it causes marked restrictive lung pathology or fibrothorax and needs surgical intervention and decortication may be required.

Empyema

It is an important complication. In this condition, there is thick pus in pleural cavity , which contains large number of *Mycobacterium*. Pleural fluid contains polymorphonuclear cells. In these cases along with standard antituberculous treatment, surgical intervention—repeated thoracocentesis, decortication, pneumonectomy, and thoracoplasty may be required. Due to availability of better chemotherapeutic agents, this condition is less frequent.

Hydropneumothorax

Sometimes, pulmonary cavity may rupture in pleural space leading to this condition. The patient presents with breathlessness and cough. This is managed with antitubercular along with intercostal drainage.

FOLLOW-UP

Regular follow-up is essential part of management: Patients must be followed up for improvement in clinical condition; in most of the cases, clinical improvement is seen after 2 weeks, and constitutional symptoms disappear by this time. As mentioned earlier, chest X-ray must be done after 8 weeks of initiation of treatment. If clinical and radiological causes are not seen by this time, we must look for causes of nonresolution, as mentioned above.

CONCLUSION

Tuberculosis is very important disease as far as morbidity and mortality are concerned. TB involves all the systems of our body. Pleural involvement is very common and presents as pleural effusion. Timely suspicion, investigation, and adequate treatment are very important, since in some of patients it resolves spontaneously, but later clinical TB occurs within 5 years. In clinical diagnoses, pleurocentesis and pleural fluid analysis remain the most important investigation and in most of the cases, it gives clue for diagnosis of pleural TB.

SUGGESTED READINGS

1. Training module on Extrapulmonary Tuberculosis, 2023.
2. Index TB guidelines.

230
CHAPTER

Management of Malignant Pleural Effusion

Nitin Jain, Nasir Hussain

ABSTRACT

Malignant pleural effusion (MPE) refers to the abnormal collection of fluid in pleural space with evidence of atypical/malignant cells in pleural fluid cytology and/or pleural tissue biopsy. It usually arises as a complication of advanced-stage cancers and virtually all cancers metastasize to pleura. Accurate diagnosis and effective management of MPE are essential to provide symptom relief, improve patient comfort and quality of life, and optimize overall treatment outcomes. Treatment options include thoracocentesis, pleurodesis, indwelling pleural catheters (IPCs), intracellular chemotherapy, and systemic cancer treatments such as chemotherapy, and immunogene therapy to address the underlying malignancy. Future advancements such as cryotherapy and radiotherapy are in the research pipeline.

INTRODUCTION

Malignant pleural effusion (MPE) is a distressing and often debilitating complication that arises in advanced stages of various cancers, impacting the quality of life and prognosis of affected individuals. The most common underlying tumors are lung cancer, breast cancer, and lymphomas. It is seen in 15% of cases of all cancer patients, which signifies an advanced stage of malignancy. The median survival is 3–12 months after diagnosis, with the shortest survival period in patients with lung cancer.

Most of the patients of MPE present with respiratory symptoms, the most common being dyspnea and chest pain. While few patients can be asymptomatic, in which MPE is detected incidentally. It usually presents with symptoms such as dyspnea due to impairment of the hemidiaphragm and collapse of the lung, localized chest pain as a result of pressure on pleural membranes, dry cough due to pleural irritation, while fatigue and weakness may occur due to reduced lung function and oxygenation. Exercise intolerance is also common and tachypnea may develop as a compensatory response to maintain adequate oxygen levels.

Diagnosis of MPE involves the patient's medical history, physical examination, pleural fluid examination with cytology, and imaging tests, such as chest X-ray and computed tomography (CT) scans. The presence of atypical cells in pleural fluid cytology or its absence or suspicion of malignancy not confirmed by cytology alone, a closed pleural biopsy or biopsy by a medical thoracoscopy can be done to establish the diagnosis, and later biomarker studies and immunohistochemistry aid in determining the presence of malignant cells and their origin.

The management of MPE is multifaceted, aiming to provide symptomatic relief, optimize patient comfort, and address the underlying cancer. There may be different treatment options including serial thoracocentesis, tube thoracostomy with or without pleurodesis, indwelling pleural catheters (IPCs), pleuroperitoneal shunt, chemotherapy (systemic and intrapleural), radiotherapy, and immunotherapy. The choice of treatment modality is determined by the patient's clinical conditions as well as the underlying disease.

TREATMENT OPTIONS

Conservative Approach

In MPE if the patient is asymptomatic and if the volume of pleural effusion is small, we should just observe the patient. Individuals under chemotherapy may experience good control of pleural effusion, especially in patients with lymphoma, small cell carcinoma, and breast cancer.

Therapeutic Thoracocentesis

Therapeutic thoracocentesis is a relatively safe and effective procedure for providing rapid relief from symptoms caused by MPE, such as shortness of breath and chest discomfort. It is recommended for all patients with MPE involving 50% of the hemithorax and patients presenting with symptoms. The main disadvantage of thoracocentesis is the recollection of pleural fluid, secondary infection, and pneumothorax. It is the treatment of choice in patients with a limited survival period of < 1 month. In patients with a life expectancy < 1 month, repeated thoracocentesis may be needed to relieve symptoms such as shortness of breath, cough, or chest pain.

Chest Tube Drainage and Chemical Pleurodesis

It is accomplished in cases of recurrent pleural effusion by draining the pleural fluid by chest tube intubation in patients with a life expectancy > 1 month. This procedure can be accompanied by instilling a chemical sclerosing agent into the pleural space, the procedure called *pleurodesis*, which causes intense inflammatory response and fibrosis leading to adhesions between parietal and visceral pleura. These adhesions cause the pleural layers to stick together, efficiently sealing the pleural space and reducing the risk of recurrent pleural effusion. Pleurodesis is not recommended in the presence of a trapped lung, or multiple pleural septa, as the apposition of the two layers of pleura will not be achieved and pleurodesis will be unsuccessful and the patient may again present with recurrent refilling of pleural fluid. Pleurodesis is still considered the mainstay treatment for recurrent MPE with a success rate of nearly 80–90% depending on the choice of sclerosing agent and in cases where it is not contraindicated.

Sclerosing Agents for Pleurodesis

- *Mineral*: Graded talc most commonly used (80–90% success rate and can be used as talc slurry via a chest drain or can be used as talc poudrage via a medical thoracoscope)
- *Antineoplastic agents*: Bleomycin (58–85% success rate), cisplatin, docetaxel, etc.
- *Antibiotics*: Tetracycline and doxycycline
- *Antiseptic*: Povidone iodine and silver nitrate
- *Bacterial products*: *Corynebacterium parvum*
- *Autologous blood*
- *Cytokine*: Interferon alpha (INF-α)-2b

Talc Pleurodesis

Talc is the most commonly used chemical agent for pleurodesis. The talc utilized for intrapleural administration is free from asbestos and can be administered in two ways (1) by thoracoscopy, using an atomizer termed "talc poudrage" or (2) via an intercostal tube in the form of a suspension termed "talc slurry."

Talc poudrage can be performed under local anesthesia using either medical thoracoscopy or video-assisted thoracoscopic surgery (VATS). Before atomizing the talc, the pleural fluid should be completely drained, and there must be complete reexpansion of the lungs. All loculation must be broken down to provide access to the entire pleural space, if possible, pleural biopsies should be taken if necessary and lung reexpansion should be confirmed.

Talc slurry is also an effective agent for pleurodesis for MPE. It is a suspension of talc in a sterile saline solution. When introduced into the pleural space, the talc particles cause inflammation and irritation of the pleura, which leads to the formation of adhesions. Povidone iodine is also been used for this procedure with a good success rate and is also economical and safe with fewer side effects mainly chest pain and fever [talc is costlier and has some reported adverse events such as acute respiratory distress syndrome (ARDS) except chest pain and fever].

Mechanical Pleurodesis

It is done through VATS or open thoracotomy. It involves physically irritating the pleural surfaces to promote adhesion. Abrasion techniques, such as thoracoscopy and thoracotomy use surgical instruments to scratch and roughen the pleura. Video-assisted thoracoscopy allows for precise visualization and manipulation, minimizing trauma. These techniques are often employed when there is a trapped lung or significant pleural rind where chemical pleurodesis is unsuitable or contraindicated.

Indwelling Pleural Catheters

It is designed to provide a long-term, outpatient-based solution for managing recurrent MPE in patients having a life expectancy > 1 month in cases with trapped lungs, where failure of chest tube drainage usually prevails and can also be a choice of management in patients of advanced cancer stage with limited life expectancy who might not benefit from more invasive interventions. Its primary function is to allow controlled and continuous drainage of pleural fluid from pleural space. Indwelling pleural catheter helps to relieve symptoms, such as shortness of breath, chest discomfort, and cough associated with MPE. Indwelling pleural catheter placement is typically performed under sterile conditions in an outpatient setting or in the hospital, depending on the patient's overall health status. The procedure involves inserting a flexible Pleurx™ catheter into the pleural space under local anesthesia, usually through a small incision. The catheter is then tunneled under the skin and sutured in place to prevent movement or dislodgment. Intermittent pleural fluid drainage can be done at home by a patient himself or a healthcare provider and trained family member. After IPC insertion, pleural fluid can be drained as and when required depending upon the patient's presenting symptoms. If a patient has three drainages that are scant (< 50 mL) and the imaging shows no fluid reaccumulation, the pleural catheter is removed as spontaneous pleurodesis has occurred. The procedure and its maneuver are well explained to patients and their caregivers to make it easy for home management.

Pleuroperitoneal Shunt

Pleuroperitoneal shunting is a surgical procedure used to manage MPE in cases of trapped lung or large effusions refractory to chemical pleurodesis. The shunt allows the excess fluid to drain from the pleural cavity into the peritoneal cavity in the abdomen, where it can be reabsorbed by the body. This procedure is typically considered when other methods of managing pleural effusion, such as thoracocentesis, chest tubes, or pleurodesis are not effective or appropriate. However, the use of a pleuroperitoneal shunt in the management of MPE can have the potential risk of peritoneal seeding of malignant cells along with complications, including infection, shunt malfunction, skin erosion, and potential damage to organs.

Chemotherapy and Targeted Therapies

The chemotherapeutic drugs commonly used in clinical practice alongside thoracic infusion mainly include cisplatin, carboplatin, docetaxel, and bleomycin.

Typically, only one chemotherapeutic agent is used clinically, but some researchers have explored combining multiple agents to enhance treatment efficacy through synergistic effects. However, it is important to note that these chemotherapeutic agents used intrapleurally have shown variable effectiveness in the literature. When administered intrapleurally there can be challenges, particularly in those with advanced tumors, patients may not tolerate these agents well and the use of these agents needs further studies.

Systemic Chemotherapy and Radiotherapy

These should be continued in conjunction with palliative therapy.

Newer Advancements

Immune gene therapy using interleukin-2 (IL-2), IFN-α, interferon beta (IFN-β), and interferon-gamma (IFN-γ), IFNα-2B, OK-432 as solely and also in conjunction with intrapleural chemotherapy is in studies. It has shown to have promising results though further studies are needed.

Cryotherapy and radiotherapy are also in the pipeline for the management of recurrent MPE.

Pleurectomy

Pleurectomy involves surgical stripping of the pleura and pericardium. It is indicated especially in cases of mesothelioma and decortication may be required if the tumor hinders lung reexpansion. Complications include empyema, hemorrhage, and cardiorespiratory failure.

This method should be reserved for those who failed to respond to other forms of treatment and when a patient has good health status and life expectancy, though rarely used because it is highly invasive and has high mortality rates.

CONCLUSION

Management of MPE is solely a palliative approach to relieve symptoms and to prevent reaccumulation of fluid by a least invasive procedure with minimal morbidity. The choice of the procedure depends on the type of malignancy, the patient's symptoms, life expectancy, functional status, quality of life, and goals of therapy. Newer advancements with treatment approaches and physical rehabilitation are in trials and present variable treatment options available are mainly focused on relieving symptoms and improving quality of life and are completely palliative.

SUGGESTED READINGS

1. Anderson CB, Philpott GW, Ferguson TB. The treatment of malignant pleural effusions. Cancer.1974;33(4):916-22.
2. Ramakant Dixit, KC Agarwal, Gokhroo A, Patil CB, Meena M, Shah NS, et al. Diagnosis and management options in malignant pleural effusions. Lung India. 2017;34(2):160-6.
3. Mierzejewski M, Korczynski P, Krenke R. Chemical pleurodesis – a review of mechanisms involved in pleural space obliteration. Respiratory Research. 2019;20:247.
4. Zahid I, Routledge T, Billè A, Scarci M. What is the best treatment for malignant pleural effusions? Interact Cardiovasc Thorac Surg. 2011;12(5):818-23.
5. Frost N, Brünger M, Ruwwe-Glösenkamp C, Raspe M, Tessmer A, Temmesfeld-Wollbrück B, et al. Indwelling pleural catheters for malignancy-associated pleural effusion: report on a single centre's ten years of experience. BMC Pulm Med. 2019;19(1):232.

231
CHAPTER

Physician's Approach to a Case of Lung Abscess

Sanjay Tandon, Arjun Tandon

ABSTRACT

Lung abscesses are localized collections of purulent material within the lung parenchyma. Aspiration is one of the most common causes of lung abscess, others being obstruction of the bronchial lumen, contagious spread from thoracic and airway sources of infection, and hematogenous spread. Patients who are at risk of developing a lung abscess secondary to aspiration include those with oral cavity and sinus infections. Isolates are primarily polymicrobial and are usually the constituents of the oral and gingival flora, most commonly microaerophilic streptococci (*Streptococcus anginosus, Streptococcus milleri, Streptococcus mitis*) and anaerobes (*Peptostreptococcus*). A case of lung abscess usually presents with features of an indolent lung infection with symptoms comprising fever, shortness of breath, sweating, bloody or putrid sputum, history of weight loss, to list a few. Fever and chills are the most common presenting symptoms and are present in four out of every five patients with lung abscess. Prompt empiric antibiotic therapy should be initiated as soon as the suspicion of lung abscess is confirmed in order to prevent its complications. The initial therapy consists of a combination of beta-lactam and beta-lactamase inhibitor or carbapenem with the most commonly used regimens being ampicillin–sulbactam 3 g intravenously QID.

INTRODUCTION

Lung abscesses are localized collections of purulent material within the lung parenchyma, usually occurring as a complication of aspiration but can also be secondary to acute infections with pyogenic bacteria. Kuhajda et al. described lung abscess as a type of liquefactive necrosis of the lung tissue and formation of cavities (>2 cm) containing necrotic debris or fluid caused by microbial infection.

CLASSIFICATION

Lung abscess can be classified as primary or secondary:

- *Primary lung abscess:*
    - Involves healthy individuals
    - Direct infection of the pulmonary parenchyma
    - *Causes:*
        - Aspiration of oral or gastric contents
        - Secondary to necrotizing pneumonia
- *Secondary lung abscess:*
    - It involves individuals with predisposing conditions.
    - *Causes:*
        - Hematogenous spread (right-sided endocarditis)
        - Bronchial obstruction (neoplasm, foreign body)
        - Surgical procedures involving the thoracic cavity
        - Immunocompromised status

PATHOGENESIS

Aspiration is one of the most common causes of lung abscess, others being obstruction of the bronchial lumen, contagious spread from thoracic and airway sources of infection, and hematogenous spread.

- *Aspiration:* Patients who are at risk of developing a lung abscess secondary to aspiration include those with oral cavity and sinus infections. Elderly patients who are usually bedridden and have impaired swallowing abilities are also at risk for recurrent aspiration, increasing their chances of developing lung abscesses. Anaerobes are the most common microorganisms that reach the lower airways with aspirated material, initiating pneumonitis, which progresses over 1–2 weeks to necrosis of the lung tissue leading to the development of an abscess. Individuals who are at a high risk of developing lung abscess include:
  - Alcoholics
  - Sedative consumers
  - Intubated patients
  - Near-drowning cases
  - Poor dental hygiene
  - Elderly age
  - Neurological deficits
  - Acid-suppressive medication consumers
- *Contagious spread from thoracic cavity infections:* Lung abscesses can result as a direct extension of an abscess present in the mediastinum, subphrenic infections, and bronchoesophageal or treacheobroncheal fistulas.
- *Obstruction to the bronchial lumen:* An obstruction to the bronchus by an inhaled foreign object can lead to collection and decreased drainage of the pulmonary secretions, leading to abscess formation. Other causes of obstruction include stenosis of the bronchus and obstruction by a bronchogenic or mediastinal mass, lymph nodes, or aneurysm.
- *Blood route:* Tricuspid valve endocarditis can lead to the formation of a lung abscess as a result of septic embolization. Septic embolization can also occur in patients having an indwelling intravascular (IV) catheter, IV drug abusers, and patients having thrombophlebitis of the jugular vein.
- *Sequelae of airway infections:* Pulmonary injuries, infarcts, and malformations can be infected, culminating into an abscess. Rarely, exacerbation of bronchiectasis can lead to abscess formation as a result of parenchymal infection.

ETIOLOGICAL AGENTS

- *Organisms implicated in aspiration as the primary pathology:* Isolates are primarily polymicrobial and are usually the constituents of the oral and gingival flora, most commonly microaerophilic streptococci (*Streptococcus anginosus, Streptococcus milleri, Streptococcus mitis*) and anaerobes (*Peptostreptococcus*, nonfragilis *Bacteroides* species, *Prevotella*, and *Fusobacterium*).
- *Organisms implicated in pyogenic pneumonia as the primary pathology:* The most common organisms in this group of etiopathogenesis include *Klebsiella pneumonia* (especially in structural lung defects), *Staphylococcus aureus, Streptococcus pyogenes, Pseudomonas aeruginosa, Burkholderia pseudomallei, Actinomyces, Nocardia, Legionella*, and *Haemophilus influenzae* type B.
- *Nonbacterial agents:*
  - Fungi: *Cryptococcus, Histoplasma capsulatum, Aspergillus*, and *Coccidioides* species, *Blastomyces dermatitidis*, mucormycosis
  - *Mycobacterium tuberculosis*, nontuberculous mycobacterium
  - Parasites: *Echinococcus, Entamoeba histolytica*, and *Paragonimus westermani*
- *In the immunocompromised group:* The most common organisms causing lung abscess in the immunocompromised group of patients include *Pseudomonas aeruginosa, Nocardia, Aspergillus*, and aerobic gram-positive bacilli.

HOW TO SUSPECT, DIAGNOSE, AND APPROACH A CASE OF LUNG ABSCESS AS A PHYSICIAN?

When to Suspect?

Clinical Features

A case of lung abscess usually presents with features of indolent lung infection with symptoms comprising fever, shortness of breath, cough with bloody or putrid sputum, history of weight loss, to list a few. Fever and chills are the most common presenting symptoms and are present in four out of every five patients with lung abscess, followed by productive cough, which is present in more than half of such patients. Other symptoms include shortness of breath, hemoptysis, and chest pain (when the pleura gets involved). These symptoms usually progress and present over a period of time, as a lung abscess is primarily a chronic pathology. However, abscesses resulting from septic embolization, infection with *Staphylococcus aureus*, and immunocompromised patients can present with acute signs and symptoms. The constitutional symptoms of a lung abscess comprise anorexia, weight loss, night sweats, and fatigue and are nonspecific. On general physical examination, one should start by examining the oral cavity and look for gingivitis, tonsillar inflammation and enlargement, teeth pathologies, halitosis, and tongue weakness followed by examination of the neck for lymphadenopathy. The patient may be febrile to touch and may have features suggestive of weight loss, decreased sensorium, alcohol intoxication or some neurological disorder, such as bulbar speech. Systemic examination that focused on the respiratory system may be completely unremarkable or may reveal features of consolidation in cases of large or subpleural abscesses.

Risk Factors

A detailed history should be obtained to identify the major risk factors for lung abscess, including neurological disorders and weaknesses, disorders of the esophagus, dental infections, pain or procedures, consumption of alcohol or illicit substance abuse, immunodeficiency disorders, history of cough, neck pain, and dysphagia.

Radiographical Features

The diagnosis of lung abscess is primarily clinched by obtaining a chest radiogram, which may reveal a fluid-filled space with an air–fluid interface. It may also show features of a nodule, mass, or consolidation. Lung abscesses are usually unilateral and located in the dependent segment of the lung, as aspiration is the most common etiology.

How to Diagnose?

History and Examination

Detailed history and examination, as mentioned above, should be done.

Blood Investigations

Routine blood investigations should be done as they may demonstrate leukocytosis and anemia of chronic disease and bring out other comorbidities.

Investigations

Investigations to rule out an immunocompromised state include HIV testing, tests to rule out tuberculosis, and vasculitis.

Microbiological Testing

The physician must send different paired sets of blood cultures for anaerobic and aerobic organisms. Sputum examination should include Gram staining and special stains for any suspected microorganisms. Sputum samples containing upper airway flora can lead to erroneous findings and clinicians must be careful in starting treatment against the same. More than half of the samples may not reveal a positive culture; hence, an empiric antimicrobial therapy is usually initiated. If suspected, the sputum sample should also be screened for *Mycobacterium tuberculosis* by acid-fast staining.

Radiography

Chest X-ray is the primary mode of radiographical investigation and may reveal findings as mentioned above. To confirm, a chest computed tomography (CT) must be performed, as it serves the dual purpose of not only confirming the lung abscess but also helping in identifying other diagnostic clues, such as lymphadenopathy or malignancies. From the diagnostic point of view, a CT scan identifies the exact location of the abscess and helps in differentiating a pleural pathology from a parenchymal one and the underlying etiology which may have led to the formation of an abscess, such as bronchial obstruction, structural lung defects, congenital lesions, cysts, and bullae. CT scan also helps the surgeon in decision-making if resection is considered as the modality of treatment. On a CT scan, the lung abscess looks like an area of consolidation surrounding an area of cavitation, apart from showing an air–fluid interface.

Special Investigations

Invasive investigations such as bronchoscopy are usually reserved for patients who are unable to produce sputum or in patients where an assessment of the airways is warranted. For those patients where a septic embolization is suspected, a 2D echocardiogram should be performed to rule out right-sided valve endocarditis. In cases where empiric antibiotic therapy fails to improve the clinical condition of the patient and sputum cultures and bronchoscopy are inconclusive, transthoracic needle aspiration or biopsy may be performed. If the chest radiograph reveals obliteration of the costophrenic space or the CT scan is suggestive of the presence of pleural fluid, thoracocentesis may have to be performed to exclude empyema.

Ruling Out Other Differential Diagnoses

If the lesion fails to improve despite intensive antimicrobial therapy or if a solitary thick-walled cavity is present without a surrounding area of consolidation, lung cancer should be ruled out. The presence of other systemic features, such as those suggestive of vasculitis, may raise concern to initiate a battery of investigations to diagnose noninfectious granulomatous diseases, such as sarcoidosis, nodular silicosis, and cavitating lung nodules. For patients living in endemic areas with *Echinococcus*, a CT scan should be carefully observed to rule out specific signs, such as the "water lily sign", which is cyst fluid containing germinative membranes. Postprimary tuberculosis may present with thin-walled cavities in the pulmonary parenchyma and hence, a history of tuberculosis should be meticulously confirmed.

How to Treat a Case of Lung Abscess?

Initial Empiric Treatment

Prompt empiric antibiotic therapy should be initiated as soon as the suspicion of lung abscess is confirmed in order to prevent its complications. The results of the investigations looking into the causative agent can be used to alter the course of the treatment as and when they are available. For patients who are not allergic to penicillin, the initial therapy consists of a combination of beta-lactam and beta-lactamase inhibitor or carbapenem, with the most commonly used regimens being ampicillin–sulbactam 3 g intravenously QID. For penicillin-allergic patients, moxifloxacin 400 mg PO OD or clindamycin 600 mg IV TDS followed by 300 mg PO QID can be used. An alternative regimen of a combination of levofloxacin 750 mg PO OD + metronidazole 500 mg PO TDS can be used.

Antibiotics in Special Cases

For cases in which a methicillin-sensitive *Staphylococcus aureus* (MSSA) infection is suspected, oxacillin (2 g IV every 4 hourly), cefazolin (2 g IV TDS), and nafcillin (2 g IV every 4 hourly) can be used whereas in cases of methicillin-resistant *Staphylococcus aureus* (MRSA), linezolid (600 mg IV BD) or vancomycin can be employed.

Follow-up of Treatment

These antibiotics should be switched to oral therapy when the patient improves clinically. The total duration of treatment varies from 3 to 6 weeks, while most clinicians use chest imaging suggesting clearance of the lesion to decide the termination of therapy.

Within 1 week of initiation of therapy, most patients start showing clinical improvement in the form of decreased body temperatures and reduced leukocyte count. Sputum clearance happens later than clinical improvement in most cases. In case of delayed improvement, the physician must look carefully for complications such as empyema or look for other differential diagnoses, such as malignancies, vasculitis, bronchus obstruction, or other causes of pyrexia of unknown origin.

Need for Intervention

A small proportion of the patients do not improve despite optimum antimicrobial therapy and may require either transthoracic catheter drainage or a transbronchoscopic catheter drainage. Surgical interventions are usually reserved for those cases who fail to respond to both catheter drainage and antimicrobial therapy.

Prognosis

According to many studies, 90–95% of patients with primary lung abscess, including those with typical aspiration-related lung abscess, improve well with adequate and optimum antimicrobial therapy. A poor prognosis is usually observed in patients who are either immunocompromised, those requiring surgery, and those having an underlying malignancy or irreversible bronchial obstruction.

SUGGESTED READINGS

1. Kuhajda I, Zarogoulidis K, Tsirgogianni K, Tsavlis D, Kioumis I, Kosmidis C, et al. Lung abscess-etiology, diagnostic and treatment options. Ann Transl Med. 2015;3(13):183.
2. Hsu-Kim C, Hoag JB, Cheng GS, Lund ME. The microbiology of postobstructive pneumonia in lung cancer patients. J Bronchology Interv Pulmonol. 2013;20(3):266-70.
3. Mukae H, Noguchi S, Naito K, Kawanami T, Yamasaki K, Fukuda K, et al. The importance of obligate anaerobes and the Streptococcus anginosus group in pulmonary abscess: a clone library analysis using bronchoalveolar lavage fluid. Respiration. 2016;92(2):80-9.

232

CHAPTER

Lungs in Thyroid Disorders

Ketan K Mehta

ABSTRACT

Thyroid hormones and disorders have a close interaction with the respiratory system. Both hypothyroidism and hyperthyroidism have an impact on the physiology of breathing as well as can manifest with respiratory symptoms. Besides that, all patients with obstructive sleep apnea (OSA) should be screened for hypothyroidism. Thyroid malignancy can also metastasize to the lungs. Hence, any patient with respiratory symptoms should be evaluated for thyroid.

INTRODUCTION

Over the past decades, modern studies have demonstrated the roles of hormones in the physiological mechanisms of respiration and the morphological maturation of the respiratory system components. Endocrine control alongside other factors implicates in the regulation or adaptation of respiration in some disorders. Some hormones such as hypothalamic neuropeptides act as neurotransmitters and neuromodulators and have central effects, while others, by acting through chemoreceptors or by direct action on the lungs and respiratory airways, have peripheral effects.

The action of hormones on the respiratory system can be stimulating or inhibiting. Testosterone appears to predispose to sleep-disordered breathing whereas estrogen and progesterone seem to protect from it. For long, progesterone and thyroxine have been known to stimulate respiration. Recently, certain hormones such as leptin and corticotropin-releasing hormone have been recognized to act as respiratory stimulants. Somatostatin, dopamine, and neuropeptide Y have been known for their depressing or inhibitory effect on breathing. Certain hormones can act on the respiratory airways, inducing bronchodilation (epinephrine) or bronchoconstriction (histamine).

Thyroid hormones through their effect on metabolism play a key role in regulating the function of different systems of the human body including cardiovascular, respiratory, renal, homeostasis, vascular tone, and central nervous system. Thyroid hormones via their complex metabolic effects interact with the complex mechanism of respiration. Significant alteration in pulmonary ventilation can occur due to thyroid hormone in patients with dysfunctional thyroid disorders. Hyperthyroidism and hypothyroidism can cause disorders of respiratory function and disturbances of ventilation. Hypothyroidism is characterized by hypoventilation, while hyperthyroidism can reflect into dyspnea and hyperventilation as typical symptoms. Under this background, this article is aimed to highlight respiratory manifestations of various thyroid disorders.

THYROID HORMONE

The thyroid hormone has a role in the metabolism of proteins, lipids, and carbohydrates, and it controls the activity of membrane-bound enzymes. The thyroid hormone enhances mitochondrial oxidation and enhances metabolic rate. This effect on metabolic rate may have a role to play in the association between the thyroid hormone and respiratory drive. Further, the thyroid hormone also regulates the transcription of many genes encoding myofibrillar and calcium-regulatory proteins in myofibers. This plays a significant role in the development of the lungs and the maturation of pulmonary surfactants.

With the help of adequate therapy, the alteration of thyroid function accompanied by sometimes life-threatening respiratory manifestations can be corrected.

HYPOTHYROIDISM

Patients with hypothyroidism clinically have expiratory dyspnea induced by partial upper airway obstruction through edema and mucopolysaccharide infiltration, and speech disorders with hoarseness of voice. Lung volume is normal unless the person is obese in which case lung volume may be slightly decreased. Respiratory functional tests may exhibit pulmonary hypoventilation and diminished ventilatory response to hypoxia and hypercapnia. As demonstrated in several studies, this major change in ventilation is of central origin, owing to reduced peripheral oxygen consumption and to a lesser extent, by an alteration of ventilatory mechanics. Some hypothyroid patients can have low carbon monoxide diffusing capacity, even in the case of nonobese individuals with normal lung volume. Measurement of muscle pressure during maximal inspiration and expiration can demonstrate reduced inspiratory and expiratory muscle tone. Myopathy is present in both types of myxedema—idiopathic as well as iatrogenic. With thyroxine replacement, myasthenia can be corrected significantly. Diaphragmatic muscle dysfunction is another muscle change in hypothyroidism. It is variable from mild with limiting effort tolerance to severe with dyspnea and hypercapnia. It is impacted by the severity of hypothyroidism, regardless of obesity or nonobesity. According to certain studies, diaphragmatic myasthenia is due to both—myopathic and neuropathic (lesions of the phrenic nerve).

Pleural collection is evidenced in 25% of patients with hypothyroidism. This should be differentiated from pleural collections caused by disorders associated with hypothyroidism, pneumonia, cardiac failure, cirrhosis with ascites, and malignant lesions. Hypothyroid pleural collection is in small amounts (less than one-third of the pleural cavity), unilateral or bilateral, serous or serosanguineous, transudate or exudate, in general noninflammatory. It is asymptomatic, and more rarely, it can induce restrictive pulmonary function. Its pathophysiological mechanism is unknown; it is thought to be developed through increased capillary permeability. Hypothyroid pleural effusion resolves by hormone replacement therapy. Hypothyroid coma, the final stage of untreated or insufficiently treated myxedema, evolves with severe respiratory failure as a result of hypoventilation, respiratory acidosis, upper airway obstruction through laryngeal edema, and infiltration, respiratory muscle asthenia, decreased pulmonary surfactant, pulmonary and airway infections, reduced lung capacity through pleural effusion, respiratory center dysfunction, dyselectrolytemia, hypoglycemia, and arterial hypotension.

Hypothyroidism and Sleep Apnea

Hypothyroidism and obstructive sleep apnea syndrome (OSAS) are closely associated. OSAS has been diagnosed in 25% of patients with hypothyroidism. On the other hand, in 3.1% of OSAS patients, thyroid hypofunction has been detected. Risk and causal factors associated with OSAS in hyperthyroidism include ventilator dysfunction, oropharyngeal, and upper airway infiltration with mucopolysaccharides and protein deposits, protein extravasations leading to edema, respiratory muscle asthenia, obesity, male sex, and advanced age. Sleep apnea of central origin can also be identified in patients with hypothyroidism, usually in younger persons, having a rapidly favorable evolution after thyroxine replacement therapy. However, in subclinical hypothyroidism, the prevalence of sleep disorders is not different from euthyroidism. Overall, contrasting data are available concerning the efficacy of thyroid replacement therapy in improving sleep apnea in patients with clinical hypothyroidism. Certain studies suggested a prompt reversal of symptoms, sleep-disordered breathing, and nocturnal hypoxia, while others reported little or no improvement in sleep apnea. Nocturnal continuous positive airway pressure (nCPAP) treatment can be necessary initially and, in some patients even after remission of clinical signs of hypothyroidism.

HYPERTHYROIDISM

Hyperthyroidism is associated with respiratory dysfunction, leading to an increase in respiratory rate, respiratory muscle weakness, and pulmonary hypertension. The mechanism responsible for reduced pulmonary compliance in patients with hyperthyroidism is not clear, but there are several proposed theories such as changes in functional residual capacity, pulmonary congestion, edema, increased intrathoracic blood volume, and changes in the recoil of alveolar septa. A significant reduction in respiratory muscle strength particularly involving the diaphragm is also common in patients with hyperthyroidism. This leads to reduced ventilation, especially during exercise. Effort and rest dyspnea are also commonly experienced by patients with hyperthyroidism. In the context of associated cardiac disorders, these clinical manifestations can be more frequent and more severe. High thyroid hormone levels induce hyperventilation and an increase in the ventilatory response to hypoxia and hypercapnia, particularly through an increase in the central ventilatory drive. Respiratory muscle asthenia results in reduced vital capacity. Several studies have identified an atopic background, with the elevation of serum immunoglobulin E in 30% of patients with Graves, hyperthyroidism. As a result, a warning should be given regarding the association of allergic bronchial asthma in hyperthyroid patients, the evolution of which can be aggravated by β-blockers administered for the control of hyperthyroidism. Clinical studies have also shown an association between Graves' disease treated with propylthiouracil and Wegener's granulomatosis.

Clinical observations have reported the association of hyperthyroidism, particularly Graves' disease, with pulmonary arterial hypertension. Its causes are not completely understood; several mechanisms could be involved: secondary to an autoimmune process, through direct thyroid hormone action, the intervention of endogenous pulmonary vasodilators/vasoconstrictors on pulmonary vessels, a decrease of pulmonary surfactant production and function, and cardiovascular stimulation by the sympathetic-adrenal system. Children born to mothers with Graves' disease may develop severe metabolic and growth disorders, usually associated with severe pulmonary hypertension and respiratory failure.

THYROID HYPERTROPHY (GOITER)

Thyroid nodules more frequently develop in an anterior position which spares the trachea from their compressive action. Unilateral, posterior location or marked hypertrophy of one lobe causes tracheal deviation and upper airway compression. Patients experience dyspnea, stridor, wheezing, and cough. A large intrathoracic/ substernal goiter determines the orthopneic position. The rapid growth of nodules accompanied by perinodular edema may induce severe acute respiratory distress.

AUTOIMMUNE HYPOTHYROIDISM

Many endocrinopathies have an underlying autoimmune component. The association between pulmonary disease and autoimmune thyroid disease has not been emphasized in the literature but there are several reports of the occurrence of lymphocytic interstitial pneumonitis in patients with thyroiditis. Lymphocytic interstitial pneumonitis might be a manifestation of underlying immune dysfunction in autoimmune thyroid disease.

Striking excess cases of treated hypothyroidism amongst a population of idiopathic chronic cough and in nonsmokers with fixed airflow obstruction have shown that idiopathic chronic cough is associated with bronchoalveolar lavage lymphocytosis. This is thought to be resulting from the homing of activated lymphocytes from the primary site of autoimmune inflammation to embryologically related structures, such as the airways. The mechanism of airway inflammation and damage in autoimmune thyroid disease may be analogous to the mechanism of airway complications of inflammatory bowel disease. It is tempting to speculate that other nonspecific symptoms as well as recognized complications of hypothyroidism such as ischemic heart disease are related to similar inflammatory mechanisms.

ASSESSMENT OF LUNG DYSFUNCTION WITH SPIROMETRY IN PATIENTS WITH THYROID DISORDERS

Assessment of pulmonary function with spirometry in patients with thyroid disorders is particularly important considering the fact that low levels of thyroid hormones can trigger bronchial hyperreactivity and obstructive pulmonary disorders. Salih Valjevac et al. 2011 conducted a study to evaluate lung ventilation in patients with thyroid disorders. According to the serum-free triiodothyronine (FT3), free thyroxine (FT4), and thyroid-stimulating hormone (TSH) values total of 60 subjects were included. After an overnight fast, all the subjects underwent full medical assessment and laboratory examinations. The results are shown in **Table 1**.

Average VC%, forced vital capacity (FVC)% and forced expiratory volume in one second (FEV_1)% values were significantly lower in subjects with hyperthyroidism and in subjects with hypothyroidism compared to euthyroid subjects. In a hyperthyroid group of subjects, a significant positive correlation between TSH and FVC% values were observed ($r = 0.51$, $p < 0.05$) (**Table 2**). In the group of subjects with hypothyroidism, a significant positive correlation between serum FT3 levels and VC% ($r = 0.54$, $p < 0.05$) was observed. There was also a negative correlation between serum TSH levels and VC% ($r = -0.627$, $p < 0.01$) and between serum TSH levels

TABLE 1: Spirometry parameters in patients with thyroid dysfunction.

	Hyperthyroid group	Hypothyroid group	Euthyroid group
VC%	94.18 ± 1.24	96.13 ± 1.09	98.54 ± 0.93*
FVC%	92.5 ± 1.47	94.08 ± 1.42	99.16 ± 1.15*
FEV_1%	90.97 ± 2.07	87.59 ± 1.4	93.48 ± 1.1*
FEV_1/FVC%	94.9 ± 2.14	92.0 ± 1.5	93.9 ± 1.25

*Significant difference between euthyroid, hyperthyroid, and hypothyroid groups.

(FEV_1: forced expiratory volume in one second; FVC: forced vital capacity; VC: vital capacity)

TABLE 2: Correlation coefficients between thyroid hormones and lung function parameters in hyperthyroid and hypothyroid groups.

	FT3		FT4		TSH	
	Hyperthyroid group	Hypothyroid group	Hyperthyroid group	Hypothyroid group	Hyperthyroid group	Hypothyroid group
VC%	$r = -0.46$	$r = 0.54$*	$r = -0.305$	$r = 0.414$	$r = 0.322$	$r = -0.627$*
FEV_1%	$r = 0.245$	$r = 0.349$	$r = -0.213$	$r = 0.313$	$r = -0.01$	$r = -0.388$
FVC%	$r = -0.218$	$r = -0.375$	$r = -0.38$	$r = -0.428$	$r = 0.51$*	$r = -0.514$*
FEV_1/FVC%	$r = 0.278$	$r = 0.122$	$r = -0.145$	$r = 0.057$	$r = -0.302$	$r = -0.011$

r = Spearman correlation coefficients.

*$p < 0.05$.

(FEV1: forced expiratory volume in one second; FVC: forced vital capacity; TSH: thyroid-stimulating hormone; VC: vital capacity)

and FVC% ($r = -0.514$, $p < 0.01$) **(Table 2)** in subjects with hypothyroidism. In a euthyroid group of subjects, there was no significant correlation between thyroid hormones, TSH, and the ventilation parameters.

This study showed a significant positive correlation between serum levels of TSH and FVC% in hyperthyroid subjects. Low TSH levels suggest a longer duration of disease, and in these subjects, FVC% was significantly lower. In hypothyroid, there was a negative correlation between serum levels of TSH and FVC%, and between TSH and VC%. In a hypothyroid group of subjects, serum TSH levels ranged from 5 to 20 mIU/L. These findings suggest that the higher levels of TSH and the longer duration of illness are associated with lower FVC% values. The results of the study therefore supported the hypothesis that the degree and the duration of thyroid disorder is associated with lower FVC% values and poor pulmonary function. In this study, the average values of VC%, FVC%, and FEV_1% in both the hyperthyroid and hypothyroid groups were within the reference value. A possible explanation for these results is the fact that the study had included patients with subclinical and clinical hyperthyroidism and hypothyroidism. Thus, this study showed that a thyroid disorder causing hyperthyroidism and hypothyroidism could cause disorders of respiratory function and ventilation.

THYROID DISORDERS AND COUGH

The most common respiratory symptoms in patients suffering from hypothyroidism are cough, shortness of breath, and increased production of sputum. Hypercapnia stimulates the respiratory center, which cannot respond to an increased need for ventilation due to the decreased levels of thyroid hormones. In addition, decreased levels of thyroid hormones lead to decreased expression of β-adrenergic receptors which often causes bronchial tree hyperreactivity. Birring et al. (2005) noted that in patients with low levels of thyroid hormone, there is an increased sensitivity of the cough reflex, increased airway hyperresponsiveness, and an increased number of inflammatory cells in sputum.

THYROID CANCER AND LUNG

Thyroid cancers are the most common endocrine malignant tumors. Papillary thyroid carcinoma (PTC) is the most common form of well-differentiated thyroid cancer constituting > 70% of thyroid malignancies. PTC commonly metastasizes to regional lymph nodes, though distant metastasis may rarely occur accounting for 5% of the patients. Common sites for distant metastasis are the lungs and the bones. The main risk factors for PTC include excess dietary iodine, radiation exposure, Gardner's syndrome, and dyshormonogenetic goiter. Asymptomatic lung metastasis can occur many years after thyroidectomy, hence warranting periodic evaluation after thyroid surgery. Their radiological size is usually < 1 cm and frequently below the spatial resolution of the chest X-ray. Chest computed tomography (CT) is preferred over chest X-rays and it enhances the diagnostic accuracy in most patients with normal chest X-ray findings.

CONCLUSION

Thyroid hormones and disorders have a close interaction with the respiratory system. Hypothyroidism predisposes the patients to hypoventilation, speech disorders, diaphragmatic muscle dysfunction, OSAS, and hypothyroid come in untreated cases of myxedema. In hyperthyroidism, patients develop hyperventilation, rest dyspnea, and respiratory muscle asthenia resulting in reduced vital capacity. Pulmonary arterial hypertension in Graves' disease may occur as a result of several mechanisms. Thyroid hypertrophy can induce compression of the upper airways causing dyspnea, stridor, and cough. Assessment of pulmonary function with spirometry in patients with thyroid disorders is very important. Symptomatic lung metastasis can occur many years after thyroidectomy, hence periodic evaluation after thyroid surgery is required. Thus, in any patient with a thyroid disorder, respiratory disorders should be timely recognized, investigated, and monitored. They are frequently severe, causing an unfavorable evolution of the association between endocrine and respiratory disease.

SUGGESTED READINGS

1. Lencu C, Alexescu T, Petrulea M, Lencu M. Respiratory manifestations in endocrine Diseases. Clujul Medical. 2016;89(4):459-63
2. Saaresranta T, Polo O. Hormones and breathing. Chest. 2002;122(6):2165-82.
3. Sadek SH, Khalifa WA, Azoz AM. Pulmonary consequences of hypothyroidism. Ann Thorac Med. 2017;12(3):204-8.
4. Valjevac S, Hadzovic-Dzuvo A, Valjevac A, Kucukalic-Selimovic E, Lepara O. Assessment of Lung Dysfunction with Spirometry in Patients with Thyroid Disorders. Act Inform Med. 2011;19(1):16-8.
5. Lanfranco F. Sleep apnea syndrome and hypothyroidism. Endocrine. 2013;44(3):551-2.
6. Khardori R, Eagleton LE, Soler NG, McConnachie PR. Lymphocytic Interstitial Pneumonitis in Autoimmune Thyroid Disease. Am J Med. 1991;90(5):649-52.
7. Birring SS. Autoimmune hypothyroidism and respiratory disease. BMJ. 2003;326:295.
8. Ali ER. Assessment of functional lung impairment in patients with thyroid disorders. Egypt J Bronchol. 2016;10:337-47.
9. Erden ES, Babayigit C, Davran R, Akin M, Karazincir S, Isaogullari N, et al. Papillary thyroid carcinoma with lung metastasis arising from dyshormonogenetic goiter: a case report. Case Rep Med. 2013;2013:813167.
10. Hameed SS, Arackal A, Poulose KP. Incidental detection of thyroid lung metastasis 20 years after thyroidectomy. Thyroid Research and Practice. 2013;10(2):83-5.
11. Song HJ, Qiu ZL, Shen CT, Wei WJ, Luo QY. Pulmonary metastases in differentiated thyroid cancer: efficacy of radioiodine therapy and prognostic factors. Eur J Endocrinol. 2015;173(3):399-408.

SECTION

19

RHEUMATOLOGY

233

CHAPTER

Rheumatologists are Becoming Preventive Cardiologists

Anand N Malaviya

ABSTRACT

Shortened lifespan and premature death in rheumatoid arthritis (RA) and other systemic immunoinflammatory rheumatic diseases (SIRDs) have been recognized for decades and confirmed by several population-based studies that have included millions of people. The cause of premature death has been established as accelerated atherosclerotic cardiovascular disease (ASCVD), specifically in coronary arteries, the severity of which is comparable to that of diabetes mellitus. Extensive studies have confirmed the causal role of a combination of atherogenic blood lipids and systemic inflammation in premature ASCVD in RA, SIRDs, as well as in the general population. Consequently, international, and national guidelines have recommended assessment of the 10-year risk for ASCVD, using appropriate 'instruments' to identify individuals at 'high risk' or 'very high risk'. After the initial assessment, statin treatment is recommended to target the level of low-density lipoprotein cholesterol (LDL-C) to < 70 mg/dL in 'high-risk' and < 55 mg/dL in 'very high-risk' individuals.

In recent times, extensive research publications by several groups of workers, led by researchers from Harvard University School of Medicine in Boston, USA, have emphasized the importance of estimating the 'level of inflammation' in the body. Using high-sensitivity C-reactive protein (hs-CRP) levels in the blood as a biomarker of systemic inflammation, it has been confirmed that inflammation could be even more important than atherogenic blood lipids in the causation of premature ASCVD. The recommended treatment for prevention and control of premature ASCVD with high-intensity or very-high intensity statin therapy has been proven to be successful. It has been confirmed that statins not only reduce the level of atherogenic blood lipids but also have an additional effect on reducing inflammation in the body, as measured by hs-CRP blood levels. More recently, Paul Ridker of Harvard Medical School has proposed the notion of 'residual inflammatory risk' (RIR) in patients taking statin therapy, which appears to be more strongly associated with future ASCVD events than 'residual cholesterol risk'. Considering RIR, the possibility of chemically reducing residual inflammation is the current research agenda in the field of ASCVD prevention. The main drugs that are under intense scrutiny from this standpoint and may become part of the treatment armamentarium for ASCVD in the future include low-dose colchicine, inhibitors of proinflammatory cytokines (e.g., interleukin-6 inhibitors), and a few others. In this regard, the appropriate use of disease-modifying anti-rheumatic drugs (DMARDs) for the treatment of RA and other SIRDs has already shown their ameliorative and preventive effects on ASCVD in these diseases. It can be confidently predicted that premature ASCVD in RA, SIRDs, and possibly in the general population is likely to become 'a problem of the past'. With the bourgeoning knowledge about premature ASCVD in RA and other SIRDs, it is obvious that rheumatologists will have to take up the mantal of 'preventive cardiologist' as well!

234

CHAPTER

Hypermobile Joints: A Boon or Bane

Anjana Pandey, Sudhanshu Pandey, PK Maheshwari

ABSTRACT

Joint hypermobility syndrome (JHS) is a connective tissue disorder characterized by a joint greater than normal range of motion. It is a dominant inherited disorder, distinct from other disorders, such as Marfan syndrome and Ehlers–Danlos syndrome (EDS). JHS is associated with neuromusculoskeletal symptoms, including significant pain, and shares some features with more serious hereditary disorders, such as osteogenesis imperfecta, EDS, and Marfan syndrome.

INTRODUCTION

Joint hypermobility syndrome (JHS) or hypermobility syndrome (HMS) or benign joint hypermobility syndrome (BJHS) is a disorder of connective tissue disease in which a joint has a range of motion greater than normal. The HMS was first described in 1967 by Kirk et al. as the occurrence of musculoskeletal symptoms in hypermobile healthy persons. HMS is a connective tissue disorder described as "generalized articular hypermobility," with or without subluxation or dislocation. It is a dominant inherited disorder. This syndrome is different from other disorders that cause local joint hypermobility and generalized joint laxity, such as Marfan syndrome and Ehlers–Danlos syndrome (EDS). Generalized joint hypermobility (GJH) may not have any adverse effects, and it can be an asset for various profession (music, dance, athletics, yoga, etc.), but in JHS, the hypermobility is associated with neuromusculoskeletal manifestations including significant pain. Less severe features of some of the serious hereditary disorders of connective tissue, such as osteogenesis imperfecta, EDS, and Marfan syndrome are seen in JHS, all of which can have joint hypermobility as a feature. JHS is synonymous with the EDS hypermobility type (formerly EDS type III).

PATHOPHYSIOLOGY

The pathophysiology is still under covers, it appears to be a systemic collagen abnormality. The ratio of collagen (type I, II, and III) is reduced in the skin. Though the diagnostic criteria include joint hypermobility but it also affects muscles of various organs, such as cardiac tissue, smooth muscle in the female genital system, and the gastrointestinal system. It can also affect the joint position sense.

PREVALENCE

The true prevalence of JHS is unknown. It ranges between 5 and 43%. Age, sex, and ethnicity are all important factors in JHS. Increased prevalence is seen in females and in non-Caucasians. Joint mobility is maximum at birth and subsequent decrease is seen at around 9-12 years of age. Decrease in joint mobility and hypermobility are generally seen with advancing age. In general, hypermobility is more common in children than adults, is more common in girls than in boys, more common in Asian, African, and middle eastern people.

CLINICAL PRESENTATION

The myriad of symptoms and signs are seen, most common symptom being joint pains in one or multiple joints.

Acute or traumatic sprains, meniscus tears, acute or recurrent dislocations or subluxations of the shoulder, patella, metacarpophalangeal joint and temporomandibular joint, bruising, traumatic arthritis, chronic or nontraumatic fractures, soft tissue rheumatism-tendinitis, epicondylitis, rotator cuff syndrome, synovitis, juvenile episodic synovitis, bursitis, chondromalacia, scoliosis, marfanoid habitus, varicose veins, rectal or uterine prolapse, thin skin, nerve compression disorders, such as carpal tunnel syndrome, tarsal tunnel syndrome, thoracic outlet syndrome, back pain, osteoarthritis, congenital hip dislocation, exercise-related/postexercise-related pains, nocturnal leg pains, and low nocturnal sleep quality. The association of BJHS with mitral valve prolapse (MVP) is a subject of controversy. Primary care physicians should refer patients with hypermobility in whom cardiac findings suggest MVP to a cardiologist for further evaluation to rule out more serious cardiac abnormalities and connective tissue disorders.

Physical examination demonstrates pain, occasionally mild effusions are seen but clinically significant inflammation is not present in patients with JHS.

DIAGNOSTIC CRITERIA

Assessment of patient on the Beighton score is essential for making the diagnosis. The first step is to calculate the Beighton score, which is a measure of generalized joint laxity. Physicians calculate this score by doing five simple maneuvers **(Fig. 1)** that can be completed in 45–60 seconds. A score of 4 or more is pointer toward generalized joint laxity. Majority of patients show symmetrical joint laxity. The Brighton criteria were developed to establish diagnostic criteria for BJHS. It helps physicians to distinguish BJHS from other connective tissue disorders.

Brighton Criteria

Major Criteria

- Beighton score of ≥4/9
- Arthralgia for >3 months in >4 joints

Minor Criteria

- Beighton score of 1–3
- Arthralgia in 1–3 joints
- History of joint dislocation
- Soft tissue lesions >3
- Marfan-like habitus
- Skin striae, hyperextensibility, or scarring
- Eye signs, lid laxity
- History of varicose veins, hernia, and visceral prolapse

For a diagnosis to be made either both of the major criteria must be present or one major and two minor or four minor.

Requirement for diagnosis of HMS:
- Two major criteria
- One major criteria + two minor criteria
- Four minor criteria
- Two minor criteria and unequivocally affected first-degree relative in family history

Beighton Score (Fig. 1)

- A passive dorsiflexion of the little finger above 90° (1 point for each hand).
- Bringing the thumb passive against the ventral side of the forearm (1 point for each thumb).
- Hyperextension of the elbow above 10° (1 point for each elbow)
- Hyperextension of the knee above 10° (1 point for each knee)
- Flexion of the trunk, whit knees straight, and the palms flat on the ground (1 point)

Benign joint hypermobility syndrome is diagnosis of exclusion. If patients present with painful or swollen joints most important differential is infective, inflammatory, or autoimmune causes. Investigations include a complete blood cell count, C-reactive protein, erythrocyte sedimentation rate, rheumatoid factor,

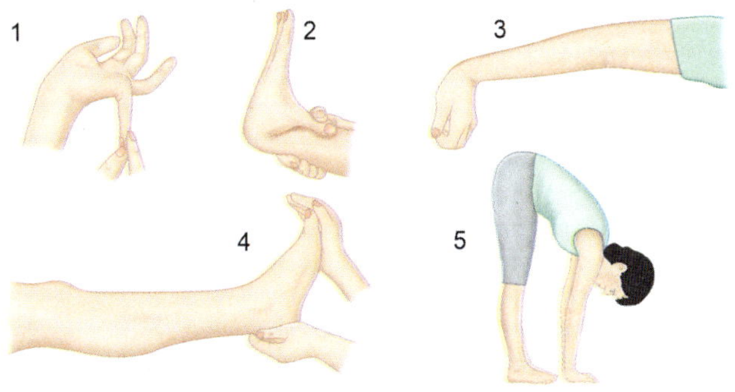

FIG. 1: Beighton and Horan criteria, generalized joint laxity is present when four or more of five tests are positive, including contralateral knee hyperextension.

antinuclear antibody test, serum complement (C3, C4, and CH50) levels, and serum immunoglobulin (IgG, IgM, and IgA) levels. Other differential diagnosis is from Marfan syndrome, EDS, and osteogenesis imperfecta. Generalized hypermobility is common to all these hereditary connective tissue disorders and share many overlapping features. Abovementioned conditions can be distinguished from each other by certain distinct features.

MANAGEMENT

Most important step in management of patient is to counsel him/her regarding the benign and nonprogressive nature of this disease. There is no specific medical treatment. Lifestyle modification, guided exercise regimen, joint protection, and proper body mechanics are effective way to achieve good outcomes. To control pain nonsteroidal anti-inflammatory drugs (NSAIDs) or acetaminophen can be used.

Long-term management typically focuses on physical therapies like modification of inciting activities. Another important step in treating HMS is education. Excessive joint movement is associated with the development of symptoms in patients. Often, vigorous and repetitive activities have been considered as aggravating factors. Patient should be educated to not go over the normal joint range because extreme joint range can cause a more unstable joint. Psychosomatic features, such as fatigue, anxiety, and depression are sometimes associated with HMS, and all these must be properly addressed to achieve good quality of life.

Over training, poor pacing, too many performances or athletic competitions, and focusing on joint flexibility rather than stability may all increase joint pain and the risk of injury. If avoidance of these activities is not an acceptable, other approaches can be tried. NSAIDs taken before performance often may reduce symptoms but best resort is to start muscle strengthening program to provide stability to both muscle and joints. Active mobilization of joints, strength training, stretching, and proprioception exercises is effective ways to reduce joint damage.

Along with physical therapy, osteopathic manipulative treatment (OMT) is a useful adjunctive treatment modality for BJHS. It helps in articular release resulting in increased joint motion, and decrease in pain as well as improved blood circulation, lymphatic drainage, and joint position sense. Current recommendation is to limit OMT not more than three times per week.

PROGNOSIS

The prognosis of BJHS is generally good because of its nonprogressive nature. However, patients need to be aware of the potential sequelae that have an increased frequency associated with BJHS.

CONCLUSION

Hypermobility is a common cause of unexplained joint pain but lack of awareness at primary level often delays the diagnosis as well as effective management. Therefore, physicians need to be aware of the clinical presentation of BJHS to enhance their diagnostic acumen. The Brighton criteria are used to make the diagnosis. Education, activity modification, and exercise therapy to improve muscular stability and proprioception at specific joints are essential to symptom management. Manual therapy (OMT) should be used judiciously. Future clinical trials are necessary to determine effective clinical management strategies for patients with BJHS.

SUGGESTED READINGS

1. Kirk JA, Ansell BM, Bywaters EG. The hypermobility syndrome. Musculoskeletal complaints associated with generalized joint hypermobility. Ann Rheum Dis. 1967;26(5):419-25.
2. Castori M, Morlino S, Celletti C, Ghibellini G, Bruschini M, Grammatico P, et al. Re-writing the natural history of pain and related symptoms in the joint hypermobility syndrome/Ehlers-Danlos syndrome, hypermobility type. Am J Med Genet A. 2013;161A(12):2989-3004.
3. Ross J, Grahame R. Joint hypermobility syndrome. BMJ. 2011;342:275-8.
4. Larsson LG, Baum J, Mudholkar GS. Hypermobility: Features and differential incidence between the sexes. Arthritis Rheum. 1987;30:1426-30.
5. Simpson MR. Benign joint hypermobility syndrome: evaluation, diagnosis, and management. J Am Osteopath Assoc. 2006;106(9):531-6.
6. Grahame R. The revised (Brighton 1998) criteria for the diagnosis of benign joint hypermobility syndrome (BJHS). J Rheumatol. 2000;27:1777-9.
7. Russek LN. Examination and treatment of a patient with hypermobility syndrome. Phys Ther. 2000;80:386-98.

235
CHAPTER

Skin and Eyes: The Windows in Clinical Rheumatology

Arup Kumar Kundu, Kaushik Basu

ABSTRACT

The skin and the eyes act as windows to underlying systemic rheumatologic diseases. Skin involvement in rheumatoid arthritis (RA) includes rheumatoid nodules, pyoderma gangrenosum (PG), Sweet's syndrome, or vasculitic skin ulcers. Nail changes in psoriasis are common and may be associated with distal interphalangeal (DIP) joint involvement in psoriatic arthritis (PsA); arthritis can precede, or copresent, or develop after the skin involvement. Skin involvement in lupus may be acute, subacute, or chronic, while the later most commonly causes scarring. In dermatomyositis heliotrope rash, shawl sign, V-sign, and Gottron's papules are the classic skin lesions, while in vasculitis skin lesions are determined by the caliber of the vessel involved. In addition to different symptoms, dermatological involvement is a source of distress and cosmesis.

Rheumatoid arthritis, ankylosing spondylitis (AS), and PsA are associated with sight-threatening inflammatory eye diseases. Other than sight loss, these are chronic, recurrent, painful and debilitating conditions, which may require long-term treatment with topical corticosteroid, ocular lubricant, systemic corticosteroid as well as immunosuppression. Uveitis may present as grittiness along with redness of eyes and diminution of vision, commonly in spondyloarthritis (SpA), or juvenile idiopathic arthritis (JIA). Scleritis is a painful condition, which may lead to blindness and may be associated with RA, systemic lupus erythematosus (SLE), or vasculitis. Retinal vasculitis may occur in SLE, antiphospholipid syndrome (APS), and Behçet's disease. Giant cell arteritis (GCA) may present with sudden-onset blindness. Ulcerative keratitis (peripheral) is common in RA or SLE vasculitis. Keratoconjunctivitis sicca is common in Sjögren's syndrome, RA, and SLE. A close liaison between ophthalmologist and rheumatologist is necessary for management of eye involvement.

INTRODUCTION

The skin, being the largest organ of the body, is frequently involved in rheumatologic diseases and since it is one of the most visible organs, often gives to certain clues for diagnoses or prognostication in various rheumatic diseases. The common rheumatological diseases with classical skin involvement are described in the following text.

Major types of skin involvement in rheumatoid arthritis (RA) include rheumatoid nodules, pyoderma gangrenosum (PG), Sweet's syndrome, or vasculitic skin ulcer. Rheumatoid nodules occurs over pressure areas such as extensor surface of forearms, olecranon process, extensor surfaces of fingers, ischial tuberosities, heels and posterior surface of the scalp. They are usually painless, firm, deeply placed, freely movable and have association with severe disease, rheumatoid vasculitis or interstitial lung disease (ILD), or presence of high-titer rheumatoid factor. Biopsy of the nodules reveals necrobiosis-fibrinoid degeneration of the connective tissue with surrounding histiocytes. Rheumatoid vasculitis occurs late in the disease, predominantly in high seropositive individuals and may be present as palpable purpura, macules, nodules, ulcers or infarcts. Neutrophilic dermatoses encompass Sweet's syndrome and PG. PG appears quickly to form a large, clean-based, well-marginated ulcer usually over the lower limbs. Sweet's syndrome appears as an erythematous lesion with small vesicles, which might be painful and associated with fever.

Psoriasis is common (2–3% of general population) but neither it is essential to co-occurrence with psoriatic arthritis (PsA), nor does the severity of the two conditions go hand in hand. Types of psoriasis include guttate, chronic plaque type, localized pustular, generalized pustular and erythrodermic variety. Nail changes (pitting, onycholysis, subungual hyperkeratosis and nail dystrophy) are common and maybe associated with distal interphalangeal (DIP) joint involvement in PsA; there may be peripheral arthritis ± sacroiliitis. Arthritis can precede (10%) or copresent (20%) with skin involvement; obtaining family history of psoriasis is important. Examination of scalp, buttocks, ears, genitalia, and body folds are important to reveal small psoriatic lesions.

Skin findings of reactive arthritis (previous Reiter's syndrome) include circinate balanitis, which are serpiginous, erosive or crusted lesions present over the glans penis. Keratoderma blennorrhagica may develop over soles and palms of patients which look exactly like psoriatic skin lesions, although, more hyperkeratotic; even biopsy cannot differentiate between the two conditions.

Patients of systemic lupus erythematosus (SLE) can develop a wide array of specific and nonspecific skin lesions. Nonspecific skin symptoms are more frequent in patients with active SLE or overlap syndromes. **Table 1** demonstrates various skin manifestations of SLE.

TABLE 1: Skin manifestations of lupus.

Subtype	Clinical presentation	Systemic association	Scarring
Acute	• "Butterfly rash" • Photosensitive erythema • Upper extremity erythematous papules/plaques **(Fig. 1)** • Palatal ulcers/cheilitis **(Fig. 2)** • Vasculitis (painful nodules on palms/soles) • TEN-like lesions	Almost always	Nil
Subacute	• Papulosquamous rash over trunk/arms • Photosensitive erythema	• 50% • Anti-Ro/La antibodies • Frequently drug induced (e.g., ACE-inhibitors)	Less common
Chronic	• Localized erythrosquamous patch/plaque with follicular plugging (in sun-exposed areas) • Commonly on face and scalp (alopecia) • Lupus profundus/ panniculitis (subcutaneous nodules) • Chilblain lupus (tender, bluish plaques/nodules in cold-exposed areas)	• 5–10% • DLE (5–10%) **(Fig. 3)** may develop into SLE over time	Recurrent

(ACE: angiotensin-converting enzyme; DLE: discoid lupus erythematosus; SLE: systemic lupus erythematosus; TEN: toxic epidermal necrolysis)

Source: Adapted from Mazzoni D, et al. (2021).

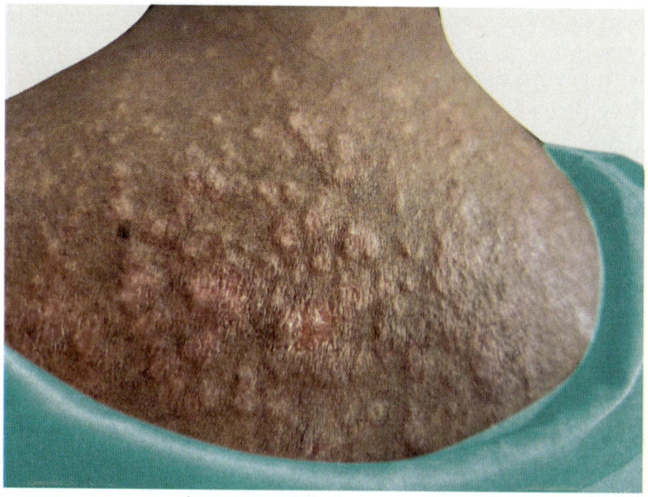

FIG. 1: Erythematous papules with recurrent cutaneous flare in systemic lupus erythematosus.

Courtesy: Dr. Bodhibrata Banerjee, SR, Medical College, Kolkata.

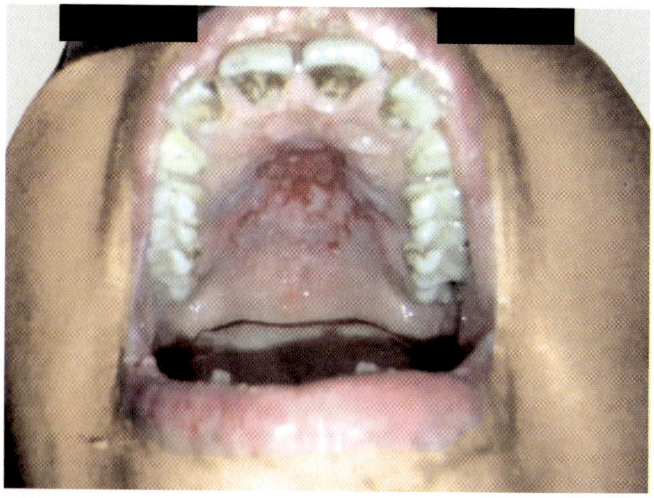

FIG. 2: Painless, active palatal ulcer in lupus.

Courtesy: Dr. Bodhibrata Banerjee, SR, Medical College, Kolkata.

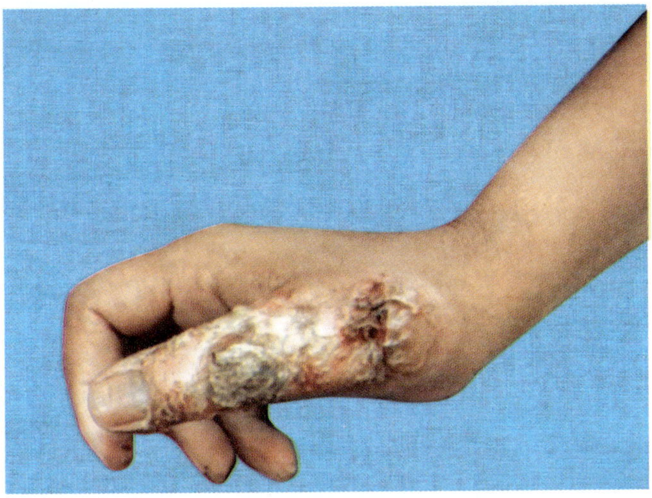

FIG. 3: Hypertrophic discoid lupus erythematosus.
Courtesy: Dr. Bodhibrata Banerjee, SR, Medical College, Kolkata.

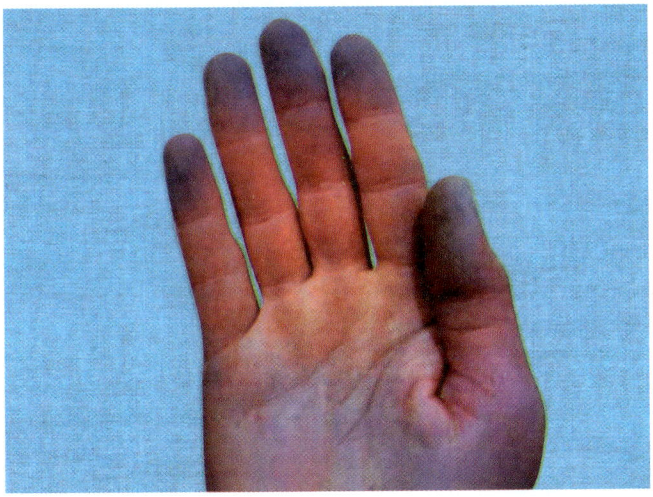

FIG. 4: Raynaud's phenomenon in systemic sclerosis.
Courtesy: Dr. Bodhibrata Banerjee, SR, Medical College, Kolkata.

Neonatal lupus includes malar rash in neonates, and may have cytopenias and hepatic diseases, and are usually associated with maternal Ro/La antibodies that have been passively transferred to the neonates; the lesions usually subside spontaneously, which have no relation with development of lupus later in life.

Frequently encountered dermatologic signs of systemic sclerosis (SSc) include Raynaud's phenomenon (RP) **(Fig. 4)** in response to cold or emotional stress, symmetric skin thickening, finger swelling, sclerodactyly, digital pits and fingertip ulcers, diffuse hyperpigmentation, telangiectasias and calcinosis cutis. Sclerosis means hardening, which is due to excessive deposition of collagenous tissue in interstitium with associated fibrosis. In limited SSc, the skin induration is limited to the face and distal extremities, associated with RP and predominant telangiectasias. Telangiectasia mostly affects the face and lips but may be found over the neck and hands. In diffuse SSc, skin indurations are more generalized and are associated with diffuse hyperpigmentation of the skin. RP may be triphasic (white, blue, and red) or biphasic (white and blue) when exposed to cold with subsequent rewarming. History of RP often predates the onset of typical symptoms of SSC. Differential diagnoses would include Morphea (generalized, linear, circumscribed, or mixed), eosinophilic fasciitis, diabetic scleredema, chronic graft-versus-host disease (GvHD) and silica exposure. Patients with digital ulcers usually develop internal organ involvement 2–3 years earlier than the patients without digital pits/ulcers. Calcinosis is key feature in CREST (calcinosis, RP, esophageal dysmotility, sclerodactyly, and telangiectasia) syndrome but may develop in other forms of systemic sclerosis. Salt-pepper appearance of the skin may be found due to a combination of hypopigmentation and hyperpigmentation side by side, predominantly found over scalp, face, neck, and upper part of the trunk.

Dermatomyositis may manifest in skin in the form of: Heliotrope rash—a violacious erythematous rash over the eyes and forehead, malar erythematous rash, Gottron's papules—plaques or papules over the metacarpophalangeal joints or interphalangeal joints, V-sign and shawl sign—which are erythematous rash over the anterior upper chest and the upper back respectively. Hyperkeratosis of the palms and lateral surface of the first 2/3 fingers (mechanic's hand) may be seen in antisynthetase syndrome (may be associated with ILD/fever/arthritis). RP and calcinosis may be associated with dermatomyositis. Various myositis specific-autoantibodies and myositis-associated autoantibodies may help in prognostication in patients with dermatomyositis.

Cutaneous vasculitis might be a skin manifestation of systemic vasculitis (palpable purpura in IgA vasculitis with renal involvement) or vasculitis limited only to the skin (cutaneous small vessel vasculitis). Important factor for determining the sign would be specific vessels involved in vasculitis. If the small-sized arteries are involved they may present as palpable purpura, urticarial rashes, or morbilliform eruptions **(Fig. 5)**. Medium-sized artery involvement would present as subcutaneous nodules, ulcers, gangrene, mononeuritis multiplex and livedo reticularis. Small-vessel vasculitis includes antineutrophil cytoplasmic antibodies (ANCA)-associated vasculitis and immune complex vasculitis though each of these may "spillover" to the medium vessels.

Erythema nodosum is common and usually self-limiting, primarily septal panniculitis without vasculitis that is secondary to some underlying disorders such

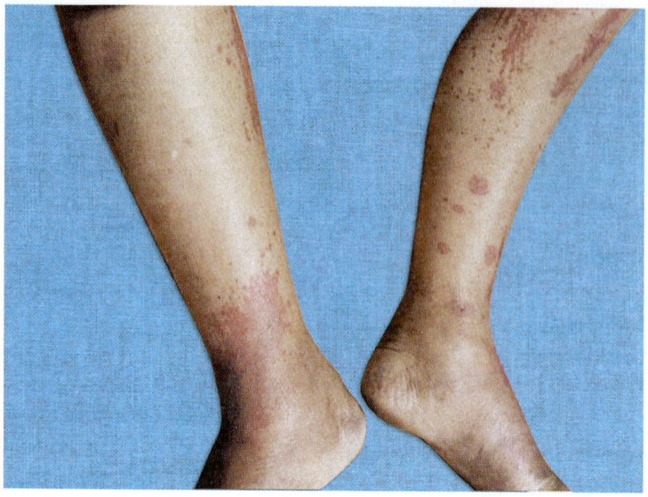

FIG. 5: Petechiae, purpura, ecchymosis in small-vessel vasculitis.
Courtesy: Dr. Bodhibrata Banerjee, SR, Medical College, Kolkata.

BOX 1: Ocular manifestations in various rheumatological diseases.

- *RA*: Scleritis, keratitis, dry eyes
- *AS*: AAU
- *Sjögren's syndrome*: Dry eyes
- *Reactive arthritis*: AAU, conjunctivitis
- *IBD*: AAU, scleritis
- *SLE*: Eyelid discoid lesion, retinal vasculitis
- *GCA*: ION, retinal vasculitis
- *Takayasu's arteritis*: Retinal arteriovenous anastomosis
- *JIA*: Acute/chronic anterior uveitis
- *Sarcoidosis*: Anterior uveitis, vitritis
- *GPA*: Orbital pseudotumor, scleritis, keratitis
- *Behçet's disease*: Anterior uveitis, retinal vasculitis
- *Kawasaki disease*: Conjunctival hyperemia
- *Polyarteritis nodosa*: Cranial nerve palsies, hypertensive retinopathy
- *Gout*: Tophi deposition in eyelids (rare)
- *IgG4-related disease*: Dacryoadenitis, proptosis

(AAU: acute anterior uveitis; AS: ankylosing spondylitis; GCA: giant cell arteritis; GPA: granulomatosis with polyangiitis; IBD: inflammatory bowel disease; IgG: immunoglobulin G; ION: ischemic optic neuropathy; JIA: juvenile idiopathic arthritis; RA: rheumatoid arthritis; SLE: systemic lupus erythematosus)

as tuberculosis, sarcoidosis, leprosy, streptococcal infections, histoplasmosis, inflammatory bowel disease (IBD), SLE, Behçet's disease or exposure to certain drugs such as penicillin or sulfonamides. In half of the cases, the cause is not detected, but due to its well-known benign and self-limiting nature, it is usually treated with nonsteroidal anti-inflammatory drugs (NSAIDs), topical applications (potassium iodide), and colchicine ± corticosteroids.

Cutaneous emergencies in rheumatology recorded are Stevens-Johnson syndrome, toxic epidermal necrolysis (TEN), erythroderma, GvHD, generalized pustular psoriasis, and autoimmune bullous diseases.

THE EYES IN RHEUMATOLOGY

The eyes are commonly affected in various rheumatologic diseases. Though there are considerable overlaps, **Box 1** shows common areas of the eye involved in certain rheumatologic diseases.

Uveitis is commonly referred to a rheumatologist by an ophthalmologist to rule out common infectious and rheumatological diseases confined to the eyes. Sometimes the referrals are to identify the underlying systemic diseases (40%), or at other times to facilitate and maintain immunosuppressive treatment.

Approximately 50% of acute anterior uveitis (AAU) is HLA-B27 positive and majority among them have other features of axial SPA **(Fig. 6)**. HLA-B27-associated AAU is usually recurrent, mostly unilateral and the attacks are of short duration. Nearly 5–10% patients having IBD and PsA may also develop uveitis, where many of them suffer bilateral diseases, which are chronic in duration. Sarcoidosis commonly presents with granulomatous uveitis, but may spillover to other parts of the eye such as choroiditis or retinal vasculitis, though florid features of sarcoidosis are absent in majority of these patients. Among the several types of JIA, in oligoarticular JIA, most commonly in girls between 2 and 8 years develop chronic anterior uveitis, while most of them are ANA (antinuclear antibody)-positive. In many instances, uveitis is silent and hence mandatory periodic eye

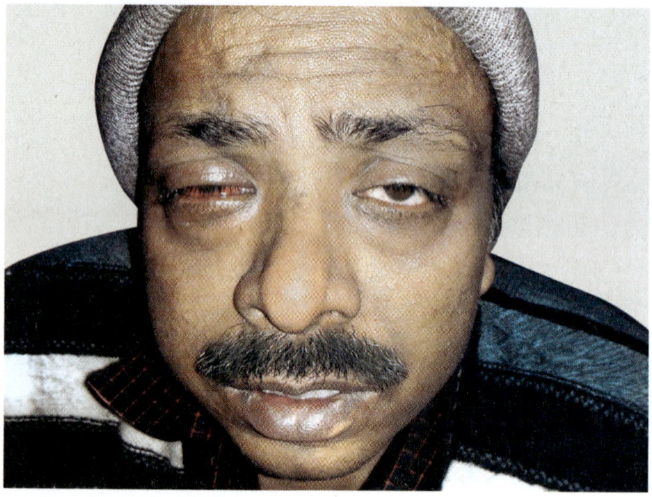

FIG. 6: Uveitis in a patient of ankylosing spondylitis.
Courtesy: Dr. Bodhibrata Banerjee, SR, Medical College, Kolkata.

examinations are required in children with JIA, especially those who are ANA-positive. Uveitis in Behçet's disease is usually bilateral, recurrent and associated with retinal vasculitis. Other rarer diseases associated with uveitis are relapsing polychondritis, Cogan syndrome, and various autoinflammatory diseases.

Scleral diseases may be scleritis or episcleritis, both of which cause redness of eyes without involving the palpebral conjunctiva; episcleritis causes more scratchy sensation rather that pain, less ocular complications and is rarely associated with systemic diseases. About 40% of patients having scleritis may have systemic diseases. Scleritis may be found in long-standing, seropositive RA, which may be associated with other extra-articular manifestations such as subcutaneous nodules, vasculitis, or pleural effusion **(Fig. 7)**. Scleritis may be the initial manifestation of granulomatosis with polyangiitis (GPA). Other causes of scleritis include IBD, relapsing polychondritis or SLE, when infections are ruled out.

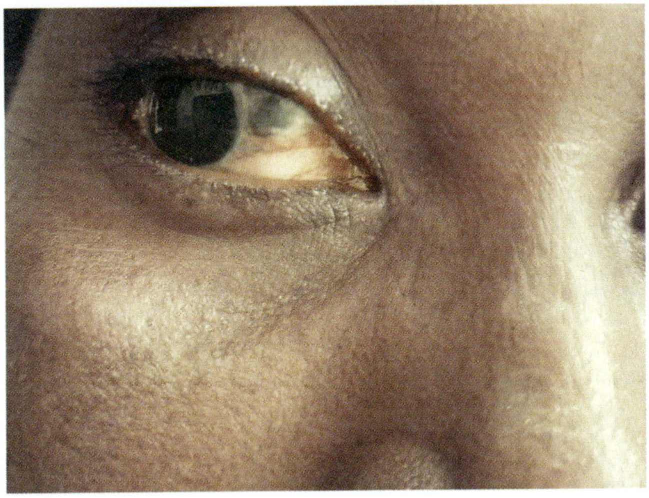

FIG. 7: Scleral thinning with choroidal staphyloma in long-standing rheumatoid arthritis.
Courtesy: Dr. Bodhibrata Banerjee, SR, Medical College, Kolkata.

Retinal vasculitis may be due to inflammation or retinal vessel occlusion. In Behçet's disease, retinal vasculitis is the most common ocular complication, which may involve both retinal veins and artery. In SLE, the retinal capillaries may be involved. Involvement may range from asymptomatic retinal vessel occlusion detected in routine eye check-up to more extensive disease, usually associated with APS or neurolupus. Lupus choroidopathy is an uncommon complication where detachments of retinal pigment epithelium occur, usually associated with a severe clinical lupus, vasculitis, or nephritis with elevated blood pressure. GCA may be complicated by central retinal artery occlusion though sudden blindness due to ischemic optic neuropathy (ION) is a more classic presentation.

Drug like hydroxychloroquine is generally safe at normal doses, but higher amounts can damage the retina and may give rise to keratopathy, ciliary body changes and retinopathy; bull's eye maculopathy, a type of retinopathy, is very rare though reported. Periodic eye checkup and fundus autofluorescence (FAF) imaging should be done yearly after consuming the drug for continuously 5 years.

Orbital inflammatory disease occurs predominantly with ANCA-associated granulomatous vasculitis and sarcoidosis, usually associated with proptosis of the involved eye with pain, diplopia, and chemosis. Corneal disease may be interstitial keratitis or peripheral ulcerative keratitis (PUK). Interstitial keratitis may be found in Cogan syndrome, characterized by nonsuppurative inflammation and pain, lacrimation, photophobia and conjunctival redness, which typically responds to local corticosteroids. PUK is reported in RA, Sjögren's syndrome, SLE, ANCA-associated vasculitis, relapsing polychondritis, and systemic sclerosis, which is identified by pain and peripheral corneal infiltrates. Keratoconjunctivitis sicca may be a presenting feature of Sjögren's syndrome, or presents late in RA or SLE; symptoms include gritty eyes, foreign body sensation, photophobia, and pain. Diagnosis is usually made with Schirmer's test showing decreased tear production, or decreased tear film breakup time.

SUGGESTED READINGS

1. Mazzoni D, Kubler P, Muir J. Recognising skin manifestations of rheumatological disease. Aust J Gen Pract. 2021;50(12):873-78.
2. Murray PI, Rauz S. The eye and inflammatory rheumatic diseases: The eye and rheumatoid arthritis, ankylosing spondylitis, psoriatic arthritis. Best Pract Res Clin Rheumatol. 2016;30(5):802-25.

236

CHAPTER

Erythema Nodosum: A Clinician's Approach

Chandan Das

ABSTRACT

Erythema nodosum is the most common form of panniculitis, primarily manifesting as tender, erythematous nodules on the lower limbs, particularly the pretibial area. While its exact cause remains elusive, it is believed to result from a hypersensitivity reaction to various antigenic triggers. While idiopathic cases are frequent, it is crucial to rule out potential underlying causes before diagnosing primary erythema nodosum. This condition can serve as an early indicator of systemic disorders such as infections, inflammatory conditions, malignancies, or medication reactions.

Common causative factors encompass streptococcal infections, tuberculosis, systemic diseases such as sarcoidosis, Behçet's disease, and inflammatory bowel disease, as well as drug reactions and pregnancy. This chapter outlines a diagnostic approach to promptly identify and manage the underlying condition. The proposed algorithm involves assessing core symptoms, conducting a systematic diagnostic work-up, considering potential differential diagnoses, and suggesting appropriate treatments. Although various treatments alleviate erythema nodosum symptoms, they do not address the root causes. An accurate diagnosis facilitates a holistic management strategy that targets the underlying processes responsible.

INTRODUCTION

Panniculitis is understood as a heterogeneous group of subcutaneous tissue inflammation, which can be broadly classified into either lobular or septal type. Erythema nodosum (EN) is the most common form of panniculitis and is the prototypic septal panniculitis but without vasculitis. In fact, it is the most common cause of inflammatory nodules seen in clinical practice.

This is a delayed-type hypersensitivity reaction which is self-limiting and benign, usually seen on the lower part of the body. It was first described by an English physician Dr Robert Willan in 1798. But the earlier records of this entity have been described in Vienna from a letter from Mozart writing about a lesion in his father which possibly was an EN. The aim of this chapter is to analyze the recent literature on the triggering factors and a simplified diagnostic and treatment algorithm.

EPIDEMIOLOGY

Though EN can occur in any age-group, it is most commonly seen in females in their second to fourth decade. Male to female ratio is 1:5 in most of the studies. Specific causes of EN vary according to the triggering factors in different geographical and ethnic differences. For example, the trigger of EN in the Indian subcontinent is usually an infection, but in the Hispanic population, it is commonly associated with sarcoidosis.

PATHOGENESIS

Erythema nodosum is generally considered a delayed-type hypersensitivity reaction from exposure to various antigenic stimuli. Though the mechanism is not completely understood, it is postulated that the deposition of immune complexes on the small venules of the septal subcutaneous fat triggers inflammation and subsequent tissue injury. Expression of certain adhesive molecules such as vascular cell adhesion molecules-1, P-selectin, and E-selectin are contributory in the pathogenesis. Increased levels of cytokines such as interleukin 6 (IL-6), IL-8, IL-12, and interferon gamma (INF-γ) lead to nutrophilic recruitment and their activation, later leading to oxidative tissue damage due to reactive oxygen species formation and tumor necrosis factor-alpha (TNF-α) production. All these factors may lead to granuloma formation. Few data also hint at genetic predisposition, especially in the TNF-α-ll allele in sarcoidosis and many established susceptibility loci in inflammatory bowel disease (IBD).

CLINICAL PICTURE

Erythema nodosum can be clinically classified as either primary (idiopathic) or secondary type. It starts as an acute-onset tender symmetrical nodule or a plaque of 1–6 cm in diameter. They are typically found on distal lower limbs in pretibial area, but they can also be seen on ankles, thighs, or even on forearms. This is characteristically a self-limiting condition, resolving in 1–6 weeks often changing its appearance from bright red to brownish to sometimes into a bruise-like lesion (erythema contusiformis). Healing of the lesions is not associated with atrophy or scarring. It does not ulcerate like other nodules and can also be recurrent.

Secondary EN is associated with systemic symptoms such as myalgia, fever, weight loss, cough, headache, arthalgia, lymphadenopathy, and gastrointestinal (GI) symptoms. Idiopathic primary EN is rarely accompanied by these symptoms and they are usually recurrent.

HISTOLOGICAL FEATURES

The characteristic histological finding of EN is septal panniculitis without vasculitis. Early stage is infiltrated with mixed inflammatory cells such as neutrophils, lymphocytes, histiocytes, and eosinophils. In the later phase, the neutrophils are replaced by multinucleated giant cells. A relatively specific finding of radial Miescher's granuloma consists of a few macrophages and histiocytes arranged around a star-shaped cleft in the center. But this is not a pathognomic finding.

SPECIFIC ETIOLOGY

Approximately, 32–73% of EN are of unknown etiology which may be considered as primary or idiopathic EN. The etiology also varies according to ethnicity, geographical area, and seasons. Among the most common identifiable causes are infections [*streptococcus* and tuberculosis (TB)], sarcoidosis, Behçet's disease, IBD, drugs, malignancy, and pregnancy. Some cases of EN have been reported post-coronavirus disease 2019 (COVID-19) infection and even after vaccination. EN has even some predictive and prognostic information, e.g., it accompanies or sometimes precedes a flare of IBD or its presence in sarcoidosis indicates a lesser aggressive form. In Behçet's disease, its presence is a very important diagnostic clue as it is found in 44% of cases and is a part of its diagnostic criteria. In sarcoidosis, it is the most common skin lesion. A lot of infections such as bacterial, fungal, viral, and protozoa are present with EN. They are the most common cause in tropical countries such as India, most notable being pharyngeal streptococcal infection. In TB-endemic areas, nearly half of the EN cases are diagnosed with TB within 1 month of their EN diagnosis. Both Mycobacterium tuberculosis and atypical mycobacteria can trigger EN. A long list of infections can cause EN; among them, fungal infections and *Salmonella* infections are notable.

Drugs also frequently give rise to EN (2.9–5%), especially oral contraceptive pill (OCP) and sulfonamides. Certain vaccines such as diphtheria–pertussis–tetanus (DPT), Bacille Calmette–Guérin (BCG), hepatitis B, and anti-rabies can also give rise to EN. The role of hormones in the development of EN has also been emphasized as it frequently appears in pregnancy (2–6%) and OCP users. Malignancy should be suspected in unexplained EN or in poor response to treatment and recurrent EN. Hematological malignancy has more association with this compared to solid neoplasms. It may indicate relapse of the parent disease. Even radiation treatment can precipitate EN.

DIAGNOSTIC APPROACH TO A CASE OF ERYTHEMA NODOSUM

Due to the extensive list of possible etiologies of EN, we need to adopt a cost-effective approach to reach a specific diagnosis and its treatment.

Good history and physical finding of acute, tender plaques or nodules on bilateral shins without ulceration strongly suggest a diagnosis of EN. Skin biopsy is not mandatory to confirm the diagnosis.

Indications of biopsy in suspected EN are cases with atypical presentation such as location other than shin of

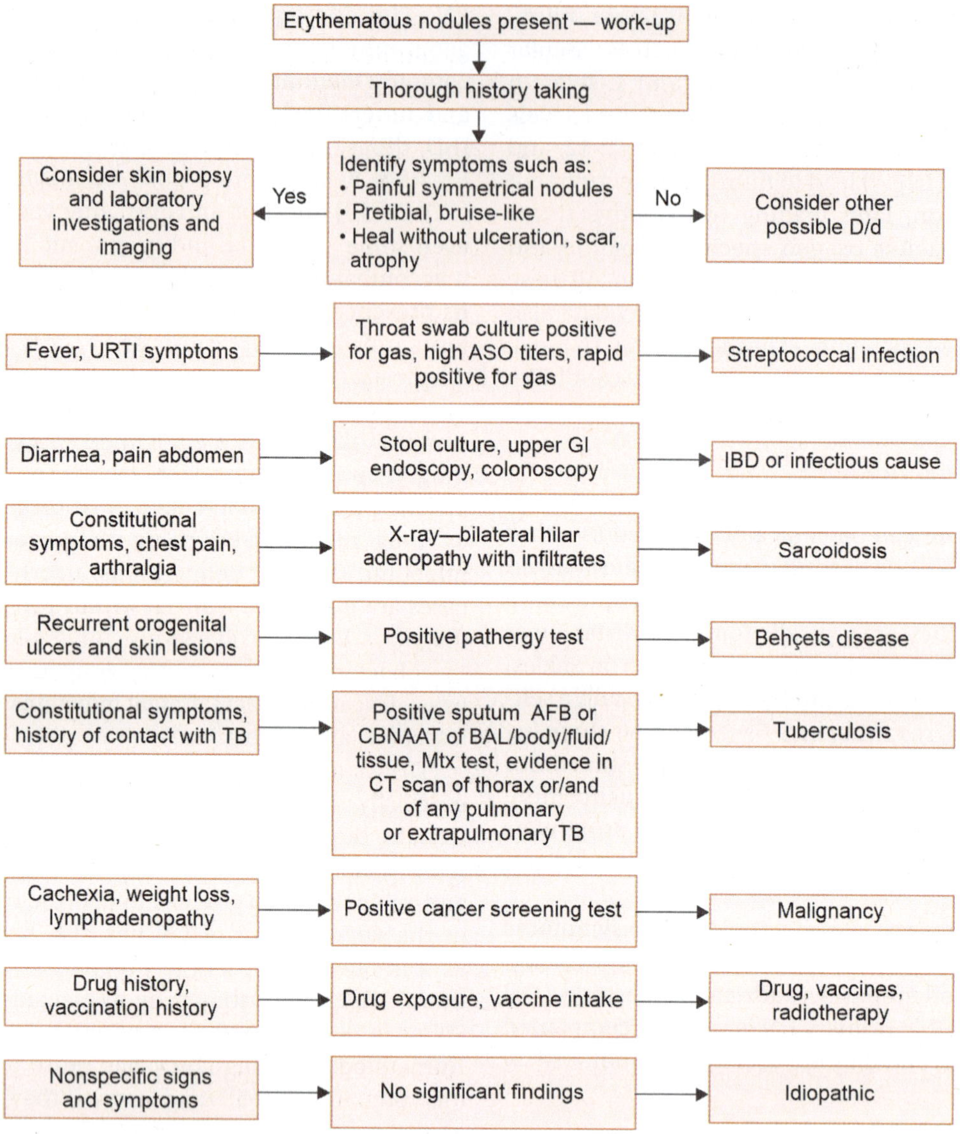

FLOWCHART 1: Diagnostic approach to a case of EN.

(AFB: acid-fast bacilli; ASO: antistreptolysin O; CT: computed tomography; EN: erythema nodosum; GI: gastrointestinal; IBD: inflammatory bowel disease; MTX: methotrexate; TB: tuberculosis; URTI: upper respiratory tract infection)

leg, ulcerations, large-sized nodule of >5 cm, associated purpuric lesions, and immunosuppressive state. No laboratory parameter or imaging finding is diagnostic of EN, but they can be a clue to the underlying secondary cause.

Based on recent literature taking account of the commonly occurring etiologies, this reasonably practical diagnostic algorithm is proposed in **Flowchart 1**.

DIFFERENTIAL DIAGNOSIS

A group of certain conditions forms the main differential diagnosis of EN. EN leprosum, a type 2 lepra reaction presents with systemic symptoms and inflamed erythematous nodules and papules on face and limbs. Tender and thickened peripheral nerves are the most conspicuous findings in this condition. Erythema induratum of Bazin, mostly associated with TB, presents as tender, erythematous nodules on the back of legs, which may lead to ulceration and scarring. Cutaneous polyarteritis nodosa (PAN), a type of vasculitis, involving medium-sized arteries, presents with tender nodules, livedo reticularis, or ulcers on extremities. Alpha-1 antitrypsin deficiency manifests as erythematous, purpuric, tender nodules/plaques that may ulcerate and heal with scarring and atrophy. It may be associated with emphysema or hepatic dysfunction. However, histopathology differentiates the conditions with great accuracy. Certain pancreatic disorders can present with nodules in shin known as pancreatic panniculitis which exactly mimics EN. Systemic lupus erythematosus (SLE) can present with panniculitic lesions on most parts of the body. T-cell lymphoma can have similar-looking nodules and plaques on the trunk and extremities. These lesions are replaced by lipoatrophy after a few days.

TREATMENT

Most cases of primary EN are self-limiting. But secondary EN may have changes in treatment. In non-debilitating, mild EN, nonsteroidal anti-inflammatory drugs (NSAIDs) are very helpful. The only contraindication of this drug is IBD as it may flare up the disease. Potassium iodide (KI) can be tried in patients who are refractory to NSAIDs. It is thought to concentrate in EN granulomas, release heparin, and inhibit chemotaxis. KI is marketed in the form of tabs, granules, or drops [supersaturated KI (SSKI)]. Dose typically for adults with EN is 300 mg (six drops of SSKI 47 mg per drop or 0.3 mL of SSKI 1,000 mg/mL thrice daily). If improvement does not occur within 2–3 weeks of its use, then it must be discontinued. Suspect iodism if symptoms such as nausea, vomiting, burning sensation of mouth, increased salivation, teeth and gum tenderness, and metallic taste devolop. KI is contraindicated in pregnant and lactating women. Caution to be taken while administering KI to TB and renal failure patients.

Most of the secondary EN associated with systemic involvement require glucocorticoids, particularly in patients with underlying IBD, where it not only improves skin manifestation but also decreases inflammation of bowel. Preferred dose is oral prednisone 20 mg for 7–10 days. Before starting steroids, infectious cause of EN must be ruled out. Intralesional steroids such as triamcinolone acetonide are still under the experimental stage but should be tried in resistant, recurrent, and recalcitrant EN. A concentration of 10–20 mg/mL can be tried in the center of the inflamed nodule. Side effects include atrophy and hypopigmentation after resolution of the lesions.

Dapsone starting at a dose of 50 mg/day with maximum dose of 100 mg/day can be tied in recurrent and recalcitrant EN. Adverse effects include hemolysis and methemoglobinemia. Prolonged treatment may cause dapsone-induced peripheral neuropathy.

Hydroxychloroquine (HCQ) is preferred in chronic and recurrent EN at a dose of 200 mg twice daily. Annual eye check-up is recommended to rule out irreversible retinopathy. Its dose should not be more than 5 mg/kg.

Colchicine 1–2 mg/day is used in patients with EN, particularly in Behçet's disease. It acts by decreasing chemotaxis and degranulation of neutrophils. Dapsone, HCQ, and colchicine are preferred in patients with recalcitrant, recurring or chronic EN, but optimum duration of treatment is not known.

Tumor necrosis factor-alpha inhibitors can be considered in severe or refractory, noninfectious causes of EN. Clinical benefits have been reported with etanercept, adalimumab, and infliximab. Use of thalidomide, methotrexate, and cyclosporine in IBD and Behçet's associated EN has been in clinical practice but lacks support of primary literature **(Flowchart 2)**.

CONCLUSION

Although EN is idiopathic, in large proportion of patients, it can be an early sign of a systemic disease. Early diagnosis is necessary for better management of systemic disease. A proper work-up of clinical and drug history, physical examination, and laboratory investigations make us arrive at a proper diagnosis and treatment. The diagnostic algorithm described in this chapter is intended to help the physician to reach an easy and early diagnosis, avoiding expensive, cumbersome investigations.

ACKNOWLEDGMENTS

My acknowledgments to Dr Nikita, Dr Vamsi Annamdevula, and Dr Vihari Jonnalagadda.

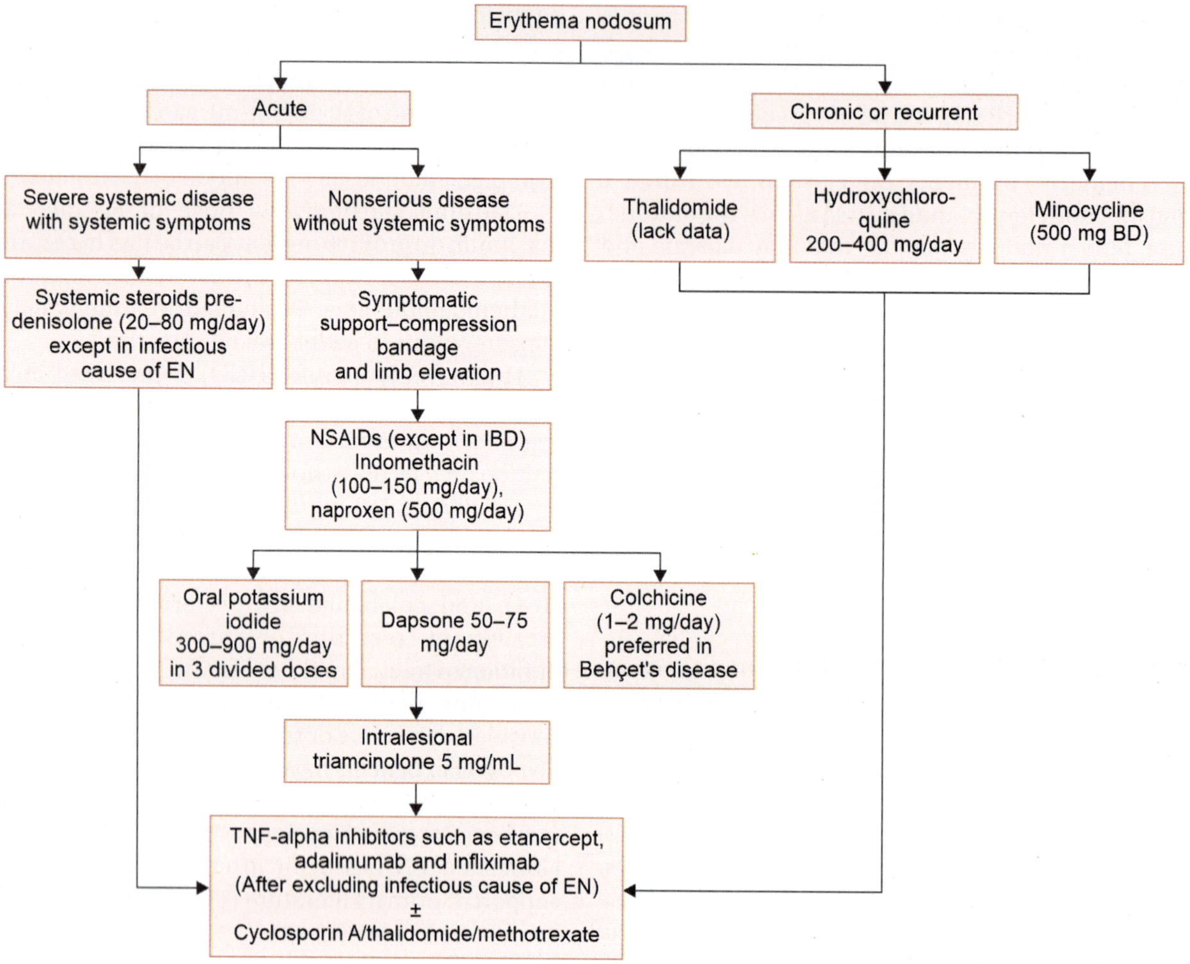

FLOWCHART 2: Algorithm on treatment of EN.

(EN: erythema nodosum; IBD: inflammatory bowel disease; NSAIDs: nonsteroidal anti-inflammatory drugs; TNF: tumor necrosis factor)

SUGGESTED READINGS

1. Molina-Ruiz AM, Requena L. Erythema nodosum. Med Clin (Barc). 2016;147(2):81-6.
2. Requena L, Sanchez Yus E. Erythema nodosum. Semin Cutan Med Surg. 2007;26(2):114-25.
3. Mert A, Ozaras R, Tabak F, Pekmezci S, Demirkesen C, Ozturk R. Erythema nodosum: an experience of 10 years. Scand J Infect Dis. 2004;36(6-7):424-7.
4. Mert A, Kumbasar H, Ozaras R, Erten S, Tasli L, Tabak F, et al. Erythema nodosum: an evaluation of 100 cases. Clin Exp Rheumatol. 2007;25(4):563-70.
5. Xu X, Liang G, Duan M, Zhang L. Acute myeloid leukemia presenting as erythema nodosum: a case report. Medicine (Baltimore). 2017;96(47):e8666.
6. Hayashi S, Ishikawa S, Ishii E, Koike M, Kaminaga T, Hamasaki Y, et al. Anti-inflammatory effects of potassium iodide on SDS-induced murine skin inflammation. J Invest Dermatol. 2020;140(10):2001-8.
7. De Coninck P, Baclet JL, Di Bernardo C, Buschges B, Plouvier B. Treatment of erythema nodosum with colchicine. Presse Med. 1984;13(11):680.
8. Clayton TH, Walker BP, Stables GI. Treatment of chronic erythema nodosum with infliximab. Clin Exp Dermatol. 2006;31(6):823-4.
9. Chavez-Alvarez S, Gomez-Flores M, Ocampo-Candiani J. Cutaneous manifestations in inflammatory bowel disease. Gac Med Mex. 2016;152(5):622-30.

237
CHAPTER

Polymyalgia Rheumatica versus Fibromyalgia

Harpreet Singh

ABSTRACT

Polymyalgia rheumatica (PMR) and fibromyalgia (FM) are both conditions of pain syndrome affecting more often the female gender but are of differing etiologies. Let us deliberate briefly on these two conditions.

POLYMYALGIA RHEUMATICA

Polymyalgia rheumatica (PMR) is almost exclusively a disease of population aged over 50 years with a prevalence that increases progressively with advancing age. Peak incidence is between ages of 70 and 80 years. Lifetime risk of PMR is 2.43% for women and 1.6% for men and is second only to rheumatoid arthritis (RA) as a systemic rheumatic disease of adults. Highest incidence is seen in people of North European descent. PMR has a strong association with giant cell arteritis (GCA).

Pathogeneses/Pathophysiology

Though the name PMR suggests myopathic process, but the muscle in PMR is histopathologically normal. Subdeltoid and subacromial bursitis is the hallmark of the disease. Both PMR and GCA are associated with specific alleles of human leukocyte antigen (HLA) DR4. Proinflammatory cytokine interleukin-6 (IL-6) is elevated in peripheral blood of patients with PMR and GCA. This is thought to be responsible for constitutional symptoms.

Diagnostic criteria for PMR are:

- Age of onset 50 years or older
- Erythrocyte sedimentation rate (ESR) > 40
- Pain persisting for >1 month involving two of these areas: Neck, shoulder, and pelvic girdles
- Morning stiffness of >1 hour and gel phenomenon.
- Absence of other diseases capable of causing similar musculoskeletal symptoms.
- Rapid response to low-dose prednisolone (<20 mg)

More than 50% of the patients have systemic features like low-grade fever, weight loss, malaise, fatigue, and depression. Onset of symptoms can be abrupt sometimes strikingly so seemingly to occur almost overnight. Bilateral shoulder pain with limited range of mobility is the main presenting manifestation in most patients. Others may complain of pain in the neck or hip girdle.

Patients of PMR are often in good health prior to disease onset which is abrupt in 50% of patients. In most patients, symptoms appear in shoulder girdle. In the remainder hip and neck are involved at the onset.

Symptoms if unilateral become bilateral within few weeks. Symptoms include pain and stiffness of shoulder and hip girdle which might last for >1 hour and come up after periods of rest (gel phenomenon).

Morning stiffness and gel phenomenon is hall mark of rheumatic diseases but notably severe in PMR. Muscle weakness is not a feature of PMR but disuse atrophy might occur.

Some patients describe distal peripheral joint swelling or more rarely edema. Carpal tunnel syndrome can occur in some patients. Cardiovascular examination should include assessment for asymmetry of blood pressure abnormalities, temporal arteritis, and vascular bruits which could point to the presence of GCA.

A clinical assessment for GCA is a key consideration in the evaluation of patients with suspected or diagnosed PMR in the following conditions:

- New-onset headache
- Visual impairment
- Jaw pain with mastication

Low-dose corticosteroids do not prevent the progression of PMR to GCA. Low-dose steroids do not seem to affect the yield of temporal artery biopsy (TAB).

Differential Diagnosis

Polymyalgia rheumatica is mainly a clinical diagnosis. It needs to be distinguished from other rheumatic conditions like elderly onset rheumatoid arthritis (EORA) and FM. PMR tends to involve shoulder or pelvic girdle. EORA primarily affects large joints such as knees, ankles, and sometimes shoulder or hip joints. Anti-cyclic citrullinated peptide (CCP) is raised in most patients of EORA and not in PMR.

Laboratory Workup

Erythrocyte sedimentation rate is elevated, usually >40, but it can exceed to 100 if there is associated GCA. C-reactive protein (CRP) is often elevated and is more specific indicator of inflammation.

Other tests usually done to rule not alternative diagnosis are:

- RA factor, anti-CCP, complete blood count (CBC), renal function test (RFT), liver function test (LFT)
- Bone profile, thyroid-stimulating hormone (TSH), antinuclear antibody (ANA), antineutrophil cytoplasmic antibody (ANCA)

Radiographs are not helpful but sonography may be useful in identifying bursitis.

Treatment

Corticosteroids are considered the treatment of choice because they produce complete or near complete resolution and reduction of inflammatory markers like ESR and CRP to normal. Starting dose is 12.5–25 mg/day. Most patients respond to 15 mg/day. Discontinuation of steroids should take a long time and it should be associated with optimal control of disease activity. Therapeutic response is characteristically brisk and complete. There is no consensus about tapering regimen and duration of treatment. But in most patients, PMR runs a self-limited course. Treatment can be stopped in 1–2 years. Maintenance dose is usually 5 mg/day. If patients do not respond to steroids within 1 week, either revisit your diagnosis or consider an association with GCA. Therapeutic goals are:

- Control painful myalgia
- Improve morning stiffness
- Resolve constitutional features

Other drugs which can prove beneficial are tocilizumab (IL-6 antagonist) and methotrexate. In patients not fit for corticosteroid therapy methotrexate can be used.

Preliminary studies on the use of 1L-6 receptor blockade (sarilumab) are encouraging. This drug has been approved for use in adults with PMR by United States Food and Drug Administration (USFDA) in February, 2023.

Nonsteroidal anti-inflammatory drugs (NSAIDS) have no role in the initial management.

Diet and Activity

Calcium and vitamin D supplementation should be started in all patients on corticosteroids therapy.

There is no use of activity restriction. Exercise program should be initiated for patients of PMR with the goal of maintaining muscle mass and function.

FIBROMYALGIA

Fibromyalgia (FM) is the most common cause of chronic widespread, musculoskeletal pain, usually accompanied by fatigue, cognitive disturbance, psychiatric symptoms, and sleep disorder present at least for 3 months and not explained by any other medical condition. Etiology and pathophysiology is uncertain. Earlier regarded as psychosomatic disorder but now it has been suggested to be a disorder of pain regulation often classified as a form of central sensitization. There is a mix of biological, psychological, and environmental variables.

Fibromyalgia usually affects younger people but can be seen in older population. Symptoms are of longer duration in contrast to PMR where symptoms are of recent, acute, or subacute onset. Patients of FM experience widespread musculoskeletal pain stiffness and fatigue.

In the blood of FM patients, excess excitatory neurotransmitter like substance P and low levels of inhibitory neurotransmitter like serotonin is found. FM is six times more common in women than men. Though it can occur at any age but usually affects women between the ages of 20 and 50 years. Some disorders like irritable bowel syndrome (IBS), migraine, and tension headache are seen in greater frequency in patients with FM.

Apart from tender points in multiple soft tissue anatomic locations, physical examination, and laboratories are normal. Tender point locations are at upper and mid trapezius, lateral epicondyle near elbow, second costochondral junction, greater trochanter, and other location. Except for painful tender points, physical examination findings are typically normal in patients of FM.

Since there are no laboratory or other markers available diagnosis rests on documenting multiple subjective symptoms and excluding other conditions that may account for these symptoms.

Fibromyalgia is a diagnosis of exclusion after thorough evaluation for the presence of other disorders like hypothyroidism, RA, PMR, and systemic lupus erythematosus (SLE).

Treatment

Fibromyalgia is a chronic relapsing condition. Entirely reversing the allodynia and hyperalgesia in patients of FM may be impossible. There is no permanent cure. education, lifestyle change, and proper medication that can help the individual to regain control and achieve significant improvement. Treatment goal is improvement in daily functioning.

Good nutrition, weight control, and vitamin supplementation is part of management plan.

Patient education, good sleep hygiene, and addressing the comorbidities that may contribute to symptoms including mood and sleep disorder should be the first approach. In one prospective study from Denmark there was tenfold increased risk of death by suicide in patients of FM. Symptoms can be significantly improved. Low impact aerobic exercises render significant improvement in pain and sleep.

Those patients who do not show any improvement with nonpharmacological measures will need medication. Patients should be started on low-dose amitriptyline (5–10 mg maximum, up to 25 mg) at bedtime or cyclobenzaprine (5–10 mg up to 30 mg) as an alternative drug. For patients showing inadequate response we can choose drugs like duoloxetine (increases level of serotonin) or pregabaline (decreases the level of substance P).

Tramadol a weak opioid antagonist with additional effects on serotonin and norepinephrine improves pain associated with FM.

Other avenues to address are stress management, aerobic exercise, sleep therapy, and behavioral therapy.

Nonsteroidal anti-inflammatory drugs and acetaminophen show little benefit.

238

CHAPTER

COVID and Rheumatological Disorders

Yogita Pendurkar, Bitukaur Sodhi

ABSTRACT

The interplay between coronavirus disease 2019 (COVID-19) infection and rheumatological disorders is complex. The scarcity of data further complicates the matter. The activation of immune pathways by severe acute respiratory syndrome coronavirus 2 (SARS-CoV-2) infection and its resemblance to the pathophysiology of various autoimmune diseases, along with the potential threat of rheumatological disease flare or new onset of autoimmune disease, makes this interplay interesting. The effectiveness of a few biological therapies in both diseases adds to this. More research and data collection are required in this domain to formulate guidelines that can help to reduce mortality and morbidity in patients with rheumatological disorders.

INTRODUCTION

The severe acute respiratory syndrome coronavirus 2 (SARS-CoV-2) infection has affected >700 million people worldwide, resulting in the deaths of over 7 million. Patients with rheumatological disorders are no exception. The interaction between coronavirus disease 2019 (COVID-19) infection and rheumatological disorders is intricate and not yet fully comprehended. The diversity of various autoimmune diseases, along with their respective therapeutics, combined with their interaction with COVID-19 infection, compounds the challenge of understanding.

PATHOGENESIS

SARS-CoV-2 is an enveloped single-stranded RNA virus. It enters human cells by binding to the angiotensin-converting enzyme (ACE)-related carboxypeptidase ACE2 receptor, which is present in the lung, brain, intestine, heart, pancreas, and kidney. After being cleaved by transmembrane protease-2, the virus enters target cells, and ACE2 is subsequently downregulated, contributing to a cytokine-mediated hyperinflammatory response.

The COVID infection is divided into three phases. The first phase is characterized by viral replication, lasting from around day 1 to 6. The second phase, known as the immune phase, begins around day 7 and continues up to day 14. The third phase involves fibrosis, marking the onset of chronic sequelae such as lung fibrosis **(Fig. 1)**.

SARS-COV-2 INFECTION IN PATIENTS WITH RHEUMATOLOGICAL DISORDERS

Susceptibility

In the early stages of the pandemic, there was a belief that patients with rheumatological disorders were more susceptible to COVID-19 infection. Although earlier studies from China and Spain have shown an increased rate of COVID infectivity in patients with rheumatological disorders, recent population-based cohort studies from Italy and Korea did not observe a definitive increase in COVID infection among patients with rheumatological disorders.

Severity

The outcome of COVID-19 infection in patients with rheumatological disorders depends on various factors, such as genetic predisposition, associated comorbid conditions such as diabetes, hypertension, ischemic

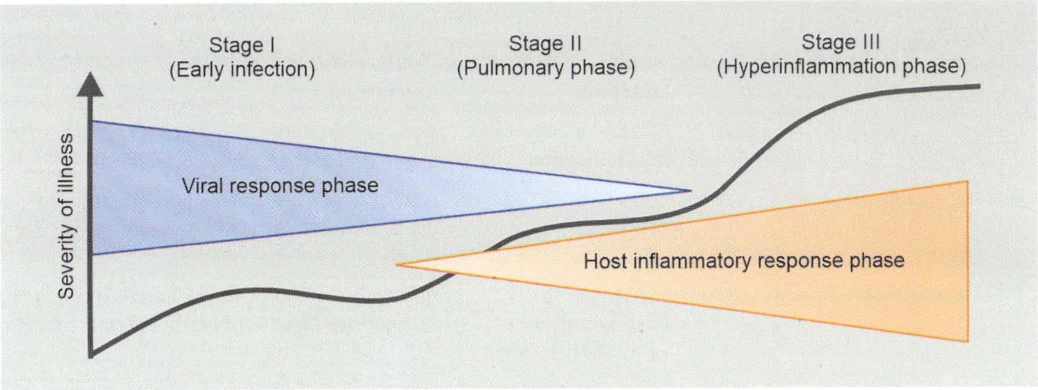

FIG. 1: Phases of coronavirus disease (COVID) infection.

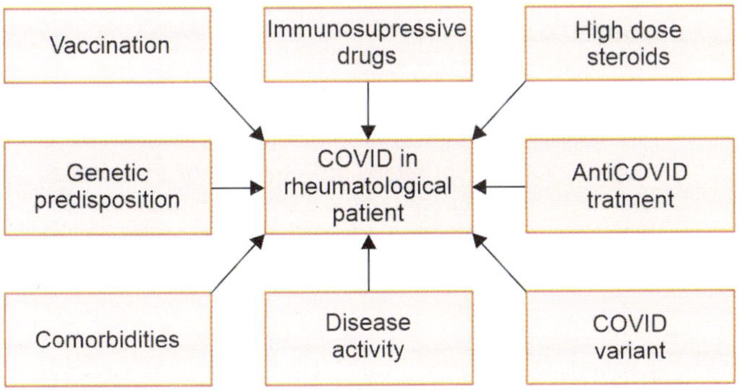

FIG. 2: Factors affecting outcome of Covid-19 infection in rheumatological disorders.

disease, chronic obstructive pulmonary disease (COPD), obesity, the patient's age, the disease activity of the rheumatological disorder, disease-modifying antirheumatic drug (DMARD) and biological therapy for the disease, the variant of the COVID-19 virus that infected them, the treatment received for COVID-19 infection, and vaccination **(Fig. 2)**.

One subset of a cohort study found a higher prevalence of severe COVID-19 infection among patients with connective tissue disease, unlike those with inflammatory arthritis. Rheumatological disorders coupled with interstitial lung disease result in more severe COVID-19 infections.

European Alliance of Associations for Rheumatology (EULAR) recommends continuing DMARDs in patients with controlled disease activity of rheumatological disorders. For patients whose disease is not well controlled, there is an increased risk of severe COVID infection and COVID-related morbidity. Medical data reveals that patients administered high doses of steroids experience more severe disease and higher mortality rates compared to other patients. Patients who were on mycophenolate, cyclophosphamide, or rituximab displayed greater morbidity and mortality than their counterparts. In such patients, the drug may be discontinued. In patients with comorbidities who are at risk of developing bacterial and fungal infections, discontinuing DMARDs may be considered. The decision to continue or discontinue DMARDs should be made in consultation with the treating rheumatologist.

Recent data have revealed similarities in immunoregulatory pathways, pro-inflammatory markers, and the progression to cytokine storms between COVID-19 infection and rheumatoid arthritis (RA). Interleukin-6 (IL-6) plays a significant role in the pathophysiology of both conditions. Furthermore, certain other pro-inflammatory markers, such as interferons (IFNs), IL-1β, along with tumor necrosis factor alpha (TNF-α)-related pathways, are also involved in similar ways. Consequently, some treatments used to manage COVID-19 patients have been adopted from rheumatologists. These treatments include hydroxychloroquine sulfate, corticosteroids, IL-1 and IL-6 inhibitors, JAK-1 (Janus kinase 1) and JAK-2 inhibitors as well as TNF-α inhibitors **(Table 1)**.

SARS-COV-2 INFECTION AND NEW-ONSET RHEUMATOLOGICAL DISORDER

The SARS-CoV-2 infection itself acts as a triggering factor for various autoimmune conditions. This infection has been shown to activate toll-like receptors and the complement system. This activation leads to NETosis and the formation of autoantibodies. Both reactive arthritis and other connective tissue disorders, such as lupus and inflammatory myositis, have been reported following COVID-19.

Additionally, post-COVID multisystem inflammatory syndrome in adults and children (MISA and MISC) crystal-induced arthritis, antineutrophil cytoplasmic antibody (ANCA) vasculitis, adult-onset still disease, or small-vessel vasculitis, endotheliitis, immunoglobulin A (IgA)-

TABLE 1: Coronavirus disease 2019 (COVID-19) Global Rheumatology Alliance studies reporting outcomes in patients with rheumatic disease.

Conditions		*n*	Outcome	Key findings
Any rheumatic disease	April, 2020	600	COVID-19 hospitalization	Age, comorbidities and dosage of glucocorticoids associated with increased risk of hospitalization
Any rheumatic disease	July, 2020	3,729	COVID-19 related death	Age, comorbidities, rituximab, sulfasalazine, glucocorticoid use and disease activity associated with COVID-19-related death
Any rheumatic disease	August, 2020	1,324	COVID-19 hospitalization, ventilation or death	African Americans, Latinos, and Asians have higher odds of hospitalization or ventilatory support than whites
Rheumatoid arthritis	April, 2021	2,869	COVID-19 outcome assessed on WHO ordinal scale	Use of JAK inhibitors and rituximab-associated with poor outcomes than TNF inhibitors
Pregnant women with any rheumatic disease	January, 2021	39	COVID-19 outcomes and pregnancy outcomes	Two women hospitalized and required supplemental oxygen, no maternal deaths; 19 of 21 had live births
Any rheumatic disease, inflammatory bowel disease, skin psoriasis	February, 2021	6,077	COVID-19 hospitalization and death	TNF inhibition plus azathioprine or 6-mercaptopurine, azathioprine or 6-mercaptopurine monotherapy, methotrexate monotherapy or JAK inhibition associated with higher risk of poor outcome than TNF inhibition alone.

(JAK: Janus kinase; TNF: tumor necrosis factor)

vasculitis, and hemophagocytic lymphohistiocytosis (HLH) have also been reported.

Chang et al. reported that approximately 50% of patients hospitalized with COVID-19 infection had autoantibodies associated with various rheumatological disorders, such as systemic sclerosis or myositis. Another study reported frequencies of anti-52 kDA SSA/Ro, anti-60 kDA SSB/Ro, and antinuclear antibodies (ANA) at 20%, 25%, and 50%, respectively among patients hospitalized with COVID-19 infection.

The question of whether the manifestation of COVID-19-induced autoimmune diseases is solely limited to genetically predisposed patients or if COVID-19 can induce such antibodies in nongenetically predisposed patients as well remains an area of research.

DRUGS USED IN COVID INFECTION IN RHEUMATOLOGICAL DISORDERS

Corticosteroids

These drugs have anti-inflammatory action. Recommendations suggest using them in patients requiring oxygen therapy or mechanical ventilation, but not in the early phase of viral replication. They should be initiated after 7 days. The recommended dose of dexamethasone is 6 mg daily for 10 days. The RECOVERY trial showed decreased mortality with dexamethasone: in noninvasive ventilation (NIV) patients, 29.3% versus 41.4%, and in those receiving oxygen, 23% versus 26.2% in general population.

ORAL ANTIVIRALS

The study findings published recently have shown that two oral antivirals—molnupiravir and nirmatrelvir/ritonavir are safe and effective among high-risk non hospitalized patients with systemic autoimmune rheumatic disease.

Favipiravir did not show promising results.

Remdesivir

This is a nucleotide analog with antiviral activity. The dosing is 200 mg intravenous (IV) on day 1, followed by 100 mg OD for 5 days up to 10 days. The ACTT-1 trial demonstrated a median recovery time of 10 days in the remdesivir group compared to 15 days with a placebo, while the Solidarity trial showed no difference in hospital death in general population. Remdesivir is recommended as the only antiviral for hospitalized patients requiring supplementary oxygen.

Tocilizumab

This is an IL-6 receptor binder that blocks signaling pathways. It is used for RA as well as for COVID-19. The dose is 8 mg/kg (maximum: 800 mg) IV over 60 minutes, repeatable after 8 hours if required.

The REMAP-CAP trial showed reduced mortality (28% vs. 36%), and the recovery trial showed reduced mortality at 28 days (29% vs. 33%). Tocilizumab is recommended for RA patients with COVID and cytokine storms who rapidly deteriorate in respiratory function.

Baricitinib

This is a JAK1/JAK2 inhibitor that blocks cytokine pathways and has in vitro antiviral activity. The dose is 4 mg daily for 14 days, with renal adjustment. ACT-T2 trial showed recovery in 10 days versus 18 days, and the COV-BARRIER trial showed a relative reduction in mortality (10% vs. 15% in the baricitinib group). Baricitinib is suitable for hospitalized patients on oxygen, not ventilated patients.

Hydroxychloroquine

There is no evidence of a therapeutic role for HCQ. The potential theoretical usefulness of HCQ could be in the context of long COVID syndrome, due to its inhibition of steroid-like receptor signaling pathways binding to their ligands and dampening proinflammatory cytokine production.

Colchicine

Colchicine is an anti-inflammatory agent that did not meet primary efficacy endpoints like reducing hospitalization or death in the COLCORONA trial, so it is not recommended but can be continued if patient is already on colchicine.

Anticoagulation

It is advised due to COVID-19's prothrombotic nature in patients with rheumatological disorder.

Monoclonal Antibodies

Monoclonal antibodies are for post-exposure prophylaxis (PEP), and act as neutralizing antibodies by targeting the spike protein of the COVID-19 virus. The panel recommends not using bamlanivimab plus etesevimab and casirivimab plus imdevimab for PEP against Omicron subvariants as they are not susceptible. For the delta variant, monoclonal antibodies can be used as they prevent the progression to severe disease.

Plasmapheresis

Plasmapheresis can be used in patients with COVID-19 and rheumatological disorders who experience severe cytokine storms.

LONG COVID SYNDROME

Persistent symptoms such as myalgia, malaise, arthralgia, generalized weakness, palpitations, fatigue, and breathlessness lasting beyond 3 months are considered indicative of long COVID syndrome. It is important to distinguish long COVID syndrome from underlying rheumatological disorders.

The mechanism of long COVID syndrome consists of viral persistence, chronic low-grade inflammation, resulting in the production of autoantibodies, endotheliopathy, and vascular complications. Tissue damage and multi-organ dysfunction may occur in patients with long COVID syndrome. COVID-19 patients may experience severe complications due to immune imbalance.

Hydroxychloroquine and low-dose steroids may have promising role in long COVID.

PREVENTION

Several associations recommend steps to reduce the contagious risk in rheumatological patients, such as hand washing, social distancing, wearing masks, and isolation.

COVID VACCINES AND RHEUMATOLOGICAL DISORDERS

Both EULAR and American College of Rheumatology (ACR) recommend COVID-19 vaccination for all patients with autoimmune disorders. It is advised to administer the vaccine when the disease is in a quiescent state. However, vaccine effectiveness appears to be suboptimal in patients who are on therapies such as rituximab, cyclophosphamide, mycophenolate, or steroids at dosages exceeding 20 mg/day. To enhance vaccine efficacy, temporarily withholding immunosuppressants for 1–2 weeks is recommended, although this approach carries a risk of disease flare. Thus, the decision to suspend immunosuppressive drugs should be made in consultation with a rheumatologist. There is potential for disease flare, and recent data suggests a 4% chance of such flares occurring in patients with rheumatological disorders following COVID-19 vaccination. However, most flares are mild, and only 1.5% of patients require adjustments to their medication. If rituximab therapy is being considered, the vaccine should be administered either 2 weeks before or 4 weeks after the rituximab dose.

Three types of vaccines are available in different countries: messenger RNA (mRNA) vaccine, adenovirus-based vaccine, and inactivated vaccine.

Vaccines Available in India

Covaxin is an inactivated virus vaccine administered in two doses 0.5 mL intramuscular spaced 4–8 weeks apart. A booster shot can be given either 4–6 months after the primary series. It is considered safe for patients with rheumatological disorders.

Corbevax, on the other hand, is a protein subunit vaccine given in a 0.5-mL intramuscular dose, with two doses administered 4 weeks apart. It is typically used for children.

Covishield is a recombinant adenoviral vector vaccine given in a 0.5-mL intramuscular dose. The second dose is administered 4–12 weeks after the first, with a booster shot recommended 6–9 months later.

The mechanisms by which a COVID-19 vaccine can trigger autoimmunity for autoimmune diseases include molecular mimicry, epitope spreading, bystander activation, and polyclonal activation. Antigens, as well as adjuvants used in the vaccine, can also induce autoimmunity through various mechanisms.

The mRNA or DNA in adenovirus-based vaccines stimulates innate immunity by activating endosomal and cytosolic pattern recognizing receptors (PRRs). This activation leads to the activation of PRRs such as toll-like receptors and RIG-1-like receptors, subsequently triggering intracellular signaling pathways that result in the activation of inflammatory genes and the production of type 1 IFNs. This production of type 1 IFNs can simulate the pathogenesis of other rheumatic diseases such as systemic lupus erythematosus (SLE), systemic sclerosis, and RA. Hence, vaccination may potentially trigger disease flares or the onset of these diseases.

Further research and data analysis are required to determine the impact of COVID-19 infection on individual rheumatological disorders in accordance with disease severity.

SUGGESTED READINGS

1. Grainger R, Kim AHJ, Conway R, Yazdany J, Robinson PC. COVID-19 in people with rheumatic diseases: risks, outcomes, treatment considerations. Nat Rev Rheumatol. 2022;18(4):191-204.
2. Antonelli A, Fallahi P, Elia G, Ragusa F, Paparo SR, Mazzi V, et al. Effect of the COVID-19 pandemic on patients with systemic rheumatic diseases. Lancet Rheumatol. 2021;3(10):e675-76.
3. Zacharias H, Dubey S, Koduri G, D'Cruz D. Rheumatological complications of Covid 19. Autoimmun Rev. 2021;20(9):102883.

239

CHAPTER

Relevant (Laboratory) Investigations and Interpretation in Rheumatic Diseases

Yojana Gokhale

ABSTRACT

Rheumatic diseases can be inflammatory or noninflammatory, systemic or predominantly arthritic, acute/chronic or "life- or organ-threatening" at presentation to a doctor. They can involve joints/soft tissue/muscles/bones/skin-mucous membranes/organs like kidneys/lungs/nervous system/heart/blood cells/eye-ear-nose-throat at presentation or during their natural course.

Most rheumatic diseases due to chronic nature and remitting relapsing course need lifelong treatment, and thus need investigations for monitoring treatment side effects, disease activity and for organ involvements. This part of investigations is not included in this write-up due to space constraints.

Thus, laboratory investigations which help in making correct diagnosis along with their interpretation are predominantly discussed. Wherever necessary, roles of imaging and other relevant investigations are mentioned. Case scenarios are included for practical application.

Two important points before we start:

1. Always include complete blood count (CBC), erythrocyte sedimentation rate (ESR) and urine examination as a part of bedside examination for patients with rheumatic complains. It helps to narrow down differential diagnosis (D/D) and categorize in one of the following groups.
2. *First step toward diagnosis*: For judicious use of investigations; after history, examination and CBC, ESR, urine test, categorize patient into one of the seven groups: (1) Articular syndrome [inflammatory arthritis or osteoarthritis (OA)], (2) Systemic syndrome, (3) Low back or neck pain (inflammatory/noninflammatory), (4) Muscle syndrome, (5) Bone pain, (6) General pain syndrome, and (7) Regional pain. Second step is to diagnose specific disease with correct interpretation of investigations.

INTRODUCTION

Investigations in Monoarthritis

For acute monoarthritis (i.e., duration <6 weeks), most likely diagnosis (after ruling out history of trauma) is ReA, i.e, reactive arthritis (young patient), gout, beginning of any chronic arthritis, septic arthritis, and flare of osteoarthritis (OA) (elderly). Most important investigation is joint fluid examination. In inflammatory conditions (like ReA) synovial fluid cell count is >2,000/mm^3. In OA flare, it will be <2,000/mm^3. In gout, synovial fluid will show needle-shaped monosodium urate crystals **(Figs. 1A and B)**. Serum uric acid can be normal during acute attack of gout. In septic arthritis, synovial fluid cell count is near to a lac, with 95% neutrophils. Do Gram stain (for choosing antibiotics) awaiting culture. Erythrocyte sedimentation rate (ESR) is raised in inflammatory arthritis. For chronic monoarthritis, tuberculosis should be considered in the differential diagnosis (D/D) and synovial fluid should be sent for mycobacterial culture (MGIT/BACTEC). X-ray of affected joint does not contribute to diagnosis in acute stage, but for ruling out fracture in a patient with doubtful history of trauma. Joint X-ray will show degenerative changes in OA flare and may show para-articular bone

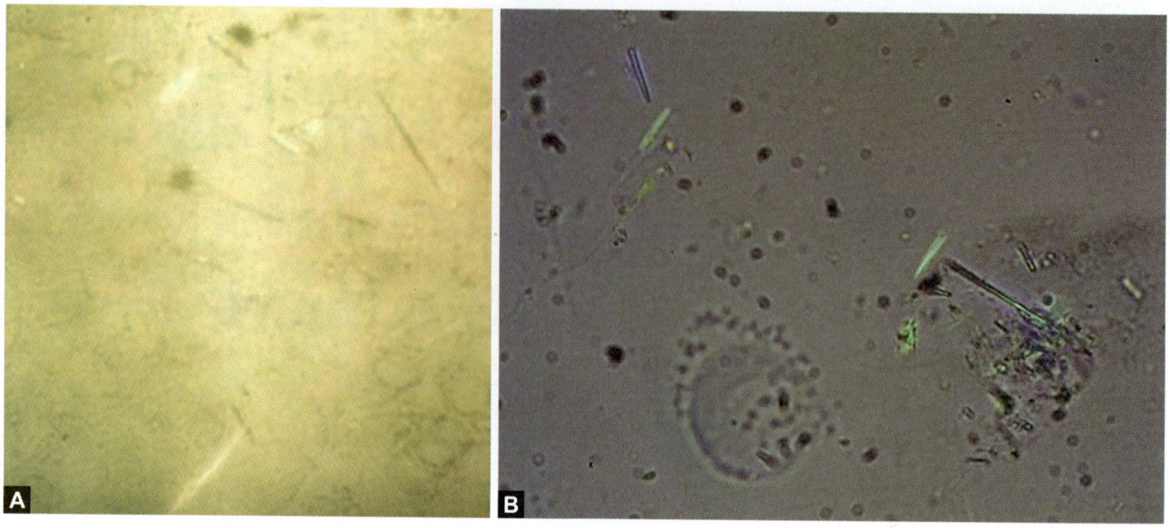

FIGS. 1A AND B: (A) Needle-shaped monosodium urate (MSU) in synovial fluid under light microscope and (B) MSU crystals (blue and green at right angle) under polarized microscope.
Courtesy: Dr Shashank Inamdar.

pathology (like osteolytic lesion due to infection or malignancy) in chronic cases.

Investigations in Polyarthritis

Four or less joints affection is called oligoarthritis, particularly seen in spondyloarthropathies. **Box 1** gives list of investigations in polyarthritis.

Complete blood count (CBC), erythrocyte sedimentation rate (ESR), and urine: Cytopenias occur in systemic lupus erythematosus (SLE) whereas leukocytosis/thrombocytosis occurs in rheumatoid arthritis (RA). Leukocytosis also occurs in vasculitis and if patient has consumed steroids in any form for relief of pain. Anemia of chronic disease (normocytic normochromic) is seen in RA patients. It improves with disease control. Low hemoglobin with positive direct Coomb test in a person with arthritis would suggest autoimmune hemolytic anemia due to lupus.

ESR is raised in inflammatory disorders like RA, SLE, vasculitis, mixed connective tissue disease (MCTD), Sjögren syndrome (SS), polymyalgia rheumatica-giant cell arteritis, polymyositis (PM) but normal in OA, fibromyalgia, hypothyroid, metabolic bone diseases like osteomalacia and scleroderma.

Another important investigation in patients with joint pain is urine examination. Presence of proteins or red cells in urine would suggest nephritis and point toward a systemic illness like SLE or vasculitis as against just arthritic conditions. RA does not affect kidneys, so if

BOX 1: Investigations in polyarthritis (including oligoarthritis, i.e., ≤4 joint arthritis).

- *CBC, ESR, CRP*: Leukocytosis—RA, infection, steroids, cytopenia—SLE
- *Urine analysis*: RBC/WBC cast, albumin—SLE, CTD, WBC—ReA

Synovial fluid examination:

- *ASO titers*: Young patient, acute migratory polyarthritis
- Chik IgM, Parvo B IgM, Hep B for acute cases only
- Rheumatoid factor (RA test), anti-CCP
- *Biochemistry*: Uric acid, creatinine, SGPT, lipids
- X-ray chest (Poncet, sarcoidosis, GPA)/HRCT chest, X-ray joint
- ANA for CTD screening in selected cases (e.g., associated features like fever, ulcer, weight loss, cytopenia, abnormal urine report, etc.)
- For oligoarthritis with or without inflammatory back pain and/or heel pain (symptom of enthesitis) investigate for SpA: HLA-B27, imaging of SI joint (MRI for IBP of short duration, X-ray if IBP for 5–7 years), ESR, CRP will be raised, synovial fluid will be inflammatory, X-ray heel lateral for calcaneal spur/USG for plantar fasciitis.
- Tm99 bone scan (SOS) or MRI in selected cases

(ANA: antinuclear antibody; ASO: antistreptolysin O; CBC: complete blood count; CCP: cyclic citrullinated peptide; CRP: C-reactive protein; CTD: connective tissue disease; ESR: erythrocyte sedimentation rate; GPA: granulomatosis with polyangiitis; HLA: human leukocyte antigen; HRCT: high-resolution computed tomography; IBP: inflammatory back pain; RA: rheumatoid arthritis; ReA: reactive arthritis; SGPT: serum glutamate pyruvate transaminase; SLE: systemic lupus erythematosus; SpA: spondyloarthropathy) patient with polyarthralgia has microscopic hematuria one should consider a systemic connective tissue disease (CTD) like lupus or vasculitis.

RHEUMATOID FACTOR AND ANTICYCLIC CITRULLINATED PEPTIDE

Rheumatoid factor (RF) is present in serum of 60–70% RA patients. It can be positive in SLE, SS, PM, leprosy and is thus less specific as compared to anti-CCP which is also present in serum of 60–70% RA patients. Anti-CCP is more specific (95%) for RA. Around 30–40% RA patients are seronegative, i.e., diagnosis is clinical (symmetric polyarthritis affecting small and large joints of upper and lower limbs of >6 weeks duration, with early morning stiffness, raised ESR, and C-reactive protein).

In ACR-EULAR 2010 classification criteria for RA-1, two points are for seropositivity and strong positivity respectively [two times upper limit of normal (ULN)].

In RA early in disease X-ray of hand and wrist is normal, later shows juxta-articular osteoporosis, with or without erosions and joint space reduction. When in doubt, MRI of hand and wrist may be used for early detection of erosions in RA.

Polyarthritis Case

A female patient, 45 years old, has painful swelling of both knees for 3 months, pain in both hands, wrists, and feet for 2 months, morning stiffness for 30 minutes, has generalized fatigue and is feverish (not recorded) for 1 month. No history of rash, oral ulcer, Raynaud disease, alopecia, and muscle weakness. No history of LBP, heel pain, psoriasis, arthritis in family. Our differential diagnosis (D/D) will be *RA, psoriatic arthritis,* postviral, e.g., Chikungunia, early CTD, e.g., *SLE.*

On examination: Eight tender and two swollen joints, GE: No abnormality, Hb: 9, ESR: 56 mm/1 h, RF and anti-CCP negative. She can be classified as RA. But, if her WBC count is 3,200/mm^3 and/or platelets are 1.2 L and/or urine examination revealed proteins or red blood cells, one would like to consider lupus and send antinuclear antibody (ANA) test as well as direct Coomb test to look for autoimmune hemolytic anemia (AIHA) due to lupus.

Whereas if her WBC is 11,500/mm^3, platelets 4.5 L/mm^3, and urine is normal one would diagnose and treat her as RA.

Child or Adolescent Patient with Joint Pain (Monoarticular or Polyarticular)

Diagnostic considerations will be juvenile idiopathic arthritis (JIA), juvenile spondyloarthropathy (JSpA), arthritis of acute rheumatic fever, postviral (parvo B), HSP, any CTD.

Investigations in children with arthritis are antistreptolysin O (ASO) titer, 2D echo, ferritin (very high in Still disease), ANA (monitor for uveitis in JIA if ANA +ve), HLA-B27 for all oligoarthrits as IBP is rare in JSpA, skin biopsy with IF for IgA deposits and urine routine in suspected HSP (prognosis and treatment depend on renal involvement).

Biochemistry

Uric acid can be raised above 7 mg/dL due to gout, drugs such as diuretics, aspirin (often elderly patients are on these drugs). Gout starts as sudden onset of episodic monoarthritis affecting first metatarsophalangeal (MTP) or ankle. In-between attacks, patient is asymptomatic. But after repeated attacks and in elderly, the disease can be polyarticular. Such patients have gouty tophi on helix and around joints. Monosodium urate (MSU) crystals can be documented in tophi or joint fluid.

Imaging in gout: Joint X-ray may reveal parrot beak-shaped gouty erosion with overhanging edge **(Fig. 2A)**. On ultrasound examination of joint "double contour sign" is seen in gout. Dual-energy CT (DECT) **(Fig. 2B)** of joint can be used to document MSU crystals. As uric acid can be raised due to many causes other than gout, documentation of MSU in join fluid or US or DECT or typical gouty erosion on X-ray is important to make diagnosis of gout.

INVESTIGATIONS IN CONNECTIVE TISSUE DISEASES AND VASCULITIS (TABLE 1): (SYSTEMIC DISEASES AND MUSCLE DISEASES)

Suspect CTD when there is in addition to joint pain/muscle pain ± skin changes ± fever ± raised APR (ESR and CRP) ± kidney (urine abnormality). Skin changes may be in the form of rashes, mucocutaneous ulcers, nodes, Raynaud's phenomenon, digital gangrene, and tight skin.

Antinuclear antibody is a screening test for CTD. It is positive in CTDs such as SLE, scleroderma, Sjögren syndrome, myositis, and MCTD. It can also be positive in RA, autoimmune thyroiditis, and malignancy. Positive ANA by immunofluorescence is highly sensitive for SLE (two negative tests by two different kits rule out SLE). If clinical suspicion of SLE and ANA +ve 1:160, order anti-ds-DNA and anti-Smith (they are more specific antibodies for SLE). Also check if there is hypocomplementemia, autoimmune hemolytic anemia, serositis by doing C3, direct Coomb test, and USG chest abdomen, respectively. If patient gives history of abortions or thrombosis do lupus

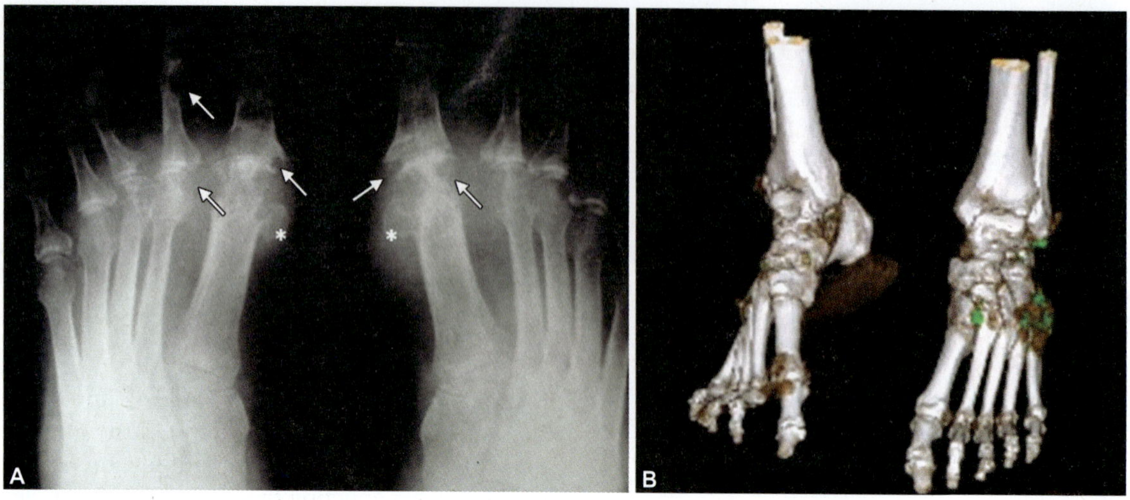

FIGS. 2A AND B: (A) Gouty erosions (arrows), gouty tophi (asterisks) and (B) Dual-energy CT (DECT) ankle green monosodium urate (MSU) crystals.
Courtesy: Dr Bavin Jhankaria.

TABLE 1: Investigations in a suspected case of vasculitis.	
CBC, ESR, urine, stool OB	Leukocytosis, eosinophilia in EGPA, raised ESR, proteinuria or microscopic hematuria, stool occult blood positive in gut involvement, e.g., in HSP, Behçet disease
Biochemistry	Creatinine raised in nephritis; SGOT/SGPT raised in chronic hepatitis
ANCA, anti-PR3, and anti-MPO	Positive in GPA, MPA, at times in EGPA
Cryoglobulins	Positive in cryoglobulinemic vasculitis. Blood sample should reach laboratory at 37°C (hold in armpit and take to laboratory)
HBsAg, anti-HCV/HCV-RNA, PCR, and HIV	In PAN Australia antigen may be positive, in cryoglobulinemic vasculitis investigates for HCV infection, as treatment of viremia which triggered vasculitis is important
RF and ANA	Positive in rheumatoid vasculitis and lupus vasculitis respectively
X-ray chest, CT-chest, PNS	DAH **(Fig. 4)**, granuloma/cavity/infiltrates can occur in ANCA-associated vasculitis
Biopsy of skin, kidney, nerve, muscle, etc.	Nerve biopsy **(Fig. 3B)**, kidney biopsy
Aortogram and angiography	In suspected Takayasu aortoarteritis **(Fig. 5)**, in PAN aneurysm in abdominal aortogram
Investigations to rule out other diagnosis	
2D echocardiography	Rule out infective endocarditis, LV clot, LA myxoma, coronary aneurysm in Kawasaki disease (age <5 years)
Blood culture (in certain patients with MSOF)	As endocarditis can mimic vasculitis, occasionally sepsis-DIC-purpura fulminance can mimic vasculitis
LA, ACLA, anti-β-2-GP1-Ab	APS can mimic vasculitis (with skin/digit/viscera gangrene or CVA)
Anti-GBM antibody	Can present with pulmonary renal syndrome (though much less often than AAV) with hemoptysis and nephritis

(AAV: ANCA-Associated vasculitides; Ab: antibody; ACLA: anticardiolipin antibody; ANA: antinuclear antibodies; ANCA: antineutrophil cytoplasmic antibody; APS: antiphospholipid syndrome; CBC: complete blood count; CVA: cerebrovascular accident; DAH: diffuse alveolar hemorrhage; EGPA: eosinophilic granulomatosis with polyangiitis; ESR: erythrocyte sedimentation rate; GBM: glomerular basement membrane; GP1: glycoprotein 1; HBsAg: hepatitis B surface antigen; HCV: hepatitis C virus; HIV: human immunodeficiency virus; HSP: Henoch–Schönlein purpura; LV: left ventricular; MPA: microscopic polyangiitis; MSOF: multiple system organ failure; OB: occult blood; PAN: polyarteritis nodosa; PCR: polymerase chain reaction; PNS: paranasal sinus; RF: rheumatoid factor; SGOT: serum glutamic-oxaloacetic transaminase; SGPT: serum glutamic pyruvic transaminase)

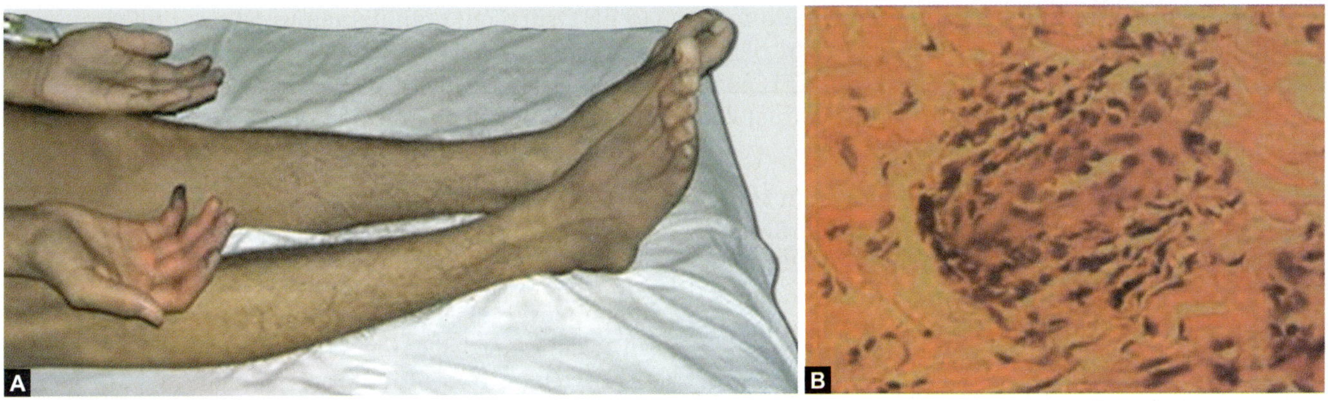

FIGS. 3A AND B: (A) Digital gangrene, left foot drop, (B) left sural nerve biopsy showing vasculitis in vasa nervosum in a patient of microscopic polyangiitis (MPA) with positive antimyeloperoxidase antibody (MPO).

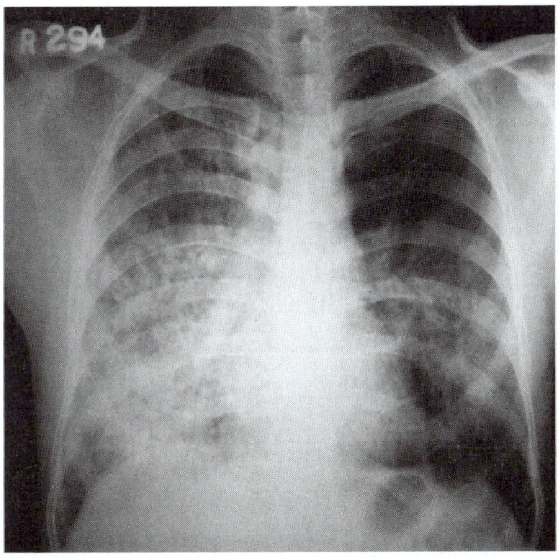

FIG. 4: Diffuse alveolar hemorrhage in a patient of granulomatosis with polyangiitis with positive antiproteinase-3 (PR3).

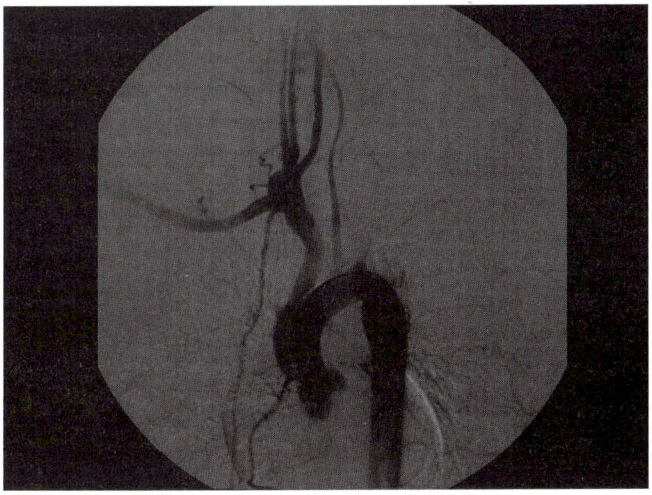

FIG. 5: Aortogram in Takayasu aortoarteritis: Stenosis of left subclavian at root, and left common carotid.

anticoagulants, anticardiolipin antibodies, i.e., ACLA (IgM and IgG) and anti-β-2 glycoprotein IgG, and IgM.

Other Investigation in Connective Tissue Diseases (Based on Clinical Suspicion)

For suspected myositis: Creatinine phosphokinase, aldolase, EMG, muscle MRI, and muscle biopsy.

For suspected Sjögren syndrome (SS): Anti-Ro, anti-La, lip salivary gland biopsy, ultrasonography of parotids, rule out drugs causing dryness on history and rule out simulators [antihepatitis C virus (HCV), human immunodeficiency virus (HIV), and angiotensin-converting enzyme (ACE)]. Generally, primary SS affects postmenopausal women.

For suspected vasculitis: Antineutrophil cytoplasmic antibodies (ANCA), antiproteinase-3 (PR3), anti-myeloperoxidase antibody (MPO), biopsy of skin rash or ulcer/kidney/muscle, angiography [digital subtraction angiography (DSA), CT-angiography, MR-angiography], hepatitis B surface antigen (HBsAg), anti-HCV, antiglomerular basement membrane (GBM), cryoglobulin, 2D echo, lupus anticoagulant (LA), anticardiolipin antibody (ACLA), anti-β-2-glycoprotein (GP)-1 in relevant cases.

Connective Tissue Disease: Case 1

In January 2011, a female patient of 25 years of age presented to family physician with high-grade fever, which was treated with antimalarials by FP (smear for malarial parasite was negative). Her fever recurred 1 month later. This time treated with antimalarials + ceftrioxone, on 4th day got rash on face, and arms, diagnosed by FP as drug reaction, and treated symptomatically.

After 3 weeks, she started getting low-grade fever, fatigue, lost 4 kg weight, CT chest: small right pleural effusion, TT: 20 × 20 mm. She was started on ATT, on 1st Mar. On 22nd April, she got rash on forearms: Dermatology opinion was obtained, who asked for ANA.

On examination: Vitals: Normal, BP: 134/80 mm Hg, she was pale, had no malar rash or palatal ulcer. Systemic examination was normal. Hb: 7.5, WBC: 3,200/mm^3, platelets: 1 L/mm^3, ESR: 80 mm, urine protein 1+, bilirubin 2 (direct-0.8), SGOT: 35, SGPT: 40, smear for MP: negative, widal: negative, ANA-1: 160 +ve, and anti-ds-DNA negative. Rheumatology opinion was asked for. Other organ involvement: Direct Coomb test positive, urine protein/creatinine ratio: 0.3, 2D echo: pericardial effusion, C3-60 (low), thyroid function test is normal. Thus, this patient has cytopenia, positive ANA, positive Coomb test, and serositis. Thus, diagnosis is SLE with AIHA.

Connective Tissue Disease: Case 2

In January 2010, a female patient of 48 years of age was admitted in surgery ward with nonhealing ulcer over right lower limb for 6 weeks. She had right lower limb swelling for 2 weeks, ultrasound Doppler revealed deep vein thrombosis (DVT). A week later in hospital she developed gangrene of left 5th toe and right index fingertip, when rheumatology opinion was asked. We got following additional history: in December of 2009, she was operated for adnexal mass in a private hospital. Its histopathology revealed inflammatory granulomas and ATT was started, but later omitted after negative mycobacterial BACTEC. She also gave history of low-grade intermittent fever and arthralgias for 1 month for which she took Ayurvedic treatment. She denied ENT complaints. Investigations revealed, Hb: 6.5, WBC: 20,000/mm^3, platelets: 1.4 L, ESR: 120 mm at 1 hour, urine proteins 2+, RBC: 8–10/hpf, creatinine: 3.2 mg/dL, chest X-ray was normal. Suspecting systemic vasculitis with rapidly progressive glomerulonephritis (RPGN), following investigations were asked for: 2D echo: normal—no vegetations or LV thrombus, ANA was negative, ANCA: 1:120 3+, anti-PR-3 positive, anti-GBM antibody negative, ACLA IgG 29 U (lab cut-off 16 U), cryoglobulins negative in serum, C3 normal, and hepatitis B and C serology was negative. CT-chest left upper lobe granuloma, on direct inquiry she gave history of sudden onset bilateral hearing loss (while speaking on phone) 6 month before current admission. Her ENT surgeon attributed it to common cold. Audiometry in our hospital in February 2010 revealed bilateral severe conductive deafness. Thus, she was a patient of Wegener granulomatosis (GPA) presenting as sudden hearing loss to ENT surgeon, granulomatous adnexal inflammation and later nonhealing leg ulcer, and digital gangrene to general surgeon. By then she had developed RPGN. After injection methyl prednisolone and cyclophosphamide 1 g within 2 weeks serum creatinine was 0.9 mg/dL. Hearing improved significantly at 1 year. She is doing well till date.

Vasculitis should be suspected when patient has multisystem affection like skin rash (gangrene, ulcer) ± kidney involvement, ± nervous system affection: mononeuritis **(Fig. 3A)**, cerebrovascular accident (CVA), alveolar hemorrhage **(Fig. 4)**, etc.

Investigations for large vessel vasculitis like Takayasu aortoarteritis include aortogram (CT, MR, or digital) **(Fig. 5)**, CT-PET will show abnormal F-18 fluorodeoxyglucose (FDG) uptake in aorta. These patients are young (<40 years) and present with hypertension or CVA or limb claudications, PUO, peripheral pulse may be absent and there may be bruit on carotids, subclavian, and aorta. Inflammatory markers are raised. For diagnosis of giant cell arteritis USG or biopsy of temporal artery, raised ESR, and CRP. Patients of GCA are in 6th decade or more. Medium vessel vasculitis (PAN) is diagnosed on angiography (e.g., celiac angiography showing aneurysms) or inflammation of medium-size vessels on surgical biopsy of skin, muscle, etc.

INVESTIGATIONS FOR BACK PAIN

Inflammatory back pain: IBP features—onset before the age of 40 years, duration > 3 months, worsens on rest, improves with activity, nocturnal pain, and good response to nonsteroidal anti-inflammatory drugs (NSAIDs).

Imaging of SI joint (for early detection of sacroiliitis MRI SI joint, as X-ray of SI joint may be normal for 7 years), HLA-B27, for documentation of enthesitis (X-ray heel, USG, and MRI), ESR, and CRP.

Patients with low back pain with history of fever in previous 6–12 months and cattle contact or consumption of unpasteurized milk or milk products (like paneer) should be investigated for Brucella spondylitis with IgG, IgM antibodies for Brucella by enzyme-linked immunosorbent assay (ELISA). MRI shows either unilateral sacroiliitis or abnormal marrow signals in one or more lumbar vertebrae (often L4). Initially X-ray lumbosacral spine is normal, but Tm99 bone scan may show uptake in affected areas.

Since low back pain is a very common complaint, investigations should be ordered when patient has red flags (fever, weight loss, elderly, history of malignancy, cannot walk or has neurologic signs symptoms, dorsal back pain, or IBP).

INVESTIGATIONS FOR DIFFUSE ACHES AND PAINS

- Erythrocyte sedimentation rate and CRP (will be normal in noninflammatory cases)
- T3, T4, thyroid-stimulating hormone (TSH) raised in hypothyroidism
- Alkaline phosphatase (ALP), Ca, P, 25-OH-D, B12, parathyroid hormone (PTH) (in some cases)

Investigations are not substitute for good history and examination (evidence of skin psoriasis, nails, and scalp), past history of heel pain, IBP, and check enthesial sites.

SUGGESTED READINGS

1. Firestein GS, Budd RC, Gabriel SE, McInnes IB, O'Dell JR, Koretzky G. Kelley's Textbook of Rheumatology, 11th edition. Amsterdam, Netherlands: Elsevier; 2020.
2. West SG, Kolfenbach J. Rheumatology Secrets, 4th edition. Amsterdam, Netherlands: Elsevier; 2019.

240 CHAPTER

New Insights into Medical Management of Rheumatoid Arthritis

Liyakat Ali Gauri, Subhita Choudhary, Ummed Singh, Nadeem Liyakat, Ambreen Liyakat

ABSTRACT

Rheumatoid arthritis (RA) is a systemic autoimmune disease characterized by persistent destructive synovitis typically of the small joints of the hands [metacarpophalangeal (MCP) and proximal interphalangeal (PIP)], wrists, and feet and extra-articular manifestations, leading to severe disability and even mortality. As rapid destruction occurs in the early phase of RA with resultant irreversible joint deformity and functional impairment, early and appropriate treatment is crucial for management of RA. Over decades, there were no such drugs which could halt the disease progression, conventional synthetic disease-modifying antirheumatic drugs (csDMARDs) were the core treatment regimen but the introduction of biologic agents, such as tumor necrosis factor alpha (TNF-α) inhibitors and other novel agents have dramatically changed the therapeutics of patients who have an insufficient response to methotrexate (MTX) and/or other csDMARDs. Despite the advent of many molecular target drugs, multiple drug resistance, and intolerance to treatment still remains an important outdaring aspect that demands appropriate obviation for the treatment of RA.

INTRODUCTION

Rheumatoid arthritis (RA) is a typical autoimmune disease with primary pathological manifestation of polyarthritis, which inevitably causes permanent structural destruction of joints leading to irreversible physical dysfunction and is often accompanied by multiple organ damage of extra-articular origin. Therefore, a prompt and appropriate diagnosis along with adequate early treatment is of utmost importance.

With the introduction of disease-modifying antirheumatic drugs (DMARDs), particularly biologic DMARDs (bDMARDs) and targeted synthetic DMARDs (tsDMARDs), in addition to conventional synthetic DMARDs (csDMARDs), clinical remission has become a realistic therapeutic goal in all RA patients. In addition, these drugs through sustained remission prevent progression of joint structural damage and physical disability in the long-term. Difficult to treat RA is still a therapeutic challenge. While prescribing a new drug, advances in therapeutic strategy to maintain balance in safety and efficacy with proper screening at treatment initiation and adequate monitoring thereafter should be one of utmost priority.

MOST COMMONLY ENCOUNTERED JOINT DEFORMITIES IN RA PATIENTS

Most commonly encountered joint deformities in RA patients are represented in **Figures 1 to 3**.

OVERVIEW OF RECENT ADVANCES AND UNMET NEEDS IN MANAGEMENT OF RA

Conventional DMARDs

The mainstay of DMARD therapy is methotrexate (MTX) both in past as well in present time, it is administered weekly, either orally or subcutaneously. Its use began for RA in the 1970s, and it has shown sustained benefits for majority of RA patients.

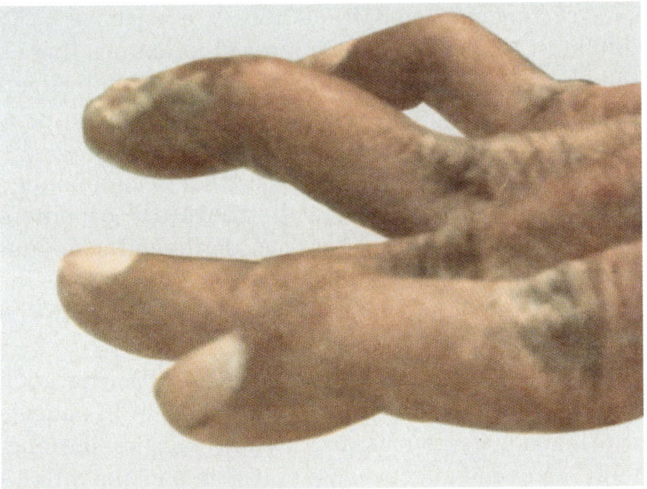

FIG. 1: Swan neck deformity.

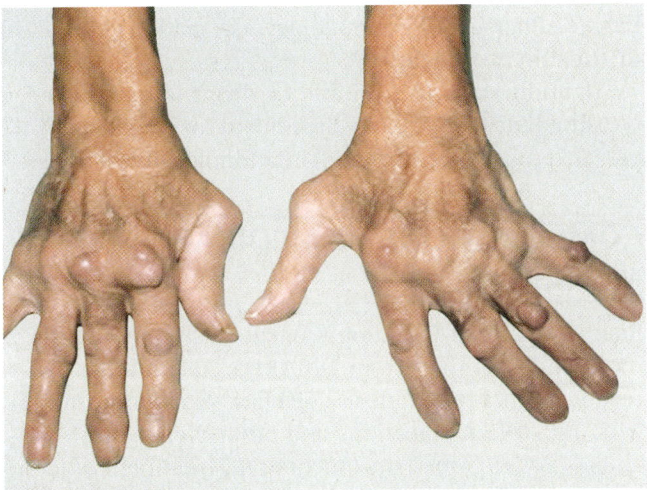

FIG. 2: Rheumatoid nodules.

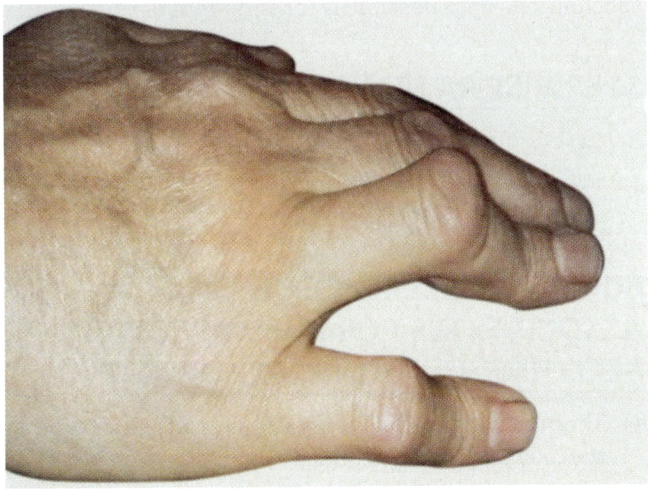

FIG. 3: Boutonnières deformity.

Other drugs approved are:

- Hydroxychloroquine
- Sulfasalazine
- Leflunomide

Biological DMARDs

Biological DMARDs are a class of drugs with inhibitory activities against specific molecular pathways implicated in the processes of inflammation in RA. The first Food and Drug Administration (FDA)-approved bDMARDs were a tumor necrosis factor alpha (TNF-α) inhibitor (TNFi). Subsequently, several other biological molecules, inhibiting different pro-inflammatory cytokines were developed.

Currently marketed biologics for management of RA include five TNF-targeting drugs, two interleukin 6 (IL-6) receptor-targeting drugs, one B-cell antigen CD20-targeting antibody, and one selective T-cell co-stimulatory modulator **(Table 1)**. They have all been demonstrated to be highly effective and acceptably safe when used in combination with MTX for the treatment of RA refractory to MTX and/or with other bDMARDs.

Sarilumab is a recently approved human monoclonal antibody directed against both soluble and membrane-bound IL-6 receptor alpha (anti-IL-6Rα). Sarilumab at dosages of 150 mg every 2 weeks and 200 mg every 2 weeks plus csDMARD(s) demonstrated clinical efficacy and improvement in physical function compared with placebo plus csDMARD(s) in patients with active, moderate-to-severe RA who had an inadequate response or intolerance to anti-TNF agents **(Table 1)**.

For MTX-refractory RA cases, monotherapy with sarilumab have been demonstrated to be as effective as monotherapy with adalimumab. Efficacy of sarilumab as monotherapy has also been demonstrated to be comparable to that of tocilizumab.

Other Biologic DMARDs Under Trial

Vobarilizumab, an anti-IL-6 receptor antibody preparation one-tenth the size of a human antibody with high affinity to the antigen, has been examined in a phase II international clinical trial which yielded significant results in RA patients and is currently in phase III trials.

Clazakizumab is an aglycosylated, humanized rabbit monoclonal antibody against IL-6 and is in phase IIb trials.

Olokizumab (OKZ), another anti-IL-6 receptor antibody, is under phase III clinical trials. In active RA inadequately controlled by TNF-α inhibitors, treatment with OKZ 64 mg q2w and 64 mg q4w plus MTX was associated with significant improvements in the signs and symptoms of RA compared with placebo plus MTX over a

TABLE 1: Currently available biologic disease-modifying antirheumatic drugs (DMARDs).

TNF-targeting drugs	• Infliximab • Adalimumab • Etanercept • Golimumab • Certolizumab
IL-6 receptor-targeting drugs	• Tocilizumab • Sarilumab
B-cell antigen CD20-targeting antibody	Rituximab
T-cell co-stimulatory modulator	Abatacept

(IL-6: interleukin 6; TNF: tumor necrosis factor)

24-week period with a safety profile similar to approved IL-6 inhibitors. Being a direct inhibitor of IL-6, less protein needs to be injected to obtain a therapeutic response, and every 4-week dosing of OKZ may be advantageous to the patients rather than the weekly or every 2-week dosing required with the two approved anti-IL-6R antibodies.

Targeted Synthetic DMARDs

Janus kinase (JAK) inhibitors have gained increasing attention recently and are categorized as tsDMARDs (also known as small molecule DMARDs). They can easily enter a cell through the plasma membrane because of their low-molecular-weight, and bind to intracellular signaling molecules to inhibit their target molecules. The rationale behind the use of JAK inhibitors is that JAKs have pivotal role in pathophysiologic mechanisms of RA such that their targeted inhibition leads to suppression of downstream signaling pathways, with resultant immunomodulatory effects eventually resulting into effective disease control.

At present, 5 JAK inhibitors such tofacitinib, baricitinib, peficitinib, upadacitinib, and filgotinib are approved by different agencies for the management of RA.

Tofacitinib is a potent inhibitor of JAK1 and JAK3, but it is less active against JAK2 and TYK2. It was the first JAK inhibitor approved for the treatment of RA. Baricitinib is a selective JAK1 and JAK2 inhibitor. Upadacitinib and filgotinib are selective JAK1 inhibitors.

In patients with RA who have an inadequate response to MTX, monotherapy with upadacitinib results in improvements in clinical and functional outcomes compared with continuation of MTX.

Filgotinib 200 mg once-daily dosage (but not 100 mg once-daily dosage) is noninferior to adalimumab. The apparent selectivity of filgotinib might have benefits in terms of safety profile with preliminary evidence of a lower incidence of herpes zoster infection and venous thrombotic events.

Deucravacitinib (BMS-986165) is a selective TYK2 inhibitor. Unlike currently approved inhibitors, that all bind to the JAK catalytic domain, deucravacitinib targets the pseudokinase or regulatory domain potentially resulting in higher selectivity.

In general, JAK inhibitors are not recommended for use in combination with bDMARDs or potent immunosuppressants such as cyclosporine and tacrolimus because these combinations might overly suppress the immune system and unacceptably increase the risk of infection and lymphoma.

Iguratimod (IGU) is a novel tsDMARD with good efficacy and tolerability as treatment for RA in patients with inadequate response to MTX and biologics. The long-term safety and effectiveness of IGU in patients with RA have been confirmed in clinical studies in Japan. Now IGU has become a new option for the treatment of RA, and is also listed as a DMARDs drug as recommended by the Asia Pacific Alliance for Rheumatology Association (APLAR) in the treatment guidelines.

In addition to JAK inhibitors, drugs targeting spleen tyrosine kinase (Syk) and Bruton's tyrosine kinase (Btk) are currently being examined in multiple clinical trials.

COMPLICATIONS OF MEDICAL MANAGEMENT

Risk of bacterial infections, particularly pneumonia is increased with the use of DMARDs. Also a huge risk of reactivation of tuberculosis (TB) has also been witnessed with anti-TNF medications and other biologic DMARDs. Thus, screening for TB exposure and treatment of latent TB prior to initiation of such agents is recommended. Hepatitis B and C reactivation have also occurred with biologic DMARDs, so screening prior to treatment and vaccination when possible is recommended.

STEPWISE RA MANAGEMENT

Remission induction (before joint damage) → *Remission maintenance* (to prevent joint damage) → *De-escalation of DMARDs* for drug holiday.

EUROPEAN ALLIANCE OF ASSOCIATIONS FOR RHEUMATOLOGY RECOMMENDATIONS 2022 UPDATE

- Therapy with DMARDs should be started as soon as the diagnosis of RA is made.
- Treatment should be aimed at reaching a target of sustained remission or low disease activity in every patient.

- Monitoring should be frequent in active disease (every 1–3 months); if there is no improvement by at most 3 months after the start of treatment or the target has not been reached by 6 months, therapy should be adjusted.
- MTX should be part of the first treatment strategy.
- In patients with a contraindication to MTX (or early intolerance), leflunomide or sulfasalazine should be considered as part of the (first) treatment strategy.
- Short-term glucocorticoids should be considered when initiating or changing csDMARDs, in different dose regimens and routes of administration, but should be tapered and discontinued as rapidly as clinically feasible.
- If the treatment target is not achieved with the first csDMARD strategy, in the absence of poor prognostic factors, other csDMARDs should be considered.
- If the treatment target is not achieved with the first csDMARD strategy, when poor prognostic factors are present, a bDMARD should be added; JAK inhibitors may be considered, but pertinent risk factors must be taken into account.
- bDMARDs and tsDMARDs should be combined with a csDMARD; in patients who cannot use csDMARDs as co-medication, IL-6 pathway inhibitors and tsDMARDs may have some advantages compared with other bDMARDs.
- If a bDMARD or tsDMARD has failed, treatment with another bDMARD or a tsDMARD should be considered.
- After glucocorticoids have been discontinued and a patient is in sustained remission, dose reduction of DMARDs (bDMARDs/tsDMARD and/or csDMARDs) may be considered.

CONCLUSION

So far, there are four classes of bDMARDs and one class of tsDMARDs approved for targeted therapy making clinical, structural, and functional remission an achievable target in RA. The latest JAK inhibitors are even effective for treating difficult-to-treat RA cases. Early diagnosis with rational use of therapeutic drugs and timely de-escalation of drugs after remission induction are very crucial. Achievement of sustained remission with a drug holiday/withdrawal regime indicates the probability of achieving a drug-free remission and cure even in the later stages of treatment.

SUGGESTED READINGS

1. Smolen JS, Aletaha D, Barton A, Burmester GR, Emery P, Firestein GS, et al. Rheumatoid arthritis. Nat Rev Dis Prim. 2018;8:18001.
2. Tanaka Y. Rheumatoid arthritis. Inflamm Regen. 2020;40:20.
3. Smolen JS, Landewé RBM, Bijlsma JWJ, Burmester GR, Dougados M, Kerschbaumer A, et al. EULAR recommendations for the management of rheumatoid arthritis with synthetic and biological disease-modifying antirheumatic drugs: 2019 update. Ann Rheum Dis. 2020;79:685-99.
4. Burmester GR, Lin Y, Patel R, van Adelsberg J, Mangan EK, Graham NM, et al. Efficacy and safety of sarilumab monotherapy versus adalimumab monotherapy for the treatment of patients with active rheumatoid arthritis (MONARCH): a randomised, double-blind, parallel-group phase III trial. Ann Rheum Dis. 2017;76:840-7.
5. Dorner T, Weinblatt M, Van Beneden K et al. Results of a phase 2B study of vobarilizumab, an anti-interleukin-6 receptor nanobody, as monotherapy in patients with moderate to severe rheumatoid arthritis [abstract]. Ann Rheum Dis. 2017;76.
6. Feist E, Fatenejad S, Grishin S, Korneva E, Luggen ME, Nasonov E, et al. Olokizumab, a monoclonal antibody against interleukin-6, in combination with methotrexate in patients with rheumatoid arthritis inadequately controlled by tumour necrosis factor inhibitor therapy: efficacy and safety results of a randomised controlled phase III study. Ann Rheum Dis. 2022;81:1661-8.
7. Smolen JS, Pangan AL, Emery P, Rigby W, Tanaka Y, Vargas JI, et al. Upadacitinib as monotherapyin patients with active rheumatoid arthritis and inadequate response to methotrexate (SELECT-MONOTHERAPY): a randomised, placebo-controlled, double-blind phase 3 study. Lancet. 2019;393:2303-11.
8. McInnes IB, Byers NL, Higgs RE, Lee J, Macias WL, Na S, et al. Comparison of baricitinib, upadacitinib, and tofacitinib mediated regulation of cytokine signaling in human leukocyte subpopulations. Arthritis Res Ther. 2019;21:183.
9. Tanaka Y, Kavanaugh A, Wicklund J, McInnes IB. Filgotinib, a novel JAK1-preferential inhibitor for the treatment of rheumatoid arthritis: An overview from clinical trials. Mod Rheumatol. 2022;32(1):1-11.
10. Burke JR, Cheng L, Gillooly KM, Strnad J, Zupa-Fernandez A, Catlett IM, et al. Autoimmune pathways in mice and humans are blocked by pharmacological stabilization of the TYK2 pseudokinase domain. Sci Transl Med. 2019;11:eaaw1736.
11. Xie S, Li S, Tian J, Li F. Iguratimod as a New Drug for Rheumatoid Arthritis: Current Landscape. Front Pharmacol. 2020;11:73. Erratum in: Front Pharmacol. 2020;11:488.

241 CHAPTER

Refractory Rheumatoid Arthritis: In Concept and Practice

Vijaya Prasanna Parimi, Vinod Ravindran

ABSTRACT

Despite the tremendous progress in the treatment of rheumatoid arthritis (RA), a significant proportion of patients continue to have inadequately controlled disease and are resistant to multiple medications with different mechanisms of action. This group of patients, who are considered refractory, presents a challenge to clinicians and carries the risk of encountering undesirable effects not only related to disease but to medicines as well. On one hand, there is a lack of clear insights into the biology of refractory RA and on the other hand, owing to limitations of composite scores used in assessing disease activity and the attendant risk of misclassification due to coexistent noninflammatory conditions, correct identification of these patients remains difficult. No precise management guidelines for refractory RA have been developed as yet.

INTRODUCTION

Rheumatoid arthritis (RA) is a chronic systemic inflammatory condition that mostly affects the joints. Early diagnosis and implementing a treat-to-target strategy, particularly in the early stages of the disease improve long-term outcomes. However, a proportion of RA patients fail to respond to treatment, despite the availability of a wide range of medications with different mechanisms of action, and deemed being refractory to treatment. This refractory RA is still under-represented in the literature and there is a knowledge gap in the identification of its real magnitude and effect. Management of these refractory patients is clinically challenging as no precise management guidelines have been developed. It is difficult to accurately estimate the prevalence of refractory RA since there is no universally accepted definition of the disorder. Depending on the criteria and research population from various studies, the prevalence of refractory RA ranges from 6 to 21%. On a positive note, in recent years, substantial advances have been made to overcome treatment failure, including the identification of biomarkers, exploring the underlying causes of loss of effectiveness, development of approaches using sequential or combined disease-modifying antirheumatic drugs (DMARDs), and the advent of some novel DMARDs.

CONCEPT OF REFRACTORY RHEUMATOID ARTHRITIS

Currently, though there is no universally accepted definition, a patient is deemed to have refractory RA when there is a failure to achieve low-disease activity (LDA) despite multiple DMARDs, of which one must be a biologic DMARD (bDMARD). In essence, it implies treatment resistant persistent joint and/or systemic inflammation.

Refractory RA and difficult to treat (D2T) RA are frequently used interchangeably. According to the EULAR Task Force 2020, patients with RA are considered to have D2T disease if they do not achieve LDA or remission and/or continue to experience symptoms despite treatment in accordance with EULAR recommendations and failure of two biologic with different mechanisms of action or targeted synthetic DMARD (tsDMARD) after failing conventional synthetic DMARD (csDMARD) therapy. Contrarily, refractory RA patients endure unabating systemic and joint inflammation along with the inefficacy of multiple agents.

According to the treat to target initiative, the refractory disease could be defined as the failure to achieve the specified goal of remission or a LDA state identified by composite disease activity scores and correspondingly increasing the intensity of therapy. For newly diagnosed patients, achievement of the clinical target within 6 months of commencing csDMARD is advocated. A primary nonresponse is defined as failure to attain remission, or at least LDA in 3–6 months while a secondary nonresponse is a loss of control following an initial response lasting months to years.

Despite using two or more biologic agents with different mechanisms of action/tsDMARD, up to 10% of all RA patients continue to have active disease. Lack of response to therapy may be caused by factors other than the inflammatory nature of the RA. There is a discrepancy between clinically assessed disease activity and validated clinical methods because the latter are occasionally overly influenced by more subjective factors. Furthermore, it is well established that secondary osteoarthritis misrepresents the state of the actual disease. Consequently, people with noninflammatory pathology could be mislabelled as having an active disease. Switching therapies in this situation is unlikely to alleviate symptoms and hence these patients may appear to be refractory to treatment.

CAUSES OF REFRACTORY RHEUMATOID ARTHRITIS

The current goal for newly diagnosed RA patients is remission, and achieving it is linked to improved short- and long-term clinical outcomes. In accordance with data from the available randomized controlled trials (RCT), RA patients experience a failure of approximately 20–40% on the first bDMARD and an additional 40% on the second bDMARD treatment. However, adequate dosage and compliance are necessary before RA can be deemed refractory. Similarly, before categorizing RA as refractory, it is crucial to determine the noninflammatory causes of pain.

Treatment resistance is influenced by factors that are both disease-specific and disease-nonspecific **(Table 1)**. Age, environmental, smoking-related genetic, and epigenetic changes may all have the potential to contribute to the development of a treatment-resistant state. Similarly, female gender, younger age at disease onset, high-disease activity at the baseline, and treatment with many DMARDs in the past are associated with poor treatment response and thereby refractoriness.

The response to therapy is also influenced by the serological status of the patient. Seropositivity for cyclic citrullinated peptide (CCP) or rheumatoid factor (RF) is associated with the severe, aggressive disease with poor outcomes, and a higher risk of developing refractory disease. For RA patients who are seropositive rituximab works better.

TABLE 1: Factors affecting the treatment response in rheumatoid arthritis.

Disease-specific	Disease-nonspecific

• Seropositivity for cyclic citrullinated peptide antibodies or rheumatoid factor or both
• High-disease severity
• Past therapy with multiple disease modifying drugs
	• Young age
	• Female gender
	• Environmental factors
	  ○ Obesity
	  ○ Smoking
	  ○ Alcohol
	  ○ Drug compliance
	  ○ Comorbidities
	  ○ Poor compliance to therapy
	  ○ Awareness regarding the disease and need for treatment

Obesity promotes an inflammatory milieu and is associated with undesirable pharmacological side effects that further reduce the efficacy of therapy. Coexisting comorbidities, poor adherence, chronic fatigue, central sensitization, and secondary damage offer yet another rationale for refractory subgroups.

TYPES OF REFRACTORY RHEUMATOID ARTHRITIS

Refractory RA may be divided into two main types and to customize treatment approaches, it is important to understand each of them.

1. *Persistent inflammatory refractory rheumatoid arthritis (PIRRA)*: It is characterized by persistent inflammation and elevated systemic inflammatory markers despite the use of drugs with different mechanisms of action.
2. *Noninflammatory refractory rheumatoid arthritis (NIRRA)*: It is characterized by little or no elevation of systemic inflammatory markers but high-composite scores of disease activity mainly due to higher weightage to tender joint count and patient reported outcome measure (PROM). Pain in NIRRA is often brought on by secondary degenerative changes, fatigue, central sensitization, fibromyalgia, depression, and other psychosocial causes rather than by active inflammation. This may result in a significant impact on their quality of life.

BIOLOGIC BASIS FOR RESPONSE TO TREATMENT IN REFRACTORY RHEUMATOID ARTHRITIS

The biological basis of refractory RA is increasingly being better understood from the research on synovial analysis which potentially would help form a useful basis of the therapeutic response. Focused therapies to modify the activity of these tissue-resident synovial cells, including fibroblasts and macrophages that variably influence particular aspects of inflammatory joint disease in RA are being studied. It helps in categorizing patients based on distinctive underlying histology patterns, and associated cytokine profiles to forecast csDMARD response and radiographic progression. Since the concept of refractory RA has not been precisely defined, there are not definite biomarkers to identify it yet. However, in a few recent investigations, the ratio of soluble intercellular adhesion molecule 1 (sICAM1) to C-X-C motif chemokine 13 (CXCL13) predicted responsiveness to anti-tumor necrosis factor (TNF) and anti-interleukin-6 (IL-6) therapy.

MANAGEMENT OF REFRACTORY RHEUMATOID ARTHRITIS

Several initiatives have been executed in recent years to address treatment failure. The best strategy to reduce refractoriness is to initiate DMARD as soon as they are diagnosed in order to minimize poor outcomes and improve the functional outcome. Treat to target strategy is always preferable to standard care. Remission is the main goal in RA, and for individuals who are unable to achieve remission, LDA state is an alternative choice. Strict disease activity monitoring by validated instruments no less than once every 3 months and periodic treatment modifications as required are the key elements in achieving better outcomes.

Methotrexate (MTX) and other csDMARD are effective in treating RA. They are associated with improvement in symptoms, a decrease in radiographic progression, and good long-term outcomes. Combination of csDMARD offers additional benefits if the patient does not respond to DMARD monotherapy. Glucocorticoids are best employed as a bridging therapy at the time of diagnosis or in refractory patients between switches for brief periods. Continuous low-dosage glucocorticoids in conjunction with other DMARD may be recommended for persistently active RA. A bDMARD or tsDMARD may be required in about two-fifths of patients who are unresponsive to aforementioned first-line therapies. The EULAR Task Force recommends initiating patients on bDMARD instead of combination csDMARD if a patient is refractory to the first csDMARD and has predictors of poor outcome.

The Food and Drug Administration (FDA) and the European Medicine Agency (EMEA) have granted their approval for the use of all TNF inhibitors (TNFi), rituximab, abatacept, and tocilizumab in DMARD-refractory patients. TNFi such as infliximab, etanercept, adalimumab, certolizumab, and golimumab are the first-line bDMARDs to be initiated following csDMARD failure and exhibit similar efficacy. The development of antidrug antibodies is reduced when MTX and TNFi are used together. While the first inadequate response or a subsequent failure upon taking TNFi occurs, increasing the dosage or reducing the interval between doses may serve to overcome the lack of efficacy in certain circumstances and, in doing so, ameliorate refractoriness. For patients who exhibit either a primary or secondary nonresponse to a TNFi, different treatment options such as switching to an alternative TNFi (cycling strategy) or changing to an agent with a different mechanism of action (swap strategy) are recommended. A major RCT had demonstrated the effectiveness of the use of different biologics such as rituximab, tocilizumab, and abatacept in managing anti-TNF refractory RA. Such an approach may also overcome the issue of antidrug antibodies. Additionally, retreatment using rituximab can boost the effectiveness of the individuals who respond, and subsequent loss of response is generally unusual.

For those in whom rituximab has failed, switching to a bDMARD that targets other immunologic pathways such as tocilizumab should be taken into consideration. The use of TNFi as a second-line b/tsDMARD has declined over time and the use of IL-6 inhibitors and JAK inhibitors as second- and third-line drugs has increased. It has been noted that between 10 and 20% of patients receiving treatment with a second biologic fail to attain remission or LDA. For these individuals, novel biological treatments are being developed, including IL-17 inhibitors and new cytokine antagonists.

Irrespective of the pharmacologic therapy, nonpharmacological interventions such as patient's education, physiotherapy, self-management training, managing modifiable lifestyle factors such as obesity and smoking, and behavioral therapies have all been shown to improve functional quality, and fatigue and alleviate the severity of pain **(Flowchart 1)**.

CONCLUSION

Refractory RA is one of the major unmet needs in rheumatology currently. Lack of consensus regarding correct labeling and identification of these individuals hampers care. Identifying at-risk individuals and implementing

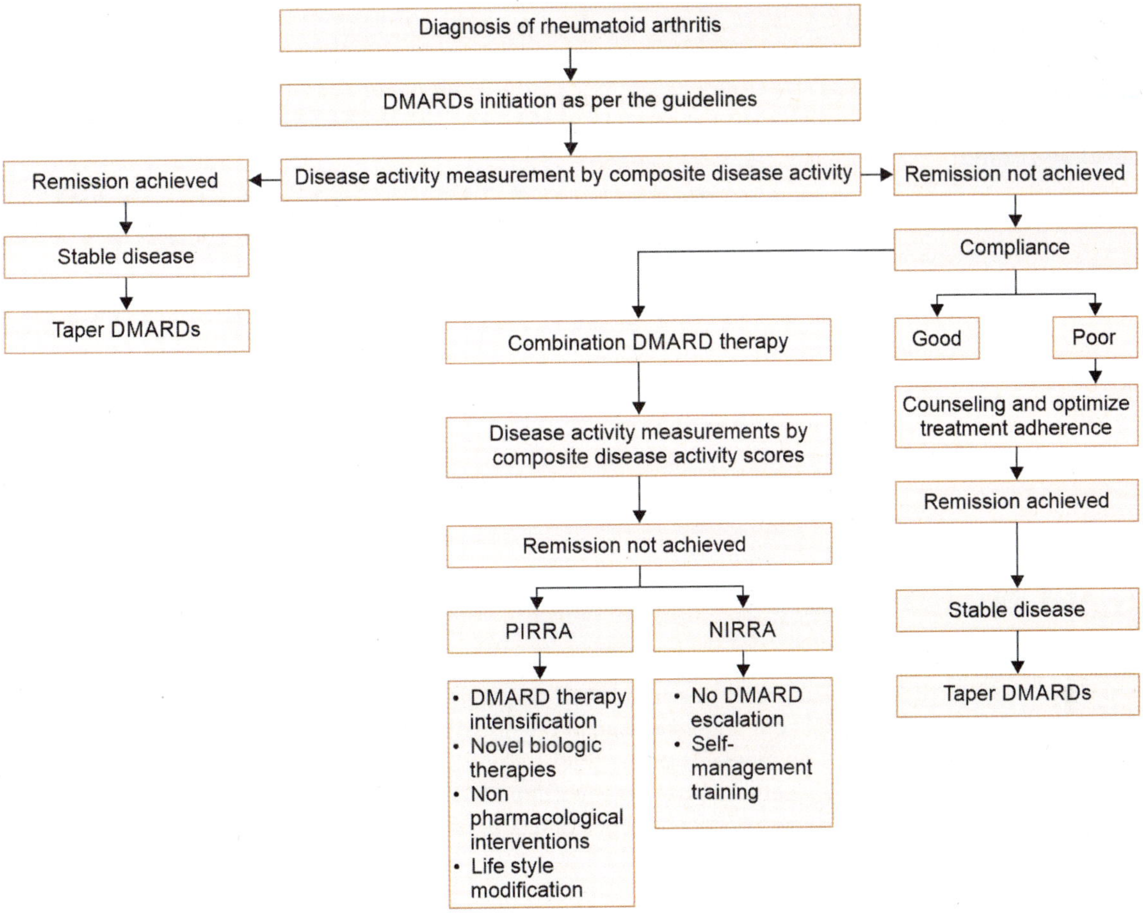

FLOWCHART 1: Algorithm of management of refractory rheumatoid arthritis (RA).
(DMARD: disease-modifying antirheumatic drug; NIRRA: noninflammatory refractory rheumatoid arthritis; PIRRA: persistent inflammatory refractory rheumatoid arthritis).

more effective strategies in the early stages of the disease mitigate refractoriness. Future research in multi-drug resistant RA may build on real-world knowledge of personalized pharmacological and nonpharmacological therapy and pave the way for useful management guidelines.

SUGGESTED READINGS

1. Melville AR, Kearsley-Fleet L, Buch MH, Hyrich KL. Understanding Refractory Rheumatoid Arthritis: Implications for a Therapeutic Approach. Drugs. 2020;80(9):849-57.
2. Zhao SS, Kearsley-Fleet L, Bosworth A, Watson K, Hyrich KL; BSRBR-RA Contributors Group. Effectiveness of sequential biologic and targeted disease modifying anti-rheumatic drugs for rheumatoid arthritis. Rheumatology (Oxford). 2022;61(12):4678-86.
3. Buch MH, Eyre S, McGonagle D. Persistent inflammatory and non-inflammatory mechanisms in refractory rheumatoid arthritis. Nat Rev Rheumatol. 2021;17(1):17-33.

242 CHAPTER

Spondyloarthritis: What a Physician Needs to Know?

Bibhuti Nath Jha

ABSTRACT

Spondyloarthritis (SpA) is a group of inflammatory arthritides that share some common clinical and pathological features. Treatment outcomes have been unsatisfactory due to delayed diagnosis based mainly on radiological changes. Over the years, there has been a paradigm shift in our understanding of the disease leading to early diagnosis and better treatment. Classifying the disease into axial and peripheral is better than sticking to the traditional classification. Early diagnosis is imperative and is facilitated by the introduction of Assessment of SpondyloArthritis International Society (ASAS) classification criteria for the two. Treatment of axial and peripheral types differs regarding the role of conventional synthetic disease-modifying agents.

INTRODUCTION

Spondyloarthritis (SpA) is the second most common, inter-related group of inflammatory arthritides seen in India after rheumatoid arthritis (RA). It is a common disease with worldwide prevalence ranging from 0.2 to 1.6% across the population. It is a diverse group of inflammatory conditions affecting primarily the spine and sacroiliac (SI) joints but has peripheral joint and extra-articular involvement as well. Early intervention is essential in mitigating the disease progression and improving quality of life.

CARDINAL FEATURES OF SPONDYLOARTHRITIS

Spondyloarthritis is characterized by features that are entirely different from RA. Clinical features include:

- Seronegativity
- Male predominance
- Asymmetrical oligoarthritis
- Inflammatory back pain (IBP)
- Human leukocyte antigen (HLA)-B27
- Enthesitis
- Dactylitis
- Psoriasis and inflammatory bowel disease (IBD)

Unlike RA, where most of the patients are seropositive, SpA patients are seronegative as rheumatoid factor and anticyclic citrullinated peptide (anti-CCP) antibodies are not detected, hence the earlier name seronegative spondyloarthritis (SSA). This was done to differentiate SpA from RA. In the past, SpA was regarded as a variant of RA itself. Later, the "seronegative" prefix was removed to emphasize that seronegative RA was different from SpA. The term spondyloarthritis was adopted in favor of spondyloarthropathy, and the plural spondyloarthritides reflected the multitude nature of the group. In contrast to RA, which usually affects middle-aged women, SpA is a disease of younger males. In SpA, mainly the spine and SI joints are affected. Peripheral joints also get involved and there is extra-articular involvement also. Peripheral joint involvement is usually oligoarticular and asymmetrical involving bigger joints of the lower limbs preferably. IBP is a common, yet not an invariable feature of the group. There is a striking association with the *HLA-B27* gene. Painful inflammation of the entheses (enthesitis) is the hallmark of the disease. Dactylitis is another important feature. It is the inflammation of an entire digit giving it a uniformly swollen appearance (sausage digit). Some of the cases are associated with psoriasis and IBD.

CLASSIFICATION

The SpA is traditionally classified into the following subtypes:

- *Ankylosing spondylitis (AS):* It is the prototype or the flagship member of the group. It has predominantly axial features like sacroiliitis and involvement of the spine. IBP is present in the majority. It is divided into two types, nonradiographic axial SpA (nr-axSpA) and its radiographic form, ankylosing spondylitis. The two are a continuum, the nonradiographic form being an early stage of the disease. The challenge for the physician is to pick the disease in its nonradiographic stage as radiographic changes take 7–10 years to appear.
- *Psoriatic arthritis (PsA):* It affects 10% of psoriasis cases. It is characterized by oligo- or polyarthritis and dactylitis. Most of the cases have typical skin and nail changes of psoriasis which help in diagnosis.
- *Reactive arthritis (ReA):* It follows infection elsewhere in the body by 1–4 weeks. The most prevalent infections are gastrointestinal or genitourinary infections. It usually presents as acute oligoarthritis involving bigger joints of the lower limbs.
- *Enteropathic arthritis:* This subtype is associated with IBD, either Crohn's disease or ulcerative colitis.
- *Peripheral SpA (pSpA):* These patients have peripheral manifestations only like peripheral arthritis, enthesitis, dactylitis, etc.
- *Juvenile SpA (jSpA):* When SpA affects children < 14 years of age, it is jSpA.
- *Undifferentiated SpA:* Cases that do not fit into any other subtype belong to this undifferentiated group.

Axial versus Peripheral SpA

Different subtypes of SpA have both axial and peripheral manifestations. Some of the subtypes have predominant axial while others have mainly peripheral joint involvement. The most common form of SpA is axial SpA, characterized predominantly by axial manifestations. It is of two types, nonradiographic axial SpA (nr-axSpA) and radiographic axial SpA (r-axSpA or AS). The less prevalent forms are PsA, ReA, IBD-related, jSpA, peripheral, and undifferentiated ones. These have predominant peripheral manifestations and are collectively designated as peripheral SpA (pSpA). Importantly, all these forms overlap among themselves sharing clinical or pathological features. So, based on the clinical presentation, SpA can be clinically classified into two groups **(Box 1)**.

BOX 1: Clinical classification of spondyloarthritis (SpA).

- *Predominantly axial SpA*:
  - Nonradiographic axial SpA
  - Ankylosing spondylitis
- *Predominantly peripheral SpA*:
  - Reactive arthritis
  - Psoriatic arthritis
  - Arthritis with inflammatory bowel disease
  - Undifferentiated SpA

Source: Assessment of SpondyloArthritis International Society.

Classifying SpA into axial and peripheral is more suitable for clinical and treatment purposes than traditionally classifying it into seven subtypes.

INVESTIGATIONS

Acute Phase Reactants

C-reactive protein (CRP) and erythrocyte sedimentation rate (ESR) are raised in almost half of the cases.

Imaging

X-ray: Plain X-ray of the SI joint shows sclerosis, erosions, and widening of the joint space, the features of sacroiliitis. Later ankylosis of SI joints follows signifying the late stage of axSpA. X-ray of the spine in axSpA shows features like squaring of vertebrae, Romanus lesions, and syndesmophytes culminating ultimately into typical bamboo spines seen in almost 40% of cases of AS. The utility of X-rays in diagnosis is limited as findings take several years to develop and are not helpful in diagnosing nr-axSpA.

MRI: It has been the real game changer as far as early diagnosis of axSpA is concerned. It detects inflammation long before definite lesions are visible on a plain X-ray. Bone marrow edema (BME) in the SI joint is indicative of active sacroiliitis. MRI evidence of sacroiliitis is used in the Assessment of SpondyloArthritis International Society (ASAS) classification of axSpA. The ASAS/OMERACT (Outcome Measures in Rheumatology) working group has proposed a definition of sacroiliitis by MRI to be used for ASAS classification of axSpA (Rudwaleit et al, 2009):

- BME on SI joints (on STIR) must be in a typical anatomical area (subchondral or periarticular bone marrow).

- If there is a solitary BME lesion, this should be present on at least two slices.
- When more than one BME lesion is seen on a slice, this is sufficient.
- Presence of synovitis, enthesitis, or capsulitis without BME/osteitis is insufficient for diagnosis.

HLA-B27: It is present in 90% of AS patients and ranges from 50 to 70% in other sub-types. However, it does not have any diagnostic value as it is found in up to 8% of healthy subjects.

DIAGNOSIS

The guiding principle of diagnosis is to 'diagnose early.' Late diagnosis is a lost opportunity as far as prevention of deformity and thus functional impairment are concerned. Deformities brought about by unabated inflammation cannot be reversed if treatment is delayed. In the early stage of AS (nr-axSpA), the patient has an IBP but sacroiliitis cannot be detected by plain X-ray. Progression from nr-axSpA to radiographic form or AS takes about 7–10 years when definite X-ray changes appear. By that time, it is too late, and an opportunity for effective treatment is lost. Hence, early diagnosis is imperative.

How to Diagnose Early?

Early diagnosis of SpA has been made possible by the introduction of ASAS classification criteria for axSpA and pSpA in 2009.

axSpA: The ASAS classification criteria for the diagnosis of axSpA can be applied to those patients who have predominantly axial features with or without peripheral manifestations. Entry criteria are that the patient should have a back pain for 3 months or more and the age at onset should be < 45 years. Once the patient has qualified for entry, he/she should fulfill the conditions of either an imaging arm or a clinical arm. For the imaging arm, the patient should have sacroiliitis on imaging plus ≥ 1 SpA feature. Sacroiliitis on imaging means definite sacroiliitis on X-ray according to the modified New York criteria or a positive sacroiliitis on MRI. For the clinical arm, the patient should be HLA-B27 positive plus have ≥ 2 SpA features. The ASAS criteria for axSpA comprise 11 features, as given in **Box 2**.

pSpA: Patients with predominant peripheral joint involvement can be diagnosed as pSpA again with ASAS classification criteria for pSpA. These patients should have a history of arthritis, enthesitis, or dactylitis in addition to SpA features **(Box 3)**.

BOX 2: ASAS classification criteria for axial spondyloarthritis.

Patients with back pain ≥ 3 months and age at onset < 45 years

- *Imaging arm*: Sacroiliitis on imaging* plus ≥ 1 SpA feature†
- *Clinical arm*: HLA-B27 plus ≥ 2 SpA features

*Sacroiliitis on imaging: Definite radiographic sacroiliitis according to the modified New York criteria or positive MRI

†*SpA features*:
- IBP
- Arthritis
- Enthesitis
- Uveitis
- Dactylitis
- Psoriasis
- Crohn's/Colitis
- Good response to NSAIDs
- Family history of SpA
- HLA-B27
- Elevated CRP

(ASAS: Assessment of SpondyloArthritis International Society; CRP: C-reactive protein; HLA-B27: human leukocyte antigen; IBP: inflammatory back pain; NSAIDs: nonsteroidal anti-inflammatory drugs)

BOX 3: ASAS classification criteria for pSpA.

Arthritis or enthesitis or dactylitis (without current back pain)

Plus ≥ 1 of the following features:
- Uveitis
- Psoriasis
- Crohn's/Colitis
- Preceding infection
- HLA-B27
- Sacroiliitis on imaging

OR

≥ 2 of the following features:
- Arthritis
- Enthesitis
- Dactylitis
- IBP (ever)
- Family history of SpA

(ASAS: Assessment of SpondyloArthritis International Society; HLA-B27: human leukocyte antigen; IBP: inflammatory back pain; pSpA: peripheral spondyloarthritis)

IBP: It is the most important clinical feature of axSpA present in more than 70% of patients. In clinical practice, most of the backpain patients (90%) have mechanical back pain caused by conditions like herniated discs, osteoarthritis, spondylolisthesis, back strain, etc. The mechanical back pain needs to be differentiated from IBP which is present in 5–10% of patients presenting with back pain. As opposed to mechanical back pain, IBP affects the younger population, is of insidious onset, improves with exercise, and does not improve but rather deteriorates with rest. Pain is maximal in the later part of the night and early morning and improves as the patient moves around after getting up.

TREATMENT

Part of the rationale behind dividing SpA into predominantly axial and predominantly peripheral lies in the different treatment options available for the two. As opposed to axSpA where conventional synthetic disease-modifying antirheumatic drugs (DMARDs) (csDMARD) are ineffective and nonsteroidal anti-inflammatory drugs (NSAIDs) are the only conventional treatment available, conventional DMARDs are effective in the treatment of peripheral manifestations of the disease.

Exercise: Physiotherapy is the most crucial nonpharmacological treatment for axSpA. It prevents deformity and helps improve pain and stiffness.

NSAIDs: These are the mainstay of pharmacological intervention. There is a remarkable reduction in pain and stiffness within 48–72 hours of its introduction. The effect is so pronounced and quick that a good response to NSAID is retained as one of the SpA features of axSpA in ASAS classification for axSpA **(see Box 1)**. To deal with the morning stiffness, it is a good idea to give a long-acting preparation at bedtime. The good efficacy of NSAIDs in SpA is quite interesting to note as other anti-inflammatory agents like glucocorticoid (GC) and csDMARD are much less effective than NSAIDs in contrast to their good efficacy in RA.

GC: Systemic use of GC has no role in the treatment of SpA. Its role is limited to intra-articular injection to an overly symptomatic joint or to an area of enthesitis. This again is quite in contrast to GC's excellent efficacy as an anti-inflammatory agent in RA.

csDMARD: It needs to be re-emphasized that as opposed to axSpA where csDMARDs are ineffective, these agents are effective in the treatment of peripheral manifestations of the disease. Maximal evidence is available for sulfasalazine; however, leflunomide and methotrexate can also be used with equal efficacy.

bDMARD: Biologics are very effective in the treatment of SpA, both axial and peripheral. In contrast to RA where a variety of agents against different cytokines are effective, till recently, in SpA only tumor necrosis factor inhibitor (TNFi) had been approved for use. In recent times, interleukin (IL) 17A blocker secukinumab and IL-12/23 inhibitor ustekinumab has been approved for AS.

tsDMARD: Tofacitinib has been approved for PsA since April 2012. In December 2021, Food and Drug Administration (FDA) approved the use of tofacitinib in AS but with a black-boxed warning for serious infections, mortality, malignancy, major adverse cardiovascular events (MACE), and thrombosis.

CONCLUSION

Spondyloarthritis is a constellation of inflammatory arthritides with overlapping features. It is better to classify them as axial and peripheral diseases for management purposes. Early diagnosis is crucial and is facilitated by ASAS classification criteria.

SUGGESTED READINGS

1. Malaviya AN. Studies of Spondyloarthritis from India: Rheumatology Clinics Spondyloarthritis. New Delhi: Evangel Publishing; 2021. pp. 16-28. [Chapter 3]
2. Stolwijk C, van Onna M, Boonen A, van Tubergen A. Global Prevalence of Spondyloarthritis: A Systematic Review and Meta-Regression Analysis. Arthritis Care Res. 2016;68:1320-31.
3. Handa R. Evolution of the Concept of Spondyloarthritis: Rheumatology Clinics. New Delhi: Evangel Publishing; 2021. pp. 1-9 [Chapter 1].

243 CHAPTER

New Biologics in Axial Spondyloarthritis (Ankylosing Spondylitis)

Ved Chaturvedi, Molly Mary Thabah

ABSTRACT

Enthesitis, dactylitis, and arthritis in ankylosing spondylitis (AS) or axial spondyloarthritis (axial SpA) are dependent upon interleukin 17 (IL-17) and IL-23 cytokines. Secukinumab is a human monoclonal antibody [IgG1κ (immunoglobulin G1 kappa)] that targets IL-17A is indicated in active AS (radiographic axial SpA) where an anti-tumor necrosis factor (TNF) agent has failed. The recommended dose of secukinumab is subcutaneous injection of 150 mg at 0, 1, 2, 3, and 4 weeks, followed by 150 mg every 4 weeks. Secukinumab may also be able to retard new bone formation. Ixekizumab is a humanized IgG4κ that targets IL-17A; it is second IL-17A monoclonal antibody to be tested in AS and axial SpA. The indication is active AS (radiographic axial SpA) which has not responded to nonsteroidal anti-inflammatory drugs (NSAIDs) or failed ≥anti-TNF agent. Ixekizumab is effective also in non-radiographic SpA who have inflammation either a positive magnetic resonance imaging (MRI) or high C-reactive protein (CRP). The safety profile related to ixekizumab is similar to those for secukinumab, with candidiasis being the most common infection reported, while nasopharyngitis was also reported. IL-23/IL-12 inhibition though effective in peripheral SpA conditions namely psoriatic arthritis (ustekinumab) and inflammatory bowel disease are ineffective in AS and axial SpA.

INTRODUCTION

Ankylosing spondylitis (AS) is the prototype disease of the spondyloarthritis (SpA) family, a group of interrelated disorders characterized by sacroiliitis, inflammation of the spine, and lower limb-predominant large joints arthritis with extraspinal manifestations that include uveitis, involvement of the skin (psoriasis), and gut inflammation. The Assessment of SpondyloArthritis International Society (ASAS), SpA classifies SpA as "predominantly axial" or "predominantly peripheral" based on clinical presentation. Axial SpA further includes non-radiographic SpA (when there are no findings on plain radiographs) and radiographic axial SpA (AS). Peripheral SpA includes SpA associated with psoriasis, inflammatory bowel disease, and reactive arthritis.

CLINICOPATHOLOGICAL BASIS OF BIOLOGICS IN ANKYLOSING SPONDYLITIS (AXIAL SPONDYLOARTHRITIS)

The disease pathology in SpA begins as enthesitis, in contrast to rheumatoid arthritis (RA) where the main pathology is in the synovium. New bone formation exemplified by the occurrence of bamboo spine in the late stages of axial SpA (AS) is another important manifestation of the SpA group of diseases. Clinically axial SpA typically presents with inflammatory back pain arising due to inflammation of the sacroiliac joints and spine and lower limb-predominant large joint arthritis, which are parts of the body that are subjected to stress and strain.

Tumor necrosis factor alpha (TNF-α) plays a central role in the pathogenesis of SpA and RA. It is found in high concentrations in the rheumatoid joints and in the sacroiliac joints of SpA patients. Monoclonal antibodies (MAb) to TNF-α are able to prevent cytokine inflammatory cascade, resulting in amelioration of inflammation and good clinical effect. Thus, TNF inhibitors (TNFi) are the cornerstone agents in the management of both axial and peripheral SpA.

Another common feature of SpA is the high prevalence of human leukocyte antigen B27 (*HLA-B27*) gene. HLA-B27 is found in up to 95% of AS, 40–50% psoriatic arthritis, and 35–75% in enteropathic arthritis when spondylitis is present. HLA-B27 is pathogenic by various mechanisms. First, HLA-B27 is involved in antigen (peptide) presentation, thus can result in cross-reactivity of the antigen with normal tissue. Secondly, HLA-B27 modulates the gut microbiome in AS. More recently, it has been shown that there can be misfolding of the HLA-B27 molecule leading to endoplasmic reticulum stress *which if unabated triggers the production of interleukin 23 (IL-23) and IL-17 by hematopoietic cells.* Genome-wide association studies show that polymorphisms of genes encoding the inflammatory cytokine of the IL-17/IL-23 axis, namely IL-23R, signal transduction and transcription factor 3 (STAT3), and *Tyk2* genes among others contribute to the genetic burden of SpA.

Clinical studies show that IL-17 positive CD4+ T cells and IL-22 positive CD4+ T cells are increased in the peripheral blood mononuclear cells from patients with AS and RA, thus giving evidence that T helper 17 (Th-17) are important contributory factors in arthritis of both AS and RA. Further, IL-23R expression in T cells from patients with AS was twofold higher as compared to healthy controls. IL-23 and IL-17 are coordinated in function and follow the same pathway in generation of inflammatory mediators that are responsible for the disease severity in SpA. Hence, they are often referred to as the IL-17/IL-23 axis.

Interleukin 17 is a proinflammatory, first described in 1993 by Rouvier and colleagues who found that they were produced by activated CD4+ T helper cells under the influence of transforming growth factor-beta (TGF-β) and IL-6. The receptor for this new cytokine was soon characterised by Yao et al. IL-17 superfamily comprises six members, namely IL-17A to IL-17F, of which IL-17A is the prototypic member and shares highest homology with IL-17F.

The IL-17 receptor (IL-17RA, IL-17RB, IL-17RC, IL-17RD, and IL-17RE) are expressed in hematopoietic tissues and mesenchymal cells such as fibroblast, epithelial cells, and bone cells. The biological function of IL-17 includes production of growth factors such as granulocyte colony-stimulating factors and cytokines, namely IL-6 and TNF-α. They also induce the expression of CXC chemokines that result in neutrophil recruitment to inflammatory sites. They promote expression and production of antibacterial peptides that help in host defense against extracellular pathogens in the mucosa and lung tissue. IL-17 also promotes production of tissue matrix metalloproteinases. In the bone IL-17 promotes bone resorption by an increase in expression of receptor activator of nuclear factor kappa B ligand (RANK-L) in osteoblasts, leading to activation of osteoclasts; bone destruction thus ensues.

Interleukin-23 a member of IL-12 family has a structure similar to IL-12, consisting of p40 and p35 subunits, whereas IL-12 contains p40 and p19 subunits. IL-23 in the IL-17/23 axis *has a major role to sustain and expand Th-17 cells.* IL-23 binds to two kinds of receptors, IL-23R and IL-12R beta-1. Binding of IL-23 to its receptor causes signal transduction by way of the Janus kinases (JAK and Tyk 2) to activate downstream STAT3 and STAT4. STAT4 induces the transcription and production of interferon-gamma essential for Th-1 differentiation, while STAT3 is vital to the upregulation of ROR-γt (retinoic acid receptor-related protein γt) and subsequent differentiation and development of Th-17 cells. *Thus, IL-23's unique function is inducing the proliferation of Th-17 cells and thus Th-17 cytokines.* IL-12, on the other hand, induces Th-1 response.

Basic and translational research utilizing *mouse models* of AS and psoriatic arthritis reveal that enthesitis, dactylitis, aortitis, and arthritis are dependent IL-17 and IL-23 cytokines. On the basis of this, IL-17A and IL-23 are considered eligible therapeutic targets in the treatment of SpA.

NEW BIOLOGICS IN SPONDYLOARTHRITIS TARGETTING THE INTERLEUKIN 23/ INTERLEUKIN 17A AXIS

Interleukin 17A inhibitors

Secukinumab

Secukinumab is a fully human immunoglobulin G1 kappa (IgG1κ) antibody that targets IL-17A. The typical indication for secukinumab in SpA is AS (radiographic axial SpA), where an anti-TNF agent has failed. The recommended dose of secukinumab is subcutaneous injection of 150 mg at 0, 1, 2, 3, and 4 weeks, followed by 150 mg every 4 weeks. However, the loading dose can be omitted. The author in his experience has found that even without the loading dose, patients response is very good [measured by the Bath Ankylosing Spondylitis Disease Activity

Index (BASDAI)]. One reason for omitting the loading dose is the anticipation of some unknown adverse effect and secondly, the high cost of the drug. In the authors' experience, it is also preferred as first-line biological disease-modifying antirheumatic drug (bDMARD) in AS when the patient has a risk of developing tuberculosis and anti-TNF is contraindicated. The most common adverse event noted from trial data is candidiasis and neutropenia; although in practice, the author has observed none of these side effects.

The efficacy of secukinumab in active AS was shown in three major trials named MEASURE 1, MEASURE 2, MEASURE 3 (**Table 1**). At 16 weeks, the ASAS20 response was achieved by 60% secukinumab patients compared to only 28% patients in the placebo group. Further, treatment with secukinumab over 3 years resulted in 60 and 80% patients achieving ASAS20 and ASAS40, respectively. A subgroup analysis of these trials also shows that it is effective in Asian patients as well.

Secukinumab may also be able to retard new bone formation. The effect of secukinumab (given for 2 years) on spinal radiographic progression has been examined by analyzing data from the MEASURE 1 trial compared to patients from the ENRADAS trial who did not receive

TABLE 1: Clinical trials that established the efficacy and safety of secukinumab in ankylosing spondylitis.

Year, trial name, participants	Dose of secukinumab	Primary efficacy endpoints and outcomes	Safety
MEASURE 1 and MEASURE 2 phase 3 trials were published in 2015. These trials included patients with AS who fulfilled modified New York criteria, who were having a BASDAI ≥ 4, spinal pain VAS ≥ 4 cm, despite undergoing treatment with NSAIDs at maximal doses. Those patients who have received anti-TNF in the past were also eligible to be included. All patients could continue sulfasalazine or methotrexate during the trial	In the MEASURE 1 trial, AS patients (n = 371) were randomized to *IV secukinumab* 10 mg/kg at 0, 2, and 4 weeks or placebo followed by *SC secukinumab* 150 or 75 mg or placebo every 4 weeks, starting at week 8	ASAS20 response at week 16 was 61%, 60%, and 29% for 150 mg, 75 mg, and placebo, respectively	Improvements were sustained till weeks 52
	In the MEASURE 2 trial, AS patients (n = 219) were randomized to *SC secukinumab* 150 or 75 mg at 0, 1, 2, 3 weeks; and every 4 weeks starting at week 4 or placebo At week 16, placebo group received *SC secukinumab* 150 or 75 mg	ASAS20 response at week 16 was 61%, 41%, and 28% for 150 mg, 75 mg, and placebo respectively, $p < 0.001$ for 150 mg vs. placebo	Infections, including candidiasis, were more common in secukinumab group. Other adverse events recorded were neutropenia and Crohn's disease
A follow-up of the MEASURE 1 was published in 2018	Of those AS patients who completed 2 years (n = 290), treatment with *SC secukinumab* 150 or 75 mg every 4 weeks for 16 weeks, 274 entered a 3-year extension study, of whom 260 completed 3 years	ASAS20/40 response was seen in 80%, 61% in 150 group, and 75%, 50% in the 75 mg group. Sustained improvements in BASDAI, BASFI, BASMI, health-related quality of life, ASAS partial remission and ASDAS-CRP were observed as well over the 3-year period	Retention rate were high
The MEASURE 3 trial was published in 2017. Active ankylosing spondylitis patients (n = 226) were included	AS patients were randomized to *IV secukinumab* 10 mg/kg at 0, 2, and 4 weeks, followed by *SC secukinumab* or placebo. The maintenance dose was SC 300 mg or SC 150 mg every 4 weeks, higher than the maintenance dose in the MEASURE 1 and 2	• ASAS20 response was 60.5%, 58.1%, and 36.8% in 300 mg, 150 mg, and placebo, respectively • Other endpoints ASAS40, ASAS 5/6, BASDAI, ASAS partial remission, and change in hs-CRP. All other endpoints were also met, except ASAS partial remission	Candidiasis and neutropenia occurred in the secukinumab group. Improvements were sustained through week 52

Note: Clinical trial endpoint measures in AS, namely the ASAS20 response, ASAS40 response, ASAS5/6, BASDAI, BASFI, BASMI, and ASDAS.

(ASDAS: Ankylosing Spondylitis Disease Activity Score; AS: ankylosing spondylitis; ASAS: assessment of SpondyloArthritis international Society; BASDAI: bath ankylosing spondylitis disease activity index; BASFI: bath ankylosing spondylitis functional index; BASMI: bath ankylosing spondylitis metrology index; hs-CRP: highly sensitive C-reactive protein; IV: intravenous; NSAIDs: nonsteroidal anti-inflammatory drugs; SC: subcutaneous; TNF: tumor necrosis factor; VAS: visual analog scale) biologics. It was found that secukinumab-treated patients had significantly lower modified stoke ankylosing spondylitis scoring system (mSASSS) scores, thus suggesting that secukinumab might be able to retard new bone formation.

Ixekizumab

Ixekizumab is a humanized IgG subclass 4-kappa (IgG4κ) that targets IL-17A; it is second IL-17A MAb to be tested in AS and axial SpA. The indication is active AS (radiographic axial SpA) who have not responded to nonsteroidal anti-inflammatory drugs (NSAIDs) (COAST-V trial) or failed ≥anti-TNF agent (COAST-W trial). Ixekizumab is effective also in non-radiographic SpA who have inflammation either a positive magnetic resonance imaging (MRI) or high C-reactive protein (CRP) (COAST-X trial).

In *bDMARD-naïve AS patients,* 50% patients achieve ASAS40 response at week 16 and up to week 52. The clinical efficacy is seen as early as the first week after the initial injection. The dose is 80 mg subcutaneous injection every 2 weeks. A similar proportion (53%) achieve ASAS40 response at week 52 with 80 mg 4 weekly dose. Thus, the recommended dose is 80 mg by subcutaneous injection every 4 weeks. The response rates with *ixekizumab* appears to be better compared with adalimumab.

In AS who have failed anti-TNF (COAST-W trial), the proportion of patients achieving ASAS40 response at week 16 was 25% and increased to 34% by week 52, with a 2-weekly injection of 80 mg. In those who received 80 mg 4 weekly, the proportion of patients achieving ASAS40 response at both week 16 and week 52 was 31%. Thus in AS with anti-TNF failure, the recommended dose of ixekizumab is 180 mg (loading), followed by 80 mg subcutaneous every 4 weeks.

The safety profile related to ixekizumab is similar to those for secukinumab, with candidiasis being the most common infection reported, while nasopharyngitis was reported in COAST-X trial. As for any other biologic trials, the common exclusion criteria for the secukinumab and ixekizumab remain active infections, active malignancy, previous treatment with B cell-depleting therapy, and total spinal ankyloses.

Brodalumab is a human IgG2 MAb that targets IL-17 receptor.

Interleukin 23/Interleukin 12 Inhibitors

The MAbs that target IL-23/IL-12 pathway are ustekinumab (IgGκ) and Briakinumab (gGλ). Both are human MAbs that target the p40 subunit of IL-23 and IL-12. Guselkumab (human IgG1λ), tildrakizumab (humanized IgG1κ), and risankizumab (humanized IgG1κ) target p19 subunit of IL-23.

Because IL-23 is a driver of IL-17 production, it was assumed that IL-23/IL-12 inhibition would also be an effective treatment for AS (axial SpA). A proof of concept trial (TOPAS) had proved the efficacy of ustekinumab in AS, but a subsequent phase 3 trial found that ustekinumab was ineffective. Both trial design related and biological factors were thought to have contributed to the negative results.

The TOPAS trial was a single-arm, open-label trial, without a placebo. At 24 weeks, 65% patients achieved ASAS40 response, 75% achieved ASAS20 response, while 30% achieved partial remission. Since the TOPAS study did not have a placebo group, it is unknown whether ustekinumab was really better than placebo. Secondly, phase 2 dose-finding study should have been explored before proceeding to phase 3 study.

On the contrary, ustekinumab is effective in psoriatic arthritis which is a predominantly peripheral SpA. IL-23 inhibition also improves inflammatory bowel disease, but IL-17 inhibitors exacerbates it. The lack of efficacy of IL-23 inhibition in predominantly axial diseases such as AS but good efficacy in peripheral SpA such as psoriatic arthritis is the differential effect of IL-17 and IL-23 on different tissues. The other biological mechanism offered is that IL-17A production in axial SpA occurs independently of IL-23. Risankizumab is also not effective in patients with active AS.

CONCLUSION

Interleukin 17A inhibitors, namely secukinumab and ixekizumab, are new biologics and have good efficacy in AS/axial SpA and are indicated in patients who have failed TNF inhibitors or who have contraindications to anti-TNF inhibitors. But *IL-23/IL-12 inhibition* though effective in peripheral SpA conditions namely psoriatic arthritis (ustekinumab) and inflammatory bowel disease, but they are ineffective in AS and axial SpA.

SUGGESTED READINGS

1. Rudwaleit M, van der Heijde D, Landewé R, Listing J, Akkoc N, Brandt J, et al. The development of Assessment of SpondyloArthritis international Society classification criteria for axial spondyloarthritis (part II): validation and final selection. Ann Rheum Dis. 2009;68:777-83.
2. Rudwaleit M, van der Heijde D, Landewé R, Akkoc N, Brandt J, Chou CT, et al. The Assessment of SpondyloArthritis International Society classification criteria for peripheral spondyloarthritis and for spondyloarthritis in general. Ann Rheum Dis. 2011;70:25-31.

3. Braun J, Sieper J. Ankylosing spondylitis. Lancet. 2007;369: 1379-90.
4. Khan MA. Update on spondyloarthropathies. Ann Intern Med. 2002;136:896-907.
5. DeLay ML, Turner MJ, Klenk EI, Smith JA, Sowders DP, Colbert RA. HLA-B27 misfolding and the unfolded protein response augment interleukin-23 production and are associated with Th17 activation in transgenic rats. Arthritis Rheum. 2009;60: 2633-43.
6. Colbert RA, Tran TM, Layh-Schmitt G. HLA-B27 misfolding and ankylosing spondylitis. Mol Immunol. 2014;57:44-51.
7. Reveille JD. Genetics of spondyloarthritis—beyond the MHC. Nat Rev Rheumatol. 2012;8:296-304.
8. Shen H, Goodall JC, Hill Gaston JS. Frequency and phenotype of peripheral blood Th17 cells in ankylosing spondylitis and rheumatoid arthritis. Arthritis Rheum. 2009;60:1647-56.
9. Kenna TJ, Davidson SI, Duan R, Bradbury LA, McFarlane J, Smith M, et al. Enrichment of circulating interleukin-17-secreting interleukin-23 receptor-positive γ/δ T cells in patients with active ankylosing spondylitis. Arthritis Rheum. 2012;64:1420-9.
10. Rouvier E, Luciani MF, Mattéi MG, Denizot F, Golstein P. CTLA-8, cloned from an activated T cell, bearing AU-rich messenger RNA instability sequences, and homologous to a herpesvirus saimiri gene. J Immunol. 1993;150:5445-56.
11. Yao Z, Fanslow WC, Seldin MF, Rousseau AM, Painter SL, Comeau MR, et al. Herpesvirus Saimiri encodes a new cytokine, IL-17, which binds to a novel cytokine receptor. Immunity. 1995;3: 811-21.
12. Xu S, Cao X. Interleukin-17 and its expanding biological functions. Cell Mol Immunol. 2010;7:164-74.
13. Stritesky GL, Yeh N, Kaplan MH. IL-23 promotes maintenance but not commitment to the Th17 lineage. J Immunol. 2008;181:5948-55.
14. Mathur AN, Chang HC, Zisoulis DG, Stritesky GL, Yu Q, O'Malley JT, et al. Stat3 and Stat4 direct development of IL-17-secreting Th cells. J Immunol. 2007;178:4901-7.
15. Sherlock JP, Joyce-Shaikh B, Turner SP, Chao CC, Sathe M, Grein J, et al. IL-23 induces spondyloarthropathy by acting on ROR-γt+ CD3+ CD4− CD8− entheseal resident T cells. Nat Med. 2012;18:1069-76.
16. Glatigny S, Fert I, Blaton MA, Lories RJ, Araujo LM, Chiocchia G, et al. Proinflammatory Th17 cells are expanded and induced by dendritic cells in spondylarthritis-prone HLA-B27-transgenic rats. Arthritis Rheum. 2012;64:110-20.
17. Lories RJ, Matthys P, de Vlam K, Derese I, Luyten FP. Ankylosing enthesitis, dactylitis, and onychoperiostitis in male DBA/1 mice: a model of psoriatic arthritis. Ann Rheum Dis. 2004;63(5):595-8.
18. Bowness P, Ridley A, Shaw J, Chan AT, Wong-Baeza I, Fleming M, et al. Th17 cells expressing KIR3DL2+ and responsive to HLA-B27 homodimers are increased in ankylosing spondylitis. J Immunol. 2011;186:2672-80.
19. Baeten D, Sieper J, Braun J, Baraliakos X, Dougados M, Emery P, et al; MEASURE 1 Study Group, MEASURE 2 Study Group. Secukinumab, an Interleukin-17A Inhibitor, in Ankylosing Spondylitis. N Engl J Med. 2015;373(26):2534-48.
20. Baraliakos X, Kivitz AJ, Deodhar AA, Braun J, Wei JC, Delicha EM, et al. MEASURE 1 Study Group. Long-term effects of interleukin-17A inhibition with secukinumab in active ankylosing spondylitis: 3-year efficacy and safety results from an extension of the Phase 3 MEASURE 1 trial. Clin Exp Rheumatol. 2018;36(1):50-5.
21. Pavelka K, Kivitz A, Dokoupilova E, Blanco R, Maradiaga M, Tahir H, et al. Efficacy, safety, and tolerability of secukinumab in patients with active ankylosing spondylitis: a randomized, double-blind phase 3 study, MEASURE 3. Arthritis Res Ther. 2017;19(1):285.
22. Landewé R, van Tubergen A. Clinical tools to assess and monitor spondyloarthritis. Curr Rheumatol Rep. 2015;17(7):47.
23. Braun J, Haibel H, de Hooge M, Landewé R, Rudwaleit M, Fox T, et al. Spinal radiographic progression over 2 years in ankylosing spondylitis patients treated with secukinumab: a historical cohort comparison. Arthritis Res Ther. 2019;21:142.
24. van der Heijde D, Cheng-Chung Wei J, Dougados M, Mease P, Deodhar A, Maksymowych WP, et al. Ixekizumab, an interleukin-17A antagonist in the treatment of ankylosing spondylitis or radiographic axial spondyloarthritis in patients previously untreated with biological disease-modifying anti-rheumatic drugs (COAST-V): 16 week results of a phase 3 randomised, double-blind, active-controlled and placebo-controlled trial. Lancet. 2018;392:2441-51.
25. Deodhar A, Poddubnyy D, Pacheco-Tena C, Salvarani C, Lespessailles E, Rahman P, et al. Efficacy and Safety of Ixekizumab in the Treatment of Radiographic Axial Spondyloarthritis: Sixteen-Week Results From a Phase III Randomized, Double-Blind, Placebo-Controlled Trial in Patients With Prior Inadequate Response to or Intolerance of Tumor Necrosis Factor Inhibitors. Arthritis Rheumatol. 2019;71:599-611.
26. Dougados M, Wei JC, Landewé R, Sieper J, Baraliakos X, Van den Bosch F, et al. Efficacy and safety of ixekizumab through 52 weeks in two phase 3, randomised, controlled clinical trials in patients with active radiographic axial spondyloarthritis (COAST-V and COAST-W). Ann Rheum Dis. 2020;79:176-85.
27. Deodhar A, van der Heijde D, Gensler LS, Kim TH, Maksymowych WP, Østergaard M, et al. Ixekizumab for patients with non-radiographic axial spondyloarthritis (COAST-X): a randomised, placebo-controlled trial. Lancet. 2020;395:53-6.
28. Poddubnyy D, Hermann KG, Callhoff J, Listing J, Sieper J. Ustekinumab for the treatment of patients with active ankylosing spondylitis: results of a 28-week, prospective, open-label, proof-of-concept study (TOPAS). Ann Rheum Dis. 2014;73:817-23.
29. Deodhar A, Gensler LS, Sieper J, Clark M, Calderon C, Wang Y, et al. Three Multicenter, Randomized, Double-Blind, Placebo-Controlled Studies Evaluating the Efficacy and Safety of Ustekinumab in Axial Spondyloarthritis. Arthritis Rheumatol. 2019;71:258-70.
30. Mease P. Ustekinumab Fails to Show Efficacy in a Phase III Axial Spondyloarthritis Program: The Importance of Negative Results. Arthritis Rheumatol. 2019;71:179-81.
31. Fieldhouse KA, Ukaibe S, Crowley EL, Khanna R, O'Toole A, Gooderham MJ. Inflammatory bowel disease in patients with psoriasis treated with interleukin-17 inhibitors. Drugs Context. 2020;9:2020-2-1.

244

CHAPTER

Glucocorticoid-induced Osteoporosis

Arun Kumar Kedia, Amit Dua

ABSTRACT

Glucocorticoid (GC)-induced osteoporosis (GIOP) is the most common cause of iatrogenic osteoporosis (OP), associated with fractures in 30–50% of patients on chronic GC therapy. While the majority of the epidemiological data associating OP risk with GC therapy are from the use of oral GCs, other disease-related factors such as chronic inflammation and immobility also need to be kept in mind. Bone remodeling is a complex process regulated by an intricate network of local and systemic factors. Differential effects of low GC dose on bone loss in different patients point toward the role of genetic factors too. All patients treated with long-term GCs should be suspected of suffering from GIOP. While routine Laboratory evaluation for GIOP is essential, the earliest changes in BMD during GC therapy can be detected by dual-energy X-ray absorptiometry (DXA). In patients under GC treatment fractures tend to occur at bone mineral density (BMD) values that are lower than the conventional threshold T-score of –2.5 and this fact accounts for incorporating GC dosage for the Fracture Risk Assessment tool (FRAX). Various International bodies have put forth guidelines for the prevention and treatment of GIOP. Prevention should start for all as soon as GCs are administered because bone loss is more rapid in the first few months of therapy and supplementation with calcium and vitamin D is a must during the treatment. Several antiresorptive and anabolic agents are available to prevent and treat GIOP.

INTRODUCTION

Glucocorticoids (GCs) are widely used agents in various medical conditions including autoimmune, rheumatological, respiratory, and neuromuscular disorders. Long-term use of GCs is associated with multiple adverse effects and one among them is glucocorticoid-induced osteoporosis (GIOP), which is also the most common cause of secondary osteoporosis (OP) worldwide. With epidemiological data suggesting almost 0.9% of the population taking GCs, a large number of patients are at significant risk of morbidity associated with GIOP-related fractures.

EPIDEMIOLOGY

Though the association between GC and OP has long been known, its importance in clinical practice remains underrecognized. Some distinct features of GIOP include the rapidity of bone loss early after initiation of therapy with the accompanying increase in fracture risk, and the combined pathology of suppressed bone formation and increased bone resorption during therapy.

There is a clear epidemiological association between GC therapy and fracture risk. Oral GC therapy is prescribed in up to 2.5% of the population for a wide range of medical disorders and fractures may occur in up to 30–50% of patients on chronic therapy. The vertebrae and femoral neck of the hip are specifically involved, sparing the forearm (predominantly consisting of cortical bone), confirming that GCs affect predominantly cancellous bone. Vertebral fractures may be asymptomatic.

The fracture incidence is also related to the dose and duration of GC exposure. No dose is considered truly safe; even 2.5 mg of prednisone equivalents per day can be a risk factor for fracture. However, the risk is greater with higher doses and chronic use. The risk of fractures increases several folds with continuous, longer, and higher doses of GCs and it declines after discontinuation although the recovery of the lost bone may be gradual and often incomplete.

The epidemiological data associating fracture risk with GC therapy majorly come from the use of oral GCs. Less is known about the risk associated with inhaled GCs. The underlying disorder for which inhaled or systemic GCs are used may also be a cause of bone loss. The systemic release of local bone-resorbing cytokines in some inflammatory autoimmune disorders can stimulate bone loss. Malabsorption of vitamin D, calcium, and other nutrients can add to the problem of inflammatory bowel disease. Chronic hypoxia, acidosis, immobilization, reduced physical activity, and smoking may all contribute to bone loss in respiratory diseases.

MECHANISMS OF BONE LOSS

Skeletal Mechanisms

Glucocorticoids accelerate bone resorption early and also inhibit bone formation. So, their use can lead to early and rapid bone loss. The early bone resorption is followed by a stable decrease in bone formation. This is explained by increased apoptosis of osteoblasts as evident from the histological changes consisting of thinning of trabeculae, increase in trabecular space, decreased osteoid width, and reduced bone turnover. GCs also indirectly affect the Wnt signaling pathway important for bone formation by enhancing the function of the dickkopf-related protein-1 (Dkk-1) and sclerostin. This results in suppression of bone morphogenetic proteins (BMP) which are critical for osteoblast differentiation.

Decreasing BMD is directly correlated with increased fracture risk. But apart from BMD, GCs-induced microarchitectural alteration of collagen peptides and cross-linking are also important in determining the fracture risk due to their adverse effects on the osteocytes.

Extraskeletal mechanisms:

- GCs decrease calcium absorption from the intestine and increase urinary calcium excretion leading to secondary hyperparathyroidism. This increases osteoclast activity and stimulates bone loss. There is also reduced tubular reabsorption of phosphate leading to phosphaturia.
- Oral GCs inhibit follicle-stimulating hormone, suppressing estrogen production in women and testosterone production in men. These effects lead to increased bone absorption.
- GC can inhibit the hypothalamic-pituitary-adrenal (HPA) axis which inhibits the levels of adrenal androgens. Reduced production of androgens decreases their positive effect on bone formation.
- High-dose and prolonged GCs can inhibit the production of gonadotropin-releasing hormone thereby decreasing the production of luteinizing hormone (LH) and causing secondary hypogonadism. This decreases testosterone production which ultimately decreases bone formation and increases bone resorption.
- GCs can also cause muscle atrophy, especially type 2a and type 1 fiber by reducing muscle protein synthesis and glycogen synthesis and interfering with fatty acid oxidation. This further leads to low bone mass and increases susceptibility to physical falls.
- GC further adds to the problem by inhibiting growth hormone (GH) secretion and reducing bone sensitivity to GH.

CLINICAL FEATURES AND RISK FACTORS

The clinical manifestations of GIOP are often insidious, with loss of BMD occurring over several months to years before any symptoms or complications become apparent. In some patients, the first sign of GIOP may be a fracture due to low trauma or even spontaneous fractures detected incidentally on a plain X-ray. The most common site of fracture is the vertebral body which may not be painful but may manifest as a loss in height or a change in posture. Sometimes it may present as a new onset back pain.

Risk factors associated with the dose and duration of GCs are well known. Other factors include advanced age, low BMI, postmenopausal status, physical inactivity, smoking, baseline low BMD, and frequent falls. The underlying disease for which the GCs are prescribed are also risk factors and it's important to control inflammation in inflammatory arthritis.

LABORATORY INVESTIGATIONS

Laboratory evaluation for GIOP should aim to exclude other common secondary causes of OP and include total blood cell count, renal and liver function tests, serum protein electrophoresis, serum, and 24-hour urine calcium, serum levels of 25-hydroxyvitamin (OH) D, alkaline phosphatase, thyroid-stimulating hormone, and parathyroid hormone, estradiol in women and total and free testosterone in men.

In patients receiving GCs, a dose-dependent decrease in serum osteocalcin may be found, indicating inhibition of osteoblastic activity. Other markers of bone formation such as total and bone-specific alkaline phosphatase and procollagen type 1 carboxy-propeptide may be diminished. Some studies of patients treated with GCs have shown elevated markers of bone resorption [such as urinary collagen N-telopeptides (NTX)]. Given such inconsistency and heterogeneity, the measurement of serum bone turnover markers is considered to be of little clinical utility and it is not currently advocated for routine use.

Assessment of the BMD by dual-energy absorptiometry (DXA) alone is not a good tool to predict fractures in GIOP. The poor bone quality induced by GCs resulting in fractures does not correlate with BMD. Similarly, Fracture Risk Assessment tool (FRAX) may underestimate the fracture risk because it does not account for the actual and cumulative dose, and the duration of GCs intake. In FRAX, GC use is considered yes if the patient is currently on oral GC or has been exposed to at least 5 mg prednisolone or equivalent for 3 months. For those taking prednisolone 7.5 mg or more, FRAX adjustments are required. FRAX also includes femoral neck BMD while GIOP preferentially affects vertebrae more. High-resolution peripheral quantitative computed tomography (HRpQCT) and TBS (trabecular bone score) are evolving modalities to assess bone microarchitecture and fracture risk associated with GCs.

MANAGEMENT OF GLUCOCORTICOID-INDUCED OSTEOPOROSIS

General Measures

Minimizing GCs dose and duration is the most important in the prevention of GIOP. Wherever possible, systemic use of GCs should be avoided and GC-sparing drugs should be used. Elderly patients and those on high doses of GCs, those with painful joints and sarcopenia especially of lower limbs, should be evaluated for the risk of falling. Physiotherapy, balanced nutrition, physical activity for strength and flexibility, and mobilization should be used for these conditions to decrease the fracture risk. The use of walking aids and better footwear can further diminish the risk of falls and subsequent fractures. Apart from physical fitness, smoking cessation and limitation of alcohol consumption should also be considered.

Calcium and Vitamin D

Adequate supplementation of calcium (1,000–1,200 mg/day) and vitamin D (600–800 IU/day) should be considered in patients with GCs, although their effect on BMD is controversial. An adequate dose of vitamin D (2,000 IU/day) is recommended for the Indian population to attain sufficient 25(OH) D levels (>30 ng/mL). For the same purpose, daily exposure to sunlight for 10–30 minutes in the morning for two to three times a week is recommended.

Pharmacotherapy

Bisphosphonates

These antiresorptive drugs are the standard therapy of GIOP management. Alendronate (weekly 35–70 mg or daily 5–10 mg, orally), Risedronate (weekly 35 mg or daily 5 mg, orally), Ibandronate (monthly 150 mg, oral or 3 mg IV once in 3 months), Zoledronic acid (5 mg IV infusion once a year) are commonly used bisphosphonates available. They are recommended for primary prevention in all patients who are taking GCs (daily dose of >7.5 mg of prednisolone) for more than three months duration, especially in postmenopausal women and elderly men. Though safe and cost-effective, these drugs are associated with rare side-effects including osteonecrosis of the jaw and atypical femoral fractures with long-term use. Bisphosphonates should be avoided in patients with an estimated glomerular filtration rate (eGFR) <35 mL/min.

Parathormone Analogs (Teriparatide and Abaloparatide)

These are anabolic agents which effectively enhance bone formation by improving the trabecular bone mass thereby reducing the fracture risk. High cost and parenteral route of administration are the major obstacles to their use. Their major adverse effects include hypercalcemia and hypercalciuria, which require regular monitoring during the therapy. Discontinuation of the therapy leads to rapid bone loss increasing the risk of fractures making. The addition of an antiresorptive agent such as a bisphosphonate or denosumab after discontinuation is therefore advisable.

Denosumab

It is a monoclonal antibody to an osteoclast-differentiating factor that binds with RANKL and interferes with osteoclasts differentiation thereby decreasing bone resorption and thus increasing BMD. Even though there is a lack of studies on denosumab use in GIOP, some data suggest that denosumab can be used in patients where bisphosphonates are contraindicated (e.g., in renal failure). Some studies point toward a higher risk of infection with denosumab when compared with bisphosphonates. There is a lack of sufficient safety data with denosumab for patients who are on multiple immunosuppressive agents including biological disease-modifying drugs and hence not recommended as first-line therapy in GIOP. Upon discontinuation, there is a rapid rate of bone loss and vertebral fracture increases rapidly, especially among patients with a previous vertebral fracture. Hence, it is advisable to start alternative antiresorptive agents such as bisphosphonates after the discontinuation of denosumab.

Other Agents

Raloxifene, a selective estrogen-receptor modulator (SERM) used in postmenopausal women is currently not widely used in GIOP. Calcitonin is no longer used to prevent and treat GIOP. Long-term use of calcitonin for OP has been associated with an increased risk of cancers. Newer agents such as Odanacatib, a Cathepsin K inhibitor, and Romosozumab, a monoclonal antibody to sclerostin are now available options for GIOP. However, their benefit and long-term safety remain to be investigated.

RECENT GUIDELINES

Patients with GIOP should be risk-stratified into low, moderate, or high-risk groups for fracture, with low risk being < 10% probability, moderate risk being 10–19%, and high risk being at least 20% probability of major osteoporotic fracture. The latest update strongly recommends treatment with oral bisphosphonates for patients with a high risk receiving long-term GCs, while the prophylactic treatments of choice for patients with a moderate risk include oral or intravenous bisphosphonates, parathyroid hormone (PTH)/parathyroid hormone-related peptide (PTHrP), and denosumab. SERMs or romosozumab can be prescribed in specific patients at low risk for cardiovascular events, thrombosis, or stroke.

The American College of Rheumatology 2022 updated guidelines also highlight the need for sequential therapy. Patients receiving denosumab, PTH, PTHrP, or romosozumab may require additional treatment with bisphosphonates after discontinuation of these medications and GCs while those receiving treatment with SERMs or bisphosphonates do not require subsequent therapy. Within 6–7 months after the last denosumab dose, patients should receive an oral or intravenous bisphosphonate for 1–2 years, or potentially be transitioned to receive PTH, PTHrP, or romosozumab to prevent rapid bone loss and vertebral compression fractures. Patients completing a course of PTH, PTHrP, or romosozumab must receive an oral or intravenous bisphosphonate or denosumab followed by bisphosphonates. Discontinuation of PTH, PTHrP, and romosozumab without bisphosphonates substitution may result in rapid bone loss and new fractures.

CONCLUSION

Glucocorticoid-induced osteoporosis is the most common cause of secondary OP and clinicians must prioritize its prevention and treatment. Despite increasing awareness of GIOP amongst healthcare professionals, its management remains suboptimal. Guidelines have contributed to increased diagnosis and treatment rates, but overall, these rates remain low. Bone loss and the resulting fracture risk start early after the initiation of GCs necessitating clinical assessment for fracture risk in all age groups within 6 months of starting GCs and repeating yearly. No dose is considered safe for OP. Bisphosphonates form the mainstay of the therapy in the absence of contraindications.

SUGGESTED READINGS

1. Ilias I, Milionis C, Zoumakis E. An Overview of Glucocorticoid-Induced Osteoporosis. South Dartmouth (MA): MDText.com, Inc.; 2000.
2. Adami G, Saag KG. Glucocorticoid-induced osteoporosis update. Curr Opin Rheumatol. 2019;31(4):388-393.
3. Buckley L, Guyatt G, Fink HA, Cannon M, Grossman J, Hansen KE, et al. 2017 American College of Rheumatology Guideline for the Prevention and Treatment of Glucocorticoid-Induced Osteoporosis. Arthritis Rheumatol. 2017;69(8):1521-37.

245 CHAPTER Osteoporosis: A Barebone Guide to Diagnosis and Management

CL Nawal, RS Chejara

ABSTRACT

Osteoporosis is a common metabolic bone disease. The imbalance in remodeling by resorption and new bone formation leads to osteoporosis.

Osteoporosis is a multifactorial disorder. Primary osteoporosis is due to aging and postmenopausal state. Secondary osteoporosis is caused by many diseases, drugs, and lifestyle. Women with postmenopausal state has progressive loss of bone mass primarily affecting trabecular part of bone while aging affects cortical part of bone.

Osteoporosis largely remains asymptomatic until a fracture occurs with fall or trauma. Pain in the affected part of the body maybe a presenting complaint. Loss of height due to compression fracture of multiple vertebrae. Fractures cause chronic pain, disability, and death by themselves or due to complications.

Careful history, physical examination, and appropriate investigations help in early recognition. Bone mineral density (BMD) measurement by dual-energy X-ray absorptiometry (DEXA) and other tools remains the mainstay in the diagnosis. World Health Organization (WHO) also recommends an algorithm-based tool like Fracture Risk Assessment Tool (FRAX) to assess future fracture risk that can be confirmed by BMD.

Adequate intake of calcium and vitamin D especially in postmenopausal period is preventive for osteoporosis. Bisphosphonates are the first-line agents used in osteoporosis. Intravenous zoledronate given every year is most potent agent. Romosozumab and denosumab are monoclonal antibodies against receptor activator of nuclear factor-kappa B (RANK) ligand (RANKL), which are being increasingly used nowadays.

INTRODUCTION

Osteoporosis is the most common metabolic bone disease especially in postmenopausal women. It is clinically characterized by bone fracture following trivial trauma, jerk, or stress over the bones that may lead to painless vertebral fractures and nerve root compression causing severe pain in the affected region.

Osteoporosis has multiple etiological factors. Age-related osteoporosis is commonly found in postmenopausal women. It is also associated with many diseases, deficiencies and drugs. Risk factors are: advancing age, female sex, ethnicity, postmenopausal state, tobacco and alcohol use, sedentary lifestyle, and smoking.

Diagnosis of osteoporosis is based on a perfect history of the patient related to demography, lifestyle, risk factors, comorbid illness, and drug intake. It is supported by appropriate laboratory investigations and radiological imaging.

Commonly used quantitative methods used are bone mineral density (BMD), dual-energy X-ray absorptiometry (DEXA), and quantitative computed tomography (QCT) at hip and vertebrae. Fracture Risk Assessment Tool (FRAX) with BMD and Garvan fracture risk calculator have shown the best performance to assess the risk of osteoporosis.

Management of osteoporosis is focused on prevention, nonpharmacological, and pharmacological treatment. Adequate calcium supplementation, vitamin D intake, and exercise are major areas for prevention.

Bisphosphonates are the most commonly used agents to retard the progression and treatment of osteoporosis. Selective estrogen receptor modulators (SERMS) are used effectively in postmenopausal women. Similarly parathyroid hormone (PTH) analogs like teriparatide are also used. Monoclonal antibodies romosozumab and denosumab a humanized monoclonal antibodies directed against receptor activator of nuclear factor-kappa B (RANK) ligand (RANKL) are being increasingly used.

ETIOPATHOGENESIS

Osteoporosis is a multifactorial disease caused by interplay of various risk factors. Physiologically, normal bone tissue is continuously modified by bone resorption and formation of new bone.

Osteoporosis can be classified into two categories: primary and secondary osteoporosis. Primary osteoporosis can be divided into two subgroups: Involutional type-1 osteoporosis also known as postmenopausal osteoporosis caused by estrogen deficiency mainly affecting the trabecular part of the bone. Involutional type-2 osteoporosis is also called senile osteoporosis related to loss of bone mass due to aging affecting cortical part of the bone. Secondary osteoporosis is due to different diseases, lifestyle, and drugs that can cause osteoporosis **(Table 1)**.

CLINICAL FEATURES AND COMPLICATIONS

Osteoporosis affects both males and females. There are multiple risk factors which may lead to osteoporosis and its complications. Detailed history and physical examination give important clues about the risk factors and association with other diseases. History of repeated fractures with minimal/trivial trauma in the weight-bearing bones may suggest osteoporosis in an otherwise healthy individual.

Pain is the most common presenting symptom for osteoporosis due to fractures. Sometimes fracture in vertebrae and other sites may go unnoticed until it is displaced and causes nerve impingement leading to pain in the affected dermatomes. Importantly, pain may be dull, poorly localized that is increased after physical activity and relieved by the rest.

Swelling in the affected area, redness over the site, difficulty in walking, or a limp may be presenting features when pain is minimal when long bones of lower limb are affected.

Loss of height may be a first complaint in case of multiple vertebral fractures. Comparison with historical height of the patients is important to suspect before any investigation. Similarly, kyphosis may be noticed in such

TABLE 1: Secondary causes of osteoporosis.

Lifestyle changes	Genetic disorders	Endocrine causes	Hematologic causes
Smoking	Cystic fibrosis	Central obesity	Hemophilia
Alcohol use	Glycogen storage disease	Cushing syndrome	Leukemia
Vitamin D deficiency	Marfan syndrome	T1DM and T2DM	Lymphoma
Immobilization	Gaucher's disease	Thyrotoxicosis	Sickle cell disease
Sedentary lifestyle	Hemochromatosis	Hyperparathyroidism	Thalassemia
Frequent falls	Osteogenesis imperfecta	Premature menopause	Monoclonal gammopathy
Low calcium intake	Porphyria	Hyperprolactinemia	Multiple myeloma
	Ehlers–Danlos syndrome	Turner's syndrome	Mastocytosis
	Homocystinuria	Klinefelter's syndrome	
Gastrointestinal causes	Rheumatological causes	Neurological causes	Others
Celiac disease	Ankylosing spondylosis	Multiple sclerosis	HIV
Gastric bypass	Systemic lupus	Epilepsy	COPD
Malabsorption	Rheumatoid arthritis (RA)	Muscular dystrophy	Amyloidosis
Pancreatic disease	Autoimmune disorders	Parkinson's disease	Sarcoidosis
Primary biliary cirrhosis		Stroke	Depression
Inflammatory bowel disease		Proximal myopathy	Congestive heart failure

(COPD: chronic obstructive pulmonary disease; HIV: human immunodeficiency virus; T1DM: diabetes mellitus; T2DM: type 2 diabetes mellitus)

patients. Multiple fracture vertebrae leading to deformity of chest can cause restriction to the lung movement, restrictive lung disease, increased pulmonary artery hypertension and right side heart failure.

Fractures cause chronic pain, disability, and death related to their complications and interventions. Fracture of hip, pelvis, and long bones require prolonged immobilization, surgical interventions, nursing care, and family support and it is also associated with pain, anxiety, and depression in many individuals.

DIAGNOSIS

There are multiple tools available for the assessment of the bone quality and strength. According to WHO osteoporosis is defined as *"BMD less than 2.5 SD or more, compared to average value of a healthy young individual"*; similarly osteopenia is defined when *"BMD is between 1 and 2.5 SD below the mean level of a young individual"*.

Various laboratory investigation are necessary to rule out causes of secondary osteoporosis that includes biochemical markers for bone turnover, which can be measured to differentiate between actual status of bone metabolism. Bone-specific alkaline phosphatase (BSAP), osteocalcin (OC), carboxy- and aminoterminal propeptide of type 1 collagen (P1CP and P1NP) are major biomarkers for bone formation. They are osteoblast products. Similarly cross-linked C-telopeptide of type-1 collagen (1-CTP), tartrate-resistant acid phosphatase 5b (TRAP-5b), N-terminal telopeptide of collagen type I (NTX-1) and C-terminal telopeptide of type 1 collagen (CTX-1) are serum markers; and hydroxyproline, pyridinoline (Pyd) and deoxypyridinoline (Dpd) CTX-1 and NTX-1 are urinary markers for osteoclastic activity. These markers can be used as aid to the diagnosis and to follow up early response to therapy for osteoporosis.

Guidelines

American Association of Clinical Endocrinology (AACE) recommends BMD testing in:

- Women age 65 or older
- Postmenopausal women with history of fracture, osteopenia identified radiographically and glucocorticoid therapy > 3 months
- Early menopause, smoking, excessive alcohol use, and secondary osteoporosis are other indications.

The 2020 update of AACE guidelines recommends evaluation of all the women age 50 years or more after a clinical fracture risk assessment by with FRAX tool.

Various other organizations including National Osteoporosis Foundation (NOF), International for Clinical Densitometry (ISCD), and US Preventive Services Task Force (USPSTF) also recommend screening programs for osteoporosis. The indications for BMD testing can be summarized as women aged 65 or older, men aged 70 years or older, younger postmenopausal women, men aged 50–69 years with clinical risk factors, adults with fragility fractures, adults with risk of secondary osteoporosis, and anyone being considered for pharmacologic therapy.

Radiography and Tools

Plain radiography is used when the patient is already suspected as osteoporosis fracture. X-ray spine and lateral chest radiography are used to assess vertebral fracture in patients with loss of height and kyphosis or scoliosis. Osteoporosis largely affects trabecular part of bone compared to cortical bone and it is not adequately visualized by plain radiographs. So, it is an insensitive tool to assess osteoporosis.

Dual-energy X-ray absorptiometry is the standard method to evaluate BMD. DEXA is easy to use and cost-effective method to assess osteoporosis in suspected patients on outpatient basis. Standard sites are vertebra, hip, and femur head. DEXA can better assess trabecular bone structure affected by osteoporosis. T-scores are used to classify osteoporosis and osteopenia in postmenopausal women and older population while Z-scores are used in others.

Quantitative computed tomography is another method to measure BMD. It accurately assesses trabecular and cortical bone structure. In fact it is the most sensitive method to assess BMD. Compared to DEXA, it is better in identifying fracture line, healing sclerosis, and callous formation areas at comparable cost and accuracy.

FRAX: Even like various modalities of BMD testing, the probability of a osteoporotic fracture remains uncertain. Recently, WHO has introduced an algorithm-based tool called fracture risk assessment tool model to estimate 10 years' risk of osteoporosis fracture. It takes consideration of various clinical risk factors including age, sex, BMD at femur neck, body mass index (BMI), smoking, alcohol intake, rheumatoid arthritis, and glucocorticoid use.

MANAGEMENT OF OSTEOPOROSIS

Approach to a patient with osteoporosis requires meticulous history-taking, physical examination, and BMD scores to assess the risk of fractures. Osteoporosis is a preventable and treatable disease when diagnosed in time to received appropriate and effective treatment. A holistic approach should be followed in the management of osteoporosis.

Nonpharmacological Intervention and Prevention

There are several interventions that are recommended to the people with high risk of osteoporosis and to prevent fractures related to osteoporosis. Adequate intake of dietary calcium and vitamin D is required to maintain calcium homeostasis. Older individuals (>50 years) and postmenopausal women have increased requirement of calcium that cannot be fulfilled by diet alone and daily intake should be increased to 1,000 mg/day in men and 1,200 mg/day in women. Many patients have high risk of vitamin D deficiency such as malabsorption syndromes, inflammatory bowel disease (IBD), gastric bypass, pernicious anemia, chronic used of proton-pump inhibitor (PPI), and renal and liver failure. Excessive intake of alcohol badly affects bone health and fractures may be due to high risk of falls, vitamin D deficiency, and chronic liver disease (CLD). It predisposes for osteoporosis. They are recommended to limit alcohol intake <7 drinks per week. Prevention of falls is most important in patients with high risk of osteoporosis and taking medications that affect alertness of the patient. These patients may require support during walking by caregivers.

Pharmacologic Management

Bisphosphonates are first-line therapy recommended for the patients of osteoporosis. Commonly used oral agents are alendronate, risedronate, ibandronate, and zoledronic acid is used as an intravenous agent. They are mainly used as antiresorptive agents.

Alendronate is used in treatment of postmenopausal women, men, and glucocorticoid-induced osteoporosis. Treatment dose of 70 mg every week is recommended taken 30 minutes before the meals with plenty of water. The patient has to maintained upright posture to reduced risk of gastroesophageal reflux disease (GERD). It can be also taken with combination with vitamin D3 to increase bone mass. It reduced risk of osteoporotic fracture by 50% in patients with established osteoporosis.

Risedronate and *ibandronate* are other orally active bisphosphonates given in osteoporosis.

Zoledronic acid is a once-yearly intravenous agent given in osteoporotic men, postmenopausal women, and glucocorticoid-induced osteoporosis. It is the most potent bisphosphonate available for the treatment of osteoporosis. It significantly reduced risk of vertebral fracture by 67%.

Complications of oral bisphosphonates include severe gastritis and GERD. Zoledronic acid may cause acute kidney injury (AKI) in patient with dehydration. A specific side effect: Osteonecrosis of jaw is seen in many patients. Patients should be screened for dental hygiene, caries and loose teeth before infusion. Hypersensitivity and acute phase reactions are seen in few patients.

Selective estrogen receptor modulators, raloxifene and bazedoxifene, are recommended in postmenopausal women. Raloxifene is given as 60 mg orally daily has shown improvement in bone loss and reduction in osteoporotic vertebral fracture by 35%. It also has beneficial effect is reducing breast cancer risk. It increases risk of deep vein thrombosis (DVT) stroke and hot flushes. A combination of bazedoxifene and estrogen is approved by Food and Drug Administration (FDA) to prevent osteoporosis in postmenopausal women.

Parathyroid hormone analogs, teriparatide and abaloparatide, are recommended in postmenopausal women and men who are intolerant to previous treatment. Teriparatide is also recommended in glucocorticoid-induced osteoporosis. Intermittent use has demonstrated increased bone mass by 13% over spine and hip.

Romosozumab is a monoclonal antibody that inhibits sclerostin, which inhibits bone morphogenetic protein (BMP)-induced bone formation, increases bone formation, and decreases bone resorption; it was recently approved for treatment of osteoporosis in postmenopausal women. It may increase the risk of myocardial infarction (MI), stroke, and cardiovascular death.

Denosumab is a humanized RANKL, which is the key mediator of bone resorption. It decreases osteoclastic activity and bone resorption. It has beneficial effect in postmenopausal women, men, and cancer patients. It reduces the incidence of vertebral and hip fractures in postmenopausal women. The recommended dosage is 60 mg subcutaneous every 6 months. When denosumab is discontinued, it is associated with an increased risk of vertebral fracture and should be continued indefinitely or followed by bisphosphonate therapy.

Calcitonin is a hormone that decreased osteoclast activity. It is recommended in patients with contraindication to bisphosphonate therapy in conjunction with vitamin D and calcium. It is not commonly used as it is associated with many side effects including allergy, irritability, and sweating.

The AACE updated guidelines 2020 and National Osteoporosis Foundation (NOF) have almost similar guidelines. They recommend pharmacologic treatment for postmenopausal women with:

- T-score between –1.0 and –2.5 in spine, femur neck, and hip with history of fragility fracture; T-score –2.5 or lower spine, femur neck, and hip or 1/3 radius with FRAX 10-year probability of osteoporotic fracture >20% or 10-year probability of hip fracture >3%; first-line agents for most high-risk patients: alendronate, risedronate, zoledronate, denosumab; first-line agents for high-risk patients unable to use oral therapy: teriparatide, zoledronate, denosumab, romosozumab; First line agents for spine-specific indications in selected patients: ibandronate, raloxifene.

The AACE guidelines currently advice against the use of combination therapy, until the effect of combination therapy on fracture is better understood.

SUGGESTED READINGS

1. Porter JL, Varacallo M. Osteoporosis. In: StatPearls [Internet]. Treasure Island (FL): StatPearls Publishing; 2023.
2. Beaudoin C, Moore L, Gagné M, Bessette L, Ste-Marie LG, Brown JP, et al. Performance of predictive tools to identify individuals at risk of non-traumatic fracture: a systematic review, meta-analysis, and meta-regression. Osteoporos Int. 2019;30(4):721-740.
3. Sözen T, Özışık L, Başaran NÇ. An overview and management of osteoporosis. Eur J Rheumatol. 2017;4(1):46-56.
4. Cosman F, de Beur SJ, LeBoff MS, Lewiecki EM, Tanner B, Randall S, et al. Clinician's guide to prevention and treatment of osteoporosis. Osteoporosis Int. 2014;25:2359-81.
5. Compston J, Bowring C, Cooper A, Cooper C, Davies C, Francis R, et al; National Osteoporosis Guideline Group. Diagnosis and management of osteoporosis in postmenopausal women and older men in the UK: National Osteoporosis Guideline Group (NOGG) update 2013. Maturitas. 2013;75:392-6.
6. Cooper C, Melton LJ 3rd. Epidemiology of osteoporosis. Trends Endocrinol Metab. 1992;3:224-9.
7. Siminoski K, Warshawski RS, Jen H, Lee K. The accuracy of historical height loss for the detection of vertebral fractures in postmenopausal women. Osteoporos Int. 2006;17:290-6.
8. Kanis JA on behalf of the World Health Organization Scientific Group. Assessment of Osteoporosis at the Primary Health-care Level. Technical Report. World Health Organization Collaborating Centre for Metabolic Bone Diseases. United Kingdom: University of Sheffield; 2007.
9. Seeman E, Delmas PD. Bone quality—the material and structural basis of bone strength and fragility. N Engl J Med. 2006;354: 2250-61.
10. Vasikaran S, Cooper C, Eastell R, Griesmacher A, Morris HA, Trenti T, et al. International Osteoporosis Foundation and International Federation of Clinical Chemistry and Laboratory Medicine position on bone marker standards in osteoporosis. Clin Chem Lab Med. 2011;49(8):1271-4.
11. Camacho PM, Petak SM, Binkley N, Diab DL, Eldeiry LS, Farooki A, et al. American Association Of Clinical Endocrinologists/American College Of Endocrinology Clinical Practice Guidelines for the Diagnosis and Treatment of Postmenopausal Osteoporosis-2020 Update. Endocr Pract. 2020;26(Suppl 1):1-46.
12. Schousboe JT, Shepherd JA, Bilezikian JP, Baim S. Executive summary of the 2013 International Society for Clinical Densitometry Position Development Conference on bone densitometry. J Clin Densitom. 2013;16(4):455-66.
13. Nayak S, Roberts MS, Greenspan SL. Cost-effectiveness of different screening strategies for osteoporosis in post-menopausal women. Ann Intern Med. 2011;155(11):751-61
14. Kulkarni AG, Thonangi Y, Pathan S, Gunjotikar S, Goparaju P, Talwar I, et al. Should Q-CT Be the Gold Standard for Detecting Spinal Osteoporosis? Spine (Phila Pa 1976). 2022;47(6):E258-E264.
15. Moyer VA. Vitamin D and calcium supplementation to prevent fractures in adults: U.S. Preventive Services Task Force recommendation statement. Ann Intern Med. 2013;158:691-6.
16. Kanis JA, Johansson H, Johnell O, Oden A, De Laet C, Eisman JA, et al. Alcohol intake as a risk factor for fracture. Osteoporos Int. 2005;16:737-42.
17. Boonen S, Orwoll E, Magaziner J, Colón-Emeric CS, Adachi JD, Bucci-Rechtweg C, et al; HORIZON Recurrent Fracture Trial. Once-yearly zoledronic acid in older men compared with women with recent hip fracture. J Am Geriatr Soc. 2011;59(11):2084-90.
18. Grady D, Cauley JA, Stock JL, Cox DA, Mitlak BH, Song J, et al Effect of Raloxifene on all-cause mortality. Am J Med. 2010;123(5): 469.e1-7.
19. Orwoll E, Teglbjærg CS, Langdahl BL, Chapurlat R, Czerwinski E, Kendler DL, et al. A randomized, placebo-controlled study of the effects of denosumab for the treatment of men with low bone mineral density. J Clin Endocrinol Metab. 2012;97(9):3161-9.

246
CHAPTER

Current Understanding of Pathophysiology of Systemic Sclerosis

Asish Mondal

ABSTRACT

Systemic sclerosis (SSc) is a rare and complex autoimmune disease. Due to unclear pathophysiology, the optimal therapeutic approach is still not available specially to halt the fibrotic process, which is responsible for high mortality and morbidity of SSc patients. In recent years, several new aspects in the pathophysiology of SSc have been discovered which enable the researcher to develop new therapeutic targets to halt the process of fibrosis.

INTRODUCTION

Systemic sclerosis (SSc) is a rare and complex autoimmune disease which is characterized by vasculopathy, inflammation, and fibrosis of skin and internal organs. Development of fibrosis may affect gastrointestinal, pulmonary, and renal systems. The widespread fibrosis is responsible for high morbidity and mortality in SSc patients. It has been found that around 75% of patients with SSc may develop moderate-to-severe pulmonary fibrosis which is a single most important mortality indicator.

Systemic sclerosis is primarily of two varieties: *Limited cutaneous* (LcSSc) and *diffuse cutaneous* (DcSSc). DcSSc is the most aggressive variety where the internal organs can be affected. A lot of efforts have been given in recent years to elucidate the events behind the pathophysiology and the risk factors of SSc, but still they are only partially understood. Due to lack of complete understanding, the targeted treatment of SSc could not be introduced successfully. In recent years, it has somehow become clear that instead of different triggering factors, the development of fibrosis usually occurs through a similar pathophysiologic pathway.

Pathophysiology of SSc is initiated with microvascular or endothelial damage, which is followed by autoimmune response and inflammation and lastly diffuse fibrosis. It has been reported that both genetic and environmental factors have key roles for the development and progression of this disease. Uninhibited fibrosis in SSc is due to excessive production, remodeling, and cross-linking of extracellular matrix (ECM) from persistent activated myofibroblasts.

GENETIC FACTORS

In an analysis of combined American cohorts involving 703 families, it has been revealed that frequency of SSc is significantly more in families with SSc (1.6%) than in the general population (0.026%). A largest SSc twin study showed that overall concordance of SSc was as low as 4.7% and was similar in monozygotic and dizygotic twins, and also this concordance rate was much lower than that in other autoimmune diseases. In early a genome-wide association study (GWAS) conducted in SSc patients, the strongest association seen was found in the human leukocyte antigen (HLA) class II region on chromosome 6 but could not locate the responsible gene. The GWAS supported not only the hypothesis regarding dysregulated autoimmune response as key events of SSc patients but also the additional role of environmental factors and epigenetic influences for the development of SSc. Dysregulation of the type 1 interferon (IFN) pathway has been evident in several autoimmune diseases including SSc.

ENVIRONMENTAL FACTORS

Increased incidence and severity of SSc have shown to be associated with exposures to silica and organic solvents. Few observational studies found that exposure to epoxy resins, asbestos, and particulate air pollution is associated with an increased incidence of SSc. Infectious agents and dysbiosis have been found to be associated with an increased incidence of SSc though the exact role has still not cleared.

MICROVASCULAR PATHOPHYSIOLOGY

Microvasculopathy is responsible for the early manifestations of SSc like Raynaud's phenomenon and nailfold capillary changes and it is also plays a key role in the development of digital ulcers, telangiectasias, pulmonary arterial hypertension (PAH), scleroderma renal crisis, gastric antral vascular ectasia (GAVE), and coronary microvascular disease. Endothelial injury is the primary event to develop microvasculopathy. Infections, autoantibodies, reactive oxygen species (ROS), and cytotoxic T cell are the factors involved for endothelial injury. Anti-endothelial cell antibodies (AECA) have been found in 28–85% of patients with SSc which induce endothelial cell apoptosis and secretion of chemotactic mediators. Anti-angiotensin II receptor antibodies (ATRA) and anti-endothelin type-A receptor antibodies (ETRA) act on their receptors on endothelium to increase vasoconstriction which is responsible for *obliterative vasculopathy*. Affected endothelial cells showed endothelial cell activated with increased leukocyte adhesion molecules [e.g., E-selectin, vascular cell adhesion molecule-1 (VCAM-1) and intercellular adhesion molecule-1 (ICAM-1)], cytoplasmic vacuolization, ballooning, cytoskeletal rearrangement, loosening of tight junctions and apoptotic changes.

Vasospasm: In patients of SSc, microvascular endothelial cells have decreased the expression of endothelial NO-synthase with reduced NO and increased endothelin 1 (ET-1) production. NO is a potent vasodilator and it also inhibits platelet aggregation, smooth muscle cell proliferation, and cytokine-induced endothelial activation. On the other hand, ET-1 is a vasoconstrictor and responsible for smooth muscle cell proliferation, fibrosis, and inflammation. Unopposed action of ET-1 in SSc leads to a chronic vasoconstrictive state.

Procoagulant state: Elevated levels of von Willebrand factor (vWF), fibrinogen, tissue plasminogen activator (tPA), and/or tPA inhibitor have been seen in patients of SSc, which results in microvascular thrombosis and fibrin deposition. vWF is positively correlated with disease severity. Oxidized-low-density lipoprotein (LDL) is elevated in SSc which may promote endothelial dysfunction.

Defective angiogenesis: Angiogenesis occurs in SSc which is trigged by chronic tissue hypoxia due to microvasculopathy, vasospasm, and microthrombosis. But this angiogenesis is dysregulated, and it happens from the differential expression of proangiogenic [e.g., vascular endothelial growth factor (VEGF), platelet-derived growth factor (PDGF), fibroblast growth factor-2 (FGF-2)] and angiostatic [e.g., endostatin, soluble endoglin (ENG), CXC chemokine ligand (CXCL) 4, 8, 9, 10] factors. Bone marrow-derived circulating endothelial progenitor cells (EPCs) may affect angiogenesis as these progenitors normally replace the damaged endothelial in ischemic and injured tissues. A lower number of ECPs has seen in SSc patients than a normal individual.

ACTIVATION OF THE ADAPTIVE AND INNATE IMMUNE SYSTEMS

Damaged and apoptotic endothelial cell release damage-associated molecular patterns (DAMPs) which activate and recruit immune cell. Altered expression of cell adhesion molecules also facilitates immune cell infiltration like T cells, monocytes, and macrophages during early SSc.

Immune cells are responsible for the secretion of interleukin 4 (IL-4), IL-13, and transforming growth factor (TGF)-β which have key roles in fibrosis. IL-4 and IL-13 are predominantly secreted by type 2 helper T (Th2) cells and both the factors stimulate TGF-β production, fibroblast proliferation and differentiation, ECM proliferation, and at the same time inhibiting the synthesis of collagenases like metalloproteinase (MMP)1 and MMP3 and enhancing tissue inhibitor of metalloproteinase (TIMP)-1. TGF-β has a pivotal role in the process of fibrosis it acts by inducing *SMAD4*-mediated gene expression, activation of mitogen-activated protein kinase (MAPK)-mediated signaling via c-Jun N-terminal kinase (JNK), p38, and extracellular signal-regulated kinases (ERK) 1 and 2. Both *M1 and M2 macrophages* are able to produce TGF-β, IL-4, and IL-13 or proinflammatory mediators like IL-6. M2 macrophages also influence crosslinking of collagen by modulating fibroblast activities.

Neutrophils also produce TGF-β, IL-6, and VEGF35 and release ROS which activate fibroblasts through the TGF-β pathway.

Dendritic cells (DCs) are known as antigen-presenting cell. In SSc, DCs activate naive T cells to present antigens, which influence the autoimmune responses. In SSc patients, an increased number of toll-like receptor-8

(TLR8) on the cell surface of plasmacytoid (p) DCs has been found that enhances signaling and causes secretion of high amounts of IFN-α and chemokine (C-X-C motif) ligand 4 (CXCL4) into the skin.

Mast cells can secrete a large number of fibrogenic mediators apart from histamine release which induces lung fibroblast proliferation. It releases platelet-activating factor which causes platelets to aggregate and release TGF-β, PDGF, and fibronectin.

Intercellular adhesion molecule 1 (ICAM1) is highly expressed in SSc lesion. It can give way the T cells that are attracted by a local increase in TGF-β levels.

In SSC, the activated *B-cell* can secrete IL-6 which induces differentiation of *M2 macrophage* and *Th2* cells and augment fibrosis through direct activation of skin fibroblast or through secretion of TGF-β. Most of the autoantibodies secreted from B cells are directed to nuclear antigens. Autoantibodies to PDGF and ET-1 were shown positive in some cases that may promote fibrosis.

Natural killer (NK) cells inhibit myofibroblast activation and differentiation by stimulating myofibroblast apoptosis as seen in liver fibrosis or by secretion of IFN-γ. In SSc patients, a reduction in both number and killing activity of CD56hi NK cells was observed that may further promote fibrosis.

DEVELOPMENT OF FIBROSIS

It has been observed that myofibroblasts are the main drivers of SSc-related tissue fibrosis. Myofibroblasts are a type of mesenchymal cells having both the ECM-synthesizing features of fibroblasts and the cytoskeletal characteristics of contractile smooth muscle cells.

Myofibroblast Location

In skin, the presence of myofibroblasts correlates well with the amount of (hyalinized) collagen and skin parameters related to fibrosis (tightness, hardness, and stiffness) and do so more significantly than inflammation.

In early lung fibrosis, it can be identified in interstitial tissue, but in advanced fibrosis it can be identified in bronchoalveolar lavage fluid of SSc patients also. Fibrosis in pulmonary vessels causes vessel narrowing. At the same time, myofibroblast expresses ET-1 leading to vasoconstriction resulting in PAH.

Myofibroblasts were also identified in the esophagus and gastric wall of patients with SSc with severe fibrosis. Fibrosis leads to decrease contractile power of smooth muscle that results in gastric acid reflux into the esophagus.

Decreased Apoptosis of Myofibroblasts

Cellular apoptosis occurs through extrinsic and intrinsic pathways. The extrinsic pathway is initiated by activation of fas cell surface death receptor (Fas). Fas ligand triggers the formation of a death-inducing signaling complex (DISC) which activates caspase 8. Caspase 8 activates caspase 3, which is the final step for apoptosis. The intrinsic pathway is triggered by the release of cytochrome c from mitochondria. Cytochrome c comes out through a pore-forming protein—BCL2-associated X protein (BAX)—and activates caspase 9 which in turn activates caspase 3. BCL2 and BCL2-X_L are two important inhibitors of BAX. The apoptosis of myofibroblast is determined by the ratio of activity of proapoptic BAX and antiapoptic BCL2/ BCL2-$X_{L.}$

Systemic sclerosis myofibroblasts express less BAX compared to myofibroblasts of a control individual. The probable cause for this is increased activity of tyrosine-protein kinase ABL1 (c-Abl). Stiffness of the ECM in SSc patients produces antiapoptic BCL2-$X_{L.}$ This stiffness induces BCL2-X_L which counteracts BAX and prevents apoptosis.

In SSc skin, phosphatidylinositol 3-kinase (PI3K)/AKT serine/threonine kinase (AKT) signaling is increased. This pathway is responsible for increased survival of myofibroblast by inhibiting apoptosis. Many growth factors including TGF-β can induce PI3K/AKT signaling. TGF-β also lowers Fas-mediated apoptosis and lowers the expression of acid sphingomyelinase (SMPD1). SMPD1 facilitates Fas-mediated apoptosis and inhibits AKT signaling. Due to high AKT signaling and low Fas-mediated apoptosis in SSc, activated myofibroblasts survived.

Lastly, micro-RNA (miRNA) also has a key role for survival of myofibroblast in SSc patients because this miRNA targets and degrades proapoptotic BAX mRNA and lowers apoptosis of myofibroblast.

Formation of Myofibroblasts in SSc

Along with decreased apoptosis, formation of myofibroblasts is increased in SSc. Myofibroblasts can originate from differentiation of fibroblasts from different pathways **(Fig. 1)**. There are four variants of PDGF which interact with homo- or heterodimers of *PDGF receptor* alpha (PDGFRα) and beta (PDGFRβ) and induce signaling by phosphoinositide 3-kinase (PI3K)/AKT serine/threonine kinase (AKT), p38 MAPK (p38 MAPK), focal adhesion kinase (FAK), and tyrosine-protein kinase ABL1 (c-ABL). Enhanced *Wnt signaling* with increased blood and tissue level of Wnt agonist has been seen in SSc. This Wnt signaling activated when a Wnt/frizzled/LRP5/6 complex formed. This complex recruits dishevelled (Dvl) to the plasma membrane, which inhibits degradation and accumulation of β-catenin. β-catenin recruits the transcriptional co-activator and acetyltransferase proteins CBP and p300 to generate a transcriptionally

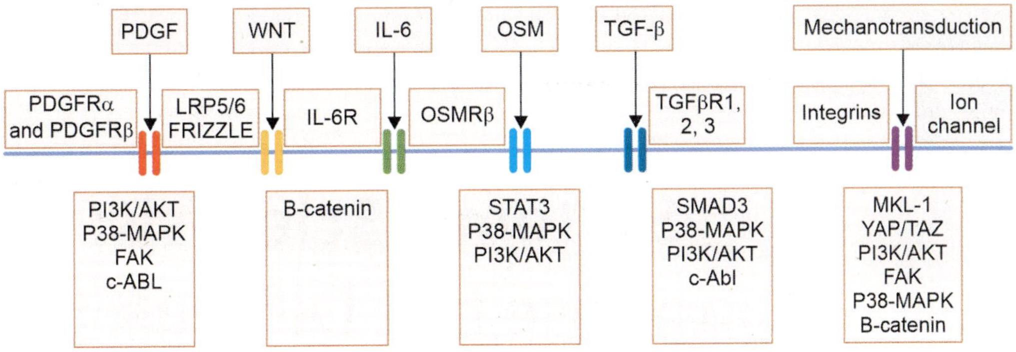

FIG. 1: Stimuli for myofibroblast formation and their intracellular pathways.

active complex. *IL-6 signaling* occurs when IL-6 binds with its receptor (IL-6R) and glycoprotein 130 (gp130) and forms a complex which activates PI3K/AKT, p38MAPK, and signal transducer and activator of transcription 3 (STAT3) signaling. *Oncostatin M* (OSM) also coupled with gp130 but together with oncostatin M receptor beta (OSMRβ). *TGF-β* induces heterotetramerization of TGF-β-receptor type I (TGFBR1) and II (TGBR2) leading to intracellular activation of SMAD3, p38 MAPK, and PI3K/AKT c-ABL. TGFBR3 and ENG regulate TGF-β availability and receptor complex formation. *Mechanotransduction* occurs through mechanosensitive ion channels. This leads to Ca ion influx, integrin complexes, and deformation of cellular structures, which can activate myocardin-like protein 1 (MLK1), β-catenin, FAK, p38 MAPK, and PI3K/AKT signaling.

Myofibroblast can differentiate not only from fibroblast, but also from adipocytes, monocytes/fibrocytes, pericytes, endothelial cells, and epithelial cells. Epithelial to mesenchymal transition (EMT) and endothelial to mesenchymal transition (EndoMT) are the two processes for epithelial and endothelial cells to form myofibroblast, respectively. Along with increased formation, activity of myofibroblasts is also markedly increased in SSc. That leads to increased fibrosis in SSc. Immune cells like mast cells, neutrophils, macrophages, and Th2 lymphocytes produce various mediators (e.g., IL-4, IL-13, and TGF-β) which can influence myofibroblast formation and function and survival.

TABLE 1: New therapeutic agents and their targets in systemic sclerosis (SSc).

Molecules	Targets
C-82	Canonical Wnt signaling pathway
Fresolimumab	TGF-β receptor
Nintedanib	PDGFR/VEGFR/FGFR
Lenabasum	CBr2
Tocilizumab, IL-31RA receptor inhibition	IL-6
Tofacitinib	JAK1/JAK3 kinase

Due to better understandings of pathophysiology of SSc, researchers are now able to develop new molecules to inhibit formation and functions of myofibroblast to halt or to reverse the process of fibrosis. **Table 1** shows some of the new molecules and their targets in the pathophysiologic process of SSc.

CONCLUSION

A lot of efforts has been given to know the events in the pathophysiology of SSc. Microvasculopathy is the initial event followed by autoimmunity and inflammation that lead to formation and persistent activation of myofibroblast, resulting in diffuse fibrosis. The therapeutic approach to inhibit autoimmunity and formation of myofibroblast can halt the process of fibrosis in SSc and hence can improve the quality of life of SSc patients.

SUGGESTED READINGS

1. Ota Y, Kuwana M. Updates on genetics in systemic sclerosis. Inflamm Regener. 2021;41:17.
2. Hummers LK, Hall A, Wigley FM, Simons M. Abnormalities in the regulators of angiogenesis in patients with scleroderma. J Rheumatol. 2009;36:576-82.
3. Saygin D, Highland KB, Tonelli AR. Microvascular involvement in systemic sclerosis and systemic lupus erythematosus. Microcirculation. 2019;26(3):e12440.
4. van Caam A, Vonk M, van den Hoogen F, van Lent P, van der Kraan P. Unraveling SSc Pathophysiology: The Myofibroblast. Front Immunol. 2018;9:2452.

247

CHAPTER

Systemic Sclerosis: Easy to Diagnose but Difficult to Treat

Renu Saigal

ABSTRACT

Systemic sclerosis (SSc) is an uncommon, connective tissue disease (CTD) with multiorgan involvement, characterized by dysregulated immune reaction, vasculopathy, and fibrosis of multiple organs. Multiorgan involvement occurs mostly, in the first 5 years of disease onset so early therapy is recommended to salvage the function of various organs, as there is no cure for SSc currently. Organ-specific screening is mandatory for timely and effective treatment.

Some immunosuppressive drugs such as mycophenolate mofetil, cyclophosphamide, methotrexate, and biological agents such as rituximab and tocilizumab have been added to the treatment regimen for this disease, especially to treat interstitial lung disease (ILD), myocarditis, and diffuse skin involvement. Drugs such as endothelin receptor antagonists (ERAs), phosphodiesterase-5 inhibitors (PDE5Is), prostacyclin analogs, and soluble guanylate cyclase stimulators (Riociguat) have been added in recent years to treat pulmonary artery hypertension (PAH). Raynaud's phenomenon (RP) and digital ulcers (DUs) can be managed by dihydropyridine calcium channel blockers (CCBs) and PDE5I and intravenous Iloprost.

In recent years, autologous hematopoietic stem cell transplantation (AHSCT) has been shown to improve the survival of rapidly progressive early diffuse cutaneous systemic sclerosis (dcSSc).

INTRODUCTION

Systemic sclerosis (SSc) is a rare, multisystem autoimmune connective tissue disease (CTD), that affects the skin (sclerosed or hardened), and various organs of the body. Initially, there is microvasculopathy, dysregulation of immunity, and later fibrosis of the skin and internal organs. Lungs, heart, blood vessels, gastrointestinal tract (GIT), kidneys, and musculoskeletal system are involved. The onset of the disease is highest in the fourth and fifth decades. The prevalence of the disease is about 30–120 cases per million. Treatment of SSc is organ-based. Interstitial lung disease (ILD) and pulmonary artery hypertension (PAH) are the main causes of death in SSc.

According to the extent of skin involvement, it is divided into:

- *Limited cutaneous SSc (lcSSc)*: Skin distal to elbows and knees, face, and neck are involved, with no truncal involvement, and vascular manifestations such as Raynaud's phenomenon (RP) and telangiectasia **(Figs. 1A to D)**, and PAH are present. The anticentromere antibody is positive in these patients. Many patients have CREST syndrome (calcinosis, Raynaud phenomenon, esophageal dysmotility, sclerodactyly, and telangiectasia).
- *Diffuse cutaneous SSc (dcSSc)*: Skin of the trunk, whole upper and lower limb is involved. Anti-Scl-30 antibody (or anti-topoisomerase 1) is present in 30% of these patients who also have ILD. Anti-RNA polymerase III is positive in patients of dcSSc who are at risk to develop, scleroderma renal crisis (SRC), and hand disability.
- *SSc sine scleroderma*: Internal organ involvement without skin thickening occurs in 1.5–8% of patients of SSc. Autoantibodies, specific for SSc are present in these patients.
- *SSc overlap syndromes*: CTD with any of the earlier-mentioned subsets of SSc are present.

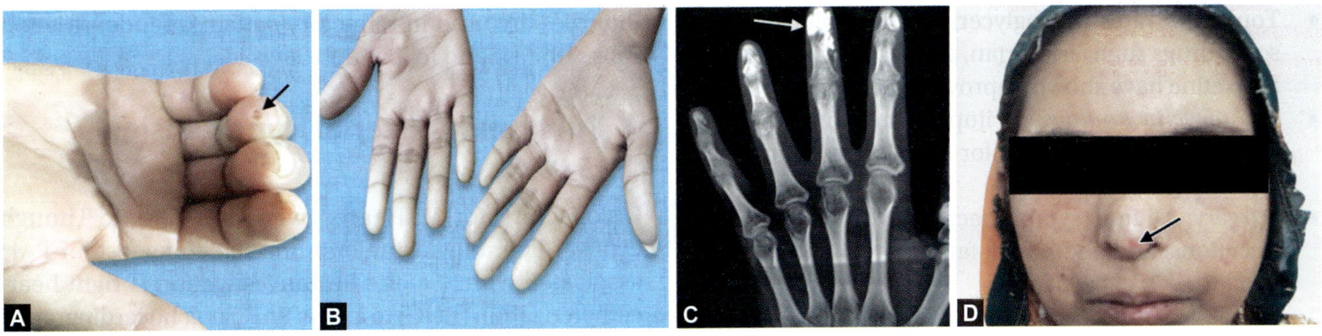

FIGS. 1A TO D: (A) Pulp pitting; (B) Raynaud's phenomenon; (C) Calcinosis; (D) Telangiectasia over tip of nose, blanches on pressing.

- The *"prescleroderma"* subset has RP, puffy fingers, capillaroscopic changes of capillary loss, and positive antinuclear antibody. Up to 50% of this subset, in the long term, develop a classifiable CTD.

Major clinical manifestations and complications of SSc are digital vasculopathy, digital contractures, acro-osteolysis, calcinosis, ILD, PAH, gastrointestinal complications, and renal and cardiac involvement.

MANAGEMENT OF VARIOUS MANIFESTATIONS OF SYSTEMIC SCLEROSIS

Major organ involvement occurs early in the disease and the disease progression can be slowed by early treatment. Systematic baseline assessment and follow-up is the most important aspect of management.

Skin Involvement

Skin is involved in most patients of SSc (except in subset 3, sine scleroderma), leading to pigmentation alone or associated depigmentation (salt and pepper appearance) pruritus, and ulceration. The extent of skin involvement can be assessed by a modified Rodnan score, the skin of 17 areas of the body is given 0–3 grading depending on how much the skin can be folded (range 0–51). Extensive skin thickening in early disease is associated with internal organ involvement and progresses usually till 4 years in most patients and regresses thereafter.

Treatment of Skin Involvement

General measures include avoidance of soaps and the use of emollients, for sclerodactyly heat, wax baths, stretching exercises, and physiotherapy should be done.

- Methotrexate (MTX) 15–25 mg per week, for diffuse and progressive skin involvement, arthritis, and myositis, without visceral involvement.
- Mycophenolate mofetil (MMF) 1.5–3.0 g per day, if associated with visceral involvement.
- Cyclophosphamide (CYC) (2 mg/kg orally, or IV pulses 15 mg/kg every month), is preferred in patients refractory to MTX, MMF, or skin involvement is associated with progressive ILD.
- Rituximab (RTX) or intravenous immunoglobulin (IVIg) may be used in patients refractory to the earlier-mentioned agents.
- Tocilizumab (TCZ) (focuSSced trial) may be used for refractory skin involvement with arthritis or ILD.

Digital Ulcer Treatment and Prevention

Pulp pitting is seen in these patients **(Fig. 1A)**, which may lead to digital ulcer (DU).

Calcium channel blocker (CCB) is the first line and various trials have shown that IV iloprost and phosphodiesterase-5 inhibitor (PDE5I) improve healing. Bosentan [endothelin receptor antagonist (ERA)] was useful in the prevention of new DUs despite CCB, PDE5I, or iloprost therapy. Antibiotics are used when there is an infection.

Raynaud's Phenomenon (100%) (Fig. 1B) and Digital Ulcers (50%)

Vasoconstriction and obliterative vasculopathy lead to RP, SRC, pulmonary hypertension, and other visceral diseases. Patients should avoid cold exposure, vibration injury, smoking, emotional stress vasoconstrictors, bleomycin, clonidine, and ergot alkaloids.

Treatment of Raynaud's Phenomenon

- *CCBs*: Most widely studied drug is nifedipine.
- PDE5I (sildenafil and tadalafil) increase levels of nitric oxide, a vasodilator. Both CCB and PDE5I reduce the severity and frequency of RP.

X-ray chest and pulmonary function tests (PFTs) including DLco and CT scans in the prone position (to detect early changes) are required to diagnose ILD, biopsy is not recommended. Screening for concomitant PAH should be done.

Disease severity is assessed at baseline and monitored every 6 months, by symptoms, 6MWD, FVC, TLC, and DLco (if FVC decreases by 10% or by 5% with a corroborative decrease of 15% in DLco, it predicts reduced survival).

Hyperpolarized xenon MRI to quantify gas exchange is a new modality.

Treatment of Interstitial Lung Disease in Systemic Sclerosis

Immunosuppression and Antifibrotic Therapy (Table 2)

Indications of immunosuppressive drugs:

- Moderate-to-severe ILD on high-resolution computed tomography (HRCT) (or >20% lung involvement)
- Less than 10% lung involvement in HRCT with abnormal PFTs
- FVC (<80%) and/or DLco below the normal lower limit, or early progressive findings on HRCT

TABLE 2: Management of pulmonary artery hypertension (PAH) and interstitial lung disease (ILD).

PAH (15–18%)	*Endothelin receptor antagonists (ERA):* • Bosentan 62.5–125 mg, BD orally • Ambrisentan 5–10 mg/day orally • Macitentan 10 mg/day orally • Adverse effects: Anemia and increased liver enzymes *Phosphodiesterase 5 inhibitors:* • Pulmonary vasodilatory and antiproliferative effects because of increased cyclic guanosine monophosphate (cGMP) levels • Sildenafil 20 mg thrice daily orally • Tadalafil 40 mg/day orally *Prostacyclin analogs—vasodilator and platelet inhibitor:* • Iloprost initial dose: 2.5 μg inhaled; if well-tolerated, then 5 μg subsequent dose 6–9 times/day as needed; not more than once every 2 hours while awake • Maintenance: 2.5–5 μg per dose; not to exceed 45 μg/day • Iloprost, IV infusion over 6 hours daily at 0.5–2.0 ng/kg/min • Epoprostenol: 1–12 ng/kg/min continuous IV infusion via a central venous catheter. Used in advanced disease. Dose titrated up every 1–2 weeks • Selexipag (prostacyclin receptor agonist) 200–1,600 μg BD orally • Treprostinil, SC 0.625–1.25 ng/kg/min continuous IV infusion via a central venous catheter or continuous subcutaneous infusion • Treprostinil, inhaled 18 μg inhaled QID *Soluble guanylate cyclase stimulator: (Increases cGMP production) antiproliferative and antiremodeling effect:* • Riociguat Initial dose: 0.5–1 mg TID orally, titrated up by 0.5 mg TID every 2 weeks to a maximum dose daily of 2.5 mg TID. (PATENT-1 study)
• ILD • Duration of immunosuppression: 4–5 years of stable spirometry then careful tapering	*Immunosuppressants:* • Oral mycophenolate mofetil (MMF) (2–3 g/day): First-line drug. Better tolerated • IV monthly pulses of cyclophosphamide (CYC) (600 mg/m^2) or oral CYC 2 mg/kg/day • Azathioprine (2 mg/kg/day) is used if ILD is mild or after CYC pulses or if MMF is not tolerated • Rituximab two IV infusions 2 weeks apart then one infusion every 6 months, better tolerated than CYC with fewer adverse events, used as second-line therapy • Tocilizumab (IL-6R antagonist) 162 mg SC once weekly or 4–8 mg/kg IV monthly, there was less decline of lung function and CT changes. It is indicated in patients with early systemic sclerosis (SSc) ILD with elevated acute-phase reactants, with adverse effects to MMF, CYC, and antifibrotics, also proposed as first-line therapy by American College of Rheumatology (ACR) recently • Corticosteroids are indicated only in ILD secondary to overlap syndromes, as they can precipitate scleroderma renal crisis (SRC) (in RNAPIII-positive patients) and other adverse effects

Continued

Continued

	Antifibrotic therapy:
	Indications:
	• If progressive [declining FVC or DLco, high-resolution computed tomography (HRCT) showing progression] ILD is present
	• Long-standing (>5 years) disease, monotherapy, if immunosuppressive therapy is not recommended
	• Add on therapy when MMF, CYC, TCZ fail, and aggressive ILD is there, i.e., FVC decline > 10% in 1 year (INBUILD trial showed the superiority of nintedanib over placebo)
	• With advanced disease at initial presentation (FVC < 50%) in combination with MMF/CYC/TCZ, it showed a beneficial effect (SENSCIS trial)
	• ILD patients with contraindication, inefficacy, intolerance, or with adverse effects to MMF/CYC/TCZ (inefficacy is defined as worsening symptoms, worsening PFTs or HRCT findings)
	  ○ Nintedanib (tyrosine kinase inhibitor) 150 mg twice a day; if not tolerated reduce to 100 mg twice a day
	  ○ Pirfenidone (fewer data) 801 mg three times per day, if not tolerated, reduce the dose

	If worsening ILD is there, the following are the options as proposed by ACR: • Change the immunomodulator • Combine immunomodulator and antifibrotic • Combine immunomodulator with rituximab or tocilizumab • Autologous hematopoietic stem cell transplantation (AHSCT) and lung transplantation

- High-risk patient viz. early rapidly progressive diffuse cutaneous disease (even when FVC > 80% and mild ILD, i.e., <10% on HRCT)
- The decline of oxygen saturation (SpO_2) on exercise or hypoxemia at rest
- Worsening HRCT with symptoms and declining PFTs

Who should not be Treated?

Long-standing disease (close to 10 years duration) with stable PFTs and stable ILD over recent years.

Other Measures in the Management of Interstitial Lung Disease

- Rigorous antireflux therapy
- Identification and treatment of concomitant PAH
- Smoking cessation
- *Vaccinations*: For influenza, coronavirus disease 2019 (COVID-19), and pneumococcal infections.
- *Oxygen*: If hypoxia or desaturation with exercise or when lying down
- Exercise program
- Pulmonary rehabilitation
- *For prevention of infection*: With immunosuppressive therapy azithromycin 250 mg three times every week (if associated with bronchiectasis) and for *Pneumocystis jirovecii* prophylaxis, Trimethoprim plus sulfamethoxazole double-strength three times a week is recommended.
- Lung transplantation

Duration of Therapy

Patients should be weaned from therapy, after stable disease for >2 years, if there is stabilization or improvement of symptoms, FVC, DLco, HRCT chest scans, 6MWD, significant reduction of NT-proBNP, and/or improvement of O_2 saturation with exercise. Oxygen saturation should be measured from forehead or ear sensors and not from fingers because of vasculopathy, false low O_2 saturation may be detected.

Tapering should be done slowly in 1–2 years and PFT should be monitored every 6 months with or without a low maintenance dose of MMF.

Renal Involvement

Mild proteinuria, elevated serum creatinine concentration, and/or hypertension may occur with renal involvement. About 50% of patients of SSc may have renal involvement on autopsy.

Scleroderma Renal Crisis

Occurs more frequently in early dcSSc (5–20%) than in lcSSc (1–2%) and it is a life-threatening condition. Blood pressure (BP) monitoring should be done at home to detect the onset of SRC in high-risk patients **(Table 1)**.

Clinical Presentation of Scleroderma Renal Crisis

- Acute kidney injury
- Moderate to marked hypertension, about 10% of SRC patients may be normotensive and have unexplained poor outcomes.

- Normal urine sediment without heavy proteinuria.
- Microangiopathic hemolytic anemia is evidenced by the presence of schistocytes, microspherocytes, and helmet cells on peripheral blood film.

Goals of Therapy of SRC

Blood pressure should be lowered to baseline within 72 hours. Angiotensin-converting enzyme (ACE) inhibitors especially captopril should be started immediately, because of its rapid onset and short duration of action, and its dose can be escalated. If BP is not controlled, CCB may be added. Beta-blockers are usually avoided as these can produce vasospasm. ACE inhibitors are not stopped despite an increase in serum creatinine as recovery eventually occurs in most cases unless the irreversible injury has occurred.

Gastrointestinal Tract Manifestations (90%)

Any part of GIT may be involved, leading to reflux, bloating, distension, constipation, diarrhea, and anorectal incontinence. The esophagus being the most commonly affected part of GIT lead to dysphagia and GERD.

Treatment of Gastroesophageal Reflux Disease

- GERD is managed by proton pump inhibitor as first-line treatment, H2 antagonist, prokinetic drugs, sucralfate, and antacids.
- Lifestyle modification by raising the head of the bed, early dinner, chewing food well, eating slowly, drinking water with eating, avoiding foods like fatty meals that trigger reflux or worsen dysphagia
- Esophageal dilations when required. Fundoplication surgery if severe reflux with aspiration.

Gastric antral vascular ectasia or watermelon stomach can cause silent anemia, weight loss, and malnutrition and may be associated with anti-RNA polymerase III autoantibodies.

For small intestinal bacterial overgrowth, intermittent, or rotating antibiotics are used.

Gastrointestinal manifestations are not considered immune responsive.

Cardiac Disease

The patient may present with arrhythmias, pericardial disease, myocardial disease, heart failure, and ischemic heart disease (IHD) due to microvascular disease. Baseline electrocardiogram (ECG), echocardiography, cardiac troponin, and cardiac catheterization should be planned. Fibrosis occurs in the myocardium, intrafascicular conducting fibers, and late gadolinium enhancement on MRI detects and confirms diffuse or focal cardiac fibrosis.

Implantable cardioverter defibrillators may prevent sudden deaths due to sudden severe arrhythmias. IHD or congestive heart failure (CHF) is treated on routine guidelines. Beta-blockers can worsen RP so is contraindicated. Treatment of myocarditis is the same as of ILD.

Other Nonlethal Manifestations of Systemic Sclerosis

These manifestations include facial changes and oral complications such as limited jaw opening, sicca symptoms, dental disease, and, might be amenable to treatment. Sexual dysfunction, depression, and osteoporosis may also occur, affecting the quality of life. Malignancy risk may be increased if anti-RNA polymerase III is positive and with the use of CYC and AHSCT.

For pruritus, a cannabinoid receptor modulator (lenabasum) is recommended.

Nutrition is very often neglected and due attention should be given to this complication.

Intensive Immunosuppression with Autologous hematopoietic Stem Cell Transplantation

Patients with early dcSSc with skin and lung fibrosis or advanced internal organ involvement or other features of poor prognosis, who fail to respond to conventional immunosuppressive therapy, have shown better outcomes with AHSCT, especially in experienced centers with proper patient selection and excluding patients with severe cardiac disease. Infection and procedure-related complications increase the mortality of this procedure.

Emerging Therapies (Flowchart 2)

Phase I and II trials are going on with these drugs.

Inflammatory targets (trials ongoing)

- JAK inhibitors—tofacitinib
- B-cell inhibitors—rituximab
- T-cell inhibitors—abatacept

Therapy for fibrotic targets (trials ongoing)

Targets	Inhibitors
TGF beta family:	Fresolimumab
Oncostatin M:	GSK233308
Thrombin:	Dabigatran
Lysophosphatidic acid (LPA):	LPA receptor 1 antagonist
B-cell activating factor (BAFF):	BAFF antagonists
Inducible T-cell costimulator (ICOS):	ICOS inhibitor
IL-4/IL-13 antibody:	Romilkimab
Cannabinoid receptor 2 agonist:	Lenabasum

FLOWCHART 2: Emerging targets for SSc.
(IL: interleukin; SSc: systemic sclerosis TGF: transforming growth factor)

CONCLUSION

Systemic sclerosis is a rare disease. Treatment should be started early as organ involvement occurs early in the course of the disease. Proper screening, monitoring, and treatment can salvage organ function and decrease morbidity and mortality.

SUGGESTED READINGS

1. van den Hoogen F, Khanna D, Fransen J, Johnson SR, Baron M, Tyndall A, et al. 2013 classification criteria for systemic sclerosis: an American College of Rheumatology/European League against Rheumatism collaborative initiative. Ann Rheum Dis. 2013;72:1747-55.
2. Denton CP, Khanna D. Systemic sclerosis. Lancet. 2017;390: 1685-99.
3. Rahaghi FF, Hsu VM, Kaner RJ, Mayes MD, Rosas IO, Saggar R, et al. Expert consensus on the management of systemic sclerosis-associated interstitial lung disease. Respir Res. 2023;24:6.
4. Pope JE, Denton CP, Johnson SR, Fernandez-Codina A, Hudson M, Nevskaya T. State-of-the-art evidence in the treatment of systemic sclerosis. Nat Rev Rheumatol. 2023;19:212-26.
5. Volkmann ER, Varga J. Emerging targets of disease-modifying therapy for systemic sclerosis. Nat Rev Rheumatol. 2019;15(4):208-24.
6. Khanna D, Lescoat A, Roofeh D, Bernstein EJ, Kazerooni EA, Roth MD, et al. Systemic Sclerosis–Associated Interstitial Lung Disease: How to Incorporate Two Food and Drug Administration–Approved Therapies in Clinical Practice. Arthritis Rheumatol. 2022;74(1):13-27.
7. Varga J, Axford JS (Ed). Clinical manifestations and diagnosis of systemic sclerosis (scleroderma) in adults. [online] Available from www.uptodate.com. [Last accessed April, 2023].

248

CHAPTER

Management of Gout

Satyabrata Ganguly, Sayonee Das, Shikhar Bansal

ABSTRACT

The frequency of gout worldwide has been steadily adding over the past several decades. Although both the physician and patient may easily recognize the acute attack of gout, significant confusion still prevails in selecting the most appropriate medication and proper doses. The clinical stages of gout include asymptomatic hyperuricemia, intermittent gouty arthritis, and chronic tophaceous gout. Treatment of gout is usually considered after the first attack of arthritis. Treatment aims to alleviate the pain and inflammation associated with acute attacks, prevent future attacks, and decrease uric acid levels. Despite time-recognized remedies for acute gout, i.e., nonsteroidal anti-inflammatory drug (NSAID), colchicine, and oral corticosteroids, 50% of patients still have acute pain after 2 days. Allopurinol and probenecid, the mainstays of urate lowering therapy, fail to bring the uric acid level to <6 mg% in 50% of patients. Moreover, in a significant proportion of patients, the drugs have to be discontinued due to toxicity.

The purpose of this management update is to provide practical advice about better and safer treatment modalities considering both therapeutic goals and patient comorbidities.

INTRODUCTION

Hyperuricemia, defined as serum uric acid (SUA) concentration over 6.8 mg/dL, is a unique feature found only in *Homo sapiens* due to the absence of enzyme uricase which degrades uric acid to more soluble allantoin and highly efficient reabsorption of uric acid in the distal tubules.

Antonie van Leeuwenhoek described gout and its relation with hyperuricemia as its key causal precursor as early as 1679. In 1848, Sir Alfred Garrod first demonstrated elevated levels of uric acid in patients with gout. Many great kings, emperors, generals, admirals, and philosophers have died of gout. Around 85% of causes of hyperuricemia are underexcretion and the rest are either uric acid overproduction or sometimes combined mechanisms. As far as treatment is concerned, mainly overproduction is addressed as these compounds are cheap and readily available. In India, the cases of gout are generally mild to moderate and respond to such treatment whereas worldwide severe cases of gout are frequently observed necessitating other treatment options that address underexcretion as well.

DIAGNOSIS

- Primarily clinical
- Demonstration of *monosodium urate (MSU)* crystals in synovial fluid—gold standard
- *X-ray*: Punched out lesion with overhanging edges—*Martel sign* or *rat bite sign*
- *Ultrasonography (USG):*
    - MSU crystals within the joint
    - Acute gouty arthritis: Snowstorm sign
    - Uric acid deposition in joint: Double-contour sign.
- *Dual-energy computed tomography (DECT)*: It is a new modality in the armamentarium of gout imaging which has received quite an applause and is increasingly being introduced and used. It is a noninvasive method of seeing MSU crystal deposits,

especially in early gout. Subclinical MSU deposits can also be detected in asymptomatic hyperuricemic patients.

MANAGEMENT

Management of hyperuricemic individuals, whether asymptomatic or with gout, aims primarily at maintaining serum urate concentrations in a subsaturating range (usually <6 mg/dL), thus preventing or reversing the clinical consequences of urate crystal formation and deposition. Managing a case of gout includes dietary and lifestyle modification, local treatment, analgesics, and approaches to lower blood and tissue uric acid levels.

Dietary and Lifestyle Modification

- Weight loss of obese—diet, exercise, medications, and bariatric surgery
- *Diet*:
    - Avoid purine-rich food. Not all foods which are high in purines cause gout; there is no risk for peas, beans, mushrooms, cauliflower, or spinach. Those having seafood are more likely to have gout. Low-fat dairy products decrease the risk of gout whereas overall protein intake has no effect.
    - Alcohol can increase the risk of gout and the risk increases with increasing intake.
    - Avoid high fructose-containing beverages
    - Higher levels of coffee consumption significantly decrease the risk of gout

Hence, diets shown to be connected to gout are the same kinds of diets linked to cardiovascular diseases.

Medications that increase the risk of gout: Thiazide, loop diuretics, cyclosporine, pyrazinamide, and low-dose aspirin.

Local Treatment

- Local therapy with ice is somewhat beneficial.
- The treatment of acute attacks of gouty arthritis with intra-articular injection of corticosteroids is a relatively recently recommended approach, i.e., triamcinolone 10 mg intra-articular injection.

Analgesics

- *Colchicine*: One tablet (0.6 mg) given hourly until relief of symptoms or gastrointestinal (GI) toxicity, i.e., diarrhea occurs. In the 18th century, Viennese physician Baron Anton Von Stoerk first used colchicum to treat gout.
- *Nonsteroidal anti-inflammatory drugs (NSAIDs)*: They are effective in 90% of patients and resolution of signs and symptoms usually occurs within 5–7 days. The most effective are indomethacin 25–50 mg TID, ibuprofen 800 mg TID, or diclofenac 50 mg TID; cyclooxygenase-2 (COX-2) inhibitors are equally effective.
- *Glucocorticoids*: Oral prednisolone 30–40 mg/day, 1 g IV methylprednisolone, and 20–40 mg of intra-articular triamcinolone are very effective.

Hyperuricemia is present in approximately 5% of the population and up to 25% of hospitalized individuals. It does not appear to have a causal role in the development of coronary heart disease or death from cardiovascular disease. Hence, asymptomatic hyperuricemia should only be treated in the case of cytolytic therapy for neoplastic disease to prevent acute renal failure.

Approaches of Lowering Blood and Tissue Urate

- *Dietary modification*: Alcohol raises the SUA by enhancing urate production and by reducing renal clearance, hence best avoided.
- *Uricostatic drugs*:
    - Allopurinol: It is the best drug to lower serum urate in overproducers, stone formers, and patients with advanced renal failure.
        - Dose: 300 mg OD
        - *Side effect*: Acute hypersensitivity syndrome (AHS)—a potentially fatal cutaneous reaction, the risk for AHS depends on the presence of HLA B5801 and this test should be done in Asian and African patients before giving allopurinol.
    - *Febuxostat*: A newly approved drug by the Food and Drug Administration (FDA), it is a specific xanthine oxidase inhibitor and less toxic than allopurinol.
        - Dose: 80 mg/daily.
- *Uricosuric drugs*: In 85–90% of patients with gout, impaired renal uric acid clearance is the major mechanism resulting in hyperuricemia. Uricosuric drugs are weak organic acids that promote uric acid clearance by inhibiting proximal tubule urate anion transporters that mediate urate reabsorption.
    - *Probenecid* is the most potent uricosuric drug with a dose of 500 mg twice daily. It is reabsorbed by the proximal convoluted tubule (PCT) instead of uric acid which is more excreted in the urine. The urate-lowering efficacy of probenecid is markedly lowered in patients with moderate-to-severe renal impairment.
    - *Losartan* and *fenofibrate* have modest uricosuric properties and can be used as an adjunct to the uric acid-lowering therapy (ULT) of patients

with gout with hypertension or hyperlipidemia, respectively.

- *Uricolytic drugs*:
  - Infusion of *uricase* to decrease uric acid was used from as early as 1957.
  - More recently, *rasburicase* has been used to prevent the development of tumor lysis syndrome in patients undergoing chemotherapy for malignancies.
  - Pegloticase: In the United States, a *polyethylene glycol* (PEG)—modified mammalian urate oxidase as a subcutaneous injection is under trial to reduce uric acid levels. Within hours of an initial 8 mg IV pegloticase infusion, plasma, or serum urate levels decrease to very low to undetectable levels and remain subsaturating for several weeks. Treatment involves a biweekly infusion of 8 mg, usually for a minimum of 6 months but with no maximum duration yet defined. It should be considered for patients with gout refractory to oral ULTs and should not be used in conjunction with other ULTs.

A combination of uricosuric and uricostatic drugs is very effective.

Mobilization Flare in Gouty Arthritis

A drop in SUA may precipitate mobilization flare (MF) in patients treated with ULT. Flare occurs when MSU crystals stimulate NLRP3 inflammasome. To prevent this, NSAID prophylaxis is to be given and continued for up to 6 months after flare or colchicine in the presence of chronic kidney disease (CKD).

Aggressive Urate-lowering Therapy

When usual ULT fails and rapid lowering is desired, i.e., before organ transplantation or before chemotherapy.

Drug: Pegloticase IV every 2 weeks.

How Long to Give Acid-lowering Therapy?

Till SUA comes to 6 mg% and there are no tophi and to 5 mg% if there are tophi either clinically or radiologically.

How Long to Give Anti-inflammatory?

Up to 6 months from the last flare. If NSAIDs are contraindicated then colchicine or prednisolone can be used as a prophylactic therapy to prevent migration flare.

DRUGS IN PIPELINE

Lesinurad (RDEA594)

About 70% of uric acid in our body is excreted via kidneys and hyperuricemic patients are mostly underexcretors.

Lesinurad is a uricosuric agent that inhibits both urate anion transporter 1 (URAT1) and organic anion transporter 4 (OAT4) in the renal tubule. Two-phase 2b trials were conducted on gout patients with lesinurad, where increased renal excretion of uric acid was demonstrated in a 200–600 mg/day dose.

Ulodesine (BCX4208)

It is an oral, once daily, novel purine nucleoside phosphorylase (PNP) inhibitor. It blocks the production of uric acid at a higher step in the purine catabolic pathway than the xanthine oxidase inhibitor.

A phase 2 placebo-controlled dose-ranging trial of the efficacy and safety of ulodesine monotherapy was done, which involved 24 gout subjects receiving a placebo and 85 gout subjects receiving ulodesine in various doses. Results were encouraging with 240 mg/day dosing.

The main side effects are diarrhea and drug rash.

Levotofisopam

It is a 2,3-benzodiazepine derivative, approved in >20 countries for the treatment of anxiety. Two-phase 1 studies were performed in the UK and Netherlands, and urate-lowering capacity was shown with reasonable safety and tolerability.

Dual-acting Anti-inflammatory and Urate-lowering therapy

While developing this peroxisome proliferator-activated receptor-γ (PPAR-γ) modulator for glycemic control, scientists of CymaBay Therapeutics noted several metabolic properties that made it suitable for the management of acute and chronic gout.

Arhalofenate was studied to have uricosuric properties and was shown to inhibit the uric acid transporters URAT1, OAT4, and OAT10. In studies on isolated mouse macrophages, arhalofenate was able to block MSU crystal-induced production of prointerleukin and other nuclear factor-dependent inflammatory mediators by PPAR-γ transrepression. Four phases 2 trials of 3–6 months duration have been carried out in healthy volunteers and diabetic subjects using 600 mg arhalofenate daily. Decreases in uric acid ranging from 20 to 40% have been noted, and, unlike probenecid, the uricosuric effect persists even after the deterioration of renal function.

Anti-inflammatory Therapy (Figs. 1 and 2)

- *Anakinra*: IL-1 inhibitor, treated with a daily injection of 100 mg for 2–3 days. More than 60% of patients reported a very satisfactory and rapid resolution of symptoms of acute gout **(Table 1)**.

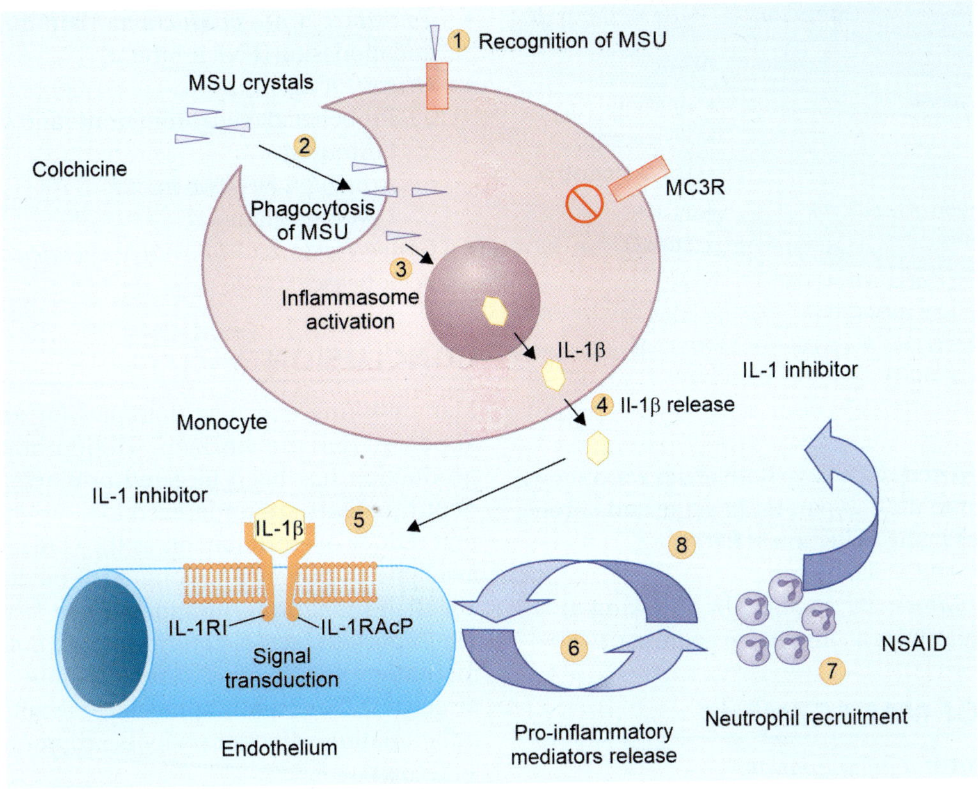

FIG. 1: Role of the NLRP3 inflammasome and IL-1β in the inflammatory cascade of acute gout.
(IL-1: interleukin 1; IL-1β: interleukin-1β; MSU: monosodium urate)

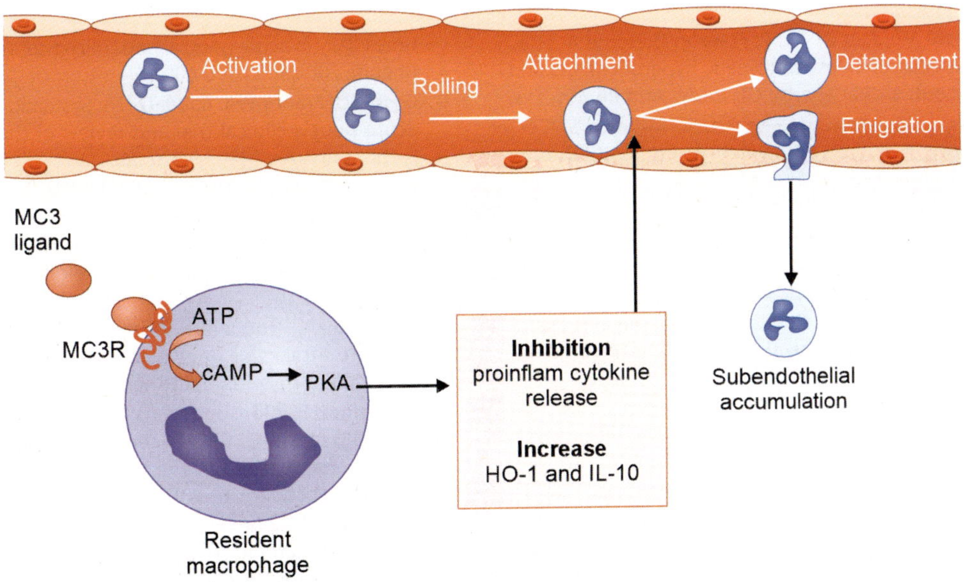

FIG. 2: Reversal of IL-1β-induced neutrophil migration in gout through MC3R activation.
(ATP: adenosine triphosphate; cAMP: cyclic adenosine monophosphate; IL-10: interleukin 10; IL-1β: interleukin-1β; PKA: protein kinase A)

TABLE 1: Drugs for treatment of gout.

Site	Action	Agent
Site 5	IL-1 inhibitor	• Anakinra • Rilonacept • Canakinumab
Site 6	Prevention of leukocyte trafficking	• ACTH • Steroid
Site 7	Prevention of prostaglandin release from leukocytes	NSAID

(ACTH: adrenocorticotropic hormone; NSAID: nonsteroidal anti-inflammatory drug)

- *Canakinumab and rilonacept*: Both drugs were shown to be superior to the comparator in acute and chronic gout as well as in the reduction of flares.
- Corticotropin and melanocortin
- *Caspase inhibitors*: By specifically blocking IL-1β secretion, it may have an impact on acute gout.

SUMMARY OF MANAGEMENT

- *To reduce pain and inflammation*:
  - First line: NSAID, colchicine, and corticosteroid
  - Second line: IL-1 inhibitor—anakinra
- *To reduce urate production*: Allopurinol, febuxostat, and ulodesine (PNP inhibitor)
- *Uricosuric agents*:
  - Probenecid, benzbromarone, and sulfinpyrazone
  - Lesinurad
  - Arhalofenate—two in one
  - Levotofisopam
- *Convert uric acid to soluble chemical*: Allantoin and pegloticase

CONCLUSION

Many exciting and new therapies for acute gout have appeared on the horizon. Diminution of uric acid production has been targeted primarily. Though most of our patients are underexcretors, we still prefer drugs that reduce overproduction as they are cheap and easily available. Adherence to long-term medication use and adequate monitoring/titration of urate-lowering therapies are important factors contributing to optimal outcomes for patients with gout. There is hope that therapies directed at the recently appreciated mechanisms of gouty inflammation will offer patients prompt relief from their sufferings.

We may dream of a day when the King of diseases and the disease of Kings will cease to be a problem!!

SUGGESTED READINGS

1. Dalbeth N, House ME, Aati O, Tan P, Franklin C, Horne A, et al. Urate crystal deposition in asymptomatic hyperuricaemia and symptomatic gout: a dual energy CT study. Ann Rheum Dis. 2015;74(5):908-11.
2. Choi HK, Atkinson K, Karlson EW, Willett W, Curhan G. Purine-rich foods, dairy and protein intake, and the risk of gout in men. N Engl J Med. 2004;350(11):1093-103.
3. Choi HK, Atkinson K, Karlson EW, Willett W, Curhan G. Alcohol intake and risk of incident gout in men: a prospective study. Lancet. 2004;363(9417):1277-81.
4. Choi HK, Willett W, Curhan G. Coffee consumption and risk of incident gout in men: a prospective study. Arthritis Rheum. 2007;56:2049-55.
5. Schlesinger N, Detry MA, Holland BK, Baker DG, Beutler AM, Rull M, et al. Local ice therapy during bouts of acute gouty arthritis. J Rheumatol. 2002;29(2):331-4.
6. Vonkeman HE, van de Laar MA. Nonsteroidal anti-inflammatory drugs: adverse effects and their prevention. Semin Arthritis Rheum. 2010;39(4):294-312.
7. Macagno A, Di Giorgio E, Romanowicz A. Effectiveness of etodolac (Lodine) compared with naproxen in patients with acute gout. Curr Med Res Opin. 1991;12(7):423-9.
8. Rubin BR, Burton R, Navarra S, Antigua J, Londoño J, Pryhuber KG, et al. Efficacy and safety profile of treatment with etoricoxib 120 mg once daily compared with indomethacin 50 mg three times daily in acute gout: a randomized controlled trial. Arthritis Rheum. 2004;50(2):598-606.
9. Groff GD, Franck WA, Raddatz DA. Systemic steroid therapy for acute gout a clinical trial and review of the literature. Semin Arthritis Rheum. 1990;19:329-36.
10. Man CY, Cheung IT, Cameron PA, Rainer TH. Comparison of oral prednisolone/paracetamol and oral indomethacin/paracetamol combination therapy in the treatment of acute goutlike arthritis: a double-blind, randomized, controlled trial. Ann Emerg Med. 2007;49(5):670-7.
11. Fernández C, Noguera R, González JA, Pascual E. Treatment of acute attacks of gout with a small dose of intraarticular triamcinolone acetonide. J Rheumatol. 1999;26(10):2285-6.
12. Perez-Ruiz F, Alonso-Ruiz A, Calabozo M, Herrero-Beites A, García-Erauskin G, Ruiz-Lucea E. Efficacy of allopurinol and benzbromarone for the control of hyperuricaemia. A pathogenic approach to the treatment of primary chronic gout. Ann Rheum Dis. 1998;57(9):545-9.
13. Becker MA, Schumacher HR Jr, Wortmann RL, MacDonald PA, Eustace D, Palo WA, et al. Febuxostat compared with allopurinol in patients with hyperuricemia and gout. N Engl J Med. 2005;353(23):2450-61.
14. Schumacher HR Jr, Becker MA, Wortmann RL, Macdonald PA, Hunt B, Streit J, et al. Effects of febuxostat versus allopurinol and placebo in reducing serum urate in subjects with hyperuricemia

and gout: a 28-week, phase III, randomized, double-blind, parallel-group trial. Arthritis Rheum. 2008;59(11):1540-8.

15. Becker MA, Schumacher HR, Espinoza LR, Wells AF, MacDonald P, Lloyd E, et al. The urate-lowering efficacy and safety of febuxostat in the treatment of the hyperuricemia of gout: the CONFIRMS trial. Arthritis Res Ther. 2010;12(2):R63.
16. Puig JG, Torres RJ, de Miguel E, Sánchez A, Bailén R, Banegas JR. Uric acid excretion in healthy subjects: a nomogram to assess the mechanisms underlying purine metabolic disorders. Metabolism. 2012;61(4):512-8.
17. Enomoto A, Kimura H, Chairoungdua A, Shigeta Y, Jutabha P, Cha SH, et al. Molecular identification of a renal urate anion exchanger that regulates blood urate levels. Nature. 2002;417(6887):447-52.
18. Anzai N, Ichida K, Jutabha P, Kimura T, Babu E, Jin CJ, et al. Plasma urate level is directly regulated by a voltage-driven urate efflux transporter URATv1 (SLC2A9) in humans. J Biol Chem. 2008;283(40):26834-8. Erratum in: J Biol Chem. 2008;283(46):32152.
19. Dalbeth N, Merriman T. Crystal ball gazing: new therapeutic targets for hyperuricemia and gout. Rheumatology (Oxford). 2009;48:222-6.
20. Sherman MR, Saifer MG, Perez-Ruiz F. PEG-uricase in the management of treatment-resistant gout and hyperuricemia. Adv Drug Deliv Rev. 2008;60:59-68.
21. Perez-Ruiz F, Sundy J, Krishnan E, Hingorani V, Welp J, Suster M, et al. Efficacy and safety of Lesinurad (RDEA594), a novel uricosuric agent, given in combination with allopurinol in allopurinol-refractory gout patients: randomized, double-blind, placebo-controlled, Phase 2B study. Ann Rheum Dis. 2011;70(Suppl 3):104.
22. Hollister AS, Becker M, Terkeltaub R, Waugh A, Lyman S, Flynt A, et al. BCX4208 shows synergistic reductions in serum uric acid in gout patients when combined with allopurinol. Ann Rheum Dis 2011;70(Suppl 3):183.
23. O'Day R, Williams KM, Graham GG. (2013). Urate-lowering therapy: uricosurics. [online] Available from https://www.futuremedicine.com/doi/10.2217/ebo.13.104 [Last accessed January, 2024].
24. Gregoire F, Zhang F, Clarke HJ, Gustafson TA, Sears DD, Favelyukis S, et al. MBX-102/JNJ39659100, a novel peroxisome proliferator-activated receptor-ligand with weak transactivation activity retains antidiabetic properties in the absence of weight gain and edema. Mol Endocrinol. 2009;23:975-88.
25. Ghosh P, Cho M, Rawat G, Simkin PA, Gardner GC. Treatment of acute gouty arthritis in complex hos- hospitalized patients with anakinra. Arthritis Care Res (Hoboken). 2013;65:1381-4.
26. Schlesinger N, Alten RE, Bardin T, Schumacher HR, Bloch M, Gimona A, et al. Canakinumab for acute gouty arthritis in patients with limited treatment options: results from two randomised, multicentre, active-controlled, double-blind trials and their initial extensions. Ann Rheum Dis. 2012;71(11): 1839-48.
27. Terkeltaub R, Sundy JS, Schumacher HR, Murphy F, Bookbinder S, Biedermann S, et al. The interleukin 1 inhibitor rilonacept in treatment of chronic gouty arthritis: results of a placebo-controlled, monosequence crossover, non-randomised, single-blind pilot study. Ann Rheum Dis. 2009;68(10):1613-7.
28. Terkeltaub RA, Schumacher HR, Carter JD, Baraf HS, Evans RR, Wang J, et al. Rilonacept in the treatment of acute gouty arthritis: a randomized, controlled clinical trial using indomethacin as the active comparator. Arthritis Res Ther. 2013;15(1):R25.
29. Mitha E, Schumacher HR, Fouche L, Luo SF, Weinstein SP, Yancopoulos GD, et al. Rilonacept for gout flare prevention during initiation of uric acid-lowering therapy: results from the PRESURGE-2 international, phase 3, randomized, placebo-controlled trial. Rheumatology (Oxford). 2013;52(7): 1285-92.
30. Schlesinger N, Mysler E, Lin HY, De Meulemeester M, Rovensky J, Arulmani U, et al. Canakinumab reduces the risk of acute gouty arthritis flares during initiation of allopurinol treatment: results of a double-blind, randomised study. Ann Rheum Dis. 2011;70(7):1264-71.
31. Getting SJ, Kaneva M, Bhadresa Y, Renshaw D, Leoni G, Patel HB, et al. Melanocortin peptide therapy for the treatment of arthritic pathologies. ScientificWorldJournal. 2009;9:1394-414.
32. Getting SJ, Christian HC, Flower RJ, Perretti M. Activation of melanocortin type 3 receptor as a molecular mechanism for adrenocorticotropic hormone efficacy in gouty arthritis. Arthritis Rheum. 2002;46(10):2765-75.
33. Wannamaker W, Davies R, Namchuk M, Pollard J, Ford P, Ku G, et al. (S)-1-((S)-2-{[1-(4-amino-3-chloro-phenyl)-methanoyl]-amino}-3,3-dimethyl-butanoyl)-pyrrolidine-2-carboxylic acid ((2R,3S)-2-ethoxy-5-oxo-tetrahydro-furan-3-yl)-amide (VX-765), an orally available selective interleukin (IL)-converting enzyme/caspase-1 inhibitor, exhibits potent anti-inflammatory activities by inhibiting the release of IL-1beta and IL-18. J Pharmacol Exp Ther. 2007;321(2):509-16.

249

CHAPTER

New and Emerging Therapies for Gout

Binoy J Paul

ABSTRACT

Twenty-first century has witnessed remarkable advances in gout therapy. This renaissance started with the development of new xanthine oxidase inhibitors, such as febuxostat or topiroxostat, pegylated uricase (pegloticase), and newer uricosuric agents such as lesinurad and dotinurad. Our understanding of the pathogenesis of hyperuricemia and gout has drastically improved in the recent years, which has resulted in the development of newer, more effective drugs. Our present armamentarium against gout includes drugs that exploit the newfound knowledge about the various mechanisms involved in the pathogenesis of gout as well as drugs used in other conditions, which are effective in gout as well. Many more drugs that promise better management of gout in the future are in the pipeline.

INTRODUCTION

Colchicine, an alkaloid derived from the autumn crocus, was first used in treatment of gout in sixth century AD. But it went out of use for more than a century for fear of gastrointestinal side effects, after which, it resurged as a therapeutic option. The use of uricosuric agents started in late 19th century with probenecid and sulfinpyrazone. But the major milestone in the treatment of hyperuricemia was the development of xanthine oxidase inhibitor (XOI), allopurinol.

But from the latter half of 20th century, gout therapeutics came to a virtual standstill. During this period, there were not much fruitful researches in the field of gout and no new drugs approved for the management of hyperuricemia. However, the incidence of gout was increasing in all these years. Often deemed a "poor sibling" of chronic joint pathologies such as rheumatoid arthritis and psoriatic arthritis, gout was never being a focus of attraction for pharmaceutical research. But the increasing incidence of gout makes it a more attractive disease for novel drug discovery programs.

Twenty-first century has witnessed remarkable advances in gout therapy. This renaissance started with the development of new XOIs such as febuxostat, the development of pegylated uricase (pegloticase) and newer uricosuric agents such as lesinurad. Our understanding of the pathogenesis of hyperuricemia and gout has drastically improved in the recent years, which has resulted in the development of newer, more effective drugs. Gout is now considered to be more of a *transportopathy*. Various urate transporters are involved in the renal and intestinal excretion as well as renal reabsorption. Urate anion transporter 1 (URAT1) is involved in renal reabsorption at the proximal convoluted tubule. ABCG2 (ATP-binding cassette transporter G2) is involved in renal urate secretion as well as in gastrointestinal urate excretion.

NEWER ANTI-INFLAMMATORY THERAPIES

Interleukin-1 Inhibitors

Conventionally in acute gouty arthritis the inflammation is treated by nonsteroidal anti-inflammatory drugs (NSAIDs), colchicine or corticosteroids. However the discovery of urate crystals causing NOD-like receptor protein 3 (NLRP3) inflammasome activation and interleukin-1β (IL-1β) production revolutionized clinicians' perception of gouty flares.

TABLE 1: Interleukin-1 (IL-1) antagonists.

Name	Anakinra	Canakinumab	Rilonacept	Gevokizumab
Structure	IL-1 receptor antagonist	Human monoclonal antibody against IL-1β	Dimeric fusion protein (IL-1 receptor combined with Fc portion of IgG)	Humanized anti-IL-1β monoclonal antibody
Dose and route of administration	100 mg S/C daily for 3 days	150 mg S/C	80–120 mg S/C weekly	60 mg intravenously monthly
Indications	Refractory gout	Refractory gout	Refractory gout	Refractory gout
Approval and usage	Approved for JIA, periodic fevers; Off-label use in refractory gout	Approved by European medical agency for refractory gout	Not freely available commercially	Approved for pyoderma gangrenosum; Ongoing clinical trials in refractory gout

(IgG: immunoglobulin G; JIA: juvenile idiopathic arthritis; S/C: subcutaneous)

Blocking IL-1 is a novel concept in the treatment of acute gout because monosodium urate (MSU) crystals stimulate the inflammasomes leading to IL-1β secretion. IL-1 inhibitors prevent IL-1β secretion via this mechanism and also block IL-1 secretion by macrophages through toll-like receptor-dependent mechanism. The anti-IL-1 drugs, such as *anakinra, canakinumab, rilonacept, and gevokizumab* have been studied in patients with acute gout **(Table 1)**. Subcutaneous injection of anakinra 100 mg daily was found to be well tolerated and very effective in acute gout flares when used in patients who were unable to take other gout medications because of renal impairment, allergies, or gastrointestinal hemorrhage. Pain decreased in 79% on average after three injections. No side effects were noted during the trial and clinical examination showed complete resolution in nine out of 10 patients on third day.

Canakinumab 150 mg subcutaneously was found to be superior to triamcinolone 40 mg intramuscularly in gouty arthritis patients in flares and approved by European medical agency for clinical use in refractory gout. Another anti-IL-1 agent is rilonacept, given as 80–120 mg subcutaneously weekly on initiation of urate-lowering therapy to prevent acute gout flares. Anti-IL-1 treatments are highly effective in terminating gout flares in those unresponsive to NSAIDs and colchicine and also reducing the risk of flares in initiation of urate-lowering therapy; the effect is long-lasting over several weeks. However, they are extremely expensive when compared with traditional agents and therefore their place in the management of gout is still to be determined. None of these IL-1 inhibitors are available in India **(Box 1)**.

Bucillamine

It is a derivative of D-penicillamine with anti-inflammatory and antioxidant action. It was approved for the treatment of rheumatoid arthritis in Japan. Studies have found that it was equally or more effective than colchicine to control acute gouty inflammation.

BOX 1: Indications of IL-1 therapy.

Indications of anti-IL-1 drugs in acute gout:
- Peptic ulcer or GI hemorrhage
- Renal impairment
- Allergies to conventional agents
- Refractory to NSAIDs/colchicine/steroids

(GI: gastrointestinal; IL-1: interleukin-1; NSAIDs: nonsteroidal anti-inflammatory drugs)

Caspase Inhibitors

They act through blockade of IL-1β secretion by inhibiting intracellular processing of pro-IL-1β. Pralnacasan, a reversible caspase-1 inhibitor and emricasan, an irreversible orally active pan-caspase inhibitor, are under clinical trials.

Selective Inflammasome Inhibitors

NOD-like receptor protein 3 (also known as cryopyrin) inflammasome activation results in secretion of IL-1β and IL-18 via caspase-1. This is a vital step in the pathogenesis of gout.

Dapansutrile is an oral β-sulfonyl nitrile molecule which selectively inhibits NLRP3 inflammasome, thereby reversing inflammatory changes. Studies demonstrate a reduction in activated caspase-1 levels by about 35%, with no effects on levels of tumor necrosis factor-alpha (TNF-α) or IL-1β and IL-18 precursors. It reduces joint pain and inflammation and hence has potential in the treatment of gout flares as well as other NLRP3-mediated diseases. Though the optimal dose of dapansutrile is yet to be determined, dose up to 2,000 mg/day has acceptable safety profile comparable to IL-1 inhibitors.

Corticotropin and Melanocortin

These drugs trigger the release of endogenous steroids and also downregulate inflammatory responses by activating melanocortin 3 receptor (MC3R) on innate immune cells like macrophages. Stimulation of MC3R was found to significantly reduce inflammatory response to MSU crystals by reducing activities of nuclear factor kappa B (NF-κB) and heme oxygenase. They also thought to exert an anti-IL-1 effect. Studies have shown that adrenocorticotropic hormone (ACTH) is an effective option for treatment of gout in patients with multiple comorbidities, especially postoperative patients and those on steroids for other conditions like postrenal transplant. A single injection of 60 IU IM is more effective than corticosteroids. Recently, γ-melanocyte-stimulating hormone (γ-MSH) is also found to be more effective than corticosteroids in acute gout flare.

NEWER URATE-LOWERING THERAPIES (TABLE 2)

New Xanthine Oxidase Inhibitors

Topiroxostat

Nonpurine selective XOI is recently available in India.

Unlike febuxostat, it is a hybrid inhibitor of XO with dual mechanisms of action of inhibiting serum urate (SU) production. Like other XOIs, topiroxostat causes a structure-based inhibition due to the common ring. It also covalently binds with the molybdenum cofactor of the XO enzyme and interacts with the amino acid residues in the substrate-binding pocket which is the reaction center of the enzyme causing additional inhibition. It is mainly inactivated by hepatic metabolism and eliminated via urine and feces. Since topiroxostat and its metabolites are unaffected by renal conditions, it is an effective option in patients with chronic kidney disease. Additionally, it decreases albuminuria in these patients. Adverse effects include nasopharyngitis, elevated transaminases and leukopenia. It has no cardiac toxicities. Dose is 40–120 mg/day.

TABLE 2: Emerging therapeutic agents in gout.

Newer agents for acute gout	Newer urate-lowering drugs
IL-1 inhibitors: • Anakinra • Rilonacept • Canakinumab *D-penicillamine derivative*: • Bucillamine *Selective inflammasome inhibitor*: • Dapansutrile *Corticotropin and melanocortin*: • γ-MSH *Caspase-1 inhibitors*: • Pralnacasan • Emricasan	*Uricostatic drugs*: • Ulodesine • Topiroxostat *Uricosuric agents*: • *Lesinurad* • *Verinurad* • *Dotinurad* • *Tranilast* • *Arhalofenate* • *Levotofisopam* • *Canagliflozin* *Uricolytic drugs (uricases)*: • Pegloticase • Pegsiticase • SEL-212 *Urate transporters in intestinal lumen*: • ABCG2 activators

(ABCG2: ATP-binding cassette transporter G2; γ-MSH: γ-melanocyte-stimulating hormone; IL-1: interleukin-1)

Newer Uricases

Pegsiticase is a pegylated recombinant uricase developed from *Candida utilis*, which is less immunogenic than pegloticase.

SEL-212 is a combination of pegadricase and ImmTOR is a biodegradable nanoparticle encapsulating rapamycin. Combination treatment will produce antigen (uricase)-specific tolerance by inducing T regulatory cells that reduce the formation of antidrug antibodies. A phase 2 clinical trial has demonstrated very low incidence of adverse drug reactions and resulting in sustained reduction of serum uric acid (SUA) with monthly dosing. It is designed to be the first nonimmunogenic version of uricase.

Newer Uricosuric Agents (Fig. 1)

Lesinurad

This drug is a potent inhibitor of URAT1 and approved by US FDA. It also inhibits organic anion transporter 4 (OAT4), which is involved in diuretic-induced hyperuricemia. It is devoid of major drug interactions as it does not interfere with OAT1 and OAT3. It is used at a dose of 200 mg daily and causes a sustained decrease in SU levels. Common side effects are renal dysfunction and nephrolithiasis. The drug should be combined with an XOI to reduce renal adverse effects. Due to the nonprofitability, the manufacturers stopped the production of this molecule recently.

Verinurad

It is a highly selective URAT1 inhibitor. It is 100 times more potent than probenecid and more selective than lesinurad. In a phase 1 trial, a 36-hour sustained decrease in serum uric acid concentrations was observed after a single dose of 40 mg orally. Currently the drug is in phase 2 trial comparing monotherapy and combination therapy with allopurinol and febuxostat are ongoing.

Dotinurad

Novel URAT1 inhibitor which was developed in Japan as a safer alternative to benzbromarone. It was structurally designed to avoid the hepatotoxicity seen with benzbromarone. It effects excellent uric acid excretion

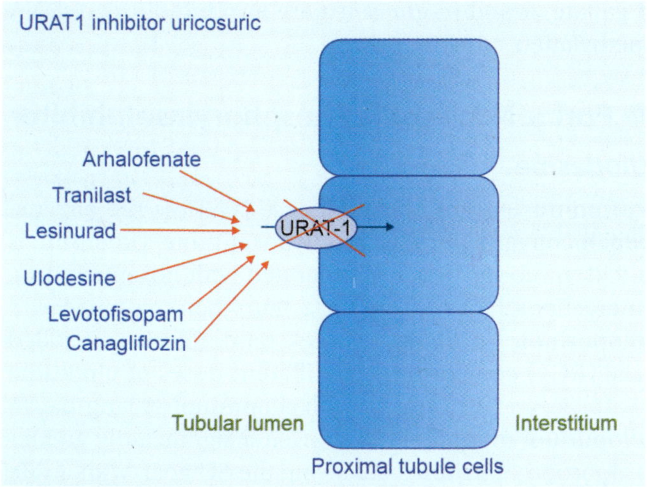

FIG. 1: Newer uricosuric agents inhibiting urate anion transporter 1 (URAT1).

without inhibiting gastrointestinal excretion and renal urate secretion. The urate-lowering effect of dotinurad is not affected by renal dysfunction and hence thought to be beneficial in hyperuricemic patients with moderate renal impairment. Daily dose of 2 mg orally is equally effective as benzbromarone 50 mg daily in Japanese hyperuricemic patients with or without gout. No serious adverse effects have been observed with dotinurad use.

Tranilast

This molecule which was originally developed as an antihistamine used for allergic rhinitis and asthma. It was found to have urate-lowering properties due to inhibitory action on URAT1 and glucose transporter 9. It has an additional benefit of reducing urate crystal-associated inflammation in vivo by suppressing leukocyte infiltration and plasma extravasation similar to colchicine. Hence has a possible role in flare prevention also. Its main side effect is headache.

Two phase 2 clinical trials evaluated the effect of tranilast, one by using a single dose of tranilast with doses ranging from 100 to 900 mg. The second study used total daily doses of 300, 600, or 900 mg daily for 7 days. The first study reported mean SU decrease of 0.17 and 0.24 mg/dL at 4 and 24 hours, respectively. In the second study, mean SU reductions of 1.1, 3.2, and 3.3 mg/dL were reported in the tranilast 300, 600, and 900 mg groups, respectively. A phase 2 clinical trial using tranilast in combination with allopurinol is in progress, no results have been published yet.

Levotofisopam

This is the S-enantiomer of the benzodiazepine derivative, tofisopam, used in anxiety and autonomic instability. It increases the fractional excretion of uric acid by its action on URAT1, though its exact mechanism of action is uncertain. Two phase 1 trials showed a reduction of SU levels in healthy individuals. In a phase 2 trial with 13 patients with hyperuricemia with gout, one day of levotofisopam 50 mg daily followed by TID doses on days 2–6 and one final single dose on day 7 showed a mean absolute SU reduction of 3.9 mg/dL (range 2.3–5.3). All patients achieved the SUA goal below 6 mg/dL with a mean treated SU of 4.1 mg/dL. No serious adverse effects were reported except 23% of patients experiencing a gout flare initially.

Canagliflozin

It is an sodium-glucose cotransporter-2 (SGLT-2) inhibitor, which acts by increasing urinary glucose excretion. It has been reported to lower SUA levels. SUA level changes were evaluated in pooled data from four randomized, phase 3, multinational, 26-week trials, where canagliflozin (100 or 300 mg) was compared with placebo as monotherapy, or dual or triple combination therapy (add-on to metformin, metformin and sulfonylurea, or metformin and pioglitazone). From mean baseline SUA levels of 5.3–5.4 mg/dL in the canagliflozin groups, both canagliflozin 100 and 300 mg reduced SUA levels by around 13% (or 0.7 mg/dL) relative to placebo at week 26 in the overall cohort.

Drugs with Dual Mechanisms

Arhalofenate

This is an emerging drug with dual action and long half-life of about 50 hours. Owing to the slow equilibration of serum levels, arhalofenate slowly reduces SUA levels by increasing urinary uric acid and the fractional excretion of uric acid. Besides the uricosuric action, it reduces gout flares by inhibiting production of IL-1β through action on peroxisome proliferator-activated receptor-gamma (PPAR-γ). This drug is thought to be an effective alternative to colchicine. Combination of arhalofenate with febuxostat was found to be synergistic, being more effective than febuxostat monotherapy while combination with allopurinol did not have any additional benefit over allopurinol monotherapy.

Arhalofenate has some additional beneficial actions in patients with other comorbidities. It retains its urate-lowering property even in the presence of renal insufficiency. Also, by its action on OAT4, it is effective in patients on diuretic therapy including thiazides, similar to lesinurad. It also has a lipid and glucose-lowering action which is advantageous in patients with diabetes and dyslipidemia.

Drugs Increasing Gastrointestinal Excretion (ABCG2 Activators)

Intestinal tract, owing to expression of high levels of xanthine oxidase and exposure to large amounts of nucleic acid is a significant site of uric acid production from exogenous purines, while liver produces uric acid from endogenous purines. ABCG2 contributes to about 40% of total elimination of uric acid. In the gut, small intestine is the major producer of uric acid and ABCG2 is expressed most abundantly in jejunum and ileum. The role of ABCG2 transporter is hence relevant. Promotion of uric acid excretion can be achieved with activation of ABCG2. This may be of benefit to those with normal ABCG2 or mutant ABCG2 with partial loss of function. ABCG2 activation may be achieved through transcription factors, such as PPAR-α, PPAR-γ, NRF2, and AhR. PPAR-α selective agonists like fibrates, originally used for dyslipidemia in diabetics, induce ABCG2 in intestine and liver. PPAR-γ agonists like pioglitazone, used as oral hypoglycemics, also induce ABCG2 in certain cell types. Fumarate esters, sulforaphane, and astemizole activate NRF2 which targets ABCG2 in liver through its action on antioxidant machinery. Drugs like omeprazole, a proton pump inhibitor and carbidopa, used in Parkinson's disease, are potent activators of AhR, which works through xenobiotic response element. As epigenetic mechanisms like promoter hypermethylation cause suppression of ABCG2, drugs preventing DNA methylation may be beneficial in that aspect. Two such drugs are decitabine and azacitidine, which are actually anticancer drugs. Laccaic acid, a natural food additive and epigallocatechin-3-gallate, found in green tea are also inhibitors of DNA methylation.

Purine Nucleoside Phosphorylase Inhibitor

Ulodesine

Purine nucleoside phosphorylase (PNP) is the enzyme which converts purines into hypoxanthine. Ulodesine is a PNP inhibitor. It is well tolerated with not much drug interactions. It has synergistic action when combined with allopurinol. An initial 12-week randomized controlled trial (RCT) comparing four different doses of ulodesine (5, 10, 20, and 40 mg/day) with allopurinol 300 mg/day to allopurinol monotherapy showed a significantly greater proportion of patients achieving the SU goal, with a safe profile and adequate tolerance to the combination.

Marine Active 10

Commercial tuna extract produced by ion-exchange purification and spray drying from a hot water extract of skipjack and yellowfin tuna, without enzymatic hydrolysis. Originally developed as an antifatigue drug, it was found to have marked urate-lowering property owing to the presence of imidazole compounds. Studies show significant increase in hypoxanthine phosphoribosyl transferase levels in the liver of those treated with tuna extract. Hypoxanthine phosphoribosyl transferase utilizes hypoxanthine and guanine for purine synthesis thereby inhibiting uric acid synthesis. Tuna extract metabolites excreted in urine stabilize urinary pH which improves solubility of uric acid and accelerates its excretion **(Fig. 2)**.

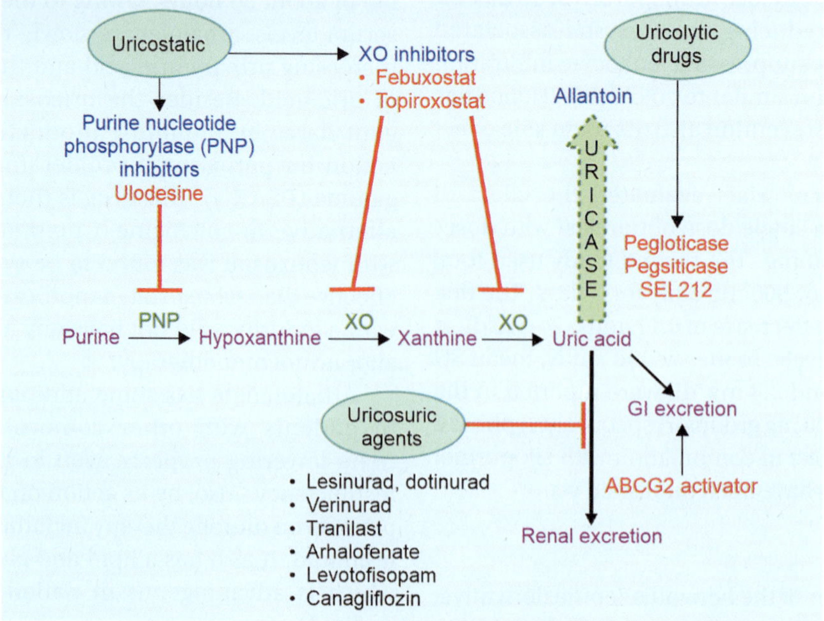

FIG. 2: Mechanism of action of newer drugs in gout.
(ABCG2: ATP-binding cassette transporter G2; GI: gastrointestinal; XO: xanthine oxidase)

SUGGESTED READINGS

1. James R, Paul BJ. New and emerging therapy of gout. Rheumatol Autoimmun. 2023;1-8.
2. Shahid H, Singh JA. Investigational drugs for hyperuricemia. Expert Opin Investig Drugs. 2015;24(8):1013-30.
3. Sebastian E. Treatment of hyperuricemia in gout: current therapeutic options, latest developments and clinical implications. Ther Adv Musculoskel Dis. 2016;8(4):145-59.

250 CHAPTER

Biologics and Biosimilars in Rheumatology

N Subramanian

ABSTRACT

Biologics and biosimilar drugs are increasingly being used in different immune-mediated diseases not only in rheumatology but also in other systemic diseases. These cytokine blockers, also called targeted therapy, have revolutionized the management of chronic rheumatological diseases and achieve early remission. While biologic drugs are expensive and can be used in affluent countries, biosimilar drugs are used more in developing countries and with equal efficacy. Physicians need to know the basics of these biodrugs and their actions. Nearly two decades have passed by since the invention of first biologic etanercept; now we are seeing newer molecules every month and more drugs are in the research pipeline, including phase 2 and 3 studies.

INTRODUCTION

Rheumatological diseases are immune-mediated, multisystem diseases affecting all age groups and in particular women of childbearing age. Recent evidence suggests a big change in the genotype, phenotype, and evolution of these diseases with increasing number of new and complex diseases. Diagnostic and therapeutic innovations also have contributed to our understanding of these and the coronavirus disease 2019 (COVID-19) pandemic has allowed more clinicians to share their research on this topics.

Biologics and biosimilar drugs are cytokine blockers specifically targeting the inflammatory mediators, thereby achieving disease remission without many complications.

SCOPE FOR NEWER DRUGS

While corticosteroids and disease-modifying drugs have no doubt helped to achieve disease control for four to five decades in 1990s, therapies and effects have been suboptimal and there exists an unmet need in managing the rheumatological diseases and comorbidities including cardiovascular risk. Hence, researchers delved into innovative new drugs which can block specific cytokines, which biologics have hit the market since 2000 not only in rheumatology but even all other specialties have specific drugs.

BIOLOGICS

Biologics are medications derived from biological sources which act by blocking or inhibiting specific molecular or cellular targets. They are highly effective in the management of rheumatoid arthritis (RA), ankylosing spondylitis, ulcerative colitis, uveitis, vasculitis, lupus, psoriatic arthritis (PsA), and many non-rheumatological diseases also. Some of the target mediators include tumor necrosis factor (TNF)-alpha, interleukin 1 (IL-1), interleukin 6 (IL-6) inhibitor, CD20, cytotoxic T lymphocyte-associated antigen-4 (CTLA-4) inhibitors, interleukin 16 (IL-16) or 23 blocker, and many more coming to the market.

■ Brief Information on the Biologic Drugs

Etanercept (ETN) was the first anti-TNF drug registered for treatment of RA. Evidence points to the combination of ETN and methotrexate (MTX) found to improve radiographic and clinical outcomes over placebo-treated patients. The PRESERVE (PREdicting the Safety and

Effectiveness of inferioR VEna cava filters) trial has shown that in patients with combined therapy of ETN and MTX, drug-free remission was possible. Subsequently, it was approved for PsA and ankylosing spondylitis.

Infliximab has similar probability of achieving remission/low disease activity, response rate, cardiovascular risk reduction, and potential to stop radiographic progressions as other TNF inhibitors (TNFis) in RA, PsA, and spondyloarthritis (SpA). Patients have shown the highest rate of drug-free remission compared to ETN or adalimumab.

Adalimumab is monoclonal antibody targeting soluble and transmembrane TNF and is used in second-line treatment preferably with MTX along with other TNFis in RA and PsA.

Certolizumab (CTZ) is another bio-originator TNFi drug. Due to its lack of transplacental transport, it has been approved in RA treatment during pregnancy. Efficacy of CTZ seems to be comparable to other TNFi in RA or PsA treatment; although in the majority of patients, neutralizing antibodies were found.

Golimumab (GOL)—fully human monoclonal antibody in comparison to other TNFi, GOL shows similar efficacy and safety. GOL also might be considered as a safe drug during lactation because its high mass might prevent its exudation to breast milk.

Tocilizumab (TCZ)—the first humanized monoclonal antibody against the IL-6 receptor (anti-IL-6R) is TCZ, approved for the treatment of RA. This drug binds to both soluble- and membrane-bound IL-6R, preventing IL-6 from interacting with both IL-6R and the signal converter glycoprotein 130 complex. This results in Janus kinase/signal transducers and activators of transcription (JAK-STAT) pathway inhibition. This was used very much in COVID-19 pneumonia too and also in systemic-onset juvenile arthritis.

Sarilumab is a human monoclonal antibody of the immunoglobulin G1 (IgG1) subclass that acts selectively on IL-6R and is being used in RA patients, based on MOBILITY and TARGET clinical trials.

Olokizumab is a humanized monoclonal antibody anti-IL-6. This antibody was tested for safety and efficacy in CREDO study in RA patients. The preliminary data show good efficacy, tolerability, and favorable safety profile of olokizumab. Clazakizumab and vobarilizumab are being studied in RA but not approved yet.

Abatacept (ABA) became the first biologic disease modifying anti-rheumatic drug (bDMARD), which modulates T-cell activation in RA. ABA is a recombinant fully human, soluble, fusion protein, and T-cell costimulation modulator that consists of the extracellular domain of human CTLA-4, which is linked to the modified fragment crystallizable (Fc) region of the IgG.

B-cell therapies can be divided into several main therapeutic mechanisms. The drugs that cause direct depletion of B-cells are peripheral pool (rituximab), indirect depletion via costimulation blockade (belimumab), plasma cell targeting (such as bortezomib), and B-cell function inhibition (such as Bruton's kinase inhibitors). Rituximab has been approved for use in RA, lupus, antineutrophil cytoplasmic antibody (ANCA) vasculitis, and scleroderma and also in non-rheumatological conditions.

Despite the ability of bDMARDs to improve the lives of many patients with rheumatic diseases, the high cost of these drugs limits widespread use and contributes to inequalities of care. Patent expiration of biologics has enabled development of lower-cost biosimilars that opens on increased market competition and price reduction.

BIOSIMILARS

A biosimilar is defined by the World Health Organization (WHO) as a biotherapeutic product which is similar in terms of quality, safety, and efficacy to an already licensed reference biotherapeutic product, with similarity defined as "*the absence of a relevant difference in the parameter of interest.*"

Biosimilar medicines contain a version of the active substance of an approved biological medicinal product, known as the reference product. They are made by or derived from a biological source. Biosimilars include monoclonal antibodies, soluble receptors, growth factors, and hormones. They do not meaningfully differ from the reference product in terms of quality, safety, and efficacy and they are more cost-effective.

Numerous studies have specifically compared the safety of biosimilars among the inflammatory arthritis patients, including biosimilars for infliximab, adalimumab, and ETN. Safety has been largely assessed by evaluating rates of adverse events among groups of patients on biosimilars as compared with originator.

DRUGS APPROVED FOR DISEASES IN RHEUMATOLOGY

There are consensus-based recommendations regarding the use of biosimilars to treat rheumatological conditions. These were developed by a group of rheumatology, dermatology, and gastroenterology specialists, pharmacologists, patients, and a regulator from 10 countries **(Table 1)**.

TABLE 1: Biologics in rheumatology and biosimilars in same indications.

Drug	Pathway	Diseases	How to give?
• Etanercept • Infliximab • Adalimumab • Golimumab • Certolizumab	Anti-TNF	• RA • Psoriatic arthritis • Ankylosing spondylitis	All subcutaneous
• Tocilizumab • Sarilumab	IL-6 blockers	• Juvenile arthritis • Still's disease • All of the above	Subcutaneous
Abatacept	Anti-CD40	RA	Intravenous
Rituximab	Anti-CD20	RA, ANCA vasculitis	Intravenous
Secukinumab, ixekizumab	Anti-IL-17	Psoriasis and arthritis	Subcutaneous
Ustekinumab	Anti-IL-12/23 drugs	Psoriatic arthritis	Subcutaneous

(ANCA: antineutrophilic cytoplasmic antibody; IL: interleukin; RA: rheumatoid arthritis; TNF: tumor necrosis factor)

INDICATIONS

- RA
- Juvenile idiopathic arthritis
- PsA
- Ankylosing spondylitis
- Crohn's disease
- Ulcerative colitis
- Plaque psoriasis
- Pediatric Crohn's disease
- Pediatric ulcerative colitis
- Lupus
- ANCA vasculitis

Screening tests include blood count, C-reactive protein (CRP), liver function test (LFT), renal function tests, hepatitis B and C screening, Mantoux, and immunoglobulins for rituximab. Electrocardiogram (ECG) and ECHO should be done when appropriate. Consider flu and pneumococcal vaccination. Consider varicella vaccine in those with negative varicella zoster virus (VZV).

CONTRAINDICATIONS

The following conditions are contraindications for use of biologics:

- Uncontrolled heart failure, active infections, and untreated cancers
- Previous septic arthritis, pregnancy, and lactation and history of multiple sclerosis
- Risk of tuberculosis (TB) has been found to be more in Asian countries.
- Hepatitis B/C and human immunodeficiency virus (HIV) relative contraindications

SIDE EFFECTS

- Infection and malignancy—skin cancer and lymphoma
- Lupus with anti-TNF, rare, most commonly manifests as rash
- Demyelinating disease
- Psoriasis may develop with anti-TNF
- Tuberculosis reactivation, nocardiosis, and listeriosis
- Fungal—invasive candidiasis and pneumocystosis
- Viral—hepatitis-B and herpes zoster reactivation

There is increasing use of biologics in pregnancy; however, uncertainty persists about increased infection risk in early neonatal life. Any planned surgery may need stopping, e.g., 2 weeks prior to surgery, but risks of flare must be weighed up.

LONG-TERM IMPLICATIONS

Evaluation of biology at both the systemic and local tissue levels is important in heterogeneous diseases such as PsA or RA. Similarly in lupus and vasculitis, genomic studies might throw more light on our understanding of specific biomarkers to assess the treatment response and the choice of specific biodrug.

With this in mind, high-throughput omics techniques (genomics, transcriptomics, proteomics, and metabolomics) are increasingly being employed. Integrative multi-omics approaches might be the way forward to increase the detection of accurate response predictors.

CONCLUSION

In summary, biosimilar medications have been in widespread use for several years now. They offer equivalent efficacy and safety profiles to the originator biologic drugs but have the added benefit of being cost-effective, which has resulted in increased access to these medications.

Several biosimilar medications have been approved for use across various fields of medicine to treat many conditions and more biosimilars are in development. The future seems bright for this new class of medicines.

Physicians need to know the benefits and side effects of these newer drugs, especially in acute medical care, when patients with comorbidities come with complex problems.

SUGGESTED READINGS

1. Fautrel B. Biologics in rheumatoid arthritis: a lifetime treatment or possibility of drug holidays? Nat Rev Rheumatol. 2023;19: 611-2.
2. Sharma SK. Use of Biologics and Biosimilars in Rheumatology. J Assoc Physicians India. 2017;65(5 Suppl):9-14.
3. Smolen JS, Landewé RBM, Bergstra SA, Kerschbaumer A, Sepriano A, Aletaha D, et al. EULAR recommendations for the management of rheumatoid arthritis with synthetic and biological disease-modifying antirheumatic drugs: 2022 update. Ann Rheum Dis. 2023;82(1):3-18.

251
CHAPTER

Clinical Pearls in Connective Tissue Diseases: What and What not to do?

Rohini Handa

ABSTRACT

Autoimmune connective tissue diseases (CTDs) comprise a broad group of conditions with overlapping clinical features and the common thread of antinuclear antibodies. Almost any organ can be involved, and being multisystem illnesses, CTDs frequently enter the domain of internists. Clinicians need to differentiate 'classification' from 'diagnosis'. The former needs 'validated criteria' while the latter requires 'clinical reasoning'. The diagnosis of CTDs is clinicoserologic. Diagnoses of CTDs based on tenuous serologic evidence bereft of robust clinical correlation are likely to be wrong. The widespread availability, and indiscriminate ordering, of sensitive tests like fluorescent antinuclear antibody (ANA) and extractable nuclear antigen (ENA) panels has spawned an epidemic of asymptomatic patients with low titer autoantibodies. Factoring in pretest probability before ordering tests and clinicolaboratory correlation are the key mantras to avoid overtreatment. The dictum is to treat the patient and not chase the serology! Glucocorticoids are invaluable but not inevitable in the treatment of CTDs. Not all patients require steroids all the time. There is a growing tendency to curtail steroid exposure both in terms of dose and duration. If required, steroid-sparing strategies like methotrexate, azathioprine, or mycophenolate mofetil are employed upfront. 'Disease activity' in CTDs needs to be differentiated from 'disease damage'. Attention to comorbidities such as hypertension, dyslipidemia, and bone heath is an integral part of treatment. Pregnancy is feasible in most patients with CTDs during periods of disease quiescence.

INTRODUCTION

The CTDs include several conditions like systemic lupus erythematosus (SLE), Sjögren's syndrome, systemic sclerosis, undifferentiated connective tissue disease, and overlap syndromes including mixed connective tissue disease (MCTD). The clinical features often overlap, and the spectrum of autoantibodies encountered can be vast. Notwithstanding this, the approach to CTDs is overwhelmingly clinical. This write up discusses some common clinical pearls.

CLINICAL PEARLS

Interpret autoimmune serology only in light of the clinical picture

In absence of pathognomonic features, connective tissue diseases (CTDs) are diagnosed on clinicoserologic grounds. The indiscriminate use of "panels" has led to a piquant situation where some clinicians base their diagnosis only on laboratory tests. With increasing use of immunofluorescence, low titer antinuclear antibodies (ANAs) are not uncommonly encountered in several nonrheumatic conditions, especially infections. It is important to interpret serology in light of clinical features. A diagnosis of CTD requires two pillars—compatible clinical profile and a supportive serology. One without the other can lead to wrong diagnosis or missed diagnosis.

Antinuclear antibody is a sensitive test but not specific while double-stranded deoxyribonucleic acid (dsDNA) is specific but not sensitive. ANA is seen in >98–99% of patients with systemic lupus erythematosus (SLE) while double-stranded DNA (dsDNA) is seen in ~60% of patients. Therefore, ANA positive and dsDNA negative situations are commonly encountered in lupus while

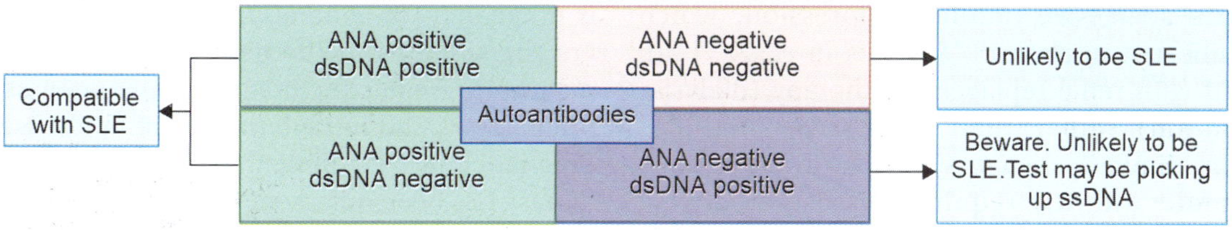

FIG. 1: Serologic combinations in systemic lupus erythematosus (SLE).
(ANA: antinuclear antibody; dsDNA: double-stranded DNA; ssDNA: single-stranded DNA)

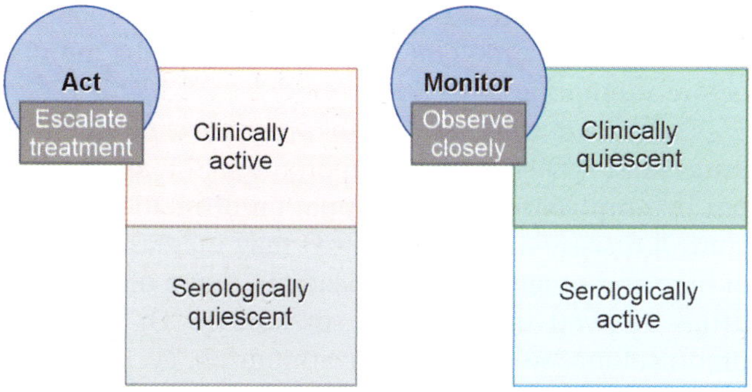

FIG. 2: Clinicoserologic dissociation in connective tissue diseases (CTDs).

the reverse is not true. Clinicians should be reluctant to accept this serologic constellation of dsDNA positivity in face of ANA negativity **(Fig. 1)**. This can happen because enzyme-linked immunosorbent assay (ELISA), the commonly used method for dsDNA detection, can detect both low avidity and high avidity dsDNA antibodies. At times, partial denaturation of dsDNA leads to the test picking up singe-stranded DNA (ssDNA) antibodies.

Clinicoserologic dissociation is also not uncommon. Clinically active, serologically quiescent disease needs treatment escalation while disease that is clinically inactive with active serology merits observation **(Fig. 2)**.

Classification is not the same as diagnosis

Connective tissue diseases lack unique clinical symptoms. Features like fever, joint pains, and Raynaud's are encountered in several conditions. Also, these clinical features may be synchronous or metachronous. This has spawned the need for criteria. Criteria are for 'classification' and not 'diagnosis'. This is a subtle yet important difference. Classification criteria are intended for research purposes, homogenize patient groups, and trade sensitivity for specificity. Most of the criteria available are classification criteria and not criteria for diagnosis. The foundation of diagnosis is a through history, complete physical examination, and integration of laboratory data with clinical parameters.

For example, the current lupus criteria mandate an ANA positivity of 1:80 as the entry point. On the bedside, a young woman with a characteristic malar rash and ANA of 1:40 would receive a "diagnosis" and treatment of lupus yet not be "classified" as SLE. Such a patient would be excluded from clinical trials, because she lacks the classification tag of SLE despite having SLE. This highlights the fact that nonfulfillment of criteria or a score below the classification threshold does not negate that diagnosis on the bedside. Classification criteria should not eclipse rational clinical judgment. Also, treatment should not be delayed pending classification.

Labels are not important—the extent of organ involvement is

Clinical features like arthritis and rash are shared by several CTDs and crossovers are not uncommon. A patient with the phenotype of Sjögren syndrome, to begin with, may down the line develop sclerodactyly, digital ulcers, and Raynaud's suggestive of scleroderma overlap. Therefore, more than the label, it is the organ involvement that will influence choice of treatment. For example, Raynaud's will be treated in broadly the same fashion no matter whether the underlying disease is systemic sclerosis or mixed connective tissue disease (MCTD). Similarly, methotrexate is a reasonable choice for the inflammatory arthritis of all CTDs—whether lupus or scleroderma or Sjögren's syndrome.

Insist on urine examination at all visits

Renal involvement is often paucisymptomatic. Urinalysis is imperative at every patient visit. Active renal involvement requires treatment escalation and is a major determinant of outcome.

Disease 'activity' is different from disease 'damage'

Disease 'activity' refers to *reversible* manifestations while 'damage' refers to *nonreversible* charges present for at least 6 months that are not related to active inflammation. Disease activity means the extent to which the immunoinflammation is contributing to the clinical setting at a particular point in time and the likelihood that it will produce related morbidity or mortality. It is analogous to the concept of 'tumor burden' in oncology. The change in disease activity helps a clinician to decide whether CTD is improving or worsening. Active disease, for example, active lupus nephritis class III and

IV, warrants aggressive immunosuppression, which is contraindicated in class VI. Patients in class VI are best treated with renal replacement therapy (dialysis/transplantation) rather than aggressive immunosuppression. Similarly, active synovitis of hand joints in rheumatoid arthritis requires disease-modifying antirheumatic drug (DMARD) initiation or escalation. In contrast, the mechanical knee pain of osteoarthritis in a patient with rheumatic arthritis (RA) will not respond to DMARDs.

Not all patients with CTDs require corticosteroids. Those who require steroids need different doses at different points of time in their disease course

Let me exemplify this using SLE as the prototype. SLE is a multisystem disorder where patients are categorized into those with *major organ* involvement and those with *minor organ* involvement. Therapy is directed accordingly. Minor involvement includes serositis, mucocutaneous, musculoskeletal, or constitutional symptoms. The major manifestations include lupus nephritis neuropsychiatric SLE, significant cytopenias, and interstitial lung disease. In general, patients with minor organ involvement of lupus can be treated with nonsteroidal anti-inflammatory drugs (NSAIDs) and hydroxychloroquine (HCQ). Corticosteroids, if needed, are given in relatively small doses (prednisolone 0.25–0.5 mg/kg/day). On the other hand, major organ involvement necessitates use of higher dose corticosteroids (prednisolone 1 mg/kg/day or higher) apart from HCQ and other drugs, such as azathioprine and mycophenolate.

Of note, patients with minor organ involvement may also require high-dose corticosteroids during disease flare. In the same vein, once the patients with major organ involvement go into quiescence, the corticosteroids can be tapered to a maintenance dose and even stopped. The current paradigm is parsimonious use of steroids—lowest dose for shortest time.

Pregnancy and fatherhood are possible in most instances

Autoimmune rheumatic diseases are plagued by nihilism and multiple social barriers. A significant issue is pregnancy. In general, fertility rates in CTD patients are the same as in the general population, but there may be a greater incidence of spontaneous abortion, prematurity, and intrauterine death in diseases like SLE. Pregnancy in CTD patients is often possible when the disease has been quiescent for at least 6 months. Relative contraindications to pregnancy include active disease, recent stroke, significant cardiac involvement, pulmonary hypertension, severe interstitial lung disease, and advanced renal insufficiency. For male patients, there are virtually no restrictions on fatherhood, except in patients on cyclophosphamide that should be stopped 3 months before attempting conception.

Continued treatment with pregnancy compatible drugs like HCQ is crucially important in SLE and cannot but be emphasized. Discontinuation of medications to control disease activity like HCQ may increase the risk of flare and pregnancy complications. Some of the other drugs allowed in pregnancy include HCQ, low-dose prednisolone, sulfasalazine, azathioprine, cyclosporine, and tacrolimus. A multidisciplinary approach ensures better outcomes.

Do not overlook comorbid conditions like hyperlipidemia, hypertension, and osteoporosis

Comorbidities need as much attention as the primary disease. Accelerated atherosclerosis is an important contributor to mortality. What hurts are the joints, what kills is the heart! Cardiac health, bone health, mental health—all are the responsibility of the treating physician. Judicious interdisciplinary consults improve results. Rheumatic diseases cannot and should not be managed in isolation.

CONCLUSION

Connective tissue diseases are multispecialty disorders that can present to any discipline. Internists are uniquely positioned to handle these diseases in a holistic fashion. Internist rheumatologist collaboration ensures better outcomes.

SUGGESTED READING

1. Handa R (Ed). Clinical Rheumatology, 1st edition. Singapore: Springer Nature Pte Ltd.; 2021.

252 CHAPTER

Recent Advances in Renal Vasculitis

Surabhi Talwar, Siwalik Banerjee

ABSTRACT

Renal involvement is a common manifestation of vasculitis which can be large, medium, or small-vessel vasculitis. The common types of vasculitis involving the kidneys include polyarteritis nodosa (PAN), cryoglobulinemic vasculitis, antineutrophilic cytoplasmic antibody (ANCA)-associated vasculitis (AAV), immunoglobulin A (IgA) vasculitis (IgAV), and anti-glomerular basement membrane (GBM) disease.

We discuss the common manifestations and evidence-based management strategies for these conditions, which are evolving with ongoing research trials.

The most common of small vessel vasculitis involving the kidneys is AAV, which includes eosinophilic granulomatosis with polyangiitis (EGPA), granulomatosis with polyangiitis (GPA), and microscopic polyangiitis (MPA). It has been the focus of many large trials in the last decade, which led to change in management strategies of AAV. The latest immunosuppressive regimens include rituximab (RTX)—a chimeric anti-CD20 monoclonal antibody and avacopan, a C5a inhibitor (administered orally). Recent trials have also helped establish that EGPA should be treated differently as compared to GPA and MPA. Other forms of vasculitis, such as anti-GBM disease, are treated with plasma exchange, and a short course of immunosuppression.

Glucocorticoids (GCs) form the mainstay of treatment in most of these conditions and steroid reduction strategies have become important. Immune-checkpoint inhibitors (ICIs), which are a group of medications being used widely in oncology, can be associated with renal vasculitis.

INTRODUCTION

Vasculitis is an inflammatory condition involving vessel walls and damaging their mural structure. This results in bleeding and obstruction of the lumen causing downstream tissue ischemia. The Chapel Hill consensus conference (2012) divides vasculitis into large-vessel vasculitis, medium-vessel vasculitis, and small-vessel vasculitis. The common types of vasculitis which affect the kidneys include medium-vessel vasculitis such as polyarteritis nodosa (PAN) and small-vessel vasculitis such as antineutrophilic cytoplasmic antibody (ANCA)-associated vasculitis (AAV), microscopic polyangiitis (MPA), granulomatosis with polyangiitis (GPA), eosinophil granulomatosis with polyangiitis (EGPA), anti-glomerular basement membrane (GBM) disease, cryoglobulinemic vasculitis, immunoglobulin A (IgA) vasculitis (IgAV), and immune complex-mediated vasculitis. We aim to discuss new advances of treatment available for these conditions causing renal vasculitis.

- *Polyarteritis nodosa:* A necrotizing vasculitis involving medium-sized arteries, including renal arteries. It can be a classic variant with systemic and constitutional symptoms, or can be "limited" to neurological or cutaneous manifestations. Frequently it is associated with hepatitis B.

  Presentations include mononeuritis multiplex, cutaneous ulceration, gonadal vasculitis, gastro-intestinal ulcerations, hypertension, and fever. Its hallmark is formation of microaneurysms in blood vessels, frequently in kidneys, resulting in hematuria, proteinuria, renovascular hypertension, thrombosis, and infarction. Characteristically ANCA is negative and there is absence of glomerulonephritis.

Treatment includes induction of remission with high-dose glucocorticoids (GCs), initiated with 500 mg–1 g methylprednisolone × 3 doses, and followed by GC taper starting at 1 mg/kg. Both oral and IV cyclophosphamide (CYC) can be used, however, intravenous CYC has the advantage of having lower cumulative dose. Efficacy of rituximab (RTX) remains questionable in PAN. Evidence of plasmapheresis in non-hepatitis B-associated PAN is unavailable.

After induction of remission, patients are maintained on azathioprine or methotrexate for at least 18 months, duration of treatment is decided individually. Mycophenolate has not been extensively studied in PAN.

- *Antineutrophilic cytoplasmic antibody-associated vasculitis:* A group of conditions presenting with inflammatory small-vessel vasculitis and presence of ANCA antibody in blood. AAV is divided clinicopathologically into three types—GPA, MPA, and EGPA. Serologically, it is divided into anti-myeloperoxidase (MPO) or anti-proteinase-3 (PR-3) positive disease. Renal involvement in the form of rapidly progressive glomerulonephritis (RPGN) is common and can affect overall morbidity and mortality. Renal involvement is classified as organ threatening disease.

  Management of MPA/GPA is different to that of EGPA and hence will be discussed separately.
- *Eosinophilic granulomatosis with polyangiitis,* formerly known as Churg–Strauss syndrome, is a necrotizing vasculitis involving the small blood vessels and is characterized by refractory asthma and eosinophilia. It predominantly causes respiratory involvement, myocarditis, and mononeuritis multiplex. It may be associated with renal necrotizing vasculitis. Though it is a variant of AAV only 30% patients are ANCA positive-predominantly MPO.

  Milder forms of EGPA can be treated with prednisolone only or in conjunction with steroid-sparing drugs such as azathioprine, methotrexate, or mycophenolate. In patients with refractory asthma, pulmonary infiltrates and pneumonitis associated with hyper-eosinophilia, mepolizumab, an anti-IL-5 agent, can be used.

  Treatment for renal disease includes induction of remission with high dose GCs along with CYC or RTX. Patients with a Five Factor Score ≥1, should be treated with CYC to reduce mortality and risk of relapse. Myocarditis is an independent risk factor of mortality in patients with EGPA.

  After six doses of CYC, patients can be switched to methotrexate, azathioprine or mycophenolate to maintain remission.

  Rituximab can also be used as an alternative for patients who have relative contraindications to CYC. The REOVAS trial including 105 patients with new or relapsing organ-threatening EGPA compared CYC and RTX as agents for induction. Patients received GCs with either nine doses of CYC or two doses of 1 g RTX. Remission rates in both groups were similar, and there was no significant difference in response to RTX in patients who were MPO positive versus MPO negative. ANCA positivity, thus, should not be the sole determinant in choosing CYC versus RTX.

  For maintenance of remission after organ-threatening disease, methotrexate, azathioprine, or Mepolizumab, can be used. Due to the relapsing nature of the disease, there is a high long-term steroid exposure and these steroid sparing agents can reduce relapses as well as cumulative steroid dose. RTX also has shown promise as an agent for maintenance of remission.
- *Granulomatosis with polyangiitis and MPA:* These conditions present with variable organ involvement and most commonly affect upper and lower respiratory tract and kidneys. Patients can present with constitutional symptoms or organ/life-threatening disease. ENT involvement (more common in GPA–90%) can manifest as nasal crusting, nasal ulcers, otitis media, hearing loss, or saddle-nose deformity. Absence of kidney involvement (seen in 85% of patients) in the form of hematuria, proteinuria or worsening creatinine, does not imply benign disease. Typically, kidney involvement occurs in the form of RPGN with creatinine worsening over days to weeks. Involvement of lungs can present as wheezing, cough, or hemoptysis. Patients may develop pulmonary hemorrhage or interstitial lung disease (ILD). ILD is associated with MPO antibody.

  A total of 30–50% of patients have skin manifestations in the form of vasculitic rash or purpura. Skin lesions also include livedo reticularis, urticaria, and skin nodules. There can be neurological involvement (mononeuritis multiplex, cranial nerve involvement, and meningeal disease) or ophthalmic involvement (episcleritis/scleritis, retinal vasculitis, and conjunctivitis).

  In GPA/MPA, induction of remission is with GCs as well as either CYC or RTX. In new-onset GPA/MPA, RTX is non-inferior to CYC for induction of remission. RTX is preferred in patients who wish to preserve their reproductive potential as CYC can cause infertility in men and women. CYC can be associated with myelodysplastic syndrome (MDS), bladder cancer and other malignancies. RTX is given at a dose of 375 mg/m^2/week for 4 weeks or in two doses (1 g dose at 0 and 2 weeks). RTX has been found to be superior in maintaining remission at 6 and 12 months in relapsing disease. RTX and CYC combination (used in RITUXVAS) has been used for induction to reduce glucocorticoid use and improve renal response, but needs investigation by randomized controlled trials (RCTs).

Glucocorticoids are started at a dose of 1 mg/kg. The PEXIVAS protocol or reduced dose protocol for GCs reduced the dose of GCs by 40% in the first 6 months and led to reduction in serious infections during first year, with equivalent response to therapy. There is no compelling evidence to use IV methylprednisolone therapy along with oral GCs and this needs further research.

Plasma-exchange (PLEX) can be considered for those with creatinine of >300 µmol/L due to renal involvement. The PEXIVAS trial, after a median follow-up of 2.9 years did not show any difference in death of any-cause or end-stage renal disease (ESRD) in patients who received PLEX or not. A meta-analysis has then confirmed no benefit to all-cause mortality from PLEX. However, it revealed that PLEX reduced the risk of ESRD at 12 months, and the benefit was maximum for those with creatinine of >300 µmol/L.

Avacopan, a C5a inhibitor, is a new drug which is recommended for use in new and relapsing GPA/MPA, to minimize glucocorticoid use. This is based on ADVOCATE trial, which included 331 newly diagnosed patients with GPA/MPA and compared the use of Avacopan (30 mg twice a day for 52 weeks), versus GCs (1 mg/kg/day to 0 by 21 weeks). Remission was similar in both groups at 6 months (72% vs. 70%). Patients with renal involvement, had a greater recovery of kidney function in the avacopan group and the glucocorticoid toxicity index was lower in the avacopan group. The rate of severe adverse events and infections was no different in both groups. Hence, avacopan is recommended to be used along with RTX or CYC, to induce remission. However, the study did not involve patients with GFR <15 mL/min and those with pulmonary hemorrhage.

After remission is achieved, maintenance therapy is continued for 24–48 months with 6 monthly doses of RTX or with Azathioprine. RTX has been shown to be associated with lower relapse rate in MAINRITSAN and RITAZAREM trials, when compared to Azathioprine, after induction therapy with GCs and CYC/RTX.

- *Cryoglobulinemic glomerulonephritis:* Mixed cryoglobulinemia can be associated with hepatitis C, or can be associated with autoimmune diseases such as SLE, rheumatoid arthritis, Sjögren's syndrome. This can also be associated with lymphoproliferative disorders, rarely idiopathic. It can cause cutaneous vasculitis, Raynaud's, and arthralgia, however, it has potential to cause severe organ-threatening disease including RPGN, polyneuropathy, mononeuritis multiplex, central nervous system vasculitis, digital infarction, and limb ischemia.

  For moderate-to-severe vasculitis, in case of hepatitis C-associated disease, immunosuppressive treatment is started first, and later antiviral treatment is added. However, if there is associated hepatitis B or HIV infection, antiviral treatment has to be initiated concomitantly. Renal vasculitis is treated with high-dose prednisolone with RTX. Recent RCTs have shown RTX is superior to CYC in inducing remission.

  Plasma-exchange has limited role in patients with high cryocrit, hyperviscosity syndrome, pulmonary hemorrhage, gastrointestinal vasculitis, and RPGN with crescents.

  Immunosuppressive treatment should be initiated along with PLEX so as to prevent the production of cryoglobulin.
- *Immunoglobulin A (IgA) vasculitis:* Formerly known as Henoch–Schönlein purpura (HSP), IgAV is more common in children. It is characterized by palpable purpura, arthritis, kidney disease, and abdominal pain. Biopsy from skin or kidneys, show leukocytoclastic vasculitis or proliferative glomerulonephritis respectively with IgA deposition.

  Renal involvement in IgAV warrants treatment with immunosuppressive therapy only if proteinuria is >1 g/day and in presence of acute worsening of renal function. These patients are treated with GCs at 0.5 mg/kg/day, tapered over 6 months. A second-line agent such as CYC or mycophenolate mofetil (MMF) can be given if patients fail to respond to GCs alone. However, evidence on use of second-line agents is limited. Patients with proteinuria of <1 g/day should receive angiotensin-converting enzyme (ACE) inhibitors or angiotensin receptor blockers (ARBs).
- *Anti-GBM disease:* This is a rare small-vessel vasculitis affecting the kidneys, lungs or both. Most patients present with RPGN which can lead to development of ESRD. Pulmonary hemorrhage is a common manifestation and its presence along with that of RPGN, was termed as Goodpasture's syndrome.

Treatment is recommended with PLEX, combined with GCs and CYC. All patients with renal disease should have a kidney biopsy, and KDIGO recommends treatment of all patients, except for those who have 100% crescents or >50% scarring on biopsy and do not have lung involvement. Treatment can be started even before confirmation of diagnosis if suspicion is strong. PLEX is recommended in all patients, to be continued till the antibody is undetectable. Treatment with GCs is started at 1 mg/kg and dose is tapered over 6 months. CYC is recommended for 2–3 months. No maintenance therapy is recommended as relapses are very uncommon (0–6%), other than in patients who are also ANCA positive.

RENAL INVOLVEMENT DUE TO IMMUNE CHECKPOINT INHIBITORS

Immune checkpoint inhibitors (ICI) are novel drugs designed for treatment of different malignancies which have been associated with multiple autoimmune manifestations. Rarely, they can be associated with acute kidney injury (AKI)—most commonly interstitial nephritis, however thrombotic microangiopathy and glomerulonephritis has also been reported. Withholding these drugs in case of AKI is a rational approach along with treatment with systemic GCs for 3–4 weeks. Once renal function normalizes, an alternative agent may be used. In an observation study, once re challenged, 84% patients did not develop AKI after the initial incidents.

SUGGESTED READINGS

1. Hellmich B, Sanchez-Alamo B, Schirmer JH, Berti A, Blockmans D, Cid MC, et al. EULAR recommendations for the management of ANCA-associated vasculitis: 2022 update. Ann Rheum Dis. 2023:ard-2022-223764.
2. Rovin BH, Adler SG, Barratt J, Bridoux F, Burdge KA, Chan TM, et al. Executive summary of the KDIGO 2021 Guideline for the Management of Glomerular Diseases. Kidney Int. 2021;100(4):753-79.

253

CHAPTER

Infectious Arthritis

Bhupen Barman, Debashis Priyadarshan Sahoo

ABSTRACT

Infectious arthritis is a condition characterized by inflammation of a joint caused by an infection. It occurs when microorganisms like bacteria, viruses, or fungi enter a joint and trigger an immune response leading to joint pain, swelling, and reduced range of motion. This form of arthritis can be caused by various infectious agents, and it often warrants meticulous medical attention to prevent further damage, complications, and disability. In this chapter, we will discuss the causes, signs, symptoms, diagnosis, treatment, prevention, and rehabilitation options, emphasizing the importance of early intervention and appropriate management to minimize the impact on joint function and overall well-being.

INTRODUCTION

Infectious arthritis is characterized by joint pain, redness, stiffness, and swelling caused by an infectious microorganism such as bacteria, virus, fungi, and other uncommon organisms.

These infections enter into joints in various ways:

- Through nearby wound
- Through bloodstream dissemination
- After surgery, an injection, or trauma

Once infectious microbes reach the joint, it results in joint inflammation. Depending on the type of infection, single or multiple joints are affected.

The most common infectious arthritis caused by bacteria is in the knee. Small joints like fingers and toes are mostly affected by viral infections and direct injury. Joints of spine and breast bones are mostly affected in people with intravenous drug use.

Symptoms of infectious arthritis include:

- Joint pain typically in the knee, hip, shoulder, ankle, finger, and wrist
- Joint stiffness
- Redness and soreness around the joint
- Fever and chills
- Skin rash
- Other symptoms vary depending upon the cause of infection as mentioned below

TYPES OF ARTHRITIS

Infections can cause several types of arthritis, including the following:

- *Septic arthritis*: This is a bacterial infection of a joint, typically caused by *Staphylococcus aureus*, *Streptococcus pyogene*, *Mycobacterium tuberculosis*, or *Neisseria gonorrhoeae*. It can cause severe joint pain, swelling, warmth, and reduced range of motion. *Staphylococcus* is a common bacterium that causes infection through breaks in skin, cuts, or contaminated food. After release into bloodstream, the bacteria spread into knee and other joint spaces, causing sudden intense pain, swelling, and immobility of the joint. It is a very serious condition, as joint destruction develops within days, if not treated properly.
    - Tubercular arthritis, caused by *M. tuberculosis*, when affects musculoskeletal system usually involves spine or larger joints, such as hips and knees. It develops slowly and progresses less dramatically as compared to other bacterial

infections. Poncet's disease, a reactive symmetrical polyarthritis, can occur especially in patients with disseminated or visceral tuberculosis.
  - Gonorrhea, caused by *N. gonorrhoeae*, is a sexually transmitted infection that involves one or more joints or tendons and sometimes along with fever and rash. About one third of patients with gonorrhea reports joint pain.
  - Syphilitic arthritis, caused by *Treponema pallidum*, occurs in different stages of syphilis. Parrot's pseudoparalysis is seen in early congenital syphilis with periarticular swelling and immobilization of involved limbs. Secondary syphilis is associated with symmetric arthritis involving large joints and sacroiliitis. Clutton's joint, a late manifestation of congenital syphilis, occurs in 8–18 years of age group, caused by painless synovitis with effusion of knees and elbows.
- *Reactive arthritis*: This is a type of acute nonpurulent arthritis caused by immune reaction to certain infections elsewhere in the body, typically in genitourinary or gastrointestinal tract. Common triggers include *Chlamydia trachomatis, Salmonella, Shigella, Yersinia*, or *Campylobacter*. It develops after weeks or months of infection. Reactive arthritis typically affects the larger joints and is characterized by the "classic triad" of arthritis, urethritis, and conjunctivitis.
- *Viral arthritis*: Certain viral infections can cause arthritis symptoms. Examples include the dengue virus and chikungunya virus, which can cause severe joint pain and swelling. Human immunodeficiency virus (HIV), hepatitis virus (B and C), mumps, rubella, and parvovirus can manifest as a combination of simultaneously affecting multiple joint pain, swelling, and systemic symptoms. Symptoms usually resemble rheumatoid arthritis; however, these usually disappear within days to weeks, if the offending organism is removed or controlled. HIV and some other hepatitis may cause chronic infections along with long-standing joint pain.
- *Fungal arthritis*: Fungal infections can also affect the joints, although they are less common. Fungi such as *Candida, Aspergillus*, or *Coccidioides* species can invade joints and cause symptoms like joint pain, swelling, and limited mobility.
- *Lyme arthritis*: Lyme disease, caused by the bacterium *Borrelia burgdorferi*, can lead to Lyme arthritis if left untreated. The liver deer ticks are transmitted through bloodstream from the site of infection. Arthritis usually develops in the later stage of the disease. It primarily affects the larger joints, especially the knees, causing swelling, pain, and stiffness.

EVALUATION OF INFECTIOUS ARTHRITIS

The diagnosis of infectious arthritis includes a combination of proper medical history, physical examination, laboratory investigations, and imaging studies.

Steps involving in diagnosing infectious arthritis are as follows:

1. *Medical history*: To inquire about the symptoms such as joint pain, swelling, redness, and reduced range of motion as well as about any recent infections, surgeries, or injuries that may have preceded the joint symptoms.
2. *Physical examination*: To perform a thorough examination of the affected joint(s) to assess for signs of inflammation, warmth, tenderness, and swelling and also check for other systemic symptoms, such as fever or skin rashes.
3. *Laboratory tests*: Various laboratory tests are to be conducted to aid in the diagnosis of infectious arthritis. These may include the following:
   - *Blood tests*: A complete blood count (CBC) can reveal leukocytosis, signifying an ongoing infection. Blood cultures can help identify the causative organism. Erythrocyte sedimentation rate (ESR), C-reactive protein (CRP), and uric acid are measured.
   - *Joint fluid analysis*: Joint fluid aspiration (Arthrocentesis) is done from the involved joint and then examined for the presence of any microorganism. Analysis of the fluid can also provide information about the inflammatory markers like white blood cell count and presence of crystals, which can help differentiate infectious arthritis from other forms of arthritis.

     If synovial fluid analysis shows a white blood cell (WBC) count 2,000/μL and Gram-stain and culture are positive, it is septic arthritis. If synovial fluid analysis shows WBC count of 2,000/μL and Gram-stain and culture are negative, then differential diagnosis will be inflammatory arthritis, Lyme arthritis, tuberculous arthritis, and fungal arthritis.
4. *Microbiological tests*: Depending on the suspected infectious agent, additional microbiological tests may be performed, such as cultures of blood, joint fluid, or other relevant samples like vaginal swab, cervical swab, urine samples for women, and penile swab and urine for men. However, some common causes of viral arthritis caused by HIV, hepatitis B, hepatitis C, mumps, and parvovirus can be detected from blood investigations. These tests help identify the specific bacteria, viruses, or fungi responsible for the infection.

5. *Imaging studies*: Joint X-rays, ultrasound, or magnetic resonance imaging (MRI) may be conducted to assess the joint structure or check for signs of erosion, soft-tissue swelling, or collections of fluid within or around the joint.

APPROACH TO AN ARTHRITIS PATIENT

Comprehensive evaluation with detailed history and musculoskeletal examination is the initial step followed by proper management of joint pain which includes a multifaceted approach, including rest, medication, lifestyle changes, physiotherapy, and, if required, surgical intervention **(Flowchart 1)**. Proper diagnosis and personalized treatment plans (precession medicine) are critical for effective pain relief and improvement of quality of life.

Treatment

The treatment of infectious arthritis involves a combination of antibiotics or antiviral medications, joint drainage, pain management, and supportive care. The causative organism and the severity of the infection lead to specific treatment. The main aspects of treatment are as follows:

- *Antibiotics or antiviral medications*: If the infectious arthritis is caused by bacteria, antibiotics are the mainstay of treatment. The choice of imperial antibiotics depends on the suspected bacteria and can be modified as per sensitivity to identified bacteria in culture. Intravenous antibiotics are often initially used to ensure a high concentration of the drug in the bloodstream. As the infection resolves, oral antibiotics may be prescribed for a prolonged period (usually 4–6 weeks).
  - If the infectious arthritis is caused by a viral infection, antiviral medications may be prescribed in cases like HIV, hepatitis B, and hepatitis C. Viral infections do not usually cause joint damage.
  - Antifungal medications are used for fungal infections.
- *Joint drainage*: If there is significant fluid accumulation in the affected joint, aspiration or arthroscopy may be performed to remove the infected fluid. This helps reduce pain, relieve pressure, and facilitate the effectiveness of antibiotics. In some cases, surgical drainage may be required.
- *Pain management*: Pain and inflammation can be managed with nonsteroidal anti-inflammatory drugs (NSAIDs), such as naproxen or ibuprofen. In more severe cases, corticosteroids can be prescribed to reduce inflammation. Analgesics can be used to manage pain, and physiotherapy should be recommended to maintain joint mobility and strength.
  - Reactive arthritis may be treated with other medications like NSAIDs, corticosteroids, methotrexate, and sulfasalazine, but only after the infection has been cured.
- *Supportive care*: It is important to provide proper rest to the affected joint, to prevent further damage and

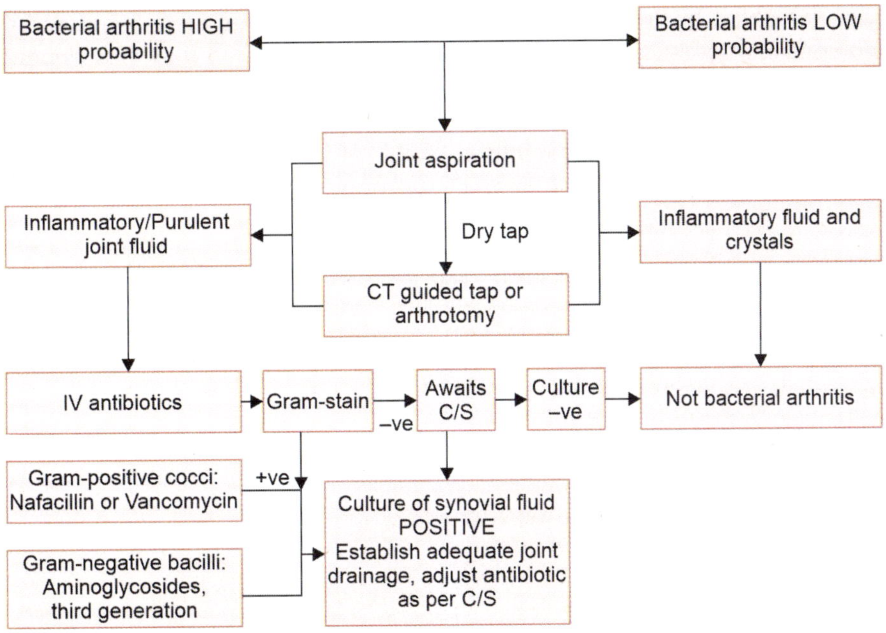

FLOWCHART 1: Approach to infectious arthritis.
(C/S: culture and sensitivity)

fasten healing. Ice pack application to reduce swelling and elevation of the joint can help alleviate symptoms. Adequate fluid intake and a healthy diet can support the body's immune response. Joint needs to be immobilized briefly with brace or splint. Exercise and physiotherapy are recommended to restore mobility.

- *Treating the underlying cause*: If the infectious arthritis is associated with an underlying infection elsewhere in the body, such as a urinary tract infection or skin abscess, that infection needs to be appropriately treated to prevent reinfection of the joint.

PREVENTION

Prevention of infectious arthritis includes obtaining steps to diminish the risk of developing an infection that can lead to joint inflammation. Some key preventive measures are as follows:

- *Practice good hand hygiene*: Maintain proper hand hygiene. Regular hand washing with soap and water, especially before handling food, after using the restroom and after coughing or sneezing is important.
- *Avoid close contact with infected individuals*: Take necessary precautions to reduce the risk of transmission of respiratory tract infections and sexual transmitted diseases. This may involve wearing masks, avoiding direct contact, and ensuring proper sanitation and practising safe sex.
- *Take precautions during healthcare procedures*: If a patient is planned for invasive procedures, such as surgery, joint injections, or dental work, the risk of infection can be reduced by following proper sterile techniques and ensuring that healthcare providers adhere to infection-control guidelines.
- *Proper wound care*: If a patient has any cuts, scrapes, or wounds, it is essential to clean and dress them appropriately to prevent infection. Regularly monitor the wound for signs of infection, such as increasing pain, redness, swelling, or pus formation, and seek medical attention if necessary.
- *Vaccinations*: Keeping up to date with recommended vaccinations, such as tetanus, pneumococcal, and influenza vaccines, can help prevent infectious illnesses that can potentially lead to infectious arthritis.
- *Safe food handling*: Maintain safe food handling procedures, such as cooking meats thoroughly, avoiding cross-contamination, and refrigerating perishable foods promptly. These measures can help reduce the risk of food-borne infections, such as Salmonella or Campylobacter, which can sometimes spread to the joints.
- *Practice safe sex*: If you are sexually active, it is important to practice safe sex to reduce the risk of sexually transmitted infections (STIs) that can lead to joint infections, such as gonorrhea or chlamydia. This includes using barrier methods of contraception, such as condoms, and getting regular STI screenings.
- *Maintain a healthy lifestyle*: A healthy lifestyle, including adequate sleep, regular exercise, and a balanced diet, can support a strong immunity, reducing the risk of infections and their potential complications.

CONCLUSION

It is crucial to suspect infectious arthritis promptly, as quick diagnosis and management can help preventing ongoing joint damage and complications. It is important to note that the diagnosis of infectious arthritis can sometimes be challenging, as the symptoms may overlap with other forms of arthritis or joint conditions. The treatment regimen may vary depending on the specific circumstances. Therefore, a multidisciplinary approach involving rheumatologists, infectious disease specialists, and orthopedic doctors is often necessary to ensure an accurate diagnosis and appropriate management.

SUGGESTED READINGS

1. Shirtliff ME, Mader JT. Acute septic arthritis. Clin Microbiol Rev. 2002;15(4):527-44.
2. Colston J, Atkins B. Bone and joint infection. Clin Med (Lond). 2018;18(2):150-4.
3. Radolf JD, Strle K, Lemieux JE, Strle F. Lyme Disease in Humans. Curr Issues Mol Biol. 2021;42:333-84.

254

CHAPTER

Adult-onset Still's Disease: An Update

Vijay Kumar, Suvarthi Ray

ABSTRACT

Recent research on the pathophysiology of adult-onset Still's disease (AOSD) classified it as a "complex" autoinflammatory disorder and placed it at the nexus of autoinflammatory and autoimmune diseases. Two phenotypes of the disease can be distinguished based on how it presents clinically at the time of diagnosis—a highly symptomatic, systemic, and feverish one that would progress to a systemic pattern; and a more lax one with arthritis in the foreground and poor systemic symptomatology that would progress to a chronic articular pattern. Despite potentially fatal complications, AOSD has a fair prognosis and a very low fatality rate. The majority of AOSD treatment is corticosteroids (0.8–1 mg/kg/day) and low-dose methotrexate. In the case of chronic polyarticular refractory AOSD, tumor necrosis factor (TNF)-blockers, particularly infliximab, may be of interest. In refractory systemic AOSD, anakinra appears to be an effective, well-tolerated, and steroid-free treatment, but it is just a suspensive one. In refractory AOSD with active arthritis, tocilizumab inhibition of the interleukin 6 (IL-6) pathway appears effective.

INTRODUCTION

An inflammatory condition known as adult-onset Still's disease (AOSD) is characterized by quotidian (daily) fevers, arthritis, and an ephemeral rash. George Still first identified systemic juvenile idiopathic arthritis in children in 1896, and since then, the condition has been referred to as "Still's disease" or "Still's disease" in its entirety. The term "adult-onset Still's disease" was first used by EG Bywaters in 1971 to describe the first group of 14 people who shared the same symptoms as those associated with pediatric Still's illness. Due to the vast variety of potential diagnoses, AOSD is still an uncommon multisystemic autoinflammatory illness with an unidentified origin. However, the prognosis might be enhanced by an early diagnosis.

EPIDEMIOLOGY AND PATHOPHYSIOLOGY

The disease is present in every country and often affects young individuals (the median age at diagnosis is 36 years, while onsets have been reported as early as 83 years). Men do not appear to be affected as frequently as women.

Due to the similar clinical characteristics of AOSD and other infectious syndromes, such as sudden onset, high fever, widespread adenopathy, splenomegaly, and leukocytosis, an infectious etiology has been hypothesized. Thus, numerous microorganisms were looked for. Rubella, measles, echovirus 7, coxsackievirus B4, cytomegalovirus, Epstein–Barr virus, human herpes-virus 6, adenovirus, influenza A, hepatitis B and C, and parvovirus B19 were among the viruses and bacteria that were found in AOSD patients, but it has never been determined with certainty how or why they caused the condition. It is hypothesized that infection might set off a cascade of interactions between host genetic variables, autoimmune mechanisms, and disease-causing antigens, ultimately contributing to the pathogenesis of the illness.

There are no genetic loci that have been definitively linked to AOSD, despite the fact that AOSD and systemic juvenile inflammatory arthritis share a similar phenotype and exhibit high levels of interleukin 6 (IL-6) and IL-18 as well as similar peripheral blood gene expression profiles. AOSD is linked to human leukocyte antigen (HLA)-B17, -B18, -B35, and -DR2.

As previously mentioned in hemophagocytic lymphohistiocytosis, malignancies such as solid cancer (60% of cases, primarily breast and lung) and hematological malignancies (40% of cases, primarily malignant lymphoma) can also cause the start of AOSD **(Fig. 1)**.

CLINICAL FEATURES

Adult-onset Still's disease is characterized by fever, rash, and arthritis or arthralgia as its main clinical manifestations. Myalgia, pharyngitis, lymphadenopathy, and splenomegaly are other symptoms. Few people experience hepatomegaly, pleurisy, pericarditis, or abdominal pain. Although rare, macrophage activation syndrome (MAS) is a condition that could be lethal.

- *Fever*: Between 60% and 100% of patients experience fever. The maximum temperatures (39°C) usually peak once or twice daily in the evening. Typically, a fever comes up before other signs. A fever of unknown origin (FUO) can also be a symptom of AOSD.
- *Arthralgia and arthritis*: Joint pain is the most prevalent symptom of arthritis and arthralgia (70–100% of the time). The wrists, knees, and ankles are typically affected by arthritis and arthralgia. Even while arthritis usually starts off being moderate and temporary, it can eventually develop into a chronic destructive symmetrical polyarthritis with a characteristic carpal ankylosis. Findings in the tissue and synovial fluid are consistent with inflammatory arthritis. The arthritis may start out mild, temporary, and oligoarticular. The knees, wrists, ankles, elbows, proximal interphalangeal joints, and shoulders are the joints most frequently affected, in that order.
- *Rash*: The typical skin rash associated with AOSD is an evanescent, salmon-colored, macular or maculopapular cutaneous eruption that is often nonpruritic, tends to emerge along with the fever, and then vanishes during afebrile times. In 60–80% of AOSD cases, it is present. The face and extremities are frequently affected, although the trunk, hands, and feet are also occasionally affected.
- *Myalgia*: Myalgia is frequent (40–50%), frequently made worse by temperature spikes and occasionally

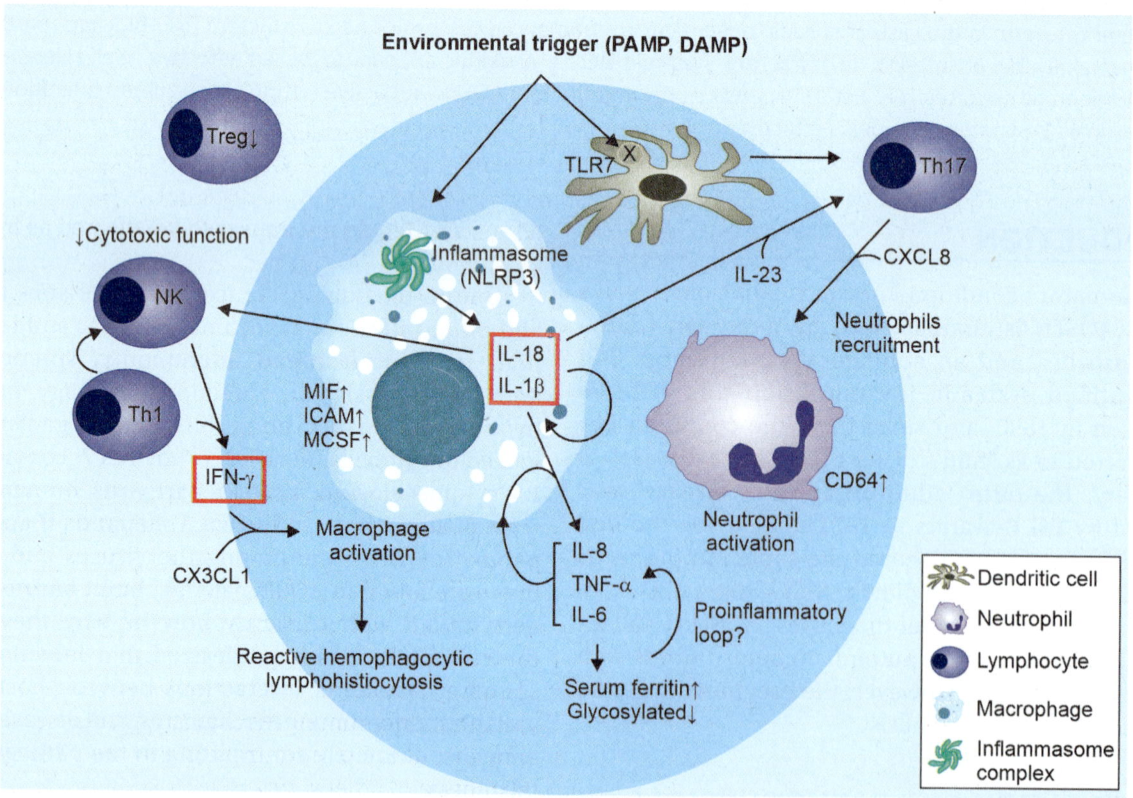

FIG. 1: Pathology of adult-onset Still's disease.

(DAMP: damage-associated molecular pattern; IFN-γ: interferon gamma; ICAM: intercellular adhesion molecule; IL: interleukin; MCSF: macrophage colony-stimulating factor; MIF: migration inhibitory factor; NK: natural killer; NLRP3: nucleotide-binding domain, leucine-rich-containing family, pyrin domain-containing-3; PAMP: pathogen-associated molecular pattern; Th1: T-helper 1; TLR7: toll-like receptor 7; TNF: tumor necrosis factor) severe and incapacitating. Although there is little muscle wasting, blood levels of aldolase and creatine kinase may be modestly increased. Muscle biopsy and electromyographic investigations typically reveal a generic myopathy or are normal.

- *Pharyngitis*: A sore throat may be an initial sign of AOSD. About 70% of patients experience it prior to or during the first month of each illness flare.

Other symptoms include weight loss (27%), lymphadenopathy (50%), splenomegaly (40%), hepatomegaly (30%), pleurisy (21%), pericarditis (16%), and abdominal pain (18%). The following manifestations are much less common—ischemic stroke, reversible posterior leukoencephalopathy syndrome, bilateral perception of deafness, aseptic meningitis or encephalitis, collapsing glomerulopathy, membranous glomerulonephritis, even necrotizing crescentic glomerulonephritis, or tubulointerstitial nephritis; conjunctivitis (local case), and intense, paracortical immunoblastic hyperplasia is frequently seen on lymph node biopsy in AOSD, which is different from the alterations seen in rheumatoid arthritis (RA), systemic lupus erythematosus (SLE), Sjögren's syndrome, or Kikuchi's disease.

Other hematologics manifestations: Other hematologic symptoms that may be related to AOSD include disseminated intravascular coagulation and microangiopathic hemolytic anemia linked to thrombotic thrombocytopenic purpura-hemolytic uremic syndrome.

LABORATORY FINDINGS

A number of laboratory findings are characteristic of AOSD as shown in **Table 1**.

TABLE 1: Laboratory tests in adult-onset Still's disease.

Laboratory tests	Percentage (%) of patients
• Elevated ESR	99
• WBC	
○ ≥10,000/mm^3	92
○ ≥15,000/mm^3	81
• Neutrophils ≥ 80%	88
• Serum albumin ≤ 3.5 g/dL	81
• Elevated liver enzymes (any)	73
• Anemia (Hb ≤ 10 g/dL)	68
• Platelets ≥ 400,000/mm^3	62
• Negative ANA	92
• Negative RF	93

(ANA: antinuclear antibody; ESR: erythrocyte sedimentation rate; Hb: hemoglobin; RF: rheumatoid factor; WBC: white blood cell)

DIAGNOSIS

The diagnosis of AOSD can generally be determined based on the presence of the distinctive clinical and laboratory features in the absence of another disease that may generate similar symptoms and findings. This is known as a diagnosis of exclusion. Although the clinical picture can vary, the following characteristics stand out:

- Daily spikes in temperature
- An evanescent salmon-pink maculopapular eruption on the skin, most frequently present during the febrile hours
- Arthritis or arthralgia
- Leukocytosis with a neutrophil predominance
- A marked elevation in serum ferritin

DIFFERENTIAL DIAGNOSIS

Due to the lack of a definitive clinical or laboratory test, the diagnosis of AOSD is still based on exclusion. Before making this diagnosis, it is important to exclude infectious, neoplastic, and autoimmune illnesses that can resemble the clinical manifestation of AOSD **(Box 1)**.

CLASSIFICATION CRITERIA

For study and diagnosis, a number of sets of classification criteria have been put forth. The Yamaguchi set of diagnostic criteria showed the best sensitivity (78.57%) and a better accuracy (87.14%) in a recent study evaluating four sets of diagnostic criteria in a Chinese population. The classification made by Fautrel was 98.5% specific and 80.6% sensitive. Nowadays, patients who fulfill Yamaguchi's **(Table 2)** and/or Fautrel's **(Table 3)** criteria are included in the majority of investigations on AOSD.

TREATMENT

The goals of therapy include:

- Reducing physical manifestations of inflammation such as fever, rash, morning stiffness, joint pain, and edema, as well as secondly, reducing laboratory manifestations of inflammation, such as increase in erythrocyte sedimentation rate (ESR) and C-reactive protein (CRP) levels.
- Prompt diagnosis and treatment of MAS, a hyperinflammatory consequence of AOSD.
- The avoidance of end-organ problems, such as joint damage and other serious organ issues.
- Reducing the possibility of treatment-related side effects, such as long-term effects of corticosteroids.

BOX 1: Differential diagnosis of adult-onset Still's disease.

- *Diseases*:
  - Infections
- *Viral infections*:
  - HIV
  - *Herpesviridae*
  - Measles
  - Rubella
  - Viral hepatitis
  - Parvovirus B19
- *Infective endocarditis*:
  - Borreliosis, brucellosis, yersiniosis
  - *Mycoplasma pneumoniae*, syphilis
  - Toxoplasmosis
- *Neoplasia*:
  - Malignant lymphoma
  - Multicentric Castleman disease
  - Angioimmunoblastic T-cell lymphoma
- *Drug reactions*:
  - Drug reaction with eosinophilia
  - Systemic symptoms
- *Autoimmune diseases*:
  - Systemic lupus erythematosus
  - Idiopathic inflammatory myositis
  - Rheumatoid arthritis
  - Systemic vasculitides
  - Autoinflammatory diseases
  - Familial Mediterranean fever
  - Mevalonate kinase deficiency
  - TNF receptor-associated periodic syndrome
  - Reactive arthritis
- *Others*:
  - Sarcoidosis
  - Neutrophilic dermatosis
  - Kikuchi–Fujimoto disease

(HIV: human immunodeficiency virus; TNF: tumor necrosis factor)

TABLE 2: Yamaguchi classification criteria for adult-onset Still's disease.

Major criteria	Minor criteria	Exclusion criteria
Fever ≥ 39°C lasting 1 week or longer	Sore throat	Infections
Arthralgia or arthritis lasting 2 weeks or longer	Recent development of significant lymphadenopathy	Malignancies (mainly malignant lymphoma)
Typical rash	Hepatomegaly or splenomegaly	Other rheumatic disease (mainly systemic vasculitides)
Leukocytosis ≥ 10,000/mm^3 with ≥80% polymorphonuclear cells	• Abnormal liver function tests • Negative tests for antinuclear antibody (IF) and rheumatoid factor [immunoglobulin M (IgM)]	

Note: Five or more criteria are required of which two or more must be major.

TABLE 3: Fautrel classification criteria for adult-onset Still's disease.

Major criteria	Minor criteria
Spiking fever ≥39°C	Maculopapular rash
Arthralgia	Leukocytosis ≥ 10,000/mm^3
Transient erythema	
Pharyngitis	
Polymorphonuclear cells ≥80%	
Glycosylated ferritin ≤20%	

Note: Four or more major criteria are required or three major + two minor criteria.

Initial Therapy: New-onset Disease

Mild-to-moderate Disease

Nondisabling fever, rash, arthralgias or mild arthritis, and the lack of MAS are the hallmarks of mild-to-moderate disease at the time of disease initiation. We advise first-line management with nonsteroidal anti-inflammatory drugs (NSAIDs) alone rather than glucocorticoids, disease-modifying antirheumatic drugs (DMARDs), or biologics for patients suspected of new-onset AOSD who only have mild-to-moderate symptoms and do not have MAS, especially while investigation for other possible causes of fever (such as infection or lymphoma) is ongoing. Ibuprofen (800 mg three times daily), naproxen (500 mg twice daily), and indomethacin (25–50 mg three times daily) are common options for NSAIDs that have an anti-inflammatory dose and schedule. There is no proof that any one NSAID is more effective for AOSD than another. The approach for patients who have not responded sufficiently to a 7- to 14-day trial of an NSAID alone during the acute phase of the illness is similar to that for patients who present with moderate-to-severe disease.

Moderate-to-severe Disease

The presence of further clinically significant serositis (such as pleurisy or peritonitis), moderate-to-severe and incapacitating polyarthritis, recurrent high fevers despite therapy with NSAIDs, or internal organ involvement may be used to identify moderate to severe illness.

Treatment Approach

We prefer to start anakinra treatment for patients with new-onset moderate-to-severe AOSD and those with milder disease for whom NSAIDs are insufficient. Although glucocorticoids are a viable choice, they have certain relative drawbacks in this situation.

Anakinra

We recommend anakinra rather than continuing with NSAIDs alone, glucocorticoids, or another DMARD (such as biologics and traditional synthetic DMARDs) for the management of new-onset moderate-to-severe AOSD and for individuals in whom 2 weeks of NSAIDs are insufficient.

Glucocorticoids

Glucocorticoids are a reasonable substitute for anakinra, especially for those who cannot get the medication. Prednisone oral starting doses for AOSD range from 20 to 60 mg per day, based on the patient's unique assessment of the disease's severity and the speed of the initial therapeutic response. Both the systemic and arthritic aspects of AOSD are treated with oral glucocorticoids. Patients often respond to glucocorticoids within a few hours to a few days, but in certain cases, a longer course of therapy may be necessary. Approximately, 70% of patients react to glucocorticoids either taken alone or in combination with NSAIDs.

Glucocorticoids are swiftly tapered to a low-maintenance dose for 2–3 months once symptom management is sustained for at least 2 weeks and laboratory indices have normalized in order to maintain control of illness signs and symptoms. Although some patients may still need up to 5 mg of glucocorticoids per day, the long-term goal is to completely stop using them.

TREATMENT OF CASES REFRACTORY TO STANDARD THERAPY (FLOWCHART 1)

When standard treatments for AOSD patients are ineffective, there are various more possibilities to take into account as follows:

- *Janus kinase (JAK) inhibitors*: Patients with AOSD who have tried conventional nonbiologic and biologic therapy without success should consider JAK inhibitors.
- *Other agents are*:
  - o Cyclosporine
  - o Rituximab
  - o Intravenous immunoglobulin
  - o Tadekinig alfa

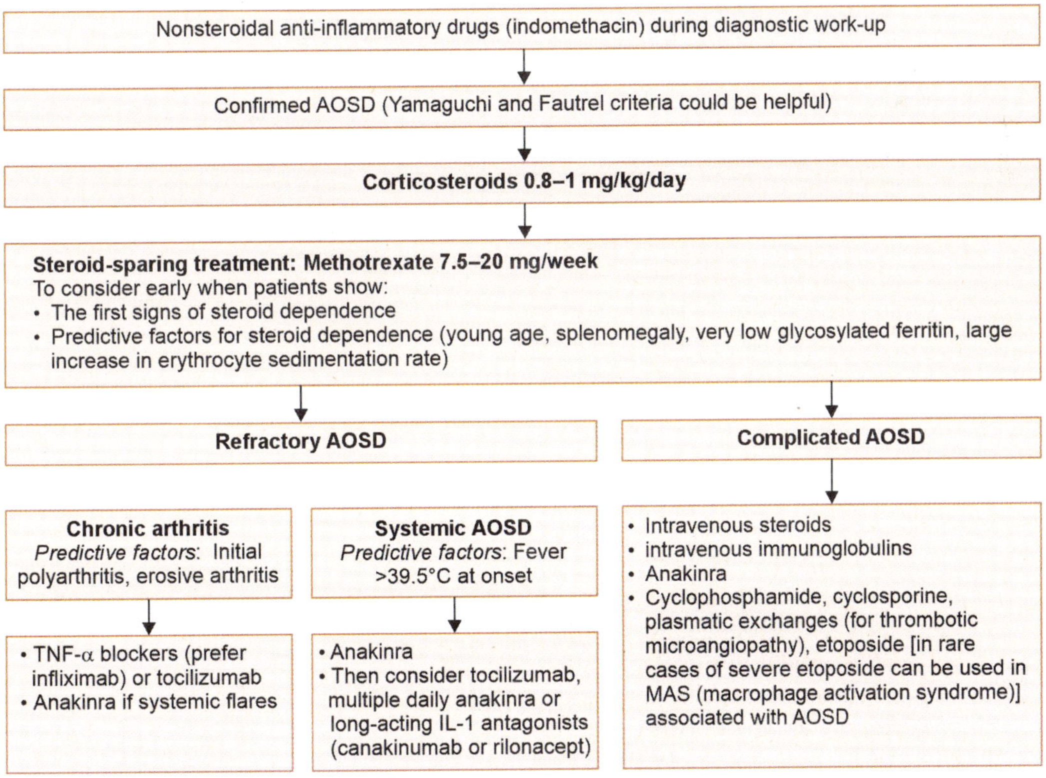

FLOWCHART 1: Therapeutic strategy in AOSD.

(AOSD: adult-onset Still's disease; IL-1: interleukin 1; TNF-α: tumor necrosis factor alpha)

- Cyclophosphamide
- Combination biologic therapy
- Allogeneic bone marrow transplantation

PROGNOSIS

Even in the presence of a chronic illness pattern, the functional level of people with AOSD is frequently good. The AOSD has documented a number of risk factors for chronic disease and adverse outcomes. A poor prognosis is also associated with the need for more than 2 years of systemic glucocorticoid therapy prior to the widespread use of biologics, as well as the development of an erosive polyarthritis during the initial presenting episode of the disease, involvement of the shoulders or hips, a history of MAS, a history of cardiac involvement, including pericarditis, and involvement of the shoulders or hips.

SUGGESTED READINGS

1. Asanuma YF, Mimura T, Tsuboi H, Noma H, Miyoshi F, Yamamoto K, et al. Nationwide epidemiological survey of 169 patients with adult Still's disease in Japan. Mod Rheumatol. 2015;25(3): 393-400.
2. Magadur-Joly G, Billaud E, Barrier JH, Pennec YL, Masson C, Renou P, et al. Epidemiology of adult Still's disease: estimate of the incidence by a retrospective study in west France. Ann Rheum Dis. 1995;54(7):587-90.
3. Efthimiou P, Kontzias A, Hur P, Rodha K, Ramakrishna GS, Nakasato P. Adult-onset Still's disease in focus: Clinical manifestations, diagnosis, treatment, and unmet needs in the era of targeted therapies. Semin Arthritis Rheum. 2021;51(4): 858-74.
4. Sugiura T, Maeno N, Kawaguchi Y, Takei S, Imanaka H, Kawano Y, et al. A promoter haplotype of the interleukin-18 gene is associated with juvenile idiopathic arthritis in the Japanese population. Arthritis Res Ther. 2006;8(3):R60.
5. Hofheinz K, Schett G, Manger B. Adult onset Still's disease associated with malignancy-Cause or coincidence? Semin Arthritis Rheum. 2016;45(5):621-6.

SECTION

20

MISCELLANEOUS

255
CHAPTER

History Taking in Clinical Medicine

Atanu Chandra

ABSTRACT

History taking in clinical medicine is a crucial aspect of patient care. It involves collecting information about a patient's medical history, symptoms, and relevant personal details to aid in diagnosis and treatment. The process usually follows a structured approach, beginning with demographic information and proceeding to the patient's chief complaint, medical history, family history, social history, and review of systems. Effective history taking requires communication skills, empathy, and the ability to ask open-ended questions. It forms the foundation for a patient-centered approach to healthcare.

INTRODUCTION

History taking in medicine is a fundamental process in patient care that involves gathering essential information about a patient's medical history, symptoms, and personal details. This structured approach assists healthcare professionals in understanding the patient's condition, making accurate diagnoses and providing appropriate treatment. The process entails establishing rapport, active listening, using open-ended questions, and being culturally sensitive to encourage patients to share their experiences. By following a systematic framework, healthcare providers can uncover vital information that forms the basis for effective patient-centered care. The patient history is a vital piece of the physician-patient encounter and helps lead to the final diagnosis about 75% of the time. Skilled history taking is reported to be declining among medical trainees, and many educators believe that current educational methods do not emphasize these skills during medical school training.

DURATION OF HISTORY TAKING

According to a study in the UK, the adequate time needed for consultation is 12 minutes (on an average) for new uncomplicated problems and follow-up patients and 30 minutes (on an average) for new, multisystem, complex problems.

GOALS OF HISTORY TAKING

The goals of history taking in clinical medicine include understanding the patient's medical history, symptoms, and concerns as well as identifying potential underlying causes of their condition. This information helps in making an accurate diagnosis, developing a suitable treatment plan, and building a strong patient-provider relationship.

The primary objectives of gathering a patient's medical history include the following:

- *Diagnosis*: Understanding the patient's symptoms, medical background, and relevant history helps in accurately planning the clinical examination process and focused investigations to diagnose their condition.
- *Treatment*: A comprehensive history aids in tailoring an effective treatment plan based on the patient's individual needs and medical history.
- *Prognosis*: Knowing the patient's medical history can sometimes help to predict the likely course and outcome of their condition. A thorough history taking often helps to identify risk factors and potential triggers of the disease.

- *Others*: Accurate history documentation serves as a legal proof of the care provided and supports decision-making. Engaging in open communication builds trust, making the patient more comfortable sharing their concerns and improving overall care. Patients can better understand their health when they are informed about their medical history and its implications. A well-documented history ensures that different healthcare providers can collaborate effectively for the patient's ongoing care.

STEPS IN HISTORY TAKING: A STRUCTURED APPROACH

History taking in clinical medicine follows a structured approach to gather relevant information. The typical steps include the following:

1. *Introduction*: To start with small sense of formalities like wishing patients and their accompanying persons, by shaking hands, introducing self and team members will definitely make the situation for the patient familiar. Begin by introducing yourself (give your name and your job: "Hello, I'm Dr AC, ward doctor"), confirming that you are speaking to the correct patient ("Are you Mr SM?" or "How can I address you?"), explaining your role, and gaining the patient's permission for the interview (confirm the reason for seeing the patient: "I am going to ask you a few questions about your problems, is that OK?"). The patient should be seated in chair approximately a meter away from the doctor, and both should be at the same level.
2. *Chief complaint (CC)*: Ask the patient about the main reason for their visit, describe their problem using open questions, duration of symptoms, encouraging them to describe their symptoms in their own words (Dr AC: "Mr SM, what brings you here today?"; Mr SM: "I have a tightness in my chest"). If possible, do not interrupt the patient's first few sentences. Try to elicit the patient's ideas, concerns, and expectations (ICE) (Mr SM: "I am worried I might have a malignancy").
3. *History of present illness (HOPI)*: Obtain a detailed account of the onset, duration, progression, and characteristics of the symptoms. Gather information about associated factors, alleviating or aggravating factors, and any attempts at self-treatment. Significant negatives have to be mentioned. (Dr AC: "Tell me more about this chest pain. When did it start? Can you describe the pain? Does it radiate to any other areas?" Mr SM: "It started suddenly two days ago while I was jogging. It's a sharp pain in the center of my chest, and it sometimes goes to my left arm.") A useful mnemonic for pain is "SOCRATES" (*S*ite, *O*nset, *C*haracter, *R*adiation, *A*lleviating factors, *T*iming, *E*xacerbating factors, *S*everity).
4. *Past medical history (PMH)*: Inquire about the patient's medical history including chronic illnesses (especially ask about any past history of myocardial infarction, stroke, jaundice, tuberculosis, rheumatic fever, epilepsy, or cancer), surgeries, hospitalizations, and significant past events (Dr AC: "Have you had any medical conditions in the past, surgeries, or hospitalizations?"). It is better to avoid the history of chronic diseases such as diabetes or hypertension in the PMH.
5. *Medications and allergies*: Document the patient's current medications, dosages, and any known allergies. A thorough search about the intake of any over-the-counter, homeopathic, ayurvedic, or alternative medicines should be done.
6. *Family history*: Ask about the medical conditions present in the patient's immediate family, as some conditions may have a genetic predisposition.
7. *Social history*: Obtain information about the patient's lifestyle, occupation, living situation, dietary habits, exercise, and substance use (e.g., smoking, alcohol, recreational drugs).
8. *Review of systems (ROS)*: Systematically go through various systems, asking about any related symptoms the patient might be experiencing. This can help identify any additional pathology. Run through major symptoms from major systems:
    - *Cardiovascular*: Chest pain (angina), exertional breathlessness, palpitation, pedal edema, paroxysmal nocturnal dyspnea (PND), orthopnea
    - *Respiratory*: Cough, shortness of breath (breathlessness), hemoptysis, expectoration (sputum production), wheezing, seasonal variation
    - *Gastrointestinal*: Abdominal pain, distension of abdomen, dysphagia, reflux symptoms, vomiting, upper gastrointestinal bleeding (hematemesis/melena), jaundice, diarrhea, constipation, bleeding per rectum
    - *Renal*: Dysuria, loin pain, oliguria, frothy urine, hematuria
    - *Neurological*: Weakness, tingling, numbness, bladder/bowel dysfunction, visual change, diplopia, drooping of eyelid, facial deviation, bulbar symptoms
    - *Psychiatric*: Depression, anxiety
    - *General review*: Unintentional weight loss, loss of appetite, lumps or bumps (nodes), rashes, joint pain.

9. *Personal and psychosocial history*: Inquire about the patient's personal relationships, emotional well-being, stressors, and any history of mental health issues.
10. *Sexual and reproductive history*: If relevant, ask about sexual activity, contraception, pregnancies, and menstrual history.
11. *Functional status*: Assess the patient's ability to perform daily activities and any limitations due to their medical condition.
12. *Closing and summary*: Summarize the information collected, address any remaining concerns, and ask if the patient has additional questions.

Remember to use open-ended questions to encourage the patient to share their experiences in their own words. Active listening, empathy, and respectful communication are essential throughout the process. This structured approach ensures that no important aspects of the patient's history are overlooked and helps guide clinical decision-making.

DIFFICULTIES THAT WE COMMONLY FACE DURING HISTORY TAKING FROM PATIENTS

During history taking from patients, healthcare professionals often encounter several common difficulties. Patients might not have complete or accurate information about their medical history, especially if they have a complex medical condition or have seen multiple healthcare providers. Patients who speak a different language or have limited proficiency in the local language may have difficulty expressing their symptoms accurately. Cultural beliefs and practices can influence how patients describe their symptoms and may impact their willingness to share certain details. Patients might hesitate to discuss sensitive topics, such as sexual health, substance abuse, or mental health issues, due to embarrassment or concerns about privacy. Elderly patients or those with cognitive impairments may struggle to remember important medical details, leading to incomplete or inaccurate information. Patients might describe their symptoms in vague terms, making it challenging for healthcare providers to pinpoint the underlying issue (patients of inferior wall myocardial infarction may often be misdiagnosed as acute gastritis if appropriate history and evaluation are not done). Some patients might provide inconsistent or exaggerated accounts of their symptoms, making it difficult to determine the actual medical history. Patients who are anxious, uncooperative, or hostile can make the history-taking process challenging and hinder effective communication. Patients might not understand medical terminology, which can lead to confusion and miscommunication during the history-taking process. Healthcare professionals often have limited time to gather all necessary information, which can result in rushed interactions and incomplete histories. Patients might omit certain details that they perceive as irrelevant or that they are uncomfortable sharing, potentially leading to a misdiagnosis. Relying on family members or friends for information can introduce biases and inaccuracies in the patient's medical history.

STRATEGIES TO FOLLOW TO OBTAIN A GOOD HISTORY FROM THE PATIENT

Obtaining a comprehensive and accurate medical history from a patient requires a combination of strategies to foster effective communication and build trust. Some key strategies to follow are given in the following text:

- *Establish rapport*: Begin by introducing yourself and creating a welcoming atmosphere. Use open body language, maintain eye contact and show empathy to put the patient at ease.
- *Active listening*: Pay close attention to the patient's words, tone, and nonverbal cues. Listen without interrupting and avoid making assumptions. Demeanor, attitude, and dress of doctors silently influence at the outset to gain confidence of the patients. Similarly using smart phone frequently, if not very urgent, while attending patients may create a impression of casualness on the part of doctor toward the patient's problem. Doctor's each attitude is being silently, attentively; and critically observed by patients and accompanying persons.
- *Open-ended questions*: Use open-ended questions to encourage patients to provide detailed information. These questions cannot be answered with a simple "yes" or "no" and allow patients to share their thoughts and experiences.
- *Use the ICE approach*: Inquire about the patient's ideas, concerns, and expectations related to their health issue. This helps you understand their perspective and tailor your approach accordingly.
- *Chronological approach*: Begin with demographic details and then proceed chronologically through the patient's medical history. This ensures a structured and organized approach.
- *Structured history taking*: It has already been discussed earlier.
- *Be culturally sensitive*: Respect cultural differences and adapt your communication style to suit the patient's cultural background.
- *Avoid medical jargon*: Use simple and understandable language, avoiding medical terminology that the patient might not be familiar with.

- *Clarify and summarize*: Repeat back the information you have gathered to ensure accuracy and understanding. This also demonstrates that you are actively engaged in the conversation.
- *Address sensitive topics*: Approach sensitive topics delicately and without judgment. Assure the patient of confidentiality to encourage open sharing.
- *Educate and involve*: Provide information about the diagnosis, treatment options, and what to expect. Involve the patient in decision-making.
- *Manage time effectively*: While being thorough, also be mindful of time constraints to ensure a balanced history-taking process.
- *Use digital tools*: Electronic health records and digital forms can help streamline the process and capture relevant information efficiently.
- *Follow-up*: If certain details are unclear or incomplete, schedule a follow-up session to gather more information.

Remember that every patient is unique, so adapt your strategies based on their individual needs and preferences. By combining these strategies, you can obtain a comprehensive and accurate medical history that forms the basis for effective diagnosis and treatment.

CONCLUSION

In conclusion, history taking is a fundamental and structured process in clinical medicine that serves as the cornerstone of patient care. Through effective communication and active listening, healthcare providers gather essential information about the patient's medical history, symptoms, concerns, and overall health status. This comprehensive approach enables accurate diagnosis, appropriate treatment planning, and the establishment of a strong patient–provider relationship. By focusing on the patient's narrative and employing a systematic approach, medical professionals can ensure that no critical details are overlooked and that patient care remains personalized, empathetic, and of the highest quality.

SUGGESTED READINGS

1. Hampton JR, Harrison MJ, Mitchell JR, Prichard JS, Seymour C. Relative contributions of history-taking, physical examination, and laboratory investigation to diagnosis and management of medical outpatients. Br Med J. 1975;2(5969):486-9.
2. Nichol JR, Sundjaja JH, Nelson G. Medical History. In: StatPearls [Internet]. Treasure Island (FL): StatPearls Publishing; 2023.
3. Ramani S. Promoting the art of history taking. Med Teach. 2004;26(4):374-6.

256

CHAPTER

Clinical Significance of the Examination of Pulse

HS Pathak, Ankan Pathak, Sudipta Modak

"The physician cannot prescribe by letter, he must feel the pulse."

—Seneca

ABSTRACT

The arterial pulse is the sudden expansion of an artery due to blood ejection into the aorta and transmission throughout the arterial system. It is crucial to assess pulse during clinical examinations as peripheral pulse contour is determined by left ventricular (LV) ejection and vascular properties.

INTRODUCTION

The arterial pulse is the abrupt expansion of an artery resulting from the sudden ejection of blood into the aorta and its transmission throughout the arterial system. The impulse that arises as a result of the left ventricular (LV) ejection is then transmitted over to the aorta at a velocity that is 20 times greater than the velocity of the blood bolus that was ejected. Systolic blood pressure refers to the peak of the arterial pulse.

HISTORICAL IMPORTANCE

The ancient Chinese physicians had the unique ability and skill to judge the state of disease—its cause, duration, and prognosis—by merely assessing the volume, strength, weakness, regularity, or interruption of the four main varieties of pulse beats, i.e., superficial, deep, slow, and quick.

Avicenna (981–1037 CE) categorized the pulse based on different characteristics and enumerated different pulse modes in each of the following categories:

- *Size of dilation*: Strong, weak, and intermediate
- *Duration of each movement*: Short, long, and intermediate
- *Duration of the pause*: Hurried, sluggish, or intermediate pulse
- *Temperature of the pulse*: Hot, cold, or intermediate
- *Compressibility of the artery*: Easily compressible, incompressible, and moderately compressible
- *Fullness or emptiness of the artery*: Full of humor, containing no humor, and intermediate, humor being blood, phlegm, yellow bile, and black bile
- The equality or inequality of force in consecutive beats
- *Regularity of the rhythm*: Regular or irregular (irregularly regular and irregularly irregular)

TECHNIQUE

One of the first and most important methods to understand the dynamism of arterial pulse is to know the correct technique of the examination of pulse. Needless to say, examination of pulse is one of the most basic questions, which is often asked in any internal medicine examination, be it undergraduate or postgraduate. As a matter of fact, pulses should be palpated when the patient is in a reclining or resting position.

Before you begin:

- Wash your hands using the seven steps of hand washing. This will help to prevent cross-infection.
- Explain in the patients' preferred language what you are about to do. This will help the patient to understand

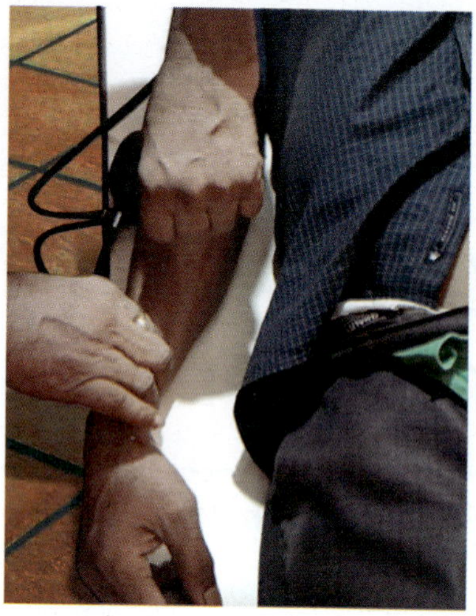

FIG. 1: Correct method of examination of the radial pulse.

what is about to happen and will make it easier for them to cooperate.
- Place the tips of your first and second fingers on the inside of the patient's wrist as illustrated in **Figure 1**.
- Make sure that you press gently against the pulse. Take your time to note if there are any irregularities in volume rate or rhythm.
- If the pulse is regular and strong, it is practically feasible to measure the pulse for 30 seconds. Double the number to give the beats per minute (e.g., 40 beats in 30 seconds means the pulse is 80 beats per minute). If you notice changes in rhythm or volume, it is imperative that you measure the pulse for 1 minute.
- The volume of the pulse is a very subjective measurement, but an experienced clinician can compare it with what has been felt previously in other patients and describe the pulse as "weak", "faint", "strong", or "bounding".
- Think about the rhythm of the pulse. Determine if it is regular. If irregular, determine if it is regularly irregular or irregularly irregular.
- Make sure that you clean and dry your hands after the procedure.

ALTERATIONS IN RATE OF PULSE

Sinus Tachycardia

Pulse rate > 100 is defined as sinus tachycardia.

Conditions: Physiologically in a child up to 5 years of age, exercise, fever, thyrotoxicosis, severe anemia, and shock

Note: Certain drugs, e.g., amlodipine, are known to cause reflex tachycardia; beta-2 agonists are also known to cause tachycardia.

Paroxysmal tachycardia implies when the pulse rate is > 160/minute. It may be paroxysmal supraventricular tachycardia (PSVT) or ventricular tachycardia (VT). PSVT may be caused due to paroxysmal atrial tachycardia or paroxysmal nodal tachycardia. VT is almost always due to organic lesions of the heart.

Bradycardia

Pulse rate < 60 beats per minute is known as bradycardia.

Conditions: Physiologically in athletes and also during sleep; pathologically in myxedema, obstructive jaundice, raised ICT, different degrees of heart block, drugs like beta blockers, and rate-limiting calcium channel blockers (CCBs) are also known to cause bradycardia.

ABNORMALITIES IN RHYTHM

Rhythm in a pulse is defined as the spacing of successive pulse waves in time. The two broad classifications in pulse are as follows:

1. *Regularly irregular*: In this type, irregularity in pulse comes at regular intervals or the irregularity may continue in a regular manner. This is usually found in second-degree heart block or bigeminy, or trigeminy.
2. *Irregularly irregular*: This suggests irregularity in two pulses in all aspects. It is commonly encountered in atrial fibrillation (AF) or multiple extrasystoles/ectopics.

Note: To differentiate between AF and multiple ectopics, pulse deficit (PD) is calculated. The difference between the heart rate and pulse rate is defined as the pulse deficit. A PD of <10 usually indicates multiple ectopics or rate-controlled AF, whereas a PD of >10 is suggestive of AF. The sequence of events is also of importance. Irregularities in all aspects of rate rhythm and volume are suggestive of AF, whereas a beat that comes earlier than expected followed by a compensatory pause is suggestive of an extrasystole.

Sinus Arrhythmia

Sinus arrhythmia is characterized by a decrease in pulse rate during expiration. It is a physiological phenomenon found in children.

Mechanism: During expiration due to the squeezing action of lungs, the excess blood comes to the left atrium. As a result, the LV stroke volume is increased, which in turn stimulates the baroreceptors leading to slowing of heart rate. It is usually abolished in autonomic neuropathies/dysautonomia.

VOLUME OF PULSE

High-volume pulse is associated with hyperkinetic circulatory states such as hyperthyroidism, exercise, severe anemia, and arteriovenous (AV) fistulas.

Low-volume pulse is found in states of low cardiac output such as shock, aortic stenosis (AS), tight mitral stenosis (MS), and constrictive pericarditis.

QUALITY OF PULSE

Abnormalities

Abnormalities include inequal pulse on two sides, may be due to anatomical variations or due to organic lesions such as thoracic inlet syndrome, subclavian coarctation, or aortic arch syndrome.

Always make it to palpate both the radial and femoral arteries. Normally, radial and femoral arteries pulsate at the same time, but the radial artery pulsation is 0.02–0.03 seconds earlier than the dorsalis pedis artery pulsation.

In coarctation, the pulsations of the lower limbs may come after the pulsations of the upper limbs. In conditions such as saddle embolism and aortic arch syndrome, femoral pulse may be absent.

SPECIAL CHARACTERS

Water Hammer Pulse

Water hammer pulse is also known as high-volume collapsing pulse. There is an abrupt and sharp fall of the pulse wave. Causes include severe aortic regurgitation (AR), severe anemia, and thyrotoxicosis.

Note: Another variation is the low-volume collapsing pulse found in mitral regurgitation.

Pulsus Parvus

In pulsus parvus, low-volume pulse is characteristically found in severe AS and tight MS. When the upstroke is delayed as in AS, it is called pulsus parvus et tardus.

Pulsus Paradoxus

In pulsus paradoxus, pulse volume decreases with inspiration and increases with expiration. In pure terms, it is nothing but an exaggerated response to a normal condition and hence sometimes also known as "pulsus normalis exaggeratus". Causes include rapidly developing pericardial effusion and cardiac tamponade, severe bronchial asthma, extreme obesity, and superior mediastinal syndrome.

Note: Total paradoxus is defined as a state of complete disappearance of the palpated pulse during inspiration, which is found in severe tamponade combined with hypovolemia.

Always remember that pulsus paradoxus may be absent in tamponade when there is an associated atrial septal defect (ASD) or associated AR.

Pulsus Alternans

In pulsus alternans, small-volume beat is delivered alternatively with a normal beat. It is characteristically found in severe acute LV failure. This can also be recorded with the help of a sphygmomanometer.

Pulsus Bisferiens

Pulsus bisferiens is a double-kicking pulse, best demonstrated in the brachial and carotid arteries. There are two distinct palpable peaks, percussion wave and tidal wave. If the percussion wave is greater than the tidal wave, AR is the dominant lesion. If it is vice versa, AS is the dominant lesion.

Pulsus Bigeminy

In pulsus bigeminy, two beats and a compensatory pause recur in a regular manner. If three beats and a pause recur regularly, it is known as pulsus trigeminus.

CONCLUSION

As peripheral pulse contour is determined by LV ejection and vascular properties, it is of vital importance that due importance is placed on the assessment of pulse during a clinical examination. It is one of the most important methods by which we can diagnose or narrow down our differentials in cases of not only cardiac but many other systemic diseases as well.

SUGGESTED READINGS

1. Marx HJ, Yu PN. Clinical examination of the arterial pulse. Prog Cardiovasc Dis. 1967;10:207-35.
2. O'Rourke MF, Avolio AP. Pulsatile flow and pressure in human systemic arteries. Studies in man and in a multibranched model of the human systemic arterial tree. Circ Res. 1980;46(3):363-72.
3. O'Rourke RA. Physical examination of the arteries and veins. In: Hurst JW (Ed). The heart, 6th edition. New York: McGraw-Hill; 1986. pp. 138-51.

257

CHAPTER

Physical Examination: The Dying Art

Payal Jain, Shilpa Gupta

ABSTRACT

History and physical examination have always been an integral part of medical practice and aid tremendously in making an accurate medical diagnosis. The recent shift in diagnostic paradigm associated with the new advances of technology in field of imaging and laboratory services is perplexing. It is a matter of concern that there has been now almost total dependence on this technology with fading of clinical skills and acumen. Various studies in recent times have mentioned and reported a decline in the art of physical examination among the clinicians worldwide.

Absent or poor examination skills endanger safety of patient as they result in missed or wrong diagnoses, which may lead to delay in administration of appropriate treatment. The blend of detail history, physical examination along with recommended investigations are indispensable for a treating clinician in making a correct diagnosis and a quick management plan. This also enhances a healthy doctor–patient relation with more trust and assurance. Considering and understanding the obvious importance of the history taking and clinical examination, the medical curriculum should be strengthened and inculcated with the same.

INTRODUCTION

The clinical skills of the history taking and physical examination which were once considered as the most crucial tool enabling the competent clinician in making a correct diagnosis, are slowly being undermined by recent technologies. The whole approach in medical field is showing drastic changes.

High-tech imaging, biochemical, and molecular diagnostic assays have simplified the tough path for physicians in diagnosing complex ailments which have unusual manifestations. But this success has been attained by paying a heavy price by gradually neglecting and loss of the art of physical examination.

EVOLUTION OF PHYSICAL EXAMINATION

Various crucial developments over the past 3,000 years lead to evolution of the art of physical examination as we know it today. Hippocrates and his colleagues declared that medicine has a rational basis and established it as a profession. Discovery of the art of percussion by Auenbrugger was perhaps the most initial thing in field of physical diagnosis in 1760 which was further expanded by Corvisart in 1808. By invention of stethoscope by Laennec in 1816, an exponential development of clinical skills was witnessed. The French school lead by Pierre Louis established systematic approach to clinical case and Johannes Mueller from German school enhanced experimental laboratory science from 1830 until 1900.

The standard bedside protocol of inspection, palpation, percussion, and auscultation were incorporated by Sir William Osler at Johns Hopkins University in 1893. He played a central role in defining the modern bedside practice of doing physical examination.

KEY ELEMENTS OF PHYSICAL EXAMINATION

The formulation and correlation of the history of the patient with the elicited clinical signs is the crux of a reliable physical examination sequence. This is best deciphered and learned bedside experience rather than from the text. An important attribute of a physical examination is that it is patient centered and demands keen observation and attention of the examiner. Consent is an integral part and is mandatory along with good communication so that patient feels comfortable during the examination. Communication skills are a key to a successful physical examination and helps to develop rapport between clinician and the patient. Respecting privacy of the patient with ritual undressing and physical contact is to be kept in mind. The physician-student relationship is also positively reinforced in a teaching institute by this bedside physical examination process.

VALUE AND SIGNIFICANCE OF PHYSICAL EXAMINATION

The value of technology and imaging tests cannot be denied because they confirm the findings of a detailed physical examination and without technology, we would never be able to see what we cannot visualize from outside. But technology fails to do so many things such as it can never detect a raised jugular venous pressure or even cannot comment on how the patient feels now. There are still many diagnoses that cannot be made in absence of an examination, e.g., confirming orthostatic hypotension. A lump found in abdominal palpation, a fixed hard cervical node metastasis discovered during a routine physical examination pointing toward a hidden malignancy is one of the few thrills which only a clinical examination can provide.

An absence of a proper physical examination was found to be major contributing reason for medical errors.

Physically examining a patient alleviates anxiety of patient to a certain extent and builds a sense of reassurance. Not only the patient, it is reassuring for the treating physician as well and imparts confidence in both the parties. It helps to convince and counsel the patients about the need for further investigations and treatment or vice versa. The use of skill is thus not always meant to find an abnormality on examination but also to make the patient feel better and building up of mutual trust. Patients usually appreciate those doctors who spend time on examining them.

For a dedicated physician, the art of physical examination is much more than mere tool of diagnosis. It is a connect, not less than meditation that brings satisfaction to the physician. This forms the foundation of physician's confidence and calmness while delivering care to the patient. In a world full of information on web and internet, physical examination is the only domain which only a trained physician can boast to acquire. Robbins et al. reported in his study that patients were found to be more satisfied when they were examined by their physician and were informed about the interventions.

Good history along with meticulous clinical examination can help in guiding which investigations need to be done. Some of the potentially harmful investigations such as exposure to undue radiation can be prevented by the judicious application of a comprehensive physical examination. This can also help by reducing the extra financial burden to the patient. This is particularly important in resource limited settings where examination guided investigations could be done judiciously and a burden on economy can be eased off. Apart from this, analyzing only the printed reports without being aware of the history and clinical scenario can lead to nowhere. As only a sound clinician interpret what is important and when to ignore and overlook the less important parameters in blood reports.

DECLINE OF CLINICAL SKILLS

There has been continuous decline in the skill of physical examination over the years and many recent studies have documented this thing. The grand rounds of any teaching medical facility which were once an essential part of bedside physical examination where each and every case was examined and discussed with all possible differentials made, are now a rarity. On the contrary, these are being replaced by passive study of the laboratory and imaging investigations from the case files without the physical presence of the patient himself.

The reason behind this decline seems to be multifactorial.

Improvements in technology and availability of modern diagnostic tests have resulted in more reliance on these tests than the physical examination. There is always a time constraint owing to the busy schedule of clinicians as well as students. This is due to the involvement of teaching faculty of medical colleges in various other activities and constant pulling in diverse directions. Another factor appears to be the disproportionate time spent at the screen and computers for one or the other reason. All these collectively result in very limited time spared forward rounds and bedside teaching. Also, a mindset that somehow clinical skills are not valued is gaining strength like why waste time in picking up a murmur with stethoscope bedside, when more sophisticated and time saving investigation such as 2D echocardiography is easily available? With time, a lack of confidence in clinical skills develops among the physicians and students which leads to further decline and resistance for this art.

A recent surge of telemedicine with virtual consultations, especially during and after pandemic of coronavirus disease-2019 (COVID-19) has added to the existing problem. Telemedicine is now a well-recognized field with many doctors and patients preferring it nowadays.

HOW TO OVERCOME THE ISSUE?

The revival of the art of physical examination depends on the emphasis on bedside teaching skills. The unfortunate trend of shifting bedside teaching to conference room due to comfort and ease should be stopped.

The foremost important thing in this regard is the actual conduct of bedside teaching in the medical schools because many a times these bedside teachings are replaced by tutorial classes. Increased exposure to these skills and spending more time with the patient help in acquiring skills and confidence. Learning by observing and then practicing under supervision are essential to develop confidence and empathy in the junior doctors and residents.

Not only the students, faculty and physician also need to be in constant touch of the clinical skills. Periodic training in clinical teaching methods can help to revive the art of physical examination among faculty. The faculty members need to observe the medical students or resident, any error thus made in examination need to be identified and corrected there itself. The teaching pattern should be able to help students acquire skills to identify common abnormalities on a physical examination. The growing notion of less utility of clinical skills should be curbed with more emphasis given to change the attitude of the students.

The new curriculum of competency-based medical education in our country has been devised after understanding the present scenario of vanishing clinical skills. The early clinical exposure, electives, directly observing, and demonstration of skills are an integral part of curriculum. But successful implementation of this program is yet to be achieved and requires constant efforts at all levels.

CONCLUSION

The debate over the superiority of technology over clinical skills or vice versa is ongoing. Physical examination has always been an integral part of medical school teachings and is in fact a powerful diagnostic tool if coupled with the judicious use of technology. Revival of the art of physical examination requires changes and implementation of those changes in existing medical curriculum, faculty skill training activities, and last but not the least, creating mindfulness among young doctors in their early learning years about the importance of clinical skills.

SUGGESTED READINGS

1. Zaman JAB. The Enduring Value of the Physical Examination. Med Clin North Am. 2018;102(3):417-23.
2. Datta A. Clinical skill: the ebbing art of medicine. Malays J Med Sci. 2021;28(1):105-8.
3. Asif T, Mohiuddin A, Hasan B, Pauly RR. Importance of Thorough Physical Examination: A Lost Art. Cureus. 2017;9(5):e1212.

258
CHAPTER

Good, Bad, and Ugly of Artificial Intelligence in Health Care

Bidita Khandelwal, Chamma Gupta

ABSTRACT

Artificial intelligence (AI) will be used more frequently in the healthcare industry owing to the intricacy and expansion of data in that industry. Payers, medical professionals, and pharmaceutical organizations currently use an assortment of AI technologies. The primary usage segments include indications for medical diagnostics and therapy, patient participation and compliance, and management of huge medical records and data. AI has been proposed to add a new dimension to healthcare facilities. However, evolution is barely devoid of unforeseen repercussions. Regarding the risks associated with AI technologies, numerous concerns have been voiced. Calls for regulation and ethical concerns associated with data security and confidentiality of the patient history are becoming steadily more vocal as technology advances quickly. While there are many situations in which AI can execute healthcare obligations equally as effectively or better than mankind, difficulties may arise with the deployment of duties of medical personnel from becoming extensively automated for an extended duration of time. With the increasing impact of AI in health care, it brings a range of consideration over potential risks and ethical concerns. So, AI has been both idolized and demonized.

INTRODUCTION

The integration of artificial intelligence (AI) into health care has been revolutionary and transformative. This has redefined the whole medical system for the diagnosis, treatment, management, and prevention of diseases, as well as ensuring healthcare supply chain. This technology is radically boosting medical investigations and consequences by delivering a more precise diagnosis and facilitating more tailored therapies. Healthcare systems can become more advanced, quicker, and more productive at delivering treatment to multitudes of individuals globally by deploying AI within medical facility and clinical settings. Is AI the best or the worst that happened in the sector of health care? The answer is that if used properly, AI is the best tool to assist, but if misused, then it can be very detrimental.

HISTORY

The journey began with the introduction of IBM's Watson AI-enabled healthcare-specific version in 2011 concentrated on natural language processing (NLP), an algorithm used to comprehend and decipher human communication was introduced in health care. The advancement continued with the development of machine learning, NLP, physical robots, and robotic process automation as specific AI technologies that are highly relevant to the healthcare industry.

WHAT IS GOOD ABOUT ARTIFICIAL INTELLIGENCE IN HEALTH CARE?

Artificial intelligence is rather promising to be the next frontier of medical care revolutionizing how patients acquire high-quality treatment while lowering expenditures for practitioners and enhancing the quality of life for patients.

- *Improving accuracy and efficiency in medical diagnosis* by analyzing medical images, laboratory results, and electronic healthcare records. AI algorithms can diagnose skin cancer with accuracy equivalent to dermatologist and analyze mammography images to diagnose breast cancer with efficiency greater than that of radiologist. IDx-DR is a Food and Drug Administration (FDA)-approved AI system for diagnosing diabetic retinopathy.

- *Providing personalized treatment* plans based on their medical condition background, clinical or prognosis data, or their outcome from therapies. The decision-making process for personalized medicine is aided by AI by considering genetic variants in addition to relevant elements of health care, such as age, gender, geographical location, race, ancestral history, immunological profile, metabolic profile, microbes, and ambient susceptibility.
- *Prediction and prevention of diseases* by identifying patterns and creating prediction model of disease or outbreaks that identifies high-risk patients thus allowing early intervention and prevention of debilitating and economically burdening diseases.
- *Decision-making* is often erroneous due to non-accessibility of medical data which though existing in the hospital information system, is not available due to lack of inter-operability and data connectivity. AI-driven digital decision system enhances decision-making by making the data accessible.
- *Streamlining and automation of administrative tasks*, such as appointment scheduling, medical coding, billing, data input, and filing of claims provides quicker and more accurate outcomes.
- *Assist patient for clinic documentation and discharge certificates*. Medico-legal adherence necessitates documentation of communication between the patient and doctor, the recording of which is time- consuming. Novel technology of NLP helps in creating generative text, e.g., a preliminary discharge summary which can be reviewed and validated by humans. This would ease the overburdened healthcare system by saving time and, at the same time, ensure completeness and accuracy of the records.
- *Creating a healthier world* is noteworthy. Wearable Health Devices (WHDs) are another integral part of personal health systems, a notion popularized in the late 1990s with the aim of implementing the typical individual at the core of the medical care procedure, coping with their own health and communicating with medical professionals. The goal was to increase the public's interest in their health state while enhancing the standard of care and utilizing new technological capabilities for monitoring of health metrics.
- *Ensuring uninterrupted healthcare supply chain* thus improving compliance to treatment was well evidenced during the Coronavirus disease (COVID) pandemic where AI ensured the maintenance of the supply chain.
- *Speeding drug discovery and developments* by analyzing large datasets of genetic and molecular information leading to identification of new drug targets and predict effectiveness of new drugs.
- *Accessibility to health care* has improved due to advancements in wireless technology and smartphones which has offered options for on-demand medical services employing health surveillance applications and search engines. This has also initiated a novel mode of delivering healthcare assistance by making remote interactions, which are accessible at all times and at geographically challenging locations.
- *AI-robotic technologies in health care have mixed expectations*. It shows promising future but one needs to be cautious regarding the over-hyped vision.

WHAT IS BAD ABOUT ARTIFICIAL INTELLIGENCE IN HEALTH CARE?

It is evident that AI has added a new dimension to healthcare facilities. However, transformations are seldom devoid of unintended consequences. Regarding the distinctive characteristics and risks associated with AI technologies, numerous concerns have been voiced.

- *Use of AI can lead to over-reliance on technology*. Critical thinking and analytical diagnostic skills are the requisites of a good healthcare provider. Intuition and human judgment are essential along with the speed and accuracy which AI can provide. So AI technology is to be used for assisting and not as a substitute for human skills.
- *Potential for errors* is inherent to any technology-based systems. Undetected errors, and if not corrected timely, can lead to serious consequences as human lives are at stake. Inaccessibility to relevant data and retraining of the machine as new data adds are the challenges.
- *Implementational cost* in terms of hardware and software as well as for training of healthcare personnel requires huge investments. The institutions or organizations, who cannot invest to that extent, may lack behind.
- *AI gap* is the difference between the clinical efficacy that has been proven in the actual world and the technical accuracy of AI tests. The metrics used to assess the efficacy of an AI model are not always transferable to clinical contexts.
- *Lack of human empathy* in AI apps. Patients' adherence to treatment, prognostication, and breaking bad news, all require clinical empathy. This is a human quality and cannot be replaced by AI as it will lead to dehumanization of health care.

WHAT IS UGLY ABOUT ARTIFICIAL INTELLIGENCE IN HEALTH CARE?

If there is a "good" and a "bad', then "ugly" also exists with it. Ethical concerns associated with AI are the reason for majority of the anti-AI petitions.

- *Discrimination and biased output* are the worst part of AI. AI assistants are based on the data on which they are trained. Thus if the data is biased or inadequate, then the output is also discriminatory and incorrect. For example, under representation of minorities due to gender and age bias in the data, leads to biased decisions and predictions, hence defeating the goal of health care for all.
- *Data privacy and security concerns* tend to be crucial because AI systems capture a great deal of sensitive private medical information that could be abused if not managed properly.
- *Decreasing effectiveness of AI* if regular updating on revised information and datasets is not done. Ongoing monitoring and rigorous testing and evaluation of an AI system are required so that it functions the way it is intended to work.
- *Accountability and transparency* of the decisions made by AI tools are a matter of concern. Deep learning algorithms are unable to provide convincing explanations for their predictions (black box problem). If the recommendation is wrong, then the machine cannot defend itself and the trust on healthcare system is shaken.
- *Creation and circulation of misinformation* is assisted by AI. AI-assisted synthetic media, for example, DeepFake, which is a combination of "deep learning" and "fake media" creates fake contents and due to the widespread use of social platforms, this misinformation is circulated widely, harming the health care.

FUTURE OF ARTIFICIAL INTELLIGENCE IN HEALTH CARE

In an ideal world, universal accessibility to high quality health care is aspired and to achieve this at such a large scale is only possible with cost-effective, and scalable innovations without compromising quality. Explainable AI or interpretable AI is gaining momentum and will enhance the accuracy and trust in the algorithms.

CONCLUSION

Artificial intelligence in health care has the potential to revolutionize the industry, paving ways for a time when recipients will receive high-quality medical attention more quickly and precisely than ever before, from discovering novel oncology cures to enhancing patient experiences. The biggest issue confronting AI in the medical field does not involve the effectiveness of the technology, but rather its acceptance into routine clinical practice. AI is a boon to supplement or eliminate redundant mechanical repetitive tasks, but it can never be a replacement for humans in health care.

The absence of standard guidelines for use of AI health care has led to vulnerability of health records being hacked. AI to be accountable, transparent, and fair, needs to be ethically governed, audited, possess model explainability and interpretability. As technology develops quickly, there are mounting calls for regulation. A High-Level Expert Group on Artificial Intelligence was established by the European Commission in April 2018 to promote the implementation of the AI plan for Europe and to address its ethical and legal ramifications. However, there has not been a lot of ethical and legal research done on the use of AI in health care.

Artificial intelligence systems can be adopted universally in health care if it is accepted as a dynamic learning experience at all levels. There is need to invest time and resources for effective integration of AI in health care with collaboration across various healthcare sectors, country councils, and industry linkage. Integration of AI in health care will require significant training and skill development of healthcare providers. The only medical professionals who may not benefit fully from AI in health care are those who choose not to align themselves with it.

ACKNOWLEDGMENTS

Dr Akash Kumar Bhoi, Adjunct Research Faculty, Directorate of Research, SMU and Mr Aryan Prasad, CSCE, KIIT-DU.

SUGGESTED READINGS

1. Davenport T, Kalakota R. The potential for artificial intelligence in healthcare. Future Healthc J. 2019;6(2):94-8.
2. ForeSee Medical. (2023). AI in Healthcare. [online] Available from https://www.foreseemed.com/artificial-intelligence-in-healthcare [Last accessed January, 2024]
3. Kirch DG, Petelle K. Addressing the Physician Shortage: The Peril of Ignoring Demography. JAMA. 2017;317(19):1947-8.
4. Schönberger D. Artificial intelligence in healthcare: a critical analysis of the legal and ethical implications. Int J Law Inf Technol. 2019;27(2):171-203.

5. Parashar G, Chaudhary A, Rana A. Systematic Mapping Study of AI/Machine Learning in Healthcare and Future Directions. SN Comput Sci. 2021;2(6):461.
6. De Togni G, Erikainen S, Chan S, Cunningham-Burley S. Beyond the hype: 'acceptable futures' for AI and robotic technologies in healthcare. AI Soc. 2023;22:1-10.
7. Montemayor C, Halpern J, Fairweather A. In principle obstacles for empathic AI: why we can't replace human empathy in healthcare. AI Soc. 2022;37(4):1353-9.
8. Capasso M, Umbrello S. Responsible nudging for social good: new healthcare skills for AI-driven digital personal assistants. Med Health Care Philos. 2022;25(1):11-22.
9. Khan B, Fatima H, Qureshi A, Kumar S, Hanan A, Hussain J, et al. Drawbacks of Artificial Intelligence and Their Potential Solutions in the Healthcare Sector. Biomed Mater Devices. 2023;8:1-8.

259

CHAPTER

Telemedicine: The Road Ahead

SS Dariya, Deepak Agarwal, Alok Modi, Lalita Verma

ABSTRACT

Since the middle of the 20th century, telemedicine has emerged as a distinctive approach to provide remote clinical services in a wide range of medical fields. It has expanded to include telehealth, mobile monitoring applications, and various other methods. The coronavirus disease 2019 (COVID-19) pandemic has greatly amplified the utilization of telemedicine. In the future, with the incorporation of artificial intelligence (AI) into healthcare systems, it is anticipated that telemedicine will continue to expand.

INTRODUCTION

What is Telehealth?

Telemedicine employs technology, encompassing electronic data and communication techniques to bolster healthcare provisions. This includes remote clinical services, public health education, awareness initiatives, and health management. Through telehealth, consultations can be facilitated between two healthcare professionals or between a physician and a patient using live chat, video conferencing, or mobile monitoring devices.

Telemedicine Yes, you are correct. Telemedicine, a subset of telehealth, involves the exchange of medical information from one site to another through electronic communication to improve a patient's health status. It includes a growing variety of applications and services using two-way video, email, smartphones, wireless tools, and other forms of telecommunications technology. This can involve providing clinical services from a distance, which can be particularly beneficial for communities in rural locations or for individuals who are physically immobile.

Wireless technologies (known as mobile health, or "mHealth") are used to provide telemedicine and telehealth services.

Telemedicine does differ from telephonic consultation. While telephonic consultation relies solely on audio for patient interaction, telemedicine utilizes both audio and visual components, providing a more comprehensive consultation experience.

- *Synchronous*: This is a live, two-way interaction between a patient and a healthcare provider using audiovisual technology. It is much like a traditional doctor's appointment, just conducted over distance. This type of telemedicine allows for real-time communication, making it useful for consultations, check-ups, or even certain types of examinations.
- *Asynchronous* or "store-and-forward" telemedicine, where medical data (like medical images and biosignals) are recorded and then transmitted to a healthcare provider for later review.

BENEFITS AND APPLICATIONS OF TELEMEDICINE

Indeed, the use of telemedicine has evolved significantly over time. Initially, it was primarily used in specific situations, such as treating acute respiratory or urinary tract infections, especially when primary care was not readily available. However, the scope of telemedicine has expanded considerably in recent times. It is now increasingly being utilized for managing chronic diseases, among other applications. This shift reflects the advancements in technology and the changing needs of healthcare delivery.

Rural versus urban population: There is a significant disparity in healthcare access between rural and urban populations in India, which can lead to lower life-expectancy among rural residents. Telemedicine has the potential to be a game changer in this regard. It can provide both primary and specialized care to rural populations, provided that internet services are made widely available in remote areas. This could help bridge the healthcare gap and improve health outcomes for rural communities. However, it is important to note that the successful implementation of telemedicine also depends on other factors, such as training healthcare providers in telemedicine practices, ensuring patient privacy and data security, and addressing potential technical issues.

Primary care: In primary care settings, main areas of telemedicine consultations may be as follows:

- Video components are suitable for many clinical conditions.
- For upper respiratory infections or urinary tract infections.
- Evaluation of dermatologic conditions.
- Medication management of chronic anxiety and depression.
- Management of chronic conditions, such as diabetes, mental health issues, heart failure, nutrition, chronic obstructive pulmonary disease (COPD), and obesity.

It may also be utilized for medicine reconciliation appointments, substance use disorder treatment (individual and group treatment), and form completion (e.g., return to work or school paperwork). In addition, various monitoring reports may be analyzed with telemedicine.

Specialty care management: Telemedicine is being used in many specialties, such as cardiology, endocrinology, hepatology, nephrology, neurology, ophthalmology, dermatology, and surgical perioperative care management.

Diabetes mellitus: Indeed, the application of telemedicine in managing chronic conditions like diabetes mellitus has been well documented. Numerous studies have underscored the advantages of telemedicine interventions for diabetes care, which can encompass a variety of care modalities, from teleconsultations to remote patient monitoring.

A meta-analysis conducted in 2016, which included 55 randomized trials and over 9,000 patients, found that the most significant improvement in A1c levels was observed in patients with type 2 diabetes mellitus, those over 40 years old, and those who received teleconsultations.

Furthermore, a systematic review in 2017 that included 111 randomized controlled trials and nearly 24,000 patients showed that telemedicine interventions modestly reduced A1c at all time intervals measured (ranging from –0.20 to –0.74%) compared to usual care. In a meta-regression analysis, the highest effect was seen in patients with higher baseline A1c as well as in trials that utilized text messaging or web portals for communication and applications that facilitated medication adjustment.

These findings highlight the potential of telemedicine in improving diabetes management and patient outcomes. However, it is important to note that the successful implementation of these interventions also depends on other factors, such as patient engagement, healthcare provider training, and the availability of necessary technological infrastructure.

Heart failure: Telemonitoring is indeed used in patients with chronic heart failure to predict and prevent episodes of acute decompensation by tracking symptoms that require therapy optimization.

While systematic reviews and meta-analyses have shown benefits of telemedicine for patients with heart failure, randomized trials have not consistently demonstrated benefits in terms of reducing hospitalization and mortality when telemedicine monitoring is used alone.

For heart failure patients with implantable cardioverter-defibrillators (ICDs), combining telemonitoring with scheduled in-person visits has been shown to reduce healthcare utilization and acute care visits. The Evolution of Management Strategies of Heart Failure Patients with Implantable Defibrillators (EVOLVO) study found that remote monitoring of intrathoracic impedance (as a marker of fluid status), atrial arrhythmias, and ICD shocks reduced emergency and unscheduled physician visits compared to usual care.

These findings underscore the potential of telemedicine in managing chronic conditions like heart failure, but also highlight the importance of integrating it with traditional in-person care for optimal results. As always, it is crucial to remember that the successful implementation of these interventions also depends on factors such as patient engagement, healthcare provider training, and the availability of necessary technological infrastructure.

Mental health: Indeed, the delivery of mental health services via telemedicine, often referred to as tele-mental health, has been a rapidly expanding field, especially in regions where there is a scarcity of in-person mental healthcare.

Individuals suffering from mental health disorders are generally capable of effectively participating in telemedicine sessions. Telemedicine appointments can be utilized for capacity evaluations and the management of mood disorders and psychosis. This approach can make mental health services more accessible and convenient for patients, potentially leading to improved outcomes.

However, it is important to note that while tele-mental health can be highly beneficial, it may not be suitable for everyone. Some individuals may prefer in-person therapy, and certain types of therapy may be more effective when conducted face-to-face. As with all healthcare services, it is crucial to consider the individual needs and preferences of each patient.

Telemedicine during coronavirus disease 2019 (COVID-19) pandemic: Absolutely, telemedicine has proven to be a vital tool in times when minimizing in-person visits is necessary. It can substitute for a variety of in-person encounters, thereby expanding the scope of virtual care.

For instance, telemedicine is being utilized to evaluate patients with known or suspected COVID-19. This remote management can prevent unnecessary in-person medical visits, including visits to primary care providers, urgent care facilities, and emergency departments. This helps avoid additional strain on an already overburdened healthcare system and preserves limited resources, such as personal protective equipment (PPE).

Moreover, telemedicine can be used for managing certain hospitalized patients where in-person hospital room visits should be limited or avoided to minimize risk to healthcare staff and conserve PPE. This can be particularly useful in managing some infectious diseases to minimize the risk of infection transmission (e.g., COVID-19 and Ebola) and other potential high-risk exposures (e.g., following I-131 ablation). An on-site assistant can act as a tele-presenter to assist with managing the video device or with physical examination maneuvers. Telemedicine interviews can be conducted with inpatients as part of scheduled rounds or on an as-needed basis.

During the COVID-19 pandemic, telemedicine has been particularly beneficial for chronic disease management by allowing continuity of care for high-risk populations while enabling social distancing and reducing the risk of exposure to infection.

In the context of serious illness and hospice care, communication regarding diagnosis, prognosis, and medical decision-making can be especially challenging when not conducted in person. However, strategies are available for conducting such conversations via telemedicine. These strategies can be applied not only in the context of COVID-19 but also other illnesses.

In conclusion, telemedicine has emerged as a critical tool in healthcare delivery, particularly during times of crisis, such as the COVID-19 pandemic. It offers a way to provide necessary care while minimizing risks associated with in-person visits.

LIMITATIONS OF TELEMEDICINE

Telemedicine visits are not a complete substitute for in-person visits, nor are telemedicine visits feasible for all patients or clinical situations.

Some limitations of telemedicine include:

- It is important to acknowledge that certain aspects of traditional doctor–patient interactions can be hindered by digital technologies. Elements such as touch, physical presence, and emotional connection, which can play a crucial role in the healing process, can be challenging to replicate in a virtual environment.
- One of the significant limitations of telemedicine is indeed the inability to conduct an in-person physical examination. While visual inspection can be effectively carried out via telemedicine, other examination techniques, such as palpation and auscultation, can be challenging or even impossible to perform remotely.

  The use of peripheral devices like digital stethoscopes can help overcome some of these barriers, but these devices are not widely available. Additionally, having a tele-presenter (an individual assisting with the examination) can be particularly useful for certain maneuvers; however, the availability of such ancillary services may be limited.

  Patients may also be able to assist with self-palpation (e.g., abdominal examination), which can not only aid in the examination but also enhance health literacy and patient engagement.
- The perceptions and experiences during a tele-medicine visit can indeed differ significantly from those during an in-person visit. For instance, during a telemedicine visit, the provider's face is likely to be more of a focus than during a typical in-person encounter. As a result, facial expressions may be perceived as more pronounced.

  Moreover, interpreting body language cues can be more challenging in a virtual setting for both the clinician and the patient. Nonverbal communication plays a crucial role in conveying information and emotions, and some of these subtle cues may be missed or misinterpreted during a telemedicine visit.

  Therefore, it is essential for both healthcare providers and patients to be aware of these potential differences and adapt their communication strategies accordingly. For healthcare providers, this might involve being more conscious of their facial expressions and verbal communication. For patients, this could mean being more explicit about their symptoms or concerns.

- The "digital divide" can indeed create potential disparities in access to telemedicine. This is particularly true for individuals living in rural areas with limited internet access, older adults, and those from diverse cultural and socioeconomic backgrounds.

  Even among individuals with adequate internet access, their comfort level with conducting a telemedicine visit is an important factor to consider. Their internet access may be limited to a public location or may incur significant monetary costs due to data charges.

  Older adults, in particular, may face challenges in accessing telemedicine services due to inexperience with technology or physical disabilities. These factors can make it difficult for them to navigate digital platforms and participate effectively in virtual consultations.

  Therefore, while telemedicine has the potential to greatly enhance healthcare accessibility, it is crucial to address these barriers and ensure that these services are accessible and user-friendly for all individuals, regardless of their location, age, or background. This might involve improving internet infrastructure in rural areas, providing training and support for older adults and others who are less familiar with technology, and ensuring that telemedicine platforms are user-friendly and accessible for individuals with disabilities.
- Technology does not always work smoothly, and technical difficulties may interfere with delivery of care.
- Some patients may prefer in-person interactions over telemedicine visits, although patients are generally equally satisfied with in-person and telemedicine encounters.
- Inaccurate dosing of weight-based drugs (e.g., chemotherapy treatments and pediatric medications) may occur due to the inability to weigh patients.
- Telemedicine visits may not be appropriate or feasible for all patients or all clinical situations; the clinician must use telemedicine services appropriately for care to be delivered effectively and accurately.

MEDICOLEGAL ASPECTS

Telemedicine is governed by laws and regulations in India. There are official guidelines laid down by the Government of India on March 25, 2020. They can be found on the link—https://www.mohfw.gov.in/pdf/Telemedicine.pdf

In short you cannot prescribe schedule C drugs or narcotics on teleconsultations.

You should verify the identity of the patient by a government-approved ID card before initiating teleconsultation.

If any point of time the physician or patient is not comfortable with teleconsultation, it should be stopped immediately and in-clinic consultation should be scheduled.

If some parts of consultations are beyond the scope of teleconsultations, they should be deferred and a physical consultation should be carried out instead like a particular part of the anatomy needs to be inspected or palpated or auscultated, etc.

Teleconsultations should preferably be recorded and a copy should be kept with the healthcare provider for medicolegal safety, with prior consent of the patient.

Teleconsultations are subject to litigation in courts, like there was a litigation against two medicos for teleconsultations by celebrity Rhea Chakravorty for prescribing narcotics to deceased Sushant Singh Rajput. The details can be found on the link—FIR Against Sushant Singh's Sisters, Doctor After Rhea's Complaint (thewire.in)

SUGGESTED READINGS

1. Dwyer TF. Telepsychiatry: psychiatric consultation by interactive television. Am J Psychiatry. 1973;130:865.
2. Mermelstein H, Guzman E, Rabinowitz T, Krupinski E, Hilty D. The application of technology to health: The evolution of telephone to telemedicine and telepsychiatry: A historical review and look at human factors. J Technol Behav Sci. 2017;2:5.
3. Weinstein RS, Lopez AM, Joseph BA, Erps KA, Holcomb M, Barker GP, et al. Telemedicine, telehealth, and mobile health applications that work: opportunities and barriers. Am J Med. 2014;127(3):183-7.
4. Humphreys J, Schoenherr L, Elia G, Saks NT, Brown C, Barbour S, et al. Rapid Implementation of Inpatient Telepalliative Medicine Consultations During COVID-19 Pandemic. J Pain Symptom Manage. 2020;60(1):e54-9.
5. Office of the National Coordinator for Health Information Technology. What is telehealth? How is telehealth different from telemedicine? [online] Available from https://www.healthit.gov/faq/what-telehealth-how-telehealth-different-telemedicine [Last accessed January, 2024].
6. Kvedar J, Coye MJ, Everett W. Connected health: a review of technologies and strategies to improve patient care with telemedicine and telehealth. Health Aff (Millwood). 2014;33:194.
7. Daskivich LP, Vasquez C, Martinez C Jr, Tseng CH, Mangione CM. Implementation and Evaluation of a Large-Scale Teleretinal Diabetic Retinopathy Screening Program in the Los Angeles County Department of Health Services. JAMA Intern Med. 2017;177(5):642-9.

8. Zakaria A, Maurer T, Su G, Amerson E. Impact of teledermatology on the accessibility and efficiency of dermatology care in an urban safety-net hospital: A pre-post analysis. J Am Acad Dermatol. 2019;81:1446.
9. Vegesna A, Tran M, Angelaccio M, Arcona S. Remote Patient Monitoring via Non-Invasive Digital Technologies: A Systematic Review. Telemed J E Health. 2017;23:3.
10. Center for Connected Health Policy. State telehealth laws and reimbursement policies report, fall 2023. [online] Available from https://www.cchpca.org/resources/state-telehealth-laws-and-reimbursement-policies-report-fall-2023-2/ [Last accessed January, 2024].
11. Calton B, Abedini N, Fratkin M. Telemedicine in the Time of Coronavirus. J Pain Symptom Manage. 2020;60:e12.
12. Benziger CP, Huffman MD, Sweis RN, Stone NJ. The Telehealth Ten: A Guide for a Patient-Assisted Virtual Physical Examination. Am J Med. 2021;134:48.
13. Laskowski ER, Johnson SE, Shelerud RA, Lee JA, Rabatin AE, Driscoll SW, et al. The Telemedicine Musculoskeletal Examination. Mayo Clin Proc. 2020;95(8):1715-31.
14. Eble SK, Hansen OB, Ellis SJ, Drakos MC. The Virtual Foot and Ankle Physical Examination. Foot Ankle Int. 2020;41:1017.
15. Wilson AM, Ong MK, Saliba D, Jamal NI. The Veterans Affairs Neuropathy Scale: A Reliable, Remote Polyneuropathy Exam. Front Neurol. 2019;10:1050.
16. Soldatova L, Williams C, Postma GN, Falk GW, Mirza N. Virtual Dysphagia Evaluation: Practical Guidelines for Dysphagia Management in the Context of the COVID-19 Pandemic. Otolaryngol Head Neck Surg. 2020;163(3):455-8.
17. Uscher-Pines L, Mehrotra A. Analysis of Teladoc use seems to indicate expanded access to care for patients without prior connection to a provider. Health Aff (Millwood). 2014;33(2):258-64.
18. Liaw WR, Jetty A, Coffman M, Petterson S, Moore MA, Sridhar G, et al. Disconnected: a survey of users and nonusers of telehealth and their use of primary care. J Am Med Inform Assoc. 2019;26(8):420-8.
19. Singh GK, Siahpush M. Widening rural-urban disparities in life expectancy, U.S., 1969-2009. Am J Prev Med. 2014;46:e19.
20. Esteban C, Moraza J, Iriberri M, Aguirre U, Goiria B, Quintana JM, et al. Outcomes of a telemonitoring-based program (telEPOC) in frequently hospitalized COPD patients. Int J Chron Obstruct Pulmon Dis. 2016;11:2919-30.
21. Bashshur RL, Shannon GW, Smith BR, Alverson DC, Antoniotti N, Barsan WG, et al. The empirical foundations of telemedicine interventions for chronic disease management. Telemed J E Health. 2014;20(9):769-800.
22. Davis AM, Sampilo M, Gallagher KS, Dean K, Saroja MB, Yu Q, et al. Treating rural paediatric obesity through telemedicine vs. telephone: Outcomes from a cluster randomized controlled trial. J Telemed Telecare. 2016;22(2):86-95.
23. Lee JY, Lee SWH. Telemedicine Cost-Effectiveness for Diabetes Management: A Systematic Review. Diabetes Technol Ther. 2018;20(7):492-500.

260 CHAPTER

Nanotechnology in Medicine

VN Mishra, Ishan Mishra

ABSTRACT

Nanotechnology refers to the design and use of technologies at 1–100 nm scale. The application of nanotechnology in medical field is often termed as '*nanomedicine*'. Nanomaterials can be engineered to have different size, shape, chemical composition, and surface, making them to interact with specific biological targets. They generally retain the mechanical, electrical, thermal, optical, and chemical properties of parent material which is very useful in their clinical applications. Nanoparticles may be organic like liposome and polymeric compounds, inorganic nanoparticles—metallic such as gold and silver, metal oxides, and ceramic and quantum dots. Carbon-based nanoparticles are fullerenes and carbon nanotubes. At present the most common use of nanoparticles is in drug delivery systems, about 15 anticancer nanomedicines are being used across the world and the number is increasing with every passing year. They are used in genetic editing, vaccine manufacturing, and free radical scavenging and are other upcoming fields. They are being tried in Alzheimer disease, skin diseases, toxic overdoses, inflammatory bowel disease, and in preventive medicine. Futuristic nanoscale sensors and devices will be able to provide a personal and cost-effective medical monitoring of patient's health. They will also enhance prediction of diseases such as cancer or inflammation at an early stage.

INTRODUCTION

There is enough evidence of use of nanotechnology in the ancient civilizations. The use of nanoparticles could be traced as far back as 4th century AD by the Roman civilization. The Lycurgus Cup is a living example of use of nanotechnology in that time. Peculiar dichroic effect seen in this cup is due to presence of silver and gold nanoparticles in the glass, and because of this the cup looks green when white light is reflected on it and a red coloring appears when white light is transmitted through it. Similar effect of use of nanotechnology is seen in phenomenon of light scattering by nanoparticles in stained glass windows of medieval churches. The elasticity and resistance noticed in the legendary Damascene sword have been attributed to nanometer-sized particles of carbon.

In the modern times the pioneering work of nanotechnology was by Richard Feynman, an American physicist and Nobel laureate. Hence, he is known as the father of *modern nanotechnology*. He introduced the concept of nanotechnology in 1959 in his famous lecture "There's plenty of room at the bottom." Gerd Binnig and Heinrich Rohrer invented the scanning tunneling microscope (STM). They manipulated xenon atoms on a nickel background using the STM to form the IBM (International Business Machines Corporation) logo. This further led to the development of atomic force microscope (AFM) and scanning probe microscope which are used in nanotech research in present days.

WHAT IS NANOTECHNOLOGY?

The prefix 'nano' is derived from Greek word meaning dwarf. It depicts one thousand millionth of meter. Nanotechnology refers to the design and use of technologies at 1–100 nm scale. The application of nanotechnology in the medical field is often termed as '*nanomedicine*'. This could broadly be defined as the use of nanomaterials for diagnosis, monitoring, control, prevention, and treatment of diseases.

NANOMATERIAL

According to the European Commission recommendation, nanomaterial refers to a natural, incidental, or manufactured material comprising particles with one or more external dimensions in the size range of 1–100 nm for ≥50% of the particles. Structures with one or more external dimensions below 1 nm, such as fullerenes, graphene flakes, and single-wall carbon nanotubes, should also be considered as nanomaterials. There are three fundamental aspects to identify the presence of a nanomaterial; these are size, particle size distribution, and surface area. United States Food and Drug Administration (FDA) has not established its own definition for 'nanomaterial', instead they have adopted the meaning commonly employed in relation to the engineering of materials that have at least one dimension in the size range of approximately 1–100 nm.

Properties of Nanomaterials

Due to their small size, nanomaterials have a high surface area in relation to the volume. Consequently, the particle surface energy is increased, making the nanomaterials much more reactive. Nanomaterials have a tendency to adsorb biomolecules, e.g., proteins and lipids when they come in contact with the biological fluids; this is known as 'corona'. that forms on the surface of colloidal nanoparticles, as the nanoparticles cross from one biological compartment to another. This dynamic change could influence the 'corona' constitution. Nanomaterials can be engineered to have different size, shape, chemical composition, and surface, making them able to interact with specific biological targets. Nanoparticles generally retain the mechanical, electrical, thermal, optical, and chemical properties of parent material, which could be beneficial when selecting a nanoparticle for applications.

Types of Nanoparticles

- *Organic*: Proteins, carbohydrates, lipids, and other organic molecules may be synthesized into organic nanoparticles with a specific dimension, such as a radius of fewer than 100 nm.
  - Liposome nanoparticles: These are spherical vesicles with a membrane composed of a lipid bilayer containing an aqueous substance. Nanoliposome technology has evolved significantly over the years in carrying active molecules to specific targets. Pegylated liposomal doxorubicin (Doxil) was the first FDA-approved nanomedicine which is used for treatment of breast cancer.
  - Polymeric nanoparticles: Most polymeric nanoparticles are known for their biodegradability and biocompatibility, constituting the most commonly used nanoparticles in drug delivery systems.
- *Inorganic*: Inorganic nanoparticles are nontoxic, hydrophilic, biocompatible, and highly stable compared to organic materials. They include the following:
  - Metallic nanoparticles: These include precious metals (gold or silver) and magnetic metals (iron oxide, cobalt and manganese doped ferrites). Metallic nanoparticles such as gold possess unique electronic and optical properties. Their surface could be modified with other biomolecules such as proteins, oligonucleotides and antibodies due to their negative charge. Metallic nanoparticles have mainly been used as imaging contrast agents.
  - Metal oxide nanoparticles: Currently the most widely used metal oxides are iron oxide, titania, zirconia, and more recently ceria. Ceria nanoparticles are useful because of their catalytic and antioxidant properties. They are being tried as antioxidant and anti-inflammatory agents.
  - Ceramic nanoparticles: They have recently emerged as vehicles for drugs. They are capable of transporting molecules such as proteins, enzymes, or drugs. For instance, cerium oxide (CeO_2)-capped mesoporous silica nanoparticles have been developed to act as vehicles for drug delivery by releasing beta-cyclodextrin into lung cancer cells.
  - Quantum dots: These are nanoparticles made of semiconductor materials with fluorescent properties. These are the most commonly used in bioimaging and biosensing strategies. However, this requires them to be conjugated to biomolecules, such as proteins, peptides, or oligonucleotides, which enables them to bind to specific sites.
- *Carbon-based nanoparticles*:
  - Fullerene is a novel carbon allotrope with a polygonal structure made up exclusively of 60 carbon atoms; it is being used in magnetic resonance imaging (MRI) to enhance contrast.
  - Carbon nanotubes: Carbon nanotubes are cylindrical molecules that consist of rolled up sheets of a single layer of carbon atoms. There are two classes of carbon nanotubes: single-walled and multiwall. Due to their high external surface area, they could be used as drug carriers. Additionally their unique optical, mechanical, and electronic properties made carbon nanotubes appealing as imaging contrast agents and biological sensors.

MEDICAL APPLICATIONS OF NANOTECHNOLOGY

Medical Diagnostics

Nanoparticles are being incorporated more and more for in vitro diagnostic devices. These devices aim to detect proteins, DNA, or other biomarkers that indirectly identify for a specific disease. These are two step devices. The first step captures a molecule that recognizes the disease biomarker and in the second step a nanoparticle transduces the capture. The most common capture molecules are antibodies, aptamers, or peptides. The transduced signal can occur in different forms by changing the color, fluorescence, and magnetic or electrical signal. Gold nanoparticle-based lateral flow immunoassays are popular examples of diagnostic assay which is commercially available for diagnosing cardiovascular diseases, diabetes, and infectious pathogens. Considerable research is being done to build devices, systems, and software for nanoparticles-based diagnostic appliances. Readout systems are being developed for nanoparticles-based assay, e.g., heat as signal generated from gold nanoparticle during lateral flow immunoassay could be picked up using near-infrared cameras, the optical emission generated from quantum dot barcodes could be detected by a smart phone camera, whereas a miniaturized superconducting quantum interference device (SQUID) system can measure the magnetism of the iron oxide nanoparticles.

Drug Delivery Systems

The common use of nanoparticles at present is in drug delivery systems. This process could be done in various forms. Drug could be encapsulated inside the nanoparticles or integrated into the material matrix; they could also be presented on the surface of nanoparticles, depending on their desired cellular interaction. Drugs when incorporated with nanomaterials could evade the immune system reaction upon intravenous injection as nanoparticles shield drugs from immune recognition. Nanoparticles can also prolong the elimination half-life of drugs. Specific polymers such as polyethylene glycol (PEG) are used for this purpose; nanoparticle size plays a significant role in determining the elimination kinetics of a drug.

Nanooncology

Use of nanoparticles-based anticancer therapy is one of the oldest and most researched areas of nanomedicine. At present about 15 anticancer nanomedicines are being used across the world and the number is increasing every year. Most of these anticancer medicines are in the form of liposomal nanoparticles. The first liposomal nanoparticles-based anticancer drug was Doxil which carries doxorubicin, few other approved examples of liposomal formulations include DaunoXome (carrying daunorubicin), Marqibo (carrying vincristine), Mepact (carrying mifamurtide), and Vyxeos (carrying cytarabine and daunorubicin in a 5:1 molar ratio). One more exciting area for anticancer treatment by nanotechnology is 'origami nanorobot'. It consists of a flat sheet of synthetic DNA which is coated in a blood clotting enzyme. This could be folded into various shapes. This nanosized DNA sheet is injected into the bloodstream on attaching with tumor cells; it injects them with the blood clotting enzyme, which starves the tumor cell of the blood thus destroying cancer cells without harming nearby healthy tissue.

Nanoparticles and their Role in Oxidative Stress

One of the important uses of nanoparticles is their use against diseases involving oxidative stress, such as atherosclerosis. Nanoparticles made from metal oxide, such as CeO_2 or yttrium oxide and those that are carbon-based, such as fullerenes, have generated much interest because of their free radical quenching and catalytic properties. Cerium nanoparticles are capable of scavenging intracellular reactive oxygen species (ROS). It appears that these types of nanoparticles could be used as ROS scavengers, thus providing a novel strategy against oxidative stress.

Genetic Editing and Vaccines

This is the most exciting emerging area of nanomedicine. First drug developed through genetic editing with nanoparticles was for the treatment of a rare hereditary disease known as transthyretin amyloidosis. In this disease, the liver produces mutant and wild type of amyloid called transthyretin, this amyloid deposit in different organs and ultimately causes polyneuropathy and cardiomyopathy leading to mortality. This drug is a lipid nanoparticles platform named ONPATTRO (patisiran); it delivers the small interfering RNA (siRNA) to liver hepatocytes and silences the transthyretin (*TTR*) gene responsible for production of TTR. In human studies ONPATTRO reduced serum transthyretin levels by 70–80% with a significant neurological status improvement compared with placebo. Use of nanoparticles in manufacturing process of vaccines has led to development of nanoparticle-based messenger RNA (mRNA) and DNA vaccines in the coronavirus disease 2019 (COVID-19) pandemic era. These newer vaccines have stood test of time and proved their worth.

Nanotechnology in Preventing Disease

Recently a team of researchers developed a technique that uses a paper chip coated in nanoparticles of a fluorescent polymer similar to Styrofoam; each particle had antibodies against the norovirus pathogen coated on the surface. When water that contains the norovirus is dropped on the chip, the viruses attach themselves to the particles, which begin to fluoresce which could be detected through a basic microscope, thus dramatically reducing the cost of detecting norovirus in water supply. Nanofibrous scaffolds are promising platforms for wound healing, especially due to their similarity to the extracellular matrix and their capability to promote cell adhesion and proliferation and restore skin integrity. When grafted into the wound site, they provide a 3D structure for the cell homing and the tissue formation. Nanotechnologies are even helping to prevent infections in wounds through smart bandages that contain nanoparticles of blood clotting agents, growth hormones, or sensors that can detect infection and release antibiotics accordingly.

FUTURE OF NANOMEDICINE

Nanotechnology promises to facilitate the development of personalized medicine, in which patient therapy will be tailored by his/her genetic and disease profile. Futuristic nanoscale sensors and devices will be able to provide a personal and cost-effective continuous medical monitoring of patient's health; they will also enhance prediction of diseases such as cancer or inflammation at an early stage. Use of nanomaterial is being tried to diagnose and treat atherosclerosis, Alzheimer disease, skin diseases, toxic overdoses, and inflammatory bowel disease. Finally, there is a significant effort in developing nanoparticle probes for MRI, computed tomography (CT), and positron emission tomography (PET) imaging. Near-infrared fluorescent imaging shows promise as a new modality for colorectal cancer and other gastrointestinal imaging. Use of nanoshells in cancer management is yet another upcoming field of nanotechnology. Nanoshells are miniscule beads coated with gold. These can carry molecular conjugates that can bind to an antigen displayed on a cancer cell surface. Subsequent application of mechanical, radiofrequency or optical energy to these nanoshells from an external source would result in energy absorption by them, as these excited nanoshells have the property of relaxing to the ground state, and without radiating the absorbed energy this will produce intense local heating, thus killing the tumor cells without harming the neighboring healthy cells.

TOXICITY CONCERNS

The properties that make nanoparticles so attractive can also contribute to their toxicological profile in biological systems. This has resulted in extensive discussions regarding their safety and health risks with their use. It has been demonstrated that low solubility nanoparticles are more hazardous and toxic on a mass-by-mass basis than larger particles. Their absorption, distribution, metabolism, and clearance have a bearing on their cellular interactions and endocytic pathway and therefore, nanoparticles can exert cytotoxicity through interference with cellular homeostasis. Nanoparticles have displayed toxicity as well as proinflammatory and pro-oxidant effects in endothelial cells. More in-depth studies are required to understand what happens to these materials inside the body. This will provide a fundamental basis for nanoparticle engineering. Combining enthusiasm and insights will be the key to advancing nanomedicine to benefit society.

CONCLUSION

The last decades, has seen translation of several applications of nanomedicine in the clinical practice, ranging from medical devices to nanopharmaceuticals. The prospect of nanotechnology lies within using the right nanomaterials and reducing any possible harmful effects. Although the expectations from nanotechnology in medicine are very high and the potential benefits are endless, the safety of nanomedicine is not yet fully defined. At present use of nanotechnology in medical therapeutics needs adequate evaluation of its risk and safety. A full lifecycle evaluation is required to more accurately ascertain the sustainability and safety of their long-term use. However, it is certain that in coming years nanomedicine would play a crucial role in treatment of human diseases and in enhancement of normal human physiology. Its utility is likely to be still more into medical diagnostics and molecular research techniques.

SUGGESTED READINGS

1. Krukemeyer MG, Krenn V, Huebner F, Wagner W, Resch R. History and Possible Uses of Nanomedicine Based on Nanoparticles and Nanotechnological Progress. J Nanomed Nanotechnol. 2015;6:336.
2. Tinkle S, McNeil SE, Mühlebach S. Nanomedicines: addressing the scientific and regulatory gap. Ann N Y Acad Sci. 2014;1313:35-56.
3. Commission Recommendation. Commission Recommendation of 18 October 2011 on the definition of nanomaterial 2011/696/EU. Off J Eur Union L. 2011;275:38-40.
4. Louro H. Relevance of physicochemical characterization of nanomaterials for understanding nano-cellular interactions. Adv Exp Med Biol. 2018:1048:123-42.

5. Saquib Q, Faisal M, Al-Khedhairy AA, Alatar AA. Cellular and Molecular Toxicology of Nanoparticles. Advances in Experimental Medicine and Biology, volume 1048. Cham: Springer; 2018. pp. 123-42.
6. Lombardo D, Kiselev MA, Caccamo MT. Smart Nanoparticles for Drug Delivery Application: Development of Versatile Nanocarrier Platforms in Biotechnology and Nanomedicine. J Nanomater. 2019;12:1-26.
7. Nie L, Liu F, Ma P, Xiao X: Applications of gold nanoparticles in optical biosensors. J Biomed Nanotechnol. 2014;10:2700-21.
8. Waters EA, Wickline SA. Contrast agents for MRI. Basic Res Cardiol. 2008;103:114-21.
9. Shi Kam NW, Jessop TC, Wender PA, Dai H: Nanotube molecular transporters: Internalization of carbon nanotube-protein conjugates into Mammalian cells. J Am Chem Soc. 2004;126:6850-1.
10. Panahi Y, Farshbaf M, Mohammadhosseini M, Mirahadi M, Khalilov R, Saghfi S, et al. Recent advances on liposomal nanoparticles: synthesis, characterization and biomedical applications. Artif Cells Nanomed Biotechnol. 2017;45(4): 788-99.
11. Sindhwani S, Chan WCW. Nanotechnology for modern medicine: next step towards clinical translation. J Intern Med. 2021;290(3):486-98.
12. Wu T, Chen X, Wang Y, Xiao H, Peng Y, Lin L, et al. Aortic plaque-targeted andrographolide delivery with oxidation-sensitive micelle effectively treats atherosclerosis via simultaneous ROS capture and anti-inflammation. Nanomedicine. 2018;14: 2215-26.
13. Adams D, Gonzalez-Duarte A, O'Riordan WD, Yang CC, Ueda M, Kristen AV, et al. Patisiran, an RNAi therapeutic, for hereditary transthyretin amyloidosis. N Engl J Med. 2018;379:11-21.
14. Javaid M, Haleem A, Singh RP, Suman R. 3D printing applications for healthcare research and development. Glob Health J. 2022;6(4):217-26.
15. Hoshyar N, Gray S, Han H, Bao G. The effect of nanoparticle size on in vivo pharmacokinetics and cellular interaction. Nanomedicine (Lond). 2016;11:673-92.

261
CHAPTER

Role of Artificial Intelligence in Medical Education

Jananee Muralidharan

ABSTRACT

Artificial intelligence (AI) has the potential to revolutionize medical education by offering precision learning and personal tutoring. Adaptive learning platforms can be used to optimize teaching methods and track student progress across the years of medical education. Educators can use data-driven insights which can help select suitable pedagogy for students. However, the risks of AI, including issues with academic integrity and diminished face-to-face interactions need to be considered when implementing an AI-driven system in medical education.

INTRODUCTION

Is there a need for artificial intelligence (AI) in medical education?

Artificial intelligence can be used as a tool in delivering quality medical education. Since August 2019, the National Medical Council's (NMC) adoption of competency-based medical education (CBME) has shifted the paradigm of medical education toward a focus on both summative and formative assessments as fundamental components of effective learning. The provision of meaningful and targeted feedback, rooted in the identification of individual knowledge gaps, emerges as a critical factor in this context. However, the task of identifying personalized knowledge gaps for each student becomes formidable within academic institutions characterized by inadequate student–faculty ratios and limited faculty time. AI emerges as a viable solution to this challenge and can offer precision learning to cater to individual student needs.

Precision learning is composed of two components: Mastery learning and personal tutoring. Mastery learning is derived from Bloom's principles where a student achieves a level of mastery in prerequisite knowledge before moving onto newer information. Personal tutoring focuses on identifying and addressing individual learning gaps. When education is delivered uniformly, the performance of a class typically follows a bell-shaped curve. However, with optimal instruction based on personalized requirements, the class's achievement curve may shift to the right, indicating enhanced learning outcomes. AI-driven medical education can help provide tailored guidance to students requiring additional support.

HOW CAN AI ASSIST IN DELIVERY OF QUALITY MEDICAL EDUCATION?

Several adaptive learning platforms exist which utilize AI as a tool in the delivery of primary school education. Much of this can be translated and applied to medical education with minimal changes. These learning platforms can track students across each year of medical education, breaking up the silos in which education is traditionally delivered. Analyzing students' mistakes over time offers insights into their learning patterns, enabling educators to address specific challenges and identify learning gaps. Furthermore, AI-driven learning platforms match teaching methods with learning outcomes, ensuring the most effective pedagogical approaches are employed for a batch of students. Such platforms also enhance accessibility for students with physical disabilities and language barriers, fostering inclusivity in medical education delivery.

ROLE OF AI IN THE DOMAINS OF MEDICAL EDUCATION

In the cognitive domain, AI-based platforms can identify knowledge gaps, reinforce learning, and recommend optimal learning methods for each student. Chatbots, for instance, can revise high-yield questions from predefined resources, fostering retention of relevant material. AI-generated case scenarios can be used to teach problem-solving skills in a simulated environment and be an engaging way of teaching clinical material. Interestingly, AI can also be used in the psychomotor domain with the use of virtual reality (VR)-based teaching. Students can practice in high-fidelity simulation laboratories, using equipment with sensors which can track movement and angulation to give feedback on their psychomotor skills. AI-powered systems can also aid in training students for patient counseling by recognizing emotions in speech, thereby refining affective domain skills.

Utility of AI for Educators

AI-based learning platforms empower educators by mapping teaching methodologies against learning outcomes. The teacher dashboard can be used to visualize data on the class performance in assessments. Granular student data can be used to generate recommendations to educators on an appropriate lesson plan and predict learning outcomes for students. Even seating plans can be generated for the class based on student learning patterns and behaviors from the data-driven insights. Integration of AI-powered personal tutoring can offer appropriate feedback, ensuring timely correction of conceptual misunderstandings.

POTENTIAL RISKS WITH AI USE

While AI holds immense promise, there are risks that need to be considered. The availability of large language models, like ChatGPT, could lead to compromised academic integrity. Both educators and students might resort to generative AI models for setting and answering question papers, undermining authentic learning. Increased reliance on AI-powered learning platforms might reduce face-to-face interactions between students and educators. The "hidden curriculum", encompassing nonacademic skills learned through observation of teachers, could be missed out. Students performing poorly may need intervention from teachers which may not happen when opportunities for interaction with teachers decrease. Moreover, the use of AI for outcome prediction may inadvertently promote determinism, prematurely judging students based on initial performances.

WAY FORWARD

Using AI-based systems in medical education requires a nuanced approach. While in-depth technical knowledge of such systems might not be needed for clinicians, it is important to that understand the capabilities and limitations of such systems. AI can help mitigate the challenges of inadequate student-teacher ratios, but its incorporation should not diminish the irreplaceable aspects of traditional teaching. In conclusion, striking a balance is important to navigate the future of medical education as we veer away from a fact-based education system.

SUGGESTED READINGS

1. Tolsgaard MG, Pusic MV, Sebok-Syer SS, Gin B, Svendsen MB, Syer MD, et al. The fundamentals of Artificial Intelligence in medical education research: AMEE Guide No. 156. Med Teach. 2023;45(6):565-73.
2. Cheng CT, Chen CC, Fu CY, Chaou CH, Wu YT, Hsu CP, et al. Artificial intelligence-based education assists medical students' interpretation of hip fracture. Insights Imaging. 2020;11(1):119.

262

CHAPTER

Building Bridges Between Mental and Physical Health

Veerendra Singh

ABSTRACT

Mental health and physical health are deeply connected. Psychological well-being reduces the risk of serious physical problems; in contrast, people with mental illness are more likely to suffer from metabolic disorders, cardiovascular diseases (CVD), asthma, or cancer. Stressful events experienced during gestation or early in life can lead to increased vulnerability to both physical and mental health. Life expectancy of patients with major psychiatric disorders is reduced by 7–24 years.

Metabolic disorders can cause stress-induced neuroendocrine changes that lead to mental disorders. Likewise, mental health disorders can trigger metabolic changes that, over time, develop into metabolic diseases. A new theory argues mental disorders as metabolic disorders of the brain. People with diabetes are at a higher risk of developing depression and vice versa.

Acute trauma leads to disruption of gastrointestinal, cardiovascular, immunological, reproductive system, musculoskeletal, and neuroendocrine functioning. During the coronavirus disease 2019 (COVID-19) pandemic, anxiety symptoms and depression in youth doubled to prepandemic state. Chronic stress can alter endocrine and immune systems and increase the risk of hypertension, coronary artery disease, diabetes, asthma, stroke, and cancer. Changing ways to mental issues, physical issues, stress reduction (SR), and behavioral interventions may reduce perceived stress. Properly selected psychotherapy and pharmacotherapy effectively improve overall health.

INTRODUCTION

In 1948, the World Health Organization defined health as a state of complete physical, mental, and social well-being and not merely the absence of disease or infirmity. A bidirectional relationship exists between mental and physical health. An improvement or decline in one can lead to improvement or decline in the other. In people with mental illness, unhealthy behaviors and antipsychotic medication side effects lead to higher morbidity and mortality. Depression has been linked to cancer, diabetes, and asthma. People with mental illness have poor access to healthcare. Life expectancy of patients with major psychiatric disorders is reduced by 7–24 years. People with multimorbidity tended to have worse mental health.

MIND–BODY CONNECTION

The brain integrates and coordinates behavioral and physiologic responses to stressful challenges through neuroendocrine, autonomic, immune, and metabolic mediators. Body reacts to stress through changes in the hypothalamic–pituitary–adrenal (HPA) axis. Adverse socioeconomic conditions, physical, emotional, or sexual abuse are well-established risk factors for mood disorders. Stressful experiences by mothers during gestation can perturb metabolic homeostasis in the offspring. Adverse stress and attenuate the neural-immune-arterial axis. Stress reduction (SR) modifies the structure and connectivity of neural centers. Its downstream effects include reduced systemic inflammation, improved blood pressure, and health behaviors (e.g., reduced smoking). SR favorably alters gene expression, insulin production, and proinflammatory pathways. Modern tools such as wearables and remote monitoring provide opportunities to better monitor these behaviors.

In individuals with depression and CVD, selective serotonin reuptake inhibitors (SSRIs) attenuate depressive symptoms and lower secondary CVD risk. Beta-blockers may decrease SNS-driven leukopoiesis. Anti-inflammatory agents (e.g., canakinumab) may also prove beneficial by directly targeting elevated proinflammatory cytokines.

HEALTH ISSUES DURING COVID-19 PANDEMIC

During the pandemic, pooled estimates for anxiety symptoms and depression in youth doubled to pre-pandemic state. Viral infection correlated strongly with mental health indices. Coronavirus 2 (CoV-2) spikes protein-induced recruitment of macrophages and monocytes that release cytokines, increasing neuroinflammation in the brain. Disruption of blood-brain barrier allows peripheral inflammatory mediators to enter the central nervous system (CNS) and damage neural tissues. Higher use of television and digital media has been linked to worsening psychological well-being.

TECHNOLOGY AND MENTAL HEALTH

Artificial intelligence (AI), combined with sensors and smartphone applications, enable increased monitoring in the community. Cognitive behavioral therapy (CBT) chatbots decreased both depression and anxiety in college students. AI techniques will help mental health practitioners redefine mental illnesses more objectively and deliver personalized treatments.

IMPROVING THE MIND-BODY CONNECTION

Changing the way to deal with mental and physical issues is the most effective way to improve overall health. CBT can change negative thinking patterns that worsen mental well-being. Taking care of the body in turn protects the mind. A healthy diet, enough sleep, and regular exercise improve well-being.

Transformation of the existing mental healthcare system toward a system that utilizes a coordinated, multidisciplinary, holistic approach not only may effectively bridge the existing gap between mental and physical health but also may save lives. Preventative strategies should focus on promoting a healthy life via safer environments at work and outside work.

SUGGESTED READINGS

1. Doan T, Ha V, Strazdins L, Chateau D. Healthy minds live in healthy bodies. Curr Psychol. 2022;42:18702-13.
2. Cirulli F. Interactions between early life stress and metabolic stress in programming of mental and metabolic health. Curr Opin Behav Sci. 2017;14:65-71.
3. Olafson K The 5-year pre- and post-hospitalization treated prevalence of mental disorders and psychotropic medication use in critically ill patients: a Canadian population-based study: Intensive Care Medicine. 2021;47:1450-61.
4. Andreas Walther Depressive disorders are associated with increased peripheral blood cell deformability: a cross-sectional case-control study (Mood-Morph): Transl Psychiatry; 2022;12(1):150.
5. Yun Gi Kim Association of Depression With Atrial Fibrillation in South Korean Adults: JAMA Netw Open. 2022 Jan 4;5(1).
6. Parveen K Garg Negative Affect and Risk of Atrial Fibrillation: MESA; J Am Heart Assoc. 2019;8(1).

263
CHAPTER

Doctor Heal Thyself

Sandeep Rai, Madhur Rai

ABSTRACT

Stress and burnout among doctors is often a neglected issue. If doctors, who are the lifesavers of the community, are themselves under stress, their efficiency is reduced. This will directly affect the lives of a large number of people whom they treat. It is appalling to see that doctors who are there to protect the health of the people, in fact themselves succumb to various stress-related health conditions and more over they do not have the necessary framework to seek timely help. Doctors have 2.5 times the risk of dying by suicide as compared to the general population. Multiple factors that have been identified to contribute to this are poor training environment in residency, trying for perfectionism in practicing the profession, taboo associated with seeking professional help for their own health or psychological issues, high-demand work profiles, lack of sleep, unregulated working hours, fear of violence and litigation, etc. We as doctors cannot avoid all these sources of stress in our professional and personal lives, but we can definitely develop healthier ways of coping with them. In fact new research studies, along with real-world experience of its practitioners globally, have revealed that *Sahaja Yoga* (SY) meditation (SYM) practiced for 15–20 minutes daily is proving to be a robust strategy for stress management.

INTRODUCTION

Being a doctor has long been considered one of the most noble and sought-after professions throughout the world. According to recent estimates, there are more than 10 lakh doctors practicing in India and each year more than 80,000 medical students graduate as doctors. However, practicing this profession also comes with a heavy price to pay. This is a highly skilled and a high-pressure profession. Doctors are not immune to stress-related illness, with between a quarter and a third reporting increased symptoms of psychological stress and burnout which has been specially heightened after coronavirus disease 2019 (COVID-19) pandemic. The modern hospitals and clinics have a stressful environment, and doctors respond differently to it; some finding it stimulating and exciting, whereas others become stressed and feel burnt out from the heavy workload. Burnout is considered as a state of psychological stress generated by occupation or in workplace and is designated as a distinct entity in the World Health Organization's International Classification of Diseases. The prevalence of burnout among doctors has been found to be as high as 75%. Workplace stress affects the brain performance, including memory, concentration, and learning **(Fig. 1)**. Although reasonable amount of stress can have positive effects on people by energizing them to attain their goals but excessive stress may negatively impact a person's health and work performance. Stress in occupation occurs when job-related demands interact with individual factors, resulting in a negative change in the individual's psychological or physiological state. Burnout among doctors has been associated with lower satisfaction in career, higher rates of work absenteeism, greater probability of quitting the profession or opting for early retirement, and greater risk of difficulties in relationships, such as with family and partners.

Stress is now becoming part of the "new normal" for doctors. This is causing a decrease in productivity and health problems in doctors which can be initially silent,

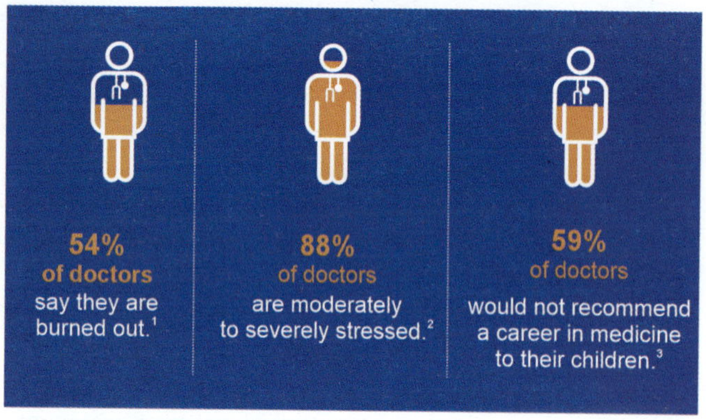

FIG. 1: Physician burnout.

Sources:

1. Mayo Clinic 2014.
2. VITAL Worklife & Cejka Search. (2015). Physician Stress and Burnout Survey. [online] Available from https://info.vitalworklife.com/download-survey-reports [Last accessed January, 2024].
3. Jackson Healthcare. (2013). Filling the Void: 2013 Physician Outlook and Practice Trends. [online] Available from https://www.kff.org/wp-content/uploads/sites/2/2014/04/2013physiciantrends-void_ebk0513.pdf [Last accessed January, 2024].

but after a while can catch up and result in morbidities such as high blood pressure, diabetes, and cardiovascular disease, all of which are made worse by chronic stress, which is an essential byproduct of medical profession. In a study by the Centers for Disease Control and Prevention in USA, it was found that about 66% of workers in America say that they lie awake at night troubled by the physical or emotional effects of stress. While stress is a normal human reaction that affects everyone from time to time, chronic stress is a killer as it is linked to health problems such as cardiovascular disease, poor sleep, digestive issues, a weakened immune system, and mental health conditions such as anxiety and depression, all of which can lead to a variety of devastating illnesses.

Healthcare workers have to deal with a lot of stress especially because they are overwhelmed with maintaining the work and life balance. Amygdala is the part of our brain that helps process the threatening situations. This is seen to appear larger in people who are chronically stressed. Researchers have also shown that the hippocampus and prefrontal cortex appear smaller in stressed individuals. When our life spins out of control, we turn on genes that cause chronic inflammation leading to a host of lifestyle-related chronic diseases. Meditation activates the parasympathetic nervous system which initiates the relaxation response, depresses heart rate, blood pressure, and respiration, and allows your body to engage in reparative and restorative functions. One of the ways described to activate the "relaxation response", is through a technique that was first described by cardiologist Dr Herbert Benson, at Harvard Medical School in 1970. The relaxation response is the exact opposite of the stress response. It is a profoundly restful state that can be elicited in numerous ways. We as medical doctors, advise our patients every day about how important it is to have a fit, healthy body, however, we forget the fact that it is equally important to have a fit and healthy mind. Through regular practice of meditation, our minds can become more relaxed and focused, enabling us to handle the stressful situations in life, in a much better way. During the process of meditation, the stress and strain which accumulated over a long period of time, are gradually eliminated and both the body and mind feel more positive and energized and thus the overall health of the individual gets positively impacted. Presently extensive research has led to the presence of robust evidence in the medical literature for the mind–body medicine practices such as *Sahaja Yoga* (SY) meditation (SYM) for invoking the relaxation response in an individual and influencing the mind and body in a positive way.

Sahaja Yoga meditation is indeed a very unique meditation technique developed by Dr Nirmala Devi Srivastava, popularly known all over the world as HH Shri Mataji Nirmala Devi. This meditation technique causes a transformation in a person by which one becomes balanced and destressed. It offers an easy method of understanding your own energy systems and teaches ways of harnessing the innate powerful energy "*kundalini*" present in all human beings, for improving one's own health. Scientific studies have now clearly shown that SYM acts by reducing the activity of the sympathetic system (stress) and increasing the parasympathetic activity (relaxation) in an individual. SYM practice for 12–16 weeks, in subjects who had never practiced any form of meditation, has shown a decrease in heart rate, a decrease in the respiratory rate, decrease in blood pressure and in the production of urinary vanillylmandelic acid (VMA), which is a breakdown product of stress hormone adrenalin and an increase of galvanic skin resistance. Physiological changes in all these parameters indicate activation of a deep parasympathetic state, indicating a physiologically relaxed state of the body and mind, and this may play a vital role in the prevention of stress-related diseases.

Detailed electrophysiological studies [electroencephalography (EEG)] and analysis on SY meditators have shown specific brain activation patterns, which indicate a relaxed state of mind, a subjective feeling of happiness, and an enhanced interconnectivity of different brain regions. In an interesting study examining emotional reactions of SY meditators compared to nonmeditators, decreased electrophysiological, physiological, and psychological reactions were seen in meditators when exposed to stressful stimuli, compared to subjects who were not meditating, thus, probably for the first time in the world, showing the neurophysiologic proof to support the hypothesis that regular practice of SYM leads to development of capability of greater resilience to deal with stressful life events. Many other randomized trials on SYM have demonstrated beneficial effects on depression and work-related stress.

In other studies conducted on SYM around the world, very good results were achieved in patients suffering from anxiety and depression, enhancing quality of life (QoL) and significant improvement in psychological health of a mixed population consisting of subjects from different countries and of different age groups. Encouraging results have also been recorded in patients with hypertension, asthma, and perceived stress in workplace, only after a couple of weeks of SYM practice. Other studies on SYM have shown significant reduction in epilepsy attacks, attacks of bronchial asthma, and improvements in control of diabetes and blood pressure.

Chronic stress in known to increase cortisol levels in body, which in turn decreases immunity and consequently impairs a person's ability to fight infections. Two randomly controlled studies, conducted in the Department of Medicine and the Department of Physiology at the MGM Institute of Health Sciences, Navi Mumbai, by the authors of this chapter, on the effect of SY on perceived stress and serum cortisol levels showed a very robust reduction in perceived stress and serum cortisol levels in SYM practitioners as compared to the healthy nonmeditating controls. They also showed that meditators had a decrease in oxidative stress and more production of nitric oxide as compared to normal nonmeditating population. An increase in heart rate variability compared to nonmeditating normal individuals, indicating a relaxed destressed mental state was also observed. Moreover an exciting new research has shown that practice of SY resulted in increase in gray matter volume of brain in many cortical and subcortical brain regions of the right hemisphere. These regions are associated with self-control, compassion, and stress modulation.

Modern medicine's understanding of the human immune system, as a complex multidimensional interaction among different organ systems, is slowly expanding, throwing its light on new facets like neuroendocrine and psychoemotional aspects governing its effective functioning. Chronic stress, although mental in origin, has many detrimental effects on the body as well as on the immunity by creating an imbalance in the neuroendocrine pathways. These chronic stressors overwhelm the immune system of our body, thus weakening the immune system's ability to mount a strong immunological response to an infectious organism and in turn making the individual more susceptible to life-threatening medical consequences.

Both health and yoga experts now firmly believe that meditating on a regular basis can help to improve the immunity of the body, thus creating a shield in fight against the infectious diseases. Scientific research has already shown that meditation produces remarkable effects on the brain and immune functions. Recent studies have now shown that the relaxation produced after meditation reduces the levels of IL-6, which is a proinflammatory cytokine which plays a major role in the pathophysiology of several diseases.

Stress in medical profession is unavoidable these days, but it is not insurmountable. Meditation is not only for eliminating stress, but it is also about how to manage it. We cannot entirely eliminate stress from our lives, but through regular meditation, we can slowly learn to reframe how we view stress to relate to it in a more accepting way. The popularity of meditation is increasing as more and more people discover its huge health benefits **(Fig. 2)**. Numerous studies have shown that meditation is an effective stress management tool, ultimately reprogramming the brain to the extent that meditators end up with more capacity to manage stress when meditation is a consistent, daily practice. Having a regular meditation practice may feel elusive and difficult, but in fact it does not have to be so. Approaching your meditation practice with a flexible attitude and experimenting what works best for you can help you make meditation a realistic and enjoyable part of your life.

Chronic stress in the long run reduces the telomerase activity and accelerates shortening of telomere which in turn accelerates premature aging. Meditation has shown to enhance the telomerase activity of chromosomes and thus promotes cell longevity. Meditation has also shown to reduce the activity of nuclear factor-kappaB (NF-κB) which is a known mediator in the generation of C-reactive protein which is increased in inflammatory conditions. Meditation has shown to boost the immunity levels especially of salivary immunoglobulin A, which is an immune mediator at mucosal surfaces, such as gastrointestinal (GI) tract, respiratory tract, and genitourinary tract.

Meditation and yoga practices positively affect gene expression. Research has shown that a program of comprehensive lifestyle changes (including vegetarian diet and stress management with meditation) improved the overall health and impacted the expression of genes in patients of prostate cancer who were not treated with surgery, radiation, or hormone therapy. This 3-month study showed changes were observed in >500 genes: 48 genes were upregulated and 453 genes were downregulated. The downregulated genes included disease-promoting genes with critical roles in tumor genesis.

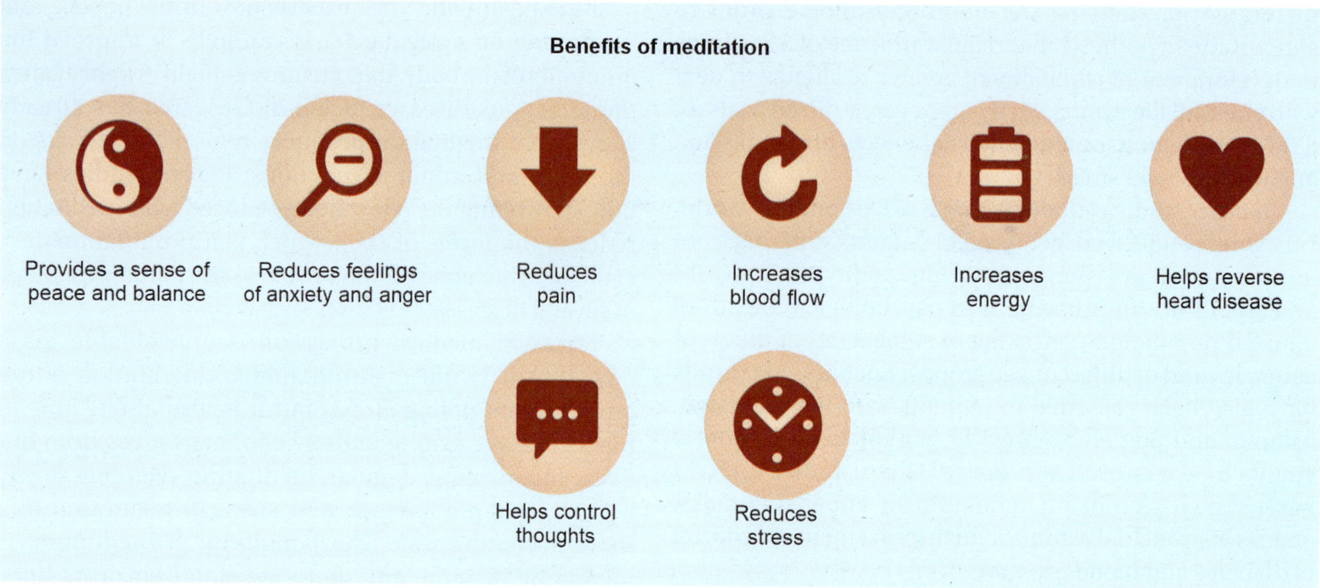

FIG. 2: Benefits of meditation.

HOW SAHAJA YOGA MEDITATION REDUCES STRESS?

Possible Mechanisms

For thousands of years, people have been meditating often as part of a spiritual practice. But in more recent years, meditation has become a popular way to help people manage their stress and improve their overall well-being. Mammals, including humans, have over millions of years evolved the ability to deal quickly and reflexively with perceived threats to their survival and this ability has conferred a robust survival advantage to this group of animals. In humans, however, the same stress response can be triggered in situations which, while they do not necessarily threaten survival, but occur fairly frequently over a prolonged period of time. The stress response gets activated repeatedly, and is thought to result in dysregulation of the immune system which hampers the body's own survival mechanisms and this in turn damages health. The changes in mind and body achieved by SYM are characterized by the relaxation response. Psychophysiological studies on SYM suggest that indeed it elicits a relaxation response. The hypothesis is that by regular practice of meditation, the innate energy, called kundalini energy described in detail in the ancient Indian Vedic scriptures, actualizes in limbic area of the brain and modulates the stress response of an individual through the limbic system **(Fig. 3)**. The limbic system has intricate connections with hypothalamus and via hypothalamus it modulates the autonomic nervous system. The limbic system by its action on the hypothalamic-pituitary-adrenal (HPA) axis modulates the release of various important hormones including cortisol which is secreted in response to stress. Practicing SYM balances the energy systems of the body for its optimum functioning.

Sahaja Yoga is now practiced in many schools, institutions, colleges, and corporate offices all over India and is an integral part of wellness programs around the world. It is also increasingly being incorporated in many youth development programs around the world. In many medical institutions around the world, researches are being conducted on the therapeutic benefits of SYM.

In 1993, Dr Nirmala Devi Srivastava, the founder of Sahaja Yoga, addressed a large gathering of doctors and scientists at the National Institute of Health (NIH), Washington DC (NIH USA), which is the apex body of research in America. She explained the scientific basis of SYM. This was followed few years later in 1998 by a scientific presentation on the physiological effects and the therapeutic benefits of SY at NIH, by the eminent physiologist of India, late Professor UC Rai, who was formerly heading of Department of Physiology at JIPMER (Pondicherry) and MAMC (Maulana Azad Medical College) and LHMC (Lady Hardinge Medical College) (New Dehi). SYM since then is practiced at NIH (USA) for 1 hour, once every week, and with the Government of India's impetus on yoga and meditation, many institutions are now adopting practice of SY for their staff and students.

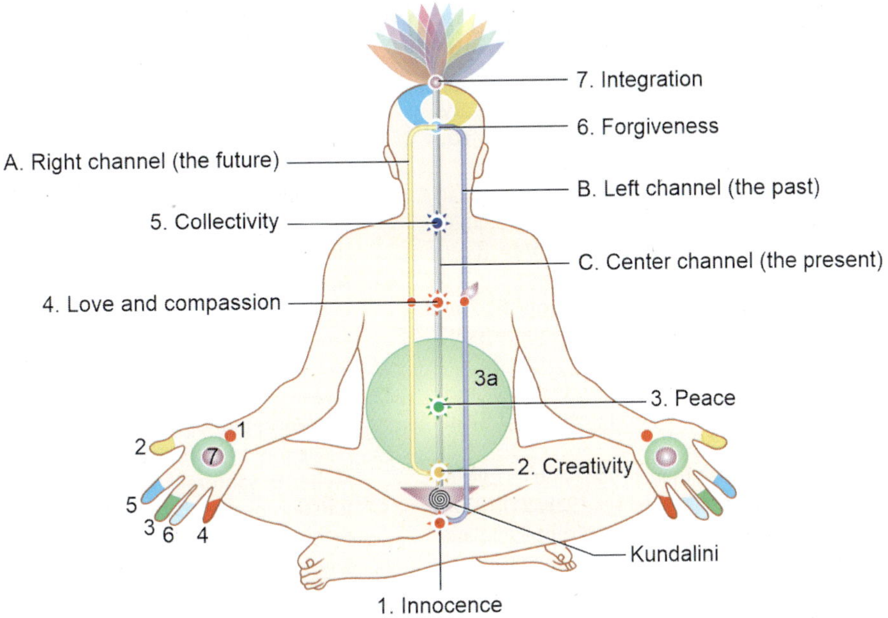

FIG. 3: The subtle system and chakras.

HH Shri Mataji Nirmala Devi has been internationally recognized for her contribution to humanity through a lifetime of work for peace and the well-being of mankind. She has received numerous awards and citations from the governments of many countries in the recognition of her selfless efforts for social improvement and for her significant contribution to the understanding of subtle energy systems of the human body. To just name a few, she was conferred the "Honorary Doctorate in Cognitive Science" from the Romanian University and the *UN Peace Medal* as a recognition for her outstanding contribution to the humanity and *world peace*. She was appointed as Honorary Member of the Petrovskaya Academy of Art and Science in Russia. In the history of the academy, only 12 people have been granted this honor, with Einstein being one of them. SY was awarded "Best Diagnosis and Therapies of Regenerative Medicine 2003" by the Ministry of Health of Russia. She had also been twice nominated for the Nobel Peace Prize.

Meditation is not about eliminating stress, but managing it. We cannot entirely eliminate stress, but through meditation we can learn to cope with stress in a better way and relate to it in a more accepting way. A number of SYM programs are now available online or through smartphone apps as well. During the COVID-19 pandemic, technology had enabled to conduct free online SY collective meditation programs, for lakhs of people in India and across the world. These online programs are still continuing today and have become hugely popular all over the world. SY is now available free of charge, to learn and practice at all the centers of SY which are present today in more than 130 countries of the world. People can be recommended to download free meditation apps or join online programs. These well researched and supported programs and are designed to help you tackle your day-to-day stress in a way that is both convenient and effective. Meditation is something everyone can do to improve their physical, mental, and emotional health. You can do it anywhere, without special equipment or memberships.

Stress in doctors may originate from personal and professional life, and is closely related to the amount of psychosocial resources that are possessed or thought to be possessed to cope with the requirements of certain demanding situations. Meditation has proved to be a robust coping mechanism to deal with day-to-day psychological stress. Incorporating stress-relieving activities like meditation and yoga in daily life, conducive working environment, and proper rest are the need of the hour for preventing and treating the stress and burnout faced by healthcare providers. For any further information on learning SYM you may visit: www.freemeditation.com, www.sahajayoga.org.in, toll-free number: 18002-700-800 or write to doctorsandeeprai@gmail.com.

SUGGESTED READINGS

1. Sahasrabuddhe AG, Suryawanshi SR, Bhandari SR. Stress among doctors doing residency: A cross-sectional study at a tertiary care hospital in the city of Mumbai. Natl J Community Med. 2015;6:21-4.
2. World Health Organization. (2016). International Statistical Classification of Diseases and Related Health Problems. [online] Available from https://icd.who.int/browse10/2016/en [Last accessed January, 2024].
3. Iacovides A, Fountoulakis KN, Kaprinis S, Kaprinis G. The relationship between job stress, burnout and clinical depression. J Affect Disord. 2003;75:209-21.
4. Willcock SM, Daly MG, Tennant CC, Allard BJ. Burnout and psychiatric morbidity in new medical graduates. Med J Aust. 2004;181:357-60.
5. Rai U, Sethi S, Singh S. Some effects of sahaja yoga and its role in the prevention of stress disorders. J Int Med Sci. 1988;2(1):1923.
6. Aftanas LI, Golocheikine SA. Human anterior and frontal midline theta and lower alpha reflect emotionally positive state and internalized attention: High resolution EEG investigation of meditation. Neurosci Lett. 2001;310(1):57-60.
7. Aftanas LI, Golocheikine SA. Linear and non-linear concomitants of Altered state of consciousness during meditation: high-resolution EEG investigation. Int J Psychophysiol. 2002;45 (1-2):158-1158.
8. Aftanas L, Golosheykin S. Impact of regular meditation practice on EEG activity at rest and during evoked negative emotions. Int J Neurosci. 2005;115(6):893-909.
9. Manocha R, Marks GB, Kenchington P, Peters D, Salome CM. Sahaja yoga in the management of moderate to severe asthma: a randomized controlled trial. Thorax. 2002;57(2):110-5.
10. Morgan D. Sahaja yoga: an ancient path to modern mental health? Transpersonal Psychol Rev. 2001;4(4):41-9.
11. Chung SC, Brooks MM, Rai M, Balk JL, Rai S. Effect of sahaja yoga meditation on quality of life, anxiety, and blood pressure control. J Altern Complement Med. 2012;18(6):589-96.
12. Rai S, Sharma RC, Singh CB, Shaunak AA, Gangawane AK. Effect of higher state of consciousness thoughtless awareness on psychological health. Neurosci Res. 2010;1(1):1-8.
13. Chugh D. The effects of sahaja yoga in bronchial asthma and essential hypertension. New Delhi Medicos. 1997;5(4):46-7.
14. Panjwani U, Selvamurthy W, Singh SH, Gupta HL, Thakur L, Rai UC. Effect of Sahaja Yoga practice on seizure control and EEG changes in patients of epilepsy. Indian J Med Res. 1996;103: 165-72.
15. Harrison L, Manosh R, Rubia K. Sahaja yoga meditation as a family treatment program for attention deficit hyperactivity disorder children. J Clin Psychol Psychiatr. 2004;9(4):479-97.
16. Peters RK, Benson H, Peters JM. Daily relaxation response breaks in a working population: II effects on blood pressure. Am J Pub Health. 1977;67(10):954-9.
17. Rubia K. The neurobiology of meditation and its clinical effectiveness in psychiatric disorders. Biol Psychol. 2009;82(1): 1-11.
18. Panjwani U, Gupta HL, Singh SH, Selvamurthy W, Rai UC. Effect of Sahaja Yoga practice on stress management in patients of epilepsy. Indian J Physiol Pharmacol. 1995;39(2):111-6.
19. Manocha R, Black D, Sarris J, Stough C. A randomized, controlled trial of meditation for work stress, anxiety and depressed mood in full-time workers. Evid Based Complement Alternat Med. 2011;2011:960583.
20. Vishesh A. RCT to Evaluate the Role Mind Body Technique of Sahaja Yoga Meditation in Stress reduction. Mumbai: MGM University of Health Sciences; 2013.
21. Hernández SE, Suero J, Barros A, González-Mora JL, Rubia K. Increased Grey Matter Associated with Long-term Sahaja Yoga Meditation: A Voxel-based Morphometry Study. PLoS One. 2016;11(3)e0150757.
22. Rivest S. Regulation of innate immune responses in the brain. Nat Rev Immunol. 2009;9(6):429-39.
23. Davidson RJ, Kabat-Zinn J, Schumacher J, Rosenkranz M, Muller D, Santorelli SF, et al. Alterations in brain and immune function produced by mindfulness meditation. Psychosomatic Medicine. 2003;65(4):564-70.
24. Smith JC. Alterations in brain and immune function produced by mindfulness meditation: three caveats. Psychosom Med. 2004;66(1):148-52; author reply 148-52.
25. Ishihara K, Hirano T. IL-6 in autoimmune disease and chronic inflammatory proliferative disease. Cytokine Growth Factor Rev. 2002;13(4):357-68.
26. Jacobs TL, Epel ES, Lin J, Blackburn EH, Wolkowitz OM, Bridwell DA, et al. Intensive meditation training, immune cell telomerase activity, and psychological mediators. Psychoneuroendocrinology. 2011;36(5):664-81.
27. Creswell JD, Irwin MR, Burklund LJ, Lieberman MD, Arevalo JM, Ma J, et al. Mindfulness based stress reduction training reduces loneliness and proinflammatory gene expression in older adults: a small randomized controlled trial. Brain Behav Immun. 2012;26(7):1095-101.
28. Malarkey WB, Jarjoura D, Klatt M. Workplace based mindfulness practice and inflammation: a randomized trial. Brain Behav Immun. 2013;27(1):145-54.
29. Pace TW, Negi LT, Adame DD, Cole SP, Sivilli TI, Brown TD, et al. Effect of compassion meditation on neuroendocrine, innate immune and behavioral responses to psychosocial stress. Psychoneuroendocrinology. 2009;34(1):87-98.
30. Hall JM, Cruser D, Podawiltz A, Mummert DI, Jones H, Mummert ME. Psychological stress and the cutaneous immune response: roles of the HPA axis and the sympathetic nervous system in atopic dermatitis and psoriasis. Dermatol Res Pract. 2012;2012:403908.
31. Saatcioglu F. Regulation of gene expression by yoga, meditation and related practices: A review of recent studies. Asian J Psychiatr. 2013;6:74-7.
32. Ornish D, Magbanua MJ, Weidner G, Weinberg V, Kemp C, Green C, et al. Changes in prostate gene expression in men undergoing an intensive nutrition and lifestyle intervention. Proc Natl Acad Sci USA. 2008;105:8369-74.
33. Shanafelt TD, Hasan O, Dyrbye LN, Sinsky C, Satele D, Sloan J, et al. Changes in Burnout and Satisfaction With Work-Life Balance in Physicians and the General US Working Population Between 2011 and 2014. Mayo Clin Proc. 2015;90(12): 1600-13.

264

CHAPTER

Wellness among Physicians

Anubha Srivastava, Anurag Varma

ABSTRACT

The ever increasing challenges of medical profession and for the physicians, who are at its pinnacle as healers, have paradoxically put them increasingly toward the risk of exhaustion and poor well-being. The pressure of dealing with illness and death and the ever increasing workload and demands of a materialistic society coupled with daily advancements and in age of information technology is bringing new challenges, in terms of hostile work environment, challenges to their professional judgment and competence as well as doctors being managed by corporates. This has thrown the profession and the medical personal in a conundrum and fine tuning yourself with the changing social structure and public expectations have increasingly brought out what we now have started realizing is physician burnout.

Traditionally, medical healthcare professional used to feel proud in working in extremely tiring hours and inconducive environment; we would also emphasize this to our colleagues, juniors, and students and expect them to do the same. News of colleagues having sudden cardiac events and sometimes jolted by physician suicide and dropouts, we are reluctantly realizing that another pandemic is fast spreading; sadly, it is still neglected topic of physicians own well-being. This is all the more important because healthy physicians will be able to promote better healthcare rather than compromised and distressed physicians. Physician burnout may have devastating effect on cost and quality of healthcare, especially in modern era of medicolegal implications, digital information, and artificial intelligence bringing more scrutiny and social and legal pressure with worsening doctor–patient relationship contributing to a vicious cycle of healers becoming health seekers.

INTRODUCTION

Wellness does not mean absence of disease. It can be defined as an individual's or a group's perception of their lives; it can be termed as presence of positive emotions and moods such as contentment and happiness along with absence of negative emotions such as depression and anxiety. It is a sense of fulfillment, satisfaction, and feeling good. The concept of well-being is always neglected and it took a pandemic for physicians to realize the serious health consequences of burnout, exacerbation of substance abuse, and depression leading even to suicide.

A cross-sectional multicenter study done by Geeta et al. in 2020 showed that overall, 52.9% of the participants had the risk of psychological distress that needed further evaluation; further, the study pointed out what we already know and have been neglecting for so long that the *risk* of psychological distress was significantly associated with longer work hours (≥ 8 hours a day and with poor income ≥ 20,000). This negative attribute may hamper heathcare delivery and harm doctor–patient interactions. A 2021 review article in Lancet highlighted physician burnout and further eluding the concept which was first described by Freudenberger and been made more widely known by Maslach. In 2019, the World Health Organization (WHO) further described burnout in the 11th revision of the International Classification of Diseases as a syndrome (not as an illness or health condition) resulting from "workplace stress that has not been successfully managed." They have described burnout as primarily a social and organizational problem, not an individual one;

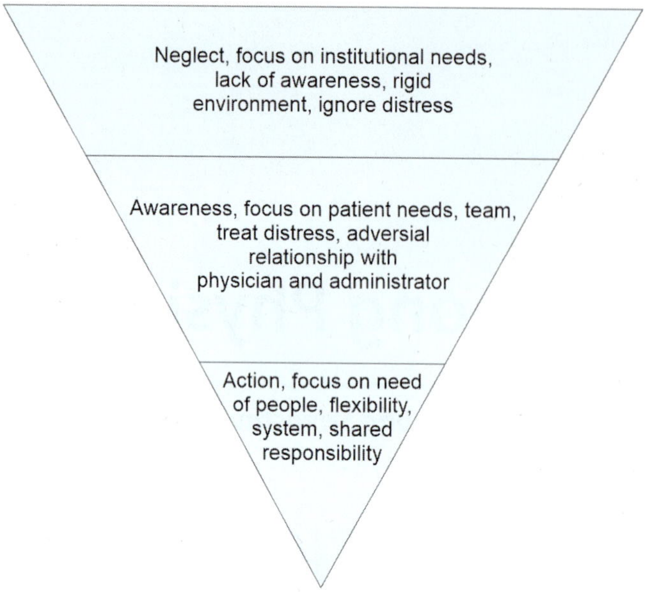

FIG. 1: Transition of awareness about well-being from neglect in past to distress in present and future interventions.

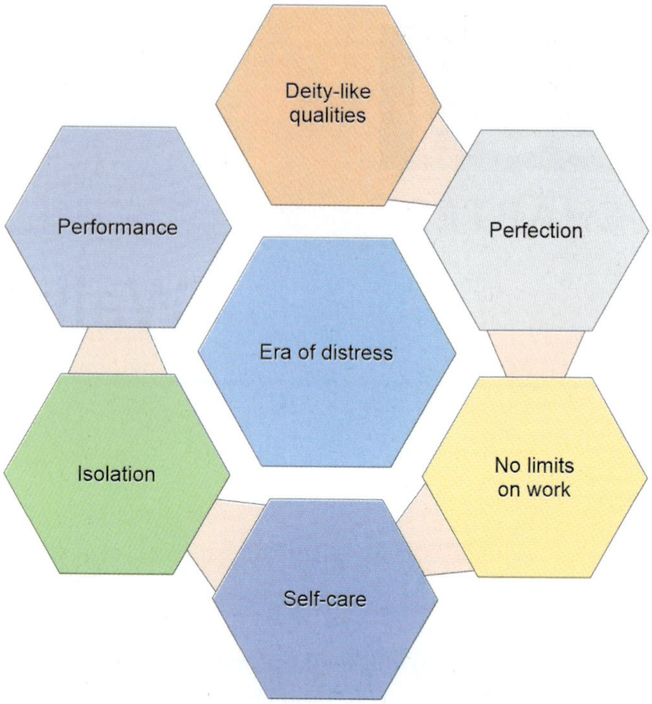

FIG. 2: Characteristics of past era.

however, it takes a collective as well as individual toll in terms of individual experiences, emotional exhaustion, cynicism, or feelings of being ineffective.

The challenges faced by physicians working in government setup may vary from the ones in private or corporate sector but moreover are similar ranging from poor infrastructure, tiring and undisciplined working hours, violence from patients and their relatives, and lack of appreciation. The pressure, especially on doctors, early in their careers of getting recognition and proving their worth makes them work harder and neglect a balanced lifestyle; this sets a template ultimately leading to array of lifestyle disorders and mental exhaustion.

Figure 1 shows the transition of awareness about well-being from neglect in past to distress in present and future interventions.

PAST TRADITION

This was a phase of lack of awareness or even deliberate neglect of physician distress and was even looked upon as weakness. The physicians were expected to go through arduous training and work environment in short work as superhumans. The medical school training was of uncompromising work environment with unlimited consecutive working hours, lack of sleep rest or breaks, and expectations to perform with unwavering excellence; those unable were labeled as uncommitted or weak. Yesteryears physicians were dedicated to their work at expense of their health and had little to do at home front and outside hospital responsibilities and recreation. It is always expected for a physician to be god like, omnipresent, omniscient, and to be able to overcome every deficiency of the healthcare delivery system to ensure optimal care for patients under any circumstance without any consideration of his own personal well-being. Institutional needs were prioritized above patients and clinician's need. **Figure 2** demonstrates characteristics of past era.

PRESENT ERA

There were increasing number of studies highlighting the concern of burnout, occupational stress, substance abuse, and even suicide among medical students. This negative wellness affected the patient care, medical errors, and led to patient dissatisfaction. The focus is on enhancement of concept of "triple aim of healthcare," i.e., better patient care, reduced cost, and health of elderly; we have not yet moved to the "quadruple aim," i.e., to include clinician's well-being along with the previous three. With more women joining healthcare force now has come a need of work–life balance, the openness, and acceptance of our personal vulnerabilities both physical and mental health and the concept of well-being and need for more and more physicians to identify and work toward it.

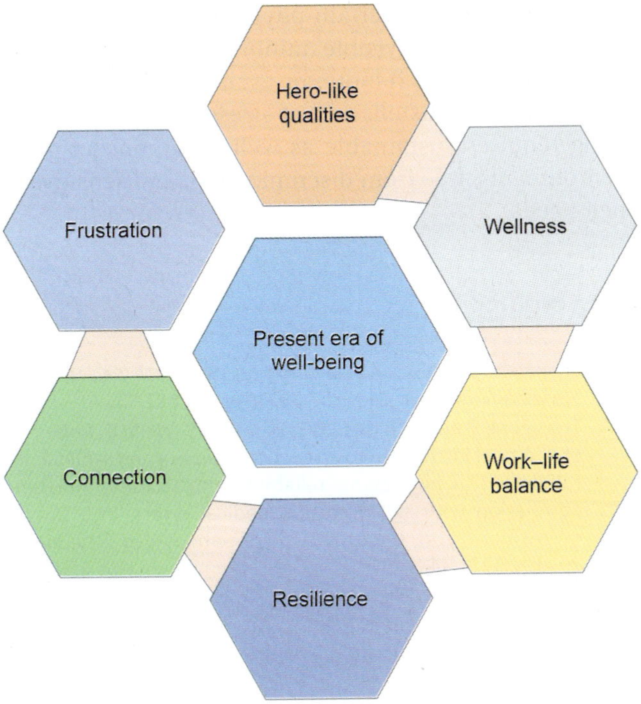

FIG. 3: The characteristics of present era.

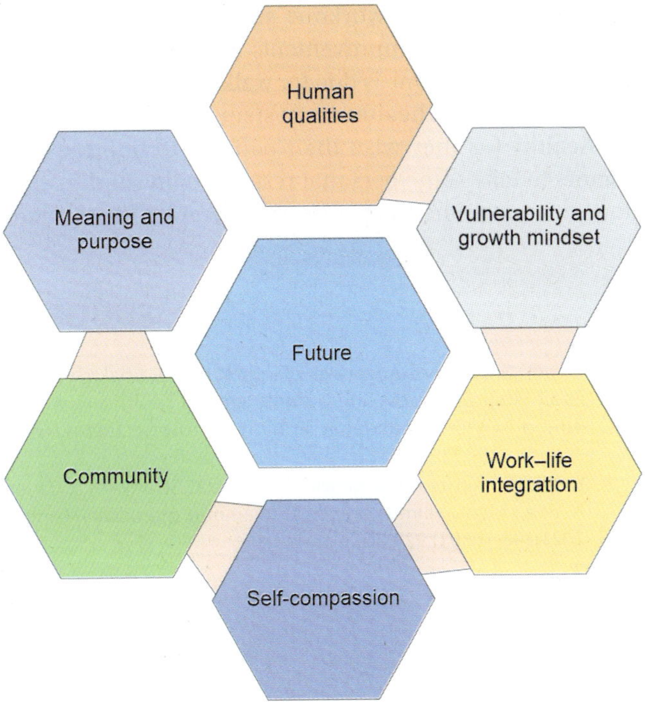

FIG. 4: Future attributes for well-being.

The enhancement of technology in healthcare has become a versatile tool for patient care, and health apps are used for healthcare and health promotion. There still lies apathy both on administrative and government levels, which needs to be changed in the near future **(Fig. 3)**.

FUTURE ERA

The loss of lives of innumerable physicians and mental stress to many in COVID-19 pandemic led to the paradigm shift in realization of occupational stress and need of conducive environment, holiday breaks, regular exercise, meditation and yoga, role of spirituality similar limitations and special requirements in addition to as in other profession for physician well-being. There is acceptance, realization and a mindset of physician well-being responsibility lies both in individuals and in the healthcare system.

The WHO has defined the term burnout and put it as distinct from depression and have now many validated measurements tools and scales for burnout which measure burnout and professional fulfillment in physicians they should be used and would be useful both at an individual and institutional level. There is administrative level change in leadership looking for wellness of physicians and preventing occupational distress.

There has been advocation of flexibility in practice environments which should help enable us to fulfill both personal and professional commitments. There is need of diversity, equity, and inclusion of wellness in our profession and to acknowledge that physicians too are human being and can make mistakes and not perfect are vulnerable and should support one another **(Fig. 4)**.

This change needs to start from early years of clinical training. The teaching of commitment to patients, needs, services, altruism along with realities of human limitation, appropriate working hours, work-life integration and attention to personal needs are part of professionalism. The effort to change professional culture from perfectionism to cultural excellence along with self-compassion and growth should be the motto.

CONCLUSION

We are now shifting from past era of ignorance and neglect to an era of awareness and insight, so leading institutions should be taking lead in implementation. Organizations as well as individuals should be committing for all healthcare workers' well-being.

Physician wellness is a shared responsibility among practitioners, organization, and administration. Promotion of wellness should be a multifaceted approach, although various researchers have found this gap and have also emphasized tools in literature but its implementation is still lacking. Addressing well-being in an organization will be instrumental, like taking transformational steps with relaxed environments, friendly working hours, better recreation facilities, workout stations, availability of nutritious food and improvements in overall quality may pave the way. The time is due for walking the talk.

The vision of a healthcare system, where the doctors are healthy (as they wish their patients to be), requires doctors to take some personal responsibility, and institutions to create nurturing environments. Also, institutions must recognize that certain physicians—women, those from visible and invisible minority groups, or those practicing in rural, remote, or even underserved areas face a unique constellation of stressors, so their well-being requires sustainable as well as supportive work environments, free from discrimination, and sensitive to their needs.

SUGGESTED READINGS

1. Menon GR, Yadav J, Aggarwal S, Singh R, Kaur S, Chakma T, et al. Psychological distress and burnout among healthcare worker during COVID-19 pandemic in India-A cross-sectional study. PLoS One. 2022;17(3).
2. Harvey SB, Epstein RM, Glozier N, Petrie K, Strudwick J, Gayed A, et al. Mental illness and suicide among physicians. Lancet. 2021;398(10303):920-30.
3. Shanafelt TD. Physician well-being 2.0: Where are we and where are we going? Mayo Clin Proc. 2021;96(10):2682-93.
4. Trockel M, Bohman B, Lesure E, Hamidi MS, Welle D, Roberts L, et al. A brief instrument to assess both burnout and professional fulfillment in physicians: reliability and validity, including correlation with self-reported medical errors, in a sample of resident and practicing physicians. Acad Psychiatry. 2018;42(1):11-24.

265

CHAPTER

Doctor versus Doctor

Jagdeep Chugh, Jyoti Chugh

ABSTRACT

We, the doctors, were and still are the most respectable people in society. With time, this respect is weaning off due to many reasons. We may not be fighting openly, but some fire is always simmering amongst ourselves. There are a number of reasons that are stopping us to be recognized as a big force. A few causes are division on many lines, open criticism and demeaning of colleagues, greed, lack of respect for seniors and juniors, and finally, power and politics. The respect, money, and resources which our counterparts enjoy in the west are much more than what we get here. Our clinical experience far exceeds the west and so, our decision-making, diagnosis, and management are much more precise.

INTRODUCTION

We, the doctors, are healers for the masses, but our profession is ailing from many diseases. The causes are external and internal. We are a divided lot and we cannot fight the external forces till we are all united. The first step for this is to identify the internal pathogens, do some introspection, and adopt remedial measures.

DOCTORS VERSUS NON-DOCTORS

Doctors are a big divided lot. They are first classified into allopathic and nonallopathic. Allopathic doctors are MBBS and above. Nonallopathic doctors are Bachelor of Ayurvedic and Homeopathic Medicine, i.e., Bachelor of Homeopathic Medicine and Surgery (BHMS), Bachelor in Unani Medicine and Surgery (BUMS), and Bachelor of Ayurveda, Medicine, and Surgery (BAMS). Then there are non-doctor doctors—these are physiotherapists, naturopaths, faith healers, quacks, chemists, etc. They prefix *doctor* in front of their names and real doctors are defamed by their misdeeds. Many a times, a few PhDs who prefix as doctors, project themselves as healers or take undue advantage by projecting themselves as clinicians. Allopathic doctors are further divided as per education status—graduates or postgraduates or divided into general practitioner, specialist, or super specialists. These are further divided as per area of specialization. Clinical or nonclinical is another subset. There is another subgroup of government or semi-government, charitable, private, or working in corporate. We are also divided as per alumnae or state. There is a vertical split group called 'ladies' doctors'. This division between doctors plays a very crucial role in many instances.

DOCTOR VERSUS DOCTOR

Interprofessional relationship or rivalry is a very controversial topic. We always feel that we doctors are a big family and always consider that giving care and respect to fellow doctors is a moral responsibility. There is always some discordance in the family and there are a few dear friends we are not happy with. Following are a few words of caution, precaution, and scope for improvement.

Criticize

There are many doctors who criticize other doctors or those who instigate patients against their colleagues openly. At times, it is seen that the cause of many litigations is the instigation by another doctor. There is generally some medical brain behind every litigation or complaint. They have a tendency to change the medicines immediately, even if medicines are rightly prescribed and no change is required.

Demeaning

A few dear friends find pleasure in saying that I have taught him or he is too junior to me. How can he write this treatment or this prescription? It cannot be him or this does not seem like his prescription. Very good treatment but he should have gone for XYZ regime or a cheaper or better option. At least, he should have done this test. Even a crooked smile is enough to cause irreparable damage. It is not graceful.

Unsolicited Calls

Some doctors call you repeatedly to enquire about the patients, especially sick patients or patients admitted to intensive care. Many of them have not even seen the face of the patient or are not aware of the complications. Moreover, at times they try to dictate the line of treatment and end up telling the doctor: 'Tell the patient that I called you'. Most irritating is that even when they are aware of the 'poor prognosis', they will ask 'when is this patient going to get discharged?' We should stop calling other doctors to know the condition of the patients we have not seen or referred or are related to us.

Free Treatment

Many doctors send all their distant relatives to a doctor and expect that relatives should be treated on priority and that too for free. Making payments should be done for all except self and dependent family members. Many doctors seek a sincere opinion about their relatives or acquaintances after posting reports on WhatsApp. It should be discouraged since the doctor has not seen the patient at any time and it is difficult to comment just on report basis. For a sincere advice, three things are essential—physical presence of patient, all investigation reports, and payments. Nothing is free in this world. Sending reports on WhatsApp and asking for opinion is a poor practice unless that is discussed among colleagues.

Professional Courtesy

Although most doctors do not charge from their colleagues, but charging or not for the consultation will be an individual choice. It again depends upon many factors such as total amount and expenses involved, time spent, proximity or closeness between the two doctors, nature of job, and the working culture. But if a senior or elderly colleague comes to the outpatient department (OPD), then preference, respect, and some extra time must be given. It is lacking many a times. There was an old school of thought which was that nothing should be charged from other doctors, the new school of thoughts says that all should be charged and we are the generation which is caught between these two thoughts. Charging your colleagues for services rendered by you can be acceptable but neglecting them whether charging or not is simply a deplorable practice.

Megalomania

Those who while climbing the ladder took professional help or seeked referrals from other doctors and now when they are established, they easily forget them. Some big doctors in big hospitals do not acknowledge other doctors. Some have a feeling that they are bigger than other doctors or bigger than the association—that "*megalomaniac*" feeling. It hurts when they charge and do not give the desired care. Some discounts on consultations and procedures should be considered positively.

It has been seen that some of the treating doctors (who are caring for one of your acquaintances) may act erratically if you attempt to reach him. If a politician, official, administrator, or another person in a position of authority calls the same treating doctor, he will behave much more humbly and tenderly.

There is a good lot of junior doctors or the general practitioners who give free consultations, home visits, and time to other colleagues, but when they go to some big consultants, they do not get their due. Here comes the role of 'empathy'.

Misuse

Some doctors tend to misuse your service on odd days or odd times or when they are in a 'soup' as if it is their birthright but refer their own patients to other doctors or your competitors. A few botch up most of their cases and expect others to bail them out every time. It is unpalatable.

Greed

Those who send you the patients expect some gains, cuts, or referrals in return. There are a few doctors who are very happy to distribute the bounty and encourage cut practice. This is the main cause of the thriving of quacks.

Power

There are our doctor colleagues who have stepped up on our shoulders and have become politicians. Another group has gone into Indian Administrative Services. Their attitude has changed toward their ex-colleagues or for doctors in general. They consider themselves above the rest and are rarely helpful. This was seen recently during confrontation with some '*guru*' or during tabulation of law against 'prevention of violence against doctors'. Hardly any doctor parliamentarian supported it.

Some doctors have become administrators or chairpersons in corporate or big hospitals. We understand they have their loyalty toward the organization and they sing their song. Their aim and goals are now only money and manipulations. They are hardly concerned about the issues and welfare of doctors working there. They can create inter-doctor rivalry, divide the medical fraternity to maintain their supremacy. Most doctors speak in hushed tones and the human resource (HR) department is loud and overbearing despite knowing nothing about medicine and its intricacies.

My Patient

Some doctors fight for the possession of patients, 'he is my patient; no he is my patient'. We all must realize that patients are never loyal to one doctor and moreover, the patients are not their property. Healthy competition between two colleagues is a good sign, but professional rivalry should be avoided.

Politics

Nowadays, the doctors are divided on lines of political parties, be it national politics or elections of our own medical associations. They look for instances to insult their colleagues on petty politics. When it comes to election of office bearers, in medical associations, the elections are not on credential basis but by hook or crook, along with internal arrangements to retain power at the secretariat level and capture office. Award distribution in conferences or otherwise has a biased approach to own favorite doctors or on the basis of 'you scratch my back and I will yours'.

The politics should not spoil your relations and politicians should not be able to divide you.

Nursing Homes

The doctors who are running their nursing homes try to fleece working and visiting doctors. They take more work, pay less, and do not provide basic facilities to their resident doctors. When it comes to visiting consultants, there is a big disparity between what is charged and what is paid. Seniors must see that their juniors should also flourish.

Medical Councils

State medical councils were built after protests by our colleagues to eradicate quacks, streamline the modern medical system and improve the overall ethical professional scenario, but the outcome was adverse for many doctors. It boomeranged and many doctors were harassed in spite of medical councils full of doctors.

Even the Medical Council of India (MCI), which was an autonomous body and governed by doctors, was dissolved due to mismanagement, internal politics, and irregularities in working. It was again our mistake and the outcome is unfortunate. Now, it became the National Medical Council (NMC) and its bill was tabled and passed by the Parliament in 3 days without any amendment. No suggestions or advice was taken from our esteemed medical associations.

Unity

There is no one platform where the doctors can unite or they can be brought under one umbrella. There is lack of young and dynamic leaders who can lead the doctors from front rather than the old leaders who have selfish interests and lack both will and energy to change the scenario. They always follow '*divide and rule*'.

The government also knows that we are a divided lot and so does not give any attention. They know that in private practice, we have become so selfish that we will never put our shutters down continuously and unitedly even for 48 hours and the doctors working in corporate or government sectors do not have the guts to revolt. We have seen recently in two states where unity among doctors was able to bend the governments and soften their tough and dictatorial attitude. Now, it is time we should act as a trade union.

We should be alert that the persons who are not MBBS should not prefix *doctor* in front of their name. If they do, it should be reported immediately to association and medical councils and strict legal action should be initiated against them.

Real change minus manipulative politics among our own colleagues and doctors is required. It is the need of the hour. We should respect our junior doctors and let them rise. We should be practical and motivate young people to bring this change and stand beside them in their struggles.

Your respect and dignity are in your hands. You always have to *earn* your respect. The world is watching us, so we will have to change and develop new equations. Sooner or later, we will have to adapt to the new rules of the game. It will be a win–win situation for all of us. Without prejudices to one and all.

SUGGESTED READINGS

1. Lehmann C. (2021). Doctors Fight Unfair Payer Tactics; Is It Working? [online] Available from https://www.medscape.com/viewarticle/965357 [Last accessed January, 2024].
2. Weiss R. (1993). Doctors who fight over patients—literally. [online] Available from https://www.washingtonpost.com/archive/lifestyle/wellness/1993/12/21/doctors-who-fight-over-patients-literally/d3b8e5ff-1402-4dc9-a2ec-6c522555dfee/ [Last accessed January, 2024].

266 CHAPTER

Common Medical Errors: How to Avoid?

Mukesh K Sarna, Nipun Goel, Sudha Sarna

ABSTRACT

Medical errors pose a significant public health concern and pose a risk to patient safety. To address these issues, healthcare personnel must identify the underlying causes, develop solutions, and assess their effectiveness. Interprofessional collaboration is crucial for safe medication use and distribution, and a culture of safety prioritizing system improvement is essential. By understanding common medical mistakes and implementing strategies, healthcare professionals can enhance patient care and overall patient experience. Remember, do no harm and prioritize safety in healthcare.

INTRODUCTION

"Primum non nocere"
(Which means *"First do no harm"* is a Latin phrase, and is an important part of Hippocratic Oath.)

Healthcare is a privileged profession that offers doctors the opportunity to provide high-quality care and affordable treatments for their patients. However, mistakes can occur, causing unintentional harm to patients. Medical errors are a taboo subject in our community, but this chapter discusses common mistakes and how to minimize or avoid them to improve practice. By understanding the most common medical mistakes and implementing strategies to minimize or avoid them, healthcare professionals can enhance their patient care and overall patient experience.

DEFINITION

A medical error is an unplanned action that can result in an unexpected outcome. The definition of a medical error specifically mentions the primary areas where error can occur i.e., (omission, commission, planning, and execution). Whether it is obvious to the patient or not, it is an unintentional negative impact of treatment ('iatrogenesis') that can be avoided.

The National Coordinating Council for Medication Error Reporting and Prevention of the United States defines a medication error as 'any preventable event that may cause or lead to inappropriate medication use or patient harm while the medication is under the control of the healthcare professional, patient, or consumer'.

STATS AND EPIDEMIOLOGY

Medical errors are one of the most serious public health problems and can pose threat to patient safety.

According to research in John Hopkins Hospital, medical error is the third leading cause of death in the US after cancer and heart disease, and a study conducted by the National Academy of Sciences' Institute of Medicine in 2000, hospital errors cause up to 98,000 deaths annually in the United States. The study found that medical errors cause more death per year than road traffic accidents, acquired immunodeficiency syndrome (AIDS), and cancer of breast combined **(Fig. 1)**.

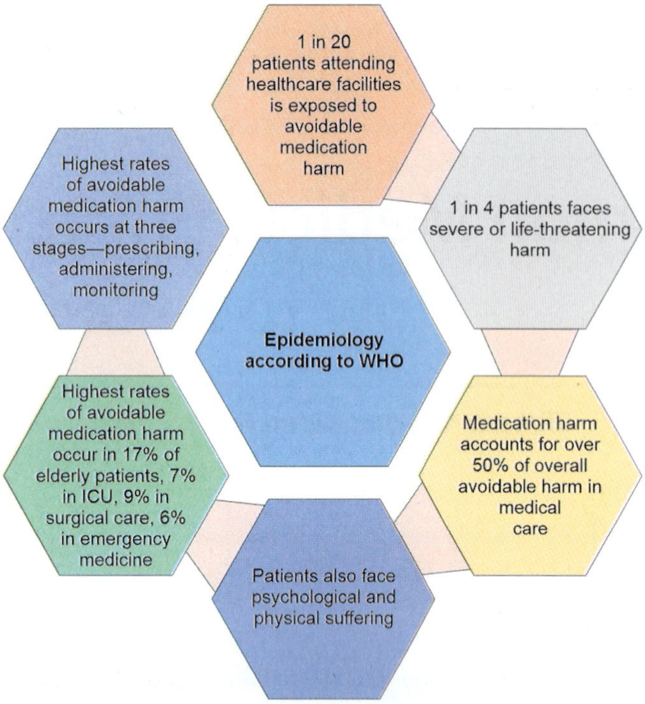

FIG. 1: Epidemiology by World Health Organization (WHO).
(ICU: intensive care unit)

CATEGORIES

Box 1 lists the categories of medical errors.

BOX 1: Categories.

- *Category A*: Event that potentially can cause error
- *Category B*: Error occurred but did not reach to the patient
- *Category C*: Error occurred and reached to the patient but did not cause any harm
- *Category D*: Error occurred and reached to the patient—requires monitoring to confirm whether it causes any harm or not
- *Category E*: Error occurred that causes temporary harm to the patient and requires intervention
- *Category F*: Error occurred that causes temporary harm to the patient resulting in initial/prolonged hospital stay
- *Category G*: Error that resulted in permanent harm to the patient
- *Category H*: Error that contributes to near death event or requires intervention to sustain life
- *Category I*: Error that resulted in patient's death

TYPES OF COMMON MEDICAL ERRORS/ FACTORS ASSOCIATED (TABLE 1)

Intensive Care Unit Errors

The goal in intensive care unit (ICU) for critically ill patients is to implement a wide range of therapies based on clinical condition of patient. Here are a few examples of typical therapeutic situations when doing more might be linked to a higher chance of unfavorable outcomes.

Fluid Overload

The basic treatment for hypovolemia, which commonly occurs due to blood loss or dehydration, is intravenous (IV) fluid therapy. Fluid overload can occur and can be dangerous because it results in edema. The most frequent negative outcomes are acute kidney injury (AKI), longer hospital stay, pulmonary edema, pleural effusion, more days spent on invasive mechanical ventilation (IMV), and higher mortality.

Over Sedation

The ICU routinely uses sedatives. Long-term sedation results in higher prevalence of delirium and prevents early recovery. Since they have been associated with worse outcomes, sedative medications like benzodiazepines are not advised as first-line drugs.

Absurd Use of Antibiotics

Sepsis is the most common diagnoses in ICU. It has been proven that receiving antibiotics quickly (within an hour) leads to greater results. However, some people do not need antibiotics since they do not have an active infection. Misuse of antibiotics can cause arrhythmias (azithromycin), seizures (carbapenems), mild-to-severe gastrointestinal problems (such *Clostridioides difficile* infection), and other consequences.

Prophylaxis of Gastrointestinal Ulcers

Proton-pump inhibitors (PPIs) and histamine 2-receptor antagonists (H2A) are commonly used in critically ill patients to prevent peptic ulcers by reducing acid production. But, reducing acid secretion could promote lung and intestinal infections because it serves as a barrier to outside germs.

Inappropriate Blood Transfusions

There are specific indications for blood transfusion in patients, such as hemorrhagic shock, severe anemia, or coagulopathy. Longer hospital stays, transfusion-

TABLE 1: Common medical errors/factors associated.

Intensive care unit	Nursing	Surgical	Medication	Technical	Communication	Patient-based issues	Work environment
• Fluid overload • Over sedation • Irrational use of antibiotics • Prophylaxis of gastrointestinal ulcers • Inappropriate blood transfusion • Abuse and misuse of laboratory test • Invasive monitoring • Malnutrition and overfeeding • Over treatment • Immobilization	• Less knowledge and training • Improper drug knowledge and lack of experience	• Wrong site surgery • Accidently leave something inside body after operation	• Similar sounding names of medicine • Labeling and packaging • Monitoring of patient (depends on doctor's practice, patient)	• Difficulty in generating first prescription (type of drug and its pick list, standard dose, regimen, missed dose alert) • Difficulty in generating correct follow-up prescription • Inaccurate patient record • Lack for proper design that promotes human error	• Lack of communication among healthcare workers and of them with attendants of patient • Limited communication with supportive care team • Not taking seriously the advice of secondary care team	• Lack of knowledge of patient • Insufficient perception of risk • Patient characteristics, i.e., personality of the patient, patient and their attendant's literacy and language barrier • Intricated clinical case	• Overworked or fatigue healthcare staff • Emotional health issue • Physical health issue • Time pressure and work overload • Distraction and cessation of work (by both staff and patient) • Insufficient resources • Lack of standardized protocols for the procedure • Issue with the work environment (temperature, ventilation)

related acute lung injury (TRALI), transfusion-associated circulatory overload (TACO), and higher mortality are all associated with unnecessary blood transfusion.

Abuse and Misuse of Laboratory Tests

Blood tests are now standard for ICU patients. Daily blood sampling is unjustified. It causes needless removal of 40–70 mL of blood every 24 hours. This causes a decrease in hemoglobin of about 1–1.2 g/day, which may lead to iatrogenic anemia.

Invasive Monitoring

To monitor the patient's macrohemodynamics (heart output, systemic vascular resistances, volume status, etc.), and respiratory status (extravascular lung water and pulmonary vascular permeability index), patient requires the insertion of a central venous line (jugular or subclavian) and an arterial line (typically femoral, brachial, or radial). It has not been proven that using these techniques can decrease mortality. In addition to the dangers of central venous catheterization, installing arterial lines has occasionally resulted in thrombosis and other vascular issues.

Malnutrition and Overfeeding

Despite this, it has been shown that extended fasting and malnutrition in hospitals are associated with poor outcomes and increased mortality.

Less protein consumption is associated with greater infection and death rates in ICU patients. The daily protein requirement (0.8–1.2 g/kg) of patients should be calculated. Intakes > 1.2 g protein/kg/day have not been proven to improve outcomes.

Overtreatment

Critically ill patients with severe pathologies complicated by irreversible organ failure or chronic terminal illnesses are frequently given supportive therapies like sedation, fluid therapy, vasopressors, inotropes, blood products, nutrition, antibiotics, and other drugs, which will not increase their chance of survival but instead lengthen their hospital stays and result in an inefficient use of resources (laboratory and imaging).

Immobilization

Patients with serious illnesses typically remain motionless. The prolonged immobility could have adverse effects. During the first 10 days, the patient starts to lose muscle mass and bone density. The patient's heart, lungs, and brain may suffer if they spend more time in bed. It could lead to venous embolism risk, pressure ulcers, bed sores, and weakness (polyneuropathy or myopathy). Early mobilization has several benefits, like increased muscle strength and increased patient independence. The technique should be carried out by trained physical therapists. Always take safety precautions and monitor the patient's vital signs as well as their cardiovascular, neurological, and pulmonary condition.

Too Long or Too Short Hospital Stay

Despite the fact that being in the hospital is unpleasant, the patient should not be discharged before he is ready. Studies show that patients who leave the hospital too quickly have a higher chance of developing serious complications later on. But patient should not stay too long either. Otherwise that is related to more infections and other problems.

Nursing Errors (Table 2)

Nursing errors can occur at various levels and due to various reasons.

Surgical Errors

Failure to get Informed Consent

This surgical error occurs most frequently. It is the surgeon's duty to inform the patient of any potential surgical issues. The surgeon should try to be upfront and honest with the patient about topics relevant to their care in order to prevent confusion and self-indiscrimination.

Malfunctioning of Medical Computers and Equipment

A surgeon cannot operate with damaged tools and equipment. It might harm the patient permanently, which would be medical malpractice.

Wrong Site Surgery

This could happen as a result of the operating room's layout, distractions, or being late. One thing that may be done is to make sure that the right mark on the patient's body is designated before the operation.

What is Left Behind?

Although unlikely, it is possible for the surgical team to unintentionally left something inside the patient's body, such as a sponge or instrument, which could lead to the emergence of a new, more serious issue, such as an abscess, infection, or inflammation.

TABLE 2: Nursing errors.

Work space	• Sense of urgency • Instructor not readily available • Increased number of patient to cover • Shortcuts by staff making it look acceptable and false vitals charting and other parameters • Intimidation by instructor • Lack of familiarity with unit or floor or other staff • Increased number of medications to give
Work culture	• Poor communication between staff and with doctor/instructor • Staff allows the undertraining staff to give medications • Reporting and correction was inconsistent • Varying leniency in following hospital protocols between units • Adequate directions were not given from instructor • Definition of medical error was not standardized and understood by staff
Education	• Staff not coached in situation where hierarchical statutes exist • Importance of self-evaluation and root cause analysis after error occur was not emphasized • Risk of multiple manifestations of shortcuts and their consequences were not reiterated • Medication error teaching does not focus on multilevel opportunity for prevention (indirect focus on blame of the individual)
Personal factor	• Not considering the legal implications of action • Physical state was abnormal (tired and emotionally distracted) • Standard protocols not followed • Doer personality, quick to act without thinking fully • Concerned about time • Not understanding the importance of pausing and critically thinking before acting

Clumsy Surgery

If the required standard of care is not properly followed, the patient could get a serious injury. Some injuries, like scarring, are essentially cosmetic, and serious infection, organ damage, and nerve damage are all possible life-threatening side effects from poor surgical outcomes. The vascular system may also be affected, leading to internal bleeding, hematomas, and possibly lethal blood clots [deep vein thrombosis (DVTs)].

Unnecessary Operations

When a patient is exposed to the risks of a procedure that is not recommended, it is considered medical malpractice.

Anesthesia Errors

- Ignoring the patient's past or present situation
- Sedation mistakes and anesthesia awareness
- Anesthesia mistakes associated with pregnancy
- Overdosage of anesthesia
- Using the incorrect anesthetic agent.

Outpatient Department Errors

Errors in Laboratory Tests

Sometimes the appropriate test is not requested or requested inaccurately or the results are misread.

Delay in Prescribing Medication/Incorrect Medications Prescribed

Medical errors could be in giving the wrong medication, or in wrong dosage, or starting treatment later than necessary. It may also occur if a prescription is given or ordered without consideration for the patient's allergies or potential drug combinations.

Misdiagnosis or Delayed Diagnosis

A delayed or incorrect identification of a medical illness may lead to harm or death. Medical negligence occurs when a doctor makes a mistake in diagnosing a problem that should have been diagnosed and the patient's condition worsens as a consequence of the incorrect treatment, delayed therapy, or no treatment at all.

Failing in Follow-up of the Patient

Medical malpractice may occur if a patient is not followed up with. If the doctor or healthcare institution (such as a hospital or doctor's office) fails to promptly communicate with the patient about appointments, orders, concerns about the patient's well-being, test results, and other information, failure to follow-up can turn into negligence.

Ignoring Patient's Symptoms or Concerns

Healthcare professionals have a duty to listen to their patients. The doctor must take patient complaints seriously and investigate the complaints and symptoms, even if they seem to be common.

Pathological Errors

Pathological errors can occur at various phases of laboratory analysis **(Table 3)**.

TABLE 3: Pathological errors can occur at various phases of laboratory analysis.

Preanalytical phase	Analytical phase	Postanalytical phase
• Delivery and registration of material/sample • Incomplete/error in registering sample • Registration details do not correspond to specimen/sample • Sample quantity does not correspond to registration details • Specimen without previous marking/ incorrect orientation • Incorrect anatomical site • Incomplete/inaccurate clinical information • No material in sample sent • Inappropriate packaging/fixing conditions • Specimen loss in laboratory • Integrity not preserved • Malfunction of equipment • Freezing error and registering error	• Quality of the slides • Repetition of coloration • Foreign tissue in the specimen • Incorrect block identification • Interpretation errors • Delayed results • Work environment (e.g., refrigeration failure and other equipment failures)	• Correlation errors of freezing biopsy with conventional histology • Specimen discarded during routine examination • Patients exchange/report exchange • Transcription errors • Delayed results • Malfunction of laboratory information systems

TABLE 4: Types of errors in pathology.

Operator and method	Machine reagent and environment	Sample	Management
• Attention of operator • Training, experience, and subspecialization • Competency and work load • Delay in report • Accuracy and report • Completeness	• Error in selecting program • Reagent—calibration, expiration, storage, preparation, degradation • Inadequate maintenance • IT problems • Dirty optics • Temperature, dust, and humidity • Water quality • Insect and rodents	• Incorrect fixation, transport and storage • Artifacts caused by procedure • Loss or change of specimen • Patient and sample identification • Bubble in slide • Fungal contamination of sample	• Inability in use of finance resources • Acquisition poor quality reagent and machines • Inappropriate management of human resources

The types of errors in pathology are given in **Table 4**.

Technical Errors

Technical glitch can involve machinery like ventilators, infusion pumps, and monitors. The main cause of technical errors is failure to maintain the equipment and improper service of it. Errors can occur in computer-generated dispensing orders and laboratory data generation and interpretation.

Medication Errors/Dispensing Errors

The various medication errors/dispensing errors are shown in **Box 2**.

BOX 2: Medication errors/dispensing errors.

Types of drug errors

- *Prescribing error*: Elements of good prescribing practice were observed and each medication prescribed was evaluated for compliance with pharmacy legislation as stipulated in good pharmacy practice, i.e., the correct name, dosage, units, route, frequency, and duration of treatment.

Preparation

- *Wrong drug*: Preparation of a drug which differs from that prescribed
- *Wrong dose/time*: Preparation of a dose that is higher than, or less than, the amount prescribed (+10%), > 1 hour difference between scheduled time and time administered

Continued

Continued

- *Wrong dosage form*: Formulation of drug deviates from that prescribed
- *Deteriorated drug*: Preparation of a drug that has the physical expired or for which or chemical dosage-form integrity has been compromised
- *Incorrect duration/frequency*: Medication administered for longer duration than was prescribed/not stopped or administered at incorrect intervals
- *Wrong preparation technique/mislabeling/failure to administer*: Inappropriate procedure or improper technique in the preparation of a drug (compared to the manufacturer's instructions or hospital policy, including wrong diluent, wrong solvent, wrong volume, possible incompatibility)

Administration

- *Omission*: Failure to administer an ordered dose to a patient
- *Unordered drug*: Administration to the patient of nonprescribed medication
- *Wrong administration technique*: Inappropriate procedure or improper technique in the administration of a drug (rate, incompatibility, route dose (+10%) if prepared with correct dose; a rate error was identified if administration took <3 or >5 minutes (for a bolus dose) or 15% shorter/longer than the required infusion time (for an infusion dose)
- *Dispensing errors*: Any unintended deviation from an interpretable written prescription or medication order, labeling errors; any unintended deviation from professional or regulatory references, or guidelines affecting dispensing procedures, is also considered as dispensing error

Communication Errors

Communication Error between Staff

Communication failure most commonly occurs when there is change of shift of the staff. The chances of medical errors increase manifold when an untrained staff gave insufficient and unclear information during transition. Poor communication may cause patients to receive wrong medication or in wrong dose or even no medication, all of which may have a detrimental result.

Poor Communication between Doctor and Staff

When patient's critical information, condition, or symptom is not properly conveyed to the doctor and the seriousness of the patient's condition is not grasped, it might result in inappropriate decision resulting in less effective treatment.

Effects of Poor Communication between Clinicians and Patients

Effective communication is important between clinician and patient. Doctor needs to know about any significant past history, personnel history, previous history of hospitalization, etc. At the same time, he has to counsel the attendants about condition of patient. Poor communication can lead to misconceptions about follow-up instructions, not understanding order written in prescription which can risk patient's life.

Inadequate Information Flow

In every healthcare setup, flow of information is important, especially between various service areas. Lack of information flow can result in inadequate communication of test results, inadequate coordination, incomplete orders for transfer, etc.

Workplace Errors/Inadequate Policies

These include risky behaviors by healthcare workers, using medication without knowing much about the medicine, reluctance to ask for help, failure to educate patients, and not communicating important information such as allergies. Understaffing, sleep deprivation and environmental factors, like facilities and air conditioning, affect patient safety.

Monitoring Errors

Monitoring errors take place when patients are not properly watched, before and after receiving a medication. It entails, ordering serum medication levels but failing to review them, failing to react to values outside of the therapeutic range, failing to order medicine levels when necessary, and providing an antihypertensive medication but neglecting to check blood pressure. A monitoring error has happened, for instance, if a patient is started on warfarin therapy but proper blood tests are not done to gauge the patient's reaction, leading to a hemorrhage that is life-threatening.

EXAMPLES OF COMMON MEDICAL ERRORS

Table 5 shows the examples of common medical errors.

TABLE 5: Common medical errors.

Rule-based mistakes		
Examples	**Level of treatment**	**Result**
Giving cardiac massage in a patient who has fainted	Decision of treatment	Can cause panic in family if not informed by someone about what has happened and what we are doing
Giving oral treatment to a patient of dysphagia	Prescription writing error	Aspiration or treatment failure
Prescribing a short course of antibacterial treatment	Cessation of treatment	Under treatment of infection
Giving amoxicillin to a patient of sore throat	Treatment error	Rash in patient of glandular fever
Not giving alendronate tablet with water	Drug administration	Esophageal damage
Giving prolonged unnecessary antibiotics	Cessation of treatment	Bacterial resistance
Giving diclofenac injection intramuscularly in thigh	Drug administration	Skin and tissue necrosis
Memory-based lapses/errors		
Examples	**Level of error**	**Result**
Overlooking that the patient is allergic to penicillin	Deciding to treat	Anaphylaxis
Forgetting to wipe the rubber of a drug vial	Preparing for administering the drug	Sepsis/Infection
Not arranging a warfarin clinic appointment	Monitoring error	Uncontrolled warfarin-induced bleeding
Omitting a date on which to stop treatment	Prescription writing	Drug poisoning or unrequired treatment
Neglecting to check the allergy wristband	Administrative error	Anaphylaxis
Action based errors/slips		
Example	**Level of error**	**Result**
Serving out the wrong drug/strength/concentration	Dispensing error	Under treatment of disease or drug toxicity
Intravenous injection given extra vascularly	Drug administration	Tissue necrosis, pain, loss of drug efficacy
Lack of knowledge to measure BP correctly	Monitoring error	Overtreatment or undertreatment
Failing to mix infusion to which potassium was added	Preparing for administration	Hyperkalemia
Mistakenly writing the wrong drug name or writing illegibly	Prescription writing error	Under treatment or toxicity
Stopping warfarin treatment after 3 months for recurrent DVT (deep vein thrombosis)	Cessation of treatment	Recurrent thromboembolism
Knowledge-based mistake		
Examples	**Level of treatment**	**Result**
Lack of knowledge of the interaction between warfarin and azapropazone	Prescription writing	Warfarin toxicity
Lack of knowledge that paraldehyde dissolves plastic syringes	Drug administration	Toxicity/Cancer
Neglecting that chloroform and chloroform water are different	Drug dispensing	Poisoning due to chloroform
Lack of knowledge of value of sodium bicarbonate in amitriptyline poisoning	Treatment decision	Death due to arrhythmia
Not aware of the course of the sciatic nerve	Drug Administration	Intramuscular injection causing sciatic nerve palsy
Giving amiodarone at the loading dose after 2 weeks	Treatment adjustment	Amiodarone-induced poisoning
Taking blood sample in a heparin tube for finding lithium concentration, not knowing that it contains lithium heparin	Monitoring error	Inaccurate lithium concentration

HOW TO AVOID ERRORS? POTENTIAL SOLUTIONS/MANAGEMENT

This section provides some possible ways to avoid medical errors that a healthcare staff can use to improve its patient safety.

Medication Reviews and Reconciliation

The practice of reviewing a patient's prescriptions in order to improve health outcomes and lessen drug-related problems is known as medication review. A clinician or a chemist should conduct the drug review.

Education

Education of patients and medical personnel is one of the most important steps to improve safety. Through educational activities, it is possible to improve the writing and dispensing of antibiotic prescriptions as well as physician behavior and adherence to guidelines.

Using Computerized Systems

Improving alert and prescription electronic systems. Computerized provider order input with decision support may concentrate on a small number of possibly inappropriate prescriptions; it is also more likely to be effective when it concentrates on clinically relevant warnings to reduce alert burden.

Prioritizing Areas for Quick Wins

Implement multifaceted approaches that combine community chemist involvement, medication reviews, health informatics, and education. When some drugs, such as warfarin, are prescribed and need ongoing monitoring, think about visiting specialized outpatient clinics.

Preventing Errors in the Intensive Care Unit

High-quality multidisciplinary management should be followed to reduce expenditures associated with treatment. Lessening or eliminating the patient's pain and suffering without resorting to useless treatments should be the aim of humanization and palliative care programs.

Focus on Making a Positive Work Environment

Strong leadership and a healthy workplace atmosphere are necessary for increasing safety of patient. To achieve this, an ecosystem must be established in which medical personnel and patients can express their worries about safety issues without fear of punishment or condemnation. We should promote a culture where risks are reported so to learn from them and stopping them from happening again. This highlights how important it is to set up feedback channels to support any improvements made in response to safety concerns. Practical steps to promote safety culture include leadership walk rounds, in which senior administrative and clinical leaders 'walk the floor' (in this example, visiting clinics and engaging with employees and patients about what is working well and what is not so well).

Use of Two-way Practice to Focus on Safety Issues

It comprises steps like audits and giving people a place to submit safety-related concerns, including frequent team meetings.

Measuring and Monitoring Safety of Patient

It includes having precise definitions of patient safety indicators that can be measured annually, setting up local or national incident reporting systems where data is regularly compiled, which can be used for further assessment and making of further policies to improve patient safety.

Maintenance of Data

High-quality data are needed to measure goals in improving patient safety. If accurate and comprehensive medical records are not maintained, it may likely result in omission and error. As health systems improve, clinical governance practices often become more sophisticated. This entails creating risk management policies and development strategies.

Focus on those at Higher Risk of Safety Incidents

In primary care, some patients are more prone to encounter safety issues. It includes young people, the elderly, those living in nursing homes or residential care facilities, and people with various illnesses. Focusing on them may improve the quality and safety of care by delivering more individualized care and promoting seamless transitions between care providers.

- Dissatisfaction on the part of physicians breeds poor clinical management as well as dissatisfaction and noncompliance among patients, and that the rapid turnover of unhappy doctors in offices and hospitals may lead to discontinuous, substandard medical care. In contrast, surveys administered within the past 10 years have shown that 30–40% of practicing physicians would not choose to enter the medical profession, if they were deciding on a career again, and an even higher percentage would not encourage their children to pursue a medical career.
- The past 30 years have witnessed both a rising trend of medical malpractice litigation and recurrent difficulties between physicians and their insurers. These events, for many practicing physicians, have merged into a single, continually escalating malpractice crisis repercussions. "Defensive medicine", a strategy of using tests and procedures primarily to thwart potential litigation rather than to advance the well-being of patients, is widely deployed as a growing blight on medical practice that raises healthcare costs, compromises the physician's professional integrity, and drives a wedge through the doctor–patient relationship. Although lawsuits have become common, doctors are not yet injured to their emotional punch. No matter what the background or outcome of the suit, physician-defendants routinely describe feelings of shame, self-doubt, and disillusion with medical practice that may persist for years.
- *Disparities in expectations*: These include the discrepancy between what patients demand from a doctor and what the doctor can actually accomplish, the discrepancy between standards set in a doctor's training and the compromises forced by practice, the discrepancy between how physicians practiced medicine 50 years ago and how physicians must practice today, and the frequent discrepancy between the wide-open promise of medical science and the limited results that individual doctors—whether hamstrung by the poverty of a developing country or by the bureaucratic tangles of a wealthy one—are able to achieve. For every failure to live up to goals and expectations, large and small, the doctors who responded to the editorial described feeling guilty, defensive, and estranged from colleagues and patients, often railing at the inadequacies of their local healthcare systems when the problems transcend those systems.
- "Doctors are assaulted from within by the impossibility of knowing everything they feel they have to know, and from without by a system that removes authority and forces adherence to conflicting allegiances." The public reacts with hostility. Says Lipp: "*Complaints about medicine...bombard the physician at every turn....Our fuzzy science isn't scientific enough, and our awkward art is not artful enough....The real world in which they function fails to support the inner sense of dedication which many doctors feel.*" Doctors who disappoint themselves, Lipp concludes, will inevitably disappoint their patients, too. Majority of doctors still take satisfaction in their work.
- Physicians muster nonprofessional sources of happiness instead, such as time with family and friends, exercise, good nutrition, and spiritual activity.
- Plethora of laws and regulations leads to red-tapeism, breed the corruption, or leads to assault on doctors and a sword always hangs on doctors' head.
- Doctors have to make quick decisions in seconds to save patients, this decision may be right/wrong. If it is wrong that is medical error in taking decisions not negligence but party always tries to prove it medical negligence.

SOCIAL DECLINE IF DOCTORS WORK UNDER PLETHORA OF RULES AND REGULATIONS

Doctors are a part of society and society too has social responsibility toward this noble profession. Unfortunately, there is a progressive loss of faith between doctors and patients which can be attributed to several factors. Especially to progressive degradation of social, moral, ethical, and cultural values in society under the hypnotizing influence of greed, consumerism, and excessive commercialization, where money has become GOD. This ultimately is leading to collapse of the healthcare system primarily affecting the doctors practicing solo or in small single doctors' hospitals, where many rural physicians have experiences of similar kind. Over years of work in a sub-taluka industrial place on a highway and district not away from a metro city, one of the authors had similar experiences, even in 2022, 4 out of 14 talukas in his district of Maharashtra did not have a resident practicing physician due to poor infrastructure, lack of support from local bodies and government authorities, pay divide, corruption, ransoms, and extortions in the name of social contributions. Society considers that doctors are the softest target. Such a situation will lead to defensive practice where no doctor will be ready to take risk and lead to increased cost, investigations, and unnecessary referrals.

These doctors are lonely warriors, their problems and fate are different than those who are working in protected, corporate, and commercialized healthcare institutions. The society and fraternity may not be actually aware of the problems faced by grassroot doctors working in rather constrained facilities. Organizations can play a big role in advocacy and generating public opinion resulting in tougher laws for violence against doctors.

CONCLUSION

As of today, time to time change and modification in laws and regulations to regulate medicine practice have made the clinical practice so difficult and doctors are unable to perform their duties or apply their skills due to the fear of litigations and started defensive practice.

PROPOSED REMEDIES

Plethora of rules and regulations must be softened as medicine practice is evidence- and situational-based. Doctors have to make quick decisions in seconds to save patients, and this decision may be right/wrong. If it is wrong that is medical error in taking decisions not medical negligence.

Ethics also requires modification as laws which makes practice safe and fearless.

MORAL

Law and ethics have made clinical practice so difficult, hence there is requirement of urgent and appropriate action to improve clinical practice so that doctors can extend their medical services/apply their skills for which they are morally bound.

SUGGESTED READINGS

1. Haas JS, Cook EF, Puopolo AL, Burstin HR, Cleary PD, Brennan TA. Is the professional satisfaction of general internists associated with patient satisfaction? J Gen Intern Med. 2000; 15(2):122-8.
2. Daugird A, Spencer D. Physician reactions to the healthcare care revolution: a grief model approach. Arch Fam Med. 1996;5(9):497-500.
3. DiMatteo MR, Sherbourne CD, Hays RD, Ordway L, Kravitz RL, McGlynn EA, et al. Physicians' characteristics influence patients' adherence to medical treatment: results from the Medical Outcomes Study. Health Psychol. 1993;12(2):93-102.
4. Kulkarni SV, Gupta VK, Basak S. "Society, Stress, and Doctor's Suicides": It is not only Dr Archana Sharma; you could be the next! J Assoc Physicians India. 2022;70(8):99.

268

CHAPTER

Role of Genomics and Transcriptomics in Patient Care

Rajiv Kumar Bandaru, Mehdi Ali Mirza

ABSTRACT

Genomic medicine contributes to improved patient outcomes by an exact diagnosis of rare disorders, prenatal diseases, cancers, and infections. Targeted pharmacogenomics therapy has a promising role in dealing with mutations and polymorphisms of metabolic enzymes pertaining to oncology, cardiovascular diseases, and diabetes. Transcriptomics support has a key role in disease biomarkers for early detection, diagnosis, monitoring of diseases, and guiding personalized treatment decisions. The substantial contributions of customized genomic medicine and transcriptomics have transformed the concept of 'one size fit all' to 'every patient as an individual'. Therefore, in this era of omics, the clinical practice approach is shifting from guidelines-based to algorithm-based treatments. Since the information of any organism is stored in the deoxyribonucleic acid (DNA) (genome) and expressed by ribonucleic acid (RNA) (transcriptome), it is known that not all genomes end up in transcribed RNA molecules. Similarly, all the transcribed RNAs will not end up in protein formation. These strategies are applied in precise diagnosis, targeted therapy selection, prognostic assessments, and therapeutic monitoring. The early identification of mutations and altered gene expressions via huge omics data derived from unconventional DNA sequencing and microarray if assisted by artificial intelligence, may bring a change in clinical care. Such a colossal approach may also be of economic significance.

INTRODUCTION

Medical genetics is involved in the diagnosis and management of hereditary disorders and genomics applies to identify mutations and the interactions between the genes and environment, to medical care. The human genome project (1990–2003) provides a virtually complete sequence of human deoxyribonucleic acid (DNA), which serves as catalogue to all human genes. Understanding of genomic structure and its regulation uncovered how genetic variation contributes to disease. Gene is a segment of DNA that codes for functional protein, whereas genome is the total DNA content in the cell of an organism. The DNA is the genetic material within the nucleus that replicates and creates new copies. Transcription of DNA forms a ribonucleic acid (RNA) which on translation produces protein; this is the central dogma of molecular biology **(Fig. 1)**.

Currently, clinical practice has evolved from intuition medicine, i.e., a signs- and symptoms-based practice to clinical trial and evidence-based medicine guidelines. In future, it is expected that medicine will be practiced according to algorithms that will take into consideration the patient's characteristics, such as their genome,

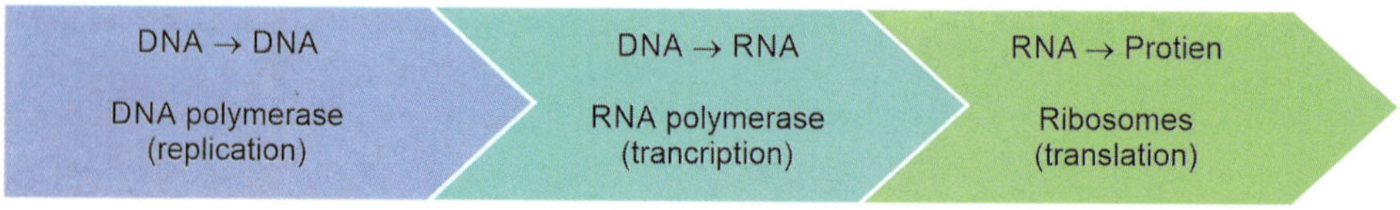

FIG. 1: The central dogma.

epigenetics, environment, and lifestyle as a tailored healthcare, constituting precision medicine. All precision medicine strategies include the use of high-throughput omics disciplines and technologies that includes genomics, transcriptomics, proteomics, metabolomics, and pharmacogenomics. In this regard, genomics and transcriptomics has made significant contributions to medical practice. Transcriptomics deals with complete set of RNA transcripts in a cell or tissue, playing a crucial role in patient care.

Deoxyribonucleic acid sequencing is fundamental to genome analysis. It is the process of determining the order of nucleotides adenine, thymidine, cytosine, and guanine along a DNA strand. The two conventional and most popular methods include Sanger-chain termination sequencing method and Maxim and Gilbert-chemical sequencing method. The next-generation sequencing (NGS) is similar to Sanger sequencing to process millions of reactions in parallel, resulting in very high speed and throughput at reduced cost. In case of transcriptomics, the techniques include hybridization-based approach microarray and RNA sequence approach through complementary DNA (cDNA), serial analysis of gene expression (SAGE), cap analysis of gene expression (CAGE), and massively parallel signature sequence (MPSS).

The roles of genomics and transcriptomics in diagnosis, prognosis, and therapeutics are discussed. Screening tests are intended for asymptomatic people, whereas diagnostic tests are intended for those showing symptoms in need of a diagnosis. Prognosis is the prospect of recovery as anticipated from the usual course of disease or peculiarities of the case. Risk predictions here are related to onset of disease, treatment complications, and untoward effects.

ROLE IN DIAGNOSIS

Cystic fibrosis (CF) is characterized by chronic respiratory problems, greasy stools, salty-tasting skin, and poor growth. It was considered to be nonexistent in Indian subcontinent. Reports in last one decade have suggested that CF occurs in India but its precise magnitude is not known. Studies on migrant Indian population in United States and United Kingdom estimate frequency of CF as 1:10,000 to 1:40,000. CF is a genetic disorder caused by mutations in the cystic fibrosis transmembrane conductance regulator (*CFTR*) gene. DNA sequencing and analysis are used to identify these mutations. Carrier screening is used to identify individuals who carry a single copy of the *CFTR* gene mutation. It is particularly relevant for family planning purposes and counseling couples about their risk of having a child with CF. Newborn screening programs to detect CF early in life involve analyzing blood samples from newborns for specific *CFTR* gene mutations. The variant analysis helps in determining the functional consequences of the mutations and their impact on disease severity. It also aids in tailoring treatment plans based on the specific *CFTR* gene variants present in an individual. CTFR modulating drugs available are ivacaftor, lumacaftor/ivacaftor, tezacaftor/ivacaftor, and elexacaftor/tezacaftor/ivacaftor.

Breast cancer is a carcinoma that occur in women and rarely in men. Its treatment depends on the stage of cancer and every patient responds differently to conventional chemotherapy. NGS is used to identify genetic alterations and mutations in breast cancer susceptibility genes, such as *BRCA1* and *BRCA2*. It helps to determine if an individual carries pathogenic mutation in these genes, which are associated with an increased risk of developing breast cancer. Genomic profiling of breast cancer can help classify tumors into distinct molecular subtypes based on their gene expression patterns. This molecular subtyping provides valuable information for predicting treatment response, prognosis, and selecting targeted therapies. Common subtypes include luminal A (HER2 negative), luminal B (Ki-67 enriched), HER2-enriched, and basal-like (triple-negative—estrogen, progesterone, and HER2) breast cancers. Genomic analysis of circulating tumor DNA (ctDNA) in the blood, known as liquid biopsy, has emerged as a noninvasive approach for diagnosing and monitoring breast cancer. Liquid biopsies can detect genetic alterations and mutations in ctDNA, providing real-time information about tumor characteristics and treatment response. This approach has the potential to complement or replace traditional tissue biopsies in certain situations. Genetic alterations, such as *HER2* gene amplification or mutations in the *PIK3CA* gene, guide the use of targeted drugs like trastuzumab or phosphoinositide 3-kinases (PI3K) inhibitors (idelalisib and alpelisib), respectively. The list of diagnostic markers and their significance in several common diseases is presented in **Table 1**.

ROLE IN PROGNOSIS

Alzheimer's disease (AD) is the most common cause of dementia in the elderly. Genetic testing can identify mutations in genes such as amyloid protein precursor (APP), presenilin-1 (PSEN1), and PSEN2 associated with familial autosomal dominant AD. The presence of these mutations can influence disease progression and prognosis. Variants in genes such as apolipoprotein E (*APOE*) have been widely studied and are associated with an increased risk of developing late-onset AD. Biomarkers related to amyloid beta (Aβ) and tau protein accumulation,

TABLE 1: Role of genomics and transcriptomics in diagnosis.

Disease	Diagnostic marker	Significance
Lung cancer	Epidermal growth factor receptor (EGFR)	Mutations predict response to EGFR inhibitors (e.g., gefitinib and erlotinib)
	Anaplastic lymphoma kinase (ALK)	Translocations indicate response to ALK inhibitors (e.g., crizotinib)
Colorectal cancer	Kirsten rat sarcoma (KRAS)	Mutations affect response to anti-EGFR therapy (e.g., cetuximab)
	Microsatellite instability (MSI)	High MSI indicates potential response to immune checkpoint inhibitors (e.g., pembrolizumab)
Prostate cancer	Prostate-specific antigen (PSA)	Elevated levels indicate the possibility of prostate cancer
	Androgen receptor (AR)	Overexpression may indicate resistance to androgen deprivation therapy
	TMPRSS2-ERG	Gene fusion used as a diagnostic marker for prostate cancer
Leukemia	BCR-ABL	Translocation associated with chronic myeloid leukemia (CML) and targeted therapy with tyrosine kinase inhibitors (e.g., imatinib)
	FLT3-ITD	Internal tandem duplication predicts poor prognosis and targeted therapy in acute myeloid leukemia (AML)
	NPM1	Mutation used for risk stratification in AML and minimal residual disease monitoring

such as Aβ42, total tau (t-tau), and phosphorylated tau (p-tau), can be detected in cerebrospinal fluid or through neuroimaging techniques. These biomarkers can help identify individuals in the early stages of AD pathology, even before clinical symptoms manifest. Genetic variations in genes involved in drug metabolism, such as cytochrome P450 (CYP2D6) enzymes, can influence the effectiveness and tolerability of certain medications (donepezil) used in the management of AD symptoms.

Lung cancer is a complex and heterogeneous disease with distinct molecular subtypes that have varying clinical behaviors, treatment responses, and prognoses. Adenocarcinoma is the most common subtype of nonsmall cell lung cancer (NSCLC) and can be further classified based on specific molecular alterations. Patients with certain molecular features, such as epidermal growth factor receptor (EGFR) mutations, anaplastic lymphoma kinase (ALK) rearrangements, ROS1 rearrangements, or *BRAF* mutations, tend to have better treatment responses and improved prognosis compared to those without these alterations. These patients may benefit from targeted therapies specific to their molecular subtype. Lung adenocarcinomas with *KRAS* mutations have been associated with a poorer prognosis and limited response to targeted therapies. STK11/LKB1 and KEAP1/NFE2L2 mutations have been linked to resistance to immunotherapy and worse prognosis in NSCLC patients. High PD-L1 expression in NSCLC tumors has been associated with a better response to immune checkpoint inhibitors, leading to improved prognosis for some patients. Squamous cell carcinoma is another subtype of NSCLC. Genomic studies have identified genomic alterations, including mutations in TP53 and alterations in fibroblast growth factor receptor 1 (FGFR1) and discoindin domain receptor 2 (DDR2), associated with squamous cell carcinoma. These alterations can influence treatment response and prognosis.

Small cell lung cancer (SCLC) is a highly aggressive subtype of lung cancer. While it has traditionally been treated as a single entity, recent studies have revealed distinct molecular subtypes within SCLC. For example, SCLC tumors can be classified based on neuroendocrine markers, such as ASCL1, NEUROD1, and POU2F3 expression. These subtypes may have differences in treatment response and prognosis, with ASCL1-high tumors being associated with a better prognosis compared to NEUROD1-high or POU2F3-high tumors. The list of prognostic markers and their significance in several common diseases is presented in **Table 2**.

ROLE IN TARGETED THERAPY AND PHARMACOGENOMICS

Targeted therapy targets proteins required for cancer growth. Monoclonal antibodies (MAbs) and small molecules, tyrosine kinase inhibitors (TKIs) are the two well-known examples. Pharmacogenomics defines the role of genome in drug response. It helps in personalized medication selection, optimal drug dosing, predicting drug response, minimizing adverse reactions, and treatment optimization. It has shown most successful impact in dealing cancers.

Cancer varies both phenotypically and genetically, even among patients with identical types and stages of

TABLE 2: Role of genomics and transcriptomics in prognosis.

Disease	Prognostic marker	Significance
Colorectal cancer, lung cancer, and pancreatic cancer	KRAS mutation	Associated with poor prognosis, resistance to certain treatments
Lung cancer	EGFR mutation	Predicts response to targeted therapies, better prognosis
Breast cancer and gastric cancer	HER2 amplification	Indicates response to anti-HER2 therapies, associated with aggressive disease
Various cancers (e.g., breast, lung, and colorectal)	TP53 mutation	Predicts poor prognosis, resistance to therapy
Melanoma, colorectal cancer, and thyroid cancer	BRAF mutation	Associated with poorer outcomes, targeted therapy options available
Glioblastoma	MGMT promoter methylation	Indicates better response to chemotherapy, improved survival
Prostate cancer and endometrial cancer	PTEN loss	Associated with poor prognosis, resistance to certain treatments
Gastric cancer and lobular breast cancer	CDH1 mutation	Indicates increased risk and poor prognosis
Alzheimer's disease	APOE ε4	Predicting faster disease progression and earlier onset
Alzheimer's disease	TOMM40	Assessing the age of onset of Alzheimer's disease

disease. Many targeted cancer therapies are active against cell surface receptors or downstream effector molecules, so that mutations in signaling pathway components can influence drug sensitivity and resistance. One major theme emerging from pharmacogenomic research in oncology is that such mutations can inform treatment decisions and predict patient outcomes. Significant advances in cancer tissue analysis techniques and patient stratification have also occurred in the past decade. Much of this progress has been based on the identification of molecular features that determine tumor classification, prognosis, targeted treatments, and treatment response. Diagnostic pharmacogenetic tests for some cancers have been developed and are now readily available. The availability of tests for nonheritable, somatic cell DNA mutations is rapidly increasing. The best known of these is the *HER2* receptor gene amplification test, which is used to guide breast cancer treatment with trastuzumab. The HER2 is overexpressed in approximately one quarter of patients with breast cancer. Overexpression of the *HER2* oncogene has been found to correlate with increased tumor formation and metastasis, a poor prognosis, and resistance to chemotherapy. Trastuzumab treatment is considered only when the patient has HER-positive cancer, defined by very high levels of HER2 protein in the tumor. Pharmacogenetic testing has become an integral part of the breast cancer treatment with trastuzumab, since variability in *HER2* receptor gene expression aids in determining degree of patient response. Pharmacogenomics has also been responsible for significant advances in treating lung cancer. Erlotinib and gefitinib are TKIs designed to target the EGFR, which has been shown to influence predisposition to lung cancer. A European study also screened patients with NSCLC for EGFR mutations to identify those who were most likely to respond to erlotinib treatment. A recent East Asian study investigated the role of an EGFR mutation as a predictor for improved progression-free survival (PFS) with gefitinib treatment compared with carboplatin–paclitaxel therapy. Results indicated that the response to gefitinib was almost entirely limited to the mutation-positive group, whereas mutation-negative patients benefited more from chemotherapy. The list of therapeutic markers and their significance in several common diseases is presented in **Table 3**.

ROLE IN COVID-19 DISEASE

Genomics and transcriptomics have played a crucial role in the study and management of coronavirus disease 2019 (COVID-19). Genomic sequencing has been used to identify and characterize the severe acute respiratory syndrome coronavirus 2 (SARS-CoV-2) virus responsible for COVID-19. Sequencing the viral genome helps in tracking its spread, identifying new variants, and understanding their potential impact on disease transmission, severity, and response to interventions. By analyzing the genomes of infected individuals, researchers aim to identify genetic variations that may influence an individual's response to the virus, providing insights into

TABLE 3: Role of genomics and transcriptomics in targeted therapy.

Disease	Therapeutic marker	Significance
Breast cancer and gastric cancer	HER2 amplification/ overexpression	Targeted therapies, such as trastuzumab, pertuzumab, and lapatinib
Lung cancer	ROS1 rearrangement	ROS1 inhibitors, such as crizotinib and entrectinib
Melanoma, colorectal cancer, and thyroid cancer	BRAF V600E mutation	BRAF inhibitors, such as vemurafenib and dabrafenib
Various cancers	NTRK fusion	TRK inhibitors, such as larotrectinib and entrectinib
Colorectal cancer and endometrial cancer	MSI-H/dMMR	Immunotherapy with immune checkpoint inhibitors, such as pembrolizumab and nivolumab
Various cancers (e.g., lung, bladder, and head and neck)	PD-L1 expression	Immunotherapy with immune checkpoint inhibitors
Colorectal cancer	RAS mutation	Anti-EGFR therapy resistance
Lung cancer	EML4-ALK fusion	ALK inhibitors, such as crizotinib and alectinib
Lung cancer	HER2 mutation	HER2 inhibitors, such as afatinib and neratinib
Lung cancer and thyroid cancer	RET rearrangement	RET inhibitors, such as selpercatinib and pralsetinib

potential host factors affecting disease susceptibility and progression. Genomic surveillance programs have been employed to monitor the genetic changes in the virus over time. This enables the detection of new variants, such as the alpha, beta, gamma, and delta variants, and provides insights into their prevalence, transmissible, and potential impact on diagnostics, therapeutics, and vaccines. In this way identifying potential drug targets and guiding the development of antiviral therapies are determined.

Transcriptomic profiling can help identify distinct molecular subtypes or clusters of COVID-19 patients based on their gene expression patterns. Transcriptomic analysis of host cells, such as respiratory epithelial cells or immune cells, infected with SARS-CoV-2, provides insights into the host response to the virus. By comparing gene expression profiles of infected and uninfected cells, specific genes and pathways involved in the immune response, inflammation, and tissue damage associated with COVID-19 may be identified. By identifying potential biomarkers that can aid in COVID-19 diagnosis, prognosis, and monitoring early detection, risk stratification, and treatment decision-making can be reached. Transcriptomic analysis can also be used to identify existing drugs that may have potential efficacy against COVID-19. This approach facilitates drug repurposing and the identification of potential therapeutic targets.

ETHICAL ISSUES

Genomic medicine raises important ethical and privacy considerations. Uncertainty, anxiety, and the potential for stigmatization are among the psychological impacts that need to be carefully addressed. This information is highly sensitive and can have implications for an individual's personal and familial well-being, insurance coverage, and employment opportunities. Safeguarding patient privacy and ensuring appropriate consent, data protection, and secure storage and transmission of genomic data are critical. Genomic testing and receiving genetic risk information can have psychological implications for individuals and families. In summary, the four cardinal principles of medical ethics, i.e., autonomy, beneficence, nonmaleficence, and justice must be weighed upon balancing conflicting demands and ethical dilemmas.

LIMITATIONS

Most common disease such as diabetes, heart disease, and psychiatric disorder are multifactorial. The interpretation of variants requires extensive knowledge databases and expertise. Distinguishing between benign and pathogenic variants can be complex. Identifying the specific genetic contributions in diseases involving complex interactions between multiple genetic and environmental factors is a challenging task. The precise mechanisms by which certain genetic variants lead to disease manifestation or treatment responses are often not fully elucidated, making it challenging to translate genomic findings into actionable clinical decisions. Our understanding of the genomic and transcriptomic basis of many diseases is still incomplete. The costs associated with genomic sequencing, data analysis, and interpretation can be a barrier to widespread adoption in clinical practice, limiting it to certain regions or healthcare settings.

With regard to transcriptomics, gene expression is a highly dynamic and complex process while transcriptomic analysis provides a snapshot of gene expression at a given time point. So, it may not capture the full complexity of gene regulation and the interactions between different regulatory mechanisms. Tissues and cell types within an organism exhibit heterogeneity, analysis on bulk tissue samples may not provide a complete picture of gene expression in specific cell types or subpopulations of interest. Variations in sample collection, processing, RNA extraction, library preparation, and sequencing can introduce bias and affect the comparability of data between various studies.

CONCLUSION

We may look upon genomics and transcriptomics as a future replacement for conventional therapy. Individualized algorithms can be created by using artificial intelligence and machine learning as complementary tools. The economic burden on the state can be reduced if precision medicine is made available going back to the old saying "prevention is better than cure".

SUGGESTED READINGS

1. Pareek CS, Smoczynski R, Tretyn A. Sequencing technologies and genome sequencing. J Appl Genet. 2011;52(4):413-35.
2. Roychowdhury S, Chinnaiyan AM. Translating cancer genomes and transcriptomes for precision oncology. CA Cancer J Clin. 2016;66(1):75-88.
3. Baronti L, Karlsson H, Marušič M, Petzold K. A guide to large-scale RNA sample preparation. Anal Bioanal Chem. 2018;410(14):3239-52.
4. Takemasa I, Hamabe A, Miyo M, Akizuki E, Okuya K. Essential updates 2020/2021: Advancing precision medicine for comprehensive rectal cancer treatment. Ann Gastroenterol Surg. 2022;7(2):198-215.
5. Gaudenzi G, Dicitore A, Carra S, aronni D, Pozza C, Giannetta E, et al. Management of Endocrine Disease: Precision medicine in neuroendocrine neoplasms: an update on current management and future perspectives. Eur J Endocrinol. 2019;181(1):R1-10.

269

CHAPTER

How Should Clinicians Evaluate Clinical Trials?

Anuj Maheshwari, Shivangi Maheshwari

ABSTRACT

Nowadays, when we see multiple new molecules are hitting the market, it becomes difficult for a clinician to make a choice. Promoters come with the backup of randomized controlled studies or sometimes with real-world studies. A plethora of studies and their presentation as per their own convenience causes confusion among prescribers. Physicians are mostly presented with a myriad of clinical data in their busy practice schedule, just to face a challenge of what is really relevant or valid. So, it is important to know how should a clinician interpret a clinical trial. Focusing on study population, their baseline characteristics, keeping an eye on drop outs, and their reasons of exit are important. Usually, a higher sample size is needed in noninferiority or equivalence studies. Noninferiority study needs 4 times larger sample size than superiority study. If a study is initially designed to test for superiority but this outcome is not found, switching to a noninferiority study would be inappropriate. Measurements and scales should be precise, reproducible and validated. Ideally, the outcome being studied should be the one in which clinicians are most interested. If the surrogate markers have inconsistent correlation with important clinical outcomes, then those markers should be viewed skeptically. While having a look over statistical analysis, it should be remembered that statistical significance does not always translate into clinical significance. A study that reports a correlation and gives a *p*-value but not a 95% confidence interval should be viewed with caution. Larger studies have more precision, which may generally lead to a smaller *p*-value without a meaningful change in effect.

INTRODUCTION

Randomized controlled trials (RCTs) evaluate social and psychological therapies and guide policy and practice decisions when feasible and appropriate. Readers need information on the design, context, conduct, analysis, outcomes, and interpretation of RCT papers to use them. RCTs, like other types of research, can produce biased estimates of intervention effects if they are not conducted properly. As a result, accurate, thorough, and transparent RCTs are critical for maximizing their usefulness, allowing replication of studies to enhance the evidence base, and facilitating the comparison and implementation of beneficial interventions in real-world scenarios.

Clinical trials are necessary for the advancement of new medical therapies and diagnostic tests. Without clinical trials, we cannot tell if novel therapies produced in the laboratory or using animal models are useful or safe or if a diagnostic test will operate properly. This is due to the fact that computer simulation and animal testing can only tell us so much about how a novel treatment may perform and are no substitute for testing in a living human body.

STUDY DESIGN

Clinical study designs vary, but they always attempt to acquire objective data to evaluate interventions in relation to an associated outcome in a specific population. The two main types of clinical studies are clinical trials and observational studies. RCTs have traditionally been regarded as the gold standard of clinical trial design, occupying the top of the hierarchy of levels of evidence in a clinical study; this is because the process of randomization can minimize differences in group characteristics that may influence the outcome, providing the most definitive evidence regarding the impact of the exposure or intervention on the outcome. Each group in an RCT is referred to as an "arm;" therefore, in a two-arm trial, the experimental treatment versus the control group would be referred to as the "treatment arm" and the "control arm," respectively.

On discussing the study design, **Figure 1** represents the levels of evidence available in the literature: The hierarchy of the pyramid progresses incrementally with higher validity of studies toward the apex of the triangle and depreciates as it progresses downward from the apex with sequential lesser validity in the order: Single-masked randomized trials, open-label randomized trials, historical control trials, and observational studies.

Description of Subtypes of Study Design

Active Control

If a well-established treatment for the disease as an investigation exists, it could be utilized as the control arm against which the innovative experimental treatment is tested. The goal of an active control trial may be to demonstrate that the experimental treatment is superior to the standard-of-care treatment *(superiority study)*, to demonstrate that the experimental treatment is similar to the standard-of-care treatment *(equivalence study)*, or to demonstrate that the experimental treatment is not significantly less effective than the standard-of-care treatment *(noninferiority study)*.

Placebo Control

In the absence of an effective treatment for an illness, the control arm may be made up of patients who receive no treatment or a sham treatment known as a placebo group.

Multiple Arm

Multiple-arm trials are classified into two kinds. The first involves comparing several dose levels or regimens of the experimental treatment to a single control arm. The second approach combines a single treatment arm with numerous control arms (e.g., active control and a placebo control arm).

Cluster Randomized

In a cluster randomized experiment, groups of subjects are randomized rather than individual subjects. Administrative convenience, ethical considerations, and ease of application at the cluster level are all reasons for randomizing clusters rather than individuals.

Adaptive Design

In adaptive designs information gathered during the trial is used to modify some part of the experiment.

Platform

Platform trials are multi-arm studies having the capacity to include control and experimental arms that can be

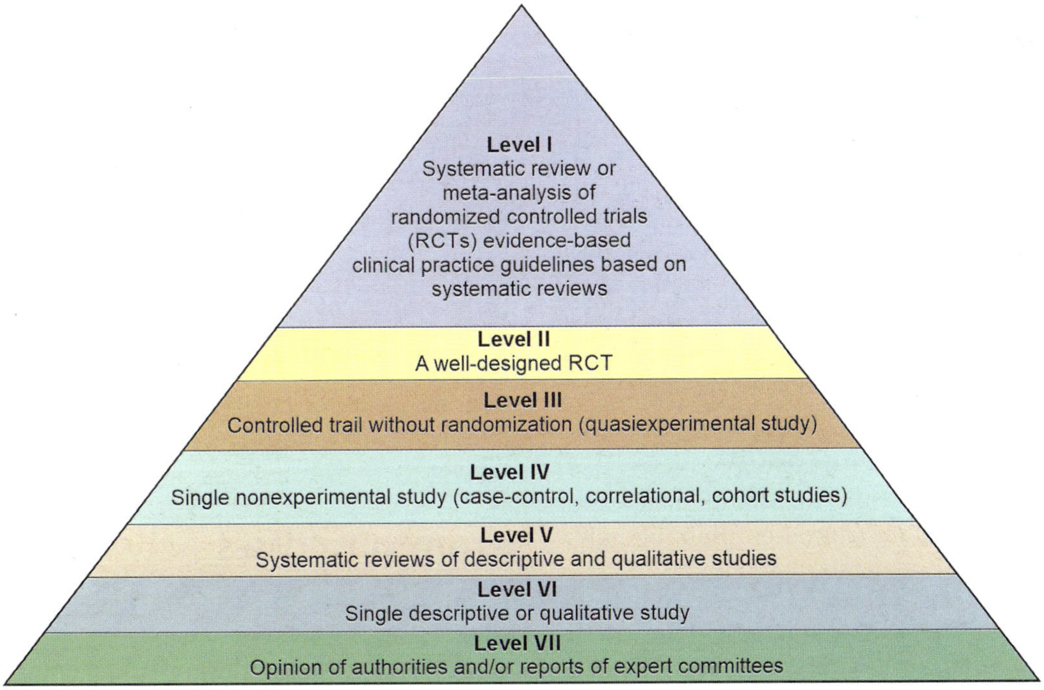

FIG. 1: Level of evidence available in the literature.

opened or closed for recruitment at any time during the trial.

Patient Population

The inclusion and exclusion criteria are an important factor in the design of an RCT. These criteria affect a range of aspects of the study's conduct and interpretability and are primarily intended to ensure patient safety. If the eligibility requirements are excessively stringent, it may be difficult to enroll the intended number of patients due to a potentially time-consuming screening process, as many screened individuals may turn out to be ineligible. Furthermore, overly rigid qualifying criteria may result in a study population not representative of the broader target population, limiting the generalizability of the study results and the ability to show treatment effectiveness.

Subjects drop out of studies for many reasons, but two of the most important reasons:

1. Lack of benefits (they were too sick to stay in the study)
2. Side effects (which made them want to leave the study)

Effect Size

After defining the endpoint, the investigators must determine the relevant difference between the groups they intend to detect. This is a clinical decision with statistical consequences for the study's design in terms of the number of patients required.

Power, Error Rates, and Sample Size

The typical statistical technique evaluates the trial's two possible outcomes. Consider a two-arm RCT in which the patient represents the treatment arm's rate of a binary outcome and the control arm's rate. Traditionally, the sample size is determined by error rates. A type I error is when a null hypothesis is rejected when it is true, while a type II error is when the null hypothesis is not rejected when it is false, in which case the alternative hypothesis is presumed true. Statistical power is defined as the complement of type II error (i.e., I-type II error). When the alternative hypothesis is correct, statistical power represents the chance of rejecting the null hypothesis.

Methods for Randomization

- *Simple randomization*: Other than the ultimate sample size, no constraints are placed on the randomized sequence in simple randomization.
- *Permuted block randomization*: To avoid imbalances with simple randomization, the permuted block design splits patients into blocks across time and balances the randomization to each arm within each block.
- *Minimization*: The assignment to a research arm is done with the goal of achieving balance among randomization groups in terms of prognostic criteria of interest.
- *Outcome adaptive randomization:* The goal of outcome adaptive randomization is to assign more patients to the more promising treatments based on the trial's accumulating data in order to minimize the expected number of treatment failures and overcome the questionable ethics of continuing to assign patients to treatment arms with evidence of lower efficacy.

Data Analysis

Two types of errors are committed when designing clinical research which should be kept in mind:

1. *Systematic error*: Due to bias in the study's design (such as selection of outcome measures) and confounding
2. *Random error*: Variations in either biology or measurement is evaluated by examining the study's outcomes with statistics.

Statistical Analysis at the End of the Trial

One method is "*intention-to-treat analysis*," in which all patients are analyzed in the group to which they were randomized, regardless of treatment adherence. In *A "per-protocol" analysis,* only patients who finished the treatment to which they were initially assigned are analyzed in this approach. A per-protocol analysis may yield a more accurate assessment of the treatment impact, but the results should be regarded with caution because bias might be introduced by the reasons individuals did not follow the scheduled treatment regimen.

Subject Categorization

The Consolidated Trial Reporting Standards Guidelines (http://www.consort-statement.org/) were developed to assist investigators in making proper decisions for reporting RCTs. These recommendations include a 25-item checklist for creating an RCT report as well as a template with a flowdiagram for inclusion in the trial report.

STUDY OUTCOMES

Ideally, the outcome being studied should be the one, clinicians are most interested in.

- *Primary outcomes:* Stronger and more meaningful than surrogate outcomes such as biomarker levels

- *Surrogate outcomes*:
  - Appear to be an easy, inexpensive, and less invasive method. But the validity of the surrogate markers should be scrutinized closely.
  - A strong *independent association* between the surrogate and the desired outcome should exist.
  - *Evidence from RCTs* in other drug classes should show that improvement in the surrogate leads to improved clinical outcomes.
- *Dichotomous outcomes:* The definitions of these endpoints are critical and should be scrutinized carefully to ensure that they are not too lenient.
- *Continuous outcome*: Provides more power to detect a difference between groups

STATISTICAL TESTING: *P*-VALUE

The goal of data collecting and analysis is to determine whether or not there is a difference between the two groups. This difference could be attributable to chance or to a genuine difference. Many statistical approaches are used to rule out differences caused by chance: One of these is the *p*-value. The *p*-value is a popular yet commonly misunderstood and misconstrued index. The *p*-value was used as a rough numerical indicator for the strength of evidence against the null hypothesis in Fisher's approach, and its value was arbitrarily set to 0.05. In a nutshell, a *p*-value of 0.05 indicates that the experiment should be repeated, whereas significance means "worthy of notice."

The *p*-value is a function of sample size, the magnitude of the differences between the tested groups, and the observations' variability. Probably best to ignore the *p*-value for correlations and instead look at the correlation itself (and its 95% confidence interval). A correlation of 90% with a confidence interval of 85–95% is impressive.

STUDY RESULTS

The *p*-value is based on the assumption that the null hypothesis is true. It gives the probability that the difference observed between the two treatment arms is due to chance alone. *P*-value serves as a combination of two measurements.

1. Effect size (the difference between the 2 groups).
2. Precision (the variation of that difference represented by the confidence interval).

A very large study will have more precision, which will generally lead to a smaller *p*-value without a meaningful change in effect size. A very small study will inherently have less precision, in which a clinically meaningful effect size may be missed due to a higher *p*-value.

Addressing the Missing Data

Common approaches for handling missing data are as follows:

- *Nonresponder imputation*: one who would have failed to meet the endpoint. It lowers success rates (and placebo rates), thus making results look less impressive.
- *The last observation carried forward*: Use the last observation at which the subject was measured in place of the missing data.
- *Imputation*: Other data are used to estimate what the missing data would have been. This approach is generally considered appealing but questionable, as it is impossible to check the accuracy of these estimates.

How Big of an Effect Is It?

To help judge the impact of a study's findings, it is worthwhile to calculate the number needed to treat (NNT). This number represents the reciprocal of the absolute risk reduction. Gives the reader an understanding of how many patients a clinician would have to treat to see the desired outcome. NNT can be used for binary outcome.

RECENT MODIFICATIONS OF THE CONSORT CHECKLIST

The original Consolidated Standards of Reporting Trials (CONSORT) 2010 statement specifies the elements that should be included when reporting the results of RCTs. However, study results are frequently presented inconsistently or incompletely. To address this need, JAMA released details of CONSORT Outcomes 2022, an extension to CONSORT 2010. The CONSORT Outcomes 2022 Extension includes 17 new outcome-specific items that should be reported for all RCTs, in addition to the original 25-item CONSORT checklist.

CONCLUSION

In conclusion, clinical trial evaluation is a critical competency for medical professionals to ensure evidence-based practice and make knowledgeable decisions about patient care. Clinicians can evaluate the reliability and relevance of clinical trial findings for their practice by taking into account multiple aspects of trial design, methodology, outcomes, and potential biases. The study design, sample size, power, blinding, randomization and allocation concealment, statistical analysis, adverse events, safety, bias and confounding, external validity and generalizability, publication bias, and conflicts of interest are important factors to consider. The reliability and applicability of trial results may be assessed by physicians through a thorough evaluation of these variables, which also makes it easier to integrate evidence-based practices into patient care. Clinicians may deliver high-quality, patient-centered treatment supported by the best available evidence by keeping up with the most recent research and regularly evaluating clinical trials.

SUGGESTED READINGS

1. Petrosino A, Boruch RF, Rounding C, McDonald S, Chalmers I. The Campbell collaboration Social, Psychological, Educational and Criminological Trials Register (C2-SPECTR) to facilitate the preparation and maintenance of systematic reviews of social and educational interventions. Eval Res Educ. 2000;14(3–4): 206-19.
2. Bristow D, Carter L, Martin S. Using evidence to improve policy and practice: the UK what works Centres. Contemp Soc Sci. 2015;10(2):126-37.
3. Social and Behavioral Sciences Team. 2015 Annual Report. Washington, DC: Executive Office of the President, National Science and Technology Council; 2015.
4. Clark ML, Thapa S. Systematic reviews in the bulletin. Bull World Health Organ. 2011;89:3.
5. Petrosino A. Reflections on the genesis of the Campbell collaboration. Exp Criminol. 2013;8(2):9-12.
6. Oliver S, Bagnall AM, Thomas J, Shepherd J, Sowden A, White I, et al. Randomised controlled trials for policy interventions: a review of reviews and meta-regression. Health Technol Assess. 2010;14(16):1-165.
7. Goodman S, Dickersin K. Metabias: A challenge for comparative effectiveness research. Ann Intern Med. 2011;155(1):61-2.
8. Moher D, Glasziou P, Chalmers I, Nasser M, Bossuyt PMM, Korevaar DA, et al. Increasing value and reducing waste in biomedical research: Who's listening? Lancet. 2016;387: 1573-86.
9. Hoffmann TC, Glasziou P, Boutron I, Milne R, Perera R, Moher D, et al. Better reporting of interventions: template for intervention description and replication (TIDieR) checklist and guide. BMJ. 2014;348:g1687.
10. Pinnock H, Epiphaniou E, Sheikh A, Griffiths C, Eldridge S, Craig P, et al. Developing standards for reporting implementation studies of complex interventions (StaRI): A systematic review and e-Delphi. Implement Sci. 2015;10(1):42
11. The periodic health examination. Canadian Task Force on the Periodic Health Examination. Can Med Assoc J. 1979;121(9):1193-254.
12. Sackett DL. Rules of evidence and clinical recommendations on the use of antithrombotic agents. Chest. 1989;95(suppl 2):2s-4s.
13. Kim ES, Bruinooge SS, Roberts S, Ison G, Lin NU, Gore L, et al. Broadening eligibility criteria to make clinical trials more representative: American Society of Clinical Oncology and Friends of Cancer Research Joint Research Statement. J Clin Oncol. 2017;35(33):3737-44.
14. US Department of Health and Human Services Food and Drug Administration. (2001). Guidance for Industry: Choice of Control Group and Related Issues in Clinical Trials. Available from https://www.fda.gov/ regulatory-information/search-fda-guidance-documents/e10-choicecontrol-group-and-related-issues-clinical-trials. [Last accessed December, 2020].
15. Hemming K, Eldridge S, Forbes G, Weijer C, Taljaard M. How to design efficient cluster randomised trials. BMJ. 2017;358:j3064.
16. Hobbs BP, Berry DA, Coombes KR. Biostatistics and bioinformatics in clinical trials. In: Niederhuber JE, Armitage JO, Doroshow JH, Kastan MB, Tepper JE, (eds). Abeloff's Clinical Oncology, 6th edition. Philadelphia, PA: Elsevier; 2020. 284-295.e2.
17. Hobbs BP, Lee JJ. Adaptive trial designs. In: Crowley J, Hoering A, (eds). Handbook of Statistics in Clinical Oncology,. 3rd edition. Boca Raton, FL: Taylor & Francis/CRC Press; 2012. pp. 265-92.
18. Renfro LA, Sargent DJ. Statistical controversies in clinical research: basket trials, umbrella trials, and other master protocols: a review and examples. Ann Oncol. 2017;28(1):34-43.
19. Woodcock J, LaVange LM. Master protocols to study multiple therapies, multiple diseases, or both. N Engl J Med. 2017;377(1):62-70.
20. Matts JP, Lachin JM. Properties of permuted-block randomization in clinical trials. Control Clin Trials. 1988;9(4):327-44.
21. Pocock SJ, Simon R. Sequential treatment assignment with balancing for prognostic factors in the controlled clinical trial. Biometrics. 1975;31(1):103-15.
22. Thall PF, Wathen JK. Practical Bayesian adaptive randomisation in clinical trials. Eur J Cancer. 2007;43(5):859-66.
23. Zabor EC, Kaizer AM, Hobbs BP. Randomized controlled trials. Chest. 2020;158(1S):S79-87.
24. Moher D, Hopewell S, Schulz KF, Montori V, Gøtzsche PC, Devereaux PJ, et al. CONSORT 2010 Explanation and Elaboration: updated guidelines for reporting parallel group randomised trials. BMJ. 2010;340:c869.
25. Goodman S. A dirty dozen: twelve P-value misconceptions. Semin Hematol. 2008;45(3):135-40.
26. Butcher NJ, Monsour A, Mew EJ, Chan A-W, Moher D, Mayo-Wilson E, et al. Guidelines for reporting outcomes in trial reports: The CONSORT-Outcomes 2022 Extension. JAMA. 2022;328(22):2252-64.

270
CHAPTER

Ethical Challenges in Undertaking Implementation Research

Prasanta Kumar Bhattacharya

ABSTRACT

Implementation research (IR) is a type of health research that aims to improve access and utilization of already existing health interventions for populations and communities in resource-limited regions. It differs from conventional clinical research (CR) in terms of study designs, consent processes, implementation, and translation in the community. It is a complex process involving multiple deviations from conventional research. Consequently, it raises various ethical issues which differ from conventional research and require specific considerations. Ethical issues in IR are usually not comprehensively covered in most international ethical guidelines on health research. It is important that ethical issues arising while carrying out IR are given due importance so that the communities who would benefit from such research outcomes are covered by the ethical guidelines that govern biomedical research in general, and IR in particular. This will ensure that the risks are minimized and the results of such research reach out to the communities for a positive and sustained outcome.

INTRODUCTION

Implement (Latin: "implere") means to fulfill or to carry something into effect. Implementation research (IR) tires to scientifically find out answers to research questions in terms of the implementation of policies, programs, and practices. The intent is to understand *"what"*, *"why,"* and *"how"* interventions do work (or do not work) in "real world" settings and to test different approaches to improve them by adapting to the local context, stakeholders, and end-users.

ETHICAL CHALLENGES IN IMPLEMENTATION RESEARCH

Implementation research is a complex research process involving multiple trade-offs from conventional clinical research (CR). It raises ethical issues at various steps of implementation, which require specific consideration. The distinction between clinical care, quality improvement, and public health research are often unclear; therefore, the relevant ethical implications are not as clear as in clinical trials, which usually occur under tight research conditions. Therefore, the application of ethical principles differs in IR from that in CR **(Table 1)**. Further, there are various lacunae in the understanding of ethical issues in IR as compared to conventional CR **(Box 1)**. These ethical issues involved in IR can be systematically grouped under the (1) planning, (2) implementation, and (3) postresearch phases **(Table 2)**.

ETHICAL CONSIDERATION IN THE PLANNING PHASE OF IMPLEMENTATION RESEARCH

Responsiveness to Local Needs and Priorities

Conventional CR focuses on the proof of principle of research, while IR addresses those research topics having local relevance in the community where the research

TABLE 1: Differences in the ethical issues between clinical research and implementation research.

Domain	Clinical research	Implementation research
Research subjects	Individuals	Nations, regions, communities, institutions, and individuals
Informed consent	Written informed consent by competent subjects, assent by minors, and consent by legally authorized representative	Informed consent difficult in various situations; CRT may require a two-level consent—from community head for randomization, from individual subjects for participation; sometimes individual consent may not be feasible
Equipoise	Clinical equipoise	Situational and/or contextual equipoise
Prerequisites	• Understanding of disease pathophysiology • Intervention aimed at disease-specific management	Identification of population health needs; understanding relative priority of need for intervention within local context; community engagement to understand community needs, ensure scalability, and sustainability
Research conditions	Ideal research environment	Real-life or pragmatic research environment
Research designs	*Conventional designs*: Cross-sectional, case-control, cohort studies, and RCT	*Nonconventional designs*: CRT, pragmatic, mixed methods, other hybrid designs, participatory action research, and quasi-experimental
Integration within health system	Usually no *a-priori* plan for health system integration	*A-priori* focus on health system strengthening; has ethical obligation for horizontal integration into health system
Boundary between research and clinical care	Usually, clear	Often unclear, because intervention is of proven efficacy

(CRT: cluster randomized trial; RCT: randomized controlled trial)

BOX 1: Lacunae in understanding ethical issues in implementation research as compared to clinical research.

- Need for comprehensive engagement of various stakeholders throughout the process of implementation research
- *A-priori* commitment to maintain sustainability if the intervention is successful
- No clear-cut guidelines about obtaining informed consent—from whom and how
- The risks and benefits of individual participants involved in research not well defined
- Concept of clinical equipoise is not applicable; rather equipoise is either situational or contextual. Ethical considerations are applicable accordingly
- Should follow local standards of care of the community
- Responsibility of researchers is to address ancillary findings, especially where existing health systems are underdeveloped
- Focus should be on appropriate dissemination of results in the community to ensure timely uptake and scale-up of successful interventions

TABLE 2: Key ethical consideration in different phases of implementation research.

Different phases of implementation research	Key ethical considerations
Planning phase	• Responsiveness to local needs and priorities • Equipoise • Study design • Stakeholder and community engagement • Balance between risks and benefits
Implementation phase	• Autonomy and informed consent • Privacy and confidentiality • Ancillary care • Community and health-system empowerment
Postresearch phase	• Dissemination of research findings • Data ownership and sharing • Translating research into public health utility • Sustainability of research outcome • Benefit sharing with the community

is undertaken. It is ethically important that IR studies be initiated by local health authorities to address the barriers in the implementation of a CR that is necessary for a particular community. However, problems that are of local priority depend on available health data, which may be lacking in resource-limited areas. The ethical concern of undertaking the particular IR will arise if the said research does not include any problem of local health importance.

Equipoise

From the ethical standpoint, equipoise is very important to identify any risk that may potentially happen to the participants in any research. The term "clinical" equipoise tries to point out the fact that prior to undertaking the particular research the researchers are unaware of whether the intervention would be superior (or inferior) to the comparator of the study. Such "clinical" equipoise usually does not arise in IR, for example, *"whether ceftriaxone is known to cure typhoid,"* but instead, the issue that would arise is, *"whether it is feasible to administer parenteral ceftriaxone to treat typhoid in such resource-limited community"* where the IR has been planned. In carrying out IR, instead of "clinical" equipoise the concept of either *"situational"* or *"contextual"* equipoise is justified, i.e., there is a definite doubt that a new intervention (already accepted scientifically) will work in a specific resource-constraint context. Therefore, to justify IR from an ethical standpoint, the "contextual" equipoise of the effect of the research process must be intact.

Study Design

Randomized controlled trial (RCT) is the gold standard in conventional CR and the ethical issues are well defined. However, in IR many other study designs, like cluster-randomized trial (CRT), often with multidisciplinary involvement are used. However, withholding intervention in the control arm of such CRT raises ethical concerns. Although step-wedge design (SWD) can be used to overcome this, in the early stages of the sequential delivery system in SWD some groups do not receive the intervention and become analogs to controls; hence, the ethical challenge persists. Here *"quasi-experimental"* designs, without a control group can be considered from an ethical standpoint, but this may not be scientifically sound. Therefore, engaging all stakeholders is crucial to develop the most practically effective study design.

Stakeholder and Community Engagement

Key stakeholders in IR may include policy-makers, healthcare providers and managers, and the community. The community further includes: (1) individuals *actually* receiving the interventions, (2) a broader community to which these individuals belong, and (3) a broader society that may eventually benefit from the outcome of such interventions. Members of the community who are actually exposed to the potential risks of such intervention should be actively consulted and engaged so that they play an active partnership role throughout the IR process. Ethical concerns for policymakers include a determination that the intervention will address a local priority health need and adequate commitment for scale-up and sustainability of an effective intervention.

Balance between Risks and Benefits

In conventional clinical trials testing the efficacy of a new vaccine or drug, the risks and benefits are borne by the individual participants. In any IR involving large-scale administration of medications in the community, the said community may stand to gain from the treatment, but the individual participants may develop drug-induced side effects from a medication that was unnecessary at a personal level. The modality of implementation may carry potential risks, for example, a successful community public health screening campaign for sexually transmitted infection (STI) in one country may carry different risks of stigmatization and social discrimination if implemented in another country having different religious and social beliefs. To weigh the risks in one group of subjects as opposed to the benefits obtained by another group is an ethical challenge for such types of IR. This requires interaction and counseling of the research participants, the community, and the stakeholders of the IR, so as to ethically justify the risk in a subset of participants vis-à-vis benefit in another subset.

ETHICAL CONCERNS IN IMPLEMENTATION PHASE OF IMPLEMENTATION RESEARCH

Autonomy and Informed Consent

While taking informed consent in IR, the issue of community agreement (consent) *versus* individual informed consent *versus* dual consent of community and individuals is important. Hence it is pertinent to identify the head of the community or *"gate-keepers"* providing the community agreement. Such person(s) should have adequate knowledge about the issue, be genuinely willing to support the subjects of research living in that community, and who is part of the society, rather than simply be the administrative head of the community. Notwithstanding, community consent cannot replace individual consent where appropriate. Challenges in implementing informed consent are to identify whether research participants are individual subjects or a population as a whole. The extent of information to be revealed to the intervention and control arms is also important, especially in behavior-change interventions because knowledge of the intervention itself may change outcomes and the implementation process.

Privacy and Confidentiality

Implementation research often requires that both healthcare facility-level and individual-level data on patient outcomes are available from health records. Confidentiality restricting access to patient data may hamper analyses of the impact of intervention on the health system. Either data obtained from the healthcare facility should be anonymized, or one should obtain consent from individuals whose data is being analyzed. If individual consent is not possible then one should obtain a waiver of consent from the concerned ethics committee and keep a mechanism to ensure that the confidentiality of patient information is respected by a patient-researcher strategy.

Ancillary Care

Ancillary care includes the provision to provide medical support for those health problems that do not fall within the ambit of the study under reference. Sometimes these can be foreseen at the design stage, otherwise it is observed while the research is ongoing. The need to provide ancillary care becomes essential when these are either serious and/or urgent in nature and fall within the capacity of the researchers to provide such care. Although it is not realistic or feasible to expect researchers to assume all ancillary care responsibilities, it is ethical that they should identify those requirements falling within their scope of responsibilities.

Community and Health-system Empowerment

It is ethically important that the IR process should try to integrate community interventions into the health system of the region, along with an attempt at capacity building and empowerment of the healthcare structure of that community. This can lead to incorporation of the research outcomes into local health policies.

ETHICAL CONCERNS IN POSTRESEARCH PHASE

Dissemination of Research Findings

Since IR has a positive impact on the health of the people in the community, it is ethically justifiable that the outcome of such research, *both positive and negative*, and the feedback should reach out to the community and stakeholders who participated in the research. This is important for other researchers planning similar research elsewhere and helps optimize and enhance resource utilization globally. Knowledge of outcomes of similar IR tested in different local contexts may help in generalizing results and obviate the need for new IR on similar lines.

Data Ownership and Sharing

It is ethical that all stakeholders should decide at the planning stage who would own the data, to ensure appropriate access to the research findings by the relevant stakeholders after the study is completed. This would help in the better utility of knowledge generated from the research. However, it is ethically vital to consider the implications of the privacy and confidentiality of the participants.

Translating Research into Community

There is an ethical responsibility of the investigators to oversee that the results of the research are properly translated for effective public health benefit. Potential barriers in such translation include a lack of coordination with policymakers, communication gaps among stakeholders, financial constraints, poor health infrastructure, and a lack of evidence-based decision-making capacity. To overcome such barriers all stakeholders should be informed at the planning stage of the research to ensure effective translation into public health policies.

Sustainability

For the sustainability of research outcomes, it is ethically important that researchers ensure thorough effective engagement of all stakeholders during the planning and conduct stages of IR so that the nonresearch stakeholders are also involved in the overall sustained implementation of the intervention. This would ensure greater public access to the outcome of the intervention and would also be ethically justified.

Benefit Sharing with the Community

There is an ethical obligation to share the research benefits with the community, which may be a direct outcome of the research or indirectly as a result of community participation and improved capacity building.

SUGGESTED READINGS

1. World Health Organization. (2019). Ethics in implementation research: Facilitator's guide. [online] Available from https://www.who.int/publications/i/item/9789241515375 [Last accessed December, 2023].
2. Gopichandran V, Luyckx VA, Biller-Andorno N, Fairchild A, Singh J, Tran N, et al. Developing the ethics of implementation research in health. Implement Sci. 2016;11(1):161.

271 CHAPTER

Noncompliance to Medications in Indian Patients

Aparna Agrawal, Prashasti Gupta

ABSTRACT

Noncompliance or nonadherence (often used synonymously) is increasingly being recognized as an important public health issue responsible for ineffective treatment worldwide, more so in the developing countries. Accurate assessment of its magnitude is crucial in monitoring and reducing it, thereby attaining the desired health outcomes. This can be done via both direct and indirect measures. It is often graded as a good (≥80%), moderate (50–80%), or poor (<50%) adherence rate based on arbitrary cutoffs. A whole range of factors could be playing a role in influencing the medication-use pattern including disease-related, drug-related, social and psychological factors, etc., with certain factors unique to India because of cultural differences. High nonadherence rates are directly associated with inadequate control of disease, increased occurrence of complications, and poorer quality of life, all causing greater economic burden on the family as well as nation. Certain practical interventions can help in greatly improving medication adherence rates, some of which include educating provider and patients alike, use of consented reminders, modifying properties of drug to better accommodate patient preferences, incentivization, reducing pill burden, addressing demand supply gaps, and efficient policy making.

INTRODUCTION

Compliance is the degree or the extent to which the prescribed recommendations on the treatment of an illness by the healthcare provider (HCP) are followed correctly by the patient with regards to the drug dosage, timing, frequency, and duration. It could also be nonmedication-related in the form of dietary advice, exercise prescription, physiotherapy, any device use, or habit modification. In simple words, it is passively following the advice and sticking to the prescription provided by HCP. Adherence [preferred term by the World Health Organization (WHO)] is slightly different from compliance in being an active process in which the patient is self-motivated and takes charge for his/her own well-being by becoming an active collaborator in the treatment process, for example, timely filling of new prescriptions. Often, the two are used interchangeably in clinical practice as well as research. Compliance is crucial, be it for curing acute illnesses or controlling chronic conditions and in general for ensuring the overall long-term health and well-being of individuals.

Noncompliance to medication by a patient is thus failure or refusal to comply with prescribed medication. It is fairly widespread, frequently goes undetected, and poses a difficult and at times tricky challenge to successful delivery of healthcare to the masses. Nonadherence can be primary, when medication is not initiated at all, or secondary, when it is initiated but prematurely discontinued. The contributory factors are often complex, may be multiple, and varied across the globe. Certain sociocultural factors and belief systems, however, may be unique to India further adding to the problem. In addition to being detrimental for the individual in the form of uncontrolled disease and its attendant complications, it has serious economic consequences for the nation too in terms of wastage of resources (loss of money and time, lack of wages/productivity, and underutilization of skilled manpower).

HOW TO CHECK FOR NONCOMPLIANCE?

Reliable and accurate estimation of medication nonadherence is imperative, because failure to do so can lead to unnecessary expenditure and dangerous scenarios like labeling therapy as ineffective, unnecessary, and often hazardous intensification of treatment regimens. In addition, from a research perspective, without determination of medication adherence while conducting trials, misrepresentation of findings may occur and wrong conclusions are drawn. Various methods are in use for measuring nonadherence. Since there is no gold standard technique, usually a combination of methods is employed. These could be classified as either subjective/objective/biochemical methods or direct/indirect, each having its own set of pros and cons.

Both the HCP and the patient are asked to give their own assessments of adherence behavior in the form of ratings. Often, however, for the fear of disapproval, patients tend to falsely overreport their adherence. Many times, physicians also tend to oversee, fostering a practice of copying the same treatment on outpatient department (OPD) slips without bothering to pay attention to whether prescriptions are really being complied with. Another way could be by evaluation of standardized patient-administered questionnaires, e.g., brief medication questionnaire, medication adherence questionnaire, eight-item Morisky Medication Adherence Scale (MMAS), and Medication Adherence Report Scale (MARS).

One objective way is counting the remaining pills or inspecting the empty drug blister packs at each clinic visit. However, counting errors may creep in and this technique does not take into account the timing of dosage. Another technique includes using an electronic monitoring device, especially the well-known medication event monitoring system (MEMS). It keeps a tab on time and date when the pill bottle is opened to take medication by virtue of a chip inserted in the bottle cap. But being expensive, it has limitations for widespread use across society. Relatively recent developments include the real-time medication monitoring system and real-time wireless electronic adherence monitor. Pharmacy databases can help in knowing about what drugs are being taken, which are being discontinued, and how frequently prescriptions are being filled, but patients may use more pharmacies than one and buying a drug does not translate into the patient taking it always. Advantages include no recall bias, records can be accessed at any time, and analysis takes less time. Two common measures being used are medication possession ratio (MPR) and proportion of days covered (PDC).

MPR: Number of days for which the medication was obtained divided by the number of days in the period between index refill and last refill.

PDC: Number of days medication was available with the patient divided by the number of days in study period.

These measures involving secondary database analysis can be used only in countries that allow prescription refilling with a centralized computerized system in place with proper upkeep of records (not yet available in India). A direct objective measure would be the act of the patient consuming medication being observed by a family member or an attendant given this responsibility.

Biochemical Estimation

Biochemical estimation is a direct measure as it includes tagging medications with nontoxic markers and then tracing their levels in blood and/or urine to ensure that the patient has indeed taken it. This can get cumbersome while taking into account dietary factors and interindividual and interdrug variation in absorption and excretion rate. Also, they are frequently invasive in nature, expensive, and tend to oversimplify results in a yes or no manner, thus failing to shed light on the pattern of nonadherence. Therapeutic drug monitoring is often done for many diseases like epilepsy to check compliance in addition to being used for drugs with a narrow therapeutic index to adjust dosage to reach serum concentrations in the target range.

HOW TO GRADE NONCOMPLIANCE?

Adherence, measured over a fixed period of time, is commonly represented in percentages, giving an idea about the patient's behavior regarding the intake of medicine against the prescribed manner. It is calculated as the number of pills being actually taken divided by the number that was prescribed and then given as a percentage. An arbitrary threshold is defined above which patients are said to be adherent and below as nonadherent. Another way is classifying the patients as having good, moderate, or poor adherence with predefined ranges.

The adherence should be ≥80% for most chronic diseases. This cutoff is based on data from past studies, both observational and randomized controlled clinical trials. Furthermore, adherence beyond this specific threshold has been linked to both intermediate and long-term outcomes. In most adherence analyses, patients were classified in arbitrarily defined categories as ≥80%, <80%, but ≥50% and <50%.

PREVALENCE OF NONCOMPLIANCE

As per the 2003 WHO report on adherence to long-term therapies, the adherence rate for chronic diseases among the developed countries averaged around 50%, with the magnitude most likely being lower in the developing countries due to limited resources and health inequity.

As per a meta-analysis conducted with eight studies in 2021 by Foley et al., pooled prevalence of nonadherence was found to be 42.6%, the range in these studies being 16.4–61.4%.

In a recent population-based survey from Jordan (2022), nonadherence rate to short-term antibiotics was found to be about 32.1%. In two meta-analyses (2015 and 2017) and a systematic review (2015), the rates of nonadherence (labeled when PDC or MPR < 80%) to medication for type 2 diabetes mellitus were found to range from 21.3 to 90.6%, 10.2 to 55.6%, and 6.9 to 61.5%. Such variation could be attributed to different populations, methodology, and study designs. Likewise, nonadherence rates to oral antidiabetic drugs were reported by various studies conducted in different countries as about 24% (Germany), 53% (Malaysia), 20% (Bangladesh), 29% (Tanzania), 83.3% (Dehradun, India), and 70% (Nagpur, India). In a systematic review and meta-analysis (2010–2021), the overall prevalence of hypertensive medication nonadherence was 65.9% (67.7%—study from Cameroon, 17%—Zambia, 95.9%—Ibadan, Nigeria, 81%—Sokoto, Nigeria, 25%—North-West Ethiopia, 45.4%—South Africa, 35.4%—North-west Ethiopia). For antihypertensives, in various separate studies, nonadherence rates were found to be 49.67% (Bengaluru, India), 18.3% (Korea), and 75.9% (Kancheepuram, South India).

In a meta-analysis of 161 studies (2010–2020) involving 27 million patients published in Journal of American Heart Association, the global nonadherence prevalence was found to range from 27 to 40%, with higher prevalence in low-middle-income countries and in non-Western countries.

FACTORS CONTRIBUTING TO NONCOMPLIANCE

Factors behind poor compliance can be better discussed under the following broad categories

Drug-related Factors

- *Polytherapy/high pill burden*: Often required when multiple comorbidities are present
- *Complexity of drug regimen*: Multiple doses in a day with premeal and postmeal specifications cause greater disruption of routine schedule
- *Side effects*: Minor as well as major side effects are an important cause of secondary nonadherence.
- *Cost*: Direct (price of medication per se) as well as indirect like special diet, transportation, etc.
- *Route of administration*: Oral route tends to have better adherence compared to inhaled or injectables
- Nonavailability due to defective supply chain or erratic supply in some dispensaries or demand–supply mismatch as in some remote areas
- Taste of medication
- *Requirements for drug storage*: As in the case of insulin, which requires refrigeration, especially when ambient temperatures rise sharply in summers
- Concerns regarding long-term use
- Change of medications may impact adherence

Disease-related Factors

- *Indefinite period of use/long use as in all chronic diseases*: Shorter therapy is associated with better adherence rates.
- *Poor perception and unawareness about diseases*: For example, epilepsy in some cultures is considered as a punishment for "sins of past life" or having gone insane or possession by evil spirit, so medications cannot help
- *Degree of behavioral change required*: Lifestyle-related noncommunicable diseases often require behavior change from the patient which is difficult to achieve, and patients become frustrated and unmotivated and may turn nonadherent
- Lack of insight, distorted reality (e.g., schizophrenia)
- Disappearance of symptoms accounts for non-adherence in a significant percentage of patients.
- Disease control status may impact adherence either way (motivating/disheartening).
- Disease complications resulting in physical handicap or effort intolerance may reduce adherence.
- Comorbidities

Social Factors

- *Impairment of function/stigmatization/job loss*: Patients feel impaired and weak, fear loss of job upon disclosure. They feel that they will get addicted to medications and will be devalued and discriminated against by the society (e.g., tuberculosis, epilepsy, HIV).
- Lack of family support/living alone
- Low socioeconomic status
- Lack of/limited insurance coverage
- *Travel*: Many times, when patients are traveling for work/leisure, they forget to take medicines.
- *Festivals*: Celebrating these with family/friends is another time when drug compliance can go for a toss, including dietary indiscretion.
- *Tobacco smoking, alcohol intake*: Those who smoke or drink alcohol are found to be less adherent.

- *Superstitious religious beliefs and faulty cultural values*: Religious fasts can impair adherence, as patients skip medications too.
- Illness/death in family
- Inability to take time off work for hospital visits or investigations or going to the pharmacy

Psychological Factors

- Change of routine
- Forgetfulness, denial, lack of self-discipline, or willful default
- Stress/anxiety/depression
- Mental stereotypes
- Negative attitudes toward health
- *Phobia*: Fear of side effects/fear of dependence
- *Felt better*: Medications are stopped since symptoms abate and patients feel that those are no longer required.
- *Felt worse/not improved*: Including patient's unrealistic expectation of getting cured

Healthcare System Factors

- *Lack of communication with HCP, doctor–patient relationship*: For example, lack of a written action plan in asthma management. Nonadherence is high when patients do not trust their physicians. Counseling by the HCP about the nature of illness, its complications, expectations from treatment, follow-up, etc., is a must. Language barriers can also hinder effective communication.
- Nonavailability of the same HCP (more common in government setups)
- *Logistics*: Distance of health facility from home, frequency of visits, long queues/waiting times
- Prefers/belief in complementary and alternative medicine or more "natural" therapy, treatment from quacks (often easier to access)
- Nonavailability/affordability of monitoring devices (e.g., glucometer, BP apparatus, peak expiratory flow meter)
- Natural disasters or epidemics

Patient-related Factors

Better adherence has been reported in married people, in those with higher educational or financial status, and in retired persons. Literature is divided on the impact of increasing age, gender, and homemakers on adherence. Obesity, addictions, absence of family history of similar disease, and occupation involving a lot of travel have been found to negatively influence adherence.

EFFECTS OF NONCOMPLIANCE

Noncompliance leads to uncontrolled disease which culminates in increased mortality, morbidity, and poorer quality of life as well as greater healthcare resource utilization. Short-term and long-term disease-related complications may set in with increase in the requirement for outpatient visits, emergency department visits, and hospitalization, and overall prognosis becomes worse. Uncontrolled disease often can also have an adverse effect on employment and income opportunities, starting a vicious cycle as the patient may not be in a position to bear the direct and indirect costs of therapy anymore. There is a loss of productivity that affects the society as much as it affects a family. In certain cases like young females suffering from epilepsy, it can impair their prospects for marriage/child bearing. Other issues like social withdrawal/isolation, souring of family ties due to high caregiver burden, high divorce rates, and stigmatization/discrimination may creep in. Noncompliance to antimicrobial drugs can result in spread of drug resistance among microbes.

INTERVENTIONS TO REDUCE NONCOMPLIANCE

Many interventions can be planned and implemented to encourage good patient adherence. Some easy and practical strategies are mentioned below:

- Educating the HCP by holding frequent hospital grand rounds, organizing continuing medical education to stay abreast of latest drug developments, team consults where everyone weighs in, judicious drug use after discussing pros and cons and other teaching activities is an important first step, since this can significantly boost the patient's will to achieve high adherence rates.
- A healthy doctor–patient relationship is at the crux of delivering effective therapy. Strong communication skills with an empathetic attitude and patient listening are equally important. Discussing options and alternatives while respecting the patient's autonomy and ultimately letting the patient choose what suits him best empower the patient to take responsibility and play an active role in managing his/her illness. Such patients are likely to stay compliant. If patients agree, they can be sent timed reminders via messages/emails/automated calls to address the problem of forgetfulness. Reminder systems using short message service (SMS) and smartphone applications with synchronization for transmitting data to physicians can keep the physician updated. It is worthwhile to

recheck the patient's understanding at every visit about the dose, timing, and duration of each medication (inform about what, why, when, how, how long). For those who cannot read, picture-based methods can help to educate them about the same. Also, inform about what side effects to expect or be wary of.

- A patient's education is equally important; they should be provided with information about the nature of disease, need for medication, regular follow-ups, and the short- and long-term consequences of not adhering to therapy. This can be done by word of mouth or handing out pamphlets in the clinic itself or by mass communication using social media applications including blogs, websites, shows on television, radio, and print media like articles in magazines or newspapers. Equally important is to shun the various myths, fraudulent treatments, and conspiracy theories abound on the internet that people tend to easily fall prey to.
- Drug regimens should be kept simple to the extent possible. Combination pills might help in reducing pill burden significantly though at the cost of less flexibility and difficulty in dose adjustment.
- Incentivization of adherent patients is another slightly more direct approach.
- Developing partnership with spiritual leaders with huge following/popular faith-based organizations to spread awareness and information among the masses could be a wise initiative.
- Modifying medication properties in a way to improve adherence rates; for example, sustained-release tablets over conventional-release ones allow less frequent dosing. Different flavors can be added to help with taste issues. Certain modifications may even help to reduce side effects.
- Steps by policymakers and concerned authorities to develop and make available cheaper yet effective generic alternatives to the branded medicines and better access to healthcare for all including outreach clinics.

CONCLUSION

Noncompliance or nonadherence is a major impediment to the realization of benefits of healthcare services and can have serious consequences. Detecting it often proves to be a challenge even for astute physicians. Its prevalence is grossly underestimated across all diseases and geographic borders. The etiology is multifactorial and complex. Its ill-effects are confined not only to an individual or a family but also affect the society and the nation as a whole. A multipronged approach with judicious and rational prescribing, an empathetic HCP with good communication skills, aware and proactive patients, good social support systems, drug research development, and conscientious policymakers is required to fight off this evil.

SUGGESTED READINGS

1. Jin J, Sklar GE, Min Sen Oh V, Chuen Li S. Factors affecting therapeutic compliance: A review from the patient's perspective. Ther Clin Risk Manag. 2008;4(1):269-86.
2. World Health Organization (2003). Adherence to long-term therapies: evidence for action. [online]. Available from https://apps.who.int/iris/handle/10665/42682 [Last accessed December, 2023].
3. Aremu TO, Oluwole OE, Adeyinka KO, Schommer JC. Medication adherence and compliance: Recipe for improving patient outcomes. Pharmacy. 2022;10:106.
4. Foley L, Larkin J, Lombard-Vance R, Murphy AW, Hynes L, Galvin E et al. Prevalence and predictors of medication non-adherence among people living with multimorbidity: a systematic review and meta-analysis. BMJ Open. 2021;11(9):e044987.
5. Almomani BA, Hijazi BM, Awwad O, Khasawneh RA. Prevalence and predictors of non-adherence to short-term antibiotics: A population-based survey. PLoS One. 2022;17(5):e0268285.

272

CHAPTER

Biological Warfare: How Real is the Threat?

Manas Das, Anupam Prakash

ABSTRACT

Biological warfare, the use of living organisms or their toxic products to harm or kill humans, animals, or plants, has long captured the imagination of writers and filmmakers. But is this threat just a product of fiction, or does it pose a genuine danger to global security? This chapter delves into the realm of biological warfare, exploring its historical roots, contemporary developments, and the factors contributing to its potential threat. While the use of biological agents in warfare has been limited, advances in biotechnology have raised concerns about the ease of weaponizing pathogens. The COVID-19 pandemic showcased the catastrophic impact of a naturally occurring pathogen, emphasizing the need for preparedness. International efforts such as the Biological Weapons Convention (BWC) aim to curb the proliferation of such weapons, but enforcement challenges persist. As technology advances and our understanding of genetics deepens, the potential for engineered pathogens with specific targets becomes a concerning reality. While the immediate threat may be debated, the importance of robust surveillance, global cooperation, and ethical considerations cannot be overstated.

INTRODUCTION

Bioterrorism is defined as the unlawful use, or threatened use, of microorganisms or toxins derived from living organisms to produce death or disease in humans, animals, or plants. The act is intended to create fear and intimidate governments or societies in the pursuit of political, religious, or ideological goals.

The idea of using disease as a weapon dates back centuries, but it was not until the 20th century that the concept of biological warfare gained scientific and military interest. The potential to inflict mass casualties without the immediate destruction associated with conventional explosives piqued the curiosity of military strategists and researchers alike. However, the real-world use of biological agents has been relatively limited, with a few notable exceptions. Despite this, advances in biotechnology and the global sociopolitical landscape have reignited concerns about the threat of biological warfare.

HISTORICAL PRECEDENTS

The use of biological agents goes as far back as antiquity, with instances of contaminating water sources with animal carcasses to spread disease **(Table 1)**. In more modern times, the deployment of smallpox-infected blankets against Native Americans during colonial conflicts and Japan's covert biological warfare program during World War II stands as chilling examples. The 1972 Biological Weapons Convention (BWC) sought to prohibit the development, production, and acquisition of biological weapons, marking a significant step toward international disarmament. However, the convention's efficacy has been hindered by verification challenges and allegations of noncompliance.

CLASSIFICATION

According to the Centers for Disease Control and Prevention (CDC), the criteria for assessing the public

TABLE 1: Examples of biological warfare during the past millennium.

Year	Event
1155	Emperor Barbarossa poisons water wells with human bodies, Tortona, Italy
1346	Mongols catapult bodies of plague victims over the city walls of Caffa, Crimean Peninsula
1495	Spanish mix wine with the blood of leprosy patients to sell to their French foes, Naples, Italy
1650	Polish fire saliva from rabid dogs toward their enemies
1675	First deal between German and French forces not to use 'poison bullets'
1763	British distribute blankets from smallpox patients to Native Americans
1797	Napoleon floods the plains around Mantua, Italy, to enhance the spread of malaria enhance the spread of
1863	Confederates sell clothing from yellow fever and smallpox patients to Union troops, USA

health impact of an event or situation are based on several factors **(Table 2)**

- *Morbidity and mortality*: The extent of illness and death caused by the event is a primary indicator. The higher the number of cases and severity of outcomes, the greater the public health impact.
- *Delivery potential*: This refers to the ability of the event to spread rapidly and widely. If the event has the potential to affect a large population in a short period, its impact on public health is considered significant.
- *Public perception (fear, civil disruption)*: The level of fear, panic, and civil disruption that an event causes within the community contributes to its overall impact. Events that lead to heightened public anxiety or disruption are assessed as having a substantial public health impact.
- *Public health preparedness needs*: If an event requires significant and immediate mobilization of public health resources, it is considered to have a notable

TABLE 2: Categories of bioterrorism agents.

	Category A	Category B	Category C
Definition	High-priority agents include organisms that pose a risk to national security because they: • can be easily disseminated or transmitted from person to person; • result in high mortality rates and have the potential for major public health impact; • might cause public panic and social disruption; and • require special action for public health preparedness	Second highest priority agents include those that: • are moderately easy to disseminate • result in moderate morbidity rates and low mortality rates; and • require specific enhancements of the CDC's diagnostic capacity and enhanced disease surveillance	Third highest priority agents include emerging pathogens that could be engineered for mass dissemination in the future because of: • availability; • ease of production and dissemination; and • potential for high morbidity and mortality rates and major health impact
Examples	• Anthrax • Botulism • Plague • Smallpox • Tularemia • *Viral hemorrhagic fevers including:* ○ Flavivirus (Ebola, Marburg) ○ Arenavirus (Lassa, Machupo)	• Brucellosis (*Brucella* species) • Epsilon toxin of *Clostridium perfringens* • Food safety threats (*Salmonella* species, *Escherichia coli* 0157:H7, *Shigella*) • Glanders (*Burkholderia mallei*) • Melioidosis (*Burkholderia pseudomallei*) • Psittacosis (*Chlamydia psittaci*) • Q fever (*Coxiella burnetii*) • Ricin toxin from *Ricinus communis* (castor beans) • Staphylococcal enterotoxin B • Typhus fever (*Rickettsia prowazekii*) • Viral encephalitis (alphaviruses, such as eastern equine encephalitis, Venezuelan equine encephalitis, and western equine encephalitis) • Water safety threats (*Vibrio cholerae*, *Cryptosporidium parvum*)	Emerging infectious diseases such as the Nipah virus and Hanta virus

impact. The strain on healthcare systems and resources indicates the seriousness of the event.

These criteria help public health authorities prioritize their responses and allocate resources efficiently to mitigate the impact of various events, including outbreaks, bioterrorism incidents, and other health-related emergencies.

IDEAL BIOTERRORISM AGENT

The concept of an ideal bioterror weapon revolves around several strategic factors that maximize its impact and potential for chaos. Such a weapon would possess characteristics that ensure its widespread transmission and devastating effects.

Firstly, it would be highly contagious, rapidly spreading among populations and amplifying its reach. Additionally, its virulence would be heightened, causing severe illness or even death in those infected. This combination of contagion and virulence would contribute to a rapid and widespread outbreak.

To enhance its resilience, the ideal bioterror weapon would be robust, capable of surviving in various environments and conditions, enabling it to maintain its potency over time. The ability to remain undetected is crucial, achieved through mechanisms that evade early detection, diagnosis, and containment efforts, enabling the pathogen to spread further before countermeasures are implemented.

Resistance to available treatments, including drugs and vaccines, would be a key trait of such a weapon, rendering conventional medical interventions ineffective and exacerbating the impact on public health. Moreover, having a certain degree of user control over the weapon's dissemination could provide a strategic advantage to the perpetrators, allowing them to manipulate its timing and distribution for maximum impact.

It is important to note that discussions about bioterrorism and potential weapons should always be approached with extreme caution and within the framework of ethical considerations, public safety, and international regulations. The focus of global efforts should remain on preventing such events and building robust response systems to mitigate their potential consequences.

TRANSMISSION

Modes of transmission play a crucial role in the spread of infectious agents. Here are the various means through which transmission can occur:

- *Ingestion and contaminated consumables*: Spread through contaminated food and water sources, leading to ingestion of harmful agents.
- *Aerial dissemination via aircraft sprayers*: Dispersal of pathogens through aircraft, potentially affecting widespread areas.
- *Pathogen distribution via vehicle sprayers*: Utilization of vehicles for releasing pathogens, influencing a broader geographic region.
- *Localized dispersion using handheld sprayers*: Discharge of agents through handheld devices, causing targeted exposure in specific areas.
- *Transmission via mail and packages*: Introduction of pathogens through mail items, risking infection for those handling contaminated packages.
- *Airborne circulation through heating, ventilation and air conditioning systems (HVAC) systems*: Movement of pathogens through air handling and ventilation systems, potentially affecting enclosed spaces.
- *Human-mediated transmission as vectors*: Infected individuals intentionally transmit pathogens through direct contact or respiratory means.
- *Animal-mediated pathogen carriers*: Use of animals as carriers, facilitating the transmission of agents to humans.

Understanding these various routes of transmission is crucial for developing effective countermeasures and response strategies in the event of a bioterror incident or an outbreak of infectious disease.

When to suspect?

Identifying potential indicators of a biological terror event is vital for timely detection and response to mitigate its impact. Several key signs can raise suspicion and prompt further investigation:

- *Unusual vector-borne disease incidence*: Detection of vector-borne diseases in regions lacking the appropriate vectors.
- *Anomalous animal mortality clusters*: Identification of abnormal groupings of sick or deceased animals, suggesting potential pathogen release.
- *Disrupted seasonal patterns*: Observing diseases appearing at atypical times of the year, indicating potential deliberate intervention.
- *Uncommon geographic disease distribution*: Noticing disease cases concentrated in specific locations contrary to natural patterns, possibly indicating intentional spread.
- *Elevated respiratory disease cases*: Increased instances of respiratory illnesses that deviate from the typical regional or temporal trends, warranting suspicion.

It is important to note that while these indicators could raise concern, they might also result from natural events or other factors. Therefore, an effective response requires the collaboration of medical professionals, public health agencies, law enforcement, and other relevant entities to investigate and accurately assess the situation.

If one suspects the presence of a bioterrorist disease, swift and effective action is imperative.

Immediate alert to relevant parties:

- *Hospital infection control*: Swiftly inform the hospital's infection control department to initiate necessary protocols.
- *Implementation of isolation*: In cases of diseases like smallpox, plague, and hemorrhagic fevers, promptly establish isolation measures.
- *Laboratory notification*: Alert the appropriate laboratory responsible for diagnostic testing to begin analysis.
- *Communication with hospital administration*: Notify hospital administrators to coordinate resources and organizational response.
- *Reporting to local public health department*: Inform the local public health department to enable coordinated efforts and guidance.

Timely communication and collaboration with relevant parties are essential to contain the potential outbreak and minimize its impact on public health.

CONTEMPORARY CONCERNS

Recent advancements in biotechnology have raised alarms about the potential for engineered pathogens to be used as weapons. Gene editing tools such as CRISPR have enabled precise modifications to genetic material, blurring the lines between natural and engineered agents. The accidental release of pathogens from research laboratories also underscores the risk of unintentional outbreaks. The advent of tools like CRISPR-Cas9 has revolutionized gene editing, offering the potential to create designer pathogens tailored for specific targets. This dual-use nature of technology presents challenges in distinguishing between legitimate research and nefarious intent. Moreover, the interconnected nature of our globalized world could exacerbate the rapid spread of a bioengineered pathogen, potentially causing a pandemic of unprecedented proportions.

Furthermore, synthetic biology has emerged as a game-changer. This field allows scientists to construct organisms from scratch, blurring the lines between naturally occurring and engineered pathogens. The capability to design organisms with specific traits or abilities could lead to unprecedented threats in the biowarfare landscape.

LESSONS FROM THE COVID-19 PANDEMIC

The COVID-19 pandemic serves as a sobering reminder of the devastating impact a naturally occurring pathogen can have on society. While not a deliberate act of biological warfare, the rapid spread of the virus showcased the vulnerabilities in global preparedness and response. The pandemic exposed the limitations of healthcare systems, the importance of timely information sharing, and the need for international cooperation in addressing health emergencies.

CHALLENGES AND CONSIDERATIONS

The Biological Weapons Convention, although a crucial step toward preventing the use of biological weapons, faces significant challenges in enforcement and verification. The covert nature of biological weapons development makes it difficult to monitor and prevent violations. States may engage in dual-use research, blurring the line between defensive and offensive capabilities. The dynamic nature of biotechnology further complicates matters, as breakthroughs in medical research can inadvertently contribute to biowarfare potential.

Disputes over interpretations of the BWC's provisions persist, with some states pursuing ambiguous paths that raise suspicions about their intentions. The everlooming threat of nonstate actors, including terrorist organizations, adds a layer of complexity. These groups may seek to exploit the vulnerabilities of the biotechnology landscape to create and deploy bioagents for their agendas.

ETHICAL AND MORAL IMPLICATIONS

The ethical dilemmas surrounding biological warfare are profound. The deliberate use of pathogens to cause suffering and death challenges the principles of human morality. The potential for unintended consequences, including environmental damage and the erosion of civilian immunity, raises questions about the long-term consequences of biowarfare. These concerns force us to question the limits of warfare and the values that underpin our actions.

Balancing scientific progress with ethical considerations is a daunting task. While scientific research drives innovation and contributes to human progress, its dual-use nature calls for responsible oversight. The global scientific community must navigate the intricate intersection of technological advancement, ethical guidelines, and national security concerns.

LOOKING AHEAD

The immediate threat of large-scale biological warfare might be debated, given the complexities and uncertainties involved. However, the potential consequences demand proactive measures. Strengthening global surveillance systems, enhancing laboratory safety protocols, and fostering international collaboration are crucial steps. The scientific community must play a responsible role by adhering to codes of conduct and actively engaging in discussions about the ethical implications of their research.

Preparation for a potential bioterrorism attack necessitates a comprehensive approach that involves multiple facets. First and foremost, it is crucial to ensure that medical personnel are well-versed in the identification and handling of various bioterrorism agents, enabling swift response and containment. Integration of these scenarios into disaster planning protocols enhances readiness. Decontamination and infection control measures must be refined to effectively manage the aftermath of an attack.

Establishing clear lines of communication with key agencies, such as governmental bodies and public health organizations, is essential for a coordinated response. Collaboration with laboratories and respective health authorities at the national-level facilitates the prompt sharing of information and resources. Building contacts to acquire stockpiled supplies such as antibiotics, immune sera, and vaccines is pivotal in securing the necessary resources for treatment and prevention.

Amidst these preparations, security measures must also be heightened to safeguard against potential threats and breaches. By holistically addressing these aspects, society can better equip itself to respond effectively to the complex challenges posed by the prospect of a bioterrorism attack.

CONCLUSION

Biological warfare is not merely a fictional trope; it is a historical reality with contemporary implications. While the threat might not be imminent, the potential for catastrophic harm cannot be ignored. As science continues to push boundaries, it is our responsibility to ensure that knowledge is used for the betterment of humanity rather than its destruction. Striking a balance between scientific progress, ethical considerations, and global security is a formidable challenge that requires the concerted efforts of governments, scientists, and societies at large. Only through collective action can we effectively mitigate the threat posed by biological warfare and safeguard the future of humanity.

SUGGESTED READINGS

1. Frischknecht F. The history of biological warfare. Human experimentation, modern nightmares, and lone madmen in the twentieth century. EMBO Rep. 2003;4Spec No(Suppl 1):S47-52.
2. Centers for Disease Control and Prevention. Biological Agents. Emergency Preparedness & Response. [online] Available from https://emergency.cdc.gov/agent/agentlist-category.asp. [Last accessed December, 2023].
3. Clark DP, Pazdernik NJ. Biological warfare: infectious disease and bioterrorism. In: Clark DP, Pazdernik NJ, editors. Biotechnology 2nd edition. MA: Academic Cell; 2016. pp. 687-719.

273

CHAPTER

Skin: What a Physician Should Know?

Avina Jain

ABSTRACT

In India, patients with common skin conditions often receive care from physicians, not dermatologists. Therefore, Indian physicians should be proficient in managing common skin conditions such as urticaria, oral ulcers, drug reactions, post herpes zoster neuralgia, fungal infections, etc. Management of acute urticaria should include oral antihistamines, avoidance of oral steroids, ruling out any infective foci, food additives, and drugs. Oral ulcers require complete physical examination of skin and mucosa. In cases of drug reactions, it must be made mandatory for the patient to carry a "Drug allergy card."

Post-herpes zoster neuralgia can be very well managed by physicians by drugs such as gabapentin, amitriptyline, and opioids. Avoid carbamazepine as a choice of drug for the same. Tinea needs proper treatment with oral and plain topical antifungal.

Fixed-drug topical combinations are banned and should be avoided as the majority of them have super potent corticosteroids such as clobetasol causing severe cutaneous side effects.

General tips for skin management for the physicians: Prescribe oral antihistamines, moisturizers, and plain antifungal creams, and avoid topical steroids to prevent side effects. The physicians should refer or discuss the case with a dermatologist if the concerns of the patients do not resolve after one consultation.

INTRODUCTION

In India, patients with common skin conditions often receive care from physicians, not dermatologists. Therefore, Indian physicians should be proficient in managing common skin conditions, such as urticaria, oral ulcers, drug reactions manifesting in the skin, herpes zoster neuralgia, fungal infections, etc. Indian dermatologists have often expressed that the management of common skin conditions at the level of physicians can be improved by understanding basic management and thus avoiding persistent suffering of patients for years altogether.

For the management of urticaria, oral steroids should be avoided. In case it is really required, oral steroids should be given for 5–7 days and then stopped without tapering. The antihistamines are gold standard treatment and can be stepped up to four times. H2 blockers and Montelukast [in case of food additive or nonsteroidal anti-inflammatory drugs (NSAIDs) induced] can be added. In uncontrolled urticaria, cyclosporine, biologicals such as omalizumab and methotrexate are needed. The physician should also rule out any infective foci, food additives, and the usage of NSAIDs and angiotensin-converting enzyme (ACE) inhibitors for acute urticaria **(Flowchart 1)**.

Recurrent oral ulcers require complete physical examination, including skin, genital, nasal mucosa and conjunctiva, which can point to the diagnosis of a systemic illness or appropriate specialist referral. Oral lichen planus, oral pemphigus vulgaris, and drug reactions are common differential. Generally, treatment by physicians with topicals, oral antibiotics, and vitamin supplements is

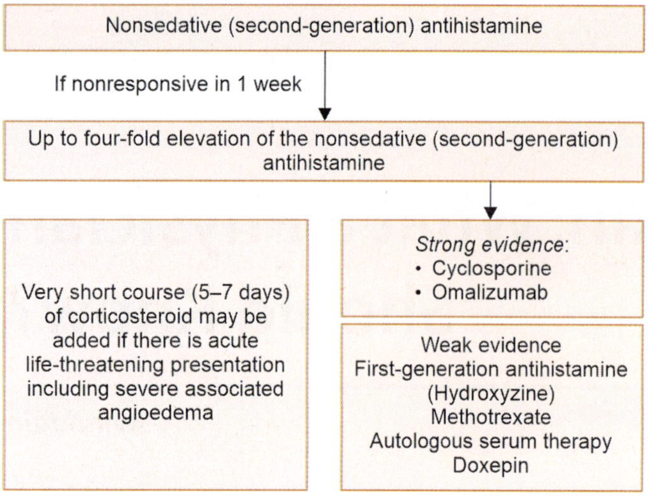

FLOWCHART 1: Management of urticaria.

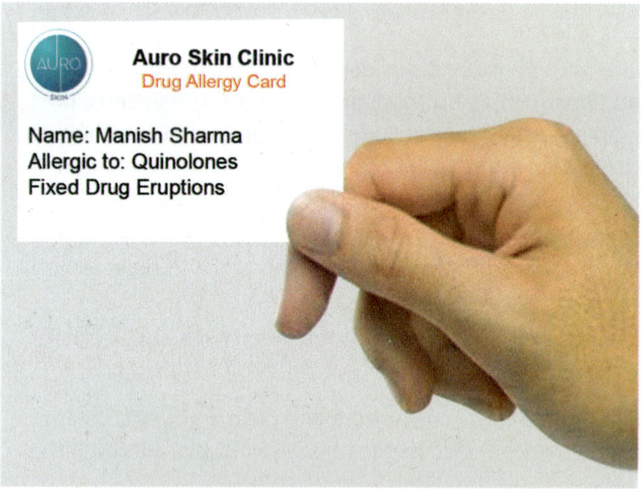

FIG. 1: Sample for a drug allergy card.

done for oral ulcers. If a patient does not respond to the above even after one to two consultations, an opinion of an ENT/dentist or dermatologist should be seeked.

In cases of drug reactions, it must be made mandatory for the patient to carry a "Drug allergy card," clearly mentioning the drugs with which the patient is allergic to. Practitioners should make the drug allergy card themselves and ask the patient to carry in their wallet and encourage the patient to inform all doctors during future consultations **(Fig. 1)**.

Exposure to the same drug after a reaction can be fatal, thus holding the necessity of the allergy card. A good history and temporal association can help delineate the drug causing reaction.

It is also very important to differentiate between different kinds of cutaneous drug reactions, e.g., Stevens-Johnson syndrome (SJS) and bullous fixed-drug eruptions (FDE). Sometimes, the lip mucosa is crusted and gives the appearance of SJS. Always examine the body to rule out any FDE patches on the body as it helps in determining the prognosis. In FDE, there is no systemic involvement so it holds a good prognosis. In SJS, involvement of two or more mucosa with skin tenderness and skin erosions are the key to diagnosis. FDE responds well to topical treatment whereas in SJS patients may need admission and injectables as the patient may go into toxic epidermal necrolysis (TEN).

Post herpes zoster neuralgia (PHN), a common complaint handled by practitioners, should be managed by oral Gabapentin or Pregabalin in upward titrating doses. If not controlled, tricyclic antidepressant (TCA) such as amitriptyline should be added and the opioids are the third line of treatment. Avoid carbamazepine for managing PHN as it is a common cause of systemic and cutaneous drug reaction.

Tinea is an epidemic in India and is often managed suboptimally using a blanket treatment and steroid-containing creams. Tinea mismanagement can lead to poor quality of life, severe cutaneous (striae, recalcitrant disease, skin ulcers, and atrophy) and rarely systemic complications such as glaucoma, and Cushing's syndrome. Physician practitioners must refrain from using steroid-containing creams completely for Tinea to prevent addiction and side effects. Another issue is regarding the resistance to topical antifungals such as miconazole and clotrimazole. The treatment of Tinea requires a full oral antifungal course of 4–6 weeks, oral antihistamines, along with plain antifungal creams only. The physicians must guide the patient and the family to avoid sweating, keep skin dry, keeping personal hygiene products such as soap and towel separate, complete the full oral course of medications, and treat all affected family members simultaneously.

The Indian pharma market is flooded with combination creams (antifungal/antibiotic/steroid). These fixed-drug topical combinations have been banned by the Govt of India but are still available in medical shops. Avoid using these combinations as the majority of them have super potent corticosteroids such as clobetasol. Others like neomycin are known causes of skin allergy so are advised by dermatologists to avoid completely in practice.

In conclusion, when in doubt, the physicians should prescribe oral antihistamines, moisturizers, and plain antifungal creams and avoid topical steroids to prevent side effects. For sending the skin biopsy, prefer a dermatopathologist or a pathologist who has a keen interest in dermatology. Leprosy and syphilis are still prevalent and should always be in high suspicion in differentials, just like how tuberculosis is always kept in the differentials by physicians. Physicians should discuss or refer the case with a dermatologist if the concerns of the patients do not resolve after one consultation.

SUGGESTED READING

1. Godse K, Patil A, De A, Sharma N, Rajagopalan M, Shah B, et al. Diagnosis and management of urticaria in Indian settings: Skin allergy research society's guideline-2022. Indian J Dermatol. 2022;67(6):732-43.

274

CHAPTER

Andropause: Myth or Reality

Ankit Shrivastav, Akash Panigrah

ABSTRACT

Aging is associated with gradual decrease in functional capacity of most organ systems, including the endocrine system. The gradual decline in testosterone level with aging is called andropause or late-onset hypogonadism (LOH). It is less discrete than menopause and possible clinical consequences of andropause are not well established. The prevalence of LOH increases with advancing age. All the symptoms and signs of androgen deficiency are nonspecific and the testosterone cut-off level to define LOH is still debated. Diagnosis of LOH is based on concurrent presence of symptoms suggestive of testosterone deficiency and demonstration of unequivocally and consistently low serum testosterone levels. Testosterone therapy should be offered to men with symptomatic testosterone deficiency after discussing the potential benefits and risks of therapy. Careful exclusion of contraindication for testosterone replacement therapy (TRT) and subsequent monitoring are of paramount importance. If poor response is observed in 3–6 months of TRT, it should be discontinued and alternate cause should be investigated.

INTRODUCTION

Aging is inevitable for all living organisms. The reproductive system, in both male and female, also undergoes various changes with aging, and the sex hormone production by the gonads gradually decreases with age.

In females, at menopause, the cessation of ovarian hormone production is precipitous and resulting clinical consequences are well established. In contrast to menopause, in males the age-related decrease in androgen production is gradual and often subtle.

Andropause is defined as a clinical and biochemical syndrome associated with advancing age, characterized by symptoms and a deficiency in serum testosterone (below the young healthy adult male reference range).

It is less discrete than menopause and possible clinical consequences of andropause are not well established.

The age-associated hypogonadism in male (andropause syndrome) has various other names, like male climacteric, androgen deficiency in the aging male (ADAM), and partial androgen deficiency in the aging male (PADAM), testosterone deficit (syndrome), adult hypogonadism, and *late-onset hypogonadism (LOH)*.

Age after which testosterone deficiency can be classified as late-onset is still debated.

According to the World Health Organization, 60 years of age was used as the cut-off to describe the segment of the older population, whereas in testosterone trials, 65 years was chosen as cut-off.

PREVALENCE

The prevalence of low testosterone increases with increasing age. In Baltimore Longitudinal Study of Aging, the percentage of subjects with low estimates of free testosterone (FT) was 40%, 70%, and 90% for men in their 60s, 70s, and 80s, respectively.

PATHOPHYSIOLOGY

Aging-associated Changes in Hypothalamic–pituitary–testicular Function

The testicular volume decreases by about 15% between 25 and 80–90 years. Production of seminal fluid decreases. Sperms become less motile, and their structure deteriorates but sperm concentration in semen remains quite constant. Sertoli and Leydig cells decrease to around half of that of the young testis. Compensatory response can minimize the decline of testicular function in most aging men.

Hormonal Changes with Aging

Testosterone levels reach maximum at around 25-30 years of age. Thereafter testosterone starts slow steady decline with aging. Total testosterone (TT) ↓ at the rate of 1%/year, but the decline is more pronounced in FT (1.2%/year) **(Fig. 1)**.

Luteinizing hormone (LH) and follicle-stimulating hormone (FSH) concentrations increase (by about 1-2% per year) with aging but do not usually rise above normal range until very old age (>70 years).

Pulsatile LH secretion becomes more irregular and disorderly and LH pulse amplitude ↓.

Middle age to older men usually have ↓ testosterone with normal LH and FSH concentrations, consistent with *secondary hypogonadism*. The gonadotropin suppression is thought to be largely related to age-related comorbidities (e.g., obesity, illness, and medications). ↓ testosterone and ↑ LH and FSH, consistent with *primary hypogonadism*, is more prevalent in very old men, particularly after 70 years of age.

CLINICAL FEATURES OF TESTOSTERONE DEFICIENCY IN AGING

Consequences of declining testosterone are not known with certainty. The evidences are mainly from young hypogonadal men. All the symptoms and signs of androgen deficiency are nonspecific and strictly depend on the age at onset, duration, severity, and the underlying pathogenesis **(Table 1)**.

Different domains may be involved including:

- Sexual (e.g., erectile dysfunction)
- Physical (e.g., gynecomastia, decreased body hair)
- Psychological (e.g., changes in mood and well-being)
- Cardiometabolic (e.g., changes in body composition and metabolic syndrome)

Questionnaires

To improve detecting hypogonadism including LOH and discriminating it from other disorders, various questionnaires are used. Mostly used questionnaires are: Aging Male's Symptoms Scale (AMS); Androgen Deficiency in the Aging Males (ADAM); Massachusetts

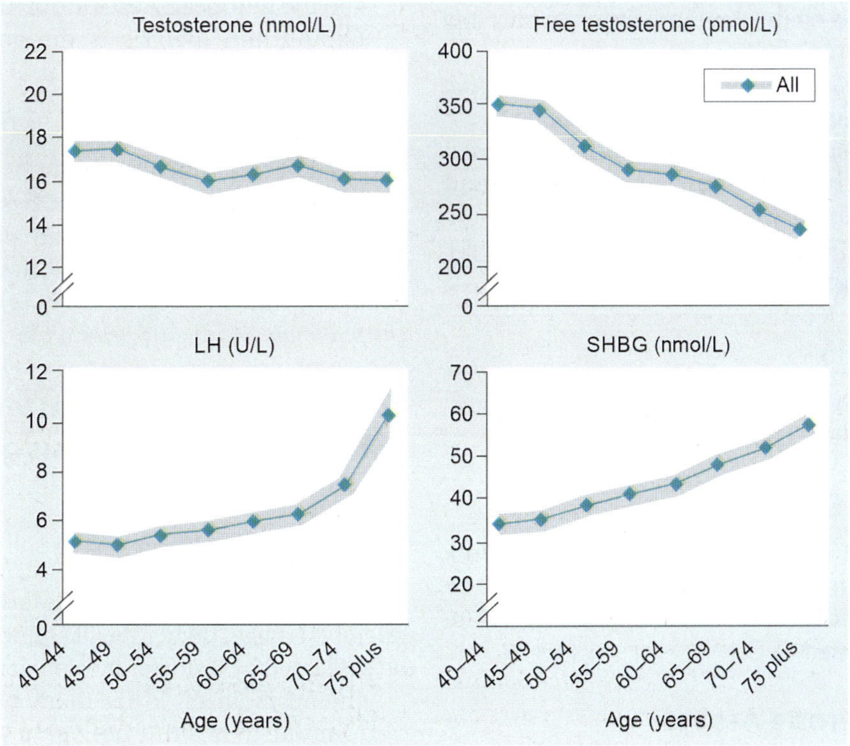

FIG. 1: Hypothalamic–pituitary–testicular axis disruptions in older men.
(LH: luteinizing hormone; SHBG: sex hormone-binding globulin)

TABLE 1: Clinical features of testosterone deficiency in aging male.

More specific symptoms	More specific signs
Reduced libido	Small or shrinking testes
Loss of morning erections	Loss of male hair
Infertility	Aspermia or azoospermia or severe oligozoospermia
Breast enlargement	Gynecomastia
Reduced shaving frequency	Low bone mineral density
Hot flashes and sweats	Unexplained reduction in prostate size or prostate-specific antigen (PSA)

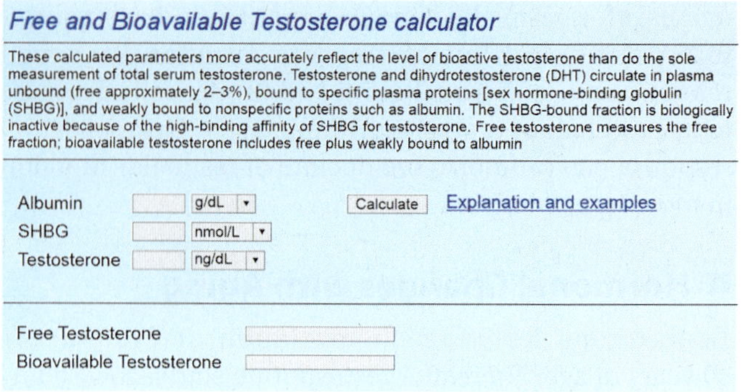

FIG. 2: Online calculator for free testosterone calculation.

Male Ageing Study questionnaire or Smith's screener questionnaire, and the Androtest.

Most societies recommend against their use for universal screening for hypogonadism due to limited diagnostic accuracy.

DIAGNOSIS OF ANDROPAUSE

It is a *diagnosis of exclusion*. Depression, hypothyroidism, chronic alcoholism, and use of medications such as corticosteroids, cimetidine, spironolactone, digoxin, opioid analgesics, antidepressants, and antifungal agents should be excluded before making a diagnosis of LOH. Diagnosis of LOH should not be made during acute illness.

Diagnosis requires characteristic symptoms plus low total (or free) testosterone on two occasions.

Minimum criteria for the diagnosis of LOH in aging men in European Male Aging Study (EMAS) include:

- Presence of at least three *sexual symptoms* (decreased sexual interest, reduced morning erections, and erectile dysfunction) *combined with*
- *Low testosterone* (TT <11 nmol/L (320 ng/dL) *or* FT <220 pmol/L (64 pg/mL)

INVESTIGATIONS

Hormonal investigations needed are: TT, FT, sex hormone-binding globulin (SHBG), FSH, and LH.

Testosterone Sampling

Testosterone should be measured in the *fasting state* between 7 and 11 am on at least two different days. In addition, measurement of testosterone during acute illness should be avoided.

Total Testosterone Assays

Liquid chromatography-tandem mass spectrometry (LC-MS/MS) is most accurate and precise, but it is not universally available, and there are financial and technical constraints.

Automated platform testosterone immunoassays, if well-standardized, can show high correlation with LC-MS/MS within the adult male testosterone range (although they offer less precision in the hypogonadal range).

Free Testosterone Assays

Free testosterone may be indicated only in:

- Conditions that alter SHBG levels, or
- TT at or near lower limit of normal {200–400 ng/dL (Endocrine Society) versus 8–12 nmol/L (231–346 ng/dL) [the British Society for Sexual Medicine (BSSM) and the European Academy of Andrology (EAA)]}

Equilibrium dialysis is the gold standard in free hormone measurement, but it is technically difficult, expensive, and seldom available to physicians.

Immunoassays do not provide reproducible results and are not recommended.

Calculated free testosterone, based on measurements of total testosterone, SHBG, and albumin correlate well with measurements by equilibrium dialysis. Different validated online calculators **(Fig. 2)** are available for use *(http://www.issam.ch/freetesto.htm)*.

Cut-off Level of Testosterone for Biochemical Diagnosis of Late-onset Hypogonadism

There is no general consensus on the cut-off level of testosterone for defining LOH and the present cut-offs are arbitrary. Lower the testosterone level below lower limit of reference range, higher the likelihood that symptoms will be explained by testosterone deficiency.

The harmonized lower limits of reference range for testosterone in healthy, nonobese young men (aged 19–39 years) were 264 ng/dL and 303 ng/dL (2.5th and 5th percentiles respectively).

There is some agreement amongst various professional bodies that the TT level >12 nmol/L (350 ng/dL) does not require substitution. Similarly, patients with serum TT levels <8 nmol/L (230 ng/dL) will usually benefit from testosterone treatment. If the serum TT level is between 8 and 12 nmol/L (230 and 350 ng/dL), repeating the measurement of TT with SHBG to calculate FT or bioavailable testosterone will benefit the patient.

Further Investigations

If organic secondary hypogonadism is suspected:

- MRI of pituitary hypothalamus, iron saturation and prolactin as well as determination of other pituitary hormones
- These patients usually have evidence of pituitary mass effects such as visual disturbances, headache or hyperprolactinemia, and testosterone concentrations <6 nmol/L (<175 ng/dL).

TESTOSTERONE REPLACEMENT THERAPY IN ANDROPAUSE

There is dilemma in deciding "which elderly man should be treated?". As benefit of testosterone replacement is not very clear in older adults, treatment has unfavorable side effect profile.

Clinical challenge is to identify individuals who will benefit from testosterone replacement therapy (TRT) **(Fig. 3)**.

Endocrine Society Clinical Practice Guideline 2018 Recommendations

The Endocrine Society Clinical Practice Guideline 2018 recommendations include:

- Not to treat asymptomatic older men with age-related decline in testosterone levels.
- Consider offering testosterone therapy on an individualized basis to older men with low testosterone levels measured on more than one occasion and clinically significant symptoms of androgen deficiency.
- Explicit discussion of uncertainty about the risks and benefits of testosterone therapy.
- Once the decision for TRT is taken, the appropriate testosterone preparation is chosen based on local availability, cost, and its sideeffect profile.
- Aim of TRT is target TT 400–500 ng/dL (mid normal range).

Lifestyle, concomitant medications, and comorbidities management:

- Lifestyle changes, including physical exercise and weight reduction, in overweight and obese men are important, since weight loss may increase testosterone concentrations.
- Similarly, withdrawal/modification of drugs (e.g., opiates, anabolic steroids, and glucocorticoids) potentially interfering with testosterone production should be attempted.
- Few experts recommended treating comorbidities first and starting TRT only in patients with persistently low testosterone levels.

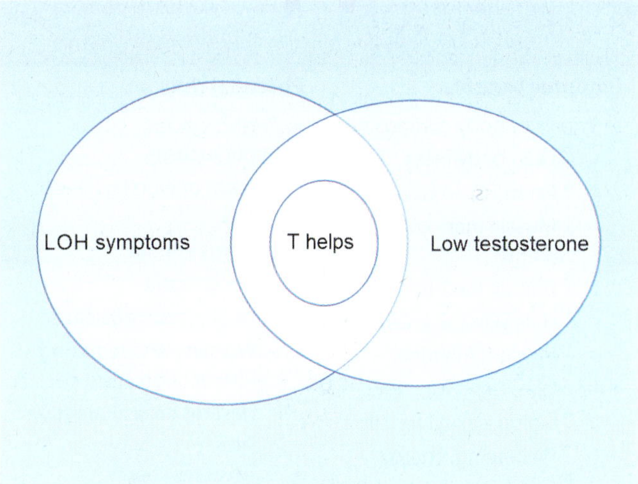

FIG. 3: Subset of patients benefiting from testosterone replacement therapy (TRT).
(LOH: late-onset hypogonadism; T: testosterone)

Various Effects of Testosterone Replacement Therapy in Late-onset Hypogonadism

Effects of TRT in LOH noted in various clinical trials **(Table 2)** are summarized here:

- Increased sexual activity, sexual desire, and erectile function
- Slightly improved mood and decreased depressive symptoms
- Increased hemoglobin in men who had anemia of either known or unknown cause
- Increased volumetric bone mineral density (BMD) and the estimated strength of the spine and hip. Despite improvements in BMD, limited evidence supports a direct effect of TRT on fractures risk.
- No changes in energy or cognitive function were found.
- Discordant results were found concerning the distance walked.
- Erythrocytosis (Hb > 17.5 g/dL) ↑ prostate-specific antigen (PSA) >1.0 ng/mL in small number of men
- There was no difference in lower urinary tract symptom (LUTS) or cardiovascular (CV) or prostate

TABLE 2: Benefits and risks of testosterone replacement therapy.

Potential benefits	Potential risks
• Improves body composition: ○ ↑ Lean body mass ○ ↑ Fat mass, ↓ visceral fat ○ ↑ Muscle mass and strength ○ ↑ BMD, ↓ fractures ○ ↑ Hair, skin thickness ○ ↑ Physical function • Improves brain function: ○ ↑ Libido, sexual function ○ ↑ Well-being, energy ○ ↑ Irritability, depression ○ ↑ Cognitive function ○ ↑ Sleep quality • Increases hematocrit • Decreases cardiovascular risk	• Erythrocytosis, hyperviscosity • Induces or worsens sleep apnea • Worsens edema • Gynecomastia • Clinical prostate disease ○ Worsens BPH requiring intervention ○ Hastens clinical prostate cancer • Suppresses sperm production • Increases cardiovascular risk

adverse events in testosterone- and placebo-treated men.

- *CV risk*: There is conflicting evidence. It increases coronary artery noncalcified plaque volume as assessed using computed tomographic angiography. Increased CV risk found only with TRT at higher dosage than those recommended or when frail men were considered. There are differences in included patients, doses, or formulations, which may explain the heterogeneity of findings.
- *Larger, long-term, randomized trials are needed* to determine balance of clinical benefits and risks (particularly prostate cancer and CV risks) associated with TRT in older men.

Before initiation of TRT in men > 40 years:

- PSA
- Digital rectal examination (DRE) of the prostate
- TRT not recommended if PSA > 4 ng/mL (or elevated PSA according to local/national guidelines) or prostate abnormalities on DRE without further evaluation and/or urological consultation.

Contraindications for Testosterone Replacement

- *Absolute contraindications*: Prostate and breast cancer
- *Relative contraindications*:
  - PSA > 4 ng/mL or 3 ng/mL in men with increased risk for prostate cancer (African descent or with first-degree relatives with a history of prostate cancer)
  - Hematocrit > 50%
  - Severe LUTSs caused by benign prostatic hypertrophy [International Prostate Symptom Score (IPSS) > 19]
  - Untreated or poorly controlled congestive heart failure
  - Untreated sleep apnea

Which Testosterone Preparation?

The preparations available in India are injections (testosterone enanthate/cypionate, testosterone undecanoate), testosterone patch, testosterone gel, testosterone solution, and oral testosterone undecanoate.

Mostly injections are used due to their easy availability and cost-effectiveness.

Adverse Effects

Adverse effects include increased hematocrit, increased prostate-related events, obstructive sleep apnea (OSA), reduced sperm count, gynecomastia, acne and oily skin, frontal balding, weight gain, stimulation of excess libido, dyslipidemia, and derangement of liver function.

MONITORING ON TESTOSTERONE THERAPY

- Most symptoms improve within 3–6 months of starting TRT.
- If no clinical improvement after 6 months of sufficient testosterone replacement, TRT should be discontinued, and alternative causes should be searched.
- If the patient shows significant clinical benefits, switching to longer acting testosterone prep considered. Clinical and laboratory follow-up at 3 and 12 months and then annually in any patient on TRT, including those with LOH.
- Both the efficacy and safety of TRT should be assessed at each visit. DRE at each assessment. TT, PSA, hematocrit, liver function test (LFT), and lipids (with or without glycemic profile) should always be evaluated.

CONCLUSION

There is gradual decline in testosterone level with age. The prevalence of LOH increases with age, and it is associated with myriad age-related diseases. The concept of late-onset hypogonadism is still developing and various aspects of it are still debatable. The symptoms are nonspecific, and its possible health consequences are not known. The decision for TRT should be individualized

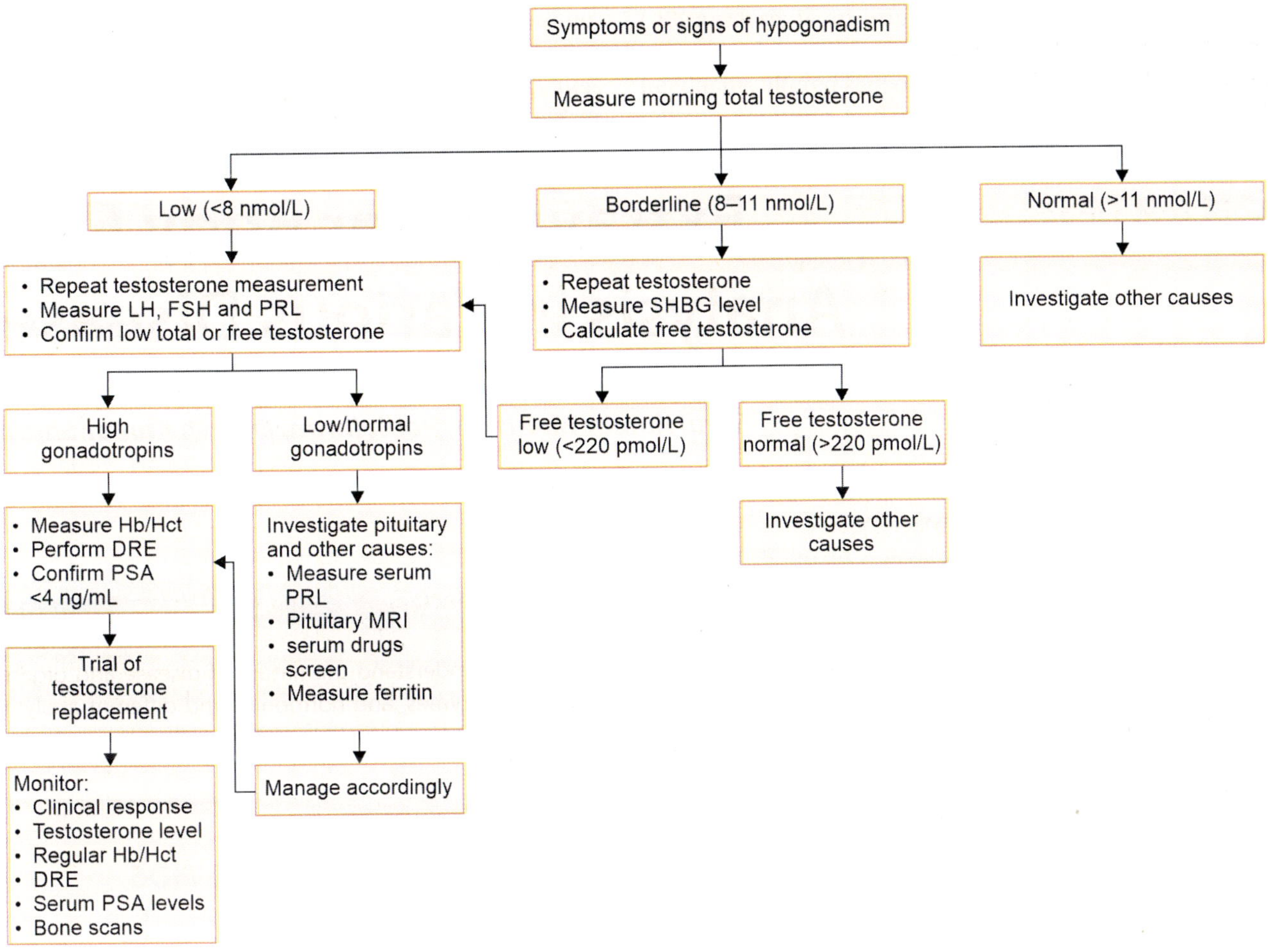

FLOWCHART 1: Approach to hypogonadism in aging males.

(DRE: digital rectal examination; FSH: follicle-stimulating hormone; Hb: hemoglobin; Hct: hematocrit; LH: luteinizing hormone; PRL: prolactin; PSA: prostate-specific antigen; SHBG: sex hormone-binding globulin)

Source: Huhtaniemi I, Forti G. Male late-onset hypogonadism: pathogenesis, diagnosis and treatment. Nat Rev Urol. 2011;8(6):335-44.

(Flowchart 1). Present indication of TRT is the presence of characteristic symptoms with low testosterone (total or free) on two occasions.

Hematocrit, screening for prostate cancer and OSA should be monitored at baseline and during therapy. Lack of benefit in sexual symptoms and energy, vitality, or mood at 6 months should lead to discontinuation of therapy. More research including larger, long-term, randomized trials is needed to understand this complex interaction between aging and androgen deficiency.

SUGGESTED READINGS

1. Bhasin S, Brito JP, Cunningham GR, Hayes FJ, Hodis HN, Matsumoto AM, et al. Testosterone therapy in men with hypogonadism: an Endocrine Society clinical practice guideline. J Clin Endocrinol Metab. 2018;103(5):1715-44.
2. Tajar A, Huhtaniemi IT, O'Neill TW, Finn JD, Pye SR, Lee DM, et al. EMAS Group. Characteristics of androgen deficiency in late onset hypogonadism: Results from European Male Aging Study (EMAS). J Clin Endocrinol Metab. 2012;97:1508-16.
3. Wang C, Nieschlag E, Swerdloff R, Behre HM, Hellstrom WJ, Gooren LJ, et al. Investigation, treatment and monitoring of late-onset hypogonadism in males: ISA, ISSAM, EAU, EAA and ASA recommendations. Eur J Endocrinol. 2008;159:507-14.
4. Bassil N. Late onset hypogonadism. Med Clin North Am. 2011;95:507-23.

TABLE 3: CSF analyses in various noninfectious CNS disorders.

CNS condition	Clinical features	CSF analysis
Transverse myelitis	• Bilateral (not necessarily symmetric) sensorimotor and autonomic spinal cord dysfunction • Clearly defined sensory level • Hyperreflexia • Babinski positive	• Signs of inflammation (pleocytosis, elevated protein concentration, oligoclonal bands, or elevated IgG index) • Elevated CSF IL-6 • PCR negative for infections • CSF sugar, pressure usually normal
Guillain–Barré syndrome	• Acute symmetrical progressive weakness, areflexia • Post infection • Autonomic dysfunction • Cranial nerve involvement • Mild sensory signs	• Normal CSF cell count • Elevated CSF protein levels • Cytoalbuminologic disassociation
Multiple sclerosis	• Loss of sensation • Muscle weakness • Visual loss • Incoordination, cognitive impairment • Fatigue, pain • Bladder and bowel disturbance	• Pleocytosis (5–50 cells/mm^3; lymphocytes) • Elevated protein • OCB may be present (highly diagnostic) • IgG index (increase CSF IgG compared to serum IgG levels)
Neuromyelitis optica	• A severe transverse myelitis • An acute unilateral or bilateral optic neuropathy • No other clinical involvement	• Nonspecific • Pleocytosis (5–50 cells/mm^3; lymphocytes) • Elevated protein • OCB may be present (most cases) • Normal glucose levels
Acute demyelinating encephalomyelitis (ADEM)	• Fever, meningeal signs, and acute encephalopathy • The level of consciousness ranges from lethargy to frank coma • Maximum progression 4–7 days • Common in children • MRI diagnostic	• Pleocytosis (5–50 cells/mm^3) and/or increased protein concentration • May be normal • CSF nondiagnostic • Presence of OCB favors diagnosis of MS

(CSF: cerebrospinal fluid; CNS: central nervous system; IgG: immunoglobulin G; IL: interleukin; OCB: oligoclonal bands; MRI: magnetic resonance imaging; MS: multiple sclerosis)

Pleural Fluid analysis

Pleural fluid is ultrafiltration of plasma and usually volume is <10 mL each pleural space. Pleural fluid accumulates in pleural cavity by different mechanism, including increased hydrostatic pressure, increased permeability, and increased production. Different etiopathogenesis causes pleural fluid accumulation like infective, inflammatory, noninflammatory, and malignant condition. Mainly differentiate in two categories, exudative pleural effusion and transudative pleural effusion. Pleural fluid analysis has bundle of different tests and markers, which include appearance, cytology, biochemistry [protein, glucose, lactate dehydrogenase (LDH), adenosine deaminase (ADA), pH, amylase, cholesterol, carcinoma markers, antinuclear antibody (ANA) titers, creatinine, procalcitonin, and N-terminal-pro-brain natriuretic peptide (NT-proBNP)], and microbiology (parasitic infections).

Gross appearance, character of the fluid (transudative or exudative), and odor help in diagnosing several conditions **(Table 4)**.

Transudate and exudate: Transudate pleural effusion produces imbalances in both hydrostatic and oncotic pressures, as in congestive heart failure (CHF), nephrotic syndrome, hepatic hydrothorax, movement of fluid from peritoneal cavity, retroperitoneal spaces, or can be iatrogenic. Exudate pleural effusion results primarily from pleural and lung inflammation such as infection (bacterial, fungal, viral, tubercular, parasitic, hepatic, or splenic abscess, etc.), malignancy, connective tissue disorder, pancreatitis, endocrine disorders (ovarian hyperstimulation syndrome, hypothyroidism), lymphatic abnormalities, and iatrogenic.

Light's criteria, originally published in 1972 and revised 2002 is used to differentiate between transudate

TABLE 4: Diagnosis based on naked eye examination of pleural fluid.

Based on gross appearance	
Pale yellow (straw)	Tubercular
Red (bloody)	Malignancy, asbestos pleural effusion, postcardiac injury or pulmonary infarction
White (milky)	Chylothorax or cholesterol
Brown	Long standing effusion, rupture of amebic liver abscess
Black	*Aspergillus niger*, metastatic melanoma, pancreaticopleural fistula, bronchogenic adenocarcinoma, chronic hemothorax, and cocaine use
Yellow-green	Rheumatoid pleurisy
Dark green	Biliothorax
Odor	
Putrid	Anaerobic empyema
Ammonia	Urinothorax

and exudate. If at least one of the three criteria is fulfilled, the fluid is exudate:

1. Pleural fluid protein/serum protein ratio >0.5, or
2. Pleural fluid LDH/serum LDH ratio >0.6, or
3. Pleural fluid LDH greater than two-thirds the upper limits of the laboratory's normal serum LDH

Light's criteria are highly sensitive but low specificity.

Biochemical analysis:

- *Protein*: Transudate fluids have proteins <3 g/dL, although diuresis in heart failure causes increased pleural fluid protein, which is differentiated from exudate by serum to pleural fluid albumin gradient >1.2 g/dL. Tubercular pleural fluid has protein concentration >3 g/dL. If protein concentration is between 7 and 8 g/dL, diagnosis of multiple myeloma or Waldenström macroglobulinemia must be considered.
- *Cholesterol*: Cholesterol > 45 mg/dL is indicative of exudative effusion and cholesterol >250 mg/dL is pseudochylothorax. Triglycerides > 110 mg/dL are diagnostic of chylothorax.
- *LDH*: Pleural fluid LDH plays diagnostic role in differentiating exudate from transudate as well as amongst various types of exudative effusions. LDH > 1,000 IU/L is characteristic of empyema, rheumatoid pleurisy, and malignancy. They are increased in both tuberculosis and synpneumonic effusions but less in tuberculosis. A pleural fluid to serum LDH ratio >1.0 is diagnostic of *Pneumocystis jirovecii*-associated effusion.
- *Glucose*: Glucose concentration equal to serum; except in a few conditions that have glucose concentration <60 mg/dL. The classic example of low glucose concentration is rheumatoid pleurisy, empyema, malignancy, lupus pleuritis, tubercular effusion, and esophageal rupture.
- *Amylase*: Most common causes of amylase-rich fluid are acute and chronic pancreatitis, esophageal rupture, and malignancy. Pancreatic effusion is rich in pancreatic isoenzyme, whereas esophageal and malignant effusion are rich in salivary isoenzyme.
- *ADA*: Differentiates tubercular (35–50 U/L) from malignancy (<40 U/L) when exudate is rich in lymphocytes. The defined threshold for diagnosis of tuberculosis is ADA levels >40 U/L. ADA has negative predictive value in regions with low tubercular prevalence.
- *pH*: Normal pH of pleural fluid is 7.6. Transudates have a pleural fluid pH 7.40–7.55, while majority of exudates range from 7.30–7.45. Pleural fluid pH < 7.20 is an indication of chest tube drainage and poor prognosis. Pleural fluid to serum creatinine ratio >1.0 is diagnostic of urinothorax.
- *Cancer biomarkers*: No single pleural fluid biomarker is accurate enough to establish diagnosis of malignancy. A meta-analysis found a combination of CEA, CYFRA 21-1, and CA19-9 to have a 95.06% sensitivity for adenocarcinoma-associated malignant effusion. Mesothelin in pleural fluid has an adjuvant diagnostic value with high specificity and low sensitivity in diagnosis of mesothelioma.
- *Cytology*: Malignant cell cytology has a sensitivity of 60% and varies highly with the histological type of the underlying malignancy (78% for adenocarcinoma, 53% for small cell carcinoma, and 25% for squamous cell carcinomas). Cell numbers are never diagnostic but may be helpful in some instances, such as pleural fluid cells counts >50,000 cells/mm^3 are indicative of empyema, cells counts >10,000 cells/mm^3 are indicative of bacterial pneumonia, acute pancreatitis, and lupus pleuritis, and chronic effusions associated with tuberculosis and malignancy have counts <5,000 cells/mm^3. Nucleated cell type also helps in diagnosis of various etiologies of effusion **(Tables 5 and 6)**.

Pericardial Fluid Analysis

Pericardial fluid is originated from visceral pericardium ultrafiltration of plasma, and approximate amount is 15–20 mL. Pericardial effusion may be acute or chronic and may have significant impact on patient clinical history. Because clinical manifestation depends on the filling pressure and amount of pericardial fluid (tamponade), acute and subacute pericardial effusions have no definitive time duration, but chronic pericardial effusion have duration >3 months. Pericardial fluid content normally includes protein, albumin, LDH, sugar, cholesterol, and nucleated cells. Most useful parameters are Gram stain, bacterial, and fungal culture, cytology, acid-fast bacilli (AFB) stain and mycobacterial culture along with ADA, interferon-gamma, or lysozyme (for tubercular pericarditis), and polymerase chain reaction (PCR). ANA must be assessed in young females with acute pericardial effusion as sometimes it can be initial presentation of lupus.

The derived normal reference values are as follows: Total protein (1.7–4.6 g/dL), pericardial fluid/serum protein ratio (0.29–0.83), LDH (141–2613 U/L), pericardial fluid/serum LDH ratio (0.40–2.99), albumin (1.19–3.06 g/dL), and pericardium to serum albumin gradient (0.18–2.37 g/dL).

Pericardial effusion has important prognostic (as in intrathoracic neoplasm), diagnostic (as in myopericarditis or acute pericarditis), or both (as in dissection of the ascending aorta) implications.

Pericardial effusion develops in various local and systemic disease, so biochemical, cytological, microbiological analyses are necessary to find out diagnosis. Major categories are of two types: Transudative and exudative. Exudative pericardial effusion has infective, inflammatory, malignant, and autoimmune diseases. Transudative effusion is mainly due to lymphatic channel obstruction. However, differentiations of biochemist tests criteria refer range same as pleural effusion criteria, so validity of this approach is uncertain. Important biochemical tests are LDH and total protein, so Light's criteria is used for differentiation.

- Pleural fluid protein/serum protein ratio >0.5, or
- Pleural fluid LDH/serum LDH ratio >0.6, or
- Pleural fluid LDH greater than two-thirds the upper limits of the laboratory's normal serum LDH

Pericardial effusion can be exudative (inflammatory, infectious, malignant, or autoimmune) or transudative (heart failure, hypoalbuminemia, postradiation therapy, and renal insufficiency). Criteria to establish exudative effusion include:

- SEAG (in patients treated with diuretics) ≤ 12/L
- Pericardial fluid/serum cholesterol ratio ≥ 0.3

Echocardiography is used to assess for the sign of pericardial effusion, presence of lemonade, and ejection fraction. Small effusion is 50–100 mL seen only posteriorly <10-mm thickness, moderate effusion is 100–500 mL, and large effusion is >500 mL.

Echocardiography findings of tamponed include diastolic right heart collapse, abnormal ventricular septal motion, exaggerated inspiratory variability in mitral inflow velocity, and inferior vena cava plethora.

Etiology of pericardial effusion varies with geographic location, and some of the common ones are:

- Acute pericarditis (viral, bacterial, tuberculous, or idiopathic in origin)
- Autoimmune
- Postmyocardial infarction or cardiac surgery
- Sharp or blunt chest trauma, including a cardiac diagnostic or interventional procedure

TABLE 5: Disorders related to neutrophilia, lymphocytosis, and eosinophilia in pleural fluid.

Neutrophilia	Lymphocytosis	Eosinophilia
• Bacterial pneumonia (parapneumonic effusion) • Pulmonary infarction • Pancreatitis • Early tuberculosis • Usually found in >10% transudates	• Tuberculosis • Viral infection • Malignancy • Chylothorax • Rheumatoid pleuritis • Usually found in >30% transudates	• Pneumothorax • Malignancy • Trauma (hemothorax) • Pulmonary infarction • Congestive heart failure • Parasitic and fungal infection

TABLE 6: Clinically relevant comparative pleural fluid analysis.

Parameters	Normal value	Tubercular	Exudative	Transudative
Protein		>4 g/dL	Pleural fluid/serum protein ratio >0.5	Below 3 g/dL
Appearance	Clear, light yellow, odorless, and nonviscous	Straw yellow colored	Cloudy, turbid, purulent, and pronounced clotting tendency	Clear, light yellow, odorless, and nonviscous
Cell type/cell count		<5,000 cells/mm^3	More than 10,000 cells/mm^3	
LDH	200 IU/L		Pleural fluid/serum LDH ratio >0.6	
Glucose			Pleural fluid/serum glucose <0.5	
pH	7.60		7.30–7.45	7.40–7.55
Cholesterol			>45 mg/dL	

(LDH: lactate dehydrogenase)

- Malignancy, particularly metastatic spread of noncardiac primary tumors
- Mediastinal irradiation
- Renal failure
- Myxedema, ovarian hyperstimulation syndrome
- Aortic dissection extending into the pericardium
- Drugs (methysergide, anticoagulants, thrombolytics, phenytoin, penicillin, phenylbutazone, and doxorubicin)

Pericardiocentesis has a diagnostic yield of only 40%. Hence, as per 2015 European Society of Cardiology (ESC) guidelines, it is performed under the following instances:

- Therapeutic in those with tamponade
- In those with purulent pericarditis, tubercular pericarditis, or neoplastic pericarditis
- In those with moderate to large effusions of unknown etiology and not rapidly responding to anti-inflammatory therapy

Autoreactive pericarditis/pericardial effusion: This is a diagnosis of exclusion and responds to steroids. ESC established guidelines in 2004 to diagnose autoreactive pericarditis using following criteria **(Table 7)**:

- Increased number of lymphocytes and mononuclear cells > 5,000/mm^3 (autoreactive lymphocytosis), or antibodies against heart muscle (antisarcolemmal) in pericardial fluid
- Signs of myocarditis on epicardial/endomyocardial biopsies (>14 cells/mm^2)
- Exclusion of active viral infection both in pericardial effusion and endomyocardial/epimyocardial biopsies (no virus isolation, no immunoglobulin M titer against cardiotropic viruses in pericardial effusion, and negative PCR for major cardiotropic viruses)
- Tuberculosis, *Borrelia burgdorferi*, *Chlamydia pneumoniae*, and other bacterial infections excluded by PCR and/or cultures
- Neoplastic infiltration absent in pericardial effusion and biopsy samples
- Exclusion of systemic, metabolic disorders, and uremia

Peritoneal/Ascitic Fluid Analysis

Accumulation of free fluid in peritoneal sac called ascites. Normal volume is 5 mL in male and 5–18 mL in female, depending on the phase of the menstrual cycle. Ascitic fluid etiopathogenesis is divided in two mainly group as exudative and transudative. Transudative fluid is produced by visceral capillary or drained by lymphatic system of diaphragm. Exudative fluid is generated by inflammation of vessels and tissue. The most common cause of ascites is portal hypertension due to cirrhosis followed by heart failure, malignancy, tubercular ascites, and others. Peritoneal fluid analysis helps to diagnose the underlying pathology **(Table 8)**.

Due to the vast etiology that underlies ascites, ascitic fluid analysis plays a major role in determining the diagnosis. Clinically, ascites is suspected in those with progressive abdominal distention with flank dullness and signs and symptoms of underlying disease (e.g., cirrhosis: jaundice, pedal edema, splenomegaly, caput medusae, spider naevi, palmar erythema; constrictive pericarditis or heart failure: elevated JVP, etc.). The presence of ascites and underlying pathology is then confirmed by imaging [ultrasound, contrast-enhanced computed tomography (CECT), or magnetic resonance imaging (MRI)], depending on clinical scenario.

TABLE 7: Pericardial fluid analysis in various disorders.

Parameters	Normal value	Bacterial pericarditis	TB pericarditis	Exudative	Transudative
Appearance	Clear	Cloudy to turbid		Cloudy, bloody or turbid	Clear to pale yellow
Glucose					
Color	Pale yellow	Pale yellow			
Protein	1.7–4.6 g/dL			>3 g/dL	
Cell type/cell count		6,000–240,000 cells/mm^3			>1,000 cells
LDH	141–2613 IU/L			>200 IU/L	
ADA			Positive in tuberculosis		
Lymphocyte/neutrophil ratio			>1		
Fluid LDH/serum LDH				>0.6	<0.6
Specific gravity				1.015	
Fluid protein/serum protein	0.29–0.83			>0.5	

(ADA: adenosine deaminase; LDH: lactate dehydrogenase)

Peritoneal fluid analysis comprises gross appearance and a battery of tests including cytology (including malignant cytology), biochemistry (protein, glucose, LDH, and amylase), serum-ascites albumin gradient (SAAG), microbiological (culture, Gram's-stain), and others [ADA, carcinoembryonic antigen (CEA), triglycerides, bilirubin, and NT-proBNP]. SAAG measured as a difference between serum albumin and ascitic fluid albumin helps differentiate transudative from exudative ascites. Peritoneal effusions with SAAG ≥ 11 g/L are classified as high albumin gradient effusions and those with SAAG <11 g/L are classified as low albumin gradient effusions and labeled as transudative and exudative, respectively **(Tables 9 and 10)**.

TABLE 8: Etiology of ascites.

Hepatic	Cardiogenic	Nephrogenic	Malignant	Infectious	Others
• Cirrhosis • Hepatic venous outflow obstruction (hepatic vein obstruction, Budd–Chiari syndrome, and veno-occlusive disease) • Portal vein occlusion • Inferior vena cava obstruction • Hepatic cancer	• Congestive cardiac failure • Constrictive pericarditis	• Nephrotic syndrome	• Ovarian • Cervical • Endometrial • Breast • Esophageal • Gastric • Pancreatic • Colorectal • Hepatobiliary • Lung • Primary peritoneal	• Tubercular • Spontaneous bacterial peritonitis • Fungal • Parasitic • Chlamydia	• Systemic lupus erythematosus • Sarcoidosis • Whipple's disease • Ovarian disease (Meig's syndrome, struma ovarii, and ovarian hyperstimulation syndrome) • Chylous ascites • Protein losing enteropathy • Myxedema

TABLE 9: Peritoneal fluid analysis.

Parameters	Inference
Gross appearance	• *Clear*: Uncomplicated, transudative, translucent, and pale yellow • *Turbid or cloudy*: Spontaneous bacterial peritonitis (SBP) • *Opalescent*: Cirrhosis, due to elevated triglycerides, and it is rare • *Milky*: Triglycerides in ascitic fluid more than serum (>200 mg/dL), >1,000 mg/dL is chylous ascites, malignancy is the most common cause of chylous ascites • *Pink or bloody*: RBC count > 10,000 cells/mm^3, in traumatic tap sample, is heterogeneously bloody with clot formation if sample is not placed in anticoagulant tube, whereas hemorrhagic ascites due to an intraperitoneal bleed is homogenously red and does not clot. Most common cause is malignancy; predominantly hepatocellular carcinoma (HCC) • *Brown*: Hyperbilirubinemia with ascitic fluid bilirubin levels 40% that of serum, if it is as dark as molasses it is due to ruptured gallbladder or perforated duodenal ulcer
Serum-ascites albumin gradient (SAAG)	*High albumin gradient (SAAG ≥ 1.1 g/dL)*: • Cirrhosis (high SAAG diagnostic of portal hypertension-related ascites) • Alcoholic hepatitis • Massive hepatic metastasis • Heart failure/constrictive pericarditis • Budd–Chiari syndrome • Portal vein thrombosis • Idiopathic portal vein fibrosis *Low albumin gradient (SAAG < 1.1 g/dL)* • Peritoneal carcinomatosis • Peritoneal tuberculosis • Pancreatitis • Serositis • Nephrotic syndrome

Continued

Continued

Parameters	Inference
Cell count and differential	Single-most useful test to establish or negate infection. Corrected neutrophil count ≥ 250 cells/mm^3, warrants infection (SBP), and need for immediate institution of antibiotics due to high associated mortality. Assessment of total protein (>1 g/dL), glucose (<50 mg/dL), and LDH (> ULN for serum) in ascites favor diagnosis of bowel perforation over SBP when ascitic fluid counts are elevated.
Others	• *Glucose*: Usually similar to serum concentration. Low in malignancy (peritoneal carcinomatosis) and bacterial infection (bowel perforation) • *LDH*: Usually, ascitic fluid to serum LDH ratio is <0.4 as it is large molecule and unable to enter ascitic fluid across peritoneal membrane. Ratio increases to >1.0 only in bowel perforation, SBP and malignancy • *Amylase*: Normal mean amylase concentration in uncomplicated ascites is ~100 IU/L and ascitic fluid to serum (AF/S) amylase ratio is ~0.4. In pancreatitis, ascitic fluid amylase is ~2,000 IU/L and AF/S amylase ratio is ~6.0 • *Adenosine deaminase (ADA)*: Useful only in high prevalence countries like India, to diagnose tuberculosis. In setting of cirrhosis with TB, the values can be falsely low. Hence, peritoneoscopy with culture of biopsy specimen is almost 100% diagnostic • *Culture*: Indicated in those who deteriorate with fever, abdominal pain, azotemia, acidosis, or confusion. 10 mL sample must be inoculated in each of the two bottles for both aerobic and anaerobic cultures • *Gram-stain*: Approximately 10,000 bacteria/mL are required for detection by Gram-stain, while the median concentration of bacteria in SBP is only one organism/mL; helpful in ruling out free perforation of the bowel • *Malignant cell cytology*: All patients (100%) have malignant cell cytology positive in peritoneal carcinomatosis, albeit only two-thirds with positive cytology have peritoneal carcinomatosis. Rest have massive hepatic metastasis, HCC, and lymphoma • *Carcinoembryonic antigen (CEA)*: Its precise utility in ascitic fluid remains undetermined • *Triglycerides*: Levels obtained in milky ascites. Chylous ascites have levels >1,000 mg/dL • *Bilirubin*: Measured in those with brown ascites. Diagnostic of ruptured gallbladder or perforated duodenal ulcer • *NT-proBNP*: Median values are higher in ascitic fluid due to heart failure and differentiates it from ascitic fluid due to cirrhosis

(LDH: lactate dehydrogenase; RBC: red blood cell; ULN: upper limit of normal)

TABLE 10: Comparative peritoneal fluid analysis in various pathological scenarios.

Parameters	Cirrhosis	Malignancy	Tuberculosis	SBP	Pancreatitis
Gross appearance	Clear straw or milky	Milky or bloody	Milky or normal	Cloudy or turbid	Milky or cloudy or turbid
Total protein	<25 g/L	≥25 g/L	≥25 g/L	≥25 g/L	≥25 g/L
SAAG	≥1.1 g/dL	<1.1 g/dL	<1.1 g/dL	<1.1 g/dL	<1.1 g/dL
LDH	Decreased	Increased	Increased or normal	Increased or normal	Increased or normal
Glucose	Normal	Decreased	Decreased	Decreased	Decreased
Amylase	Normal	Increased or normal			Increased
ADA	Decreased or normal	Decreased or normal	Increased		
Cell counts	≥250/μL or normal		≥250/μL or normal	≥250/μL	
Bacterial culture	Positive or negative		Positive or negative	Positive or negative	
Viscosity	<1.03 cP	≥1.03 cP	≥1.03 cP	≥1.03 cP	≥1.03 cP
^{1}H NMR spectroscopy	Increased or decreased				
VEGF	Decreased	Increased	Decreased	Decreased	Decreased
Tumor markers	Increased or normal	Increased	Increased or normal		Increased or normal

(ADA: adenosine deaminase; LDH: lactate dehydrogenase; SAAG: serum-ascites albumin gradient; SBP: spontaneous bacterial peritonitis; VEGF: vascular endothelial growth factor)

Synovial Fluid Analysis

Synovial fluids have the characteristic of colorless or light yellow, egg white consistency, highly viscous, unclotted, and found in joint cavity spaces. Synovial fluid is secreted by ultrafiltration of plasma across the plasma membrane and give nutrition supply to cartilage, carries away waste product, and provide lubrication to joint surface. Etiopathogenesis of synovial fluid effusion majorly includes noninflammatory (osteoarthritis, neuro-arthritis) septic arthritis or fungal infection, inflammatory (rheumatoid arthritis, gout), and hemorrhagic (hemophilia and trauma).

After arthrocentesis string test will be performed for viscosity. Normal synovial fluid dropped from syringe 10–15 cm string appears but in inflammatory condition fluid dropped as water.

Synovial fluid analysis comprises gross appearance, cytology and differential cytology, polarizing microscopy, cultures, and Gram-staining. If the joint aspirate is small, then polarizing microscopy and cultures are prioritized **(Tables 11 and 12)**.

TABLE 11: Synovial fluid analysis.

Parameters	Inference
Gross appearance	• *Opaque milky white*: Lipids in fat necrosis, chyle droplets, or numerous monosodium urate (MSU) crystals from gouty tophi • *Yellow or yellow green*: Inflammatory or septic arthritis • *Bright red, chocolate, or rustic brown*: Hemarthrosis or traumatic

Crystal analysis **(Fig. 1)**	Synovial fluid is examined for crystals by using polarizing microscopy and a quarter-wave plate by the phenomenon of "*birefringence*".
	• *MSU crystals*: Brightly birefringent and needle shaped, negatively birefringent and appear yellow. Sensitivity of crystal analysis for MSU crystals ranges from 63 to 78%, specificity ranges from 93 to 100%, and positive likelihood ratio is 14 for a diagnosis of gout
	• *Calcium pyrophosphate deposition disease (CPPD)*: Rhomboid or rectangular shaped, positively birefringent and appear blue. Many CPPD crystals are not birefringent, thus make diagnosis difficult.
	  ○ *Sensitivity*: 12–83%
	  ○ *Specificity*: 78–96% and positive likelihood ratio is 2.9 for diagnosis of CPPD-associated arthritis
	• *Other crystals*:
	  ○ *Cholesterol crystals*: Seen in chronic gout as notched polygonal crystals. Lipid droplets in synovial fluid appear as "*maltese crosses*" under polarizing microscopy and are seen in fracture at joints
	  ○ *Hydroxyapatite crystals*: Light microscopy with alizarin red or Von Kossa stains, detects calcium-containing crystals

Cytology and differential cytology	Cells counts increase dramatically in cases of septic arthritis (range from 50,000 to 150,000 cells/mm^3). In cases of purulent septic arthritis, a lower cut off count (25,000 cells/mm^3) has been shown to be better predictor rather than 50,000 cells/mm^3. However, in some cases of septic arthritis in immunocompromised individuals, some cases of *Neisseria* and *Mycobacterium* have lower cell counts. Septic arthritis has ≥75% neutrophils. Eosinophilia in synovial fluid is seen in parasitic infection, allergy, neoplasm, or Lyme disease
Gram-stain	• Provides rapid information on infecting organism in cases of septic arthritis • Sensitivity varies from 29 to 50% and many at times it may be negative, especially in cases of *Mycobacterium*, *Mycoplasma*, and fungi
Bacterial culture	Synovial fluid should be sent for cultures immediately after arthrocentesis in sterile tubes, prior to institution of empirical antibiotics to increase the yield of positive cultures

TABLE 12: Comparative Synovial fluid analysis in various pathological states.

Parameters	Normal	Noninflammatory	Inflammatory	Septic	Hemorrhagic
Clarity	Transparent	Transparent or slightly cloudy	Cloudy, turbid, and milky	Opaque, turbid, and purulent	Bloody or turbid
Color	Clear, Straw-yellow	Light yellow	Yellow-white	Dirty/yellow or yellow-green	Red or chocolate brown or Xanthochromic
Viscosity	High	High	Low	Low	Variable

Continued

Continued

Parameters	Normal	Noninflammatory	Inflammatory	Septic	Hemorrhagic
WBC (cells/mm^3)	<200	200–2,000	• 2,000–50,000 • Up to 100,000	>50,000	200–2,000
Polymorphonuclear (%)	<25%	<25%	>50%	>75%	50–75%
Crystals	None	Calcium hydroxyapatite	• MSU (gout) • CPPD (CPPD arthropathy)	None	None
Possible diagnosis	None	Osteoarthritis, traumatic arthritis	Gout, pseudogout, SLE, and rheumatoid arthritis	Bacterial, fungal, and mycobacterial	Traumatic, hemophilia, joint prosthesis, tumor, and anticoagulant therapy

(CPPD: calcium pyrophosphate deposition disease; MSU: monosodium urate; SLE: systemic lupus erythematosus)

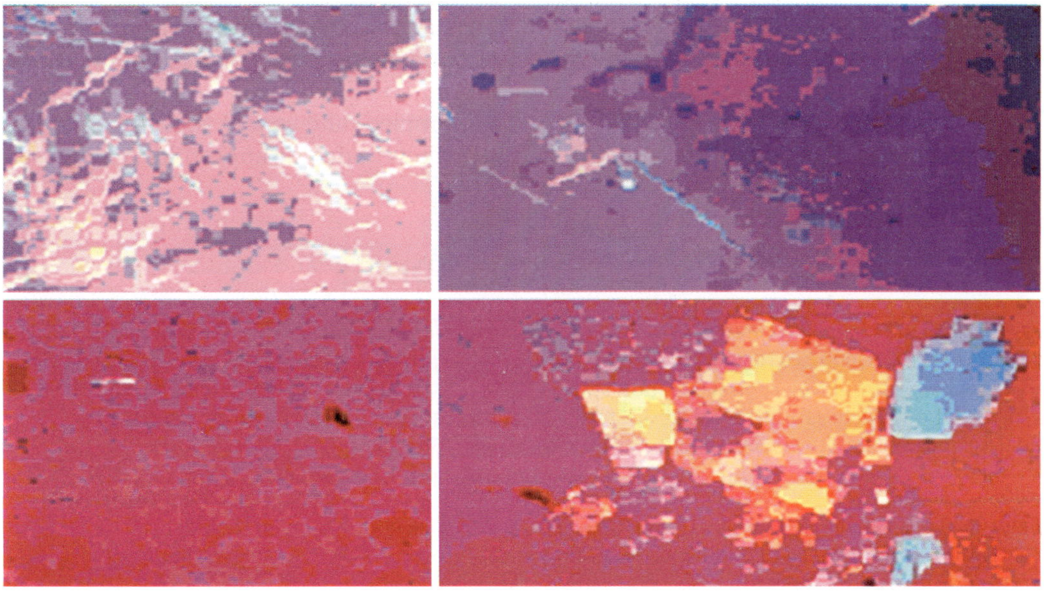

FIG. 1: Crystals in synovial fluid.
Courtesy: Michael A Becker, MD.

Sweat Analysis

Sweat is watery secretion secreted by eccrine and apocrine sweat gland to regulate body temperature. Sweat is regulated through hypothalamic thermoregulation center via sympathetic cholinergic nerves. Sweat is produced by isotonic ultrafiltration of plasma, which contains salt, urea, fatty acids, sodium, and potassium ions.

Cystic fibrosis (CF) is a disease of mutation in *CFTR* (cystic fibrosis transmembrane conductance regulator), but mostly chloride channels are affected. Along with chloride channel reabsorption sodium channels are also affected not only in sweat but also fluid secretions in lungs and pancreas. Normal sodium and chloride concentration is 5–40 mm/L. Sample is collected from pilocarpine iontophoresis provocative tests through sodium chloride filter paper pad.

Sweat chloride	<40 mm/L	40–60 mm/L	>60 mm/L
	Normal	Suggestive CF	Diagnosis of CF

Contraindication: Generalized edema, use of systemic corticosteroid, and eczematous skin lesion.

Saliva

Saliva content includes a salivary gland secretion, hormones, food debris, and cellular material. Salivary secretion mainly affected by systemic disease, Sjögren's syndrome, infection, malignancy, and endocrinopathy. Saliva is primarily used testing for toxicology analysis, infection, noninfectious disease, and endocrinological disease. Some advantages of saliva examination include easily collection, storage, and noninvasive method. Saliva tests is done for infectious disease, antibody detection, Lyme disease, *pylori*, measles, HIV, and mumps. Hormones profile such as cortisol and testosterone measures nonprotein bound level or free form level, so saliva has significant role in diagnosis of disease.

Hormones enter saliva by passive diffusion into the acinar cells of the salivary gland. Cortisol hormones have significant role in saliva secretion, because in saliva cortisol change to cortisone, which may have specific diagnostic value. Salivary testosterone may be a useful test in male hypogonadism or in sport medicine. For toxicology analysis, saliva analysis is diagnostic because unbound fraction of drugs are available in saliva. Saliva can be used to detect or monitor cotinine, codeine, diazepines, cannabinoids, opioids, and ethanol. Laboratory saliva collector contains absorbent pads, which are left in the mouth for 2–3 minutes. On thawing and centrifugation, the glycoprotein precipitate out leaving a nonviscous fluid that is easier to analyze.

CONCLUSION

This chapter includes most of the body fluid but amniotic and seminal fluids are left due to the restriction of words. Most of the body fluids have been explained briefly as fluid content, etiopathogenesis, analysis, and correlation with specific disease. Specific fluid has more specificity to pathology compared to the blood, because blood has multiple ion, protein, hormones, toxic substance, etc.

The increased accumulation as well as alteration in composition as analyzed by various imaging and a battery of assays of the aspirated fluid aid in establishing definitive diagnosis of a wide range of pathologies day in and day out. Hence, it is imperative that physicians must have a thorough knowledge of the methodology of sampling of appropriate fluid, the battery of assays to be ordered for the sampled fluid as well as an accurate interpretation of the results under the appropriate clinical settings.

SUGGESTED READINGS

1. Leinonen V, Vanninen R, Rauramaa T. Cerebrospinal fluid circulation and hydrocephalus. Handb Clin Neurol. 2017;145:39.
2. Hasbun R. Cerebrospinal fluid in central nervous system infections. In: Scheld WM, Whitley RJ, Marra CM (Eds). Infections of the Central Nervous System, 4th edition. Lippincott Williams; 2014. p. 4.
3. Bijlsma MW, Brouwer MC, Kasanmoentalib ES, Kloek AT, Lucas MJ, Tanck MW, et al. Community-acquired bacterial meningitis in adults in the Netherlands, 2006-14: a prospective cohort study. Lancet Infect Dis. 2016;16(3):339-47.
4. Horowitz ML, Schiff M, Samuels J, Russo R, Schnader J. *Pneumocystis carinii* pleural effusion. Pathogenesis and pleural fluid analysis. Am Rev Respir Dis. 1993;148(1):232-4.
5. Sturges S, Brown M. Polypsychopharmacy. Bull Menninger Clin. 1975;39:274.
6. Porcel JM, Esquerda A, Vives M, Bielsa S. Etiology of pleural effusions: analysis of more than 3,000 consecutive thoracenteses. Arch Bronconeumol. 2014;50:161.

276

CHAPTER

Resistance Exercise: Role in Lifestyle Management

Dinesh Kumar, Harshita Lachhwani

ABSTRACT

Physical inactivity significantly influences lifestyle diseases such as obesity, diabetes, hypertension, and cardiovascular diseases (CVDs). Adipose tissue inflammation leads to impaired insulin response, causing decreased glucose absorption and storage. This results in dyslipidemia, type 2 diabetes mellitus (T2DM), and cardiovascular illnesses. While drugs are prescribed to treat chronic diseases, routine exercise can offset age-related decline in physical mobility and reduce the risk of developing chronic diseases.

INTRODUCTION

Lifestyle diseases such as overweight/obesity, diabetes mellitus/insulin resistance, hypertension, and cardiovascular diseases (CVDs) are all significantly influenced by physical inactivity. For everyone at risk of such diseases, intensive lifestyle changes are advised as the first line of treatment.

As a person gains weight and approaches obesity, macrophages invade adipose tissue and change its endocrine and metabolic functions to produce aberrant levels of cytokines and adipokines such as leptin and interleukin 6 (IL-6). This leads to widespread inflammation, which in turn leads to reduced ability of liver, muscle, and adipose tissues to respond to cellular actions of insulin. A deficiency in insulin action in these tissues leads to decreased glucose absorption and storage because liver, muscles, and adipose tissue are crucial for maintaining glucose homeostasis. Dyslipidemia, type 2 diabetes mellitus (T2DM), and cardiovascular illnesses are all effects of disturbed glucose homeostasis.

To treat or stop the progression of serious chronic diseases, physicians routinely prescribe drugs, but they are not without unfavorable side effects. Routine exercise, however, can occasionally offset the age-related decline in physical mobility and significantly lower the chance of developing chronic diseases.

EXERCISE: DEFINITION

Physical activity is defined as any bodily movement caused by the contraction of skeletal muscles that increases energy expenditure. Exercise is defined as physical activity that is planned, structured, and repetitive. Physical activity and exercise are cornerstone in the prevention of chronic diseases.

EXERCISE MODE

Exercise mode refers to the type of exercise. Aerobic exercise (AE), which includes walking, jogging, cycling, swimming, and rowing, is the most studied type of exercise in patients with obesity and related metabolic disorders. Resistance exercises (RE) include shoulder presses, squats, lunges, and deadlifts performed using progressive resistance equipment, free weights, bands, or bodyweight. The basic principles of resistance exercise training (RET) involve repeated overloading of a group of muscles, typically by contracting the muscles under heavy resistance and returning to the start position for several repetitions until failure. The basic method of resistance training uses the principle of progressive overload, in which the muscles are overloaded by working against a resistance. They respond by growing larger and stronger. RE and AE are exercise modalities that have traditionally been considered to exist at opposite ends of the exercise continuum in terms of the phenotypes they produce. A common misconception is that RET and AE training (AET) also offer different health benefits. However, there is growing evidence that RET may be as effective as AET in reducing the risk of chronic disease.

Recent studies have shown that the effects of AET are enhanced when combined with RET. This was previously not recommended for overweight people. In a 14-year study, Shiroma et al. reported that RET reduced the incidence of diabetes and CVD by 30 and 17%, respectively. This may be because, unlike AET, RET maintains free fat mass (FFM) and resting energy expenditure (REE), which are key factors in weight management.

EXERCISE VOLUME AND INTENSITY

Exercise volume and intensity refer to the amount and effort required to exercise.

Aerobic Exercise Training

Exercise intensity (moderate, vigorous, or high) is characterized by objective and subjective measures such as percentage of heart rate reserve (HHR) and rate of perceived exertion [Borg's 6–20 rate of perceived exertion (RPE)] respectively. Exercise training at 40–60% of HHR or 12–13 RPE is considered moderate-intensity training (MIT). Vigorous intensity exercise is performed at 60–85% of HHR or RPE > 14 while high-intensity training (HIT) is performed at near maximal to maximal efforts 19–20 on the RPE scale.

Resistance Exercise Training

The intensity of resistance training is represented as the weight lifted in relation to an individual's maximal strength for a single repetition of that exercise (RM). The intensity of exercise determines the volume needed to achieve the therapeutic effect. High load low volume (heavy weights but less repetitions) RET is traditionally considered to produce superior physiological adaptations including skeletal muscle hypertrophy when compared with low load high volume (low weights but a greater number of repetitions). However, a recent study by Morton et al. found comparable increases in the lean muscle mass in the two groups.

RESISTANCE EXERCISE TRAINING AND TYPE 2 DIABETES MELLITUS

The underlying pathophysiology behind T2DM is insulin resistance, resulting in delayed suppression of hepatic glucose production and impaired peripheral glucose uptake by skeletal muscle. Given that 80% of glucose is stored in skeletal muscle after a meal, loss of muscle metabolic activity is one of the triggers for insulin resistance and T2DM. Lifestyle considerations are probably the most effective treatment strategy when it comes to diabetes prevention and treatment. In fact, the Diabetes Prevention Program (DPP) showed that lifestyle changes were associated with a significant reduction in his T2DM incidence compared with metformin (58% vs. 31%).

The DPP emphasized on AET without considering the beneficial effects of RET on glycemic control. The data from Davy et al. showed that after only twice-weekly progressive, supervised, whole-body RET (1 set at 70–80% 1RM) for 3 months, 34% of overweight/obese prediabetic older adults achieved normal glucose tolerance. A study of 32,000 men between the ages of 40 and 75 years from the Health Professionals Study demonstrated that men engaging in at least 150 min/weeks of RET had a 34% lower risk of developing diabetes over an 18-year period.

People living with T2DM may benefit from the inclusion of RET in their lifestyle to control glycemia as an add-on to antidiabetic drugs. In a meta-analysis of 360 older patients with T2DM, RET for 8 weeks was also associated with clinically significant improvements in glycated hemoglobin (HbA1c).

Evidence from a systematic review (Gordon et al. 2009) suggests that exercise is an important variable, with high-intensity RET (≥ 70 1RM) performance leading to the greatest improvement in glycemic control. Another study in T2DM patients showed that there was no significant difference in glycemic control between high-intensity and low-intensity RET (75% vs. 50% of 1RM) when training volume was adjusted. Going forward, people with prediabetes or T2DM should focus on doing RET, regardless of exercise intensity. Resolving hyperglycemia and hyperinsulinemia in metabolically compromised adults with exercise prevents not only the development of T2DM but also associated microvascular complications.

RESISTANCE EXERCISE TRAINING AND CARDIOVASCULAR DISEASE

Aerobic exercise training mitigates the risk of CVD and mortality and has been the considered the cornerstone of lifestyle change needed to target these diseases. This belief comes as no surprise given that improved cardiorespiratory fitness is inversely associated with CVD risk and mortality. To add to it, Ruiz et al., Srikanthan et al., and Kim et al. showed that muscle mass and strength are also independently associated with reduced CVD risk and mortality. Despite the above evidences, RET is still considered way less as an exercise modality that reduces CVD risk.

A follow-up from the health professional's study showed that 30 min/week of RET was associated with a similar risk reduction compared to brisk walking of 2.5 hours as far as cardiovascular events are concerned (Tanasescu et al., 2002). An analysis of the Women's Health Study found that women who did 60–120 minutes of RET per week had a similar risk reduction of incident CVD as women doing 60–120 minutes of AET per week (Shiroma et al. 2017). Smutok et al. (1993) did a comparison of older men at risk of developing CVD between those who did whole-body RET (2 sets at 60–70% 1RM) and those who did treadmill walking/jogging (75–85% heart rate). The results were similar in both groups. It is clear from the above studies that the results from AET and RET are comparable when it comes to the reduction in cardiovascular risk.

The benefits of RET are also seen in risk factors associated with CVD and to the same degree as AET (i.e., blood pressure, blood lipids, insulin sensitivity, and vascular function).

Meta-analyses of population in general show that RET helps in reduction of systolic blood pressure (SBP) by 5–6 mm Hg and diastolic blood pressure (DBP) by 3–4 mm Hg which is finally associated with an 18% reduction of major cardiovascular events. The benefits by RET also apply to persons living with hypertension. In fact, hypertensive individuals get the better benefit in blood pressure reduction following RET.

Resistance exercise training is rarely advised by the doctors, primarily because AET is considered safer and possibly easier to perform in patients with CVD. It has been contemplated that high pressure loading of the heart by RET may result in mild cardiac hypertrophy and an increased risk of death (Kamada et al., 2017). However, excessive blood pressure elevation is only observed with high-intensity RET (>70% of 1RM) and is generally not an issue with low-to-moderate-intensity RET (30–69% of 1RM). Holdings et al. (2017) analyzed data from five studies that investigated adverse events during RET of low-to-moderate intensity (30–69% of 1RM) in older adults with CVD and found that the incidence of adverse cardiovascular events was lower than with AET. Acute bouts of RE appear to be more protective against ischemic changes than bouts of AE because of decreased heart rate and increased diastolic perfusion pressure. These physiological changes make myocardial oxygenation more favorable during RE. There is no significant evidence that RET is less safe than AET in physically or metabolically high-risk individuals.

RESISTANCE EXERCISE TRAINING AND CANCER

Cancers (most of them), T2DM, and CVD have common risk factors and are associated with a sedentary lifestyle. Regular physical activity is associated with a reduced incidence of cancer, death from cancer, and better cancer prognosis (Keum et al. 2016).

Stamatakis et al., using data from the England and Scottish Health Survey of 80,000 adults aged 30 years and more, found in 2018 that doing regular RET (at least twice a week) was found to be associated with a 34% reduction in cancer mortality, whereas adherence to the AET provided no statistical advantage. Additionally, cancer patients who participated in RET at least once a week had a 33% reduction in all-cause mortality.

Although the above studies were merely observational and inference regarding causation cannot be concluded, they do support the hypothesis that regular use of RET reduces cancer risk, cancer mortality, and cancer recurrence.

CONCLUSION

There is ample of evidence to show the beneficial effects of RET in reducing chronic disease risk. Based on these evidences, RET-induced benefits in chronic disease risk are similar if not superior in magnitude to AET. Regular performance of RET improves muscles mass, strength, and function and can have direct effects on the primary prevention of a number of chronic diseases. In spite of that, several agencies endorse performing 150 minutes of AET per week to mitigate age-related chronic disease risk, whereas the role of RET on the overall health is not appreciated.

Based on the evidence presented here, we propose that RET may serve as another armamentarium for individuals to remain physically active and combat chronic disease risk. It is true that there is some knowledge gap such as the optimal dose and intensity of RET required to achieve those health benefits and there are no head-to-head trials between RET and AET to demonstrate the superiority of either, and further investigations are needed.

SUGGESTED READINGS

1. Peterson MD, Sen A, Gordon PM. Influence of resistance exercise on lean body mass in aging adults: a meta-analysis. Med Sci Sports Exerc. 2011;43:249-58.
2. Shiroma EJ, Cook NR, Manson JE, Moorthy MV, Buring JE, Rimm EB, et al. Strength training and the risk of type 2 diabetes and cardiovascular disease. Med Sci Sports Exerc. 2017;49(1):40-6.
3. Morton RW, Oikawa SY, Wavell CG, Mazara N, McGlory C, Quadrilatero J, et al. Neither load nor systemic hormones determine resistance training-mediated hypertrophy or strength gains in resistance-trained young men. J Appl Physiol. 2016;121(1):129-38.
4. Gordon BA, Benson AC, Bird SR, Fraser SF. Resistance training improves metabolic health in type 2 diabetes: a systematic review. Diabetes Res Clin Pract. 2009;83:157-75.
5. Tanasescu M, Leitzmann MF, Rimm EB, Willett WC, Stampfer MJ, Hu FB. Exercise type and intensity in relation to coronary heart disease in men. JAMA. 2002;288:1994-2000.
6. Stamatakis E, Lee IM, Bennie J, Freeston J, Hamer M, O'Donovan G, et al. Does strength-promoting exercise confer unique health benefits? A pooled analysis of data on 11 population cohorts with all-cause, cancer, and cardiovascular mortality endpoints. Am J Epidemiol. 2018;187:1102-12.
7. Davy BM, Winett RA, Savla J, Marinik EL, Baugh ME, Flack KD, et al. Resist diabetes: a randomized clinical trial for resistance training maintenance in adults with prediabetes. PLOS ONE. 2017;12(2):e0172610
8. Srikanthan P, Horwich TB, Tseng CH. Relation of muscle mass and fat mass to cardiovascular disease mortality. Am J Cardiol. 2016;117(8):1355-60.
9. Ruiz JR, Sui X, Lobelo F, Morrow JR, Jr., Jackson AW, Sjöström M, et al. Association between muscular strength and mortality in men: prospective cohort study. BMJ. 2008;337(7661):a439.
10. Kim Y, Wijndaele K, Lee DC, Sharp SJ, Wareham N, Brage S. Independent and joint associations of grip strength and adiposity with all-cause and cardiovascular disease mortality in 403,199 adults: the UK Biobank study. Am J Clin Nutr. 2017;106(3):773-82.
11. Keum N, Bao Y, Smith-Warner SA, Orav J, Wu K, Fuchs CS, et al. Association of physical activity by type and intensity with digestive system cancer risk. JAMA Oncol. 2016;2(9):1146-53.
12. Smutok MA, Reece C, Kokkinos PF, Farmer C, Dawson P, Shulman R, et al. Aerobic versus strength training for risk factor intervention in middle-aged men at high risk for coronary heart disease. Metabolism. 1993;42(2):177-84.
13. Kamada M, Shiroma EJ, Buring JE, Miyachi M, Lee IM. Strength training and all-cause, cardiovascular disease, and cancer mortality in older women: a cohort study. J Am Heart Assoc. 2017;6(11):1-9.
14. Hollings M, Mavros Y, Freeston J, Fiatarone Singh M. The effect of progressive resistance training on aerobic fitness and strength in adults with coronary heart disease: a systematic review and meta-analysis of randomised controlled trials. Eur J Prev Cardiol. 2017;24(12):1242-59.

277

CHAPTER

Patient Experience: A Vital Sign for Health Organization: A Review

Sidhartha Gautam Senapati, Amit Ghosh

ABSTRACT

Patient experience (PE) is defined as range of interaction that patients have with the healthcare system while they seek and receive care. To assess PE, it is required to find out if something that should happen (such as clear communication) happened and how often it happened, while patient satisfaction is whether patients' expectations were met. Understanding PE is a cornerstone in moving toward patient-centered care. Some of the factors that impact PE include effective communication, convenience in receiving healthcare, wait time, clinical atmosphere, and transparency. Evaluation of PE along with other components such as effective healthcare delivery and safety would give us a complete picture of the healthcare quality. HCAHPS (Hospital Consumer Assessment of Healthcare Providers and Systems), also known as CAHPS, hospital survey is the most widely used tool for assessing PE. With the healthcare industry becoming extremely competitive and patients and family actively making choices that impact their healthcare experience, it is becoming evident that the future of the healthcare industry concentrates around PE. Studies have shown that improved PE leads to better clinical outcomes, less physician burnout, increased financial success of healthcare organizations, and higher patient satisfaction scores. Our chapter describes the best evidence-based methods to improve PE.

INTRODUCTION

While the exact definition of patient experience (PE) remains elusive, it has been defined as the "sum of all interactions, shaped by an organization's culture that influence patient perceptions across the continuum of care" by the Beryl Institute. PE is formed by everyone with whom the patient interacts along the journey starting from the front desk. "Patient satisfaction" can be defined as what people think of their healthcare provider based on preconceived notions often formed through marketing materials. However in the outpatient and hospital's context, PE could be seen as a collective business process where healthcare providers deliver care and information flows between patient, people, and systems across various touchpoints **(Fig. 1)**. Since patient plays a key role in connecting each step of the journey, understanding each patient's experience becomes vital for the healthcare providers to improve the quality of service. Improving PE could lead to more satisfied patients by strengthening the patient-physician bond, while improving the patient compliance, better reputation of the organization, and better patient flow, improving the clinical productivity.

The first and foremost step is identifying all the important aspects of PE; second is finding a way to improve in those areas. Measuring PE routinely can help in quality improvement initiatives in patient care. For instance, a primary care physician might have lower patient satisfaction if potential new patients find it difficult to book an appointment online or they call repeatedly only to be told that there's no availability for weeks. But if those patients get access to teleconsultation that could address their concerns, this would result in improvement of both patient satisfaction and experience. Understanding individual patient's experience could help in addressing certain innovation at the point of care, guide toward further research, and provide directions for quality improvement.

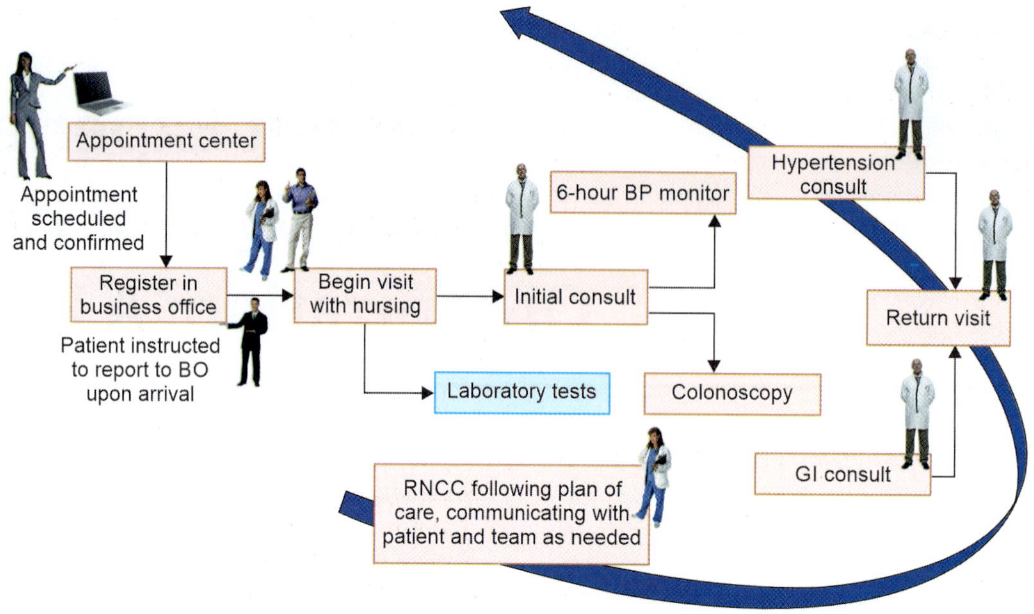

FIG. 1: The process for patient's services in an outpatient clinic.
(BO: business office; BP: blood pressure; GI: gastrointestinal; RNCC: registered nursing care contribution)

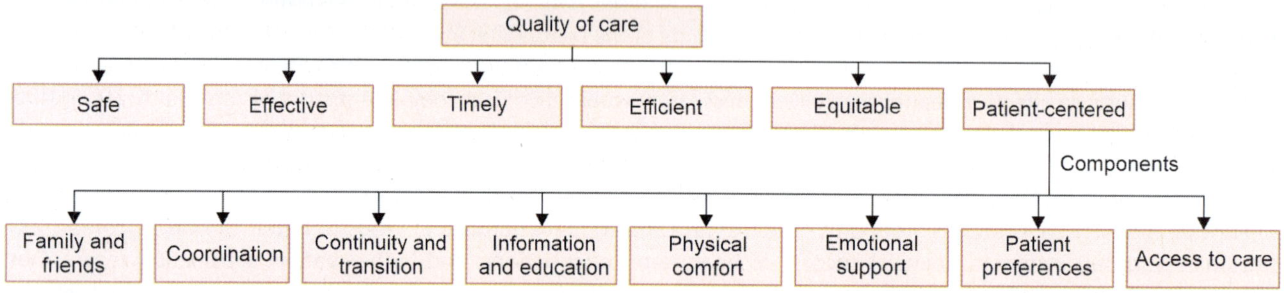

FLOWCHART 1: Domains of "quality care" and patient-centered care.
Source: Defined by Institute of Medicine (2001).

Patient experience in a complex hospital setting is affected by multiple factors that traditional questionnaire and static observation may not be able to evaluate patients' perception. The use of unstructured diaries in which patients could write their entire hospital-stay experience in their own words is unclear as it cannot help in differentiating real-time experiences in relation to high-emotional situations or clinical activities that can affect patient's willingness to write. Many tools are being used currently to record PE, thereby evaluating the quality and safety of various clinical processes, for example, Hospital Consumer Assessment of Healthcare Providers and Systems (HCAHPS), National Health Service Inpatient Survey (NHSIP), Picker Patient experience Questionnaire (PPE-15), Patient Experience Questionnaire (PEQ), Quality from the Patients' Perspective (QPP), QPP Shortened (QPPS), and Patient Experience with Inpatient Care (I-PAHC). Many hospitals have a new administrative position titled "Chief Experience Officer (CXO)" who is in-charge of overseeing, improving, and implementing best practices in PE.

In the current chapter, we describe the 2001 Institute of Medicine attributes of quality care, factors affecting PE, potential benefits of PE, summarizing the evidence on the strategies of various interventions to improve PE. Though the evidence is evolving, we use a consensus approach to recommend which interventions could be most effective.

ATTRIBUTES OF QUALITY CARE

Patient-centered care is one of the six domains of "Quality care" and has shown to be associated with clinical benefits and healthcare cost reduction **(Flowchart 1)**. The components of patient-centered care includes:

- *Family and friends*: Involving friends and family in the decision-making process, providing them accommodation and supporting them as caregivers could help in addressing their role in PE.

- *Coordination*: Proper coordination between all the stakeholders involved in the patient care can help in alleviating feeling of vulnerability and powerless.
- *Continuity and transition*: Proper planning of ongoing treatment and coordination following discharge
- *Information and education*: Educating patients about their condition can facilitate autonomy and health promotion
- *Physical comfort*: Pain management and assistance with daily living needs can have a significant impact on the experience during the hospital stay.
- Emotional support
- *Patient preferences*: Recognizing the individuality of each patient and involving them in the decision-making process
- *Access to care*: Assuring patients that they could access the care when needed

Improvement efforts in healthcare services through patient feedback, participation of healthcare professionals, and support organization are needed to achieve a good quality care.

FACTORS AFFECTING PATIENT EXPERIENCE

Patients characteristics, such as age, gender, race, and educational background, all play an important role in PE. In the United States (US), racial minority groups such as Asians and native Americans had less-positive experience with inpatient care compared to Hispanics. Similarly, English-speaking patients had positive care experiences than the non-English speakers. Some studies have shown that patients who are non-Hispanic white, female, with lower educational level, and better mental health tend to give more positive rating to the hospital. Similarly, teaching hospitals, with lower Medicare-Medicaid proportions and use electronic health record (EHR) also have positive PE.

A systematic qualitative assessment of online surveys found positive PE when physicians cared about them and listened to them, corroborating the development of patient–physician trust. Similarly, another study on outpatient plastic surgery patients showed significant association between positive PE and physician's mannerisms, interpersonal skills, and clear communication. Similarly, empowering staff members of the hospitals can help foster strong interpersonal connections between patients and staff of the hospital, thereby adding on to a positive PE.

IMPROVING THE PATIENT EXPERIENCE—POTENTIAL BENEFITS

Positive PE are associated with better clinical outcomes—lower rates of postoperative mortality, failure to rescue, and minor complications. Wang DE et al. showed that higher centers for Medicare and Medicaid services (CMS) rating is associated with lower patient mortality and readmissions. In patients with chronic illnesses, there exists a significant relationship between patient satisfaction and adherence to medical advice in patients. Similar findings were also reported in oncology patients on treatment. Patient satisfaction positively correlates with short-term outcomes after major cancer surgery, lower 30-day mortality rates, 30-day admission rates, and failure to rescue. Satisfied patients later lead to loyal healthcare consumers.

Online patient reviews could provide an honest rating of experience of quality of care delivered. Potential patients are provided with a "social proof," giving them an opportunity to base choices on what others are saying. A satisfied patient will share his/her experience with five others, leading to quick publicity of quality of care, drawing attention of more potential patients. As per an industry estimate, loss of a patient due to dissatisfaction may lead to lifetime practice loss of $200,000. According to a survey by Rush University Medical Center in Chicago, higher patient satisfaction can generate additional revenue of $2.3 million annually. Delivering excellent care to existing patients will help in patient retention, thereby reducing turnover, increased loyalty, and extended lifetime value. Patients' willingness to pay more to get a consultation with a physician of their choice gives a command to the medical practices to charge higher prices for the superior service without losing the profit or market share.

STRATEGIES TO IMPROVE PATIENT EXPERIENCE

Strategies to improve PE include both individual and systems-based efforts.

Patients' Autonomy and Shared Decision-making Process

Patient–physician relationship plays an important role in the patient's decision-making capacity. They may not be able to make decisions if they do not trust their healthcare provider. It is important for the patient to feel as an individual and healthcare professionals should know their patients well enough to ensure that their decisions are not misunderstood. Shared decisions enable patients to understand all the alternative choices in their healthcare management and make decisions that are in their best interest. Being involved in the decision-making process improves the patient's quality of life, feeling of self-worth, so that they are more satisfied with the care received.

Shared decision-making (SDM) is a three-step process. First step, the healthcare practitioner provides them with the "choices" of viable treatment options. Second step, patients are provided with adequate "information" to make an informed decision. Third step, helping patients to explore the treatment options before making an informed decision. Decision aids for the patients may be given in the form of booklet, a video, or Internet-based tool; studies have shown decision aids to be effective in making an informed decision, reducing decisional conflict and regret.

High-quality Communication

A high-quality communication between patients and doctors has manifold advantages. Apart from improving treatment adherence and diagnostic accuracy, it helps in building trust that helps in positive and productive relationship and psychological benefits for patients. A quality communication is influenced by emotions, health literacy, and last but not the least, personal and cultural values. Since verbal communication is the most common form of interaction, clarity and being explicit are two key components of a high-quality communication. Using a comprehensible and reducing the use of medical jargon or complex terminologies are some ways to ensure that verbal communication is able to provide the information and meets the desire of the patients. Sometimes doctors to avoid their own discomfort rely on euphemistic language, making patients overtly optimistic about their prognosis.

Physicians' verbal communication choices greatly impact patients' participation in the healthcare process. Using questions that entail submissive responses (Do you understand?) may result in disempowering the patient. Verbal communication also plays an important role in building emotional connection between patients and healthcare providers. Some of the strategies that have proven to be effective are use of first-person plural pronoun "we" and hearer-oriented language choices such as tag questions, colloquial language, and sharing personal stories.

Approach to Breaking Bad News

In the context of healthcare, bad news refers to the information which can negatively affect the future of the patient. Healthcare professionals face an ethical dilemma of "do no harm" at the same time respect patients' autonomy. Reactions to bad news may be intensified in case of lack of detailed discussion, inadequate training of physician in end-of-life discussions, and other factors related to patients such as faith, culture, past experiences, age, and family responsibilities. Some of the elements that have been shown to be helpful in delivering bad news are good therapeutic relationship, reading cues to assess patients' readiness to know more, use of appropriate language (describe in their own words a less use of medical jargon), and choosing appropriate time/place for end-of-life discussions. Healthcare personnel are required to be compassionate, empathetic, nonjudgmental, sensitive, kind, and comfortable while assessing patient's distress. Patients' fear and anxiety can become a barrier toward decision-making and may require recurring conversations. An honest and open discussion about the illness will allow them to exercise their autonomy and make informed decisions.

Adopting eHealth Technology

An example of systems-based approach to improving PE could be early adoption and improvement of health technology. The coronavirus disease 2019 (COVID-19) pandemic forced healthcare providers to shift from in person visits to virtual visits and incorporation of technology in the healthcare industry. Patient- and family-centered care interventions are being widely implemented in various settings with the primary aim to improve the patient. For example, the electronic food service management, for food preparation, meal ordering, and delivery, leading to positive patient and organizational outcome. Electronic bedside meal ordering system (eBMOS) allows the patients to order meals using bedside television/computers or their own phone. This model has an advantage over the traditional paper menu methods of meal ordering, making the real-time data on diet and patient allergies available at the time of ordering. It also gives patients the liberty of ordering food when they feel like eating, resulting in increased dietary intake, with an added advantage of increased patient interaction with the meal ordering system and improved patient satisfaction.

Another area of focus which can negatively impact the PE is appointment wait time and scheduling. It also has detrimental effect on access to care, patient safety, and organizational reputation. Self-scheduling offers the convenience the patients seek, with an added advantage to the healthcare organizations in the form of labor saving, information transparency, operational cost reduction, and improved patient satisfaction. With patient surge during the COVID-19 pandemic, many organizations implemented providing evidence of adaptability and tribality. Studies have shown that there had been a 300% increase in self-scheduling appointments. It also gives the patients the flexibility to schedule an appointment after office hours.

Even though it has helped in overcoming the difficulties during the pandemic, some of the challenges that are usually encountered are issues with implementation, patient acceptance, regular maintenance by technology experts, language barriers, issues with privacy, reliability, and cultural and societal restrictions.

Studies from Saudi Arabia have revealed that there exists a significant association between female gender, stable Internet connection, type of medical specialty (cardiology and orthopedic clinic had highest agreement among patients), and patient satisfaction toward telemedicine services. Higher patient satisfaction has been seen with services with the ease of use, ability to communicate and engage, and simultaneously increasing accessibility and cost reduction. Expansion of telemedicine services to other departments/specialties with long waiting list or in cases where patients have to travel long to attend could help in improving patient satisfaction.

Adoption of Newer Technology—Example of Minimally Invasive Surgical Techniques and Robotic Surgery

An effort toward promoting comfort and improving surgical experience plays an important role in strengthening patient–physician relationship. Minimal invasive surgery (MIS) whether robotics or laparoscopic surgery has recently gained a lot of popularity because of better short-term clinical outcomes, reduced risk of soft tissue injuries (reduced blood loss and postoperative drainage), increased accuracy, and improved clinical outcomes promoting positive PE.

Adoption of enhanced recovery after surgery (ERAS) guideline is an evidence-based multimodal approach to accelerate recovery and rehabilitation post-surgery, without increasing mortality and readmission rates **(Box 1)**.

BOX 1: Guidelines in enhanced recovery after surgery (ERAS).

- Preoperative counseling
- Preoperative carbohydrate loading
- Perioperative nutrition
- Avoidance of bowel preparation
- No routine use of surgical drain
- Thromboembolism prophylaxis
- Antibiotic prophylaxis
- Minimally invasive approach
- Intraoperative fluid restriction
- Multimodal analgesia
- Glycemic control
- Prevention of delayed gastric emptying
- Stimulation of bowel movement
- Early mobilization
- Prevention of postoperative nausea and vomiting
- Fluid management
- Systematic audit
- Prevention of hypothermia
- Early oral fluid and normal diet intake

Honesty and Transparency in Patient Care

Honesty, transparency, and family-centered approach prioritizing patient and family forms indispensable part of the clinical mission. In case of any harm, the sea of uncertainty fans out in all directions, draining them physically, emotionally, and financially. Not just patients, even health professionals also experience their own trauma/powerful mix of emotions because of unexpected patient outcome. Seldom they have the time to process what happened. In case a patient is harmed, rather than stonewalling and defensiveness, a comprehensive approach to respond to the unintended harm, with a strong emphasis on honesty and transparency will reinforce the patient–physician relationship **(Fig. 2)**.

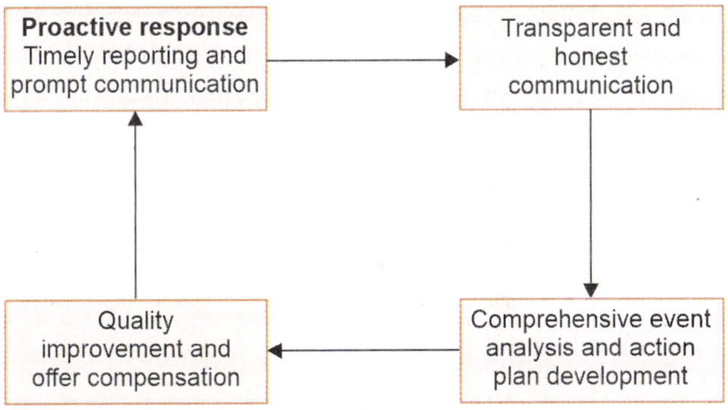

FIG. 2: Approach toward dealing with a medical error.

Quality Nursing Care and Patient Outcomes

Quality healthcare and patient outcomes are the measures of success of an organization. Nurses who are in constant interaction with the patient play an important role in achieving quality nursing care (QNC) provision and positive patient outcomes. Behavior of nursing leaders influences the behavior of the nurses whom they are responsible for. Reduced incidences of adverse events have been reported when nurses' decision-making processes are managed by experienced nurses. An interactive nursing leadership is associated with increased patient satisfaction and lower patient mortality rates.

Discharge Planning and Follow-up Plan—Best Practices

Inability to communicate with the providers between the appointments can be extremely frustrating for the patients. Through technological intervention, making the communication between the patients and physician can strengthen patient–physician relationship and improve better patient outcomes. Telephone follow-up could be a low-cost intervention, which gives an opportunity to discuss and address problems and complications in between the appointments, clarify the discharge instructions, and ensure treatment adherence and psychosocial well-being of the patients.

Attention to Patient Feedback

In the old days, individuals used to ask their friends and families about their experiences with a particular procedure, but with this conversation moving online, patients use the Internet to obtain health information. It provides them with a dual advantage by providing them with reliable medical information from sources such as Mayo Clinic and content created by healthcare consumers giving them advice, recommendations, and warnings on various social media platforms, websites dedicated for recording online patient reviews about various medical procedures, facilities, and practitioners. However, majority of the online patient reviews are in the form of unstructured data such as Facebook comments, tweets on twitter, and posts on blogs and forums.

In an increasingly digitalized society, online patient feedback **(Table 1)** is a low-cost convenient way to capture PEs of healthcare, providing an opportunity to incorporate PE data in healthcare monitoring and delivery, focusing on patient centeredness, quality improvement, and cost-effectiveness. A positive association has also been between online positive feedback and lower hospital standardized mortality rate, lower readmission rate, lower healthcare-associated infections, and better hospital cleanliness. A study based on patient web-based ratings showed a positive correlation between overall rating of PE and "willingness to recommend the hospital to a friend."

Building up a dedicated patient testimonial section on the website and sharing patients' success stories would be a great way to show how satisfied patients are, attracting more potential patients.

Effective patient education enhances patient satisfaction post-healthcare delivery, attracting positive patient outcome. Positive reviews are often a result of high-quality interaction with staff and postoperative care.

TABLE 1: Reviewer anonymity and patient verification on different review websites.

Review website	Reviewer anonymity	Verified patient
Facebook	Only if reviewer's account is set up under a pseudonym	No
Google	Only if reviewer's account is set up under a pseudonym	No
Healthgrades	Yes, the patient is offered a choice of a display name	No, but email is verified
Vitals	Yes	No, but uses an IP verification system to stop same person leaving multiple reviews
Vizium360	Yes	Yes
Yelp	Only first name and initials of last name shown	No

Emerging Role of Artificial Intelligence

Artificial intelligence (AI) is being widely used in interpretation of radiology data and image analysis. AI is an umbrella term that encompasses various disciplines such as machine learning (ML) and deep learning (DL). ML comprises both supervised and unsupervised learning methods. Supervised learning includes prediction of labeled outputs focusing primarily on classifying data into specific subgroups for prediction of quantitative outcomes. Latest advances in AI in gastroenterology and hepatology have helped in various aspects of clinical care such as detection of neoplastic lesions on endoscopic assessment and improving current survival methods on predicting treatment response.

Artificial intelligence-enabled decision aid technology by incorporating patient-reported outcome measurements (PROMs), patient education, and preference assessment has shown to improve quality of decision, SDM, patient satisfaction, and functional outcomes. New technologies such as IBM Watson's natural language processing software, which analyzes the content and converts the unstructured online reviews into quantified data that later can be used for statistical analysis. There are similar other content analysis tool such as LIWC (Linguistic Inquiry and Word Count), T-lab, and DICTION that are also gaining popularity nowadays. Similarly, a nursing quality platform based on the experience of patients has been designed to analyze the quality of patient care across 1,300 healthcare facilities in China, which has shown potentials for improvement in patient care quality.

OPTIMIZING PATIENT EXPERIENCE—3Ps

Patients experience a range of experiences in their emotional and physical state while undergoing healthcare procedure. It becomes essential to optimize the PE to achieve wellness in patients' social and mental health. Needham et al. proposed 3Ps—personalized medicine, partner with patients, and empower employees.

P1—Personalized Medicine

Personalized medicine has been one of the primary objectives of the medical field. However, owing to complex human physiology and many complex factors related to genes, it has been difficult to achieve its goal. Healthcare consumers are often categorized into a common group "patient," without taking into consideration individual patients' composition and preference. Moreover, discharge instructions are containing information irrelevant to the patient. Advancement in personalized medicine technology would allow us tracking health records of each patient and studying individual patients' physiologic characteristics for personalized delivery of healthcare services. Richardson et al. reported 100% improvement in chances of survival with 20% increase in medication compliance. It becomes critical that personalizing PEs would improve health outcomes.

P2—Partner with Patients

Building up partnerships with patients has shown to improve decision quality, improve knowledge about the disease, decrease rates of hospitalization, and enhance loyalty, leading to better clinical outcomes. However, in patients with depression, due to complexity of mental health and lack of decision-making capacity, SDM is less often seen in this field of medicine. Stigma associated with mental illness and shame creates additional hinderance. While organizations are focusing on improving and adopting connection-building strategies.

P3—Empowering Employees

Physicians, nurses, receptionists, and other staff members of the hospital who are constantly interacting with the patients in one way or the other play an important role in PE. Empowering every staff member of the hospital would serve as a fuel to build personal connections. They can act as a help in identifying current trends and gaps in healthcare delivery, creating a scope for improvement. Concurrently, attention should also be given on employee stress and burnout. Reduce the sitting time near computer, implementation of internal communication strategies, and making them feel ensured about mental health being the top priority would help in promoting a positive culture in the workplace and achieve overall stability. Free and easy communication between employees and leaders and appreciative feedback would make staff feel like they are playing an important role in the organization. Orientation programs, training sessions, coaching on personal and professional development would help in educating them, making them feel valued and promote staff enrichment.

CONCLUSION

There exists a large amount of scope for the hospitals to understand individual patients journey and improve the quality of service provided to the patients. Each patient's feedback can help in delving into a problem and provide guidance toward next step for improvement, enabling to create a distinct value both for the patient and organization. Following 3Ps—personalizing medicine, partnering with patients, and empowering employees shall help in improving health outcomes and promote physical, mental, and social well-being of the patients and employees.

SUGGESTED READINGS

1. Park S, Xu J, Smith FS, Otani K. What Factors Affect Patient Perceptions on Their Hospital Experience? Hosp Top. 2020;98(3):127-34.
2. Adler-Milstein J, Everson J, Lee SY. EHR Adoption and Hospital Performance: Time-Related Effects. Health Serv Res. 2015;50(6):1751-71.
3. Trbovich P, Vincent C. From incident reporting to the analysis of the patient journey. BMJ Qual Saf. 2019;28(3):169-71.
4. Glickman SW, Schulman KA. The mis-measure of physician performance. Am J Manag Care. 2013;19(10):782-5.
5. Oben P. Understanding the Patient Experience: A Conceptual Framework. J Patient Exp. 2020;7(6):906-10.
6. Gualandi R, Masella C, Viglione D, Tartaglini D. Exploring the hospital patient journey: What does the patient experience? PLoS One. 2019;14(12):e0224899.
7. Tsianakas V, Maben J, Wiseman T, Robert G, Richardson A, Madden P, et al. Using patients' experiences to identify priorities for quality improvement in breast cancer care: patient narratives, surveys or both? BMC Health Serv Res. 2012;12:271.

8. Beattie M, Murphy DJ, Atherton I, Lauder W. Instruments to measure patient experience of healthcare quality in hospitals: a systematic review. Syst Rev. 2015;4:97.
9. Anhang Price R, Elliott MN, Zaslavsky AM, Hays RD, Lehrman WG, Rybowski L, et al. Examining the role of patient experience surveys in measuring health care quality. Med Care Res Rev. 2014;71(5):522-54.
10. McMillan SS, Kendall E, Sav A, King MA, Whitty JA, Kelly F, et al. Patient-centered approaches to health care: a systematic review of randomized controlled trials. Med Care Res Rev. 2013;70(6):567-96.
11. Stoelwinder JU. Final report of the National Health and Hospitals Reform Commission: will we get the health care governance reform we need? Med J Aust. 2009;191(7):387-8.
12. Doyle C, Lennox L, Bell D. A systematic review of evidence on the links between patient experience and clinical safety and effectiveness. BMJ Open. 2013;3(1):e001570.
13. Mead N, Bower P. Patient-centred consultations and outcomes in primary care: a review of the literature. Patient Educ Couns. 2002;48(1):51-61.
14. Figueroa JF, Reimold KE, Zheng J, Orav EJ. Differences in Patient Experience Between Hispanic and Non-Hispanic White Patients Across U.S. Hospitals. J Healthc Qual. 2018;40(5):292-300.
15. Quigley DD, Elliott MN, Hambarsoomian K, Wilson-Frederick SM, Lehrman WG, Agniel D, et al. Inpatient care experiences differ by preferred language within racial/ethnic groups. Health Serv Res. 2019;54(S1):263-74.
16. Al-Amin M, Schiaffino MK, Park S, Harman J. Sustained Hospital Performance on Hospital Consumer Assessment of Healthcare Providers and Systems Survey Measures: What Are the Determinants? J Healthc Manag. 2018;63(1):15-28.
17. Xiao H, Barber JP. The effect of perceived health status on patient satisfaction. Value Health. 2008;11(4):719-25.
18. Golda N, Beeson S, Kohli N, Merrill B. Recommendations for improving the patient experience in specialty encounters. J Am Acad Dermatol. 2018;78(4):653-9.
19. Sacks GD, Lawson EH, Dawes AJ, Russell MM, Maggard-Gibbons M, Zingmond DS, et al. Relationship Between Hospital Performance on a Patient Satisfaction Survey and Surgical Quality. JAMA Surg. 2015;150(9):858-64.
20. Wang DE, Tsugawa Y, Figueroa JF, Jha AK. Association Between the Centers for Medicare and Medicaid Services Hospital Star Rating and Patient Outcomes. JAMA Intern Med. 2016;176(6):848-50.
21. Bakar ZA, Fahrni ML, Khan TM. Patient satisfaction and medication adherence assessment amongst patients at the diabetes medication therapy adherence clinic. Diabetes Metab Syndr. 2016;10(2 Suppl 1):S139-43.
22. Kaye DR, Richardson CR, Ye Z, Herrel LA, Ellimoottil C, Miller DC. Association Between Patient Satisfaction and Short-Term Outcomes After Major Cancer Surgery. Ann Surg Oncol. 2017;24(12):3486-93.
23. Furnas HJ, Korman JM, Canales FL, Pence LD. Patient Reviews: Yelp, Google, Healthgrades, Vitals, and RealSelf. Plast Reconstr Surg. 2020;146(6):1419-31.
24. Luecke RW, Rosselli VR, Moss JM. The economic ramifications of "client" dissatisfaction. Group Pract J. 1991;40:8-18.
25. Kuosmanen L, Hupli M, Ahtiluoto S, Haavisto E. Patient participation in shared decision-making in palliative care—an integrative review. J Clin Nurs. 2021;30(23-24):3415-28.
26. Elwyn G, Frosch D, Thomson R, Joseph-Williams N, Lloyd A, Kinnersley P, et al. Shared decision making: a model for clinical practice. J Gen Intern Med. 2012;27(10):1361-7.
27. Stoll K, Jackson J. Supporting Patient Autonomy and Informed Decision-Making in Prenatal Genetic Testing. Cold Spring Harb Perspect Med. 2020;10(6):a036509.
28. Zolnierek KB, Dimatteo MR. Physician communication and patient adherence to treatment: a meta-analysis. Med Care. 2009;47(8):826-34.
29. Forsey J, Ng S, Rowland P, Freeman R, Li C, Woods NN. The Basic Science of Patient–Physician Communication: A Critical Scoping Review. Acad Med. 2021;96(11s):S109-18.
30. Ubel PA, Scherr KA, Fagerlin A. Empowerment Failure: How Shortcomings in Physician Communication Unwittingly Undermine Patient Autonomy. Am J Bioeth. 2017;17(11):31-9.
31. Harres A. 'But basically you're feeling well, are you?': tag questions in medical consultations. Health Commun. 1998;10(2):111-23.
32. Gafaranga J, Britten N. "Fire away": the opening sequence in general practice consultations. Fam Pract. 2003;20(3):242-7.
33. Manning P, Ray GB. Setting the agenda: an analysis of negotiation strategies in clinical talk. Health Commun. 2002;14(4):451-73.
34. Beste J. Instilling hope and respecting patient autonomy: reconciling apparently conflicting duties. Bioethics. 2005;19(3):215-31.
35. Mostafazadeh-Bora M, Zarghami A. Breaking and Sharing Bad News in End of Life: The Religious and Culture Matters. J Relig Health. 2017;56(5):1655-7.
36. Anderson WG, Kools S, Lyndon A. Dancing around death: hospitalist-patient communication about serious illness. Qual Health Res. 2013;23(1):3-13.
37. Millar C, Reid J, Porter S. Refractory cachexia and truth-telling about terminal prognosis: a qualitative study. Eur J Cancer Care (Engl). 2013;22(3):326-33.
38. Mishelmovich N, Arber A, Odelius A. Breaking significant news: The experience of clinical nurse specialists in cancer and palliative care. Eur J Oncol Nurs. 2016;21:153-9.
39. Miller EM, Porter JE, Barbagallo MS. The experiences of health professionals, patients, and families with truth disclosure when breaking bad news in palliative care: A qualitative meta-synthesis. Palliat Support Care. 2022;20(3):433-44.
40. Moro Visconti R, Morea D. Healthcare Digitalization and Pay-For-Performance Incentives in Smart Hospital Project Financing. Int J Environ Res Public Health. 2020;17(7):2318.
41. Maunder K, Lazarus C, Walton K, Williams P, Ferguson M, Beck E. Energy and protein intake increases with an electronic bedside spoken meal ordering system compared to a paper menu in hospital patients. Clin Nutr ESPEN. 2015;10(4):e134-9.
42. MacKenzie-Shalders K, Maunder K, So D, Norris R, McCray S. Impact of electronic bedside meal ordering systems on dietary intake, patient satisfaction, plate waste and costs: A systematic literature review. Nutr Diet. 2020;77(1):103-11.
43. Mazaheri Habibi MR, Abadi FM, Tabesh H, Vakili-Arki H, Abu-Hanna A, Eslami S. Evaluation of patient satisfaction of the status of appointment scheduling systems in outpatient clinics: Identifying patients' needs. J Adv Pharm Technol Res. 2018;9(2):51-5.
44. Zhang M, Zhang C, Sun Q, Cai Q, Yang H, Zhang Y. Questionnaire survey about use of an online appointment booking system in one large tertiary public hospital outpatient service center in China. BMC Med Inform Decis Mak. 2014;14:49.

45. Volk AS, Davis MJ, Abu-Ghname A, Warfield RG, Ibrahim R, Karon G, et al. Ambulatory Access: Improving Scheduling Increases Patient Satisfaction and Revenue. Plast Reconstr Surg. 2020;146(4):913-9.
46. Abdulwahab SA, Zedan HS. Factors Affecting Patient Perceptions and Satisfaction with Telemedicine in Outpatient Clinics. J Patient Exp. 2021;8:23743735211063780.
47. Mancino F, Cacciola G, Malahias MA, De Filippis R, De Marco D, Di Matteo V, et al. What are the benefits of robotic-assisted total knee arthroplasty over conventional manual total knee arthroplasty? A systematic review of comparative studies. Orthop Rev (Pavia). 2020;12(Suppl 1):8657.
48. Brenner MJ, Hickson GB, Rushton CH, Prince MEP, Bradford CR, Boothman RC. Honesty and Transparency, Indispensable to the Clinical Mission-Part II: How Communication and Resolution Programs Promote Patient Safety and Trust. Otolaryngol Clin North Am. 2022;55(1):63-82.
49. Akbiyik A, Akin Korhan E, Kiray S, Kirsan M. The Effect of Nurses' Leadership Behavior on the Quality of Nursing Care and Patient Outcomes. Creat Nurs. 2020;26(1):e8-18.
50. van Loon-van Gaalen M, van Winsen B, van der Linden MC, Gussekloo J, van der Mast RC. The effect of a telephone follow-up call for older patients, discharged home from the emergency department on health-related outcomes: a systematic review of controlled studies. Int J Emerg Med. 2021;14(1):13.
51. Ferguson SL, Pitt C, Pitt L. Using artificial intelligence to examine online patient reviews. J Health Psychol. 2020;26(13):2424-34.
52. Liang B, Scammon DL. E-Word-of-Mouth on health social networking sites: An opportunity for tailored health communication. J Consum Behav. 2011;10(6):322-31.
53. Kozinets R. Netnography: Radical participative understanding for a networked communications society. In: Willig C, Rogers WS (Eds). The SAGE Handbook of Qualitative Research in Psychology. London: SAGE Publications Ltd; 2017. pp. 374.
54. Weinberg BD, Davis L, Berger PD. Perspectives on big data. J Market Anal. 2013;1:187-201.
55. Greaves F, Pape UJ, King D, Darzi A, Majeed A, Wachter RM, et al. Associations between Internet-based patient ratings and conventional surveys of patient experience in the English NHS: an observational study. BMJ Qual Saf. 2012;21(7):600-5.
56. Greaves F, Pape UJ, King D, Darzi A, Majeed A, Wachter RM, et al. Associations between Web-based patient ratings and objective measures of hospital quality. Arch Intern Med. 2012;172(5):435-6.
57. Kröner PT, Engels MM, Glicksberg BS, Johnson KW, Mzaik O, van Hooft JE, et al. Artificial intelligence in gastroenterology: A state-of-the-art review. World J Gastroenterol. 2021;27(40):6794-824.
58. Jayakumar P, Moore MG, Furlough KA, Uhler LM, Andrawis JP, Koenig KM, et al. Comparison of an Artificial Intelligence-Enabled Patient Decision Aid vs Educational Material on Decision Quality, Shared Decision-Making, Patient Experience, and Functional Outcomes in Adults With Knee Osteoarthritis: A Randomized Clinical Trial. JAMA Netw Open. 2021;4(2):e2037107.
59. Belk R, Fischer E, Kozinets RV (Eds). Qualitative Consumer and Marketing Research. London: SAGE; 2012. pp. 1-240.
60. Humphreys A, Wang RJ-H. Automated text analysis for consumer research. J Consum Res. 2018;44(6):1274-306.
61. Wang Z, Zhao QH, Yang JL, Zhou F. Enhancing Quality of Patients Care and Improving Patient Experience in China with Assistance of Artificial Intelligence. Chin Med Sci J. 2020;35(3):286-8.
62. Needham BR. The truth about patient experience: what we can learn from other industries, and how three Ps can improve health outcomes, strengthen brands, and delight customers. J Healthc Manag. 2012;57(4):255-63.
63. Ho D, Quake SR, McCabe ERB, Chng WJ, Chow EK, Ding X, et al. Enabling Technologies for Personalized and Precision Medicine. Trends Biotechnol. 2020;38(5):497-518.
64. Richardson JL, Shelton DR, Krailo M, Levine AM. The effect of compliance with treatment on survival among patients with hematologic malignancies. J Clin Oncol. 1990;8(2):356-64.
65. Lachman P, Batalden P, Vanhaecht K. A multidimensional quality model: an opportunity for patients, their kin, healthcare providers and professionals to coproduce health. F1000Res. 2020;9:1140.

278

CHAPTER

Point-of-care Ultrasound for Physicians

Lalatendu Mohanty, Amit Jajodia

ABSTRACT

Point-of-care ultrasound or POCUS is the bedside application of ultrasonographic technique for diagnostic and therapeutic purposes in a variety of clinical settings. It is a radiation-free tool and provides noninvasive immediate bedside diagnosis and guides definitive clinical decision-making. It has been used for assessment and monitoring of cardiorespiratory, hemodynamic, abdominal or other organ function status of patients. It is economical and cost-effective. Lack of standardization or generalizability of recommendations due to heterogeneity of its areas, applications, and patient populations is an unanswered question. Formulation of structured course designs or training programs for expertise in its usage for clinicians is in process. It therefore becomes pertinent for clinicians to be aware and familiar with its usage as it possibly can become standard of care and so is the need of the times ahead.

INTRODUCTION

Point-of-care ultrasound (POCUS) is use of portable ultrasound at patient's bedside by treating clinician for diagnostic and therapeutic purposes. It involves acquiring, interpreting, and simultaneous clinical correlation of ultrasonographic imaging by the clinician rather than by a radiologist or cardiologist.

Introduction of smaller, portable, and economical ultrasound machines has allowed the imaging technique to reach patient's bedside which has proven to serve uses in many clinical settings from screening, diagnosis, monitoring to procedural guidance thus pioneering POCUS. Rapid cardiac, pulmonary, hemodynamic, vascular, neurological, and gastrointestinal assessment of patients has been possible with POCUS. It has hastened the recognition of life-threatening clinical situations, decision-making process and timely delivery of emergency and life-saving measures.

A recent study has showed that in up to 50% of cases, it has aided confirmation of the suspected clinical diagnosis and in 23% of cases, supported a change in the initial diagnosis. In this chapter, we attempt to discuss the uses and applications of POCUS in commonly encountered clinical settings and emergencies including critical care and present a perspective to physicians to acquaint with this emerging concept.

PULMONARY ASSESSMENT

Use of thoracic ultrasonography in an acutely dyspneic or hypoxemic patient provides an immediate assessment of the state of the lung and guides therapeutic decisions. It employs BLUE (Bedside Lung Ultrasound in Emergency) protocol which involves examination of three well-defined points on the thorax (anterior, lateral, and posterolateral) bilaterally. It helps in identifying underlying etiology in majority of cases.

Ultrasound of lung relies on the principle that fluid accumulates in dependent areas while gases collect superiorly. Accordingly, probe is placed posterior and inferior for detection of fluid and anterior and superior for detecting air. Visualizing the diaphragm is one of the initial steps in performing lung ultrasound, which appears hyperechoic and descends with every breath.

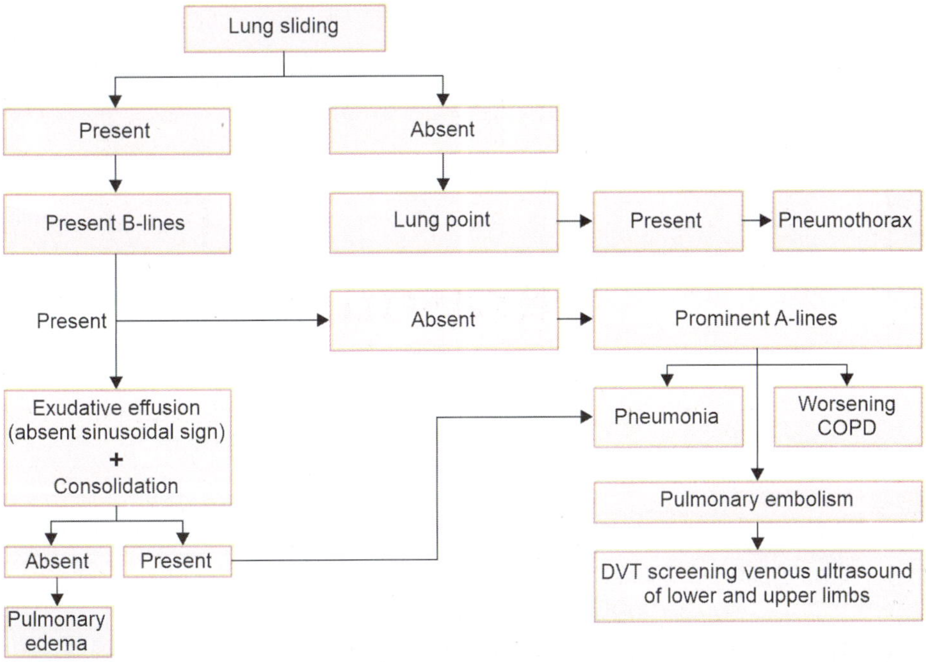

FLOWCHART 1: Approach to identify common pathologies in lung ultrasonography (USG).
(COPD: chronic obstructive pulmonary disease; DVT: deep venous thrombosis)

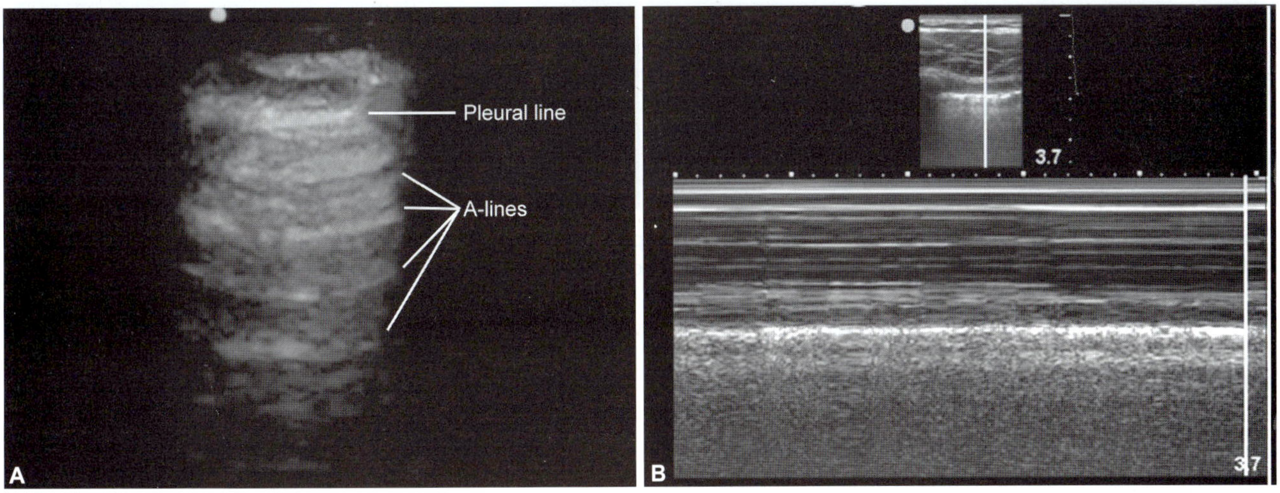

FIGS. 1A AND B: (A) Normal lung ultrasound; (B) Seashore sign in M mode.

A normal lung ultrasound has following features **(Flowchart 1, and Figs. 1 and 2)**:

- *Lung sliding*: It refers to the to and fro movement of visceral pleura moving against parietal pleura as the lung inflates or deflates. It is more prominent at bases than apex. It is absent in presence of fluid (pleural effusion) or air (pneumothorax) in the pleural cavity. In the M mode, it is best visualized with muscle and parietal pleura represented by static horizontal lines above the to and fro movement of visceral pleura and lung which appear granular (*seashore sign*).
- *A-lines*: Motionless horizontal artifacts arising from the pleural line at regular intervals which are equal to the skin-pleural interface distance indicative of physiologic air.
- *B-lines*: Ultrasonic equivalent of radiologic Kerley B-lines are also known as ultrasound lung comets. They are artifacts of water-thickened interlobular septa and indicate extravascular pulmonary edema. They arise from pleural lining, have hyperechoic signals, associated with disappearance of A-lines, move with lung sliding, and have a pattern of indefinite spreading in a cephalad direction.

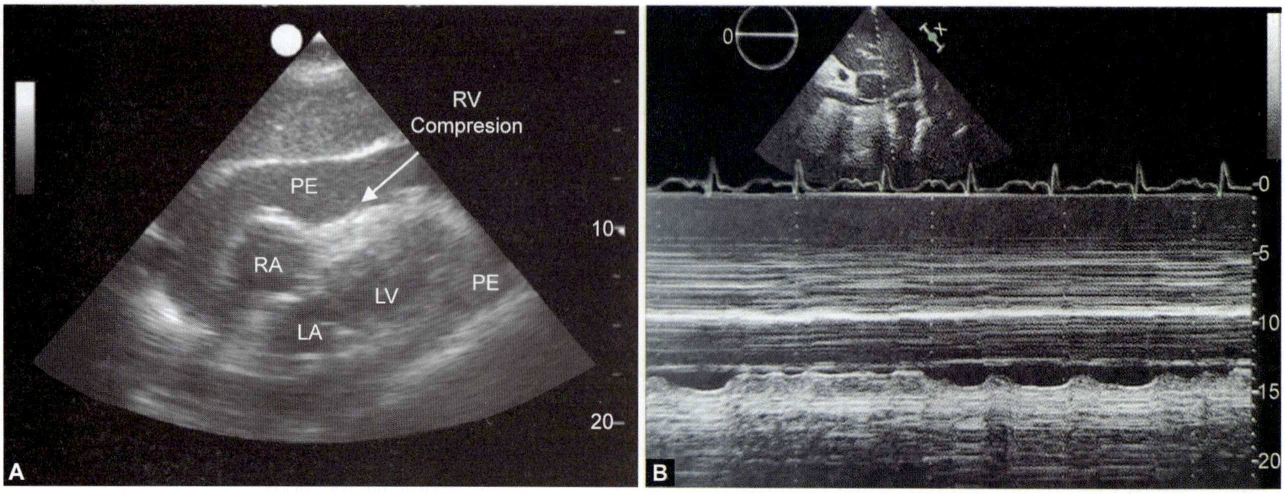

FIGS. 3A AND B: (A) Cardiac tamponade (B) Inferior vena cava (IVC) velocities in hypovolemia; an IVC < 1.5 cm with >50% respiratory collapse indicates intravascular hypovolemia.

(LA: left atrium; LV: left ventricle; PE: pulmonary embolism; RA: right atrium; RV: right ventricle)

VASCULAR ASSESSMENT

It involves use of ultrasound for evaluation of deep venous thrombosis (DVT) in the upper and lower limbs, advanced vascular access, and assessment of abdominal aortic syndromes.

Compression ultrasound is performed in transverse direction wherein a firm, rapid compression with the probe is applied without causing distortion of the neighboring artery. Veins which are compressible are patent and devoid of thrombus, while veins having thrombus cannot be compressed. Compression is not required if visible thrombus is within the vein. In lower limbs, vein compressibility is usually assessed at proximal common femoral vein, saphenofemoral junction, and bifurcation of the common femoral and popliteal veins.

Ultrasound has proven to reliably aid in central and peripheral venous catheterizations and placement of intraarterial catheters with increased success rates and decreased risks of complications.

It also helps in identifying abdominal aortic syndromes including ruptured aneurysms and dissections and is the imaging modality of choice in hemodynamically unstable patients. Enlarged aortic diameter in the abdomen may be seen with or without any fluid collection **(Fig. 4)**.

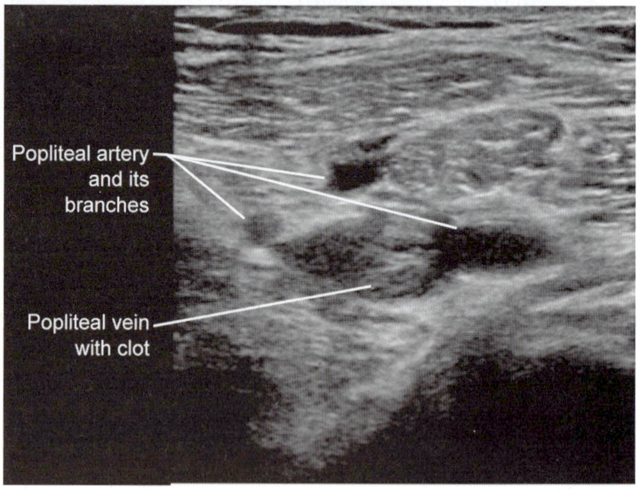

FIG. 4: Ultrasonography (USG) showing clot in popliteal vein.

ABDOMINOPELVIC ASSESSMENT

Bedside ultrasonography of the abdomen and pelvis is commonly used for detection of abdominal free fluid or air, evaluation of acute undifferentiated abdominal pain, localization of possible source of sepsis and urinary obstructions or retention.

Focused Assessment with Sonography for Trauma (FAST) is ultrasonography done during the initial examination and resuscitation of a trauma patient. When views are added for pneumothorax evaluation, the term used is extended FAST (E-FAST).

It is done to detect pathological free fluid in pericardial, thoracic, or peritoneal cavities or pneumothorax.

The order of evaluation is pericardial, right flank (hepatorenal view or Morrison's pouch), left flank (perisplenic view), pelvic (retrovesical views) including paracolic gutters, rectovesical and rectouterine pouches, and evaluation of pneumothorax and hemothorax **(Fig. 5)**.

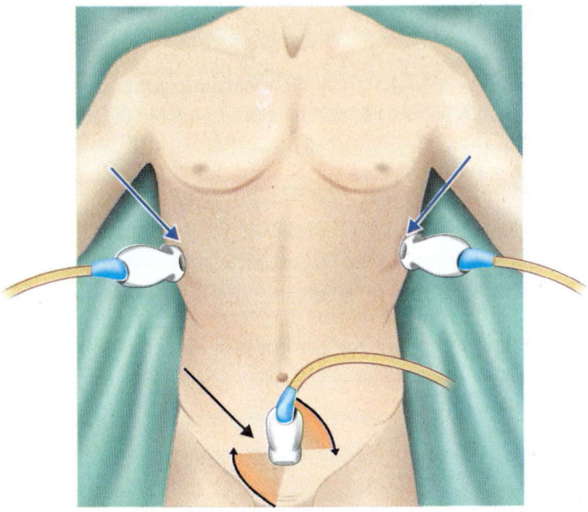

FIG. 5: Probe positions in right and left hypochondria and suprapubic area during Focused Assessment with Sonography for Trauma (FAST) examination.

Free fluid due to blood (traumatic or ruptured abdominal aortic aneurysm) is detected as described in FAST protocol.

Noncomplicated collections of fluid appear anechoic. Complicated accumulations appear as complex non-septated or septated collections. Free fluid from ascites due to liver cirrhosis, for example, is also detected and guides paracentesis if required.

Free intraperitoneal air is detected over ventral aspect of liver in supine or semi-left lateral decubitus position. With more free air, multiple layers of air bubbles create reverberation artifacts referred to as "comet tails" and "ring-downs". Identification of abdominal organs and bowel structures rules out pneumoperitoneum at the site of the probe position as air blocks transmission of sound waves. Intraluminal free air (air in portal vein due to bowel necrosis) or intraparenchymal free air (emphysematous pyelonephritis) is also detected and interpreted according to clinical context.

Assessment of the kidneys for hydronephrosis (dilated pelvicalyceal system) and bladder for distension can be performed for evaluation of urinary obstruction. Bladder distension is assessed by position of bladder dome with respect to the umbilicus. Its extension at least till half the distance to the umbilicus signifies urinary retention.

MUSCULOSKELETAL ASSESSMENT

Point-of-care ultrasound is also used to detect and treat many joint and soft tissue pathologies. It is useful in differentiating cellulitis (scattered fluid collections) from abscess (definite fluid collection in subcutaneous plane) and reducing inappropriate incision and drainage by 20% compared with clinical examinations besides guiding the procedure. It helps in detection of joint effusions and diagnostic and therapeutic arthrocentesis with less chances of periprocedural complications.

ADVANTAGES

Besides being handy, portable and radiation-free, it has been shown that POCUS is cheaper and quicker than routine ultrasonography in yielding information that may decrease emergency department stays so that definitive procedures can be initiated. Its usage for a wide range of clinical situations in practice of medicine has reduced number of planned referrals. It can also be used in patients receiving palliative care to address symptoms such as severe dyspnea due to malignant pleural effusions and is beneficial in terms of triage (helps in prioritizing patients depending on urgency of clinical setting) and patient satisfaction.

LIMITATIONS (OR AREAS UNEXPLORED)

Given its variety of applications in different settings, it is difficult to evaluate its impact on patients' functional status, morbidity, or mortality due to the heterogeneity of patients, the lack of standardized scanning protocols or therapeutic decisions, the confounding effect of various multiple therapeutic interventions and interpersonal variation in skill levels related to POCUS and the difficulty in finding clinicians with exposure and familiarity to POCUS. More information is needed to identify duration and structure of training programs required to achieve expertise with respect to skills of acquisition and interpretation of images especially for clinicians who are new to this world of radiology.

CONCLUSION

Point-of-care ultrasound is an evolving concept which has brought ultrasonography to patient's bedside, thus providing the treating clinician with real-time diagnostic and monitoring information and enhancing the safety of standard procedures. It finds wide variety of applications encompassing specialities, protocols, or organ systems. Introduction of courses and training programs for the same at various medical educational levels is upcoming and with the increasing amount of evidence of its benefits in clinical practice coupled with technological advances, it can become a frontline standard of patient care and pertinent tool for physicians.

SUGGESTED READINGS

1. Kendall JL, Hoffenberg SR, Smith RS. History of emergency and critical care ultrasound: the evolution of a new imaging paradigm. Crit Care Med. 2007;35(5 Suppl.):S126-130.
2. Díaz-Gómez JL, Mayo PH, Koenig SJ. Point-of-Care Ultrasonography. N Engl J Med. 2021;385(17):1593-602.
3. Baker DE, Nolting L, Brown HA. Impact of point-of-care ultrasound on the diagnosis and treatment of patients in rural Uganda. Trop Doct. 2021;51:291-6.
4. Seif D, Perera P, Mailhot T, Riley D, Mandavia D. Bedside ultrasound in resuscitation and the rapid ultrasound in shock protocol. Crit Care Res Pract. 2012;2012:503254.
5. Kratzert WB, Mahajan A. Echocardiography. In: Vincent JL, Abraham E, Moore FA, Kochanek PM, Fink MP (Eds). Textbook of Critical Care,1st edition. Haryana: Elsevier; 2017. pp. 138-51.
6. Singh R. Point of care ultrasound. In: Vincent JL, Abraham E, Moore FA, Kochanek PM, Fink MP (Eds). Textbook of Critical Care, 1st edition. Haryana: Elsevier; 2017. pp. 132-7.
7. Barbic D, Chenkin J, Cho DD, Jelic T, Scheuermeyer FX. In patients presenting to the emergency department with skin and soft tissue infections what is the diagnostic accuracy of point-of-care ultrasonography for the diagnosis of abscess compared to the current standard of care. BMJ Open. 2017;7(1):013688.

279

CHAPTER

Presenting Like a Pro in Your Journal Clubs

(Maj) Gowri Shanker R

ABSTRACT

Standard textbooks are a reliable source of medical knowledge, but they are updated every 3–5 years. Journals can help stay current, but it is important to verify the source and authenticity of the article.

Presenting effectively in journal clubs is crucial for academic growth. This guide outlines key strategies to enhance presentation skills and captivate your audience. Before presenting, thoroughly understand the research paper, creating a structured outline.

Engage your audience with a compelling introduction, summarizing the background, and clearly explaining what the article is all about. Emphasize key results, discuss limitations, and relate findings to real-world implications.

During the presentation, focus on clear communication, maintain eye contact, and use visuals judiciously. Encourage questions for interactivity. Post-presentation, welcome feedback and facilitate a discussion. This comprehensive approach ensures a polished and impactful journal club presentation.

INTRODUCTION: WHY TO READ JOURNALS?

We all learnt medicine by reading the standard textbooks. When our textbooks, many of which have lasted a century and are supported by reputed authors and editorial teams, can teach us so much, why should we spend extra time reading journals?

The textbooks are revised every 3–5 years, and if we depend on only textbooks as the source of updates, we might need to catch up in our current knowledge.

Portals like UpToDate are current and stay ahead and evidence-based in the current era. However, when the added information is being passed, we need to know the source and authenticity of the article which brings these changes. The article can be a case control study, cohort study, randomized controlled trial (RCT) or meta-analysis.

Trainees in cardiac imaging reading 40 papers a day, 5 days a week, would take over 11 years to bring themselves up to date with the specialty. Nevertheless, by the time they had completed that task, another 82,000 relevant papers would have been published, requiring another 8 years of reading—Fraser and Dunstan: BMJ.

WHERE CAN WE FIND THE GEM IN THE WORLD OF INFORMATION TSUNAMI?

The prominent four journals which carry the top hits are NEJM, BMJ, JAMA, and Annals of Internal Medicine. The best way to access these journals is to subscribe to their E-mail alerts. E-mail alert exists for all these journals and other reputed journals too.

Lancet and Nature also should be added to the list. Each specialty branch of medicine has its list of Journals to follow. For example, the field of diabetes journals that one can follow are Diabetes Care, JCEM, Diabetologia, Lancet Diabetes and Endocrinology, and Nature Reviews Endocrinology.

ACCESSING THE ARTICLE IS A COSTLY AFFAIR: HOW SHOULD WE GO ABOUT IT?

The E-mail alert gives an idea of the abstract of the article. If the article interests us, try to have access to the original article. Most of the time, it may be a paid version.

- Portals like *sci-hub.ren* (the domain extension may keep varying for the sci-hub website, but the latest one can easily be accessed by googling) may give access to the article.
- The central library of most academic institutes in various countries has access to these articles. Find a friend who can get it for you; it is not that difficult.
- The scientific team of pharmaceutical industries will have access to these articles. Know the key person and ask them directly.
- If nothing works, send a request mail to the corresponding author of the article, and they will always be happy to share it with you.

NOW THAT WE HAVE THE ARTICLE, HOW SHOULD ONE GO ABOUT IT?

Always start the presentation with what attracted you to present this article. It could be a clinical problem, a concept one want to challenge, a concept one may seek more clarity on, an innovative drug (or otherwise) or for whatever reasons you choose to present the article.

Let there be a good prelude. The prelude is the key component which most presenters generally miss. Let the prelude be nonacademic but succeed in starting with a good introduction.

An intro can go like this "I was moderating a session on management challenges in Diabetic Kidney Disease. The floor was divided when a question was asked about using RAAS blockers in stage IV–V DKD to the panellists comprising Endocrinologist, Nephrologist, and Cardiologist. The subsequent literature search yielded this article."

Renin–Angiotensin System Inhibition in Advanced Chronic Kidney Disease

Sunil Bhandari

N Engl J Med. December 1, 2022

PS: This article is the reference article for further discussion. The article is available for free download at NEJM website.

DESCRIBE THE STUDY AND THE RESEARCH QUESTION?

Study

When presenting an article, we can broadly look at the phenotype of the study.

- Does the study look at the etiology, efficacy, therapeutics, cost-effectiveness, or outcome
- What type of study method was used—a Cohort study, case-control, RCT, meta-analysis, or a review article on a subject.
- Where was the study done—a single center, country, or multiple continents involved?
- Race, ethnicity, and gender difference being adequately addressed.
- Any other distinguishing feature like the first study of its kind or the research center/author group is well recognized for its authority on the subject.

Research Question

The most essential part of an article is the hypothesis or the research question which is evaluated. PICO questionnaire helps in formulating the research questionnaire in a structured manner.

- *P—population*: This includes characteristics such as age, gender, health status, and relevant medical conditions.
- *I—intervention or exposure*: This could be a medication, therapy, procedure, or any other intervention being studied.
- *C—comparison*: This could be a different therapy, placebo, standard care, or no intervention.
- *O—outcome*: This can include clinical outcomes, patient-reported outcomes, quality-of-life measures, adverse events, or any other relevant outcome.

Adults above 18 years of age with stage 4 or 5 chronic kidney disease (CKD) [estimated glomerular filtration rate (eGFR), <30 mL/min] were not on dialysis and had not undergone renal transplantation. Patients were screened at 39 centers in the United Kingdom. It is a multicenter, open-label trial and was funded by the National Institute for Health Research and the Medical Research Council; no industry support was provided.

About 410 patients were randomly assigned either to discontinue or to continue therapy with renin–angiotensin system (RAS) inhibitors. The eGFR was monitored every 3 months for the next 3 years.

ANSWER THE CRITICAL APPRAISAL QUESTION ON VALIDITY

Once the study is briefly described, further discussion can be taken based on *JAMA users' guides to the medical literature*, third edition. This book is a must-read book for every one of us who wants to embrace evidence-based medicine. Chapter 6 of the book addresses Randomized Controlled Trial and Users' Guides for an article about therapy. For a better understanding of the article, the following heads in the book will help us to dissect the article properly:

- How serious was the risk of bias?
- Did intervention and control groups start with the same prognosis?
- Were patients randomized?
- Was randomization concealed?
- Were patients in the study groups similar with respect to known prognostic factors?
- Was prognostic balance maintained as the study progressed?
- To what extent was the study blinded?
- Were the groups prognostically balanced at the study's completion?
- Was the follow-up complete?
- Were patients analyzed in the groups to which they were randomized?
- Was the trial stopped early?

In the study, the patients were randomized, but it was an open-label study. In the RAS inhibitor discontinued arm, the blood pressure (BP) was slightly higher in the first year, but the study allowed them to choose any other antihypertensive, and in both arms, the BP was < 140/80 mm Hg or less. The analysis was based on the intention to treat principle and included all the patients who were randomized.

LET STATISTICS NOT BAFFLE YOU AND THE AUDIENCE TOO!

Not to get lost in the analysis of data and statistics section. "Statistics are a tool while study methods rule!".

Medical Statistricks and Clinical Trials–a serious fun book for the Clinicians by Dr Tiny Nair is a small but great ready reckoner and highly recommended.

FINALLY, THE RESULTS

After the descriptors and research question, one can discuss the study results. The summary of the primary outcome is most important.

The secondary outcomes can be presented if they are relevant.

Bring the audience's attention to the chart/image/line diagram or figure and expose them to what happened to the results.

Discuss limitations, shortcomings, and future directions. Acknowledge the limitations and shortcomings of the study and discuss the potential areas for future research. This shows a comprehensive understanding of the topic and critical thinking.

Though there were a few trials before this study which assessed the role of RAS inhibitors in stage 4–5 CKD, this study is the largest study which assessed the utility of continuation versus discontinuation and showed that continuation of RAS inhibitors did not lead to a significant change in GFR. The rate of decline of eGFR is a valid predictor of the development of end-stage kidney disease (ESKD). Preservation of eGFR by >0.75 mL/min/year predicts a clinically reasonable delay in the progression of CKD. The study also reinforced that the choice of antihypertensive is not essential. Instead, the control of BP is more important in stage 4–5 CKD. The incidence of hyperkalemia was not mentioned in the entire study population.

CAN I APPLY THE STUDY TO MY PATIENTS?

The study's external validity can be checked by extrapolating the facts to your practice. Summing up how it is relevant to your current practice is the best way to finish the presentation.

The results may be beneficial to our patients, or they may be irrelevant, or one may need some adjustments and modifications.

Patients with non-White ethnic backgrounds were not included in the study questioning the relevance to our study population.

CONCLUDING REMARKS

Now conclude the presentation with the case or the story that prompted you to look for this article. Circulate a one-page, preferably physical summary with all the relevant information, including PICO, brief discussion, necessary diagram, or relevant graphs, and three important carry-home messages. Let the listeners get a sense of closure.

The session I moderated led me to find this article; the panelists argued that the RAS blockers in stage 4–5 CKD are for cardio protection, not nephroprotection. This article points out that there is no difference in cardio-protection whether one continues or discontinues the RAS inhibitor in stage 4–5 CKD.

B

C

G

H

I

J

K

L

M

N

W

X

Y

Z

Clinical to Digital Medicine

Medicine Update 2024

An Official Publication of
Association of Physicians of India

1

Clinical to Digital Medicine

Medicine Update 2024

Volume 34 | 2024

An Official Publication of
Association of Physicians of India

Editor-in-Chief

Milind Y Nadkar MD FICP FACP
President-Elect
Association of Physicians of India
Professor and Head
Department of Medicine and
Chief of Rheumatology Services
Seth GS Medical College and KEM Hospital
Mumbai, Maharashtra, India

Foreword

KK Pareek

JAYPEE

JAYPEE BROTHERS MEDICAL PUBLISHERS
The Health Sciences Publisher
New Delhi | London

Dedication

To my honorable grandmother
Late Smt Saraswati Vinayak Nadkar

And my parents
Late Shri Yeshwant V Nadkar and
Smt Pramodini Y Nadkar
for all the values they taught me.

My wife Mrs Jayshree Nadkar
for being so tolerant and supportive all the life.

My son Gaurav Nadkar
for making me so proud of him

And
My respected teachers and beloved patients
who taught me the Science and Art of Medicine.

CONTRIBUTORS

Aaliya Jabbar MBBS
Junior Resident
Department of Medicine
Era's Lucknow Medical College
Lucknow, Uttar Pradesh, India

Aarathy Kannan MD (Dip Diab) MBA
Consultant Physician and Diabetologist
Sundaram Arulrhaj Hospitals
Tuticorin, Tamil Nadu, India

Aayushi Rathi DNB
Resident (Final Year)
Department of Respiratory Medicine
Apollo Gleneagles Hospital
Kolkata, West Bengal, India

Abdul Haroon Shah MBBS
PG Student (3rd Year)
Sardar Patel Medical College
Bikaner, Rajasthan, India

Abha Gupta MD
Professor and Head
Department of Medicine
Lala Lajpat Rai Memorial Medical College
Meerut, Uttar Pradesh, India

A Bhagwati MD(Medicine) FICP FICCM ADHA(Hospital Administration)
Honorary Physician and Intensivist
Department of Internal Medicine and Critical Care
Bhatia Hospital
Honorary Physician
Saifee Hospital
Wockhardt Hospital
Smt Motiben Dalvi Hospital
Mumbai, Maharashtra, India

Abhishek Borkotoky MBBS
Junior Resident
Department of General Medicine
Institute of Medical Sciences
Banaras Hindu University
Varanasi, Uttar Pradesh, India

Abhishek Kumar MD(General Medicine) FICP FIACM
Consultant Medicine, Avni Care
Patna, Bihar, India

Abhishek Kumar Tiwari MD
DM Resident Cardiology
Coimbatore Medical College and Hospital
Coimbatore, Tamil Nadu, India

Abhishek Singhai MD(Medicine)
Associate Professor
Department of Medicine
All India Institute of Medical Sciences
Bhopal, Madhya Pradesh, India

Aditi Aggarwal MBBS
Junior Resident (DNB)
Nemcare Hospital
Guwahati, Assam, India

Aditya Chakravorty MBBS
Post Graduate Student
Department of General Medicine
School of Medical Sciences and Research
Sharda University
Greater Noida, Uttar Pradesh, India

Aditya Prakash Misra MD FICP
Senior Consultant
Department of Internal Medicine
Fortis Flt Lt Rajan Dhall Hospital
Medeor (Rockland) Qutab Hospital
New Delhi, India

AG Unnikrishnan MD DM(Endocrinology) DNB MNAMS
CEO and Chief Endocrinologist
Chellaram Diabetes Institute
Pune, Maharashtra, India

Aishwarya N Udupa MBBS
Resident of General Medicine
Jawaharlal Nehru Medical College
KLE Academy of Higher Education and Research
Belagavi, Karnataka, India

Ajay K Pandey MD(Medicine) DM(Cardiology) FACC FESC FSCAI(USA)
Consultant Interventional Cardiologist and Head (Cardiology)
Galaxy Hospital
Varanasi, Uttar Pradesh, India

Ajaypal Singh MBBS
PG Student (3rd Year)
Sardar Patel Medical College
Bikaner, Rajasthan, India

Ajeet Singh Chahar MD(General Medicine)
Associate Professor in Medicine
PG Department of Medicine
SN Medical College and Hospital
Agra, Uttar Pradesh, India

Ajoy Tewari MD FRCP FACP FICP
Director Consultant Diabetologist
Jai Clinic and Diabetes Care Centre
Lucknow, Uttar Pradesh, India

A Kader Sahib MD MRCP DNB
Consultant Cardiologist
Apollo and Ayesha Hospital
Trichy, Tamil Nadu, India

Akanksha Gautam MS(Obstetrics and Gynecology)
Senior Resident
Department of Gynaecology
Eternal Hospital
Jaipur, Rajasthan, India

Akashkumar Navinprakash Singh MD(Internal Medicine) MSc(Diabetes) FACP FICP FIACM FRSSDI Fellow Diabetes India
Consultant Physician
Spandan Multispeciality Hospital
Vadodara, Gujarat, India

Akash Panigrahi DM(Endocrinology)
Consultant Endocrinologist
Tata Main Hospital
Jamshedpur, Jharkhand, India

Akhani S Krupa MBBS
PG Resident
Department of Medicine
American International Institute of Medical Sciences
Udaipur, Rajasthan, India

Akhilesh Kumar Singh MD(Medicine)
Professor of Medicine
SN Medical College
Agra, Uttar Pradesh, India

Akshat Taneja MD
Anesthetist, ESI Hospital
Gurugram, Haryana, India

Akshaykumar Chhallani DNB(General Medicine) FNB(CCM) FICP FCPS(Medicine) MNAMS
Medical Adviser and Critical Care Expert, Apollo Hospital
Navi Mumbai, Maharashtra, India

AK Singh MD FICP FGSI Fc Card
Former Head
Department of Medicine
SSPG Hospital
Varanasi, Uttar Pradesh, India
President, Geriatric Society of India
President, Indian College of Hematology and Oncology Society of India

Alok Modi MD FISH FIACM (India) FACP (USA) PGDL(UK)
Senior Consultant
Kevalya Hospita, Thane
Jupiter Hospital, Mumbai
Ex-Associate Professor of Medicine
Rajiv Gandhi Medical College and Chhatrapati Shivaji Hospital
Mumbai, Maharashtra, India

Alpana Raizada MD
Professor
Department of Medicine
University College of Medical Sciences
New Delhi, India

Amal Kumar Banerjee MD DM FACC FESC FACP FAPSC FICC FCSI FICP
Consultant and Interventional Cardiologist
Formerly
Institute of Cardiovascular Sciences
IPGMER and SSKM Hospital
Kolkata, West Bengal, India

Aman Singh MD
Resident
Department of General Medicine
Institute of Medical Sciences
Banaras Hindu University (IMS-BHU)
Varanasi, Uttar Pradesh, India

Brig Ambika P Mohanty VSM MD DNB FICP FISG
Professor in Medicine
Kalinga Institute of Medical Sciences
KIIT Deemed to be University
Bhubaneswar, Odisha, India

Ambika Tyagi MD(Medicine)
Assistant Professor
Mahatma Gandhi University of Medical Sciences and Technology
Jaipur, Rajasthan, Inda

Ambreen Liyakat MD(Radiodiagnosis)
Director
The Galaxy Ultrasound and Diagnostic Centre
Jaipur, Rajasthan, India

Amita Diwaker MD
Associate Professor
Department of Obstetrics and Gynecology
Institute of Medical Sciences, Banaras Hindu University (IMS-BHU)
Varanasi, Uttar Pradesh, India

Amit Aggarwal DNB MNAMS FIACM FICP
Senior Specialist
Department of Medicine
ABVIMS and Dr Ram Manohar Lohia Hospital
New Delhi, India

Amit A Saraf MD FRCP(London, Edinburgh, Glasgow) FACP(Philadelphia) FICP FCPS
Director
Department of Internal Medicine
Jupiter Hospital
Mumbai, Maharashtra, India

Amitav Mohanty MD FICP FDiab India
Advisor and Senior Consultant
DNB Course Director and Faculty
Department of Medicine
Apollo Hospital
Bhubaneswar, Odisha, India

Amit Dua DNB(Medicine)
Consultant Rheumatologist
Dua's Clinic
Rheumatology and Arthritis Care
Bilaspur, Chhattisgarh, India

Amit Ghosh MD DM FACP FRCP
Professor of Medicine
Mayo Clinic College of Medicine and Sciences
Rochester, Minnesota, USA

Amit Gupta DNB(General Medicine) MNAMS FACE FICP FRCP(Glasgow, Edinburgh) FACP(USA) FRSSDI PGD-Diab (Cardiff UK) DFID(CMC Vellore)
Director
Centre for Diabetes Care
Greater Noida, Uttar Pradesh, India

Amit Jajodia MBBS
Postgraduate Resident
Department of Medicine
Kalinga Institute of Medical Sciences
Bhubaneswar, Odisha, India

Amit Kumar Das MD(Medicine) FICP FISH FDI FICCMD FIACM
Assistant Professor of Medicine
Shree Krishna Medical College and Hospital
Muzaffarpur, Bihar, India

Amrish Agrawal MD DM(Cardiology) FACC FRCP(Glasgow) FRCP(Edinburgh) MRCP(UK) Fellow Cardiology(Australia)
Senior Consultant Cardiologist
Associate Professor of Medicine
Fujairah Hospital, Emirates Health Services (EHS)
Fujairah, UAE

Ananda Bagchi MD(Medicine) MRCPS(Glasgow) FACP(USA) FICP FCSI FIAMS
Senior Consultant Physician
Dum Dum Specialised Hospital and ILS Hospital
Kolkata, West Bengal, India

Anand N Malaviya MD FRCP(London) 'Master'-ACR & APLAR FACP FICP FAMS FNASc
Head (Retired)
Department of Medicine
Chief of Clinical Immunology and Rheumatology Services
All India Institute of Medical Sciences
Consultant Rheumatologist
A&R Clinic
Visiting Senior Consultant Rheumatologist
ISIC Superspeciality Hospital
New Delhi, India

Anand P Ambali MD PGDGM MSc FGSI FICP FIACM FRCPE
Professor and Head
Department of Geriatric Medicine
BLDE Deemed to be University
Shri BM Patil Medical College Hospital and Research Centre
Vijayapura, Karnataka, India

Anchin Kalia DNB(Medicine) FICP
Professor and Unit Head
Mahatma Gandhi Hospital
Jaipur, Rajasthan, India

Anil Kumar Kulshreshtha MD(Medicine) FICP FIACM
Director
Anubhuti Medical and Gynec Hospital
Thalthej, Ahmedabad, Gujarat, India

Anil Mahla MBBS
Resident
Mahatma Gandhi Medical College and Hospital
Jaipur, Rajasthan, India

Anil Samaria MD(Medicine)
Unit Head and Senior Professor
JLN Medical College and Hospital
Ajmer, Rajasthan, India

Anish Kumar Gupta M Pharm (PP)
Consultant (Research and Development)
Faculty of Medicine and Health Sciences, Shree Guru Gobind Singh Tricentenary University
Gurugram, Haryana, India

Anita Nambiar MD(General Medicine) FICP FRCP (Edinburgh)
Senior Consultant
VPS Lakeshore Hospital
Ernakulam,, Kerala, India

Anjana Pandey MD(General Medicine)
Professor
Department of Arthritis and Autoimmune Unit
Arogya Laxmi Health Care
Agra, Uttar Pradesh, India

Anju Bharti MD
Associate Professor
Department of Pathology
Institute of Medical Sciences
Banaras Hindu University
Varanasi, Uttar Pradesh, India

Ankan Pathak MD(Medicine) DNB(Cardiology)
Postdoctoral Trainee, Department of Interventional Cardiology
Apollo Multispeciality Hospitals
Kolkata, West Bengal, India

Ankita Kabi MD DNB
Associate Professor in Anesthesiology
All India Institute of Medical Sciences
Gorakhpur, Uttar Pradesh, India

Ankit Shrivastav DM(Endocrinology)
Consultant Endocrinologist
Arogya Diabetes and Endocrine Centre
Ranchi, Jharkhand, India

Ankur Gupta MD DM FRACP
Consultant Nephrologist
Palmerston North Hospital
Roslyn, New Zealand

Antarleena Ray MBBS
Junior Resident
Department of General Medicine
Medical College
Kolkata, West Bengal, India

Anubha Srivastava MD(Medicine) MMSc(Endocrinology) FRCPE FACP FISH Fellow Diabetes India FUPDA FISMN
Professor Medicine
MLN Medical College
Prayagraj, Uttar Pradesh, India

Anu Goswami MD DNB
Ex-Assistant Professor
Department of Obstetrics and Gynecology
Subharti Medical College
Meerut, Uttar Pradesh, India

Anuj Maheshwari MD FICP FACP FACE FRCP(London, Edinburgh)
Professor
Department of Medicine
Hind Institute of Medical Sciences
Lucknow, Uttar Pradesh, India

Anuj Sharma MBBS
1st Year PG Student of Medicine
Shree Krishna Medical College and Hospital
Muzaffarpur, Bihar, India

Anu Maheshwari MD
Professor
Department of Pediatrics
Lady Hardinge Medical College and Associated Hospitals
New Delhi, India

Anupama YJ MD(Medicine) DNB(Nephrology)
Consultant Nephrologist
Nanjappa Hospital
Shivamogga, Karnataka, India

Anupam Dey MD FICP FACP
Professor and Head
Department of General Medicine
All India Institute of Medical Sciences
Bhubaneswar, Odisha, India

Anupam Prakash MD(General Medicine)
Director Professor
Department of Medicine
Lady Hardinge Medical College
New Delhi, India

Anup Kumar Das MD FICP
Professor of Medicine
Assam Medical College
Dibrugarh, Assam, India

Anurag DM(Gastroenterology)
Resident Doctor
JLN Medical College and Hospital
Ajmer, Rajasthan, India

Anurag Varma MD(Psychology) FIPS FIACAM
Consultant Psychiatrist
MLN Medical College
Prayagraj, Uttar Pradesh, India

Anusha Yadav MBBS
PG Student (3rd Year)
Sardar Patel Medical College
Bikaner, Rajasthan, India

Anushka Deogaonkar MBBS
Intern, Bharti Vidyapeeth
Pune, Maharashtra, India

Anyam Borpuzari MBBS
Medical Officer
Government of Assam
Sivasagar, Assam, India

Aparna Agrawal MD
Director Professor of Medicine
Lady Hardinge Medical College
New Delhi, India

Aparna Tewari MD(Anesthesiology and Critical Care Medicine)
Postgraduate Trainee
Kolkata Medical College
Kolkata, West Bengal, India

Appandraj Jain MD(General Medicine)
Professor and Head
Department of Internal Medicine
Melmaruvathur Adhiparasakthi Institute of Medical Sciences and Research (MAPIMS)
Melmaruvathur, Tamil Nadu, India

Aqsa Jafri MD(General Medicine Student)
Junior Resident
PG Department of Medicine
SN Medical College and Hospital
Agra, Uttar Pradesh, India

Aradhana Singh MD(Medicine)
Professor and Founder Head
Department of Clinical Immunology and Rheumatology
SMS Medical College and Hospital
Jaipur, Rajasthan, India

Aradhya Sekhar Bagchi MD(Medicine)
Consultant Physician
Nil Ratan Sircar Medical College
Kolkata, West Bengal, India

Arathi Darshan MD FICP
Professor of Medicine
KLE Academy of Higher Education and Research
Jawaharlal Nehru Medical College
Belagavi, Karnataka, India

Arghya Chattopadhyay
MD(Medicine) DM(Clinical Immunology and Rheumatology)
Assistant Professor
Department of Rheumatology
North Bengal Medical College and Hospital
Siliguri, West Bengal, India

Arijit Sinha MD DNB(General Medicine) FICP
Professor, Department of General Medicine, NRS Medical College
Kolkata, West Bengal, India

Arjun Tandon MD(Medicine)
Senior Resident
Department of Cardiology
Banaras Hindu University
Varanasi, Uttar Pradesh, India

Arkadip Choudhury MD(Medicine)
Assistant Professor
Department of General Medicine
Tripura Medical College and Dr BRAM Teaching Hospital, Hapania
Agartala, Tripura, India

Arpit Jain MD(Radiation Oncology) DrNB(Medical Oncology)
Consultant
Department of Medical Oncology
Rajiv Gandhi Cancer Institute and Research Centre
New Delhi, India

Arun Kumar Kedia MD(Medicine)
Consultant Physician
Lifeworth Hospital
Raipur Chhattisgarh, India

Arup Kumar Kundu MD FRCP FICP MNAS
Ex-Professor of Medicine and In-Charge, Division of Rheumatology
Department of Medicine
RG Kar Medical College
Kolkata, West Bengal, India

Ashee Verma MBBS
Locum Resident
Government Medical College
Kota, Rajasthan, India

Ashima Katyal MD
Assistant Professor
Kalpana Chawla Government Medical College
Karnal, Haryana, India

Ashish Goel MD
Professor and Head
Department of Medicine
Dr BR Ambedkar State Institute of Medical Sciences (AIMS)
Mohali, Punjab, India

Ashok K Taneja MD DipCARD FRCP FACP FICP FIAE FDI
Director
Taneja Heart Diabetes Centre
Gurugram, Haryana, India

Ashok Kumar MD
Professor and Head
Department of Medicine
Santosh Medical College and Hospital
Ghaziabad, Uttar Pradesh, India

Ashutosh Kumar Karn MD DM(Neurology)
Chief Medical Officer
Department of Medicine
ABVIMS and Dr Ram Manohar Lohia Hospital
New Delhi, India

Ashwini Nigam MD(Medicine)
Professor of Medicine
PG Department of Medicine
SN Medical College
Agra, Uttar Pradesh, India

Asish Mondal MD(Internal Medicine)
Assistant Professor
Kolkata Medical College
Kolkata, West Bengal, India

AS Mohan MD FICP
Retired Professor and Head (Medicine)
Tirunelveli Medical College
Tirunelveli, Tamil Nadu, India

AS Senthilvelu MD
Managing Trustee
Erode Diabetes Foundation
Physician, Diabetologist and Medical Superintendent
Maaruthi Medical Centre and Hospitals
Erode, Tamil Nadu, India

Aswin Sasikumar MBBS
Resident of General Medicine
Jawaharlal Nehru Medical College
KLE Academy of Higher Education and Research
Belagavi, Karnataka, India

Atanu Chandra MD(Internal Medicine) DNB(Internal Medicine) MRCP (UK)
Assistant Professor
Department of Internal Medicine
Bankura Sammilani Medical College
Bankura, West Bengal, India

Atanu Thakur MD(Medicine)
Associate Professor
Department of Medicine
Veer Surendra Sai Institute of Medical Science and Research (VIMSAR)
Burla, Odisha, India

Atul Bhasin DNB(Internal Medicine, Army Hospital R&R) MNAMS FIACM FICP FACP(USA) FRCP(London)
Senior Director
Department of Internal Medicine
BLK-MAX Super Speciality Hospital
New Delhi, India

Atul Gupta MBBS
Junior Resident 3rd Year
Department of Medicine
GSVM Medical College
Kanpur, Uttar Pradesh, India

Atul Kumar MD
Consultant, Dr Prasad Diabetes and Hypertension Care Clinic
Patna, Bihar, India

Atul Mehrotra DTCD MD(Medicine) FICP FISC FACP PGDDM
Consultant Physician
Mehrotra Family Clinic
Lucknow, Uttar Pradesh, India

Ashutosh Chaturvedi MD(Medicine) Certified in Diabetes(Chennai)
Assistant Professor
Department of Medicine
Mahatma Gandhi Medical College
Jaipur, Rajasthan, India

Avik Chakraborty MD(Medicine) FICP FIACM
Professor
Department of General Medicine,
Tripura Medical College and Dr BRAM Teaching Hospital, Hapania
Agartala, Tripura, India

Avina Jain MD(Dermatology, Venereology and Leprosy)
Chief Dermatologist
Auro Skin Clinic
Mumbai, Maharashtra, India

Balakrishnan Kannan MD DM(Neurology)
Consultant Neurologist
Sundaram Arulrhaj Hospitals
Tuticorin, Tamil Nadu, India

Balbir Singh Kohli MD DNB(Medicine) AFIH FAIMS
Head
Department of Critical Care and Emergency
Hira Mongi Navneet Hospital
Consultant Physician
Fortis and Jupiter hospital
Mumbai, Maharashtra, India

Basabbijay Sarkar MD
Consultant Physician and Head
Department of Internal Medicine
Fortis Hospitals
Kolkata, West Bengal, India

BD Goswami MD(Medicine) PhD(Gastroenterology, Russia) FISG FACG(USA) AGAF(USA) FSGEI FRCP(Edinburgh, Glasgow)
Senior Consultant Gastroenterologist
Dispur Hospital
Former Professor and Head
Department of Gastroenterology
Gauhati Medical College and Hospital
Guwahati, Assam, India

Bharat Bhushan Sharma MD(Internal Medicine)
Senior Professor and In-Charge
Respiratory Allergy Clinic
Department of Medicine
SMS Medical College
Jaipur, Rajasthan, India

Bharath HR MD
Senior Resident
Department of Gastroenterology
Dr SN Medical College,
Jodhpur, Rajasthan, India

Bharat Panigrahy MD FICP FACP FIMAMS
Senior Consultant in Medicine and Rheumatology
LVPEI, CARE and AMRI
Bhubaneswar, Odisha, India

Bhaskar Kanti Nath MD FICP
Associate Professor
Department of Medicine
Dhubri Medical College and Hospital
Dhubri, Assam, India

Bhupen Barman MD(General Medicine)
Additional Professor and Head
Department of General Medicine
All India Institute of Medical Sciences
Guwahati, Assam, India

Bibhuti Nath Jha DTM&H MD(Medicine)
Physician, Rheumatologist
Private Practice
Sitamarhi, Bihar, India

Bidita Khandelwal MD(Medicine)
Professor and Former Head
Department of Medicine
SMIMS, Sikkim Manipal University
Tadong, Sikkim, India

Bijender Singh MD
Consultant, Positron Multispeciality and Cancer Hospital
Rohtak, Haryana, India

Binod Prusty MD
DM Endocrinology Resident
Kalinga Institute of Medical Sciences
Bhubaneswar, Odisha, India

Binoy J Paul MD PhD DNB FRCP
Professor of Medicine and Chief of Rheumatology
KMCT Medical College
Kozhikode, Kerala, India

Biranchi Narayan Mohapatra MD FICP
Professor of Medicine, Dean and Principal
DRIEMS Institute of Health Sciences and Hospital
Cuttack, Odisha, India

Birata Debbarma MD(Medicine)
Assistant Professor
Department of Medicine
Tripura Medical College
Agartala, Tripura, India

Bitukaur Sodhi DNB(Medicine)
Clinical Associate
Department of Internal Medicine
Jupiter Hospital
Mumbai, Maharashtra, India

Biva Bhakat MD(General Medicine)
Postdoctoral Trainee
Department of Neurology
Medical College and Hospital
Kolkata, West Bengal, India

BK Singh MD FICP
Associate Professor
Department of Medicine
Narayan Medical College and Hospital
Sasaram, Bihar, India

BK Sundar MD MRCP(UK) FRCP(UK) FICP
Consultant Physician
BKS Hospital
Ballari, Karnataka, India

Bobby Mitrolia MD
Senior Resident
SN Medical College
Jodhpur, Rajasthan, India

CBK Mohanty MD
Professor of Medicine
Pro VC, KIMS
Bhubaneswar, Odisha, India

Chamma Gupta MSc(Medical Biotechnology)
Tutor, Department of Medical Biotechnology
SMIMS, Sikkim Manipal University
Tadong, Sikkim, India

Chandan Das MD FICP
Professor
Postgraduate Department of Medicine
Institute of Medical Sciences and SUM Hospital
Bhubaneswar, Odisha, India

Chennakesavulu Dara MD DNB(General medicine) FGID(CMC Vellore) FRSTM&H(London)
Professor of General Medicine
ESIC Medical College
Hyderabad, Telangana, India

Chilaka Rajesh MD DNB DM(Nephrology)
Assistant Professor
Department of Nephrology
Christian Medical College
Vellore, Tamil Nadu, India

CL Nawal MD FACP(USA) FICP FRCP(Edinburg, Glasgow)
Senior Professor and Former Head
Department of Medicine
SMS Medical College
Jaipur, Rajasthan, India

Col Sambhu Dutta DNB(Internal Medicine) FICM FICP FACP
Head
Department of Medicine
RCU and ICU, St Ann's JM Hospital
Visakhapatnam, Andhra Pradesh, India

DC Thirupathi Rao MD(Internal Medicine)
Retired Professor of Medicine
Prathima Institute of Medical Sciences
Karimnagar, Telangana, India

Debaprasad Chakrabarti MD(Medicine) FICP FIAMS FIACM FIMSA
Professor and Head
Department of Medicine
Tripura Medical College
Agartala, Tripura, India

Debashis Priyadarshan Sahoo MD(General Medicine)
Senior Resident Doctor
Department of General Medicine
All India Institute of Medical Sciences
Guwahati, Assam, India

Deepak Agarwal MD(General Medicine) DHM PGJMC
Senior Faculty, Department of General Medicine, Central Hospital, NWR
Jaipur, Rajasthan, India

Deepak Jain MD FIACM FICP FRCP(Edinburgh)
Senior Professor and Unit Head
Department of Medicine
Pandit Bhagwat Dayal Sharma Post Graduate Institute of Medical Sciences
Rohtak, Haryana, India

Deepak Sharma MD(Medicine)
Assistant Professor
Department of Medicine
Government Institute of Medical Sciences
Greater Noida, Uttar Pradesh, India

Deepti Sharma MD
Professor and Head
Department of Medicine
Government Medical College
Kota, Rajasthan, India

Devendra Gupta MD(Medicine)
Resident
Department of Medicine
College of Medicine and Sagore Dutta Hospital
Kolkata, West Bengal, India

Devendra Prasad Singh MD DTCD FICP FICS FCSI FIACM FRCP(Edinburgh, Glasgow, London)
Head, Department of Medicine
Angika Hospital and Research Centre
Former Professor and Head
Department of Respiratory Medicine
Jawahar Lal Nehru Medical College
Bhagalpur, Bihar, India

Dhanashri Atre Singh MD(Medicine) FRCP(UK) FICC(Australia)
Consultant Physician
Jupiter Hospital
Mumbai, Maharashtra, India

Dheeraj Kapoor MD DM FACE FRCP(Edinburgh, Glasgow) FACP FICP FRSSDI FDiab FIACM FGSI FISH
Chief of Endocrinology
Artemis Hospitals
Gurugram, Haryana, India

Dhiraj Kishore MD FICP FACP FISH
Professor
Department of General Medicine
Institute of Medical Sciences, Banaras Hindu University (IMS-BHU)
Varanasi, Uttar Pradesh, India

Dhruvi Hasnani MD FRCP FACP
Chief Diabetologist - HOD Clinical Research
Rudraksha Institute of Medical Sciences
Ahmedabad, Gujarat, India

Diksha Goyal DNB CCIDM
Senior Resident
Artemis Hospitals
Gurugram, Haryana, India

Dinesh Khullar MD DM(Nephrology)
Chairman and Head
Department of Nephrology and Renal Transplant Medicine
Max Super Speciality Hospital
Saket, New Delhi, India

Dinesh Kumar MD
Consultant
Harsha Clinic and Diabetes Care Centre Alambagh
Lucknow, Uttar Pradesh, India

Dinesh Kumar Sharma MD(General Medicine)
Director
Porwal Hospital
Bhilwara, Rajasthan, India

Dinesh Sharma MD(General Medicine) FICP FRSSDI
Senior Consultant Physician
Imperial Hospital
Jaipur, Rajasthan, India

Divendu Bhushan MD FACP
Associate Professor and Head
Department of Emergency Medicine
All India Institute of Medical Sciences
Patna, Bihar, India

Divyansh Mathur MBBS
PG Resident, Geetanjali Medical College
Udaipur, Rajasthan, India

Divya Taneja MD
Oncohistopathologist
Medanta—The Medicity
Gurugram, Haryana, India

D Nageshwar Reddy MD DM DSc FAMS FRCP FACG MWGO MASGE AGAF FJGES FAAAS
Chairman, Asian Institute of Gastroenterology and AIG Hospitals
Hyderabad, Telangana, India

D Selvaraj MD FRCP(Glasgow)
Chairman, SRRA Hospital and Research Institute Pvt Ltd
Thoothukudi, Tamil Nadu, India

Durga Prasad Chakraborty MD FICP DIPCard
Consultant Physician, Cardiologist and Diabetologist
Apollo Hospital Kolkata
Kolkata, West Bengal, India

Dwijen Das MD FACP(USA) FRCP(Glasgow, Edinburgh) FICP FIACM
Professor and Head
Department of Medicine
Tezpur Medical College Hospital
Tezpur, Assam, India

Eish Kumar Dalla MD(Psychiatry)
Consultant Psychiatrist
JLN District Hospital
Rudrapur, Uttarakhand, India

Gagan Gunjan MD(General Medicine)
Assistant Professor
Rajendra Institute of Medical Sciences
Ranchi, Jharkhand, India

Garv Gupta MBBS
2nd Year Postgraduate
Department of Medicine
Government Medical College
Kota, Rajasthan, India

Gaurav Singh MD(Medicine)
Senior Resident
Department of Medicine
Narayan Medical College and Hospital
Sasaram, Bihar, India

Gautam Bhandari MD
Senior Consultant
Manidhari Hospital
Jodhpur, Rajasthan, India

GC Khilnani MD FCCP(USA) FAMS FICCM FICP FNCCP FISDA
Chairman
PSRI Institute of Pulmonary
Critical Care and Sleep Medicine
PSRI Hospital
New Delhi, India

GD Ramchandani MD FICP FRCP(London, Ireland, Glasgow, Edinburg) FACE FACP FRSSDI FIACM FDI FGSI
Professor
Department of Internal Medicine
Daswani Dental College
Senior Physician and Consultant Diabetologist
Ramchandani Diabetes Care and Research Center
Kota, Rajasthan, India

Geeta Kampani MD(General Medicine) FICP
Professor and Consultant
Department of Medicine
ABVIMS and Dr RML Hospital
New Delhi, India

Girish Mathur MD(Medicine) FICP FIACM FACP(USA) FRCP(Glasgow, London, Edinburgh)
Senior Consultant Physician
Alka Diagnostic Centre
Kota, Rajasthan, India
President- API

Girish Verma MD(Medicine) FRCP(Edinburgh) FICP FIACM FIAE F.Diab. India FRSSDI
Professor of Medicine
Geetanjali Medical College and Hospital
Udaipur, Rajasthan, India

Gopika Dineshan MBBS
Postgraduate in Geriatric Medicine
Bangalore Medical College and Research Institute
Bengaluru, Karnataka, India

(Maj) Gowri Shanker R MB DA PG(DipDiab) FCD
Physician, IIT Madras
Chennai, Tamil Nadu, India

G Prakash MD DDiab FICP
Professor and Head
Department of Diabetology
Government Mohan Kumaramangalam Medical College Hospital
Salem, Tamil Nadu, India

Gurinder Mohan MD(Medicine)
Professor and Head
Department of Medicine
Sri Guru Ramdas University of Medical Sciences and Research
Amritsar, Punjab, India

G Usha MD(General Medicine)
Consultant Physician
Fernandez Hospital
Hyderabad, Telengana, India

Harbir Kaur Rao MD FICP FGSI FIMSA
Professor and Head (Retired)
Medicine and Cardiology
Government Medical College
Patiala, Punjab, India
Professor and Head (Retired)
Medicine
MM Institute of Medical Sciences and Research
Mullana, Haryana, India

Hardik Rughwani MD DM
Consultant Gastroenterologist
AIG Hospitals
Hyderabad, Telangana, India

Harikishan Boorugu MD
Consultant Physician
Fernandez Hospital
Hyderabad, Telangana, India

Harpreet Singh MD
Associate Professor Medicine
Unit In-Charge
Government Medical College
Amritsar, Punjab, India

Harshita Lachhwani MBBS
Intern
Shri Ram Murti Institute of Medical Sciences
Bareilly, Uttar Pradesh, India

Hemshanker Sharma MD FICP FIAMS MACP FICCD
Professor of Medicine
Department of Postgraduate Medicine
JLN Medical College
Bhagalpur, Bihar, India

HK Aggarwal MD FIACM FICP FRCP(Edinburgh, London)
Senior Professor and Head
Department of Medicine
Pandit Bhagwat Dayal Sharma Post Graduate Institute of Medical Sciences
Rohtak, Haryana, India

HS Pathak MD(Medicine) DBMS FICP FIACM
Retired Professor and Head
Department of Medicine
College of Medicine and JNM Hospital
Kalyani, West Bengal, India

Iman Kalyan Sarkar DNB(Medicine)
Senior Resident
Department of Medicine
College of Medicine and JNM Hospital, WBUHS
Kalyani, West Bengal, India

Ishan Mishra MBBS
Area Medical Advisor
Pfizer Oncology
Bhopal, Madhya Pradesh, India

ISM Giridhar MD
Senior Resident
Department of Neurology
MS Ramaiah Medical College
Bengaluru, Karnataka, India

Jacquiline D Shira MD
Assistant Professor of Medicine
Nagaon Medical College Hospital
Nagaon, Assam, India

Jagdeep Chugh MD(Medicine) FICP
Senior Consultant
Department of Internal Medicine and Diabetes, Satyam Medical Centre, Gujranwala Town
Fortis Hospital, Shalimar Bagh
New Delhi, India

Jaisuresh K DM(Nephrology)
Consultant Nephrologist and Transplant Physician
Assured Best Care Hospital
Tiruchirappalli, Tamil Nadu, India

Jalees Fatima MD(Medicine) FACP FICP FRSSDI FIMSA
Professor and Head
Department of Medicine
Era's Lucknow Medical College
Lucknow, Uttar Pradesh, India

Jananee Muralidharan MD MRCP(UK)
Assistant Professor
Department of Medicine
Faculty
Department of Medical Education
St John's Medical College and Hospital
Bengaluru, Karnataka, India

Javal Bhatt DNB(Medicine)
Consultant Physician, Jupiter Hospital
Thane, Maharashtra, India

Jaya Bhanu Kanwar MD(General Medicine) DM(Endocrinology)
Professor and Head
Department of Endocrinology
Institute of Medical Sciences and SUM Hospital
Bhubaneswar, Odisha, India

Jayanta K Panda MD(Internal Medicine) FACP(USA) FICP FRSSDI FIMAMS
Consultant in Diabetes, Metabolic and Critical Care Medicine
Professor, Department of General Medicine, SCB Medical College
Cuttack, Odisha, India

Jayanta Sharma MD FICP FIACM FIAMS FCCS FCSI FGSI FACP FRCP(Glasgow) FRCP(Edinburgh)
Senior Consultant
Department of Internal Medicine
Apollo Multispeciality Hospitals
Kolkata, West Bengal, India

Jay Tewari MBBS
Final Year Student
King George's Medical University
Lucknow, Uttar Pradesh, India

Jeevan Prakash MD(Medicine)
Head (Critical Care Medicine)
Era's Lucknow Medical College
Lucknow, Uttar Pradesh, India

Jitendra Singh MD(General Medicine) CCCKD(Kidney Disease) PGDC(Cardiology) PGDRM(Diabetes and Renal Management) Postgraduate Diploma in Advanced Diabetes Care & Clinical Endocrinology FICN FIACM FICP
Co-Incharge of Emergency and Assistant Professor
Department of General Medicine
Institute of Medical Sciences, Banaras Hindu University
Varanasi, Uttar Pradesh, India

Jothydev Kesavadev MD FACE(USA) FRCP(London, Glasgow, Edinburgh) FACP(USA)
Chairman and Managing Director
Jothydev's Diabetes Research Centers
Kerala, India

Joydeep Samanta MD(Medicine) DM(Clinical Immunology and Rheumatology)
Assistant Professor
Rheumatology Unit
Department of Internal Medicine
All India Institute of Medical Sciences
Raipur, Chhattisgarh, India

Jugal Kishor Sharma MD(Medicine) FICP FRCP(London, Ireland, Glasgow and Edinburgh) FACP FACE FICN FRSSDI FGSI FISH FIACM FIMSA FDiab(India)
Medical Director
Central Delhi Diabetes Centre
New Delhi, India

Jyoti Chugh MD DNB
Senior Consultant (Obstetrics and Gynecology)
Satyam Medical Centre, Gujranwala Town
Fortis Hospital, Shalimar Bagh
New Delhi, India

Jyoti Kiran DM PDT(Neurology)
Neurologist
Calcutta National Medical College and Hospital
Kolkata, West Bengal, India

Kamal Garg MD
Postgraduate
Maulana Azad Medical College
New Delhi, India

Kanupriya Goel DM(Cardiac Anesthesia)
2nd Year
Dr Ram Manohar Lohia Hospital
New Delhi, India

Karandeep Kaur MBBS
Junior Resident
Department of Medicine
Sri Guru Ramdas University of Medical Sciences and Research
Amritsar, Punjab, India

Karnati Prudhveer Reddy MBBS
Postgraduate
Department of General Medicine
JSS Hospital
Mysuru, Karnataka, India

Kashish Gupta MD(Medicine)
Senior Resident
SMS Medical College and Hospital
Jaipur, Rajasthan, India

Kauser Usman MD FIMSA FIACM FICP FACP(USA) FRCP(Edinburgh)
Professor
Department of Medicine
Officiating Head
Department of Geriatric Medicine
King George's Medical University
Lucknow, Uttar Pradesh, India

Kaushik Basu MD DM(Rheumatology and Clinical Immunology)
Associate Professor
Department of Rheumatology
Medical College
Kolkata, West Bengal, India

Kaushik Hazra DTCD MD(General Medicine)
Associate Professor of Medicine
Jagannath Gupta Institute of Medical Sciences and Hospital (JIMSH)
Budge Budge, West Bengal, India

Kaushik Sen MD DM(Endocrinology)
Associate Professor
Department of General Medicine
Barasat Government Medical College
Kolkata, West Bengal, India

Kaustubh Dilip Salagre MD(Medicine)
Associate Professor
Department of Medicine
Seth GS Medical College and
KEM Hospital
Mumbai, Maharashtra, India

Ketan K Mehta MD FCPS FICP FISE FGSI
Consulting Physician
Asian Heart Institute
Mumbai, Maharashtra, India

K Nagesh MD FICP FCCP
Consultant Physician and Director
Nagesh Hospital
Hassan, Karnataka, India

Krishna Pawan Jaldu MBBS
Resident
Department of Medicine
Santosh Medical College and Hospital
Ghaziabad, Uttar Pradesh, India

Krunal Patel MD(General Medicine)
2nd Year PG Resident
Mahatma Gandhi Hospital
Jaipur, Rajasthan, India

Kshitija Gadekar MD DM
Professor and Head
Department of Nephrology
MGM Medical College
Aurangabad, Maharashtra, India

Kuldeep Gurjar MBBS
3rd Year Post graduate Student
Department of Medicine
Maulana Azad Medical College
New Delhi, India

Kunal Ahuja DNB
Associate Consultant
PSRI Institute of Pulmonary
Critical Care and Sleep Medicine
PSRI Hospital
New Delhi, India

Kushal Markanday MD(Medicine)
Assistant Professor
Department of Medicine
Maharishi Markandeshwar Institute of Medical Sciences and Research
Mullana, Haryana, India

Lalatendu Mohanty MD
Professor and Head
PG Department of Medicine
Kalinga Institute of Medical Sciences
Bhubaneswar, Odisha, India

Lalita Verma MD(Microbiology)
Senior Demonstrator
Department of Microbiology
SMS Medical College
Jaipur, Rajasthan, India

LH Ghotekar MD MNAMS FIACM FIMSA
Director-Professor and Head
Department of Medicine
Head, Department of Neurology
Lady Hardinge Medical College
and SSKH
New Delhi, India

Liyakat Ali Gauri MD(General Medicine)
Senior Professor
Department of General Medicine
Sarder Patel Medical College
Bikaner, Rajasthan, India

LP Meena MD
Professor
Department of General Medicine
Institute of Medical Sciences
Banaras Hindu University
Varanasi, Uttar Pradesh, India

Madhulata Agarwal MD(Internal Medicine)
Assistant Professor
Department of Medicine
SMS Medical College
Jaipur, Rajasthan, India

Madhuri Matta MD(Medicine)
Head
Department of Medicine
INHS Kalyani
Visakhapatnam, Andhra Pradesh, India

Madhur Rai MD(Physiology)
Associate Professor
Postgraduate Department of Physiology
MGM Institute of Health Sciences
Navi Mumbai, Maharashtra, India

Mahabir Thakur MD(General Medicine) DTM&H
Consultant
Department of Internal Medicine
Cardiac Care and Research Centre
Sitamarhi, Bihar, India

Mahesh Choudhary DNB(Medicine)
Trainee, Jupiter Hospital
Thane, Maharashtra, India

Manabendra Nayak MD PhD FICP MRCP FRCP(Edinburgh, Glasgow, London) FACP(USA) FCCP(USA)
Head, Department of Medicine
Down Town Hospital
Guwahati, Assam, India
Postgraduate Teacher of Medicine
NBEMS

Manab Narayan Baruah MD(Pediatrics)
Associate Professor
Department of Paediatrics
Jorhat Medical College and Hospital
Jorhat, Assam, India

Manas Das MD(General Medicine)
Senior Resident
Department of Medicine
Lady Hardinge Medical College
New Delhi, India

Manas Thakur MD(Internal Medicine)
Resident (DM Cardiology)
Mahatma Gandhi Medical College
Jaipur, Rajasthan, India

Manikandan DNB(General Medicine)
DNB Post Graduate
Sundaram Arulrhaj Hospitals
Tuticorin, Tamil Nadu, India

Manisha MBBS
PG Student (3rd Year)
Sardar Patel Medical College
Bikaner, Rajasthan, India

Manish Kumar MD DTM&H(UK) FICP FIACM FIAMS Certified Echocardiologist (IAE) Fellow Royal Society of Tropical Medicine(UK)
Consultant Physician and Chief
Noninvasive Cardiac Lab
Department of Medicine
Arc Hospital
Bhagalpur, Bihar, India

Manish Pahariya MD
Professor of Medicine
Mahatma Gandhi Medical College and Hospital
Jaipur, Rajasthan, India

Manish Sharma MBBS
Third Year Postgraduate Student
Department of Medicine
ABVIMS and Dr RML Hospital
New Delhi, India

Manjari Saha MD(General Medicine)
Associate Professor
Department of Internal Medicine
Kolkata Medical College
Kolkata, West Bengal, India

Manoj Khanal MD DM(Neurology)
Associate Director and Head
Department of Neurology
Max Super Speciality, Shalimar Bagh
New Delhi, India

Manoj K Srivastav MD(Medicine)
Professor
Department of Medicine
Narayan Medical College and Hospital
Sasaram, Bihar, India

Manoranjan Behera MD FICP
Professor and Head
Department of Medicine
Bhima Bhoi Medical College
Balangir, Odisha, India

Masum Talesara MD(Medicine)
Junior Resident
Department of Medicine
RD Gardi Medical College
Ujjain, Madhya Pradesh, India

Mathew Thomas MD FRCP(London) FRCP(Edinburgh) FICP FISHTM
Professor of Internal Medicine and Hematology and Senior Consultant
KIMS Hospital
Thiruvananthapuram, Kerala, India

Mayank Gupta MD(Internal Medicine)
Assistant Professor, Department of Medicine, NIMS Medical College
Jaipur, Rajasthan, India

Meenakshi MS(Obstetrics and Gynaecology)
Professor
JLN Medical College and Hospital
Ajmer, Rajasthan, India

Meenaxi Sharda MD(Medicine) DCH FIAE FICP
Senior Professor of Medicine
Head Geriatric Medicine
Government Medical College
Kota, Rajasthan, India

Meghna Aggarwal MD(Medicine)
Senior Resident
Department of Nephrology
Government Medical College
Kota, Rajasthan, India

Meghna Dutta DNB(Family Medicine)
Junior Consultant
Department of Internal Medicine
Apollo Multispeciality Hospitals
Kolkata, West Bengal, India

Mehdi Ali Mirza MD DM
Assistant Professor
Department of Pharmacology
ESIC Medical College and Hospital
Hyderabad, Telangana, India

ME Yeolekar MD(General Medicine and Therapeutics) MNAMS(Medicine) FICP
Senior Consultant Physician (Internal Medicine)
Ex-Professor and Head (Medicine)
Sion Hospital
Past Dean LTMG/KEM Hospital
Former DMER (MCGM)
Mumbai, Maharashtra, India

M Gunasekaran MD FICP
Senior Consultant Physician
Dravidian Speciality Hospital
Pattukkottai, Tamil Nadu, India

Minal Harde MD DNB(Anesthesia)
Associate Professor
Department of Anaesthesia
Topiwala National Medical College and BYL Nair Charitable Hospital
Mumbai, Maharashtra, India

M Jawahar Farook DNB(Medicine) DNB(Cardiology) MNAMS FNB(Interventional Cardiology) FESC FCSI FSCAI
Senior Interventional Cardiologist
Meenakshi Mission Hospital and Research Centre (MMHRC)
Madurai, Tamil Nadu, India

ML Patel MD MNAMS FIACM FICP FACP
Professor
Department of Medicine
King George Medical University
Lucknow, Uttar Pradesh, India

Molly Mary Thabah MD FRCP(Edinburgh)
Professor
Department of Clinical Immunology
Jawaharlal Institute of Postgraduate Medical Education and Research
Puducherry, India

Monica Gupta MD(Medicine) DNB(Medicine) FICP
Professor
Department of General Medicine
Government Medical College and Hospital
Chandigarh, India

Monika Maheshwari DNB MD PhD DM(Cardiology) FACC FRCP(Glasgow, Edinburgh) FESC FAPSC FEAC FCSI FISE FIAE FICP FIACM MAMS FICA
Former Professor of Medicine and Assistant Professor
Department of Cardiology
Jawahar Lal Nehru Medical College
Ajmer, Rajasthan, India

MPS Chawla MD FACP FRCP FICP FIACM FISC FIMSA
Professor and Head
Department of Medicine
ABVIMS and Dr Ram Manohar Lohia Hospital
New Delhi, India

MP Sharma DM(Gastroenterology)
Head
JLN Medical College and Hospital
Ajmer, Rajasthan, India

M Raveendran MD(General Medicine)
Professor of Medicine and Dean
Government Medical College and ESI Hospital
Coimbatore, Tamil Nadu, India

Mrinal Kanti Roy MD DM(Neurology) FIACM FICP FRCP(Glasgow) FACP(USA)
Retired Professor, Calcutta National Medical College and Hospital
Kolkata, West Bengal, India

Mritunjay Kumar MBBS
Junior Resident
Department of General Medicine
Institute of Medical Sciences
Banaras Hindu University
Varanasi, Uttar Pradesh, India

M Sabir MD(General Medicine)
Senior Consultant Physician and Pulmonologist, Kothari Medical and Research Institute
Retired Professor and Head
Respiratory Division
Department of Medicine
SP Medical College
Bikaner, Rajasthan, India
Former President: Indian Chest Society

MS Prasad MS
Consultant Surgeon
MedIndia Hospitals
Chennai, Tamil Nadu, India

Mukesh K Sarna MD FACP FRCP(London, Edinburgh, Glasgow) FICP FISH FRSSDI FIACM FDI
Professor and Unit Head
Department of General Medicine
Mahatma Gandhi Medical College and Hospital
Jaipur, Rajasthan, India

Mukulesh Gupta MD(General Medicine) PG Diploma in Diabetes (Cardiff, UK) FICP FRSSDI FUPDA FInSH FISCM FIACM FISMN Fellow Diabetes, India FACP(USA)
Director
Udyan Health Care Pvt Ltd
Lucknow, Uttar Pradesh, India

Murugesh Pastapur MD
Consultant Physician
Ex-Professor of Medicine
MR Medical College
Kalaburagi, Karnataka, India

Nadeem Liyakat MD(Radiodiagnosis)
Senior Resident
Department of Radiodiagnosis
SP Medical College
Bikaner, Rajasthan, India

Nalini Humaney MD(General Medicine) FICP
Professor in Medicine
NKPSIMS & RC and LMH
Nagpur, Maharashtra, India

Narayan Deogaonkar MD FRCP(London) FICP
Director
Deogaonkar Hospital
Nashik, Maharashtra, India

Narayan Prasad MD DM FRCP
Professor and Head
Department of Nephrology
Sanjay Gandhi Postgraduate Institute of Medical Sciences
Lucknow, Uttar Pradesh, India

Naresh Kumar Midha MD(Medicine)
Associate Professor
Department of Medicine
All India Institute of Medical Sciences
Jodhpur, Rajasthan, India

Narinder Pal Singh MD MBA
Dean Research
Eternal University
Baru Sahib, Himachal Pradesh, India
Consultant
Academic Program in Nephrology
Max Super Speciality Hospital
Saket, New Delhi, India

Nasir Hussain MBBS
Medical Officer
Jain Chest Care Center
Jaipur, Rajasthan, India

Naween Kumar MD
Assistant Professor
Department of Medicine
Darbhanga Medical College
Darbhanga, Bihar, India

Neeti Agrawal MD DM
Senior Resident
Department of Endocrinology and Metabolism
Medical College Superspeciality Block (SSB)
Kolkata, West Bengal, India

Niharika Sinha MBBS PG Diploma in Rheumatology EULAR
Consultant Rheumatologist
Joint Pain and Arthritis Clinic
Patna, Bihar, India

Nikita Srivastava MD
Ex-Senior Resident
Department of Medicine
Lady Hardinge Medical College and SSKH
New Delhi, India

Nilanjan Mal MBBS
PGT-3
Department of General Medicine
Rajendra Institute of Medical Sciences
Ranchi Jharkhand, India

Nilesh Kumar MD(General Medicine)
Associate Professor and
Co-Nodal Officer
COE for Hemoglobinopathies and
Bleeding Disorder
Department of General Medicine
Institute of Medical Sciences
Banaras Hindu University
Varanasi, Uttar Pradesh, India

Nipun Goel MBBS
PG Resident
Department of General Medicine
Mahatma Gandhi Medical College
and Hospital
Jaipur, Rajasthan, India

Niraj Lodha MD FICP PGD in Clinical Endocrinology and Diabetes
Senior Consultant Physicians and
Diabetologist, Lodha Hospital and
Test Tube Baby Center
Pali, Rajasthan, India

Nirmal Das Vaishnav MD
DrNB Resident (Medical Oncology)
Bhagwan Mahaveer Cancer Hospital
and Research Center
Jaipur, Rajasthan, India

Nirupam Prakash MD(Medicine) FICP PGCC(Diabetes) PGCC(Cardiology)
Consultant Physician, CGHS
Lucknow, Uttar Pradesh, India

Niteesh Singh MD
Junior Resident III
PG Department of Medicine
SN Medical College
Agra, Uttar Pradesh, India

Nitin Jain MD(Respiratory Medicine)
Consultant and Director Intervention
Jain Chest Care Center
Jaipur, Rajasthan, India

Nitin Sinha MD(Medicine) PGDHHM(IGNOU)
Professor, Department of Medicine
ABVIMS and Dr RML Hospital
New Delhi, India

Nitu Chauhan MD(Pathology)
Associate Professor and Head
Department of Transfusion Medicine
SN Medical College and Hospital
Agra, Uttar Pradesh, India

N Subramanian MD MRCP(UK) MRCP CCT(Rheumatology) FRCP FICP
Consultant Rheumatologist
Rosemary Mission Hospitals,
Tirunelveli
Assistant Professor of Rheumatology
and Medicine
Velammal Medical College Hospital
and Research Institute
Madurai, Tamil Nadu, India

Om Prakash Sharma MD FICN FICP FIAMS FCGP FGSI FACM FIMSA FRCP(Edinburgh) FGAPIO
Senior Consultant Geriatric Medicine
Indraprastha Apollo Hospitals
Sarita Vihar, New Delhi, India
Emeritus Clinical Tutor
Apollo Hospitals Educational and
Research Foundation

Paila Deepika MBBS
Resident
Department of Medicine
Lady Hardinge Medical College
New Delhi, India

Pankaj Manoria MD DM FACC FESC
Director
Manoria Heart and Critical Care
Hospital
Bhopal, Madhya Pradesh, India

Pankaj Nand Choudhry MD(Medicine) FICP FIACM
Senior Consultant and Academic
Head
Department of Internal Medicine
Max Super Speciality Hospital
Ghaziabad, Uttar Pradesh, India

Pankaj R Jawandhiya MD DM DNB
Nephrologist
NewEra Hospital
Nagpur, Maharashtra, India

Pankaj Verma MD(Medicine)
Assistant Professor
Department of Medicine
Dr Ram Manohar Lohia Institute of
Medical Sciences
Lucknow, Uttar Pradesh, India

Paramita Bhattacharya DNB(Medicine)
Assistant Professor
Department of Medicine
College of Medicine and JNM
Hospital, WBUHS
Kalyani, West Bengal, India

Partha Karmakar MD(Medicine) DNB(Medicine) Dip Cardiology FICP FACP
Professor
Department of Medicine
College of Medicine and Sagore Dutta
Hospital
Kolkata, West Bengal, India

Partha Pratim Chakraborty MD DM DNB MNAMS FRCP FACE FICP
Assistant Professor
Department of Endocrinology and
Metabolism
Medical College Superspeciality
Block (SSB)
Kolkata, West Bengal, India

Parth Deogaonkar MD(Medicine) DNB(Nephrology)
Consultant
Deogaonkar Hospital
Nashik, Maharashtra, India

Pawan Suri MD DM FRCP FESC FSCAI FCSI
Director and Chief Cardiologist
Global Super Speciality Hospital
Jalandhar, Punjab, India

Payal Jain MD(General Medicine) FIACM FICP FIMSA
Professor
Department of General Medicine
Government Institute of Medical
Sciences
Greater Noida, Uttar Pradesh, India

PC Manoria MD DM FACC FESC FCAPSC
Director
Manoria Heart and Critical Care Hospital
Bhopal, Madhya Pradesh, India

Pearl Samaria MBBS(Student)
Mahatma Gandhi University of Medical Sciences and Technology (MGUMST)
Jaipur, Rajasthan, India

Pinaki Mukhopadhyay DM FICP FASN FRCP(London)
Head, Department of Nephrology
Nil Ratan Sircar Medical College
Kolkata, West Bengal, India

Piyush Manoria DTCD MD(Medicine) DM(Gastroenterology)
Chief Gastroenterologist and Hepatologist
Manoria Hospital
Bhopal, Madhya Pradesh, India

PK Maheshwari MD DM(Neurology) MAMS FFIACM FRCP(Edinburgh) FIAN FICP
Professor and Head
Department of Neurology
Superspeciality Block
SN Medical College
Agra, Uttar Pradesh, India
President, Agra Academy of Neurology

P Paranthaman MD DTCD FICP FRCP(Glasgow) FACP FIMSA MHSc(Diabetology)
Professor of Medicine and Head
Department of General Medicine
Government Kilpauk Medical College
Chennai, Tamil Nadu, India

Prabhakar K MD(General Medicine) FICP MNAMS
Principal and Dean
Sri Devaraj Urs Medical College
Kolar, Karnataka, India

Prabhat Pandey MD(Medicine) MIP FCCP FICA FICP FCSI FCGP FIAMS PG Dip(Diabetology) FDiab India
Professor and Head
Department of Medicine
DNB Faculty
Chandulal Chandrakar Memorial Superspeciality Hospital
Bhilai, Chhattisgarh, India

Prakhar Gupta MBBS
Practitioner
Osmo Kidney Care Centre
Varanasi, Uttar Pradesh, India

Pramod Kumar Agrawal MD(Medicine) FICP FRCP(Glasgow)
Professor and Head
Department of Medicine
Katihar Medical College
Katihar, Bihar, India

Pramod Kumar Sinha MD(Medicine) FICP FCSI Dip(Echocardiography)
Associate Professor and Head
Department of Medicine
Anugrah Narayan Magadh Medical College and Hospital
Gaya, Bihar, India

Prasanta Kumar Bhattacharya MD PhD FACP FICP
Senior Professor (HAG) and Head
Department of General Medicine
Member Secretary, Institutional Ethics Committee
North Eastern Indira Gandhi Regional Institute of Health and Medical Sciences
Shillong, Meghalaya, India

Prashant Prakash MD(Medicine) MD(Chest) MAMS FICP FIACM
Professor and Head
Super Specialty Department of Pulmonary Medicine
SN Medical College
Agra, Uttar Pradesh, India

Prashasti Gupta MD
Assistant Professor of Medicine
Lady Hardinge Medical College
New Delhi, India

Preeti Sarma MD
Registrar
Department of Gastroenterology
Gauhati Medical College and Hospital
Guwahati, Assam, India

Pritam Gupta MD(Medicine) FRCP FICP FIMS
Senior Consultant
Fortis Hospital, Shalimar Bagh
New Delhi, India

Priyank Rastogi MD
Associate Professor
Department of Medicine
ESI Post Graduate Institute of Medical Sciences and Research
Basaidarapur, New Delhi, India

Priyanshu Shah MD
Assistant Professor
Medical ICU
Department of Medicine
LTM Medical College and General Hospital, Sion
Mumbai, Maharashtra, India

Puneet Rijhwani MD FICP FRCP(Edinburgh) FACP FIACM FDI
Professor and Head
Department of Medicine
Mahatma Gandhi University of Medical Sciences and Technology
Jaipur, Rajasthan, India

Radha TR MD(General Medicine) MD(Pediatrics) DNB(Pediatrics)
Professor and Head
Department of Medicine
Government Medical College
Kottayam, Kerala, India

Rahul Ramchandani MBBS
Final Year Resident
Department of Internal Medicine
Institute of Medical Sciences and
SUM Hospital
Bhubaneswar, Odisha, India

Rahul T Chakor MD(Medicine)
DM(Neurology)
Professor and Head
Department of Neurology
TN Medical College
BYL Nair Hospital
Mumbai, Maharashtra, India

Rajat Chaudhary MD(Medicine)
Senior Resident
Department of Cardiology
GIPMER
New Delhi, India

Rajinder Singh Gupta MD FICP FGSI
FIMSA
Professor and Head (Retired)
Medicine
Government Medical College
Patiala, Punjab, India
Professor (Retired)
Medicine
MM Institute of Medical Sciences
and Research
Mullana, Haryana, India

Rajiv Kumar Bandaru MD(General
Medicine)
Associate Professor
Department of General Medicine
ESIC Medical College and Hospital
Hyderabad, Telangana, India

Raj Kamal Choudhary MD(Medicine)
FICP
Associate Professor
Department of Post Graduate
Medicine
Jawaharlal Nehru Medical College
Bhagalpur, Bihar, India
Former SRTL, WHO
Former Consultant, CDC

Rajneesh Sachan MD
Resident
Department of General Medicine
Institute of Medical Sciences
Banaras Hindu University (IMS-BHU)
Varanasi, Uttar Pradesh, India

Rakesh Bhadade MD(Internal Medicine)
FICP FRCP(London)
Associate Professor
Department of Medicine and
In-Charge EMS
Topiwala National Medical College
and BYL Nair Charitable Hospital
Mumbai, Maharashtra, India

Rakesh Kumar Goel MD(Medicine)
PG Dip(Public Health) PG Dip(Hospital
Administration)
Senior Professor and Head
Department of Medicine
Maharaja Agrasen Medical College
(MAMC), Agroha
Hisar, Haryana, India

Rakesh M Parikh FCPS(Medicine)
Dip. Diabetology
Consultant Diabetologist
CKS Hospital Jaipur and Diabecity
Jaipur, Rajasthan, India

Raman Sharma MD
Professor of Medicine
Mahatma Gandhi Medical College
and Hospital
Jaipur, Rajasthan, India

Ramesh Aggarwal MD FRCP(Edinburgh)
FICP
Professor
Department of Medicine
Lady Hardinge Medical College
New Delhi, India

Ramesh Duraisamy MD
Assistant Professor of Medicine
Coimbatore Medical College and
Hospital
Coimbatore, Tamil Nadu, India

Ramesh Mundle MD
Professor
Department of Medicine
NKP Salve Institute of Medical
Sciences
Nagpur, Maharashtra, India

Ranjan Kumar MD
Chief Consultant
Ranjan Heart Clinic
Patna, Bihar, India

Ranjit Mohan Anjana MD DipDiab(UK)
PhD FACP FICP FRCP(Glasgow Edinburgh,
London) FACE
Managing Director
Dr Mohan's Diabetes Specialities
Centre
President
Madras Diabetes Research
Foundation
Chennai, Tamil Nadu, India

Rashi Maheshwari MD
DM(Rheumatology and Clinical
Immunology)
Assistant Professor
Department of Clinical Immunology
and Rheumatology
SMS Medical College and Hospital
Jaipur, Rajasthan, India

Raveendran AV MD FRCP(Edinburgh)
Assistant Professor of Medicine
(Former)
Government Medical College
Kottayam, Kerala, India

Ravikeerthy M MD(Medicine)
FRCP(Glasgow) FICP PGDM(London)
Professor of Medicine
Meenakshi Medical College and
Research Centre
Kanchipuram, Tamilnadu, India

Ravindra Kumar Modi MD FICP
Senior Consultant
Modi's Diabetes Research Centre
Purnea, Bihar, India

R Dharini DNB(General Medicine)
Consultant Physician
Chellaram Diabetes Institute
Pune, Maharashtra, India

Renu Saigal MD FICP MAMS FRCP FACP
Consultant Rheumatologist
Former Senior Professor and Head
Department of Medicine
SMS Medical College
Jaipur, Rajasthan, India

Ripun Borpuzari MD(Medicine) FICP
Retired Joint Director
Health and Family Welfare
Government of Assam
Senior Physician
Sivasagar, Assam, India
Chairperson, RSSDI Assam 2022–2023

Rishabh Kochar MD(General Medicine)
Senior Resident (DM fellow)
Department of Pulmonary Medicine
All India Institute of Medical Sciences
Jodhpur, Rajasthan, India

Ritu Karoli MD(Medicine) FICP MAMS
Additional Professor
Department of Medicine
Dr Ram Manohar Lohia Institute of Medical Sciences
Lucknow, Uttar Pradesh, India

RK Singal MD FACP(USA) FRCP(Glasgow) FICP FIAMS
Principal Consultant and Head
Department of Internal Medicine
BLK-MAX Super Speciality Hospital
New Delhi, India

R Lakshmi Narasimhan
DM(Neurology) DNB(Neurology) PhD FAAN FRCP(London, Glasgow) FIAN FEBN
Director and Professor of Neurology
Institute of Neurology
Madras Medical College
Chennai, Tamil Nadu, India

RM Chhabra MD(Medicine) FIMSA FICP FDI FRCP(Edinburgh)
Senior Consultant Physician
Department of Medicine
Max Super Speciality Hospital, Shalimar Bagh
Saroj Super Speciality Hospital
New Delhi, India

Rohini Handa MD DNB FAMS FICP FACR FRCP(Glasgow)
Professor and Senior Consultant Rheumatologist
Apollo Indraprastha Hospitals
New Delhi, India

Rohith Velusamy DNB
Postgraduate of Internal Medicine
Sundaram Arulrhaj Hospitals
Tuticorin, Tamil Nadu, India

Rohit Ihran MD
Assistant Professor
Department of General Medicine
SMS Medical College and Hospital
Jaipur, Rajasthan, India

Rohit Ram Kumar MD(General Medicine)
Senior Resident (DM Neurology)
Government Medical College
Kottayam, Kerala, India

Rosemarie de Souza MD(Internal Medicine)
Professor and Head,
Department of Medicine
Topiwala National Medical College and BYL Nair Charitable Hospital
Mumbai, Maharashtra, India

RS Chejara MD
Associate Professor of Medicine
Department of Medicine
SMS Medical College
Jaipur, Rajasthan, India

Ruchi Kapoor MD
National Head – Lab Clinical Excellence and Quality Assurance
TATA 1mg Labs
Gurugram, Haryana, India

Rupa Kasaraneni MBBS
Junior Resident
Sri Devaraj Urs Medical College
Kolar, Karnataka, India

Sahil Langde MD
Postgraduate Student (Medicine)
Seth GS Medical College and KEM Hospital
Mumbai, Maharashtra, India

Sahubar Sadiq MD DM
Consultant Physician and Neurologist
Ramnad Neuro Care Center
Ramanathapuram, Tamil Nadu, India

Saibal Chakravorty MD(Medicine) FRCP FICP FIACM Diploma in Diabetes(UK)
Senior Consultant Physician and Unit Head
Department of Internal Medicine
Diabetology and Critical Care
Metro Multispeciality Hospital
Noida, Uttar Pradesh, India

Sajid Ansari MD(Medicine) FACP(USA) FICP FISC FISH FEAC FIAE FCSI
Director
SS Heart Care Centre
Lucknow, Uttar Pradesh, India

Sambit Das MD(Medicine) DM(Endocrinology)
Professor
Department of Endocrinology
Kalinga Institute of Medical Sciences
Bhubaneswar, Odisha, India

Sameer Gulati MD FICP FIACM FIMSA
Professor
Department of Medicine
Lady Hardinge Medical College and Associated Hospitals
New Delhi, India

Samir Sahu MD(Medicine) FICP
Professor and Head
PG Department of Medicine
Institute of Medical Sciences and SUM Hospital
Bhubaneswar, Odisha, India

Sandeep Garg MD(Medicine)
Director Professor
Department of Medicine
Maulana Azad Medical College
New Delhi, India

Sandeep Rai DNB(Medicine) PG DipDiab MNAMS FACP(USA) FRCP(UK)
Senior Professor and Unit Head
Postgraduate Department of Medicine
MGM Institute of Health Sciences
Navi Mumbai, Maharashtra, India

Sandeep Suri MD(Medicine)
Consultant Physician and Diabetologist
Holy Help Hospital
Hisar, Haryana, India

Sanjay Bandyopadhyay MD DNB DM(Gastrology) MNAMS FRCP
Head
Department of Gastroenterology
ILS Hospitals Dumdum
Kolkata, West Bengal, India

Sanjay Gupta MD(Medicine) DNB FRCP(Edinburgh)
Senior Consultant
SG Diabetes Centre
New Delhi, India

Sanjay Kumar MD
Chief Consultant, Chest Clinic
Patna, Bihar, India

Sanjay Mehndiratta MD(Medicine)
Consultant Physician
MRG Hospital
Jaipur, Rajasthan, India

Sanjay Tandon MD(Medicine) FICP FISC FACP FACC FRCP
Director
Tandon Clinic
Lucknow, Uttar Pradesh, India

Sanjay V Patane MD AFIH PGDMT
Professor and Head
Department of Emergency Medicine
Indian Institute of Medical Science (IIMSR)
Jalna, Maharashtra, India

Santosh Salagre MD MBA FAIMER Fellow
Professor of Medicine
Seth GS Medical College and KEM Hospital
Mumbai, Maharashtra, India

Sarabmeet Singh Lehl MD(Medicine) FIACM FAIMER Fellow
Professor
Department of General Medicine
Government Medical College and Hospital
Chandigarh, India

S Arulrhaj MD PhD FRCP(Glasgow and London) MBA
Chairman, Chief Physician and Intensivist
Sundaram Arulrhaj Hospitals
Tuticorin, Tamil Nadu, India

Satyabrata Ganguly MD(General Medicine)
Emeritus Professor
Apollo Multispeciality Hospital
Kolkata, West Bengal, India

Saumik Datta MD DM(Endocrinology) FICP FISH
Professor and Head
Department of General Medicine
Burdwan Medical College and Hospital
Bardhaman, West Bengal, India

Saumitra Ray MD FRCP FCSI FICP FESC FACC FSCAI
Ex-Professor
Vivekananda Institute of Medical Sciences
Director, Invasive Cardiology
Advanced Medical Research Institute
Kolkata, West Bengal, India

Saumitra Singh MBBS
Medical Officer
Spandan Multispeciality Hospital
Vadodara, Gujarat, India

Saurabh Puri DNB(General Medicine) DNB SS(Nephrology)
ILBS Hospital
New Delhi, India

Saurabh Srivastava MD(General Medicine) FRCP(Edinburgh, Glasgow) FACP FICP FIMSA FIACM FIAMS FGSI FISH FUDA FDI MAMS
Professor and Head
Department of Medicine
Government Institute of Medical Sciences
Greater Noida, Uttar Pradesh, India

Sayan Kar DNB(General Medicine)
Junior Resident
Department of General Medicine
Medica Superspecialty Hospital
Kolkata, West Bengal, India

Sayantani Bhattacharya MBBS
Associate Physician
Urban Healthcare Hospital
Kolkata, West Bengal, India

Sayonee Das MD(General Medicine, Gold Medal)
Resident (DrNB Nephrology)
Apollo Multispeciality Hospital
Kolkata, West Bengal, India

SB Gupta MD FACC FISE FCSI FICP FICC
Ex-Head, Medicine and Cardiology
Central Railway HQ Hospital
Ex-Consultant Physician Cardiologist
Asian Heart Institute
Mumbai, Maharashtra, India

S Chiranth MBBS
Postgraduate 3rd Year
Department of Medicine
VMMC and Safdarjung Hospital
New Delhi, India

Shaibal Guha MD
Director
Positive Health Center
Patna, Bihar, India

Shailendra Kumar MD
Associate Professor and Head
Department of TB and Chest
SK Medical College
Muzaffarpur, Bihar, India

Sharad N Deshmukh MD MNAMS
Former Associate Professor of Medicine
IGMC Nagpur, NKPSIMS
Nagpur, Maharashtra, India

Shashidhara KC MD
Professor
Department of General Medicine
JSS Medical College
Mysuru, Karnataka, India

Sheila Nainan Myatra MD FCCM FICCM
Department of Anaesthesiology, Critical Care and Pain
Tata Memorial Hospital
Parel, Mumbai, India

Shikhar Bansal MD(General Medicine)
Resident (DM Cardiology)
IPGMER and SSKM Hospital
Kolkata, West Bengal, India

Shikhar Garg MD
Senior Resident (1st Year DM)
Department of Cardiology
Dr Ram Manohar Lohia Institute of Medical Sciences
Lucknow, Uttar Pradesh, India

Shilpa Gupta MD(General Medicine)
Senior Physician
Punjab Cancer Care and Multispeciality Hospital
Bhathinda, Punjab, India

Shivangi Maheshwari MBBS
Clinician
Sri Hari Kamal Diabetes and Heart Clinic
Lucknow, Uttar Pradesh, India

Shiv Ghodasara MD(Medicine)
Resident (DM Oncology)
Geetanjali Medical College and Hospital
Udaipur, Rajasthan, India

Shouvik Datta MBBS
Post Graduate (JR-3)
Department of General Medicine
SRMS Institute of Medical Sciences
Bareilly, Uttar Pradesh, India

Shrivarthan Radhakrishnan MD(Medicine) DM(Neurology) DrNB(Neurology)
Associate Consultant
Department of Neurology
MGM Healthcare
Chennai, Tamil Nadu, India

Shubha Laxmi Margekar MD
Professor
Department of Medicine
Lady Hardinge Medical College and SSK Hospital
New Delhi, India

Shubham MD(Medicine)
Resident Doctor
JLN Medical College and Hospital
Ajmer, Rajasthan, India

Shubhransu Patro MD(General Medicine) FICP
Professor
Postgraduate Department of General Medicine
Kalinga Institute of Medical Sciences
KIIT Deemed to be University
Bhubaneswar, Odisha, India

Shuchita Mundle MD
Professor
Department of Obstetrics and Gynecology
All India Institute of Medical Sciences
Nagpur, Maharashtra, India

Shweta Saxena MD(Obstetrics and Gynecology)
Consultant Gynecologist
Lucknow, Uttar Pradesh, India

Sidhartha Gautam Senapati MBBS
Research Fellow
Mayo Clinic College of Medicine and Sciences
Rochester, Minnesota, USA

Simi Patoa MD(Medicine)
Registrar
Silchar Medical College and Hospital
Silchar, Assam, India

Sirshendu Pal MD(Medicine) FRCP(Glasgow, Edinburgh)
Senior Consultant Physician and Diabetologist
Mitra's Multi Speciality Hospital
Siliguri, West Bengal, India

Siwalik Banerjee MD
Consultant Rheumatologist
Department of Rheumatology
University Hospitals Coventry and Warwickshire NHS Trust
Coventry, UK

SK Gautam MD(Medicine) FACP(USA) FICP FIACM FInSH
Professor of Medicine
GSVM Medical College
Kanpur, Uttar Pradesh, India

S Meenakshi-Sundaram MD(General Medicine) DM(Neurology)
Associate Professor of Neurology
Department of Neurosciences
Apollo Speciality Hospitals
Madurai, Tamil Nadu, India

Smita Gupta DNB(General Medicine) MNAMS
Professor and Head
Department of General Medicine
SRMS Institute of Medical Sciences
Bareilly, Uttar Pradesh, India

Smit Shrivastava MD PGDHHM DM (Cardiology) FACC FSCAI FESC FICP FIMSA FICN FISE
Professor and Head
Advance Cardiac Institute
PT JNM Medical College and Dr BRAM Hospital
Raipur, Chhattisgarh, India

SM Mishra MD FICP
Head
Department of Respiratory Medicine
Bhagwan Mahavir Institute of Medical Sciences, Pawapuri
Nalanda, Bihar, India

Sneha Modi MBBS
DNB Trainee Medicine
Sri Balaji Action Medical Institute
New Delhi, India

Somnath SM MD DNB(Medicine) FICP FRCP
Consultant Physician
Sanjana Diabetes and Eye Care
Ballari, Karnataka, India

Sonam Spalgais DNB(Pulmonary Medicine) MNAMS
Assistant Professor
Department of Pulmonary Medicine
Vallabh Bhai Patel Chest Institute
New Delhi, India

Sourav Paul MBBS
Junior Resident
Department of Internal Medicine
Kolkata Medical College
Kolkata, West Bengal, India

SP Sondhi MD
Guest Faculty
Department of Medicine
Subharti Medical College
Director
Omnibus Healthcare India Pvt Ltd
Meerut, Uttar Pradesh, India

Sreelakshmi R PhD
Research Scientist
Jothydev's Diabetes Research Center
Thiruvananthapuram, Kerala, India

Srina Ray MBBS(Cal)
Clinical Assistant
Heart Clinic
Kolkata, West Bengal, India

SS Dariya MD(Medicine) FACP FGSI FDI FIPA
Senior Consultant Physician
SMS Hospital
Jaipur, Rajasthan, India

S Sreenivas MD DM(Neurology)
Consultant Neurologist and Professor
Department of Medicine/Neurology
GSL Medical College
Chairman
Sri Padma Madhav Super Speciality Hospital
Rajahmundry, Andhra Pradesh, India

Subhita Choudhary MD(General Medicine)
Assistant Professor
Department of General Medicine
Shri Kalyan Government Medical College
Sikar, Rajasthan, India

Sudhanshu Pandey BPT MPT
Consultant Physical Therapist
Department of Physiotherapy and Rehabilitation
CISF Hospital
New Delhi, India

Sudha Sarna MD(Anesthesia)
Professor and Head
Department of Palliative Medicine
Mahatma Gandhi Medical College and Hospital
Jaipur, Rajasthan, India

Sudhir Bhandari MD DNB MNAMS FRCP (London, Edinburgh) DSc
Vice-Chancellor
Rajasthan University of Health Science (RUHS)
Professor Emeritus
SMS Medical College and Attached Group of Hospitals
Jaipur, Rajasthan, India

Sudhir Chandra Jha MD(Medicine) DNB(Medicine)
Associate Professor
Department of Medicine
Darbhanga Medical College
Darbhanga, Bihar, India

Sudhir Kulkarni MD DM
Emeritus Professor
Department of Nephrology
MGM Medical College
Aurangabad, Maharashtra, India

Sudhir Mehta MD(Internal Medicine)
Senior Professor and Head
Department of Medicine
SMS Medical College
Jaipur, Rajasthan, India

Sudipta Modak MD
Retired Associate Professor
Department of Chemistry
Calcutta University
Kolkata, West Bengal, India
Chairman BMC, CMC

Sugandha Sharma MS(Obstetrics and Gynecology)
Consultant Gynecologist
Global Heart and General Hospital
Jaipur, Rajasthan, India

Sujoy Ghosh DM FRCP FACE
Professor
Department of Endocrinology
Institute of Post Graduate Medical Education and Research
Kolkata, West Bengal, India

Sumbul Mazhar MD
Resident
Department of General Medicine
Institute of Medical Sciences
Banaras Hindu University (IMS-BHU)
Varanasi, Uttar Pradesh, India

Sumita Chaudhry MD
Consultant and Clinical Incharge, BMT
Department of Hematology
Safdarjung Hospital & VMMC
New Delhi, India

Sunil K Dadhich MD DM
Senior Professor and Head
Department of Gastroenterology
Dr SN Medical College
Jodhpur, Rajasthan, India

Sunil Kumar Bakshi MD(Medicine) FIAMS FGSI
Senior Consultant Physician
Department of Medicine
Metro Multispeciality Hospital
Noida, Uttar Pradesh, India

Sunil Kumar Mahavar MD
Professor
Department of General Medicine
SMS Medical College and Hospital
Jaipur, Rajasthan, India

Sunita Aggarwal MD(Medicine) FACP FRCP FICP FIACM FIMSA
Director Professor
Maulana Azad Medical College
New Delhi, India

Supriya Sarkar MD(Respiratory Medicine) FICP FCCP
Professor and Head
Department of Respiratory Medicine
College of Medicine and Sagore Dutta Hospital
Kolkata, West Bengal, India

Surabhi Talwar MD
Consultant Nephrologist
Department of Nephrology, University Hospitals Coventry and Warwickshire NHS Trust
Coventry, UK

Suraj S Yadav PhD
Assistant Professor
School of Pharmacy
National Forensic Sciences University
Gandhinagar, Gujarat, India

Surendra Kumar MD(General Medicine) Fellowship in Clinical Endocrinology PG Dip(Diabetology) AMU FACP FRCP FIACM FICP
Senior Professor and Unit Head
Department of Medicine
Sardar Patel Medical College
Bikaner, Rajasthan, India

Suryasnata Rath MS FRCS
Network Director—Operations
Ophthalmic Plastic Surgery Services
LV Prasad Eye Institute
Bhubaneswar, Odisha, India

Suvarthi Ray MBBS
Postgraduate Trainee
Department of General Medicine
All India Institute of Medical Sciences
Patna, Bihar, India

SV Ramanamurty MD FICP FIACM FACP
Professor
Academic Director—PG Education
Department of General Medicine
GSL Medical College
Rajahmundry, Andhra Pradesh, India

Swaroop Kumar Baruah MD(Medicine) MCA FICP
Senior Consultant Physician
Nemcare Hospital, Guwahati
Former Professor and Head
Department of Medicine
Gauhati Medical College
Guwahati, Assam, India

Swati Srivastava MD FACE FACP FICP
Senior Professor and Unit Head
SMS Medical College and Hospital
Jaipur, Rajasthan, India

Tanuja Manohar MD(Internal Medicine)
Professor and Head
Department of Medicine
NKPSIMS & RC and LMH
Nagpur, Maharashtra, India

Tanushree Debgupta MD(Medicine)
Assistant Professor
Silchar Medical College and Hospital
Silchar, Assam, India

Tapas Bandyopadhyay MD(Medicine) FICP FDI
Senior Consultant
Department of General Medicine
Medica Superspecialty Hospital
Kolkata, West Bengal, India

Tapas Kannu Vyas MBBS
Resident, Mahatma Gandhi Medical College and Hospital
Jaipur, Rajasthan, India

T Geetha MD
Professor of Medicine
Coimbatore Medical College and Hospital
Coimbatore, Tamil Nadu, India

Thair Al Jumaily Arab Board of Medicine Arab Board of Cardiology
Consultant, Interventional Cardiologist
Fujairah Hospital, Emirates Health Services (EHS)
Fujairah, UAE

Tribhuwan Gupta DM(Nephrology)
Director, Osmo Kidney Care Centre
Varanasi, Uttar Pradesh, India

Triven Sagar Sandepogu MD(General Medicine) FGID(CMC Vellore)
Professor
Department of General Medicine
Malla Reddy Institute of Medical Sciences and Hospital
Hyderabad, Telangana, India

TR Sirohi MD
Professor of Medicine
Subharti Medical College
Meerut, Uttar Pradesh, India

Trupti Trivedi MD
Professor of Medicine, Medical ICU
Department of Medicine
LTM Medical College and General Hospital, Sion
Mumbai, Maharashtra, India

TS Chandrasekar MD DM DSc FRCP(Edinburg, Glasgow, Ireland and London) FASGE FACG AGAF MWGO
Founder, Chairman and Chief Interventional Gastroenterologist
MedIndia Hospitals
Chennai, Tamil Nadu, India

Tuhina Gupta MS(Obstetrics and Gynecology) FMAS DMAS
Assistant Professor
SGT Medical College and Hospital
Gurugram, Haryana, India

Udas Chandra Ghosh MD(General Medicine) DNB(General Medicine) DNB(Respiratory Diseases) DTCD FICP FRCP(Glasgow)
Professor
Department of Medicine and In-Charge of Rheumatology Division
Medical College Kolkata
Kolkata, West Bengal, India

Umar Faruque MD
Registrar
Department of Medicine
Dhubri Medical College and Hospital
Dhubri, Assam, India

Ummed Singh MD(General Medicine)
Associate Professor
Department of General Medicine
Shri Kalyan Government Medical College
Sikar, Rajasthan, India

Upal Sengupta MD(General Medicine) DM(Nephrology)
Associate Professor
Department of Nephrology
KPC Medical College and Hospital
Kolkata, West Bengal, India

Upendra Sharma MD(General Medicine) DM(Clinical Hematology)
Senior Consultant Hematologist and Hemato-oncologist
Bhagwan Mahaveer Cancer Hospital and Research Center
Jaipur, Rajasthan, India

Utkarash Mishra MD DM(Nephrology)
Assistant Professor
Department of Nephrology
Christian Medical College
Vellore, Tamil Nadu, India

Uttam Kr Nath MD(Medicine) DFID(Diabetology)
Associate Professor
Department of Medicine
Jorhat Medical College and Hospital
Jorhat, Assam, India

Vaibhav Shukla MD(Medicine) FRCP(Edinburgh) FICP
Professor
Department of Medicine
Era's Medical College
Lucknow, Uttar Pradesh, India

VA Kothiwale MD PhD
Professor of General Medicine
Jawaharlal Nehru Medical College
KLE Academy of Higher Education and Research
Belagavi, Karnataka, India

Vamsi Krishna Annamdevula MD(Medicine)
Senior Resident
PG Department of Medicine
Institute of Medical Sciences and SUM Hospital
Bhubaneswar, Odisha, India

Vanita Arora MD DNB(Cardiology) MNAMS FRCP(Edinburgh) FESC FHRS
Senior Consultant
Apollo Hospital
New Delhi, India

Varun Vinayak Prakash Rao MD
MS Ramaiah Medical College
Bengaluru, Karnataka, India

Vasantha Kamath MD(Medicine) FICP
Professor Emeritus
Department of Medicine
MVJ Medical College and Research Hospital
Bengaluru, Karnataka, India

(Lt Gen) Ved Chaturvedi MD DM
Senior Consultant Rheumatologist
Sir Ganga Ram Hospital
New Delhi, India

Veerendra Singh MD(Internal Medicine) FICP FIACM FDI FUPDA
Director
GSSM Cardiorespiratory Centre
Ayodhya, Uttar Pradesh, India

Vibha Sharma MBBS MD
Postgraduate Resident (Medicine)
Department of General Medicine
Kalinga Institute of Medical Sciences
KIIT Deemed to be University
Bhubaneswar, Odisha, India

Vidita Kalra MD(Medicine)
Final Year Postgraduate Student
Mahatma Gandhi University of Medical Sciences and Technology
Jaipur, Rajasthan, India

Vijaya Prasanna Parimi MD DM(Rheumatology)
Consultant Rheumatologist
Department of Clinical Immunology and Rheumatology
ESIC Medical College and Hospital
Hyderabad, Telangana, India

Vijay Budhwar DM(Endocrinology) PDT
Department of Endocrinology
Institute of Post Graduate Medical Education and Research
Kolkata, West Bengal, India

Vijay Garg MD FIAE FICP FCSI FICA(USA) FISE FACC(USA) FACP(USA) FIMSA FISC FESC(EUROPE)
Professor
Department of Medicine
RD Gardi Medical College
Ujjain, Madhya Pradesh, India

Vijaykumar G Warad MD(General Medicine)
Professor, Department of Medicine
BLDE Deemed to be University
Shri BM Patil Medical College Hospital and Research Centre
Vijayapura, Karnataka, India

Vijay Kumar MD(General Medicine) FICP FDI FIACM PGDHM
Additional Professor
Department of General Medicine
All India Institute of Medical Sciences
Patna, Bihar, India

Vikash Khandelia DM(Nephrology)
Professor and Head
Department of Nephrology
Government Medical College
Kota, Rajasthan, India

Vineet Behera MD DM FACP FASN FICP
Professor of Medicine and Nephrologist
INHS Kalyani
Visakhapatnam, Andhra Pradesh, India

Vineet Talwar MD(Medical Oncology) FRCP(UK) DNB FICP FIMSA MNAMS
Director
Department of Medical Oncology
Rajiv Gandhi Cancer Institute and Research Centre
New Delhi, India

Vinod Ravindran MD MRCP(UK) CCT(Rheumatology, UK) FRCP(Edinburgh)
Consultant Rheumatologist
Centre for Rheumatology
Kozhikode, Kerala, India
Adjunct Professor
Department of Medicine
Kasturba Medical College
Manipal, Karnataka, India

Vipul Chavda MD FRCP FACP
Chairman and Endocrine Physician
Rudraksha Institute of Medical Sciences
Ahmedabad, Gujarat, India

Virendra Kumar Goyal MD FICP FACP FIACM FDI FRCP(Edinburgh, Glasgow, London)
Professor and Head
Department of Medicine
American International Institute of Medical Sciences
Udaipur, Rajasthan, India

Vishwanath Krishnamurthy MD FICP
Professor of Medicine
MS Ramaiah Medical College
Bengaluru, Karnataka, India
Honorary Secretary API Karnataka Chapter

Vishwas Galav MD(Medicine)
Second Year DM(Cardiology)
Resident
Department of Cardiology
Jawahar Lal Nehru Medical College
Ajmer, Rajasthan, India

Viswanathan Mohan MD PhD DSc FRCP(London, Edinburgh, Glasgow and Ireland) DSc(Honoris Causa) FAMS FNASc FASc FNA FAMS FACE FTWAS MACP FRS (Edinburgh)
Chairman
Dr Mohan's Diabetes Specialities Centre and Madras Diabetes Research Foundation
Chennai, Tamil Nadu, India

VK Katyal MD FACC(USA)
Head
Department of Medicine
Positron Multispeciality and Cancer Hospital
Rohtak, Haryana, India

VN Mishra MD(Medicine) FACP FICP FIACM FIAOG
Professor, Department of Medicine
All India Institute of Medical Sciences
Bhopal, Madhya Pradesh, India

V Palaniappan MD FICP FRCP(London)
Managing Director
Sri Sakthi Vinayaga Multispeciality Hospital and Dr V Palaniappan's Diabetes Specialities Center
Guziliamparai, Tamil Nadu, India

V Palanikumaran MD DDiab(MMC)
Senior Assistant Professor
Madurai Medical College
Madurai, Tamil Nadu, India

Wesley Hannah BDS MPH PhD
Research Associate
Dr Mohan's Diabetes Specialities Centre (IDF Centre of Excellence in Diabetes Care) and
Madras Diabetes Research Foundation (ICMR Centre for Advanced Research on Diabetes)
Chennai, Tamil Nadu, India

Yashasvi Gautam MD FICP FIACM
Honorary Senior Consultant Physician
Sudha Hospital and Jaiswal Hospital
Kota, Rajasthan, India

Yogesh Kumar Govil MD FACP FACG AGAF MRCP(E)
Senior Consultant
Department of Gastroenterology
Einstein Jefferson Medical Centre
Philadelphia, Pennsylvania, USA

Yogita Pendurkar DNB(Medicine)
Consultant Physician
Department of Medicine
Jupiter Hospital
Thane, Maharashtra, India

Yojana Gokhale MD
Professor of Medicine and In-Charge of Rheumatology
Lokmanya Tilak Municipal Medical College
Mumbai, Maharashtra, India

Zairemliana Chenkual MBBS
Post Graduate Trainee
Department of Emergency Medicine
All India Institute of Medical Sciences,
Patna, Bihar, India

FOREWORD

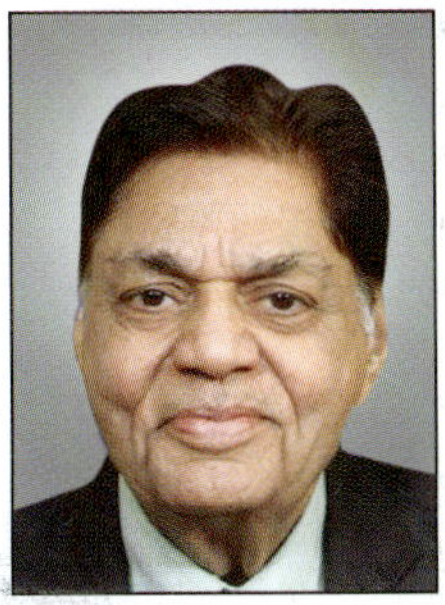

KK Pareek MD FICP FRCP
Past President API
Past Dean API
Immediate Past President IACM
Chairman API House Committee

It is both a privilege and an honor to contribute the foreword for "*Medicine Update 2024*", the annual publication of the *Association of Physicians of India (API)*. As we come together to celebrate the wealth of knowledge encapsulated within these pages, we pay tribute to the visionary physicians who, in 1944, laid the foundation for API with the noble aim of fostering collaboration, sharing experiences, and advancing medical science in our diverse and dynamic nation on one platform.

In the ever-evolving landscape of healthcare, where learning is a perpetual journey, the Medicine Update plays a pivotal role. In a country like India, with its vast expanse and varied healthcare challenges, disseminating knowledge becomes a necessity to stay updated with the cutting-edge developments in medicine. API has been at the forefront of this mission, providing a common platform for physicians across the nation to converge, exchange ideas, and stay abreast of the latest advancements.

Dr Milind Nadkar, the Scientific Chairman for APICON 2024 and the President-Elect of the API, stands as a beacon of leadership in the physician community. His wealth of experience, dedication to academic pursuits, and dynamic approach to healthcare have been instrumental in shaping its annual scientific program. Dr Nadkar's expertise has been evident through his tenure as the Chief Editor of the Journal of API and as the Honorary Secretary of API.

Medicine, as a field, is undergoing a transformative journey, and the theme of APICON 2024, "Clinical to Digital Medicine," reflects this paradigm shift. We are witnessing the integration of traditional clinical practices with cutting-edge digital technologies, promising to revolutionize patient care, diagnostics, and medical research. This forward-looking theme demonstrates a commitment to not only addressing current clinical challenges but also embracing the potential of digital interventions to shape the future of medicine in India.

The substantial undertaking of crafting the extensive scientific program for APICON 2024 spanning over 3½ days and featuring >500 lectures is a testament to the unwavering dedication of Dr Nadkar and his editorial team. Medicine Update 2024 serves as a tangible manifestation of their commitment to delivering a comprehensive and enlightening experience for conference delegates and readers alike, with each chapter authored by experts in their respective fields.

Dr Nadkar's meticulous curation ensures that the content is tailored to meet the diverse needs of practicing physicians, adeptly translating theoretical concepts into practical applications for the benefit of our patients.

I extend my heartfelt appreciation and congratulations to Dr Milind Nadkar and his editorial team for their exceptional work in creating this invaluable resource.

May *Medicine Update 2024* persist as a guiding beacon of knowledge, supporting physicians on their journey of lifelong learning.

Wishing all the delegates of APICON 2024 an enriching and enlightening experience.

PREFACE

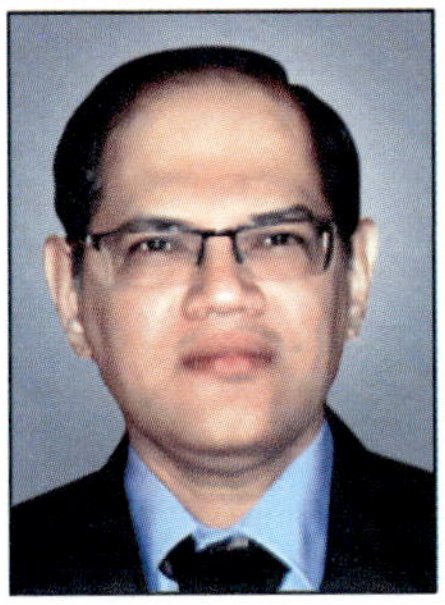

Milind Y Nadkar MD FICP FACP
President-Elect
Association of Physicians of India
Professor and Head
Department of Medicine and
Chief of Rheumatology Services
Seth GS Medical College and KEM Hospital
Mumbai, Maharashtra, India

With immense pleasure, I present before you the two volumes of "*Medicine Update 2024*" on the occasion of the 80th Annual Conference of the Association of Physicians of India—APICON 2024—being held at New Delhi from February 22 to 25, 2024.

I first go down to the memories of my mentor, Late Dr Siddhrath N Shah, who has guided me throughout my API career. His teachings and insights have greatly helped me in formulating the Scientific Program for APICON 2024 and also in editing of this book "Medicine Update 2024". Without his hand-holding over the years, I could not have moved a step further.

Truly, it was a herculean task to put up such a huge Scientific Program and to publish Medicine Update 2024. I thank my entire Scientific Committee and the Editorial Board for their relentless support in this venture.

Internal medicine and all its subspecialties are undergoing a tremendous transformation with new research every day. A lot of research is published every day. It is extremely difficult for a physician to update his knowledge by reading the literature in their busy schedule. The Scientific Program of APICON 2024 attempts to breach the gap in the knowledge of physicians. During the scientific program, we have planned interactive lectures, scientific celebrations, orations, panel discussions, and workshops.

The theme of this year's scientific program is "*clinical to digital*". On these lines, the Scientific Committee has tried to strike a balance between clinical medicine, laboratory medicine, and therapeutic advances. The scientific content of the program is published in this book with over 281 Chapters that will be a ready reference for future use.

There will be 12 workshops with hands-on training in the subjects of Ventilator Management, Biological and Nuclear Warfare, Communication Skills, Sleep, Intraarticular Injections, etc. A quiz has been organized for the interest of PG students.

There are over 1,500 research papers that will be presented on the platform or as e-posters which will give an opportunity to young physicians and postgraduate students to showcase their research.

I hope that the readers will find "Medicine Update 2024" worth our efforts and help in enhancing their knowledge and clinical skills.

ACKNOWLEDGMENTS

It was an enormous responsibility to compile and publish a book of the magnitude of "*Medicine Update 2024*" and I find myself absolutely short of words to thank enough all who have helped and guided me in executing this mammoth task.

I would express my deep appreciation and indebtedness to all the authors from across the country for their outstanding contribution and sharing their learnings and knowledge through the chapters of this book.

I extend a very special gratitude to Dr Yash Pal Munjal, stalwart of the Association of Physicians of India (API), for being on my side ever guiding me. Dr KK Pareek needs a special mention and gratitude for the support I received from him and for his kind words for me in the "Foreword" of the book.

It was not possible to successfully complete the task of publishing this book without the support and help of the members of the Scientific Committee and the members of the Editorial Board. I am grateful to them for providing timely inputs which were crucial in bringing everything together.

I express my very sincere thanks to my friend and close associate Dr Rakesh Bhadade for his constant support and standing shoulder to shoulder with me. I extend my special thanks to Dr Anupam Prakash for his tireless help in formulating this book.

I express my sincere gratitude and appreciation to the efforts of Shri Jitender P Vij (Group Chairman), Mr MS Mani (Group President), and Mr Ankit Vij (Managing Director), Jaypee Brothers Medical Publishers (P) Ltd, New Delhi, India, for their sincere efforts in publishing this book. Furthermore, I am thankful to Ms Chetna Malhotra (Senior Director—Professional Publishing, Marketing and Business Development), Ms Pooja Bhandari (Director—Production), Ms Nedup Bhutia Pillai (Team Leader—Print Publishing), Ms Tamali Deb (Manager—Copyediting), Mr Ajay Kumar Sharma (DGM—Production), Mr Sunil Dogra [Assistant Manager Production (Designing Department)], Mr Keshav Kumar (Assistant Manager—Production), Mr Manoj Kumar (Team Leader—Production), Ms Seema Dogra (Cover Visualizer), and Mr Varun Rajoria (Senior Graphic Designer) and the entire team of M/s Jaypee Brothers Medical Publishers (P) Ltd, New Delhi, India, who have been instrumental in giving the final shape to this book. Their sincere efforts are truly praiseworthy.

I extend my very sincere thanks and deep sense of appreciation to the members of the editorial office Mr Aniruddha Sapatnekar, Director, OneMD, for all his help. He has worked tirelessly and diligently at every step of giving final shape to this book.

I also express my very sincere thanks to the members of the Governing Body, API; Faculty Council, Indian College of Physicians (ICP); and Members of Board of Directors, Physicians Research Foundation (PRF), for helping me with their valuable suggestions, inputs, and guidance.

I appreciate the help and cooperation of API office members, especially Mrs Sunita Shukla and Mr Rajanikant Parmar.

I am grateful to all the honorable members of API who gave me the opportunity to publish this book as Chairman Scientific Committee APICON 2023 and President-Elect of the elite organization, API.

The compilation of this book would not have been possible without the participation and assistance of so many people whose names may not all be enumerated, but their contribution is sincerely appreciated and gratefully acknowledged.

In the end, I would like to thank the Almighty God for his blessings without which I would not have been able to do any of this.

Milind Y Nadkar

CONTENTS

VOLUME 1

SECTION 1: CARDIOLOGY

SECTION 2: CRITICAL CARE

SECTION 3: DIABETES

SECTION 4: ENDOCRINE

SECTION 5: GASTROENTEROLOGY

SECTION 6: GERIATRICS

SECTION 7: HEMATOLOGY

SECTION 8: HEPATOLOGY

SECTION 9: HYPERTENSION

SECTION 10: IMMUNOLOGY

VOLUME 2

SECTION 11: INFECTIONS

SECTION 18: PULMONOLOGY

SECTION 19: RHEUMATOLOGY

SECTION 20: MISCELLANEOUS

SECTION

1

CARDIOLOGY

1

CHAPTER

Current Scenario of Rheumatic Heart Disease in India

Prabhat Pandey

ABSTRACT

The rheumatic heart disease continues to be an important cause of disease burden in India, affecting the population in their prime and productive phase of the life. The prevalence of rheumatic heart disease is varied in different Indian studies, because of the inclusion of different populations at different point of times and using different screening methods for the diagnosis. The data on incidence and prevalence on a nationally represented sample are lacking. There is a need for establishing a population-based surveillance system in the country for monitoring trends, management practices, and outcomes to formulate informed guidelines for initiating contextual interventions for prevention and control of rheumatic heart disease.

INTRODUCTION

Rheumatic fever (RF)/rheumatic heart disease (RHD) is caused due to the triggering of the autoimmune response by group A beta-hemolytic streptococcal pharyngitis which leads to immune-inflammatory injury and then to cardiac valves. The injury of the pericardium and myocardium is transient and self-limiting. One of the main cause of the acute and long-term morbidity in acute rheumatic fever (ARF) patients and mortality in patients with RHD is the valvular injury. The risk of the RHD is usually determined by the factors such as host, agent, and environmental factors.

Poverty is considered to be the physical manifestation for RHD. The distribution of the human development index (across various regions, states, nations, and globally) corresponds with the burden of RHD. There are important determinants for the burden of RHD such as socioeconomic state, access, and quality of healthcare. The incidence of RHD has practically disappeared in developed countries. However, RF/RHD continues to be a major cause of disease burden in developing countries affecting especially children, adolescents, and young adults in low-income countries and even in high-income countries with socioeconomic inequalities.

Acute rheumatic fever and its long-term sequel, RHD is a major health problem in children, adolescents, and young adults. Despite the tremendous progress made in cardiology, the menace of morbidity and mortality due to ARF and its consequences remain very high in India. Because of the preoccupation of the cardiologist with adult cardiac disease like ischemic heart disease, the problems of ARF/RHD have been sidelined and studies on prevalence, treatment, and prevention receive only scant attention and only exotic palliative methods such as balloon mitral valvotomy, valve/replacement have become the center stage in India.

Precise diagnosis of ARF has presented problems since Hippocrates, who provided the first written description of arthritis in man in 400 BC. Lack of specific criteria had led to diagnostic chaos until the Jones criteria in 1944. Despite the Jones criteria and four revisions and modifications, ARF is either under diagnosed leading to nearly 50% of established RHD not receiving prophylaxis or over diagnosed by depending on traditional characteristic auscultatory findings for diagnosing carditis. Unfortunately modern facility like echocardiography is not included in Jones criteria, despite the fact that echocardiography can help to diagnose carditis more frequently than auscultatory findings. Early diagnosis of ARF though difficult is very important to prevent the serious consequences in young.

Worldwide, past few decades has witnessed, disturbing figures of 40 million people affected by RHD and its antecedent RF. It is often found predominantly in poverty-stricken children, adolescents, and young adults and thus affects the productive years of life despite our understanding of the preventable nature of the disease. Following untreated and repeated infection of the pharynx with group A beta-hemolytic *Streptococcus* (Strep A) may lead to an immune-mediated inflammatory response, namely ARF and follow on ARF-associated carditis with likely permanent damage to at least one of the four heart valves, long-term sequelae of RHD may include stroke, heart failure, and premature mortality.

Acute rheumatic fever is a diffuse inflammatory disease of the joints, heart, blood vessels, brain, and subcutaneous tissue. Carditis is the most serious major manifestation of RF. The heart valves are the most commonly affected structures. The presence or absence of carditis is an important determinant of the course and prognosis of ARF. The prognosis worsens with increasing severity of the initial carditis and with recurrences. Hence, the treatment of ARF is not just about relieving fever and joint pain but also to reduce the cardiac damage and prevent the recurrence. Although the prevention of ARF and the management of recurrences are well established, the optimal management of active rheumatic carditis is still unclear. Hence, there are both consensus and controversies in the management of various affections of ARF.

EPIDEMIOLOGICAL TRENDS OF BURDEN OF RHEUMATIC HEART DISEASE IN INDIA

The burden of RHD is not only variable among countries; with in the country but also within the states. This discrepancy depends on two factors, i.e., the socioeconomic status and state of health systems. The major determinant of the persistent burden of RHD in developing countries is because of the poor standards of living conditions, overcrowding, and lack of strong population-based surveillance system for pharyngitis, RF, and RHD for effective implementation of primary and secondary preventive interventions. The Indian Council of Medical Research has initiated a project named Jai Vigyan Mission Mode Project (2000–2010) which was based on the community control and prevention of RF/RHD through hospital-based passive surveillance and implementation of secondary prophylaxis at a national level, there is no structured program for prevention and control of RHD. However, with the changing conditions in the country after adopting a policy of economic liberalization and globalization since 2000 with respect to the socioeconomic state, living conditions and connectivity and healthcare centers, it has expected to have translated into a decline in the burden of RF/RHD in India.

The burden of RF/RHD has been estimated and reported since 1960s from hospital-based, population-based, and school-based survey studies, using different case definitions and screening methods. There are no survey studies estimating the burden of RF/RHD based on national- and state-representative sample using uniform screening method at the different timeline to evaluate the trends of the burden of RF/RHD in India.

DISEASE BURDEN

In India, RF is endemic and remains one of the major causes of cardiovascular disease, accounting for nearly 25–45% of the acquired heart disease. The annual incidence of RF is 100–200 times greater than that observed in developed countries and fluctuates between 100 and 200 per 100,000 children of school age (from 5 to 17 or 18 years depending on the study). India is in the phase of "epidemiological transition". On one hand there is a substantial burden due to RHD for the treatment of which enormous money is spent, on the other hand the government resources are scarce to treat and prevent the disease.

The publication from the Global Burden of Disease (GBD) study reported the trends and current estimates of RHD worldwide is decreasing overall by as much as 47.8% in the period 1990–2015. However, there is broad difference noticed in endemic versus nonendemic rates with 3.4/100,000 in nonendemic regions of the world compared to 444/100,000 in endemic countries. The regions at highest prevalence and disability-adjusted life years (DALYs) are those in Oceania, South Asia, and Central Sub-Saharan Africa. In the other disconcerting finding, India is home to 40% of all global RHD population. This finding might be going largely unnoticed as prevalence of RHD is also not systematic in all regions of our country. Some initiatives have been taken by the government in states such as Kerala, Assam, and Chhattisgarh to strengthen the primary healthcare infrastructure which accounted for over RHD burden than other states. In the last decade, school-based clinical surveys conducted and estimate that the prevalence of RHD to be between 0.5 and 1.47 per 1,000 children in age group of 5–15 years. However, this may not be a representative sample and the trend of prevalence would be greater in underdeveloped states of India. Therefore, results are variable but studies showing declining trends of RHD over time and it is a difficult question to answer and cannot be extrapolated to the whole of the country.

India is home to 40% of all people living with RHD. Of the estimated 33 million people with RHD, 13.2 million live in India. Likewise, in the year 2015, of the 347,000 deaths due to RHD worldwide, nearly 120,000 (over a third) are estimated to have occurred in India. The other disconcerting finding is below the average pace of reduction in prevalence and mortality. During the 25-year period from 1990 to 2015, the age standardized mortality due to RHD worldwide fell from 9.2 to 4.8 per 100,000 population, a reduction of nearly 48%. However, the reduction for India is a mere 18% (from 15.5 to 12.7 per 100,000 population). By contrast, China showed a 71% reduction from 18.8 to 5.4 per 100,000 population over this period. North Africa and Southeast Asia have now achieved age-standardized mortality rates due to RHD that are similar to those in nonendemic countries (about 2 per 100,000 population).

EPIDEMIOLOGY OF RHEUMATIC HEART DISEASE

Emerging Genetic Susceptibility in Rheumatic Heart Disease

The role of genetic susceptibility in reemergence of streptococcal disease is driven by microbial evolution and mechanisms of genetic exchange. Long way back, unexplained susceptibility to RHD among certain individuals in the population suggests a genetic contribution to the condition. In the 1980s and 1990s, several reports inked the disease to the human leukocyte antigen (HLA) locus on chromosome 6, followed in the 2000s by reports suggesting additional candidate regions elsewhere in the genome. Subsequently, the search for susceptibility loci has been rejuvenated by the use of genome-wide association studies (GWAS) which provide the best approach to compare the frequency of variants or traits associated with complex disease (autoimmune etiology and infectious) in a population.

Nongenetic Risk Factors

It is accepted RHD influenced by combination of group A *Streptococcus* (GAS) and RF risk factors. Risk factors include poverty, overcrowding, malnutrition, and maternal educational level and employment. Henceforth, an interaction between GAS infections, such as streptococcal pharyngitis, the socioeconomic status of the patient and community, access to primary healthcare, and genetic susceptibility are defined as likely to develop RHD.

METHODS OF DETECTION AND EVALUATION

Evaluation Methods

The economic evaluations conducted so far have been focused on the interventions for the prevention of RF. However, RHD has more important long-term consequences. The high costs associated with a usually lifelong secondary prophylaxis for the prevention of RF recurrence, and associated with the medical management and surgical interventions required to manage the complications of RHD.

Methods of Detection

The detection of RF/RHD in the population is challenging. The RF and RHD are detected based on symptoms, audible murmurs, and echocardiography evidence of structural and functional abnormalities of the affected valves. The ability to detect murmurs and differentiating functional from pathological murmurs depends upon clinical skills of the physician, settings of auscultation, and so on. Thus, auscultation-based methods of screening RF/RHD have their limited sensitivity and specificity. The morphological and Doppler-based detection of RHD in echocardiography study has high sensitivity and specificity in detection being more objective and subject to validation. The echocardiography detects RHD in patients without being clinically evident called subclinical RHD. The prevalence of subclinical RHD is about seven to ten times higher than clinically evident RHD. However, the clinical significance of subclinical RHD needs to be validated in future long-term follow-up studies.

The severity and nature of valvular dysfunction in RHD is variable from patient to patient. The hemodynamically insignificant valvular dysfunctions may be asymptomatic and may not be evident on clinical examination, thus escapes detection. Thus, the variable prevalence of RHD reported may be partly related to differences in the methodology adopted for screening.

CLINICAL PROFILE

The major manifestations of ARF are: (1) Carditis, (2) polyarthritis, (3) chorea, (4) erythema marginatum, and (5) subcutaneous nodules. The clinical profile of acute RF seems to be changing. Clinical diagnosis of carditis was noted in at least 50% of acute RF in the past. There seems to be a declining incidence of carditis. The diagnosis of carditis that is considered a major criteria in ARF depends on the clinical and traditional auscultatory findings.

Diagnosis of Carditis: Auscultation versus Echocardiography

All the diagnostic guidelines on ARF/RHD give emphasis on auscultatory findings. The auscultation is not recognized by any current guidelines due to which it is becoming outdated.

RHEUMATIC FEVER DIAGNOSTIC CRITERIA

The diagnosis of ARF is made using the modified Jones criteria. The main changes in the latest 2015 update include that a low, medium, and high-risk population was identified based on the disease endemic and inclusion of subclinical carditis as on major basis. Lower thresholds for joint manifestations, fever, etc., are adopted for the high-risk population. These modifications are made to advance the sensitivity of the criteria in moderate/high-risk population **(Table 1)**.

DECLINE OF RHEUMATIC HEART DISEASE: IS IT REAL?

Systematic review of available data on epidemiological studies of RF/RHD conducted in different points of time using clinical screening followed by echocardiography confirmation as the methods of detecting RF/RHD, across the country by individual authors and the Indian Council of Medical Research (ICMR) lead multicentric survey studies, suggest declining trends, especially after 2000 onward **(Fig. 1)**.

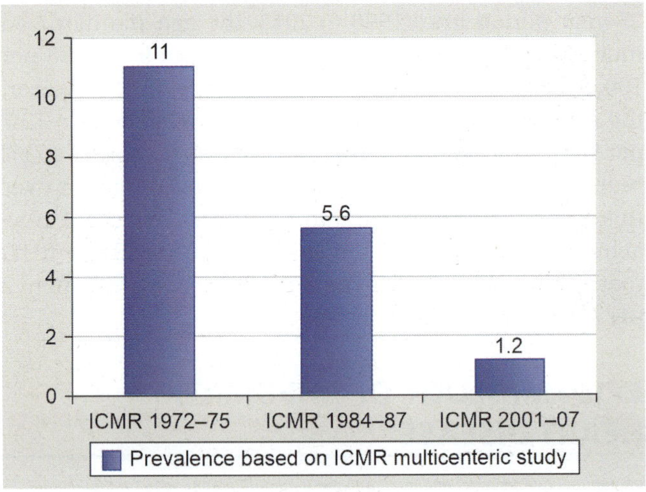

FIG. 1: Trends of change in prevalence of RF/RHD in ICMR-led multicentric survey studies across the country over a period of 40 years.

(ICMR: Indian Council of Medical Research; RF: rheumatic fever; RHD: rheumatic heart disease)

TABLE 1: Summary of the 2015 updates of Jones criteria.

	Low-risk population	Moderate/high-risk population
Definition	Annual incidence of ARF ≤ 2 per 100,000 school-aged children or all age prevalence of RHD ≤ 1 per 1,000	Those not fulfilling criteria for low risk
Major manifestations		
Joint manifestations	Polyarthritis	• Polyarthritis and/or **polyarthralgia** • **Monoarthritis**
Carditis	• Clinical and/or subclinical chorea • Erythema marginatum • Subcutaneous nodules	• Clinical and/or subclinical chorea • Erythema marginatum • Subcutaneous nodules
Minor manifestations		
Carditis	PR prolongation (age adjusted)	PR prolongation (age adjusted)
Arthralgia	Polyarthralgia	**Monoarthralgia**
Fever	≥ 38.5°C	≥ 38°C
Inflammatory markers	ESR ≥ 60 mm in first hour and/or CRP ≥ 3.0 mg/dL	**ESR ≥ 30 mm in first hour** and/or CRP ≥ 3.0 mg/dL
Supporting evidence of antecedent GAS infection: • Increased or rising antistreptolysin O titer or other streptococcal antibodies (anti-DNase B) • Positive throat culture for GAS or positive rapid GAS carbohydrate antigen First episode of ARF: Two major or one major plus two minor (in the presence of supporting evidence). *Recurrence*: Two major or one major plus two minor or three minor (in the presence of supporting evidence).		

Note: Changes compared with the previous 1992 revision are highlighted in bold. Subclinical carditis: Only detected by echocardiography, no audible murmur.

(ARF: acute rheumatic fever; CRP: C-reactive protein; ESR: erythrocyte sedimentation rate; GAS: group A *Streptococcus*; RHD: rheumatic heart disease)

CONCLUSION

For past several decades, we had been following the dictates of the Jones committee with regard to diagnosis and management of RF and RHD although the disease has always been more prevalent in India than the West, and today more than ever before it has become imperative that we have our own guidelines for management of RF/RHD, as this disease has practically been eradicated in the developed countries of the world.

Valvular heart disease is more common in India than the rest of the world, the leading cause being RF.

Rheumatic fever/RHD is the disease of poverty. India, having >1.3 billion population with wide social and economic disparities RF/RHD, will continue to be a major public health problem. Although data on incidence and prevalence on a nationally represented sample are lacking, there is an indication of declining trends, especially after 2000 mirroring with improving economic growth of the country. There is a need for establishing population-based surveillance system in the country for monitoring trends, management practices, and outcomes to formulate informed guidelines for initiating contextual interventions for prevention and control of RF/RHD.

SUGGESTED READINGS

1. Sanyal SK, Thapar MK, Ahmed SH, Hooja V, Tewari P. The initial attack of acute rheumatic fever during childhood in North India; a prospective study of the clinical profile. Circulation. 1974;49:7-12.
2. Padmavathi S. Present status of rheumatic fever and rheumatic heart disease in India. Indian Heart J. 1995;47:395-8.
3. Vijayalakshmi IB. Rheumatic fever, rheumatic heart disease registry and control program. In: Vijayalakshmi IB (Ed). Acute Rheumatic Fever and Chronic Rheumatic Heart Disease, 1st edition. New Delhi: Jaypee Brothers Medical Publishers (P) Ltd.; 2011. pp. 324-36.
4. Mishra TK, Acute Rheumatic Fever and Rheumatic Heart Disease: Current Scenario. Indian Acad Clin Med. 2007;8:324-30.
5. Karthikeyan K. Rheumatic heart disease in India: Declining, but not fast enough. Natl Med J India. 2017;30(5):247-8.
6. Lalchandani AD, Vijayalakshmi IB. Consensus and Controversies in the management of acute rheumatic fever. In: Vijayalakshmi IB (Ed). Acute Rheumatic Fever and Chronic Rheumatic Heart Disease, 1st edition. New Delhi: Jaypee Brothers Medical Publishers (P) Ltd.; 2011.
7. Negi PC, Sondhi S, Asotra S, Mahajan K, Mehta A. Current status of rheumatic heart disease in India. Indian Heart J. 2019;71:85-90.

2

CHAPTER

Rheumatic Fever: What's New in Diagnosis and Management?

Monika Maheshwari, Vishwas Galav

ABSTRACT

Acute rheumatic fever (ARF) is an immune-mediated disease caused by group A *Streptococcus* (GAS) infection, causing pharyngitis in children and adults. Repeated or severe ARF can lead to rheumatic heart disease (RHD), causing high morbidity and mortality. ARF and RHD are prevalent in regions with low income and limited healthcare access. The pathogenesis of ARF and RHD is poorly understood, and no immune-modulating therapies exist. Pro-inflammatory cytokines and chemokines, such as interleukin 6 (IL-6), IL-8/CXCL8, and tumor necrosis factor alpha (TNF-α), are implicated in ARF and RHD pathogenesis.

INTRODUCTION

Acute rheumatic fever (ARF) is an immune-mediated disease that occurs as a late sequelae to group A *Streptococcus* (GAS) infection. It accounts for 15–30% cases of pharyngitis among children and 10% cases among adults. Repeated or severe ARF leads to rheumatic heart disease (RHD), with high morbidity and mortality. ARF and its complication RHD cause a large burden of morbidity and mortality with an estimate 40.5 million people living with RHD and causing 3.06 lakhs deaths annually. In many high-income countries, improvements in living conditions and the introduction of antimicrobial drugs to treat GAS pharyngitis have nearly eliminated ARF. High prevalence rates of ARF and RHD continue to be reported from several geographic regions around the world with low income and limited access to healthcare such as Southeast Asia, the Western Pacific, and Africa.

The pathogenesis of ARF and RHD is poorly understood, and there are currently no immune-modulating therapies available to stop the progression of ARF to RHD. Cytokines and chemokines are immune-signaling molecules that are critical to the development of autoimmune diseases. Several studies point to a role for pro-inflammatory cytokines and chemokines in ARF and RHD pathogenesis, in particular interleukin (IL)-6, IL-8/CXCL8, and tumor necrosis factor alpha (TNF-α), which are elevated in circulation in both ARF and RHD patients. Histological studies also implicate T helper 1 (Th1)- and Th17-associated proinflammatory cytokines, chemokine CXCL9, and the fibrosis-associated cytokine Transforming growth factor beta (TGF-β) in progressive cycles of inflammatory damage and fibrotic repair. All of this suggests immune molecules contribute to both the acute inflammatory disease stage of ARF as well as cardiac remodeling and valve dysfunction in RHD.

DIAGNOSIS OF RHEUMATIC FEVER

The Jones criteria have been used for guidance in the diagnosis of ARF since 1944 and were modified by the American Heart Association (AHA) in 1992. The prominent role played by echocardiography in the diagnosis of heart disorders which have evolved over the past two decades which lead to identification of newer entity called 'subclinical carditis'. All these changes lead to further revision of Jones criteria in 2015 for the diagnosis rheumatic fever (RF). The 2020 Australian guideline for prevention, diagnosis, and management of ARF and RHD takes into consideration the 2015 revised Jones criteria, but it is more specific for Australian population.

2015 AHA-REVISED JONES CRITERIA FOR DIAGNOSIS OF ARF

For all patient population with evidence of preceding GAS infection **(Table 1)**

Diagnosis: Initial ARF—2 major manifestations *or* 1 major plus 2 minor

Diagnosis: Recurrent ARF—2 major *or* 1 major and 2 minor *or* 3 minor

To differentiate between low-risk and high-risk population the following criteria may be utilized:

- If a person comes from an environment or group where low rates of ARF or RHD are known to occur, it is reasonable to assume that they are at low risk for ARF (class IIa; level of evidence C).
- It is reasonable that low risk be defined as having an all-age prevalence of RHD of ≤ 1 per 1,000 population per year or an ARF incidence of < 2 per 100,000 school-aged children (typically 5–14 years old) each year where trustworthy epidemiological data are available (class IIa; level of evidence C).
- Depending on their reference population, children who are not obviously from a low-risk demographic are at moderate to high risk (class I; level of evidence C).

TABLE 1: American Heart Association (AHA)-revised Jones criteria 2015 for diagnosis of acute rheumatic fever (ARF).

Low-risk populations	Moderate- and high-risk populations
Major criteria	
Carditis (clinical or subclinical)	Carditis (clinical or subclinical)
• Arthritis (polyarthritis only) • Chorea	Arthritis (including polyarthritis, monoarthritis, or polyarthralgia)
Erythema marginatum	Chorea
Subcutaneous nodules	• Erythema marginatum • Subcutaneous nodules
Minor criteria	
Polyarthralgia	Monoarthralgia
Fever (≥ 38.5°C)	Fever (≥ 38°C)
ESR ≥ 60 mm in the first hour and/or CRP ≥ 3.0 mg/dL	ESR ≥ 30 mm in the first hour and/or CRP ≥ 3.0 mg/dL
Prolonged PR interval, after accounting for age variability (unless carditis is a major criterion)	Prolonged PR interval, after accounting for age variability (unless carditis is a major criterion)

(CRP: C-reactive protein; ESR: erythrocyte sedimentation rate)

ADVANCES IN UNDERSTANDING OF RF/RHD PATHOGENESIS

The precise mechanisms that underlie this intricate process are still not fully understood. According to what we know, the immune responses ARF and RHD are brought on by GAS pharyngitis. But more recently, RHD has been linked to other superficial streptococcal diseases such pyoderma and impetigo. Additionally, there is growing evidence that suggests the pathophysiology of RHD may involve group C and group G *Streptococcus*.

Molecular mimicry is the most widely accepted theory regarding the pathogenesis of RF/RHD; however, more recent research points to a more intricate series of events, including the possibility of collagen-associated neoantigens and additional mechanisms that may contribute to pathology, such as epitope spreading and T cell receptor (TCR) degeneration. Furthermore, some natural killer (NK) cells, CD4- CD8- T cells, and CD4+ T cells may also have a significant role in the destruction of tissue in RHD.

ADVANCES IN UNDERSTANDING OF THE GENETIC PREDISPOSITION TO ARF

Acute rheumatic fever occurs in about 3–6% in GAS-endemic populations, and the genetic risk for RHD is thought to be complex. This theory has been validated by historical research on RHD twins, and more recently, genetic investigation has provided fresh insights into the etiology and propensity of RHD.

Human leukocyte antigen (HLA) molecules, which are encoded by genes on chromosome 6, have been linked to a predisposition to develop RF/RHD through genetic connections in RHD. Class II *HLA* genes have been extensively documented, with most of them being associated with HLA-DR7 and HLA-DR4.

There is evidence linking polymorphisms in the *IL-2*, *IL-4*, *IL-6*, and *IL-10* genes to clinical illness, and IL-4 has been proven to have value in differentiating between latent and clinical RHD. Higher levels of IL-10 and IL-4 indicated unfavorable clinical outcomes, while IL-4, IL-8, and IL-1RA also appeared to predict the transition from latent to clinical disease. In people with advanced RHD, co-regulated production of IL-6 and TNF-α is associated with severe valvular dysfunction.

Genome-wide association studies (GWAS) have been the most significant development in the field of RHD genetics. When single-nucleotide polymorphism (SNP) distributions in patients and selected controls are compared, GWAS can evaluate a large number of gene variants in complicated disorders.

Group A carbohydrate, N-acetyl-β-D-glucosamine-specific immunoglobulin G2 (IgG2) may be an important autoantibody in initial stages of the pathogenesis of streptococcal sequelae, emerging as a future candidate for a biomarker in early disease stages.

ADVANCES IN MANAGEMENT

Primordial Prevention

A number of factors, including ventilation, wetness, and home quality, are linked to a 1.7–3.6-fold greater risk of infection. These factors include household crowding. First-degree relatives of people with clinical RHD may be more likely to have RHD because of their similar socioeconomic circumstances. Primordial prevention approach is being tried in Australia.

Multivalent M protein-based vaccines, M protein vaccines with conserved C-repeat epitopes, cell wall carbohydrate vaccines, and non-M protein multi-component vaccines are possible options for vaccination against GAS, but none have shown encouraging results so far.

Primary Prevention

Nucleic acid amplification tests (NAATs) like illumigene assay for GAS pharyngitis have been explored and their sensitivity and specificity are estimated to be in excess of 99%, but their use is restricted by high cost.

Electrochemical detection which uses DNA is an affordable and effective method for diagnosing GAS; its results are available in 30 minutes and specificity is nearly 100%.

The Strepic® device (under development), has been especially developed as an effective, affordable, and commercially feasible autofluorescence-based diagnostic test.

Treatment of Group A Strep Pharyngitis

Benzathine Penicillin G is the gold standard for treatment of group A streptococcal infection. Streptococcal carriers are found in many communities, therefore, treatment is recommended only for acute streptococcal infection.

Secondary Prevention

The modified Jones criteria 2015 addressed two significant features: (1) distinguished criteria between low-risk and moderate-to-high risk populations based on ARF incidence or RHD prevalence; and (2) recommending echocardiography to suspected cases of ARF and incorporating subclinical carditis as evidenced by echocardiography as a major criteria.

The GOAL study demonstrated that subsequent antibiotic prophylaxis lowers the risk of disease progression at 2 years in children with latent RHD aged 5–17. This shows that echo screening and active case detection is an effective method for the management of RHD **(Table 2)**.

TABLE 2: Drug treatment of acute rheumatic fever.

Indication	Drug options listed in order of preference	Comment
Eradication of inciting streptococcal infection	• Benzathine benzylpenicillin G 1,200,000 units (child < 20 kg: 600,000 units, ≥ 20 kg: 1,200,000 units) intramuscularly, single dose, OR • Phenoxymethylpenicillin 500 mg (child: 15 mg/kg up to 500 mg) orally, every 12 hours for 10 days, OR • For patients with penicillin hypersensitivity (nonsevere): cefalexin 1 g (child: 25 mg/kg up to 1 g) orally, every 12 hours for 10 days, OR • For patients with immediate penicillin hypersensitivity: azithromycin 500 mg (child: 12 mg/kg up to 500 mg) orally, daily for 5 days	• Streptococcal infection may not be evident by the time acute rheumatic fever manifests (e.g., cultures often negative), but eradication therapy for possible persisting streptococci is recommended • Intramuscular penicillin is preferred as streptococcal eradication therapy due to better adherence and its subsequent ongoing use in secondary prophylaxis • Between 3 and 30% of group A *Streptococcus* isolates internationally are resistant to macrolide antibiotics (e.g., azithromycin)
Initial analgesia while awaiting diagnostic confirmation: • Mild-to-moderate pain • Severe pain	• Paracetamol 1,000 mg (in children: 15 mg/kg) orally, every 4 hours as needed up to a maximum of 60 mg/kg/day or 4,000 mg/day	• Initial analgesia is preferred during diagnostic uncertainty to avoid the masking effect that anti-inflammatory use can have on migratory joint symptoms, fever, and concentrations of inflammatory markers

Continued

Continued

Indication	Drug options listed in order of preference	Comment
	• Tramadol immediate-release 50–100 mg (in children: 1–2 mg/kg) orally, every 4 hours as needed up to a maximum of 400 mg/day	• Tramadol (or codeine) is usually avoided in children < 12 years of age due to variable metabolism. Use only when strong analgesia is essential and cautious monitoring is available
Symptomatic management of arthritis/arthralgia after confirmation of acute rheumatic fever diagnosis	• Naproxen immediate-release 250–500 mg (in children: 10–20 mg/kg/day) orally twice daily, up to a maximum of 1,250 mg daily, OR • Ibuprofen 200–400 mg (in children: 5–10 mg/kg) orally three times daily, up to a maximum of 2,400 mg daily, OR • Aspirin 50–60 mg/kg/day orally, in 4–5 divided doses in adults and children; dose can be escalated up to a maximum of 80–100 mg/kg/day in 4–5 divided doses	• Naproxen may be safer than aspirin and convenient due to twice-daily dosing and the availability of oral suspension • Ibuprofen is well-tolerated and readily available, but there are less data and experience with its use for acute rheumatic fever than those associated with naproxen • The dose of NSAIDs needed for acute rheumatic fever is generally higher than the dose recommended for other conditions; therefore, it may be appropriate to start at the higher dose range • Due to the rare possibility of Reye's syndrome in children, aspirin may need to be discontinued during intercurrent acute viral illness; thus, influenza vaccination is strongly recommended to reduce the likelihood of this case
Symptomatic management of moderate to severe chorea	• Carbamazepine 3.5–10 mg/kg per dose orally twice daily • Sodium valproate 7.5–10 mg/kg per dose orally twice daily	Treatment of Sydenham chorea should be considered if movements interfere substantially with normal activities
Symptomatic management of very severe chorea or chorea paralytica	In addition to an anticonvulsant drug, consider adding a corticosteroid: • Prednisolone 1–2 mg/kg up to a maximum of 80 mg orally once daily	
Symptomatic management of carditis	Pediatric dosing: • Furosemide (frusemide) 1–2 mg/kg orally as a single dose, then 0.5–1 mg/kg (to a maximum of 6 mg/kg) orally every 6–24 hours • Spironolactone 1–3 mg/kg (initially) up to 100 mg orally in divided doses daily; round dose to a multiple of 6.25 mg (a quarter of a 25 mg tablet)	Treatment of heart failure may be required for severe, acute carditis. Seek advice from a specialist cardiologist
	Enalapril 0.1 mg/kg orally in 1 or 2 divided doses daily, increased gradually over 2 weeks to a maximum of 1 mg/kg orally in 1 or 2 divided doses daily; alternative ACE inhibitors: captopril, lisinopril	The choice of ACE inhibitor will vary depending on the clinical situation. Seek advice from a specialist cardiologist
	Adult dosing: • Furosemide (frusemide) 20–40 mg orally or intravenously as a single dose followed by 20–40 mg orally or intravenously every 8–12 hours. Ongoing dose adjustment is based on clinical progression and renal function • Spironolactone may be added for patients with limited or no response to loop diuretic; 12.5–200 mg orally once daily with dose escalation based on clinical and electrolyte responses	The management of acute carditis follows the same principles as those for the management of acute heart failure. This table provides a guide to the initial management of acute heart failure due to acute carditis in adults. Seeking advice from a specialist cardiologist early is strongly recommended

Continued

Continued

Indication	Drug options listed in order of preference	Comment
	• Nitrate therapy may be added for patients with limited or no response to diuretic therapy and systolic blood pressure greater than 90 mmHg. Intravenous or topical glyceryl trinitrate may be used • ACE inhibitor therapy with perindopril or ramipril is recommended in patients with moderate or severe left ventricular systolic dysfunction, unless contraindicated	
Disease-modifying (immunomodulatory) treatments	Prednisolone 1–2 mg/kg up to a maximum of 80 mg orally, once daily	Considered for use in selected cases of severe carditis, despite meta-analyses in which the overall benefit was not evident
Secondary prophylaxis	• Benzathine benzylpenicillin G by deep intramuscular injection 1,200,000 units (≥20 kg) or 600,000 units (<20 kg), OR • Phenoxymethylpenicillin (penicillin V) 250 mg orally twice daily, OR • For patients with penicillin hypersensitivity (nonsevere) or immediate penicillin hypersensitivity: erythromycin 250 mg orally twice daily	• Every 28 days • Every 21 days for selected groups • Intramuscular penicillin is preferred due to greater effectiveness in head-to-head trial and better adherence

(ACE: angiotensin-converting enzyme; NSAIDs: nonsteroidal anti-inflammatory drugs)

SUGGESTED READINGS

1. Carapetis JR, Beaton A, Cunningham MW, Guilherme L, Karthikeyan G, Mayosi BM, et al. Acute rheumatic fever and rheumatic heart disease. Nat Rev Dis Primers. 2016;2:15084.
2. Pandey M, Langshaw E, Hartas J, Lam A, Batzloff MR, Good MF. A Synthetic M Protein Peptide Synergizes with a CXC Chemokine Protease To Induce Vaccine-Mediated Protection against Virulent Streptococcal Pyoderma and Bacteremia. J Immunol. 2015;194:5915-25.
3. Parks T, Smeesters PR, Steer AC. Streptococcal skin infection and rheumatic heart disease. Curr Opin Infect Dis. 2012;25:145-53.
4. Sikder S, Williams NL, Sorenson A, Alim A, E Vidgen M, Moreland N, et al. Group G Streptococcus Induces an Autoimmune Carditis Mediated by Interleukin 17A and Interferon γ in the Lewis Rat Model of Rheumatic Heart Disease. J Infect Dis. 2017;218:324-35.
5. O'Sullivan L, Moreland N, Webb RH, Upton A, Wilson NJ. Acute Rheumatic Fever After Group A Streptococcus Pyoderma and Group G Streptococcus Pharyngitis. Pediatr Infect Dis J. 2017;36:692-4.
6. Sikder S. (2018). Determination of the Role of Group G Streptococcus in the Pathogenesis of Rheumatic Heart Disease Using a Rat Model. Ph.D. Thesis, James Cook University, Douglas, Australia. [online] Available from https://researchonline.jcu.edu.au/56013/ [Last accessed December, 2023].
7. Dooley LM, Ahmad TB, Pandey M, Good MF, Kotiw M. Rheumatic heart disease: A review of the current status of global research activity. Autoimmun Rev. 2020;20:102740.
8. Dinkla K, Talay SR, Mörgelin M, Graham RM, Rohde M, Nitsche-Schmitz DP, et al. Crucial role of the CB3-region of collagen IV in PARF-induced acute rheumatic fever. PLoS One. 2009;4:e4666.
9. Guilherme L, Köhler KF, Kalil J. Rheumatic heart disease: Mediation by complex immune events. Adv Clin Chem. 2011;53:31-50.
10. Guilherme L, Kalil J. Rheumatic Fever and Rheumatic Heart Disease: Cellular Mechanisms Leading Autoimmune Reactivity and Disease. J Clin Immunol. 2010;30:17-23.
11. Auckland K, Mittal B, Cairns BJ, Garg N, Kumar S, Mentzer AJ, et al. The Human Leukocyte Antigen Locus and Rheumatic Heart Disease Susceptibility in South Asians and Europeans. Sci Rep. 2020;10:1-9.
12. Akkaya E, Berkowitsch A, Rieth A, Erkapic D, Hamm CW, Neumann T, et al. Clinical outcome and left atrial function after left atrial roof ablation using the cryoballoon technique in patients with symptomatic persistent atrial fibrillation. Int J Cardiol. 2019;292:112-8.
13. Nascimento B, Beaton A, Guilherme L, Sampaio R,. Rheumatic fever 21st century: clinical and experimental insights. Front Cardiovasc Med. 2023;10:1190372.
14. Wyber R, Noonan K, Halkon C, Enkel S, Cannon J, Haynes E, et al. Ending rheumatic heart disease in Australia: The evidence for a new approach. Med J Aust. 2020;213:S3-S31.
15. Thompson TZ, McMullen AR. Group A streptococcus testing in pediatrics: The move to point-of-care molecular testing. J Clin Microbiol. 2020;58:e01494-19.
16. Malinowska N, Białobrzeska W, Łęga T, Pałka K, Dziąbowska K, Żołędowska S, et al. Antibody Modified Gold Electrode as an Impedimetric Biosensor for the Detection of Streptococcus pyogenes. Sensors. 2020;20:5324.
17. Beaton AZ, Okello E, Rwebembera J, Grobler A, Engelman D, Carapetis J, et al. A Randomized Controlled Trial of Secondary Antibiotic Prophylaxis for Latent Rheumatic Heart Disease. Circulation. 2021;144:A12503.
18. Ralph AP, Currie BJ. Therapeutics for rheumatic fever and rheumatic heart disease. Aust Prescr. 2022;45:104-12.

3

CHAPTER

Evaluation of Chest Pain: Cardiologist's View

Amal Kumar Banerjee

ABSTRACT

Chest pain is one of the most common reasons, for which people seek medical care. It is the most challenging condition to evaluate and to rapidly identify the small number of patients who have acute coronary syndrome (ACS) or other life-threatening conditions among the large number who have more benign conditions, many of which are noncardiac. The electrocardiography (ECG) is critical for the initial assessment. Patients with a nonischemic ECG should undergo rapid risk assessment and exclusion of ACS and patients classified as low risk based on high-sensitive cardiac troponin T (hs-cTn) assay, can generally be discharged directly from the emergency department (ED) without additional testing. Patients with substantially elevated initial hs-cTn values or those who have significant dynamic changes over 1–3 hours are stratified as abnormal/high-risk category and should be further classified. High-risk patients should usually be admitted to an inpatient setting for further evaluation and treatment. Intermediate-risk group should undergo additional observation with repeat hs-cTn measurements at 3–6 hours and risk assessment, and noninvasive tests should be considered.

INTRODUCTION

Chest pain is a common complaint and encompasses a broad differential diagnosis that includes several life-threatening causes, and it is one of the most common reasons for emergency department (ED) visits. An urgent workup must focus on ruling in the small number of patients who have acute coronary syndrome (ACS) or other life-threatening conditions among the large number who have more benign conditions, many of which are noncardiac.

CAUSES OF ACUTE CHEST PAIN

Most common causes of acute cardiovascular chest pain with important distinguishing clinical features have been shown in **Table 1**.

INITIAL EVALUATION

The initial clinical evaluation **(Flowchart 1)** of a patient with acute chest pain should focus on rapid identification and treatment of patients with life-threatening conditions such as ACS, aortic dissection, and pulmonary embolism. Patients who are hemodynamically unstable, have significant arrhythmias, or have evidence of significant heart failure should be evaluated and treated appropriately.

The term chest pain is embedded in clinical use, but chest discomfort is more accurate.

Clinical assessment should include the chest pain description and associated symptoms, onset, duration, location, radiation, and precipitating and relieving factors. In addition, a detailed assessment of cardiovascular risk factors and medical, family, and social history should complement the assessment of presenting symptoms. There are no physical examination findings specific for coronary ischemia; thus, the examination should be targeted to identify findings associated with high risk for morbidity and mortality in ACS, or to the presence of potential alternative diagnoses. High-risk examination findings include signs of low cardiac output such as tachycardia, hypotension, cool extremities, low urine output, and altered mental status; heart failure with

TABLE 1: Common causes of acute cardiovascular chest pain.

System	Syndrome	Clinical features	Distinguishing features
Cardiac	Angina	Retrosternal chest pressure, burning or heaviness; radiating occasionally to neck, jaw, epigastrium, shoulders, and left arm	Precipitated by exercise, cold or emotional stress lasting for 2–10 minutes
	Rest or unstable angina	Same as angina, may be more severe	Typically, <20 minutes, lower tolerance for exertion; crescendo pattern
	AMI	Same as angina, may be more severe	Sudden onset, usually lasting ≥20 minutes; often associated with shortness of breath, weakness, nausea, and vomiting
	Pericarditis	Sharp pleuritic pain aggravated by changes in position, highly variable duration	Pericardial friction rub
Vascular	Aortic dissection	Excruciating ripping pain of sudden onset in anterior aspect of chest, often radiating to back	Marked severity of unrelenting pain usually occurs in hypertension or underlying connective tissue disorder such as Marfan syndrome
	Pulmonary embolism	Sudden onset of dyspnea and pain, usually pleuritic with pulmonary infarction	Dyspnea, tachypnea, tachycardia signs of right-sided heart failure
	Pulmonary hypertension	Substernal chest pressure, exacerbated by exertion	Pain associated with dyspnea and signs of pulmonary hypertension

pulmonary edema, elevated jugular venous pressure, and peripheral edema, and a new systolic murmur concerning for acute mitral regurgitation or a ventricular septal defect. Clues to non-ACS cause for the patient's symptoms include fever (endocarditis, pneumonia), pulse differential in aortic dissection, abnormal lung findings in pneumonia, pneumothorax; and abnormal cardiac findings such as a pericardial friction rub (pericarditis) or other murmurs (aortic stenosis, outflow tract obstruction, and endocarditis).

A chest X-ray should be performed in almost all patients with possible ACS, given the potential to identify high-risk findings such as pulmonary edema and potential noncardiac causes.

An electrocardiography (ECG) is the key for the initial assessment and management of patients with potential ACS and should be performed and interpreted within 10 minutes of arrival at the ED. In patients with chest pain in which an initial ECG is nondiagnostic, serial ECGs to detect potential ischemic changes should be performed. The ECG should also be examined for subtle changes that are also consistent with ACS as well as for other findings that could suggest a non-ACS cause for their symptoms.

In patients presenting with acute chest pain, serial cardiac troponin (cTn) I or T levels are useful to identify abnormal values and a rising or falling pattern indicative of acute myocardial injury. In patients presenting with acute chest pain, high-sensitivity cTn (hs-cTn) is the preferred biomarker because it enables more rapid detection or exclusion of myocardial injury and increases diagnostic accuracy. Clinicians should be familiar with the analytical performance and the 99th percentile upper reference limit that defines myocardial injury for the cTn assay used at their institution. In patients with chest pain and nonischemic ECG, myocardial infraction (MI) is ruled out if initial hs-cTnI < 5 ng/L or hs-cTnT < 6 ng/L (if >3 hours from symptom onset) or if change from initial to 3-h hs-cTn is <3 ng/L and remains below sex-specific 99th percentile upper reference level (URL). Detectable values represent a continuum of risk for adverse events; thus, no detectable cTn level can be considered normal. Sex-specific 99th percentile cutoffs are endorsed to increase sensitivity for diagnosis of MI among women and specificity among men.

Many risk scores have been used for ED chest pain evaluation. The HEART score and EDACS pathway **(Table 2)**, which use readily available clinical data and the clinician's interpretation of the history, to risk stratify patients. Suspected ACS patients with serial conventional cTn values < the 99th percentile URL and nonischemic ECGs, a low HEART score ≤ 3 or EDACS < 16 can identify patients eligible for discharge without a requirement for further diagnostic testing. Patients with intermediate- or high-risk scores, elevated cTn concentrations, ischemic ECGs, or high suspicion for unstable angina should undergo further diagnostic testing. The EDACS and the HEART score are the best validated strategies and identify the largest number of patients as low risk using conventional cTn assays.

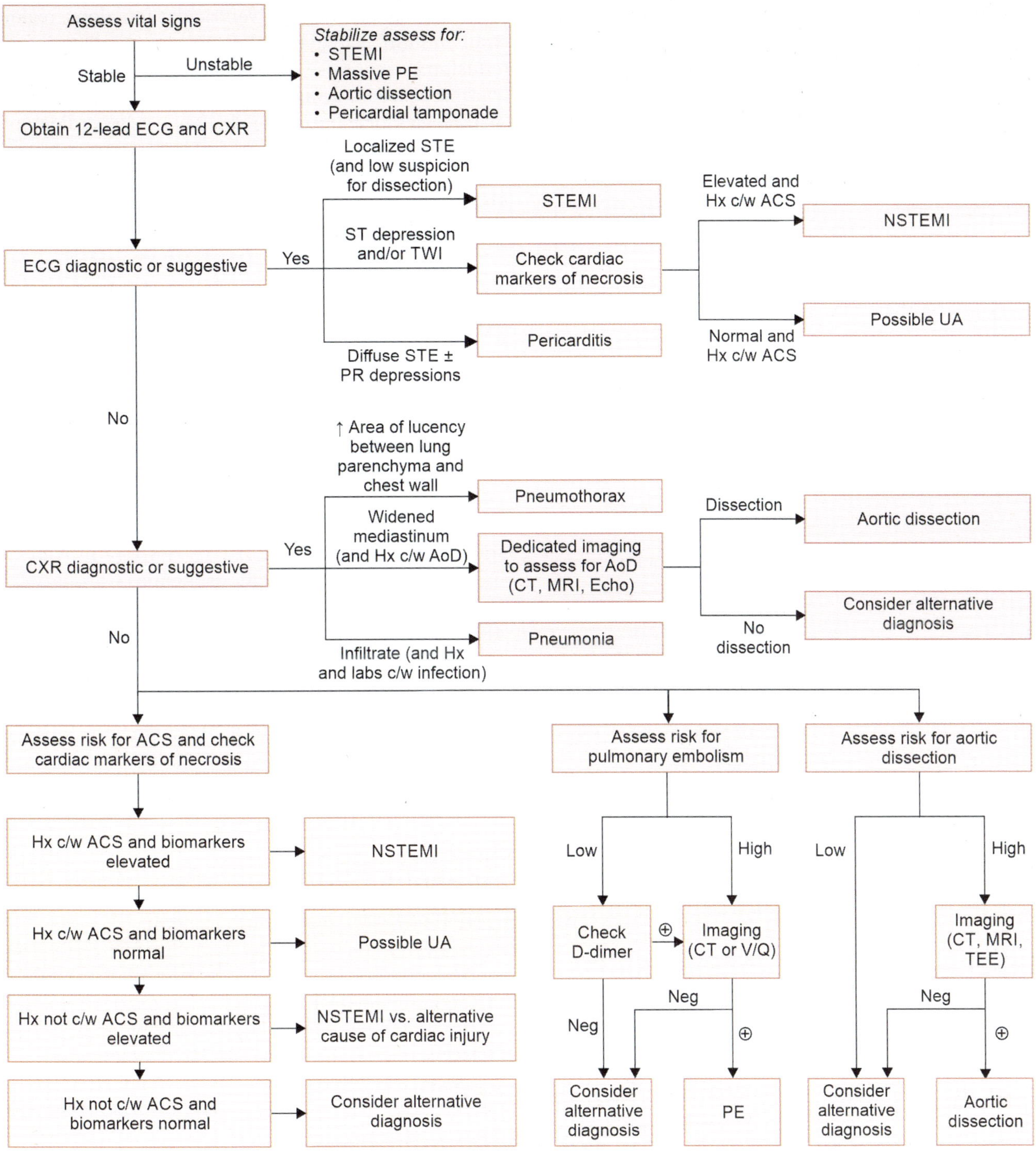

FLOWCHART 1: The initial diagnostic approach to a patient with chest pain.

(ACS: acute coronary syndrome; AoD: aortic dissection; c/w: consistent with; CXR: chest X-ray; CT: computed tomography; ECG: electrocardiography; Hx: history; MRI: magnetic resonance imaging; NSTEMI: non-ST-elevation myocardial infarction; PE: pulmonary embolism; STE: ST-segment elevation; TEE: transesophageal echocardiography; TWI: T-wave inversion; UA: unstable angina; V/Q : ventilation perfusion scan)

The intermediate risk patients have minimally elevated hs-cTn or hs-cTn above the 99th percentile URL but below the abnormal/high-risk threshold, with no or only minor changes in the cT concentration over the serial measurements. Given the increased risk for an index MI diagnosis and 30-day major adverse cardiac events in the intermediate risk group, further monitoring is recommended, and diagnostic testing may be needed.

TABLE 2: HEART scores and EDACS data components.

HEART score components ***Low risk*: 0–3 points** ***Non-low risk*: ≥4 points**		**EDACS components** ***Low risk*: 0–15 points** ***Non-low risk*: ≥16 points**	
History		*Age, years*	
High suspicion	2	18–45	2
Moderate suspicion	1	46–50	4
Low suspicion	0	51–55	6
ECG		56–60	8
ST-segment deviation	2	61–65	10
Paced, LBBB, RBBB, or LVH	1	66–70	12
Normal or nonspecific changes	0	71–75	14
Age, years		76–80	16
>65	2	81–85	18
45–65	1	86+	20
<45	0	Male sex	6
Cardiac risk factors		Age 18–55 and either ≥3 cardiac risk factors or known CAD	4
≥3 or known CAD	2	Diaphoresis	3
1–2	1	Pain radiating to arm or shoulder	5
	00	Pain worsened with inspiration	–4
		Pain reproduced by palpation	–6

(CAD: coronary artery disease; ECG: electrocardiography; LBBB: left bundle branch block; LVH: left ventricular hypertrophy; RBBB: right bundle branch block)

FURTHER EVALUATION: NONINVASIVE CARDIOVASCULAR DIAGNOSTIC TESTING

The diagnostic evaluation of patients with acute chest pain is the accurate risk stratification into low-, intermediate-, or high-risk groups to allow for appropriate diagnostic and therapeutic treatments. Low-risk patients have a very low event rate and can usually be discharged directly from the ED without additional in-hospital testing. The high-risk patients should usually be admitted, and appropriate therapies should be initiated for STEMI/NONSTEMI. The primary role of further noninvasive cardiac testing is for the evaluation of patients stratified as at intermediate risk.

Transthoracic Echocardiography

Bedside transthoracic echocardiography (TTE) can aid in the diagnostic evaluation of patients with acute chest pain by assessing left and right ventricular functions, regional wall motion, valvular abnormalities, and pericardial effusion. Prompt use of TTE allows for an evaluation of cardiac cause for symptoms and evaluation of alternative pathologies for acute chest pain. Rapid echocardiographic assessment may facilitate imaging of patients while they are symptomatic. Point-of-care echocardiograms performed by properly trained clinicians and technicians may be particularly useful.

CORONARY COMPUTED TOMOGRAPHY ANGIOGRAPHY

Coronary computed tomography angiography (CTA) is an accurate, noninvasive method for the diagnosis of coronary artery disease (CAD). It can visualize and help to diagnose the extent and severity of nonobstructive and obstructive CAD, as well as atherosclerotic plaque composition and high-risk features such as positive remodeling and low attenuation plaque. Calculation of fractional flow reserve with CT (FFR-CT) provides an estimation of lesion-specific ischemia. Coronary CTA is also effective as a gatekeeper to invasive coronary angiography in patients with inconclusive ischemia tests. Coronary calcium scoring may be performed. Nonobstructive CAD, identified by CTA, may be unrelated to the patient's presentation but carries important long-term prognostic and preventive treatment implications, identifying patients with unsuspected atherosclerosis who would benefit from aggressive risk factor modification and treatment.

ISCHEMIA TESTING

Tests that assess myocardial ischemia as a marker of clinically relevant CAD include exercise ECG testing without imaging and exercise or pharmacologic rest/stress ECG combined with imaging, using echocardiography, single-photon emission computed tomography, positron emission tomography, and cardiac magnetic resonance imaging. Majority of patients with acute chest pain at intermediate risk are likely to require stress testing with imaging, given the high frequency of known coronary disease, heart failure, and other comorbidities that limit the diagnostic utility of exercise ECG alone.

Assessment of coronary artery calcium (CAC) burden using the Angaston calcium score or visual description like none, mild, moderate, severe, should be included in nuclear stress test reports such as single-photon emission computed tomography, positron emission tomography, if CT attenuation testing or dedicated CAC scoring is routinely performed by nuclear testing laboratories. Such information may assist in risk stratification, decision-making in the case of equivocal stress test findings or artifacts, and post-testing use of preventive therapies.

Invasive Coronary Angiography

Invasive coronary angiography (ICA) defines the presence and severity of a luminal obstruction of an epicardial coronary artery, including its location, length, and diameter, as well as coronary blood flow. For ICA, the primary goal is the characterization and detection of a high-grade obstructive stenosis to define feasibility and necessity of percutaneous or surgical revascularization. The use of physiologic indices (IFR and FFR) provides complementary functional information.

CONCLUSION

A systematic approach is essential to achieve optimal outcomes for patients presenting with chest pain to the ED. Although, most patients will not have a cardiac cause, the evaluation of all patients should focus on the early identification or exclusion of life-threatening causes. Early evaluation includes careful ECG review. hs-cTns are the preferred standard to rule-in or rule-out myocardial injury. For appropriate patients, combination of hs-cTn measurements with risk assessment and selective use of noninvasive testing are necessary.

SUGGESTED READINGS

1. Gulati M, Levy PD, Mukherjee D, Amsterdam E, Bhatt DL, Birtcher KK, et al. 2021 AHA/ACC/ASE/CHEST/SAEM/SCCT/SCMR Guideline for the evaluation and diagnosis of chest pain: A report of the American College of Cardiology/American Heart Association Joint Committee on Clinical Practice Guidelines. J Am Coll Cardiol. 2021;78: e187-285.
2. Writing Committee; Kontos MC, de Lemos JA, Deitelzweig SB, Diercks DB, M Gore O, Hess EP, et al. 2022 ACC Expert Consensus Decision Pathway on the Evaluation and Disposition of Acute Chest Pain in the Emergency Department. A Report of the American College of Cardiology Solution Set Oversight Committee. J Am Coll Cardiol. 2022;80(20):1925-60.

4

CHAPTER

Metabolic Modulation in Management of Angina: What is New?

Sajid Ansari

ABSTRACT

Ischemic heart disease (IHD) and chronic stable angina significantly impact patients' prognosis, quality of life, and healthcare costs. Despite the availability of conventional medications, research is focusing on improving IHD management through metabolic modulation. This approach is particularly promising due to its involvement in the disease's progression through energy metabolism alterations. Traditional treatments, such as beta-blockers, calcium channel blockers, and nitroglycerin, have been ineffective in treating this subgroup of patients. Emerging research suggests that myocardial ischemia, a key factor in IHD, can be triggered by various mechanisms, such as coronary stenosis, coronary vasospasm, microvascular dysfunction, and mitochondrial dysfunction. A comprehensive approach targeting multiple mechanisms, such as targeting cardiac myocytes, protecting them from ischemic damage, and modulating myocardial metabolism, may be more effective in enhancing cardiac efficiency and improving long-term outcomes. Metabolic agents can be considered as a complementary or alternative therapy when conventional antianginal medications are not suitable due to intolerance or contraindications.

INTRODUCTION

While cardiovascular mortality has been on a progressive decline in developed nations, the impact of ischemic heart disease (IHD) and chronic stable angina on patients' prognosis, quality of life, and healthcare costs remains significant. Despite the availability of conventional medications, their limitations and the presence of medication-refractory patients have prompted ongoing scientific research aimed at advancing IHD management. These endeavors hold great promise for the development of improved treatment modalities that can enhance patients' quality of life. Among the strategies being explored, metabolic modulation stands out as a particularly promising approach due to its involvement in the disease's progression through energy metabolism alterations. Thus, the objective of this review is to draw attention to the use of metabolic modulators in the management of angina and provide an overview of the current understanding of cardiac energy metabolic pathways.

The traditional approach to treating IHD focused on improving symptoms by increasing oxygen supply and reducing oxygen demand. Current guidelines recommend the use of pharmacological agents such as beta-blockers, calcium channel blockers, and nitroglycerin alone or in combination, in addition to percutaneous coronary intervention (PCI). However, despite the success of PCI and medical therapy, clinical trial data reveal that approximately one-third of individuals continue to experience angina. This subgroup of patients either does not qualify for or does not respond to conventional treatments. Additionally, numerous experiments focused on the treatment of chronic stable angina and revascularization have not demonstrated advantages in terms of primary outcomes such as survival, cardiovascular death, or all-cause mortality. Furthermore, there is no evidence of significant improvements in symptom relief or echocardiographic parameters in these trials.

New research indicates that myocardial ischemia, a critical element in IHD, may be initiated by diverse mechanisms, including coronary stenosis, coronary vasospasm, microvascular dysfunction, and mitochondrial dysfunction. Consequently, a holistic approach to treating IHD, addressing multiple mechanisms such as safeguarding cardiac myocytes from ischemic damage and regulating myocardial metabolism, could emerge as a more effective treatment strategy. This approach has the potential to enhance cardiac efficiency and improve long-term outcomes. Metabolic modulation emerges as a promising approach in the management IHD, as a compromised energy supply to the heart not only hampers its energy sources but also plays a pivotal role in progression of the disease. This approach assumes a pivotal role in the acute phase of ischemic events, impacting the results of immediate interventions and shaping the subsequent development of heart failure (HF), as well as the conditions of stunned and hibernated myocardium, alongside chronic stable angina.

Shifting cardiac metabolism from reliance on free fatty acids (FFAs) to glucose presents a promising therapeutic approach for individuals with stable angina, regardless of the specific underlying disease, whether it involves macrovascular, microvascular, or a combination of both. The use of metabolic modulators for the heart contributes to a deeper understanding of IHD and its prevalent clinical manifestations. This perspective frames the condition as an energy-related disorder rather than just an imbalance between the demand and supply of oxygen and metabolites.

Metabolic agents offer a practical recommendation, either in conjunction with or as an alternative to traditional antianginal agents, particularly when challenges arise due to intolerance or contraindications. Clinical trials consistently demonstrate their effectiveness in patients experiencing refractory angina, chronic IHD, and those subjected to ischemia–reperfusion injury. Furthermore, in individuals with HF, metabolic agents play a pivotal role in slowing the progression of the disease and improving overall prognosis. Given that both failing and ischemic hearts operate as energy-starved organs relying on inefficient fatty acid oxidation, these metabolic agents facilitate a crucial transition in substrate utilization, optimizing the heart's efficiency in oxygen consumption.

HEART METABOLISM IN HEALTH AND DURING ISCHEMIA

The heart has a high energy demand but little energy reserves and therefore continually produces a large amount of adenosine triphosphate (ATP). It uses FFAs mainly and carbohydrates to some extent as energy sources. Alterations in cardiac metabolism are a major contributor to a number of heart diseases, and optimizing energy metabolism in the heart is an important approach to treatment.

Cellular function heavily depends on the consumption of oxygen by mitochondria to generate energy. Under normal physiological conditions, mitochondria maintain a homeostatic balance of metabolic and cellular ions, which is crucial for ensuring proper functioning. However, any deviation from this balanced state can result in an accumulation of mitochondrial Ca^{2+} and increased oxidative stress. This oxidative stress can cause damage to mitochondrial membranes, enzymes, and components of the electron transport chain (ETC), ultimately impairing ATP production. Additionally, it can trigger the opening of permeability transition pores, leading to cellular apoptosis and necrosis. The myocardium, in particular, requires a substantial and continuous supply of ATP derived from the breakdown of carbohydrates and fatty acids to meet its energy demands.

A healthy heart primarily obtains majority of its energy through the FFA pathway, accounting for approximately two-thirds of ATP production. The remaining energy is derived from glucose oxidation (via the glycolysis pathway) and lactate. A healthy heart possesses the capability to dynamically adjust substrate usage, a process influenced by factors such as substrate availability, overall nutritional status, and levels of physical activity. In instances of mild-to-moderate cardiac ischemia, myocardial cells respond by increasing glucose uptake to generate sufficient ATP, ensuring the preservation of ionic gradients and calcium homeostasis. Paradoxically, during prolonged and severe ischemia, the myocardium continues to primarily use beta-oxidation for energy production, even with an elevated rate of lactate production. In this state, heightened rates of fatty acid oxidation impede glucose oxidation through a competitive interaction, known as the Randle mechanism. Although the complete oxidation of fatty acids produces more ATP than the complete oxidation of glucose, it requires a greater amount of oxygen. Consequently, for a given oxygen consumption, glucose metabolism is considered 'oxygen sparing' compared to fatty acid metabolism, yielding approximately 15% more ATP. Consequently, in scenarios with limited oxygen availability, fatty acid oxidation imposes an adverse effect on cells by necessitating more oxygen, producing less ATP, and elevating reactive oxygen species (ROS) levels. This amplifies the compromise in mitochondrial respiratory efficiency. These metabolic shifts contribute to the overall metabolic, morphological, and functional changes in the myocardium, ultimately culminating in arrhythmias and contractile failure. **Figure 1** illustrates the healthy heart's energy generation process, while **Figure 2** portrays the metabolic disruptions occurring during ischemia.

The connection between glycolysis and glucose oxidation is significant due to the correlation between these enzymes and the activity of two survival-promoting membrane-bound pumps: The sodium–potassium ATPase

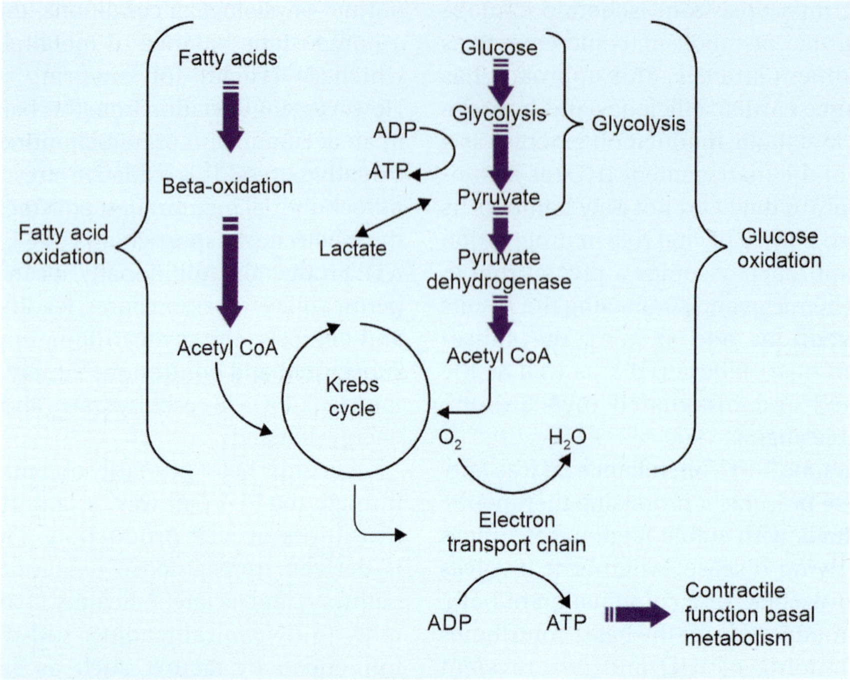

FIG. 1: Cardiac metabolism in normal conditions.

Note: The heart drives most of its energy from the oxidation of fatty acids, but nutritional status (e.g., fasting, substrate availability) as well as exercise and hormones can modify fuel selection.

(ADP: adenosine diphosphate; ATP: adenosine triphosphate; CoA: coenzyme A)

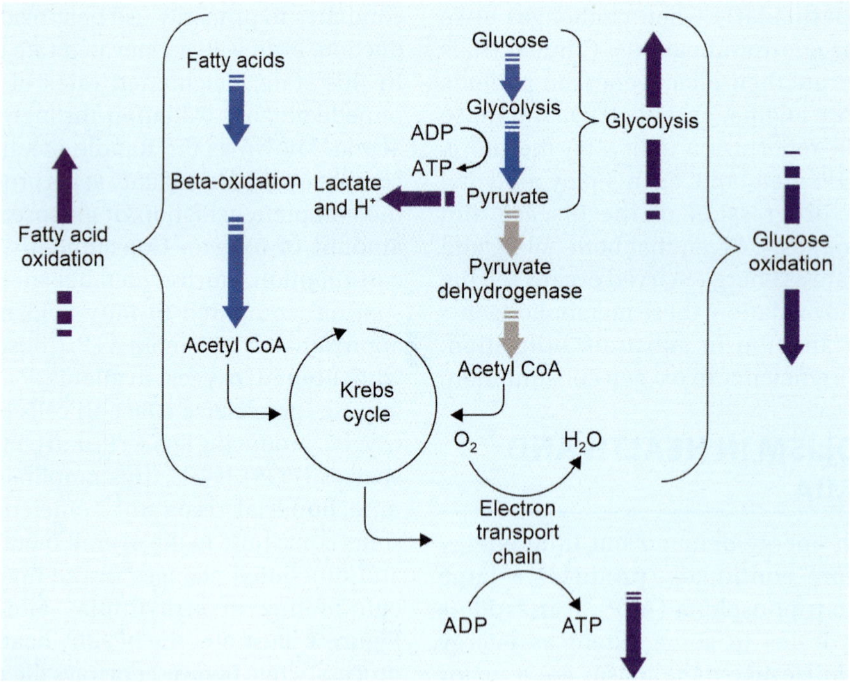

FIG. 2: Metabolic alterations during sustained period of ischemia.

Note: Glycolysis is the main catabolic pathway during ischemia, whereas fatty acid oxidation is enhanced in this period. As a consequence, less ATP is generated at the expense of more protons production, which are ultimately responsible for myocardial acidosis and the accumulation of ions (mainly calcium). Purple arrows: enchanced pathway; pale blue arrows: almost abolished pathways.

(ADP: adenosine diphosphate; ATP: adenosine triphosphate; CoA: coenzyme A) and the calcium uptake pump of the sarcoendoplasmic reticulum (SERCA). This complex interplay underscores the effectiveness of anti-ischemic fatty acid inhibitors, such as trimetazidine (TMZ) and ranolazine (RNZ). Consequently, considerable progress has been achieved in the treatment of stable angina through metabolic therapy, particularly with the introduction of direct inhibitors of myocardial fatty acid oxidation, namely TMZ and RNZ.

CARDIAC METABOLIC MODULATORS

Addressing ischemia, which is fundamentally a metabolic disorder, necessitates a metabolic therapy approach. Since its recognition in 1999, remarkable advancements have occurred. Recognizing the interplay between fatty acid and glucose oxidation, the optimization of energy substrate utilization can be achieved through metabolic modulation therapy. This involves three major strategies: Directly enhancing glucose oxidation, reducing circulating levels of fatty acids and/or their uptake by cardiac myocytes or mitochondria, and directly inhibiting the enzymes involved in fatty acid oxidation.

STRATEGIES TO ENHANCE GLUCOSE OXIDATION

Dichloroacetate

The pyruvate dehydrogenase (PDH) complex, comprising PDH, PDH kinase (PDK), and PDH phosphatase (PDHP) enzymes, regulates the rate-limiting step in glucose oxidation. PDH flux responds to increased glycolysis and heightened pyruvate generation, decreasing in the presence of elevated ratios of mitochondrial nicotinamide adenine dinucleotide ($NADH/NAD^+$) and acetyl-coenzyme A (acetyl CoA/CoA). PDHP dephosphorylates to activate PDH, while PDK phosphorylates to inhibit it. Dichloroacetate improves the coupling of glycolysis and glucose oxidation, reducing proton production by inhibiting PDK activity, and stimulating mitochondrial PDH.

STRATEGIES TO REDUCE CELLULAR/MITOCHONDRIAL FATTY ACID UPTAKE

Carnitine Palmitoyltransferase Inhibitors: Perhexiline

The direct optimization of fatty acid metabolism focuses on the mitochondrial entry of fatty acids. Carnitine palmitoyltransferase 1 (CPT1) is a key enzyme targeted by various pharmacological agents, as it catalyzes the crucial step in the uptake of long-chain fatty acids into mitochondria. Inhibitors of CPT1, such as etomoxir, oxfenicine, and perhexiline, decrease its activity, thereby impeding fatty acid oxidation while promoting glucose oxidation. Another approach to inhibit CPT1 activity and reduce fatty acid uptake involves targeting malonyl CoA decarboxylase (MCD), an enzyme involved in the degradation of malonyl CoA—an influential endogenous reversible inhibitor of CPT1.

Malonyl CoA Decarboxylase Inhibitors

Malonyl CoA serves as a potent endogenous inhibitor of CPT1, effectively decreasing the entry of fatty acids into the mitochondria and subsequently reducing mitochondrial fatty acid beta-oxidation. MCD plays a role in breaking down malonyl CoA, leading to an increase in fatty acid oxidation. Consequently, inhibiting MCD results in a significant elevation of malonyl CoA levels, causing a substantial reduction in fatty acid oxidation rates and, in turn, an increase in glucose oxidation rates.

STRATEGIES TO REDUCE FATTY ACID OXIDATION

Metabolic protection for the ischemic myocardium has attracted increased attention and is supported by clinical studies that affirm the positive effects of fatty acid oxidation inhibitors, such as TMZ and RNZ. These inhibitors are capable of coupling glycolysis to glucose oxidation, contributing to the preservation of metabolic function in the ischemic heart.

3-ketoacyl-CoA Thiolase Inhibitors (Trimetazidine)

Inhibitors of 3-ketoacyl-CoA thiolase (3-KAT), a novel category of metabolic drugs, can induce a rise in glucose and lactate oxidation while partially inhibiting fatty acid oxidation. This mechanism has demonstrated consistent clinical benefits in patients with IHD.

Trimetazidine functions by specifically inhibiting the long-chain activity of the enzyme acetyl CoA C-acyltransferase, also known as 3-KAT. This enzyme catalyzes the terminal step of fatty acid beta-oxidation, utilizing long-chain 3-ketoacyl CoA as a substrate to generate acetyl CoA. The inhibition of 3-KAT by TMZ implies a release of the inhibition on PDH in the mitochondrial matrix, leading to an increased rate of glucose oxidation. In animal studies, TMZ has been shown to significantly enhance the rate of glucose oxidation while only modestly reducing the rate of fatty acid oxidation.

Numerous clinical studies have demonstrated that TMZ, either alone or in combination with calcium channel blockers, effectively improves symptoms, quality of life, and markers of ischemia on stress tests in patients with chronic stable angina and ischemic cardiomyopathy when used in addition to conventional treatment. Generally, treatment-related adverse effects are mild and well-tolerated, mostly comprising gastrointestinal disturbances such as nausea, vomiting, and minor headaches.

Ranolazine

Ranolazine, a piperazine analog, is a relatively recent anti-ischemic drug that inhibits fatty acid oxidation while promoting the partial oxidation of glucose. Its likely molecular mechanism is associated with the inhibition of the late inward Na^+ channel, which pathologically remains open during adverse stimuli to the myocardium, such as myocardial ischemia, hypertrophy, or oxidative stress. The accumulation of Na^+ inside the cell can lead to significant metabolic, contractile, and electrophysiological issues. The regulation of PDH activity involves PDH kinase and PDHP. PDH kinase phosphorylates the active form of PDH to its inactive form, while PDHP dephosphorylates the inactive form of PDH to its active form. RNZ does not directly affect PDH kinase or phosphatase; instead, it inhibits the beta-oxidation of fatty acids. By inhibiting fatty acid beta-oxidation, there is a reduction in the amount of acetyl-CoA, leading to an increase in the active form of PDH. This, in turn, facilitates carbohydrate oxidation, ultimately shifting myocardial substrate utilization from fatty acids to carbohydrates. This metabolic shift reduces the oxygen requirements of the heart while maintaining cardiac work. An additional benefit of RNZ is that glycolysis remains coupled to pyruvate oxidation, minimizing lactate accumulation. The glucose pathway requires less oxygen for a given level of myocardial work, enhancing oxygen efficiency, which may contribute to its anti-ischemic action. In its immediate-release formulation, RNZ significantly reduces episodes of angina, nitroglycerin usage, and demonstrates notable improvements in exercise duration and time to exercise-elicited myocardial ischemia in patients with stable coronary disease.

Indeed, randomized clinical trials have provided evidence of improved exercise capacity and a reduction in angina episodes in patients with chronic stable angina treated with RNZ. Additionally, in patients undergoing elective coronary angioplasty, RNZ has shown efficacy in reducing periprocedural myocardial infarction (MI). These findings underscore the potential benefits of RNZ in enhancing cardiovascular outcomes and mitigating ischemic events in specific patient populations.

CONCLUSION

Metabolic agents provide a practical recommendation, either in combination with or as an alternative to traditional antianginal agents, particularly when there are issues with tolerability or contraindications. Clinical trials have confirmed their effectiveness, especially in patients with refractory angina, chronic IHD, and those facing ischemia-reperfusion injury. Additionally, in individuals with HF, metabolic agents have shown the ability to slow down the progression of the disease and improve prognosis. Both failing and ischemic hearts experience energy deficiency, relying on inefficient fatty acid oxidation. Metabolic agents facilitate a transition in substrate utilization, making the heart more efficient in oxygen consumption. This shift contributes to improved oxygen efficiency in the heart, a crucial aspect for both ischemic and failing hearts. IHD and HF patients require multifactorial approach to improve their symptoms and quality of life. Metabolic agents such as TMZ and/or RNZ offer an attractive option to improve symptoms and quality of life. Addition of such metabolic drugs needs to be initiated early to provide optimal benefits, including quality and quantity of life of patients.

SUGGESTED READINGS

1. Guarini G, Huqi A, Morrone D, Capozza PFG, Marzilli M. Trimetazidine and Other Metabolic Modifiers. Eur Cardiol. 2018;13(2):104-11.
2. Yehualashet AS, Belchew TF, Kifle ZD, Abebe AM. Targeting Cardiac Metabolic Pathways: A Role in Ischemic Management. Vasc Health Risk Manag. 2020;16:353-65.
3. Pradhan AK. Metabolic management of heart disease. J Pract Cardiovasc Sci. 2016;2(3):157-62.
4. Ferrari R, Camici PG, Crea F, Danchin N, Fox K, Maggioni AP, et al. A 'diamond' approach to personalized treatment of angina. 2018;15:120-32.

5

CHAPTER

Coronary Physiology in Management of Coronary Artery Disease

M Jawahar Farook, Sahubar Sadiq

ABSTRACT

Coronary angiography remains common mode of quantifying coronary arterial stenosis. However, it is limited by two-dimensional assessment of a three-dimensional structure. Intravascular imaging provides the estimation of atheroma burden. There is usually a disconnect between anatomical appearance and flow limitation. Physiological indices not only determine flow limitation caused by stenosis but also provide potential value of revascularization. Coronary flow is major determinator of ischemia and measuring coronary flow by coronary flow reserve (CFR), fractional flow reserve (FFR), instantaneous wave-free ratio (IFR), and index of microvascular resistance (IMR) is the ultimate aim of all physiological indices in the management of coronary artery disease (CAD). FFR measured noninvasively using computed tomography (CT) coronary angiography also provides physiological information about lesion specific ischemia similar to invasive techniques.

INTRODUCTION

Coronary circulation represents 5% of the total cardiac output. Due to its constant work resting oxygen demand is high and extraction of oxygen by myocardium is close to its maximum to reduce venous saturation up to 20%. Coronary circulation can only meet oxygen demand by fine tuning of myocardial flow. Coronary autoregulation occurs by mechanism of hyperemia in improving the coronary perfusion pressure depending on myocardial oxygen demand. Stenosis alters the pressure and flow. Severity of perfusion defect depends on pressure, volume, and microvascular resistance in the coronary circulation. There is constant relationship between coronary pressure gradient and coronary flow velocity which can be measured to assess myocardial ischemia in the management of coronary artery disease (CAD).

INDICES OF MYOCARDIAL ISCHEMIA

- Coronary flow reserve (CFR)
- Fractional flow reserve (FFR)
- Instantaneous wave-free ratio (IFR)
- Index of microvascular resistance (IMR)
- Newer indices

Coronary Flow Reserve

Coronary flow reserve is derived from ratio of maximum hyperemic flow (Q_{max}) to baseline coronary blood flow ($Q_{baseline}$)

$$\text{CFR Doppler} = Q_{max}/Q_{baseline}$$

Volumetric blood flow in a given vessel can be derived from the product of the vessel surface area and blood flow velocity. As a result Q can be substituted for the vessel surface area and velocity.

$$\text{CFR Doppler} = (SA \times V_{max})/(SA \times V_{baseline})$$

Assuming a constant surface area CFR can be measured from ratio of hyperemic blood flow to baseline blood flow velocity.

$$\text{CFR Doppler} = V_{max}/V_{baseline}$$

Coronary flow reserve also can be measured by indicator thermodilution techniques

$$\text{CFR thermo} = \text{Baseline Tmn}/\text{Maximal Tmn}$$
(mean transit time)

Normal CFR is 2 and below which major adverse cardiovascular event (MACE) rate increases by 6–9%.

However, flow is difficult to assess in daily practice and there is no definite cut of value. It does not differentiate between the relative contribution of epicardial and microvascular compartment toward change in blood flow, susceptible to hemodynamic influences and it has poor reproducibility.

Fractional Flow Reserve—Pressure as a Surrogate of Flow

Fractional flow reserve is the ratio of maximal myocardial flow in the presence of stenosis to normal myocardial flow.

$$\text{Pressure gradient} = \text{Blood flow} \times \text{Resistance}$$

$$\text{Delta P} = Q \times R$$

If resistance is constant,

$$\text{Pressure} = \text{Flow}$$

By using pharmacological hyperemia,

$$\text{FFR} = Pd/Pa$$

Fractional flow reserve is well-defined with normal value of 1.0, well-defined ischemic threshold of 0.8 take in to account collateral flow. It accounts for the extent of the effective perfusion territory and is extremely reproducible. It is not influenced by hemodynamic changes. Valued in almost all clinical conditions and lesion subsets, it has unsurpassed spatial resolution. FFR has constant relationship to clinical outcomes to decide and defer percutaneous coronary intervention (PCI) in management of CAD. There is 35–96% discordance between angio and FFR.

The DEFER trial has shown that we can safely defer PCI when FFR is >0.75. FAME 1 (Fractional Flow Reserve Versus Angiography for Multivessel Evaluation 1) trial has shown that treating lesion with FFR > 0.8 with drug-eluting stent (DES) is harmful. FAME 2 trial has shown that when FFR is <0.8 deferring PCI is harmful. Between 0.75 and 0.8 is gray zone. FAME 3 has shown that in multivessel disease coronary artery bypass grafting (CABG) is superior to FFR-guided PCI. **(Figs. 1 to 3)**. DEFER trial 15 years' outcome data and FAME trial 5 years' outcome data has shown that FFR-guided PCI has long-term safety in management of CAD.

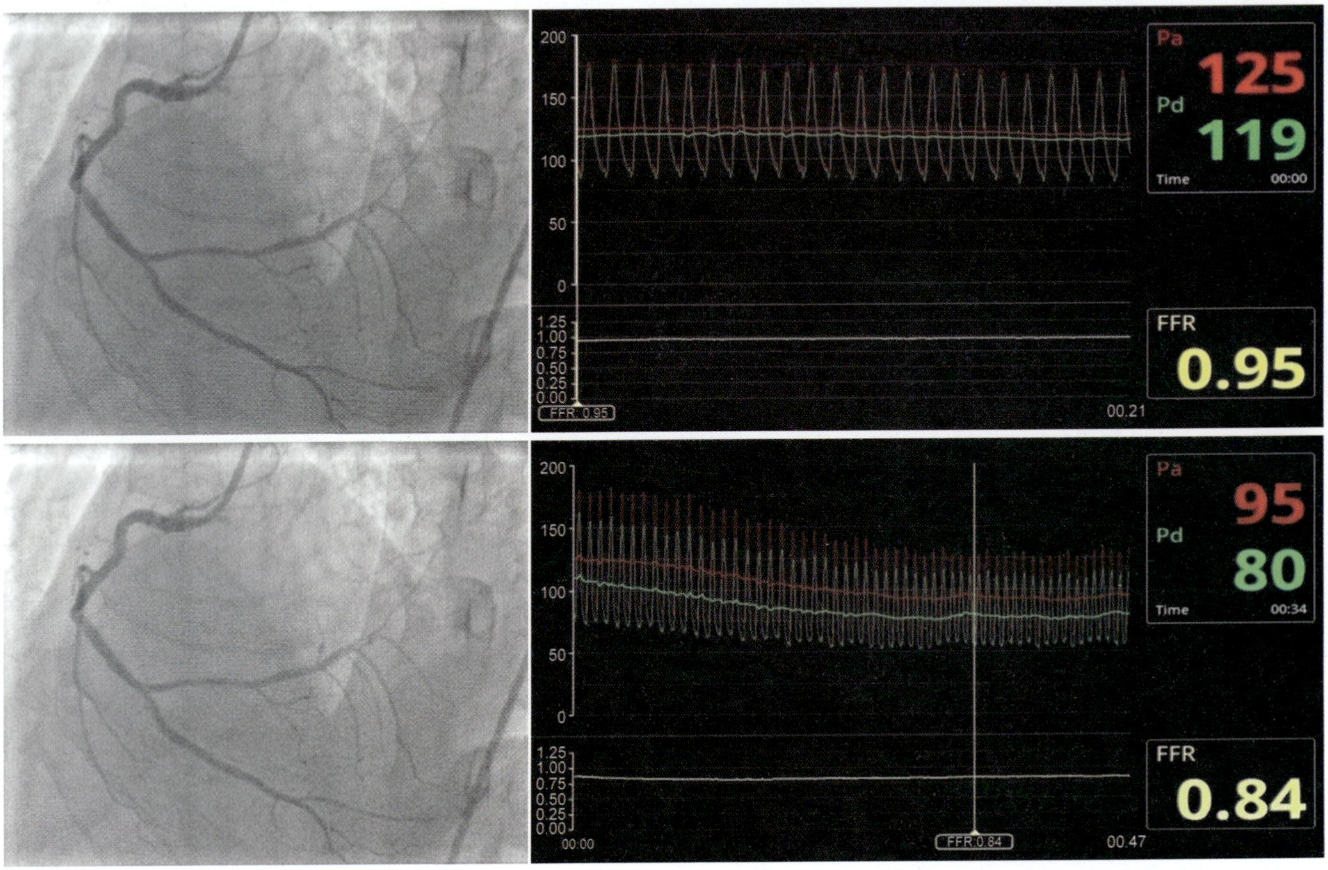

FIG. 1: Right coronary artery (RCA) angio shows 80% stenosis and fractional flow reserve (FFR) negative.

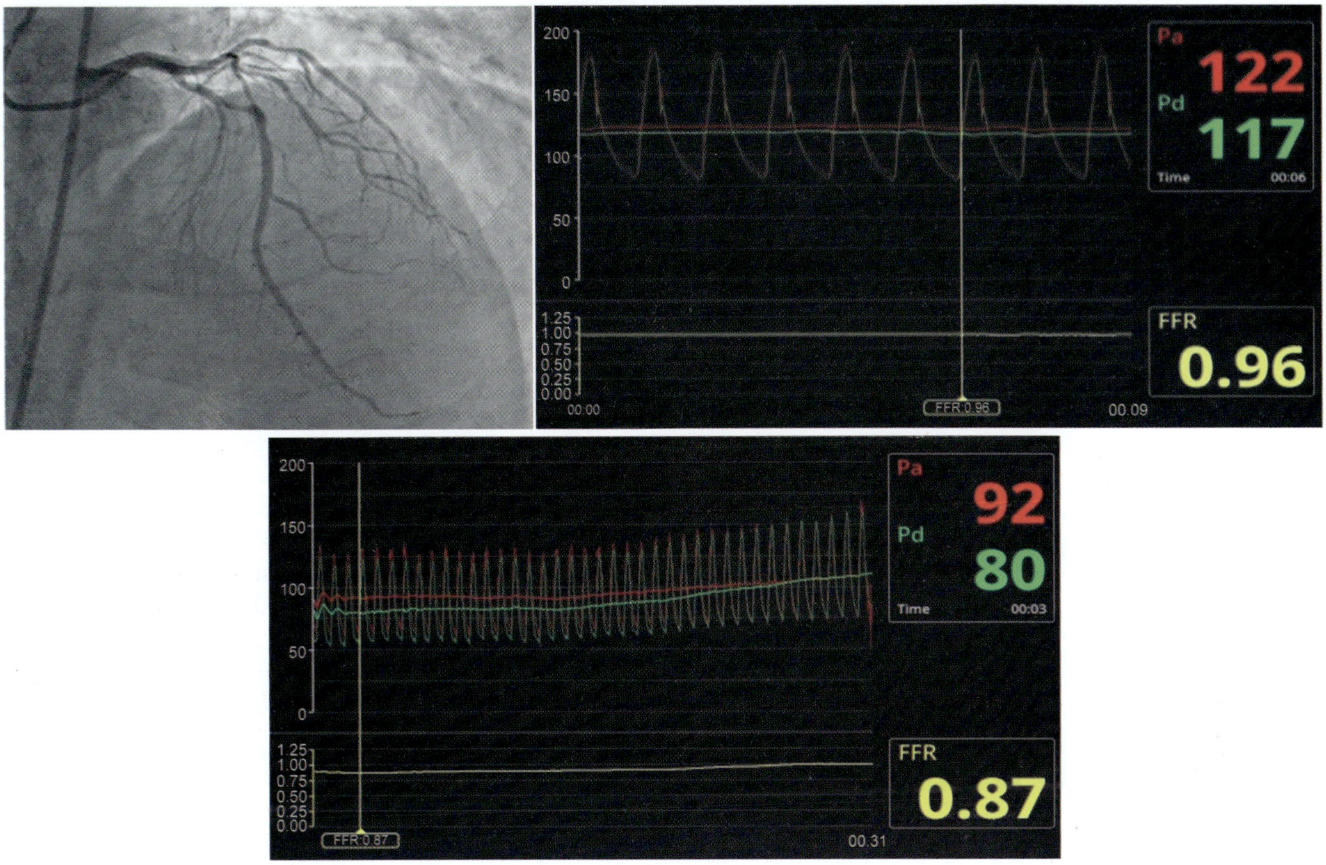

FIG. 2: Left anterior descending (LAD) angio shows 70% stenosis and fractional flow reserve (FFR) negative.

Resting Index of Coronary Physiology

Instantaneous Wave-free Ratio

IFR = Pd wave-free period/Pa wave-free period

where, Pd is pressure distal to stenosis and Pa is the aortic pressure. Wave-free period during which resistance is negligible.

The FFR and IFR use the pressure as a surrogate of flow. IFR is noninferior to FFR and it is resting index of coronary blood flow. IFR results in less frequent revascularization with similar MACE rate. IFR is associated with less incidence of patient discomfort and short procedure time. IFR may better predict ischemia in nonculprit acute coronary syndrome (ACS) lesion and *tandem* lesions. IFR may reflect flow better than FFR. Microvascular resistance may be the main determinant of IFR and FFR discordance.

The SWEDHEART and DEFINEFLAIR trials have shown that IFR is noninferior to FFR and better tolerated with no side effects. IFR with angio co-registration is called virtual angioplasty and it is possible to get better long-term outcome related to stents and devices leaving nonischemic coronary segments for medical management (**Figs. 4 to 6**).

Index of Microvascular Resistance

Index of microvascular resistance is a quantitative evaluation of coronary microcirculatory function which provides significant reference for prediction, diagnosis, treatment, and prognosis of CAD.

IMR = Pd × Tmn at maximal hyperemia which is measured by thermodilution technique.

Index of microvascular resistance of <20 is normal and >30 is elevated. Elevated IMR predicts early and late mortality in stable and unstable CAD.

Multivariate analysis has shown that IMR >40 was only independent predictor of infarct size >25% on cardiovascular magnetic resonance (CMR) at 6 months. Higher mortality at long-term follow-up is predicted by elevated IMR after ST-segment elevation myocardial infarction (STEMI).

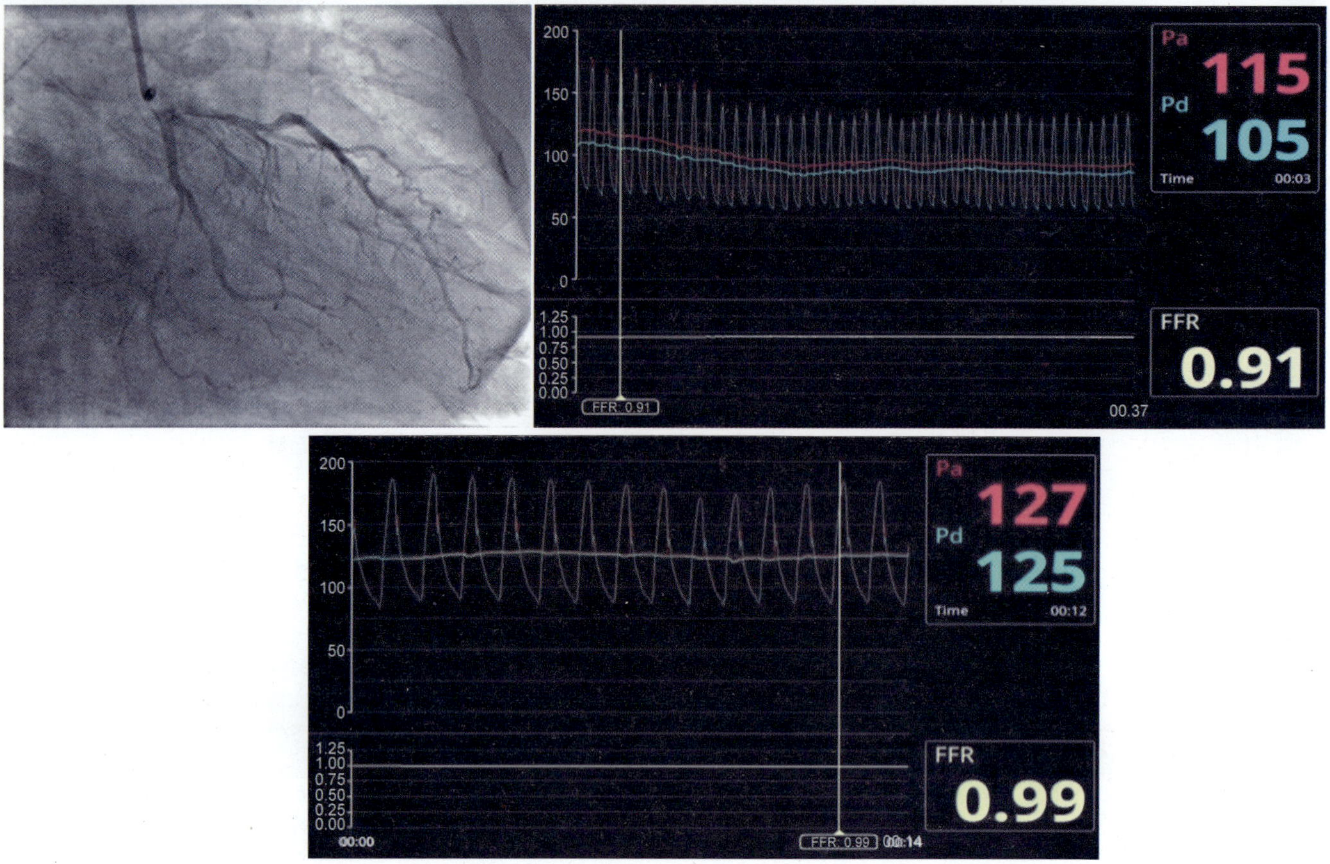

FIG. 3: Left circumflex (LCX) angio shows 90% stenosis and fractional flow reserve (FFR) negative.

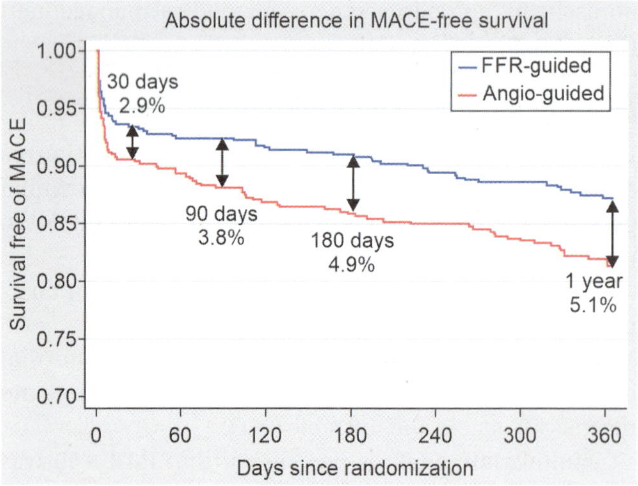

FIG. 4: FAME 1 trial shows FFR-guided PCI outcome is better than angio-guided PCI.

(FAME: Fractional Flow Reserve Versus Angiography for Multivessel Evaluation; FFR: fractional flow reserve; MACE: major adverse cardiovascular event; PCI: percutaneous coronary intervention)

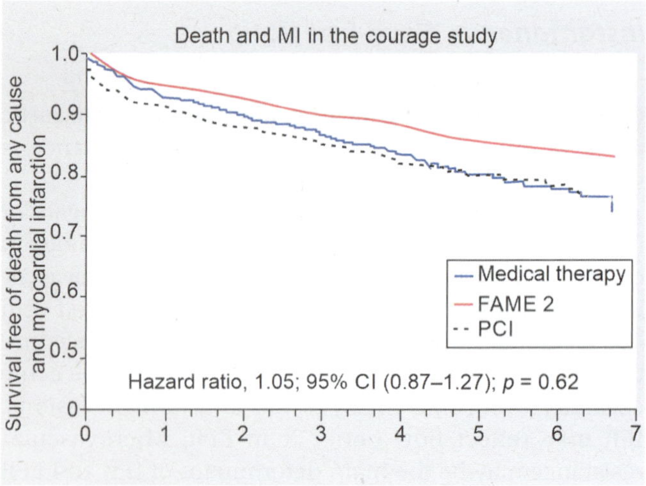

FIG. 5: FAME 2 trial shows functional percutaneous coronary intervention (PCI) is better than medical therapy.

(CI: confidence interval; FAME: Fractional Flow Reserve Versus Angiography for Multivessel Evaluation)

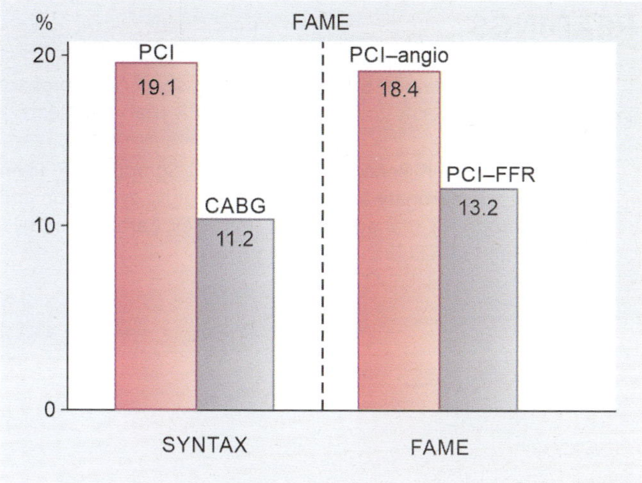

FIG. 6: FAME 3 trial shows CABG outcome is better than physiologically guided PCI in multivessel CAD.

(CABG: coronary artery bypass grafting; CAD: coronary artery disease; FAME: Fractional Flow Reserve Versus Angiography for Multivessel Evaluation; FFR: fractional flow reserve; PCI: percutaneous coronary intervention)

Nonhyperemic Pressure Ratios—Newer Indices

- Resting whole cycle Pd/Pa
- IFR
- dFR (diastolic pressure ratio)
- RFR (resting full cycle ratio)
- DFR (diastolic hyperemia-free ratio)

Resting whole cycle Pd/Pa is average of Pd/Pa during entire cardiac cycle. IFR is average Pd/Pa during wave-free period. dFR has average Pd/Pa during entire diastole. RFR has lowest instant Pd/Pa recorded during entire cardiac cycle. DFR has average Pd/Pa during the period between Pa less than mean Pa and downsloping Pa.

The IRIS FFR (Interventional Cardiology Research In-cooperation Society Fractional Flow Reserve) registry has shown that there is a strong correlation between hyperemic and resting physiological indices in defining the long-term outcome in management of CAD. IFR of 0.89 predicts FFR of 0.8 is applicable to all physiological indices. It is safe to defer PCI-based on negative resting indices like FFR. Prognostic performance of resting indices are also similar compared to FFR.

COMPUTED TOMOGRAPHY-DERIVED PHYSIOLOGICAL ASSESMENT

Cardiac computed tomography (CT) angiogram is the best noninvasive technique to asses CAD and characterize atherosclerotic plaque. FFR can be measured noninvasively by CT angiography-derived technique (CT-derived FFR) or FFRCT and physiological information gained about lesion specific ischemia is similar to invasive technique. CCTA and FFRCT have broad application including simple and complex plaque characterization, assessment of ischemia in a patient with stable CAD, with acute chest pain in emergency department, preoperative evaluation, and planning of revascularization strategies. CCTA and FFRCT will likely to become the gatekeeper to the cardiac catheterization laboratory. These can be used to determine the anatomical and functional SYNTAX score to plan approach to myocardial revascularization in appropriate management of CAD.

FUTURE TRENDS

The use of pre- and post-percutaneous interventional physiology are both key in improving the long-term clinical outcome and the parametric assessment is prognostically relevant. Functional coronary angiography is emerging as a clinically useful method of physiological assessment of coronary arterial stenosis with emerging data supporting the use of these indices pre- and post-PCI with prognostic guidance.

LIMITATIONS

Although FFR and IFR are widely used to evaluate the hemodynamic significance of coronary lesions both have important limitations in variety of clinical scenarios that operator should be cognizant of. Aortic stenosis and atrial fibrillation are major limitations and one should know to interpret data based on elevated filling pressure and beat-to-beat variation in heart rate etc.

CONCLUSION

Unwanted revascularization can be avoided so as to achieve favorable outcome using coronary physiology in management of CAD. Numerous clinical trial and applications refocused PCI from anatomical revascularization to functional revascularization.

All resting pressure-derived indices of coronary physiology showed similar diagnostic performance to predict FFR accurately 83–85% and IFR accurately 94–96%. They showed similar prognostic performance to predict the clinical outcome in CAD. These results suggest class effect among nonhyperemic indices. And hence, guidelines and clinical recommendations can therefore be applied in the similar manner.

SUGGESTED READINGS

1. Dangas GD, Mario CD, Kipshidze NN, Barlis P, Addo T. Interventional Cardiology: Principle and Practice, 2nd edition. United Kingdom: Wiley; 2017.
2. Topol EJ. Textbook of Interventional Cardiology, 1st edition. United Kingdom: W.B. Saunders; 1990.
3. Zimmerman FM, Ferrara A, Johnson NP, van Nunen LX, Escaned J, Albertsson P, et al. Deferral vs. performance of percutaneous coronary intervention of functionally non-significant coronary stenosis: 15-year follow-up of the DEFER trial. Eur Heart J. 2015;36:3182-3.
4. Habibi SE, Shah R, Berzingi CO, Melchior R, Sumption KF, Jovin IS. Left main coronary artery stenosis: severity evaluation and implications for management. Expert Rev Cardiovasc Ther. 2017;15(3):157-63.

6

CHAPTER

Management of ST Elevation Myocardial Infarction in Special Situations

A Kader Sahib

ABSTRACT

ST elevation myocardial infarction (STEMI) is the most common and dramatic presentation of acute coronary syndrome (ACS). Timely diagnosis and treatment will help save many lives.

INTRODUCTION

Anything which occludes the coronary artery completely can cause ST elevation myocardial infarction (STEMI). A plaque rupture leading to thrombus formation is the most common cause, but it is not the only cause. STEMI can also occur in conditions such as coronary artery dissection and coronary artery anomalies.

The general principle of management of STEMI involves opening the occluded coronary artery as early as possible either by pharmacological measures (thrombolysis) or mechanical means [percutaneous coronary intervention (PCI)]. However, there are certain situations where both modalities may not be applicable or one is preferred over the other. Certain special situations where the routine STEMI treatment must be modified and treatment must be individualized according to the special condition are discussed in this chapter. Criteria to diagnose STEMI is described in **Table 1**.

TABLE 1: Criteria to diagnose ST elevation myocardial infarction (STEMI).

Lead	Men < 40 years	Men > 40 years	Women (all ages)
In lead V_2 and V_3	ST ≥ 2.5 mm	≥2 mm	≥1.5 mm
All other leads	≥1 mm	≥1 mm	≥1 mm

ST ELEVATION MYOCARDIAL INFARCTION IN PEDIATRIC AGE GROUP (BOX 1)

Diagnosis of STEMI in pediatric age group is difficult due to two reasons: (1) Unlike adults, there is no definite criteria in children and (2) children present with atypical symptoms such as fatigue, irritability, reduced feeding, and nausea.

Management includes treatment of underlying causes such as cardiac surgery in anomalous left coronary artery from the pulmonary artery (ALCAPA) and intravenous (IV) immunoglobulin with high-dose aspirin in Kawasaki disease.

BOX 1: Common causes of ST elevation myocardial infarction (STEMI) in pediatric population.

- Coronary artery anomalies [anomalous left coronary artery from the pulmonary artery (ALCAPA)] is the most common anomaly
- Cardiomyopathies an myocarditis
- Hematological conditions like prothrombotic states
- Kawasaki disease
- Neonatal causes such as asphyxia, sepsis, lung pathologies, metabolic causes, and toxins

ST ELEVATION MYOCARDIAL INFARCTION IN ADOLESCENTS (BOX 2)

Important to consider acute myocardial infarction (MI) as a potential diagnosis in adolescents with chest pain. Prompt diagnosis of acute MI at a young age is mainly hampered by a paucity in understanding of the different potentially underlying pathophysiological mechanisms. Insight into the potential operational mechanisms of the coronary artery incident may have a major impact on the clinical course following admission.

Management

Premature Atherosclerosis

Treatment includes prompt recognition and treatment of MI with primary PCI. Thrombolysis should be considered when PCI cannot be done. Aggressive risk factor modification is necessary for secondary prevention because all these patients will have persistent residual risk.

Nonatherosclerotic Cause

Treatment of underlying mechanism. This involves abstinence from substance abuse, immunoglobulins/ aspirin for Kawasaki disease, corrective surgery for congenital anomalies, etc.

ST ELEVATION MYOCARDIAL INFARCTION IN VERY ELDERLY

With increasing human lifespan, the incidence of STEMI above the age of 80 years is increasing.

Unique features of STEMI in very elderly:
- Crushing chest pain which is the classical feature decreases with age and they present with dyspnea, worsening heart failure, fatigue, and confusional states.
- They are often precipitated by a concurrent illness.
- Patients are usually frail, with multiple comorbidities and often on multiple medicines.
- Electrocardiogram (ECG) diagnosis of STEMI is challenging, frequently complicated by an abnormal baseline ECG, often reflecting left ventricular hypertrophy, prior MI, conduction system disease, and at times the presence of atrial fibrillation.

Management of STEMI in elderly:
- Loading dose of clopidogrel is 75 mg only for patients >75 years. Loading dose of aspirin remains the same
- Thrombolysis is associated with increased risk of myocardial rupture and increased cerebral bleed. If thrombolysis remains the only option, tenecteplase should be used.
- Primary PCI is the preferred reperfusion strategy because of a decrease in risk of ischemic events, less bleeding risk, and a decreased need for subsequent target vessel revascularization.
- If angiogram reveals multivessel disease, revascularization of infarct related artery alone may be enough and probably lifesaving in many situations.
- Postprocedure recommendation include early ambulation and deep venous thrombosis (DVT) prophylaxis.

BOX 2: Common causes of ST elevation myocardial infarction (STEMI) in adolescents.

Premature atherosclerosis:
- Conventional risk factors such as smoking and diabetes
- Familial hyperlipidemia
- Genetic disorders such as antiphospholipid antibody (APLA) and metabolic abnormalities

Nonatherosclerotic causes:
- Kawasaki disease and vasculitis
- Myocarditis and cardiomyopathies
  - Substance abuse, coronary anomalies, post cardiac surgery

ST ELEVATION MYOCARDIAL INFARCTION IN PREGNANCY

Myocardial infarction is an uncommon event in women of childbearing age. However, as the birth rate for women older than 40 years has increased in recent years, MI in pregnant women may become more common. The average estimated incidence is one acute MI for every 16,000 deliveries.

Etiology (Table 2)

Several hemodynamic changes that occur during pregnancy serve as precipitating factors for spontaneous coronary artery dissection (SCAD) in the presence of an underlying predisposition. These include an increase in plasma volume by 40% and cardiac output by 50%, and an increase in heart rate which increases myocardial oxygen consumption.

It is helpful to classify the causes based on the trimester of presentation. It is important to understand this is not a strict iron clad classification and every cause can occur during any trimester, however, it provides a useful framework.

- *First trimester*: Atherosclerotic MI, especially in the presence of vascular risk factors
- *Second trimester*: Atherosclerotic MI and thrombosis

TABLE 2: Causes of acute (MI) during pregnancy.

Pathophysiological causes of MI in pregnancy	Percentage of cases
Spontaneous coronary artery dissection	43%
Atherosclerosis	27%
Thrombosis	17%
Spasm	2%

BOX 3: Medical management of the pregnant MI patient.

- Pregnancy-associated MI carries a grave prognosis with a mortality rate significantly higher than that in the general population
- Thrombolysis is risky and should be used only as a last resort because of the risk of worsening if MI is due to a SCAD
- PCI is the preferred option to know the coronary anatomy and possible etiology
- Statins are contraindicated in pregnancy
- Only aspirin and clopidogrel should be used as antiplatelets
- Heparin is the safest anticoagulant

(MI: myocardial infarction; PCI: percutaneous coronary intervention; SCAD: spontaneous coronary artery dissection)

- *Third trimester*: SCAD, rarely spasm
- *Postpartum*: SCAD; rarely due to thrombosis and spasm

Management (Box 3)

STEMI in pregnancy

↓

Avoid thrombolysis/shift to the nearest catheterization laboratory

↓

Angioplasty: Atherosclerosis → stent

(Choose a bare metal stent if antiplatelets must be stopped soon)

↓

Angioplasty: SCAD → PCI if proximal vessels are involved; success rate is very low. Conservative management for distal vessel involvement.

In our opinion, conservative management is a reasonable option for management of SCAD-related MI in pregnancy due to the lack of suitable revascularization techniques, high rate of recurrence, and favorable outcomes with spontaneous healing in most patients, particularly in relatively stable patients with a small myocardial area at risk. Most studies have documented the safety of this strategy in SCAD presenting with distal lesions involving small branches with thrombolysis in myocardial infarction (TIMI) 2–3 flow and/or no ongoing ischemia. Revascularization should be considered in the presence of proximal lesions with TIMI 0–1 flow, presenting with ongoing ischemia and or in STEMI/shock/cardiac arrest settings.

BOX 4: Challenges faced.

- Increased bleeding risk
- Underlying anemia, electrolyte abnormalities
- Preexistent LV dysfunction
- Readjustment of drug dosing
- Suboptimal PCI results (calcified vessels)/contrast issues
- Multiple comorbidities
- Difficulty in performing routine dialysis if BP is low

(BP: blood pressure; LV: left ventricular; PCI: percutaneous coronary intervention)

END-STAGE RENAL DISEASE

Compared to non-end-stage renal disease (ESRD) patients, ESRD patients have two-fold increased risk to die from STEMI. The increased risk with worsening glomerular filtration rate (GFR) can be partly explained by factors associated with renal decline such as anemia, oxidative stress, and derangements in calcium-phosphate homeostasis, inflammation, and conditions promoting coagulation, all of which are associated with accelerated atherosclerosis and endothelial dysfunction **(Box 4)**.

Management

Although decisions on reperfusion in patients with STEMI must be made before any assessment of renal function is available, it is important to estimate the GFR as soon as possible. The following are guideline directed strategies in STEMI with renal failure:

- Aspirin and clopidogrel can be used in all stages of chronic kidney disease (CKD). Ticagrelor and prasugrel is not recommended in stage 5 CKD (GFR < 15 mL/min).
- Heparin is the recommended anticoagulant; enoxaparin must not be given if GFR is < 15 mL/min.
- Primary PCI can be safely done in ESRD patients who are on regular dialysis. For other patients with CKD, the choice of reperfusion strategy (lysis vs. PCI) must be individualized.

- Ensuring proper hydration during and after primary PCI and limiting the dose of contrast agents, preferentially low-osmolality contrast agents, are important steps in minimizing the risk of contrast-induced nephropathy.
- GP IIb/IIIa inhibitors are best avoided in stage 5 CKD.

COAGULATION/BLEEDING DISORDERS (BOX 5)

Guideline directed approach in managing high bleeding risk patients are as follows:

- Primary PCI is the preferred mode of reperfusion
- Radial approach is preferable
- Choice of antiplatelet is aspirin along with clopidogrel
- Patients in whom dual antiplatelet therapy (DAPT) cannot be continued, bare metal stent is a good option instead of the routine drug eluting stent
- In rare case scenarios, where the bleeding risk is extremely high; simple plain balloon angioplasty (without stenting) can be done to the culprit vessel alone
- Tenecteplase must be used if fibrinolytic therapy is used; dose can be halved if risk is very high
- An international normalized ratio (INR) of > 1.7 is a contraindication for thrombolysis
- Loading dose of clopidogrel is only 75 mg for patients > 75 years receiving fibrinolysis
- Enoxaparin should be chosen over unfractionated heparin

For Patients on Oral Anticoagulation

Primary PCI is the treatment of choice. Ticagrelor and prasugrel are not recommended. Post PCI, aspirin, and clopidogrel must be continued along with oral anticoagulation for 1–6 months depending on bleeding risk. After 6 months, it is recommended to give one antiplatelet along with the oral anticoagulant. After 1 year, it is preferable to continue oral anticoagulant only.

Increased Coagulation Risk

Patients with increased coagulation risk:

- Inherited conditions such as factor V Leiden, protein C and S deficiency, and antithrombin deficiency
- Acquired conditions such as cancer, chemotherapy, polycythemia vera, antiphospholipid syndrome, smoking, and hormone replacement therapy

Management

There is no specific recommendation. However, triple therapy (DAPT and oral anticoagulant) can be given for few months till the risk persists.

ST ELEVATION MYOCARDIAL INFARCTION IN CANCER/CHEMOTHERAPY PATIENTS (BOX 6)

- With the improving survival of cancer patients, it is common to see acute STEMI in cancer survivors or in patients with active cancer.

BOX 5: Conditions associated with increased bleeding risk.

- Age > 75 years, females, and low body weight
- Diabetes, hypertension, and obesity
- CKD, anemia, and sepsis
- Genetic conditions (hemophilia and von Willebrand disease)
- Anemia and previous UGI bleed
- Chronic oral anticoagulation use
- Heart failure or shock

Hypertension poses the biggest hazard of intracranial hemorrhage with an incremental risk beginning at SBP > 160–170 mm Hg.

(CKD: chronic kidney disease; SBP: systolic blood pressure; UGI: upper gastrointestinal)

BOX 6: Unique features of STEMI in cancer patients.

- Patients are older, suffer more frequently from triple vessel disease, had more frequent atrial arrhythmias, chronic kidney disease, chronic heart failure, cerebrovascular disease, and PAD
- The following four serious independent risk factors for death in a study were advanced PAD, lung cancer, an existing metastasis, and stroke
- Concurrent cancer more often leads to a conservative medical management strategy and worse clinical outcomes in STEMI
- New specific cancer therapies such as immunotherapy improve cancer survival and quality of life, but sometimes carry the risk of myocardial ischemia. Thus, more patients with malignancies achieve a temporary or indefinite remission of the tumor growth—and are at risk of suffering a myocardial infarction
- Treatment will be influenced by many factors such as stage of cancer, its prognosis, and survival rate
- Primary PCI is always better; limited revascularization may be a better option in many patients. Bare metal stents must be used if the cancerous bleeding is anticipated

(PAD: peripheral artery disease; PCI: percutaneous coronary intervention; STEMI: ST elevation myocardial infarction)

- There are not much studies in this subgroup of patients
- Because of chemotherapeutic agents, there may be higher chance that these patients may have a prior myocardial dysfunction.

ST ELEVATION MYOCARDIAL INFARCTION IN POSTOPERATIVE PATIENTS

- Noncardiac surgery poses a significant circulatory stress and may trigger a cardiovascular event like STEMI.
- Ischemic ECG changes may be subtle and clinical signs are masked by strong analgesia.
- Acute coronary syndrome (ACS) in postoperative patients may be due to demand ischemia (most patients) and due to plaque rupture in some cases, a few are due to stress-induced cardiomyopathy.
- Thrombolysis is contraindicated in postoperative patients
- Angiogram is likely to reveal the cause and dictate further treatment plan.
- Primary angioplasty should be done in obstructive lesions secondary to plaque rupture.
- If antiplatelets cannot be given due to surgical site bleeding risk; plain balloon angioplasty alone must be done to tide over the crises and elective complete revascularization must be done subsequently.
- If the angiogram shows nonobstructive CAD, the likely mechanism for ACS is demand ischemia.
- Stress-induced cardiomyopathy must be treated with beta blockers and renin-angiotensin-aldosterone system (RAAS) inhibitors.
- Strategies that reduce myocardial oxygen demand (e.g., beta-blocker therapy and adequate pain control) and increase myocardial oxygen supply [e.g., adequate oxygenation and coronary blood flow; correction of anemia (if hemoglobin <8 g/dL); adequate intravascular volume status; and correction of hypotension] will likely have the biggest impact in preventing and treating ACS in patients undergoing noncardiac surgery.

CONCLUSION

More lives are lost due to STEMI than any other disease. Proper insight and understanding of the pattern of STEMI presentation including age, background history, and comorbidities will help us to choose the right revascularization strategy and subsequent optimization of medicines.

SUGGESTED READINGS

1. Thygesen K, Albert JS, Jaffe AS, Chaitman BR, Bax JJ, Morrow DA, et al. Fourth universal definition of myocardial infarction (2018). Eur Heart J. 2019;40(3):237-69.
2. Towbin J, Bricker JT, Carson A, McNamara DG. Myocardial infarction in children. Pediatr Res. 1987;21:195.
3. van der Schoot GGF, Anthonio RL, Jessurun GAJ. Acute myocardial infarction in adolescents: reappraisal of underlying mechanisms. Neth Heart J. 2020;28(6):301-8.
4. Edupuganti MM, Ganga V. Acute myocardial infarction in pregnancy: current diagnosis and management approaches. Indian Heart J. 2019;71(5):367-74.
5. Lawton JS, Tamis-Holland JE, Bangalore S, Bates ER, Beckie TM, Bischoff JM, et al. 2021 ACC/AHA/SCAI Guideline for Coronary Artery Revascularization: A Report of the American College of Cardiology/American Heart Association Joint Committee on Clinical Practice Guidelines. Circulation. 2022;145(3):e18-e114.

7

CHAPTER

Pros and Cons of Computed Tomography Coronary Angiography

Ankan Pathak, Aparna Tewari

ABSTRACT

Coronary artery disease (CAD) continues to be the leading cause of cardiovascular death throughout the world. There have been various innovations over the last few decades as far as cardiovascular imaging is considered, enabling the physicians and cardiologists gain insights into CAD. While invasive coronary angiography remains the gold standard in the diagnosis of CAD, computed tomography coronary angiography (CTCA) has increasingly become a more feasible noninvasive alternative. CTCA avoids the risks which are associated with any invasive procedure. In addition, it provides a more faster and possibly more cost-effective means of assessing a patient at low or intermediate risk for CAD.

INTRODUCTION

Coronary artery disease (CAD) remains an important subset of cardiovascular disease that requires time-bound, accurate, and cost-effective diagnostic methods. Patients with CAD can be classified into low, intermediate, and high pretest probability of ischemic heart disease groups based on presenting symptoms, family history, addiction history, physical exam findings, ECG changes, and cardiac enzyme profiles. After ruling out acute coronary syndrome (ACS) as a potential diagnosis, the clinician has a vast array of diagnostic options to choose from when aiming to determine the presence or absence of CAD and quantify its extent in such groups of patients. Computed tomography coronary angiography (CTCA) is an anatomic test that can be used in intermediate-risk patients to provide a diagnostician with these answers quickly. Multiple studies have reported that CTCA shows a high sensitivity and high negative predictive value for detecting significant CAD.

PATIENT PREPARATION

Informed consent should be obtained as is the norm. The patient should have nothing to eat for 4 hours before the exam and no caffeine for 12 hours before the test specifically to not precipitate tachycardia. Intravenous (IV) access with an 18-gauge catheter is preferred. This minimizes streak artifact during image acquisition and also allows the rapid infusion of contrast. Central lines should not be used unless rated for power injection.

The ideal heart rate for CTCA image acquisition is typically 60 beats per minute or less. An oral beta-blocker is typically administered 1 hour before the test, and this can be supplemented with intravenous beta-blocker administration just before the test commences.

Nitrates vasodilate coronary arteries and are usually given 5 minutes before CTCA image acquisition improves visualization of coronary arteries and stenoses. Typically, 400–800 μg of sublingual nitroglycerin are used for this effect.

Coronary Artery Motion

To image the coronary arteries, one of the paramount important facts is that it requires high spatial, motion-free resolution images. These images should be taken during breath holding, and hence a regular heart rate coupled with a slow heart rate is of utmost importance. However, with the advent of more than 64 multislice and dual-source CT scanners coupled with high spatial and temporal resolution, there has been a marked increase in improvement of image quality and also in patients with higher heart rates or in patients with irregular heart rates like atrial fibrillation or multiple extrasystoles. Spatial resolution refers to the smallest distance across which two points can be differentiated. Temporal resolution refers to how quickly images of a moving structure can be acquired.

Types of Cardiac Computed Tomography

Depending on the area of interest, cardiac CT can be ECG gated or non-ECG gated.

ECG-gated cardiac CT is primarily used for coronary artery assessment (native coronaries/grafts/stent evaluation).

Other indications of cardiac CT are valvular assessment, congenital heart disease evaluation, functional cardiac assessment, and evaluation of a cardiac mass.

Nongated scans are used for morphological assessment of pulmonary artery and veins and pericardial assessment and anatomical assessment of congenital heart disease and valves where functional indices are not required.

Method of Gated Cardiac Computed Tomography

It is an established fact that the least amount of cardiac movement is during the end systole and end diastole of a particular cardiac cycle. Hence, without doubt, motion-free imaging is best acquired during this phase.

Specific Artery Selection

Each artery suffers from motion artifacts at different phases; hence, the following intervals are the best windows to prevent movement of different arteries.

- *Right coronary artery*: 40% of R-R interval
- *Left anterior descending artery*: 60–70% of R-R interval
- *Left circumflex artery*: 50–60% of R-R interval

Coronary Artery Calcium Score

Calcification of coronary arteries occurs by means of an active process of mineralization with deposition of hydroxyapatite crystals as atherosclerosis is the major driving factor for the development of overt CAD. It is now a proven fact that coronary artery calcium (CAC), determined by CT, is equivalent to the measure of atherosclerotic burden. Traditional scorings methods for CAC include the Agatston score, volume score, mass score, and visual score.

Agatston Score and CAD

- *0*: No evidence of CAD
- *1–10*: Minimal evidence of CAD
- *11–100*: Mild evidence of CAD
- *101–400*: Moderate evidence of CAD
- *>400*: Extensive evidence of CAD

CLINICAL CONSIDERATIONS

Which patients should undergo a CTCA examination is a question that is frequently asked. The answer to this lies in determining the pretest probability of the patient having a CAD. *CTCA is most beneficial in patients with a low to intermediate pretest probability of obstructive CAD.* According to the latest guidelines, in patients with high pretest probability of CAD, the appropriateness of CTCA is classified as either uncertain or not recommended. The ACCURACY study, conducted by Budoff et al. in 2008, investigated the diagnostic performance of 64-multidetector row CTCA in symptomatic patients having suspected coronary heart disease who had been referred for elective invasive coronary angiography. The results demonstrated that CTCA had a high sensitivity for the detection of stenosis at both 50 and 70% thresholds with a negative predictive value touching around 99. Hence, it can be concluded from the above study that CTCA holds greatest value in the reliable exclusion of CAD, particularly in low- or intermediate-risk patients.

ROLE OF COMPUTED TOMOGRAPHY CORONARY ANGIOGRAPHY IN PATIENTS OF CHEST PAIN

By virtue of being a modality with high sensitivity and negative predictive value, CTCA is primarily used to rule out significant CAD in patients who have a low-to-intermediate pretest probability of suffering from CAD. CTCA is also beneficial in patients who have a noninterpretable ECG or the patient cannot exercise.

Computed Tomography Coronary Angiography in Patients with Acute Chest Pain

Computed tomography coronary angiography can be used in patients presenting with acute chest pain whose diagnosis is uncertain with normal ECG and normal cardiac enzymes with a low pretest probability of obstructive CAD.

Computed Tomography Coronary Angiography in Evaluation of Patency of Bypass Grafts and Stents

In patients with a history of coronary artery bypass graft (CABG), there remain two methods by which the patency of bypass grafts can be assessed with the help of CTCA.

First, in patients who are acutely symptomatic with a previous history of CABG, CTCA can be a potent modality to exclude graft occlusion.

Computed tomography coronary angiography can also be used for follow-up of asymptomatic patients with a history of CABG performed more than 5 years back.

Computed tomography coronary angiography can also be a useful investigation for the evaluation of coronary stents. In patients who have a stent diameter >3 mm, CTCA can be an excellent investigation to judge the patency of the stent. However, smaller stent diameter with increased strut thickness has limitations as far as imaging with CTCA is concerned.

PLAQUE CHARACTERIZATION WITH COMPUTED TOMOGRAPHY CORONARY ANGIOGRAPHY

Computed tomography coronary angiography is a useful tool to assess and characterize coronary atherosclerotic plaques, which unfortunately in coronary angiography is not possible. Features suggestive of increased chances of rupture include positive remodeling, presence of spotty calcification, lipid-rich core, and a thin cap fibroatheroma (suggested by the napkin ring sign).

OTHER NEWER MODALITIES

One of the drawbacks of CTCA is that various lesions which are considered anatomically obstructive according to imaging may not cause ischemia. Computed tomography fractional flow reserve (CT-FFR) uses computational fluid dynamics to calculate the three-vessel FFR which are acquired from coronary CTA images. The advantages of CT-FFR are that in addition to revealing the site of blockage, it also gives us an information on the flow and hemodynamics and therefore can help guide treatment, all this being noninvasive.

COMPUTED TOMOGRAPHY CORONARY ANGIOGRAPHY FOR ASSESSMENT OF SURGICAL RISK

In patients awaiting surgery, who have risk factors of CAD, if the pretest probability of CAD is low or intermediate, then CTCA can be an ideal choice for risk stratification.

CONTRAINDICATIONS

Contraindications for CTCA are similar to those encountered during any routine contrast-enhanced CT scan. Absolute contraindications are a patient history of severe or anaphylactic reaction to iodinated contrast, inability to cooperate with standard scan protocols, hemodynamic instability, acute decompensated heart failure, acute myocardial infarction, renal impairment, and patients not capable of adequate breath holding. Relative contraindications include pregnancy, inability to tolerate heart rate-slowing medications or nitroglycerine, recent phosphodiesterase inhibitor use, severe aortic stenosis, and bronchospastic disease.

CONCLUSION

Computed tomography coronary angiography is one of the preferred noninvasive modalities for the evaluation of CAD. However, for making the best use of CTCA, it is important that we identify the ideal patient and ideal situation at which CTCA will yield the best possible result. Analyzing the pretest probability of the patient harboring CAD is the most vital step.

SUGGESTED READINGS

1. Neurauter E, Leschka S, Wildermuth S, Ehl NF, Joerg L, Rickli H, et al. Use of coronary computed tomography angiography in clinical practice - single centre experience in Switzerland in light of current recommendations based on pretest probability considerations. Swiss Med Wkly. 2019;149:w20010.
2. Budoff MJ, Dowe D, Jollis JG, Glitter M, Sutherland J, Halamert E, et al. Diagnostic performance of 64-multidetector row coronary computed tomographic angiography for evaluation of coronary artery stenosis in individuals without known coronary artery disease: results from the prospective multicenter ACCURACY (Assessment by Coronary Computed Tomographic Angiography of Individuals Undergoing Invasive Coronary Angiography) trial. J Am Coll Cardiol. 2008;52(21):1724-32.

8

CHAPTER

Management of Heart Failure with Preserved Ejection Fraction

Ajeet Singh Chahar, Aqsa Jafri, Nitu Chauhan

ABSTRACT

Heart failure with preserved ejection fraction (HFpEF) includes patients with ejection fraction (EF) > 50%. The prevalence of HFpEF increases with age and is much more common in females than in males. The clinical manifestations of heart failure (HF) are similar regardless of EF. Till today, no specific treatment for HFpEF is available, and hence, management is aimed at treating associated comorbid states. Diuretics should be used for relief of symptoms due to volume overload. In various trials β-blocker, angiotensin receptor blocker (ARB), angiotensin-converting enzyme (ACE) inhibitor, and digitalis treatments have not been successful in HFpEF. But in recent trials, aldosterone antagonist, empagliflozin, and angiotensin receptor-neprilysin inhibitor (ARNI) have reduced heart failure hospitalization. But, still effective therapy having significant mortality benefit is still lacking. Hence, novel and effective management strategies for HFpEF should be developed.

INTRODUCTION

Heart failure (HF) is a clinical syndrome due to structural and functional impairment of ventricular systolic and diastolic functions. Heart failure with reduced ejection fraction (HFrEF) is defined as ejection fraction (EF) < 40%. The term heart failure with preserved ejection fraction (HFpEF) refers to patients who have EF > 50%. A score is proposed to diagnose HFpEF is given in **Table 1**. It ranges between 0 and 9. Score < 2 indicates low, between 2 and 5 indicates intermediate, and ≥ 6 indicates high likelihood of HFpEF.

TABLE 1: H2FPEF score for diagnosis of HFpEF.

	Clinical variable	Values	Points
H2	Heavy	BMI > 30 kg/m^2	2
	Hypertensive	≥ 2 antihypertensives	1
F	Atrial fibrillation	Paroxysmal or persistent	3
P	Pulmonary hypertension	PASP > 35 mm Hg	1
E	Elder	Age > 60 years	1
F	Filling pressure	E/e' > 9 (Echocardiography)	1

(BMI: body mass index; HFpEF: heart failure with preserved ejection fraction)

EPIDEMIOLOGY AND NATURAL HISTORY

The HFpEF accounts for 50% of patients of HF and the HFrEF accounts for rest 50%. The prevalence of HFpEF increases with age and is much more common in females than in males at any age. The prevalence of HFpEF is increasing because of aging population and increasing recognition of HFpEF.

Studies have shown that irrespective of EF, 5 years survival for patients of HF lies below 50%. Due to the development of recent guideline directed medical therapy for patients of HFrEF, their overall mortality has improved considerably but unfortunately this has not been the case with patients of HFpEF. In some trials, all-cause mortality for HFpEF is equal to that of HFrEF, but some trials report a slightly lower all-cause mortality in HFpEF than in HFrEF. Most common cause

(50–70%) of death in HFpEF is due to cardiovascular causes which includes sudden cardiac death (35%) and HF (20%). The noncardiovascular causes account for 30–40% of deaths in HFpEF which is higher than that in HFrEF (15%).

DIAGNOSIS

The clinical manifestations of HF are similar regardless of EF. The diagnosis of HFpEF is made using a combination of clinical and laboratory parameters. The presence of signs and symptoms of HF is the first diagnostic step and then objective assessment of exercise intolerance and increased pulmonary extravascular fluid is done. In the second step, there should be EF > 50% and a normal left ventricular end-diastolic volume (LVEDV). In the third step, expected antecedent or comorbid conditions, such as hypertension, diabetes, advanced age, chronic kidney disease (CKD), and atrial fibrillation should be present and noncardiac causes of symptoms and signs should be excluded. The presence of these findings is sufficient to make a preliminary diagnosis of HFpEF. However, if ambiguous or borderline findings are present, then further diagnostic confirmation can be obtained with a fourth step. This entails noninvasive and invasive workup for evidence of cardiac dysfunction.

COMORBID CONDITIONS AFFECTING PATIENTS OF HFpEF

Comorbid states commonly affect patients of both HFpEF and HFrEF. Some of these conditions precede the development of HF and often contribute in acute decompensation. Because of the higher age strata of patients with HFpEF, an increased proportion of these patients are afflicted with these conditions, such as hypertension, obesity, diabetes mellitus, coronary artery disease, atrial fibrillation and other rhythm disturbances, CKD, sleep apnea, anemia, and pulmonary hypertension. And as no specific treatment for HFpEF is available, treatment per se is aimed at treating these comorbid states predominantly. However, even after taking age, sex, body size, and comorbidities into consideration, patients with HFpEF usually have a larger left ventricular (LV) mass, greater degree of systolic and diastolic dysfunction, more left atrial (LA) enlargement, and increased arterial stiffness. And also in view of recent trials, the prognosis with HFpEF is much worse than that expected with a specific comorbidity alone. Thus, targeting the comorbid diseases while might delay the development of HFpEF but may not be a sufficient therapy.

CLINICAL EVALUATION OF CARDIOVASCULAR STRUCTURE AND FUNCTION

Nearly all patients of HFpEF have some characteristic structural and functional variation which can be evaluated most commonly using echocardiography, computed tomography (CT), and magnetic resonance imaging (MRI).

Left Ventricular Volume

Normal LV chamber dimension, area and volume are seen in 90% of patients of HFpEF. One of the guideline-based diagnostic criteria for HFpEF is LV volume < 75 mL/m^2.

Left Ventricular Mass

In 30–50% of patients of HFpEF, LV hypertrophy is present. These patients are associated with a worse prognosis.

Left Ventricular Geometry

Left ventricular geometry comprises the ratio between LV mass to volume (m/v), or of LV wall thickness to LV internal dimension, i.e., the relative wall thickness. When either of the parameters is increased out of proportion to volume or dimension that is known as concentric remodeling, and is seen in 20–30% of patients of HFpEF and has a higher risk of HF.

Left Ventricular Diastolic Function

Patients with HFpEF have changes in every aspect of diastolic function, i.e., a delayed and slow relaxation, slow and incomplete early filling, decreased recoil, decreased distensibility, and increased filling during atrial contraction. Echocardiography is employed to characterize a diastolic function grade of 0 (normal), 1 (abnormal relaxation), 2 (pseudonormalized), 3a (reversible restrictive), or 3b (irreversible restrictive). This is the most common investigation for assessing severity of diastolic dysfunction.

Systolic Properties

Patients with HFpEF have > 50% EF and at rest have normal dp/dt max, stroke volume, stroke work, and preload recruitable stroke work.

MANAGEMENT OF PATIENTS OF HFpEF

Evidence-based medical therapy has been developed for patients with HFrEF in light of the benefit shown by many prospective randomized controlled trials (RCTs). However, no such evidence is there for patients with HFpEF. And at present, no treatment has yet shown convincingly to reduce morbidity or mortality in patients with HFpEF. Therapies that are having mortality and morbidity benefit in HFrEF including drugs, such as angiotensin-converting enzyme (ACE) inhibitors, angiotensin receptor blockers (ARBs), β-blockers, or hydralazine/nitrates as well as device therapy, such as cardiac resynchronization and implantable defibrillators, have not demonstrated any clear benefits in HFpEF.

There are three main components in the management of HFpEF. The first part is reduction of pulmonary and peripheral venous congestion. This can be achieved by fluid and sodium restriction, adequate use of diuretics and nitrates, and neurohormonal modulation. The second part is aggressive management of comorbid diseases. It includes controlling blood pressure, treating and preventing ischemic damage especially to myocardium, controlling blood sugar, maintaining adequate renal function, weight loss using drugs, surgical techniques, and exercise training. The third aspect of management is optimization of cardiac performance status to match heart rate and metabolic demand, to maintain normal sinus rhythm, and to limit ventricular response rate during atrial arrhythmias.

The DIG (Digitalis Investigators Group) trial registers patients with HFpEF in normal sinus rhythm and showed no benefit in mortality and HF-related hospitalization.

In the CHARM (Candesartan in Heart Failure-Assessment of Reduction in Mortality and Morbidity) trial, the ARB candesartan is given in HFpEF patients. There is no benefit in primary endpoint of cardiovascular death and HF hospitalization.

The NEAT-HFpEF (Nitrate's Effect on Activity Tolerance in HFpEF) trial registers HF patients with EF >50% and evaluated nitrate's response. It found no significant benefits in exercise tolerance, quality of life, and N-terminal pro-brain natriuretic peptide (NT-proBNP) levels.

In the Study of the Effects of Nebivolol Intervention on Outcomes and Rehospitalization in Seniors with Heart Failure (SENIORS) trial, the nebivolol was given to HFpEF patients. There is no mortality benefit, but a significant reduction was observed in the hospitalization.

The TOPCAT (Treatment of Preserved Cardiac Function Heart Failure with an Aldosterone Antagonist) trial was done to assess the role of spironolactone in HFpEF patients. There was no mortality benefit, but there was significant reduction in hospitalization with HF. Mineralocorticoid receptor antagonists improve diastolic function and exercise capacity in HFpEF patients by reducing both preload and afterload and also reduce myocardial fibrosis.

The Empagliflozin Outcome Trial in patients with Chronic Heart Failure with Preserved Ejection Fraction (EMPEROR-preserved) showed significant benefit of empagliflozin [sodium-glucose cotransporter-2 (SGLT-2) inhibitor] in HFpEF patients. It caused significant decrease in HF hospitalizations, modest improvement in quality of life, and reduced natriuretic peptide levels regardless of presence of diabetes.

The PARAMOUNT HF [Prospective Comparison of angiotensin receptor-neprilysin inhibitor (ARNI) with ARB on Management of Heart Failure with Preserved Ejection Fraction] is a phase 2 trial showed that sacubitril-valsartan resulted in reduction in value of NT-proBNP after 12 weeks of treatment.

In PARAGON HF trial (Prospective Comparision of ARNI with ARB Global Outcomes in HFpEF), there was no mortality benefit, but it showed benefit in HF hospitalizations.

For the management of HFpEF several novel approaches are being developed and some of them are in phase II and III trials. These include ARNI sacubitril/valsartan, soluble guanylate cyclase agonists, serelaxin, oral and inhaled nitrites, and placement of atrial septostomy device.

Sensor-based Strategies

Multiple sensor-based novel strategies are being developed using remote monitoring-based tailored therapy that facilitates management of HFpEF. These include both implantable hemodynamic monitors (IHMs), non-invasive monitors (to assess measures of volume status, subcutaneous and cutaneous sensors, rhythm, heart rate, sympathetic tone, and activity), and serum measured biomarkers.

Remote Monitoring Systems to Help Tailor Management

The COMPASS-HF (Chronicle Offers Management to Patients with Advanced Signs and Symptoms of Heart Failure) trial showed that data provided by IHM demonstrated that patients with HFpEF have significantly increased filling pressures even when they were stable clinically and these pressures increased further when patients decompensated. It was hypothesized that treatment in accordance with data obtained through remote monitoring using an IHM would cause a decline

TABLE 2: Summary of results of various trials in the management of heart failure.

Treatment	HFrEF	HFpEF	HFpEF trial
β blocker	Yes	No	SENIORS
ACE-inhibitor/ARB	Yes	No	CHARM, I-PRESERVE, PEP-CHF
Digitalis	Yes	No	DIG-PEF
PDE-V I	ND	No	RELAX
Aldosterone antagonist	Yes	Yes	TOPCAT
Hydralazine/N2	Yes	No	NEAT-HFpEF
Endothelin antagonist	No	Yes PII	SITAXSENTAN
Sacubitril/valsartan	Yes	Yes PII	PARAMOUNT, PARAGON
CRT/ICD	Yes	ND	
Vagal spinal cord stimulators	No	ND	
Baroreceptors	Yes PII	ND	HOPE4HF, BEAT-HF
Exercise	Yes	Yes	META-ANALYSIS,
IHM	Yes	Yes	CHAMPION

(ACE: angiotensin-converting enzyme; ARB: angiotensin receptor blocker; CRT: cardiac resynchronization therapy; HFpEF: heart failure with preserved ejection fraction; HFrEF: heart failure with reduced ejection fraction; ICD: implantable cardioverter defibrillator; IHM: implantable hemodynamic monitor; PDE-V I: phosphodiesterase V I)

in baseline pressure, prevent an increase in pressure, and also lower HF events. This was tested in the CHAMPION trial, which concluded that patients receiving active treatment demonstrated a 152% decline in pulmonary artery both diastolic and systolic pressures and also a 52% decline in HF-related hospitalizations and ultimately a decreased cardiovascular mortality rate. The summary of results of various trials in HFpEF patients is given in **Table 2**.

NONPHARMACOLOGIC THERAPY

The management of HFpEF includes modification of diet and lifestyle, avoidance of obesity, regular exercise, compliance to management strategies, regular monitoring of weight, patient education, and close medical follow-up. Sodium intake of < 2 g/day is seen to be effective. Excessive fluid volume intake should be balanced with respect to renal function. Exercise training in patients with HFpEF results in improvement of exercise tolerance.

TREATMENT OF COMORBID CONDITIONS

Patients with HFpEF commonly have significant underlying comorbid diseases, which often contribute to the development of HFpEF, and not only affect its clinical severity, but also precipitate decompensation. The most frequently prevalent comorbid conditions include hypertension, diabetes mellitus, obesity, CKD, obstructive sleep apnea, and anemia.

Hypertension is prevalent in about 85% of patients with HFpEF and hypertension if untreated or uncontrolled, becomes an important risk factor for the development of HF. And hence treatment and control of systolic hypertension especially in elderly population (who are at maximum risk for development of HFpEF) cause > 50% reduction in incidence of HF. Therefore evidence-based therapy for HFpEF includes control of systolic hypertension. The target is systolic blood pressure < 140 mm Hg and diastolic blood pressure < 90 mm Hg. However, evidence from recent large RCTs conducted on hypertension suggests that lowering blood pressure to targets < 120 mm Hg systolic pressure may further reduce the incidence of development of HFpEF.

Diabetes and obstructive sleep apnea, if present alongside HFpEF, are together associated with worse outcomes. The available data from multiple RCTs points that treatment of diabetes and sleep apnea leads to improved diastolic function in patients with HFpEF.

One of the highly prevalent conditions in patients of HFpEF is obesity. The large ADHERE registry found that half of the patients weigh > 172 pounds, and one quarter weigh > 213 pounds. Weight loss, reduction in daily caloric intake, and regular exercise improve diastolic function. Weight reduction by any means like diet or bariatric surgery or even appetite-suppressant drugs represents an important strategy for these patients.

Chronic kidney disease is commonly seen with HFpEF and is an important contributor in the development of acute decompensated heart failure (ADHF). Therefore, in patients of HFpEF, low glomerular filtration rate (GFR) is associated with poor prognosis and increased events are seen with falling GFR. The presence of anemia in HFpEF is associated with a poor prognosis. **Table 3** shows the ACC/AHA/HFSA (American College of Cardiology/American

TABLE 3: ACC/AHA/HFSA guidelines for treatment of patients with stage C HFpEF.

Class indication		Level of evidence
I	Systolic and diastolic blood pressure should be controlled in accordance with published clinical practice guidelines to prevent morbidity	B
	Diuretics should be used for relief of symptoms due to volume overload	C
IIa	Coronary revascularization is reasonable in patients with coronary artery disease in whom symptoms (angina) or demonstrable myocardial ischemia is judged to be having an adverse effect on symptomatic heart failure	C
	Management of atrial fibrillation according to published clinical practice guidelines is reasonable to improve symptomatic heart failure	C
	The use of β-blocking agents, ACE inhibitors, and ARBs in patients with hypertension is reasonable to control blood pressure	C
IIb	In appropriately selected patients with HFpEF (with EF ≥ 45%, elevated BNP levels or heart failure admission within 1 year, estimated glomerular filtration rate > 30 mL/min, creatinine < 2.5 mg/dL, and potassium < 5.0 mEq/L), aldosterone receptor antagonists might be considered to decrease hospitalizations	B-R
IIb	The use of ARBs might be considered to decrease hospitalizations	B
III	The routine use of nitrates or phosphodiesterase-5 inhibitors to increase activity or quality of life in patients with HFpEF is ineffective	B-R
III	Routine use of nutritional supplements is not recommended	C

(AHA: American Heart Association; ACC: American College of Cardiology; HFSA: Heart Failure Society of America; ACE: angiotensin-converting enzyme; ARBs: angiotensin receptor blockers; BNP: brain natriuretic peptide; EF: ejection fraction; HFpEF: heart failure with preserved ejection fraction)

Heart Association/Heart Failure Society of America) guidelines for the treatment of patients with stage C HFpEF.

CONCLUSION

Till today, use of β-blocker, ARB, ACE inhibitor, and digitalis treatments have not been successful in HFpEF. But in recent trials, aldosterone antagonist, empagliflozin, and ARNI reduced HF hospitalization. IHMs also showed reduction in HF-related hospitalization and cardiovascular deaths. But still the effective therapy having significant mortality benefit is still lacking. Hence, novel and effective management strategies for HFpEF should be developed. These include treatments that alter LV myocardial, cellular/extracellular, and molecular structure and function. For example, treatments that aim to normalize natriuretic peptide levels restore calcium homeostasis, reduce extracellular matrix (ECM) fibrosis, and change the phosphorylation state of titin. Each of these may contribute to improved outcomes in HFpEF. The comprehensive treatment will require the use of multiple drugs and devices that will individually target multiple independent mechanisms. This multifaceted approach is necessary because each mechanism independently contributes to disease progression.

SUGGESTED READINGS

1. Yancy CW, Jessup M, Bozkurt B, Butler J, Casey DE Jr, Colvin MM, et al. 2017 ACC/AHA/HFSA Focused Update of the 2013 ACCF/AHA Guideline for the Management of Heart Failure: A Report of the American College of Cardiology/American Heart Association Task Force on Clinical Practice Guidelines and the Heart Failure Society of America. Circulation. 2017;136(6):e137-61.
2. Fonarow GC, Stough WG, Abraham WT, Albert NM, Gheorghiade M, Greenberg BH, et al. Characteristics, treatments, and outcomes of patients with preserved systolic function hospitalized for heart failure: a report from the OPTIMIZE-HF Registry. J Am Coll Cardiol. 2007;50(8):768-77.
3. Butler J, Fonarow GC, Zile MR, Lam CS, Roessig L, Schelbert EB, et al. Developing therapies for heart failure with preserved ejection fraction: current state and future directions. JACC Heart Fail. 2014;2(2):97-112.
4. Solomon SD, Janardhanan R, Verma A, Bourgoun M, Daley WL, Purkayastha D, et al. Effect of angiotensin receptor blockade and antihypertensive drugs on diastolic function in patients with hypertension and diastolic dysfunction: a randomised trial. Lancet. 2007;369(9579):2079-87.

9

CHAPTER

Does Ejection Fraction Still Hold Relevance in 2024?

Amrish Agrawal, Thair Al Jumaily

ABSTRACT

Left ventricular ejection fraction (LVEF) is the most commonly used parameter in cardiology and is a valuable tool used for many diagnostic and therapeutic decisions in the current guidelines and practice. LVEF is relatively easy to obtain by many cardiac imaging techniques, commonly echocardiography, but also on cardiac magnetic resonance (CMR) and nuclear imaging. However, there are limitations, such as LVEF does not correlate with patient symptoms, a normal LVEF does not exclude nor imply diastolic dysfunction, and there are issues regarding variability and reproducibility of the ejection fraction (EF). It is a reflection of radial contraction of the ventricle and does not account for both longitudinal and torsional contraction nor the speed of contraction. This is an important point when EF is preserved. A variety of new parameters, especially global longitudinal strain (GLS) by speckle tracking echocardiography, is emerging and taking its place alongside EF in the field of echocardiography, especially when EF appears to be normal such as cardio-oncology, amyloidosis, or hypertrophic cardiomyopathy where GLS is inherently superior.

INTRODUCTION

Ejection fraction (EF) is a measurement, expressed as a percentage or fraction, of the amount of blood pumped by the left ventricle for each contraction and hence provides an easily interpretable impression of cardiac performance. It has become the leading feature used by clinicians to characterize the left ventricular (LV) function. Around three decades back, Bartle proposed the term "ejected fraction" to describe the ratio of stroke volume (SV) to end-diastolic volume (EDV). The left ventricular ejection fraction (LVEF) value, therefore, correlates inversely with left ventricular end-diastolic volume (LVEDV). Therefore, for the same SV, LVEF will be greater if EDV is smaller and vice versa. A low EF may be due to low SV or increased LV diastolic volume, which is the denominator in the calculation. Hence, these variables may influence the calculation of EF without any change in cardiac contractility.

In heart diseases, where both systolic and diastolic ventricular volumes may be increased, such as heart failure with reduced EF (HFrEF) and coronary artery disease (CAD), even though SV is preserved, LVEF can be reduced. On the other hand, LV remodeling in athletes means that a normal SV originating from an enlarged ventricle can lead to the calculation of an impaired LVEF at rest. Similarly, in a small heart with a normal EF, SV may be low, insufficient to generate a significant gradient across a stenotic aortic valve, even though this lesion is physiologically significant.

IS EJECTION FRACTION RELIABLE AND WHAT DOES EJECTION FRACTION HIDE?

The parameter of EF by itself is an artificial construct, an expressed percentage, and therefore does not truly represent any physiological measurement. All imaging modalities can provide an EF measurement, and normal ranges of EF are different among different modalities as well as age and sex **(Table 1)**. The pitfalls of putting too much reliance on values of EF are as follows:

- *Variability and reproducibility of the EF*: Previous studies have reported a high intraobserver variability of

TABLE 1: Different methodology of EF calculation and weighted lower limits of normal in recent reports.

Empty cell	Advantage	Disadvantage	Men	Women
2D echo	Accessible, inexpensive, quick, easy, online hemodynamic information	• Dependent on image quality, may be controlled with contrast LV opacification but this is underused • High interobserver and intraobserver variability Requires geometric assumptions	0.52	0.54
3D echo	Overcomes concern about foreshortening, test–retest variation, and geometric assumptions	Very dependent on image quality	0.50	0.53
CMR	High contrast resolution; excellent discrimination of LV wall and cavity	Access, cost Multibeat protocols are susceptible to RR variation	0.57	0.59
Gated SPECT	High feasibility of gathering EF data	Radiation exposure, low temporal resolution may lead to undersampling	0.52	0.55
radionuclide ventriculography			0.46	0.46
Computed tomography	High feasibility of gathering EF data	Radiation exposure, low temporal resolution may lead to undersampling	0.47	0.53

(EF: ejection fraction; LV: left ventricular; SPECT: single-photon emission computed tomography)

both EDV and end-systolic volume (ESV) (11–15% and 15–25%, respectively) and of EF (7–10%), regardless of the methods used (area-length, Simpson's rule). This variability increases in dilated ventricles and for the lowest EF values (<20%).

- EF is a parameter of chamber function (expressing the emptying of the left ventricle) rather than a real index of LV contractile function. Thus, it is strongly affected by LV geometry and load. The relationship between EDV (mL/m^2) and the EF is inverse and is regulated by LV geometry. In the initial phase of heart failure and volume overload of the left ventricle, LV preload and afterload tend to increase, acting in opposite directions. Thus, EF remains normal despite the development of eccentric hypertrophy and dilatation, tending to stay stable for progressive volume increases as expressed by the Starling principle.
- Further, EF is mainly an index of radial contraction of the ventricle and does not account for both longitudinal and torsional contraction. Many studies in patients with preserved LVEF have shown significant longitudinal global function impairment, despite preserved EF.
- Another issue for error is due to inconsistencies in the tracing of the LV cavity leading to lack of uniformity in the measurement of LV volumes and EF. The guidelines for echocardiography suggest that LV is segmented from the cavity at the junction of the compacted myocardium (i.e., trabeculae and papillary muscles are included in the cavity).
- LVEF does not account for the speed of contraction. An alternative that takes into account the speed of contraction is the velocity of circumferential fiber shortening, as well as more modern and sophisticated markers such as strain rate.
- *Intraventricular synchrony*: Features of disturbed LV activation such as left bundle branch block (LBBB) can be noted on 2 dimensional echocardiography (2D E) but need high temporal resolution and sampling throughout the RR interval, rather than just frames frozen in end-systolic and end-diastolic used for measurement of EF. Modern machines can calculate the difference in time to peak contraction in various cardiac segments and allow to calculate dyssynchrony index; however, clinical trials for use of this index for cardiac resynchronization therapy have given mixed results.

APPROPRIATE USE

Despite the pitfalls, the use of EF and assessment of ventricular volumes are considered appropriate in diverse conditions such as HF, cardiomyopathy, myocardial infarction (MI), and valvular heart disease. Testing is appropriate with multiple different modalities **(Table 2)**, although echocardiography is the most widely used. The most commonly used method of measurement is by echocardiography, using the biplane Simpson calculation, which has a good relationship to the angiography measurement. EF is so important to

TABLE 2: Limitations of EF as a marker of LV function.

	Circumstances of inaccuracy	Potential solution
Physiological limitations	Load dependent	Pressure volume loops
	Difficult at high and low HR	High frame-rate imaging
	Mitral regurgitation (unloading, typical fall of EF after MV repair)	Pre-ejection markers
	Small LV (LVH and small cavity leads to overestimation)	Consider another marker (e.g., GLS)
Technical considerations	Image quality	LV opacification
	Geometry dependent	3D imaging, geometry-independent techniques
	LBBB (regional systole and diastole are not simultaneous)	No ready solution
	Irregular RR intervals (e.g., AF)	Single-beat imaging
	LV hypertrophy	Mid-myocardial shortening
	Hyperdynamic areas remote to myocardial infarction lead to a higher EF than might be expected for a given infarct size	Use of a sum of regional function (e.g., wall motion score index)
Clinical considerations	Prognosis—close to EF 0.50	Consider another marker (e.g., GLS)
	Subclinical LVD	

(AF: atrial fibrillation; EF: ejection fraction; HR: heart rate; GLS: global longitudinal strain; LBBB: left bundle branch block; LV: left ventricular; LVD: left ventricular dysfunction; LVH: left ventricular hypertrophy)

decision-making that steps should be taken to ensure the accuracy of the data acquired. When EF is obtained from echocardiography, suboptimal image quality, especially endocardial border delineation, may not be uniform in all segments and LV opacification with contrast should be considered. Use of LV opacification produces LV volumes which are quite close to those obtained with cardiac magnetic resonance (CMR). The use of echo contrast has improved the accuracy and reliability of 2DE.

NEW PARAMETERS BEYOND EJECTION FRACTION

A variety of new parameters have become available and tested for the LV function assessment. Among them, indices of myocardial deformation, such as strain and strain rate, have been proposed as adjunctive parameters to LVEF. The clinical adoption of this modality has been slow, related to measurement variations between vendors, which have now been reduced. Myocardial strain rate has a linear relationship with LV dP/dt and currently is among the most feasible clinical markers of contractility.

Global longitudinal strain (GLS) **(Fig. 1)** by speckle tracking echocardiography utilizes 2D gray-scale images to identify the movement of speckles to assess both global and regional functions of the left ventricle. Peak GLS has better intra- and interobserver reproducibility in post-hoc analysis compared to LVEF. There is a huge volume of data to suggest that GLS and segmental strain had better ability than LVEF to predict infarct size and segmental viability in patients with myocardial infarction (MI), characterize subclinical LV dysfunction when EF is preserved, predict risk of ventricular arrhythmias, guide treatment with chemotherapeutic agents in cardio-oncology, and predict the need for valvular intervention in valvular heart diseases.

Global circumferential strain is much more closely associated with EF than GLS. More importantly, conditions such as increased LV wall thickness or reduced LV diameter which can lead to preserved EF are noted to have reduced longitudinal strain as well as circumferential fiber shortening.

WHAT IS THE CURRENT STATUS OF EJECTION FRACTION IN CARDIOLOGY?

Heart Failure

The most important use of EF is stratification into distinct phenotypes of heart failure (HF) subtypes. HF with reduced LVEF is defined as ≤40%, and that with EF between 41% and 49% have mildly reduced LV systolic function (HFmrEF). Lastly, those with a diagnosis of HF and LVEF ≥50% are characterized as having HF with preserved EF (HFpEF).

Considering the fact that 95% confidence intervals (CIs) of repeated measures of EF are >10%, it is inevitable that some of the patients move into and out of cutoff levels on subsequent echocardiograms.

In addition, a number of patients improve from being in the category of HFrEF (EF ≤40%) to a higher category of EF and categorized into HF with recovered

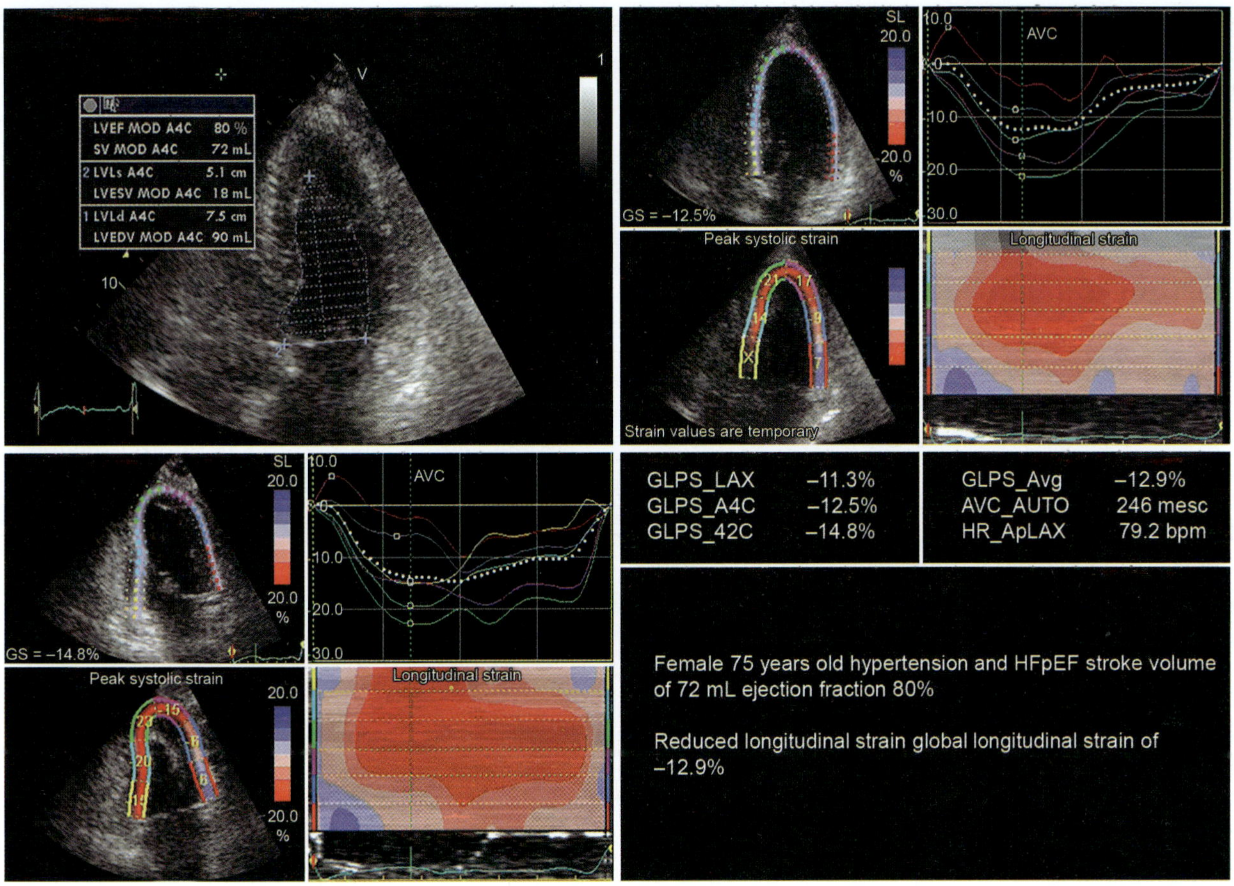

FIG. 1: A female, 75 years old, with hypertension and heart failure with preserved ejection fraction (HFpEF), stroke volume of 72 mL, ejection fraction of 80%, reduced longitudinal strain, and global longitudinal strain of −12.9%.

EF (HFrecEF) or improved EF. These patients could be classified as HFpEF on a single initial echocardiogram, so the lack of information regarding the trajectory of EF is an important limitation of the current EF criteria. The relative insensitivity of EF to minor changes makes the separation of HFpEF versus HFrecEF difficult, and further work is needed to characterize patients with true myocardial recovery.

It is important to note that in HF patients with EF >40%, there may be some benefit in considering other contractile markers, such as GLS. Impairment of GLS provides prognostic information across the spectrum of LV function and provides the greatest incremental information when the EF is relatively preserved.

In that experience, EF < 35% and GLS less than −12% were analogous. The categorization of HFrEF, HFmrEF, and HFpEF was recently compared with mildly (GLS more than −12.6%), moderately (GLS −8.1% to −12.5%), and severely (GLS less than −8.0%) reduced strain in a series of 4,172 consecutive acute HF patients. Reduced GLS provided better gradation of 5-year mortality of 49%, 38%, and 34% in severely, moderately, and mildly reduced GLS, respectively ($p < 0.001$) than the classification of HFrEF, HFmrEF, and HFpEF (5-year mortality 41%, 38%, and 39%, respectively; $p = 0.03$).

Ejection Fraction in Coronary Artery Disease

The prognostic value of EF in the setting of CAD has been known for over 40 years. However, there are measurement and temporal issues. The assessment is complicated by compensatory hyperkinesis in the noninfarct territory and the irregular shape of LV in CAD, making use of geometric assumptions inherent in 2D imaging difficult if not impossible. This can be partially mitigated by the use of 3D imaging. In the initial phase of acute MI, EF may be low due to stunned and hibernating residual viable myocardium, which may lead to spontaneous improvement of LV function in over 50% of post-MI patients.

Improvement in EF post-MI has an impact and an important clue in optimizing the timing of implantable cardioverter-defibrillator (ICD) implantation. An important measurement of this was made in 100 patients with LVEF 31% ± 6% after MI, 10% of whom had life-threatening arrhythmias over the next couple of months. Sequential echocardiograms showed that the main improvement in LVEF was at 1 month (at which stage 55% no longer had an indication for ICD insertion due to an LVEF > 0.35), but the mean EF change between 1 and 3 months was only 2%.

Ejection Fraction and Arrhythmias

The current European Society of Cardiology (ESC) guidelines for HF of 2019 give a class IIa recommendation for ICD to reduce the risk of sudden death and all-cause mortality in patients with symptomatic HF [New York Heart Association (NYHA) class II–III] of a nonischemic etiology and an LVEF ≤ 35% despite ≥3 months of optimal medical treatment (OMT). Cardiac resynchronization therapy (CRT) should be considered for sinus rhythm and LVEF ≤ 35% and LBBB morphology to improve symptoms and reduce morbidity and mortality as class I for QRS ≥ 150 ms and class IIa with a QRS duration of 130–149 ms. In case of non-LBBB, it is class IIa if QRS ≥150 ms.

This is due to the fact that LVEF ≤35% is significantly associated with malignant ventricular arrhythmias and sudden cardiac death. The strongest evidence in favor of ICD is in setting of ischemic cardiomyopathy and a recent large study showing no benefit from ICD implantation in nonischemic patients with EF < 0.35. Overall, <50% of patients of HF experiencing sudden cardiac death have EF < 30–35% and one-half of ICD implants with EF < 30% do not derive survival benefit; the use of EF seems an inexact approach to the selection of primary prevention ICDs at least in nonischemic LV dysfunction. Alternative and perhaps superior testing strategies include the quantification of LV fibrosis using CMR, and its analog mechanical dispersion at strain imaging could be of use.

Ejection Fraction in Valvular Heart Disease

Patients with critical aortic stenosis (AS) may have impaired EF due to high wall stress owing to afterload mismatch and are likely to recover from EF following aortic valve replacement. Hence, though reduced EF may be a contributor to perioperative risk, it should not be used as a criterion to deny intervention. In fact, reduced LVEF has been used as a rationale for valve replacement in asymptomatic AS. Further, the aging of the population and the impact of hypertension can have effects on the LV independently and incremental to AS. As in HFpEF, EF is not a good marker of LV function, and an alternative parameter such as GLS is attractive for this purpose. A basal longitudinal strain <13% is predictive of the need for aortic valve replacement in asymptomatic patients over 2 years of follow-up, and other observational data have proposed an increased risk with GLS <16%.

Similarly, in severe aortic regurgitation (AR), volume load associated with AR eventually leads to LV decompensation and impaired EF and LV dysfunction precede symptom onset in >25% of patients. Till the time EF is preserved, GLS has been shown to provide independent and incremental information. Presence of GLS < 18% in asymptomatic medically treated AR has been associated with disease progression, evidenced by symptom onset, >15% increase in LV ESV index, and >10% EF reduction.

In the setting of asymptomatic mitral regurgitation (MR), surgical decisions are based on LV geometry and function, and due to LV unloading due to the regurgitant volume, the presence of EF 60% is considered abnormal. Similar to above, reduced resting GLS can identify patients who are likely to demonstrate LV dysfunction in follow-up. Several studies have associated GLS of <18% to 20% as a predictor of postoperative LV dysfunction and therefore an indicator which needs to be taken into consideration for making decisions regarding surgical interference timing.

WHAT IS THE FUTURE OF EJECTION FRACTION?

There can be few parameters in the field of cardiology that have had such a ubiquitous role in the characterization and management of diseases. No doubt, EF offers practical advantages due to its ease of use, the short scan time, wide acceptability, and wide application in clinical practice. Further, EF can be calculated easily, and it can be assessed visually, even without specific expertise. Advances are continuing in the field of alternative methodologies, such as CMR where protocols are shorter, as well as improvements in 3DE, where echo acquisitions can be performed using a single beat. Automation is already being available in the process of tracing the endocardium, though technology is still in evolution, and caution is necessary.

However, there is a gap in patients with preserved or mildly reduced contractile function. This is related due to intrinsic mechanistic, methodological limitations and hemodynamic variables that do not really describe the real contractile performance. There is an increasing and expanding role of use of GLS alongside EF in the field of echocardiography. GLS has the ability to identify subclinical LV dysfunction and pick the disease at an early stage. This is especially true in conditions where EF is preserved such as HFpEF with EF > 50% and the recognition of amyloidosis and hypertrophic cardiomyopathy.

Hence, the future of EF lies in its retaining due to its wide availability and acceptance, its historical role, and to couple it with new and more sensitive markers of LV dysfunction, especially GLS, which should be used when EF appears to be normal or when particular diagnoses are sought where EF is unsuitable.

SUGGESTED READINGS

1. Marwick TH. Ejection Fraction Pros and Cons: JACC State-of-the-Art Review. J Am Coll Cardiol. 2018;72:2360-79.
2. ACCF/ASE/AHA/ASNC/HFSA/HRS/SCAI/SCCM/SCCT/SCMR 2011 Appropriate Use Criteria for Echocardiography. J Am Coll Cardiol 2011;57:1126-66.
3. Potter E, Marwick TH. Assessment of left ventricular function by echocardiography: the case for routinely adding global longitudinal strain to ejection fraction. J Am Coll Cardiol Imaging. 2018;11:260-74.
4. Sengelov M, Jorgensen PG, Jensen JS, Bruun NE, Olsen FJ, Fritz-Hansen T, et al. Global longitudinal strain is a superior predictor of all-cause mortality in heart failure with reduced ejection fraction. JACC Cardiovasc Imaging.2015;8:1351-9.

10

CHAPTER

Medical Therapy and Quality of Life in Heart Failure

Vishwanath Krishnamurthy, Varun Vinayak Prakash Rao

ABSTRACT

Heart failure (HF) raises the risk of mortality and hospitalization while simultaneously decreasing function and health-related quality of life (HRQOL). The prevailing approach to pharmacological therapy of HF relies on the progressive addition and titration of drugs that have been shown to lower the risk of mortality and hospitalization and revolves around the famed 'four pillars of HF', i.e., beta-blockers, angiotensin receptor–neprilysin inhibitors (ARNi), sodium-glucose cotransporter-2 (SGLT-2) inhibitors, and mineralocorticoid receptor antagonists (MRA), with additional therapies supporting these pillars. With the recent reclassification of HF based on ejection fraction (EF) into HF with reduced ejection fraction (HFrEF), HF with preserved ejection fraction (HFpEF), and HF with midrange ejection fraction (HFmrEF), the therapeutic approach to each of these entities of HF varies based on the available evidence. Studies have demonstrated that among patients with HFpEF, comorbidities are more prevalent, there is associated higher mortality risk and more physical impairment than patients with HFrEF. Various tools have been designed and validated to measure the quality of life (QOL) in these set of patients. The tools include the Kansas City Cardiomyopathy Questionnaire (KCCQ), the Minnesota Living with Heart Failure Questionnaire (MLHFQ), and the Chronic Heart Failure Questionnaire, among others. The various therapies for medical management of HF have shown an objective improvement in QOL indicators after their addition, in addition to mortality and cardiovascular (CV) benefit.

INTRODUCTION

Heart failure (HF) is a chronic illness characterized by signs and symptoms that impair the patient's quality of life (QOL). QOL was observed to be associated to several characteristics, including age, gender, New York Heart Association (NYHA) functional class, hospitalizations, fragility, and many novel HF medications, among others, from the beginning of utilizing QOL questionnaires in HF.

The World Health Organization defines QOL as an individual's view of their position in life in relation to their objectives, aspirations, standards, and concerns in the context of the culture and value systems in which they live. It is a wide notion that is influenced in a variety of ways by a person's physical health, psychological condition, social interactions, and relationship to conspicuous characteristics of the environment.

Heart failure is a complex clinical syndrome with symptoms and signs that result from any structural or functional impairment of ventricular filling or ejection of blood.

MEDICAL THERAPY—FOUR PHARMACOLOGICAL PILLARS IN HEART FAILURE MANAGEMENT

Sodium-glucose Cotransporter-2 Inhibitors

- Sodium-glucose cotransporter-2 (SGLT-2) inhibitors significantly reduce the risk of hospitalization for HF and cardiovascular (CV) death across all ejection fraction (EF) subgroups therefore, SGLT-2 inhibitors should be initiated in all individuals with HF lacking contraindications.

- The DELIVER trial with dapagliflozin and the EMPEROR-Preserved study with empagliflozin on clinical outcomes in people with HF with left ventricular ejection fraction (LVEF) ≥40% demonstrated a substantial reduction in HF hospitalization in patients with HF with preserved ejection fraction (HFpEF).
- *DAPA-HF and EMPEROR-reduced trials*: SGLT-2 inhibitor therapy was associated with a reduction in all-cause mortality (17%) and CV death (18%) in patients with HF with reduced ejection fraction (HFrEF).
- The benefits in the trials were seen irrespective of baseline diabetes status.

Mineralocorticoid Receptor Antagonists

- Mineralocorticoid receptor antagonists (MRAs), including spironolactone, significantly improve metrics of diastolic function in those with HFpEF, potentially lowering the risk of hospitalization for HF in certain subgroups of people with HFpEF.
- RALES, EPHESUS, and EMPHASIS-HF study suggest a benefit of MRA across the spectrum of HFrEF, inclusive of a wide range of etiologies and disease severities.
- The starting dose of spironolactone, eplerenone is 25 mg orally daily, increased to 50 mg daily orally after a month.
- Dose reduction to half for estimated glomerular filtration rate (eGFR) 31–49 mL/min/1.73 m^2.
- Monitoring of potassium and kidney function are required and done at approximately 1 week, then 4 weeks, and then every 6 months after initiating or intensifying MRA to reduce the risk of hyperkalemia and worsening kidney function.
- Although they have not been proved to enhance QOL or exercise tolerance in people with HFpEF, MRAs will help the majority of people by providing balanced diuresis with sequential nephron blockade, controlling hypertension, and reducing HF hospitalizations.

Angiotensin Receptor–Neprilysin Inhibitors

- Sacubitril inhibits neprilysin, an enzyme that inactivates several important vasoactive peptides that contribute to the pathogenesis and progression of HF, including natriuretic peptides, bradykinin, and substance P.
- Neprilysin inhibition increases angiotensin levels, which offsets the vasodilatory effect of sacubitril unless also inhibited, hence combined with valsartan. Sacubitril/valsartan provides additional benefit compared with valsartan in individuals with HFpEF and serum creatinine elevations and hyperkalemia occur less frequently with angiotensin receptor–neprilysin inhibitors (ARNi) therapy; however, hypotension and angioedema, albeit rare, occur more frequently with ARNi.
- PARADIGM-HF study showed that symptomatic patients with HFrEF tolerated an adequate dose of either angiotensin-converting enzyme (ACE) inhibitor or angiotensin receptor blocker (ARB), and sacubitril–valsartan significantly reduced the composite endpoint of CV death or HF hospitalization by 20%
- PIONEER-HF trial showed that ARNi reduced NT-proBNP (N-terminal prohormone of brain natriuretic peptide) levels in patients hospitalized for acute decompensated HF (ADHF) without increasing rates of adverse events.
- ARNi should be initiated de novo in patients hospitalized with acute HFrEF before discharge in the absence of contraindications.
- Patients with chronic stable HFrEF who tolerate ACE inhibitor and ARB should be transitioned to ARNi with a minimum of 36-hour interval between ACE inhibitor and ARNi doses.

Beta-blockers

- Bisoprolol, sustained-release metoprolol succinate, and carvedilol have been demonstrated to be useful in lowering the risk of mortality in individuals with HFrEF, with other beta-blockers not recommended for usage.
- Even when asymptomatic, or when symptoms are mild or improve with other therapies, beta-blockers therapy is important and should not be delayed.
- Beta-blocker therapy lowers the risk of mortality and the combined risk of death or hospitalization in patients with HFrEF in addition to improving the LVEF, lessening the symptoms of HF, and improving clinical status.
- Even if symptoms/LVEF improve, long-term treatment with beta-blockers and use of target doses should be maintained to reduce the risk of progression in left ventricular (LV) dysfunction or major adverse cardiac events (MACE).
- Abrupt withdrawal of beta-blocker therapy can lead to clinical deterioration and should be avoided.

Other Supportive Therapy

- *Diuretics*:
  - Loop diuretics: Preferred diuretic agents for use in most patients with HF
  - Treatment goal of diuretic use: To eliminate clinical evidence of fluid retention, using the lowest dose possible
  - OPTIMIZE-HF registry: Reduced 30-day all-cause mortality and hospitalization for HF with diuretic use compared with no diuretic use after hospital discharge for HF.
  - Initiated with low doses; dose is increased until urine output increases and weight decreases by 0.5–1 kg daily.
  - DOSE study found no significant difference in symptoms or changes in renal function with bolus dose versus continuous infusion of intravenous (IV) furosemide or with a low-dose approach against a high-dose strategy in patients with ADHF with moderate-to-high diuretic needs.
  - Metolazone or chlorothiazide may be added to loop diuretics in patients with refractory edema unresponsive to loop diuretics alone.
- *Ivabradine*:
  - It is a sinoatrial node modulator that selectively inhibits the If current.
  - The SHIFT trial demonstrated the efficacy of ivabradine—reduced the endpoint of CV death or HF hospitalization in patients with HF.
- *Digoxin*:
  - It is reserved for those who remain symptomatic despite optimization of guideline-directed medical therapy (GDMT).
  - The benefit of digoxin in patients with HF remains controversial.
  - Narrow therapeutic index
  - Digoxin is usually initiated at a low dose because higher doses are rarely required in the management of HF and are potentially detrimental.
- *Soluble guanylyl cyclase (sGC) stimulators—Vericiguat*:
  - VICTORIA trial showed a relative risk reduction of 10% in CV death or HF hospitalization.
  - These new therapeutic drugs may have a function in patients with HFrEF progression despite GDMT.
  - An oral soluble guanylyl cyclase stimulator (e.g., vericiguat) binds to and activates sGC, increasing cyclic guanosine monophosphate (cGMP) synthesis.
  - cGMP has multiple potentially positive effects, including vasodilation, improved endothelial function, and a reduction in fibrosis and cardiac remodeling.
  - Vericiguat has a dual mode of action:
    - sGC stimulator directly stimulates sGC via a different binding site, independently of nitric oxide (NO).
    - sGC stimulator sensitizes sGC to endogenous NO by stabilizing the NO–sGC binding
  - Vericiguat may be considered in patients in NYHA class II–IV who have had worsening HF despite treatment with an ACE inhibitor (or ARNi), a beta-blocker and an MRA to reduce the risk of CV mortality or HF hospitalization. It is off late being dubbed as the fifth pillar in treatment of HF.

NONPHARMACOLOGICAL MANAGEMENT IN HEART FAILURE

- In a meta-analysis of randomized controlled trials (RCTs) on fluid restriction in HF, restricted fluid intake compared with free fluid consumption did not result in reduced hospitalization or mortality rates, changes in thirst, duration of IV diuretic use, improvement in serum creatinine, or serum sodium levels.
- Fluid restriction has limited-to-no effect on clinical outcomes or diuretic use.

Additional therapies like IV iron have been demonstrated to be marginally beneficial.

The GDMT described above is mostly explored and used in HFrEF. There are few treatment choices for people with HFpEF. MRAs and SGLT2 inhibitors have demonstrated a degree of benefit in a subset of patients.

END-STAGE HEART FAILURE

This term indicates an extremely advanced condition where no improvement with conventional HF treatment is possible and where palliative care, ventricular assist devices or heart transplantation are indicated.

End-stage HF should be distinguished from acute HF in which a certain degree of reversibility can be achieved.

REFRACTORY HEART FAILURE

Refractory HF is similar to end-stage HF and is observed in clinical practice when patients continue to be symptomatic at rest or develop recurrence of HF despite optimal contemporary pharmacotherapy that has been proven to be of benefit in clinical trials. Physical examination, laboratory testing, multimodality imaging, and cardiopulmonary exercise testing are pivotal for the definition of refractory HF. These patients commonly have rapid clinical deterioration and may require inotropic agents to augment cardiac performance.

QUALITY OF LIFE IN PATIENTS WITH HEART FAILURE

Improvement in functional ability and QOL as well as symptom reduction, are typically stated goals for a patient with HF. All of the major guidelines for the management of HF prescribe medications that impact the course of the illness and focus on mortality, hospitalization, and measuring changes in EF or ventricular remodeling, with very few emphasizing the improvement of QOL.

Different physical and mental complications such as fatigue, depression, anxiety, edema, shortness of breath, and therapeutic processes have a serious and negative impact on the QOL. Lower health-related quality of life (HRQOL) correlate with increased hospitalization occupancy and mortality rates, and higher costs imposed on health systems, families, and patients.

The International Consortium for Health Outcomes Measurement (ICHOM) established a 17-item set that addressed selected functional, psychosocial, burden of care, and survival outcome domains, which was designed to compare and improve care for HF with relevance for patients and clinicians worldwide.

The measurement tools included the Kansas City Cardiomyopathy Questionnaire (KCCQ), the Minnesota Living with Heart Failure Questionnaire (MLHFQ), and the Chronic Heart Failure Questionnaire. KCCQ-12, after having been shown to preserve the favorable parameters of the original instrument, was ultimately included to maximize efficiency.

The regular assessment of a patients' QOL and health promotion are key measures in increasing their survival rates.

IMPACT OF DRUGS ON QUALITY OF LIFE

Two trials compared ARBs to a placebo. Valsartan improved the main result in Val-HeFT (Valsartan Heart Failure Trial), although the smaller study by Houghton et al. was equivocal. In Val-HeFT, valsartan provided a marginally significant increase in HRQOL over placebo.

In random-effects meta-analyses, differences between beta-blockers and placebo as well as between carvedilol and other beta-blockers, were equivocal.

The SGLT-2 inhibitors improved the main outcome in a random-effects meta-analysis, resulting in a mean 2.0-point improvement in KCCQ at 3–12 months.

Addition of hydralazine–nitrate considerably improved the main outcome in A-HeFT (African-American Heart Failure Trial), resulting in a mean MLHFQ improvement of 4.5.

IMPACT OF IRON REPLACEMENT ON HEALTH-RELATED QOL

Five trials compared IV iron to placebo, and one trial comparing oral iron to placebo had 225 patients. IV iron enhanced the primary outcome in random-effects meta-analyses, resulting in a mean 8.8-point improvement in KCCQ at 6 months, but oral iron did not.

In FAIR-HF, considerably more patients receiving IV iron improved their HRQOL compared to placebo.

CONCLUSION

Heart failure management involves the goal-directed medical therapy with the famed four pillars of treatment. Newer exciting drugs like vericiguat are being added to expand the current armamentarium of therapy. Supplementing them are various nonpharmacological therapies like IV iron. In addition to altering the coursed of disease through these drugs emphasis should also be placed on assessing and improving the QOL in these patients.

SUGGESTED READINGS

1. Moradi M, Daneshi F, Behzadmehr R, Rafiemanesh H, Bouya S, Raeisi M. Quality of life of chronic heart failure patients: A systematic review and metaanalysis. Heart Fail Rev. 2020;25: 993-1006.
2. Tarekegn GE, Gezie LD, Birhan TY, Ewnetu F. Health-Related Quality of Life Among Heart Failure Patients Attending an Outpatient Clinic in the University of Gondar Comprehensive Specialized Hospital Northwest, Ethiopia, 2020: Using Structural Equation Modeling Approach. Patient Relat Outcome Meas. 2021;12:279-90.
3. Heidenreich PA, Bozkurt B, Aguilar D, Allen LA, Byun JJ, Colvin MM, Deswal A, et al. 2022 AHA/ACC/HFSA Guideline for the Management of Heart Failure: A Report of the American College of Cardiology/American Heart Association Joint Committee on Clinical Practice Guidelines. J Am Coll Cardiol. 2022;79(17): e263-421
4. Kittleson MM, Panjrath GS, Amancherla K, Davis LL, Deswal A, Dixon DL, et al. 2023 ACC expert consensus decision pathway on management of heart failure with preserved ejection fraction: A Report of the American College of Cardiology Solution Set Oversight Committee. J Am Coll Cardiol. 2023;81(18): 1835-78.
5. Metra M, Ponikowski P, Dickstein K, McMurray JJ, Gavazzi A, Bergh CH, et al; Heart Failure Association of the European

Society of Cardiology. Advanced chronic heart failure: A position statement from the Study Group on Advanced Heart Failure of the Heart Failure Association of the European Society of Cardiology. Eur J Heart Fail. 2007;9:684-94.
6. Hunt SA, Abraham WT, Chin MH, Feldman AM, Francis GS, Ganiats TG, et al. ACC/AHA 2005 guideline update for the diagnosis and management of chronic heart failure in the adult summary article. A report of the American College of Cardiology/American Heart Association Task Force on Practice Guidelines (Writing Committee to Update the 2001 Guidelines for the Evaluation and Management of Heart Failure). J Am Coll Cardiol. 2005;46:1116-43.
7. Ahmad T, Patel CB, Milano CA, Rogers JG. When the heart runs out of heartbeats: treatment options for refractory end-stage heart failure. Circulation. 2012;125:2948-955.
8. Burns DJ, Arora J, Okunade O, Beltrame JF, Bernardez-Pereira S, Crespo-Leiro MG, et al. International Consortium for Health Outcomes Measurement (ICHOM): Standardized Patient-Centered Outcomes Measurement Set for Heart Failure Patients. JACC Heart Fail. 2020;8(3):212-22.
9. Spertus JA, Jones PG. Development and validation of a short version of the Kansas City Cardiomyopathy Questionnaire. Circ Cardiovasc Qual Outcomes. 2015;8(5):469-76.
10. Binanay C, Califf RM, Hasselblad V, O'Connor C, Shah M, Sopko G, et al; ESCAPE Investigators and ESCAPE Study Coordinators. Evaluation study of congestive heart failure and pulmonary artery catheterization effectiveness: the ESCAPE trial. JAMA. 294(13):1625-33.
11. Rodríguez-Artalejo F, Guallar-Castillón P, Pascual CR, Otero CM, Montes AO, García AN, et al. Health-related quality of life as a predictor of hospital readmission and death among patients with heart failure. Arch Intern Med. 165(11):1274-9.
12. Turgeon RD, Barry AR, Hawkins NM, Ellis UM. Pharmacotherapy for heart failure with reduced ejection fraction and health-related quality of life: a systematic review and meta-analysis. Eur J Heart Fail. 2021;23(4):578-89.

11

CHAPTER

Life-threatening Arrhythmia in Systemic Disorders

Vijay Garg, Masum Talesara

ABSTRACT

Inflammation plays a predominant role in three factors which potentially increase the risk of arrhythmia—structural changes, parameters of ventricular dynamics, and vascular changes. Inflammation and arrhythmia are correlated in their pathogenesis and influence each other reciprocally. Systemic or local inflammation is triggered by acute infections, chronic diseases, and autoimmune disorders. Hyperthermia or acute infections, releases stress hormones and stimulates the sympathetic system, thereby accelerating cardiac rate. Studies prove that infection-associated hyperthermia is related to an increased risk of life-threatening ventricular arrhythmia. Chronic diseases such as chronic obstructive pulmonary disease, chronic kidney disease, and diabetes mellitus (DM), etc., create a constant increase in inflammatory markers, such as C-reactive protein (CRP), tumor necrosis factor-alpha and cytokines including interleukin (IL)-1, IL-6, and IL-8. CRP is hypothesized to have a direct proarrhythmic effect or indicate subclinical inflammation that consequently damages the heart, provokes myocardial fibrosis and thus triggers ventricular arrhythmias. Autoimmune diseases (ADs) are associated with arrhythmogenesis. Chronic inflammation forms the pathophysiological connection between AD and autonomic dysfunction, consisting of sympathetic over-activation and decreased parasympathetic function. Autoantibody-mediated and drug-induced arrhythmias commonly occur among AD patients. For resolution of the arrhythmia in a patient, diagnosis and treatment of the primary infection/disease is as important as management of the arrhythmia.

INTRODUCTION

Arrhythmias pose significant challenges in cardiovascular medicine due to their potential life-threatening consequences. In addition to cardiac causes, numerous noncardiac factors can precipitate arrhythmias. Understanding the impact of these noncardiac causes is vital for optimal patient care. This chapter aims to review the diverse noncardiac conditions and factors linked to arrhythmias, shedding light on their prevalence, pathophysiology, and clinical implications.

To elucidate the occurrence of arrhythmia in a systemic disease or condition, it is important to focus on the link between inflammation and arrhythmia in the body. Inflammation plays a predominant role in three factors which potentially increase the risk of arrhythmia—structural changes, parameters of ventricular dynamics, and vascular changes. Inflammation causes fluctuations in the membrane potential of cardiac cells and is therefore labelled as a proarrhythmic. The development of structural changes over a time beginning with fibrosis, scarring, as well as hypertrophy and atrophy may lead ectopic pacemaker activity, late potentials, and re-entry tachyarrhythmias. Increased wall tension, increased oxygen consumption by the heart and diminished coronary reserve favoring ischemia and gradually arrhythmias; comprises the second factor of ventricular dynamics. The last factor, vascular changes consist of interruptions in the micro- and macrovascular perfusion of inflamed heart tissue, also contributing to ischemic effects **(Fig. 1)**.

Life-threatening arrhythmias are a common symptom in patients with cerebral infarction and myocardial infarction. *Extreme bradycardia (EB), extreme tachycardia (ET), ventricular tachycardia (VT), and ventricular flutter (VF)* are the four common types of life-threatening arrhythmias.

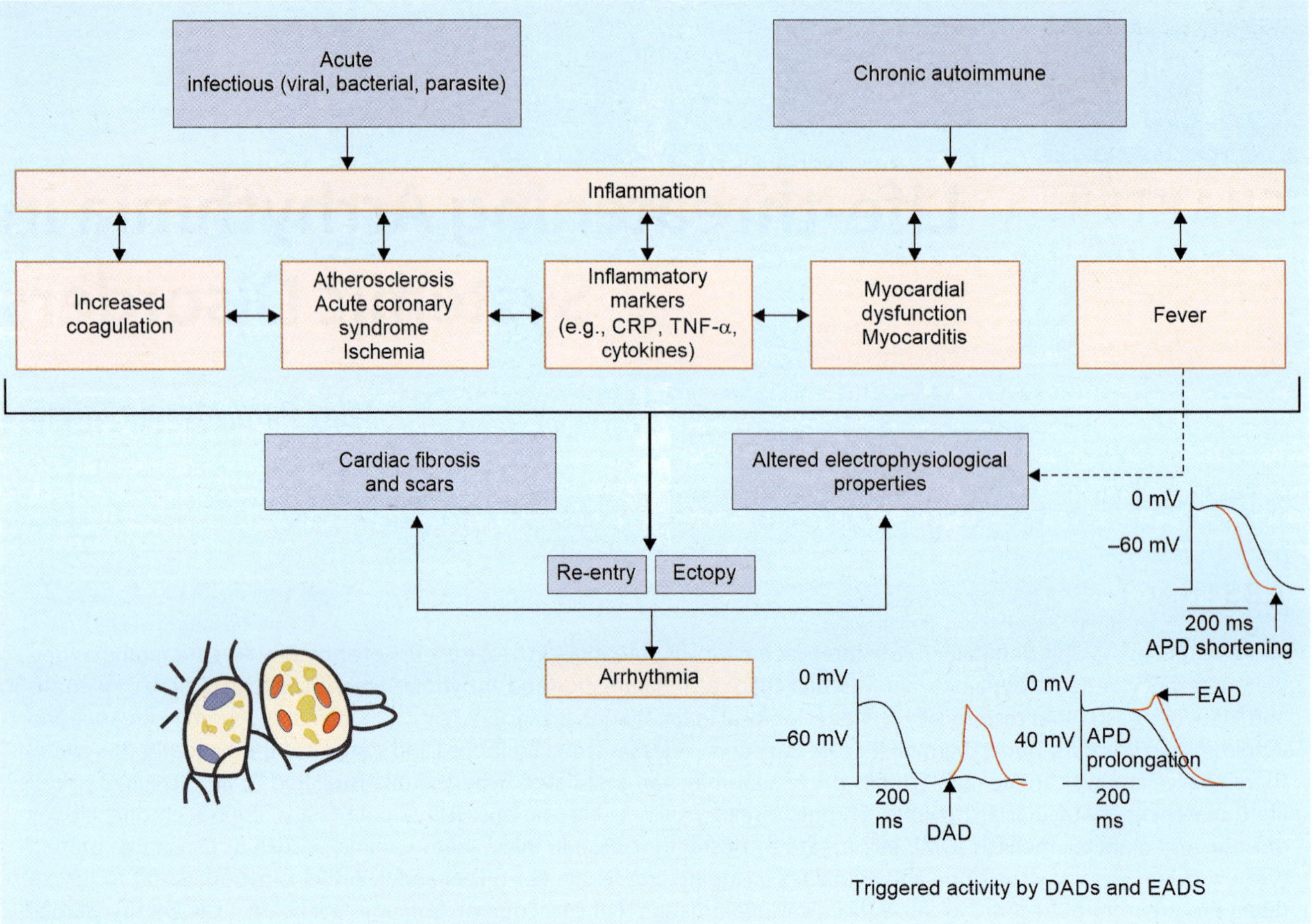

FIG. 1: Overview of association between inflammation and arrhythmia.
(CRP: C-reactive protein; TNF-α: tumor necrosis factor alpha)

ARRHYTHMIAS IN CRITICAL CARE AND IN ACUTE CONDITIONS

Atrial fibrillation (AF) [most common sustained arrhythmia in general population and occurs in 31% of intensive care unit (ICU) patients].

In the critically ill patient, arrhythmias can be caused or potentiated by:

- Increased catecholamine levels (endogenous or exogenous)
- Hypoxia
- Hypercarbia
- Severe acidosis
- Gross electrolyte disturbance and
- Pain or anxiety

INCIDENCE AND IMPACT OF ARRHYTHMIA IN INTENSIVE CARE UNIT

The incidence and impact of arrhythmia in an intensive care unit are discussed in **Table 1**.

MECHANISM OF ARRHYTHMIA

The mechanism of arrhythmia is depicted in **Flowchart 1**.

TABLE 1: Incidence and impact of arrhythmias in patients in the intensive care unit.

	Sustained supraventricular arrhythmias %	Sustained ventricular arrhythmias %	Conduction abnormalities %	No arrhythmias %
Incidence	8	2	2	88
Unadjusted in-hospital death rates	29	73	60	17
Neurological sequelae among survivors	15	38	17	6

After adjustment for prognostic factors and propensity scores, only ventricular arrhythmias increased mortality (odds ratio 3.53; 95% confidence interval 1.19–10.42).

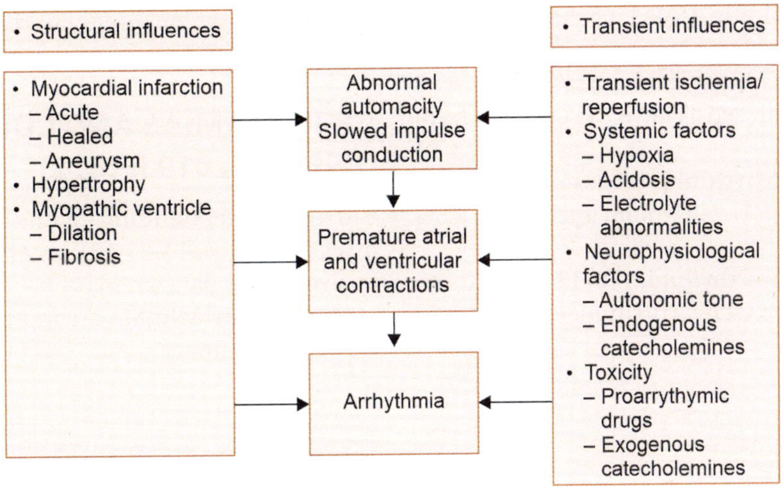

FLOWCHART 1: Mechanism of arrhythmias.

DETERMINANTS OF URGENCY IN CRITICAL CARE

- Hypotension
- Ischemia
- Heart failure (HF)
- Altered mentation
- Other signs of hypoperfusion—hypoxia, decreased urine output

Pneumonia

- Atrial fibrillation is the most common arrhythmia in the setting of critically ill patients.
- Pneumonia, and in particular community acquired pneumonia, is one of the most common causes of illness and hospital admission world.
- Even though the relationship between pneumonia and AF has been known for years, it was once considered a transient bystander.
- In recent years there has been growing knowledge on the clinical significance of this arrhythmia in acute clinical settings, in which it holds a prognostic role which is not so different as compared to that of the so called "primary" AF.
- Atrial fibrillation is a distinct entity even in the setting of pneumonia and it should therefore be managed with a guidelines-oriented approach, including prescription of anticoagulants in patients at thromboembolic risk, always considering patients' individuality.

ARRHYTHMIAS IN ACUTE RESPIRATORY FAILURE

- Metabolic abnormalities associated with respiratory failure cause arrhythmias.
- Alteration of the transmembrane action potential of cardiac conducting tissue, causing electrophysiologic phenomenon known to trigger arrhythmias.
- Cardiogenic pulmonary edema and acute respiratory insufficiency in postsurgical patients are also known to develop due to tachycardia and arrhythmias.

Sepsis

Supraventricular arrhythmia (SVA) occurred in 31% patients with a major infection.

Infection = Major precipitant in 26% cases of SVA. 33% of critically ill patients with sepsis have AF, and 10% have new-onset AF.

Supraventricular arrhythmia is associated with bacterial pneumonia in 7.5%, and wound infection in 8.5% cases.

Supraventricular tachyarrhythmias (8–13.6%) is more prevalent than ventricular tachyarrhythmias (prevalence around 2%) in sepsis.

ARRHYTHMIA IN ACUTE BRAIN INJURY

- Cardiac arrhythmias occur in 28% and 37.5% patients with acute stroke and subarachnoid hemorrhage (SAH), respectively.
- *Reasons of arrhythmia*: Catecholamine secretion
- Cushing reflexes are accounted for causing arrhythmias.
- Degeneration of the hypothalamus, insular, or brainstem due to trauma.
- Atrial fibrillation is the most common arrhythmia among patients with acute stroke and SAH.
- Prolongation of QT interval (QTc > 470 ms) and decreased heart rate in SAH patients have been found as the independent risk factors for ventricular arrhythmia.

ARRHYTHMIAS AND CORONAVIRUS DISEASE-2019 (FIG. 2)

Current understanding of the impact of coronavirus disease 2019 (COVID-19) on arrhythmias continues to evolve as new data emerge.

Cardiac arrhythmias are more common in critically ill COVID-19 patients.

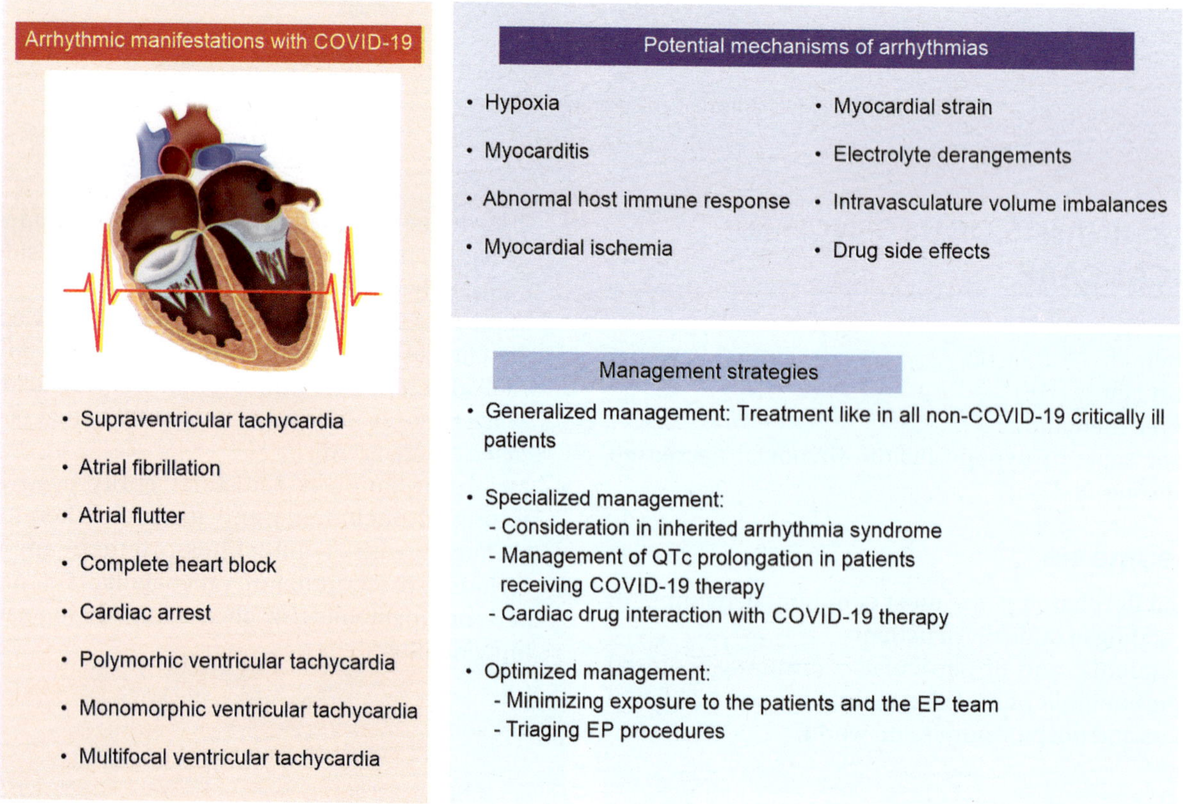

FIG. 2: Arrhythmias and COVID-19.
(EP: electrophysiology)

To manage these arrhythmias, it is imperative to increase the awareness of potential drug-drug interactions, to monitor QTc prolongation while receiving COVID therapy and provide special considerations for patients with inherited arrhythmia syndromes.

Certain drugs are responsible in acute settings for arrhythmia.

CAUSES FOR ACQUIRED LONG QTC (FIG. 3)

Cardiac

Quinidine, disopyramide, procainamide, sotalol, ibutilide, amiodarone, and bepridil.

Noncardiac

Erythromycin, grepafloxacin, moxifloxacin, pentamidine, amantadine, chloroquine, trimethoprim-sulfamethoxazole, phenothiazines, haloperidol, tricyclic antidepressants, terfenadine, astemizole, ketoconazole, itraconazole, ketanserin, cisapride, papaverine, tacrolimus, and arsenic trioxide.

Life-threatening arrhythmias in various cardiac and noncardiac conditions cause cardiac arrest in critical care settings **(Table 2)**.

ARRHYTHMIA IN CHRONIC DISEASES AND LIFESTYLE DISORDERS

Chronic diseases such as chronic obstructive pulmonary disease, chronic kidney disease (CKD), and diabetes mellitus (DM), etc., cause a constant increase in inflammatory markers, such as C-reactive protein (CRP), tumor necrosis factor-alpha and cytokines including interleukin (IL)-1, IL-6, and IL-8.

Chronic obstructive pulmonary disease (COPD): Subclinical systemic inflammation accompanying airflow obstruction has been associated with increased risk of cardiac injury. Disease mechanisms underlying COPD and also linking arrhythmias include—hyperinflation, hypoxemia, pulmonary hypertension (PH), systemic inflammation and oxidative stress, exacerbations, shared risk factors and genetics, as well as COPD phenotype. PH, usually prevalent in severe COPD, can cause right HF, which gradually leads to left HF. COPD patients may present with altered cardiac repolarization which can be traced back to hypoxemia, potentially increasing the risk of ventricular arrhythmias and sudden cardiac death (SCD).

Obstructive sleep apnea (OSA): It is a common respiratory sleep disorder affecting approximately 10% of population, and is associated with cardiac mortality and morbidity. The Sleep Heart Health Study reported a 4-fold higher prevalence of AF in OSA patients (OR 4.02; 95% CI 1.03–15.74). The risk of AF increases with the severity of OSA. In addition, OSA is more prevalent among patients with AF than in general population. A prospective study reported a strong association between these two conditions (adjusted OR 2.19; 95% CI 1.40–3.42; $p = 0.0006$). With respect to AF treatment, the presence of OSA significantly reduces the efficacy of pharmacological and non-pharmacological therapies for AF.

Type 2 diabetes mellitus (T2DM): The pathogenic factors associated with DM—glycemic fluctuations, oxidative stress, and inflammation, are also responsible for increasing the risk of AF. Studies have found that glycemic fluctuations, rather than hyperglycemia alone, as the reason of AF in diabetes. Elevated oxidative stress levels can also aggravate inflammation, leading

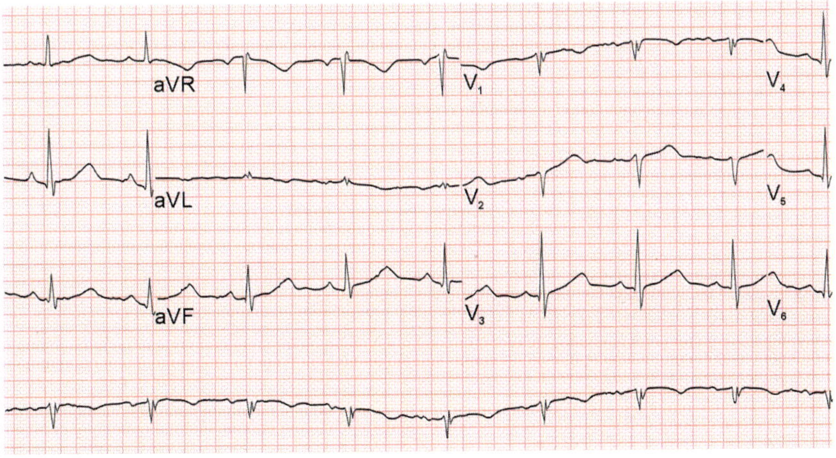

FIG. 3: Evaluation.

TABLE 2: Life-threatening arrhythmias in various cardiac and noncardiac conditions.

Cause	Pathophysiologic substrate	Rhythm presentation
Cardiac causes		
Coronary artery disease: Atherosclerotic, coronary spasm, congenital anomalies	• Acute myocardial ischemia/infarction, ventricular rupture, tamponade • Ventricular scar from healed infarction	• Polymorphic VT/VF • Bradyarrhythmia • Pulseless electrical activity • Ventricular tachycardia • Ventricular fibrillation
Cardiomyopathies: Dilated, hypertrophic, ARVC, infiltrative disease, valvular disease with LV failure	• Ventricular scar • Ventricular hypertrophy • Pump failure	• Ventricular tachycardia • Polymorphic VT/VF • Pulseless electrical activity • Bradyarrhythmia
Congenital heart disease (tetralogy of Fallot, VSD, others)	• Ventricular scar from surgical repair • Hypertrophy	• Ventricular tachycardia • Bradyarrhythmias • Polymorphic VT/VF
Aortic stenosis	• Obstruction to outflow • Ventricular hypertrophy	• Bradyarrhythmia • Pulseless electrical activity • Polymorphic VT/VF
Mitral valve prolapse/mitral regurgitation	• Pump failure • Ventricular scar	• Ventricular tachycardia • Polymorphic VT/VF

Arrhythmia syndromes without structural heart disease:
• Genetic:
  ○ Long QT
  ○ Brugada
  ○ CPVT
• Idiopathic VF, early repolarization
• Drug toxicities (acquired long QT, others)
• Electrolyte abnormalities (severe hypokalemia)
	Abnormal cellular electrophysiology	Polymorphic VT/VF

Wolff–Parkinson–White Syndrome	Accessory atrioventricular connection	Pre-excited AF/VF
Noncardiac causes of cardiovascular collapse		
Pulmonary embolism		PEA
Stroke		PEA, bradyarrhythmia
Aortic dissection		PEA, VF
Exsanguination		PEA
Tension pneumothorax		PEA
Sepsis		PEA
Neurogenic		PEA, bradyarrhythmia
Drug overdose		PEA, bradyarrhythmia

(ARVC: arrhythmogenic right ventricular cardiomyopathy; VF: ventricular fibrillation; VSD: ventricular septal defect; VT: ventricular tachycardia)

to proarrhythmic structural remodeling. Inflammatory markers are significantly elevated in diabetic patients, resulting in an increased incidence of AF. A meta-analysis found that, diabetic patients were at 34% higher risk of AF.

Pathophysiology of diabetes and AF is shown in **Flowchart 2**.

Chronic kidney disease: According to a study, it is suggested that CKD stimulates inflammasome nucleotide-binding domain, leucine-rich-containing family, pyrin domain-containing 3 (NLRP3) in cardiomyocytes and promotes arrhythmias. The risk of arrhythmias may be aggravated by CKD, which is a pro-arrhythmic in itself. The major

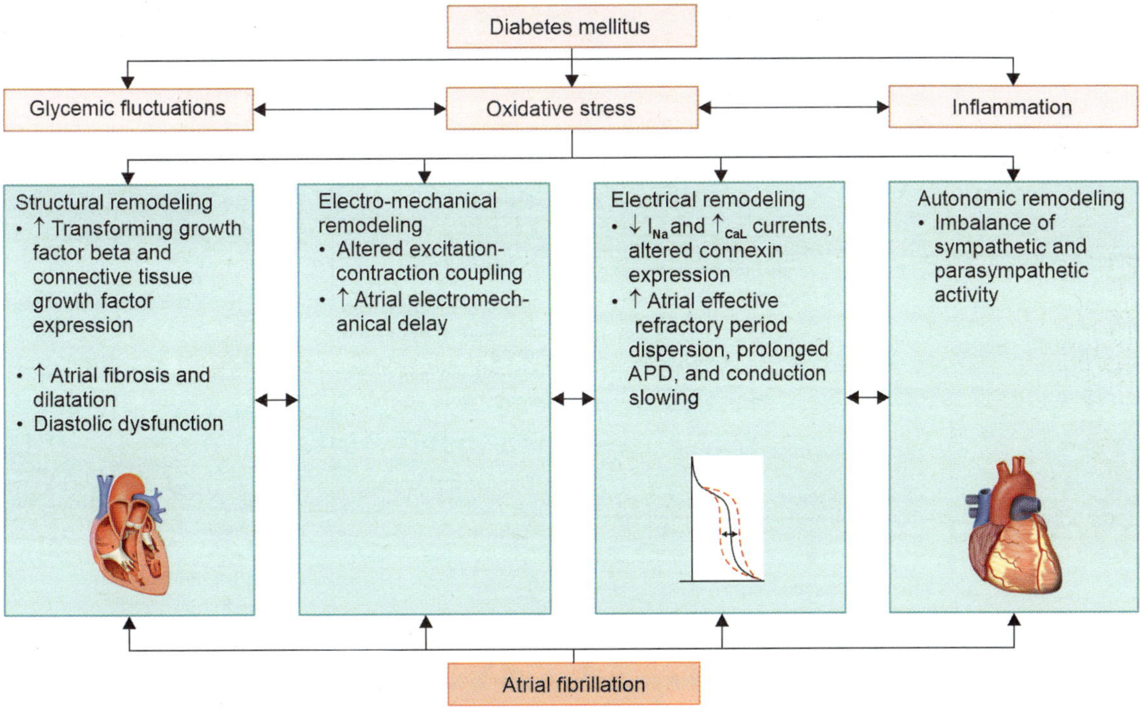

FLOWCHART 2: Pathophysiology of diabetes and atrial fibrillation.
(APD: action potential duration)

cause of death in these patients is SCD due to ventricular tachyarrhythmias or bradyarrhythmias **(Fig. 4)**.

Various electrolytes abnormalities and their electrocardiogram (ECG) changes lead to various arrhythmias **(Fig. 5)**.

Obesity: The dysregulated state of adipose tissue, which is a characteristic of obesity increases the pro-inflammatory adipokines (i.e., leptin) and decreases anti-inflammatory adipokines (i.e., adiponectin), placing the body in a chronic inflammatory state which has been related to occurrence of arrhythmia **(Fig. 6)**

Dyslipidemia: *Hypercholesterolemia* is proatherogenic, autonomic imbalance, alteration of the contractile properties of the myocardium, increased oxidative stress, and ventricular electrophysiological remodeling are the three prolonged action potential durations, longer QTc (heart rate corrected QT interval durations), conduction slowing and increased repolarization dispersion.

Hypertension (HTN): Hypertensive patients have twice the risk of AF occurrence compared to non-hypotensive patients. Blood pressure (BP) and AF share a bidirectional, complex relationship which involves both left atrium and ventricle. Atrial cardiomyopathy—the underlying process—triggers ectopic focal firing, forming reentry cycles, and interrupting atrial conduction. The pathophysiology of AF in hypertensive patients includes various coexisting processes such as structural, hemodynamic, and neuroendocrine changes **(Fig. 7)**.

Metabolic dysfunction-associated steatotic liver disease (MASLD) (NAFLD: nonalcoholic fatty liver disease): Studies prove that patients with NAFLD have a higher occurrence of permanent (chronic) AF and are predisposed to incident AF. Low-grade systemic inflammation plays is an important contributor to the progression of cardiomyopathy and cardiac arrhythmias associated with NAFLD. Proinflammatory factors associated with NAFLD have the potential to alter the electrophysiology and the structural substrates of the myocardium, which leads to a higher risk of arrhythmias.

Cancer: Presence of a strong correlation between cancer and cardiac arrhythmias, can be due to previous heart disease or tumor and its complications or of chemotherapies. Many agents used for chemotherapy, such as anthracyclines or monoclonal antibodies are known to cause cardiotoxicity. Oncological patients presenting with electrolytic abnormalities, cachexia, and systemic or local inflammation have a higher incidence of arrhythmia. Exposure of the heart during radiation therapy (RT) can potentially cause arrhythmias, including SV, VA, and AV node dysfunction. Several chemotherapeutic agents and supportive drugs (opioids, antidepressants, antiemetics, and antibiotics) can cause torsade de pointes by prolonging the QT interval. Occurrence of postoperative AF after lung resection is another common finding.

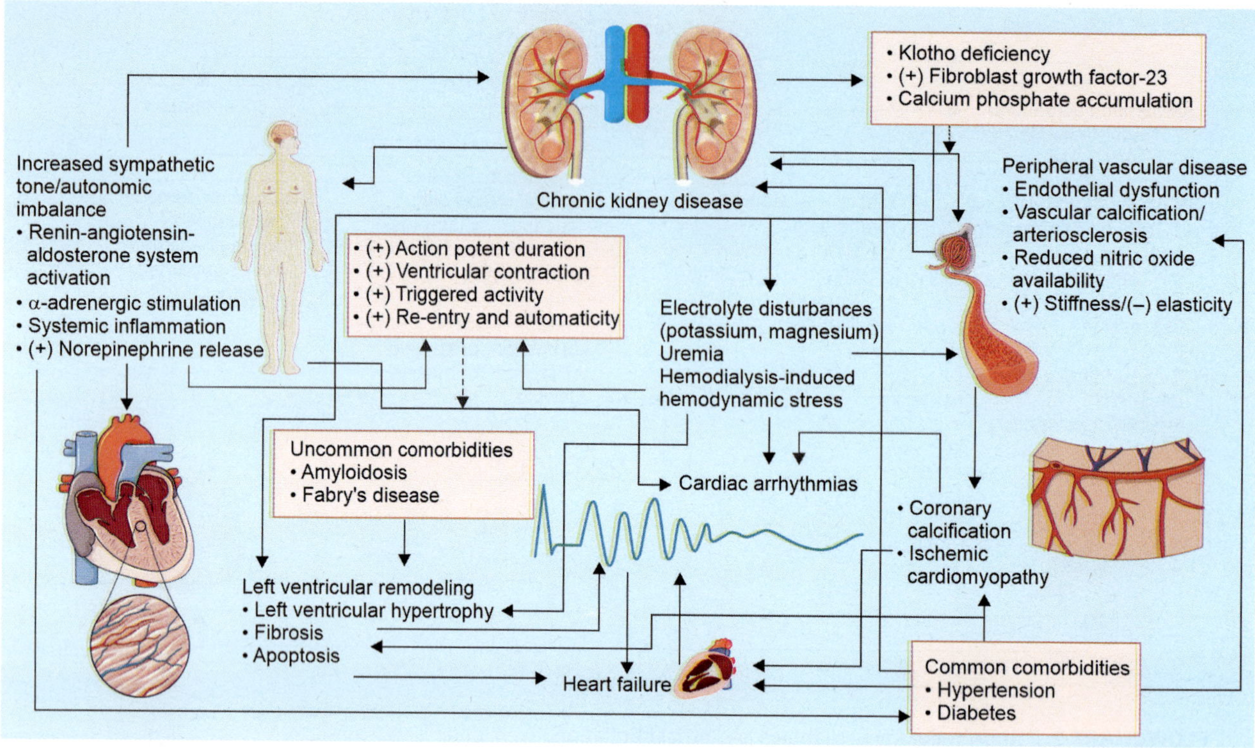

FIG. 4: Chronic kidney disease with arrhythmia.

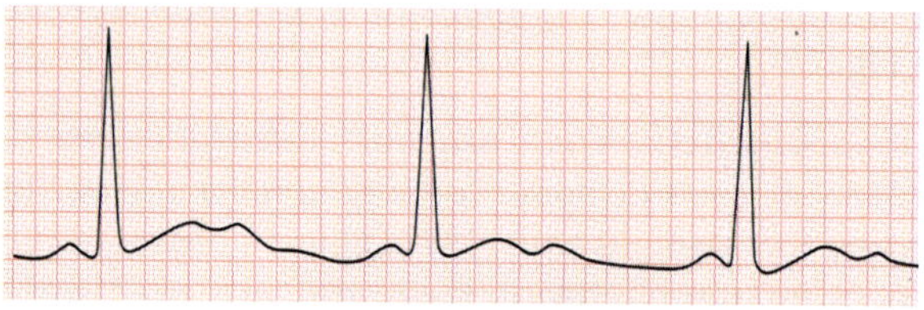

ECG S/O HYPOKALEMIA

Calcium

Hypercalcemia: This causes shortening of the QT interval due to shortening of the ST segment. This gives an abrupt slope to the proximal limb of the T wave

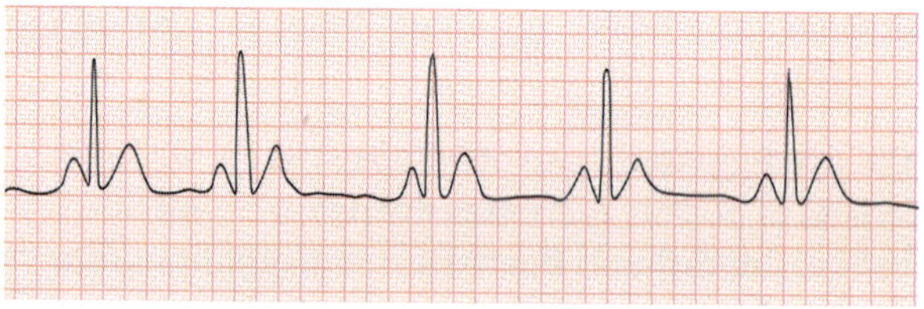

Hypercalcemia showing short QT interval

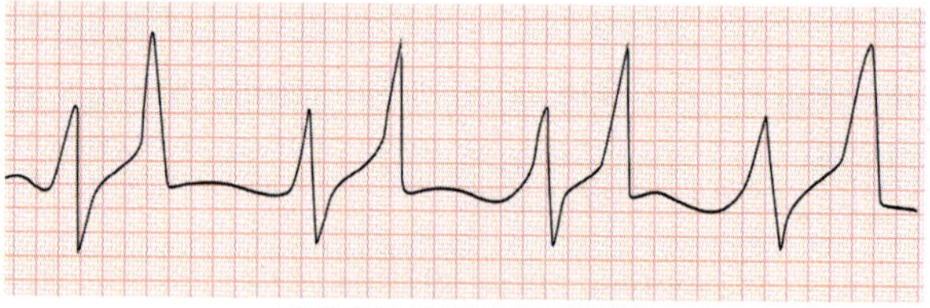

ECG S/O HYPERKALEMIA

Hypocalcemia: This causes a prolonged QT interval due to lengthening of the ST segment. In some patients, there is, in addition, terminal T wave changes some leads. These changes may also occur in hypomagnesemia

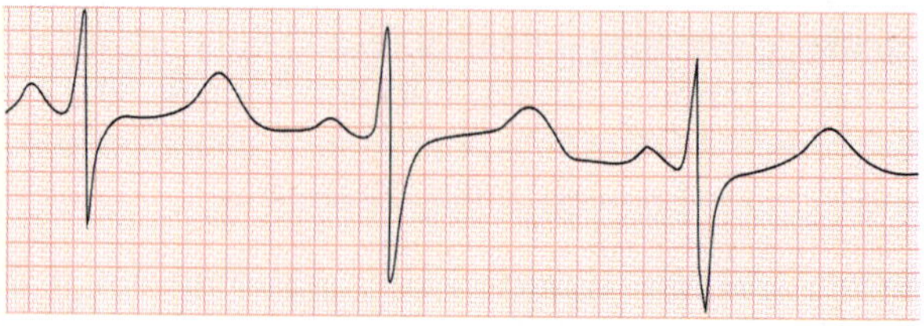

Hypocalcemia showing prolonged QT interval

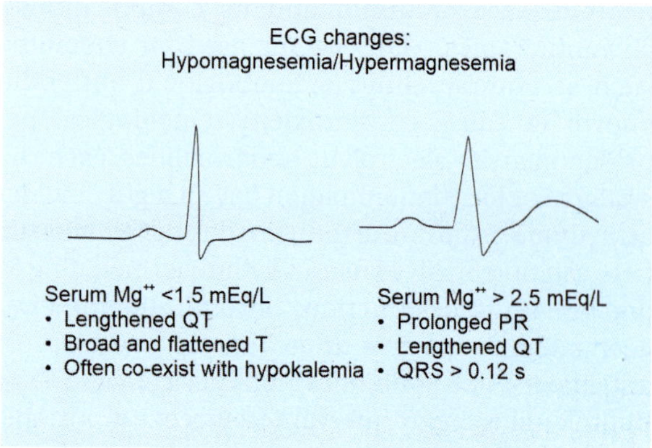

FIG. 5: Various electrolytes abnormalities and their electrocardiogram (ECG).

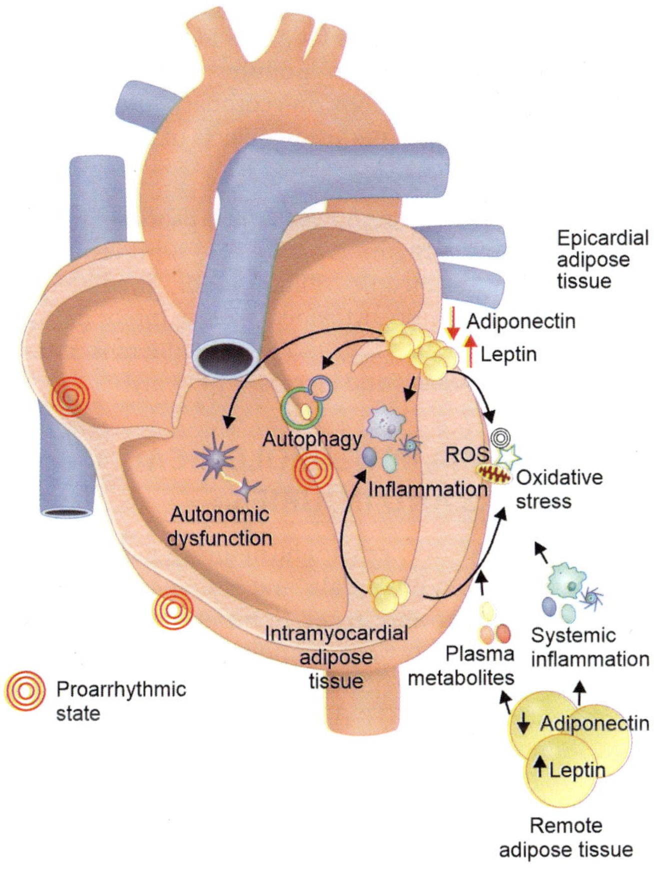

FIG. 6: Proposed mechanisms of obesity in pathogenesis of arrhythmia.

Coronary heart disease (CHD): A strong correlation between CHD and AF because the many common risk factors they share may play prominent roles in their development. CHD directly promotes the AF progression by affecting reentry formation, focal ectopic activity, and neural remodeling. AF also affects CHD through three aspects: 1. atherosclerosis, 2. the mismatch of blood supply and oxygen consumption, and 3. thrombosis. CHD and AF can aggravate each other and form a vicious loop along with other comorbidities such as DM, HTN, CKD, obesity, etc.

ARRHYTHMIA IN DISORDERS OF THE GASTROINTESTINAL SYSTEM

Gastroesophageal reflux disease (GERD): The pathological mechanisms underlying GERD, which can trigger AF include—autonomic activation, inflammation, comorbidities such as obesity and sleep-disordered breathing. Acid refluxes produce local inflammation that may directly alter the autonomic innervations of the esophageal mucosa, stimulating the adjacent vagal nerves by penetrating the esophageal wall. This cardio-esophageal reflex is assumed to trigger AF. Transmission of the local inflammatory processes through the esophageal wall to the left atrium may also cause local pericarditis or atrial myocarditis.

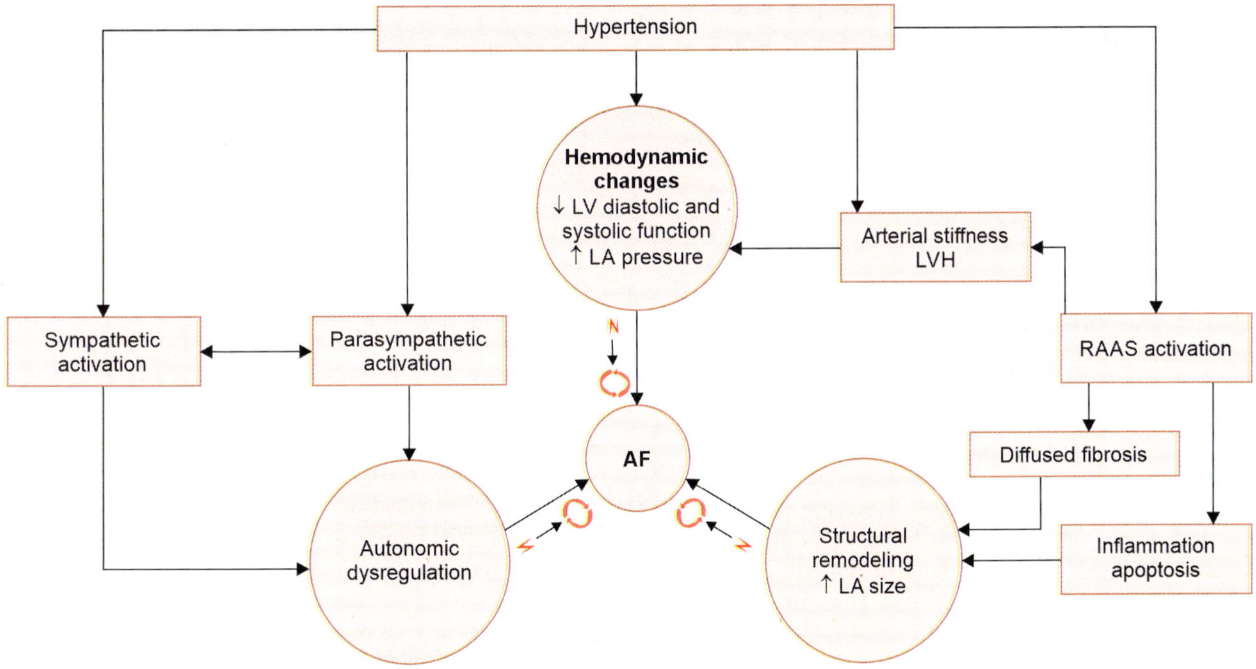

FIG. 7: Potential mechanisms of association between hypertension and AF.

(AF: atrial fibrillation; LA: left atrium; LV: left ventricle; LVH: left ventricle hypertrophy; RAAS: renin–angiotensin–aldosterone system)

Inflammatory bowel disease (IBD): A predominant pathophysiological feature of IBD, i.e., systemic inflammation is known to trigger the development of AF. Systemic inflammation is associated with negative factors such as oxidative stress, apoptosis, and fibrosis of cardiomyocytes, responsible for structural and electrical remodeling of the atria, thereby, encouraging the development of AF. Elevated CRP and IL-6 are strong predictors of AF in patients of IBD.

Celiac disease: AF is the most common arrhythmia with an occurrence rate 30% higher than in the general population. An elevated risk of VA has been also reported. Inflammation and fibrosis, the coexistence of other autoimmune conditions (T1D, RA, and thyroid disease) and hyperhomocysteinemia, resulting from vitamin B deficiency, increase the risk of AF.

ARRHYTHMIA IN AUTOIMMUNE DISORDERS

Sarcoidosis: VT (23%) is most commonly found in sarcoidosis while atrial arrhythmias (15–17%) are less common. The pathological processes of sarcoidosis, triggering AF include—active inflammation and enhanced automaticity. Atrial dilatation or pulmonary involvement can potentially lead to atrial arrhythmias.

Systemic lupus erythematosus (SLE): The most prevalent arrhythmias in systemic lupus erythematous patients are sinus tachycardia (15–50%), AF, and atrial ectopic beats. Initial inflammatory cell infiltration and, with advancing SLE, myocardial necrosis and fibrotic replacement are the disease processes that cause arrhythmias in SLE. Many small areas of fibrosis can affect atrial and ventricular repolarization and conduction, triggering cardiac rhythm disorders.

Scleroderma: Premature ventricular contractions (PVC; 20–67%) and VT (7–28%) are the most common. Supraventricular tachycardia (SVT) (32–66%) is also frequently present in scleroderma patients. The most usual pathogenesis of cardiac rhythm disorders in scleroderma patients is myocardial fibrosis, which disrupts the normal electrical connectivity of cardiac tissue. Secondary LA and RV dilation due to PH, more severe mitral and tricuspid regurgitation, and terminal renal failure can also be the reasons behind onset of arrhythmia in scleroderma.

Graves' disease: AF is the most common cardiac rhythm disorder in gestational diabetes (GD) patients. The development of AF in hyperthyroid patients can be reasoned to decreased atrial refractory period, increased sympathetic tone with decreased heart rate variability (HRV), and automaticity in the pulmonary vein.

Rheumatoid arthritis (RA): AF is most prevalent among RA patients. The mediators for AF include diffuse cardiac involvement (rheumatoid nodules or inflammatory lesions), coronary vasculitis, and coronary atherosclerotic disease, which causes perfusion defects of the heart with proarrhythmic effects.

Psoriasis: AF is most commonly found in psoriasis patients. Other common arrhythmias are single supraventricular beats and VA. Chronic inflammation mediated by systemic inflammatory cytokines, such as tumor necrosis factor alpha (TNF-α), IL-6, and IL-17, is the most crucial link between psoriasis and increased rates of AF.

ARRHYTHMIA IN NEUROLOGICAL DISORDERS AND INJURIES

Epilepsy: Conductive cardiac and neuronal tissue, cardiac and neural action potentials, and Na^+ and K^+ channels both in the heart and in the brain are all involved in the association between epilepsy and arrhythmia. Prolonged or short QT, increased QT dispersion (QTd), increased corrected QT dispersion (QTcd), and heart rate abnormalities can be observed in epilepsy patients. Patients on antiseizure medications present increased atrioventricular block, bradycardia, arrhythmia, increased QT and QTc durations, and increased QTd and QTcd on ECG. FTQ angle has been recently proved to predict the risk of cardiac arrhythmia in epileptic patients.

SUPRAVENTRICULAR AND VENTRICULAR ARRHYTHMIAS IN THE PREGNANT PATIENTS

Pregnancy is a risk factor for both supraventricular and ventricular arrhythmias due to:

- Neurohormonal changes that occur with pregnancy
- Increased sympathetic outflow
- Increased renin–angiotensin–aldosterone system activation
- Amniotic fluid embolus, obstetrical hemorrhage, and obstetrical infection can cause ventricular arrhythmias.
- In patients with ventricular tachyarrhythmia, the management is similar to the nonpregnant patient.
- Patients can be electrically cardioverted with little risk to the fetus as very little energy reaches the fetus.

HEMATOLOGIC DISEASES

There are associations between arrhythmia and anemia. In patients of anemia several electrocardiographic changes were previously seen, including prolonged QT intervals, ST segment depression, inverted T waves, increased R amplitude after stress test. Anemia was associated with prolonged QT intervals in hypertensive and end stage renal disease patients, as well.

In patients with *sickle cell anemia*, it was reported a blunted autonomic cardiovascular response to changes in posture. Left ventricular systolic and diastolic dysfunction, increased QTc intervals and QT dispersions and late ventricular potentials were found in patients with *beta-thalassemia*, a genetic cause of anemia, due to reduced synthesis of beta-globin chains. It was seen that packed red blood cells (PRBCs) *transfusions* were independently associated with an increased risk of new onset cardiac arrhythmias and conduction abnormalities in patients with acute myocardial infarction. A significant correlation was found between QT dispersion and *platelet count* in healthy centenarians, hypothesizing that a reduced number of platelets and the maintenance of normal QT dispersion may contribute to the extreme longevity and protects centenarians from cardiovascular events **(Table 3)**.

MANAGEMENT OF ARRHYTHMIAS

Diagnosis, Detection, and Management of Life-threatening Arrhythmias

Hospital admissions, high morbidity, and mortality are significantly associated with arrhythmias.

TABLE 3: Mechanisms of ventricular arrhythmias and methods used to assess sudden cardiac risk in some extracardiac diseases.

Disease	Mechanisms	Methods and arrhythmia
Obesity	Parasympathetic withdrawal, conduction abnormalities, cardiomyopathy of obesity, lipotoxicity of the myocardium induced by free fatty acids, structural heterogeneity due to fatty infiltration of the heart, focal myocardial disarray, fibrosis, and mononuclear cell infiltration	• SAECG • QTd • QT • PVCs
Hypercholesterolemia	Autonomic imbalance, endothelial dysfunction, oxidative stress, and impaired functionality of ion channels	• QTc • QTd • LVPs • PVCs
Anorexia nervosa, bulimia nervosa	Electrolyte imbalances (hypokalemia)	QT, LVPs
Diabetes mellitus	Autonomic imbalance, oxidative stress, increased cytosolic calcium, increased Na^+ current, hyperinsulinemia, insulin resistance, and hypokalemia	QT, QTd, LVPs
Liver cirrhosis	Cirrhotic cardiomyopathy, cardiac ion channel remodeling, electrolyte imbalances, impaired autonomic function	QT
Stroke, subarachnoid hemorrhage	Cardiac autonomic imbalance, neural interventions, norepinephrine, calcium influx, myocytolysis, hypokalemia, concomitant myocardial ischemia and heart failure, risk factors for coronary heart disease, aging, inflammation, and Takotsubo cardiomyopathy	• QT • QTd • VT, R/T, VF, Vf Holter monitoring
Intracranial hemorrhage	Intraventricular blood, hydrocephalus	• QTc • PVCs, TdP
Neuromuscular disorders	Cardiomyopathy, diffuse cardiac fibrosis and fatty acid infiltration, and myocyte degeneration	• QTcd, JTcd • QTc, LVPs
Parkinson's disease	Autonomic disturbance (intrinsic or iatrogenic), cardiovascular comorbidities, electrolyte imbalances, and degeneration of cardioselective neurons	QT
Epilepsy	Sympathovagal imbalance, impaired cardiac repolarization, dysfunction of cortical networks, ictal hypoxemia and hypercapnia, stress hormones, cardiorespiratory interactions, and fibrosis (perivascular, interstitial)	• QT • QTd, LVPs, PVCs
Anemia	Left ventricular hypertrophy, sympathetic nervous system activation, oxidative stress, chronic inflammation, and decreased myocardial oxygen supply	• QT • QTd • LVPs

Sudden onset of the arrhythmias could be suggestive of systemic problems due to hypoxia, acid-base disturbances, and multiple organ dysfunction.

The clinical presentation, 12-lead surface electrocardiogram and response to vagal maneuvers or drugs are helpful in *diagnosing the underlying causes of the arrhythmia* and in determining the appropriate management, particularly in the emergency settings.

Life-threatening tachyarrhythmia mainly presents as palpitations together with syncope, dizziness, or near syncope.

Management of life-threatening arrhythmia can be incredibly challenging in advanced health systems.

Published data shows that in acute conditions—cardioversion—commonly electrical cardioversion and pacemaker implantation are offered to terminate and treat the arrhythmias respectively.

Long-term therapy includes antiarrhythmic drugs-commonly amiodarone, permanent transvenous pacemaker implantation, and percutaneous coronary intervention are common therapies.

PRINCIPLES OF MANAGEMENT OF ACUTE ATRIAL FIBRILLATION (FLOWCHART 3)

- Determine if AF is the primary concern ("primary AF") or secondary to another acute medical illness ("secondary AF").
- Evaluate hemodynamic stability, defined as AF causing hypotension, acute coronary syndrome, or pulmonary edema.
- Establish an arrhythmia management strategy, defined as rate versus rhythm control.
- Assess the need for hospitalization.
- Determine of the need for oral anticoagulation.
- Schedule early follow-up sessions.

MANAGEMENT OF TACHYARRHYTHMIAS

The **Figure 8** provides an overview of the management of tachyarrhythmias.

POLYMORPHIC VENTRICULAR TACHYCARDIA–TORSADES DE POINTES (FIG. 9)

- *Reasons of acquired QT prolongation*: Drugs (most notably type IA or type III antiarrhythmic agents, tricyclic antidepressants, non-sedating antihistamines, erythromycin, and antifungal agents), electrolyte abnormalities and other conditions as hypothyroidism and CVA.
- Risk factors for QT prolongation and torsades de pointes (TdP) tachycardias in ICU/critical care unit (CCU) admitted patients include—elderly age, renal and hepatic dysfunction, and electrolyte abnormalities.

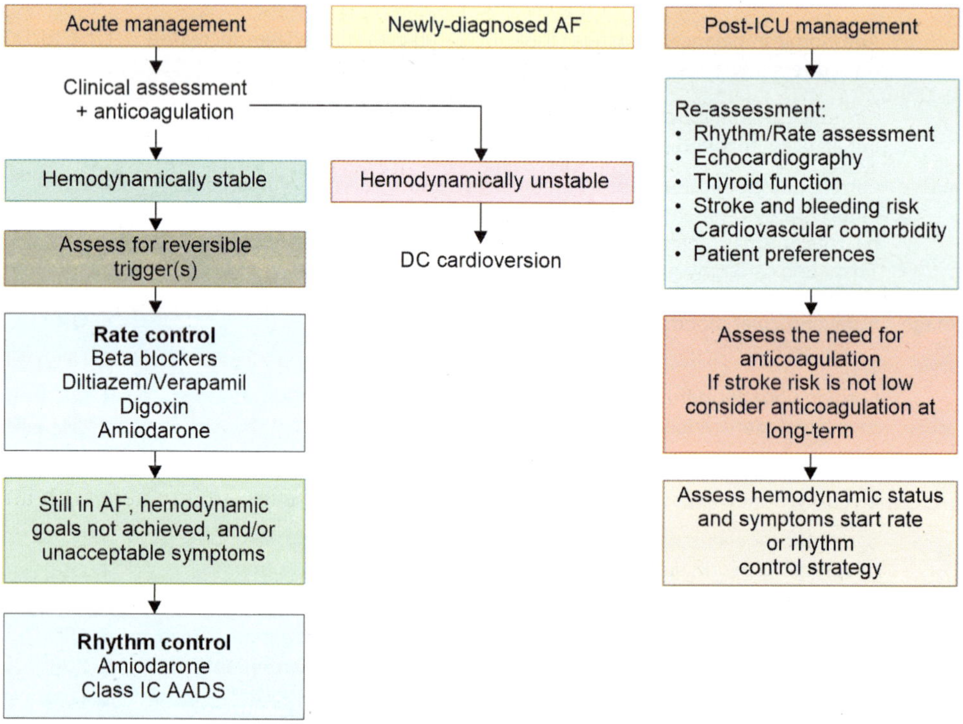

FLOWCHART 3: Management of arrhythmias.

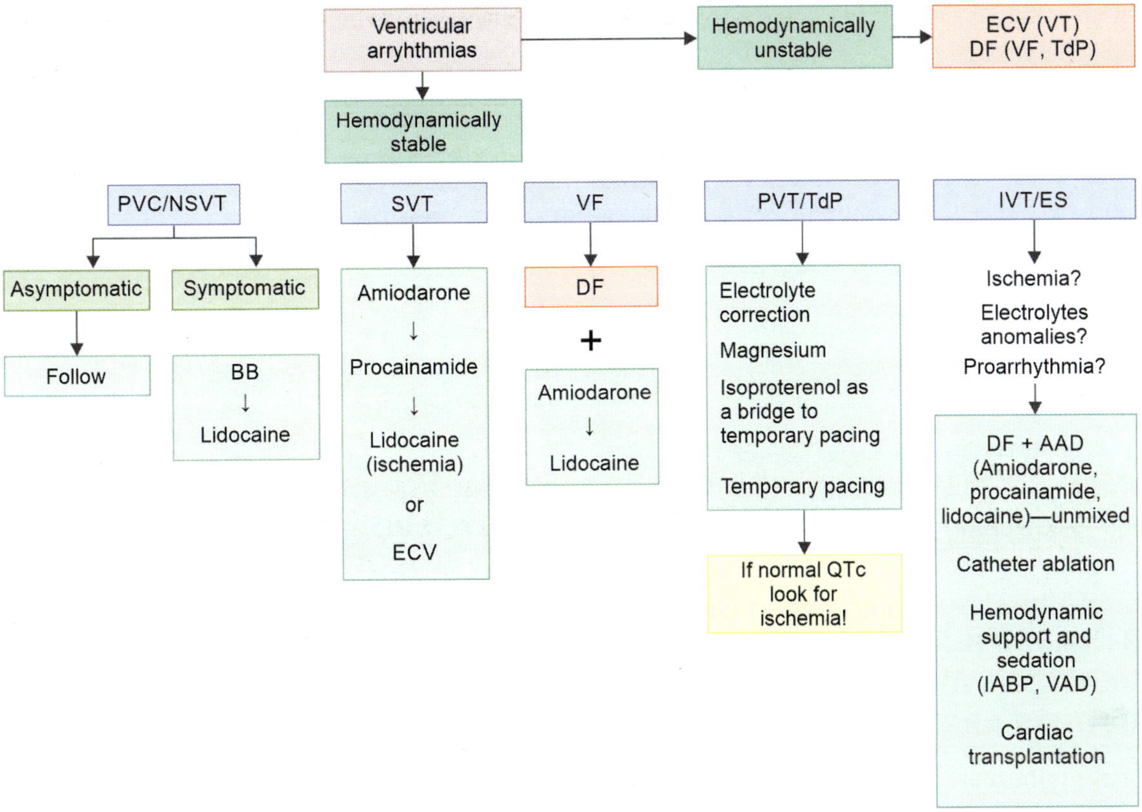

FIG. 8: Management of tachyarrhythmias.

(AAD: antiarrhythmic drug; ECV: electrical cardioversion; DF: defibrillation; ES: electrical storm; VF: ventricular fibrillation; IABP: intra-aortic balloon pump; IVT: incessant ventricular tachycardia; PVC: premature ventricular tachycardia; TdP: Torsade de pointes; SVT: sustained ventricular tachycardia; VAD: ventricular assist device)

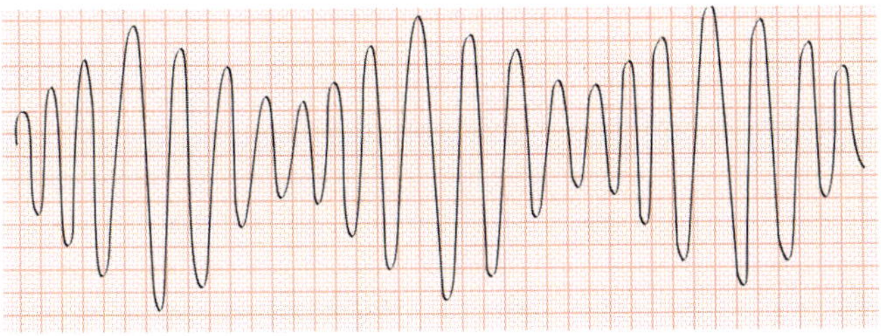

FIG. 9: Electrocardiogram (ECG)—polymorphic ventricular tachycardia–torsades de pointes (TdP).

- The management of TdP differs markedly from other forms of VT.
- Stopping of all QT prolonging drugs and correcting of electrolytes are crucial.
- These patients may also benefit from use of isoproterenol.

MANAGEMENT OF BRADYARRHYTHMIAS (FLOWCHART 4)

Medical conditions, medications, or respiratory status results in bradyarrhythmia in ICU settings.

Lots of causes of bradycardia or heart block are anticipated to be reversible in the ICU setting.

However, temporary pacing may be required in situations where recurrent bradycardia is compromising the patient or impeding care.

For few episodes of symptomatic pauses or if a definite need for transvenous pacing has not been established, external transcutaneous pacing is available.

Another indication for transcutaneous pacing might be during right heart manipulation (e.g., placement of right heart catheter) in a patient with an underlying left bundle branch block.

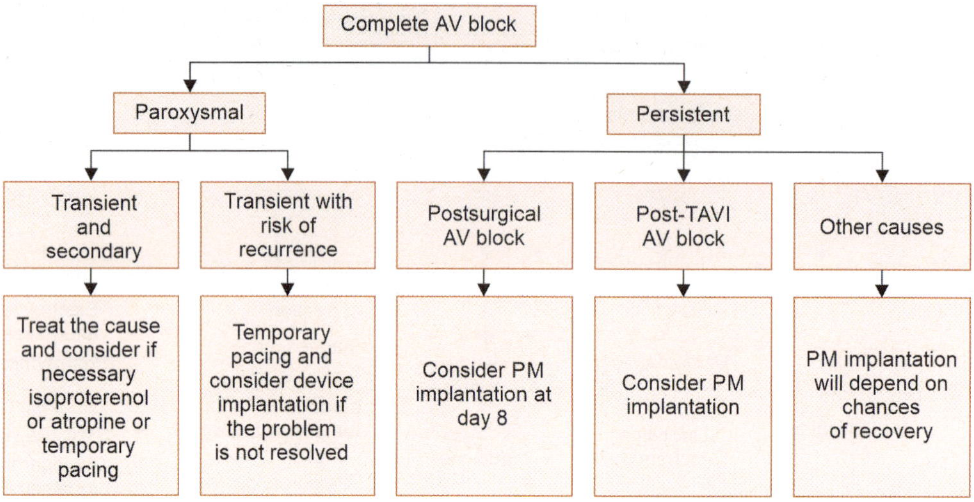

FLOWCHART 4: Management of bradyarrhythmias.
(PM: pacemaker)

MAJOR CLASSIFICATIONS OF INTERVENTIONS AVAILABLE FOR VENTRICULAR ARRHYTHMIAS

Table 4 presents the major classifications of interventions available for ventricular arrhythmias.

TABLE 4: Major classifications of interventions available for ventricular arrhythmias.

Interventions for VA	Description
Electrical	Cardioversion or defibrillation for sustained VA and SVA. First-line therapy for unstable patients
Pharmacological	Use antiarrhythmic medications which are guided by the substrate and mechanism of the rhythm, according to the Singh–Vaughan–Williams classification
Percutaneous	• Ablation can be performed both in the left and right atria and ventricles as well as on the epicardial and endocardial surfaces • Ongoing ischemia can be corrected with percutaneous coronary intervention
Surgical	Extracorporeal membrane oxygenation, biventricular assist device, or biventricular impella (BiPella) can be considered

FIRST STEP IN ARRHYTHMIA IS TO RESUSCITATE

The first step in the evaluation of an arrhythmia is to assess the hemodynamic status of the patient, BP, evidence of myocardial ischemia and/or congestive cardiac failure (chest pain, breathlessness) and cerebral perfusion (confusion or reduced consciousness level).

If the patient is in cardiac arrest, follow Advance Cardiac Life Support (ACLS) guidelines suggested by American Heart Association (AHA) and European Resuscitation Council (ERC).

In the presence of arrhythmias with significant hemodynamic instability, prompt restoration to sinus rhythm is the priority—cardioversion for tachyarrhythmias and pacing for bradyarrhythmias is indicated.

VARIOUS CORRECTABLE CAUSES OF ARRHYTHMIA

- Electrolyte disturbances—hypo and hyperkalemia, hypomagnesemia, and hypocalcemia
- Structural or ischemic heart disease
- Acute pulmonary conditions—pneumothorax, pulmonary embolism
- Medication—vasopressors and inotropes
- Intoxication—TCA, digitalis, drug producing prolongation of QT interval
- Mechanical stimulation—central venous or pulmonary artery catheter, myocardial injury
- Hypo and hyperthermia
- Metabolic acidosis or acid base imbalance
- Hypo and hyperthyroidism
- Hypoxemia or hypercarbia

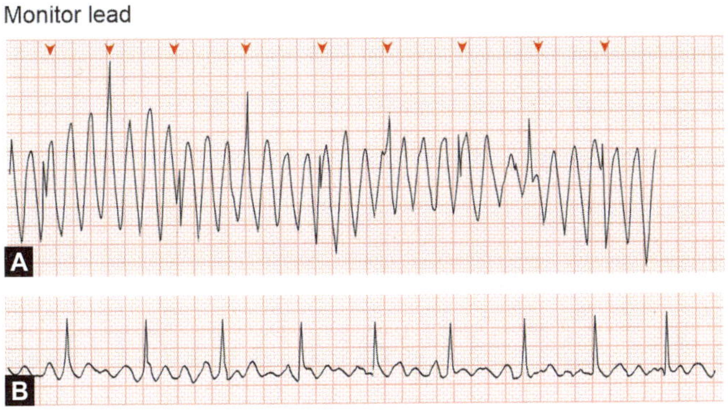

FIGS. 10A AND B: Electrocardiogram (ECG)—differentiate artefact from ventricular tachycardia.

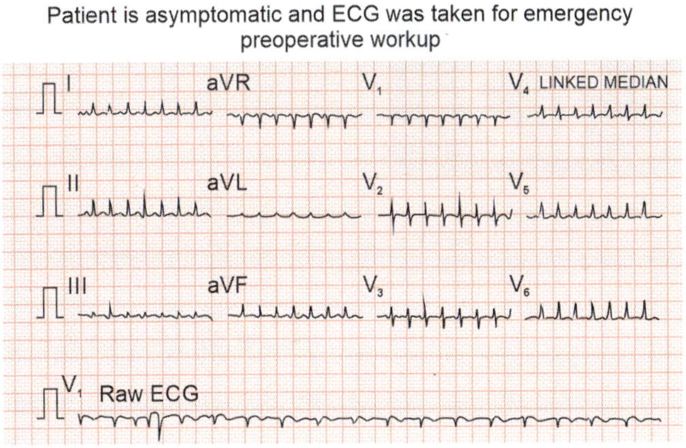

FIG. 11: Linked and raw electrocardiogram (ECG) of the same patient.

POINTS TO BE REMEMBERED

Ventricular Mimics

- Apparently the most common mimic in real world scenario is artefact.
- Such artefacts have increased over the last decade with the advent of recording devices, such as smart phones and watches, various types of long-term ambulatory monitors, loop recorders, pacemakers, and device logs.
- Artefacts have been found to be misdiagnosed as monomorphic or polymorphic VT or even VF in awake conscious humans!
- Artefacts have been found to be misdiagnosed as monomorphic or polymorphic VT or even VF in awake conscious humans!

Characteristics that may differentiate artefact from VT, over and above the common sense of the attending clinician, include the absence of hemodynamic deterioration or symptoms during the event, interspersed normal QRS complexes within the event, nonphysiologic RR intervals, an unstable baseline before the event, after the event, or both, lack of a pause after the artefactual tachyarrhythmia; and association with body movement **(Fig. 10)**.

IMPORTANCE OF RAW ELECTROCARDIOGRAM

Figure 11 shows the significance of the RAW electrocardiogram.

CONCLUSION

Systemic inflammation, a common factor in numerous acute and chronic diseases can trigger a variety of arrhythmias. Attention should be paid not only to the characteristics and mechanisms of the existing arrhythmias, but also to the upstream pathophysiology underlying the occurrence of those arrhythmias. Identification of at-risk patients along with diligent monitoring is important for prevention and early detection of life-threatening arrhythmias. The focus of the medical management should be on correction of the potential triggers as, treating the root cause may help resolve arrhythmias completely in certain cases.

Never diagnose the cause for a wide QRS complex tachycardia based on the ECG in isolation; clinical correlation is must.

SUGGESTED READINGS

1. Vonderlin N, Siebermair J, Kaya E, Köhler M, Rassaf T, Wakili R. Critical inflammatory mechanisms underlying arrhythmias. Herz. 2019;44(2):121-9.
2. Boriani G, Fauchier L, Aguinaga L, Beattie JM, Blomstrom Lundqvist C, Cohen A, et al. European Heart Rhythm Association (EHRA) consensus document on management of arrhythmias and cardiac electronic devices in the critically ill and post-surgery patient, endorsed by Heart Rhythm Society (HRS), Asia Pacific Heart Rhythm Society (APHRS), Cardiac Arrhythmia Society of Southern Africa (CASSA), and Latin American Heart Rhythm Society (LAHRS). Europace. 2019;21(1):7-8.
3. Bernardi J, Aromolaran KA, Aromolaran AS. Neurological disorders and risk of arrhythmia. Int J Mol Sci. 2021;22(1):188.

12

CHAPTER

Evaluation of Bradyarrhythmia

Ajay K Pandey

ABSTRACT

Bradyarrhythmia is a group of conditions where resting heart rate is below 60 beats/minute in adults, it is most common in sinus bradycardia. Causes include age-related degeneration, heart diseases, medications, electrolyte imbalances, autoimmune disorders, and hypothyroidism. Symptoms include fatigue, dizziness, shortness of breath, chest discomfort, confusion, and reduced exercise tolerance. Accurate evaluation is crucial for diagnosis and management.

INTRODUCTION

Bradyarrhythmia is a group of conditions in which resting heart rate is below 60 beats/minute in adults. Sinus bradycardia is the most common type of bradyarrhythmia where the heart's natural pacemaker [sinoatrial (SA) node] generates electrical signals at slower rate.

Important causes include:

- Age-related degeneration
- Certain heart diseases
- Certain medications
- Electrolyte imbalances
- Autoimmune disorders
- Medical conditions like hypothyroidism

Symptoms may include fatigue, dizziness, syncope, shortness of breath, chest discomfort, confusion, and reduced exercise tolerance. Severity of symptoms depends on the cause, heart rate reduction, and overall health; timely evaluation is crucial.

Evaluation of bradyarrhythmia plays a crucial role in establishing the causes, assessing symptom's severity, identifying risk factors, planning suitable treatment approaches, and monitoring the effect of management. Accurate evaluation is essential for diagnosing, effectively managing, and improving the overall prognosis for individuals with bradyarrhythmia to maintain optimal cardiac functions.

This chapter provides an overview of the fundamental elements of bradyarrhythmia and covers the various evaluation criteria for this condition.

CARDIAC CONDUCTION SYSTEM—ANATOMY AND PHYSIOLOGY

The cardiac conduction system is a network of specialized cells that generates, coordinates, and regulates the electrical signals responsible for the heart's rhythm and cardiac muscles contractions.

Its components are SA node, atrioventricular (AV) node, bundle of His, and Purkinje fibers. The electrical impulses generated in the SA node travel through the atria to reach the AV node; pause briefly and then rapidly spread down the bundle of His and Purkinje fibers.

This coordinated activity causes the ventricles to contract synchronously from the bottom upward, ejecting blood from the ventricles, and completing one cardiac cycle.

Any disruption in the cardiac conduction system leads to various arrhythmias including bradyarrhythmia (slow heart rate) or tachyarrhythmia (fast heart rate).

CLASSIFICATION AND ETIOLOGY OF BRADYARRHYTHMIA

Bradyarrhythmia can be classified according to its distinctive features and the factors contributing to its development. Classification aids in comprehending the root causes and facilitating suitable approaches for their management. Both intrinsic and extrinsic factors can cause bradycardia.

Intrinsic causes of bradycardia are conditions that directly impact the heart's electrical conduction system or the sinus node, which serves as the heart's natural pacemaker. These underlying factors encompass:

- *Bradycardia attributable to sinus node dysfunction (SND):* Sinus node dysfunction involves diverse pathophysiology including complex remodeling of the heart's electrical and structural properties. Age-related increase in collagen content leads to heightened fibrosis, resulting in slower heart rate and SA conduction times. SND may manifest as sinus bradycardia, sinus arrest, or SA exit block.
  Symptoms of SND ranges from mild fatigue on one hand to severe syncope on other and their severity increasing with slower heart rate. Syncope is usually observed in 50% of patients receiving pacemakers for SND. Other symptoms include exertional dyspnea, dizziness, and chronic fatigue.
- *Bradycardia attributable to atrioventricular block*: Atrioventricular block affects the conduction system between the atria and ventricles and can be congenital or acquired. Acquired causes include infections, inflammation, degeneration, ischemia, and medical interventions. Symptoms vary based on the degree of block, ventricular rate, and frequency. Significant first-degree AV block can cause fatigue or exertion intolerance where the prolonged PR interval disrupts AV synchrony, resulting in reduced cardiac output and increased pulmonary capillary wedge pressure ("pseudopacemaker syndrome" with PR interval >300 ms). Asymptomatic second-degree AV block type I (Wenckebach) is usually seen in active, healthy individuals. Still, frequent occurrences or exercise-related episodes can lead to symptoms like exertion intolerance or dizziness.
- *Conduction diseases*: Conduction diseases can have various causes including developmental factors, hereditary/genetic factors, metabolic disorders, infections, inflammation, infiltrative conditions, trauma, ischemia, malignancy, or degenerative processes. Isolated fascicular and bundle branch blocks are usually asymptomatic but may indicate underlying structural heart disease. Symptoms can occur when left bundle branch block (LBBB) presents with cardiac dyssynchrony and reduced left ventricular function. Evaluation of patients with fascicular or bundle branch block depends on the presence or absence of symptoms associated with intermittent bradycardia.

TABLE 1: Medical conditions related to bradycardia and conduction disorders.

Intrinsic	Extrinsic
• Cardiomyopathy (ischemic or nonischemic) • Congenital heart disease • Degenerative fibrosis • Infection or inflammation • Infiltrative disorders • Ischemia or infarction • Rheumatological conditions • Surgical or procedural trauma (cardiac procedures, ablation, or cardiac catheterization)	• Autonomic perturbation (carotid sinus hypersensitivity, cough, micturition, and vomiting) • Sleep (with or without sleep apnea) • Metabolic (acidosis, hyperkalemia, hypokalemia, and hypothermia)

Source: Adapted from Kusumoto FM, et al. (2019).

Extrinsic causes of bradycardia include medication side effects (e.g., β-blockers and calcium channel blockers), hypothyroidism, electrolyte imbalances, obstructive sleep apnea, vagal stimulation, and hypothermia. Medical conditions related to bradycardia and conduction disorders are summarized in **Table 1**.

DIAGNOSTIC EVALUATION OF BRADYARRHYTHMIAS

History and Physical Examination

While evaluating patients suspected of bradycardia or conduction disorders, a comprehensive medical history and physical examinations are essential. The patient's medical history should be systematically obtained, focusing on symptoms associated with these conditions. Specific details such as frequency, timing, duration, and triggers of symptoms should also be enquired. Additionally, assessment of the relationship between the symptoms and various factors, such as medications, meals, medical interventions, emotional distress, physical exertion, positional changes, and specific triggers, like urination, defecation, and coughing are important.

Medication history including prescription and over-the-counter drugs should also be reviewed for potential contributors to bradyarrhythmias.

13

CHAPTER

Conduction System Pacing: A Natural Path to Cure

Smit Shrivastava

ABSTRACT

The pacemakers have saved billions of lives since the first implant in 1958; however, the quest for improving long-term quality of the saved lives still continues. The conventional right ventricular apical pacing is associated with aberrant myocardial activation with long-term adverse consequences of increased left ventricular dysfunction, atrial fibrillation, hospitalization, and possibly mortality. The strategies to minimize right ventricular apical pacing or promote biventricular pacing have effectively subdued these afflictions. The conduction system pacing can be the next step to deliverance as it reestablishes the physiological ventricular electromechanical activation. His bundle pacing, despite being the most physiological method, is deprived of its popular application due to high pacing thresholds, lead dislodgement rates, and a steep learning curve. The left bundle branch area pacing attempts to overcome the shortcomings of His bundle pacing with higher implant success rates, better pacing parameters, and shorter procedure time; however, it awaits consolidation of evidence for a wider acceptability and applicability. The conduction system pacing by employing the intrinsic conduction tissues is fast evolving as a nonesuch panacea that bears promises to unify the implantable cardiac defibrillation, resynchronization, and antitachycardia therapies.

INTRODUCTION

The implanted cardiac pacemakers have saved billions of lives since Senning and Elmqvist implanted the first pacemaker in Sweden on October 8, 1958. The year 2023 is estimated to witness 1.43 million permanent pacemaker implantations worldwide, most of which will be a right ventricular apical implantation. The unavoidable electrical and mechanical dyssynchrony results from pre-excitation of the interventricular septum (IVS) and delayed activation of the lateral left ventricular (LV) wall by right ventricular apical pacing (RVAP). There is mounting data concerning the safety of RVAP that bestows prejudicial effects on myocardial structure and LV function resulting from a pathological electrical activation sequence and subsequent unnatural mechanical activation of the ventricles. Biventricular (BiV) alternative pacing sites including the right ventricular septum or outflow tract were explored for attaining a more profiting activation than the RVAP. These sites failed to demonstrate a significant upgrade over the RVAP as they also induced pacing-induced cardiomyopathy (PICM) due to myocardial cell-to-cell conduction. The paragon cardiac pacing to be physiological mandates a sustained pacing in the vicinity of the intrinsic cardiac conduction system to preserve normal or even compact QRS complexes in preexisting bundle branch blocks (BBB). Direct conduction system pacing (CSP), therefore, is evolving as the final frontier of cardiac pacing that promises to preserve the natural path to cure.

HISTORICAL LANDMARKS

The evaluation of slow pulse in 68-year-old patient Edmund Butler in February 1846 by William Stokes of Dublin initiated a new chapter in clinical electrocardiography. Robert Adams in 1819 had imputed a similar clinical condition to "fatty degeneration of the heart" upon autopsy. The documentation started with the first published electrocardiographic tracing of the normal heartbeat by Willem Einthoven in 1902. Mark C

Lidwill in September 1929 described the use of an external pacemaker to drive a sick infant heart to its revival. Paul M Zoll in 1952 used a bedside device to deliver electrical pulses to the heart to keep alive a patient with recurring episodes of ventricular standstill. Rune Elmqvist and cardiac surgeon Åke Senning in Stockholm implanted the first pacemaker in Sweden on October 8, 1958, on Arne Larsson to help him survive with 26th pacemaker revisions in 43 years till his death in December 28, 2001.

In 1969, Narula recorded and paced the His bundle (HB). Deshmukh used a modified stylet to pace for the first time the HB in 12 patients of atrial fibrillation (AF). Vijayaraman from Geisinger Heart Institute, USA, demonstrated the use of the 4.1 Fr Select Secure 3830 (Medtronic, USA) leads for His bundle pacing (HBP). Huang in 2017 actuated left bundle branch (LBB) pacing when HBP failed to correct left bundle branch block (LBBB) in a patient even at the highest pacing stimulus.

ANATOMICAL CONSIDERATION FOR NORMAL CONDUCTION

In 1893, Sir Wilhelm His Jr reported a yarn of specialized fibers connecting the atria and ventricles. Tawara in 1906 uncovered conduction properties of these strands between the atrioventricular (AV) node and the HB **(Fig. 1)**. The HB divides into three components: (1) Penetrating part across the fibrous membranous septum or the central fibrous body close to the mitral ring and runs anteriorly and inferiorly, (2) nonbranching portion that extends to a variable course at the muscular ventricular septal crest, and (3) branching portion in close proximity to the aortic ring to divide into the LBB and right bundle branch (RBB). The LBB, a thick band-like structure, arises beneath the membranous septum between the right and noncoronary aortic cusps. The LBB divides in a trifascicular pattern into septal, anterior, and posterior fascicles. The septal fascicles supply the mid-septal area, The left anterior fascicle travels toward the anterolateral papillary muscle, while the left posterior fascicle transits toward the posteromedial papillary muscle. The fascicles radiate into an extensive network of Purkinje fibers to supply the LV endocardium.

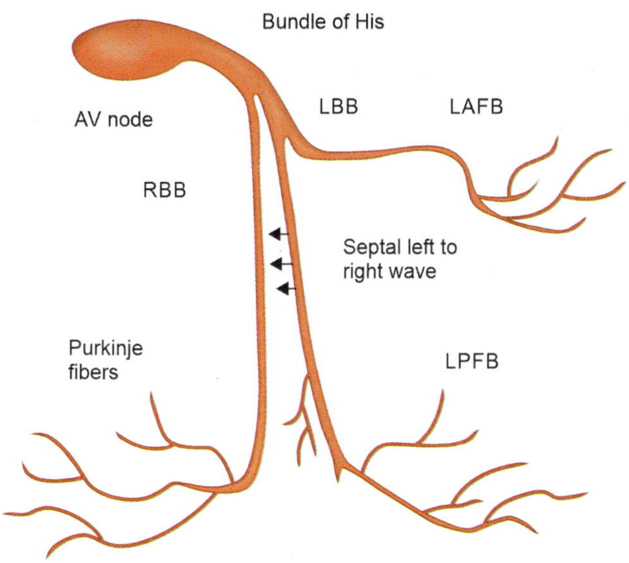

FIG. 1: Physiological initial left to right septal conduction.
(AV: atrioventricular; LBB: left bundle branch; LAFB: left anterior fascicular block; LPFB: left posterior fascicular block; RBB: right bundle branch)

PHYSIOLOGICAL CONSIDERATION FOR NORMAL CONDUCTION

The His–Purkinje system (HPS) commences from the LBB in endocardial areas on the left IVS surface to proceed from the left to the right septum in a noteworthy manner **(Fig. 1)** toward the apicobasal ventricular direction to the Purkinje system ramifications beneath the endocardium.

PACING-INDUCED CARDIOMYOPATHY

The chronic RVAP reverses the initial left to right interventricular septal activation and the sequence of ventricular depolarization. The potential benefit from CSP comes from the natural and physiological septal activation through the conduction fibers rather than slow myocardial conduction. This prevents and reverses the adverse cardiac remodeling that occurs in 20% RVAP in the form of PICM defined as:

- More than 10% reduction in left ventricular ejection fraction (LVEF) irrespective of baseline LVEF in the absence of an identifiable cause other than RV pacing
- An absolute LVEF decrease to ≤40% if the baseline LVEF was ≥50%
- An absolute reduction in LVEF ≥ 5–10% if the baseline LVEF was <50%
- New-onset HF
- Requirement for cardiac resynchronization therapy (CRT) upgrade

CONDUCTION SYSTEM PACING

Biventricular synchronized pacing (BiVP) by CRT is at the pinnacle for heart failure (HF) treatment in reduced ejection fraction and electromechanical ventricular dyssynchrony due to LBBB. Though BiVP has secured significant improvement and survival in numerous studies, it remains essentially a nonphysiological pacing through the unification of two stimuli from the LV epicardium and RV endocardium **(Fig. 2)**. The BiVP reaps no benefits in one-third of its implants. The CSP can be restorative in such complex cases for establishing physiological ventricular electromechanical activation. The CSP includes either HBP or left bundle branch area pacing (LBBAP). These two intended pacing sites encompass multiple sites **(Fig. 3)**.

The HBP includes:
- Selective (without capture of local myocardium: S-HBP)
- Nonselective (with capture of local myocardium: NS-HBP)

Similarly, LBBAP also embraces:
- Selective (S-LBBP)
- Nonselective (NS-LBBP) LBB pacing
- *LV septal pacing (LVSP*: capture of the left side of the septum without capture of the LBB)
- LBBP with anodal capture of the RBB is sometimes observed, resulting in LBBAP without RBBB morphology.

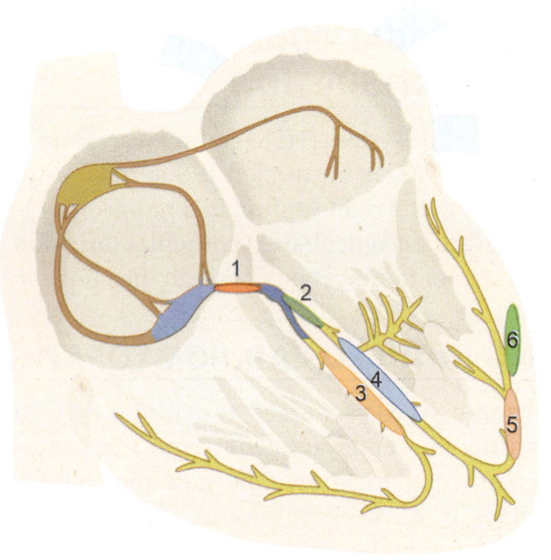

FIG. 2: Locations of the permanent lead placement for ventricular pacing along with strategies for physiological pacing. 1—His bundle pacing, 2—left bundle branch pacing, 3—left septal pacing, 4—right septal pacing, 5—epicardial left ventricular pacing, 6—endocardial left ventricular pacing.

The concept of "physiological pacing" evolved over the last 3 decades after realization of the need to achieve AV synchrony, chronotropic competence, and rate-responsive pacing. Multiple studies revealed that though the atrial-based pacing did not achieve mortality benefits, it had a 20% lower risk of incident AF and a 19% lower risk of stroke, improvements in exercise capacity, quality of life, and device diagnostic function compared to ventricular-based pacing. In the cardiac-defibrillator-implanted patients requiring pacing, the accession of atrial lead has additional ease in differentiating the mechanisms of tachyarrhythmia, though it was not associated with a reduction in inappropriate shocks. The CSP employs longitudinal fascicular dissociation of the HPS histologically and electrophysiologically that diverges early for more distal locations with very few transverse connections **(Fig. 3)**. Therefore, a more distal pacing to the predicted level of block can overcome the disruption.

HIS BUNDLE PACING

The initial studies demonstrated elevated pacing thresholds, acutely high rates of lead dislodgement, poor capture of HB, and a procedural success rate < 70%, due to nonlocalization of HB. With the development of dedicated sheaths and leads, small observational studies

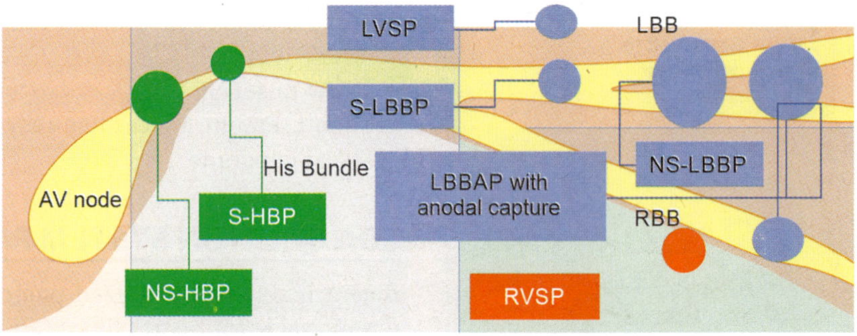

FIG. 3: Types of conduction system pacing.

(AV: atrioventricular; LBB: left bundle branch; LBBAP: left bundle branch area pacing; LVSP: left ventricular systolic pressure; NS-LBBP: nonselective left bundle branch pacing; NS-HBP: nonselective His bundle pacing; RVSP: right ventricular systolic pressure; S-HBP: selective His bundle pacing; S-LBBP: selective left bundle branch pacing) demonstrated a low complication rate and strength of HBP. The HBP system implantations then exhibited the acute beneficial hemodynamic and echocardiographic effects compared to RVAP with the abbreviated ventricular activation time, decreased interventricular dyssynchrony, and reduced mitral valve regurgitation. The tricuspid valve regurgitation was also reduced after replacing CRT with HBP. These mechanistic effects transformed into clinical outcomes in nonrandomized registry studies demonstrating a reduction of the combined endpoint of mortality and HF hospitalizations during long-term follow-up compared to RV pacing. HBP improved New York Heart Association (NYHA) functional class by QRS shortening and improvement of the LVEF in CRT-indicated subjects. Two randomized trials comparing HBP to CRT in an on-treatment fashion (His-SYNC and His-Alternative) showed that the HBP pacing was even superior to CRT in QRS narrowing and echocardiographic response rates. In the largest observational multicenter cohort study of 844 patients for bradycardia indications, HBP decreased the need for CRT to 1.7% of subjects. The device upgrade from RVAP to HBP for PICM was systematically reviewed by Zheng from 144 patients in 6 studies to demonstrate improved LV function and NYHA functional class. Many randomized controlled trials have favored HBP over ventricular resynchronization with CRT. Though the HBP group demonstrated a statistically greater reduction in QRS duration, there was no difference in LVEF improvement, CRT response, hospitalization, or death between the groups. CSP has been also proposed as an alternative to BiV pacing in the right bundle branch block (RBBB). Sharma in a prospective observational study measured RBBB with QRS duration to reduce significantly with HBP, along with improvement in LVEF and NYHA functional class. In meta-analyses that compared HBP versus BiV pacing for CRT, HBP had shorter QRS duration, LV activation time (LVAT), and LV dyssynchrony index, without any significant difference in echocardiographic parameters, functional test, quality of life, HF hospitalizations, or mortality. The present evidences have established a class IIa recommendation for CSP in the latest European pacing guidelines that when coronary sinus lead implantation is unsuccessful, HBP lead implantation emerges as an alternative.

His bundle pacing ascends as the most physiologic pacing, yet it possesses major limitations. There is a significant learning curve of initial 100 plus lead implantations. Furthermore, the His-SYNC trial showed that a crossover to BiV CRT was necessary in nearly half of the intended HBP group, and a quarter of the BiV pacing group to HBP, indicating that the two methods are more complementary than competitive. The success rate is just over 50% even with experienced implanters in the presence of BBB or a complete AV block. Patients with HBP were less likely to experience death or HF hospitalization compared to high burden RV pacing, yet the need for lead revision and generator change are higher in the HBP group as the specialized leads become defunct and the pacing thresholds remain higher. The HB encapsulated in electrically inert fibrous tissue subscribes a low R-wave amplitude resulting in oversensing atrial or His signals and undersensing of ventricular signals.

LEFT BUNDLE BRANCH AREA PACING

In 2017, the first case of LBBP was described by Huang after the failure to amend LBBB in a 72-year-old female with nonischemic dilated cardiomyopathy having LV dysfunction and LBBB. This was soon followed by the earliest observational studies by Zhang and subsequently by Vijayaraman demonstrating successful reduction in QRS duration, NYHA class, cardiac biomarkers, and improvement in echocardiographic parameters. In spite of a more distal pacing with LBBAP, QRS is not significantly prolonged and a more complete and easy rectification of a LBBB is achieved compared to HBP.

The long learning curve and hurdles of transseptal LBBAP lead implantation remain despite the larger target area for lead implantation. The initial experience of over 150 lead implantations is necessary for acquiring an optimal implantation skillset. In comparison to RVAP, the implantation duration and fluoroscopy time are longer. The 4% intraoperative benign perforations across the IVS and long-term extractability of deep-seated LBBAP lead still occupy concerns. The true full LBBP capture (not including fascicular pacing or LV septal pacing) may be achieved in less than half of cases, though successful implantation rates of over 90% for conventional bradycardia indications and over 80% for HF indications were witnessed in European multicenter registry (MELOS).The possible septal myocardial or arterial scathe remains a theoretical threat on multiple attempts at lead emplacement within the septum. The LVSP showed better interventricular synchrony with prolonged LV lateral wall depolarization than LBBP and comparable short-term hemodynamic and electromechanical outcomes to BiVP and HBP. The advantage of LVSP over LBBAP remains to be explored as it alone can improve the clinical outcomes of candidates for CRT without employing additional electrophysiological maneuvers to achieve LBBAP. The nascent LBBAP awaits fortification of the evidence base to consolidate its place in the latest European and American pacing guidelines **(Table 1)**.

TABLE 1: Advantages and disadvantages of His bundle pacing (HBP) versus left bundle branch area pacing (LBBAP).

HBP	LBBAP
Most physiological—total conduction system recruited	Lacks evidences to define capture
Small target zone	Wide area of LBB fibers to target
Long procedure time	Short procedure time
High capture threshold at implant or follow-up	Long and durable low thresholds
More lead revisions	Less lead revisions
Premature battery depletion	Stable battery life
Low sensed R waves	No significant sensing issues
Oversensing of atrial and His signals	No significant sensing issues
Undersensing of ventricular signals	No significant sensing issues
Limitation with infra-Hisian blocks	Suitable for distal conduction disease treatment

LIMITATIONS, CONTROVERSIES, AND FUTURE PERSPECTIVES

The studies on CSP for CRT were carried out in non-ischemic cardiomyopathy; the applicability needs to be validated in scarred fibrotic areas of CSP implant in ischemic, genetic, or acquired cardiomyopathies. CSP-CRT applicabilities beyond LBBB into treating intraventricular conduction delay (IVCD) and RBBB morphologies. CSP has demonstrated high success in small randomized clinical trials and observational studies with remarkable clinical and echocardiographic outcomes in different clinical scenarios such as advanced AV blocks, chronic AF, and CRT indications.

The HBP is seen as the most physiological pacing to restore electrical and mechanical synchrony by simultaneously activating both ventricles through the natural path; however, it suffers poor localization, high pacing thresholds, and lead dislodgement along with a steep learning curve. The counterpart LBBAP directly captures the widespread LBB to preserve the physiological activation of the LV with the advantage of a significantly lower pacing threshold and a higher R-wave amplitude. The LBBAP also boasts of higher implant success rates, better pacing parameters, and shorter procedure time. With trials looking into adding defibrillation capability to LBBAP lead in the future, it can unify the implantable cardiac defibrillation, resynchronization, and anti-tachycardia therapies.

CONCLUSION

The present clinical evidence for BiV pacing exceeds in a staggering manner than for CSP. However, newfangled hardware solutions for CSP are making it grow in popularity and applicability. The future still holds that CSP can evolve to be the new panacea for antibradycardia pacing, intracardiac defibrillation, and cardiac resynchronization therapy. While the evidence is gaining base, patient-specific counseling and individualized treatment decisions are advisable.

SUGGESTED READINGS

1. Larsson B, Elmqvist H, Rydén L, Schüller H. Lessons from the First Patient with an Implanted Pacemaker. Pacing Clin Electrophysiol. 2003;26(1 Pt 1):114-24
2. Statista. (2022). Pacemakers market volume worldwide in units 2023 forecast. [online] Available from https://www.statista.com/statistics/800794/pacemakers-market-volume-in-units-worldwide/#:~:text=Global%20number%20of%20pacemakers%20in%202016%20and%202023&text=As%20of%202016%2C%20it%20was,increase%20to%201.43%20million%20units [Last accessed December, 2023].
3. Tops LF, Schalij MJ, Bax JJ. The effects of right ventricular apical pacing on ventricular function and dyssynchrony. JACC. 2009;54(9):764-76.
4. Ng ACT, Allman C, Vidaic J, Tie H, Hopkins AP, Leung DY. Long-term impact of right ventricular septal versus apical pacing on left ventricular synchrony and function in patients with second- or third-degree heart block. American J Cardiol. 2009;103(8):1096-101.
5. Naqvi TZ, Chao C-J. Adverse effects of right ventricular pacing on cardiac function: prevalence, prevention and treatment with physiologic pacing. Trends Cardiovasc Med. 2023;33(2):109-22.
6. Jeffrey K. Machines in Our Hearts. Maryland: Johns Hopkins University Press; 2001.
7. Narula OS, Javier RP, Samet P, Maramba LC. Significance of His and Left Bundle Recordings from the Left Heart in Man. Circulation. 1970;42(3):385-96.
8. Deshmukh P, Casavant DA, Romanyshyn M, Anderson K. Permanent, Direct His-Bundle Pacing. Circulation. 2000;101(8):869-77.
9. Vijayaraman P, Dandamudi G. How to Perform Permanent His Bundle Pacing: Tips and Tricks. Pacing Clin Electrophysiol. 2016;39(12):1298-304.
10. Huang W, Su L, Wu S, Xu L, Xiao F, Zhou X, et al. A novel pacing strategy with low and stable output: pacing the left bundle branch immediately beyond the conduction block. Can J Cardiol. 2017;33(12):1736.e1-1736.e3.

11. Padala SK, Cabrera J, Ellenbogen KA. Anatomy of the cardiac conduction system. Pacing Clin Electrophysiol. 2021;44(1):15-25.
12. Khurshid S, Epstein AE, Verdino RJ, Lin D, Goldberg LR, Marchlinski FE, et al. Incidence and predictors of right ventricular pacing-induced cardiomyopathy. Heart Rhythm. 2014;11(9):1619-25.
13. Glikson M, Nielsen JC, Kronborg MB, Michowitz Y, Auricchio A, Barbash IM, et al. 2021 ESC Guidelines on cardiac pacing and cardiac resynchronization therapy: Developed by the Task Force on cardiac pacing and cardiac resynchronization therapy of the European Society of Cardiology (ESC) with the special contribution of the European Heart Rhythm Association (EHRA). Revista Española de Cardiología (English Edition). 2022;75(5):430.
14. Ploux S, Eschalier R, Whinnett ZI, Lumens J, Derval N, Sacher F, et al. Electrical dyssynchrony induced by biventricular pacing: Implications for patient selection and therapy improvement. Heart Rhythm. 2015;12(4):782-91.
15. Bressi E, Grieco D, Luermans J, Burri H, Vernooy K. Conduction system pacing for cardiac resynchronization therapy: State of the art, current controversies, and future perspectives. Front Physiol. 2023;14:1124195.
16. Ballantyne B, Chew D, Vandenberk B. Paradigm Shifts in Cardiac Pacing: Where have We been and What Lies Ahead? J Clin Med. 2023;12(8):2938.
17. Zaidi SMJ, Sohail H, Satti DI, Sami A, Anwar M, Malik J, et al. Tricuspid regurgitation in His bundle pacing: A systematic review. Noninvasive Electrocardiol. 2022;27(6):e12986.
18. Sharma PS, Dandamudi G, Herweg B, Wilson D, Singh R, Naperkowski A, et al. Permanent His-bundle pacing as an alternative to biventricular pacing for cardiac resynchronization therapy: A multicenter experience. Heart Rhythm. 2018;15(3):413-20.
19. Haeberlin A, Canello S, Kummer A, Seiler J, Baldinger SH, Madaffari A, et al. Conduction System Pacing Today and Tomorrow. J Clin Med. 2022;11(24):7258.
20. Zhang J, Li F, Zhang Z-Y, Yang F, Kong Q, Chen J-Y, et al. Conduction system pacing is superior to biventricular pacing in patients with heart failure: Insights from the pooled clinical studies. Front Physiol. 2023;14:1125340.
21. Baroni M, Preda A, Varrenti M, Vargiu S, Carbonaro M, Giordano F, et al. Left Bundle Branch Area Pacing over His Bundle Pacing: How Far have We Come? J Clin Med. 2023;12(9):3251.
22. Jastrzębski M, Kiełbasa G, Cano O, Curila K, Heckman L, De Pooter J, et al. Left bundle branch area pacing outcomes: the multicentre European MELOS study. Eur Heart J. 2022;43(40):4161-73.
23. Tun HN, Khan H, Chernikova D, Mareev Y, Chakrabarti S, Thant M, et al. Conduction system pacing: promoting the physiology to prevent heart failure. Heart Fail Rev. 2023;28(2):379-86.

14

CHAPTER

Management of Cardiogenic Shock: An Update

Pawan Suri, Vanita Arora

ABSTRACT

Cardiogenic shock (CS) is a complex multifactorial clinical syndrome with a 30-day mortality of 30–50% even in patients who receive appropriate treatment. It develops as a continuum and progresses from the initial insult (underlying cause) to the subsequent occurrence of organ failure and death. The recommendations and actual treatments are often based on registry data and as each phenotype of CS has a clinical impact on management, the successful management of CS is based on the early identification and treatment of the underlying cause, accurate staging, hemodynamic/respiratory stabilization and the management of multi-organ failure. Although several consensus-driven algorithms have been proposed, CS management remains challenging and outcome of substantial investments in research and development have not yielded proof of efficacy and safety for most of the therapies tested. The prognosis of these patients continues to be poor despite the efforts made to improve the care, including the development of mechanical circulatory support (MCS). Future studies should consider the identification of new pathophysiological targets, and high-quality translational research should facilitate incorporation of more targeted interventions in clinical research protocols, aimed to improve individual patient outcomes.

INTRODUCTION

Cardiogenic shock (CS) is a hemo-metabolic syndrome characterized by a state of tissue hypoperfusion in presence of an adequate intravascular volume. The tissue hypoperfusion is secondary to cardiac dysfunction, either due to an acute cardiac insult [as in acute coronary syndrome (ACS) or myocarditis] or acute decompensation of chronic heart failure (HF). Although other causes of CS are on rise, acute myocardial infarction (AMI) with left ventricular (LV) dysfunction remains the most frequent cause of CS and currently it accounts for 3–15% of AMI cases. Despite the introduction of myocardial revascularization therapy and an overall improvement in mechanical reperfusion strategies, CS remains the leading cause of death in patients with AMI, with an inhospital and 1-year mortality rate of 40% and 50%, respectively. The increased mortality rate is related to the difficulty in identifying reliable risk factors, varied clinical presentation and phenotypes, associated comorbidities, changes in the mean age, and delay in the identification and treatment of an underlying cause.

DEFINITION AND CLASSIFICATION

The diagnosis of CS is made on the basis of clinical criteria such as persistent hypotension [systolic blood pressure (SBP) < 90 mm Hg for > 30 minutes] in the presence of adequate intravascular volume along with the clinical and/or laboratory signs of hypoperfusion. The clinical signs of hypoperfusion include cold extremities, oliguria, mental confusion, dizziness, and narrow pulse pressure while the laboratory signs of hypoperfusion include metabolic acidosis, elevated lactate and newly elevated creatinine. Although not mandatory in clinical practice, objective hemodynamic parameters, such as reduced cardiac index ≤ 2.2 L/min/m^2 and elevated pulmonary capillary wedge pressure (PCWP) ≥ 15 mm Hg, are useful for a correct diagnosis. The definitions applied in selected major randomized clinical trials (RCTs) and guidelines are shown in **Table 1**.

Based on the clinical severity and response to treatment, the spectrum of CS can be divided into pre-CS, CS, and refractory CS **(Fig. 1)**. The presence of clinical signs of peripheral hypoperfusion even with

TABLE 1: Definition of cardiogenic shock in clinical trials and guidelines.

SHOCK	IABP-SHOCK II	CULPRIT-SHOCK	ESC Heart Failure Guidelines	ORBI Risk Score
• SBP < 90 mm Hg for > 30 minutes • Support to maintain SBP > 90 mm Hg • Endorgan hypoperfusion (urine output < 30 mL/h or cool extremities and heart rate > 60 beats/min) • Hemodynamic criteria*: ○ CI of < 2.2 L/min/m^2 ○ PCWP > 15 mm Hg	• SBP < 90 mm Hg for > 30 minutes or catecholamines to maintain SBP > 90 mm Hg • Clinical pulmonary congestion • Impaired endorgan perfusion with at least one of the following criteria: ○ Altered mental status ○ Cold/clammy skin and extremities ○ Urine output < 30 mL/h ○ Lactate > 2.0 mmol/L	• Planned early revascularization by PCI • Multivessel coronary artery disease defined as > 70% stenosis in at least two major vessels (> 2 mm diameter) with identifiable culprit lesion ○ SBP < 90 mm Hg for > 30 minutes ○ Catecholamines required to maintain SBP > 90 mm Hg • Pulmonary congestion • Impaired organ perfusion with at least one of the following criteria: ○ Altered mental status ○ Cold/clammy skin and extremities ○ Urine output < 30 mL/h ○ Lactate > 2.0 mmol/L	• SBP < 90 mm Hg with adequate volume and clinical or laboratory signs of hypoperfusion • Clinical hypoperfusion: Cold extremities, oliguria, mental confusion, dizziness, and narrow pulse pressure • Laboratory hypoperfusion: Metabolic acidosis ○ Elevated lactate ○ Elevated creatinine	SBP < 90 mm Hg for > 30 minutes following exclusion of hypovolemia, with clinical evidence of hypoperfusion, inotrope dependence, or mechanical left ventricular support to correct this situation

*Not required in anterior infarction or if pulmonary congestion in chest X-ray

(CI: cardiac index; CULPRIT-SHOCK: ulprit Lesion Only PCI vs Multivessel PCI in Cardiogenic Shock; ESC: European Society of Cardiology; IABP: intra-aortic balloon pump; ORBI: Observatoire Régional Breton sur l'Infarctus; PCI: percutaneous coronary intervention; PCWP: pulmonary capillary wedge pressure; SBP: systolic blood pressure; SHOCK: SHould we emergently revascularise Occluded Coronaries for cardiogenic shocK)

preserved SBP is referred as "preshock" and precedes overt CS. Preshock may occur in severe acute heart failure (AHF), which can also be associated with clinical signs of tissue hypoperfusion but without compromising cellular basal metabolism and having normal lactate. This state should be differentiated from "normotensive CS", which represents an entity of CS with all features of hypoperfusion and cellular alterations (including cellular hypoxia and elevated lactate) but without hypotension. At the end of the spectrum of severity, "refractory CS" has been defined as CS with ongoing evidence of tissue hypoperfusion despite administration of adequate doses of two vasoactive medications and treatment of the underlying etiology.

The recently published Society for Cardiovascular Angiography and Interventions (SCAI) classification describes five evolutive stages of CS, from A (at risk of CS) to B (beginning CS), C (classic CS), D (deteriorating CS), and finally to E (extremis) **(Fig. 1)**. The SCAI classification utilizes bedside clinical assessment of hypoperfusion, measurement of lactate level and invasive hemodynamic evaluation. Recently, the SCAI classification has been validated in a large cohort of unselected intensive cardiac care unit (ICCU) and the strong association between SCAI shock stages and mortality in a heterogeneous ICCU population, even after adjustment for known predictors of mortality, emphasizes the robustness of this classification system.

PATHOPHYSIOLOGY

Although etiologies vary widely, the pathophysiology of CS comprises several unique yet overlapping components to be considered: an initial cardiac insult that decreases cardiac output (CO), central hemodynamic alterations including changes in the relation between pressure and volume with increase in LV and right ventricular (RV) filling pressures, microcirculatory dysfunction, renal hypoperfusion triggering the activation of renin-angiotensin-aldosterone system and vasoconstriction of the splanchnic bed resulting in translocation of bacteria or bacterial toxins and possible subsequent septic reaction. In other words, a systemic inflammatory response syndrome, characterized by the activation of various inflammatory cascades (generation of free radicals, complement formation, cytokine release) and cellular components (leukocytes, platelets, monocytes and endothelial cells), has been described which results in pathological vasodilation followed by multi-organ dysfunction **(Fig. 2)**. Although these mechanisms might

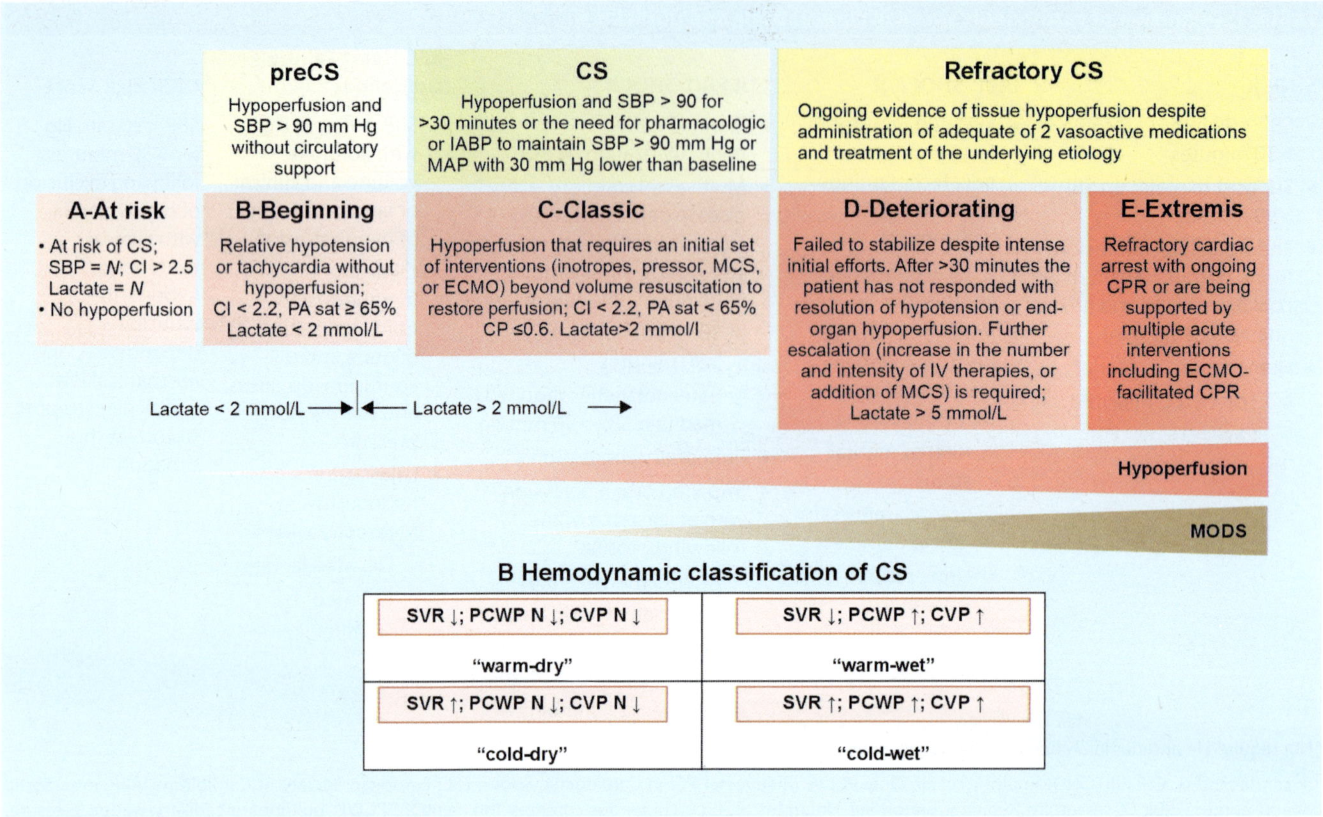

FIG. 1: Classification of cardiogenic shock (CS).

(CI: cardiac index; CPR: cardiopulmonary resuscitation; CVP: central venous pressure; ECMO: extracorporeal membrane oxygenation; IV: intravenous; MODS: multiorgan dysfunction syndrome; MCS: mechanical circulatory support; PA sat: pulmonary artery saturation; PCWP: pulmonary capillary wedge pressure; SBP: systolic blood pressure; SVR: systemic vascular resistance)

be considered as temporal stages of CS, each may occur simultaneously, the magnitude of the initial cardiac insult and/or early application of interventions may either mask or delay some of these stages.

There are also other pathophysiologic reasons, such as acute mitral regurgitation, ventricular septal defect or predominant RV infarction with CS. RV infarction and failure are associated with increased RV and right atrial pressure. The classical triad is: hypotension, elevated jugular venous pressure, and tachycardia in the presence of normal oxygen saturation. Due to ventricular interdependence, RV failure may also impair LV filling, resulting in reduced CO.

CLINICAL ASSESSMENT AND DIAGNOSIS

The clinical presentation is marked by signs of hypoperfusion, such as cool or mottled extremities, altered mental status, and low urine output, generally associated with hypotension and tachycardia as well as signs of elevated filling pressure, such as turgor of the jugular veins, orthopnea, and pulmonary rales. Moreover, low CO can cause organ damage, leading to kidney or liver failure up to multi-organ failure and death. Elevation in serum lactate is a sensitive laboratory marker of hypoperfusion, and serial assessments are of utmost importance to evaluate the response to the therapy. Since AMI is the leading cause of CS, an electrocardiogram should be carried out as soon as possible. Besides laboratory testing and chest X-ray, it is essential to perform an echocardiogram in order to exclude mechanical complications and to rapidly evaluate biventricular and valvular function. Although not essential to the diagnosis, right heart catheterization (RHC) may be important in select cases to confirm the diagnosis, identify the causes of shock, provide prognostic information, and guide vasoactive therapy. Some recent retrospective observational studies suggest a reduction in the mortality rate correlated with the use of RHC in patients with AMI-related CS treated with MCS. Even so, there is a lack of evidence and the only randomized trial addressing this issue, in which patients with CS were excluded, showed that RHC did not affect overall mortality and hospitalization in decompensated HF.

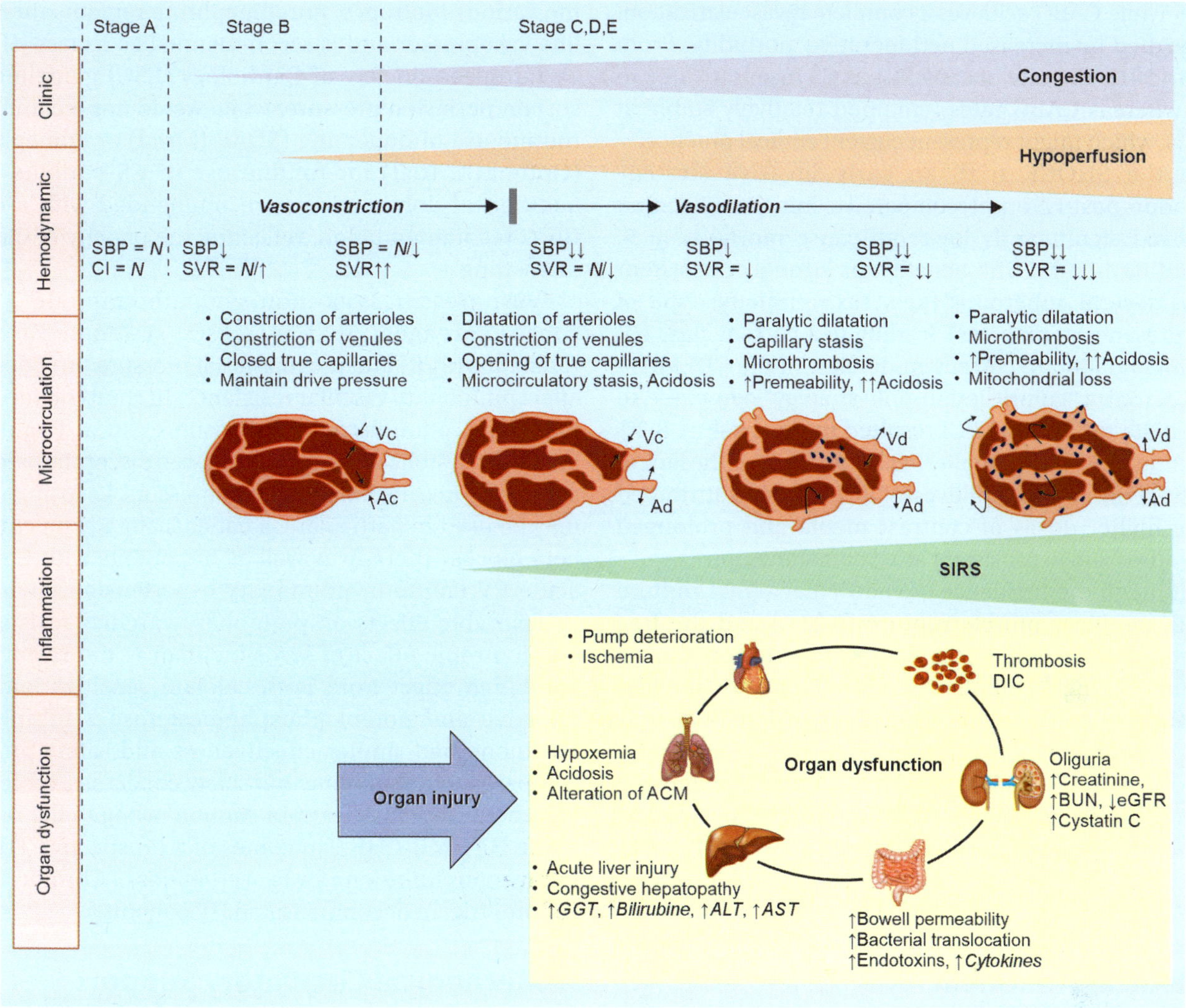

FIG. 2: Pathophysiology of cardiogenic shock with staged abnormalities of clinic examination, hemodynamics, microcirculatory dysfunction, and organ failure.

(ACM: alcoholic cardiomyopathy; ALT: alanine transaminase; AST: aspartate transaminase; BUN: blood urea nitrogen; CI: cardiac index; DIC: disseminated intravascular coagulation; eGFR: estimated glomerular filtration rate; GGT: gamma-glutamyltransferase; SBP: systolic blood pressure; SIRS: systemic inflammatory response syndrome; SVR: systemic vascular resistance)

MANAGEMENT

Management of CS should start as early as possible and a model analogous to primary percutaneous coronary intervention (PCI) pathways has been proposed by the American Heart Association to facilitate optimal care coordination and to minimize time delay. This model consists of a network between several satellite centers (type II and III) and a central "CS-center" (type I). CS centers should be high-volume centers (>107 cases/year) with highly experienced multidisciplinary team (MDT), and availability of on-site operating rooms, short- and long-term MCS, other end-organ supports, and provision of safe transfer by a mobile MCS team. A nurse to patient ratio of 1:1 is recommended and full integration into the post-ICU pathways.

Management of the Underlying Cause

In CS, early identification and treatment of the underlying cause is potentially beneficial in improving outcomes. Since AMI remains the most common cause of CS, early revascularization strategy represents the cornerstone in the management of patients presenting with CS complicating ACS. Although there are no direct randomized comparisons between PCI and coronary artery bypass grafting (CABG) in AMI-CS patients, a subanalysis from the SHOCK (SHould we emergently revascularise Occluded Coronaries for cardiogenic shocK) trial suggested similar 1-year mortality between PCI and CABG (48% vs. 53%) and a similar finding was found in a subsequent meta-analysis. The benefit of PCI is related to its early performance, but usually limited to the culprit lesion, while CABG achieves a complete revascularization, outweighed by increased perioperative morbidity. From 2003 to 2010, the rate of early PCI in CS rose from 26% to 54%, whereas CABG rates remained relatively stable at 5%–6%, which might represent current clinical practice.

In the SHOCK trial, an early invasive strategy (< 12 hours post-CS onset) compared to initial stabilization conferred significantly lower all-cause mortality at 6, 12, and 60 months. The benefit was strongly consistent across several subgroups (age, sex, ethnicity, type of ACS, presence of diabetes), leading to a current class I/B recommendation in current guidelines. In the CULPRIT-SHOCK trial, a "culprit-lesion-only strategy" compared to immediate multivessel PCI resulted in an absolute 8.2% reduction in 30-day mortality (43.3% vs. 51.5%). The lack of benefit of immediate multivessel PCI has been attributed to the higher doses of contrast media and prolonged procedures and is consistent at 1-year follow-up.

Although the incidence of ventricular septal rupture (0.2%), papillary muscle rupture (0.25%) and the free wall rupture has reduced in the post reperfusion era, yet these mechanical complications exponentially increase the mortality rate in CS patients. Early use of MCS may allow to bridge patients to a decision of delayed repair, transplantation, or palliative options, which remains the key and current guidelines recommend that mechanical complications should be treated as early as possible after heart team discussion and that intra-aortic balloon pump (IABP) may be considered (IIa/C) as interim support.

Medical Treatment

Although one-third of patients presenting with CS are "euvolemic", yet most of them respond to fluid administration by increasing stroke volume. Fluid administration in CS is mainly based on pathophysiological considerations and a fluid challenge with infusion of normal saline or Ringer's lactate 250 mL over 15–30 minutes should be considered as first-line treatment, if there are no signs of congestion (I/C). Careful administration of fluid boluses, and only used in conjunction with noninvasive or invasive assessment of CO, is recommended in patients with CS and RV dysfunction, since excessive volume overload overdistends the right ventricle and increases ventricular interdependence, impairs LV filling, and reduces systemic CO.

More than 80–90% of patients with CS receive inotropes and/or vasopressors that might restore hemodynamics, but at the cost of increasing myocardial oxygen consumption and arrhythmogenic burden. Therefore, the general recommendation is to avoid their use when tissue perfusion is restored and limit the dose and the duration of infusion to the lowest possible. Among the various inotropes, norepinephrine remains the first-line vasopressor and is recommended as a class (IIb/B) by European Society of Cardiology (ESC) guidelines to sustain perfusion pressure, while we do not recommend routine use of dopamine (SOAP II trial) or epinephrine (OptimaCC trial) for routine use in CS patients. The addition of dobutamine is recommended with a class IIb/C recommendation, reflecting the paucity of data in this setting.

Vasopressin is a non-sympathomimetic vasoconstrictor agent that increases systemic vascular resistance (SVR) and mean arterial pressure but does not affect pulmonary vascular resistance. In combination with milrinone, administration of vasopressin at low doses increased systolic pressure and allowed discontinuation or a decrease in catecholamine vasopressors. Levosimendan may be used in particular CS patients already on chronic beta blocker therapy as well as in patients with CS and acute RV failure or pulmonary hypertension, owing to its favorable effects on pulmonary vascular resistance. The inotropic effect of levosimendan is the result of a combined effect from both calcium sensitization and selective and potent phosphodiesterase 3 inhibition. Milrinone had similar effectiveness and safety profiles compared to dobutamine but safety concerns over its use in ischemic etiology warrant caution owing to the results of the OPTIME-CHF (Outcomes of a Prospective Trial of Intravenous Milrinone for Exacerbations of Chronic Heart Failure) trial in decompensated HF patients.

Mechanical Circulatory Support

Temporary MCS **(Table 2)** has an emerging role in CS. Current guidelines recommend the early use of MCS in patients with CS refractory to fluid load and inotropes/vasopressors (IIb/C), as a bridge either to recovery, re-evaluation, transplantation or a permanent implanted left ventricular assist device (LVAD). However, MCS is associated with significant complications **(Table 2)**, requires specialist multidisciplinary expertise for implantation and management, and high-quality evidence regarding outcomes is largely absent.

The IABP produces a modest increase in CO of 0.5–1 L/min and may have even less benefit in patients with tachycardia and irregular rhythms. A meta-analysis including 12 RCTs and 15 registries showed no survival benefit after IABP in AMI-CS, and has further called into question the utility of IABP therapy. Therefore, the ESC STEMI (ST-segment elevation myocardial infarction) guidelines gave III/B recommendation for the routine use of the IABP in CS but still consider IABP only in patients with mechanical complications (IIa/C) or to stabilize for transfer for higher levels of MCS. IABP still remains the

TABLE 2: Technical features of current percutaneous mechanical support devices for cardiogenic shock.

	IABP	Impella	TandemHeart	ECMO
Structure	Pneumatic pump	Axial pump	Centrifugal pump	Centrifugal pump
Cannula size	7–8 Fr	• 14 Fr (Impella CP) • 21 Fr (Impella 5.0)	• 21 Fr venous (inflow) • 12–19 Fr arterial (outflow)	• 17–21 Fr venous (inflow) • 14–19 Fr artery (outflow)
Insertion/placement	Femoral artery	• Femoral artery (CP) • Transaortic/transubclavian (for Impella 5.5)	• Femoral artery • Femoral vein for left atrial access	• Femoral artery • Femoral vein
Cardiac output	0.5–0.8 L/min	3.7–5 L/min	4.5 L/min	>4.5 L/min
Maximum number of implantation days	Weeks	5–7 day (up to 30 days for Impella 5.5)	14 days	Weeks
Complexity of insertion	Low	Medium (high for Impella 5.0)	High	Medium
Risk of hemolysis	Low	Moderate	Moderate	Moderate
Risk of complications:				
Ischemic	Low	Moderate (high for Impella 5.0)	High	High
Hemorrhagic	Low	Moderate	High	High
Infectious	Low	Low (moderate for Impella 5.0)	Moderate	Moderate

(ECMO: extracorporeal membrane oxygen; IABP: intra-aortic balloon pump)

most commonly used MCS, and in the light of new data showing more vascular and bleeding complications and possible higher mortality with other devices, the class III indication of IABP probably needs to be reconsidered.

Impella is a microaxial pump giving only left-sided support that unloads the left ventricle by expelling blood flow from the left ventricle into the aorta and may provide up to >5 L/min of blood flow depending on the device used as well as on afterload. Impella 2.5 and Impella CP can rapidly be implanted percutaneously in the catheterization laboratory while Impella 5.0 requires surgical cannulation. Unlike IABP, Impella does not require electrocardiographic or arterial waveform triggering, facilitating stability even in the setting of tachyarrhythmias or electromechanical dissociation. The ISAR-SHOCK (Impella LP2.5 vs. IABP in Cardiogenic SHOCK) was the first study to test this technology in a randomized manner and aimed to test the hypothesis that Impella LP2.5 provides superior hemodynamic support compared with IABP in patients with CS caused by AMI. A large randomized trial, the DanGer Shock study is ongoing and evaluating the benefits of preprocedural implantation of Impella LP 2.5 in STEMI patients complicated by CS patients undergoing percutaneous intervention. The results of this trial will hopefully provide more conclusive data on the use of the Impella LP 2.5 device and more generally, on mechanical circulatory support (MCS) in this population. High-quality evidence regarding Impella in other causes of CS is also lacking; however, in the RECOVER I study, including patients with post-cardiotomy CS (PCCS), the Impella 5.0 was associated with 94%, 81%, and 75% survival at 30 days, 6 months, and 1 year, respectively.

The TandemHeart provides a continuous flow (4 L/min) via a centrifugal pump. The venous cannula is inserted through the femoral vein and is advanced via transseptal puncture into the left atrium, and the arterial cannula provides oxygenated flow into the abdominal aorta or iliac arteries. In two randomized studies, including AMI-CS patients, TandemHeart significantly improved hemodynamic indexes as compared to IABP, but 30-day mortality did not differ between the two groups.

Venous-arterial extracorporeal membrane oxygenation (VA-ECMO) provides cardiopulmonary support by draining venous blood from the right atrium and returning it after oxygenation to the ascending aorta (central cannulation) or to the iliac artery (peripheral cannulation). VA-ECMO provides high levels of biventricular cardiac (V-A) and respiratory support [venovenous (V-V)] in a large spectrum of clinical settings, including CS patients with malignant arrhythmias and CA. Some studies indicated an improvement in microcirculation as measured by sidestream dark field imaging. The improvement in the oxygenator membranes permitted low resistance and improved blood compatibility characteristics. The modern centrifugal pumps generate less heat and are less thrombogenic, allowing extended duration of support.

In the event of very poor LV function, peripheral VA-ECMO can be associated with progressive LV distension and pulmonary congestion, potentially resulting in impaired myocardial recovery. When cardiac recovery precedes pulmonary recovery, ejection of deoxygenated blood flow into the ascending aorta results in upper body hypoxia ("Harlequin syndrome"), requiring reducing cardiac ejection or reconfiguration [veno-veno-arterial (VVA) or veno-arterial-venous (VAV)] until the lungs recover.

CONCLUSION

Cardiogenic shock is a complex multifactorial clinical syndrome with extremely high mortality, developing as a continuum, resulting from the initial insult (underlying cause) to the subsequent occurrence of organ failure and death. Substantial investments in research and development have not yielded proof of efficacy and safety for most of the therapies tested, and outcome in this condition remains poor. Future studies should consider delivering pathophysiological appropriate therapies in a timely manner, in appropriately selected population, while avoiding iatrogenic harm. High-quality translational research should facilitate incorporation of more targeted interventions in clinical research protocols, aimed to improve individual patient outcomes.

SUGGESTED READINGS

1. van Diepen S, Katz JN, Albert NM, Henry TD, Jacobs AK, Kapur NK, et al. Contemporary Management of Cardiogenic Shock: A Scientific Statement From the American Heart Association. Circulation. 2017;136:e232-68.
2. De Luca G, Navarese EP, Suryapranata H. A meta-analytic overview of thrombectomy during primary angioplasty. Int J Cardiol. 2013;166:606-12.
3. Zeymer U, Bueno H, Granger CB, Hochman J, Huber K, Lettino M, et al. Acute Cardiovascular Care Association position statement for the diagnosis and treatment of patients with acute myocardial infarction complicated by cardiogenic shock: A document of the Acute Cardio-vascular Care Association of the European Society of Cardiology. Eur Heart J Acute Cardiovasc Care. 2020;9:183-97.
4. Furer A, Wessler J, Burkhoff D. Hemodynamics of cardiogenic shock. Interv Cardiol Clin. 2017;6:359-71.
5. Lawler PR, Mehra MR. Advancing from a "hemodynamic model" to a "mechanistic disease-modifying model" of cardiogenic shock. J Heart Lung Transplant. 2018;37:1285-8.
6. De Backer D, Creteur J, Dubois MJ, Sakr Y, Vincent JL. Microvascular alterations in patients with acute severe heart failure and cardiogenic shock. Am Heart J. 2004;147:91-9.
7. Binanay C, Califf RM, Hasselblad V, O'Connor CM, Shah MR, Sopko G, et al. Evaluation Study of Congestive Heart Failure and Pulmonary Artery Catheterization Effectiveness. JAMA. 2005;294:1625-33.
8. Samsky MD, Morrow DA, Proudfoot AG, Hochman JS, Thiele H, Rao SV. Cardiogenic Shock After Acute Myocardial Infarction. JAMA. 2021;326:1840-50.
9. Nalluri N, Patel NJ, Atti V, Kumar V, Basir MB, O'Neill WW. Temporal Trends in Utilization of Right-Sided Heart Catheterization Among Percutaneous Ventricular Assist Device Recipients in Acute Myocardial Infarction Complicated by Cardiogenic Shock. Am J Cardiol. 2018;122:2014-7.
10. Rab T, Ratanapo S, Kern KB, Basir MB, McDaniel M, Meraj P, et al. Cardiac shock care centers: JACC review topic of the week. J Am Coll Cardiol. 2018;72:1972-80.
11. Thiele H, Desch S. CULPRIT-SHOCK (Culprit Lesion Only PCI versus Multivessel Percutaneous Coronary Intervention in Cardiogenic Shock): implications on guideline recommendations. Circulation. 2018;137:1314-16.
12. Hochman JS, Sleeper LA, Godfrey E, McKinlay SM, Sanborn T, Col J, et al. SHould We Emergently Revascularize Occluded Coronaries for Cardiogenic shocK: an international randomized trial of emergency PTCA/CABG–trial design. The SHOCK Trial Study Group. Am Heart J. 1999;137:313-21.
13. Thiele H, Ohman EM, de Waha-Thiele S, Zeymer U, Desch S. Management of cardiogenic shock complicating myocardial infarction: an update 2019. Eur Heart J. 2019;40:2671-83.
14. Maack C, Eschenhagen T, Hamdani N, Heinzel FR, Lyon AR, Manstein DJ, et al. Treatments targeting inotropy. Eur Heart J. 2018;40:3626-44.
15. Felker GM, Benza RL, Chandler AB, Leimberger JD, Cuffe MS, Califf RM, et al; OPTIME-CHF Investigators. Heart failure etiology and response to milrinone in decompensated heart failure: Results from the OPTIME-CHF study. J Am Coll Cardiol. 2003;41: 997-1003.
16. Ahmad Y, Sen S, Shun-Shin MJ, Ouyang J, Finegold JA, Al-Lamee RK, et al. Intra-aortic balloon pump therapy for acute myocardial infarction: a meta-analysis. JAMA Intern Med. 2015;175:931-9.
17. Ouweneel DM, Eriksen E, Sjauw KD, van Dongen IM, Hirsch A, Packer EJ, et al. Percutaneous Mechanical Circulatory Support Versus Intra-Aortic Balloon Pump in Cardiogenic Shock After Acute Myocardial Infarction. J Am Coll Cardiol. 2017;69:278-87.
18. Møller JE, Gerke O; DanGer Shock Investigators. Danish-German cardiogenic shock trial-DanGer shock: Trial design update. Am Heart J. 2023;255:90-3.
19. Kapur NK, Alkhouli M, DeMartini TJ, Faraz H, George ZH, Goodwin MJ, et al. Unloading the Left Ventricle Before Reperfusion in Patients With Anterior ST-Segment–Elevation Myocardial Infarction. Circulation. 2019;139:337-46.
20. Guglin M, Zucker MJ, Bazan VM, Bozkurt B, El Banayosy A, Estep JD, et al. Venoarterial ECMO for Adults: JACC Scientific Expert Panel J Am Coll Cardiol. 2019;73:698-716.
21. Ostadal P, Rokyta R, Karasek J, Kruger A, Vondrakova D, Janotka M, et al. Extracorporeal Membrane Oxygenation in the Therapy of Cardiogenic Shock: Results of the ECMO-CS Randomized Clinical Trial. Circulation. 2023;147:454-64.

15

CHAPTER

Preventing Hospitalization due to Heart Failure: The ARNI + SGLT-2i Story

Vipul Chavda, Dhruvi Hasnani

ABSTRACT

The key pathways implicated in heart failure (HF) include the autonomic nervous system, the renin–angiotensin–aldosterone system (RAAS) and the natriuretic peptide (NP) system. Hence, pharmacological development of neprilysin inhibition has been developed in combination with simultaneous inhibition of the RAAS. Sacubitril/valsartan is the first of the class of dual angiotensin receptor-neprilysin inhibitors (ARNIs). Sodium-glucose cotransporter-2 inhibitors (SGLT-2i) and ARNI demonstrate similar effects, and the combination of SGLT-2i and ARNI could result in improved cardiovascular protective effects. Currently, with an evolving understanding of HF and the development of new drug classes, the four pillars of HF therapy include SGLT-2i, ARNI, beta-blockers (BBs), and mineralocorticoid receptor antagonists (MRAs). This chapter aims to present current evidence that favors the early use of a combination of SGLT-2i + ARNIs in patients with HF to prevent hospitalization due to HF.

INTRODUCTION

Heart failure (HF) with reduced ejection fraction (HFrEF) is a disease associated with significant morbidity and reduced survival which is worse than some cancers. About 40% of hospitalized HF patients have concomitant diabetes. Both diabetes and HF are closely linked, and have a negative impact on prognosis. HF is ranked as the second most common cardiovascular presentation of diabetes after peripheral arterial disease and it is an important cause of mortality in this patient population. HF is characterized dyspnea or limited exertion due to impaired cardiac ventricular filling and/or blood ejection.

Patients with HFrEF have improved outcomes today due to the widespread implementation of disease-modifying pharmacological therapies. An improved understanding of the pathogenesis of HF has led to the development of new treatment options for HF. The key pathways implicated in HF include the autonomic nervous system, the renin–angiotensin–aldosterone system (RAAS), and the natriuretic peptide (NP) system. In patients with HF, the RAAS is overactivated, causing vasoconstriction, hypertension, elevated aldosterone levels and sympathetic tone, and eventually cardiac remodeling. However, an endogenous compensatory mechanism, the NP system is also activated, albeit insufficiently to counteract the RAAS effects. NPs are degraded by the enzyme neprilysin, but inhibition of neprilysin alone results in reflex activation of the RAAS. Hence, pharmacological development of neprilysin inhibition has been developed in combination with simultaneous inhibition of the RAAS. Sacubitril/valsartan is the first of the class of dual angiotensin receptor-neprilysin inhibitors (ARNIs).

Heart failure guidelines recommend inhibition of the renin–angiotensin and sympathetic nervous systems, the two fundamental pathways that are implicated in the pathophysiology of HFrEF using angiotensin-converting enzyme (ACE) inhibitors (ACEi) and beta-blockers (BBs). Currently, with an evolving understanding of HF and the development of new drug classes, the four pillars of HF therapy include sodium-glucose cotransporter-2 inhibitors (SGLT-2i), ARNI, BBs, and mineralocorticoid receptor antagonists (MRAs). These drugs are called the foundational quadruple therapy for HFrEF **(Table 1)**.

Treatments in Heart Failure with Mildly Reduced and Preserved Ejection Fraction: Systematic Review and Network Meta-analysis. JACC Heart Fail. 2023;S2213-1779(23)00410-9.

13. Jariwala P, Jadhav K, Punjani A, Boorugu H, Mari AR. ADDition of DAPAgliflozin, Sodium-glucose Cotransporter-2 Inhibitor to Angiotensin Receptor Blocker-Neprilysin Inhibitors Non-Responders in Patient with Refractory Heart Failure with Reduced Ejection Fraction (ADD DAPA trial). Indian Heart J. 2021;73(5):605-11
14. Younes AM, Salem M, Maraey A, Nomigolzar S, Sewell K, Khalil M, et al. Safety outcomes of SGLT2i in the heart failure trials: A systematic review and Meta-analysis. Int J Cardiol. 2022;366: 51-6.
15. Sharma A, Verma S, Bhatt DL, Connelly KA, Swiggum E, Vaduganathan M, et al. Optimizing Foundational Therapies in Patients with HFrEF: How do We Translate These Findings into Clinical Care? JACC Basic Transl Sci. 2022;7(5):504-17.
16. Jiménez-Blanco Bravo M, Valle A, Gayán Ordás J, Del Prado Díaz S, Cordero Pereda D, Morillas Climent H, et al. Safety and Efficacy of the Combination of Sacubitril/Valsartan and SGLT2i in HFrEF Patients (SECSI Registry). J Cardiovasc Pharmacol. 2021;78(5):e662-e668.
17. Mc Causland FR, Lefkowitz MP, Claggett B, Anavekar NS, Senni M, Gori M, et al. Angiotensin-Neprilysin Inhibition and Renal Outcomes in Heart Failure With Preserved Ejection Fraction. Circulation. 2020;142(13):1236-45.

16

CHAPTER

Prosthetic Valve Thrombosis

SB Gupta

ABSTRACT

Valvular heart disease having significant morbidity and mortality, affects >100 million persons worldwide. Though the incidence of rheumatic heart disease has gone down significantly, but on the other hand degenerative valve diseases are on the rise. Valve replacement is the most common therapeutic strategy for moderate to serious valve dysfunction. Prosthetic valve thrombosis (PVT) though rare, is a serious complication in patients who have undergone prosthetic valve (PV) replacement with suboptimal anticoagulation. Intensification of anticoagulation, thrombolytic therapy, and surgery are the options for the management of PVT.

INTRODUCTION

In the general population of the US, currently, the age-adjusted prevalence of mitral and aortic valve diseases is approximately 2.5% and exceeds 10% in persons above the age of 75 years. Surgical valve replacement is the usual strategy for the treatment of moderate to severe valvular heart diseases. In childhood, aortic valvuloplasty has been tried and in certain cases of mitral valve disease, mitral valve repair has worked. In the last decade, a lot of trans-catheter interventions have developed as an alternative to surgery, especially in persons with high-surgical risk.

Mechanical and bioprosthetic heart valves (BHVs) are the options based on the leaflet material. Mechanical heart valves though more durable, are more thrombogenic in comparison to BHVs. Mechanical heart valves (MHVs) are caged ball type (Starr–Edwards) or single or bileaflet tilting disc type (Bjork–Shiley or St Jude Medical Regent respectively). Caged-ball valves are the most thrombogenic, followed by single-leaflet and then bi-leaflet tilting disc valves. Similarly, BHVs are stented or stentless, and stented BHVs have more risk of thrombosis in comparison to stentless BHVs.

The annual incidence of prosthetic valve thrombosis (PVT) for MHVs ranges from 0.5 to 6.0%. In a meta-analysis of 5,837 BHV patients with a total follow-up of 31,874 patient-years reported an annual incidence rate of 0.03% for PVT and 0.38% for thromboembolic (TE) complications. PVT and TE complications have also been reported after transcatheter aortic valve replacement (TAVR) and the risk is highest in the first 3 months after the replacement. In a series from 12 centers, 4,266 patients undergoing TAVR between January 2008 and September 2013, 26 cases (0.61%) of PVT were reported in a median of 181 days of implantation.

The incidence of PVT varies on the location of the prosthesis. PVT is maximum in the tricuspid position than at the mitral position and the least at the aortic position, up to 20% for right-sided valves and 0.5–8.0% for left-sided valves per patient-year. PVT is almost 20 times more common with the tricuspid valve as compared to the mitral valve and 2–3 times more frequent at the mitral valve in comparison to the aortic valve.

Suboptimal anticoagulation is the major reason for PVT. Atrial fibrillation (AF) and severe left ventricular (LV) dysfunction are the important risk factors. There are certain hypercoagulable states such as chronic kidney disease, obesity, pregnancy, smoking, and anemia which may predispose the patients to PVT.

Patients with PVT may be asymptomatic or may present with a gradual onset of symptoms over days to weeks with shortness of breath on exertion, chest pain, or embolic events or may present acutely with heart failure or cardiogenic shock. Examination reveals loss of prosthetic click in MHVs and, the appearance of new murmurs or signs of heart failure.

Cinefluoroscopy is a quick and good screening tool to look for decreased leaflet motion. Transthoracic echocardiography (TTE) is the preferred choice of investigation for the diagnosis of PVT in most of the centers because of its ready availability. Transesophageal echocardiography (TEE) if available shall be performed for the confirmation of diagnosis and to rule out other causes of valve obstruction, such as pannus or subacute bacterial endocarditis. Doppler-derived gradients are high in obstructed PVT and a mean gradient of > 6 mm Hg and valve area of < 1.3 cm^2 of MV prosthesis and a mean gradient of > 30 mm at aortic prosthesis are suggestive of PVT and a mean gradient of > 8 mm Hg at mitral prosthesis and > 45 mm Hg at aortic prosthesis are indicative of PVT.

Four independent predictors of MHV thrombosis have been suggested by Lin et al.:

1. Aortic $P_{max} \geq 50$ mm Hg
2. Mitral $P_{mean} \geq 10$ mm Hg
3. Presence of an occlusive mass on the prosthetic valve (PV)
4. An international normalized ratio (INR) ≤ 2.5

Egbe et al. described five factors that were independently associated with BHV thrombosis:

1. > 50% increase in mean echo-Doppler gradient from baseline within 5 years
2. Paroxysmal AF
3. Suboptimal INR
4. Abnormal cusp mobility
5. Increased valve cusp thickness

If all the five risk factors were present, the specificity was 93%, the positive predictive value 85%, and the negative predictive value 89%.

Bioprosthetic heart valve thrombosis can present as isolated stenosis, isolated regurgitation, or mixed stenosis-regurgitation.

When TEE is also inconclusive, multidetector computed tomography (MDCT) is a useful tool in evaluating PV structure and functional status and can differentiate PVT from fibrotic pannus ingrowth as well as PV dysfunction because of prosthetic mismatch.

It is suggested that baseline TTE or TEE should be performed after valve replacement and prehospital discharge, thereafter 1–3 months later than annual echocardiographic screening to pick up PV dysfunction at an early stage. In cases of high risk for valve-related complications, more frequent follow-up is suggested.

The mainstay in the prevention of PVT is the proper anticoagulation and the intensity and duration of anticoagulation depend upon (1) the type of prosthesis, (2) the TE risk, and (3) the hemorrhagic risk. Various scoring systems have been quoted in the literature for TE and hemorrhagic risks. Though congestive heart failure, hypertension, age ≥ 75 years (doubled), diabetes mellitus, prior stroke or TIA or thromboembolism (doubled), vascular disease, age 65–74 years, sex category (CHA_2DS_2-VASC) score has been described to identify the risk of stroke in AF setting, it can be used to identify the risk of stroke for PVs also, especially for BHVs. Similarly, hypertension, abnormal liver/renal function, stroke, bleeding history or predisposition, labile INR, elderly, drugs/alcohol concomitantly (HAS-BLED), anticoagulation and risk factors in atrial fibrillation (ATRIA), and $HEMORR_2HAGES$ scores can predict the bleeding risk for the individuals. These scores can help the physician to titrate and balance the dose of anticoagulants for the prevention of thrombosis and avoiding major bleeds.

Lifelong anticoagulation for MHVs with vitamin K antagonists (VKA) plus aspirin 75–100 mg daily, to maintain an INR of 2.5 for aortic valve replacement (AVR) with no risk factors and INR of 3.0 for AVR with risk factors and MVR (class I) is recommended. For BHVs, anticoagulation with VKA plus aspirin 75–100 mg daily for 3 months (maintaining an INR of 2.5) followed by aspirin 75–100 mg daily for lifelong has been recommended (class IIa/IIb). For TAVR, clopidogrel 75 mg plus aspirin 75–100 mg daily for the first 6 months followed by aspirin 75–100 mg alone lifelong is advocated (class IIb).

TREATMENT OF PROSTHETIC VALVE THROMBOSIS

Literally, three options are exercised for the treatment of PVT:

1. Intensification of anticoagulant therapy
2. Thrombolytic therapy
3. Emergency surgery

The therapy depends upon:

- Hemodynamic stability
- Size of thrombus
- New York Heart Association Class (NYHA)

If the patient is hemodynamically unstable, or in NYHA class I or II status, or the size of the thrombus is small (< 0.8 cm^2), intravenous heparin is started as early as possible. Thrombolytic therapy is recommended if the thrombosis persists. In case of a large thrombus (≥ 0.8 cm^2)

and/or a patient in NYHA class III or IV, usually emergency surgery is advocated. Thrombolytic therapy carries a risk of thromboembolism, especially with large thrombus and left-sided PVT leading to serious stroke or arterial block.

For right-sided obstructed PVT, thrombolytic therapy is the treatment of choice with a high success rate and low complication rate. Thromboembolism to pulmonary circulation in comparison to cerebral circulation is less serious. In case of failure of thrombolytic therapy or contra-indication to thrombolysis, surgery is recommended.

For left-sided non-obstructive PVT, for small-size thrombus heparin therapy and/or thrombolytic therapy is recommended. For large nonobstructive thrombus, whether to use thrombolytic therapy or send the patient for surgery remains controversial. 2012 European Society of Cardiology and the European Association of Cardio-Thoracic Surgery guidelines recommended surgery for large thrombus and fibrinolysis if surgery is at high risk. However, Nagy and coworkers reported similar outcomes as far as success and complications are concerned when the patient is treated with thrombolytic therapy irrespective of thrombus size.

The TROIA study from 1993 to 2009, a single-center, prospective cohort study involving 182 patients with 220 episodes of PVT, having five arms for thrombolysis:

1. *Group I*: Rapid infusion of streptokinase (SK)
2. *Group II*: Slow infusion of SK
3. *Group III*: Full-dose tissue of tissue plasminogen activator (t-PA)—100 mg
4. *Group IV*: Half-dose of t-PA (50 mg)-–slow infusion
5. *Group V*: Low-dose of t-PA (25 mg)—very slow infusion

All patients with obstructed PVT, nonobstructed PVT with recent systemic TE, asymptomatic nonobstructed PVT with thrombus diameter of ≥ 10 mm, and PVT patients with ischemic stroke were included in the study, and patients with asymptomatic nonobstructed PVT without a history of recent systemic TE and with a thrombus diameter of < 10 mm were excluded. Overall successful thrombolysis was achieved in 83.2% of cases with no significant difference between intergroup protocols (68.8, 85.4, 75.0, 81.5, and 85.5% respectively; $p = 0.46$). Complication rates were significantly less in Group V vis-à-vis other groups (37.5, 24.4, 33.3, 29.6, and 10.5% respectively). The study concluded that low-dose t-PA (25 mg infused over 6 hours) was an effective thrombolytic regimen with very low complications.

So far, surgery has remained the mainstay for the treatment of obstructed PVT. Mortality mainly depends upon the NYHA Class and is reported as 4.7% for Class I to Class III and up to 60% in Class IV. Roudat et al. reported almost similar mortality rates (surgery 10% and thrombolysis 11%) from their nonrandomized, single-center study on 210 patients with 263 episodes of PVT, however they recommended surgery over thrombolysis as the embolic and major bleeding rates were higher in the thrombolytic group (15% vs. 0.7% and 4.7% vs. 0.7% respectively) and complete hemodynamic success rates were higher in the surgery group as compared to thrombolytic group (89% vs. 70%).

A lot of recent trials have shown higher success rates with thrombolytic therapy with lesser complication rates, even superior to surgery in all classes of patients. A recent meta-analysis of 17 studies, comprised 756 patients with 801 episodes of obstructed PVT, in whom 35% of cases were in NYHA Class I and II and 65% of cases in Class III and IV. 81% and 74% complete success were achieved in Class I/II and Class III/IV respectively with 14% thromboembolism and 8% overall 30-day mortality and suggested that the thrombolytic therapy shall be the treatment of choice in all cases unless contraindicated.

Low-dose t-PA with slow infusion with repeated doses is an effective therapy for PVT in pregnant women and safer as compared to surgery. In 25 pregnant women with 28 episodes of PVT from the year 2004–2012, 15 obstructed and 13 nonobstructed PVT with a mean age of 29 ± 6 years received thrombolytic therapy under TEE guidance and the mean dose of t-PA was 48.7 ± 29.5 mg (range 25–100 mg). All episodes resulted in complete resolution of thrombus with placental hemorrhage in one patient and minor bleeding in one patient.

CONCLUSION

Prosthetic valve thrombosis is a life-threatening complication in patients who have undergone heart valve replacement and depends on the type of valve, its location, and suboptimal anticoagulation. Right-sided PVT is commoner than left-sided PVT. Till late, surgery was the preferred option for the treatment of PVT, especially with large thrombus, obstructed PVT, and left-sided PVT. However, in the last 10–15 years, thrombolysis has become an attractive alternative for the treatment of PVT with good success and fewer complications, especially when t-PA low-dose slow infusion is chosen. Even in pregnant women, thrombolytic therapy with t-PA has been found effective.

SUGGESTED READINGS

1. Lung B, Vahanian A. Epidemiology of valvular heart disease in the adult. Nat Rev Cardiol 2011;8(3):162-72.
2. Lin SS, Tiong IY, Asher CR, Murphy MT, Thomas JD, Griffin BP. Prediction of thrombus-related mechanical prosthetic valve dysfunction using transesophageal echocardiography. J Am Coll Cardiol. 2000;86(10):1097-101.
3. Puvimanasinghe JP, Steyerberg EW, Takkenberg JJ, Eijkemans MJ, van Herwerden LA, Bogers AJ. Prognosis after aortic valve replacement with a bioprosthesis: predictions based on meta-analysis and microsimulation. Circulation. 2001;103(11): 1535-41.
4. Latib A, Naganuma T, Abdel-Wahab M, Danenberg H, Cota L, Barbanti M, et al. Treatment and clinical outcomes of transcatheter heart valve thrombosis. Circ Cardiovasc Interv. 2015;8(4):e001779.
5. Roudaut R, Serri K, Lafitte S. Thrombosis of prosthetic heart valves: diagnosis and therapeutic considerations. Heart. 2007;93(1):137-42.
6. Krishnan S. Prosthetic valve thrombosis: Diagnosis and newer thrombolytic regimes. J Pract Cardiovasc Sci. 2016;2:7-12.
7. Egbe AC, Pislaru SV, Pellikka PA, Poterucha JT, Schaff HV, Maleszewski JJ, et al. Bioprosthetic valve thrombosis versus structural failure: clinical and echocardiographic predictors. J Am Coll Cardiol. 2015;66(21):2285-94.
8. Dangas GD, Weitz JI, Giustino G, Makkar R, Mehran R. Prosthetic Heart Valve Thrombosis. J Am Coll Cardiol. 2016;68(24):2670-89.
9. Duran NE, Biteker M, Ozkan M. Treatment alternatives in mechanical valve thrombosis. Turk Kardiyol Dern Ars. 2008;36(6): 420-5.
10. Nagy A, Denes M, Lengyel M. Predictors of the outcome of thrombolytic therapy in prosthetic mitral valve thrombosis: a study of 62 events. J Heart Valve Dis. 2009;18(3):268-75.
11. Ozkan M, Gunduz S, Bitekar M, Astarcioglu MA, Çevik C, Kaynak E, et al. Comparison of different TEE-guided thrombolytic regimens for prosthetic valve thrombosis: the TROIA trial. JACC Cardiovasc Imaging. 2013;6(2):206-16.
12. Roudaut R, Lafitte S, Roudaut MF, Reant P, Pillois X, Durrieu-Jaïs C, et al. Management of prosthetic heart valve obstruction: fibrinolysis versus surgery. Early results and long-term follow-up in a single-centre study of 263 cases. Arch Cardiovasc Dis. 2009;102(4):269-77.
13. Huang G, Schaff HV, Sundt TM, Rahimtoola SH. Treatment of obstructive thrombosed prosthetic heart valve. J Am Coll Cardiol. 2013;62(19):1731-36.
14. Ozkan M, Cakal B, Karakoyun S, Gürsoy OM, Çevik C, Kalçık M, et al. Thrombolytic Therapy for the Treatment of Prosthetic Heart Valve Thrombosis in Pregnancy with Low-Dose, Slow Infusion of Tissue-Type Plasminogen Activator. Circulation. 2013;128(5):532-40.

17

CHAPTER

Atrial Hypertension including Left Atrial Dysfunction and Remodeling

VK Katyal, Ashima Katyal, Bijender Singh

ABSTRACT

Left ventricle (LV) size and its functions contribute to cardiovascular (CV) disorders is well known and investigated. Little is known of left atrial (LA) abnormalities of function, size, and remodeling toward outcome in CV diseases. Recent studies do suggest a contribution of LA hypertension (diastolic dysfunction) toward the occurrence of atrial fibrillation, stroke, CV, and all-cause mortality. Several factors such as LA size, older age, hypertension, LV dilation, and measures of obesity associated with larger LA volume and consequent LA remodeling, have been found to adversely affect outcomes in patients with established CV disease. Left atrial hypertension plays a key role in the pathophysiology of heart failure and is generally caused by poor LV relaxation and increased chamber stiffness. Two-dimensional (2D) echocardiography utilizing basic TTE, tissue Doppler imaging (TDI), and LA strain imaging have revolutionized the understanding of LA function and its abnormalities and are becoming routine during echocardiographic examination in most centers. This review; therefore, looks into the functions of LA, and its remodeling causing LA hypertension largely by echocardiography.

INTRODUCTION

Changes in the left atrium have interested researchers since 1980 when the size of normal left atrial (LA) was determined. Subsequently, LA has been extensively used in imaging techniques to determine abnormalities and prognosis of various cardiovascular (CV) disorders. Recently combined evaluation of LA size and functions has been studied to add to the prognosis of various CV diseases. LA is not considered now a simple conduit but is a highly dynamic chamber that helps in restoring hemodynamic balance by secreting natriuretics affecting vasodilation, and inhibition of sympathoadrenal and renin-angiotensin axis. LA enlargement and LA remodeling (abnormal LA pathophysiological functions) are predictors of adverse CV outcomes. LA structural and functional remodeling represents pathophysiological changes contributing to LA hypertension and include changes in ionic/genomic channels, cellular energy balance, inflammatory expressions (apoptosis and fibrosis), and hormonal imbalance. Measure to reverse remodeling are now known to affect prognosis in heart failure patients.

PATHOPHYSIOLOGY OF ATRIAL HYPERTENSION AND LEFT ATRIAL REMODELING

There are three phases of the LA function. First, it stores blood from the pulmonary venous system during the left ventricle (LV) systole, secondly, it rapidly fills the LV during early diastole and finally, it contracts and contributes 15–30% of LV stroke volume. The function of LA depends on LV filling pressures (compliance). LA afterload is the net result of compliance and filling pressures of LV and increases exponentially with an increase in LV diastolic dysfunction. Its preload on the other hand is largely volume-dependent. LA size is dependent on its volume and pressure. After progressive dilation, the contractile function of LA begins to decline similar to LV resulting in atrial hypertension. This is also affected by heart rate (HR). Neurohumoral regulation controls HR, blood pressure, cardiac output, and regional blood flow. Its persistent activation in heart failure especially results in a negative influence on LV and atrial function due to increases in atrial natriuretic peptide, brain natriuretic peptide, angiotensin II, aldosterone, and other neurohormonal factors which promote LA remodeling due to inflammatory, profibrotic, proarrhythmic, and prothrombotic actions affecting atrial contraction. The resultant atrial fibrillation is associated with significant morbidity and mortality. Atrial cardiomyopathy, a multifactorial disease, results due to fibrosis of the LA myocardium which decreases LA mechanical function, progressively slows down intra-atrial conduction, and elevates LA pressure with decreased LA compliance causing a vicious cycle promoting further LA remodeling.

LEFT ATRIAL APPENDAGE VIS-A-VIS LEFT ATRIAL FUNCTION

Atrial natriuretic peptide and brain natriuretic peptide are produced in the LA appendage. It is a more sensitive gauge of pressure changes due to its geometry and numerous myocardial stretch receptors. The left atrial appendage (LAA) is important for its role in thromboembolism and the persistence of atrial fibrillation. Low flow velocities, spontaneous echo-contrast, and thrombus have been identified in the LAA among those who sustained thromboembolic episodes. Patients presenting with AF demonstrate atrial appendage flow velocities are often, 50 cm/s, and this feature has been linked to thrombus formation and stroke.

ETIOLOGIES OF ATRIAL HYPERTENSION

Following are the etiologies that can affect LA structure and function:
- Hypertension
- Aortic valve diseases
- Mitral valve (MV) stenosis
- MV regurgitation
- Diastolic dysfunction in the LV in diverse CV disorders
- Left ventricular failure
- Ventricular septal defect
- Patent ductus arteriosus
- Mass or tumor in your left atrium
- Arteriovenous fistulas
- Athlete's heart

ASSESSMENT OF LEFT ATRIAL FUNCTIONS

A combination of flow velocities across MV, MV annular velocities, LA volume, and measurement of systolic pulmonary pressures is recommended to assess left ventricular filling pressures (LVFP) in clinical practice.

Volumetric Assessment of Left Atrial Function

LA volume assessment by 2D echocardiography is cheap, reproducible, and can be used for risk assessment and follow-up. It is a noninvasive method that has minimal difference in estimation vis-à-vis Cardiac magnetic resonance imaging (MRI) which is clinically irrelevant. LA volume measurement by Biplane Area length or Modified Simson's methods in LA four-chamber and two-chamber views are simple and accurate (maximal LA volume is 22 + 5–6 mL/m^2; minimal LA volume is 11 + 4 mL/m^2). Three-dimensional (3D) echocardiography does not provide any incremental value.

Doppler Echocardiography Evaluation of Left Atrial Function

Transmitral measurement of LA function at MV tips assesses early (mitral E) and late (mitral A) diastolic filling. These measurements are the basis of LV diastolic functions estimation **(Fig. 1)**. Additional help for estimating raised left ventricular end-diastolic pressure (LVEDP) in the absence of pulmonary arterial hypertension is systolic pulmonary artery pressure calculated from tricuspid regurgitation (TR) velocity of >2.8 m/s + right atrial (RA) pressure.

Tissue Doppler Imaging

The tissue Doppler imaging (TDI) at the mitral annulus level depicts three major waveforms; (1) peak ventricular systolic velocity (S'), (2) peak early ventricular diastolic velocity (E'), and (3) atrial contraction (A'). Mitral annulus A' velocity demonstrates excellent correlation with LA ejection fraction, LA ejection force, and LA kinetic energy in patients with various degrees of LV diastolic dysfunction. Three averaged readings of the mitral annulus were obtained with the sample placed on the atrial side of the MV annulus at the basal interatrial septum. TDI A' assesses global LA function. In healthy individuals, there is an age and HR-related increase in A' velocity and it increases also in relaxation abnormality of LV and decreases in restrictive abnormalities.

Left Ventricular Filling Pressures

Left ventricular filling pressures can be evaluated by several echocardiographic parameters including TDI assessing transmitral flow velocities and MV annular velocities, LA volumes, strain, and estimated systolic pulmonary pressures. Mitral valve velocities are determined by the transmitral flow gradient. Peak E velocity

Patients with normal EF and no known cardiac disease	
Parameter	Abnormal cut-off value
Average E/e'	> 14
Septal or lateral e'	Septal < 7 cm/s or lateral < 10 cm/s
TR velocity	> 2.8 m/s
LA volume index	> 34 mL/m^2

Number of abnormal parameters	Diastolic function
1 Abnormal value	Normal diastolic function
2 Abnormal values	Indeterminate diastolic dysfunction
3+ Abnormal values	Diastolic dysfunction

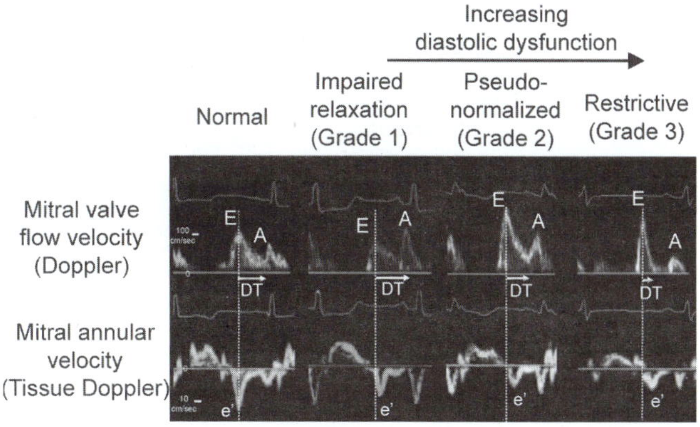

FIG. 1: Left ventricular diastolic dysfunction tissue Doppler early diastolic mitral annular velocity.

(LA: left atrial; TR: tricuspid regurgitation)

Source: Little WC, Oh JK. Echocardiographic Evaluation of Diastolic Function can be Used to Guide Clinical Care. Circulation. 2009;120(9):802-9.

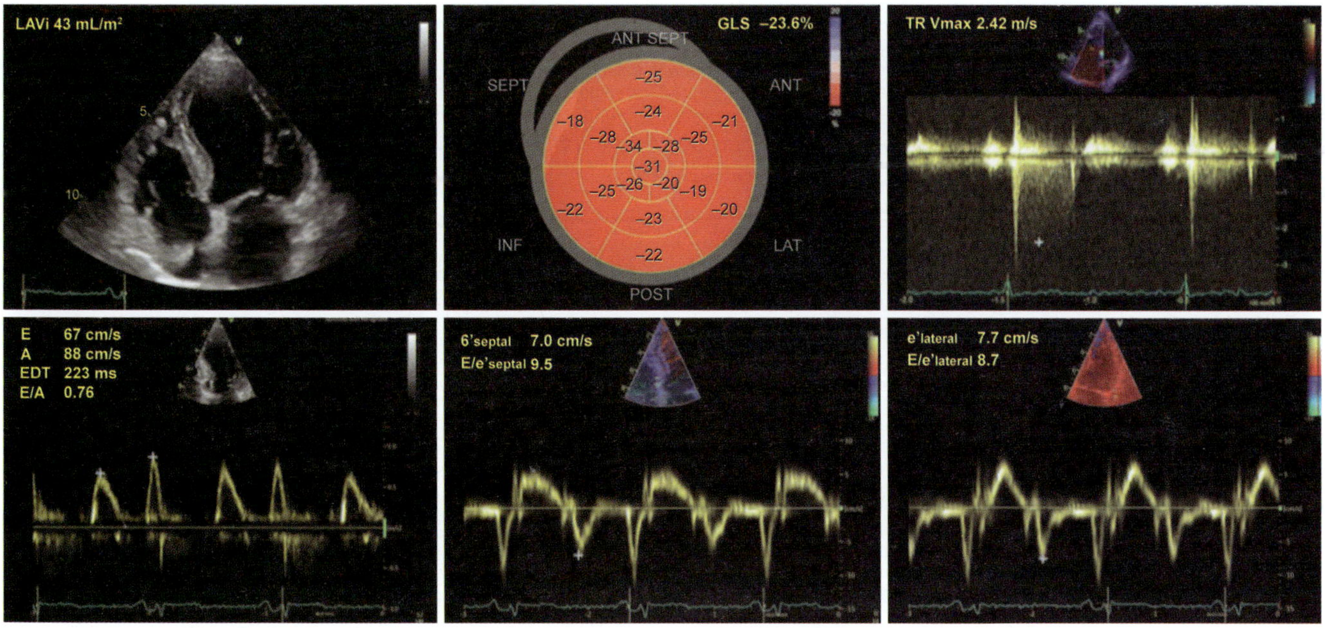

FIG. 2: Components of LA evaluation including LA strain imaging.

and its ratio of early E velocity and late A velocity ratio E/A are important determinants of LA pressure. Combining E velocity (increases with the extent of LV diastolic dysfunction) with TDI imaging e' velocity (decreases with LVDD) determines the E/e' ratio which is directly related to LV filling pressures. E/e' ratio < 8 and > 14 is associated with normal and elevated LV filling pressures respectively. It is less age-dependent and can be used in the presence of atrial fibrillation. Left atrial size and its function can be used in conjunction with other LA parameters for determining LA pressure elevation. LA volume index (>34 mL/m^2) is an accurate marker of LV elevated pressure if other conditions are absent.

Left Atrial Strain Imaging

Two-dimensional speckle tracking echocardiography in apical 4C view of LA is <19–23% and strain <18% predicts LVEDP better than LA volume **(Fig. 2)**.

ALGORITHM OF LEFT ATRIAL DIASTOLIC DYSFUNCTION (LEFT ATRIAL HYPERTENSION)

As shown in **Flowchart 1**, the European Association of Cardiovascular Imaging recommended this algorithm to evaluate LA hypertension which indirectly evaluates

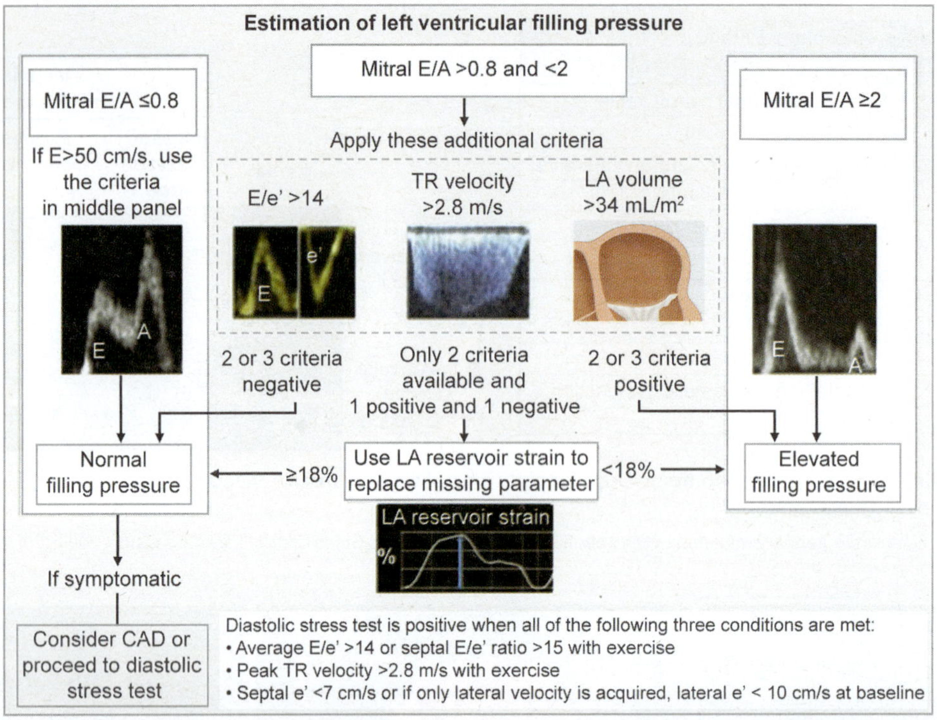

FLOWCHART 1: Algorithm of LA diastolic dysfunction tissue Doppler early diastolic mitral annular velocity .
(CAD: coronary artery disease; LA: left atrial; TR: tricuspid regurgitation)

the filling pressure of LV. They also recommend careful evaluation of clinical, echocardiographic, and Doppler data to decide LA diastolic dysfunction. This determination should start with delineation of clinical risk factors [presence of hypertension, coronary artery disease (CAD), diabetes, etc.], structural cardiac disease viz; LVH, LA hypertrophy cum dilatation, with or without LV systolic dysfunction (reduced LVEF) followed by application of various imaging data shown in **Flowchart 1**. Diastolic stress testing is also recommended in individuals with normal resting LA pressures. The European Association of Cardiovascular Imaging (EACVI) algorithm has been validated against invasive evaluation which is the gold standard.

CONCLUSION

Left atrial dysfunction (LA hypertension) plays an important part in the outcome of CV diseases associated with various types of heart failure. Its evaluation is cost-effective and reproducible in most echocardiography labs. It can be used clinically in the diagnosis, management (to reverse remodeling), and prognosis of patients with CV diseases.

SUGGESTED READINGS

1. Blume GG, Mcleod CJ, Barnes ME, Seward JB, Pellikka PA, Bastiansen PM, et al. Left atrial function: physiology, assessment, and clinical implications. Eur J Echocardiogr. 2011;12(6):421-30.
2. Popescu BA, Beladan CC, Nagueh SF, Smiseth OA. How to assess left ventricular filling pressures by echocardiography in clinical practice? Eur Heart J Cardiovasc Imaging. 2022;23(9):1127-9.

18

CHAPTER

Thyrocardiovascular Medicine: Emerging Science

S Arulrhaj, Aarathy Kannan, Manikandan, Rohith Velusamy

ABSTRACT

The association between thyroid hormones and cardiovascular conditions has been well studied, specifically, the effects of hypothyroidism on cardiomyopathy, and hyperthyroidism with arrhythmias. It is rare for patients with hyperthyroidism to remain in a chronic hyperthyroid state, making it difficult to analyze subsequent long-term effects on the cardiovascular system. Related to heart failure, some studies have demonstrated no change in ejection fraction, while others have shown an acute change along with diastolic dysfunction, with or without an underlying rhythm abnormality.

INTRODUCTION

Thyroid gland is an important organ which produces thyroid hormones responsible for maintaining body metabolism. Disease of thyroid gland causes symptoms either due to *overfunctioning* or *underfunctioning* of the gland. Both hyperthyroidism and hypothyroidism produce changes in:

- Cardiac contractility
- Myocardial oxygen consumption
- Cardiac output
- Blood pressure
- Systemic vascular resistance (SVR)

THYROID DYSFUNCTION: A MULTI-SYSTEM DISEASE (FIGS. 1 AND FLOWCHART 1)

Types of Thyroid Dysfunction

Hypothyroidism (Flowchart 2)

- *Primary hypothyroidism: Low levels of blood thyroid hormone* due to destruction of the thyroid gland
- *Secondary hypothyroidism*: Pituitary damage, and results in insufficient production of thyroid-stimulating hormone (TSH)
- *Tertiary hypothyroidism*: The hypothalamus is unable to produce sufficient levels of thyrotropin-releasing hormone (TRH).

It can be classified as clinical (overt) or subclinical.

- *Clinical hypothyroidism: Clinical features***,** consisting of mental slowing, depression, weight gain, constipation, dry skin, hair loss, cold intolerance, and irregular

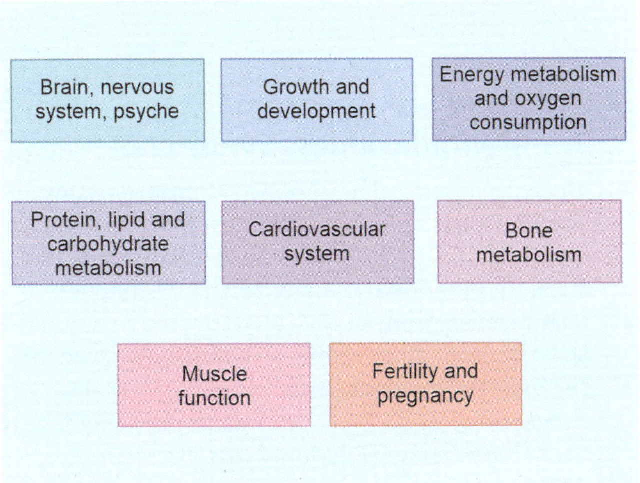

FIG. 1: Thyroid: Multisystem disease.

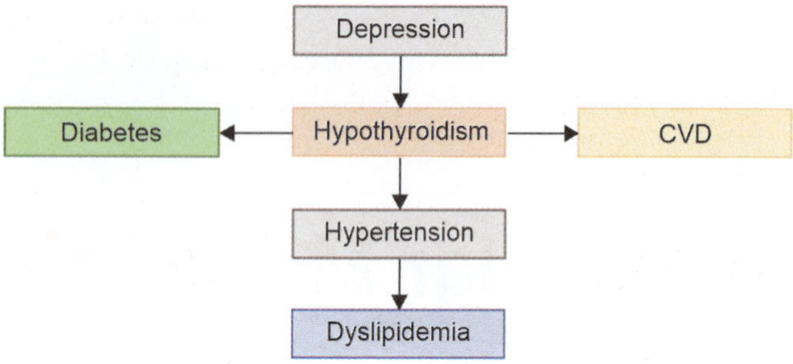

FLOWCHART 1: Links of hypothyroidism with other disorders.

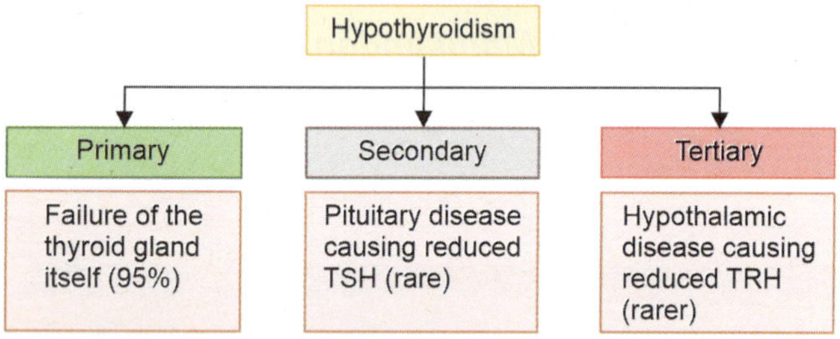

FLOWCHART 2: Types of hypothyroidism.

(TRH: thyrotropin-releasing hormone; TSH: thyroid-stimulating hormone)

Source: https://images.app.goo.gl/x3efCHEJy6m9uBWi9. [Last accessed December 2023].

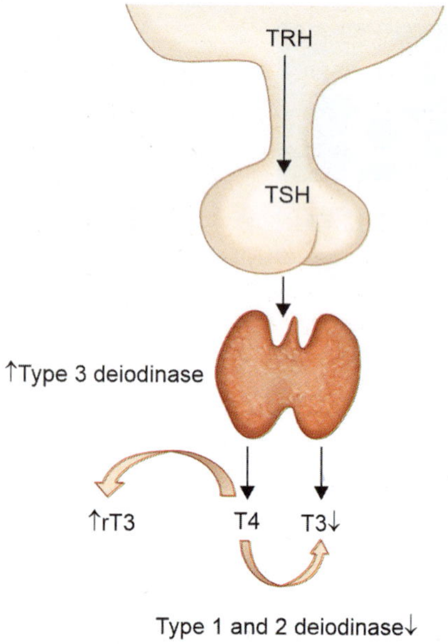

FIG. 2: Thyroid axis and changes in nonthyroidal illness. Direction of arrows (↑, ↓) indicates increase or decrease, respectively.

(rT3: reverse triiodothyronine; T4: thyroxine; TRH: thyrotropin-releasing hormone; TSH: thyroid-stimulating hormone)

menstruation, infertility. Triiodothyronine (T3), thyroxine (T4), and TSH may be abnormal.

- *Overt hypothyroidism*: A raised blood level of TSH (serum TSH levels > 12 mU/L), and a low serum T4 level (serum T4 < 60 nmol/L).

Subclinical Hypothyroidism

- Serum thyroid hormones are within their reference range in the presence of raised serum TSH concentrations.
- Subclinical hypothyroidism (SCH) can be classified as:
  - Grade 1 (TSH > 4.0 or 4.5, but < 10 mU/L)
  - Grade 2 (TSH > 10 mU/L).

Euthyroid Sick Syndrome (Nonthyroidal Illness Syndrome)

- It can be described as abnormal findings on thyroid function tests that occur in the setting of a nonthyroidal illness (NTI), without preexisting hypothalamic-pituitary and thyroid gland dysfunction
- After recovery from an NTI, these thyroid function test result abnormalities should be completely reversible.
- *The most prominent alterations are low serum T3 an elevated reverse T3 (rT3)*, leading to the general term "*low T3 syndrome.*"**(Fig. 2 and Box 1)**

BOX 1: Prevalence of thyroid disorders.

- 42 million people in India have thyroid disorders
- Hypothyroidism is the most common of the thyroid disorders in India, affecting 1 in 10 adults
- The prevalence of hypothyroidism in India is 11%, compared with only 2% in the UK and 4–6% in the USA

Source: Bagcchi S. Hypothyroidism in India: more to be done. Lancet Diabetes Endocrinol. 2014;2(10):

INCIDENCE

Global

Current estimates suggest that thyroid disease affects as many as 9–15% of the adult female population and a smaller percentage of adult males hypothyroidism affects between 4 and 10% of the population, and the prevalence of SCH is reported to be as high as 10% in various studies. The prevalence of SCH is approximately 1%.

In India

The prevalence of hypothyroidism was reported at 10.95% with significantly higher proportion of females *SCH* was observed in *8.02%* of the population in India.

HYPERTHYROIDISM

- *Hyperthyroidism*: Too much thyroid hormone produced in the body.
- *Thyrotoxicosis*: High thyroid hormone levels in the blood stream, irrespective of their source.
- *SCH*: Low (or undetectable) TSH level with a normal serum free T4 and normal serum total T3 levels.
- *Overt hyperthyroidism* occurs when the TSH level is low (or undetectable) and the free T4 level and/or total T3 level is elevated.

CLINICAL PRESENTATIONS OF THYROCARDIAC DISEASE

Clinical presentations of thyrocardiac disease is given in **Table 1**.

EFFECTS OF THYROID HORMONE ON CARDIOVASCULAR HEMODYNAMICS (FIG. 3)

Direct Effect of Thyroid Hormone on Heart (Fig. 4)

- Thyroid hormone is an important *regulator of cardiac gene expression* and, many of the cardiac manifestations of thyroid dysfunction are associated with alterations in T3-mediated gene expression
- Several components of the cardiac myocyte β-adrenergic system are regulated by thyroid

TABLE 1: Clinical presentations of thyrocardiac disease.

	Hyperthyroidism	Hypothyroidism
Symptoms	• Palpitations • Exercise intolerance • Exertional dyspnea • Angina	• Fatigue • Exercise intolerance • Palpitations
Signs	• Sinus tachycardia • Systemic hypertension • Atrial fibrillation • Hyperdynamic precordium Peripheral edema • Cardiac hypertrophy • Cardiac heart failure (CHF)	• Diastolic hypertension (Arterial elasticity ↓) bradycardia • Atherosclerosis and cholesterol↑ • QT prolongation • Torsades de pointes • Periorbital edema • Pleural and pericardial effusion • Systolic and diastolic heart failure • Cardiomyopathy

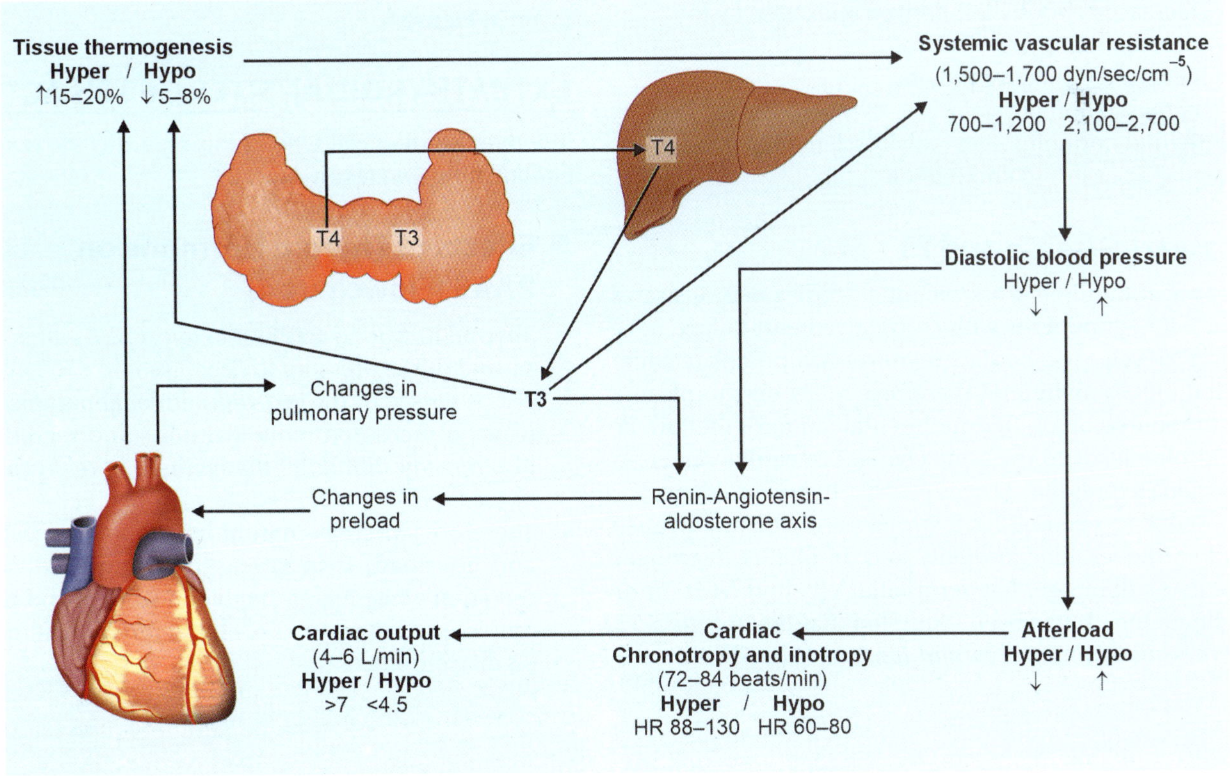

FIG. 3: Effects of thyroid hormone on cardiovascular hemodynamics.

Source: https://images.app.goo.gl/uYmMVpR73tErFBjh9. [Last accessed December 2023].

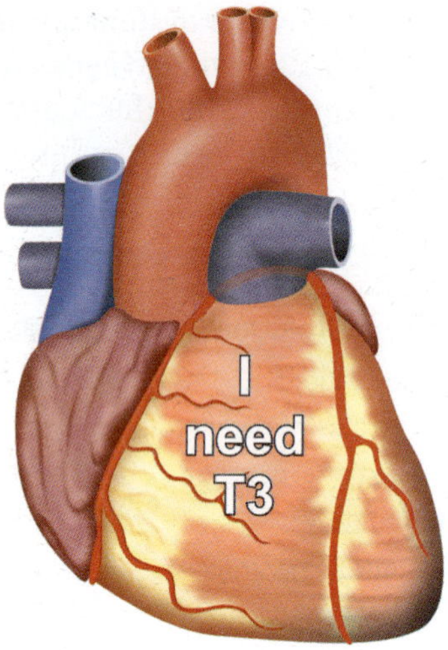

FIG. 4: Direct effect of thyroid hormone on Heart.

hormone, such as the β1-adrenergic receptor, guanine nucleotide regulatory proteins, and adenylate cyclase.
- *T3 has both genomic and nongenomic effects on the cardiac myocyte.*

Cardiovascular Risks Associated with Hypothyroidism

- Impaired cardiac contractility and diastolic function
- Increased SVR
- Decreased endothelial-derived relaxation factor
- Increased serum cholesterol
- Increased C reactive protein
- Increased homocysteine

Thyroid hormone is anti-atherosclerotic that decreases vascular disease and cholesterol.

Heart Disease and T3

Review of multiple cross-sectional studies demonstrates that ≈30% of patients with congestive heart failure have low T3 levels. The cardiac myocyte has no appreciable deiodinase activity and therefore, relies on the plasma as the source of T3. In experimental animals, the low T3 syndrome leads to the same changes in cardiac function and gene expression as does primary hypothyroidism.

Reduced serum T3 is a strong predictor of all-cause and cardiovascular mortality and, in fact, is a stronger predictor than age, left ventricular ejection fraction or dyslipidemia. It has been suggested that *physiological T3 therapy might improve cardiac function* **(Fig. 5)**.

T3-regulated Cardiac Genes

T3-regulated cardiac genes are given in **Table 2**.

Effects of Thyroid Hormone on Cardiovascular Hemodynamics

- Thyroid hormone effects on the heart and peripheral vasculature include *decreased SVR and increased resting heart rate, left ventricular contractility, and blood volume.*
- Thyroid hormone causes *decreased resistance in peripheral arterioles* through a direct effect on *vascular smooth* muscles (VSM) and decreased mean arterial pressure, which, when sensed in the kidneys, *activates the renin-angiotensin-aldosterone system* and increases renal sodium absorption.
- T3 also *increases erythropoietin synthesis,* which leads to an increase in red cell mass.
- In *hyperthyroidism*, these combined effects increase cardiac output 50–300% higher than in normal individuals.
- *In hypothyroidism, cardiac output may decrease by 30–50%.*

Thyroid Hormone Effects on Cardiovascular System

Thyroid hormone effects on cardiovascular system is given in **Figure 6**.

EXTRATHYROIDAL SITES OF TSH ACTION

The most studied cell type in this regard is the *adipocyte, endothelium and* **(Flowchart 3)**.

Effects of Thyroid Hormone on RAAS (Flowchart 4)

- Thyroid hormone acts first *to lower SVR* which causes mean arterial pressure to decrease.
- This is sensed by the juxtaglomerular apparatus, which leads to increased renin synthesis and secretion. *T3 also directly stimulates the synthesis of renin substrate in the liver.*
- Therefore, whereas thyroid hormone decreases SVR and afterload, it increases renin and aldosterone secretion while increasing blood volume and preload and contributes to the characteristic increase in cardiac output.

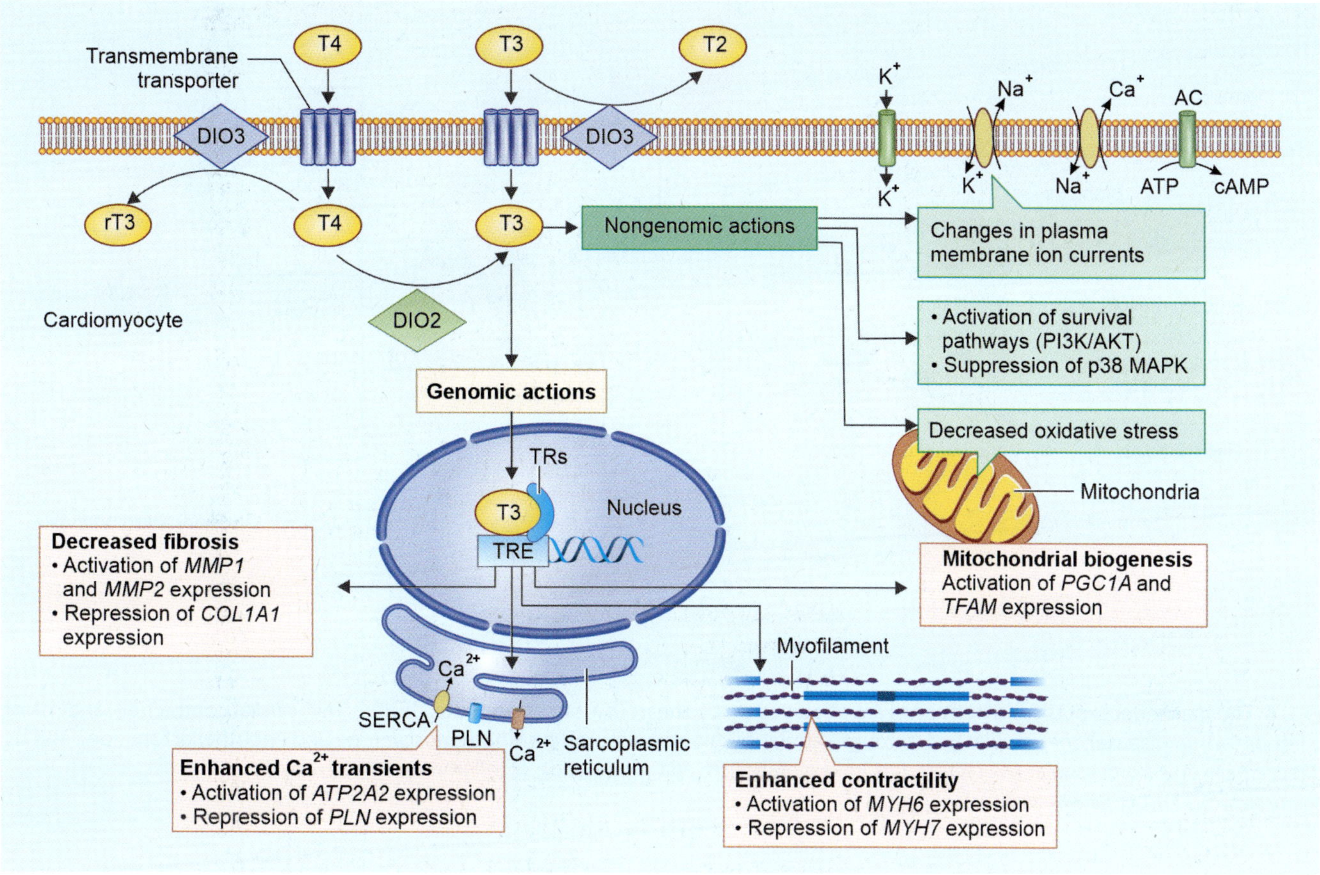

FIG. 5: Effect of Thyroid Hormones on the cardiomyocyte via genomic and nongenomic actions.
(DIO: iodothyronine deiodinase; rT3: reverse triiodothyronine; T3: Triiodothyronine; T4: thyroxine)

TABLE 2: T3-regulated cardiac genes.

Positively regulated transcriptional activation	Negatively regulated transcriptional repression
α-MHC	β-MHC
Voltage-gated K^+ channels (Kv1.5, Kv4.2)	Na^+/Ca^{2+}exchanger (NCX1)
SERCA2	Phospholamban
Na^+/K^+ ATPase	Adenylyl cyclase types V, VI
β1-adrenergic receptor	Thyroid hormone receptor α1
Adenine nucleotide translocase (ANT1)	Thyroid hormone transporters (MCT8, 10)

(ATPase: adenosine triphosphatase; Ca^{2+}: calcium; K^+: potassium; Na^+: sodium; MHC: myosin heavy chain; SERCA: sarcoplasmic reticulum adenosine triphosphatase; T3: triiodothyronine)

Diabetes, Dyslipidemia, Thyroid Disorder and Cardiovascular Risk (Fig. 11)

The role of diabetes, dyslipidemia, thyroid disorder and cardiovascular risk has been given in **Figures 7 and 11**.

THYROID AND HYPERTENSION

- Ever since Thompson et al. in 1931 observed a high incidence of hypertension in myxedema, hypothyroidism has been identified as a common form of so-called secondary hypertension.
- 20–40% patients with hypothyroidism have hypertension
- Diastolic blood pressure is increased more than systolic blood pressure—primarily due to increase in SVR. T3 may act as direct vasodilator therefore, vascular tone may increase in its absence. *Blood pressure in these patients is less sensitive to variations in salt intake.*

Thyroid Hormone Effects on Blood Pressure Regulation

- Asvold et al. reported a *linear correlation between TSH and both systolic and diastolic blood pressure.*
- A *widened pulse pressure is characteristic of hyperthyroidism.* Recent reports have shown that arterial

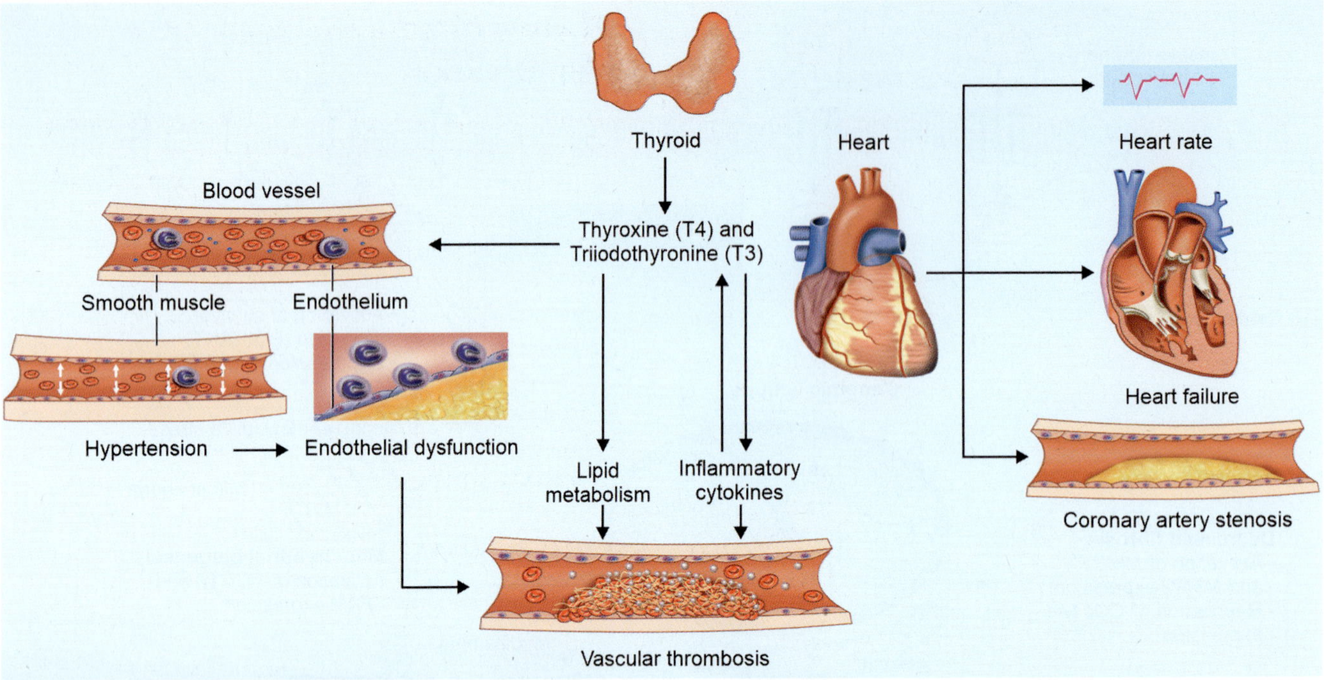

FIG. 6: The main effects of thyroid hormones are observed on the heart (by influencing rate, rhythm, myocardial contraction, and risk of coronary artery disease), *the vascular tree* (through regulating blood pressure via smooth muscle tone and endothelial function), and by *direct effects* on cardiovascular risk factors (via lipid metabolism and modulation of inflammatory pathways).

Source: Razvi S. J Am Coll Cardiol. 2018;71(16):1781-96.

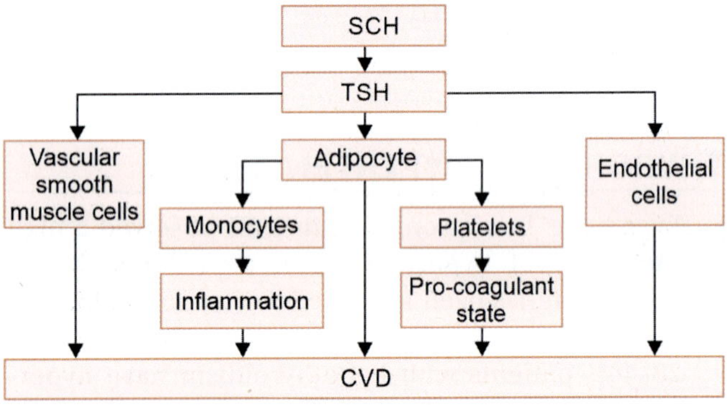

FLOWCHART 3: Effect of thyroid on smooth muscle cells, adipocytes, and endothelial cells.

(SCH: Subclinical hypothyroidism; TSH: thyroid-stimulating hormone)

stiffness is increased in hyperthyroidism despite the low SVR.

- *In hypothyroidism, endothelial dysfunction and impaired VSM relaxation lead to increased SVR.* These effects lead to diastolic hypertension in ≈30% of patients, and *thyroid hormone replacement therapy restores endothelial-derived vasorelaxation and blood pressure to normal in most.*

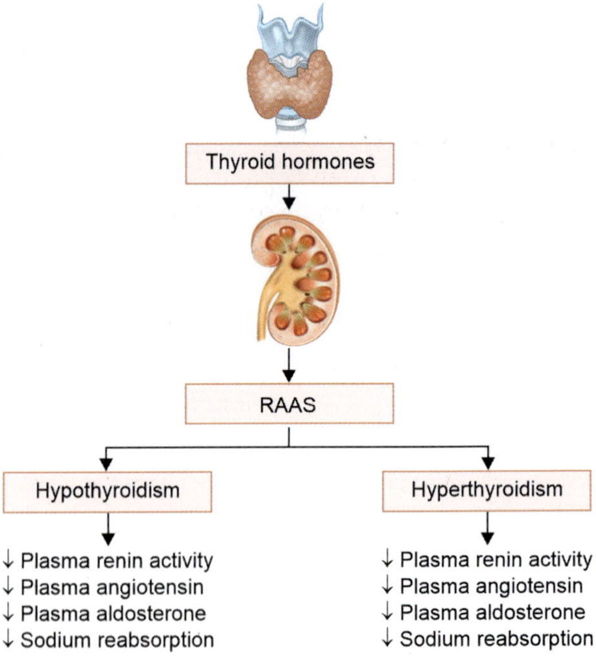

FLOWCHART 4: Effects of Thyroid Hormone on renin–angiotensin–aldosterone system (RAAS).

Source: https://images.app.goo.gl/ogRZKk2CN5U5F94M7. [Last accessed December, 2023].

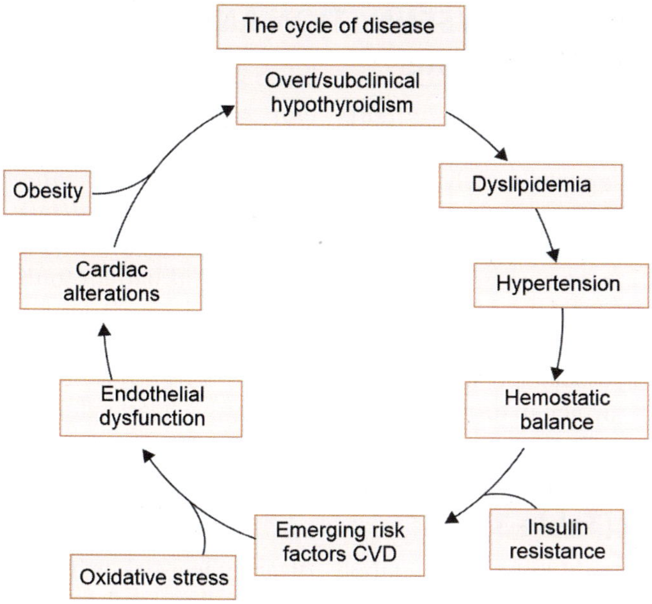

FIG. 7: Cycle of the disease.

■ Thyroid Dysfunction and Hypertension

Overt and subclinical hyper- and hypothyroidism can both lead to hypertension. In a study Saito et al. found a three-fold *higher prevalence of diastolic hypertension in hypothyroidism.* A couple of type II iodothyronine deiodinase *(DIO2) gene mutations* were found to cause hypertension in middle-aged patients with euthyroidism.

A *mutation in the TRH receptor gene* was characterized to be associated with an increased risk of essential high blood pressure. In a recently published meta-analysis, after levothyroxine therapy, systolic blood pressure was reduced significantly.

■ Hypothyroidism and Hypertension

The role of hypothyroidism and hypertension is given in **Flowchart 5**.

■ Thyroid Disease and Pulmonary Hypertension

- Pulmonary hypertension has been associated with thyroid dysfunction, *but primarily with hyperthyroidism.*
- In a recent study of 23 consecutive patients with hyperthyroidism caused by Graves' disease, 65% of patients had pulmonary hypertension. Almost all patients normalized the increased pulmonary artery pressure with definitive treatment of the Graves' disease.
- Some evidence exists that autoimmune disease may play a role in both hypothyroid- and hyperthyroid-linked cases of primary pulmonary hypertension.

THYROID HORMONE EFFECTS ON LIPID METABOLISM

- *Overt hypothyroidism* is characterized by *hypercholesterolemia* and a *marked increase in low-density lipoproteins (LDL) and apolipoprotein B.*
- Lipid profile changes are *also evident in subclinical hypothyroidism.* Mechanisms include decreased fractional clearance of LDL by a reduced number of LDL receptors in the liver in addition to decreased receptor activity **(Flowchart 6)**.

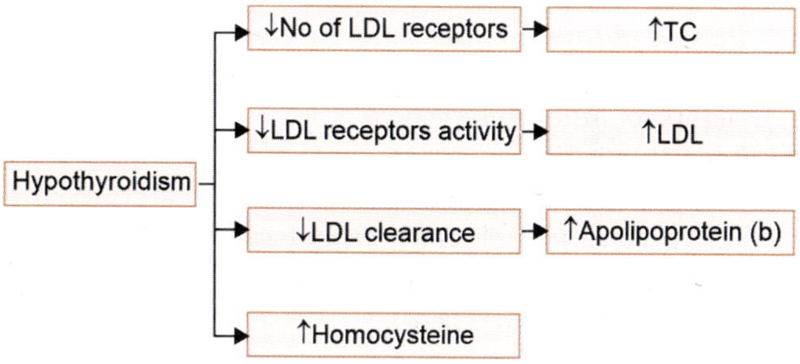

FLOWCHART 6: Effect on lipid metabolism.
(LDL: low-density lipoprotein; TC: total cholesterol)

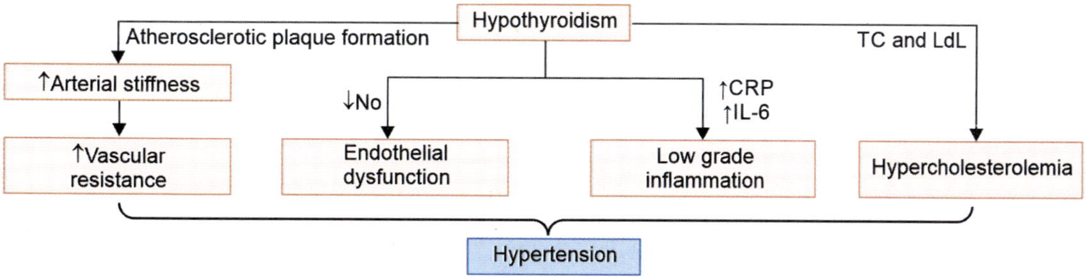

FLOWCHART 5: Hypothyroidism and hypertension.

ARRHYTHMIA IN THYROID DYSFUNCTION

- It is well known that *hyperthyroidism is associated with sinus tachycardia and atrial fibrillation (AF). Hyperthyroidism: Rate-related phenomenon*
- Similarly, *hypothyroidism* is associated with bradycardia and increased cardiovascular risk factors
- The *QT interval is often prolonged* in hypothyroidism due to prolonged ventricular action potential. This is indicative of increased ventricular irritability and in turn can lead to acquired Torsades de pointes.
- *Varying degrees of atrioventricular block and low QRS complexes* are also seen in patients with hypothyroidism.

HYPOTHYROIDISM AND PERICARDIAL EFFUSION (FLOWCHART 7)

- Several cases of cardiac tamponade due to hypothyroidism have also been described.
- Majority of effusions are *asymptomatic due to slow fluid accumulation.*
- The fluid will be *exudative due to high protein content*

THYROID DYSFUNCTION AND ATHEROSCLEROSIS

- *Thyroid hormone inhibits atherogenesis* through direct effects on the vasculature as well as modifying risk factors for atherosclerosis.
- Recent studies suggest that hypothyroidism is associated with the emerging risk factors for atherosclerosis such as *hyperhomocysteinemia* and an *increase in C-reactive protein level. Thyroid hormone is antiatherosclerotic* **(Fig. 8)**.

THYROID DYSFUNCTION AND HEART FAILURE

- *Hypothyroid patients can often present with heart failure,* and its prevalence increases from approximately *13% in New York Heart Association (NYHA) class I–II to 30% in NYHA class III–IV. Preexistent ischemic or hypertensive heart disease* may also predispose the hyperthyroid patient to the development of heart failure.
- Among *people >60 years of age,* a low TSH level is associated with increased risk for *atrial fibrillation,* which in turn could lead to congestive heart failure.

Pathogenesis and Clinical Presentation (Table 3)

Thyroid hormone metabolic disarray is a risk factor for progression development of heart failure and of heart disease.

Low T3 Syndrome and Ejection Fraction

A recent study associated low T3 syndrome with ejection fraction as shown in **Figure 9**.

Mechanism of Heart Failure in Thyroid Dysfunction

The mechanism of heart failure in thyroid dysfunction is described in **Flowchart 8**.

Management of Heart Failure in Thyroid Dysfunction

Management of heart failure in thyroid dysfunction is described in **Flowchart 9**.

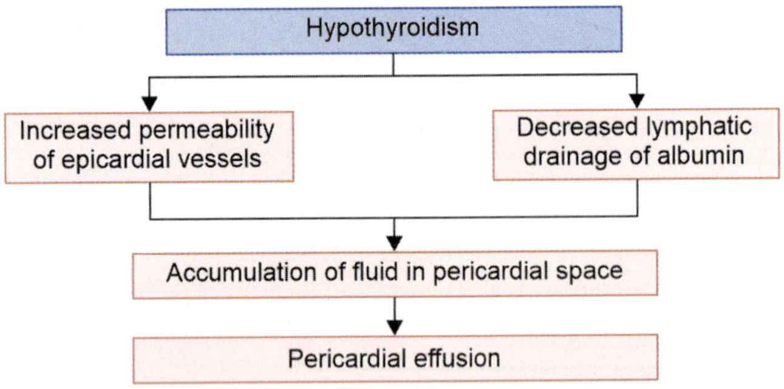

FLOWCHART 7: Hypothyroidism leading to pericardial effusion.

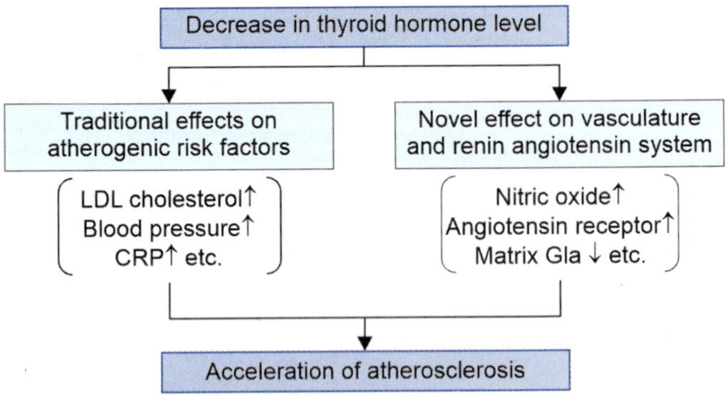

FIG. 8: The atherogenic effects of hypothyroidism.
(LDL: low-density lipoprotein; CRP: c-reactive protein)

TABLE 3: Pathogenesis and clinical presentation.

'High-output' HF (HFpEF) in hyperthyroidism	'Low-output' HF in hyperthyroidism	HF in hypothyroidism
Congestive circulation may occur with increased cardiac output in the absence of underlying heart disease due to the effects of: • Persistent tachycardia • Increased cardiac preload • Reduced systemic vascular resistance • Elevated ventricular filling pressure • Increased pulmonary arterial pressure	HF with low cardiac output may occur especially in elderly patients and in patients with underlying heart disease due to the effects of: • Increased cardiac preload • Impaired left ventricular filling • Loss of atrial contribution to atrial fibrillation • Rapid ventricular rate • Increased systemic vascular resistance decreased contractile reserve	HF may occur in patients with overt hypothyroidism and in elderly patients with subclinical hypothyroidism with TSH 10 mU/L due to the effects of: • Bradycardia • Impaired systolic function (HFrEF) • Impaired left ventricular diastolic filling • Increased systemic vascular resistance • Diastolic hypertension • Increased arterial stiffness • Endothelial dysfunction

(HF: heart failure; HFpEF: heart failure with preserved ejection fraction; HFrEF: heart failure with reduced ejection fraction; TSH: thyroid-stimulating hormone)

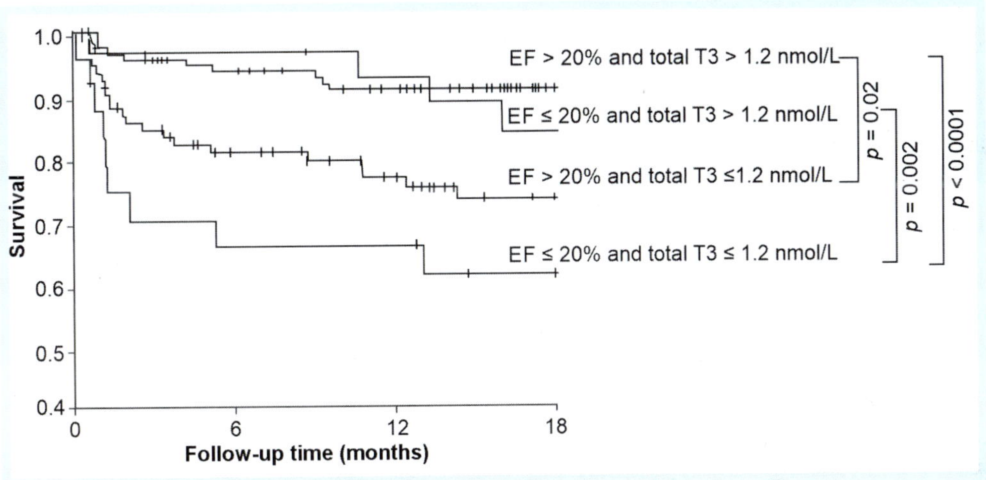

FIG. 9: Low T3, low EF—poor prognosis in heart failure.

Source: https://www.sciencedirect.com/science/article/pii/S0019483220300778. [Last accessed December, 2023].

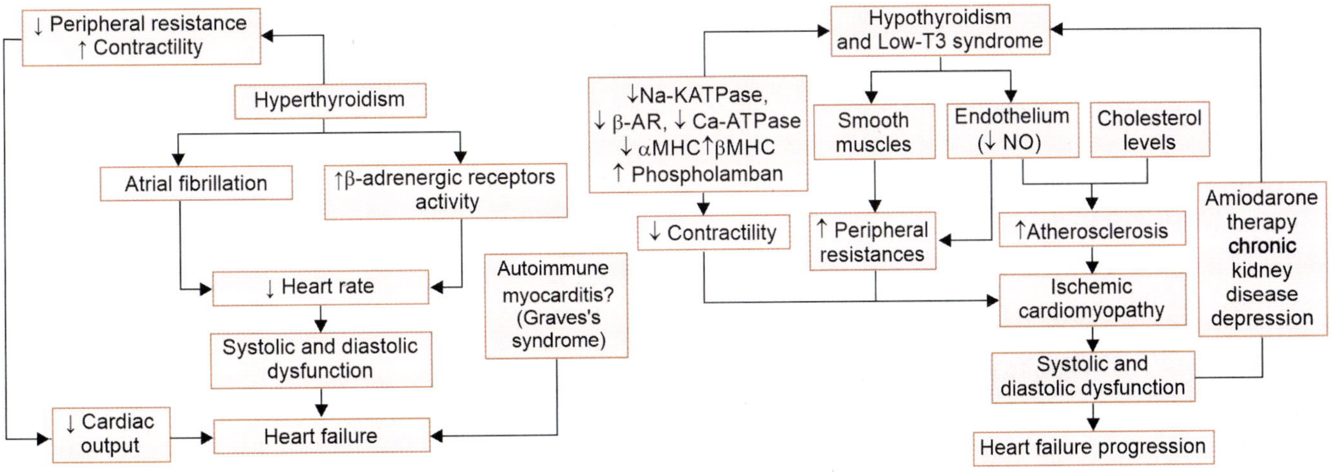

FLOWCHART 8: Mechanism of heart failure in thyroid dysfunction.

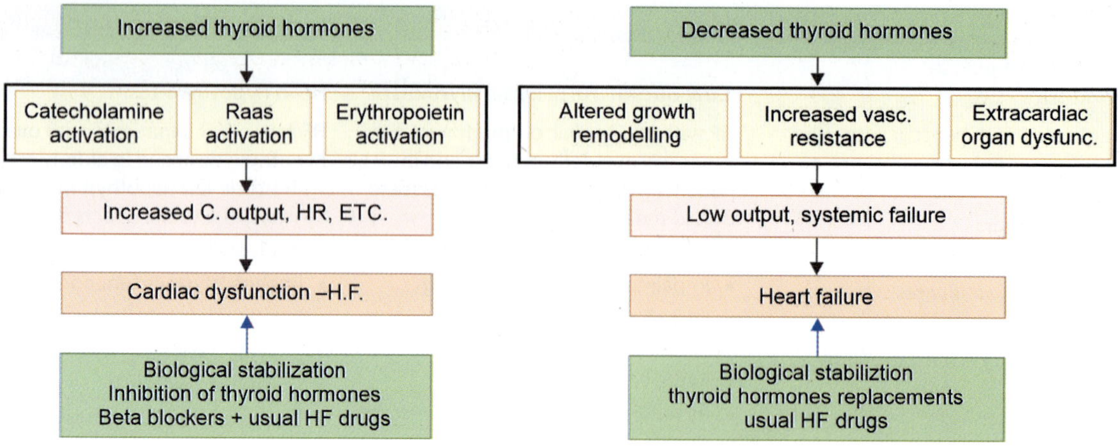

FLOWCHART 9: Management of heart failure in thyroid dysfunction.

TABLE 4: Role of thyroid hormone in cardiovascular disease and monitoring.

Condition	Recommendation
Atrial fibrillation	• Thyroid testing for a first episode and when ventricular rate is difficult to control • Beta-blocker to control ventricular rate when complicating thyrotoxicosis
Heart failure	Thyroid testing at initial presentation
Dilated cardiomyopathy	Thyroid testing at initial presentation
Amiodarone use	• Thyroid testing before, within 3 months of initiation, and every 3–6 months • Thyroid testing before, at land 3 months after initiation, and every 3–6 months • Amiodarone to be monitored with TSH
Subclinical hyperthyroidism	• If cardiac risk factors or cardiac disease, treat if TSH persistently < 0.1 mIU/L • If cardiac disease, consider treatment if TSH persistently 0.1–0.4 mIU/L
Overt hypothyroidism	• With known CAD, start low-dose levothyroxine and increase dose slowly • If unable to tolerate full dose, additional measures to treat CVD are indicated
Subclinical hypothyroidism	• Treat all patients or consider treatment with TSH level persistently > 10 mIU/L • Consider treatment: ○ For patients with TSH levels 4.5–10 mIU/L with ASCVD, heart failure, or associated risk factors for these diseases ○ For patients with TSH levels 4.5–10 mIU/L, for those patients younger than 65 years with increased CV risk (e.g., previous CVD, diabetes, dyslipidemia, hypertension, metabolic syndrome), particularly with TSH level persistently > 7 mIU/L

(CAD: coronary artery disease; CV: cardiovascular; CVD: cardiovascular disease; TSH: thyroid-stimulating disease)

Source: https://www.slideshare.net/magdyelmasry1422/thyroid-hormones-and-cardiovascular-function-and-diseases. [Last accessed December, 2023].

Role of Thyroid Hormone in CVD and Monitoring

Role of thyroid hormone in CVD and monitoring is described in **Table 4**.

A TWO-WAY STREET: RELATIONSHIP BETWEEN SCH AND HEART DISEASES

- *Heart diseases may also alter the metabolism of thyroid hormones.* Numerous reports from clinical and animal studies have documented altered thyroid hormone metabolism with low serum T3, T4, FT3, and FT4 levels.
- Congestive heart failure and major heart surgical procedures, such as cardiopulmonary bypass surgery, MI can also change thyroid function leading to "*euthyroid sick syndrome*." Pronounced low serum T3 and T4 levels have been shown to correlate with a higher mortality rate and poor prognosis in patients after MI.

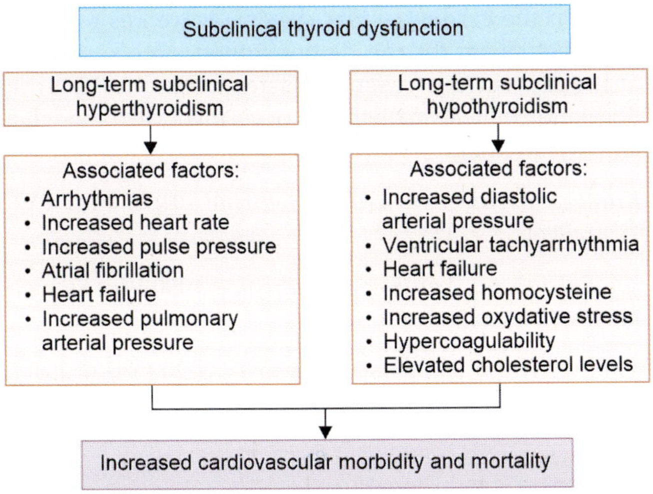

FLOWCHART 10: Subclinical thyroid dysfunction.

Source: https://www.slideshare.net/magdyelmasry1422/thyroid-hormones-and-cardiovascular-function-and-diseases. [Last accessed December, 2023].

SUBCLINICAL THYROID DYSFUNCTION AND INCREASED CARDIOVASCULAR MORBIDITY AND MORTALITY

Subclinical thyroid dysfunction causing increased cardiovascular morbidity and mortality is described in **Flowchart 10**.

CARDIOVASCULAR RISK IN ELDERLY HYPOTHYROID PATIENTS

Population studies such as NHANES III and NHANES 1999–2002 found that TSH values are higher with advancing age; however, these studies also indicate that older patients may have higher TSH values in the absence of thyroid disease. Overt hypothyroidism (OH) and SCH are frequently found in the elderly.

Overt hypothyroidism is associated with several functional cardiovascular abnormalities and increased risk of atherosclerosis resulting from hypertension associated to atherogenic lipid profile. The decision to treat elderly people is still an unresolved clinical challenge:

- Due to a lack of appropriately powered randomized controlled trials of L-T4 in sHT patients, examining cardiovascular hard endpoints in various classes of age because of the negative effects of possible overtreatment.

HYPOTHYROIDISM AND DIABETES

Prevalence of hypothyroidism in type 2 diabetes mellitus (T2DM) in India **(Fig. 10)**:

- In a cross-sectional observational study, adult patients with an established or newly diagnosed T2DM (n = 500) and T2DM + hypertension (n = 502)
- Among new hypothyroid cases, SCH were more prevalent than that of OH:
  - T2DM: 2.4% (OH) and 5.2% (SCH)
  - T2DM + hypertension: 5.2% (OH) and 6.4% (SCH)

CARDIOVASCULAR RISKS ASSOCIATED WITH HYPOTHYROIDISM

The cardiovascular risks associated with hypothyroidism have been described in **Figure 11**.

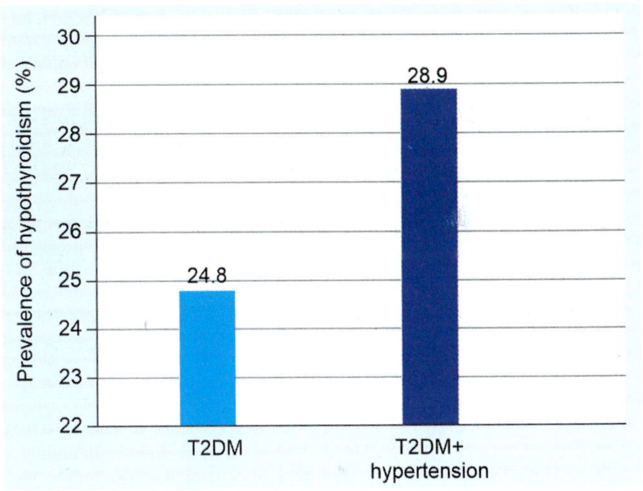

FIG. 10: Prevalence of hypothyroidism in type 2 diabetes mellitus (T2DM) and hypertension.

Source: https://www.xiahepublishing.com/2572-5505/JERP-2019-00001. [Last accessed December, 2023].

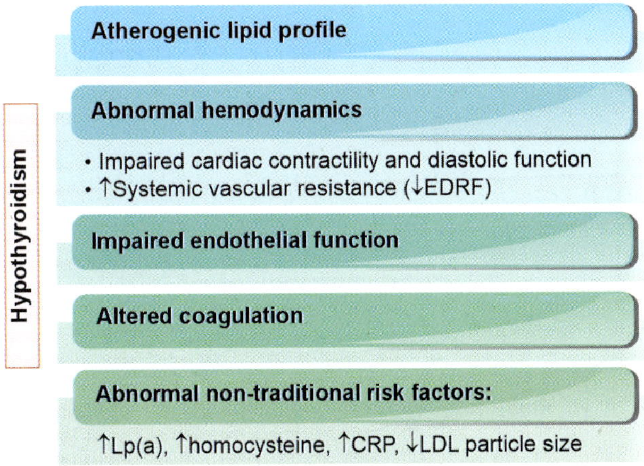

FIG. 11: Cardiovascular risks associated with hypothyroidism.

[CRP: c-reactive protein; EDRF: endothelium-derived relaxing factor; LDL: low-density lipoprotein; Lp(a): lipoprotein (a)]

CONCLUSION

Guidelines for heart failure produced by the American College of Cardiology and the American Heart Association support conducting thyroid function tests in patients with heart failure to determine if thyroid dysfunction may be a primary contributor to heart failure. In patients with a hyperthyroid state, the importance of prompt diagnosis and treatment of cardiac dysfunction is vital. Antithyroid medications are often indicated for the management of thyroid function; however, it may require several weeks to induce a euthyroid state. Further research is warranted to elucidate the long-term implications of a hyperthyroid state on the cardiovascular system, as well as to clarify the mechanism for the demonstrated effects, whether indirectly via the vascular system, directly by atrial fibrillation or tachyarrhythmia, or via myocyte remodeling and dysfunction.

Know Syphilis, You Know Medicine—1970 Prof PVR, Tirunelveli.

Know Diabetes, You Know Medicine—1990 Prof Sam GP Moses, Chennai.

Know Thyroid, You Know Medicine—2020 Prof Arulrhaj, Tuticorin.

SUGGESTED READINGS

1. Klein I, Danzi S. Thyroid disease and the heart. Circulation. 2007;116(15):1725-35.
2. Thompson EA, Ferraris S, Gress T, Ferraris V. Gender differences and predictors of mortality in spontaneous coronary artery dissection: a review of reported cases. J Invasive Cardiol. 2005;17(1):59-61.
3. Berta E, Lengyel I, Halmi S, Zrínyi M, Erdei A, Harangi M, et al. Hypertension in thyroid disorders. Front Endocrinol (Lausanne). 2019:10:482.
4. Ref: Paran Y, Nimrod A, Goldin Y, Justo D. Pulmonary hypertension and predominant right heart failure in thyrotoxicosis. Resuscitation. 2006;69:339-41.
5. Ma RC, Cheng AY, So WY, Hui DS. Thyrotoxicosis and pulmonary hypertension. Am J Med. 2005;118:927-92.
6. Pasqualetti G, Tognini S, Polini A, Caraccio N, Monzani F. Is subclinical hypothyroidism a cardiovascular risk factor in the elderly? J Clin Endocrinol Metab. 2013;98(6):2256-66.
7. Mariotti S, Cambuli VM. Cardiovascular risk in elderly hypothyroid patients. Thyroid. 2007;17(11):1067-73.
8. Talwalkar P, Deshmukh V, Bhole M. Prevalence of hypothyroidism in patients with type 2 diabetes mellitus and hypertension in India: a cross-sectional observational study. Diabetes Metab Syndr Obes. 2019;12:369-76.

19

CHAPTER

Palliative Care Dimensions in Cardiology

Kaustubh Dilip Salagre

ABSTRACT

In the era of modern medicine, the approach of treating doctors has typically medicalized patient mortality. While we need to focus more on a patient-centric holistic approach, early integration of palliative care is well recognized and has been included in guidelines of various cardiovascular societies.

Heart failure (HF) is a progressively symptomatic disease with patients experiencing a host of symptoms. Many times, patients report psychological and other noncardiac symptoms that cause more significant distress than traditional cardiac symptoms. The initiation of palliative care should therefore, be governed exclusively on palliative needs such as symptom burden. Optimizing HF management using diuretics and judicious use of oxygen therapy to improve cardiac performance is the key. Specialist palliative care can then be reserved for the management of more refractory symptoms and to assist with care near the end of life and when there is a conflict between patients and staff or patients and families. Palliative sedation is reserved for patients in advanced stage of the disease suffering from symptoms like refractory breathlessness/terminal breathlessness or overwhelming pain crisis.

Policy initiatives by state and central governments and the inclusion of palliative care in the National Health Policy of 2017 offer hope for the future.

INTRODUCTION

At the beginning of the 19th century, patients were attended to by spiritual advisors in India with only few having access to healthcare professionals and many preferring to die home than in a healthcare setting. After decades of medical advances, patients with advanced cardiovascular disease who are initiated on optimal medication regimens have options such as implantable defibrillators and cardiac resynchronization pacing systems. Currently available advanced heart failure (HF) therapies are focused on extending life and improving function. Palliative care has a multidimensional approach, thereby alleviating symptoms while addressing patients' psychosocial as well as spiritual needs. Unfortunately, very few cardiac patients get access to palliative care and hospice care. Modern medicine has effectively "medicalized our mortality".

Although there are studies demonstrating improved quality of life, better symptom control, and perhaps prolonged life expectancy with introduction of palliative care in cancer populations, it was in the mid 1990s when clinicians started looking more closely at introducing palliative care to cardiac patient populations. Attitudes have significantly changed, and the importance of palliative care for the cardiac patient population is now well recognized, with various cardiovascular societies including palliative care in their guidelines.

NEED FOR PALLIATIVE CARE

In 2016, the estimated prevalence of cardiovascular diseases (CVDs) in India was estimated to be 54.5 million. With a sedentary lifestyle, these diseases are more commonly affecting the economically productive age group resulting in catastrophic social and economic consequences. HF is a progressively symptomatic disease causing general clinical decline with rapid deteriorations in between. HF patients experience a host of symptoms in addition to dyspnea, including pain, fatigue, nausea, poor appetite, anxiety, depression, and an overall decreased sense of well-being. Patients with advanced HF have higher symptom burdens; caregivers of patients with advanced HF face and report that psychological and other noncardiac symptoms cause more significant distress than traditional cardiac symptoms. Recognition of HF worsening in the form of recurrent refractoriness of symptoms despite optimum therapy is a key and also an opportunity to initiate advance care directives and consider early palliative care involvement.

BARRIERS TO THE INTEGRATION OF CARDIAC AND PALLIATIVE CARE

According to the World Health Organization (WHO) and the Worldwide Palliative Care Alliance, there are over 7 million people with CVD worldwide who would benefit from palliative care. Several barriers have been identified in this regard. In reviewing these barriers, several main themes emerge: (1) "prognostic paralysis" secondary to unpredictable disease trajectories, (2) challenges with advance care planning, and (3) misunderstanding with respect to what palliative care represents (patients and clinicians) and also with respect to prognosis and treatment efficacies (patients). Prognostication challenges will not be overcome anytime soon. The initiation of palliative care should therefore be governed exclusively on palliative needs such as symptom burden.

Integrating Cardiac and Palliative Care

Specialist palliative care is ideally provided by a multidisciplinary team which includes physicians, nurses, pharmacists, social workers, and others who work collaboratively with the patient's baseline care team. Physicians already involved with patient care can provide many elements of palliative care such as basic symptom management, initial discussions about prognosis and treatment goals, and advance care planning. Specialist palliative care can then be reserved for the management of more refractory symptoms and to assist with care near the end of life and when there is a conflict between patients and staff or patients and families **(Fig. 1)**. Palliative care also provides counseling to reduce caregiver burden and emotional support in bereavement. Cardiac patients nearing the end of life are a special population

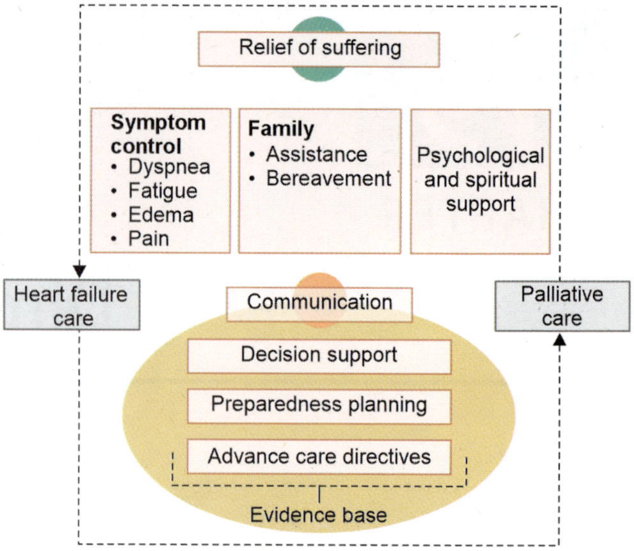

FIG. 1: Integrated model of palliative care.

of which some patients may be candidates for advanced mechanical circulatory support or transplant, while rest may be referred to hospice as an option if further decline is observed.

USE OF MEDICATIONS IN THE PALLIATIVE PATIENT POPULATION

Dyspnea, fatigue, decreased exercise capacity, pain, depression, anxiety, insomnia, and worsened cognitive function are commonly seen in patients with HF and are the strongest predictor of health-related quality of life. Assessment tools for symptom measures [Edmonton Symptom Assessment Scale (ESAS), Memorial Symptom Assessment Scale (MSAS)], disease-specific health status measures [Kansas City Cardiomyopathy Questionnaire (KCCQ), Minnesota Living with Heart Failure Questionnaire (MLWHF)], and general health status measures (EQ-5D) can be used for prognostication and management of patients with HF. Optimizing HF management using diuretics and judicious use of oxygen therapy to improve cardiac performance is the key as symptoms are mostly due to volume overload or reduced cardiac output .

Dyspnea

Breathlessness in advanced disease is a common problem with 65% of people experiencing breathlessness in the weeks before death. However, many patients requiring palliative care have multiple comorbidities, and sometimes breathlessness is not the primary problem. The sense of having dyspnea leads to anxiety, and being anxious can provoke dyspnea (dyspnea-anxiety cycle). While use of home oxygen therapy is recommended in chronic hypoxemia, if the person is breathless but not hypoxic, oxygen is generally not indicated. Alternative ways of dealing with breathlessness include the moving of air across the dermatomes of the trigeminal nerve ("fan therapy"). Oral morphine in low doses 2.5–5 mg, PO q6hr PRN is the drug of choice for breathlessness.

Pain

Paracetamol/acetaminophen can be given for mild-to-moderate pain while *opioids* remain the first line of management for moderate to severe pain. Adjuvant analgesics like gabapentin, pregabalin, selective serotonin reuptake inhibitors (SSRIs), and low-dose steroids are used for the management of other components of pain. Various nonpharmacological measures like massage, acupuncture, distraction techniques, and heat therapy are also used.

Fatigue/Cachexia

Fatigue is most common and often distressing symptom of HF as it severely hampers day-to-day work of the patient. Polikandrioti et al. in their study found that levels of fatigue in HF patients range from mild-to-severe, with fatigue being higher in hospitalized patients compared to those stable and at home. Therefore, patients with advanced HF should be systematically screened specifically for fatigue so that those at higher risk can be identified and additional supports put in place.

Psychological Symptoms

Identification of anxiety and depression and treating the underlying causes like pain and dyspnea are the first step. Palliative care is provided by a multidisciplinary team and includes an openness to conversations with patients about their fears and concerns regarding their illness and prognosis, in order to develop a plan of care that attends to the wishes and preferences of the patients and their caregivers. SSRIs are first-line pharmacological therapy owing to their general effectiveness and limited side effects. Nonpharmacological measures including exercise, psychotherapy, cognitive behavioral therapy, and distraction techniques are other effective modalities.

Constipation

In progressive HF patients, continued use of medications, such as anticholinergics, diuretics, and opioids for symptom management is likely to increase the prevalence of constipation. A thorough patient assessment with focus on history and physical examination is an essential component to understand the normal bowel routine and ascertain if patients are currently using nonpharmacological measures (i.e., increased dietary fiber, or over-the-counter products) or taking prescribed medicinal products for constipation.

PALLIATIVE SEDATION

Palliative sedation is reserved for patients in an advanced stage of the disease suffering from symptoms like refractory breathlessness/terminal breathlessness or overwhelming pain crisis. The aim is to relieve the patient's fear of suffocating to death and give a positive approach to the patient, family, and caregivers about relief of terminal symptoms. However, it will neither hamper nor hasten the process of dying.

When to Initiate Palliative Sedation?

- Repeated episodes of HF symptoms over the last 6 months despite optimal management
- Occurrence of malignant refractory arrhythmias
- Frequent use of intravenous drugs and repeated emergency admissions
- Long-term poor quality of life and inadequate symptom control despite aggressive management
- Refractory New York Heart Association (NYHA) class IV symptoms and signs of cardiac cachexia

FUTURE OF PALLIATIVE CARE IN INDIA

Policy initiatives by state and central governments and the inclusion of palliative care in the National Health Policy of 2017 offer hope for the future. Moreover, it is time for clinicians to broaden its horizon and scope by integrating palliative care in other subspecializations, spreading its awareness, with focuses on a robust evidence-based approach and research grounded in the Indian practice context.

ACKNOWLEDGMENT

I extend my sincere thanks to Dr Shamali Poojari, Assistant Professor, Department of Palliative Care, Tata Memorial College, for giving inputs while preparing this writeup.

SUGGESTED READINGS

1. Slawnych M. New dimensions in palliative care cardiology. Can J Cardiol. 2018;34(7):914-24.
2. India State-Level Disease Burden Initiative CVD Collaborators. The changing patterns of cardiovascular diseases and their risk factors in the states of India: the Global Burden of Disease Study 1990–2016. Lancet Glob Health. 2018; 6:e1339-51.
3. Abdul-Aziz AA, Desikan P, Prabhakaran D, Schroeder LF. Tackling the burden of cardiovascular diseases in India: The essential diagnostics list. Circ Cardiovasc Qual Outcomes. 2019;12(4):e005195.
4. Ezekowitz JA, O'Meara E, McDonald MA, Abrams H, Chan M, Ducharme A, et al; Cardiovascular Society Guidelines for the Management of Heart Failure. 2017 Comprehensive Update of the Canadian Cardiovascular Society Guidelines for the Management of Heart Failure. Can J Cardiol. 2017;33(11):1342-433.
5. Connor SR, Bermedo MCS (Eds). Global Atlas of Palliative Care at the End of Life. Geneva: World Health Organization; 2014.
6. Kassianos AP, Ioannou M, Koutsantoni M, Charalambous H. The impact of specialized palliative care on cancer patients' health-related quality of life: a systematic review and meta-analysis. Support Care Cancer. 2018;26:61-79.
7. Solano JP, Gomes B, Higginson IJ. A comparison of symptom prevalence in far advanced cancer, AIDS, heart disease, chronic obstructive pulmonary disease and renal disease. J Pain Symptom Manage. 2006;31(1):58-69.
8. John Fardy H. Oxygen therapy in palliative care. NPJ Prim Care Respir Med. 2016:26:15073.
9. Polikandrioti M, Kalafatakis F, Koutelekos I, Kokoularis D. Fatigue in heart failure outpatients: Levels, associated factors, and the impact on quality of life. Arch Med Sci Atheroscler Dis. 2019;28:e103-12.
10. Connolly M, Ryder M. Consideration of Symptom Management in Advanced Heart Failure. Int J Environ Res Public Health. 2022;19:15160.

20

CHAPTER

Cardiac Amyloidosis: An Update

Ananda Bagchi, Aradhya Sekhar Bagchi

ABSTRACT

Cardiac amyloidosis (CA) is an uncommon, underappreciated, and a serious disorder where there is progressive extracellular deposition of amyloid fibrils (as beta-pleated sheets) in cardiac tissues. It may be due to some rare genetic disorders or may also be due to some acquired conditions. In recent times, due to availability of latest imaging techniques and noninvasive modalities, the diagnosis of CA has become more frequent and also the availability of newer modalities of treatment has improved the recognition, treatment, and prognosis of this potentially serious disease.

INTRODUCTION

Cardiac amyloidosis (CA) is a rare disease caused by the buildup of clumps of abnormally folded protein (known as amyloid fibrils) in the heart muscle. This impairs its ability to function normally. CA can cause *restrictive cardiomyopathy* ultimately leading to heart failure with preserved ejection fraction (HFpEF) and its related symptoms, such as shortness of breath, pedal edema, and irregular heart beat (arrhythmia), and it can lead to reduced life expectancy.

Because the amyloid fibrils that build up in the heart muscle can also accumulate in other organs and tissues in the body, such as the liver, kidneys, gastrointestinal tract, and nerve tissue, people with CA may also have amyloidosis in other organs.

ETIOPATHOGENESIS OF CARDIAC AMYLOIDOSIS

Proteins are found throughout the body, where they perform a range of critical functions. Proper functioning requires that the proteins retain their specific shape. If the protein "misfolds" or changes from its normal shape, it does not function properly. In amyloidosis, certain proteins misfold, binding together to form amyloid clumps or fibrils.

The body usually breaks down and recycles misfolded proteins, but this does not happen with amyloid fibrils. Instead, they get deposited in organs and tissues, where they accumulate and impair the functioning of those organs and tissues.

When amyloid fibrils accumulate in the heart, they cause a disease known as cardiac amyloidosis. This causes the heart muscle to thicken and become stiff, which diminishes its ability to pump blood effectively and efficiently throughout the body, leading to various cardiac complications.

The etiopathogenesis of amyloid deposits can be explained by three processes: (1) Excess protein production; (2) abnormality or mutation of the native protein; and (3) an intrinsic tendency to form amyloid. The elective deposit site and consequently clinical features depend on which "amyloidogenic" protein is misfolded. Hence, numerous organs can be involved, but cardiac localization is a major determinant for survival. Although traditionally considered a rare disease, recent advances in imaging and noninvasive diagnostic tools have led some to consider that CA is an underdiagnosed and often an unacknowledged cardiac disorder.

What are the Types of Amyloidosis that affect the Heart?

There are several types of amyloidosis, each caused by a different protein that forms amyloid fibrils. Two proteins, in particular, are responsible for over 95% of cases of cardiac amyloidosis:

1. *Amyloid light-chain amyloidosis (AL amyloidosis)*: It is the most common form of CA.

   Plasma cells are primarily found in bone marrow and it produces a large variety of antibodies which are composed of both heavy and light chains. When a plasma cell becomes clonal (essentially malignant) then it produces a light chain which is prone to misfold into beta-pleated sheets which are then circulated in the bloodstream and also deposited in the heart leading to AL amyloidosis. There occurs extracardiac deposits also which are found in the kidney, liver, gastrointestinal (GI) tract, nerves, and tongue causing various symptoms. AL amyloidosis generally occurs in people over the age of 40 years but most people diagnosed with this condition are above the age of 65 years.
2. *Transthyretin amyloidosis (ATTR amyloidosis):* In this form of amyloidosis, transthyretin, a protein produced in the liver, misfolds and forms amyloid fibrils and is circulated in monomeric form. This monomeric form of transthyretin is deposited in the heart as amyloid deposits and also in other sites, such as tissues in the wrist or neck, or in the nerves. This means that people with cardiac ATTR amyloidosis may have cardiac problems, as well as carpal tunnel syndrome or cervical stenosis and/or neuropathy.

There are two types of ATTR amyloidosis **(Fig. 1)**:

1. *Wild-type ATTR amyloidosis (wtATTR)* is the most common type of ATTR amyloidosis. It is not inherited and is associated with aging. It usually occurs in people over the age of 70 years and affects more men than women. Here the transthyretin protein is the normal and nonmutated protein which is deposited as amyloid deposits primarily in the heart and also in the soft tissue (causing carpal tunnel syndrome) and vasculature.
2. *Hereditary ATTR amyloidosis (hATTR),* also known as mutant ATTR amyloidosis, is caused by an inherited genetic mutation in the *TTR* gene that predisposes the transthyretin protein to misfold at an accelerated rate. This form of CA can affect people as young as 30 years old and can affect the nervous system as well. In USA, by far the most common mutation encountered is the V1221 mutation, it is present in 3–3.5% individuals of African descent and causes severely underdiagnosed form of heart failure (HF) in the AfroAmerican population.

SYMPTOMS OF CARDIAC AMYLOIDOSIS (TABLE 1)

Cardiac amyloidosis can cause a range of symptoms. These symptoms are due to:

1. Congestive cardiac failure
2. Heart rhythm abnormalities
3. Valvular heart disease
4. Carpal tunnel syndrome (bilateral)
5. Lumbar spinal canal stenosis
6. Peripheral and autonomic neuropathy
7. Orthostatic hypotension
8. Poor appetite, diarrhea, or constipation
9. Purple discoloration around eyelids (specific to AL amyloidosis)
10. Easy bruising or bleeding
11. Enlarged tongue (specific to AL amyloidosis)

DIAGNOSTICS (FLOWCHART 1)

Along with a detailed history and physical examination, the diagnostic evaluation of cardiac amyloidosis includes laboratory studies and cardiac imaging.

Electrocardiography

A 12-lead Electrocardiography (ECG) is abnormal in 90% of cases and classically shows low-voltage QRS complexes across the precordial leads. A discordance between low-voltage on the ECG and left ventricular hypertrophy on cardiac imaging is suggestive of CA.

Echocardiography

Echocardiography is a central diagnostic imaging tool for CA using modern techniques such as deformation analyses by means of the automatic tracking of myocardial acoustic markers [speckle tracking echocardiography (STP)]. It shows an echogenic left ventricular wall thickening (>12 mm) with granular sparkling. Moreover, it may involve the right ventricle as well as the atria. A small pericardial effusion is often observed without signs of hemodynamic relevance. The left ventricular ejection fraction is often preserved.

By evaluating the shortening of cardiomyocytes regionally and globally, global longitudinal strain is a noninvasive method to detect left ventricular function impairment.

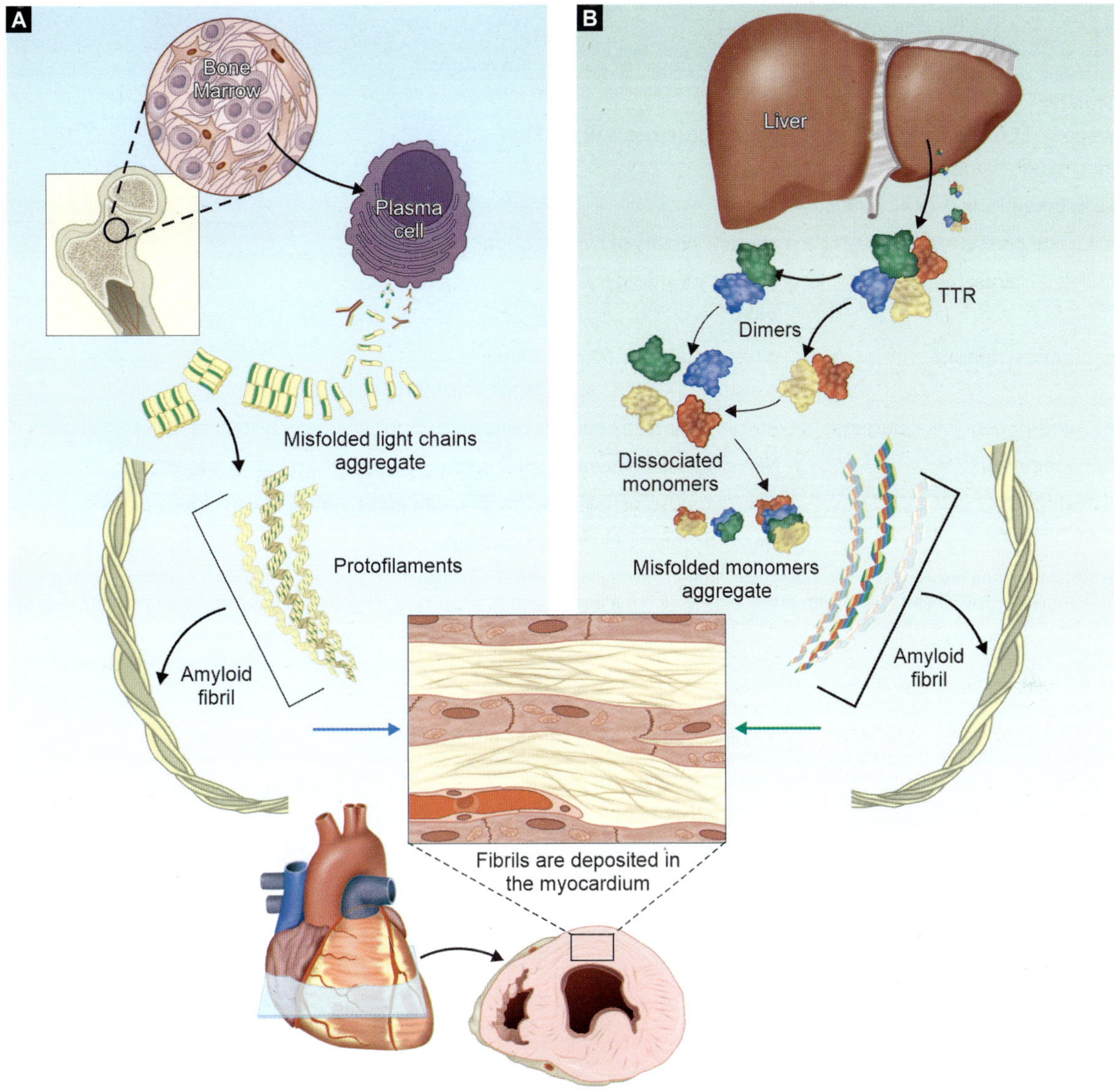

FIGS. 1A AND B: The two main types of amyloidosis that affect the heart. (A) Immunoglobulin light-chain amyloidosis (AL) results from aberrant plasma cell production of monoclonal light chains that misfold. (B) Transthyretin amyloidosis (ATTR) results from transthyretin (TTR) produced by the liver that dissociates into monomers and misfolds. The misfolded proteins aggregate to form oligomers, protofilaments, and mature amyloid fibrils that deposit extracellularly in the interstitial space of the myocardium.

Cardiac Magnetic Resonance Imaging

Cardiovascular magnetic resonance (CMR) imaging is an important tool for the diagnosis of CA and for differentiating CA from other cardiomyopathies. However, it is costlier and less widely available than echocardiography. At an early stage, the deposits of amyloid proteins lead to an increase in the extracellular volume. It is identified in the late gadolinium enhancement (LGE) sequences of the left ventricle and atria, represented by generalized subendocardial LGE-foci. Cardiovascular magnetic resonance has proven to be a key diagnostic tool when the clinical and cardiac echocardiographic presentations are suggestive of CA.

The measurement of extracellular volume is emerging as a potential measure to track the progression of CA over time and its response to therapy.

In 3–7% of patients, a biopsy is needed to prove CA. Therefore, a normal CMR cannot allow the diagnosis of CA

Radionuclide Imaging

Technetium-99m (^{99m}Tc)-phosphate-radionuclide scintigraphy is currently considered as the cornerstone diagnostic tool for ATTR cardiac amyloidosis. The tracers used are: 3,3-diphosphono-1,2-propano-dicarboxylic acid (DPD); pyrophosphate (PYR), and methylenediphosphonic acid (MDP).

TABLE 1: Symptoms that raise suspicion of cardiac amyloidosis.

Red flags for cardiac amyloidosis	
Echocardiography: • Low voltage on ECG and thickening of the septum/posterior wall > 1.2 cm • Thickening of right ventricle free wall, valves	
Intolerance to beta-blockers or ACE inhibitors	
Low normal blood pressure in patients with a previous history of hypertension	
History of bilateral carpal tunnel syndrome, often requiring surgery	
AL	**ATTR**
HFpEF + nephrotic syndrome	White male age ≥ 60 with HFpEF + history of carpal tunnel syndrome and/or spinal stenosis
Macroglossia and/or periorbital purpura	African American age ≥ 60 years with HFpEF without a history of hypertension
Orthostatic hypotension	New diagnosis of hypertrophic cardiomyopathy in an elderly patient
Peripheral neuropathy	New diagnosis of low flow, low-gradient aortic stenosis in an elderly patient
MGUS	Family history of ATTRm amyloidosis

[ACE: angiotensin-converting enzyme; AL: immunoglobulin light-chain amyloidosis; ATTR: transthyretin amyloidosis; ATTRm: hereditary mutant variant ATTR; ECG: electrocardiogram; HFpEF; heart failure with preserved ejection fraction ("diastolic heart failure"); MGUS: monoclonal gammopathy of undetermined significance]

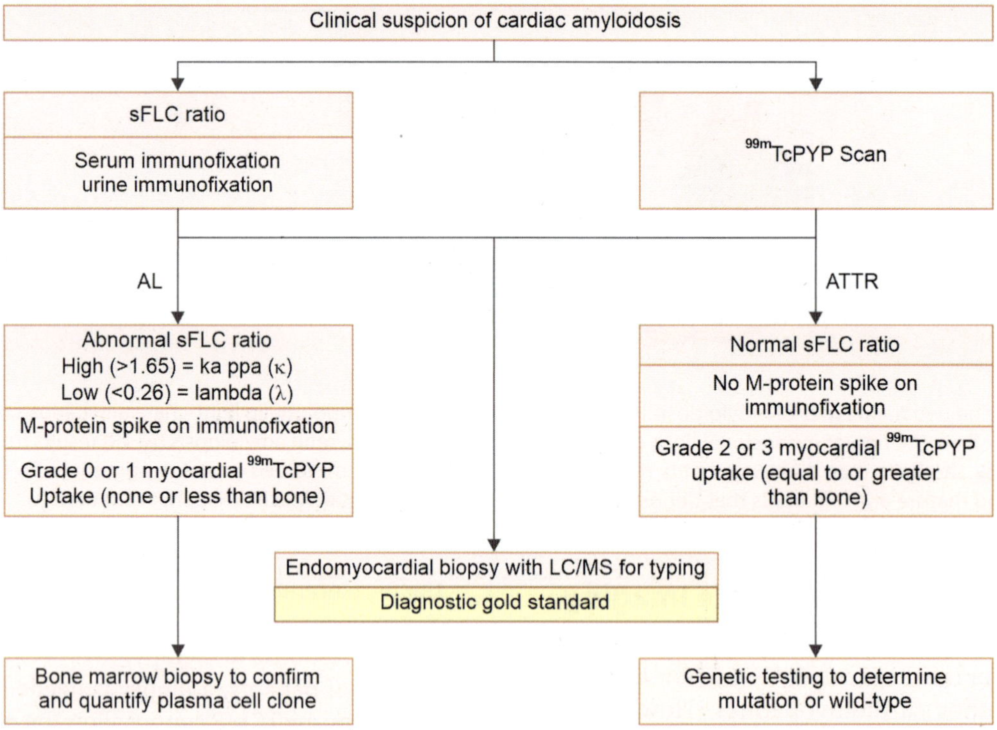

FLOWCHART 1: Diagnostic algorithm for cardiac amyloidosis (CA). Serum free light chain (sFLC) assay and serum/urine immunofixation are ordered to workup immunoglobulin light chain amyloidosis (AL). Technetium-99m pyrophosphate (^{99m}Tc-PYP) scan is ordered to workup transthyretin amyloidosis (ATTR). Normal serum free-light chains and normal immunofixation with a strongly positive ^{99m}Tc-PYP scan is diagnostic of ATTR-CA. Abnormal sFLC assay or immunofixation is suggestive but not diagnostic of AL-CA, and should prompt a bone marrow biopsy.

(LC/MS: liquid chromatography/mass spectrometry)

The ATTR-CA has an increased affinity compared with AL-CA. Nowadays, simple visual scoring and semi-quantitative visual indices are applied using the Perugini 4-point scale (0 = no cardiac and normal bone uptake, 1 = mild cardiac uptake less than bone uptake, 2 = moderate cardiac uptake and relatively equal bone uptake, and 3 = high cardiac uptake and only mild or absent bone uptake).

Consequently, different societal guidelines recommend the noninvasive diagnosis of ATTR-CA using ^{99m}Tc-phosphate radionuclide bone scintigraphy, while highlighting its use in the appropriate clinical context after ruling out AL-CA. Physicians should pay attention to the fact that about 10% of patients may have a high Perugini score (>2) in authentic cases of AL-CA.

Laboratory Testing

Routine laboratory parameters are mandatory to screen for impairment of affected organs (e.g., kidney, liver, and bone marrow). The assessment of cardiac parameters should be determined in patients with suspected amyloidosis. Brain natriuretic peptide (BNP), the N-terminal prohormone of BNP (NT-proBNP), and troponin T (TnT) are the most commonly used biomarkers of cardiac involvement for the diagnosis of CA. Normal measurement of these tests excludes the presence of CA.

Biopsy

Although the examination of endomyocardial biopsies remains the gold standard for the diagnosis of CA with a sensitivity of 100%, multimodal noninvasive tools have declined this procedure.

Amyloid deposits are confirmed using thioflavin T and most commonly Congo red stains **(Fig. 2)**. On light microscopy, Congo red-stained amyloid deposits will appear red or salmon-pink. The confirmation test is the appearance of characteristic birefringence under cross polarized light when the amyloid deposits look apple green. The experts highlight that the term "amyloid fibril" should be used for any cross β-sheet fibril. **Figure 2** shows amyloid deposits on a lip biopsy using Congo red staining.

HOW IS CARDIAC AMYLOIDOSIS TREATED?

Treatment of Cardiac Amyloidosis

While there is no cure for cardiac amyloidosis but we can successfully delay or stop the progression of the disease. Treatment of cardiac amyloidosis requires a two-pronged approach. Some therapies aim to alleviate cardiac symptoms and complications, while others treat the underlying condition. *Treatment modalities include chemotherapy, immunotherapy, and organ transplantation.*

Treatment of the Underlying Condition

Therapies that treat the underlying amyloid disorder aim to reduce the number of amyloid fibrils, which results in less buildup of amyloids in the heart tissue. The treatment for the two most frequent types of cardiac amyloidosis differs because they are caused by different abnormal proteins.

Management of Heart Failure in Cardiac Amyloidosis

The main treatment of heart failure revolves around sodium restriction and diuretics to relieve congestion.

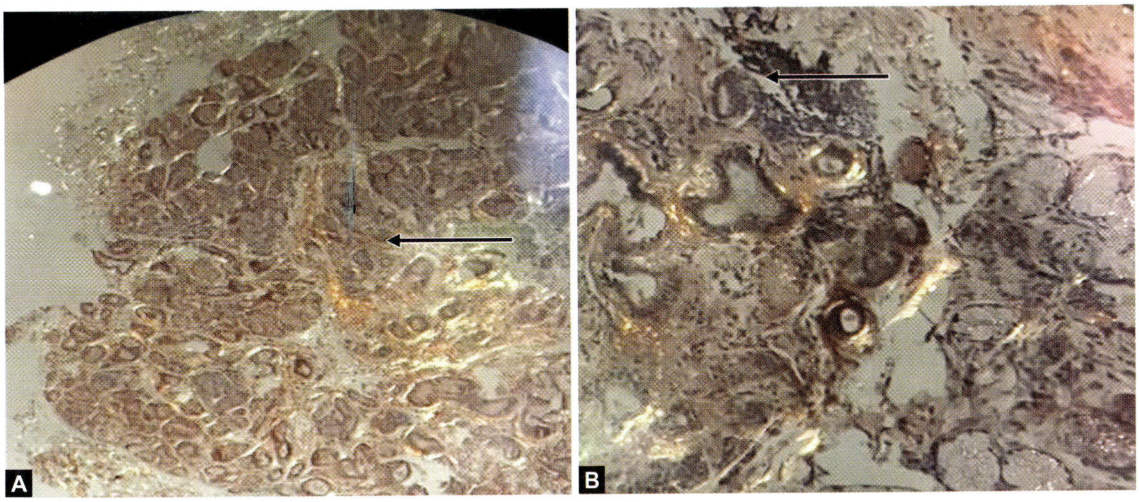

FIGS. 2A AND B: Amyloid deposits on a lip biopsy using Congo red staining. Black arrow shows the amyloid deposits.

This can prove challenging in many patients due to the narrow window between too high or too low filling pressures. A combination of loop diuretics and an aldosterone antagonist is most effective. Torsemide is preferred over furosemide due to its superior bioavailability and longer duration of action, particularly since these patients have issues with gut edema and GI absorption. Due to dependence of the cardiac output on heart rate and the tendency for orthostatic hypotension, traditional neurohormonal antagonists including beta blockers and angiotensin-converting enzyme inhibitors are neither effective nor well tolerated. However, in patients with atrial fibrillation, beta blockers may need to be used for rate control. Non-dihydropyridine calcium channel blockers bind avidly to amyloid fibrils and are contraindicated due to risk of profound hypotension and syncope. Digoxin is usually avoided in CA due to concerns of increased risk of toxicity; however, it may be used with caution for rate control in atrial fibrillation given its lack of negative inotropy. Maintenance of normal sinus rhythm is preferable due to the importance of atrial contribution to cardiac output.

Anticoagulation in patients with atrial fibrillation and even in patients with normal sinus rhythm and poor atrial function is important due to the high risk of thrombo-embolic complications. Pacemakers are indicated for heart block or symptomatic bradycardia. *The role of intracardiac defibrillators or patisiran and inotersen is controversial, but may be warranted in selected patients with AL-CA.*

Treatment for ATTR Cardiac Amyloidosis (Table 2)

In this case, the goal of treatment is to stabilize the protein once it is produced to prevent misfolding. These treatments include following:

Tafamidis: This medication [first US Food and Drug Administration (FDA)-approved drug in 2019] stabilizes the transthyretin protein and prevents it from misfolding, reducing the levels of the amyloid fibrils that build up in the heart. Tafamidis does not cure or reverse ATTR, but it has been shown to slow disease progression, reduce the frequency of heart-related hospitalization and also reduce the risk of cardiac death by 30%.

Tolcapone: These medications alter the liver's production of the transthyretin protein, thereby reducing the amount of transthyretin that can misfold and accumulate in organs.

Vutrisiran (AMVUTTRA): The US FDA has approved this drug, an RNAi therapeutic agent, for the treatment of polyneuropathy of hereditary transthyretin-mediated amyloidosis in adults.

Organ transplantation: For people with hereditary ATTR cardiac amyloidosis, *cardiac transplantation* may be an option. Some patients may also receive a liver trans-plant in certain situations. *Multiorgan transplantation including liver, heart, and kidney* has been successful in some specialized centers in slowing the natural course of the disease.

TABLE 2: Amyloid-specific pharmacotherapies.

AL			ATTR		
Anti-plasma cell therapies	Alkylating agents	Melphalan	TTR silencers	siRNA	Patisiran
		Cyclophosphamide		ASO	Inotersen (IONIS-TTRx)
	Proteasome inhibitors	Bortezomib	TTR stabilizers	Diflunisal	
		Ixazomib		Tafamidis	
	Immunomodulators	Pomalidomide		Tolcapone	
	Anti-CD38 monoclonal antibody	Daratumumab		AG10	
Anti-amyloid antibody	NEOD001		Fibril disruptors	Doxycycline + TUDCA	
				Green tea extract	
				Curcumin	
				Anti-amyloid antibody	PRX004
Ubiquitous anti-amyloid fibril antibody					
Monoclonal IgG1 anti-SAP antibody					

[AL: immunoglobulin (Ig) light chain amyloidosis; ASO: antisense oligonucleotide; ATTR: transthyretin amyloidosis; SAP: serum amyloid P component; siRNA: small interfering RNA; TTR: transthyretin protein; TUDCA: tauroursodeoxycholic acid]

Treatment for AL Cardiac Amyloidosis

Treatment for this form of amyloidosis targets the plasma cells. The goal is to reduce or prevent production of abnormal light-chain proteins.

Chemotherapy/Stem Cell Transplant

Chemotherapy medications work by reducing the number of plasma cells, which in turn reduces the number of light-chain proteins produced. These medications are often combined with steroids and other drugs. Patients may also be candidates for stem cell transplantation.

Treatment of Cardiac Symptoms and Complications

Diuretics

These medications increase the amount of urine to help remove excess fluid and salt from the body. If someone has substantial swelling in their legs, abdomen, or elsewhere, intravenous diuretics (in a hospital) may be required.

Reduce Salt Intake

A low-salt diet can help keep fluid from building up, thus reducing swelling (edema). Patients should also monitor their weight regularly; rapid weight increases may be a sign of excessive fluid accumulation.

Anticoagulants

People with cardiac amyloidosis are at increased risk for blood clots, particularly if they have abnormal rhythms like atrial fibrillation. They may be treated with antiplatelets, or anticoagulants, a type of medication that reduces blood clot formation.

Cardiac Transplantation

Some patients with cardiac amyloidosis may require Cardiac transplantation.

Monoclonal Antibodies in the Management of AL-CA

In CA, monoclonal antibodies (mAbs) may potentially be used to target misfolded amyloidogenic precursors, plasma cell clones or amyloid fibrils, thus, inducing amyloid removal through different mechanisms depending on the specific target. Among them, antibody-dependent cellular toxicity (ADCC), opsonization, and neutralization of the amyloid burden have been found. Studies suggest that mAbs against cardiac amyloid mainly activate immune response with subsequent clearance by phagocytic cells. Daratumumab is one such mAb, which has shown promising efficacy both as monotherapy and as combination therapy in the treatment of AL Amyloidosis. Based on the result of ANDROMEDA trial in 2021, the US FDA has granted accelerated approval to Daratumumab in combination with cyclophosphamide, bortezomib, and dexamethasone (CyBorD) for the treatment of AL amyloidosis.

What is the Outlook for People with Cardiac Amyloidosis?

The life expectancy and degree of cardiac impairment depend on the type and amount of amyloidosis. Because AL cardiac amyloidosis has a more serious impact on the body, early diagnosis and treatment are important and are associated with better outcomes. For those with ATTR cardiac amyloidosis, drugs that reduce the level of the proteins responsible for the condition have recently been developed and have helped people with the disease live longer, healthier lives.

CONCLUSION

Cardiac amyloidosis is an underestimated cause of infiltrative cardiomyopathy. Its incidence is rising amongst the aging population and because of the development of noninvasive diagnostic tools. It is no longer considered a rare and undiagnosed disease. A compilation of workup consisting of imaging examinations (echocardiography, cardiovascular magnetic resonance imaging, and nuclear scintigraphy) and immunological assessment can lead to a precise diagnosis of AL-CA or ATTR-CA. Therefore, a methodical approach is mandatory for a rapid diagnosis and the initiation of etiopathogenic treatment as well as the symptomatic management of the cardiovascular manifestations. With the availability newer therapeutic agents, the prognosis of CA is bound to improve in the near future.

SUGGESTED READINGS

1. Yale Medicine. Cardiac amyloidosis. [online] Available from https://www.yalemedicine.org/conditions/cardiac-amyloidosis. [Last accessed December, 2023].
2. Kittleson MM, Maurer MS, Ambardekar AV, Bullock-Palmer RP, Chang PP, Eisen HJ, et al. Circulation. 2020;142:e7-22.
3. Belfeki N, Ghriss N, Monchi M, Moini C. State of the art of cardiac amyloidosis. Biomedicines. 2023;11:1045.
4. Donnelly JP, Hanna M. Cardiac amyloidosis: An update on diagnosis and treatment. Cleve Clin J Med. 2017;84(12 Suppl 3): 12-26.

SECTION

2

CRITICAL CARE

21

CHAPTER

Expectations of Patient's Relatives in Emergency Department

M Raveendran

ABSTRACT

The emergency department (ED) deals with critically ill patients either due to accidents or acute disorders like acute coronary syndrome (ACS), stroke, poison, and snakebite. The problems arise in managing these patients in diagnosis and treating effectively and in time, communicate the status accurately to the relatives, and to meet out the expenses incurred by the relatives without any heart burn.

The relatives expect the hospital to update the status of the patient regularly, the quality of care provided inside the intensive care unit (ICU) and the cost of the treatment expected. The availability of adequate staff and facilities in the hospital forms important part in providing high-quality care. The relatives have to be counseled regularly on the progress of the patients' clinical status and the cost to be met out by them. Late referral, death of the patient, and high fees charged are some of the common issues to be addressed and dealt in this chapter.

INTRODUCTION

The emergency department (ED) is an important unit of any Multispecialty Hospital where critical cases, such as trauma, acute coronary syndrome (ACS), strokes, shock, poison, and snakebites, and has to be diagnosed and treated quickly. Unfortunately, these clinical situations impact patients' and family members' quality of life negatively and seriously due to stress and uncertainty of the unexpected situations resulting in considerable anxiety and depression. Treatment of these severely ill patients is an accurate indicator of the ED quality of service and is important in terms of the satisfaction of patients' relatives. Increased duration of stay of the patients in ED and decreased quality of care lead to patient's dissatisfaction.

Not providing accurate information on patient's clinical status and wrong attitude and behavior of the hospital staff in handling relatives lead to a crisis situation in the ED. Therefore, assessing the needs and expectations of the relatives will reduce relatives' stress while increasing the patients' recovery and improving the staff-relatives relations. If the functional environment is pleasant and clean, this will enable to shift the focus of the medical team on the patient's treatment and improve the quality of service.

COUNSELING ROOM

Counseling room may be called 'relatives room', 'visitors room' or 'waiting room' is an important part of every intensive care unit (ICU) just outside the ICU for the use of relatives, parents, friends of the patients. The waiting room can range from a fairly small and basic room to comfortable space with tea/coffee facilities, kitchen and a wash room with good ambience, ventilation and well lit. It is often while they were waiting in this room, they can interact with other visitors. Some may recall their observations, the highs and lows other visitors went through as the patients improve or deteriorate, relate their emotion, and share the empathy for another crisis.

QUALITY OF INFORMATION SHARED (CONTENT)

The highest designated person among the hospital staff should meet the relatives in his/her chamber and explain in detail about the nature of the illness, medications received with their effects, and the details of various procedures performed and their relevance and results. ED staff should explain what to eat/drink and whether one is allowed to move around. The diagnostic criteria of the disease and protocols of the treatment started can be conveyed to their family physician and update him on the clinical status of the patient, thereby involving him/her also in the management. This will increase the confidence level of the relatives on the hospital ED and the staff.

AMOUNT OF COUNSELING/ COMMUNICATION SKILLS

The doctor or nursing staff should address illness-related issues, examinations performed, care procedures undertaken, postdischarge care related to illness and information on medications received. The relatives especially family members should be taken into confidence as far as the risk involved while taking care of them and be given written instructions wherever possible and the contact numbers of the health providers to contact in emergency situation or to clarify their doubts.

The doctor or nursing staff has to clarify the patient's status clearly with no undue false hope and explain the factual situation on current status of the patient. The staff should not rush up the clarification and should maintain his/her calm posture while explaining to the relatives. If they are not satisfied with the explanation, the next higher hierarchy staff should render the same to satisfy the relatives' doubts.

The communication skill of the ED staff should be improved in such a way to handle the emotional situation in the counseling room. Enough time should be given to discuss the situation and comfort the relatives adequately. All the possible outcomes of the disease can be informed to the relatives, so that they will be prepared to face any eventuality.

EXPECTATIONS AND NEEDS OF RELATIVES

The expectations of the relatives are specific facts pertaining to patients' progress, what is being done in ICU and what will be the outcome. The relatives want their questions to be answered honestly and to be assured that best care possible is being rendered. They should feel that the hospital staff are taking care of their patient in a focused manner. Giving undue hope to the relatives may backfire if any untoward happens. Relatives also want them to be informed about the transfer plans, to see the critically ill patients as early as possible and about what is happening to their patients. The approximate cost of the treatment should be informed before admission, so that the financial part can be arranged in advance to meet out expenses or they can shift the patient to any government-sponsored free health facilities.

EXPERIENCES OF FAMILY MEMBERS OF THE COUNSELING SITUATION/COMFORT AND SUPPORT

Relatives expect a private place to wait and feel accepted by hospital staff, to be assured of patient's comfort, food and refreshments availability and toilet facilities near the waiting room.

Relatives expect to be informed about the patient's condition in understandable terms before being asked to sign papers, to be updated regularly by the doctor or nurse, to be included when decision are to be made, and to spent some time with the patient on and off if permissible. Relations expect doctor or nurse to meet them on arrival of the patients and one designated person to take care of family and to share their emotions.

DISCUSSION

While focusing on the management and taking care of the patient which is essential in the ED, meeting the expectations and needs of relatives is also an important part and indicator of providing overall services. Addressing these needs will give a positive impression about the hospital and its services.

Hence, there should be a regular program in fundamental medical education and in-service training to meet the expectations and needs of the relatives. The relatives should feel that hospital staff is taking care of the patients and be assured that the patient is receiving best care possible.

The relatives should be physically close to the patients on and off to alleviate their feelings of desperation and lack of control. Whenever discharge is impossible/ICU beds not available/treatment not provided due to inadequate staff or equipment, the patient should be transferred to another higher speciality hospital. Unfortunately, this transfer to a distant hospital causes stress and uncertainty, especially among poor patients. To overcome this, the physician should regularly inform the relatives regarding the patient's condition and the possibility of transfer to another hospital for appropriate care.

Providing physical comfort and providing a feel of acceptance to meet their emotional needs will go a long way in their satisfaction. If a doctor or nurse meets them on arrival, the level of satisfaction rate is high among the patients and relatives. One designated person to take care of the family is another important need to satisfy the relatives. Presence of important family members and friends among the attenders' group is another important factor to increase the rating of quality of ED care.

Educational status of the relatives count in understanding the condition of patient and will reduce their uncertainty and anxiety, thus increasing the trust on the hospital staff. The detailed and accurate communication by the hospital staff to the relatives will facilitate recovery of the patient by their absolute cooperation during the treatment.

CONCLUSION AND IMPLICATIONS FOR NURSING

To develop ED care, the education of nurses pertaining to content of counseling has to be improved. The improvement in quality of counseling will improve the experiences of relatives in ED. Nurses should be educated to listen to the patients and their family members which is important to control the situation in ED and to motivate for home care. Nurses should counsel on medications and their effects and patients' care at home.

BEYOND TREATMENT: FINANCIAL IMPLICATIONS

Financial details for the treatments to be incurred have to be discussed with the patient and relatives prior to admission to confirm their capability to meet out the hospital expenses. Huge medical bills is an important factor for the dissatisfaction among the relatives.

BEYOND TREATMENT: VIOLENCE IN HOSPITALS

Nowadays, we see a lot of violence in the hospitals by the relatives due to the following reasons:

- *Bad news*, if any, is broken all of a sudden, to the surprise of the family members, before preparing them for the information through counseling
- *Giving false hope* to the relatives about the outcome of the disease without telling the exact situation; once the clinical conditions worsens, the staff will not be able to explain what went wrong.
- *Exorbitant hospital bills* which was not informed to relatives before admission.
- *Referring the patient* to the other medical facilities and patient is mortally sick at the time of referral (late referral).
- *Not admitting the patients* who are poor, even for an emergency resuscitation or primary care, thereby, losing the golden hours to revive the patient.

CONCLUSION

Satisfaction of relatives is the main quality indicator for service provided in the ED. The personal needs of the patients is secondary compared to the relatives' expectations of patient-focused needs in ED. The ED physicians should develop methods to satisfy patients' and families' satisfaction when improving the ED service quality. This becomes important when ED physicians try to improve the service and consider this component to relieve anxious and stressful relatives and to provide high-class care to the patients.

SUGGESTED READINGS

1. Paavilainen E, Salminen-Tuomaala M, Leikkola P. Counselling for patients and family members: A follow-up study in the Emergency Department. ISRN Nurs. 2012;2012:303790.
2. Ocak U, Avsarogullari L. Expectations and needs of relatives of relatives of critically ill patients in the emergency department. 2018;26(6).

22 CHAPTER

The ABCDEF Bundle for the Intensive Care Management of Pain, Agitation, Delirium, Immobility, and Sleep Disturbance

Rakesh Bhadade, Minal Harde, Rosemarie de Souza

ABSTRACT

Intensive care unit (ICU) distress caused by pentad of pain, agitation, delirium, immobility, and sleep disturbance (PADIS) is detrimental for immediate and long-term recovery and outcomes of critically ill patients. This chapter provides update on prevention, management of PADIS in adult ICU patients using an integrated, evidence-based, multidisciplinary ICU protocol—the ABCDEF bundle. ABCDEF bundle incorporates assessment, prevention, and management of pain; both spontaneous awakening trial (SAT) and spontaneous breathing trial (SBT); choice of sedation and analgesia; delirium—assessment, prevention, and management; early mobility and exercise; family involvement and empowerment (ABCDEF) together as a PADIS care bundle.

INTRODUCTION

Mortality of critically ill patients has decreased due to the advanced and high quality intensive critical care, however, the long-term morbidity of intensive care unit (ICU) survivors due to acquired weakness with cognitive, physical, mental, and emotional symptoms is on the rise. These are due to the distress experienced by ICU patients mainly caused by the pentad of pain, agitation, delirium, immobility, and sleep disturbance (PADIS). To optimize recovery and outcomes of critical illnesses survivors, prevention, and management of PADIS using an integrated ABCDEF bundle is recommended. ABCDEF bundle incorporates assessment, prevention and management of pain; both spontaneous awakening trial (SAT) and spontaneous breathing trial (SBT); choice of sedation and analgesia; delirium—assessment, prevention and management; early mobility and exercise; family involvement and empowerment (ABCDEF).

This is a goal-directed multidimensional bundle aimed at improving ICU care by liberating patients from pain, oversedation, delirium, immobility, and isolation, as well as from long-term consequences and minimization of iatrogenic injury. Goal of ABCDEF is to have a calm, pain-free, well rested with normal sleep and awake cycle, calm, and comfortable patient who is cooperative with ICU procedures, nursing care, weaning trials, and exercise. This chapter provides an up-to-date information and step-by-step approach for implementation of ABCDEF bundle in ICU patients. Shared care of the critically ill by multidisciplinary clinicians, ICU staff and families for accomplished patient care, and optimal resource utilization is emphasized for early ICU liberation.

A: ASSESS, PREVENT, AND MANAGE PAIN

Pain is an unpleasant sensory, emotional experience, and a major clinical symptom in ICU patients which needs systematic diagnosis, severity scoring, prevention, and treatment. Critically ill patients experience moderate-to-severe pain during provision of standard care such as position change, chest tube removal, and endotracheal tube suction. Severe pain leads to neuroendocrine hormone release and stress responses causing tachycardia, increased oxygen consumption, cardiorespiratory compromise, hypercoagulation, increased catabolism, and immunosuppression resulting in multisystem complications.

Regular pain assessments and evaluation of responses to pain treatment using reproducible and valid scales are highly recommended. The assessment of pain should specify the characteristics of pain such as site, type, aggravating or relieving factors, and intensity. Pain evaluation should be done using reliable and validated tools, such as patient's self-report, behavioral pain scales, etc. Patient's self-report of pain using a 0–10 numerical rating scale (NRS) in verbal or visual format showing intensity of pain from 0 (no pain) to 10 (worst pain) is considered to be effective, feasible, and gold standard method and is highly recommended **(Flowchart 1)**. Patient's self-report of pain intensity is a reference standard for evaluation and treatment of pain and the 0–10 NRS is recommended for pain assessment. The Verbal Descriptor Scale (VDS) is a descriptive pain assessment scale using a series of descriptive phrases "no pain," "very severe pain," or "extremely severe pain" and Faces Pain Scale showing facial expressions referring to different levels of pain intensity are also validated and easy to use scales.

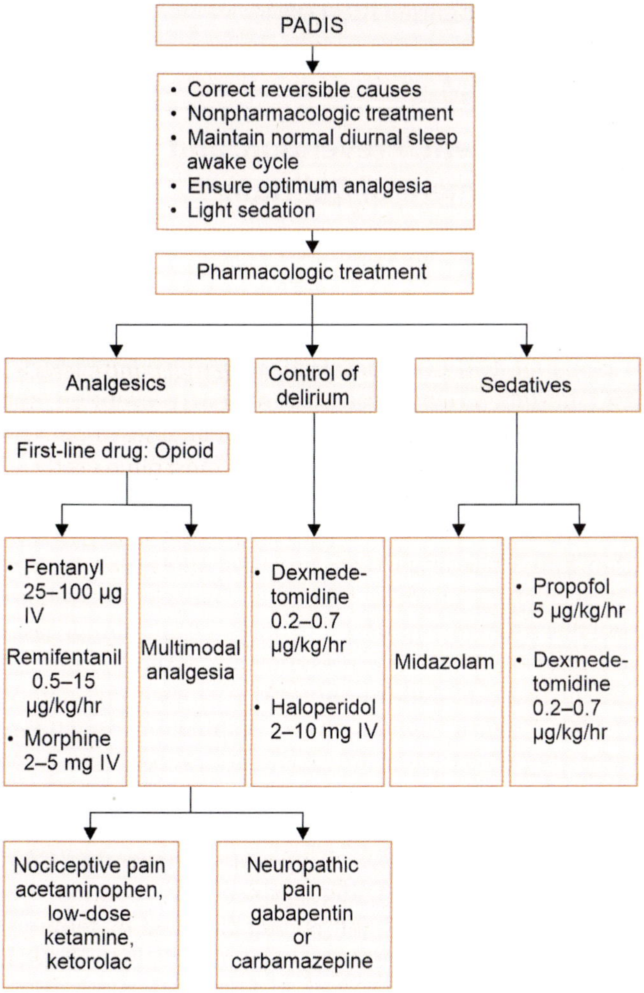

FLOWCHART 1: Management options for PADIS-ABCDEF bundle.
(PADIS: pain, agitation, delirium, immobility, and sleep disturbance)

The Behavioral Pain Scale (BPS) and the Critical-Care Pain Observation Tool (CPOT) are used in ICU patients who are unable to communicate and cannot self-report, they are the most valid and reliable behavioral pain scales. The BPS is composed of facial expression, movement of the upper limbs, and compliance with mechanical ventilation (MV), each scored from 1-4 and a BPS score of 5 or higher is considered as unacceptable pain. The CPOT has four components—facial expression, body movements, muscle tension, and compliance with the ventilator for intubated patients or vocalization for extubated patients. Each component is scored from 0 to 2 with a possible total score ranging from 0 to 8. A CPOT ≥3 is indicative of significant pain. Guidelines recommend pain medications should be routinely administered in the presence of significant pain (i.e., NRS >4, BPS >5, or CPOT >3) and prior to performing painful, invasive or any ICU procedures.

Management of pain should be by multimodal technique and should always precede sedation so as not to mask pain. Both nonpharmacologic and pharmacological therapy should be considered. Nonpharmacologic therapy can reduce the use of analgesia and maximize the patients' comfort. Ensure comfort through a proper body posture, injury stabilization, fixation of fractures, removal of physical stimuli, massage, heat/cold therapy, and relaxation therapy. In pharmacological methods parenteral opioids are the first-line agents for treating acute pain in critically ill patients. Gabapentin, carbamazepine, and pregabalin can be added with an opioid for neuropathic pain management. Nonopioid analgesics, such as nonsteroidal anti-inflammatory drugs (NSAIDs), acetaminophen, or ketamine, should be used to reduce opioid necessities as an adjunctive pain medication. Pain should be managed by "multimodal analgesia" strategy with step ladder pattern of adding analgesics for synergistic effect.

B: BOTH SPONTANEOUS AWAKENING TRIALS AND SPONTANEOUS BREATHING TRIALS

Both SAT and SBT are the core features of the ABCDEF bundle involving coordination for spontaneous awakening and breathing trials. For successful SAT and SBT to be performed during the day-time patient requires optimum analgesia, adequate rest at night, and normal sleep rhythm. Both SAT and SBT help in earlier weaning from mechanical ventilation, liberation from ICU, and discharge. It emphasizes on accurate narcotic and sedation titration, use of sedation scales for maintaining correct light level of sedation. Once pain is taken care of it has to be ensured that normal sleep cycle is maintained otherwise sleep disturbances lead to agitation and delirium. Minimal conscious sedation relieves patients' anxiety, stress, helps normal sleep pattern, compliance with catheters, tubes, mechanical ventilations and help facilitate safe and comfortable ICU stay. Hence, patient's sedation levels must be assessed and regularly re-evaluated with the help of valid scales. Guidelines recommend the use of the Richmond Agitation-Sedation Scale (RASS) and the Riker Sedation-Agitation Scale (SAS). Objective sedation monitoring which includes auditory-evoked potentials, the bispectral index (BIS), and state entropy is useful during deep sedation or use of muscle relaxants. Aim is to maintain light sedation (score of –2 RASS) where patient is calm, easily arousable and briefly awakens with eye contact to voice.

Break in the sedation with sedation holiday and awakening after normal sleep and rest is crucial for appropriate diurnal variation. Medications used for sleep induction and sedation include benzodiazepines, propofol, central α2-agonists (dexmedetomidine), melatonin, etc. Light level of sedation, daily interruption in sedation, SAT, and SBT has been effectively associated with shorten duration of mechanical ventilation, the ICU length of stay (LOS) and better outcome. Deep sedation should be avoided as it has been associated with increased duration of mechanical ventilation, delayed extubation, worse ICU outcomes. Spontaneous awakening trial when successful should be followed by SBT with breathing coordination, synchronization and trial of weaning modes of ventilation, and T-piece. Daily SBT has been proven to be effective and superior to other techniques for ventilator weaning. Breathing exercises to improve respiratory muscle strength are recommended when patients successfully perform SAT and SBT.

C: CHOICE OF ANALGESIA AND SEDATION

The pharmacological choices available for pain management are opioids and nonopioid analgesics. Parenteral opioids are first-line agents and foundation of pain management in critically ill patients. However, multimodal analgesia is recommended to reduce opioid consumption. To minimize adverse effects in critically ill patients, changes in pharmacokinetics and pharmacodynamics, the appropriate agent, dose, and route of administration should be considered. Neuropathic pain in critically ill patient should be treated with use of gabapentin or carbamazepine, along with opioids. Non-opioid analgesics, such as NSAIDs, acetaminophen, ketamine, should be used to reduce opioid necessities as an adjunctive pain medication **(Flowchart 1)**. Pain should be managed by "multimodal analgesia" strategy with step ladder pattern of adding analgesics for synergistic effect. For rapid pain management for patients with acute pain, fentanyl or remifentanil is beneficial. For patients with hemodynamic instability or renal failure hydromorphone, fentanyl, or remifentanil can be used.

The medications used for sedation include benzodiazepines, propofol, and central α2-agonists. Various studies have been conducted on sleep-inducing drugs (melatonin, dexmedetomidine, and propofol) in critically ill patients. Dexmedetomidine, has recently been used extensively in ICUs, can increase stage 2 sleep and preserve the day-night sleep cycle. Propofol is short acting and useful in patients requiring rapid and frequent awakening for neurologic evaluations or extubation. Midazolam is recommended for short duration and for alcohol withdrawal syndrome **(Flowchart 1)**. Daily awakening of patients from sedation can effectively manage normal diurnal cycle, lessen total opioid consumption, decrease the duration of mechanical ventilation, and curtail ICU LOS.

D: DELIRIUM

Assessment, Prevention, and Management of Delirium

Delirium is brain dysfunction commonly observed in ICU and characterized by disturbance in attention and awareness that has fluctuating time course. Delirium is a strong prognosticator of longer time of mechanical ventilation, ICU LOS, long-lasting cognitive impairment, and mortality. Hence, early assessment, prevention, and management of delirium is crucial. For assessment and diagnosis of delirium in ICU patients, most often used and validated tools are the Confusion Assessment Method for the intensive care unit (CAM-ICU), and the Intensive Care Delirium Screening Checklist (ICDSC). Altered level of consciousness, anything other than "normal wakefulness and fluctuating symptoms" are observed and simple tasks are given and random questions are asked to come to the diagnosis of delirium in CAM-ICU. Delirium can be characterized as hyperactive or hypoactive depending on psychomotor behavior. Hyperactive delirium (CAM positive, RASS positive range) which has a better overall prognosis presents as restlessness, agitation, irritability and emotional liability. Hypoactive delirium (CAM positive, RASS negative range), which is very common but remains undiagnosed and is characterized by lethargy, decreased responsiveness, somnolence, withdrawal, and apathy and has long-term consequences. Common symptoms are altered sleep-wake cycle, inattention, impaired short-term memory, and hallucinations.

Several risk factors associated with high occurrence of delirium should be identified, and managed. They are advanced age, medical comorbidities, trauma, transfusion, emergency surgery prior to ICU admission, mechanical ventilation, and sepsis. A multicomponent, nonpharmacologic intervention for delirium with essential focus on alleviating modifiable risk factors, early screening, promoting adequate hydration and optimum sleep, minimizing sedation, and early mobilization is highly recommended. The only strategy strongly recommended to reduce the incidence and duration of ICU delirium and to improve functional outcomes, is promoting sleep hygiene, to prevent sleep disruption and the use of early and progressive mobilization. Haloperidol prophylaxis in certain high-risk group of patients may show reduction in the severity and duration of delirium. However, their routine use is not recommended for delirium prevention. Pharmacological options for delirium are haloperidol, atypical antipsychotics, 3-hydroxy-3-methylglutaryl coenzyme A reductase inhibitors (statins), or dexmedetomidine. Atypical antipsychotics are preferred than haloperidol as they have a lower risk of extrapyramidal symptoms, however, are not recommended in patients at risk of torsades de pointes (e.g., those with a prolonged QT interval, use of drugs that prolong the QT interval, or arrhythmias). In patients on mechanical ventilation in whom delirium, agitation delays weaning from mechanical ventilation or extubation, dexmedetomidine may be useful. Although benzodiazepines can induce delirium, they can be used in patients with secondary delirium related to alcohol or benzodiazepine withdrawal. The use of haloperidol or an atypical antipsychotic in critically ill patients is not associated with a reduced incidence of delirium or an improved prognosis.

E: EARLY MOBILITY AND EXERCISE

Early mobility and intensive care rehabilitation is an integral and essential part of the ABCDEF bundle. During ICU stay, peripheral muscle weakness sets in very early in critically ill patients and they lose significant muscle mass in the initial period of immobilization. This physical dysfunction in critical illness is associated with numerous short-term and long-term consequences with significant reduction in functional status. Early mobility and intensive care rehabilitation treatment strengthens limb and respiratory muscle strength, improve physical function and quality of life, reduce the duration of delirium and mechanical ventilation, and shorten the ICU LOS.

There are apprehensions in the ICU staff about early mobilization, as critically ill patients have a variety of devices such as ventilator, central venous line, arterial line, etc. There is risk of disconnection, accidental line removal, associated hemodynamic instability, or worsening patient's condition during rehabilitation. Studies have reported that rehabilitation can be safely applied to patients on ventilators, receiving continuous renal replacement therapy (RRT) or extracorporeal membrane oxygenation (ECMO) and no serious harm has been reported during ICU rehabilitation.

The approach to early mobility starts with daily sedation breaks and awakening with coordinated physical activity, with aim of getting up and out of bed. The focus on rehabilitation of critically ill patients should begin in the ICU and continue all the way to recovery at home. Explaining, communicating and reassurance to the patient, involving them and their family is essential for better outcome. The close collaboration and coordination among ICU staff and physical therapists and patient caregivers as well are essential for an effective and safe approach. It is imperative to have standard protocol and measures for the implementation of rehabilitation management appropriate for the characteristics of each ICU. Commonly used early ICU mobilization and rehabilitation techniques are active and passive movements including limbs exercising, moving or rolling in bed, sitting on the edge of the bed, sitting in chair, walking with support, breathing exercises, etc. Physical and occupational therapy assessment along with gradual progress through range of active and passive mobilization followed by sitting, standing, walking, etc., should be initiated as early as possible. Rehabilitation treatment should be done under close monitoring and safety criteria for stopping mobilization and physical activity should be followed. These criteria are dyspnea, cyanosis, desaturation, dizziness, tachycardia, medical device disconnection, fall, patient discomfort, etc.

F: FAMILY ENGAGEMENT AND EMPOWERMENT

The ABCDE bundle has included family involvement and empowerment as an important part of bundle. For the optimal ICU treatment plan, incorporation of the family's wishes, addressing their concerns and questions, and their active participation in care is essential. Improved communication among patients, ICU staff, and relative's assist's rehabilitation avoids isolation and confusion.

Family presence on ICU rounds is helpful, and it is highly emphasized that detailed explanations about diagnosis, management, and prognosis are done on daily basis with compassion and reassurance with them. With education and communication process families have reported improved inclusion, respect, and having a better consideration of their patients care and empowerment in decision making. Evidence shows that engaging family during mobilization and intensive care rehabilitation along with ICU family conferences, palliative care consultation, can reduce hospital length of stay. Hence, a holistic approach to ICU liberation by involving family and preserving human dignity for a loving humane ICU care is recommended.

CONCLUSION

The ABCDEF bundle for pain, agitation, delirium, immobility, and sleep disturbance (PADIS) includes: Assessment, prevention, and management of pain, both spontaneous awakening trials (SAT) and spontaneous breathing trials (SBT), choice of analgesia and sedation medications, delirium—assessment, prevention, and management, early mobility and exercise, along with family involvement and empowerment. Each component of the bundle is easy to apply and flexible to implement. It is focused on timely assessment of pain, agitation and delirium, early screening, prevention and management with nonpharmacological methods for anxiolysis, natural sleep, and comfort complemented with balanced pharmacological interventions. The most valid and reliable tools and scoring system are used for assessment, multimodal analgesia strategy and maintaining a light level of sedation ensuring sleep, break in the sedation and breathing trials and early mobilization. It is essential to have regular staff education, training, routine checklist in the ICUs and performance outcome data as these have improved A–F bundle compliance with sustained performance. Having flexible and adjustable A–F bundle according to individual and institutional preferences can be incorporated to improve bundle implementation and performance.

SUGGESTED READINGS

1. Ely EW. The ABCDEF Bundle: Science and philosophy of how ICU liberation serves patients and families. Crit Care Med. 2017;45(2):321-30.
2. Armstrong RA, Kane AD, Cook TM. Decreasing mortality rates in ICU during the COVID-19 pandemic. Anaesthesia. 2021;76 (Suppl 3):10.
3. Marra A, Ely EW, Pandharipande PP, Patel MB. The ABCDEF Bundle in Critical Care. Crit Care Clin. 2017;33(2):225-43.
4. Devlin JW, Skrobik Y, Gélinas C, Needham DM, Slooter AJ, Pandharipande PP, et al. Clinical practice guidelines for the prevention and management of pain, agitation/sedation, delirium, immobility, and sleep disruption in adult patients in the ICU. Crit Care Med. 2018;46:e825-73.
5. Seo Y, Lee HJ, Ha EJ, Ha TS. 2021 KSCCM clinical practice guidelines for pain, agitation, delirium, immobility, and sleep disturbance in the intensive care unit. Acute Crit Care. 2022;37(1):1-25.
6. Balas MC, Weinhouse GL, Denehy L, Chanques G, Rochwerg B, Misak CJ, et al. Interpreting and implementing the 2018 pain, agitation/sedation, delirium, immobility, and sleep disruption clinical practice guideline. Crit Care Med. 2018;46:1464-70.
7. Vargas M, Buonanno P, Kotfis K, Marra A. Editorial: The ABCDEF bundle: Laying the foundations for long term wellness in ICU survivors. Front Med (Lausanne). 2022;9:1056056.
8. Reade MC, Finfer S. Sedation and delirium in the intensive care unit. N Engl J Med. 2014;370(5):444-54.
9. Chanques G, Viel E, Constantin JM, Jung B, de Lattre S, Carr J, et al. The measurement of pain in intensive care unit: comparison of 5 self-report intensity scales. Pain. 2010;151(3):711-21.
10. Payen JF, Bosson JL, Chanques G, Mantz J, Labarere J, DOLOREA Investigators. Pain assessment is associated with decreased duration of mechanical ventilation in the intensive care unit: a post Hoc analysis of the DOLOREA study. Anesthesiology. 2009;111(6):1308-16.
11. Chanques G, Constantin JM, Devlin JW, Ely EW, Fraser GL, Gélinas C, et al. Analgesia and sedation in patients with ARDS. Intensive Care Med. 2020;46:2342-56.
12. Hughes CG, Girard TD, Pandharipande PP. Daily sedation interruption versus targeted light sedation strategies in ICU patients. Crit Care Med. 2013;41(9 Suppl 1):S39-45.
13. Wong IMJ, Thangavelautham S, Loh SCH, Ng SY, Murfin B, Shehabi Y. Sedation and delirium in the intensive care unit: a practice-based approach. Ann Acad Med Singap. 2020;49(4): 215-25.
14. Morandi A, Piva S, Ely EW, Myatra SN, Salluh JIF, Amare D, et al. Worldwide Survey of the "Assessing Pain, Both Spontaneous Awakening and Breathing Trials, Choice of Drugs, Delirium Monitoring/Management, Early Exercise/Mobility, and Family Empowerment" (ABCDEF) Bundle. Crit Care Med. 2017;45(11): e1111-22.
15. Mart MF, Williams Roberson S, Salas B, Pandharipande PP, Ely EW. Prevention and management of delirium in the intensive care unit. Semin Respir Crit Care Med. 2021;42(1): 112-26.
16. Ely EW, Margolin R, Francis J, May L, Truman B, Dittus R, et al. Evaluation of delirium in critically ill patients: validation of the Confusion Assessment Method for the Intensive Care Unit (CAM-ICU). Crit Care Med. 2001;29(7):1370-9.
17. Rangappa R. Delirium in Ventilated Patients: Is ABCDEF Bundle the Solution? Indian J Crit Care Med. 2021;25(7):743-4.
18. Kim W. Rehabilitation in intensive care unit. J Acute Care Surg. 2018;8:2-6.
19. Davidson JE, Powers K, Hedayat KM, Tieszen M, Kon AA, Shepard E, et al. Clinical practice guidelines for support of the family in the patient-centered intensive care unit: American College of Critical Care Medicine Task Force 2004–2005. Crit Care Med. 2007;35(2):605-22.

23

CHAPTER

Hyponatremia in Intensive Care Unit

Trupti Trivedi, Priyanshu Shah

ABSTRACT

Hyponatremia is the most common electrolyte disorder amongst intensive care unit (ICU) patients and is associated with prolonged duration of stay, increased ICU cost, and higher mortality. It is more common in elderly patients with comorbid conditions and fluid imbalance. Clinical features of hyponatremia can overlap with symptoms of underlying etiology in ICU patients. Classification and identification of the cause needs extensive investigations if it is not evident clinically. Treatment has to be planned after considering duration, severity, risk factors for rapid correction, and volume status of the patient. Precise therapy with frequent monitoring of serum sodium (Na^+) levels is needed to prevent life-threatening complications related to cerebral edema and prevention of complications due to rapid sodium correction for a successful outcome.

INTRODUCTION

Hyponatremia, defined as serum sodium (Na^+) levels of < 135 mEq/L, is one of the most common electrolyte disturbances. Prevalence of hyponatremia in hospitalized patients is reported to range from 3.5 to 35% in various studies, and it is even higher in the intensive care unit (ICU). Hyponatremia can also develop in 15% of the patients with initial normal sodium levels, within 48 hours of ICU admission, especially among those with fluid imbalance and renal failure. Elderly patients and those with cardiac failure, malignancy, and cirrhosis are more prone to have hyponatremia. It contributes to higher mortality, increased cost, and duration of ICU stay. Numerous etiologies, varied presentations, and the need to correct it accurately using precise formulas make this subject challenging in clinical practice.

CLASSIFICATION AND ETIOLOGY

It is important to differentiate true hyponatremia from pseudohyponatremia and translocational hyponatremia. Serum osmolality ranges from 280 to 295 mOsm/kg. It is calculated using Smithline-Gardner formula as "2(Na) + glucose/18 + blood urea nitrogen (BUN)/2.8" with plasma concentrations measured in mmol/L. In "pseudohyponatremia", there is presence of marked hyperlipidemia or paraproteinemia, making the plasma water fraction lower than the usual 93%. Hence, measured plasma sodium is low despite normal osmolality. These patients do not need treatment for low sodium levels as plasma osmolality and sodium concentration of plasma that is water are unchanged. In patients of renal failure with hyponatremia, though elevated urea maintains serum osmolality, patients are symptomatic as urea is an ineffective osmole. Translocational hyponatremia results from presence of osmotically active solutes such as glucose, mannitol, or radiological contrast agents. Hyponatremia should be corrected by adding 1.6 mEq/L to measured sodium for each 100 mg/dL rise in blood glucose levels above normal.

In true hyponatremia, serum osmolality is reduced and it is further classified as hypovolemic, euvolemic, and hypervolemic depending on the volume status of patient. Common etiologies of hyponatremia are summarized in **Table 1**. Hypovolemia is diagnosed clinically by history of volume loss in the form of diarrhea, vomiting, diuretic use and physical examination findings of tachycardia, orthostatic hypotension, dry mucosa, and loss of skin turgor. When the clinical findings are equivocal or there

TABLE 1: Causes of hyponatremia.

Hypovolemic hyponatremia	
• Diuretic-induced GI loss • Exercise associated • Burns • Cerebral salt wasting • Mineralocorticoid deficiency	• Common with thiazide group, elderly females, associated hypochloremia and metabolic alkalosis • History usually evident, associated hypokalemia • May be euvolemic or hypovolemic, sweat sodium loss, elevated AVP • Third space loss • Higher urinary sodium • In setting of SAH, brain injury, SOL, TBM • Normal/high urine output compared to SIADH • Associated with hypotension and hyperkalemia
Euvolemic hyponatremia	
• SIADH • Glucocorticoid deficiency • Hypothyroidism • Postoperative irrigation • Beer drinker potomania • Primary polydipsia • Recreational drugs (ecstasy-MDMA)	• High urinary osmolality, normal renal and thyroid functions, low uric acid • Low 8 AM cortisol • Associated bradycardia, cold intolerance • Post TURP • Low solute intake, very low urine osmolality • Psychiatric disorder, craniopharyngioma • Sudden severe hyponatremia often noncardiogenic pulmonary edema
Hypervolemic hyponatremia	
• Cardiac failure • Cirrhosis • Acute and chronic kidney failure • Nephrotic syndrome	• Nonosmotic release of AVP • Renal vasoconstriction, water retention • Low GFR • Intravascular hypovolemia, nonosmotic AVP stimulation

(AVP: arginine vasopressin; GFR: glomerular filtration rate; GI: gastrointestinal; SAH: subarachnoid hemorrhage; SIADH: syndrome of inappropriate antidiuretic hormone secretion; SOL: space-occupying lesion; TBM: tuberculous meningitis; TURP: transurethral resection of the prostate)

is preexisting cardiac or liver disease, hemodynamic monitoring, investigations, or even fluid challenge with 500–1,000 mL of normal saline (NS) may be needed to confirm hypovolemic hyponatremia. Elevated BUN and uric acid (UA), low urinary spot Na^+ <20 mmol/L are important clues for hypovolemia. Patients without obvious volume loss or edema are considered to be euvolemic. Low BUN, UA, and spot urinary Na^+ >20 mmol/L are suggestive of euvolemia. Patients with subcutaneous edema, pulmonary rales, or ascites are considered to be hypervolemic. These patients usually have elevated brain natriuretic peptide (BNP) and low spot urinary sodium. In clinically doubtful cases, hemodynamic measurements are required.

PATHOPHYSIOLOGY

Sodium is the most abundant cation in the extracellular fluid and plays a crucial role in maintaining osmotic balance, cell membrane potentials, and overall fluid distribution. The pathophysiology of hyponatremia involves disruptions in the body's water and electrolyte balance, primarily affecting the concentration of sodium in the blood secondary to either excessive water retention due to increased antidiuretic hormone (ADH) release or impaired renal water excretion, gastrointestinal or renal loss of sodium, and dilution effect. The regulation of serum Na^+ in the body is primarily controlled by two hormones—aldosterone and ADH also known as vasopressin, these play essential roles in maintaining the body's fluid balance and blood pressure.

Aldosterone

Aldosterone is a steroid hormone produced by the adrenal glands. Its main function is to regulate the balance of sodium and potassium ions in the blood and tissues. Aldosterone acts on the distal tubules and collecting ducts of the kidneys, promoting reabsorption of sodium and excretion of potassium and hydrogen ions. This reabsorption of sodium results in an increase in blood volume and blood pressure.

When there is a fall in blood sodium levels or a drop in blood pressure, the renin-angiotensin-aldosterone system (RAAS) is activated. The activation of RAAS stimulates the release of aldosterone, which in turn, helps to conserve sodium in the kidneys and prevent its loss in urine. Thus, it helps to maintain blood sodium levels and blood pressure within the normal range.

Antidiuretic Hormone or Vasopressin

Antidiuretic hormone is produced in the hypothalamus, stored and released by the posterior pituitary gland. Its primary function is to regulate water balance in the body. When the body's fluid levels decrease (resulting in increased blood sodium concentration or high osmolality), the hypothalamus senses this change and stimulates the release of ADH into the bloodstream. ADH acts on the vasopressin receptor 2 (VR2) in the collecting ducts of the kidneys, increasing their permeability to water. As a result, more water is reabsorbed from the filtrate and less water is lost in urine. This process helps to concentrate the urine and retain water in the body, leading to a decrease in blood sodium concentration and a restoration of fluid balance.

CLINICAL PRESENTATION

Clinical features of hyponatremia not only depend on the degree of hyponatremia (mild: 130–134 mEq/L, moderate: 125–129 mEq/L, and severe: <125 mEq/L), but, also on the rate of development of hyponatremia. In acute hyponatremia, onset of symptoms is within 48 hours, hence, neurological symptoms such as impaired mental status with obtundation, seizures, and death due to respiratory arrest tend to develop from cerebral edema. In chronic hyponatremia, onset is >48 hours and there is scope for adaptation of brain to hyponatremia and brain edema does not occur. These patients may be asymptomatic or may have mild gastrointestinal symptoms such as nausea, vomiting, muscle cramps, loss of appetite, or neurological symptoms such as headache, confusion, forgetfulness, and gait disturbances. In elderly, loss of balance and frequent falls are common symptoms. In ICU patients, symptoms of hyponatremia may overlap with symptoms of presenting illness responsible for causing hyponatremia such as pneumonia, meningitis, subarachnoid hemorrhage, and brain surgery. Patients with acute severe unexplained hyponatremia and noncardiogenic pulmonary edema should be evaluated for possible use of recreational drugs like ecstasy (MDMA) or training for endurance sports.

INVESTIGATIONS AND DIAGNOSIS

The diagnosis of hyponatremia involves a series of investigations aimed at identifying the cause, determining the severity and assessing the overall health of the individual. The specific investigations conducted may vary depending on the patient's clinical presentation, medical history, and physical examination findings.

The initial step is to measure the serum Na^+ concentration followed by measurement of serum osmolality, which is essential to classify hyponatremia as hypotonic, isotonic, or hypertonic. Measuring urine osmolality helps assess the kidney's ability to concentrate or dilute urine appropriately. It aids in distinguishing between different causes of hyponatremia, such as syndrome of inappropriate antidiuretic hormone secretion (SIADH), primary polydipsia, or renal causes. Evaluating urine sodium levels can differentiate between renal and extrarenal causes of hyponatremia when it is not clinically evident. In SIADH, the urine sodium level is typically high, while in volume depletion states, the urine sodium level is usually low.

Routine investigations done in ICU patients such as blood glucose levels, lipid profile, and renal and liver function tests can identify distributive hyponatremia. Specialized tests such as thyroid function tests, serum cortisol level, serum vasopressin level, and imaging studies are needed in selected cases to determine cause. **Flowchart 1** describes approach to hyponatremia based on these investigations.

TREATMENT

Patients with severe hyponatremia, neurological symptoms, and multiple organ dysfunction are likely to be treated in a critical care unit. The treatment of hyponatremia depends on the duration of hyponatremia, presence of severe neurological symptoms, initial level of hyponatremia, presence of identifiable and rapidly correctable cause, volume status of the patient and presence of intracranial lesions. There is a risk of serious neurologic sequelae if hyponatremia is inappropriately treated. Patients with hypovolemic hyponatremia are treated with infusion of NS, treating the underlying cause and stopping the drugs that cause hyponatremia.

Patients with acute hyponatremia with euvolemia and severe neurological symptoms are at greater risk of life-threatening complications of raised intracranial pressure and respiratory arrest and need rapid correction of sodium with bolus of 3% NS. The goal of therapy in such patients is to prevent further fall in serum Na^+ levels, reducing the elevated intracranial pressure and correction of symptoms of hyponatremia while avoiding osmotic demyelination syndrome.

Treatment of hyponatremia in patients with acute life-threatening complications and severe hyponatremia (serum Na^+ <120 mEq/L) is achieved by intravenous administration of 100 mL bolus of 3% saline over 10 minutes. Coexisting hypoxia should be treated by oxygen supplementation and hyperventilation to prevent brain herniation due to cerebral edema. Ultimate goal is to correct severe hyponatremia symptoms by elevating serum Na^+ by 4–6 mEq/L in the first 6 hours. Bolus of 3% saline can be repeated two to three times with serial sodium level monitoring to achieve this goal.

Patients with acute hyponatremia of moderate grade (serum Na^+ 120–129 mEq/L) should be infused with 3% saline at a rate of 0.5 mL/kg/hour till target correction of 4–6 mEq/L from baseline is achieved to prevent brain herniation.

Patients with severe hyponatremia, but, due to a chronic cause without life-threatening symptoms should be treated with 3% saline at a rate of 0.5 mL/kg/hour. Some of these patients, who are at a risk of rapid correction (adrenal insufficiency, drug, or pain-induced SIADH) will also require concomitant desmopressin (dDAVP 1–2 µg IV 8 hourly) to prevent rapid correction of hyponatremia. Vasopressin acts by preventing aquaresis.

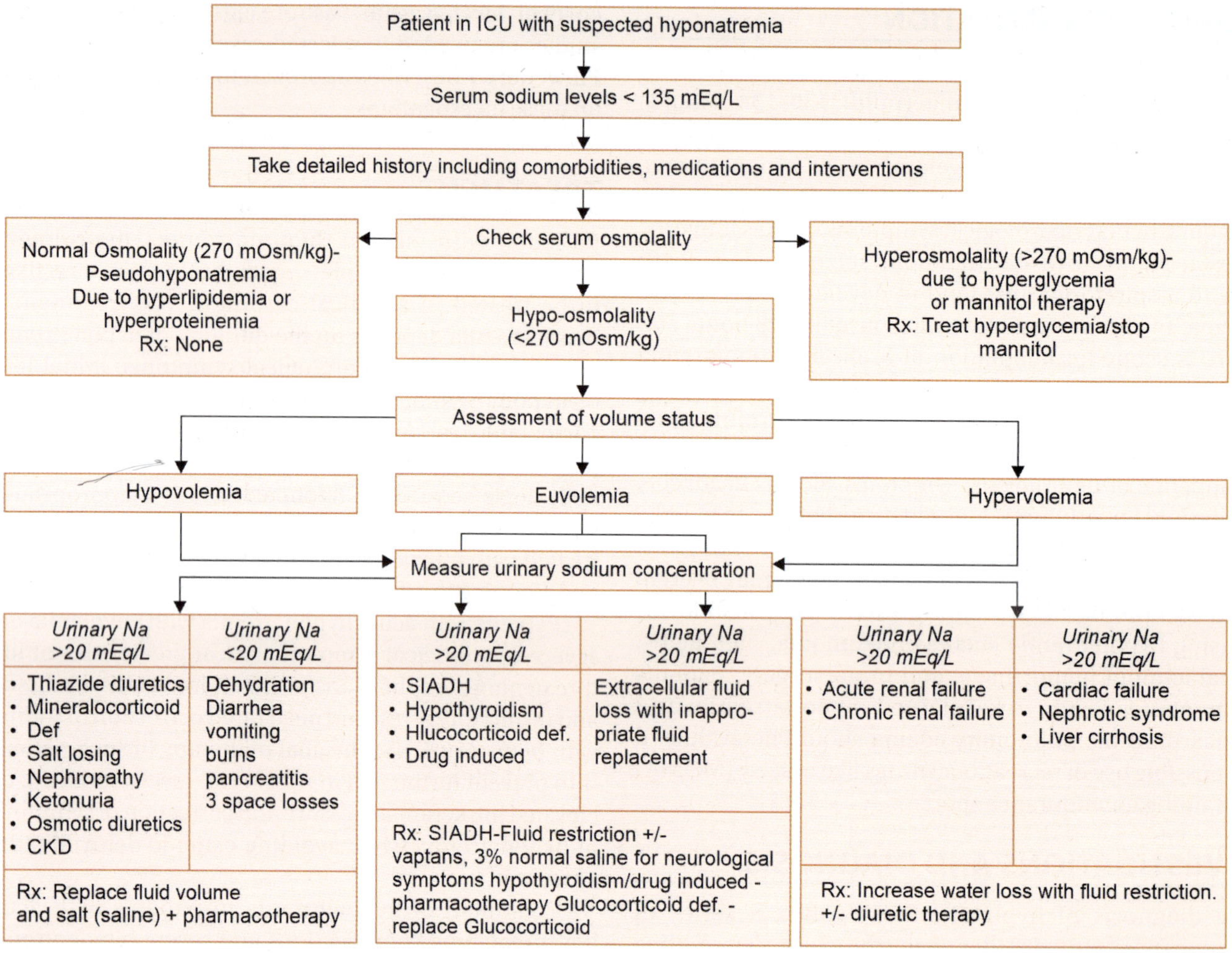

FLOWCHART 1: Algorithm for diagnosis and management of hyponatremia.

(CKD: chronic kidney disease; ICU: intensive care unit; SIADH: syndrome of inappropriate antidiuretic hormone secretion)

Once serum Na^+ is increased by 8–10 mEq/day, hypertonic saline should be stopped and other measures such as fluid restriction (below urine output) in SIADH and loop diuretics in hypervolemia should be continued. Whenever the cause for hyponatremia is identified, it should be treated. Concomitant hypokalemia should also be corrected. Electrolytes should be measured every 4 hourly and if there is rapid correction above the daily target of 10 mEq/day, relowering of sodium should be done with dextrose infusion or hypotonic saline with or without desmopressin to prevent osmotic demyelination syndrome (ODS). Intravenous infusion of 5% dextrose at a rate of 6 mL/kg over 2 hours is expected to lower serum Na^+ by 2 mEq/L. Patients with initial serum Na^+ level < 105 mEq/L or with malnutrition, cirrhosis, hypokalemia, and alcoholism are at a higher risk for development of ODS.

Central pontine myelinolysis (CPM) was first described in 1959 by Adams and Victor in alcoholic and malnourished patients. As extrapontine sites such as basal ganglia, thalamus, and cerebral white matter were later identified to be affected, the terminology was changed to ODS. Apart from rapid correction of chronic hyponatremia (47%), it can also result from acute hypernatremia, hypophosphatemia, refeeding syndrome, hyperglycemia, and hypokalemia. With rapid correction of hyponatremia, brain astrocytes are unable to regain the organic osmolytes (taurine, glutamine, glutamate, and myo-inositol) that were lost during adaptation to hyponatremia. This leads to cell shrinkage and myelin loss with manifestations of acute encephalopathy and seizures followed by dysarthria, dysphagia, spastic quadriparesis, and psychomotor manifestations within 3–5 days of rapid correction of sodium. Once symptoms develop, they are usually irreversible. Relowering of sodium followed by gradual correction should be attempted if initial sodium level was below 120 mEq/L. Plasmapheresis has been tried with some success in few cases.

For patients with chronic euvolemic hyponatremia, fluid restriction below urine output is the main therapy. Patients with lower urine output and concentrated urine are less likely to respond to fluid restriction. Patients with ratio of urine Na + K/serum Na^+ of > 1, need fluid restriction below 1 L/day. Long-term therapy with selective V2 receptor antagonist, tolvaptan is indicated in patients with chronic symptomatic hyponatremia due to SIADH or hypervolemia which is refractory to fluid restriction. This agent causes selective water diuresis–aquaresis. If initiated, it should be started ideally while the patient is in hospital, so that frequent monitoring can be done to prevent rapid correction. It is advisable to start with the smallest dose of 15 mg and increase with serial monitoring as per requirement. It is not recommended to continue this drug beyond 30 days and is avoided in patients with chronic liver disease. Patients with chronic hyponatremia due to nephrogenic SIADH or dilutional hyponatremia can be treated with oral urea therapy (15–60 g/day) or salt tablets along with loop diuretics.

Prognosis of hyponatremic patient depends on prognosis of underlying cause. Patients with lower initial serum Na^+ level, low Glasgow Coma Scale (GCS) score on admission, and correction of < 5 mEq/L on day 1 of ICU admission tend to have prolonged ICU stay and poor outcome.

In summary, though hyponatremia is the most common electrolyte disorder in ICU patients, majority patients only require treatment of the cause. Only severely symptomatic patients with risk of brain herniation need treatment with hypertonic saline. Care should be taken to achieve a correction of 4–6 mEq/L in the initial few hours to relieve neurological symptoms and subsequent correction should be restricted to 10 mEq/L per day. Vasopressin should be simultaneously used in patients at risk of rapid correction to prevent a rare but, dreadful complication of ODS.

SUGGESTED READINGS

1. Verbalis JG, Goldsmith SR, Greenberg A, Korzelius C, Schrier RW, Sterns RH, et al. Diagnosis, evaluation, and treatment of hyponatremia: expert panel recommendations. Am J Med. 2013;126(10 Suppl 1):S1-42.
2. Adrogué HJ, Tucker BM, Madias NE. Diagnosis and Management of Hyponatremia: A Review. JAMA. 2022;328(3):280-91.

24

CHAPTER

Blood Glucose Management in ICU/HDU: Challenges

Sambhu Dutta

ABSTRACT

Patients in intensive care unit/high-dependency unit (ICU/HDU) may have preexisting or de novo hyperglycemia or hypoglycemia secondary to preexisting diabetes or stress-induced hyperglycemia which significantly increases morbidity, mortality, and length of stay (LOS).

Meta-analyses of randomized controlled trials (RCTs) suggested no survival benefit of tight glycemic control and a significantly increased incidence of hypoglycemia. Studies have shown a J- or U-shaped relationship between average glucose values and mortality; maintaining glucose levels between 100 and 150 mg/dL was likely to be associated with the lowest mortality rates.

Blood glucose targets of patients with hyperglycemia admitted in critical care units are based on the NICE-SUGAR study in which it was recommended that blood glucose targets of noncritical patients is 80–180 mg/dL and for critical patients is 140–180 mg/dL.

Tight blood–glucose control without early parenteral nutrition in the ICU did not affect the length of time that ICU care was needed or mortality in multicenter RCT conducted as latest as 2023 with 9,230 patients.

The result of point-of-care (POC) glucometer differs from laboratory glucose values, especially in critically ill patients with unstable hemodynamic status while receiving some drugs.

INTRODUCTION

The occurrence of hyperglycemia in acute patients in the intensive care unit (ICU) has been seen in 83% of patients. Hyperglycemia in critical illness may occur due to stress-induced rise in counter-regulatory hormones, preexisting diabetes, prediabetes, and insulin resistance. Although it is a condition requiring urgent intervention and a marker of disease severity, hyperglycemia also has been shown to be an independent risk factor for increased mortality in the critical care department. Despite this association, tight glycemic control (TGC) has not been shown to usually improve patient outcomes and amazingly may, in some cohorts, cause more unfavorable outcomes.

For many years, hyperglycemia in the critically ill was considered a stress adaptation mechanism and was untreated. In fact, some early ICU practitioners recognized insulin resistance and believed that raised glucose levels (160–200 mg/dL) would promote cellular glucose uptake. In 2001, Van den Berghe demonstrated a statistically significant mortality benefit with TGC in surgical ICU patients. Subsequently, many professional bodies including the Surviving Sepsis Campaign (SSC) in 2004 endorsed TGC. The Leuven (Van den Berghe et al.) medical trial in 2006, Efficacy of Volume Substitution and Insulin Therapy in Severe Sepsis (VISEP, Brunkhorst et al.) trial in 2008, and Normoglycemia in Intensive Care Evaluation—Survival Using Glucose Algorithm Regulation (NICE-SUGAR, Finfer et al.) and Glucontrol (Preiser et al.) trials published in 2009 have contributed most to the continuously evolving issue of glucose management in the critically ill patients.

Risk factors for the development of hyperglycemia include preexisting diabetes mellitus, advanced age, infusion of catecholamine pressors, glucocorticoids, obesity, excessive dextrose resuscitation, sepsis, hypothermia, hypoxia, uremia, and cirrhosis. These proven risk factors highlight the multifactorial pathophysiologic mechanisms underlying ICU hyperglycemia.

The American Diabetes Association defines hypoglycemia as a blood glucose (BG) level below 70 mg/dL and classifies it as follows:

- *Level 1*: 70 to ≥54 mg/dL
- *Level 2*: <54 mg/dL
- *Level 3*: A clinical event characterized by altered mental or physical status requiring assistance for treatment of hypoglycemia.

Hypoglycemia has been independently associated with increased risk of death in critically ill patients. In randomized controlled trials (RCTs), a pooled analysis of the NICE-SUGAR study and the study by Meyfroidt et al. showed that hypoglycemia increased the odds of mortality. In one study, mild hypoglycemia (defined as <70 mg/dL) was associated with increased mortality regardless of diabetes status and diagnosis of conditions (medical, surgical, or trauma).

Guidelines of the Society of Critical Care Medicine suggest a BG value of 150 mg/dL or greater to trigger the use of insulin therapy, with the goal of maintaining a glucose level below 150 mg/dL for most critically ill patients and maintaining the glucose level absolutely below 180 mg/dL.

The American Diabetes Association, citing the NICE-SUGAR trial results, recommends that insulin therapy be started for persistent hyperglycemia (>180 mg/dL) with a target glucose range of 140–180 mg/dL in most critically ill patients and notes that more aggressive goals (110–140 mg/dL) may be more appropriate for specific groups of patients (e.g., postsurgical patients or patients with cardiac surgery) if these targets can be achieved without significant hypoglycemia. On the other hand, glucose concentrations above 180 mg/dL may be acceptable in terminally ill patients, in patients with severe comorbid conditions, and in inpatient care settings where frequent glucose monitoring or close nursing supervision is not feasible.

BLOOD GLUCOSE MONITORING IN ICU/HDU

Blood glucose management needs frequent blood sampling and insulin dose adjustment. BG monitoring in critically ill patients by plasma-based central laboratory methods using venous or arterial samples is considered standard. However, due to the long turnaround time and convenience associated with a point of care testing (POCT); currently, glucometers and arterial blood gas (ABG) analyses are being frequently used. Bedside capillary BG monitoring arguably remains the most commonly used method, even in critically ill patients. However, its accuracy may be questionable in patients with subcutaneous edema, shock, and hypoxemia, which is common in ICU patients, leading to highly variable results and higher bias (overestimation) for finger-stick sampling than arterial or venous BG monitoring, which can significantly affect clinical decision-making. Hence, arterial blood is preferred but requires repeated arterial punctures or an invasive arterial line. It can be inferred that arterial blood should be preferred over capillary blood for glucose monitoring, irrespective of the method used, provided standards of calibration are being followed. Although capillary glucose serves well in hospitalized patients, caution should be exercised in patients with shock, insulin infusion, vasopressors/inotropes, coma, and other critically ill adult patients.

INTRAVENOUS INSULIN PROTOCOL

There are multiple intensive insulin protocols that have been developed and are in vogue; however, no single protocol has been universally accepted as The Standard of Care Protocol and further, there is a protocol which is being practiced in many of the ICUs of this subcontinent including our hospital ICU (**Table 1**).

Several studies comparing computerized and paper-based protocols have found improved protocol

TABLE 1: Standard of care protocol.

Criterion	Methodology and recommendations
Preparation	50 units of regular insulin dissolved in 50 mL NS in a 50 mL disposable syringe
Mode of administration	IV infusion with an electronic syringe pump/infusion pumps
Primary target	To maintain BG level within a predefined target 140 mg/dL
Control methodology	BG to be controlled gradually in case of severe hyperglycemia by titrating the dose of IV insulin
Prerequisites	Initially, 15–20 mL of solution should be flushed through plastic tubing to saturate the insulin-binding sites in the tubing
Targets	Dose should be adjusted as per BG
Monitoring	Either by capillary BG or from the venous site/central line

(BG: blood glucose; ICU: intensive care unit; IV: intravenous; NS: normal saline)

adherence, improved glycemic control, and less hypoglycemia with computerized protocols. It is worth noting that evaluations of computerized glucose control programs have used glycemic targets that are tighter than currently recommended and although the percentages of BG readings within the target range were higher than with paper protocols, they still were not optimal in most studies. It is still not clear how computerized glucose control programs when compared to paper-based protocols when currently recommended targets are used.

TAKE-HOME MESSAGE

The optimal BG target for patients in the ICU remains unknown, but a target of 140–180 mg/dL is the most acceptable for critically ill patients. We believe that future studies investigating the optimal target for ICU patients should do the following:

- Include other glycemic metrics
- Take into account preadmission diabetes diagnosis and premorbid glycemic control [based on the glycated hemoglobin (HbA1c)]
- Use accurate BG monitoring methods combined with a standardized validated insulin algorithm.

This will enable studies to shed light on appropriate glycemic targets and may lead to a more individualized approach for the critically ill patient rather than a universal approach.

CONCLUSION

Although the past decade has seen great controversy regarding optimal glycemic targets for inpatients, it is clear that extremes of BG lead to poor outcomes and continuous intravenous (IV) protocols are the preferred treatment modality for glycemic control in the critical care setting. In addition, insulin infusion can be an effective treatment modality in other acute care settings with appropriate glycemic targets, monitoring, and education. The safety of insulin infusion protocols hinges on appropriate BG monitoring and titration. Using a computerized infusion protocol and a continuous BG sensor may allow for tighter glycemic control without increasing hypoglycemia and mortality rates.

SUGGESTED READINGS

1. Egi M, Bellomo R, Stachowski E, French CJ, Hart GK, Hegarty C, et al. Blood glucose concentration and outcome of critical illness: the impact of diabetes. Crit Care Med. 2008;36(8):2249-55.
2. Hsu CW. Glycemic control in critically ill patients. World J Crit Care Med. 2012;1(1):31-9.
3. Finfer S, Chittock DR, Su SY, Blair D, Foster D, Dhingra V, et al.; NICE-SUGAR Study Investigators. Intensive vs. conventional glucose control in critically ill patients. N Engl J Med. 2009;360(13):1283-97.
4. Gunst J, Debaveye Y, Güiza F, Dubois J, De Bruyn A, Dauwe D, et al. Blood glucose concentration and outcome of critical illness. N Engl J Med. 2023;389(13):1180-90.
5. Mahmoodpoor A, Hamishehkar H, Shadvar K, Sanaie S, Iranpour A, Fattahi V. Validity of bedside blood glucose measurement in critically ill patients with intensive insulin therapy. Indian J Crit Care Med. 2016;20:653-7.

25

CHAPTER

In-hospital Management of Hyperglycemia in Critical Care Settings

Narayan Deogaonkar, Anushka Deogaonkar, Parth Deogaonkar

ABSTRACT

Hyperglycemia is common in critically ill patients, and its management is crucial in improving patient outcomes. This chapter provides an overview of the in-hospital management of hyperglycemia in critical care settings, focusing on the principles of glycemic control, monitoring strategies, and therapeutic options. The goal is to maintain blood glucose levels within a target range while minimizing the risk of hypoglycemia. Various insulin protocols including continuous intravenous infusion and subcutaneous regimens are discussed, along with their advantages and limitations. The use of technology, such as continuous glucose-monitoring systems, is explored as a tool to optimize glycemic management. Finally, potential challenges and strategies to overcome them are addressed, emphasizing the need for individualized treatment approaches. By following evidence-based guidelines and implementing a comprehensive approach, healthcare providers can effectively manage hyperglycemia in critical care settings, leading to improved patient outcomes and reduced morbidity and mortality rates.

INTRODUCTION

Hyperglycemia is a common complication of critical illness. Hyperglycemia is associated with increased mortality and morbidity. Hyperglycemia itself does not cause poor clinical outcome. It is a marker of severity of disease. Insulin resistance is an important factor. It is observed in majority of critically ill patients. Critical illness leads to activation of the hypothalamic–pituitary–adrenal (HPA) axis, which results in the release of cortisol. Cortisol stimulates gluconeogenesis and decreases glucose utilization. Other counter-regulatory hormones (glucagon, catecholamines, and growth hormone) are also released. These hormones stimulate insulin resistance through lipolysis of adipose tissue, skeletal muscle proteolysis, and hepatic gluconeogenesis. All these processes lead to impaired glucose utilization in peripheral tissues, increased circulating free fatty acids, and stimulation of gluconeogenesis and glycogenolysis. Exogenous factors (parenteral and enteral nutrition, vasopressors, glucose infusions, and corticosteroids) further exacerbate hyperglycemia.

Hyperglycemia, if not treated, may lead to osmotic diuresis causing dehydration, which may impair renal function and worsen hyperglycemia. It further causes mitochondrial damage, endothelial dysfunction, and immune suppression, which lead to an increased risk for infection.

Several factors may increase the risk of developing hyperglycemia in critical care settings. Release of proinflammatory mediators during an immune response can contribute to hyperglycemia. The administration of certain exogenous drugs such as corticosteroids, vasopressors, and ascorbic acid can disrupt glucose regulation in the body. Parenteral solutions containing dextrose, often used in medical settings, can also elevate blood sugar levels. Stress-induced hyperglycemia can be a contributing factor, as stress can trigger the release of stress hormones and affect insulin sensitivity. Another potential risk factor is the use of commercial dietary feeds or supplements that may contain high amounts of sugars or carbohydrates, which can impact blood glucose levels. It is important to be aware of these risk factors

26

CHAPTER

Managing Fever in Intensive Care Unit Settings

Smita Gupta, Shouvik Datta

ABSTRACT

Temperature is one of the vital signs in the patients admitted to the hospital and commonly occurring problem in patients admitted in the intensive care unit (ICU). Early recognition of fever by an appropriate method is of utmost importance to prevent the mortality and also to reduce the ICU stay. Many causes have been documented for the etiology of fever in the ICU mostly because of sepsis and sometimes because of noninfectious causes. Appropriate and early laboratory investigations are required to detect the etiology of sepsis and also to rule out if the noninfectious causes. Various methods are used in ICU to reduce the temperature along with appropriate antipyretic doses. Also early initiation of right choice of empirical antibiotic in correct doses is required to control sepsis initially and later on to be replaced as per the culture sensitivity.

INTRODUCTION

Temperature is an important vital sign in all the patients admitted to the hospital, be it nonintensive care unit (non-ICU) or ICU area. It is a part of routine assessment in hospital admitted patients. In ICU, it usually denotes the infectious because, especially ventilator-associated conditions and also used to calculate APACHE 11 score. Normal body temperature is between 36 and 37.5°C with 0.5–1°C variability, depending on diurnal variation. Any temperature above this is termed as pyrexia or hyperpyrexia. Pyrexia commonly called as fever is a tightly regulated response to any exogenous stress via endogenous pathways.

In ICU, the definition of fever defers from usual definition. The American College of Critical Care Medicine (ACCCM) and the Infectious Disease Society of America (IDSA) have defined fever as a single core body temperature of >38.3°C. Hyperpyrexia also called hyperthermia is a condition when the temperature usually exceeds 41°C and is not associated with increase in hypothalamic set point. This condition is usually not very commonly encountered in ICU settings. In immunocompromised and neutropenic patients, a lower threshold of temperature is kept for the diagnosis. These patients are weak enough not to mount an appropriate febrile response. So in such patients, fever is usually considered as single temperature >38.3°C or if the temperature of >38°C is sustained for >1 hour in patients having absolute neutrophil count (ANC) of <500 cells/mm.

ETIOLOGY

Incidence

Fever is seen in up to 70% of all ICU patients. It is usually due to an infective or noninfective cause. While on one hand, fever may be an appropriate adaptation to an underlying infective process; in other situations, fever may be harmful. For example, patients who have high core body temperatures (i.e., 39–39.4°C) had significantly decreased mortality (in hospital) in comparison with patients who had peak core body temperatures between 36.5° and 36.9°C. In noninfectious fever, mortality increases with rising core body temperature. Core body temperature between 38.3° and 38.8°C can result from both infectious cause and noninfectious cause. Fevers >38.9°C (102°F) and <41°C are usually infectious **(Table 1)** in origin, and fever ≥41.1°C (105.8°F) is mostly noninfectious in etiology **(Table 2)**.

TABLE 1: Infectious causes of fever.

Most common cause	Other causes
• Bacteremia • Intravascular catheter-related infection • Surgical site infection • Ventilator-associated pneumonia • Urinary tract infection	• Cellulitis • Cholangitis • Diverticulitis • Empyema • Endocarditis • Intra-abdominal abscess • Meningitis • Myonecrosis • Necrotizing fasciitis • Pseudomembranous colitis • Septic arthritis • Sinusitis • Suppurative thrombophlebitis

TABLE 2: Noninfectious causes of fever.

Most common causes	Other causes
• Acalculous cholecystitis • Adrenal insufficiency • Benign postoperative fever • Drug fever • Pancreatitis • Thyroid storm • Transfusion reaction	• Acute respiratory distress syndrome (late) • Burns • Drug overdose (e.g., aspirin anticholinergic drugs) • Drug withdrawal • Heat stroke • Gout • Intracranial hemorrhage • Ischemic colitis • Malignancy • Malignant hyperthermia • Myocardial infarction • Neuroleptic malignant syndrome • Pheochromocytoma • Seizures • Serotonin syndrome • Thromboembolic disease • Vasculitis

PATHOPHYSIOLOGY OF FEVER

Fever occurs due to cytokines mostly interleukin-1 (IL-1), interleukin-6 (IL-6), and tumor necrosis factor-alpha (TNF-α), which is produced by white blood cells (WBCs) due to external stimuli. Receptors in Organum Vasculosum (of the lamina terminalis) are then stimulated by these cytokines, resulting in more production of prostaglandins E2 (PGE2). This PGE2 then increases cyclic adenosine monophosphate (AMP), which in turn raises the core body temperature.

TABLE 3: Methods to record temperature.

Core temperature	Peripheral temperature
More accurate	Less accurate
Less commonly used • Pulmonary artery catheter • Intravesicular • Rectal	More commonly used • Oral • Axillary • Temporal artery • Tympanic site • Chemical dot monitors

How to measure temperature in ICU?

In the ICU patients, temperature of body can be measured at:

- Peripheral site
- Core sites

Some are more accurate methods and some are less accurate **(Table 3)**.

Regardless of the methods chosen, single method and same site should be used repeatedly. The gold standard test is an Intravascular Thermistor.

INVESTIGATIONS

In most patients, we perform the following initial tests. Such testing is considered inexpensive, easy to perform, and targeted at the common and more serious etiologies of fever in the ICU patient.

- *Blood cultures*: Blood should be drawn from two different sites (aerobic and anaerobic) before initiation of antimicrobials. Blood cultures from the central intravascular catheter should also be drawn when central intravascular catheters are present. If infection with fungus is suspected, blood should be sent for fungal culture.
- *Respiratory tract sampling*: If the patient is intubated, endotracheal aspirate/sputum Gram-stain culture should be sent.
- *Urinalysis and urine culture*: Urine R/M and urine culture are indicated for febrile patients in the ICU, particularly those who are catheterized, have renal pathology (e.g., obstructing stones, trauma), or are immunosuppressed.
- *Chest imaging*: A chest radiograph usually detects a new infiltrate or progressive pulmonary infiltrate. It also distinguishes pneumonia from tracheobronchitis and identifies respiratory sources of fever other than pneumonia and tracheobronchitis that would otherwise be missed as it is not associated with cough or sputum production (e.g., development of a pleural effusion/empyema in a patient with community-acquired pneumonia).

- *Cultures (from infection site)*: ICU patients have several potential sites for infection including catheters, wounds, sinuses, fluid collections—ascitic and pleural bedsore, joint swelling, stool (e.g., for *Clostridium difficile*). If fever occurs during blood transfusion, the blood bag and its contents are usually sent for culture.
- *Laboratory studies*: Routine complete blood count (CBC) and chemistries including lactate should be obtained. For example, leukocytosis, left shift, and elevated serum lactate indicate sepsis. hyperkalemia, hyponatremia, and hypoglycemia usually indicate adrenal insufficiency, and increased serum urea and serum creatinine are suggestive of a urinary tract infection (UTI) or any obstruction. We also obtain serum glutamate pyruvate transaminase (SGPT) serum glutamic-oxaloacetic transaminase (SGOT), serum bilirubin, and serum alkaline phosphatase (for acalculous cholecystitis or any biliary pathology) as well as amylase and lipase (to look for pancreatitis) in pain abdomen patients.
- *Radioimaging of abdomen*: Radioimaging is necessary in patients with signs and symptoms of any intra-abdominal complications such as distension, tenderness, and absent bowel sounds. It is also done for patients where no other source of the fever is found.
- *Other laboratory tests*:
    - Suspected thyroid storm—perform thyroid-stimulating hormone (TSH), T3 (triiodothyronine) and T4 (thyroxine) levels.
    - Suspected acute hemolytic transfusion reaction—perform direct antiglobulin test, plasma-free hemoglobin, haptoglobin, and repeat blood type and cross-match.
    - Suspected adrenal insufficiency: Random cortisol level or cosyntropin test if necessary.

Procalcitonin (PCT) is a diagnostic indicator of infection, but it is not routinely used. Some studies report that the diagnostic value of PCT in critically ill patients is unproven. However, some studies do agree that PCT level plays a role in deciding when to discontinue antibiotics.

TREATMENT

Antibiotics

After sending the cultures, empirical antibiotic therapy has to be started in patients with all suspected sepsis cases, especially in patients with septic shock. The selection of antibiotics depends on the pathogens suspected, sepsis source, the site of infection, and the risk of developing drug resistance. Antibiotics should be given for the appropriate duration with a correct dose. De-escalation involves replacing the ongoing antibiotic with a relatively narrow-spectrum antibiotic (depending on the reports of culture) and converting intravenous (IV) antibiotics to oral antibiotics, and finally stopping the antibiotic. De-escalation combats increasing antibiotic resistance in ICUs.

Deciding to Remove Catheters

To remove an intravascular catheter in a febrile patient is challenging. The decision to remove an intravascular catheter includes the severity of illness, duration of the catheter placed, probability of catheter being the source of fever, e.g., in a patient with sepsis, removal of an intravascular catheter where the insertion site looks infected is appropriate while removal may not be necessary if the insertion site is clean and the catheter has only recently been inserted. Removal is also appropriate if the catheter (intravascular devices, urinary catheters, and drainage of empyema/abscesses) is known to be infected or patients have evidence of metastatic infection or persistent bacteremia or fungemia from the catheter (e.g., endocarditis), particularly with pathogens including *Staphylococcus aureus*, *Pseudomonas aeruginosa*, drug-resistant organisms, and *Candida* species.

Treatment of Fever

There is variation in practice regarding the routine treatment of fever. While we do not routinely treat every fever, some clinicians treat fever with an antipyretic (e.g., acetaminophen) on initial presentation and follow the course of the fever over the next 6–12 hours while investigations and cultures are pending. While a paucity of data exists, protocols that systematically prevent and treat fever in the ICU appear to offer no benefit. Most experts agree that aggressive or prolonged cooling with external cooling blankets or ice packs and use of such mechanical methods to prevent fever recurrence is not generally necessary unless the fever itself is considered harmful (e.g., patients with increased intracranial pressure) or excessively high [e.g., fever ≥41°C (≥105.8°F)]. For example, if core body temperature exceeds the limit of "critical thermal maximum" which is thought to be between 41.6° and 42°C (106.9–107.6°F), life-threatening complications can occur (e.g., Rhabdomyolysis). The management of severe hyperthermia includes external cooling, and targeted temperature management following cardiac arrest. When treating fever, acetaminophen is better than nonsteroidal anti-inflammatory drugs (NSAIDs) or aspirin. Enteral (oral) administration is preferred, when feasible. According to few studies hypotension [systolic blood pressure (SBP) ≤ 90 mm Hg or ≥20% decrease from baseline] was higher after parenteral administration of acetaminophen when it is compared with oral administration.

Treatment of Some Specific Illness

Acalculous cholecystitis: When patient is unstable, treatment is endoscopic retrograde cholangiopancreatography (ERCP) with stent placement in the gall bladder with percutaneous drainage for decompression. Definitive treatment is cholecystectomy.

Nosocomial sinusitis: It is usually missed as a source of infections. Predisposing factors—nasogastric (NG tube) or nasotracheal tubes, fractures of face, epistaxis with nasal packing and use of steroids. Treatment includes antibiotics, removal of NG tube, and nasal vasoconstrictors.

Nosocomial diarrhea: ***Clostridioides*** (previously, *Clostridium*) *difficile* infection is the most common cause for febrile diarrhea. It is seen in patients who have recently been treated for infection with antibiotics. Clindamycin is the most common antibiotic associated with *C. difficile* infection. Treatment is stopping the antibiotic which has caused the disease. Add antibiotics for C. *difficile* (e.g., metronidazole, fidaxomicin, oral vancomycin).

Drug fever: Drug-induced fever is a diagnosis of exclusion, affecting 3–5% of patients in ICU. Drugs-causing fever are—antibiotics (Beta-lactams); antiepileptic drugs (phenytoin); antiarrhythmic drugs (quinidine, procainamide); heparin, diuretics, and allopurinol. The usual time between the drug initiation and the appearance of fever is around 7–10 days, and fever generally subsides after drug withdrawal (and by 72 hours of stopping the drug).

Hyperthermia: It is defined as raise in core body temperature > 41°C. Here core body temperature is mostly elevated above the thermoregulatory set point. It does not respond to medical or pharmacological therapy. These include:

- Heat stroke
- Malignant hyperthermia (antidote: dantrolene),
- Neuroleptic malignant syndrome (drugs used are: dantrolene, bromocriptine, amantadine, and benzodiazepines).
- Serotonin syndrome (antidote: cyproheptadine, olanzapine and chlorpromazine). Endocrine conditions such as thyrotoxicosis (thionamides with beta-blockers, radioiodine, surgery)
- Adrenal crisis and pheochromocytoma also cause hyperthermia.

SUGGESTED READINGS

1. Achaiah NC, Bhutta BS, Ajith Kumar AK. Fever in the Intensive Care Patient. In: StatPearls [Internet]. Treasure Island (FL): StatPearls Publishing; 2023.
2. Chamorro C, Romera MA, Balandin B. Fever in critically ill patients. Crit Care Med. 2008;36(11):3129-30.
3. Coburn B, Morris AM, Tomlinson G, Detsky AS. Does this adult patient with suspected bacteremia require blood cultures? JAMA. 2012;308:502.

27

CHAPTER

Central Line-related Bloodstream Infection

Javal Bhatt, Mahesh Choudhary

ABSTRACT

Catheter-related bloodstream infection (CRBSI) is a laboratory confirmed bloodstream infection (BSI) not related to an infection at any other site that develops within 48 hours of central line placement.

Although preventable these infections are major causes of morbidity and mortality in critically ill patients. CRBSI and central line-associated bloodstream infection (CLABSI) are interchangeable terms but have different definitions in the clinical context. Host- and catheter-related risk factors along with the causative organisms (gram-negative, gram-positive and fungi) are responsible for CRBSI. Skin contamination, hub contamination, hematogenous seeding, and infusate contamination are the major pathophysiology involved in CRBSI. It manifests clinically as fever, hypotension, and other local signs of infection. Clinical examination plays an important role in the diagnosis of CRBSI along with the help of laboratory investigations. In the suspected cases paired blood cultures should be ideally obtained before the start of empirical treatment which is decided based on many factors. Gram-positive, gram-negative, and fungal coverage should be given empirically till the antimicrobial susceptibility results are available after which de-escalation to specific treatment can be done. Removal of catheters also forms an important role in the treatment of CRBSI. For prevention, adequate measures should be taking during, at, and after the insertion of invasive venous catheters.

INTRODUCTION

Modern healthcare employs many types of invasive devices and procedures to treat patients and help in their recovery, but they also lead to many complications with bloodstream infection (BSI) being one of them. Catheter-related bloodstream infection (CRBSI) is a laboratory confirmed BSI not related to an infection at any other site that develops within 48 hours of central line placement. With proper aseptic techniques, surveillance, and management strategies, most of these cases can be prevented. Central venous catheters (CVCs) are associated with greater risk of device-related infections as compared to any other medical devices. Although necessary in critically ill patients for various uses, intravascular catheterization causes nosocomial bacteremia and significant morbidity and mortality. CRBSI and central line-associated bloodstream infection (CLABSI) terms are often used interchangeably even though the meanings differ. CRBSI is a clinical definition while CLABSI is a definition typically used for surveillance purposes.

EPIDEMIOLOGY

Catheter-related bloodstream infection incidence reported varies from country to country and even hospital to hospital. According to the National Nosocomial Infections Surveillance (NNIS) system of the Centers for Disease Control and Prevention (CDC), the median rate of CRBSI in intensive care units (ICUs) of all types of ranges from 1.8 to 5.2 per 1,000 catheter-days with the rate of about 25.6%. There are limited Indian studies on CRBSI which have found the incidence of these infections to be around 27%.

ETIOLOGY

- *Risk factors*:
  - Host Factors:
    - Chronic illnesses [hemodialysis (HD), malignancy, gastrointestinal tract disorders, pulmonary hypertension]
    - Immune suppressed states (organ transplant, diabetes mellitus, malnutrition, total parenteral nutrition, extremes of age, loss of skin integrity/ burns)
    - Prolonged hospitalization before line insertion
  - Catheter-related factors:
    - Type of catheter—non-tunneled catheters (temporary CVC) are responsible for more cases than the tunneled catheters (HD catheter)
    - Site of insertion—femoral CVCs are associated with the highest risk of CLABSI, followed by internal jugular and subclavian catheters.
    - Others—duration of catheterization, type of catheter material, insertion condition, catheter site care, and skills of operator
- *Causative organism*: Prior to the 1980s, gram-negative aerobes were the predominant organisms associated with nosocomial BSIs. Since then, gram-positive aerobes (e.g., coagulase-negative staphylococci, *Staphylococcus aureus*, and *Enterococcus*) and *Candida* species have increased in relative importance. The following distribution of pathogens was noted in the United States CDC's National Healthcare Safety Network between 2011 and 2014:
  - Coagulase-negative staphylococci—16.4%
  - *S. aureus*—13.2%
  - Enterococci—15.2%
  - *Candida* species—13.3%
  - *Klebsiella* species—8.4%
  - *Escherichia coli*—5.4%
  - *Enterobacter* species—4.4%
  - *Pseudomonas* species—4%

PATHOPHYSIOLOGY

There are four important sources of CRBSI mentioned as follows:

1. *Skin contamination*: Within 7–10 days of CVC placement, bacteria on the skin surface migrate along the external surface of the catheter from the skin exit site toward the intravascular space.
2. *Hub contamination*: CLABSIs that occur beyond 10 days are usually caused by contamination of the hub (intraluminal), typically from a healthcare provider's contaminated hands but rarely from a host and often due to a breach of standard aseptic precautions to access the hub.
3. Hematogenous seeding
4. Infusate contamination

CLINICAL MANIFESTATIONS

Clinical features depend on the severity of illness which includes:

- Fever and chills are the most common manifestations. They may be masked in immunocompromised patients or in extreme age group patients.
- *Local signs*: Pain, swelling, or discharge from the exit site and redness surrounding or along the subcutaneous track when exit site or tunnel infections are present; local signs observed in the first 7 days following insertion are highly predictive of CRBSI.
- Hemodynamic instability/ hypotension
- Lethargy/fatigue
- Altered mental status
- For long-term catheters, difficulty drawing blood or poor flow are considered risk factors and manifestations of CLABSI.

Complications

- *Septic thrombophlebitis*: This refers to venous thrombosis associated with inflammation in the setting of bacteremia. It should be suspected in patients with CRBSI and persistent bacteremia after 72 hours of appropriate therapy.
- *Infective endocarditis (IE)*: IE should be suspected in patients with CRBSI or bacteremia >48–72 hours with a pathogen associated with IE.
- *Metastatic musculoskeletal infection (such as septic arthritis, osteomyelitis, orthopedic hardware infection)*: Bacteremia may be associated with seeding of joints, bone, or orthopedic hardware.

DIAGNOSIS/CLINICAL EVALUATION

- The diagnosis of CRBSI should be suspected in patients with fever, chills, or hypotension in the setting of a catheter placed at least 48 hours prior to development of symptoms.
- Clinical examination plays an important role in the diagnosis of CRBSI along with the help of laboratory investigations. Exit site examination to look for signs of inflammation of tunneled catheters with inspection and palpation of the subcutaneous track is essential.

- *Role of blood culture*: In suspected cases paired blood cultures (one from peripheral line while the other from central line) should be obtained ideally prior to initiation of antibiotic therapy. In the case of poor peripheral access or when unable to obtain a peripheral sample, two or more samples must be drawn from different lumens of a multi-lumen central line. Catheter tip cultures are no longer recommended for CRBSI diagnosis, given low positive predictive value.

The following definitions help in arriving at a diagnosis:

- *CRBSI*: *IDSA* (*Infectious Diseases Society of America*) *definition*: CRBSI is the preferred term used by IDSA.
  The definite diagnosis of CRBSI requires one of the following:
  - Isolation of the same pathogen from a quantitative blood culture drawn through the central line and from a peripheral vein with the single bacterial colony count at least threefold higher in the sample from the central line as compared to that obtained from a peripheral vein
  - Same organism recovered from percutaneous blood culture and from quantitative (>15 colony-forming units) culture of the catheter tip
  - A shorter time to positive culture (>2 hours earlier) in the central line sample than the peripheral sample [differential time to positivity (DTP)]
- *CLABSI*: *CDC definition*—CLABSI is a surveillance definition used by the CDC and defined as the recovery of a pathogen from a blood culture (a single blood culture for an organism not commonly present on the skin and two or more blood cultures for organism commonly present on the skin) in a patient who had a central line at the time of infection or within 48 hours before the development of infection. The infection cannot be related to any other infection the patient might have and must not have been present or incubating when the patient was admitted to the facility.

TREATMENT

- *Role of antibiotic therapy*: When CRBSI is suspected, empirical antibiotic therapy should be started based on:
  - Severity of infection
  - Host factors
  - Organisms responsible
  - Local prevalence and antimicrobial susceptibility patterns in institutional antibiograms
- *Gram-positive coverage*: If methicillin-resistant *Staphylococcus aureus* (MRSA) is prevalent parenteral vancomycin is preferred over penicillin or cephalosporins such as nafcillin or cefazolin. Daptomycin is preferred in cases of MRSA isolates with minimum inhibitory concentration (MIC) >2 mg/mL for vancomycin and vancomycin-resistant enterococci (VRE).
- *Gram-negative coverage*: If risk of *Pseudomonas* infection is high or in the critically ill patients (neutropenia, sepsis, and prior colonization) cefepime or carbapenem with or without an aminoglycoside is preferred otherwise a third-generation cephalosporin (ceftriaxone) is sufficient if the risk is low.
- *Role of antifungal*: Antifungals must be considered in femoral catheterization, total parenteral nutrition (TPN), prolonged administration of broad-spectrum antibiotics, hematological malignancy or solid organ or bone marrow transplant recipients. Intravenous (IV) fluconazole or echinocandins (micafungin, caspofungin, anidulafungin) in cases where azole resistance is suspected (prior azole use or non-*albicans Candida* such as *Candida glabrata* or *Candida krusei*)

Once antimicrobial susceptibility results are available, de-escalation to specific and appropriate therapy is recommended.

- *Removal of catheters*:
  - Non-tunneled catheters: They should be removed promptly if there is high clinical suspicion of CRBSI. Salvage therapy can be practiced [systemic therapy coupled with antimicrobial lock (heparin + high concentration of antimicrobial agent that is selected based on susceptibility results)] can be attempted in limited instances such as:
    - Uncomplicated CLABSI is caused by organisms other than *S. aureus*, *Pseudomonas aeruginosa*, *Bacillus*, *Micrococcus* species, propionibacteria, fungi, or mycobacteria.
    - The patients with limited vascular access sites or the ones who are solely dependent on central access for survival.
  - Tunneled catheters (HD catheters): Indications for removal of HD catheters are the following:
    - Persistent symptoms >36 hours or severe sepsis, hemodynamic instability (shock), and metastatic infection
    - Blood cultures that remain positive >72 hours of appropriate antimicrobial therapy.
    - Difficult to clear organisms (*S. aureus*, *Pseudomonas*, or fungi).
    - Recurrence of uncomplicated CLABSI (any nonvirulent organism) when salvaged for difficult access.

- *Duration of therapy*: For patients with uncomplicated CRBSI (e.g., no endocarditis, or metastatic infection), in the absence of risk factors for hematogenous spread (e.g., hardware, immunosuppression) and negative blood cultures 72 hours of catheter removal, following approach for IV antimicrobial therapy is recommended:
  - *S. aureus*—14 days in the absence of endocarditis
  - Coagulase-negative staphylococci—7 days
  - Enterococci and gram-negative bacilli—10-14 days
  - *Candida*—14 days in the absence of retinitis

PREVENTION

The following are some key components of a prevention program, abstracted from an extensive list provided by the CDC and IDSA, sponsored by the Society for Healthcare Epidemiology of America (SHEA).

Before Insertion

- Provide easy access to an evidence-based list of indications for CVC use to minimize unnecessary CVC placement
- Require education and competency assessment of heathcare personnel (HCP) involved in insertion, care and maintenance of CVCs about CLABSI prevention
- Bathe ICU patients aged >2 months with a chlorhexidine preparation on a daily basis

At Insertion

- In ICU and non-ICU settings, a facility should have a process in place, such as a checklist, to ensure adherence to infection prevention practices at the time of CVC insertion
- Perform hand hygiene prior to catheter insertion or manipulation
- The subclavian site is preferred to reduce infectious complications when the catheter is placed in the ICU setting.
- Use an all-inclusive catheter cart or kit
- Use ultrasound guidance for catheter insertion
- Use maximum sterile barrier precautions during CVC insertion
- Use an alcoholic chlorhexidine antiseptic for skin preparation

After Insertion

- Ensure appropriate nurse-to-patient ratio and limit use of float nurses in ICUs
- Use chlorhexidine-containing dressings for CVCs inpatients over 2 months of age
- For non-tunneled CVCs in adults and children, change transparent dressings and perform site care with a chlorhexidine-based antiseptic at least every 7 days or immediately if the dressing is soiled, loose, or damp. Change gauze dressings every 2 days or earlier if the dressing is soiled, loose, or damp
- Disinfect catheter hubs, needle less connectors, and injection ports before accessing the catheter
- Remove nonessential catheters
- Routine replacement of administration sets not used for blood, blood products, or lipid formulations can be performed at intervals up to 7days.
- Perform surveillance for CLABSI in ICU and non-ICU settings

SUGGESTED READINGS

1. National Healthcare Safety Network. (2024). Bloodstream Infection Event (Central Line-associated Bloodstream Infection and Non-central Line-associated Bloodstream Infection) Device-associated Module BSI. [online]. Available fromhttps://www.cdc.gov/nhsn/pdfs/pscmanual/4psc_clabscurrent.pdf [Last accessed December, 2023].
2. Centers for Disease Control and Prevention. (2015). Background Information: Terminology & Estimates of Risk. Guidelines for the Prevention of Intravascular Catheter-Related Infections (2011). [online] Available from https://www.cdc.gov/infectioncontrol/guidelines/bsi/background/terminology.html [Last accessed December, 2023].
3. Magill SS, Edwards JR, Bamberg W, Beldavs ZG, Dumyati G, Kainer MA, et al; Emerging Infections Program Healthcare-Associated Infections and Antimicrobial Use Prevalence Survey Team. Multistate point-prevalence survey of health care-associated infections. N Engl J Med. 2014;370:1198-208.
4. Patil HV, Patil VC, Ramteerthkar MN, Kulkarni RD. Central venous catheter-related bloodstream infections in the intensive care unit. Indian J Crit Care Med. 2011;15:213-23.
5. Weiner LM, Webb AK, Limbago B, Dudeck MA, Patel J, Kallen AJ, et al. Antimicrobial-Resistant Pathogens Associated With Healthcare-Associated Infections: Summary of Data Reported to the National Healthcare Safety Network at the Centers for Disease Control and Prevention, 2011-2014. Infect Control Hosp Epidemiol. 2016;37(11):1288-301.
6. Centers for Disease Control and Prevention. (2015). Strategies for Prevention of Catheter-Related Infections in Adult and Pediatric Patients. Guidelines for the Prevention of Intravascular Catheter-Related Infections (2011). [online] Available from https://www.cdc.gov/infectioncontrol/guidelines/bsi/background/prevention-strategies.html [Last accessed December, 2023].
7. Baker CC, Petersen SR, Sheldon GF. Septic phlebitis: a neglected disease. Am J Surg. 1979;138(1):97-103.

8. Washington JA 2nd, Ilstrup DM. Blood cultures: Issues and controversies. Rev Infect Dis. 1986;8(5):792.
9. Mermel LA, Allon M, Bouza E, Craven DE, Flynn P, O'Grady NP, et al. Clinical practice guidelines for the diagnosis and management of intravascular catheter-related infection: 2009 Update by the Infectious Diseases Society of America. Clin Infect Dis. 2009;49(1):1-45; Corrections can be found in Clin Infect Dis. 2010;50(3):457; Clin Infect Dis. 2010;50(7):1079. Commentary can be found in Clin Infect Dis. 2009;49(11):1770.
10. Buetti N, Marschall J, Drees M, Fakih MG, Hadaway L, Maragakis LL, et al. Strategies to prevent central line-associated bloodstream infections in acute-care hospitals: 2022 Update. Infect Control Hosp Epidemiol. 2022;43(5):553-69.

28

CHAPTER

Invasive Fungal Infections in the Intensive Care Unit

Dhanashri Atre Singh, Bitukaur Sodhi

ABSTRACT

Invasive fungal infections in critically ill patients pose a challenge to the clinicians at every step right from diagnosing to treating. Maintaining a high index of suspicion is necessary in order to diagnose it and initiate early therapy because the mortality of these infections remains high. With the changing spectrum of pathogens, advent of new diagnostic modalities, and availability of newer antifungals, being up to date about these infections is crucial to ensuring a better outcome for the patient.

INTRODUCTION

The advances in critical care and contemporary medicine have, on one hand, managed to add to the survival of critically ill patients; however, on the other hand, they have also increased the incidence of opportunistic infections, especially fungal, in such patients. There are multiple causal factors for this rising incidence—invasive procedures, central venous catheters, ventilators, prolonged antibiotics disrupting the normal flora, breach in the natural protective barriers, and the underlying medical or surgical conditions responsible for the prolonged stay in the intensive care unit.

Because invasive fungal infections were considered to be more common in immunocompromised patients—malignancies, solid organ transplant, neutropenic patients—diagnosing them in patients who do not have these risk factors remains challenging and requires a high index of suspicion.

EPIDEMIOLOGY AND DEFINITIONS

The most common invasive fungal infection seen in the critical care unit is invasive candidiasis. This could be either candidemia or disseminated tissue candidiasis, resulting from hematogenous dissemination or the direct inoculation of *Candida* into a sterile site during an invasive procedure. While earlier, most of the cases of invasive candidiasis were because of *Candida albicans*, over the years, the nonalbicans group has also emerged as a causative agent for it, namely *C. parapsilosis, C. glabrata, C. tropicalis,* and *C. krusei*.

The second most common invasive fungal infection is aspergillosis. Believed to be common in neutropenic patients or post-transplant patients, now it is being seen in non-neutropenic patients as well, particularly those with chronic pulmonary and liver conditions. It predominantly affects the lungs and sinuses in an immunocompetent patient, while in immunocompromised, it can result not only in cavitation but also in aggressive angioinvasive disease. The species most commonly isolated are *Aspergillus fumigatus,* followed by *Aspergillus flavus* and *Aspergillus terreus*.

Mucormycosis is the third most common invasive fungal infection seen in the critical care unit. The pathogens implicate here are *Rhizopus, Mucor, Rhizomucor, Absidia,* and *Apophysomyces*. This is usually seen in patients who have prolonged acidosis, diabetic patients with uncontrolled sugars, or patients suffering massive injuries due to road traffic accidents, disasters, or complex combat trauma.

The European Organization for Research and Treatment of Cancer (EORTC)/Invasive Fungal Infections Cooperative Group and the National Institute of Allergy and Infectious Diseases Mycoses Study Group (MSG) published the first standardized definitions for invasive fungal diseases (IFDs) in 2002, revised them in 2008, and finally came up with the latest definition in 2020. As per these definitions, IFD can either be a "proven" IFD or a "probable" IFD.

For labeling the IFD as proven, the fungus needs to be detected either by blood culture or by histopathology/culture of the tissue specimen. For a probable IFD, three components are taken into consideration: (i) Risk factor, (ii) clinical characteristics of the disease entity, and (iii) mycological evidence [cultures, polymerase chain reaction (PCR), and antigen detection, microscopy].

CLINICAL FEATURES

In neutropenic patients, patients with malignancies, or post-transplant patients, suspecting an IFD is relatively easier as compared to suspecting it in an immunocompetent patient. The physician needs to have a high index of suspicion to be able to make an early diagnosis and initiate antifungal treatment at earlier stages.

The clinical features depend on the site and the organ involved. However, certain common features include:
- Persistent fever despite ongoing antibiotic therapy
- Cough, hemoptysis, pleuritic chest pain, and dyspnea
- Sinus tenderness and congestion
- Skin ulceration, nodules, and abscesses
- Abdominal pain, diarrhea, gastrointestinal bleeding, and hepatosplenomegaly
- Headache, altered sensorium, seizures, focal neurological deficits, visual disturbances, and redness of the eyes.

DIAGNOSIS

The diagnostic approach for invasive fungal infections involves first and foremost having a high index of suspicion, evaluating the risk factors, taking into consideration the clinical and radiological signs, and prescribing the appropriate laboratory investigations including specialized assays.

For diagnosing invasive candidiasis, though blood culture forms an important part, the sensitivity unfortunately is suboptimal. Additionally, the cultures may be negative in deep-seated tissue candidiasis or in patients already taking azole prophylaxis. Apart from cultures, the serological markers, namely beta-D-glucan, mannan, and anti-mannan antibodies, can be used. Nucleic acid-based detection methods, with sensitivity comparable to blood cultures, have been developed for *Candida*. They have an advantage of being able to detect deep-seated tissue candidiasis and remain unaffected by azole prophylaxis.

Latest diagnostic tools include:
- Matrix-assisted laser desorption ionization—time of flight mass spectrometry (MALDI-TOF MS)
- Commercial assays based on fluorescence in situ hybridization (FISH) and the ones that allow molecular detection of fungi in blood

In order to guide the initiation of antifungal treatment, the "*Candida* Score" is used in non-neutropenic patients which takes into consideration the presence of total parenteral nutrition, severe sepsis, initial surgery, and multifocal *Candida* colonization. A score of < 3 suggests a 2.3% risk of developing invasive candidiasis without treatment.

In cases of invasive aspergillosis, the clinical features that should alert the clinician include, but are not limited to, fever unresponsive to antibiotics, neutropenia, thrombocytopenia, development of pneumonia, and at times neurological symptoms in cases of dissemination to the brain.

An important thing to keep in mind is that chest radiographs might be normal or might show some nonspecific findings in the early and at times even in the late stages of aspergillosis. CT chest might show diffuse infiltrates or the classical "halo" sign (zone of low attenuation with a translucent ground glass halo around). The gold standard for diagnosis remains histopathological identification of the species in specimens obtained by invasive procedures. Cultures of bronchial secretions or secretions obtained by bronchoalveolar lavage (BAL) can be used for the detection of *Aspergillus*. Nonculture-based tests include the detection of two fungal wall components—galactomannan in serum and BAL samples and beta-D-glucan.

Diagnosing *Mucor* requires careful and meticulous examination of the skin, sinuses, and palate to look for black eschar followed by debridement and then staining of the tissue sample with hematoxylin and eosin, periodic acid-Schiff (PAS), and visualization of broad nonseptate, irregularly branched hyphae.

TREATMENT

The following classes of antifungal can be used for the management of invasive fungal infections in critically ill patients.
- Polyenes
- Azoles

- Echinocandins
- Pyrimidine analogs

The key factor determining the outcome in invasive candidiasis is the time of treatment initiation. A delay of even 24–48 hours can have a negative impact on the outcome of the patients. An empirical antifungal is chosen based on the local resistance patterns, the clinical status of the patient, prior use of fluconazole, associated comorbidities, and risk factors.

The antifungals that are usually preferred for invasive candidiasis include fluconazole and echinocandins.

In cases of documented *Candida* infection, a fundoscopic examination is warranted and treatment is immediately started. Echinocandins (caspofungin 70 mg loading dose followed by 50 mg/day, micafungin 100 mg/day, and anidulafungin 200 mg loading dose followed by 100 mg/day) are preferred in patients with hemodynamic instability whereas in hemodynamically stable patients, fluconazole (3–6 mg/kg/day) can be used, provided there is no prior history of fluconazole usage and infection with nonalbicans species is not suspected.

Because the mortality of invasive pulmonary aspergillosis is high, treatment should be initiated the moment a clinical suspicion arises. The drug of choice is voriconazole. The recommended dosage is 6 mg/kg BD on day 1 and thereafter 4 mg/kg TDS. The duration of treatment can be months and needs to be tailored as per the patient's response.

Salvage therapy options for refractory cases include echinocandins (caspofungin), posaconazole (200 mg), and liposomal amphotericin B (3–5 mg/kg/day).

The treatment of mucormycosis is a challenging one because, in addition to antifungal therapy, it requires aggressive surgical intervention and management of the underlying predisposing conditions. The drug of choice remains liposomal amphotericin B at a dose of 5–10 mg/kg/day with the maximal dose being used in case of cerebral involvement. The second-line agent that can be used is posaconazole at a dose of 400 mg BD. It can either be added to liposomal amphotericin B or used as a long-term monotherapy.

The newer drugs being studied for invasive fungal infections are ravuconazole and albaconazole and a monoclonal antibody: Mycograb-NeuTec Pharma that is being considered in combination with amphotericin B.

SUGGESTED READINGS

1. Paramythiotou E, Frantzeskaki F, Flevari A, Armaganidis A, Dimopoulos G. Invasive fungal infections in the ICU: how to approach, how to treat. Molecules. 2014;19(1):1085-119.
2. Bassetti M, Azoulay E, Kullberg B-J, Ruhnke M, Shoham S, Vazquez J. et al. EORTC/MSGERC Definitions of Invasive Fungal Diseases: Summary of Activities of the Intensive Care Unit Working Group. Clin Infect Dis. 2021;72(Suppl 2):S121-7.

29

CHAPTER

Altered Sensorium in the Intensive Care Unit: An Approach

T Geetha, Ramesh Duraisamy

ABSTRACT

Altered sensorium is a very common presentation in the intensive care unit (ICU). The causes of altered sensorium are myriad. Initial hemodynamic stabilization is essential irrespective of the cause. Good history and thorough clinical examination is extremely important, before investigations are undertaken. A multidisciplinary approach may be needed in many of the cases of altered sensorium.

INTRODUCTION

Altered sensorium or altered mental status is a frequent presentation in the intensive care unit (ICU). The causes are enormous, ranging from easily reversible (e.g., hypoglycemia) to permanent (e.g., stroke) and from relatively benign (e.g., ethanol intoxication) to life-threatening conditions [central nervous system (CNS) infections]. A systematic approach is essential for a prompt diagnosis and appropriate management **(Table 1)**.

TABLE 1: Causes of altered mental status—mnemonic: AEIOU TIPS.

A	Alcohol	Abuse/withdrawal
	Acidosis	Diabetic ketoacidosis, respiratory acidosis, hyperchloremic acidosis, lactic acidosis
	Arrhythmias	Tachy/bradyarrhythmias, atrial fibrillation, and ventricular fibrillation
E	Electrolytes	Hypernatremia, hyponatremia, hypercalcemia, and hypocalcemia
	Endocrine	Adrenal insufficiency and thyroid disease
	Encephalopathy	Hepatic, chronic traumatic, Hashimoto's, mitochondriopathy, and Wernicke's
I	Insulin	Hypo/hyperglycemia
O	Oxygen	Hypoxia
	Overdose	Overdosage, opiates, and other drug abuse
U	Uremia	Renal failure and urinary obstruction
	Underdose	Insufficient dose of medications
T	Trauma	Concussion, traumatic brain injury, raised ICT, and organ failure
	Tumor	Brain tumor
	Temperature	Heat stroke, hyperthermia, and hypothermia
I	Infection	Meningitis, encephalitis, meningoencephalitis, liver abscess, pneumonia, sepsis, and urinary tract infection

Continued

Continued

P	Poisoning	Carbon monoxide, gases, iron, lead, and snakebite
	Psychogenic	Conversion disorder and psychosis
S	Stroke	Hemorrhagic/ischemic and transient ischemic attack (TIA)
	Seizures	Epileptic seizure and psychogenic nonepileptic seizure
	Shock	Cardiogenic, hypovolemic, and neurogenic
	Syncope	Temporary loss of consciousness due to various causes
	Shunt	Ventriculoperitoneal (VP) shunt malfunction

INITIAL ASSESSMENT AND ACUTE MANAGEMENT

The aim of initial assessment is to identify the reversible causes of altered mental status and life-threatening situations which require rapid intervention.

The goal of acute management is to ensure that blood, oxygen, and glucose reach the brain and to protect the brain from further damage.

Always start with the ABCDEF approach and continuous cardiac monitoring and venous access must be established as early as possible.

A (Airway)

- Hypoxia is one of the reversible causes of altered mental status.
- Ensure the airway is open and protected. If not, secure the airway and supplement oxygen if oxygen saturation (SpO_2) < 94%.

B (Breathing)

- Inadequate ventilation may cause hypercarbia.
- If the respirations are inadequate (apneustic or ataxic) or hyperventilation perform bag-mask ventilation and/or endotracheal intubation

C (Circulation)

- Hypoperfusion causes altered mental status due to decreased supply of oxygen and glucose to the brain.
- Check the distal pulses, blood pressure, cardiac rhythm, capillary refill time, skin color, and temperature.
- If the patient is hypotensive, administer intravenous (IV) fluids and investigate the cause.
- Presence of hypertension may have the possibility of a raised intracranial tension and an impending herniation, and should be treated immediately.

D (Disability) (Mini Neurological Evaluation)

- Assess Glasgow Coma Scale (GCS) or alert, verbal, painful, and unresponsive (AVPU) score, pupillary size, and reaction (to rule out space occupying lesions), motor power in the limbs (stroke), involuntary movements (seizures), and brainstem reflexes.
- If GCS < 8 may need urgent intubation and mechanical ventilation.
- Administer benzodiazepines in case of ongoing seizure activity.
- Cervical stabilization should be provided if trauma is suspected.

E (Exposure)

Perform a quick head to foot examination to look for signs of trauma, petechiae, bite marks, stings, infectious sources such as indwelling catheters, needle pricks in intravenous drug abuse, or transdermal drug patches.

F (Finger Stick Glucose)

- Bedside finger stick glucose is performed in all patients to exclude hypoglycemia.
- If the blood glucose is <70 mg/dL, administer 50 mL of 50% dextrose IV along with thiamine 100 mg IV to prevent the precipitation of acute Wernicke's encephalopathy (in chronic alcoholics and malnourished patients).

BASIC BEDSIDE INVESTIGATIONS

- While managing the airway, breathing, and circulation (ABC), an intravenous access is established and blood to be sent for investigations simultaneously [serum chemistries include renal function test (RFT) and liver function test (LFT), glucose, electrolytes, basic hematologic panel, arterial blood gas, ammonia, and toxicology screens].

- Electrocardiogram (ECG) should be performed.
- Bedside ultrasound [extended focused assessment with sonography for trauma (eFAST) protocol for trauma or rapid ultrasound for shock and hypotension (RUSH) protocol for nontrauma] should be done in patients with shock or trauma.

CLINICAL HISTORY (TABLE 2)

- Use SAMPLE approach to elicit history from the patient and/or family.
- If the patient is unable to provide the proper history details, ask a family member, caregiver, or medical personnel and also check for previous treatment records.
- Get details about surrounding environment (i.e., living house, alcohol bottles, drug strips, etc.).

TABLE 2: Clinical history.

	History/Finding	Diagnostic clue
S: Signs and symptoms	Baseline mental status	
	Rapid onset	Infection, inflammation, bleeding, or drugs/toxic exposures
	Gradual onset	SOL, such as a tumor or slow bleeding in the brain
	Episodic with normal intervals between episodes	Seizures/convulsions or psychiatric disease
	History of fever	CNS infections and other sepsis such as UTI and pneumonia
	Neck pain or stiffness	Meningitis and encephalitis
	Is there any weakness, gait disturbances, imbalance, and sensory deficit?	Stroke or tumor
	Headache and vomiting	Raised ICT-CNS infection, stroke, tumor
	Dizziness or fainting	Hypoperfusion of brain
	Shortness of breath	Hypoxia/hypercarbia
	Dehydration	Shock, electrolyte imbalance, and hypoglycemia
	History of trauma or fall	• Intracranial bleed • Chronic alcohol—slow bleeding even several days after fall • Consider unwitnessed trauma—if patient found unconscious
	Depression or behavior changes	Alcohol/drug abuse or psychiatric problems and suicidal attempt
	Other people with similar illness	Gaseous poisoning, e.g., CO poisoning
A: Allergic history	Any allergic history of or recent exposure to medication/known allergen?	Anaphylaxis
M: Medications history	Current medications history	Gives clue for current illness/side effect/interaction, especially for seizures/convulsions, pain, and sleeping
P: Past history	Diabetes	Hypoglycemia/DKA/HHS
	Heart disease	• Hypoperfusion • Increased risk for stroke
	Stroke	Recurrent stroke/scar seizures
	Hypertension	Stroke/HT encephalopathy
	Seizure disorder	Convulsive/postictal state
	HIV disease	Meningitis and encephalitis
	Tuberculosis (TB)	TB meningitis/tuberculoma
	History of liver or kidney failure?	Hepatic/uremic encephalopathy
	History alcohol abuse?	Alcohol intoxication and alcohol withdrawal/hypoglycemia/head injury
	Any drug abuse?	Opioids, sedatives, and stimulants
	History of pregnancy with HT	Eclampsia (or seizures/convulsions and high blood pressure)

Continued

Continued

	History/Finding	Diagnostic clue
L: Last intake of oral feeds	History of last meal or drink	Hypoglycemia/dehydration/electrolyte imbalance
E: Events during illness	Recent trauma	Head injury/blunt injury abdomen/hypoperfusion
	Recent travel history	Malaria/scrub typhus, etc.
	Recent exposures-contact with a sick person, recent bites, chemical exposures, hot or cold environments, etc.	• *Sick contacts*: Infectious cause • *Chemical exposures*: Pesticides • *Bites*: Snakebite • Hypothermia/heat stroke
	Recent alcohol or drug use?	• Alcohol intoxication/withdrawal • Methamphetamines and cocaine causes agitation • Heroin and other opioids causes lethargy and coma

(CNS: central nervous system; CO: carbon monoxide; DKA: diabetic ketoacidosis; HHS: hyperglycemic hyperosmolar state; HIV: human immunodeficiency virus; HT: hypertension; UTI: urinary tract infection)

VITAL SIGNS

Vital signs are given in **Table 3**.

CENTRAL NERVOUS SYSTEM EXAMINATION

- Assessment of consciousness can be done with using the following assessment scales: GSC (in trauma), AVPU score (in medical emergency settings), or FOUR (full outline of UN responsiveness) score (in intubated patients)
- *Type of breathing*: Hyperventilation (pons/midbrain lesions), apneustic or ataxic (medullary lesion), Cheyne-Stokes (raised ICT and CO poisoning).
- Pinpoint pupils—pontine lesions and opioid overdose
- Dilated pupils—3rd cranial nerve palsy and midbrain lesions
- Nystagmus—cerebellar lesions and alcoholism
- Gaze deviation—seizures and hemispheric/pontine lesions
- Papilledema—raised ICT
- *Motor system examination*: To be done to rule out hemi/paraparesis/plegia.

NEUROIMAGING

- *CT brain*: Indicated in trauma and acute stroke
- *MRI brain*: For better studying of cortical and subcortical structures, white matter lesions, acute infarcts, perilesional edema, and enhancement of leptomeninges
- *CT/MR angiography*: Indicated in basilar artery strokes

TABLE 3: Vital signs.

Variable	Finding	Diagnostic clue
Pulse rate	Bradycardia	Raised ICT and drugs (e.g., clonidine/barbiturates)
	Tachycardia	Intracranial hemorrhage, sepsis, and drugs (e.g., ketamine)
Blood pressure	Hypotension	Sepsis, drug overdosage (e.g., clonidine, tricyclic antidepressants, and sedative-hypnotics)
	Hypertension	Raised ICT, hypertensive encephalopathy, drugs like ketamine, etc.
Respiratory rate	Bradypnea	Brainstem lesions, drugs like opioids, etc.
	Tachypnea	Sepsis, acidosis, and drug overdose
Temperature	Hypothermia	Frostbite, severe sepsis, hypothyroidism, hypoglycemia, sedative-hypnotic drug overdose
	Hyperthermia	Sepsis, heat stroke, subarachnoid hemorrhage, hypothalamic injury, and drugs like salicylates

OTHER INVESTIGATIONS

- Electroencephalogram (EEG)—indicated in seizures and to rule out nonconvulsive status epilepticus
- *Lumbar puncture and cerebrospinal fluid (CSF) analysis*: Indicated in acute CNS infection.

MANAGEMENT

- Treatment of a patient with altered sensorium is mainly based on the initial assessment and underlying etiology.
- Adequate hemodynamic stabilization must be done irrespective of etiology.
- Secure the airway, ensure adequate oxygenation if needed intubate and provide mechanical ventilation.
- In trauma cases, immobilize the patient/body parts to avoid further neurovascular damage.
- Resuscitate with IV fluids and vasopressors in the setting of shock. Blood products may be needed in active bleeding/trauma cases.
- Appropriate antibiotics to be initiated within one hour if sepsis/acute CNS infection suspected.
- Benzodiazepines to be given in case of active seizures and alcohol withdrawal. Magnesium sulfate is the drug of choice in eclampsia.
- In patients with metabolic encephalopathy, the treatment target is to achieve homeostasis, e.g., hypoglycemia to be corrected completely with dextrose, hyponatremia to be corrected partially as per the protocol.
- Follow poison management protocols and give specific antidote in case of any intoxication.
- Intravenous thrombolysis ± endovascular thrombectomy may be indicated in thrombotic stroke.
- Neurosurgical intervention may be needed in raised ICT/structural neurological causes.
- Treat the other causes and comorbidities.

CONCLUSION

Altered sensorium in the ICU is very common and etiologies are numerous, ranging from reversible to irreversible, medical, or surgical causes. Systematic approach is needed to identify the cause and manage appropriately. This can reduce morbidity and mortality. All cases presenting with altered sensorium should be managed with initial hemodynamic stabilization, followed by the treatment of underlying etiology and comorbidities.

SUGGESTED READINGS

1. World Health Organization. WHO-ICRC Basic Emergency Care: Approach to the Acutely Ill and Injured. Geneva: World Health Organization and the International Committee of the Red Cross; 2018.
2. Singhal V. Clinical Approach to Acute Decline in Sensorium. Indian J Crit Care Med. 2019;23(Suppl 2):S120-3.
3. Cetin M, Oktem B, Canakci ME. Altered Mental Status. [online] Available from https://iem-student.org/altered-mental-status/. [Last accessed December, 2023].
4. Morrissey T. (2008). Approach to Altered Mental Status. [online] Available from https://www.saem.org/about-saem/academies-interest-groups-affiliates2/cdem/for-students/online-education/m4-curriculum/group-m4-approach-to/approach-to-altered-mental-status. [Last accessed December, 2023].

30

CHAPTER

Critical Care Nephrology: Role of Nephrologist in ICU

Jaisuresh K, V Palaniappan

ABSTRACT

Critical care nephrology or intensive care nephrology is a core subspecialty in the practice of nephrology. The advent of advanced critical care units and multiorgan transplant programs has expanded the role of nephrologist in intensive care units (ICU). Critically ill patients with or without preexisting renal disease may require nephrology consultation for renal protection, renal support and/or renal replacement therapy (RRT). This chapter summarizes the various scenarios where the renal system needs to be monitored and intervened appropriately.

INTRODUCTION

Nephrologist in a critical care team contributes to establishing vascular access, fluid electrolyte management, correction of acid–base abnormalities, detection and management of acute kidney injury (AKI), selection of medications, dosing of medications, removal of toxins through extracorporeal therapies, and administering renal replacement therapy (RRT).

ACUTE KIDNEY INJURY IN INTENSIVE CARE UNIT

The most common causes of AKI in intensive care unit (ICU) include: (1) sepsis, (2) postcardiac surgery, (3) acute liver failure, (4) intra-abdominal hypertension, (5) hepatorenal syndrome, (6) malignancy, and (7) cardiorenal syndrome. In most of the scenarios, more than one factor may contribute to the occurrence of AKI (Multifactorial AKI). A detailed history must be obtained to enumerate all the possible antecedent triggers (drugs, toxins, and dehydration), preexisting systemic ailments, history of any AKI in the past and/or preexisting chronic kidney disease. Often, removal and treatment of inciting agent is the most important step in avoiding renal injury as well as achieving renal recovery.

- Sepsis-associated AKI is defined as AKI that occurs within 7 days of sepsis onset. Sepsis-associated AKI is a multifactorial AKI due to sepsis, other contributing causes of AKI (hypovolemia, drugs, and cardiac failure) and its therapeutic measures. Sepsis-induced AKI is defined as AKI due to immunopathological changes caused "directly" by sepsis. Sepsis-induced AKI is a subset of sepsis-associated AKI. Almost 50% percent of AKI In ICU is due to sepsis. AKI occurs in 10–20% of patients with sepsis and 50–70% of patients with septic shock. The pathophysiology involves microvascular injury, endothelial dysfunction, inflammation, complement activation, renin–angiotensin–aldosterone system (RAAS) dysfunction, oxidative stress, and ischemia.
    - Postcardiac surgery AKI is usually multifactorial. Extracorporeal circuit-related hemolysis may contribute to AKI in these situations.
    - In acute liver failure, renal hypoperfusion, renal vasoconstriction, and direct tubular injury (drugs and toxins) contribute to the occurrence of AKI.
    - Intra-abdominal hypertension is defined as intra-abdominal pressure >12 mm Hg. The causes could be trauma, postabdominal surgeries, massive ascites, ileus, and acute pancreatitis. Excessive

abdominal pressure leads to renal venous pressure elevation and renal parenchymal pressure elevation causing AKI.
- Hepatorenal syndrome is due to intrarenal vasoconstriction without structural renal damage.
- Malignancy-associated AKI is often multifactorial. Cast nephropathy, thrombotic microangiopathy, chemotherapy-associated nephrotoxicity, and lymphomatous infiltration of kidneys are specifically seen causes of AKI in patients with malignancy.
- Cardiorenal syndrome type 1, 3, and 5 presents as AKI. Type 1 is acute cardiac dysfunction leading to AKI. Type 3 is cardiac dysfunction secondary to acute decrease of kidney function and type 5 is systemic process like sepsis resulting in cardiac and kidney dysfunction. Reduced systolic function leads to renal hypoperfusion and venous congestion.

Acute kidney injury-induced complications including volume overload, acidemia, hyperkalemia, hyperphosphatemia and hypocalcemia must be anticipated and appropriately managed. Volume overload is an independent marker of poor patient outcomes. In addition, patient may have uremia-related complications such as encephalopathy and pericarditis, which can confound with the presentation of underlying primary disease.

When patients require dialysis the mode of RRT must be based on clinical scenario, anticoagulants which can be used and the expertise of the technical team available. It is essential to ensure that adequate solute clearances are achieved, adequate volume removal is done, filter-circuit patency is maintained, and hemodynamic stability is maintained through-out the dialysis sessions.

FLUID AND ELECTROLYTE BALANCE

Intravenous (IV) fluids can be used as resuscitation fluids (correct intravascular volume deficit), replacement fluids (correct deficits that cannot be treated by oral replacement alone) or maintenance fluids (provide daily requirements in hemodynamically stable patients with poor oral intake). "Fluid creep" refers to fluids administered as drug diluents and catheter patency maintaining solutions. In AKI patients, fluid creep must also be considered during evaluation of volume status.

Fluids with electrolyte composition close to plasma are called as "balanced" solutions (Ringer's lactate, Hartmann's solution and Plasmalyte). Administration of 0.9% sodium chloride in large volumes leads to hyperchloremic metabolic acidosis. Hyperchloremia in critically ill patients is associated with AKI, metabolic acidosis, increased morbidity, and mortality. Balanced solutions with low chloride content can avoid the occurrence of these complications.

Hemodynamic management of sepsis-associated AKI is same as the sepsis recommendations given by surviving sepsis guidelines. The initial resuscitation fluid recommended is 0.9% saline. Further choice of fluid can be based on the need for electrolyte and acid-base correction. Albumin and sodium bicarbonate are administered for correction of volume status and acidosis. The ALBIOS study showed that correction of serum albumin to >30 g/L has survival benefit in septic shock patients. Diuretics are recommended for volume overload states. Noradrenaline is the preferred vasopressors in AKI patients. Certain special situations may warrant the use of vasopressin, midodrine, terlipressin, or octreotide.

Cumulative positive fluid balance is detrimental to critically ill patients. Deresuscitation or de-escalation refers to aggressive and active fluid removal using diuretics or ultrafiltration (RRT). De-escalation of IV fluid therapy after initial resuscitation and stabilization has been shown to be associated with better outcomes.

OPTIMIZING ANTIMICROBIAL DOSING IN ACUTE KIDNEY INJURY

Optimal dose of antimicrobials in critically ill patients is a challenging task. Achieving therapeutic blood levels is vital with the understanding that supra and sub-therapeutic levels can lead unfavorable outcomes. In the first 48 hours of admission, fluid replacements lead to increased volume of distribution. The creatinine clearance calculations are validated only in patients with stable renal functions. Hence, it is recommended that antibiotic dosing need not be changed in the first 48 hours of ICU admission. Recommended full dose of IV antibiotics on admission includes aminoglycosides (amikacin 15 mg/kg, gentamicin 5 mg/kg), beta-lactams (IV piperacillin/tazobactam 4.5 g IV three times a day, amoxicillin/clavulanate 1.2 g three times a day, meropenem 1–2 g three times a day) and fluoroquinolones in their usual doses. After 48 hours, dose modification is done based on renal function, volume of distribution (edema), and RRT. Whenever possible, drug level monitoring is the ideal method to decide appropriate dosage.

TOXICOLOGY

Alkalinization of urine can enhance renal excretion of salicylates. IV sodium bicarbonate is administered 1–2 mEq/kg over a period of 3–4 hours with a target urine pH of ≥7.5. Serum potassium needs to be monitored and corrected during alkalinization therapy. Established renal failure is a contraindication to urine alkalinization.

Extracorporeal therapies include hemodialysis, hemofiltration, hemoperfusion, continuous RRTs and therapeutic plasma exchange. Hemodialysis is used to remove toxins such as salicylates, lithium, methanol, ethylene glycol, and isopropanol. Significant neurological symptoms, severe acidosis, and cardiovascular instability are the most common indications to start hemodialysis.

Plasma exchange uses hemodialysis machine coupled with plasma filter. The filtered plasma is replaced with fresh frozen plasma, albumin, or other fluids. Plasma exchange is used to remove high molecular weight hydrophilic and lipophilic substances such as amatoxins (mushroom type), plant toxins (ricin), heavy metals, and highly protein-bound drugs. Hemoperfusion cartridges fitted to dialysis circuits are used to adsorb specific lipid soluble drugs or toxins such as phenobarbital, phenytoin, carbamazepine, and paraquat.

VASCULAR ACCESS

Before placing vascular access, nephrologist must consider the required blood flows, size of dialysis catheter (length, diameter), lumens (double or triple) available for use, and choose appropriate site for dialysis catheter placement. Internal jugular and femoral veins are the preferred sites for placement of dialysis catheters. Subclavian vein is avoided due to increased incidence of central venous stenosis. The nephrologist should also guide the nursing team on appropriate ways to handle the catheter for maintaining patency and life of catheters. After each dialysis session, the catheter needs to be locked with heparin or trisodium citrate solution to maintain patency. It is essential to follow the standard protocols for prevention of dialysis catheter-related blood stream infections.

RENAL REPLACEMENT THERAPY

In critically ill patients, RRT helps to restore fluid, electrolyte, and acid–base balance. RRT is used in the form of renal support to maintain edema-free state, allows large-volume replacements, rapid correction of electrolyte abnormalities, and toxin removal. Administration of RRT involves a multidisciplinary team involving nephrologist, critical care consultants, dialysis technicians, and ICU nurses. Effective coordination is required to choose the best modality of RRT and to administer it appropriately **(Table 1)**. Nephrologist shall ensure adequate fluid removal, electrolyte correction,

TABLE 1: Summary of RRT options in ICU.

Modality	Duration	Principle	Clearance	Flow rates	Advantages	Disadvantages
IHD	3.5–4.5 hours	Diffusion ultrafiltration	Small molecules (<500 Da)	QB > 300 ml/min QD > 500 mL/min	Rapid solute and volume removal Rapid correction of acidosis and hyperkalemia	Hypotension CNS disequilibrium
SCUF	Up to 24 hours per day	Ultrafiltration	No solute clearance	QB 50–200 mL/min	Removes fluid only	No solute removal
SLED	6–8 hours	Diffusion Ultrafiltration	Small molecules	QB 100–200 ml/min QD 100–200 mL/min	Cost effective than CRRT Patient mobility Excellent toxin removal	Higher starting cost than IHD
CRRT: Three types 1. CVVH 2. CVVHD 3. CVVHDF	Continuous		Small and Middle molecules (500–15,000 Da)	QB 50–200 mL/min	Hemodynamic stability is better Middle molecule clearance	Larger dose of anticoagulation in all forms of CRRT Cost Trained personnel required Restricts patient mobility
CRRT-CVVH	Continuous	Convection ultrafiltration		---		Needs replacement fluid
CRRT-CVVHD	Continuous	Diffusion		QD < 50 mL/min		
CRRT-CVVHDF	Continuous	Diffusion Convection		QD < 50 mL/min		Needs replacement fluid

(CRRT: continuous renal replacement therapy; CVVH: continuous venovenous hemofiltration; CVVHD: continuous venovenous hemodialysis; CVVHDF: continuous venovenous hemodiafiltration; CNS: central nervous system; ICU: intensive care unit; IHD: intermittent hemodialysis; QB: blood flow rate, QD: dialysis flow rate; RRT: renal replacement therapy; SCUF: slow continuous ultrafiltration; SLED: sustained low-efficiency dialysis) filter-circuit life, and correction of uremic parameters. Further, it is important to decide the type and dose of anticoagulant depending on the clinical profile of the patient. Apart from initiation, nephrologist shall also decide on maintenance and discontinuation of RRT procedures. It is recommended that RRT units have a review process for recording and analysis of safety events.

CONCLUSION

The role of nephrologist in an ICU includes risk assessment, recognition of renal problems, staging of renal ailments, providing renal support, renal replacement, and rehabilitation. As part of critical care team, nephrologist shall understand the renal perspectives of critical care literature and collaborate with all healthcare personnel involved in treatment of critically ill patients.

SUGGESTED READINGS

1. Zarbock A, Nadim MK, Pickkers P, et al. Sepsis-associated acute kidney injury: consensus report of the 28th Acute Disease Quality Initiative workgroup. Nat Rev Nephrol. 2023;19:401-17.
2. Hughes S, Heard KL, Mughal N, Moore LSP. Optimization of antimicrobial dosing in patients with acute kidney injury: a single-centre observational study. JAC Antimicrob Resist. 2022;4(4).

31

CHAPTER

Nutrition in Critically Ill Patients

Gagan Gunjan, Nilanjan Mal

ABSTRACT

The nutritional requirements of critically ill patients are not well comprehended and can vary depending on the stage of critical illness. The occurrence of malnutrition in critically ill patients has been observed to be between 38 and 78%. The critical illness has three phases: (i) Acute, (ii) postacute, and (iii) rehabilitation/chronic phase. The acute phase has an early and late stage, with great possibility of fatality. There are two main modes of providing nutrition, namely enteral and parenteral. Enteral nutrition (EN) is typically initiated when patients are relatively stable in terms of hemodynamics. Parenteral mode involves providing early nutritional support through intravenous (IV) administration to patients who are unable to receive EN due to absolute or relative contraindications. Providing appropriate nutrition support is crucial for critically ill patients in order to influence the trajectory and outcome of their critical illness. It is important to regularly monitor and adjust the nutritional interventions based on the patient's condition and response.

INTRODUCTION

The nutritional requirements of critically ill patients are not well comprehended and can vary depending on the stage of critical illness. Although randomized trials have not provided sufficient evidence regarding outcomes, the primary objective of nutrition support is to influence the trajectory and outcome of the critical illness.

Carbohydrates are considered the preferred source of energy during this period due to impaired fat mobilization. Protein prescriptions are based on the aim of reducing the breakdown of muscle proteins into amino acids, which subsequently serve as substrates for gluconeogenesis, leading to a favorable nitrogen balance.

EVALUATION OF NUTRITIONAL STATUS

The occurrence of malnutrition in critically ill patients has been observed to be between 38 and 78%, and it is linked independently to extended intensive care unit (ICU) stays, higher rates of ICU readmission, increased infection incidence, and elevated hospital mortality. Various approaches exist to assess nutritional status, including the nutrition risk in critically ill (NUTRIC) score, nutrition risk screening (NRS) 2002, and subjective global assessment (SGA). However, it is important to note that none of these methods are flawless or perfect in their assessment.

Adapting to Phases of Critical Illness

The critical illness has three phases: (i) Acute, (ii) postacute, and (iii) rehabilitation/chronic phase. The acute phase has an early and late stage, with the possibility of fatality. The postacute phase is a recovery phase lasting over 7 days, where macronutrient supply is crucial. Patients may not meet their calorie requirements orally and may need a combination of oral, enteral, and parenteral feeding. After recovery, there is a rehabilitation phase lasting months to repair initial metabolic damage. Alternatively, the post acute phase can merge into a chronic phase with persistent organ dysfunction and an uncertain prognosis.

ASSESSMENT OF ENERGY REQUIREMENT

When determining the appropriate caloric and protein intake for enteral or parenteral nutrition (PN) in critically ill patients, it is crucial to establish the dosing weight. This can be achieved by considering the individual's resting energy expenditure (REE) or body weight. Indirect calorimetry and predictive equations are commonly used to estimate the REE in this population.

Here are some recommendations based on different scenarios:

- *Underweight patients [body mass index (BMI) < 18.5 kg/m²]*: For patients who are underweight, it is suggested to use their current weight as the initial dosing weight. Calculating caloric intake based on ideal body weight (IBW) could result in excessive initial calories, potentially triggering refeeding syndrome. Once the patient stabilizes, calories may be increased to promote weight gain.
- *Normal or overweight patients (BMI 18.5–29.9 kg/m²)*: For patients with a normal weight or who are overweight, using their current weight as the dosing weight is recommended. Efforts should be made to estimate and subtract the weight of any peripheral edema.
- *Obese patients (BMI ≥ 30 kg/m²)*: Guidelines suggest using the current weight and the Penn State University 2010 predictive equation for dosing weight determination. If neither expertise with this equation nor calorimetry is available, adjusting the dosing weight is suggested. The most commonly used method involves adding 0.4 times the difference between the IBW and the actual body weight (ABW) to the IBW. An alternative method is to use 110% of the IBW.

Calories Requirements

In the critically ill patient receiving appropriate treatment, energy expenditure is generally equivalent to REE. A conservative starting point for caloric intake in most critically ill patients is around 8–10 kcal/kg/day. After 1 week, it is reasonable to aim for a target of 25–30 kcal/kg of dosing weight per day for stable patients. This progressive increase in calorie intake allows for adaptation and adjustment as the patient's condition stabilizes. Associated non-nutritional calories should also be counted to improve accuracy.

MACRONUTRIENT REQUIREMENTS

Carbohydrates

The recommended daily energy intake from carbohydrates is approximately 45–65%. When carbohydrates are oxidized, they provide 4 kcal/g, while intravenous (IV) dextrose monohydrate provides 3.4 kcal/g. To maintain proper central nervous system function, it is necessary to provide around 120 g/day of exogenous glucose. It is recommended to administer glucose at a rate of 3–4 mg/kg/min or approximately 50–60% of the total energy requirements in critically ill patients.

Measurement of respiratory quotient (RQ) using indirect calorimetry can provide insights into macronutrient utilization. An RQ value > 1 indicates lipogenesis and excessive carbohydrate administration. Currently, it is recommended to maintain blood glucose levels between 140 and 180 mg/dL.

Protein

In critically ill patients, catabolism is highest in the early phase and gradually decreases, but the optimal timing of protein intake remains uncertain. Recent clinical practice guidelines generally suggest higher protein intake (> 1.2 g/kg of ABW per day) for critically ill patients compared to healthy individuals. Higher protein intake is typically recommended in the later phase of illness. For metabolically stressed patients with a BMI < 30 kg/m², protein requirements should range from 1.2 to 2 g/kg of ABW per day. Patients with severe sepsis and burns often require up to 2.5–3 g/kg of protein per day. Protein plays a crucial role in the synthesis of enzymes involved in wound healing, cell proliferation, collagen formation, and connective tissue formation.

Lipids

Fat should contribute to approximately 15–30% of the total calorie intake. Essential fatty acids should account for 2–4% of the total calories. The recommended maximum amount of fat is 2.5 g/kg/day or < 60% of the total calories. Fat serves as a significant fuel source, providing 9 cal/g. Intravenous lipid emulsions (IVLEs) contain an emulsifier that adds extra calories (10 cal/g).

MICRONUTRIENTS AND ANTIOXIDANTS

There have been numerous studies on micronutrient therapy in critically ill patients. Deficiencies in micronutrients are common in this population. However, recent studies have not shown significant benefits. For instance, in the REDOXS trial, antioxidants did not affect 28-day mortality or other secondary outcomes. As per the 2018 European Society of Enteral and Parenteral Nutrition (ESPEN) recommendation, high-dose antioxidants such as copper, selenium, and zinc, and electrolytes such as potassium, magnesium, and phosphate should be monitored at least once a day during the first 7 days. In patients with refeeding hypophosphatemia (phosphate

TABLE 1: Micronutrients and antioxidants role in nutrition of critically ill.

Substrate	DGEM	ESPEN	ASPEN
Micronutrients	A patient should receive vitamins and trace elements, if EN cannot meet daily needs, and if supplemental PN is required	To enable substrate metabolism, micronutrients (i.e., trace elements and vitamins) should be provided daily with PN	N/A
Vitamin D	Patients may receive a pharmacotherapy with vitamin D if they have a severe deficiency (25-hydroxy-vitamin D ≤ 30 nmol/L corresponding to 12 ng/mL)	In critically ill patients with low plasma levels (25-hydroxy-vitamin D < 12.5 ng/mL, or 50 nmol/L), a high dose of vitamin D3 can be administered within a week	N/A
Antioxidants/ selenium	Patients shall not receive a pharmacotherapy with selenium	Patients should not routinely receive a pharmacotherapy with zinc, alpha-tocopherol, vitamins A and C, or a combination of those	We suggest providing a combination of antioxidant vitamins and trace minerals to patients who require therapy. We cannot make a recommendation regarding selenium supplementation in sepsis due to conflicting studies

(ASPEN: American Society for Parenteral and Enteral Nutrition; DGEM: German Society for Nutritional Medicine; EN: enteral nutrition; ESPEN: European Society of Enteral and Parenteral Nutrition; PN: parenteral nutrition)

< 0.65 mmol/L), electrolyte levels should be measured two to three times a day and supplemented as necessary **(Table 1)**.

MODES OF PROVIDING NUTRITION

There are two main modes of providing nutrition, namely enteral and parenteral.

Enteral Nutrition

This mode of nutrition is typically initiated when patients are relatively stable in terms of hemodynamics, including those who are being weaned off or receiving modest vasopressor support.

Access

Enteral nutrition (EN) is commonly delivered into the stomach (gastric feeding), but it can also be administered into more distal parts of the digestive tract (postpyloric) for patients who are intolerant to gastric EN, such as those with delayed gastric emptying or gastric outlet obstruction.

Amount and Rate

The daily amount of EN is tailored to meet the nutritional and fluid needs of each patient. A reasonable initial calorie goal is in the range of 18–25 kcal/kg/day for critically ill patients of normal weight. Typically, enteral feeding is initiated at a rate of 10–30 mL/hour (for standard enteral formulations), known as "trophic" feeding, for 6 days, and then gradually increased to reach the target rate. It is common practice to initiate feeds at 25–30% of the estimated goal rate.

Contraindications

According to the European Society of Intensive Care Medicine (ESICM) clinical practice guidelines, contraindications for EN include hemodynamic instability (escalation of or high vasopressor medication and increased lactate) and gastrointestinal (GI) intolerance, ranging from minor to major symptoms such as gastric residual volume (GRV) exceeding 500 mL/6 h or acute GI injury grade higher than 2.

Parenteral Nutrition

This mode involves providing early nutritional support through IV administration to patients who are unable to receive EN due to absolute or relative contraindications.

The ESPEN guideline suggests that PN should only be initiated after all efforts to maximize EN tolerance have been attempted. In patients who cannot tolerate full-dose EN during the first week in the ICU, the decision to initiate PN should be carefully evaluated on a case-to-case basis, considering the safety and potential benefits. According to the guidelines, patients at low nutrition risk should not receive PN during the first 7 days following ICU admission unless EN is contraindicated. However, in severely malnourished or high-risk patients, early and progressive PN should be considered if EN is not feasible. Malnourished patients often experience GI dysfunctions, making PN a preferred route of nutrition in such cases, as stated in the guidelines.

Access

When PN is administered for an extended period, it requires a central venous catheter for delivery due to its high osmotic load, known as central parenteral nutrition (CPN). However, if the solution is significantly more dilute (< 900 mOsm), it can be delivered through a peripheral vein, referred to as peripheral PN.

Timing

The optimal timing for initiating PN in critically ill patients is uncertain. However, recent evidence suggests that earlier initiation of PN during the ICU stay is safe **(Table 2)**.

NUTRITION IN SPECIFIC SITUATIONS

Hepatic Disease

In dietary intervention trials for liver cirrhosis, a calorie intake of at least 35 kcal/kg actual body weight (ABW) per day is commonly recommended. Using genuine body weight corrected for ascites is considered safe. Frequent feeding, such as having a protein-containing breakfast and a late-night snack, is advised to prevent increased hunger and associated proteolysis. Normal to high protein intake does not precipitate hepatic encephalopathy (HE) and may even benefit mental health.

Renal Diseases

Acute kidney injury (AKI) is characterized by increased protein catabolism where protein synthesis and amino acid transport into skeletal muscle are impaired, leading to a hypercatabolic state. Renal replacement therapy (RRT) further contributes to protein loss and the breakdown of body proteins due to inflammatory mediators. Caloric intake for patients with renal diseases should be around 25–30 kcal/kg/day. Specialized formulas low in potassium and phosphate are recommended.

Central Nervous System Diseases

Critically ill patients with central nervous diseases, such as head trauma, stroke, and spinal trauma, require specific nutritional support. Stroke patients are at risk of malnutrition, dehydration, and aspiration pneumonia due to impaired swallowing and cognitive deficits. Postpyloric tubes, elevated head position and prokinetics should be considered for patients at risk of aspiration. PN is an option for patients with preexisting malnutrition or inadequate EN.

Cardiac Diseases

Critically ill patients with cardiac diseases often suffer from malnutrition, cachexia, and sarcopenia. Regular

TABLE 2: Enteral versus parenteral nutrition.

Enteral nutrition	Parenteral nutrition
When patients have problems with eating or digestion, it is sometimes necessary to provide nutrition via an alternative route with food which is specially formulated to provide the right balance of fats, proteins, sugars, vitamins and minerals. Enteral feeding is the delivery of a special liquid food mixture through a feeding tube into the stomach or small intestine	It is generally preferrable to use enteral nutrition, but there are times when that is not possible. When a person is not able to receive enough calories or cannot adequately absorb nutrients through the gut, nutrition can be given directly into the bloodstream. Parenteral nutrition is a sterile liquid chemical formula given directly into the bloodstream through an intravenous (IV) catheter
Delivery location: Enteral nutrition can be given through different types of tubes. Tubes can be placed through the nose, into the stomach, or even directly into the small intestine	*Delivery location*: Parenteral nutrition can be irritating to small veins, therefore, it is often delivered through a central catheter. A central catheter is a long tube which may be inserted in the arm ar chest. The end of the catheter is located in the large blood vessel above the heart
Delivery mechanism: Enteral nutrition can be delivered using gravity drip bags, syringes, enternal feeding pumps, or even by using a combination of methods	*Delivery mechanism*: Parenteral nutrition requires slow and controlled delivery using either a pole mounted or ambulatory infusion pump
Who gets enteral nutrition? People of all age, from infants, to young children, to adults, can be given enteral nutritions. Enteral nutrition can be administered as long as it is needed. When it is no longer needed, the patient's feeding tube is removed	*Who gets parenteral nutrition*? Parenteral nutrition is administered to People of all ages, infants through adults. People can live on parenteral nutrition for as long as necessary, and it is discontinued when no longer medically necessary
Statistics: According to Nationwide Inpatient Survey (NIS) statistics, patents received enteral feeding in over 250,000 hospital stays. It estimated that over 400,000 patients receive enteral nutrition at home	*Statistics*: According to the 2014 National Inpatient Survey data, patients received short-term parenteral nutrition in over 290,000 hospital stays. It is estimated that about 25,000 patients receive parenteral at home

nutritional screenings are necessary for high-risk patients. Energy-dense formulas are recommended due to fluctuations in volume status. For patients with mechanical assist devices, EN is preferred if hemodynamically stable.

Respiratory Diseases

Critically ill patients with respiratory diseases may benefit from formulas with increased fat content and reduced carbohydrates to influence CO_2 production. However, evidence for their use in acute respiratory failure is lacking. Hyperalimentation should be avoided to prevent increased CO_2 production. EN is contraindicated in patients with life-threatening hypoxia, hypercapnia, and acidosis but can be initiated in stable respiratory failure. EN can be given to patients in prone position, and a 30° head elevation may improve tolerance and prevent aspiration.

Shock and Acute Gastrointestinal Injury

Enteral nutrition may not be suitable for patients with shock on high-dose vasopressors or severe GI injury (e.g., severe ileus, vomiting, high GRV, and intra-abdominal hypertension) as it can potentially cause harm. Therefore, EN should be delayed in these conditions.

CONCLUSION

In conclusion, providing appropriate nutrition support is crucial for critically ill patients in order to influence the trajectory and outcome of their critical illness. The nutritional requirements can vary depending on the stage of illness, and it is important to assess the nutritional status using various methods. Determining the appropriate caloric and protein intake requires considering the patient's weight status and avoiding complications associated with excessive or inadequate nutrition support.

Enteral nutrition is commonly initiated when patients are relatively stable, while PN is used when EN is not feasible. Overall, providing appropriate nutrition support tailored to the specific needs of critically ill patients can contribute to improved outcomes and recovery. It is important to regularly monitor and adjust the nutritional interventions based on the patient's condition and response.

SUGGESTED READINGS

1. Maday KR. The importance of nutrition in critically ill patients. JAAPA. 2017;30:32-7.
2. Lew CCH, Yandell R, Fraser RJL, Chua AP, Chong MFF, Miller M. Association between malnutrition and clinical outcomes in the intensive care unit: a systematic review. JPEN J Parenter Enteral Nutr. 2017;41(5):744-58.
3. Lee ZY, Heyland DK. Determination of nutrition risk and status in critically ill patients: what are our considerations? Nutr Clin Pract. 2019;34(1):96-111.
4. Kondrup J, Rasmussen HH, Hamberg O, Stanga Z; Ad Hoc ESPEN Working Group. Nutritional risk screening (NRS 2002): a new method based on an analysis of controlled clinical trials. Clin Nutr. 2003;22(3):321-36.
5. Detsky A, McLaughlin JR, Baker J, Johnston N, Whittaker S, Mendelson RA, et al. What is subjective global assessment of nutritional status? J Parenter Enteral Nutr. 1987;11(1):8-13.
6. Gonzalez-Granda A, Schollenberger A, Haap M, Riessen R, Bischoff SC. Optimization of Nutrition Therapy with the Use of Calorimetry to Determine and Control Energy Needs in Mechanically Ventilated Critically Ill Patients: The ONCA Study, a Randomized, Prospective Pilot Study. JPEN J Parenter Enteral Nutr. 2019;43:481-9.
7. McClave SA, Taylor BE, Martindale RG, Warren MM, Johnson DR, Braunschweig C, et al. Guidelines for the provision and assessment of nutrition support therapy in the adult critically ill patient: Society of Critical care Medicine (SCCM) and American Society for Parenteral and Enteral Nutrition (A.S.P.E.N.). JPEN J Parenter Enteral Nutr. 2016;40:159-211.
8. Charriere M, Ridley E, Hastings J, Bianchet O, Scheinkestel C, Berger MM. Propofol sedation substantially increases the caloric and lipid intake in critically ill patients. Nutrition. 2017;42:64-8.
9. National Heart, Lung, and Blood Institute Acute Respiratory Distress Syndrome (ARDS) Clinical Trials Network; Rice TW, Wheeler AP, Thompson BT, Steingrub J, Hite RD, Moss M, et al. Initial trophic vs full enteral feeding in patients with acute lung injury: the EDEN randomized trial. JAMA. 2012;307:795-803.
10. Ferrie S, Allman-Farinelli M, Daley M, Smith K. Protein Requirements in the Critically Ill: A Randomized Controlled Trial Using Parenteral Nutrition. JPEN J Parenter Enteral Nutr. 2016;40:795-805.
11. US Food and Drug Administration. (2013). FDA approves Clinolipid for intravenous nutrition. [online] Available from http://www.fda.gov/NewsEvents/Newsroom/PressAnnouncements/ucm370740.htm. [Last accessed December, 2023].
12. Mueller C. The A.S.P.E.N. Adult Nutrition Support Core Curriculum, 2nd edition. Silver Spring, Maryland, US: American Society for Parenteral and Enteral Nutrition; 2012.
13. Weimann A, Braga M, Carli F, Higashiguchi T, Hubner M, Klek S, et al. ESPEN practical guideline: Clinical nutrition in surgery. Clin. Nutr. 2021;40:4745-61.
14. Yang S, Wu X, Yu W, Li J. Early enteral nutrition in critically ill patients with hemodynamic instability: An evidence-based review and practical advice. Nutr Clin Pract. 2014;29:90-6.
15. McClave SA, Taylor BE, Martindale RG, Warren MM, Johnson DR, Braunschweig C, et al. Guidelines for the provision and assessment of nutrition support therapy in the adult critically ill patient: Society of Critical care Medicine (SCCM) and American Society for Parenteral and Enteral Nutrition (A.S.P.E.N.) JPEN J Parenter Enteral Nutr. 2016;40:159-211.

16. Reintam Blaser A, Starkopf J, Alhazzani W, Berger MM, Casaer MP, Deane AM, et al. Early enteral nutrition in critically ill patients: ESICM clinical practice guidelines. Intensive Care Med. 2017;43:380-98.
17. Elke G, Hartl WH, Kreymann KG, Adolph M, Felbinger TW, Graf T, et al. Clinical Nutrition in Critical Care Medicine—Guideline of the German Society for Nutritional Medicine (DGEM) Clin Nutr ESPEN. 2019;33:220-75.
18. Singer P, Blaser AR, Berger MM, Alhazzani W, Calder PC, Casaer M, et al. ESPEN guideline on clinical nutrition in the intensive care unit. Clin Nutr. 2018;38:48-79.
19. Amodio P, Bemeur C, Butterworth R, Cordoba J, Kato A, Montagnese S, et al. The nutritional management of hepatic encephalopathy in patients with cirrhosis: International Society for Hepatic Encephalopathy and Nitrogen Metabolism Consensus. Hepatology. 2013;58(1):325-36.
20. Nielsen K, Kondrup J, Martinsen L, Stilling B, Wikman B. Nutritional assessment and adequacy of dietary intake in hospitalized patients with alcoholic liver cirrhosis. Br J Nutr. 1993;69:665-79.
21. Ikizler TA, Burrowes JD, Byham-Gray LD, Campbell KL, Carrero JJ, Chan W, et al. KDOQI Clinical Practice Guideline for Nutrition in CKD: 2020 Update. Am J Kidney Dis. 2020;76:S1-S107.
22. Volkert D, Bauer JM, Frühwald T, Gehrke I, Lechleitner M, Lenzen-Großimlinghaus R, et al. Leitlinie der Deutschen Gesellschaft für Ernährungsmedizin (DGEM) in Zusammenarbeit mit der GESKES, der AKE, der DGN und der DGG. Aktuelle Ernährungsmedizin. 2013;38:e1-e48.

32
CHAPTER

Risk Assessment of Pulmonary Embolism in Critically Ill

Akshaykumar Chhallani, Sheila Nainan Myatra

ABSTRACT

Pulmonary embolism (PE) is a potentially fatal form of venous thromboembolic disease in intensive care unit (ICU) patients. A few risk factors have been associated with PE in the critically ill. It is crucial to identify specific factors which may predict the occurrence of PE. It will help in early detection and well-timed prompt treatment. Mechanical ventilation, blood transfusion, sepsis, emergency admission, inotropes, and vasopressor requirements seem to be the risk factors for PE in ICU. Rapid and accurate risk stratification is, therefore, of paramount importance to ensure the highest quality of care. Appropriately assessing these factors in timely manner will help the clinicians to predict, change the strategies, and treat PE.

INTRODUCTION

Pulmonary embolism (PE) is the leading cause of cardiovascular death in the United States of America (USA). Annually, approximately 10,000-180,000 deaths occur in the USA as per estimates from Surgeon General. PE is said to be the most common cause of in-hospital preventable deaths.

Venous thromboembolism (VTE) represents one of the most common unsuspected autopsy findings in critically ill. Delay in thromboprophylaxis is associated with increased morbidity and mortality in intensive care unit (ICU) patients. Inadequate risk assessment predicts the VTE events, highlighting the need for rapid and near-accurate risk assessment; hence, it is imperative to identify the subset of critically ill patients who had risk of developing VTE.

SCORING AND IMPORTANCE

Scoring in critically and noncritically ill is not the same. Critically ill patients on mechanical ventilation or with cardiorespiratory failure will decompensate very fast once they have VTE events. It may be life-threatening.

Varied scoring systems are used to assess the risk of VTE in a patient.

Padua Prediction Score, the Geneva Risk Score, Improve Risk Score, and Wells score had been studied in medical patients but still do not cover all the risk factors of critically ill patients **(Table 1)**.

Various risk factors for VTE such as CVC (central venous catheter), sepsis, septic shock, mechanical ventilatory support, and need for blood transfusion, which is commonly seen in critically ill patients, were not considered in the above scoring systems. The coronavirus disease 2019 (COVID-19) appears to be a risk factor for deep venous thrombosis (DVT) and PE. Although part of the risk may be due to reduced mobility associated with illness, it is thought that severe acute respiratory syndrome coronavirus 2 (SARS-CoV-2) infection is a prothrombotic condition.

In addition, all these scores help to guide thromboprophylaxis, but it does not take into account hemorrhagic risk.

Due to the complex heterogenicity (medical, surgical, cardiac, and respiratory) of ICU patient population, it is not easy to identify exactly which critically ill patients are at risk of VTE. There are no risk stratification scores that

TABLE 1: Scoring system.

Factors	Padua Prediction Score	The Geneva Risk Score (revised)	Improve and IMPROVEDD Risk score
Previous VTE	✓	✓	✓
Malignancy	✓	✓	✓
Mobility	✓		✓ Paralysis
Thrombophilia	✓		✓
Age	✓ 70	✓ 65	✓
Hemoptysis	✓	✓	
Surgery or fracture within 1 month	✓	✓	
Unilateral lower limb swelling	✓	✓	
Obesity	✓ BMI > 30		
Ongoing hormonal treatment	✓		
Pain on palpitation	✓	✓	
Heart/respiratory failure	✓		
D-dimer			✓
ICU admission			✓
Heart rate		✓ 75–94 bpm	
Mechanical ventilation	×	×	×
Blood /Blood product transfusion	×	×	×
Vasopressor/ Inotropes	×	×	×
Acute kidney injury	×	×	×

(BMI: body mass index; ICU: intensive care unit; VTE: venous thromboembolism)

are specifically designed and validated for critically ill patients.

The complex 30-item Caprini model applied in PROF-ETEV trial (Garcia-Olivarez et al, 2014) for risk stratification of 777 ICU patients, calculated that 83% of these patients fell into the "very high-risk" category (8.5–11.6% in-hospital incidence of VTE).

This was not critically ill or ICU specific, but has relatively good validity in the ICU population so far as lower scores are associated with a lower risk of VTE, and higher risks are associated with higher risk, but still, it does not serve the purpose as there are many more risk factors of VTE in ICU such as invasive lines, mechanical ventilation, shock, blood and blood product transfusion which were not considered. Cook et al. (2000) did an Observational Study in a Medical-Surgical Intensive Care Unit—Out of 93 patients they studied a total of eight patients had thromboembolic episodes, 5 had DVT and PE before admission, 1 had DVT on day 2 and PE on day 3, and 1 had PE.

Mechanical ventilation, immobility, femoral venous catheter, sedatives, and paralytic drugs were the risk factors or PE, while heparin prophylaxis, aspirin, and thromboembolic disease stockings were associated with a lower risk.

Following four risk factors were identified for ICU-acquired DVT prophylaxis:

1. Personal or family history of VTE
2. End-stage renal failure
3. Platelet transfusion
4. Vasopressor use

Patients with DVT had a longer duration of mechanical ventilation, ICU stay, and hospitalization than the patients without DVT.

In both the above-mentioned studies in majority of the admissions, primary diagnosis was other than sepsis.

In initial study by Cook et al., 93.5% of admissions were for noninfectious reasons, and in later study 94.6% had primary diagnosis other than sepsis.

Kaplan et al. studied 113 patients with severe sepsis with 77% of them on mechanical ventilation, 54% required vasopressor and average APACHE II score was 18.2. Overall, 80.5% of patients were on VTE chemoprophylaxis, 2.7% were on warfarin and 19.5% received were prescribed sequential compressive devices (SCDs). The primary outcome was DVT, while symptomatic PE was observed in 3.5% of cases. Though the real cause of such high incidence in septic patient is not known, it was attributed to sepsis induces a marked proinflammatory and prothrombotic systemic milieu **(Table 2)**.

The Indian Society of Critical Care Medicine (ISCCM) recommends all critically ill patients in ICU should be considered moderate-to-high risk for DVT.

Due to the heterogeneity of ICU patients and varied other risk factors in ICU patients, the ISCCM does not recommend the use of any specific scoring system for risk stratification of DVT. The ISCCM consensus statement suggests to consider the following risk factors for thromboembolic phenomenon:

- Mechanical ventilation
- Need for vasopressors
- Platelet transfusion
- Septic shock
- Use of CVC
- Use of sedatives and paralytic agents
- Prolonged immobilization

TABLE 2: Deep venous thrombosis (DVT) and pulmonary embolism trials.

Study	Design	Patients	Aim/Objective	Risk factors for DVT	Conclusion	Limitations
PROF-ETEV trial (Garcia-Olivarez et al., 2014)	Single-day point prevalence	777 total 62% medical 30% surgical and 7% trauma	High risk/moderate/low risk of DVT	• Vasopressor • Acute cardiac and respiratory pathology • Mechanical ventilation	High risk of DVT but low rate of appropriate prophylaxis	Limited factors studied
Cook et al. (2005)	Prospective cohort	261	Prevalence of incidence and risk factors for proximal DVT	Personal/family history • ESRD • Platelet Transfusion • Vasopressor	Medical-surgical critically ill are at risk of DVT	Trauma and orthopedic patients not involved
Kaplan et al. (2015)	Multicenter and pros-pective	113	Sepsis is risk factor for DVT?	• Presence of CVC • ICU-Stay • Age • Mechanical ventilation needs	Severe sepsis and septic shock have high incidence of VTE	• Small size • Previous history of DVT not included • Severe sepsis is outdated now
Validation of the Caprini Venous Thromboembolism Risk assessment model in critically ill surgical patients Andrea T Obi	Retrospective cohort	4,844 adults	Validity of Caprini VTE risk in Critically ill surgical	• Age • Surgery • Trauma • Sepsis • COAD • Congestive heart failure	The Caprini VTE risk assessment model is Valid	Only surgical patients

(COAD: chronic obstructive airway disease; CVC: central venous catheter; ESRD: end-stage renal disease; ICU: intensive care unit)

- End-stage renal disease
- longer length of stay in ICU
- Age > 60 years
- Past history of any DVT

Patients having any of the above factors should be considered at risk for DVT and more the factors the greater the risk.

A prediction score (the ICU-Venous Thromboembolism score) was derived from independent risk factors identified using multivariable logistic regression.

The ICU-Venous Thromboembolism score can identify patients at increased risk for VTE. This may be a very important tool to identify those patients at particularly high risk for VTE in order to more aggressively mitigate modifiable risk factors and more closely monitor for development of VTE.

In this study of 37,050 patients who met the eligibility criteria, 529 patients (1.4%) developed symptomatic VTE, the ICU-Venous Thromboembolism score consists of six independent predictors. Each risk factor is allotted a specific point/points depending upon the severity of the risk factor.

- CVC (5 points)
- Immobilization ≥ 4 days (4 points)
- Prior history of VTE (4 points)
- Mechanical ventilation (2 points)
- Lowest hemoglobin during hospitalization ≥ 9 g/dL (2 points)
- Platelet count at admission > 250,000/μL (1 point)

In this study population, patients with higher scores had high risk of VTE and vice versa.

COMORBIDITIES AND HOST FACTORS RESOLUTION OF COMMUNITY-ACQUIRED PNEUMONIA

The comorbidities and host factors most commonly associated with CAP that affect the rate of resolution include chronic obstructive pulmonary disease, alcoholism, diabetes mellitus, neurological disorders, ischemic heart disease, malignancy, renal failure, immunosuppression, human immunodeficiency virus (HIV) infection, and primary immune deficiencies. Without comorbidities there is clearing of radiographic infiltrates by 4 weeks, whereas only 20–30% of patients with these comorbidities will clear by 4 weeks. The rest persist to have infiltrates in the chest films for a longer duration.

INFECTIOUS ETIOLOGIES

If the initial suspect of an infectious etiology is the actual cause, then factors that can lead to a progressive or nonresolving pneumonia need to be further assessed. These factors include those associated with the pathogen, the host, or the therapy.

Pathogen Factors

Additive alternate or unusual pathogens need to be considered in the patient who fails to respond to treatment. The most important are *Mycobacterium tuberculosis*, fungi, *Nocardia* and *Actinomyces*, *Coxiella burnetii*, and *Pneumocystis carinii*. In addition, the possibility of a relatively 'common' pathogen with drug resistance needs to be considered too.

Tuberculosis

The clinical presentation of tuberculosis as a cause of nonresolving pneumonia is often 'atypical', especially in the elderly. The classic presentation of a cavitary lesion in the apical or posterior segments of one or both upper lobes may not always be present. In such scenario, the diagnosis of tuberculosis may be arduous. Tuberculin testing may be negative in 10–20% of patients even with active disease, and in an even higher percentage of the elderly and patients with acquired immunodeficiency syndrome (AIDS). Sputum acid-fast cultures are positive in up to 80% of cases, but ideal sputum sample is not always obtained for testing, especially in the elderly.

Fungi

Both opportunistic as well as endemic fungi are mimickers of bacterial pneumonia. Of all other opportunistic fungi, *Aspergillus* is the most important. The spectrum of pulmonary *Aspergillus* infections ranges from benign mycetomas, chronic necrotizing aspergillosis, to invasive pulmonary aspergillosis. Of these various forms, it is the chronic necrotizing and invasive forms of disease that are most likely to be for bacterial pneumonia. Invasive aspergillosis is being increasingly found in neutropenic patients on multiple antimicrobials, and chronic obstructive pulmonary disease (COPD) patients on corticosteroids and AIDS.

Other Atypical Organisms

Legionella, Nocardia, Actinomyces, C. burnetii, and P. carinii have all been implicated in causing nonresolving pneumonias. Thus, a strong clinical suspicion should be exercised during the treatment of refractory pneumonias.

Resistant Pathogens

An important consideration and drawback in the management of any pneumonia is the possibility of antibiotic resistance. In particular, the possibility of penicillin-resistant *Streptococcus pneumoniae* (PRSP) must be considered when evaluating patients with nonresolving pneumonia.

In patients with nonresolving pneumonia who have by definition survived the initial 5 days, the possibility of drug resistance must be evaluated as a contributing factor. The suspicion of PRSP should be especially high in cases of nonresolving pneumonia associated with risk factors, which include prior therapy with beta lactams within 6 months, pneumonia within 1 year, hospitalization in the prior 3 months, and nosocomial infections.

Therapy-related Factors

When pneumonia does not respond to treatment, certain aspects related to therapy need to be considered, including possible medication errors as well as the concentrations of antibiotics used. If intermediate-level resistant PRSP is present, higher doses of penicillin will be required. Similarly, if *Pneumocystis carinii* pneumonia (PCP) is suspected, higher doses of trimethoprim-sulfamethoxazole will be required. When aminoglycosides are used, it is important to check levels and adjust the dosing regimen accordingly. Similarly, based on renal function, drug doses may require readjustment. In addition, aminoglycosides do not penetrate the lung well, so it may be necessary to aim for higher peak concentrations when using a traditional dosing regimen, especially when treating pseudomonal pneumonia. The effect of decreased pulmonary penetration on aminoglycoside efficacy using a once-daily dosing regimen has not yet been studied for pneumonia. It is also important to ensure that adequate levels of drug are reaching the site of infection by ruling out sequestered foci of infection, such as empyemas and lung abscesses.

NONINFECTIOUS ETIOLOGIES

Other diseases with acute involvement of the pulmonary parenchyma may mimic CAP and therapeutic failure. This group includes:

- Neoplasms
- Pulmonary hemorrhage
- Inflammatory diseases [bronchiolitis obliterans and organizing pneumonia (BOOP), acute interstitial pneumonitis, eosinophilic pneumonia, hypersensitivity pneumonitis, etc.].

The frequency of noninfectious etiologies is not well established. Neoplasms are the most common, with Feinsilver et al. observing 10% of lung cancers in adults with nonresolving pneumonia.

EVALUATION OF NONRESOLVING AND PROGRESSIVE PNEUMONIA

Clinical Evaluation

In a patient with nonresponding or progressive pneumonia, a complete reevaluation of the anamnesis and a full physical examination is required in order to rule out the probable causes(infectious and noninfectious). This evaluation includes important epidemiologic keys, which may reveal unusual microorganisms (*Coxiella, Nocardia, Legionella,* etc.), risk factors for resistant microorganisms, or immunocompromised due to HIV infection.

Laboratory Investigations

Microbiologic investigation may begin with studies of noninvasive samples, such as sputum with special conventional and modified Ziehl staining for *M. tuberculosis* and *Nocardia*, methenamine silver for *P. carinii*, urinary antigens detection. Blood cultures and serum antibody studies are done to detect the microorganism in circulation. Also, nowadays blood and urine polymerase chain reaction (PCR) allow identification of *Streptococcus pneumoniae, Legionella,* and *Chlamydia pneumoniae*, and *Mycoplasma pneumoniae*. PCR of pharyngeal swabs is also done.

ROLE OF FIBROBRONCHOSCOPY

Respiratory tract samples may be obtained with fibrobronchoscopy and simultaneously the permeability of the airway may be inspected at the site of disease. The diagnostic yield for some bacterial microorganisms may be reduced because of previous antibiotic administration, thereby decreasing their usefulness, being around 41–42% in nonresolving pneumonia, and 72% in nosocomial pneumonia in the intensive care unit (ICU). Bronchoalveolar lavage (BAL) fluid and protected specimen brush (PSB) are recommended prior to changes in therapy in order to avoid the masking of unusual microorganisms. In a group of pneumonias with bad therapeutic response in ICUs, Jacobs et al. were able to orient the diagnosis toward a noninfectious etiology in 19% of cases, with the study of cytocentrifuged BAL fluid.

Possible diseases depending on differential cell count in BAL fluid:

- *Polymorphonuclear leukocytes*:
  - Bacterial infection
  - BOOP
- *Lymphocytes*:
  - Tuberculosis
  - Hypersensitivity pneumonitis
  - Sarcoidosis
  - Idiopathic pulmonary fibrosis
  - Hemosiderin-laden macrophages
  - Alveolar hemorrhage
- *Eosinophils*:
  - Eosinophilic pneumonia
  - Fungal infection
  - *P. carinii* systemic disease
  - Drug-induced disease

Additional studies recommended for macrophages with hemosiderin or blood in BAL fluid:

- *Autoantibodies*: Perinuclear neutrophil cytoplasmic antibody (pANCA) and cytoplasmic ANCA
- Antibodies against basement membrane
- Renal function with biochemical and sediment tests
- Bronchial and/or transbronchial biopsy

ROLE OF RADIOLOGIC STUDIES

The follow-up by chest radiograph in resolving pneumonia is not indicated for sequential treatment or hospital discharge. Repeat chest X-ray after 4 weeks of discharge is sufficient. In progressive pneumonia, the clinical deterioration and the extension of the chest radiograph lesions may appear prior to the first 3 days after starting of treatment. In nonresolving pneumonia, the chest radiographs with posteroanterior and lateral views may show pleural effusion, appearance of cavitation, and/or new infiltrates. These findings are more evident on CT scan that also allows detailed study of the parenchyma, interstitium, pleurae, and the mediastinum.

Pulmonary CT findings may be characteristic of some microorganisms. For example, nodular areas with a halo sign (nodules surrounded by a halo of ground-glass attenuation) or pleura-based wedge-shaped areas of consolidation is suggestive of pulmonary aspergillosis and/or mucor. Nodular appearance is also described in *Candida*, cytomegalovirus (CMV) infection, Wegener's granulomatosis, Kaposi's sarcoma, and hemorrhagic metastases. Ground-glass opacity or images of interstitial pneumonia are characteristic features of pneumonia by *P. carinii*. Bacterial infection with nodules or multiple masses with or without cavitation may be caused by *Nocardia* species, *M. tuberculosis*, or Q fever. Diffuse or mixed interstitial infiltrates may be due to viral infection or *M. pneumoniae*. High-resolution CT (HRCT) is helpful for distinguishing between an infectious and noninfectious etiology.

OTHER STUDIES

Other imaging studies are performed according to the initial examination and suspicion. Investigations such as *perfusion ventilation scintigraphy* is done to exclude pulmonary embolism, which is highly suspected in the absence of microorganisms and in patients with risk factors like recent surgery, prolonged immobilization, or signs of deep vein thrombosis or right ventricular failure. *Spiral CT* and *pulmonary angiography* complement this diagnosis. In cases with suspicion of endocarditis, pericarditis, or congestive cardiac failure, an *echocardiogram* should be performed. *Open biopsy* is indicated when other diagnostic methods have not yielded any results.

EMPIRIC THERAPEUTIC CHANGES IN NONRESPONDING PNEUMONIA

The most frequently observed in nonresponding pneumonia are infections, and the results of microbiologic studies may be delayed up to 48 hours. Thus, after acquisition of samples, an empiric therapeutic change is indicated. This is done by reviewing initial microbiologic results and treatment should be adjusted with the determination of positive results.

The treatment of nonresponding CAP patients should include combined therapy, and coverage should be extended to cover anaerobes, *Pseudomonas aeruginosa,* and *Staphylococcus aureus* and maintain therapy toward usual microorganisms, such as *S. pneumoniae* and *Legionella,* with antipseudomonal *beta-lactam drugs* (piperacillin/tazobactam, imipenem, meropenem, and cefepime) and intravenous antipneumococcal *fluoroquinolones* (trovafloxacin or levofloxacin) or an intravenous *macrolide* (azithromycin or clarithromycin). If suspicion of *P. aeruginosa* is very high, the antimicrobial should include at least two antipseudomonal agents: Antipseudomonal beta-lactam (piperacillin/tazobactam, imipenem, meropenem, and cefepime) plus intravenous ciprofloxacin or aminoglycosides and intravenous macrolide (azithromycin or clarithromycin). In non-responding nosocomial pneumonia, combinations up to three antibiotics may be required to cover *P. aeruginosa*, methicillin-resistant *S. aureus* (MRSA), and according to the local flora of each hospital as well as *Acinetobacter* species.

CONCLUSION

Nonresponding pneumonia has increased mortality by threefold in CAP and fivefold in nosocomial pneumonia as compared to global mortality in hospitalized patients. Empiric therapeutic changes are presently aimed at broadening the bacteriologic spectrum in order to cover drug-resistant or atypical microorganisms.

SUGGESTED READING

1. Menendez R, Torres A. Evaluation of nonresolving and progressive pneumonia. In: Vincent JL (Eds). Intensive Care Medicine. New York, NY: Springer; 2003.

SECTION

3

DIABETES

35

CHAPTER

How to Prevent or Delay Onset of Type 2 Diabetes Mellitus?

Girish Verma, Ashee Verma, Shiv Ghodasara

ABSTRACT

Individuals having prediabetes [fasting plasma glucose 100–126 mg/dL, impaired glucose tolerance test (IGT), plasma glucose 140–199 mg/dL, glycated hemoglobin (HbA1c) 5.7–6.4%] are prone to be converted into type 2 diabetes mellitus (T2DM) and its complications. Various studies have shown that we can delay or prevent the onset of T2DM by lifestyle modifications (low-calorie diet plan plus exercise) and by giving metformin which has ample evidence in its favor. The details are described in the chapter.

INTRODUCTION

Prevention is better than cure is an old saying that also holds true for diabetes mellitus (DM). As type 2 diabetes mellitus (T2DM) cases are more as compared to type 1 diabetes mellitus (T1DM), it is logical to prevent or delay the onset of T2DM so as to help an individual, society, and nation stay away from economic loss, manpower loss, and national health loss.

Levels of prevention in T2DM may be as follows:

1. *Primordial prevention*: In the preconceptional stage
2. *Primary prevention*: Preventing the onset of T2DM
3. *Secondary prevention*: Early diagnosis and treatment of T2DM so as to prevent its complications
4. *Tertiary prevention*: Limiting the physical disability as a result of T2DM and rehabilitation measures

A state of prediabetics, i.e., impaired fasting glucose (IFG) (plasma glucose 100–125 mg/dL) and impaired glucose tolerance (IGT) (plasma glucose 140–199 mg/dL), and glycated hemoglobin (HbA1c) 5.7–6.4% can be prevented to develop as an overt T2DM. This prevention, i.e., prevention of prediabetes into T2DM is primary prevention or in other words prevention of onset or delaying the onset of T2DM from the prediabetes state.

WHY IS IT NECESSARY TO PREVENT OR DELAY THE ONSET OF TYPE 2 DIABETES MELLITUS?

According to the International Diabetes Federation (IDF) Diabetes Atlas (9th edition, 2019), 700 million adults will have DM by 2045 throughout the world. India ranks number 2 in the list of countries with the largest number of adults with diabetes in 2019 and is anticipated to remain so in 2030 and 2045 as well.

Hence, it is logical and important to prevent or delay the onset of T2DM in Indian population so as to curb the epidemic of T2DM by creating awareness for T2DM, and thereby helping the people of the country to enjoy good health without economic and work loss.

WHY INDIANS ARE DIFFERENT AND AT RISK THAN OTHER POPULATIONS OF THE WORLD?

Approximately, 50% of beta-cell function is lost at diagnosis of prediabetes. This happens in Indians as they have earlier on set of DM, considerably thinner (particularly in the limbs) but more centrally obese than Caucasians and despite being lean, Indians are more insulin resistant and hyperinsulinemic.

The number of vehicles (two wheelers and four wheelers) are increasing day by day, resulting in decreasing trend of physical activity. At the same time, there is increasing trend of spending more time in front of screen (TV, laptop, mobile, etc.) throughout the world. This holds true for India, especially after coronavirus disease 2019 (COVID-19) (work from home distant education), leading to marked decrease in physical activities. Thus, all these factors predispose Indian population to prediabetes, which should be prevented from being converted into DM.

IN WHOM SHOULD WE TRY TO PREVENT OR DELAY THE ONSET OF TYPE 2 DIABETES MELLITUS?

It is very difficult to screen everyone or whole population for DM; thus, asymptomatic individuals who are at risk of having DM or prediabetes should be screened for the purpose of prevention of DM. The following category asymptomatic adults should be screened **(Box 1)**.

BOX 1: Criteria for screening for diabetes or prediabetes in asymptomatic adults.

- Testing should be considered in adults with overweight or obesity (BMI ≥ 25 kg/m^2 or ≥23 kg/m^2 in Asian American individuals) who have one or more of the following risk factors:
  - First-degree relative with diabetes
  - High-risk race/ethnicity (e.g., African American, Latino, Native American, Asian American, Pacific Islander)
  - History of CVD
  - Hypertension (≥130/80 mm Hg or on therapy for hypertension)
  - HDL cholesterol level < 35 mg/dL (0.90 mmol/L) and/or a triglyceride level 250 mg/dL (2.82 mmol/L)
  - Individuals with polycystic ovary syndrome
  - Physical inactivity
  - Other clinical conditions associated with insulin resistance (e.g., severe obesity, acanthosis nigricans)
- People with prediabetes [HbA1c ≥ 5.7% (39 mmol/mol), IGT, or IFG] should be tested yearly
- People who were diagnosed with GDM should give a lifelong testing at least every 3 years
- For all other people, testing should begin at the age of 35 years
- If results are normal, testing should be repeated at a minimum of 3-year intervals, with consideration of more frequent testing depending on initial results and risk status
- People with HIV

(BMI: body mass index; CVD: cardiovascular disease; GDM: gestational diabetes mellitus; HbA1c: glycated hemoglobin; HDL: high-density lipoprotein; HIV: human immunodeficiency virus; IGT: impaired glucose tolerance; IFG: impaired fasting glucose)

HOW TO PREVENT OR DELAY THE ONSET OF TYPE 2 DIABETES MELLITUS?

Many major randomized controlled trials including the Diabetes Prevention Program (DPP) trial, the Finnish Diabetes Prevention Study (DPS), and Da Qing Diabetes Prevention Study (Da Qing Study) demonstrated that lifestyle/behavioral intervention with an individualized reduced calorie meal plan is highly effective in preventing or delaying the T2DM and improving cardiometabolic markers (such as blood pressure, lipids, and inflammation). The DPP demonstrated that intensive lifestyle and intervention could reduce the risk of incident of T2DM by 58% over 3 years.

The Indian Diabetes Prevention Program (IDPP) shows that lifestyle modification and metformin prevent T2DM in Asian Indian subjects with IGT.

In view of these scientific facts, we can prevent or delay the onset of T2DM by planning the following strategies:

- Diet alteration/diet plan
- Exercise
- Pharmacological intervention

This remains individualized when prevention of T2DM is planned.

Diet Plan

Good nutrition is an important part of a healthy lifestyle. Emphasis on whole grains, legumes, fruits, and vegetables and minimum refined and processed foods are associated with lower risk of developing T2DM. Studies have shown that vegetarian, plant-based (may include some minimal animal products), and dietary approach to stop hypertension (DASH) eating pattern are associated with a lower risk of developing T2DM.

There is not an ideal percentage of calories derived from carbohydrates, proteins, and fats for all the people to prevent diabetes. Therefore, distribution of protein, fat, and carbohydrate percentage should be based on an individualized assessment of eating patterns, preferences, and metabolic goals.

Indian diet by and large contains major portion of carbohydrates, that too having a high glycemic index (consuming sweets with meals). This is associated with less satiety, which increases voluntary energy intake and contributes to weight gain that predisposes an individual to development of diabetes in future. Thus, simple carbohydrates (such as carbonated cold drinks, cookies, juices, etc.) should be avoided.

Saturated fats (butter, ghee, red meat, coconut oil, etc.) should be in a very minor part of daily diet and trans-fats (bakery products, *vanaspati/dalda, samosa, jalebi, bhajia*, French fries, chips, etc.) should be avoided in routine and prediabetics.

In DPP, the goal of 7% of loss of initial weight was decided to decrease the risk of T2DM. However, further analysis suggested maximum prevention of diabetes with at least 7–10% weight loss. To achieve this goal, recommended pace of weight loss was 1–2 lb/week. Reduction of this much of weight in terms of calories was estimated by calculating daily calorie needed to maintain the participants' initial weight and subtracting 500–1,000 calories/day (depending on initial weight).

Exercise

The goal is to achieve and maintain at least 7% weight reduction from initial weight, reducing calorie diet, and >150 minutes per week of moderate intensity of physical activity such as brisk walk, jogging, cycling, and swimming is required. Thus, the moderate physical activity along with reduced-calorie diet plan can prevent T2DM in patients who are at risk. As specified by the DPP study, high-risk individuals are aged 25–59 years with [body mass index (BMI) > 35 kg/m^2], higher fasting plasma glucose (>110 mg/dL), higher HbA1c (>6%), and individuals with prior gestational diabetes mellitus (GDM).

It has also been found that moderate physical activity has been shown to improve insulin sensitivity and reduce abdominal fat in children in young adults. In addition to aerobic activity, a physical activity plan designed to prevent diabetes may include resistance training. Breaking up prolonged sedentary time (sitting on the office chair for hours together) is associated with lowering of postprandial glucose level. Physical activity also appears to prevent gestational diabetes.

Pharmacological Intervention

Weight loss through behavior change in diet and physical activity may be difficult to maintain in the long term. People at high risk of diabetes may be benefitted by pharmacological intervention. However, no pharmacological agent has been approved by the US FDA (United States Food and Drug Administration) for a specific indication of T2DM prevention.

Various drugs used for prevention of T2DM such as metformin, alpha-glucosidase inhibitors, glucagon-like peptide-1 receptor agonist (GLP-1 RA) (liraglutide and semaglutide), thiazolidinediones, testosterone, and insulin have been shown to lower the incidence of diabetes in specific population, whereas prevention was not seen with nateglinide.

One prospective randomized controlled trial showed no significant benefit of vitamin-D versus placebo on the progression to T2DM in individuals at high risk.

Metformin has the longest history of safety data as a pharmacological agent for the prevention of diabetes. American Diabetes Association (ADA) 2023 has class A recommendation in high-risk adults using metformin to prevent T2DM (as specified by DPP), especially in those aged 25–59 years of age with BMI 35 kg/m^2, higher fasting plasma glucose (e.g. >110 mg/dL), and higher HbA1c (e.g., >6%) and in individuals with prior GDM. In individuals with a history of GDM in DPP, metformin and intensive lifestyle modification led to 50% reduction in diabetes risk.

The IDPP shows that lifestyle modification and metformin prevent T2DM in Asian Indian subjects with IGT. In IDPP, metformin was used in the doses of 250 mg twice per day. The Indian Council of Medical Research (ICMR) guidelines for the management of T2DM 2018 also mention to target people who are in the stage of prediabetes to prevent the onset of diabetes (primary prevention). The guidelines also state that when lifestyle alone is not sufficient and especially in those with combined IFG and IGT, where the progression appears imminent; use of metformin in addition to lifestyle measures may be considered. The RSSDI-ESI (Research Society for the Study of Diabetes in India and Endocrine Society of India) clinical practice recommendation for the management of T2DM 2020 mentions that people with prediabetes failing to achieve any benefit of lifestyle modifications after 6 months may initiate metformin in younger individuals with one or more risk factors for diabetes regardless of BMI if they are overweight/obese and having IFG + IGT or IFG + HbA1c > 5.7%. Recommendations of metformin in 500 mg twice daily dose is advisable.

SUGGESTED READINGS

1. Arun N, Chamukuttan S, Ramachandran A. Strategies for prevention of type-2 DM evidences from Indian studies. In: Joshi SR (Ed). RSSDI Textbook of Diabetes Mellitus, 4th edition. New Delhi: Jaypee Brothers Medical Publishers; 2020. pp. 805-14.
2. Kristian R, Gottwald-Hostalek U. Understanding Prediabetes: Definition, prevalence, burden and treatment options for an emerging disease. Curr Med Res Opin. 2019;35(9):1529-34.
3. Isharwal S, Misra A, Wasir JS, Nigam P. Diet and insulin resistance a review & Asian Indian perspective. Indian J Med Res. 2009;129(5):485-99.
4. ElSayed NA, Aleppo G, Aroda VR, Bannuru RR, Brown FM, Bruemmer D, et al. Classification and diagnosis of diabetes. Diabetes Care. 2023;46(Suppl 1):519-40.

5. Knowler WC, Barret Conor E, Fowler EC, Hamman RF, Lachin JM, Walker EA, et al. Reduction in the incidence of type-2 diabetes with lifestyle intervention or metformin. N Eng J Med. 2002;346:393-403.
6. Lindström J, Ilanne-Parikka P, Peltonen M, Aunola S, Eriksson JG, Hemiö K, et al. Finnish Diabetes Prevention Study Group. Sustained reduction in the incidence of type-2 diabetes by lifestyle intervention; follow-up of the Finnish diabetes prevention study. Lancet. 2006;368:1673-69.
7. Li G, Zhang P, Wang J, An Y, Gong Q, Gregg EW, et al. Cardiovascular mortality, all-cause mortality, and diabetes incidence after lifestyle intervention for people with impaired glucose tolerance in the Da Quing Diabetes prevention study: A 23-year follow-up study. Lancet Diabetes Endocrinol. 2014;2:474-80.
8. Nathan DM, Bernett PH, Crandall JP, Edelstein SL, Goldberg RB, Kahn SE, et al.; DPP research group. Does diabetes prevention translate into reduced long term vascular complication of Diabetes? Diabetologia. 2019;62(8):1319-28.
9. Ramchandran A, Snehlata C, Mary S, Mukesh B, Bhaskar AD, Vijay V; Indian Diabetes Prevention Programme. The Indian Diabetes Prevention Programme shows that lifestyle modification and metformin prevent type 2 diabetes in Asian Indian subjects with impaired glucose tolerance (IDPP-1). Diabetologia. 2006;49:289-97.
10. ElSayed NA, Aleppo G, Aroda VR, Bannuru RR, Brown FM, Bruemmer D, et al. Prevention or Delay of Type 2 Diabetes and Associated Comorbidities: Standards of Care in Diabetes-2023. Diabetes Care. 2023;46(Suppl 1):S41-8.
11. Hu FB, van Dam RM, Liu S. Diet and risk of type-2 diabetes: the role of type of fat and carbohydrate. Diabetologia. 2001;44(7):805-17.
12. Hamman RF, wing RR, Endelstein S, Lachin JM, Bray GA, Delahanty L, et al. Effect of weight loss with lifestyle intervention on risk of diabetes. Diabetes Care. 2006;29:2102-7.
13. Fedeva MV, Gist NH, Evans EM, Dishman RK. Exercise and insulin resistance in youth: a meta-analysis. Pediatrics. 2014;133:e163-74.
14. Davis CL, Pollocl NK, Waller JL, Allison JD, Dennis BA, Bassali R, et al. Exercise dose and diabetes risk in overweight and obese children: A randomized control trial. JAMA. 2012;308:1103-12.
15. Russo LM, Nobles C, Ertel KA, Chasan-Taber L, Whitcomb BW. Physical activity intervention in pregnancy and risk of gestational diabetes mellitus: a systemic review and meta-analysis. Obstet Gynecol. 2015;125:576-82.
16. Wittert G, Bracken K, Robledo KP, Grossmann M, Yeap BB, Handelsman DJ, et al. Testosterone treatment to prevent or revert type-2 diabetes in men enrolled in a lifestyle programme (T4DM): Randomized double blind, placebo controlled, 2 years phase 3-b trial, Lancet Diabetes Endocrinol. 2021;9:32-45.
17. Pittas AG, Dawson Huges B, Sheehan P, Ware JH, Knowler WC, Aroda VR, et al. D2d research group vitamin D supplementation and prevention of type-2 diabetes. N Eng J Med. 2019;381:520-30.
18. Diabetes prevention program research group. Long term safety, tolerability and weight loss associated with metformin in the diabetes prevention program outcomes study. Diabetes Care. 2012;35:731-7.
19. Ranter RE, Christophic A, Metzger BE, Dabelea D, Bennett PH, Pi-Sunyer X, et al. Diabetes prevention program research group. Prevention of diabetes in women with a history of gestational diabetes: Effects of metformin and lifestyle interventions. J Clin Endocrinol Metab. 2008;93:4774-9.

36

CHAPTER

Diabetes in Young—Beyond Type 1 Diabetes Mellitus

Rakesh M Parikh, Sanjay Mehndiratta

ABSTRACT

Diabetes in young individuals extends beyond the traditional type 1 diabetes mellitus (T1DM). This chapter explores the different types of diabetes that affect young individuals, their etiology, clinical features, management strategies, and long-term implications. The prevalence of type 2 diabetes mellitus (T2DM) in the young is rising due to increasing obesity rates and sedentary lifestyles. The diagnosis of T2DM in young individuals is often made during routine screening or with mild symptoms. Monogenic forms of diabetes, known as maturity-onset diabetes of the young (MODY), are caused by single gene mutations affecting pancreatic beta cell function and insulin secretion. Different subtypes of MODY are discussed, along with their specific clinical features and management options. Genetic testing plays a crucial role in confirming the diagnosis of MODY. Other genetic forms of diabetes in the young, including neonatal diabetes mellitus, Wolfram syndrome, Alström syndrome, and Prader–Willi syndrome, are also discussed.

Gestational diabetes mellitus (GDM), defined as diabetes diagnosed during pregnancy, is explored in terms of its diagnosis and management strategies. GDM is largely due to insulin resistance caused by placental hormones. Lifestyle changes and, if necessary, insulin therapy are used to achieve glycemic control during pregnancy. Secondary types of diabetes, such as cystic fibrosis-related diabetes, drug-induced diabetes, pancreatic diabetes, and diabetes associated with endocrinopathies such as Cushing's syndrome, acromegaly, and hyperthyroidism are also addressed. Proper diagnosis and management of these secondary types of diabetes are crucial, often involving treatment of the underlying condition.

Understanding the various types of diabetes that can present in young individuals is essential for accurate diagnosis, appropriate management, and optimal long-term outcomes. This chapter provides a comprehensive overview of these different types of diabetes, aiding clinicians in their approach to young patients with diabetes.

INTRODUCTION

Diabetes is a chronic metabolic disorder characterized by elevated blood glucose levels. Although diabetes is a multifactorial disease with varying etiologies, diabetes in children and young adults is traditionally labeled as type 1 diabetes mellitus (T1DM). While T1DM is often associated with the onset of diabetes in young individuals, there are various other forms of diabetes that can affect this population. With the rising prevalence of type 2 diabetes mellitus (T2DM), its prevalence in adolescents and young individuals is also rising. With ongoing research several new variants of diabetes affecting young individuals are identified. Detailed history and examination is usually sufficient to differentiate T1DM from the other variants, while serological and genetic tests may be needed for confirmation. Before labeling a child as T1DM, it is important to exclude the other causes as it may significantly impact the treatment and prognosis of the patient. This chapter aims to explore the different types of diabetes beyond T1DM in young individuals, their etiology, clinical features, management strategies, and long-term implications.

TYPE 2 DIABETES MELLITUS IN YOUNG

The prevalence of T2DM in children and adolescents has been increasing due to rising rates of obesity and sedentary lifestyles. Genetic predisposition and ethnicity also play a role. Those with strong family history, childhood obesity, and features of insulin resistance such as acanthosis nigricans, skin tags, and polycystic ovarian syndrome are at a higher risk. T2DM in young individuals often presents with features similar to adult-onset T2DM. Unlike T1DM, they are diagnosed during routine screening or with mild symptoms. Diagnosis is based on clinical criteria and confirmed by laboratory tests. Lifestyle modifications, including diet and physical activity, are key components of managing T2DM in young individuals. Children with T2DM respond very well to oral antidiabetic drugs. Regular monitoring and follow-up are crucial for optimal glycemic control.

Type 2 diabetes mellitus in young is associated with an increased risk of long-term complications, including cardiovascular disease, nephropathy, and retinopathy. Close monitoring, early intervention, and comprehensive care are essential to mitigate these risks. Unlike elderly individuals with comorbidities, intensive glycemic control with glycated hemoglobin (HbA1c) target of below 6.5% should be advised to all young individuals with T2DM. Females in reproductive age group also need to be counseled to observe strict contraception and plan pregnancy only after achieving good glycemic control and shifting to insulin under supervision of healthcare provider.

MONOGENIC FORMS OF DIABETES (MATURITY-ONSET DIABETES OF THE YOUNG)

Monogenic forms of diabetes, also known as maturity-onset diabetes of the young (MODY), are caused by single gene mutations that are transmitted in an autosomal dominant manner. These mutations affect pancreatic beta cell function and insulin secretion. MODY typically presents with mild hyperglycemia at a young age, often before the age of 25 years. Unlike T1DM, they rarely have a severe presentation with ketoacidosis and weight loss and are negative for islet autoantibodies. They can be differentiated from T2DM by absence of obesity and features of insulin resistance. The clinical features may vary depending on the specific gene mutation involved. Genetic testing plays a crucial role in confirming the diagnosis. There are several subtypes of MODY, each associated with a different gene mutation.

- *MODY 1 (HNF4A):* HNF4A is a transcription factor involved in regulation of genes that are required for glucose transport and metabolism. This subtype accounts for approximately 5–10% of MODY cases and is characterized by impaired insulin production and progressive beta cell failure. These patients have higher birth weight and higher chances of macrosomia. They respond well to sulfonylureas.
- *MODY 2 (glucokinase):* Glucokinase is glycolytic enzyme that catalyzes conversion of glucose to glucose-6-phosphate. It controls the glucose-mediated insulin release from beta cells. MODY 2 is characterized by a defect in this glucose sensing mechanism, leading to chronic mild fasting hyperglycemia from birth. The patients are usually asymptomatic and are diagnosed through screening usually during pregnancy. These patients usually do not require any treatment.
- *MODY 3 (HNF1A):* This subtype is the most common form of MODY and is associated with impaired insulin secretion and progressive beta cell failure. The hyperglycemia is severe and progresses over time exposing the patients to risk of microvascular and macrovascular complications in long-term. MODY 3 patients respond very well to sulfonylureas and meglitinides initially. With progressive beta cell failure eventually most of them require insulin for achieving good glycemic control.
- *MODY 4 (PDX1):* PDX1, also known as insulin promoter factor 1 (IPF1), is a transcription factor involved in development of pancreas and insulin gene expression. This rare form of MODY is characterized by impaired pancreatic development and beta cell dysfunction. Homozygous mutation may lead to pancreas agenesis and present with permanent neonatal diabetes.
- *MODY 5 (HNF1B):* This subtype is associated with renal abnormalities, genital malformations, and pancreatic dysfunction. These patients may not respond well to oral antidiabetic medicines and require insulin.
- *MODY 6 (NEUROD1):* This subtype is characterized by impaired beta cell development and function. This mutation might affect neuronal development as well and patients usually require insulin.
- *Other rare subtypes:* MODY 7 (KLF11), MODY 8 (CEL), MODY 9 (PAX4), MODY 10 (INS), MODY 11 (BLK), MODY 12 (ABCC8), and MODY 13 (KCNJ11).

Management of MODY involves personalized treatment strategies based on the specific gene mutation and individual patient characteristics. Lifestyle modifications and oral antidiabetic drugs are sufficient in most of the patient, although some patients may require insulin. The prognosis for MODY is generally favorable, with a milder course compared to other forms of diabetes. However, long-term complications such as diabetic nephropathy and retinopathy can still occur. Genetic counseling is important to assess the risk of diabetes in family members and to guide reproductive decisions.

OTHER FORMS OF GENETIC DIABETES IN THE YOUNG

There are several other types of genetic diabetes that can affect young individuals. These include:

- *Neonatal diabetes mellitus:* Neonatal diabetes mellitus is a monogenic form of diabetes that presents within the first 6 months of life. It can be transient or permanent, with different genetic etiologies, including mutations in the *KCNJ11*, *ABCC8*, and *INS* genes. Genetic testing is crucial for diagnosis and appropriate management, which may include sulfonylureas as a treatment option.
- *Wolfram syndrome:* Wolfram syndrome, also known as diabetes insipidus, diabetes mellitus, optic atrophy, and deafness (DIDMOAD), is a rare genetic disorder characterized by the early-onset of insulin-dependent diabetes mellitus, optic atrophy, hearing loss, and diabetes insipidus. Genetic testing can help confirm the diagnosis, and management involves addressing the different clinical manifestations in a multidisciplinary approach.
- *Alström syndrome:* Alström syndrome is a rare autosomal recessive disorder that can present with childhood-onset obesity, insulin resistance, and progressive insulin-dependent diabetes. Genetic testing aids in the diagnosis, and management involves a multidisciplinary approach addressing the various organ system involvement.
- *Prader–Willi syndrome:* Prader–Willi syndrome is a complex genetic disorder characterized by neonatal hypotonia, hyperphagia leading to obesity, intellectual disability, and multiple endocrine abnormalities, including an increased risk of developing diabetes. Early diagnosis, close monitoring, and addressing the underlying metabolic abnormalities are crucial for managing diabetes in individuals with Prader–Willi syndrome.
- *Others:* There are several other rare genetic forms of diabetes, including neonatal syndromic diabetes associated with genetic syndromes such as Down syndrome and Turner syndrome, as well as mitochondrial diabetes caused by mutations in mitochondrial deoxyribonucleic acid (DNA). Genetic testing and individualized management are essential in these cases.

GESTATIONAL DIABETES MELLITUS

Gestational diabetes mellitus is defined as diabetes diagnosed during second or third trimester of pregnancy which is not clearly overt diabetes prior to gestation. Various organizations recommend oral glucose tolerance test (OGTT) based one-step and two-step approaches for diagnosis of GDM.

The mild hyperglycemia in GDM is largely due to insulin resistance because of placental hormones. If left untreated it can cause macrosomia, difficult labor and perinatal complications. If lifestyle changes fail to achieve strict glycemic control recommended during pregnancy, insulin is often the treatment of choice. Most of the patients usually become euglycemic immediately postpartum as soon as the placenta is out.

SECONDARY DIABETES

There are several secondary types of diabetes that can present in young adults. While MODY and GDM are the most common forms other than T1DM and T2DM, there are other less prevalent but important secondary types to consider. Here are a few examples:

- *Cystic fibrosis-related diabetes (CFRD):* Individuals with cystic fibrosis (CF) are at risk of developing CFRD due to the impact of the disease on the pancreas. CF affects the ability of pancreas to produce sufficient insulin, leading to high blood sugar levels. CFRD often occurs in young adults with CF and requires careful monitoring and treatment to manage blood glucose levels effectively.
- *Drug-induced diabetes:* Certain medications can induce diabetes as a side effect. For example, long-term use of corticosteroids, such as prednisone, which are prescribed for various conditions like asthma or autoimmune disorders, can cause drug-induced diabetes. This type of diabetes usually resolves once the medication is discontinued, but it requires close monitoring and management in the meantime.
- *Pancreatic diabetes:* This form of diabetes occurs when the pancreas is damaged or removed due to disease, injury, or surgery. Pancreatitis, pancreatic cancer, or surgical removal of the pancreas can lead to a loss of insulin-producing cells, resulting in diabetes. Pancreatic diabetes typically presents in young adults who have undergone pancreatic surgery or have pancreatic diseases. Fibrocalculous pancreatic diabetes (FCPD) is a specific subtype prevalent in tropical regions including India. Pancreatic calcification can often be seen on X-ray abdomen in these patients. This should be suspected in patients who have history of recurrent admissions for pain abdomen and history of steatorrhea. Most of the patients require insulin for achieving good glycemic control.
- *Endocrinopathies:* Endocrinopathies such as Cushing's syndrome, acromegaly, and hyperthyroidism may present with diabetes. The basic pathophysiology is

insulin resistance due to increased levels of hormones such as cortisol, growth hormone, and thyroid hormones. Diabetic patients presenting with clinical features suggestive of any of these endocrinopathies should be investigated further. Treatment approaches may involve addressing the underlying endocrine disorder, managing insulin resistance, and implementing lifestyle modifications to optimize blood sugar control. This type of diabetes is usually reversible once the primary pathology is addressed.

CONCLUSION

Diabetes presenting at younger age is not necessarily T1DM. Children and young adults presenting with diabetes should be thoroughly evaluated before labeling them as T1DM. Detailed history and thorough clinical examination is usually sufficient to raise clinical suspicion and the accurate diagnosis is possible with investigations. Diagnosing the exact etiology might significantly impact the treatment and long-term prognosis of patient.

SUGGESTED READINGS

1. ElSayed NA, Aleppo G, Aroda VR, Bannuru RR, Brown FM, Bruemmer D, et al. Classification and Diagnosis of Diabetes: Standards of Care in Diabetes—2023. Diabetes Care. 2023;46(Suppl. 1):S19-40.
2. Naylor R, Johnson AK, del Gaudio D, Adam MP, Feldman J, Mirzaa GM, et al. Maturity-Onset Diabetes of the Young Overview. Seattle (WA): University of Washington; 2018.

37

CHAPTER

Diabetic Dyslipidemia and Nonalcoholic Steatohepatitis

AS Senthilvelu

ABSTRACT

India is the global hub for chronic metabolic conditions like diabetes and dyslipidemia, due to a higher prevalence of insulin resistance (IR). A high level of IR also contributes to more deposition of fat in liver causing nonalcoholic fatty liver disease (NAFLD) and inflammation, called nonalcoholic steatohepatitis (NASH). All metabolic conditions are associated with a higher risk of cardiovascular (CV) events. Currently, multiple therapeutic options are available. However, saroglitazar is the first molecule approved by the Drug Controller General of India (DCGI) in India for elevated triglyceride in diabetes mellitus (DM) patients and NAFLD as well.

INTRODUCTION

India accounts for 21% of the world's global burden of disease, where noncommunicable diseases (NCDs) are responsible for two-thirds of the total morbidity burden and about 53% of total deaths in India. Two out of four leading NCDs in India are cardiovascular diseases (CVDs) and diabetes mellitus (DM). DM is one of the major risk factors for the development of dyslipidemia and CVD. As per the International Diabetes Federation (IDF) 2021, India is ranking 2nd globally in the incidence of DM with a patient population of 74.2 million. The major associated comorbid condition of diabetes is dyslipidemia, and it is known as diabetic dyslipidemia (DD). As per ICMR–INDIAB (Indian Council of Medical Research–India Diabetes) study 2014, 79% of Indian population had dyslipidemia and more importantly 9 out 10 Indian DM patients were dyslipidemic. Unlike western population, the most common dyslipidemia pattern in India was low high-density lipoprotein (HDL)—72.3%, high triglycerides (TG)—29.5% and followed by high low-density lipoprotein (LDL)—11.8%. This study showed significant evidence of high prevalence of low HDL and high TG in India.

DIABETIC DYSLIPIDEMIA

Diabetic dyslipidemia consists of specifically mild to marked elevation of TG-rich lipoproteins, very low-density lipoprotein-cholesterol (VLDL-C) and VLDL-C remnants, and low levels of HDL. In addition, LDL particles are converted to smaller, perhaps more atherogenic, lipoproteins termed "small dense LDL-C" (sd-LDL-C). This combination of hypertriglyceridemia, low HDL-C and high levels of sd-LDL-C, better addressed as atherogenic diabetic dyslipidemia (ADD), is particularly seen in Asian Indians. Krishnamurthy et al. showed that in Indian DM patients, the prevalence of ADD was seen in 34.2% and raised non-HDL-C in 73.3%, which was significantly more associated with poor glycemic control [glycated hemoglobin (HbA1c) > 8%]. Although the precise reason for such dyslipidemia is unknown, genetic predisposition and characteristic body composition (excess intra-abdominal fat) may be important contributors. A common outcome of such a body composition and dyslipidemia in Asian Indians is the tendency to develop insulin resistance (IR). This condition is majorly responsible for the development of coronary artery disease (CAD), which is 2–4 times higher in diabetic subjects, and in Indians,

CAD occurs prematurely, i.e., one to two decades earlier than in the West.

Diabetic Dyslipidemia Including Elevated Triglycerides and Increased Cardiovascular Risk

Several large trials and meta-analyses have investigated the effects of lipid-lowering statin therapy and have consistently demonstrated that statin therapy significantly reduces LDL-C levels and the incidence of cardiovascular (CV) events. In spite of the efficacy of statin therapy in these studies, statins did not eliminate CV risk. Rather, significant residual CV risk remains after treatment with statins, especially in high-risk patients such as those with DM. Residual CV risk stems, at least partially, from low HDL-C and elevated TG. With elevated TG levels, a combination of LDL-C with VLDL-C in the measure of non-HDL-C may be a better predictor of CV risk than LDL-C alone. Recently, international guidelines by the European Society of Cardiology (ESC) and European Atherosclerosis Society (EAS) recommended that hypertriglyceridemia in high-risk patients be managed with TG-lowering agents. ESC/EAS 2019 guidelines on the management of dyslipidemia recommended no goal for TG level, but <1.7 mmol/L (<150 mg/dL) indicates lower risk and higher levels indicate a need to look for other risk factors. In high-risk (or above) patients with TG levels between 1.5 and 5.6 mmol/L (135–499 mg/dL) despite statin treatment, TG-lowering drugs [n-3 PUFAs (icosapent ethyl 2 × 2 g/day)] should be considered in combination with a statin. In primary prevention patients who are at LDL-C goal with TG levels > 2.3 mmol/L (>200 mg/dL), TG-lowering drugs (fenofibrate or bezafibrate) may be considered in combination with statins.

NONALCOHOLIC FATTY LIVER DISEASE

Nonalcoholic fatty liver disease (NAFLD) is a clinicopathologic entity, being increasingly recognized as a major health burden in developed countries. It includes a spectrum of liver damage ranging from simple steatosis to nonalcoholic steatohepatitis (NASH), advanced fibrosis, and, rarely, progression to cirrhosis. As per guideline recommendations, alcohol intake should be limited up to 30 g/day for men and 20 g/day for women. Pathogenesis of NAFLD and metabolic syndrome seems to have common pathophysiological mechanisms, with focus on IR as a key factor. NAFLD prevalence is around 9–32% of the general population globally and in India with a higher prevalence of approximately 40% in those who are overweight or obese and those with DM or prediabetes. NAFLD is extremely common in people with type 2 diabetes mellitus (T2DM) with nearly 7 out of every 10 T2DM patients being affected by it. Overweight/obesity and IR have been strongly linked with NAFLD. NAFLD is an asymptomatic disease which starts with fatty liver and then progresses to NASH, cirrhosis, and hepatocellular carcinoma and is detected either accidentally or incidentally. Initial assessment in high-risk patients, such as DM, obese, and dyslipidemia, done through liver enzymes and USG may give information about the presence of disease. To evaluate further progression of disease and risk of fibrosis, the noninvasive indices like FIB 4 and NFS scores can be used, these scores use routine blood parameters and other simple indices to predict the presence of advanced fibrosis. Transient elastography is currently recommended to observe liver stiffness along with presence of fat, but the gold standard test is liver biopsy.

MANAGEMENT OF DIABETIC DYSLIPIDEMIA AND NASH

Along with lifestyle modifications, statins are being considered as first-line therapy for DD. Statins are capable of decreasing the LDL-C levels by as much as 50%. They may have additional benefits on HDL-C and TG levels. These medications may be used in monotherapy or they may need to be used in combination for the patient with multiple lipid abnormalities in addition to high LDL-C, like high TG and low HDL-C. The mainstay of management interventions is lifestyle changes with diet and exercise with a target weight loss of at least 7–10%. As per various studies, 7–10% weight reduction may be able to improve fibrotic stage, while 3–5% weight reduction can reduce liver fat content in NAFLD patients. Reducing calorie intake by 700–1,000 kcal/day may help in weight reduction. But a major challenge here is to maintain sustained weight loss for a prolonged period of time.

Role of Dual PPAR-α/γ Agonists in NASH and DD

Peroxisome proliferator-activated receptor (PPAR)-α/γ agonists can play a vital role in the management of ADD poststatin therapy. Dual PPAR receptor agonism leads to improvement of insulin sensitivity in adipose tissue and increases fatty acid (FA) uptake in liver and adipose tissue, resulting in reduction of elevated triglyceride.

Saroglitazar: A First Novel Dual PPAR-α/γ Receptor Agonist

Peroxisome proliferator-activated receptors are nuclear lipid-activated transcription factors that regulate the expression of genes involved in the control of lipid and lipoprotein metabolism, glucose homeostasis, and inflammatory processes. PPAR-α is implicated in the uptake and oxidation of FAs and lipoprotein metabolism, while PPAR-γ agonism has beneficial effects on glucose homeostasis by increasing insulin sensitivity and glucose disposal and prevent the loss of beta-cell mass in the pancreas. PPAR-α agonists like fibrates are effective in managing lipids and PPAR-γ agonists are insulin sensitizers that control hyperglycemia in T2DM; by using dual PPAR-α/γ agonists, one can control both the lipid and the glucose levels simultaneously. Saroglitazar is non-TZD and nonfibrate molecule, belongs to the glitazar class compound, is designed as a dual PPAR-α/γ agonist, and has a strong PPAR-α effect with moderate PPAR-γ effect. Saroglitazar is a potent and predominantly PPAR-α agonist with moderate PPAR-γ agonistic activity. PPARs are nuclear lipid-activated transcription factors that regulate the expression of various genes involved in the control of lipid and lipoprotein metabolism, glucose homeostasis, and inflammatory processes. The pharmacological effects of saroglitazar were extensively evaluated in various preclinical models. Saroglitazar showed both anti-dyslipidemic and anti-diabetic effects mainly mediated via activation of both PPAR receptors, respectively.

Saroglitazar has been investigated in various indications such as hypertriglyceridemia in T2DM, NAFLD, T2DM, etc. In a euglycemic clamp study of saroglitazar, insulin sensitivity and glucose metabolism were increased in T2DM patients with high TG, which supports saroglitazar as an insulin sensitizer agent. In phase III clinical trials of PRESS V and PRESS VI, saroglitazar showed significant reduction of elevated TG up to 45% from baseline after 3–6 months of therapy. As per recently published Saroglitazar Integrated Review Analysis of approximately 5,800 DD patients by Kaul et al., saroglitazar has shown reduction in TG in the range from 45 to 62%, HbA1c from 0.7 to 1.6%, and sd-LDL by 20.3%. In phase-III clinical trials and observational studies, saroglitazar is found to be safe with minor side effects in patients with T2DM. In 2020, saroglitazar biopsy-driven study in NAFLD was published, wherein it has shown significant improvement in liver fat, liver enzymes, and fibrotic conditions. Based on this clinical data, saroglitazar has become the world's first approved drug for NAFLD management in India by the Drug Controller General of India (DCGI).

CONCLUSION

Diabetes mellitus is a widely prevalent condition and steadily growing as well. Indian T2DM patients have a higher amount of TG and atherogenic lipid sd-LDL. Atherogenic DD is associated with a higher residual CV risk and should be treated with statin as first-line agents. To control TG after statin therapy, currently many options are available, including saroglitazar as an efficacious and a safe option.

SUGGESTED READINGS

1. World Health Organization. Global status report on noncommunicable diseases 2010. Chapter 1 – Burden: Mortality, Morbidity and Risk Factors. Geneva: World Health Organization; 2010.
2. International Diabetes Federation. IDF Diabetes Atlas, 10th edition. Brussels: International Diabetes Federation; 2021. [online] Available from https://www.diabetesatlas.org [Last accessed December, 2023].
3. Joshi SR, Anjana RM, Deepa M, Pradeepa R, Bhansali A, Dhandania VK, et al; ICMR-INDIAB Collaborative Study Group. Prevalence of dyslipidemia in urban and rural India: the ICMR-INDIAB study. PLoS One. 2014;9(5):e96808.
4. Muačević-Katanec D, Reiner Z. Diabetic dyslipidemia or 'diabetes lipidus'? Expert Rev Cardiovasc Ther. 2011;9(3):341-8.
5. Krishnamurthy V, Kerekoppa AR, Prabhakar B. Cross-sectional study of pattern of dyslipidemia and prevalence of atherogenic diabetic dyslipidemia in newly detected diabetic patients. Asian J Med Sci. 2019;10(6):45-9. .
6. Misra A, Luthra K, Vikram NK. Dyslipidemia in Asian Indians: determinants and significance. J Assoc Physicians India. 2004;52:137-42.
7. Cziraky MJ, Watson KE, Talbert RL. Targeting low HDL-cholesterol to decrease residual cardiovascular risk in the managed care setting. J Manag Care Pharm. 2008;14(8 Suppl):S3-28.
8. Catapano AL, Graham I, De Backer G, Wiklund O, Chapman MJ, Drexel H, Hoes AW, et al. 2016 ESC/EAS Guidelines for the Management of Dyslipidaemias. Eur Heart J. 2016;37(39):2999-3058.
9. Handelsman Y, Jellinger PS, Guerin CK, Bloomgarden ZT, Brinton EA, Budoff MJ, et al. Consensus Statement by the American Association of Clinical Endocrinologists and American College of Endocrinology on the Management of Dyslipidemia and Prevention of Cardiovascular Disease Algorithm – 2020 Executive Summary. Endocr Pract. 2020;26(10):1196-224.
10. Mach F, Baigent C, Catapano AL, Koskinas KC, Casula M, Badimon L, et al; ESC Scientific Document Group. 2019 ESC/EAS Guidelines for the management of dyslipidaemias: lipid modification to reduce cardiovascular risk. Eur Heart J. 2020;41(1):111-88.
11. Duseja A, Singh SP, De A, Madan K, Rao PN, Shukla A, et al. Indian National Association for Study of the Liver (INASL) Guidance Paper on Nomenclature, Diagnosis and Treatment of Nonalcoholic Fatty Liver Disease (NAFLD). J Clin Exp Hepatol. 2023;13(2):273-302.

12. Barakat L, Jayyousi A, Bener A, Zuby B, Zirie M. Comparison of Efficacy and Safety of Rosuvastatin, Atorvastatin and Pravastatin among Dyslipidemic Diabetic Patients. ISRN Pharmacol. 2013;2013:146579.
13. Sosale A, Saboo B, Sosale B. Saroglitazar for the treatment of hypertriglyceridemia in patients with type 2 diabetes: current evidence. Diabetes Metab Syndr Obes. 2015;8:189-96.
14. Rubenstrunk A, Hanf R, Hum DW, Fruchart JC, Staels B. Safety issues and prospects for future generations of PPAR modulators. Biochim Biophys Acta. 2007;1771(8):1065-81.
15. Jain N, Bhansali S, Kurpad AV, Hawkins M, Sharma A, Kaur S, et al. Effect of a Dual PPAR α/γ agonist on Insulin Sensitivity in Patients of Type 2 Diabetes with Hypertriglyceridemia – Randomized double-blind placebo-controlled trial. Sci Rep. 2019;9(1): 19017.
16. Pai V, Paneerselvam A, Mukhopadhyay S, Bhansali A, Kamath D, Shankar V, et al. A Multicenter, Prospective, Randomized, Double-Blind Study to Evaluate the Safety and Efficacy of Saroglitazar 2 And 4 mg Compared to Pioglitazone 45 mg in Diabetic Dyslipidemia (PRESS V). J Diabetes Sci Technol. 2014;8(1):132-41.
17. Jani RH, Pai V, Jha P, Jariwala G, Mukhopadhyay S, Bhansali A, et al. A multicenter, prospective, randomized, double-blind study to evaluate the safety and efficacy of Saroglitazar 2 and 4 mg compared with placebo in type 2 diabetes mellitus patients having hypertriglyceridemia not controlled with atorvastatin therapy (PRESS VI). Diabetes Technol Ther. 2014;16(2):63-71.
18. Kaul U, Parmar D., Manjunath K. Shah M, Parmar K, Patil KP, et al. New dual peroxisome proliferator activated receptor agonist—Saroglitazar in diabetic dyslipidemia and non-alcoholic fatty liver disease: integrated analysis of the real world evidence. Cardiovasc Diabetol. 2019;18:80.

38

CHAPTER

Waist–height Ratio vis-à-vis Body Mass Index for Prediction of Cardiovascular Complications in People with Diabetes

Ajoy Tewari, Jay Tewari

ABSTRACT

In individuals with diabetes, there is a significant correlation between central obesity and the risk of cardiovascular disease (CVD). The measurement of body mass index (BMI) alone does not accurately reflect the fat distribution in specific regions of the body. Other anthropometric indicators, such as waist circumference (WC) and waist–hip ratio (WHR), which are indicative of central obesity, are influenced by factors, such as age, gender, and ethnicity. However, a measurement called waist–height ratio (WHtR), which takes central obesity into account, demonstrates superior performance compared to BMI in predicting the risk of cardiometabolic disorders. WHtR provides a valuable screening tool for obesity in population-based settings by utilizing a universal threshold of 0.5, regardless of variations in age, gender, and ethnicity.

INTRODUCTION

According to the recent International Diabetes Federation (IDF) atlas, there are 537 million adults living with diabetes. In India, there are more than 101 million individuals with diabetes, accounting for 11.4% of the total population, which is an increase of 44% over 4 years since 2019. Additionally, approximately 136 million people or 15.3% of the population have been identified as having prediabetes. Generalized obesity affects 28.6% of the population, while 39.5% demonstrate abdominal obesity.

When evaluating adiposity, it is important to recognize that the commonly used measurement, body mass index (BMI), does not fully capture the entire range of fat distribution patterns including normal-weight central obesity and metabolically healthy obesity. Hence, it may not accurately reflect the proportion of adipose tissue and lean body mass, particularly among young children and adolescents, potentially leading to misclassification. Moreover, it is not a true index in the mathematical sense, as a true index is dimensionless. Furthermore, its limitations include the fact that increases in mass are measured in cubic increments rather than the square of height, as outlined by Futter et al. in 2011.

ADVANTAGES OF WAIST–HEIGHT RATIO OVER OTHER MARKERS OF CENTRAL OBESITY

The waist-hip ratio (WHR) is not practical for effective risk management since both waist and hip measurements can decrease with weight loss, resulting in an unchanged ratio. Furthermore, measuring waist circumference (WC) without adjusting for height can lead to an overestimation of fat mass in taller individuals and an underestimation in shorter individuals, as noted by Schneider in 2010. It is worth mentioning that WC requires specific values tailored to each population according to the World Health Organization (WHO) Consultation on Obesity in 1997.

In contrast, waist–height ratio (WHtR) has been proposed as a reliable method for assessing abdominal obesity by incorporating an individual's height into the measurement of WC. This is particularly important considering the inverse correlation between cardiovascular disease (CVD) and height, making it essential to adjust for height in anthropometric evaluations, as emphasized by various studies. Unlike other indices like WHR, WHtR is less sensitive to changes in body size, as it primarily reflects changes in waist measurement rather than proportional adjustments in both waist and hip.

Central adiposity is a major contributor to adverse outcomes in individuals with type 2 diabetes mellitus, with adverse cardiovascular effects being a significant factor contributing to mortality in this population. WHtR has shown promise as a superior indicator compared to BMI for assessing obesity, particularly in Southeast Asians, due to the high prevalence of central adiposity and susceptibility to coronary artery disease, as noted by Misra et al. in 2009. For an anthropometric index to be suitable as a public health screening tool, it should have well-defined thresholds applicable across different ethnicities, ages, and genders. WHtR meets this criterion as it remains unaffected by usual factors such as age, sex, and race, and does not require the use of scales, as mentioned by Ashwell and Hsieh in 2005. The simplicity of reporting WHtR, with a threshold value of <0.5 or >0.5 defining obesity, allows for a straightforward public health message of "keeping the waist less than half of the height," as highlighted by Browning et al. in 2010.

The concept of WHtR predicting coronary heart disease originated from Japanese researchers in 1995, as noted by Hsieh and Yoshinaga. WHtR has demonstrated a strong correlation with abdominal fat measured using imaging techniques, similar to WC, as observed by Soto González et al. in 2007. In the general population, WHtR is a more effective predictive marker for "early health risk" compared to BMI, as reported by Schneider et al. in 2010 and Ashwell and Gibson in 2016.

SOME REPRESENTATIVE STUDIES IN THE LAST 10 YEARS COMPARING WHTR WITH OTHER MARKERS OF CENTRAL OBESITY TO PREDICT ADVERSE CARDIOVASCULAR OUTCOMES IN PEOPLE WITH DIABETES

The study by Moazzeni et al. found no significant association between BMI and sudden cardiac death in both individuals with and without type 2 diabetes mellitus. However, they did observe a significant association between WHR in people with diabetes and WHtR in individuals without type 2 diabetes mellitus.

A study conducted by Aleksandra Markova et al. aimed to investigate the association between obesity indices (WC, WHtR, and WHR) and body composition parameters (body fat percentage, fat mass, fat-free mass, and total body water) with markers of cardiovascular risk. They found that BMI, followed by WHtR and body fat percentage, had the strongest associations with calculated cardiovascular risk estimates. Fat mass, fat-free mass, and total body water showed weaker associations and were mainly associated with the risk of stroke. Levels of N-terminal pro-brain natriuretic peptide (NT-proBNP) were not related to any measure of obesity, while asymmetric dimethylarginine (ADMA) showed links to WHtR, fat-free mass, total body water, and endothelin-1 (ET-1) to BMI and fat mass only.

Gomez-Sanchez L et al. utilized the cardio-ankle vascular index (CAVI) and brachial-ankle pulse wave velocity (baPWV) to assess cardiovascular risk. They found a statistically significant negative association between both BMI and WHtR and other adiposity markers, indicating that higher values of these indices were associated with a lower cardiovascular risk. The association between CAVI variability and BMI, WHtR, and other adiposity indicators was more pronounced in people with diabetes.

Guasch-Ferré M et al. conducted a cross-sectional study to examine the correlation between adiposity markers and hypertension, atherogenic dyslipidemia, and metabolic syndrome (MetS). They found that the area under the curve (AUC) values for WHtR and WC were significantly higher than the AUC values of BMI for atherogenic dyslipidemia and MetS. Conversely, BMI was the strongest predictor of hypertension.

The results from the ADVANCE ON trial, a randomized controlled trial primarily conducted in people with type 2 diabetes mellitus, demonstrated that one standard deviation higher WHtR was associated with a hazard ratio of 1.16 for significant major macrovascular events. BMI had a hazard ratio of 1.09, with a more substantial effect observed in individuals aged 66 years or older. WHtR marginally outperformed BMI and WHR in predicting major cardiovascular events.

Christian Obirikorang et al. examined the correlation between adiposity indicators and hypertension, high total cholesterol (TC), high triglycerides (TG), low high-density lipoprotein cholesterol (HDL-C), and MetS according to the International Diabetes Federation (MetS-IDF) criteria. They found that both WHtR and BMI were significantly associated with hypertension and MetS according to MetS-IDF criteria.

Lim RBT et al. conducted a prospective cohort study to assess the correlation between adiposity markers and all-cause and cardiovascular mortality. They found that while BMI was not positively associated with short-term mortality, the fourth and highest quintiles of WHtR were significantly associated with an increased risk of all-cause or cardiovascular mortality.

Ping Li et al. conducted a cross-sectional study and found that as WHtR, WC, and BMI increased, the likelihood of achieving therapeutic goals for blood pressure, glucose, and lipid levels decreased. Individuals with WHtR >0.59 had a lower likelihood of attaining all three targets.

Simone F Tonding et al. conducted a cross-sectional study and found no significant association between WHtR and cardiovascular risk scores. However, they did find a significant association between the conicity index and body adiposity index. This suggests that WHtR may not be a strong predictor of cardiovascular risk in this particular study, but other indices of body adiposity showed a relationship.

Shayesteh Khalili et al. conducted a prospective cohort study and found that WHtR, independent of cofounders, was marginally associated with incident CVD in both genders. They reported that a 1 standard deviation increase in WHtR led to a 19% increase in the risk of CVD in men and an 18% increase in women. This indicates that WHtR may have some predictive value for CVD risk, although the association was only marginally significant in this study.

Hossein Mozafar Saadati, et al. designed a prospective cohort study to examine the association of BMI and central obesity with the risk of stroke in both diabetics and nondiabetic patients. They used the targeted maximum likelihood estimation (TMLE) method and adjusted for various covariates. The results showed that the effect of BMI on stroke risk was more attenuated in people with diabetes compared to those without diabetes. The effects for other obesity indices, except for WHtR, were marginally significant. Interestingly, WHtR had a protective effect but was not significant. This suggests that BMI may have a stronger association with stroke risk compared to WHtR in this study population.

Ashwell and Hsieh presented a narrative review supporting the use of WHtR as a rapid and effective global indicator of the health risks of obesity. They listed six reasons to support their argument including: (1) WHtR being more sensitive than BMI as an early warning of health risks, (2) a boundary value of WHtR indicating increased risk for men and women, (3) the potential for WHtR to indicate an increased risk in different ethnic groups, (4) the cost-effectiveness and ease of measurement of WHtR compared to BMI, (5) the potential for using the same boundary values for children and adults, and (6) the conversion of WHtR boundary values into a consumer-friendly chart. These points highlight the advantages of using WHtR as a simple and practical tool for assessing obesity-related health risks.

Several systematic reviews have been conducted to evaluate the association of WHtR with various health outcomes. Schneider et al. (2010) investigated the association of WHtR with coronary artery disease and found that WHtR outperformed BMI in predicting this outcome. Savva et al. (2013) conducted a systematic review of the general population and found that WHtR was a better predictor than BMI for MetS, diabetes, cardiovascular risk, and cardiovascular and all-cause mortality with stronger predictive power observed in the Asian population. Corrêa et al. (2016) focused on the elderly population and found an association between WHtR and diabetes, MetS, and cardiovascular risk compared to BMI and other parameters. These systematic reviews support the use of WHtR as a potentially superior indicator compared to BMI for assessing various health risks, particularly in specific populations.

Further, a systematic review by the author found that WHtR outperforms BMI to predict cardiovascular outcomes in people with diabetes.

CONCLUSION

The simplicity of the WHtR and its conversion into the easily remembered public health message "keep your WC to less than half your height" is its key strength. This straightforward guideline eliminates the need for age, sex, and ethnic-specific cut-offs, making it a practical and universal tool for assessing abdominal obesity and related health risks. The use of a single cut-off value of 0.5 for WHtR, irrespective of demographic variations, supports its ease of implementation and interpretation.

In the context of CVD and related risk factors in people with diabetes, WHtR as a predictor can be particularly valuable. The use of WHtR as an index in these settings can help overcome the challenges associated with obtaining precise measurements and utilizing population-specific cut-offs. By relying on a single cut-off value, WHtR simplifies the process and allows for a more practical adoption in various healthcare settings.

Overall, the practicality and universality of WHtR, along with its potential as a predictor of CVD and related risk factors, make it an appealing index, particularly in resource-constrained environments, countries with high burdens on health infrastructure, and populations with diverse ethnic backgrounds.

SUGGESTED READINGS

1. IDF. (2019). IDF Diabetes Atlas, Ninth edition 2019. [online] Available from https://www.diabetesatlas.org/upload/resources/material/20200302_133351_IDFATLAS9e-final-web.pdf [Last accessed January, 2024].
2. Anjana RM, Unnikrishnan R, Deepa M, Pradeepa R, Tandon N, Das AK, et al. Metabolic non-communicable disease health report of India: the ICMR-INDIAB national cross-sectional study (ICMR-INDIAB-17). Lancet Diabetes Endocrinol. 2023;11(7):474-89.
3. Futter JE, Cleland JGF, Clark AL. Body mass indices and outcome in patients with chronic heart failure. Eur J Heart Fail. 2011;13(2):207-13.
4. Schneider HJ, Friedrich N, Klotsche J, Pieper L, Nauck M, John U, et al. The predictive value of different measures of obesity for incident cardiovascular events and mortality. J Clin Endocrinol Metab. 2010;95(4):1777-85.
5. World Health Organization. Obesity: preventing and managing the global epidemic: report of a WHO Consultation. Geneva: World Health Organization; 1997.
6. Langenberg C, Shipley MJ, Batty GD, Marmot MG. Adult socioeconomic position and the association between height and coronary heart disease mortality: findings from 33 years of follow-up in the Whitehall Study. Am J Public Health. 2005;95(4):628-32.
7. McCarron P, Okasha M, McEwen J, Smith GD. Height in young adulthood and risk of death from cardiorespiratory disease: a prospective study of male former students of Glasgow University, Scotland. Am J Epidemiol. 2002;155(8):683-7.
8. Misra A, Chowbey P, Makkar BM, Vikram NK, Wasir JS, Chadha D, et al. Consensus statement for diagnosis of obesity, abdominal obesity and the metabolic syndrome for Asian Indians and recommendations for physical activity, medical and surgical management. J Assoc Physicians India. 2009;57:163-70.
9. Ashwell M, Hsieh SD. Six reasons why the waist-to-height ratio is a rapid and effective global indicator for health risks of obesity and how its use could simplify the international public health message on obesity. Int J Food Sci Nutr. 2005;56(5):303-7.
10. Browning LM, Hsieh SD, Ashwell M. A systematic review of waist-to-height ratio as a screening tool for the prediction of cardiovascular disease and diabetes: 0.5 could be a suitable global boundary value. Nutr Res Rev. 2010;23(2):247-69.
11. Hsieh SD, Yoshinaga H. Abdominal fat distribution and coronary heart disease risk factors in men-waist/height ratio as a simple and useful predictor. Int J Obes Relat Metab Disord. 1995;19(8):585-9.
12. Soto González A, Bellido D, Buño MM, Pértega S, De Luis D, Martínez-Olmos M, et al. Predictors of the metabolic syndrome and correlation with computed axial tomography. Nutrition. 2007;23(1):36-45.
13. Ashwell M, Gibson S. Waist-to-height ratio as an indicator of "early health risk": simpler and more predictive than using a "matrix" based on BMI and waist circumference. BMJ Open. 2016;6(3):e010159.
14. Moazzeni SS, Tamehri Zadeh SS, Asgari S, Azizi F, Hadaegh F. Anthropometric indices and the risk of incident sudden cardiac death among adults with and without diabetes: over 15 years of follow-up in The Tehran Lipid and Glucose Study. Diabetol Metab Syndr. 2021;13(1):82.
15. Markova A, Boyanov M, Bakalov D, Tsakova A. Body Composition Indices and Cardiovascular Risk in Type 2 Diabetes. CV Biomarkers are not Related to Body Composition. Open Med. 2020;15:309-16.
16. Gomez-Sanchez L, Garcia-Ortiz L, Patino-Alonso MC, Recio-Rodriguez JI, Rigo F, Martí R, et al. Adiposity measures and arterial stiffness in primary care: the MARK prospective observational study. BMJ Open. 2017;7(9):e016422.
17. Guasch-Ferré M, Bulló M, Martínez-González MÁ, Corella D, Estruch R, Covas MI, et al. Waist-to-height ratio and cardiovascular risk factors in elderly individuals at high cardiovascular risk. PLoS One. 2012;7(8):e43275.
18. Rådholm K, Chalmers J, Ohkuma T, Peters S, Poulter N, Hamet P, et al. Use of the waist-to-height ratio to predict cardiovascular risk in patients with diabetes: Results from the ADVANCE-ON study. Diabetes Obes Metab. 2018;20(8):1903-10.
19. Obirikorang C, Obirikorang Y, Acheampong E, Anto EO, Toboh E, Asamoah EA, et al. Association of Wrist Circumference and Waist-to-Height Ratio with Cardiometabolic Risk Factors among Type II Diabetics in a Ghanaian Population. J Diabetes Res. 2018;2018:1838162.
20. Lim RBT, Chen C, Naidoo N, Gay G, Tang WE, Seah D, et al. Anthropometrics indices of obesity, and all-cause and cardiovascular disease-related mortality, in an Asian cohort with type 2 diabetes mellitus. Diabetes Metab. 2015;41(4):291-300.
21. Li P, Chen K, Nie Y, Guo LL, Wang HB, Wang SS, et al. Association of obesity with glucose, blood pressure, and lipid goals attainment in patients with concomitant diabetes and hypertension. Curr Med Res Opin. 2015;31(9):1623-31.
22. Tonding SF, Silva FM, Antonio JP, Azevedo MJ, Canani LHS, Almeida JC. Adiposity markers and risk of coronary heart disease in patients with type 2 diabetes mellitus. Nutr J. 2014;13(1):124.
23. Khalili S, Hatami M, Hadaegh F, Sheikholeslami F, Azizi F. Prediction of cardiovascular events with consideration of general and central obesity measures in diabetic adults: results of the 8.4-year follow-up. Metab Syndr Relat Disord. 2012;10(3):218-24.
24. Mozafar Saadati H, Mehrabi Y, Sabour S, Mansournia MA, Hashemi Nazari SS. Estimating the effects of body mass index and central obesity on stroke in diabetics and non-diabetics using targeted maximum likelihood estimation: Atherosclerosis Risk in Communities study. Obes Sci Pract. 2020;6(6):628-37.
25. Savva SC, Lamnisos D, Kafatos AG. Predicting cardiometabolic risk: waist-to-height ratio or BMI. A meta-analysis. Diabetes Metab Syndr Obes. 2013;6:403-19.
26. Corrêa MM, Thumé E, De Oliveira ERA, Tomasi E. Performance of the waist-to-height ratio in identifying obesity and predicting non-communicable diseases in the elderly population: A systematic literature review. Arch Gerontol Geriatr. 2016;65:174-82.
27. Tewari A, Kumar G, Maheshwari A, Tewari V, Tewari J. Comparative Evaluation of Waist-to-Height Ratio and BMI in Predicting Adverse Cardiovascular Outcome in People With Diabetes: A Systematic Review. Cureus. 2023;15(5):e38801.

39

CHAPTER

Atypical Diabetes: Physician's Role

V Palanikumaran

ABSTRACT

Atypical diabetes is increasingly recognized but is often poorly defined and may masquerade as type 1 diabetes mellitus (T1DM) or type 2 diabetes mellitus (T2DM). Recognition of an atypical diabetes phenotype is important in facilitating timely work-up and often leads to referral for confirmation of the specific diagnosis, prognosis, and treatment plans. The growing recognition of these atypical cases underscores the importance of considering and diagnosing rare forms of diabetes accurately and expeditiously in a cost-effective manner.

INTRODUCTION

Classification of diabetes includes a long list of common, rare, and not-so-rare conditions characterized by hyperglycemia of variable degrees. The majority of patients with diabetes are easily classified as having type 1 diabetes mellitus (T1DM) or type 2 diabetes mellitus (T2DM), whereas the other forms of diabetes, in aggregate, account for approximately 10% of diabetes cases. These cases may be grouped under the umbrella of rare forms of diabetes or "atypical diabetes." Cases of atypical diabetes are not only challenging from the diagnostic perspective, but more often than not, they demand distinct therapeutic approaches, emphasizing that "one size does not fit all" in clinical medicine. This chapter will give an overall view about atypical diabetes with more emphasis on more common forms.

COMMON FORMS OF ATYPICAL DIABETES

- *Monogenic forms of diabetes*:
  - Various forms of maturity onset of diabetes in young (MODY), especially MODY 3, MODY 2, MODY 1, and MODY 5
  - Neonatal diabetes: Permanent and transient neonatal diabetes
  - Wolfram syndrome
  - Mitochondrial diabetes
- *Diabetes secondary to pancreatic disorders (type 3c diabetes mellitus)*: Including diabetes due to hemochromatosis, cystic fibrosis-related diabetes
- *Hybrid forms of diabetes (diabetes 1.5)*:
  - Ketosis-prone diabetes (KPD)
  - Latent autoimmune diabetes in adults (LADA)
- Diabetes secondary to endocrinopathies
- Diabetes secondary to drugs
- *Rare forms of severe insulin resistance (IR) syndromes*:
  - Type A IR syndrome
  - Type B IR syndrome
  - Type C IR syndrome
  - Lipodystrophy syndromes
- Diabetes secondary to certain genetic syndromes

Maturity Onset of Diabetes in Young

Monogenic diabetes is a heterogeneous group of uncommon but important causes of diabetes, accounting for 1–2% of all diabetes worldwide. The identified genes that lead to MODY encode transcription factors important for β-cell function and regulation and an enzyme that allows the β-cell to respond to changes in glycemia. The *glucokinase* (*GCK*) gene was the first gene to be subsequently identified in 1992, shortly followed by the discovery of hepatic nuclear factor 1 alpha (HNF1α) and HNF4α in 1996. These three genes along with HNF1β account for > 90% of all MODY with a known genetic diagnosis. Altogether, there are at least 13 MODY genes that affect insulin secretion.

Clinical Presentation and Diagnosis

Maturity onset of diabetes in young is classically defined as autosomal dominant, nonketotic, noninsulin-dependent diabetes with onset typically before 25 years of age with two to three consecutively affected generations. Patients typically lack significant obesity or metabolic features and pancreatic autoantibodies **(Table 1)**.

Neonatal Diabetes

- Presentation of diabetes within the first 6 months of life—neonatal diabetes. Between 6 months and 1 year—infantile-onset diabetes
- Nonautoimmune in nature in contrast to T1DM, which usually does not present before the first year.
- Neonatal diabetes mellitus (NDM) is stratified as transient NDM (TNDM) and permanent NDM (PNDM).
- TNDM—temporary insulinization
- PNDM—lifelong treatment

Transient Neonatal Diabetes Mellitus

- Neonates with TNDM present with intrauterine growth retardation, hyperglycemia, macroglossia, umbilical hernia, and absence of ketosis. The response of oral sulfonylurea (SU) is uncertain.
- Genetic testing alone helps in differentiating the TNDM and PNDM children in the early age as the clinical differentiation is not possible.

Permanent Neonatal Diabetes Mellitus

- Mutations in the adenosine triphosphate-sensitive potassium (K_{ATP}) channels encoded by the *KCNJ11* and *ABCC8* genes are common causes of PNDM.
- Activating mutations in the K_{ATP} channel complex lead to increased K_{ATP} channel opening, resulting in a suppression of insulin secretion and subsequent hyperglycemia.
- Identification of *KCNJ11* and *ABCC8* mutations becomes important for clinical management as most of these children with K_{ATP} mutations are responsive to oral SU drugs.
- SU drugs bind to sulfonylurea receptor 1 (SUR1) subunit of K_{ATP} channel, which leads to the closure of the channel independent of ATP, with subsequent release of insulin.
- The dose of SU required in children with neonatal diabetes—0.5–1.5 mg/kg/day (relatively larger dose compared to adults)
- Improvement in motor and cognitive function with SU drugs has also been reported in children with developmental delay, epilepsy, and neonatal diabetes (DEND)/intermediate DEND (iDEND) syndrome as SUs could act on mutated K_{ATP} channels in the central nervous system.
- Children diagnosed with autoantibody-negative hyperglycemia below 1 year of age should be considered for genetic testing to identify the underlying genetic defect.

Wolfram Syndrome—Diabetes Insipidus, Diabetes Mellitus, Optic Atrophy, and Deafness Syndrome

- Confirmed by genetic testing, wolframin gene mutation—Wolfram syndrome-1 (*WFS1*) gene
- Lack of wolframin leads to Wolfram syndrome

TABLE 1: Clinical features and treatment of the common subtypes of MODY.

Monogenic diabetes phenotype and clinical features	First-line therapy
HNF1α-MODY (MODY 3): Progressive insulin secretory defect with presentation in adolescence or early adulthood; lowered renal threshold for glucosuria; large rise in 2-hour glucose level on OGTT (>90 mg/dL; >5 mmol/L)	Sulfonylureas (frequently low doses) GLP-1 agonists may be considered for adjunctive therapy
HNF4α-MODY (MODY 1): Progressive insulin secretory defect with presentation in adolescence or early adulthood; may have large birth weight and transient neonatal hypoglycemia	Sulfonylureas (frequently low doses)
HNF1β-MODY (MODY 5): Developmental renal disease (typically cystic); genitourinary abnormalities; hypoplasia, atrophy of the pancreas; hyperuricemia; gout; HNF1β mutations often cause renal disease without diabetes	Variable type 1 diabetes mellitus (around 30%)
GCK-MODY (MODY 2): Lifelong stable, elevated fasting blood glucose with minimal age-related progression	Treatment is not needed for isolated GCK-MODY except during pregnancy with an unaffected fetus

(GCK: glucokinase; GLP-1: glucagon-like peptide 1; MODY: maturity onset of diabetes in young; OGTT: oral glucose tolerance tests)

- Chronic endoplasmic reticulum (ER) stress-mediated apoptosis of β-cells of pancreas and neurons
- An autosomal recessive disorder
- Autoimmunity negative
- Diabetes and optic atrophy needed for diagnosis
- Other components—diabetes insipidus, deafness, and neurological manifestations may be present.
- Death due to neurological complications

Mitochondrial-inherited Diabetes and Deafness (Mitochondrial Diabetes)

- Confirmed by detection of mitochondrial deoxyribonucleic acid (DNA) mutation m.3243A>G in patient's urinary epithelial cell DNA sample
- Mitochondrial dysfunction in the highly metabolically active pancreatic islets leads to progressive deterioration of β-cells.
- Strong familial clustering of diabetes and maternal transmission
- Usually no diabetic ketoacidosis (DKA)
- High-frequency hearing impairment precedes the onset of diabetes.
- Autoimmunity negative
- Other features—pigmentary retinopathy, renal disorders, neurological manifestations—MELAS (mitochondrial encephalomyopathy, lactic acidosis, and stroke-like episodes) and psychiatric manifestations
- Death due to lactic acidosis and renal failure
- Because of progressive insulin deficiency, exogenous insulin is the mainstay of treatment.
- Metformin is contraindicated because of the risk of lactic acidosis.
- Coenzyme Q10 and carnitine have been used in the treatment of patients with mitochondrial myopathies.

Diabetes Secondary to Pancreatic Disorders (Type 3c Diabetes Mellitus)

Refer to **Box 1**.

BOX 1: Causes.

- *Pancreatitis*:
  - Acute
  - Chronic calcifying
  - Chronic noncalcifying
- Pancreatic carcinoma
- *Pancreatectomy*:
  - Total
  - Partial
- Trauma
- *Infiltrative disorders*:
  - Hemochromatosis
  - Primary (common)
  - Secondary
  - Amyloidosis and sarcoidosis
- Cystic fibrosis

Diagnostic Criteria for Type 3c Diabetes Mellitus

Major criteria (all must be fulfilled):
- Presence of exocrine pancreatic insufficiency (according to monoclonal fecal elastase—one or direct function tests)
- Pathological pancreatic imaging [by endoscopic ultrasound, magnetic resonance imaging (MRI), or computed tomography (CT)]
- Absence of T1DM-associated autoimmune markers

Minor criteria:
- Impaired β-cell function [as measured by Homeostasis Model Assessment (HOMA)-B, C-peptide/glucose ratio]
- No excessive IR (measured by HOMA-IR)
- Impaired incretin [e.g., gastric inhibitory polypeptide (GIP)] or pancreatic polypeptide secretion
- Low serum levels of lipid-soluble vitamins (A, D, E, and K)

Peculiarities

- Ketosis rare
- Prolonged hypoglycemia
- Less macrovascular complications (chronic malabsorption undernutrition)
- Brittle diabetes

Ketosis-Prone Diabetes

Refer to **Table 2**.

Latent Autoimmune Diabetes in Adults

Refer to **Tables 3 and 4**.

Diabetes Secondary to Endocrinopathies

Refer to **Flowcharts 1 to 3**.

Drug-induced Diabetes

- *Reduce insulin secretion—β-cell toxin*:
  - Pentamidine
  - Streptozotocin

TABLE 2: Clinical and laboratory features of ketosis-prone diabetes.

Clinical considerations	Laboratory features
• Unprovoked ketoacidosis often occurs; may be new-onset diabetes • Afro-Caribbean or Hispanic ancestry • Periods of insulin independence interspersed with periods of acute insulin deficiency and diabetic ketoacidosis • Type 2 diabetes mellitus phenotype common (obesity, insulin resistance, and metabolic syndrome) • Fluctuating glycated hemoglobin (HbA1c) pattern consistent with β-cell failure and recovery • Male predominance among patients with unprovoked diabetic ketoacidosis (male–female ratio 2.6:1) • Insulin should always be initial therapy, with reduction of cardiovascular risk factors	• β-cell antibodies present in up to 28% of patients • C-peptide often low or undetectable during diabetic ketoacidosis; recovery expected in >60% • Ratio of fasting C-peptide (nmol/L) to glucose (mmol/L) >11 may be used as reliable predictor of insulin discontinuation • Presence of human leukocyte antigen (HLA) alleles for type 1 diabetes associated with insulin dependence within 1–2 years

TABLE 3: Clinical and laboratory features of latent autoimmune diabetes of adulthood.

Clinical considerations	Laboratory features
• Age > 30 years • Patients may be overweight, but typically leaner than those with T2DM • Patients may have mild-to-moderate insulin resistance • Occurs in people of various ethnicities • Progression to insulin therapy slower than for patients with T1DM, but quicker hand for those with T2DM • Avoid β-cell stressors such as secretagogues • May be treated initially with oral antihyperglycemic agents, but insulin should be introduced early if glycemic control cannot be maintained	• GAD and ICA antibodies present • Insulin antibodies often absent • Autoimmune markers may show subtle differences from those of childhood T1DM but are more similar to antibodies seen in adult-onset T1DM

(GAD: glutamic acid decarboxylase; ICA: islet cell antibodies; T1DM: type 1 diabetes mellitus; T2DM: type 2 diabetes mellitus)

TABLE 4: Compares the clinical characteristics of HNF1α diabetes, T2DM, T1DM, ketosis-prone diabetes, and latent autoimmune diabetes of adulthood.

Characteristic	T2DM	T1DM	HNF1α diabetes (monogenic)	Ketosis-prone diabetes	Latent autoimmune diabetes of adulthood
Mode of inheritance	Polygenic, with environmental interaction	Polygenic, class II HLA	Monogenic, autosomal dominant	Polygenic; increased frequency of HLA alleles associated with type 1 diabetes mellitus	Polygenic, with environmental interaction
Age at presentation	Variable (usually adulthood)	Young	Young (often <25 years)	Variable (usually adulthood)	>30 years (adult, by definition)
Penetrance (%)	Variable (10–40)	Incomplete (<25)	High (80–96)	Variable (<50)	Similar to T1DM
Body habitus	Obese	Nonobese	Nonobese	Typically obese	Nonobese
Ethnicity	High prevalence worldwide	White	White, European ancestry	Afro-Caribbean or Hispanic, with strong family history of phenotypic T2DM	Similar to T1DM
β-Cell antibodies (%)	<10	>85	<1	<30	100 (by definition)
First-line therapy	Metformin in most patients	Insulin	Low-dose sulfonylurea	Insulin during acute presentation; up to 60% of patients require insulin by 10 years after diagnosis	Insulin independence for at least 6 months, progressing to insulin dependence over time

(HLA: human leukocyte antigen; HNF1α: hepatic nuclear factor 1 alpha; T1DM: type 1 diabetes mellitus; T2DM: type 2 diabetes mellitus)

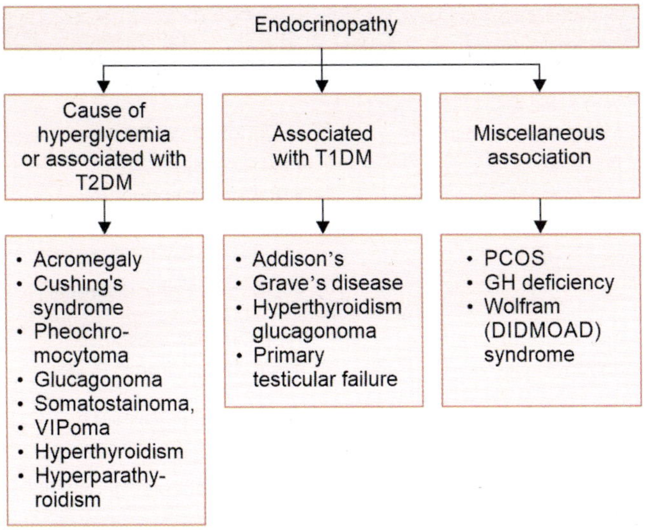

(DIDMOAD: diabetes insipidus, diabetes mellitus, optic atrophy, and deafness; GH: growth hormone; PCOS: polycystic ovary syndrome; T1DM: type 1 diabetes mellitus; T2DM: type 2 diabetes mellitus)

FLOWCHART 1: Endocrinopathies.

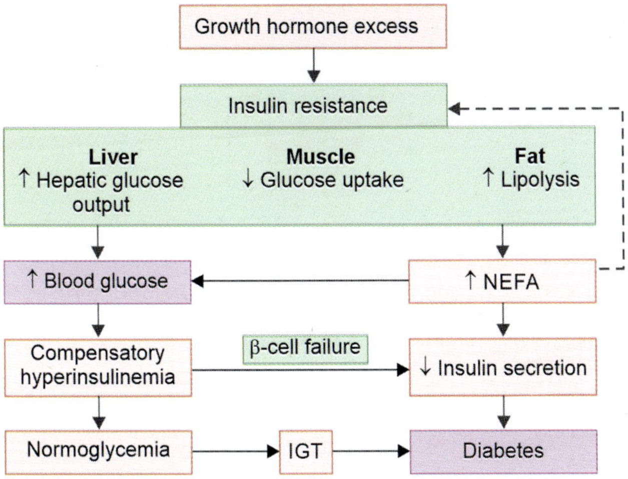

FLOWCHART 2: Acromegaly.
(IGT: impaired glucose tolerance; NEFA: non-esterified fatty acid)

- *Reduce insulin release*:
  - Thiazides
  - Diazoxide
  - Somatostatin
- *Reduce insulin action*:
  - Glucocorticoids
  - Estradiol, levonorgestrel
  - Glucagon
  - Growth hormone (GH)
  - Thiazides

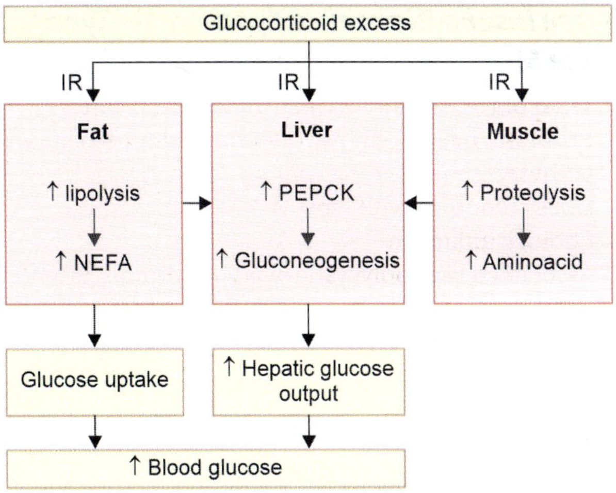

FLOWCHART 3: Cushing's syndrome.
(IR: insulin resistance; NEFA: non-esterified fatty acid; PEPCK: phosphoenolpyruvate carboxykinase)

Rare Forms of Severe Insulin Resistance Syndromes

Severe Insulin Resistance Syndrome—Type A

Features of severe IR include acanthosis nigricans (AN), hyperandrogenism (HA), mostly lean patients, in the absence of autoantibodies to insulin receptors. This occurs mainly due to mutations in the insulin receptor gene.

- Adolescent onset, mostly lean
- Frequently females
- Triglyceride level (TGL) unusually normal or low (in contrast to metabolic syndrome)
- High adiponectin
- Other rare variants include Rabson-Mendenhall syndrome and leprechaunism—Donohue syndrome

Severe Insulin Resistance Syndrome—Type B

- Due to autoantibodies to insulin receptor
- Common in middle-aged women, mostly lean
- AN involving periocular, perioral, and labial regions giving a characteristic facial appearance
- Commonly associated with systemic lupus erythematosus (SLE) and other autoimmune disorders, as a part of paraneoplastic syndrome associated with multiple myeloma or Hodgkin's disease
- Glycemic manifestation may range from extreme IR with or without hyperglycemia to fasting hypoglycemia.
- Low fasting TGL

Severe Insulin Resistance Syndrome—Type C (Table 5)

- Triad of HA, IR, and AN—HAIR-AN syndrome
- Problem occurs in postinsulin receptor-signaling pathways
- Obese (contrast with type A)
- Etiology unknown
- Associated with polycystic ovary syndrome (PCOS)

Lipodystrophy Syndromes (Figs. 1A to F)

Loss of adipose tissue with severe hypertriglyceridemia and low adiponectin

- *Familial*:
  - Congenital generalized lipodystrophy (Berardinelli-Seip syndrome)
  - Partial lipodystrophy (Dunnigan syndrome)

TABLE 5: Etiology and clinical syndrome.

Etiology	Clinical syndrome
Mutations of the insulin receptor	• Donohue syndrome (leprechaunism) • Rabson–Mendenhall syndrome • Type A insulin resistance • Lipodystrophic disorders
Post-binding defects in insulin action	Type C insulin resistance (HAIR-AN syndrome; PCOS)
Anti-insulin receptor antibodies	Type B insulin resistance

(HAIR-AN: hyperandrogenism insulin resistance-acanthosis nigricans; PCOS: polycystic ovary syndrome)

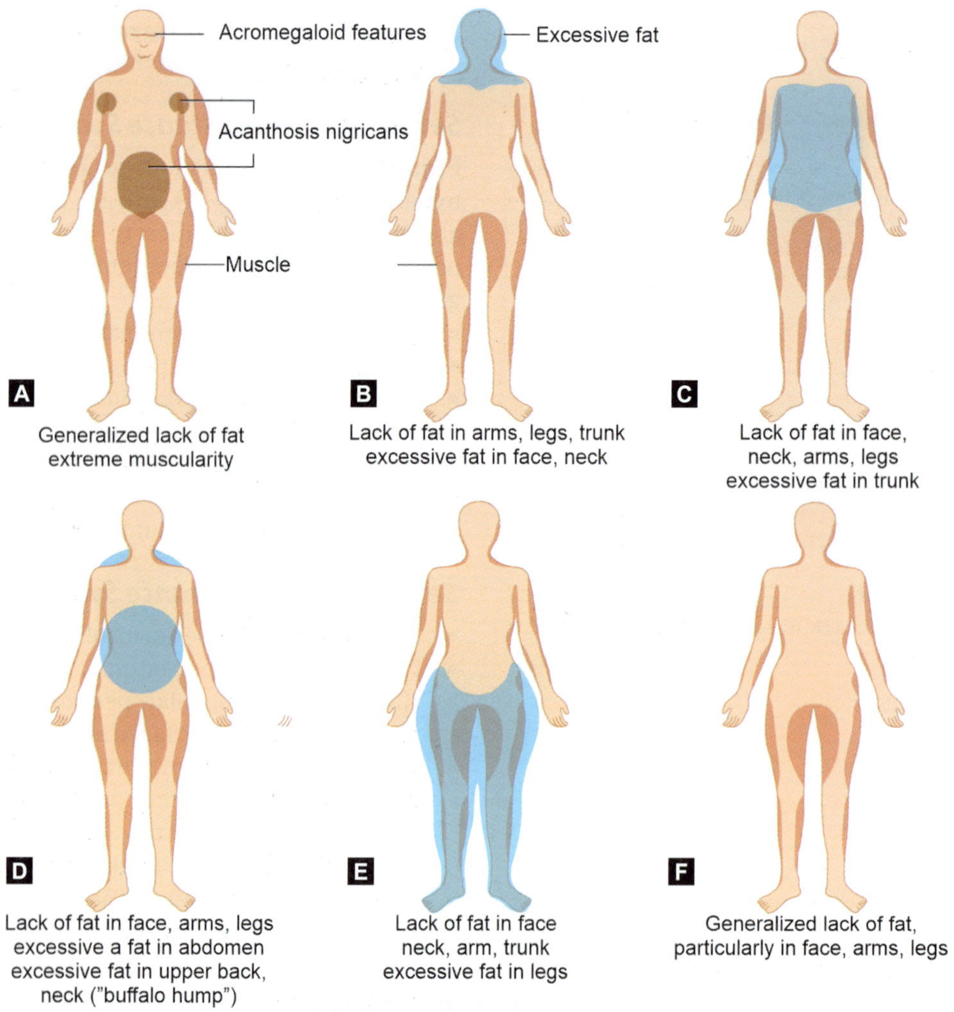

FIGS. 1A TO F: (A) Congenital generalized lipodystrophy 1/2; (B) Familial partial lipodystrophy (Dunnigan variety); (C) Familial partial lipodystrophy; (D) Retroviral therapy-associated lipodystrophy; (E) Acquired partial lipodystrophy; and (F) Acquired generalized lipodystrophy.

Acquired:
- Generalized (Lawrence syndrome)
- Partial (Barraquer-Simons syndrome)
- *Pseudo acromegaly*: GH-insulin-like growth factor 1 (IGF-1) axis normal
- Alstrom's syndrome
- Myotonic dystrophy
- Congenital fiber-type disproportion myopathy (CFTDM)
- Werner syndrome

Diabetes Secondary to Certain Genetic Syndromes

- *Chromosomal abnormality syndromes*:
  - Down syndrome
  - Klinefelter syndrome
  - Turner syndrome
- *Base pair repeat syndromes*:
  - Friedreich's ataxia
  - Huntington's disease
  - Myotonic dystrophies
- *Severe obesity syndromes*:
  - Bardet-Biedl syndrome
  - Laurence-Moon syndrome
  - Prader-Willi syndrome

CONCLUSION

Although the various forms of atypical diabetes are relatively uncommon, it is important that they must be accurately diagnosed, as diagnosis may have a substantial impact on the prognosis and management of individual patients and their families.

SUGGESTED READINGS

1. Fajans SS, Bell GI, Polonsky KS. Molecular mechanisms and clinical pathophysiology of maturity-onset diabetes of the young. N Engl J Med. 2001;345:971-80.
2. Carmody D, Støy J, Greeley SAW, Bell GI, Philipson LH. A clinical guide to monogenic diabetes. In: Weiss RE, Refetoff S (Eds). Genetic Diagnosis of Endocrine Disorders, 2nd edition. United Kingdom: Academic Press; 2016. pp. 21-30.
3. Støy J, Greeley SAW, Paz VP, Ye H, Pastore AN, Skowron KB, et al. Diagnosis and treatment of neonatal diabetes: a United States experience. Pediatr Diabetes. 2008;9:450-9.
4. Murphy R, Turnbull DM, Walker M, Hattersley AT. Clinical features, diagnosis, and management of maternally inherited diabetes and deafness (MIDD) associated with the 3243A>G mitochondrial point mutation. Diabet Med. 2008;25:383-99.
5. Steenkamp DW, Alexanian SM, Sternthal E. Approach to the patient with atypical diabetes. CMAJ. 2014;186(9):678-84.
6. Tsoukas MA, Mantzoros CS. Lipodystrophy syndromes. In: Jameson JL, DeGroot LJ (Eds). Endocrinology: Adult and Pediatric, 7th edition. Philadelphia: Elsevier; 2016. pp. 648-61.

40

CHAPTER

Gestational Diabetes: Newer Perspectives

Aarathy Kannan, Rohith Velusamy

ABSTRACT

Gestational diabetes mellitus (GDM) is a long-standing complication of obstetrics and neonatology, mainly related to high infant birth weight. It occurs in about six out of every 100 pregnancies. It should not be confused with likely preexisting diabetes/glucose intolerance. Diagnosis of GDM is a separate entity that occurs in the second half of pregnancy. American College of Obstetricians and Gynecologists (ACOG) supports insulin as the first-line treatment for GDM and recommends that oral hypoglycemic agents should be reserved for women who are unable or unwilling to receive insulin. A multidisciplinary plan and approach is needed to manage GDM and long-term follow-up of the mother and baby is essential.

INTRODUCTION

Gestational diabetes mellitus (GDM) refers to abnormal glucose tolerance with onset or first recognition during pregnancy. GDM is a long-standing complication of obstetrics and neonatology, mainly related to high infant birth weight. GDM is becoming more and more associated with future cardiovascular disease in both mothers and offspring. The significant role of GDM in the worldwide epidemic of intergenerational cardiovascular disease emphasizes the need to identify GDM as early risk factor in type 2 diabetes/cardiovascular disease. This broadens the current clinical approach to long-term maternal and progeny complications after GDM diagnosis. Diagnosis of GDM is a separate entity that occurs in the second half of pregnancy. It should not be confused with likely preexisting diabetes/glucose intolerance.

PREVALENCE

Gestational diabetes mellitus in India ranges from 3.8 to 21% depending on the geographical location and diagnostic techniques used. GDM is more common in urban areas than rural areas. It occurs in about six out of every 100 pregnancies. Pregnant women >35 years of age are more likely to develop GDM than women <25 years of age. Indian women are 11 times more likely to develop glucose intolerance during pregnancy.

NEW NOMENCLATURE

Refer to **Flowchart 1**.

DIAGNOSTIC CRITERIA

Overt diabetes in pregnancy is diagnosed if any of the following apply:

- Fasting blood glucose level (BGL) ≥ 126 mg/dL
- Glycated hemoglobin (HbA1c) values ≥6.5%
- Diabetic retinopathy is certainly present
- Casual blood glucose ≥200 mg/dL or 2-hour 75 g oral glucose tolerance test (OGTT) value ≥200 mg/dL

PATHOPHYSIOLOGY (FLOWCHART 2)

Increased Insulin Resistance

- Increased insulin resistance is due to hormones secreted by the placenta that are "diabetogenic":
    - Human placental lactogen (HPL)

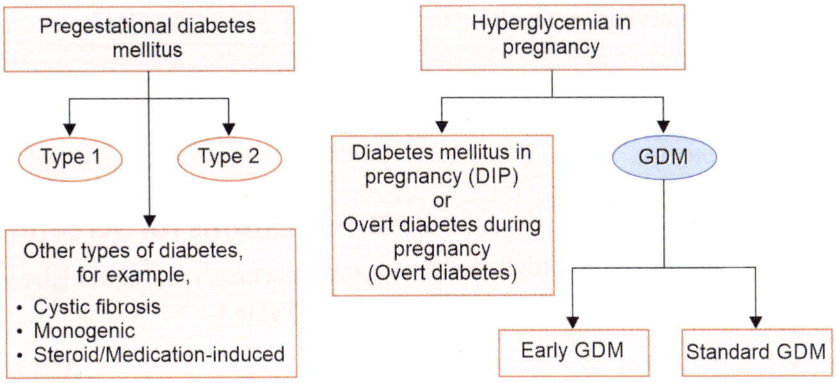

FLOWCHART 1: New nomenclature of gestational diabetes mellitus (GDM).

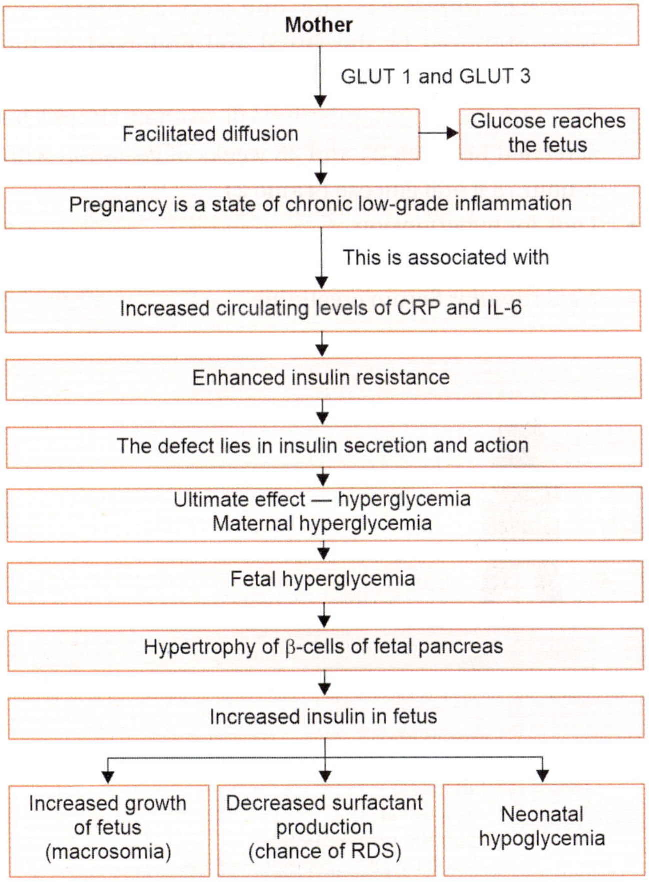

FLOWCHART 2: Pathophysiology of GDM.

(CRP: C-reactive protein; GDM: gestational diabetes mellitus; GLUT1: glucose transporter 1; IL-6: interleukin-6; RDS: respiratory distress syndrome)

- Progesterone and estrogen
- Corticotropin-releasing hormone

- Transient maternal hyperglycemia occurs after meals because of increased insulin resistance
- Mainly seen in 24–28 weeks of pregnancy

Relative Baseline Hypoglycemia

Increased pancreatic β-cell proliferation results in increased insulin secretion. Pregnant women have higher fasting insulin levels than nonpregnant women. Postprandial and fasting insulin levels are higher than normal. Continuous fetal drawing results in hypoglycemia. BGLs are reduced by 10–20% between meals. Hypoglycemia is also common at night.

Before conception, the 24-hour insulin requirement is about 0.6 unit/kg. The insulin requirement increases to about 0.7 unit/kg of pregnant weight during the first 3 months of pregnancy. During the first 3 months, glycemia tends to be more unstable, with low fasting glucose levels and high postpregnancy excursions and nighttime hypoglycemia. During the second and third trimesters, insulin requirement increases to 0.8 unit/kg. By the 24th month, insulin requirement has increased steadily and glycemia has stabilized. By the third trimester, insulin requirement is between 0.9 and 1.0 units/kg/day. During the last month of pregnancy, insulin requirement may decrease and hypoglycemia may occur, especially nocturnal.

GESTATIONAL DIABETES MELLITUS—RISK FACTORS AND PATHOGENESIS

Gestational Diabetes Mellitus is Driven by Microbiota-induced Inflammation Months before Diagnosis

The gut microbiome and inflammatory markers were studied in 394 pregnant women during their first trimester. The gut microbiome plays a role in inflammation-induced GDM pathogenesis. Interleukin-6 may play a role in the pathogenesis of GDM. Potential GDM markers including microbiota can be targeted for

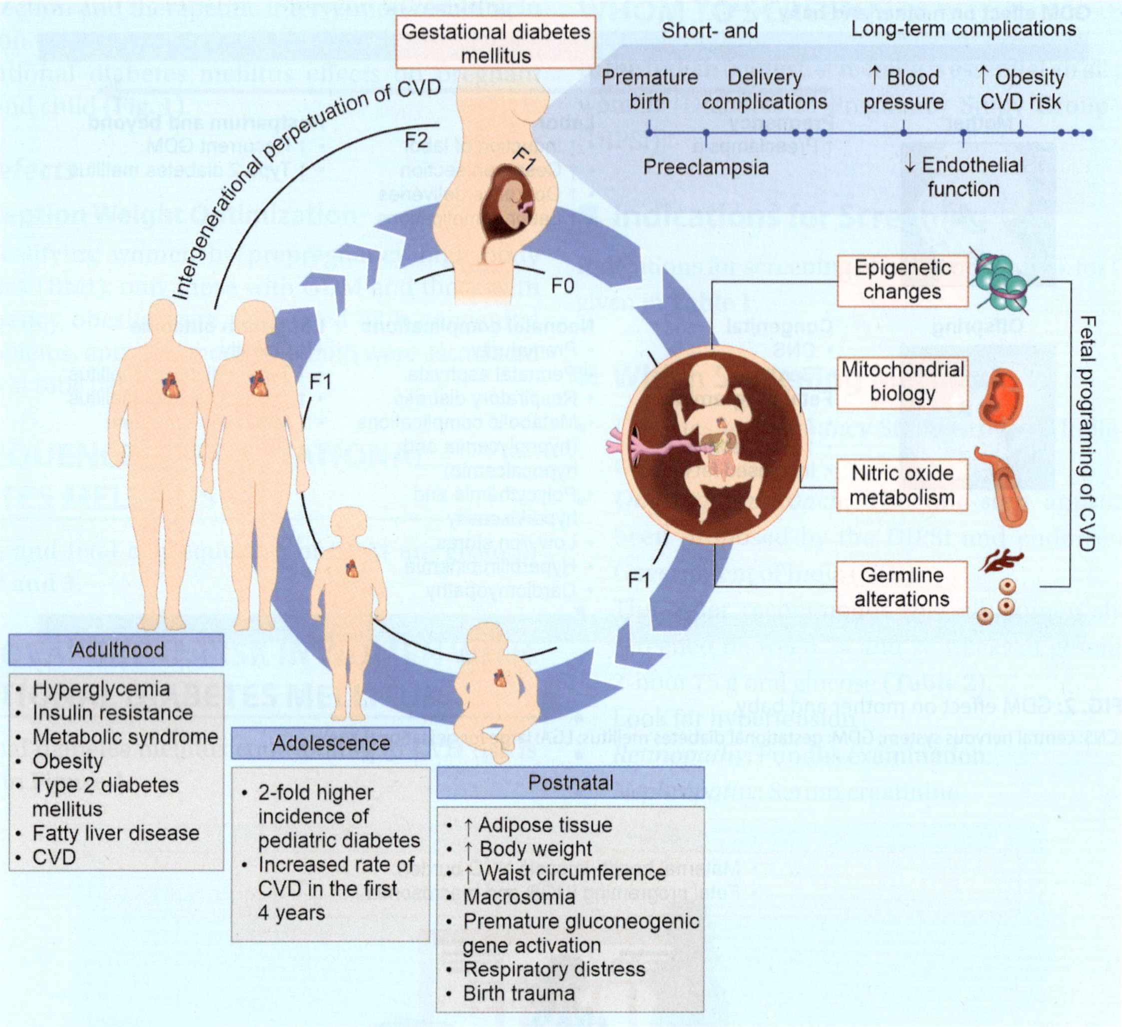

FIG. 4: GDM and CVD.

(CVD: cardiovascular disease; GDM: gestational diabetes mellitus)

Source: Tocantins C, Diniz MS, Grilo LF, Pereira SP. The birth of cardiac disease: Mechanisms linking gestational diabetes mellitus and early onset of cardiovascular disease in offspring. WIREs Mech Dis. 2022;14(4):e1555.

TABLE 1: Indications for screening of high and low risk for gestational diabetes mellitus (GDM).

High risk for GDM	Low risk for GDM
• Family history of diabetes	• Age <25 years
• Glucose in second fasting urine sample	• Weight normal before pregnancy
• History of unexplained perinatal loss	• No known diabetes in first-degree relatives
• History of large for gestational age infant	• No history of abnormal glucose intolerance
• History of congenitally malformed infant	• No history of poor obstetric outcome
• Maternal obesity	

TABLE 2: Oral glucose tolerance test (OGTT) interpretation.

With 75 g oral glucose tolerance test		
Plasma glucose	**In pregnancy**	**Nonpregnant**
2 hours > 200 mg/dL	Diabetes	Diabetes
2 hours >140 mg/dL and <199 mg/dL	Gestational diabetes	Impaired glucose tolerance
2 hours >120 mg/dL and <139 mg/dL	Gestational glucose intolerance	–
2 hours <120 mg/dL	Normal	Normal

MANAGEMENT OF GESTATIONAL DIABETES MELLITUS

- Medical nutrition therapy
- Gestational weight management
- Physical activity
- Self-monitoring of glucose
- Pharmacotherapy
- Fetal/maternal health surveillance

Target Weight Gain in Gestational Diabetes Mellitus

Target weight gain in GDM is given in **Table 3**.

Nutrition Recommendations and Management in GDM (Table 4)

Cooking oil: Sesame oil/groundnut oil/sunflower oil—10 g or two teaspoon daily
Skimmed milk amount in daily—620 mL
1 cup—120 mL, 1 bowl—150 mL

Glycemic Management during Pregnancy

Glycemic targets during pregnancy are given in **Box 1**.

Time-in-range TARGETS

- Help to achieve A1c targets in diabetes and pregnancy
- Reduce macrosomia and neonatal hypoglycemia in pregnancy complicated by type 1 diabetes mellitus (T1DM)

Exercise

- Reduce insulin requirement by as much as 50%
- 1 hour after mealtime
- For 20–30 min/day walking
- ACOG recommends—benefits in the postpartum period, reducing recovery time postpartum and preventing postpartum depression, risk reduction for gestational diabetes, cesarean section, and operative vaginal delivery.

TABLE 3: Target weight gain in GDM.

Weight category	BMI (kg/m²)	Calorie requirement in kcal/kg/day	Total weight gain (kg)
Underweight	<18.5	Up to 40 kcal	12.5–18 kg
Normal weight	18.5–24.9	30	11.5–16 kg
Overweight	23–24.9	22–25	7–11.5 kg
Obese	>25	12–14	5–9 kg

Pharmacotherapy

When medical nutrition therapy (MNT) does not work, pharmacological therapy should be used.

The American Association of Clinical Endocrinology (AACE) guidelines suggest insulin as the best approach to treating T1DM. Insulin therapy is necessary to treat T1DM in pregnancy. Metformin and sulfonylurea (glyburide) are the two most frequently prescribed oral hypoglycemic agent (OHA) medications during pregnancy. The American Diabetes Association (ADA) and the Diabetes in Pregnancy Study Group India

TABLE 4: Nutrition recommendations and management in GDM.

Dietary component	Recommendations
Energy	• Optimize growth and development of the fetus • 30 kcal/kg desirable body weight in first trimester + 300 kcal/day in second and third trimester are recommended
Carbohydrates	Minimum 175 g/day; 20–30 g of dietary fiber per day (50–55% of calories) (not <200 g)
Protein	Normal adult RDA + 10 g/day (20%)
Fat	Percentage based on nutritional assessment and treatment (<30% of calories)
Sodium/alcohol	Should be avoided
Vitamins and minerals	Ferrous iron 30 mg/day, folic acid 400 µg/day, calcium and magnesium requirement is increased
Sweeteners	• Sweeteners for pregnancy in moderation (sucralose) • Saccharin is contraindicated
Dietary adjuvant therapy	Pregnant women should not take any herbs and botanical products

(BMI: body mass index; GDM: gestational diabetes mellitus; RDA: recommended dietary allowance)

BOX 1: Target glucose values in pregnancy.

Target glucose values:
- Fasting plasma glucose (PG) <95 mg/dL
- 1-hour postprandial PG <140 mg/dL
- 2-hour postprandial PG <120 mg/dL
- A1c target 6–7%

(DIPSI) do not recommend OHA in pregnancy for GDM or preexisting T2DM due to efficacy and safety issues.

Insulin versus Metformin as First-line Therapy

The ACOG supports insulin as the first-line treatment for GDM and recommends that oral hypoglycemic agents should be reserved for women who are unable or unwilling to receive insulin.

PHARMACOLOGICAL TREATMENT—INSULIN

Pharmacological treatment with insulin is given in **Tables 5 and 6**.

- *Total daily dose (TDD)*: 50% for basal insulin, 50% for premeal rapid-acting insulin boluses.
- Lactating women should reduce their nighttime basal insulin by 50% (to avoid severe hypoglycemia).
- Patients with T1DM go through a period of increased sensitivity between 10 and 14 weeks of pregnancy; insulin dosage might need to be decreased accordingly.
- From weeks 14 to 35 of pregnancy, insulin requirements tend to increase gradually.
- After 35 weeks, insulin requirements may decrease or even plateau.
- Patients with obesity may require higher insulin doses than nonobese people.

Management of pregnant women with GDM for initiation and titration of insulin is shown in **Flowchart 3**.

POSTPARTUM FOLLOW-UP

Immediate Postpartum Care—GDM on OHAs

- Most women's glucose tolerance will return to normal right after delivery.
- Keep prepregnancy BGL QID for 24 hours.
- If prepregnancy BGL is 72–126 mg/dL, stop monitoring.
- If BGL is >126 mg/dL, seek medical advice and continue monitoring.
- 1–8% of women may still have glucose intolerance and require insulin hydrochloride (OHAs).
- Metformin is safe to use during breastfeeding.
- Breastfeeding should be encouraged to avoid newborn hypoglycemia.

Immediate Postpartum Care—GDM on Insulin

- Preprandial BGL monitoring QID for 24 hours
- If BGL >126 mg/dL, medical review and start OHAs
- Insulin therapy is generally not indicated unless marked fasting hyperglycemia (200–250 mg/dL)
- Encourage breastfeeding to prevent neonatal hypoglycemia

Benefits of Postpartum Follow-up

- Early detection of DM and prediabetes
- Lifestyle changes
- Recognition of CV risk factors
- Early intervention
- Planned pregnancy
- Prevention of future GDM and DM
- Prevention or delaying complications of diabetes

Weight Loss

The risk of developing T2DM is increased by 1.7% for mothers with a gain of 1–2 kg/m^2 and by 80% for those with a gain of >2 kg/m^2. It is not only postpartum weight gain that is clinically important, but also postpregnancy weight gain. For example, Peters et al. showed that for every additional 4.5 kg of postpartum weight gained, the risk for developing T2DM was doubled.

TABLE 6: Insulin dosing guidelines during pregnancy and postpartum.

Weeks' gestation	Total daily dose (TDD) of insulin
1–13 weeks	(0.7 × weight in kg) or [0.30 × weight (lbs)]
14–26 weeks	(0.8 × weight in kg) or [0.35 × weight (lbs)]
27–37 weeks	(0.9 × weight in kg) or [0.40 × weight (lbs)]
38 weeks to delivery	(1.0 × weight in kg) or [0.45 × weight (lbs)]
Postpartum (and lactation)	(0.55 × weight in kg) or [0.25 × weight (lbs)]

TABLE 5: Insulin options shown to be safe during pregnancy.

Insulin name	Type	Onset	Peak effect	Duration	Dosing interval
Aspart	Rapid acting	15 minutes	60 minutes	3–5 hours	At start of each meal
Lispro	Rapid acting	15 minutes	60 minutes	3–5 hours	At start of each meal
Regular	Short acting	60 minutes	2–4 hours	6–8 hours	60–90 minutes before meal
Insulin detemir	Long acting	2 hours	-	24 hours	Every 24 hours

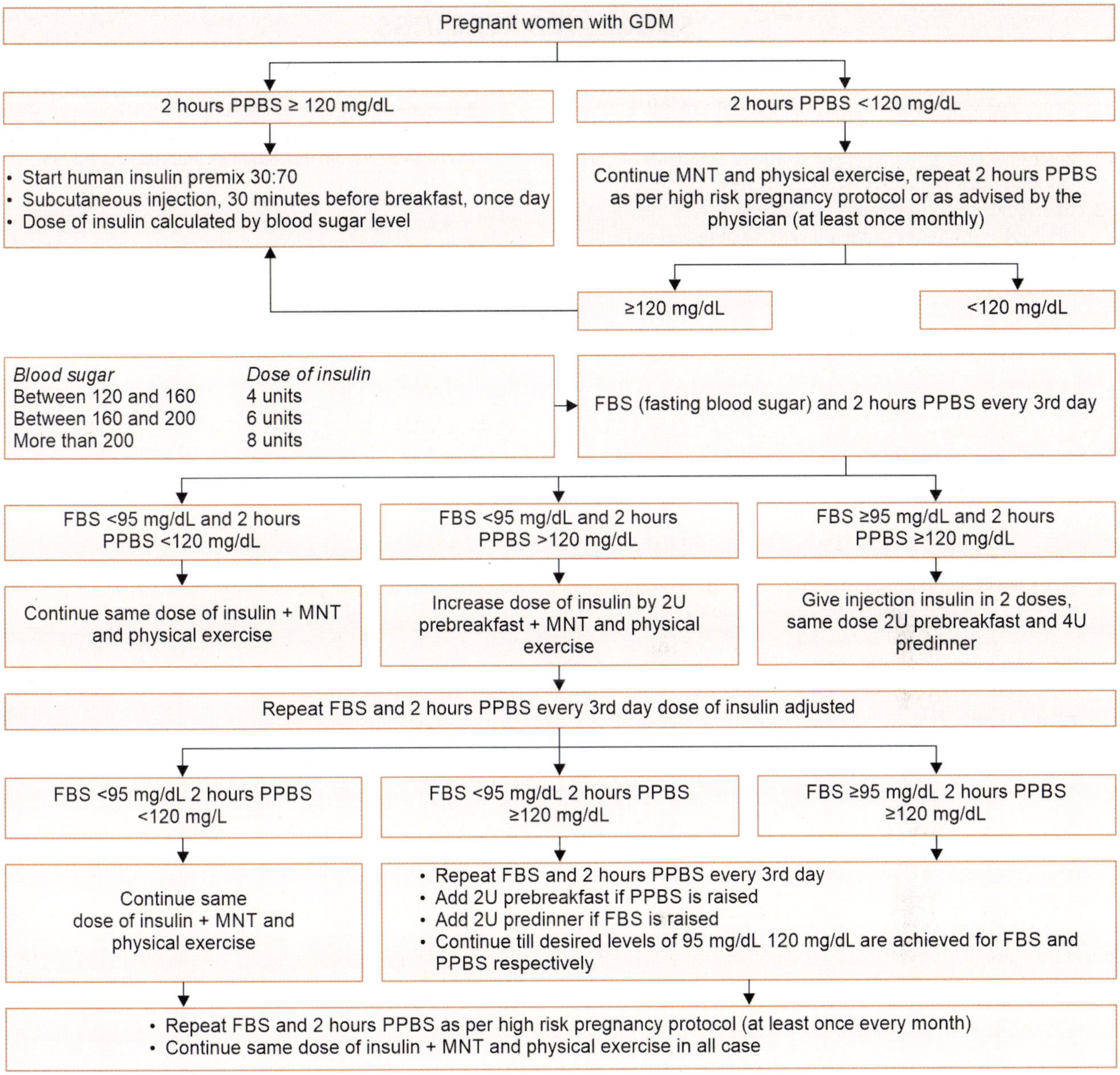

FLOWCHART 3: Management of pregnant women with GDM for initiation and titration of insulin.

(FBS: fasting blood sugar; GDM: gestational diabetes mellitus; MNT: medical nutrition therapy; PPBS: postprandial blood sugar)

Source: Chawla R. RSSDI Textbook of Diabetes Mellitus, 5th edition. New Delhi; Jaypee Brothers Medical Publishers (P) Ltd.; 2022.

TAKE HOME MESSAGES

- GDM is a common problem in India.
- Universal testing of all pregnant women for GDM.
- DIPSI/WINGS criteria are followed in India.
- Metformin and glyburide can be used but ADA does not recommend it, ADA recommends insulin.
- Neonatal monitoring for hypoglycemia and other complications.
- Postpartum evaluation of glycemic status by a 75 g OGTT at 6–12 weeks after delivery.
- A multidisciplinary plan and approach is needed.
- Long-term follow-up of the mother and baby is essential.

SUGGESTED READINGS

1. Chawla R. RSSDI Textbook of Diabetes Mellitus. 5th edition. New Delhi: Jaypee Brothers Medical Publishers (P) Ltd.; 2022.
2. ElSayed NA, Aleppo G, Aroda VR, Bannuru RR, Brown FM, Bruemmer D, et al. Summary of Revisions: Standards of Care in Diabetes-2023. Diabetes Care. 2023;46(Suppl 1):S5-S9.
3. Guariguata L, Linnenkamp U, Beagley J, Whiting DR, Cho NH. Global estimates of the prevalence of hyperglycaemia in pregnancy. Diabetes Res Clin Pract. 2014;103(2):176-85.
4. ElSayed NA, Aleppo G, Aroda VR, Bannuru RR, Brown FM, Bruemmer D, et al. Classification and Diagnosis of Diabetes: Standards of Care in Diabetes-2023. Diabetes Care. 2023;46(Suppl 1):S19-S40. Erratum in: Diabetes Care. 2023;46(9):1715.

41 CHAPTER

Latent Autoimmune Diabetes of Adults: An Underdiagnosed Entity

Somnath SM

ABSTRACT

Latent autoimmune diabetes (LAD) is a type of diabetes that evolves slowly, similar to both type 1 diabetes mellitus (T1DM) and type 2 diabetes mellitus (T2DM). It is often overlooked in daily practice due to age, body mass, or rapid insulin requirement. Early diagnosis and treatment are crucial for better outcomes. Latent autoimmune diabetes of adults (LADA) is heterogeneous, with some patients progressing faster to insulin therapy due to high antibody titers and low body mass index (BMI). The disease's nomenclature varies regionally, with Japan referring to it as slowly progressive insulin-dependent type 1 diabetes mellitus (SPIDDM), the American Diabetes Association (ADA) as T1DM, and the World Health Organization as "slowly evolving immune-related diabetes".

INTRODUCTION

Latent autoimmune diabetes of adults (LADA) is a steady evolving diabetes mellitus (DM) that exhibits clinical features similar to both type 1 diabetes mellitus (T1DM) and type 2 diabetes mellitus (T2DM) and is sometimes referred to as 1.5 DM and leaving behind diagnostic dilemmas to the treating physician.

In daily practice among adult patients, we by and large encounter T2DM patients but occasionally run into patients who deviate from routine because of age, body mass, or rapid progression to insulin requirement which should ring a bell about LADA.

It is important to recognize the entity for early prognostication, optimal management, and in turn leading to better outcome. The prospect of precise treatment and the forehand knowledge of the disease leads us to better counseling of the patient. India being a high-burden country for diabetes, precision of diagnosis and focused approach on treatment would go a long way in achieving set goals.

Latent autoimmune diabetes (LAD) of adults being a heterogeneous disease by itself in presentation, where some patients having high antibody titers and a low body mass index (BMI), progress to insulin therapy faster and few others having antibody titers low, insulin resistance high with higher BMI, progressing more slowly to insulin requirement.

The nomenclature for LADA is different in various regions. In Japan, it is labeled slowly progressive insulin-dependent type 1 diabetes mellitus (SPIDDM). The American Diabetes Association (ADA) has christened LADA as T1DM that evolves more slowly than the classic disease and does not place it as a different form of DM. The World Health Organization considers LADA as "slowly evolving immune-related diabetes". The early recognition of LADA gains precedence so that appropriate strategies are employed to delay beta-cell destruction and thereby reduce complications.

MAGNITUDE OF THE PROBLEM

The prevalence of LADA has been variable in different sections of the globe. The tools for diagnosis may be contributing for more accurate estimation.

Prevalence of LADA in Global Studies

The prevalence in Asia of LADA has been put at 2–12% of all cases of T2DM. Western studies estimate it to be around 2.8–10%. A Chinese study in Tianjin found it to be 7% **(Table 1)**.

TABLE 1: Prevalence of latent autoimmune diabetes of adults (LADA) in global studies.

Study	Country	Age range	Number of subjects	Autoantibodies	Positivity
UKPDS	UK	25–65	3,672	GAD/ICA	12%
ADOPT	US/Europe	30–75	4,357	GAD/IA2	4.2%
Tianjin	China	>15	8,109	GAD	9.2%
NIRAD	Italy	30–75	5,330	GAD/IA2	4.5%
Ehime	Japan	>20	4,980	GAD	3.8%
Action LADA	Europe	30–70	6,810	GAD/IA2, ZnT8	9.7%

(GAD: glutamic acid decarboxylase; ICA: islet cell antibodies; NIRAD: Non-Insulin Requiring Autoimmune Diabetes; UKPDS: United Kingdom Prospective Diabetes Study)

ETIOPATHOGENESIS

Latent autoimmune diabetes of adults first coined by Tumol et al. in 1993 with phenotypic features of T1DM and immunologic features of T1DM. A combination of environmental and genetic factors has been attributed to LADA. A number of lifestyle factors have been reported, including *Enterovirus* exposure, many dietary factors, gain in body weight, and psychological stress but unfortunately have not been replicated in different studies. The risk for getting LADA increases in people of certain human leukocyte antigen (HLA) haplotypes.

Analysis using immunochemistry and polymerase chain reaction (PCR) in model of rat mimicking LADA and pancreatic tissue from humans with LADA showed infiltration of predominant macrophage [cluster of differentiation 68 (CD68)] in islet cells as opposed to T1DM which showed CD8 T lymphocytes infiltration.

The risk of faster progression to beta cell failure is related to presence of multiple diabetes-associated antibodies (DAA). The sensitivity of using glutamic acid decarboxylase (GAD) in predicting insulin requirement decreases in older patients markedly. A variant of the IA2A antibody (256–760) being characteristic, when present is more frequently found in LADA and may help detect the same.

The factors promoting insulin resistance and T2DM such as obesity, sedentary lifestyle, smoking, low birth weight, sweetened beverage intake, moderate alcohol consumption (protective) is associated with risk of LADA and is corroborated by many studies published till date. The studies also found potential effects on autoimmunity exerted by intake of coffee (harmful) and fatty fish (protective). The above findings support the concept of LADA as being a hybrid form of diabetes with an etiology associated with both autoimmunity and insulin resistance among others.

The patients with LADA display higher levels of C-peptide on a consistent basis, indicative of insulin secretion, which points out the autoimmune process being milder and beta cell failure progression slower. The production of insulin in LADA patients being more than patients with T1DM at the time of diagnosis which indicate mechanisms other than autoimmune destruction of the beta cells playing a role in the pathogenesis. It is reinforced by the fact that LADA patients have insulin resistance.

The following factors are indicative:
- Presence of one or more islet-specific antibodies including GAD, protein tyrosine phosphotase (IA-2A) and isoform (IA-2)
- Rapid progression to insulin requirement
- Age at diagnosis > 35 years

Slowly progressive beta cell destruction leading to diabetes has also been described in children and is referred to as latent autoimmune diabetes in the young (LADY).

Patients with LADA show a positive corelation between BMI and interleukin-17, a peripheral B lymphocytes proinflammatory cytokine which has been found in T2DM and obesity.

T-cell immunoreactivity modulation may be a prospective therapeutic option which is showing promise in research.

PRESENTATION/HISTORY

Patients with LADA may not differ much in presentation. The symptoms may be:
- Polyuria
- Nocturia
- Neuropathy
- Polydipsia
- Visual disturbances
- Weight loss
- Patients may also be asymptomatic.

Autoimmune history in family or patient with hyperglycemia should raise suspicion of LADA or T1DM.

A screening tool for LADA diagnosis was used in diabetic patients above 50 years of age. This tool has sensitivity to detect 75% of patients with LADA.

- A fasting blood glucose >270 mg/dL, glycated hemoglobin (HbA1c) 10% or greater despite good compliance.
- BMI being low or normal
- Weight loss in spite of constant calorie diet.

Alternatively, another tool for diagnosis includes:

- Age <50 years
- Symptomatic hyperglycemia
- BMI of <25 kg/m^2
- Family or personal history of autoimmune disease

The presence of two or more criteria yielded a sensitivity of 90% and specificity of 71% while less than two virtually excluded LADA. Patients with LADA are usually ketosis-resistant at diagnosis.

DIAGNOSTIC ASSESSMENT

Clinical: Adults with hyperglycemia who need no insulin for 6 months suspect LADA.

Tests:

- Fasting blood sugar (FBS)
- HbA1c
- Lipid profile
- Creatinine
- Urinalysis
- Continuous glucose monitoring (CGM) for glycemic variability
- C-peptide
- Autoantibodies
- GADA (GAD antibodies)
- IA-2A
- IA2
- Stimulation C peptide test
- Glucagon stimulation test
- Mixed meal tolerance

TREATMENT/MANAGEMENT

The treatment options include non-pharmacological and pharmacological.

Non-pharmacological therapy includes a diet with carbohydrate and calorie restriction and exercise which forms a part in all forms of DM. The goal is to achieve good glycemic control and delay or prevent complications.

Since LADA is a heterogeneous disease, it is essential to customize pharmacologic option to get maximum therapeutic advantage. Therapies to preserve beta cell function should be a priority. Insulin remains the cornerstone of treatment.

Sulfonylureas:

- Poor choice, as they deplete beta cell function and early progression to insulin.
- Metformin may help initially in glycemic control but little role in preserving beta cell function.

Thiazolidinediones: These have anti-inflammatory effects on beta cells, may increase their survival, and may be useful in early stages. The only glitazone studied in LADA, rosiglitazone has cardiovascular (CVS) risk which has limited its use in the past. Long-term studies with pioglitazone may be required to start using it.

Dipeptidyl peptidase 4 (DPP-4) inhibitors: DPP-4 inhibitors alone or in combination with insulin to preserve beta cell function have shown promise. They affect metabolic control by prolonging levels of glucagon-like peptide 1 (GLP-1) and other peptides. Vitamin D addition to insulin or DPP-4 inhibitors shows improvement in glycemic control and preserving beta cells

GLP-1 agonist: Dulaglutide a GLP-1 receptor agonist usage has shown to reduce HbA1c levels and also beta cell function improvement in patients with LADA with results comparable to T2DM.

Sodium-glucose cotransporter-2 (SGLT-2) inhibitors: SGLT-2 inhibitors have not been well-studied in LADA and some reports of euglycemic ketosis have been reported which prevent their use.

A Chinese herbal decoction in combination with insulin has shown positive results.

Th use of an immunomodulating treatment with recombinant human GAD65 formulated with alum is being tried. The administration of three injections of 4 μg each into a lymph node in the groin, along with daily oral vitamin D, has shown promise in phase II of GAD in LADA trials.

Bariatric surgery: Some patients having T2DM presumably and obesity, in reality, have LADA. In such patients, bariatric surgery causes successful weight loss, little success with glycemic control postsurgery and the remission of diabetes often seen in T2DM are absent pointing to beta cell failure.

DIFFERENTIAL DIAGNOSIS (TABLE 2)

A mistaken diagnosis a of T1DM, T2DM, or LADA may be made in a young adult with maturity-onset diabetes of the young (MODY). Though relatively rare, MODY presents with strong family history with residual C-peptide. The humoral and cellular immunity to islet cell antigens is absent and can thereby be distinguished from LADA. The line of management makes it imperative to differentiate LADA from T1DM or T2DM.

COMPLICATIONS

Neuropathy

Patients with LADA have early onset of small fiber neuropathy (SFN) and with increased frequency compared

TABLE 2: Comparison between the features of type 1 diabetes mellitus (T1DM) and type 2 diabetes mellitus (T2DM) and latent autoimmune diabetes of adults (LADA).

	T1DM	LADA	T2DM
Autoantibodies	>1	GAD commonly may have more	Absent
C-peptide	Absent or very low	Levels between T1DM and T2DM	High normal Increased fasting levels
Insulin requirement	From diagnosis	May not need for at least 6 months after diagnosis	No insulin for extended period of time
Oral hypoglycemics	Little role for oral drugs	Sulfonylurea metformin Sodium-glucose cotransporter 2 (SGLT2) inhibitors no role	Lifestyle management pharmacologic therapy

to T2DM due to poor glycemic control and higher HbA1c. SFN if detected early, treatment of hyperglycemia may reverse SFN.

Vascular

Patients with LADA show lower risk in the first 9 years but a higher risk in later years for microvascular complications when compared to T2DM when followed up on long term. Carotid artery atherosclerosis in patients with LADA is very similar as in T1DM and T2DM despite a better vascular risk. LADA, like T1DM and T2DM, is associated with both microvascular and macrovascular complication.

CONCLUSION

Latent autoimmune diabetes of adults because of its infrequent occurrence and complexity of presentation has been relatively missed and under diagnosed. Some observations to be kept in mind are as follows:

- LADA has features common to both T1DM and T2DM, which can be easily missed.
- Early diagnosis is important for initiating correct treatment and preventing complications.
- A C-peptide test after a mixed-meal or basal may be used as an initial, cost-effective test to screen patients with LADA. This may help to choose patients who need confirmatory testing for islet autoantibodies.
- Sulfonylureas may not have a role in treatment and conversely lead to faster progression to insulin usage
- Insulin, DPP-4 inhibitors with or without insulin, gliptins, and GLP-1 analogs remain mainstay of treatment for preserving B cell function.
- GAD65 injected into lymph node, a novel immunomodulatory treatment is undergoing trial and holds lot of promise.
- It becomes imperative to recognize LADA early for better therapeutic options and one should have a high index of suspicion to diagnose LADA.

SUGGESTED READINGS

1. Carlsson S. Etiology and Pathogenesis of Latent Autoimmune Diabetes in Adults (LADA) Compared to Type 2 Diabetes. Front Physiol. 2019;10:320.
2. D'Alessio DA, Denney AM, Hermiller LM, Prigeon RL, Martin JM, Tharp WG, et al. Treatment with the dipeptidyl peptidase-4 inhibitor vildagliptin improves fasting islet-cell function in subjects with type 2 diabetes. J Clin Endocrinol Metab. 2009;94(1):81-8.
3. O'Neal KS, Johnson JL, Panak RL. Recognizing and Appropriately Treating Latent Autoimmune Diabetes in Adults. Diabetes Spectr. 2016;29(4):249-52.
4. Rajkumar V, Levine SN. Latent Autoimmune Diabetes. In: StatPearls [Internet]. Treasure Island (FL): StatPearls Publishing; 2023.
5. Maddaloni E, Coleman RL, Agbaje O, Buzzetti R, Holman RR. Time-varying risk of microvascular complications in latent autoimmune diabetes of adulthood compared with type 2 diabetes in adults: a post-hoc analysis of the UK Prospective Diabetes Study 30-year follow-up data (UKPDS 86). Lancet Diabetes Endocrinol. 2020;8(3):206-15.

42

CHAPTER

Exocrine Deficiency in Type 2 Diabetes Mellitus

SP Sondhi, TR Sirohi

ABSTRACT

Type 2 diabetes mellitus is a disease of endocrine functions of pancreas, which has many micro and macrovascular complications. This chapter discusses one of the less appreciated complications involving the exocrine function, resulting in exocrine pancreatic deficiency (EPD), which is seen in approximately 27% type 2 diabetic patients. It usually presents with milder symptoms like bloating, abdominal discomfort rather than steatorrhea, fat-soluble vitamin deficiency, and weight loss. The various pathophysiological mechanisms are discussed. Fecal elastase is the most practical way to diagnose EPD. Chronic pancreatitis with ductal distortion and calcifications needs to be excluded. The treatment consists of pancreatic enzyme replacement therapy (PERT) other than some general measures like avoidance of alcohol and some medicines capable of diarrhea and small frequent meals.

INTRODUCTION

Pancreas is a unique gland, which has both endocrine and exocrine functions. It remained anatomically hidden for centuries because of its peculiar location behind stomach. Herophilus, Ruphos, and Galen brought some focus on pancreas during 16th century, but it was Claude Bernard who underlined its exocrine role in 1850. It took another 72 years for Banting and Best to make a crude pancreatic extract to treat diabetes in dogs and subsequently in humans, underlining its endocrinal role in maintaining euglycemia. The patent was given to Eli Lilly, which named this pancreatic extract "iletin". With the explosion of *diabetes* all over the world, importance of pancreas is finally fully recognized. Langerhans had first noticed that 1–2% pancreas looks differently from the rest and it came to be known as islets of Langerhans. These islets have alpha, beta, and delta cells, producing hormones like insulin and glucagon, which are the backbone of glucose homeostasis in human. Type 2 diabetes mellitus (T2DM) occurs as a result of dysfunction of these hormones and for a long time it was felt that only endocrine dysfunction occurs in diabetes while exocrine functions remain intact (except in pancreatic diabetes/type 3c diabetes mellitus). Exocrine function impairment as a part of complications of T2DM is now being increasingly appreciated. In the current chapter, we describe its prevalence, pathophysiology, diagnosis, and treatment.

PREVALENCE

In the past, it was neither easy nor practical to assess exocrine functions of pancreas in a large population of diabetics, as the diagnostic tests to detect these were cumbersome, unreliable, and invasive. In the last decade, fecal elastase-1 (FE-1) estimation in a spot stool specimen has simplified the diagnosis of exocrine deficiency, which made the prevalence studies to be feasible in type 1 diabetic patients and type 2 diabetic patients. In a study by Softeland E et al., 12.7% of diabetic patients had exocrine pancreatic deficiency (EPD) defined by FE-1 level of <200 μg/g of stool. In this study, the prevalence was higher in type 1 diabetic patients than type 2 diabetic patients. It was also found to be related to duration of diabetes. Other studies by Hardt et al. and Larger et al. showed different prevalence rates. In a meta-analysis of 17 studies involving >3,500 patients, EPD was present in 40% (range 26–74%) type 1 diabetic patients and 27% (range 10–56%) type 2 diabetic patients. In some of the studies FE-1 was correlated with fecal fat and not all patients with low FE-1 had high fecal fat content.

PATHOPHYSIOLOGY

Human body has huge reserves, thus functional impairment of 60–70% of any organ goes unnoticed. Exocrine dysfunction of pancreas becomes symptomatic only when the enzyme production is decreased to < 10% of normal. How does the endocrine cells, which constitutes < 2% of pancreas decrease of exocrine functions (which constitutes 90% of pancreas), remains an enigma and till recently was not well appreciated. The following mechanisms may be involved in its pathophysiology:

- *Islet-acinar axis (trophic effect of hormone on exocrine cells)*: It is believed that hormones secreted in pancreas directly affect the health of exocrine cell. Though many hormones including glucagon and somatostatin are involved, most important of all remains insulin. Insulin levels around islets is very high and exocrine cells around islets receive blood with this high insulin level (two times the systemic levels). Insulin is hypothesized to keep exocrine cells healthy and its deficiency, which worsens with the duration of T2DM, can result in exocrine deficiency. In some diabetics who have EPD, histopathology revealed that the exocrine cells around the atrophied islets show the maximum effect (acinar atrophy: halo effect). Vice versa is also true.
- *Steatosis of pancreas*: Pancreas may have fat deposition like fatty liver.
- *Microvascular complication*: T2DM peculiarly affect small vessels which results in nephropathy, retinopathy, and neuropathy. Exocrine deficiency could occur as a result of microvascular changes.
- *Autonomic neuropathy*: This could also affect exocrine functions.
- *Inflammatory changes*: Autoantibodies against exocrine cells are present not only in type 1 diabetes mellitus (T1DM) but also in T2DM, albeit rarely.
- It needs to be mentioned here that some of the diabetics who undergo Roux-en-Y surgery for obesity along with diabetes have EPD.

PRESENTATION

Classically, EPD presents with steatorrhea as dietary fats are not absorbed and lost in the stools. Diarrhea with oily and foul smelly stools is the result. Along with this, fat-soluble vitamin (A, D, E, K) are also lost in the stools resulting in their deficiency with related symptoms like night blindness. Patients can lose weight as a result of losing calories in unabsorbed fats. The symptoms in T2DM are usually not that obvious. They present with milder symptoms like bloating of abdomen, mild pain in abdomen, cramping, increased flatulence and abdominal discomfort. Thus, high index of suspicion is important to suspect and diagnose EPD in T2DM.

DIAGNOSIS

The gold standard in diagnosing EPD, remains stimulated (by secretin cholecystokinin or secretin cerulein) pancreatic enzymes estimation in pancreatic fluid collected from pancreatic duct. It is a good test for research, but being invasive, is not feasible in general practice. Fecal fat estimation substituted as a practical test to diagnose EPD in the past. Fecal fat estimation is a cumbersome test, requiring standardized fat intake (100 g/day for 5 days) and collection of stool for 3 days and keeping the stool sample in refrigerator till assessed. Fecal fat of > 7 g/day is suggestive of malabsorption, but it does not diagnose the cause of malabsorption.

The most promising test which is revolutionizing the diagnosis of EPD is FE-1. Elastase is secreted along with other enzymes by pancreas and passes unmetabolized in stools. Low levels of FE-1 is suggestive of EPD. It is done in a spot stool sample and normal values are > 200 µg/g stool. Values between 100 and 200 µg/g are seen in mild to moderate deficiency and < 100 µg/g in severe deficiency. It has a better sensitivity and specificity when it is measured by ELISA (enzyme-linked immunosorbent assay) as compared to direct measurement.

Why is FE-1 the Preferred Test of EPD?

- It is cost-effective, easy to do, noninvasive indirect test of pancreatic function.
- Day-to-day variation < 15%
- Sample can be stored for 1 week at room temperature
- Does not require special diet
- It is not affected by enzyme use, thus can be employed for diagnosing EPD, even if the patient is taking enzymes. For the same reason it cannot be used for monitoring effect of treatment.
- It does not require timed stool collection.
- Sensitivity of this test is 63%, 100%, and 100% for mild, moderate, and severe exocrine pancreatic insufficiency, respectively.
- It has a specificity of 93%.

It should be remembered that watery diarrhea from nonpancreatic diseases and some medicines may produce false-positive results by diluting the stool specimen.

Differential Diagnosis

The list of differential diagnosis depends on the presentation of patient.

Weight loss: Uncontrolled diabetes, diabetic drugs causing weight loss, cancers, steatorrhea.

Malabsorption: Type 3c diabetes mellitus (chronic pancreatitis, pancreatectomy, pancreatic cancer) celiac disease, tropical sprue.

The hallmark of chronic pancreatitis are ductal irregularities and calcifications, which are not seen in EPD in T2DM. Thus, when diagnosing EPD in T2DM, computed tomography (CT) pancreas is required to rule out chronic pancreatitis.

Magnetic resonance imaging (MRI) and CT scan studies in diabetes have shown that they have smaller pancreas than controls. In at least one study, the reduced pancreas size in T1DM or T2DM was found to be associated with EPD. Histopathology specimens done in some of the EPD patients among diabetics revealed lymphocytes infiltration (more so in T1DM), fibrosis, and fat deposition. It is unclear whether pancreatic steatosis is a cause or result of EPD.

TREATMENT

This can be divided into: (1) general measures and (2) pancreatic enzyme replacement therapy (PERT).

General Measures

- Stop voglibose if the patient is receiving.
- Decreased or stop metformin, especially if the dose is high.
- Alcohol (decreases lipase activity) and smoking should be avoided.
- Patients are encouraged to have small frequent meals with normal fat content.

Fat-soluble vitamin supplements should be added to the diet to correct their deficiency.

Proton-pump inhibitors can be added, if pancreatic enzymes are not enteric-coated, to protect pancreatic enzymes from degradation by acid.

Pancreatic Enzyme Replacement Therapy

The aim of PERT is to provide the deficient pancreatic enzymes, so that malabsorption and its related symptoms can be corrected. Pancreatic enzyme preparations are available in various forms. Most are derived from pork. Usually, these are enteric-coated to protect it from acid in stomach. The microsphere formulations are theoretically better as these mix properly.

Cost is an important consideration as these preparations are costly.

Each capsule has a standardized lipase activity, e.g., 10k, 25k, 50k.

Dose: 30–40k with each meal (10% of normal secretion) of lipase should eliminate steatorrhea (preferably half dose at the first bite and the rest half during the meal).

Smaller dose (15–20k) can be given with snacks.

Common causes of failure:
- Inadequate doses (increase the dose)
- Noncompliance (cost is an issue)
- Deactivation of enzymes by acid in stomach (add PPI)

DOES PERT IN A PATIENT OF TYPE 2 DIABETES MELLITUS WITH EXOCRINE PANCREATIC DEFICIENCY IMPROVE DIABETIC CONTROL TOO?

There is no clear answer to this question as there are no large-scale studies looking at this aspect. In a small eight patients' study in type 3 diabetes mellitus PERT improved the glucose-dependent insulinotropic polypeptide (GIP) and glucagon-like peptide (GLP) after meals but not blood glucose. Another small study in insulin-dependent 39 patients with type 1/2 diabetics, PERT failed to improve glycated hemoglobin (HbA1c) and glucose profile. More studies are needed in this field as well as in the area of effects of antidiabetic drugs including glucagon-like peptide 1 agonists (GLP-1A) on EPD.

TAKE-HOME POINTS

- Exocrine deficiency is not a very uncommon complication in T2DM.
- It needs to be kept in mind when a type 2 diabetic patient complains of (c/o) diarrhea, weight loss and fat-soluble vitamins' deficiencies.
- It frequently presents with much milder symptoms like bloating, mild abdominal pain, and flatulence.
- FE-1 remain the most practical test to diagnose EPD.
- Treatment includes general measures, e.g., small frequent meals, avoidance of smoking and alcohol, stopping voglibose and stopping/reducing metformin.
- Pancreatic enzyme replacement is the specific treatment.

SUGGESTED READING

1. Søfteland E, Poulsen JL, Starup-Linde J, Christensen TT, Olesen SS, Singh S, et al. Pancreatic exocrine insufficiency in diabetes mellitus—prevalence and characteristics. Eur J Intern Med. 2019;68:18-22.

43

CHAPTER

Continuous Glucose Monitoring System in Clinical Practice

G Prakash

ABSTRACT

The importance of glycemic control in preventing the development of complications that occur due to diabetes mellitus was highlighted in various trials, including the landmark trials [Diabetes Control and Complications Trial (DCCT) and the UK Prospective Diabetes Study (UKPDS)]. The glucose assessment was done with urine sugar in olden days to continuous glucose monitoring (CGM) in recent days. Continuous glucose monitoring system (CGMS) is continuous subcutaneous sensing of interstitial glucose since late 1990. Glucose monitoring still remains a cornerstone in the management of diabetes mellitus. CGM is currently a valuable tool for assessing glucose fluctuations due to its accuracy, convenience, and in-software advancement. Although glycated hemoglobin (HbA1c) still remains the key surrogate marker for glycemic control, CGMS helps in therapeutic decision-making.

INTRODUCTION

Glycemic assessment is essential for effective management of diabetes mellitus. There are various methods of monitoring blood sugar levels. Hypoglycemia still remains barrier in achieving target glycemic control and is also a common complication in the management of diabetes mellitus. The ACCORD (Action to Control Cardiovascular Risk in Diabetes) trial was permanently terminated due to increase in all-cause mortality with severe hypoglycemia in intensive treatment arm. Glycemic variability is now being focused as an important risk factor for the development of complications such as cardiovascular disease in diabetes mellitus. Self-monitoring of blood glucose (SMBG) measures blood sugar at a single point of time and cannot detect nocturnal or asymptomatic hypoglycemia and glycemic variability. Continuous glucose monitoring system (CGMS) helps by indicating the rate of change of blood sugar levels or glucose trends. Continuous glucose monitoring (CGM) provides information on excursions of glucose levels in a day or between days. It also exposes the glucose levels that occur over overnight fasting, 2–4 hours of postprandial state, and schedule of insulin and drugs. CGMS is useful in minimizing glycemic variability by reducing hypoglycemia risk and maintaining glycemic stability. Glycated hemoglobin (HbA1c) does not reflect inter- and intra-glucose excursions that occur due to hypoglycemia or postprandial state. CGM technology can be successfully utilized to measure day-to-day glycemic excursions and glucose variability in achieving glycemic goals. CGM improves treatment decisions to achieve glycemic targets.

MECHANISM

Continuous glucose monitoring system is continuous, subcutaneous quantification of interstitial glucose levels. It consists of a small disposable sensor which is inserted into the subcutaneous tissue, a transmitter, and receiver. The sensor inserted may be either transcutaneous or implantable. The transmitter attached to the sensor wirelessly transmits glucose values at 1- and 5-minute intervals to a reader, an application, or an automated insulin delivery device. Currently, the transcutaneous system has sensors of wear time from 6 to 14 days after which a new sensor should be inserted. Implantable systems can transmit glucose levels for up to 180 days

TABLE 1: Types of CGM.

Type of CGM	Description
rt-CGM (real-time CGM)	Measures and displays glucose levels continuously
is-CGM—with or without alarm (intermittently scanned CGM)	Measures glucose levels continuously but requires scanning for visualization and storage of glucose values
Professional CGM	These devices are clinic based and not owned by the person with diabetes mellitus. The device is worn for a desirable period of time (7–14) days. Data may be blinded or visible to the person who wear the device
I-CGM (integrated CGM)	A higher standard set by the FDA where the device can be integrated with other digitally connected devices

(CGM: continuous glucose monitoring; FDA: Food and Drug Administration)

before replacement. CGM sensors that are available now are mostly factory calibrated. The receiver provides with trends in glucose levels and alert the user as well when glucose levels exceed or fall below the predetermined thresholds.

TYPES OF CONTINUOUS GLUCOSE MONITORING (TABLE 1)

Real-time CGM systems are also classified as adjunctive where user has to perform self-glucose monitoring and nonadjunctive where devices are authorized by regulators to replace SMBG.

TIME IN RANGE

The time spent by the individual within the target range of glucose levels is time in range (TIR). It is the key metric currently used in various current clinical trials. The evidence from the Data of Diabetes Control and Complications Trial (DCCT) showed that the intensive treatment group had substantially higher TIR when compared to the conventional treatment. TIR measurement helps in evaluation and comparing intervention of various glucose-lowering agents. The TIR of 70–180 mg was demonstrated as target from quarterly seven point blood glucose testing of DCCT data. The TIR had a strong association with the risk of micro-albuminuria and retinopathy development and its progression. TIR correlates well with A1c in most of the studies. The goal of TIR of 70% align with HbA1c of 7%. Time below range (TBR < 70 mg and < 54 mg) and time above range (TAR > 180 mg) are useful parameters for adjustment of insulin dose and modification of treatment plan. The clinical targets for CGM from International Consensus on TIR is depicted in **Figure 1**.

Clinical Targets for Continuous Glucose Monitoring Data Interpretation: Recommendations from the International Consensus on Time in Range

AVAILABLE CONTINUOUS GLUCOSE MONITORING DEVICES (TABLE 2)

The available CGM devices are given in **Table 2**.

SIDE EFFECTS

Contact dermatitis (both irritant and allergic) due to devices that attach to the skin had been reported.

SUBSTANCES INTERFERING WITH CONTINUOUS GLUCOSE MONITORING DEVICES

It is necessary to review medications for the person with diabetes mellitus to identify interfering substances and advice to use additional blood glucose monitor (BGM) values if sensor values are unreliable **(Table 3)**.

QUANTIFYING CONTINUOUS GLUCOSE MONITORING ACCURACY

The established statistic used is mean absolute relative difference (MARD) to assess the accuracy of CGM devices. MARD is derived by averaging the absolute values of the relative differences between a CGM measured and the corresponding simultaneous value obtained by the reference system. MARD value range between 8% and 14% for the currently available CGM devices.

INDICATIONS

- Person with type 1 diabetes mellitus for achieving glycemic targets
- Person with diabetes mellitus and pregnancy to maintain strict control
- Person with type 2 diabetes mellitus, who are on multiple doses on insulin
- Person with diabetes mellitus having hypoglycemia unawareness
- Person with diabetes mellitus on insulin pump therapy

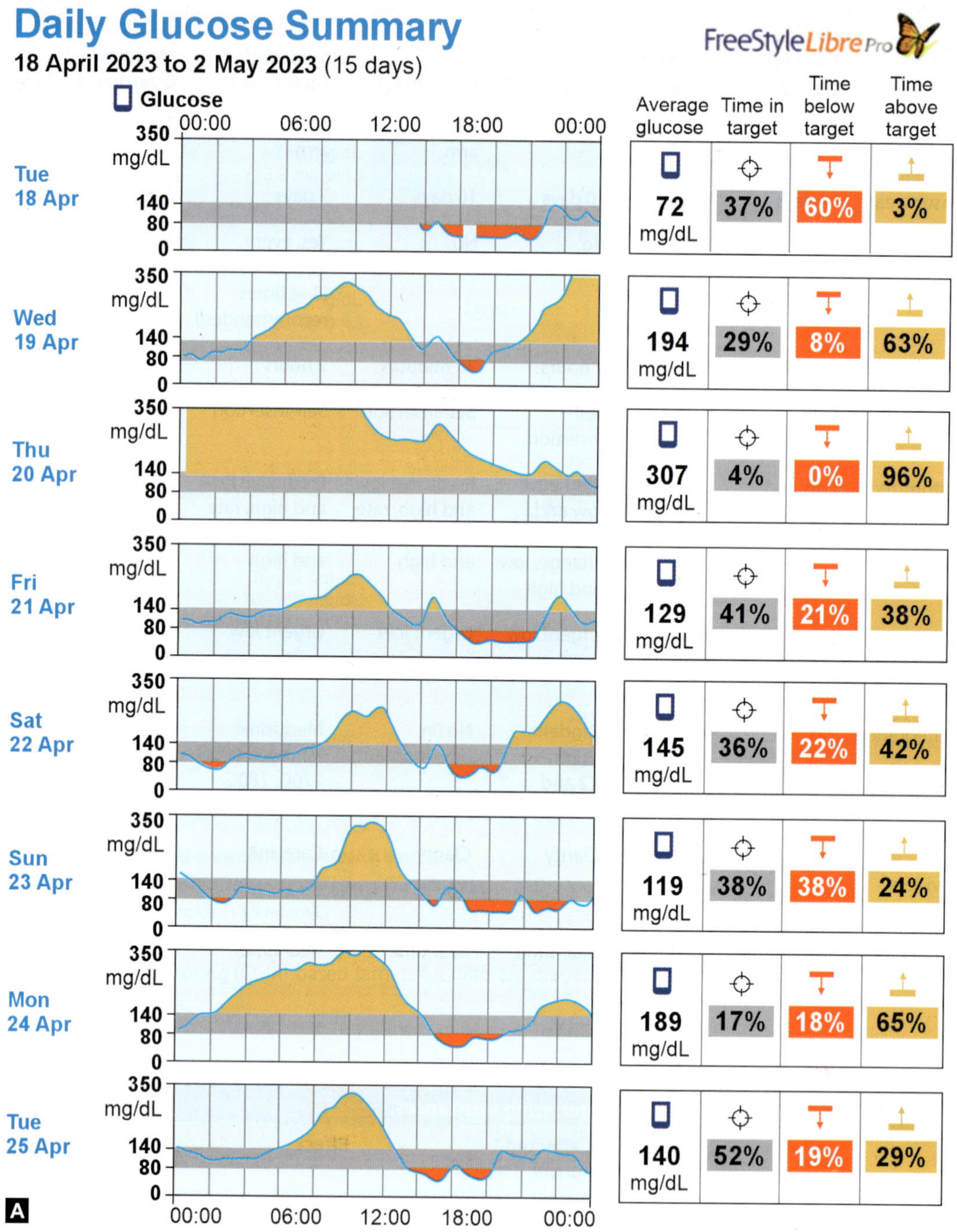

FIGS. 2A AND B: *Continued.*

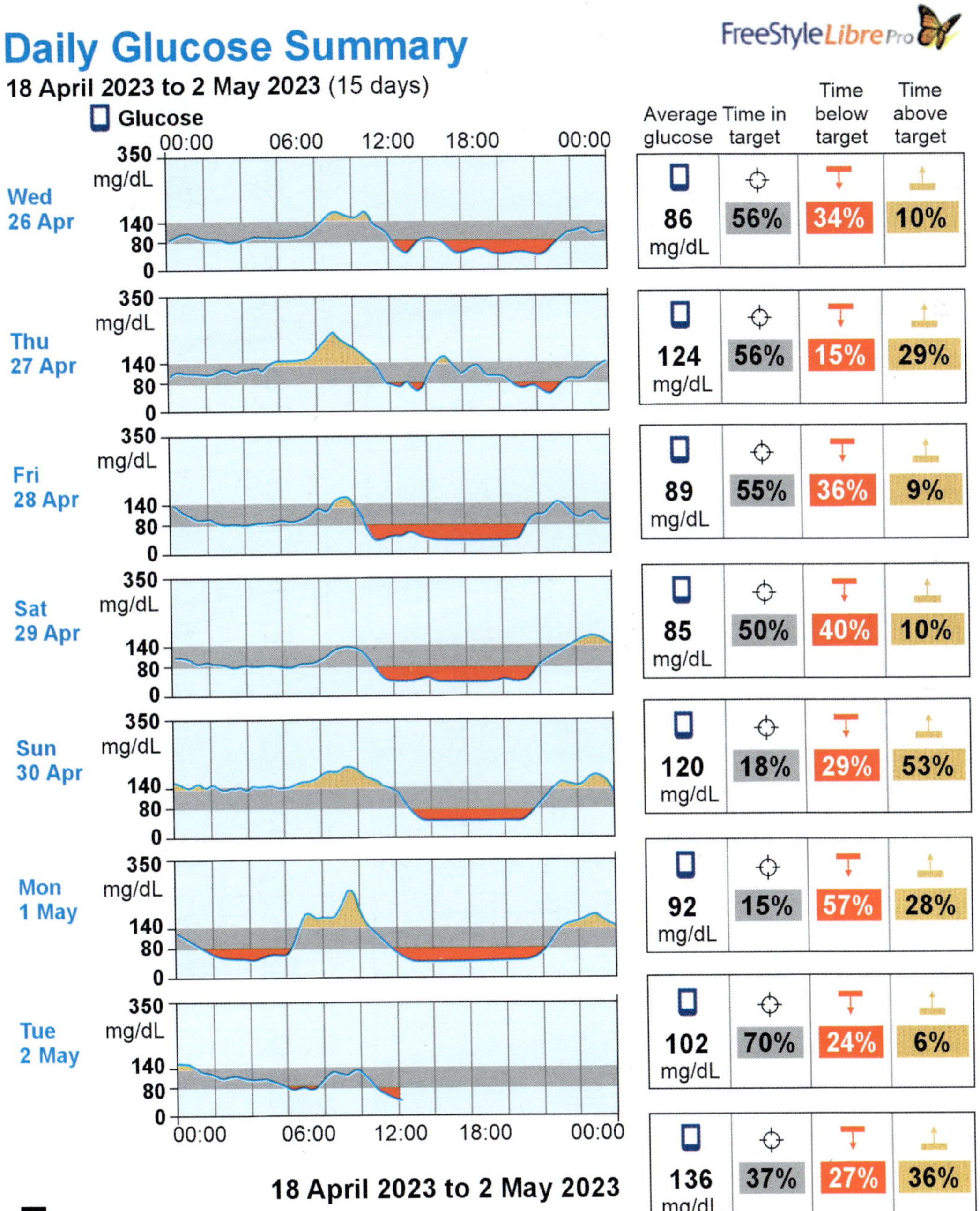

B

FIGS. 2A AND B: Case 1: Continuous glucose monitoring report of person with type 1 diabetes mellitus.

Source: Adapted from FreeStyle Libre Pro.

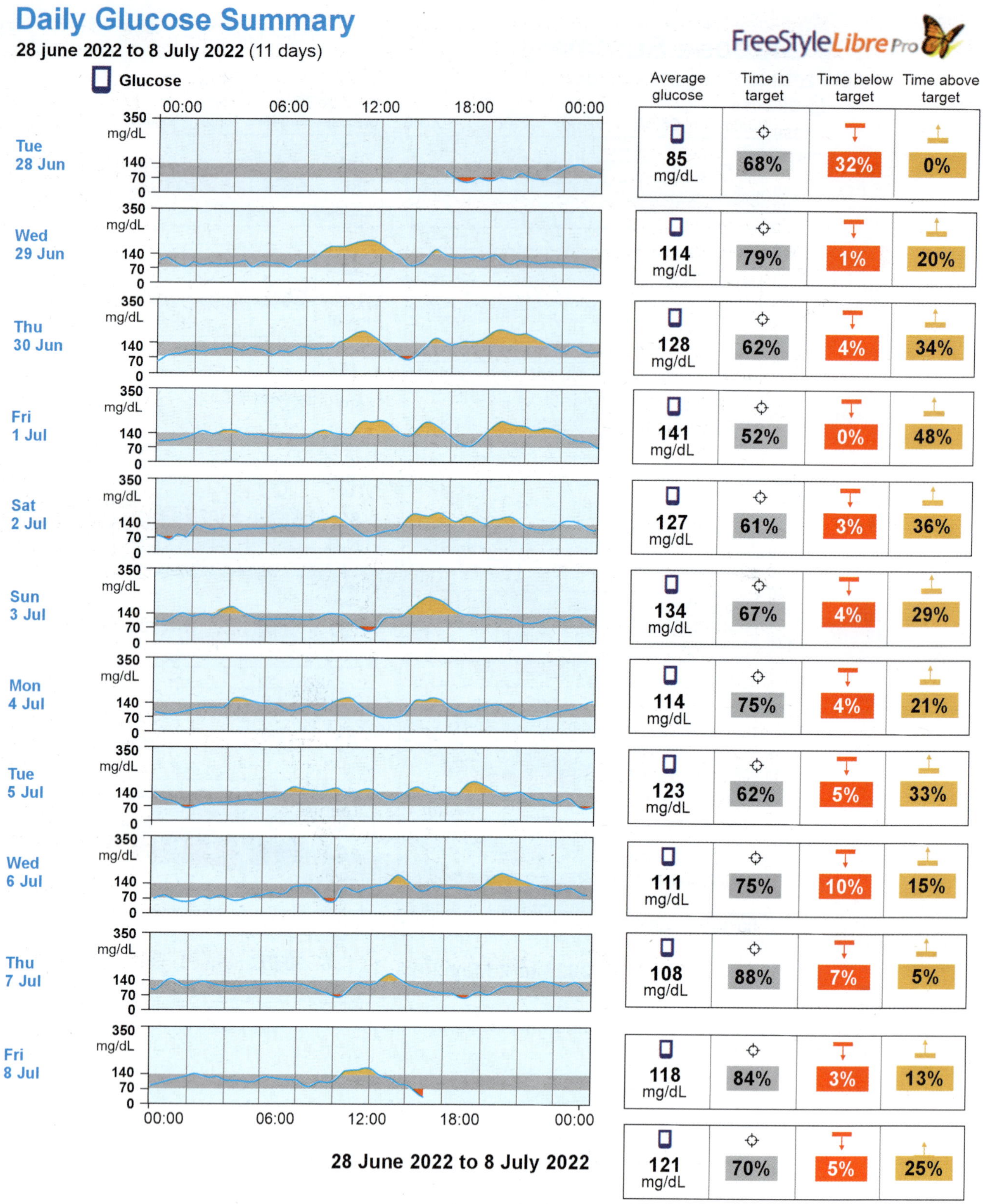

FIG. 3: Case 2: Continuous glucose monitoring report of person with pregestational diabetes mellitus.

Source: Adapted from FreeStyle Libre Pro.

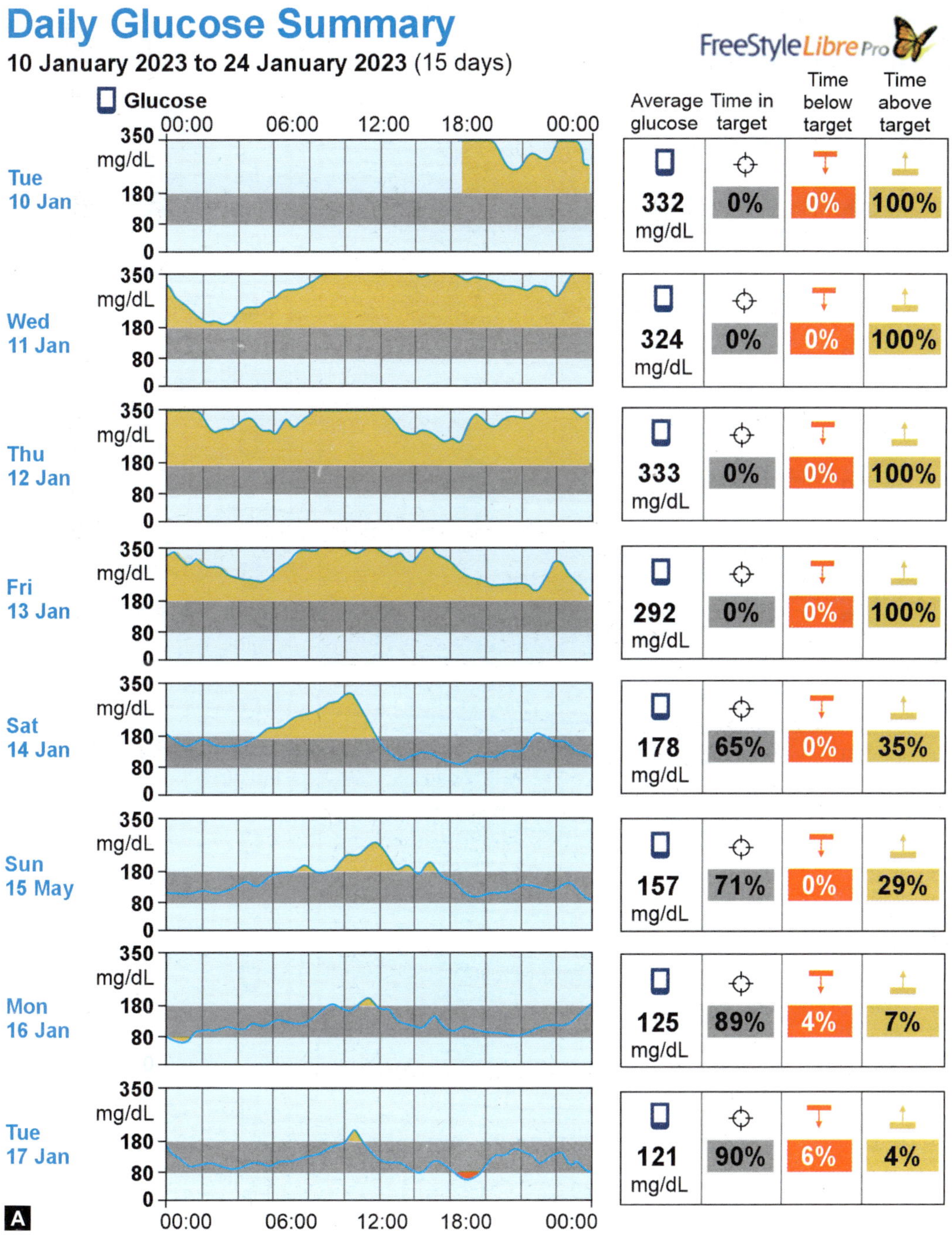

FIGS. 4A AND B: *Continued.*

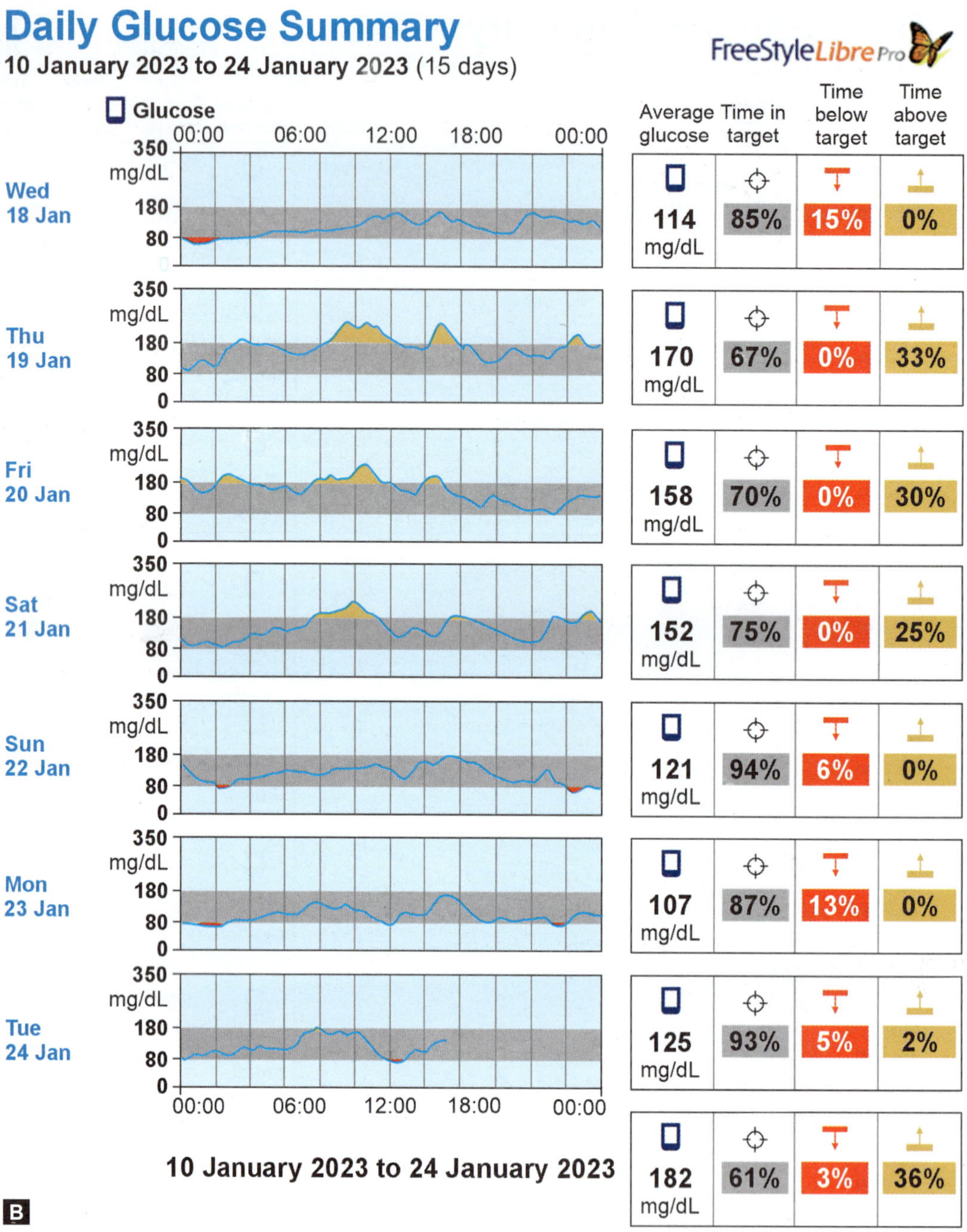

B

FIGS. 4A AND B: Case 3: Continuous glucose monitoring report of person with type 2 diabetes mellitus on insulin therapy.
Source: Adapted from FreeStyle Libre Pro.

CONCLUSION

Continuous glucose monitoring system is emerging as an invaluable tool in comprehensive diabetes care. It is rapidly evolving is both affordability and accuracy with advances in newer technologies. CGMS use is associated with increased time in glycemic target range with reduced time in hyperglycemia and hypoglycemia. Persons with diabetes mellitus who use CGMS devices have lower glucose variability and better quality of life with fewer hospital admissions. Prospective current clinical studies are also using CGMS devices for evaluation of glycemic profile in the study participants.

SUGGESTED READINGS

1. Gerstein HC, Miller ME, Byington RP, Goff DC Jr, Bigger JT, Buse JB, et al.; Action to Control Cardiovascular Risk in Diabetes Study Group. Effects of intensive glucose lowering in type 2 diabetes. N Engl J Med. 2008;358(24):2545-59.
2. Monnier L, Mas E, Ginet C, Michel F, Villon L, Cristol JP, et al. Activation of oxidative stress by acute glucose fluctuations compared with sustained chronic hyperglycemia in patients with type 2 diabetes. JAMA. 2006;295(14):1681-7.
3. Rodbard D, Bailey T, Jovanovic L, Zisser H, Kaplan R, Garg SK. Improved quality of glycemic control and reduced glycemic variability with use of continuous glucose monitoring. Diabetes Technol Ther. 2009;11(11):717-23.
4. Danne T, Nimri R, Battelino T, Bergenstal RM, Close KL, DeVries JH, et al. International Consensus on Use of Continuous Glucose Monitoring. Diabetes Care. 2017;40(12):1631-40.
5. Freckmann G, Pleus S, Grady M, Setford S, Levy B. Measures of Accuracy for Continuous Glucose Monitoring and Blood Glucose Monitoring Devices. J Diabetes Sci Technol. 2019;13(3):575-83.
6. Battelino T, Alexander CM, Amiel SA, Arreaza-Rubin G, Beck RW, Bergenstal RM, et al. Continuous glucose monitoring and metrics for clinical trials: an international consensus statement. Lancet Diabetes Endocrinol. 2023;11(1):42-57.
7. Alva S, Bailey T, Brazg R, Budiman ES, Castorino K, Christiansen MP, et al. Accuracy of a 14-Day Factory-Calibrated Continuous Glucose Monitoring System With Advanced Algorithm in Pediatric and Adult Population With Diabetes. J Diabetes Sci Technol. 2022;16(1):70-7.
8. ElSayed NA, Aleppo G, Aroda VR, Bannuru RR, Brown FM, Bruemmer D, et al.; on behalf of the American Diabetes Association. Diabetes Technology: Standards of Care in Diabetes-2023. Diabetes Care. 2023;46(Suppl 1):S111-27.
9. US Food and Drug Administration. Product classification (database). [online] Available from https://www.accessdata.fda.gov/scripts/cdrh/cfdocs/cfpcd/classification.cfm [Last accessed January, 2024].
10. Aleppo G, Ruedy KJ, Riddlesworth TD, Kruger DF, Peters AL, Hirsch I, et al.; REPLACE-BG Study Group. REPLACE-BG: A Randomized Trial Comparing Continuous Glucose Monitoring With and Without Routine Blood Glucose Monitoring in Adults With Well-Controlled Type 1 Diabetes. Diabetes Care. 2017;40(4):538-45.
11. Beck RW, Bergenstal RM, Riddlesworth TD, Kollman C, Li Z, Brown AS, et al. Validation of Time in Range as an Outcome Measure for Diabetes Clinical Trials. Diabetes Care. 2019;42(3):400-5.
12. Lu J, Ma X, Zhou J, Zhang L, Mo Y, Ying L, et al. Association of Time in Range, as Assessed by Continuous Glucose Monitoring, With Diabetic Retinopathy in Type 2 Diabetes. Diabetes Care. 2018;41(11):2370-6.
13. Vigersky RA, McMahon C. The Relationship of Hemoglobin A1C to Time-in-Range in Patients with Diabetes. Diabetes Technol Ther. 2019;21(2):81-5.
14. Battelino T, Danne T, Bergenstal RM, Amiel SA, Beck R, Biester T, et al. Clinical Targets for Continuous Glucose Monitoring Data Interpretation: Recommendations From the International Consensus on Time in Range. Diabetes Care. 2019;42(8):1593-603.
15. Pleus S, Ulbrich S, Zschornack E, Kamann S, Haug C, Freckmann G. Documentation of Skin-Related Issues Associated with Continuous Glucose Monitoring Use in the Scientific Literature. Diabetes Technol Ther. 2019;21(10):538-45.
16. Heinemann L. Interferences With CGM Systems: Practical Relevance? J Diabetes Sci Technol. 2022;16(2):271-4.
17. Garg SK, Kipnes M, Castorino K, Bailey TS, Akturk HK, Welsh JB, et al. Accuracy and Safety of Dexcom G7 Continuous Glucose Monitoring in Adults with Diabetes. Diabetes Technol Ther. 2022;24(6):373-80.
18. Boyne MS, Silver DM, Kaplan J, Saudek CD. Timing of changes in interstitial and venous blood glucose measured with a continuous subcutaneous glucose sensor. Diabetes. 2003;52(11):2790-4.

44

CHAPTER

Continuous Glucose Monitoring: An Update

Samir Sahu, Vamsi Krishna Annamdevula

ABSTRACT

The use of continuous glucose monitoring (CGM) has nowadays become more important in the treatment of diabetes mellitus and is poised to revolutionize its treatment in future. CGM devices are minimally invasive, using subcutaneous sensor coated with an enzyme to measure interstitial glucose level. Various commercially available CGM systems are available in the market with features which have been improving over the years to meet the patient's requirement. Several key metrics are used for CGM data analysis and reporting, such as glycemic variability and percentage of time spent in range, hyperglycemia, and hypoglycemia. Use of these data goes a long way in identifying the cause and managing hypoglycemia and hyperglycemia, guide mealtime insulin dose, monitoring overall improvement of glycemic status, etc.

INTRODUCTION

For determining long-term glycemia in diabetes, glycated hemoglobin (HbA1c) has been long since considered the gold standard. However, HbA1c partially expresses the glycemic variability (GV). Since people with the same HbA1c level may have markedly different glucose patterns, it is encouraged to self-monitor blood glucose (SMBG) by finger prick glucose measurement, in addition to HbA1c evaluation. Self-monitoring, on the other hand, is uncomfortable and time-consuming and only offers snapshots of glucose levels with only little knowledge of glucose trends over time. The advent of continuous glucose monitoring (CGM), which provides real-time and ongoing glucose level information, has revolutionized the management of diabetes. CGM provides a thorough view of glucose changes, unlike conventional techniques such as finger-stick testing, allowing people with diabetes to make educated decisions regarding their food, lifestyle, and insulin administration. In order to improve glycemic control, lower the risk of hypoglycemia and hyperglycemia, and enhance general quality of life, it has grown to be an essential tool.

CONTINUOUS GLUCOSE MONITORING

Continuous glucose monitoring devices **(Table 1)** being minimally invasive use tiny sensors placed beneath the skin to monitor interstitial fluid glucose levels. To identify and measure glucose concentrations, these sensors make use of cutting-edge technologies such as enzymatic or fluorescence-based glucose sensing components. The wirelessly transmitted glucose readings are subsequently processed, examined, and shown in real-time on a receiver or smartphone. CGM sensors are calibrated using a number of techniques in order to guarantee accuracy and dependability. While some systems require extra calibration by the user using finger-stick blood glucose readings, factory calibration involves initial calibration conducted by the manufacturer. Calibration increases accuracy by bringing the sensor's readings into line with the actual blood glucose level. CGM devices measure the glucose content of interstitial field (which correlates well with plasma glucose, with a 10–15-minute delay when blood glucose values are changing rapidly). Glucose levels are measured every 5–15 minutes, depending on the device.

TABLE 1: Personal continuous glucose monitoring (CGM) devices.

	FreeStyle Libre 2	FreeStyle Libre 3	Dexcom G6	Dexcom G7	Medtronic Guardian 3	Medtronic Guardian 4	Eversens
Insertion site	Arm	Arm	Abdomen	Arm or abdomen	Arm or abdomen	Arm or abdomen	Arm
Duration of sensor wear	14 days	14 days	10 days	10 days	7 days	7 days	180 days
Calibration required	No	No	No	No	Yes every 12 hours	No	Yes every 12 hours
Warm-up time	1 hour	1 hour	2 hours	30 minutes	2 hours	2 hours	24 hours
Method of insertion	Self	Self	Self	Self	Self	Self	Office based
Optional or customized alarms for glucose values	Low and high	Low and high	Predictive low and high, rate of change, low and high	Predictive low and high, rate of change, low and high	Predictive low and high, rate of change, low and high	Predictive low and high, rate of change, low and high	Predictive low and high, rate of change, low and high
Insulin pump integration	No	No	Tandem t:slim X2 and Omnipod 5	No	Medtronic MiniMed 670G, 770G, 780G	Medtronic MiniMed 780G	No
Intermittent scanning (flash) or real time	Intermittent scanning	Real-time	Real-time	Real-time	Real-time	Real-time	Real-time

Mainly there are two types of CGM systems: 'Real time' and devices that require intermittent scanning. Real-time CGM devices measure and transmit glucose values every 5 minutes. Most of the real-time CGM devices alert for hypoglycemia or hyperglycemia. Glucose value can be automatically and securely shared with a clinician, friends, and families via a mobile medical glucose monitoring application downloaded onto a mobile device, such as a smartphone and web-based diabetes management software.

Warm-up period is the duration after the device is placed on the arm, it cannot be used for blood glucose readings. Integration of some CGM devices with insulin pumps to create closed-loop system is another key development. People taking medications containing acetaminophen or treated with high-dose vitamin C may experience falsely elevated CGM glucose values with some but not all CGM devices.

INDICATION OF CONTINUOUS GLUCOSE MONITORING

- Type 1 diabetes mellitus (T1DM)
- Gestational diabetes or diabetes in pregnancy
- Type 2 diabetes mellitus (T2DM) requires intensive insulin therapy, including multiple daily injections and continuous subcutaneous insulin infusion therapy
- T2DM patients who use hypoglycemic treatment but still experience one of the following situations—repeated hypoglycemia or severe hypoglycemia, asymptomatic or nocturnal hypoglycemia, large blood glucose excursions, and diabetic patients who continue in a state of hyperglycemia due to the fear of hypoglycemia
- Where it is required to use CGM to educate patients that blood glucose changes results from exercise, diet, stress, and hypoglycemic treatment.

ADVANTAGES OF CONTINUOUS GLUCOSE MONITORING

Continuous glucose monitoring has a number of benefits over conventional glucose monitoring techniques. First of all, it offers real-time glucose data, enabling people to choose their food, level of exercise, and insulin dosage wisely. This results in better glucose regulation, lower HbA1c levels, and a decreased risk of long-term complications from diabetes. Secondly, by sending out prompt alarms when blood glucose levels get dangerously low, CGM aids with the recognition and prevention of hypoglycemia episodes, particularly nocturnal. Additionally, CGM enables more effective postprandial glucose control, permitting individualized modifications to insulin administration. Furthermore, sharing CGM data with healthcare professionals enables remote monitoring and prompts actions.

LIMITATIONS OF CONTINUOUS GLUCOSE MONITORING

Continuous glucose monitoring has certain drawbacks despite its many benefits. The accuracy of CGM readings can be impacted by problems, such as sensor calibration mistakes and inaccuracies in blood glucose and interstitial fluid measurements. Accuracy can be affected by sensor wear time and calibration methods. CGM systems may be expensive with a limited coverage by insurance plans. Local site discomfort and irritation may arise from the insertion and usage of sensors. Being a recent technology, it requires an adequate knowledge about the data interpretation and intervention on the part of the persons concerned, including healthcare professionals.

DOWNLOADED DISPLAY

The data from CGM devices can be downloaded and patterns of hyperglycemia and hypoglycemia examined. For example, hyperglycemia after breakfast would suggest the need to either administer more insulin with breakfast or reduce carbohydrate content of breakfast. Standardization of glucose reporting has been recommended in the form of an ambulatory glucose profile **(Fig. 1)**. This display contains graphics as well as glucose metrics.

TIME IN RANGES (FIG. 2)

Three key CGM measurements are used according to the 2019 International Consensus on CGM metrics **(Table 2)**—the percentage of readings and the amount of time each day spent within the target in range (TIR), the amount of time spent below the target below range (TBR), and the amount of time spent over the target above range (TAR).

Studies have demonstrated that data collected from 14 days for mean glucose levels, TIR, hypoglycemia, and hyperglycemia, closely correspond with those from 3 months.

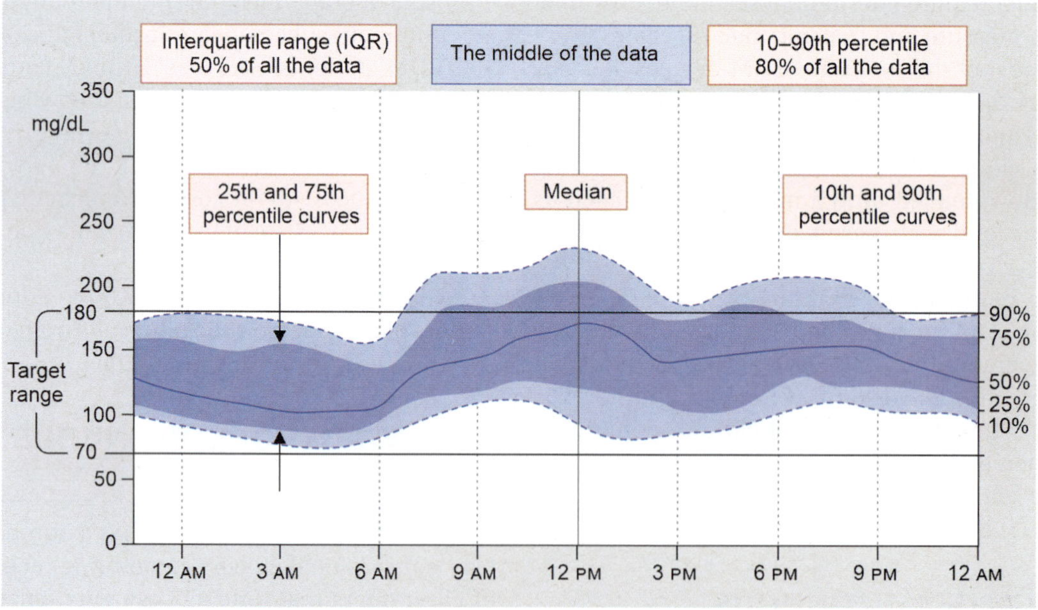

FIG. 1: An example of ambulatory glucose profile (AGP) report, which represents 14 daily glucose profiles integrated to create a single AGP visual display. The solid line is the median or 50% line; half of all glucose values are above and half are below this value. The interquartile range, or 50% of all data, is represented by the 25th and 75th percentile curves, which are shaded in dark blue. These curves are an excellent visual representation of the degree of glycemic variability (GV). The dashed outer lines (10th and 90th percentile curves) indicate that only 10% of glucose readings were above or below these values over 2-week period.

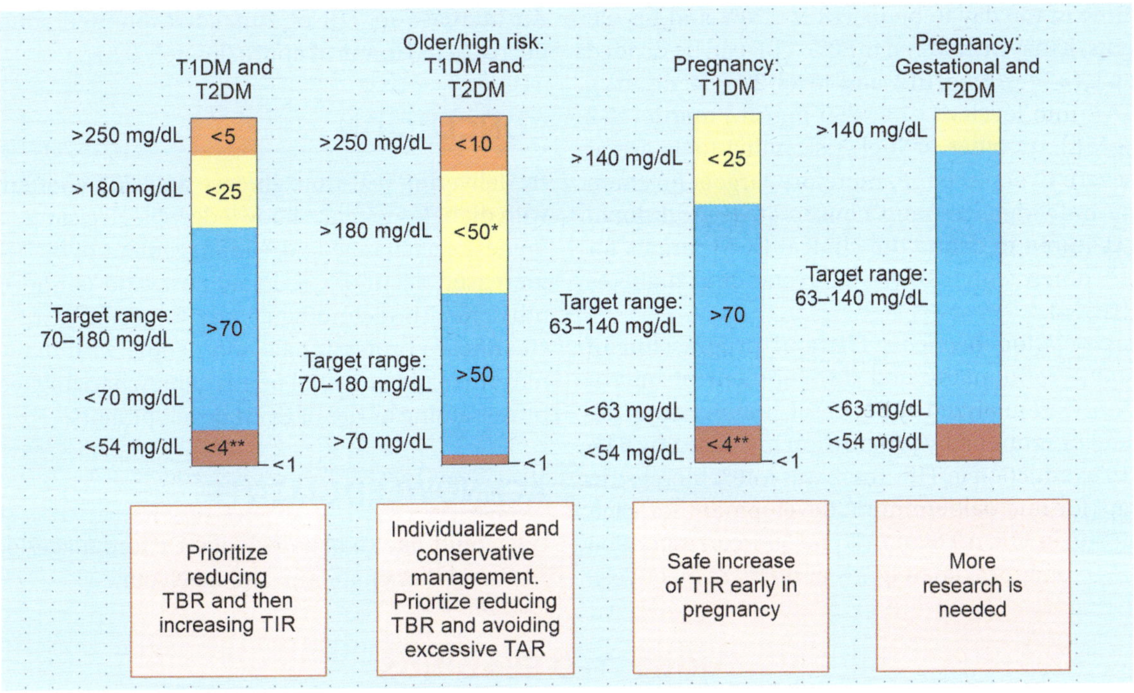

Notes:
1. Numbers inside the box indicate percentage of time spent per day.
2. Improvement of 5–10% in TIR can deliver significant glycemic benefits.

FIG. 2: Guidance on targets for assessment of glycemic control for various groups of adult type 1 diabetes mellitus (T1DM) and type 2 diabetes mellitus (T2DM) patients.
(TAR: time above range; TBR: time below range; TIR: time in range)

TABLE 2: Standardized CGM metrics for clinical care—2019 International Consensus on CGM metrics.

1. Number of days CGM worn (recommend 14 days)	
2. Percentage of time CGM is active (recommend 70% of data from 14 days)	
3. Mean glucose	
4. Glucose management indicator (GMI)	
5. Glycemic variability (% CV) target ≤ 36%	
6. *Time above range (TAR)*: % of readings and time > 250 mg/dL	Level 2
7. *Time above range (TAR)*: % of readings and time 181–250 mg/dL	Level 1
8. *Time in range (TIR)*: % of readings and time 70–180 mg/dL	In range
9. *Time below range (TBR)*: % of readings and time 54–69 mg/dL	Level 1
10. Time below range (TBR): % of readings and time < 54 mg/dL	Level 2

(CGM: continuous glucose monitoring; CV: coefficient of variation)

Glucose management indicator (GMI) is a new measure that estimates HbA1c from mean CGM glucose. It can be calculated from at least 10 days of CGM data (preferably 14 days). The GMI-estimated HbA1c uses a conversion formula based on updated clinical trials and modern-day CGM devices. It may be similar, higher, or lower than laboratory HbA1c values.

The degree of fluctuation in blood glucose readings during a specific time period is known as GV. Intraday variability measurements can be used to describe these oscillations in the short term. The coefficient of variation (% CV) is currently regarded as the preferred metric to describe intraday GV. As advised by international agreement, patients with CV > 36% are classified as having high GV and patients with these values are unstable. According to an additional research, a value of CV < 34% is ideal for reducing hypoglycemia occurrences below 54 mg/dL.

The proposed TIR in T1DM and T2DM is 70-180 mg/dL, which can be changed for a specific population group like pregnancy, where it is 63-140 mg/dL. The target percent time of the day to be in TIR is ≥70% and for old frail patients, it may be lowered to 50%. TBR can be divided into level-1 (<54–70 mg/dL) and level-2 (<54 mg/dL), so also TAR into level-1 (>180–250 mg/dL) and level-2 (>250 mg/dL). As older or high-risk individuals are at risk for severe hypoglycemia, therefore targets for them should be individualized and conservative. Additional data are required to define the clinical CGM targets for pregnant women with T2DM and gestational diabetes mellitus (GDM).

The association between TIR and progression of both diabetic retinopathy and development of microalbuminuria were analyzed by Beck et al. It showed that the hazard rate for retinopathy progression increased by 64% for each 10% reduction in TIR. There was a 40% increase in hazard rate for microalbuminuria development for each 10% reduction in TIR. A TIR of 70% and 50% corresponded to an HbA1c of approximately 7% and 8%, respectively. An increase in TIR of 10% corresponded roughly to a decrease in HbA1c of approximately 0.5%.

CONCLUSION

By delivering real-time glucose data and enabling people with diabetes to make knowledgeable decisions, CGM has made a sea change in the management of diabetes. With increased accuracy, reduced cost, and connection with other health technologies, the future of CGM is bright. Healthcare professionals and people with diabetes may maximize the potential of this game-changing technology by remaining aware of CGM developments.

ACKNOWLEDGMENTS

We would like to acknowledge Dr Jonnalagadda Vihari, Dr Rahul Ramchandani, and Dr Nikita.

SUGGESTED READINGS

1. Maahs DM, DeSalvo D, Pyle L, Ly T, Messer L, Clinton P, et al. Effect of acetaminophen on CGM glucose in an outpatient setting. Diabetes Care. 2015;38(10):e158-9.
2. Beck RW, Bergenstal RM, Riddlesworth TD, Kollman C, Li Z, Brown AS, et al. Validation of time in range as an outcome measure for diabetes clinical trials. Diabetes Care. 2019;42:400-5.

45

CHAPTER

Intermittent Fasting and Diabetes

Shaibal Guha, Atul Kumar

ABSTRACT

Most of the presently available medicines for treating type 2 diabetes mellitus (T2DM) have effects on metabolism of glucose, but not on the etiology of T2DM. Conversely, lifestyle interventions including exercise and dietary modifications do affect the underlying pathological mechanisms. Since loss of bodyweight reduces glycated hemoglobin (HbA1c), blood pressure (BP), and lipid levels, calorie restriction has been demonstrated to be effective in taming diabetes. Imbalance of levels of adiponectin and leptin is crucial to the pathophysiology of metabolic syndrome, of which T2DM is a major component.

In fasting beyond 12–24 hours, due to unavailability of glucose, lipase breaks down the triglycerides (TG) into glycerol and fatty acids by β-oxidation. A number of different dietary modification strategies have been tried, which can be either fasting-mimicking diet (FMD), or intermittent fasting (IF). Since loss of bodyweight reduces HbA1c, blood pressure, and lipid levels, IF patients have a better glucose profile. For people with insulin resistance, prediabetes, and diabetes, there has been weight loss and improved metabolic profile. IF has also been seen to reduce BP, TG, HbA1c, and low-density lipoprotein cholesterol (LDL-C).

INTRODUCTION

Type 2 diabetes mellitus (T2DM) is a metabolic disease, pathogenesis of which is a result of interplay of genes and environmental factors. An imbalance of dietary quantity and quality leads to positive energy balance, leading to accumulation of excessive carbohydrates and obesity, along with insulin resistance due to hitherto less understood factors, ultimately resulting in β-cell fatigue and impaired insulin secretion and resultant hyperglycemia.

Most of the presently available medicines for treating T2DM have effects on metabolism of glucose, but not on the etiology of T2DM. Conversely, lifestyle interventions including exercise and dietary modifications do affect the underlying pathological mechanisms. Intermittent fasting (IF) leads to metabolic reprogramming, leading to increased utilization of fatty acids and ketones, and also leads to reduction of body fat and body weight, and improvement in the levels and sensitivity of adipokinin.

OBESITY, CALORIE RESTRICTION, AND DIABETES

Since loss of bodyweight reduces glycated hemoglobin (HbA1c), blood pressure, and lipid levels, calorie restriction has been demonstrated to be effective in taming diabetes. In fact, just 1 kg of weight loss can reduce the risk of diabetes to the tune of 16%. Further, continuous caloric restriction has shown to even cause remission of diabetes mellitus in several studies.

Obesity is very closely associated with T2DM. Excessive lipid deposition, and at abnormal sites in the body due to chronic inflammation, is supposed to be one of the causes of insulin resistance in obesity. These abnormal fat deposits start secreting adipokines like adiponectin, which is anti-inflammatory, and leptin, which is proinflammatory. These chemicals have shown to have their effect on satiety center in hypothalamus and influence food intake and energy expenditure. Leptin resistance has often been seen to be associated with insulin resistance and high body mass index (BMI) in diabetic individuals. Conversely, adiponectin, the anti-inflammatory molecule which increases glucose uptake by the liver and reduces gluconeogenesis, is seen to decrease in the presence of accumulation of excessive fat.

Scientists postulated that imbalance of levels of adiponectin and leptin is crucial to the pathophysiology of metabolic syndrome, of which T2DM is a major component. For reasons still not clear, reduced levels of leptin and increased levels of adiponectin are often found in subjects doing IF even if there was no fat loss.

Over the years, it has been known that metabolic health can be improved, and weight reduction achieved simply by restricting intake of calories, possibly by improvement in insulin sensitivity. Studies have shown that the body starts using fatty acids and ketones in preference to glucose while in the fasting state after 12–24 hours. However, it is very difficult to continue calorie restriction for a long period of time. In this situation, IF methods are more practical and doable, and hence have a better compliance.

WHAT HAPPENS DURING FASTING?

The benefits of IF are twofold. Firstly, it leads to metabolic reprogramming, leading to increased utilization of fatty acids and ketones. Secondly, the negative calorie balance leads to reduction of body fat and body weight, and improvement in the levels and sensitivity of adipokinin, thus reducing both, appetite as well as level of chronic inflammation.

The human body normally derives its energy supply almost entirely from glucose during the nonfasting state. Till about 12–24 hours of abstinence from food, glucagon-induced glycogenolysis in liver and skeletal muscle supplies the glucose required for maintaining the serum levels. Beyond this, due to unavailability of glucose, hormone-sensitive lipase breaks down the triglycerides (TG) into glycerol and fatty acids by β-oxidation to provide the requisite calories, and subsequently, to acetyl-coenzyme A (acetyl-CoA), and then to ketones.

To attain this loss of weight in the long-term goal to reduce or revert diabetes, a number of different dietary modification strategies have been tried, which can be mainly classified into:

- Fasting-mimicking diet (FMD)
- Intermittent fasting

Fasting-mimicking diets: These provide a small amount of calories and try to replicate the hormonal and metabolic effects of complete fasting. FMDs basically consist of low protein levels, complex carbohydrates, and healthy fats, preferably from plant sources, and virtually no (or, minimal) refined sugar.

Intermittent fasting: A broad heading encompassing various types of timed eating and limited fasting, with the aim of restricting calorie intake, improve body composition and overall health.

TYPES OF INTERMIITENT FASTING

1. *Complete alternate day fasting:* Alternating fasting days (without consuming high-energy food and drinks) with eating days (eating and drinking ad libitum)
2. *Alternate day fasting:* It allows consumption from 20 to 25% of energy demand on scheduled fasting days. This scheme forms the basis of the popular 5:2 diet, which is associated with severe energy restriction for 2 uninterrupted days a week and eating ad libitum for the remaining 5 days.
3. *Time-restricted feeding:* Eating meals with a certain energy value during the "food window," which lasts several hours. The most common modification is eating for 8 hours, followed by fasting for the next 16 hours. The hours of fasting and eating can be shortened and extended.
4. *Periodic fasting:* Up to 24 hours fasting, once or twice a week with normal food intake on the remaining days.
5. *The 5:2 diet:* Done by restricting caloric intake (not complete fasting) on 2 nonconsecutive days a week (500 kcal for women and 600 kcal for men), and normal calorie diet on the remaining days.
6. *Religious fasting:* A wide range of fasts is undertaken for religious or spiritual purposes.

BENEFITS OF INTERMITTENT FASTING

For people with insulin resistance, prediabetes and diabetes, there has been weight loss and improved metabolic profile. IF has also been seen to reduce BP, TG, HbA1c, and low-density lipoprotein cholesterol (LDL-C).

Randomized controlled trials (RCTs) with IF have not been conclusive about the reduction of inflammatory markers, but they have shown decrease in markers of oxidative stress, which might be associated with improved insulin sensitivity.

Intermittent fasting can also alter the gut microbiome composition and the host biological clock or circadian rhythm, enhancing cardiometabolic health in the process.

PHYSIOLOGY BEHIND THE BENEFITS

Intermittent fasting has shown beneficial effects in animal studies on immune system, metabolism, atherosclerosis, cognitive functions, and also has shown to extend the lifespan. Weight loss of up to 8–10%, and significant reductions in LDL-C, TG, and C-reactive protein (CRP) have been seen with IF compared to the control group.

It is postulated that these metabolic benefits occur through three main pathways:

1. *Path 1:* Reduced intracellular adenosine triphosphate (ATP) increases adenosine monophosphate (AMP), leading to stimulation of AMP-activated protein kinase (AMPK).
2. *Path 2:* Mammalian target of rapamycin (mTOR), the intracellular energy sensor, is inhibited due to the reduced levels of circulating glucose and amino acids.
3. *Path 3:* As a result of the energy deficit, glycolysis starts in the liver, along with a fatty acid release from adipose tissue. There is also decrease in oxidative stress and increased autophagy. These mechanisms ultimately lead to weight loss, an improvement in insulin sensitivity with reduction in insulin levels and blood glucose, and a decrease in blood pressure and serum lipid levels.

INTERMITTENT FASTING VERSUS STARVATION

Intermittent fasting and starvation are not the same. Since IF is done in a controlled fashion, there is no period of undue severe or prolonged calorie restriction, unlike starvation, which is a purely catabolic state, and hence, is more severe and prolonged. Therefore, symptoms such as diarrhea, delirium, weight loss, emancipation, and anemia, commonly seen in starvation, are not found associated with IF.

HOW TO ADVISE INTERMITTENT FASTING IN DIABETICS?

The pregnant and breastfeeding women, frail people, and the elderly should be advised against IF. Also, if the patient has recovered from severe disease or complications, or has had severe hypoglycemia in past, or is poorly oriented, he is not an ideal subject for IF.

All patients planning to start IF are given due instructions under the guidance of their physician and dietician, trained to check their blood sugar levels and identify hypoglycemia, and their medicine doses are adjusted. They are initially made to fast for fewer times per week, and for a shorter duration than intended, and then shifted to the actual regimen once acclimatized. Most patients are suggested to follow a 16:8 diet on at least 2 days a week, and some follow the same on a daily regimen. After few weeks, the patients are followed up for symptoms of hypoglycemia episodes, loss of weight, and decrement in blood sugar and lipid levels. Quite a few do complain of malaise and headache. All of them are cautioned against self-medication and tweaking the dietary and fasting advice, being influenced by suggestions on social media and internet, or from friends.

CONCLUSION

If one goes through the details of the animal studies, epidemiological studies, RCTs, and their own clinical experiences, one can definitely claim that IF is beneficial for a diabetic patient. Having said that, there are still not too many studies with robust evidence to recommend IF as a part of regular treatment in a diabetic patient. For interested patients, if found clinically fit, a short-term supervised IF regimen can be tried. This would be even more fruitful in an obese diabetic. However, as mentioned earlier, which regimen to follow, and how frequently, and for how much duration needs to be individualized. Needless to say, prior information regarding the complications such as hypoglycemia, hypotension, electrolyte imbalance, and dehydration, and about the precautions needed to prevent those has to be imparted.

SUGGESTED READING

1. Patterson RE, Laughlin GA, LaCroix AZ, Hartman SJ, Natarajan L, Senger CM, et al. Intermittent fasting and human metabolic health. J Acad Nutr Diet. 2015;115(8):1203-12.

46

CHAPTER

Prediabetes and Cardiovascular Disease Risk

Akashkumar Navinprakash Singh, Saumitra Singh

ABSTRACT

Prediabetes is a condition in which blood glucose levels are higher than normal but not high enough to be considered diabetes. People with prediabetes are more prone to progress to diabetes, while diabetes is known to cause serious health conditions such as cardiovascular diseases (CVDs), stroke, and kidney problems. Prediabetes is known to be associated with an increased risk of all-cause mortality and CVDs in the general population and in patients with atherosclerotic CVD. Screening and proper management of prediabetes might contribute to primary and secondary prevention of CVDs. It is well-known that lifestyle interventions in people with prediabetes can reduce the risk of cardiovascular events and all-cause mortality. It is also important to determine the risk of heart failure in individuals with prediabetes who are undergoing lifestyle interventions.

INTRODUCTION

Prediabetes is a precursor of type 2 diabetes mellitus (T2DM) and is described as a continuum from normal glucose tolerance (NGT) through worsening dysglycemia. It is often referred to as "intermediate hyperglycemia" involving conditions such as impaired fasting glucose (IFG) and/or impaired glucose tolerance (IGT), and includes people with glycated hemoglobin (HbA1c) between 39 and 47 mmol/mol (5.7–6.4%). Reports estimate that >470 million people will have prediabetes by 2030. Prediabetes is an asymptomatic progressive condition which may lead to onset of T2DM with yearly conversion rate of 5–10% and is associated with high-risk rate of developing various macrovascular and microvascular complications. The principal pathophysiological defects such as obesity, metabolic syndrome (MetS), insulin resistance (IR), and systemic inflammation that underlie T2DM have now been increasingly recognized in patients with prediabetes as well. These factors impart a significant risk for development of atherogenesis and cardiovascular disease (CVD) as most patients with prediabetes also have coexisting and well-recognized risk factors such as dyslipidemia, hypertension, and a prothrombotic state. Over the last 10–15 years, a significant wealth of evidence has uncovered the link between prediabetes with macrovascular CVD and related mortality and morbidity. Management of prediabetes includes lifestyle changes and pharmacotherapy which have shown beneficial effects in delaying the progression of prediabetes to overt T2DM and have also been useful in mitigating CVD risk in these patients.

DIAGNOSTIC CRITERIA AND THEIR CLINICAL SIGNIFICANCE

The diagnostic criteria for prediabetes have evolved over time and the "cut offs" that are used may vary as per different organizations. **Table 1** shows the criteria used by the American Diabetes Association (ADA) and the World Health Organization (WHO).

The most important clinical implication of IGT and IFG has been to primarily identify individuals who are at risk of developing T2DM. However, although both IGT and IFG are associated with IR and impaired insulin secretion; their significance with respect to progression of disease and development of CVD complications may not be the

TABLE 1: The ADA and WHO definitions for IFG and IGT.

Parameter	Organization	FPG	2-h OGTT with 75 g oral glucose load levels
Isolated IFG (iIFG)	ADA	100–125 mg/dL (5.6–6.9 mmol/L)	<140 mg/dL (<7.8 mmol/L)
	WHO	110–125 mg/dL (6.1–6.9 mmol/L)	<140 mg/dL (<7.8 mmol/L)
Isolated IGT (iIGT)	ADA	<100 mg/dL (<5.6 mmol/L)	140–199 mg/dL (7.8–11 mmol/L)
	WHO	<110 mg/dL (<6.1 mmol/L)	140–199 mg/dL (7.8–11 mmol/L)
Combined IFG+IGT	ADA	100–125 mg/dL (5.6–7.0 mmol/L)	140–199 mg/dL (7.8–11 mmol/L) or HbA1c of 39–47 mmol/mol (5.7–6.4%)
	WHO	110–125 mg/dL (6.1–6.9 mmol/L)	140–199 mg/dL (7.8–11 mmol/L)

(ADA: American Diabetes Association; HbA1c: glycated hemoglobin; IFG: impaired fasting glucose; IGT: impaired glucose tolerance; FPG: fasting plasma glucose; OGTT: oral glucose tolerance test; WHO: World Health Organization)

same. There is adequate available data to suggest that IGT is associated with several other clinical events other than progression to T2DM which establishes the clinical significance of IGT beyond being a simple diagnostic criterion. In the Whitehall study, amongst 18,403 patients who were followed up for 7 years, the risk of CVD-related mortality was twice in the IGT group in comparison to patients with NGT.

On the contrary, the correlation of IFG with macrovascular events has not been well established. Well-known studies such as the DECODE (Diabetes Epidemiology: Collaborative analysis of Diagnostic criteria in Europe) and ARIC (Atherosclerosis Risk in Communities) could not identify significant association between IFG with future CVD events though DECODE investigators did find an increased risk of mortality for IFG compared with NGT using the 110 mg/dL (6.1 mmol/L) threshold. Although, association of IFG with CVD risk remains uncertain, its association with other features of IR and MetS, including dyslipidemia, hypertension, abdominal obesity, microalbuminuria, endothelial dysfunction (ED), and markers of inflammation and hypercoagulability remains clear, which are often associated with progression of prediabetes to overt T2DM, CVD risk, and increased mortality.

HOW DOES PREDIABETES INCREASE CVD RISK?

The disturbances in glucose homeostasis in IFG and IGT are very distinct as the process of insulin secretion, insulin sensitivity, and resistance vary widely among these two conditions. Individuals with IFG/IGT also have IR and associated MetS which play an important role in the development of atherosclerotic cardiovascular disease (ASCVD). Individuals with prediabetes have a similar state of IR as lean patients with T2DM and obese patients with NGT. IR among individuals with prediabetes also primarily affects the glycogen synthesis pathway and promotes atherogenesis via multiple mechanisms such as advanced glycation end products (AGEs) activation, decrease in nitric oxide (NO) production, protein kinase C (PKC) activation, platelet and coagulation system activation, and peroxisome proliferator-activated receptors (PPAR) activation. It also causes hypertension, obesity, and dyslipidemia [characterized by hypertriglyceridemia, reduced high-density lipoprotein cholesterol (HDL-C) and elevated low-density lipoprotein cholesterol (LDL-C)], which are major risk factors of CVD. Several large meta-analyses have shown that MetS raises the CVD risk and macrovascular complications by approximately two-fold in individuals with prediabetes. There are several cross-sectional and interventional studies as well that have tried to explore whether IFG/IGT increases the risk of CVD or not and define the risk of CVD, CAD, stroke, and all-cause mortality among individuals with prediabetes. Studies have shown that IGT is associated with increased risk of CVD; however, the association of IFG and the risk of CVD is far more unclear.

SCREENING STRATEGY FOR PREDIABETES

It is highly imperative to identify and screen individuals for prediabetes especially who are at high risk for developing diabetes **(Box 1)**.

The screening strategy for prediabetes should include the following patients.

Individuals having more than one of the above risk factors are eligible for screening for prediabetes and should be screened at repeated intervals which may be

BOX 1: Screening strategy for prediabetes.

- Physically inactive
- First-degree relative or second-degree relative with diabetes
- *High-risk race/ethnicity*: African American, Latino, Native American, Asian American, Pacific Islander, etc.
- Women with polycystic ovarian disease (PCOD) or who delivered a baby weighing >9 lb or were diagnosed with gestational diabetes
- Hypertension (≥140/90 mm Hg or on therapy for hypertension)
- HDL-C < 35 mg/dL and/or a
- TG > 250 mg/dL
- HbA1c ≥ 5.7%, IGT, or IFG on previous testing
- Overweight or obesity (BMI ≥ 25 kg/m^2)
- History of CVD, etc.
- MetS and IR

(BMI: body mass index; CVD: cardiovascular disease; HbA1c: glycated hemoglobin; HDL-C: high-density lipoprotein cholesterol; IGT: impaired glucose tolerance; IFG: impaired fasting glucose; IR: insulin resistance; MetS: metabolic syndrome; TG: triglycerides)

biannual, annual, or every 2 years based on the initials results and risk status. However, in individuals with none of the risk factors, screening should begin no later than age 45 and repeated at ≥3-year intervals at a minimum or more often based on the initials results and risk status. According to the ADA, children and adolescents also need to be screened for prediabetes, especially those who are overweight [defined as a body mass index (BMI) >85th percentile for age and gender]; weight-for-height defined as >85th percentile or weight >120% of ideal body weight for height; ethnic diversity, low birth weight compared to gestational age, and maternal history of diabetes of gestational diabetes mellitus (GDM) during child's gestation, etc. Screening should begin at the age of 10 years or early onset of puberty, whichever occurs earlier and repeated every 3-year intervals at a minimum or more often based on the initials results and risk status. The most preferred test recommended by the ADA for prediabetes among children and adolescents is HbA1c, except in rare cases such as cystic fibrosis and hemoglobinopathies. The screening tools are same as the diagnostic tools for prediabetes or T2DM which include HbA1c, FPG, and 75-g 2 hours post-oral glucose tolerance test (OGTT).

MANAGEMENT OF PREDIABETES

The effective measures of treating prediabetes include prevention of progression to diabetes and its potential consequences. The majority of the studies have focused on lifestyle changes, which should be the cornerstone for diabetes prevention whereas, pharmacotherapy and bariatric surgery can also be chosen in selected individuals. The primary aim of lifestyle interventions is to prevent or delay the development of T2DM and its complications by targeting obesity and physical inactivity, the two most important modifiable risk factors of diabetes development. The two largest diabetes prevention studies, the United States DPP and the Finnish Diabetes Prevention Study (DPS) have both shown beneficial effects of intensive lifestyle interventions (ILS). Several groups of antidiabetic drugs such as biguanides, thiazolidinediones, alpha-glucosidase inhibitors, glucagon-like peptide-1 (GLP-1) analogs have shown to be effective in managing the progression of prediabetes. Metformin has been used for several decades for treatment of prediabetes especially in individuals with high-risk (age <60 years, BMI >30, HbA1c >6.0%). Available literature data on treating subjects with prediabetes with lifestyle and drug-based interventions showed that these interventions resulted in reduction in stroke risk but did not result in any risk reduction for all-cause mortality, cardiovascular death, or myocardial infarction. Therefore, there remains a need of systematic evaluation of the health outcomes of prediabetes and benefits with its early treatment. Antiplatelet therapy is advocated in patients with this condition who are at high risk for CVD. Also, Aspirin therapy is recommended among individuals with a history of CVD.

DISCUSSION AND CONCLUSION

In conclusion, CVD is the leading cause of morbidity and mortality in patients with dysglycemia. The progression of normoglycemia to prediabetes and then to overt diabetes is a disease continuum as the underlying pathophysiological mechanisms that impart IR and impair insulin secretion, and sensitivity is similar and tends to deteriorate over time. Moreover, in association with other vascular risk factors, it augments the risk of CVD and related mortality. Early identification and interventions are needed in patients with prediabetes to prevent progression overt diabetes and to mitigate chances of development of macrovascular disease and its related complications.

ACKNOWLEDGMENT

The author acknowledges the writing support provided by Tatineni Swathi from Arkus Research Pvt. Ltd.

SUGGESTED READINGS

1. Wu J, Liang D, Xie Y. Prediabetes and risk of heart failure: the link grows stronger. Cardiovasc Diabetol. 2021;20:112.
2. Huang Y, Cai X, Mai W, Li M, Hu Y. Association between prediabetes and risk of all cause mortality and cardiovascular disease: updated meta-analysis. BMJ. 2020;370:m2297.
3. American Diabetes Association. Classification and diagnosis of diabetes: Standards of medical care in diabetes-2019. Diabetes Care. 2019;42 (Suppl 1):S13-28.
4. Makaroff LE. The need for international consensus on prediabetes. Lancet Diabetes Endocrinol. 2017;5(1):5-7.
5. Faerch K, Vistisen D, Johansen NB, Jørgensen ME. Cardiovascular risk stratification and management in prediabetes. Curr Diab Rep. 2014;14(6):493.
6. Sussman JB, Kent DM, Nelson JP, Hayward RA. Improving diabetes prevention with benefit based tailored treatment: risk-based reanalysis of Diabetes Prevention Program. BMJ. 2015;350:h454.

47

CHAPTER

C-peptide and its Clinical Implications

Amit Kumar Das, Anuj Sharma

ABSTRACT

Impaired beta-cell function is a fundamental aspect of the pathophysiology of diabetes. Estimations regarding the capacity of insulin secretion serve as valuable tools in informing clinical practice, as they aid in the classification of diabetes types, stratification of risk for complications, and facilitation of treatment decisions. C-peptide secretion has appeared as a clinically significant biomarker, particularly in diabetes (autoimmune) and specifically in cases of adult-onset diabetes. In order to address the heterogeneity and intricacy of diabetes, there is a need for dependable, straightforward, and cost-effective clinical indicators. These markers should provide clinicians with valuable insights into the likely pathophysiology and progression of the disease. This chapter provides a comprehensive overview of the existing body of evidence regarding the possible utility of C-peptide in management of diabetes, namely autoimmune diabetes and type 2 diabetes mellitus. The objective is to elucidate how C-peptide levels measurement may contribute to improving daily clinical practice, while also shedding light on the current limitations and areas of uncertainty that necessitate further investigation in future research.

INTRODUCTION

The identification of proinsulin, a compound consisting of a connecting peptide and insulin known as C-peptide, was made by Steiner. This breakthrough facilitated the quantification of C-peptide, separate from insulin, as demonstrated by Heding and Rubenstein. The potential role of the connecting peptide of proinsulin, commonly referred to as C-peptide, has been the subject of investigation in relation to addressing certain gaps in the understanding of the pathogenesis of complications associated with type 1 diabetes mellitus (T1DM). The 31-amino-acid sequence serves as a physiological linkage between the A and B chains of proinsulin. The hormone folding and assembly within islet vehicles is facilitated by this factor, which is subsequently cleaved by endoproteases.

The amino acid sequence exhibits interspecies variability, with certain amino acid residues remaining conserved among mammals, while others undergo alteration within a single species. C-peptide is released into the circulatory system in equimolar quantities relative to insulin and serves as a marker for the endogenous production of the latter hormone.

Several researchers have reported the introduction of C-peptide in rodents (diabetic) resulted in notable enhancements in glomerulosclerosis, along with reductions in, albumin in the urine, basement membrane thickening, and excessive filtration. Therefore, the potential of C-peptide as a clinical therapeutic agent for the management and prevention of diabetic kidney disease has been acknowledged. It is being explored as a supplementary option to the existing therapeutic protocols, which encompass angiotensin-converting-enzyme inhibitors and angiotensin II receptor blockers. However, up until recent times, the utilization of C-peptide in the clinical setting has been infrequent. The present article provides a comprehensive evaluation of the clinical significance of C-peptide, focusing on the resurgence of interest in its measurement and its potential utility in guiding healthcare professionals in the treatment of individuals diagnosed with type 2 diabetes mellitus (T2DM) or autoimmune diabetes, which are the most commonly observed types of diabetes. Additionally, this chapter underscores the limitations of C-peptide measurement and identifies areas of uncertainty that exist in current medical knowledge.

METHODS

The references were extracted by conducting searches on PubMed, encompassing articles published until November 2021. The search strategy involved the utilization of specific keywords either independently or in conjunction. These keywords included "proinsulin," "C-peptide," "insulin," "T1DM," "beta-cell," "T2DM," "autoimmune diabetes," "retinopathy," "complications," "cardiovascular," and "nephropathy." The inclusion criteria for this study encompassed solely articles that were published in the English language **(Flowchart 1)**.

Why to measure C-peptide and not insulin?

C-peptide is a commonly employed and valuable technique for evaluating the functionality of pancreatic beta cells. Following proinsulin cleavage, both C-peptide and insulin are generated in equivalent quantities. The utilization of C-peptide testing is generally favored over insulin as a means of assessing beta-cell functionality. The breakdown rate of C-peptide in humans is comparatively slower than the breakdown rate of insulin, resulting in a more consistent and reliable timeframe for assessing the fluctuating response of beta cells. The plasma concentration of C-peptide ranges from 0.3 to 0.6 nmol/L during the fasting state among healthy patients. However, after consuming a meal, there is an observed rise in C-peptide levels to a range of 1–3 nmol/L. The liver is responsible for metabolizing around 50% of the insulin produced by pancreas in a process known as first-pass metabolism. In contrast, the clearance of C-peptide by the liver is considered to be insignificant. C-peptide is consistently eliminated from the peripheral circulation, while the clearance of insulin exhibits variability, resulting in less reliable direct measurement. In individuals with diabetes who are receiving insulin treatment, the inclusion of C-peptide measurement in assessments helps to circumvent the issue of assay cross-reaction between endogenous and exogenous insulin.

MEASUREMENT OF C-PEPTIDE LEVEL AND REFERENCE LEVELS

C-peptide in whole blood is often collected using potassium ethylenediaminetetraacetic acid (EDTA) as an anticoagulant, as opposed to the more frequently employed serum gel. The measurement of C-peptide is conducted using contemporary immunoassay analyzers, and it has been observed that the stability of C-peptide at room temperature extends for a minimum duration of 24 hours. C-peptide can be quantified in both urine and blood samples **(Table 1)**.

CLINICAL SIGNIFICANCE

Measurement of C-peptide in clinical scenario has of late been picked up due to some promising research studies. C-peptide assessment in clinical practice can be grouped as following:

- *As a diagnostic tool*: The plasma concentration of C-peptide ranges from 0.3 to 0.6 nmol/L during the fasting state among healthy patients. However, after consuming a meal, there is an observed rise in C-peptide levels to a range of 1–3 nmol/L.

 The cut-off values obtained by various methods of estimation has already been defined, when there

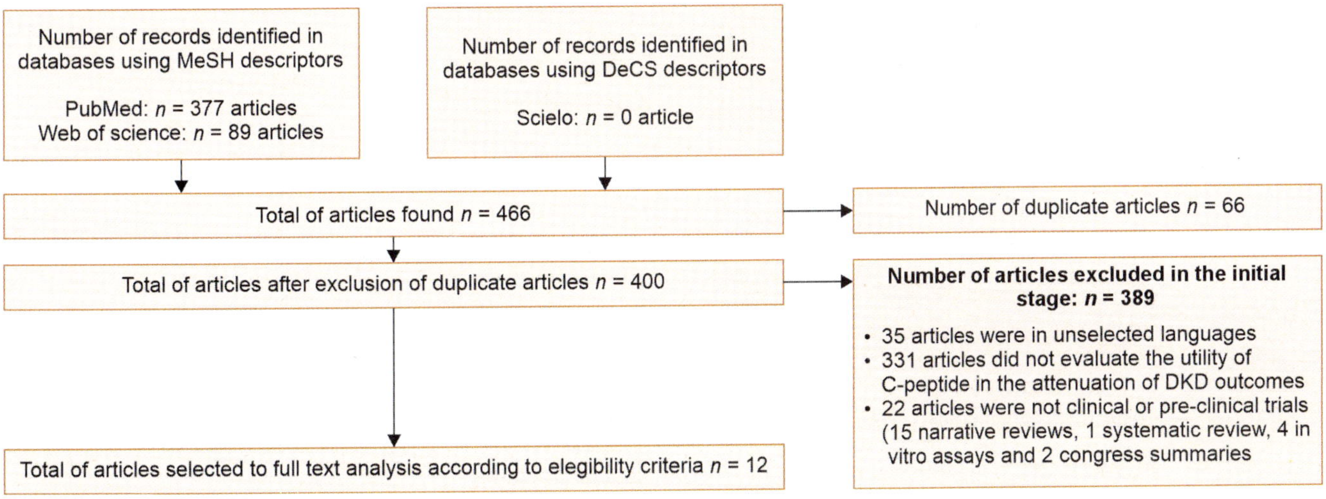

FLOWCHART 1: Paper selection.

is absolute deficiency of insulin like 3–5 years of diagnosis of T1DM the C-peptide level would be at its nadir in blood and urine. A stimulated test would also not be sufficient enough to cause release of insulin or C-peptide in blood.

A stimulated blood C-peptide < 0.2 nmol/L, fasting < 0.08 nmol/L and or postmeal urinary C-peptide: Creatinine ratio (UCPCR) < 0.2 nmol/mmol) in the presence of hyperglycemia confirms absolute insulin deficiency. These are the patients who require insulin as valid therapeutic tool and are at the highest risk of ketoacidosis. A higher value than these can be seen in T1DM patients when some amount of insulin release is seen in early part of T1DM (Honeymoon phase). Serial measurement of C-peptide in this subset can solve the diagnostic confusion **(Flowchart 2)**.

TABLE 1: C-peptide measurement.

Blood	Urine
Fasting C-peptide (fCP)	Urinary C-peptide (UCP)
Non fasting or random C-peptide (rCP)	Urinary C-peptide to creatinine ratio (UCPCR)
Stimulated C-peptide tests • Mixed meal tolerance test (MMTT) • Oral glucose tolerance test (OGTT) • Tolbutamide tolerance test (tCP) • Glucagon stimulation test (GST)	24-hour urinary collection C-peptide (24-h UCP)

Differentiating maturity-onset diabetes of young (MODY) from T1DM: MODY is monogenic diabetes with autosomal dominant inheritance pattern and usually presents in nonobese children, adolescents, and young adults. This is a nonketotic type of diabetes and does not have pancreatic autoantibodies. Because of similarity in age of presentations and BMI, most of the MODY patients are wrongly diagnosed as T1DM and treated with insulin. C-peptide estimation is one tool which can differentiate T1DM from MODY.

A proposed criterion for considering MODY testing is a random blood C-peptide level of 0.2 nmol/L in individuals diagnosed with diabetes before the age of 30 years and with a duration of >3 years. The UCPCR of 0.2 nmol/mmol, after 5 years of diagnosis, demonstrates 97% sensitivity and 96% specificity in distinguishing between HNF1A/4A MODY and T1DM. C-peptide testing is unlikely to be useful in differentiating MODY from T2DM.

- *As a prognostic tool:* It is well established that poor glycemic control in any type of diabetes is associated with both short-term complications and myriad of long-term complications. Absolute deficiency of insulin in both T2DM and T1DM places the person at highest risk of ketoacidosis, hypoglycemia, high glycemic variability, and microvascular deficiency.

  The Diabetes Control and Complications Trial (DCCT) observed that those with post-mixed-meal tolerance test C-peptide levels exceeding 0.2 nmol/L exhibited a reduction of 10 mmol/mol in baseline screening glycated hemoglobin (HbA1c) levels. Furthermore, these participants saw a notable decrease in the occurrence of retinopathy, nephropathy, and

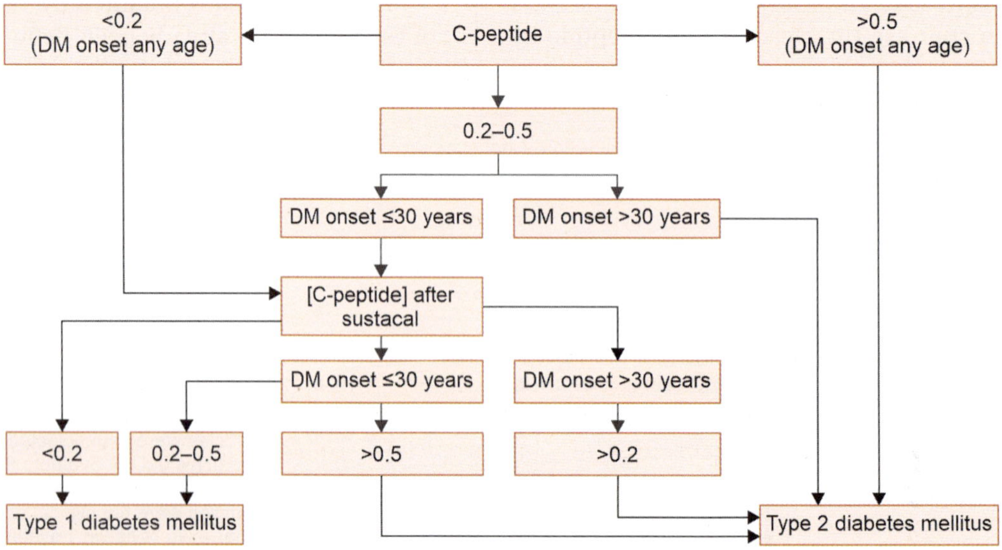

FLOWCHART 2: Algorithm showing serial measurement of C-peptide.
(DM: diabetes mellitus)

hypoglycemia. Elevated C-peptide levels are found to potentially correlate with the presence of metabolic syndrome characteristics and an augmented risk of macrovascular problems in T2DM individuals. Several studies have reported a potential association between microvascular problems in T2DM individuals and C-peptide, while contrasting findings have also been reported.

- *As marker of therapeutic response*: C-peptides help in distinguishing insulin-treated individuals with beta-cell function, enabling the safe substitution of insulin with alternative hypoglycemia treatments. Previous studies demonstrated a range of stimulated C-peptide levels (between 0.3 and 0.8 nmol/L), can effectively distinguish between those with diabetes who require insulin treatment and those who do not. T2DM patients who are on insulin and once glycemic targets have been achieved may be switched over to oral antidiabetics (OADs) if the stimulated C-peptide level is >0.8 nmol/L.

Absolute deficiency of insulin as predicted by C-peptide assays could clear the way of starting insulin in late stage of T2DM. Even insulin regimens can well be predicted now in both T1DM and T2DM. C-peptide level has been found to be inversely proportional to glycemic variability and post prandial peaks. Therefore a high C-peptide level in T2DM patients planning to be started on insulin may fair well on long-acting insulin alone but a low-to-very low C-peptide level may warrant one to multiple doses of prandial insulin then(Basal bolus regimen). C-peptide's clinical function in predicting response to specific hypoglycemic agents is poorly supported. There is evidence that insulin-resistant patients with higher C-peptide levels respond better to thiazolidinediones. Metformin, sulfonylureas, and dipeptidyl peptidase-4 (DPP-4) inhibitors do not appear to exhibit this characteristic.

C-peptide measurement may assist in identifying adult patients presenting with diabetic ketoacidosis without classic T1DM and who may not require long-term insulin treatment. Preoperative C-peptide assessment has been associated with remission of T2DM following bariatric surgery in an Asian population. Remission rates were 55% in patients with preoperative fasting C-peptide levels of 1 nmol/L versus 90% in those with fasting C-peptide levels of >2 nmol/L. In the subgroup that underwent bypass surgery, these disparities were less pronounced. C-peptide can be used to aid in patient selection for islet cell transplantation and post-transplant surveillance. C-peptide 0.1 nmol/L (fasting and/or mixed-meal tolerance test) has been utilized as a criterion for islet cell transplantation and to define graft failure **(Table 2)**.

TABLE 2: C-peptide measurement indication.

Diagnostic	Prognostic	Therapeutic response
Defining T1DM	Marking diabetes duration	Low baseline level with insulin increase
Acceptance criteria for CSII	Low levels with T1DM microvascular complication risk	Low baseline level with short insulin treatment
Determining T1DM or T2DM	Glycemic variability/HbA1c level	High level in patients responding to metformin and glibenclamide combination
MODY diagnostic test	Low levels with greater hypoglycemia risk	High levels in thiazolidinediones response
LADA diagnostic testing, and antibody testing		Correlation with HbA1c reduction after GLP-1 agonist therapy initiation

(GLP-1: glucagon-like peptide 1; HbA1c: glycated hemoglobin; LADA: latent autoimmune diabetes in adults; MODY: maturity-onset diabetes of young; T1DM: type 1 diabetes mellitus; T2DM: type 2 diabetes mellitus)

CONCLUSION

C-peptide is a valuable biomarker for assessing the functionality of beta cells, enabling the differentiation between individuals with diabetes who have sufficient insulin production and those who are lacking in insulin. Due to its sensitivity, repeatability, and ease, we would suggest the utilization of glucagon stimulation testing in clinical settings. Previous studies have demonstrated a significant association between C-peptide levels and many factors related to diabetes, including the specific type of diabetes, the duration of the condition, and the age at which it was diagnosed. It is noteworthy that C-peptide has been shown to exhibit an association with microvascular problems. Additional research is necessary; however, initial findings indicate that in the future, with HbA1c, the inclusion of C-peptide sampling may serve as a crucial diagnostic and monitoring method.

SUGGESTED READINGS

1. Heding LG. Radioimmunological determination of human C-peptide in serum. Diabetologia. 1975;11(6):541-8.
2. Horwitz DL, Starr JI, Mako ME, Blackard WG, Rubenstein AH. Proinsulin, insulin, and C-peptide concentrations in human portal and peripheral blood. J Clin Invest. 1975;55(6):1278-83.
3. Ludvigsson J. Lise G. Heding, 1936–2008. Diabetologia. 2009;52(10):2245-6.
4. Taylor SW, Clarke NJ, McPhaul MJ. Quantitative amino acid analysis in insulin and C-peptide assays. Clin Chem. 2016;62:1152-3.
5. Zhou A, Webb G, Zhu X, Steiner DF. Proteolytic processing in the secretory pathway. J Biol Chem. 1999;274:20745-8.
6. Wahren J, Larsson C. C-peptide: New findings and therapeutic possibilities. Diabetes Res Clin Pract. 2015;107:309-19.
7. Hills CE, Brunskill NJ, Squires PE. C-peptide as a therapeutic tool in diabetic nephropathy. Am J Nephrol. 2010;31:389-97.
8. Xu S, Jiang Y, Wang H, Wang Z, Liu H, Peng L, et al. C-peptide ameliorates renal injury in type 2 diabetic rats through protein kinase A-mediated inhibition of fibronectin synthesis. Biochem Biophys Res Commun. 2015;458:674-80.
9. Maezawa Y, Yokote K, Sonezaki K, Fujimoto M, Kobayashi K, Kawamura H, et al. Influence of C-peptide on early glomerular changes in diabetic mice. Diabetes Metab Res Rev. 2006;22:313-22.
10. Samnegård B, Jacobson SH, Jaremko G, Johansson BL, Sjöquist M. Effects of C-peptide on glomerular and renal size and renal function in diabetic rats. Kidney Int. 2001;60:1258-65.
11. Antão CF, Gallego R, Caldeira J. Complicações renais da diabetes Mellitus. Rev Port Clin Geral 2007;23:577-94.
12. Hope SV, Knight BA, Shields BM VH Anita, C Pratik, GJ Angus, et al. Random non-fasting C-peptide testing can identify patients with insulin-treated type 2 diabetes at high risk of hypoglycaemia. Diabetologia. 2018;61(1):66-74.
13. Dario T, Riccardo G, Silvia P, Mikiko W, Daria M, Andrea P, et al. The utility of assessing C-peptide in patients with insulin-treated type 2 diabetes: a cross-sectional study. Acta Diabetol. 2020;58:411-7.
14. Wod M, Yderstræde KB, Halekoh U, Beck-Nielsen H, Højlund K. Metabolic risk profiles in diabetes stratified according to age at onset, islet autoimmunity and fasting C-peptide. Diabetes Res Clin Pract. 2017;134:62-71.
15. Foteinopoulou E, Clarke CAL, Pattenden RJ, Ritchie SA, McMurray EM, Reynolds RM, et al. Impact of routine clinic measurement of serum C-peptide in people with a clinician-diagnosis of type 1 diabetes. Diabet Med. 2021;38(7):e14449.
16. Thivolet C, Marchand L, Chikh K. Inappropriate glucagon and GLP-1 secretion in individuals with long-standing type 1 diabetes: effects of residual C-peptide. Diabetologia. 2019;62(4):593-7.
17. Marren SM, Hammersley S, McDonald TJ, Shields BM, Knight BA, Hill A, et al. Persistent C-peptide is associated with reduced hypoglycaemia but not HbA1c in adults with longstanding type 1 diabetes: evidence for lack of intensive treatment in UK clinical practice? Diabet Med. 2019;36(9):1092-9.
18. Zenz S, Mader JK, Regittnig W, Brunner M, Korsatko S, Boulgaropoulos B, et al. Impact of C-peptide status on the response of glucagon and endogenous glucose production to induced hypoglycemia in T1DM. J Clin Endocrinol Metab. 2018;103(4):1408-17.
19. Willemsen RH, Burling K, Barker P, Ackland F, Dias RP, Edge J, et al. Frequent monitoring of C-peptide levels in newly diagnosed type 1 subjects using dried blood spots collected at home. J Clin Endocrinol Metab. 2018;103(9):3350-8.
20. Jacobsen LM, Bocchino L, Evans-Molina C, DiMeglio L, Goland R, Wilson DM, et al. The risk of progression to type 1 diabetes is highly variable in individuals with multiple autoantibodies following screening. Diabetologia. 2020;63(3):588-96.
21. Landgraf W, Owens DR, Frier BM, Zhang M, Bolli GB. Fasting C-peptide, a biomarker for hypoglycaemia risk in insulin-naïve people with type 2 diabetes initiating basal insulin glargine 100 U/mL. Diabetes Obes Metab. 2019;22:315-23.
22. Sokooti S, Kieneker LM, de Borst MH, Kobold AM, Kootstra-Ros JE, Gloerich J, et al. Plasma C-peptide and risk of developing type 2 diabetes in the general population. J Clin Med. 2020;9(9):3001.
23. Buzzetti R, Tuomi T, Mauricio D, Pietropaolo M, Zhou Z, Pozzilli P, et al. Management of latent autoimmune diabetes in adults: a consensus statement from an international expert panel. Diabetes. 2020;69(10):2037-47.
24. Cotter MA, Ekberg K, Wahren J, Cameron NE. Effects of proinsulin C-peptide in experimental diabetic neuropathy: Vascular actions and modulation by nitric oxide synthase inhibition. Diabetes. 2003;52:1812-7.
25. Eckelman WC, Kilbourn MR, Joyal JL, Labiris R, Valliant JF. Justifying the number of animals for each experiment. Nucl Med Biol. 2007;34:229-32.
26. Alves MT, Chaves AC, Almeida APM, Silva ACS, Araújo SDA, Mota APL, et al. Anti-inflammatory effects of C-peptide on kidney of type 1 diabetes mellitus animal model. Mol Biol Rep. 2020;47:721-6.
27. Wahren J. C-peptide and the pathophysiology of microvascular complications of diabetes. J Intern Med. 2017;281(1):3-6.
28. Vasic D, Walcher D. C-peptide: a new mediator of atherosclerosis in diabetes. Mediators Inflamm. 2012;2012:1-8.
29. Thanabalasingham G, Pal A, Selwood MP, Dudley C, Fisher K, Bingley PJ, et al. Systematic assessment of etiology in adults with a clinical diagnosis of young-onset Type 2 diabetes is a successful strategy for identifying maturity-onset diabetes of the young. Diabetes Care. 2012;35:1206-12.
30. Besser RE, Shepherd MH, McDonald TJ, Shields BM, Knight BA, Ellard S, et al. Urinary C-peptide creatinine ratio is a practical outpatient tool for identifying hepatocyte nuclear factor 1-a/ hepatocyte nuclear factor 4-a maturity-onset diabetes of the young from long-duration type 1 diabetes. Diabetes Care. 2011;34:286-91
31. Winter WE, Schatz DA. Autoimmune markers in diabetes. Clin Chem. 2011;57:168-75.
32. Jones AG, Besser RE, Shields BM, McDonald TJ, Hope SV, Knight BA, et al. Assessment of endogenous insulin secretion in insulintreated diabetes predicts postprandial glucose and treatment response to prandial insulin. BMC Endocr Disord. 2012;12:6.
33. Trischitta V, Italia S, Raimondo M, Guardabasso V, Licciardello C, Runello F, et al. Efficacy of combined treatments in NIDDM patients with secondary failure to sulphonylureas. Is it predictable? J Endocrinol Invest. 1998;21:744-7.
34. Lee WJ, Chong K, Ser KH, Chen JC, Lee YC, Chen SC et al. Cpeptide predicts the remission of Type 2 diabetes after bariatric surgery. Obes Surg. 2011;22:293-8.
35. Ryan EA, Paty BW, Senior PA, Lakey JR, Bigam D, Shapiro AM. Beta-score: an assessment of beta-cell function after islet transplantation. Diabetes Care. 2005;28:343-7.

48

CHAPTER

Mitochondrial Diabetes

BK Singh

ABSTRACT

Mitochondrial diabetes is one of the rare forms of genetic disorder. Malfunction of mitochondria may lead to hyperglycemia due to defective insulin secretion from beta cells or insulin resistance due to decreased adenosine triphosphate (ATP) generation. Mitochondrial diabetes may be due to mutation or deletion of mitochondrial or nuclear deoxyribonucleic acid (DNA). Mostly mitochondrial DNA is affected. Most common mitochondrial mutation is m.3243A>G mutation. Mitochondrial DNA is inherited from mother only. Diagnosis is suspected by history, clinical features, and multiorgan involvement. Diagnosis is confirmed by genetic testing. No definite treatment is available. Supportive treatment and control of blood sugar are important. Metformin should be avoided due to increased risk of lactic acidosis.

INTRODUCTION

Mitochondrial disease is the most common form of genetic disorder. Malfunction of mitochondria may produce wide variety of diseases; mitochondrial diabetes is one of them and it is the most common among mitochondrial diseases. The main function of mitochondria is oxidative phosphorylation to produce adenosine triphosphate (ATP). If it affects beta cells of pancreas, it may cause defective insulin production and release leading to diabetes. Similarly, if it affects liver, muscle, and fat cells, it may cause insulin resistance. So, mitochondrial diabetes may be defined as poor functioning of beta cells of pancreas and/or insulin resistance due to defective function of fat, muscle and liver cells. The m.3243A>G mutation is the most common heteroplasmic mitochondrial deoxyribonucleic acid (mtDNA) mutation causing mitochondrial diabetes.

PREVALENCE

Mitochondrial disease is one of the most common groups of genetic disorder with prevalence of 1 in 5,000 adults. Diabetes mellitus is the most common endocrinopathy reported in mitochondrial diseases. Exact prevalence is not known. The American Diabetes Association (ADA) classifies mitochondrial diabetes under the category of "Other; genetic defects of the beta cell" and is thought to account for up to 3% of all diabetes cases. In India, <1% of total diabetic may be mitochondrial diabetes.

PATHOPHYSIOLOGY

Mitochondria are double membrane-bound organelles present in the cytoplasm of cell. Main functions are oxidative phosphorylation to produce ATP, cell signaling, calcium store, and cell fate (Releasing cytochrome C which activates caspase). It is a unique structure contains DNA called mitochondrial DNA. Mitochondrial DNA always comes from their mothers only. Mitochondrial disorders are caused by mutation of either mitochondrial DNA or nuclear DNA.

Mitochondrial diabetes is a genetic disorder. Mutation or deletion of mitochondrial or nuclear DNA may cause diabetes. Mitochondrial DNA mutations are more common occurring in 20 per 100,000 adults and are transmitted from maternal inheritance. Highest prevalence detected in those with the m.3243A>G mutation (replacement of adenosine by guanine). Nuclear DNA mutations are less common occurring in 2.9 per 100,000 adults and are inherited in autosomal dominant or recessive pattern. Sometimes, it may be caused by spontaneous gene mutation (de novo mutations) and not inherited. Environmental toxins can also trigger mitochondrial disease. Clinical symptoms correlate poorly with mutation load in the blood. Mitochondrial DNA contains nearly 17,000 base pairs and 37 genes. More than 100 mutations are linked with mitochondrial disorders. Classification of mitochondrial diseases is dependent on the mutation and organ involved. High energy requiring structures such as muscles, kidney, retina, pancreas, brain, and nerves are affected most.

CLINICAL FEATURES

Mitochondrial diabetes present as ketone-positive, insulin-dependent diabetes, like type 1 diabetes mellitus (T1DM); however, they are autoantibodies negative. Presentation may vary from ketone-positive insulin-dependent diabetes to noninsulin-dependent diabetes. Most common presentation is like type 2 diabetes mellitus (T2DM), but they are rarely obese. They usually develop insulin dependency in 2–4 years. Autoantibodies, which is the hallmark of T1DM, are usually absent. The m.3243A>G mutation can give rise to several different syndromes:

- *Maternally inherited diabetes and deafness (MIDD)*: MIDD is suspected when there is maternal heritability of diabetes with sensorineural deafness, myopathy, particularly proximal and macular dystrophy, particularly pigmentary retinal dystrophy. Renal focal segmental glomerular sclerosis may also be present.
- *Mitochondrial encephalomyopathy, lactic acidosis, and stroke-like episodes (MELAS)*: MELAS is mitochondrial disease characterized by stroke-like episodes, especially below the age of 40 years, encephalopathy with seizure or dementia, myopathy with/without red ragged fibers, recurrent headache and vomiting, and lactic acidosis due to impaired glucose oxidation.
- *Chronic progressive external ophthalmoplegia (CPEO)*: CPEO is a form of hereditary myopathies affecting extra ocular muscle.

When to Suspect?

Following are the features which will indicate to suspect that the patient may have mitochondrial disease:

- Multiorgan involvement mostly high-energy requirement organs such as muscles, fat, and liver
- Raised serum lactate level
- More rapid progression to insulin therapy
- Earlier onset of diabetes-related complications in comparison to individuals with T2DM

SCREENING OF PATIENTS

Annual screening is recommended to all who have mitochondrial disease or the person who have increased risk of developing mitochondrial disease due to known carrier state or they are first-degree relative of mitochondrial disease patient. Mitochondrial diseases increase the risk of gestational diabetes; so, screening should be done at first antenatal visit.

DIAGNOSIS

Genetic testing is the only way to confirm the diagnosis of clinically suspected patients. History of patient is particularly important to detect maternal heritability. Characteristic clinical features are also important. mtDNA mutation usually detected in white blood cells. Due to heteroplasmy, other tissue samples are important particularly urine epithelial cell sediment. Where diagnosis is not confirmed by DNA testing, tissue biopsy of vastus lateralis muscle is gold standard.

Diabetes can be detected by the World Health Organization (WHO) criteria—fasting plasma sugar ≥126 mg/dL, postprandial ≥ 200 mg/dL, random sugar ≥200 mg/dL, and glycated hemoglobin (HbA1c) > 6.4%.

DIFFERENTIAL DIAGNOSIS

- *Kearns–Sayre syndrome*: Chronic progressive external opthalmoplegia, atypical retinitis pigmentosa, and cardiac manifestation help to distinguish it.
- *Myoclonus epilepsy associated with ragged red fibers (MERRF)*: Characteristic myoclonus
- Leigh syndrome

MANAGEMENT

- Control of blood sugar (glycemic control)
- Supportive measures

Control of Blood Sugar

- *Lifestyle modification*: Diet, exercise, yoga, and avoidance of sedentary habits
- *Pharmacological therapy*:
    - Oral hypoglycemic agent (OHA): If the patient is asymptomatic, ketone bodies are absent and C-peptides are in normal range than OHAs should be tried.
        - Metformin should be avoided due to risk of lactic acidosis.
        - Sulfonylureas can be given, but due to risk of hypoglycemia and fluctuating blood sugar level,

short-acting sulfonylurea should be given with small dose and uptitrated according to response.

- Sodium-glucose cotransporter-2 (SGLT-2) inhibitors are well tolerated and often prescribed drug in mitochondrial diabetes. Mitochondrial diabetes patient are increased risk rapid progression of insulin deficiency, so regular check of ketone bodies and renal function is very important.
- Dipeptidyl peptidase-4 (DPP-4) inhibitors are well tolerated but it should be avoided if there is history of pancreatitis. Glucagon-like peptide-1 (GLP-1) analogs are useful if patient have obesity and fatty infiltration.
- Pioglitazone may cause cardiac dysfunction in mitochondrial diabetes, so pioglitazone should be used with care and better should be avoided with insulin.

○ Insulin therapy: Mitochondrial diabetic patients are nonobese and usually insulin dependent. Basal insulin should be started first, then according to need, basal bolas or premixed insulin can be given.

Supportive Management

There is no definite treatment of mitochondrial diabetes. Low levels of nitric oxide detected, so nitric oxide precursors such as arginine and citrulline have been tried and they have been observed to reduce lactate levels.

If the patient is suffering from MELAS syndrome, intravenous (IV) arginine may be tried to decrease severity and frequency of stroke-like episodes. Folinic acid can correct cerebral folate deficiency and improve hypomyelination. Coenzyme-Q and L-carnitine may be beneficial in some patients. Idebenone is experimental manmade drug similar to Coenzyme Q10 is in different phase of trials.

Females with mitochondrial disease may utilize "three-parent in vitro fertilization (IVF)" in which father sperm combined with mitochondria and cytoplasm from donated healthy ovum and nuclear DNA from mother ovum.

CONCLUSION

Mitochondrial diseases are rare affecting organ depend on high aerobic metabolism. Multiorgan involvement and maternal inheritance should prompt consideration. MELAS and MIDD are the most common mitochondrial diabetes caused by mutation in m.3243A>G in 80% of cases. Metformin should be avoided due to risk of lactic acidosis. There is rapid progression of insulin requirement and higher prevalence of complications. Diagnosis leads to family screening, education, and surveillance for future complications.

SUGGESTED READINGS

1. Takano C, Ogawa E, Hayakawa S. Insulin resistance in mitochondrial diabetes. Biomolecules. 2023;13(1):126.
2. Maassen JA, M 'T Hart L, Van Essen E, Heine RJ, Nijpels G, Tafrechi RSJ, et al. Mitochondrial diabetes: Molecular mechanisms and clinical presentation. Diabetes. 2004:53 (Suppl 1):S103-9.
3. Wellcome Trust Centre for Mitochondrial Research. Clinical Guidelines. [online] Available from https://www.newcastle-mitochondria.com/clinical-professional-home-page/clinical-publications/clinical-guidelines/. [Last accessed December, 2023].

49

CHAPTER

Basal Insulin and its Initiation

D Selvaraj

ABSTRACT

Basal insulin is the insulin of choice for initiation of insulin in those patients with diabetes who are not reaching targets of glucose value with 2 or 3 oral antidiabetic drugs and basically an ideal basal insulin should have a long duration of action, flexibility and low risk of hypoglycemia. The evolution of basal insulin from neutral protamine Hagedorn (NPH) to glargine U-100, detemir, glargine U-300, and degludec is evident from its efficacy. The advantage of newer insulin basal analog is its once-daily dosing, better targeting fasting blood glucose (FBG) control, lower glycemic variability, and overall hypoglycemia and nocturnal severe hypoglycemic risk and flexibility 8–40 hours along with cardiovascular (CV) safety.

INTRODUCTION

The International Diabetes Federation (IDF) estimates that there are currently 336 million people worldwide who have diabetes. The IDF Diabetes Atlas (2021) reports that 10.5% of the adult population (20–75 years), with almost half unaware that they are living with diabetes. By 2045, IDF projection show that one in eight adults, approximately 78.3 million will be living with diabetes, an increase in 46%. The prevalence of diabetes in India stands at 11.4% while 35.5% of Indian suffer from hypertension, additionally abnormal obesity stands at 40% across the population and female abnormal obesity stands at 50%.

The rapid rise in rate of type 2 diabetes mellitus (T2DM) echoes a similar rise in the rate of obesity, which causes insulin resistance and places an increased insulin secretary demand on pancreatic beta cells. Interventions that reduce body fat or that changing fat biology provide the best evidence for slowing or arresting the deterioration of beta cell function that causes T2DM. T2DM results from an interaction between genetic and environmental factors that impact beta cell function and insulin action. Patients with impaired glucose tolerance have < 50% of normal beta cell function and patients with T2DM have <15% of normal beta cell function for their degree of insulin resistance.

INFLUENCE OF PLASMA GLUCOSE LEVELS ON INSULIN SECRETION

Ambient fasting plasma glucose influences the action of insulin response to a great extend as has been shown in several studies. The higher the fasting plasma glucose above its normal level, the greater the attenuation of insulin response to any rise in blood glucose concentration. Bunzell et al. measured insulin secretion and glucose disappearance rate in subjects with a wide range of fasting plasma glucose level. The degree and duration of the insulin response relation to an intravenous glucose load were compared in a series of 66 patients with a wide range of fasting plasma glucose levels. The immediate rise in glucose secretion is referred to as first-phase response and the slow return to baseline as the second-phase response **(Fig. 1)**.

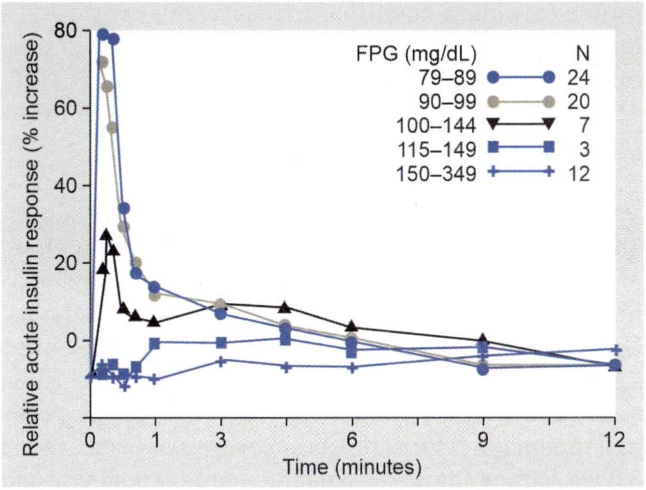

FIG. 1: Effect of fasting plasma glucose (FPG) on the acute insulin response.

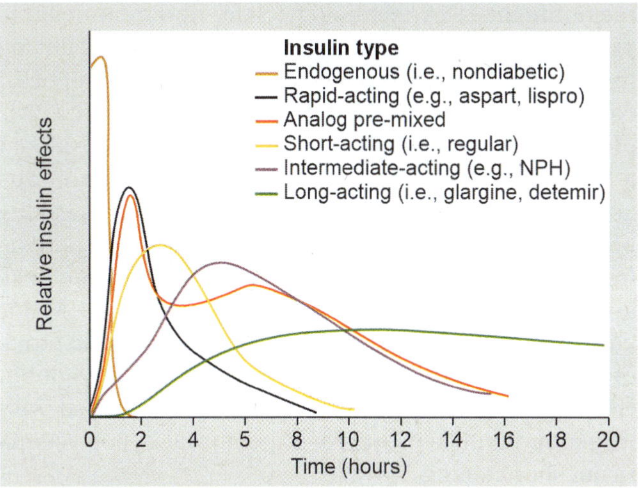

FIG. 2: Temporal pattern of insulin action.

(NPH: neutral protamine Hagedorn)

Source: Wong J, Tabet E. The introduction of insulin in type 2 diabetes mellitus. Aust Fam Physician. 2015;44(5):278-83.

The acute first-phase insulin response was present in subjects with fasting blood glucose (FBG) < 115 mg/dL and absent in those with higher value. This study demonstrated that hyperglycemia is associated with a defect in the release of insulin from the pancreas. It also supports epidemiological data indicating 115 mg/dL as an upper limit of normal for fasting plasma glucose levels. Thus, beta cell dysfunction—or inability of beta cells to secrete insulin in proportion to the need for glucose disposal, lipid storage, and maintaining endothelial nitric oxide synthase (eNOS) activity in the vascular endothelium—is an innate feature of the diabetic state.

Management of diabetes mellitus started with the discovery of insulin on 1921 by Banting and Best. Few years after its first use, need for long-acting insulin was felt; subsequently, neutral protamine Hagedorn (NPH) and zinc protamine insulin became available. Up to 1980s, bovine and porcine insulin were mainstay of insulin therapy. Around 1982, recombinant human insulin was produced by recombinant technology and a new turn came in the history of insulin.

TYPES OF INSULIN

The types of insulin came under the heading of prandial and basal insulin **(Fig. 2)**.

Prandial Insulin

This is used before meal to control postprandial level of plasma glucose. These are either regular or rapid-acting insulin.

Regular Insulin

It is a short-acting human insulin, which is a crystalline zinc insulin which makes a clear solution. It starts to act 50–60 minutes after subcutaneous administration. Regular insulin reaches peak effect 2–4 hours after injection and action lasts for 5–8 hours. Its profile does not mimic physiological one. It should be given 30–45 minutes before meal to match its profile with food absorption.

Rapid-acting Insulin

There are three types of rapid-acting analog insulins: lispro, aspart, and glulisine. They are rapidly absorbed from the injection site. Onset of action is with 15 minutes. It reaches peak around 1 hour, and action lasts for 3–5 hours.

Basal Insulin

Intermediate-acting Insulin

- Basal insulin analog
- Insulin glargine
- Insulin detemir
- Insulin degludec
- Insulin glargine 300 U/mL

Isophane/Neutral Protamine Hagedorn

It was originally discovered in 1936. The process used in its production has evolved greatly. Today with the use of recombinant DNA technology, safe, nonimmunogenic preparations are ubiquitous. Prior to the advent of analog insulin, it served a vital role in providing a degree of basal cover. However, considering its pharmacokinetic (PK)/pharmacodynamic (PKD) profile, it cannot be considered a true peakless insulin. Following subcutaneous administration, onset of action is seen at 2 hours, peaking between 6 and 14 hours, with a duration of action ranging from 10 to 16 hours, with larger doses delaying the peak and prolonging the overall duration of action. Major advantage of this formulation includes its efficacy in terms of glycemic control deflected by glycated hemoglobin (HbA1c) reduction, however, the peak associated with its action is subsequent risk of nocturnal hypoglycemia major shortcoming.

Detemir

Administered subcutaneously, the onset of action is seen with 2 hours, with persistence seen for 20 hours. Among the available basal insulin, detemir causes less weight gain. Despite being candidate for single-day use, twice-daily regimen are common.

Glargine

Formulated at an acidic pH of 4, glargine is neutralized by the physiologic pH of subcutaneous tissue. When administered the resulting microprecipitate acts as a depot, releasing small amounts of insulin steadily. Glargine should not be mixed with other formulations. Following administration, the onset of action is seen with 2 hours with a duration ranging from 20 to 24 hours and usually no peak.

Although it is suitable for once-daily administration at doses routinely used, its profile changes as dose increases. At high doses, typically exceeding 50 units, it may no longer act as peakless insulin and thus it may be preferable to administer the required quantity in two divided doses, 12 hours apart. Commercially available preparation of glargine includes U-100 (100 U/mL) and U-300 (300 U/mL). The U-300 formulation has been designated as a "*concentrated insulin*". The EDITION studies have shown comparable efficacies in terms of HbA1c lowering efficacy, but suggest better safety profile (avoiding nocturnal hypoglycemia) with U-300 for both T1DM and T2DM. Glargine has also been used in conjunction with oral dipeptidyl peptidase 4 (DPP-4) inhibitors, exhibiting an efficacy comparable to the standard basal-bolus regimen.

Degludec

This is an ultra-long-acting modified human insulin. Onset of action is usually in <2 hours and with a half-life of 24 hours, the period over which clinical efficacy is 42 hours. Once injected into the subcutaneous tissue, degludec forms a multi-hexamer depot. Gradual dissociation of insulin monomers into the blood stream accounts for its steady and prolonged action. Steady state levels are achieved in 3 days, with minimal subsequent interday variability and less nocturnal hypoglycemia **(Flowchart 1)**.

COMPARISON ACROSS AGENTS

Numerous studies have been conducted comparing various basal insulin formulations with one another. Summarized below are certain key features described across various studies:

- The risk of nocturnal hypoglycemia with the use of the true peakless insulins is approximately half that associated with the use of NPH.
- Efficacy in terms of reaching HbA1c targets remain similar across all available basal formulations, including NPH.
- Glargine is currently considered as the gold standard basal formulation and as such is used as reference standard for all comparative trials.
- The SWITCH 1 and 2 studies establish the safety of insulin degludec in T1DM and T2DM, respectively, with overall rates of symptomatic hypoglycemia compared to glargine U-100.

CONCLUSION

The introduction of safe and effective biosimilars seems to be the need of the hour, and further research in this regard is likely to engender keen interest globally.

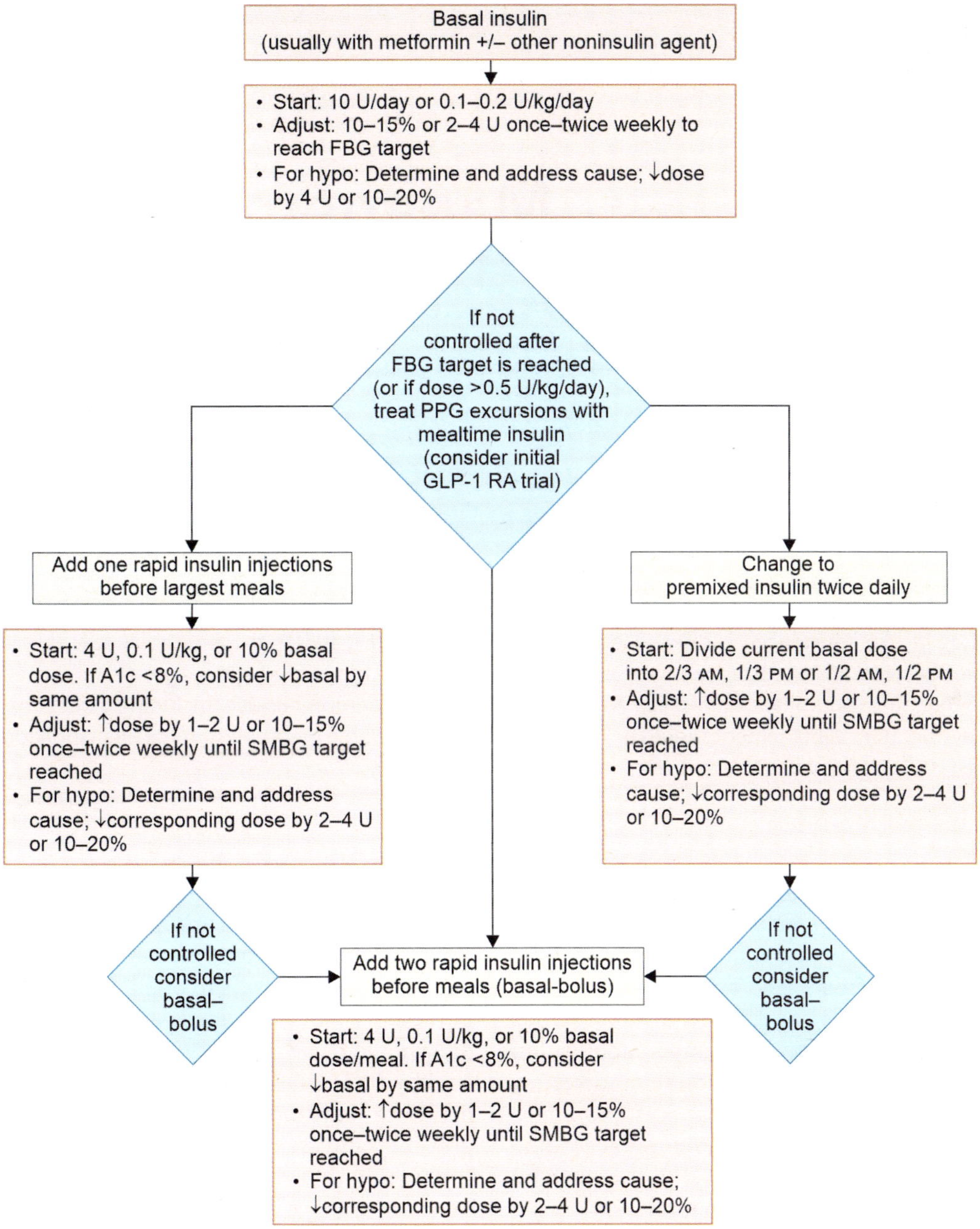

FLOWCHART 1: American Diabetes Association (ADA) 2016 recommended protocols for insulin intensification.
(FBG: fasting blood glucose; GLP-1 RA; glucagon-like peptide-1 receptor agonist; PPG: postprandial glucose; SMBG: self-monitoring of blood glucose)

SUGGESTED READINGS

1. Standl E, Owen DR. New long-acting basal insulins: Does benefit outweigh cost? Diabetes Care. 2016;39 Suppl 2:S172-9.
2. Dalal MR, Kazemi M, Ye F, Xie L. Hypoglycemia after initiation of basal insulin in patients with type 2 Diabetes in the United States: implications for treatment discontinuation and healthcare costs and utilization. Adv Ther. 2017;34(9): 2083-92.
3. Fonseca V. Clinical significance of targeting postprandial and fasting hypoglycemia in managing type 2 diabetes mellitus. Curr Med Res Opin. 2003;19(7):635-41.

50

CHAPTER

Management of Type 2 Diabetes Mellitus in Elderly

DC Thirupathi Rao

ABSTRACT

Aging increases insulin resistance, leading to glucose intolerance and diabetes in genetically susceptible individuals. As population ages and life expectancy increases, diabetes becomes a disease of older age, characterized by multiple comorbidities, geriatric syndromes, and frailty. Assessments should be comprehensive, including screening for cognitive and physical dysfunction. Management should be individualized, with variable metabolic targets for fit individuals and focus on improving nutrition and physical activity for frail older people.

INTRODUCTION

The prevalence of diabetes is increasing in older people because of increased life expectancy. The phenotype of diabetes in old age is characterized by multiple comorbidities, geriatric syndromes, and frailty. Diabetes has strong emphasis on cost-effectiveness and simplification of management strategies. Motivational counseling, cognition enhancement, and social support should be essential tools. Treatment should be tailored according to individual needs. Improving subjective well-being and quality of life is an essential care component.

GERIATRIC SYNDROMES

Many geriatric syndromes such as dementia, frailty, depression, falls, urinary incontinence, arthritis, osteoporosis, and poor vision compromise the abilities of older diabetics to self-manage their disease. Older diabetics should undergo screening for early detection of neurocognitive impairment and dementia annually. Older diabetics should undergo screening for early detection of frailty, so that its progress can be arrested or reversed. Comorbidities should be screened and managed accordingly.

LIFESTYLE MANAGEMENT

Indian diet is high in carbohydrates and low in protein which promotes weight gain and central obesity on one hand and muscle loss (sarcopenia) and frailty on the other. Low calorie, low carbohydrate, balanced, and nutritious diet should be advised.

Physical activity and exercise lower blood glucose, promote cardiac function, improve muscle mass, prevent frailty, strengthen bone mass, and elevate mood. Independent and fit older diabetics can engage in 150 minutes of brisk walking per week, roughly 30 minutes of walking each day for 5 days a week. On average, they should also be advised to perform muscle strengthening exercises three times a week. However, all exercises should be tailored under medical advice, and the extent and type of physical activity recommended should consider cardiorespiratory reserve and the status of joints, bones, vision, nerves, muscles, etc.

Stress management and promoting good sleep in older diabetics can be achieved by de-stressing mechanisms such as meditation, music, social networking, and befriending grandchildren. Sleep hygiene includes going to bed at least 1–2 hours after dinner, avoiding daytime naps, keeping the room free from noise and bright light, avoiding TV, coffee, tea, and alcohol, and drinking excess water before sleep.

Older diabetics should be subjected to periodic health checkups as a thorough medical examination, including necessary laboratory tests. Checking and monitoring all medications, assessment of teeth, nutrition, urinary problem, depression, and physical and mental disabilities such as impaired vision, mobility, hearing, and memory should be a part of health checkup. The need for any vaccination, especially the pneumococcal and flu vaccination, is also important.

Miscellaneous steps include avoiding excess alcohol, self-medication, exposure to pollution, smoke, dust, and weather extremes. House should be well-ventilated, and inside the house, there should not be any poor lighting, slippery and wet floors, loose fitting carpets, cluttering of furniture, any stairs without railings, or toilets without support grips because all of these make the elderly vulnerable to falls, injuries, and fractures.

MEDICAL NUTRITION THERAPY

- In elderly diabetics with obesity, medical nutrition therapy plays a significant role.
- Foods with a low glycemic index, complex carbohydrates, and high fiber are advised.
- Food supplements rich in protein and fiber and fortified with vitamins and minerals may be used.
- Carbohydrate content should be limited to 50–60% of total calorie intake. Complex carbohydrates and high fiber diet should be advised.
- Fiber intake should be about 25–30 g/day.
- Protein intake should be maintained at about 15% of total calorie intake. The quantity of protein intake depends on age, sarcopenia, and renal dysfunction.
- Fat intake should be limited (<30% of total calorie intake). Avoid consumption of foods with high amounts of saturated fats (butter, coconut oil, margarine, and ghee). Saturated fatty acids (SFAs) intake should be <10% of total calories/day.
- A diet rich in fruits, leafy vegetables, nuts, fiber, whole grains, and unsaturated fat should be recommended.
- The diet should include pulses, legumes, unprocessed vegetables, and low-fat dairy products.
- Overall salt consumption should be <5 g/day.

ORAL ANTIDIABETIC AGENTS

Elderly diabetics are to be treated with tailor-made therapy. Polypharmacy should be avoided. Oral antidiabetic drugs (OADs) which do not cause hypoglycemia, osteoporosis, weight gain, and fluid retention should be selected. Fixed-dose combinations (FDCs) are preferred.

Recommendations for the use of OADs in elderly diabetic patients are as follows:

- *Metformin*: First line of drug, especially in obese diabetics
- *Sulfonylureas*: First/second line of drug
- *Alpha-glucosidase inhibitors*: May be given
- *Pioglitazone*: May be used in low doses
- *DPP-4 inhibitors*: Good drug, weight neutral, renal and cardiac friendly, and no hypoglycemia
- *Glucagon-like peptide-1 (GLP-1) receptor agonist*: In obese diabetics
- *Sodium-glucose cotransporter-2 (SGLT-2) inhibitors*: Recommended for up to 70 years of average weight/obese elderly
- GLP-1 receptors and SGLT-2 inhibitors are good for cardiorenal protection and heart failure

INJECTABLES THERAPIES

- Injectable therapies such as insulin and GLP-1 receptor agonist offer reasonable glycemic control in elderly diabetics if used with caution, and the appropriate patient selection is made judiciously.
- Starting low and going slow should be the mantra to avoid adverse effects.
- Patient and caregiver education, monitoring, and regular follow-ups are the key to the success of injectable therapies in elderly diabetics.
- Ultra-long-acting insulins such as degludec and glargine U300 are the insulins of choice in elderly diabetics.
- Newer ultra-short-acting prandial insulins are preferable to cover prandial peaks.
- In case of frequent hypoglycemic events, especially nocturnal hypos, the nighttime prandial insulin should be stopped.
- The type of insulin and the insulin regimen (e.g., basal only, basal plus, basal-bolus, or premix) should be chosen based on individual patient characteristics.
- Self-monitoring of blood glucose (SMBG) and individualized insulin titration charts are the keys to sustained euglycemia.
- GLP-1 receptor agonist, such as dulaglutide, lixisenatide, and liraglutide, offers the same pleiotropic benefits even in elderly diabetics. Starting with the lowest dose possible and slow up-titration will allow for better tolerability of these agents in elderly diabetics.

HYPOGLYCEMIA IN ELDERLY

Hypoglycemia and its unawareness is more common among older diabetics than young diabetics and is fraught with dreadful consequences.

Hypoglycemia in the elderly is defined as any blood sugar level below 70 mg/dL, and a glucose value of 70–100 mg/dL should raise the alarm of the need to change or adjust the regimen. Although hemoglobin A1c (HbA1c) alone should not be the sole criteria for glycemic control, HbA1c <7.0 should also be taken as a warning for overtreatment.

Liberal relaxation of glycemic targets is essential to avoid hypoglycemia among older diabetics who are functionally dependent or/and are under long-term or end-of-life care. Even functionally independent older patients are vulnerable to hypoglycemia if tight blood glucose control is attempted. Oral hypoglycemic agents (OHAs) can also be withdrawn among them if there is a high risk of hypoglycemia.

An individualized care plan is required, including the desired blood glucose range to minimize the risk of hypoglycemia. This includes both pharmacological and nonpharmacological treatment.

Among OHAs, sulfonylureas are not the preferred class of drugs as they can cause hypoglycemia. Still, if at all, shorter-acting sulfonylureas such as gliclazide and glipizide should be used, but the longer-acting ones such as glibenclamide and chlorpropamide should not be used. Glinides group of OHAs are to be avoided. Glitazones have a low risk of causing hypoglycemia, yet it is better to avoid in the elderly for the risk of fluid retention, increased incidence of bone fractures, and bladder cancer. Metformin and DPP-4 inhibitors are relatively safe in older diabetics. SGLT-2 inhibitors do not cause hypoglycemia but should be used cautiously in frail older populations for the risk of further weight loss.

Among the injectables, insulin should be prescribed only after evaluation of administering abilities, regular glucose monitoring, and understanding of hypoglycemia. GLP-1 agonists may not increase hypoglycemia risk, but their cost and weight loss limit their use in the elderly diabetic population.

The nonpharmacological approach comprises proper nutrition therapy, immediate control of fever if present, and training of carers for recognition and treatment of hypoglycemia.

TREATMENT GOALS

Although glycemic targets are based on HbA1c, in the uncommon instances of anemia, polycythemia, hemoglobinopathies, hemodialysis, or recent blood loss or transfusion, this parameter may be misleading.

Elderly diabetics should be regularly assessed for physical function, cognitive impairment, microvascular complications, frailty, and comorbidities to set the glycemic targets.

Elderly diabetics and their caregivers should be assessed for disease managing skills for diabetes care and be given education.

Elderly diabetics with good quality of life with either none or very mild microvascular complications with a life expectancy of at least 10–15 years should have an A1c target of 7–7.5%.

Those with diabetes with moderate cognitive impairments, microvascular complications, and comorbid conditions should have an A1c target of 7.5–8.5%.

The elderly with advanced microvascular complications and/or major comorbid illness and/or life expectancy of fewer than 5 years may have an A1c target of >8.5%. Such people should be treated only to prevent osmotic symptoms, infection control, or modify cardiovascular risk factors.

For older adults with type 1 diabetes mellitus (T1DM), continuous glucose monitoring should be considered mainly for those at risk of hypoglycemia, including insulin deficiency necessitating insulin therapy, progressive renal insufficiency, etc.

For patients receiving palliative and end-of-life care, the focus should be on avoiding hypoglycemia and symptomatic hyperglycemia while reducing the burden of glycemic management. Thus, as organ failure develops, several agents will have to be de intensified or discontinued. For the dying patient, most agents for type 2 diabetes mellitus (T2DM) may be removed.

TREATMENT SIMPLIFICATION REGIMENS

Timely simplification and deintensification of complex treatment regimens in elderly diabetics go a long way in reducing adverse events, improving the compliance, and quality of life of an individual. Implementing the available screening tools to access the safety of polypharmacy will help the clinician in selecting a regimen which is simple, safe, and most beneficial to an elderly diabetic. Based on the overall health status of an elderly patient, the appropriate treatment simplification or deintensification should be done.

In an elderly diabetic, the overall medications being used should be thoroughly checked and their safety and drug-drug interactions should be assessed using the screening tools. Preventing adverse events such as hypoglycemia and reducing polypharmacy are the two important goals for simplification of therapy regimens in elderly diabetics.

Fixed-dose combination can be used to decrease the pill burden and improve compliance. The FDC should be cost-effective and have a synergistic effect without causing any adverse events. Choice of OHAs should depend on the functional status of the older diabetic patient. Simplification of insulin regimen should be carried out according to accepted protocols.

Tailor-made simplification or deintensification of treatment regimen should be done based on overall individual health status and regular follow-up must be done. Proper education of the caregiver is vital for the success of therapy in elderly diabetics, especially patients with complex/poor health status and those receiving end-of-life care.

CONCLUSION

Aging is associated with increased insulin resistance, due to decreased muscle mass, increased visceral fat, and decreased insulin secretion, because of diminished beta cell mass and function, leading to glucose intolerance and diabetes in genetically susceptible individuals. Through population aging and increased life expectancy, diabetes is increasingly becoming a disease of older age. The phenotype of diabetes in old age is characterized by an increased prevalence of multiple comorbidities, geriatric syndromes, and frailty. Therefore, the assessment of older people with diabetes on diagnosis and annually thereafter should be comprehensive and include screening for these syndromes, especially cognitive and physical dysfunction. Older people are a highly heterogeneous population ranging from a fit person living in the community to a frail individual with multiple comorbidities living in a care home. Management should therefore be individualized with variable metabolic targets from tight control in fit individuals to a conservative approach in frail ones. More attention should be focused on optimal management of undernutrition in frail older people by improving nutrition and physical activity to maintain muscle mass and improve overall function, quality of life should be at the center of the management plans.

SUGGESTED READINGS

1. International Diabetes Federation. Diabetes: facts and figures; 2015 [cited Jan 16, 2016]. Available from: https://idf.org/worlddiabetesday/toolkit/gp/facts-figures.
2. Sinclair A. Diabtes and Primary Care. 2011;13:29-38.
3. Diabetes UK. National diabetes audit 2012-2013. Report 2. Complication and mortality. [Last accessed Jan, 2016]. Available from: https://www.diabetes.org.uk/Upload/NDA%20Report%202%20Complications%20and%20Mortality%20Audit_interative.pdf
4. Harding JL, Shaw JE, Peeters A, Guiver T, Davidson S, Magliano DJ. Mortality trends among people with type 1 and type 2 diabetes in Australia: 1997–2010. Diabetes Care. 2014;37:2579-86.
5. Gregg EW, Cheng YJ, Saydah S, Cowie C, Garfield S, Geiss L. Trends in death rates among U.S. adults with and without diabetes between 1997 and 2006: findings from the National Health Interview Survey. Diabetes Care. 2012;35(6):1252-7.

51

CHAPTER

Ceramides: A New Target to Improve Insulin Sensitivity

Dhiraj Kishore, Amita Diwaker, Aman Singh, Rajneesh Sachan, Sumbul Mazhar

ABSTRACT

Understanding how insulin works and the molecular abnormalities that cause insulin resistance has made great strides in recent years. Sphingolipids play a distinct function in insulin resistance in skeletal muscle, the liver, and the fat pad, according to scientific studies conducted on humans and animals over the past 20 years. Ceramides have received special attention as the primary suspects in the emergence of insulin resistance A number of different enzymes involved in various pathways of ceramide metabolism, such as serine palmitoyl transferase (SPT), ceramide synthase enzymes (CerS) family, or glycerol-3-phosphate acyltransferases (GPATs), are being looked as potential targets to manipulate ceramide generation. In the treatment of obesity-related disorders, genetic inhibition of the enzymes governing global ceramide synthesis is increasingly being considered as a promising therapeutic aim. It is important to remember that because ceramides are involved in a number of cellular functions, inhibiting systemic sphingolipid formation carries a risk of adverse effects. Determining whether, enzymes in the ceramides pathway are involved in the development of metabolic diseases appears to be of utmost importance.

INTRODUCTION

N-acetylsphingosine and a fatty acid combine to form the waxy lipid molecule known as a ceramide. Sphingomyelin, one of the important lipids in the lipid bilayer of the cell membrane of eukaryotic cells, is made up of ceramides. Ceramides have been recently discovered to have a variety of different physiological functions in addition to being a structural component of cell membranes (bioactive lipid).

PHYSIOLOGICAL ROLES

- Ceramides create lipid rafts in biological membranes, which stabilize the shape of the cell membrane and control the distribution of receptors and signaling molecules.
- They form the lipid mortar, a water-impermeable barrier that stops evaporative water loss from skin, along with cholesterol and free fatty acids.
- The outer membrane of the mitochondria is traversed by structured channels made of ceramide. Proteins leave the intermembrane gap through these channels.
- Apoptosis, cellular senescence, differentiation, and cell growth arrest
- Migration and adhesion of cells
- Control the activity of several enzymes, such as kinases and phosphatases
- Change the transcription factors' activity

PATHOLOGICAL ROLES

Ceramides are implicated in the pathophysiology of:

- Cancers
- Neurodegeneration
- Diabetes and insulin resistance (in liver, skeletal muscles, and adipose tissues)
- Obesity
- Nonalcoholic fatty liver disease (NAFLD)
- Atherosclerosis and endothelial dysfunction increasing the risk of major adverse cardiovascular events

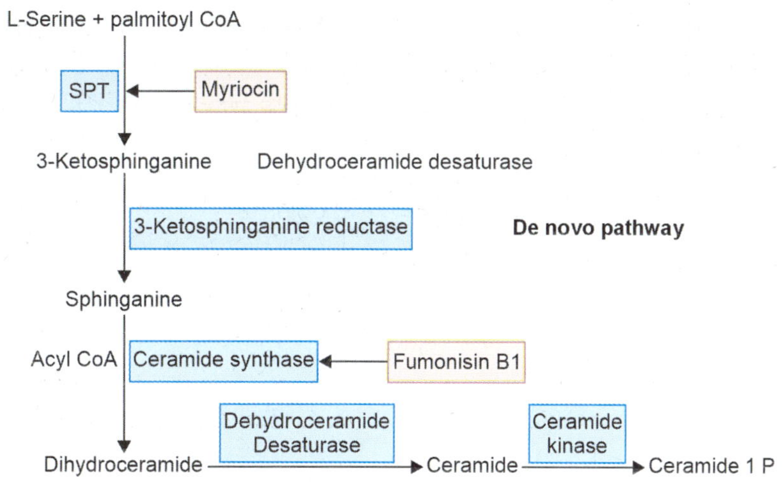

FIG. 1: De novo pathway.
(SPT: serine palmitoyl transferase)

CERAMIDE SYNTHESIS PATHWAYS

De Novo Pathway (Fig. 1)

- The endoplasmic reticulum produces ceramides de novo, and the pace at which they are produced largely depends on the availability of long-chain saturated fatty acids.
- Serine palmitoyl transferase (SPT) catalyzes the rate-limiting step by causing the condensation of serine and palmitoyl-CoA to yield 3-ketosphinganine.
- Sphinganine is created by additional processes and is acylated to dihydroceramide by six ceramide synthase enzymes (CerS1–6), which is subsequently converted to ceramide by dihydroceramide desaturase.
- The ceramide transfer protein (CERT) or vesicular trafficking is then used to carry ceramide to the Golgi apparatus. Ceramide can undergo further metabolism in the Golgi apparatus to produce other sphingolipids including sphingomyelin and complex glycosphingolipids.
- Exogenous fatty acids, cytokines [such interleukin 1 (IL-1)], and even ultraviolet B (UVB) light have been shown to increase ceramide, according to recent studies by increasing SPT expression.

Sphingomyelin Hydrolysis (Fig. 2)

- The sphingomyelinase enzyme, occurring as neutral and acid sphingomyelinases (nSMase and aSMase), catalyze the hydrolysis of sphingomyelin.
- TNF, Fas ligand, TLR4 activation, or oxidative stress cause an upregulation of this stress-activated pathway for ceramide production.

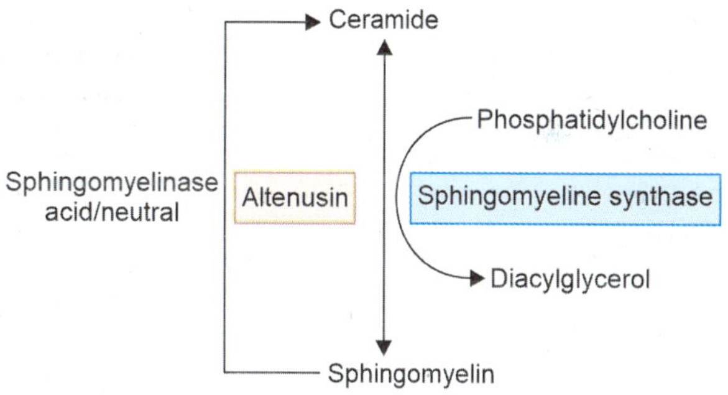

FIG. 2: Sphingomyelin hydrolysis.

- According to certain studies, ionizing radiation that induces death in some cells also activates the sphingomyelinase enzyme in the cell membrane, which results in the production of ceramide which triggers apoptosis.

Salvage Pathway (Fig. 3)

- Through the activity of ceramide synthase, the salvage route recycles long-chain sphingoid bases to create ceramide.
- Ceramide synthase converts sphingosine into ceramide, and glucosylceramide is broken down into ceramide by glucosylceramidase. Ceramide and complex sphingolipids cycle between one another, thanks to the recycling route.
- In the acidic subcellular compartments (lysosomes and late endosomes), sphingolipids and glycosphingolipids undergo constitutive breakdown with the aim of creating sphingosine.

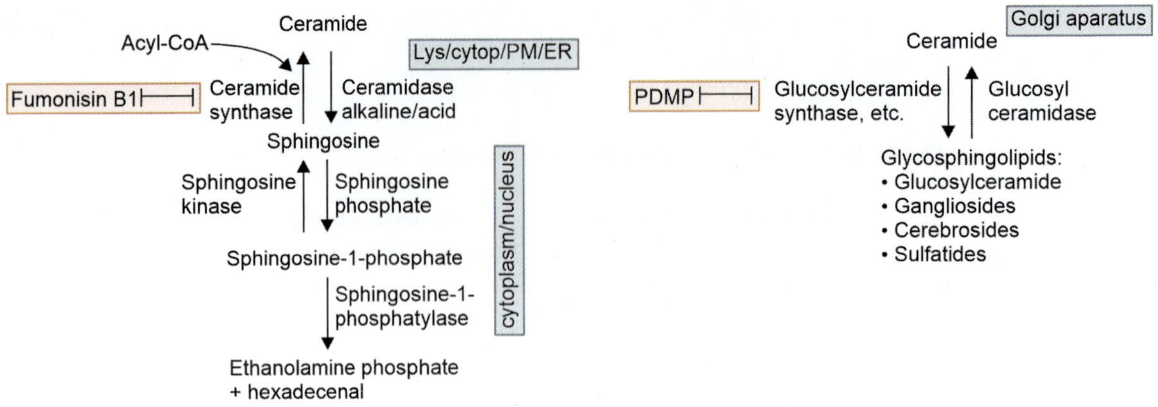

FIG. 3: Salvage pathway.

- Acid ceramidase can further hydrolyze ceramide to produce sphingosine and a free fatty acid, both of which, unlike ceramide, are able to exit the lysosome. Once freed from the lysosome, the long-chain sphingoid bases may re-enter pathways for the production of ceramide and/or sphingosine-1-phosphate (S1P).

INSULIN

The transmembrane, heterotetrameric insulin receptor (IR), which is a member of a wide family of tyrosine kinase receptors, is responsible for the action of insulin. Lipid phosphatidylinositol 3-kinase (PI3K), which in turn activates the Akt kinase/protein B (PKB), is one of the intracellular effector enzymes that are activated when the IR is engaged. PKB controls transcriptional regulation, nutrition metabolism, cell growth, and proliferation of cells, among other biological processes. PKB also controls cell survival and proliferation. Akt/PKB also promotes the movement of the insulin-dependent glucose transporter (GLUT 4) from the depot inside the cell to the cell membrane in muscle and fat tissue.

Insulin Resistance

- Insulin resistance is characterized by impaired postprandial nutrition storage, primarily in skeletal muscle and the liver, as a result of diminished peripheral tissue response to insulin activity. When blood glucose levels are high, pancreatic islets oversecrete insulin, which causes them to enlarge and become necrotic. Peripheral tissues grow resistant to this hormone as a result of chronic hyperinsulinemia. One of the metabolites suspected of acting as an insulin antagonist is ceramide.
- Stroke, NAFLD, asthma, cancer, polycystic ovary syndrome, Alzheimer's disease, hypertension, and atherosclerosis are all conditions that are influenced by insulin resistance and obesity.
- Adipocytes store extra fatty acids to provide energy during fasting periods. Neutral lipids build up in nonadipose tissues such the liver, heart, pancreas, and skeletal muscle after exceeding the capacity of adipose tissue to act as a buffer, leading to organ damage known as lipotoxicity.
- Oversupply of nutrients that circulate in the blood and are taken up by cells leads to metabolic overload, which affects the function of enzymes associated with the mitochondria and endoplasmic reticulum, reduces the accumulation of acetyl coenzyme A in cells, and inhibits glycolysis by inhibiting the activity of crucial Krebs cycle enzymes.
- Insulin resistance is thought to be induced by intramuscular lipid buildup, specifically diacylglycerols (DAG), ceramide (Cer), and long-chain acyl-CoAs (LCACoA) (which are substrates in the de novo synthesis of both ceramide and DAG).
- Nuclear receptor peroxisome proliferator-activated receptors (PPAR) family dysfunction, alterations in the release of adipokines (leptin, adiponectin, and resistin), and proinflammatory cytokines [IL-6, tumor necrosis factor alpha (TNF-α)] are also linked to decreased tissue sensitivity to insulin.

Ceramides and Insulin Resistance

- Ceramides interfere with insulin signaling by preventing the PI3K enzyme from transmitting signals and by preventing the anabolic enzyme Akt/PKB from being activated. As a result, ceramides inhibit the storage of nutrients including triglycerides and glycogen, activate protein phosphatase 2A (PP2A), and stimulate proinflammatory cytokines.
- Additionally, these sphingolipids interfere with lipid metabolism, notably in the liver, by preventing

oxidation and promoting fatty acid uptake. Ceramides also promote cell death by activating the enzymes cathepsin D, protein kinase C, caspase, and serine/threonine protein phosphatase 1 (PP1).

- Negative impact on pancreatic cells by triggering the stress-induced apoptotic pathway (i.e., release of cytochrome C and formation of free radicals)
- Children with obesity, diabetic adults, or nonhuman primates who were fed a Western diet all had greater plasma ceramide levels. It has been demonstrated that pioglitazone treatment results in a decrease in plasma ceramides, that ceramide production is inhibited (by myriocin or fumonisin B1), or that ceramide breakdown is stimulated (by acid ceramidase overexpression), all of which improve insulin signaling. Furthermore, PKB activity and insulin-stimulated glucose transport were largely conserved when SPT inhibitors (myriocin or L-cycloserine) were added to muscle cell lines L6 (rat normal skeletal muscle myoblasts).
- In contrast to a diet high in polyunsaturated fatty acids (PUFA), a diet high in saturated fats (SAT) causes ceramide levels to rise.

OVERPRODUCTION OF CERAMIDES

- The availability of long-chain saturated fatty acids, which are involved in de novo ceramide synthesis inside the endoplasmic reticulum, has a major impact on the rate of ceramide production.
- Increases in muscle ceramides have been linked to muscle insulin resistance in people with general or abdominal obesity. There are also observed associations between adipose ceramides and fatty liver disease and liver ceramides and hepatic insulin resistance.
- TNF is injected intraperitoneally into C57BL/6J mice, which increases the activity of neutral and acidic sphingomyelinases and results in an overproduction of ceramide.

TISSUE CERAMIDES AND THEIR EFFECTS

Skeletal Muscles

- Responsible for 70–80% of the glucose absorption induced by insulin in the entire body
- Increased intracellular levels of ceramides directly inhibit insulin-stimulated glucose uptake in L6 myotubes, decrease GLUT4 translocation, and are followed by a decrease in levels of activated Akt/PKB through several pathways in the muscles of insulin-resistant, overweight adults.
- Atypical PKC isoforms (/λ) are first activated by ceramides, which favor their combination with PKB/Akt and further suppress PKB/Akt activation in response to insulin. Ceramides also stimulate PP2A, which in turn indirectly suppresses PKB/Akt activity.
- Skovbro et al. did, however, show that the main predictor of muscle sensitivity to insulin is not the amount of ceramides present in human skeletal muscle. In a related investigation, Straczkowski et al. discovered a considerable discrepancy between the level of ceramide in skeletal muscle and the degree of insulin resistance in humans following injection of a lipid infusion.

Adipose Tissue

- Increased ceramide can inhibit insulin-stimulated GLUT4 expression and glucose uptake in 3T3-L1 (Cell line) and brown adipocytes, and it may also mediate the action of TNF-α on GLUT4 messenger ribonucleic acid (mRNA) levels.
- TNF-α affects insulin action in brown adipocytes by de novo ceramide synthesis, whereas in 3T3-L1 adipocytes, ceramide generated by sphingomyelin hydrolysis inhibits GLUT4 expression.
- The hyperinsulinemia and increased TNF-α associated with obesity cause nSMase, aSMase, and SPT, three important enzymes involved in ceramide production in adipose tissue, to express themselves at higher levels in leptin-deficient, genetically obese (ob/ob) mice. The higher ceramide level in the adipocytes of obese individuals is likely due to the increased activity of the ceramide-producing enzymes SPT and nSMase.
- Holland et al. demonstrated that elevated levels of circulating adiponectin, an adipocyte secretory factor, lowers ceramide levels in various organs in mice. Adiponectin promotes ceramide catabolism from sphingosine by increasing the activity of ceramidase related to its two receptors, AdipoR1 and AdipoR2. The formation of S1P, a key bioactive antiapoptotic sphingolipid molecule, occurs in the next phase by phosphorylation.

THERAPEUTIC WINDOWS

Dietary Interventions

- Diets that limit calories, exercise, or bariatric surgery can decrease levels of muscle ceramide and increase muscle insulin sensitivity.
- Consuming SAT reduces insulin sensitivity. Palmitate, a type of SAT, is particularly damaging because it triggers the buildup of ceramide, which interferes with insulin's ability to activate and signal PKB/Akt, a downstream mediator of the IR.
- Contrary to a diet high in PUFA, a diet high in SAT causes ceramide levels to rise.

52

CHAPTER

Semaglutide for Treatment of Obesity in People with Type 2 Diabetes Mellitus

Sudhir Bhandari

ABSTRACT

The use of glucagon-like peptide-1 receptor agonists (GLP-1 RAs) is a common practice in managing various aspects of type 2 diabetes mellitus (T2DM), which includes weight loss and glycemic control and reducing cardiovascular risks. Semaglutide is one of the well-established GLP-1 RAs approved for managing T2DM and weight loss, which has shown significant efficacy in achieving the desired outcomes. The American Diabetes Association (ADA) recommends a comprehensive approach to managing T2DM, with weight control being a crucial aspect of achieving positive patient outcomes. Semaglutide has been identified as a highly effective drug for glucose lowering and weight loss in T2DM treatment. It has well-established safety and tolerability profiles and some countries have approved it to reduce cardiovascular risk in specific T2DM populations. Therefore, semaglutide is a highly recommended therapeutic option that aligns with the guidelines for T2DM management, with a particular emphasis on weight control and addressing other cardiometabolic risk factors.

INTRODUCTION

Obesity is characterized as the excessive accumulation of adipose tissue over an extended period of time, resulting from a chronic interplay between genetic predisposition and environmental factors. The most commonly used means of measuring obesity are through body mass index (BMI). The international classification for BMI defines a normal range as >18.5 to <25 kg/m^2, preobesity falls between >25 and <30 kg/m^2, and obesity is considered when BMI is >30 kg/m^2. Conversely, the Asian classification for BMI defines a normal range as >18 to <23 kg/m^2, preobesity falls between >23 and <25 kg/m^2, and obesity is established when BMI > 25 kg/m^2.

With the escalating prevalence of overweight and obesity, there has been a growing interest in the consequences of this health issue and its association with diabetes. This link between diabetes and obesity is often referred to as "diabesity," a term first coined by Sims et al. in 1973. The term describes a condition where diabetes and obesity are interconnected, leading to severe public health issues. Sedentary lifestyles and unhealthy dietary habits are the main contributors to the increasing incidences of both diabetes and obesity. Patients who are overweight or obese tend to accumulate fat around their abdominal region, leading to insulin resistance and putting them at risk of developing diabetes.

PREVALENCE OF OBESITY AND DIABETES IN INDIA

The prevalence of overweight and obesity has seen a rapid increase in recent years, with projections indicating that by 2030, approximately 27.8% and 5% of Indians will be overweight and obese, respectively. Furthermore, it is projected that 20% of rural India will also be affected by this issue by 2030. These projections suggest that by 2030, 29.1% of men and 29.9% of women in India will be either overweight or obese based on current demographics. Obesity, characterized by a BMI of >30 kg/m^2, is a major risk factor for type 2 diabetes mellitus (T2DM). Currently, approximately 25.2 million Indian adults are expected to have T2DM, with this number expected to increase to

35.7 million by 2045. It is estimated that between 60 and 90% of diabetic patients are overweight or obese, with a BMI of >25 kg/m^2.

RAMIFICATIONS OF DIABESITY

Metabolic syndrome is a common occurrence in patients with diabesity, which is characterized by a combination of cardiovascular risk factors such as hypertension, hyperlipidemia, abdominal obesity, and insulin resistance. The presence of metabolic syndrome has a direct correlation with T2DM. Furthermore, diabesity is often associated with various complications related to T2DM, such as micro- and macrovascular events (cardiovascular diseases and stroke), renal (nephropathy), or ocular disease (retinopathy). Conversely, obesity is associated with a multitude of chronic diseases such as T2DM, hypertension, hyperlipidemia, stroke, and various cancers. Tan and his colleagues have reported that diabesity increases the risk of cardiovascular complications such as atherosclerosis, myocardial infarction, and stroke. Furthermore, Sung and his colleagues have reported that nonalcoholic fatty liver disease (NAFLD) is prevalent in 30–40% of men and 15–20% of women with obese diabetic patients. Patients with NAFLD may progress to nonalcoholic steatohepatitis (NASH), which is characterized by liver inflammation and injury, leading to cirrhosis and hepatocellular carcinoma.

IMPORTANCE OF WEIGHT MANAGEMENT IN DIABETES

There is strong evidence to suggest that obesity management can delay the progression from prediabetes to diabetes. The American Diabetes Association (ADA) 2023 guidelines suggest that patients with T2DM who are overweight or obese have shown to improve glycemic control with modest and sustained weight loss. It also mentions that a weight loss of ≥5% in T2DM patients with obesity have shown benefits with improved cardiovascular outcomes, improved blood glucose, minimizing the use of oral hypoglycemic drugs and improved quality of life and comorbidities.

EVIDENCE WITH SEMAGLUTIDE IN THE MANAGEMENT OF OBESITY IN DIABETES

Glucose-lowering medication that causes weight loss, such as glucagon-like peptide-1 receptor agonists (GLP-1 RAs) and sodium glucose cotransporter-2 inhibitors (SGLT-2i), can be the preferred antidiabetic agents in people with overweight or obesity.

Semaglutide is a potent, long-acting GLP-1 RA developed for the treatment of T2DM and weight management and is also being evaluated for NASH. It is a close analog of native human GLP-1, a hormone of the incretin system. Semaglutide has 94% homology to human GLP-1 and a half-life of approximately 1 week, enabling once-weekly administration.

Semaglutide selectively binds to and activates the GLP-1 receptor, the target for native GLP-1. In nonclinical studies, semaglutide exhibits GLP-1-mediated effects (i.e., stimulates insulin secretion, lowers inappropriately high glucagon secretion, and improves beta-cell function in a glucose-dependent manner), which results in lowering of fasting and postprandial glucose. Furthermore, animal studies have demonstrated that semaglutide can access brain regions that are critical to the regulation of energy intake, leading to decreased food intake and weight loss mediated by increased satiety and reduced hunger. In animal studies, semaglutide also attenuates the development of atherosclerosis, an effect which was believed to be mediated by anti-inflammatory mechanisms.

Semaglutide was initially developed as a once-weekly subcutaneous (SC) injection in the SUSTAIN program and later as a daily oral option in the PIONEER program. During the SUSTAIN trials, the change in body weight was assessed as secondary confirmatory outcomes. The results showed that weight loss with the 1.0 mg dose of semaglutide was greater than with comparators, with up to 6.5 kg weight loss observed after 40 weeks and around 63% of trial participants achieving a clinically meaningful weight reduction of at least 5%. In the SUSTAIN FORTE trial, which tested a higher dosage level of 2.0 mg for T2DM, weight losses of 6.9 kg and 6.0 kg were observed with 2.0 and 1.0 mg once-weekly semaglutide SC, respectively. In the PIONEER program, oral semaglutide at up to 14 mg also produced clinically significant weight loss **(Table 1)**. In the PIONEER PLUS trial, which lasted for 68 weeks and involved people with T2DM, once-daily oral semaglutide at 25 and 50 mg led to weight losses at week 52 of up to 7.0 and 9.2 kg, respectively, from a baseline body weight of 96.4 kg. These results were superior to the weight loss observed for oral semaglutide 14 mg (4.5 kg).

The phase 3a STEP development program played a key role in securing regulatory approval for semaglutide 2.4 mg for once-weekly SC injection as a weight management therapy in people with comorbidities associated with overweight (BMI > 27 kg/m^2) or obesity (BMI > 30 kg/m^2). The program consisted of several phase 3a trials designed to evaluate the efficacy and safety

TABLE 1: Key trials and results with semaglutide in people with T2DM.

	SUSTAIN 1 Monotherapy 30 weeks	SUSTAIN 7 H2H Dula 40 weeks	SUSTAIN FORTE Higher dose SC 40 weeks	PIONEER 1 Monotherapy 26 weeks	PIONEER PLUS Higher dose oral 68 weeks	STEP 2 Obesity and T2DM 68 weeks
Population	388 adults with T2DM	1,201 adults with T2DM	961 adults with T2DM on metformin	703 adults with T2DM	1,606 adults with T2DM	1,210 adults with overweight or obesity and T2DM
Semaglutide	0.5 and 1.0 mg OW SC	0.5 and 1.0 mg OW SC	2.0 mg OW SC	3, 7, and 14 mg OD oral	25 and 50 mg OD oral	2.4 mg OW SC
Comparator	Placebo	Dula 0.75 and 1.5 mg	Sema 1.0 mg OW SC	Placebo	Sema 14 mg OD oral	Sema 1.0 mg OW SC placebo
Body weight from baseline in kg (mean)	*Sema 0.5 mg*: –3.7* *Sema 1.0 mg*: –4.5* *Placebo*: –1.0	*Sema 0.5 mg*: –4.6* *Sema 1.0 mg*: –6.5* *Dula 0.75 mg*: –2.3 *Dula 1.5 mg*: –3.0	*Sema 2.0 mg*: –6.9* *Sema 1.0 mg*: –6.0	*Sema 14 mg*: –4.1* *Sema 7 mg*: –2.5* *Sema 3 mg*: –1.7 *Placebo*: –1.5	*Sema 50 mg*: –9.2* *Sema 25 mg*: –7.0* *Sema 14 mg*: –4.5	*Sema 2.4 mg*: –10.6* *Sema 1.0 mg*: –7.5 *Placebo*: –3.1
≥5% weight loss% of participants	*Sema 0.5 mg*: 37# *Sema 1.0 mg*: 45# *Placebo*: 7	*Sema 0.5 mg*: 44# *Sema 1.0 mg*: 63# *Dula 0.75 mg*: 23 *Dula 1.5 mg*: 30	*Sema 2.0 mg*: 59.2# *Sema 1.0 mg*: 51.3	*Sema 14 mg*: 44# *Sema 7 mg*: 29# *Sema 3 mg*: 21 *Placebo*: 16	*Sema 50 mg*: 76# *Sema 25 mg*: 63# *Sema 14 mg*: 44	*Sema 2.4 mg*: 73.2# *Sema 1.0 mg*: 59.2 *Placebo*: 27.6
≥10% weight loss% of participants	*Sema 0.5 mg*: 8# *Sema 1.0 mg*: 13# *Placebo*: 2	*Sema 0.5 mg*: 14# *Sema 1.0 mg*: 27# *Dula 0.75 mg*: 3 *Dula 1.5 mg*: 8	*Sema 2.0 mg*: 28.4# *Sema 1.0 mg*: 22.6	*Sema 14 mg*: 15.4# *Sema 7 mg*: 8.7# *Sema 3 mg*: 2.7 *Placebo*: 1.5	*Sema 50 mg*: 44# *Sema 25 mg*: 32# *Sema 14 mg*: 16	*Sema 2.4 mg*: 49.9# *Sema 1.0 mg*: 29.7 *Placebo*: 7.1

*Estimated change from baseline, statistically significantly different ($p < 0.05$) from change with comparator(s).

#Estimated odds of achieving ≥5%/10% weight loss at end of treatment was statistically significantly higher than with comparator(s). Results at study end are estimates based on the trial product estimand (estimates based on data collected while on treatment with study medication and before any initiation of rescue medication).

(Dula: dulaglutide; H2H: head-to-head; OD: once-daily; OW: once-weekly; SC: subcutaneous; sema: semaglutide; T2DM: type 2 diabetes mellitus)

of semaglutide 2.4 mg compared to placebo and other comparators across various populations and treatment regimens relevant to weight management. Semaglutide treatment was administered alongside supervised lifestyle changes. All the STEP trials except for STEP 2 enrolled adult participants without T2DM but with overweight or obesity and at least one weight-associated complication. In contrast, the STEP 2 participants had both T2DM and overweight or obesity and this trial evaluated semaglutide at dose levels of 1.0 and 2.4 mg compared to placebo. In STEP 2, participants achieved an average weight loss of up to 10.6 kg at the end of the 68-week treatment period with semaglutide 2.4 mg. In comparison, weight loss in those treated with semaglutide 1.0 mg or placebo was 7.5 and 3.1 kg, respectively. Thus, semaglutide 2.4 mg provided superior weight loss compared to both comparators in this population ($p < 0.0001$) and was also statistically significantly, more likely than placebo in enabling participants to achieve a ≥5% or ≥10% weight loss. Currently, a higher semaglutide SC dose level of 7.2 mg once weekly is being tested in the ongoing STEP UP and STEP UP T2DM studies in people with obesity, with or without T2DM, respectively. Additionally, data from the OASIS clinical development program suggest that once-daily oral semaglutide 50 mg can provide weight loss comparable to that observed with once-weekly semaglutide 2.4 mg in the STEP program, although this was not tested in people with T2DM in addition to obesity/overweight.

SAFETY AND TOLERABILITY OF SEMAGLUTIDE

The safety and tolerability profiles of semaglutide have been established through various development programs, including SUSTAIN and PIONEER for SC semaglutide at doses of 0.5, 1.0, and 2.0 mg and oral semaglutide at doses of 3, 7, 14, 25, and 50 mg for people with T2DM. Similarly, the safety and tolerability profiles of semaglutide SC 2.4 mg once weekly for weight management were established through the STEP program. Real-world clinical data, with over 9.5 million person-years of exposure (Novo Nordisk, data on file), have also confirmed the safety and tolerability profiles of semaglutide across all indications. The use of this evidence, along with any future data collected, will aid in further comprehending the long-term benefits and risks of semaglutide.

CONCLUSION

Diabesity is a term which is used to describe the combined effect of diabetes and obesity. The incidences for diabesity are growing at a rapid rate. The consequences of diabesity may lead to constellation of problems such as hypertension, hyperlipidemia, and stroke The ADA recommends a meaningful weight loss of ≥5% with the use of GLP-1 RA/SGLT2i and physical activity for patients who are obese or overweight with diabetes. GLP-1 RAs generally, and semaglutide in particular, as arguably the most effective compound of the drug class, provide an opportunity to lower body weight and reduce cardiometabolic risk in people with T2DM.

SUGGESTED READINGS

1. Ortega MA, Fraile-Martínez O, Naya I, García-Honduvilla N, Álvarez-Mon M, Buján J, et al. Type 2 diabetes mellitus associated with obesity (Diabesity). The central role of gut microbiota and its translational applications. Nutrients. 2020;12(9):1-29.
2. Malnick SDH, Knobler H. The medical complications of obesity. QJM. 2006;99(9):565-79.
3. Misra A, Chowbey P, Makkar BM, Vikram NK, Wasir JS, Chadha D, et al. Consensus statement for diagnosis of obesity, abdominal obesity and the metabolic syndrome for Asian Indians and recommendations for physical activity, medical and surgical management. J Assoc Physicians India. 2009;57:163-70.
4. Kinlen D, Cody D, O'Shea D. Complications of obesity. QJM. 2018;111(7):437-43.
5. Kumar N, Puri N, Marotta F, Dhewa T, Calabro S, Puniya M, et al. Diabesity: An epidemic with its causes, prevention and control with special focus on dietary regime. Funct Foods Heal Dis. 2017;7(1):1-16.
6. Luhar S, Timæus IM, Jones R, Cunningham S, Patel SA, Kinra S, et al. Forecasting the prevalence of overweight and obesity in India to 2040. PLoS One. 2020;15(2):e0229438.
7. Siddiqui S. Obesity and diabetes: Interrelationship. Adv Obes Weight Manag Control. 2018;8(2):155-8.
8. Elabbassi WN, Haddad HA. The epidemic of the metabolic syndrome. Saudi Med J. 2005;26(3):373-5.
9. Colagiuri S. Diabesity: therapeutic options. Diabetes Obes Metab. 2010;12(6):463-73.
10. Tan BK, Adya R, Randeva HS. Omentin: A novel link between inflammation, diabesity, and cardiovascular disease. Trends Cardiovasc Med. 2010;20(5):143-8.
11. Sung KC, Lee MY, Kim YH, Huh JH, Kim JY, Wild SH, et al. Obesity and incidence of diabetes: Effect of absence of metabolic syndrome, insulin resistance, inflammation and fatty liver. Atherosclerosis. 2018;275:50-7.
12. ElSayed NA, Aleppo G, Aroda VR, Bannuru RR, Brown FM, Bruemmer D, et al. Obesity and Weight Management for the Prevention and Treatment of Type 2. Diabetes: Standards of Medical Care in Diabetes—2023. Diabetes Care. 2023;46 (Suppl 1):S128-9.
13. Wilding JPH. Medication use for the treatment of diabetes in obese individuals. Diabetologia. 2018;61(2):265-72.
14. Lau J, Bloch P, Schaffer L, Pettersson I, Spetzler J, Kofoed J, et al. Discovery of the once-weekly glucagon-like peptide-1 (GLP-1) analogue semaglutide. J Med Chem. 2015;58(18):7370-80.
15. Knudsen LB, Lau J. The discovery and development of liraglutide and semaglutide. Front Endocrinol (Lausanne). 2019;10:155.
16. Kapitza C, Nosek L, Jensen L, Hartvig H, Jensen CB, Flint A. Semaglutide, a once-weekly human GLP-1 analog, does not reduce the bioavailability of the combined oral contraceptive, ethinylestradiol/levonorgestrel. J Clin Pharmacol. 2015;55(5): 497-504.
17. Marbury TC, Flint A, Jacobsen JB, Derving Karsbøl J, Lasseter K. Pharmacokinetics and tolerability of a single dose of semaglutide, a once-weekly human GLP-1 analog, in subjects with and without renal impairment. Clin Pharmacokinet. 2017;56(11):1381-90.
18. Marso SP, Holst AG, Vilsbøll T. Semaglutide and cardiovascular outcomes in patients with type 2 diabetes. N Engl J Med. 2017;376(9):891-2.
19. Ahmann AJ, Capehorn M, Charpentier G, Dotta F, Henkel E, Lingvay I, et al. Efficacy and safety of once-weekly semaglutide versus exenatide ER in subjects with type 2 diabetes (SUSTAIN 3): A 56-week, open-label, randomized clinical trial. Diabetes Care. 2018;41(2):258-66.
20. Ahrén B, Masmiquel L, Kumar H, Sargin M, Karsbøl JD, Jacobsen SH, et al. Efficacy and safety of once-weekly semaglutide versus once-daily sitagliptin as an add-on to metformin, thiazolidinediones, or both, in patients with type 2 diabetes (SUSTAIN 2): a 56-week, double-blind, phase 3a, randomised trial. Lancet Diabetes Endocrinol. 2017;5(5): 341-54.
21. Aroda VR, Bain SC, Cariou B, Piletič M, Rose L, Axelsen M, et al. Efficacy and safety of once-weekly semaglutide versus once-daily insulin glargine as add-on to metformin (with or without sulfonylureas) in insulin-naïve patients with type 2 diabetes (SUSTAIN 4): a randomised, open-label, parallel-group, multicentre, multinational, phase 3a trial. Lancet Diabetes Endocrinol. 2017;5(5):355-66.
22. Capehorn MS, Catarig A, Furberg JK, Janez A, Price H, Tadayon S, et al. Efficacy and safety of once-weekly semaglutide 1.0 mg vs once-daily liraglutide 1.2 mg as add-on to 1–3 oral antidiabetic drugs in subjects with type 2 diabetes (SUSTAIN 10). Diabetes Metab. 2020;46(2):100-9.
23. Frías JP, Auerbach P, Bajaj HS, Fukushima Y, Lingvay I, Macura S, et al. Efficacy and safety of once-weekly semaglutide 2.0 mg versus 1.0 mg in patients with type 2 diabetes (SUSTAIN FORTE): a double-blind, randomised, phase 3B trial. Lancet Diabetes Endocrinol. 2021;9(9):563-74.

24. Ji L, Dong X, Li Y, Li Y, Lim S, Liu M, et al. Efficacy and safety of once-weekly semaglutide versus once-daily sitagliptin as add-on to metformin in patients with type 2 diabetes in SUSTAIN China: A 30-week, double-blind, phase 3a, randomized trial. Diabetes Obes Metab. 2021;23(2):404-14.
25. Kaku K, Yamada Y, Watada H, Abiko A, Nishida T, Zacho J, et al. Safety and efficacy of once-weekly semaglutide vs additional oral antidiabetic drugs in Japanese people with inadequately controlled type 2 diabetes: A randomized trial. Diabetes Obes Metab. 2018;20(5):1202-12.
26. Kellerer M, Kaltoft MS, Lawson J, Nielsen LL, Strojek K, Tabak Ö, et al. Effect of once-weekly semaglutide versus thrice-daily insulin aspart, both as add-on to metformin and optimized insulin glargine treatment in participants with type 2 diabetes (SUSTAIN 11): A randomized, open-label, multinational, phase 3b trial. Diabetes Obes Metab. 2022;24(9):1788-99.
27. Lingvay I, Catarig AM, Frias JP, Kumar H, Lausvig NL, le Roux CW, et al. Efficacy and safety of once-weekly semaglutide versus daily canagliflozin as add-on to metformin in patients with type 2 diabetes (SUSTAIN 8): a double-blind, phase 3b, randomised controlled trial. Lancet Diabetes Endocrinol. 2019;7(11):834-44.
28. Pratley RE, Aroda VR, Lingvay I, Lüdemann J, Andreassen C, Navarria A, et al. Semaglutide versus dulaglutide once weekly in patients with type 2 diabetes (SUSTAIN 7): A randomised, open-label, phase 3b trial. Lancet Diabetes Endocrinol. 2018;6(4):275-86.
29. Rodbard HW, Lingvay I, Reed J, de la Rosa R, Rose L, Sugimoto D, et al. Semaglutide added to basal insulin in type 2 diabetes (SUSTAIN 5): A randomized, controlled trial. J Clin Endocrinol Metab. 2018;103(6):2291-301.
30. Seino Y, Terauchi Y, Osonoi T, Yabe D, Abe N, Nishida T, et al. Safety and efficacy of semaglutide once weekly vs sitagliptin once daily, both as monotherapy in Japanese people with type 2 diabetes. Diabetes Obes Metab. 2018;20(2):378-88.
31. Sorli C, Harashima SI, Tsoukas GM, Unger J, Karsbøl JD, Hansen T, et al. Efficacy and safety of once-weekly semaglutide monotherapy versus placebo in patients with type 2 diabetes (SUSTAIN 1): a double-blind, randomised, placebo-controlled, parallel-group, multinational, multicentre, phase 3a trial. Lancet Diabetes Endocrinol. 2017;5(4):251-60.
32. Zinman B, Bhosekar V, Busch R, Holst I, Ludvik B, Thielke D, et al. Semaglutide once weekly as add-on to SGLT-2 inhibitor therapy in type 2 diabetes (SUSTAIN 9): a randomised, placebo-controlled trial. Lancet Diabetes Endocrinol. 2019;7(5):356-67.
33. Aroda VR, Rosenstock J, Terauchi Y, Altuntas Y, Lalic NM, Morales Villegas EC, et al. PIONEER 1: Randomized clinical trial of the efficacy and safety of oral semaglutide monotherapy in comparison with placebo in patients with type 2 diabetes. Diabetes Care. 2019;42(9):1724-32.
34. Rodbard HW, Rosenstock J, Canani LH, Deerochanawong C, Gumprecht J, Lindberg SØ, et al. Oral semaglutide versus empagliflozin in patients with type 2 diabetes uncontrolled on metformin: The PIONEER 2 trial. Diabetes Care. 2019;42(12):2272-81.
35. Rosenstock J, Allison D, Birkenfeld AL, Blicher TM, Deenadayalan S, Jacobsen JB, et al. Effect of additional oral semaglutide vs sitagliptin on glycated hemoglobin in adults with type 2 diabetes uncontrolled with metformin alone or with sulfonylurea: The PIONEER 3 randomized clinical trial. JAMA.2019;321(15):1466-80.
36. Pratley R, Amod A, Hoff ST, Kadowaki T, Lingvay I, Nauck M, et al. Oral semaglutide versus subcutaneous liraglutide and placebo in type 2 diabetes (PIONEER 4): A randomised, double-blind, phase 3a trial. Lancet. 2019;394(10192):39-50.
37. Mosenzon O, Blicher TM, Rosenlund S, Eriksson JW, Heller S, Hels OH, et al. Efficacy and safety of oral semaglutide in patients with type 2 diabetes and moderate renal impairment (PIONEER 5): A placebo-controlled, randomised, phase 3a trial. Lancet Diabetes Endocrinol. 2019;7(7):515-27.
38. Husain M, Birkenfeld AL, Donsmark M, Dungan K, Eliaschewitz FG, Franco DR, et al. Oral semaglutide and cardiovascular outcomes in patients with type 2 diabetes. N Engl J Med. 2019;381:841-51.
39. Pieber TR, Bode B, Mertens A, Cho YM, Christiansen E, Hertz CL, et al. Efficacy and safety of oral semaglutide with flexible dose adjustment versus sitagliptin in type 2 diabetes (PIONEER 7): a multicentre, open-label, randomised, phase 3a trial. Lancet Diabetes Endocrinol. 2019;7(7):528-39.
40. Zinman B, Aroda VR, Buse JB, Cariou B, Harris SB, Hoff ST, et al. Efficacy, safety, and tolerability of oral semaglutide versus placebo added to insulin with or without metformin in patients with type 2 diabetes: The PIONEER 8 trial. Diabetes Care. 2019;42(12):2262-71.
41. Yamada Y, Katagiri H, Hamamoto Y, Deenadayalan S, Navarria A, Nishijima K, et al. Dose-response, efficacy, and safety of oral semaglutide monotherapy in Japanese patients with type 2 diabetes (PIONEER 9): A 52-week, phase 2/3a, randomised, controlled trial. Lancet Diabetes Endocrinol. 2020;8(5):377-91.
42. Yabe D, Nakamura J, Kaneto H, Deenadayalan S, Navarria A, Gislum M, et al. Safety and efficacy of oral semaglutide versus dulaglutide in Japanese patients with type 2 diabetes (PIONEER 10): an open-label, randomised, active-controlled, phase 3a trial. Lancet Diabetes Endocrinol. 2020;8:392-406.
43. Aroda VR. Aberle J, Bardtrum L, Christiansen E, Knop FK, Gabery S, et al. Efficacy and safety of once-daily oral semaglutide 25 mg and 50 mg compared with 14 mg in adults with type 2 diabetes (PIONEER PLUS): a multicentre, randomised, phase 3b trial. Lancet, 2023;402(10403):693-704.
44. Wilding JPH, Batterham RL, Calanna S, Davies M, Van Gaal LF, Lingvay I, et al. Once-weekly semaglutide in adults with overweight or obesity. N Engl J Med. 2021;384(11):989-1002.
45. Davies M, Færch L, Jeppesen OK, Pakseresht A, Pedersen SD, Perreault L, et al. Semaglutide 2.4 mg once a week in adults with overweight or obesity, and type 2 diabetes (STEP 2): A randomised, double-blind, double dummy, placebo-controlled, phase 3 trial. Lancet. 2021;397:971-84.
46. Wadden TA, Bailey TS, Billings LK, Davies M, Frias JP, Koroleva A, et al. Effect of subcutaneous semaglutide vs placebo as an adjunct to intensive behavioral therapy on body weight in adults with overweight or obesity: The STEP 3 randomized clinical trial. JAMA. 2021;325(14):1403-13.
47. Rubino D, Abrahamsson N, Davies M, Hesse D, Greenway FL, Jensen C, et al. Effect of continued weekly subcutaneous semaglutide vs placebo on weight loss maintenance in adults with overweight or obesity: The STEP 4 randomized clinical trial. JAMA. 2021;325(14):1414-25.
48. Garvey WT, Batterham RL, Bhatta M, Buscemi S, Christensen LN, Frias JP, et al. Two-year effects of semaglutide in adults with overweight or obesity: the STEP 5 trial. Nat Med. 2022;28(10):2083-91.

49. Kadowaki T, Isendahl J, Khalid U, Lee SY, Nishida T, Ogawa W, et al. Semaglutide once a week in adults with overweight or obesity, with or without type 2 diabetes in an east Asian population (STEP 6): a randomised, double-blind, double-dummy, placebo-controlled, phase 3a trial. Lancet Diabetes Endocrinol. 2022;10(3):193-206.
50. Rubino DM, Greenway FL, Khalid U, O'Neil PM, Rosenstock J, Sørrig R, et al. Effect of weekly subcutaneous semaglutide vs daily liraglutide on body weight in adults with overweight or obesity without diabetes: The STEP 8 randomized clinical trial. JAMA. 2022;327(2):138-50.
51. Weghuber D, Barrett T, Barrientos-Pérez M, Gies I, Hesse D, Jeppesen OK, et al. Once-weekly semaglutide in adolescents with obesity. N Engl J Med. 2022;387(24):2245-57.
52. Knop FK, Aroda VR, do Vale RD, Holst-Hansen T, Laursen PN, Rosenstock J, et al. Oral semaglutide 50 mg taken once per day in adults with overweight or obesity (OASIS 1): a randomised, double-blind, placebo-controlled, phase 3 trial. Lancet. 2023;402(10403):705-19.
53. Kurtzhals P, Flindt Kreiner F, Singh Bindra R. The role of weight control in the management of type 2 diabetes mellitus: Perspectives on semaglutide. Diabetes Res Clin Pract. 2023;203:110881.

53 CHAPTER

GLP-1 Analogs versus SGLT-2 Inhibitors in Diabetic Patients with CVD

Dinesh Sharma, Jugal Kishor Sharma

ABSTRACT

Cardiovascular complications such as myocardial infarction (MI), stroke, and heart failure are very high and are the leading cause of death in patients with type 2 diabetes mellitus (T2DM). The novel glucose-lowering agents such as glucagon-like peptide 1 (GLP-1) receptor agonist (GLP-1 RA) and sodium-glucose cotransporter-2 (SGLT-2) inhibitors have shown a significant and robust reduction in major adverse cardiovascular events (MACE) and additional benefits such as reduced hospitalization for heart failure; this has been proved in multiple cardiovascular outcome trials (CVOT). This evidence has resulted in major change in treatment of diabetes as both cardiologist and diabetologist included strong recommendation to use these two agents in diabetic patients with high risk of CV complications independent of glucose control. The magnitude of CV benefits of SGLT-2 inhibitor and GLP-1 RA on MACE are equal which ranges from 12 to 14% risk reduction; however, GLP-1 RA may reduce the stroke risk. The difference between these two classes of drugs on improvement in hospitalization for heart failure is three times more in SGLT-2 inhibitors as compared to GLP-1 RA. GLP-1 RA also has significant benefit in heart failure which can be used where SGLT-2 inhibitors are contraindicated. However, the difference between these two classes on renal outcome is very less.

INTRODUCTION

Diabetes is a "cardiovascular disease (CVD)" as stated by the American Heart Journal in 1999. In spite of major decline in CVD, patients with diabetes have higher rates of major adverse cardiovascular events (MACE). The overall prevalence of CVD in diabetic patients is 32% and all-cause mortality is twice more in diabetic patients than nondiabetic patients. Diabetic patients with history of prior heart failure, cardiovascular (CV) events, peripheral arterial disease, older age, and kidney disease are at higher risk of mortality and are benefited by treatment of risk factors and newer glucose-lowering agents. Glucagon-like peptide 1 receptor agonist (GLP-1 RA) and sodium-glucose cotransporter-2 (SGLT-2) inhibitors can reduce the MACE and its individual components such as myocardial infarction (MI), CV death, and stroke. This beneficial effect is independent of previous CV disease. There are some differences in two class of drugs in prevention of cardiovascular events. GLP-1 RA has major effect on atherosclerotic CVD while SGLT-2 inhibitor have major effect on prevention of hospitalization for heart failure. Both the classes of drugs have beneficial effect on CV mortality and reduce the risk of kidney disease. Despite similar benefits both the classes of drugs differ in mechanism of action, safety, tolerability administration, and side effects. These differences results in preference to choose the agents according to patients need.

GLUCAGON-LIKE PEPTIDE 1 RECEPTOR ANALOGS

Glucagon-like peptide 1 is a small peptide hormone which is released from gastrointestinal L cells after ingestion of food nutrients. It exhibits incretin effect after binding to GLP-1 receptors. This effect leads to glucose-dependent insulin secretion from beta cells of pancreas, inhibition of glucagon release from alpha cells of pancreas, and prolongation of gastric emptying. All these actions cause reduction in blood glucose and improvement in postprandial glucose metabolism. It also has an effect on hypothalamic neurons which induces satiety and leading to weight loss. GLP-1 has its half-life only few minutes because its cleavage by dipeptidyl peptidase-4 (DPP-4) enzyme.

Eight cardiovascular outcome trials (CVOTs) of benefits of GLP-1 RA have been published; the meta-analysis of these trials shows 14% reductions in three MACE components (cardiovascular death, nonfatal MI, and non-fatal stroke) which suggests these beneficial effects are due to reduced atherosclerotic events and are independent of presence of established CV disease at baseline. GLP-1 RA leads to reduction of 2–6 mm Hg blood pressure which leads to CV event reduction. In previous meta-analysis, 10 mm Hg BP reduction was associated with 20% reduction in MACE. GLP-1 RAs have shown modest reduction of total cholesterol, triglycerides, low-density lipoprotein (LDL) causing beneficial effect on CV risks. GLP-1 RA reduces 0.8–1.5% HbA1c and 2.5–4 kg weight, which contribute to reduced CV events. Different mechanisms have been proposed for these results. GLP-1 RA has its effect on pancreas, gut, stomach, liver, adipose tissue, skeletal muscle, kidney, heart, vessels, and the immune system **(Fig. 1)**. Dedicated studies on efficacy and safety of GLP-1 RA are not there. CVOTs included only a limited number of patients on GLP-1 RA with history of heart failure (HF) and had a neutral effect on risk of hospitalization for heart failure (HHF). On kidney outcomes, many GLP-1 RAs have shown to reduce albuminuria to 21–22% which is a parameter of worsening kidney functions. Analysis of SUSTAIN 6 trial and LEADER trial suggests semaglutide and liraglutide may have kidney-protective effect, which is more in patients with preexisting chronic kidney disease (CKD). The CV benefits of GLP-1 RA in high-risk patients with diabetes are a combination of vascular, metabolic, antithrombotic, and anti-inflammatory effects. The recommendation of the American Diabetes Association (ADA) Standard Care 2021 states that patients with T2DM with established CVD or multiple risk factors for CVD, GLP-1 RA is recommended, which shows cardiovascular benefits to reduce the risk of MACE.

SODIUM-GLUCOSE COTRANSPORTER-2 INHIBITORS

Sodium-glucose cotransporter-2 inhibitors are new class of glucose-lowering drugs, which block the SGLT-2 protein present in proximal convoluted tubules of nephron. This protein reabsorbs 90% of filtered glucose

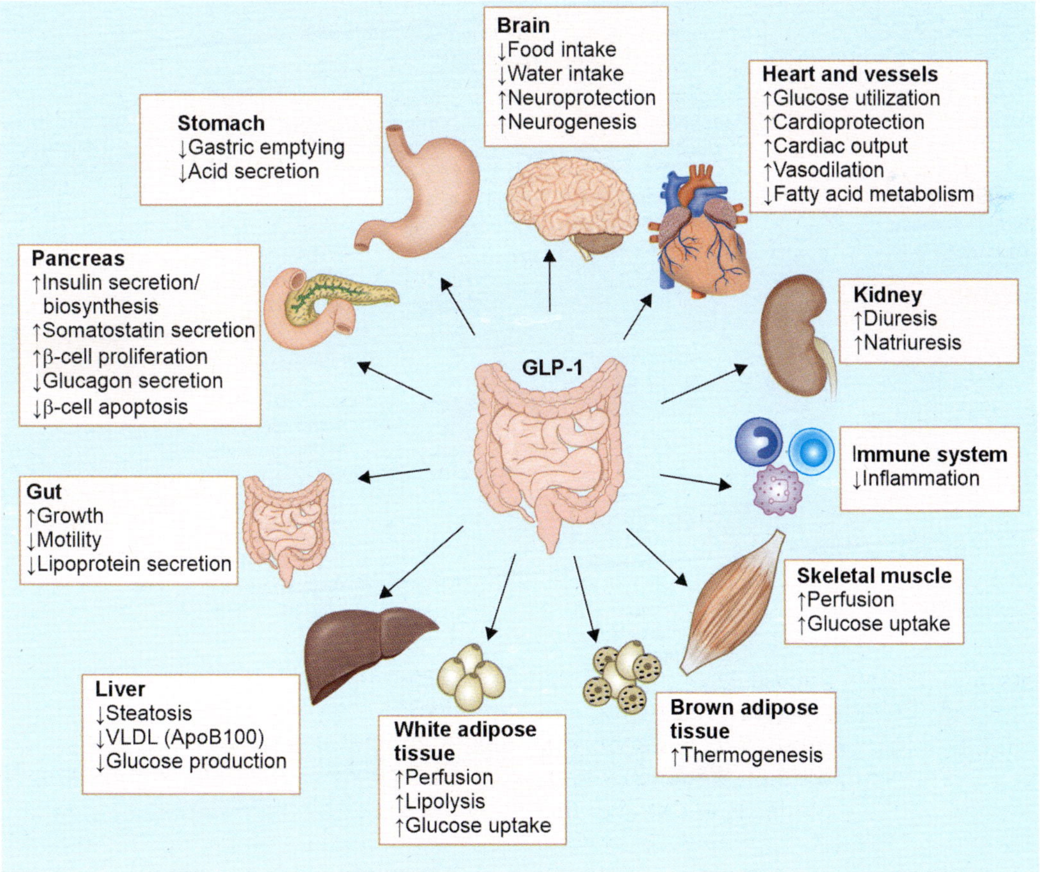

FIG. 1: Glucagon-like peptide 1 (GLP-1) and the kidney from physiology to pharmacology and outcomes in diabetes.

and remainder by SGLT-1 in distal part of convoluted tubule. SGLT-2 inhibitor cause glycosuria thereby causing decreased plasma glucose concentration; this is independent of insulin or incretin pathway. In recent CVOT, SGLT-2 inhibitor shows 30–35% lower risk of HF, which is preserved even at lower estimated glomerular filtration rate (eGFR). In DAPA-HF (Dapagliflozin and Prevention of Adverse Outcomes in Heart Failure) trial, the efficacy of SGLT-2 inhibitor in patients with heart failure and reduced ejection fraction regardless of diabetes was evaluated. This trial showed 26% risk reduction of worsening heart failure or death from CVD, which is independent of glucose-lowering effect. EMPEROR-Reduced (Empagliflozin Outcome Trial in Patients with Chronic Heart Failure and a Reduced Ejection Fraction) trial also showed that empagliflozin treatment is associated with the composite risk reduction of CV death and heart failure hospitalization in patients with heart failure with reduced ejection fraction irrespective of diabetes status. After the results of both DAPA-HF and EMPEROR-R, the Food and Drug Administration (FDA) has approved empagliflozin and dapagliflozin in patients of HF and reduced ejection fraction to reduce the risk of CV death or hospitalization for HF regardless of presence of diabetes. Many other trials have been conducted in patients with diabetes with established CVD, CV risk factors and renal insufficiency and in patients with established heart failure and reduced ejection fractions with or without diabetes. Results from EMPA-REG OUTCOME (Empagliflozin Cardiovascular Outcome Event Trial in Type 2 Diabetes Mellitus Patients), CANVAS (Canagliflozin Cardiovascular Assessment Study), CREDENCE (Canagliflozin and Renal Events in Diabetes with Established Nephropathy Clinical Evaluation), and DECLARE-TIMI (Dapagliflozin Effect on Cardiovascular Events–Thrombolysis in Myocardial Infarction) also showed reduction in all-cause death, CV death, hospitalization for heart failure, and decline in renal functions.

The mechanism of cardiovascular benefits with SGLT2 inhibitor is multifactorial **(Fig. 2)**. The actual mechanism for these beneficial effects is not clear. Several mechanisms have been proposed for the cardioprotective effect of SGLT-2 inhibitor. Antihypertensive and diuretic effects of SGLT-2 inhibitor improve cardiovascular outcomes, which is due to osmotic diuresis as a result of glycosuria and natriuresis. Antihypertensive effect may be due to improvement in endothelial functions, reduced arterial stiffness, and changes in sympathetic

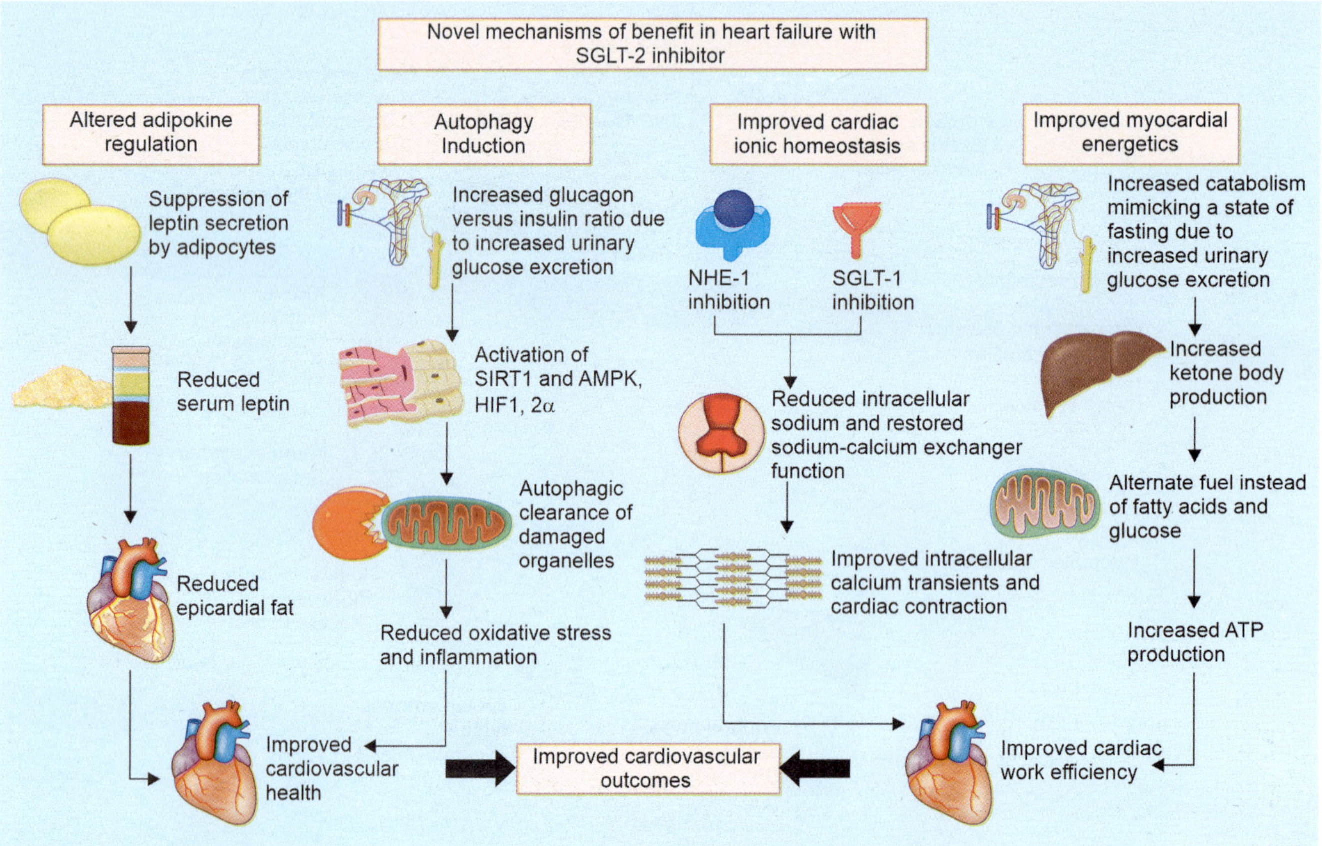

FIG. 2: Schematic diagram showing proposed novel mechanisms of action of SGLT-2 inhibitors in heart failure.

(AMPK: adenosine monophosphate-activated protein kinase; HIF: hypoxia-inducible factor; sodium-hydrogen exchanger; SGLT-2: sodium-glucose cotransporter-2; SIRT: sirtuin)

nervous activity. Weight reduction and glycemic control have been postulated the CV benefits of SGLT-2 inhibitor treatment. Weight loss is due to an increased glucagon:insulin ratio leading to increased lipid metabolism causing reduction in heart failure. Around 2.7 kg weight loss was seen in SGLT-2 inhibitor therapy. This also increases renal erythropoietin production, red cell mass, and hematocrit, reversal of adverse cardiac remodeling, improved cardiac energy metabolism, inflammation reduction, sympathetic nervous system inhibition, prevention of ischemia, reperfusion injury, inhibition of Na^+/H^+ exchanger, SGLT-1 inhibition, decrease in hyperuricemia, decreased epicardial fat mass, increasing autophagy, and lysosomal degradation, decrease oxidative stress, and improved vascular functions.

CARDIOVASCULAR OUTCOME TRIALS

Nearly 18 CVOTs have been published regarding these newer antidiabetes drugs **(Fig. 3)**. The World Health Organization (WHO) has demonstrated the hazard ratio (HR) < 1.8 **(Fig. 4)** for MACE by enrolling T2DM patients with established CVD or at high risk of CVD. In 2015, EMPA-REG OUTCOME showed reduced 3P-MACE and CV death in patients of T2DM with established CVD by empagliflozin. Also hospitalization for heart failure, progression to kidney disease, and all-cause mortality was reduced. There was paradigm shift in evidence for improvements in CV, HHF, and renal outcomes by treatment with these medications in subsequent CVOTs. These trials now updated the treatment guide lines and insights for diabetes management.

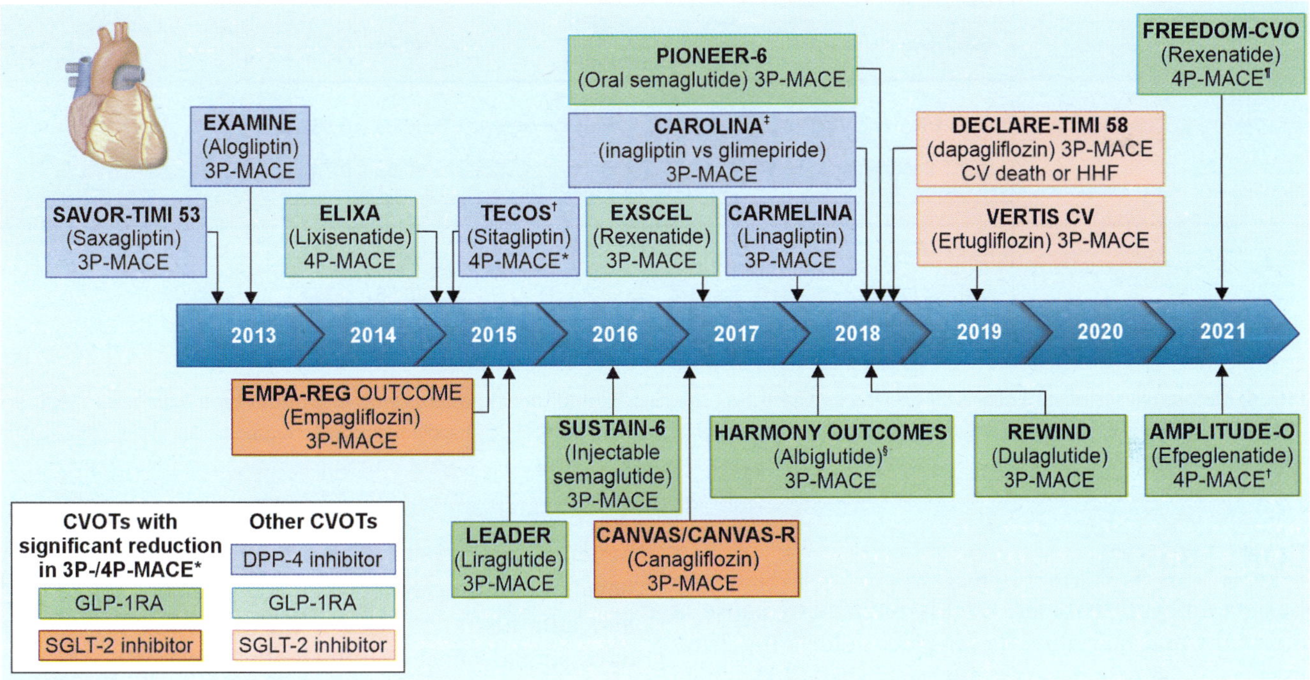

*3P-MACE is a composite of CV death, nonfatal myocardial infarction and nonfatal stroke. 4P-MACE is an expanded composite of 3P-MACE plus either hospitalization for unstable angina (ELIXA, TECOS and FREEDOM-CVO) or death from undetermined causes (AMPLITUDE-O).

†TECOS and FREEDOM-CVO included 3P-MACE as a secondary outcome.

‡CAROLINA was conducted in addition to regulatory requirements, as an active-controlled CVOT complementary to the core placebo-controlled CVOT CARMEUNA.

§Albiglutide is no longer a licensed treatment.

#Efpeglenatide is not a currently licensed treatment.

¶FREEDOM-CVO (exenatide subcutaneous implant; not a currently licensed treatment) was completed in 2016, but the primary outcome (4P-MACE) was reported in 2022.

FIG. 3: A timeline of published diabetes CVOTs. The comparator in all trials was placebo, unless otherwise stated. Primary endpoints for each trial are listed.

(3/4P-MACE: 3/4-point major adverse CV event; CV: cardiovascular; DPP-4: dipeptidyl peptidase-4; GLP-1 RA: glucagon-like peptide-1 receptor agonist; HHF: hospitalization for heart failure; SGLT-2: sodium-glucose cotransporter-2)

Source: clinicaltrials.gov.

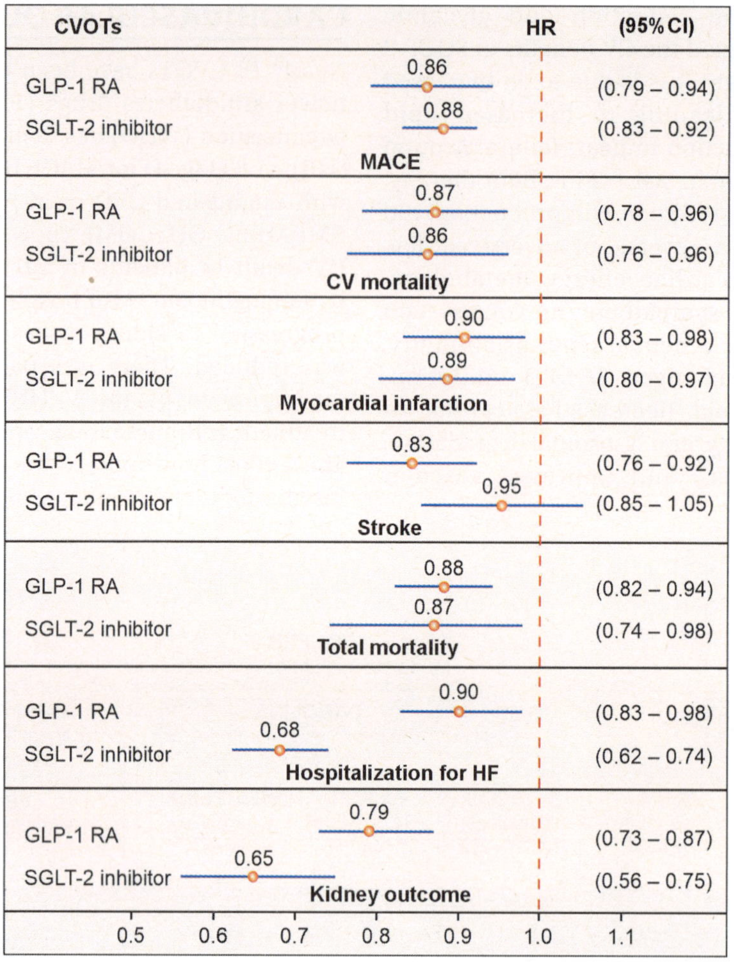

FIG. 4: Meta-analyses of cardiocervical exerted by GLP-1 RA and SGLT-2 inhibitors in patients with or without type 2 diabetes mellitus.
(CV: confidence interval; GLP-1 RA: glucagon-like peptide-1 receptor agonist; HR: hazard ratio; SGLT-2: sodium-glucose cotransporter-2)

CONCLUSION

In patients with diabetes, CVD is the leading cause of morbidity and mortality. Newer glucose-lowering drugs having CV safety in patients with established CVD or high risk of CVD led to the introduction of CVOT. GLP-1 RA and SGLT-2 inhibitor have shown cardio protective effect in patients who have established CVD or high risk of CVD. In many CVOTs, reductions in 3-point MACE (3P-MACE) and CV deaths have been shown with additional effect on reduced risk of HHF, progression to renal disease and all-cause mortality. These data have resulted in a paradigm shift in treatment of diabetes with international guidelines keeping SGLT-2 inhibitor and GLP-1 RA as first-line treatment in patients with CV risk. In spite of similar benefits on CV risk, SGLT-2 inhibitor and GLP-1 RA have different mechanisms of action, safety, tolerability and administration. GLP-1 RA and SGLT-2 inhibitor have similar effect to reduce atherosclerotic MACE in patients with established atherosclerotic CVD; however, SGLT-2 inhibitor have more effect on preventing HHF and progression to kidney disease independent of diabetes status. This opens new possibilities for use of these classes of drugs in patients at risk of CVD or established CVD or kidney disease. A coordinated action is to be taken to treat the T2DM patients with CV disease, HF, and CKD. There is urgent need to incorporate multiple care systems in high-risk patients, who may be benefited from this class of drugs.

SUGGESTED READINGS

1. Grundy SM, Benjamin IJ, Burke GL, Chait A, Eckel RH, Howard BV, et al. Diabetes and cardiovascular disease: a statement for healthcare professionals from the American Heart Association. Circulation. 1999;100:1134-46.
2. Einarson TR, Acs A, Ludwig C, Panton UH. Prevalence of cardiovascular disease in type 2 diabetes: a systematic literature review of scientific evidence from across the world in 2007-2017. Cardiovasc Diabetol. 2018;17:83.
3. Bragg F, Holmes MV, Iona A, Guo Y, Du H, Chen Y, et al. Association between diabetes and cause-specific mortality in rural and urban areas of China. JAMA. 2017;317:280-9.
4. American Diabetes Association. Pharmacologic approaches to glycemic treatment: standards of medical care in diabetes. Diabetes Care. 2021;44(Supplement 1):111-24.
5. Zinman B, Wanner C, Lachin JM, et Fitchett D, Bluhmki E, Hantel S, et al. Empagliflozin, cardiovascular outcomes, and mortality in type 2 diabetes. N Engl J Med. 2015;373:2117-28.
6. Neal B, Perkovic V, Mahaffey KW. Canagliflozin and cardiovascular and renal events in type 2 diabetes. N Engl J Med 2017;377:644-57.
7. Wiviott SD, Raz I, Bonaca MP. Dapagliflozin and cardiovascular outcomes in type 2 diabetes. N Engl J Med. 2019;380:347-57.
8. Cannon CP, Pratley R, Dagogo-Jack S. Cardiovascular outcomes with ertugliflozin in type 2 diabetes. N Engl J Med. 2020;383: 1425-35.
9. McMurray JJV, Solomon SD, Inzucchi SE. Dapagliflozin in patients with heart failure and reduced ejection fraction. N Engl J Med. 2019;381:1995-2008.
10. Packer M, Anker SD, Butler J. Cardiovascular and renal outcomes with empagliflozin in heart failure. N Engl J Med. 2020:NEJMoa2022190.
11. Cherney DZ, Perkins BA, Soleymanlou N, Har R, Fagan N, Johansen OE, et al. The effect of empagliflozin on arterial stiffness and heart rate variability in subjects with uncomplicated type 1 diabetes mellitus. Cardiovasc Diabetol. 2014;13:28.
12. Pfeifer M, Townsend RR, Davies MJ, Vijapurkar U, Ren J. Effects of canagliflozin, a sodium glucose co-transporter 2 inhibitor, on blood pressure and markers of arterial stiffness in patients with type 2 diabetes mellitus: a post hoc analysis. Cardiovasc Diabetol. 2017;16:29.
13. Zinman B, Wanner C, Lachin JM, Fitchett D, Bluhmki E, Hantel S, et al. Empagliflozin, cardiovascular outcomes, and mortality in type 2 diabetes. N Engl J Med. 2015;373:2117-28.

54

CHAPTER

Cardiorenal Metabolic Risk Continuum Approaching Holistic Care in Type 2 Diabetes Mellitus

V Palaniappan

ABSTRACT

This manuscript discusses the high prevalence of diabetes in India and associated cardiometabolic risks, emphasizing the need for personalized, evidence-based treatment. It highlights the role of sodium-glucose cotransporter-2 inhibitors (SGLT-2i) in managing these risks, including their impact on comorbidities, such as chronic kidney disease (CKD) and cardiovascular disease (CVD). The paper underscores the need for early intervention and multifactorial control to prevent disease progression. It also points out the global inertia in adopting new cardioprotective therapies, urging for improved patient education to enhance adoption and adherence. The manuscript concludes by advocating for holistic care in managing diabetes and associated risks.

INTRODUCTION

Despite advancements in diabetes care, there are still unmet needs to address patient-centric goals. The prevalence of diabetes as per a recent Indian Council of Medical Research–India Diabetes (ICMR-INDIAB) study was estimated to be 11.4% (>100 million in India as of 2021). We know that poor glycemic control and other risk factor control lead to micro- and macrovascular complications. South Asian phenotype adds oil to the fire, i.e., high carb diet, poor lifestyle, earlier beta-cell dysfunction, insulin resistance, and dysfunctional adiposity make people more vulnerable to diabetes. The cost burden to individuals with diabetes not only comes from medicine but mainly from other associated costs.

CARDIOMETABOLIC RISK FACTORS AND ITS EPIDEMIOLOGY

The presence of multiple risk factors such as hyperglycemia, hypertension, and obesity often leads to end-organ damage if not managed appropriately. Currently, the interventions must be focused toward cardiometabolic risk factor control with evidence-based and goal-directed approach for every individual patient.

Insulin resistance primarily, with other risk factors plays a critical role in early atherogenesis, even before 5–7 years prior to diagnosis of diabetes. Presence of subclinical atherosclerosis may be evident in people with normal glucose levels. A study published in 2021 assessed the risk of early atherosclerosis in people without diabetes and showed that as glycated hemoglobin (HbA1c) increases, the atherogenic markers also proportionately increase in those people. Not only that, Nurse's health study also has shown that there's a 3.6 times increased risk for cardiovascular (CV) events in people even 10 years prior to diagnosis of diabetes relative to a person without diabetes.

CARDIOMETABOLIC COMORBID CONDITIONS

Diabetes per se does not persist usually as a single entity but rather with many other comorbid conditions. Approximately one out of every two people with diabetes have chronic kidney disease (CKD) and diastolic dysfunction and one out of four patients have nonalcoholic fatty liver disease (NAFLD). Nearly one in five patients with diabetes may have cardiac autonomic neuropathy (CAN).

Promising Hypothesis Generating Evidence from Sodium-glucose Cotransporter-2 Inhibitors

Let us see the impact of relatively newer therapies on all these comorbidities, especially with sodium-glucose cotransporter-2 inhibitors (SGLT-2i).

Cardiac autonomic neuropathy is a definite and independent predictor of mortality in type 2 diabetes mellitus (T2DM). In South Asians, although polyneuropathy is less common, the prevalence of CAN is as high as in Caucasians. Approximately 1 of 20 patients develop CAN annually in T2DM (4.6–6%/year). In patients with T2DM, vasovagal syncope (VVS) recurrence could be due to the alteration of autonomic system function. Non-sodium-glucose cotransporter-2 inhibitors (non-SGLT-2i) users compared to SGLT-2i users had alterations of the autonomic nervous system, with a higher rate of VVS recurrence at 1 year of follow-up.

Sodium-glucose cotransporter-2 inhibitors are believed to exert promising mechanisms that aim to reduce lipo, glucotoxicity, oxidative stress, and inflammation in adipose tissues particularly. Some of the postulated mechanisms include modulating the adiponectin-leptin pathway, reducing T-cell accumulation, and improving fat utilization in peripheral tissues.

A study published in 2021, has shown the prevalence of clinically relevant liver fibrosis in T2DM individuals with NAFLD to be 28.2%. More than one out of four T2DM patients with NAFLD were suffering with liver disease of clinical relevance. Sodium-glucose cotransporter-2 inhibitors reduce liver fat content in people with T2DM and NAFLD. E-LIFT study (with empagliflozin)—a randomized controlled trial (RCT) in 42 patients with T2DM and NAFLD; empagliflozin versus standard treatment control for 20 weeks.

About 4.0% placebo-corrected reduction in liver fat achieved with empagliflozin ($p < 0.001$). A RCT in around 30 patients with T2DM and NAFLD; dapagliflozin versus standard treatment control for 8 weeks was conducted. About 3.74% placebo corrected reduction in liver-fat achieved with dapagliflozin ($p < 0.01$).

Sodium-glucose cotransporter-2 inhibition in people with nonalcoholic steatohepatitis and T2DM has demonstrated possible histological improvement in NASH at 6 months of treatment. Improvements were seen in fibrosis and hepatocellular ballooning aspects.

Meta-analysis of 27 echocardiography-based studies in people with T2DM has shown that early one out of two people with T2DM have left ventricular diastolic dysfunction.

Progression of diabetic kidney disease (DKD) varies depending on the duration of diabetes unlike with other causes of CKD. In the initial stages of DKD, there may be no symptoms or signs. Usually, it starts as a silent DKD without any signs or symptoms in people and progresses to ESRD (full-blown overt kidney disease).

Sodium-glucose cotransporter-2 inhibition may reduce the risk of new-onset obstructive sleep apnea. This was evident from the subanalysis of EMPA-REG OUTCOME trial. There was a 52% lowered risk of new-onset OSA with empagliflozin compared to placebo in people with T2DM and atherosclerotic cardiovascular disease (ASCVD).

We had discussed about various comorbid conditions associated with diabetes.

CARDIOVASCULAR DISEASE BURDEN IN TYPE 2 DIABETES MELLITUS SETTING

Now in this section, we will discuss specifically on the prevalence of cardiovascular disease (CVD) in people with T2DM. One out of three patients have any CVD. One out of five patients approximately have coronary artery disease and one out of every seven T2DM patients suffers from heart failure. Ever since the rosiglitazone controversy in 2008, global regulatory bodies such as the Food and Drug Administration (FDA) and the European Medicines Agency (EMA) have mandated the long-term CV safety requirements of newer antidiabetic drugs for their marketing authorization. In the last one and a half decades, newer classes of antidiabetic agents came into the market with their respective CV outcome trials (CVOTs). Dipeptidyl peptidase 4 (DPP-4) inhibitors that have undergone CVOTs, in general, have demonstrated its CV safety baring the increased risk for hypertensive heart failure (HHF) with saxagliptin. Sodium-glucose cotransporter-2 inhibitors as a class on the other hand have not only demonstrated its CV safety but also benefits in reducing HHF and renal outcomes. However, major adverse cardiovascular events (MACE) benefit was observed in CVOTs of both empagliflozin/canagliflozin and CV mortality benefit in people with T2DM and ASCVD was demonstrated with Empagliflozin only. But we know that there are no credible, CV outcome-based head-to-head trials amongst SGLT-2is to compare between each other.

Major renal outcome studies with SGLT-2i agents were CREDENCE, DAPA-CKD (Dapagliflozin and Prevention of Adverse Outcomes in Chronic Kidney Disease), and EMPA-KIDNEY (The Study of Heart and Kidney Protection With Empagliflozin). Credence had included people with

DKD and estimated glomerular filtration rate (eGFR) ≥30 to <90 mL/min/1.73 m^2 and urine albumin-creatinine ratio (UACR) > 300 mg/g DAPA-CKD included patients with or without DKD and eGFR > 25 to <75 mL/min/1.73 m^2 and UACR ≥ 200 to ≤5,000 mg/g. EMPA-KIDNEY; EMPA included patients with or without DKD and eGFR ≥20 to <45 mL/min/1.73 m^2 or eGFR ≥45 to <90 mL/min/1.73 m^2 and UACR ≥200 mg/g.

There was a 38% lowered risk for kidney disease progression in T2DM patients with SGLT-2is in a meta-analysis published recently in 2022.

Kidney disease progression: Sustained decrease in eGFR (≥50%) from randomization, a sustained low eGFR, end-stage kidney disease, or death from kidney failure in all trials.

With the approval of these newer agents, the treatment of patients with CKD has evolved to involve a multifactorial approach.

This multifactorial approach has a positive effect on kidney outcomes.

Early initiation of combination treatment with SGLT-2i and finerenone, together with traditional multifactorial intervention, including blood pressure control, use of angiotensin-converting enzyme (ACE) inhibitors or angiotensin receptor blockers (ARBs), and reduction of traditional CV and kidney risk factors, might slow the decline of eGFR to levels commonly observed in healthy individuals > 50 years of age.

However, important questions remain over the use of these newer agents in combination with each other and their efficacy and safety in CKD patients.

Unlike it was believed, SGLT-2is does not increase the risk of acute kidney injury and a meta-analysis published recently in 2022 has shown. In fact, there was a lowered risk of AKI compared to placebo.

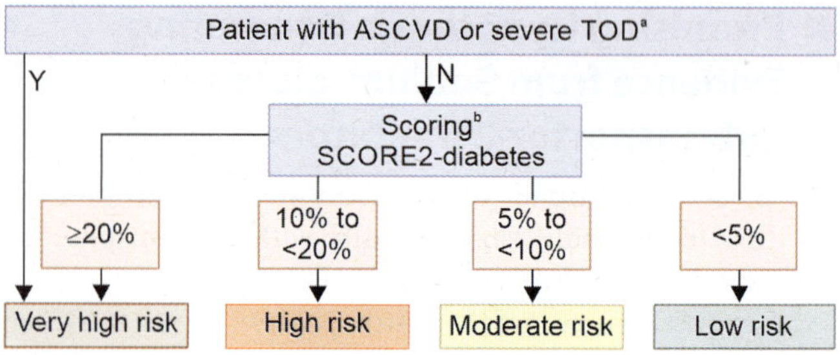

[a]Severe TOD defined as eGFR < 45 mL/1.73 m^2 irrespective of albuminuria; or eGFR 45–59 mL/min/1.73 m^2 and microalbuminuria (UACR 30–300 mg/g; stage A2); or proteinuria (UACR > 300 mg/g; stage A3), or presence of microvascular disease in at least three different sites [e.g., microalbuminuria (stage A2) plus retinopathy plus neuropathy].

[b]The thresholds (10-year CVD risk) suggested are not definitive but rather designed to prompt joint decision-making conversations with patients about intensity, as well as additional interventions. SCORE2-Diabetes refers to patients aged ≥ 40 years.

FLOWCHART 1: Cardiovascular risk categories in patients with type 2 diabetes mellitus.

(ASCVD: atherosclerotic cardiovascular disease; CVD: cardiovascular disease; eGFR: estimated glomerular filtration rate; TOD: target-organ damage; UACR: urine albumin-to-creatinine ratio)

Source: Marx N, Federici M, Schütt K, Müller-Wieland D, Ajjan RA, Antunes MJ, et al. 2023 ESC Guidelines for the management of cardiovascular disease in patients with diabetes. Eur Heart J. 2023;44(39):4043-140.

WHAT DO THE GUIDELINES SAY?

European Society of Cardiology 2023 guidelines recommend screening of patients with diabetes for the presence of severe target organ damage (TOD) (class 1A recommendation) and to estimate the 10-year ASCVD risk in T2DM patients without severe TOD or symptomatic ASCVD (class 1B recommendation).

SCORE2 algorithm for CVD risk assessment **(Flowchart 1)**.

NEED OF THE HOUR

Holistic cardiorenal metabolic risk management is relevant at every stage of cardiorenal risk continuum in people with T2DM. Evidence-based interventions should be directed at prevention, regression, and even retardation of CRM disease progression.

There is global inertia on the adoption of new cardioprotective therapies, in patients with T2DM and CVD.

In the CAPTURE study, the prevalence of CVD was reported to be 34.8% (based on data of close to 10,000 patients with T2DM from 13 countries. It is surprising to know from the study that only one out of five patients (21.5%) with CVD either had received glucagon-like peptide-1 receptor agonists (GLP-1 RA) or SGLT-2is.

CONCLUSION

- Indian people with T2DM have increased cardiorenal metabolic risk, which may begin at younger ages.
- It is possible to prevent the occurrence of diseases, events, and complications, with early and intensive multifactorial control.
- Beyond control of glycemia, personalized approaches for cardio-vascular and kidney protection are relevant early in T2DM.
- Evidence-based therapy facilitated by optimum patient education, can improve adoption, adherence, and outcomes for holistic care.

SUGGESTED READINGS

1. Anjana RM, Unnikrishnan R, Deepa M, Pradeepa R, Tandon N, Das AK, et al. Metabolic non-communicable disease health report of India: the ICMR-INDIAB national cross-sectional study (ICMR-INDIAB-17). Lancet Diabetes Endocrinol. 2023;11(7):474-89.
2. Nuffield Department of Population Health Renal Studies. SGLT2 inhibitor Meta-Analysis Cardio-Renal Trialists' Consortium. Impact of diabetes on the effects of sodium glucose co-transporter-2 inhibitors on kidney outcomes: collaborative meta-analysis of large placebo-controlled trials. Lancet. 2022;400(10365):1788-801.
3. Fernández-Fernandez B, Sarafidis P, Soler MJ, Ortiz A. EMPA-KIDNEY: expanding the range of kidney protection by SGLT2 inhibitors. Clin Kidney J. 2023;16(8):1187-98.
4. Vaduganathan M, Docherty KF, Claggett BL, Jhund PS, de Boer RA, Hernandez AF, et al. SGLT-2 inhibitors in patients with heart failure: a comprehensive meta-analysis of five randomised controlled trials. Lancet. 400(10354):757-67.
5. Marx N, Federici M, Schütt K, Müller-Wieland D, Ajjan RA, Antunes MJ, et al. 2023 ESC Guidelines for the management of cardiovascular disease in patients with diabetes. Eur Heart J. 2023;44(39):4043-140.

55

CHAPTER

Glycemic Variability versus HbA1c as Predictor of Cardiovascular Outcome

Harbir Kaur Rao, Rajinder Singh Gupta

ABSTRACT

Diabetes mellitus is one of the most common noncommunicable diseases which affect humans all over the world. Glycosylated hemoglobin (HbA1c) is currently the gold standard for assessment of long-term glycemic control and response to treatment in patients with diabetes. However, it does not address the oscillations throughout the day and between days. Recently clinicians have focused their studies on the effect of glycemic variability (GV) which is equally responsible for cardiovascular disease (CVD). Clinically GV can be measured by different parameters. Recent clinical data indicate that GV is associated with increased risk of hypoglycemia, microvascular and macrovascular complications and mortality in diabetes independently of HbA1c levels. In clinical practice, availability of continuous glucose monitoring (CGM) devices has markedly facilitated the assessment of GV and hypoglycemia. Here we review the current concepts on the definition and assessment of GV and its association with CV complications.

INTRODUCTION

Diabetes is a chronic disease with a world-wide prevalence. Global projections show an increase of 50% in the next 25 years. India is ranked second in total number of diabetic patients and is fast emerging as the world capital of diabetes. Diabetic patients have two to three times morbidity and mortality because of cardiovascular disease (CVD) and other complications.

For assessment of blood sugar control and response to therapy, glycosylated hemoglobin (HbA1c) is the gold standard investigation in patients with type 1 or 2 diabetes mellitus. Based on various epidemiological studies during the last three decades, high HbA1c is considered an important risk indicator of complications in diabetes. There are other studies which support that reduction in HbA1c is associated with significant reduction in cardiovascular risk, microvascular complications, and mortality. Recently the attention has been drawn to blood sugar variability as an independent risk factor in addition to hyperglycemia for CVD.

High glycemic variability (GV) has been associated with more risk of hypoglycemia, reduced patient quality of life, reduced patient psychological well-being, and increased risk of CVD and death in type 2 diabetic patients. Although the underlying pathogenesis is not completely understood, but the available evidence suggests that daily fluctuations in blood glucose are associated with endothelial dysfunction, inflammation, and oxidative stress. Self-monitoring of blood glucose (SMBG) and continuous glucose monitoring (CGM) are useful tools to assess GV.

Glycemic variability is defined by variation in blood glucose and related parameters over a certain time interval.

- *Short-term variability*: Short-term GV is represented by both within a day and between day-to-day GV.
- *Long-term variability*: Usually based on serial determination using HbA1c over a longer period or SMBG and CGM data.

Glycemic variability has emerged as important tool than average glucose or HbA1c in the evaluation of glycemic control and prediction of complications. GV has been associated with microvascular complications as well as increased risk of adverse cardiovascular outcomes in diabetic patients.

Continuous glucose monitoring has revolutionized blood sugar monitoring. The main CGM metrics reported with CGM use are:

- Glycemic target range/time in range (TIR) of 70–180 mg/dL
- Time spent below range or hypoglycemia (<70 mg/dL)
- Coefficient of variation (CV)—standard deviation (SD)/mean glucose
- SD is the rate of dispersion from average glycemia.

$$\text{CV (\%)} = \left(\frac{\text{Standard deviation}}{\text{Mean}}\right) \times 100$$

Present-day recommendations recommend a CV of 36% or less and is considered a marker of stable blood glucose concentration.

GLYCEMIC VARIABILITY AND CLINICAL IMPLICATIONS

Although several epidemiological investigators have identified chronic hyperglycemia as a risk factor for diabetic complications and CVD, but recently GV has been reported as an independent risk factor and predictor of bad cardiovascular outcomes. These glucose variations are independent of blood glucose and HbA1c. Thus, the gold standard HbA1c only reflects the long-term blood glucose control and not these variations. There are studies to show that the patients with same HbA1c levels have different risk of development or progression of microvascular and macrovascular complications. According to these studies, mean blood glucose and preprandial and postprandial blood glucose were significantly correlated with risk of cardiovascular complications and not HbA1c. Even there are studies which provide evidence that HbA1c variability is an independent risk factor for CVD in type 2 diabetes mellitus even when their HbA1c falls within the range recommended by the available guidelines.

Nowadays there are many indexes applied for GV measurement **(Table 1)**.

ROLE OF GLYCEMIC VARIABILITY IN SUBCLINICAL ATHEROSCLEROSIS

In subclinical atherosclerosis before plaque formation, GV leads to increased carotid intimal medial thickness (IMT). Latest meta-analysis indicates that GV reduction is accompanied by IMT decline leading to a decreased risk of acute myocardial infarction (AMI) and stroke.

Glycemic Variability and Stable Coronary Artery Disease

In stable coronary artery disease (CAD) patients, preprocedural GV was found to correlate with myocardial and renal damage markers. GV measured by mean amplitude glycemic excursion (MAGE) before percutaneous coronary intervention (PCI) was associated with increased coronary neointimal growth after 9 months of follow-up. In addition patients who were taken up for coronary artery bypass grafting (CABG) surgery, postoperative GV was associated with increased risk of postoperative atrial fibrillation (AF), cardiac arrest pneumonia, renal failure, stroke, and mortality.

TABLE 1: Glycemic variability (GV) index.

GV index	Definition
Average daily risk range (ADRR)	The sum of daily peak risks for hyperglycemia and hypoglycemia
Continuous overlapping net glycemic action (CONGA)	Intraday (within-day) glycemic variation; the SD of the differences of glucose readings for a defined period of hours
Mean and standard deviation (SD)	The amount of variation or dispersion of a data set; the SD of the data set is the square root of its variance
Coefficient of variation (CV)	The extent of variability in relation to the mean population; 100 × SD/mean of observations
Mean of daily difference (MODD)	Interday (between-day) glycemic variation; the absolute value of difference between glucose values taken on 2 consecutive days at the same time
Time in range (TIR)	The amount of time that glucose is in the target ranges between 3.9 and 10.0 mmol/L within 24 hours
Low blood glucose index (LBGI)/high blood glucose index (HBGI)	Implemented by converting glucose values into risk scores; if the risk score is below 0, then the risk is labeled LGBI; if it is above 0, then HGBI
Mean absolute glucose (MAG)	Absolute differences between sequential readings divided by the time between the first and last blood glucose measurement
Mean amplitude glycemic excursion (MAGE)	Average of all blood glucose excursions or swings (peak to trough) that are >1 SD of all measures for a glucose profile

Glycemic Variability and Coronary Plaque Vulnerability

Blood GV is also related to coronary plaque vulnerability with resultant risk of developing AMI. Higher GV was closely linked with markers of oxidative stress and inflammation. As per recent data there is evidence to show relationship of GV with vulnerability of coronary plaque because of alteration of fibrous and necrotic plaque volume in acute coronary syndrome (ACS).

Glycemic Variability and Acute Coronary Syndrome

Greater GV in patients with AMI undergoing primary PCI was independently associated with composite major adverse cardiovascular events (MACE). Other studies suggest that higher GV in ACS patients have a greater evidence of acute kidney injury, AF, longer hospital stay, and MACE for 30 days' follow-up.

PHARMACOLOGICAL TREATMENT TO CONTROL HIGH GLYCEMIC VARIABILITY

Newer antidiabetic drugs introduced during the last 15 years have a potential to stabilize the glycemic fluctuations. These include glucagon-like peptide-1 receptor (GLP1-R) agonist, sodium-glucose cotransporter 2 (SGLT-2) inhibitors, and dipeptidyl peptidase 4 (DPP-4) inhibitors. These agents alleviate GV with a low risk of hypoglycemia. Several studies have indicated an effect of DPP-4 inhibitors on GV reduction, of course with a neutral effect on cardiovascular events. SGLT-2 inhibitors and GLP-1R agonists are effective not only on attenuation of GV but also reduction of MACE. According to Mathieu et al. treatment with Dapagliflozin over 24 weeks improved TIR, mean glucose, and GV without increasing the time spent in the hypoglycemic range.

Glargine and the new long-acting insulin analogs like degludec have also been proven to be effective strategies for reducing GV. The main strategy to control GV is represented by proper CGM strategy, patient education, and use of effective GV reducing drugs.

CONCLUSION

Glycemic variability is measured by fluctuations in glycemic metrics, either short-term (within day and day-to-day variability), or long-term GV which usually involves HbA1c as well as fasting and postprandial plasma glucose values. During the past three decades HbA1c has been the main target to assess the response to diabetes treatment and reduction in HbA1c leads to lower rates of diabetes complications. Various experimental as well as clinical studies have demonstrated that glucose fluctuations are associated with oxidative stress, endothelial dysfunction, and inflammation. However, clear data confirming GV as an independent risk factor of diabetic complications is lacking. Thus in clinical practice, antidiabetic strategy should be aimed at minimizing the different components of dysglycemia including HbA1c, fasting and postprandial glucose, and GV. Future prospective randomized clinical trials using CGM are needed to evaluate the role of GV in development of CV complications.

SUGGESTED READINGS

1. Martinez M, Santamarina J, Pavesi A, Musso C, Umpierrez GE. Glycemic variability and cardiovascular disease in patients with type 2 diabetes. BMJ Open Diabetes Res Care. 2021;9(1):e002032.
2. Alfieri V, Myasoedova VA, Vinci MC, Rondinelli M, Songia P, Massaiu I, et al. The Role of Glycemic Variability in Cardiovascular Disorders. Int J Mol Sci. 2021;22(16):8393.
3. Jang JY, Moon S, Cho S, Cho KH, Oh CM. Visit-to-visit HbA1c and glucose variability and the risks of macrovascular and microvascular events in the general population. Sci Rep. 2019;9(1):1374.

56

CHAPTER

Sodium-glucose Cotransporter-2 Inhibitors for Renal Protection

Sharad N Deshmukh

ABSTRACT

Diabetes is an important cause of chronic kidney disease (CKD). Cardiovascular (CV) safety trials of sodium-glucose cotransporter-2 (SGLT-2) inhibitors demonstrated potential for renal benefits in diabetic patients. This chapter has a focus on use of SGLT-2 inhibitors in diabetic kidney disease (DKD) and non-DKD.

The CREDENCE (Canagliflozin and Renal Events in Diabetes with Established Nephropathy Clinical Evaluation) trial compared canagliflozin versus placebo in patients with DKD. In 4,401 patients with diabetes and proteinuria with urinary albumin creatinine ratio (UACR) 300–5,000 mg/g, the trial showed 30% relative risk reduction (RRR) in renal-specific end points with canagliflozin versus placebo.

The DAPA–CKD (Dapagliflozin and Prevention of Adverse Outcomes in Chronic Kidney Disease) trial recruited 4,304 patients of CKD and tried dapagliflozin against placebo. Trial recruited 58% diabetic patients and 42% nondiabetic patients with CKD. All patients had UACR from 200 to 5,000 mg/g and estimated glomerular filtration rate (eGFR) from 25 to 75 mL/min. Trial showed 39% RRR in renal-specific outcomes, in both diabetic and nondiabetic patients.

The EMPA-KIDNEY trial recruited 6,609 patients, 54% of which had DKD. This trial tried empagliflozin versus placebo. About 20% subjects had UACR below 30 mg/g and 35% subjects had eGFR below 30 mL/min. There was 28% RRR in renal endpoints with empagliflozin compared to placebo. Benefits were there even in patients with eGFR below 30 mL/min. Mechanism of renal benefits with SGLT-2 inhibitors is possibly inhibition of tubuloglomerular feedback mechanism.

INTRODUCTION

Diabetes mellitus has a prevalence of 6.9–10.2% in developed countries and almost over 7% in developing countries. Recently published ICMR-INDIAB (Indian Council of Medical Research-India Diabetes) study revealed a prevalence rate of diabetes mellitus in India as 11.3% and prevalence of prediabetics above 15%.

International Society of Nephrology's Kidney Disease Data Center Study reported 17% prevalence of chronic kidney disease (CKD) in India. A study by Rajesh Rajput et al. found 48.4% prevalence of CKD in type 2 diabetes mellitus (T2DM) patients in India.

STAGES OF DIABETIC NEPHROPATHY

The mortality and morbidity of diabetic patients is linked to microvascular and macrovascular complications associated with diabetes. Most patients at the commencement of diabetes have intraglomerular hypertension and hyperfiltration. This stage lasts for a few years. After about 5 years, patients start showing microalbuminuria which is defined as urinary albumin creatinine ratio (UACR) from 30 to 300 mg/g. Uncontrolled diabetes and hypertension results in further progression of proteinuria to macroalbuminuria defined a UACR above 300 mg/g. This is labeled as overt diabetic nephropathy. Following this there is gradual decline in estimated glomerular filtration rate (eGFR) and gradual rise in creatinine levels. Patient can progress to end-stage renal disease (ESRD) over several years.

Chronic kidney disease in diabetic patients is defined as elevated urinary albumin excretion >30 mg/g or persistent reduction in eGFR below 60 mL/min/1.73 m^2.

RECOMMENDED STEPS TO PREVENT PROGRESSION OF DIABETIC NEPHROPATHY

- Tight glycemic control during the entire course of diabetes. Both DCCT (Diabetes Control and Complications) and UKPDS (United Kingdom Prospective Diabetes Study) demonstrated reduction in microvascular events in type 1 and type 2 diabetic patients, respectively.
- *Good control of blood pressure*: Recommended targets of blood pressure control are below 130/80 mm Hg.
- *Angiotensin-converting enzyme (ACE) inhibitors or angiotensin receptor blockers (ARBs)*: Both ACE inhibitors and ARBs have been shown to reduce the surrogate end points like albuminuria by reducing the intraglomerular pressure. Though these hard renal end points are not adequately studied.
- Sodium-glucose cotransporter-2 (SGLT-2) inhibitors' use has been shown to benefit the diabetic patents in recent trials.
- *Finerenone*: This is a nonsteroidal mineralocorticoid receptor antagonist which has been shown in FIDELIO-DKD (Finerenone in Reducing Kidney Failure and Disease Progression in Diabetic Kidney Disease) trial to significantly protect the kidneys.

JOURNEY OF SGLT-2 INHIBITORS TOWARD NEPHROPROTECTION

The SGLT-2 inhibitor came into clinical use in 2013 as an antidiabetic drug. By blocking SGLT-2 receptors in proximal convoluted tubules, it prevents glucose reabsorption and sodium reabsorption and promotes excretion of glucose in urine and reduces glycemia. This is a mechanism independent of insulin secretion by pancreas. In compliance with the United States Food and Drug Administration (USFDA) guidelines, the drug underwent a cardiovascular (CV) safety trial which was mandatory for any new oral hypoglycemic drug in clinical use. EMPA-REG was the first trial in which empagliflozin was tried against placebo in diabetic patients with coronary artery disease (CAD). The drug was found to be, not only CV safe, but also offered cardioprotection by causing significant 14% RRR in 3P-MACE (3-point major adverse cardiovascular events) consisting of nonfatal myocardial infarction (MI), nonfatal strokes, and CV deaths as compared to placebo. CANVAS and DECLARE-TIMI 58 soon followed. In these CV safety trials subjects with significant kidney disease were not recruited considering the potential renal injury which SGLT-2 inhibitors may cause by virtue of its action of promoting glucose loss in urine. In these trials, SGLT-2 inhibitors were shown to be not only renally safe but were also found to be beneficial. The subsequent trials, hence, recruited patients with diabetic kidney disease (DKD) and reduced eGFR to find out efficacy of SGLT-2 inhibitors in more advanced renal disease.

CREDENCE TRIAL

CREDENCE (Canagliflozin and Renal Events in Diabetes with Established Nephropathy Clinical Evaluation) was a double-blind, randomized placebo-controlled trial in which canagliflozin 100 mg daily was tried against placebo. The trial recruited 4,401 patients, all diabetics above 30 years age, with eGFR 30–90 mL/min/1.73 m^2, UACR 300–5,000 mg/g and on a stable dose of ACE inhibitor or ARB. The primary end points were doubling of serum creatinine from baseline, reaching ESRD, needing dialysis or transplant or renal or CV death. In 2.6 years of average follow-up, trial showed 30% RRR in primary end points in patients treated with canagliflozin compared to placebo. There was a significant reduction in secondary end points namely CV deaths, heart failure hospitalization, and composite of nonfatal MI, nonfatal strokes, or CV deaths.

DAPA–CKD TRIAL

CREDENCE data showed renal benefits of canagliflozin in DKD. In CREDENCE, all patients were diabetic. This trial results also convincingly showed that renal benefits were irrespective of the glycemic control in these subjects.

DAPA-CKD (Dapagliflozin and Prevention of Adverse Outcomes in Chronic Kidney Disease) was again a double-blind randomized placebo controlled trial in which 10-mg dapagliflozin was tried against placebo. There were 4,304 subjects, above 18 years age, with eGFR > 25 mL/min and <75 mL/min/1.73 m^2, and UACR 200–5,000 mg, on stable dose of ACE inhibitor or ARB, with or without diabetes.

Median follow-up was of 2.4 years. The primary end points were sustained decline in eGFR > 50 mL/min, ESRD, or renal or CV death. The trial showed 39% RRR in patients treated with dapagliflozin versus placebo; which

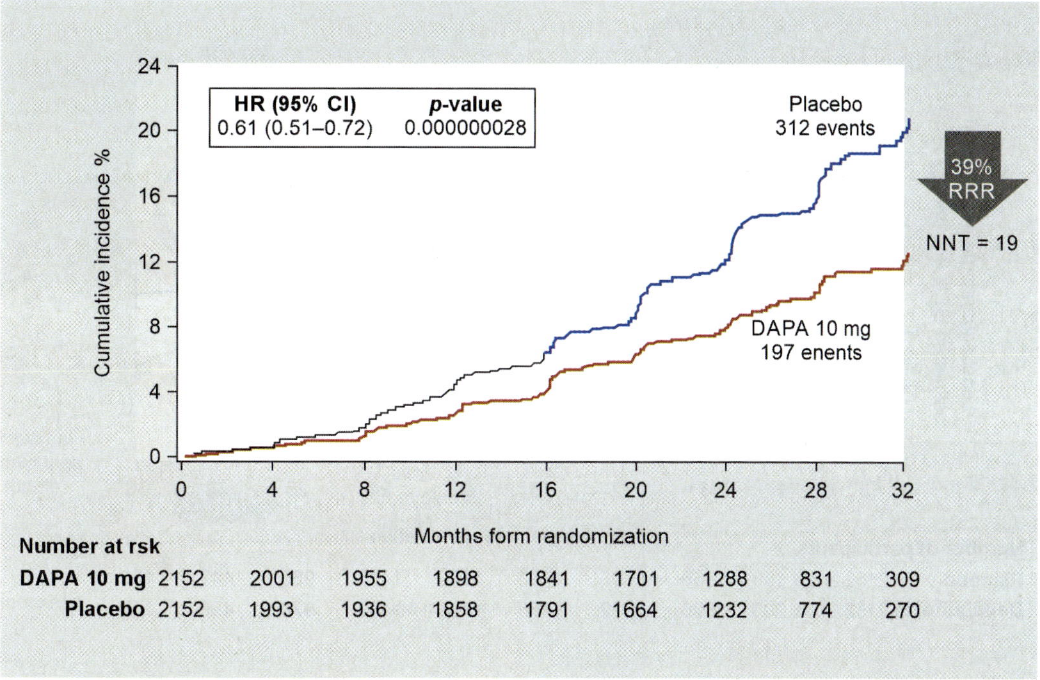

*ESKD defined as the need for maintenance dialysis (peritoneal or hemodialysis) for at least 28 days and renal transplantation or sustained eGFR < 15 mL/min/1.73 m^2 for at least 28 days. Renal death was define as death due to ESKD when dialysis treatment was deliberately withheld for any reason.

FIG. 1: Primary composite outcome: sustained ≥50% estimated glomerular filtration rate (eGFR) decline, end-stage kidney disease (ESKD), renal or cardiovascular (CV) death*.

(CI: confidence interval; DAPA: dapagliflozin; HR: hazard ratio; NNT: number needed to treat; RRR: relative risk reduction)

Sources:

1. Heerspink H. DAPA-CKD—Dapagliflozin in Patients with Chronic Kidney Disease. Presented at: ESC Congress 2020—The Digital Experience, 2020 August 29 to September 1.
2. Heerspink HJL, Stefansson BV, Chertow GM, Correa-Rotter R, Greene T, Hou FF, et al. DAPA-CKD Investigators. Rationale and protocol of the Dapagliflozin And Prevention of Adverse outcomes in Chronic Kidney Disease (DAPA-CKD) randomized controlled trial. Nephrol Dial Transplant. 2020;35(2):274-82.

was statistically significant. The secondary end points both CV-specific and renal-specific were significantly reduced **(Fig. 1)**.

It was also observed that during first 2 weeks, there was a greater reduction in eGFR in dapagliflozin-treated patients than in placebo group (–3.97 vs. –0.82 mL/min/1.73 m^2). It recovered in dapagliflozin treated patients in subsequent few months. Thereafter the rate of annual decline was smaller with dapagliflozin than placebo (–1.67 and –3.59 mL/min/1.73 m^2, respectively) **(Fig. 2)**.

When effects of dapagliflozin were studied in diabetic versus non-DKD the RRR of primary end points versus placebo was 36% in DKD and 50% in non-DKD. Even renal-specific secondary end points were significantly reduced in both DKD and non-DKD (RRR 43% and 49% respectively). The non-DKD patients were benefitted more in numbers. Thus it was clear that the renal benefits were not due to glycemic control and some other mechanism was possible.

EMPA-KIDNEY TRIAL

The EMPA-KIDNEY trial was published in January 2023 and it has widened the scope of renal benefits of SGLT-2 inhibitors. This was double-blind randomized placebo controlled trial in CKD patients. Trial recruited 6,609 patients. There were two groups of CKD patients; group with eGFR 20–45 mL/min/1.73 m^2 and group with eGFR 45–90 mL/min/1.73 m^2. The second group was with UACR above 200 mg/g. This trial included 54% patients who were nondiabetic patient.

About 20% patients had UACR below 30 mg/g. Patients received empagliflozin 10 mg or placebo and followed over 2 years. The primary endpoints were sustained reduction of eGFR > 40% or to 10 mL/min/1.73 m^2, ESRD or renal cause of death. The secondary endpoints were all hospitalizations, first occurrence of hospitalization for heart failure or CV death and all-cause mortality.

There was 28% RRR in primary composite outcome compared to placebo which was significant. Subgroup

SUGGESTED READINGS

1. Perkovic V, Jardine MJ, Neal B, Bompoint S, Heerspink HJL, Charytan DM, et al; CREDENCE Trial Investigators. Canagliflozin and Renal outcomes in Type 2 Diabetes and Nephropathy. N Engl J Med. 2019;380:2295-306.
2. Heerspink HJL, Stefánsson BV, Correa-Rotter R, Chertow GM, Greene T, Hou FF, et al; DAPA-CKD Trial Committees and Investigators. Dapagliflozin in patients with chronic kidney disease. N Engl J Med. 2020;383:1436-46.
3. The EMPA-KIDNEY Collaborative Group; Herrington WG, Staplin N, Wanner C, Green JB, Hauske SJ, Emberson JR, et al. Empagliflozin in patients with chronic kidney disease. N Engl J Med. 2023;388:117-27.

57

CHAPTER

Early Gestational Diabetes: What are the Clinical Implications?

Wesley Hannah, Ranjit Mohan Anjana, Viswanathan Mohan

ABSTRACT

Gestational diabetes mellitus (GDM) refers to glucose intolerance of any severity first diagnosed during pregnancy. Based on the trimester of pregnancy at which GDM is diagnosed, GDM can be of two types—conventional (or classical) GDM (cGDM) which is usually diagnosed between 24 and 28 weeks' gestation and early GDM (eGDM) which is diagnosed in early pregnancy, i.e., in the first trimester of pregnancy. The prevalence of eGDM varies widely in different studies because of different diagnostic criteria used to diagnose it. Very little is known about eGDM with respect to its treatment, prognosis, and outcomes. The recent ToBOGM (Treatment of BOoking Gestational diabetes Mellitus) study has shown the benefit of early diagnosis and treatment of eGDM. However, the protocol and timing for early pregnancy screening and the diagnostic criteria for eGDM are still a matter of debate. Despite this, the importance of early pregnancy screening to diagnose eGDM is now agreed upon by most professional bodies. This chapter deals with our current knowledge about eGDM with a focus on the results of the ToBOGM study.

INTRODUCTION

Gestational diabetes mellitus (GDM) is defined as *"any degree of glucose intolerance with onset or first recognition during pregnancy."* Deleterious effects of GDM on the mother and the offspring during the intrapartum and postpartum periods are well established. Hence, screening to identify women with GDM to initiate prompt management is necessary to achieve optimal glucose control. Traditionally, screening for GDM is recommended during the second or third trimester of pregnancy. Recent evidence suggests that GDM can also occur in the first trimester of pregnancy. Hence, based on which trimester GDM is diagnosed, it can be classified into two types: conventional GDM (cGDM) which is GDM diagnosed between 24 and 28 weeks' gestation and early GDM (eGDM), where the GDM occurs earlier in pregnancy, i.e., in the first trimester of pregnancy.

DIAGNOSTIC CRITERIA FOR GESTATIONAL DIABETES MELLITUS

The diagnostic criteria recommended for cGDM and eGDM are given further.

- *cGDM*: The World Health Organization (WHO) and other bodies have adopted the International Association of Diabetes in Pregnancy Study Group (IADPSG) criteria to diagnose cGDM using the following diagnostic thresholds: Fasting plasma glucose (FPG) ≥ 92 mg/dL (5.1 mmol/L) or 1-hour plasma glucose (PG) ≥ 180 mg/dL (10.0 mmol/L) or 2-hour PG 153 mg/dL (8.5 mmol/L) at 24–28 weeks' gestation.
- *eGDM*: In the first trimester of pregnancy, the International Association of Diabetes and Pregnancy Study Groups (IADPSG) earlier recommended an FPG threshold of 92–125 mg/dL (5.1–6.9 mmol/L) as a diagnostic of eGDM.

WHAT DO WE KNOW ABOUT EARLY GESTATIONAL DIABETES MELLITUS?

There are several reports on eGDM and these studies have reported on different aspects of eGDM and a brief summary is given further. For further details, refer to reference 1 which is a systematic review of eGDM published by us from which some snippets are mentioned further.

Prevalence of Early Gestational Diabetes Mellitus

The global prevalence of eGDM ranges from 0.7 to 36.8%. This wide variation is due to inconsistency in diagnostic thresholds used to diagnose eGDM.

Risk Factors for Early Gestational Diabetes Mellitus

Clinically, women diagnosed with eGDM present with unique maternal characteristics such as higher age, higher body mass index (BMI) (preconception and at booking), higher waist circumference, history of GDM in previous pregnancy, family history of diabetes, and multiparity, previous history of macrosomia or fetal loss.

Intrauterine Growth and Offspring Health in Early Gestational Diabetes Mellitus

According to the concept of fetal origins of adult disease, fetal nutrition in early pregnancy permanently programs organ development, structure, and metabolism. Studies demonstrate intrauterine growth restriction followed by catch-up growth during infant life, is associated with glucose intolerance, insulin resistance, increased blood pressure, dyslipidemia, type 2 diabetes mellitus (T2DM), cardiovascular disease (CVD), and nonalcoholic fatty liver disease. Thus, maternal hyperglycemia in early pregnancy could imprint metabolic programming on the fetus, which may lead to metabolic disorders in their adulthood.

Management of Early Gestational Diabetes Mellitus

An increased need for medical management (insulin and/or metformin) has been observed in eGDM. Earlier initiation of insulin and requirement of a higher dosage of insulin has also been reported in women with eGDM compared to cGDM. Gestational weight gain through pregnancy was observed to be higher in women with eGDM compared to cGDM.

Pregnancy Outcomes

Occurrence of adverse pregnancy outcomes such as the need for cesarean delivery, large for gestational age baby, neonatal hypoglycemia, gestational preterm delivery, congenital anomaly, gestational hypertension, perinatal death, preeclampsia, need for neonatal intensive care unit (NICU) admission, shoulder dystocia, and need for induction of labor have been reported as adverse outcomes associated with eGDM in various papers.

Postpartum Maternal Health and Early Gestational Diabetes Mellitus

Some studies have reported on the occurrence of postpartum glucose intolerance in women diagnosed with eGDM. Studies have shown that the occurrence of T2DM was higher in women diagnosed with eGDM compared to those with cGDM. However, long-term postpartum follow-up of women diagnosed with eGDM is needed.

WHO TO SCREEN FOR EARLY GESTATIONAL DIABETES MELLITUS?

In countries such as India where the prevalence of GDM is high, screening of all pregnant women for eGDM is advocated. The Australian Diabetes in Pregnancy Study Group (ADIPS) recommends selective early pregnancy screening with factors such as previous GDM, BMI ≥ 90 kg/m^2, first-degree relative with diabetes, previous macrosomia, polycystic ovary syndrome, or non-European ancestry (Asian, Indian subcontinent, Aboriginal, Torres Strait Islander, Pacific Islander, Māori, Middle Eastern, and nonwhite African). It is to be noted that even ADIPS recommend universal early pregnancy screening to identify eGDM in Indians. Most Western bodies including the American Diabetes Association (ADA) recommend selective screening for GDM, i.e., only in high-risk women. The IADPSG's oral glucose tolerance test (OGTT) thresholds were adopted by the ADIPS, the WHO, and the International Federation of Gynecology and Obstetrics (FIGO) for early pregnancy screening. The ADA recommends an FPG threshold or a glycated hemoglobin (HbA1c) threshold to diagnose early abnormal glucose metabolism. Hence, it can be seen that there is a discrepancy in the diagnostic criteria to be used for eGDM screening.

BENEFITS OF EARLY TREATMENT

A pivotal factor in advocating early screening is the potential benefit of treating those women diagnosed to have eGDM. The impact of early screening and immediate treatment on fetal, neonatal, and maternal health is being studied extensively. Earlier studies were small randomized controlled trials (RCTs) which failed to show any benefits of early treatment. However, a recent multiethnic RCT showed improvement in composite primary outcomes, including preterm birth, birthweight, birth trauma, respiratory distress, need for phototherapy, stillbirth/neonatal death, and shoulder dystocia. This is the ToBOGM (Treatment of BOoking Gestational diabetes Mellitus) study and will be described in some detail because it is a path-breaking trial.

PROTOCOL OF TREATMENT OF BOOKING GESTATIONAL DIABETES MELLITUS STUDY

The ToBOGM study is a RCT aiming to elucidate the role of early treatment in women diagnosed with hyperglycemia before 20 weeks' gestation in terms of improved obstetric outcomes. The protocol registered with Australian New Zealand Clinical Trials Registry (ACTRN12616000924459) had the following four groups:

- *Group 1—intervention group (n = 400)*: Women with eGDM randomized to early treatment formed the intervention group. Early treatment included lifestyle modification (diet and physical activity) and initiation of self-monitoring of capillary blood glucose. If required, as per the local guidelines, these women were initiated on insulin or metformin.
- *Group 2—control participants (n = 400)*: Women with eGDM randomized to the no-treatment arm formed the control group. However, they were screened again to identify cGDM between 24 and 28 weeks.
- *Group 3—decoy participants (n = 800)*: Women with a normal early OGTT who were screened at 24–28 weeks and provided the standard of care formed the decoy group. They served as a point of reference in comparing the pregnancy outcomes between the intervention and control groups mainly to eliminate a possible placebo effect.
- *Group 4—nonactive participants (n = 2,400)*: Women with a normal early OGTT who were followed by medical record review and provided the standard of care formed the nonactive group.

It was planned to recruit 4,000 women and to follow them through delivery to collect details of maternal and neonatal outcomes as given further.

- *Composite primary outcome*: Birth at <37 weeks' gestation, birth trauma, birth weight of ≥4,500 g, respiratory distress, phototherapy, stillbirth or neonatal death, or shoulder dystocia
- *Other primary outcomes*: Pregnancy-related hypertension (preeclampsia, eclampsia, or gestational hypertension) and neonatal lean body mass
- *Secondary maternal outcomes*: Total gestational weight gain, cesarean delivery, induction of labor, perineal injury, quality of life, and maternal hypoglycemia
- *Secondary neonatal outcomes*: Birth weight, large-for-gestational-age, small-for-gestational-age, mean upper-arm circumference, neonatal fat mass, severe neonatal hypoglycemia, and number of days in the NICU.

IMPLEMENTATION OF TOBOGM STUDY AND INDIAN PARTICIPATION IN THE STUDY

In the ToBOGM study, 43,721 pregnant women were approached before 20 weeks' gestation from 17 sites across Australia, Sweden, Austria, and India [the Madras Diabetes Research Foundation, Chennai (MDRF) represented India in the trial]. A total of 4,537 women consented to risk-based early screening using an OGTT as part of this study, finally at a mean gestational age of 15.6 ± 2.5 weeks (*range*: 4 to 19 weeks 6 days), 3,681 women were screened. The IADPSG OGTT thresholds—fasting glucose ≥ 92 mg/dL (≥5.1 mmol/L) or 1-hour glucose level of ≥180 mg/dL (≥10.0 mmol/L), or 2-hour glucose level of ≥153 mg/dL (≥8.5 mmol/L) were used to diagnosed eGDM. A total of 802 women were diagnosed with eGDM and they were randomized to the intervention group (*n* = 406) and control group (*n* = 396). These women were followed through pregnancy and delivery data was available in 98.9% (*n* = 793) women.

KEY FINDINGS OF THE TOBOGM STUDY

The occurrence of composite primary outcomes was reported in 24.9% (94/378) in the intervention group and 30.5% (113/370) in the control group. Thus, a clear beneficial effect was observed with a significant adjusted risk difference [–5.6 percentage points; 95% confidence interval (CI) –10.1 to –1.2; $p = 0.02$]. Greater benefits of early treatment were observed in women in the 'higher glycemic band' compared to those women in the 'lower glycemic band.' The threshold used for the 'higher glycemic band' is FPG 95–109 mg/dL (5.3–6.0 mmol/L), 1-hour > 191 mg/dL (≥10.6 mmol/L), and 2-hour glucose 162–199 mg/dL (9.0–11.0 mmol/L) and that for 'lower glycemic band' is FPG 92–94 mg/dL (5.1–5.2 mmol/L), 1-hour ≤ 190 mg/dL (10.0–10.5 mmol/L), and 2-hour 153–161 mg/dL (8.5–8.9 mmol/L). The ToBOGM study proved early treatment of women in the higher glycemic band had more beneficial results. It was also seen that women screened before 14 weeks of pregnancy had more favorable results compared to those who were screened later.

CONCLUSION

Early gestational diabetes mellitus is a growing public health problem, influencing the health of the offspring and the mother through this pregnancy and beyond. Hence, there is a need for early screening and prompt treatment of eGDM. In India, universal screening of all pregnant women for eGDM should be done in the first trimester of pregnancy. The ToBOGM study shows that women in the higher glycemic band and those screened before 14 weeks of pregnancy fared the best. These findings have widespread policy implications and it is likely that the guidelines for diagnosing and treating GDM will undergo significant changes soon.

SUGGESTED READINGS

1. Hannah W, Bhavadharini B, Beks H, Deepa M, Anjana RM, Uma R, et al. Global burden of early pregnancy gestational diabetes mellitus (eGDM): A systematic review. Acta Diabetol. 2022;59(3):403-27.
2. Immanuel J, Simmons D. Screening and Treatment for Early-Onset Gestational Diabetes Mellitus: a Systematic Review and Meta-analysis. Curr Diab Rep. 2017;17(11):115.
3. Bhattacharya S, Nagendra L, Krishnamurthy A, Lakhani OJ, Kapoor N, Kalra B, et al. Early Gestational Diabetes Mellitus: Diagnostic Strategies and Clinical Implications. Med Sci (Basel). 2021;9(4):59.
4. Raets L, Beunen K, Benhalima K. Screening for Gestational Diabetes Mellitus in Early Pregnancy: What Is the Evidence? J Clin Med. 2021;10(6):1257.
5. Simmons D, Immanuel J, Hague WM, Teede H, Nolan CJ, Peek MJ, et al.; TOBOGM Research Group. Treatment of Gestational Diabetes Mellitus Diagnosed Early in Pregnancy. N Engl J Med. 2023;388(23):2132-44.
6. Bhavadharini B, Anjana RM, Deepa M, Pradeepa R, Uma R, Saravanan P, et al. Association between number of abnormal glucose values and severity of fasting plasma glucose in IADPSG criteria and maternal outcomes in women with gestational diabetes mellitus. Acta diabetol. 2022;59(3):349-57.

58

CHAPTER

Assessment of Silent Coronary Artery Disease in Diabetes

Ashok K Taneja, Akshat Taneja, Divya Taneja

ABSTRACT

Cardiovascular and cerebrovascular diseases are the leading cause of morbidity and mortality in diabetes, accounting for a significant fraction of death index. Type 2 diabetes mellitus is a stronger risk factor for silent ischemia and infarction, with a 10× higher risk of developing a first myocardial infarction (MI). High mortality in these patients is due to coexisting diseases. Early detection and management of silent MIs are crucial for reducing cardiovascular (CV) events. Combining clinical and investigational approaches can yield good results.

INTRODUCTION

Cardiovascular and cerebrovascular diseases are the leading cause of morbidity and mortality in diabetes and this accounts for large fraction of death index. The situation is compounded if the event occurrence is in silent zone, i.e., without exhibiting signs and symptoms. Type 2 diabetes mellitus (T2DM) is recognized as a stronger risk factor for silent ischemia and infarction. Among patients of T2DM the 7-year risk of developing a first myocardial infarction (MI) is 10 fold and akin to recurrent MI in normal persons who had a previous MI. High mortality in such patients is due to clustering effect of other coexisting diseases such as Dyslipidemia/Hypertension/Genetic factors/Obesity, etc. Diabetes is considered a 'coronary artery disease (CAD) equivalent because patients with diabetes without known CAD have a similar cardiac event rate to patients without diabetes who had a prior MI.

PREVALENCE OF SILENT CORONARY ARTERY DISEASE

The prevalence of CAD especially the multi vessel CAD is 10 times greater amongst diabetics than age-sex matched nondiabetic persons. The reason, thereof, is the fact that T2DM is considered as an accelerated atherosclerosis state and poses a considerable risk for development of cardiovascular-metabolic disease. Prevalence of silent ischemia or significant cardiovascular (CV) event varies widely due to different parameters used by different investigators. Framingham study, initiated in 1948, also calculated the CV risk in asymptomatic diabetic individuals and found that at least 25% of diabetic individuals (followed for 30 years) had MIs, previously having normal electrocardiogram (ECG). Hence, the various protocols used have serious limitations. ADA in 1998 and 2008 and American Endocrine Society (2010) proposed a screening module based on age, gender, hypertension, and dyslipidemia for early detection of CAD in T2DM patients. However, subsequent studies have shown that the traditional risk factors do not accurately predict the risk for cardiovascular events in T2DM patients. This led to the developing a rationale module for an aggressive screening approach for CAD in asymptomatic patients with T2DM, independent of other risk factors. Nevertheless, there is no uniform policy regarding CAD screening in patients with T2DM, reflecting the statistical challenges of screening patients at low risk and the decisions to be made per se. In November 2013, the American College of Cardiology (ACC) and American Heart Association (AHA) released new guidelines on assessment of CV risk based on a new tool, the Race and Sex Specific Pooled Cohort Equations. These are comprehensive multivariable, multiethnic population (age 40–70 years) based risk analysis equations to predict 10 tear CV risk. In these calculations 10-year risk is defined as the risk of developing a first atherosclerotic cardiovascular disease (CVD) event (nonfatal or fatal MI and nonfatal or fatal stroke) over a 10-year period amongst people not having any previous CVD. Indian guidelines are also not evaluated or updated any protocol. Larger cohort studies confirmed that a glycemic control with hemoglobin A1c (HBA1c) of 7% resulted in approximately 50% reduction in incidence of CVD. With further tight control, the risk reduction may further be expected. Hence, a comprehensive approach that recognizes and controls multiple risk factors is the most effective management strategy in diabetics. Many associations, the world over, suggested that a risk factor-guided screening protocol be developed to identify such diabetic persons who are having asymptomatic CAD. Because delayed identification of CAD in such patients unquestionably worsens their prognoses. Thus, there should be a clear need to identify T2DM patients who are at risk for cardiovascular events before the onset of symptoms. Unfortunately, the protocols used for screening patients with T2DM for asymptomatic coronary atherosclerosis remain debatable.

Individuals, however, we can develop their own protocol. Suggested one is:

Proposed Methodology

Many protocols are in vogue but the most useful and practical is the one which is easy to implement, easy to analyze and cost effective. Following are the various parameters being used:

- *Clinical evaluation*: A detailed history and complete general physical examination (including weight, height, and waist circumference) will be performed for each subject following which they will be investigated for routine investigations (hemoglobin, total and differential leukocyte count, erythrocyte sedimentation rate, fasting and postprandial blood sugar, fasting serum lipid profile, blood urea, serum creatinine, serum bilirubin and serum liver enzymes, urine routine and microscopy, and ECG).
- *Risk factor assessment:*
    - *Age:* 40–79 years. But in India take 35–75 years of age
    - *Gender:* Higher male preponderance. After menopause male-female ratio is equal
    - Smoking/tobacco/alcohol/other addictions
    - *Body mass index:* Obesity as indicated by BMI >27 kg/m^2
    - *Waist circumference*: Central obesity as indicated by WC > 90 cm in males and > 80 cm in females
    - *Blood pressure*: Routine check and 24 hour ambulatory BP monitoring (ABPM). Hypertension evidenced by BP ≥ 140/90 mm Hg. Intense lowering of BP to < 130 mm may not be required. As per ACCORD trial, the reduction of systolic BP to 120 mm instead of 140 mm, did not yield any further benefit in CV outcome. The ADVANCE trial also indicated that intense lowering of glycemia with adequate control of BP reduced the risk of CV events.
    - *Fasting serum lipid profile*: Hypercholesterolemia ≥ 200 mg/dL, hypertriglyceridemia ≥ 150 mg/dL, high low-density lipoprotein (LDL) cholesterol ≥ 100 mg/dL and low HDL-cholesterol < 40 mg/dL in males and < 50 mg/dL in females. In the lipid arm of the ACCORD trial, the control of dyslipidemia along with HBA1c to < 7.0 was associated with reduction in CV events. Hence, it is very important to measure the lipid levels and control it by life style change and medication.
    - *Electrocardiogram:* Abnormalities of ischemia/ infarction/left ventricular hypertrophy. Also look for pathological Q waves, left bundle block (in men), trifascicular block or deep T inversion. Framingham study evidenced very clearly that over a follow-up period of 30 years, with the baseline ECG normal, the chances of getting CV events are reduced to almost 25%, by controlling lipids and glycemic parameters.
    - *6-minute walking test (6 MWT):* The 6-minute walk test (6 MWT) is a submaximal exercise test that calculates the distance walked over a span of 6 minutes. The 6-minute walk distance test provides a measure for integrated response of multiple cardiopulmonary and musculoskeletal systems involved in exercise. The 6 MWT provides information regarding functional capacity, response to therapy, and prognosis of chronic cardiopulmonary conditions. Main strengths of the 6 MWT are—it is simple to perform, very low cost, repeatable multiple times, and easy interpretation.
    - *Echocardiography:* Evidence of regional wall motion abnormality (in all 16 segments), diastolic dysfunction, or low ejection fraction. Routine calculation of LA volumes (s/o DDF) and Tie Index should be encouraged among the investigators. Strain rate imaging is very useful echocardiography mode to evaluate myocardial functioning. The high sensitivity of both TDI-derived and 2D speckle tracking derived strain and strain rate are good for the early detection of myocardial dysfunction.
    - *Stress testing-TMT:* ST segment variation, HR, BP response to exercise and origin of ventricular arrhythmias (Gr III and above).
    - *Stress/dobutamine echocardiography:* Look for evidence of stress induced hyperkinesia (assess all 16 segments); newer regurgitation in mitral or

aortic valve or area of dyskinesia. Calculate E:A ratio or LA volumes (s/o diastolic dysfunction) in pre-exercise and post-exercise phase. It is a good marker of ischemia if DDF appears afresh or increases in post-exercise phase.

- *Serum homocysteine* levels: Suggest the high likelihood prevalence of CV events in future. Exact usefulness is unclear.
- *High sensitivity troponin (hs-cTnT) and amino terminal pro-brain natriuretic peptide (NT-proBNP)* are useful in indicating to detect cardiac injury or failure. But the sensitivity and specificity of these tests to detect silent myocardial ischemia in T2DM is unknown at present.
- *Carotid intima-media thickness (CIMT):* The carotid intima-media thickness test (CIMT) is a measure used to diagnose the extent of carotid atherosclerotic vascular disease. The test measures the thickness of the inner two layers of the carotid artery the intima and media when patients are still asymptomatic. Early detection may indicate the need for a more aggressive approach to managing the risk factors associated with heart disease and stroke.
- *Calcium scoring on cardiac CT:* Since the calcium is a marker of CAD, the amount of calcium detected on a cardiac CT scan is a helpful diagnostic and prognostic tool. The findings on cardiac CT are expressed as a calcium score as it calculates the amount of calcium in atherosclerotic plaque which gives a clue to the extent of atherosclerosis in coronaries in asymptomatic individual.
- *Gadolinium enhanced cardiac magnetic resonance imaging (MRI)*: Cardiovascular magnetic resonance (CMR) study with images on LV long and short axis should be performed wherever possible. Gadolinium enhanced CMR yields better results. Analyzing endocardial and epicardial contours drawn on longitudinal and short axis of all chambers, peak global longitudinal strain, systolic strain rate and early and late diastolic strain rates provide useful information on the presence of silent myocardial ischemia.
- *Prevalence of metabolic syndrome* as determined by the National Cholesterol Education Program Adult Treatment Panel III (NCEP ATP III) criteria (with South Asian cut-offs).
- *Atherosclerotic cardiovascular disease (ASCVD) risk score* (ACC) charts.

CONCLUSION

The prevalence of silent MI is found to be 17% on detailed evaluation in diabetics. Earlier the detection, earlier the management and better the good results in reducing CV events. We should adopt an approach which should be clinical (clinical evaluation) and investigational. Combining the two with an economical protocol (India) shall yield good results. Practically clinical examination, ECG, echocardiography, stress testing, constraint-induced movement therapy (CIMT) should give us a clear picture. For more clarity one can add calcium scoring strain imaging (echocardiography) and NT-pro BNP.

SUGGESTED READINGS

1. Kannel WB, Abbott RD. Incidence and prognosis of unrecognized myocardial infarction. An update on the Framingham study. N Engl J Med. 1984;311:1144-7.
2. Prevalence of unrecognized silent myocardial ischemia and its association with atherosclerotic risk factors in noninsulin-dependent diabetes mellitus Milan Study on Atherosclerosis and Diabetes (MiSAD) Group. Am J Cardiol. 1997;79(2):134-9.
3. Wackers FJ, Young LH, Inzucchi SE, Chyun DA, Davey JA, Barrett EJ, et al. Detection of silent myocardial ischemia in asymptomatic diabetic subjects: the DIAD study. Diabetes Care. 2004;27(8):1954-61.
4. Faerman I, Faccio E, Milei J, Nunez R, Jadzinsky M, Fox D, et al. Autonomic neuropathy and painless myocardial infarction in diabetic patients. Histologic evidence of their relationship. Diabetes. 1977;26:1147-58.
5. Ambepityia G, Kopelman PG, Ingram D, Swash M, Mills PG, Timmis AD. Exertional myocardial ischemia in diabetes: a quantitative analysis of anginal perceptual threshold and the influence of autonomic function. J Am Coll Cardiol. 1990;15:72-7.
6. Langer A, Freeman MR, Josse RG, Armstrong PW. Metaiodobenzylguanidine imaging in diabetes mellitus: assessment of cardiac sympathetic denervation and its relation to autonomic dysfunction and silent myocardial ischemia. J Am Coll Cardiol. 1995;25:610-8.
7. Gottlieb SO, Gottlieb SH, Achuff SC, Baumgardner R, Mellits ED, Weisfeldt ML, et al. Silent Ischemia on Holter Monitoring Predicts Mortality in High-risk Postinfarction Patients. JAMA. 1988;259(7):1030-5.
8. Guyatt GH, Sullivan MJ, Thompson PJ. The 6-minute walk: a new measure of exercise capacity in patients with chronic heart failure. Can Med Assoc J. 1985;132:919-23.
9. Young LH, Wackers FJ, Chyun DA, Davey JA, Barrett EJ, Taillefer R, et al. Cardiac outcomes after screening for asymptomatic coronary artery disease in patients with type 2 diabetes: the DIAD study: a randomized controlled trial. J Am Med Assoc. 2009;301:1547-55.
10. Frye RL, August P, Brooks MM, Hardison RM, Kelsey SF, MacGregor JM, et al. A randomized trial of therapies for type 2 diabetes and coronary artery disease. N Engl J Med. 2009;360(24):2503-15.
11. American Diabetes Association. Standards of medical care in diabetes--2011. Diabetes Care. 2011;34(Suppl 1):S11-61.

59

CHAPTER

Peculiar Infections in Diabetes

Manoranjan Behera, Jayanta K Panda

ABSTRACT

Diabetes mellitus is a secondary immune deficiency state predisposing patients to various infections. Many specific and some exclusive peculiar infections are seen in patients with diabetes contributing to high morbidity and mortality. These peculiar infections are uncommon and usually found in subjects with uncontrolled glycemic status. They are rapidly progressive and potentially lethal. They need early recognition, hemodynamic stabilization, good glycemic control with insulin, broad-spectrum antibiotics, and surgical intervention/multidisciplinary approach as and when necessary. Despite best of management the mortality rate is alarming.

INTRODUCTION

Diabetes mellitus (DM) is considered as a secondary immune deficiency disorder by World Health Organization (WHO) as the disease is characterized by frequent, severe, prolonged, and recurrent infections due to alteration of at least one of the immune response mechanisms and elimination of underlying cause leads to resolution. This immunocompromised state predisposes the patient to increased risk of infection and sepsis which are contributing factors for increasing rate of morbidity and mortality in diabetic subjects. Several factors contribute to increased propensity for infection in patients of diabetes which includes, importantly, an altered immunity. The innate immunity is predominantly affected manifesting as dysfunction of polymorphonuclear neutrophil (PMN) cells which include dysfunction in adhesion, impaired migration, altered chemotaxis, reduced phagocytosis, oxidative burst, and capacity of microbial killing. Abnormalities in monocyte/macrophage chemotaxis and phagocytic function have also been found. Diabetes has direct inhibitory effect on the adaptive immune system as well. Certain infections associated with increased incidence in DM are genitourinary tract infections, respiratory tract infections, skin and soft tissue infections, and gastrointestinal infections. Some peculiar infections are exclusively associated with DM are rhino-orbital-cerebral-mucormycosis (ROCM), invasive malignant otitis externa, emphysematous cholecystitis (EC), emphysematous pyelonephritis (EPN), emphysematous cystitis (EC), necrotizing fasciitis (NF), and Fournier's gangrene (FG) as shown in **Box 1**.

BOX 1: Peculiar infections associated with diabetes.

- Emphysematous pyelonephritis
- Emphysematous cystitis
- Emphysematous cholecystitis
- Necrotizing fasciitis
- Fournier's gangrene
- Malignant otitis externa
- Rhinocerebral-mucormycosis

These infections are peculiar in the sense they occur most commonly or exclusively in uncontrolled diabetic patients, uncommon or rare, rapidly progressive, potentially fatal, needs high index of suspicion for early diagnosis, and aggressive multimodality treatment. Despite best of treatment the mortality is high.

EMPHYSEMATOUS PYELONEPHRITIS

Emphysematous pyelonephritis is an acute severe necrotizing infection of the renal parenchyma and its surrounding tissues resulting in accumulation of gas in the renal parenchyma, collecting system, or perinephric tissue. Uncontrolled DM is the single most common underlying associated factor found in up to 95% of patients with EPN. *Escherichia coli* is the most common causative organism, isolated from urine or pus cultures in about 70% of the reported cases. Other organisms reported are *Proteus, Klebsiella,* Enterobacteriaceae spp., group D *Streptococcus,* and coagulase-negative *Staphylococcus.*

Various postulated factors responsible for pathogenesis of EPN in diabetes are high level of glucose within the renal tissues, presence of gas-forming microorganisms, impaired blood supply due to microvascular angiopathy and deranged host immunity. A high level of tissue glucose along with vasculopathy associated ischemia of the kidneys facilitates the process of anaerobic metabolism. Gram-negative organisms like *E. coli* behave as facultative anaerobes (in absence of oxygen) and produce gas via the fermentation of glucose and lactates, resulting in accumulation of high levels of carbon dioxide and hydrogen at the site of inflammation. The air is a combination of various gases, such as carbon dioxide, hydrogen, nitrogen, oxygen, and traces of ammonia. Gas may extend from site of inflammation to the subcapsular, perirenal, and pararenal spaces.

The presenting clinical features are like those of acute pyelonephritis such as fever with chills/rigors, dysuria, hematuria, nausea, vomiting, and flank pain or pneumaturia. Other clinical manifestations may be acute renal dysfunction, altered sensorium, and rapid progression to septic shock. Loin tenderness is the most common sign and in some cases crepitus around the renal area and the scrotum may be found. Laboratory investigations may show neutrophilic leukocytosis in 70–80% cases, thrombocytopenia in 15–20% cases, hyperglycemia, acute renal failure, microscopic/macroscopic hematuria and severe proteinuria.

Emphysematous pyelonephritis is a radiological diagnosis as most of the clinical and laboratory investigations will indicate sepsis of renal origin. A plain X-ray of abdomen shows an abnormal gas shadow in the renal area raising suspicion, whereas an ultrasonography (USG) or computerized tomography (CT) of abdomen will confirm the presence of intrarenal gases **(Fig. 1)**. CT scan is the diagnostic procedure of choice as it is more sensitive and shows the extent of EPN.

Patients of DM with acute pyelonephritis and fail to respond to standard medical therapy should always be subjected to CT scan to exclude the possibility of emphysematous complications of genitourinary tract.

Emphysematous pyelonephritis is a life-threatening condition and requires urgent attention. Most of the mortality from EPN is attributable to septic complications. The bad prognostic factors are systolic blood pressure (SBP) <90 mm Hg, altered sensorium, increased serum creatinine, thrombocytopenia, and bilateral EPN.

Management includes basic resuscitation, judicious antibiotic, and glycemic control with insulin. It is necessary to maintain SBP >100 mm Hg. As gram-negative bacteria are the most common pathogen, it is prudent to start an empirical broad-spectrum antibiotic along with an aminoglycoside till culture and sensitivity report is available. Antibiotics are usually required for 6–8 weeks. The mortality from EPN is 70–80% with medical management (MM) alone. Over last few years, there is a nephron saving approach with percutaneous drainage (PCD), with or without elective nephrectomy at a later stage has reduced the mortality significantly to 21%. PCD is the procedure of choice in patients who have localized collection of gas and having functional renal tissue. Recent treatment strategies include MM alone, MM plus

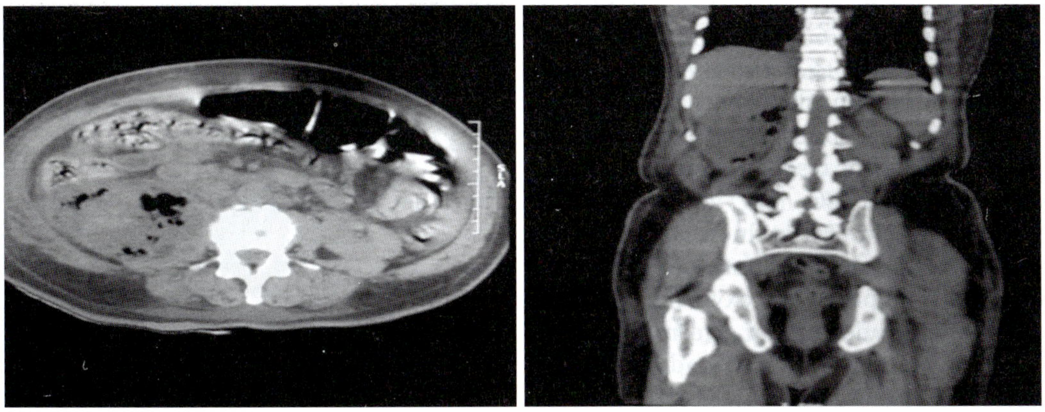

FIG. 1: Computed tomography (CT) scan of abdomen showing emphysematous pyelonephritis of right kidney.

much of the research has revolved around the role of glucotoxicity, which is the direct effect of hyperglycemia in producing damage to the beta cell and the insulin signaling pathway. People with KPD are especially prone to glucose toxicity, which triggers ketoacidosis. Despite insulin therapy, glucotoxicity takes time to resolve. This explains the gradual process that is required for recovery from ketosis and the gradual and careful process of reducing and stopping insulin. Ketosis in ketosis prone β+ diabetes is from a defective mitochondrial oxidation of ketone bodies. This makes the pathophysiology distinct from β– diabetes, where ketogenesis results from excess free fatty acid delivery to the liver following beta cell dysfunction. In addition to this reversible beta cell dysfunction, there is defective alpha cell function too, as evidenced by excess glucagon production. This alpha cell dysfunction aspect of KPD is similar to T2DM. The natural history of A–β+ KPD appears to be marked by chronic but varying dysregulation of branched chain amino acid metabolism. These branched-chain amino acids, via a peptide called B chain amino acid 9–23 related peptide, may result in immunoreactivity and beta cell dysfunction. The role of genetic factors, especially X-linked glucose-6-phosphate dehydrogenase (G6PD) deficiency in males, has been postulated as a pathogenic mechanism. There seems to be a correlation between beta cell functional reserve and erythrocyte G6PD activity. Clearly, pathophysiology of KPD requires further elucidation via research.

CLASSIFICATION OF KETOSIS PRONE DIABETES

Ketosis prone diabetes is categorized based on four different classification schemes **(Box 1)**.

Balasubramanyam et al. concluded that Aβ classification is the most accurate classification of KPD.

BOX 1: Classification of ketosis prone diabetes.

- *American Diabetes Association (ADA) system*
  - Type 1a-antibody positive type 1 diabetes mellitus
  - Idiopathic type 1 diabetes mellitus or type 1b diabetes mellitus-antibody negative type 1 diabetes mellitus
- *Modified ADA system*
  - Type 1a-antibody positive type 1 diabetes mellitus
  - Insulin-dependent ketosis prone diabetes
  - Noninsulin-dependent ketosis prone diabetes
- *Body mass index (BMI) system*
  - Lean (BMI < 28 kg/m^2)
  - Obese (BMI > 28 kg/m^2)
- *Aβ classification*
  - A+β+ (antibody positive with preserved beta cell function)
  - A+β– (antibody positive without preserved beta cell function)
  - A–β– (antibody negative without preserved beta cell function)
  - A–β+ (antibody negative with preserved beta cell function)

A+β+

A+β+ KPD group of patients have antibodies positive in the serum and have preserved beta cell function. This group of patients represent 7% of newly diagnosed cases of diabetes mellitus presenting with diabetic ketoacidosis. They are classified as having slowly progressive T1DM or latent autoimmune diabetes of the adult/one and a half diabetes. A higher incidence rate is reported in Northern Europe and parts of China. Few of the patients do not require insulin until a much later stage indicating preservation of beta cell function over a prolonged period, but most of the patients slowly progress to T1DM and require insulin supplementation for about 6 months to 3 years after the diagnosis. The decline in C-peptide levels in these patients is much slower than in T1DM. Positivity for GAD-65 antibodies is most frequently seen, and other less commonly associated antibodies such as islet antibody-2 and zinc transporter-8 antibodies are also seen. These patients are younger at the time of diagnosis and have a strong family history of autoimmunity. They are probably misdiagnosed as T2DM and emerge as clearly defined cases of T1DM over a period of time.

A+β–

This group of patients are positive for serum antibodies but does not have preserved beta cell function. Antibody positive or autoimmune diabetes, also termed type 1a diabetes mellitus is the insulin-dependent diabetes in which autoantibodies such as GAD-65 antibodies, islet antigen-2 antibodies, and zinc transporter-8 antibodies are positive, which leads to beta cell destruction and complete insulin dependency.

A–β–

In this subgroup of patients, antibodies in the serum are negative, and beta cell function is not preserved. Idiopathic T1DM or type 1b diabetes mellitus is the category of diabetes that belongs to this subgroup. The strong family history of diabetes among relatives of most A–β– KPD patients suggests a familial trait and the possibility that genes required for beta cell development, regeneration, or function may be defective.

A–β+

In this subgroup of patients, antibodies in the serum are negative, and the beta cell function is preserved.

This category is further subdivided into:

- Provoked KPD
- Unprovoked KPD

Provoked KPD is when there is a precipitating factor (such as dehydration, intercurrent infections, and noncompliant with antidiabetic treatment) leading to the development of diabetic ketoacidosis.

Unprovoked A–β + is labeled as ketosis-prone T2DM, which is a rare form of diabetes, however, it is commonly seen in African, African American, Hispanic, and some Asian populations. This entity was also termed Flatbush diabetes/atypical diabetes. They represent more than half of newly diagnosed African and Hispanic patients presenting with diabetic ketoacidosis.

Ketosis prone T2DM patients are usually males and are generally overweight with a strong family history of T2DM. This is an entity in which patients who are GAD-65 and islet autoantibodies negative present with ketoacidosis and do not have any *HLA* gene association.

MANAGEMENT

Management of Acute Ketoacidosis

Diabetic ketoacidosis is a fatal crisis that leads to increased morbidity and mortality. Therefore, timely intervention and effective management is the key. The goal of therapy in diabetic ketoacidosis is to correct the volume status, and correction of hyperglycemia. It is managed with aggressive hydration and insulin therapy, identification and treatment of precipitating factors, correction of electrolytes, and transition from intravenous to subcutaneous insulin.

Patients are discharged on a basal-bolus insulin regimen with the total dose calculated from the previous 2 days, with 50% as basal and 50% as prandial insulin.

Insulin is continued for a period of at least 2 weeks after discharge from the hospital to tide over the glucotoxic phase, especially in classic, ketosis prone T2DM. When in doubt about the diagnosis, or where there is a high risk of relapse of ketosis, insulin treatment may be needed long-term.

Glycemic Management in the First 2–10 Weeks Following Discharge

About 2–3 weeks after an acute episode, testing for beta cell function and a C-peptide level is recommended to assess the beta cell function. In all β– patients and most of the β+ patients, insulin therapy is continued.

Long-term Management

Assessing for Insulin Independence

After achieving the target levels, the insulin dose is reduced by 50% and continued. If the blood glucose levels are at the target level for two consecutive visits, the insulin is gradually withdrawn over a period of 10–14 weeks. These patients are then monitored closely, and lifestyle modification is advised. If these patients maintain their blood glucose levels at the target range without pharmacological intervention, they are advised strict diet, and weight reduction is encouraged. In case of rising blood sugars without the development of ketosis, the use of drugs like metformin is encouraged. If the blood glucose levels do not achieve target values within 8 weeks, the use of oral antidiabetic drugs like sulfonylureas, dipeptidyl peptidase-4 (DPP-4) inhibitors, glucagon-like peptide-1 (GLP-1) agonists, and alpha-glucosidase inhibitors are considered. The use of sodium-glucose cotransporter-2 (SGLT-2) inhibitors in these patients is not recommended due to the propensity to cause ketoacidosis.

Patients with unprovoked diabetic ketoacidosis have a higher chance of restoration of beta cell function and discontinuation of insulin rather than patients with provoked diabetic ketoacidosis.

In case of recurrence of ketoacidosis after withdrawing insulin, then the insulin regimen should be intensified and switching to oral antidiabetic agents is not an option even in unprovoked cases of diabetic ketoacidosis.

Some patients are able to discontinue insulin after a few months of therapy. These patients are advised lifestyle modification and weight reduction. Regular follow-up with a dietician is advised. At least 150 minutes of physical activity per week is recommended.

Assessment of Beta Cell Reserve

Beta cell reserve is assessed by measuring the fasting C-peptide levels. A low fasting C-peptide level is suggestive of poor beta cell reserve and these patients require lifelong insulin therapy. Wherever the beta cell response is improving, the dose of insulin may be reduced or even stopped.

Clinical Pointers toward Management

While it is mentioned that careful follow-up and tapering or stopping insulin is possible in many cases, the feasibility of monitoring in Indian settings has to be considered. In India, patients travel long distances to meet the diabetes specialist and regular follow-up may be difficult. In these cases, an adequate insulin prescription, either basal-bolus or at least a basal insulin (preferably an ultra-long-acting basal insulin like glargine-U-100 or degludec) is important to offer a 24-hour insulin coverage and prevent ketosis. In case the patient is on SGLT-2 inhibitors, stopping the same and observing for recurrence or careful monitoring is important to conclude whether the previous episode of ketosis was due to SGLT-2 inhibitor use or whether it was a classic case of KPD. With careful follow-up, appropriate insulin treatment, anticipating ketosis early and taking preventive steps, people with KPD, especially ketosis prone T2DM can lead a healthy life.

SUGGESTED READINGS

1. Banerji MA, Chaiken RL, Huey H, Tuomi T, Norin AJ, Mackay IR, et al. GAD antibody negative NIDDM in adult black subjects with diabetic ketoacidosis and increased frequency of human leukocyte antigen DR3 and DR4: Flatbush diabetes. Diabetes. 1994;43:741-5.
2. Balasubramanyam A, Garza G, Rodriguez L, Hampe CS, Gaur L, Lernmark Å, et al. Accuracy and predictive value of classification schemes for ketosis-prone diabetes. Diabetes Care. 2006;29:2575-9.

61

CHAPTER

Management of Diabetic Foot in Physician's Office

Ravindra Kumar Modi, Sneha Modi

ABSTRACT

Diabetic foot (DF) is a common, serious, yet a preventable problem and awareness in this field is the greatest challenge. Both patient and clinician have to participate equally to reduce the burden to save a limb. Triad of neuropathy, ischemia, and infection are the three pathological components which give rise to a wide spectrum of foot diseases that may lead to amputation at the end if ignored. Saving a limb will not only decrease morbidity and increase productivity but also reduce economic loss and mortality. Time is precious in DF disease (DFD) and early recognition and timely management can change the scenario.

INTRODUCTION

Diabetes is a major global health problem which is increasing day by day due to longer life expectancy, sedentary lifestyle, economic revolution, and changing dietary patterns. As a consequence, diabetic foot (DF) or DF disease (DFD) is also increasing and sometimes ends in the most devastating consequence such as amputation. The prevalence of DFD in India is 12–14% in urban areas and 2–3% in rural areas. DF is the result of either neuropathy or vasculopathy or from its combination and DFD is a result of complex interplay between neuropathy, peripheral arterial disease (PAD), foot deformities, and infection.

Diabetic foot disease does not spontaneously occur on its own and there are multiple messages sent by the body to alert us in the form of warning signs and symptoms so that we can predict, take action, and prevent foot at risk. In the words of Dr Elliott Joslin who recognized this long back "diabetic gangrene is not heaven sent but earth born."

SPECTRUM OF DISEASE

Diabetic foot disease may present as subjective symptoms such as dysesthesia (unpleasant sensation of burning, pain, tingling, and numbness) or may be combined with one or more objective signs which include dry skin, loss of protective sensation (LOPS), dermatophytosis of web space, blister and bullae, callosity and corn, cellulitis, foot deformities, DF ulcer (DFU), diabetic gangrene, and neuro-osteoarthropathy (Charcot's foot).

Diabetic Neuropathy

Peripheral nerve dysfunction in diabetes is called diabetic neuropathy (DN) after excluding all other possible causes of peripheral neuropathy (alcohol, B12 deficiency, neurotoxic medications, malignancies, hypothyroidism, and renal disease). Both myelinated and unmyelinated fibers are affected. Small fiber dysfunction results in pain and dysesthesia (sensory neuropathy) and large fiber involvement results in loss of proprioception, vibration, and sensory ataxia (sensorimotor neuropathy). Sensory neuropathy presents as LOPS. Motor neuropathy produces muscle weakness and intrinsic muscle atrophy, leading to functional anatomical changes due to imbalance between the flexors and extensors of toes, loss of normal plantar arch, hammer-toe formation, and development of high-pressure zones on the plantar surface of the foot at the metatarsal heads. Autonomic neuropathy is characterized by anhidrosis and altered superficial blood flow responsible for dry skin and fissure formation. Disordered proprioception and abnormal weight bearing lead to callus formation and later ulceration. Up to 50% of DN may be asymptomatic. To conclude, all forms of neuropathy make the foot vulnerable to trauma both intrinsic and extrinsic which can result in DFU.

Peripheral Arterial Disease

Atherosclerosis causes narrowing of large- and medium-sized arteries, resulting in sluggish flow of blood, causing reduced delivery of oxygen (ischemia) and nutrients in distal parts of limb, as well as deficient availability of cells and antibodies that fight against infection. Apart from diabetes, other risk factors for PAD are smoking, hypercholesterolemia, hypertension, and renal disease. PAD in diabetes commonly affects the tibial and peroneal arteries of the calf and their branches in foot.

Foot Deformities

Foot deformities may be congenital or acquired as in diabetes due to neuropathy. Sensorimotor neuropathy leads to abnormal foot muscle mechanics and structural changes in the foot. Hammer toes, hallux valgus, claw toe, prominent metatarsal heads, and Charcot's joint are a few examples. Deformities are surrogate markers of raised plantar pressure, leading to ulceration.

Infection

Hyperglycemic environment depresses the immune system and bacterial and fungal infection is common in DF. The presence of pain, erythema, fever, and leukocytosis points toward an infected wound, but these pointers may sometimes be absent in diabetic patients. Gram-positive cocci are typically the most common pathogen (superficial), but they may be polymicrobial including gram-negative rods and anaerobes (deep-seated).

Diabetic Foot Ulcer

Sixty percent of DFU are due to neuropathy. It results from mechanical trauma unnoticed due to LOPS most commonly in forefoot. Ulcer develops at sites of high-pressure zone (causing tissue ischemia) on either side planter or dorsal surface caused by bony prominence, ill-fitting footwear, and limited joint mobility (LJM) and toe deformity. Bony deformity and callus are the markers of elevated planter pressure **(Table 1)**.

Osteomyelitis

Practically in all chronic, nonhealing ulcer, osteomyelitis must be ruled out, especially when it lies over a bony prominence or if the bone can be palpated and if erythema and induration present. Plain X-ray should be done as well as probing bone by sterile probe.

TABLE 1: Wagner ulcer classification.

Grade	Lesion
0	Intact skin
1	Superficial ulcer of skin or subcutaneous tissue
2	Ulcer extends into tendon, bone, or capsule
3	Deep ulcer with osteomyelitis or abscess
4	Gangrene of toes or forefoot
5	Midfoot or hindfoot gangrene

Limb Amputation

Limb amputation is a global burden; in every 20 seconds, one limb is lost and 85% of all amputations are preceded by DFU or minor lesion.

RISK FACTORS FOR DIABETIC FOOT DISEASE

Poor glycemic control, smoking, barefoot walking, diabetic peripheral neuropathy (DPN) with LOPS, PAD, foot deformity, chronic kidney disease (CKD), callus or corn, past history of DFU or amputation, and visual impairment all are important risk factors. Foot is more commonly affected because of attainment of erect posture (tetrapod to bipedal), change in weight bearing on foot, and less care taken by the body being the distant part. Lastly, neuropathy and vasculopathy affect peripheral parts classically in diabetes.

PATHOPHYSIOLOGY

In India, neuropathy causes 75–90% of the primary foot pathology associated with diabetes. Pathological basis of neuropathy is hyperglycemia-induced metabolic abnormalities (polyol pathway, increased intracellular sorbitol and fructose, increased oxidative stress, glycation of nerve cell protein, etc. All types of neuropathies (sensory/motor/autonomic) with or without PAD super-added by infection account for the pathophysiology of majority of DF lesions. This damage may be increased in the presence of plantar callus, foot deformity, and LJM. Pathophysiology of DFU is not different. Studies have shown that a diabetic patient has 25% lifetime risk of developing a foot ulcer.

EXAMINATION

- *Inspection* for dry skin cracks, fissure, callosity, corn, fungal infection of toes, cellulitis, and ulceration.

Hot and turgid feet indicate autonomic neuropathy, cold and pale feet indicate vasculopathy, and neuropathic feet have a special appearance. There is atrophy of the intrinsic foot muscles, which allow the strong flexor muscles to draw up the toes in a "clawed" position and new pressure points emerge at the tips of the toes and the prominent metatarsal heads.

- *Neuropathy detection* or LOPS detection by 10 g nylon monofilament, 256 Hz tuning fork, pinprick, and examination of ankle jerk.
- *Vasculopathy detection*: By palpation of dorsalis pedis and posterior tibial arteries and measurement of ankle-brachial index (ABI) by vascular Doppler.
- *Footwear examination*: Good footwear can prevent many complications of DFD, so examination of footwear is an integral part of foot examination and management. Improper footwear can cause repetitive friction and may result in a sore and ulceration because a neuropathic foot can easily get injured. Impression on insole and worn-out outer sole are pointers to high plantar pressure. A rigid outsole, soft insole (microcellular rubber), roomy toe box, wide mouth, and extra depth of shoe with a counter are the features of good footwear **(Fig. 1)**.
- *Off-load devices*: Off-loading devices not only improve in healing of foot ulcers, but they can also prevent ulceration by reducing friction and ischemia. Plantar pressure reduction can be achieved by casting, removable walker, and customized footwear. Surgical off-loading is employed for forefoot pressure reduction by metatarsal head resection **(Figs. 2A to F)**.

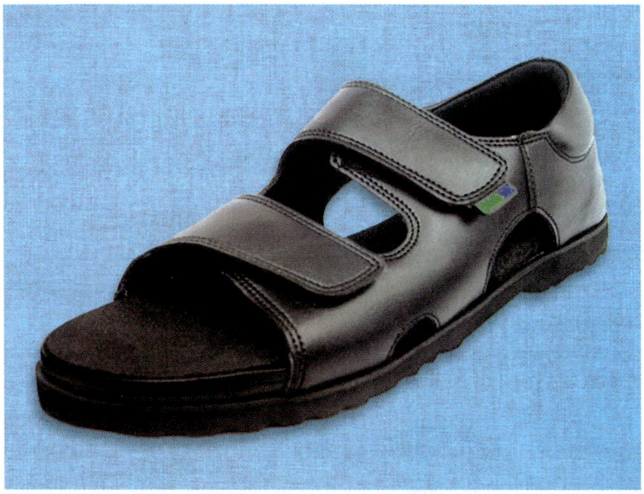

FIG. 1: Footwear.

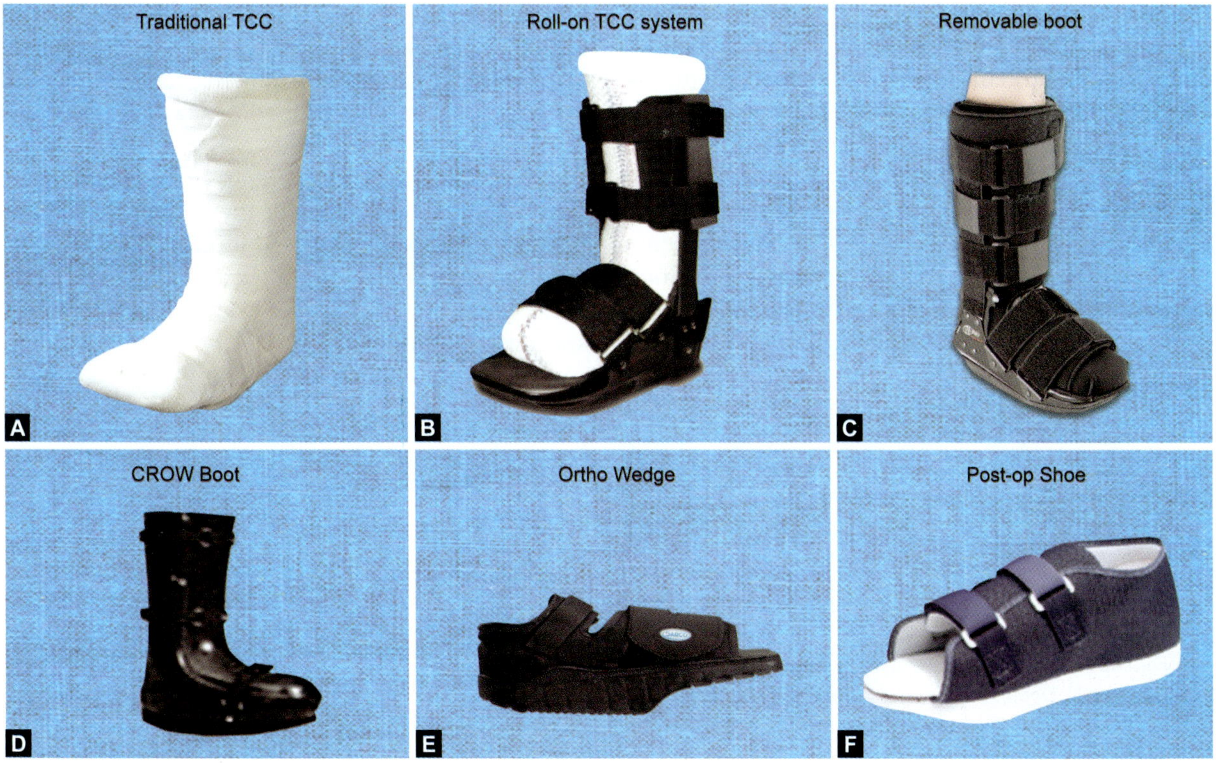

FIGS. 2A TO F: Off-load devices.

(CROW: charcot restraint orthotic walker; TCC: total contact casting)

MANAGEMENT

It requires teamwork and a multidisciplinary approach to combat this menace. The role of a physician or diabetologist is crucial. A DF can be saved with the help of a surgeon, nutritionist, diabetic nurse, foot care worker, diabetic educator, and a diabetic cobbler, among other team members; all are important for salvaging a DF.

First step is to establish nature of pathology neuropathic, ischemic, or neuroischemic. Strict metabolic control is a rule.

Second step is to classify DFD—it may be one of the three types: (1) Nonlimb-threatening (uninfected/infected), (2) limb-threatening, and (3) life-threatening (metabolic instability).

Nonlimb-threatening conditions such as callosity and corn; dermatophytosis of web space; deformities such as hallux valgus, hammer toes, fissures and cracks, and hypertrophic bursitis can be managed on outpatient basis by giving proper advice regarding foot care and footwear; minor procedures for callus and corn removal; antifungal drugs for dermatophytosis; moisturizing lotions for cracks and fissures; and advice regarding customized preventive footwear for foot with structural deformity and foot at risk (foot with LOPS). In mild infection, empirical antibiotics such as moxifloxacin, cefdinir, linezolid, cephalexin, and azithromycin can be used in usual doses for a period till infection has resolved. Limb and life-threatening conditions need indoor admission and help from a surgeon for proper management. So, identification of such conditions is important for early referral. Common indications are severe infection, metabolic instability, critical foot ischemia, need for continuous observation, and need for surgical procedure. Physicians must consult with the surgeons to discuss the management strategy for correcting dehydration with the appropriate intravenous fluid, the insulin infusion schedule for correcting hyperglycemia, and the choice of empirical antibiotics in consideration of renal status before the results of culture sensitivity comes.

In limb-threatening conditions, preferred intravenous antibiotics are cefoperazone/sulbactam (2g 12 hourly) + metronidazole (500 mg 8 hourly), or moxifloxacin (400 mg OD) + metronidazole (500 mg 8 hourly).

For life-threatening or severe infection, piperacillin/tazobactam (4.5 g 8 hourly) + amikacin (15 mg/kg OD) or meropenem (1 g 8 hourly) or clindamycin (600 mg 8 hourly) + amikacin (15 mg/kg OD). Intravenous tigecycline, vancomycin, and ciprofloxacin can be added if required.

Best dressing material for DF is normal saline and use of Savlon, betadine, and hydrogen peroxide (H_2O_2); eusol is not suitable for diabetic wounds because they have direct cytotoxic effect on fibroblast and keratinocytes. Other dressing materials are hydrogel, hydrocolloid, alginates, collagen, and growth factors. Use of topical antibiotics is good for keeping the wound moist ideal for healing of diabetic wounds. Ointments such as metrogyl, silver sulfadiazine, mupirocin [gram-positive cocci MRSA (methicillin-resistant *Staphylococcus aureus*)], nadifloxacin (gram-positive cocci, anaerobes, and gram-negative bacteria), ensamycin (pseudomonas). Always remember that the final choice of antibiotics depends on the results of culture sensitivity. Clindamycin, azithromycin, and moxifloxacin can be safely used for patients with impaired renal function, but for rest mentioned antibiotics, dose adjustment is necessary. So to conclude, tight metabolic control, extensive debridement, appropriate antibiotics, and off-loading of wounds are pillars of management of DF.

Preventive care and awareness are imperative not just for the clinician but also for the patient. Daily foot inspection, use of appropriate footwear, use of moisturizing lotion, patient education—all bear importance. Clinicians must conduct periodic foot examinations while paying special attention to LOPS, PAD, deformities, history of ulcers, and amputation.

SUGGESTED READINGS

1. Abbas ZG, Viswanathan V. The diabetic foot in Africa and India. Int Diab Monit. 2007;19:8-12.
2. Joslin EP. The menace of diabetic gangrene. N Engl J Med. 1934;211:16-20.
3. Katsilambros N. Who is the patient at risk for foot ulceration? In: Katsilambros N, Dounis E, Tsapogas P, Tentolouris N (Eds). Atlas of the Diabetic Foot. Chichester; Hoboken, NJ: Wiley; 2003. pp. 1-21.
4. Powers AC, Stafford JM, Rickels MR. Diabetes Mellitus: Complications. In: Jameson J, Fauci AS, Kasper DL, Hauser SL, Longo DL, Loscalzo J (Eds). Harrison's Principles of Internal Medicine, 20th edition. USA: McGraw Hill; 2018.
5. Simmons Z, Feldman E. Update on diabetic neuropathy. Curr Opin Neurol. 2002;15:595-603.
6. Singh N, Armstrong DG, Lipsky BA. Preventing foot ulcers in patients with diabetes. JAMA. 2005;293:217-28.
7. Bowering CK: Diabetic foot ulcers: pathophysiology, assessment, and therapy. Can Fam Phys. 2001;47:1007-16.
8. Wagner F. A classification and treatment program for diabetic, neuropathic, and dysvascular foot problems. Instr Course Lect. 1979;28(1):143-65.

62

CHAPTER

Male Sexual Dysfunction in Diabetes

Raveendran AV

ABSTRACT

Sexual dysfunctions are common in people with diabetes. Commonly reported sexual dysfunctions in people with diabetes include erectile dysfunction (ED), premature ejaculation (PE), low desire disorder, and retrograde ejaculation (RE) or anejaculation (AE). Proper knowledge about sexual dysfunction helps in the management of such conditions.

INTRODUCTION

Sexual dysfunctions are common, but least addressed in day-to-day clinical practice. Sexual dysfunction leads to inability to engage in satisfactory sexual activities resulting in relationship issues and psychological stress. Diabetes mellitus (DM) is a common metabolic disorder characterized by chronic hyperglycemia and is associated with various short- and long-term complications. The prevalence of diabetes is increasing worldwide. It has got a significant impact on the sexual health of both men and women leading to various sexual dysfunctions.

MALE SEXUAL DYSFUNCTION IN DIABETES

Common sexual dysfunctions in people with diabetes include erectile dysfunction (ED), premature ejaculation (PE), low desire disorder, and retrograde ejaculation (RE) or anejaculation (AE).

Erectile dysfunction is common in people with diabetes and the risk is threefold higher compared to people without diabetes. ED can be a presenting symptom of diabetes. ED occurs 10–15 years earlier in men with diabetes and it is a strong indicator of underlying atherosclerotic vascular illness. People with ED may be having underlying coronary artery disease (CAD) or develop CAD within 3–5 years after the onset of ED. Hence, in people with diabetes presenting with ED, cardiac evaluation is indicated and it will help to prevent the future development of acute coronary syndrome.

Erectile dysfunction is a clinical diagnosis. In people presenting with ED look for risk factors like diabetes, hypertension, dyslipidemia, and metabolic syndrome. Look for evidence of atherosclerotic vascular disease, especially CAD.

Control of blood sugar and other risk factors is important in the treatment of ED. Phosphodiesterase-5 (PDE5) inhibitors revolutionized the treatment of ED. Sildenafil and tadalafil are commonly prescribed PDE5 inhibitors. Treatment options in PDE5 inhibitor non-responders include intracavernous injection therapy, vacuum constriction device, combination therapy, or penile prosthesis.

Sexual desire or interest is complex and influenced by various factors like biological, psychological, and social factors. Hormones and neurotransmitters like testosterone, estrogen, dopamine, and oxytocin influence sexual desire. Usually, people with diminished desire present with decreased interest in any type of sexual activities including masturbation, sexual thoughts, and fantasies. The presence of other sexual dysfunction like ED and PE can lead to low sexual desire.

Premature ejaculation or early ejaculation is also quite commonly reported in people with diabetes. Diagnosis of PE is a challenge due to subjective and various vague terminology in the case definition. Our proposed diagnostic criteria help clinicians to make a diagnosis. People with PE present with a history suggestive of early ejaculation which is usually associated with psychological distress and relationship issues.

The exact mechanism of PE in people with diabetes is still not clear. The proposed mechanism includes diabetic autonomic neuropathy, neurotransmitter dysfunction, psychogenic factors, diabetes distress, performance anxiety, and depression. In people with diabetes, PE is associated with increased duration of diabetes and poor glycemic control. The treatment of PE in people with DM includes metabolic control, non-pharmacological measures like "stop-start" and "squeeze" techniques, pelvic floor exercise, and medications like selective serotonin reuptake inhibitor (SSRI), tramadol, and dapoxetine.

Retrograde ejaculation is a condition associated with the abnormal passing of ejaculate into the urinary bladder after deposition into the posterior urethra following orgasm in contrast to normal antegrade ejaculation, where ejaculate comes out of the external urethral meatus. It is also described with increased frequency in people with diabetes. Dysfunction of the internal urethral sphincter mechanism due to diabetic autonomic neuropathy leads to RE. People with RE notice cloudy urine following orgasm and post ejaculatory urine examination shows spermatozoa. RE is also associated with fertility issues. Sympathomimetics with alpha-1 adrenergic action like imipramine and pseudoephedrine are useful in the treatment of RE.

Delayed ejaculation (DE) or AE is associated with marked delay or absence of ejaculation is also seen commonly in people with diabetes. Cabergoline, bupropion, and pseudoephedrine are the agents used in the treatment of DE/AE.

People with diabetes have various changes in semen quality. In people with diabetes low testosterone levels are seen which is due to impaired Leydig cell function. All these can result in fertility issues in people with diabetes.

CONCLUSION

Sexual dysfunction is common in people with diabetes. ED is a marker of atherosclerotic vascular disease. Ejaculatory dysfunction is associated with diabetes autonomic neuropathy. A proper understanding of sexual dysfunction helps to formulate treatment strategies.

SUGGESTED READINGS

1. Defeudis G, Mazzilli R, Tenuta M, Rossini G, Zamponi V, Olana S, et al. Erectile dysfunction and diabetes: A melting pot of circumstances and treatments. Diabetes Metab Res Rev. 2022;38(2):e3494.
2. Raveendran AV. Premature Ejaculation: Proposed Diagnostic Criteria, A Letter to Editor. Mens Health J. 2022;6(1):e9.
3. Raveendran AV, Agarwal A. Premature ejaculation—current concepts in the management: A narrative review. Int J Reprod Biomed. 2021;19(1):5-22.

63

CHAPTER

Diabetes and Nuts

SK Gautam, Atul Gupta

ABSTRACT

Diabetes is a continuously growing global concern affecting > 10% of adults, which may be mitigated by modifiable lifestyle factors. Lifestyle changes, related to nutrition, reduce the risk of developing diabetes and help in management of diabetes. Current diabetes guidelines recommend Mediterranean and vegetarian dietary patterns, which encourage the consumption of nuts. Nuts, classified by tree nuts (almonds, Brazil nuts, cashews, hazelnuts, macadamias, pecans, pine nuts, pistachios, and walnuts) and peanuts (technically a legume, but sharing a similar nutritional and culinary profile to tree nuts, so they are kept under the "nuts" classification). Nuts are nutrient-dense foods with complex matrices providing unsaturated fatty acid, bioactive compounds, plant protein, phenolic compound, nonsodium minerals. Findings suggest higher nut consumption may have beneficial effects on diabetes prevention and management. Studies have demonstrated reductions in postprandial glucose levels, and long-term trials have indicated modest positive effects on blood glucose control, as shown by reductions in HbA1c and fasting blood glucose. Although inability to determine the causation and lack of ability to establish a temporal relationship between exposure and outcome are limited by cross-sectional and prospective cohort study design. So, further meta-analysis with large sample size is required to establish the role of nuts in prevention and management of diabetes.

INTRODUCTION

Type 2 diabetes mellitus (T2DM) is one of the challenging and prevalent metabolic disorders affecting around 10.5% of adult population worldwide. Within last 2 years, prevalence has increased by an alarming rate of 16%. As per the IDF Diabetes Atlas 10th edition 2021 diabetes worldwide projections, there are currently 537 million people of working age (20–64 years) with diagnosed or undiagnosed diabetes in 2021. If current trends continue, 783.2 million adults will have diabetes by 2045.

India ranks number two in the list of countries with the largest numbers of adults with diabetes in 2021 and is anticipated to remain so in 2030 and 2045 as well. Around 11% of adults across the world are have impaired glucose tolerance and are the risk of developing T2DM.

Lifestyle modification including nutrition intake is an important approach in prevention and management of diabetes. Recent guidelines recommend Mediterranean diet which includes high consumption of nuts. As per the various guidelines for dietetic management of diabetes, consumption of nuts and their inclusion in diet are beneficial for health; however, specific recommendations related to nuts for prevention and management of diabetes have been limited.

NUTS AND GLUCOSE METABOLISM

Few epidemiological studies have evaluated the relation between nut consumption and markers of glycemic control. One such prospective population-based study, Tehran Lipid and Glucose Study (TLGS), concluded a lower fasting serum glucose with higher intake of nuts.

In one cross-sectional study, National Health and Nutrition Examination Survey (NHANES, 2005–10), higher nut intake was found to be significantly related to lower fasting blood glucose, plasma insulin, homeostasis model assessment-insulin resistance (HOMA-IR), glycated hemoglobin (HbA1c), and oral glucose tolerance test (OGTT).

Based on the clinical trial evidence, when high glycemic index (GI) foods are consumed with the nuts alone, it show a lower postprandial glycemia compared to high GI foods alone. Several clinical trials have studied the effect of almond consumption on management of postprandial hyperglycemia. In nondiabetic individuals, the consumption of almonds with high carbohydrate diet (white bread) was shown to significantly decreases the postprandial area under the insulin concentration versus time curve when compared to a high GI meal and significantly lower the glucose peak height when compared with white bread.

Several systematic reviews and meta-analyses (SRMAs) of randomized controlled trials (RCTs) of various durations conducted to see the effect of a tree nut(s) on markers of glycemic control in people with different health statuses (the effect of tree nuts on markers of glycemic control in T2DM). In 2014, SRMA of 49 RCTs was conducted to assess the effect of tree nuts on metabolic syndrome criteria including fasting glucose. Twenty-six trials were included for fasting glucose, which showed tree nuts significantly lowered fasting glucose compared with the control group **(Table 1)**.

Nuts

It is advisable to consume certain nuts every day for healthy life. But if you have diabetes, then consuming all types of nuts might not be a good idea for you. Some nuts are better than others for people suffering from diabetes. Nuts, classified by tree nuts (almonds, Brazil nuts, cashews, hazelnuts, macadamias, pecans, pine nuts, pistachios, and walnuts) and peanuts (technically a legume, but sharing a similar nutritional and culinary profile to tree nuts, hence, they are kept under the "nuts" classification). Nuts are nutrient-dense foods with complex matrices providing unsaturated fatty acid, bioactive compounds, plant protein, phenolic compound, and nonsodium minerals **(Table 2)**.

TABLE 1: Association between nut consumption and markers of glycemic control.

Findings	Level of evidence	
Epidemiological evidence		
Fasting blood glucose	↓	+
Plasma insulin	↓	+
HOMA-IR	↓	+
HOMA-β	↓	+
HbA1c	↓	+
OGTT	↓	+
Diabetes incidence	↓/↔	+
Diabetes prevalence	↓/↔	+
CVD incidence in participants with T2DM	↓	+
Diabetes mortality	↓	++
Clinical trial evidence		
Acute trial evidence		
In participants free of T2DM:		
Postprandial glycemia	↓	++
Postprandial insulinemia	↓/↔	+
In participants with T2DM:		
Postprandial glycemia	↓	+
Postprandial insulinemia	↓/↔	+
Glucose metabolic clearance rate	↑	+
Longer-term trial evidence:		
In participants free of T2DM at baseline:		
Diabetes incidence	↓/↔	+
In participants with T2DM at baseline:		
Fasting glucose	↓	+
Fasting insulin	↔	+
HbA1c	↓	+

(CVD: cardiovascular disease; HbA1c: glycated hemoglobin; HOMA-β: homeostasis model assessment of β-cell function; HOMA-IR: homeostasis model assessment-insulin resistance; OGTT: oral glucose tolerance test; T2DM: type 2 diabetes mellitus)

POSSIBLE MECHANISM OF ACTION OF NUTS IN DIABETES PREVENTION AND MANAGEMENT

There are several proposed effects of the constituents of nuts which may act together in prevention and management of T2DM.

The macro, micro, and other bioactive compounds present in the nuts to regulate postprandial glycemic and insulinemic levels. In addition, they aid in body weight management, have anti-inflammatory and antioxidant properties, control cellular membrane fluidity and protect β-cells against glucose toxicity, microRNAs (miRNAs), and pancreatic insulin secretion.

Related to Macronutrients

Nuts have *low GI*, have low amount of carbohydrates, and do not contribute to postprandial glycemia. When they are added with high glycemic foods, they demonstrate dose-dependent reduction in GI or relative glycemic response of the composite meal.

TABLE 2: Macro- and micronutrient composition of 1 ounce (28 g) of whole natural nuts.

	Almonds	Walnuts	Hazelnuts	Pistachios	Macadamias
Nutrient					
Water (g)	1.5	1.2	1.5	1.1	0.4
Energy (kcal)	163.9	185.4	178.0	157.9	203.6
Protein (g)	6.0	4.3	4.2	5.9	2.2
Total lipid (g)	14.4	18.5	17.2	12.6	21.5
Carbohydrates, by difference, (g)	5.6	3.9	4.7	7.9	3.9
Fiber, total dietary, (g)	3.3	1.9	2.8	2.9	2.4
Sugars, total, (g)	1.4	0.7	1.2	2.2	1.3
Minerals (mg)					
Calcium	70.3	27.8	32.3	30.3	24.1
Iron	1.2	0.8	1.3	1.2	1.0
Magnesium	78.0	44.8	46.2	34.3	36.9
Phosphorus	134.4	98.1	82.2	138.9	53.3
Potassium	206.4	125.0	192.8	290.6	104.3
Sodium	0.3	0.6	0.0	0.3	1.4
Zinc	1.0	0.9	0.7	0.6	0.4
Copper	0.3	0.5	0.5	0.4	0.2
Manganese	0.7	1.0	1.8	0.3	1.2
Selenium	1.2	1.3	1.1	2.0	1.0
Nutrient					
Selenium	1.2	1.3	1.1	2.0	1.0
Vitamins (mg)					
Vitamin C	0.0	0.4	1.8	1.4	0.3
Thiamin	0.1	0.1	0.2	0.2	0.3
Riboflavin	0.2	0.0	0.0	0.0	0.0
Niacin	1.1	0.6	0.5	0.4	0.7
Pantothenic acid	0.1	0.2	0.3	0.1	0.2
Vitamin B6 (µg)	0.0	0.2	0.2	0.5	0.1
Folate, total, (µg)	8.2	27.8	32.0	14.5	3.1
Vitamin B12 (µg)	0.0	0.0	0.0	0.0	0.0
Vitamin A	0.8	3.5	3.4	47	0.0
Vitamin E	7.4	0.8	4.3	1.3	0.2
α-tocopherol	7.3	0.2	4.3	0.7	0.2
Lipids					
SFA	1.1	1.7	1.3	1.5	3.4
MUFA	9.1	2.5	12.9	6.6	16.7
PUFA	3.5	13.4	2.2	3.8	0.4
Phytosterols	34.0	20.4	27.2	60.7	32.9
Amino acids					
Lysine	0.2	0.1	0.1	0.3	0.0
Arginine	0.7	0.6	0.6	0.6	0.4

(MUFA: monounsaturated fatty acid; PUFA: polyunsaturated fatty acid; SFA: saturated fatty acid)

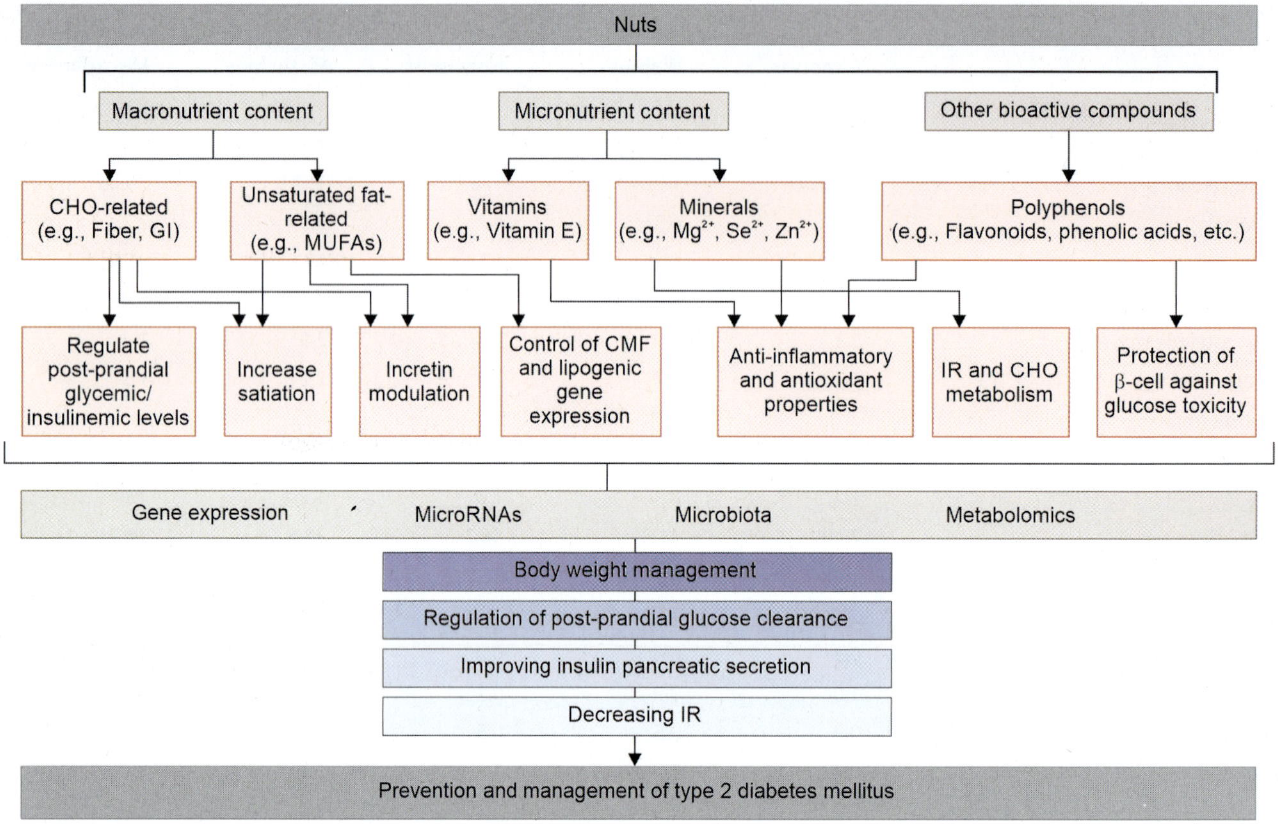

FLOWCHART 1: Mechanisms of action of nuts in diabetes prevention and management.
(GI: gastrointestinal; IR: insulin resistance; MUFAs: monounsaturated fatty acids)

Studies have shown an increase in energy density from high fat-protein foods and decrease gastric emptying, which can cause feelings of satiety and would decrease postprandial glycemic response.

Dietary fiber in nuts contributes to low postprandial spike by increase the viscosity of the food thereby slow down the absorption of the food. They are also resistant by gut enzymes; therefore, undergo fermentation in colon by gut bacteria leads to the production of short-chain fatty acids (SCFAs) **(Flowchart 1)**.

Short-chain fatty acids have been found to have the property to reduce the glucose output by the liver and stimulate the secretion of incretin hormone glucagon like peptide-1 (GLP-1) which in turn has positive impact on glucose metabolism.

Nuts have *high unsaturated fat* and many studies conclude that its substitution from carbohydrate and saturated fats are found to be beneficial for insulin sensitivity. Insulin sensitivity can be affected by quality of dietary fat which affects the composition of membrane and function.

Gene expression and enzyme activity are also affected by the quality of dietary fat. Omega-6 and Omega-3 polyunsaturated fatty acids (PUFAs) found to suppress lipogenic genes and induce the genes involves in fatty acid oxidation, which in turn may reduce hepatic insulin resistance. Several RCTs have shown that the supplementation with omega-3 fatty acid to people with T2DM causes significant lowering in HbA1c, fasting glucose, and HOMA-IR.

Related to Vitamins and Minerals

While direct evidence is not available about the micronutrient present in the nuts and its impact on prevention and management of T2DM, there are evidences from oral supplementation studies about the benefits of the vitamin and minerals present in nuts. When oral supplementation of antioxidant and vitamins like vitamin E (200–800 IU/day) and minerals like zinc (30–660 mg/day) were given to people with T2DM, reduction in HbA1c and fasting blood sugar were found, respectively.

Oral magnesium supplementation equivalent to just over half cup of nuts significantly improved glycemic control indicators. Low magnesium levels in the body have been shown to inhibit glucose transporter type 4 (GLUT-4), increase insulin resistance, affect lipid metabolism, and cause oxidative stress. However, when magnesium is consumed as a constitute of nuts, it responds differently than the oral supplement, so the further investigation is required to establish its role in T2DM prevention and management.

Phenolics and Other Bioactive Compounds

Polyphenols have anti-inflammatory and antioxidant properties and radical scavenging activity. These ways may reduce the risk of developing diabetes and its complication. They may also protective by modifying gut microbiota.

Cellular and Molecular Mechanism

Bioactive compounds in nuts prevent the diabetes through various mechanisms including modification of gut microbiota, modifying gene expression, or mediating gene expression through miRNAs.

Gut Microbiota

Nuts content like fibers and polyphenols are not digested by the gut enzymes and reach the colon, interact with gut microbials, and change their composition. Fermentation of fibers by the colonic microbes leads to the production of metabolites like SCFA, which acts as prebiotics and has good effect on homeostasis of gut microbes. SCFA reduces motility of gut and appetite stimulating peptide YY, also triggers GLP-1, which maintains glucose homeostasis by lowering glucagon and increases insulin secretion.

Undigested polyphenols exert prebiotic effect by promoting growth of some specific bacteria like *Bifidobacterium* which has been associated with improved glucose tolerance and diminished inflammatory markers.

Gene Expression

Modulation of the gene expression may be one of the ways by which components of the nuts or their metabolites affect the insulin resistance, carbohydrate metabolism, and adiposity. Expression of interleukin-6 and resistin is significantly reduced in pistachio consumption in comparison to control as shown by gene expression data. Also, the consumption of pistachio facilitates glucose transporter gene as assessed by *SLC2A3* and *SLC2A4*. In patient with T2DM and impaired glucose metabolism, increased expression of *SLC2A4* protein on the lymphocyte surface has been described and it suggests how the pistachio could improve systemic inflammatory profile increasing insulin sensitivity.

MicroRNAs

Nuts may modulate the expression of genes related to glucose metabolism through the mediatory effect of nutrients on miRNAs, defined as small noncoding RNAs of 20–25 nucleotides that post-transcriptionally and negatively regulate the expression of the genes.

In 8 weeks of following a PUFA-enriched (achieved via daily intake of 30 g of almonds and walnuts) normal caloric diet resulted in significant modifications to several common miRNAs like changes in circulating PUFAs were associated with changes of plasma miRNA-106a, changes in plasma miRNA-130b and miRNA-221 were associated with changes in plasma C-reactive protein, and changes in plasma miRNA-125a-5p were associated with changes in plasma fasting triglycerides and adiponectin levels.

EPIRDERM study shows that seven human circulating miRNAs were selected for analysis, which are considered widely related to glucose metabolism, insulin resistance status, prediabetes status, and biomarkers of T2DM. After pistachio intervention, circulation of miRNA-192 and miRNA-375 is significantly reduced. Lowering in their circulation is positively associated with insulin, plasma glucose level, and insulin resistance. Increase in these miRNAs is associated with the insulin resistance.

Results from trials have shown that PUFA-enriched nuts significantly change the various miRNAs. Changes in C-reactive protein level is linked with plasma miRNA-106a, miRNA-130b, and miRNA-221.

LIMITATIONS

Inability to determine the causation and lack of ability to establish a temporal relationship between exposure and outcome are limited by cross-sectional and prospective cohort study design. Most of the studies have collected the data by food frequency questionnaires (FFQs) which have the inherent property of recall bias and measurement error. These FFQs involve the question which assesses the combination of nuts, not the specific type of nut. It also does not provide the data about their preparation that whether they are raw, roasted, or salted. Only the few cohort studies include the repeated measure of nuts and other dietary factors. Sample size of the various studies is also small which questions about its generalization over all the population. The effects still to be confirmed by the updated SRMAs study individuals without diabetes and with diabetes separately and without mixing the nuts with the nut extracts.

CONCLUSION

Findings suggest that higher nut consumption may have beneficial effects on diabetes prevention and management. Studies have demonstrated reductions in postprandial glucose levels, and long-term trials have indicated modest positive effects on blood glucose control as shown by reductions in HbA1c and fasting blood glucose. More understanding about mechanism of action of various constituents in nuts (micro and macro) will provide future role of nut consumption in prevention and management of diabetes.

SUGGESTED READINGS

1. Park SK, Oh CM, Jung JY. The Association between Insulin Resistance and the Consumption of Nut Including Peanut, Pine Nut and Almonds in Working-Aged Korean Population. Public Health Nutr. 2022; 25:1904-11.
2. Becerra-Tomás N, Paz-Graniel I, Hernández-Alonso P, Jenkins DJA, Kendall CWC, Sievenpiper JL, et al. Nut consumption and type 2 diabetes risk: a systematic review and meta-analysis of observational studies. Am J Clin Nutr. 2021;113(4):960-71.
3. Pan A, Sun Q, Manson JE, Willett WC, Hu FB. Walnut consumption is associated with lower risk of type 2 diabetes in women. J Nutr. 2013;143(4):512-8.
4. Micek A, Godos J, Cernigliaro A, Cincione RI, Buscemi S, Libra M, et al. Total Nut, Tree Nut, and Peanut Consumption and Metabolic Status in Southern Italian Adults. Int J Environ Res Public Health. 2021;18(4):1847.
5. Muley A, Fernandez R, Ellwood L, Muley P, Shah M. Effect of tree nuts on glycemic outcomes in adults with type 2 diabetes mellitus: a systematic review. JBI Evid Synth. 2021;19(5):966-1002.

64

CHAPTER

Artificial Sweeteners in Diabetes: Must Know

Jitendra Singh, Mritunjay Kumar

ABSTRACT

Artificial sweeteners (AS), also known as very low-calorie sweeteners (LCS), non-nutritive sweeteners (NNS), noncaloric sweeteners, and intense sweeteners are by definition sweeter per gram than caloric sweeteners such as sucrose, corn syrups, and fruit juice concentrates. NNS are a common ingredient in hundreds of foods and beverages in our present food supply, including diet soft drinks, yoghurt, sweets, and gum. Food makers frequently combine NNS with sugar or other ingredients to make NNS more palatable. Reviewing the literature is the primary purpose of this chapter to ascertain whether there were sufficient data to offer recommendations for using NNS.

INTRODUCTION

Artificial sweeteners (AS) also called non-nutritive sweeteners (NNS), represent the sweetness of sugar but contain neither calories nor carbohydrates. Simply said, AS do not raise blood sugar levels.

Worldwide, obesity is a significant public health concern, and over the past few decades, its incidence has increased. It is regarded as the primary contributor to comorbidities that result in diabetes mellitus, heart disease, hypertension, several malignancies, and other health issues. Since sugar increases the caloric content of meals, it is well-known to be one of the main risk factors for obesity. To tackle the problem of obesity and associated comorbidities, regulatory authorities around the world have suggested lowering sugar consumption. Due to the increasing prevalence of the disease, the WHO has also recommended that the total amount of added sugars be kept to < 10% (preferably 5%) of total calorie intake. Due to their sweetness, palatability, and addition of no or few calories to meals, NNS are one of the most important approaches in preventing and managing obesity and related disorders by substituting sugar. The current chapter discusses the uses of numerous NNS in people and discusses difficulties with their safety and varied health effects.

JOURNEY OF NON-NUTRITIVE SWEETENERS

Today, AS are utilized all over the world. Since more than a century ago, NNS have been used without harm in food and beverages all across the globe. Due to their greater sweetness than sugar, these agents are used only in small amounts. In 1879, Remsen and Fahlberg discovered saccharin. It served as the first NNS. Following this, stevia, cyclamate, aspartame, acesulfame potassium (Ace-K), sucralose, and neotame were found.

TYPES/CLASSIFICATION

Non-nutritive sweeteners can be either synthetic (artificial) or naturally occurring plant-derived compounds (natural). Plant-derived NNS are chemically glycoside and nonglycoside compounds in nature. The first generation of polyols, such as sorbitol, xylitol, and erythritol, as well as stevia glycosides and luo han guo fruit (monk fruit) extract, are examples of glycosides. Nonglycoside, second-generation polyols include maltitol. Whereas synthetic (artificial) NNS include neotame, aspartame, advantame, alitame, cyclamate, and potassium acesulfame.

VARIOUS NON-NUTRITIVE SWEETENERS

This section briefly discusses the various artificial sweetener types and their characteristics. **Table 1** shows a few key characteristics of various AS.

Saccharin

It is the earliest synthetic sweetener, frequently found as an organic acid sodium salt. After consumption, saccharin is not metabolized and is eliminated unchanged through the kidneys. Saccharin is heat stable as well. When compared to sugar equivalent consumption, saccharin is more prevalent, yet its primary usage is in pharmaceuticals. It has a bitter aftertaste. Soft drinks, fruit juices, chewing gum, baked foods, and canned fruits all contain saccharin.

Aspartame

Its chemical composition consists of methanol and two amino acids, aspartate, and tryptophan. Under heat, aspartame becomes unstable. Unlike other AS, aspartame is metabolized into methanol, aspartic acid, and tryptophan. Aspartame is metabolized to provide 4 kcal of energy per gram, but the amount required to produce a sweet taste is so little that its caloric contribution is minimal. Aspartame is present in various products, including tabletop sweeteners, chewing gum, instant coffee, puddings, and soft drinks. It should be avoided or restricted in persons with the genetic condition phenylketonuria (PKU).

Neotame and Advantame

These are aspartame analogs. Neotame is metabolized by esterase into deesterified neotame and methanol. Within 72 hours, it is excreted in the feces and urine. Advantame is originally a secondary amine created from aspartame and 3-(3-hydroxy-4-methoxyphenyl)propanal (HMPA). Interestingly, advantame improves the flavors of chewing gum, dairy products, fruit, citrus, and mint.

Acesulfame Potassium

It is the potassium salt of 6-methyl-1,2,3-oxathiazine-4(3H)-one 2,2-dioxide. Like saccharin, a bitter aftertaste can be detected when Ace-K is used in large quantities. It is a heat-stable sweetener. It is blending with other sweeteners has actually demonstrated synergistic effects on sweetness. Ace-K is eliminated unaltered through the kidney since it is not metabolized in vivo. Ace-K is used as a food additive in processed fisheries products, dairy products, baked goods, ice cream, tabletop sweets, soups, and sauces.

Sucralose

One of the most popular AS, whose chemical name is (1,6-dichloro-1,6-dideoxy-β-D-fructofuranosyl-4-chloro-4-deoxy-α-D-galactopyranoside). Sucralose is a trichlorinated derivative of sucrose produced by the chlorination of sucrose. It is heat stable and water-soluble. Sucralose is minimally metabolized in the body and excreted unchanged. Feces primarily eliminate sucralose, with 11–27% absorbed and removed through urine. Tabletop sweeteners, baked foods, frozen desserts, fruit juices, chewing gum, and dairy items all contain sucralose.

Cyclamate

It is cyclohexylsulfamic acid salt. The calcium salt comparable to sodium cyclamate is employed specifically in low-sodium diets as a NNS. It has a bitter aftertaste. However, cyclamate exhibits relatively low toxicity but is metabolized by the gut bacteria to cyclohexylamine, which exhibits higher toxicity.

TABLE 1: Characteristics of individual artificial sweeteners.

AS	Discovery (year)	Sweetness*	Calories (kcal/g)	ADI**	Status of approval	US FDA approval	Indian approval
Saccharin	1879	300–500	0	5	>90 countries	Before 1958	Permitted
Aspartame	1965	200	4	40	>100 countries	1981	Permitted
Neotame	1992	7,000–13,000	0	2	>40 countries	2002	Permitted
Advantame		20,000	0			2014	
Acesulfame potassium (Ace-K)	1967	130–200	0	15	>100 countries	1988	Permitted
Sucralose	1976	600	0	15	>80 countries	1999	Permitted
Cyclamate	1937	30	0	11	>100 countries	Not accessible	Not allowed

* Comparative value when the sweetness of sucrose is 1.

** As per JECFA in (mg/kg BW/day)

(ADI: average daily intake; AS: artificial sweeteners; JECFA: Joint FAO/WHO Expert Committee on Food Additives; US FDA: United States Food and Drug Administration)

SAFETY STANDARDS AND SAFE LIMITS

The Joint FAO/WHO Expert Committee on Food Additives (JECFA), the US Food and Drug Administration (FDA), the European Food Safety Authority (EFSA), Food Standards Australia/New Zealand (FSANZ), and the Food Safety and Standards Authority of India (FSSAI) have all conducted extensive reviews on the use of NNS. NNS have undergone rigorous testing to ensure their safety, and all available data from scientific research shows that everyone over the age of one, including children, pregnant women, and breastfeeding mothers, can ingest NNS. According to the JECFA, average daily intake (ADI) is "an estimate of the amount of a food additive, expressed on a bodyweight basis, that can be ingested over a lifetime without appreciable health risk". It is usually expressed in mg/kg body weight/day.

NON-NUTRITIVE SWEETENERS IN SPECIAL CONSIDERATION

Children

According to studies, aspartame is metabolized similarly in adults and children, with no effects on learning or behavior. Various groups of people, including normal children, hyperactive children, children with PKU, aggressive school boys, and sugar sensitive children, have participated in human clinical trials. These studies collectively demonstrate no impact on childhood malignancies. NNS are, therefore, safe for children (> 1 year).

Pregnancy and Lactation

It is essential to stop gaining too much weight during pregnancy, especially if you have gestational diabetes. This can be achieved safely by using low-calorie sweetener (LCS), and they can keep eating other, more nutritious items to balance out their calorie intake. Actually, according to the American Cancer Society, being overweight poses a much greater risk for having cancer than LCS. The risk of developing cancer is reduced when LCS consumption results in lower calorie intake and decreases in overweight and obesity.

Renal Toxicity

Regarding the debate, several research studies have found no connection between chronic kidney disease (CKD) and these beverages. However, the National Kidney Foundation's guidance, planning for emergencies, a suggestion for people with CKDs, suggests including an artificial sweetener as part of an emergency food plan due to the advantages of these substances.

NON-NUTRITIVE SWEETENERS AND GUT MICROBIOTA

Animal models have shown evidence that NNS change the gut microbiome. Sucralose allegedly affects intestinal flora and may result in liver inflammation in mice. According to a study on mice, saccharin and aspartame intake was linked to changes in the gut flora and glucose intolerance.

Studies were conducted to determine the veracity of this assertion. Test animals were given high dosages of sucralose. It was found that changes in the microflora in the control group were comparable to those in the treatment group. Thus, well-done studies provide no evidence of NNS side effects brought on by changes in the gut microbiome. A recent randomized trial using saccharin on humans revealed no change in the diversity and composition of the microbiome at any taxonomic level of humans and did not cause glucose intolerance.

NON-NUTRITIVE SWEETENERS AND BODY WEIGHT

To keep the enjoyment of sweet flavor and cut back on energy intake, obese subjects frequently switch caloric sweeteners with NNS. Although evidence points to weight loss or otherwise, the impact of NNS on weight increase and loss is controversial. Several epidemiological studies using rat models and human observational studies concluded that NNS contribute to weight gain by increasing appetite, hunger, and sweets cravings while lowering satiety. Instead, randomized controlled trials (RCTs) and human interventional or experimental trials have shown that NNS help with weight management by encouraging weight loss and maintenance by decreasing the consumption of sugar-containing foods, hence reducing the net calorie intake. Optimizing for more conclusive outcomes requires RCTs with the highest degree of evidence. A news report published by the WHO on May 15, 2023, states that the suggestion is based on research showing that using NSS does not have any long-term benefits for lowering body fat in either adults or children. This also implies that prolonged usage of NSS can have unfavorable effects.

NON-NUTRITIVE SWEETENERS AND DIABETES

The American Diabetes Association, in a 2013 position statement and a 2019 consensus report, stated that "the use of NNS has the potential to reduce overall calorie and carbohydrate intake if substituted for caloric sweeteners and without compensation by intake of additional calories from other food sources." The committee continued by stating that "substituting low-calorie sweetened beverages for sugar-sweetened beverages may help to reduce increases in blood glucose levels associated with high intakes of sugar-sweetened beverages in people with diabetes mellitus." The American Heart Association (AHA) and the 2018 Medical Care Standards for Diabetes agreed with this assertion. According to the AHA committee, "for adults who are habitually high consumers of sugar-sweetened beverages, switching to low-calorie sweetened beverages may be a useful replacement strategy to reduce intake of sugar-sweetened beverages." Additionally, according to clinical data, using LCS is also not linked to an increase in glycated hemoglobin (HbA1c), fasting and postprandial glucose, or insulin levels in people with or without diabetes. However, there are some inconsistencies because some research link consumption of NNS to a higher risk of obesity, type 2 diabetes mellitus, hypertension, and cardiovascular events.

NON-NUTRITIVE SWEETENERS AND DENTAL HEALTH

It is widely recognized that frequent ingestion of free sugars is linked to the emergence of dental caries. Limiting free sugar to < 10% of daily energy intake lowers the risk of dental caries throughout a person's life, according to research on the association between free sugar intake and the development of dental caries across age groups. Similarly, the usage of NNS has been shown to affect the microbial composition of the oral mucosa, which may be used to lower the risk of developing dental caries. Additionally, aspartame, saccharin, and sucralose have been shown in in vitro experiments to exhibit antibacterial action against typical periodontal infections.

NON-NUTRITIVE SWEETENERS AND ASSOCIATION WITH CARDIOVASCULAR DISEASE AND MORTALITY

In research by the Women's Health Initiative, consuming more artificially sweetened drinks was linked to a higher risk of stroke, coronary heart disease, and all-cause mortality; however, hemorrhagic stroke was unrelated to artificial sweetener consumption. A just-released study assessed aspartame, Ace-K, and sucralose using 103,388 members of the online NutriNet cohort. The total amount of AS consumed was linked to an elevated cardiovascular risk. Different AS have distinct risks of heart disease and cerebrovascular illness, which is extremely intriguing and important. These findings imply that the outcome of cardiovascular disease (CVD) is not improved by replacing added sugar with AS.

NON-NUTRITIVE SWEETENERS AND CANCER

The US FDA's 1970 decision to withdraw cyclamate from the market owing to concerns that it may have caused cancer in laboratory animals was the first known instance of NNS-induced cancer. However, other countries kept using cyclamates. The WHO, the Cancer Assessment Committee of the Centre for Food Safety and Applied Nutrition of the FDA, and the Scientific Committee for Foods of the European Union all conducted additional assessments of cyclamate's toxicity. They concluded it is not a carcinogen, allowing it to be reintroduced to the food supply. Earlier human epidemiological research found a link between extremely high saccharin dosages and an elevated risk of bladder cancer.

However, further epidemiological investigations on humans could not confirm these results. A few research suggested that higher aspartame usage was linked to an increased risk of breast cancer and brain cancer. The largest case-control study analyzed these findings and showed no connection between using AS and cancer risk. Finally, according to reports from the USFDA (2014) and the American Cancer Society (2020), NNS are safe for the general population when used under certain conditions and in moderation.

CONCLUSION

Non-nutritive sweeteners are still being debated not only for increased risk for cerebrovascular, CVD, cancer incidence, and mortality but also for their potential to cause health problems such as renal toxicity, genotoxicity, neurotoxicity, and disruption of the gut flora. Though, subsequent studies debunked these myths. Since they are beneficial and safe, AS need much more evaluation to understand more individual information, including gut bacteria, genetic traits, epigenetics, etc.

SUGGESTED READINGS

1. Tiwaskar M, Mohan V. Clearing the Myths around nonnutritive/noncaloric Sweeteners: An Efficacy and Safety Evaluation. J Assoc Physicians India. 2022;70(7):11-2.
2. International Life Sciences Institute-India. (2017). Sweetness: Role of Sugar and Low Calorie Sweeteners. [online] Available from http://www.ilsi-india.org/PDF/Monograph_on_Sweetness_Role_of_Sugar_Low_Calorie_Sweeteners.pdf. [Last accessed December, 2023].
3. Iizuka K. Is the Use of Artificial Sweeteners Beneficial for Patients with Diabetes Mellitus? The Advantages and Disadvantages of Artificial Sweeteners. Nutrients. 2022;14(21):4446.
4. Chattopadhyay S, Raychaudhuri U, Chakraborty R. Artificial sweeteners—a review. J Food Sci Technol. 2014;51(4):611-21.

65

CHAPTER

Is Reversing Insulin Resistance a Myth or Reality?

LH Ghotekar, Nikita Srivastava, Anu Goswami

ABSTRACT

Diabetes and insulin resistance (IR) are slowly shaping a global pandemic on an unprecedented scale. According to International Diabetes Federation data (2021), 537 million adults are living with diabetes and another 547 million adults are at increased risk of developing type 2 diabetes mellitus (T2DM). IR has various metabolic effects on human body in the form of hyperglycemia, dyslipidemia, hypertension, hepatic steatosis, polycystic ovary, atherosclerotic events, and obesity-related cancers like endometrial cancer. This chapter is meant to recall what we know so far, but more importantly it focuses on evidence-based recent advances in both lifestyle interventions and pharmacotherapy that may help turn back the clock on resistance.

INTRODUCTION

Diabetes and insulin resistance are causing a global pandemic, with 537 million adults living with diabetes and 547 million at increased risk of developing T2DM. Since IR plays a vital role in the pathogenesis of what is now popularly being called diabesity, this chapter is about revisiting what we know so far and how to reverse IR.

Insulin resistance is defined as a lower than expected response to insulin action from target tissues, resulting in the impairment of both glucose and lipid metabolism at different levels and predisposing to the development of T2DM.

In other words, it is the inability of insulin to increase glucose uptake and utilization in insulin-sensitive cells chiefly adipocytes, skeletal muscle and hepatocytes, leading to a myriad of metabolic complications. Thus, failure to dispose glucose results in compensatory increase in endogenous insulin which in due course will lead to weight gain, progression to diabetes, polycystic ovaries, nonalcoholic steatohepatitis (NASH), hypertension, atherosclerotic events and obesity related cancers **(Table 1)**.

MECHANISM OF INSULIN ACTION AND RELEASE

Insulin is a peptide hormone which is secreted by pancreatic beta cells in response to raised plasma glucose levels. The hormone is first produced as preproinsulin which is cleaved into proinsulin and stored in secretory granules after which mature insulin gets acted upon by proteases and released by exocytosis. Release of insulin is primarily controlled by entry of glucose into the hepatic beta cells via glucose transporter 2 (GLUT2). After entry, glucose gets phosphorylated to glucose 6 phosphate by glucokinase activity which then acts as the glucose sensor controlling the rate of release of insulin. Once insulin is released, it primarily acts through transmembrane insulin receptor (IR) tyrosine kinase having alpha and beta chains. Insulin, insulin-like growth factor 1 (IGF-1) and IGF-2, bind to alpha chain and cause structural changes in beta chain by inducing autophosphorylation in tyrosine residues followed by recruitment of adaptor proteins and insulin receptor substrates (IRSs). Activated IRS triggers subsequent signal transduction by binding to phosphoinositide 3-kinase (PI3K) and activating it, which catalyzes the conversion of phosphatidylinositol

4,5-bisphosphate (PIP2) to phosphatidylinositol 3,4,5-trisphosphate (PIP3). PIP3 is a potent inducer of various protein kinases, chiefly protein kinase B which then facilitates glucose entry into cells by translocation of GLUT4 **(Fig. 1)**.

PATHOPHYSIOLOGY OF INSULIN RESISTANCE

The chief pathophysiology behind IR is defect in signal transduction.

Skeletal Muscle

In healthy individuals, in fed state, glucose is taken up by skeletal muscle via GLUT4 and phosphorylated to glucose 6-phosphate which is either used in tricarboxylic acid (TCA) pathway to produce energy or stored as glycogen.

- In an insulin-resistant state, there is an impaired phosphorylation of IRS-1, leading to a reduced translocation of GLUT4 and subsequently reduced glucose uptake by the muscle.

TABLE 1: Etiology of insulin resistance (IR).

Inherited causes	Acquired causes
• Type A insulin resistance • Type B insulin resistance • Rabson–Mendenhall syndrome • Leprechaunism • Lipodystrophies • Donohue syndrome • Alstrom syndrome • Werner syndrome	• Obesity, lipotoxicity from excess circulating free fatty acids • Inactivity • Drugs (glucocorticoids, oral contraceptives, antiretrovirals, protease inhibitors, atypical antipsychotics, and calcineurin inhibitors, etc.) • Stress (due to increase in counterregulatory hormones—trauma, sepsis, surgery, diabetic ketoacidosis) • Pregnancy (due to placental lactogen) • Puberty • Endocrine disorders • Acromegaly, glucagonoma, thyrotoxicosis, Cushing's syndrome, pheochromocytoma • Anti-insulin antibodies • Human immunodeficiency virus (HIV)-associated lipodystrophy • Pseudoresistance—poor administration technique, incorrect storage of insulin, malingering for secondary gain

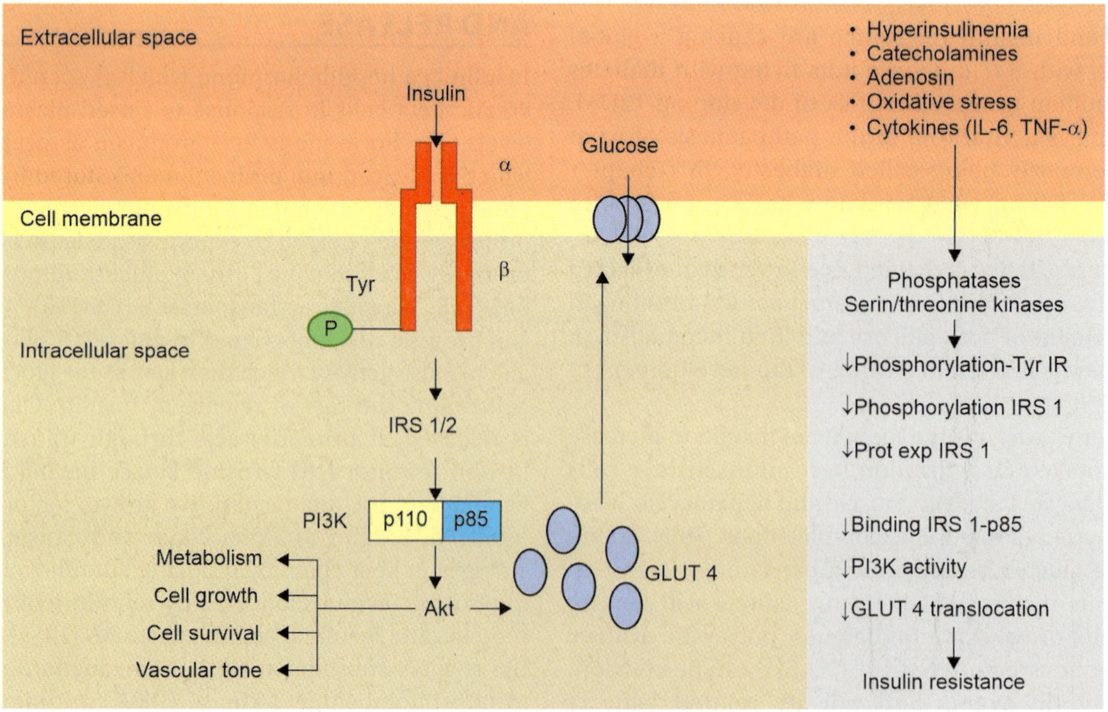

FIG. 1: Schematic representation of early steps of insulin signaling, and the principal mechanisms that account for insulin resistance (IR).
(IL-6: interleukin 6; P: phosphorylation; Pro Exp: protein expression; TNF-α: tumor necrosis factor alpha; Tyr: tyrosine; IR: insulin resistance)

- Also, reduced activity of glycogen synthase is an early defect in IR, leading to deranged glycogen synthesis, followed by reduced glucose oxidation.
- Chronic inflammation in IR also leads to upregulation of chemokines tumor necrosis factor alpha (TNF-α) and interleukin 1β (IL-1β) which activate protein kinase C and IKK–NFκB pathways which lead to defective insulin signaling.

Hepatocytes

- Increased efflux of free fatty acids (FFA) due to inadequate suppression of lipolysis as a result of impaired inhibition of protein kinase A.
- De novo lipogenesis (DNL) is increased by regulation of the mTOR (mammalian target of rapamycin) and SREBP-1c (sterol regulatory element binding protein 1c) pathways.
- Lipid overload leads to activation of the protein kinase C pathway, disrupting insulin signaling and promoting gluconeogenesis through the upregulation of FoxO1.

Adipocytes

Normal role of insulin in adipocytes is stimulation of lipoprotein lipase resulting in increased fatty acid uptake, suppression of lipolysis, and promotion of triglyceride storage.

- Several proinflammatory factors such as TNF-α and IL-6 and IL-1β are over expressed in enlarged adipocytes linking obesity to IR. TNF-α promotes the serine phosphorylation of IRS-1, decreasing its association with PI3K, thus disrupting insulin signaling.
- Obesity is a state of chronic inflammation which can lead to endoplasmic reticulum's (ER) stress, adiponectin reduction, leptin elevation, adipocytes death, macrophage infiltration and lipolysis.

Miscellaneous Mechanisms

Insulin receptor antibodies leading to increased insulin degradation, free radical injury, and mitochondrial dysfunction are other mechanisms of IR.

CLINICAL FEATURES

The clinical features are shown in **Box 1**.

DIAGNOSIS (TABLE 2)

- There can be a constellation of metabolic syndrome features in the form of hyperglycemia, dyslipidemia, abdominal obesity, and hypertension which point toward a clinical diagnosis of IR.
- In order to quantify IR, the following methods are used as mentioned in **Table 2**.

BOX 1: Clinical features.

- *Metabolic*: Diabetes, polyuria, polydipsia, polyphagia, weight gain, *obesity*
- *Musculoskeletal*: Muscle hypertrophy, pseudoacromegaly, muscle cramps
- *Hypertension*: Headache
- *Nonalcoholic fatty liver*
- *Cutaneous*: *Acanthosis nigricans* (darkening of arm pits, neck, groin); skin tags; xanthomas and xanthelasmas due to dyslipidemia; alopecia
- *Reproductive (features of PCOS)*: *Amenorrhea*, hirsutism, infertility

(PCOS: polycystic ovary syndrome)

TABLE 2: Diagnosis.

In clinical setting	In research setting
Triglycerides (TG), TG:HDL ratio, fasting insulin (cutoff values 130 mg/dL, 3 and 15.7 μU/mL respectively)	Euglycemic clamp/gold standard
• Insulin-to-glucose ratio (higher ratio in IR) • Valid only in early stage	HOMA-IR or HOMA (Homeostasis Model Assessment of Insulin Resistance)
Serum sex hormone-binding globulin (SHBG) (low in IR)	–

(HDL: high-density lipoprotein; ITT: insulin tolerance test; IVGTT: intravenous glucose tolerance test)

MANAGEMENT APPROACH

The management of reversing IR is a complex and widely debated topic in the field of medicine and nutrition.

First step is to stop or replace medication known to cause IR. Poor medication-taking behaviors or "pseudo-resistance" should be ruled out before modifying or intensifying therapy **(Fig. 2)**.

Intensive Lifestyle Modification

- *Dietary recommendations*:
  - *What to eat?* American Diabetes Association (ADA) emphasizes on consumption of nonstarchy vegetables, preference of whole foods to processed foods, and minimal use of added sugars and refined grains. Low-carbohydrate diets and diets rich in fiber, whole grains, and lean proteins are particularly beneficial.

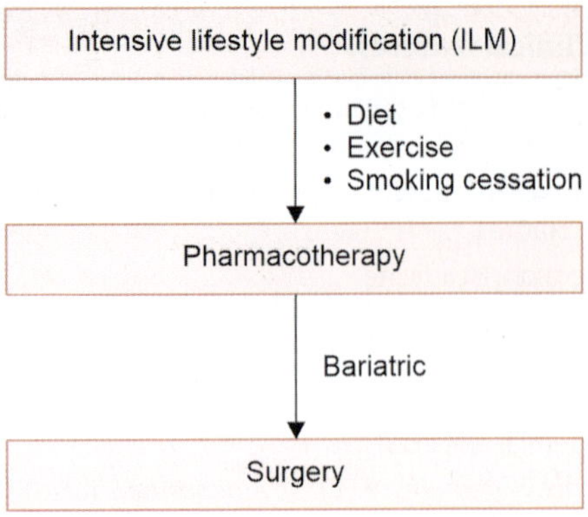

FIG. 2: Management approach.

  - *How to eat?* Mediterranean style eating pattern led to more favorable changes in glycemic control and coronary risk factors and delayed the need for antihyperglycemic drug therapy in overweight patients with newly diagnosed T2DM compared with a low-fat, low-carbohydrate diet. In this study, the group following a low-carbohydrate Mediterranean style eating pattern experienced greater rates of partial diabetes remission, with rates of 14.7% at year 1 and 5% at year 6 compared with 4.7% and 0%, respectively, in the group following a low-fat eating plan (PREDIMED trial).
- *Weight loss—How much to lose?* According to ADA recommendations, weight loss should be 7%–10% for preventing progression to T2DM. Even a modest weight loss of 5%–10% of body weight can have a positive impact on IR. Lifestyle interventions producing < 5% weight loss had less effect on A1c, lipids, or blood pressure compared with studies achieving weight loss of ≥ 5%. Even a modest weight loss of 5%–10% of body weight can have a positive impact on IR.
- *Exercise*: Exercise can dramatically reduce IR in both the short- and long-terms.

How to exercise? Resistance exercise training (RET) is preferred to aerobic exercise training (AET) which includes squats, lunges, shoulder press, and deadlifts. People who performed RET reduced their risk of diabetes and cardiovascular diseases (CVDs) by 30% and 17%, respectively. RET when compared to AET maintains fat-free mass (FFM) and resting energy expenditure (REE), factors that are pivotal in weight loss and weight maintenance.

How much to exercise? Three sets of 20-second sprint interval training 3/week produced comparable improvements in cardiorespiratory fitness, insulin sensitivity, and mitochondrial content as 45 minutes of medium intensity training (MIT) exercise despite the fivefold lower exercise volume.

- *Stress management*: Chronic stress can contribute to IR. Practice stress reduction techniques such as meditation, yoga, or deep breathing exercises.
- *Adequate sleep*: Poor sleep habits can affect insulin sensitivity. Aim for 7–9 hours of quality sleep per night.
- *Avoiding smoking and excessive alcohol*: Smoking and excessive alcohol consumption can worsen IR and should be avoided or minimized.

Pharmacotherapy

Metformin: Metformin chiefly acts by reducing hepatic glucose production and increasing glucose uptake by skeletal muscles. It is indicated in individuals with impaired fasting glucose, impaired glucose tolerance or glycated hemoglobin (HbA1c) between 5.7 and 6.4% on lifestyle modification with the following: <60 years of age, body mass index (BMI) > 35 kg/m^2, and/or history of gestational diabetes. The recommended initial dosing is 850 mg BD.

Orlistat: Orlistat reversibly inhibits gastric and pancreatic lipases thus reduce FFA production. Its use is limited in those with a BMI > 28 kg/m^2 in who fasting plasma glucose or HbA1c show deterioration, as part of an overall strategy to reduce weight which helps in IR [recommended by (NICE) National Institute for Health and Care Excellence].

Glitazones: Pioglitazone is a TZD which has been shown to be effective in glycemic control by lowering IR. Pioglitazone also has beneficial effects on lipid metabolism and cardiovascular risk.

Glucagon-like Peptide-1 Receptor Agonist

- *Semaglutide*: Across the SUSTAIN 1 to 3 clinical trials, a significant decrease was found in IR in semaglutide-treated subjects compared with that in exenatide extended-release (ER) treated subjects.
- *Exenatide*: It ameliorates IR-induced inflammation and nonalcoholic fatty liver disease (NAFLD).
- *Liraglutide*: It significantly reduces metabolic dysfunction, hepatic lipogenesis, hepatic and adipose IR, and adipose inflammation in patients with NASH. The American Heart Association, American College of Cardiology, and The Obesity Society recommend its use in individuals having a BMI > 30 or 27 kg/m^2 and associated comorbid conditions such as T2DM, hypertension, dyslipidemia, or obstructive sleep apnea.

- *Pramlintide*: Pramlintide is usually given after other diabetes medicines have been tried without success in patients using insulin.
- *Tirzepatide*: Glucagon-like peptide-1 (GLP-1) receptor agonist—by decreasing IR, tirzepatide likely reduces metabolic demand for insulin secretion from pancreatic beta cells, diminishing ongoing beta cell stress. Improvements in IR with tirzepatide 10-mg and 15-mg doses were only partially attributable to weight loss, suggestive of additional mechanisms by which tirzepatide improved insulin sensitivity to achieve substantial reductions in HbA1c. Tirzepatide 10 and 15 mg significantly decreased fasting insulin ($p \leq 0.033$) and tirzepatide 10 mg significantly decreased HOMA2-IR (Homeostasis Model Assessment of Insulin Resistance) ($p = 0.004$) compared with placebo and dulaglutide. By both improving pancreatic beta cell function and reducing IR through dual activation of GLP-1 and glucose-dependent insulinotropic polypeptide (GIP) receptors, tirzepatide has the potential to confer not only glucose control and weight loss but also to reduce disease severity to improve metabolic health. Wilson et al. concluded in their study that tirzepatide improves lipoprotein biomarkers associated with IR and cardiovascular risk in patients with T2DM.
- *U-500* (500 units/mL) is sometimes used in patients with severe IR. I am not in favor of giving insulin as hyperinsulinemia per se aggravates IR.

Landmark Trials (Table 3)

- Other currently available drugs include phentermine, phentermine/topiramate extended release (ER), lorcaserin, and naltrexone ER/bupropion ER.
    - Lorcaserin can restrain patients' appetite and improve insulin sensitivity and hyperinsulinemia mainly through activating 5-hydroxytryptamine 2C receptor (5-HT2CR) in the hypothalamus.
    - Study indicated that intermittent phentermine therapy resulted in greater decrease in waist circumference while continuous phentermine therapy produced greater reduction in fasting insulin, HOMA-IR, and high-sensitivity C-reactive protein (hsCRP).
    - Low-dose naltrexone rescues inflammation and IR.
- *Surgery*: Surgical intervention in the form of gastric sleeves, banding, and bypass is available for qualified individuals with obesity. The excess fat loss associated with bariatric surgery improves insulin sensitivity. The results of the STAMPEDE trial provide good evidence of the benefit of bariatric surgery on T2DM, but to be considered only if there is morbid obesity not responding to other therapy.

TABLE 3: Landmark trials.

Trial	Drug	Results
STOP NIDDM trial (1998)	Acarbose	Reversion of impaired glucose tolerance to normal glucose tolerance in treatment arm ($p < 0.0001$)
ACE trial (2009–2015)	Acarbose	13.3% in acarbose group developed diabetes as compared to 15.8% in placebo ($p = 0.0005$)
DPP trial (1996–2001)	Metformin	Metformin group had a 31% lower chance of developing diabetes
DPPOS (2002–ongoing)	Metformin	Prevention/delay of diabetes with Li or metformin can persist for at least 10 years
STEP 1 trial (2021)	Semaglutide	Participants who received semaglutide were more likely to lose > 5%, >10%, > 15% and > 20% of baseline body weight at week 68 as compared to placebo ($p < 0.001$ except for > 20% loss)

(DPP: Diabetes Prevention Program; DPPOS: Diabetes Prevention Program Outcomes Study; Li: lifestyle intervention)

Newer Approaches

- *Fetal microbiota transplantation*: Salamone et al. proposed *Faecalibacterium prausnitzii,* both as a biomarker for the development of different gut pathologies and as a potential treatment of insulin metabolism disturbances, due to its production of anti-inflammatory metabolites linked with toll-like receptors and nuclear factor kappa B (NF-κβ) signaling.
- *Metreleptin*: It is indicated in patients with congenital or acquired generalized lipodystrophy (leptin deficiency). It is in phase II trial for the treatment of IR.
- *Silymarin*: Additive effect of silymarin in metformin therapy can mitigate fatty liver development in prediabetic states and before the onset of IR due to positively affected transcription factors involved in lipogenesis.
- *Berberine and quercetin*: As per the experimental studies on animals evidence suggest that both substances modulate IR and there is a need to investigate the therapeutic potential of these in human pathology.

COMPARISON OF ILM VERSUS PHARMACOTHERAPY (TABLE 4)

Managing IR is a long-term commitment to a healthy lifestyle, and ongoing vigilance is often necessary to

TABLE 4: Intensive lifestyle modification (ILM) versus pharmacotherapy.

Trial	ILM	Metformin
DPP (1996–2001) Follow-up period = 3 years	Cerebrovascular and peripheral neurologic complications	Lowered chances of developing T2DM by 31% compared with participants who took a placebo
DPPOS (2002–ongoing) Follow-up period = 10 years	Reduced rate of developing T2DM by 34%, delayed T2DM by about 4 years, and reduced cardiovascular risk factors, hemoglobin A1c, and fasting glucose when compared with placebo	Reduced rate of developing diabetes by 18%, delayed diabetes by 2 years, and reduced hemoglobin A1c and fasting glucose when compared with placebo

(DPP: Diabetes Prevention Program; DPPOS: Diabetes Prevention Program Outcomes Study; T2DM: type 2 diabetes mellitus)

maintain improved insulin sensitivity Hence, the above studies prove that lifestyle interventions play an upper hand over pharmacotherapy in reversing IR.

Team approach: The management of IR is best done with multidisciplinary team. Early and aggressive management should be done in consultation with the specialist for obesity (obesity medicine specialist), T2DM, hyperlipidemia, and PCOS (endocrinology), cardiovascular complications (cardiology and cardiac surgery), cerebrovascular and peripheral neurologic complications (neurologist). Team should also comprise nurse, diabetic educator, dietician, physical therapist, pharmacist, social worker, and psychologist.

CONCLUSION

Though reversing IR is no longer a myth but it is not correct that IR can be fully reversed. But for sure it can often be effectively managed and improved. Lifelong lifestyle changes such as diet, exercise, and weight loss can significantly enhance insulin sensitivity and should be considered as first line of therapy. Thus lifestyle changes can increase insulin sensitivity and decrease IR, not all causes are reversible. Recent studies have customized the lifestyle interventions in such a way that time is no longer an excuse to incorporate the modifications. Also, advances in clinical trials might just turn back the clock on resistance. Finally, while the complete reversal of IR may be challenging, personalized lifestyle changes can significantly improve insulin sensitivity and reverse IR even due to genetic causes. However, IR in some patients can be reversed completely while in others it can be partially reversed while in a few it cannot be reversed at all. It is essential for individuals with IR to work with healthcare professionals to develop a personalized plan for their specific need.

TAKE HOME MESSAGE

Do not give up. As per ADA there are effective tactics to combat IR. Losing weight, exercising more, or taking an insulin-sensitizing medication can help you get back to good blood glucose control and better health.

Resilience, not hesitance, is what will help us in insulin resistance.

SUGGESTED READINGS

1. Petersen MC, Shulman GI. Mechanisms of insulin action and insulin resistance. Physiol Rev. 2018;98:2133-223.
2. Angelidi AM, Filippaios Á, Mantzoros CS. Severe insulin resistance syndromes. J Clin Invest. 2021;131(4):e142245.
3. White BA. Hormonal regulation of energy metabolism. In: Koeppen BM, Stanton BA (Eds). Berne and Levy Physiology, 7th edition. Philadelphia: Elsevier; 2018. pp. 704-5.
4. Rutter GA, Pullen TJ, Hodson DJ, Martinez-Sanchez A. Pancreatic β-cell identity, glucose sensing and the control of insulin secretion. Biochem J. 2015;466(2):203-18.
5. Ho CK, Sriram G, Dipple KM. Insulin sensitivity predictions in individuals with obesity and type II diabetes mellitus using mathematical model of the insulin signal transduction pathway. Mol Genet Metab. 2016;119(3):288-92.
6. Abdul-Ghani MA, DeFronzo RA. Pathogenesis of insulin resistance in skeletal muscle. J Biomed Biotechnol. 2010;2010: 476279.
7. Shulman GI, Rothman DL, Jue T, Stein P, DeFronzo RA, Shulman RG. Quantitation of muscle glycogen synthesis in normal subjects and subjects with non-insulin-dependent diabetes by 13C nuclear magnetic resonance spectroscopy. N Engl J Med. 1990;322(4):223-8.
8. Wu H, Ballantyne CM. Skeletal muscle inflammation and insulin resistance in obesity. J Clin Invest. 2017;127(1):43-54.
9. O-Sullivan I, Zhang W, Wasserman DH, Liew CW, Liu J, Paik J, et al. FoxO1 integrates direct and indirect effects of insulin on hepatic glucose production and glucose utilization. Nat Commun. 2015;6:7079.
10. Rui L, Aguirre V, Kim JK, Shulman GI, Lee A, Corbould A, et al. Insulin/IGF-1 and TNF-α stimulate phosphorylation of IRS-1 at inhibitory Ser 307 via distinct pathways. J Clin Invest. 2001;107(2):181-9.
11. Ye J, McGuinness OP. Inflammation during obesity is not all bad: evidence from animal and human studies. Am J Physiol Endocrinol Metab. 2013;304(5):E466-E477.
12. Yaribeygi H, Farrokhi FR, Butler AE, Sahebkar A. Insulin resistance: Review of the underlying molecular mechanisms. J Cell Physiol. 2019;234(6):8152-61.

13. Esposito K, Maiorino MI, Petrizzo M, Bellastella G, Giugliano D. The effects of a Mediterranean diet on the need for diabetes drugs and remission of newly diagnosed type 2 diabetes: follow-up of a randomized trial. Diabetes Care. 2014;37(7):1824-30.
14. Franz MJ, Boucher JL, Rutten-Ramos S, VanWormer JJ. Lifestyle weight-loss intervention outcomes in overweight and obese adults with type 2 diabetes: a systematic review and meta-analysis of randomized clinical trials. J Acad Nutr Diet. 2015;115(9):1447-63.
15. Shiroma EJ, Cook NR, Manson JE, Moorthy MV, Buring JE, Rimm EB, et al. Strength training and the risk of type 2 diabetes and cardiovascular disease. Med Sci Sports Exerc. 2017;49(1): 40-6.
16. Gillen JB, Martin BJ, MacInnis MJ, Skelly LE, Tarnopolsky MA, Gibala MJ. Twelve weeks of sprint interval training improves indices of cardiometabolic health similar to traditional endurance training despite a five-fold lower exercise volume and time commitment. PLoS One. 2016;11(4):e0154075.
17. National Institute for Health and Care Excellence. (2017). Type 2 diabetes: Prevention in people at high risk. Public health guideline [PH38]. [online] Available from https://www.nice.org.uk/guidance/ph38/chapter/Recommendations#orlistat [Last accessed January, 2024].
18. Desouza CV, Shivaswamy V. Pioglitazone in the treatment of type 2 diabetes: safety and efficacy review. Clin Med Insights Endocrinol Diabetes. 2010;3:43-51.
19. Wilding JP, Batterham RL, Calanna S, Davies M, Van Gaal LF, Lingvay I, et al. STEP 1 Study Group. Once-weekly semaglutide in adults with overweight or obesity. New Engl J Med. 2021;384(11):989-1002.
20. Lule KO, Akarsu E, Sayiner ZA, Lule NO, Balci SO, Demirel C, et al. The effects of metformin, pioglitazone, exenatide and exercise on fatty liver in obese diabetic rats: The role of IRS-1 and SOCS-3 molecules. Inflammopharmacology. 2022;30:243-50.
21. Thomas MK, Nikooienejad A, Bray R, Cui X, Wilson J, Duffin K, et al. Dual GIP and GLP-1 Receptor Agonist Tirzepatide Improves Beta-cell Function and Insulin Sensitivity in Type 2 Diabetes. J Clin Endocrinol Metab. 2021;106(2):388-96.
22. Wilson JM, Nikooienejad A, Robins DA, Roell WC, Riesmeyer JS, Haupt A, et al. The dual glucose-dependent insulinotropic peptide and glucagon-like peptide-1 receptor agonist, tirzepatide, improves lipoprotein biomarkers associated with insulin resistance and cardiovascular risk in patients with type 2 diabetes. Diabet Obes Metab. 2020;22:2451-9.
23. Chiasson JL, Josse RG, Gomis R, Hanefeld M, Karasik A, Laakso M; STOP-NIDDM Trial Research Group. Acarbose treatment and the risk of cardiovascular disease and hypertension in patients with impaired glucose tolerance: the STOP-NIDDM trial. JAMA. 2003; 290(4):486-94.
24. Holman RR, Coleman RL, Chan JC, Chiasson JL, Feng H, Ge J, et al. Effects of acarbose on cardiovascular and diabetes outcomes in patients with coronary heart disease and impaired glucose tolerance (ACE): a randomised, double-blind, placebo-controlled trial. Lancet Diabetes Endocrinol. 2017;5(11):877-86.
25. Diabetes Prevention Program (DPP) Research Group. The Diabetes Prevention Program (DPP) description of lifestyle intervention. Diabetes care. 2002;25(12):2165-71.
26. Salamone D, Rivellese AA, Vetrani C. The relationship between gut microbiota, short-chain fatty acids and type 2 diabetes mellitus: The possible role of dietary fibre. Acta Diabetol. 2021;58:1131-8.
27. MacDonald-Ramos K, Michán L, Martínez-Ibarra A, Cerbón M. Silymarin is an ally against insulin resistance: A review. Ann Hepatol. 2021;23:100255.
28. Bellavite P, Fazio S, Affuso F. A descriptive review of the action mechanisms of berberine, quercetin and silymarin on insulin resistance/hyperinsulinemia and cardiovascular prevention. Molecules. 2023;28(11):4491.

66

CHAPTER

Automated Insulin Delivery Devices (Artificial Pancreas)

Jothydev Kesavadev, Sreelakshmi R

ABSTRACT

Automated insulin delivery (AID) devices have been a breakthrough in optimizing treatment for diabetes in those individuals on insulin, prone to hypoglycemia and with significant glucose variability. Typically, an AID consists of an insulin pump, a real-time continuous glucose monitoring (CGM) and a control algorithm, wirelessly connected to each other. This chapter explores their evolution from early insulin pumps to sophisticated closed-loop systems. However, the time lag for commercial availability of trouble-free automation has led to the emergence of do-it-yourself artificial pancreas system (DIY-APS) within the type 1 diabetes community.

This chapter delves into various facets of employing AID for diabetes management. Despite therapeutic advancements, maintaining glucose levels in the physiological range while avoiding hypoglycemia remains a challenge. Most recent developments in CGM and AID systems are discussed. Currently available systems worldwide such as MiniMed™ 780G, Omnipod® 5 AID System, Tandem t:slim X2, and DBLG1 (Diabeloop) advanced hybrid closed-loop system are reviewed for their features optimizing insulin delivery and glucose control.

INTRODUCTION

Since the landmark discovery of insulin in 1921, there has been a relentless pursuit to refine insulin therapy. The goal has always been clear: to administer insulin in a manner that mimics the body's natural processes while preventing the perilous lows of hypoglycemia. This endeavor, once a distant aspiration, has seen remarkable strides in the last three years with the advent of automated insulin delivery (AID) devices. These innovative systems, a synthesis of technology and medicine, are revolutionizing diabetes management. They are categorized into two main streams: Commercially available AIDs, which represent the forefront of medical technology, and open-source AIDs, which embody a collaborative, patient-driven approach to healthcare technology. The chapter shed insights into the currently available artificial insulin delivery devices.

AUTOMATED INSULIN DELIVERY SYSTEMS

Automated insulin delivery is a system that incorporates an insulin infusion device, a glucose sensor, and a control algorithm.

WORKING PRINCIPLE OF AUTOMATED INSULIN DELIVERY SYSTEMS

Automated insulin delivery systems consist of three components:

1. *Continuous glucose monitor*: CGM monitors glucose levels every few minutes, using a tiny sensor inserted subcutaneously. The sensor measures the glucose in the interstitial fluid and sends the information wirelessly to the user's smartphone or on an insulin infusion

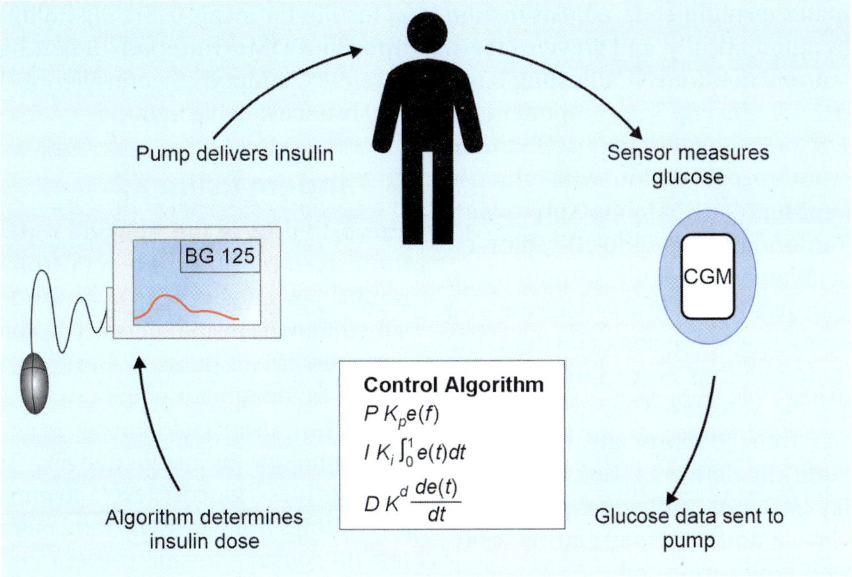

FIG. 1: Automated insulin delivery systems.

Source: Pauley ME, Berget C, Messer LH, Forlenza GP. Barriers to uptake of insulin technologies and novel solutions. Med Devices (Auckl). 2021;14:339-54.

pump. CGM continuously displays an estimate of glucose levels, their trends and rate of change of these estimates. Some of the currently available sensors globally include Guardian Connect (Medtronic), G6, G7 (Dexcom), FreeStyle Libre (Abbott), Eversense, etc.

2. *Control algorithm*: The control algorithm calculates the required dose of insulin and signals the insulin infusion pump when insulin needs to be delivered.
3. *Insulin infusion pump*: The insulin infusion pump adjusts the insulin delivery based on the control algorithm and the glucose readings from the CGM **(Fig. 1)**.

EVOLUTION OF AUTOMATED INSULIN DELIVERY SYSTEMS

The evolution of AID can be traced back to 50 years ago, when trials in people with type 1 diabetes mellitus (T1DM) demonstrated the possibility of external glucose regulation. In the early 1960s, an intravenous insulin pump delivering insulin and glucagon to counteract hypoglycemia was reported by Dr Arnold Kadish. Kadish designed the first insulin pump in 1963, which was worn on the back and was huge in size. Following this was the introduction of the "Biostator", a device featuring the characteristics for closed-loop intravenous insulin infusion and intravenous CGM, commercialized in 1977 by Dr Ernst Friedrich Pfeiffer. Further works by Keen and Pickup, and Tamborlane et al., on subcutaneous insulin infusion had led to the introduction of insulin pump therapy and new-generation insulin pumps in the subsequent years.

The first wearable insulin pump, known as the "blue brick" and later the "autosyringe", was designed by Dean Kamen in 1976. The 43 years of inventive research by SOOIL led to the introduction of DANA Diabecare IIS insulin pump designed for the subcutaneous delivery of insulin in 2006.

In 2006, MiniMed™ introduced the MiniMed™ Paradigm Real-Time System consisting of insulin pump and CGM. The introduction of real-time, sensor-augmented insulin pump is considered a major step toward the development of "closed-loop" insulin delivery or an artificial pancreas (AP). The sensor-augmented pump (SAP) therapy provided room for potential innovations, particularly focusing on fully "closed-loop systems". In 2009, Medtronic launched the MiniMed™ Veo System, with a low glucose suspend feature that automatically halts insulin delivery when sensor glucose levels hit a preset low threshold. This device has been considered as the first stepping stone to an AP system. In 2015, Medtronic introduced the MiniMed™ 640G system, with SmartGuard® feature offering predictive low glucose suspension.

CURRENTLY AVAILABLE AUTOMATED INSULIN DELIVERY SYSTEMS

MiniMed™ 780G

MiniMed™ 780G or advanced hybrid-closed loop (AHCL) system is the most advanced AID system from Medtronic approved by the Food and Drug Administration (FDA) for use in individuals with T1DM, aged 7 years and above.

It continuously anticipates insulin needs, adjusts insulin delivery, corrects highs automatically, and prevents lows. It has SmartGuard™ automation for self-adjusting basal delivery with autocorrection dosing. The components of 780G include MiniMed™ 780G insulin pump, Guardian 4 sensor (does not require calibration with glucose meter) and transmitter, MiniMed™ Mobile App to view glucose levels, pump information, and insulin data on their phone or Apple Watch. CareLink Connect app can be used by care partners for all-in-one viewing and customizable alerts of patient's pump and CGM data. The sensor measures the glucose levels every 5 minutes and sends the information to the waterproof pump. The pump gathers glucose readings from the sensor and accordingly the transmitter automatically delivers a variable rate of insulin, 24 hours a day based on individualized needs. 780G tracks glucose levels and provides alarms, real-time glucose trends, and notifications on the connected smartphone *via the* CareLink Connect app. The system requires user-initiated meal announcements for optimal glycemic results. The 780G system includes an AHCL algorithm, which provides both basal and correction bolus AID. The system uniquely features SmartGuard technology to prevent highs and lows and is proven for its efficacy in achieving a time-in-range of >70%. The MiniMed™ 780G pump is available in India since 2022. The Indian experience with 780G exploring its merits and demerits has been recently published. Though automated, it still requires user intervention at various levels.

Omnipod® 5 Automated Insulin Delivery System

Omnipod® 5 is the first wearable, tubeless, and hybrid closed-loop insulin delivery system to integrate with the Dexcom G6 CGM. The device is approved by the FDA for use in people with T1DM aged 2 years and older. This system, which eliminates the need to carry a separate control unit, is the first of its kind that gets FDA approval for mobile app controls and insulin dosing directly through user smart phones. Omnipod® 5 comprises of three parts: (1) A tubeless, waterproof, wearable pod, (2) Dexcom G6 CGM system, and (3) Omnipod® 5 mobile app. The pod delivers insulin using the built-in SmartAdjust™ technology, according to the values communicated to the pod by the CGM. When in automated mode with Dexcom G6, it adjusts insulin delivery every 5 minutes depending on the user's current CGM value, glucose values anticipated to occur 60 minutes in the future, glucose trend, and previous insulin delivery in order to bring glucose to a user-defined target. The user is responsible for delivering bolus doses of insulin for meals using the bolus settings programmed into the PDM. Omnipod® 5 can be controlled with the wireless Omnipod® 5 controller or Omnipod® 5 App. This AID is not available in India.

Tandem t:slim X2

The t:slim X2 is the first interoperable hybrid closed-loop system (alternate controller-enabled infusion pump), which got the FDA authorization in 2019 for the subcutaneous insulin delivery in children and adults with diabetes. It can be used either as a stand-alone pump, or can be integrated with Dexcom G6 CGM. When used with CGM, users can choose either Control-IQ or Basal-IQ technology for insulin delivery. The Control-IQ system predicts blood glucose levels 30 minutes in advance based on readings from the CGM, and automatically adjust basal insulin delivery, to help prevent highs and lows. Control-IQ delivers an automatic correction bolus up to once per hour, if required. Users are still required to bolus for meals, which can be done from the touch screen pump or from a compatible phone with the t:connect app. This device is yet to be available in India.

DBLG1 Hybrid Closed-loop System

The DBLG1 hybrid closed-loop system (Diabeloop) comprises of the Dexcom G6 CGM, Kaleido's patch insulin pump, and the Diabeloop decision-making algorithm. The DBLG1 algorithm developed by Diabeloop is hosted on a handset is connected to a CGM and an insulin pump. The glucose measurement is transmitted every 5 minutes via Bluetooth to the handset. The DBLG1 artificial intelligence analyzes data in real time considering the patient's physiology, history, and data entries (meals or exercise) for insulin dose determinations. This device has not hit the Indian market.

Do-it-yourself Artificial Pancreas System

The DIY-APS is an initiative from the highly motivated and tech-savvy members of the diabetes community who gathered online under the hashtag "#WeAreNotWaiting" to share knowledge of the open-source hardware and software solutions for better glycemic management. The tech-savvy diabetes enthusiasts primed the designing of their own HCL systems from commercially available insulin pumps, CGM devices, and open-source algorithms. Online social networking resources such as GitHub, CGM in the Cloud, and Twitter have been used for sharing open-source technologies and user experiences. Observational studies, anecdotal evidence, and real-world patient stories revealed significant improvements in time-in-range (TIR), time in hypoglycemia, glycated hemoglobin (HbA1c) levels, and quality of life (QoL) after the initiation of DIY-APS. Kesavadev et al., in their study had provided the real-world experience of the first successful patient from India on DIY-APS which highlighted better TIR, negligible time spent in hypoglycemia, and superior QoL. However, healthcare professionals, regulatory authorities, and device manufacturers view this approach with extreme caution, making users the ultimate risk-takers. It has been of great fret that regularized CGM and insulin pumps when combined with unauthorized algorithms makes them off-label. In addition to these, impediments to the widespread embrace of these systems among patients include a lack of safety evidence, funding or insurance coverage, ethical, and legal concerns.

CONCLUSION

AID systems represent a significant breakthrough in the management of type 1 and other challenging types of diabetes, seamlessly integrating CGM, advanced algorithms, and insulin infusion. Despite challenges and the need for user intervention, the evolution from basic insulin pumps to sophisticated systems like MiniMed™ 780G, Omnipod® 5, Tandem t:slim X2, and DBLG1 highlights a future where diabetes management is more intuitive, less invasive, and closely aligned with the physiological needs of individuals. The rise of DIY-APS underscores the community's role in driving innovation and optimizing care. As we look ahead, the ongoing refinement of AID systems promises to make diabetes a less burdensome condition to manage..

SUGGESTED READINGS

1. Kesavadev J, Saboo B, Krishna MB, Krishnan G. Evolution of Insulin Delivery Devices: From Syringes, Pens, and Pumps to DIY Artificial Pancreas. Diabetes Ther. 2020;11(6):1251-69.
2. Kesavadev J, Saboo B, Kar P, Sethi J. DIY artificial pancreas: A narrative of the first patient and the physicians' experiences from India. Diabetes Metab Syndr. 2021;15(2):615-20.
3. Kesavadev J, Basanth A, Krishnan G, Shankar A, Sanal G, Jothydev S. Real-World User and Clinician Perspective and Experience with MiniMed™ 780G Advanced Hybrid Closed Loop System. Diabetes Ther. 2023;14(8):1319-30.

67

CHAPTER

Vaccination in Diabetic Adults

Nirupam Prakash, Shweta Saxena, Jeevan Prakash

ABSTRACT

Cardiovascular disease (CVD) and chronic kidney disease (CKD) are major causes of morbidity and mortality in diabetes, however, infections still remain a major cause of hospital visits and admissions in diabetic individuals. In spite of all the progress in medicine, discovery of antimicrobials and improved diagnostics, infections are a challenge to treat in diabetic individuals, due to the impaired host immunity, drug-related adverse events, comorbidities leading to compromised hemodynamic, and metabolic status. The relationship between infections and hyperglycemia is bi-directional and they complement each other. Chronic inflammatory state in diabetes is characterized by a hyperglycemia-induced dysfunctional innate and adaptive immunity which predisposes them to infections on one hand and a nonspecific hyperinflammatory response on the other. Diabetic individuals are more susceptible to skin, soft tissue, respiratory, and genitourinary infections. The incidence and severity of vaccines preventable diseases (VPDs) is greater in diabetes and therefore it is pertinent to implement vaccination in adults with diabetes. Infectious disease prevention also lowers the incidence of cardiovascular (CV) events and deterioration in diabetic individuals. Vaccination provides for specific protection for diseases of public health importance in diabetes and can serve as a major tool to reduce morbidity and mortality in the long term.

INTRODUCTION

Diabetes is a chronic lifestyle disorder with multisystem affections. While microvascular and macrovascular complications are well known and regularly monitored, the implications of uncontrolled diabetes on increased risk and complications of infections are often missed and so is the greater need of diabetic subjects for vaccination. With rising population and a greater rise in diabetic population in both rural and urban India the challenges are increased manifolds. Herein we discuss the increased risk of diabetic patients to infections and role of vaccination in adult diabetics.

WHY INFECTION PREVENTION IS ESSENTIAL IN DIABETIC PATIENTS?

Infections of skin, bone, ear, eyes, urinary tract, gut, and respiratory tract in diabetes are more common and severe requiring hospitalizations. Severe infections and associated inflammation can in turn precipitate diabetic ketoacidosis and systemic complications. The odds of infection-related hospitalization or deaths in diabetic patients are 3.7 and 2.39 times higher compared to nondiabetic patients. During the 2009 H1N1 influenza epidemic the hospitalization were six times greater in diabetic patients compared to nondiabetic patients. The risk is higher in obese, elderly, type 1 diabetic patients (HR 3.71 vs. 1.88 in comparison to controls), uncontrolled diabetic patients and diabetic subjects with chronic kidney disease (CKD) and coronary artery disease (CAD).

DIABETES, IMMUNITY, AND PREDISPOSITION TO INFECTIONS

Diabetes is characterized by hyperglycemia and impaired host defense **(Box 1)** which predisposes to increased risk of infections, severity, and complications. Infection, associated inflammation, and release of stress hormones

BOX 1: Causes of immune dysfunction in diabetes.

- Hyperglycemia impairs neutrophil chemotaxis, phagocytosis, and opsonization
- Elevated glucose and FFA activates kinases (IKKβ and JNK1)
- DAG, ceramide, IL-6, TNF-α, ROS, hypoxia activate kinases (IKKβ and JNK1 mediators of stress and inflammation) in adipose tissue and liver which induce IRS1 inhibition and transcription of genes related to inflammatory response through NF-κβ
- TNF-α inhibits PPAR-γ
- Hyperglycemia induces impaired cytokine production to infections
- Impaired recruitment of CD45+ leukocyte and CD8+ T cells in diabetic subjects
- Hyperglycemia induces reduced expression of TLR on neutrophils and macrophages responsible for defective pathogen recognition
- Hyperglycemia inhibits neutrophil ROS generation, degranulation, opsonization, phagocytosis and extracellular traps generation
- Hyperglycemia inhibits macrophage phagocytic and antibacterial activity and expression of complement and Fcγ receptors and similarly the natural killer cells
- Inhibition of antibodies and classical complement pathway

(DAG: diacylglycerol; FFA: free fatty acid; IKK: I kappa B kinase; IL-6: interleukin-6; JNK: c-Jun N terminal Kinase; NF-κB: nuclear factor kappa B; PPAR-γ: peroxisome proliferator-activated receptor gamma; ROS: reactive oxygen species; TLR: toll-like receptor; TNF-α: tumor necrosis factor-alpha)

in turn worsens glycemic control, setting up a vicious cycle of worsening prognosis. Persistent dysfunctional chronic systemic inflammation of diabetes results in an exhausted, weak, nonspecific and misdirected immune response to infections. The host defense system including the first barrier of skin, local macrophages, cellular, and humoral immunity are impaired in diabetic subjects which is aggravated further by a hyperglycemic local and systemic milieu, micro and macroangiopathic changes and autonomic neuropathy responsible for poor wound healing, dermopathy, decreased antibacterial activity in urine, impaired gut barrier function and dysbiosis.

VACCINATION IN DIABETES

With the surge in community burden of noncommunicable diseases, the importance of infectious diseases is often forgotten. Diabetes itself provides a confluence of metabolic disorder with high cardiovascular (CV) risk and risk of infectious diseases and consequent complications. Infectious diseases account for 25% cases of mortality in adult population. 95% of mortality due to vaccine preventable diseases occur in adulthood. Influenza and pneumococcal infections are two common vaccine preventable diseases accounting for high morbidity and mortality in diabetic individuals. Similarly with increasing age and waning immunity, there is greater incidence of herpes zoster infections. Diabetes is a risk factor for both herpes zoster and post herpetic neuralgias. Frequent needle pricks for glycemic assessment; need for intravenous iron supplementation and blood transfusions in anemic diabetic CKD and dialysis in diabetics with CKD puts them at greater risk of parenterally transmitted infections such as hepatitis B. Therefore, vaccination can serve as an effective means of prevention of infections in diabetes. However, lack of awareness, confidence in vaccination measures, cost, hesitation, and physician inertia are few impediments to the implementation of preventive vaccination in diabetic adults. Hospital visits or admission serves as the most opportune time for implementation and spreading awareness of need and effectiveness of vaccination in diabetic patients.

VACCINE RESPONSIVENESS IN DIABETES

Humoral immunity is not affected in diabetes and antibody levels and response to vaccination such as hepatitis B and influenza vaccine is similar to reference control individuals. In contrast during the coronavirus disease 2019 (COVID-19) epidemic, correction of obesity and hyperglycemia, improved response rates to COVID-19 vaccination. Other independent confounding factors noted were hypertension, increased waist circumference, smoking, and dyslipidemia. Therefore, it is preferable to maintain euglycemia and encourage weight loss for better response rates to vaccination.

VACCINATION RECOMMENDATIONS IN DIABETES

Vaccination of an adult should be planned in continuation to the universal immunization program and carried forward throughout life. The vaccination strategy for an adult diabetic individual should be in accordance to the age appropriate existing guidelines for adult vaccination schedule and past vaccination status of the individual. If any dose is missed in between or if there is a gap additional dosage should be administered. Vaccination in young diabetic individuals should be ensured as per schedule provided in **Table 1**.

In later life there is age-related deterioration in immune status (immunosenescence) further aggravated by long duration of diabetes and associated hyperglycemia. Common infections in later life in diabetic individuals are very similar to nondiabetics viz. influenza, pneumococcal pneumonia, invasive pneumococcal disease, and herpes zoster. But the presentation is severe and associated

TABLE 1: Vaccination schedule for young diabetic adults.

Organism/Disease	Vaccine	Age of administration and dosage recommendations
Diphtheria, pertussis, tetanus	(Tdap/Td) 0.5 mL IM	• Immunize with Tdap once at 10–18 years; then Td 10-yearly (IMA, API, CDC); if nonimmune three doses two doses 4 weeks apart followed by third at 6–12 months and then every 10 yearly • Give additional doses in pregnancy or post injury
Measles, mumps, and rubella	MMR 0.5 mL SC	Two doses 1 month apart (ACIP); one dose if previously immunized. Pregnancy should be deferred for 3 months after immunization
Human papilloma virus	• 0.5 mL IM • Merck4 strain	• 9–14 years two doses 0 day and 6 months (IMA) • 15–45 years three doses 0 day, 1 and 6 months, defer if pregnancy

(ACIP: Advisory Committe on Immuniztion Practices; API: Association of Physicians of India; CDC: Association of Physicians of India; IMA: Indian Medical Association; MMR: measles, mumps, and rubella; Td: diphtheria-tetanus toxoid; Tdap: tetanus, diphtheria, and pertussis)

TABLE 2: Vaccination recommendation for diabetic individuals in later life.

Organism/Disease	Vaccine	Age of administration and dosage recommendations
Influenza	Trivalent/Quadrivalent	0.5 mL IM one dose annually in all diabetic patients especially those >50 years of age
Streptococcus pneumoniae	• PCV 13 • PPSV23	AACE recommends vaccination in >19 years of age with underlying medical condition including DM. PCV13 followed by PPSV23 at 1 years
Herpes zoster	0.5 mL SC	Individuals >50 years (AACE) including those with prior episode of zoster. Adults >19 year with weak immune system. Two doses 2–6 months apart.
COVID vaccine	0.5 mL SC	All individuals; primary dose and booster doses as per recommendations

(AACE: American Association of Clinical Endocrinology; DM: diabetes mellitus; IM: intramuscular; PCV13: pneumococcal vaccine 13-valent; PPSV23: pneumococcal polysaccharide vaccine)

with greater morbidity and mortality. The presence of comorbidities such as CKD, CAD, and heart failure further worsens the prognosis and limits the therapeutic options and dose. For instance use of tricyclic antidepressant (TCA), nonsteroidal anti-inflammatory drugs (NSAIDs), antivirals, antibiotics, and gamma-aminobutyric acid (GABA) analogues is dose limited in patients with CAD, heart failure, action potential duration (APD) and CKD. Use of certain OHAs is postulated to increase the risk of infections such as dipeptidyl peptidase-4 (DPP-4) inhibition of CD26 present on macrophages, T and B lymphocytes is theorized to inhibit cell mediated immunity. A timely vaccination strategy would not only prevent the occurrence of disease but also avoid the occurrence of drug-related side effects and in turn worsening of CVD/CKD. The vaccination schedule to be implemented in later life in diabetics is as provided in **Table 2**.

With increasing duration and progression of diabetes, renal and cardiovascular functioning may be compromised. Vaccination should be planned timely considering the future need for hemodialysis or renal transplant, immunosuppressants, deteriorating immune responsiveness in renal disease and coexisting CAD/heart failure. In advanced kidney disease the vaccine response rates are reported to be lower 50–60% in comparison to 90% in normal individuals.

Hepatitis B vaccination was incorporated in universal immunization schedule in India in 2010 and most of adult diabetic individuals on date are therefore unimmunized. AACE (American Association of Clinical Endocrinology) recommends hepatitis B immunization in all diabetic individuals <59 years of age. For those above 60 years of age, decision should be based on risk and quality of immune response. Hepatitis B vaccine should be administered as per schedule of 0, 1, and 6 months till stage 3 CKD diabetic individuals. Higher vaccine dose and increased number of doses are recommended for CKD subjects with estimated glomerular filtration rate (eGFR) <30 mL/min. Vaccine should be given intramuscularly in double dose (40 μg) intramuscularly in deltoid region at 0, 1, 2, and 6 months. Anti-HBs titers should be monitored 1–3 months after completion of schedule and annually thereafter. Booster or adjuvants be administered accordingly.

No live vaccine should be administered to transplant recipients. If a live vaccine has been administered a minimum time of 4 weeks should elapse before transplantation or starting immunosuppressants. Vaccine response in terms of protective antibody levels should be monitored for individuals on immunosuppressants. Vaccination should be avoided for the first 3–6 months following transplant, which is the period of intense immunosuppression.

Key points to drive home for implementing a successful vaccination strategy are:

- Vaccination is not a one time but a life-long process and needs to be emphasized at each clinic visit.
- Appropriate vaccination regimen for each individual needs to be reassessed at periodic life stages.
- Vaccine schedule for a diabetic individuals should be planned comprehensively and individualized taking cognizance of his age, prior vaccination status, presence of comorbidities (CKD, CAD), and immune status.
- Vaccination is not an all or none phenomenon and a diligent and persistent attempt to instill confidence in vaccination measures should be made.
- The vaccination schedule should be restructured considering the individual's travel needs and attendance to mass gatherings.
- Preventive measures such as protective clothing and masks, safe and potable drinking, hygienic food, nutritious food, and personal hygiene are neither foolproof nor alternatives but adjuvant to vaccination which provides specific protection against VPDs.
- There is greater need for spreading vaccination awareness and confidence amongst diabetic individuals and physicians alike.

SUGGESTED READINGS

1. Erener S. Diabetes, infection risk and COVID-19. Mol Metabol. 2020;39:1-10.
2. Berbudi A, Rahmadika N, Tjahjadi AI, Ruslami R. Type 2 Diabetes and its Impact on the Immune System. Curr Diabetes Rev. 2020;16(5):442-9.
3. Prakash N, Saxena S, Prakash J. Adult Vaccination: Need of the Hour. In: Mathur G (Ed). Medicine Update 2023. New Delhi: Jaypee Brothers Medical Publishers Pvt. Ltd.; 2023. Volume 33 (1), pp. 819-22.
4. Lohan L, Cool C, Viault L, Cestac P, Renard E, Galtier F, et al. Impact of hospitalization in an endocrinology department on vaccination coverage in people living with diabetes: a real-life study. Medicina (Kaunas). 2022;58(2):219.
5. Trivedi S, Trivedi R, Trivedi A. Influence of diabetes and metabolic risk factors on the outcomes of COVID-19 Vaccination: Scoping Review of the Observational Studies. Diabetes, Obesity, Metabolism and Nutrition. Endocr Abstr. 2022;81:588.
6. Prakash N, Mittra H, Prakash J. Adult Vaccination. In: Tewari K (Ed). Evangel's Medicine Update 2021. 2021. Volume 31, pp. 1137-40.
7. Papagianni M, Metallidis S, Tziomalos K. Herpes Zoster and Diabetes Mellitus: A Review. Diabetes Ther. 2018;9:545-50.
8. Prasad N, Chaudhuri AR, Gopal B, Bhadauria D, Sahay M, Sethi S, et al. Guidelines for vaccination in patients with chronic kidney disease. Indian J Nephrol. 2016;26 (Supplement 1):S15-18.

68

CHAPTER

Health Apps in Diabetes Management

M Gunasekaran

ABSTRACT

Diabetes is a complex, chronic illness requiring continuous medical care with multifactorial risk-reduction strategies beyond glycemic control. In patients with diabetes, mobile health-monitoring facility proves to play a significant role in providing significant assistance toward personal management. With >90% of individuals worldwide using mobile phones, m-Health interventions can reach numerous populations to promote healthcare and encourage behavioral change. Mobile phone-based interventions with clinical feedback improve glycemic control [glycated hemoglobin (HbA1c)] compared to standard care. India too is witnessing a digital revolution in healthcare, aided by its growing smartphone and internet penetration. At present, more than hundreds of apps for diabetes self-management are commercially available. Diabetes apps vary in the functions they provide, including tracking blood glucose measurements, nutrition database and carbohydrate tracking, physical activity and weight tracking, sharing data with clinicians or peers, social support, messaging, and reminders. The use of these features could help patients adhere to diet, exercise, and medication management plans, which could lead to improved diabetes-related outcomes. It is crucial for Physicians, general practitioners, nurse practitioners, and allied health professionals who may integrate apps into a holistic care strategy that considers techniques outside the clinical environment, given that self-management is a substantial element in glycemic control.

INTRODUCTION

India has *the second largest diabetes population* worldwide. Approximately 77 million people in India live with diabetes, and the number is estimated to almost double to approximately 134 million by the year 2045.

India shows a wide range of prevalence of diabetes ranging from 2 to 40%, depending on the region. Data suggests that every sixth person with diabetes in the world is an Indian.

Management of diabetes in India remains a major challenge due to the following reasons:

- Glycemic target in India is supposed to be ≤7% as suggested by the current Indian Council of Medical Research (*ICMR*) guidelines; however, data suggests that, diabetes control in India is far from ideal with a mean glycated hemoglobin (*HbA1c*) of *9.0%*, which is at least 2.0% higher than global standards.
- Targets for metabolic control too are not achieved in nearly 40% of the patients.
- Data also suggests that over 50% of diabetes cases in rural India and about 30% in urban areas go undiagnosed.

DIGITAL TECHNOLOGY IN DIABETES

Technological advancements in digital healthcare designed to improve healthcare efficiency hold extraordinary promise for a better future in diabetes care.

The *4D* approach of diabetes treatment consists of:

1. *D*iagnosis
2. *D*iet and daily exercise
3. *D*rug therapeutics
4. *D*igital technology

Digital technology help to *minimize risk*, *maximize benefit*, are *effective* and *efficient for users, convenient for users*, and time as well as *cost-efficient*.

Both behavior change and treatment models of intervention, as well as *interventions delivered via digital modes* have a larger effect on diabetes management.

M-HEALTH (MOBILE APP) IN DIABETES CARE

m-Health interventions use mobile technology to deliver real-time health and metabolic information, to engage patients in their diabetes management and help them achieve better health outcomes.

m-Health interventions can utilize texting to remind patients of glycemic goals set in the clinic, to enable patients to contact providers, or to provide diabetes education.

Smartphone applications bring even greater sophistication and customizability to patients' self-monitoring regimens than texting. Patients can have options when deciding which self-management behaviors are most suitable for their goals. Smartphones can serve as an interface between blood glucose-monitoring (BGM) devices, patients, and healthcare providers.

With >90% of individuals worldwide using mobile phones, m-Health interventions can reach numerous populations to promote healthcare and encourage behavioral change **(Fig. 1)**.

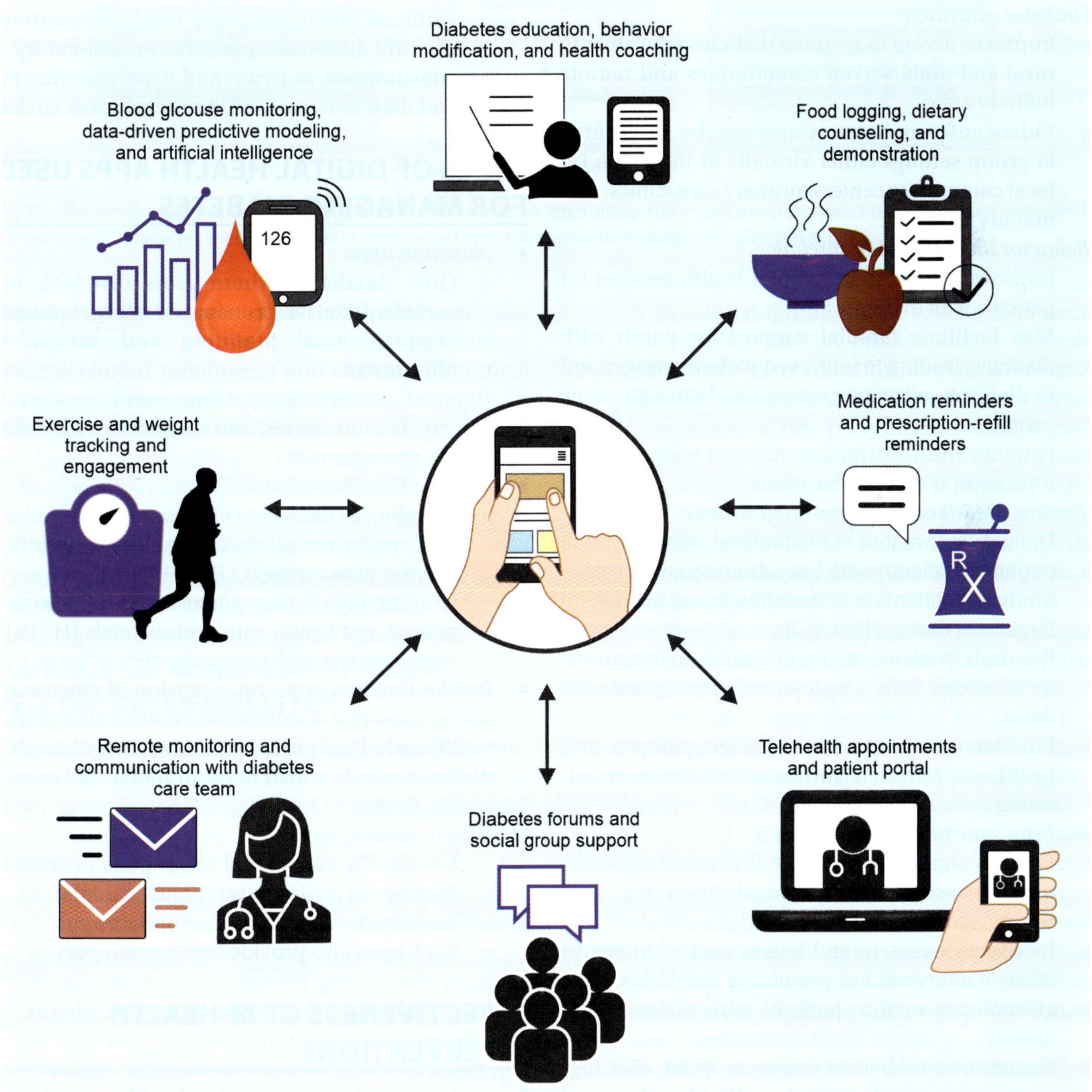

FIG. 1: The figure on the slide depicts a *digital ecosystem of diabetes care* that uses innovative means to support patients through all aspects of the day in the holistic management of diabetes.

Cushing's Syndrome

Cushing's syndrome is a complex disease arising from chronic hypercortisolemia due to any cause. Cushing's disease (CD) is hypercortisolemia caused by an adrenocorticotropic hormone (ACTH)-secreting pituitary tumor. Untreated hypercortisolemia is associated with an increase in mortality rate, ranging from 3 to 5 times higher than individuals without this condition. Subclinical CS may have a higher prevalence than clinically evident CS, although ongoing debate surrounds its precise definition, diagnostic criteria, and optimal treatment strategies. The clinical manifestations of CS encompass a range of symptoms, such as the presence of a moon-shaped face, a complexion that appears flushed and red, the occurrence of spontaneous ecchymoses (bruises), weakness in the muscles located near the center of the body, and the early onset of bone fractures, specifically those that are not caused by trauma, such as fractures in the ribs or vertebrae. Additionally, individuals affected by this syndrome may experience weight gain and a reduction in growth rate, particularly in pediatric patients.

The primary insulin antagonistic hormones are glucocorticoids such as growth hormone (GH). They have a variety of metabolic effects on the liver, adipose tissue, and muscle. Short-term increases in plasma cortisol levels in normal humans result in just a minor increase in glucose levels, mediated by hepatic and extrahepatic actions, but produce a considerable increase in ketone and branched-chain amino acid levels. In normal humans, insulin resistance caused by continuous administration of moderate dosages of glucocorticoids is usually compensated for by increased insulin secretion, resulting in minor changes in glucose levels. Thus, the range of glucose intolerance in CD or exogenous steroid use is largely determined by endogenous beta-cell reserve, as in acromegaly. Glucose intolerance affects 75–80% of CD patients, while only 10–15% develop diabetes. However, nearly all individuals have both basal and induced hyperinsulinemia as well as insulin resistance.

Primary Aldosteronism

Primary aldosteronism is described as excessive aldosterone synthesis in the presence of low plasma renin. PA was once thought to be a rare cause of secondary hypertension, but it is now known to be the most common cause, with a prevalence of 20% among patients with resistant hypertension, 10% in those with severe hypertension [systolic blood pressure (SBP) 180 mm Hg, diastolic blood pressure (DBP) 110 mm Hg], and 6% in those with otherwise uncomplicated hypertension. Only a small percentage of PA patients are diagnosed and treated. Even when controlling for the degree of blood pressure elevation, data suggests that PA increases cardiovascular morbidity and mortality beyond basic hypertension. As a result, early detection and treatment of PA are critical; nonetheless, PA remains underrecognized by both internists and specialists. PA screening is straightforward and easy to do, and it should be done routinely in individuals with resistant hypertension, hypertension with hypokalemia, or early-onset hypertension.

Moderately severe hypertension develops, which is frequently resistant to standard treatment. Left ventricular hypertrophy may be disproportionate. Asymptomatic hypokalemia is common. Patients with severe hypokalemia may manifest with tetany, myopathy, polyuria, and nocturia (hypokalemic nephrogenic diabetic insipidus).

Pheochromocytoma and Paraganglioma

Pheochromocytomas are tumors that produce adrenomedullary catecholamines. Paragangliomas are cancers that develop from extra-adrenal medullary neural crests derivatives, such as the organ of Zuckerkandl (sympathetic) or carotid body, aorticopulmonary, intravaginal, or jugulotympanic (parasympathetic) aorta. They are typically found in the head and neck, and only 25% of them are secretory. These uncommon tumors account for <0.1% of all causes of hypertension. Tumors typically appear in the third and fourth decades, with an equal gender distribution. Up to 50% of cases can be diagnosed postmortem.

Approximately 15–20% are malignant, with local invasion or distant metastases rather than capsular invasion. Differentiating benign from malignant tumors is challenging and is primarily predicated on the existence of metastases. However, chromosomal ploidy may be informative. Paragangliomas have a higher risk of being malignant and recurring. The retroperitoneum, lymph nodes, bone, liver, and mediastinum are common locations for metastases.

Sweating and heat intolerance >80%, pallor and flushing, apprehension, pyrexia, headache, paresthesia, visual impairment, seizures, and other symptoms are common in pheochromocytoma and paraganglioma.

Acromegaly

Acromegaly is a model for diabetes and glucose intolerance caused by endocrinopathy. Excess GH secretion before puberty causes gigantism, whereas acromegaly appears in adulthood. Many glucose metabolism problems are caused by excessive GH secretion. GH boosts insulin secretion in the first phase, which increases insulin-like growth factor 1 (IGF-1) synthesis in the liver and is implicated in insulin receptor activation. Insulin antagonism is a late consequence of GH. As a result, adipocyte glucose utilization is disrupted, and insulin resistance rises. The clinical characteristics result from the somatic and metabolic repercussions of long-term excess GH/IGF-1 exposure. After the oral glucose tolerance test, approximately 60% of patients with acromegaly show glucose tolerance issues. The majority of these patients have normal fasting glucose levels. Endogenous insulin levels are elevated in around 20% of people with acromegaly and normal glucose tolerance. After successful surgical or radiation treatment, most patients' glucose intolerance and insulin resistance disappear or dramatically diminish. Despite normal blood glucose, GH, and IGF-1 levels, about a third of individuals with acromegaly had unusually high insulin secretion during the oral glucose tolerance test for up to 2 years after surgical therapy. It could be linked to the onset of T2DM. A tiny subset of acromegaly patients has poor basal insulin secretion and an inappropriate response to stimulation, resulting in severe hyperglycemia and exogenous insulin needs.

Somatostatinoma

Somatostatinomas are extremely rare neuroendocrine tumors that can develop in both the pancreas and the duodenum. It is responsible for < 1% of all gastroenteropancreatic (GEP) endocrine tumors. The annual incidence is predicted to be 1 in 40 million, with a median age at onset of 54 years (range 24–84 years). More than 60% are big tumors in the pancreas's head or body. When metastatic dissemination to local lymph nodes and the liver has already occurred, the clinical syndrome may be detected late in the disease's progression. Glucose intolerance or frank diabetes mellitus may have been present for many years previous to diagnosis and is frequently the initial clinical indicator. It is most likely owing to somatostatin's inhibitory influence on insulin production. A significant incidence of gallstones has been reported, which is similar to the negative effect seen with long-term somatostatin analog therapy. Diarrhea, steatorrhea, and weight loss appear to be consistent clinical symptoms and may be related to somatostatin's suppression of the exocrine pancreas. Small duodenal somatostatinomas have been linked to neurofibromatosis type 1 (NF1) (43%). Although they rarely induce the inhibitory clinical condition, they do present with obstructive biliary disease due to tumor localization. Somatostatinomas are only 7% of the time associated with multiple endocrine neoplasia type 1 (MEN1).

Most patients (92.7%) have symptoms from these tumors, which are caused by the suppression of insulin, glucagon, gastrin, secretin, somatotrophin, thyrotropin, stomach inhibitory peptide, vasoactive intestinal polypeptide (VIP), pancreatic polypeptide (PP), and cholecystokinin. Diabetes mellitus, diarrhea/steatorrhea, and cholelithiasis are all symptoms of this 'inhibitory' condition, which is more common in pancreatic somatostatinomas than in duodenal tumors due to higher quantities of somatostatin secreted by pancreatic tumors. Dyspepsia, weight loss, anemia, and hypochlorhydria are among the additional symptoms that have been identified.

Glucagonoma

Glucagonomas are neuroendocrine tumors that often originate from pancreatic alpha cells and cause the glucagonoma syndrome by secreting glucagon and other peptides produced from the preproglucagon gene. The vast majority of glucagonomas are malignant, yet they are also slow-growing tumors that can lie undetected for years. At the time of presentation, up to 90% of patients will have lymph node or liver metastases. They are commonly linked with a rash called necrolytic migratory erythema. The annual incidence is predicted to be 1 per 20 million people.

The characteristic rash, necrolytic migratory erythema, appears in >70% of cases and begins as a well-demarcated region of erythema in the groin before spreading to the limbs, buttocks, and perineum. Stomatitis, glossitis, vaginitis, and urethritis are common symptoms of mucous membrane involvement. Glucagon counteracts the actions of insulin, notably on hepatic glucose metabolism, and glucose intolerance is a common (>90%) relationship. Sustained gluconeogenesis also produces amino acid shortages and protein catabolism, which is linked to unrelenting weight loss in >60% of patients. Glucagon has a direct suppressive impact on the bone marrow, resulting in almost all patients having normochromic normocytic anemia. MEN1 may be present in up to 20% of glucagonoma patients.

CONCLUSION

Treatment of underlying cause is of paramount importance in secondary diabetes. The treatment must be adjusted according to the pathogenesis of the condition. It is critical to properly question patients who exhibit the earliest signs of glucose metabolism problems. Subsequently, proper investigations may be required to confirm the diagnosis. Early diagnosis may be of vital importance to execute suitable treatment at the early stage of the disease to give the maximum benefit to the patient.

SUGGESTED READINGS

1. World Health Organization. (2023). Diabetes. [online] Available from http://www.who.int/mediacentre/factsheets/fs312/en/ [Last accessed December, 2023].
2. Rouiller N, Jornayvaz FR. Diabète sucré secondaire à une endocrinopathie: quand y penser? [Diabetes mellitus secondary to an endocrine pathology : when to think about it ?]. Rev Med Suisse. 2017;13(565):1158-62.
3. Borges-Martins L, Betea D, Daly A, Beckers A. Diabètes secondaires à une endocrinopathie [Secondary forms of diabetes mellitus associated with endocrine diseases]. Rev Med Liege. 2005;60(5-6):442-7.
4. Vila G, Gessl AW, Riedl M, Luger A. Other specific types of diabetes. Wien Klin Wochenschr. 2016;128:S208-11.
5. Borges-Martins L, Betea D, Daly A, Beckers A. Secondary forms of diabetes mellitus associated with endocrine diseases. Rev Med Liege. 2005;60:442-7.
6. Krysiak R, Rudzki H, Okopień B. Diabetes and prediabetes in endocrine disorders. Wiad Lek. 2012;65:187-98.
7. Rogowicz-Frontczak A, Majchrzak A, Zozulińska-Ziółkiewicz D. Insulin resistance in endocrine disorders—treatment options. Endokrynol Pol. 2017;68:334-51.
8. Hannon AM, Thompson CJ, Sherlock M. Diabetes in Patients With Acromegaly. Curr Diab Rep. 2017;17:8.
9. Mercado M, Ramírez-Rentería C. Metabolic Complications of Acromegaly. Front Horm Res. 2018;49:20-8.

SECTION

4

ENDOCRINE

71

CHAPTER

Vitamin D Deficiency and Bone Disease

Niraj Lodha

ABSTRACT

Vitamin D is crucial for bone mineralization and bone development, as it stimulates calcium absorption from the gut. Deficiency in vitamin D negatively impacts calcium metabolism, osteoblastic activity, matrix ossification, bone remodeling, and bone density. Prolonged deficiency can lead to rickets in children and osteomalacia in adults. Suboptimal vitamin D status is especially concerning in old age, as it reduces calcium absorption, causing bone turnover, and resorption, increasing fracture risk. The relationship between vitamin D and bone mineralization is direct, and optimal vitamin D status is essential for reducing fracture risk. Vitamin D may also enhance muscle strength, reducing fall risk, especially when used in combination with calcium.

INTRODUCTION

Vitamin D is an essential vitamin for normal development and maintenance of the skeleton. It is a secosteroid hormone necessary for calcium absorption and bone mineralization which is positively linked with bone mineral density (BMD). The principal effect of the active vitamin D metabolite 1,25(OH)2D is to stimulate the absorption of calcium from the gut. The active vitamin D metabolite 1,25(OH)2D opens the calcium channels present in the gut, also stimulates the development of calcium binding protein in the intestinal cell, and thereby stimulates the absorption of calcium and phosphate from the gut. By this way, optimal environment for bone mineralization is created. Deficiency of vitamin D negatively affects calcium metabolism, osteoblastic activity, matrix ossification, bone remodeling, and bone density as well. It is well-established that prolonged and severe deficiency of vitamin D leads to rickets in children and osteomalacia in adults. Suboptimal vitamin D status is reported in many populations, but it is a particular concern in people with old age. The reduction in calcium absorption because of vitamin D deficiency results in release of calcium from the bones to maintain the levels of circulating calcium concentrations. Continuous bone turnover and resorption makes the architecture of bones weak and increases the risk of fracture through secondary hyperparathyroidism eventually leading to the development of osteomalacia and osteoporosis.

There is a direct relationship between BMD and fracture risk. Considering the relationship between vitamin D and bone mineralization, optimal vitamin D status is essential for reducing the risk of fracture. Even though the potential benefits of vitamin D on fracture incidence may be at least partly credited to beneficial effects on BMD, vitamin D may also impart advantages by reducing fracture occurrence through enhancing muscle strength and thereby decrease the risk of falls which is one of the largest contributors to fracture. The incidence vitamin D appears to be more effective in reducing the risk of falls when it is used in combination with calcium **(Fig. 1)**.

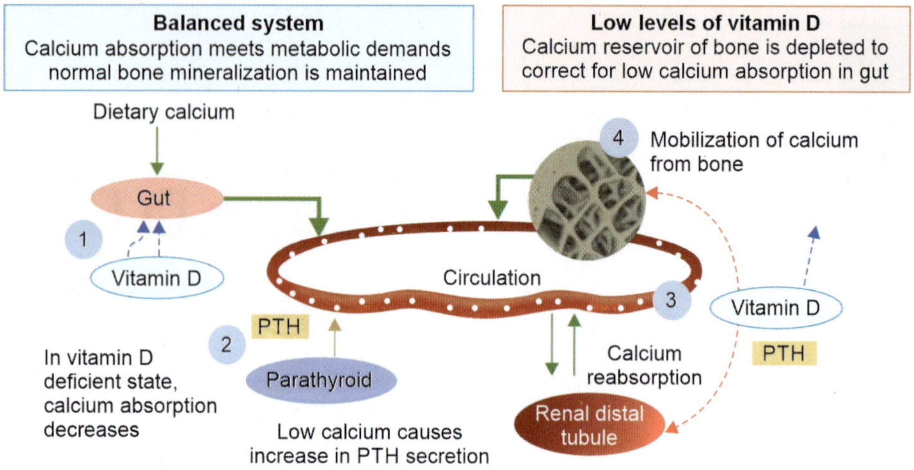

FIG. 1: Vitamin D and bone metabolism.

(PTH: parathyroid hormone)

Sources: Adapted from:

1. Hollick M. Vitamin D: the underappreciated D-lightful hormone that is important for skeletal and cellular health. Curr Opin Endocrinol Diabetes. 2002;9:87-98.
2. DeLuca HF. Overview of general physiologic features and functions of vitamin D. Am J Clin Nutr. 2004;80(6 suppl):1689S-96S.
3. Lips P. Vitamin D deficiency and secondary hyperparathyroidism in the elderly: consequences for bone loss and fractures and therapeutic implications. Endocr Rev. 2001:22:477-501.
4. Hollick MF. The vitamin D epidemic and its health. Consequences. J Nutr. 2005;135:2739-48S.

VITAMIN D DEFICIENCY AND HEART DISEASES

Various research unveiled new dimensions of vitamin D deficiency and potential involvement in cardiovascular disease (CVD). Deficiency of vitamin D is a widespread concern affecting approximately 30–50% of the global population, irrespective of ethnicity or age (CVD). Numerous epidemiological and clinical investigations have shed light on a compelling link between low vitamin D levels and significant CVDs such as coronary artery disease, heart failure, and atrial fibrillation. Strikingly, vitamin D deficiency appears to magnify the risk of adverse outcomes, including heightened morbidity, mortality, and recurrent cardiovascular events. Despite this mounting evidence, the use of vitamin D supplementation in patients either at risk of or afflicted by CVD remains a topic of debate **(Fig. 2)**.

The relationship between vitamin D deficiency and cardiovascular risk factors has garnered substantial attention. Vitamin D deficiency can instigate a cascade of detrimental effects, including increased renin and angiotensin II production, resulting in elevated levels of reactive oxygen species (ROS) and G protein RhoA. This, in turn, leads to the inhibition of intracellular glucose transporter pathways, paving the way for insulin resistance and the development of metabolic syndrome. Furthermore, vitamin D's direct influence on smooth muscle calcification and proliferation could further contribute to its impact on cardiovascular health.

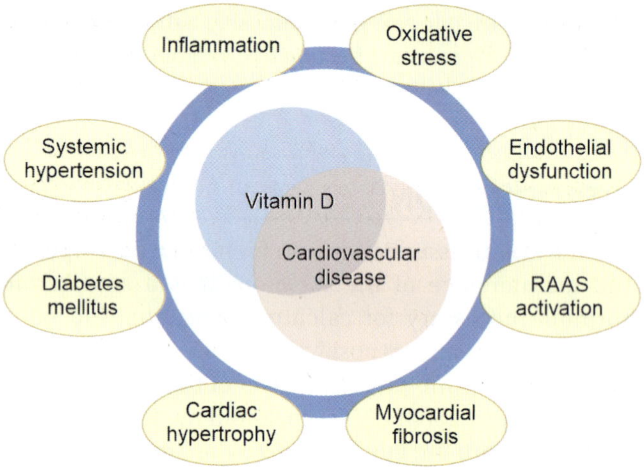

FIG. 2: Major hypothetical mechanisms underlying the association between vitamin D and cardiovascular disease.

A significant study involving 6,784 participants, known as the Inter99 study, revealed that higher vitamin D levels were associated with a favorable lipid profile and a reduced incidence of metabolic syndrome. The connection between vitamin D deficiency and CVDs and their risk factors has been examined extensively in both animal and human studies. However, the outcomes of studies and trials investigating the effects of vitamin D supplementation on cardiovascular risk factors and hypertension have been inconsistent and contradictory. Consequently, there is an urgent need for large-scale, well-designed randomized controlled trials to provide clarity on this matter.

Should these trials yield positive results, the widespread and cost-effective availability of vitamin D supplementation could potentially revolutionize our approach to cardiovascular health. The implications of such a discovery would extend far beyond conventional treatments, offering a simple yet powerful tool in our ongoing battle against CVDs. As we develop deeper understanding into the intricate relationship between vitamin D and heart health, the potential to enhance the well-being of individuals at risk of CVD becomes an exciting and promising avenue for future research.

VITAMIN D DEFICIENCY AND DIABETES

Type 2 diabetes mellitus (T2DM) is a prevalent noncommunicable disease that causes a high mortality rate worldwide. Vitamin D deficiency has become a growing pandemic, and it has been linked to obesity and insulin resistance. A study found that every 3 out of 4 diabetic patients in India is suffering from vitamin D deficiency.

Vitamin D is essential for the secretion of insulin from pancreatic beta cells, as reported by in vitro and in vivo studies. The mechanisms of how vitamin D acts on insulin secretion are believed to be direct and indirect. The direct effect of vitamin D on insulin synthesis and secretion is suggested by the binding of the active form of vitamin D to the vitamin D receptor (VDR) on beta cells, the identification of vitamin D response elements in the human insulin gene promoter, and the transcriptional activation of the human insulin gene caused by vitamin D. The indirect effects of vitamin D on beta-cell secretory function seem to be mediated by changes in calcium flux through the beta-cell membrane.

There is mounting evidence that suggests vitamin D deficiency may contribute to the development of diabetes. This is supported by the discovery that polymorphisms of the VDR have been linked to diabetes.[] Studies indicate that taking vitamin D supplements may help prevent the onset of T2DM. It will be argued later that vitamin D helps control several processes that initiate the onset of diabetes, such as the formation of Ca^{2+} and ROS. Essentially, vitamin D regulates the expression of genes that ensure the levels of Ca^{2+} and ROS are kept at their normal low levels. Another important function of vitamin D is to maintain normal mitochondrial control of cellular bioenergetics. Previous intervention studies evaluating the effect of vitamin D supplementation on glycemic control have produced conflicting findings. A meta-analysis found that vitamin D supplementation may be beneficial for the reduction of fasting plasma glucose (FPG), glycated hemoglobin (HbA1c), and homeostasis model assessment of insulin resistance (HOMA-IR) in patients with T2DM and deficient vitamin D status.

VITAMIN D AND AUTOIMMUNE DISEASE

Vitamin D not only enhances calcium absorption but also has an impact on the immune system by activating vitamin D in immune cells. Immune cells such as macrophages, T cells, dendritic cells, monocytes, and B cells express the VDR and harbor the enzyme 1-α-hydroxylase, allowing them to respond to and activate vitamin D. Vitamin D plays a role in regulating both innate and adaptive immunity. Vitamin D is a regulator of the innate immune system and has been used for over 150 years to treat infections, particularly those caused by mycobacteria such as tuberculosis and leprosy.

Autoimmunity is a condition where the immune system attacks the body's own cells and tissues, and its natural history is not fully understood. However, it is believed that both genetic susceptibility and environmental factors contribute to the development of autoimmune diseases. Vitamin D has been found to have immunomodulatory effects on various immune cells, including T and dendritic cells. These immune cells express VDR and produce enzymes that allow them to locally produce active 1,25(OH)2D3, which is the active form of vitamin D. Activation of CD4+ T cells leads to an increase in VDR expression, which enables the regulation of many genes responsive to 1,25(OH)2D3. These also directly inhibit Th1 cells and may modulate a skewing toward a Th2 response. Vitamin D has been found to suppress the Th17 response, a subset of CD4+ T cells involved in organ-specific autoimmunity, thereby inhibiting autoimmunity and tissue destruction. Vitamin D also has a direct effect on B cells, when exposed to 1,25(OH)2D3, the differentiation of B cells is interrupted, which may be beneficial in autoimmune diseases, where the immune system mistakenly attacks the body's own tissues.

Overall, the effects of vitamin D on B cells and dendritic cells suggest that it may play a crucial role in the development and progression of autoimmune diseases. Low levels of vitamin D are associated with an increased risk of infections and autoimmune diseases, while high levels have immune regulatory effects on NK cell cytotoxicity and cytokine secretion. Studies have shown that treatment with active vitamin D is effective in modulating immune function and ameliorating autoimmune disease **(Figs. 3 and 4)**.

VITAMIN D AND CANCER

Beyond its role in calcium homeostasis, bone metabolism, heart disease, diabetes, and autoimmune disease. Vitamin D deficiency has been found to be positively associated with a variety of cancers such as breast, multiple myeloma, colon, and prostate. Various studies shown that

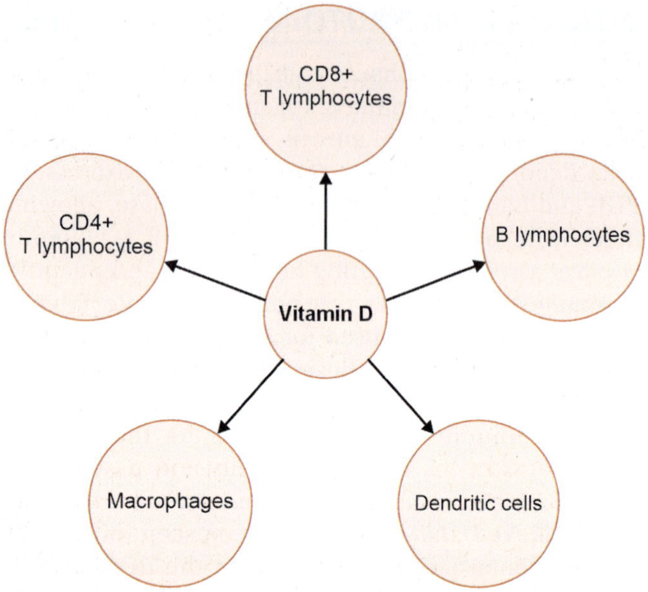

FIG. 3: Cells of the immune system regulated in part by vitamin D.

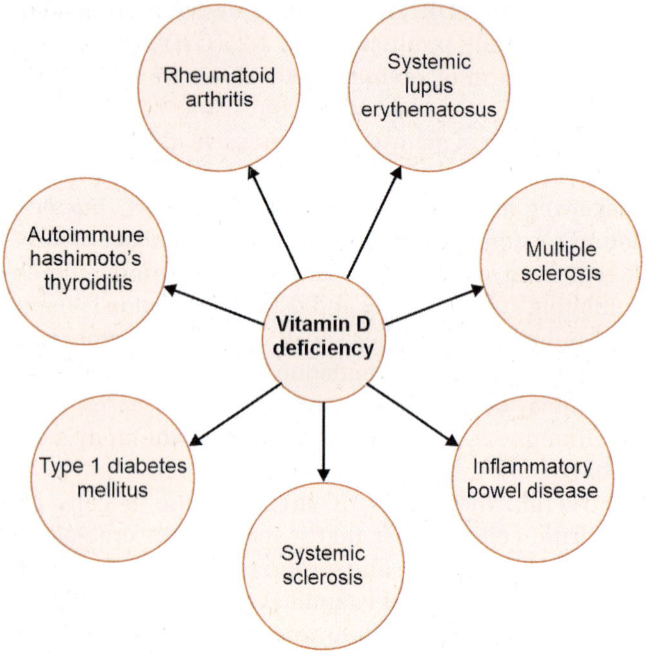

FIG. 4: Autoimmune diseases related to vitamin D deficiency.

levels of vitamin D to have an inverse relation with cancer mortality while others have considered it a potential risk factor. Low levels of vitamin D, as well as an increase in the enzyme vitamin D 24-hydroxylase (CYP24A1), are linked to a poor prognosis in cancer patients. Vitamin D and its metabolites reduce the incidence of many types of cancer by inhibiting tumor angiogenesis stimulating mutual adherence of cells and enhancing intercellular communication through gap junctions thereby strengthening the inhibition of proliferation that results from tight physical contact with adjacent cells within a tissue (contact inhibition). Metabolites of vitamin D maintain a normal calcium gradient in the colon epithelial crypts, and high serum levels of 25(OH)D are associated with markedly decreased proliferation of noncancerous but high-risk epithelial cells in the colon. Actions of the active metabolite 1,25(OH)2D are mediated by its binding to the VDRVDR in turn, regulate multiple genes in a cell-specific manner. However, certain cancers such as human esophageal squamous cell carcinoma have less expression of VDR than the normal tissues. Among the most widely studied VDR single-nucleotide polymorphism (SNP) is the rs731236 (TaqI) polymorphism. In a meta-analysis, this SNP was associated with increased risk of prostate cancer, particularly in Asians. Supplementation of vitamin D in high dose will help in suffice the serum 1,25(OH)2D levels that in turn will suppress the proliferation of cancer cells. Chandler PD et al. reported in his study that high-dose vitamin D supplementation for 5 years daily reduced the incidence of advanced (metastatic or fatal) cancer.

CONCLUSION

Vitamin D is a prohormone that has multiorgan system interaction. It has a pivotal role in various disease condition. Vitamin D deficiency positively associated with disease of bone as well as other system such as cardiovascular (heart disease), metabolic (diabetes), and immune system (autoimmune disease and cancers). Supplementation of vitamin D in high dose would help in mitigating the deficiency for prevention of multiorgan malfunctioning.

SUGGESTED READINGS

1. Christodoulou S, Goula T, Ververidis A, Drosos G. (2013). Vitamin D and Bone Disease. [online] Available from: https://www.hindawi.com/journals/bmri/2013/396541/ [Last accessed January, 2024].
2. Laird E, Ward M, McSorley E, Strain JJ, Wallace J. Vitamin D and bone health; Potential mechanisms. Nutrients. 2010;2(7):693-724.
3. Lips P, Van Schoor NM. The effect of vitamin D on bone and osteoporosis. Best Pract Res Clin Endocrinol Metabol. 2011;25(4):585-91.
4. Lips P. Vitamin D deficiency and secondary hyperparathyroidism in the elderly: consequences for bone loss and fractures and therapeutic implications. Endocr Rev. 2001;22(4):477-501.

5. Cummings SR, Black DM, Nevitt MC, Browner W, Cauley J, Ensrud K, et al. Bone density at various sites for prediction of hip fractures. The Study of Osteoporotic Fractures Research Group. Lancet. 1993;341:72-5.
6. Consentino N, Campodonico J, Milazzo V, De Metrio M, Brambilla M, Camera M, et al. Vitamin D and Cardiovascular Disease: Current Evidence and Future Perspectives. Nutrients. 2021;13(3603):1-14.
7. Kheiri B, Abdalla A, Osman M, Ahmed S, Hassan M, Bachuwa G. Vitamin D deficiency and risk of cardiovascular diseases: a narrative review. Clin Hypertens. 2018;24(9):1-9.
8. Anjana RM, Unnikrishnan R, Deepa M, Pradeepa R, Tandon N, Das AK, et al. Metabolic non-communicable disease health report of India: the ICMR-INDIAB national cross-sectional study (ICMR-INDIAB-17). Lancet Diabetes Endocrinol. 2023;11(7): 474-89.
9. Vijay GS, Ghonge S, Vajjala SM, Palal D, Vijay GS. Prevalence of Vitamin D Deficiency in Type 2 Diabetes Mellitus Patients: A Cross-Sectional Study. Cureus. 2023;15(5):e38952.
10. Hyppönen E, Power C. Vitamin D status and glucose homeostasis in the 1958 British birth cohort: the role of obesity. Diabetes care. 2006;29(10):2244-6.
11. Cade C, Norman AW. Vitamin D3 improves impaired glucose tolerance and insulin secretion in the vitamin D-deficient rat in vivo. Endocrinology. 1986;119(1):84-90.
12. Pittas AG, Lau J, Hu FB, Dawson-Hughes B. The role of vitamin D and calcium in type 2 diabetes. A systematic review and meta-analysis. J Clin Endocrinol Metabol. 2007;92(6):2017-29.
13. Maestro B, Dávila N, Carranza MC, Calle C. Identification of a Vitamin D response element in the human insulin receptor gene promoter. J Steroid Biochem Molec Biol. 2003;84(2-3):223-30.
14. Maestro B, Molero S, Bajo S, Dávila N, Calle C. Transcriptional activation of the human insulin receptor gene by 1, 25-dihydroxyvitamin D3. Cell Biochem Funct. 2002;20(3):227-32.
15. Mezza T, Muscogiuri G, Sorice GP, Prioletta A, Salomone E, Pontecorvi A, et al. Vitamin D deficiency: a new risk factor for type 2 diabetes. Ann Nutr Metabol. 2012;61(4):337-48.
16. Scragg R, Sowers M, Bell C. Serum 25-hydroxyvitamin D, diabetes, and ethnicity in the Third National Health and Nutrition Examination Survey. Diabetes care. 2004;27(12): 2813-8.
17. Mathieu C, Gysemans C, Giulietti A, Bouillon R. Vitamin D and diabetes. Diabetologia. 2005;48:1247-57.
18. Palomer X, González-Clemente JM, Blanco-Vaca F, Mauricio D. Role of vitamin D in the pathogenesis of type 2 diabetes mellitus. Diabetes, Obes Metabol. 2008;10(3):185-97.
19. Sentinelli F, Bertoccini L, Barchetta I, Capoccia D, Incani M, Pani MG, et al. The vitamin D receptor (VDR) gene rs11568820 variant is associated with type 2 diabetes and impaired insulin secretion in Italian adult subjects, and associates with increased cardio-metabolic risk in children. Nutr, Metabol Cardiovasc Dis. 2016;26(5):407-13.
20. Berridge MJ. Vitamin D deficiency and diabetes. Biochem J. 2017;474(8):1321-32.
21. Calton EK, Keane KN, Soares MJ. The potential regulatory role of vitamin D in the bioenergetics of inflammation. Curr Opin Clin Nutr Metabol Care. 2015;18(4):367-73.
22. Farahmand MA, Daneshzad E, Fung TT, Zahidi F, Muhammadi M, Bellissimo N, et al. What is the impact of vitamin D supplementation on glycemic control in people with type-2 diabetes: a systematic review and meta-analysis of randomized controlled trails. BMC Endocr Dis. 2023;23(1):15.
23. Kostoglou-Athanassiou I, Athanassiou L, Athanassiou P. (2019). Vitamin D and autoimmune diseases. [online] Available from https://www.intechopen.com/chapters/69633 [Last accessed January, 2024].
24. Cervantes JL, Oak E, Garcia J, Liu H, Lorenzini PA, Batra D, et al. Vitamin D modulates human macrophage response to Mycobacterium tuberculosis DNA. Tuberculosis (Edinburgh, Scotland). 2019;116s:S131-7.
25. Singh I, Lavania M, Pathak VK, Ahuja M, Turankar RP, Singh V, et al. VDR polymorphism, gene expression and vitamin D levels in leprosy patients from North Indian population. PLoS Negl Trop Dis. 2018;12(11):e0006823.
26. Yang CY, Leung PS, Adamopoulos IE, Gershwin ME. The implication of vitamin D and autoimmunity: a comprehensive review. Clin Rev Allergy Immunol. 2013;45(2):217-26.
27. Murdaca G, Tonacci A, Negrini S, et al. Emerging role of vitamin D in autoimmune diseases: An update on evidence and therapeutic implications. Autoimmun Rev. 2019;18(9):102350.
28. Gupta D, Vashi PG, Trukova K, Lis CG, Lammersfeld CA. Prevalence of serum vitamin D deficiency and insufficiency in cancer: Review of the epidemiological literature. Exp Ther Med. 2011;2(2):181-93.
29. Feldman D, Krishnan AV, Swami S, Giovannucci E, Feldman BJ. The role of vitamin D in reducing cancer risk and progression. Nat Rev Cancer. 2014;14(5):342-57.
30. Garland CF, Garland FC, Gorham ED, Lipkin M, Newmark H, Mohr SB, et al. The role of vitamin D in cancer prevention. Am J Public Health. 2006;96(2):252-61.
31. Holt P, Arber N, Halmos B, Forde K, Kissileff H, McGlynn KA, et al. Colonic epithelial cell proliferation decreases with increasing levels of serum 25-hydroxy vitamin D. Cancer Epidemiol Biomarkers Prev. 2002;11(1):113-9.
32. Young MRI, Xiong Y. Influence of vitamin D on cancer risk and treatment: Why the variability? Trends Cancer Res. 2018;13: 43-53.
33. Kang S, Zhao Y, Wang L, Liu J, Chen X, Liu X, et al. Vitamin D receptor Taq I polymorphism and the risk of prostate cancer: a meta-analysis. Oncotarget. 2017;9(6):7136-47.
34. Chandler PD, Chen WY, Ajala ON, Hazra A, Cook N, Bubes V, et al. Effect of vitamin D3 supplements on development of advanced cancer: A secondary analysis of the vital randomized clinical trial. JAMA Netw Open. 2020;3(11):e2025850.

72

CHAPTER

Fibrocalculous Pancreatic Diabetes

Vijay Budhwar, Sujoy Ghosh

ABSTRACT

Fibrocalculous pancreatic diabetes (FCPD) is a rare variant of diabetes, secondary to chronic nonalcoholic calcific pancreatitis that is seen almost exclusively in developing countries of the tropical world. The novel characteristics of FCPD include exocrine and endocrine pancreatic insufficiency, brittle glycemic control, and insulin-requiring, ketosis-resistant diabetes. Etiopathogenesis is multifactorial and not yet well determined, with malnutrition, cassava intake, micronutrient deficiencies, genetic mutations like serine protease inhibitor Kazal type 1 (*SPINK1*) gene variations being implicated. In contrast to the initial belief that, end-organ damage (microvascular and macrovascular complications) is uncommon in FCPD; recent reports have suggested the increased occurrence of such complications in FCPD. Though the diagnosis can be easily made in a patient with characteristic triad of pain abdomen, steatorrhea, and diabetes with pancreatic calcifications on imaging, management is challenging. Holistic care including glycemic management with insulin, nutritional support, adequate pain management, and high index of suspicion for pancreatic malignancy during follow-up is required for satisfactory outcome.

INTRODUCTION

Type 2 diabetes mellitus and type 1 diabetes mellitus (T2DM and T1DM, respectively) are the most common forms worldwide. However, approximately 1–5% of patients present with diabetes that may be secondary to other disorders. In this group, disorders of the pancreas are the most common. Various pancreatic disorders can cause diabetes, including pancreatic infections, inflammation, neoplasms, cystic fibrosis, and hemochromatosis. However, most common pancreatic disorder associated with diabetes is chronic pancreatitis and worldwide alcoholism is the most common cause of chronic pancreatitis. However, in many tropical countries such as India, the etiology frequently includes so-called "tropical chronic pancreatitis" and the diabetes associated with the condition has been termed "fibrocalculous pancreatic diabetes".

Pancreatic pathology leading to diabetes was published >200 years ago by Cawley who described the presence of pancreatic calcification in a patient with diabetes. The first description of tropical pancreatitis (TCP) was made by Zuidema in 1959 from Indonesia in a case series of 45 patients. Subsequently, it was reported from many parts of tropical Asia and Africa, but primarily from India and the Indian states of Tamil Nadu and Kerala in particular. Indeed, the largest series of patients with fibrocalculous pancreatic diabetes (FCPD) was collected from Kerala in the 1960s by Geevarghese, father of pancreatic diabetes. After being classified as a subtype of malnutrition-related diabetes mellitus (MRDM) by the World Health Organization (WHO) in 1985, FCPD was later included as an exocrine pancreas disease under other specific forms of diabetes, as suggested by a workshop held in Cuttack, India, in 1995 **(Figs. 1 and 2)**.

EPIDEMIOLOGY

Epidemiological data suggest that the prevalence of FCPD, a rare form of diabetes, is declining over time. According to a retrospective analysis conducted in Chennai, the prevalence of FCPD as a percentage of all cases of diabetes decreased from 1.6% in 1991–1995 to 0.2% in 2006–2010. Although the cause for same is unknown, better nutrition brought about by socioeconomic growth may be one of them.

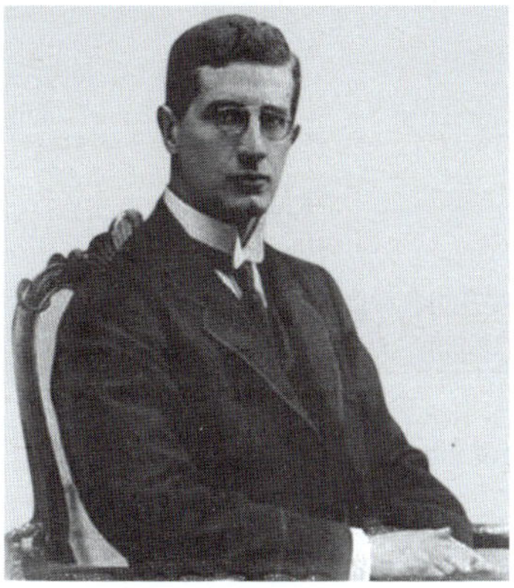

FIG. 1: *Sir Thomas Cawley*: First described diabetes secondary to pancreatic disease in 1788.

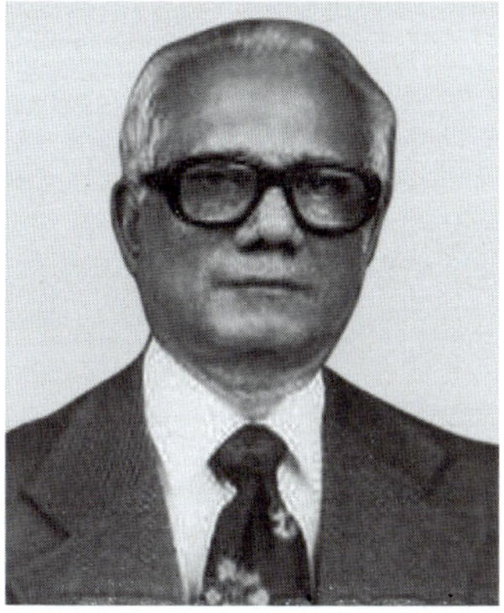

FIG. 2: Dr PJ Geevarghese (1925–2002) Father of pancreatic diabetes.

ETIOLOGY

The exact etiology remains unclear in spite of FCPD having been known to medical science for >75 years. Preliminary studies showed malnutrition as the cause of FCPD which was refuted by later studies which showed that it is the effect rather than the cause. The McMillan and Geevarghese cassava hypothesis linking two cyanogenic glycosides, linamarin and lotaustralin, which in the setting of malnutrition do not get detoxified and lead to pancreatic damage and diabetes have been refuted by recent epidemiological and experimental studies. Another controversial hypothesis is that deficiencies of trace elements and antioxidants may impair the body's ability to detoxify free radicals, leading to excess oxidative stress and tissue damage in FCPD. Some authors have also reported the presence of beta-cell autoantibodies in the serum of patients with FCPD, however, the individual autoantibody frequencies were low. It is much more likely that the presence of autoantibodies represents the body's response to widespread pancreatic damage rather than playing a role in the pathogenesis of disease.

GENETIC SUSCEPTIBILITY

Despite the fact that FCPD has been observed to recur within families, the illness is not heritable. Nonetheless, recent research has linked the likelihood of developing TCP and FCPD to variations in specific genes linked to exocrine pancreatic function. The *SPINK type 1* gene has been the subject of the most research out of all of these genes. This gene produces a protein called pancreatic secretory trypsin inhibitor (PSTI), which cleaves trypsinogen into inactive metabolites to stop premature activation of the pancreas. Therefore, recurring episodes of pancreatitis may result from a deficiency or impaired function of this protein. Studies from Bangladesh and southern India have observed 33–55% association of SPINK1 with FCPD. The cationic trypsinogen gene (*PRSS1*), which has been thoroughly investigated in relation to hereditary pancreatitis, and cathepsin B are two more genes that have been linked to the development of TCP. According to some authors, the main process leading to the development of TCP is the inappropriate activation of trypsinogen caused by mutations in the *PRSS1* gene. Defects in *SPINK1* (as well as other unknown genes) are thought to play a modulatory role in this process by preventing the inactivation of the prematurely activated trypsinogen. This is termed as "two-hit" hypothesis **(Figs. 3A and B)**.

PATHOGENESIS

The epithelial cells of the pancreatic ducts and interlobular ductules are the main injury targets in FCPD, which impairs watery alkaline secretions and fails the flushing mechanism. The enzymes released by the acini stagnate as a result, and the pressure inside the acini and ductules increases. Following pressure atrophy, the acinar cells die and there is localized fibrosis which consequently leads to exocrine insufficiency. Insufficient secretion of soluble lithostathine S and its conversion to more lithogenic lithostathine H2 are also caused by damage to the ductular epithelium. The viscid intraductal secretion, combined with increased intraluminal pressure and intraductal calculi, causes metaplastic alterations in the ductular epithelium, resulting in decreased beta-cell neogenesis from ductal progenitor cells. Fibrosis of the acinar cells and surrounding parenchyma obstructs intrapancreatic insulin circulation and its access to blood vessels. Diabetes may be caused by damage to endocrine tissue, as well as poor beta-cell neogenesis and decreased insulin supply to draining microvessels **(Flowchart 1)**.

Capillary plexus arising out of major arteries supply the islets and acini separately. Outflow of blood coming out of islets drain the acinar cells thus acinar cells receive high concentration of islets hormone. Trophic role of insulin

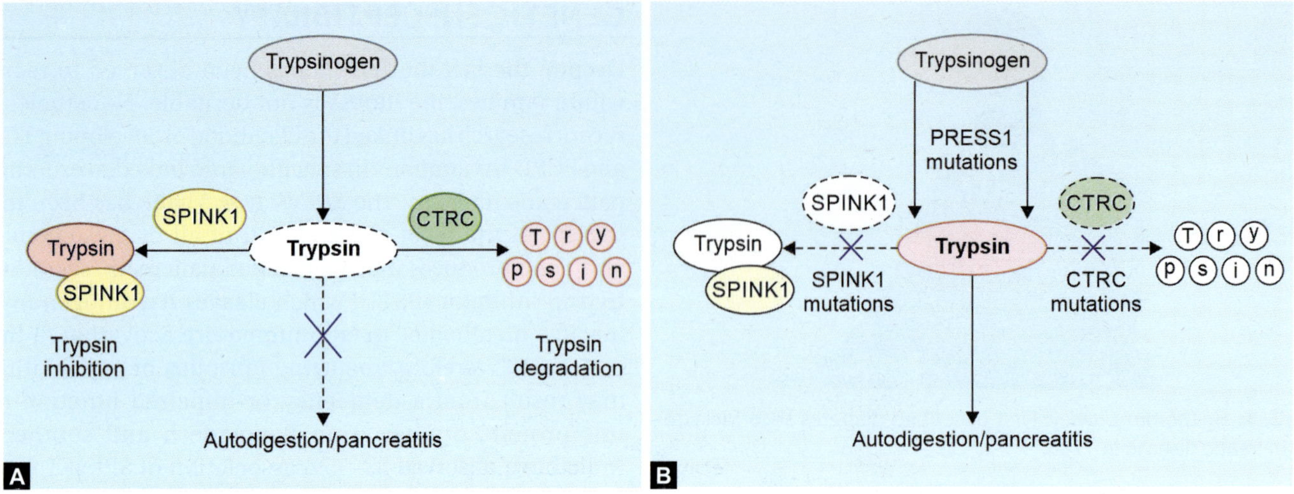

FIGS. 3A AND B: Postulated mechanism of *SPINK1*, *PRSS1*, and *CTRC* mutations in pancreatitis pathogenesis.

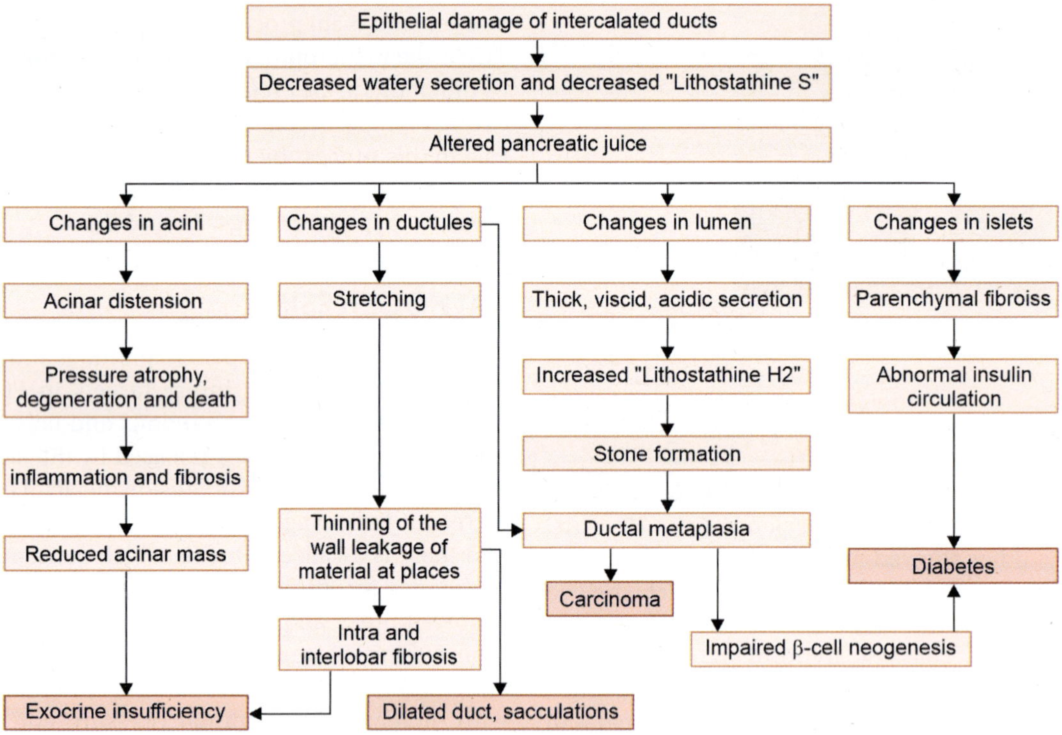

FLOWCHART 1: Pathogenesis of fibrocalculous pancreatic diabetes.

on acinar cells influences exocrine pancreas functioning. In diabetes patient, pancreatic insufficiency occurs due to loss of this trophic action. Other important mechanism is autonomic neuropathy associated with diabetes. Autonomic neuropathy impairs the enteropancreatic reflexes, which mediate up to 50% of pancreatic response after a meal. Furthermore, in the presence of intestinal autonomic neuropathy, gastric emptying and nutrition delivery to the proximal small intestine are delayed. As a result, cholecystokinin (CCK) secretion is lesser stimulated and exocrine pancreatic secretion is inhibited **(Figs. 4A and B)**.

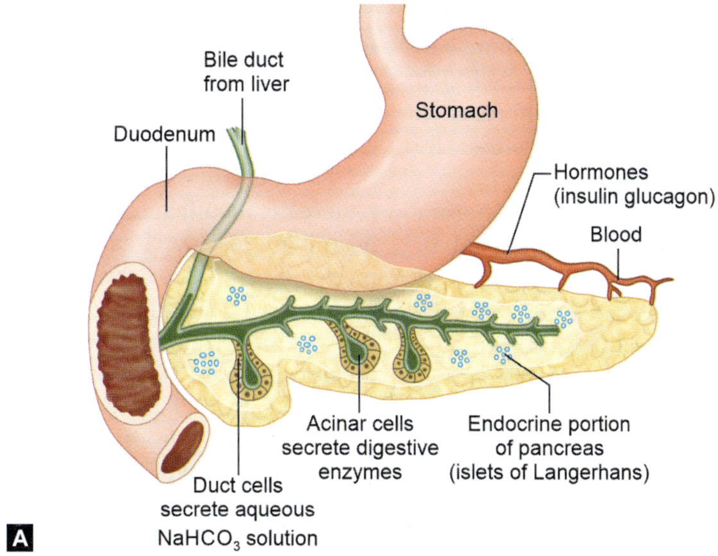

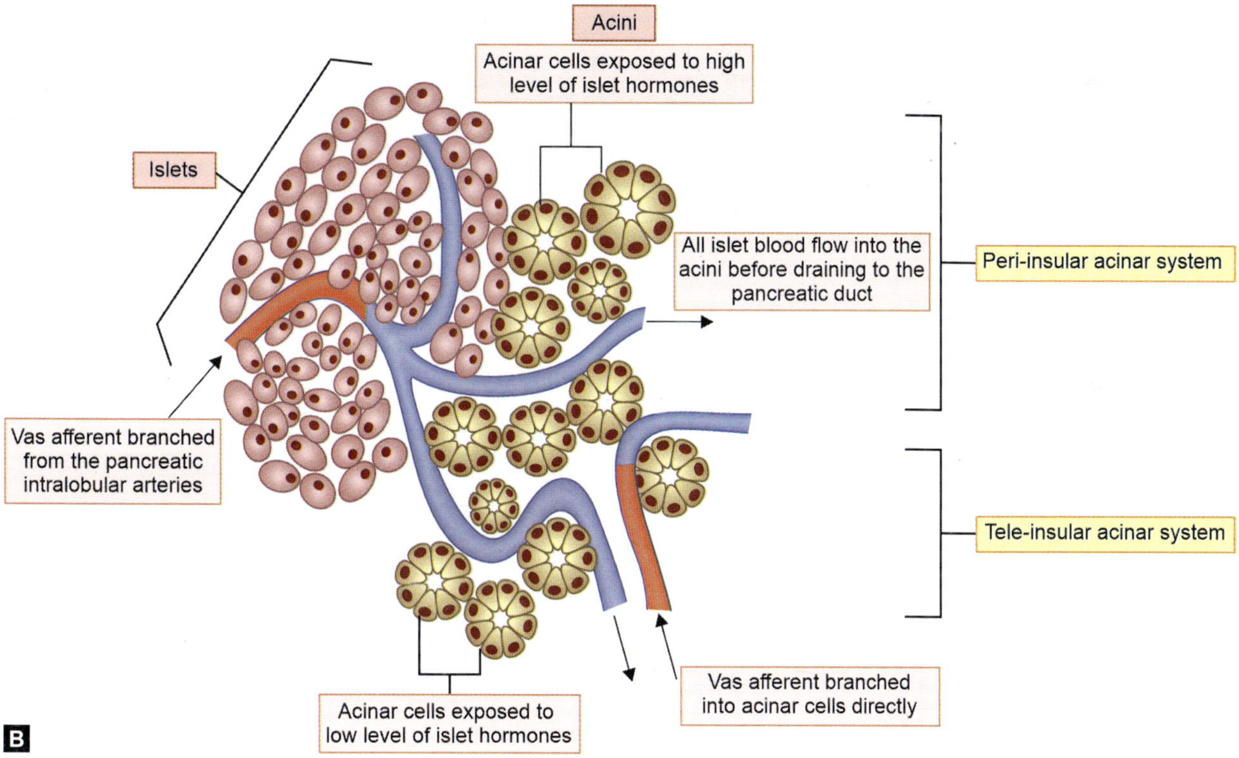

FIGS. 4A AND B: Endocrine—exocrine crosstalk and insulin-acinar axis.

Hyperglycemia in Fibrocalculous Pancreatic Diabetes

Insulin deficiency due to the pancreatic islet destruction in TCP is the most predominant reason for the development of diabetes in FCPD. Study involving 101 FCPD, 41 T1DM, 40 T2DM, and 40 non-DM control at our institute showed that beta-cell reserve is lowest in T1DM followed by FCPD than T2DM.

Pancreatogenic diabetes is associated with exocrine pancreas insufficiency. This may lead to decreased nutritional entry due to malabsorption, which can eventually lead to a lack of or a muted incretin response to meals and reduced postprandial insulin secretion. However, a study from our institute found that active glucagon-like peptide 1 (GLP-1) levels were two times higher in the FCPD group compared to controls and one and a half times higher than in T2DM group in both fasting and postglucose state. In our study, all groups showed a significant increase in GIP level in response to glucose; however, increment was most robust in the FCPD group. Furthermore, there was no significant difference in the GIP level between the other groups during either the fasting or postglucose state. The dipeptidyl peptidase-4 (DPP-4) levels in the three groups were not different in fasting state, and they dramatically increased in both FCPD and control following the glucose load. This demonstrates that the significantly elevated incretin level in FCPD is not caused by preferentially more reduced DPP-4 levels in FCPD, but rather by enhanced secretion or resistance at the effector level. This might be due to an exaggerated secretion of GLP-1 from the L cells in face of target organ failure analogous to negative feedback control of other endocrine systems. Variable outcomes were obtained while using the pancreatic enzyme replacement therapy (PERT) with mixed meals to assess changes in the glycemic state as well as incretins, insulin, and glucagon. Thus, the impaired incretin response may actually be a consequence of diabetes rather than its cause. Our results unequivocally elucidate that, though FCPD is included in the general category of pancreatogenic diabetes, its incretin response differs from that of other types of pancreatogenic diabetes. Our research further indicates that, in contrast to other types of pancreatogenic diabetes (particularly chronic pancreatitis), PERT is unlikely to result in an improvement in glycemic control in FCPD. Additionally, incretin-based therapies for FCPD are unwarranted based on findings of our study. Previous study showed that in response to glucose load, the glucagon levels decreased in controls, increased in T2DM and did not show any change in FCPD. Hence increased glucagon is not the reason for hyperglycemia in FCPD.

Few studies have suggested role of insulin resistance (IR) in development of hyperglycemia in FCPD, however, in two studies conducted at our institute, IR measured by indices using serum insulin and C peptide [Homeostatic model assessment (HOMA)-IR and HOMA-C peptide) did not reveal increased IR in FCPD patients.

CLINICAL PICTURE

"Pain in childhood, diabetes mellitus by puberty and death in prime of life"(Dr PJ Geevarghese)

The classic patient with FCPD is a lean young adult of either sex belonging to the lower socioeconomic stratum from a tropical country with the triad of recurrent abdominal pain, steatorrhea, and diabetes. However, the condition is now also found in people from more affluent groups, and some patients are not lean either. In the natural course of the illness, each of these basic triad symptoms often predominates at a distinct stage.

The presenting feature in the early stage (typically in the first decade of life) is abdominal pain (indistinguishable from that in other forms of acute pancreatitis). Throughout childhood and adolescence, pain episodes can reoccur at varied intervals.

The patient then develops symptoms of exocrine pancreatic insufficiency, with steatorrhea being the most prominent feature. Steatorrhea may not be prominent in many cases (particularly in India) because the diet is low in fat. Prolonged fat malabsorption can result in deficiency of fat-soluble vitamins and essential fatty acids with the development of corresponding disease syndromes.

In the third stage, which typically occurs in the initial years of adulthood, the patient exhibits glucose intolerance; "prediabetes" phase similar to T2DM. The abdominal pain usually subsides or gets less severe before endocrine insufficiency sets in, but the symptoms of exocrine pancreatic insufficiency persist.

Due to severe insulin deficiency, FCPD patients typically have severe diabetes. Even within a single day, it exhibits considerable glycemic fluctuation and brittleness; patients frequently experience unpredictable hypoglycemia spells. Ketosis is uncommon in FCPD despite frequently having very high glucose levels. The following theories have been put forth to explain the phenomena of ketosis resistance in FCPD:

- Partial preservation of beta-cell function; enough endogenous insulin to prevent ketogenesis, but not to sustain euglycemia.
- Decreased glucagon reserve; alpha cells are also get involved in the destructive process.
- As there is less subcutaneous fat, there is less availability of nonesterified fatty acids (NEFA), the substrate for ketogenesis.
- Deficiency of carnitine, an important fatty acid transporter that shifts fatty acids into the mitochondria for beta-oxidation has also been postulated by some authors.

Very rarely, some patients become truly "insulin dependent" and may develop ketoacidosis on withdrawal of insulin.

DIAGNOSIS

Diagnostic criteria for FCPD by Mohan et al.:

- Patient from a tropical country
- Presence of DM
- *Evidence of chronic pancreatitis*: Abdominal imaging revealing pancreatic calculi or at least three of the following:
    1. Abnormal pancreatic morphology on ultrasound abdomen or computed tomography (CT) scan
    2. History of recurrent abdominal pain since childhood

3. Steatorrhea
4. Abnormal pancreatic function tests

- Absence of other causes of chronic pancreatitis (e.g., alcohol abuse, hypercalcemia, and hypertriglyceridemia)

INVESTIGATIONS

Investigation of choice: Plain abdominal X-ray may indicate presence of the distinctive pancreatic calculi that cross the midline at the first lumbar vertebral level **(Fig. 5)**.

An abdominal ultrasound examination is also helpful in detecting pancreatic duct dilatation in addition to calcification and calculi **(Fig. 6)**. While not recommended in routine practice, other imaging tests such as endoscopic retrograde cholangiopancreatography (ERCP) and CT or magnetic resonance imaging (MRI) scans can be helpful in ruling out problems (such pancreatic cancer) or as a component of therapeutic intervention.

Assessment of exocrine insufficiency is difficult and controversial. The gold standard is the examination of stool collected over 72 hours after ingesting 100 g of oral fat daily, however, the process is laborious, time-consuming, and might not be acceptable due to dyspepsia and worsening steatorrhea. Pancreatic elastase remains stable during intestinal transit and can be measured in fecal elastase by an enzyme-linked immunosorbent assay (ELISA). Subjects with fecal elastase concentration (FEC) <200 µg/g are considered to have pancreatic exocrine insufficiency (when FEC is <100 µg/g, insufficiency is considered severe). In a study from our institute, all 31 FCPD patients had severe exocrine insufficiency. The prevalence of pancreatic insufficiency in T2DM was 37.5% (severe deficiency in 25) and in T1DM was 37.9% (severe deficiency in 16.7%).

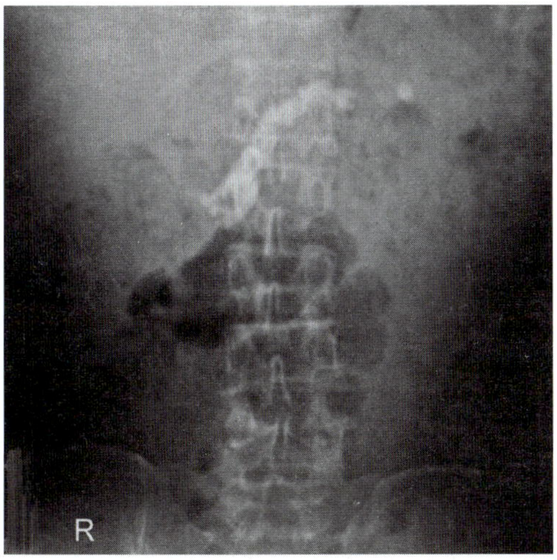

FIG. 5: Plain X-ray abdomen showing pancreatic calculi in fibrocalculous pancreatic diabetes (FCPD).

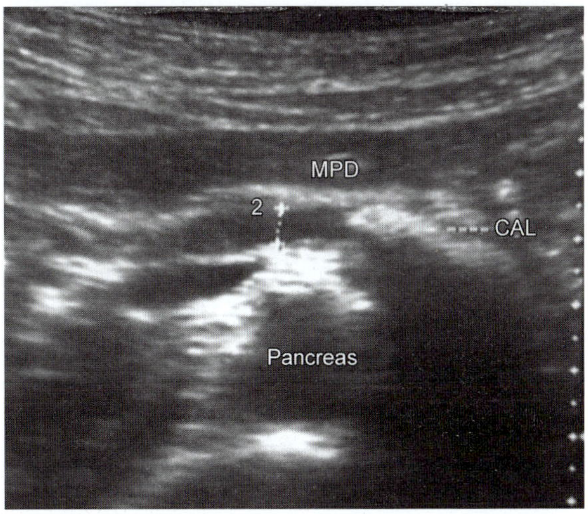

FIG. 6: Ultrasound showing features of chronic calcific pancreatitis [main pancreatic duct (MPD) dilatation, intraductal calculus].

TABLE 1: Differences between tropical chronic pancreatitis and alcoholic chronic pancreatitis.

Alcoholic chronic pancreatitis	Tropical chronic pancreatitis
Occur in all socioeconomic strata	Mainly restricted to less affluent sections of society
Males almost exclusively affected	Male preponderance (~70%)
Occurs later in life (fourth and fifth decades)	Occur earlier in life (second and third decades)
Diabetes occurs in around 50%	Diabetes occurs in around 70%
Calculi are small, speckled, and restricted to smaller ducts	Calculi are large and found in larger ducts
Fibrosis and duct dilatation less common	Fibrosis and duct dilatation more common
Increased risk of pancreatic cancer	Markedly increased risk of pancreatic cancer

Diabetes secondary to alcoholic chronic pancreatitis (ACP) is the main differential diagnosis of FCPD. The major differences between these two conditions are outlined in **Table 1**.

COMPLICATIONS

Although, it was initially thought that complications associated to diabetes were rare in FCPD, it being a secondary type of diabetes; however, subsequent reports defied this opinion. As the longevity of these patients increased due to better pain and diabetes management, diabetes-related vascular complications have been reported. While individuals with FCPD have the same risk of microvascular complications (retinopathy and nephropathy) as T2DM patients with comparable levels

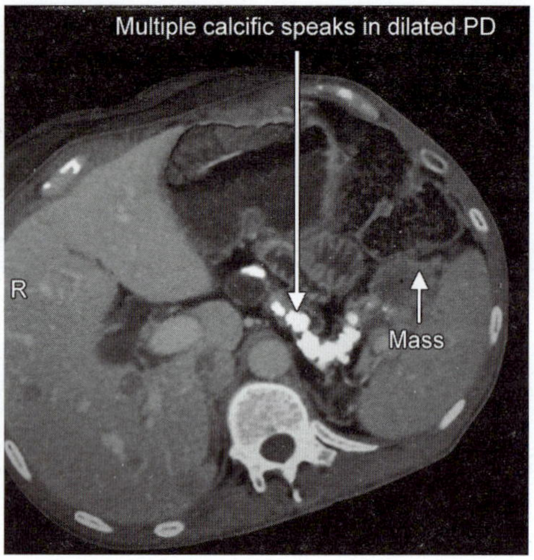

FIG. 7: Computed tomography abdomen of patient-1 showing atrophic pancreas, dilated main pancreatic duct with multiple calculi in the head, body, and tail of pancreas with a 38 mm × 38 mm × 32 mm mass in the tail of pancreas. Multiple target lesions can also be seen in liver suggestive of metastasis.

of glycemic control, their risk of macrovascular (cardiovascular) disease is substantially lower. When compared to people with T2DM, it appears that these lean patients had fewer risk factors for CVD, such as dyslipidemia and hypertension. Study from our institute has shown about 40% of FCPD patients had cardiac autonomic neuropathy (CAN) while 13.33% had borderline CAN. Isolated parasympathetic dysfunction was the most common (66.67%) among them.

Patients with FCPD are at risk for malnutrition in addition to the complications of diabetes because of fat malabsorption. This may manifest as deficiency syndromes of fat-soluble vitamins A, D, E, and K (coagulopathy, night blindness, etc.).

Most dreaded complication of FCPD is pancreatic adenocarcinoma. It has been suggested that the risk of developing pancreatic cancer is the highest in patients with FCPD as compared to all other forms of pancreatitis and is believed to be 100-fold greater than those without FCPD. Even in the absence of the classic symptoms of pancreatic cancer, such as obstructive jaundice, palpable gallbladder, and abdominal pain; patients with FCPD who exhibit anorexia, weight loss, or worsening glycemic control should be taken seriously as warning signs and evaluated for any occult pancreatic malignancy. There is no consensus on screening patients with FCPD for cancer using tumor markers (e.g., Ca-19.9) or serial imaging at present **(Fig. 7)**.

MANAGEMENT

The management of FCPD focuses on symptoms alleviation and achieving the best feasible glycemic control in order to prevent the development of complications.

■ Glycemic Control

The majority of patients requires insulin to control their diabetes, however, for varied lengths of time, some may be adequately managed with oral antidiabetic medications or even only lifestyle changes. There are probably no contraindications to any class of medicines in FCPD, with the exception of those that can potentially cause pancreatitis (incretin-based therapy). Agents that cause weight loss and catabolic effects, on the other hand, should be avoided.

■ Nutrition Support

Pancreatic enzyme supplements have been found to alleviate abdominal pain by inhibiting endogenous pancreatic secretion and thereby lowering intraductal pressure. They may also help with steatorrhea and nutritional status. Furthermore, the use of these supplements may promote improved glycemic control by encouraging patients to eat better and therefore allowing the administration of adequate amounts of insulin, however, the results are conflicting. Supplementation of fat-soluble vitamins (A, D, E, and K) is needed. To combat the negative effects of malnutrition, patients with FCPD, high-protein diet is recommended. Smoking and drinking should be severely discouraged.

■ Analgesic Management

Nonopioid analgesics are the treatment of choice. Severe and resistant to medical management warrants surgical intervention such as sphincterotomy, endoscopic removal of pancreatic calculi, and drainage procedures such as lateral pancreaticojejunostomy.

CONCLUSION

The FCPD should be considered in the differential diagnosis of any young person with diabetes, especially from tropical regions with a history of acute pancreatitis or exocrine pancreatic insufficiency. A plain X-ray of the abdomen can aid in the diagnosis. While diabetes care in this disease is challenging, a holistic strategy combines symptomatic therapy, nutritional assistance, and glycemic control (which primarily requires insulin). Potential of pancreatic cancer development should always be kept in mind if a patient exhibit unexplained worsening of glycemic control, anorexia, and weight loss; even in the absence of the classic symptoms of pancreatic cancer, such as obstructive jaundice, palpable gallbladder, and abdominal pain.

SUGGESTED READINGS

1. Chakraborty PP, Chowdhury S. A Look Inside the Pancreas: The "Endocrine-Exocrine Cross-talk". Endocrinol Metab Synd. 2015;4:160.
2. Anne B, Ghosh S, Ghosh I, Ray S, Chowdhury S, Dutta D. Prevalence of end-organ damage, beta cell reserve, and exocrine pancreas defect in fibrocalculous pancreatic diabetes: An Eastern India perspective. Indian J Endocr Metab. 2019;23:438-45.
3. Ghosh I, Mukhopadhyay P, Das K, Anne MB, Ali Mondal S, Basu M, et al. Incretins in fibrocalculous pancreatic diabetes: A unique subtype of pancreatogenic diabetes. J Diabetes. 2021;13(6):506-11.
4. Ghosh I, Basu M, Beatrice A, Mukhopadhyay P, Ghosh S. Exocrine pancreatic dysfunction in diabetes: An observational study. Indian J Endocr Metab. 2021;25:67-8.
5. Chakraborty PP, Dutta D, Biswas K, Sanyal T, GhoshS, Mukhopadhyay S, et al. Pancreatic carcinoma in fibrocalcificpancreatic diabetes: An eastern India perspective. Indian J Endocr Metab. 2012;16:S486-8.
6. Unnikrishnan R, Mohan V. Fibrocalculous pancreatic diabetes. Curr Diab Rep. 2020;20(6):19.

73

CHAPTER

Unusual Patterns of Thyroid Function Tests: Diagnosis Made Easier

Swati Srivastava

ABSTRACT

Though the interpretation of thyroid function tests (TFTs) is usually simple, sometimes they may not correlate with the clinical scenario or have an unusual pattern. Thyroid-stimulating hormone (TSH) is considered to be a sensitive indicator to gauge the variations occurring in the thyroid levels. In spite of TSH being a highly sensitive indicator for evaluation of thyroid status, there are conditions where TSH alone may not be adequate and my give misleading directions to the diagnosis. In such situations, thyroid hormone levels T3 and T4 are important in making diagnosis. Pregnancy, levothyroxine therapy, concomitant medications, nonthyroidal illness (NTI), assay interference, antithyroid treatment, and thyroid hormone resistance are some factors which may lead to discordant thyroid function tests. When thyroid tests are interpreted, the clinical status of patient and diagnosis should be kept in mind. On encountering discordant thyroid tests, re-evaluating the clinical condition will help to guide further management. Insufficient attention to clinical profile may lead to confusion and unnecessary investigations in patients.

INTRODUCTION

Unusual patterns of thyroid function tests (TFTs) may cause misdiagnosis and not correlate with the clinical scenario. Reassessment of the clinical background and proper understanding of such unusual patterns is helpful in avoidance of misdiagnosis. Inability to recognize discordant TFTs may lead to inappropriate line of treatment and complications.

REGULATION OF THYROID HORMONE SYNTHESIS

The thyroid hormones bear a log-linear alliance with the thyroid-stimulating hormone (TSH). A minor change in the levels of thyroxine may not be obvious as it would still be within the normal range. However, this minor change will lead to a marked excursion in the level of TSH. A two times reduction in free-thyroxine level may result in a rise of TSH by hundredfold.

CONDITIONS IN WHICH MEASUREMENT OF THYROID-STIMULATING HORMONE ALONE IS NOT ADEQUATE

Conditions in which measurement of TSH alone is not adequate are seen in:

- Secondary and tertiary hypothyroidism
- Nonthyroidal illness (NTI)
- Patients who were thyrotoxic and have recently begun treatment for thyrotoxicosis may also show change in thyroid hormone levels to the normal range, but TSH may persist to remain suppressed for long duration. If this is not perceived, the treating physician may continue to increase the dose of antithyroid medication leading to drug-induced hypothyroidism
- Resistance of thyroid hormone

Subclinical Thyroid Disorders

The reference levels for normal thyroid hormones are wide-ranged in proportion to the small changes occurring in them in normal individuals.

This means that though the changes in thyroid hormone levels which are significant enough to result in hypothyroidism or hyperthyroidism in an individual, have occurred, still due to the normal ranges of these hormones being quite wide, numerically the values may still fall in normal limits.

Hence, in spite of numerically normal T4 and T3 levels, one may have evidence of mild thyroid hypo- or hyperfunction. In such individuals, the changes are seen in TSH values. Hence, changes in TSH without abnormal T3 and T4 levels are termed subclinical thyroid disorders.

IMPORTANT CONSIDERATIONS PRIOR TO EVALUATION OF THYROID TESTS

Pregnancy

The thyroid tests undergo physiological changes during pregnancy. The high human chorionic gonadotropin (hCG), particularly in the first trimester of pregnancy, having structural similarity with TSH, results in simultaneous reduction in TSH and increase in T3 and T4. Also, the effect of estrogen on thyroid hormone-binding proteins, the effect of placental deiodinases and alteration in immune status during pregnancy result in changes during pregnancy. Trimester-specific thyroid ranges should be taken into consideration while evaluating thyroid tests during pregnancy, if available. Also, while treating thyroid disorders in pregnancy, target levels of TSH, T3, and T4 are different than in general population.

Levothyroxine Therapy

Patients on thyroxine treatment may present with anomalous reports of thyroid tests. Inappropriate administration, malabsorption, increased thyroid hormone metabolism following interaction with other drugs, increased thyroxine binding, change in drug formulation, poor compliance, and TSH-assay interference are some of the causes where the tests may be discordant in patients on thyroxine treatment.

Medications

Many drugs prescribed commonly can cause thyroid dysfunction. Drugs can also effect thyroid assays, causing interference. Drugs affecting thyroid function are amiodarone, lithium, tyrosine kinase inhibitors, and some immune modulators. Commonly used medications such as heparin, dopamine, estrogens, androgens, and corticosteroids can also affect thyroid tests. A careful treatment history is important in patients with thyroid abnormalities.

Nonthyroidal Illness

Nonthyroidal illness refers to intercurrent illness, usually critical in nature, leading to abnormalities in thyroid levels without any features of preexisting intrinsic thyroid or hyperparathyroidism (HPT) disorder. Intensive care unit (ICU) patients may present with low T3 levels with increased rT3. Simultaneously, the TSH may be low, normal, or mildly suppressed. Sometimes, a low T4 may also be encountered, which if significantly low may correlate with a poor prognosis. The thyroid abnormalities are adaptive changes to the critical illness and usually return to reference ranges upon correction of primary illness and recovery of patient. Thyroid tests should be advised only if primary thyroid or hypothalamic–pituitary disease is suspected in critically ill patients and not otherwise.

Assay Interference

Sometimes, when we get discordant thyroid reports not explained by clinical presentation, errors by laboratories should also be kept in mind. There are some genetic and acquired causes which may interfere with assays of thyroid hormones or TSH tests. Heterophile antibodies, anti-animal immunoglobulins, and anti-iodothyronine antibodies are few antibodies which may cause interference. These assay interference may not necessarily be identified by sending to another laboratory for testing but may require specialist laboratory or endocrine advice.

Thyroid Hormone Resistance

Thyroid-stimulating hormone resistance is a relatively uncommon condition where there is resistance to TSH action at the TSH receptor level. There is thyroid receptor (TR) β-gene mutation which is responsible for thyroid hormone resistance. These patients have elevated TSH levels but no goiter. The patients may be euthyroid or hypothyroid.

DIFFERENT PATTERNS OF ABNORMAL THYROID FUNCTION TESTS

Normal thyroid function patterns have normal TSH along with T3 and T4 within normal range. The various abnormal patterns which can be observed are mentioned further.

Increased Thyroid-stimulating Hormone with Reduced Thyroid Hormone Levels, T3, and T4

Increased TSH with reduced thyroid hormone levels, T3, and T4 is one of the most common patterns of thyroid abnormality encountered in clinical practice. Elevated TSH with reduced levels of thyroid hormones indicates overt primary hypothyroidism.

- This may occur due to Hashimoto's thyroiditis or other causes of hypothyroidism.
- Atrophic or congenital primary hypothyroidism
- Hypothyroid phase of subacute thyroiditis
- Postsurgical removal of thyroid gland will also lead to this clinical picture.
- Postradiotherapy and neck irradiation may also lead to overt hypothyroidism.
- Iodine deficiency or excess availability also may lead to primary hypothyroidism.
- Some drugs such as amiodarone have a large content of iodine and produce thyroid abnormalities. Other drugs which may impact thyroid function, resulting in primary hypothyroidism are lithium, tyrosine kinase inhibitors, and antithyroid drugs.
- Riedel's thyroiditis and thyroid infiltration with amyloid or tumor cells are some less often causes of primary hypothyroidism

Increased Thyroid-stimulating Hormone, with Normal T3 and T4

Such a situation is seen in mild thyroid insufficiency also termed subclinical hypothyroidism. In this condition, the TSH is mildly elevated, usually below 10 mIU; however, the thyroid hormone levels are still within normal range.

- Patients with poor compliance to treatment with thyroxine may also have similar pattern of TFT. The patient who is irregular in treatment or misses doses may have this pattern of TFT.
- Malabsorption of thyroxine may also present in similar picture. If patient takes food or other medications immediately after the thyroxine administration, he/she may also show mildly increased TSH.
- Some drugs may also result in such a pattern of TFT. Drugs such as amiodarone and lithium may be associated with thyroid profile of this pattern.
- *Assay interference*:
    - Sometimes when we get discordant thyroid reports not explained by clinical presentation, errors by laboratories should also be kept in mind. There are some genetic and acquired causes which may interfere with assays of thyroid hormones or TSH tests. These assay interference may not necessarily be identified by sending them to another laboratory for testing but may require specialist laboratory or endocrine advice.
- *Recovery phase of NTI*:
    - NTI, also termed sick euthyroid illness, indicates effect of intercurrent illness on thyroid function. This is usually seen in ICU and hence, it is advised to test for thyroid function only in those patients where primarily thyroid or HPT axis disorder is being suspected.
- *TSH resistance*:
    - TSH resistance is a relatively uncommon condition where there is resistance to TSH action at the TSH receptor level. These patients have elevated TSH levels but no goiter. The patients may be euthyroid or hypothyroid.

Reduced Thyroid-stimulating Hormone with Increased Thyroid Hormones, T3 and T4

This biochemical profile of TFTs is also often encountered in clinical practice.

This indicates a state of primary hyperthyroidism, where the thyroid hormones are increased and lead to negative feedback suppression of the TSH from the pituitary.

Causes of primary hyperthyroidism leading to this pattern of biochemical thyroid profile are seen:

- Graves' disease
- Toxic multinodular goiter
- Toxic adenoma
- Thyroiditis (postviral and postpartum)
- Drugs (amiodarone); excess iodine intake
- Excess thyroxine ingestion
- Pregnancy-related (hyperemesis, molar pregnancy, and gestational thyrotoxicosis)
- Congenital hyperthyroidism

Reduced Thyroid-stimulating Hormone, with Normal T3 and T4 Levels

Many times reduced TSH levels with normal thyroid hormone levels create confusion in treating physicians. This pattern can occur in many situations as listed further **(Flowchart 1)**.

- *Subclinical hyperthyroidism*: In subclinical hyperthyroidism, the TSH is below normal; however, the thyroid hormones, T3, and T4 would be normal. This usually indicates a state of mild hyperthyroidism.
- *Recent treatment for hyperthyroidism*: Patients who have started treatment for thyrotoxicosis by antithyroid drugs may initially for few weeks present

such a pattern of TFT. The thyroid drugs begin to control the excess thyroid levels and bring the high thyroid levels down. However, the TSH may remain suppressed for a longer duration. This pattern has to be kept in mind by clinicians treating hyperthyroidism to avoid unnecessary escalation of doses where actually patients are adequately responding as indicated by falling levels of T3 and T4. The TSH may take longer time to normalize and the treatment should be directed by the thyroid hormone levels.

- *Drugs*: Some drugs also may be associated with decrease in TSH levels alone. Steroids and dopamine can result in this pattern of TFT.
- Assay interference
- *NTI*: Sometimes NTI may be associated with low TSH; however, T3 and T4 may be normal. Correction of the primary disorder should be done and thyroid tests may be repeated when patient is free from the disorder.

Reduced T3 and T4, with Normal or Reduced Thyroid-stimulating Hormone

- *Hypothalamic-pituitary disease*: In conditions of primary pituitary disorder leading to reduction in TSH or primary hypothalamic disorder leading to reduced thyrotropin-releasing hormone (TRH), the thyroid hormones would be decreased. However, the decreased thyroid hormones will fail to have feedback increase in TSH due to disease affecting the pituitary or hypothalamus. Hence, the TSH may be reduced or inappropriately normal.
- *NTI*: Acute illnesses may result in low T3 levels. Sometimes, low T4 may also be seen and usually indicates poor prognosis.
- *Isolated TSH deficiency*: Assay interference
- *Recently treated Grave's disease*: Treatment of Grave's disease may sometimes be associated with lowering thyroid hormone levels to even lower than normal. Occasionally, the TSH may also persist to be suppressed as it takes longer time to normalize. In such situations, care should be taken to monitor and adjust the dose of antithyroid medications on the basis of T3 and T4 levels, rather than TSH levels, which may be misguiding.

Increased/Normal Thyroid-stimulating Hormone and Increased Levels of T3 and T4

- *TSH-secreting pituitary adenoma*: Centrally excess production of TSH by a TSH-secreting adenoma can produce high levels of TSH along with increased thyroid hormone levels.
- *Neonatal period*: In this time, such pattern may be observed.
- Effect of drugs such as heparin and amiodarone
- *Thyroxine replacement therapy*: In patients having poor compliance to thyroxine treatment may have such picture. These patients would not be regular in treatment; hence, TSH would be high. But in attempt to rapidly control, they may get started on higher dose than required, leading to high T3 and T4. In such patients, proper counseling of good compliance along with a correct thyroid dosing will bring back the TFT levels to normal.
- *Assay interference—familial dysalbuminemic hyperthyroxinemia (FDH)*: FDH is an inherited condition where there is increased binding of mutant

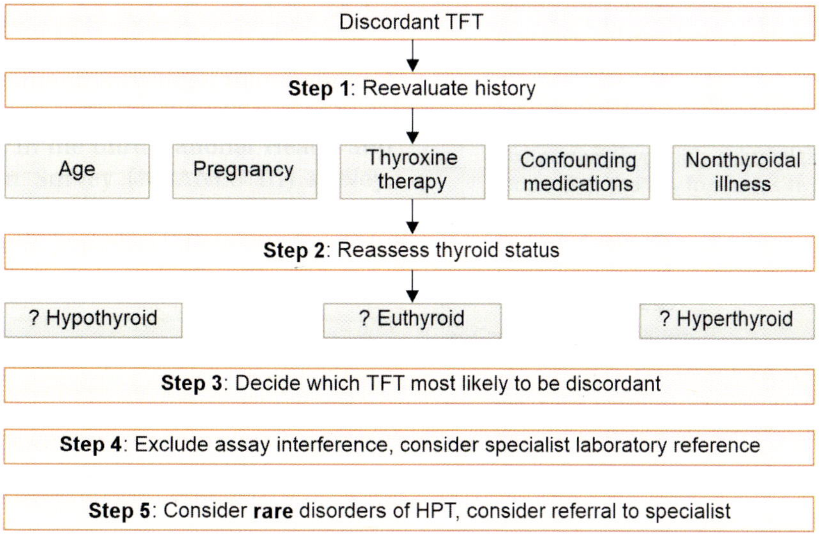

FLOWCHART 1: Approaching the discordant TFTs.

(HPT: hyperparathyroidism; TFT: thyroid function test)

managed with serial monitoring of TFTs. Besides this, the monitoring of TFTs for dose titration of levothyroxine is of utmost importance as different varieties of patients have different targets. Whenever in doubt, an expert consultation with an endocrinologist can go a long way in improving patient care.

SUGGESTED READINGS

1. Koulouri O, Moran C, Halsall D, Chatterjee K, Gurnell M. Pitfalls in the measurement and interpretation of thyroid function tests. Best Pract Res Clin Endocrinol Metab. 2013;27(6):745-62.
2. Ross DS. (2022). Diagnosis of and screening for hypothyroidism in nonpregnant adults. [online] Available from https://pro.uptodatefree.ir/Show/7893 [Last accessed January, 2024].
3. Soh S-B, Aw T-C. Laboratory Testing in Thyroid Conditions - Pitfalls and Clinical Utility. Ann Lab Med. 2019;39(1):3-14.
4. Jonklaas J, Bianco AC, Bauer AJ, Burman KD, Cappola AR, Celi FS, et al. Guidelines for the Treatment of Hypothyroidism: Prepared by the American Thyroid Association Task Force on Thyroid Hormone Replacement. Thyroid. 2014;1670-751.

75

CHAPTER

Subclinical Hypothyroidism: When to Treat?

Arathi Darshan

ABSTRACT

Subclinical hypothyroidism (SCH) is a common disorder characterized by elevated serum thyroid stimulating hormone (TSH) levels. This condition occurs in 3–8% of general population. The most important implication of SCH is high likelihood of progression to overt hypothyroidism. SCH is associated with adverse maternal and fetal outcomes that may improve with treatment. Current guidelines recommend, routine levothyroxine therapy for individuals with a persistent serum TSH more than 10 mU/L and individualized therapy for those with a TSH of <10 mU/L.

INTRODUCTION

Primary hypothyroidism can be classified as overt hypothyroidism when TSH values exceeds >10 mU/L (non pregnant individuals) and SCH when TSH values are between 4.5 and 10 mU/L.

Subclinical hypothyroidism (SCH), also called mild thyroid failure, is diagnosed when serum thyroid-stimulating hormone (TSH) is elevated in the presence of normal serum free thyroxine (T4) concentration. It is a common disorder in day-to-day practice. There is a higher prevalence of SCH in women, elderly individuals, and those with thyroid autoimmunity. Appropriate treatment of SCH may prevent its progression to overt hypothyroidism. SCH is associated with adverse cardiovascular events, adverse maternal and fetal outcomes, neuromuscular and cognitive abnormalities

Current guidelines recommend routine treatment with L-thyroxine for individuals with a persistent rise in serum TSH of >10 mU/L, in nonpregnant patients. Management of SCH with serum TSH values between 4 and 10 mU/L is controversial. Treatment in such patients, should be individualized depending on the age, clinical features, presence of goiter, presence of antibodies to thyroid peroxidase (TPO), pregnancy status, individuals with infertility and comorbid states like CVD.

DEFINITION OF SUBCLINICAL HYPOTHYROIDISM

Subclinical hypothyroidism is a condition in which there is a persistent elevation of TSH (12 weeks or longer) in the setting of a normal free T4/T4 concentration, which are repeatedly found within the reference interval.

DIAGNOSIS OF SCH?

By definition SCH is asymptomatic. SCH is primarily a laboratory diagnosis. The most accepted initial screening test for SCH and overt hypothyroidism is serum TSH. TSH levels typically range between 0.4–4 mU/L, according to American Thyroid Association (ATA).

The ATA recommends screening for hypothyroidism starting at the age of 35 years with repeat screening every 5 years.

Definition of Elevated Levels of Thyroid-stimulating Hormone?

Controversies exist on the upper limits of TSH. TSH values depend on age, gender, ethnicity, body mass index (BMI), and pregnancy status. In the United States National Health and Nutrition Examination Survey 111 (NHANES 111), which enrolled 16,533 people without thyroid disease, the upper limit of TSH reference value was 4.2 mU/L. There is a physiological rise in TSH values in elderly individuals. The upper limit of TSH in individuals above 80 years of age is 6–8 mU/L. Age-specific reference ranges for TSH interpretation are recommended.

A transient rise in TSH should be ruled out, before the diagnosis of SCH. Repeat thyroid function test is recommended after 2 months, for the confirmation of diagnosis of SCH. Most common causes of transient elevation in TSH values are nocturnal measurement of TFT and physiological rise in TSH values with ageing.

Other causes are recovery phase of nonthyroid illness, severe obesity, medications like amiodarone and chronic lithium therapy, assay variability, presence of heterophile antibodies interfering with TSH assay, untreated Addison's disease, central hypothyroidism, and thyroid hormone resistance.

PREVALANCE OF SUBCLINICAL HYPOTHYROIDISM

Prevalence of SCH varies from 4 to 20% in general population. Higher prevalence is seen in women, older individuals and in individuals with suboptimal iodine status. However, the prevalence is determined by the upper limit of TSH values **(Table 1 and Box 1)**.

CLINICAL FEATURES OF SUBCLINICAL HYPOTHYROIDISM

About 70% of patients with SCH are asymptomatic. Symptoms may be vague and nonspecific. Symptoms are similar to overt hypothyroidism. Fatigue, weakness, cramps, weight gain, constipation, impaired concentration, depression, anxiety, and poor quality of life have been frequently reported. Fatigue is one of the symptoms which is considered as an indication to start treatment in SCH.

TABLE 1: Epidemiology of subclinical hypothyroidism (SCH) in India.

Reference	*n*	SCH (%)
Unnikrishnan et al. (2013)	5,370	8
Unnikrishnan et al. (2011)	971	9.4
Rohil et al. (2010)	1,741	2.6
Abraham et al. (2009)	505	9.5
Sahu et al. (2009)	633	6.4

CONSEQUENCES OF SUBCLINICAL HYPOTHYROIDISM

Progression to Overt Hypothyroidism

The natural history of SCH is that it can either progress to overt hypothyroidism or have a spontaneous recovery. The annual rate of progression to overt hypothyroidism is approximately 3–18%. The underlying disease and patient characteristics are the major factors determining the risk of conversion to overt hypothyroidism.

The risk factors for progression to overt hypothyroidism include older individuals, female gender, and elevated titers of thyroid peroxidase antibodies TPOAb.

The underlying disease may also determine the progression. Patients who have received radioiodine ablation for Graves' disease, history of external radiation therapy for non-thyroid malignancies and those who have received chronic lithium treatment are likely to convert to overt hypothyroidism

Spontaneous recovery and normalization of TSH are more likely to occur in patients with initial TSH values of <10 mU/L and with negative antithyroid antibodies. In a study of 422,242 individuals without a known thyroid disease, serum TSH was elevated (>5–10 mU/L) in 3% of individuals. During a 5-year follow up-period, TSH values became normal without treatment in 62% of patients, within the first 2 years of diagnosis.

BOX 1: Causes of subclinical hypothyroidism (SCH).

- Chronic autoimune thyroiditis
- Persistent TSH increase—in subacute thyroiditis, postpartum thyroiditis, painless thyroiditis
- Thyroid injury—partial thyroidectomy or other neck surgery, radioactive iodine therapy, external radiotherapy for head and neck
- Drugs impairing thyroid function—iodine and iodine-containing medications (amiodarone, radioactive contrast agents), lithium, cytokines (especially interferon alpha), sulfonamides, sulfonylureas
- Inadequate replacement therapy for overt hypothyroidism—inadequate dosage, noncompliance, drug interactions
- Thyroid infiltration—amyloidosis, sarcoidosis, Reidel's thyroiditis, AIDS
- Central hypothyroidism
- Toxic substances, industrial and environmental agents
- TSH receptor gene mutations

(AIDS: acquired immunodeficiency syndrome; TSH: thyroid-stimulating hormone)

Source: Biondi B, Cooper DS. The clinical significance of subclinical thyroid dysfunction. Endocr Rev. 2008;29(1):76-131.

Cardiovascular Disease

Meta-analysis of several prospective cohort studies have reported, a significant increase in the risk of coronary heart disease and heart failure in patients with overt hypothyroidism (Serum TSH >10 mU/L).

Large number of studies support an association between subclinical hypothyroidism and cardiovascular events like CVD and heart failure. This association was strongly seen in patients of less than 65 years of age.

Increased CV risk may be explained due to the presence of atherogenic lipid profile [elevated total cholesterol and low-density lipoprotein (LDL) cholesterol levels], higher systolic and diastolic blood pressure, and increased carotid intima-media thickness. The most consistent cardiac abnormality reported in SCH is impaired left ventricular (LV) diastolic function. In overt and SCH, there is reduced peripheral action of thyroid hormone, thus leading to altered intracellular calcium handling. This results in slowed myocardial relaxation and impaired LV filling. LV systolic dysfunction with exercise, impaired endothelial function, increased vascular tone at rest, increased systemic vascular resistance, and arterial stiffness has been reported.

Reproductive Abnormalities and Pregnancy Outcome

Thyroid screening is important in women with reproductive abnormalities. There is an increased risk of pregnancy loss in women with SCH. This risk is more in the presence of positive anti-TPO antibodies. Data from various observational studies have demonstrated improved fertility outcomes after initiation of treatment. 44–84% of women treated with levothyroxine successfully conceived after initiation of treatment.

Undetected SCH in pregnancy is a risk factor for poor pregnancy outcomes in mother and fetus. Spontaneous abortion, preeclampsia, gestational hypertension, gestational diabetes, premature birth, low birth weight, and poor developmental outcomes in offspring have been reported.

Nonalcoholic Fatty Liver Disease

Studies have shown an association between TSH levels and nonalcoholic fatty liver disease (NAFLD). 30–36% of individuals with SCH and overt hypothyroidism had ultrasonographic findings of NAFLD (vs. 20% of controls), 20–26% had abnormal liver enzymes, nonalcoholic steatohepatitis (NASH) was seen in 58%, and fibrosis was reported in 26% of patients.

Neuromuscular Dysfunction

Studies have reported fatigue, weakness, paresthesias, and cramps in patients with SCH, which can be reversed with L-thyroxine therapy.

Psychiatric and Cognitive Dysfunction

In a large population-based study, SCH was associated with depression, cognitive dysfunction, and bipolar disease.

WHEN TO TREAT SUBCLINICAL HYPOTHYROIDISM?

Treatment of SCH depends on the following factors:

- *TSH values:* <10 or >10 mU/L
- *Age of the patient:* >65 years or <65 years
- *Patient clinical profile:* Clinical features, presence of goiter, TPOAb, pregnancy or intention of pregnancy
- *Comorbidities:* Presence of CVD, heart failure, dyslipidemia, obesity

Recommendations Depending on Thyroid-stimulating Hormone Values

TSH > 10 mU/L (in Nonpregnant Patients)

There is a strong recommendation from American Thyroid Association and Endocrine society of India, to treat all patients of overt hypothyroidism with TSH values > 10 mU/L.

Recommendations Depending on Age

Elderly patients > 65 years of age with TSH value < 10 mU/L

Treatment of SCH in this group of patients is not recommended, due to the absence of benefit. Since there is a physiological rise of TSH with ageing, unintended overtreatment can lead to complications in elderly. Treatment in older patients is indicated only in those who have convincing symptoms of hypothyroidism.

For younger patients < 65 years of age with TSH < 10 mU/L

Treatment is recommended in younger individuals with TSH <10 mU/L, in view of increased CV mortality and an increase risk of progression to overt hypothyroidism **(Box 2)**.

MANAGEMENT OF SCH

Management of subclinical hypothyroidism is shown in **Flowchart 1**.

BOX 2: Factors favouring levothyroxine treatment for patients < 65 years of age with TSH levels of 5–10 mU/L.

- Degree of TSH raised (2 TSH levels >8 mU/L)
- Progressive TSH increase
- Presence of goiter
- Presence of antithyroid antibodies
- Therapeutic trial for clinical symptoms
- Patient preference
- Young age of the patient
- Cardiovascular risk factors or prevalent CHD
- Smoking
- Dyslipidemia
- Bipolar disorder, depression
- Pregnancy or intention of pregnancy
- Infertility, ovulatory dysfunction
- Childhood and adolescence

Source: Javed Z, Sathyapalan T. Levothyroxine treatment of mild subclinical hypothyroidism: a review of potential risks and benefits. Ther Adv Endocrinol Metab. 2016;7(1):12-23.

TREATMENT OF SUBCLINICAL HYPOTHYROIDISM

Before initiating the treatment of SCH with L-thyroxine, conditions causing transient and physiological rise in serum TSH should be ruled out. Confirmation with repeat testing of TSH and free T4 is recommended after 8–12 weeks, before initiating therapy. Therapy should not be delayed, when there are compelling indications of benefit of immediate therapy, like pregnancy or infertility.

Dosage

Factors to be considered before starting therapy are age of the patient, severity of the condition, and presence of comorbid conditions like CVD. Guidelines recommend initiating therapy with the lowest dose necessary to normalize serum TSH. Typically, 25–50 µg of L-thyroxine is recommended in patients with SCH. This approach is most appropriate to avoid overtreatment in elderly patients and with underlying CVD.

Goals of Therapy

The goal of therapy is to achieve euthyroid status, resolution of symptoms, and avoid over- or undertreatment. A TSH target of 0.5–2.5 U/L in young and middle-aged patients is recommended. In elderly patients beyond

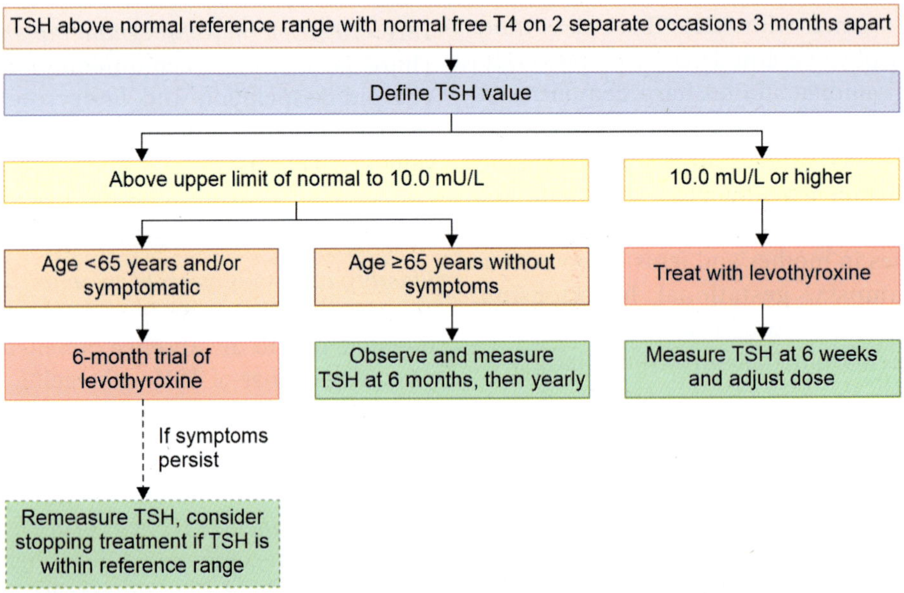

FLOWCHART 1: Approach to management of subclinical hypothyroidism (SCH).

(TSH: thyroid-stimulating hormone)

Source: NICE 2019 Guidelines: Thyroid disease: Assessment and management.

65 years of age, a higher TSH target of 3–5 mU/L is recommended.

Monitoring of Therapy

Serum TSH should be repeated 8–12 weeks after initiation of therapy. If the target TSH is not achieved, the dose of L-thyroxine should be increased with a minimum dosage of 12.5–25 μg. If serum TSH is low, the dosage should be decreased accordingly. Once normal TSH values has been achieved, TSH should be repeated after 6 months and then annually.

For untreated patients of SCH who are not on treatment, repeat TSH is recommended after 6 months and thereafter annually.

SUBCLINICAL HYPOTHYROIDISM IN PREGNANCY

Diagnosis of SCH differs slightly in pregnant women. Diagnostic thresholds are different in pregnancy and trimester-specific references are recommended by the American Thyroid Association. The dosage of L-thyroxine in pregnant women is 1.2 μg/kg/day.

CONCLUSION

SCH is usually asymptomatic and is primarily a laboratory diagnosis. Transient rise in TSH levels should be ruled out, before initiating treatment. SCH is associated with increased risk of CV events, poor pregnancy outcomes and has a high risk of progression to overt hypothyroidism. Treatment is strongly recommended for all non-pregnant patients, with persistent elevation of TSH > 10 mU/L. However, routine treatment of patients with serum TSH between 4.5 and 10 mU/L remains controversial. In elderly individuals above 65–70 years of age with TSH < 10 mU/L, treatment is routinely not recommended. For individuals below 65 years of age with TSH < 10 mU/L, treatment decisions are based on individual patient profile and co-morbid states.

SUGGESTED READINGS

1. Jayakumar RV. (2015). Consensus Statement on the Management of Subclinical Hypothyroidism. Elsevier India. [online] Available from https://www.indianthyroidsociety.in/pdf/SCH_Guidelines.pdf [Last accessed December, 2023].
2. Ross DS, Cooper D, Mulder J. (2023). Subclinical hypothyroidism in non-pregnant adults. UpToDate. [online] Available from https://www.uptodate.com/contents/subclinical-hypothyroidism-in-nonpregnant-adults [Last accessed December, 2023].
3. Biondi B, Cooper DS. The clinical significance of subclinical thyroid dysfunction. Endocr Rev. 2008;29(1):76-131.
4. Unnikrishnan AG, Kalra S, Sahay RK, Bantwal G, John M, Tewari N. Prevalence of hypothyroidism in adults: An epidemiological study in eight cities of India. Indian J Endocrinol Metab. 2013;17(4):647-52.
5. Unnikrishnan AG, Menon UV. Thyroid disorders in India: An epidemiological perspective. Indian J Endocr Metab. 2011;15: 78-81.
6. Rohil V, Mishra AK, Shrewastawa MK, Mehta KD, Lamsal M, Baral N, Majhi S. Subclinical hypothyroidism in eastern Nepal: A hospital based study. Kathmandu Univ Med J. 2010;8:231-7.
7. Abraham R, Murugan VS, Pukazhvanthen P, Sen SK. Thyroid disorders in women of Puducherry. Indian J Clin Biochem. 2009;24:52-9.
8. Sahu MT, Das V, Mittal S, Agarwal A, Sahu M. Overt and subclinical thyroid dysfunction among Indian pregnant women and its effect on maternal and fetal outcome. Arch Gynaecol Obstet. 2010;281:215-20.
9. Javed Z, Sathyapalan T. Levothyroxine treatment of mild subclinical hypothyroidism: a review of potential risks and benefits. Ther Adv Endocrinol Metab. 2016;7(1):12-23.
10. Chelsea Simon et al, Subclinical hypothyroidism: To treat or not to treat? Journal of American Academy of Physician Assistants 2020.

76

CHAPTER

Adrenal Incidentaloma

Neeti Agrawal, Partha Pratim Chakraborty

ABSTRACT

The purpose of evaluating an incidentally detected adrenal mass, termed adrenal incidentaloma (AI), is to characterize the lesion as benign or malignant, and functional or nonfunctional, based on their imaging characteristics and hormone secretory profile. Noncontrast computed tomography (CT) scan is the initial investigation of choice. Washout percentages following intravenous contrast administration are useful in certain cases. Endocrine work-up aims at determining adrenocortical (cortisol, dehydroepiandrosterone sulfate, and mineralocorticoid, only in presence of hypertension) and adrenomedullary hormone secretion from the mass. Overnight dexamethasone suppression test should be performed in all, and cortisol value of > 1.8 μg/dL suggests autonomous cortisol secretion (ACS). Diagnosis of pheochromocytoma is established by elevated urinary/plasma metanephrines, and should be measured in all AIs with noncontrast Hounsfield unit of > 10. Primary adrenal insufficiency needs to be ruled out in bilateral AIs. Nonfunctional, homogenous AIs, measuring < 4 cm and having noncontrast attenuation of < 10 HU do not require further imaging and long term follow-up, while pheochromocytoma and most of the functional AIs, irrespective of size, warrant surgical resection. Management of AIs with ACS depends on clinical features and underlying comorbidities. AIs with ACS warrants glucocorticoid replacement during and after surgery. Management of bilateral AIs depends on underlying etiology.

INTRODUCTION

Adrenal incidentaloma (AI) is a clinically inapparent adrenal mass measuring at least 1 cm in maximum diameter, which is detected on imaging, performed for indications other than suspected adrenal disorder. Lesions smaller than 1 cm are not classically termed as AI, and do not require additional work-up, unless clinical evidences of adrenal dysfunction coexist. Adrenal mass(s) discovered during routine whole body screening of patients with underlying hereditary syndromes or extra-adrenal malignancy is not considered as AI.

EPIDEMIOLOGY

With the widespread use of computed tomography (CT) and magnetic resonance imaging (MRI) scans in current day clinical practice, the prevalence of AI has been on the rise. Incidence of AI has increased by almost 10-fold over the past two decades in parallel to the increase in prescription of such abdominal scans. Prevalence of AI varies widely across studies, depending largely on nature of the study (autopsy or radiology or surgery), patient selection (general population or special groups) and inclusion criteria (age of the study population) among others. In adults, the overall prevalence is about 1% in relatively young individuals, and about 6% at fifth decade of life; it increases further with advancing age. Majority of these AIs are nonfunctional, and only about 14% of them seem to secrete one or more of the adrenocortical or adrenomedullary hormones. However, recent data suggest that up to half of the adrenocortical adenomas (ACAs) are associated with some degree of autonomous cortisol secretion (ACS).

ETIOLOGY

Various underlying etiologies in incidentally detected adrenal mass(s) have been summarized in **Table 1**.

TABLE 1: Etiology of adrenal incidentaloma (AI).

Unilateral (Fig. 1)	Bilateral (Fig. 2)
Adrenocortical adenoma	Infections (histoplasmosis, tuberculosis, others)
Pheochromocytoma	Metastases
Adrenocortical carcinoma	Hemorrhage
Myelolipoma	Lymphoma
Adrenal cyst	Myelolipoma*
Nerve cell tumors (ganglioneuroma, ganglioneuroblastoma, neuroblastoma, and schwannoma)	Pheochromocytoma* Cyst*
Hemangioma	Primary bilateral macronodular adrenocortical hyperplasia
Adrenal hemorrhage	Extramedullary hematopoiesis in chronic hemolytic anemia
Adrenal infections*	
Adrenal metastasis*	
Teratoma	

*Relatively rare as far as laterality is concerned.

EVALUATION

The important issues that need to be addressed while evaluating any AI are: (1) nature of the mass (benign or malignant), (2) documentation of autonomous hormone secretion, if any, (3) primary adrenocortical insufficiency (PAI) in bilateral adrenal involvement, and (4) plan of management (surgical or conservative).

Imaging

Computed Tomography Scan

Adrenal CT is very much useful to identify the nature of the adrenal mass, hence, is considered the initial investigation of choice during evaluation of AI. Noncontrast CT of the adrenals should be ordered first, which can easily identify calcification and hemorrhage. Pheochromocytoma, adrenocortical carcinoma (ACC), myelolipoma and teratoma often are heterogeneous with areas of calcification, necrosis and even hemorrhage **(Figs. 1B, D, and F)**. Calcification is rare in primary adrenal lymphoma and adrenal metastases. A homogeneous, smooth and well-marginated mass with an attenuation value of <10 Hounsfield unit (HU) indicates lipid-rich ACA **(Fig. 1C)**, and does not require further evaluation with intravenous contrast administration or by any other imaging procedure. Adrenal myelolipoma contains varying amount of extra-cellular macroscopic fat (triglyceride) having noncontrast attenuation value ranging between –20 and –150 HU. The hypodense areas, easily identified on noncontrast CT scan, are characteristic of these tumors and further imaging work-up is also not required **(Fig. 1B)**. The appearance of the contralateral adrenal gland should always be noted in unilateral AI; atrophy of the opposite gland suggests ACS by the mass.

On the other hand, attenuation value of ≥10 HU is encountered in a wide variety of lesions including lipid-poor ACA, ACC, pheochromocytoma, metastases, neurogenic tumors, and infections. A dedicated adrenal protocol with measurement of the HUs in three different phases following intravenous contrast administration is often required to differentiate lipid-poor ACA from ACC. The three phases include early arterial phase (EAP), early venous phase (EVP, also known as portal venous phase) and delayed venous phase (DVP), acquired about 20 seconds, 60–90 seconds, and 10–15 minutes postcontrast administration, respectively. Average HU in each phase is measured by placing a circular region of interest (ROI) tool over a relatively homogeneous area within the central part of the mass, ideally at the same point in each phase, including at least two-third of the lesion while excluding areas with calcification and necrosis. The absolute and relative washout percentages are then to be calculated by the following formulae: Absolute washout % (AW): $[(HU_{EVP} - HU_{DVP})/(HU_{EVP}) - HU_{Unenhanced})] \times 100$; relative washout % (RW): $[(HU_{EVP} - HU_{DVP})/HU_{EVP}] \times 100$. AW of ≥60% and RW ≥40% have been widely accepted as thresholds for differentiating lipid-poor ACAs from ACCs. One recent study has modified the AW and RW cut-offs to >83% and >58%, respectively. None of these thresholds, however, can characterize adrenal masses with absolute certainty, and current guideline has emphasized on the need of further validation of such washout characteristics. Metastases from renal cell carcinoma and hepatocellular carcinoma may display washout patterns similar to ACA.

In patients without extra-adrenal malignancy, a noncontrast HU of 10 has long been recommended as the threshold to separate malignant adrenal masses from the benign ones with a sensitivity of 100% and specificity of 58%, necessitating additional work-up and subsequent surgery for a large number of benign lesions (like lipid-poor ACA). Raising the cut-off to 20 HU increases the specificity (80%) for malignancy without significant decrement in overall sensitivity (97%). Recent data suggest that attenuation of <20 HU on unenhanced CT scan effectively rules out ACC in an adrenal mass having a maximum diameter of <4 cm. The likelihood of ACC in a mass with a diameter of 4 cm or more is also very low if the unenhanced HU is <20, and virtually nil if <10. The best way to diagnose ACC preoperatively seems to be a combination of tumor diameter of ≥4 cm, unenhanced CT attenuation >20 HU, and urine steroid metabolomics indicating a high risk of ACC [positive predictive value (PPV): 76·4%; negative predictive value (NPV): 99·7%].

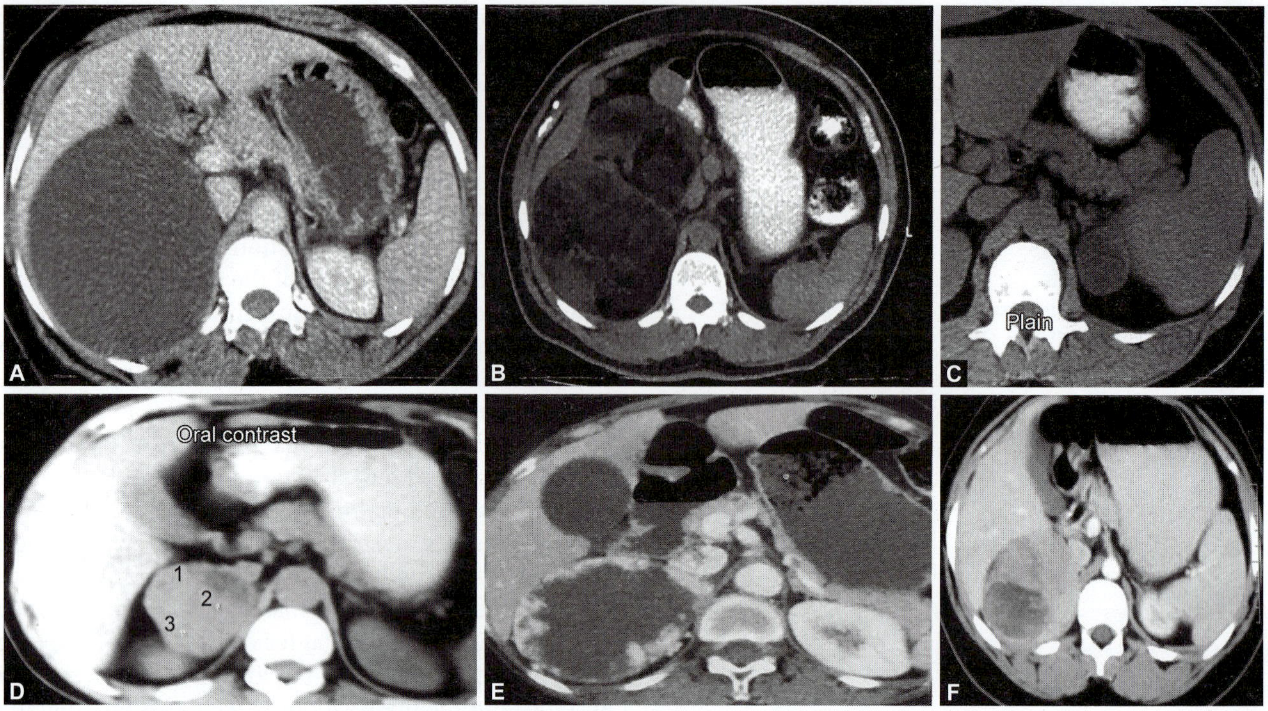

FIGS. 1A TO F: CT appearance of unilateral adrenal incidentalomas. (A) Benign adrenal cyst (right); (B) Myelolipoma (right) (note the heterogeneous appearance and areas with marked hypodensity within the lesion, suggestive of macroscopic fat); (C) Lipid-rich ACA (left) (noncontrast HU is 3 indicating intracellular fat); (D) Pheochromocytoma (right) (note the heterogeneous appearance with noncontrast HU ranging between 32–39; (E) Cystic pheochromocytoma (right) (note the thick rim and rim enhancement unlike A); (F) ACC (right) (note the heterogeneous appearance).

Pheochromocytomas demonstrate variable washout percentages, hence, these are not required for diagnosis. EAP, at times, can discriminate norepinephrine secreting pheochromocytomas from ACCs and adrenal metastases. Maximum enhancement of the mass in EAP, HU of ≥100 in EAP and percentage arterial enhancement $[(HU_{EAP} - HU_{Unenhanced})/HU_{Unenhanced}]$ of ≥100% have a specificity of 100% to differentiate norepinephrine secreting pheochromocytomas from other malignant adrenal lesions. Contrast enhancement patterns are also helpful in certain other conditions. Neurogenic tumors such as adrenal ganglioneuroma and schwannoma may show wash-in pattern where gradual and progressive contrast enhancement leads to maximum attenuation in the DVP. Adrenal hemorrhage appears as hyperdense mass having noncontrast HU between 50–90 along with adjacent retroperitoneal fat stranding and without appreciable contrast enhancement. Adrenal hemorrhage of recent onset may exhibit "train-track" appearance following contrast enhancement due to preserved peripheral enhancement of normal adrenal tissue with central area of low attenuation. Peripheral discontinuous nodular enhancement with central fill-in pattern following contrast administration is suggestive of adrenal hemangioma.

Adrenal infections such as histoplasmosis and tuberculosis, during the early phase of the disease, usually present with bilateral adrenal masses with heterogeneous appearance in both noncontrast and postcontrast scans. The adreniform shape of the glands is often preserved in histoplasmosis. The adrenals may remain enlarged for a prolonged period and areas of dystrophic calcification and gland atrophy may become evident in later stage.

Magnetic Resonance Imaging Scan

Magnetic resonance imaging is performed only if CT is contraindicated. Chemical shift MRI often reliably identifies lipid-rich ACAs. Lipid-rich ACA contains intracellular lipid (cholesterol ester) and shows loss of signal intensity (i.e. hypointense) on out-of-phase compared to in-phase sequences.

Hormonal Evaluation

Endocrine evaluation in AI depends on the imaging characteristics and clinical background. Functional lesion may be clinically silent, but detection of underlying hormone excess has immense diagnostic and therapeutic implications. For an instance, though ACS is seen both in ACA and ACC, cosecretion of cortisol and adrenal androgen or estrogen increases the likelihood of ACC by manyfold. In tumors with underlying ACS, the hypothalamic-pituitary-adrenal (HPA) axis often remain suppressed for many months postadrenalectomy. Such patients should be operated under hydrocortisone coverage and replaced with glucocorticoid postsurgery to avoid life-threating adrenal crisis. Patients with pheochromocytoma needs adequate preparation before surgery and strict monitoring during the perioperative period. In suspected ACC, the operating surgeon should ensure complete removal of the mass with intact capsule and locoregional lymph node dissection to avoid future recurrence. Dehydroepiandrosterone sulfate (DHEAS), if elevated at baseline, may be used as a tumor marker during follow-up of ACC. All necessary precautions should be strictly adopted during hormonal evaluation of AIs.

Evaluation for Autonomous Cortisol Secretion

One milligram overnight dexamethasone suppression test (ONDST) should be performed in all patients with AI unless the imaging characteristics are unequivocally suggestive of benign adrenal cyst or myelolipoma **(Figs. 1A and B)**. Post-ONDST cortisol of >1.8 µg/dL is suggestive of ACS. A single cut-off cortisol value is not sufficient for diagnosis of ACS. Hence, the test should be repeated after about 1 week. Low DHEAS concentration (compared to age and sex-specific reference range), particularly in those younger than 60 years, indicates suppressed adrenocorticotrophic hormone (ACTH) drive due to ACS from the mass. Low/low-normal ACTH is another marker of ACS. Such patients should be thoroughly evaluated for clinical signs of cortisol excess, hypertension, diabetes, dyslipidemia, and asymptomatic vertebral fracture.

Evaluation for Catecholamine Excess

All AIs with unenhanced HU of at least 10 (possibly except those with unequivocal features of benign adrenal cyst) should be screened for pheochromocytoma. Urine should be collected for 24 hours for measurement of metanephrine and normetanephrine along with creatinine. Urine creatinine of ≥15 mg/kg/day in males and ≥10 mg/kg/day in females ensures adequate collection. Estimation of plasma metanephrine and normetanephrine is an effective alternative. Patient should undergo overnight fasting and avoid tea, coffee, alcohol, tobacco, and strenuous exercise for at least 24 hours before the test. Sample should be collected after being supine for at least 30 minutes.

Evaluation for Adrenal Androgen Excess

While elevated DHEAS is highly suggestive of ACC, normal level does not exclude the condition.

Evaluation for Mineralocorticoid Excess

All hypertensive patients with AI, ACA in particular, should undergo plasma/serum aldosterone and plasma renin activity (PRA)/direct renin concentration (DRC) measurements to calculate aldosterone to renin ratio (ARR).

Detection of Primary Adrenocortical Insufficiency

Patients with bilateral adrenal masses **(Fig. 2)** should be evaluated with early morning (8–9 AM) cortisol, ACTH and PRA/DRC. A combination of low cortisol (<5 µg/dL) and high ACTH (>2 times of the upper limit of reference range) with/without high PRA/DRC is suggestive of PAI. Patients with evolving or subclinical PAI often have elevated ACTH and serum cortisol higher than 5 µg/dL, and may require cosyntropin stimulation test. However, an ACTH value >300 pg/mL denotes maximum stimulus for cortisol secretion obviating the need for such stimulation test. High PRA/DRC suggests poor mineralocorticoid reserve. In addition, early morning 17-hydroxyprogesterone (17-OHP) should be measured to rule out congenital adrenal hyperplasia (CAH) in all patients with bilateral adrenal myelolipoma **(Fig. 2D)** or unilateral adrenal myelolipoma and bilaterally enlarged adrenal glands **(Fig. 2E)**.

Urine Steroid Metabolomics

This noninvasive test (24-hour urine steroid excretion analysis) is being tested to detect functional status and malignant potential of adrenal masses. Recent data suggest that this has immense potential in management of AI with indeterminate imaging characteristics.

Adrenal Biopsy/Fine Needle Aspiration Cytology

There is a very limited role of adrenal biopsy/fine needle aspiration cytology (FNAC) in evaluation of adrenal masses. It cannot differentiate between ACA and ACC; moreover, it increases the risk of tumor dissemination and may reduce overall survival in stage 1 and 2 ACC. Adrenals should be biopsied only in suspected infective and infiltrative processes (lymphoma, metastases), particularly if tissue diagnosis is likely to alter management protocol. Adrenal biopsy/FNAC should strictly be performed once pheochromocytoma is reliably excluded by relevant biochemical tests. However, patients with bilateral adrenal masses and documented PAI may not necessarily be evaluated for catecholamine excess before the procedure.

The suggested approach to unilateral and bilateral AIs has been summarized in **Flowcharts 1 and 2**, respectively.

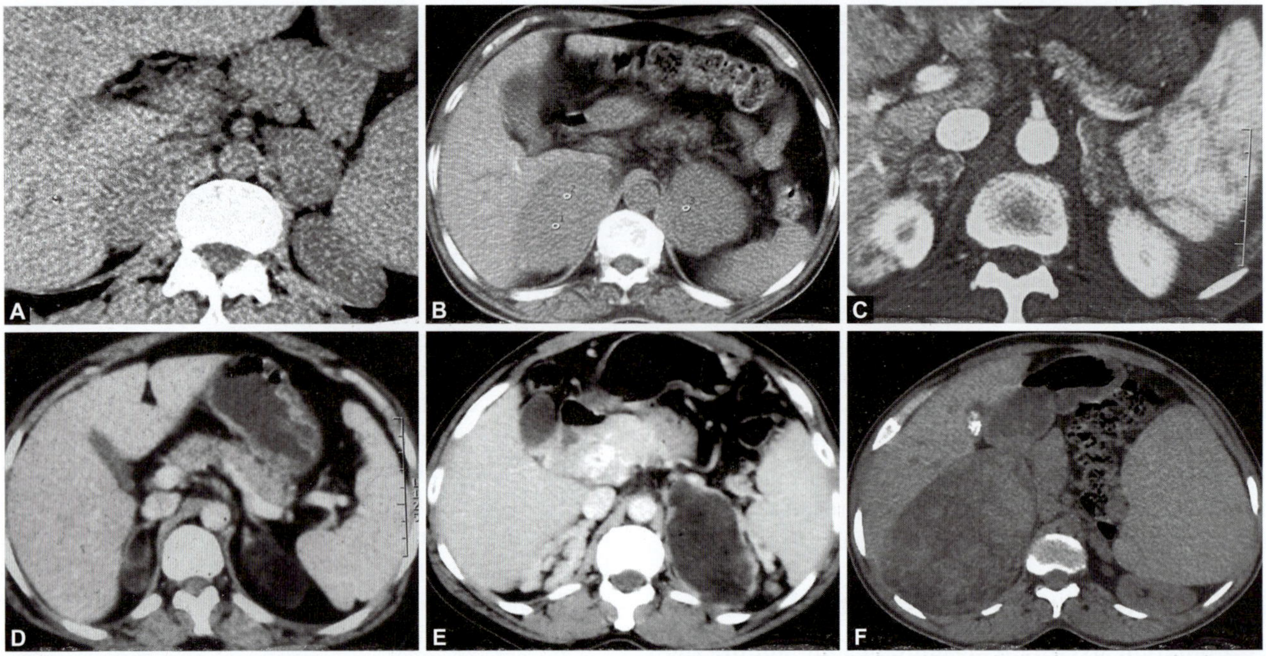

FIGS. 2A TO F: CT appearance of bilateral adrenal incidentalomas. (A) Adrenal histoplasmosis; (B) Primary adrenal lymphoma; (C) Adrenal metastases in bronchogenic carcinoma; (D) Bilateral myelolipoma in CAH; (E) Unilateral myelolipoma (left) and markedly enlarged right adrenal gland in CAH (the patient also had a small right adrenal myelolipoma, visible in a separate section); (F) Extramedullary hematopoiesis in transfusion dependent thalassemia (right adrenal is much bigger than the left one).

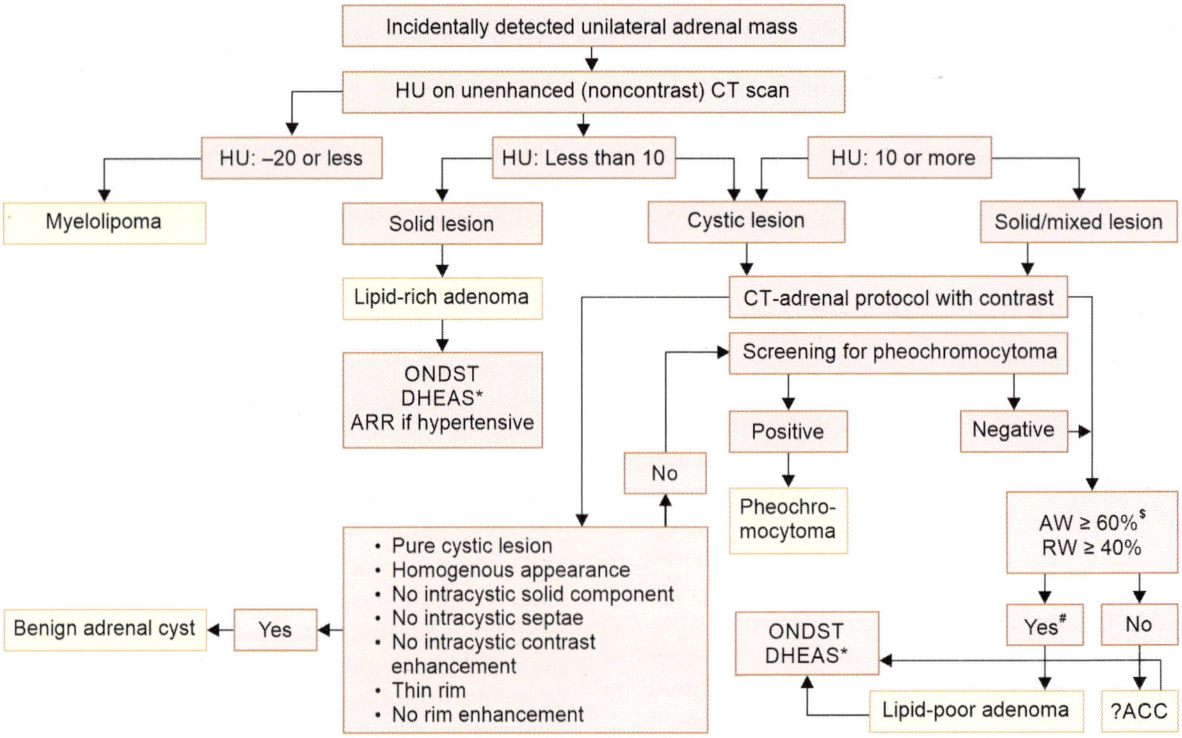

*Low DHEAS in ACA (lipid-rich and lipid-poor) suggests ACS from the mass. High DHEAS suggests underlying ACC and serves as a tumor marker during follow-up.

$Recent data suggest that AWO of >83% and RWO of >58% rule out malignant lesion.

#ACC should be considered if unenhanced HU is between 10 and 19 and size of the mass is 4 cm or more.

FLOWCHART 1: Diagnostic approach to unilateral adrenal incidentaloma.

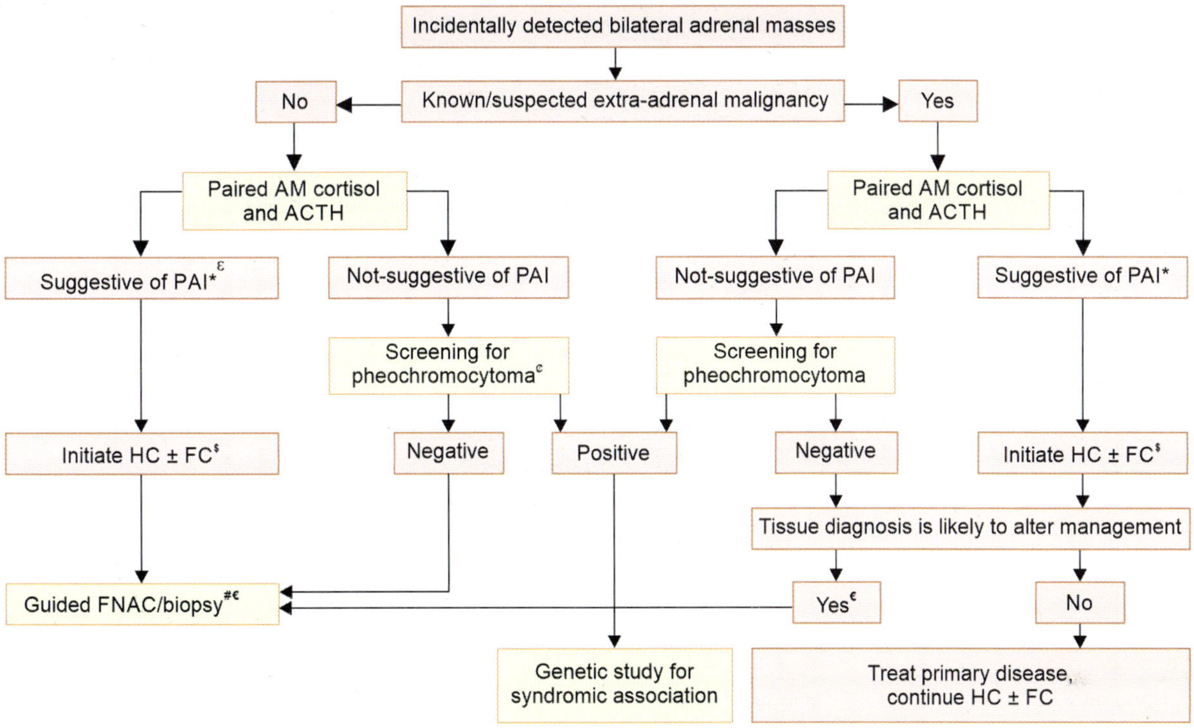

*Patients with PAI should tested for serum potassium and PRA/DRC.

εPatients with PAI and bilateral myelolipoma/unilateral myelolipoma and enlarged contralateral gland should be tested for AM 17-hydroxyprogesterone.

¢Screening for pheochromocytoma is not needed if CT features are suggestive of myelolipoma.

$Fludrocortisone (FC) is indicated in patients with high potassium and/or elevated PRA/DRC.

€Whole body ^{18F}FDG-PET in selected patients.

#Not indicated if CT features are suggestive of myelolipoma or hemorrhage.

FLOWCHART 2: Approach to bilateral adrenal incidentaloma.

MANAGEMENT

Once the diagnosis of pheochromocytoma is confirmed by hormonal evaluation, the mass should be surgically removed. The management protocol in other unilateral adrenal masses has been summarized in **Flowchart 3**. Nonfunctional lipid-rich ACAs (noncontrast HU: < 10) of <4 cm (possibly larger ones also) are to be left alone, and repeat hormonal work-up is needed only if clinical signs of hormone excess develop. Those with ACA and signs of cortisol excess (i.e., adrenal Cushing's) should undergo unilateral adrenalectomy. Patients with ACA having post-ONDST cortisol of >1.8 μg/dL and without obvious features of Cushing's syndrome is divided into two groups—mild autonomous cortisol secretion (MACS) (those with relevant comorbidities such as diabetes, hypertension, dyslipidemia, and low bone mass) and silent autonomous cortisol secretion (SACS) (those without comorbidities). Patients with MACS and suppressed DHEAS and/or low/low normal ACTH should also be operated. Patients with SACS may be monitored periodically for possible progression to MACS. Nonfunctional AIs having noncontrast HU of 10–19 and size of <4 cm may undergo surgery or may be kept under observation. All functioning adrenal mass except those with isolated SACS should be removed irrespective of its size.

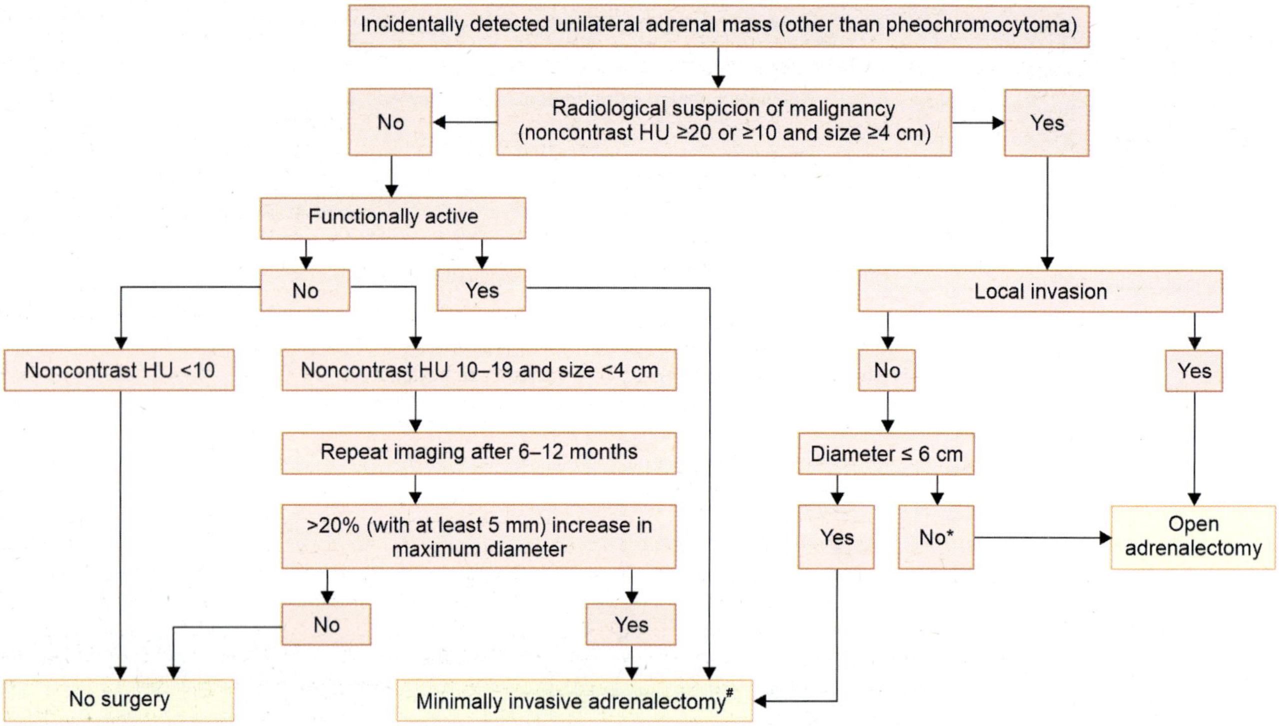

*In centers with experienced high volume (≥4 surgeries/year) adrenal surgeon minimally invasive adrenalectomy may be tried.
#Mass with SACS (ONDST-cortisol >1.8 μg/dL without comorbidities) may be followed up without adrenalectomy.

FLOWCHART 3: Management algorithm in unilateral adrenal incidentaloma (other than pheochromocytoma).

SUGGESTED READINGS

1. Schloetelburg W, Ebert I, Petritsch B, Weng AM, Dischinger U, Kircher S, et al. Adrenal wash-out CT: moderate diagnostic value in distinguishing benign from malignant adrenal masses. Eur J Endocrinol. 2022;186(2):183-93.
2. Fassnacht M, Arlt W, Bancos I, Dralle H, Newell-Price J, Sahdev A, et al. Management of adrenal incidentalomas: European Society of Endocrinology Clinical Practice Guideline in collaboration with the European Network for the Study of Adrenal Tumours. Eur J Endocrinol. 2016;175(2):G1-G34.
3. Kebebew E. Adrenal Incidentaloma. N Engl J Med. 2021;384(16):1542-51.
4. Bancos I, Prete A. Approach to the Patient with Adrenal Incidentaloma. J Clin Endocrinol Metab. 2021;106(11):3331-53.

77

CHAPTER

Approach to Cushing's Syndrome

Ritu Karoli, Pankaj Verma

ABSTRACT

Cushing's syndrome (CS) is characterized by chronic exposure to excess glucocorticoids. Early detection is uncommon due to various overlapping nonspecific clinical features common in the general population. The diagnostic evaluation of a suspected Cushing's syndrome is a challenging task. Two measurements of urinary free cortisol or late-night salivary cortisol or 1 mg overnight dexamethasone suppression test and low-dose dexamethasone suppression test are the initial screening biochemical tests followed by plasma adrenocorticotrophin hormone (ACTH), high-dose dexamethasone suppression test, inferior petrosal sinus sampling and various imaging studies including high-resolution computed tomography (CT), positron emission tomography CT (PET-CT), and magnetic resonance imaging (MRI) of pituitary/adrenals help in resolving the issue whether Cushing's syndrome is ACTH dependent or independent. Treatment includes transsphenoidal pituitary adenoma removal, radiotherapy, unilateral/bilateral adrenalectomy, adenoma, or tumor removal depending upon the cause.

INTRODUCTION

Cushing's syndrome (CS) is a clinical entity that results from chronic exposure of the body to excessive circulating glucocorticoids. More than a century ago, in 1912, Dr Harvey Cushing first time reported clinical features of CS due to a pituitary adenoma. When CS presents with all overt signs and symptoms, diagnosis is easy, but because of the overlapping, highly prevalent nonspecific clinical features such as obesity, hypertension, glucose intolerance, muscle weakness, and depression often delays the diagnostic suspicion and it becomes one of the most intriguing problems for the most senior endocrinologists.

PATHOPHYSIOLOGY

Adrenal gland is the part of hypothalamic–pituitary–adrenal (HPA) axis. The excess glucocorticoids are secreted from zona fasciculata of adrenal glands under stimulus of adrenocorticotrophin hormone (ACTH) secreted by pituitary gland, that in turn is stimulated by corticotrophin-releasing hormone (CRH) secreted by hypothalamus. The secretion of cortisol follows diurnal variation, having peak in the morning 8–9 AM and nadir around midnight. The clinical features of CS are the result of continuous excessive exposure to hypercortisolism which is the result of loss of normal negative feedback mechanism and loss of diurnal variation in cortisol secretion.

ETIOLOGY

Exogenous glucocorticoid administration should be excluded.

The etiologic causes of CS can be divided into two: ACTH dependent and ACTH independent.

Adrenocorticotrophin Hormone-dependent Causes

- Pituitary tumors (Cushing's disease)
- Ectopic CS (ACTH secreting nonpituitary tumors)—small cell lung carcinoma, neuroendocrine tumor (bronchial, pancreatic, gastrointestinal, thymic)
- CRH-producing tumors

Adrenocorticotrophin Hormone-independent Causes

- Adrenal adenoma
- Adrenal carcinoma
- Bilateral macronodular adrenal hyperplasia
- Primary pigmented nodular adrenocortical disease associated with Carney complex or sporadic
- McCune–Albright syndrome

CUSHING'S DISEASE

Pituitary corticotroph adenoma or ACTH-producing pituitary tumors constitute 10–15% of all pituitary tumors and are the most common cause of endogenous CS, comprising more than two-thirds of all the patients diagnosed with CS. Cushing's disease is 5–10 times more frequent in females than males. Pituitary macroadenoma can present with bitemporal hemianopsia with central visual field defects because of compression at optic chiasma.

The typical Cushing's phenotype consists of moon facies, facial plethora, and fat redistribution, leading to truncal obesity, buffalo hump, supraclavicular fat deposition, signs of hyperandrogenism in the form of temporal recession, acne, hirsutism, menstrual irregularities, loss of libido, impotence, thinning of the skin, and thick (>1cm) violaceous striae. Other metabolic alterations are hyperglycemia, glucose intolerance, hypertension, osteoporotic vertebral fractures leading to loss of height, avascular necrosis of femoral neck, mental changes including depression, mania, insomnia, poor cognition, increase in suicidal tendency, and proximal muscle weakness. The frequency of clinical features have been shown in **Table 1**.

TABLE 1: Clinical features of Cushing's syndrome according to prevalence.

Clinical features	Frequency (%)
Obesity	80
Thin skin	80
Moon facies	80
Hypertension	75
Violaceous striae	75
Acne and hirsutism	65
Menstrual alterations	65
Glucose intolerance	50
Proximal muscle weakness	50
Impotence	50
Easy bruisability	50
Mental changes	45
Hyperpigmentation	25
Hypokalemia	25
Osteoporosis	25
Pedal edema	25

Hypercortisolism results in immunosuppression due to decreased cell-mediated immunity. It causes delayed wound healing and increased propensity for opportunistic particularly bacterial and fungal infections. There is recent evidence that humoral immune responses can also be dysregulated. Hematologic parameters are altered in the form of polymorphonuclear leukocytosis, lymphopenia, and eosinopenia. CS is a hypercoagulable state associated with a high risk of venous thromboembolic events.

Ectopic CS is characterized by rapid development of clinical features. There is marked muscle weakness, no weight gain, hypokalemia, alkalosis, hyperglycemia, hypertension, and peripheral edema. The combination of rapid clinical deterioration and signs of mineralocorticoid excess, anorexia, and hyperpigmentation lead to suspicion of small cell lung carcinoma.

Patients with adrenal carcinoma also have rapid course and may have palpable abdominal mass associated with pain. There is excess androgen secretion and mineralocorticoid along with hypercortisolism in contrast to adrenal adenoma which only secretes cortisol.

Hypercortisolism is associated with an increase in cardiovascular events (myocardial infarction), cerebrovascular events (stroke) and usually a cause of death. It is associated with three to five times increased mortality risk compared with the general population.

CYCLICAL CUSHING'S SYNDROME

Cyclical CS is when there are rhythmic fluctuations in cortisol levels that alter the clinical and biochemical results. Diagnosis of cyclical Cushing is sometimes difficult and requires demonstration of at least three peak levels and two trough levels in cortisol production on prolonged testing. The cortisol values above the baseline can be seen in these patients before and after the peaks, indicating that cortisol levels were rising over a few days. It is more commonly seen in patients with ACTH-producing pituitary tumors, although cyclical Cushing's can also be encountered in patients with adrenal and ectopic ACTH-driven CS.

PSEUDO-CUSHING'S SYNDROME

One diagnostic challenge in the evaluation of endogenous hypercortisolism is differentiating neoplastic CS from pseudo-CS. Pseudo-CS, or hypercortisolism due to non-neoplastic causes, can occur in many medical disorders such as chronic alcoholism, chronic kidney disease, type 2 diabetes mellitus, and psychiatric conditions. Hypercortisolism in these conditions is mainly mediated by activation of the HPA axis through neural pathways. There is decreased negative feedback in most of these conditions which results in increased circulatory cortisol. This chronic glucocorticoid exposure can result in pathologic features of hypercortisolism. A detailed history and physical examination can reveal the underlying clinical condition.

DIAGNOSIS

Evaluation of suspected CS as has been (shown in **Flowchart 1**) is very challenging. Diagnosis of CS has two steps:

1. To establish the status of pathological hypercortisolism
2. To determine the etiology of CS

Step 1: To Establish the Status of Pathological Hypercortisolism

Indications of Screening

The clinical signs and symptoms of CS are variable, depending on patient's age, gender, etiology, and duration of hypercortisolism. The nonspecific features and metabolic abnormalities such as obesity, hypertension, glucose intolerance, and muscle weakness are so common in general population that it is challenging to suspect and diagnose CS at early stage. Following are the situations for recommended screening:

- Detection of adrenal incidentaloma
- Presence of Cushingoid features at uncommon age
- Presence of multiple relatively specific clinical features
- Children who have disproportionate weight gain but decrease in height

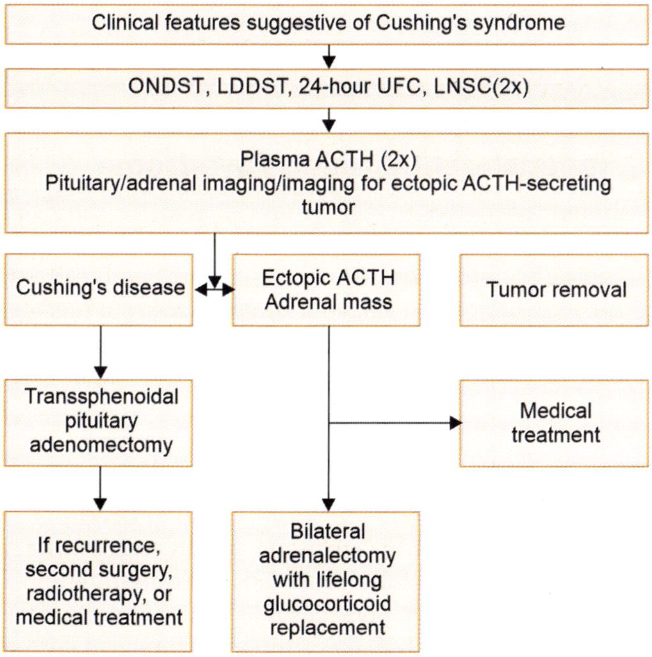

FLOWCHART 1: Approach to Cushing's syndrome.

(ACTH: adrenocorticotrophin hormone; LDDST: low-dose dexamethasone suppression test; LNSC: late-night salivary cortisol; ONDST: overnight dexamethasone suppression test; UFC: urine free cortisol)

The commonly used screening tests are: Glucocorticoid excess in the circulation which is in suppressible due to loss of circadian rhythm and negative feedback has to be demonstrated by any of the three screen tests. Morning cortisol levels may remain in normal range in most of the Cushing patients.

1. *Overnight 1 mg dexamethasone suppression test (DST)*: This test has a high sensitivity in which 1 mg of dexamethasone is given at 11 PM and cortisol sample is collected next morning at 8 AM. The cortisol levels normally suppress to <50 nmol/L.
2. *24-hour urinary free cortisol (UFC)*: A commonly performed test. The limitation is inadequate collection of 24-hour urine or cross reactivity of certain drugs such as carbamazepine or exogenous steroids which may give false positive results.
3. *Late-night salivary cortisol (LNSC) test*: This is good test that provides estimate of plasma free cortisol as cortisol-binding globulin is not present in saliva. It is a convenient test that can be performed at home. The salivary cortisol is stable at room temperature. The cortisol to creatinine ratio in first urine sample of the day can be useful in diagnosis of cyclical Cushing.

There is no specific sequence of these tests. There are advantages and limitations of these tests and depending upon patients' characteristics, they can be chosen. The two tests, 24-hour UFC and late-night salivary cortisol should be performed at two occasions to rule the presence of CS to address day-to-day variation in cortisol secretion.

Low-dose DST (LDDST): The specificity of this 48 hours test is higher, so it is used for confirmation of CS. In this, 0.5 mg dexamethasone is administered every 6 hourly and serum cortisol <50 nmol/L after 48 hours confirms the presence of Cushing's.

In problematic cases, some second-line tests can be performed. An awake midnight cortisol level >207 nmol/L is a good documentation of hypercortisolism. A single-sleeping serum cortisol < 50 nmol/L effectively rules out presence of Cushing's. Sometimes, it is difficult to differentiates Cushing's from other pseudo-Cushing's states such as critically ill, acute infection, heart failure, obesity, alcoholism, and depression.

A 48-hour 2 mg/day DST or secondary tests can be performed after referral to endocrinologist, including DDAVP (1-deamino-8-D-arginine vasopressin) stimulation and dexamethasone–CRH testing.

Dexamethasone CRH test: This test is based on the fact that some patients with CS will show suppression of cortisol after dexamethasone and will also respond to CRH with a rise in ACTH and cortisol.

Step 2: To Differentiate between ACTH-Dependent and ACTH-Independent Cushing's Syndrome

Plasma Adrenocorticotrophin Hormone Levels

After the establishment of hypercortisolism status, plasma ACTH concentrations can help determine whether the etiology is ACTH dependent or ACTH independent. Because of decreased glucocorticoid negative feedback effects, plasma ACTH levels will be inappropriately normal or elevated (generally >20 pg/mL) in ACTH-dependent causes and low (generally <10 pg/mL) in ACTH-independent causes of CS. It is recommended that plasma ACTH estimation should be done twice by two different methods to exclude false positive or false negative results. In intermediate values (ACTH levels between 10 and 20 pg/mL), CRH stimulation can help in the diagnosis.

High-dose Dexamethasone Suppression Test

High-dose dexamethasone suppression test (HDDST) can be done to determine different causes of hypercortisolism. The test is performed by oral administration of dexamethasone 2 mg 6 hourly for 2 days, followed by measuring serum cortisol the next morning. Pituitary tumors usually retain the responsiveness to dexamethasone, so there will be suppression of <50% of the basal cortisol to mark as positive test, while in ectopic ACTH-secreting tumors or adrenal tumors, it will not.

Dynamic testing with CRH test and desmopressin testing can also be used to help differentiate between ACTH-dependent and ACTH-independent Cushing's disease on the same principle that corticotroph adenoma will show positive response and ectopic tumors will not be responsive as they lack CRH receptors.

Bilateral Inferior Petrosal Sinuses Sampling

Bilateral inferior petrosal sinuses sampling (BIPSS) is the gold standard test to differentiate between Cushing's disease and ectopic ACTH-secreting tumors. It is invasive procedure in which catheters are placed in bilateral inferior petrosal sinuses. The sampling for ACTH is done simultaneously from the two sinuses and from peripheral vein basal and after administration of intravenous (IV) 100 μg CRH. The central to peripheral difference in ACTH ratio basal 2:1 and after CRH 3:1 confirms presence of Cushing's disease. The difference of ACTH > 1.84 times on one side helps in lateralization of the corticotroph tumor. Prolactin levels can be measured to confirm the proper position of the catheters in this procedure.

IMAGING STUDIES

Pituitary imaging by 3 Tesla magnetic resonance imaging (MRI) T1-weighted spin echo and spoiled gradient recalled acquisition techniques.

High-resolution abdomen computed tomography (CT) to assess adrenal masses > 1 cm and evaluation of contralateral adrenal gland.

High-resolution MRI will help in differential diagnosis of adrenal mass. Adrenal adenomas are homogenous and hypointense in T1-weighted images. Large size, necrosis, hemorrhage and calcification favor carcinoma.

Ectopic ACTH-secreting tumors can be detected by high-resolution CT of thorax or with MRI, if CT is nonrevealing.

Most of the ectopic tumors are from neuroendocrine origin, so they may have expression of somatostatin receptors. Radiolabeled somatostatin analogue scintigraphy can help in localization and to know functional status.

TREATMENT

Adrenocorticotrophin Hormone-independent Cushing's Syndrome

Adrenal adenoma or carcinoma has to be removed surgically. Ectopic Cushing has to be treated by surgical removal of the tumor. If tumor could not be localized, then other options are bilateral adrenalectomy or medical antisteroid therapy. After adrenalectomy, patient needs lifelong steroid replacement with proper education. Oral agents with established efficacy in CS are metyrapone and ketoconazole, which inhibit the steroid synthesis.

Cushing's Disease

Adrenocorticotrophin hormone-producing pituitary tumors are successfully removed by transsphenoidal endoscopic approach and selective microadenectomy is done. In majority, up to 80%, initial biochemical cure is achieved. In some patients, recurrence is observed which can be treated by second surgery, radiotherapy, stereotactic surgery, or bilateral adrenalectomy by individualized approach. Development of Nelson's syndrome is common in patients with ACTH-secreting tumors, which occurs due to adrenalectomy as a treatment of Cushing's disease. There is rapid growth in pituitary residual corticotrophs and hyperpigmentation due to excess ACTH secretion.

For Cushing's disease, the subcutaneous administration of pasireotide, a somatostatin receptor agonist, is another therapeutic option, if surgical cure cannot be achieved.

PROGNOSIS

The ectopic ACTH syndrome shows the best recovery rate (80%) and adrenal Cushing's has the lowest (40%), with Cushing's disease being intermediate (60%).

SUGGESTED READINGS

1. Lacroix A, Feelders RA, Stratakis CA, Nieman LK. Cushing's syndrome. Lancet. 2015;386:913-27.
2. Pappachan JM, Hariman C, Edavalath M, Waldron J, Hanna FW. J Clin Pathol. 2017;70:350-9.

78

CHAPTER

Adrenal Crisis: An Update

Jaya Bhanu Kanwar

ABSTRACT

Adrenal crisis is an acute life-threatening emergency, which occurs when the glucocorticoid production by the adrenal glands is insufficient in response to an increased demand. Adrenal glands secrete glucocorticoids and mineralocorticoids; and these steroids play major role in energy, salt, and fluid homeostasis. Adrenal insufficiency can be due to impaired function of adrenal glands itself (primary adrenal insufficiency) or due to disruption of hypothalamic–pituitary–adrenal (HPA) axis leading to inadequate synthesis and secretion of adrenocorticotropic hormone (ACTH) (secondary adrenal insufficiency). Adrenal crisis is a condition where acute adrenal insufficiency or failure occurs, which may be the first presentation of adrenal insufficiency as in patients with adrenal or pituitary hemorrhage or infarction, or in patients already on glucocorticoid replacement with preexisting adrenal insufficiency, or can occur in patients with previously undiagnosed adrenal insufficiency in times of stress. Prevalence of adrenal crisis ranges from 5.2 to 8.3 per 100 patient years. Every year almost 8% patients with adrenal insufficiency may have an episode of adrenal crisis. There is mortality of almost 6% in adrenal crisis events.

INTRODUCTION

There is no universally accepted definition of an adrenal crisis, also called acute adrenal insufficiency or Addisonian crisis. The Endocrine Society guideline on primary adrenal insufficiency defines adrenal crisis as a medical emergency associated with hypotension, abdominal symptoms, and laboratory abnormalities like hyponatremia which may or may not be associated with hyperkalemia. Rushworth et al. define an acute deterioration in health that is associated with absolute [systolic blood pressure (BP) < 100 mm Hg] or relative (systolic BP < 20 mm Hg lower than the patients' usual BP) hypotension, the features of which resolve following parenteral glucocorticoid administration (demonstrated by a marked resolution of hypotension within 1 hour and improvement of clinical symptoms over 2 hours). Bruno Allolio proposed criteria-based definition depending on clinical and biochemical parameters of adrenal insufficiency and introduced a grading system depending on the settings required for treatment **(Box 1)**.

BOX 1: Definition and grading of adrenal crisis.

Definition:
- Major impairment of general health with at least two of the following signs/symptoms:
  - Hypotension (systolic blood pressure < 100 mm Hg)
  - Nausea or vomiting
  - Severe fatigue
  - Fever
  - Somnolence
  - Hyponatremia or hyperkalemia
  - Hypoglycemia
- Parenteral glucocorticoid (hydrocortisone) administration followed by clinical improvement

Grading:
- Grade 1: Outpatient care only
- Grade 2: Hospital care (general ward)
- Grade 3: Admission to intensive care unit
- Grade 4: Death from adrenal crisis (with or without parenteral glucocorticoid administration)

Source: Adapted from Allolio B. (2015).

PATHOPHYSIOLOGY

Adrenal crisis results due to an absolute or a relative deficiency of cortisol. The physiological consequences of cortisol deficiency are due to the loss of the normal suppressive action of endogenous glucocorticoids on inflammatory cytokines levels [interleukin 1 (IL-1), interleukin 6 (IL-6) and tumor necrosis factor alpha (TNF-α)]; which result in increased cytokine levels causing fever, malaise, anorexia, and bodily pain. Animal experiments have also shown that there is enhanced sensitivity of TNF-α and there is a state of relative glucocorticoid resistance state induced by inhibition of glucocorticoid receptors by TNF-α. Glucocorticoids also known to have permissive action on adrenergic receptors as well as plays important role in the conversion of norepinephrine to epinephrine by phenylethanolamine N-methyltransferase (PNMT). In patients with adrenal insufficiency, the decrease in intra-adrenal cortisol concentrations leads to a decrease in catecholamine. So, a lack of the permissive action of glucocorticoids on adrenergic receptors and reduced catecholamine levels lead to hypotension, which may be further exacerbated by volume depletion caused by a lack of sodium and fluid retention due to missing mineralocorticoid activity. Cortisol deficiency leads to reduced hepatic gluconeogenesis, which may occasionally lead to hypoglycemia.

CLINICAL FEATURES

Patients with adrenal crisis typically present with most severe manifestation of adrenal insufficiency like hypotension and clinical evidence of hypovolemia (particularly in those with mineralocorticoid deficiency which is predominantly present in primary adrenal insufficiency). Hypotension (particularly postural hypotension) occurs secondary to hypovolemia as well as due to hypocortisolism. Hence, if adrenal crisis is not suspected and not appropriately treated, hypotension may be refractory to parenteral fluids and inotropes. However, they also manifest symptoms of mild hypoadrenal state like anorexia, nausea, vomiting, fatigue, postural dizziness, abdominal pain, and limb and back pain. In patients with undiagnosed adrenal insufficiency, there is usually history of gradual decline in physical wellbeing over the week, months, and even years together, associated with fatigue, anorexia, weight loss. They often appear exhausted and depressed. Hence, it needs diligent clinical suspicion to diagnose adrenal insufficiency as in many instances, these symptoms are attributed to psychiatric illness, acid peptic disorder or age-related decline in health. Fever may also be a presenting feature as adrenal crises are often precipitated by infection. At a later stage, they may develop impaired sensorium. Finding of hyperpigmentation of mucosa, skin, or nails characteristically present in primary adrenal insufficiency.

BIOCHEMICAL ABNORMALITIES ON ROUTINE TESTING

Hyponatremia is the common biochemical abnormality found in adrenal crisis. Hyperkalemia is associated with hyponatremia in adrenal crisis when pathological abnormalities involve adrenal glands (primary adrenal insufficiency) as because of deficiency of mineralocorticoids. Hyponatremia in secondary adrenal insufficiency (defect in pituitary and hypothalamus) is primarily because of hypocortisolism leading to reduction in the osmolar threshold, which stimulates vasopressin secretion resulting in reduction in free water excretion. The hyponatremia occurs in secondary adrenal insufficiency indistinguishable clinically from the syndrome of inappropriate antidiuretic hormone (SIADH). Other biochemical features that can present in an adrenal crisis include renal impairment secondary to hypovolemia, hypoglycemia and, rarely, hypercalcemia, which is due to decreased renal excretion of calcium and increased bone resorption.

FACTORS PRECIPITATING ADRENAL CRISIS

Various pathophysiological states precipitate adrenal crisis if body fails to increase endogenous cortisol secretion in response to precipitating events, or replacement dose of steroid is not increased adequately in patients with diagnosed adrenal insufficiency at the time of stress. Infection is the most common etiology which precipitates adrenal crisis. Bacterial infections are common precipitants of crisis in adults, whereas viral infections are more common cause in pediatric population. Gastroenteritis is the most common infection precipitating adrenal crisis, and it is often troublesome for treatment with oral steroid in view of associated vomiting and diarrhea which impair absorption of oral medications. It is prudent to realize that abdominal symptoms may also be due to adrenal crisis itself rather than because of gastroenteritis. Other events like serious injury, e.g., road traffic accidents and major surgeries are common precipitants; even minor medical procedures like dental procedures, vaccinations, injection zoledronic acid administration or chemotherapy can precipitate crises. Noncompliance to glucocorticoid replacement in known adrenal insufficiency; and undiagnosed coexisting thyrotoxicosis or the initiation of thyroxine therapy in a patient with undiagnosed hypoadrenalism, may precipitate an adrenal crisis. Cytochrome P-450 inducers such as carbamazepine, rifampicin, and phenytoin may increase cortisol metabolism, necessitating an increase in the replacement glucocorticoid dose in patients with adrenal insufficiency or may induce an adrenal crisis in patients with undiagnosed adrenal insufficiency.

TREATMENT

Treatment of adrenal crisis is quite effective if glucocorticoid treatment started very promptly. Even in patients with undiagnosed adrenal insufficiency if diagnosis is suspected, then treatment should be started with glucocorticoid after taking serum samples for cortisol and adrenocorticotropic hormone (ACTH), rather than waiting for the investigation results to come. Hydrocortisone (cortisol) is the drug of choice for treatment of an adrenal crisis because of its physiological glucocorticoid pharmacokinetics, plasma protein binding, tissue distribution, and balanced glucocorticoid-mineralocorticoid effects. Hydrocortisone is administered intravenously as a 100-mg bolus, followed by 200 mg every 24 hours (administered as a continuous infusion or as frequent intravenous or intramuscular boluses of 50 mg every 6 hours). Subsequent doses adapted according to the clinical response. If hydrocortisone is unavailable, another parenteral glucocorticoid, such as dexamethasone (4 mg every 24 hours), methylprednisolone (40 mg every 24 hours), or prednisolone (25 mg every 8 hourly with total dose of 75 mg in the first 24 hours; thereafter, 50 mg every 24 hours) may be used. In children, hydrocortisone should be administered as a parenteral bolus of 50 mg/m^2 of body-surface area, followed by 50–100 mg/m2 every 24 hours (administered as a continuous intravenous infusion, or as intravenous or intramuscular boluses every 6 hours). Fludrocortisone is not required if hydrocortisone doses exceed 50 mg given every 24 hours. In patients with primary adrenal insufficiency, fludrocortisone therapy is usually resumed once the adrenal crisis has resolved and oral steroid replacement is feasible.

During an ongoing adrenal crisis in an adult, intravenous normal saline should be administered (1,000 mL within the first hour), with crystalloid fluids (e.g., 0.9% isotonic sodium chloride) given according to standard resuscitation guidelines and with adjustment for the circulatory status, body weight, and relevant coexisting conditions. Intravenous 5% dextrose solution is given for hypoglycemia (i.e., when the glucose values are < 70 mg/dL). In children, a bolus of normal saline is given at a dose of 20 mL/kg of body weight, with repeated doses at up to 60 mL/kg the first hour. If there is hypoglycemia, dextrose at a dose of 0.5–1 g/kg is administered.

Concomitant therapy of the precipitating illness should be started along with steroid and intravenous fluid. Appropriate antibiotics for infection are initiated. After successful management of an adrenal crisis, hydrocortisone doses should be tapered over a period of few days based on the clinical response, and oral glucocorticoid treatment is to be instituted before discharge of the patient. Then patient should continue replacement doses of steroid, which is 20–25 mg of hydrocortisone or 5–7.5 mg of prednisolone.

PREVENTION

Adrenal crisis prevention in patients with diagnosed adrenal insufficiency on steroid replacement is based on effective patient education about "sick day" rules. Patients should be explained the need to double or triple the daily replacement dose of steroids, depending on the intensity of the stress. If mild fever is present then doubling the dose of steroid may be sufficient, whereas in case of severe illness with higher temperatures ≥38.5°C, tripling of steroid dose is advised till the illness resolves. Especially in patients with vomiting or diarrhea, parenteral hydrocortisone is recommended. In patients undergoing various medical procedures steroid dose to be adjusted according to the need for achieving the expected cortisol levels during stress of surgical intervention. **Table 1** provides an outline of steroid dose adjustment as recommended by UK Addison's Disease Self-Help Group.

Suppression of the hypothalamic-pituitary-adrenal (HPA) axis by systemic steroids leading to adrenal insufficiency and crisis is expected with steroid doses ≥5 mg prednisolone equivalent for >4 weeks. Abrupt discontinuation of steroids without gradual tapering may precipitate adrenal crisis. In order to avoid this, patients receiving exogenous steroids should be counseled regarding the side effect of HPA axis suppression and advised not to discontinue steroids abruptly but to taper the dose of steroids gradually before stopping steroid therapy. Awareness regarding the problem of adrenal crisis and its preventative strategies can mitigate this catastrophic complication. Emergency steroid wallet card (credit card size) mentioning urgent treatment of adrenal crisis should be provided to all adrenal insufficiency patients, so that healthcare providers can provide appropriate treatment.

TABLE 1: Outline of steroid dose adjustments for medical procedures.

Procedure	Preoperative needs	Postoperative needs
Major surgery	Start hydrocortisone infusion 100 mg over 12 hours just before anesthesia	Continue hydrocortisone infusion (100 mg over 12 hours) until able to eat and drink; then double oral dose for 48 hours, then taper to normal dose
Labor and vaginal birth	• Start hydrocortisone infusion (100 mg hydrocortisone over 12 hours) at onset of labor • Continue hydrocortisone infusion until delivery (100 mg over 12 hours)	Double oral dose for 24–48 hours after delivery, then taper to normal dose
Minor surgery and major dental surgery	100 mg hydrocortisone before anesthesia given as a bolus IM or SC or as hydrocortisone infusion for the duration of surgery	Double oral dose for 24 hours, then return to normal dose
Invasive bowel procedures requiring laxatives	Hospital admission overnight with 100 mg hydrocortisone IM or SC and fluid (isotonic saline), repeat dose before start of procedure	Double oral dose for 24 hours, then return to normal dose
Dental procedure	Extra morning dose 1 hour prior to surgery	Double oral dose for 24 hours, then return to normal dose
Minor procedure	Usually not required	Extra dose (e.g., 20 mg hydrocortisone) if symptoms

(IM: intramuscular; SC: subcutaneous)

Source: Adapted from Allolio B. (2015).

CONCLUSION

Diagnosis of adrenal crisis is straightforward in patients with diagnosed adrenal insufficiency and needs good clinical suspicion in undiagnosed cases. Treatment is very rewarding with steroid and intravenous fluid supplementation. However, adrenal crisis remains a significant cause of mortality, despite availability of steroid for more than half a century. Patient education on compliance of steroid replacement, increasing the steroid dose at the time of stress, and parental hydrocortisone administration at the time of its requirement are particularly important strategies for prevention of these crises.

SUGGESTED READINGS

1. Hahner S, Loeffler M, Bleicken B, Drechsler C, Milovanovic D, Fassnacht M, et al. Epidemiology of adrenal crisis in chronic adrenal insufficiency: the need for new prevention strategies. Eur J Endocrinol. 2010;162:597-602.
2. Bornstein SR, Allolio B, Arlt W, Barthel A, Don-Wauchope A, Hammer GD, et al. Diagnosis and Treatment of Primary Adrenal Insufficiency: An Endocrine Society Clinical Practice Guideline. J Clin Endocrinol Metab. 2016;101:364-89.
3. Rushworth RL, Torpy DJ, Falhammar H. Adrenal crises. N Engl J Med. 2019;381(9):852-61.
4. Allolio B. Extensive expertise in endocrinology. Adrenal crisis. Eur J Endocrinol. 2015;172:R115-24.
5. Turnbull AV, Rivier CL. Regulation of the hypothalamic-pituitary-adrenal axis by cytokines: actions and mechanisms of action. Physiol Rev. 1999;79:1-71.
6. Yatagai T, Kusaka I, Nakamura T, Nagasaka S, Honda K, Ishibashi S, et al. Close association of severe hyponatremia with exaggerated release of arginine vasopressin in elderly subjects with secondary adrenal insufficiency. Eur J Endocrinol. 2003;148:221-6.

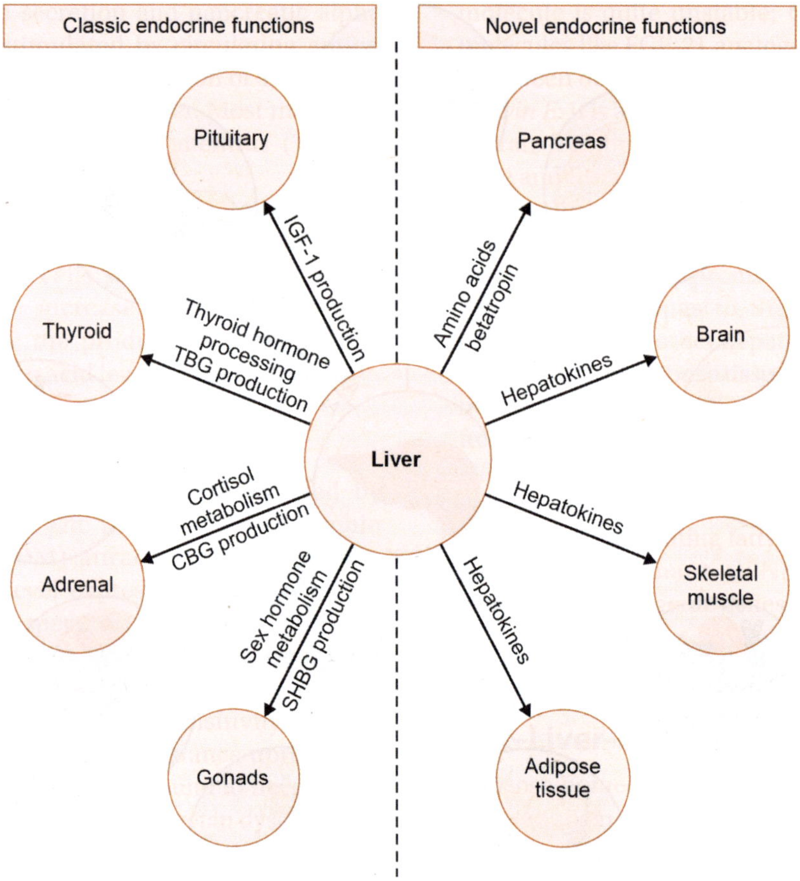

FIG. 2: Classic and endocrine functions of liver. Right: Classical functions of the liver. Left: Novel endocrine functions of the liver.

Many more organ intercommunications have been discussed in various researches as in liver-kidney, liver-spleen, liver-skin, and liver-eye which have time and again reemphasized the role of liver as a true endocrine organ.

In summary, the liver is an endocrine organ producing several molecules with multiple actions, and whose actions are only partly revealed. Several emerging hepatokines are involved in the regulation of liver and adipose tissue homeostasis in obesity. In the last 10 years, many new endocrine functions have been discovered. Betatrophin and other hepatokines such as fetuin A and FGF-21 play a significant role in moderating insulin sensitivity, lipid metabolism, and body fat weight. More endocrine functions of the liver shall be discovered in the near future but at present we should also maintain caution while interpreting newer findings **(Fig. 2)**.

SUGGESTED READINGS

1. Watt MJ, Miotto PM, DeNardo W, Montgomery MK. The Liver as an endocrine organ-Linking NAFLD and Insulin resistance. Endocr Rev. 2019;40:1367-93.
2. Rhyu J Yu R. Newly discovered endocrine functions of the liver. World J Hepatol. 2021;13(11):1611-28.
3. Karsenty G, Olson EN. Bone and muscle endocrine functions: Unexpected paradigms of interorgan communication. Cell. 2016;164:1248-56.
4. Wang PY, Caspi L, Lam CK, Chari M, Li X, Light PE, et al. Upper intestinal lipids trigger a gut-brain-liver axis to regulate glucose production. Nature. 2008;452(7190):1012-6.

80

CHAPTER

Female Health in Endocrinology Perspective

Dhruvi Hasnani, Vipul Chavda

ABSTRACT

Endocrine issues have a significant impact on women's health and well-being. Additionally, the typical variations in sex hormone levels that affect a woman's quality of life and risk of chronic disease throughout her lifetime, beginning in pregnancy and continuing during menopause and adolescence, also have an impact. For instance, changes in sex hormone levels during the menopausal transition can cause severe vasomotor symptoms in some women, such as hot flashes and night sweats, and declining estrogen levels have been associated with an increased risk of cardiovascular disease (CVD) and osteoporosis. Women are disproportionately more likely to experience endocrine disorders such as hypothyroidism and obesity, while conditions such as polycystic ovary syndrome (PCOS) and gestational diabetes mellitus (GDM) are specific to women. Major global public health threats such as osteoporosis and diabetes also present different clinical outcomes in women in terms of risk factors, drivers, and outcomes. This chapter provides a concise overview of key areas within female health that intersect with endocrinology.

INTRODUCTION

Women have traditionally been underrepresented in scientific studies, and many essential health issues for women have been largely disregarded by medical research. Women's health is already a major concern on a worldwide scale, and in the post-pandemic world, it is likely to become even more important and urgent. However, it has been customary to only consider how women's health relates to their sexual and reproductive systems. Through this chapter we seek to further explore gender as a factor influencing health and shed light on all facets of women's health, with a particular emphasis on endocrinology and metabolic illnesses.

MENSTRUAL CYCLE AND THE HORMONES

The menstrual cycle is hormonally controlled, usually lasting 28 days, with estrogen and progesterone from the ovaries regulating follicle growth, ovulation, and uterine lining preparation for implantation. Variations in duration are common. The hypothalamus releases gonadotropin-releasing hormone (GnRH), stimulating the pituitary gland to release follicle-stimulating hormone (FSH) and luteinizing hormone (LH), which then act on the ovaries to induce follicle growth and ovulation.

POLYCYSTIC OVARY SYNDROME

Polycystic ovary syndrome (PCOS) is a common endocrine disorder in reproductive-age females, causing hormonal imbalances, irregular menstrual cycles, excess androgen production, and ovarian cysts. It is linked to insulin resistance (IR), leading to fertility problems, weight gain, and long-term health concerns.

Therapy for PCOS focuses on the patient's main concerns, aiming to reduce hyperandrogenism symptoms, restore menstrual regularity, and improve fertility. Treatment should be tailored to the patient's phenotype, symptoms, and desire for conception. Letrozole, an aromatase inhibitor, has shown greater efficacy than clomiphene citrate for PCOS-related infertility. A multidisciplinary approach is vital, providing integral care to support lifestyle changes, reduce body fat, and restore metabolic and reproductive health.

FERTILITY AND REPRODUCTIVE HEALTH

Understanding the menstrual cycle and its variations is crucial for family planning and addressing fertility issues since fertility is closely connected to hormonal regulation. When trying to conceive, monitoring ovulation and maintaining proper hormone levels are vital. Fertility issues and other reproductive health concerns can arise due to hormonal imbalances.

PREGNANCY AND HORMONAL CHANGES

Pregnancy triggers notable changes in the endocrine system to support fetal development. Essential hormones such as human chorionic gonadotropin (hCG), estrogen, and progesterone play key roles in sustaining pregnancy and preparing for childbirth.

HORMONAL CONTRACEPTIVES

A range of hormonal contraceptives, including pills, patches, injections, and intrauterine devices (IUDs), prevent pregnancy by modifying hormone levels to inhibit ovulation and thicken cervical mucus, hindering sperm movement. Selecting the most appropriate option should consider individual health requirements.

MENOPAUSE

Menopause, typically at 45–55 years old, signifies the end of a woman's reproductive years. Ovaries produce fewer hormones, leading to decreased estrogen and progesterone levels. This hormonal shift causes symptoms such as hot flashes, mood changes, and heightened risks of osteoporosis and cardiovascular disease (CVD). Hormone replacement therapy (HRT) is commonly utilized to address conditions like menopause or hormonal imbalances.

HYPOTHYROIDISM AND HYPERTHYROIDISM

Women are more likely to develop autoimmune illnesses; hypothyroidism appears to affect them nearly exclusively. Due to their increased prevalence of obesity, propensity for autoimmune illnesses, and usage of lower thyroid-stimulating hormone (TSH) cutoffs for infertility management, preconception care, and pregnancy, women are also frequently burdened with a diagnosis of subclinical hypothyroidism. The aim of treatment is to alleviate symptoms and minimize untreated hypothyroidism-related consequences. The recommended treatment for hypothyroidism is levothyroxine monotherapy.

Hyperthyroidism, unlike hypothyroidism, is marked by an overproduction of thyroid hormones, resulting in symptoms such as weight loss, anxiety, and irregular menstrual cycles. Ensuring effective management is essential to avoid potential long-term complications.

OBESITY

Obesity is a worldwide epidemic with substantial implications for morbidity and mortality. Women are more susceptible to obesity than men, possibly due to a lower basal metabolic rate. Additionally, obesity is increasingly prevalent in girls, potentially leading to greater reproductive impacts as they reach reproductive age.

Numerous endocrine changes connected to obesity might result from variations to the hypothalamic-pituitary hormone axis. These include growth hormone deficiency, hypogonadism, Cushing's disease, Prader–Willi syndrome and hypothyroidism. Hyperinsulinemia is the main etiological component for PCOS, which also frequently manifests as obesity. The risk of obesity in women is increased by reproductive hormonal changes seen during pregnancy and menopause. The degree of obesity, health concerns, prior weight loss attempts, and individual differences in motivation and treatment readiness should all be taken into account while treating obesity in women.

DIABETES

Type 1 Diabetes Mellitus

Type 1 diabetes mellitus (T1DM) is an autoimmune disorder in which the immune system targets and eliminates insulin-producing beta cells in the pancreas. It is commonly diagnosed in childhood or adolescence but can manifest at any age. Women with T1DM may face difficulties in controlling blood glucose levels during menstruation, pregnancy, and menopause due to hormonal variations affecting insulin sensitivity.

Type 2 Diabetes Mellitus

Type 2 diabetes mellitus (T2DM) is identified by IR, where the body's cells have reduced responsiveness to insulin. This diabetes type is commonly linked to lifestyle factors such as obesity and lack of physical activity.

The management of T1DM and T2DM in women involves similar approaches, including monitoring blood sugar levels, embracing a healthy lifestyle, and effectively managing medications. Close collaboration with their healthcare team is crucial for women with both T1DM and T2DM to create a personalized management plan that caters to their unique needs and objectives.

GESTATIONAL DIABETES MELLITUS

Pregnancy can reveal preexisting metabolic problems, leading to the diagnosis of gestational diabetes mellitus (GDM), which seems to be the most significant risk factor for women's development to T2DM. The physiological changes associated with pregnancy, such as IR, prenatal weight gain, and changes in body composition, make managing diabetes even more difficult. Women with a history of GDM after pregnancy are at a higher risk of developing T2DM due to both preexisting (often undiagnosed) baseline abnormalities and further, progressive beta cell dysfunction after the index GDM pregnancy, which are linked to issues like the retention of excessive gestational weight gain and an increase in IR.

If a woman is diagnosed with GDM, not only does her current pregnancy require optimal hyperglycemia control, but she also needs to receive counseling regarding the significance of preconception care and making plans for future pregnancies. The necessity of strict glycemic management in ensuring a complication-free pregnancy and improved maternofetal outcomes must also be emphasized to all females with preexisting diabetes, both T1DM and T2DM, beginning in adolescence.

BONE HEALTH

Women's bone health is particularly vulnerable during the menopause transition, when dramatic reductions in bone strength and mass take place over a 3-year timeframe surrounding the end of the last menstrual cycle. Estrogen controls the metabolism of bones as it encourages the activity of osteoblasts and is crucial for bone health. Loss of bone density when estrogen levels fall, as happens during menopause, for instance leads to an increased possibility of fractures by making their bones brittle and fragile. The commencement of the rapid bone loss phase is preceded by significant changes in sex steroid hormones, and measures of these hormones may be therapeutically helpful in anticipating the onset of the rapid loss phase. Moreover, in postmenopausal women, variations in thyroid function are linked to altered bone mineral density (BMD) and fracture risk.

The management of osteoporosis in women typically involves a multifaceted approach. This includes lifestyle modifications, such as regular weight-bearing exercise, a balanced diet rich in calcium and vitamin D, and avoiding smoking and excessive alcohol consumption. Additionally, pharmacological interventions may be recommended, such as bisphosphonates, selective estrogen receptor modulators (SERMs), or monoclonal antibodies targeting specific pathways involved in bone metabolism.

HORMONAL INFLUENCE ON MENTAL HEALTH

In women's health and emotions, estrogen, progesterone, and testosterone play significant roles. Estrogen, specifically, affects serotonin, dopamine, and norepinephrine in the brain. Decreases in estrogen and progesterone levels can lead to feelings of irritability and anxiety. Hormone dysregulation happens when the endocrine system releases either excessive or insufficient amounts of a hormone. Mood and mental health can be affected by hormonal changes during the menstrual cycle, pregnancy, and menopause. Some women may encounter premenstrual syndrome (PMS) symptoms, while others may experience mood swings during pregnancy or menopause. Recognizing these effects is crucial in offering the right support and care.

NEUROENDOCRINE TUMORS AND FEMALE HEALTH

Neuroendocrine tumors (NETs) are uncommon tumors arising from the hormone-producing neuroendocrine system. Although affecting both genders, specific types, such as ovarian and breast NETs, are more prevalent in females. NET symptoms can differ based on their location and hormone production. Typical signs may comprise abdominal pain, diarrhea, flushing, wheezing, and weight loss.

Ovarian Neuroendocrine Tumors

These originate from neuroendocrine cells in ovaries and can manifest with hormonal symptoms. The symptoms often include irregular menstrual cycles, altered hair growth, and abnormal vaginal bleeding. Early detection and treatment are crucial for effective management of ovarian NETs.

Breast Neuroendocrine Tumors

These tumors are uncommon and distinct from typical breast cancers. They arise from neuroendocrine cells in the breast and can produce hormones, resulting in specific symptoms such as nipple discharge or hormonal imbalances.

The management of NETs relies on multiple factors, such as tumor location, stage, and grade. Treatment choices can encompass surgery, radiation therapy, chemotherapy, targeted therapy, and somatostatin analogs.

ENDOCRINE-DISRUPTING CHEMICALS

Endocrine-disrupting chemicals (EDCs) are substances found in specific environmental elements, such as certain plastics, pesticides, and household items. They can imitate or disrupt natural hormones, posing potential health risks. These substances are linked to a broad range of health problems, including issues with reproduction, cognitive functions, metabolic disorders, several types of cancers, and obesity. Minimizing exposure to EDCs is vital for preserving female endocrine well-being.

IMPORTANCE OF EARLY DETECTION AND AWARENESS

Detecting and being aware of diabetes, osteoporosis, and NETs early on is essential for effective management. Routine screenings such as bone density tests for osteoporosis and blood tests for diabetes can aid in identifying problems before they escalate. Furthermore, increasing awareness among healthcare providers and the public about symptoms and risk factors associated with these conditions can improve outcomes.

IMPORTANCE OF RESEARCH AND EDUCATION

As an endocrine researcher, the author acknowledges the significance of ongoing research and education to comprehend female health and manage endocrine disorders efficiently. Progress in medical science and technology has facilitated the creation of targeted treatments, enhancing the quality of life for numerous women.

SUMMARY

Women's health is a major concern on a worldwide scale, and in the post-pandemic world, it is likely to become even more important. The interplay between a woman's hormones, gender, sex, genetics, biology, and sociocultural environment ultimately determines her health. By emphasizing on women, their specific problems, and their demands throughout their life cycles, endocrinologists, and diabetologists hold the key to reducing the burden of serious chronic diseases.

SUGGESTED READINGS

1. Sriram U. Applying a women's health lens to endocrine and metabolic disorders. Indian J Endocrinol Metab. 2021;25(3):171-5.
2. Hawkins SM, Matzuk MM. Menstrual Cycle: Basic Biology. Ann N Y Acad Sci. 2008;1135:10-8.
3. Singh S, Pal N, Shubham S, Sarma KD, Verma V, Marotta F, et al. Polycystic Ovary Syndrome: Etiology, Current Management, and Future Therapeutics. J Clin Med. 2023;12, 1454.
4. Akre S, Sharma K, Chakole S, Wanjari MB. Recent Advances in the Management of Polycystic Ovary Syndrome: A Review Article. Cureus. 2022;14(8):e27689.
5. Rocha AL, Oliveira FR, Azevedo RC, Silva VA, Peres TM, Candido AL, et al. Recent advances in the understanding and management of polycystic ovary syndrome. F1000Res. 2019;8:F1000 Faculty Rev-565.
6. Emokpae MA, Brown SI. Effects of lifestyle factors on fertility: practical recommendations for modification. Reprod Fertil. 2021;2(1):R13-26.
7. Kumar P, Magon N. Hormones in pregnancy. Niger Med J. 2012;53(4):179-83.
8. InformedHealth.org. (2017). Contraception: Hormonal contraceptives. [online] Available from https://www.ncbi.nlm.nih.gov/books/NBK441576/. [Last accessed December, 2023].
9. Lee SR, Cho MK, Cho YJ, Chun S, Hong SH, Hwang KR, et al. The 2020 Menopausal Hormone Therapy Guidelines. J Menopausal Med. 2020;26(2):69-98.
10. Dunn D, Turner C. Hypothyroidism in Women. Nurs Womens Health. 2016;20(1):93-8.
11. Mathew P, Kaur J, Rawla P. Hyperthyroidism. Treasure Island (FL): StatPearls Publishing; 2023.
12. Metwally M, Ledger WL, Li TC. Reproductive Endocrinology and Clinical Aspects of Obesity in Women. Ann N Y Acad Sci. 2008;1127(1):140-6.
13. Ylli D, Sidhu S, Parikh T, Burman KD. Endocrine Changes in Obesity. South Dartmouth (MA): MDText.com, Inc.; 2000.
14. Azarbad L, Gonder-Frederick L. Obesity in Women. Psychiatr Clin North Am. 2010;33(2):423-40.
15. Toor S, Yardley JE, Momeni Z. Type 1 Diabetes and the Menstrual Cycle: Where/How Does Exercise Fit in? Int J Environ Res Public Health. 2023;20(4):2772.
16. Olokoba AB, Obateru OA, Olokoba LB. Type 2 Diabetes Mellitus: A Review of Current Trends. Oman Med J. 2012;27(4):269-73.
17. Tagliente I, Digilio G, Ullmann N, Solvoll T, Trieste L, Murgia F, et al. Management and Treatment of Type 1 and 2 Diabetes: State of Art. Gen Med (Los Angeles). 2016;4:3.
18. Kautzky-Willer A, Leutner M, Harreiter J. Sex differences in type 2 diabetes. Diabetologia. 2023;66(6):986-1002.
19. Alfadhli EM. Gestational diabetes mellitus. Saudi Med J. 2015;36(4):399-406.
20. Plows JF, Stanley JL, Baker PN, Reynolds CM, Vickers MH. The Pathophysiology of Gestational Diabetes Mellitus. Int J Mol Sci. 2018;19:3342.
21. Karlamangla AS, Shieh A, Greendale GA. Hormones and bone loss across the menopause transition. Vitam Horm. 2021:115:401-17.

22. Solimon M. How does estrogen affect osteoporosis? [online] Available from https://www.medicalnewstoday.com/articles/estrogen-and-osteoporosis. [Last accessed December, 2023].
23. Keen MU, Reddivari AKR. Osteoporosis in Females. Treasure Island (FL): StatPearls Publishing; 2023.
24. Wieczorek K, Targonskaya A, Maslowski K. Reproductive Hormones and Female Mental Wellbeing. Women. 2023;3(3):432-44.
25. Handy AB, Greenfield SF, Yonkers KA, Payne LA. Psychiatric Symptoms Across the Menstrual Cycle in Adult Women: A Comprehensive Review. Harv Rev Psychiatry. 2022;30(2):100-17.
26. Raphael MJ, Chan DL, Law C, Singh S. Principles of diagnosis and management of neuroendocrine tumours. CMAJ. 2017;189(10):E398-E404.
27. Pang L, Guo Z. Primary neuroendocrine tumors of the ovary: Management and outcomes. Cancer Med. 2021;10(23):8558-69.
28. Sun H, Dai S, Xu J, Liu L, Yu J, Sun T. Primary Neuroendocrine Tumor of the Breast: Current Understanding and Future Perspectives. Front Oncol. 2022;25:12:848485.
29. Kandarakis ED, Bourguignon JP, Giudice LC, Hauser R, Prins GS, Soto AM, et al. Endocrine-Disrupting Chemicals: An Endocrine Society Scientific Statement. Endocr Rev. 2009;30(4):293-342.

81

CHAPTER

Obesity in Adolescent and Childhood

GD Ramchandani, Sugandha Sharma, Rahul Ramchandani

ABSTRACT

Obesity is the most prevalent nutritional disorder among children and adolescents in the United States. Approximately 21–24% of American children and adolescents are overweight, and another 16–18% is obese; the prevalence of obesity is highest among specific ethnic groups.

Childhood obesity predisposes to insulin resistance and type 2 diabetes mellitus, hypertension, hyperlipidemia, liver and renal disease, and reproductive dysfunction. This condition also increases the risk of adult-onset obesity and cardiovascular disease.

Obesity in children is a complex disorder. Its prevalence has increased so significantly in recent years that many consider it a major health concern of the developed world. The National Health and Nutrition Examination Survey (NHANES) indicates that the prevalence of obesity is increasing in all pediatric age groups, in both sexes, and in various ethnic and racial groups.

Many factors, including genetics, environment, metabolism, lifestyle, and eating habits, are believed to play a role in the development of obesity. However, > 90% of cases are idiopathic; < 10% are associated with hormonal or genetic causes.

INTRODUCTION

Operational definitions of obesity in adults are derived from statistical data that analyze the association between body mass and the risk of acute and long-term morbidity and mortality. Because acute medical complications of obesity are less common in children and adolescents than in adults, and because longitudinal data on the relation between childhood weight and adult morbidity and mortality are more difficult to interpret, no single definition of obesity in childhood and adolescence has gained universal approval.

Some investigators have used the terms overweight, obese, and morbidly obese to refer to children and adolescents whose weights exceed those expected for heights by 20%, 50%, and 80–100%, respectively. The body mass index (BMI) has not been consistently used or validated in children younger than 2 years. Because weight varies in a continuous rather than a stepwise fashion, the use of these arbitrary criteria is problematic and may be misleading. Nevertheless, children and adolescents defined as overweight or obese according to published criteria are highly likely to maintain this ponderal status as adults.

BODY MASS INDEX

The BMI is a continuous, although imperfect, measure of body fatness. Calculated as weight (kg) divided by height (m^2), BMI corrects for body size and can be readily and reliably quantified in clinical settings. The BMI correlates closely with total body fat (TBF), which is estimated using dual-energy X-ray absorptiometry (DEXA) scanning in children who are overweight and obese.

Normal values for BMI vary with age, sex, and pubertal status, and standard curves representing the 5th through the 95th percentiles for BMI in childhood and adolescence were generated using data from the 1988 to 1994 the National Health and Nutrition Examination Survey (NHANES). Consensus committees have recommended that children and adolescents be considered overweight or obese if the BMI exceeds the 85th or 95th percentiles, on curves generated from the 1963 to 1965 and 1966 to 1970 NHANES, or exceeds 30 kg/m^2 at any age.

McGavock et al. demonstrated that low cardiorespiratory fitness and reductions in fitness over time are significantly associated with weight gain and the risk of being overweight in children aged 6–15 years. Analysis on a cohort of 902 schoolchildren showed higher waist circumference and disproportionate weight gain over a 12-month follow-up period in those children with low cardiorespiratory fitness. The 12-month risk of overweight classification was 3.5-fold higher in youth with low cardiorespiratory fitness, relative to fit peers. Reductions in cardiorespiratory fitness were significantly and independently associated with increasing BMI. Low levels of cardiorespiratory fitness have also been associated with elevated depressive symptoms in obese adolescents.

ETIOLOGY AND PATHOPHYSIOLOGY

Genetic syndromes associated with childhood obesity include the following:
- Prader–Willi syndrome
- Pseudohypoparathyroidism
- Laurence–Moon–Biedl (Bardet–Biedl) syndrome
- Cohen syndrome
- Down syndrome
- Turner syndrome

Hormonal disorders associated with childhood obesity include the following:
- Growth hormone deficiency
- Growth hormone resistance
- Hypothyroidism
- Leptin deficiency or resistance to leptin action
- Glucocorticoid excess (Cushing syndrome)
- Precocious puberty
- Polycystic ovary syndrome (PCOS)
- Prolactin-secreting tumors

Medications that may cause weight gain in children and adolescents include the following **(Fig. 1)**:
- Cortisol and other glucocorticoids
- Megace
- Sulfonylureas
- Tricyclic antidepressants (TCAs)
- Monoamine oxidase inhibitors (MAOIs), such as phenelzine
- Oral contraceptives
- Insulin (in excessive doses)
- Thiazolidinediones
- Risperidone
- Clozapine

ENERGY IMBALANCE

During childhood and adolescence, excess fat accumulates when total energy intake exceeds total energy expenditure. This energy imbalance can result from excessive energy intake and/or reduced energy expenditure, the latter is usually a consequence of a sedentary lifestyle. This is particularly associated with excessive television viewing, excessive computer use, and insufficient physical activity. In infancy, excess fat deposition occurs when excess energy is provided, especially when the protein-to-energy ratio is altered. This is often seen when feedings are supplemented with additives such as carbohydrates or fat and protein content remains the same. In addition, one study reported an increased incidence of obesity at age 3 years in infants weaned to solid foods by 4 months.

GHRELIN/LEPTIN HORMONAL PATHWAY DYSFUNCTION

In individuals who are obese, dysfunction in the gut-brain-hypothalamic axis via the ghrelin/leptin hormonal pathway has been suggested to have a role in abnormal appetite control and excess energy intake **(Fig. 1)**.

Studies indicate that dysfunction in this hormonal axis may be the causative factor in as many as 10% of obese subjects, with emphasis particularly on those individuals who appear to manifest familial morbid obesity. In these families, several reports have shown a dramatic, weight loss response to hormone replacement therapy in patients with leptin deficiency.

Reductions in energy expenditure characterize other hormonal deficiency states, including hypothyroidism and growth hormone deficiency. Increases in energy intake are observed in genetic syndromes, such as Prader-Willi syndrome, Cushing syndrome, and drug-induced obesity.

WEIGHT GAIN FACTORS

Despite observations of an etiologic role for genetic and hormonal disorders, these factors alone do not explain the excess weight gain observed in most patients who have obesity and are referred to physicians for evaluation and treatment.

Although most overweight children have a familial form of obesity, with one or two obese parents, excess weight gain in obese children clearly depends on both genetic and environmental factors. Correlations between parent and child habitus likely reflect, at least in part, the familial patterns of food intake, exercise, and selection of leisure activity (including amount of television watching), as well as familial and cultural patterns of food

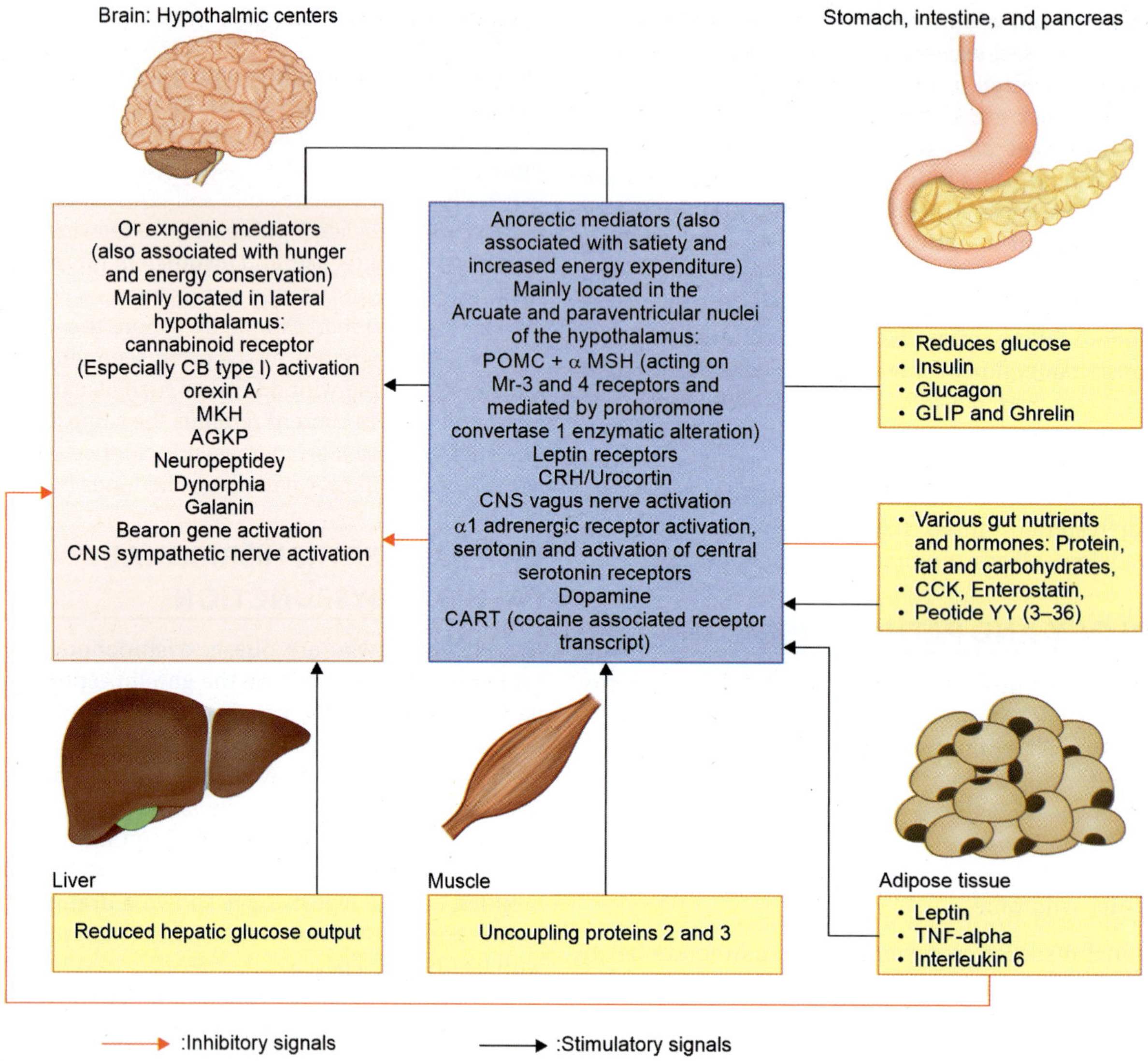

FIG. 1: Neurocircuits related to the pathogenesis of obesity and the feeding satiety cycles.

(AGRP: agouti-related protein; α-MSH: alpha-melanocyte-stimulating hormone; CB: cannabinoid; CCK: cholecystokinin; CNS: central nervous system; CRH: corticotropin-releasing hormone; GLIP: glucagon-like peptide; Mc-3 and 4: melanocortin-3 and 4; MCH: melanin-concentrating hormone; POMC: pro-opiomelanocortin; TNF: tumor necrosis factor)

selection. Nevertheless, evidence from twin, adoption, and family studies suggests that genetic factors also play a considerable role in the development of childhood obesity.

GENETICS

Concordance rates for obesity and type 2 diabetes mellitus (T2DM) are higher in monozygotic twins than in dizygotic twins, and measures of TBF correlate nearly as strongly in monozygotic twins reared apart as in monozygotic twins reared together. Still, genetic factors cannot explain the increased prevalence of obesity observed among American adolescents over the past generation.

INSULIN RESISTANCE, DYSLIPIDEMIA, AND HYPERTENSION

The accumulation of body fat, particularly in a visceral distribution, reduces the sensitivity to insulin in skeletal muscle, liver tissue, and adipose tissue; this 'insulin resistance' predisposes to glucose intolerance and hypertriglyceridemia. Low levels of high-density lipoprotein (HDL), observed both genetically and in association with a sedentary lifestyle, likely contribute to the increase of premature coronary artery disease (CAD) observed in adults with obesity. Increases in circulating levels of insulin and insulin-like growth factor may increase blood pressure (BP) and may stimulate the production of androgens from ovarian and adrenocortical cells. Excess androgens lead to menstrual irregularities, including amenorrhea and oligomenorrhea.

Aromatization of adrenal androgens to estrone leads to gynecomastia in males. The insulin resistance, dyslipidemia, and hypertension predispose to T2DM and cardiovascular disease, reducing life expectancy.

In a study by D'Adamo et al. that evaluated the role of fatty liver in the alteration of insulin sensitivity and β-cell function in obese patients, the investigators concluded that fatty liver, independent of visceral fat, and intramyocellular lipid content (ICML) have a central role in insulin resistance in obese adolescents. Patients were divided into two groups: 23 obese adolescents with and 20 obese adolescents with low hepatic fat fraction (HFF) were matched for age, Tanner stage, BMI score, and percentage of body fat, visceral fat, and IMCL. The group with a high HFF had lower whole-body insulin sensitivity index and lower estimates of insulin secretion, as well as a significantly lower glucose disposal rate, than the group with low HFF.

While insulin resistance represents an important associated finding in adolescents with steatosis, a recent study reported that in younger children with fatty liver, markers for oxidative stress (e.g., oxidized glutathione) were the most significant and independent risk factors.

EPIDEMIOLOGY

United States Statistics

Using BMI criteria, the most recent national surveys demonstrate that 21–24% of American children and adolescents are overweight and that another 16–18% are obese. A 2012 study noted a 16.9% prevalence of obesity in children and adolescents in 2009–2010, which is comparable to the prevalence rates reported in 2007–2008. These findings indicate that the prevalence of overweight (BMI ≥ 85th percentile) children and adolescents in the US has increased by 50–60% in a single generation, and the prevalence of obesity has doubled. The prevalence of obesity in American Indians, Hawaiians, Hispanics, and blacks is 10–40% higher than in whites.

International Statistics

International data reporting regarding childhood obesity varies, and accuracy may be less than optimal; however, Eneli and Dele Davies reported that in 77% of the countries analyzed the prevalence rate for children who were overweight was at least 10%. Notably, the highest rates for children at risk for obesity were found in Malta (25.4%) and the United States (25.1%). Lithuania (5.1%) and Latvia (5.9%) had the lowest rates. A recent European Youth Heart Study suggests Swedish children have a lower risk of becoming overweight or obese in adolescence compared with Estonian children.

Racial, Sexual, and Age Differences in Incidence

Race and ethnicity are associated with increased rates of obesity in children and adolescents. Puerto Rican, Cuban American, and Native American preschoolers have an increased incidence of obesity; black, Native American, Puerto Rican, Mexican, and native Hawaiian school-aged children have the highest rates of obesity in this age group. Approximately 25% of black adolescents are obese. Rosen reported that obstructive sleep apnea/hypoventilation (OSA/H) is more commonly seen in black children than in Hispanic or white children. Tonsils and adenoids are at their peak size, relative to the size of the oropharynx, when children are aged 2–7 years.

During the second decade of life, females are more likely to be obese than males, except for black teenagers, among whom males are more likely to be obese than females. Although the male sex is associated with an increased incidence of OSA in adults, no differences have been identified in children before puberty.

Adolescent obesity is predictive of adult obesity, with 80% of teenagers who are obese continuing on to be obese as adults. Obesity is more likely to occur during specific periods of life, such as when children are aged 5–7 years and during adolescence. A recent European Youth Heart Study suggests male sex confers a higher risk of obesity in adolescence.

PROGNOSIS

For many years, complications arising from obesity were considered unusual in childhood. However, a plethora of minor and major problems may arise in children and adolescents with obesity; most of these problems have considerable impact on quality of life, and some may reduce life expectancy.

Childhood and, especially, adolescent obesity is predictive of adult obesity, which is associated with an increased incidence of diabetes, hypertension, gallstones, and hypercholesterolemia. Pulmonary consequences observed in children and adolescents include an increased frequency of reactive airways, poor exercise tolerance, increased work of breathing, and increased oxygen consumption. The few people who develop obesity-hypoventilation syndrome experience right-sided heart failure with right ventricular hypertrophy.

From an analysis of four prospective cohort studies, data suggest that overweight or obese adults who were also obese as children are at increased risk of T2DM, hypertension, dyslipidemia, and carotid-artery atherosclerosis. However, obese children who achieved a normal BMI by adulthood realized similar risks of these outcomes to individuals who were never obese.

The results from one study suggest that dieting and unhealthy weight-control behaviors in adolescence are associated with greater weight and BMI increases into young adulthood.

A study by Parker et al. observed that compared with those who maintained a healthy weight, children and adolescents who became obese or maintained obesity had a more than threefold increased risk of incident hypertension.

ACUTE COMPLICATIONS OF CHILDHOOD OBESITY

Acute complications of childhood obesity include T2DM, hypertension, hyperlipidemia, accelerated growth and bone maturation, ovarian hyperandrogenism and gynecomastia, cholecystitis, pancreatitis, and pseudotumor cerebri. Fatty liver is common; rarely, patients develop cirrhosis and renal disease (focal glomerulosclerosis). Sleep apnea and sleep-disordered breathing are common in children and adolescents with obesity; in some cases, the apnea is accompanied by neurocognitive dysfunction. Tonsillectomy and adenoidectomy and/or BiLevel positive airway pressure/continuous positive airway pressure (BiPAP/CPAP) may be beneficial in patients with reduced oxygenation or carbon dioxide retention.

Orthopedic Disorders

Numerous orthopedic disorders, including genu valgum, slipped capital femoral epiphysis, and tibia vara, are observed more commonly in children with obesity. Excess weight in young children can cause bowing of the tibia and femurs; the resulting overgrowth of the proximal tibial metaphysis is called Blount disease.

A study by Perry et al. that included BMI data from 597,017 children reported that children 5–6 years of age with severe obesity had almost six times the risk for slipped capital femoral epiphysis and children 11–12 years of age with severe obesity had 17 times the risk compared to children with normal BMI.

Liver and Gallbladder Dysfunction

Evidence of liver dysfunction [nonalcoholic fatty liver disease (NAFLD)], with elevated plasma concentrations of transaminases, is observed in 20% of children with obesity; the liver dysfunction most commonly reflects hepatic steatosis. Increasingly, hepatic steatosis may progress to steatohepatitis, hepatic fibrosis, and cirrhosis. The prevalence of NAFLD is particularly high in individuals of Hispanic descent, because of a single nucleotide polymorphism in the *PNPLA3* gene. Vitamin E supplements may be effective in reversing steatohepatitis in some patients, suggesting that the disorder reflects, at least in part, a relative state of vitamin E deficiency. Cholelithiasis is more common in adults with obesity than in adults with normal weight. Although gallstones are unusual in childhood, nearly one half of all cases of cholecystitis in adolescents are associated with obesity. Cholecystitis may be even more common during rapid weight loss, particularly with very controlled energy diets.

PSYCHOLOGICAL COMPLICATIONS

Emotional and psychosocial sequelae are widespread. Anecdotal evidence suggests that depression and eating disorders are common in children and adolescents referred to obesity clinics. Prejudice and discrimination against individuals with obesity are ubiquitous within US culture; even young children have been found to regard their peers who have obesity in negative ways. Social isolation, peer problems, and lower self-esteem are frequently observed.

CARDIOVASCULAR AND ENDOCRINE COMPLICATIONS

Obesity during childhood and adolescence is associated with numerous cardiovascular risk factors, including hyperinsulinism and insulin resistance, hypercholesterolemia, hypertriglyceridemia, reduced levels of HDL, and hypertension. A hallmark of insulin resistance is acanthosis nigricans, the presence of which indicates an increased risk of T2DM. Adolescent girls with obesity also demonstrate a hyperandrogenic profile, consisting of elevated serum concentrations of androstenedione, dehydroepiandrosterone-sulfate (DHEA-S), and testosterone, as well as reduced levels of sex hormone-binding globulin. The clinical picture resembles that of PCOS. The excess androgens are of adrenal and ovarian origin and may be related, at least in part, to increased serum concentrations of insulin and insulin-like growth factor 1 (IGF-I).

Among sexually mature adolescents, changes in serum lipids and androgens seem to correlate more strongly with body fat distribution than with absolute weight. Thus, adolescents with central obesity (i.e., android or abdominal fat pattern) are more likely to manifest these cardiovascular risk factors than individuals with peripheral obesity (i.e., gynoid or gluteal pattern). In prepubertal children, however, the cardiovascular risk factors correlate better with body weight than with body fat distribution. The increasing prevalence of obesity in childhood and adolescence, accompanied by insulin resistance, appears to explain the increasing incidence of T2DM in adolescents, particularly in minority populations.

Studies indicate that obese children with NAFLD may be at increased risk for atherosclerosis.

LONG-TERM COMPLICATIONS

Obesity during childhood and adolescence is associated with an increased risk of obesity during adulthood, with its attendant long-term health risks. This increased risk appears most pronounced for adolescent males with moderate to severe obesity. The long-term implications of obesity during infancy and early childhood on subsequent health are less clear. In general, the proportion of children with obesity who have obesity as adults increases with increased age at onset of obesity, such that 26–41% of preschoolers with obesity have obesity as adults, compared with 42–63% of school-aged children. Additionally, the higher the degree of obesity during childhood, the higher the risk of adult obesity.

Individuals aged 18 years with a BMI at or above the 95th percentile have a 66–78% risk of being overweight at age 35 years. A recently published study reported that at age 18 years, a BMI of 35 or greater was independently associated with an increased risk of lower extremity edema, walking limitation, PCOS, abnormal kidney function, asthma, OSA, and T2DM.

A study by Lang et al. that included the data from 507,496 children reported that approximately 23–27% of new pediatric asthma cases are directly caused by obesity.

Diabetes

Epidemiologic data, although limited, indicate that adolescent obesity is associated with increased morbidity and mortality in later life. Accordingly, the dramatic increase in the prevalence of T2DM among adolescents with obesity is likely to be accompanied by a host of diabetic-related complications in adulthood and a reduction in life span. Although obesity, per se, is associated with a heightened risk of morbidity related to abnormalities in glucose homeostasis, recent data indicate that the rate of increase in BMI during adolescence may also represent a significant risk factor for diabetes.

Cardiovascular Disease

An increased risk of death from all causes and from CAD has been consistently observed in males, but not in females, who had obesity during adolescence. In a follow-up of the Harvard Growth Study, the risk of morbidity from CAD and atherosclerosis was increased among men and women who had been overweight (BMI >75th percentile) as teenagers. The trend toward higher BMI values among adolescents in the US has also been associated with increases in left ventricular (LV) mass, when compared to similar cohorts in earlier generations, further suggesting that early obesity increases the long-term risk for development of cardiac disease.

Mangner et al. conducted a study to assess geometric and functional changes of the heart in obese compared with nonobese children and adolescents. The authors found thicker LV walls and an increased LV mass, as well as impaired measures of systolic function, among the obese children when compared with nonobese children. The authors also reported no difference in ejection fractions between the obese and nonobese children, but the average LV strain, strain rate, and displacement, which are markers of LV longitudinal function assessed by 2D speckle-tracking echocardiography (2D-STE), were significantly impaired among the obese children. The results of this study demonstrate that childhood obesity is associated with significant changes in myocardial geometry and function, indicating an early onset of potentially unfavorable alterations in the myocardium.

Gout and Colorectal Cancer

Gout and colorectal cancer increased among men who had obesity as adolescents, and arthritis increased among women who had obesity as adolescents. Many of these adverse health outcomes appear to be independent of adult weight, suggesting a direct effect of adolescent obesity on adult health and mortality.

Psychosocial Dysfunction

Psychosocial dysfunction in individuals who have obesity in childhood and adolescence is a serious concern. Among teens and young adults who were tracked after 7 years, overweight females were found to have completed less schooling, were less likely to have married, and had higher rates of household poverty compared with their nonoverweight peers. For overweight males, the only adverse outcome was a decreased likelihood of being married.

PREVENTION

In the absence of a clear, organic etiopathogenesis (e.g., leptin deficiency and other hormonal abnormalities), the long-term management of moderate or morbid obesity in adulthood is highly problematic and rarely successful. Preventing the development of obesity in childhood and adolescence is more likely to reduce long-term complications than treatment of obesity in adults (see long-term complications of childhood obesity under prognosis).

Further studies are needed to achieve the following:

- Identify young children who are predisposed to adolescent and adult obesity
- Identify interventions that prevent the development of obesity in children at risk
- Assess the long-term risks of obesity in prepubertal children
- Identify measures that prevent further weight gain in children and adolescents with obesity

In 2008, the Endocrine Society released guidelines for the prevention and treatment of childhood obesity.

In 2010, the American Heart Association/American Stroke Association (AHA/ASA) issued guidelines for the primary prevention of stroke. A few of the recommendations were as follows:

- *Diet and nutrition*: A diet that is low in sodium and high in potassium is recommended to reduce BP; diets that promote the consumption of fruits, vegetables, and low-fat dairy products such as the Dietary Approaches to Stop Hypertension (DASH)–style diet help lower BP and may lower risk of stroke.
- *Physical inactivity*: Increasing physical activity is associated with a reduction in the risk of stroke; the goal is to engage in at least 30 minutes of moderate intensity activity on a daily basis.
- *Obesity and body fat distribution*: Weight reduction among overweight and obese persons is recommended to reduce BP and risk of stroke.

Learning lifelong habits that incorporate exercise and healthy eating is essential and research is emerging regarding various methods of educating youth.

In a systematic review and meta-analysis to determine the effect of school-based physical activity interventions on BMI in children, Harris et al. concluded that current population-based policies that mandate increased physical activity in schools are unlikely to have a significant effect on the increasing prevalence of childhood obesity. Meta-analysis showed that BMI did not improve with physical activity interventions.

In contrast, a Swedish study by Marcus et al. determined that school-based intervention can reduce obesity in children aged 6–10 years and may affect home-based eating habits. The study of 3,135 boys and girls found a 3.2% decrease in prevalence of obesity and overweight at schools where intervention was attempted. A German study also concluded that school-based intervention was effective, after noting that intervention resulted in 31% reduction in the risk of overweight, and a Dutch study reported beneficial effects of a Dutch Obesity Intervention program.

The results of another study suggest that school wellness policies, mandated by the 2004 Child Nutrition and WIC Reauthorization, can significantly reduce the risk of adolescent obesity.

Specifically, wellness policies related to diet were significantly associated with lower BMI, while those related to physical activity were significantly associated with lower odds of severe obesity only.

A Cochrane Database of Systemic Reviews study notes that child obesity prevention programs implemented in the health, education and care systems and targeted to children aged 6–12 years may have a positive effect on BMI.

A European Youth Heart Study confirms that improving fitness habits in children correlates with a lower incidence of obesity in adolescence.

MANAGEMENT

The glucagon-like peptide-1 (GLP-1) agonists liraglutide (Saxenda) and semaglutide (Wegovy) have gained the Food and Drug Administration (FDA) approval for adjunctive therapy to a reduced calorie diet and increased physical activity for chronic weight management in adolescents meeting criteria for obesity. Studies of liraglutide or semaglutide plus lifestyle intervention results in greater reduction in BMI than lifestyle intervention alone.

Orlistat (Alli and Xenical), a pancreatic lipase inhibitor, is approved for long-term obesity management in patients aged 12 years and older in the United States. Remaining available weight loss products in the US for short-term use in adults include phentermine (Adipex-P) and diethylpropion.

Setmelanotide (Imcivree) is a melanocortin-4 agonist. It was approved by the US FDA in November 2020 for patients aged 6 years and older for weight control caused by rare genetic conditions [e.g., pro-opiomelanocortin (POMC), proprotein convertase subtilisin/kexin type 1 (PCSK1), and leptin receptor (LEPR) deficiencies]. Phase 3 clinical trials observed 80% of patients with obesity owing to POMC or PCSK1 deficiency achieved >10% weight loss and 45.5% of patients with obesity due to LEPR deficiency achieved >10% weight loss after 1 year of treatment. Additionally, hunger scores improved from baseline to 1 year.

SUGGESTED READINGS

1. Ogden CL, Yanovski SZ, Carroll MD, Flegal KM. The epidemiology of obesity. Gastroenterology. 2007;132:2087-102.
2. Fiore H, Travis S, Whalen A, Auinger P, Ryan S. Potentially protective factors associated with healthful body mass index in adolescents with obese and nonobese parents: a secondary data analysis of the third national health and nutrition examination survey, 1988-1994. J Am Diet Assoc. 2006;106(1):55-64.
3. Flegal KM, Ogden CL, Wei R, Kuczmarski RL, Johnson CL. Prevalence of overweight in US children: comparison of US growth charts from the Centers for Disease Control and Prevention with other reference values for body mass index. Am J Clin Nutr. 2001;73(6):1086-93.
4. McGavock JM, Torrance BD, McGuire KA, Wozny PD, Lewanczuk RZ. Cardiorespiratory fitness and the risk of overweight in youth: the Healthy Hearts Longitudinal Study of Cardiometabolic Health. Obesity (Silver Spring). 2009;17(9):1802-7.
5. Shomaker LB, Tanofsky-Kraff M, Zocca JM, Field SE, Drinkard B, Yanovski JA. Depressive symptoms and cardiorespiratory fitness in obese adolescents. J Adolesc Health. 2012;50(1):87-92.
6. Carter PJ, Taylor BJ, Williams SM, Taylor RW. Longitudinal analysis of sleep in relation to BMI and body fat in children: the FLAME study. BMJ. 2011;26:342:d2712.
7. Archbold KH, Vasquez MM, Goodwin JL, Quan SF. Effects of Sleep Patterns and Obesity on Increases in Blood Pressure in a 5-Year Period: Report from the Tucson Children's Assessment of Sleep Apnea Study. J Pediatr. 2012;161(1):26-30.
8. Mosli RH, Kaciroti N, Corwyn RF, Bradley RH, Lumeng JC. Effect of Sibling Birth on BMI Trajectory in the First 6 Years of Life. Pediatrics. 2016;137(4):e20152456.
9. Garcia J. (2016). Birth of a Sibling May Decrease Obesity. [online] Available from http://www.medscape.com/viewarticle/860298. [Last accessed December, 2023].
10. Huh S, Rifas-Shiman S, Taveras E, Oken E, Gillman M. Timing of solid food introduction and risk of obesity in preschool-aged children. Pediatrics. 2011;127(3):e544-51.
11. D'Adamo E, Cali AM, Weiss R, Santoro N, Pierpont B, Northrup V. Central role of fatty liver in the pathogenesis of insulin resistance in obese adolescents. Diabetes Care. 2010;33(8):1817-22.
12. Ruiz-Extremera A, Carazo A, Salmerón A, León J, Casado J, Goicoechea A, et al. Factors associated with hepatic steatosis in obese children and adolescents. J Pediatr Gastroenterol Nutr. 2011;53(2):196-201.
13. Ogden CL, Carroll MD, Kit BK, Flegal KM. Prevalence of obesity and trends in body mass index among US children and adolescents, 1999-2010. JAMA. 2012;307(5):483-90.
14. Eneli I, Dele Davis H. Epidemiology of childhood obesity. Dele Davis H (Ed). Obesity in Childhood and Adolescence. Westport, Connecticut: Praeger Publishers Inc; 2008. pp. 3-19.
15. Ortega FB, Labayen I, Ruiz JR, Kurvinen E, Loit HM, Harro J, et al. Improvements in fitness reduce the risk of becoming overweight across puberty. Med Sci Sports Exerc. 2011;43(10):1891-7.
16. Rosen CL. Clinical features of obstructive sleep apnea hypoventilation syndrome in otherwise healthy children. Pediatr Pulmonol. 1999;27(6):403-9.
17. Juonala M, Magnussen CG, Berenson GS, Venn A, Burns TL, Sabin MA, et al. Childhood adiposity, adult adiposity, and cardiovascular risk factors. N Engl J Med. 2011;365(20):1876-85.
18. Neumark-Sztainer D, Wall M, Story M, Standish AR. Dieting and unhealthy weight control behaviors during adolescence: associations with 10-year changes in body mass index. J Adolesc Health. 2012;50(1):80-6.
19. Parker ED, Sinaiko AR, Kharbanda EO, Margolis KL, Daley MF, Trower NK, et al. Change in Weight Status and Development of Hypertension. Pediatrics. 2016;137(3):1-9.
20. Brown T. Obesity, High BMI Raise Hypertension Risk in Kids, Teenagers. [online] Available from http://www.medscape.com/viewarticle/859416. [Last accessed December, 2023].
21. Perry DC, Metcalfe D, Lane S, Turner S. Childhood Obesity and Slipped Capital Femoral Epiphysis. Pediatrics. 2018;142(5): e20181067.
22. Mann JP, Anstee QM. NAFLD: PNPLA3 and obesity: a synergistic relationship in NAFLD. Nat Rev Gastroenterol Hepatol. 2017;14:506-7.
23. Di Sario A, Candelaresi C, Omenetti A, Benedetti A. Vitamin E in chronic liver diseases and liver fibrosis. Vitam Horm. 2007;76:551-73.
24. Akin L, Kurtoglu S, Yikilmaz A, Kendirci M, Elmali F, Mazicioglu M. Fatty liver is a good indicator of subclinical atherosclerosis risk in obese children and adolescents regardless of liver enzyme elevation. Acta Paediatr. 2013;102:e107-13.
25. Inge TH, King WC, Jenkins TM, Courcoulas AP, Mitsnefes M, Flum DR, et al. The effect of obesity in adolescence on adult health status. Pediatrics. 2013;132(6):1098-104.
26. Lang JE, Bunnell T, Hossain J, Wysocki T, Lima JJ, Finkel TH, et al. Being Overweight or Obese and the Development of Asthma. Pediatrics. 2018;142(6): e20182119.
27. Frellick M. One Quarter of New Pediatric Asthma Cases Tied to Obesity. [online] Available from https://www.medscape.com/viewarticle/905558. [Last accessed December, 2023].
28. Tirosh A, Shai I, Afek A, Dubnov-Raz G, Ayalon N, Gordon B, Derazne E, et al. Adolescent BMI trajectory and risk of diabetes versus coronary disease. N Engl J Med. 2011;364(14):1315-25.
29. Crowley D, Khoury P, Urbina E, Ippisch H, Kimball T. Cardiovascular Impact of the Pediatric Obesity Epidemic: Higher Left Ventricular Mass is Related to Higher Body Mass Index. J Pediatr. 2011;158(5):709-714.e1.
30. Mangner N, Scheuermann K, Winzer E, Wagner I, Hoellriegel R, Sandri M, et al. Childhood obesity: impact on cardiac geometry and function. JACC Cardiovasc Imaging. 2014;7(12):1198-205.
31. O'Riordan M. Obesity in Kids Affects Heart Shape, Functional Impairments. [online] Available from http://www.medscape.com/viewarticle/832982. [Last accessed December, 2023].
32. August GP, Caprio S, Fennoy I, Freemark M, Kaufman FR, Lustig RH, et al. Prevention and treatment of pediatric obesity: an endocrine society clinical practice guideline based on expert opinion. J Clin Endocrinol Metab. 2008;93(12):4576-99.
33. Goldstein LB, Bushnell CD, Adams RJ, Appel LJ, Braun LT, Chaturvedi S, et al. Guidelines for the primary prevention of stroke: a guideline for healthcare professionals from the American Heart Association/American Stroke Association. Stroke. 2011;42(2):517-840.
34. Harris KC, Kuramoto LK, Schulzer M, Retallack JE. Effect of school-based physical activity interventions on body mass index in children: a meta-analysis. CMAJ. 2009;180(7):719-26.
35. Marcus C, Nyberg G, Nordenfelt A, Karpmyr M, Kowalski J, Ekelund U. A 4-year, cluster-randomized, controlled childhood obesity prevention study: STOPP. Int J Obes (Lond). 2009;33(4): 408-17.

36. Muckelbauer R, Libuda L, Clausen K, Toschke AM, Reinehr T, Kersting M. Promotion and provision of drinking water in schools for overweight prevention: randomized, controlled cluster trial. Pediatrics. 2009;123(4):e661-7.
37. Singh AS, Chin A Paw MJ, Brug J, van Mechelen W. Dutch obesity intervention in teenagers: effectiveness of a school-based program on body composition and behavior. Arch Pediatr Adolesc Med. 2009;163(4):309-17.
38. Coffield JE, Metos JM, Utz RL, Waitzman NJ. A multivariate analysis of federally mandated school wellness policies on adolescent obesity. J Adolesc Health. 2011;49(4):363-70.
39. Waters E, de Silva-Sanigorski A, Hall BJ, Brown T, Campbell KJ, Gao Y, et al. Interventions for preventing obesity in children. Cochrane Database Syst Rev. 2011;12:CD001871.
40. Kelly AS, Auerbach P, Barrientos-Perez M, Gies I, Hale PM, Marcus C, et al; NN8022-4180 Trial Investigators. A Randomized, Controlled Trial of Liraglutide for Adolescents with Obesity. N Engl J Med. 2020;382(22):2117-28.
41. Weghuber D, Barrett T, Barrientos-Pérez M, Gies I, Hesse D, Jeppesen OK, et al; STEP TEENS Investigators. Once-Weekly Semaglutide in Adolescents with Obesity. N Engl J Med. 2022;387(24):2245-57.
42. Clément K, van den Akker E, Argente J, Bahm A, Chung WK, Connors H, et al; Setmelanotide POMC and LEPR Phase 3 Trial Investigators. Efficacy and safety of setmelanotide, an MC4R agonist, in individuals with severe obesity due to LEPR or POMC deficiency: single-arm, open-label, multicentre, phase 3 trials. Lancet Diabetes Endocrinol. 2020;8(12):960-70.
43. Rhythm Pharmaceuticals. (2020). IMCIVREE® (setmelanotide) injection, for subcutaneous use Initial US Approval. [online] Available from https://www.accessdata.fda.gov/drugsatfda_docs/label/2022/213793s001lbl.pdf. [Last accessed December, 2023].

82
CHAPTER

Ectopic Fat: Pathophysiology and Consequences

Mukulesh Gupta, Tuhina Gupta

ABSTRACT

Ectopic fat refers to the accumulation of triglycerides within nonadipose tissues, such as the liver, skeletal muscle, heart, and pancreas, which normally contain minimal fat deposits. This ectopic fat deposition can impair cellular functions and organ performance, and it is closely associated with insulin resistance. Various methods are available to quantify ectopic fat, including invasive techniques like histomorphology and chemical analyses, as well as noninvasive imaging methods such as ultrasound, MRI, CT scan, and MRS scan.

In the context of cardiac health, ectopic fat accumulation around the heart or within the pericardium can lead to obesity-related cardiomyopathy. Lipid oversupply to cardiomyocytes causes mitochondrial dysfunction, inflammation, and compromised cardiac function, ultimately contributing to heart failure. Understanding the impact of obesity on cardiac metabolism is crucial for preventing heart disease and developing targeted metabolic therapies.

Epicardial adipose tissue (EAT) and perivascular adipose tissue (PVAT) have distinct roles in cardiac health. EAT provides mechanical support and serves as an energy depot for the myocardium, while PVAT exhibits both anti-inflammatory and proinflammatory characteristics, depending on obesity status. Both tissues have the potential to serve as markers of cardiometabolic risk and therapeutic targets.

In the context of hepatic health, ectopic fat accumulation in the liver can lead to nonalcoholic fatty liver disease (NAFLD) and its progressive stages, including nonalcoholic steatohepatitis (NASH) and cirrhosis. Insulin resistance and altered glucose and fat metabolism contribute to hepatic steatosis. NAFLD is closely linked to metabolic syndrome and affects diabetic, obese, and dyslipidemic populations. Lifestyle interventions and certain medications have shown promise in reducing hepatic fat and improving glycemic control in NAFLD patients.

Skeletal muscle adiposity, including intermuscular and intramuscular fat, correlates with insulin resistance and can impact cardiometabolic risk. Renal lipid accumulation and lipotoxicity play a crucial role in the development and progression of chronic kidney disease (CKD). Pancreatic fat accumulation can lead to nonalcoholic fatty pancreatic steatosis (NAFPD), which may contribute to inflammation and β-cell dysfunction.

The role of ectopic fat in type 2 diabetes mellitus (T2DM) is complex and remains debated. Some evidence suggests that ectopic fat causes organ-specific insulin resistance, while others demonstrate a more nuanced relationship between fat distribution and insulin sensitivity.

The mineralocorticoid receptor (MR) is involved in adipocyte differentiation and adipocyte dysfunction in obesity. Hepatokines, hormone-like proteins secreted by hepatocytes, play a central role in metabolism, and their altered secretion in NAFLD can lead to systemic metabolic dysregulation.

Ectopic fat accumulation has profound implications for various organ systems, including the heart, liver, skeletal muscle, pancreas, and kidneys. Understanding the mechanisms underlying ectopic fat accumulation and its metabolic consequences is essential for developing targeted therapies to mitigate the adverse effects of obesity-related ectopic fat deposition and associated diseases. Further research is needed to explore potential therapeutic strategies and their impact on reducing the prevalence of obesity-related cardiovascular and metabolic disorders.

INTRODUCTION

Ectopic fat, defined as the deposition of triglycerides (TGs) within nonadipose tissues (like liver, skeletal muscle, heart, and pancreas), interferes with cellular and organ function and can cause insulin resistance.

QUANTIFICATION OF ECTOPIC FAT

Ectopic fat can be assessed invasively through histomorphology or chemical analysis of tissue biopsies. However, noninvasive methods like ultrasound, MRI, CT scan, and MRS scan offer advantages like intact regions of interest, large tissue volume examination, and repeated measurements during interventions.

ECTOPIC FAT AND DISEASE CONDITIONS

Ectopic Fat in the Cardiac Health

Cardiac fat accumulates around the heart (pericardial fat) or within the pericardium (epicardial fat), with varying capacities and metabolic effects. Cardiomyopathy brought on by obesity changes the energetics and metabolism of the heart, causing cardiac dysfunction. Over 70% of the adenosine triphosphate (ATP) needed by the heart is produced by fatty acid oxidation. Only a minor quantity of TG is present in the heart due to the close coupling between the oxidation and absorption of fatty acids. When the rate of fatty acid intake exceeds that of oxidation, lipids build up in the cardiomyocytes, which can contribute to cardiac fat accumulation, causing mitochondrial dysfunction, reactive oxygen species, inflammation, and compromised cardiac function. Insulin resistance and impaired glucose utilization further increase fatty acid uptake and accumulation in the myocardium **(Figs. 1A and B)**.

Future Implications

Understanding how obesity affects cardiac metabolism and function is crucial for preventing cardiovascular-related morbidity and mortality. Advanced imaging techniques can help study the relationship between adiposity, cardiac fat depots, cardiac metabolism, and the risk of obesity-related heart diseases. Future research can reveal the independent and combined effects of different fat depots on cardiac metabolism. Identifying high-risk patients and developing targeted therapies can prevent various obesity-related cardiac diseases. Further studies are needed to determine if correcting cardiac metabolic disturbances through metabolic therapies can reduce the prevalence of heart failure in this population **(Figs. 2 and 3)**.

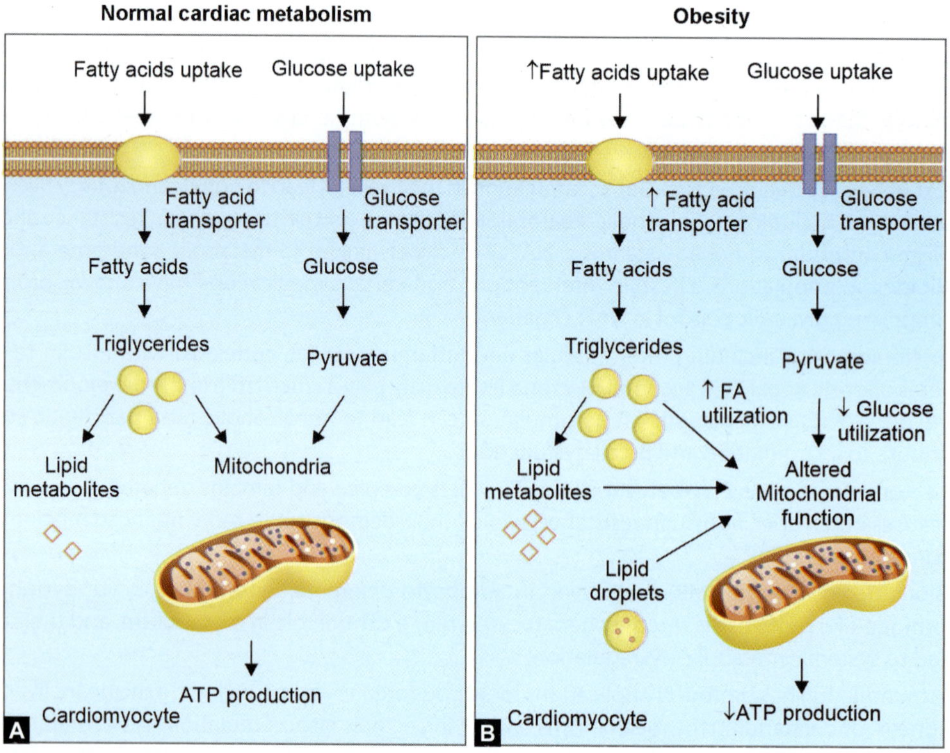

FIGS. 1A AND B: Cardiac metabolism in normal and obese conditions.
(ATP: adenosine triphosphate; FA: fatty acid)

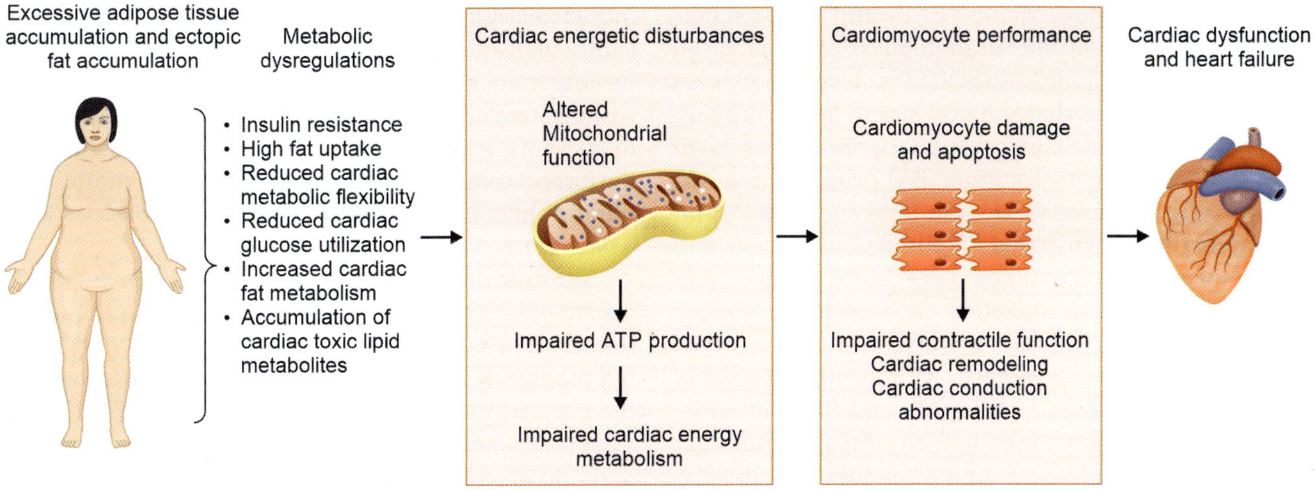

FIG. 2: Accumulation of ectopic fat and cardiac dysfunction: The pathophysiological link.

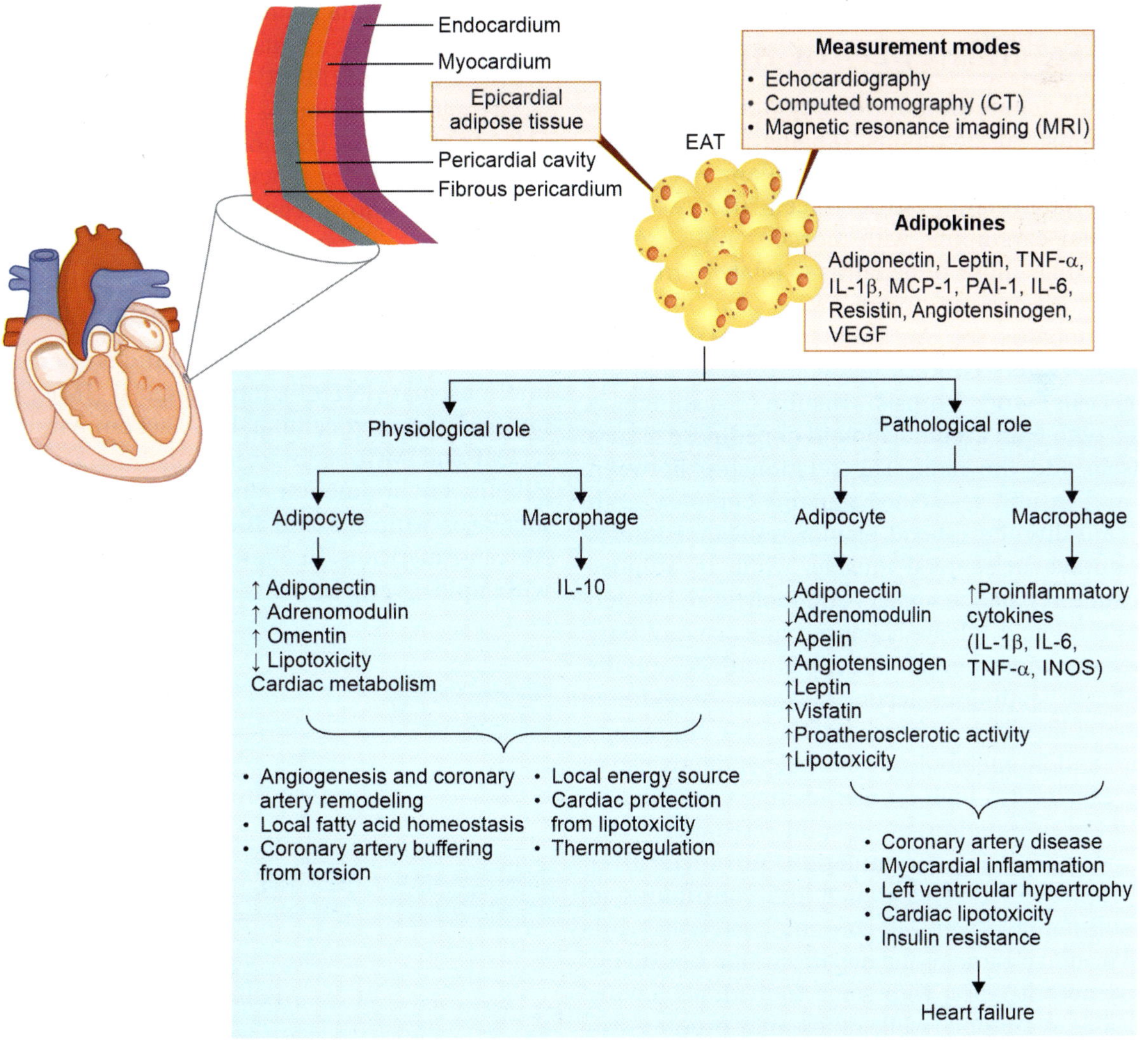

FIG. 3: Epicardial adipose tissue: Physiological and pathophysiological roles.

Epicardial adipose tissue (EAT) and perivascular adipose tissue (PVAT) differ in anatomical, embryological, and biochemical characteristics. EAT is closely connected to the myocardium, shares blood supply with coronary arteries, provides mechanical support, and serves as an energy depot for the myocardium. EAT provides up to 50–70% of the energy used for myocardium contraction, and its dysfunction is associated with impaired glucose and lipid uptake, causing conditions like obesity, diabetes, and heart failure. EAT accumulation can lead to myocardial steatosis and lipotoxic cardiomyopathy. It also exhibits a specific secretome pattern with proinflammatory mediators, causing atherosclerosis and inflammation. PVAT surrounding arteries has an anti-inflammatory role but can become proinflammatory in obesity. PVAT expansion is linked to adverse vascular function, neointimal formation, and hypertension. While further research is needed, EAT and PVAT have potential as markers of cardiometabolic risk and therapeutic targets.

ECTOPIC FAT IN THE HEPATIC HEALTH

Excess lipid accumulation in hepatocytes causes various histological alterations, ranging from steatosis to nonalcoholic steatohepatitis (NASH) and eventually cirrhosis. NASH-related cirrhosis can also result in hepatocellular carcinoma, with mortality rates similar to or worse than those of hepatitis C-related cirrhosis. NAFLD is characterized by the presence of fat (TGs) in >5% of hepatocytes. An imbalance in TG storage and release triggers NAFLD, leading to inflammation, steatonecrosis, and fibrosis. Insulin resistance is associated with lipid accumulation in nonadipose tissues like muscle and the liver. The relationship between NAFLD and insulin resistance remains complex, with unclear causality. Peripheral insulin resistance affects glucose uptake in skeletal muscle, while in adipose tissue, insulin resistance impairs antilipolytic action and increases fatty acid release. Elevated glucose and fatty acid levels promote hepatic fatty acid and TG uptake and synthesis, leading to hepatic steatosis. In addition to peripheral insulin resistance, intrahepatic alterations in glucose and fat metabolism can independently cause steatosis. Short-term high-fat diet feeding can result in hepatic fat accumulation and insulin resistance, even without peripheral fat accumulation. Advanced liver disease reduces insulin clearance and contributes to hyperinsulinemia. Liver fat content correlates with impaired insulin clearance and hepatic insulin sensitivity. NAFLD symptoms vary, with some individuals having no noticeable symptoms, while others may present with hyperglycemia and classic diabetes symptoms. Also, fatty liver disease is an independent predictor of a higher heart rate and early cardiac remodeling associated with reduced ventricular volumes. South Asian men and women appear to store more ectopic fat in the liver compared with their white European counterparts with similar body mass index (BMI) levels. Given the emerging understanding of the importance of liver fat in diabetes pathogenesis, these findings help explain the greater diabetes risks in South Asians **(Figs. 4 and 5)**.

Multiple factors contribute to NAFLD, including oxidative stress, mitochondrial dysfunction, endoplasmic reticulum (ER) stress, hypoxia, adipocytokine imbalance, hypothalamic signaling alterations, and changes in the gut microbiota. Lifestyle interventions focusing on weight loss are the first-line treatment for NAFLD, with bariatric surgery showing significant benefits. Vitamin E is recommended for nondiabetic patients, while glucagon-like peptide-1 receptor agonists (GLP-1 RAs) and sodium-glucose cotransporter-2 (SGLT-2) inhibitors are beneficial for diabetic patients. Statins may reduce cardiovascular risk in dyslipidemia patients with NAFLD or NASH. Also, several antifibrotic agents [like peroxisome proliferator-activated receptor (PPAR) agonists, Farnesoid X receptor (FXR) agonists, apoptosis signal-regulating kinase 1 (ASK-1) inhibitors, chemokine receptor 2 (CCR2)/CCR5 chemokine receptor blockers, galectin antagonists, and siRNA targets downregulating heat shock protein] are being tested.

Ectopic Fat in Skeletal Muscle

Skeletal muscle adiposity includes perimuscular, intermuscular (INTMF), intramuscular (IM), para-osseal fat, and intramyocellular lipid accumulation (IMCL). INTMF and IMCL are more identifiable and correlate with genetic, environmental, and metabolic factors. INTMF increases with age and BMI and is more common in African-Americans. In obese individuals, IMCL increases with lipid overflow, causing incomplete β-oxidation,

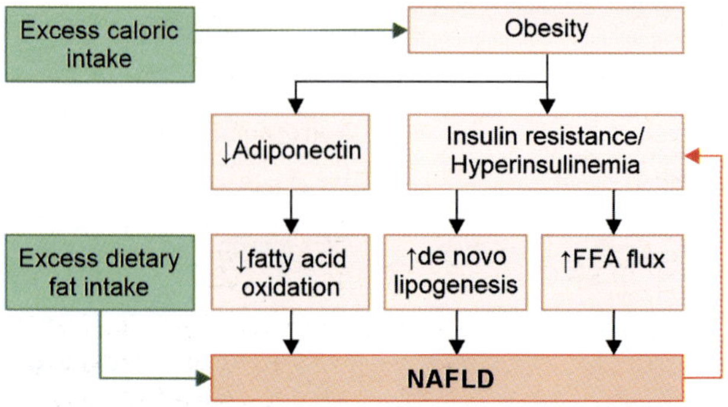

FIG. 4: Excess calorie intake, insulin resistance, and NAFLD: The vicious cycle.
(FFA: free fatty acid; NAFLD: nonalcoholic fatty liver disease)

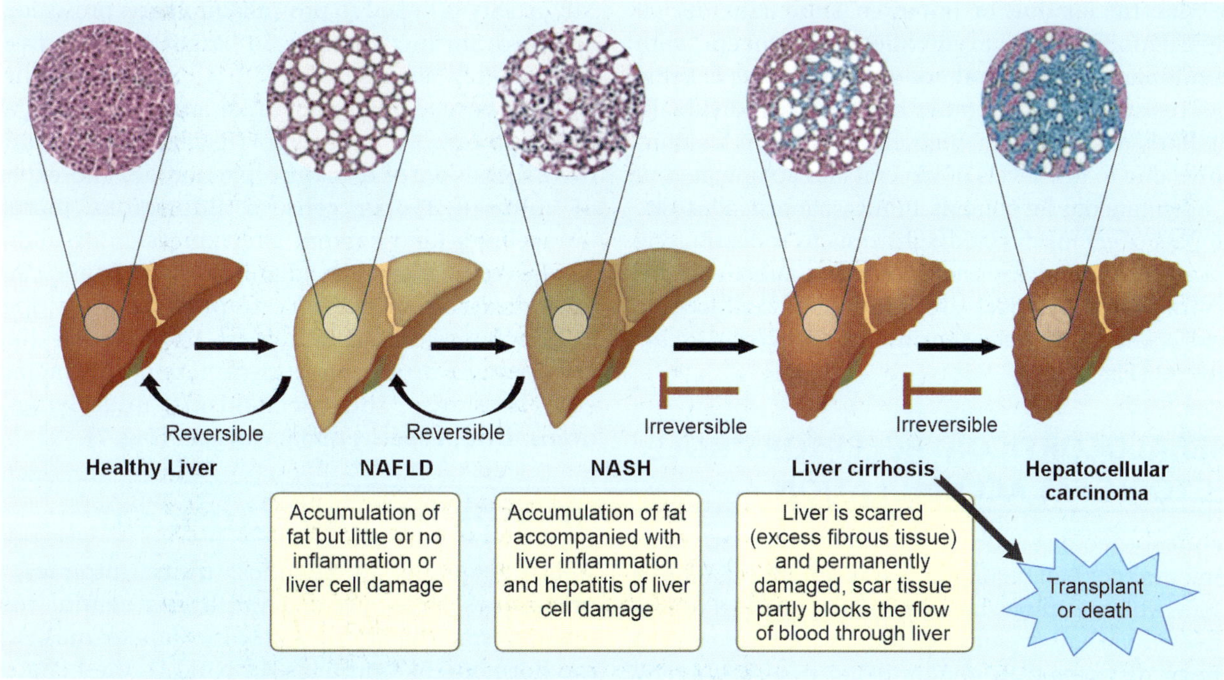

FIG. 5: NAFLD progression: Spectrum of pathological changes.
(NAFLD: nonalcoholic fatty liver disease; NASH: nonalcoholic steatohepatitis)

reactive oxygen species (ROS) formation, and insulin resistance, while trained athletes with comparable IMCL levels are insulin sensitive, known as "the athlete's paradox". INTMF and IMCL correlate with fasting glucose and insulin resistance independent of subcutaneous fat tissue. Skeletal muscle fat may have a direct clinical impact on the cardiometabolic risk. A preliminary artificial intelligence (AI)-based profiling of body composition from routine abdominal CT scans identified myosteatosis as a key predictor of mortality risk in asymptomatic adults.

Ectopic Fat in Renal Metabolism

Renal lipid accumulation plays an important role in the development and progression of CKD. Obese mice show lipid accumulation in glomerular and tubulointerstitial cells, causing a characteristic proteome signature with upregulated sterol regulatory element-binding protein and related genes. Renal insulin resistance also causes lipotoxicity, as observed in diabetic mice where specific insulin receptor deletion causes glomerulosclerosis. Podocytes are vulnerable to nonesterified fatty acid (NEFA) accumulation, while mesangial cells' scavenging function is reduced by lipid overload, causing lipid accumulation, apoptosis, and foam cell formation. In tubular cells, TG accumulation disrupts mitochondrial function, triggering autophagy, renal gluconeogenesis, tubulointerstitial fibrosis, and lipoapoptosis. These mechanisms cause obesity-related glomerulopathy, a form of focal segmental glomerulosclerosis with early glomerular hyperfiltration, mesangial proliferation, and lipid deposition in mesangial and tubular cells. Therapeutic approaches targeting lipid overload hold promise in preventing kidney injury.

Ectopic Fat in Pancreas Health

Pancreas volume decreases with age, while pancreatic adipose content increases. Nonalcoholic fatty pancreatic steatosis (NAFPD) prevalence varies (higher rates in males and obese individuals). NAFPD is mainly due to pancreatic fatty infiltration, leading to nonalcoholic steatopancreatitis (NASP) which may contribute to atherosclerosis and β-cell dysfunction. Unsaturated fatty acids released from peripancreatic fat might worsen acute pancreatitis. Weight loss through a Mediterranean diet and physical activity reduces pancreatic fat, but its effect is lower than on other fat deposits. Bariatric surgery and certain drugs show promising effects in reducing pancreatic fat and improving glycemic control.

Ectopic Fat and Diabetes

Ectopic fat may cause organ-specific insulin resistance, termed "lipotoxicity." Some individuals with type 2 diabetes mellitus (T2DM) predisposition accumulate more visceral fat due to impaired subcutaneous fat storage. Lipodystrophy exemplifies this concept, with fat accumulation in visceral and ectopic tissues causing insulin resistance. On the other hand, some individuals, particularly women with high BMIs, remain insulin-sensitive due to low levels of visceral and ectopic fat but high subcutaneous fat content. PPAR-γ agonists illustrate the impact of ectopic fat on dysglycemia by redistributing fat away from the liver and increasing subcutaneous fat. Transplanting adipose tissue into lipoatrophic mice normalizes hepatic insulin sensitivity by removing excess hepatic fat **(Fig. 6)**.

MINERALOCORTICOID RECEPTORS' ROLE IN ECTOPIC FAT ACCUMULATION

Mineralocorticoid, a nuclear receptor, binds to aldosterone and cortisol, acting as a transcription factor. It regulates volume status, blood pressure, and electrolyte balance in various tissues, including the kidney. MR has been discovered in nonepithelial tissues, thereby extending MR's role beyond electrolyte homeostasis. MR activity is linked to pro-inflammatory, pro-oxidative, and pro-fibrotic changes in target tissues, causing cardiometabolic diseases. MR is expressed in brown adipose tissue (BAT) and white adipose tissue (WAT) and has a key role in preadipocyte differentiation, driving the acquisition of a mature phenotype. The exposure of cultured 3T3-L1 cells to aldosterone increased intracellular lipid content and expression of adipocyte conversion markers like adiponectin and leptin, causing an increased white adipocyte phenotype. In obesity, MR is overexpressed in adipose tissue, suggesting its involvement in adipocyte dysfunction and metabolic complications. The mechanisms underlying MR overactivity in obesity remain unclear **(Fig. 7)**.

HEPATOKINES AND ECTOPIC FAT

ssAdvancements in genetics, transcriptomics, and proteomics have revealed the liver's central role in metabolism. Hepatocytes release hepatokines, which are hormone-like proteins. In NAFLD, the hepatokine secretory profile is disturbed, and NAFLD often precedes

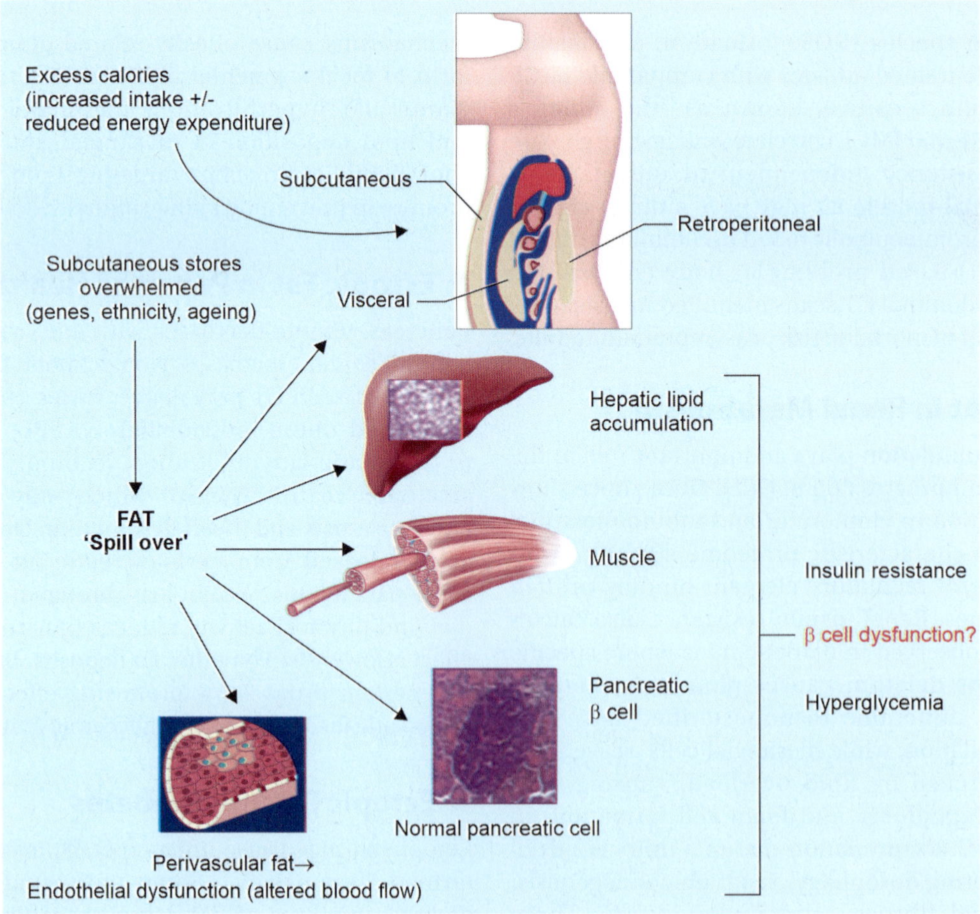

FIG. 6: Ectopic fat distribution and insulin resistance.

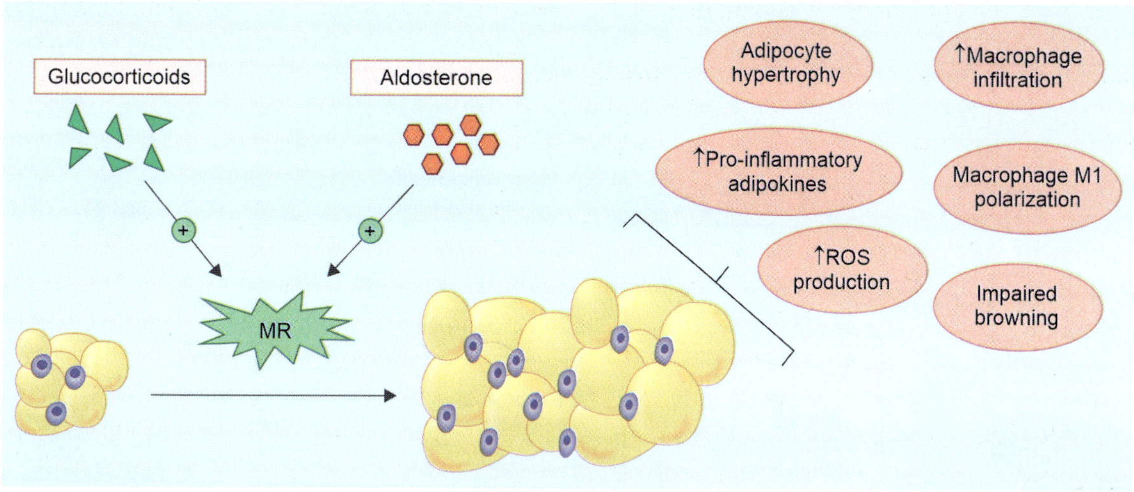

FIG. 7: Mineralocorticoid (MR) signaling and adipocytes hypertrophy.
(ROS: reactive oxygen species)

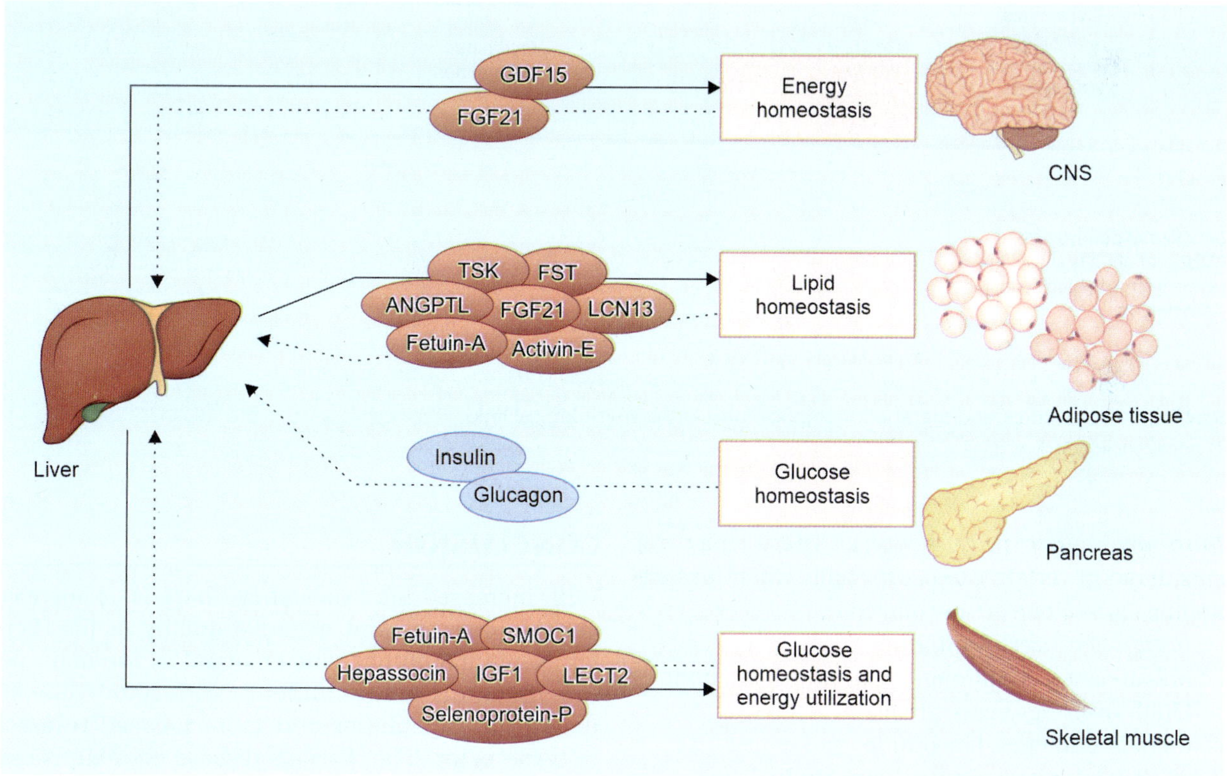

FIG. 8: Hepatokines and their roles.

dysfunction in other organs during the pathogenesis of systemic metabolic diseases. This altered hepatokines' secretion disrupts interorgan signaling, leading to complex metabolic dysregulation. More than 20 hepatokines have been identified and studied to establish their hepatic expression in the fatty liver and their metabolic effects **(Figs. 8 and 9)**.

ECTOPIC FAT: MANAGEMENT

Key approaches for managing ectopic fat are as follows:

- *Lifestyle modifications:*
  - A balanced diet and regular exercise are the foundation of ectopic fat management.
  - Aim to promote a healthy body weight and reduce ectopic fat deposition.

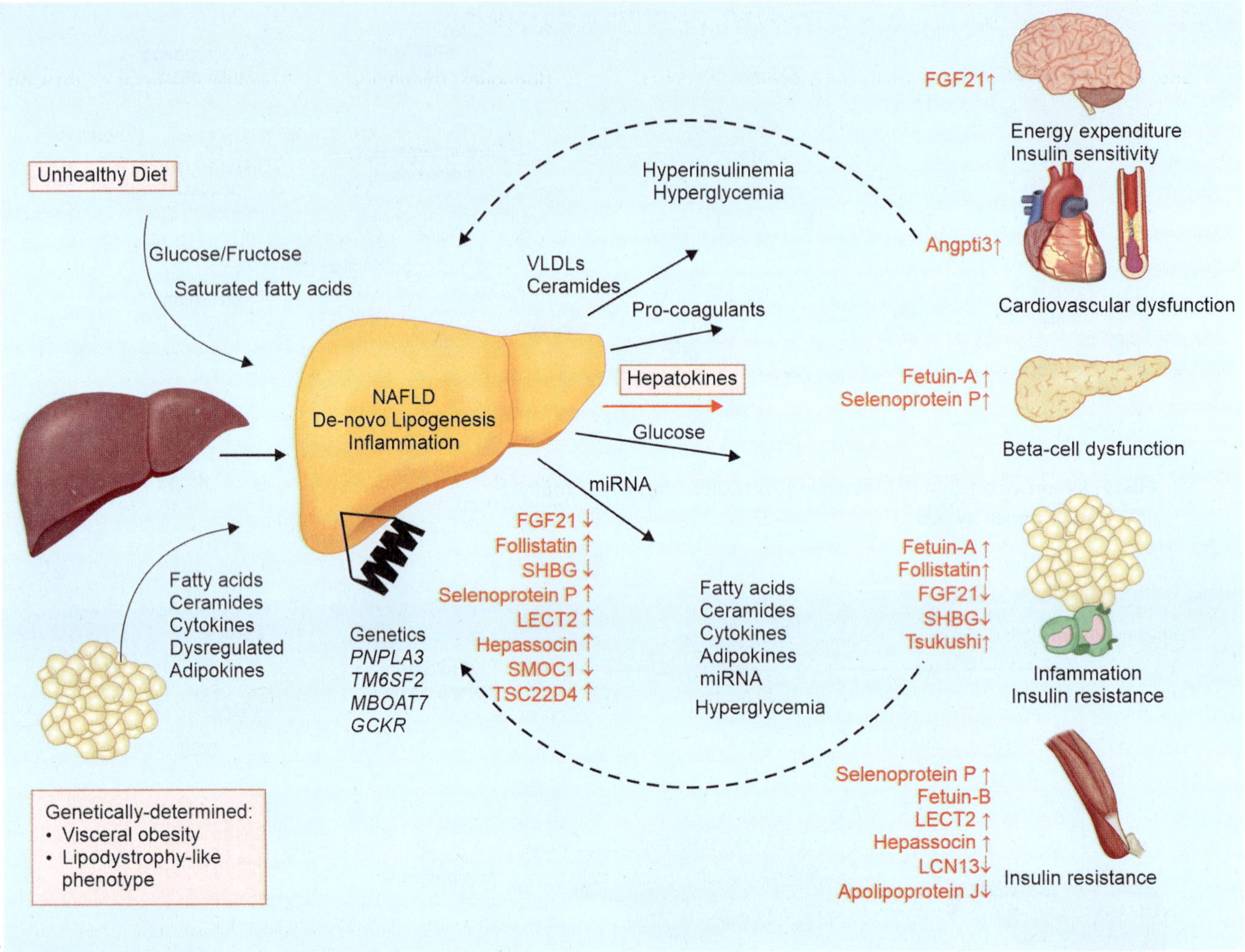

FIG. 9: NAFLD, hepatokines, and metabolic complications: Pathophysiological link.
(NAFLD: nonalcoholic fatty liver disease)

- *Pharmacological interventions:* These may be considered in certain cases, especially when lifestyle modifications alone are insufficient.
  - *Insulin sensitizers*: Metformin
  - MR antagonists: Spironolactone and eplerenone
  - Lipid-lowering agents: Statins
  - Incretin mimetics: Liraglutide
  - SGLT-2 inhibitors are also being studied.
  - Saroglitazar, vitamin E, and PPAR-γ agonists have shown promising results in NAFLD.
- *Surgical interventions:*
  - Bariatric surgery
  - Can also be considered in severe cases of ectopic fat deposition in critical organs

CONCLUSION

With increased life expectancy, there is an increase in chronic diseases and negative quality of life. Ectopic fat accumulation has now emerged as the main player in various disease conditions. With improvements in diagnostic capabilities and more focused research to mitigate ectopic fat, various disease conditions can be prevented, managed, and even cured. More research targeting adipocyte conversion, angiogenesis, and epigenetic modulations can pave the way to halt the "ectopic endemic". While the roles of mineralocorticoid receptors and hepatokines are promising, further research is needed to identify them as potential targets for the management of ectopic fat.

SUGGESTED READINGS

1. Snel M, Jonker JT, Schoones J, Lamb H, de Roos A, Pijl H, et al. Ectopic fat and insulin resistance: pathophysiology and effect of diet and lifestyle interventions. Int J Endocrinol. 2012;2012:983814.
2. Lettner A, Roden M. Ectopic fat and insulin resistance. Curr Diab Rep. 2008;8:185-91.
3. Piché M-E, Poirier P. Obesity, ectopic fat and cardiac metabolism. Expert Rev Endocrinol Metab. 2018;13(4):213-21.
4. Lu Z, Jiang Z, Tang J, Lin C-P, Zhang H. Functions and origins of cardiac fat. FEBS J. 2023;290(7):1705-18.
5. Aeddula NR, Cheungpasitporn W, Thongprayoon C, Pathireddy S. Epicardial adipose tissue and renal disease. J Clin Med. 2019;8(3):299.
6. Ferrara D, Montecucco F, Dallegri F, Carbone F. Impact of different ectopic fat depots on cardiovascular and metabolic diseases. J Cell Physiol. 2019;234(12):21630-41.
7. Liu Q, Bengmark S, Qu S. The role of hepatic fat accumulation in pathogenesis of non-alcoholic fatty liver disease (NAFLD). Lipids Health Dis. 2010;9:42.
8. Jamialahmadi O, Tavaglione F, Rawshani A, Ljungman C, Romeo S. Fatty liver disease, heart rate and cardiac remodelling: Evidence from the UK Biobank. Liver Int. 2023;43(6):1247-55.
9. Wang J, He W, Tsai P-J, Chen P-H, Ye M, Guo J, et al. Mutual interaction between endoplasmic reticulum and mitochondria in nonalcoholic fatty liver disease. Lipids Health Dis. 2020;19(1):72.
10. Nachit M, Horsmans Y, Summers RM, Leclercq IA, Pickhardt PJ. AI-based CT Body Composition Identifies Myosteatosis as Key Mortality Predictor in Asymptomatic Adults. Radiology. 2023;307(5):e222008.
11. Sattar N, Gill JMR. Type 2 diabetes as a disease of ectopic fat? BMC Med. 2014;12:123.
12. Parasiliti-Caprino M, Bollati M, Merlo FD, Ghigo E, Maccario M, Bo S. Adipose tissue dysfunction in obesity: Role of mineralocorticoid receptor. Nutrients. 2022;14(22):4735.
13. Infante M, Armani A, Marzolla V, Fabbri A, Caprio M. Adipocyte mineralocorticoid receptor. In: Litwack G (Ed). Vitamins and Hormones, 109th edition. Philadelphia: Elsevier B.V.; 2019. pp. 189-209.
14. Kim TH, Hong D-G, Yang YM. Hepatokines and non-alcoholic fatty liver disease: Linking liver pathophysiology to metabolism. Biomedicines. 2021;9(12):1903.
15. Stefan N, Schick F, Birkenfeld AL, Häring H-U, White MF. The role of hepatokines in NAFLD. Cell Metab. 2023;35(2):236-52.
16. Jensen-Cody SO, Potthoff MJ. Hepatokines and metabolism: Deciphering communication from the liver. Mol Metab. 2021;44:101138.
17. Hens W, Taeyman J, Cornelis J, Gielen J, Gaal L Van, Vissers D. The Effect of Lifestyle Interventions on Excess Ectopic Fat Deposition Measured by Noninvasive Techniques in Overweight and Obese Adults: A Systematic Review and Meta-Analysis. J Phys Act Heal. 2016;13(6):671-94.
18. Wang C, Liu F, Yuan Y, Wu J, Wang H, Zhang L, et al. Metformin suppresses lipid accumulation in skeletal muscle by promoting fatty acid oxidation. Clin Lab. 2014;60(6):887-96.
19. Hulse JL, Habibi J, Igbekele AE, Zhang B, Li J, Whaley-Connell A, et al. Mineralocorticoid Receptors Mediate Diet-Induced Lipid Infiltration of Skeletal Muscle and Insulin Resistance. Endocrinology. 2022;163(11):bqac145.
20. Zhou M, Wang H, Chen J, Zhao L. Epicardial adipose tissue and atrial fibrillation: Possible mechanisms, potential therapies, and future directions. Pacing Clin Electrophysiol. 2020;43(1): 133-45.
21. He F, Chen W, Xu W, Liu D, Xiao Z, Tang Y, et al. Safety and efficacy of liraglutide on reducing visceral and ectopic fat in adults with or without type 2 diabetes mellitus: A systematic review and meta-analysis. Diabetes, Obesity and Metabolism. 2023;25(3):664-74.
22. Angelini G, Gissey LC, Corpo G Del, Giordano C, Cerbelli B, Severino A, et al. New insight into the mechanisms of ectopic fat deposition improvement after bariatric surgery. Sci Rep. 2019;9(1):17315.

of sarcopenia and muscle quality. *Example*: Hand grip dynamometers to measure isometric strength.

The hand grip strength records the mean value (in kilograms) of three consecutive measurements of the dominant arm gripping a dynamometer, <26 kg for men and <18 kg for women are the standard cut off values among the Asian population.

- Physical performance: The Short Physical Performance Battery based on gait speed, chair stands, and balance tests are among the widely used and validated measures to assess physical performance. It consists of the following three tests: Balance test, gait speed test, and chair stand test. The total score calculated from the three tests is 12 and patients will be categorized as sarcopenic based on below written scores.
  - Score <2 = Sarcopenia
  - Score 3–9 = Possible sarcopenia
  - Score >10 = No sarcopenia

- *Anthropometric measurements:* Anthropometric measurements provide additional information about body composition and distribution of body fat. These measurements include waist circumference, hip circumference, and waist-to-hip ratio, which can indicate central obesity and the risk of metabolic disorders.
- *Medical history and physical examination:* A comprehensive medical history review and physical examination can help identify potential underlying causes or contributing factors for sarcopenic obesity. This may involve assessing hormonal imbalances, chronic diseases, medication use, and lifestyle factors.

DO SARCOPENIA AND OBESITY HAVE A SYNERGISTIC INFLUENCE ON EACH OTHER?

Yes, sarcopenia and obesity can have a synergistic influence on each other, meaning they can interact and exacerbate each other's effects. The combination of these two conditions, known as sarcopenic obesity, creates a unique set of challenges that can contribute to a negative spiral of worsening health outcomes. Here are some of the ways in which sarcopenia and obesity can synergistically influence each other:

- *Muscle loss and fat accumulation:* Sarcopenia involves the progressive loss of muscle mass, while obesity is characterized by excessive accumulation of body fat. As muscle mass decreases, the body's ability to burn calories and regulate metabolism diminishes. This can result in a lower resting metabolic rate, making it easier to gain weight, and further contribute to obesity.
- *Insulin resistance and muscle function:* Obesity is often associated with insulin resistance, which impairs the body's ability to efficiently use insulin to regulate blood sugar levels. Insulin resistance can negatively affect muscle function and impair muscle protein synthesis, further contributing to muscle loss in individuals with sarcopenia.
- *Inflammation:* Both sarcopenia and obesity are associated with chronic low-grade inflammation. Inflammatory molecules released by adipose tissue in obesity can promote muscle catabolism and contribute to muscle wasting in individuals with sarcopenia. In turn, muscle loss can further exacerbate inflammation, creating a vicious cycle.
- *Functional limitations:* The combination of reduced muscle mass and increased body weight in sarcopenic obesity can lead to functional limitations and difficulties in performing daily activities. The excess body fat can place additional strain on weakened muscles, making movements and mobility more challenging.
- *Metabolic abnormalities:* Sarcopenia and obesity both contribute to metabolic abnormalities, such as dyslipidemia, insulin resistance, and impaired glucose metabolism. These shared metabolic disturbances can increase the risk of cardiovascular disease, T2DM, and other chronic conditions.

Overall, sarcopenia and obesity interact synergistically, with each condition worsening the effects of the other. The presence of sarcopenia in obesity amplifies the metabolic and functional impairments associated with obesity, while obesity exacerbates the muscle loss and functional limitations seen in sarcopenia.

MANAGEMENT OF SARCOPENIC OBESITY

Managing sarcopenic obesity involves addressing both components to improve overall health and quality of life.

Nutritional Intervention

- *Caloric intake:* Caloric intake for the treatment of sarcopenic obesity should be carefully managed to achieve a balance between weight loss (reducing body fat) and preserving muscle mass. Aim for a gradual and sustainable weight loss of around 0.5–1 kg (1–2 pounds) per week. Rapid weight loss can lead to muscle loss and other health issues.
- *Protein intake:* Encourage a higher protein intake to support muscle protein synthesis and preserve muscle mass. Aim for about 1.2–1.5 g of protein per kilogram of body weight. Distributing protein intake evenly across meals throughout the day can be beneficial for

maximizing muscle protein synthesis. High-quality protein sources, such as lean meats, poultry, fish, eggs, dairy products, legumes may be beneficial.

- *Micronutrients:* Address any deficiencies in vitamins and minerals that might affect muscle health, such as vitamin D, calcium, and magnesium.

Hormone Replacement Therapy

Hormone replacement therapy (HRT) is a medical treatment that involves replacing hormones in the body, often to address deficiencies or imbalances. While HRT can play a role in addressing certain aspects of sarcopenic obesity, it is important to note that its use should be carefully considered. Some other hormones which may find use in treatment of sarcopenia with obesity include testosterone replacement therapy, estrogen therapy, growth hormone therapy, and dehydroepiandrosterone (DHEA) therapy.

Also lifestyle modifications are the cornerstone in the management of sarcopenic obesity like resistance exercises which is a crucial component of the management of sarcopenic obesity. It is an effective way to counteract muscle loss and promote muscle growth. Additionally aerobic exercises such as walking or cycling can help with weight management and overall cardiovascular health.

SUGGESTED READINGS

1. Scott D, Sanders KM, Aitken D, Hayes A, Ebeling PR, Jones G. Sarcopenic obesity and dynapenic obesity: 5-year associations with falls risk in middle-aged and older adults. Obesity. 2014;22:1568-74.
2. Zamboni M, Rubele S, Rossi AP. Sarcopenia and obesity. Curr Opin Clin Nutr Metab Care. 2019;22(1):13-9.

SECTION 5

GASTROENTEROLOGY

84

CHAPTER

Abdominal Distension and Bloating Management

Anil Kumar Kulshreshtha, Yogesh Kumar Govil

ABSTRACT

Abdominal bloating is a personal experience characterized by gassiness, trapped gas, or pressure without external signs. It can increase abdominal girth and resemble a balloon or pregnancy. Diagnosis is extensive, and organic causes should be considered. Treatment involves investigating the predominant complaint, symptom timing, dietary habits, medications, supplements, and other medical comorbidities. A systematic approach is essential for diagnosis and treatment.

INTRODUCTION

Abdominal distension and bloating are common presenting complaint. The sensation of abdominal bloating is a personal experience characterized by feelings of gassiness, trapped gas, or a sense of pressure and distension without apparent external signs. Patients often articulate a feeling of fullness or pressure across different areas of the abdomen (such as epigastric, mid, lower, or general). The objective manifestation of abdominal distension is an increase in abdominal girth. Patients frequently liken their appearance to that of a balloon or describe feeling pregnant. The differential diagnosis is extensive, and it is crucial to consider and rule out organic causes when managing patients. The approach involves investigating and identifying the predominant complaint, noting symptom onset timing, reviewing dietary habits, medications, and supplements, and exploring other medical comorbidities. There are various therapeutic options available, and their application should target the underlying mechanism, symptom, or cause. A systematic approach is essential for diagnosing and a systematic approach is essential for diagnosing and addressing patients presenting with abdominal distension and bloating.

Diagnostic criteria: The prevalence of bloating affects 16–19% of the general population. Criteria for diagnosing functional abdominal bloating and/or distension include:

- Recurrent bloating and/or distension occurring at least once a week on average.
- Bloating and distension should be the predominant gastrointestinal (GI) symptoms.
- Patients should not meet criteria for irritable bowel syndrome, functional constipation, functional diarrhea, or postprandial distress syndrome.
- Symptom onset should have occurred at least 6 months prior to diagnosis.
- Symptoms should have been active within the preceding 3 months.

Pathophysiology: The complex and often multifactorial nature of the pathophysiology of abdominal distension and bloating is not fully understood **(Fig. 1)**. While a majority of patients attribute their symptoms to an increased volume of "gas" within the GI tract, this explanation accounts for symptoms in only a minority of cases. Computed tomography (CT) imaging has revealed that luminal gas increases in only 25% of patients with functional gastrointestinal disorders (FGIDs) during spontaneous episodes of abdominal distension or after consuming a "high-flatulence" diet.

Etiology of abdominal distension and bloating: This includes both organic and functional disorders. See **Table 1** below.

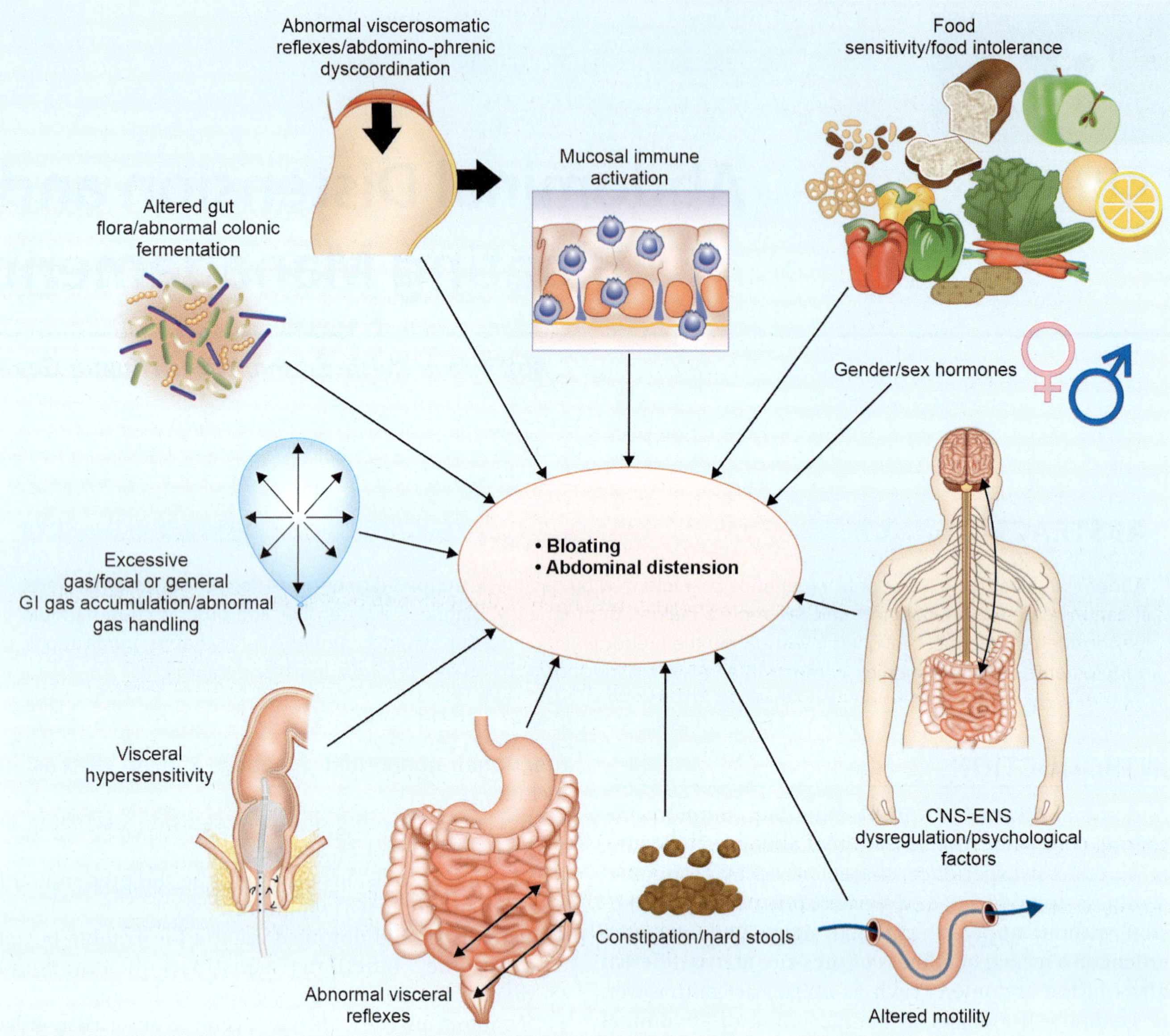

FIG. 1: Pathophysiology of abdominal distension and bloating.
(CNS-ENS: central nervous system–enteric nervous system)

TABLE 1: Etiologies of abdominal distension and bloating.

Organic/pathologic etiologies	Disorders of gut-brain interaction
• Small intestinal bacterial overgrowth • Lactose, fructose, and other carbohydrate intolerances • Celiac disease • Pancreatic insufficiency • Prior gastroesophageal surgery (e.g., fundoplication, bariatric surgery) • Gastric outlet obstruction • Gastroparesis • Ascites • Gastrointestinal or gynecologic malignancy • Hypothyroidism • Adiposity • Small intestine diverticulosis • Chronic intestinal pseudo-obstruction	• Irritable bowel syndrome • Chronic idiopathic constipation • Pelvic floor dysfunction • Functional dyspepsia • Functional bloating

COMMON CAUSES OF ABDOMINAL BLOATING AND DISTENSION

Small Intestinal Bacterial Overgrowth

Small intestinal bacterial overgrowth (SIBO) can induce symptoms through the fermentation of carbohydrates, leading to the subsequent production of gas and the stretching and distension of the small intestine. While altered sensation and abnormal viscerosomatic reflexes may contribute to these symptoms, their role remains inadequately explored in SIBO patients. A meta-analysis revealed a prevalence of SIBO ranging from 0 to 20% in healthy controls, in contrast to 4 to 78% in individuals with irritable bowel syndrome (IBS).

- *Carbohydrate intolerance:* Symptoms of bloating and distension arising from carbohydrate intolerance result from an increased osmotic load, excessive fluid retention, and heightened fermentation in the colon. The prevalence of food intolerance, exhibiting similar symptoms, approaches 20% in the general population (as indicated by data from FGIDs and IBS studies). The actual prevalence of carbohydrate intolerance remains unclear, as it does not necessarily align with carbohydrate malabsorption according to breath tests. Prospective studies involving various FGIDs have reported lactose intolerance and malabsorption rates of 51% and 32%, respectively, and fructose intolerance and malabsorption rates of 60% and 45%, respectively.
- *Lactase deficiency:* Lactase deficiency alone may not result in malabsorption, as not all individuals with lactase deficiency experience symptoms after consuming lactose. This suggests that additional factors, such as genetic predisposition or visceral hypersensitivity, may be necessary for symptom development in some patients.
- *Intestinal microbiota:* Quantitative and qualitative disparities in the intestinal microbiota have been observed when comparing IBS patients with healthy controls. Notably, one study identified significant reductions in specific taxa from the Ruminococcaceae and Eubacteriaceae families among IBS patients without bloating, as opposed to those with bloating and healthy control subjects.
- *Dysmotility:* Bloating is prevalent in patients with gastroparesis (occurring in over 50% of cases) and those with small bowel dysmotility, such as chronic intestinal pseudo-obstruction and scleroderma. A prospective study involving >2,000 patients with functional constipation and IBS-C revealed that over 90% reported bloating symptoms. In IBS-C patients, prolonged colonic transit was associated with increased abdominal distension compared to those with normal transit. Individuals with anorectal motor dysfunction may experience bloating and distension due to impaired evacuation of both flatus and stool. Prolonged balloon expulsion is correlated with distension symptoms in constipated patients, and pelvic outlet obstruction has been linked to delayed colonic transit.

Paradoxical Abdominophrenic Response

Also called abdominophrenic dyssynergia, develops in some patients with chronic bloating and distension **(Fig. 2)**. The physiological response to increased intraluminal gas the normal response is diaphragm relaxation (ascends) and the anterior abdominal muscles contract in order to increase the craniocaudal capacity of the abdominal cavity without abdominal bloating. However, in patients with abnormal physiologic response the diaphragm contracts (descends) and the anterior abdominal wall muscles relax leading to abdominal bloating.

In a sophisticated CT scan investigation, individuals experiencing functional bloating exhibited noticeable protrusion of the abdominal wall and descent of the diaphragm, accompanied by relatively modest increases in intraluminal gas. Contrastingly, subjects with bloating and intestinal dysmotility displayed substantial elevations in intraluminal gas content, leading to diaphragmatic ascent. Abdominophrenic dyssynergia has been recognized in patients with functional dyspepsia (FD) who present symptoms of postprandial bloating.

- *Disruptions in brain-gut interaction:* The conscious perception of intraluminal content and abdominal distension may contribute to the symptomatic experience of bloating. This perception can be magnified by intricate brain-gut neural pathways, influenced further by factors such as anxiety, depression, somatization, and hypervigilance.
- *Approach to management:* A comprehensive clinical history and thorough physical examination are essential for unraveling the root cause of bloating and distension. Key details include the onset and timing of these symptoms, their correlation with food intake or bowel movements, any surgical history (e.g., Nissen fundoplication), and a meticulous review of medications (e.g., narcotics), supplements, and dietary habits. In cases of constipation, a rectal examination should be conducted to identify potential evacuation disorders. See **Flowcharts 1, 2,** and **Table 2** for a simplified approach to narrow down the underlying cause of abdominal distension and bloating.

disease or colon cancer. Although symptoms may wax and wane, most individuals can effectively manage their condition through lifestyle modifications and appropriate medical treatments.

Support and Self-care Strategies

Living with IBS can be challenging, but several self-care strategies can help individuals cope, such as:

- *Building a strong support system*: Seek understanding and support from family, friends, or support groups.
- *Educating oneself*: Learning more about IBS and its management can empower individuals to take an active role in their care.

In recent years, there have been notable advancements in the understanding and management of IBS. Some of the significant developments are as follows:

- *Microbiome research*: There has been a growing emphasis on studying the gut microbiome and its role in IBS. Research has identified alterations in the composition and diversity of gut bacteria in individuals with IBS. This has led to investigations into the use of probiotics, prebiotics, and fecal microbiota transplantation (FMT) as potential treatment options for IBS.
- *Emerging therapies*: Advances in understanding the underline mechanism of IBS have paved the way for targeted therapies [(i) Tenapanor is a drug that acts on sodium hydrogen exchanger. At a dose of 50 mg twice daily. It appears to be beneficial in IBS-C in terms of its effect on a composite increase in stool frequency and improvement in abdominal pain. (ii) Ibodutant, a neurokinin receptor-2 antogonist which may be beneficial in motility in IBS-D. At a dose of 10 mg once daily has shown satisfcatory relief of global symptoms and improvement in abdominal pain] **(Flowchart 2)**.
- *FMT*: FMT, the process of transferring fecal matter from a healthy donor to the gastrointestinal tract of

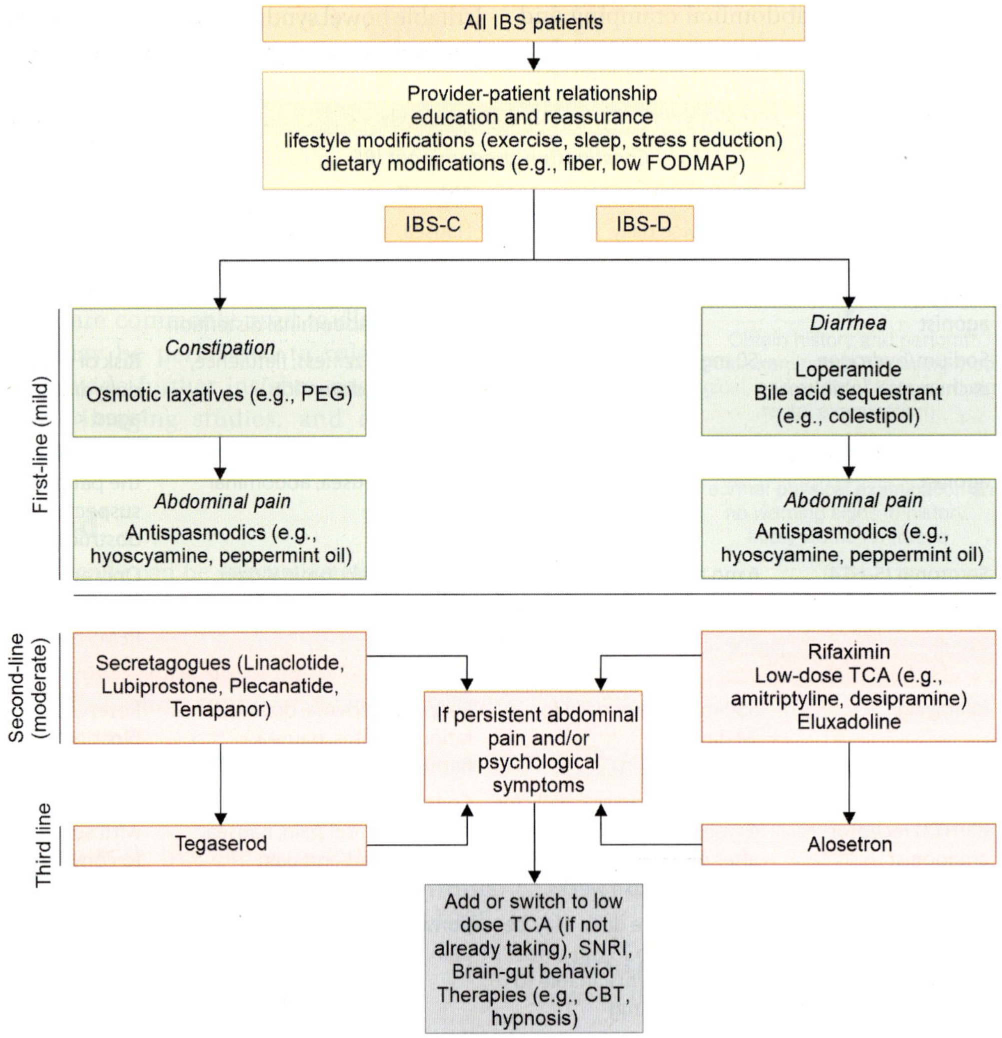

FLOWCHART 2: Clinical decision support tool in IBS treatment.
(CBT: cognitive behavioral therapy; IBS: irritable bowel syndrome; PEG: polyethylene glycol; TCA: tricyclic antidepressant)

a recipient, has shown promising results in certain cases of IBS. This procedure aims to restore a healthier balance of gut bacteria and improve symptoms. However, further research is needed to determine its long-term efficacy and safety **(Fig. 4)**.

- *Personalized medicine*: The recognition that IBS is a heterogeneous condition has led to the concept of personalized medicine. By understanding individual factors such as genetic predisposition, gut microbiome composition, and specific symptom patterns, healthcare providers can tailor treatment plans to meet the unique needs of each patient. This approach may involve a combination of dietary modifications, stress management techniques, and targeted medications.

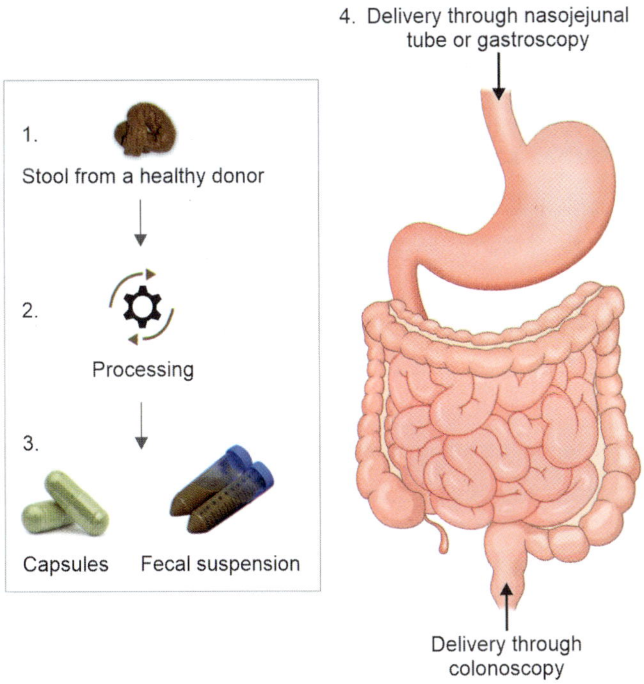

FIG. 4: Fecal microbiota transplantation.

- *Psychological interventions*: Psychological factors, such as stress and anxiety, can significantly impact IBS symptoms. As a result, psychological interventions, such as cognitive-behavioral therapy (CBT), mindfulness-based stress reduction (MBSR), and gut-directed hypnotherapy, have gained attention as complementary therapies for IBS. These interventions aim to reduce stress levels and improve coping mechanisms, leading to symptom relief.
- *Telemedicine and digital health*: The COVID-19 pandemic has accelerated the adoption of telemedicine and digital health platforms, providing new avenues for managing IBS. Virtual consultations and remote monitoring enable individuals to access healthcare services conveniently. Additionally, mobile applications and online resources offer educational materials, symptom tracking tools, and support communities to help individuals manage their condition.

It is important to note that while these recent developments offer promising avenues for improved understanding and management of IBS, further research and clinical trials are needed to validate their effectiveness and long-term outcomes. Individuals with IBS should work closely with their healthcare providers to determine the most appropriate treatment approach based on their specific needs and symptoms.

- *Prioritizing self-care*: Engage in activities that promote relaxation, stress reduction, and overall well-being.

CONCLUSION

Irritable bowel syndrome is a common gastrointestinal disorder that can significantly impact an individual's quality of life. While the exact cause remains elusive, understanding the symptoms, triggers, and management strategies can empower individuals to effectively cope with IBS. By implementing lifestyle modifications, utilizing appropriate medical treatments, and practicing self-care, individuals with IBS can take control of their symptoms and improve their overall well-being.

SUGGESTED READINGS

1. Mearin F, Lacy BE, Chang L, Chey WD, Lambo AJ, Simren M, et al. Bowel disorders. Gastroenterology 2016;150:1393-407.
2. Holtmann GJ, Ford AC, Talley NJ. Pathophysiology of irritable bowel syndrome. Lancet Gastroenterol Hepatol. 2016;1:133-46.
3. Canavan C, West J, Card T. The economic impact of the irritable bowel syndrome. Aliment Pharmacol Ther. 2014;40:1023-34.
4. Lovell RM, Ford AC. Global prevalence of and risk factors for irritable bowel syndrome: a meta-analysis. Clin Gastroenterol Hepatol. 2012;10(7):712-21.e4.
5. Everhart JE, Ruhl CE. Burden of digestive diseases in the United States part I: overall and upper gastrointestinal diseases. Gastroenterology. 2009;136:376-86.

6. Ford AC, Moayyedi P, Lacy BE, Lambo AJ, Saito YA, Schiller LR, et al. American College of Gastroenterology monograph on the management of irritable bowel syndrome and chronic idiopathic constipation. Am J Gastroenterol. 2014;109(Suppl 1): S2-S26.
7. Spiegel BM, Farid M, Esrailian E, Talley J, Chang L. Is irritable bowel syndrome a diagnosis of exclusion? A survey of primary care providers, gastroenterologists, and IBS experts. Am J Gastroenterol. 2010;105:848-58.
8. Sucampo Pharmaceuticals Inc. (2012). Lubiprostone: Package Insert. Bethesda, MD.
9. Forest Pharmaceuticals Inc. (2012). Linaclotide: Package Insert. St. Louis, MO.
10. Salix Pharmaceuticals Inc. (2020). Plecanatide: Package Insert. Bridgewater, NJ.
11. Ardelyx Inc. (2019). Tenapanor: Package Insert. Fremont, CA.
12. Druken T. FDA approves the reintroduction of Zelnorm (tegaserod) for irritable bowel syndrome with constipation (IBS-C) in women under 65. Finanzen.ch. 2019.
13. Novartis Pharmaceutical Coproration. (2002). Tegasorod: Package Insert. East Hanover, NJ.
14. Salix Pharmaceuticals Inc. (2010). Rifaximin: Package Insert. Morrisville, NC, USA: Food and Drug Administration.
15. GlaxoSmithKline. (2002). Alosetron: Package Insert. Research Triangle Park, NC.
16. Barshop K, Staller K. (2017). Eluxadoline in irritable bowel syndrome with diarrhea: rationale, evidence, and place in therapy. Ther Adv Chronic Dis.;8(11):153-60.
17. Axcan Scandipharm Inc. (2006). Dicyclomine: Package Insert. Birmingham, AL.
18. Ford AC, Lacy BE and Talley NJ. (2017). Irritable Bowel Syndrome. N Engl J Med 376; 26.

86

CHAPTER

Approach to a Patient with Chronic Constipation

Atul Mehrotra, Anita Nambiar

ABSTRACT

Constipation is one of the most common problems presenting in outpatient and inpatient settings with a prevalence rate of 14–16% in the general population being higher in women and those above 60 years. The most widely used definition is based on Rome IV criteria with fewer than three bowel movements in a week being a practical one. Careful history and a thorough physical examination may identify the cause in most, but no underlying cause is identified in some. Treatment involves lifestyle measures and use of pharmacotherapeutic agents like bulk, osmotic, or stimulant laxatives or other agents like prokinetics or opioid receptor antagonists. Bio-feedback therapy may be tried as well as sacral nerve stimulation in some. Surgical treatment is usually tried in patients with refractory constipation with delayed transit.

INTRODUCTION

Constipation cannot be defined objectively. While three times a day to three times a week may be normal for an individual, a patient usually defines it as difficulty with defecation, straining or hard stools with a sense of incomplete evacuation or a nonproductive urge. A healthcare provider defines constipation as bowel movement less than three times a week. Chronic constipation is a common and heterogeneous condition having a prevalence of 14–16% in the general population with a higher prevalence in women and above the age of 60 years. Over the last few years, both old and new mechanisms of treatment with different mechanisms of action have proved to be effective. It has a significant impact on quality of life and productivity at work.

Definition

Constipation is defined in various ways with apparently small differences between them that need to be acknowledged to understand potentially distinct responses to treatment. The most widely used definition for constipation is one based on Rome IV criteria which is characterized by the presence of two or more of the following symptoms for >25% of the defecations for the last 3 months:

- Straining
- Lumpy or hard stools
- Sensation of incomplete evacuation
- Sensation of anorectal obstruction/blockage
- Manual maneuvers to facilitate evacuation
- Fewer than three spontaneous bowel movements per week

It is pertinent to add that loose stools are rarely present without the use of laxatives and that the criteria for irritable bowel syndrome (IBS) are not met.

Alternatively, constipation may be defined based on a patient's dissatisfaction with the frequency of defecation and stool passage. This lacks objectivity; however, we can stick to the one used in clinical trials of less than three bowel movements per week. Another important thing to keep in mind is that chronic constipation and IBS with constipation often overlap.

CAUSES AND PATHOPHYSIOLOGY

Majority of the cases of chronic constipation are primary or idiopathic. However, it is necessary to know that a few may be secondary to several medications or diseases.

SUGGESTED READINGS

1 Basilico G, Colleta MC. Chronic constipation: A critical review. Dig Liver Dis. 2013:45:886-93.

2 Milosavljevic T, Popovic DD, Mijac DD, Milovanovic T, Krstic S, Krstic MN. Chronic Constipation: Gastroenterologist's Approach: Dig Dis. 2022;40:175-80.

3 McQuaid KR. Gastrointestinal disorders. In: Papadakis MA, McPhee SJ, Rabow MW (Eds). Current Medical Diagnosis and Treatment, 62nd edition. India: Mc Graw Hill Education (India) Pvt Ltd; 2023. pp. 585-8.

87

CHAPTER

Management of Refractory Gastroesophageal Reflux Disease

BD Goswami, Preeti Sarma

ABSTRACT

Patients who do not respond to 8 weeks of double-dose proton-pump inhibitor (PPI) (symptoms present at least 3 times per week) with objective evidence of gastroesophageal reflux disease (GERD) are called refractory GERD. The cause may be multifactorial such as poor drug compliance, polymorphism of CYP2C19 group enzymes, persistent weakly acid reflux or weakly alkaline reflux, and bile reflux. The 24-hour impedance pH monitoring is the gold standard for the diagnosis of GERD. In patients with alarm feature, upper gastrointestinal (GI) endoscopy is to be done early. Otherwise, pharmacotherapy is to be started with a PPI along with avoidance of trigger factors, lifestyle changes, and elevation of the head end of the bed. Optimization of PPI treatment along with counseling of the patient is the key to correct approach.

INTRODUCTION

Gastroesophageal reflux disease (GERD) is defined as reflux of gastric contents into the esophagus leading to significant symptoms/complications. Some amount of reflux is physiological, but to be considered a disease, the symptoms need to be significant and complications may be associated. Sour regurgitations and heartburn are the cardinal symptoms for diagnosis (at least once a week for at least 1 month).

In majority of situations, GERD is diagnosed by history and clinical examination alone with a sensitivity of 67% and specificity of 70%. Many a times, functional dyspepsia symptoms (post prandial fullness, early satiety, epigastric pain, and epigastric burning) may overlap with GERD and that is why it is important to identify such cases early. Patients with difficult-to-treat asthma, chronic cough, noncardiac chest pain (recurrent episodes of retrosternal chest pain in the absence of cardiac abnormalities), and sleep disturbances must be evaluated for GERD. Notably, *Helicobacter pylori* has a negative association with GERD.

As this chapter will specifically deal with *refractory GERD* and its management, we shall proceed for the same.

REFRACTORY GASTROESOPHAGEAL REFLUX DISEASE

Patients not responding to 8 weeks of double-dose PPI (symptoms present at least 3 times per week) with objective evidence of GERD are categorized as refractory GERD. Multiple studies have demonstrated that 10–40% patients do not respond to standard proton-pump inhibitor (PPI) dosage.

Possible causes of refractory GERD:

- *Poor compliance*: Not taking PPI in correct dose or wrong timing
- *PPI metabolism*: PPIs are metabolized by the liver enzyme complex cytochrome P450 (CYP2C19, CYP3A4) and in the population there may be *rapid metabolizers, intermediate metabolizers, and slow metabolizers*. Studies are still ongoing regarding the role of polymorphisms in this group of liver enzymes and resultant non response or slow response to certain PPIs.
- *Difference in PPIs?* There are no studies to demonstrate that one particular PPI is superior to the other, but sometimes, in clinical practice, we have all noted that

switching PPI from one variant to another does make some difference in particular patients. Recent studies have asserted the superiority of Esomeprazole 40 mg over the other PPIs for treatment of esophagitis.

- *Persistent weakly acidic reflux (WAR-pH between 4 and 7) or weakly alkaline reflux (WalkR-pH >7)*: There may be distension of the esophagus due to reflux volume and also presence of esophageal hypersensitivity that causes symptoms. Especially, if there is WAR, pepsin may migrate into the esophagus and cause some proteolytic activity. Also, mucosal healing may be affected.
- *Bile reflux*: Seen in some cases, especially after gastrectomy. Bilirubin and bile can cause damage to the esophageal mucosa.

PATHOGENESIS

- *Weak antireflux barrier*: The normal *antireflux barrier* is made up of the lower esophageal sphincter (LES) attached to the crural diaphragm via the esophageal ligament. Due to various factors such as presence of hiatus hernia and transient relaxation of the LES that cause weakening of the antireflux barrier, there may be increase in the volume of reflux and also increase in the exposure time thereby causing disturbing symptoms to the patient.
- *Delayed esophageal clearance*: Lower basal esophageal clearance, especially noted in refractory GERD, may cause delayed clearance of acid and bolus thereby causing symptoms. It may also be associated with alterations in secretions from salivary glands, esophageal glands, and peristaltic dysfunction of the esophagus .
- *Delayed gastric emptying*: Although not very conclusive, it has been hypothesized that delayed gastric emptying may cause gastric distension and increased number of transient relaxation of LES events thereby leading to refractory GERD.
- *Esophageal hypersensitivity and hypervigilance*: There is increased perception of certain stimuli such as temperature, acid, mechanical distension, and electric stimulation in some persons due to central and peripheral sensitization. Stress can cause increased intestinal epithelial permeability leading to visceral hyperalgesia. Keefer et al. introduced the concept of esophageal hypervigilance—cognitive affective process that results from overawareness of the discomfort, as a possible pathogenesis of refractory GERD.

MANAGEMENT

- If the patient presents with alarming symptoms–such as dysphagia, odynophagia, gastrointestinal (GI) bleed, weight loss, anemia and new onset of symptoms beyond 55 years of age, then we have to send the patient for upper GI endoscopy immediately.
- In the absence of alarm features, the triggers for the symptoms of GERD, if identifiable, need to be avoided at all costs. There are no generalized recommendations for diet in GERD, but avoidance of certain food items such as carbonated beverages, chocolate, mint, fatty food, spicy food, and citrus fruits may be of some benefit to patients.
- It is very important to make some lifestyle changes. Several studies have shown a decline in GERD symptoms following reduction in body mass index (BMI) and maintenance of an active lifestyle. Infact, dietary advice to reduce weight may be given and dietary fibers such as Psyllium 15 g/day can be added to increase LES resting pressure along with meals based on vegetable proteins. Smoking is to be absolutely avoided.
- It is important to advice patients with nocturnal symptoms to elevate the head end of the bed as it decreases the reflux of gastric contents into the esophagus. They should be advised to go for early dinner and not to lie down within 2 hours of a meal.
- The pharmacotherapy of GERD starts with a PPI. The PPI challenge test is both useful for diagnosis and treatment. For sustained acid suppression, PPIs need to be administered daily 30-60 minutes before meal. Especially in refractory GERD, it is pertinent on the part of the physician to talk to the patient whether he/she is taking the medicine correctly and to counsel them about the correct usage. PPIs are more effective than histamine type-2 receptor (H2R) antagonists in relieving the symptoms of GERD and also support the healing of erosive disease.

Despite all these measures, when refractory GERD is suspected, we need to go for the following:

- These type of patients should be sent for detailed evaluation including a detailed check of associated comorbidities (need to look for obesity, cardiological abnormality, respiratory illness, psychiatric disorders, and gut-brain axis issues) and whether the patient is on concomitant medication that may cause symptoms of GERD.
- An upper GI endoscopy is essential to differentiate whether, it is a case of erosive disease or nonerosive reflux disease (NERD).

- In case *erosive disease* is found, these patients will need prolonged use of PPI for healing and symptom control and also for maintenance therapy to prevent relapse. Some studies have also suggested that increasing the duration of PPI therapy to 12–16 weeks may have an incremental effect on healing. Remission at 1-year time period was found to be higher with PPI in comparison to H2R antagonists. In case of erosive disease and nocturnal acid breakthrough, dexlansoprazole has been studied that can be administered, irrespective of time of day or food intake.
- On the other hand, in case NERD is suspected, it is important to send the patient for 24-hour pH-metry to find out whether the symptoms are truly due to GERD or not. Patients with GERD symptoms but without erosions on endoscopy are categorized as NERD. For long-term maintenance, these patients benefit from on-demand PPI therapy but not intermittent therapy.
- The 24-hour multichannel intraluminal impedance pH monitoring is a very important aid in diagnosing cases with refractory GERD. This test is carried out after stopping all types of acid-suppressing medication for at least 7 days. The 24-hour multichannel intraluminal impedance pH monitoring when carried out in patients who are already taking PPI is usually done in a situation wherein the patient is already a known case of GERD and we need to know the cause of treatment failure. The 24-hour impedance pH monitoring is the gold standard for the diagnosis of GERD. It can detect both anterograde and retrograde refluxate and can also do chemical characterization of the refluxate. Ambulatory pH monitoring involves inserting a probe 5 cm above the LES and then recording the pH exposure data for 24 hours. A fall in pH to <4 is considered to be an acid reflux. We can find the esophageal acid exposure time (AET), both acid and nonacid reflux events. The symptom index (SI) and the symptom association probability (SAP) help to differentiate reflux from functional heartburn.
- Another concern in refractory GERD is polymorphisms of CYP2C19 that may cause nonresponsiveness to PPI. Hence, physicians may opt to switch from CYP2C19-dependent PPI (omeprazole and lansoprazole) to CYP2C19-independent PPI (rabeprazole and esomeprazole).
- In those cases where GERD has been excluded (negative endoscopy findings and normal pH-metry), it is important to rule out non acid reflux, eosinophilic esophagitis, esophageal dysmotility, functional heartburn, and functional chest pain. For this, multiple other tests such as upper GI endoscopy with or without biopsy, high-resolution esophageal manometry, scintigraphy, or breath test to look for gastric emptying may be required.
- GERD is the most common cause of noncardiac chest pain. Hence, such patients, after ruling out cardiac issues may be given once or twice daily PPI according to symptom response.
- In patients presenting with disturbing nocturnal symptoms, the PPI therapy has to be optimized by adding an evening dose of PPI as per necessity. There might still be a group of patients who present with nocturnal acid breakthrough (gastric pH <4 for more than one continuous hour at night despite being on PPI) who might need an additional bedtime H2R antagonist dose over and above the twice daily PPI. Histamine is an important factor for nighttime acid secretion and hence H2R antagonist work better in such cases. Titration should be started after 2–3 months to bring down the dose of PPI to the lowest possible dose, so as to avoid unnecessary adverse effects.
- Prokinetics do not have much role in management of GERD. They may be added to PPI regimens only in cases that have delayed gastric emptying and overlapping functional dyspepsia.
- Baclofen may be tried in some cases of refractory GERD. It is a gamma-aminobutyric acid type B (GABA-B) agonist that can relieve GERD symptoms by decreasing the transient LES relaxations. It decreases both the number and length of reflux episodes; however, its use is limited by the central nervous system and abdominal side effects.
- In those patients who experience recurrence, the lowest possible dose of PPI or H2R antagonist should be given for maintenance.
- Mucosal protective agents, alginates, and sucralfate may be added as adjunctive therapy in selected group of patients. Alginates form a viscous gel that forms a physical barrier to the acid pocket. Sucralfate acts as a mucosal protective agent and also stimulates mucosal growth factors.
- After a patient experiences relief of symptoms on PPI, the complete course should be done and the patient needs to be counseled for maintaining positive lifestyle changes (weight loss, stopping smoking, and tobacco use), avoiding triggers and also the risks of using unnecessary long term PPIs. It is of utmost importance to counsel the patient regarding compliance, proper dosing, and administration of the PPI as well as explain its side effects on prolonged use.
- Physicians need to periodically reassess the need of PPI in those cases who are on long-term maintenance therapy.
- *Potassium competitive acid blockers (PCABs) Vonoprazan, and Tegoprazan*: These drugs bind reversibly to the potassium ions and block the work of the H^+K^+ATPase thereby reducing acid production. However, because of their hepatic toxicities, these

drugs are still under trial and have not been widely used.

- *IW-3718*: This is a novel bile acid sequestrant that binds with the bile present in the refluxate. When used as an adjunct to PPIs, this drug reduced heartburn and regurgitation in study models. But it failed to demonstrate statistically significant effects.
- Patients who are suspected to be suffering from esophageal hypersensitivity and hypervigilance may benefit from use of *selective serotonin reuptake inhibitors* and *serotonin norepinephrine reuptake inhibitors*.
- Some cases of refractory GERD who have associated functional issues may benefit from cognitive behavioral therapy involving diaphragmatic breathing, esophageal directed hypnotherapy, and biofeedback therapy

Need for Surgery

Indications:

- Proven GERD not responding to medical therapy
- Patients having volume reflux
- Large hiatus hernia
- Patients with complications such as Barrett's and peptic stricture
- Some cases of extraesophageal complications

Multiple studies have demonstrated that long-term remission is more in medication group while regurgitation symptoms are considerably reduced in the surgical group. Types of surgery may be—Nissen fundoplication (complete 360° wrap), Dor procedure (anterior 180° wrap), Toupet (posterior 270° wrap), magnetic sphincter augmentation, radiofrequency therapy, and ultrasonic surgical endostapler procedure.

Endoscopic antireflux therapies can be offered to patients with refractory GERD. They are minimally invasive but treatment response varies from 16 to 82%, which is rather unpredictable. However, in those patients in whom these procedures actually work, it has been seen that there is considerable improvement in the quality of life with marked reduction of GERD symptoms. Endotherapy candidates need to be carefully selected—patients with mild esophagitis, small hiatus hernia, and absence of Barrett's.

In all cases, who are put up for surgery, it is pertinent to confirm the diagnosis of GERD and rule out other causes that may create similar symptoms.

SUGGESTED READINGS

1. Bhatia S, Pareek KK, Kumar A, Upadhyay R, Tiwaskar M, Jain A, et al. API-ISG Consensus Guidelines for management of gastroesophageal reflux disease. J Assoc Physicians India. 2020;68(10):69-80.
2. Yadlapati R, Gyawali CP, Pandolfino JE; CGIT GERD Consensus Conference Participants. AGA Clinical Practice Update on the personalized approach to the evaluation and management of GERD: Expert Review. Clin Gastroenterol Hepatol. 2022;20(5):984-94.e1.
3. Rettura F, Bronzini F, Campigotto M, Lambiase C, Pancetti A, Berti G, et al. Refractory gastroesophageal reflux disease: A management update. Front Med (Lausanne). 2021;8:765061.

88

CHAPTER

Approach to Chronic Pancreatitis

Hardik Rughwani, D Nageshwar Reddy

ABSTRACT

Chronic pancreatitis (CP) is a progressive fibroinflammatory disease. It is mainly idiopathic in India. Pancreatic stellate cell activation and progressive fibrosis are pathological hallmarks. Majority of patients (90%) present with recurrent abdominal pain. The other major features are malnutrition due to pancreatic exocrine insufficiency (PEI) and diabetes mellitus (type 3c) due to beta cell dysfunction.

The mechanism of pain in CP is due to multiple different but overlapping mechanisms like pancreatic neuropathy, neuroplasticity, and nociception. PEI results from progressive loss of pancreatic parenchyma. Type 3c diabetes mellitus results from beta cell dysfunction in the early stage and structural destruction because of inflammation and fibrosis in the later stage.

The initial evaluation should include a detailed history of pain, nutritional evaluation, and assessment of glycemic control. Cross-sectional imaging to evaluate the location of calculi, ductal morphology, presence of mass, and parenchymal volume assessment is important to plan optimal treatment modality. Long-term medical management includes methionine-based antioxidant drugs and neuromodulators. Ductal interventions for calculi include extracorporeal shock wave lithotripsy (ESWL), endoscopic retrograde cholangiopancreatography (ERCP) and pancreatic duct (PD) stenting, and surgical drainage procedures.

INTRODUCTION

Chronic pancreatitis (CP) is challenging for the treating physician and the patient. It is a progressive fibroinflammatory disease manifesting pancreas-specific symptoms and some extrapancreatic involvement of cardiovascular, neurologic, and musculoskeletal systems. Malnutrition and diabetes are frequently manifested. The disease demographics of CP in India are different from those in the west. About 70% of CP in India is idiopathic compared to alcohol is the most common etiology in the west. Diabetes appears early in the disease course in Indian CP patients, compared to west ones. Also, the time lag between the onset of CP and diabetes in Indian patients is relatively shorter compared to that in the west.

The natural history consists of recurrent inflammation with clinical or subclinical episodes of acute pancreatitis, progressive fibrosis, and eventual development of morphological changes. The disease sets in much earlier than the appearance of features such as pancreatic atrophy, calcifications, strictures, and masses.

MANIFESTATIONS

The most common symptom of CP is recurrent, debilitating, intractable abdominal pain. It is proposed that the pain of CP has four different patterns which are: (1) pain attacks without pain between them, (2) pain attacks with pain between them, (3) persistent pain with pain attacks, and (4) persistent pain with slight fluctuation. These patterns of pain could change from one to the other during the natural progression of CP. The other important manifestations of CP are pancreatic exocrine insufficiency (PEI) and type 3c diabetes mellitus. Other manifestations include musculoskeletal problems such as osteopenia/osteoporosis and cardiovascular ailments.

MECHANISMS AND TREATMENT TARGETS

Pain in CP is multifactorial and mainly results from broadly three mechanisms namely nociception, neuropathy, and neuroplasticity, resulting in genesis of pain. PEI is a progressive deterioration of pancreatic exocrine function. Overt steatorrhea and signs of malnutrition appear once the pancreatic exocrine function comes down by 80–90%. Main reasons for PEI are either due to loss of pancreatic parenchyma or obstruction of pancreatic duct (PD) due to calculi or both. In the early stages of the disease, glycemic abnormalities result from insulin secretory defect. Later on in advanced CP development of type 3c diabetes mellitus is ascribed to islet cell apoptosis resulting from pancreatic inflammation and fibrosis.

ASSESSMENT OF A PATIENT WITH CHRONIC PANCREATITIS

Assessment of a patient with CP should not be restricted to only evaluation of the morphologic aspects of the disease. They should undergo and holistic evaluation including detailed history, nutritional workup, endocrine dysfunction evaluation, and mental health assessment. **Boxes 1 to 3** show the assessments of different manifestations of CP.

TREATMENT OF PAIN

Identification of the predominant pain mechanism of CP at a given point in time is important.

Short-term Pain Management

Acute exacerbations of CP should be treated as any other acute pancreatitis episode. Short-term pain relief can be achieved following the World Health Organization (WHO) pain ladder. Based on this, an on-demand administration of nonsteroidal anti-inflammatory drugs (NSAIDs) can be initiated as the first line. However, a substantial proportion of patients with CP usually will not respond satisfactorily to NSAIDs and needs to be treated with an opiate-based analgesic. In NSAID nonresponsive pain, escalation should be done to low-potency narcotic agents such as tramadol

BOX 1: Pain assessment in patients with chronic pancreatitis.

History:
- Pain character, origin and radiation, trigger, change in character, involvement of new areas

(Semi) quantitative/subjective evaluation:
- Visual analog scale (VAS)
- Pain detect tool

Objective evaluation for neural sensitization:
- Pinprick testing for temporal summation
- Pressure algometer-based testing for pain detection and tolerance threshold (PDT and PTT)
- Cold pressor test
- Conditional pain modulation (CPM)

BOX 2: Evaluation of nutritional status of patients with chronic pancreatitis.

History:
- Dietary history including 24 hours recall
- Objective measurement of calorie, protein, carbohydrate and fat intake
- History of adherence to PERT

Physical examination:
- Anthropometry
- Dynamic hand grip strength
- Measurement of percent of weight loss
- Examination of signs of vitamin and micronutrient deficiency

Laboratory evaluations:
- Biochemical markers for PEI and protein malnutrition-related nutrient deficiencies (vitamin D, vitamin B12, prealbumin, transferrin) (repeat at least once in a year)
- Fecal elastase assay

Imaging:
- CECT abdomen for sarcopenia
- DEXA scan for osteopenia/osteoporosis (repeat at least 2 yearly for those who develop osteopenia)

(CECT: contrast-enhanced computed tomography; DEXA: dual-energy X-ray absorptiometry; PEI: pancreatic exocrine insufficiency; PERT: pancreatic enzyme replacement therapy)

BOX 3: Evaluation of diabetes in patients with chronic pancreatitis.

For diagnosis and assessment of glycemic control:
- Fasting and 2 hours postprandial blood glucose
- Glycosylated hemoglobin (HbA1c)

For evaluation of beta cell reserve:
- Fasting and 2 hours postprandial plasma C-peptide

To differentiate type 3c from other types of diabetes (in case of ambiguity):
- Pancreatic polypeptide response to mixed meal (under research)

To evaluate hepatic insulin resistance:
- Pancreatic polypeptide response to mixed meals (under research)

hydrochloride and tapentadol. Tramadol hydrochloride is a low-potency selective μ-opiate receptor agonist, which has been shown to have comparable efficacy as higher potency narcotics but with a significantly better safety profile. Tapentadol is another recently available safer option. Occasionally, the other option that can be resorted to is transdermal fentanyl or epidural buprenorphine. Looking at the side effect profile of the above medications, specially NSAIDs, these agents should be used for a short duration under strict monitoring.

Long-term Pain Management

For long-term pain management in CP, it is essential to target the pathophysiological mechanisms such as oxidative stress, nociception, and neuropathic changes.

Antioxidants

Even though several studies have tested antioxidants, single and in combination, for treating pain in CP, the most useful have been with the use of a cocktail of methionine, organic selenium, alpha-tocopherol, ascorbic acid, and beta-carotene. The rationale for using methionine and vitamin C in the antioxidant cocktail is to provide methyl and thiol moieties for the deranged transsulfuration pathway in the acinar cells. It is, however, important to select the appropriate kind of patients to achieve the maximum benefit of antioxidant therapy. Observations from studies have shown us that a methionine-containing antioxidant cocktail will benefit the majority of Indian patients with CP since these are young individuals, approximately 70% are idiopathic, and long-term high-potency narcotics are still not routinely used for CP in this country.

It has been suggested that the daily dose of methionine should be at least 2 g for optimal efficacy. There has not yet been a consensus on the duration of therapy. However, from the published studies, this antioxidant cocktail can be used safely for 6 months. After this, the dosage can be reduced or treatment can be stopped based on the patient's response and then restarted if required. Even though the combination is safe in the short term, its long-term efficacy, especially in high doses of methionine and selenium, needs to be evaluated.

Pancreatic Duct-directed Modalities

These modalities are primarily meant to manage the intraductal calculi, PD strictures, or dilated ducts. Currently, the European Society of Gastrointestinal Endoscopy (ESGE) recommends endotherapy as the first line of treatment for painful PD stones. Obstructing PD stones larger than 5 mm and located in the head and body that are associated with pain should be subjected to extracorporeal shock wave lithotripsy (ESWL). This is the most frequently used modality even though other modalities such as electrohydraulic lithotripsy (EHL) and laser lithotripsy are also used in a few centers. The goal of pancreatic lithotripsy is to pulverize the stones to a size smaller than 3 mm which can then be cleared after pancreatic sphincterotomy with or without sphincteroplasty using balloon trawl, mini basket, or saline flush.

A PD stent should be placed if there is partial stone clearance or if there are concomitant PD strictures. PD stents, if placed, can be removed after 3–6 months, or replaced if there is persistence of ductal obstruction with associated pain. The clinical efficacy and safety profile is best when ESWL is done for ductal stones located in the head, neck, and proximal body of the pancreas. ESWL for pancreatic stones should ideally be performed with a dual-focus higher generation lithotripter with 5,000–6,000 shocks with an intensity of 15–16 kV at a rate of 90 shocks per minute. While either general or epidural anesthesia can be used, in our experience epidural anesthesia provides better results. Efficacy-wise, it was demonstrated in a recent meta-analysis of 22 studies ($n = 3,868$, included 636 Indian patients) that there was complete stone fragmentation in 86.3% [95% confidence interval (CI) 76.0–94.0] patients, complete duct clearance in 69.8% (95% CI 63.8–75.5), and complete absence of pain during follow-up in 64.2% (95% CI 57.5–70.6). 4.0% (95% CI 2.5–5.8) of patients developed postprocedural acute pancreatitis. Other minor side effects as reported in a recent series of over 5,000 patients include mild pain at the site of contact of the cushion of the lithotripter in 13.5% and ecchymosis in 19% of patients.

Even though endoscopic therapy is the recommended first line of treatment for painful obstructive PD stones, if the patient has large stones all along the duct, or if there are associated multiple strictures in the PD, or local complications such as gastric outlet/duodenal obstruction, pancreatic head mass with or without distal biliary obstruction, surgical modalities should be resorted to as the first choice. The most common surgical options in these situations are lateral pancreaticojejunostomy (LPJ), Frey's operation, and Whipple's pancreaticoduodenectomy, based on the disease morphology.

Nerve-directed Modalities

So far, the only drug that has been tested for pancreatic neuropathic pain in randomized controlled trials (RCTs) is pregabalin. This drug is a pharmacologically active S-enantiomer of a racemic 3-isobutyl gamma-aminobutyric acid (GABA) analog that acts supraspinally by binding to the alpha2-delta subunit of voltage-gated calcium channels, thereby reducing the synaptic transmission of several neurotransmitters. It activates the descending inhibitory noradrenergic pathways that inhibit central sensitization, thereby alleviating neuropathic pain. It was demonstrated in an RCT that there was a 12% reduction in the pain score over a period of 3 weeks with a starting dose of 150 mg/day of pregabalin that was progressively escalated to 600 mg.

Modalities Directed toward Pain Relapse

A substantial proportion of patients with CP develop pain relapse after initial success with medical and interventional therapies. If no structural changes that could explain pain recurrence are found, treatment should be directed against the mechanistic targets. It was shown in an RCT that an initial combination of methionine-containing antioxidant cocktail with pregabalin (maximum dose of 150 mg twice a day) for 2 months followed by continuation of the antioxidant preparation till the end of 6 months resulted in significant and sustained pain relief.

Potential Newer Approaches

Recent studies have shown a high prevalence of anxiety and depression in patients with CP. This and pain were linked with metabolomic changes in the hippocampus and the basal ganglia. Modalities such as cognitive behavioral therapy (CBT), antianxiety/antidepressants, and spinal cord stimulation could be of potential benefit but require high-quality data before incorporating these into routine treatment.

TREATMENT OF EXOCRINE INSUFFICIENCY AND NUTRITIONAL DEFICIENCIES

The mainstay of treatment of PEI is pancreatic enzyme replacement therapy (PERT). Even though several guidelines exist on PERT, the ideal dose and duration of therapy is still speculative. Patients with CP without evidence of substantial parenchymal loss and measurable nutrient depletion need not be started on PERT. Those with steatorrhea and/or overt malnutrition and/or substantial pancreatic atrophy and/or PD obstruction should be treated with PERT. Use of fecal elastase should be done cautiously in view of its wide range of sensitivity and specificity and limited utility in advanced CP, since other signs of suggestive PEI will be evident from clinical and imaging parameters.

Pancreatic enzyme replacement therapy should be taken ideally along with food and an ideal preparation of PERT should be an enteric-coated micro- or minimicrosphere. The rationale for this is the easy passage of the supplemented enzyme into the duodenum through the pyloric channel along with the food chyme, which would ensure the release of the enzymes in the duodenum and adequate mixing with food. Even though the recommended dose in different guidelines ranges from 25,000 to 50,000 units of lipase with each meal and 24,000–25,000 with snacks, from a practical Indian standpoint, 25,000–40,000 units appear to be optimum. In case the patient has an occasional heavier-than-usual meal, he can increase the dosage of the enzymes according to his meal size. Addition of a proton-pump inhibitor could be helpful for a subgroup of patients since the supplemented pancreatic enzymes get activated at a pH of around 5.5 and there is a significant reduction in ductal bicarbonate in advanced CP (which would reduce the duodenal pH).

Like the dosage of PERT, the duration of PERT is also not clearly defined. This will have implications for Indian patients with CP due to the cost of therapy of PERT. From a practical standpoint, in patients with gross pancreatic atrophy and overt malnutrition, PERT needs to be considered for a very long duration. On the other hand, for instance, for those with a preserved pancreatic volume and ductal obstruction, PERT can be withdrawn after ductal clearance with an expectation that pancreatic secretion would resume optimally after ductal clearance. If the nutritional status of the patient continues to improve even without PERT, then it need not be restarted. Similarly in other situations, the duration of PERT can be customized to the extent of pancreatic morphologic changes, clinical manifestations, and the socioeconomic status of the patients.

In addition to optimal PERT therapy, it is extremely important to advise the patients to have a balanced and inclusive diet. There should not be fat restriction especially when on PERT and a medium-chain triglyceride-based diet need not be mandatorily advised. However, high amounts of dietary fiber should be avoided as it could compromise the action of pancreatic enzymes.

Dietary assessment by a trained dietitian is mandatory. These patients should be fed small-volume, high-protein, and high-energy meals at frequent intervals (5–6 meals/day). Those with severe malnutrition and unable to tolerate orally due to pain, persistent nausea, and vomiting, and delayed gastric emptying should be fed enterally via a nasojejunal tube. The other nondietary factors that contribute to malnutrition should also be concomitantly managed. It is essential to replenish micronutrients (e.g., prealbumin, retinol-binding protein, transferrin, vitamin C, selenium, zinc) in addition to PERT and a normal diet.

TREATMENT OF ENDOCRINE DYSFUNCTION

A detailed description of the management of endocrine dysfunction is out of the scope of this chapter. However, since now it is understood that initially there is beta cell dysfunction rather than beta islet destruction, and is accompanied by hepatic insulin resistance, treatment should be started with metformin provided the baseline glycemic control is not grossly deranged. Once metformin ceases to work optimally, a switchover to insulin or combination can be resorted to. Follow-up and evaluation for complications should be done in a similar manner that is done for type 1 diabetes mellitus and type 2 diabetes mellitus.

The effect of pancreatic interventions on diabetes in CP has been debatable, with some studies reporting an improvement while others showing no change. In a recent 5 years' follow-up study, it was shown that ductal clearance delayed the development of diabetes by nearly 4 years in patients with idiopathic CP with obstructive ductal calculi. However, for those who already developed diabetes before the ductal intervention, there was not much difference in glycemic control post intervention.

Since gut microbial dysbiosis has been associated with diabetes in CP, gut microbial manipulation could be a potential add-on to the armamentarium of therapeutic modalities for CP in the future.

CONCLUSION

Even though studies over the past decade have provided important understanding of CP, we still do not have a curative or durable palliative treatment. The primary pathophysiology of CP is in the pancreatic parenchyma and the ductal changes. Hence, it is essential that more parenchyma-directed therapies be tested with an intent to reduce the inflammation and slow the progression of the disease.

SUGGESTED READINGS

1. Balakrishnan V, Unnikrishnan AG, Thomas V, Choudhuri G, Veeraraju P, Singh SP, et al. Chronic pancreatitis. A prospective nationwide study of 1,086 subjects from India. JOP. 2008;9(5):593-600.
2. Rajesh G, Veena AB, Menon S, Balakrishnan V. Clinical profile of early-onset and late-onset idiopathic chronic pancreatitis in South India. Indian J Gastroenterol. 2014;33:231-6.
3. Talukdar R, Reddy DN. Pain in chronic pancreatitis: managing beyond the pancreatic duct. World J Gastroenterol. 2013;19(38):6319.
4. Duggan SN, Smyth ND, Murphy A, MacNaughton D, OKeefe SJ, Conlon KC. High prevalence of osteoporosis in patients with chronic pancreatitis: a systematic review and meta-analysis. Clin Gastroenterol Hepatol. 2014;12(2):219-28.
5. Talukdar R, Sasikala M, Kumar PP, Rao GV, Pradeep R, Reddy DN. T-helper cell–mediated islet inflammation contributes to β-cell dysfunction in chronic pancreatitis. Pancreas. 2016;45(3):434-42.
6. Talukdar R, Murthy H, Reddy DN. Role of methionine containing antioxidant combination in the management of pain in chronic pancreatitis: a systematic review and meta-analysis. Pancreatology. 2015;15(2):136-44.
7. Bhardwaj P, Garg PK, Maulik SK, Saraya A, Tandon RK, Acharya SK. A randomized controlled trial of antioxidant supplementation for pain relief in patients with chronic pancreatitis. Gastroenterology. 2009;136(1):149-59.e2.
8. Dumonceau JM, Delhaye M, Tringali A, Arvanitakis M, Sanchez-Yague A, Vaysse T, et al. Endoscopic treatment of chronic pancreatitis: European Society of Gastrointestinal Endoscopy (ESGE) guideline–updated August 2018. Endoscopy. 2019;51(2):179-93.
9. van Huijgevoort NCM, Veld JV, Fockens P, Besselink MG, Boermeester MA, Arvanitakis M, et al. Success of extracorporeal shock wave lithotripsy and ERCP in symptomatic pancreatic duct stones: a systematic review and meta-analysis. Endosc Int Open. 2020;8(08):E1070-E1085.
10. Tandan M, Reddy DN, Talukdar R, Vinod K, Kiran S, Santosh D, et al. ESWL for large pancreatic calculi: report of over 5000 patients. Pancreatology. 2019;19(7):916-21.
11. Talukdar R, Lakhtakia S, Reddy DN, Rao GV, Pradeep R, Banerjee R, et al. Ameliorating effect of antioxidants and pregabalin combination in pain recurrence after ductal clearance in chronic pancreatitis: Results of a randomized, double blind, placebo-controlled trial. J Gastroenterol Hepatol. 2016;31(9):1654-62.
12. Talukdar R, Unnisa M. Optimizing nutrition in chronic pancreatitis. Curr Opin Gastroenterol. 2022;38(5):495-500.
13. Singh S, Midha S, Singh N, Joshi YK, Garg PK. Dietary counseling versus dietary supplements for malnutrition in chronic pancreatitis: a randomized controlled trial. Clin Gastroenterol Hepatol. 2008;6(3):353-9.
14. Talukdar R, Reddy DN, Tandan M, Gupta R, Lakhtakia S, Ramchandani M, et al. Impact of ductal interventions on diabetes in patients with chronic pancreatitis. J Gastroenterol Hepatol. 2021;36(5):1226-34.

89

CHAPTER

Metabolic Pancreatitis: What a Physician Should Know?

Piyush Manoria, Abhishek Singhai

ABSTRACT

Acute pancreatitis is a commonly encountered medical emergency with varied etiologies. Alcohol and gallstones are the most common causes of it. Metabolic causes of pancreatitis are underestimated causes of pancreatitis and it includes hypertriglyceridemia, hypercalcemia, diabetes mellitus, porphyria, Wilson disease, and glycogen storage disease. It is important to identify the exact metabolic cause of pancreatitis because over the standard routine management of pancreatitis, specific treatment of the underlying metabolic conditions will reduce the morbidity and mortality.

INTRODUCTION

Acute pancreatitis is a common gastrointestinal disorder that occurs due to inflammation of pancreas. It is a common indication for hospital admission and its severity varies from mild disease requiring only conservative treatment to severe disease with high morbidity and mortality. The most common causes of pancreatitis are gallstones and alcohol accounting for 60–75% of cases. Metabolic causes of pancreatitis constitute less common but important and treatable causes of pancreatitis. It includes hypertriglyceridemia, hypercalcemia, diabetes mellitus (DM), porphyria, Wilson disease, and glycogen storage disease.

HYPERTRIGLYCERIDEMIA-INDUCED PANCREATITIS

Hypertriglyceridemia is a well-established but underestimated cause of acute pancreatitis. It is the third most common cause of acute pancreatitis after gall stones and alcohol and is the most common metabolic cause of pancreatitis and accounts for around 10% of all cases. It typically occurs in persons with preexisting dyslipidemia (Fredrickson type I, IV, and V) with secondary precipitating factors such as uncontrolled diabetes, excessive alcoholism, pregnancy, or use of some medications such as estrogen therapy, tamoxifen, protease inhibitors, isotretinoin and olanzapine. Serum triglyceride level >1,000 mg/dL is an established risk factor in causing acute pancreatitis. Clinical features of hypertriglyceridemia-induced acute pancreatitis is similar that of any other cause of acute pancreatitis but its associated with increase severity and more complications.

Chylomicrons, which are the triglyceride-rich lipoprotein are the key molecules causing pancreatic inflammation. There are two theories explaining the pathophysiology of hypertriglyceridemia-induced acute pancreatitis which is shown in **Flowchart 1**.

Hypertriglyceridemia-induced acute pancreatitis present in a similar fashion as of any other causes of acute pancreatitis. Pancreatic enzymes levels in serum in it are falsely low due to interference of lipemic serum with the calorimetric method assay used. Serial dilution of the serum leads to reduced interference of the lipids in the transmission of light and it leads to detection of real value of pancreatic enzymes. Serum triglyceride levels should be assessed immediately when the patient comes because with fasting state, its level started falling rapidly as its primary source is the food which we take. In fasting state, the supply of chylomicrons from intestinal absorption is stopped and triglyceride level started normalizing in 24–48 hours. Triglyceride level should be > 1,000 mg/dL to be a causative factor in acute pancreatitis. Modest elevation of triglyceride can be an epiphenomenon in alcoholic pancreatitis but it does not causes acute pancreatitis. Lipemic or milky serum **(Fig. 1)** is the most rapid and important clue that pancreatitis is due to hypertriglyceridemia. In any case of suspected hypertriglyceridemia-induced acute pancreatitis, serum of patient should be checked for its milky color.

No fixed treatment guidelines exist for the treatment of hypertriglyceridemia-induced pancreatitis. Initial treatment of it is similar like that of any other etiology and it includes keeping patient nil orally, bowel rest, intravenous fluids, and appropriate analgesia. Though triglyceride and chylomicron level will fall rapidly with fasting state, ways to accelerate their removal has been tried. Various treatment modalities include plasmapheresis, intravenous insulin, intravenous heparin, lipid lowering agents, fish oil, omega-3 fatty acids, and antioxidants **(Table 1)**. In severe pancreatitis, plasmapheresis can be used for quickly removing the triglyceride and chylomicrons from the serum, though this procedure is costly and has limited availability. Also there is scarce evidence that it will reduce the severity or improve the outcomes in terms of morbidity and mortality in these patients. Lipid lowering agent fibrates such as fenofibrate, which binds the peroxisome proliferator-activated receptor-alpha (PPAR-α) are the drug of choice for lowering triglyceride. Niacin is the second-line agent which can be used to lower triglyceride level. Its side effects such as flushing, hyperuricemia, and increase of hepatic transaminases precludes its use. Recently a new drug, saroglitazar, which is a dual agonist of PPAR-α/γ, has been used to treat hypertriglyceridemia in diabetic patients. Lowering the triglyceride level to < 500 mg/dL can prevent further attacks of acute pancreatitis. At the time of discharge patient should be advised for strict alcohol abstinence, strict control of diabetes, weight reduction, dietary restriction of fat, and discontinuation of any drug causing hypertriglyceridemia.

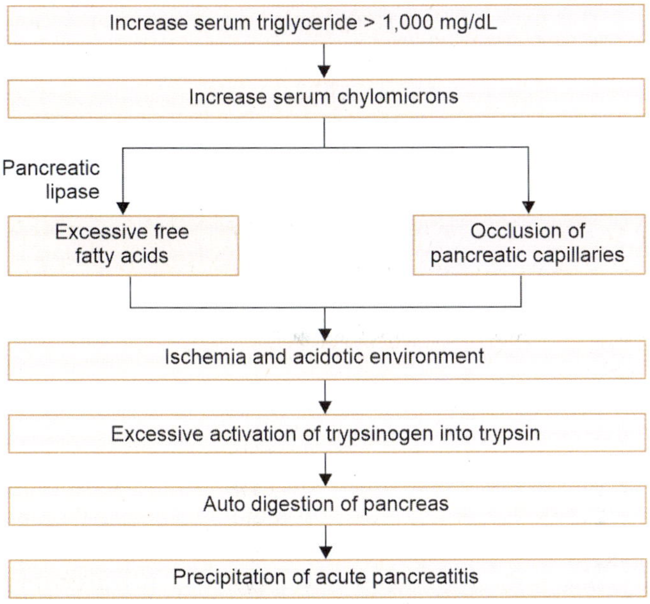

FLOWCHART 1: Pathogenesis of hypertriglyceridemia-induced pancreatitis.

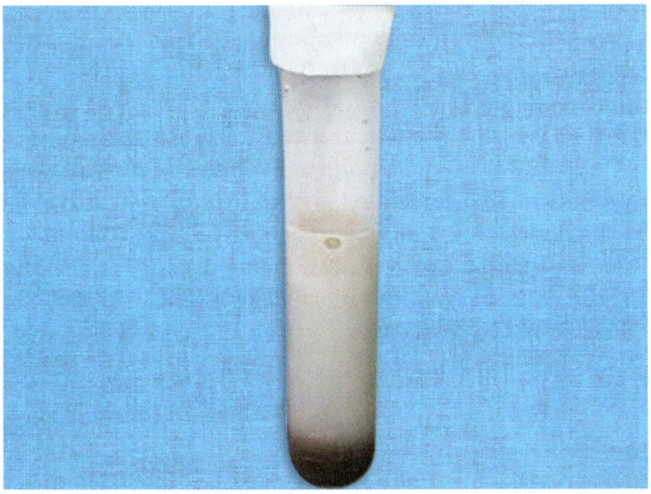

FIG. 1: Milky serum in hypertriglyceridemia-induced pancreatitis.

HYPERCALCEMIA

Acute pancreatitis can result from hypercalcemia. Hypercalcemia is caused by hyperparathyroidism, paraneoplastic syndrome, multiple myeloma, vitamin D toxicity, sarcoidosis, familial hypocalciuric hypercalcemia, and total parenteral nutrition.

Prevalence of pancreatitis in primary hyperparathyroidism (PHPT) ranges from 1.5 to 13%. This association's description dates back to 1940. Smith and Cooke suspected pancreatitis in a patient of hyperparathyroidism who died suddenly. The focus of later reports has been on patients who have surgery for hyperparathyroidism developing pancreatitis. Four individuals in Muthukrushnan et al.'s series of 51 cases of PHPT exhibited pancreatic calcification with a prior medical history suggestive of acute pancreatitis.

According to one center in North India, in 6.8% of PHPT patients, clinical deterioration was suspected due to unexplained pancreatic disease. According to data from a different South Indian series, pancreatic illness affected 12% of PHPT patients. Males predominated in the distribution of sexes, with a male:female ratio of about 2:1. In contrast, the PHPT without concomitant pancreatic illness has a female preponderance. The

TABLE 1: Specific treatment modalities in hypertriglyceridemia-induced pancreatitis.

Modality	Mechanism of action	Dose	Limitations/ADR
Plasmapheresis	Removal of TG and chylomicrons in plasma	-	• Costly • Limited availability • Transfusion reactions
Intravenous insulin	Activates LPL enzymes	0.1–0.4 unit/kg/hours with dextrose infusion*	Hypoglycemia
Intravenous UF heparin	Release of LPL enzyme from endothelial cells	18 unit/kg 4–6 hourly*	• Transient effect • Bleeding tendency
Fibrates	PPAR-α agonist: Increase LPL synthesis and decrease hepatic TG synthesis	Fenofibrate 100–300 mg/day	• Myalgia • Elevated hepatic transaminases • Rarely rhabdomyolysis and cholelithiasis
Niacin	Reduce hepatic secretion of TG	3–6 g/day	• Flushing • Hyperuricemia • Elevated hepatic transaminases • Pruritis • Glucose intolerance
Saroglitazar	Dual PPAR-α/γ agonist	4 mg OD	• Used only in diabetic hypertriglyceridemia • Dyspepsia • Pyrexia • Asthenia
Fish oil supplement	Decrease in concentration of TG rich lipoprotein	3–4 g/day	• Weight gain • Bleeding tendency

*No fixed protocol exist.

(ADR: adverse drug reaction; LPL: lipoprotein lipase; PPAR: peroxisome proliferator-activated receptor; TG: triglyceride; UF: unfractionated)

history of recurring upper abdomen pain was the most typical sign of pancreatic illness with PHPT.

The four key categories in which pancreatic disease is presented in PHPT are acute pancreatitis, acute recurrent pancreatitis without signs of chronic pancreatitis, chronic pancreatitis with or without pancreatic calcification, acute pancreatitis complicating PHPT in the postoperative period.

Hypercalcemia causes pancreatitis through a variety of mechanisms. Hypercalcemia leads to de novo activation of trypsinogen to trypsin, causing injury to acinar cells, pancreatic autodigestion, and pancreatitis. Other additional risk factors such as alcoholism, ductal hypertension, ischemia, hyperlipidemia, and viral infections may worsen pancreatitis by elevating intracytoplasmic calcium levels.

Cellular injury brought on by hypercalcemia has many harmful effects. The entire zymogen activation cascade is started by intracellular trypsin; subsequent steps include the fusion of the lysosomal and zymogen granule compartments and the extrusion of secretory vesicles through the basolateral membrane into the interstitium, where molecular fragments serve as chemoattractants for inflammatory cells.

The issue is then made worse by activated neutrophils producing superoxide or proteolytic enzymes. Finally, macrophages release cytokines including interleukin-6, interleukin-8, and platelet-activating factor, which further drive local (and, in extreme circumstances, systemic) inflammatory responses. These mediators of inflammation enhance the permeability of the pancreatic arteries, resulting in hemorrhage, edema, and ultimately pancreatic necrosis. Recurrent acute pancreatitis can develop into chronic pancreatitis.

According to a study from South India, preclinical and subclinical illnesses may become apparent in people who are sensitive to tropical chronic pancreatitis, a type of chronic calcific nonalcoholic pancreatitis. This is because hypercalcemia is linked to PHPT in these patients.

Pancreatic calculi are formed by hypercalcemia, which may also cause protein plug development by altering pancreatic output. Subsequent bouts of acute or chronic pancreatitis may arise from the resulting ductal blockage.

Genetic risk factors may also play some role in acute pancreatitis due to hypercalcemia. To treat the pancreatitis brought on by hypercalcemia, the underlying cause of hypercalcemia must be treated, and the proper surgical procedures must be performed if required.

DIABETES MELLITUS

Pancreatic involvement can occur in DM of both types 1 and 2 (T1DM and T2DM). The most frequent contributing factors to inflammation and damage are the acute hyperglycemic states of diabetic ketoacidosis and hyperglycemic hyperosmolar coma. Pancreatic damage is also attributed to the associated acidosis, dehydration, and temporary hypertriglyceridemia in DM. Damage and dysfunction of the exocrine system can result from persistently elevated glucagon and somatostatin levels in diabetic patients.

Pancreatic exocrine tissue damage can also occur by immune system in T1DM. In a study by Taniguchi T et al., 77% of individuals with T1DM had antibodies against carbonic anhydrase or lactoferrin which are directed against exocrine glands.

Diabetic autonomic neuropathy, which causes abnormal pancreatic secretion and ensuing insufficiency of the pancreatic exocrine pancreas may also be a contributing factor to pancreatitis. An autonomic neuropathy may impair 50% of the exocrine pancreatic response to a meal by interfering with the enteropancreatic reflexes.

PORPHYRIA

Pancreatic involvement can occasionally be seen in cases of porphyria, notably acute intermittent porphyria and erythropoietic protoporphyria. The described pancreatic conditions linked to porphyria include transient macroamylasemia, acute pancreatitis, chronic pancreatitis, and chronic pancreatitis with cystadenocarcinoma. Pancreatitis may also occur due to spastic contraction of the sphincter of Oddi caused by autonomic neuropathy in porphyria. The etiology of pancreatitis is aggressively influenced by fasting and calorie restriction.

WILSON DISEASE

Copper accumulates intracytoplasmically as a result of inflammatory diseases like Wilson disease. These metals are hazardous to different parts of the cell and excessive concentrations cause membrane disintegration, increased permeability, and lysosomal degeneration. The pancreatic proteolytic enzymes are activated by these alterations, which results in autodigestion and inflammation.

GLYCOGEN STORAGE DISORDER

Acute pancreatitis, hemorrhagic pancreatitis, chronic pancreatitis, and pancreatic pseudocyst formation can all be caused by glycogen storage abnormalities, most specifically type 1 (Von Gierke disease). Excessive glycogen buildup that causes pancreatic duct blockage and the ensuing hypertriglyceridemia are thought to be responsible for pancreatitis' etiology.

CONCLUSION

Metabolic factors constitute a significant proportion of the causes of pancreatitis, after alcohol and gallstones. They cause recurring episodes of pancreatitis and its related comorbidities if they are not treated appropriately. Early detection and effective treatment lead to recovery and the avoidance of adverse effects.

SUGGESTED READINGS

1. Valdivieslo P, Ramirez-Brueno A, Ewald N. Current knowledge of hypertriglyceridemic pancreatitis. Eur J Intern Med. 2014;25: 689-94.
2. Yadav D, Pitchumoni CS. Issues in Hyperlipidemic pancreatitis. J Clin Gastroenterol. 2003;36:54-62.
3. Uysal E, Acar YA, Gokmen E, Kutur A. Hypertriglyceridemia induced pancreatitis (Chylomicronemia syndrome) treated with supportive care. Case Rep Crit Care. 2014;2014:767831.
4. Kota SK, Kota SK, Jammula S, Krishna SVS, Modi KD. Hypertriglyceridemia-induced recurrent acute pancreatitis: A case-based review. Indian J Endocrinol Metab. 2012;16:141-3.
5. Jacob JJ, John M, Thomas N, Chacko A, Cherian R, Selvan B, et al. Does hyperparathyroidism cause pancreatitis? A South Indian experience and a review of published work. ANZ J Surg. 2006;76:740-4.
6. Smith FB, Cooke RT. Acute fatal hyperparathyroidism. Lancet. 1940;2:650-1.
7. Agarwal A, George RK, Gupta SK, Mishra SK. Pancreatitis in patients with primary hyperparathyroidism. Indian J Gastroenterol. 2003;22:224-5.
8. El Newihi H, Dooley CP, Saad C, Staples J, Zeidler A, Valenzuela JE. Impaired exocrine pancreatic function in diabetics with diarrhea and peripheral neuropathy. Dig Dis Sci. 1988;33:705-10.
9. Kikuchi M, Hasegawa K, Handa I, Watabe M, Narisawa K, Tada K. Chronic pancreatitis in a child with glycogen storage disease type 1. Eur J Pediatr. 1991;150:852-3.

90

CHAPTER

Artificial Intelligence in Gastroenterology

TS Chandrasekar, MS Prasad

ABSTRACT

Once a buzzword, "artificial intelligence (AI)" has gradually attained a mainstream application status to rapidly evolve and usher in organizational change and digital transformation in every conceivable field including healthcare. With its analytical capabilities, AI in gastroenterology has a great deal of potential to transform diagnostic endoscopy and enable precise diagnosis. AI can be trained to detect even the most minute mucosal changes in precancerous lesions, with an accuracy and sensitivity of 92%, matching or even outperforming a skilled gastroenterologist. AI-assisted improved adenoma detection rate is a boon to the screening colonoscopy for colorectal cancer (CRC) detection. AI with computer-aided detection (CADe) system merged with optical biopsy may altogether eliminate the need for biopsy in future, saving on the costs of screening. In the surveillance of patients with inflammatory bowel disease (IBD), AI can play a role in the objective assessment of mucosal healing, the sole objective of the clinician for deciding treatment strategy. Although AI is still in its infancy, it has great potential to develop and break many barriers clinicians currently face in managing patients. However, AI cannot substitute human clinical reasoning.

INTRODUCTION

The progress of medical practice happened in phases. Tumultuous developments in medical sciences occurred from the mid-19th century through the 20th century following epoch-making discoveries and inventions in physical sciences. With the thrust provided by the latter, the progress of medicine occurred in four stages. The development of antisepsis by Joseph Lister (1867), which swiftly led to the development of asepsis, the introduction of anesthesia by Morton, and the discovery of microorganisms, all set the foundation for the future of surgery. The discovery of X-rays (Roentgen 1895) put into motion the second stage, and the dawn of the antibiotic era with the introduction of penicillin (Fleming 1940s) gave the third spurt. The breakthroughs in optoelectronics in the 1980s that brought forth contemporary endoscopic and laparoscopic surgery that rocked the world gave the fourth surge. We have now entered the fifth stage of evolution, known as the *"AI renaissance"* thanks to the availability of unprecedented processing power **(Fig. 1)**.

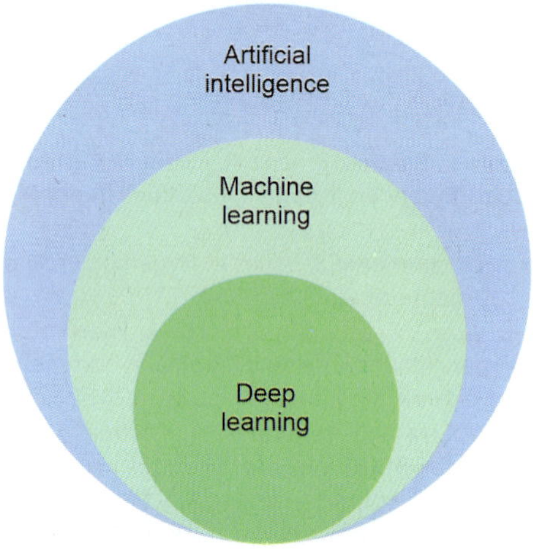

FIG. 1: Artificial intelligence.

WHAT IS ARTIFICIAL INTELLIGENCE?

The term artificial intelligence (AI) is not entirely new. It was coined in 1956 by John McCarthy at the Dartmouth Conference, Massachusetts Institute of Technology (MIT).

Artificial intelligence is the simulation of human intelligence by a machine to perform any intellectual task that a human being can do successfully. In simple words, AI is instilling human senses in machines. For this to be accomplished, the machine-computer system goes through a process of learning (the acquisition of information and rules for applying the data), reasoning (following the rules to reach approximate or definite conclusions), and self-correction by deep learning (DL). AI is an umbrella term that includes anything from robotic process automation to pattern recognition, including the identification of faces and objects. With the availability of incredible computer power and massive amounts of data, AI has recently acquired popularity and significance due to its diverse uses spanning from crime investigation, marketing, finance, and military gadgets to healthcare.

Machine Learning

A subfield of AI that allows computers to learn without being explicitly programmed. Machine learning (ML) uses algorithms trained on gathered data to identify patterns in a particular situation and perform various complex tasks like humans **(Fig. 2)**.

Deep learning is a subset of ML that uses *convolutional neural networks (CNNs)* similar to the human brain, which can learn and make decisions independently through the automation of predictive analytics. The accuracy of image recognition using AI with DL has dramatically progressed in recent times. The availability of an enormous number of digital images and accumulated data in this computer age allowed several DL models to develop, and CNN showed outstanding performance in image analysis.

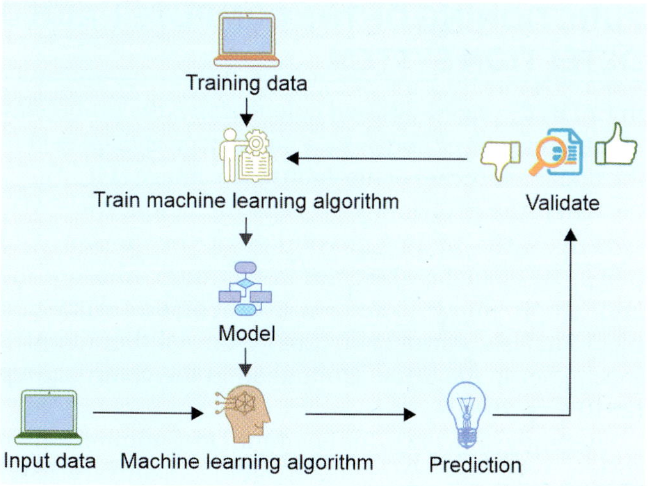

FIG. 2: Machine learning algorithm.

Though AI entered the medical arena three decades ago, the progress in the medical field to tap into the physician's expertise has been tardy to start with but picked up momentum with entries into genomics, electronic health records (EHRs), and robotic surgery. Diagnostic GE being mostly image dependent, AI is useful for faster, cheaper and more accurate diagnosis, thus improving patient outcomes and reducing costs. The application of AI in gastroenterology (GE) has been gradually increasing from its earlier fledgling status in research laboratories to becoming a mainstream application in clinical practice.

CONSTRUCTING ARTIFICIAL INTELLIGENCE SYSTEM—MACHINE LEARNING

The machine must first learn to analyze patterns and diligently flag them to perform human-like tasks. The device needs to be taught appropriately to carry out such intelligent tasks. In order to train the computer to learn and analyze patterns in the images, the gathered project-related data is manipulated to fit a desired model of algorithms. In one of the projects for the application of AI in diagnostic endoscopy to identify early gastric cancer, thousands of endoscopic images of gastric cancer were retrospectively obtained to develop an algorithm to detect gastric cancer during endoscopy. The inclusion criteria were images with standard white light, chromoendoscopy using indigo carmine spraying, and narrow-band imaging (NBI). The exclusion criteria were any images that were magnified and poor-quality images. After selection, 2,639 histologically proven gastric cancer lesions were collected from 13,584 images. For data marking, all images of gastric cancer lesions were marked manually by an expert on gastric cancer. The AI system automatically extracted features of gastric cancer and learned about analyzing patterns of gastric cancer. These model algorithms were tested for accuracy in patients with gastric cancers independently following the same inclusion and exclusion criteria. The final test data set of 2,296 images were manually marked by AI and an expert endoscopist. AI diagnosed 232 lesions—71 gastric cancer (71/77) with a sensitivity of 92.2% and 161 noncancerous lesions with a positive predictive value (PPV) of 30.6% to turn malignant.

WHY DO WE NEED ARTIFICIAL INTELLIGENCE?

Typical videoendoscopy is an operator-dependent procedure. The interpretation of endoscopic imaging depends on the endoscopist's training and keen eye to discern fine nuances in morphology, which matter a lot in identifying early lesions and their correct interpretation. Due to the repetitive nature of the work and inevitable fatigue, the endoscopist may fail to give the same attentiveness all the time and can miss fine details of an evolving sinister condition like gastric cancer. Sometimes, early gastric cancer lesions show only subtle morphological changes and are difficult to detect for even experts. The false negative rate for detecting early gastric cancer with esophagogastroduodenoscopy (EGD) is about 5–26%. Such misses can be minimized with a well-developed AI model with DL to provide greater insight and accuracy of the diagnosis to detect what a physician may not identify routinely. Imagine the embarrassment of missing polyps that have gone undetected during colonoscopy but present as malignant tumors later. Such examples are not uncommon in our practice. The miss rate is estimated to be as high as 20% on high-definition (HD) colonoscopy. In contrast, an AI-supported endoscopy has the potential to provide automated detection of colorectal polyps and reduce polyp misdetection.

ARTIFICIAL INTELLIGENCE IN DIAGNOSTIC GASTROINTESTINAL ENDOSCOPY

Esophagus

It is now a settled matter that Barrett's esophagus (BE) is a premalignant condition with a risk of progression to esophageal adenocarcinoma, albeit slowly. Though the incidence of such progression is only 0.3% per year, it tends to occur gradually from low-grade to high-grade dysplasia and esophageal adenocarcinoma. Given its slow progression, periodic surveillance becomes necessary. The objective is to identify premalignant and malignant lesions at an early stage. Many studies have confirmed that computer-aided diagnosis (CAD) systems score over even expert endoscopists in detecting and delineating dysplastic lesions system with an accuracy of 88% versus 73%, respectively. Similarly, sensitivity and specificity in the detection are superior to conventional endoscopy. Thus, CAD can potentially improve the endoscopic surveillance of BE by nonexpert endoscopists.

The recently introduced volumetric laser endomicroscopy (VLE) that uses optical coherence tomography to produce high-resolution scans of 6-cm segments of the esophagus throws up a lot of data on numerous gray-shade images. Interpreting such vast data is complex and time-consuming, even for experts. CAD systems have been developed that proved better than VLE experts at identifying early BE neoplasia in ex vivo VLE images.

Artificial Intelligence-assisted Computer-aided Detection System in Colonoscopy

There is an inverse relationship between the adenoma detection rate (ADR) and the risk of interval colorectal cancer (CRC) or advanced-stage CRC. Therefore, the importance of a meticulous, high-quality colonoscopy cannot be overemphasized. However, the undetection of adenomas (up to 30%) does happen because of "blindspots" or human error in paying attention to detail. To overcome this shortcoming and accomplish consistent high-quality colonoscopies during screening, AI-assisted computer-aided detection (CADe) comes to the rescue. CADe is based on DL, which attempts to mitigate this problem. In a meta-analysis, Vivek et al. concluded that incorporating AI as an aid for the detection of colorectal neoplasia results in a significant increase in the detection of colorectal neoplasia, and such an effect is independent of main adenoma characteristics. AI in colonoscopy helps to increase the ADR by picking up polyps that endoscopists are likely to miss.

Development of a Convolutional Neural Network Model for Diagnosing *Helicobacter pylori* Infections

A CNN model for diagnosing *Helicobacter pylori* infection performed exceptionally well, with notable accuracy, sensitivity, and specificity. This DL model could aid gastroenterologists in identifying the *H. pylori* infection status and making better decisions (Gastrointest Endosc. 2023;97:880-8).

FUNCTIONING OF THE COMPUTER-AIDED DETECTION SYSTEM

In CADe, during AI-assisted colonoscopy, the probability of the presence of polyps as a percentage is displayed in the upper left corner of the endoscopic image **(Fig. 3)**.

When the probability exceeds the cutoff, the CADe system warns of the possibility of the presence of polyps by changing the color in the four corners of the endoscopic image to red. In a systematic review and meta-analysis, Barua et al. (2021) showed that the ADR was higher in the CADe group than in the control group (29.01% vs. 20.91%).

Recently (July 2023), the Food and Drug Administration (FDA), USA has approved AI-guided software (SW) "Magentiq Colo" to detect lesions in real time. According to the company, the ADR rate improved by 26% relatively (7% in absolute value).

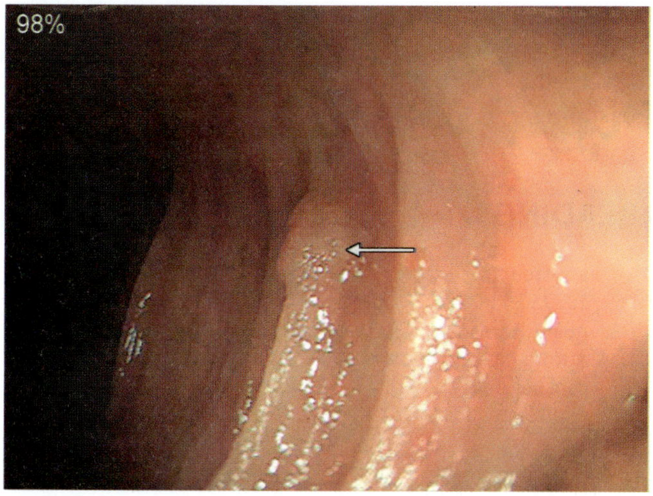

FIG. 3: Computer-aided detection (CADe)-assisted detection of polyps.

ARTIFICIAL INTELLIGENCE IN THE HISTOLOGICAL CHARACTERIZATION OF COLORECTAL POLYPS

The diminutive polyps (≤5 mm) are commonly encountered during colonoscopy. Excision and histopathological examination (HPE) of such polyps involve high costs with financial implications that affect the efficacy of CRC surveillance. A "diagnose-and-leave" strategy is appropriate to reduce the costs of screening. To achieve that, an optical biopsy of diminutive polyps supported by image-enhanced endoscopy may be sufficient in 90% of cases of polyps of ≤5 mm size. However, the optical diagnosis of colorectal polyps is not yet widely available. The dilemma of deciding whether the polyp in view has any malignant portends or is benign can be overcome by computer-aided diagnostic (CADx) that helps predict the histology.

Endocytoscopy (EC) is a new technique that can differentiate between diminutive neoplastic and non-neoplastic colorectal polyps in combination with NBI. EC in combo with CAD (EC-CAD) was used to classify the histology of colorectal polyps. According to Mori et al., this technology achieved a sensitivity of 92%, a specificity of 79.5%, and an accuracy of 89.2%. The performance was comparable to the EC image evaluation by experts and superior to the assessment by trainees for identifying neoplastic polyps.

ARTIFICIAL INTELLIGENCE IN INFLAMMATORY BOWEL DISEASE

The therapeutic goals in the current management of ulcerative colitis (UC) have changed over the last decades such that the objective now is toward mucosal healing, not merely freedom from symptoms. Endoscopic evaluation assesses mucosal healing to assess inflammatory activity and determine therapeutic and follow-up strategies. To overcome the limitations of subjective bias in visual interpretation and the costs and time involved in mucosal biopsy for real-time decision-making, Takenaka et al. have used AI for the macroscopic and histological characterization of colonic mucosa in UC. They developed a deep neural network to evaluate UC to predict endoscopic remission and a UC endoscopic index of severity score. The AI system identified patients with endoscopic remission with 90.1% accuracy and histologic remission with 92.9% accuracy. This suggests that CAD can reliably assist endoscopic and histologic disease activity in UC without the need for mucosal biopsies. The potential benefit of AI in the assessment of disease activity in Crohn's disease is still lacking.

HEPATOBILIARY SYSTEM

Hepatology is another fertile ground for applying AI for the early detection of nonalcoholic fatty liver disease (NAFLD) and assessing the severity of alcoholic hepatitis. There are reported studies of CNN-based DL models for pattern recognition in HPE and ultrasonographic images of focal liver lesions. AI is also used in the selection of liver transplant candidates.

ARTIFICIAL INTELLIGENCE IN CAPSULE ENDOSCOPY

Capsule endoscopy, a marvel of technology, involves the manual reading of videos, a time-intensive and error-prone process. AI-assisted DL, computerized algorithms can automate this tedious process. As discussed earlier, CNN enabled AI detects multiple lesions simultaneously with increasing accuracy and sensitivity. Validation of CNN performance in accurately reading unique characteristics of images in capsule endoscopy is a work in progress. Still, it holds great promise to elevate it from its preclinical level to routine clinical application to reduce reading time effectively.

CONCLUSION

Artificial intelligence has ushered in revolutionary endoscopic diagnostic processes equaling human diligence. GE is an ideal field for adopting AI since the diagnostic methods in GE are primarily image-dependent. Time-consuming mass colonoscopy screenings and the interpretation of innumerable images thrown out by capsule endoscopy can be ably assisted by AI-assisted technologies to improve the diagnostic accuracy and quality of patient care. Precision medicine is at hand, with AI-assisted treatment regimes in inflammatory bowel disease (IBD) becoming tailor-made. The availability of vast amounts of clinical data from large patient datasets has made it possible for AI to prognosticate response to treatment more accurately and reliably. However, it must be remembered that AI cannot substitute human clinical reasoning.

SUGGESTED READINGS

1. Hashimoto R, Requa J, Dao T, Ninh A, Tran E, Mai D, et al. Artificial intelligence using convolutional neural networks for real-time detection of early esophageal neoplasia in Barrett's esophagus (with video). Gastrointest Endosc. 2020;91:1264-1271.e1.
2. Lui TKL, Guo CG, Leung WK. Accuracy of artificial intelligence on histology prediction and detection of colorectal polyps: a systematic review and meta-analysis. Gastrointest Endosc. 2020;92:11-22.e6.
3. Aoki T, Yamada A, Aoyama K, Saito H, Tsuboi A, Nakada A, et al. Automatic detection of erosions and ulcerations in wireless capsule endoscopy images based on a deep convolutional neural network. Gastrointest Endosc. 2019;89:357-63.e2.

SECTION

6

GERIATRICS

Firmicutes, butyrate-producing bacteria like *Clostridium* cluster XIVa (*Roseburia intestinalis, Ruminococcus obeum, Eubacterium ventriosum, E. rectale, E. hallii*), *Clostridium* cluster IV (*Faecalibacterium prausnitzii, Papillibacter cinnamovorans, Anaerotruncus colihominis*), *Clostridium* cluster XV *(E. limosum*), lactobacillus, mucin-degrading bacteria Akkermansia muciniphila of Planetomycetes, Verrucomicrobia, Chlamydiae (PVC) superphylum, etc.

FORMATION AND DEVELOPMENT

The formation of gut microbiota starts with birth when a fetus comes in contact with mother's fecal, vaginal and skin microbiota and after that its development depends upon hygiene and feeding. In infancy, *Bifidobacterium* is dominant strain with limited diversity especially in breastfed children where it utilizes human milk oligosaccharides (HMO) and converts them into lactate and SCFA acetate, whereas the gut of formula-fed children is colonized by a diverse microbial population. In the beginning, it is unstable. It became stable and progressively diverse at the age of 3 years when children consume more solid food. This is the time when core microbiota is formed. In adults, dominant phyla are Firmicutes and Bacteroidetes with smaller proportion of Actinobacteria, Proteobacteria, and Verrucomicrobia.

The microbial concentration is maximum in colon as compared to other parts of gut. It may be due to increased pH, availability of nutrients, mucin secretion, gastrointestinal transit time, etc.

The composition of gut microbiota of elderly differs with that of younger or middle-aged people. This alteration in gut microbiota (dysbiosis) is characterized by reduced Firmicutes/Bacteroidetes ratio, decreased richness of microflora with reduced diversity and reduction in butyrate producing bacteria, diminished SCFA production with increase in pathobionts, and LPS production. This alteration was consistent in various studies done in different parts of the world. This decrease in beneficial and increase in proinflammatory microbiota is probably intrinsic to the aging process. Progressively with aging, carbohydrate fermentation reduces resulting in lower levels of SCFAs and protein fermentation increases resulting in higher levels of branched fatty acids, ammonia, and phenols.

FUNCTIONS

The gut-microbiota performs many beneficial functions. These are the only source of production of SCFAs which constitute and promote intestinal barrier integrity, strengthen intestinal epithelial tight junctions. This in turn inhibit leakage or bypass of intestinal pathogens, their toxins, byproducts (LPS, etc.) into blood stream (endotoxemia) and reduces chances of inflammation which is the leading cause of aging, inflammageing, metabolic syndrome, cardiovascular, neurovascular and neurodegenerative disorders, frailty, and ill health in elderly. Microbiota also helps in digestion and absorption of food and production of vitamins and nutrients from them. These are the master regulator of immune homeostasis. They improve gut immunity by inducing secretion of IgA and B cells, which suppress pathogens. They also suppress pathogens by competitively metabolizing nutrients which are mandatory for the existence of the pathogens. Gut microbiota produces a low-grade physiological inflammation (by continuously stimulating immune system) which is also a quick and effective way in fighting against pathogens.

Primary bile acids are formed in the liver and are converted into secondary bile acids by enzymatic actions of gut microbiota. These secondary bile acids are associated with regulation of insulin sensitivity through activation of farnesoid X receptor (FXR) and Takeda G protein-coupled receptor 5 (TGR5). FXR activation induces increased secretion of Fibroblast growth factor 19 (FGF-19) which improves glucose tolerance and insulin resistance. Activation of TGR receptor stimulates intestinal L cells to secrete glucagon-like peptide 1 (GLP-1), thereby improving insulin sensitivity.

A plethora of studies are there which shows association between changes in gut microbiota (dysbiosis) and different diseases and unhealthy aging. In many studies, severity of dysbiosis was associated with severity of the disease and its restoration by modulation of gut microbiota [by prebiotic, probiotic and symbiotic supplementation or fecal microbiota transplantation (FMT)] was also associated with improvement in symptoms and disease progression. Even though, our knowledge regarding the subject is still incomplete. Preclinical and animal model studies are promising and show direct effect of certain bacteria on certain metabolic and clinical parameters of various diseases and unhealthy aging but there are only a few clinical trials in human model with less promising and inconsistent results.

Certain beneficial microbiota needs special consideration.

Faecalibacterium prausnitzii: This is a major and most important member of Firmicutes phylum. It is a gram-negative, strict anaerobic bacteria which cannot sustain ambient air for ≥2 minutes. It is an acetate-consuming and butyrate-producing bacterium. Its anti-inflammatory effects are related to butyrate production. In abundance, it improves diabetes and its complications such as nephropathy, neuropathy, and cerebrovascular and cardiovascular diseases. It also reduces inflammageing and delay aging. It is proposed as a biomarker for the development of gut diseases and also for assessing dietary interventions in intestinal inflammatory conditions.

Akkermansia muciniphila: It is very important and well-studied beneficial microbiota belonging to Verrucomicrobia. It is an aerotolerant anaerobic gram-ve bacterium, which colonizes at the mucus layer of intestine. It is a mucin-degrading bacterium and also stimulates mucin production. Intestinal mucin is the main source of carbon and nitrogen for them. They adhere to intestinal epithelium and strengthen intestinal barrier. Its membrane protein Amuc_1100 binds to toll-like receptor 2 (TLR2) and participates in the protective mechanism of intestinal barrier. This protein is also responsible for immunomodulatory properties of this bacterium. This protein also improves glucose tolerance and decreases body weight and fat mass gain. Its abundance reduces hepatic steatosis, inflammation, cholesterol level, and atherosclerosis; improves insulin sensitivity; restores gut barrier function; improves endotoxemia; ameliorate insulin resistance and metabolic syndrome; reduces inflammageing; and delays aging. It provides energy to other butyrate- and propionate-producing bacteria and hence, increases butyrate and propionate production. It increases hydrogen sulfide production which has anti-inflammatory, muscle relaxing, and antioxidant properties. It improves lipid and glucose metabolism. It is also being used as diagnostic tool for dietary interventions. This single bacterium can be used as a probiotic to reduce the incidence of diabetes. This fact underscores the capability and importance of *A. muciniphila*.

Short-chain Fatty Acids

The gut microbiota converts indigestible dietary fibers and starch into SCFAs (acetic acid, butyric acid and propionic acid) and nutrients. Their production reduces pH of gut which stimulates growth of Firmicutes and reduces overgrowth of pathogens like *E. coli*. They also promote growth of beneficial bacteria by directly providing energy to them. Butyric acid has a protective effect on intestinal barrier as it induces mucin synthesis, reduces intestinal permeability and hence prevents bacteria from passing through it. Butyrate also acts on colonic epithelium reducing oxidative stress and inflammation. Acetate reduces frequency of autoimmune T cells in lymphoid tissue and butyrate increases number and function of regulatory T cells. SCFAs modulate intestinal transit time and insulin resistance and can reduce metabolic syndrome, obesity and type 2 diabetes mellitus (T2DM). They inhibit inflammation by promoting IL-10 production (anti-inflammatory cytokine) and inhibiting tumor necrosis factor alpha (TNF-α), interleukin 6 (IL-6), and nitric oxide (NO) (proinflammatory cytokines) production. SCFAs, by inhibiting inflammatory cytokines, are very important in keeping microglial integrity and hence inhibiting cognitive decline with aging. By reducing inflammation and resultant atherosclerosis they are also effective in reducing vascular dementia in elderly. They up regulate 5-adenosine monophosphate (5-AMP) activated in muscle and liver tissue and the protein kinase signaling pathway which are related to insulin resistance and inflammation and oxidative stress. By reducing inflammation, they also reduce inflammageing, which is the key factor behind unhealthy aging.

Lipopolysaccharides

These are produced in gut by cell wall of gram-negative bacteria. LPS in huge amount (produced by dysbiosis) may destroy the integrity of intestinal barrier. When breach in intestinal barrier occurs, then LPS bypass it and enter into blood stream and induce inflammatory cytokines through immune cells and adipocytes and produce low-grade inflammation, which is responsible for insulin resistance, metabolic syndrome, atherosclerosis, cognitive impairment, cardiovascular neurovascular and neurodegenerative disorders (Alzheimer's disease, Parkinson's disease), frailty and ill health in elderly and aging itself. LPS are strongly amyloidogenic and its excess may be related with Alzheimer's disease.

Increased levels of butyrate in intestine of centenarians and supercentenarians of different parts of the world were observed in many studies showing its importance in longer life. Dysbiosis was associated with unhealthy and premature aging whereas its preservation was associated with healthy aging and overall good health.

GUT MICROBIOTA MODULATION

From the very beginning, reversal of aging was the dream of mankind and remained in center of many scientific researches and gut microbiota modulation is also among one of them. The modulation of gut microbiota can be done either by prebiotic, probiotic, and symbiotic supplementation or by FMT. In vitro and in vivo studies are very promising and results in formation of next-generation probiotics (NGPs).

Next-generation Probiotic

These are the specific bacteria which possesses enhanced functional characteristic against specific disease or metabolic effect or complication. The primary candidates of this group are *A. muciniphila, F. prausnitzii, Roseburia intestinalis, Ruminococcus bromii, Anaerobutyricum hallii,* etc.

CONCLUSION

Gut microbiota has a great impact upon health and diseases. Dysbiosis is the primary cause of premature aging and pathologies associated with it. There modulation by prebiotic, probiotic, and symbiotic supplementation or FMT may reverse these pathologies and may delay aging.

SUGGESTED READINGS

1. Mangiola F, Nicoletti A, Gasbarrini A, Ponziani FR. Gut microbiota and aging. Eur Rev Med Pharmacol Sci. 2018;22:7404-13.
2. Ragonnaud E, Biragyn A. Gut microbiota as the key controllers of "healthy" aging of elderly people. Immun Ageing. 2021;18(1):2.
3. Ghosh TS, Shanahan F, O'Toole PW. The gut microbiome as a modulator of healthy aging. Nat Rev Gastroenterol Hepatol. 2022;19(9):565-84.

92

CHAPTER

Antiaging Medications

Kauser Usman, Rajat Chaudhary, Suraj S Yadav

ABSTRACT

The search for antiaging medications has intensified as the world's population ages. In this chapter, the idea, how it works, and problems with antiaging medications are examined. Senescence, deoxyribonucleic acid (DNA) damage and other variables play a role in the complex process of aging. Antiaging medications aim to extend healthy lifetime by concentrating on these systems. Telomere maintenance, protein homeostasis, nutrition sensing, DNA repair, and cellular senescence are a few crucial systems. Hormonal changes, inflammation, and immunosenescence also play important role. Promising area of management include hormone replacement, exercise, and calorie restriction. The antiaging drug classes that have the most potential include senolytics, nicotinamide adenine dinucleotide (NAD^+) precursors, and calorie restriction mimetics. Natural chemicals including vitamins, spermidine, and curcumin are the subject of investigation. Enhancing healthspan as well as lifespan should be the objective of longevity research, which calls for rigorous study design and regulatory guidance. However, in longevity research there are obstacles to overcome, such as unanticipated effects, legal restrictions, and moral dilemmas. As research advances, it is critical to strike a balance between safety, efficacy and equal access to everyone. The pursuit for antiaging medicines has enormous promise for improving quality of life on an aging world if ethical, scientific, and regulatory issues are resolved.

INTRODUCTION

Aging is an inevitable biological process that leads to a gradual decline in physical and cognitive abilities. Age is one of the strongest independent risk factors for many chronic diseases, such as Alzheimer's disease, cancer, and ischemic heart disease. As life expectancy continues to rise globally, the pursuit of slowing down or even reversing the aging process has become a focus of scientific research. Antiaging medicine, an evolving branch of medical sciences, aim to extend healthy lifespan and enhance the quality of life for older individuals. This chapter explores into the concept of antiaging medications, their potential mechanisms, current research, and the ethical considerations surrounding their development.

UNDERSTANDING THE AGING PROCESS

Cellular aging is the result of a progressive decline in cellular function and viability caused by genetic abnormalities and the accumulation of cellular and molecular damage due to the effects of exposure to exogenous influences **(Fig. 1)**. Multiple mechanisms, both intrinsic to cells and triggered by external factors contribute to the aging process.

Unrepaired deoxyribonucleic acid (DNA) damage, telomere shortening, altered protein homeostasis, and dysregulated nutrient sensing play important role in the aging process. The decline of certain hormones, such as growth hormone (GH) and sex hormones such as estrogen and testosterone, is closely linked to the aging process. These hormonal changes contribute to a reduction in muscle mass, bone density, and skin elasticity.

INFLAMMATION, IMMUNOSENESCENCE, AND AGING

Inflammation is crucial for fighting infections and promoting tissue repair; however, chronic low-grade inflammation contributes to the aging process. The

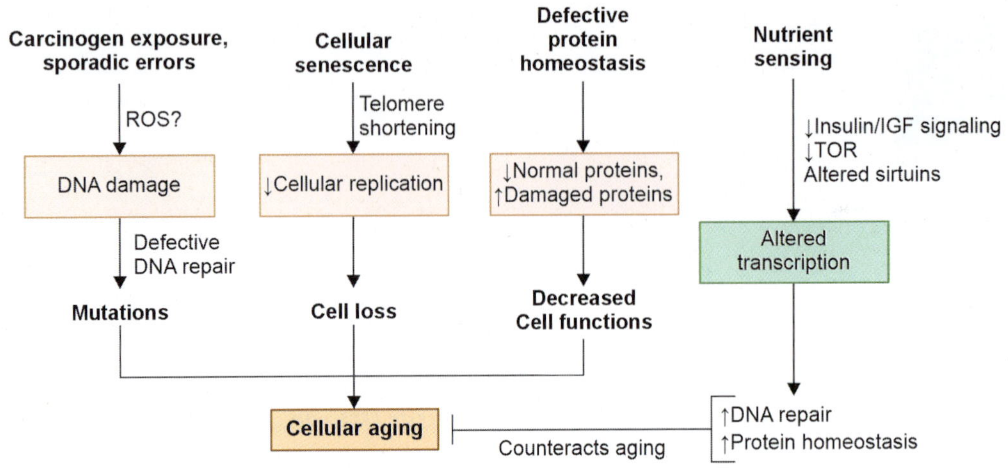

FIG. 1: Mechanisms that cause and counteract cellular aging.
(DNA: deoxyribonucleic acid; IGF: insulin-like growth factor; ROS: reactive oxygen species; TOR: target of rapamycin)

term inflammaging has been coined to emphasize that many major age-related disabilities, including cancers, susceptibility to infections, and dementia have immunopathogenic components.

Immunosenescence is characterized by decline in immune function and an increased susceptibility to infections and age-related diseases. This decline is accompanied by chronic inflammation, which fuels a cycle of tissue damage and dysfunction.

MOLECULAR TARGETS FOR ANTIAGING

Insulin and Insulin-like Growth Factor 1 Signaling Pathway

Insulin-like growth factor 1 (IGF-1) is produced in many cell types in response to GH secretion by the pituitary gland. IGF-1 mimics intracellular signaling by insulin and thereby informs cells of the availability of glucose, promoting an anabolic state as well as cell growth and replication. The IGF-1 signaling cascade has two kinases: AKT (protein kinase B), and its downstream target, mammalian target of rapamycin (mTOR). Out of its two complexes, mTORC1 drives protein synthesis and cell growth, while its inhibition hinders growth and triggers stress response pathways such as autophagy. Several regulators that transmit signals through the AKT pathway, such as insulin and IGFs, incite mTORC1 activity. Human IGF-1 receptor gene polymorphisms are associated with exceptional longevity **(Fig. 2)**.

Sirtuins

Sirtuins are a family of NAD-dependent protein deacetylases. They are believed to enhance the expression of multiple genes that contribute to lifespan extension. Elevated levels of sirtuins, particularly sirtuin-6, have a dual role: Firstly, they aid in the metabolic adaptation linked to caloric restriction, and secondly, they support the integrity of the genome by activating DNA repair enzymes through a deacylation process.

ANTIAGING MEDICINE

Antiaging medicine strives to maintain or achieve youthful vitality regardless of actual age for the purpose of overall health and optimal biological functioning. The objective of this field is to decelerate, halt, or even reverse the aging process and its consequent effects, such as disability and frailty.

Nonpharmacological Therapies

Calorie Restriction

Caloric restriction has displayed the greatest potential in counteracting the aging process which is achieved by reducing the signaling strength of the IGF-1 pathway and bolstering sirtuin activity. It offers protection against conditions such as obesity, heart disease, hypertension, and cancer. Promising outcomes are emerging from studies involving prolonged and intermittent fasting in human subjects.

Exercise

Exercise is a promising lifestyle intervention that has antiaging effects. It decreases overall risk of death, prevents age-associated muscle degeneration, improves cardiopulmonary outcome, reduces physical disability, reduces sarcopenia, improves muscle endurance,

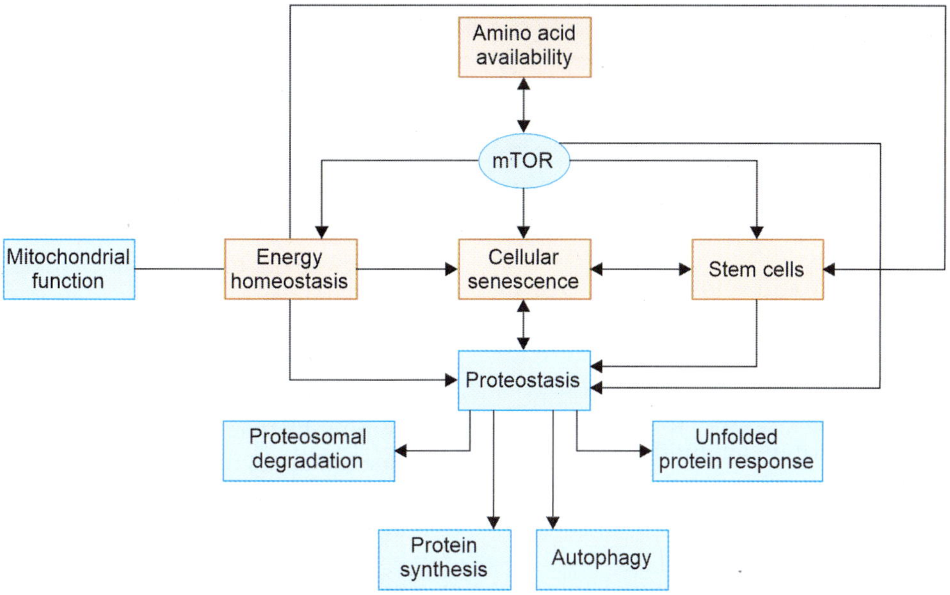

FIG. 2: Mammalian target of rapamycin (mTOR) regulates several hallmarks of aging which are also interconnected, suggesting that aging is a coordinated process in which mTOR plays a significant role.

enhances balance, efficient motor coordination, and decreases osteoporosis. Exercise also increases insulin sensitivity.

Dietary Preferences

Foods supposed to escalate aging such as baked foods, alcohol, and energy drinks are mainly implicated in their high sugar content which is proven to be proinflammatory. Conversely foods supposed to have antiaging effects such as turmeric, nuts, avocado, blueberries, seaweed derivatives, dark chocolate, green tea, mushrooms, and salmon as they are mainly attributed to their antioxidant property.

Natural Products as Antiaging Agents

Carotenoids

It quenches free radicals or neutralizes other oxidants and prevents DNA damage and decreases inflammatory markers. They also has a role in improving vision.

Curcumin (Curcuma Longa)

It has demonstrated antiaging, anti-inflammatory, and potential anticancer properties on in vivo studies. Curcumin appears to impact the gut microflora, which is linked to various chronic illnesses.

Spermidine

Spermidine, the most prevalent polyamine in human tissues, decreases with natural aging. It is found in high amounts in sperm, where it counters cellular aging, promoting germ cell line longevity.

Ursolic Acid

Ursolic acid, present in apples, prunes, and papaya, triggers AMPK activation, affecting cellular energy levels by modifying adenosine diphosphate (ADP) and adenosine triphosphate (ATP) concentrations.

Coenzyme Q10

Coenzyme Q10 is crucial for mitochondrial electron transport system. It is explored for conditions like Parkinson's disease, showing potential to slow its progression.

Pharmacological Therapies

Antiaging medications target underlying mechanisms of aging, aiming to delay age-related diseases and extend healthy lifespan. Several classes of drugs have shown promise in preclinical studies, which are discussed here.

Senolytics

These drugs remove the senescent cells which accumulate with age and contribute to inflammation and tissue dysfunction, potentially improving tissue function and reducing age-related diseases, e.g., *fisetin*, a flavonoid found in strawberries, apples, grapes, and onion.

Nicotinamide Adenine Dinucleotide Precursors

Nicotinamide adenine dinucleotide (NAD^+) can raise the activity of sirtuins. NAD^+ precursors, such as nicotinamide riboside, could improve mitochondrial function and cellular health.

Caloric Restriction Mimetics

These compounds aim to activate cellular pathways that promote longevity. They might enhance cellular stress responses and improve metabolic health.

Activators of the AMPK Pathway

These agents improve insulin sensitivity, promoting glucose uptake in skeletal muscles while reducing hepatic glucose production and enhancing fatty acid oxidation in various tissues. Certain Food and Drug Administration (FDA)-approved drugs such as metformin, thiazolidinediones, glucagon-like peptide-1 receptor agonists, salicylates, and resveratrol possess AMPK-activating properties. Metformin, an antidiabetic agent, has potential for preventing age-related degeneration and cancer by extending lifespan in organisms like *Caenorhabditis elegans* and mice.

Inhibitors of Growth Hormone/IGF-1 Axis

It is perhaps the most validated and consistent genetic intervention to extend mouse lifespan and healthspan. *Pegvisomant* is unique as it does not suppress GH secretion but blocks its action by binding to the GH receptor. Additionally, it is an insulin sensitizer that blocks the diabetogenic action of GH. Therefore, it could have positive effects on both longevity and healthy aging by lowering serum IGF-1 and increasing insulin sensitivity. Somatostatin analogs also decrease serum IGF-1 levels but significant adverse events unwarrant their use. Under research are monoclonal antibodies targeted at inhibiting the GH/IGF-1 axis.

Rapamycin and mTOR Inhibitors

These drugs by inhibiting mTOR might slow down the aging process and promote longevity.

Activators of the Sirtuin Pathway

The first potent sirtuin-activating compounds (STACs) were initially found in various types of plant-derived compounds such as flavones, stilbenes, chalcones, and anthocyanidins. Among these, *resveratrol* (3,5,40-trihydroxystilbene) remains the most potent natural activator identified so far. It is found in grape skin, blueberries, raspberries, mulberries, and red wine. They also address health issues such as cancer, type 2 diabetes mellitus, cardiovascular disease, stroke, and hepatic steatosis.

Inhibitors of Glycolysis

Inhibiting glycolysis through a nutraceutical derived from *unripened avocados* containing mannoheptulose, a sugar that inhibits hexokinase, has shown potential antiaging activity.

Inhibitors of Inflammatory Pathways

Chronic, low-grade inflammation is recognized as a major characteristic of aging. Anti-inflammatory drugs such as nordihydroguaiaretic acid (NDGA) and aspirin have displayed potential to somewhat extend lifespan.

Modulators of Epigenetic Pathways

Epigenetics refers to heritable changes in traits caused by modifications to chromatin after DNA replication, rather than traditional genetic mutations. *Spermidine*, a naturally occurring polyamine, directly inhibits enzymes called histone acetyltransferases (HATs), thereby maintaining histone H3 in a hypoacetylated state. This outcome enhances resistance to heat and oxidative stress and significantly lowers the occurrence of cell death as the cells age.

■ Miscellaneous Drugs used as Antiaging

Acarbose

It is an alpha-glycosidase inhibitor used in diabetes treatment. Its lifespan-extending effects may involve increased short-chain fatty acids due to influence on gut microbiota.

Deprenyl

An inhibitor of monoamine oxidase B (MAO-B), upregulates the activity of antioxidant enzymes superoxide dismutase (SOD) in the dopaminergic region of the brain.

Minocycline and Doxycycline

These antibiotics, also have antioxidant and anti-inflammatory properties as they may counteract aging processes by inhibiting kynurenine formation (upregulation of kynurenine pathway of tryptophan was suggested as one of the mechanisms of aging).

Vitamin C

A powerful antioxidant that protects cells from oxidative damage. It plays important role in immune function and healthy aging. Rich sources are citrus fruits, Indian gooseberry, kiwi, and broccoli.

BIOTECHNOLOGICAL ADVANCES IN ANTIAGING RESEARCH

■ Gut Microbiota

The digestive system holds particular significance as the body's largest immune organ, housing trillions of bacteria capable of releasing inflammatory substances into the bloodstream. Modifying the healthy gut microbiota via prebiotics, probiotics, or fecal microbiota transplantation holds significant potential in the field of antiaging medicine.

Stem Cells

Stem cells have demonstrated utility in treating certain autoimmune and cardiovascular conditions. Their regenerative capabilities are being explored for rejuvenating or repairing aged or damaged tissues.

Biotechnological Therapies in Antiaging

Recombinant DNA therapy, proteomics (protein expression and modifications), therapeutic cloning where stem cells are used to generate specific tissues or organs for transplantation or regenerative purposes, and gene therapy are some of the effective options to prevent disease and aging.

CONCLUSION

In almost all animals, aging is a systemic and evolutionarily conserved phenomenon. It is clearly a very challenging endeavor to conduct clinical trials to examine the antiaging potential of conventional medications. This is related to the fact that older people frequently take several drugs at a time due to the comorbidities. Another significant issue is the lack of accurate and measurable biomarkers to judge the success of antiaging therapies. In order to make sure that any developments in this subject are both helpful and available to everyone, ethical, scientific, and regulatory issues must be carefully observed in continuing the research work.

SUGGESTED READINGS

1. Longo VD, Antebi A, Bartke A, Barzilai N, Brown-Borg HM, Caruso C, et al. Interventions to Slow Aging in Humans: Are We Ready? Aging Cell. 2015;14(4):497-510.
2. Papadopoli D, Boulay K, Kazak L, Pollak M, Mallette F, Topisirovic I, et al. mTOR as a central regulator of lifespan and aging. F1000Res. 2019;8:F1000 Faculty Rev-998.
3. Argyropoulou A, Aligiannis N, Trougakos IP, Skaltsounis AL. Natural compounds with anti-ageing activity. Nat Prod Rep. 2013;30(11):1412-37.
4. Ok SC. Insights into the Anti-Aging Prevention and Diagnostic Medicine and Healthcare. Diagnostics (Basel). 2022;12(4):819.
5. Liu JK. Antiaging agents: safe interventions to slow aging and healthy life span extension. Nat Prod Bioprospect. 2022;12:18.
6. Arora BP. Anti-aging medicine. Indian J Plast Surg. 2008;41(Suppl):S130-3.
7. Kumar V, Abbas AK, Aster JC. Cell injury, cell death and adaptations. In: Kumar V, Abbas AK, Aster JC (Eds). Robbins and Cotran Pathologic Basis of Disease, 10th edition. Amsterdam, Netherlands: Elsevier; 2020.

93 CHAPTER

Human Immunodeficiency Virus and Noncommunicable Diseases: Challenges in Elderly

Meenaxi Sharda

ABSTRACT

The world presently and in coming decades will be witnessing a dual disease epidemic of human immunodeficiency virus (HIV) and noncommunicable diseases (NCDs), especially in low- and middle-income group countries (LMIC). HIV care, treatment programs, and unprecedented expansion in coverage have increased longevity in people living with HIV (PLHIV). It has led to a changing population pyramid of HIV-infected persons with an increasing prevalence of older people.

A triad of HIV, antiretroviral therapy (ART), and traditional risk factors increase the risk of NCDs among PLHIV. HIV-associated immune activation and inflammation are associated with faster aging, atherosclerosis, cardiovascular diseases (CVDs), and cancer. Some ARTs increase low-density lipoprotein (LDL) and decrease insulin sensitivity, aggravating the risk of CVD and diabetes. Mental health illness also increases due to social stigma and neglect.

Aging with HIV poses a challenge in NCDs and in the ongoing treatment of HIV itself. Hence, a strong rationale for the integration of HIV and NCD services has been proposed by the United Nations Program on HIV/AIDS (UNAIDS) in 2016.

Approaches and strategies pioneered for HIV, focus on prevention, care, and treatment services for NCDs also. It is pivotal in reducing morbidity, mortality, and the burden of NCDs among PLHIV.

INTRODUCTION

Human immunodeficiency virus (HIV), once a life-threatening illness, has now become a manageable chronic condition. Noncommunicable diseases (NCDs) are a growing problem in people living with HIV (PLHIV), as they live longer on successful antiretroviral therapy (ART). The life expectancy of HIV patients is reaching up to the life expectancy of non-HIV patients. NCDs increase in frequency with age. A triad of HIV, ART, and traditional risk factors of aging increase the prevalence of NCDs in HIV.

EPIDEMIOLOGY

The proportion of older PLHIV has increased globally. One-third of the share is from India. New infection in older adults has also shown an increase. The proportion of PLHIV aged 50 years and above will increase from 28% in 2010 to 73% in 2030.

The HIV-related morbidity and mortality trend has shown significant change over the decades shifting from opportunistic infections, acquired immunodeficiency syndrome (AIDS)-related mortality, and hepatitis B and C to non-AIDS defining illnesses. 2004 onward NCDs are a prime cause of morbidity and mortality.

PATHOGENESIS

Aging and Human Immunodeficiency Virus

Human immunodeficiency virus accelerates the aging process. Both have drastic effects on the immune system leading to a phase of chronic immune activation. Also, the system recovery after ART is slow in older individuals because the rise in CD4 count in the aging population is less rapid compared to young adults. Low CD4 is associated with increased risk.

Aging and Noncommunicable Diseases

The trimodal pathways for prevalence of NCDs in HIV are as follows:

- HIV infection itself increases the risk of developing NCDs.
- Some antiretroviral drugs (particularly older agents) have side effects that increase cardiovascular risk factors and the risk of comorbid disease. Decreased metabolism in older adults may lead to more toxicity of the drug.
- The increased life expectancy due to ART suggests that PLHIV reaches the age with an increased risk of developing age-related NCDs.

PATHOGENETIC MECHANISM

Several determinants are involved in the pathogenesis of NCDs in HIV. A high prevalence of traditional risk factors such as hypertension, type 2 diabetes mellitus (T2DM), dyslipidemia, obesity, genetic factors, and poor socioeconomic conditions pose an increased threat. HIV infection causes persistent inflammation, immune activation, endothelial damage, and hypercoagulability. It leads to the activation of several pathways, causing the release of cytokines and increased proinflammatory mediators such as interleukin-6 (IL-6) and tumor necrosis factor-alpha (TNF-α). Monocyte activation plays a central role in the development of atherosclerosis. Coinfection with other viruses and a late diagnosis predispose the individual to more metabolic derangements. Antiretroviral therapy can produce endothelial dysfunction and oxidative stress and promote an inflammatory response. Polypharmacy causes increased drug interactions and potential deleterious effects.

INTEGRATION OF HUMAN IMMUNODEFICIENCY VIRUS AND NONCOMMUNICABLE DISEASES

For the control of this enormously progressive syndemic, approaches and strategies pioneered for HIV care are now integrated for the care of other chronic ailments simultaneously, especially NCDs to provide prevention and treatment of these conditions. Different types of integration models are suggested.

HUMAN IMMUNODEFICIENCY VIRUS AND NONCOMMUNICABLE DISEASES

People living with HIV at risk for NCDs are those:

- Who has a delay in the diagnosis of HIV infection
- Those on older ART regimens as effectivity and safety differ from new drugs
- Who do not achieve optimal immune recovery, like elderly patients

Human immunodeficiency virus-associated NCDs include cardiovascular diseases (CVDs), T2DM, dyslipidemia, hypertension, chronic kidney disease (CKD), poor bone mineral health, frailty, and mental health illnesses.

HUMAN IMMUNODEFICIENCY VIRUS AND CARDIOVASCULAR DISEASES

People living with HIV have a 1.5–2-fold risk of CAD and a 4.5-fold risk of sudden cardiac death. Other CVDs occurring in HIV infection are dilated cardiomyopathy, arterial aneurysm, pericarditis/tuberculosis (TB), and pulmonary hypertension.

Prolonged HIV viremia, delayed initiation of ART, HIV treatment failure/nonadherence, metabolic syndrome, and hepatitis coinfection are HIV-related CVD risk-enhancing factors leading to chronic inflammation immune activation and hypercoagulability. Screening of CVD requires the calculation of the atherosclerotic CVD (ASCVD) risk score and the identification of CVD risk-enhancing factors. Low-risk approach treatment is lifestyle modification and yearly reassessment of risk. A high-risk approach for CVD includes lipid-lowering drug therapy in addition to lifestyle modification. Patients should be started on lipid-safe ART. Metabolic syndrome and diabetes are kept under control. Abacavir is not used in patients with an elevated risk of CVD.

HUMAN IMMUNODEFICIENCY VIRUS AND HYPERTENSION

About 25.2% is the overall prevalence of hypertension, 34.7% for ART-experienced, and 12.7% for ART-naïve participants. Hypertension among PLHIV shows an increasing trend since 2010 and is associated with older age and those on ART.

All patients should be screened for hypertension at the time of ART registration and followed up once in 6 months after initiation of ART or whenever the patient is symptomatic.

Ace inhibitors and thiazides have no interactions with ART. The blood level of calcium channel blockers increases when used with protease inhibitors (PIs) and decreases when used with non-nucleoside reverse transcriptase inhibitor (NNRTI). Therefore, necessary dose adjustments and drug selection are advisable for optimal target blood pressure (BP) control.

HUMAN IMMUNODEFICIENCY VIRUS AND LIPID METABOLISM

The natural history of HIV infection is associated with characteristic changes in lipid levels. A low CD4 count and high HIV RNA level are independently associated with these changes.

Treatment requires lifestyle modification and lipid-lowering drugs. Statins reduce cardiovascular events by 44%. European AIDS Clinical Society (EACS) recommends initiating statins if total cholesterol (TC) > 190 mg/dL and/or low-density lipoprotein cholesterol (LDL-C) > 115 mg/dL to achieve optimal levels. Starting dose of atorvastatin 10 mg OD and a maximum of 20 mg can be given if the patient is on a PI ritonavir, and up to 80 mg once daily if the patient is not on this drug. Simvastatin and lovastatin are contraindicated in the presence of PIs. Fenofibrate is added when triglyceride (TG) is >400 mg/dL. In PLHIV on ART with a known impact on lipid metabolism **(Table 1)**, a single drug substitution to a lipid-friendly drug is recommended **(Table 2)**.

TABLE 1: Lipid unsafe antiretroviral therapy (ART).

Group	Drug	Change in lipid levels
Protease inhibitor	Lopinavir/ritonavir Fosamprenavir/ritonavir	Increase triglyceride and total cholesterol Increase triglyceride and total cholesterol
Nucleoside reverse transcriptase inhibitor (NRTI)	Zidovudine Stavudine	Increase total cholesterol and low-density lipoprotein (LDL) Increase total cholesterol/triglyceride (TC/TG)
Non-nucleoside reverse transcriptase inhibitor (NNRTI)	Efavirenz	Increase lipids

TABLE 2: Lipid safe antiretroviral therapy (ART).

Group	Drug	Changes in blood lipid levels
Protease inhibitor	Atazanavir Darunavir	Decrease low-density lipoprotein (LDL) and total cholesterol Decrease total cholesterol
Nucleoside reverse transcriptase inhibitor (NRTI)	Tenofovir Abacavir	Decrease total cholesterol (TC)/LDL No change in TC and high-density lipoprotein (HDL)
Non-nucleoside reverse transcriptase inhibitor (NNRTI)	Nevirapine Etravirine	Increase HDL No change
Integrase inhibitor	Dolutegravir	Less change
CK receptor antagonists	Maraviroc	No change

HUMAN IMMUNODEFICIENCY VIRUS AND DIABETES

The relative risk of T2DM in HIV-infected patients is 1.2–2. The prevalence of T2DM and impaired glucose tolerance is 10 and 18–35%, respectively.

Screening for T2DM is initiated at ART registration, 3 monthly, and whenever ART is changed. The diagnosis and management of T2DM are the same as non-HIV patients except that glycated hemoglobin (HbA1c) underestimates glycemia in HIV-infected persons and NNRTI and PI reduce sulfonylurea level whereas dolutegravir limits the use of metformin up to 1 g only.

HUMAN IMMUNODEFICIENCY VIRUS AND BONE MINERAL METABOLISM

There is a 6.4-fold increased risk of low bone mineral density (BMD) and a 3.7-fold increased risk of osteoporosis in PLHIV. In India, the prevalence of low BMD in ART naïve patients is 67% and 80.4% in ART experienced. In addition to virus-induced inflammation, immune activation, and ART, traditional risk factors (menopause, smoking, alcohol, vitamin D deficiency, and hypothyroidism) are responsible for derangement in bone metabolism.

Screening guidelines should be strengthened using Fracture Risk Assessment Tool (FRAX) score and dual energy X-ray absorptiometry (DEXA) monitoring. The treatment includes vitamin D, calcium supplementation, and bisphosphonates such as alendronate and zoledronic acid. ART regardless of regimen leads to reductions in BMD, especially in the first 48 weeks of therapy.

HUMAN IMMUNODEFICIENCY VIRUS AND RENAL DISEASE

Screening for CKD should be done at the initial diagnosis using urine protein to creatinine ratio, urine analysis, estimated glomerular filtration rate (eGFR), and ultrasound kidney, ureter, and bladder (KUB), if required. Patients should then be followed up once in 6 months if risk factors for CKD are present or if clinically indicated otherwise.

In high-risk patients with eGFR < 70, urine protein-to-creatinine ratio (uPCR) > 500, age > 60 years with uncontrolled T2DM, hypertension (HTN), and CVD, or with hepatitis C, avoid nephrotoxic ART such as tenofovir, atazanavir/ritonavir, lopinavir/ritonavir, and nonsteroidal anti-inflammatory drugs (NSAIDs). Abacavir is safe for these individuals.

HUMAN IMMUNODEFICIENCY VIRUS AND CANCER

Older adults with HIV are at greater risk of developing cancer. There is an increased prevalence of non-AIDS-defining malignancies such as anal, rectal, colon, gastric, liver, and lung cancer.

For HIV males >50 years of age with anemia, a fecal occult blood test is done for screening. Sigmoidoscopy and colonoscopy can be done if indicated. In ages 50–79 years and heavy smokers, low-dose CT chest is done, however, there is no role of prostate-specific antigen (PSA) in screening for prostatic malignancy.

HUMAN IMMUNODEFICIENCY VIRUS AND FRAILTY

Frailty is an independent risk factor for morbidity and mortality. Frailty is more in HIV infected person than non-HIV infected.

HUMAN IMMUNODEFICIENCY VIRUS AND POLYPHARMACY

As the age advances, the number of comedications increases. In the Swiss HIV Cohort study, 5.2% of patients aged 50–64 years and 14.2% of patients >65 years received more than four comedications other than ART.

HUMAN IMMUNODEFICIENCY VIRUS AND MENTAL HEALTH

Older adults with HIV and on ART are more susceptible to depression (efavirenz), dementia, and Alzheimer's disease. Social stigma, rejection by the family, financial insecurity, dependence, and fear of disease and death increases depression. Up to 50–75% of older patients with HIV show depression. Depression can exacerbate immune dysfunction, nonadherence to all medications including ART, and an increase in the suicide rate.

CONCLUSION

Addressing and integrating NCDs in HIV care is important as the burden of NCDs is increasing globally. People now living longer with good ARTs and HIV care will experience more age-related NCDs with the interplay of traditional risk factors. HIV and NCDs pose more challenges in older persons due to immune dysfunction, polypharmacy, drug-drug interactions, ART toxicity, depression, and frailty. These challenges can be met by:

- Widening of management focus
- Strengthening of screening guidelines
- Enforcement of lifestyle modification strategies
- Use of statins and bisphosphonates when needed
- Close watch over comorbidities with the initiation of highly active antiretroviral therapy (HAART)
- Individualizing a suitable alternative regimen, if needed
- Giving some extra time to them

SUGGESTED READINGS

1. Smit M, Brinkman K, Geerlings S, Smit C, Thyagarajan K, van Sighem A, et al. Future challenges for clinical care of an aging population infected with HIV: a modeling study. Lancet Infect Dis. 2015;15(7):810-8.
2. Duffy M, Ojikutu B, Andrian S, Sohng E, Minior T, Hirschhorn LR. Noncommunicable diseases and HIV care and treatment: models of integrated service delivery. Trop Med Int Health. 2017;22(8):926-37.
3. Casper C, Crane H, Menon M, Money D. HIV/AIDS comorbidities: impact on cancer, noncommunicable diseases, and reproductive health. In: Holmes KH, Bertozzi S, Bloom BR, Jha P (Eds). Major Infectious Diseases, 3rd edition. Washington (DC): The International Bank for Reconstruction and Development/The World Bank; 2017.
4. Ledergerber B, Egger M, Opravil M, Telenti A, Hirschel B, Battegay M, et al. Clinical progression and virological failure on highly active antiretroviral therapy in HIV-1 patients: a prospective cohort study. Swiss HIV Cohort Study. Lancet. 1999;353(9156):863-8.

94

CHAPTER

Geriatric Nephrology: Whose Time has Come

Narinder Pal Singh, Dinesh Khullar, Anish Kumar Gupta

ABSTRACT

The aging population in India presents numerous healthcare challenges, with kidney disease emerging as a prominent concern due to its substantial burden, significant cost implications, and limited awareness. A significant proportion of individuals with chronic kidney disease (CKD) also contend with multiple concurrent medical conditions. In the field of geriatric nephrology, geriatric syndromes add further complexities for nephrologists. The shortage of adequately trained geriatricians compounds this issue, often requiring nephrologists to take on roles akin to internists or geriatric specialists. Geriatric nephrology is a complex and multifaceted field that necessitates a coordinated and comprehensive care approach. Both geriatricians and nephrologists in a single platform are crucial for optimal healthcare delivery. Geriatricians can contribute by conducting comprehensive geriatric assessments, assisting in long-term care planning, and engaging in discussions about palliative care. On the other hand, nephrologists play a vital role in addressing and managing medical conditions, preparing and delivering dialysis when needed. This collaborative approach not only enhances treatment strategies but also has the potential to reduce healthcare costs. This article emphasizes the necessity of integrating geriatrics into nephrology, highlighting its critical role in providing the best possible patient care and ultimately leading to improved healthcare outcomes.

INTRODUCTION

The aging of our population is an undeniable reality, and nephrologists must prepare for the consequences of this demographic shift. The projected increase in the elderly population (those over 65) in the coming decades presents significant challenges for the healthcare system. Globally, life expectancy is rising, with an average of 76.5 years in developed countries and 65.4 years in developing ones. However, these numbers vary across different developing countries. To illustrate, India is home to approximately 138 million elderly citizens, with 67 million being males and 71 million females. The proportion of the elderly population in India has already risen to 10.1% in 2021 and is projected to reach 13.1% by 2031. This shift in the age pyramid is reshaping healthcare needs, especially in fields like nephrology, giving rise to the specialized discipline of geriatric nephrology. Nephrologists are increasingly encountering older patients with unique challenges, from diagnosing and treating diseases with comorbidities to balancing quality of life with aggressive treatment options. This demographic change presents nephrologists with unprecedented epidemiological, research, and clinical challenges, as nephrology training traditionally lacks geriatric medicine components.

HISTORY OF GERIATRIC NEPHROLOGY

The demographic composition of the global population has undergone substantial changes since the term "geriatrics" was first coined in 1909. In recognition of the anticipated demands associated with an increasingly elderly population in the 21st century, the field of geriatric nephrology was formally established as a specialized discipline in 1980. Notably, in 1985, the inaugural international symposium on geriatric nephrology convened in Toronto, Canada, culminating in the establishment of the International Society of Geriatric Nephrology and the launch of its dedicated journal. Despite these initiatives, interest among nephrologists in the field of geriatric nephrology did not witness significant growth and, if anything, experienced a decline. However, since 2002, the American Society of Nephrology and various other nephrology societies have joined forces with the association of specialty professors to provide grants aimed at training the next generation of scholars and leaders specializing in the geriatric aspects of nephrology.

CHALLENGES OF AN AGING INDIAN POPULATION

The elderly population, especially those in the very elderly category, is anticipated to experience the most significant growth in the coming century, making kidney disease an increasingly prevalent issue among the geriatric population. Aging leads to age-related changes in the function and structure of the kidneys, contributing to the overall prevalence of kidney diseases. Multiple studies have highlighted that CKD predominantly affect the elderly. Managing renal diseases in older patients presents challenges not only to internists but also to geriatric-trained physicians due to various factors. It is crucial to differentiate between age-related decline in kidney function and intrinsic renal diseases in this age group. Furthermore, predicting the progression of kidney disease in older adults is a complex task, and the formulas used for categorizing kidney disease, such as the Modification of Diet in Renal Disease (MDRD) equation, have their limitations. The CKD Epidemiology Collaboration equation has been suggested as an alternative with improved accuracy.

The elderly CKD population often presents with concurrent medical conditions such as atherosclerotic cardiovascular disease, congestive heart failure, hypertension, diabetes, cognitive impairments, and functional limitations. Managing drug therapy in elderly patients is intricate, and this complexity escalates when renal disease is involved. Approximately one-third of prescription drugs are consumed by geriatric patients, but there is a lack of comprehensive clinical data on drug dosing for elderly individuals with kidney disease. Adverse events occur at a significantly higher rate in elderly patients with kidney disease, posing challenges for internists and geriatricians in terms of effectively managing drug dosages, mitigating side effects, and addressing complications. Moreover, the management of fluid and electrolytes may necessitate a different approach in this population when compared to adults.

GERIATRIC SYNDROMES IN NEPHROLOGY

Geriatric syndromes refer to clinical health conditions that are distinct to the elderly population and do not fall under disease-specific categories. Examples include cognitive impairment, falls, dizziness, incontinence, and frailty. Renal disease and dialysis can exacerbate geriatric syndromes, leading to poor outcomes. Dialysis, in particular, can worsen cognitive function, increase hospitalizations, and pose risks of falls due to dialysis-related complications. The risk is further elevated by anorexia, depression, and nutritional losses during dialysis.

THE NEED FOR COLLABORATION BETWEEN GERIATRICS AND NEPHROLOGY

The absence of a geriatric curriculum in nephrology training and the scarcity of geriatricians underscore the critical importance of collaboration and care coordination between geriatricians and nephrologists. It is imperative to establish comanagement teams at an early stage in the disease process to tailor patient care according to their specific goals and needs. Geriatricians play a pivotal role by conducting comprehensive geriatric assessments, encompassing evaluations of cognitive, functional, and psychosocial aspects. This assessment aids in the identification of potential issues and the provision of appropriate treatments as the disease advances. Nephrologists, on the other hand, can actively contribute to managing fluid and electrolyte balance, addressing anemia, managing bone mineral diseases, and ensuring appropriate drug monitoring and dosing right from the initial stages of the disease. Complex decisions regarding issues like dialysis in the geriatric population should be made with input from multiple perspectives, including patients, caregivers, families, and the collaborative geriatrician-nephrologist team.

CHALLENGES FOR NEPHROLOGISTS IN GERIATRIC PATIENT CARE

Several challenges specifically affect nephrologists caring for geriatric patients, including knowledge gaps in understanding the pathogenesis, diagnosis, and therapy of kidney disease in the elderly. Critical research questions remain unanswered, such as whether CKD in elderly patients is distinct from CKD in younger patients and how age-related kidney changes influence CKD progression. Additionally, age-related clinical variations exist, affecting the diagnosis and treatment of conditions such as hypertension, glomerular diseases, diabetes, cardiovascular disease, and acute kidney injury. For example, age-related changes in the renin–angiotensin–aldosterone system may impact the efficacy of certain drugs.

Nephrologists often find themselves assuming the roles of primary care physicians for patients on maintenance dialysis, despite lacking specific geriatric training. This responsibility includes addressing issues such as fall risk, frailty, dementia, delirium, depression, polypharmacy, and urinary incontinence, all of which are common in elderly patients. Changes in dialysis reimbursement may further affect the management of these comorbid conditions. Nephrologists must also consider the physiological changes in the kidneys, such as the decline in estimated glomerular filtration rate (eGFR) with age, when assessing kidney function in the elderly. Additionally, pharmacokinetics and pharmacodynamics of drugs differ in the elderly, making drug prescribing more complex.

THE ROLE OF NEPHROLOGISTS IN GERIATRIC PATIENT CARE

With the increasing demand for geriatric care and a potential decrease in physicians seeking geriatric medicine training, nephrologists must address the challenges of aging patients with kidney disease. Elderly CKD patients often experience medical complexity, chronic conditions, coordination challenges, and administrative burdens. Nephrologists are tasked with managing complications such as cardiovascular disease, anemia, hypertension, malnutrition, and bone disease in elderly CKD patients. As primary care physicians seek assistance in managing these patients, nephrologists must understand the interactions between aging and kidney disease to provide effective care.

Nephrologists also play a crucial role in patients on maintenance dialysis, taking on responsibilities that resemble those of primary care physicians. This role involves addressing issues such as fall risk, frailty, dementia, delirium, depression, polypharmacy, and urinary incontinence in patients they follow over time. Changes in dialysis reimbursement, such as bundled payments for services, may impact the management of these comorbid conditions. Nephrologists need education in geriatrics, particularly in addressing quality of life issues and making informed decisions about dialysis for patients aged over 85 and their families.

Additionally, nephrologists must consider age-related anatomical and physiological changes in the kidneys, such as the gradual decline in GFR **(Fig. 1)**. These changes can lead to mislabeling of elderly patients with moderate CKD, even when their age-adjusted GFR is normal. Serum creatinine levels may not accurately reflect kidney function in older adults due to factors like loss of lean body mass.

In terms of therapeutics, nephrologists must account for the altered pharmacodynamics and pharmacokinetics of drugs in the elderly, as well as the potential for polypharmacy and its associated risks. Nephrologists should also be mindful of the socioeconomic burden that medication costs may impose on fixed-income elderly patients.

Ultimately, the goal of geriatric nephrology is to preserve or enhance the quality of life for elderly patients. Palliative care plays a crucial role in managing symptoms, optimizing well-being, and preserving dignity in advanced kidney disease patients. Advance care planning and open discussions about end-of-life decisions are integral components of holistic care for this vulnerable population.

GOVERNMENT INITIATIVES ON ELDERLY HEALTHCARE IN INDIA

The Government of India has taken significant steps to address the healthcare needs of senior citizens. Initiatives like the National Program for the Health Care of Elderly, formulated in 2011, aim to provide elderly individuals with access to a wide range of healthcare services, including preventive, promotive, curative, and rehabilitative care. This program also emphasizes specialized training for healthcare professionals to meet the growing health needs of the elderly. Health and Wellness Centers under the Ayushman Bharat program further enhance healthcare access for the elderly at primary healthcare settings.

CONCLUSION

Geriatric nephrology is emerging as an essential subspecialty equipped to address the evolving healthcare landscape characterized by an aging population. This multifaceted discipline encompasses epidemiology, clinical presentation, diagnosis, treatment, prevention, palliative care, and research. As the world grapples with the challenges of kidney disease in an aging society, the time for geriatric nephrology has undoubtedly arrived. There is a growing body of literature and increasing attention devoted to geriatric issues within nephrology, reflecting the increasing importance of this field.

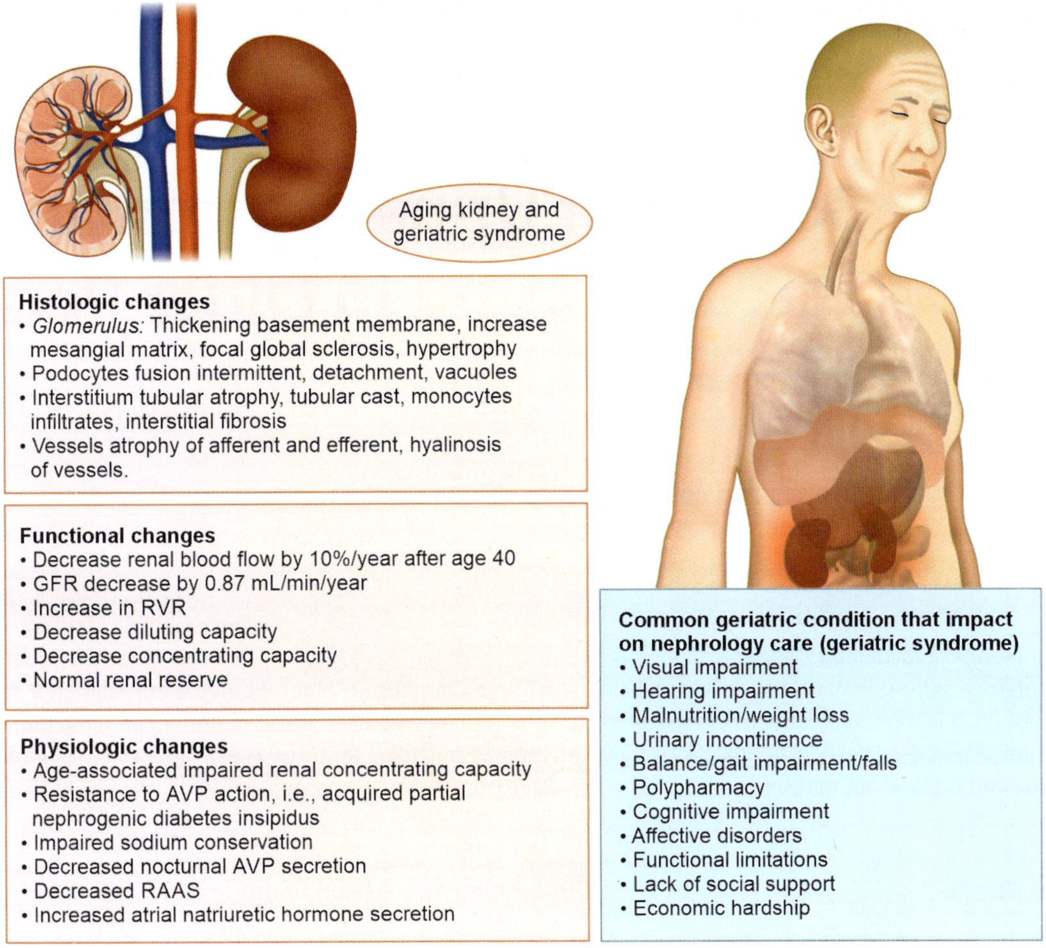

FIG. 1: Addressing multifaceted issues encompassing age-related changes in the kidney and geriatric syndrome.
(AVP: arginine vasopressin; RAAS: renin–angiotensin–aldosterone system)

SUGGESTED READINGS

1. Online curricula: Geriatric Nephrology. [online] Available from https://www.asn-online.org/education/distancelearning/curricula/geriatrics/ [Last accessed December, 2023].
2. Ahmed FA. Kidney Disease in Elderly: Importance of Collaboration between Geriatrics and Nephrology. Aging Dis. 2018;9(4):745-7.
3. Schlanger LE, Bailey JL, Sands JM. Geriatric nephrology: old or new subspecialty. Clin Geriatr Med. 2009;25(3):311-24.
4. Rosner M, Abdel-Rahman E, Williams ME; ASN Advisory Group on Geriatric Nephrology. Geriatric nephrology: responding to a growing challenge. Clin J Am Soc Nephrol. 2010;5(5):936-42.

95

CHAPTER

Burden of Urinary Incontinence in Older Persons

Alpana Raizada, Ashish Goel

ABSTRACT

Urinary incontinence or involuntary leakage of urine is a common problem in older patients impacting their independence, mobility, autonomy, self-esteem, and social acceptance. It is more common in older women especially after multiple or difficult parturition. It is commonly underreported and often inadequately treated. Stress incontinence is the most common type seen in clinical practice. Lifestyle modifications, behavior therapy, and mechanical devices in addition to pharmacological therapy are the cornerstone of treatment.

INTRODUCTION

Involuntary leakage of urine is a problem commonly perceived by the older persons as a part of aging. The prevalence of the condition has been variably estimated depending upon the definition used and the population being studied. Some studies have even reported a prevalence as high as 55% among older persons more so in women and those in long-term care facilities. Incontinence of urine, unlike many other medical conditions, impacts not only the physical life of the individual but also results in social isolation, poor hygiene, and considerable stigma. While most patients experience minor and occasional leakage during periods of increased stress, some may experience more severe leakage and dribbling.

PRESENTATION

Patients often tend to ignore leakage of urine and are embarrassed to discuss this problem with family or peers. They are hesitant to approach the healthcare systems for issues related to incontinence unless it becomes severe. A typical patient with urinary incontinence would be an obese older female with multiple child births and often with comorbid conditions. Female sex, older age, and obesity have been found to be associated with increased risk for incontinence. Other risk factors that have been associated with incontinence include drugs such as diuretics, psychotropics, and narcotics besides substance abuse.

While evaluating a patient presenting with urinary incontinence it is important to elicit the *history* of frequency, quantity, urgency, hesitancy, nocturia, enuresis, post-void dribbling, incomplete voiding, poor urine stream, and leakage with cough. It is important to elicit the history of medication history, caffeine intake, and substance abuse. A history of surgical procedures in the past involving catheterization, dilation, etc., may be helpful in identifying the appropriate cause for incontinence. It is important to remember that incontinence may merely be a presentation of another unrelated illness in the older persons where the disease pathways overlap resulting in common symptoms. A search for stroke or pneumonia may be reasonable in an older person presenting with acute onset of symptoms of leakage of urine when no clear cause is identified. While evaluating a patient presenting with incontinence who complains of leakage happening during coughing, sneezing or other actions where intra-abdominal pressure may be increased, it may be helpful to perform a stress test where the individual is asked to cough while observing the urethral meatus for minimal amounts of leakage. This is helpful in identifying minor degrees of incontinence.

Standardized assessment tools are available for evaluation of incontinence in the form of a urogenital distress inventory developed to determine how troubling the symptoms are. It includes questions around frequency, urgency, physical activity, amount, straining, and pain. The incontinence impact questionnaire includes questions around ability to participate in household chores, physical recreation, entertainment (movies), travel, social activities besides exploring the individual's mental health, and frustration.

Types of Urinary Incontinence (Table 1)

Several types of incontinence have been described and can be differentiated on clinical assessment:

- *Stress incontinence* involves leakage of small amounts of urine with episodes of increase in intra-abdominal pressure while coughing, sneezing, etc. This is often due to sphincter damage or prolapse of pelvic structures in women. It has been found to be associated with genetic factors, multiple and/or difficult childbirth leading to poor pelvic tone, smoking, and obesity.
- *Urge incontinence* occurs when there is a delay in voiding resulting in an inability to hold urine after an urge is perceived. This is often seen in central nervous system conditions resulting in uninhibited bladder contractions such as stroke, Parkinson's disease, dementia, multiple sclerosis, prostatic obstruction, and following prostatectomy.
- *Overflow incontinence* is the leakage of small amounts of urine without the urge to void when the bladder is full. This is often seen in obstructive lesions such as benign hyperplasia of prostate, urethral stricture or in patients with hypotonic bladder seen in diabetes, syphilis or spinal cord compression. This is typical of a lower motor neuron involvement.
- *Functional incontinence* occurs when the patient is unable to void due to medical or psychosocial conditions limiting his mobility or access to a toilet. This may be seen in conditions such as arthritis.
- *Reflex incontinence* occurs when contractions occur with little amounts of urine reaching the bladder. This occurs due to impaired neurological control. The patient feels no urge and often the volume is small.
- *Transient incontinence* may occur due to acute and reversible medical conditions. The symptoms recover with the correction of the underlying problem. One in three of all presentations are transient and will recover. Acute confusional states, drug or toxin intake, electrolyte imbalance, and other medical conditions may cause transient incontinence.
- *Mixed incontinence* is seen when the symptoms suggest a combination of more than one type of incontinence above.

TABLE 1: Types of incontinence.

Type	Pathology	Presentation	Test	Management
Stress	Pelvic floor muscle dysfunction and poor urinary sphincter function	Activity related Leakage occurs during cough, sneezing, laughing, lifting, walking, or bending Volume small; No urge	*Cough test*: Patient is asked to cough and any leakage of urine is directly observed	• Kegel exercises to improve pelvic floor strength • Duloxetin in older women
Urge: Overactive bladder	• Detrusor hyperactivity or instability • LOCAL – Inflammation or irritation of bladder (malignancy, calculus, infection, or vaginitis/urethritis) • CNS – Loss of central inhibition (stroke, PD or AD)	Frequent need to pass urine, inability to control Volume maybe large; Urge +	Post-void residual (PVR) urine measurement by bladder scan or catheterization	• Reduce caffeine and fluid intake • Weight loss if obese • Pelvic floor exercises • Bladder training • Anticholinergic drugs
Overflow	• Obstruction (BPH) • Contractile bladder—diabetic neuropathy, spinal cord injury • Neurogenic bladder—MS • Drugs (sedatives, ACEI, etc.) • LMN lesion	Poor stream of urine, incomplete voiding, constant dribbling of urine Volume small; No urge	Digital rectal examination and pelvic scanning	• Alpha blockers (tamsulosin, alfuzosin, silodosin, doxazosin) • Remove obstruction (surgical/pharmacological) • Intermittent self-catheterization

Continued

Continued

Type	Pathology	Presentation	Test	Management
Reflex: • Unaware incontinence • Unconscious incontinence	• Spasm of bladder after spinal (injury/trauma) or supraspinal reflex (MS, stroke, AD, PD) • UMN lesion	Volume small or large; No urge	Urine analysis	• Reduce caffeine and fluid intake • Weight loss if obese • Pelvic floor exercises • Bladder training • Anticholinergic drugs
Mixed		Combination of stress and urge incontinence Volume small to large; Urge +		An individualized treatment approach is needed
Functional	• Cognitive impairment • Limited physical functioning • Environmental barriers	Leakage of urine before patient can get up and reach the toilet Volume large; Urge +	Patient is asked to get up from a sitting position with arms crossed to test for balance, gait, and mobility	Treatment involves attention to underlying cause
Transient	Reversible medical condition such as acute confusional state, UTI, hyperglycemia, hypercalcemia, constipation, or increased intake of fluids	Causes of transient incontinence can be remembered using the acronym DIAPPERS (Delirium, Infection, Atrophic vaginitis, Pharmacological intake, Psychological factors, Excessive fluids, Restricted mobility, Stool impaction)		Treatment should include attention to the underlying cause

[ACEI: angiotensinogen converting enzyme blocker (may worsen stress incontinence); AD: Alzheimer's dementia; MS: multiple sclerosis; PD: Parkinson's disease; UTI: urinary tract infection]

MANAGEMENT OF URINARY INCONTINENCE

The management of incontinence of urine is always challenging and needs to be individualized according to the patient's lifestyles, social expectations, and needs. Nonpharmacological approaches to optimize quality of life while living with incontinence are as important as drugs and medications to control symptoms where the cause cannot be identified or alleviated.

Nonpharmacological Interventions

- *Lifestyle modification* involving regulating the amount and frequency of fluid intake while reducing the use of caffeinated beverages is important to improve incontinence. Attention to diet while avoiding bladder irritants such as spices, artificial sweeteners, and citrus fruits is important. Similarly, maintaining a regular physical activity schedule, reducing obesity, and avoiding smoking are helpful in controlling symptoms.
- *Absorbent pads* have been used for enuresis in children as well as older adults. Similarly, diapers can be used during the day to allow mobility and flexibility in day-to-day activities.
- *Pelvic floor muscle exercise training* involving strengthening exercises for pelvic muscles has been found to reduce frequency of leakage episodes and improve quality of life. Kegel exercises are beneficial in both men and women. Vaginal weight training with graded cones of different weights is helpful in improving muscle tone and reducing leakage.

> *Kegel exercises* involve sustained contraction of pelvic muscles. To identify the right muscles, one needs to try to stop passage of flatus by contracting the muscles around the anal sphincter. Once correctly identified, the patient tries to hold the contraction for a count of ten. While the recommendations on the number of repeats in each performance and the number of performances differ in literature, the patient could be advised to perform three to four sets of exercises at one time and repeat ten times during the day. Three to five repetitions performed three times a day have shown improvement after 2–6 months in 50–80% individuals.

- *Bladder training* includes maintenance of voidance diaries, following a scheduled voiding pattern while trying to postpone micturition to improve bladder capacity and sphincter strength. The individual is advised to delay voiding each time there is an urge and void at specific times and intervals. The patients are

advised to focus on deeper breathing while taking the mind away from the urge. They are in turn encouraged to void once the urge has been successfully controlled. Prompted and scheduled voiding may be effective in cases where bladder training is not helpful in order to control incontinence in cognitively impaired individuals. It is initiated by giving regular verbal reminders by caregivers while supporting the patient to the bathroom while providing positive reinforcement and encouragement if voiding occurs. This reduces episodes of incontinence.
- *Sacral neuromodulation* and *tibial nerve stimulation* are other novel approaches that have been tried, but with variable response.

Pharmacological Interventions

Several therapeutic agents are available for control of symptoms:

- *Anticholinergic agents* are useful in cases of urge incontinence due to an overactive bladder and help in suppressing excessive detrusor muscle contractions. Agents such as oxybutynin, tolterodine, darifenacin, solifenacin, and trospium have been used. Anticholinergic agents often cause dryness which may further cause dysphagia for older persons in addition to cognitive impairment which limits their use. Presence of glaucoma, constipation, and gastroesophageal reflux in older persons may often limit their use.
- β_3 agonist Mirabegron has been tried as an alternative to anticholinergic drugs and has been found to be free of major side effects in initial studies.
- *Botulinum toxin type A* injection in the detrusor muscle just below the bladder mucosa has been used with some therapeutic benefit in patients with detrusor-sphincter dyssynergia and incontinence due to neurogenic detrusor over-activity.
- *Serotonin reuptake inhibitor*, duloxetine has been found to be effective in reducing incontinence in older women with stress incontinence.
- *Local application of estrogen* has been tried with some benefit in postmenopausal women.
- *Stem cell therapy* has been found helpful in preclinical models and their role is being explored, although this has not been licensed for clinical use at the present time.

Surgical Interventions

The role of surgery in management of urinary incontinence remains limited but has proven to be of benefit especially in stress incontinence in women. Intermittent or indwelling self-retaining *catheterization* may be needed where symptoms are not controlled after lifestyle changes and pharmacological therapy of when these are not possible. *External collection systems* may be used in men. *Mid urethral sling procedures* have gained acceptance due to relative ease. *Urethral bulking agents* increase urethral wall thickness and urethral closing pressure. Autologous fat and other inert substances have been tried. However, the results are poor and often repeat procedures are required. *Artificial urinary sphincters* have been used with success in severe stress incontinence. Future research involving automated control systems may result in significant improvement in the life of people living with incontinence.

Appropriate, timely and repeated attention to skin care is important in all patients with incontinence in order to prevent pressure sores especially in bed bound patients with limited mobility.

Urinary Incontinence in Older Adults

Recognized as one of the traditional *Geriatric Giants,* incontinence of urine is more common and more severe in older persons and is often associated with significant comorbidity. Association with falls, pressure ulcers, urinary tract infection, and fractures is well known. It is often more difficult to manage in frail older persons in institutional settings especially when associated with severe dementia. It is associated with an increased risk of falls. A personalized multicomponent therapeutic approach is often required.

APPROACH TO INCONTINENCE

- *Step 1:* Identify the type of incontinence
  - Is there an urge before incontinence of urine?
  - What is the frequency of incontinence?
  - Is it related to coughing, sneezing, straining, or another event that causes increase in intra-abdominal pressure?
  - What is the amount of urine passed with each episode of incontinence?
  - Is there burning, pain, or dysuria associated with incontinence?
- *Step 2:* Elicit the associated features with the type of incontinence identified
  - Stress
  - Overflow
  - Reflex
- *Step 3:* Can the cause be removed/repaired/corrected? Is it transient? If a transient cause is found, this should be corrected?
- *Step 4:* Is the condition treatable or reparable?
- *Step 5:* Optimization of quality of life with non/pharmacological interventions.

CONCLUSION

While literature around the occurrence of incontinence of urine remains limited, its impact is under-recognized. The stigmatic social isolation impacts not only autonomy and self-respect but also quality of life in older adults. A scientific approach helps in identifying the pathophysiology and cause of incontinence as the management of these individuals often continues to be challenging.

SUGGESTED READINGS

1. United Kingdom: National Institute for Health and Care Excellence. (2019). Urinary incontinence and pelvic organ prolapse in women: management. [online] Available from: https://www.nice.org.uk/guidance/ng123. [Last accessed January, 2024].
2. The American College of Clinical Pharmacy. (2013). Urinary Incontinence in the older adult 2013. [online] [Available from: https://www.accp.com/docs/bookstore/psap/p13b2_m1ch.pdf. [Last accessed January, 2024].
3. Gallo F, Ninotta G, Schenone M, Cortese P, Giberti C. Advances in stem cell therapy for male stress urinary incontinence. Expert Opin Biol Ther. 2019;19(4):293-300.
4. McDonnell B, Birder LA. Recent advances in pharmacological management of urinary incontinence. F1000Res. 2017;6:21-48.

96

CHAPTER

Uses of Anticoagulants in Geriatric Clinical Practice

Jayanta Sharma, Meghna Dutta

ABSTRACT

In our daily clinical practice, we encounter large number of elderly people with multiple comorbidities. It is often not feasible to apply the existing guidelines, which must sometimes be amended to the patient we are treating, especially the elder ones. With age the risk of thrombosis and bleeding increases, as well as the prevalence of geriatric syndromes. This can have undesirable implications on the efficacy and safety of anticoagulant therapy.

The arrival of non-vitamin K oral antagonists heralded a major advancement in anticoagulant therapy, principally for the elderly age group, as they are safer than conventional vitamin K antagonists (VKAs), such as warfarin. Direct oral anticoagulants (DOACs), commonly known as novel oral anticoagulants (NOACs), are often administered in lower doses than those recommended by the guidelines, because of increased risk or fear of bleeding. Inadequate treatment in older patients contribute significantly toward preventable morbidity and mortality. Treating physicians should target their efforts on avoiding concomitant therapies that augment bleeding. Close clinical follow-up of those receiving anticoagulation therapy can help extract maximum benefits and prevent adverse outcomes.

INTRODUCTION

The risk of falls increases with age. Anticoagulants may augment the risk of intracranial hemorrhage associated with falling, but the absolute risk is comparatively low compared to the probability of ischemic stroke and venous thromboembolism (VTE).

Addressing preventable risk factors for falls and bleeding can make anticoagulant therapy safer. Atrial fibrillation (AF) is asymptomatic in large number of cases and may be identified at a later date incidentally or once the patient has a stroke, leading to delay in initiation of anticoagulation therapy in those cases. Although these agents are less likely to be avoided in people with VTE, we need to consider the risk of recurrence of such events and the risk of bleeding when deciding regarding extension of treatment with these molecules.

Anticoagulants are used prophylactically against VTE in situations where mobility is reduced for a considerable period of time, and lifelong following replacement of a mechanical heart valve and when a bioprosthetic heart valve has been implanted. Patients who have successfully undergone ablation, anticoagulation therapy is required for at least 8 weeks postprocedure, otherwise lifelong uses are recommended in reducing the risk of stroke in patients with AF.

The CHA_2DS_2-VASc score is widely accepted and recommended to determine the possibility of stroke and whether treatment with anticoagulation therapy is required or not. In elderly, the benefit of anticoagulation is mainly observed in those having moderate to high risk of stroke. The risk of stroke is then weighed against the chances of bleeding with different guidelines recommending various scores. The National Institute for Health and Care Excellence (NICE) guidelines recommended the Outcomes Registry for Better Informed Treatment (ORBIT) score to discriminate between high versus low risk of bleeding, whereas the European Society of Cardiology (ESC) advocates the use of HAS-BLED score to assess major bleeding. International nationalized ratio (INR) is a dynamic variable used to determine the dose of vitamin K antagonists (VKAs), which are less frequent in use now, hence HAS-BLED has lost its significance; ORBIT can be used for both novel oral anticoagulants (NOACs) and VKAs. The main objective of these scores is to ascertain potentially modifiable risk factors for bleeding including control of hypertension, uses of other medications, consumption of alcohol, etc.

In deep venous thromboembolism (DVT) or pulmonary embolism (PE), anticoagulation therapy is recommended for all patients for at least 3 months duration and for a maximum of up to 6 months for patients with active malignant disease. Long-term uses of anticoagulants are needed in people with history of recurrent VTE that have irreversible risk factors and those having antiphospholipid syndrome.

CHOOSING THE RIGHT ANTICOAGULANT

When VKAs were discovered in the early 1940s, they were the only oral anticoagulants available for use. However, in 2008 a new class of drugs were licensed, the NOACs. The NOACs outweighed the VKAs in many aspects such as the availability of fixed dosage regimens, lesser number of drug-drug interactions and drug-food interactions, and not requiring frequent blood tests. Thereby the newer group of drugs ensured better compliance from the elderly patients and better feasibility of monitoring on part of the physicians.

Several randomized control trials proved NOACs to be equally effective as warfarin in the prevention of cerebrovascular accidents in the geriatric population having AF. NOACs were associated with significantly decreased chances of intracranial hemorrhages. Observational studies on the population aged ≥75 years showed that the resultant clinical benefit after considering both the stroke risk reduction and the tendency to bleed, was more in favor of NOACs than warfarin.

PARENTERAL ANTICOAGULANTS

Parenteral anticoagulant agents are used for prevention and treatment of thromboembolism. Three types of molecules are present in this group, namely, unfractionated heparin (UFH), low molecular weight heparin (LMWH), and synthetic heparin such as fondaparinux.

Heparin is the preferred agent for inpatient anticoagulation. Side effects with this molecule include complications from bleeding and heparin-induced thrombocytopenia (HIT). Therefore, close monitoring of platelet count needs to be done on patients who are on parenteral anticoagulants such as heparin **(Table 1)**.

Unfractionated heparin is the anticoagulant of choice in elderly patients who are prone to blood loss, critically ill, or need surgical intervention. This is because of its short half-life that ranges from 30 to 90 minutes, leading to rapid onset and offset of its effects within hours of intravenous discontinuation. Besides, owing to its unique metabolism and clearance through the reticuloendothelial system, it is a favorable option for subjects with impaired or unstable renal function. Also, due to the absence of cytochrome p450 activity in the liver, drug interactions with UFH are limited to elevated risk of bleed when used simultaneously with antiplatelet agents

Low molecular weight heparin offer the advantage of uniform anticoagulant effect when administered via subcutaneous route and after dose adjustment according to body weight. It is the anticoagulation of choice in pregnancy and malignancy. The risk of HIT is low with LMWH as compared to UFH.

For reversal of UFH and LMWH associated bleeds, protamine sulfate is the recommended reversal agent. With LMWH, only partial reversal is noted with protamine, since binding exclusively occurs with long and large molecular weight heparin molecules.

Treatment guidelines are different in management of PE in special populations. Patients having malignancy, pregnancy, obesity, renal impairment, hepatic impairment, coronavirus infection, etc. LMWH is recommended over therapy with VKAs.

Prophylaxis against PE in inpatients involves use of either LMWH, or low-dose UFH which may be administered at an interval of 12 or 8 hours, or synthetic heparin. In cases with a PE triggered by an operative procedure, anticoagulation is recommended for a minimum of 3 months. On the contrary, in cases where the PE has occurred unprovoked, the risk of blood loss determines the duration of therapy. However, in cases

TABLE 1: Classification of anticoagulants.

Anticoagulants	Parenteral	Indirect		• Unfractionated heparin • Low molecular weight heparin • Fondaparinux • M118
Anticoagulants	Parenteral	Direct	Thrombin inhibitors	• Hirudin • Bivalirudin • Argatroban
Anticoagulants	Parenteral	Direct	Factor Xa inhibitors	Otamixaban
Anticoagulants	Oral	Indirect		Vitamin K antagonists
Anticoagulants	Oral	Direct	Thrombin inhibitors	Dabigatran
Anticoagulants	Oral	Direct	Factor Xa inhibitors	• Rivaroxaban • Apixaban • Edoxaban

with high tendency to bleed, the duration of treatment is confined to 90 days. In situations where patients are at low to moderate risk of bleeding, the duration of therapy becomes undefined.

NOVEL ORAL ANTICOAGULANTS

Also known as direct oral anticoagulants (DOACs) or non-VKA oral anticoagulants, NOACs have a marked advantage over warfarin in that they can be given in fixed doses without routine coagulation monitoring, hence simplifying patient management and increasing adherence, leading to their mention in globally recommended guidelines.

This class of drugs include direct thrombin inhibitors such as dabigatran and factor Xa inhibitors namely, rivaroxaban, apixaban, betrixaban, and edoxaban.

Factor Xa inhibitors apixaban and rivaroxaban are the NOACs that are most often in use. Modified doses of NOACs have been recommended by international guidelines for patients with preexisting risks of drug accumulation, such as older age, low body weight, impaired renal function, or parallel use of other drugs which may interact with the prescribed anticoagulant.

The highest prevalence of comorbid conditions is witnessed in the very elderly patients. This inclines them to drug accumulation and hence they are amongst those at the maximum risk of bleeding complications. No wonder, doctors are quite hesitant to prescribe anticoagulants or to use the recommended dose of NOACs in later decades of life. Real-world data including community-based registries have regularly revealed that up to 50% of very elderly patients with AF who match guideline indications for oral anticoagulation remain untreated, while many of those treated with a NOAC received suboptimal dose. It may also be noted that these geriatric AF patients symbolize a clinically complex phenotype, which is associated with a significantly higher risk of stroke and bleeding, as well as a greater risk of anticoagulant interruption.

Apixaban and rivaroxaban are cleared via predominantly extra-renal pathways, there is minimal effect on the variability in drug levels in the setting of advanced age and impaired renal function. Both these drugs can be safely administered in advanced age and kidney disease. Guidelines endorse regular monitoring of kidney function in patients who are on these drugs.

Major bleeding in comparison to thromboembolic events at 6 months in very elderly patients with AF may prompt physicians to doubt the net advantage of anticoagulant therapy, advanced age itself is a major risk factor for thromboembolism in subjects with AF, and randomized studies with both warfarin and very low-dose edoxaban have established the supremacy of anticoagulant therapy over lack of prophylactic therapy for stroke prevention in the very elderly.

Reduced incidence rates of thromboembolism with apixaban and rivaroxaban may be justified by the efficacy of these agents since both the drugs are expected to decrease the risk of stroke by approximately 67%.

CONCLUSION

Medication review and falls prevention strategies need to be implemented before initiation of anticoagulants. Despite of the raised incidence rates for major bleeding events, the best tactic to diminish morbidity and mortality in the very aged population with AF is to prescribe NOACs using the dosage regimens mentioned by the guidelines.

Deprescribing should be considered in severe frailty, limited life expectancy, and increased risk of bleeding (e.g., cerebral microbleeds). Shared decision making with the patients and their caregivers is pivotal as patient and prescriber views often differ.

SUGGESTED READINGS

1. National Institute for Health and Care Excellence. (2021). Atrial fibrillation: diagnosis and management. [online] Available from https://www.nice.org.uk/guidance/ng196. [Last accessed December, 2023].
2. Karamichalakis N, Georgopoulos S, Vlachos K, Liatakis I, Efremidis M, Sideris A, et al. Efficacy and safety of novel anticoagulants in the elderly. J Geriatr Cardiol. 2016;13:718-23.
3. Van Ganse E, Danchin N, Mahe I, Hanon O, Jacoud F, Nolin M, et al. Comparative safety and effectiveness of oral anticoagulants in nonvalvular atrial fibrillation: the NAXOS study. Stroke. 2020;51:2066-75.

97

CHAPTER

Perioperative Assessment in Geriatric Patients

Ravikeerthy M, Gopika Dineshan

ABSTRACT

The number of elderly patients undergoing elective and emergency surgeries is increasing, necessitating risk assessment and stratification. Excessive preoperative tests can lead to complications and delays. Postoperative care should support physiologic and social needs. Aging affects organ systems, necessitating assessment of functional reserve. Geriatric specialty care is crucial for achieving high-quality surgical care.

INTRODUCTION

There is an increase in the number of elderly patients undergoing elective and emergency surgeries. Risk assessment and stratification are important to devise proper management strategies. However, excessive and indiscriminate preoperative tests can lead to many consequences like unintentional delay in surgery, harm from additional workups and additional cost to the patient. Postoperative complications were more common with increasing age, with 20% of those ≥80 years old experiencing one or more complications compared with 12.1% in those <80 years of age. Perioperative care for older adults should be formulated in such a way that it supports their unique physiologic and social needs.

PREOPERATIVE CARE OF OLDER ADULTS

Preoperative care of older adults is directed at assessment of functional reserve to minimize any complications along with screening for common geriatric syndromes. Comprehensive geriatric assessment (CGA) is being increasingly used in the preoperative setup to meet this need.

Approach to preoperative assessment:
- History
- Assessment of functional reserve and review of organ systems
- Investigations based on assessment of functional reserve

History

History should be directed at general health, any comorbidities, especially drug use and compliance and allergies to any medications.

Assessment of Functional Reserve

There are two systems for assessment of functional reserve:
1. Metabolic equivalence
2. ASA (American Society of Anesthesiologists) status

Metabolic Equivalence

Surgery can lead to systemic inflammatory response which is often accompanied by a rise in oxygen requirement. Elderly patients with low cardiorespiratory reserve are unable to meet this rise during postoperative

TABLE 1: Duke Activity Status Index.

Metabolic equivalent	Common activities—are you able to:
1.75	Walk around the house/no stairs
2.70–2.75	Light housework (dusting, dishes); self-care (eating, bathing); walk two blocks slowly on flat ground
3.5	Moderate housework (vacuuming, carrying groceries)
4.5	Moderate yardwork (raking leaves, weeding)
5.5	Climb a flight of stairs or a short hill
6.0	Moderate recreation activities (doubles tennis, bowling, dancing)
7.5	Strenuous sports (singles tennis, basketball, vigorous swimming)
8.0	Heavy housework (scrubbing floors, moving furniture, shoveling snow); run a short distance

period creating oxygen debt. This functional limitation is assessed preoperatively as the number of metabolic equivalents (METS) that a patient can achieve. METS can be measured by objective tests like electrocardiogram (ECG) exercise testing or with the help of questionnaires like Duke Activity Status **(Table 1)**.

American Society of Anesthesiologists Status

The ASA physical status classification is based on identification of significant organ system dysfunction and severity of functional impairment.

- *ASA I*: Healthy patient; no organic disorder
- *ASA II*: Systemic disease that is well-controlled, either by the condition that is being treated or by another pathologic process [e.g., controlled hypertension, acute sinusitis, treated hypothyroidism, obesity [30 < body mass index (BMI) < 40]
- *ASA III*: Severe systemic disturbance from any cause or causes (e.g., complicated or uncontrolled diabetes mellitus, morbid obesity (BMI > 40), end-stage renal disease undergoing regular hemodialysis)
- *ASA IV*: Extreme systemic disturbance that is a constant threat to life (e.g., end-stage renal disease without regular dialysis; recent myocardial infarction or cerebrovascular accident)
- *ASA V*: Condition in which the patient will not survive without surgery (e.g., dissecting aortic aneurysm, massive trauma)
- *ASA VI*: A person who is brain-dead who is presenting for organ donation

The ASA status is a very good predictor of outcome in elderly patients. However, it does not include age of the patient, type of surgery, and physical and mental activities, all of which can affect the outcome in elderly patients.

Review of Organ Systems

Cardiovascular System

Age-related changes in cardiovascular system and high prevalence of comorbid conditions like hypertension, diabetes, and coronary artery disease increases the incidence of cardiovascular complications in elderly patients. ECG remains the most useful investigation.

Preoperative ECGs should be done in patients with cardiac risk factors or a history of cardiac disease and in those undergoing intermediate-risk or high-risk surgery. Echocardiography is another modality useful in assessing the function of myocardium.

Cerebrovascular disease especially of vertebral and carotid arteries should be assessed in patients undergoing carotid endarterectomy and surgeries where flexion and extension of neck is likely. Autonomic dysfunction is assessed to identify risk of reflex dysfunction. Exercise testing for ischemia is also a useful modality and in cases where there is limitation of movement, inotrope-induced stress test can be done.

Patients taking drugs for heart failure, hypertension, and ischemic heart disease should continue their medications in the perioperative period and should take the drugs on the day of surgery. Sudden withdrawal may be harmful, especially cessation of beta blockers. Only exception to this is angiotensin-converting enzyme (ACE) inhibitors which should be omitted on the day of surgery.

There is significant controversy regarding preoperative blood pressure control and the decision to treat or postpone a surgery. In a study done by Weksler et al. in patients with poorly controlled hypertension presenting for elective surgery, patients were randomized to a control group, in which surgery was delayed to allow blood pressure therapy, or a treatment group, who received acute treatment to bring the diastolic blood pressure to <110 mm Hg. However, results showed that there was no difference in adverse cardiac events between the two groups. A systematic review and meta-analysis of association of hypertensive disease and perioperative complications also was unable to show the clear relationship between hypertension and adverse cardiac events.

Respiratory System

Age-related changes in the respiratory system can reduce pulmonary reserve, increasing the risk of perioperative pulmonary complications. In routine investigations, arterial blood gas analysis and chest X-ray do provide useful information. A "6-minute walk test" is a good predictor of the patient's ability to withstand a major surgery. Pulmonary function testing for peak flow rate, forced expiratory volume in 1 second (FEV_1), and forced vital capacity (FVC) also helps in the estimation of physiological reserve.

Nervous System

Age-related changes in the brain increases the vulnerability to systemic stressors such as surgery. Developing delirium in the early postoperative period is associated with long-term consequences, including increased mortality, prolonged hospitalization, discharge to an institution, long-term cognitive decline and dementia. Postoperative cognitive dysfunction has also been associated with higher mortality, and inability to return to previous function and dementia.

History should be sought regarding any recent surgeries with particular emphasis on the incidence of interval delirium or confusion, which indicates a very high risk for postoperative cognitive impairment. Commonly used cognitive screening tools include the Mini Mental Status Evaluation, Animal Fluency Test, the Montreal Cognitive Assessment, and the Mini-Cog.

Hepatic System

Liver dysfunction is usually suspected on the basis of history or routine preoperative liver function tests, and usually indicates a poor surgical outcome. Preoperative measures which can be taken include correction of coagulation abnormalities using vitamin K or blood products.

Renal System

Aging is accompanied by a progressive loss of renal mass. Loss of nephrons is accompanied by nearly 50% reduction in functioning glomeruli for individuals in their 70s compared to younger adults.

Renal insufficiency also increases the surgical risk. Prerenal azotemia can be corrected by intravenous (IV) fluids. Hemodialysis may be required in some cases to reduce uremia. Dosages of renally excreted drugs should be adjusted in patients with impaired creatinine clearance.

TABLE 2: Geriatric syndromes.

Domain	Assessment	Follow-up/implication of low scores
Cognition	• Mini Mental Status Evaluation • Mini-Cog • Montreal Cognitive Assessment	• Delirium risk • Decision-making potential • Increased risk of nonhospital discharge • Increased length of stay
Functional	• Basic activities of daily living (ADL) • Instrumental ADL • Timed up and go test • Walking speed	• Increased risk of postoperative complications • Increased mortality • Delirium • Preoperative exercise
Behavioral	• Alcohol history • Depression screening	• Delirium risk • Quality of life • Decision-making
Polypharmacy	• Medication list • Screen for inappropriate medications	• Delirium • Readmission • Morbidity/Mortality
Nutritional	• Albumin/ Prealbumin levels • Mini Nutritional Assessment	• Preoperative nutrition supplements • Increased risk of postoperative complications
Frailty	• Unintentional weight loss • Grip strength • Exhaustion • Gait speed • Low physical activity	• Preoperative nutrition supplements • Increased risk of postoperative complications • Prehabilitation opportunity • Treatment decisions

COMMON GERIATRIC SYNDROMES (TABLE 2)

Aging is often accompanied by increased incidence of common geriatric syndromes like cognitive impairment, frailty, immobility, and polypharmacy.

COMPREHENSIVE GERIATRIC ASSESSMENT

Comprehensive geriatric assessment is a multidimensional diagnostic approach to identify deficits in physical, functional, and psychosocial domains resulting in an individualized but evidence-based management plan. The effectiveness of preoperative CGA has been studied in a single-site randomized control trial in elective vascular surgical patients showing a 40% reduction in length of stay ($p < 0.001$) when compared to standard care. In another study done in hip fracture patients, CGA was found to reduce mortality rates, financial costs and incidence of postoperative institutionalization.

PREOPERATIVE BLOOD TESTS

Routine investigations include complete hemogram, liver function tests, renal function tests, serum electrolytes, serology, and coagulation profile.

INTRAOPERATIVE CARE OF OLDER ADULTS

The intraoperative care of older adults does not differ much from that of other adults. Specific management strategies for older adults include:

- During positioning of the patient, extra care in padding should be done to prevent skin breakdown and nerve atrophy.
- Use of pre-emptive non-narcotic pain management strategies before the incision to decrease anesthesia medications during the surgery.
- High-risk mediations to be avoided in the immediate preoperative and intraoperative phase of care.

POSTOPERATIVE CARE OF OLDER ADULTS

Interprofessional Collaborative Practice

Interprofessional collaborative practice is defined as multiple health workers from different professional backgrounds working together with patients and families. This helps to focus on issues central to optimal recovery in the postoperative period like functional preservation, prevention of delirium, nutritional support, and planning of discharge. The multidisciplinary team may include surgery, geriatrics, social work, physical therapy, occupational therapy, nutrition, and pharmacy.

Functional Preservation

Reduced ambulation during the period of hospital stay is associated with loss of independent ambulation in geriatric patients. To prevent this, early ambulation by physical therapy protocols is needed. Early mobilization is associated with improved functional status of the patient at the time of discharge, decreased likelihood of discharge to an institution, reduction in the length of hospital stay and cost, and also reduces the incidences of other preventable complications like inpatient falls and pressure ulcers.

Prevention of Delirium

Delirium is the most common complication seen in hospitalized older adults during the postoperative period. Risk factors for developing delirium include sensory and sleep deprivation, polypharmacy, and use of psychoactive drugs.

Perioperative pain control is important in the prevention of delirium, as higher baseline and postoperative pain scores are associated with increased incidence of postoperative delirium. Opioids are the mainstay in the management of postoperative pain, but may be deliriogenic. Multimodal opioid-sparing pain regimens and regional anesthesia are other alternatives. Multicomponent, nonpharmacologic prevention protocols include: (1) frequent orientation, (2) calm environment, (3) decreased use of restraints, (4) removal of catheters, (5) use of assistive devices like hearing aids and glasses, and (6) continuity of caregiver support.

Appropriate Medication Usage (Box 1)

Polypharmacy is another source of adverse events in hospitalized older adults during the postoperative period. Aging is associated with increased sensitivity to benzodiazepines and opioids because of decreased number and affinity of receptors for neurotransmitters. Aging is also associated with decreased cardiac output, decreased hepatic and renal outflow, and decrease in lean body mass with increase in fat, all of which can affect drug redistribution, metabolism, and clearance. Polypharmacy is also associated with increased drug–drug interactions.

BOX 1: Common perioperative medications with high risk of adverse events in older adults.

Pain medications:

- *Meperidine*: Related to postoperative delirium
- *Indomethacin*: NSAID with most CNS side effects
- *Pentazocine*: Associated with hallucinations and confusion
- *Ketorolac*: Increased risk of GI bleeding and peptic ulcer disease

GI stress ulcer prophylaxis:

- *Cimetidine*: Anticholinergic properties predispose to delirium
- *Famotidine*: Anticholinergic properties predispose to delirium
- *Ranitidine*: Anticholinergic properties predispose to delirium

Nausea medications:

- *Scopolamine*: Anticholinergic properties predispose to delirium
- *Promethazine*: Anticholinergic properties predispose to delirium

Insomnia medications:

- *Benzodiazepines*: CNS toxicity, increase fall risk and fractures
- *Zolpidem*: Increase risk of delirium and falls

Other medications:

- *Diphenhydramine*: Anticholinergic properties predispose to delirium
- *Cyclobenzaprine*: Drowsiness, confusion
- *Metoclopramide*: Extrapyramidal effects

(CNS: central nervous system; NSAID: nonsteroidal anti-inflammatory drug; GI: gastrointestinal) make them prone to infections such as hepatitis B. The immunocompromised state makes them prone to herpes zoster infection. Considering all these factors, the older people should be immunized against hepatitis B, tetanus, and herpes zoster. Recently, the mass immunization program to prevent coronavirus disease 2019 (COVID-19) has been carried out successfully, which itself is a testimony that vaccines do prevent infections.

The response to vaccination, requiring cell-mediated adaptive immune function, is often impaired among older people.

Despite this, we must immunize the older people, so that the immune response is stimulated and provides a protective response.

Following the infections and recovery, there is a drastic reduction in quality of life among older people; hence, preventive measures such as immunization will help reduce the severity of disease and better recovery.

INDICATIONS

The World Health Organization, Centre for Disease Control and Prevention (CDC), Advisory Committee on Immunization Practices (ACIP), Indian Council of Medical Research 2017 (ICMR 2017), Association of Physicians of India, and the Geriatric Society of India (GSI) have recommended that older people should receive the vaccines are per immunization schedule laid out by them.

- All the older people above 60 years of age irrespective of having comorbidities are eligible to receive vaccines.
- The other common indications are diabetes mellitus, chronic kidney disease, cirrhosis of liver, heart failure, chronic obstructive lung disease, bone marrow transplantation, multiple myeloma, malignancy, patient having undergone splenectomy, and traveling to jathas and melas.

TABLE 1: Vaccines for older people.

Disease against	Frequency
Influenza	Annual (once every year), 1 month before onset of winter season
Pneumococcal	One dose at age of 60 years of age—PCV 13
Pneumococcal	First give PCV 13, followed by PPSV 23 after 1 year. Repeat PPSV 23 every 5 years in special situations
Hepatitis B	Three doses, one each in 3 consecutive months (0, 1, 2 or 0, 1, 6)
Tetanus/ diphtheria	One dose every 10 years
Herpes zoster	Two doses separated by 2–6 months
COVID-19	Three doses

(COVID-19: coronavirus disease 2019; PCV: pneumococcal conjugate vaccine; PPSV: pneumococcal polysaccharide vaccine)

VACCINES RECOMMENDED FOR OLDER PEOPLE

The Vaccine Adverse Event Reporting System (VAERS) is a national early warning system to detect possible safety problems in vaccines used in the United States. VAERS accepts and analyzes reports of adverse events (AEs) after a person has received a vaccination. Anyone can report an adverse event to VAERS. Healthcare professionals are required to report certain adverse events and vaccine manufacturers are required to report all adverse events that come to their attention **(Table 1)**.

CONTRAINDICATIONS

The older people who have severe hypersensitivity reaction to vaccine in past or egg and severe allergic reactions to vaccines should not receive the vaccines.

The specific contraindications for Varicella Zoster vaccine are immunocompromised states such as leukemia, lymphoma, active pulmonary tuberculosis, patients receiving chemotherapy, radiotherapy, and large doses of corticosteroids.

INDIVIDUAL VACCINES

- *Td (tetanus and diphtheria) or Tdap (tetanus, diphtheria, and whooping cough)*: For people who were never vaccinated against tetanus, a primary series of three doses is recommended, after which a booster dose is recommended every 10 years.

Dose: 0.5 mL

Route: Intramuscular on deltoid

Revaccination: After 10 years

- *Pneumococcal vaccine*: There are two kinds of pneumococcal vaccines available:
  a. Pneumococcal conjugate vaccines (PCV13)
  b. Pneumococcal polysaccharide vaccine (PPSV23)

  Dose: 0.5 mL

  Route: Intramuscular on deltoid

  Revaccination is required after 5 years in immunosuppressed individuals.

  PCV13 should be given first, followed by a dose of PPSV23 after 1-year gap.

  Brand name: Pneumovax 23 and Prevnar 13

- *Influenza vaccine*: The constantly evolving nature of influenza viruses across hemispheres requires continuous global monitoring and frequent reformulation of influenza vaccines. Hence every year, new strain is used and the vaccine has to be administered every year.

  A quadrivalent influenza (flu) vaccine is designed to protect against four different flu viruses, including two influenza A viruses and two influenza B viruses. To improve the efficiency of vaccine, the elderly should be administered vaccine every year.

  The healthcare workers, and nurses looking after elderly in hospital and long-term care facilities for elderly, should also receive the influenza vaccine which helps to reduce patient mortality.

  Dose: 0.5 mL

  Route: Intramuscular on deltoid. Also available for intranasal use, but not recommended in elderly.

  Frequency: Every year before the onset of winter season

  Brand name: Vaxigrip or Fluzone quadri

  Contraindication: Past history of Guillain-Barré syndrome following previous dose

- *Hepatitis B vaccine*: The elderly people should be immunized against hepatitis B as they are likely to undergo surgeries.

  Schedule: 0, 1, and 6 months

  Dose: 0.5 mL

  Route: Intramuscular on deltoid

  Number of doses: Three doses

  Name of brand: Hepavax or Recombivax HB

- *Shingrix for herpes zoster*: It is a recombinant adjuvanted vaccine used to prevent shingles and the complications from the disease in older people irrespective of whether they had episode of herpes zoster in past or not. It reduces the incidence of herpes zoster, post-herpetic neuralgia, and reduces the pain burden of illness.

  Dose: 0.5 mL each dose

  Route of administration: Intramuscularly on deltoid

  Number of doses: Two, A first dose at month 0, followed by a second dose administered 2–6 months later.

  Brand name: Shingrix

  Contraindicated in known severe immunodeficiency, (e.g., from hematologic and solid tumors, receipt of chemotherapy, congenital immunodeficiency, untreated tuberculosis, long-term immunosuppressive therapy or patients with HIV infection who are severely immunocompromised), patients on prednisolone more than 20 mg/day, and active stage of herpes infection.

  Special precaution: Avoid salicylates for 6 weeks after administration of this vaccine to prevent Reye's syndrome.

- *COVID-19 vaccine:* It is an inactivated vaccine

  Schedule: 0, 2, and precautionary all three doses should be of same brand.

  Covishield®: Two doses, an interval of 12–16 weeks (84–112 days)

  Covaxin®: Two doses at an interval of 4–6 weeks (28–42 days)

  Dose: 0.5 mL

  Route: Intramuscular

  Number of doses: Three doses

  Brand name: Covaxin/Covishield

STORAGE

- All vaccines are stored in refrigerator. Should not freeze
- Cold chain has to be maintained throughout process.

ADVERSE EVENTS

The adverse events following vaccination are rare and mild in older people. Though the vaccines are costly but is very meager compared to the cost of treatment of the disease when it occurs. The adverse effects can occur within minutes to years after administration of vaccine. They are:

Local reaction: Pain at injection site

Systemic reaction: Lymphadenopathy, fever, muscle aches, headache, vomiting, and diarrhea

Allergic reaction: Anaphylaxis

Neurological events: Seizure and Guillain-Barré syndrome

Others: Very rarely syncope

Reporting of adverse effect: The VAERS stands for Vaccine Adverse Event Reporting System

This is a surveillance system that collects reports of adverse events following vaccination across the world. It is established in the United States by the Food and Drug Administration (FDA) and CDC in 1990.

Any person who comes across adverse event following vaccination can file a report to VAERS online in a format provided by them.

IMMUNIZATION FOR OLDER PEOPLE TRAVELING ABROAD

The older people traveling within and outside the country is rising every year. They are also participating in mega events such as *melas* and *jathas* which makes them prone for infections. The vaccines are recommended by respective countries that they are traveling to and should be taken at least 4–6 weeks before the trip. The Haj committee has made it mandatory to get pneumococcal vaccine for all the pilgrims before traveling. Meningococcal vaccine is recommended for travelers to North American countries.

SETTING UP AN IMMUNIZATION CLINIC

The vaccines can be given in the existing clinic of the clinicians. It must be ensured that they have facilities to treat the major and rare complications such as anaphylaxis. Emergency medicines, oxygen support, and adequate staff are mandatory in immunization clinic. A immunization schedule card should be prepared and provided to the elderly and inform them of their next due dates.

CONCOMITANT USAGE OF VACCINES

- Pneumovax and influenza vaccines can be given on same day in different sites preferably deltoid, whereas Pneumococcal 23 and Pneumococcal 13 should not be given concomitantly.
- Shingrix and pneumococcal vaccine can be administered at the same visit if the person is eligible for both.
- Tdap and inactivated influenza vaccine can be administered simultaneously.
- The quadrivalent meningococcal conjugate vaccine (MCV4)-D and PCV13 should not be administered simultaneously in patients with asplenia or HIV infection.

CONCLUSION

Preventing the infectious diseases in older people should be the priority among clinicians. The immunization schedule is in place and vaccines are available. All the doctors should be made aware regarding immunization in older people. They should also immunize their older parents first and then older patients so that they will have active aging. This will also improve quality of life of the older people.

The elderly deserve a good quality of life and the clinicians have a larger responsibility toward them in preventing the communicable diseases by administering vaccines. The vaccines have least side effects and are safe. The vaccines will definitely help improve immune status to larger extent.

"An ounce of prevention is worth a pound of cure."

SUGGESTED READINGS

1. Centers for Disease Control and Prevention. (2022). Vaccines & Immunizations: Glossary. [online] Available from https://www.cdc.gov/vaccines/terms/glossary.html [Last accessed January, 2024].
2. Pawelec G. Immunosenescence: impact in the young as well as the old? Mech Ageing Dev. 1999;108:1-7.
3. Weinberger B, Weiskopf D, Grubeck-Loebenstein B. Immunology and aging. Hazzard's Geriatric Medicine and Gerontology, 6th edition. New York: McGraw-Hill, Columbus; 2009. pp. 23-6.
4. Gavazzi G, Krause KH. Ageing and infection. Lancet Infect Dis. 2002;2(11):659-66.
5. Berger R, Florent G, Just M. Decrease of the lymphoproliferative response to varicella-zoster virus antigen in the aged. Infect Immun. 1981;32(1):24-7.
6. Potter JM, O'Donnel B, Carman WF, Roberts MA, Stott DJ. Serological response to influenza vaccination and nutritional and functional status of patients in geriatric medical long-term care. Age Ageing. 1999;28(2):141-5.
7. Matanock A, Lee G, Gierke R, Kobayashi M, Leidner A, Pilishvili T. (2019). Use of 13-Valent Pneumococcal Conjugate Vaccine and 23-Valent Pneumococcal Polysaccharide Vaccine Among Adults Aged ≥65 Years: Updated Recommendations of the Advisory Committee on Immunization Practices. [online] Available from https://www.cdc.gov/mmwr/volumes/68/wr/mm6846a5.htm [Last accessed January, 2024].
8. Ministry of Health and Family Welfare. (2017). Seasonal Influenza: Guidelines for vaccination with influenza vaccine. Available from https://main.mohfw.gov.in/sites/default/files/30580390001493710612.pdf [Last accessed January, 2024].
9. Expert Group of the Association of Physicians of India on Adult Immunization in India. The Association of Physicians of India Evidence-Based Clinical Practice Guidelines on Adult Immunization. J Assoc Physicians India. 2009;57:345-56.
10. Sharma OP. Indian Recommendations for Vaccination in Older adults. Delhi: Geriatric Society of India; 2015.
11. Centre for Disease Control and Prevention (CDC). (2023). Adult Immunization Schedule by Age: Recommendations for Ages 19 Years or Older, United States, 2024. [online] Available from https//www.cdc.gov/vaccines/schedules/hcp/imz/adult.html [Last accessed January, 2024].

12. World Health Organization. Global Influenza Programme: Vaccines. [online] Available from https://www.who.int/teams/global-influenza-programme/vaccines [Last accessed January, 2024].
13. Centre for Disease Control and Prevention (CDC). (2023). Quadrivalent Influenza Vaccine. [online] Available from https://www.cdc.gov/flu/prevent/quadrivalent.htm [Last accessed January, 2024].
14. Carman WF, Elder AG, Wallace LA, McAulay K, Walker A, Murray GD, et al. Effects of influenza vaccination of health-care workers on mortality of elderly people in long-term care: a randomised controlled trial. Lancet. 2000;355:93-7.
15. Muruganathan A, Guha S, Munjal YP, Agarwal SS, Parikh KK, Jha V, et al. Recommendations for Vaccination Against Seasonal Influenza in Adult High Risk Groups: South Asian Recommendations. J Assoc Physicians India. 2016;64(7 Suppl):3-11.
16. Centre for Disease Control and Prevention (CDC). (2023). Shingles Vaccination. [online] Available from https://www.cdc.gov/vaccines/vpd/shingles/public/shingrix/index.html [Last accessed January, 2024].
17. MoHFW. FAQs on COVID-19 vaccines vaccination program. [online] Available from https://www.mohfw.gov.in/pdf/FAQsCOVID19vaccinesvaccinationprogramWebsiteupload27Sep.pdf [Last accessed January, 2024].
18. https://vaers.hhs.gov/index.html. Last accessed 01/7/2023
19. Centre for Disease Control and Prevention (CDC). (2012). Use of 13-valent pneumococcal conjugate vaccine and 23-valent pneumococcal polysaccharide vaccine for adults with immunocompromising conditions: Recommendations of the Advisory Committee on Immunization Practices (ACIP). [online] Available from https://www.cdc.gov/mmwr/preview/mmwrhtml/mm6140a4.htm [Last accessed January, 2024].
20. Centre for Disease Control and Prevention (CDC). (2022). Administering Shingrix. [online] Available from https://www.cdc.gov/vaccines/vpd/shingles/hcp/shingrix/administering vaccine.html [Last accessed January, 2024].
21. Kretsinger K, Broder KR, Cortese MM, Joyce MP, Ortega-Sanchez I, Lee GM, et al. Preventing tetanus, diphtheria, and pertussis among adults: use of tetanus toxoid, reduced diphtheria toxoid and acellular pertussis vaccine recommendations of the Advisory Committee on Immunization Practices (ACIP) and recommendation of ACIP, supported by the Healthcare Infection Control Practices Advisory Committee (HICPAC), for use of Tdap among health-care personnel. MMWR Recomm Rep. 2006;55(RR-17):1-37.
22. Centre for Disease Control and Prevention (CDC). Recommendation of the Advisory Committee on Immunization Practices (ACIP) for use of quadrivalent meningococcal conjugate vaccine (MenACWY-D) among children aged 9 through 23 months at increased risk for invasive meningococcal disease. MMWR Morb Mortal Wkly Rep. 2011;60(40):1391-2.

99

CHAPTER

Chronological Age versus Vascular Age: How can We Reverse Vascular Age?

Durga Prasad Chakraborty

ABSTRACT

Use of antiplatelets in high-risk bleeding patients has always been concern regarding their risk of complications that is Chronological age is amount of time that has been elapsed from birth to a given date and is the main way of defining age that's why it is also known as birthday age. On the contrary, biological age or vascular age occurs as result of gradually accumulation of various damaged vascular or biological cells. We cannot modify our chronological age but on the contrary, we can modulate our biological or vascular age.

Vascular age is nothing but time gap between birth and the moment of observation of physical fitness. It varies substantially among individual and it is based on biological growth indicators or on senescence for adults and it is strongly affected by individual living conditions and lifestyle changes. Hence, biological or vascular age stands reliable statistical link in between life stage and chronological age.

INTRODUCTION

Our chronological age and vascular (or biological) age might not be the same. Chronological age has been defined the number of the years, we have been alive, it is also known as birthday age. Vascular age refers to how old your biological cells and tissue, if we are healthy and fit for our age, our biological age may well be lower, compared to our stated chronological age. On the other hand, if we are sedentary, have chronically ill health, or in poor physical condition our vascular age may be even higher. Recent studies and researches show that vascular age is more accurate than chronological age for predicting onset of diseases of death. With just a few generations the mean is at puberty has decreased and growth processes have accelerated in response to recent improvement in diet, hygiene lifecare changes, and medical care.

It has been reported that tumor microenvironment (TME) plays an important role in aging and this is a complex processes involving epithelial cells and inflammatory cells. It has been observed that aging in characterized inflammation and intern inflammation lists to cell death and aging. It has been observed that certain medication and agents can halt vascular age progression (e.g., metformin), although there is no such hard data supporting this hypothesis.

CHRONOLOGICAL VS. BIOLOGICAL AGE

Our chronological age is unchangeable. We were born on a particular day and had spent a certain amount of time on the planet, and this is fixed and we cannot change our chronological age that is birthday age.

However, we are sometimes observing some people whose chronological age surprises us because they look much older or younger than there chronological age; this is the different between chronological age and biological age, because biological age may be significantly different from the chronological age. Our chronological age cannot be changed and it is beyond our control. However, our biological age can be altered by various external and internal factors, including:

- Diet
- Exercise
- Stress
- Smoking
- Sleeping habits
- Physical environment (where you live, work, etc.)

Biological age also called vascular age is influenced by this factors and our DNA (genetic material) is a reflection of all those factors. Among the difference between chronological and biological age regarding our longevity of life, development of diseases, etc., is that our biological age may predict things like whether we will develop diabetes or dementia or how soon we will die. Likely we have some control over our biological/vascular aging and can even get *younger* by making positive changes in our day-to-day life, and hence, knowing your biological/vascular age may provide an incentive to lead a healthier lifestyle.

Determination of Chronological and Vascular Age

Chronological age is a measurement of how many days you will remain alive, i.e., no. of birthday ceremonies; on the contrary, while biological age/vascular age is a measurement of how much life you likely have left, and it is based on our physiology at any given time.

How biological/vascular age is determined?

Vascular disease onset and mortality are highly variable among individuals. Biological/vascular age should be used to select individuals for early prevention of cardiovascular and other degenerative diseases. Biological/vascular aging can be targeted by various behavioral and pharmacological measures **(Fig. 1)**.

RISK FACTORS OF BIOLOGICAL AGE

- *Aging*: Aging is the main risk factor for vascular and other emerging diseases such as cardiovascular, cerebrovascular, and renal diseases. Vascular aging entails arterial degeneration and hardening that impairs vascular function and ultimately causes end organ damage, predominantly in the heart, brain, and kidney. Age-dependent arterial diseases typically manifest clinically after the 5th or 6th decade of life; however, there is a high interindividual variability in vascular disease onset and associated mortality.
- *Presence of chronic illness:* e.g., diabetes mellitus, chronic bronchial asthma, and hypertension.
- *Early death in family*: Presence of neurodegenerative disorder.
- *Diet*: Various studies on diet and biological age suggest the ideal should be:
  - Low-calories diets
  - Plant-based
  - High-fiber diet
  - A Mediterranean diet
  - Education status
  - Obesity and other sedentary habitus
- *Excessive stress and strain:* Both physical and mental stress increase in a reversible manner. A 2022 study monitor the effects of stressors such as pregnancy, COVID-19 infection, trauma, and surgery and they found that biological age increases rapidly (measured by DNA methylation) while on round-the-clock stress. However, it back to based line with in a few days. In 2021, study on psychological stress and biological aging revealed that people who are emotionally stressed and cannot regulate their emotions live shorter period of life.
- *Smoking and drinking*: Smoking is said to cause serious health problems and shortens our life span. Smoking

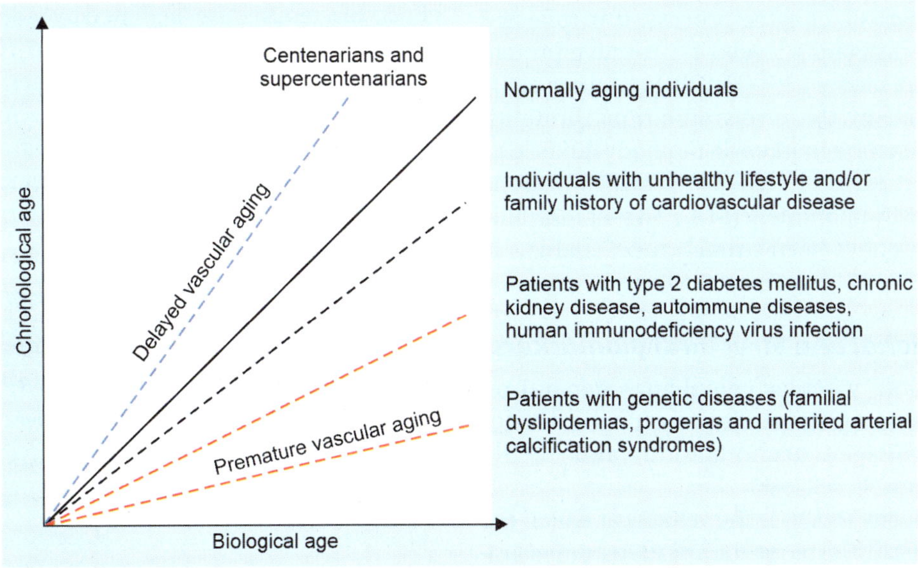

FIG. 1: Risk factors.

also increases our biological/vascular age, proved by various studies and trials.

- *Poor sleep quality*: Poor sleep quality has a negative impact on our vascular age; one may be able to improve sleep duration or quality by making simple changes such as going to bed earlier, switching off your mobile phone at list 1 hour before going to bed or reducing distraction in the bed room.
- *Physical environment:* Our physical environment includes where we live, work, and span significant amount of time. Our environmental toxins can speed up our biological age.
- *Sex difference*: Various clinical studies found a sex-based difference of biological age according to this studies females live little bit longer than males.
- *Less exercises*: A 2022 study showed that changing the dietary style and addition of more exercises lower our vascular age. A 2020 study revealed good aerobic exercises were almost 5.5 years younger than people who were sedentary.

Calculating and Assessment of Our Risk Factors for Biological/Vascular Age

Molecular and Cellular Biomarkers

Our DNA sequences are bounded by telomeres, specific nucleoproteins, and protecting chromosome ends. Whenever these telomeres shorten, our lifespan also decreases. This age-dependent telomere shortening is strongly correlated with coronary artery disease (CAD) and predicts both all-cause and CVD-related mortality.

Another major factor for regulating gene expression is DNA methylation, a major epigenetic mechanism.

A chronic low-grade inflammation is another important characteristic of aging process. It is reflected and measured by circulating levels of C-reactive protein (CRP) and high-sensitivity CRP (HsCRP). Another aging process is reflected by the levels of various proteins, metabolites, and other biomarkers in our body fluids, e.g., insulin-like growth factor 1 (IGF-1),, growth hormone (GH), and low-density lipoprotein (LDL). Higher mortality and morbidity rates have been strongly meet changes in above molecules.

Vascular Functional and Structural Biomarkers

Arterial stiffness and vascular compliance depend on structural changes in aging arteries resulting in elastin fragmentation, collagen accumulation, and media vascular smooth muscle cell loss.

Pulse-wave velocity (PWV) is the velocity at which the blood pressure wave moves alone the arterial tree measure arterial stiffness. Carotid-to-femoral PWV is accepted and standardized. High PWV increases risk of CVD and all-cause mortality.

Hypertension and atherosclerosis follow arterial stiffness and they are associated with increased cardiovascular events and mortality. Intravascular ultrasound reflects endothelial dysfunction, a major driver of atherogenesis.

Carotid intima medial thickness (IMT), picked up vascular ultrasound, indicates subclinical atherosclerotic burden in large arteries.

Carotid IMT increases with age and is responsible for high incidence and prevalence of CVD mortality and morbidity. Vascular aging is also characterized by the addition and deposition of calcium phosphate crystals in both the arterial intima and media (called Monckeberg medial sclerosis) **(Table 1)**.

Composite Biomarker Predictors

All previous biomarkers mentioned earlier often fail to predict and reflect the complexity of aging processes and they are totally suboptimal assessments of biological age; therefore, better aging estimates are sought out.

Many other novel biomarkers are trying to develop by adding physical physiological and biochemical parameters, e.g., Klemera–Doubal method biological age index is based on 10 biomarkers **(Flowchart 1)**.

DIET AND EXERCISE AND HEALTHY LIFESTYLE STRATEGIES

Regular aerobic exercises are to be considered as pivot in reversing vascular age. Regular exercise in various forms is the most effective overall approach in reversing biological/vascular aging. Exercises also reduce vascular endothelial dysfunction, large arterial stiffness, etc. The beneficial effects of exercises are mediated by reduced inflammation and oxidative stress and increased NO bioavailability. Broad dietary pattern places another important role in reversing biological/vascular age. Amount the diets, various fruits (e.g., apple, berries whole greens, low-fat dairy products, increase dietary fiber sea fish). Various Dietary plans (e.g., Ketogenic , Mediterranean, and DASH diets) **(Figs. 2 and 3)**.

TABLE 1: Grading of coronary artery disease (based on total calcium score).

Calcium score	Presence of CAD
0	No evidence of CAD
1–10	Minimal evidence of CAD
11–100	Mild evidence of CAD
101–400	Moderate evidence of CAD
Over 400	Extensive evidence of CAD

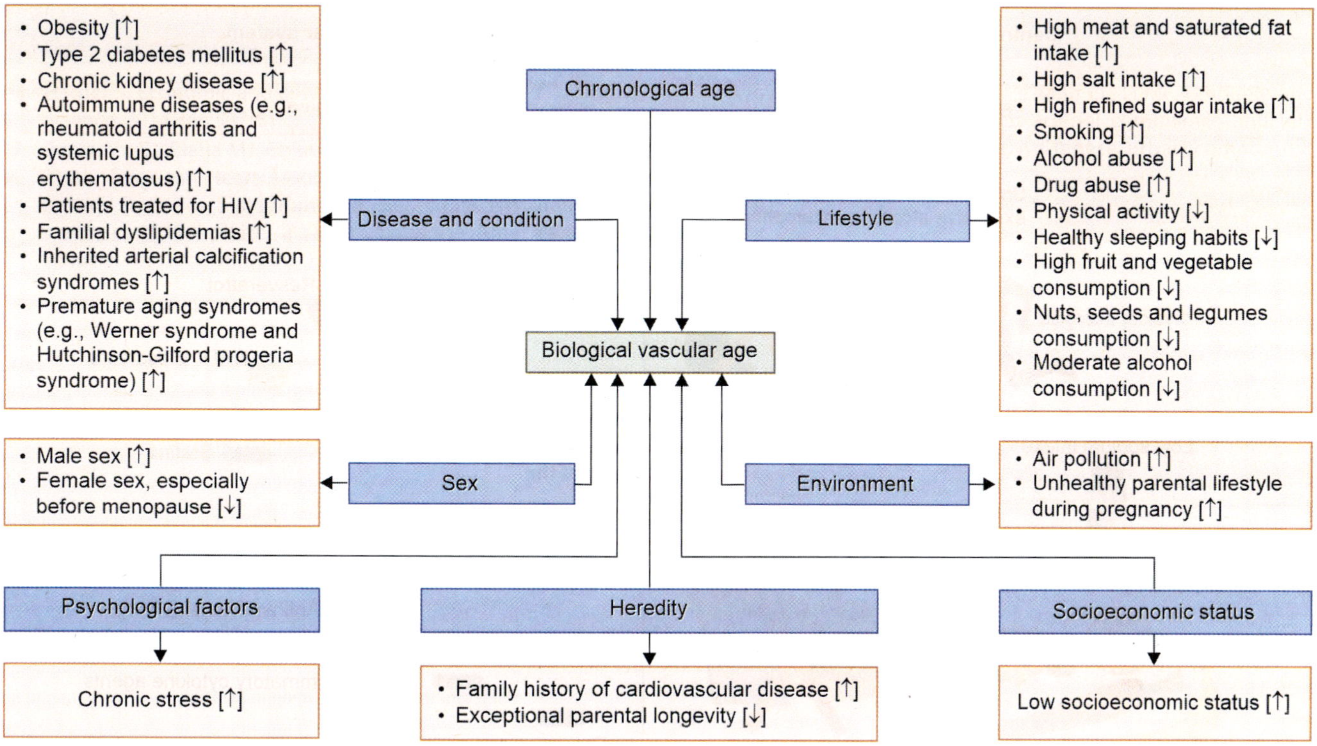

FLOWCHART 1: Reversal of biological/vascular age.

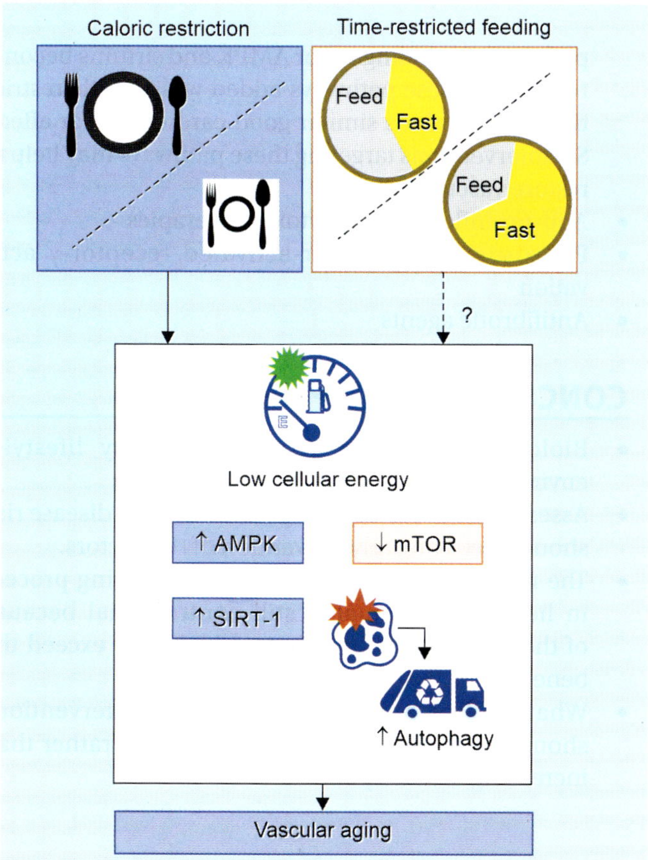

FIG. 2: Diet and lifestyle modification strategies.

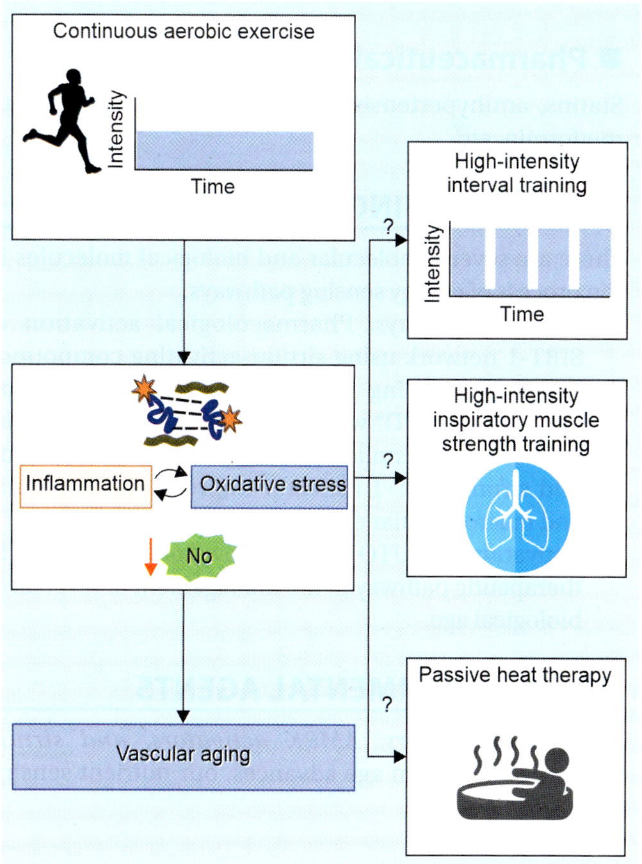

FIG. 3: Exercise strategies.

100

CHAPTER

Inflammaging

Om Prakash Sharma, Anand P Ambali

ABSTRACT

Inflammaging is a recently evolved concept in the understanding of process of aging and age-related diseases. Attempts have been made to explain aging by various processes besides genetics. The role of environment and nutrition affecting aging has been a matter of research. Ever since immunosenescence, a process based upon immunity is being understood, inflammation and aging are being related to each other. The thinking is the control of environmental factors and the beneficial effects of proper elements of nutrition may herald the process of aging. Therefore, attempts are being made to slow down the process of inflammaging; various medications and the role of minerals, vitamins, flavonoids in foods and vegetables, and senolytics have been part of various studied and have shown promising results. Further researches in this direction continues.

INTRODUCTION

Aging is a physiological process which continues throughout the lifespan. There is a difference between the chronological aging and biological aging. The biological aging, a genetically controlled process is also affected by many factors which include diseases as well as environment. The factors other than genetics are among the modifiable factors affecting the process of aging and hence have an important role in slowing down the process of aging.

Inflammation is a body response to any kind of injury. It is because of this response that there occur many changes. However, inflammaging is a chronic sterile process, which has low-grade inflammation that develops during the process of aging and contributes to the pathogenesis of age-related diseases. The term inflammaging was coined by Franceschi et al. in the year 2000. It is an asymptomatic process but comes under the control of immune system. It plays an important role in the process of aging and age-related diseases. It affects the functions of body at all levels ranging from cells, various tissues, organs, organ systems, and the body as a whole. It is associated with diseases such as Alzheimer's, heart disease, atherosclerosis, diabetes mellitus, endothelial dysfunctions, and cancers.

The understanding of pathogenesis of process of inflammaging and to know about the factors which could slow it down is a matter of research. This understanding will not only herald the process of aging but will also slow down the process of atherosclerosis and other tissue functions which contribute in the development of various diseases.

PATHOPHYSIOLOGY

As we grow old, though the number of neutrophils remains constant but their functions related to phagocytic activity and power to kill the pathogens comes down. The macrophages also lose their ability to kill pathogens and their antigen presentation function is affected.

During the process of aging, the adaptive immunity declines which leads to immunosenescence (a term coined by Roy Walford). Meanwhile innate immunity is also activated which leads to rise in proinflammatory state and is called inflammaging. The immunosenescence and inflammaging coexist.

When inflammation occurs and resolves over time, it is called resolving inflammation. Whereas, when inflammation that does not resolve is called inflammaging. This means that the inflammaging is a continuous process occurring in human beings.

Innate immune system is affected in the process. The cells involved are neutrophils, monocytes, macrophages, natural killer and natural killer T (NKT) cells, and dendritic cells.

It triggers morphological and functional changes, most prominently endothelial dysfunction, diffuse intimal-medial thickening, and arterial stiffness.

It is caused by chronic stimulation of the innate immune system by products of degradation processes and/or by the partial inability of the aged immune system to eliminate certain pathogens this leads to chronic and less efficient innate immune response.

The chronic inflammatory mediators induce pathophysiologic changes in multiple physiologic systems and contribute to multiple disease states.

This makes older people susceptible for infections, cancer, and autoimmune disease, which leads to increase in mortality and morbidity with decrease in quality of life.

The factors that precipitate inflammaging are autophagy and reduced proteasome activity. Autophagy is elimination of debris; reactive oxygen species (ROS) and products of cellular metabolism are not recognized and lead to inflammation while reduced proteasome activity in aging activates inflammatory pathway.

BIOMARKERS OF INFLAMMAGING

Inflammaging is a progressive proinflammatory state in older people with elevated plasma concentrations of interleukin 6 (IL-6), IL-10, IL-18, IL-1β, tumor necrosis factor alpha (TNF-α), microRNAs (miRNAs), and C-reactive protein (CRP).

STAGES OF INFLAMMAGING

There are five stages, they are:

1. Low-grade
2. Controlled
3. Asymptomatic
4. Chronic
5. Systemic

The inflammation process during inflammaging is not in a controlled inflammatory state. This belongs to nonresolving inflammation.

INFLAMMAGING AND DISEASES PROCESS

Inflammaging perse will not cause disease. It either triggers or worsens the existing damage. The common diseases associated with it are cancer, cardiovascular disease, depression, dementia, anemia, neurodegenerative disease, metabolic diseases such as diabetes mellitus and obesity, sarcopenia, and osteoporosis. All these lead to frailty, increased disability and mortality.

IMPACT ON HEALTH STATUS

Inflammaging leads to several changes in major organs physiology and reduces its activity. The changes are:

- Decline in physiologic systems
- Development and exacerbations of disease states
- Decline in skeletal muscle strength which in turn contributes to frailty and sarcopenia.
- Reduced grip strength by 40% over 3 years
- Stimulates anorexic proteins such as leptin, orexin, and melanocortin which suppressed hunger.
- The overall outcome will be frailty, disability, and high mortality.

POSSIBLE INTERVENTIONS IN INFLAMMAGING AND ITS EFFECTS ON HEALTH

The research so far has been able to interfere with the process of inflammaging leading to beneficial effects on health and diseases. Following are the few examples.

- *Use of metformin enhance longevity*: It acts by inhibiting action of NF-κB (nuclear factor-kappa B). It also inhibits the senescence-associated secretory phenotype (SASP). It helps in alleviating several age-related conditions and chronic diseases.
- *Use of rapamycin*: It inhibits mammalian target of rapamycin (mTOR) and declines the autophagy pathway. It helps reduce the incidence of infection and promote expression of antiviral genes. This is also found to enhance response to a vaccine against influenza among older people.

- *Tocilizumab in COVID-19*: Decreased serum levels of the miR-146a are associated with nonclinical response to tocilizumab in COVID-19 patients.
- *Cytomegalovirus (CMV) infection*:
  - CMV infection induces the production of IL-6 and IL-8 in old age. Lifelong infection with CMV may contribute to age-related inflammatory processes. CMV infection affects many cell types and has wide-ranging direct and indirect effects on innate immune mechanisms.
  - In response to influenza vaccination, a high proportion of potentially senescent CD8+ T cells do not coexpress granzyme B (GrzB) and perforin. The level of bGrzB increases with age and is higher in CMV positive. It also affects the outcome in patients with organ transplantation.
- *Use of gliflozins/SGLT-2 inhibitors*: It is recommended in ischemic heart disease with heart failure because of its antiremodeling and antisenescent effect on the heart. It is used even in nondiabetics. It helps prevent deterioration of heart function. The drugs available are dapagliflozin and canagliflozin.
- *Megestrol*: It is a hormone that blocks IL-6 transcription has been to show to improve cachexia related to HIV and cancer. It has not shown beneficial effects in stimulation appetite in older people.

Can it be Halted or Delayed?

- The interventions that halt progress of inflammaging are calorie restrictions.
- Intake of zinc, resveratrol, flavonoids, icariin, and metformin
- The quercetin which is abundant in tomato, blueberry, cherries, in layer and peels of fruits have been beneficial in delaying the immune response.
- *Senolytics*: The drugs that selectively clear senescent cells has led to promising strategies for preventing or treating multiple diseases and age-related conditions in humans, e.g., dasatinib.

Is Inflammaging Beneficial for Aging?

Inflammaging is a driving force for longevity in super semicentenarians. It has been observed that the Infection did not impact the longevity of the elderly especially in octogenarians. If immunosenescence and inflammaging do not exist, our life would be shortened. Why and how these changes happen is still unanswered.

CONCLUSION

The longevity is on rise and so are the diseases. Our body immune mechanism has a dual role to play. One is to nullify the effects of pathogens on our immune system and second is to enhance and sustain the effects of immune system in older people. The efficiency of vaccines is also affected because of poor and delayed immune response. Much of the research is happening to know whether inflammaging is beneficial to the human body and should we halt or let it be in a silent phase. The role of nutrition, physical activity, and stress management on inflammaging is also being studied. Coming days will bring out results of the research happening across the globe and provide answers.

SUGGESTED READINGS

1. Hazzard WR. Ways to make 'usual' and 'successful' ageing synonymous: Preventive gerontology. West J Med. 1997;167(4):206-15.
2. Lee KA, Flores RR, Jang IH, Saathoff A, Robbins PD. Immune Senescence, Immunosenescence and Aging. Front Aging. 2022;3:900028.
3. Teissier T, Boulanger E, Cox LS. Interconnections between inflammageing and immunosenescence during ageing. Cells. 2022;11:359.
4. Fulop T, Larbi A, Pawelec G, Khalil A, Cohen AA, Hirokawa K, et al. Immunology of aging: the birth of inflammageing. Clin Rev Allergy Immunol. 2023;64(2):109-22.
5. Fulop T, Witkowski JM, Olivieri F, Larbi A. The integration of Inflammageing in age-related diseases. Semin Immunol. 2018;40:17-35.
6. Walford Roy L. The 120-year diet. New York: Pocket Books; 1986.
7. Ferrucci L, Fabbri E. Inflammageing: Chronic inflammation in ageing, cardiovascular disease, and frailty, Nat Rev Cardiol. 2018;15(9):505-22.
8. Duggal NA. Reversing the Immune Ageing Clock: Lifestyle Modifications and Pharmacological Interventions. Philadelphia: Springer; 2018.
9. Franceschi C, Bonafe M, Valensin S, et al. Inflamm-aging. An evolutionary perspective on immunosenescence. Ann NY Acad Sci.2000;908:244-54.

SECTION

7

HEMATOLOGY

101

CHAPTER

New Insights into Autoimmune Hemolytic Anemia

Nilesh Kumar, Abhishek Borkotoky

ABSTRACT

Autoimmune hemolytic anemia (AIHA) is defined as immune-mediated destruction of red blood cells with increased red blood cell (RBC) turnover, an estimated incidence of 0.8–3 per 10^5/year in adults, and a prevalence of 17 per 100,000. Reports of autoimmune hemolytic anemia date back to 13th century Byzantine era, when court physician Johannes Actuarius observed black color urine of his patient after cold exposure, probably a case of paroxysmal cold hemoglobinuria (PCH). In 1930s, Dameshek and Schwartz drew a line between autoimmune and congenital hemolytic anemia, which in later years was postulated to be due to hemolysin in the sera. With the entry of the millennium, we saw a diverse run in workup along with a growing number of therapies tailored to individualized patient conditions.

INTRODUCTION: ETIOPATHOGENESIS OF AUTOIMMUNE HEMOLYTIC ANEMIA

The characteristic feature of autoimmune hemolytic anemia (AIHA) is the interplay between pathologic autoantibodies attaching to RBC at specific temperatures leading to its immune-mediated destruction, which is identified by detecting autoantibodies and byproducts of red blood cell (RBC) consumption along with its increased turnover. **Figure 1** shows the development of autoimmunity (autoimmune antibodies) and the close interrelationship between central and peripheral tolerance.

Warm Autoimmune Hemolytic Anemia

Accounts for about 70% of all AIHA cases, antibodies in this spectrum are mostly polyclonal, directed against erythrocytes antigens of Rh system **(Figs. 2A and B)**, optimally binding at a temperature of 37°C. Most immunoglobulins (Ig) are immunoglobulin G (IgG) type, but occasional instances have been found where other antibodies are also involved, mainly immunoglobulin A (IgA) or warm reactive immunoglobulin M (IgM) alone or in combination with IgG subclasses. The severity and persistence of hemolysis depend on the ability of the IgG antibody to initiate the complement pathway and its ability to bind to the fragment crystallizable (Fc) binding receptor portion. The antibodies opsonized RBCs are phagocytosed by macrophages in the spleen, which is the major factor for extravascular hemolysis and complement-mediated hemolysis, accounting for 50% of patients. Warm-autoimmune hemolytic anemia (w-AIHA) occurs as a primary disease in <50% of the cases; the bulk of the cases are secondary to other disorders or underlying associated disease pathogenesis, as listed in **Box 1**. It increases the risk of thrombosis, which contributes to its increased mortality rates in addition to the risk of infection. Recently warm AIHA has been reported with a certain class of drugs; immune checkpoint inhibitors are used for cancer patients.

Cold-antibody Autoimmune Hemolytic Anemia

- *Cold agglutinin disease (CAD):* It is responsible for 20–30% cased mediated by monoclonal cold agglutinin leading to clumping of RBC at temperature below 37°C

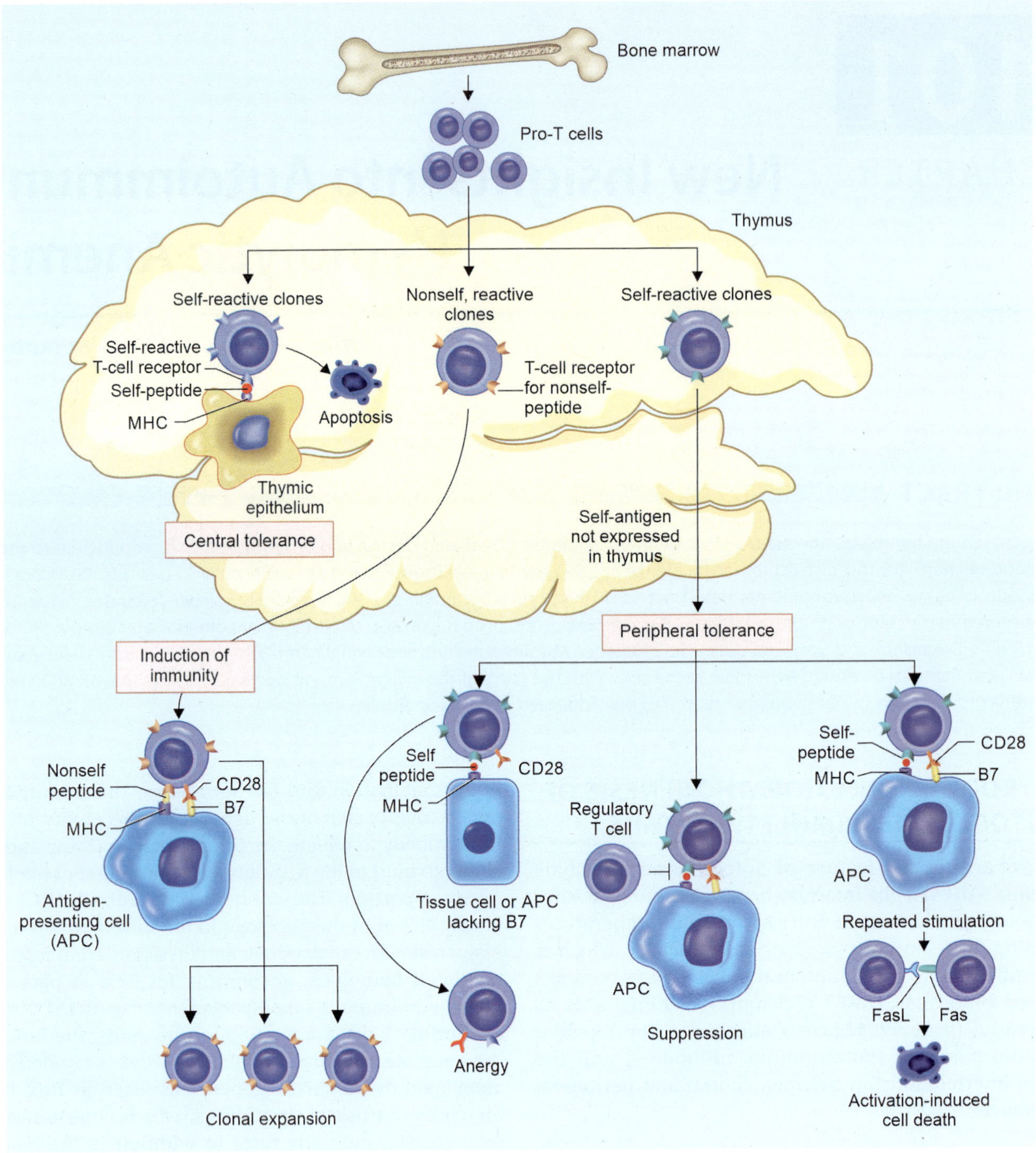

FIG. 1: Schematic illustration of the mechanisms involved in central and peripheral tolerance; the principal mechanisms of tolerance in CD4+ T-cells are shown.

(APC: antigen-presenting cell)

Source: Abbas AK, Diseases of immunity. In: Kumar V, Abbas A, Fausto N (Eds). Robbins and Cotran Pathologic Basis of Disease, 7th edition. Philadelphia, PA: Elsevier Saunders; 2005. pp. 223-5.

(Fig. 2B), predominantly in peripheral limbs with cold extremities. They are usually of IgM class with Kappa light chain restriction, and it is being recognized as a distinct nonmalignant clonal B cell lymphoproliferative neoplasm by World Health Organization (WHO) classification for hematolymphoid neoplasm.

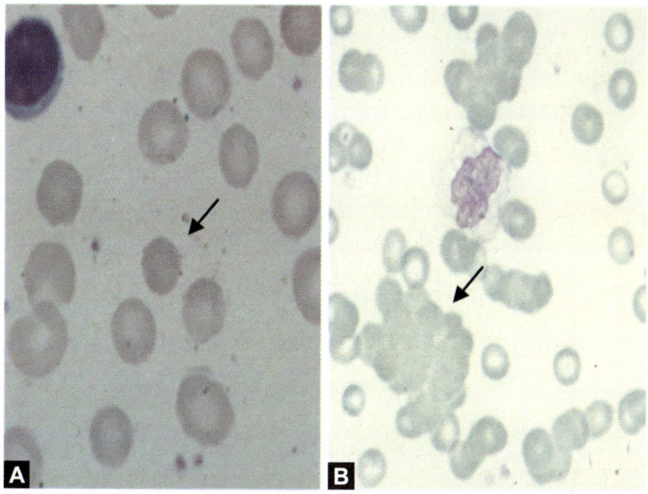

FIGS. 2A AND B: Blood film appearances in patients of AIHA, both using May–Grünwald–Giemsa (MGG) stain; (A) Spherocyte in a patient of w-AIHA; (B) Red cell agglutination in patient of Cold agglutinin disease (CAD).

Source: Hill A, Hill QA. Autoimmune hemolytic anemia. Hematology Am Soc Hematol Educ Program. 2018;2018(1):382-9.

Hemolysis is usually complement-mediated, leading to extravascular hemolysis (predominantly liver). It is important to note that peripheral symptoms such as the Raynaud-like phenomenon and acrocyanosis are not complement-mediated. The soluble splits of complement pathways C3a and C5a also contribute to these patients' chronic fatigue by being proinflammatory. The disease severity and hemolysis have been negatively correlated with hemoglobin (Hb) levels rather than IgM levels.

- *Paroxysmal cold hemoglobinuria:* Paroxysmal cold hemoglobinuria (PCH) is mediated by polyclonal, biphasic (Donath–Landsteiner antibody), which is usually IgG type, fixes the RBC at temperature below 37°C followed by an intense initiation of complement activation (classical below 37°C and terminal after rewarming) along with intravascular hemolysis of RBCs. The course is somewhat transient, causing anemia in children, which follows a viral infection. Still, even though very rare, the adult counterpart has a more chronic course, usually associated with tertiary syphilis, hematological malignancies, or idiopathy.

BOX 1: Classification of autoimmune hemolytic anemia.

Warm-autoantibody (active at 37°C):
- Primary [idiopathic warm autoimmune hemolytic anemia (w-AIHA)]
- *Secondary w-AIHA:*
  - Lymphoproliferative disorder
  - Associated with rheumatologic disorders (e.g., SLE—systemic lupus erythematosus)
  - Nonlymphoid neoplasm's (e.g., ovarian tumors)
  - Drug related (e.g., methyldopa)
  - Chronic inflammatory states (e.g., ulcerative colitis)
  - Allogeneic stem cell transplant

Cold-autoantibody type (optimally active temperature <37°C):
- *Mediated cold agglutinins:*
  - Idiopathic chronic cold agglutinin disease (clonal B lymphocyte proliferation)
  - Secondary cold agglutinin hemolytic anemia (mycoplasma, associated malignant B cell lymphoproliferative disorder)
- *Mediated cold hemolysins:*
  - (Primary) paroxysmal cold hemoglobinuria
  - (Secondary) Donath–Landsteiner hemolytic anemia, congenital tertiary syphilis

Mixed cold and warm autoantibodies:
- Idiopathic mixed AIHA
- Secondary mixed AIHA (SLE)

Drug-immune hemolytic anemia:
- Hapten (drug adsorption)
- Ternary immune complex
- True antibody mechanism

Source: Lichtman MA, Kaushansky K, Prchal JT, Levi MM, Burns LJ, Armitage JO. Williams Manual of Hematology. 9th edition. McGraw Hill Professional; 2017.

Atypical Autoimmune Hemolytic Anemia

- *Mixed warm and cold AIHA:* Mixing of two separate entities yet the treatment is governed, or more so in line with w-AIHA, this variant of AIHA runs a particular chronic course (without Raynaud-like symptoms or acrocyanosis) with exacerbations (not due to cold exposure) leading to drop in Hb level <5 g/dL. Laboratory workup reveals a direct antiglobulin test (DAT) positive with monospecific DAT reactivity toward IgG, C3d and cold agglutinins. Compared to the separate diseases, this variant's autoantibody interplay attribute is significantly difficult in cross-match and antibody screens. Because of technical difficulties, cross-match incompatible units must be transfused in severely anemic and symptomatic patients.
- *DAT-negative AIHA* amounts to 3–10% of AIHA with polyspecific DAT being negative; the possible reasons may be due to low antibody titer, low-affinity autoantibodies, IgA, and IgM. This entity remains a diagnosis of exclusion when a picture of immune-mediated hemolysis is present, indicating its strong suspicion.

AUTOIMMUNE HEMOLYTIC ANEMIA DIAGNOSTIC LANDSCAPES

The onset of AIHA is usually of a dramatic sense, with clinical features rolling in the scenario of generalized weakness and easy fatigability abruptly, marked changes in body physiology which can be seen sometimes in Hb levels dropping up to 4 g/dL, removal of such RBC mass leads to rise of jaundice and resulting splenic enlargement, persistent associations have been seen with high lactate dehydrogenase (LDH). AIHA associated with EVANS syndrome carries a high-risk disease course, a typical presentation of common variable immune deficiency. Common predictors of relapse include severe anemia (<6 g/dL), acute renal failure, secondary infection, and involvement of specific class of antibody.

Well, the myriad and varied presentation of AIHA, which can be summed in a background of the autoimmune process yet going into its depth, is beyond the scope of this chapter. In contrast, the ever-entailing workups which help us land on a deal with the diagnosis are very specific, with ever-changing dimensions involved in its management; the detailed line of workup, as shown in **Flowchart 1**, adapted from Frontiers' immunology journal.

The fundamental laboratory diagnostic test used is the direct Coombs test, whose sensitivity depends on the techniques used. The conventional ones require at least 400 molecules of an antibody of Ig and complement on each red cell; recent methods have a lower threshold for detecting up to 30–40 antibody molecules per red cell (flow cytometry).

AUTOIMMUNE HEMOLYTIC ANEMIA: THE CURRENT STANDARDS, NEWER AVENUES

A presentation of a severe acute AIHA is always a medical emergency. The immediate treatment always involved is blood transfusion; the old anecdote "transfusing the least incompatible" holds still. However, newer methods in phenotyping the RBC can lead to better cross-match results. However, time-consuming; the avenues for more unique autoadsorption techniques in CAD have made it easy, but transfusion in patients of CAD is only done in severely symptomatic with the use of inline blood warmer, keeping the extremity undergoing transfusion warm.

- *Warm-AIHA:* The selection of a line of therapy is still dynamic, but recent practices have shown the use of biological with the simultaneous addition of high-dose corticosteroids. The line delineating such role play is the characterization of patients based on severity as such, Hb (<8 g/dL), transfusion-dependent, IgA type, Evans syndrome necessitating the role of rituximab (350 mg/m^2 weekly for 4 weeks or 1,000 mg/m^2 for 1st and 15th day) with the addition of prednisolone 1 mg/kg /day for 2 weeks followed by tapering of prednisolone over 2 weeks if responses are sustained prednisolone under slow tapering within 6 months, well nonsevere types can be managed with prednisolone alone with gradual taper slowly within 6 months. During the course, it is recommended to add rituximab if response or relapse or hauling into severe anemia is met while on treatment if

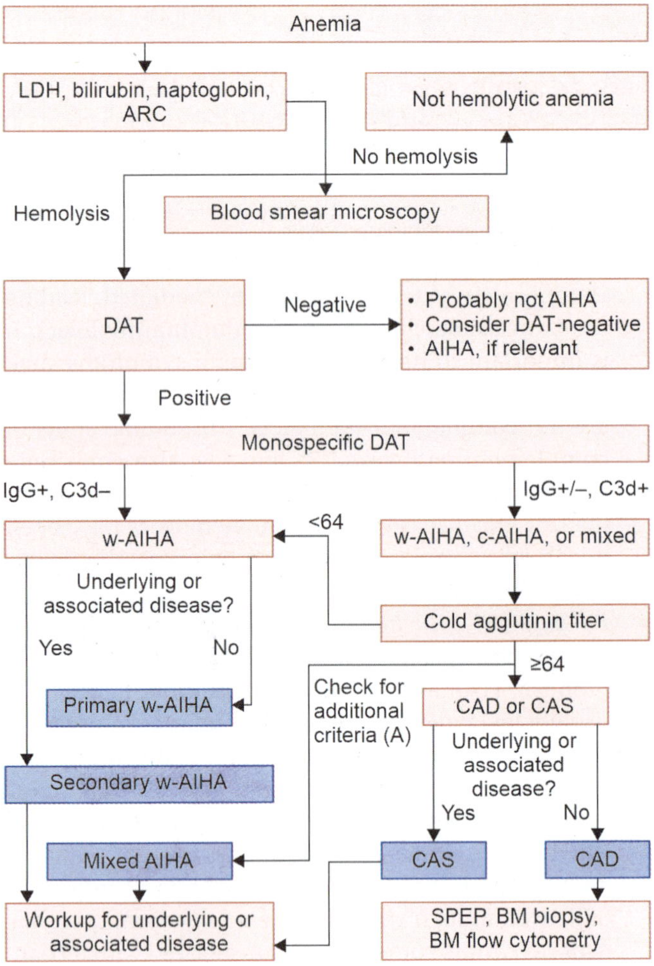

Diagnostic workup in AIHA. A, additional criteria for mixed AIHA (DAT strongly positive for both IgG and C3d, cold agglutinin titer ≥64, indirect antiglobulin test positive for IgG at 37°C).

FLOWCHART 1: Diagnostic workup for autoimmune hemolytic anemia (AIHA).

(CAD: cold agglutinin disease; DAT: direct antiglobulin test; LDH: high lactate dehydrogenase; w-AIHA: warm-autoimmune hemolytic anemia; c-AIHA: cold-autoimmune hemolytic anemia)

Source: Berentsen S, Fattizzo B, Barcellini W. The choice of new treatments in autoimmune hemolytic anemia: how to pick from the basket? Front Immunol. 2023.

not added initially. It is worth noting that the role of unspecific immunosuppression (azathioprine, cyclophosphamide, and mycophenolate) along with splenectomy has taken a seat back as 3rd line, limited to 1st failure. The upcoming role of proteasome inhibitor bortezomib has been reported in studies with relatively low toxicities. Newer avenues are opening for relapse and loss, suggesting using erythropoietin stimulating agents (ESA) and low-dose corticosteroid (prednisolone <10 mg/day) in transfusion dependent. Regarding more recent approaches in emergency settings, the role of c1 inhibitors and c1 serine proteases inhibitor target monoclonal antibody (sutimlimab) are still in study awaiting validation, though rationalistically has a valid course in its use. The use of splenectomy, partial splenic embolization, intravenous immunoglobulin (IVIg), and plasma exchange in patients who are severely anemic with mild or no response to prednisolone have been studied but have documented success in single cases that need review since they are very old.

- *Cold agglutinin disease:* The selection of therapy in cold agglutinin disease rests on whether bothersome symptoms, circulatory symptoms (not complement-mediated) or symptomatic anemia is present, directing the role of B cell targeted therapy; by use of bendamustine with rituximab or rituximab alone which has shown overall complete response, time-limited treatment, effect on circulatory symptoms and prolong duration response with fewer drawbacks related with the time needed to respond, the toxicity profile of bendamustine. The role of the newly studied drug sutimlimab c1 directed inhibitor has risen due to high faster response rates, longer duration of remission, and overall low toxicity profile. However, its effect on circulatory symptoms is yet to be established. Worthwhile mentioning its availability. The cost pulls it over from the role or uses it as a first line. There is no based algorithm as of now. Still, it can be directed when the above-pertaining indications occur, as mentioned before, with the role of sutimlimab coming in for need in rapid onset because of severity, rapidity of onset and failure to respond on rituximab and bendamustine. However, in emergencies, the role of plasma exchange still holds with albumin in settings where sutimlimab is limited, with case studies showing increase survival but short duration of remission and response rates yet to be established. Coming years will see the role of ibrutinib, rituximab with fludarabine, and bortezomib in the second line; current trials are being held to include patient individualization for trials and C3 inhibitor pegcetacoplan.

CONCLUSION

The ever-changing dynamics of w-AIHA still pursue the role of steroids. Still, the addition of rituximab has slowly developed importance due to its class action in cases of severe w-AIHA. At the same time, therapies in CAD, B cell-directed therapy, and complement inhibition have taken a front seat. The last two decades have seen the rise of evidence-based medicine, which has caused conventional strategies to take a back seat. At the same time, a review of the underlying etiology and targeted therapies has an upcoming role in future. Therefore more clinical trials will be of foremost importance along with the availability of better laboratory diagnostics helping us build better insights into AIHA.

SUGGESTED READINGS

1. Gehrs BC, Friedberg RC. Autoimmune hemolytic anemia. Am J Hematol. 2002;69(4):258-71.
2. Fadlallah J, Michel M, Crickx E, Limal N, Costedoat N, Malphettes M, et al. Bortezomib and dexamethasone, an original approach for treating multi-refractory warm autoimmune hemolytic anemia. Br J Haematol. 2019;187(1):124-8.
3. Barcellini W, Fattizzo B. The changing landscape of autoimmune hemolytic anemia. Front Immunol. 2020;11:946.
4. de Boer ECV, Jalink M, Delvasto-Nuñes L, Meulenbroek EM, Baas I, Janssen SR, et al. Peritransfusional C1-inhibitor in patients with severe complement-mediated autoimmune hemolytic anemia: an open-label phase 2 trial. Presented at the European Hematology Association 2022 Congress. Hema Sphere. 2022;6(S3):2690.

102

CHAPTER

Sickle Cell Disease and its Complications

Atanu Thakur

ABSTRACT

Sickle cell disease (SCD) is an autosomal codominant hemoglobinopathy. The global burden of SCD is increasing. Sickle cell occurs due to the substitution mutation leading to the change of glutamic acid to valine at the sixth position of the β-globin chain. It is the key point of formation of HbS polymer in hypoxic conditions and leads to distorted sickle RBC. Sickle cell is diagnosed by slide test, Hb electrophoresis, high-performance liquid chromatography, and mutation confirmation by polymerase chain reaction (PCR) methods. The hallmarks of pathogenesis are vaso-occlusion and intra and extravascular hemolysis; these lead to acute life-threatening crises and also chronic organ damage. With the increasing global burden of SCD, premarital counseling and prenatal and antenatal diagnosis hold promising results in early intervention and prevention of mortality. Therapeutic measures like hydroxyurea and repeated blood transfusion reduce mortality. Newer drugs under study like inhalation of NO, Crizanlizumab, and Vepoloxamer are hopefully better treatments and may reduce the complication and mortality.

INTRODUCTION

Sickle cell disease (SCD) is an autosomal codominant hemoglobinopathy. This is caused by a transversion mutation on the sixth codon (GAG>GTG) of the β-globin gene leading to a change in the amino acid from glutamic acid to valine. Individuals with heterozygous for the HbS allele are known as the sickle cell trait (HbAS), whereas individuals with homozygous for the HbS allele are known as sickle cell anemia (SCA). The compound heterozygote forms of the HbS with other Hb variants are known as sickle cell disease. SCD patients show a pleiotropic clinical feature, with a wide variable in clinical presentation. High fetal Hb (HbF) and coinheritance of α-thalassemia were modulators of clinical presentation in SCD patients.

EPIDEMIOLOGY

The global burden of SCA is increasing, with the annual number of SCA newborns expected to increase from ~300,000 to more than ~400,000 between 2010 and 2050. In India, it was observed that the prevalence of sickle gene was more in central India (1–40%), while it was 1.40% in southern India and 0.18% in North-eastern India. The Odisha state (eastern state of India) has shown a higher prevalence of sickle cell gene, about 21–40%. There were more than 28,400 SCD death cases globally in 2000, which increased by 20.8% of 34,400 (25,000–45,000) in 2021.

PATHOGENESIS

In sickle cell, the substitution mutation of glutamic acid to valine at the sixth position of the β-globin chain is the key point of formation of HbS polymer in hypoxic condition and leads to distorted sickle RBC. Deoxy Hb polymer in the cell exists from a single individual fiber to a highly ordered aggregate. Upon oxygenation, these polymers dissolve or melt and the sickled erythrocyte loses all the pathologic properties. If the concentration of HbS is >30 g/dL, a semisolid gel is formed. The equilibrium of HbS between its liquid and solid phase is determined by four variables: (1) O_2 tension, (2) HbS concentration, (3) temperature, and (4) presence of Hb variant other than HbS. An increase in the 2,3-diphosphoglycerate (DPG) decreases the affinity of HbS to O_2 which enhances the gelation. The presence of HbA and HbF has an inhibitory effect on gelation.

Pathogenesis of Hemolysis

Intravascular hemolysis results from hemolysis of complement-sensitive red cells and shear-induced membrane fragmentation. Extravascular hemolysis occurs due to monocyte and macrophage recognition and phagocytosis of red cells that have undergone sickling or oxidation-induced membrane changes and physical entrapment of the compromised red cells.

Pathogenesis of Vaso-occlusion

Possible risk factors for the development of vaso-occlusion include HbS polymerization, sickle cell deformability, sickle blood viscosity, sickle RBC-endothelial cell adherence, endothelial cell activation, vascular tone, and contribution from WBC and platelets. Abnormal interaction between sickle RBC and vascular endothelium may be of greater relevance for vaso-occlusive events than the alteration of red cell morphology, viscosity, and vascular flow. Specific ligands that may mediate adhesion of sickle cell endothelium include von Willebrand factors, fibronectin, fibrin, thrombospondin, vitronectin, and certain vasoconstrictor-like prostaglandin I2 (PGI2), prostaglandin D2 (PGD2), and endothelin. Infection may exacerbate erythrocyte endothelial adhesion by TNF.

CLINICAL FEATURES

Although disease attributable to HbS has been observed in early infancy, this can be modulated by the production of sufficient HbF to limit clinically significant sickling. Dactylitis and acute chest syndrome have the highest incidence during the first year of life. Among clinical features of SCA, vaso-occlusion is the most common clinical presentation than anemia.

ACUTE EVENTS

Vaso-occlusive Crises or Painful Crisis

The vaso-occlusive crisis (VOC) is the hallmark clinical presenting symptom of SCD. It is a qualitative term and may be termed the period of pain which may last up to 4 hours and analgesics are needed to be administered for pain relief when other causes might not explain the symptoms. Although VOC is a complex mechanism, HbS polymerization is the key factor for its occurrence. HbS polymerization changes the properties and shape of the sickle-RBCs leading to obstruction in blood flow in micro- and macrovasculature. Polymerization of HbS, cellular adhesion, and inflammation are complex interactions, which lead to VOC in SCD.

Hand-foot Syndrome

The initial episodes in young children often involve the small bones hand and feet. Typically, the dorsum of the hand and feet are swollen, erythematous, and painful with radiological evidence of cortical thinning and destruction of metacarpals, metatarsals, and phalanges.

Central Nervous System

Stroke is a catastrophic complication. It affects 6% of children and 17% of young adults. Infarction is quite frequent in children, while hemorrhagic stroke is frequent in the age group of 20–29 years. The mortality is 20–29% after hemorrhagic stroke and 0% after infarct. Transient ischemic attack, anemia, recurrent acute chest syndrome, and hypertension are the independent risk factors for ischemic stroke. Transcranial Doppler (TCD) predicts the risk of stroke in SCD.

Acute Chest Syndrome

Acute chest syndrome (ACS) is characterized by fever, tachypnea, chest pain, leukocytosis and pulmonary infiltrate. It is a common cause of morbidity and mortality in SCD patients. Infection and vascular occlusion are the predominant cause of sickle cell ACS. Mostly infection in children and pulmonary vascular infarction in adults are cause of ACS. Infection and vascular infraction are interrelated and concurrent. Chlamydia, mycoplasma, and respiratory syncytial virus are the common organisms implicated in ACS.

Hematologic Crises

Aplastic Crises

Aplastic crises are the most common complication seen among children caused due to parvovirus B19 infection. Aplasia is due to the direct toxicity of the parvovirus on the erythroid cell mainly the colony-forming unit.

Splenic Sequestration Crisis

Splenic sequestration is characterized by the sudden trapping of blood in the spleen. It is more documented in infants and children. There is evidence of compensatory erythropoiesis and splenic enlargement. Sometimes, it may lead to hypovolemic shock and death.

Hemolytic Crises

Hemolytic crises result from a sudden acceleration of the hemolytic process. They have been associated with mycoplasma infection. Increased lipid peroxidation of the sickle cell by reactive O_2 species derived from activated neutrophils is another mechanism of hemolysis.

Megaloblastic Crises

Megaloblastic crises result from sudden arrest of erythropoiesis by folate depletion. They are precipitated by conditions imposing increased folate requirements like pregnancy, alcoholism, and any chronic illness. It is a common practice to prescribe 1 mg daily of folic acid to patients with SCD.

Infection

Sickle cell patients are in a state of immune-depression condition. As a result, different microbial agents attack these patients. *Streptococcus pneumoniae* is the usual infecting organism that causes 70% of meningitis in children with sickle cell disease. At 5 years of age, gram-negative bacteria, mostly *Escherichia coli*, cause urinary tract infection. Osteomyelitis is caused by *Salmonella*. Bloodstream infection in SCD is mostly *Staphylococcus aureus* in adults. Among all these, malaria and tuberculosis are the most common types of infections.

CHRONIC ORGAN DAMAGE

Growth and Development

The height and weight of the children with SCD are delayed by 2 years. The magnitude of the growth spurt is substantially less than the healthy children, puberty is delayed, and menarche occurs 2–3 years later than the normal population. It has been hypothesized that chronic hemolysis leads to a state of high protein turnover and increased basal metabolic rate. The resting energy expenditure is 15–20% greater in HbS patients.

Bone and Joints

In addition to acute episodes of skeletal pain, chronic and progressive destruction of bones and joints may take place in SCD patients. The cumulative effect of recurrent small ischemia and infarct results in the weakening of bones; further weight bearing may collapse the femoral head causing osteonecrosis.

Central Nervous System

Children of SCD with overt stroke have significant cognitive impairment-reduced language function and problems in adjustment. They also have diminished performance in areas of visual-motor integration, attention and concentration arithmetic, memory, and reading.

Cardiovascular System

Cardiac enlargement, particularly the left ventricular dimension and mass, has got an early occurrence in childhood due to chronic anemia and an increase in cardiac output. Physical examination reveals cardiomegaly and hyperdynamic precordium. Pulmonary arterial hypertension is found in 58% of adult patients. Adults with SCD may have acute myocardial infarction in the absence of atherosclerosis; this could be due to fat embolism.

Pulmonary System

Chronic pulmonary disease probably due to recurring pulmonary infarction and infection is characterized by a decrease in radiolucency and moderate-to-severe pulmonary function. In a recent study, 32% of patients with HbS had pulmonary arterial hypertension which was associated with a 10-fold increase in death and a mortality rate.

Hepatobiliary and Gastrointestinal System

Hepatomegaly is present from 1 year of life and persists through life. Hyperbilirubinemia seen in this state. This episode may be affected by intercurrent infection with hepatitis B and C and intrahepatic sickling or choledocholithiasis.

Kidney

A variety of defects in renal function have been described. Renal cortical infarct, hemosiderin deposits in the epithelium of the PCT, glomerular arteriolar congestion, and dilatation symmetrical enlargement of kidneys occur. Hematuria and nephrotic syndrome are common in adolescent pathological lesions.

Eye

Vaso-occlusive disease of retina is responsible for both nonproliferative and proliferative retinopathy. Nonproliferative changes include "salmon patch" due to small intraregional hemorrhages; the iridescent spot is the coloration of iron-loaded retinal macrophages; schisis cavity is left over after the resolution of blood.

Leg Ulcer

The leg ulcer typically forms a shallow depression with a smooth and slightly elevated margin with a surrounding area of edema, exudation, and ground lesion at the base. Secondary infection is common. Healing is done by leg elevation, wet-to-dry dressing, and systemic antibiotics.

DIAGNOSIS

The basic laboratory techniques for the diagnosis of sickle are the sickling slide test, Hb electrophoresis, and high-performance liquid chromatography (HPLC). Molecular methods of diagnosis include amplification refractory mutation system-polymerase chain reaction (ARMS-PCR) and deoxyribonucleic acid (DNA) sequencing. Neonatal SCD is diagnosed by reverse transcription PCR (RT-PCR) and prenatal diagnosis requires fetal DNA samples obtained from chorionic villus analysis performed at 9 weeks of gestation and diagnosed by RT-PCR.

MANAGEMENT

Sickle cell disease is a complex multisystem affected state characterized by acute and chronic complications. Advances in medical care, early diagnosis, and comprehensive treatment have led to substantial improvements in life expectancy. Routine and emergency care of individuals with SCD is needed along with substantial psychological and social impact.

THERAPIES

Three therapies modify the disease course of SCD: (1) Hydroxycarbamide, (2) erythrocyte transfusion, and (3) hematopoetic stem cell transplantation.

Hydroxycarbamide

Hydroxycarbamide or hydroxyurea is a ribonucleotide reductase inhibitor. It increases HbF expression and reduces leukocyte count, hospitalization, and mortality. The drug significantly reduces the incidence of vaso-occlusive crises; up to 63% of SCA may be on hydroxycarbamide. A study in India suggests that a minimum dose of 10 mg/kg/day is an effective dose in the improvement of clinical and hematological parameters.

Erythrocyte Transfusion

Treatment with this therapy improves microvascular flow by decreasing the number of circulating sickle RBCs and decreasing endothelial injury and inflammatory damage. Chronic transfusion therapy can prevent strokes and vaso-occlusive crises. Adverse effects of chronic transfusion are iron overload and allogenic immunization.

Hematopoietic Stem Cell Transplantation

Hematopoietic stem cell transplantation in SCD is curative and should be considered in symptomatic patients, with a human leukocyte antigen (HLA)-matched family donor. The survival exceeds more than 90% in USA and European studies. The average rate of chronic graft versus host reaction is 14% and the rate of graft failure is 2%.

MANAGEMENT OF ACUTE COMPLICATION

Acute Pain

Pain assessment and initiation of analgesics should be undertaken promptly. The treatment should be individualized with the degree of pain. Oral analgesics can be used in patients who can tolerate, but most recommendations suggest I/V or S/C morphine in doses from 0.05 to 0.01 mg/kg every 2–4 hours. Close monitoring of vital signs like O_2 saturation and pain assessment should be done.

Acute Chest Syndrome

The severity of acute chest syndrome increases with age and more than 10% are fatal. Early X-ray imaging and O_2 monitoring with any pulmonary events are necessary. Hospitalizations with broad-spectrum antibiotics, bronchodilators, O_2 supplementation and red blood transfusion are the mainstay of treatment. Exchange transfusion with steroids can modify the course of the disease.

Acute Stroke

An acute stroke including ischemia and hemorrhage needs emergency management. Rapid exchange transfusion is the standard treatment. Chronic transfusion decreases stroke recurrence. The importance of subsequent monthly transfusion to prevent secondary stroke has been reaffirmed. Imaging and angiography could reveal a treatable aneurysm. An individual with vasculopathy who tends to bleed is corrected by a method called encephaloduroarteriosynangiosis (EDAS).

Acute Anemia

Fifty percent of SCA patients experience acute anemic events in the form of sequestration crises, hemolytic crises, and aplastic crises. Transfusion with early splenectomy is helpful in sequestration crises.

Cholelithiasis

Cholelithiasis results from a chronic accelerated rate of erythrocyte destruction. About 20% of patients of SCA suffer from acute complications of cholelithiasis as cholecystitis, which often necessitates cholecystectomy.

PREVENTION OF COMPLICATION

The prevention strategy has changed long-term outcomes in SCD more than any other approach. Prophylactic penicillin in children up to 5 years of age has remained safe and beneficial. There is a 93.4% reduction in pneumococcal infection by giving the conjugated pneumococcal vaccine. TCD screening to detect children with high risk of stroke can be prevented by early transfusion therapy. Early detection of pulmonary hypertension by echocardiogram and treatment can prevent a cardiac event.

Newer Therapy

- *Crizanlizumab*: The cell–cell interactions of endothelial and platelet by P-selection involve in the pathogenesis of vaso-occlusive crisis in patients with SCD. The Crizanlizumab therapy resulted in a significantly lower rate of VOC than the placebo study.
- *Vepoloxamer (P-188)*: The Vepoloxamer or Poloxamer-188 therapy is used to decrease the VOC episodes by increasing the oxygenation of tissue and leads to a reduction in pain, inflammation, and also duration of painful episodes in SCD patients.
- *CRISPR/Cas9 nuclease system*: The CRISPR/Cas9 nuclease system can cleave bacteriophage or plasmid DNA and enables targeting of insertions or deletions at a specific genomic DNA site. It restores γ-globin synthesis by inhibiting or deletion of inhibitors like BCL11.

CONCLUSION

With the increasing global burden of SCD, premarital counseling and prenatal and antenatal diagnosis hold promising results in early intervention and prevention of mortality. Therapeutic measures like stem cell transplantations and CRISPR technology are newer hopes in the treatment. Newer drugs under study like inhalation of NO, Crizanlizumab, and Vepoloxamer are hopefully better treatments and may reduce the complication and mortality.

ACKNOWLEDGMENT

The author would like to thank the staff of the Multi-Disciplinary Research Unit (MRU) of Veer Surendra Sai Institute of Medical Science and Research (VIMSAR), Burla, Sambalpur for their support in manuscript preparation.

SUGGESTED READINGS

1. Thomson AM, McHugh TA, Oron AP, Teply C, Lonberg N, Tella VV, et al. Global, regional, and national prevalence and mortality burden of sickle cell disease, 2000–2021: a systematic analysis from the Global Burden of Disease Study 2021. Lancet Haematol. 2023. [online] Available from https://doi.org/10.1016/S2352-3026(23)00118-7 [Last accessed December, 2023].
2. Kato GJ, Piel FB, Reid CD, Gaston MH, Ohene-Frempong K, Krishnamurti L, et al. Sickle cell disease. Nat Rev Dis Primers. 2018;4(1):1-22.
3. Onimoe G, Rotz S. Sickle cell disease: A primary care update. Cleve Clin J Med. 2020;87(1):19-27.
4. Ataga KI, Kutlar A, Kanter J, Liles D, Cancado R, Friedrisch J, et al. Crizanlizumab for the Prevention of Pain Crises in Sickle Cell Disease. N Engl J Med. 2017;376(5):429-39.
5. Orringer EP, Casella JF, Ataga KI, Koshy M, Adams-Graves P, Luchtman-Jones L, et al. Purified poloxamer 188 for treatment of acute vaso-occlusive crisis of sickle cell disease: a randomized controlled trial. JAMA. 2001;286(17):2099-106.
6. Frangoul H, Altshuler D, Cappellini MD, Chen YS, Domm J, Eustace BK, et al. CRISPR-Cas9 gene editing for sickle cell disease and β-thalassemia. New England J Med. 2021;384(3):252-60.

103

CHAPTER

Thalassemia: Iron Chelation and Monitoring

LP Meena, Anju Bharti

ABSTRACT

Thalassemia is one of the most common inherited hereditary disorders which results from quantitative defects in hemoglobin. The estimated prevalence of hemoglobinopathies in India is 1.2/1,000 live birth and the annual birth is estimated at around 27.72 million. On the basis of the globin chain, thalassemia is classified into alpha- and beta-thalassemia. Overall, the prevalence of beta-thalassemia is much higher than alpha-thalassemia. Therefore, in this chapter, we will discuss beta-thalassemia only. Depending on the extent of reduction in beta-chain synthesis, there are three types of beta-thalassemia: Beta-thalassemia major (homozygous form), beta-thalassemia intermedia, and beta-thalassemia minor (trait). Patients with beta-thalassemia minor/trait remain asymptomatic, so they do not require treatment. Unlike thalassemia minor, patients with thalassemia intermedia require blood transfusion intermittently after an age. Treatment of beta-thalassemia major is largely supportive. In majority of children with beta-thalassemia major, iron chelation is required before 6 years of age (sometimes as early as 2–4 years). For those with beta-thalassemia intermedia, the requirement for iron chelation depends on whether (or when) chronic transfusion is started and the indications are written above; often, this is in the second or third decade.

INTRODUCTION

Thalassemia is one of the most common inherited hereditary disorders which results from quantitative defects in hemoglobin. The estimated prevalence of hemoglobinopathies in India is 1.2/1,000 live birth and the annual birth is estimated at around 27.72 million. On the basis of the globin chain, thalassemia is classified into alpha- and beta-thalassemia. Overall, the prevalence of beta-thalassemia is much higher than alpha-thalassemia. Therefore, in this chapter, we will discuss beta-thalassemia only. Beta-thalassemia arises from different types of mutations of the beta-globin gene. The symbol beta^0 indicates the complete absence of beta-globin chain synthesis while beta$^+$ denotes the partial synthesis of the beta-globin chain. Depending on the extent of reduction in beta-chain synthesis, there are three types of beta thalassemia:

1. *Beta-thalassemia major (homozygous form)*: It is the most severe form, which is further subclassified into two types:
    i. Beta^0 thalassemia major: It is characterized by a complete absence of beta chain.
    ii. Beta$^+$ thalassemia major: It has incomplete suppression of beta-chain synthesis.
2. *Beta-thalassemia intermedia*: It is beta-thalassemia of an intermediate degree of severity that does not require regular blood transfusions. These cases are genetically heterozygous (b^0/b or b^+/b).
3. *Beta-thalassemia minor (trait)*: It is a mild asymptomatic form in which there is moderate suppression of beta-chain synthesis. Besides beta-thalassemia minor,

a few uncommon globin chain combinations resulting in the beta-thalassemia trait are as follows:

a. db-thalassemia minor in which there is a total absence of both b- and d-chain synthesis and is characterized by an elevated HbF level but unlike beta-thalassemia minor, there is a normal or reduced HbA2 level.
b. Hb Lepore syndrome is characterized by a nonhomologous fusion of *b* and *d* genes forming an abnormal hemoglobin called Hb Lepore (named after a family called Lepore). There is a total absence of normal beta-chain synthesis. An individual may inherit one beta-chain gene from each parent and produce heterozygous, homozygous, or double heterozygous state. Statistically, 25% of offspring born to two heterozygotes (i.e., beta-thalassemia trait) will have the homozygous state, i.e., beta-thalassemia major. It has been estimated that 2 million units of packed red cells would be needed annually for transfusion of thalassemia patients in the country. In India, the blood components are provided free of cost without a donor to all thalassemic patients, but these facilities are not available in the peripheral regions of the country. Along with the blood transfusion, patients with thalassemia also require iron-chelating agents which are very costly. Although the treatment of thalassemia is provided free of cost in India, for the healthcare system, these treatment options are enormously expensive causing a huge drain on the health resources of the nation.

TREATMENT

Patients with beta-thalassemia minor/trait remain asymptomatic, so they do not require treatment. However, they should be explained about the genetic implications of the disorder, particularly those of child-bearing age. Unlike thalassemia minor, patients with thalassemia intermedia require blood transfusion intermittently after an age. Treatment of beta-thalassemia major is largely supportive. Thalassemia major and some beta-thalassemia intermedia phenotypes are now designated as transfusion-dependent thalassemia (TDT). These patients usually require chronic and frequent transfusions. Patients with thalassemia major and a subset of those with thalassemia intermedia will in due course develop iron overload, which in turn can cause end-organ damage and even death. Iron stores are monitored on a regular basis in these thalassemic patients **(Table 1)**.

TABLE 1: Assessment of iron overload in adults.

Parameters	Duration/Indication
Total volume of RBCs transfused	Assess every 6–12 months
Serum ferritin	Every 3 months
Iron, TIBC, transferrin saturation	As clinically indicated (e.g., if the ferritin level is higher than expected)
Liver ultrasound	Biannually in those with severe liver disease, iron overload
Liver iron by MRI	Upon increases in ferritin or changes in clinical condition that suggest increased iron burden
Cardiac MRI	Upon significant increases in ferritin

(MRI: magnetic resonance imaging; RBCs: red blood cells; TIBC: total iron-binding capacity)

INDICATION OF IRON CHELATION THERAPY

Iron chelation is generally initiated in one or more of the following settings:

- After the serum ferritin exceeds 1,000 ng/mL (1,000 μg/L)
- After the liver iron concentration (LIC) exceeds 3 mg iron per gram of dry weight
- After transfusion of approximately 20–25 units of red blood cells (RBCs)

In majority of children with beta-thalassemia major, iron chelation is required before 6 years of age (sometimes as early as 2–4 years). For those with beta-thalassemia intermedia, the requirement for iron chelation depends on whether (or when) chronic transfusion is started and the indications are written above; often, this is in the second or third decade. In patients with beta-thalassemia intermedia, serum ferritin may underestimate the total body iron stored. MRI appears to be more useful and superior to the measurement of serum ferritin for estimating the total body iron burden in these patients, especially in individuals with beta-thalassemia intermedia.

OBJECTIVES OF IRON CHELATION THERAPY

- *Primary objective*: The primary objective of chelation therapy is the prevention of toxic iron burden and the maintenance of safe iron levels. This can be achieved by using chelator doses that balance iron intake from transfusions with iron excretion by chelation.

- *Rescue iron chelation therapy*: When toxic levels of iron have developed, the objective of iron chelation is not only the iron maintenance therapy but is instead iron rescue therapy, which requires a more intensive and aggressive approach to iron chelation.

Iron chelation therapy must be given over a prolonged time in patients with iron overload and must be strictly followed. The choice of a chelating therapy should be based on the ability of the patient to tolerate and pursue the chosen regimen with high adherence and to be in regular follow-ups to evaluate the efficacy and safety of the provided agent.

CHOICE OF INITIAL THERAPY

Presently, there are three iron chelating agents in wide use and numerous ways in which iron chelation therapy can be given to patients. None of the agents or any combination of agents is considered the "gold standard" of therapy for all patients. There are no universal gold standard guidelines in iron chelation treatment. There are consensus recommendations from the experts and thalassemia organizations that share the same approaches in most of the cases. The three approved chelating agents are (1) deferasirox, (2) deferiprone, and (3) deferoxamine (DFO).

Deferasirox

Deferasirox is approved as a first-line monotherapy in most countries because of its oral formulation, long half-life, and fewer side effects. The dose of this chelating agent is 20 mg/kg once a day. The dose may be increased by 5–10 mg based on the level of serum ferritin. If the disorder does not get controlled at 30 mg/kg/day, it may be raised up to 40 mg/kg/day along with monitoring of the toxicity of a higher dose.

The long half-life allows once-daily dosing. Deferasirox is the most common choice for initiating chelation therapy in the United States.

Deferoxamine

This iron chelating agent has been available since the time of the late 1970s and is considered a first-line therapy for young children by many organizations including the Thalassaemia International Federation (TIF), particularly in children < 2 years of age. The efficacy of this drug is equal to deferasirox, but it is given parenterally. It is given by slow subcutaneous infusion of a 10% solution over 8–12 hours for a minimum of 5 days/week. The usual daily dose in children is around 20 mg/kg/day, but it can be increased up to 40 mg/kg/day. In adults, the DFO dose can be increased up to 60 mg/kg/day.

Deferiprone

Deferiprone has been available in an oral form worldwide since the 2000s. It is given three times a day, but twice-daily dosing is also acceptable which may improve adherence. Although it has fewer gastrointestinal (GI) side effects (GI toxicity) than deferasirox, it has the risk of developing agranulocytosis. Because of its low cost and ease of administration, it is widely used in resource-poor settings.

To date, there are no randomized controlled trials (RCTs) that guide the preference of chelating agents for starting therapy. That is why the choice is predominantly dependent on the availability and cost of drugs, where it is not in government supply, route of administration, local experience, age of the patient, adverse effects, comorbidities, and patient preference.

MONITORING IRON OVERLOAD

The following tests should be advised routinely in these patients for iron load monitoring:

- *Serum ferritin level*: It should be performed at baseline before starting the chelation therapy and should be repeated every 3 months at least.
- *Cardiac T2* by MRI*: If the child has been well chelated, then cardiac MRI can be deferred until 8–10 years of age to determine the cardiac iron overload. However, this test can be done earlier in the child if significant degrees of iron overload are present and/or when levels of serum ferritin and/or LIC are worsening with chelation treatment. If the thalassemic patient has had stable levels of serum ferritin and LIC and a previous normal cardiac MRI, then this test should be repeated every 2 years, otherwise in patients with significant iron overload, this test should be repeated yearly. At any time, if the cardiac MRI value falls below 15 ms, the test should be advised immediately and additional cardiac monitoring should be started.
- *Other monitoring*: Depending upon the type of chelating agent(s) given, some other monitoring (e.g., growth retardation, renal and hepatic function, complete blood count, absolute neutrophil count) is also needed.

Dose Adjustments and Monitoring of Treatment

The dose of the chelating agent should be adjusted to attain serum ferritin levels < 1,000 µg/L, LIC < 7 mg Fe/g dry weight, and a cardiac T2* by MRI > 20 ms. The same dose is continued if the above levels remain stable or are improving with time and therapy is stopped or if the ferritin is <300–500 µg/L, or LIC becomes < 3 mg/g dry weight. The iron chelation treatment is stopped or reduced when the serum ferritin level falls to <300–500 μg/L and/or LIC falls to <3 mg/g dry weight.

INTENSIFICATION OF CHELATION THERAPY

Intensification of therapy is required if:

- LIC > 15 mg Fe/g, serum ferritin > 2,500, cardiac T2* MRI < 15 ms *or*
- A fall in the left ventricular ejection fraction (LVEF) because of cardiac iron overload
- Cardiac failure or arrhythmia indicates inadequate chelation

Options include:

- Increasing the dose to the maximum allowed dose
- Switching to other agents, if adherence with the present agent has been inadequate, or
- Use of combined chelating agents

Some prospective RCTs have confirmed the superiority of deferiprone, either alone or in combination with DFO, compared with DFO alone, for the treatment of established cardiac disease due to iron overload. Increments in doses are appropriate when ferritin and LIC levels are raised when averaged over a minimum period of 6 months. Expert guidance on this issue is not available, but it is reasonable to accelerate the dose only when significant alterations in serum ferritin and LIC have developed. Some experts suggest that the development of acute decompensated heart failure is the major cause of death in these patients and is a medical emergency. In this subgroup of patients, treatment can be initiated with high-dose continuous IV DFO along with oral deferiprone.

CONCLUSION

Iron chelation therapy must be given over a prolonged time in patients with iron overload and must be strictly followed. The choice of a chelating therapy should be based on the ability of the patient to tolerate and pursue the chosen regimen with high adherence and to keep in regular follow-ups to evaluate the efficacy and safety of the provided agent.

SUGGESTED READINGS

1. Mohan H. Textbook of Pathology, 7th edition. New Delhi: Jaypee Brothers Medical Publishers; 2015.
2. Musallam KM, Cappellini MD, Wood JC, Motta I, Graziadei G, Tamim H, et al. Elevated liver iron concentration is a marker of increased morbidity in patients with β thalassemia intermedia. Haematologica. 2011;96(11):1605-12.
3. http://www.thalassaemia.org.cy/uploads/1466152679tifguidelinesformanagementfinalmerged.pdf [Last accessed].
4. Angelucci E, Barosi G, Camaschella C, Cappellini MD, Cazzola M, Galanello R, et al. Italian Society of Hematology practice guidelines for the management of iron overload in thalassemia major and related disorders. Haematologica. 2008;93(5): 741-52.
5. Taher A, El Rassi F, Isma'eel H, Koussa S, Inati A, Cappellini MD. Correlation of liver iron concentration determined by R2 magnetic resonance imaging with serum ferritin in patients with thalassemia intermedia. Haematologica. 2008;93(10): 1584-6.
6. Cappellini MD, Farmakis D, Porter J, Taher A (Eds). Guidelines for the Management of Transfusion Dependent Thalassaemia (TDT), 4th edition. Nicosia: Thalassaemia International Federation; 2021.
7. Hoffbrand AV, Taher A, Cappellini MD. How I treat transfusional iron overload. Blood 2012;120:3657.
8. Elalfy MS, Saber MM, Adly AA, Ismail EA, Tarif M, Ibrahim F, et al. Role of vitamin C as an adjuvant therapy to different iron chelators in young β-thalassemia major patients: efficacy and safety in relation to tissue iron overload. Eur J Haematol. 2016;96(3):318-26.
9. Musallam KM, Angastiniotis M, Eleftheriou A, Porter JB. Cross-talk between available guidelines for the management of patients with beta-thalassemia major. Acta Haematol. 2013;130(2):64-73.
10. Pennell DJ, Porter JB, Cappellini MD, El-Beshlawy A, Chan LL, Aydinok Y, et al. Efficacy of deferasirox in reducing and preventing cardiac iron overload in beta-thalassemia. Blood. 2010;115(12):2364-71.
11. Maggio A, Vitrano A, Capra M, Cuccia L, Gagliardotto F, Filosa A, et al. Improving survival with deferiprone treatment in patients with thalassemia major: a prospective multicenter randomised clinical trial under the auspices of the Italian Society for Thalassemia and Hemoglobinopathies. Blood Cells Mol Dis. 2009;42(3):247-51.
12. Rachmilewitz EA, Giardina PJ. How I treat thalassemia. Blood. 2011;118(13):3479.

104

CHAPTER

Immune Thrombocytopenia: Advances in Management

Sumita Chaudhry

ABSTRACT

Immune thrombocytopenia (ITP) is isolated thrombocytopenia characterized by autoimmune-mediated destruction of platelets caused by immunoglobulin G (IgG) antibodies directed against platelet glycoproteins mainly glycoprotein IIb/IIIa (GPIIb/IIIa). Recent studies have demonstrated that in addition to enhanced destruction of platelets opsonized by antiplatelet antibodies, T-cell cytotoxicity, and impaired megakaryopoiesis are additional factors in its pathophysiology.

INTRODUCTION

Immune thrombocytopenia (ITP) characterized by autoimmune destruction of platelets presents as isolated thrombocytopenia. It is classified as *primary* in the absence of an identifiable underlying disorder or *secondary* to drugs, autoimmune disorders, or infections [e.g., hepatitis C virus (HCV) and human immunodeficiency virus (HIV)]. International working group on ITP in 2009 classified primary ITP into *newly diagnosed* (from diagnosis till 3 months), *persistent* (3–12 months from diagnosis), and *chronic* (>12 months from diagnosis). It tends to follow a chronic course in 70–80% of adults whereas most children achieve remission in 1 year. The bleeding severity in ITP can be classified as *critical* (bleeding into a critical anatomical site/that causing hemodynamic instability/respiratory compromise, e.g., intracranial, intraspinal, intraocular, retroperitoneal, or pericardial), severe (bleeding causing a fall in hemoglobin of 2 g/dL or requiring > 2 units of transfusion but not meeting criteria for critical) and minor bleeding. *The risk of bleeding* is highest in those older than 60 years, with platelet counts < 10,000 /mm^3, or those with a history of prior bleeding.

TREATMENT

The treatment aims to maintain a platelet count of ≥ 20–30,000/mm^3 which is generally regarded as a safe count. *The goal of treatment* is to treat bleeding episodes and prevent bleeding while maintaining the quality of life, especially in chronic ITP. British Society of Hematology (2019) recommends no treatment if the patient has a platelet count >20,000/mm^3 while the American Society of Hematology in its 2019 guidelines recommends treatment only at a platelet count of <30,000/mm^3. There is no benefit in treating patients maintaining platelet counts > 20–0,000/mm^3 because of the risk of treatment-related toxicity with little or no reduction in bleeding risk. However, in patients with a high bleeding risk (peptic ulcer, liver disease, need for anticoagulation or antiplatelet therapy, and surgery) or those with a high probability of falls or professions with a high chance of injury higher thresholds may be acceptable as clinically indicated.

RESPONSE DEFINITIONS

- *Complete response (CR)*: Platelet count ≥ 100,000/mm^3
- *Partial response (PR)*: Platelet response 30,000–100,000/mm^3
- *Refractory*: Disease requiring treatment that persists or recurs after splenectomy or for which splenectomy is not an option

FIRST-LINE THERAPIES

Steroids, intravenous immunoglobulin (IVIg), and anti-D are the first-line therapeutic options. Steroids [time to response (TTR) 2–14 days] and IVIg (TTR 1–3 days) may be used as monotherapy or combined for an augmented effect in critical bleeding considering their different mechanism of action and TTR. In critical and severe bleeding, pulse steroids in the form of dexamethasone 40 mg IV or oral for 4 days or Methylprednisolone 1 g IV for 3 days may be given. Thereafter, oral Prednisolone 1 mg/kg for 3 weeks is to be given followed by taper. IVIg 1 g/kg/day for 1–2 days is the usual dose. Day 2 dose of IVIg may be omitted if the patient achieves a platelet count >50,000/mm^3 after the first dose. Patients with contraindications to steroids such as uncontrolled diabetes and psychosis may be given IVIg or second-line options.

SECOND-LINE THERAPIES

While the majority of ITP patients respond to first-line treatment, a number of patients require second-line treatment to achieve/maintain long-term responses. Before starting second-line agents rule out alternative diagnoses such as drug-induced thrombocytopenia, myelodysplastic syndrome (MDS), or inherited thrombocytopenias. Options for second-line treatment may be medical [thrombopoietin receptor agonist (TPO-RA) and rituximab] or surgical (splenectomy).

Splenectomy offers the greatest chance of a durable response [objective response rate (ORR): 88–90%] but is associated with operative risk, venous thromboembolism, and long-term immunosuppression. Splenectomy should ideally be planned after 1 year of diagnosis to allow for rare cases of spontaneous remission.

Rituximab, an anti-cluster of differentiating 20 (anti-CD20) monoclonal antibody (Ab), acts by reducing the production of anti-platelet antibodies. Dosed at 375 mg/m^2/week for 4 weeks, it has an ORR of 40–60%. Low-dose rituximab (100 mg or 100 mg/m^2/week for 4 weeks) has also been studied to avoid treatment-related adverse events. Rituximab is also associated with prolonged immunosuppression and may need to be repeated as effects may be short-lived.

Thrombopoietin Receptor Agonists

It binds and activates the TPO receptor thereby stimulating the production of megakaryocytes by the bone marrow. About 80% of the patients will respond to these agents but long-term remissions after stopping these agents have been seen only in around 15% of cases. Prolonged maintenance therapy is therefore required as most patients lose their response on stopping these agents and may even have worse counts than baseline (rebound thrombocytopenia). However, in a recent study reported in Blood 2023, Guillet et al. reported a treatment-free remission (TFR) of 56.2% which suggested an immunomodulatory effect of these agents. Currently, there are three agents (eltrombopag, romiplostim, and avatrombopag) that are approved for the treatment of chronic ITP of which only the first two are available in India at present. Since there are no randomized controlled trials comparing the three TPO-RAs, the choice of agent depends on patient choice, cost, and comorbidities. Romiplostim [1–10 μg subcutaneous (SC) once weekly] is the preferred agent in those with liver dysfunction when Eltrombopag is best avoided. Eltrombopag (25–75 mg/day) offers the advantage of once-daily oral administration but the food interactions mandate staggering as regards meals. Avatrombopag is approved by the United States Food and Drug Administration (USFDA); its efficacy is similar to eltrombopag but has the advantage of having no food interactions. Other TPO-RAs undergoing investigation include lusutrombopag, hetrombopag, and human recombinant thrombopoietin (rhTPO). These agents can be of value in the treatment of patients in whom surgery/immunosuppression are contraindicated or patient wants to avoid them.

Third-line options include dapsone, danazol, mycophenolate mofetil, azathioprine, cyclophosphamide, and vincristine, and their use is restricted to patients who have failed the first two lines because of a lack of large clinical series.

Novel treatments are needed in case of patients who fail the available options. Spleen tyrosine kinase (Syk) and Bruton tyrosine kinase (BTK)are involved in the phagocytosis of opsonized platelets; thus inhibitors of these kinases are being investigated as therapeutic targets.

Fostamatinib, a Syk inhibitor, was approved by the USFDA in 2018 for ITP patients who have failed first- or second-line therapy, or are intolerant to these therapies. Given in a dose of 100 mg twice a day (with an increase to 150 mg BD if needed), trials demonstrated an ORR of 43%. Responses were quick with a median TTR of 2 weeks. Posthoc analysis of the phase three trials showed higher benefits if the drug was used as second-line therapy. Since sustained responses can be seen in multidrug refractory patients it is an encouraging option. Hypertension and diarrhea are important side effects and need monitoring.

Rilzabrutinib, an oral, reversible, covalent, highly selective *BTK inhibitor* that increases platelet counts in ITP by decreasing macrophage-mediated platelet destruction and reducing the production of pathogenic autoantibodies. Ongoing phase 1/2 study in adults with relapsed/refractory ITP revealed that rilzabrutinib given in a dose of 400 mg twice a day produced a rapid rise in platelet count (median TTR of 8.5 days) in 42% of patients who had failed a median of six prior lines of therapy. The ongoing, randomized phase III LUNA 3 trial will further elucidate rilzabrutinib's clinical benefit in ITP. In contrast to the presently available BTK inhibitors, rilzabrutinib does not have inhibitory effects on platelet aggregation.

Long-lived plasma cells are implicated as a cause of failure of B cell-depleting therapies. Hence *plasma cell targeting therapies* such as proteasome inhibitor *bortezomib* and anti-CD38 monoclonal Ab *daratumumab* are undergoing trials for their potential role in autoimmune disorders including ITP. Thrombocytopenia secondary to bortezomib as seen in multiple myeloma is a concern while treating ITP cases. *Mezagitamab*, another anti-CD38 monoclonal Ab is also undergoing trials.

Neonatal Fc Receptor (FcRn) is a homeostatic receptor that increases the half-life of IgG. Its blockers will cause the clearance of autoreactive antibodies. *Rozanolixizumab*, a neonatal Fc receptor blocker, approved in 2023 for myasthenia gravis, permits the reduction of pathologic IgG and, consequently, may increase the platelet counts in ITP. In a recent multicenter, open-labeled phase 2 trial including 66 adult ITP patients, the response (platelet count $\geq 50 \times 10^9$/L) was achieved in 66.7 and 54.5% of patients receiving a single SC infusion at 15 and 20 mg/kg, respectively. It showed a favorable safety profile. *Efgartigimod (APGX-113)* is another neonatal Fc receptor (FcRn) inhibitor that showed an ORR of 46% versus 25% with placebo and a stable response in 38% versus 0% with placebo in a phase 2 trial. Stable response (platelet count $\geq 50 \times 10^9$/L for at least 10 consecutive days) was achieved in 38% on efgartigimod as compared to none in the placebo.

Platelet desialylation has been identified as a novel mechanism of Fc-independent platelet clearance by the Ashwell- Morell receptors in the liver in ITP. *Oseltamivir*, a desialidase inhibitor, along with dexamethasone showed a higher platelet response of 86% versus the dexamethasone alone group (ORR: 66%) in a phase 2 multicenter trial on newly diagnosed ITP patients. A 6-month sustained response rate (53% vs. 30%) was also higher in the combination arm.

Classical complement pathway is activated in ITP with complement deposition on platelet surface seen in >50% of patients. *Sutimlimab* is a humanized monoclonal anti-C1s immunoglobulin G4 (IgG4) antibody, that decreases C3b deposition and formation of membrane attack complex. Phase 1 trial on 12 chronic ITP patients showed an ORR and stable response in 42 and 33.3% respectively. The median TTR was 2 days and there were no adverse events. However, since complement is not activated in all patients more studies are needed to identify potential biomarkers for use of this agent in routine practice.

PLATELET TRANSFUSION IN IMMUNE THROMBOCYTOPENIA

Platelet transfusion in the form of apheresis platelets or random pooled platelets may be given in case of critical bleeding along with other therapies to increase platelet count as the transfused platelets will be immunologically destroyed within 1 hour of transfusion. Administration of IVIg along with platelets may potentiate the response of transfused platelets.

CONCLUSION

Most patients respond to first- and second-line therapies for chronic ITP. However, there is a lacuna in the treatment of patients with an inadequate response. Newer agents targeting different pathogenetic mechanisms are being developed. However, the long-term efficacy and safety profiles of these drugs need to be proven through randomized controlled trials.

SUGGESTED READINGS

1. Neunert C, Terrell DR, Arnold DM, Buchanan G, Cines DB, Cooper N, et al. American Society of Hematology 2019 guidelines for immune thrombocytopenia. Blood Adv. 2019;3(23):3829-66.
2. Al-Samkari H, Kuter DJ. An alternative intermittent eltrombopag dosing protocol for the treatment of chronic immune thrombocytopenia. Br J Clin Pharmacol. 2018;84(11):2673-7.
3. Iino M, Sakamoto Y, Sato T. Treatment-free remission after thrombopoietin receptor agonist discontinuation in patients with newly diagnosed immune thrombocytopenia: an observational retrospective analysis in real-world clinical practice. Int J Hematol. 2020;112(2):159-68.
4. Wang J, Li Y, Wang C, Gao C, Lang H, Chen H. Efficacy and safety of the combination treatment of rituximab and dexamethasone

for adults with primary immune thrombocytopenia (ITP): a meta-analysis. Biomed Res Int. 2018;2018:1316096.

5. Bussel J, Arnold DM, Grossbard E, Mayer J, Treliński J, Homenda W, et al. Fostamatinib for the treatment of adult persistent and chronic immune thrombocytopenia: results of two phase 3, randomized, placebo-controlled trials. Am J Hematol. 2018;93(7):921-30.
6. Robak T, Kaźmierczak M, Jarque I, Musteata V, Treliński J, Cooper N, et al. Phase 2 multiple-dose study of an FcRn inhibitor, Rozanolixizumab, in patients with primary immune thrombocytopenia. Blood Adv. 2020;4(17):4136-46.
7. Newland AC, Sánchez-González B, Rejtő L, Egyed M, Romanyuk N, Godar M, et al. Phase 2 study of Efgartigimod, a novel FcRn antagonist, in adult patients with primary immune thrombocytopenia. Am J Hematol. 2020;95(2):178-87.
8. Sun L, Wang J, Shao L, Yuan C, Zhao H, Li D, et al. Dexamethasone plus oseltamivir versus dexamethasone in treatment-naive primary immune thrombocytopenia: a multicentre, randomised, open-label, phase 2 trial. Lancet Haematol. 2021;8(4):e289-98.
9. Broome CM, Röth A, Kuter DJ, Kuter DJ, Scully M. Long-term safety and efficacy of Sutimlimab in patients with chronic immune thrombocytopenia. Blood. 2020;136(Suppl 1):14-5.

105

CHAPTER

Hemophilia Current Diagnosis and Treatment

Manoj K Srivastav, Gaurav Singh

ABSTRACT

Hemophilia is an X-linked recessive hemorrhagic disease due to mutation in the *F8* gene leading to factor VIII deficiency (hemophilia A) and mutation in *F9* gene characterized by deficiency of factor IX (hemophilia B). X-linked disorder, females carry gene, and males are affected. Up to 30% are due to spontaneous mutation. Deficiency results in recurrent bleeds into joints and muscles, leading to hemophilic arthropathy and contractures. Incidence of hemophilia A is 1 in 5,000 and hemophilia B is 1 in 30,000 live male births. All races and socioeconomic groups are equally affected. Hemophilia C (factor XI deficiency) generally occurs in 1 in 100,000 people.

INTRODUCTION: DIAGNOSIS

Screening

Blood investigations (with reference ranges) for any child with suspected bleeding disorder include platelet count (150–450 × 103/μL); prothrombin time (PT) (11–15 seconds), and activated partial thromboplastin time (aPTT) (29–35 seconds). In hemophilia, screening tests reveal a prolonged aPTT with a normal PT and platelet count. Mixing study is a simple test performed by mixing plasma from the patient with pooled normal plasma in 1:1 proportion and repeating aPTT after incubating for 30–60 minutes. Correction of aPTT after mixing suggests deficiency in any of the factors in intrinsic pathway. Prolonged aPTT may not get corrected with mixing study in case of presence of antibodies to factor VIII or IX, lupus anticoagulant, or heparinized sample. Specific factor assays for factor VIII or IX should be done for specific diagnosis and ascertaining its severity.

The diagnosis of hemophilia B in neonatal period and infancy may be challenging as the normal factor IX level is low in neonatal period, and age-specific cut-off levels should be used. While a diagnosis of moderate and severe cases is still possible, a suspected mild hemophilia B requires confirmation at 3–6 months of age.

Genetic Analysis

It helps in genetic counseling for the family and provides prenatal diagnosis. During pregnancy of carrier females, it is advisable to perform chorionic villous sampling at 11–14 weeks, gestation. Identification of mutation also helps in preimplantation genetic diagnosis (PGD) that is legal in India if carried out under strict conditions and criteria. In case the fetus is affected, the family is counseled regarding the diagnosis and options of continuing the pregnancy or medical termination. In patients with severe hemophilia A, inversions of intron 22 (reported in 40–45%) and intron 1 (reported in 1–6%) of factor VIII (*FVIII*) gene are the most common mutations. If these two variations are not identified, Sanger sequencing of the gene identifies other mutations.

In hemophilia B, majority are point mutations (commonly missense mutations). Specific gene defects are thought to contribute to about 40% risk of inhibitor formation. Large deletions and nonsense mutations carry the highest risk, whereas missense and splicing mutations carry the lowest risk for inhibitor formation. There are >2,000 identified mutations in hemophilia A and >1,000 in hemophilia B. Mutation may not be identifiable in a small proportion of hemophilia patients.

In a patient with acquired hemophilia, the bleeding time, PT, and platelet count are normal. However, the aPTT typically shows a prolongation that is not reversed on a correction study. Heparin and lupus anticoagulant must be screened for. FVIII levels must be measured and evidence of FVIII inhibitor sought. Other factor levels should be determined to establish inhibitor specificity **(Flowchart 1)**.

MANAGEMENT

A person with hemophilia is born with it and has it all his life. The amount of factor VIII or IX in blood usually stays the same throughout his life (exception factor IX Leyden). With appropriate management, it can lead near normal life. Avoid injuries, intramuscular injections, and nonsteroidal anti-inflammatory drugs (NSAIDs). Vaccination to be given subcutaneously. First-aid treatment for bleeds. For minor bleeds, antifibrinolytics (tranexamic acid) can be used topically or systemically (oral/intravenous). Desmopressin (DDAVP): It boosts plasma level of FVIII in mild-to-moderate cases. There is no effect on factor IX. A single dose (0.3 µg/kg IV infusion/SC) increases FVIII levels by three-to-sixfold **(Table 1)**.

Calculation of dose of factors: Calculation of the doses in individual episodes for different patients to achieve a desired factor level is based on the formulae given below:

- *Factor VIII (IU per dose) = U/dL desired rise (%) × Body weight (kg) × 0.5*; (1 U/kg of FVIII increases the body level by 2%; half-life of FVIII is 8–12 hours)
- *Factor IX (IU per dose) = U/dL desired rise (%) × Body weight (kg);* (1 U/kg of factor IX increases the body level by 1%; half-life of FVIII is 18–24 hours).

Because recovery of recombinant factor IX activity is less than that of therapeutic plasma-derived factor IX, 1.2–1.5 times the dose should be administered if using recombinant factor IX.

The frequency of doses should be 12 hourly in hemophilia A and 24-hourly in hemophilia B. For example, if a 25 kg severe hemophilia A patient had a hemarthrosis and the targeted factor level is 20% (in view of resource constraints), requirement of FVIII (IU per dose) = 20 × 25 × 0.5 = 250 IU per dose. The child should receive 250 IU of FVIII as a slow intravenous injection every 12 hourly till the desired duration (say 2 days in this case). In case of hemophilia B, the same dose of factor IX is given every 24 hourly. It is a good practice to carefully round off the dose to nearest vial strength without any treatment compromise in order to avoid wastage of factors.

Continuous infusion is preferable in life-threatening bleeds. It avoids peaks and troughs. It may lead to reduction in total factors consumed (cost-effective). Factor levels should be monitored and doses adjusted accordingly. Pump failure is a concern and should be monitored.

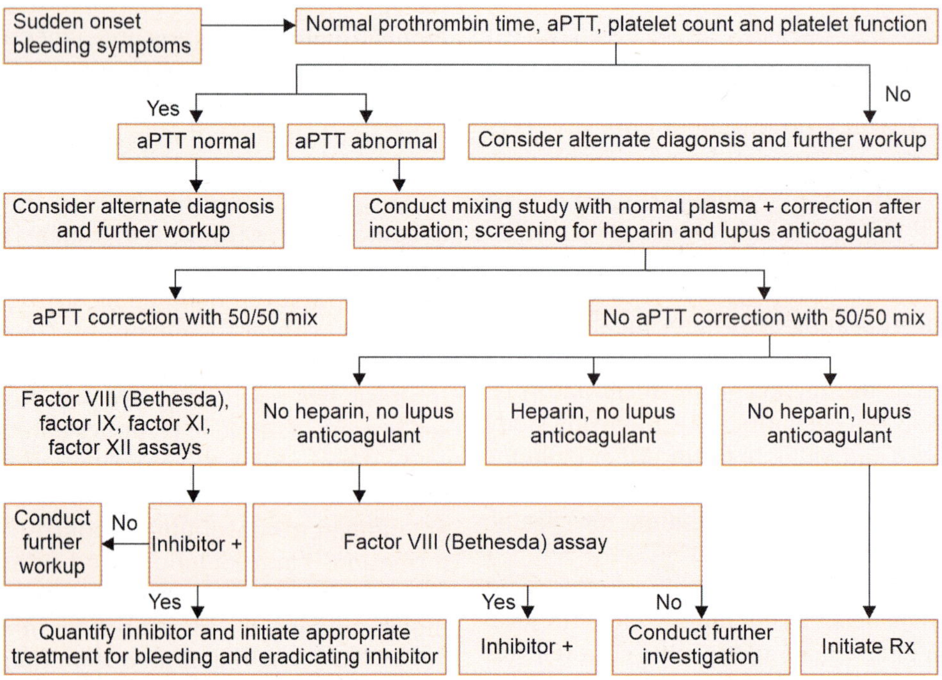

FLOWCHART 1: Workup for acquired hemophilia.
(aPTT: activated partial thromboplastin time)

TABLE 1: Factor replacement for major bleed.

	Hemophilia A		Hemophilia B	
Hemorrhage type	**Desired level**	**Duration (days)**	**Desired level**	**Duration (days)**
Joint	40–60%	1–2; longer if inadequate response	40–60%	1–2; longer if inadequate response
Muscle (except iliopsoas)	40–60%	2–3; longer if inadequate response	40–60%	2–3; longer if inadequate response
Iliopsoas:				
• Initial	80–100%	1–2	60–80%	1–2
• Maintenance	30–60%	3–5 (sometimes longer as secondary prophylaxis during physiotherapy)	30–60%	3–5 (sometimes longer as secondary prophylaxis during physiotherapy)
CNS/Head:				
• Initial	80–100%	1–7	60–80%	1–7
• Maintenance	50%	8–21	30%	8–21
Throat and neck:				
• Initial	80–100%	1–7	60–80%	1–7
• Maintenance	50%	8–14	30%	8–14
Gastrointestinal:				
• Initial	80–100%	1–6	60–80%	1–6
• Maintenance	50%	7–14	30%	7–14
Renal	50%	3–5	40%	3–5
Deep laceration	50%	5–7	40%	5–7
Surgery (major):				
• Preoperative	80–100%		80–100%	
• Postoperative	60–80%	1–3	60–80%	1–3
	40–60%	4–6	40–60%	4–6
	30–50%	7–14	30–50%	7–14

Source: Srivastava A, Santagostino E, Dougall A, Kitchen S, Sutherland M, Pipe SW, et al. WFH Guidelines for the Management of Hemophilia, 3rd edition. Haemophilia. 2020:26(Suppl 6):1-158.

Choice of factor replacement products: In the 1950s and 1960s, bleeding episodes were treated with fresh frozen plasma (FFP). Modern treatment started in 1965 with identification of the cryoprecipitate fraction. Subsequently, plasma-derived factor VIII and IX concentrates were introduced. The recombinant FVIII and recombinant factor IX were introduced in 1992 and 1997, respectively. The salient features of various products containing FVIII are compared in **Table 2**.

PROPHYLAXIS

- Prophylaxis prevents bleeding and joint destruction
- Aim of prophylaxis is to keep factor VIII/IX levels > 1% all the time.
- *Principle of prophylaxis*: Convert bleeding pattern of severe hemophilia into milder bleeding pattern of moderate hemophilia.
- *Long-term goals*: Improvement in quality of life and reduction in long-term social costs.
- Prophylaxis can be started at any age.
- Types of prophylaxis **(Table 3)**.

Development of Inhibitors

Approximately 33% patients with severe hemophilia A, 13% with mild-moderate hemophilia A and 3% with hemophilia B develop neutralizing alloantibodies (inhibitors) directed against factor VIII or IX. In mild-to-moderate hemophilia, inhibitor formation is common with intense immune stimulation with high doses of factors in a short period (like in postoperative cases). In a recent study of 1,285 Indian patients with hemophilia A, 6% had inhibitors, with incidence being higher in patients from Southern India (13%) and highest in Chennai (21%).

Severe allergic reactions are known to occur in patients with inhibitors, especially in hemophilia B. Risk factors

TABLE 2: Comparison of salient features of various products containing factor VIII.

Feature	Plasma-derived factor concentrates	Recombinant factor concentrates	Cryoprecipitate	Fresh frozen plasma
Contents	Factor VIII and vWF	Factor VIII only	Factor VIII, vWF, fibrinogen, factor XIII	All coagulation factors
Risk for TTI	Screened for TTIs. Viral inactivation (heat/solvent) done. Risk of prion mediated diseases exists	No risk for TTIs (free of viral contamination)	Screened for TTIs, but viral inactivation not done	Screened for TTIs, but viral inactivation not done
Risk of allergic reactions	More with lower purity preparations	Rare	More common than factor concentrates	More common than factor concentrates
Uses	Hemophilia A, vWD	Hemophilia A	Used only if specific factor concentrates not available (hemophilia A, vWD, factor XIII deficiency, not in hemophilia B)	Used in DIC, coagulopathy of unknown cause, liver failure. Used in factor deficiencies (including hypofibrinogenemia, hemophilia B), only if factor concentrates not available
Strengths	*Vials*: 250 IU, 500 IU, 1,000 IU, 1,700 IU	*Vials*: 250 IU, 500 IU, 1,000 IU, 1,500 IU, 2,000 IU, 3,000 IU	1 bag = 70–80 IU of factor VIII	1 mL = 1% factor activity

(DIC: disseminated intravascular coagulation; TTI: transfusion transmitted infection; vWD: von Willebrand disease; vWF: von Willebrand factor)

TABLE 3: Types of prophylaxis.

Primary prophylaxis	Regular continuous treatment initiated in the absence of documented osteochondral joint disease, determined by physical examination and/or imaging studies, and started before the second clinically evident large joint bleed
Secondary prophylaxis	Regular continuous treatment started after two or more bleeds into large joints and before the onset of joint disease, documented by physical examination and imaging studies
Tertiary prophylaxis	Regular continuous treatment started after the onset of joint disease, documented by physical examination and plain radiographs of the affected
Intermittent prophylaxis	Treatment given to prevent bleeding for periods not exceeding 45 weeks in a year

include early age at exposure, presence of the common inversion mutation, large deletions of *FVIII* gene, and a sibling with hemophilia and an inhibitor. Majority of inhibitors develop early in the treatment trajectory (after a median exposure of 10 exposure days and less common after 150 exposure days). Initially, if feasible, inhibitor screen should be performed once in every 5 exposure days until 20 exposure days, every 10 exposure days between 21 and 50 exposure days, at least two times a year until 150 exposure days, and later annually.

Later, inhibitor should be screened in the following situations:
- Prior to and after any surgery or invasive procedure
- Before and after a switch of products
- Whenever clinically indicated (bleeding episodes while on prophylaxis, response to factor therapy in acute bleeds is suboptimal).

Nijmegen Bethesda Assay

It is used to quantify inhibitors. One Bethesda unit (BU) is the amount of antibody that neutralizes 50% of factor activity. High titer inhibitors have ≥5 BU/mL and low titers have 0.6 to <5 BU/mL. Low titer patients who have rapid anamnestic response upon exposure to factors are termed high responders and those without anamnestic response are low-responders.

Eradicating inhibitors: Immune tolerance induction (ITI) remains the mainstay of treatment to eradicate the inhibitors. ITI refers to regular, frequent, and prolonged exposure of the patient to specific factor concentrates thereby inducing peripheral tolerance. Various regimens with regard to dosage and duration of factor exposure are available and are beyond the scope of this guideline.

Again, high cost involved in this treatment precludes its routine use. Bleeding episodes need treatment with bypassing agents for patients on ITI (especially with titers > 10 BU).

If ITI alone fails, it can be tried again in combination with various drugs like rituximab, cyclophosphamide, and intravenous immunoglobulin (IVIG). In a phase II trial, RICH (Rituximab for the Treatment of Inhibitors in Congenital Hemophilia A) study, rituximab monotherapy (375 mg/m^2/dose weekly for 4 weeks) was administered to 16 hemophilia A patients with inhibitor level > 5 BU. Three patients (18.8%) had a major response (i.e., inhibitor level < 5 BU). The role of rituximab monotherapy needs further investigation **(Table 4)**.

TABLE 4: Agents used in inhibitor management.

	Recombinant FVIIa	aPCC (FEIBA)
Mechanism of action	Activates FX on the surface of platelets	Action of FXa and FII
Half-life	2–3 hours	8–12 hours
Dosing and frequency		
Acute bleeding	90–120 μ/kg every 2–3 hourly	50–100 U/kg 2–3 times daily (maximum dose is 200 U/kg/day)
Prophylaxis	90 μg/kg/day	85 U/kg three times/week

(aPCC: activated prothrombin complex concentrate)

SUGGESTED READINGS

1. Jameson J, Fauci AS, Kasper DL, Hauser SL, Longo DL, Loscalzo J (Eds). Harrison's Principle of Internal Medicine, 20th edition. New York: McGraw-Hill Education; 2018. p. 830.
2. Mannucci PM, Tuddenham EG. The hemophilias—from royal genes to gene therapy. N Engl J Med. 2001;344(23):1773-9.
3. Kamal AH, Tefferi A, Pruthi RK. How to interpret and pursue an abnormal prothrombin time, activated partial thromboplastin time, and bleeding time in adults. Mayo Clin Proc. 2007;82(7): 864-73.
4. Bagnall RD, Waseem N, Green PM, Giannelli F. Recurrent inversion breaking intron 1 of the factor VIII gene is a frequent cause of severe hemophilia A. Blood. 2002;99(1):168-74.
5. Peyvandi F, Garagiola I, Young G. The past and future of haemophilia: diagnosis, treatments, and its complications. Lancet. 2016;388(10040):187-97.
6. Cohen AJ, Kessler CM. Acquired inhibitors. Baillieres Clin Haematol. 1996;9(2):331-54.
7. Srivastava A, Santagostino E, Dougall A, Kitchen S, Sutherland M, Pipe SW, et al. WFH Guidelines for the Management of Hemophilia, 3rd edition. Haemophilia. 2020:26(Suppl 6):1-158.
8. White GC 2nd, Beebe A, Nielsen B. Recombinant factor IX. Thromb Haemost. 1997;78:261-5.
9. Gouw SC, van den Berg HM, Oldenburg J, Astermark J, de Groot PG, Margaglione M, et al. F8 gene mutation type and inhibitor development in patients with severe hemophilia A: Systematic review and meta-analysis. Blood. 2012;119:2922-34.
10. Kempton CL, Meeks SL. Toward optimal therapy for inhibitors in hemophilia. Blood. 2014;124:3365-72.
11. Pinto P, Shelar T, Nawadkar V, Mirgal D, Mukaddam A, Nair P, et al. The epidemiology of FVIII inhibitors in Indian haemophilia A patients. Indian J Hematol Blood Transfus. 2014;30:356-63.
12. De Moerloose P, Fischer K, Lambert T, Windyga J, Batorova A, Lavigne-Lissalde G, et al. Recommendations for assessment, monitoring and follow-up of patients with haemophilia. Haemophilia. 2012;18:319-25.
13. Kempton CL, White GC 2nd. How we treat a hemophilia A patient with a factor VIII inhibitor. Blood. 2009;113:11-7.
14. Leissinger C, Josephson CD, Granger S, Konkle BA, Kruse-Jarres R, Ragni MV, et al. Rituximab for treatment of inhibitors in haemophilia A. A Phase II study. Thromb Haemost. 2014;112: 445-58.

106
CHAPTER

Hematological Malignancies: Recent Advances in Management

Manjari Saha, Sourav Paul

ABSTRACT

Hematological malignancies, comprising 8–9% of all cancers and the fourth most common cancer in developed nations, are a significant burden worldwide. Advancements in immunotherapy have significantly improved care options and fewer relapsing/resistant hematological malignancies in the past decade. With more drugs being licensed, the future may see a decrease in the number of these diseases.

INTRODUCTION

Hematological malignancies are one of the most burdensome disorders not only in India or at any part of the world. Previously there were only limited options for the treatment of various disorders such as myeloproliferative neoplasms (MPNs), lymphoma, and leukemia.

The hematological malignancies comprise 8–9% of all cancers, fourth most common cancer in developed nations. In 2019, it was found that the incidence of leukemia, multiple myeloma, non-Hodgkin lymphoma, and Hodgkin lymphoma were 116.18, 23.55, 103.62, and 10.29 in 1 lac population in 204 countries across the world.

There is a rising concern about increasing resistance against common drugs due to mutations in the gene expressions, drug efflux mechanisms, overcame by the new drug designing and widespread clinical trials for efficacy safety of new drugs.

Among the newer aspects in the treatment are:
- Hematological cell transplant
- Natural killer (NK) cell stimulation
- T cell immunotherapy
- Immune check point inhibitor
- Monoclonal antibodies
- Bispecific T cell engager
- Immune modulatory drugs
- Immune therapeutic vaccines

Also there are newer options being opened as part of palliative care management. So together with increased early diagnostic scopes and ever improving therapeutic strategies, mortality and morbidity of these diseases expected to reduce in near future.

ADVANCEMENTS IN MOLECULAR DIAGNOSIS

The development of molecular biology tools has led to the disclosure of genetic or targeted therapy schemes with cytotoxic, as well as the individual molecular diagnosis of hematological cancers with immunomodulatory or antimetabolic properties.

Karyotyping, newer techniques of polymerase chain reaction (PCR), chromosomal microarray (CMA), new-generation sequencing (NGS), and fluorescence in situ hybridization (FISH) all these methods have came up to help identify the diseases early and also to check for any epigenetic modifications, and deoxyribonucleic acid

(DNA) alterations. These help in identifying the minimally residual disease after treatment.

Several molecular markers which are commonly associated with the common hematological malignancies are as follows:

- *Acute myeloid leukemia (AML)*: FLT3-ITD, CEBPA, RUNX1, NPM1, PML-RARA, ASXL1, IDH1, IDH2, DNMT3A, TET2, and BCR-ABL1
- *Acute lymphocytic leukemia (ALL)*: IKFZ1, CDKN2A/B, BCR-ABL1, BCR-ABL1-like, NOTCH1, ETV6, and RUNX1
- *MPN*: CAL-R, MPL, JAK2, SRSF2, SETBP1, TP53, CSF3R, and ASXL1
- *Myelodysplastic syndrome (MDS)*: RUNX1, JAK2, EZH2, SF3B1, IDH1/2, N-RAS, TP53, TET2, KIT, SRSF2, and ASXL1
- *Chronic lymphocytic leukemia (CLL)*: ATM, TP53, BIRC3, del11q, SF3B1, and NOTCH1 mutation
- *Chronic myeloid leukemia (CML)*: BCR-ABL1
- *B cell lymphoma*: MYC/BCL2, MYC/BCL2/BLC6, and SOX11
- *T cell lymphoma*: TP63, IRF4, DUSP22, and ALK
- *Multiple myeloma*: KRAS, CCND1, CCND2, CCND3, TP53, DI53, NRAS, MAF, FAM46C, and BRAF

CURRENT TARGETED AND NOVEL THERAPIES IN HEMATOLOGICAL MALIGNANCIES

Invention of the monoclonal antibodies paved the path of providing optimum therapy to majority of patients not only just for malignancies but also for certain rheumatological disorders. Monoclonal antibodies have been suggested to be able to destroy cancer cells by a variety of mechanisms, such as apoptosis, cell growth inhibition, and cellular cytotoxicity.

The current novel therapies for the hematological malignancies are listed in **Table 1.**

Examples of newer advancements are given in **Table 2.**

CHIMERIC ANTIGEN RECEPTOR T-CELL THERAPY

It is one of the most promising therapeutic option that have emerged in the past decade. Chimeric antigen receptors (CARs) are artificial receptors that help T lymphocytes identify and destroy cells by expressing their specific ligands. The same patient's autologous T cells are purified, genetically altered to express a CAR that is specific to tumor-associated antigen (TAA) amplified, and injected. By recognizing particular TAAs in a major histocompatibility complex (MHC)-independent manner, T cells expressing CARs enable the combination of their cytotoxic capabilities with a high degree of antibody specificity **(Fig. 1)**.

Chimeric antigen receptor T cells that are directed against CD19, which is expressed by a variety of B cells (pro to memory B cells), have been employed in preliminary clinical trials. A prime CAR target, CD19 has been shown to be expressed in a variety of B cell malignancies, including acute lymphoblastic leukemia (ALL), CLL, and B cell lymphoma and absence of other hematologic

TABLE 1: Novel therapies.

Diseases	Therapies
Acute myeloid leukemia (AML) subtypes	Lintuzumab, midostaurin, gemtuzumab, ulocuplumab, sorafenib, navitoclax, panobinostat, vorinostat, Dr383-IL3, and lestaurtinib
Acute promyelocytic leukemia (APML)	All-trans-retinoic acid, arsenic trioxide, gemtuzumab, and ozogamicin
Acute lymphoblastic leukemia (ALL)	Tyrosine kinase inhibitors, rituximab, inotuzumab ozogamicin, nelarabine, blinatumomab, and CAR T-cell
Myelodysplastic syndrome (MDS)	Azacitidine, decitabine, and lenalidomide
Chronic myeloid leukemia (CML)	Imatinib, nilotinib, dasatinib, and ponatinib
Chronic lymphatic leukemia (CLL)	Rituximab, idelalisib, ibrutinib, venetoclax obinutuzumab, and duvelisib
Chronic myeloproliferative neoplasms (MPN)	Ruxolitinib, busulfan, and chlorambucil
Hodgkin's lymphoma (HL)	Brentuximab vedotin, nivolumab, rituximab, and everolimus
B cell lymphoma	Tositumomab, rituximab, ibritumomab tiuxetan, and CAR T-cells
T cell lymphoma	Romidepsin, alemtuzumab, epratuzumab, denileukin, and nelarabine
Multiple myeloma (MM)	Bortezomib, carfilzomib, lenalidomide, pomalidomide, daratumumab milatuzumab, and ixazomib
Hairy cell leukemia (HCL)	Vemurafenib

CONCLUSION AND FUTURE PERSPECTIVES

As the day progresses newer advances are always appear to come and provide new set of options to the care givers and often circumvent the drawbacks of the previous treatments. This topic is an ever changing topic since every single day newer drugs are being licensed for the use. In the past decade, a significant advancements has been seen in the domain of immunotherapy and lots of promising results have come up. In the newer future it is well established fact that there might be very less number of relapsing/resistant hematological malignancies with the advent of more number of drugs.

SUGGESTED READINGS

1. Smith A, Howell D, Patmore R, Jack A, Roman E. Incidence of haematological malignancy by sub-type: a report from the Haematological Malignancy Research Network. Br J Cancer. 2011;105(11):1684-92.
2. Zhang N, Wu J, Wang Q, Liang Y, Li X, Chen G, et al. Global burden of hematologic malignancies and evolution patterns over the past 30 years. Blood Cancer J. 2023;13(1):82.
3. Bowman RL, Busque L, Levine RL. Clonal hematopoiesis and evolution to hematopoietic malignancies. Cell Stem Cell. 2018;22(2):157-70.
4. Braggio E, Egan JB, Fonseca R, Stewart AK. Lessons from next-generation sequencing analysis in hematological malignancies. Blood Cancer J. 2013;3:e127.
5. Prakash G, Kaur A, Malhotra P, Khadwal A, Sharma P, Suri V, et al. Current role of genetics in hematologic malignancies. Indian J Hematol Blood Transfus. 2016;32(1):18-31.
6. Miles RR, Shah RK, Frazer JK. Molecular genetics of childhood, adolescent and young adult non-Hodgkin lymphoma. Br J Haematol. 2016;173:582-96.
7. Cazzola M. Introduction to a review series: The 2016 revision of the WHO classification of tumors of hematopoietic and lymphoid tissues. Blood. 2016;127(20):2361-4.
8. Benjamin H, Yiping Y. New developments in immunotherapy for lymphoma. Cancer Biol Med. 2018;15(3):189-209.
9. Olsen E, Duvic M, Frankel A, Kim Y, Martin A, Vonderheid E, et al. Pivotal phase III trial of two dose levels of denileukin diftitox for the treatment of cutaneous T-cell lymphoma. J Clin Oncol. 2001;19:376-88.
10. Passamonti F, Mora B, Maffioli M. New molecular genetics in the diagnosis and treatment of myeloproliferative neoplasms. Curr Opin Hematol. 2016;23(2):137-43.
11. Shih LB, Lu HH, Xuan H, Goldenberg DM. Internalization and intracellular processing of anti-B-cell lymphoma monoclonal antibody, LL2. Int J Cancer. 1994;56:538-45.
12. Moss P. BTK inhibition saunters to the front of the line in CLL. Hematologist. 2017;14:1.
13. The ASCO Post. (2018). Enasidenib in IDH2-Mutant Relapsed or Refractory Acute Myeloid Leukemia. [online] Available from http://ascopost.com/issues/february-10-2018/enasidenib-in-idh2-mutant-relapsed-or-refractory-acute-myeloid-leukemia/. [Last accessed December, 2023].
14. Stone RM, Fischer T, Paquette R, Schiller G, Schiffer CA, Ehninger G, et al. Phase IB study of the FLT3 kinase inhibitor midostaurin with chemotherapy in younger newly diagnosed adult patients with acute myeloid leukemia. Leukemia. 2012;26(9):2061-8.
15. Glennie MJ, French RR, Cragg MS, Taylor RP. Mechanisms of killing by anti-CD20 monoclonal antibodies. Mol Immunol. 2007;44:3823-37.
16. Ginaldi L, De Martinis M, Matutes E, Farahat N, Morilla R, Dyer MJ, et al. Levels of expression of CD52 in normal and leukemic B and T cells: Correlation with in vivo therapeutic responses to Campath-1H. Leuk Res. 1998;22:185-91.
17. Russ A, Hua AB, Montfort WR, Rahman B, Riaz IB, Khalid MU, et al. "Don't eat me" signal of CD47-SIRPα in hematological malignancies, an in-depth review. Blood Rev. 2018;32:480-9.
18. Carnahan J, Stein R, Qu ZX, Hess K, Cesano A, Hansen HJ, et al. Epratuzumab, a CD22-targeting recombinant humanized antibody with a different mode of action from rituximab. Blood Rev. 2018;32(6):480-9.
19. Kantarjian HM, DeAngelo DJ, Stelljes M, Martinelli G, Liedtke M, Stock W, et al. Inotuzumab ozogamicin versus standard therapy for acute lymphoblastic leukemia. N Engl J Med. 2016;375:740-53.
20. Dreyling M, Santoro A, Mollica L, Leppa S, Follows GA, Lenz G, et al. Abstract CT149: Copanlisib in patients with relapsed or refractory indolent B-cell lymphoma: Primary results of the pivotal Chronos-1 study. Cancer Res. 2017;77(13 Suppl):49.
21. Miklos D, Cutler CS, Arora M. Ibrutinib for chronic graft-versus-host disease after failure of prior therapy. Blood. 2017;130(21):2243-50.
22. Rafiq S, Hackett CS, Brentjens RJ. Engineering strategies to overcome the current roadblocks in CAR T cell therapy. Nat Rev Clin Oncol. 2020;17(3):147-67.
23. Feins S, Kong W, Williams EF, Milone MC, Fraietta JA. An introduction to chimeric antigen receptor (CAR) T-cell immunotherapy for human cancer. Am J Hematol. 2019;94(S1):S3-9.
24. Khalil DN, Smith EL, Brentjens RJ, Wolchok JD. The future of cancer treatment: immunomodulation, CARs and combination immunotherapy. Nat Rev Clin Oncol. 2016;13(5):273-90.
25. Ghorashian S, Pule M, Amrolia P. CD19 chimeric antigen receptor T cell therapy for haematological malignancies. Br J Haematol. 2015;169(4):463-78.
26. Xie G, Dong H, Liang Y, Ham JD, Rizwan R, Chen J. CAR-NK cells: a promising cellular immunotherapy for cancer. EBioMedicine. 2020;59:102975.
27. Mack M, Riethmuller G, Kufer P. A small bispecific antibody construct expressed as a functional single-chain molecule with high tumor cell cytotoxicity. Proc Natl Acad Sci USA. 1995;92(15):7021-5.
28. Armand P, Chen YB, Redd RA, Joyce RM, Bsat J, Jeter E, et al. PD-1 blockade with pembrolizumab for classical Hodgkin lymphoma after autologous stem cell transplantation. Blood. 2019;134(1):22-9.

29. Ansell SM, Minnema MC, Johnson P, Timmerman JM, Armand P, Shipp MA, et al. Nivolumab for relapsed/refractory diffuse large B-cell lymphoma in patients ineligible for or having failed autologous transplantation: a single-arm, Phase II study. J Clin Oncol. 2019;37(6):481-9.
30. Herrera AF, Moskowitz AJ, Bartlett NL, Vose JM, Ramchandren R, Feldman TA, et al. Interim results of brentuximab vedotin in combination with nivolumab in patients with relapsed or refractory Hodgkin lymphoma. Blood. 2018;131(11):1183-94.
31. Galustian C, Meyer B, Labarthe MC, Dredge K, Klaschka D, Henry J, et al. The anti-cancer agents lenalidomide and pomalidomide inhibit the proliferation and function of T regulatory cells. Cancer Immunol Immunother. 2009;58(7):1033-45.
32. Jackson GH, Davies FE, Pawlyn C, Cairns DA, Striha A, Collett C, et al. Lenalidomide maintenance versus observation for patients with newly diagnosed multiple myeloma (Myeloma XI): a multicentre, open-label, randomised, Phase III trial. Lancet Oncol. 2019;20(1):57-73.
33. Morschhauser F, Le Gouill S, Feugier P, Bailly S, Nicolas-Virelizier E, Bijou F, et al. Obinutuzumab combined with lenalidomide for relapsed or refractory follicular B-cell lymphoma (GALEN): a multicentre, single-arm, Phase II study. Lancet Haematol. 2019;6(8):e429-37.
34. Shah NJ, Najibi AJ, Shih TY, Mao AS, Sharda A, Scadden DT, et al. A biomaterial-based vaccine eliciting durable tumour-specific responses against acute myeloid leukaemia. Nat Biomed Eng. 2020;4(1):40-51.
35. Gratwohl A, Baldomero H, Horisberger B, Schmid C, Passweg J, Urbano-Ispizua A; Accreditation Committee of the European Group for Blood and Marrow Transplantation (EBMT). Current trends in hematopoietic stem cell transplantation in Europe. Blood. 2002;100:2374-86.

107
CHAPTER

Management of Multiple Myeloma in 2024

Upendra Sharma, Nirmal Das Vaishnav

ABSTRACT

Multiple myeloma (MM) is a hematological malignancy characterized by uncontrolled proliferation of immature plasma cells causing destructive bone lesions, kidney injury, anemia, and hypercalcemia. Three drug regimens consisting of a combination of an injectable proteasome inhibitor, oral immunomodulatory agent, and dexamethasone have become the standard first-line for the management of myeloma. This induction therapy combined with autologous hematopoietic stem cell transplant (AHSCT) followed by maintenance (lenalidomide) is the standard of care for transplant-eligible patients. Myeloma remains an incurable disease and patients will ultimately relapse. Recent advances in the management of MM have improved patient survival. These advances will influence the management of myeloma in 2024 and the future. Immunotherapy, with the development of anti-cluster of differentiation 38 monoclonal antibodies (anti-CD38 mAb), is a milestone in the treatment of myeloma across all categories of patients. Drugs targeting B-cell maturation antigen (BCMA) have recently been approved and are a new ray of hope for patients who have progressed or are unresponsive to CD38 mAbs. These include BCMA bispecific drugs such as teclistamab and two anti-BCMA chimeric antigen receptor (CAR)-T cell therapies. Talquetamab a new bispecific targeting G protein-coupled receptor, class C, group 5, member D (GPRC5D) and a cluster of differentiation 3 (CD3) receptors has recently been approved in relapsed myeloma. These new drugs though currently approved for relapsed myeloma, in the future have the potential to challenge the current strategies in early lines of treatment.

INTRODUCTION

Multiple myeloma (MM)is a type of blood cancer that accounts for 1% of all cancers and approximately 10% of all hematologic malignancies. It is more common in men than in women. The median age of patients at the time of diagnosis is around 65 years. Incidence in India is lower than in the Western world (1.1/100,000/year). As per the recent Global Cancer Observatory (GLOBOCAN) data in India 14,641 new cases of myeloma are reported with 12,556 deaths and, the 5-year prevalence is 30,640 cases.

Unexplained bone pain is the most common presenting feature of patients with MM (almost 80%). Other major clinical manifestations are anemia, hypercalcemia, renal insufficiency, and increased risk of infections. Approximately 1–2% of patients have extramedullary disease (EMD) at the time of initial diagnosis, while 8% develop EMD later in the disease course.

The treatment of MM has greatly evolved over time, and the recent history of MM has been marked by the advent of multiple novel agents. From conventional regimens, based mainly on chemotherapy, to the emergence of immunotherapy, treatment options are expanding, and patient survival has improved. The current drugs used in the management of MM are mentioned in **Table 1**. Three drug regimens consisting of a combination of any injectable proteasome inhibitor, oral immunomodulatory agent, and dexamethasone have become the standard first-line for the management of myeloma. This induction therapy combined with autologous hematopoietic stem cell transplant (AHSCT) followed by maintenance (lenalidomide) is the standard of care for transplant-eligible patients. Treatment selection is often based on drug resistance patterns and performance status.

TABLE 1: Current drugs used in the management of multiple myeloma.

Immunomodulatory drugs	Proteasome inhibitors	Steroids	Monoclonal antibodies	Chemotherapy alkylators	XPO-1 inhibitor	Histone deacetylase inhibitor
Thalidomide (PO)	Bortezomib (SC)	Dexamethasone (IV and PO)	Daratumumab (IV or SC)	Cyclophosphamide (IV and PO)	Selinexor (PO)	Panobinostat (PO)
Lenalidomide (PO)	Carfilzomib (IV)	Prednisone (PO)	Isatuximab (IV)	Bendamustine (IV)		
Pomalidomide (PO)	Ixazomib (PO)		Elotuzumab (IV)	Melphalan (IV and PO)		

(IV: intravenous; PO: per os; SC: subcutaneous)

Several novel therapies are available for the management of MM. In this chapter, we will go through the different novel therapy approach which has the potential to revolutionize the management of MM in 2024.

CLUSTER OF DIFFERENTIATION 38 ANTIBODIES

Cluster of differentiation 38 (CD38) is a glycoprotein that is overexpressed on malignant plasma cells. Anti-cluster of differentiation 38 monoclonal antibodies (anti-CD38 mAb), whose impact is seen across all groups of patients, are possibly the greatest evolution in the field of myeloma so far. Daratumumab a first-in-class anti-CD38 mAb, is now widely integrated into MM treatment algorithms. Isatuximab is another CD38 mAb that received approval by the United States Food and Drug Administration (US FDA) in March 2021. New anti-CD38 mAbs, such as MOR2021 and TAK-0792 are still under early phases of drug development. MOR2021 is different from other CD38 antibodies as it does not activate complement-dependent cytotoxicity mainly responsible for the infusion-related reaction. TAK-0792 on the other hand is as highly selective of targeted cells, thus reducing off-target adverse events experienced with the use of other CD38 antibodies.

There is increasing evidence for support of the role of CD38 antibodies in the front-line management of MM patients. The MAIA trial compared daratumumab in combination with lenalidomide and dexamethasone to lenalidomide and dexamethasone combination. At a median follow-up of 56.2 months median progression-free survival was not reached in the daratumumab group versus 34.4 months in the control group. Median OS was not reached in either group. Another study the ALCYONE trial studied the combination of daratumumab, bortezomib, melphalan, and prednisone (D-VMP) versus Velcade melphalan-prednisone (VMP). At a median follow-up of 40 months, the study showed the median progression-free survival (mPFS) was 36.4 months in the D-VMP arm and 19.3 months in the VMP arm.

In the first-line setting for transplant-eligible newly diagnosed MM patients, the phase III multicenter CASSIOPEIA trial demonstrated that daratumumab in combination with bortezomib, thalidomide, and dexamethasone (Dara-VTd) could improve the depth of response and PFS in comparison with VTd alone. CASSIOPEIA part 2 studied the use of daratumumab monotherapy in maintenance every 8 weeks for 2 years as compared to observation. At a median follow-up of 35.4 months from the second randomization, daratumumab significantly improved PFS as compared to observation. Median PFS was not reached with daratumumab versus 46.7 months with observation.

After the encouraging results of the phase II GRIFFIN trial [42.4% of stringent complete response (sCR) rate with daratumumab plus bortezomib, lenalidomide, and dexamethasone (D-VRd) by the end of consolidation], the phase III PERSEUS study will further investigate the association with D-VRd. VRd is still a standard of care in most countries worldwide. Data from D-VRd therefore will be highly anticipated.

The phase III ICARIA trial demonstrated the activity of isatuximab in association with pomalidomide and dexamethasone (Isa-Pd) for patients with relapsed refractory MM (mPFS of 11.5 months). The phase III IKEMA trial has investigated the association of isatuximab, carfilzomib (K), and dexamethasone (isa-Kd) versus Kd (median PFS of 35.7 months with isa-Kd versus 19.15 months with Kd, $p = 0.0007$).

The most recent developments with anti-CD38 are based on the objective to combine anti-CD38 with other novel drugs and mechanisms of action to improve the depth of response and particularly the minimal residual disease (MRD)-negative rate and the focus on MRD to tailor the treatments. The MASTER trial is such an example. It uses MRD by next-generation sequencing

(NGS) to inform the use and duration of daratumumab, carfilzomib, lenalidomide, dexamethasone (Dara-KRd) postautologous hematopoietic cell transplantation, and treatment cessation in patients with two consecutive MRD-negative assessments.

Daratumumab has also been approved by the US FDA in a subcutaneous formulation.

B-CELL MATURATION ANTIGEN ANTIBODIES

B-cell maturation antigen (BCMA) (tumor necrosis factor receptor family) is highly expressed in myeloma cells, thus offering an encouraging potential target for novel treatments. Evolving concepts of BCMA-targeted therapy have different mechanisms of action, currently, there are three types of BCMA-targeted treatment options that are available: Antibody-drug conjugates (ADCs), BCMA bispecific T-cell engagers (BiTEs) and anti-BCMA chimeric antigen receptor (CAR)-T-cell-mediated treatments.

Antibody-drug Conjugate

Antibody-drug conjugate consists of a mAb-directed against a tumor-antigen and a cytotoxic agent inducing cell death. After binding to the antigen on the tumor cell, the ADC is internalized and then the linker is hydrolyzed inside of the lysosomes or endosomes and the payloads are released to cause cell death. Auristatin is used as a payload for MM.

Belantamab Mafodotin

Belantamab mafodotin (Bel) is a humanized immunoglobulin G1 (IgG1) ADC, first-in-class, originally approved by the US FDA as monotherapy in relapsed myeloma patients treated with four prior therapies including a proteasome inhibitor, anti-CD38 mAb, and an immunomodulatory agent. Bel is formed by an antibody directed to BCMA and covalently linked to the microtubule inhibitor monomethyl auristatin F (MMAF). Bel binds to BCMA on malignant plasma cell, and is internalized and MMAF is released, leading to cell-cycle arrest and apoptosis. In November 2022 Bel was withdrawn from the market as the DREAMM-3 trial which was the confirmatory phase III trial did not meet the requirements for the FDA accelerated approvals regulation.

B-cell Maturation Antigen Bispecific

Bispecific T cell engagers (BiTEs) are engineered proteins with two different antigen-binding fragments that bind to MM cells and T cells, thus creating an immunological synapse with direct plasma cell killing by T-cells. The two common antigens targeted are a cluster of differentiation 3 (CD3) and a cluster of differentiation 16 (CD16) for T cells and BCMA for MM plasma cells. Many studies with BITEs utilizing BCMA showed great efficacy with moderate toxicity, such as cytokine-release syndrome (CRS) and associated neurotoxicity syndrome (ICANS).

Teclistamab

It is a bispecific antibody targeting both CD3 expressed on the surface of T cells and BCMA expressed on the surface of myeloma cells, thus mediating T-cell activation and subsequent lysis of BCMA-expressing myeloma cells. On 25th October 2022, the US FDA granted accelerated approval to teclistamab for adults with relapsed refractory myeloma who have received at least four prior lines of therapy including a proteasome inhibitor, an immunomodulatory agent, and an anti-CD 38 mAb.

The approval was based on the results of the phase 1/2 MajesTEC-1 trial. The most common adverse reactions (≥20%) were pyrexia, CRS, musculoskeletal pain, injection-site reaction, fatigue, upper respiratory tract infection, nausea, headache, pneumonia, and diarrhea.

B-cell Maturation Antigen Chimeric Antigen Receptor-T Cell

Chimeric antigen receptor T-cell therapy involves genetic modification of a patient's autologous T-cells to express a CAR-specific for a tumor antigen, this is followed by ex vivo cell expansion and reinfusion back to the patient. CAR which are versatile synthetic receptors composed of an antigen-targeting domain, mostly derived from the single-chain variable fragment (scFv) of a mAb, fused to an intracellular T-cell activation signaling domain and one or two costimulatory domains. It functions as a specific antigen receptor that enables the identification of a particular antigen directly without any need for a major histocompatibility complex (MHC). CAR strategy targeting BCMA is a novel therapy with the characteristics of combining the target specificity of mAbs and the cytotoxicity of T cells.

Currently, two BCMA-directed CAR-T cell therapies have been approved by the US FDA for patients of MM and several trials for the use of CAR-T cell therapy in MM are underway.

Idecabtagene Vicleucel

Idecabtagene vicleucel (ide-cel) is a second-generation CAR-T that targets BCMA. Ide-Cel includes a CD3 signaling domain and a scFv, a costimulating domain. On March 26, 2021, the US FDA approved ide-cel for the treatment of adult patients with relapsed refractory MM after four or more prior lines of therapy, including an immunomodulatory agent, proteasome inhibitor, and an anti-CD38 mAb. This was the first cell-based gene therapy for MM approved by the FDA.

The approval was based on the results of the pivotal phase 2 KarMMa trial. The ide-cel label carries a boxed warning for CRS, neurologic toxicities, hemophagocytic lymphohistiocytosis/macrophage activation syndrome, and prolonged cytopenias. The most common side effects of ide-cel include CRS, infections, lethargy, muscle and skeletal pain, and hypogammaglobulinemia.

Ciltacabtagene Autoleucel

Ciltacabtagene autoleucel differs from ide-cel in that it entails CARs with two BCMA-targeting single-domain antibodies that detect two epitopes of BCMA expressed on the malignant MM cells. It was approved by the FDA on 22nd February 2022 for the treatment of adult patients with relapsed or refractory MM after four or more prior lines of therapy, including a proteasome inhibitor (PI), an immunomodulatory agent (IMiD), and an anti-CD38 mAb. It induces early, deep, and long-lasting responses with a tolerable safety profile in relapsed refractory MM. The approval was based on the results of the phase 1a/2b CARTITUDE-1 trial.

The most common adverse reactions were pyrexia, CRS, hypogammaglobulinemia, musculoskeletal pain, fatigue, infections, diarrhea, nausea, encephalopathy, headache, coagulopathy, constipation, and vomiting.

■ Non-B-cell Maturation Antigen Targeting Bispecific

Talquetamab

G protein-coupled receptor, family C, group 5, member D (GPRC5D) is an orphan receptor that is primarily expressed in plasma cells, with low expression in normal human tissue. Talquetamab is a bispecific immunoglobulin G4 (IgG4) antibody which binds to both GPRC5D and CD3 to induce the killing of GPRC5D-expressing myeloma cells by means of T-cell recruitment and activation.

On August 9, 2023, the US FDA granted accelerated approval to talquetamab for adults with relapsed or refractory MM who have received at least four prior lines of therapy.

Efficacy was evaluated in MonumenTAL-1 a single-arm, open-label, and multicenter study.

CONCLUSION

The future of therapies of MM is bright as many new treatments are emerging providing newer and novel treatment options to patients. Immunological agents (CD38 mAbs) have revolutionized the treatment of MM however the optimal sequencing of these agents so that the best management options are available to the patients is of utmost importance. BCMA bispecific and CAR-T cell therapies are promising new treatment options and are currently critical in patients who are unresponsive to or relapsed on CD38 MAbs.

SUGGESTED READINGS

1. Rajkumar SV. Multiple myeloma: 2022 update on diagnosis, risk stratification, and management. Am J Hematol. 2022;97(8): 1086-107.
2. Bobin A and Leleu X. Recent advances in the treatment of multiple myeloma: a brief review. Fac Rev. 2022;11:28.
3. Cowan AJ, Green DJ, Kwok M, Lee S, Coffey DG, Holmberg LA, et al. Diagnosis and Management of Multiple Myeloma: A Review. JAMA. 2022;327(5):464-77.

108

CHAPTER

Current Update on Thrombotic Thrombocytopenic Purpura

Mathew Thomas

ABSTRACT

Thrombotic thrombocytopenic purpura (TTP) is an uncommon but life-threatening hematological disorder with an incidence of about 3 per million in a year. The catch word in TTP is the "high degree of suspicion" which the physician should have when he comes across certain type of clinical setting, clinical findings, and investigations.

Thrombotic thrombocytopenic purpura is included in a larger group of diseases called thrombotic microangiopathy (TMA). In TMA, changes in the small blood vessels like the arterioles produce microthrombi rich in platelets. These changes in the arterioles produce a characteristic microangiopathic hemolytic anemia (MAHA) with severe thrombocytopenia. In TTP, ADAMTS13 a metalloprotease enzyme which cleaves the large sized molecule Von Willebrand factor (VWF) into smaller molecules, is deficient. As a result, the uncleaved large VWF produces mechanical destruction of red blood cells leading to MAHA. The platelets get attached to the large VWF and form microthrombi obstructing the small arterioles producing ischemia in different organs. This also leads to severe thrombocytopenia due to consumption of platelets.

There are two types of TTP, i.e., (1) immune TTP (iTTP) where auto antibodies are formed against ADAMTS 13 leading to its deficiency and (2) hereditary TTP (hTTP) which is due to congenital deficiency of ADAMTS13. iTTP forms about 95% of cases of TTP.

The patients may present acutely with fever, severe tiredness, fatigue, history of dark urine, superficial bleeding manifestations, and neurological symptoms. If the initial investigations show evidence of MAHA with negative anti globulin test AGT (old name Coombs test) and severe thrombocytopenia usually below 30,000/cuL, TTP should be strongly suspected, and a presumptive diagnosis should be made by PLASMIC score. If PLASMIC score is also high, presumptive treatment with therapeutic plasma exchange (TPE) should be started. The diagnosis should be confirmed by ADAMTS13 activity <10% and positive ADAMTS13 inhibitor/antibodies. Glucocorticoids should be started with TPE to reduce antibodies. TPE is done by removing patient's plasma and replacing it by donor plasma. TPE clears the antibodies to ADAMTS13 and provides donor ADAMTS13. Rituximab is given to prevent relapse and clear antibodies. Caplacizumab is given in severe cases and cases where platelet increment is not quick enough. Platelets get attached to the drug and reduces VWF platelet interaction thereby increasing the platelet count.

Hereditary TTP which is seen more in children and during pregnancy is diagnosed by low activity of ADAMTS13 and absence of antibodies. The treatment of hereditary TTP is plasma infusion on demand or prophylactic. Recombinant ADAMTS13 is a recently researched drug and could be very useful in TTP, especially hereditary TTP (hTTP). Now it is available only on compassionate use. It is recommended that all patients with TTP should have a lifelong follow-up.

INTRODUCTION

Thrombotic thrombocytopenic purpura (TTP) is an uncommon but life-threatening hematological disorder (incidence of about 3 per million in a year). When it was not diagnosed and treated early, the mortality was very high. But with early diagnosis and proper treatment, about 90% of the patients with TTP do well and improve. TTP belongs to a larger group of diseases termed thrombotic microangiopathy (TMA). TMA is a pathological diagnosis where there are changes in the small blood vessels (arterioles and capillaries) leading to microthrombi which are rich in platelets. Many such conditions have microangiopathic hemolytic anemia (MAHA) and thrombocytopenia. The important primary (major) TMAs are:

- Immune TTP (iTTP)
- Hereditary TTP (hTTP)
- Shiga toxin-mediated hemolytic uremic syndrome (ST-HUS)
- Complement mediated HUS
- Drug-induced TMA (DITMA)

There are two main types of TTP, i.e., (1) immune TTP which is an autoimmune disease where autoimmune antibodies are directed against ADAMTS13 and (2) hTTP where there is a deficiency of ADAMTS13 from birth due to a genetic deficiency. The immune TTP is the common type (95%) and hTTP is uncommon (5%).

PATHOGENESIS OF IMMUNE THROMBOTIC THROMBOCYTOPENIC PURPURA (iTTP)

Von Willebrand factor (VWF) produced by the endothelial cells and the liver, helps in platelet adhesion to the injured endothelial cells of the blood vessels. ADAMTS13 is a metalloprotease enzyme which cleaves the large molecular weight VWF into smaller molecules for their proper functions.

In TTP (both types) this enzyme—ADAMTS13—is deficient. This enzyme deficiency leaves the VWF uncleaved and remain as large molecular particles. The red blood cells (RBCs) as they traverse this large VWF gets destroyed mechanically producing the classical MAHA. The destroyed or fragmented RBCs thus formed are named *schistocytes*. This is a very important finding in TTP which can be seen in the peripheral blood smear. The platelets get attached to the parts of the large VWF forming microthrombi, obstructing the small blood vessels leading to ischemia in different organs, especially the nervous system. This will result in neurological deficits and dysfunction of organs such as the heart and gastrointestinal system. Uniquely TTP does not produce severe kidney dysfunction. Many platelets get consumed in this process and the patient develops *severe thrombocytopenia*. Unlike immune thrombocytopenia (ITP) and Evans syndrome, the platelets and red cells are destroyed by nonimmune mechanism **(Fig. 1)**.

CLINICAL FEATURES AND LABORATORY FINDINGS OF IMMUNE THROMBOTIC THROMBOCYTOPENIC PURPURA

The median age of presentation is about 40 years. The patients may present acutely with fever, severe tiredness, fatigue, history of dark urine, and superficial bleeding manifestations for the first time in their life. Uncommonly they may present with neurological manifestations (seizures, neurological deficits, and altered level of consciousness) and abdominal complaints (abdominal pain and diarrhea). Older patients are likely to have more comorbidities. A careful drug history and history of other autoimmune diseases like systemic lupus erythematosus (SLE) are important. Physical examination may reveal severe pallor, icterus, superficial bleeding manifestations such as purpura and ecchymoses, and sometimes neurological features.

The initial laboratory results should make one suspect an underlying TTP. Common findings are moderate to severe normocytic anemia and moderate or severe thrombocytopenia (usually < 30,000/cuL). The further workup of anemia will show that it is a *hemolytic anemia* with increase in reticulocyte count, lactate dehydrogenase (LDH), unconjugated bilirubin and decrease in the haptoglobin. The direct antiglobulin test direct and indirect (AGT or old name—Coombs test) is negative which again makes one to suspect TTP. The examination of the peripheral blood smear shows the typical schistocytes which is again a positive clue for a MAHA and TTP.

DIAGNOSIS OF IMMUNE THROMBOTIC THROMBOCYTOPENIC PURPURA

Initially TTP should be suspected when investigations reveal an antiglobulin test (AGT) negative hemolytic anemia (MAHA), with schistocytes in the peripheral blood smear and severe thrombocytopenia. Further tests such as ADAMTS13 activity levels and inhibitor/antibody titer are necessary for more confirmation. With the clinical setting, available clinical findings and investigations a provisional or presumptive diagnosis of TTP should be made and treatment should be started with therapeutic plasma exchange (TPE). This presumptive diagnosis of immune TTP is made by *PLASMIC score*.

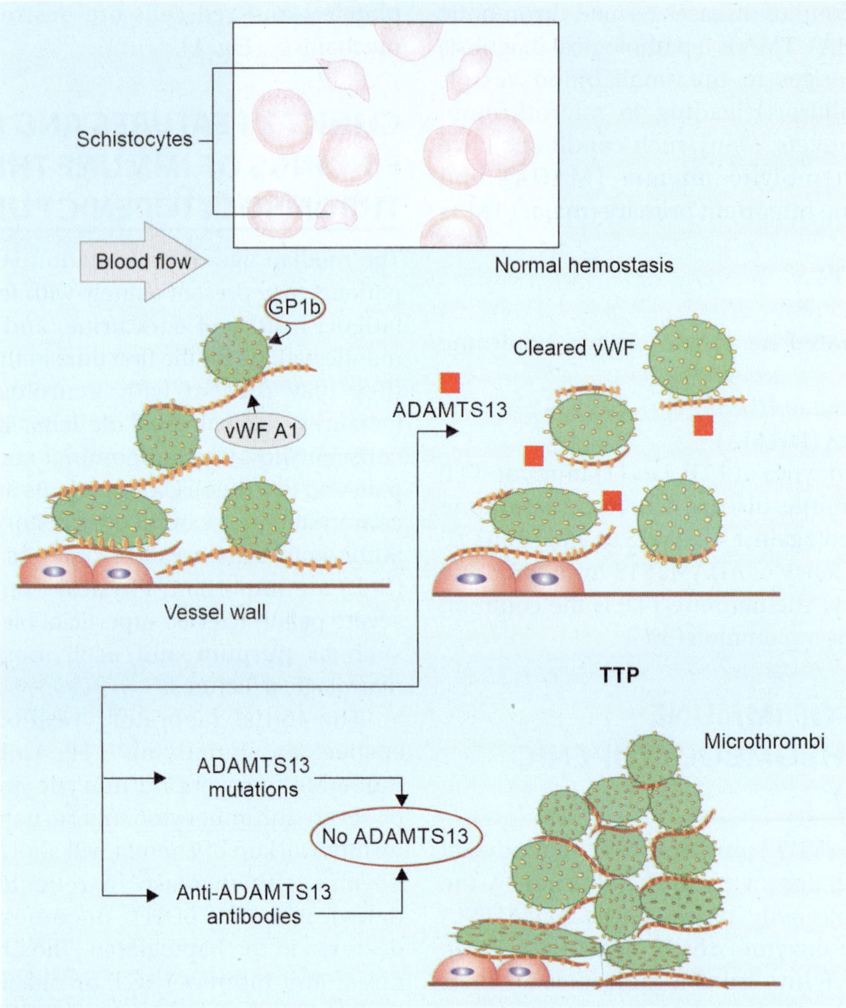

FIG. 1: Pathogenesis of immune thrombotic thrombocytopenic purpura (TTP).

One point is given for each of the following features:

- A platelet count of <30,000/mm^3
- Hemolysis (reticulocyte percentage >2.5%, very low haptoglobin, or increase in indirect bilirubin >2 mg/dL)
- There should be no solid organ or stem cell transplant
- There should be no cancer
- International normalized ratio (INR) < 1.5
- Mean corpuscular volume (MCV) < 90 fL
- Creatinine < 2 mg/dL

If there are 6–7 points indicate—high possibility of TTP, 5 points—intermediate possibility of TTP, and 0–4 points—low possibility of TTP.

The normal ADAMTS13 activity is >60%. Activity of <10% confirms the diagnosis of immune TTP in an appropriate setting. A definite diagnosis of immune TTP is confirmed when the very low activity of ADAMTS13 is combined with a high inhibitor/antibody level against ADAMTS13.

DIFFERENTIAL DIAGNOSIS OF IMMUNE THROMBOTIC THROMBOCYTOPENIC PURPURA

The differential diagnosis of immune TTP is very vast encompassing many diseases. Space permits only a mention of the important conditions and not a detailed description.

Differential diagnosis includes other primary TMAs which are hTTP, complement-mediated TMA, ST-HUS, drug-induced TMA and coagulation and metabolism-mediated TMAs.

Another group includes systemic disorders with MAHA and thrombocytopenia, e.g., disseminated intravascular coagulation (DIC), systemic infections, malignancy, pregnancy [hemolysis, elevated liver enzymes, and low platelets (HELLP) and preeclampsia], systemic hypertension, SLE and hemopoietic cell transplant.

TREATMENT OF IMMUNE THROMBOTIC THROMBOCYTOPENIC PURPURA

Therapeutic Plasma Exchange

The initial treatment for presumptive or confirmed diagnosis of immune TTP is therapeutic plasma exchange (TPE) since TTP is a medical emergency is TPE. Patient's plasma is removed (about 40 mL/kg) and this is replaced through a central venous catheter. The donor plasma contains a good quantity of normal ADAMTS13. When patient's plasma is removed the inhibitors of ADAMTS13 and the large molecules of VWF (uncleaved) are also cleared and removed. Usually, TPE is necessary daily at least for a week by which there will be clinical improvement as well as platelet increment.

Glucocorticoids

Steroids act as immune suppressive agent and reduce the inhibitors against ADAMTS13. Oral prednisone in a dose of 1 mg/kg or pulse intravenous (IV) methylprednisolone 1 g (for 3 days in severe cases) is started along with TPE. After the pulse dose, oral prednisone is continued. Oral steroids are gradually tapered and stopped after a period of 4–6 weeks.

Rituximab

Most of the hematologists use rituximab upfront after confirming the diagnosis. This drug targets the CD20 B cells and possibly reduces the antibodies. The dose is 375 mg/m^2 once a week for 4 weeks if there are no contraindications or other active infections. In addition to being immunosuppressive this drug is proved to prevent relapses in immune TTP. It must be administered after TPE.

Caplacizumab (Anti-von Willebrand Factor)

This is a monoclonal antibody against VWF. It acts by attaching to the uncleaved VWF and preventing its interaction with the platelets. As a result, the platelets are not consumed and recover very fast reducing the microthrombi. But it does not reduce the antibodies which is the main culprit in immune TTP. It may not be used for all patients with TTP. The best indication is severe illness with neurological deficits and who is not showing a fast platelet recovery. The dose is 10 mg IV for the first time and then 10 mg subcutaneous after the TPE (two doses on the first day) to be continued for 30 days after stopping TPE. The duration depends on improvement. Bleeding is one of the complications, but it is found to be only mild **(Fig. 2)**.

Hereditary Thrombotic Thrombocytopenic Purpura

This is a hereditary disease due to a congenital deficiency of ADAMTS13 activity. The deficiency is due to an abnormally functioning *ADAMTS13* gene. This disease is transmitted by an autosomal recessive inheritance trait and is also called congenital TTP (cTTP). hTTP is very uncommon accounting for only <5% of all TTP patients. This is seen more common in neonates, children, and during pregnancy. The diagnosis of hTTP is confirmed when a patient has all the features of TTP such as MAHA, severe thrombocytopenia, and a low ADAMTS13 activity without any inhibitor/antibody level.

The patients mostly have minor symptoms such as headache, abdominal pain, lethargy, and loss of concentration. During exacerbations (when disease become severe) the patient is ill with features of severe microangiopathic hemolysis and thrombocytopenia. If there is severe neonatal thrombocytopenia and increased bilirubin hTTP should be suspected. Some patients remain without any symptoms till adulthood. Severe preeclampsia, kidney injury, and fetal death (intrauterine) may complicate pregnancy in addition to severe hemolysis and thrombocytopenia. Greatest risk periods are neonatal period and pregnancy.

Diagnosis is confirmed by low levels of ADAMTS13 activity with no inhibitor/antibody on testing. Genetic tests for ADAMTS13 abnormalities reconfirm the diagnosis. The ADAMTS13 activity level is low throughout the life of the patients even during the remissions.

The treatment of choice in hTTP is infusion of plasma to replace the deficient ADAMTS13. This is either given on demand when they have the exacerbations or prophylactic to prevent the exacerbations. During pregnancy it is always given as a prophylactic treatment. It is started when pregnancy is diagnosed and continued once in 2 weeks during the early period and once weekly later.

There is a new hope for patients with hTTP and possibly for immune TTP with the discovery of recombinant ADAMTS13-rADAMTS13 (apadamtase alpha). At present it is not available for routine clinical use but can be accessed by compassionate program. A randomized trial comparing plasma infusion and rADAMTS13 has been completed.

atrophic gastritis, celiac disease, and autoimmune hemolytic syndrome. In hypothyroidism due to thyroid hormone deficiency, there is decreased stimulation of the development of erythroid colony, causing reduction in oxygen distribution to tissues and associated diminution of EPO production, leading to normocytic anemia which responds to thyroid hormone replacement therapy alone. In hypothyroid patients, iron-deficiency anemia is mostly due to menorrhagia which occurs as a result of hormonal instability and malabsorption that leads to microcytic anemia. Iron plays a significant role in the normal functioning of thyroid peroxidase (TPO) enzyme, a heme-dependent protein. Deficiency of iron decreases the activity of TPO enzyme and therefore may contribute to the decreased function of thyroid gland. Combination of treatment with both oral iron and levothyroxine results in superior improvement in hemoglobin when compared with levothyroxine alone. Macrocytic anemia is caused due to malabsorption of vitamin B12 and folic acid, associated pernicious anemia, and inadequate nutrition. Therefore, anemia in hypothyroidism needs proper evaluation because treatment depends on the cause of anemia.

Anemia and Adrenal Disorders

Adrenal Insufficiency

Anemia in primary adrenal insufficiency is normocytic normochromic anemia. Though the exact mechanism is not established, anemia in Addison's disease can be masked due to associated decrease in plasma volume, which is common for this disease. Patients with Addison's disease after initiation of hormone replacement therapy may develop transient anemia, secondary to an increased plasma volume. In animals, post-adrenalectomy mild anemia may occur, which responds to glucocorticoids. Pernicious anemia can occur in patients with type 1 autoimmune polyglandular syndrome due to autosomal recessive mutation of the autoimmune regulator gene.

Anemia and Gonadal Disorders

In older age group, the prevalence of anemia is approximately 10% and in one-third, the cause is not known. Testosterone deficiency may be one of the possible cause of unexplained anemia in elderly and treatment with testosterone in men with very low testosterone increases their hemoglobin levels. In a population of males aged 30–94 years, it is seen that there is a direct correlation between hemoglobin and testosterone levels. In men on testosterone treatment for hypogonadism, there is increase in mean hematocrit from 38.0 to 43.1% within 3 months. A meta-analysis of 11 randomized controlled trials involving 1,570 patients showed an increased risk of erythrocytosis with testosterone replacement therapy [relative risk 8.14, 95% confidence interval (CI) 1.87, 35.40]. The mechanism of testosterone is a complex process; it acts by stimulating EPO secretion and it has a direct effect on the bone marrow. Patients with nonmetastatic prostate cancer deprived of androgen therapy showed a significant decrease in hemoglobin and hematocrit levels and an increase in hepcidin concentration, but there was no associated decrease in serum iron levels, suggesting that hepcidin is not the primary driver of the anemia.

Anemia in Parathyroid Disorders

Donald Hunter and Fuller Albright were the first who described anemia in primary hyperparathyroidism (PHPT). The most common type of anemia in PHPT is generally normocytic and normochromic, characteristic of chronic disease. The anemia in PHPT is due to various causes; it may be due to parathyroid hormone (PTH)-induced marrow fibrosis, associated occult gastrointestinal bleeding, renal failure, and malnutrition due to decreased appetite. Serum levels of calcium, PTH and alkaline phosphatase, and severity of bone disease has a direct correlation with severity of anemia. PTH acts through PTH/PTH-related protein (PTHrP) receptors on extraosseous tissues, thus inducing the secretion of tumor necrosis factor alpha (TNF-α), which in turn stimulates platelet-derived growth factor alpha (PDGF-α), leading to marrow fibrosis. Due to ongoing marrow fibrosis, erythropoietic cell line is more significantly affected than the myeloid or megakaryocytic cell lines. PTH-mediated secretion of interleukin 6 (IL-6), inhibits the hypoxia-mediated secretion of EPO, thereby affecting RBC production. Lastly, EPO resistance due to severe bone marrow fibrosis may be one of the other possible causes of anemia in severe PHPT.

Anemia in Pituitary Disorders

Anemia in hypopituitary patients is usually normochromic normocytic with RBC life span being normal. It is hypothesized that anemia is related to deficiencies of various adenohypophyseal hormones and their target organ hormones, which in turn modulate the renal EPO production. Growth hormone (GH) and insulin-like growth factor 1 (IGF-1) have a direct stimulatory effect on erythroid cells and/or EPO secretion, possibly by anabolic action. In patients with multiple pituitary hormone deficiency, correction of anemia occurs by replacement of combination of deficient hormones such as thyroid, adrenal, and gonadal hormones.

Anemia in Diabetes Mellitus

Anemia in diabetes aggravates the progression of diabetes-associated complications and increase the mortality in patients with diabetes. The prevalence of anemia in diabetes mellitus (both type 1 and type 2) ranges from 14 to 45%. The risk of anemia in diabetes is estimated to be two to three times higher than that of patients without diabetes. In patients with diabetes and chronic kidney disease (CKD), anemia is more commonly seen and it greatly affects the patient outcomes. Anemia increases the risk for progression of diabetic kidney disease and cardiovascular morbidity and mortality; its severity worsens with more advanced stages of CKD and in those with proteinuria.

The pathogenesis of anemia in type 1 diabetes mellitus (T1DM) and type 2 diabetes mellitus (T2DM) is multifactorial.

Type 1 Diabetes Mellitus

In T1DM, autoimmune gastritis and pernicious anemia are the two major attributable causes of anemia. Iron deficiency anemia is more commonly seen in patients with autoimmune gastritis that may precede pernicious anemia. The prevalence of iron deficiency anemia and pernicious anemia in autoimmune gastritis is observed to be 20–40% and 15–25%, respectively. In autoimmune gastritis, there is reduced absorption of iron due to hypochlorhydria as a result of destruction of H^+/K^+ ATPase-containing parietal cells, leading to iron-deficiency anemia. Pernicious anemia in autoimmune gastritis is due to vitamin B12 deficiency caused by loss of parietal cells, leading to poor intrinsic factor production and prevention of vitamin B12-intrinsic factor complex formation, thus resulting in malabsorption of vitamin B12. T1DM is often associated with other autoimmune diseases such as celiac disease and autoimmune thyroiditis, causing hypothyroidism. Celiac disease is a malabsorption disorder associated with villous atrophy in intestinal mucosa, causing impaired absorption of iron and vitamin B12, thus leading to iron-deficiency anemia.

Type 2 Diabetes Mellitus

The major causes of anemia in T2DM having normal or abnormal glomerular filtration rates are due to deficiency of iron and decreased response to EPO. The production of EPO is mediated by sympathetic nervous system. Thus in patients with diabetes, there is impaired production of EPO by the peritubular fibroblasts due to sympathetic denervation of kidney because of autonomic neuropathy. Long-standing hyperglycemia could also lead to increased apoptosis of renal tubular cells and tubular ischemia. In addition, EPO synthesis is impaired due to underlying interstitial fibrosis, as well as disruption of interstitial and vascular architecture due to chronic hyperglycemia which worsens the function of HIF-1. Several other factors that contribute to the chronic hypoxic environment that decreases EPO secretion include diabetic nephropathy, chronic inflammation, increased levels of advanced glycation end products, low testosterone levels, and associated nutritional deficiency of iron, folic acid, and vitamin B12. Diabetes mellitus is also characterized by decreased responsiveness to EPO due to increased glycosylation, lower levels of EPO, reduced functional EPO, and EPO resistance because to glycation of EPO receptors. Diabetes mellitus is a chronic inflammatory state characterized by increased concentrations of proinflammatory cytokines such as IL-1, IL-6, TNF-α, transforming growth factor beta (TGF-β), and interferons (IFNs) in the circulation. These inflammatory cytokines are thought to regulate apoptosis of erythroid progenitor cells. Persistent hyperglycemia and formation of advanced glycation end products lead to oxidative stress by generation of free-oxygen radicals which reduce the life span of RBC, thus causing decrease in hemoglobin in the peripheral circulation. Other possible proposed mechanism for anemia in diabetes is hyporeninemia and urinary loss of EPO.

THERAPIES LEADING TO ANEMIA

- *Metformin:* Prolonged use of metformin for more than 3 years increase the risk of development of anemia. Treatment with metformin is associated with megaloblastic anemia due to malabsorption of vitamin B12. But patients usually manifest metformin-induced anemia after 5–10 years after depleting hepatic stores of vitamin B12.
- *Thiazolidinediones*: Anemia in thiazolidinedione therapy is due to expansion of plasma volume and also due to fat deposits in the bone marrow, thus causing impairment of erythrocytosis. Fall in hemoglobin to 10 g/L and hematocrit levels by 3.3% has been reported in few studies.
- *Angiotensin-converting enzyme (ACE) inhibitors and angiotensin receptor blockers (ARBs)*: Angiotensin II is an important factor for regulation of erythropoiesis and plays a key role in the growth of erythroid precursors. The use of ACE inhibitors or ARBs causes anemia by altering the action of angiotensin on erythropoiesis.
- Dipeptidyl peptidase 4 (DPP-4) and sodium-glucose cotransporter-2 (SGLT-2) inhibitors by improving the EPO level has a better outcomes in patients with anemia.

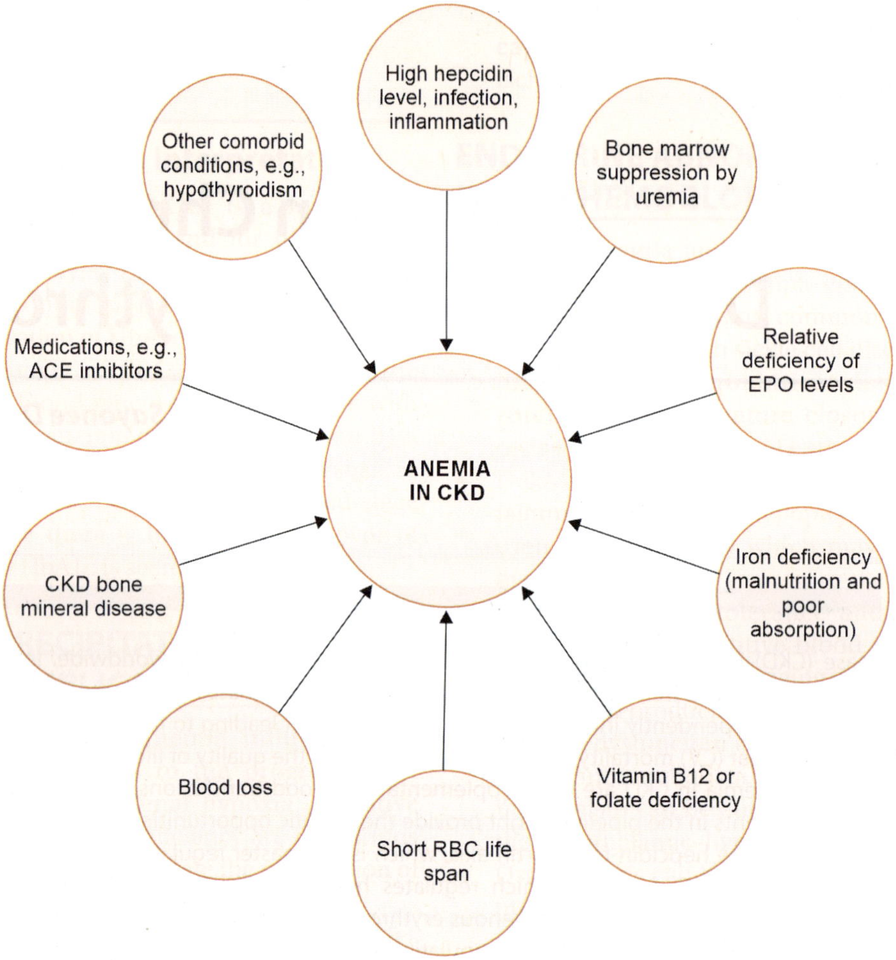

FIG. 1: Causes of anemia in chronic kidney disease (CKD).
(ACE: angiotensin-converting enzyme; EPO: erythropoietin; RBC: red blood cell)

severe cases, when patients require blood transfusions, it exposes them to human leukocyte antigen (HLA) sensitization which later reduces the chances of successful transplantation.

Therefore, standing in the 21st century there is a need for better agents beyond EPO which will not only increase Hb levels but will also reduce the risk of adverse CV events seen with the present ones.

ERYTHROPOIESIS-STIMULATING AGENTS

The term ESA encompasses short-acting rHuEPO *epoetin* (t1/2 6.8–19.4 hours, 50–100 µg/kg/week dosing), medium-acting *darbepoetin alfa* (t1/2 25.3–48.8 hours, 0.45 µg/kg/week to every 2–4 weeks dosing), long-acting *epoetin beta pegol* (t1/2 130 hours, 0.6 µg/kg every 2–4 weeks), and their biosimilars. Apart from stimulating erythropoiesis, ESAs, by inducing erythroferrone, also act as hepcidin suppressors. Hepcidin levels are frequently raised in patients with CKD due to impaired renal clearance, inflammatory state, and iron supplementation contributing to functional iron deficiency and interfering with hematopoiesis. They are started on an individual basis and to most hemodialysis patients with Hb < 10 g/dL who are not iron deficient. The target Hb level in patients on ESAs is 11.5–12.5 g/dL. However, patients treated with ESAs are exposed to supraphysiologic EPO concentrations, potentially leading to adverse CV and thromboembolic events and also enhancing thrombogenicity and tumor growth in patients with malignant disease. Furthermore, hyporesponsiveness which is defined as a continued need for >300 IU/kg/week of EPO or 1.5 mg/kg/week of darbepoetin administered SC, affecting 10% of patients with CKD represents another major clinical challenge in ESAs therapy.

Overall *darbepoetin alfa* has a better efficacy and safety profile by having a longer half-life allowing less frequent dosing, no antibody formation and lesser incidence of fistula thrombosis and hypertension thereby conferring the clinical advantage over rHuEPO.

Peginesatide is an EPO-mimetic peptide that is an effective treatment for anti-EPO antibody-mediated pure

RBC aplasia because of a lack of cross-reactivity with anti-EPO antibodies. It was also shown to be equivalent to epoetin and darbepoetin in raising Hb concentrations in dialysis and nondialysis (ND) patients, respectively, but in ND patients, a higher rate of CV events was observed. After a year of its introduction, it had to be withdrawn from the market because of severe hypersensitivity reactions.

IRON SUPPLEMENTATION

Dysregulation of iron homeostasis in cases with CKD is multifactorial, including diminished renal clearance of hepcidin, inflammation, and absolute and functional iron insufficiency **(Table 2)**.

Iron therapy is used to replenish iron stores, increase Hb level to the desired level, and decrease the need for ESA. Adult CKD patients with anemia or on ESA therapy should receive a trial of IV iron (or a 1–3 months trial of oral iron therapy in ND CKD) if transferrin saturation (TSAT) is <30% and ferritin is <500 µg/L and an increase in Hb concentration or a decrease in ESA dose are desired.

Ferric carboxymaltose (FCM), iron isomaltose (IIM), and *ferumoxytol* are among new IV iron preparations. *Ferric pyrophosphate citrate (FPC)* is a water-soluble iron salt that can be administered via dialysate, supplying the iron directly to transferrin.

Excessive iron supplementation may promote oxidative stress and potentially contribute to CV disease risk, CKD progression, and other organ damage in CKD patients. IV iron administration may cause injection site complications and consume venous capital for future access, and infections. An increasingly recognized side effect of FCM and IIM is hypophosphatemia. The need for future trials focusing on long-term effects and optimal dosing strategies of novel oral iron preparations remains.

HYPOXIA-INDUCIBLE FACTOR INHIBITORS

Hypoxia-inducible factor prolyl hydroxylase inhibitors (HIF-PHIs) represent a novel approach to the treatment of anemia in patients with CKD. These are oral drugs that mimic the natural response to hypoxia independent of cellular oxygen levels. HIF-PHIs undergoing clinical trials include *roxadustat, daprodustat, desidustat, enarodustat, molidustat, and vadadustat.* The Nobel Prize in Physiology or Medicine for 2019 was awarded to William Kaelin Jr, Sir Peter Ratcliffe, and Gregg Semenza for their work in HIF transcription factor.

The HIF-PHIs are transcription factors that inhibit the prolyl hydroxylase domain (PHD) proteins (PHD1, PHD2, and PHD3), which sense oxygen and control HIF activity. By decreasing prolyl hydroxylase activity, HIF-PHIs lead to the stabilization of HIF-α in the liver and kidney resulting in upregulation of the endogenous EPO. HIF is a heterodimer complex having 3 isoforms, HIF-1, HIF-2, and HIF-3, each of which contains an oxygen-sensitive α-subunit unique to the isoform and a common β-subunit. The controlling isoform for EPO production is HIF-2 which also stimulates iron absorption in the duodenum. HIF-1 augments the transcription of additional genes that encode proteins involved in iron mobilization, including ceruloplasmin and transferrin.

During normoxia, the enzyme prolyl hydroxylase (PHD1, PHD2, and PHD3) hydroxylate prolyl residues in the alpha subunit of HIF. Hydroxylation leads to recognition by von Hippel–Lindau (VHL) ubiquitin E3 ligase and subsequent proteasomal degradation of HIF. During hypoxic conditions, the PHDs are inactive and this leads to dimerization of α and β subunits of HIF and target gene expression. *HIF-2α* regulates erythropoiesis. It binds to hypoxia response elements of genes encoding proteins such as duodenal cytochrome B and ferroportin enabling iron absorption and also suppresses hepcidin levels which are elevated in chronic inflammatory states such as end-stage renal disease (ESRD) **(Flowcharts 1 and 2)**.

The HIF activation increases the expression of EPO and transferrin receptors on erythroblasts and decreases apoptosis of erythroid progenitors in the bone marrow.

TABLE 2: Iron deficiency.

Absolute iron deficiency	Transferrin saturation (TSAT) ≤ 20% and serum ferritin concentration ≤ 100 ng/mL in nonhemodialysis patients and ≤200 ng/mL among hemodialysis patients
Functional iron insufficiency	TSAT ≤ 20% and elevated ferritin levels

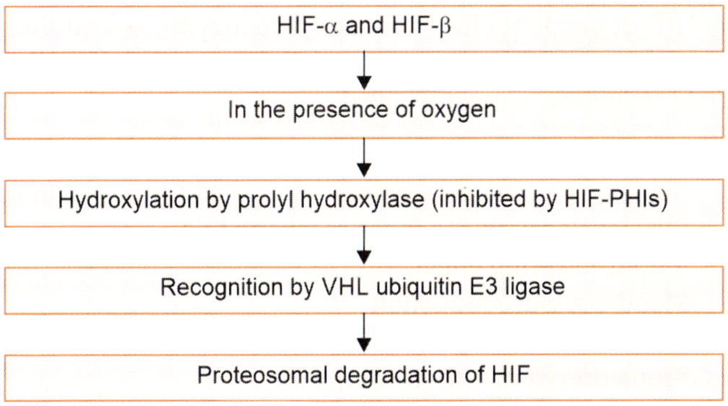

FLOWCHART 1: Mechanism of HIF-PHIs.
(HIF-PHIs: hypoxia-inducible factor–prolyl hydroxylase domain inhibitors; VHL: von Hippel–Lindau)

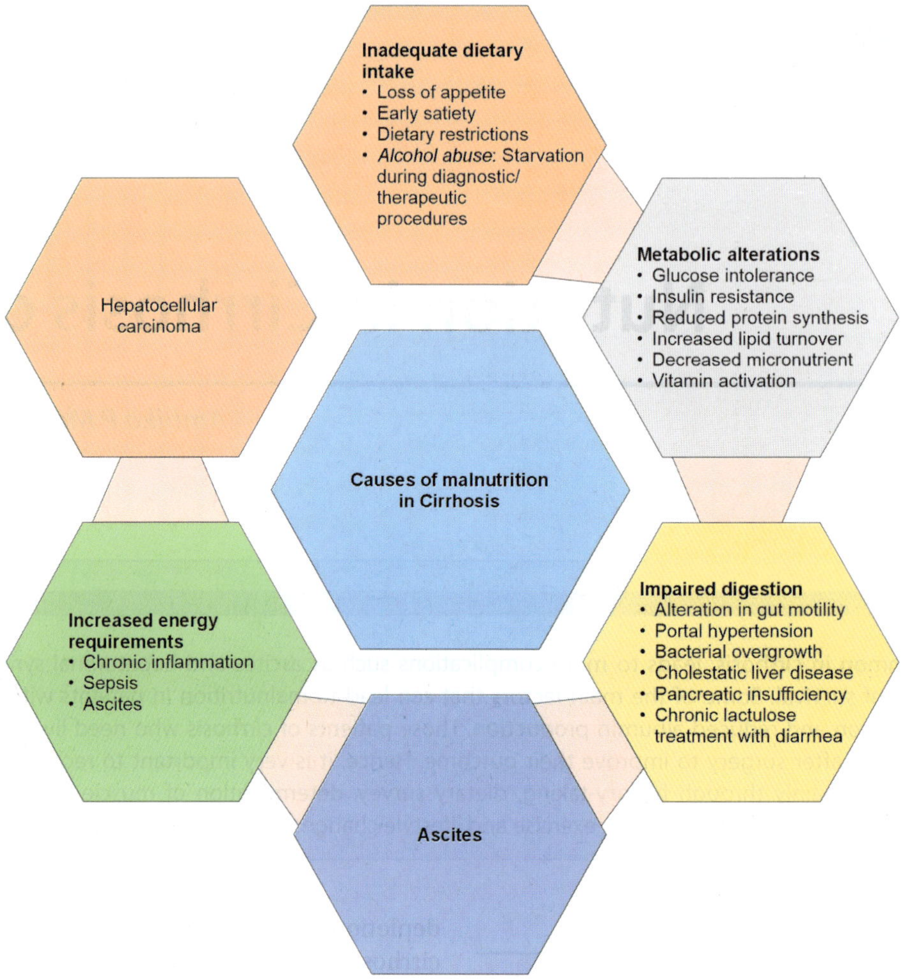

FIG. 1: Factors contributing to malnutrition and sarcopenia in liver cirrhosis.

ASSESSMENT OF NUTRITIONAL STATUS

Assessment of nutritional status in cirrhosis is complex and there is no accepted gold standard. Malnutrition is easily recognized in cachectic patients with decompensated cirrhosis but it is more difficult to identify in early stages. Body weight and Body Mass Index (BMI) are fallacious because of water and salt retention resulting in edema and ascites. While calculating BMI, the water accumulation in body has to be considered. The serum albumin level and prothrombin time are also altered because of impaired synthesis. The erythrocyte, lymphocyte, or platelet counts are lower because of hypersplenism and are not useful to assess malnutrition. The best way to assess nutritional status is to perform a complete clinical examination and to take a dietary survey daily for of at least 2 days and one at the weekend to detect micronutrient and vitamin deficiencies. An anthropometry, measurement of skinfold thickness and measurement of arm muscle circumference, is used to determine the amount of muscle mass and finally, a global subjective assessment. There are several tools to classify patients at risk of malnutrition, but most have not been validated in cirrhotic patients and are biased by salt and water retention. The predictive role of skeletal muscle mass assessed by computed tomography (CT) in liver transplant candidates has also been studied, but is rarely used in routine clinical practice. The Nutritional Screening and Assessment in Liver Cirrhosis is given in **Flowchart 1**.

SUBJECTIVE GLOBAL NUTRITIONAL ASSESSMENT AND TOOLS

Computed Tomography/Magnetic Resonance Imaging at L3 Vertebra Level

Measuring the muscle area at 3rd lumbar vertebra level in a CT or magnetic resonance imaging (MRI) is a good predictor of muscle wasting and development of complications and death. At this level, multiple muscles are easily identified and the most relevant is the psoas muscle. These muscles have advantage of being unaffected

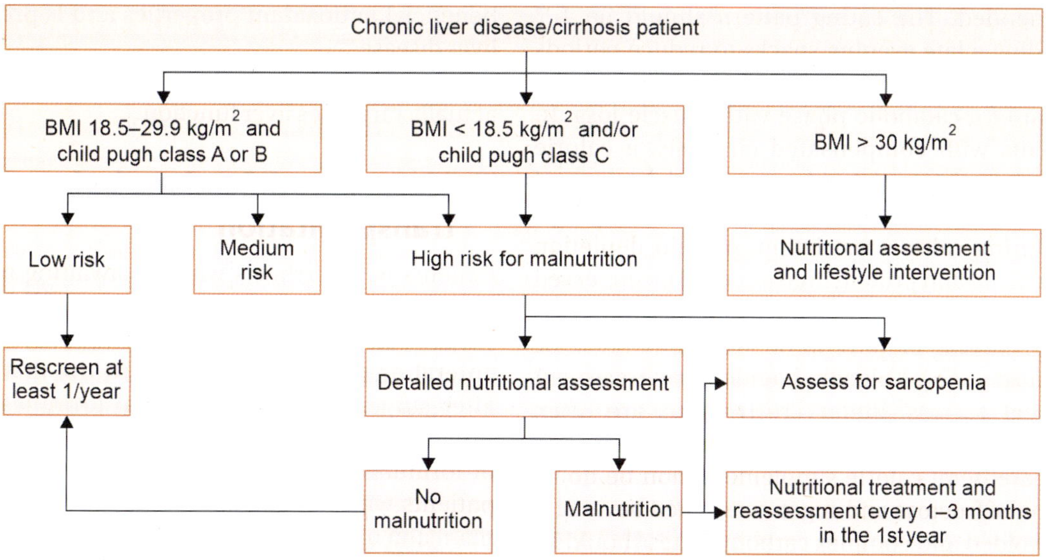

FLOWCHART 1: Algorithm for nutritional screening and assessment in liver cirrhosis.
(BMI: body mass index)

by physical activity in the same way as the dominant upper limbs and their measurement is unaffected by water retention.

Bioelectric Impedance Analysis

Bioelectric impedance analysis (BIA) has been evaluated in cirrhotic patients with controversial results. Studies have shown that it can provide a good estimate of body cell mass.

Dual-energy Exchange Absorptiometry

This can measure fat, fat free mass, and bone compartment. It shows a good correlation with anthropometry and is very accurate for fat mass and mineral contents.

Handgrip Strength

Measurement of handgrip strength is an easy and cost-effective method and rapid evaluation can be performed in outpatient. Though the sensitivity and specificity of this test are controversial in end-stage liver disease (ESLD), it is an early marker of malnutrition in mild disease, even before the muscle atrophy occurs.

Mid-arm Muscle Circumference and Triceps Skinfold

Mid-arm muscle circumference (MAMC) and triceps skinfold (TSF) are usually performed at bedside or outpatient by a measuring tape and skin calipers and is easy and reliable. MAMC correlates well with survival of these patients.

TABLE 1: Parameters in SGA and RFH-SGA.

Subjective Global Nutritional Assessment (SGA)	Royal Free Hospital Subjective Global Nutritional Assessment (RFH-SGA)
• Weight change	• Body mass index
• Loss of fat and muscle wasting	• Muscle wasting
• Change in diet	• Amount of calorie intake
• Nausea, vomiting and diarrhea	
• Functional capacity	
• Disease severity	
• Edema	
• Ascites	

Six-minute Walk or Get up and Go Test

Other functional tests like "Six-minute walk test" or "Get up and go" tests are promising but cannot be performed in severely ill patients and normal values are not available. The parameters in Subjective Global Nutritional Assessment (SGA) and Royal Free Hospital Subjective Global Nutritional Assessment (RFH-SGA)are given in **Table 1**.

TREATMENT OF MALNUTRITION IN CIRRHOSIS OF LIVER

Calorie and Protein

A dietary calorie intake of 35–40 kcal/kg body weight and a daily protein intake of 1.2–1.5 g/kg of body weight

112

CHAPTER

An Update on Alcoholic Liver Disease

Shubha Laxmi Margekar, Ashok Kumar, Anupam Prakash

ABSTRACT

Alcohol-related liver disease (ALD) is a prevalent global health issue linked to excessive drinking. ALD is linked to various clinical illnesses, including steatosis, steatohepatitis, cirrhosis, and alcoholic cirrhosis (AC) worsened by hepatocellular carcinoma (HCC). Risk factors for ALD include dangerous drinking, genetic factors, body mass index, quantity, iron overload, and social class. Co-existing liver disorders, cigarette smoking, and hepatitis B or C coinfections also contribute to the risk.

Diagnosis involves evaluating alcohol intake and assessing advanced liver disease. Noninvasive examinations like FibroTest have been developed for liver fibrosis and steatosis showing high diagnostic accuracy. Management involves achieving total abstinence from alcohol consumption, managing cirrhosis-related problems, and managing extrahepatic consequences. Alcoholic hepatitis (AH) is a severe form of ALD, characterized by rapid onset of jaundice and liver-related problems. Acute-on-chronic liver failure (ACLF) is a condition characterized by sudden decline in liver function, multiple organ failures, and a higher likelihood of near-term mortality in cirrhosis-diagnosed patients. The efficacy of corticosteroids in improving survival among patients with ACLF and ALD is still debated. ALD is the second most common reason for liver transplantation (LT) worldwide. Future therapeutics for ALD include targeting inflammation, gut permeability, dysbiosis, and hepatoprotective agents. More research is needed to understand risk factors for ALD development and to find a biomarker for alcohol use.

INTRODUCTION

One of the most common types of liver disease that is once again receiving attention worldwide is alcohol-related liver disease (ALD). Any consumption of alcohol or any other form of beverage is linked to a risk to one's health, which can range in intensity from mild to severe. Alcohol is the most often consumed substance, despite the fact that people are aware of its potential for addiction and its negative bodily and societal effects.

ALCOHOL USE DISORDER

Alcohol use disorder (AUD) is a chronic disorder in which a patient's drinking habits cause symptoms and other effects, and the patient is unable to stop drinking even though it negatively impacts his personal, professional, or health aspects. It can take a mild, moderate, or severe form and relapses are possible. There are several different clinical illnesses linked with ALD, including steatosis, alcoholic steatohepatitis (ASH), alcoholic hepatitis (AH) of varying degrees of severity, alcoholic cirrhosis (AC), and AC worsened by hepatocellular carcinoma (HCC).

A standard drink contains 355 mL (12 oz) of ordinary beer, 150 mL (5 oz) of wine, or 45 mL (1.5 oz) of distilled spirits, totalling about 14 g of pure alcohol. The National Institute on Alcohol Abuse and Alcoholism (NIAAA) defines excessive drinking as having >4 standard drinks per day (or >14 per week) for males and >3 standard drinks per day (or >7 per week) for women.

Burden: The liver damage caused by alcohol consumption receives 10 times less attention than it should. There are 3.0 million fatalities annually, or 5.3% of all deaths globally, are attributed to alcohol's negative effects, according to the WHO. According to DALYs (disability-adjusted life years), alcohol-related disease and injury account for 5.1% of all global burden.

RISK FACTORS

Hazardous drinking: ALD's cornerstone is hazardous drinking. Early heavy drinking raises the possibility of developing severe liver disease later in life.

Genetic factors: The genetic disposition is likely polygenic and the heritability for AC is widely documented.

Body mass index: Being overweight or obese and drinking alcohol, both increase the chance of developing liver disease or increasing the severity of fibrosis.

Quantity: According to a new report from the "global burden of disease" report, there is no safe lower level of consumption and that the risk of all-cause mortality increases with consumption levels.

Iron overload: Even in the absence of a specific iron overload disease, iron overload is frequently prevalent. But as hemochromatosis is one of the most prevalent hereditary disorders, it must always be considered as a cofactor for ALD.

Social class: Social class is a very robust predictor of both the health risks and the rates of alcohol-related hospitalization or fatalities.

Coexisting liver disorders: Synergistic relationship between alcohol consumption and the risk of HCC has been documented. The exact mechanism is unknown, but may be related to the numerous systemic inflammatory pathways induced by adipose tissue.

Cigarette smoking (CS): There is a substantial correlation between alcohol misuse and CS and obesity. Heavy CS is more common in patients who abuse alcohol and it worsens the harmful effects of alcohol excess in humans and that CS may exacerbate the pathogenic effects of alcohol on the liver.

Hepatitis B and C coinfection: Alcohol use has been linked to accelerated disease progression and premature mortality in those with chronic hepatitis B or C virus infections.

In addition, a prospective analysis from the atherosclerosis risk in communities study found that coffee drinkers may be at lower risk for liver-related hospitalization.

Factors responsible for escalating the risk of alcohol-related liver damage:

- Alcohol intake beyond the daily limit of one drink for women and two for men
- Daily drinking, drinking during fasts, and binge drinking are examples of consumption patterns.
- Cigarette smoking
- Women compared to men.
- *PNPLA3, TM6SF2, MBOAT7,* and *HSD17B13*—genetics.
- Increased BMI
- Concomitant illnesses present, including hemochromatosis, chronic viral hepatitis, nonalcoholic fatty liver disease (NAFLD), and nonalcoholic steatohepatitis (NASH)

DIAGNOSIS OF ALCOHOLIC LIVER DISEASE

The initial step in diagnosing ALD entails evaluating alcohol intake in all patients including alcohol levels and patterns and assessment of advanced liver disease. ALD is typically suspected in individuals who engage in habitual alcohol consumption over 20 g/day for females and 30 g/day for males. This suspicion is based on the presence of clinical and/or biochemical abnormalities that indicate liver injury. The AUDIT, also known as the Alcohol Use Disorders Inventory Test, is widely regarded as the preeminent questionnaire for assessing the presence of hazardous drinking patterns and alcohol dependency. Natural progression of liver disease in alcohol use disorder should also be noted **(Flowchart 1)**.

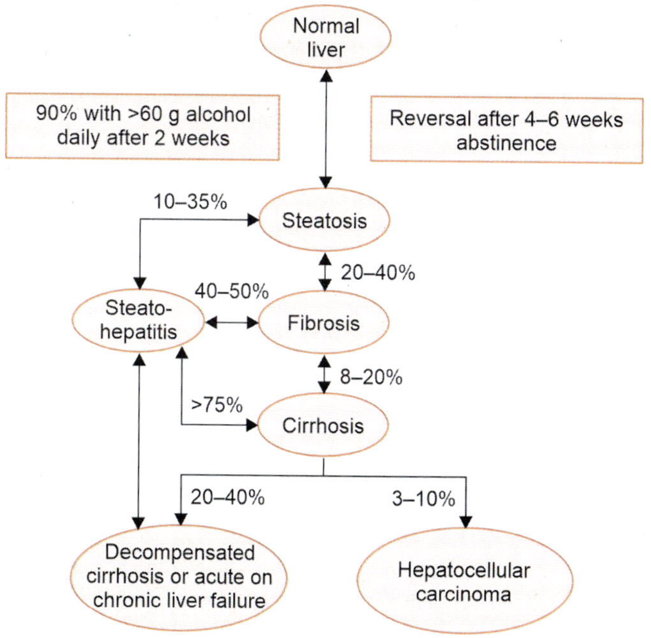

FLOWCHART 1: Natural history of alcohol-associated liver disease.

Serum markers utilized for the detection of alcohol intake encompass carbohydrate deficient transferrin and gamma-glutamyl transferase (GGT). These markers have undergone validation procedures to ascertain their efficacy in identifying alcohol consumption over 50 g/day during a timeframe of 2–3 weeks prior to testing. Nevertheless, the diagnostic usefulness of these markers in detecting heavy drinking is diminished in liver disease due to the presence of liver injury, which acts as a confounding factor.

The gold standard for definitively diagnosing and evaluating the fibrosis stage of ALD remains liver biopsy. However, due to its invasive nature and associated side effects, its recommendation is not universal. Over the past few decade, noninvasive examinations have been devised for the evaluation of liver fibrosis and steatosis, by measuring liver stiffness by transient elastography (TE), or a biological approach including the identification of serum biomarkers.

In a recent prospective study examining 10 markers of liver fibrosis, it was observed that both FibroTest and Enhanced Liver Fibrosis (ELF) had a same high level of diagnostic accuracy in identifying advanced fibrosis in patients with ALD. Ultrasound remains a viable modality for screening purposes in the identification of steatosis and portal hypertension.

MANAGEMENT OF ALCOHOLIC LIVER DISEASE

Alcoholic liver disease is characterized by impaired alcohol metabolism and the consequent inability to effectively remove alcohol from the body. The management entails the attainment of total abstinence from alcohol consumption, the effective handling of problems arising from cirrhosis, and the appropriate management of extrahepatic consequences such as neuropathy, proximal myopathy, and pancreatic exocrine insufficiency. The issue of dietary shortage in protein and calories, which is frequently linked to sarcopenia, should be given due attention and remedied accordingly. Patients with a dependency on alcohol should be provided with appropriate therapeutic interventions.

ALCOHOLIC HEPATITIS

Alcoholic hepatitis is a severe form of ALD, distinguished by the insidious onset of jaundice and liver-related problems in individuals with chronic and excessive alcohol consumption. The assessment of the severity of AH is conducted using either the Maddrey's discriminant function (mDF) of 32 or higher or the Model for End-Stage Liver Disease (MELD) score exceeding 20 **(Flowchart 2)**.

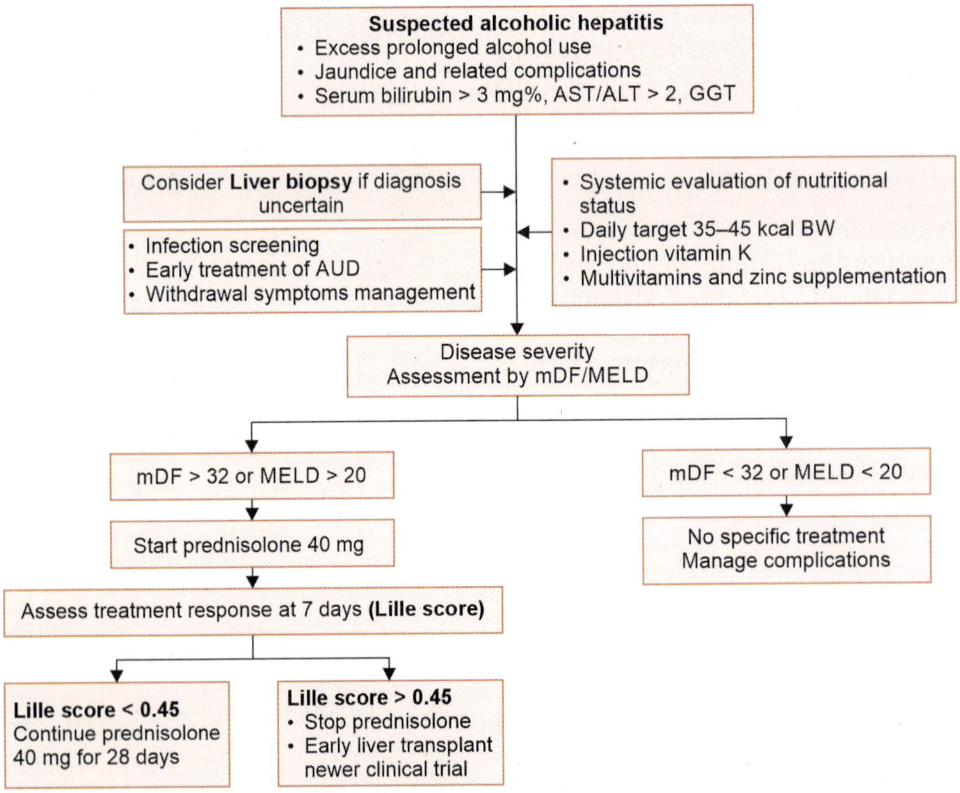

FLOWCHART 2: Approach to management of alcoholic hepatitis.

(ALT: alanine transaminase; AST: aspartate transaminase; AUD: alcohol use disorder; GGT: gamma-glutamyl transferase; mDF: Maddrey's discriminant function; MELD: model for end-stage liver disease)

The management of alcohol hepatitis includes sufficient caloric and protein consumption, administering vitamins, and mitigating the risk of withdrawal syndrome in those with alcohol dependency.

Corticosteroids are presently employed in individuals diagnosed with severe alcoholic hepatitis (SAH), but their efficacy in terms of short-term survival is limited and temporary.

The efficacy of pentoxifylline in individuals who do not exhibit a response to corticosteroids has been found to be lacking. Furthermore, the levels of lipopolysaccharide (LPS) in the serum and the baseline hepatic gene expression of a patient have been identified as potential indicators for predicting the response to corticosteroids.

Complete alcohol abstinence is considered the primary factor influencing the long-term prognosis of patients. Early LT is advocated in cases of AH where medical therapy has proven ineffective.

ACUTE-ON-CHRONIC LIVER FAILURE

Acute-on-chronic liver failure (ACLF) is a clinical state marked by the sudden decline of liver function, multiple organ failures, and a significantly elevated likelihood of near-term mortality in individuals diagnosed with cirrhosis. The diagnostic criteria for ACLF were proposed by the European Association for the Study of the Liver (EASL)-Chronic Liver Failure (CLIF) consortium, drawing from the findings of the CANONIC (Chronic Liver Failure Acute-on-Chronic Liver Failure in Cirrhosis) trial focused on patients who had decompensated cirrhosis. The prevalence of ACLF can be attributed to active alcohol consumption in approximately 25% of patients. Patients diagnosed with alcoholic cirrhosis (AC) who engage in ongoing alcohol drinking exhibit a higher propensity for developing ACLF of grades 2 and 3 compared to patients without these characteristics.

Existing knowledge on the efficacy of corticosteroids in enhancing short-term survival among patients with SAH and ACLF is limited. Corticosteroid response, as determined by the Lille model, was diminished in patients with ACLF. The chance of response to corticosteroids decreased gradually with increasing ACLF grades. Nevertheless, the efficacy of corticosteroids in improving survival remains consistent among those who respond positively to the treatment, irrespective of the severity of ACLF.

LIVER TRANSPLANTATION

The second most frequent reason for LT worldwide, accounting for about 30% of all primary transplants in Europe and roughly 25% in the USA, is ALD. The use of LT as a treatment for ALD is still a subject of debate. Leading to concerns about the possibility of alcohol relapse after LT and its potential detrimental effects on the transplanted organ is the stem of the controversy.

Most of the transplant programs enforce a strict abstinence of alcohol for 6 months in order to assess a patient's eligibility for LT and to evaluate the risk variables associated with alcohol relapse following the LT.

The prevalence of alcohol relapse varied between 11.5 and 49%, although this aspect was seldom taken into account as contributing factor to transplant failure. Data suggest a correlation between a shorter duration of prelisting abstinence and reduced interval preceding posttransplant relapse. However, the optimal duration of abstinence prior to transplantation remains a subject of ongoing scholarly discourse.

Liver Transplantation for Severe Alcoholic Hepatitis

There is growing evidence that early LT is a successful treatment for SAH that is not responding to medicinal therapy when it is administered to carefully chosen patients.

Liver Transplantation in Patients with Acute-on-chronic Liver Failure

Patients with ACLF frequently consider LT as a potential treatment option, particularly in cases classified as grades 2 and 3. Further research is required for establishing the rigorous criteria for selecting liver transplant recipients.

The long-term outcomes following LT for HCC associated with ALD are generally favorable. HCC is a prominent contributor to cancer-related mortality with its global incidence on the rise.

MECHANISM AND POSSIBLE TARGET OF THE ALCOHOLIC LIVER DISEASE

Alcohol-induced liver disease is a complex disease characterized by the direct effects of ethanol and its metabolites on the liver and other organs, as well as immune cell activation and inflammation triggered by alcohol's effects. High concentrations of alcohol result in acetaldehyde which has cellular toxic effects and produces reactive oxygen species that disrupt mitochondrial energy transport and intracellular signaling pathways. This disrupts cellular homeostasis, causing endoplasmic reticulum (ER) stress, unfolded protein response, mitochondrial, Golgi, and lysosomal stress responses, and injuries. Innate immune-system activation is a central driver in ALD, particularly in acute liver disease, where proinflammatory cell activation and proinflammatory cytokine production contribute to disease severity, clinical symptoms, and prognosis.

GUT MICROBIOTA IN ALCOHOLIC LIVER DISEASE

Alcohol-induced liver disease is linked to changes in the gut microbiota with intestinal dysbiosis playing a significant role in its development. Bacterial overgrowth of luminal and mucosa-associated microbiota in the small intestine occurs in patients with early stages of ALD. Changes in bacterial taxa are dependent on the stage of liver disease, early disease having a different microbiota composition compared to those with AC or AH.

Dysbiosis is not occurring in all patients with AUD, but taxonomic changes in fungi are largely characterized by a decrease in fungal diversity and overgrowth of *Candida* species in patients with AUD and AH. Dysbiosis-induced intestinal immune dysregulation connects the gut microbiota and translocation of microbial products in preclinical models. Alcohol affects intestinal permeability by other mechanisms, including disruption of the circadian rhythm and a direct effect of the ethanol metabolite acetaldehyde on tight junctions.

Bile acid homeostasis is disrupted in patients with ALD, with systemic total bile acids elevated in 40% of precirrhotic ALD and increased serum bile acids in 81% of patients with AC.

IMMUNE SYSTEM IN LIVER DISEASE

Chronic alcohol use and intestinal inflammation lead to increased gut permeability, allowing pathogen-associated molecular patterns (PAMPs) like LPS and bacterial DNA to enter the liver. These PAMPs are sensed by various pattern recognition receptors, activating proinflammatory innate immune activation pathways. Toll-like receptors (TLR) recognize these PAMPs, leading to the activation of nuclear factor kappa-light-chain-enhancer of activated B-cells activation, chemokines, and proinflammatory cytokines. The intracellular inflammasome complex, particularly nucleotide-binding oligomerization domain-like receptor P3, leads to caspase-1 activation, secreting bioactive interleukin (IL)-1ß. This amplification loop increases proinflammatory cytokine production, promoting hepatocyte damage, fibrosis, and inhibiting regeneration.

FUTURE THERAPEUTICS FOR ALCOHOLIC LIVER DISEASE

Future therapeutics for ALD have emerged due to advancements in understanding the molecular mechanisms of ALD. Preclinical studies have identified therapeutic targets, such as targeting inflammation, gut permeability, dysbiosis, and hepatoprotective agents. Strategies that interrupt inflammatory cascade activation may have benefits in ALD and acute liver disease. For example, the administration of the IL-1 pathway antagonist anakinra attenuated alcohol-induced steatosis, liver damage, inflammation, and early fibrosis in mice.

Another potential target is spleen tyrosine kinase (SYK), which has been proven to reduce steatosis liver damage, inflammation, and fibrosis in a mouse model of ALD. Targeting TLR 7/8 improves host anti-infective response in AC. miRNAs and extracellular vesicles play a role in the pathomechanisms of ALD, with chronic alcohol reducing liver and hepatocyte expression of miRNA-122, the most abundant microRNA essential for hepatocyte functions. Replacement of miR-122 in hepatocytes in vivo alleviated alcohol-induced liver injury, steatosis, and fibrosis.

Hepatoprotective agents, such as cytokine IL-22, can provide benefits in ALD, protecting against cell damage and improving liver regeneration. Another excellent target for therapy is intestinal dysbiosis, which can be addressed through transfer of human microbiomes from patients with ALD or healthy controls.

Other targeted approaches might include restoring intestinal eubiosis using prebiotics, probiotics, synbiotics, antibiotics, or restoring the function of altered microbial metabolism using bioengineered bacteria or supplementing metabolites. Precision editing the intestinal microbiota with bacteriophages may also represent a promising therapeutic approach. Administration of *E. faecalis*-specific bacteriophages abolished ethanol-induced liver injury in humanized mice.

Finally, the farnesoid X receptor (FXR)-bile acid axis/FXR agonists may be a promising therapeutic target for ALD, as demonstrated in mouse models of liver disease. However, more studies are needed to further examine different approaches in alcohol-induced hepatotoxicity and steatosis.

CONCLUSION

Alcohol-related liver disease is a significant health risk. Experimental models of ALD have been refined, but they do not accurately represent advanced ALD. More research is needed to understand risk factors for ALD development and progression, and to find a biomarker for alcohol use. Focus on diagnosing nonsevere acute liver failure, and the optimal therapeutic strategy for patients with severe AH and ACLF needs further investigation. Novel targets for treatment and new therapeutic approaches are also needed. Physicians should be trained in "alcohol use disorder" identification and management, and collaboration with de-addiction specialists is crucial. Governments should also come up with strict regulations and policies to reduce alcohol-related harm in the population at large.

SUGGESTED READINGS

1. Han S, Yang Z, Zhang T, Ma J, Chandler K, Liangpunsakul S. Epidemiology of Alcohol-Associated Liver Disease. Clin Liver Dis. 2021;25(3):483-92.
2. Crabb DW, Im GY, Szabo G, Mellinger JL, Lucey MR. Diagnosis and Treatment of Alcohol-Associated Liver Diseases: 2019 Practice Guidance from the American Association for the Study of Liver Diseases. Hepatology. 2020;71:306-33.
3. Avila MA, Dufour JF, Gerbes AL, Zoulim F, Bataller R, Burra P, et al. Recent advances in alcohol-related liver disease (ALD): summary of a Gut round table meeting. Gut. 2020;69:764-80.
4. Agrawal A, Gupta P. Alcoholic Hepatitis: The Growing Burden and the current management. In: Mathur G (Ed). Medicine Update 2023. New Delhi: Jaypee Brothers Medical Publishers (P) Ltd.; 2022. pp. 631-5.

113

CHAPTER

Malnutrition in Chronic Liver Disease: Challenges, Assessment, and Management

Puneet Rijhwani, Vidita Kalra, Ambika Tyagi

ABSTRACT

Malnutrition is a significant concern in chronic liver disease (CLD), adversely affecting patient outcomes. This chapter explores malnutrition's assessment, challenges, and management in CLD patients. Assessment methods, such as subjective global assessment and nutritional risk index, are crucial for early identification. Challenges include altered metabolism, gastrointestinal symptoms, and inadequate dietary intake. Management entails optimizing macronutrient balance, providing essential amino acids, and addressing micronutrient deficiencies. Individualized dietary plans, nutritional supplements, and enteral nutrition play pivotal roles. Liver transplantation candidates may require preoperative nutritional support. Collaborative efforts among healthcare professionals are essential to address the complexities of malnutrition in CLD effectively and improve patients' overall quality of life.

INTRODUCTION

Malnutrition is a frequent complication of liver cirrhosis, especially in patients with obesity-related nonalcoholic steatohepatitis. It is linked to the progression of liver failure and an elevated risk of complications. Depletion of both muscle and fat tissue is possible, with females more likely to lose muscle than males. Reduced appetite and food intake, gastrointestinal dysfunction, hepatic encephalopathy, ascites and edema, hypermetabolism, nutritional losses, modified nutrient metabolism, chronic alcohol abuse, inflammation and cytokine imbalance, and coexisting conditions such as diabetes and cardiovascular disease are just a few of the mechanisms that cause malnutrition in chronic liver disease (CLD). In order to effectively manage CLD, nutrition monitoring, and intervention are essential.

TERMINOLOGIES AND DEFINITIONS

Malnutrition

A nutrition-related disorder marked by inadequate nutrient intake or absorption that affects clinical outcomes, changes in body composition, and both physical and mental function.

Undernutrition

This condition, which is another name for malnutrition, is characterized by inadequate nutrition intake or uptake, altering body composition, and impairing both physical and mental function.

Muscle Wasting

The gradual loss of muscle mass is caused by a variety of conditions, including inflammatory illnesses, malnutrition, and increased catabolism, which eventually results in muscle atrophy.

Sarcopenia

The general decline in muscle mass and function, is primarily brought on by aging (primary sarcopenia) or by acute or chronic illness (secondary sarcopenia), including CLD.

Frailty

A state of vulnerability caused by the loss of functional, cognitive, and physiological reserve. One kind of disorder connected to nutrition is fragility.

Immunonutrition

The use of particular nutrients to modify the immune system's activity in order to enhance general health, is not always in the presence of malnutrition. Nucleotides, arginine, glutamine, and nutritional formulas enhanced with omega-3 fatty acids are a few examples.

Deconditioning

The decline in muscle function is brought on by inactivity and chronic illnesses that impair function.

MECHANISMS CONTRIBUTING TO MALNUTRITION IN CHRONIC LIVER DISEASE

- Reduced appetite and food intake
- Gastrointestinal dysfunction
- Hepatic encephalopathy (HE)
- Ascites and edema
- Hypermetabolism
- Nutritional losses
- Modified nutrient metabolism
- Chronic alcohol use
- Inflammation and cytokine imbalance

SCREENING AND ASSESSMENT OF MALNUTRITION IN CHRONIC LIVER DISEASE (FLOWCHART 1)

Nutrition Screening Tools

- Being underweight with a body mass index (BMI) of 18.5 kg/m^2 and having advanced decompensated cirrhosis (Child–Pugh C patients) are two criteria that can help identify high-risk patients for malnutrition in CLD.
- A number of scoring tools are available to determine the risk of malnutrition in CLD patients, but the majority have not been validated for this group.

The liver disease undernutrition screening tool and the Royal Free Hospital-Nutritional Prioritizing Tool (RFH-NPT) score are two instruments specific to liver disease.

Detailed Nutritional Assessment

- Imaging, anthropometric measurements, dual-energy X-ray absorptiometry (DEXA), and bioelectrical impedance analysis (BIA) are a few of the techniques that can be used to measure muscle mass.
- Measures of handgrip strength and frailty can also be used to identify malnutrition in cirrhotic patients and forecast complications and mortality.
- Global assessment tools like the subjective global assessment (SGA) and the Royal Free Hospital-Global Assessment (RFH-GA) are used.
- Dietary interviews are essential to understanding patient's food intake and identifying specific nutrient deficiencies.

Obesity in Cirrhosis: Assessment and Interpretation

- Sarcopenia obesity (muscle loss with increased adipose tissue) is common, and obesity can coexist with malnutrition in cirrhotic patients.
- To ensure complete care, obese cirrhotic patients should regularly have their malnutrition assessed and treated.

NUTRITIONAL MANAGEMENT PRINCIPLES IN PATIENTS WITH LIVER CIRRHOSIS

Energy and Protein Requirements in Cirrhosis

- Cirrhotic patients who receive frequent feedings, along with a late-evening snack and a protein-rich breakfast, have better metabolic outcomes and a higher quality of life.
- To prevent muscle loss and reverse sarcopenia, cirrhotic patients should consume 1.2–1.5 g/kg body weight (BW) of protein/day.
- Dietary advice can be given to cirrhotic subjects at the bedside and outpatient department (OPD) visits; protein intake does not result in HE and may even improve mental status.
- Practical dietary advice for bedside or outpatient clinic use:
  - Distribute your daily caloric intake among three meals—breakfast, lunch, and dinner; and three snacks, i.e., (1) midday, (2) midafternoon, and (3) late at night. A late-night snack is essential to bridge the gap between dinner and breakfast.

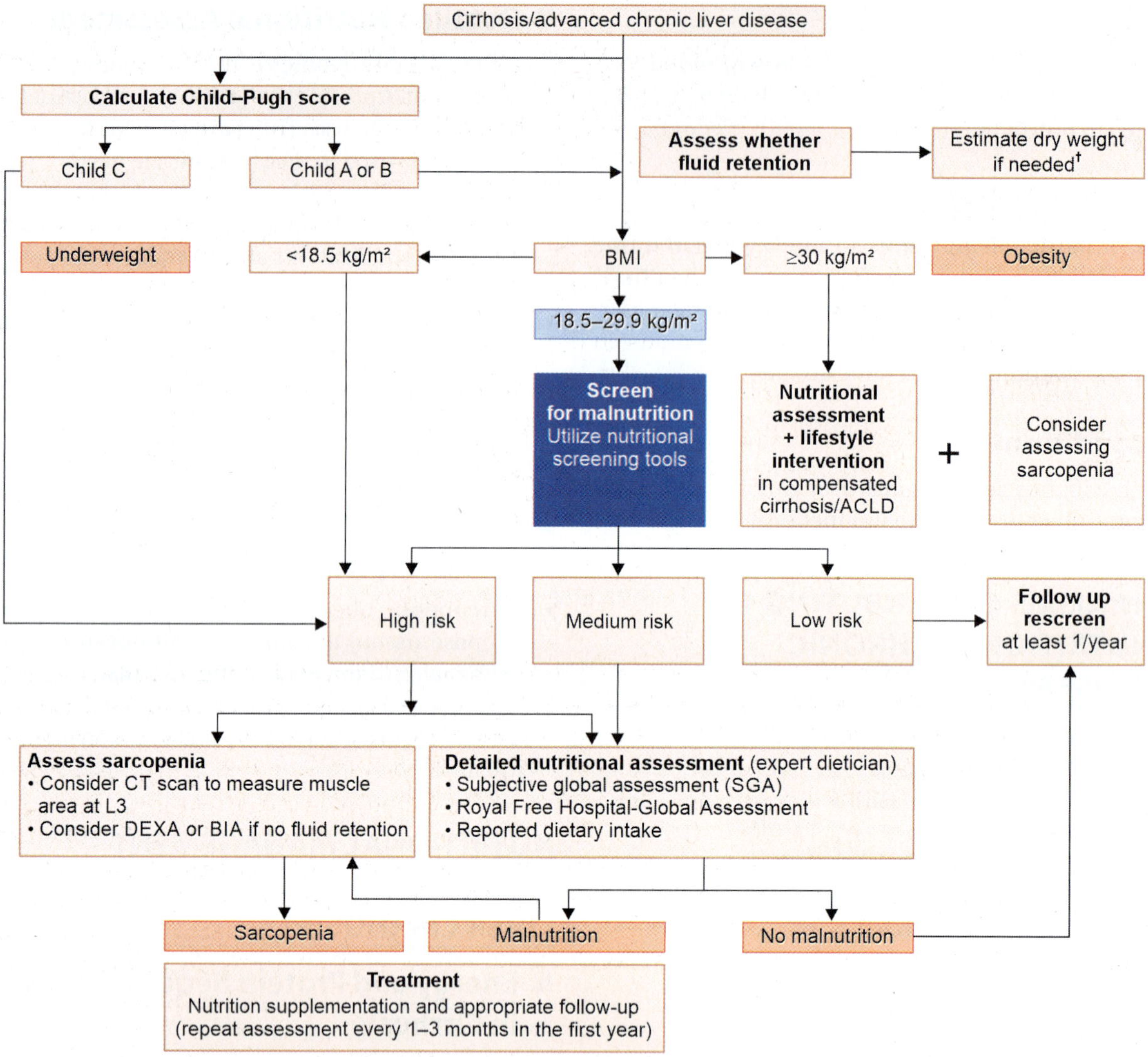

†When a patient has fluid retention, their body weight should be adjusted by weighing them dry using postparacentesis measurements, if available, or by deducting a percentage of their weight based on the severity of their ascites (mild = 5%; moderate = 10%; severe = 15%). If bilateral pedal edema is present, an additional 5% of their weight should be deducted.

FLOWCHART 1: Rapid nutritional screening is crucial for patients with cirrhosis, including fluid retention. A liver-specific tool, RHF-NPT, is advisable for high-risk patients. A detailed nutritional assessment is recommended, and supplementation or regular follow-up should be provided. Correcting fluid retention involves evaluating dry weight, BMI, CT, and DEXA.

(ACLD: advanced chronic liver disease; BIA: bioelectrical impedance analysis; BMI: body mass index; CT: computed tomography; DEXA: dual-energy X-ray absorptiometry)

- Make an effort to eat a lot of fruits and vegetables. Consult your physician or a dietician if you experience bloating or a decrease in appetite.
- Limit the amount of salt in your diet. Even though it might take some getting used to, cutting back on salt is beneficial. Inform your doctor or dietician if it makes your food unpleasant or decreases your appetite.
- Let your doctor know if you have any additional health issues, such as diabetes and obesity, as they might call for dietary changes.

– A sarcopenia approach for individuals with liver cirrhosis
– Factors related to sarcopenia in individuals with cirrhosis **(Fig. 1)**:
  - There are conflicting findings from studies on protein turnover in cirrhosis, with some suggesting unchanged levels, increased synthesis, or decreased synthesis and breakdown.
  - Gender, age, ethnicity, and the severity and cause of liver disease are some of the

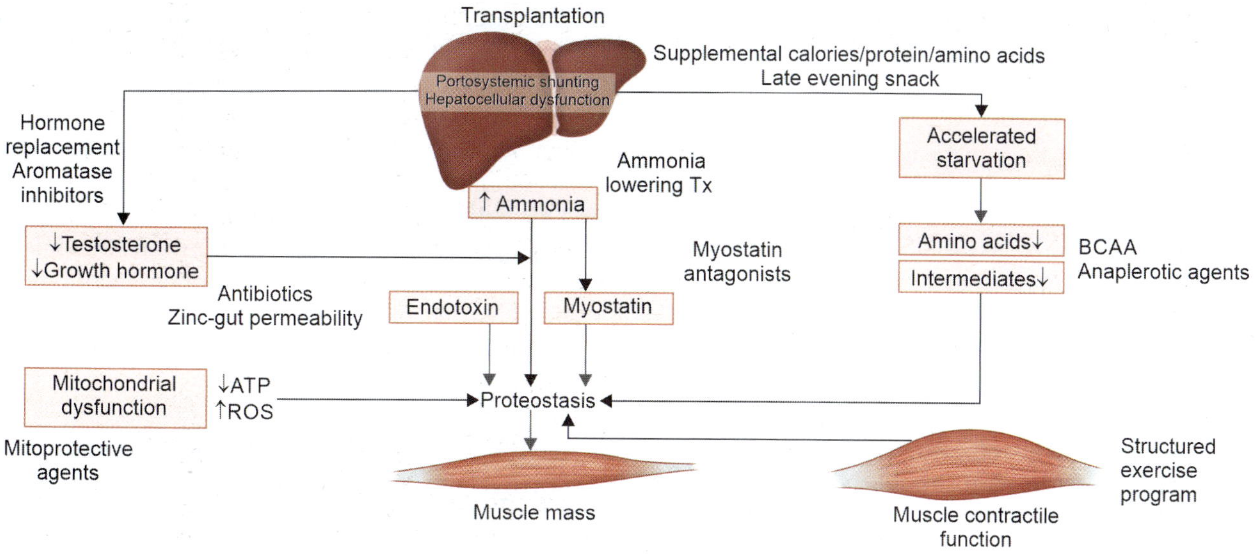

FIG. 1: Factors associated with sarcopenia.
(ATP: adenosine triphosphate; BCAA: branched-chain amino acids; ROS: reactive oxygen species)

variables that can affect muscle mass. The cholestatic and alcoholic liver disease frequently results in significant muscle loss.

- Hepatocellular dysfunction, portosystemic shunting, increased skeletal muscle ammonia, hormonal imbalances, endotoxemia, and decreased nutrient intake all contribute to sarcopenia (muscle loss) in cirrhosis.
- In addition to a decrease in the amino acid chain L-leucine, sarcopenia in cirrhosis is linked to impaired global protein synthesis and amino acid imbalances.
- It has been discovered that myostatin, a protein that inhibits protein synthesis and encourages proteolysis, is elevated in cirrhosis.

– Muscle mass improvement strategies in cirrhosis nutritional supplementation:
  - It may be difficult for malnourished sarcopenic individuals with severe liver disease to eat adequate calories and protein.
  - For addressing the challenge of attaining sufficient consumption, clinical trials have demonstrated some benefits for oral nutritional supplements and branched-chain amino acid (BCAA) supplements.
  - If malnourished cirrhotic individuals are unable to get enough calories through diet or supplements, short-term enteral, or parenteral nutrition should be considered.
  - Parenteral nutritional supplementation may be beneficial when oral intake is insufficient for prolonged periods of time due to ailments including encephalopathy, gastrointestinal hemorrhage, reduced gut motility, or ileus.
  - There are some indications that supplemental nutrition can increase lean body mass and enhance the quality of life, despite the fact that there is not much direct research on sarcopenia.

Exercise and Physical Activity

- Although there is a lack of long-term data, increased physical activity and exercise can improve muscle mass and function in cirrhosis.
- Aerobic or endurance training increases skeletal muscle capacity but may not result in a significant increase in muscle mass.
- Resistance training encourages the growth of skeletal muscle mass.
- Exercise may have negative effects on cirrhotic patients by increasing muscle ammonia production and portal pressure.
- Exercise has been shown to benefit cirrhosis patients despite possible negative reactions.
- Combining resistance and endurance training may be useful and appropriate to treat muscle atrophy and reduced contractile function in cirrhosis.

Nutritional Approach and Management of Obesity in Individuals with Liver Cirrhosis

- Patients with cirrhosis have a higher risk of disease progression and complications when their BMI is higher.
- In obese patients with compensated cirrhosis, lifestyle interventions such as nutritional therapy and moderate-intensity exercise, have produced favorable results.
- A 5–10% weight loss target is thought to be adequate and can slow the rate at which the disease progresses.
- Although resistance training is generally safe, patients with portal hypertension should avoid exercises that put pressure on the abdomen.
- Consistent exercise over a long period of time is advised for best results.

Recommendations

- Moderate-intensity exercise tailored to the individual's ability is recommended.
- It is important to maintain adequate protein intake during weight loss interventions to prevent muscle loss.
- For the greatest benefits, consistent exercise over a long period of time is advised.
- For decompensated cirrhotic patients who have trouble getting enough nitrogen through their diet, leucine-enriched amino acid supplements and amino acid chain (BCAA) supplements can be taken into consideration.
- For malnourished cirrhotic patients who are unable to meet their nutritional needs through oral intake and supplements, enteral nutrition (feeding through a tube) is advised.
- Obese cirrhotic patients with a BMI of 30 kg/m^2 or higher should adhere to a dietary and lifestyle plan for gradual weight loss (5–10% of body weight), taking water retention into consideration.

Micronutrients

- All patients with CLD should have their plasma vitamin D levels checked; if the levels are <20 ng/mL, supplementation is advised.
- Thiamine (B1) deficiency, in particular, is common in cirrhosis and may necessitate parenteral supplementation.
- Dietary sodium reduction is advised for individuals with ascites as hyponatremia (low sodium levels) is common in cirrhosis and should be monitored.
- Calcium, magnesium, iron, zinc, and selenium deficiencies can occur in cirrhosis and should be treated as needed.
- Stay away from nutritional supplements containing manganese due to the possibility of basal ganglia accumulation in cirrhosis.
- The palatability of the diet should be taken into consideration when managing cirrhotic patients with ascites on a sodium-restricted diet (recommended intake of 80 mmol/day), as it may reduce caloric intake. There should be improvements made to the restricted diet's flavor and appeal.

Nutritional Treatment Methods for Hepatic Encephalopathy

- To identify deficiencies and muscle loss, evaluate the nutritional status and sarcopenia in patients with HE.
- Restricting protein should be avoided in HE patients, unless necessary for brief periods due to severe overt HE or gastrointestinal bleeding.
- Make sure that patients with HE consumes enough protein and calories each day to meet the general guidelines for cirrhotic patients. The intake should not fall below the suggested limits.
- Vegetables and dairy proteins may be better tolerated by HE patients than meat proteins, so promote their consumption.
- To enhance neuropsychiatric performance and fulfill the advised nitrogen intake, think about taking BCAAs as a supplement. Taking BCAA supplements can be an alternative to eating less protein overall.
- Give patients with HE who can tolerate it the highest priority for oral dietary intake. However, if a patient has grade III–IV encephalopathy and is unable to eat, nutrition should be administered parenterally or through a nasogastric tube (if the airways are protected).

Options for Nutritional Therapy in Cirrhotic Subjects with Bone Diseases (Flowchart 2)

- Measure bone mineral density (BMD) in patients with cirrhosis, cholestatic liver disease, and those on long-term corticosteroid therapy before liver transplantation.
- Use lumbar and femoral densitometry (DEXA) to identify osteoporosis and osteopenia, and do lateral spine X-rays to identify vertebral fractures.
- After 2–3 years, patients with normal BMD should have another DEXA scan. Patients who are at a high

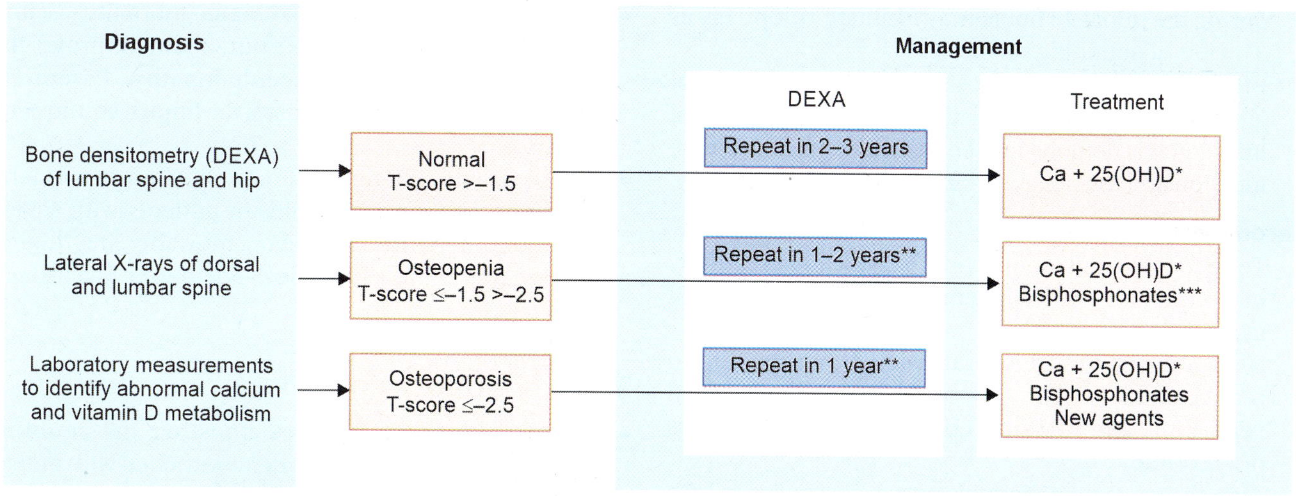

*Calcium (1,000–1,500 mg/d) and 25(OH)D (400–800 IU/d or 260 lg every two weeks) to preserve normal levels.
**According to the severity of liver disease and cholestasis, and in patients taking corticosteroids.
***Depending on additional risk factors. 25(OH)D, 25-hydroxyvitamin D. DEXA; dual-energy X-ray absorptiometry.

FLOWCHART 2: Diagnosis and management of bone disease in chronic liver disease.
(DEXA: dual-energy X-ray absorptiometry)

risk of losing bone quickly might consider redoing their DEXA in a year.

- Give vitamin D and calcium supplements to individuals with CLD and T-scores below –1.5 (400–800 IU/day or 260 mg every 2 weeks).
- Patients with cirrhosis who are waiting for liver transplants and have osteoporosis should consider bisphosphonates.
- Consider venesection and testosterone supplementation as potential therapies for men with hemochromatosis and hypogonadism.

Special Consideration Clinical Scenario

Malnutrition in Individuals Undergoing Liver Transplantation and Liver Surgery

Preoperative

- Severe malnutrition and extreme obesity have been found to be associated with increased rates of mortality and morbidity prior to liver transplantation.
- Cirrhotic patients undergoing liver transplantation exhibit elevated levels of morbidity and mortality as a result of protein malnutrition, sarcopenia, and frailty.
- Oral nutritional supplements (ONS) and nutritional counseling increase the muscle mass and grip strength of cirrhosis patients, but no appreciable difference in mortality was found.
- Various interventions, including the parenteral or enteral administration of glutamine or omega-3 fatty acids, have been found to have a generally favorable effect on morbidity and liver function. However, these interventions do not appear to have a significant impact on overall survival.
- Enhanced-recovery after surgery (ERAS) protocols have demonstrated notable advancements in morbidity reduction and decreased hospitalization duration for liver surgery. These protocols encompass early initiation of feeding and mobilization as key components.

Recommendations

- Sarcopenia can be treated before surgery, improving body protein status and producing better clinical results.
- Prior to surgery, decide on the target nutritional status. Plan an intake of 30 kcal/kg of total energy if maintenance is the goal × BW/day and 1.2 g of protein/kg × BW/day. Plan a 35 kcal/kg total energy intake if improvement is the goal × BW/day and 1.5 g of protein/kg × BW/day.

Postoperative

- Enteral nutrition is advantageous, shortening time on the ventilator, bacterial infections, intensive care unit (ICU) stay, and complications with the bile duct.
- Standard amino acid solutions are just as effective as BCAA-enriched solutions for addressing nitrogen loss after liver transplantation, ranging from 1.0 to 1.5 g/kg × BW/day.
- Like other individuals undergoing surgery, it is important to regulate glucose metabolism and blood glucose levels. Additionally, providing lower energy

during the initial 48 hours may facilitate autophagy as a means of obtaining substrate.

- In individuals with cirrhosis, the administration of glutamine and human growth hormone via parenteral nutrition has demonstrated enhancements in immune function and the preservation of gut mucosal integrity.

Recommendations

- To reduce the risk of infection, begin eating regularly or using an enteral feeding tube within 12–24 hours of surgery.
- Use parenteral nutrition rather than not feeding to reduce complications, time spent on mechanical ventilation, and ICU stay if oral or enteral nutrition is not possible.
- After the acute postoperative phase, give patients 1.5 g of protein and 35 kcal of energy/kg of body weight/day.
- For patients with CLD undergoing other surgical procedures, take into account adhering to the ERAS protocol.
- If enteral nutrition is not possible or is inappropriate for patients with compromised cough and swallow reflexes or hepatic encephalopathy, think about parenteral nutrition.
- Use parenteral nutrition and/or enteral tube feeding with a reduced energy intake target of 25 kcal/kg for obese patients × BW/day and a 2.0 g/kg target for increased protein intake × BW/day.

Nutrition in Critically Ill Cirrhotic Patients

- Regardless of their specific condition or the environment in which they are receiving care, critically ill cirrhotic patients require adequate nutritional support.
- To precisely assess the energy needs of these patients, direct measurement of resting energy expenditure (REE) through indirect calorimetry is advised.
- In critically ill cirrhotic patients, maintaining strict glucose control is essential to preventing both hyperglycemia and hypoglycemia.
- In order to meet the nutritional needs of critically ill cirrhotic patients, nutrition is frequently required.

Severe/Acute Alcoholic Hepatitis and Alcoholic Liver Disease

- It has been discovered that nutritional supplements, such as intravenous amino acids and a diet rich in calories and protein, are safe and associated with lower mortality rates in patients with alcoholic hepatitis.
- Low protein intake can make the symptoms of HE worse in people with alcoholic hepatitis and hepatic encephalopathy.
- Nutritional support did not change mortality, ascites, or laboratory parameters, but it did improve the resolution of clinical encephalopathy. Parenteral nutrition showed a propensity for improved nitrogen balance.
- There was no difference in mortality between enteral nutrition and corticosteroids in patients with severe alcoholic hepatitis. However, mortality was higher when caloric intake was low—below 21.5 kcal/kg × BW/day.

Immunonutrition

- Immunonutrition involves boosting the immune system with dietary supplements enriched with omega 3 fatty acids, arginine, and nucleotides.
- The administration of oral omega 3 fatty acids as part of immunonutrition did not enhance renal function in the case of cirrhotic patients with ascites and renal failure. Regarding its suitability for use in cirrhotic patients, it was linked to increased bleeding time and arterial blood pressure.

Nutritional Intervention for Gastrointestinal Hemorrhage

- In a random research, 22 subjects with liver cirrhosis who were bleeding suddenly from esophageal varices participated.
- The patients were split into two groups, one of which received enteral nutrition through a nasogastric tube and the other of which did not consume any food or liquids for the first four days following the bleeding event.
- The study found no statistically significant differences between the two groups in terms of rebleeding, liver function, nutritional status, length of hospital stays, or mortality after a follow-up period of 35 days.
- In spite of these results, specialists typically advise delaying enteral nutrition for 48–72 hours following acute bleeding from esophageal varices.
- This advice is based on the knowledge that enteral nutrition may increase splanchnic blood flow, which may increase portal pressure and raise the risk of variceal rebleeding.

Recommendations

- Make sure that critically ill cirrhotic patients get at least 35–40 kcal/kg × BW/day, or 1.3 times their measured REE, in energy.
- Ensure that critically ill cirrhotic patients consume 1.2–1.3 g/kg.BW/day of protein daily.

- To help with resolution in critically ill cirrhotic patients with HE, consider using BCAA-enriched solutions.
- Give patients with cirrhosis and severe/acute alcoholic hepatitis nutritional hold to encourage the resolution of HE and increase endurance.

SUGGESTED READINGS

1. European Association for the Study of the Liver. Electronic address: easloffice@easloffice.eu; European Association for the Study of the Liver. EASL Clinical Practice Guidelines on nutrition in chronic liver disease. J Hepatol. 2019;70(1):172-93.
2. Cederholm T, Bosaeus I, Barazzoni R, Bauer J, Van Gossum A, Klek S, et al. Diagnostic criteria for malnutrition - An ESPEN Consensus Statement. Clin Nutr. 2015;34(3):335-40.
3. Carey EJ, Lai JC, Wang CW, Dasarathy S, Lobach I, Montano-Loza AJ, et al. A multicenter study to define sarcopenia in patients with end-stage liver disease. Liver Transpl. 2017;23(5):625-33.
4. Yoshida T, Muto Y, Moriwaki H, Yamato M. Effect of long-term oral supplementation with branched-chain amino acid granules on the prognosis of liver cirrhosis. Gastroenterol Jpn. 1989;24(6):692-98.
5. Berzigotti A, Albillos A, Villanueva C, Genescá J, Ardevol A, Augustín S, et al. Effects of an intensive lifestyle intervention program on portal hypertension in patients with cirrhosis and obesity: The SportDiet study. Hepatology. 2017;65(4):1293-305.
6. Everhart JE, Lok AS, Kim HY, Morgan TR, Lindsay KL, Chung RT, et al. Weight-Related Effects on Disease Progression in the Hepatitis C Antiviral Long-Term Treatment Against Cirrhosis Trial. Gastroenterology. 2009;137(2):549-57.
7. Dasarathy J, Varghese R, Feldman A, Khiyami A, McCullough AJ, Dasarathy S. Patients with nonalcoholic fatty liver disease have a low response rate to vitamin D supplementation. J Nutr. 2017;147(10):1938-46.
8. Menon KV, Angulo P, Weston S, Dickson ER, Lindor KD. Bone disease in primary biliary cirrhosis: independent indicators and rate of progression. J Hepatol. 2001;35(3):316-23.

TABLE 1: Indicators on history and physical examination to identify etiology of ascites.

History	Physical examination
Presence of risk factors for cirrhosis: • Injection drug abuse • Significant alcohol intake • Obesity • Diabetes *History of prior decompensation*: • Jaundice • Upper gastrointestinal bleed • Hepatic encephalopathy • Prior ascites *Ruling out nonliver causes of ascites*: • Heart disease—chest pain, orthopnea, syncope, and paroxysmal nocturnal dyspnea • Renal disease—oliguria and frothuria • Pancreatic disease—upper abdominal pain radiating to back *History suggestive of malignancy*: • Significant weight loss • History of lump *History suggestive of tuberculosis*: • Fever • Night sweats • Weight loss	Shifting dullness or fluid thrill *Signs of liver cell failure*: • Icterus • Spider angiomas • Paper money skin • Gynecomastia • Splenomegaly • Testicular atrophy • Loss of secondary sexual characters • Caput medusae • Parotid swelling • Palmar erythema • Purpura • Edema • Fetor hepaticus *Signs of heart failure or constrictive pericarditis*: • Elevated jugular venous pressure • Pulmonary edema • Pericardial rub • Pedal edema *Signs of pancreatitis*: • Cullen's sign • Grey Turner sign *Signs of malignancy*: • Lymphadenopathy • Abdominal mass

TABLE 2: SAAG evaluation.

Routine	Optional	Unusual	Unhelpful
• Cell count • Sugar • Protein • Albumin • SAAG	• Amylase • Culture • Gram stain • LDH • ADA • Malignant cytology	• Bilirubin • TB smear, culture • PCR test • Triglyceride	• Cholesterol • Fibronectin • Lactate • pH

(ADA: adenosine deaminase; LDG: lactate dehydrogenase; PCR: polymerase chain reaction; SAAG: serum ascites albumin gradient; TB: tuberculosis)

combination with a loop diuretic. Spironolactone appears to be more effective than furosemide (response rate of 95% vs. 52%) in nonazotemic patients with cirrhosis and ascites. Spironolactone has a long half-life, allowing once a day dosing, dose changes should occur no more frequently than every 3–4 days. In patients, who are intolerant to spironolactone, amiloride can be used. Loop diuretics are added if patient have moderate to severe ascites or ascites with pedal edema. Ratio of loop diuretics and antimineralocorticoids should be maintained as 1:4.

Adverse Reactions to Diuretics

All patients on diuretics should be monitored for adverse events, the prevalence of which ranges from 19 to 33%. In hospitalized patients treated with diuretics, hepatic encephalopathy is seen in up to 25% and renal impairment in 14–20%, especially in the absence of peripheral edema. Renal impairment is reversible on discontinuing diuretics. Other adverse effects include hyponatremia (8–30%), hyperkalemia (11%), and hypokalemia. Gynecomastia is commonly seen with spironolactone, especially with higher doses.

Response Assessment to Diuretics

The aim of diuretic therapy is to ensure that urinary sodium excretion exceeds 78 mmol/day. A random spot urine sodium: potassium ratio of >1 has a sensitivity of 90.9% and specificity of 56% in predicting urinary Na^+ excretion of >78 mmol/day **(Flowchart 3)**.

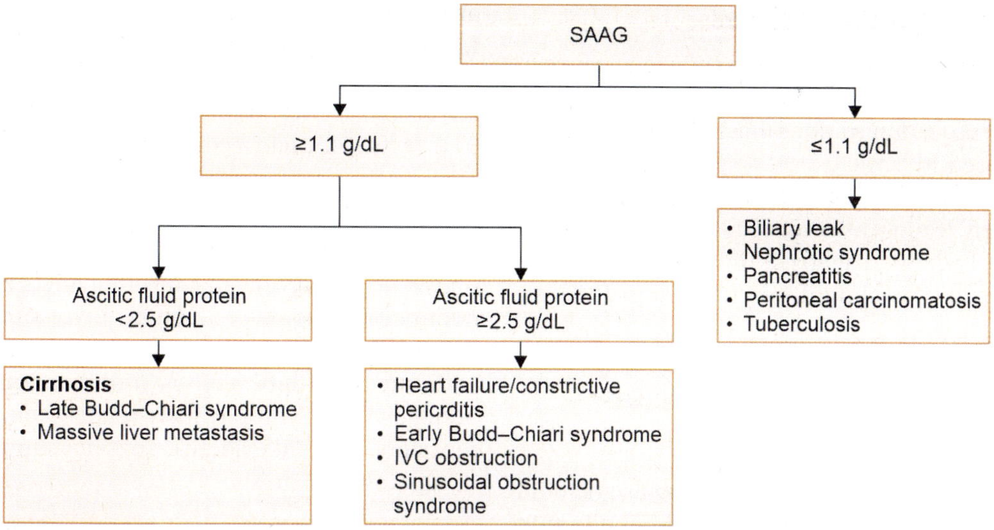

FLOWCHART 2: Diagnostic evaluation and differential diagnosis of ascites.
(IVC: inferior vena cava; SAAG: serum ascites albumin gradient)

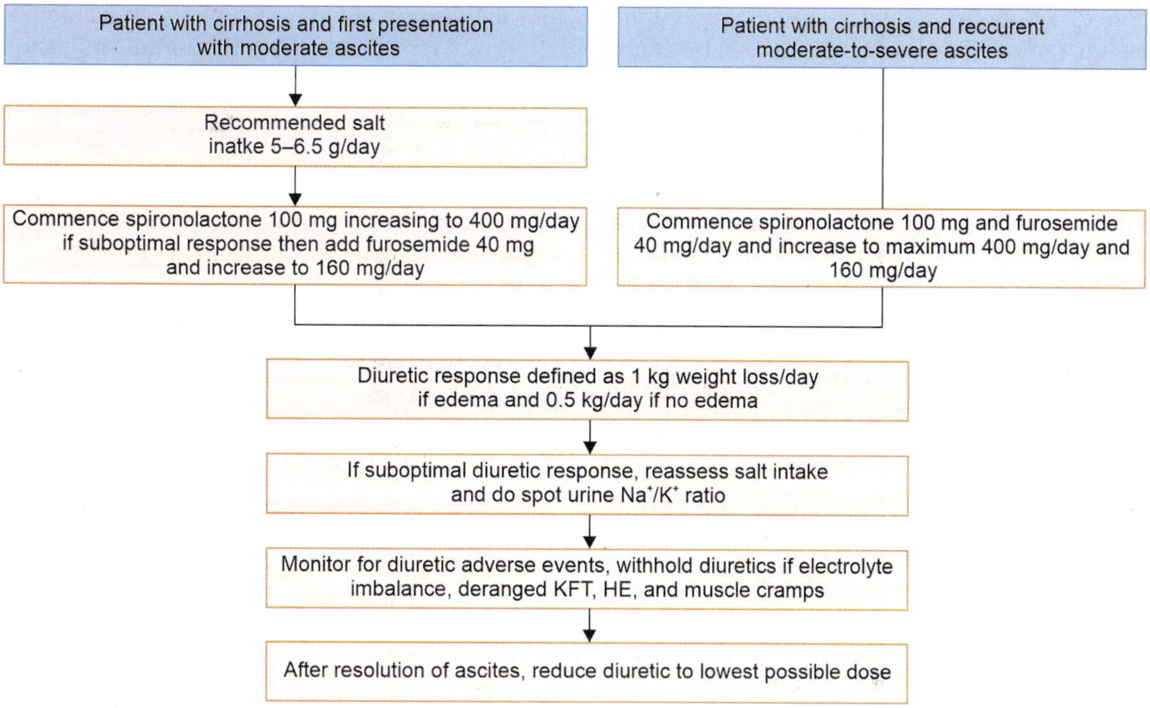

FLOWCHART 3: Approach to diuretic use in cirrhotic ascites.
(HE: hepatic encephalopathy; KFT: kidney function test)

REFRACTORY ASCITES

Ascites that cannot be mobilized or the early recurrence of which cannot be satisfactorily prevented by medical treatment. It occurs in nearly 10% of cirrhotic patients. This includes two different subgroups.

Diuretic-resistant Ascites

Ascites that cannot be mobilized or the early recurrence of which cannot be prevented because of a lack of response to sodium restriction and diuretic treatment.

Diuretic-intractable Ascites

Ascites that cannot be mobilized or the early recurrence of which cannot be prevented because of the development of diuretic-induced complications that preclude the use of an effective diuretic dosage.

Median survival of patients with refractory ascites is approximately 6 months. Mortality occurs in 70% of patients within 1 year of diagnosis. Therefore, all patients with refractory ascites should be considered for liver transplant.

Management of Refractory Ascites

Large-volume Paracentesis

Large-volume paracentesis (LVP) (removing ascitic fluid >5 L) with plasma volume expansion with IV albumin is considered the first-line treatment for patients with refractory ascites. It relieves ascites immediately but associated with recurrence and does not improve survival. LVP is associated with paracentesis-induced circulatory dysfunction (PICD). To prevent PICD, administer albumin @ 8 g/L of fluid removed; avoid diuretics and beta blocker (BB) on the day of tapping. Midodrine can be used if albumin not available and found to be equally effective.

Diuretics

Once refractory ascites develops, diuretics should be stopped to prevent adverse events, because no beneficial effects of diuretics have been demonstrated in these patients.

However, in patients who maintain a urinary sodium excretion >30 mEq/day on diuretics, diuretic therapy can be continued, if tolerated, in order to delay ascites formation and increase the interval between LVPs.

Transjugular Intrahepatic Portosystemic Shunt

Transjugular intrahepatic portosystemic shunt (TIPS) create an artificial connection between the portal and hepatic vein, which causes decompression of the portal system and reduces portal pressures. TIPS will increase preload leading to increased cardiac output. As a result, there is increase in effective arterial volume causing improved renal blood flow and increased urinary sodium excretion. Ascites will resolve slowly over 4–6 months in approximately 80% of patients, and a salt-restricted diet should be continued until ascites resolves. Most common side effect of TIPS is hepatic encephalopathy which occurs in around 50% of patients.

Midodrine

It is an α1-adrenergic agonist which improve circulatory and kidney function by causing splanchnic vasoconstriction in patients with cirrhosis and ascites. It is an oral drug therefore can be used for long-term treatment. In a randomized controlled trial (RCT) [midodrine vs. standard medical treatment (SMT)] in patients with refractory ascites, midodrine showed that at 3 months 94% versus 50% had a complete/partial ascites control.

Vaptans

Vaptans are selective V2 receptor antagonists that act on the principal cells in collecting ducts in nephron and enhance free water excretion. Two meta-analyses on vaptans in cirrhotic patients reported improved serum sodium levels and ascites mobilization, but without beneficial effect on cirrhosis-related complications and mortality. Current evidence does not support routine use of vaptans in cirrhosis.

Automated Low-flow Ascites Pump (Alfapump®)

The Alfapump® is a battery-powered pump implanted subcutaneously in the abdominal wall that aspirates and transports ascitic fluid through a subcutaneous catheter into the urinary bladder. Patients with loculated ascites, active infection or severe abdominal adhesions from previous surgery are not candidates for Alfapump® placement.

Liver Transplant

Liver transplant is the treatment of choice for patients with refractory ascites. Liver transplant can radically reverse portal HTN and survival rates are remarkable.

TREATMENT OF ASCITES DUE TO OTHER CAUSES

Tubercular Ascites

Tuberculosis is a serious infectious disease in India. Incidence of extrapulmonary TB (EPTB) is on the rise along with pulmonary TB. TB ascites is one of the clinical signs of abdominal TB. The diagnosis of TB ascites is difficult because of nonspecific symptoms. Therefore, diagnosis relies on clinical symptoms, radiological imaging, and detection of *Mycobacterium tuberculosis* (MTB) in ascitic fluid by either acid-fast bacillus (AFB) staining or culture.

Ascitic fluid analysis in tubercular ascites consists of low SAAG, high protein, lymphocytic predominant high cell count and raised adenosine deaminase (ADA).

Treatment include 6–8 months of antitubercular therapy and LVP if tense ascites.

Pancreatic Ascites

Pancreatic ascites is a rare entity. It results from persistent leakage of pancreatic secretions in the peritoneal cavity from pancreatic ductal injury. The severity of this condition depends on the location and degree of ductal injury. Minor pancreatic duct injuries cause peripancreatic fluid collection and are common in acute severe pancreatitis. Necrotizing pancreatitis can cause major pancreatic duct injury.

Diagnostic paracentesis should be performed, and fluid amylase and protein measurements should be measured along with cell count, culture, Gram stain, and cytology. Pancreatic ascites is characterized by an amylase level over 1,000 IU/L, protein level ≥ 3 g/dL and low SAAG.

The mainstay of treatment is diverting pancreatic fluid away from the leakage to the small bowel, allowing the leak to heal. Adjunct treatment includes medical therapy to decrease pancreatic exocrine secretions and salvage treatment with surgery.

Malignant Ascites

Malignant ascites is a sign of peritoneal carcinomatosis and occurs commonly in ovarian, colorectal, pancreatic, uterine, lung, and breast carcinoma. Malignant ascites accounts for approximately 10% of all cases of ascites. The presence of malignant ascites is a grave prognostic sign.

Ascitic fluid analyses can diagnose malignant causes of ascites in most cases, but laparoscopic tissue sampling may be necessary. In patients with peritoneal carcinomatosis, the ascites fluid has positive cytology, elevated protein concentrations and a low SAAG.

Traditional therapies, including paracentesis, peritoneovenous shunt placement, and diuretics, are successful and effective in varying degrees.

Heart Failure-related Ascites

Cardiac disease causing right heart failure can lead to ascites formation. Common causes include constrictive pericarditis and mitral stenosis. Ascitic fluid analysis will have high SAAG and high protein. Treatment includes salt restriction, diuretics, and therapy for underlying illness.

SUGGESTED READINGS

1. Moreau R, Delègue P, Pessione F, Hillaire S, Durand F, Lebrec D, et al. Clinical characteristics and outcome of patients with cirrhosis and refractory ascites. Liver Int. 2004;24:457-64.
2. Morali GA, Sniderman KW, Deitel KM, Tobe S, Witt-Sullivan H, Simon M, et al. Is sinusoidal portal hypertension a necessary factor for the development of hepatic ascites J Hepatol. 1992;16:249-50.
3. Pérez-Ayuso RM, Arroyo V, Planas R, Gaya J, Bory F, Rimola A, et al. Randomized comparative study of efficacy of furosemide versus spironolactone in nonazotemic cirrhosis with ascites. Relationship between the diuretic response and the activity of the renin-aldosterone system. Gastroenterology. 1983;84:961-8.
4. Angeli P, Fasolato S, Mazza E, Okolicsanyi L, Maresio G, Velo E, et al. Combined versus sequential diuretic treatment of ascites in non-azotaemic patients with cirrhosis: results of an open randomised clinical trial. Gut. 2010;59:98-104.

115

CHAPTER

Complications of Acute Viral Hepatitis

Manabendra Nayak

ABSTRACT

Acute viral hepatitis is inflammation of the liver, generally meaning inflammation by infection with one of the five hepatitis viruses. In most people, the inflammation begins suddenly and lasts only a few weeks. Acute viral hepatitis is common throughout the world. Most cases of acute viral hepatitis resolve on their own, but some persist and progress to chronic hepatitis and some develop serious complications. The hepatitis A virus (HAV) is the most common of acute hepatitis, followed by the hepatitis B virus (HBV). Other viruses can also cause acute viral hepatitis. Fulminant hepatitis can occur in people with hepatitis A, but it is more likely to develop in people with hepatitis B, particularly if they also have hepatitis D. Fulminant hepatitis can progress very quickly, usually within days or weeks, and can lead to acute liver failure. Acute viral hepatitis can develop some extrahepatic complications, such as acute kidney injury, cholestatic jaundice, coagulopathy, myocarditis, and rarely some neurological manifestation.

INTRODUCTION

Acute viral hepatitis can cause anything from a minor flu-like illness to fatal liver failure. The most common causes of acute hepatitis are viral hepatitis (hepatitis A and E) and nonviral causes such as drug-induced liver injury, autoimmune hepatitis, and toxins. Hepatotropic viruses cause classic acute viral hepatitis. These are hepatitis A virus (HAV), hepatitis B virus B (HBV), hepatitis C virus C (HCV), hepatitis D virus (HDV), and hepatitis E virus (HEV). Acute hepatitis generally does not lead to any long-term concern. Liver failure is a common complication of acute viral hepatitis which results in a build-up of fluid in the abdomen, bleeding disorders, kidney failure, increased blood pressure in the liver's portal veins, and hepatic encephalopathy. A viral infection that is not well managed can lead to damage to the liver and total failure. Other conditions causing secondary injury from extrahepatic and nonhepatic etiologies should also be considered in the differential diagnosis which includes choledocholithiasis, biliary or pancreatic malignancies, liver metastasis, systemic hypertension, hepatic artery thrombosis, congestive heart failure.

COMPLICATION OF ACUTE VIRAL HEPATITIS

Acute Liver Failure

The most severe complication of acute viral hepatitis is acute liver failure (ALF). In India, hepatitis virus(es) is the most frequent cause of ALF and encephalopathy occurs in all patients within 4 weeks of jaundice. The American Association for the Study of Liver Diseases (AASLD), however, defines ALF if encephalopathy ensues within 26 weeks of onset of acute hepatitis symptoms. Indian National Association of the Study of Liver (INASL) consensus statement on ALF published recently defines ALF as "a clinical syndrome characterized by encephalopathy, jaundice, and prolonged prothrombin time (PT) [international normalized ratio (INR) >1.5] developing in a patient without preexisting liver disease within 4 weeks of the onset of symptoms. Globally, hepatitis A, B, and E probably cause most cases of acute liver failure reported as 50% of cases in Japan, 68% of cases in India, and 91% of cases in Bangladesh. The various viral etiologies in order of frequencies those reported in published studies include, non-A to non-E in about 40%, HEV in approximately one third; whereas, HBV and HAV causing ALF is less frequent.

About <1% of acute HAV infections result in ALF. Hepatitis A-related ALF has a spontaneous survival rate of 69%, the remaining 31% require an emergency liver transplant (ELF) or die. The reasons why HAV infection may progress frequently to ALF are poorly understood. Underlying host factors such as age and even minor pre-existing damage may play a role. Moreover, viral factors including low viral load and higher rate of substitutions in the five untranslated regions of the viral genome are also thought to increase the likelihood of a fulminant course. In contrast, there is some evidence that cytolytic T cells may play an important role in the pathogenesis of HAV infection and in determining the course.

Hepatitis B viral infection can lead to both acute and chronic liver disease. The mechanisms whereby HBV induces ALF are not well known. There are several studies showing that HBV care promoter mutations have been implicated in the pathogenesis of fulminant hepatitis B. Enhanced viral replication may result in a stronger immune response and extended infection. Consequently, this could be an important factor in driving the disease toward a fulminant course. Another possible factor with a major impact on HBV-related ALF could be the overwhelming activation of humoral immunity. Hepatitis D infection may occur in conjunction with acute hepatitis B. Hepatitis D virus superinfection of a chronic HBV patient can also result in ALF. Acute HEV infection rarely proceeds to ALF as per the report. There is no evidence that hepatitis C alone appears to cause ALF.

Acute Renal Failure

Acute hepatitis A in rare cases can lead to severe complications like acute renal failure (ARF). In >80% of patients with fulminant hepatitis with massive hepatic necrosis can develop ARF as reported by a study done by Wilkinson. Hepatocyte growth factor (HGF) is a predictive factor for acute liver failure. High serum HGF is an important factor in accelerating tissue regeneration of injured organs including the kidney. Alteration of HGF in acute hepatitis can lead to ARF. Jung and his team in an analysis of 208 hepatitis A patients, found that fulminant patients were complicated with ARF. The mechanism of hepatitis A-associated ARF is uncertain, and several possible mechanisms have been considered. Activation of the renin–angiotensin system may induce prerenal failure in severe acute viral hepatitis A. Immune complex-mediated nephritis, and endotoxemia induced by acute hepatitis may cause renal injury which can proceed to ARF. Renal vasoconstriction, release of cytokines, and activation of neutrophils may all contribute to the development of renal injury from endotoxemia of acute viral hepatitis. Endotoxemia is often observed within 10 days of onset in patients with acute hepatitis A. The deposition of an immune complex containing hepatitis B surface antigen to glomeruli is the key pathological process of diffuse membranous glomerulonephritis which can lead to ARF. Deposition of immune complexes involving HCV and anti-HCV immunoglobulin G (IgG) is also important in HCV-related renal failure. Complications with ARF in acute viral hepatitis can have a negative impact on recovery.

Pancreatitis

Several viral infections have been implicated as an etiological factor of acute pancreatitis, which includes the hepatitis virus. Viral antigens have also been detected in pancreas tissues and gallbladder. Acute pancreatitis has been reported very rarely in acute viral hepatitis. It has been reported with HAV, HBV, and HEV infection. Most cases of acute pancreatitis due to hepatitis viruses had been reported in association with acute liver failure in the autopsy series of Ham and Fitzpatrick where 33% of patients with acute liver failure had acute pancreatitis. The mechanism of pancreatitis in patients with acute viral hepatitis (nonfulminant) is unknown, and it may be multifactorial. There is no direct evidence for the routes by which hepatitis viruses reach the pancreas, however, the proposed routes are most likely blood or bile. The hepatitis viruses might injure the pancreatic acinar cell membrane, resulting in the leakage of intracellular enzymes, and or precipitate a network of intracellular events culminating in cell death by a mechanism analogous to hepatocyte necrosis. A more plausible mechanism for viral-associated acute pancreatitis is direct inflammation and destruction of pancreatic acinar cells by the virus. Intrapancreatic hemorrhage due to hypoprothrombinemia may result in pancreatic damage and subsequent pancreatitis. Conservative treatment leads to recovery for all the patients.

Cholestasis

Prolonged cholestasis is one of the complications of acute viral hepatitis, particularly hepatitis A infection. Prolonged cholestasis is defined as increased total bilirubin >5 mg/dL for >4 weeks following diagnosis. Patients with acute hepatitis and cholestatic hepatitis experience intrahepatic cholestasis, persistent jaundice appetite loss, itching, dark-colored urine, and gray-colored feces. Cholestasis is caused by a variety of mechanisms, such as diminished bilirubin absorption, coagulation malfunction, bilirubin excretion dysfunction, and biliary blockage. Cholestasis occurs in hepatitis A due to an inflammatory process. The liver secretes endotoxin and proinflammatory cytokines, leading to a systemic reaction. Proper diagnosis and treatment of this manifestation are necessary because it can increase morbidity and health costs.

Cryoglobulinemia

There have not been many reported cases showing a relationship between hepatitis A and cryoglobulinemia. Cryoglobulinemia presents via continuous active stimulation to produce immunoglobulins and can result in vasculitis and other various cryoglobulinemia-related symptoms. Cryoglobulinemia has been reported as being present during the acute phase of hepatitis A and resolves as the liver disease regresses. Different intrinsic mechanisms of the virus have been proposed. One theory is that the host's immune system is unable to produce the necessary antibodies to neutralize the virus in which case the cryoglobulins are the result of interactions between the virus and the host.

Coagulopathy

The exact mechanism of coagulopathy in acute hepatocellular injury is a very complex subject. A significant alteration to the hemostatic system between procoagulant and anticoagulant pathways in acute liver failure results in a delicate balance that scales toward either thrombotic or bleeding complications. Acute hepatocellular injury by the hepatitis virus leads to a considerable reduction in coagulation factor levels, as reflected by the prolonged PT/INR values. Hepatocytes synthesize most coagulation factors including fibrinogen and factors II, V, VII, IX, X, XI, and XII which are altered by hepatitis viral antigen. In addition to the decreased levels of coagulant and anticoagulant factors, fibrinogen is affected qualitatively and quantitatively in acute hepatocellular injury. Platelet dysfunction is routinely observed in ALF. Thrombocytopenia in ALF results from impaired platelet production and thrombin-mediated platelet consumption, though the exact mechanism is not yet known. Initially, it was hypothesized that the decreased synthesis of thrombopoietin (TPO) was responsible for thrombocytopenia in ALF because TPO is produced by the liver. Overall, there is an overwhelming amount of evidence to suggest that the hemostasis in ALF is complex and rebalanced.

OTHER EXTRAHEPATIC MANIFESTATIONS

Acute viral hepatitis has long been reported to be associated with manifestations of extrahepatic tissue injury. The best documented extrahepatic syndromes associated with viral hepatitis are the serum sickness-like prodrome of acute viral hepatitis, the glomerulonephritis seen mainly in children, and some cases of systemic vasculitis accompanying hepatitis B. Other syndromes for which some evidence of association is available include myocarditis, and certain neurological disorders, including Guillain–Barré syndrome.

CONCLUSION

Acute hepatitis generally does not lead to any long-term concerns. Rarely, fulminant hepatitis develop. Acute liver failure is another complication that results in a build-up of fluid in the abdomen, bleeding disorders, kidney failure, increased blood pressure in the liver portal veins, and hepatic encephalopathy. If this happens patients will be hospitalized and monitored very carefully. A viral infection that is not well managed can lead to further damage to the liver and total failure.

SUGGESTED READINGS

1. Montrief T, Koyfman A, Long B. Acute liver failure: A review for emergency physicians. Am J Emerg Med. 2019;37(2):329-37.
2. Acharya SK, Panda SK, Saxena A, Gupta SD. Acute hepatic failure in India: a perspective from the East. J Gastroenterol Hepatol. 2000;15(5):473-9.
3. Shalimar, Acharya SK, Lee W. Worldwide differences in acute liver failure. Future Medicine; 2013. pp. 33-46.
4. Bernae W, Wenden J. Acute liver failure. N Eng J Med. 2013;369(26):2525-34.
5. Wasley A, Fiore A, Bell BP, Hepatitis A in the era of vaccination. Epidomiol Rev. 2006;28:101-21.
6. Taylor RM, Davern T, Han SH, McGuire B, Larson AM, et al. Fulminant hepatitis A virus infection in the United States: incidence, prognosis, and outcomes. Hepatology. 2006; 44(6):1589-97.
7. Brown GR, Persley K. Hepatitis A epidemic in the elderly. South Med J. 2002;95(8):826-33.
8. Razende G, Roque-Afonso AM, Samuel D, Gigou M, Nicand E, Ferre V, et al. Viral and Clinical factors associated with the fulminant course of hepatitis A infection. Hepatology. 2003;38(3):6130-8.
9. Vallbracht A, Gabriel P, Maier K, Hartmann F, Steinhardt HJ, Müller C, et al. Cell-mediated cytotoxicity in hepatitis A virus infection. Hepatology. 1986;6(6):1308-14.
10. Shukla NB, Poles MA. Hepatitis B virus infection: co-infection with hepatitis C virus, hepatitis D virus, and human immunodeficiency virus. Clin Liver Dis. 2004;8(2):441-60.

11. Cuthbert JA. Hepatitis A: old and new. Clin Microbiol Rev. 2001;14(1):38-58.
12. Wilkinson SP, Davies MH, Portmann B, Williams R. Renal failure in otherwise uncomplicated acute viral hepatitis. Br Med J. 1978;2(6133):338-41.
13. Ido A, Moriuchi A, Numata M, Murayama T, Teramukai S, Marusawa H, et al. Safety and pharmacokinetics of recombinant human hepatocyte growth factor (rh-HGF) in patients with fulminant hepatitis: a phase I/II clinical trial, following preclinical studies to ensure safety. J Transl Med. 2011;9:55.
14. Jung YJ, Kim W, Jeong JB, Kim BG, Lee KL, Oh KH, et al. Clinical features of acute renal failure associated with hepatitis A virus infection. J Viral Hepat. 2010;17(9):611-7.
15. Lin CC, Chang CH, Lee SH. Acute renal failure in non-fulminant hepatitis A. Nephrol Dial Transplant. 1996;11:2061-66.
16. Parenti DM, Steinberg W, Kang P. Infectious causes of acute pancreatitis. Pancreas. 1996;13(4):356-71.
17. Hoefs JC, Renner IG, Askhcavai M, Redeker AG. Hepatitis B surface antigen in pancreatic and biliary secretions. Gastroenterology. 1980;79(2):191-4.
18. Mishra A, Saigal S, Gupta R, Sarin SK. Acute pancreatitis associated with viral hepatitis: a report of six cases with review of literature. Am J Gastroenterol. 1999;94(8):2292-5.
19. Ham JM, Fitzpatrick P. Acute pancreatitis in patients with acute hepatic failure. Am J Dig Dis. 1973;18(12):1079-83.
20. Davis TV, Keefte EB. Acute pancreatitis associated with acute hepatitis A. Am J Gastroenterol. 1992;87(11):1648-50.
21. Lever AM. Mechanism of virally induced liver damage. J Hepatol. 1987;4(3):399-403.
22. Yoon EL, Yim HJ, Kim SY, Kim JH, Lee JH, Lee YS, et al. Clinical courses after administration of oral corticosteroids in patients with severely cholestatic acute hepatitis A; three cases. Korean J Hepatol. 2010;16(3):329-33.
23. Shali M, Wollner S, Levo Y. Cryoglobulinemia in acute type A hepatitis. Clin Exp Immunol. 1982;47(3):613-6.
24. Nassih H, Bourrahouat A, Sab IA. Hepatitis A virus infection associated with cryoglobulinemic vasculitis. Indian Pediatr. 2020;57(1):71-2.
25. Lisman T, Stravitz RT. Rebalanced hemostasis in patients with acute liver failure. Semin Thromb Hemost. 2015;41(5):468-73.
26. Pluta A, Gutkowski K, Hartleb M. Coagulopathy in liver diseases. Adv Med Sci. 2010;55(1):16-21.
27. Herrick S, Blanc-Brude O, Gray A, Laurent G. Fibrinogen. Int J Biochem Cell Biol. 1999;31(7):741-6.
28. Munoz SJ, Stravitz RT, Gabriel DA. Coagulopathy of acute liver failure. Clin Liver Dis. 2009;13(1):95-107.

116
CHAPTER

Advances in Management of Autoimmune Hepatitis

Manish Sharma, Nitin Sinha

ABSTRACT

Autoimmune hepatitis (AIH) is an uncommon, but significant chronic autoimmune disease. This condition occurs when body's immune system identifies liver as a threat and attacks it. Females are affected more than males with wide range of symptoms ultimately leading to fibrosis and cirrhosis. Timely diagnosis and intervention can lead to a favorable prognosis. This chapter provides a compact understanding of AIH. Recent advances and potential future aspects on management are also discussed in this chapter.

INTRODUCTION

As the reader finishes reading this chapter, he/she should become aware about:

- Etiology and pathophysiology of autoimmune hepatitis (AIH).
- Clinical manifestations of AIH.
- Diagnostic criteria and challenges associated with accurate diagnosis of AIH.
- Pharmacological and immunosuppressive treatment options for AIH, according to latest guidelines.
- Exploring ongoing research and future directions in the field of AIH, including emerging therapies and novel diagnostic methods.

ETIOLOGY AND PATHOPHYSIOLOGY OF AUTOIMMUNE HEPATITIS

The exact etiology of AIH is still unclear but it is believed to be a combination of genetic predisposition and environmental triggers. Certain human leukocyte antigen (*HLA*) gene variants along with some infections, medications, or exposure to certain toxins are the triggering factors.

Immune cells, primarily T cells, infiltrate the liver tissue causing inflammation and damage. B cells produce autoantibodies that target liver specific antigens. This ongoing immune-mediated liver damage leads to fibrosis and if left untreated, leads to cirrhosis.

CLINICAL PRESENTATION

Clinical spectrum of AIH is very wide.

- *Asymptomatic presentation:* More than half of the patients are asymptomatic. Disease may be first detected by abnormal liver enzymes on routine blood test done or done for some other cause.
- *Acute presentation:* Acute icteric hepatitis is the initial disease presentation in approximately one-third of cases. Generalized malaise, fatigue mild-to-moderate arthralgia, and abdominal discomfort are the common symptoms. Patient may have history of previous attacks of spontaneously recovering jaundice. Severe life-threatening acute presentations are more common in early age and are rare beyond 30 years of age. But acute icteric hepatitis as clinical presentation of AIH can occur in all age groups with similar frequency.
- *Chronic presentation:* Sign and symptoms such as fatigue, jaundice, abdominal pain, hepatomegaly, dark urine, and joint pain may develop gradually into chronic disease and are often associated with extrahepatic manifestations such as arthralgia, skin rash, palmer erythema, and leukonychia.

- *Cirrhosis:* AIH may manifest first time with decompensated cirrhosis. One-third of patient may have cirrhosis at the time of diagnosis. Few patients who were labelled as cryptogenic cirrhosis may turn out to be suffering from AIH in later life.
- *Hepatocellular carcinoma (HCC):* HCC development in AIH does exist and it is associated with cirrhosis but it is less common than HCC due to other causes of liver diseases.

INVESTIGATIONS

Diagnosis of autoimmune hepatitis involves combination of clinical, biochemical, serological, and histological criteria.

- *Clinical:* Detailed history pertaining to involvement of liver and extrahepatic manifestations along with physical examination pertaining to liver diseases is a must.
- *Laboratory testing:*
  - Liver function tests (LFTs)*:* Any degree of transaminases elevation can be observed (acute presentations >300 IU/mL, fulminant cases >1,000 IU/mL). Alkaline phosphatase (ALP) level is generally two times the upper normal limit. If ALP level is >5 times, consider other diseases also. Increased level of gamma-glutamyl transpeptidase (GGTP) is a good predictor for steroid responsiveness.
  - *Immunoglobulin levels:* Total proteins are increased; globulins are increased but albumin decreases. A:G ratio reversal is seen. Elevated immunoglobulin G (IgG) level (>90% of cases) showing polyclonal gamma globulinemia is observed.
  - *Autoantibodies:* Autoantibodies are a characteristic hallmark of AIH and can be found in almost all patients. Detailed information on antibodies is available in **Table 1**.

TABLE 1: Detailed information on antibodies found in autoimmune hepatitis (AIH).

Autoantibody	Role in AIH
ANA (antinuclear antibody)	• Reflects on immunofluorescence testing as fine speckled or homogenous pattern • Fine speckled pattern is more common • Higher are the titers more will be then specificity • ELISA testing has much false positive levels • Present in 80% of patients with AIH
Anti-SMA (smooth muscle antibody)	• Target antigen (F and G-actin) • High titers are more specific (mildly raised titers can be seen in normal individuals) • Positivity for both ANA and anti-SMA is highly suggestive of AIH in context of raised transaminases
Anti-SLA (soluble liver antigen)	• Target antigen—SEPSECS • Highly specific for diagnosis of AIH, but less sensitive • Related with more severe disease and severe relapse on drug withdrawal • Elisa estimation is necessary (if not required)
Anti-LKM-1 (liver kidney microsome antibody)	• Target antigen—(a cytochrome P450 isoenzyme, CYP2D6) • LKM-1 antibodies in absence of hepatitis C are highly suggestive of type 2 AIH • Mainly present in children
Anti-LC-1 (liver cytosol type 1)	• Target antigen—(formiminotransferase cyclodeaminase) • Similar pattern as anti-LKM-1 antibodies • Specific for type 2 AIH (less sensitive) • It has a bad prognosis if drug withdrawal is there
Atypical p-ANCA (perinuclear anti-neutrophil cytoplasmic antibody)	• Perinuclear staining pattern detected in up to one-third of patients with AIH • Present in 50–92% patients of AIH • Associated with PSC and UC
Anti-actin antibodies	Marker of severe disease

■ Noninvasive Fibrosis Assessment

- *By serum biomarkers:* Fibro test, serum aspartate aminotransferase (AST)/platelet ratio index (APRI), the fibrosis-4 (FIB-4) index, and the enhanced liver fibrosis test are the ones that can be used.
- *By measurement of liver stiffness:* **Table 2** shows various methods to assess liver stiffness.

■ Liver Biopsy

Liver biopsy is often necessary to confirm the diagnosis and assess degree of liver damage. Liver biopsy can also be used to assess the response to treatment if liver enzymes continue to remain elevated but IgG level becomes normal and vice versa.

Typical features of AIH on liver biopsy are:

- Interface hepatitis at portal parenchymal interface is the hallmark of AIH.
- Emperipolesis—active penetration by lymphocytes into hepatocytes.

symptoms such as fatigue, jaundice, abdominal pain or discomfort, and loss of appetite. Azathioprine-mediated hepatotoxicity will have only increase in AST/ALT levels. IgG levels remain same. Relapse requires a prompt identification and reinstitution of original treatment and then subsequent transition to a long-term maintenance regimen.

NOVEL TREATMENT APPROACHES

Patient not sufficiently responding to standard therapy needs alternative immunosuppressive therapy.

- *Mycophenolate mofetil:* Purine antagonist, teratogenic, and contraindicated in pregnancy.
- *6-mercaptopurine:* Used in azathioprine intolerance. Not used in case of azathioprine related injury/ pancreatitis.
- *Calcineurin inhibitors:* Cyclosporine (2–5 mg/kg) and tacrolimus (0.5–1 mg daily). Advantages of using these as first-line therapy are uncertain and hence, their use as a first-line agent has not been endorsed.
- *Anti-TNF monoclonal antibodies:* Infliximab showed encouraging results, was able to induce a stable remission along with improvement in liver histology including fibrosis regression.
- *Anti-CD20:* Rituximab (less role).

SPECIAL SITUATIONS

- *Autoimmune hepatitis in pregnancy:* Pregnancy is an immune-tolerant state. Disease activity is usually milder during pregnancy. Azathioprine taking patients should continue it in pregnancy. Steroids should be tapered down to 20 mg/day. Acute flare is more common after delivery and after cessation of breast feeding as there is immune reconstitution in both cases. So steroid dose should be increased by 10 mg/ day in these cases.
- *Autoimmune hepatitis with overlapping primary sclerosing cholangitis:* This condition received the term autoimmune sclerosing cholangitis. This condition required ursodeoxycholic acid (UDCA)—15 mg/ day along with immunosuppression. These patients require liver transplant after 20–25 years despite adequate immunosuppression.
- *Autoimmune hepatitis with overlapping biliary cholangitis:* Two approaches—
  i. Start UDCA treatment and assess biochemical response after 3–6 months then add immunosuppression to the nonresponders.
  ii. Use histological scoring: Hepatitis activity index
     - If HAI score—≥ 6—give immunosuppression to all patients.
     - If HAI score—4–5—use UDCA monotherapy trial if not responding then add immunosuppression.

LIVER TRANSPLANTATION

Indications for liver transplantation in AIH are:

- No response to steroid therapy
- Acute liver failure
- MELD score > 16

Recurrence rate is around 10% in 1 year and 50% in 5 years following transplantation.

LEARNING POINTS

- Autoimmune hepatitis is a liver disease which can be asymptomatic. Sometimes, elevated transaminases is the only finding.
- Clinical, laboratory and serological and histological investigations are helpful in making the diagnosis.
- Treatment is with corticosteroids and immunosuppressives. Treatment has to be individualized.
- Novel treatment options are being explored.

SUGGESTED READINGS

1. Boyer TD, Lindor KD. Zakim and Boyer's Hepatology: A textbook of liver disease. In: Sanyal AJ, Terrault NA (Eds). 7th edition. Philadelphia, PA: Elsevier-Health Sciences Division; 2021.
2. Mack CL, Adams D, Assis DN, Kerkar N, Manns MP, Mayo MJ, et al. Diagnosis and management of autoimmune hepatitis in adults and children: 2019 practice guidance and guidelines from the American association for the study of liver diseases. Hepatology. 2020;72(2):671-722.
3. Wang G, Tanaka A, Zhao H, Jia J, Ma X, Harada K, et al. The Asian Pacific Association for the Study of the Liver clinical practice guidance: the diagnosis and management of patients with autoimmune hepatitis. Hepatol Int. 2021;15(2):223-57.
4. European Association for the Study of the Liver. EASL Clinical Practice Guidelines: Autoimmune hepatitis. J Hepatol. 2015; 63(4):971-1004.

117

CHAPTER

Management of Hepatitis B from Conception to Labor

Deepti Sharma, Garv Gupta

ABSTRACT

Hepatitis B virus (HBV) infection management is a challenge for both mother and fetus during pregnancy. Global efforts to reduce the burden of chronic HBV are centered on reducing mother-to-child transmission. Acute HBV infection during pregnancy is usually not severe. Treatment of acute infection is mainly conservative. In chronic hepatitis patients, hepatic flares can be seen and are associated with various maternal and fetal complications which include gestational hypertension (HTN), postpartum hemorrhage (PPH), prematurity, and intrauterine growth restriction (IUGR). Antiviral therapy is indicated in chronic hepatitis patients depending on hepatitis B e-antigen (HBeAg), HBV deoxyribonucleic acid (DNA) titers, alanine aminotransferase (ALT) levels, and presence or absence of cirrhosis. Tenofovir disoproxil fumarate (TDF) is antiviral of choice. Breastfeeding can be done safely once neonate has received first dose of hepatitis B vaccine and hepatitis B immune globulin (HBIG).

Mother-to-child transmission has been reported as high as 90% without adequate vaccination. HBV DNA level should be monitored at 26–28 weeks' gestation and antiviral therapy should be started at 28 weeks in those with HBV DNA levels $> 2 \times 10^5$ IU/mL. Prevention can be done by administering passive and active immunization by hepatitis B vaccine and HBIG within 12 hours of delivery and giving antiviral therapy to women with high viral load.

INTRODUCTION

Hepatitis B virus (HBV) infection management is a challenge for both mother and fetus during pregnancy. HBV has effects on both maternal and child health.

Global efforts to reduce the burden of chronic HBV are centered on reducing mother-to-child transmission, as vertical transmission is responsible for approximately one-half of chronic infections worldwide.

Transmission has been productively reduced by maternal screening programs and vaccination **(Fig. 1)**.

ACUTE HEPATITIS B VIRUS INFECTION

The most common cause of jaundice in antepartum females is hepatitis B.

Acute HBV infection during pregnancy is usually not severe and is not associated with teratogenicity. Thus, termination of pregnancy is not done. However, the incidence of low birth weight and prematurity has been seen.

The perinatal transmission rate is 10% in acute HBV occurring in early pregnancy which increases as high as 60% in infection occurring at or near delivery.

Treatment of acute infection is mainly conservative. Antiviral therapy may be used in cases of acute liver failure or protracted severe hepatitis.

Tenofovir disoproxil fumarate (TDF) (300 mg daily) or lamivudine (100 mg daily) is safe in pregnancy, and the risk of resistance is low because of short duration of treatment. However, TDF is preferred as there is less risk of resistance.

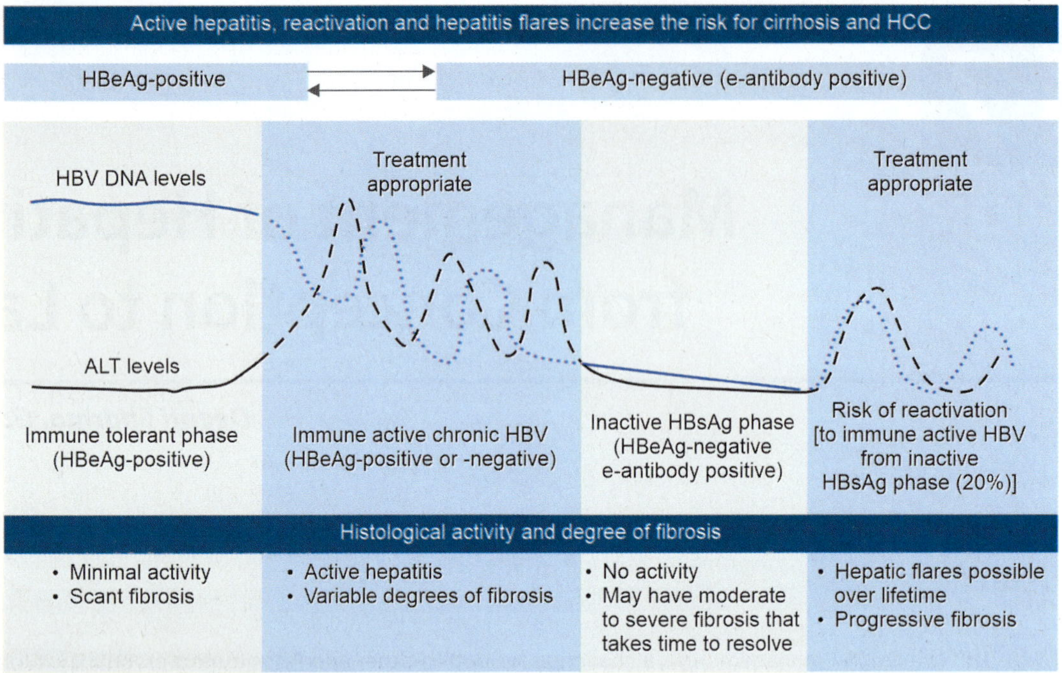

FIG. 1: Natural history of chronic HBV infection.
(ALT: alanine aminotransferase; DNA: deoxyribonucleic acid; HBV: hepatitis B virus; HCC: hepatocellular carcinoma)

CHRONIC HEPATITIS B VIRUS INFECTION

Natural Course of Chronic HBV in Pregnancy

Pregnancy is usually not affected in females with chronic HBV infection who do not have advanced liver disease. However, the following clinical manifestations may be expected due to the immune-tolerant state and high level of corticosteroids:

- *Hepatic flares*: Serious clinical sequelae in flare are usually not seen. A flare of HBV infection is typically defined as a greater than two- to three-fold rise in the alanine aminotransferase (ALT) that is at least three to five times above the reference range. Flares appear to be more common in women who are hepatitis B e-antigen (HBeAg)-positive although predictors of HBV flares during pregnancy have not been confirmed. However, it can be difficult to assess the progression of liver disease during pregnancy because of normal physiologic changes that can mimic clinical features of chronic liver disease. To be precise, alpha-fetoprotein and ALP levels are on a higher side while hematocrit and serum albumin levels are on the lower side. Similarly, spider angiomata, palmar erythema, and lower limb edema may be normally seen in pregnancy.
- *HBV deoxyribonucleic acid (DNA)*: Most studies have found that HBV DNA levels remain steady during pregnancy. However, immunologic changes associated with pregnancy also have the potential to increase HBV viremia.

Effect of Chronic HBV on Pregnancy Outcomes

Cirrhosis is a significant risk factor of maternal and fetal complication **(Box 1)**.

BOX 1: Effect of chronic hepatitis B virus on pregnancy outcomes.

Maternal complications:
- Gestational hypertension
- Placenta abruptio
- PPH
- Hepatic decompensation (15% in cirrhosis)

Fetal complications:
- IUGR
- Prematurity
- Increased mortality (2.1% vs. 5.2%)

(IUGR: intrauterine growth restriction; PPH: postpartum hemorrhage)

TABLE 1: Indications for antiviral therapy.

HBeAg-positive	HBeAg-negative
HBV DNA > 20,000 IU/mL and ALT > 2 times	HBV DNA ≥ 2,000 IU/mL and ALT > 2 times

(ALT: alanine aminotransferase; HBeAg: hepatitis B e-antigen; HBV: hepatitis B virus)

MANAGEMENT

Who are Pregnant?

Patients who become pregnant while receiving antiviral therapy—monitoring should be done to ensure viral suppression. Antivirals may be discontinued in women without cirrhosis if the patient has achieved therapeutic levels.

Indications for antiviral therapy: Initiation of therapy depends upon the occurrence of cirrhosis, HBeAg and hepatitis B e antibody (anti-HBe), HBV DNA titers, and aspartate transaminase (AST) levels.

The indications for therapy in pregnant women and nonpregnant are generally similar **(Table 1)**.

However, for those without cirrhosis, some scenarios may differ. For example:

- During pregnancy, antiviral therapy may be deferred until after delivery if there is only evidence of mild disease activity, such as aminotransferase levels just above the treatment threshold.
- On contrary, therapy should be initiated in the third trimester if a viral load > 2×10^5 IU/mL is seen even if the aminotransferase levels are normal. In this case, the target is to prevent transmission to the child.
- In pregnancy, TDF is the preferred antiviral agent.

Monitoring

- Liver function test (LFT) should be ordered every 3 months during pregnancy and for up to 6 months postpartum. Thereafter, monitoring should be done every 6 months for HBeAg-positive patients in the immune-tolerant phase and every 6–12 months for those who are confirmed to be the inactive carrier which is the same as other hepatitis B patients.
- HBV DNA can be tested simultaneously or when there is ALT elevation. The HBV DNA should be measured at 26–28 weeks to determine if antiviral therapy should be offered.

Patients with cirrhosis: Variceal screening with endoscopy and management of cirrhosis is the same as nonpregnant women, but the use of beta-blockers is associated with a small increase of IUGR, neonatal bradycardia, hypoglycemia, and respiratory distress.

Octreotide can cause uterine ischemia; therefore, it should not be used during management of acute variceal bleeding.

Patients with childbearing potential: There are important considerations in women of child-bearing potential:

- Antivirals may be deferred in mild liver disease and close monitoring should be done until completion of pregnancy.
- Pegylated interferon (because of finite duration—48 weeks) may be preferred by those patients who prefer to complete treatment before pregnancy while ensuring contraception use during treatment. However, if the patient chooses treatment with a nucleos(t)ide analog, TDF is preferred because it has been shown to be safe in pregnancy, and the risk of drug resistance is low.

Breastfeeding

- Complete vaccination with HBV is recommended. Infants receiving hepatitis B immune globulin (HBIG) and the first dose of HBV at birth can be breastfed. Precautions should be taken to avoid bleeding from cracked nipples. HBsAg-positive mothers should not participate in donating breast milk.
- The safety data on the use of HBV antiviral therapy during breastfeeding is ambiguous. The decision to breastfeeding should be based upon patient preference.
- Drug labels recommend that nucleos(t)ide analogs be avoided during breastfeeding. TDF is present in very low levels in breastmilk; hence, chances of adverse effects in infants are slim.

MOTHER-TO-CHILD TRANSMISSION

Mother-to-child transmission accounts for most of the burden of chronic HBV.

The World Health Assembly adopted the Global Health Sector Strategy (GHSS) on viral hepatitis in 2016, aiming elimination of viral hepatitis B and C by 2030.

Risk of transmission: There is a 90% risk of mother-to-child transmission in the absence of active and passive immunization. Transmission can occur intrauterine, partum, or postpartum.

Risk Factors for Transmission

Positive HBeAg and/or a high HBV DNA level $>2 \times 10^5$ IU/mL or 10^6 copies are most important risk factors for mother-to-child transmission, despite proper administration of prophylaxis.

Obstetrical procedures are less likely to cause vertical transmission. In addition, the benefit of cesarean delivery has not shown clear benefits in vertical transmission protection. Thus, HBV status has no role in deciding an obstetrical approach.

Transplacental Transmission

The villous capillary endothelial cells and the trophoblasts of the placenta harbor HBV. Therefore, HBV transmission may occur in preterm labor and spontaneous abortion.

Prevention of Mother-to-child Transmission

Preventing mother-to-child transmission involves screening pregnant women, providing antiviral therapy to women with high HBV DNA levels, and administering passive active immunization to newborns of mothers who are HBsAg positive.

Maternal screening: Testing should be performed regardless of vaccination status and history of prior testing. At the first prenatal visit, all should undergo HBV screening.

HBsAg, anti-HBc, and anti-HBs screening is done for primigravida. For subsequent pregnancies, HBsAg alone is sufficient.

- Vaccination of patients without evidence of prior HBV infection or exposure (negative for anti-HBs and anti-HBc) should be done. High-risk patients [e.g., history of sexually transmitted disease (STD), IV drug use, sexual or household contact with chronic HBV, multiple sexual partners in the last 6 months] should have HBsAg repeated late in pregnancy (approximately 28 weeks).
- For those who have evidence of prior infection (HBsAg-negative, anti-HBc-positive, anti-HBs-positive) or immunity due to vaccination (HBsAg-negative, anti-HBc-negative, anti-HBs-positive), no further intervention is needed.
- However, a booster dose of vaccine maybe given to anti-HBc positive patients to see if anti-HBs titers can increase to >10 million IU/mL, although the clinical importance of this is unclear.

Maternal Antiviral Therapy to Prevent Transmission

- *General approach*: The HBV DNA level should be monitored at 26–28 weeks' gestation and recommend antiviral therapy at 28 weeks in those with HBV DNA levels $> 2 \times 10^5$ IU/mL or $>10^6$ copies/mL.
- *Drug of choice*: TDF is preferred. A newer formulation of tenofovir, tenofovir alafenamide (TAF), is available which is associated with decreased bone and kidney toxicity, but TAF has not been routinely recommended due to lack of safety data. However, other agents are not preferred due to higher rates of antiviral resistance. Lamivudine may be a reasonable alternative.
- *Duration of antiviral therapy*: Women who start antiviral therapy during pregnancy for the sole purpose of preventing mother-to-child transmission may stop antiviral therapy immediately after delivery, especially if they want to breastfeed.

Newborn Active–passive Immunization

One dose of HBIG (200 IU IM) within 12 hours of delivery and the first dose of hepatitis B vaccine should be administered at different sites. Infants should then complete the HBV series.

Other potential adverse events of antivirals: A number of adverse events of nucleos(t)ide analogs have been described, including mitochondrial damage, lactic acidosis, acute fatty liver, and possibly bone abnormalities.

Patients Who are HBsAg Positive Males

Partners of hepatitis B positive males should be advised to get all three doses of hepatitis B vaccine (0, 1, 6 months) before planning to conceive to prevent horizontal as well as vertical transmission.

Studies have also shown that hepatitis B is associated with poor sperm quality **(Flowchart 1)**.

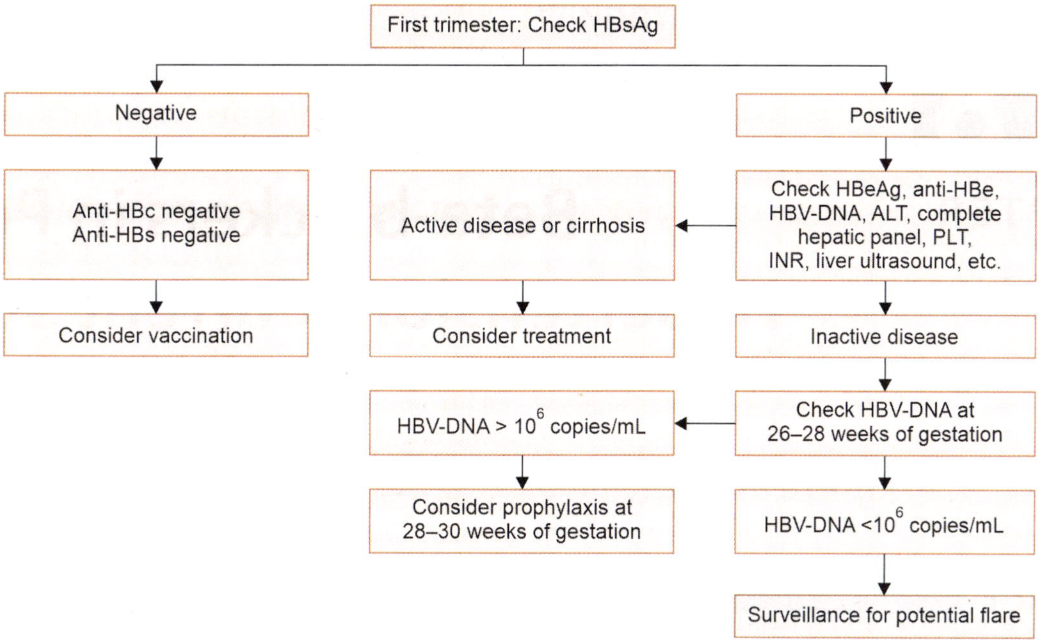

FLOWCHART 1: Algorithm for management of hepatitis B virus infection during pregnancy.

(ALT: alanine aminotransferase; anti-HBc: anti-hepatitis B core antigen; anti-HBe: antibody to hepatitis B e antigen; anti-HBs: antibodies to hepatitis B surface antigen; HBV: hepatitis B virus; INR: international normalized ratio; PLT: platelet count)

SUGGESTED READINGS

1. World Health Organization. Global health sector strategy on viral hepatitis, 2016–2021: towards ending viral hepatitis. Geneva: World Health Organization; 2016.
2. Conners EE, Panagiotakopoulos L, Hofmeister MG, Spradling PR, Hagan LM, Aaron M Harris, et al. Screening and Testing for Hepatitis B Virus Infection: CDC Recommendations—United States, 2023. MMWR Recomm Rep. 2023;72:1-25.

Acetaldehyde is a direct hepatotoxin and also a carcinogen. HCC can occur by its effects on altered immune function, hepatocyte DNA damage, oxidant injuries, and altered gene expression (*ALDH1C*1 and ALDH2*2*). The definition of AH is sudden rise of bilirubin due to recent heavy alcohol intake with raised transaminases (<500 IU) with or without ascites and hepatic encephalopathy. Many (up to 80%) heavy drinkers do not develop AH because of genetic and environmental factors and is an area of interest. Further, screening >45-year-old healthy population in France has found that 7.5% had increased LS and 36% of them had an ALD. The National Institute of Alcohol Abuse and Alcoholism (NIAAA) Consortium Criteria are:

- Appearance of jaundice in preceding 8 weeks
- Active ongoing drinking, (Males 60 g/day, Females 40 g/day or more)
- Less than 2 months of abstinence
- AST > 50 IU, AST/ALT of 1.5, but not >400 IU
- Serum bilirubin > 3 mg/dL
- Confirmatory histology by liver biopsy (Definite AH and excludes other etiologies)

Although liver biopsy is indicated, due to obvious reasons clinicobiochemical criteria are sufficient, provided other etiologies are ruled out. The various characteristics of AH are shown in **Table 1**. In diagnosing AH and ALD, staging by liver ultrasound is recommended. Recent imaging modalities such as magnetic resonance imaging (MRI) spectroscopy and Controlled Attenuation Parameter (CAP) have been shown to be very accurate to detect steatosis. Early detection of steatosis is important; within 5 years, it usually progresses to cirrhosis in heavy drinkers (>60 g alcohol/day). Liver stiffness (LS) measurement by Fibroscan [Transient Elastography (TE)] is reliable to detect fibrosis (F3 or F4 Metavir stage) and a cut-off point of 12.5 kPa usually correlates well with histological stages. LS has been shown to correlate with bilirubin and aspartate aminotransferase (AST) levels in asymptomatic or non-severe AH. Other biological noninvasive serum markers like ELF (Enhanced Liver Fibrosis panel), Fibrotest, APRI (AST to platelet ratio) are also efficient to pick up significant hepatic derangements.

The treatment goals in ALD are:

- Reducing hazardous drinking (females > 35 unit/week, males > 50 unit/week)
- Abstinence and prevent relapse
- Assessment of extent of liver disease by noninvasive bio markers by TE and biochemical tests, especially in primary care and community setting

Prednisolone is the cornerstone of therapy although not optimal or universally effective. Nutrition and control of infections/sepsis if present need intervention. On 0 and 7th day Lille model score determines the response to steroid. However, there are individual variations in steroid responsiveness. *Complete responders (91% survival at 28 day) Lille score being < 0.16, Partial responders (79% survival) with score 0.16–0.56 and Nonresponders (53% survival) with score > 0.56.* In nonresponders, liver transplant (LT) is indicated while in partial responders add-on therapy by NAC infusion or Metadoxine is started along with correction of malnutrition and antibiotics in bacterial/fungal infections if any. In steroid intolerance/contraindications (ongoing variceal bleed, active/uncontrolled infection/septicemia, multiple organ failure, AKI, uncontrolled diabetes and Maddrey's score >90) very few treatment options are available other than salvage LT. In chronic liver disease, *(compensated cirrhosis)* binge drinking (> 5 standard units of alcohol within 2 hours) can precipitate ACLF (acute-on-chronic liver failure). This has a poor prognosis since the impaired gut permeability, endotoxemia, and systemic inflammatory response syndrome (SIRS) occur frequently and rapid deterioration is common. Whether severe AH with ACLF warrants corticosteroids is controversial, especially with ACLF-3. They are candidates for rescue LT.

NEWER THERAPEUTIC OPTIONS

Modulation of gut microbiome is presently being investigated as a therapeutic option in severe AH. Acetaldehyde acts as a direct hepatotoxin and also damages the intestine (GUT-LIVER-AXIS). Healthy gut flora is important for maintaining gut barrier integrity, maturation of host immunity, synthesis of B vitamins, and neurological and intestinal functions. This concept is being increasingly focused upon all emerging targets in pathogenesis of AH. AUD with dysbiosis results in immune suppression, steatohepatitis, and altered bacterial metabolites. Translocation of bacterial products can also stimulate Kupffer cells, Stellate cells, and hepatocyte injury leading to inflammation and hepatic fibrosis. Alcohol and acetaldehyde possibly alter the intestinal barrier integrity which facilitates translocation of dysbiotic microbiomes. Ethanol also interferes with fatty acid production by microbes, which are needed to counter increased gut permeability. Gut flora changes with progressive hepatic damage and good bacteria (e.g., *Lactobacilli, Bacteroides*) are decreased, while bad bacteria (e.g., *Enterobacteria, Fusobacteria, Bifidobacteria*) increase. The net result is damaging intestinal permeability, sepsis, and neuropsychiatric derangement. Modulation of gut bacteria has become an exciting avenue because the microbes play an important role in genesis of AH. The different interventions for the same are shown in **Table 2**. Net effects are reduced inflammation, improvement of

TABLE 2: Future management modalities in AH (mostly experimental).

Effects on lipid pathways	Factors responsible	Possible targets for Intervention	Possible beneficial effects on liver	Target chemokines and cytokines	Gut microbiota modulation
Dysregulated fatty acid uptake and efflux in liver	Fatty acid transports like CD36/FA translocase and upregulation of *SLC27A1* gene	• Recombinant adiponectin, • Downregulation of CD36/FAT by genetic ablation	Reduced steatosis	IL- 1β block leads to reduced hepatic inflammation	High-fiber plant-based diet instead of animal meat and fatty diet
	Proinflammatory lipin 1β protein	Replaced by Lipin α anti-inflammatory	Reduced inflam-mation reduced cytokines	• IL-22 • Administration of recombinant IL-22 can be useful in severe AH	Pro-, Pre- and Synbiotics
	TNF-α, IL1, IL6	Pro-inflammatory	Reduced inflammation	CXCL1 block reduces inflammation	Selective gut decontamination by antibiotics by Promamycin, Quinolones and Rifaximin for short period to avoid resistance development
	High PPAR-γ	By PPAR-γ agonists	Reduced steatosis		FMT (fecal microbial transplantation) by producing Bacteriocins produced by good bacteria. Maybe useful in AH which is noneligible steroid therapy
	Low-protein kinase AMPK	Upregulation of this anti-lipogenic protein	Reduced steatosis		Bioengineering of bacteria to produce anti-inflammatory IL-22
	High heat shock protein (Hsp90)	Inhibition of Hsp90 by medication	Reduced steatosis		
	Low Adiponectin	Elevation of hepatic adiponectin receptors	Reduced steatosis		

(AH: alcoholic hepatitis; AMPK: adenosine monophosphate-activated protein kinase; CXCL1: chemokine (C-X-C motif) ligand 1; IL: interleukins; PPAR-γ: peroxisome proliferator-activated receptor-gamma; TNF-α: tumor necrosis factor alpha) gut barrier function, local production of antimicrobial agents, improving immune system and improvement in hepatic encephalopathy. Hepatic injury has been shown to regress after prebiotic (*Bacteroides)* therapy. Fecal microbiota transplantation (FMT) is an evolving therapy to improve survival in AH and showing encouraging results. It can also help as a bridging therapy before LT. It may improve encephalopathy, lower infections, control portal hypertension and its complications. Research is also going on in *bioengineering bacteria* (*E. coli, Lactobacillus reuteri*) to produce antioxidants or anti-inflammatory cytokines such as IL-22 to counter acetaldehyde-mediated intestinal barrier dysfunction or inflammation are showing encouraging results.

Targeted experimental therapies are in evolution and most of them are either experimental or very small RCTs. They have been examined as adjuvants to steroid therapy in AH.

- LPS stimulates TLR4 receptor to trigger inflammation. Purified hyperimmune bovine colostrums can neutralize LPS by secreting IgG anti-TLR antibodies
- Correction of zinc deficiency (to improve intrahepatic function)
- Anakinra acts against IL-1 (proinflammatory cytokine)
- Obeticholic acid (FXR or Farnesoid X receptor agonist) shown to have anti-inflammatory and antioxidant effects in AH by controlling bile acid and lipid metabolism.
- Emricasan (Caspase inhibitor), Selonsertib (oral agent to inhibit Apoptosis signal regulating kinase or ASK)
- Recombinant fusion protein IL-22 to increase liver regeneration
- Recruiting CD34 positive hematopoietic stem cell by granulocyte colony-stimulating factor (G-CSF) for enhancing anti-inflammatory activity and hepatocyte regeneration
- Antioxidant action N-acetyl cysteine infusion and Metadoxine. New antioxidant, mitoquinone, has a mitochondrial specificity and can be effective in near future.

Alcohol-related harms are dose related and abstinence is important and should be addressed by a team of Psychologist, Physicians, Psychiatrists, and trained nurses. Raising public awareness, screening to identify high-risk group of alcoholics, and political efforts (pricing and availability of alcohol, regulating advertising by manufacturers) are measures which need to be taken up in our country. Anticraving drugs such as Naltrexone, Disulfiram, Baclofen, Acamprosate or Nalmefene can be used with psychiatry consultation for at least 6 months to prevent relapse. Community-level screening for ALD has been initiated in some European countries.

CONCLUSION

Presently, AH is a significant global health concern. Available therapy of AH is not uniformly effective and future efforts will concentrate on possibly personalized medicine by genetic markers to improve early diagnosis and prognostication in AH since the long-term survival is unknown. Intervention in Gut–Liver axis leading to immune-modulation is going on. Holistically, it needs to be addressed by the government regulatory liquor policies and a multidisciplinary team. Future research is needed in AH to define and implement not only therapeutic measures, but also primary prevention formulated carefully by competent authorities in association with clinicians and researches and NGOs. More clinical trials of newer treatment options as well as research in genomic studies in AH are required in future.

SUGGESTED READINGS

1. Hydes T, Gilmore W, Sheron N. Treating alcohol-related liver disease from a public health perspective. J Hepatol. 2019;70: 223-36.
2. World Health Organization. (2018). Global status report on alcohol and health. [online] Available from https://iris.who.int/bitstream/handle/10665/274603/9789241565639-eng.pdf?sequence=1. [Last accessed December, 2023].
3. Li W, Amet T, Xing Y, Liangpunsakul S, Puri P, Kamath PS, et al. Alcohol abstinence ameliorates the dysregulated immune profiles in patients with alcoholic hepatitis: a prospective observational study. Hepatology. 2017;66:575-90.

120 CHAPTER

Vascular Thrombosis in Liver Abscess

Monica Gupta, Sarabmeet Singh Lehl

ABSTRACT

Liver abscesses are accompanied by numerous local complications like pleural effusion and rupture into the pleural, peritoneal, or pericardial cavities. Rarely, regional thrombosis of vessels may be recognized. Evidence from the current literature indicates that the thrombosis of the portal and hepatic veins may present in the form of asymptomatic incidental findings or as life-threatening pulmonary thromboembolism. These vascular complications are presumed to be caused by factors like localized inflammation, mechanical compression, and complement-coagulation system activation. Vascular complications have not been specifically studied, and there is a scant literature available on this important facet.

INTRODUCTION

The liver is unique by virtue of its twin perfusion from the portal vein (~75%) and the hepatic artery (~25%). It acts as an important buffer between the portal and systemic circulation. A liver abscess is a collection of pyogenic material with the destruction of liver parenchyma. The most common etiology is an amebic liver abscess (ALA), but it includes other protozoan as well as bacterial, fungal, or mixed infection. Suppuration of the liver generally occurs through biliary tree, hepatic artery, and portal vein. About two-thirds of abscesses in developing countries are ALA while three-fourths of cases in developed countries are pyogenic liver abscesses (PLA). Around 60% of abscesses are solitary with a predilection for the right lobe. This is due to the streaming of portal and superior mesenteric vein blood to the right lobe, and also given that the right lobe has a larger hepatic volume. Risk factors for liver abscess constitute male gender, diabetes mellitus, alcoholism, immunosuppressive conditions, and travel to specific endemic areas.

VASCULAR COMPLICATIONS

Complications described in the literature are systemic inflammation response syndrome, septic shock, acute kidney injury, encephalopathy, acute respiratory distress syndrome, and distant dissemination of infection. Distant spread of disease is reported to the brain, meninges, and lungs. Septic shock is a significant factor contributing to 27% of deaths in ruptured liver abscesses. Local complications include pleural effusion and rupture of abscess into body cavities leading to empyema, pyopericardium, and peritonitis. Complications such as portal and hepatic vein thrombosis or inferior vena cava (IVC) compression or thrombosis often go unnoticed since they are neither suspected nor have any apparent clinical manifestations.

CLINICAL FEATURES

Classical clinical features of a liver abscess include fever and upper-right quadrant abdominal pain. Few patients with ALA have a simultaneous or recent history of diarrhea. Jaundice is predominantly seen in PLA patients. Other less frequent symptoms include nausea, fatigue, and loss of weight and appetite. Clinical examination of the patient may include tender hepatomegaly, intercostal tenderness, tachypnea, shock, decreased air entry in the right side of the chest, pedal edema, and ascites. Patients with pylephlebitis or vascular thrombosis may have

121

CHAPTER

Hepatopulmonary Syndrome: An Overview

Balbir Singh Kohli

ABSTRACT

Hepatopulmonary syndrome (HPS) is a pulmonary vascular complication of advanced liver disease characterized by dilated pulmonary vasculature and shunts, leading to hypoxemia in the presence of advanced liver disease with or without portal hypertension. A complex interaction between lung, gut, and liver is responsible for the pulmonary alteration seen in HPS. Medical therapy has not been proven to be effective. Liver transplant is the only therapeutic option that drastically improves mortality of patients with HPS.

INTRODUCTION

Hepatopulmonary syndrome (HPS) is a progressive disease seen in patients with liver cirrhosis, leading to portal hypertension, thereby causing dysfunction of pulmonary vasculature. The alteration in pulmonary vasculature includes microvascular dilatation leading to hyperdynamic circulation, causing HPS or less common fibro-obliteration of the vascular bed, thereby vasoconstriction causing portopulmonary hypertension (POPH). HPS is associated with worsened prognosis, and patients often benefit from a liver transplant. HPS was coined by Kennedy and Knudson in 1977 after performing multiple autopsies that showed pulmonary vasculature dilatation in cirrhotic patients without any obvious lung parenchymal disease.

DEFINITION

Hepatopulmonary syndrome is a clinical disorder characterized by hypoxemia due to dilated pulmonary vasculature in the presence of advanced liver disease with or without portal hypertension.

DIAGNOSTIC CRITERIA FOR HEPATOPULMONARY SYNDROME

- Liver disease and/or portal hypertension
- Partial pressure of oxygen (PaO_2) < 80 mm Hg or alveolar-arterial oxygen gradient (A-a O_2) ≥ 15 mm Hg (or > 20 mm Hg in case of ≥65 years of age) while breathing in room air
- Intrapulmonary vascular dilatation (IPVD) confirmed by positive contrast-enhanced echocardiography or radioactive lung perfusion, showing a brain shunt fraction > 6%

INCIDENCE/PREVALENCE

Hepatopulmonary syndrome is most commonly seen in 4–35% of patients with cirrhotic portal hypertensive with severe hepatic dysfunction. It is more common in whites compared to blacks or Hispanics. It is also equally seen in both genders in the middle-aged group, less commonly in smokers, and rarely in children. HPS is also seen rarely in patients with noncirrhotic portal hypertension, Budd-Chiari syndrome, fulminant hepatitis A, and ischemic hepatitis.

PATHOPHYSIOLOGY

The pathophysiology underlying HPS is under intense investigation. The hypoxemia associated with HPS has been attributed to widespread pulmonary vascular dilatation due to an imbalance between vasodilators and vasoconstrictors, leading to ventilation-perfusion (V/Q) mismatch, diffusion limitation, and arteriovenous (AV) shunting, creating an increased A-a gradient.

- V/Q mismatch results from overperfusion of the alveolar capillary bed while ventilation remains unchanged.
- Diffusion limitation occurs due to the increased diameter of pulmonary microvessels (15–500 mm) compared to normal (8–15 mm), which increases the distance oxygen must travel from the alveolus to equilibrate with hemoglobin in red cells in alveolar capillaries. This creates a functional diffusion barrier to oxygen exchange that is further exacerbated by hyperdynamic circulation, causing rapid blood transit and a large amount of blood passing through pulmonary vasculature without undergoing gas exchange. Supplemental oxygen raises partial pressure by increasing oxygen diffusion across dilated arteries.
- True AV shunts, if present, cause mixed venous blood to flow into the pulmonary veins, bypassing the alveoli.

The exact mechanism of vasodilatation is unclear. Evidence suggests that loss of pulmonary capillary vascular tone and suppression of pulmonary vasoconstrictors may cause it. Pulmonary endothelial nitric oxide synthase (eNOS) stimulation occurs in the lungs due to increased hepatic synthesis of endothelin-1 (ET-1). This, in turn, leads to increased expression and activation of pulmonary endothelin B (ETB) receptors, in conjunction with sheer stress in the lung. Thus, eNOS activation increases nitric oxide (NO) generation, a potent pulmonary vascular smooth muscle vasodilator.

Bacterial translocation from the gut in the setting of liver disease with portal hypertension along with endotoxemia caused lung macrophage and monocyte buildup. These macrophages produce tumor necrosis factor-alpha (TNF-α) in pulmonary vasculature, activating inducible nitric oxide synthase (iNOS) and increasing NO production.

Bacterial growth and NO boost heme oxygenase synthesis, which degrades heme and produces carbon monoxide (CO). Both NO and CO are potent lung vasodilators.

Certain studies suggest that vascular endothelial growth factor (VEGF), stimulated by monocytes, macrophages, and TNF-α, may enhance pulmonary vascular angiogenesis **(Fig. 1)**.

Pulmonary vasodilatation is most distinct in the lung bases, causing symptoms like platypnea and orthodeoxia in HPS. These symptoms are caused by gravity-dependent diversion of blood flow to dilated pulmonary arteries in the lung bases in an upright posture, which worsens underlying V/Q mismatch, further creating a physiologic shunt and venous blood mixing **(Fig. 2)**.

TYPES OF HEPATOPULMONARY SYNDROME

Depending on the location of dilated pulmonary vessel (IPVDs), HPS is of two types:

- *Type 1 HPS*: Vascular dilatation at precapillary level near gas exchange units of lungs. Supplemental oxygen increases PaO_2 in this type.
- *Type 2 HPS*: Larger vessels dilate causing AV shunts that may be distant from the gas exchange unit of the lungs. Supplemental oxygen is not helpful.

CLINICAL PRESENTATIONS

Hepatopulmonary syndrome is frequently asymptomatic. Clinical symptoms raise the suspicion of HPS along with associated signs and symptoms of chronic liver disease:

- *Dyspnea*: Gradually progressive worsening breathlessness, but may be a nonspecific feature as it can be due to POPH, anemia, ascites, coexisting respiratory cause, or hepatic hydrothorax
- *Platypnea*: Worsening of dyspnea in an erect position and improvement in the supine position
- *Orthodeoxia*: Defined as increase in hypoxia and hypoxemia, when changing from supine to upright position, detected by arterial blood gas analysis (ABG analysis) or pulse oximetry documented by decrease in PaO_2 by >5% or > 4 mm Hg from baseline and or decrease in SpO_2 by > 5%
- *Cyanosis*: Seen in late stages due to hypoxemia
- Digital clubbing
- *Diffuse telangiectasia*: Spider naevi are more likely associated with HPS.
- Presence of other features of chronic liver disease like ascites, splenomegaly, asterixis, palmar erythema, caput medusae, gynecomastia, and testicular atrophy
- Extrapulmonary complications rarely seen due to left-to-right shunts in pulmonary vasculature, such as intracranial hemorrhage, polycythemia, and cerebral hemorrhages

The European Respiratory Society (ERS) task force has proposed the classification to stage the severity of HPS **(Table 1)**.

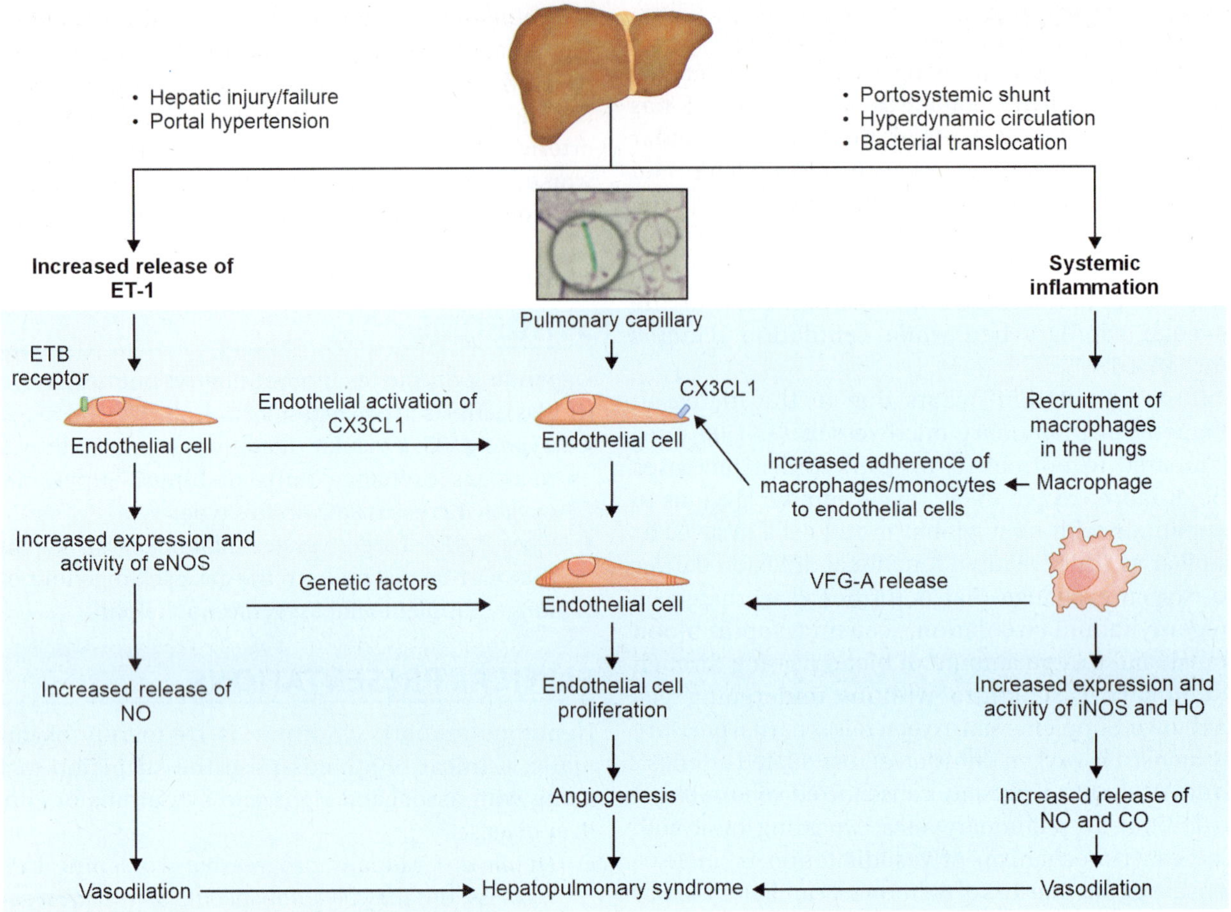

FIG. 1: Pathogenesis of hepatopulmonary syndrome.

(CO: carbon monoxide; ET-1: endothelin 1; ETB: endothelin B; eNOS: endothelial nitric oxide synthetase; HO: heme oxygenase; iNOS: inducible nitric oxide synthase; NO: nitric oxide; VFG-A: vascular endothelial growth factor A)

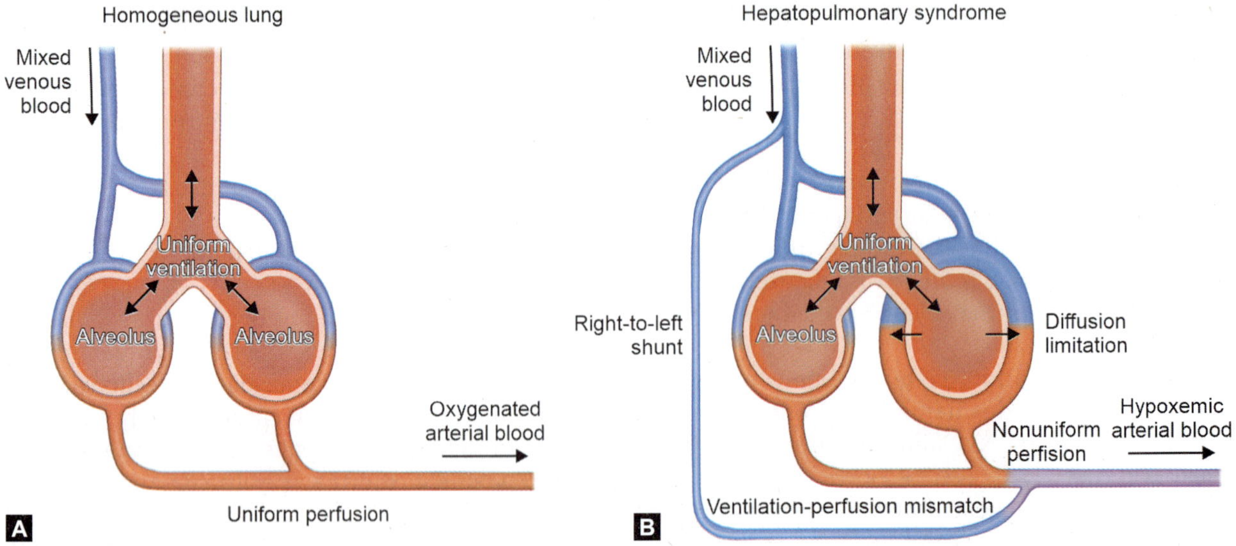

FIGS. 2A AND B: Pathophysiology of hypoxemia in hepatopulmonary syndrome (HPS). Ventilation and perfusion are balanced in the homogenous (healthy) lung (A), whereas ventilation-perfusion mismatch occurs in HPS (B).

Source: Adapted from Rodriguez-Roisin R, Krowka MJ. Hepatopulmonary syndrome—a liver-induced lung vascular disorder. N Engl J Med. 2008;358(22):2378-87.

TABLE 1: Classification based on European Respiratory Society (ERS).

Stage	PaO_2 and A–a O_2 gradient
Mild	PaO_2 > 80 mm Hg with A–a O_2 ≥ 15 mm Hg while breathing room air
Moderate	PaO_2 ≥ 60 to < 80 mm Hg, with A–a O_2 ≥ 15 mm Hg while breathing room air
Severe	PaO_2 ≥ 50 to < 60 mm Hg with A–a O_2 ≥ 15 mm Hg while breathing in room air
Very severe	PaO_2 < 50 mm Hg with A–a O_2 ≥ 15 mm Hg while breathing in room air or PaO_2 < 300 mm Hg while breathing 100% oxygen

Note: The P(A–a) O_2 gradient is calculated: [(Patm – PH_2O) × 0.21 – $PaCO_2$/0.8] – PaO_2.

DIAGNOSIS

The diagnosis is considered in all patients with:

- *Chronic liver disease*: It usually complicated by portal hypertension and complaints of dyspnea, platypnea, and orthodeoxia, along with signs of clubbing, cyanosis, spider nevi.
- *Pulse oximetry*: It is the initial screening tool to evaluate oxygen saturation in both supine and erect positions. Peripheral oxygen saturation (SpO_2) < 96% signifies PaO_2 < 70 mm Hg and is considered a positive screen.
- *Arterial blood gas (ABG)*: It is done in case of a positive screen which helps to determine PaO_2 and A–a O_2.
- *Conventional chest radiography*: Findings are very subtle and infrequent with few bibasilar nodular opacities and increased interstitial markings, probably due to IVPDs.
- *High-resolution CT chest*: Peripherally dilated pulmonary vessels and an increased pulmonary-to-bronchus ratio imply IPVDs and rule out pulmonary pathology.
- *Pulmonary function test (PFT)*: It may show a decrease in diffusing capacity of the lungs for carbon monoxide (DLCO) and rule out coexisting pulmonary disorders.
- *Transthoracic contrast echocardiography (TTCE)*: It is the most sensitive test for the diagnosis of IPVD. Normal saline is agitated to create microbubbles larger than 10 μm in diameter and then injected into the arm's peripheral vein. TTCE is done concurrently. Normally, microbubbles created by agitated saline move from the right ventricle to the lungs through the pulmonary artery, where they are trapped in the alveolar capillary bed (5–8 μm) in diameter and are also absorbed by the alveoli. The presence of IVPD and AV shunts allows microbubbles to bypass the pulmonary artery and reach the left ventricles. Pulmonary vasodilatation is indicated by the appearance of microbubbles between the 4th and 6th cardiac cycles, and intracardiac shunting [atrial septal defect (ASD), etc.] before the 3rd cycle.
- *Transesophageal echocardiography*: It is superior at identifying pulmonary dilatation and intracardiac shunting than transthoracic echocardiography. However, this test is invasive and carries a substantial risk of bleeding from esophageal varices.
- *Macroaggregated albumin (MAA) perfusion lung scan*: It is highly specific but less sensitive than contrast echo for detecting and measuring intrapulmonary dilatation; thus, it is useful in diagnosing HPS in a patient with coexisting respiratory disorder. However, it lacks in differentiating between IPVDs from intracardiac shunts. Technetium-99m-labeled MAA particles of 20 μm are administered into the peripheral vein. These particles are normally retained in the pulmonary capillaries, and absorbed scintigraphy shows practically full absorption in the lungs. In the presence of intracardiac or intrapulmonary shunts, some MAA is shunted to the brain and kidneys, which the Tc-MAA scan quantifies. 6% of brain shunt fraction is pathological.
- Contrast pulmonary angiography is costly, invasive, and infrequently used to identify type 1 and type 2 HPS and in patients with suspected AV malformation **(Flowchart 1)**.

DIFFERENTIAL DIAGNOSIS

- *Portopulmonary hypertension*: It is due to medial and intimal hypertrophy along with endothelial proliferation leading to plexogenic arteriopathy and in situ thrombosis and is histopathologically like primary pulmonary hypertension. Criteria for diagnosing POPH are based on right heart catheterization measurement.
  - Mean pulmonary artery pressure (MPAP) > 25 mm Hg + pulmonary capillary wedge pressure (PCWP) < 15 mm Hg
  - Pulmonary vascular resistance (PVR) > 120 dynes/cm^5 symptomatic of pulmonary hypertension
  - Advanced hepatic dysfunction with portal hypertension

Screening for POPH includes chest radiography, ECG, and transthoracic Doppler echocardiography to evaluate pulmonary artery systolic pressure, which if > 50 mm Hg, strongly suggests POPH.

Treatment: Intravenous epoprostenol, a prostaglandin (PGI2) analog, provides significant pulmonary arterial vasodilation and antiplatelet action. Liver transplant may aggravate pulmonary hypertension with right heart failure post transplant, thus increasing mortality.

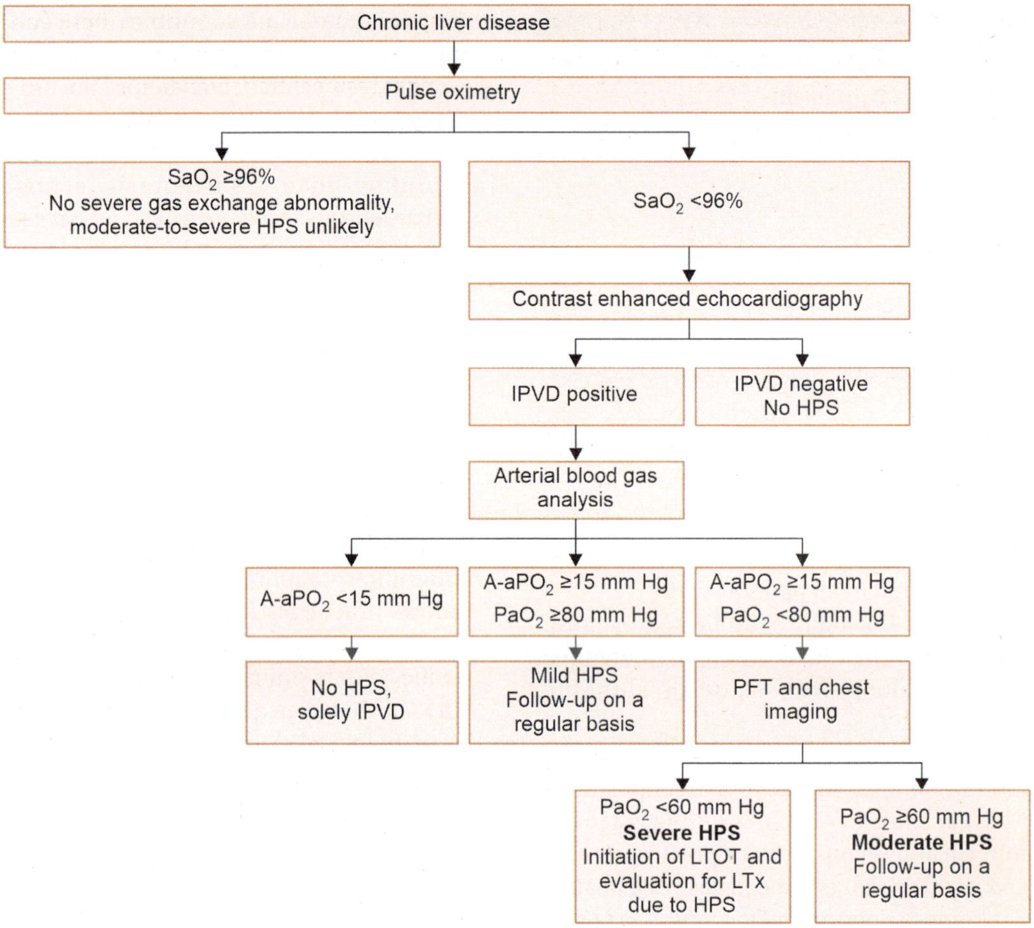

FLOWCHART 1: Hepatopulmonary syndrome (HPS) diagnosis.
(IPVD: intrapulmonary vascular dilatation; LTOT: long-term oxygen therapy; LTx: liver transplantation; PFT: pulmonary function test)

- *Hepatic hydrothorax*: Fluid accumulates in the pleural space due to peritoneal-to-pleural fluid flow through a minor diaphragmatic defect, causing lung compression, basal atelectasis, and physiological shunting. Transjugular intrahepatic portosystemic shunt (TIPS) is useful in these cases; chest tube pleurodesis or thoracic diaphragmatic defect correction are alternatives.

TREATMENT

- *Medical therapy*: Currently, no medical therapy is conclusive and approved.
- Oxygen supplementation is recommended for symptomatic relief in patients with severe hypoxemia. NO antagonists such as NG-nitro-L-arginine-methyl ester (L-Name) and methylene blue inhibit NO causing vasoconstriction and decreasing angiogenesis, which may enhance oxygen exchange, but lack evidence.
- *Almitrine bismesylate*: It is a selective pulmonary vasoconstrictor. Although initially it was found to be a promising agent in HPS as it lowered physiological shunting, the magnitude of response was small.
- *Pentoxifylline*: It is a nonspecific phosphodiesterase inhibitor and a TNF-α blocker that improved intrapulmonary vasodilatation with antiangiogenesis, and showed variable result in oxygenation improvement in HPS.
- *Garlic*: It has allicin. It is a potent vasodilator and anti-angiogenesis. In a short research, garlic powder capsules daily for 6 months were found to improve arterial blood oxygenation.
- *Sorafenib*: It is a tyrosine kinase inhibitor that reduces angiogenesis but lacks benefit in patients with HPS.
- Norfloxacin decreases bacterial translocation, to lower endotoxemia, but without improvement in gas exchange.
- Other medications include inhaled Iloprost (vasodilator), paroxetine (NO synthase inhibitor), and cyclooxygenase inhibitors like aspirin and indomethacin. Somatostatin analogs and immunosuppressive agent like mycophenolate mofetil (MMF),

cyclophosphamide, and beta blockers have been tried without any clear benefit.

- *Transjugular intrahepatic portosystemic shunt*: Clinical outcomes have showed mixed short-term effectiveness in improving pulmonary gaseous exchange. TIPS increases the risk of hepatic decompensation and encephalopathy.
- *Pulmonary artery coil embolization*: It is used only in selected cases where there are large AV communications and has shown improvement in oxygen with varying result.

Liver transplantation is the only proven and effective therapy for HPS, which resolves the condition and improves gaseous exchange in 95% of patients. Large studies found 78% mortality in HPS patients who did not have liver transplantation compared to 21% in those who did. Thus, HPS patients with $PO_2 < 60$ are prioritized for transplants before others. Several retrospective studies have shown that hypoxemia improves after 6–12 months while PaO_2 and A–a O_2 reverse rapidly in 6 months; intrapulmonary shunts take longer. Some patients' DLCO also improves post transplant.

Patients with HPS and MELD (Model for End-stage Liver Disease) score ≥ 15 are prioritized for liver transplantation. Liver transplantation is contraindicated for very severe hypoxemia (PaO_2 < 50 mm Hg), which raises the risk of complications such as pulmonary arterial hypertension, cerebral embolism, and immediate postoperative respiratory failure necessitating long-term support.

PROGNOSIS

Most studies indicate that patients with HPS have two times higher mortality than cirrhotic patients without HPS and worse functional and quality of life. Average lifespan being 11 months. Long-term survival is worse in patients with PaO_2 < 50 mm Hg.

SUGGESTED READINGS

1. Gandhi KD, Taweesedt PT, Sharma M, Surani S. Hepatopulmonary syndrome: An update. World J Hepatol. 2021;13(11):1699-706.
2. Bansal K, Gore M, Mittal S. Hepatopulmonary syndrome. StatPearls publishing; 2023.
3. Krowka MJ, Fallon MB, Kawut SM, Fuhrmann V, Heimbach JK, Ramsay MAE, et al. International Liver Transplant Society Practice Guidelines: Diagnosis and Management of Hepatopulmonary Syndrome and Portopulmonary Hypertension. Transplantation. 2016;100(7):1440-52.
4. Abrams GA, Jaffe CC, Hoffer PB, Binder HJ, Fallon MB. Diagnostic utility of contrast echocardiography and lung perfusion scan in patients with hepatopulmonary syndrome. Gastroenterology. 1995;109(4):1283-8.
5. Swanson KL, Wiesner RH, Krowka MJ. Natural history of hepatopulmonary syndrome: Impact of liver transplantation. Hepatology. 2005;41(5):1122-9.

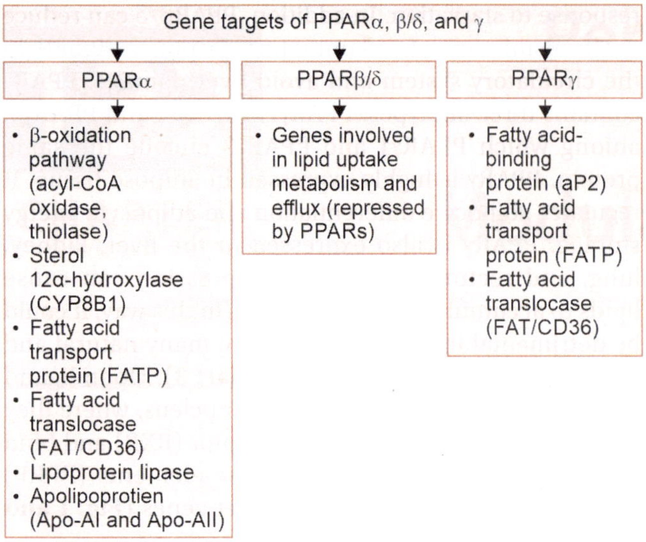

FLOWCHART 4: Peroxisome proliferator-activated receptors (PPAR) and their target genes.

ROLE OF PPAR IN THE PATHOGENESIS OF NAFLD

All the three PPARs are involved in the process of lipid handling and the attenuation of inflammation/oxidative damage in the body, and thus have a role to play in the evolution of NAFLD and NASH. The role of individual PPAR is described below.

PPARα

- Activated PPARα stimulates all three pathways of FA oxidation in the liver. This activation and increased sensing of PPARα in the liver result in increased energy burning and reduced fat storage. Thus, PPARα functions as a lipid sensor and controls energy combustion.
- Leukotriene B4 (LTB4) is a leukotriene substance produced by leukocytes and acts as a chemotactic agent. When this LTB4 binds as an endogenous ligand to PPARα, the binding promotes self-degradation of LTB4 and inhibits inflammation.
- PPARα activation inhibits the formation of macrophage-derived foam cells and thus inhibits the formation of atherosclerotic plaque.
- PPARα induces increased expression of Apo-AI and Apo-AII messenger ribonucleic acid (mRNA) and cause increased high-density lipoprotein (HDL) in the circulation.
- PPARα leads to increased lipoprotein lipase (LPL) activity and accelerates the catabolism of TG-rich lipoproteins [such as chylomicrons and very low-density lipoprotein (VLDL)].
- PPARα increases the enzyme lipoprotein esterase activity in the liver.
- PPARα mediates the transportation of FA from peripheral tissues to the liver. It weakens the FA-induced inhibition for skeletal muscle glucose metabolism, thereby increasing insulin sensitivity.
- PPARα induces the expression of base-excision DNA repair genes which remove oxidatively damaged DNA.
- PPARα increases the binding of insulin receptor to insulin and thus improves insulin sensitivity.

PPARβ/δ

- PPARβ/δ activation promotes the proliferation of adipocyte precursor cells.
- In skeletal muscles, there is an increase in FA catabolism, cholesterol efflux, and energy consumption caused by PPARβ/δ activation.

PPARγ

- As a natural ligand of PPARγ, oxidized low-density lipoprotein (Ox-LDL) can enhance the activity of scavenger receptor (SAR) and CD36 and is closely related to macrophage activation and foam cell formation.
- PPARγ promotes lipolysis by inducing the expression of LPL and thus reduces TG and low-density lipoprotein cholesterol (LDL-C) levels.
- PPARγ can activate diacylglycerol (DAG) kinase and inhibits protein kinase C (PKC) activity.
- PPARγ promotes disposal of cholesterol to the liver through the adenosine triphosphate (ATP) binding cassette protein A1 (ABCA1)/liver X receptor (LXR) pathway.
- PPARγ expression has anti-inflammatory effects by suppressing iNOS secretion, nuclear factor-kappa B (NF-κB) activation, STAT1 activation, and AP-1 signal transduction.
- PPARγ reduces the secretion of interleukin 6 (IL-6), monocyte chemoattractant protein (MCP-1), and tumor necrosis factor-alpha (TNF-α) and other cytokines by monocytes.
- PPARγ reduces the expression of vascular cell-adhesion molecule 1 (VCAM-1).

AVAILABLE PPAR AGONISTS AND THEIR ROLES IN NAFLD

Several experimental and clinical studies have reported the use of PPAR agonists in the treatment of NAFLD which will be reviewed below.

PPARα Agonists

Fibrates (as PPARα agonist) are lipid-lowering agents used in clinical practice to treat hypertriglyceridemia and atherogenic dyslipidemia. In rodent models of NAFLD, fibrates have demonstrated beneficial effects on hepatic steatosis, inflammation, and fibrosis, though no such effects have been observed in humans. In EFFECT-I trial, 12 weeks of fenofibrate caused a reduction in plasma TG levels but increased liver fat content and liver volume in overweight or obese patients with NAFLD. Thus, fibrates have a complex effect on human hepatic lipid metabolism that requires further investigation. Another PPARα agonist, gemfibrozil, has shown beneficial effects on liver enzymes but not on liver histology in a human trial.

PPARβ/δ Agonists

Current PPARβ/δ agonists, including Sedalpar, have shown encouraging results in experimental models of NAFLD, but clinical studies are lacking.

PPARγ Agonists

Thiazolidinediones (pioglitazone, rosiglitazone) are synthetic compounds that act as ligands of PPARγ and are used in the treatment of T2DM as insulin sensitizers. Though the exact molecular mechanism underlying the action of pioglitazone is not completely understood, it effectively improves hepatic steatosis in humans. Pioglitazone improves the histological features of NAFLD, including steatosis and inflammation, and a recent meta-analysis reported that pioglitazone therapy is associated with an improvement in advanced fibrosis in NAFLD, even in nondiabetic patients. This meta-analysis also indicated that weight gain and limb edema are associated with pioglitazone treatment. The Indian National Association for the Study of Liver (INASL) has, in March 2023, recommended the use of pioglitazone (30 mg/day) in both diabetic and non-diabetic NASH with fibroscan values between 8.2 and 13.6 kPa for a period up to 2 years.

In FLIRT (Fatty Liver Improvement with Rosiglitazone Therapy) trial, treatment with rosiglitazone (another PPARγ agonist) for 1 year increased adiponectin levels and reduced insulin resistance in most patients, and reduced hepatic steatosis in half of patients, but did not improve liver inflammation or fibrosis.

Novel PPAR Agonists

Novel PPAR agonists, called selective PPAR modulators (SPPARMs), aim to maximize the beneficial effects and minimize the adverse effects of current agonists. As PPARs in the liver and other organs have multiple and distinct effects, targeting two or three isotypes has emerged as a promising novel therapeutic strategy for treating NAFLD **(Table 1)**.

TABLE 1: Overview of novel peroxisome proliferator-activated receptor (PPAR) agonists.

Compound	PPAR agonists	Description
Elafibranor	α and β/δ	• High activity on PPARα, moderate activity on β/δ • More safety data needed • Currently on phase 3: Effect on fibrosis
Saroglitazar	α and γ	• High activity on PPARα, moderate activity on PPARγ • Clinical application for dyslipidemia • Safety profile in meta-analysis established • Currently in phase 3: Effect on fibrosis compared to pioglitazone and vitamin E
Lanifibranor	α, β/δ and γ	• Moderate and balanced activity on PPARα, PPARβ/δ, and PPARγ • Currently in phase 3: Effect on fibrosis

Elafibranor is a combined PPARα and PPARδ agonist in development for the treatment of NASH. It has shown a modest effect in a phase 2 trial on the histological resolution of inflammation, but not on the histological improvement of fibrosis. Elafibranor has also shown small reversible creatinine elevations in the safety results raising concerns because of known association of chronic kidney disease with NASH. The results on the efficacy and safety of the dedicated RESOLVE-IT phase 3 trial and the phase 3 trials on combinations with other developmental drugs will decide if elafibranor has a role to play in the future.

Saroglitazar has predominant activity on PPARα and moderate activity on PPARγ, reducing the adverse effects associated with sole PPARγ activation (as occurs with pioglitazone). Therapeutic usage in patients with diabetic dyslipidemia resulted in improved glucose parameter, reduction in plasma TG levels, and improved whole-body insulin sensitivity. In 2013, it was approved by the Drug Controller of India to treat diabetic dyslipidemia. A systematic review and meta-analysis that included results of two randomized controlled trials (RCTs), one single-arm interventional study, and seven observational studies in NAFLD/NASH have shown that treatment with adjunct 4 mg saroglitazar for 12–52 weeks resulted in improvements in liver function and metabolic parameters

SECTION 9

HYPERTENSION

123
CHAPTER

Hypertension and Insulin Resistance: What is New?

Ashutosh Chaturvedi, Naresh Kumar Midha, Divyansh Mathur, Girish Mathur

ABSTRACT

Insulin resistance and hypertension, often referred to as "diseases of civilization," have become increasingly prevalent in India due to rapid urbanization and lifestyle changes. Insulin resistance plays a main role in the development of type 2 diabetes mellitus (T2DM) and is also associated with hypertension. Insulin, apart from its role in metabolism, exerts various effects on inflammation, oxidative stress, and vascular function. It promotes the release of nitric oxide (NO), inhibits adhesion molecules, and suppresses oxidative damage within the vasculature. Insulin resistance arises from abnormalities in insulin signaling, particularly in the insulin receptor (IR) and its substrates. This resistance contributes to elevated blood pressure through multiple mechanisms including dysregulation of angiotensin II, aldosterone, sympathetic nervous system activity, endothelial dysfunction, and oxidative stress. Insulin resistance and hypertension also involve neurohormonal interactions such as renin–angiotensin and sympathetic nervous systems, leading to further disruption of insulin signaling. These conditions can cause end-organ damage, including left ventricular hypertrophy (LVH), carotid atherosclerosis, and kidney dysfunction. Simple surrogate indexes such as Model Assessment of Insulin Resistance (HOMA-IR), Quantitative Insulin Sensitivity Check Index (QUICKI) and Adipose Tissue Insulin Resistance Index (Adipo-IR) are used to estimate insulin resistance in clinical practice. They aid in identifying individuals at high risk for metabolic disorders and help in personalized treatment and monitoring. However, these indexes have limitations and should be interpreted alongside clinical judgment, considering factors such as age, obesity, and pregnancy.

INTRODUCTION

Insulin resistance and hypertension are commonly referred to as exemplary "diseases of civilization," which emerge in the contemporary setting characterized by abundant food availability and a sedentary lifestyle. Diabetes and hypertension pose a significant epidemiological burden in India. With the rapid urbanization and lifestyle changes, the prevalence of these conditions has risen alarmingly. Insulin resistance is defined as a diminished biological response to its specific concentration, occupies a central position in the development of type 2 diabetes mellitus (T2DM), exerting a crucial role in its pathogenesis. Clinical studies have revealed that approximately 50% of individuals with hypertension exhibit hyperinsulinemia or glucose intolerance, while up to 80% T2DM patients also have hypertension. Nowadays, it is widely recognized that insulin resistance encompasses a multifaceted and intricate syndrome that extends its influence beyond glycemic control, encompassing the regulation of blood pressure homeostasis as well. The presence of insulin resistance in individuals without diabetes is positively correlated with both systolic and diastolic blood pressure, implying that it can have detrimental effects on the vasculature even before the onset of hyperglycemia. Moreover, this association appears to be more pronounced in women compared to men.

FUNCTIONS OF INSULIN: BEYOND THE METABOLISM

Insulin, as a pleiotropic hormone, demonstrates a wide range of effects on glucose, lipid, and protein metabolism,

TABLE 1: The pleiotropic actions of insulin.

Actions	Remark
Metabolism	Insulin regulates the glucose, protein, and lipid metabolism
Cell cycle	Insulin plays crucial role in cell cycle regulation, proliferation, and differentiation
Vascular function	Insulin inhibits reactive oxygen species (ROS) synthesis and enhance NO production
Vascular inflammation	Insulin prevents endothelial injuries and inhibit atherosclerosis
Neurohormonal regulation activity	Insulin resistance is associated with enhanced RAS and SNS activity
Ion and amino acid transport	Insulin regulates sodium reabsorption, amino acid transports and calcium influx

(RAS: renin–angiotensin system; SNS: sympathetic nervous system)

as well as on cell cycle regulation, proliferation, differentiation, and even the synthesis of nitric oxide (NO) **(Table 1)**. Insulin inhibits NADPH oxidase (nicotinamide adenine dinucleotide phosphate oxidase) expression within the macrophages and inhibits the synthesis of oxygen free radicals. These reactive oxygen radicals initiate the cascade of endothelium injury and responsible for inflammation, fibrosis, and vascular damage. In the context of diabetes and hypertension, increased oxidative stress within the vasculature exacerbates the post-translational oxidative modification of proteins, leading to cellular harm and vascular dysfunction.

Insulin promotes the production of endothelial nitric oxide synthase (eNOS) within endothelial cells, which leads to the release of NO and subsequent vasodilation. Moreover, insulin acts to suppress the activation of endothelial nuclear factor-kappa-B (NF-κB), a key factor responsible for initiating the expression of adhesion molecules like E-selectin and intercellular adhesion molecule 1 (ICAM-1) in endothelial cells. As these adhesion molecules are implicated in the development of atherosclerosis, insulin's inhibitory effect directly contributes to the prevention of atherosclerosis.

MOLECULAR MECHANISM OF INSULIN RESISTANCE

Insulin resistance arises from the abnormalities in insulin signaling. Insulin interacts with the insulin receptor (IR) found on target cell membranes. The IR consists of two α subunits located extracellularly, serving as the binding sites for insulin, and two β subunits bridged by the membrane, which house a tyrosine kinase domain. By binding to the α subunit of the receptor, insulin triggers the activation of the β subunit's tyrosine kinase. This activation sets in motion a cascade of events, including autophosphorylation and subsequent tyrosine phosphorylation of various insulin receptor substrates (IRS), such as IRS-1 and IRS-2.

As a result of these phosphorylations, the translocation of the GLUT4 to the plasma membrane is facilitated, enabling glucose uptake. IR dysfunction can potentially cause insulin resistance through various mechanisms, including structural abnormalities, alterations in receptor quantity, compromised binding affinity, and impaired signaling capacity. IR or IRS signaling plays a systematic role in the development of hypertension that is distinct from glucose homeostasis and plasma insulin levels. This suggests that insulin resistance plays a significant part in the pathogenesis of hypertension.

INSULIN RESISTANCE AND BLOOD PRESSURE REGULATION

Insulin resistance exerts a substantial influence on the increase in blood pressure, through various mechanisms. These include enhanced angiotensin II and aldosterone activities within tissues, increased sympathetic nervous system activity, endothelial dysfunction, and increased oxidative stress. The robust correlation between hypertension and insulin resistance has been substantiated by evidence demonstrating the presence of hypertension-related organ damage, including left ventricular hypertrophy (LVH) and atherosclerosis of carotid arteries in the patients with essential hypertension.

INSULIN RESISTANCE AND NEUROHORMONAL INTERPLAY IN HYPERTENSION

Hypertension involves various kinds of pathophysiological mechanisms that collectively impair insulin signaling. These include enhanced renin–angiotensin and sympathetic nervous systems, as well as oxidative stress. The disturbance of neurohumoral and neuroimmune systems influences the pathophysiology of both insulin resistance and hypertension **(Flowchart 1)**.

Renin–angiotensin System

The dysregulation of the renin–angiotensin system (RAS) in hypertensive patients is well observed. Insulin signaling abnormality and development of insulin resistance are also associated with RAS activation. By activating the angiotensin type 1 receptor, Ang II hampers insulin's effects through the generation of free oxygen

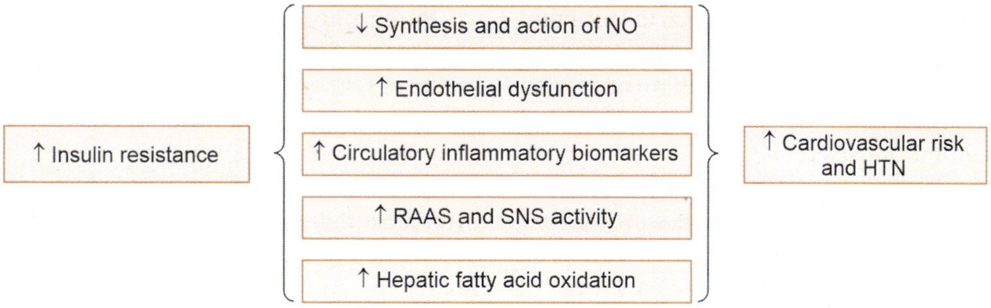

FLOWCHART 1: Impact of insulin resistance.
(HTN: hypertension; NO: nitric oxide; RAAS: renin–angiotensin–aldosterone system; SNS: sympathetic nervous system)

radicals via NADPH oxidase. Angiotensin II contributes to the generation of oxidative stress, inflammation, and apoptosis specifically of pancreatic β-cells. ACE inhibitors have the potential to enhance insulin sensitivity, while Ang II receptor blockers (ARBs) regulate the activity of peroxisome proliferator-activated receptor (PPAR)-γ. PPAR-γ, a transcription factor which demonstrates a crucial role in glucose metabolism.

Sympathetic Nervous System

Insulin is having bidirectional relationship with sympathetic nervous system. Insulin resistance is associated with overactivation of the sympathetic nervous system due to enhanced stimulation of β-adrenergic receptors. Enhanced sympathetic system leads to myocyte hypertrophy, interstitial fibrosis, diminished contractile function, and increased myocyte apoptosis. It has been established that overactive sympathetic system leads to abnormal stimulation of the β subunits of IR which can induce insulin resistance by activating various serine/threonine kinases that impede insulin signaling through phosphorylation of the IR. Sympathetic activation contributes to weight gain, exacerbates insulin resistance, and leads to subsequent hyperinsulinemia, thereby extending a vicious cycle of weight gain, insulin resistance, sympathetic activation, and further weight gain.

TARGET ORGAN DAMAGE IN INSULIN RESISTANCE AND HYPERTENSION

Hypertension leads to various forms of target organ damage, including LVH, carotid atherosclerosis, and renal dysfunction. Furthermore, insulin resistance contributes to the progression of LVH, carotid atherosclerosis, and chronic kidney disease.

Left Ventricular Hypertrophy

Insulin resistance is associated with hemodynamic and metabolic disturbances that increase the susceptibility to LVH. Insulin amplifies the hypertrophic response of the left ventricle to arterial hypertension through insulin-like growth factor 1 (IGF-1). Insulin-resistant hypertensive individuals often exhibit mononuclear cell infiltration in their myocardium; this is linked with increased risk of LVH and cardiac arrhythmia.

In the patients of hypertension with diabetes, myocardial cell growth stimulation and sympathetic nervous system activation are potential factors that could predominantly contribute to the development of LVH due to volume overload because of underlying sodium and water retention.

Carotid Atherosclerosis

Numerous mechanisms have been postulated to describe the association of insulin resistance in the progression of atherosclerosis. Two important pathogenic factors are endothelial dysfunction on the arterial walls and disturbed lipid as well as glucose metabolism. Activation of IR in the endothelium triggers insulin signaling, which enhances the production of NO. NO exerts a range of beneficial effects, including anti-inflammatory and antithrombotic properties which are antiatherogenic. Insulin-induced antithrombotic effects decrease the platelet adhesion by increasing prostacyclin production.

Low-grade inflammation is a common characteristic observed in both atherosclerosis and insulin resistance. Tumor necrosis factor-alpha (TNF-α and interleukin-6 (IL-6) are the major proinflammatory cytokines, which are associated with early atherosclerosis in diabetic patients with underlying insulin resistance. TNF-α promotes the synthesis of endothelin-1 and angiotensinogen, also inhibits insulin function by reducing the tyrosine kinase activity of the IR.

Renal Dysfunction

Hypertension and diabetes with coexistence of insulin resistance are the primary contributors to the development of chronic kidney disease. Renal dysfunction is significantly influenced by hypertension, which inflicts harm upon the nephrons through mechanisms such as elevated glomerular capillary pressure, endothelial dysfunction, and glomerulosclerosis.

Insulin resistance demonstrates a close association with the activation of both the RAS and sympathetic nervous system, which collectively impact renal function. This interplay gives rise to increased reabsorption of sodium in the kidneys, leading to fluid retention and subsequent hypertension development.

Inadequate management of insulin resistance and its associated hemodynamic and metabolic abnormalities can contribute to renal injury, causing both functional and structural loss of nephrons. This loss of nephrons further exacerbates hypertension, thereby intensifying the ongoing renal injury.

SIMPLE SURROGATE INDEXES FOR INSULIN RESISTANCE

Simple surrogate indexes, such as the Homeostatic Model Assessment of Insulin Resistance (HOMA-IR), Quantitative Insulin Sensitivity Check Index (QUICKI) and Adipose Tissue Insulin Resistance Index (Adipo-IR), have gained popularity as practical tools for estimating insulin resistance in clinical practice.

By employing these surrogate indexes, healthcare providers can quickly assess insulin sensitivity/ resistance in a cost-effective and time-efficient manner. This enables early identification of individuals at high risk for metabolic disorders, facilitates personalized treatment strategies, and aids in monitoring therapeutic interventions. However, it is essential to recognize the limitations of these surrogate indexes and interpret the results in conjunction with clinical judgment. These indexes may not capture the full spectrum of insulin resistance in diverse populations. Furthermore, factors such as age, obesity, and pregnancy can also influence the performance of these indexes.

CONCLUSION

Clinical studies have shown a strong association between insulin resistance and hypertension, with approximately 50% of hypertensive individuals exhibiting hyperinsulinemia or glucose intolerance. Insulin resistance affects blood pressure regulation through mechanisms such as increased angiotensin II and aldosterone activities, enhanced sympathetic nervous system activity, endothelial dysfunction, and oxidative stress. Target organ damage, including LVH, carotid arteries atherosclerosis, and kidney dysfunction are exacerbated by insulin resistance and hypertension.

SUGGESTED READINGS

1. Zhou MS, Wang A, Yu H. Link between insulin resistance and hypertension: What is the evidence from evolutionary biology? Diabetol Metab Syndr. 2014;6(1):12.
2. Mancusi C, Izzo R, di Gioia G, Losi MA, Barbato E, Morisco C, et al. Insulin resistance the hinge between hypertension and type 2 diabetes. High Blood Press Cardiovasc Prev. 2020;27(6):515-26.
3. Haeusler R, McGraw TE, Accili D. Biochemical and cellular properties of insulin receptor signalling. Nat Rev Mol Cell Biol. 2018;19:31-44.
4. Tagi VM, Mainieri F, Chiarelli F. Hypertension in patients with insulin resistance: etiopathogenesis and management in children. Int J Mol Sci. 2022;23(10):5814.
5. Nurun Nabi AHM, Ebihara A. Diabetes and Renin-Angiotensin-Aldosterone System: Pathophysiology and Genetics. London, UK: IntechOpen; 2021.
6. Valensi P. Autonomic nervous system activity changes in patients with hypertension and overweight: role and therapeutic implications. Cardiovasc Diabetol. 2021;20(1):170.
7. Ormazabal V, Nair S, Elfeky O, Aguayo C, Salomon C, Zuñiga FA, et al. Association between insulin resistance and the development of cardiovascular disease. Cardiovasc Diabetol. 2018;17:122.
8. Fischer HJ, Sie C, Schumann E, Witte A-K, Dressel R, van den Brandt J, et al. The insulin receptor plays a critical role in T cell function and adaptive immunity. J Immunol. 2017;198:1910-20.

124
CHAPTER

Clinical Utility of Ambulatory Blood Pressure Monitoring: Indian Perspectives

Santosh Salagre, Sahil Langde

ABSTRACT

Ambulatory blood pressure monitoring (ABPM) is useful for measuring the fluctuations in an individual's blood pressure (BP) during the activities of daily living over a period of 24–48 hours. It is an internationally recommended modality for diagnosis, treatment, and determining prognosis of hypertensive patients. ABPM consists of measuring parameters, such as systolic BP (SBP), diastolic BP (DBP), pulse pressure (PP), and pulse rate, which is followed by calculating indices like hyperbaric impact (HBI), morning surge, diurnal index, mean SBP/DBP, and percentage time elevation (PTE). These measurements are performed at a regular interval of 30–60 minutes. Nocturnal dipping patterns are determined, which if abnormal would herald a poorer prognosis and a higher risk of end-organ damage. Hypertension is diagnosed by ABPM if, the 24-hour average BP is ≥ 130/80 mm Hg or the daytime average BP is ≥ 135/85 mm Hg or the night-time average BP is ≥ 120/70 mm Hg. ABPM helps not only in diagnosis but for the monitoring of treatment in hypertensives. It can detect white-coat hypertension, masked hypertension, and alarming reactions. Its use is limited in settings like extremes of arm circumference, arrhythmias, and movement disorders. Utilization of this modality should be actively sought by every physician for better treatment of hypertension.

INTRODUCTION

Hypertension is one of the most commonly faced diseases by doctors all over the world. In the ever-expanding knowledge about the pathophysiology and treatment of hypertension, ambulatory blood pressure monitoring (ABPM) has proven its quintessential role as a diagnostic modality. Being a physician of the 21st century, it is of utmost importance to have knowledge of ABPM in the management of hypertension.

What is ambulatory blood pressure monitoring?

Ambulatory blood pressure monitoring is a serial noninvasive measurement of an individual's blood pressure (BP) at regular intervals, performed over an extended period of 24–48 hours. It is done by measuring blood pressure during activities of daily life by applying a digital BP monitor close to an individual's body.

INTERNATIONAL CONSENSUS

All the international guidelines highlight the use of ABPM in diagnosing and managing patients with hypertension. ABPM has been recommended as a method of choice for 24-hour monitoring of BP in the routine schedule and activity of a patient. This is particularly attributable to improvements in 24-hour BP monitoring methods and the use of cutting-edge devices that are more appropriate, easy to use, affordable, validated by strict international protocols, automatic, and electronically sophisticated, providing reliable performance.

A BRIEF HISTORY OF AMBULATORY BLOOD PRESSURE MONITORING

The idea for ABPM found its roots in the late 20th century. The initial report on the use of ABPM was published in

1962 by Hinman et al. in American Heart Journal which was followed by a study by Kain et al. in 1964. This ushered in a new era in hypertension diagnosis and thousands of studies have been published to date for use of ABPM in the diagnosis and management of hypertension.

RATIONALE BEHIND USING AMBULATORY BLOOD PRESSURE MONITORING

A single OPD-based measurement of BP is affected by many internal as well as external factors, like stress levels, activity, meals, time of the day, white coat phenomenon, etc. This limits the use of single or static measurements in diagnosis and management of hypertension. Instead, serial measurements taken at regular time intervals in patient's routine surroundings and schedule can help us to understand the trend of BP over time, with respect to the activities of daily living. This is helpful in the diagnosis of hypertension, determining the prognosis as well as for choosing the appropriate therapy options and their timings.

AMBULATORY BLOOD PRESSURE MONITORING MACHINE COMPONENTS

The components of ABPM machine are illustrated in **Figure 1**.

PROCEDURE OF AMBULATORY BLOOD PRESSURE MONITORING

- The procedure starts by entering the vital data of patient in the ABPM software.
- The recording intervals are programmed usually at 30 minutes in the daytime (active period as per the patient) and 60 minutes in the nighttime. This also involves entering of start time as well as duration of examination. After entering the data, the machine is placed in a reservoir provided.
- The examination is usually started at early morning before patient commences his/her work.
- Patient is explained about the procedure, machine, and care to be taken of the machine.
- The cuff is applied to the nondominant hand without any intervening clothing items. If there is a difference of >20/10 mm Hg between the upper limbs, then the machine is applied to a hand with higher readings.
- The connecting tube is attached to the ABPM device and the device with its reservoir is tied snuggly around the waist of the patient.
- A static BP reading is taken to check the working of ABPM machine. Patient is explained that this type of activity would occur at every 30–60 minutes interval. Patient is asked to avoid using that arm during the recording to prevent erroneous readings.
- After completion of predetermined duration, the patient is asked to return with the machine. The machine is unloaded and the data is extracted by ABPM software.
- ABPM should be repeated if following requirements are *not* met:
  - 24-hour measurements >70% of expected
  - At least 20 valid daytime readings
  - At least 7 valid nighttime readings
  - For research purposes, at least 2 valid daytime and 1 valid nighttime measurements per hour.

PARAMETERS STUDIED IN AMBULATORY BLOOD PRESSURE MONITORING

Ambulatory blood pressure monitoring records different BP parameters over a specific duration, typically over 24–48 hours. It includes mean BP, pulse, BP variability, diurnal variation of BP, and diurnal index with nocturnal BP dipping patterns. The software of ABPM devices is validated with international standards like the International Protocol of the European Society of Hypertension (ESH). Parameters are then displayed graphically for better understanding.

Ambulatory Blood Pressure Monitoring Parameters

- *Number of successful readings*: The number of times the machine was able to record the BP successfully. It is calculated separately for daytime and nighttime.
- *24 hours average*: It is the arithmetic average of all the recordings done over 24 hours. It is calculated separately for systolic BP (SBP), diastolic BP (DBP), mean arterial pressure, pulse pressure (PP), and pulse rate.
- *Daytime average*: It is the arithmetic average of all the recordings done in the daytime. It is calculated separately for SBP, DBP, mean arterial pressure, PP, and pulse rate.
- *Nighttime average*: It is the arithmetic average of all the recordings done at nighttime. It is calculated separately for SBP, DBP, mean arterial pressure, PP, and pulse rate.
- *Percentage time elevation*: It is the proportion of time during which BP values are higher than considered to be normal. It compares the period with elevated BP to the total time.
- *Hyperbaric index*: It provides information on how long BP is higher than normal and how much it is higher than the upper limit of normal ambulatory BP during ABPM.

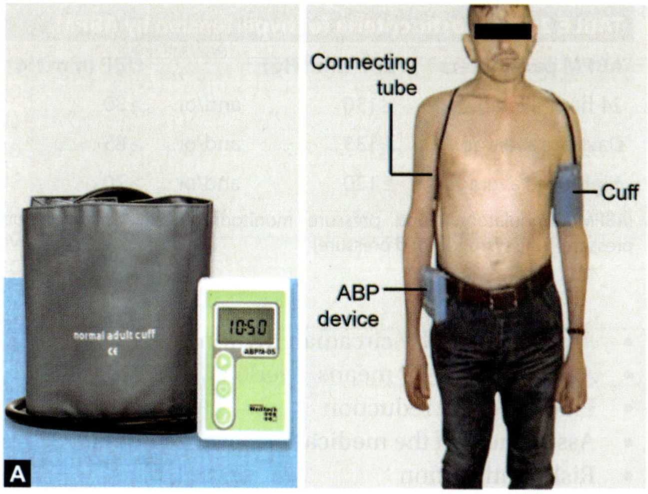

A

Examination			
Start:	14-12-2022 13:18	Start of statistics:	14-12-2022 13:18
Length:	24 hours	Length of statistics:	24 hours
No.of measurements /successful:	41/38 (93%)	Active period	07:00-00:00
ABPM-05:	519756,5.03	Programme:	EasyABPM 1.1.1.0

B

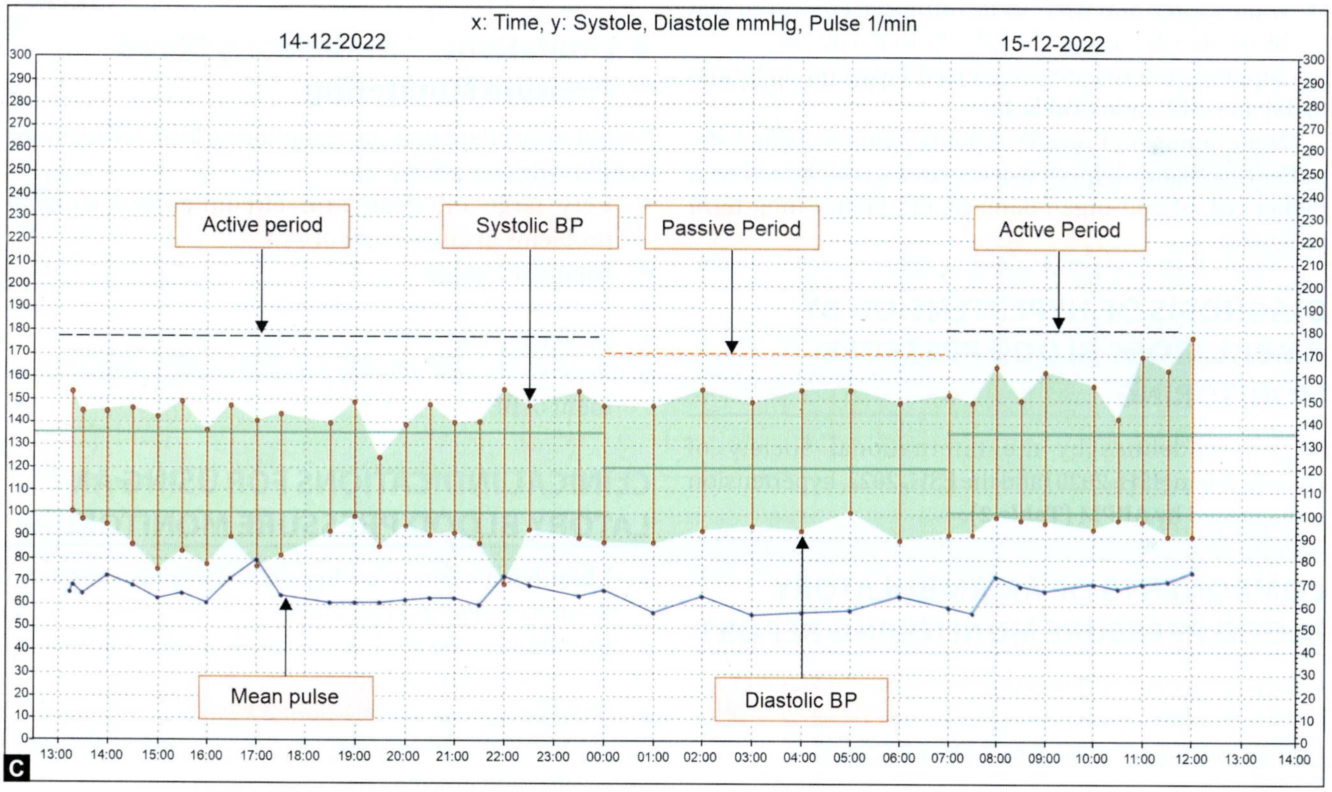

C

Statistics						
All 23:11:47	Systole mm Hg	Diastole mm Hg	MAP mm Hg	PP mm Hg	Pulse 1/min	Double product
Hypertension	130	80				
Mean	149	90	110	60	64	9,529
Maximum	177	100	120	87	79	13,098
Minimum	124	69	97	39	55	7,440
SD	10	7	7	10	6	1,258
PTE	98	29	52			
Hyperbaric impact	457	80	150			
Diurnal index	–1	–3	–2			
Morning surge						

D

FIGS. 1A TO D: (A) Ambulatory blood pressure monitoring (ABPM) machine with its components and the correct method of application; (B) The length, start time, active period, and number of successful measurements of an ABPM examination; (C) The graphical representation of ABPM parameters with respect to active and passive periods; (D) Tabular recording of ABPM parameters over 24-hour duration.

(ABPM: ambulatory blood pressure monitoring; BP: blood pressure; MAP: mean arterial pressure; PP: pulse pressure; PTE: percentage time elevation; SD: standard deviation) determined by the change in percentage in nighttime BP as compared to daytime BP.

Excessive dipping, nondipping, and inverse dipping/rising patterns are the patterns of circadian BP. If the decrease in BP is >20%, it is mentioned as excessive dipping, if it is between the range of 11 and 20%, it is mentioned as dipping, 1–10% range is considered as nondipping, and 0% is the inverse pattern. However, an increase in nighttime BP compared to daytime BP is called rising/reverse pattern.

The dipping pattern in BP is usually not seen in conditions such as sleep disorder, obstructive sleep apnea, high salt intake, obesity, orthostatic hypotension, autonomic dysfunction, diabetic nephropathy, chronic kidney disease, and advanced age (**Box 1**).

MECHANISMS OF NOCTURNAL HYPERTENSION

As salt sensitivity and sleeping in the supine posture causes increase in the circulatory volume and also the vascular damage decreases baroreflex functions, it may lead to increase in nighttime BP.

Increase in volume in night leads to kidney damage by increasing intraglomerular pressure. In addition, this increase in volume leads to heart failure by increasing left ventricular preload and wall stress.

Decrease in baroreflex functions may trigger stroke, myocardial infarction, and vascular dementia. The variation in hormonal changes on diurnal basis which usually affects the autonomic nervous system, such as the sympathetic nervous system, parasympathetic nervous system, cortisol, insulin secretion, and renin–angiotensin–aldosterone system (RAAS), leads to circadian BP changes.

The increased activity of the RAAS, increased sympathetic nervous system activity, retention of sodium, obstructive sleep apnea syndrome, deranged renal function, age, obesity, diabetes, heart failure, secondary hypertension, decreased physical activity, insomnia, and work stress can lead to NH (**Figs. 1 and 2**).

TREATMENT

Increase in the activity of sympathetic nervous system, RAAS, and increase in circulatory volume are the mechanisms which lead to NH. Multiple treatment modalities such as restriction in the intake of salt, angiotensin-converting enzyme (ACE) inhibitors, diuretics, angiotensin receptor blockers (ARBs), combination of ACE with diuretic or combination of ACE inhibitor with calcium channel blockers (CCBs) can be used in the treatment of NH. Aliskiren, a direct renin inhibitor, can be used in NH. CCBs can control BP in patients with reverse dipping or excessive dipping patterns.

According to the American guideline, the first target of treatment is morning hypertension. If the morning BP is < 130/80 mm Hg, the second goal is passed. The second goal is uncontrolled NH with a mask. Restriction in salt

BOX 1: Definition and associated conditions of nocturnal hypertension.

- Definition
- *Nocturnal hypertension*: Average of night-time BPs* > 110/65 mm Hg
- *Clinic BP-masked nocturnal hypertension*: Nocturnal hypertension with clinic BP < 130/80 mm Hg
- *Morning BP-masked nocturnal hypertension*: Nocturnal hypertension with morning home BP < 130/80 mm Hg
- Isolated masked nocturnal hypertension
- Nocturnal hypertension with both clinic and morning home BPs < 130/80 mm Hg
- Determinants
- *Environmental condition*: Summer (hot temperature)
- *Behavioral factors*:
  - High salt intake
  - Reduced physical activity
  - Poor sleep quality and nocturia
  - Shift-working
- *Risk factor*:
  - Aging
  - Asians
  - Obesity
  - Stress
  - Hypertension
  - Diabetes mellitus
- Salt sensitivity
- *Autonomic nervous dysfunction*: Orthostatic hypotension
- *Secondary hypertension*: Obstructive sleep apnea
- *Endocrine disease (primary aldosteronism, renovascular hypertension, Cushing syndrome, and pheochromocytoma)*: Chronic kidney disease
- *Disease*:
  - Heart failure
  - CNS disease (stroke, cognitive dysfunction, and depression)
  - Restless leg syndrome

*Nighttime BPs measured from bedtime to rising (at least three readings/night)

(BP: blood pressure; CNS: central nervous system)

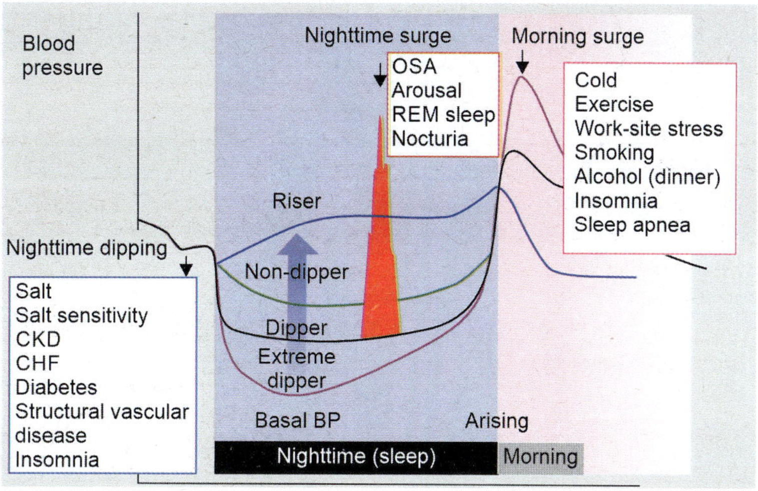

FIG. 1: Components of nocturnal hypertension and determinants—nighttime dipping status and surge in BP.
(BP: blood pressure; CHF: chronic heart failure; CKD: chronic kidney disease; OSA: obstructive sleep apnea; REM: rapid eye movement)

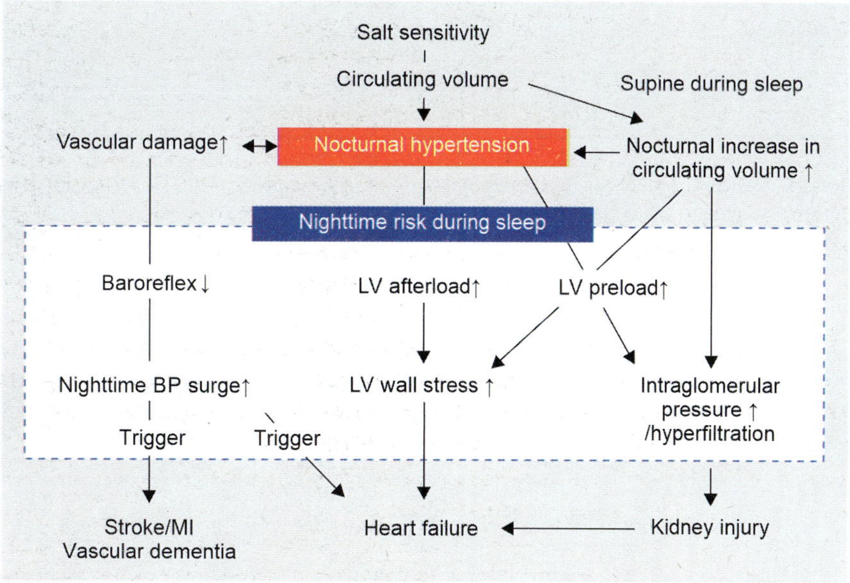

FIG. 2: Mechanism of the effects of nocturnal hypertension on cardiovascular risk.
(BP: blood pressure; LV: left ventricular; MI: myocardial infarction).

intake, diuretics, mineralocorticoid receptor antagonist, sacubitril/valsartan, or sodium-glucose cotransporter-2 (SGLT-2) inhibitors can be used in reducing the circulating volume. CCBs can be used in vascular diseases.

Sympatholytics, renal denervation, or continuous positive airway pressure (CPAP) can be used in obstructive sleep apnea syndrome and increase in sympathetic activity.

In insomnia, melatonin, melatonin receptor antagonists, and orexin receptor blockers can be used.

The benefit of beta blockers in NH significantly has not been demonstrated. In one study, intake of the antihypertensive drug at night resulted in better BP control as compared to morning. CV disease risk are found to be low if antihypertensive drugs are taken at night as combination therapy **(Fig. 3)**.

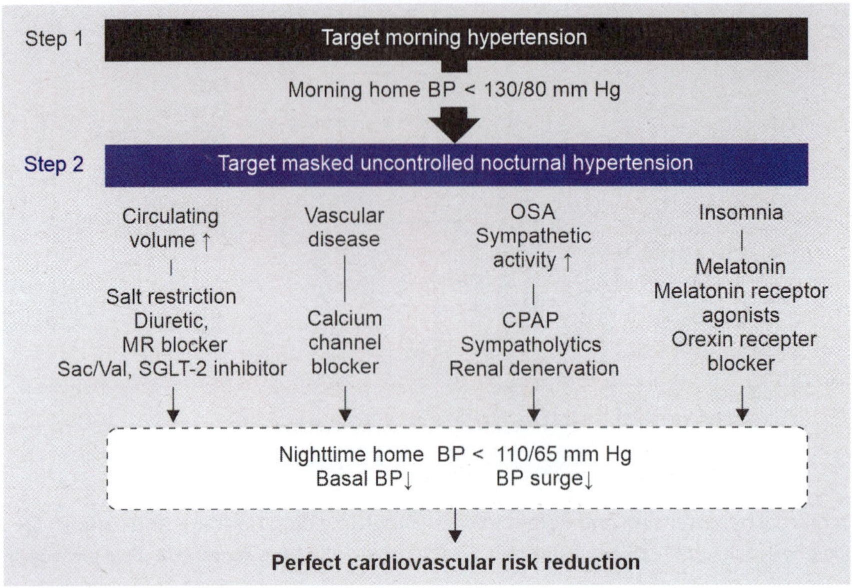

FIG. 3: Possible management strategy of nocturnal hypertension.

(BP: blood pressure; CPAP: continuous positive airway pressure; MR: mineralocorticoid receptor; OSA: obstructive sleep apnea; Sac/Val: sacubitril/valsartan; SGLT-2: sodium-glucose cotransporter-2)

SUGGESTED READINGS

1. Tadic M, Cuspidi C, Grassi G, Mancia G. (2020) Isolated Nocturnal Hypertension: What Do We Know and What Can We Do? Integr Blood Press Control. 2020;13:63-9.
2. Palatini P, Verdecchia P, Beilin LJ, Eguchi K, Imai Y, Kario K, et al. Association of extreme nocturnal dipping with cardiovascular events strongly depends on age. Hypertension. 2020;75:324-30.
3. De la Sierra A, Gorostidi M, Banegas JR, Segura J, de la Cruz JJ, Ruilope LM. Nocturnal hypertension or nondipping: which is better associated with the cardiovascular risk profile? Am J Hypertens. 2014;27:680-7.
4. Kario K. Nocturnal Hypertension. Hypertension. 2018;71:997-1009.
5. Williams B, Mancia G, Spiering W, Rosei EA, Azizi M, Burnier M, et al. 2018 ESC/ESH Guidelines for the management of arterial hypertension. Eur Heart J.2018;39:3021-104.
6. Carey RM, Calhoun DA, Bakris GL, Brook RD, Daugherty SL, Dennison-Himmelfarb CR, et al. Resistant hypertension: Detection, evaluation and management: A Scientific Statement from the American Heart Association. Hypertension. 2018;72:e53-90.

126

CHAPTER

Morning Surge of Blood Pressure

Pritam Gupta, Kamal Garg, Ankur Gupta, Sunita Aggarwal

ABSTRACT

Hypertension is a highly prevalent noncommunicable disease and one of the leading causes of morbidity and mortality in the country. Despite control in office blood pressure (BP), there is risk of masked nocturnal or morning surge of blood pressure (MSBP) which increases the risk of complications and requires appropriate treatment. MSBP is associated with cardiovascular events and has emerged as the strongest predictor of stroke and other complications, independent of the average 24-hour level.

INTRODUCTION

According to the American Heart Association (AHA), morning surge of blood pressure (MSBP) is defined by either "sleep through morning surge" or "prewakening morning surge" or "rising BP surge."

- Sleep through morning surge is defined as the difference between the average morning BP during the first 2 hours after awakening and the average of the lowest nighttime BP.
- Prewakening morning surge is defined as the difference between the average morning BP during the first 2 hours after awakening and the average BP during the last 2 hours before awakening.
- Rising BP surge is defined as morning BP measured on rising minus the BP in a supine position <30 minutes before rising.

An increase in systolic BP by approximately 3 mm Hg/h or diastolic BP by 2 mm Hg/h or an absolute value of >135/85 mm Hg is defined as MSBP **(Table 1)**.

TABLE 1: Criteria for hypertension based on single office blood pressure (BP) measurement, ambulatory blood pressure monitoring (ABPM), and home-based blood pressure monitoring (HBPM), morning surge of blood pressure (MSBP).

Office BP	≥140 and/or >90
ABPM	
24-hour average	≥130 and/or ≥80
Nighttime average	≥120 and/or ≥70
MSBP	≥135 and/or ≥85
Daytime average	≥135 and/or ≥85
HBPM	≥135 and/or ≥85

(DBP: diastolic blood pressure; SBP: systolic blood pressure)

TRIGGERS FOR MORNING SURGE

Triggers for MSBP include:

- Extreme dippers
- Non dippers or risers
- Evening time alcohol intake or smoking
- Insomnia or obstructive sleep apnea (OSA)
- Cold weather, exercise, or stress

Peak MSBP is due to an abnormal increase in renin-angiotensin system (RAS) activity, while the basal morning BP rise is generally attributed to the circulating volume and structural vascular disease with negligible sympathetic tone.

NIGHTTIME DIPPING

Normally during the night, the systolic blood pressure (SBP) usually falls by 10–20% of the daytime SBP which is known as dipping. The following dipping patterns are based on the variation in ambulatory SBP during the night and comparison with typical daytime values:

- *Extreme dippers*: >20% fall in SBP
- *Dippers*: 10–20% fall in SBP
- Nondippers: 0–10% fall in SBP
- *Risers*: No fall or overall rise in SBP

NOCTURNAL HYPERTENSION

- It is defined as nighttime BP of ≥120/70 mm Hg.
- Masked nocturnal hypertension is defined as daytime BP of <130/80 mm Hg (with or without medication) with an increase in nighttime BP during non-rapid eye movement (non-REM) three-fourths.
- This is generally due to increased circulatory volume, salt sensitivity, sympathetic hyperactivation, and vascular damage.
- Nocturnal and MSBP is a blind spot for monitoring as well as drug effectiveness.
- Based on dipping, it predisposes to MSBP which is a strong risk factor for various complications.

PATHOPHYSIOLOGY

There are several pathogenic mechanisms associated with MSBP **(Flowchart 1)**.

Salt sensitivity is increased due to:

- Baseline RAS activation
- Sympathetic overactivity
- Renal dysfunction

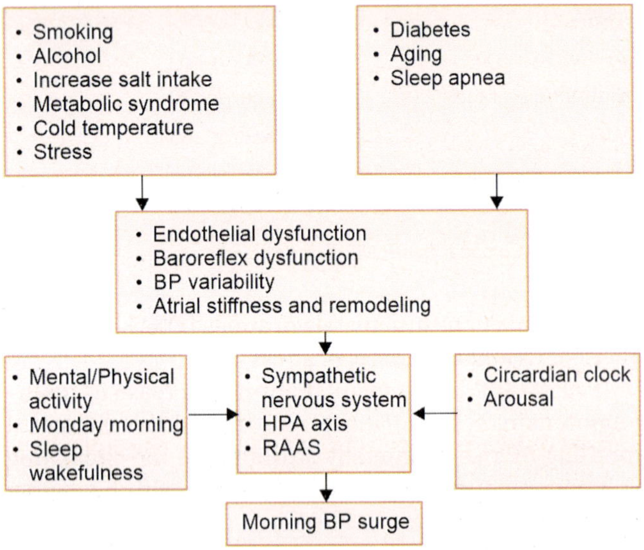

FLOWCHART 1: Pathogenesis of morning surge of BP.

(BP: blood pressure; HPA: hypothalamic-pituitary axis; RAAS: renin–angiotensin–aldosterone system)

There are multiple other factors that cause disturbances in the blood flow and circadian rhythm leading to MSBP. The raised tendency of platelet aggregation secondary to high levels of reactive oxygen species, low nitrous oxide, physiological cortisol peak, and high ubiquitin-proteasome activity also cause MSBP. Advancing age and hypertension are the two major determinants of MSBP. Normally, during sleep sympathetic activity decreases as compared to daytime leading to a slight fall in BP during nighttime. As sleep advances, the proportion of rapid eye movement (REM) sleep increases which is characterized by higher sympathetic activity. Also, there is raised activity of glucocorticoids and mineralocorticoids during the morning hours leading to higher BP during morning hours. As the individual wakes up, sympathetic activity increases further due to the activity of midbrain and basal ganglia nuclei and the circadian rhythm controlled by suprachiasmatic nucleus of the hypothalamus.

These lead to nocturnal hypertension characterized by nondipping or a rise in BP readings. Due to autonomic dysfunction, there is an increased fall in nocturnal BP, eventually increasing stress hormones and higher MSBP readings.

MONITORING

Traditionally, 24-hour ambulatory blood pressure monitoring (ABPM) is considered gold standard to measure MSBP and nocturnal hypertension. It generally measures BP every 20–30 minutes and is considered adequate when >10 day-time readings and >5 night-time readings are collected. It demonstrates BP fluctuation, variability with meals and activity and the target interval required for therapy.

Recently, the use of home-based blood pressure monitoring (HBPM) has been introduced for the measurement. The Japan Morning Surge-Target Organ Protection (J-TOP) study was conducted on MSBP using this device. The device was used to measure 24-hour HBPM at designated intervals and then it was correlated with various parameters such as left ventricular (LV) mass index, interleukin-6 (IL-6), interleukin-18 (IL-18), high-sensitivity C-reactive protein (hs-CRP), urinary albumin/creatinine ratio, peak pulse wave velocity, cardiac troponin, etc. These parameters respond equally with control in ABPM and HBPM with a difference of ~1.5 mm Hg with p value of <0.001. The simple examination of orthostatic BP change using HBPM can detect "home-orthostatic-hypertension" with high reproducibility without a white-coat effect. An increase in the Standard deviation of HBP self-measured in the morning was an independent risk for future cardiovascular events.

Information and communication technology-based night-time home BP monitoring system is a new advancement that directly sends BP measured during the last sleep period at the time of morning readings. Supplementation with pulse rate and oximetry, are particularly more useful in repeated assessments in real-time in conditions associated with triggered BP measurements such as in OSA, arousal, REM sleep, nocturia, etc. Wearable beat-to-beat pressure continuous surge monitoring (WSP) is currently being tested to measure the absolute values of maximum peaks of beat-to-beat pressure. A combined approach of WSP with triggered monitoring is also under development.

With advances in technology, there are patients unmasking these abnormalities which can be potentially dangerous.

Limitations in Monitoring

Just as every other technology, it also comes with its own limitations:

- The day-to-day reproducibility of ABPM affected by physical activity is less than that of HBP self-measured in the sitting position.
- The timing of arising may not be accurate.
- The measurement varies with the physical activity of the patient in the past 12–24 hours.
- The variation may be minimal if the patient remains supine after awakening.

Due to these limitations, the MSBP reactivity could be used as a new measure of MSBP. Using the ABPM data with physical activity simultaneously, we previously calculated the slope of daytime ABP against physical activity measured during the 6-minute period just before each ABP recording as an ambulatory BP reactivity index. This index has a diurnal variation with the morning peak, indicating that the pressors effect of physical activity is augmented more extensively in the morning than at any other period of time.

COMPLICATIONS

Morning surge of hypertension is an independent and strong risk factor for various cardiovascular and noncardiovascular conditions.

It virtually affects every organ of the body. The most important ones are described in **Flowchart 2**.

Cardiac

The heart and the vessels are severely affected with an increased risk of plaque rupture at the peak of hypertension leading to coronary artery disease, ST-T wave flattening, and depression. Even normotensives with clinic BPs < 140/90 mm Hg and 24-hour BPs < 130/80 mm Hg, sleep-trough surge was significantly correlated with left-ventricular myocardial infarction (LV-MI) explained by MSBP.

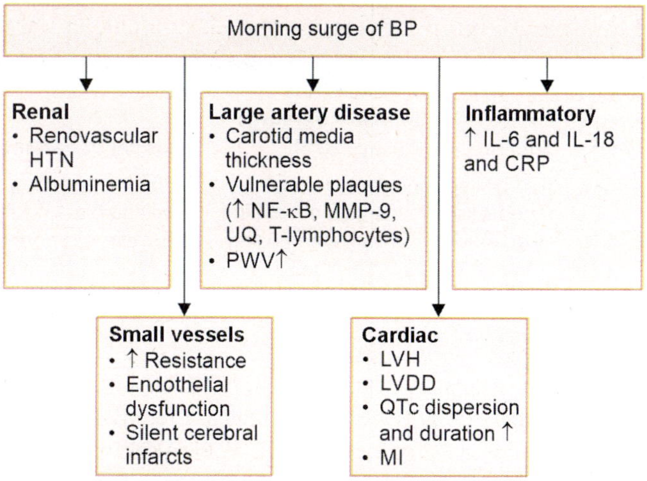

FLOWCHART 2: Complication of morning surge of BP.

[BP: blood pressure; CRP: C-reactive protein; HTN: hypertension; LVH: left-ventricular hypertrophy; LVDD: left ventricular diastolic dysfunction; NF-κB: nuclear factor kappa B (a central transcription factor regulating inflammatory genes); MI: myocardial infarction; MMP-9: matrix metalloproteinase-9 (an important enzyme in plaque rupture); PWV: pulse wave velocity; QTc: corrected QT interval; IL: interleukin; UQ: ubiquitin-proteasome activity]

Autonomic Dysfunction

Arterial baroreflex, which buffers the fluctuations in BP not only through its parasympathetic-mediated action on the heart rate (cardiac baroreflex) but also through modulating the sympathetic outflow to the vasculature (sympathetic baroreflex) is hampered. The parasympathetic tone of the vessels and sympathetic tone of the splanchnic circulation is affected leading to further worsening of ongoing situations. These autonomic variations also alter the circadian rhythm.

Renal

Nocturnal hypertension causes microalbuminuria leads to morning surge, which eventually leads to raised intra-glomerular pressure and also disruption of autoregulation of afferent arteriole.

Hemostasis

Deranged BP readings and raised inflammatory response cause platelet dysfunction and aggregation. This eventually increases the chance of thrombosis and further plaque formation.

With regard to pathophysiology and complications, MSBP is also known as "systemic hemodynamic athero-thrombotic syndrome." Various studies done over the years have shown morning BP surge to be an independent risk factor of various complications **(Table 2)**.

TABLE 2: Seven prospective studies demonstrating the association between morning surge in BP (based on ABPM) and cardiovascular events.

Year	Source	Definition of morning surge by ABPM	Number of patients	Mean follow-up	Cardiovascular end-point	Main findings
2000	Booth III et al. (The Jackson Heart study)	Sleep-trough surge, prewaking surge, and rising morning SBP surge	5,306 community-dwelling black adults ≥20 years old from three countries (mean: 59 years)	14 years	Cardiovascular events and all-cause mortality	For all of the cardiovascular, and all-cause mortality, the hazard ratios in the top decile of the systolic sleep-through surge (62 mm Hg) were 1.25 and 1.43 respectively
2003	Kario et al. (JMS-ABPM study)	Sleep-trough surge and prewaking surge	519 elderly Japanese nondedicated hypertensives (mean: 72 years)	3.4 years	Stroke	Those with a sleep-trough surge of 55 mm Hg (the highest decile) had a higher stroke incidence than those with a surge of 55 mm Hg (19.0% vs. 7.3%; $p = 0.004$) with RR of 2.7
2004	Gosse et al. (Bordeaux Cohort)	Rising surge	507 untreated hypertensives (mean: 49 years)	7.7 years	Cardiovascular events	The rate of cardiovascular events increased significant across all quartiles (maximum: 11% in Q4)
2006	Metoki et al. (Ohasama study)	Prewaking surge and sleep-trough surge	1,430 community-dwelling subjects aged 40 years (mean: 61 years)	10.4 years	Stroke	Those with a prewaking surge of 25 mm Hg (Q5) had a higher hemorrhagic stroke risk (hazard ratio: 4.0) and those with a sleep-trough surge of 40 mm Hg (Q5) had a higher hemorrhagic stroke risk (hazard ratio: 8.9)
2008	Dolan et al. (Dublin Outcome study)	Prewaking surge	11,291 referred hypertensive patients off-medicated (mean: 55 years)	5.3 years	Cardiovascular mortality, stroke mortality, and cardiac mortality	The hazard ratios for a 10 mm Hg increase in morning surge for total cardiovascular, stroke and cardiac mortality were 1.38 (1.31–1.45), 1.37 (1.23–1.51), and 1.39 (1.30–1.49), respectively
2009	Amici et al.	Sleep-trough surge	10 normotensive and 32 well-controlled hypertensive elderly outpatients 135/85 mm Hg of 24-hour BPs (mean: 66 years)	5 years	Cardiovascular events	Those with a sleep-trough surge of 34 mm Hg (the highest tertile: T3) had a higher cardiovascular risk than those with a surge of 34 mm Hg
2010	Li et al. (IDACO)	Sleep-trough surge and prewaking surge	5,645 subjects from 8 populations (mean: 53 years)	11.4 years	Cardiovascular, cardiac, coronary, and cerebrovascular events	For all of the cardiovascular, cardiac, coronary, and cerebrovascular events, and all-cause mortality, the hazard ratios in the top decile of the systolic sleep-through surge (37 mm Hg) were 1.30, 1.52, 1.45, 0.95, and 1.32, respectively

(IDACO: International Database on Ambulatory BP in Relation to Cardiovascular Outcome; RR: relative risk; SBP: systolic blood pressure)

The stroke risk is >2.2 times more in the morning hours (6 AM to 12 PM) compared to the rest of the duration. There is increased LV strain with an eventual increase in MI risk by 34% as per TIMI-2 trials and 8.8% of all infarctions are directly attributable to the morning surge. Also, there is a 2.4-fold increase in the risk of sudden cardiac death. The exogenous factors such as stress, exercise, smoking, and postural change after awakening are found to increase oxygen demand, compensated by raised cardiac output and BP, and are considered as more potent triggers of ischemia.

TREATMENT

According to the 2017 AHA guidelines for the management of hypertension, the goal of a morning BP of <130/80 mm Hg is recommended. A normal morning BP surge is a physiological phenomenon, but an exaggerated MSBP is a cardiovascular risk. Thus, the association between the degree of morning BP surge and cardiovascular risk is not linear but rather has a threshold. This should be addressed by the physician and treatment should be initiated promptly.

The ultimate goal in the management of hypertension is to achieve good 24-hour BP control which includes:

- Lowering 24-hour BP
- Maintaining the nocturnal BP and dipping
- Maintain MSBP
- Suppressing exaggerated variability in blood pressure

The main strategy is to target the mechanisms causing the morning surge of BP given in **Flowchart 1** and directed treatment strategies in **Flowchart 3**.

Longer half-lives and a greater peak-to-trough ratio are associated with most of the frequently used drugs. The ability of calcium channel blockers (CCBs) to lower BP rely on the patient's baseline BP level; the lower nocturnal BP does not decline as much, and the highest ABP levels do. As a result, MSBP is greatly reduced, hence these are the ones preferred. The most popular and initial regimen is amlodipine, which has a half-life of about 40 hours.

When morning hypertension is treated with diuretics, overnight BP levels are primarily decreased compared to daytime blood pressure, and nondippers change toward dipper status and are therefore favored in those patients.

There is also a lot of testing and utilization of other therapies. The lisinopril/angiotensin II receptor blocker olmesartan medoxomil and the CCB amlodipine were found to have equal angiotensin-converting enzyme inhibitor effectiveness. Candesartan and valsartan are additional prominent medications in this group.

Due to the sympathetic nervous system (SNS)'s participation in the morning surge, the function of beta blockers in the early morning is intriguing.

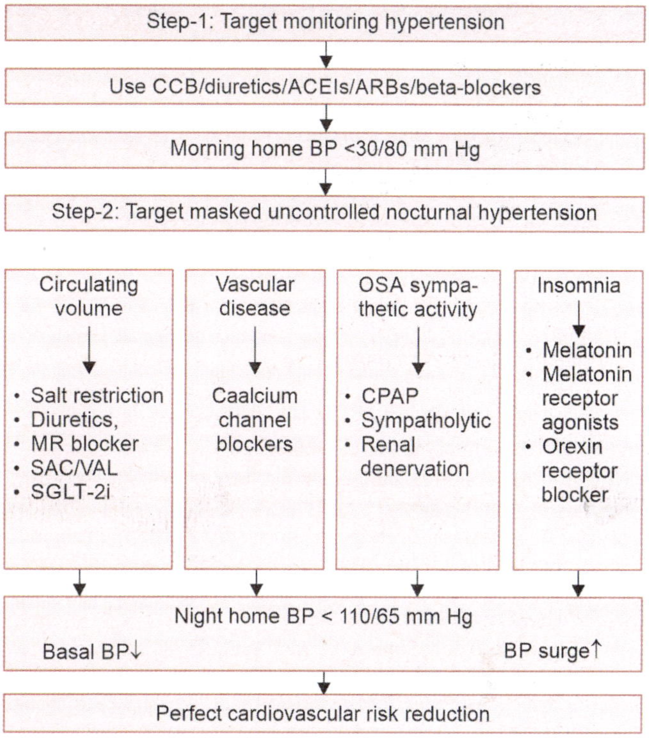

FLOWCHART 3: Directed treatment strategies.

(ACEIs: angiotensin-converting enzyme inhibitors; ARBs: angiotensin receptor blockers; BP: blood pressure; CCB: calcium channel blockers; CPAP: continuous positive airway pressure; OSA: obstructive sleep apnea; SAC/VAL: sacubitril/valsartan; SGLT-2i: sodium-glucose cotransporter-2 inhibitors)

For drugs with shorter half-lives, intake timing should be monitored according to the chronobiological cycle. These drugs are generally given during evening hours in order to maintain nocturnal and morning surge. Various other pharmacological aspects should be taken into concern. Benefits from anti-inflammatory treatment using statins, RAS inhibitors, and thiazolidinediones, have also been found promising.

The association of MSBP with adverse cardiovascular events suggests that a strict treatment schedule targeting this phenomenon is needed.

CONCLUSION

In the present scenario, management of hypertension should be better, earlier, and with minimal variability, especially during morning and nocturnal periods. We should aim at maintaining a normal circadian rhythm and MSBP management by monitoring ABPM, 24-hour HBPM is very important as it can prevent or decrease the risk of both future cardiovascular and noncardiovascular events. Therapies with longer half-lives are used to cover nocturnal and MSBP.

To make precise anticipation, more research and development is needed in regard to making new devices and therapies for the betterment of mankind.

SUGGESTED READINGS

1. Booth JN 3rd, Jaeger BC, Huang L, Abdalla M, Sims M, Butler M, et al. Morning Blood Pressure Surge and Cardiovascular Disease Events and All-Cause Mortality in Blacks: The Jackson Heart Study. Hypertension. 2020;75(3):835-43.
2. Kario K. Morning surge in blood pressure and cardiovascular risk evidence and perspectives. Hypertension. 2010;56(5):765-73.
3. Unger T, Borghi C, Charchar F, Khan NA, Poulter NR, Prabhakaran D, et al. 2020 International Society of Hypertension Global Hypertension Practice Guidelines. Hypertension. 2020;75(6):1334-57.
4. Kario K. Nocturnal hypertension: new technology and evidence. Hypertension. 2018;71(6):997-1009.
5. Linsell CR, Lightman SL, Mullen PE, Brown MJ, Causon RC. Circadian rhythms of epinephrine and norepinephrine in man. J Clin Endocrinol Metab. 1985;60(6):1210-5.
6. Kimura G. Kidney and circadian blood pressure rhythm. Hypertension. 2008;51(4):827-8.
7. Kario K. Proposal of RAS-diuretic vs. RAS-calcium antagonist strategies in high-risk hypertension: insight from the 24-hour ambulatory blood pressure profile and central pressure. J Am Soc Hypertens. 2010;4(5):215-8.
8. Kario K, Hoshide S, Shimizu M, Yano Y, Eguchi K, Ishikawa J, et al. Effect of dosing time of angiotensin II receptor blockade titrated by self-measured blood pressure recordings on cardiorenal protection in hypertensives: the Japan Morning Surge-Target Organ Protection (J-TOP) study. J Hypertens. 2010;28(7):1574-83.
9. Jones H, Atkinson G, Leary A, George K, Murphy M, Waterhouse J. Reactivity of ambulatory blood pressure to physical activity varies with time of day. Hypertension. 2006;47(4):778-84.
10. Gosse P, Lasserre R, Minifié C, Lemetayer P, Clementy J. Blood pressure surge on rising. J Hypertens. 2004;22(6):1113-8.
11. Metoki H, Ohkubo T, Kikuya M, Asayama K, Obara T, Hashimoto J, et al. Prognostic significance for stroke of a morning pressor surge and a nocturnal blood pressure decline: the Ohasama study. Hypertension. 2006;47(2):149-54.
12. Dolan E, Stanton A, Thijs L, Hinedi K, Atkins N, McClory S, et al. Superiority of ambulatory over clinic blood pressure measurement in predicting mortality: the Dublin outcome study. Hypertension. 2005;46(1):156-61.
13. Amici A, Cicconetti P, Sagrafoli C, Baratta A, Passador P, Pecci T, et al. Exaggerated morning blood pressure surge and cardiovascular events. A 5-year longitudinal study in normotensive and well-controlled hypertensive elderly. Arch Gerontol Geriatr. 2009;49(2):e105-9.
14. Li Y, Thijs L, Hansen TW, Kikuya M, Boggia J, Richart T, et al. Prognostic value of the morning blood pressure surge in 5645 subjects from 8 populations. Hypertension. 2010;55(4):1040-8.
15. Feit F, Mueller HS, Braunwald E, Ross R, Hodges M, Herman MV, et al. Thrombolysis in Myocardial Infarction (TIMI) phase II trial: outcome comparison of a "conservative strategy" in community versus tertiary hospitals. The TIMI Research Group. J Am Coll Cardiol. 1990;16(7):1529-34.
16. Kario K, Pickering TG, Umeda Y, Hoshide S, Hoshide Y, Morinari M, et al. Morning surge in blood pressure as a predictor of silent and clinical cerebrovascular disease in elderly hypertensives: a prospective study. Circulation. 2003;107(10):1401-6.

127

CHAPTER

Hypertension Management: The Role of Circadian Rhythm

Amit A Saraf, Bitukaur Sodhi

ABSTRACT

The regulation of blood pressure by the circadian rhythm is an intricate process which is not completely understood till date. Understanding the various abnormalities in the blood pressure rhythm caused due to disruption of the circadian rhythm and utilizing this understanding in developing a treatment plan to efficiently control the blood pressure and reduce the morbidity and mortality are daunting tasks. With multiple clinical trials and knowledge of an individual's blood pressure pattern with the help of ambulatory blood pressure monitoring, we are now a step closer to applying the benefit of chronotherapy in the management of hypertension and improving the overall health status of the patient.

INTRODUCTION

Circadian rhythm is an endogenous biorhythm comprising a 24-hour cycle, the driving force for which is an intrinsic molecular clock that responds to the external environmental changes by bringing about adjustments in behavior and physiological activities. The master pacemaker, suprachiasmatic nucleus, resides in the hypothalamus and exerts control over all the peripheral clocks maintaining synchrony.

Figure 1 represents the anatomic organization of the circadian clock network.

This feedback loop is synchronized with sunrise each day by photosensitive melanopsin-expressing neurons present in the retina. The impulses are transmitted via the retinohypothalamic tract to the suprachiasmatic nucleus, thereby allowing mammals to maintain the intrinsic rhythms in accordance with the external light-dark cycle. The suprachiasmatic nucleus sends output to different regions of thalamus and hypothalamus, thereby regulating the sleep-wake cycle, feeding, temperature, hormonal rhythms, and the autonomic system. It also signals the pineal gland and regulates secretion of melatonin. The output from suprachiasmatic nucleus also reaches the peripheral clocks—liver, adrenals, pancreas, etc.

Under normal light-dark cycles, the circadian system is entrained daily, thus producing diurnal rhythms of 24 hours. Light, meals, and activity patterns act as zeitgebers for the circadian clock.

As per the latest American Heart Association (AHA) guidelines, a systolic blood pressure of ≥130 mm Hg or a diastolic blood pressure ≥80 mm Hg is defined as hypertension. The global burden of hypertension is estimated to be around 1.4 billion, which represents 31% of the total population. The effect of circadian rhythm on blood pressure is evident on measuring the pressure at different times of the day—surge in the morning, plateau in the afternoon, and dip at night. In patients with hypertension, this blood pressure variation gets disrupted and is associated with adverse outcomes. Abnormal blood pressure rhythms include reverse dipping (nocturnal rise in the blood pressure), extreme dipping (more than 20% drop in the nocturnal blood pressure in comparison to daytime blood pressure), nondipping (<10% drop in the nocturnal blood pressure as compared to daytime), and isolated nocturnal hypertension (nighttime systolic blood pressure ≥120 mm Hg and diastolic blood pressure ≥70 mm Hg with daytime <135/85 mm Hg). The last two patterns are associated with an increased risk of hypertension-induced organ damage and an overall worst outcome.

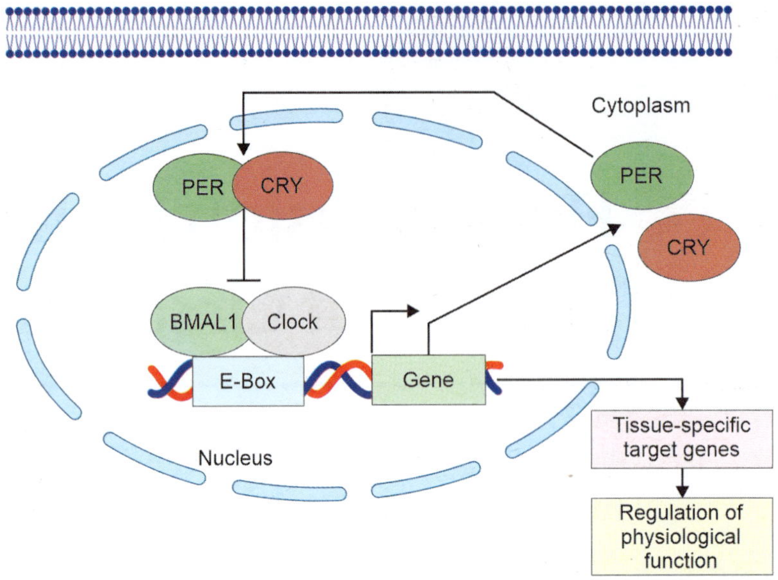

FIG. 1: Core components of the circadian clock. CLOCK and BMAL1 heterodimerize and bind E-box response elements within promoter regions of target genes, including period and cryptochrome (encoding PER1/2/3 and CRY1/2, respectively). In the negative feedback loops, PER and CRY heterodimerize and repress the activity of BMAL1 and CLOCK. This clock mechanism regulates tissue-specific target genes to regulate many physiological processes.

CIRCADIAN RHYTHM AND BLOOD PRESSURE REGULATION

The circadian pattern of blood pressure is affected by various factors. Melatonin released from the pineal gland at night is responsible not only for improving sleep but also for reducing nocturnal blood pressure. Atrial natriuretic peptide, an important regulator of the 24-hour blood pressure pattern, is released in an out-of-phase manner with respect to the blood pressure rhythm. Hormones contributing to the blood pressure pattern include renin, angiotensin-converting enzyme, angiotensin II, aldosterone, and thyroid hormone. Nitric oxide, released by the endothelial cells, also contributes to the blood pressure regulation by exerting its effects on the vascular tone.

The peripheral clocks playing a role in regulating the blood pressure rhythm include smooth muscles, liver, perivascular adipose tissue, adrenal glands, and kidney. The exact mechanisms of regulation are poorly understood, but studies have shown that the *BMAL1* gene seems to be of great significance. In smooth muscles, *BMAL1* is responsible for the diurnal variations in phenylephrine and serotonin-induced vasoconstriction of renal and mesenteric arteries. *BMAL1* exerts its effects on the perivascular adipose tissue indirectly by regulating the transcription of angiotensinogen and thereby angiotensin II levels which ultimately determine the contractility of the perivascular adipose tissue and thus the vascular tone. In the kidneys, *BMAL1* acts on the distal portions of the nephron and regulates renal sodium excretion. The exact role of liver and adrenal glands in the regulation is still under study.

Recent studies have brought to light the relationship between circadian clock and gut microbiota, demonstrating that both of them exert an effect on each other and that gut microbiota dysbiosis is a contributing factor in the development of hypertension **(Fig. 2)**.

In addition to the humoral, endocrine, and neural regulatory factors, sleep pattern, timing of food intake, temperature, noise, and other environmental factors are also found to play a role in regulating the blood pressure.

MANAGEMENT

The disruption in the circadian variation of the blood pressure rhythm, especially the presence of nondipping pattern, increases the morbidity and mortality risk associated with cardiovascular diseases. In addition, it also leads to rapid progression of renal damage and increased risk of nephropathy. In such a scenario, antihypertensives acting on the renin–angiotensin–aldosterone system, namely the angiotensin converting enzyme (ACE) inhibitors and angiotensin receptor blockers (ARBs), take on a crucial role in reducing the risk.

Chronotherapy has demonstrated relevance in the management of rheumatoid arthritis and certain malignancies. Now its effects are being studied extensively

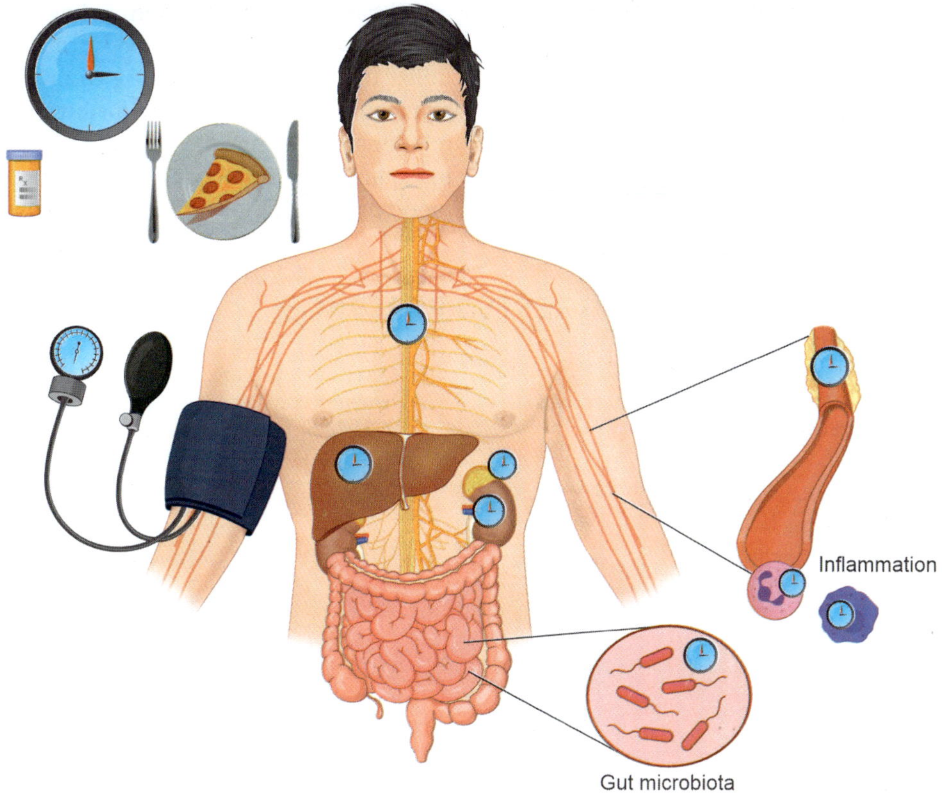

FIG. 2: Cellular circadian clocks throughout the body, entrained by food cues, contributing to the circadian rhythm of blood pressure (BP). BP has a 24-hour cycle, peaking during the day and dipping by 10–20% during the night. Studies in rodents and humans suggest that peripheral clocks within the vasculature, liver, adrenal glands, kidneys, microbiota in the gut, immune system, and autonomic nervous system contribute to regulation of the circadian rhythm of BP. These peripheral clocks can be entrained by food cues; therefore, time-of-day feeding could be important for BP rhythm. Dysregulation of the circadian rhythm of BP is associated with adverse cardiorenal outcomes and increased risk of cardiovascular mortality. There are ongoing clinical trials to determine if chronotherapy will be beneficial for hypertension management, and this should be expanded to whether it can correct any losses of BP rhythm.

in the management of hypertension in a bid to help specifically the group of patients with the nondipping pattern of hypertension since this pattern is the one associated with relatively worse outcomes as compared to the other ones.

Studies carried out with multiple ACE inhibitor—trandolapril, enalapril, ramipril, a combination of captopril and hydrochlorothiazide, spirapril, and quinapril—showed that with bedtime administration of these medications, there was a better and more effective control of blood pressure.

Studies have shown that administration of the ARB valsartan at bedtime caused a 6% increase in the difference between nocturnal and daytime blood pressure, thereby causing the blood pressure pattern to turn more similar to a "dipper" pattern rather than a nondipper. Addition of the calcium channel blocker amlodipine to valsartan at nighttime helped with the management of not only nocturnal blood pressure but also daytime blood pressure, thereby providing an efficient 24-hour control. Results similar to valsartan were seen with telmisartan and olmesartan.

Administration of nifedipine at bedtime not only resulted in a more efficient blood pressure management but also lowered the incidence of edema and other side effects associated with it.

However, the opinions on nighttime administration of medications are still divided, thanks to the contradicting results of clinical trials. On one hand, the Hygia trial showed reduced nighttime systolic blood pressure, lower prevalence of nondipping blood pressure, and 45% reduction in primary cardiovascular disease outcome in bedtime ingestion patients, compared with morning dosing, but on the other hand the HARMONY trial showed no significant differences in 24-hour, daytime, or nighttime systolic blood pressure between morning and evening administration of antihypertensive medication.

The TIME trial, a randomized UK-based trial, demonstrated that the antihypertensives can be taken at any time of the day as per the preference of the patient. The BedMed-Frail trial is currently ongoing and it will most likely shed more light on the relationship between the timing of administration of the medicine and blood pressure control.

Circadian rhythm definitely has an important role to play in the regulation of blood pressure, but how do we utilize this relation for tailoring antihypertensive therapy is still a question mark. Maybe further studies exploring this relationship and the effect of antihypertensives will help us in expanding our knowledge and formulating an efficient blood pressure management control plan for the patients.

SUGGESTED READINGS

1. Zhang J, Sun R, Jiang T, Yang G, Chen L. Circadian blood pressure rhythm in cardiovascular and renal health and disease. Biomolecules. 2021;11(6):868.
2. Costello HM, Gumz ML. Circadian rhythm, clock genes, and hypertension: Recent advances in hypertension. Hypertension. 2021;78(5):1185-96.

128

CHAPTER

Early End-organ Protection in Hypertension

Saibal Chakravorty, Aditya Chakravorty

ABSTRACT

Hypertension, or high blood pressure (BP), is a significant risk factor for the development and progression of chronic kidney disease (CKD). In fact, hypertension is the second leading cause of CKD, with diabetes being the first. Early end-organ protection is essential in patients with hypertension and CKD to prevent or delay the onset of end-stage renal disease (ESRD) and cardiovascular events. Use of various biomarkers for risk stratification and early assessment of end-organ damage along with administration of various cardio- and nephroprotective agents can prevent morbidity and mortality.

INTRODUCTION

One of the main goals of hypertension management is to reduce blood pressure (BP) to target levels, which may differ based on the presence of comorbidities like chronic kidney disease (CKD). Several guidelines recommend a BP target of < 130/80 mm Hg in patients with hypertension and CKD, particularly those with albuminuria or proteinuria. This target can be achieved through lifestyle modifications and pharmacologic interventions including angiotensin-converting enzyme (ACE) inhibitors and angiotensin receptor blockers (ARBs) .

Angiotensin-converting enzyme inhibitors and ARBs are first-line agents for the management of hypertension in patients with CKD, particularly those with albuminuria or proteinuria. These medications have renoprotective effects beyond their BP-lowering effects including reducing proteinuria and slowing the progression of CKD. Several large randomized controlled trials have demonstrated the benefits of ACE inhibitors and ARBs in patients with hypertension and CKD. For example, the REIN (Ramipril Efficacy In Nephropathy) study showed that ramipril, an ACE inhibitor, reduced proteinuria and slowed the progression of CKD in patients with type 1 diabetes and nephropathy. The RENAAL (Reduction of Endpoints in NIDDM with the Angiotensin II Antagonist Losartan) study showed that losartan, an ARB, reduced the risk of end-stage renal disease (ESRD), cardiovascular events, and death in patients with type 2 diabetes mellitus (T2DM) and nephropathy.

In addition to BP control and renoprotective medications, early end-organ protection in hypertension and CKD should include lifestyle modifications, such as a healthy diet, regular exercise, and smoking cessation. Several studies have shown that a healthy diet, such as the DASH (Dietary Approaches to Stop Hypertension) diet, can lower BP and reduce the risk of cardiovascular events and CKD progression. Regular exercise can also lower BP and improve cardiovascular and renal function.

USE OF BIOMARKERS TO PREDICT ORGAN DAMAGE

Biomarkers have become an important tool for predicting and monitoring the development of organ damage in hypertension and CKD. One of the most commonly used biomarkers for predicting organ damage in hypertension is high-sensitivity cardiac troponin (hs-cTn). Hs-cTn is a marker of myocardial injury and has been shown to be predictive of adverse cardiovascular outcomes in patients with hypertension. A recent study by Kawasaki et al. (2013)

found that hs-cTn was associated with left ventricular hypertrophy and myocardial fibrosis in patients with hypertension.

Another biomarker that has been studied in the context of hypertension and CKD is urinary albumin-to-creatinine ratio (UACR). UACR is a marker of kidney damage and has been shown to be predictive of the development of CKD in patients with hypertension. A recent meta-analysis by He et al. (2022) found that UACR was a significant predictor of the progression of CKD in patients with hypertension. This highlights the importance of UACR as a biomarker for identifying patients with hypertension who are at high risk of developing CKD.

In addition to hs-cTn and UACR, other biomarkers have been studied for their ability to predict organ damage in hypertension and CKD. These include serum creatinine, cystatin C, and brain natriuretic peptide (BNP). A study by Lin et al. (2020) found that serum cystatin C was a significant predictor of the development of CKD in patients with hypertension. Meanwhile, a study by Sakuma et al. (2010) found that BNP was a significant predictor of the development of heart failure in patients with CKD.

In a subanalysis of the BIOSTAT-CHF study, Ferreira et al. (2020) found that elevated hs-Tn levels were associated with an increased risk of all-cause mortality and cardiovascular death in patients with chronic heart failure and hypertension. These findings suggest that hs-Tn may be a useful biomarker for risk stratification and the early detection of cardiovascular damage in hypertensive patients.

Finally, BNP has been proposed as a biomarker for the prediction of cardiovascular events in hypertensive patients. BNP is a marker of cardiac dysfunction that has been shown to predict adverse cardiovascular events in patients with CKD and hypertension. In a prospective study, left atrial diameter (LAD), left ventricular ejection fraction (LVEF), ultrafiltration rate (UFR), age, and sex were utilized to ascertain the levels of B-type natriuretic peptide. A positive association was observed between BNP and LAD, indicating that BNP could serve as a valuable means of estimating the presence of left atrial enlargement. Additionally, the combination of BNP and LVEF proved to be a significant risk factor in predicting both all-cause mortality and cardiovascular events in patients undergoing hemodialysis.

RISK STRATIFICATION AND ASSESSMENT OF EARLY ORGAN INVOLVEMENT IN HYPERTENSION

Risk stratification involves evaluating a patient's overall risk for cardiovascular disease (CVD) and other hypertension-related complications. Several factors may be considered, such as age, sex, family history, smoking status, BP levels, and the presence of other medical conditions, such as diabetes or high cholesterol.

One of the most widely used biomarkers for the assessment of early organ damage in hypertension is albuminuria. Several studies have shown that albuminuria is a strong predictor of cardiovascular and renal events in hypertensive patients.

In addition to albuminuria, several other biomarkers have been proposed as predictors of cardiovascular and renal events in hypertension. Cystatin C is a marker of glomerular filtration rate (GFR) that has been shown to predict the development of CKD in hypertensive patients. In a prospective study of nondiabetic patients, Spanaus et al. (2010) found that elevated serum cystatin C levels were associated with an increased risk of CKD development. The ability to detect even slight decline in kidney function is well demonstrated by the diagnostic accuracy of serum creatinine, cystatin C, or BNP. These markers offer dependable risk assessment for the advancement of kidney disease in individuals with CKD.

ASSESSMENT OF EARLY ORGAN INVOLVEMENT

In addition to risk stratification, early detection of organ damage is also important in hypertension management. Townsend et al. (2015) discuss the use of pulse wave analysis to assess arterial stiffness, which can be an early sign of hypertension-related organ damage. The article recommends using pulse wave analysis in conjunction with other tests such as echocardiography and urinalysis to assess organ damage in hypertensive patients.

Blood tests such as creatinine and electrolyte levels may be used to assess kidney function, while blood glucose and lipid levels may be used to evaluate overall cardiovascular risk. A fundoscopy is done to assess changes in the blood vessels of the eye.

Mancia et al. (2013) provide evidence for the importance of risk stratification and early detection of organ damage in hypertension management. The 2013 European Society of Hypertension/European Society of Cardiology (ESH/ESC) guidelines and the 2017 American College of Cardiology (ACC) Expert Consensus Decision Pathway both recommend using risk stratification to guide hypertension management. Additionally, the 2009 article by Mancia et al. emphasizes the importance of individualized treatment plans based on risk stratification and organ damage assessments, particularly in elderly patients.

USE OF CYSTATIN C, LIPOPROTEIN AS INDICATORS OF EARLY ORGAN DAMAGE

Cystatin C is a small protein produced by all nucleated cells and is freely filtered by the glomerulus. A study followed elderly individuals and found that higher levels of cystatin C, a marker of renal function, were associated with an increased risk of death and cardiovascular events. The study concluded that cystatin C may be a better marker of renal function than creatinine, particularly in older adults.

Lipoprotein abnormalities have also been implicated in the pathogenesis of hypertension and CKD. Elevated low-density lipoprotein (LDL) levels have been shown to be associated with increased risk of cardiovascular morbidity and mortality. Guidelines from the American Association of Clinical Endocrinologists and American College of Endocrinology recommend using lipoproteins, specifically low-density lipoprotein cholesterol (LDL-C) as indicators of cardiovascular risk. The guidelines suggest that LDL-C levels should be measured in all adults with hypertension, and that aggressive lipid-lowering therapy should be considered for those at high risk of cardiovascular event.

A study examined the association between lipoprotein(a) [Lp(a)] levels and subclinical atherosclerosis in patients with hypertension. The study found that higher levels of Lp(a) were associated with an increased risk of subclinical atherosclerosis, even after adjusting for traditional cardiovascular risk factors.

NUTRITIONAL MEASURES AS PREVENTION OF ORGAN DAMAGE

Nutritional measures have emerged as a potential strategy to prevent organ damage in hypertension and CKD. One of the nutritional measures that have been extensively studied is the reduction of salt intake. Moreover, a meta-analysis of randomized controlled trials showed that a modest reduction in salt intake leads to a significant reduction in cardiovascular events including stroke and myocardial infarction. These findings suggest that reducing salt intake is an effective strategy to prevent organ damage in hypertension and CKD.

Another nutritional measure that has been investigated is the consumption of fruits and vegetables. Fruits and vegetables are rich in vitamins, minerals, and antioxidants, which have been shown to have a protective effect on cardiovascular health. In addition, a randomized controlled trial showed that increasing fruit and vegetable intake led to a significant reduction in BP and proteinuria in patients with CKD.

Omega-3 polyunsaturated fatty acids (PUFAs) have been shown to have a beneficial effect on lipid metabolism, inflammation, and endothelial function. Several randomized controlled trials have demonstrated that omega-3 PUFA supplementation leads to a reduction in BP, proteinuria, and cardiovascular events in patients with hypertension and CKD. These findings suggest that omega-3 PUFA supplementation may prevent organ damage in hypertension and CKD.

PHYSICAL ACTIVITY AND EARLY ORGAN PROTECTION IN HYPERTENSION AND CKD

Physical activity is an important lifestyle modification that can provide early organ protection in patients with hypertension and CKD. In a randomized controlled trial, Kokkinos (2012) and Seligman et al. (2011) evaluated the effects of a 12-week exercise program on BP, arterial stiffness, and renal function in patients with hypertension and early-stage CKD. The exercise group showed significant improvements in BP, arterial stiffness, and estimated glomerular filtration rate (eGFR), compared to the control group. These findings suggest that regular physical activity can provide early renal protection in patients with hypertension and CKD.

WEIGHT REDUCTION AND EARLY ORGAN PROTECTION WITH HYPERTENSION AND CKD

Weight reduction is an essential component of lifestyle modification for the prevention and management of hypertension and CKD. Studies have shown that weight loss can improve BP control, reduce proteinuria, and slow the progression of CKD. A randomized controlled trial conducted by Navaneethan et al. (2009) demonstrated that weight loss through a low-calorie diet and exercise in overweight and obese individuals with CKD resulted in significant reductions in BP and proteinuria, as well as improvements in kidney function. Another study by Bhavsar et al. (2011) found that in hypertensive patients with obesity and T2DM, weight loss through a lifestyle intervention program led to significant reductions in BP and albuminuria, which are key markers of kidney damage. These findings highlight the importance of weight reduction as a therapeutic approach to early organ protection in hypertension and CKD.

SMOKING AND END-ORGAN DAMAGE WITH EVIDENCE AND PREVENTION

Smoking is a well-established risk factor for various end-organ damage including CVD, stroke, and CKD. Hypertension is another significant risk factor for these conditions, and when combined with smoking, the risk for end-organ damage increases significantly. Smoking leads to vasoconstriction, platelet activation, and endothelial dysfunction, ultimately resulting in an increased risk of atherosclerosis and vascular damage.

The impact of smoking on end-organ damage in hypertension and CKD is well established. A study by Sauriasari et al. (2010) found that smoking was associated with an increased risk of cardiovascular events, stroke, and all-cause mortality in patients with hypertension. Similarly, a meta-analysis by Jo et al. (2020a) showed that smoking was associated with an increased risk of CKD development and progression in patients with hypertension. The study also found that smoking cessation could significantly slow the progression of CKD.

GUIDELINES FOR INITIATING NEPHROPROTECTIVE AGENTS EARLY

Nephroprotective agents are drugs that have been shown to have a beneficial effect on kidney function and are recommended for patients with CKD. Several nephroprotective agents have been identified that have been shown to slow the progression of CKD and reduce the risk of ESRD.

Sodium-glucose cotransporter-2 (SGLT2) inhibitors are a relatively new class of drugs that have been shown to have a nephroprotective effect in patients with diabetes and CKD. These drugs work by reducing glucose reabsorption in the kidneys, which lead to a reduction in proteinuria and a slower decline in GFR. The DAPA-CKD (Dapagliflozin and Prevention of Adverse Outcomes in Chronic Kidney Disease) study demonstrated that dapagliflozin reduced the risk of kidney failure or death from kidney or cardiovascular causes in patients with CKD, regardless of whether they had diabetes or not. It showed significant benefits in terms of preserving kidney function and reducing the risk of adverse outcomes.

The CREDENCE study demonstrated that canagliflozin reduced the risk of kidney failure, ESRD, and cardiovascular events in patients with T2DM and CKD. Similar to the DAPA-CKD study, this trial provided strong evidence for the use of SGLT-2 inhibitors as a beneficial treatment option for patients with CKD. Both the DAPA-CKD and CREDENCE studies have shown promising results in improving kidney outcomes in patients with CKD, highlighting the potential of SGLT-2 inhibitors in the management of this condition.

Mineralocorticoid receptor antagonists (MRAs): MRAs have been shown to have a beneficial effect on kidney function in patients with heart failure and CKD. These drugs work by blocking the action of aldosterone, which leads to a reduction in proteinuria and a slower decline in GFR. MRAs are recommended for patients with heart failure and CKD who have an eGFR ≥ 30 mL/min/1.73 m^2 and albuminuria.

Hydroxymethylglutaryl-coenzyme A (HMG-CoA) reductase inhibitors (statins): Statins are commonly used to manage dyslipidemia in patients with CKD. These drugs have been shown to have a beneficial effect on kidney function by reducing proteinuria and slowing the decline in GFR. Statins are recommended for patients with CKD who have dyslipidemia or a high risk of CVD.

The early initiation of these agents is crucial in the management of CKD to slow the decline in kidney function and prevent the development of ESRD. The guidelines for initiating nephroprotective agents in CKD management include ACE inhibitors and ARBs, SGLT-2 inhibitors, MRAs, and statins.

■ ACE/ARB—RENAAL and IDNT Innovation

Angiotensin-converting enzyme inhibitors and ARBs are commonly prescribed medications for the management of CKD due to their renoprotective benefits. The landmark clinical trials, RENAAL and IDNT (Irbesartan Diabetic Nephropathy Trial), evaluated the effects of these medications on renal outcomes in patients with diabetic nephropathy and hypertensive nephrosclerosis, respectively.

The RENAAL study showed that the ARB losartan significantly reduced the risk of ESRD and death in patients with T2DM and nephropathy, compared to placebo. In this study, losartan also reduced proteinuria and BP, highlighting the importance of these factors in the progression of CKD.

The IDNT study compared the effects of the ACE inhibitor benazepril, the ARB irbesartan, and a combination of both medications on renal outcomes in patients with hypertension and nephrosclerosis. Both irbesartan and the combination therapy significantly reduced the risk of ESRD compared to benazepril, while also reducing proteinuria and BP.

More recently, the INNOVATION study evaluated the effects of the ACE inhibitor lisinopril combined with the ARB valsartan compared to valsartan alone on renal outcomes in patients with T2DM and CKD. The combination therapy did not significantly reduce the risk of ESRD compared to valsartan alone, but did reduce proteinuria and BP. Close monitoring of renal function, BP, and adverse effects is also necessary when using these drugs.

CONCLUSION

Hypertension in CKD should be managed aggressively in order to prevent end-organ damage. ACE inhibitors, ARBs, and SGLT-2 inhibitors play a significant role in controlling BP in CKD along with reduction of proteinuria and delaying progression to ESRD. These medications reduce the risk of ESRD and improve renal outcomes in patients with diabetic nephropathy and hypertensive nephrosclerosis, but individual patient factors should be considered when making treatment decisions. Several newly discovered biomarkers including hs-cTn, UACR, cystatin C, BNP, and lipoproteins play an important role in risk stratification and early assessment of end-organ damage in CKD. Nutritional measures, physical activity, weight reduction, and cessation of smoking are important lifestyle modifications for prevention of end-organ damage in diabetes, hypertension, and CKD.

SUGGESTED READINGS

1. Kidney Disease: Improving Global Outcomes (KDIGO) Blood Pressure Work Group. KDIGO 2021 Clinical Practice Guideline for the Management of Blood Pressure in Chronic Kidney Disease. Kidney Int. 2021;99(3S):S1-S87.
2. Kidney Disease: Improving Global Outcomes (KDIGO) CKD-MBD Update Work Group. KDIGO 2017 Clinical Practice Guideline Update for the Diagnosis, Evaluation, Prevention, and Treatment of Chronic Kidney Disease-Mineral and Bone Disorder (CKD-MBD). Kidney Int Suppl (2011). 2017;7(1):1-59.
3. Kidney Disease Outcomes Quality Initiative (K/DOQI) Group. K/DOQI clinical practice guidelines for management of dyslipidemias in patients with kidney disease. Am J Kidney Dis. 2003;41(4 Suppl 3):I-IV, S1-91.
4. Heerspink HJL, Jongs N, Chertow GM, Langkilde AM, McMurray JJV, Correa-Rotter R, et al. Effect of dapagliflozin on the rate of decline in kidney function in patients with chronic kidney disease with and without type 2 diabetes: a prespecified analysis from the DAPA-CKD trial. Lancet Diabetes Endocrinol. 2021;9(11):743-54. Erratum in: Lancet Diabetes Endocrinol. 2022;10(10):e10.
5. Botdorf J, Chaudhary K, Whaley-Connell A. Hyper-tension in cardiovascular and kidney disease. Cardiorenal Med. 2011;1(3):183-92.
6. Gansevoort RT, Correa-Rotter R, Hemmelgarn BR, Jafar TH, Heerspink HJL, Mann JF et al. Chronic kidney disease and cardiovascular risk: epidemiology, mechanisms, and prevention. Lancet. 2013;382(9889):339-52.
7. Whelton PK, Carey RM, Aronow WS, Casey Jr DE, Collins KJ, Dennison Himmelfarb C et al. 2017ACC/AHA/AAPA/ABC/ACPM/AGS/APhA/ASH/ASPC/NMA/PCNA guideline for the prevention, detection, evaluation, and management of high blood pressure in adults: executive summary: A report of the American College of Cardiology/American Heart Association task F. Circulation, 2018.
8. Kario K, Sun N, Chiang FT, Supasyndh O, Baek SH, Inubushi-Molessa A, et al. Efficacy and safety of LCZ696, a first-in-class angiotensin receptor neprilysin inhibitor, in Asian patients with hypertension: a randomized, double-blind, placebo-controlled study. Hypertension. 2014;63(4):698-705.
9. Lewis EJ, Hunsicker LG, Clarke WR, Berl T, Pohl MA, Lewis JB, et al. Renoprotective effect of the angiotensin-receptor antagonist irbesartan in patients with nephropathy due to type 2 diabetes. N Engl J Med. 2001;345(12):851-60.
10. Brenner BM, Cooper ME, de Zeeuw D, Keane WF, Mitch WE, Parving HH et al. Effects of losartan on renal and cardiovascular outcomes in patients with type 2 diabetes and nephropathy. N Engl J Med. 2001;345(12):861-9.
11. Dickinson HO, Mason JM, Nicolson DJ, Campbell F, Beyer FR, Cook JV et al. G.A. Lifestyle interventions to reduce raised blood pressure: a systematic review of randomized controlled trials. J Hypertens. 2006;24(2):215-33.
12. Seligman BG, Polanczyk CA, Santos AS, Foppa M, Junges M, Bonzanini L et al. Intensive practical lifestyle intervention improves endothelial function in metabolic syndrome independent of weight loss: a randomized controlled trial. Metabolism. 2011;60(12):1736-40.
13. Ndanuko RN, Tapsell LC, Charlton KE, Neale EP, Batterham MJ. Dietary patterns and blood pressure in adults: A systematic review and meta-analysis of randomized controlled trials. Adv Nutr. 2016;7(1):76-89.
14. Zhang L, Wang Y, Xiong L, Luo Y, Huang Z, Yi B. Exercise therapy improves eGFR, and reduces blood pressure and BMI in non-dialysis CKD patients: evidence from a meta-analysis. BMC Nephrol. 2019;20(1):398.
15. Jo W, Lee S, Joo YS, Nam KH, Yun HR, Chang TI et al. Association of smoking with incident CKD risk in the general population: A community-based cohort study. PLOS ONE. 2020b;15(8):e0238111.
16. Kokkinos P. Physical activity, health benefits, and mortality risk. ISRN Cardiol. 2012;2012:718789.
17. Bjurman C, Petzold M, Venge P, Farbemo J, Fu ML, Hammarsten O. High-sensitive cardiac troponin, NT-proBNP, FABP and copeptin levels in relation to glomerular filtration rates and a medical record of cardiovascular disease. Clin Biochem. 2015;48(4-5):302-7.
18. Filusch A, Giannitsis E, Katus HA, Meyer FJ. High-sensitive troponin T: a novel biomarker for prognosis and disease severity in patients with pulmonary arterial hypertension. Clin Sci (Lond). 2010;119(5):207-13.
19. Hallan SI, Ritz E, Lydersen S, Romundstad S, Kvenild K, Orth SR. Combining GFR and albuminuria to classify CKD improves prediction of ESRD. J Am Soc Nephrol. 2009;20(5):1069-77.
20. Lin YL, Chen SY, Lai YH, Wang CH, Kuo CH, Liou HH, et al. Serum creatinine to cystatin C ratio predicts skeletal muscle mass and strength in patients with non-dialysis chronic kidney disease. Clin Nutr. 2020;39(8):2435-41.
21. Spanaus KS, Kollerits B, Ritz E, Hersberger M, Kronenberg F, von Eckardstein A, et al. Serum creatinine, cystatin C, and beta-trace protein in diagnostic staging and predicting progression of primary nondiabetic chronic kidney disease. Clin Chem. 2010;56(5):740-9.
22. Ishigami J, Iimori S, Kuwahara M, Sasaki S, Tsukamoto Y. Diagnostic value of B-type natriuretic peptide for estimating left

atrial size and its usefulness for predicting all-cause mortality and cardiovascular events among chronic haemodialysis patients. Nephrology (Carlton). 2014;19(12):777-83.
23. Kawachi K, Kataoka H, Manabe S, Mochizuki T, Nitta K. Low HDL cholesterol as a predictor of chronic kidney disease progression: a cross-classification approach and matched cohort analysis. Heart Vessels. 2019;34(9):1440-55.
24. Kawasaki T, Sakai C, Harimoto K, Yamano M, Miki S, Kamitani T. Usefulness of high-sensitivity cardiac troponin T and brain natriuretic peptide as biomarkers of myocardial fibrosis in patients with hypertrophic cardiomyopathy. Am J Cardiol. 2013;112(6):867-72.
25. He P, Yang Y, Tian J, Yang M, Lin Z, Li H, et al. Urinary albumin-to-creatinine ratio and the risk of first stroke in Chinese hypertensive patients treated with angiotensin-converting enzyme inhibitors. Hypertens Res. 2022;45(1):116-24.
26. Mancia G, Fagard R, Narkiewicz K, Redon J, Zanchetti A, Böhm M, et al. 2013 ESH/ESC guidelines for the management of arterial hypertension: the Task Force for the Management of Arterial Hypertension of the European Society of Hypertension (ESH) and of the European Society of Cardiology (ESC). Eur Heart J. 2013;34(28):2159-219.
27. Townsend RR, Black HR, Chirinos JA, Feig PU, Ferdinand KC, Germain M et al. Clinical use of pulse wave analysis: Proceedings From a Symposium Sponsored by North American Artery. Proceedings of the From a Symposium Sponsored by North American Artery. J Clin Hypertens (Greenwich). 2015;17(7): 503-13.
28. Shepherd J, Kastelein JJ, Bittner V, Deedwania P, Breazna A, Dobson S et al. Intensive lipid lowering with atorvastatin in patients with coronary heart disease and chronic kidney disease: the TNT (Treating to New Targets) study. J Am Coll Cardiol. 2008;51(15):1448-54.
29. Shlipak MG, Katz R, Sarnak MJ, Fried LF, Newman AB, Stehman-Breen C et al. Cystatin C and prognosis for cardiovascular and kidney outcomes in elderly persons without chronic kidney disease. Ann Intern Med. 2006;145(4):237-46.
30. Nishikura T, Koba S, Yokota Y, Hirano T, Tsunoda F, Shoji M et al. Elevated small dense low-density lipoprotein cholesterol as a predictor for future cardiovascular events in patients with stable coronary artery disease. J Atheroscler Thromb. 2014;21(8): 755-67.
31. Wanner C, Tonelli M, Kidney Disease: Improving Global Outcomes Lipid Guideline Development Work Group Members. KDIGO Clinical Practice Guideline for Lipid Management in CKD: summary of recommendation statements and clinical approach to the patient. Kidney Int. 2014;85(6):1303-9.
32. Kronenberg F. HDL in CKD-the devil is in the detail. J Am Soc Nephrol. 2018;29(5):1356-71.
33. Wang X, Ouyang Y, Liu J, Zhu M, Zhao G, Bao W, et al. Fruit and vegetable consumption and mortality from all causes, cardiovascular disease, and cancer: systematic review and dose-response meta-analysis of prospective cohort studies. BMJ. 2014;349:g4490.
34. Rebholz CM, Crews DC, Grams ME, Steffen LM, Levey AS, Miller ER, et al. DASH (Dietary Approaches to Stop Hypertension) diet and risk of subsequent kidney disease. Am J Kidney Dis. 2016;68(6):853-61.
35. Miller ER, Juraschek SP, Anderson CA, Guallar E, Henoch-Ryugo K, Charleston J, et al. The effects of n-3 long-chain polyunsaturated fatty acid supplementation on biomarkers of kidney injury in adults with diabetes: results of the GO-FISH trial. Diabetes Care. 2013;36(6):1462-9.
36. Sosnowska B, Penson P, Banach M. The role of nutraceuticals in the prevention of cardiovascular disease. Cardiovasc Diagn Ther. 2017 Cardiovasc. Diagnosis Ther. (Advances Cardiovasc. Dis. Prev.;7;Suppl 1:S21-31.
37. Chang Y, Ryu S, Suh BS, Yun KE, Kim CW, Cho SI. Impact of BMI on the incidence of metabolic abnormalities in metabolically healthy men. Int J Obes (Lond). 2012;36(9):1187-94.
38. Lloyd-Jones DM, Morris PB, Ballantyne CM, Birtcher KK, Daly DD, DePalma SM et al. Focused update of the 2016 ACC Expert Consensus decision pathway on the role of non-statin therapies for LDL-cholesterol lowering in the management of atherosclerotic cardiovascular disease risk: A report of the American College of Cardiology task Fo. J Am Coll Cardiol. 2017;70(14):1785-822.
39. Heerspink HJ, Perkins BA, Fitchett DH, Husain M, Cherney DZ. Sodium glucose cotransporter 2 inhibitors in the treatment of diabetes mellitus: cardiovascular and kidney effects, potential mechanisms, and clinical applications. Circulation. 2016;134(10):752-72.
40. Jardine MJ, Mahaffey KW, Neal B, Agarwal R, Bakris GL, Brenner BM et al. The canagliflozin and renal endpoints in diabetes with established nephropathy clinical evaluation (CREDENCE) study rationale, design, and baseline characteristics. Am J Nephrol. 2017;46(6):462-72.
41. Bakris GL, Agarwal R, Anker SD, Pitt B, Ruilope LM, Rossing P et al. Effect of finerenone on chronic kidney disease outcomes in Type 2 diabetes. N Engl J Med. 2020;383(23):2219-29.
42. Pitt B, Remme W, Zannad F, Neaton J, Martinez F, Roniker B et al. Eplerenone, a selective aldosterone blocker, in patients with left ventricular dysfunction after myocardial infarction. N Engl J Med. 2003;348(14):1309-21.
43. Remuzzi G, Ruggenenti P, Perico N. Chronic renal diseases: renoprotective benefits of renin-angiotensin system inhibition. Ann Intern Med. 2002;136(8):604-15.
44. Parving HH, Lehnert H, Bröchner-Mortensen J, Gomis R, Andersen S, Arner P et al. The effect of irbesartan on the development of diabetic nephropathy in patients with type 2 diabetes. N Engl J Med. 2001;345(12):870-8.
45. Makino H, Haneda M, Babazono T, Moriya T, Ito S, Iwamoto Y et al. Prevention of transition from incipient to overt nephropathy with telmisartan in patients with type 2 diabetes. Diabetes Care. 2007;30(6):1577-8.

129

CHAPTER

Blood Pressure Variability

Pankaj R Jawandhiya, Ankur Gupta

ABSTRACT

Blood pressure (BP) is a dynamic parameter, which undergoes fluctuations due to many internal and external factors interacting with it. There are pathological conditions impacted by enhanced BP variability (BPV) such as impaired cardiovascular regulation associated with coronary artery disease (CAD), stroke, heart failure, dementia, chronic kidney disease (CKD) causing an increase in all-cause and cardiovascular mortality. There are knowledge gaps within the available heterogeneous studies and clinical evidences with limited standardization of methods for BPV assessment. This chapter aims to summarize the current measurement techniques for BPV along with its clinical implications and future scope.

INTRODUCTION

Hypertension (HTN) affects large population and enhances the risk of other comorbidities such as stroke and other cardiovascular disease (CVD). HTN poses threat to rapidly ageing and densely populated Asian countries. BP is not static; there are constant fluctuations due to various extrinsic and intrinsic factors as listed in **Figure 1**. The change in value of arterial blood pressure (BP) in a definite timeframe is termed as BP variability (BPV). It has been demonstrated by several studies that BPV is a potent and distinct risk factor for CVDs, chronic kidney disease (CKD), dementia, and stroke, as well as morbidity and mortality linked to HTN.

Extrinsic factors
- Environmental factors
- Behavioral factors
- Emotional stimuli
- Antihypertensive treatment factor
- Other treatments
- Inappropriate BP monitoring

Intrinsic factors
- Neural mechanisms
- Humoral mechanism
- Vascular mechanism
- Cardiac function
- Rheological mechanisms
- Metabolic activity
- Respiratory activity
- Renal mechanisms
- Genetic susceptibility
- Diseases affecting the autonomic function

FIG. 1: Factors affecting blood pressure variability (BPV).

Currently, taking a patient's BP at the doctor's office (office BP) is undoubtedly the most frequent process. However, BP's inherent dynamic character continues to be unappreciated. BP levels can vary from 24 to 33 mm Hg on beat-to-beat basis due to various behavioral and external factors. Amongst individuals, the degree of BPV differs in the short and long term. There are numerous guidelines suggesting using standardized office BP approach to reduce variability in BP results. Despite the well-known dynamic nature of BP, HTN guidelines advise utilizing the average values of static BP readings (taken in or out of the office), with the goal of reducing the peaks and fluctuation in BP readings. The current measurement techniques have reduced reproducibility due to constant changes in BP making it a challenge to diagnose HTN correctly.

Various evidences from large registries, meta-analyses, and clinical trials suggest that cardiovascular outcomes can be predicted by BPV independent of average BP values. So far, BPV has been overlooked and has limited clinical application probably due to various complex and nonstandard methods. For instance, BPV has been shown to be an independent risk factor for dementia, stroke, CKD, cardiovascular events, and mortality. BP measurements are critical in the diagnosis and management of HTN and heart failure; the potential importance of BPV, alone or in tandem with heart rate variability (HRV), has not been assessed due to a lack of convenient, wearable, continuous BP monitor. It is suggested that increase in media/lumen ratio, compromised vasodilation, and decreased lumen diameter of large artery and its stiffness, activation of inflammatory cascade, sympathetic nervous system and renin-angiotensin aldosterone system may be the probable reasons for BPV as the underlying process remains a grey area.

CURRENT BLOOD PRESSURE MONITORING METHODS

Many assessments of the adequacy of HTN treatment are determined by the last recorded BP reading. This does not consider the dynamic nature of BP. The measurements of office BP will continue to be crucial for detection, treatment, and monitoring of HTN; however, precision is needed. The most unreliable feature of this measurement is the necessity for an observer which will be eliminated by devices that take automatic measures in triplicates and present the average of the most recent two or all three readings, as suggested by current recommendations. The most practical and effective option for long-term self-monitoring in people with HTN appears to be home BP monitoring (HBPM) devices. They are low cost and likely to be a primary method for managing HTN in near future.

By collaborating with chemists and other healthcare professionals, ambulatory BP monitoring (ABPM) may be significantly more affordable and its setup, calibration, reporting, and interpretation processes can be standardized and made simpler. Even though ABPM is currently recommended as the best method for diagnosing HTN, given the costs involved and the potential for patient discomfort (especially with repeated use), it is unlikely that this method will play a significant role in screening or long-term follow-up of patients who have received treatment in the future.

There are other methods developing in clinical practice to assess the effectiveness of HTN therapy taking into account the BPV over an extended time frame. One such method is time in therapeutic range (TTR) assessment, which was initially used to study the role of warfarin as an anticoagulant. TTR is represented as percentage of the time a patient's BP is in the desired range for measuring HTN.

CLINICAL IMPLICATIONS OF BLOOD PRESSURE VARIABILITY

Blood pressure variability can be classified as very short-term (beat-to-beat), short-term (within 24 hours, minute-to-minute, hour-to-hour and day-to-night), mid-term (day-to-day) and long-term (visit-to-visit over weeks, months, and years) as shown in **Table 1**. The ongoing dynamic interactions exist between intrinsic (cardiovascular and neurohormonal) and extrinsic (environmental and behavioral) factors, which are crucial for maintenance of BP equilibrium for sufficient perfusion to vital organs under various circumstances. Various pathological conditions are associated with enhanced BPV.

The evidences from clinical trials, large registries, and meta-analyses of population research suggest that elevated BPV is predictive of cardiovascular outcomes, irrespective of the average BP readings. These conclusions have been supported by all known types of BPV. An investigation of the 24-hour ambulatory BPV (Average real variability-ARV) data from the International Database on Ambulatory Blood Pressure in Relation to Cardiovascular Outcome (IDACO) database regarding short-term BPV revealed a substantial predictive value for total and cardiovascular mortality. The Ambulatory Blood Pressure International Study found a similar association between a greater risk of cardiovascular and all-cause mortality and a nocturnal systolic BP standard deviation of ≥12.2 mm Hg.

The International Database of Home blood pressure in relation to Cardiovascular Outcome (IDHOCO) accounting for all indices of systolic and diastolic

TABLE 1: Classification of blood pressure variability (BPV). Key features of measurement methodology and duration are summarized.

	Very short term	Short term	Mid term	Long term
Interval	Beat to beat	Q 15–30 minutes	Day by day in a week	Visit to visit
Methods	• Intra-arterial • Tonometry (noninvasive)	ABPM	HBPM	• Office • HBPM
Duration	5–60 min	24 hours	3–7 days	Weeks to years

(ABPM: ambulatory blood pressure monitoring; HBPM: home blood pressure monitoring)

BPV calculated from day-to-day morning HBPM was associated to cardiovascular and all-cause mortalities. However, mortality was significantly increased only in the highest BPV decile suggesting that the association might not be linear.

Post-hoc analysis of clinical trials with large patient cohorts showed substantial relationships between visit-to-visit BPV (primarily quantified as standard deviation) and cardiovascular endpoints, providing the strongest support for the predictive utility of long-term BPV. Increased long-term systolic BP was linked to a higher risk of cardiovascular events, coronary heart disease, stroke, and all-cause and cardiovascular death, according to a 2016 meta-analysis of data from prospective cohort studies and clinical trials. Similar relationships were also seen in the limited data for mid-term and short-term BPV.

It should be noted that most of the participants in these trials were from Europe and East Asia and had a higher risk of CVD. The BPV indices employed in the papers included in the meta-analysis also showed significant heterogeneity, with standard deviation being the most frequent metric. The relationships between BPV and cardiovascular outcomes across various patient subgroups exhibit significant heterogeneity as well. In the VALUE study, patients with HTN who had higher visit-to-visit systolic BPV had a higher risk of cardiovascular events regardless of their baseline cardiovascular risk. This link was stronger in younger patients and those who had lower systolic BP levels.

Additionally, the primary cardiovascular outcome was linked to visit-to-visit BPV in the ACCORD trial, but this correlation was reliant on baseline BP levels; a greater link was more pronounced in patients with low and high baseline systolic and diastolic BP levels. A pathophysiological mechanism of lower myocardial perfusion during diastole in patients with diastolic BPV may be indicated by the substantial association between diastolic BPV and coronary heart disease, particularly in patients with a history of cardiovascular illness and low baseline BP.

A poor prognosis was predicted in patients with acute intracerebral hemorrhage by a high systolic BP value. Furthermore, BPV has been linked to glaucomatous visual neuropathy even in people without HTN, most likely due to the optic nerve's hypoperfusion. In comparison to mean BP values, BPV had a greater connection with dementia and cognitive impairment, according to a 2021 meta-analysis involving 7.8 million individuals. An independent relationship between dementia and cognitive decline and greater long-term, visit-to-visit BPV, independent of average BP and antihypertensive medication use, was seen in older persons without major cognitive impairment. This conclusion was supported by a randomized experiment. Together, these results lend credence to the idea that decreasing BPV might be a future goal for dementia prevention.

The correlation between the indices of various types of BPV, as well as their agreement in identifying people with high BPV, is noted to be moderate, even though all types of BPV have a certain amount of clinical relevance and prognostic value. All BPV measurement techniques should therefore be seen as complementing rather than interchangeable or rival. It is generally known that drug-mediated BP lowering has positive cardiovascular effects. Different antihypertensive medication classes have varying effects on BPV. In 257 individuals with HTN and other cardiovascular risk factors, the ASCOT study compared the beta-blocker atenolol with the calcium-channel blocker amlodipine. The results showed that amlodipine lowered BPV more than atenolol, which may account for the discrepancy between the observed effects on stroke risk and the effects predicted by the mean BP change. In comparison to other antihypertensive medications, calcium-channel blockers and diuretics have been shown to reduce BPV in favorable ways in previous research. An inter-individual variance in systolic BP (used as a proxy for within-individual BPV) was decreased to the greatest extent by calcium-channel blockers in a meta-analysis of data from various randomized clinical trials. Additionally, drug-class effects on inter-individual BPV appeared to explain for variations in how antihypertensive medications affected stroke risk without taking into consideration their effects on average systolic BP. With amlodipine, compared to other medications, a higher decrease in the coefficient of intra-individual systolic BPV was achieved, showing a trend toward larger reductions in odds ratios for many end outcomes (including stroke) across multiple randomized clinical studies. All of these conclusions were, however, inferred from post-hoc analyses; randomized cardiovascular outcome trials have not yet been carried out to precisely evaluate the impact of different antihypertensive medication classes on BPV.

FUTURE DIRECTIONS

Hypertension is the major burden globally causing increased mortalities hence emphasis should be laid on frequent, accurate, and broad assessment of alterations in BP levels. However, medical requirements and technological advancements will determine how BP measurement is used in the future. Our history in development of BP monitoring methods and devices has been crucial to evaluate drawbacks in current technology and unmet needs to be fulfilled. The main issue is that all currently used clinically available methods only provide snapshot measures, which are insufficiently representative of BP, a continuous dynamic variable. Therefore, rather than taking snapshots, the pulsatile function of the circulation necessitates continuous high-definition video capture.

The goal of enhancing cardiovascular risk prediction with current out-of-office BP monitoring technologies or BPV measurement methods, however, remains a challenge given that snapshot office BP readings have been particularly effective in predicting cardiovascular risk. We need a novel approach that can collect more BP data (more recording days rather than more readings per day), can collect readings throughout all typical daily activities (rather than just under static conditions), is comfortable for the user over an extended period (the user should preferably not be aware when a measurement is taken), and is appropriate for repeated long-term use.

In order to be effective in enhancing patient care beyond what is now possible, novel technologies must have their accuracy confirmed using recognized worldwide standards, have well-defined diagnostic thresholds, and have a track record of innovation. The next steps will be to make sure that the enormous amount of data obtained from these technologies is effectively exploited and transformed into a straightforward format for clinical decision-making. Accurate recording of BP levels with novel technologies can improve risk prediction and patient care beyond that given by standard BP monitoring methods. Due to the widespread availability and low cost of traditional office BP devices, particularly in low-resource areas, adoption of these types of novel techniques may encounter pushback from the medical profession.

The currently used methods need to be improved until more novel, accessible, and accurate technologies are created. Technologies for cuffless wearable BP monitoring have a lot of promise for enhancing HTN screening, diagnosis, control, and long-term follow-up. Continuous BP monitoring may, in fact, offer a more comprehensive BP profile than current techniques and may open the door to a more efficient and effective integration of BPV data into clinical practice. Once their accuracy and clinical use have been proven, cuffless devices are expected to displace all existing techniques.

SUGGESTED READINGS

1. Parati G, Kollias A, Pengo M, Pengo M, Ochoa JE, Castiglioni P, et al. Blood pressure variability: methodological aspects, clinical relevance and practical indications for management - a European Society of Hypertension position paper. J Hypertens. 2023;41:527-44.
2. Stevens SL, Wood S, Koshiaris C, Law K, Glasziou P, Stevens RJ, et al. Blood pressure variability and cardiovascular disease: systematic review and meta-analysis. BMJ. 2016;354:i4098

130

CHAPTER

Renovascular Hypertension: What is New?

HK Aggarwal, Deepak Jain

ABSTRACT

Hypertension in a young patient is often due to narrowing of blood vessels of kidney leading to renovascular hypertension (RVH), which is a major and possibly amenable cause of secondary hypertension. RVH is to be suspected in severe or refractory hypertension in previously normotensive individuals or hypertension in young individuals with no prior family history. Patients of secondary hypertension after excluding other secondary causes should be evaluated for renovascular cause. If diagnosed early, RVH is often reversible or improved in young individuals who otherwise would have been subjected to lifelong therapy. RVH could be associated with multiple etiologies most common being renal artery stenosis (RAS). Arterial compromise could be corrected with renal revascularization by endovascular procedures or surgeries. Previous consensus had been to control the blood pressure (BP) while limiting the expenses on diagnosis and management. A subset of population with underlying hypertension, congestive heart failure, diabetic nephropathy and other conditions with proteinuria received renin–angiotensin–aldosterone system (RAAS) inhibitors and RVH remained undiagnosed unless they presented with acute or refractory hypertension or renal dysfunction. Major advances in noninvasive vascular imaging, effective medical management with antihypertensive medications, and evolution of surgical interventions might help overcome the challenges associated with RVH.

INTRODUCTION

Renovascular hypertension (RVH) is the most important but potentially reversible cause of secondary hypertension. It involves a group of syndromes associated with increased systemic blood pressure (BP) secondary to decreased renal perfusion leading to activation of hormonal or neuronal responses raising BP to restore the renal artery perfusion.

Primarily renal hypoperfusion causes renin-angiotensin-aldosterone system (RAAS) activation. Renal baroreceptors detect the reduced perfusion, macula densa sense the low sodium chloride levels which along with beta adrenergic stimulation increase the renin secretion from juxtaglomerular cells. Increased recruitment of juxtaglomerular cells during constant ischemia also help to achieve hyperreninemic state which acts on angiotensinogen released from liver cleaving it to angiotensin I, and which is then acted upon by angiotensinogen-converting enzyme (ACE) secreted from vascular endothelium of lungs and kidney to convert it into angiotensin II. Angiotensin II raises BP by vasoconstriction of blood vessels of heart, kidney, and smooth muscles, sympathetic nervous system activation with presynaptic release of norepinephrine, and increased aldosterone secretion from adrenal cortex causing sodium and water retention. The absence of nitric oxide or increased endothelin release, oxidative stress, or mitochondrial damage and hypertensive microvascular renal injury are also important triggers for RVH. Individuals might remain asymptomatic with maintained intrarenal oxygenation till 30–40% reduction of renal blood flow but constant and severe ischemia induces overt tissue hypoxia, inflammatory injury, and eventually irreversible kidney fibrosis.

PREVALENCE AND CAUSES

Renovascular hypertension constitutes <1% of hypertension in patients with mild elevations of BP but its prevalence is significantly higher (10–40%) in hypertension which is acute, severe, or of refractory nature. Renal artery stenosis (RAS) is the most common cause of RVH with atherosclerotic RAS being the most common etiology in patients above 50 years of age. Takayasu vasculitis is the most common cause of RAS in young patients in India while fibromuscular dysplasia (FMD) is the most prevalent cause of RAS in young patients worldwide **(Box 1)**.

Renal artery stenosis is due to occlusion of unilateral or bilateral renal artery or its branches leading to impaired blood flow to the kidneys and RAAS activation. FMD is a noninflammatory, nonatherosclerotic arteriopathy arising from smooth muscle cell proliferation and fibrosis of renal vasculature. It is more common in children and young adults with a female predilection of 90%. Patient may present with hypertension, stroke, transient ischemic attack, or amaurosis fugax. Atheroembolic renal disease arising from unstable atheromatous plaques in large vessels like aorta can slough off and occlude the renal arteries.

BOX 1: Causes of renovascular hypertension.

- Atherosclerotic renal artery stenosis
- *Fibromuscular disease*:
  - Medial fibroplasia
  - Medial hyperplasia
  - Intimal fibroplasia
- Atheroembolic renal disease
- Renal artery aneurysm, embolism, dissection, thrombosis, and infarction
- Aortic dissection or embolus
- *Renal trauma*:
  - Arterial dissection
  - Segmental renal infarction
- Congenital vascular malformations
- *Miscellaneous*:
  - Hypercoagulable states with renal infarction (e.g., lupus anticoagulant)
  - Autoimmune diseases (e.g., Takayasu's arteritis, polyarteritis nodosa)
  - Malignancy encircling the renal artery (e.g., renal cell carcinoma, pheochromocytoma)

CLINICAL FEATURES

The clinical manifestations depend on acuity of disease and functional status of the kidneys. Renovascular diseases may coexist with primary hypertension and thus are difficult to differentiate clinically. RVH is usually associated with early activation of RAAS, hypertension either at an early age (<30 years) or late onset (>60 years), or presence of secondary hyperaldosteronism with hypokalemia and metabolic alkalosis. Absence of nocturnal fall in BP, accelerated organ damage manifesting as left ventricular hypertrophy (LVH) or nephrotic range proteinuria or significant albuminuria and microvascular disease are more commonly associated with RVH than essential hypertension. RVH is usually asymptomatic but a systolic–diastolic bruit might be present in up to 50% of patients with FMD in the epigastric region radiating to upper quadrants or back.

Renovascular hypertension should be suspected if diastolic hypertension develops abruptly in patients <30 or >60 years and/or rapid worsening of new-onset or previously controlled hypertension occurs within 6 months. Systolic BP > 180 mm Hg at the time of diagnosis, hypertension refractory to medications, acute or unexplained worsening of renal function, recurrent flash pulmonary edema, significant atherosclerosis of other vasculature, abdominal bruit or unilateral small kidney with >1.5 cm discrepancy in renal size suggest high likelihood of RVH.

DIAGNOSIS

Renovascular hypertension because of its variable presentations, affecting individuals of different age groups is difficult to diagnose clinically alone. The conventional diagnostic modalities available were invasive, expensive, and had low specificity or sensitivity. Hence individuals were subjected to RVH screening only if intervention was planned on diagnosis. The newer noninvasive and sensitive diagnostic modalities lead to diagnosis of a large fraction of undiagnosed renovascular diseases.

Duplex Doppler Ultrasonography

This is a screening method with sensitivity 82% and specificity 90% for direct visualization of renal arteries along with measurement of systolic and end diastolic flow velocity which increases as the artery becomes stenotic. Peak systolic velocity above 200 cm/s is suggestive of greater than 60% stenosis. Renal resistive index (RI) is directly proportional to amount of intrinsic renal damage. RI > 0.7 is suggestive of pathological resistance to flow and >0.8 indicates extensive atherosclerotic disease of the smaller vessels predicting poor response to revascularization treatments.

Peripheral Venous Plasma Renin Activity

Peripheral venous plasma renin activity (PRA) which is increased in RVH is of limited utility as it is elevated in only 50–80% of patients. Use of 20–50 mg captopril, an ACE inhibitor, 1 hour prior to the measurement of PRA can increase the sensitivity of the method.

Computed Tomography Angiography

Computed tomography angiography (CTA) is an excellent, noninvasive method with high sensitivity (96%) and specificity (99%) to diagnose RAS (>50%) with good tissue reconstruction and resolution and minimal contrast exposure. It can also discover compression of renal arteries by surrounding structures and arterial dissection. The drawback is its inability to detect FMD as it usually involves the distal arteries.

Magnetic Resonance Angiography

Magnetic resonance angiography (MRA) uses magnetic field, radio waves, and intravenous gadolinium to visualize renal vasculature. It has nearly 97% sensitivity and 92% specificity in detecting RAS. Radiation exposure and allergic reactions are less with MRA as compared to the iodinated contrast used in CTA.

Nuclear Medicine ACE Inhibitor Renography

This uses radioactive material, a special camera, and a computer to evaluate RVH. It involves the administration of ACE inhibitor, usually captopril which causes decline in glomerular filtration rate in the stenotic kidney and concomitant increase in the contralateral kidney due to absence of angiotensin II-mediated vasoconstriction. This method has poor sensitivity of around 74–94% and specificity between 59 and 95%. Radionuclide renogram is noninvasive and a relatively safe method to estimate the function of both kidneys and determine if the cause of hypertension is due to narrowing of the renal arteries.

Catheter Angiography or Digital Subtraction Angiography

This is the gold standard test for RAS. It is an invasive method performed when suspicion for RAS and RVH is high and other tests prove inconclusive.

MANAGEMENT

The chances of getting RVH can be prevented by cessation of smoking, regular physical activity, and weight reduction. RAS can be managed with medical therapy or invasive therapy like percutaneous transluminal renal angioplasty (PTRA) with or without stent placement or surgical revascularization along with medications.

The American College of Cardiology and the American Heart Association (ACC/AHA) accepted *medical therapy* with antihypertensive medications as first-line treatment. Renal hypoperfusion activates RAAS which can be inhibited with ACE inhibitor or angiotensin II receptor blocker (ARB) which forms class Ia indication. They can be combined with other drugs like calcium channel blocker (CCB), diuretics, or beta blockers for maintaining BP.

Renovascular hypertension due to atherosclerotic RAS or FMD is treated with *percutaneous angioplasty* when hypertension cannot be controlled with pharmacological therapy. The ACC/AHA guidelines indicated revascularization of renal artery in:

- Patients with hemodynamically significant RAS and recurrent, unexplained congestive heart failure or sudden, unexplained pulmonary edema (Class Ia)
- Hemodynamically significant RAS and accelerated hypertension, resistant hypertension, malignant hypertension, or hypertension with an unexplained unilateral small kidney, and hypertension with intolerance to medication (Class IIa)
- Patients with bilateral RAS and progressive chronic kidney disease or an RAS to a solitary functioning kidney (Class IIa)
- Patients with hemodynamically significant RAS and unstable angina (Class IIa)
- Asymptomatic bilateral or solitary viable kidney with hemodynamically significant RAS (Class IIb)
- Patients with RAS and chronic renal insufficiency with unilateral RAS (Class IIb)
- In addition to angioplasty, renal stent placement is indicated for patients with ostial atherosclerotic lesions (Class I)

Percutaneous angioplasty along with stent placement is class Ib recommendation in ostial atherosclerotic RAS according to current European Society of Cardiology (ESC) guidelines. Data from multiple studies states that stent placement has higher patency, lower restenosis rate, better reduction in BP, improved renal perfusion and decreased chances of heart failure in comparison with PTRA alone.

The combined results of Essar Multicentric Medicaments versus Angioplasty (EMMA) study, the Scottish and New castle Renal Artery Stenosis trial and the Dutch Renal Artery Stenosis Intervention Cooperative

(DRASTIC) trial observed small BP reduction in patients who underwent angioplasty over medical therapy alone with nonsignificant change in creatinine value. However, the more recent randomized controlled trials like the ASTRAL (Angioplasty and stenting for Renal Atherosclerotic Lesions) trial and the CORAL (Cardiovascular Outcomes in Renal Atherosclerotic Lesions) trial have failed to record significant benefit in BP or renal function with angioplasty over medical therapy. The STAR (STent placement and blood pressure and lipid-lowering for the prevention of progression of renal dysfunction caused by Atherosclerotic ostial stenosis of the Renal artery) trial, observed no difference in glomerular filtration rate (GFR) on medical treatment or PTRA with medical therapy also supported the above findings.

Surgical revascularization or renal bypass surgery involves use of a vein or synthetic tube to create alternate route of blood supply from aorta to the kidney bypassing the blocked artery. This is a tedious procedure used only in case of recurrent RAS or hypertension refractory to medications and/or angioplasty. The indications for surgical revascularization according to ACC/AHA guidelines include:

- Patients with RAS secondary to FMD, especially those with complex disease and/or those having micro aneurysms
- Patients with atherosclerotic RAS involving multiple vessels or involvement of early primary branch of the main renal artery
- Patients with atherosclerotic RAS who require pararenal aortic reconstructions (such as with aortic aneurysms or severe aortoiliac obstruction)

CONCLUSION

Renovascular hypertension being the most common cause for secondary hypertension must be suspected in any patient with history of severe or refractory hypertension uncontrolled on antihypertensive medications associated with rapid decline in renal function. Only on high degree of clinical suspicion with intention to treat, the patient should be subjected to diagnostic methods. Trials have proven medical therapy with intensive BP control, along with smoking cessation, weight reduction, lifestyle modifications, antiplatelet agents, and statin to be equally efficacious as interventional therapy like PTRA with stenting or surgical revascularization. RVH if controlled early has high chances of halting the disease process and further deterioration of renal function especially in young patients.

SUGGESTED READINGS

1. Hicks CW, Clark TWI, Cooper CJ, de Bhaills AM, De Carlo M, Green D, et al. Atherosclerotic Renovascular Disease: A KDIGO (Kidney Disease: Improving Global Outcomes) Controversies Conference. Am J Kidney Dis. 2022;79:289-301.
2. Bhalla V, Textor SC, Beckman JA, Casanegra AI, Cooper CJ, Kim ESH, et al. American Heart Association Council on the Kidney in Cardiovascular Disease; Council on Hypertension; Council on Peripheral Vascular Disease; and Council on Cardiovascular Radiology and Intervention. Revascularization for Renovascular Disease: A Scientific Statement From the American Heart Association. Hypertension. 2022;79:e128-e143.
3. Nair R, Vaqar S. Renovascular Hypertension. In: StatPearls [Internet]. Treasure Island (FL): StatPearls Publishing; 2023.

131 CHAPTER

Hemodynamic and Metabolic Characteristics of Hypertension in Diabetes

Ripun Borpuzari, Anyam Borpuzari

ABSTRACT

Essential hypertension (HTN) and type 2 diabetes mellitus (T2DM) often coexist together in the same individual, as observed worldwide. Epidemiological studies have proved that there is high incidence of T2DM in hypertensive people and vice versa. Both share some common etiological factors including genetic predisposition. One disease increases the risk of developing the other by two- to five-folds and existing together double or triples the risk for cardiovascular (CV) events. The key link between HTN and T2DM is the insulin resistance (IR). The fundamental hemodynamic abnormality is the impaired nitric oxide (NO) synthesis and subsequent vasodilatation induced by insulin in presence of IR followed by series of changes such as renin–angiotensin–aldosterone system (RAAS) activation, increased sympathetic drive, and altered sodium homeostasis. The basic metabolic abnormality is the altered fuel surfeit from glucose to fatty acids/ketones in the smooth muscles and the myocardium that leads to altered energy balance, advanced atherosclerosis, and cardiac and skeletal maculopathy. This review is expected to shower some light in our understanding on these dual deadly diseases.

INTRODUCTION

Essential hypertension (HTN) and type 2 diabetes mellitus (T2DM) often coexist together in the same individual, as observed worldwide. HTN is approximately twice as frequent in patients with diabetes as in those without diabetes and accounts for up to 85% of the cardiovascular disease (CVD) risk. The risk for end-stage renal disease (ESRD) is also increased by five to six times compared to hypertensive patients without hyperglycemia. Over 50% of patients with diabetes, either type 1 or type 2, ultimately develop HTN in some course of time. HTN in a patient of type 1 diabetes mellitus (T1DM) almost always indicates renal impairment unless proved otherwise. This association is not observed in secondary HTN.

Epidemiological studies have proved that there is high incidence of T2DM in hypertensive people and vice versa. One disease increases the risk of developing the other by two- to five-folds and existing together double or triples the risk for cardiovascular (CV) events. The Women's Health Study (Eur Heart J, 2007) documented that presence of HTN and its progression is a strong predictor of future T2DM in middle aged women. Similarly, Augsburg Cohort Study (2008; J Hypertens) revealed that both high normal blood pressure (BP) and HTN are independent predictor of T2DM in men. Several studies thereafter reinforced the concept that HTN increases the risk of future T2DM; a mere 10 mm increase in systolic BP and 5 mm in diastolic BP could increase the risk by 13 and 5%, respectively (the Rancho Bernardo Study, 2010). Another recent study, the "Strong Heart Study" (Cardiovascular Diabetology, 2017) strongly confirms that the risk of developing T2DM is further intensified by presence of target organ diseases such as left ventricular hypertrophy or carotid atherosclerosis and microalbuminuria. In India too, in a recent study, the overall prevalence of HTN in T2DM patients was found to be as high as 39% (the urban and rural prevalence are 63.2 and 36.8%, respectively [Tharker et al., Diab Res Clin Pract. 2010;89(3)].

The common link between these two is "insulin resistance (IR)" meaning loss of desired physiological action of insulin with respect to its relatively higher concentration in blood compared to normal situation which we call hyperinsulinemia. Studies revealed higher amount of both fasting and prandial insulin levels in untreated patients of essential HTN compared to normotensive individuals and that both HTN and T2DM share common genetic mutations at the level of adrenergic receptors, insulin, leptin sequencing, etc. Another important issue is increased salt sensitivity (SS), especially in Asian Indians and African Americans. Both IR and SS playing together trigger the pathogenesis of HTN through increased tubular sodium absorption, volume expansion, RAAS stimulation, sympathetic over drive, oxidative stress, and endothelial dysfunction. Both HTN and T2DM are leading components of metabolic syndrome (MS) with features of advanced atherosclerosis. They do have some common phenotypic similarities such as higher waist girth, higher body mass index (BMI) (as per specified BMI standard in Indian subcontinent), higher heart rate, and increased pulse pressure.

INSULIN, THE OMNIPOTENT HEMODYNAMIC, AND METABOLIC AND ENDOTHELIAL REGULATOR

The physiological action of insulin is multifaceted **(Fig. 1)**. The basic vascular function of insulin is mediated by its vasodilating potential through nitric oxide (NO) synthesis resulting in good tissue perfusion and cellular metabolism. In the context of IR, NO synthesis is reduced. The resultant peripheral vascular resistance (PVR) is augmented followed by poor tissue perfusion, activation of tissue renin–angiotensin–aldosterone system (t-RAAS), sympathetic overdrive. A state of increased oxidative stress is been created paving the way for production of reactive oxygen species (ROS) and a low-grade vascular inflammation with rise of inflammatory markers such as interleukin-1 (IL-1), IL-6, tumor necrosis factor-alpha (TNF-α), and vasopressor substances like endothelin-1. This is also termed by some experts as *"endothelial IR"*. In the context of metabolic changes, firstly there is fuel surfeit shifting from free fatty acids (FFAs) and glucose to entirely FFAs and this change gradually jeopardizes the energetic efficiency of both the skeletal and the smooth musculature.

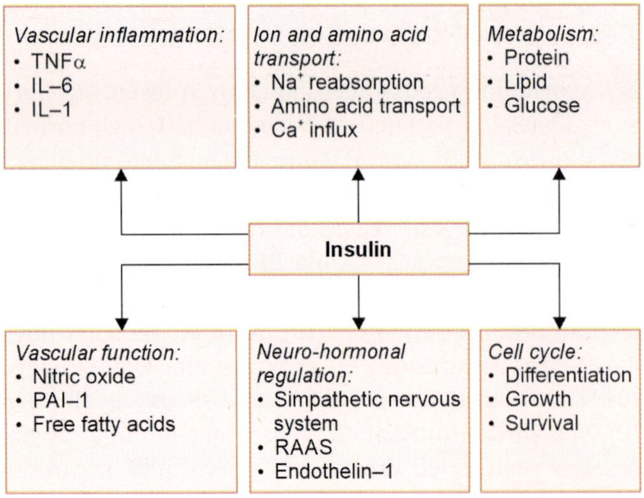

FIG. 1: The pleotropic action of insulin regulating different physiological processes.

(IL-1: interleukin-1; IL-6: interleukin-6; PAI-1: plasminogen activator inhibitor-1; RAAS: renin–angiotensin–aldosterone system; TNF-α: tumor necrosis factor-alpha)

Source: With permission from Mancusi C, et al. (2020).

HEMODYNAMIC CHANGES ON COMBINED HTN AND T2DM

Salt Sensitivity and Augmented Sodium Absorption

The first and foremost is the increased SS. It is the paradoxical response of the body to salt intake in a susceptible individual. The risk factors for increased SS are IR and T2DM, female sex, elderly age, South Asian or African American ethnicities, renal insufficiency, etc. A recent study confirms that Asians are likely to have a genetic predisposition to salt-sensitive gene polymorphism of the renin–angiotensin system (The HOPE Asia Network study).

Increased salt intake causes plasma volume expansion and normally this is combated with reflex suppression of neuroendocrine activity [RAAS and sympathetic nervous system (SNS)] and peripheral vasodilatation to increase glomerular filtration with resultant natriuresis. On the contrary in the settings of IR and increased SS, overdrive of neuroendocrine activity, endothelial dysfunction, and reduced NO synthesis coupled with higher expression of sodium-glucose cotransporter-2 (SGLT-2) receptors and hyperinsulinemia-induced overstimulation of different sodium exchange systems in renal tubules for unrestricted sodium reabsorption **(Fig. 2)**. Hyperinsulinemia-induced by IR directly stimulates Na-hydrogen exchange system 3 (NHE3), Na-chloride channel (NCC), Na-K cotransporter channel (NKCC2), and Na-bicarbonate channels in renal tubules resulting high amount of sodium absorption. Even increased secretion of epinephrine and norepinephrine due to sympathetic drive negatively affect the regulation of the NCC in distal convoluted tubule by with-no-kinin 4 (WNK4) protein **(Fig. 2)**.

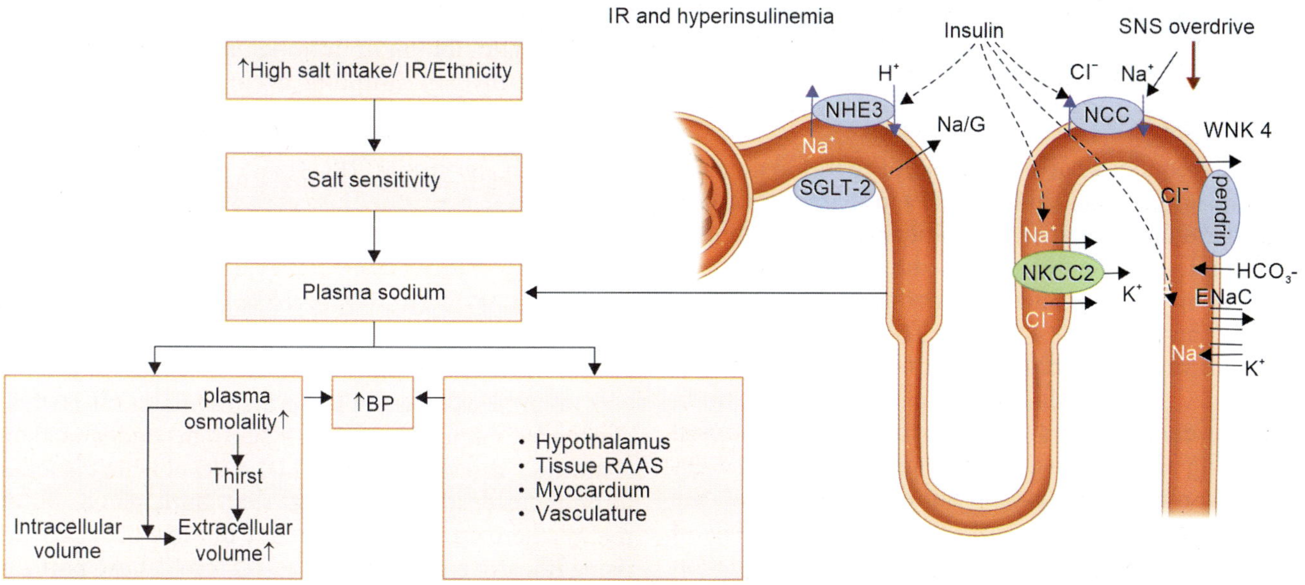

FIG. 2: Impact of SS and IR on blood pressure rise and increased Na absorption in renal tubules.
(BP: blood pressure; IR: insulin resistance; RAAS: renin–angiotensin–aldosterone system; SNS: sympathetic nervous system; SS: salt sensitivity)

Loss of Nocturnal Dipping of BP and Pulse in T2DM

Normally BP, both systolic and diastolic, falls by 10–20% during sleep, a pattern called "nocturnal dipping". Patients with diabetes are found to have lost this dipping as measured by round the clock ambulatory monitoring of BP (AMBP). They may be either *"nondippers"* who fail to show >10% fall or *"reverse dippers"* who show rather a paradoxical rise of BP nocturnally. When the BP is raised above 120/70 mm Hg, this is termed *"nocturnal hypertension (NHTN)"*. People with diabetes, obesity with obstructive sleep apnea, chronic kidney disease (CKD), and Asian Ethnicity are prone to have NHTN. Experts comment that night BP is like a basal BP status of an individual; and NHTN should always be considered abnormal and investigated properly *(Hypertension. 2007;49(4):769-70)* as people having this, are always at a higher risk of CV catastrophe.

Isolated Systolic Hypertension

Advanced atherogenesis in combined diabetes and HTN; coupled with gradual loss of elasticity and reduced expansibility of the arteries for any given volume of systolic output give rise to isolated systolic hypertension (ISH). It is a usual phenomenon observed in elderly people. In diabetes it occurs in younger age group. ISH is defined in clinical situation where systolic BP is >140 mm Hg and the diastolic is below <90 mm Hg. There is always increased risk for stroke and CKD in these people.

Orthostatic Hypotension and Supine Hypertension

When a person is detected to record a fall of the systolic pressure by >20 mm Hg or the diastolic by >10 mm Hg, the person is said to have orthostatic hypotension (OH). Many medications can cause OH namely overzealous treatment with diuretics, calcium entry blockers such as nifedipine, tricyclic antidepressants, and alpha-adrenoreceptor blockers. Few reports are also seen with SGLT-2 inhibitors use. But outside the association of drugs as a causative factor in a diabetic person with or without symptomatic hypotension, it is always indicative of autonomic neuropathy (AN). Most of the time OH due to AN may be associated with *supine HTN* where the BP goes up to 150/90 mm Hg or more. OH, with supine HTN, is much challenging to treat a case of combined T2DM and THN.

Masked Hypertension

Diabetic patients show increased incidence of *masked HTN* where outside the clinic measurement the measured BP is above >135/85 mm Hg. Asian ethnicity, poor lifestyle, and excessive salt intake predispose to masked HTN.

METABOLIC CHARACTERISTICS OF HYPERTENSION IN DIABETES

Altered Fuel Surfeit

The heart requires a constant source of energy in the form of adenosine 5' triphosphate (ATP) to maintain cardiac output and different energy dependent ionic exchanges. In normal situation, 40–60% of the total energy need (TEN), come from fatty acid β oxidation by mitochondria. Glucose contributes 20–40% of the TEN through glycolysis and then mitochondrial glucose oxidation. The heart can utilize ketones, lactate, and amino acids when situation demands and in fact ketones serves the best in a failing and/or ischemic heart producing more ATPs amidst compromised oxygen supply. The chronic use of FFAs leads to a state of reduced work efficiency of the myocardium and oxidative stress as FFA oxidation consumes more oxygen. The factors responsible for reduced cardiac efficiency are multiple such as increased PVR and afterload, trophic effect of insulin excess, myocardial ischemia, RAAS and SNS hyperactivity, effects of glycation end products, oxidative stress and ongoing inflammation, and cardiac autonomic neuropathy (CAN). Series of pathogenetic changes follow thereafter in all smooth muscle cells (SMCs) of the vascular system and skeletal muscle cells finally going to senescence and death.

Defective Calcium Handling in Sarcolemma

Myocardial contractility is a complex mechanism that involves few energy-dependent calcium exchange systems; sodium (Na^+)/calcium (Ca^{2+}), Na^+/potassium (K^+) exchanger, sarcoplasmic reticular Ca^{2+} ATPase pump (SERCA), and membrane Ca^{2+} ATPase systems. With the onset of action potential, the activated systems permit influx of Ca^{2+} into the cell which further stimulate SERCA to release calcium from sarcoplasmic reticulum (SR) to bind to troponin C (TN-C). Once Ca^{2+} binding is completed, inhibition from troponin I (TN-I) is retreated and actin-myosin coupling occurs. Abnormalities in this excitation coupling process, predispose a diabetic person to high risk of fatal arrhythmias, development of cardiomyopathies, and eventually heart failure **(Fig. 3)**.

Accelerated Atherogenesis

Combined HTN and hyperglycemia create a state of accelerated atherogenesis with abundance of triglycerides (TG), low-density lipoprotein cholesterol (LDL-C) along with lowered high-density lipoprotein cholesterol (HDL-C) concentrations in blood. With hypertriglyceridemia, there is always a discordance with LDL-C level which is found to be reciprocally much lower than anticipated. But in reality, there are innumerable tiny dot like LDL particles rising linearly corresponding to TG level. These particles are notoriously atherogenic and remain undetected by usual laboratory procedures.

Increased Propensity to Proteinuria

Hypertension augments the propensity to proteinuria in diabetic patients and vice versa. Microalbuminuria (>30 mg/g) predicts both impending renal impairment and fatal CV outcome.

CONCLUSION

Both T2DM and essential HTN frequently coexist together with higher prevalence of CV and renal outcomes. Whenever feasible AMBP measurement should be ordered to rule out masked and nocturnal HTN. Periodic assessments of the urinary protein-creatinine ratio (UPCR), fundoscopy, and lipid parameters are essential part of holistic management. Programmed lifestyle modification should always be advised right from the day of diagnosis.

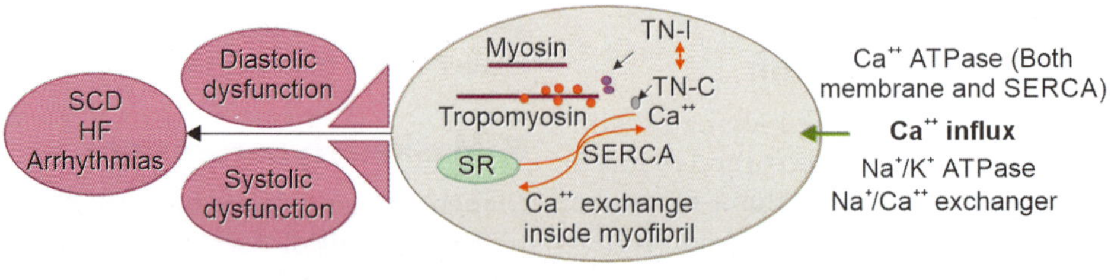

FIG. 3: Abnormalities in calcium exchange.

(HF: heart failure; SCD: Sickle cell disease; SERCA: sarcoplasmic reticular Ca^{2+} ATPase pump)

SUGGESTED READINGS

1. Kahn CR, Weir GC, King GL, Moses AC, Smith RJ, Jacobson AM. Joslin's Diabetes Mellitus, 14th edition. Philadelphia: Lippincott Williams & Wilkins; 2007. pp. 969-74.
2. Mancusi C, Izzo R, di Gioia G, Losi MA, Barbato E, Morisco C. Insulin Resistance the Hinge between Hypertension and Type 2 Diabetes. High Blood Press Cardiovasc Prev. 2020;27(6):515-26.
3. Karwi QG, Sun Q, Lopaschuk GD. The Contribution of Cardiac Fatty Acid Oxidation to Diabetic Cardiomyopathy Severity. Cells. 2021;10(11):3259.

132 CHAPTER

Measurement of Blood Pressure: Is it that Simple?

Sanjay Gupta, Kashish Gupta

ABSTRACT

High blood pressure (BP) is the most prevalent modifiable cause of cardiovascular disease, stroke, and death. Error in BP measurement can lead to incorrect hypertension status classification and mismanagement. While BP measurement apparently looks simple and easy but it is largely executed in an incorrect fashion that can inappropriately alter management decisions in 20–45% of cases. Classical sphygmomanometer BP measurement needs a standard protocol which is mostly not followed resulting in variability in BP values. Incorrect BP estimation may happen due to patient, environment, instrument, procedure, and operator factors. Many measurement errors can be minimized by following appropriate patient preparation and standardized techniques. Era of mercury sphygmomanometer and aneroid device is largely over giving way to semiautomated and automated BP measurement devices using mostly oscillometric techniques. While previous prognostic and therapeutic studies in the field of hypertension were done using classical sphygmomanometer and auscultatory techniques, all recent trials have mostly used automated office blood pressure (AOBP) measurement. Oscillometric techniques are also susceptible to measurement errors and need standardization of procedure. Out of office measurement of BP like home BP monitor and ambulatory blood pressure monitoring (ABPM) are becoming standard procedures and have been incorporated in guidelines. Cuffless BP measurement, sensor-based static and ambulatory devices, and use of artificial intelligence (AI) will provide new directions in BP measurement in future.

INTRODUCTION

Hypertension affects an estimated 1.4 billion adults globally and is a leading modifiable risk factor of heart disease, stroke, and chronic kidney disease. With an overall global adult prevalence of 31%, high blood pressure (BP) accounts for a staggering 10 million deaths per year. Accurate and reliable BP measurement is essential for the proper diagnosis and management of hypertension.

The effect of a 5 mm Hg error in BP measurement could lead to the incorrect classification of hypertension status in 84 million individuals worldwide.

While BP measurement apparently looks simple and easy but it is largely executed in an incorrect fashion that can inappropriately alter management decisions in 20–45% of cases. Classical sphygmomanometer BP measurement needs a standard protocol which is mostly not followed resulting in variability in BP values. In this chapter, we will delve into the multifaceted world of BP measurement, exploring the current practices, guidelines set by organizations like the European Society of Hypertension (ESH), and the challenges associated with ensuring accuracy in clinical settings. We will also look at the future of BP measurement, where innovation and technology are shaping a more accessible and patient-centric approach to monitoring this vital health parameter.

How to measure blood pressure?

Accurate BP measurement relies on adhering to specific principles. Indirect BP measurement is safe, painless, and reliable. The process typically involves the use of a sphygmomanometer, which includes an inflatable cuff, a pressure gauge, and a means to measure blood flow sounds (auscultation) or, in some cases, digital display. The procedure begins by placing the cuff around the upper arm and inflating it to temporarily occlude the brachial artery. This process measures the pressure at which blood flow is obstructed (systolic pressure) and the point at which normal flow resumes (diastolic pressure). These two measurements provide the systolic/diastolic blood pressure values, usually expressed in millimeters of mercury (mm Hg).

The traditional sphygmomanometer, which has been the primary tool for measuring BP in clinical settings since the inception of noninvasive BP monitoring, typically relies on a mercury manometer. However, due to significant environmental concerns regarding mercury pollution, this method has already been phased out in several countries and is expected to be discontinued for BP measurements in all countries in the near future. Furthermore, manual auscultatory BP measurement is susceptible to errors or biases introduced by the observers. Therefore, automated techniques are progressively replacing manual BP measurement for these reasons.

Currently, the most widely used mercury-free devices are automated oscillometric BP monitors.

Regardless of the type of devices employed, it is crucial to maintain a routine calibration schedule. When automated BP monitors are utilized, it is essential to undergo a validation process. While mercury column-based sphygmomanometers are gradually being phased out in clinical BP measurements, they remain indispensable for assessing the precision of electronic devices that rely on algorithm-based measurements.

Blood pressure measurement should strictly follow the current recommendations or guidelines. Adhering to these guidelines is essential to ensure that healthcare professionals and individuals obtain precise and consistent BP readings. The ESH guidelines encompass a range of recommendations and best practices for accurate BP measurement. These guidelines are widely recognized and adopted in the medical field to maintain consistency and reliability in BP readings. These guidelines include several essential recommendations for BP measurement:

- *Proper rest*: Patients should rest for at least 5 minutes in a quiet and comfortable environment before BP measurement. This period of rest helps ensure that the patient's BP has stabilized.
- *Cuff selection*: Selecting the appropriate cuff size is vital. An incorrectly sized cuff can lead to erroneous results. The cuff should encircle about 80% of the upper arm's circumference, fitting snugly but not too tight.
- *Cuff placement*: The cuff should be placed at heart level on the upper arm, typically aligned with the brachial artery. Proper cuff positioning ensures that measurements are taken at the same height as the heart.
- *Multiple readings*: To enhance accuracy, it is recommended to take multiple readings, spaced at least 2–3 minutes apart. These readings can then be averaged to provide a more reliable assessment of BP.
- *Use of validated devices*: Healthcare providers should use validated and regularly calibrated BP measurement devices. Regular calibration ensures that the equipment remains accurate over time

A recent study by Chen et al. analyzed data from 36 milestone hypertension trials and came up with the following recommendations for accurate BP measurement:

- Observers should possess adequate training and experience.
- The device used for BP measurement should be an automated electronic BP monitor, previously validated and regularly calibrated.
- On each occasion, BP should be taken 2–3 times, and the average of two or three readings should be recorded.
- There should be a time interval of 30–60 seconds between successive measurements.
- Prior to measurement, there should be a resting period of at least 5 minutes in the supine or seated position while awake and 1–3 minutes when standing.
- Blood pressure should generally be measured in the seated position, and under specific circumstances, in the supine or standing position.
- The higher arm side for measurement should be selected and noted.
- It is important to choose an appropriately sized cuff, and the cuff size should be documented.

Table 1 shows the sources of errors while BP measurements are tabulated.

TABLE 1: Sources of error during blood pressure measurement.

Patient related	Procedure related
• Acute meal ingestion • Acute caffeine intake • Acute nicotine use • Bladder fullness	• Insufficient rest • Legs crossed at knees • Arm lower than heart level • Talking during measurement • Fast deflation rate • Back not supported • Feet not on the floor
Equipment related	**Observer related**
• Instrument not calibrated • Automated device variability • Too small a cuff • Too large cuff • Cuff tied too loose • Cuff improperly placed	• Terminal digit preference for zero (rounding off) during auscultatory measurements • Reliance on a single measurement • Hearing deficit

Implementing BP measurement guidelines in clinical practice faces challenges. Time constraints are significant, with limited appointment time for patients, making it challenging to allow proper rest before measurements. Equipment availability varies, affecting the quality of readings. Not all healthcare professionals receive sufficient training in measurement techniques, impacting consistency. Addressing white-coat syndrome may be hindered by time and resource limitations.

Additionally, patient compliance poses a challenge. Some may not arrive early for rest or understand cuff placement. Clinical environments vary, influencing guideline adherence due to factors like noise and distractions.

These multifaceted challenges necessitate ongoing education for patients and healthcare providers to improve guideline adherence and measurement accuracy.

ADVANTAGES OF AUTOMATED BLOOD PRESSURE MEASUREMENT

The utilization of automated BP measurement is endorsed by numerous fundamental studies in the field of hypertension, both for predicting and treating the condition. A significant benefit of this approach is its capacity to minimize errors associated with human observation, as it automates the BP measurement procedure. Consequently, less expertise is demanded from the observer, obviating the need for specific auscultatory training.

Examples of such enhancements include step-by-step instructions displayed electronically to guide observers in maintaining proper technique, as well as automated initiation sequences that require a predetermined rest period before the initial BP reading is taken. An additional, though critically important, advantage of automated BP measurement is its ability to facilitate multiple measurements in the out-of-clinic setting within the individual's natural environment.

Automated office blood pressure (AOBP) allows for 3–5 unattended, sequential BP measurements, with an automatic calculation of the mean result.

The use of AOBP, particularly when the patient is alone in the room, promotes a more standardized measurement process (e.g., no talking, multiple automated measurements taken sequentially), leading to a reduction in the white-coat effect. However, it is important to note that AOBP requires more space, time, and comes at a higher cost.

OUT-OF-CLINIC BLOOD PRESSURE MEASUREMENT

Out-of-clinic measurements encompass a 24-hour ambulatory blood pressure monitoring (ABPM) and home blood pressure monitoring (HBPM), offering a significantly more accurate assessment of an individual's usual BP. This approach not only eliminates observer-related errors but also helps identify the 'white-coat effect' (elevated BP in a clinical setting but normal elsewhere) and 'masked hypertension' (normal clinic readings but high BP outside the clinic), which affect a substantial proportion of untreated and treated individuals. In fact, due to the presence of these phenomena, even meticulously performed standardized office BP measurements may not accurately represent an individual's typical BP.

Current guidelines recommend the confirmation of hypertension diagnoses through out of office BP measurements. Treatment is recommended for individuals with masked hypertension but not for those with white-coat hypertension. In terms of predicting cardiovascular events, both 24-hour ABPM and HBPM methods far surpass the reliability of clinic measurements. 24-hour BP monitoring is considered the gold standard for diagnosing hypertension, and HBPM is ideal for ongoing monitoring of treated hypertensive patients. It is essential to note that both out-of-clinic measurement techniques require proper execution, and healthcare professionals should recognize that patient training is vital for the effectiveness of HBPM in improving clinical decision-making.

FUTURE OF BLOOD PRESSURE MEASUREMENT

Innovations on the Horizon

The future of BP measurement holds exciting possibilities. Emerging technologies are reshaping how we can monitor and manage hypertension.

Cuffless Blood Pressure Measurement

Novel cuffless BP measuring devices, which use sensors, signal processing, machine learning and other technologies embedded in wearable devices are already available on the market. However, there are several issues that need to be addressed before these devices can be recommended for clinical use. A major concern is that the AAMI/ESH/ISO Universal Standard protocols which are used for validating cuff BP devices are inadequate for cuffless devices which mean that their accuracy remains unproven. Furthermore, there is still no agreed standard of performance for these novel technologies.

Personalized monitoring: Advances in wearable technology and artificial intelligence (AI)-driven solutions offer the potential for personalized BP monitoring. These systems can adapt to an individual's unique physiology and provide real-time feedback and alerts.

Big data and AI: The integration of big data and AI allows for more sophisticated data analysis. AI can identify trends and patterns in BP data, aiding in early detection and tailored interventions.

Empowering Patients

The future of BP measurement is not only about technology but also about empowering patients to take an active role in their health. With accessible monitoring tools and personalized feedback, individuals can make informed decisions and work closely with healthcare providers to manage their BP.

SUGGESTED READINGS

1. GBD 2017 Risk Factor Collaborators. Global, regional, and national comparative risk assessment of 84 behavioural, environmental and occupational, and metabolic risks or clusters of risks for 195 countries and territories, 1990-2017: a systematic analysis for the Global Burden of Disease Study, 2017. Lancet. 2018;392:1923-94.
2. Benjamin EJ, Virani SS, Callaway CW, Chamberlain AM, Chang AR, Cheng S, et al. American Heart Association Council on Epidemiology and Prevention Statistics Committee and Stroke Statistics Subcommittee. Heart disease and stroke statistics—2018 update: a report from the American Heart Association. Circulation. 2018;137:e67-e492.
3. Mills KT, Bundy JD, Kelly TN, Reed JE, Kearney PM, Reynolds K, et al. Global disparities of hypertension prevalence and control: a systematic analysis of population-based studies from 90 countries. Circulation. 2016;134:441-50.
4. Pickering TG, Hall JE, Appel LJ, Falkner BE, Graves J, Hill MN, et al. Recommendations for blood pressure measurement in humans and experimental animals: Part 1: blood pressure measurement in humans: a statement for professionals from the subcommittee of professional and public education of the American Heart Association Council on High Blood Pressure Research. Circulation. 2005;111:697-716.
5. Stergiou GS, Parati G, Asmar R, O'Brien E; European Society of Hypertension Working Group on Blood Pressure Monitoring. Requirements for professional office blood pressure monitors. J Hypertens. 2012;30:537-42.
6. O'Brien E, Asmar R, Beilin L, Imai Y, Mancia G, Mengden T, et al. Practice guidelines of the European Society of Hypertension for clinic, ambulatory and self blood pressure measurement. J Hypertens. 2005;23:697-700.
7. Mancia G, Kreutz R, Brunström M, Burnier M, Grassi G, Januszewicz A, et al. 2023 ESH Guidelines for the management of arterial hypertension The Task Force for the management of arterial hypertension of the European Society of Hypertension: Endorsed by the International Society of Hypertension (ISH) and the European Renal Association (ERA). J Hypertens. 2023;41(12):1874-2071.
8. Chen Y, Lei L, Wang JG. Methods of Blood Pressure Assessment Used in Milestone Hypertension Trials. Pulse (Basel). 2018;6(1-2):112-23.
9. Ettehad D, Emdin CA, Kiran A, Anderson SG, Callender T, Emberson J, et al. Blood pressure lowering for prevention of cardiovascular disease and death: a systematic review and meta-analysis. Lancet. 2015;387:957-67.
10. Giorgini P, Weder AB, Jackson EA, Brook RD. A review of blood pressure measurement protocols among hypertension trials: implications for 'evidence-based' clinical practice. J Am Soc Hypertens. 2014;8:670-6.
11. Myers MG. Eliminating the human factor in office blood pressure measurement. J Clin Hypertens (Greenwich). 2014;16:83-6.
12. Roerecke M, Kaczorowski J, Myers MG. Comparing automated office blood pressure readings with other methods of blood pressure measurement for identifying patients with possible hypertension. JAMA Intern Med. 2019;179(3):351-62.
13. Jegatheswaran J, Ruzicka M, Hiremath S, Edwards C. Are automated blood pressure monitors comparable to ambulatory blood pressure monitors? A systematic review and meta-analysis. Can J Cardiol. 2017;33:644-52.
14. Ringrose JS, Cena J, Ip S, Morales F, Hamilton P, Padwal R. Comparability of automated office blood pressure to daytime 24-Hour ambulatory blood pressure. Can J Cardiol. 2018;34:61-5.
15. Drawz PE, Pajewski NM, Bates JT, Bello NA. Effect of intensive versus standard clinic-based hypertension management on ambulatory blood pressure: novelty and significance. Hypertension. 2017;69:42-50.
16. Fagard RH, Cornelissen VA. Incidence of cardiovascular events in white-coat, masked and sustained hypertension versus true normotension: a meta-analysis. J Hypertens. 2007;25:2193-8.
17. Williams B, Mancia G, Spiering W, Agabiti Rosei E, Azizi M, Burnier M, et al. 2018 ESC/ESH guidelines for the management of arterial hypertension: The Task Force for the management of arterial hypertension of the European Society of Cardiology and the European Society of Hypertension. J Hypertens. 2018;36:1953-2041.
18. O'Brien E, Parati G, Stergiou G, Asmar R, Beilin L, Bilo G, et al., European Society of Hypertension Working Group on Blood Pressure Monitoring. European Society of Hypertension position paper on ambulatory blood pressure monitoring. J Hypertens. 2013;31:1731-68.
19. Stergiou GS, Bliziotis IA. Home blood pressure monitoring in the diagnosis and treatment of hypertension: a systematic review. Am J Hypertens. 2009;24:123-34.
20. Cloutier L, Daskalopoulou S, Padwal RS, Lamarre-Cliché M, Bolli P, McLean D, et al. A new algorithm for the diagnosis of hypertension in Canada. Can J Cardiol. 2015;31:620-30.

21. Parati G, Stergiou G, O'Brien E, Asmar R, Beilin L, Bilo G, et al. European Society of Hypertension practice guidelines for ambulatory blood pressure monitoring. J Hypertens. 2014;32:1359-66.
22. Milot JP, Birnbaum L, Larochelle P, Wistaff R, Laskine M, Van Nguyen P, et al. Unreliability of home blood pressure measurement and the effect of a patient-oriented intervention. Can J Cardiol. 2015;31:658-63.
23. Stergiou GS, Mukkamala R, Avolio A, Kyriakoulis KG, Mieke S, Murray A, et al., European Society of Hypertension Working Group on Blood Pressure Monitoring and Cardiovascular Variability. Cuffless blood pressure measuring devices: review and statement by the European Society of Hypertension Working Group on Blood Pressure Monitoring and Cardiovascular Variability. J Hypertens. 2022;40:1449-60.
24. Mukkamala R, Yavarimanesh M, Natarajan K, Hahn JO, Kyriakoulis KG, Avolio AP, et al. Evaluation of the accuracy of cuffless blood pressure measurement devices: challenges and proposals. Hypertension. 2021;78:1161-7.
25. Stergiou GS, Alpert B, Mieke S, Asmar R, Atkins N, Eckert S, et al. A universal standard for the validation of blood pressure measuring devices: Association for the Advancement of Medical Instrumentation/European Society of Hypertension/International Organization for Standardization (AAMI/ESH/ISO) Collaboration Statement. J Hypertens. 2018;36:472-8.

133 CHAPTER

Isolated Systolic Hypertension: A Divorce between Systolic and Diastolic Pressures in Elderly

Hemshanker Sharma, Abhishek Kumar Tiwari

ABSTRACT

Cumulative vascular distress caused by chronic hypertension has been known to predispose to an array of adverse cardiovascular outcomes. Age-related arterial stiffness results in systolic rise in blood pressure (BP), which during yesteryears was earmarked as a physiological attribute, not warranting attention. There are multiple evidences [including the landmark, HYVET (Hypertension in the Very Elderly Trial) and SPRINT (Systolic Blood Pressure Intervention Trial)] to downturn this hypothesis, leading to revision of BP target of < 130 mm Hg in all the recently published guidelines. Thiazide-like diuretics along with calcium channel blockers are given the first bench in the class of treatment, unless compelled by other indications warranting drugs acting on RAAS (renin–angiotensin–aldosterone system) pathway. In pursuit of buckling the systolic BP (SBP), care should be taken to maintain the diastolic pressure above at least 70 mm Hg to sustain the organ perfusion [although VALISH (Valsartan in Elderly Isolated Systolic Hypertension) trial suggested that treating SBP should be the primary target). Isolated systolic hypertension in young (ISHY) is a different subset of mostly young, obese, male patients who need careful evaluation of central BP and arterial distensibility for proper risk stratification as they have tendency to develop systolic–diastolic hypertension with associated cardiovascular risks.

INTRODUCTION

Hypertension holds the medal for being most notorious cardiovascular disease risk factor for the elder individuals of both sexes. Almost 70% of those above 75 years of age are said to be having hypertension. Hypertension appears to have the highest population attributable risk for coronary artery disease, cerebrovascular disease, and peripheral arterial diseases among the older adults. 7 out of 10 elderly with acute myocardial infarction (MI), stroke, acute aortic emergencies, and heart failure have preexisting hypertension. Glancing into the background of heart failure (especially heart failure with preserved ejection fraction) and chronic kidney disease, hypertension is found as the culprit forerunner in most of the cases.

DANGEROUS IN ISOLATION

In the early 1980s, the age associated rise of systolic blood pressure (SBP) in elderly was considered a physiological attribute not calling for any medical attention. The visibly relentless hike in SBP with increasing age garnered the view that this was nothing but an adaptation needed to sustain the perfusion of end organs, so much so that an empiric formula— "age + 100" was frequently advocated to estimate the apt SBP. Now, there are a healthy number of studies which are in notion of negating this idea and they suggest an incremental association of hypertension and cardiovascular morbidity and mortality. Isolated systolic hypertension (ISH) defined as a SBP of > 140 mm Hg and a diastolic blood pressure (BP) < 90 mm Hg, accounts for > 90% of hypertensive patients beyond 70 years of age. Diagnosis of ISH have been establish more in obese and women, and the cardiovascular outcomes and mortality are found to be elevated in subset of patients with orthostatic hypertension. Against the popular belief, trials have suggested benefits of hypertension control in this cohort. There is enough evidence to prove that hypertension control in these subset of patients has substantial effect in reducing the stroke and heart failure, although only two of them have claimed reduction in total mortality.

LESSONS FROM HYVET AND SPRINT

Hypertension in the Very Elderly Trial (HYVET) was a landmark trial which showed a 21% reduction in all-cause mortality, 64% reduction in heart failure, and a 39% fall in stroke over a 18 months of mean follow-up in >80-year-old, 3,845 patients with SBP of > 160 mm Hg. Thiazide-like diuretic (indapamide) was studied against placebo in the trial. The SPRINT (Systolic Blood Pressure Intervention Trial) showed a 34% reduction in cardiovascular events and a significant fall in mortality by a third in 2,636 patients >75 years old with SBP above target of >130 mm Hg who were randomized to a target SBP of 140 mm Hg versus 120 mm Hg. The results of these trials, in part formed the basis of the 2017 update of the hypertension guidelines which recommended a target SBP of ≤130 mm Hg irrespective of being elderly.

PATHOLPHYSIOLOGICAL STORY

Aging leads to accelerated deposition of calcium and collagen in the arterial wall, downplaying the elasticity of the arterial tree, this in turn leads to reduction in compliance of the arterial vessels, smaller lumen to wall ratio, and inversely increased fibrosis, thickening and remodeling of the vascular intima and media. The stiffened arterial conduit associated with crosslinking and degradation of elastin fibers, results in an increased pulse wave velocity and pulse pressure clinically manifesting as a falling diastolic BP and an elevated SBP **(Fig. 1)**. The various chronic conditions like thyroid disorders, arteriovenous fistula, chronic kidney disease, peripheral vascular disease, diabetes mellitus, aortic insufficiency, anemia, Paget's disease, renal artery stenosis, and obstructive sleep apnea secondarily accelerate the pathological process of deposition of calcium and collagen to the arterial tree and leads to fibrotic remodeling of vessel wall anatomy. Dietary factors like low potassium and high sodium have been linked with arterial stiffness and systolic hypertension. Mutation in gene encoding Cullin-3 present in vascular smooth muscle appear to be responsible for an early rise of arterial aging and stiffness **(Fig. 2)**.

THE 2023 ESH GUIDELINES—INSIGHTS

The 2023 ESH (European Society of Hypertension) guidelines for the management of arterial hypertension, endorsed by the European Renal Association (ERA) and the International Society of Hypertension address and state that inadvertent white-coat effect and lofty BP variability characteristic in elderly make the ISH a diagnostic challenge inviting the use of ambulatory BP monitoring or out-of-office BP monitoring. The central BP monitoring has a role in this, as it paves way for detection of ISH in individuals who have less marked aortic SBP elevation. There are ample evidence to support early commencement of antihypertensive treatment in patients with ISH. The aggregate of data favored thiazide-like diuretics and calcium channel blockers over angiotensin-converting enzyme (ACE) inhibitors/angiotensin receptor blockers (ARBs) as first-line management for ISH and indicated that the ACE inhibitors/ARBs should be considered only if there are other secondary compelling indications like heart

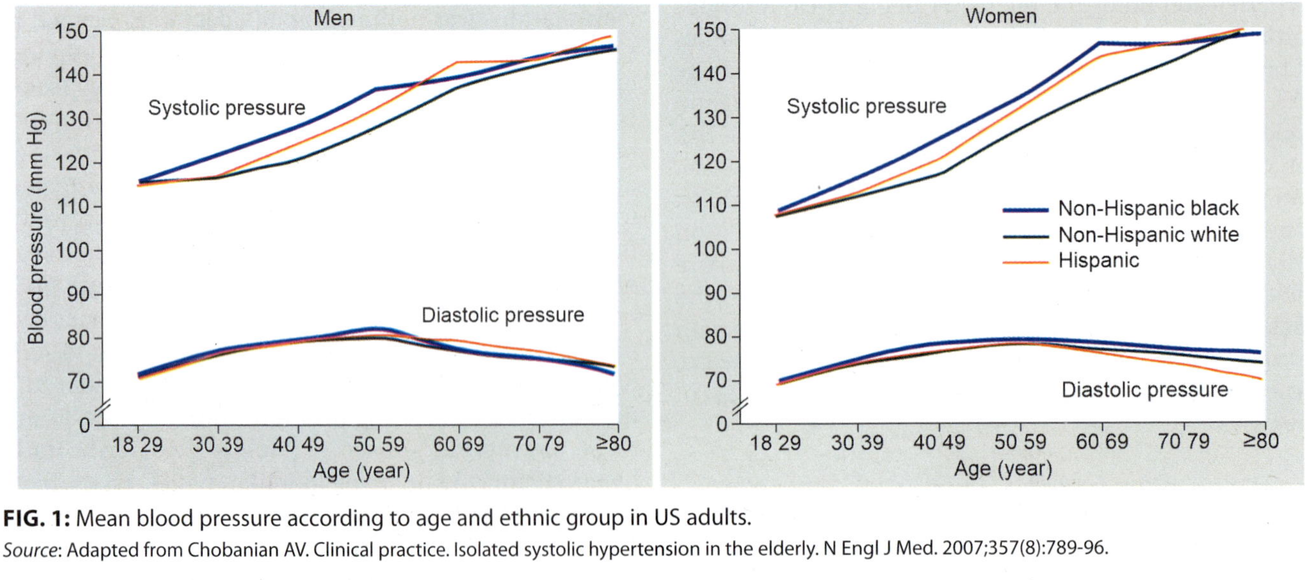

FIG. 1: Mean blood pressure according to age and ethnic group in US adults.

Source: Adapted from Chobanian AV. Clinical practice. Isolated systolic hypertension in the elderly. N Engl J Med. 2007;357(8):789-96.

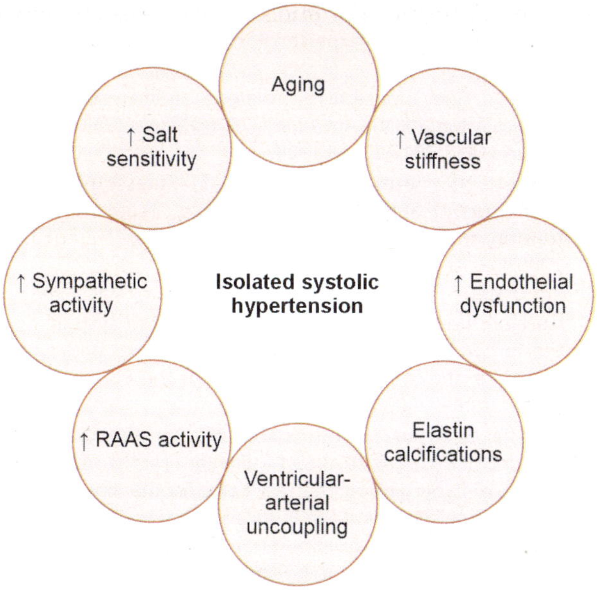

FIG. 2: Pathophysiology of isolated systolic hypertension (ISH). (RAAS: renin–angiotensin–aldosterone system)

failure, coronary artery disease, or diabetes. In non-frail individuals, it is advocated to commence with two-drug combination for adequate BP control as monotherapy is less likely to achieve fruitful BP targets. The BP targets in elderly has been a subject of passionate debate but a recent meta-analysis of 23 randomized clinical trials targeting the effect of SBP targets below 140 mm Hg have shown significant favorable outcomes. A SBP of < 140 mm Hg was earmarked as well within the safety margin in the ISH patients of VALISH (*Valsartan in Elderly* Isolated Systolic Hypertension) trial. Nonetheless, relentless reduction in diastolic BP should not be tried in these subgroups of patients as the benefit of SBP control would be blunted by reduced coronary perfusion, specially in patients with atherosclerosis. To avoid hypoperfusion diastolic pressure should be kept above 70 mm Hg. This makes treating ISH a tricky affair as in an attempt to curtail SBP, the diastolic pressure tends to go below set strict boundary. This calls for an individualized treatment regimen keeping in account the patient profile, risks and comorbidities. Despite of the aforementioned restrains, the primary aim should continue to be the reduction of SBP, as shown in SHEP (Systolic Hypertension in the Elderly Program) trial which cleared that a treatment-induced reduction in SBP was accompanied by fall in major cardiovascular outcomes despite of being slipped below the diastolic BP target (an average value of 68 mm Hg).

ISHY—THE YOUNG WITH ELDERLY VESSELS?

Isolated systolic hypertension is found not only in elderly but at times can be diagnosed in children, adolescents, and young individuals (more so in male, obese individuals)—ISHY (isolated systolic hypertension in young). Whether ISHY is associated with worse clinical outcomes and needs medical attentions remains to be answered. Technically, predominant hemodynamic attributes in ISHY are an increased heart rate, stroke volume, and hence cardiac output (hence more common in athletes). Some studies came to the conclusion that one-fifth of the ISHY patients have a normal stroke volume with higher pulse wave velocity indicating premature arterial stiffening. Contradicting this, some researchers identified subset of patients who had coexistent amplified pulse pressure and a normal central BP (so-called spurious systolic hypertension). A large multicentric population-based study showed that people with ISHY had pulse wave velocity and central SBP lower than those with arterial hypertension and ISH but similar to those with high normal BP. This contradictory information suggests that ISHY is a heterogeneous situation that may take in account individuals with varying pathophysiological and genetic backgrounds as well as clinical eccentricity. Assessment of central BP, arterial distensibility has to be applied to extract additional information and better categorize and prognosticate ISHY patients. As in elderly, white coat effect has to be dealt with appropriate out of office BP monitoring or ambulatory BP monitoring in these cohort also. Individuals with diagnosed ISHY should be advised with positive lifestyle changes including weight management, smoking cessation, and low salt diet. These people need to be kept in follow-up loop because they have a tendency to plunge into diagnosis of systolic–diastolic hypertension with time. Those who have the triad of high central BP, high out-of-office BP, and other risk factors should be subjected to pharmacological therapeutics.

SUGGESTED READINGS

1. Aronow WS, Fleg JL, Pepine CJ, Artinian NT, Bakris G, Brown AS, et al. ACCF Task Force. ACCF/AHA 2011 expert consensus document on hypertension in the elderly: a report of the American College of cardiology Foundation Task Force on clinical expert consensus documents. Circulation. 2011;123(21): 2434-506.
2. Whelton PK, Carey RM, Aronow WS, Casey DE Jr, Collins KJ, Dennison Himmelfarb C, et al. 2017 ACC/AHA/AAPA/ABC/

ACPM/AGS/APhA/ASH/ASPC/NMA/PCNA guideline for the prevention, detection, evaluation, and management of high blood pressure in adults: executive summary: a report of the American College of cardiology/American heart association Task Force on clinical practice guidelines. Circulation. 2018;138(17):e426-e483.

3. Fleg JL, Aronow WS, Frishman WH. Cardiovascular drug therapy in the elderly: benefits and challenges. Nat Rev Cardiol. 2011;8(1):13-28.
4. Beckett NS, Peters R, Fletcher AE, Staessen JA, Liu L, Dumitrascu D, et al; HYVET Study Group. Treatment of hypertension in patients 80 years of age or older. N Engl J Med. 2008;358(18):1887-98.
5. Williamson JD, Supiano MA, Applegate WB, Berlowitz DR, Campbell RC, Chertow GM, et al; SPRINT Research Group. Intensive vs standard blood pressure control and cardiovascular disease outcomes in adults aged ≥75 Years: a randomized clinical trial. JAMA. 2016;315(24):2673-82.
6. AlGhatrif M, Lakatta EG. The conundrum of arterial stiffness, elevated blood pressure, and aging. Curr Hypertens Rep. 2015;17(2):12.
7. Chobanian AV. Clinical practice. Isolated systolic hypertension in the elderly. N Engl J Med. 2007;357(8):789-96.
8. Mancia G, Giannattasio C. Diagnostic and therapeutic problems of isolated systolic hypertension. J Hypertens. 2015;33(1): 33-43.
9. Bavishi C, Goel S, Messerli FH. Isolated Systolic Hypertension: An Update After SPRINT. Am J Med. 2016;129(12):1251-8. Erratum in: Am J Med. 2017;130(9):1128.
10. Beckett NS, Peters R, Fletcher AE, Staessen JA, Liu L, Dumitrascu D, et al. HYVET Study Group. Treatment of hypertension in patients 80 years of age or older. N Engl J Med. 2008;358(18):1887-98.
11. Perry HM Jr, Davis BR, Price TR, Applegate WB, Fields WS, Guralnik JM, et al. Effect of treating isolated systolic hypertension on the risk of developing various types and subtypes of stroke: the Systolic Hypertension in the Elderly Program (SHEP). JAMA. 2000;284(4):465-71.
12. Mancia G, Kreutz R, Brunström M, Burnier M, Grassi G, Januszewicz A, et al. 2023 ESH Guidelines for the management of arterial hypertension The Task Force for the management of arterial hypertension of the European Society of Hypertension: Endorsed by the European Renal Association (ERA) and the International Society of Hypertension (ISH). J Hypertens. 2023;41(12):1874-2071.

134

CHAPTER

Hypertension in Young Adults

Abhishek Kumar, Niharika Sinha

ABSTRACT

Hypertension among young people is common, affecting 1 in 8 adults aged between 20 and 40 years. It is commonly essential hypertension and is on the rise because of rapid urbanization, increasing stress, addictions (tobacco and alcohol), and changing lifestyles. However, being remediable with appropriate management, secondary causes must be ruled out. It is imperative that a holistic approach is adopted while evaluating the young hypertensive and nonpharmacological as well as pharmacological measures should be adopted while managing these patients. Renin–angiotensin system (RAS) activity and sympathetic tone are heightened in young. Drug usage should therefore be chosen to inhibit the RAS, have long-term control, and minimize side-effects.

INTRODUCTION

Prevalence of hypertension is rapidly increasing in the community and it is estimated that the world will have about 1.5 billion adult hypertensives by end of this decade. Currently, hypertension is a major public health issue in India, causing over 1.6 million annual deaths accounting for 10.8% of the total mortalities and 4.6% of the disability-adjusted life years. The situation is alarming as its prevalence is about 33% in urban part and about 27% in rural area. Above all only 10% of rural and about 15% of urban hypertensives have good control.

Hypertension among young people is common, affecting 1 in 8 adults aged between 20 and 40 years. Weight gain, obesity, and physical inactivity are important risk factors for development of hypertension in young adults. These patients are more likely to respond to lifestyle changes and weight management but they less likely believe that they have disease. In Indians hypertension develops relatively early in life. In individuals aged between 15 and 49 years the prevalence is about 18% with variations between rural/urban and among different regions of country.

DEFINITION AND CLASSIFICATION

Definition of "young adults" for hypertension is not defined but age between 20 and 49 years may be taken as in Framingham offspring study. European guidelines and Indian guidelines for hypertension IV defines hypertension as systolic blood pressure (SBP) of ≥ 140 mm Hg and/or diastolic blood pressure (DBP) of ≥ 90 mm Hg. The same definition of hypertension applies in young adults. Classification is for adults > 18 years of age, who are not on antihypertensive medication and have no acute illness. It is based on the average of two or more office blood pressure (BP) readings taken at least on two occasions **(Table 1)**.

Also, clinicians should specify presence or absence of target organ disease and additional risk factors. The screening for hypertension in all adults is recommended. All adults (18 years or older) should have their office BP measured at every point of contact with health professionals or allied health staff. This screening will enable people with high normal BP to be identified, so that they can be prevented from developing hypertension by use of appropriate lifestyle modifications.

TABLE 1: Classification of blood pressure for adults age 18 and older.

Category	Systolic (mm Hg)		Diastolic (mm Hg)
Optimal	<120	*and*	<80
Normal	<130	*and*	<85
High-normal	130–139	*and/or*	85–89
Hypertension			
Stage 1	140–159	*and/or*	90–99
Stage 2	160–179	*and/or*	100–109
Stage 3	≥180	*and/or*	>110
Isolated systolic hypertension			
	≥140	*and*	<90
Isolated diastolic hypertension			
	<140	*and*	≥90

RISK FACTORS OF HYPERTENSION IN YOUNG ADULTS

The proposed ominous octet of "S," a constellation of risk factors starting with the letter "S," leading to development of noncommunicable diseases are sex, salt, sugar, sleep, smoking, stress, sunlight and sedentary behavior. These become more prominent in today's technology savvy young adults. Risk factors such as physical inactivity, weight gain, obesity, metabolic syndrome, and obstructive sleep apnea are more common in these patients. Smoking, alcohol, illicit drug intake, and psychosocial stress are becoming more common in this age group. High sodium intake, low potassium, and calcium in diet are the other factors responsible. Psychosocial stress is a major contributor to development of hypertension in young. This group has enormous work, travel related, and domestic pressure leading to busy and erratic schedule. The top three risk factors for hypertension in young were perceived to be smoking, mental stress, and obesity.

CAUSES OF HYPERTENSION IN YOUNG ADULTS

Most of the hypertension in young are essential hypertension having no identifiable cause. Secondary cause of hypertension should be ruled out if BP is very high at first presentation, episodic rise in BP, nonresponding hypertension, or poorly responding hypertension despite good adherence and resistant hypertension. Some endocrine disorders causing hypertension have their obvious signs and symptoms at presentation. Special enquiry of illicit drug use, oral contraceptive pills, and other medications must be made in these groups of patients. The important etiologies of hypertension are enumerated in **Table 2**.

TABLE 2: Causes of hypertension in adults.

Essential hypertension: 80–95%	
Secondary hypertension: 5–20%	
Renal	Parenchymal disease, polycystic kidney disease, renal tumor, obstructive uropathy
Renovascular	Fibromuscular dysplasia, atherosclerotic
Adrenal	Primary aldosteronism, Cushing's syndrome, pheochromocytoma
Neurogenic	Psychogenic, raised intracranial tension (acute)
Miscellaneous	Obstructive sleep apnea, thyroid disorders, acromegaly, preeclampsia/eclampsia
Medications	Estrogens, adrenal steroids, appetite suppressants, cyclosporine, tricyclic antidepressants, decongestants, nonsteroidal anti-inflammatory drugs (NSAIDs), cocaine, herbal medicines

APPROACH TO THE PATIENT

The key elements of evaluation of a patient of hypertension are accurate measurement of BP, focused medical history, physical examination, and laboratory investigations. Baseline investigations are urine dipstick, blood urea, and electrolytes +/- estimated glomerular filtration rate (eGFR), 12-lead electrocardiogram (ECG), fundoscopy, blood glucose, and serum lipid profile. A judicious search for secondary causes warrants in this age group. A secondary etiology may be suggested by symptoms like flushing and sweating in pheochromocytoma, by clinical findings; a renal bruit in renal artery stenosis, or laboratory abnormalities, e.g., hypokalemia suggestive of aldosteronism. There may be rapid onset of BP, even hypertensive crisis, or resistant hypertension. In young women, renal artery stenosis caused by fibromuscular dysplasia is one of the most common secondary etiologies. It can be detected by abdominal magnetic resonance imaging or computed tomography. For aldosteronism, the recommended initial diagnostic test is an aldosterone/renin ratio. Obstructive sleep apnea can be a secondary cause of or contribute to hypertension. The standard diagnostic test is polysomnography, but clinical assessment tools (e.g., Epworth Sleepiness Scale, Sleep Apnea Clinical Score) with nighttime pulse oximetry may be used to get initial clue particularly in places of limited availability.

In absence of comorbid conditions in patients with stage 1 hypertension at first visit lifestyle modifications should be started and BP reading should be repeated within 2–3 weeks. Drug treatment may need to be started after 1 month. For stage 2 hypertension shorter repeat interval is desirable. And in stage 3 hypertension, BP should be repeated after few hours to start pharmacological management. The target BP should be 130/80 mm Hg.

MANAGEMENT OF HYPERTENSION IN YOUNG PATIENTS

Nonpharmacological Therapy

The young hypertensives are better responders to nonpharmacological measures. Regular physical activity, weight loss, avoidance of tobacco and excessive alcohol, and stress management are important component of such therapy. 50–60 minutes of exercise 3–4 times a week since physical activity is more beneficial in hypertension control in Indians than dietary interventions. Daily physical activity like covering short distance by foot, taking staircase instead of lift and use of cycle for nearby activities, avoidance of prolonged sitting in the office, and practice of leaving the chair hourly and walk for 5 minutes, reduction of the screen time to <30 min/day, and less use of mobile and electronic gazettes are useful tips in young adults.

The patient should be encouraged to adapt DASH-type dietary plan rich in fruits, vegetables, and low-fat dairy products with reduced content of saturated and total fat. The total salt intake is to be restricted to <6 g/day. Young working person are more habituated to outside food. Avoidance of fast food, excessive tea, coffee, and aerated drinks are key components of dietary advice. Adequate sleep, yoga, and meditation have proven to be beneficial in stress management.

Pharmacological Management

A patient centered approach should be followed while choosing drug for BP management. Patients counseling is must, as many of young are unwilling to take medicines. Various classes of medicine may be associated with side effects such as increased micturition, fatigue, sexual dysfunction, and peripheral edema. Many young working patients may find these inconvenient and troublesome. Side effects must not reduce the work capability of these young achievers. All these should be discussed prior to prescription and drug should be tailored accordingly. This will increase acceptability and adherence of medicines. Any of the first line medicines, viz., diuretics, calcium channel blockers, and RAS blockers; angiotensin-converting enzyme inhibitors (ACEIs)/angiotensin receptor blockers (ARBs) may be used first. Young persons are having higher sympathetic tone and RAS. So ACEIs/ARBs are the preferred agents in young. However, in young females who may be planning conception, alternative antihypertensive agent like β-blockers, calcium channel blockers may be given. A long half-life medicine with once daily dosing is preferred. Combination therapy in single pill is encouraged for better compliance **(Box 1)**.

BOX 1: Clinical pearls: hypertension in young adults.

- Uncontrolled blood pressure (BP) is one of the main risk factors for cardiovascular diseases (CVDs) such as heart attacks and stroke and is responsible for one-third of total deaths in India
- Young-onset hypertension is common, up to 18% in age under 40 years
- Lifestyle modifications to improve risk profile including physical activity should begin in early age
- BP threshold to consider for intervention at 140/90 mm Hg
- Advice intense lifestyle changes, weight loss, dietary intervention, stress management, and yoga
- Assess lifetime cardiovascular risk/heart age
- Ensure joint decision making and personalized approach
- Consider drug treatment if BP > 140/90 mm Hg or evidence of organ damage or increased cardiovascular CV risk due to comorbidities
- Consider ARBs, ACEI, or β-blockers if young fertile female
- If appropriate, start with a single pill combination therapy to ensure control and compliance

(ACEI: angiotensin-converting enzyme inhibitor; ARBs: angiotensin receptor blockers; CV: cardiovascular)

A HOLISTIC APPROACH

Significant number of young patients having hypertension have other components of metabolic syndrome like diabetes/prediabetes, dyslipidemia, and obesity. Targeting other components of metabolic syndrome is an opportunity in these patients. Lifestyle changes like diet control and physical activity should be targeted to achieve good control of other components. Even modest weight loss may lead to reduction of BP. The selected medicines should help to other metabolic risk factors or at least it must be neutral. The initial combination therapy in a single pill is now advocated as it is difficult to control BP by a single medicine in most of the cases. A long half-life medicine with once daily dosing is preferred.

YOUNG AND TECHNOLOGY

On an average a young patient is more technology savvy than their older counterparts. There are gadgets and mobile applications available in market which monitors diet, physical activity, and acts as reminder to support adherence to the treatment. Online counseling, telehealth projects, and related services are easily accessible and offer help in management of hypertension. However, they have their own limitations.

CONCLUSION

Hypertension in the young is commonly essential hypertension and is on the rise because of rapid urbanization, increasing stress and addictions (tobacco and alcohol), and changing lifestyles. However, secondary hypertension also needs to be ruled out as it is remediable and appropriate management can obviate the need for lifelong treatment. It is imperative that a judicious approach is adopted while evaluating the young hypertensive and pharmacological as well as nonpharmacological measures are adopted while managing these patients. Anxiety levels are high in young patients, and RAS activity also is heightened. Drug usage should therefore be chosen to inhibit the RAS, have long-term control, and minimize side-effects.

SUGGESTED READINGS

1. Anchala R, Kannuri NK, Pant H, Khan H, Franco OH, Di AE, et al. Hypertension in India: a systematic review and meta-analysis of prevalence, awareness, and control of hypertension. J Hypertens. 2014;32:1170-7.
2. Prenissl J, Manne-Goehler J, Jaacks LM, Prabhakaran D, Awasthi A, Bischops AC, et al. Hypertension screening, awareness, treatment, and control in India: A nationally representative cross-sectional study among individuals aged 15 to 49 years. PLoS Med. 2019;16(5):e1002801.
3. AoPo I. Indian guidelines on hypertension-IV (2019). J Assoc Physicians India. 2019;67(Suppl 2):8-46.
4. Williams B, Mancia G, Spiering W, Agabiti Rosei E, Azizi M, Burnier M, et al. 2018 ESC/ESH Guidelines for the management of arterial hypertension. Eur Heart J. 2018;39(33):3021-104.
5. Sharma R, Kumar KH, Kalra S. The ominous octet of "S" in noncommunicable disease. J Soc Health Diabetes. 2017;5:12-5.
6. Jadhav U, Tiwaskar M, Khan A, Kalmath BC, Ponde CK, Sawhney J, et al. Hypertension in Young Adults in India: Perspectives and Therapeutic Options amongst Clinician's in a Cross Sectional Observational Study. J Assoc Physicians India. 2021;69(11): 11-2.
7. Kumar V, Agarwal S, Saboo B, Makkar B. RSSDI Guidelines for the management of hypertension in patients with diabetes mellitus. Int J Diabetes Dev Ctries. 2022;42(4):576-605.
8. Manchanda SC, Madan K. Yoga and hypertension. Hypertens J. 2015;1(1):28-33.
9. Ajay VS, Jindal D, Roy A, Venugopal V, Sharma R, Pawar A, et al. Development of a Smartphone-Enabled Hypertension and Diabetes Mellitus Management Package to Facilitate Evidence-Based Care Delivery in Primary Healthcare Facilities in India: The mPower Heart Project. J Am Heart Assoc. 2016;5(12):e004343.

135

CHAPTER

Hypertension in Elderly

Pramod Kumar Agrawal

ABSTRACT

Hypertension is prevalent in older adults, with isolated systolic hypertension (ISH) being common. Antihypertensive medications such as long-acting calcium channel blockers (CCBs) and thiazide diuretics effectively reduce cardiovascular events and mortality. Age-specific blood pressure targets are crucial. A personalized approach, considering patient characteristics and side effects, is vital for successful management. This chapter emphasizes addressing hypertension in the elderly to improve outcomes and quality of life.

INTRODUCTION

Among older individuals, hypertension, or high blood pressure, is a common cause for concern. In individuals over the age of 60–65 years, the prevalence of hypertension can increase from 70 to >80%. For instance, a staggering 76% of adults in the United States between the ages of 65 and 74 years and 82% of adults over the age of 75 years were found to have hypertension. However, compared to younger individuals, elderly patients had worse rates of hypertension control.

In this extensive guide to hypertension in the elderly, we shall discuss isolated systolic hypertension (ISH) and the effectiveness of antihypertensive medication therapy. We will go through the examination and diagnosis of over hypertension, as well as suggestions for senior people's target blood pressure levels.

PATHOPHYSIOLOGY OF HYPERTENSION IN ELDERLY

Arterial stiffness is a major physical change with age, affecting elastic arteries and causing aortic stiffness. The aorta and proximal elastic arteries dilate by 10% with each heartbeat, while the muscular arteries expand by only 3%. Rupture of elastic lamellae in the aorta with age can account for both dilatation and stiffening. Arterial stiffness is caused by structural changes in the arterial wall, endothelium-derived vasoactive mediators, and decreased bioavailability of nitric oxide. Aortic stiffness is a strong indicator for future cardiovascular events and all-cause mortality.

Neurohormonal and autonomic dysregulation also add to aging, with plasma renin activity decreasing at age of 60 years. Decreased baroreflex sensitivity with age causes orthostatic hypotension, while orthostatic hypertension is common among the elderly. The aging kidney is marked by progressive development of glomerulosclerosis and interstitial fibrosis, a decline in Glomerular filtration rate (GFR) and other homeostatic processes. Age-associated decrease in membrane sodium/potassium and calcium adenosine triphosphate pumps leads to an excess of intracellular calcium and sodium, increasing vasoconstriction and vascular resistance. Increased salt sensitivity is found in older and obese subjects due to their limited renal ability to excrete sodium overload.

ISOLATED SYSTOLIC HYPERTENSION

A typical type of hypertension that typically affects older individuals is ISH. It is characterized as having a systolic blood pressure (SBP) of >160 mm Hg and a diastolic blood pressure (DBP) of <90 mm Hg. Although a SBP of 130 mm Hg is regarded as the upper limit of normal at all ages, according to the 2017 American College of Cardiology/American Heart Association Blood Pressure Guideline, this is not the case.

Isolated systolic hypertension is responsible for 60–80% of occurrences of hypertension in older persons, according to research from the Framingham Heart Study and the National Health and Nutrition Examination Survey (NHANES). Systolic and pulse pressures have also been found to be important indicators of coronary artery disease in older individuals. The main cause of the increase in pulse pressure in ISH patients is reduced arterial compliance. Anemia, hyperthyroidism, aortic insufficiency, arteriovenous fistula, and Paget's disease of the bones are additional conditions that might cause ISH. The risk of cardiovascular events, such as myocardial infarction, left ventricular hypertrophy, renal disease, stroke, and cardiovascular mortality, is enhanced by ISH. SBP is more closely connected with cardiovascular risk in ISH patients than DBP.

DIASTOLIC PRESSURE'S VALUE

Systolic and pulse pressures affect elderly people's risk of coronary artery disease (CAD) directly, but diastolic pressure has the opposite effect. Lesser diastolic pressures are linked to a higher risk of negative cardiovascular events. It is crucial to remember that these findings are based on population studies or the blood pressure at baseline in clinical trials rather than the results of the actual treatment.

For instance, despite having relatively modest attainable diastolic pressures, patients in the SHEP (Systolic Hypertension in the Elderly Program) trial experienced considerably improved outcomes, including fewer CHD events. Similar results were shown in the HYVET (hypertension in the very elderly trial), where participants likewise attained lower diastolic pressures but experienced enhanced cardiovascular outcomes.

Although there may be a threshold DBP below which adverse cardiovascular outcomes might increase, the evidence points to poor health being associated with lower blood pressure as the likely cause of the association between lower diastolic pressures and adverse outcomes rather than an unfavorable side effect of antihypertensive therapy.

SPECIAL SITUATIONS IN HYPERTENSION IN THE ELDERLY POPULATION

According to a report published in JAPI 2019, hypertension is becoming more common among the elderly population, with projections indicating 76 million people in India over the age of 65 years in 2020. Systolic hypertension is the most prevalent type, and it is a greater predictor of cardiovascular and cerebrovascular events, end-stage renal disease, and all-cause mortality. To manage hypertension in the elderly, lifestyle changes such as weight loss and salt restriction can reduce or eliminate the need for blood pressure drugs. Treatment of hypertension in older patients is recognized as a highly successful medical procedure, with a review of five randomized trials demonstrating a reduction in 12–14 mm Hg SBP and 5–6 mm Hg DBP, a 34% reduction in stroke, a 19% reduction in CHD, and a 23% reduction in vascular deaths. Drug therapy should be progressively reduced, with no more than an initial 25% fall.

Long-acting dihydropyridine calcium channel blockers (CCBs), particularly amlodipine, are considered the best option for patients over the age of 80 years. Low-dose hydrochlorothiazide, chlorthalidone, or indapamide can be used with Angiotensin converting enzyme (ACE) Inhibitor or Angiotensin 2 receptor blockers (ARBs) when indicated. Both the HYVET and the HYVET extension provide additional evidence of the value of decreasing blood pressure in extremely elderly individuals and the significance of commencing and maintaining antihypertensive medication.

According to the joint recommendation on pharmacologic treatment of hypertension in adults aged 60 years or older to a higher versus lower blood pressure target from the American College of Physicians (ACP) and American Academy of Family Physicians (AAFP).

Recommendation 1: To lower the risk of mortality, stroke, and cardiac events, the ACP and AAFP advise clinicians to begin treatment in adults 60 years of age or older whose SBP is consistently at or above 150 mm Hg. Strong recommendation, excellent backing (grade) ACP and AAFP advise clinicians to select treatment goals for patients 60 years of age or older after regularly speaking with them about the benefits and drawbacks of various blood pressure targets.

Recommendation 2: To lower the risk of recurrent stroke and achieve a target SBP of < 140 mm Hg, the ACP and, AAFP advise clinicians to consider beginning or intensifying pharmacologic treatment in adults 60 years of age or older with a history of stroke or transient ischemic attack. (Grade: Inadequate recommendation, moderate-quality evidence) ACP and AAFP advise clinicians to select treatment goals for patients 60 years of age or older after regularly speaking with them about the benefits and drawbacks of various blood pressure targets.

Recommendation 3: To lower the risk of stroke or cardiac events, the ACP and AAFP advise clinicians to consider commencing or intensifying pharmacologic treatment for some adults 60 years of age or older who are at high cardiovascular risk. This suggestion is supported by a unique evaluation. The recommendation is weak, and the supporting evidence is of low quality. ACP and AAFP advise clinicians to select treatment goals for patients 60 years of age or older after regularly speaking with them about the benefits and drawbacks of various blood pressure targets.

According to European Heart Journal

Hypertension in the elderly is defined as office SBP ≥140 mm Hg and/or office DBP values ≥90 mm Hg, irrespective of age. The threshold SBP and target blood pressure may need to be adjusted in elderly patients. A study showed that SBP only increases cardiovascular risk and mortality after exceeding 152 mm Hg, and a lower DBP (<65.1 mm Hg) increases this risk. Frailty and activities of daily living (ADL) should be considered in decision-making regarding blood pressure management in the elderly. Both hypertension and frailty contribute to death and cardiovascular complications, so frailty/ADL should be measured and implemented in decision-making similar to blood pressure. Patients with ISH should be identified as a group that may potentially benefit the most from antihypertensive treatments. Patients with orthostatic hypotension and/or excessive blood pressure decline in response to treatment should be identified and managed cautiously as they are at the highest risk. In cases of advanced frailty and decreasing blood pressure accompanied by frailty progression, the discontinuation of antihypertensive agents should be considered.

MANAGEMENT OF HYPERTENSION IN ELDERLY

A combination of lifestyle adjustments and antihypertensive medication therapy is used to manage hypertension in older adult patients. In older persons with hypertension, lifestyle changes such as dietary salt limitation and weight reduction can reduce blood pressure. For instance, it has been demonstrated that reducing dietary sodium intake to 100–120 mEq/day is beneficial for lowering blood pressure.

Treatment of hypertension in senior citizens, particularly those above the age of 80 years, beneficial in several randomized trials. Antihypertensive medication has been associated with a decrease in cardiovascular events and mortality.

In particular, the SHEP investigation showed that older adult patients receiving antihypertensive medication experienced a substantial decrease in the risk of stroke. The trial also discovered that the treated group had superior cardiovascular outcomes and a lower left ventricular mass index.

Other studies have also demonstrated the advantages of antihypertensive medication for elderly people, including the Systolic Hypertension in Europe (Syst-Eur) study and the Medical Research Council (MRC) trial. According to the Syst-Eur study, antihypertensive medication substantially lowers the risk of cardiac and stroke events. The MRC trial showed that the use of a diuretic decreased the incidence of stroke, coronary events, and all cardiovascular events.

Antihypertensive medication decreased the incidence of fatal stroke and all-cause mortality, according to the results of the HYVET study, which exclusively examined exceedingly old patients (mean age 84 years). These findings corroborate that blood pressure lowering is effective in the extremely elderly group.

ELDERLY HYPERTENSION MEDICATION THERAPY

Several considerations should be taken into account while choosing antihypertensive medications for the treatment of hypertension in older individuals. To reduce the likelihood of adverse effects, smaller starting doses should be utilized, and blood pressure should be reduced progressively over the course of over 2–4 months. All older adult patients with hypertension should also start making lifestyle adjustments.

Antihypertensive medication selection should be based on unique patient characteristics and the existence of certain indications. Due to their proven ability to lower mortality and morbidity, long-acting dihydropyridine CCBs are frequently regarded as the medication of choice for elderly adult patients with hypertension. For seniors, for instance, amlodipine is a frequently given CCB.

In elderly adult patients, thiazide diuretics such as hydrochlorothiazide and chlorthalidone can also be utilized as first-line therapy. If necessary, these diuretics may be coupled with ACE inhibitors or ARBs, which limit the action of the enzyme that converts nitric oxide into angiotensin II. It has been demonstrated that combining an ACE inhibitor or ARB with a long-acting dihydropyridine CCB substantially lowers the risk of cardiovascular events.

Unless there is a specific indication, such as cardiac failure or myocardial infarction, beta blockers are typically not advised as first-line therapy for hypertension in older persons.

OPTIMAL BLOOD PRESSURE IN ELDERLY PERSONS

Age, the existence of substantial cardiovascular and kidney disease risk factors, and general health status are just a few of the variables that influence the objective blood pressure targets for older persons. For individuals between the ages of 55 and 79 years, a SBP goal of < 140/80 mm Hg is often advised. However, a SBP target of 140–145 mm Hg is seen as suitable for individuals 80 years of age and older. The benefits of more intensive blood pressure lowering in older individuals were shown by the Systolic Pressure Intervention Trial (SPRINT).

In comparison to less extensive blood pressure lowering, the trial found that attaining a mean SBP of 123 mm Hg resulted in a lower incidence of cardiovascular events and all-cause death. These advantages were seen in frail and fit older individuals. Blood pressure control in older individuals needs to be done carefully, taking into account the unique patient characteristics and any potential side effects, including orthostatic hypotension. It is essential to gradually lower blood pressure and closely monitor patients' therapeutic responses.

CONCLUSION

Especially in older persons with ISH, hypertension in the elderly is a widespread and significant health risk. ISH is linked to a higher risk of cardiovascular problems and mortality.

It has been demonstrated that antihypertensive medication therapy works well to lower blood pressure and enhance cardiovascular outcomes in older adult patients. Thiazide diuretics and long-acting dihydropyridine CCBs are frequently utilized as first-line treatments, although beta blockers are typically not advised.

Age and general health status should be taken into account when setting blood pressure targets, with an emphasis on achieving the best blood pressure control while minimizing side effects. Healthcare professionals can effectively address hypertension in the elderly population and enhance patient outcomes by applying the appropriate management measures.

SUGGESTED READINGS

1. Muntner P, Carey RM, Gidding S, Jones DW, Taler SJ, Wright JT Jr, et al. Potential US population impact of the 2017 ACC/AHA High Blood Pressure Guideline. Circulation. 2018;137(2):109-118.
2. Whelton PK,Carey RM, Aronow WS, Casey DE Jr, Collins KJ, Dennison Himmelfarb C, et al. 2017 ACC/AHA/AAPA/ABC/ACPM/AGS/APhA/ASH/ASPC/NMA/PCNA Guideline for the Prevention, Detection, Evaluation, and Management of High Blood Pressure in Adults: A Report of the American College of Cardiology/American Heart Association Task Force on Clinical Practice Guidelines. Hypertension. 2018;71(6):1269-324.
3. Bundy JD, Mills KT, Chen J, Li C, Greenland P, He J. Estimating the Association of the 2017 and 2014 Hypertension guidelines with cardiovascular events and deaths in US Adults: an analysis of national data. JAMA Cardiol. 2018;3(7):572-81.
4. Vasan RS, Larson MG, Leip EP, Kannel WB, Levy D. Assessment of frequency of progression to hypertension in non-hypertensive participants in the Framingham Heart Study: a cohort study. Lancet. 2001;358(9294):1682-6.
5. Vasan RS, Beiser A, Seshadri S, Larson MG, Kannel WB, D'Agostino RB, et al. Residual lifetime risk for developing hypertension in middle-aged women and men: The Framingham Heart Study. JAMA. 2002;287(8):1003-10.
6. Staessen JA, Gasowski J, Wang JG, Thijs L, Den Hond E, Boissel JP, et al. Risks of untreated and treated isolated systolic hypertension in the elderly: meta-analysis of outcome trials. Lancet. 2000;355(9207):865-72.
7. National High Blood Pressure Education Program Working Group Report on Hypertension in the Elderly. National High Blood Pressure Education Program Working Group. Hypertension. 1994;23:275.
8. National Institute for Health and Clinical Excellence. (2009). Hypertension: management of hypertension in adults in primary care (NICE clinical guideline update). [online] Available from http://www.nice.org.uk. [Last accessed December, 2023].
9. Franklin SS, Gustin W 4th, Wong ND, Larson MG, Weber MA, Kannel WB, et al. Hemodynamic patterns of age-related changes in blood pressure. The Framingham Heart Study. Circulation. 1997;96:308-15.
10. Franklin SS, Jacobs MJ, Wong ND, L'Italien GJ, Lapuerta P. Predominance of isolated systolic hypertension among middle-aged and elderly US hypertensives: analysis based on National Health and Nutrition Examination Survey (NHANES) III. Hypertension. 2001;37(3):869-74.
11. Kannel WB. Blood pressure as a cardiovascular risk factor: prevention and treatment. JAMA.1996;275(20):1571-6.
12. Franklin SS, Larson MG, Khan SA, Wong ND, Leip EP, Kannel WB, et al. Does the relation of blood pressure to coronary heart disease risk change with aging? The Framingham Heart Study. Circulation. 2001;103(9):1245-9.
13. Chobanian AV. Clinical practice. Isolated systolic hypertension in the elderly. N Engl J Med.2007;357(8):789-96.
14. Izzo JL Jr, Levy D, Black HR. Clinical Advisory Statement. Importance of systolic blood pressure in older Americans. Hypertension. 2000;35:1021.
15. Young JH, Klag MJ, Muntner P, Whyte JL, Pahor M, Coresh J. Blood pressure and decline in kidney function: findings from the Systolic Hypertension in the Elderly Program (SHEP). J Am Soc Nephrol. 2002;13(11):2776-82.
16. Neaton JD, Wentworth D. Serum cholesterol, blood pressure, cigarette smoking, and death from coronary heart disease.

Overall findings and differences by age for 316,099 white men. Multiple Risk Factor Intervention Trial Research Group. Arch Intern Med. 1992;152:56.

17. Pastor-Barriuso R, Banegas JR, Damián J, Appel LJ, Guallar E. Systolic blood pressure, diastolic blood pressure, and pulse pressure: an evaluation of their joint effect on mortality. Ann Intern Med.2003;139(9):731-9.
18. Protogerou AD, Safar ME, Iaria P, Safar H, Le Dudal K, Filipovsky J, et al. Diastolic blood pressure and mortality in the elderly with cardiovascular disease. Hypertension. 2007;50(1):172-80.
19. Prevention of stroke by antihypertensive drug treatment in older persons with isolated systolic hypertension. Final results of the Systolic Hypertension in the Elderly Program (SHEP). SHEP Cooperative Research Group. JAMA. 1991;265(24):3255-64.
20. Beckett NS, Peters R, Fletcher AE, Staessen JA, Liu L, Dumitrascu D, et al. Treatment of hypertension in patients 80 years of age or older. N Engl J Med. 2008;358(18):1887-98.
21. Somes GW, Pahor M, Shorr RI, Cushman WC, Applegate WB. The role of diastolic blood pressure when treating isolated systolic hypertension. Arch Intern Med. 1999;159(17):2004-9.
22. Vokó Z, Bots ML, Hofman A, Koudstaal PJ, Witteman JC, Breteler MM. J-shaped relation between blood pressure and stroke in treated hypertensives. Hypertension. 1999;34(6):1181-5.
23. Messerli FH, Mancia G, Conti CR, Hewkin AC, Kupfer S, Champion A, et al. Dogma disputed: can aggressively lowering blood pressure in hypertensive patients with coronary artery disease be dangerous? Ann Intern Med. 2006;144(12):884-93.
24. Boutitie F, Gueyffier F, Pocock S, Fagard R, Boissel JP; INDANA Project Steering Committee. J-shaped relationship between blood pressure and mortality in hypertensive patients: new insights from a meta-analysis of individual-patient data. Ann Intern Med. 2002;136(6):438-48.
25. Appel LJ, Espeland MA, Easter L, Wilson AC, Folmar S, Lacy CR. Effects of reduced sodium intake on hypertension control in older individuals: results from the Trial of Nonpharmacologic Interventions in the Elderly (TONE). Arch Intern Med. 2001;161(5):685-93.
26. Whelton PK, Appel LJ, Espeland MA, Applegate WB, Ettinger WH Jr, Kostis JB, et al. Sodium reduction and weight loss in the treatment of hypertension in older persons: a randomized controlled trial of nonpharmacologic interventions in the elderly (TONE). TONE Collaborative Research Group. JAMA. 1998;279(11):839-46.
27. Staessen JA, Richart T, Verdecchia P. Reducing blood pressure in people of different ages.BMJ. 2008;336:1080.
28. Staessen JA, Fagard R, Thijs L, Celis H, Arabidze GG, Birkenhäger WH, et al. Randomised double-blind comparison of placebo and active treatment for older patients with isolated systolic hypertension. The Systolic Hypertension in Europe (Syst-Eur) Trial Investigators. Lancet. 1997;350(9080):757-64.
29. Liu L, Wang JG, Gong L, Liu G, Staessen JA. Comparison of active treatment and placebo in older Chinese patients with isolated systolic hypertension. Systolic Hypertension in China (Syst-China) Collaborative Group. J Hypertens. 1998;16(12 Pt 1): 1823-9.
30. Staessen JA, Richart T, Birkenhäger WH. Less atherosclerosis and lower blood pressure for a meaningful life perspective with more brain. Hypertension. 2007;49:389.
31. Chaudhry SI, Krumholz HM, Foody JM. Systolic hypertension in older persons. JAMA. 2004;292:1074.
32. Kostis JB, Davis BR, Cutler J, Grimm RH Jr, Berge KG, Cohen JD, et al. Prevention of heart failure by antihypertensive drug treatment in older persons with isolated systolic hypertension. SHEP Cooperative Research Group. JAMA. 1997;278(3):212-6.
33. Ofili EO, Cohen JD, St Vrain JA, Pearson A, Martin TJ, Uy ND, et al. Effect of treatment of isolated systolic hypertension on left ventricular mass. JAMA. 1998;279(10):778-80.
34. Franse LV, Pahor M, Di Bari M, Somes GW, Cushman WC, Applegate WB. Hypokalemia associated with diuretic use and cardiovascular events in the Systolic Hypertension in the Elderly Program. Hypertension. 2000;35(5):1025-30.
35. Staessen JA, Fagard R, Thijs L, Celis H, Birkenhäger WH, Bulpitt CJ, et al. Subgroup and per-protocol analysis of the randomized European Trial on Isolated Systolic Hypertension in the Elderly. Arch Intern Med. 1998;158(15):1681-91.
36. Tuomilehto J, Rastenyte D, Birkenhäger WH, Thijs L, Antikainen R, Bulpitt CJ, et al. Effects of calcium-channel blockade in older patients with diabetes and systolic hypertension. Systolic Hypertension in Europe Trial Investigators. N Engl J Med. 1999;340(9):677-84.
37. Forette F, Seux ML, Staessen JA, Thijs L, Birkenhäger WH, Babarskiene MR, et al. Prevention of dementia in randomised double-blind placebo-controlled Systolic Hypertension in Europe (Syst-Eur) trial. Lancet. 1998; 352(9137):1347-51.
38. Medical Research Council trial of treatment of hypertension in older adults: principal results. MRC Working Party. BMJ. 1992;304(6824):405-12.
39. Khan N, McAlister FA. Re-examining the efficacy of beta-blockers for the treatment of hypertension: a meta-analysis. CMAJ. 2006;174:1737.
40. Messerli FH, Grossman E, Goldbourt U. Are beta-blockers efficacious as first-line therapy for hypertension in the elderly? A systematic review. JAMA. 1998;279:1903.
41. Julius S, Kjeldsen SE, Weber M, Brunner HR, Ekman S, Hansson L, et al. Outcomes in hypertensive patients at high cardiovascular risk treated with regimens based on valsartan or amlodipine: the VALUE randomised trial. Lancet 2004; 363(9436):2022-31.
42. Mariampillai JE, Eskås PA, Heimark S, Kjeldsen SE, Narkiewicz K, Mancia G. A Case for Less Intensive Blood Pressure Control: It Matters to Achieve Target Blood Pressure Early and Sustained Below 140/90mmHg. Prog Cardiovasc Dis. 2016; 59(3):209-18.
43. Mancia G, Fagard R, Narkiewicz K, Redon J, Zanchetti A, Böhm M, et al. 2013 ESH/ESC Guidelines for the management of arterial hypertension: the Task Force for the management of arterial hypertension of the European Society of Hypertension (ESH) and of the European Society of Cardiology (ESC). J Hypertens. 2013;34(28):2159-219.
44. Vanhanen H, Thijs L, Birkenhäger W, Tilvis R, Sarti C, Tuomilehto J, et al. Associations of orthostatic blood pressure fall in older patients with isolated systolic hypertension. Syst-Eur Investigators. J Hypertens. 1996;14(8):943-9.
45. Applegate WB, Davis BR, Black HR, Smith WM, Miller ST, Burlando AJ. Prevalence of postural hypotension at baseline in the Systolic Hypertension in the Elderly Program (SHEP) cohort. J Am Geriatr Soc. 1991;39(11):1057-64.
46. Gangavati A, Hajjar I, Quach L, Jones RN, Kiely DK, Gagnon P, et al. Hypertension, orthostatic hypotension, and the risk of falls in a community-dwelling elderly population: the maintenance of balance, independent living, intellect, and zest in the elderly of Boston study. J Am Geriatr Soc. 2011;59(3):383-9.

47. Tinetti ME, Han L, Lee DS, McAvay GJ, Peduzzi P, Gross CP, et al. Antihypertensive medications and serious fall injuries in a nationally representative sample of older adults. JAMA Intern Med. 2014;174(4):588-95.
48. Butt DA, Mamdani M, Austin PC, Tu K, Gomes T, Glazier RH. The risk of hip fracture after initiating antihypertensive drugs in the elderly. Arch Intern Med. 2012;172(22):1739-44.
49. Benetos A, Labat C, Rossignol P, Fay R, Rolland Y, Valbusa F, et al. Treatment With Multiple Blood Pressure Medications, Achieved Blood Pressure, and Mortality in Older Nursing Home Residents: The PARTAGE Study. JAMA Intern Med. 2015;175(6):989-95.
50. Odden MC, Peralta CA, Haan MN, Covinsky KE. Rethinking the association of high blood pressure with mortality in elderly adults: the impact of frailty. Arch Intern Med. 2012;172:1162.
51. Rosendorff C, Lackland DT, Allison M, Aronow WS, Black HR, Blumenthal RS, et al. Treatment of hypertension in patients with coronary artery disease: a scientific statement from the American Heart Association, American College of Cardiology, and American Society of Hypertension. Circulation. 2015;9(6): 453-98.
52. Blood Pressure Lowering Treatment Trialists' Collaboration, Turnbull F, Neal B, Ninomiya T, Algert C, Arima H, et al. Effects of different regimens to lower blood pressure on major cardiovascular events in older and younger adults: meta-analysis of randomised trials. BMJ. 2008;336(7653):1121-3.
53. Law MR, Morris JK, Wald NJ. Use of blood pressure lowering drugs in the prevention of cardiovascular disease: meta-analysis of 147 randomised trials in the context of expectations from prospective epidemiological studies. BMJ. 2009;338:b1665.
54. ALLHAT Officers and Coordinators for the ALLHAT Collaborative Research Group. The Antihypertensive and Lipid-Lowering Treatment to Prevent Heart Attack Trial. Major outcomes in high-risk hypertensive patients randomized to angiotensin-converting enzyme inhibitor or calcium channel blocker vs diuretic: The Antihypertensive and Lipid-Lowering Treatment to Prevent Heart Attack Trial (ALLHAT). JAMA. 2002;288:2981.
55. Hansson L, Lindholm LH, Ekbom T, Dahlöf B, Lanke J, Scherstén B, et al. Randomised trial of old and new antihypertensive drugs in elderly patients: cardiovascular mortality and morbidity the Swedish Trial in Old Patients with Hypertension-2 study. Lancet. 1999;354(9192):1751-6.
56. Wright JT Jr, Probstfield JL, Cushman WC, Pressel SL, Cutler JA, Davis BR, et al. ALLHAT findings revisited in the context of subsequent analyses, other trials, and meta-analyses. Arch Intern Med. 2009;169(9):832-42.
57. Jamerson K, Weber MA, Bakris GL, Dahlöf B, Pitt B, Shi V, et al. Benazepril plus amlodipine or hydrochlorothiazide for hypertension in high-risk patients. N Engl J Med. 2008;359(23): 2417-28.
58. Wing LM, Reid CM, Ryan P, Beilin LJ, Brown MA, Jennings GL, et al. A comparison of outcomes with angiotensin-converting-enzyme inhibitors and diuretics for hypertension in the elderly. N Engl J Med. 2003;348:583.
59. Davis BR, Furberg CD, Wright JT Jr, Cutler JA, Whelton P; ALLHAT Collaborative Research Group. ALLHAT: setting the record straight. Ann Intern Med. 2004;141(1):39-46.
60. Frohlich ED. Treating hypertension - what are we to believe? N Engl J Med. 2003;348:639.
61. Lindholm LH, Carlberg B, Samuelsson O. Should beta blockers remain first choice in the treatment of primary hypertension? A meta-analysis. Lancet. 2005;366:1545.
62. Bradley HA, Wiysonge CS, Volmink JA, Mayosi BM, Opie LH. How strong is the evidence for use of beta blockers as first-line therapy for hypertension? Systematic review and meta-analysis. J Hypertens. 2006;24(11):2131-41.
63. Rosendorff C, Black HR, Cannon CP, Gersh BJ, Gore J, Izzo JL Jr, et al. Treatment of hypertension in the prevention and management of ischemic heart disease: a scientific statement from the American Heart Association Council for High Blood Pressure Research and the Councils on Clinical Cardiology and Epidemiology and Prevention. Circulation. 2007;115(21): 2761-88.
64. James PA, Oparil S, Carter BL, Cushman WC, Dennison-Himmelfarb C, Handler J, et al. 2014 evidence-based guideline for the management of high blood pressure in adults: report from the panel members appointed to the Eighth Joint National Committee (JNC 8). JAMA. 2014;311(5):507-20.
65. Williams B, Mancia G, Spiering W, Agabiti Rosei E, Azizi M, Burnier M, et al. 2018 Practice Guidelines for the management of arterial hypertension of the European Society of Cardiology and the European Society of Hypertension. Blood Press. 2018;27(6): 314-40.
66. Egan BM, Li J, Shatat IF, Fuller JM, Sinopoli A. Closing the gap in hypertension control between younger and older adults: National Health and Nutrition Examination Survey (NHANES) 1988 to 2010. Circulation. 2014;129(20):2052-61.
67. Egan BM, Bland VJ, Brown AL, Ferdinand KC, Hernandez GT, Jamerson KA, et al. Hypertension in African Americans aged 60 to 79 years: statement from the international society of hypertension in blacks. J Clin Hypertens. 2015;17(4):252-9.
68. Egan BM, Li J, Wagner CS. Systolic Blood Pressure Intervention Trial (SPRINT) and Target Systolic Blood Pressure in Future Hypertension Guidelines. Hypertension. 2016;68:318.
69. Egan BM, Zhao Y, Axon RN, Brzezinski WA, Ferdinand KC. Uncontrolled and apparent treatment resistant hypertension in the United States, 1988 to 2008. Circulation. 2011;124(9): 1046-58.
70. Williamson JD, Supiano MA, Applegate WB, Berlowitz DR, Campbell RC, Chertow GM, et al. Intensive vs Standard Blood Pressure Control and Cardiovascular Disease Outcomes in Adults Aged ≥75 Years: A Randomized Clinical Trial. JAMA. 2016;315(24):2673-82.

136

CHAPTER

Future of Hypertension Management

Saumitra Ray, Srina Ray

ABSTRACT

Hypertension is an ever-evolving field of clinical and epidemiological research. Though being the most common disease in the adult with a prevalence of about 30% in India (by older definition; newer definition of hypertension will put the figure much higher), it is incompletely understood and often not given its due importance. But researchers are fully aware of the huge potential of new discoveries and inventions in the field of hypertension and exciting work is being done in the different aspects of hypertension management. The strategy of initial management of hypertension and the timing of the drugs are getting revised. The role of artificial intelligence (AI) is rapidly explored in the management of hypertension. Newer pathological mechanisms, like role of inflammation, immunological activation, gut microbiomes, and genetic manipulation, are being investigated actively. New drugs are being developed as well as the existing drugs are being tested for efficacy in hypertension. Here, is a brief glimpse of what is going on in the field of hypertension.

INTRODUCTION

Historically high blood pressure had been considered as normal physiological adaptation with aging and trying to reduce it might cause harm. But when President Roosevelt of the USA died of stroke with excessive blood pressure, scientific and political pressure started looking at the prospects of reducing blood pressure to attain clinical benefits. Large trials were designed, but focusing on diastolic blood pressure (DBP) reduction. First few Joint National Committees on Prevention, Detection, Evaluation and Treatment of high blood pressure (JNC) also addressed only DBP. Only from the 4th JNC the systolic blood pressure (SBP) came to limelight and subsequently took the center stage of attention.

The ideal blood pressure levels for maximum clinical benefit keep on changing. Similarly, the life-style intervention is open to newer recommendations. The ideal pharmacotherapy to start with and the subsequent additions are also subject to changes all the time.

Device therapy and renal denervation (RDN) therapy are being developed and sophisticated over last two decades. But the real changes are coming in the fields of newer understanding of the pathogenic mechanisms of high blood pressure and to target therapy accordingly, precision medicine and use of artificial intelligence (AI) in the management of hypertension.

TARGET VALUES OF BLOOD PRESSURE THERAPY

The European Society of Cardiology (ESC) set a threshold for blood pressure treatment of 140/90 mm Hg and the American College of Cardiology (ACC) set this at 130/80 mm Hg. As per ESC, the ideal SBP is 120–130 mm Hg, whereas, by ACC, the lower the better, if tolerated. In chronic renal disease patients the ESC advocates to keep the SBP between 130 and 140 mm Hg, whereas, the other major guidelines set the goal below 130 mm Hg. Further trials are needed in future to settle these discrepancies among major international guidelines to help the clinicians in general.

NUMBER OF DRUGS TO INITIATE TREATMENT

The ESC recommends to start with a two-drug fixed-dose combination in most patients whenever pharmacotherapy is needed, whereas ACC advocates monotherapy to start with in mild hypertension. However, the majority of hypertension trials had to use 2–3 drugs to achieve a control of SBP to the tune of 130–140 mm Hg. If the threshold is taken as 130 mm Hg for SBP, then three drugs may be needed in majority of patients to attain the goal. There are trials to support this view. Even, QUARTET trial showed benefit by starting four drugs in one-fourth of their maximal dose compared to full dose of a single agent.

TIMING OF DRUG INTAKE

Traditionally, the antihypertensive drugs are taken with the breakfast as this practice suits the lifestyle of the majority of the patients. However, the chronotherapy concept has emerged whereby the drugs were administered as per the biological clock to have the maximum effect. The HYGIA trial showed huge clinical benefits in terms of myocardial infarction (MI), stroke, heart failure (HF), and cardiovascular and all-cause mortality, if the antihypertensive medication is taken at bedtime rather than in the morning. However, the subsequent TIME trial annulled these findings showing exactly same results irrespective of the time of blood pressure medications. Even, the night time doses did not produce excess falls in the early morning.

ROLE OF RENAL DENERVATION THERAPY AND OTHER DEVICES

Renal denervation has long been an appealing concept to control resistant hypertension and in hypertensive patients who cannot tolerate most of the antihypertensive medications. But the dubious long-term efficacy and complications of the procedure did not allow RDN for general application. However, the recent Global SYMPLICITY Registry using Spyral devices and keeping long-term follow-up data shows promise of RDN for future.

Other newer technologies aimed at modulating the peripheral nervous system, include baroreflex activation therapy, endovascular baroreflex amplification therapy, carotid body ablation, and pacemaker-mediated programmable hypertension control.

Effective utilization of emerging technologies, such as noninvasive, continuous blood pressure monitoring technology, could improve hypertension awareness.

EXTENSION OF PHARMACOTHERAPY

As currently recommended, the first-line medicines for hypertension are renin–angiotensin–aldosterone (RAAS) inhibitors, dihydropyridine calcium channel blockers (DHP-CCBs), and thiazide-like diuretics. Beta blockers are reserved for specific indications like ischemic heart disease (IHD), atrial fibrillation (AF), HF with reduced ejection fraction (HFrEF), and hypertension during or planned pregnancy. However, the recently published guideline of the European Society of Hypertension (ESH) extended the indication of use of beta blockers in hypertension in another 19 conditions, including, interestingly, chronic obstructive pulmonary disease (COPD).

The sacubitril–valsartan is the established therapy in HFrEF, but recent trials show promise in resistant hypertension in presence of HF with preserved ejection fraction (HFpEF). In many other clinical settings of hypertension like Asian patients with hypertension, elderly with isolated systolic hypertension, hemodialysis patients with resistant hypertension, salt-sensitive hypertension, elderly Asian patients, hemodialysis patients, etc., its role is being explored and may be recommended in near future.

Sodium-glucose cotransporter-2 (SGLT-2) inhibitors are a first-line therapy in HF of any ejection fraction and chronic kidney disease, with or without diabetes, along with being the preferred antidiabetic agent in diabetic patients with high risk of IHD.

NEW DRUGS

There are a number of other new potential drug therapies for hypertension, including inhibitors of aldosterone synthase, soluble guanylate cyclase stimulators, inhibitors of phosphodiesterase-5, and xanthine oxidase, and advanced glycation end-product breakers, which are being developed.

PRECISION MEDICINE

As hypertension is a multipathological process, it may be conceptually helpful to detect the predominant pathological mechanism of hypertension in an individual and to target therapy accordingly. The fundamental two pathological processes of hypertension are absolute or relative intravascular volume excess and renin–angiotensin system overactivity. A diuretic or CCB is most effective in the former situation and a RAAS inhibitor including beta blocker in the latter situation. This was shown long ago that plasma renin activity (PRA)-based treatment allows monotherapy for effective blood pressure control.

The new Precision Hypertension trial with six different regimens of four antihypertensive drugs proves the point of a scope of precision medicine in hypertension. Future trials are needed to fully explore this exciting area.

ROLE OF ARTIFICIAL INTELLIGENCE

Artificial intelligence is coming in a big way in different fields of clinical medicine. Hypertension is no exception. As hypertensive patients need frequent clinic visits, adjustment of doses of medicines, biochemicals and tests and the data interpretation, AI is particularly useful in hypertension management. Preliminary trials have shown the benefit and new algorithms and softwares are being developed for the clinicians.

The successful convergence of digital data, AI, and biomedical sciences accompanied by their implementation in healthcare delivery and the effective strategy for population health will be the future in hypertension management.

NOVEL APPROACHES TO HYPERTENSION MANAGEMENT

Many new avenues are opening up to understand the mechanism of hypertension and to develop therapy accordingly. Following are a few examples of these newer approaches.

- Genome-wide association studies (GWAS) identified genes involved in the development of hypertension and in predicting responses to different antihypertensive agents.

  Uromodulin is a protein exclusively expressed by the epithelial cells of the thick ascending limb of the loop of Henle in the kidney. The *UMOD* gene, located on chromosome 16, encodes for the translation of uromodulin and studies have demonstrated an association between single-nucleotide polymorphisms in the region of the *UMOD* gene and renal function and hypertension.
- Within the RAAS, cleavage of angiotensinogen (AGT), a serum globulin produced in the liver is the fundamental process which produces the whole amount of angiotensin in the body. Suppression of AGT can be achieved by interfering at the RNA level with antisense oligonucleotides (ASO) and small interfering RNA (siRNA). Animal studies have demonstrated that both ASOs and siRNAs effectively lower blood pressure in spontaneously hypertensive rats with long-lasting effects.
- Chronic overactivation of immune cells, especially T cells, influences tissue damage, and development of hypertension and therapies targeting to suppress T cells hold future promise to control hypertension.

  Utilizing an individual's immune response to components of key pathways implicated in hypertension, such as the RAAS system, has the potential to improve adherence and supersede oral therapy.

  Phase 1 trials for a conjugate vaccine against angiotensin II (Ang II) and CYT006-AngQb (AngQb) demonstrated a mean SBP reduction of up to 21 mm Hg in hypertensive rat models and the vaccine was identified to be immunogenic and well-tolerated in healthy human volunteers.
- Alteration of gut microbiome flora by various factors is central to the immune responses contributing to blood pressure elevation. Strategies targeting the microbiome are being researched.
- Adipose tissue undergoing expansion and remodeling produces adipokines, vasoactive peptides and inflammatory mediators that contributes to the development of hypertension, endothelial dysfunction, and vascular stiffness. Modification and reduction of adipose tissue, especially the visceral fat, may help controlling the blood pressure, especially the resistant hypertension.
- Oxidative stress is fundamental to many of the cell stressors in hypertension. Importance of endoplasmic reticular stress and mitochondrial oxidative stress as emerging field of oxidative redox proteomics in hypertension is being evaluated.
- The Rho-kinase activity is the main modulator of Ca^{2+} sensitivity that changes with age. Interestingly, this relationship leads to modified adrenergic arterial pressure responses. Manipulation of this pathway holds promise for future treatment of hypertension.
- Recent updates highlight that measurement of the arterial stiffness should be a keystone in hypertension management and cardiovascular prevention and the potential impact of antihypertensive therapy on reversing vascular remodeling and improving cardiovascular health is suggested.
- Intake of inorganic nitrate, which is predominantly found in green leafy vegetables and beets, has a variety of favorable cardiovascular effects, and the mechanisms underlying blood pressure reduction by dietary inorganic nitrate are being reviewed.
- Albumin-induced modulation of the tone of the afferent arterioles is mediated by the increased osmolarity and nitric oxide scavenging. This is a potential area of future research.
- Drug-induced hypertension with anticancer drugs, especially VEGF (vascular endothelial growth factor) requires collaborative clinical care between

cardiologists and oncologists. Evidence-based information is needed so that anticancer effects of novel chemotherapies are maximized while minimizing cardiovascular risk.

CONCLUSION

Though hypertension is the most common disease in the adult population and the most important attributable cause of mortality, its pathology, mechanism and optimization are still incompletely understood. Thus, there are huge scopes of development and future research in the fields starting from the ideal levels of blood pressure to the way of treatment, personalized treatment, utilization of AI, roles of device therapy, and newer areas of pathological exploration and subsequent development of therapies. It is sensible to keep oneself updated with the new research findings and latest guidelines.

SUGGESTED READINGS

1. Touyz RM, Schiffrin EL. A Compendium on Hypertension: New Advances and Future Impact. Circ Res. 2021;128(7):803-7.
2. Mrowka R. Recent advances in hypertension research. Acta Physiol (Oxf). 2019;226(4):e13295.
3. Mancia G, Kreutz R, Brunström M, Burnier M, Grassi G, Januszewicz A, et al. 2023 ESH Guidelines on Management of Arterial Hypertension The Task Force for the management of arterial hypertension of the European Society of Hypertension: Endorsed by the International Society of Hypertension (ISH) and the European Renal Association (ERA). J Hypertens. 2023;41(12):1874-2071.

SECTION

10

IMMUNOLOGY

137

CHAPTER

Adult Primary Immunodeficiency

Joydeep Samanta, Arghya Chattopadhyay

ABSTRACT

Primary immunodeficiencies (PID) are a group of disorders characterized by impaired function of the immune system and increased susceptibility to various infections. It was first described almost 70 years back by Colonel Ogden Bruton. Although initially it was considered mostly as an increased susceptibility to infections, with time other spectrums like predisposition to autoimmunity, inherited nature of these conditions, etc., were recognized. Due to this improvement in knowledge in the field of immunodeficiency, the name PID has now been replaced by Inborn errors of immunity (IEI). Although initially it was considered predominantly a disease of childhood, with improvement in the diagnostics and increased awareness, it is increasingly being diagnosed in adult age too. A judicious clinical approach with careful assessment of the suggestive clinical clues like the age of presentation, the pattern of infection, the organ system involved, family history, and associated clinical manifestations can help in clinching the diagnosis.

INTRODUCTION

Primary immunodeficiencies (PIDs) are a group of diseases which affect the normal function and development of the immune system with resultant increased susceptibility to various infections. It usually occurs due to some inherited genetic defects affecting the immune system and due to its strong inherited nature, it is nowadays also known as inborn errors of immunity (IEI). The first PID described was X-linked agammaglobulinemia (XLA) by Colonel Ogden Bruton. Since then, almost 70 years passed with a vast increase in knowledge in the field of immunodeficiency disorders. Initially, PIDs were considered predominantly as a disease of the pediatric population. However, it has become clear now that although it is more common in pediatric populations, PIDs can present in adults too.

BURDEN OF PRIMARY IMMUNODEFICIENCIES IN ADULTS

Studies conducted over the last decade have given an idea about the status of PID in adults. Although previously PIDs were considered a rare disease, a telephonic survey conducted in the United States (US) estimated that 1/1,200 of the living population may have a PID. Lack of awareness and diagnostic facilities is the major reason for the presumed rarity of the condition. Two large population-based studies from the US showed that PID can be as common as diseases like leukemia. These population-based studies have also shown that more than 50% of cases of these PIDs are diagnosed in adults >18 years of age. In data published by the European Society for Immunodeficiency registry, among the patients of immunodeficiency around 8% are aged more than 65 years. Even there is the report of a new diagnosis of common variable immunodeficiency (CVID), a PID in a patient of 92 years of age, thus showing that although PIDs are traditionally considered a disease of the pediatric population, these can present in any age.

Primary immunodeficiencies in adults can be seen usually in two different settings. Children diagnosed with PID can progress to adult age as a case of adult PID. Besides, PIDs can be diagnosed in the adult age for the first time. Amongst the PIDs diagnosed in adults,

PIDs due to antibody deficiency are the most common type. Besides this, autoimmune lymphoproliferative syndrome, or hypomorphic form, many severe PIDs can also be present in adulthood. Also, due to improvements in PID diagnostics and therapeutics, many children with severe forms of PIDs can survive into adulthood. In a retrospective chart review of an adult immunodeficiency center in Canada, humoral immunodeficiency was the most common subtype observed followed by defects in T cells, natural killer (NK) cells, and phagocytic defects. In another study from Iran conducted over a 7-year period amongst adult patients with a diagnosis of PID, humoral immunodeficiency was the most common etiology followed by phagocytic defects, cell-mediated immune deficiency, and complement defects.

TABLE 1: Conditions causing predisposition to recurrent infection in absences of primary immunodeficiencies.

Location	Condition
Skin	Burn, nonhealing ulcer, eczema
Respiratory tract	Smoking, bronchiectasis, cystic fibrosis, Kartagener's syndrome, allergy
Intestinal tract	Proton-pump inhibitor therapy, prolonged antibiotic therapy
Urinary tract	Reflux, ureteric stenosis, renal calculi, indwelling urinary catheter
Systemic diseases	Diabetes mellitus, chronic liver disease, chronic kidney disease, HIV infection, sickle cell disease, multiple myeloma

(HIV: human immunodeficiency virus)

CLINICAL PRESENTATIONS OF PRIMARY IMMUNODEFICIENCIES IN ADULTS

Normally, skin and mucous membranes provide a natural barrier to invading pathogens. These are the most common site of infection even in immunocompetent individuals. However, in the event of any atypical features like the prolonged duration of infection or unusual type of pathogen, suspicion of underlying immunodeficiency should be considered. For example, a prolonged, complicated, or recurrent course of infection by a common organism like *Pneumococcus*, staphylococci, or *Klebsiella* should be investigated. Similarly, infection by atypical pathogens like *Cryptococcus* and *Candida* should also be investigated for possible immunodeficiency disorders.

However, there are certain caveats. Some abnormalities in the natural barrier can also predispose a person to recurrent infection. For example, conditions causing breaches in skin integrity and mucous membrane integrity like burns, atopic eczema, and some diseases like cystic fibrosis, etc., can predispose to recurrent infection. Also, certain systemic diseases like diabetes mellitus, chronic kidney disease, and chronic liver diseases can predispose to recurrent infection even in the absence of PIDs. Details of these conditions enumerated in **Table 1** should be kept in mind.

Although recurrent and prolonged infections are the main features of PIDs, there are certain patterns which raise the index of suspicion for an underlying PID. These features can be summarized by a mnemonic CLINO.

- *Course*: A protracted course of infection, unusual complications, and unsatisfactory response to antibiotic therapy should raise the index of suspicion.
- *Localization*: Atypical sites of infection like fungal brain abscess, cerebral toxoplasmosis, cryptococcal meningitis, pneumococcal osteomyelitis, etc., in the absence of any predisposing conditions, as enumerated in **Table 1**, should ring the alarm.
- *Intensity*: An unusually severe infection with inadequate response to antibiotic therapy is another feature of infections associated with PID.
- *Number of infections*: Although four or more ear infections/year and two or more severe sinus infections or pneumonia/year are considered abnormal in children, it is slightly different in adults. Usually, three or more bacterial infections/year in an adult with each episode lasting more than 4 weeks should be investigated for underlying immunodeficiency.
- *Organism*: Infections by unusual organisms like *Cryptococcus, Pneumocystis jirovecii, Toxoplasma gondii*, and *Lophomonas* should raise concern about possible immunodeficiency states.

Although infections are the hallmark features of PIDs, there are some associated manifestations too. These include associated lymphoproliferative disorders, autoimmunity, or some other conditions. These can also be described by a mnemonic GAPRIEL.

- *Granulomas*: In skin, lung, lymph nodes, or other organs
- *Autoimmunity*: Autoimmune cytopenia, arthritis, alopecia, enteropathy, or other autoimmune features
- *Pulmonary involvement*: Interstitial lung disease (ILD), especially in the form of granulomatous and lymphocytic lung disease (GLID)
- *Recurrent fever*: Periodic fever, hemophagocytosis
- *Inflammatory bowel disease*: Refractory to therapy, at a young age
- *Eczema*: Recurrent, atypical, unresponsive to therapy
- *Lymphoproliferation*: Splenomegaly, lymphadenopathy

Except for these associated manifestations, some manifestations can develop because of complications.

For example, some PIDs are associated with the risk of developing malignancies. Particularly, an increased risk of malignancy like gastric carcinoma and lymphoma has been recognized in patients with CVID. Also, complications like bronchiectasis due to repeated infection and respiratory failure due to long-standing ILD are well recognized.

OVERVIEW OF THE COMMON PRIMARY IMMUNODEFICIENCIES ENCOUNTERED IN ADULTS

Common PIDs observed in adults are PIDs due to predominant humoral immunodeficiency like CVID, specific immunoglobulin deficiency, especially IgA deficiency, combined cellular and humoral immunodeficiency like late-onset combined immunodeficiency (LOCID), Good's syndrome, and predominant cell-mediated immunodeficiency like idiopathic CD4+ lymphocytopenia and GATA2 deficiency. Other PIDs which can be seen in adults include some newly discovered entities like caspase B deficiency and terminal deletion of 11q. Also, certain PIDs which are common in childhood can rarely present in an adult age too, like chronic granulomatous disease (CGD), autoimmune polyendocrinopathy candidiasis ectodermal dystrophy (APECED), complement deficiency, familial hemophagocytic lymphohistiocytosis (familial HLH), and XLA. Details of the major PIDs encountered in adults are enumerated in **Table 2**.

TABLE 2: Major primary immunodeficiencies encountered in adults.

Diseases	Genes affected	Components of immunity being affected	Functions affected	Key clinical features
PIDs classically presenting in adulthood				
Common variable immune deficiency (CVID)	*TACI* (most common), *NFκB1*, *STAT3*, *CTLA4*, *PIK3CD*, *IKZF1*	Humoral immunity	Severely low IgG level with low IgA and/ or IgM	Recurrent infection (in 94% cases—upper and lower respiratory tract infection, gastrointestinal infection, unusual/ opportunistic infection), hematological/ organ-specific autoimmunity (29%—immune thrombocytopenia, autoimmune hemolytic anemia, rheumatoid arthritis, pernicious anemia, autoimmune thyroiditis, vitiligo), chronic lung disease (29%—obstructive disease, ILD, granulomatous-lymphocytic ILD), gastrointestinal disease (15%—IBD, protein-losing enteropathy, bacterial overgrowth), granulomatous disease (10%—sarcoid-like granuloma), bronchiectasis (11%), malabsorption, lymphoma (both Hodgkin and non-Hodgkin's) and other cancers like gastric cancers
Selective IgA deficiency (sIgAD)	*TACI*, *IFIH1*, *CLEC16A*	Humoral immunity	Isolated deficiency of IgA with normal serum IgM and IgG	Majority asymptomatic, less than one-third symptomatic—recurrent infections (sinopulmonary, gastrointestinal), anaphylactic reactions to transfusion of blood products, celiac disease, IBD, autoimmune disorder (SLE, RA, Grave's disease, vitiligo, myasthenia gravis, etc.)
IgG subclass deficiency	*Cγ-1*, *Cγ-2*, *Cγ-4*	Humoral immunity	Isolated deficiency of one of the subclasses of IgG	• Majority asymptomatic • Symptomatic— recurrent sinopulmonary infections • Associated with sIgAD, atopy, chronic airway diseases

Continued

Continued

Diseases	Genes affected	Components of immunity being affected	Functions affected	Key clinical features
Late-onset combined immunodeficiency (LOCID)	Genetic basis poorly understood, some harbor hypomorphic *RAG* mutation	Combined (humoral and cell-mediated) deficiency	Severely low IgG with low IgM and/or IgA, marked reduction in T, B, and NK cells	• Infections (upper and lower respiratory tracts, gastrointestinal), autoimmune cytopenia, granulomatous disease, splenomegaly, lymphoma • History of consanguinity, prevalence of gastrointestinal disease, granulomatous disease, splenomegaly, and risk of lymphoma more common in LOCID compared to CVID
GATA2 deficiency	Partial deficiency of *GATA2*	Defects in innate immunity	Monocytopenia, NK-cell cytopenia, B-cell lymphopenia	Mycobacterial infection (usually disseminated nontubercular mycobacterial infection), viral (human papilloma virus, molluscum contagiosum, herpes virus family, EBV, CMV), and fungal (histoplasmosis, aspergillosis) infections, lymphedema, myelodysplasia, leukemia
Good's syndrome	Pathogenesis not clear	Combined B- and T-cell immunodeficiency	Hypogammaglobulinemia, reduced to absent peripheral B cell, CD4+ T lymphopenia	Recurrent infection (encapsulated bacteria, viral and fungal), autoimmune diseases (myasthenia gravis, diabetes mellitus, aplastic anemia, pure red cell aplasia, hemolytic anemia, polymyositis), thymoma
Idiopathic CD4 lymphocytopenia	*RAG*, *Unc119*, *ITK*, *STK4*	Predominant cell-mediated immunodeficiency	CD4+ T-cell lymphocytopenia, reduced T-cell receptor repertoire, occasionally B-cell and NK-cell lymphopenia	Recurrent infection (viral, fungal, bacterial), autoimmune manifestations (SLE, psoriasis, Grave's disease, vitiligo, Sjögren's syndrome), malignancies (malignancies related to HPV, Kaposi's sarcoma, lymphoma)
PID occasionally presenting in adulthood				
Chronic granulomatous disease	*CYBB* (two-thirds of cases), *NCF1* (20% cases), CYBA, NCF2, NCF4	Deficiency of innate immunity	Functional impairment of NADPH oxidase complex in neutrophilic granulocytes and monocytes with defective pathogen killing	Recurrent infections (bacterial—usually catalase-positive organisms, fungal), dysregulated inflammatory manifestations with often granuloma formation (GI tract, lungs, urogenital tract, eyes), autoimmune manifestations
Familial hemophagocytic lymphohistiocytosis (HLH)	*PRF1* mutation usually in adults	Predominant cell-mediated immunity	Sustained inflammatory reaction causing cytokine storm	Fever, hepatitis, with multiorgan dysfunction involving spleen, kidney, lung, intestine, and occasionally nervous system
Autoimmune polyendocrinopathy-candidiasis-ectodermal dystrophy (APECED)	*AIRE* gene mutation	Have effective innate and adaptive immune response to exogenous stimuli	Defect in regulatory T cells	Autoimmune polyendocrinopathy (hypoparathyroidism, Addison's disease, premature ovarian failure, testicular failure, thyroid disease, type 1 diabetes mellitus), chronic mucocutaneous candidiasis, pernicious anemia, celiac disease, autoimmune hepatitis, vitiligo, alopecia, ectodermal dystrophy

Continued

Continued

Diseases	Genes affected	Components of immunity being affected	Functions affected	Key clinical features
Complement deficiency	Complement genes	Innate immunity	Defective classical or alternate complement pathway	Recurrent bacterial infections (meningitis most common, also pneumonia, bone/joint infection, salpingitis, ear infection), autoimmune disease like SLE in some patients (C1, C4 deficiency)
Partial adenosine deaminase (ADA) deficiency-related severe combined immunodeficiency (SCID)	Mutation in *ADA* gene	Combined (humoral and cell-mediated) immunodeficiency	Lymphopenia (T-cell, B-cell, and NK-cell deficiency)	Recurrent infections (bacterial, viral, fungal), chronic lung disease, autoimmune manifestations (autoimmune hypothyroidism, diabetes mellitus, hemolytic anemia), lymphoma
Hyper-IgM syndrome	*AICDA, UNG, INO80, MSH6*	Humoral immunodeficiency	Normal/elevated serum IgM with low serum IgG and IgA	Recurrent infections, noninfectious manifestations (diarrhea, aphthous ulcer, anemia, airway disease, arthralgia/arthritis)

(CMV: cytomegalovirus; EBV: Epstein–Barr virus; GI: gastrointestinal; HPV: human papillomavirus; IBD: inflammatory bowel disease; ILD: interstitial lung disease; NK: natural killer; PIDs: primary immunodeficiencies; RA: rheumatoid arthritis; SLE: systemic lupus erythematosus)

DIAGNOSING PRIMARY IMMUNODEFICIENCIES IN ADULTS

Usually, the clinical presentation of a patient with recurrent infection raises the suspicion of underlying PID. The first step in investigating a suspected immunodeficiency includes ruling out local or anatomic abnormalities and systemic predisposing conditions enumerated in **Table 1**. A judicious clinical approach can help in clinching the diagnosis. The suggestive clinical clues include the age of presentation, the pattern of infection (causative organism, severity, frequency), the organ system involved, family history (affected siblings or history of consanguinity), and associated clinical manifestations like the presence of autoimmunity, endocrinopathies, skeletal abnormalities, etc.

History of similar illness in male siblings or unexplained death due to infection in infancy or early childhood on the maternal side indicates X-linked inheritance. On the other hand, the history of consanguinity suggests autosomal-recessive inheritance. Recurrent mucosal infections like respiratory or gastrointestinal tract infections suggest antibody deficiency or opsonization defect. Abscesses of the skin, lymph node, or internal organs suggest a phagocytic defect or antibody deficiency. Recurrent candidiasis, stomatitis, gingivitis, and oral ulcerations occur in T-cell and phagocytic cell disorders. Recurrent sinopulmonary infections with encapsulated organisms (*Pneumococcus, Haemophilus influenzae* type b) are seen in B-cell abnormalities.

Recurrent pneumococcal disease is usually seen in agammaglobulinemia or complement defect. *P. jirovecii* pneumonia is the hallmark of severe combined immunodeficiency (SCID) and other primary or secondary T-cell immunodeficiencies. Infection by organisms like *Burkholderia cepacia, Serratia marcescens, Nocardia, Staphylococcal aureus*, and *Aspergillus* are usually seen in CGD. Meningococcal infection is a characteristic feature of terminal complement defects.

Baseline evaluation includes a complete blood count, peripheral blood smear, microbiological test in the form of microbiological culture, polymerase chain reaction (PCR)-based assay, etc., and radiological tests like chest radiograph and CT chest (in patients with a history of recurrent pulmonary infection). Findings in routine investigations can give clues about an underlying disease. For example, neutrophilia is seen in leukocyte adhesion deficiency and monocytopenia is seen in GATA2 deficiency. Similarly, eosinophilia in hyper-IgE syndrome, lymphopenia in combined immunodeficiency, and large platelets with thrombocytopenia in Wiskott–Aldrich syndrome are some other suggestive clues.

Amongst specific immunological tests, estimation of serum immunoglobulin levels (IgG, IgA, IgM) is very important for suspected antibody deficiency. If more than one of them is low or serum IgG is < 3 g/L, then it is suggestive of immunodeficiency. B-cell numbers (both absolute number and percentage) and B-cell immunophenotyping are also important for further diagnosis. In patients with T-cell lymphopenia, lymphocyte subset analysis (T cell, B cell, NK cell) should be performed. Complement levels (C3, C4) and functions (CH50, AH50) are sometimes assessed in suspected complement deficiency. Dihydrorhodamine (DHR) and nitroblue tetrazolium (NBT) tests are performed in suspected phagocytic defects like CGD. Another aspect of the diagnosis of PIDs is the recent advances in the next-generation sequencing (NGS). Tools like whole exome/clinical exome sequencing can help in identifying specific genetic abnormalities and thus clinching the diagnosis.

TREATMENT AND OUTCOMES OF THE PRIMARY IMMUNODEFICIENCIES

Gone are the days when there was no effective treatment for the PIDs with often the diagnosis of PID bearing a grim prognosis. Due to the availability of intravenous immunoglobulin (IVIG) replacement, which is one of the mainstays of therapy, the prognosis has significantly improved. Besides, increased awareness leading to early diagnosis has also improved the outcome. Another therapeutic modality for PIDs is hematopoietic stem cell transplantation (HSCT). Although previously HSCT was mainly used for childhood PIDs, it is now also being used in adult PIDs. Currently, there are more than 15 centers where HSCT for PIDs is routinely performed. However, there is still a lack of adequate data regarding the use of HSCT in adult PIDs in Indian settings. Also, the cost of HSCT and the risk of infection in the post-HSCT period are the other major hindrances.

CONCLUSION

Primary immunodeficiencies were traditionally considered a disease of children. However, it is increasingly being recognized that lack of awareness was the major reason behind it. However, the situation has changed over the last decade. In 2010, the Foundation for Primary Immunodeficiency Diseases (FPID) was established. Currently, there are eight established PID centers spread across India which is helping in increasing disease awareness and improving treatment outcomes. With improvements in diagnostics, an increased awareness amongst the internists will help in diagnosis of the adult PIDs more often.

SUGGESTED READINGS

1. Rosenberg E, Dent PB, Denburg JA. Primary Immune Deficiencies in the Adult: A Previously Underrecognized Common Condition. J Allergy Clin Immunol Pract. 2016;4(6):1101-7.
2. Gupta S, Madkaikar M, Singh S, Sehgal S. Primary immunodeficiencies in India: a perspective. Ann N Y Acad Sci. 2012;1250:73-9.

138

CHAPTER

Autoinflammatory Diseases in Adults

Shubhransu Patro, Vibha Sharma

ABSTRACT

Systemic autoinflammatory diseases (SAIDs) are uncommon yet severe conditions marked by mutations in fundamental regulators of innate immune responses. Significant progress in molecular genetics and next-generation sequencing over the past decade has facilitated the discovery of new mutations central to the mechanistic pathways of inflammation. They share common phenotypic manifestations such as recurrent fever episodes, skin-related symptoms, chest or abdominal pain, lymphadenopathy, vasculopathy, and musculoskeletal issues. Inflammasome, the transcription factor nuclear factor kappa-light-chain enhancer of activated B cells (NF-κB), and the proinflammatory cytokines, the key components of the innate immune system are involved in this leading to episodes of seemingly spontaneous inflammation. While these disorders are frequently diagnosed in childhood, there is an increasing recognition of adult patients, including those with adult-onset disease. Advanced understanding of innate immune mechanisms, combined with significant progress in genomics and a growing number of clinical cases, has resulted in the classification of more disorders as autoinflammatory or having autoinflammatory components. Biologic therapies targeting specific elements of the innate immune system have not only offered significant clinical benefits, but have also contributed a lot for a better understanding of the role of innate immunity in autoinflammatory disorders.

INTRODUCTION

Autoinflammatory diseases (AIDs) are a group of hereditary conditions characterized by recurring attacks of fever, often accompanied by inflammatory symptoms affecting skin, mucous membranes, serous membranes, the joints and in some cases, muscles, small, medium, and large vessels also. Some patients may develop systemic amyloidosis. The concept came when tumor necrosis factor receptor-associated periodic fevers (TRAPS) was discovered as a recurrent, spontaneous inflammation, all without the presence of increased titer of autoantibodies or antigen-specific T-lymphocytes. In 1999, Michael McDermott and Daniel Kastner coined the term 'autoinflammation' to describe a group of disorders characterized by unprovoked localized or systemic inflammation, in the absence of the key features of autoimmunity, such as autoreactive lymphocytes and increased titer of antibodies. The innate immune system, a nonspecific, genetically encoded defense, rapidly responds to danger signals through pattern recognition receptors (PRRs), mainly in myeloid immune cells, triggering the release of proinflammatory cytokines like interleukin (IL)-1, IL-18, tumor necrosis factor-alpha (TNF-α), and type-1 interferons (IFNs) and initiating downstream immune responses. This process is essential for countering various threats and becomes exaggerated in 'autoinflammation', leading to sporadic, spontaneous inflammation affecting multiple organs, and causing tissue damage.

The key components of the innate immune system involved in this are the inflammasome, the transcription factor nuclear factor kappa-light-chain enhancer of activated B cells (NF-κB), and the proinflammatory cytokines.

In contrast, 'autoimmunity' which usually encompasses disorders of the adaptive immune system, driven mainly by lymphocytes, featuring increased serum autoantibodies and varying IL activation. While autoimmune and autoinflammatory disorders are traditionally distinct, recent evidences suggest that aberrant signaling through innate mechanisms may be critical in initiating or perpetuating systemic autoimmune processes. Further, ongoing researches into the various complex pathways of innate immunity has resulted in the further classification of several diseases, originally autoimmune or unclassified, as having autoinflammatory components.

While initially thought to primarily affecting the young, over time autoinflammatory diseases have increasingly emerged in adult patients, often milder and more treatable, especially in monogenic cases mostly influenced by low-penetrance mutations or somatic mosaicism, sometimes differing from childhood characteristics **(Fig. 1)**.

CLASSIFICATION OF AUTOINFLAMMATORY DISEASES

Clinical Classification

- *Episodic and multisystemic*:
  - NLRP12-associated disease
  - Mevalonate kinase deficiency (MKD)
  - Periodic fever syndrome, aphthous stomatitis, pharyngitis, and adenitis (PFAPA)
  - Tumor necrosis factor receptor-associated periodic fever syndrome (TRAPS)
- Episodic and affecting the joints—gout
- Episodic and affecting bone—chronic recurrent multifocal osteomyelitis (CRMO)
- *Persistent and multisystem*:
  - Schnitzler syndrome
  - Crohn disease
  - Deficiency of interleukin-1 receptor antagonist (DIRA)
- *Persistent and affecting the skin*:
  - Interleukin-36-receptor antagonist deficiency (DITRA)
  - Sweet syndrome
  - Neutrophilic panniculitis

Molecular Mechanism of the Origin

- *Inflammasome activation*: MKD/Muckle-Wells syndrome
- *NF-κB activation*: NLRP12-associated disease, Crohn disease, Blau syndrome
- *IL-1β pathway dysregulation*: PFAPA, Schnitzler syndrome, DIRA or DITRA
- Impaired efficacy of cytotoxic T lymphocytes with compensatory macrophage activation—familial hemophagocytic lymphohistiocytosis (HLH)
- Inactivation of IL-10 signaling (early onset of enterocolitis)
- Multiple (TRAPS) and uncharacterized (CRMO or Behçet disease)

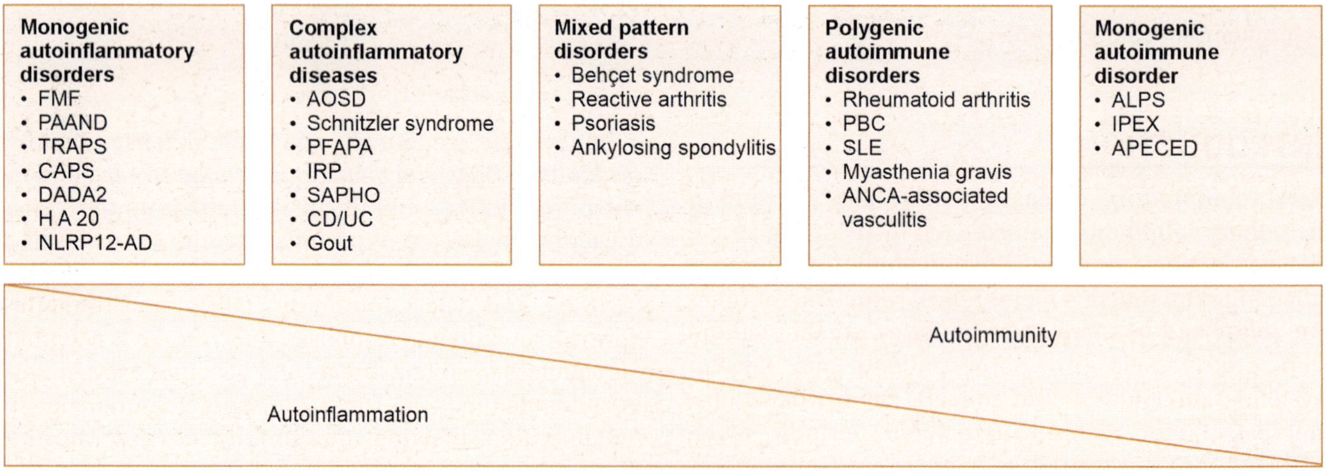

FIG. 1: Schematic representation of the immunological disease continuum.

(ALPS: autoimmune lymphoproliferative syndrome; AOSD: adult-onset Still's disease; APECED: autoimmune polyendocrinopathy-candidiasis-ectodermal dystrophy; CAPS: cryopyrin-associated periodic syndromes; CD: Crohn disease; DADA2: deficiency of ADA2; FMF: familial Mediterranean fever; HA20: haploinsufficiency A20; IPEX: immune dysregulation polyendocrinopathy enteropathy; IRP: idiopathic recurrent pericarditis; NLRP12-AD: NLRP12-associated autoinflammatory disease; PAAND: pyrin-associated autoinflammation with neutrophilic dermatosis; PBC: primary biliary cirrhosis; PFAPA: periodic fever syndrome, aphthous stomatitis, pharyngitis, and cervical adenitis; SAPHO: synovitis, acne, pustulosis, hyperostosis, osteitis; SLE: systemic lupus erythematosus; TRAPS: tumor necrosis factor receptor-associated periodic fever syndrome)

TABLE 1: Monogenic autoinflammatory diseases.

Monogenic autoinfla-mmatory disease	Gene	Mode of inheritance	Cardinal features	In adults
Familial Mediterranean fever (FMF)	*MEFV*	AR	Recurrent self-limiting attacks of fever, abdominal pain, thoracic pain, and arthritis	Less erythema and arthritis. Better response to treatment
Tumor necrosis factor receptor-associated periodic syndrome (TRAPS)	*TNFRSF1A*	AD	Arthromyalgia, fasciitis, rash, conjunctivitis and periorbital edema, splenomegaly	Milder clinical presentation, less chronicity
NLRP3-AID	*NLRP3*	AD	Fever, urticarial rash, sensorineural hearing loss, lymphadenopathy, splenomegaly, myalgia, arthropathy	No major differences
A20 haploinsufficiency (HA20)	*TNFRSF1A*	AD	Fever, recurrent oral and genital ulcers, abdominal pain, skin rash, and arthritis	No major differences
Mevalonate kinase deficiency (MVK)	*MVK*	AR	Abdominal pain, diarrhea, hepatosplenomegaly, and lymphadenopathy	Cases mainly due to diagnostic delay
VEXAS (vacuoles, E1 enzyme, X-linked, autoinflammatory, somatic) syndrome	*UBA1*	–	Fever, cutaneous vasculitis, neutrophilic dermatosis, ear and nose chondritis, pulmonary infiltrates, and bronchial vasculitis	–

Simplified Classification by the Predominant Cytokine or Pathway

- IL-1 mediated
- IFN-mediated
- Increased activation of NF-κB

MONOGENIC VERSUS POLYGENIC AUTOINFLAMMATORY DISEASES

Autoinflammatory diseases can be categorized as either monogenic or multigenic (polygenic). Monogenic autoinflammatory syndromes involve specific genetic mutations, primarily associated with innate immune system errors.

In contrast, multigenic autoinflammatory syndromes do not stem from a single identified genetic mutation, and their genetic characterization is intricate due to the involvement of multiple genes.

Monogenic Autoinflammatory Diseases

Monogenic autoinflammatory diseases encompass a group of inherited disorders resulting from specific genetic mutations, primarily associated with innate immune system errors, including inflammasome assembly, NF-κB activation, cytokine secretion, ubiquitination, and type I IFN signaling.

Table 1 outlines the most prevalent and thoroughly studied monogenic autoinflammatory diseases, with a particular focus on their manifestations in adult patients.

Multifactorial Autoinflammatory Diseases

Unlike monogenic autoinflammatory diseases, multigenic autoinflammatory syndromes are a group of disorders characterized by dysregulated myeloid activation and autoinflammation and do not stem from a single identified genetic mutation, hence their genetic characterization is intricate due to the involvement of multiple genes.

As these conditions are mostly diagnosed in adulthood, these should be included in the list of potential diagnoses when evaluating adult patients with recurrent fever of unknown origin **(Table 2)**.

CLINICAL FEATURES

These clinical features are characteristic of autoinfla-mmatory diseases; however, may vary in severity and presentation among different individuals and specific syndromes.

- *Recurrent fever:* Patients typically experience recurrent episodes of fever, often without an obvious infection.
- *Cutaneous symptoms:* These may include skin rashes, hives, or other skin manifestations.
- *Mucosal involvement:* Some individuals may have inflammation in mucous membranes, leading to symptoms in the mouth, eyes, or genital areas.
- *Serosal involvement:* Inflammation may affect serous membranes that line body cavities, such as the lining of the abdomen (peritoneum) or the lungs (pleura).

TABLE 2: Potential diagnoses.

Disease	Inheritance pattern/most common age at presentation	Systemic features (along with fever)
Adult onset still disease (AOSD)	Acquired; no known genetic link 3–35 years	Polyarthritis, polyarthralgia, myalgia, prodromal sore throat, serositis, and lymphadenopathy
Periodic fever with aphthous stomatitis, pharyngitis, and adenitis (PFAPA)	• Unknown • 5–35 years	Aphthous ulcerations and abdominal pain
Schnitzler syndrome	50 years	Bone or joint pain especially over the ilium or tibia, lymphadenopathy, and hepatosplenomegaly
Synovitis, acne, pustulosis, hyperostosis, and osteitis (SAPHO) syndrome	15–35 years	Osteoarticular conditions often accompanied by neutrophilic dermatosis.
Nucleotide-binding oligomerization domain containing 2 (NOD2)–associated autoinflammatory disease	Mutations in *NOD2* gene	Dermatitis, inflammatory arthritis, and gastrointestinal symptoms

- *Osteoarticular manifestations:* Joint pain and inflammation can be common, often mimicking symptoms of arthritis.
- *Other symptoms:* Additional symptoms can include muscle pain, fatigue, and, in some cases, more severe systemic manifestations.

DIAGNOSIS

Diagnosing autoinflammatory diseases may be very cumbersome and may require a combination of thorough clinical evaluation, laboratory tests, and sometimes genetic testing.

- Clinical evaluation to look for any recurring symptoms, including fever, rash, joint pain, and other signs of inflammation and family history of similar symptoms.
- Laboratory tests to assess inflammation and which may include:
    - Complete blood count (CBC) to check for elevated leukocyte count.
    - Acute-phase reactants such as C-reactive protein (CRP) and erythrocyte sedimentation rate (ESR).
    - Serum amyloid A (SAA) levels, which may be found elevated in some autoinflammatory diseases.
- *Genetic testing:* In few cases, genetic testing is essential to identify specific mutations associated with autoinflammatory diseases. It can confirm the diagnosis and help to guide treatment decisions.
- *Exclusion of other conditions:* As autoinflammatory diseases can share symptoms with many other clinical conditions; like autoimmune diseases, infections or other inflammatory conditions, it is crucial to rule out these potential causes of symptoms before confirming diagnosis.
- *Response to therapy:* Sometimes, a diagnosis is confirmed if the patient responds well to treatment with medications that target specific cytokines such as IL-1 or IL-6 inhibitors, which are characteristic of autoinflammatory diseases.
- Because of varied symptoms and genetic variations, diagnosing a case of autoinflammatory disease is very complex, hence demanding a collaboration among medical specialists for precise identification and management.

Last but not the least, in diagnosing autoinflammatory diseases, several clinical features play a crucial role, including:

- Age of onset
- Details about fever
- Duration of episodes of attacks
- Urticaria or rashes
- Distinguishing clinical features suggestive of any systemic or organ involvement
- Ethnicity
- Family history of similar illness

TREATMENT

Traditional Drugs

- *Colchicine:* In addition to inhibition of microtubule polymerization and disruption of cell mitosis in various cell types; including neutrophils, recent evidences suggest additional supplementary anti-inflammatory mechanisms that involve modifying the expression of adhesion molecules and chemotactic factors.
  Dosage: <0.5 mg/day for children under 5 years, 0.5–1.0 mg/day for children aged 5–10 years, and 1.0–1.5 mg/day for children over 10 years and adults.
- *Nonsteroidal anti-inflammatory drugs (NSAIDs):* Alone or in combination with baseline therapy, NSAIDs are used symptomatically in monogenic autoinflammatory diseases, but they do not address

the disease's root cause, offering symptomatic relief and benefits in only around half of the cases.

- *Glucocorticoids*: Glucocorticoids are used in the management of various autoinflammatory diseases. They are effective in FMF when colchicine alone is inadequate and short-term use benefits individuals with TRAPS, MKD, and cryopyrin-associated periodic syndrome (CAPS). For PFAPA syndrome, glucocorticoids are the preferred treatment.

Biologic Agents

- *Interleukin-1 blockers*:
  - Anakinra
  - Rilonacept
  - Canakinumab
- *TNF-blockers:* They generally exhibit lower efficacy when compared to IL-1 blockers and should only be used after excluding latent tuberculosis.
  - Etanercept
  - Infliximab
  - Adalimumab
- *Anti-IL-6 agents:* Tocilizumab, an anti-IL-6 agent, has been used in patients who are not responding to other biologic agents and has shown some success in management of FMF, TRAPS, and MKD.
- *Janus kinase (JAK) inhibitors:* In several monogenic autoinflammatory diseases mediated by type I IFN, JAK inhibitors have shown positive results. These conditions include chronic atypical neutrophilic dermatosis with lipodystrophy and elevated temperature/proteasome-associated autoinflammatory syndrome, STING-associated vasculopathy with onset in infancy, familial chilblain lupus, and Aicardi–Goutières syndrome.

CONCLUSION

Autoinflammatory disorders result from uncontrolled activation of the innate immune system and possess a clinical challenge for diagnosis, particularly in adults, because of the varied range of clinical symptoms they exhibit. The primary approach while treating autoinflammatory diseases (AIDs) involves mitigating the inflammatory response. While autoinflammatory disorders are typically diagnosed in childhood, there is a rising recognition of adult patients. Despite advancements in diagnostic methods including genetic testing, diagnosing of this group of disorders often relies on a profound understanding of the clinical presentation. Hence, knowledge about unique clinical features of autoinflammatory disorders is crucial for maintaining a high index of suspicion in patients experiencing unexplained episodes of fever or inflammation, accompanied by manifestations affecting various body systems.

SUGGESTED READINGS

1. Rodolfi S, Nasone I, Folci M, Selmi C, Brunetta E. Autoinflammatory manifestations in adult patients. Clin Exp Immunol. 2022;210(3):295-308.
2. Betrains A, Staels F, Schrijvers R, Meyts I, Humblet-Baron S, De Langhe E, et al. Systemic autoinflammatory disease in adults. Autoimmun Rev. 2021;20(4):102774.
3. Grateau G, Hentgen V, Stojanovic KS, Jéru I, Amselem S, Steichen O. How should we approach classification of autoinflammatory diseases? Nat Rev Rheumatol. 2013;9(10):624-9.
4. Vineetha M, Palakkal S, Skaria L, Jose N, Philomina D, Nithin A. Autoinflammatory syndromes: A review. J Skin Sex Transm Dis. 2020;2(1):5-12.

139

CHAPTER

Approach to Autoinflammatory Syndrome

Sameer Gulati, Anu Maheshwari

ABSTRACT

Autoinflammatory syndromes comprise rare diseases which are characterized by unregulated activation of inflammatory pathways without any antigenic stimulation. This is distinct from autoimmunity and concerns innate immunity disorders. The recurrent, episodic/periodic clinical presentations with phases of generalized well-being in between make them difficult to diagnose. Adult presentations with milder and atypical clinical features are well known. A high index of suspicion is required to diagnose them after ruling out commoner differentials such as infections, malignancy, and autoimmune diseases. Many of these diseases are being diagnosed with increased awareness among physicians and availability of better genetic diagnostic facilities. Response to specific therapeutic modalities may also aid in differentiating these conditions from each other. The present review aims to provide a practical approach to autoinflammatory diseases.

INTRODUCTION

The term autoinflammation was introduced recently in the year 1999 by McDermott and Kastner while describing tumor necrosis factor (TNF) receptor-associated periodic syndrome (TRAPS). It was later defined by Kastner et al. in 2010 as a persistent or recurrent hyperinflammatory syndrome mediated by the innate immune system, which leads to excessive secretion of proinflammatory cytokines, notably in the absence of infection, malignancy, and/or autoimmunity. The European Society for Immunodeficiencies (ESID) working group has categorized systemic autoinflammatory diseases (SAIDs) into group VII. This is distinct from autoimmunity because of the absence of autoantibodies, no female predisposition, and absence of immunological memory. Since the innate immune system does not learn, every recurrence is of the same severity and unlike autoimmunity does not escalate quickly in a shorter time. Besides recurrent fever, this SAID may lead to a widely distributed tissue damage and a multisystemic involvement. Hence, it may be difficult to diagnose SAID clinically because of a wide range of possible clinical presentations. Besides these disorders may present without fever and the inflammation may be persistent rather than episodic. Adult presentations, even though rare, are possible and should be considered in appropriate clinical scenarios. Improved awareness and better availability of genetic diagnostic techniques can help us to diagnose these syndromes early. The present review presents an approach to systemic autoinflammatory disorders with focus on the hereditary recurrent fevers.

CLASSIFICATION

The SAIDs have been classified according to the number of genes involved (monogenic/polygenic) and the monogenic disorders are further classified depending on the immunological deficit. This classification system may lead to considerable overlap of symptoms among these disorders.

The monogenic disorders involve a single gene and follow Mendelian inheritance patterns. They typically present in childhood and usually have first-degree or second-degree relatives with similar features. On the contrary, systemic juvenile idiopathic arthritis (JIA), periodic fever aphthous stomatitis pharyngitis adenitis (PFAPA) syndrome, adult-onset Still's disease (AOSD), Schnitzler's syndrome, idiopathic recurrent pericarditis, gout, Crohn's disease/ulcerative colitis, Behçet's disease, chronic nonbacterial osteomyelitis/chronic recurrent multifocal osteomyelitis (CNO/CRMO), and synovitis acne pustulosis hyperostosis osteitis syndrome (SAPHO) are examples of polygenic/complex autoinflammatory syndrome. The 2019 International Union of Immunological Societies (IUIS) Expert Committee further classifies monogenic SAID into three major groups as enumerated further.

1. *Type 1 interferonopathies*: This group is characterized by an increased expression of type I interferons which in turn leads to a surge in inflammatory mediators, e.g., Aicardi–Goutières syndrome (AGS), STING-associated vasculopathy with onset in infancy (SAVI), chronic atypical neutrophilic dermatosis with lipodystrophy and elevated temperature (CANDLE).
2. *Defects affecting the inflammasome*: This group is characterized by involvement of the interleukin 1 (IL-1) pathway. The inflammasome complex activates caspase-1, which in turn cleaves the pro-IL-1β to inflammatory cytokines such as IL-1β, IL-18, TNF-α, IL-6, IL-17, interferon alpha (IFN-α), IFN-β, etc., for example, familial Mediterranean fever (FMF), cryopyrin-associated periodic syndrome (CAPS), hyper-immunoglobulin D (IgD) syndrome/mevalonate kinase deficiency (HIDS/MKD).
3. *Non-inflammasome-related conditions*: For example, TRAPS, deficiency of the IL-1 receptor antagonist, ubiquitination defects (otulipenia), nuclear factor κβ activation-mediated disorder (Blau syndrome), and proteasome-related disorder (pyogenic arthritis, pyoderma gangrenosum, and acne)

STATUS OF SYSTEMIC AUTOINFLAMMATORY DISEASE IN INDIA

A nationwide cohort of SAID patients comprising 78 patients was evaluated by Suri et al. These patients presented with diverse clinical manifestations. The authors stressed upon a delay in diagnosis which often happens due to overlap of clinical features with other common rheumatological diseases. Hence, an emphasis was laid upon an emergent need to increase awareness of SAID among healthcare professionals. The spectrum of SAID in India comprised noninflammasomes-related conditions (41%), disease-affecting inflammasomes (26%), and type I interferonopathies (15%). Since this cohort comprised just six centers, this profile may not be representative of the entire nation. Jain et al. performed the genetic epidemiology of autoinflammatory syndrome in India. Their analysis revealed 20 pathogenic and likely pathogenic variants with significant differences in the allele frequency compared with the global population. The cumulative carrier frequency of the autoinflammatory syndrome was determined to be 3.5% in India which was higher than reported earlier. These findings highlight that the prevalence of SAID may be much higher than anticipated in our country. Better awareness and diagnostic facilities in the country may lead to detection of more cases. Even with genetic analysis, we may be missing a few cases because of different pathogenic/likely pathogenic variants in our country as highlighted by Jain et al. Importantly various Indian authors have also stressed upon the need for strengthening genetic diagnostic services in our country. The unavailability of anakinra to manage these SAIDs is also a matter of concern.

SYSTEMIC AUTOINFLAMMATORY DISEASE IN ADULTS

The childhood-onset disease may be diagnosed in adulthood due to delayed diagnosis. These patients may have a long-standing history of unexplained recurrent fever since childhood. Many times, individuals with milder phenotype get used to their symptoms and do not report to medical centers for an evaluation. At times, their symptoms are dismissed as recurrent infections. A diagnosis of a SAID in a child/infant may trigger a diagnosis in one of the parents with a milder phenotype which was hitherto missed. Due to variable expressivity of clinical manifestations, development of a new symptom at an older age and the subsequent connecting dots with earlier clinical features facilitates a diagnosis of SAID.

However, SAIDs may also manifest for the first time in adulthood. For instance, patients with Schnitzler syndrome may have their first clinical manifestation at a mean age of 51 years. A delayed onset of monogenic SAID may be due to low penetration germline mutation with a variable clinical phenotype. Hypomorphic mutations such as missense mutations, small deletions in the coding sequence, splice donor or acceptor site mutations that flank exons, and mutations in promoter/noncoding transcriptional regulatory regions may all lead to adult onset of disease. Availability of better genetic tools such as amplicon-based deep sequencing may help in detecting somatic mosaicism and consequent identification of monogenic autoinflammatory diseases in adulthood. Significantly mosaicism increases with age and hence may lead to adult presentations. Both epistasis and epigenetics may also explain adult presentations of SAIDs.

APPROACH TO SYSTEMIC AUTOINFLAMMATORY DISEASES

These SAIDs may present with variable presentations with significant overlap of clinical features. Typically, they present as recurrent febrile episodes, with a standard duration, along with ophthalmological, mucocutaneous, serosal, and/or musculoskeletal manifestations. There are periods of generalized well-being in between attacks, and symptoms in between fever episodes point toward an alternate diagnosis, such as an autoimmune disease or a malignancy. Worsening of generalized well-being and organ systems over time also is not characteristic of monogenic autoinflammatory diseases. The pattern of febrile episodes may help in differentiating these monogenic SAIDs from other differential diagnoses and from each other. The duration of episodes in each recurrence may help in differentiating these clinical syndromes. For instance, recurrent episodes of FMF, HIDS, and TRAPS may last for 1–3 days, 3–7 days, and 1–2 weeks, respectively. Usually, the fever episodes are episodic rather than periodic. Typical periodicity may only be seen in cyclical neutropenia and PFAPA syndrome. The associated typical features, which remain fairly constant for each recurrence, further help us in classifying these SAIDs **(Table 1)**. The atypical presentations may include various heterogeneous presentations which may include features such as enterocolitis, interstitial lung disease, vasculitic rash, stroke, cerebrovascular hemorrhage, and basal ganglia calcifications. The cutaneous manifestations may be characteristic such as an erysipeloid rash seen in FMF or may present as urticaria, pustules, maculopapular rash, oral ulcers, generalized pustular psoriasis, pyoderma gangrenosum, and Sweet's syndrome such as lesions. Musculoskeletal manifestations, if typical, may also help to differentiate the monogenic autoinflammatory diseases. FMF characteristically presents with monoarthritis, usually involving the lower limbs. In contrast, TRAPS usually presents with myalgia/arthralgia along with a migratory rash and arthritis is not very characteristic. Long-standing disease may cause secondary amyloidosis, which may occasionally be a presenting manifestation. The inflammatory episodes may get triggered by emotional stress, infections, menstruation, exercise, and fatigue. Some of the SAIDs may have typical triggers, such as HIDS/MKD may get triggered by childhood vaccinations or cold that may precipitate episodes of Muckle-Wells syndrome/familial cold autoinflammatory syndrome (MWS/FCAS). The expressivity of the clinical features may change over time with worsening or improving of the symptoms. Hence, the clinical features may be different in childhood and adult presentations. Signs of chronic inflammation such as anemia, hepatomegaly, and splenomegaly may also be appreciable. The suggestive clinical features are associated with elevated acute phase reactants such as neutrophilia, serum amyloid levels, erythrocyte sedimentation rate (ESR), and C-reactive protein (CRP). The discordant values CRP and procalcitonin (high CRP and normal procalcitonin) point toward the possibility of PFAPA and FMF. Lack of high titers autoantibodies will also point toward a possibility of IL-1-mediated disease.

The serum IgD levels are usually slightly increased in a number of autoinflammatory disorders; however, they are

TABLE 1: Eurofever/PRINTO clinical classification criteria based on typical clinical features.

SAID	Presence of	Absence of	Requirement for classification
Periodic fever with aphthous stomatitis, pharyngitis and adenitis (PFAPA)	Pharyngotonsillitis, duration of episodes 3–6 days, cervical lymphadenitis, periodicity	Diarrhea, chest pain, skin rash, arthritis	At least 7 out of 8
Cryopyrin-associated periodic syndrome (CAPS)	Urticarial rash, cold/stress-triggered sensorineural hearing loss, chronic aseptic meningitis, skeletal abnormalities (epiphyseal overgrowth/frontal bossing)		At least 2 out of 5
Familial Mediterranean fever (FMF)	• Eastern Mediterranean ethnicity, duration of episodes—1–3 days • Chest pain, abdominal pain, arthritis	Aphthous stomatitis, urticarial rash, maculopapular rash, painful lymph nodes	At least 6 out of 9
Tumor necrosis factor receptor-associated periodic fever syndrome (TRAPS)	• Fever ≥ 7 days (2 points) • Fever 5–6 days (1 point) • Migratory rash (1 point) • Periorbital edema (1 point) • Myalgia (1 point) • Positive family history (1 point)	• Aphthous stomatitis (1 point) • Pharyngotonsillitis (1 point)	Score ≥ 5 points
Mevalonate kinase deficiency/hyper-IgD syndrome (MKD/HIDS)	Age of onset < 1 year, gastrointestinal symptoms, painful lymph nodes, aphthous stomatitis, triggers, maculopapular rash		Presence of at least 3 out of 6

(SAID: systemic autoinflammatory disease)

markedly increased in HIDS/MKD. Increased mevalonic acid activity in urine may be appreciable during an inflammatory attack. The diagnosis is usually confirmed with the help of a molecular genetic evaluation. However, the genetic evaluation may throw occasional clinical challenges when low penetrance variants, oligogenic or digenic presentations, somatic mosaicism, variants of unknown significance, and mutation negative profiles are detected. All of these difficult genetic situations may present with atypical clinical profile and may respond differently to standard therapeutics. Hence occasionally, these patients may need individual personified management protocols. At times, patients with a distinct recurrent autoinflammatory clinical profile may have a negative genetic profiling. In these circumstances, patients are classified to be having undifferentiated SAID. Response to therapeutics may also provide clues to probable diagnosis in case of recurrent fevers. Response to antibiotics is usually not appreciable in SAIDs. Steroids will usually show a good response in systemic-onset JIA (SoJIA), AOSD, and PFAPA. Response to steroids is usually not very good in HIDS/MKD and classical FMF attacks. In contrast, many SAIDs show a very good response to IL-1 inhibitors. Significantly, a dramatic response to adequate colchicine therapy may confirm FMF **(Box 1)**.

Certain groups of SAID may present predominantly with fever, rash, musculoskeletal, or various organ involvements. These distinct phenotypes may also aid in identifying and diagnosing these autoinflammatory diseases **(Table 2)**. The work-up should be systematically planned to rule out the more common differential diagnosis since the primary autoinflammatory syndromes are rare entities. It is imperative to rule out infections, malignancy, autoimmune diseases, primary immunodeficiencies, inflammatory bowel disease, chronic osteomyelitis, etc. by effective utilization of investigative modalities. Many rheumatological diseases may form important differential diagnoses for SAID as outlined further.

- *Rheumatoid arthritis*: Coatomer-associated protein alpha (COPA) syndrome
- *Early-onset sarcoidosis, JIA, granulomatous uveitis*: Blau syndrome
- *Systemic lupus erythematosus*: AGS
- *Polyarteritis nodosa*: Deficiency of adenosine deaminase-2 (DADA-2)
- *Generalized pustular psoriasis*: Deficiency of IL-1 receptor antagonist (DIRA); deficiency of IL-36 receptor antagonist (DITRA); pustular psoriasis (AP1S3); CAMPS (CARD 14)
- *Behçet's*: Haploinsufficiency A20 (HA20)

BOX 1: Approach to differential diagnosis of recurrent fever ("at least two episodes of fever separated by a symptom-free interval of at least 2 weeks").

- At what age did symptoms first appear?
- What is the duration of individual fever episodes?
- What other symptoms are associated with the fever episodes?
- What is the time interval in between these episodes?
- What can trigger or alleviate a fever episode?
- How have symptoms developed over time?
- Which treatments have been used and what was the response?
- Is there a family history; does the patient come from a specific ethnicity?

TABLE 2: Distinct phenotypes of SAID may aid in identifying the autoinflammatory diseases.

Autoinflammatory diseases predominantly presenting as fever	FMF, HIDS, TRAPS
Autoinflammatory disease presenting predominantly as fever and urticarial rash	CAPS, FCAS, MWS, CINCA, FCAS2, SoJIA
Syndromes of predominant rash	CAMPS (CARD14), ADAM 17 deficiency, H syndrome (SLC29A3), ORAS/otulipenia, pustular psoriasis (AP1S3), SAVI, CANDLE/PLAID, APLAID, HA20, DITRA
Syndrome of predominant musculoskeletal	Predominant arthritis, Blau syndrome, COPA syndrome, PAPA, predominant osteitis, Majeed syndrome, DIRA
Syndromes with organ involvement	CNS (DADA2 and AGS), uveitis (Blau syndrome, HA20), reticuloendothelial system (PFAPA), hematological (PFIT, SFID, and NLRC4-MAS), immunodeficiency (PFIT, SFID, and APLAID)

(AGS: Aicardi–Goutières syndrome; APLAID: autoinflammation with phospholipase Cγ2-associated antibody deficiency and immune dysregulation; CANDLE/PLAID: chronic atypical neutrophilic dermatosis with lipodystrophy, and elevated temperature/phospholipase Cγ2-associated antibody deficiency and immune dysregulation; CAPS: cryopyrin-associated periodic syndrome; CINCA: chronic infantile neurological cutaneous and articular; CNS: central nervous system; COPA: coatomer-associated protein alpha; DADA-2: deficiency of adenosine deaminase 2; DIRA: deficiency of IL-1 receptor antagonist; DITRA: deficiency of IL-36 receptor antagonist; FCAS: familial cold autoinflammatory syndrome; FMF: familial Mediterranean fever; HA20: haploinsufficiency A20; HIDS: hyper-immunoglobulin D syndrome; MAS: macrophage activation syndrome; MWS: Muckle–Wells syndrome; PAPA: pyogenic arthritis, pyoderma gangrenosum, and acne; PFAPA: periodic fever aphthous stomatitis pharyngitis adenitis; PFIT: periodic fever, immunodeficiency, and thrombocytopenia; SAID: systemic autoinflammatory disease; SAVI: STING-associated vasculopathy with onset in infancy; SFID: sideroblastic anemia with B-cell immunodeficiency, periodic fevers, and developmental delay; SoJIA: systemic-onset juvenile idiopathic arthritis; TRAPS: tumor necrosis factor receptor-associated periodic syndrome)

MANAGEMENT

The goal of therapy is to achieve control of disease progression and prevention of organ damage along with normalization of acute phase reactants such as CRP and serum amyloid. 'Treat to target' approach helps to achieve this goal just like in other autoimmune diseases. Further, the management algorithm might need to be individualized for any given patient. Autoinflammatory disease activity index (AIDAI) is a valid and reliable tool for assessment of disease activity for the hereditary recurrent fever syndromes. It is easy to use wherein patients collect all the desired variables in a diary for about 3 months. A cutoff score of 9 helps to accurately differentiate patients with active disease from inactive disease.

Treatment is focused on diminishing the inflammatory pathway. Steroids and nonsteroidal anti-inflammatory drugs (NSAIDs) have a supportive role in management of these SAIDs. Colchicine has a remarkable therapeutic effect on FMF, idiopathic recurrent pericarditis, gout, and Behçet's disease. Steroids are not very efficient besides SoJIA and AOSD. Interleukin 1 blockade is effective in conditions such as inflammasomopathies, DIRA, and TRAPS. The TNF blockade works well in TRAPS, CNO, and DADA-2. Finally, diseases mediated by interferons respond well to Janus kinase inhibitor (JAK) inhibitors.

TABLE 3: Approach to systemic autoinflammatory diseases (SAID).

When to suspect	Patients who present with inflammatory episodes that recur or persist over months or years in absence of another cause should be evaluated for autoinflammatory diseases
Rule out differentials	Malignancy, infections, autoimmune diseases, inflammatory bowel disease, chronic osteomyelitis should be ruled out
Assess family history	A family history of a similar syndrome suggests a heritable disorder such as monogenic autoinflammatory disease (recessive and de novo mutation will lack such a history)
Identify a clinical pattern	Identify a clinical pattern consistent with one of the major autoinflammatory disorders

CONCLUSION

As SAIDs are challenging to diagnose, a high index of suspicion should be maintained in appropriate clinical settings. A simplified approach to identify these autoinflammatory diseases is summarized in **Table 3**. The other common differential diagnosis should always be ruled out before considering the rarer possibility of SAIDs. These autoinflammatory diseases are being diagnosed more often because of increased awareness among physicians and better genetic diagnostic facilities. They do occur in adults but more often with milder and atypical clinical features. Therapeutic armamentarium includes biological agents which control specific inflammatory pathways. However, availability of anti-IL-1 (anakinra) in India remains a concern.

SUGGESTED READINGS

1. Kışla Ekinci RM, Balcı S, Erol AH, Karagöz D, Ufuk Altıntaş D, Bisgin A. Differentiating children with familial Mediterranean fever from other recurrent fever syndromes: The utility of new Eurofever/PRINTO classification criteria. Arch Rheumatol. 2021;36(4):493-8.
2. Kallinich T, Gattorno M, Grattan CE, de Koning HD, Traidl-Hoffmann C, Feist E, et al. Unexplained recurrent fever: when is autoinflammation the explanation? Allergy. 2013;68(3):285-96.
3. Suri D, Rawat A, Jindal AK, Vignesh P, Gupta A, Pilania RK, et al. Spectrum of Systemic Auto-Inflammatory Diseases in India: A Multi-Centric Experience. Front Immunol. 2021;12:630691.
4. Jain A, Bhoyar RC, Pandhare K, Mishra A, Sharma D, Imran M, et al. Genetic epidemiology of autoinflammatory disease variants in Indian population from 1029 whole genomes. J Genet Eng Biotechnol. 2021;19(1):183.

140

CHAPTER

Immunomodulators in Medicine

Prabhakar K, Rupa Kasaraneni

ABSTRACT

Immunomodulators are revolutionary in the field of medicine. These agents either stimulate or suppress the immune system. These are classified based on the activation of the type of immune-responsive cells and the site of action. They are used in various infections, autoimmune conditions, connective tissue disorders, vaccines, cancers, etc. They were widely used during the crisis of coronavirus disease 2019 (COVID-19). Their use is now being studied in multiple myeloma and various other tumors with their increasing incidence. In this chapter, we describe and discuss various immunomodulators with their action, uses, and side effects.

INTRODUCTION

Drugs known as immunomodulators change how the human immune system responds. Immunomodulators are divided into two categories based on whether they stimulate or reduce the body's generation of serum antibodies, respectively.

Immune stimulators are often prescribed for enhancing the immune response against immunodeficiency disorders, infections, tumors, and alterations in antibody transfer, etc.

Immunosuppressants suppress the immune response which are useful in various autoimmune disorders and post-transplantation.

Thus, immunotherapy is defined as the treatment of disease by either stimulating/suppressing the immune system using various substances.

MECHANISM OF ACTION

Immunomodulators regulate the immune system at several levels. There are numerous medications available that can specifically suppress or promote certain immune cell types, such as macrophages and lymphocytes (cytotoxic and helper T lymphocytes), natural killer (NK) cells, and neutrophils. Immunomodulators affect the soluble mediators that signal the immune system for further action like cytokines.

Immune stimulants augment the immune response in conditions like immunodeficiency disorders, infections, and cancers. Immunosuppressants prevent the immune system from responding to ailments such as autoimmune disorders, post-transplantation.

For a drug that causes significant alterations in immune function, the term "immunomodulator" is used in lieu of "immune stimulator". They are divided into specific and nonspecific based on activity.

When an inducement results in an immunological reaction to one or more antigens, such as with adjuvants or therapeutic vaccinations, specific action immunomodulators, which modify the immune response selectively, work on the immune system.

New-generation antigens and other synthetic antigens in vaccines are strengthened by immunological adjuvants. In order to obtain monoclonal antibodies and polyclonal antisera for use in vaccines, these are also utilized in immunization probing.

Immunomodulators that are nonspecific either drive or halt the immune response without pointing the activity of activated cells toward a specific antigen. Based on the sort of immune system they affect, they are divided into three categories:

- *Type 1*: Acts on the normal immune system; e.g., bladder cancer—Intravesical BCG (bacillus Calmette-Guérin)
- *Type 2*: Acts on the immunosuppressed immune system; e.g., interleukins, cytokines, interferons
- *Type 3*: Acts on the operational and immunosuppressed immune system; e.g., colony-stimulating factors **(Tables 1 and 2)**.

IMMUNOSTIMULANTS

Recombinant Cytokines

- Interleukin 2 (IL-2) activates proliferation of Th (T helper) lymphocytes. The drug also called Aldesleukin is used in renal cell carcinoma and trials for other cancer therapy.
- IL-1 activates Tc (cytotoxic T cell) and B lymphocytes.
- It is one of the critical mediators of intestinal inflammation in inflammatory bowel disease (IBD). A recombinant IL-1 receptor antagonist, anakinra is used in cancer therapy, rheumatoid arthritis (RA), psoriasis, sepsis, and granulomatous pulmonary disease.
- IL-12 activates Th lymphocytes and is used in central nervous system (CNS) autoimmune diseases and multiple sclerosis.
- Interferon-gamma (IFN-γ) activates the propagation of monocytes, stimulation of lymphocytes, macrophages, and NK cells, and enhances the countenance of major histocompatibility complex (MHC) II. Actimmune is a recombinant IFN-γ1b used in tuberculosis (TB), hepatitis, chronic granulomatous disease, osteopetrosis, and scleroderma. Bropirimine is an oral interferon inducer used in transitional cell carcinoma.

TABLE 1: Immunostimulants.

Family	Drug	Pharmacological effect
Recombinant cytokines	• Interleukin 2 • Interleukin 1 • Interleukin 12 • Interferon gamma • Colony stimulating factors (CSF) • G-CSF (granulocyte CSF) • M-CSF (monocyte CSF) • GM-CSF (granulocyte–monocyte CSF)	• Activation of lymphocytes Th (proliferation) • Activation of Tc B cells • Activation of Th cells • Stimulation of lymphocytes, NK cells, and macrophages; enhance the expression of MHC II • Proliferation of monocytes • Proliferation and differentiation of macrophage, monocyte
Monoclonal antibodies	CD27, CD137, etc.	Triggers specific immunity (effector phase) counters the antigen
Polyclonal antibodies	Digoxin immune Fab, etc.	Triggers specific immunity (effector phase) counter multiple antigens
Synthetic drugs	• Levamisole • Isoprinosine	• Activation as well as the maturation of T cells, chemotaxis, and phagocytosis • Propagation of T cells, stimulation of Th, Tc, NK, chemotaxis, and phagocytosis
Vaccines	Antigens	Trigger specific immunity (the phases of recognition activation, effector)
Bacterial and fungal products	• Bacillus Calmette Guerin (BCG) • Muramyl dipeptide (MDP) • L-MTP-PE • Lipopolysaccharides (LPS) • *Propionibacterium* species • Glucan	• Stimulation of macrophages (antigen-presenting cells), natural killer cells, B cells • Stimulation of macrophages (antigen-presenting cells), phagocytosis • Stimulation of macrophages and B cells • Stimulation of Tc and B cells, phagocytosis • Phagocytosis
Thymic factors	Thymosins	Evolution of thymocytes into T cells

(Fab: fragment of polyclonal antibody; L-MTP-PE: liposomal muramyl tripeptide phosphatidyl ethanolamine; MHC: major histocompatibility complex; NK: natural killer; Tc: cytotoxic T cell; Th: T helper)

TABLE 2: Immunosuppressants.

Family	Drug	Pharmacological effect
Glucocorticoids	Prednisone dexamethasone	Hindrance of transcription of cytokines into T cells and macrophages
Dings that bind to immunophilins	• Cyclosporine A • Tacrolimus, sirolimus	• Hindrance of gene transcription of cytokines (e.g., IL-2) to T cells (block propagation) • Hindrance of transcription of cytokines to T cells
Cytostatics	• Azathioprine • Leflunomide • Cyclophosphamide, mycophenolate mofetil	• Hindrance of cell propagation • Hindrance of propagation of T and B cells
Monoclonal antibodies	• Muromonab (OKT3) • Anticytokines and antireceptors	• Demolition of CD3+ T lymphocytes • Neutralization or demolition of mediators of the immune system
Antilymphocyte antibodies	• Polyclonal antibodies • Antithymocytes	Trigger effector phase of specific immunity counter multiple lymphocytes
Hyposensitization	Allergens	• Switching from IgE to IgC response (or from Th2 to Th1) • Decreased sensitivity to the allergen

(IgE: immunoglobulin E; IL-2: interleukin 2; Th2: T helper 2)

- *Colony-stimulating factors (CSF)*:
    - G-CSF is a granulocyte CSF used after bone marrow transplantation.
    - M-CSF is a monocyte CSF used in antitumors, anti-infection, and myelosuppression.
    - GM-CSF is a granulocyte-monocyte CSF used in the stimulation of antigen-presenting cells (APC) for immunotherapy and recruitment of peripheral blood stem cells.

Monoclonal Antibodies

These are specific antibodies that act by triggering the effector phase of specific immunity to counter various antigens, e.g., cancers.

CD27—Varlilumab is an anti-CD27 agonist antibody used in hematological malignancies like refractory Hodgkin lymphoma, acute lymphoblastic leukemia (ALL), and Burkitt's lymphoma.

Anti-CD40 agonist antibodies are used in the treatment of melanoma and gastroesophageal neoplasms.

CD137—Utomilumab—diffuse large B-cell lymphoma.

Polyclonal Antibodies

Polyclonal antibodies are the specific antibodies that trigger the effector phase of specific immunity to counter multiple antigens.

Digoxin immune Fab (fragment of polyclonal antibody)—Digoxin toxicity reversal.

Synthetic Drugs

These help in the propagation of T lymphocytes, stimulation, and maturation of activation of Th cells, Tc cells, NK cells, chemotaxis, and phagocytosis.

For example, levamisole is an anthelmintic that can be used infrequently relapsing steroid-dependent idiopathic nephrotic syndrome and RA due to its ability to restore depressed immune function via T cell activation.

Isoprinosine is used in herpes simplex, sclerosing pan encephalitis.

Vaccines

Vaccines are the antigens that trigger specific immunity at various phases of recognition, activation, and effector; e.g., Tdap (tetanus, diphtheria, and pertussis), Hep A (hepatitis A).

Bacterial and Fungal Products

- BCG activates macrophages (APC), B cells, and NK cells used as vaccines for *Mycobacterium*.
- Muramyl dipeptide (MDP) and L-MTP-PE (liposomal muramyl tripeptide phosphatidyl ethanolamine)—activate macrophages (APC) and phagocytosis.

  For example, MDP derivatives like murabutide and polimuramil are used in skin infections and respiratory tract infections.

  Threonyl MDP is used as an adjuvant in the acquired immunodeficiency syndrome (AIDS) vaccine.

- Lipopolysaccharides (LPS) activate macrophages and B lymphocytes, e.g., PS-K protein-bound polysaccharide used in various infections.
- *Propionibacterium* species activates macrophages, phagocytosis, and activation of Tc and B lymphocytes, used in infections.
- Beta-glucan acts by phagocytosis.

For example, peptidoglycan, yeast glucan (*Saccharomyces cerevisiae*) are used in infections and cancer therapy. These can be used as dietary supplements for heart disease.

Thymic Factors

Thymic factors including thymosins help in the maturation of thymocytes into T lymphocytes **(Fig. 1)**.

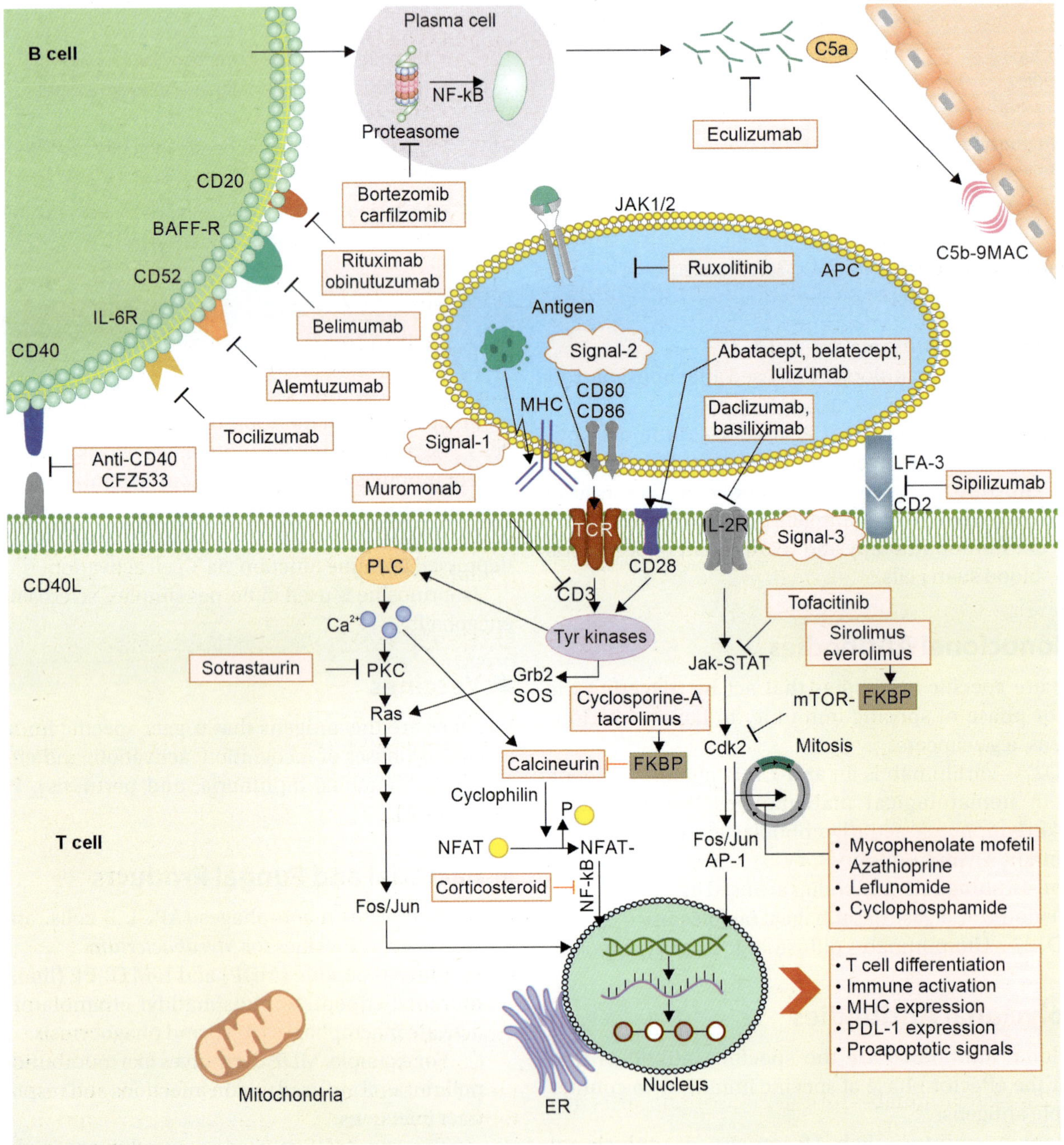

FIG. 1: B and T lymphocyte activation with various drugs interrupting the pathway at specific receptor sites.

(APC: antigen-presenting cells; BAFF-R: B-cell activating factor receptor; CD: cluster differentiation; ER: endoplasmic reticulum; FKBP: factor K506 binding proteins; IL: interleukin; mTOR: mammalian target of rapamycin; NFAT: nuclear factor of activated T cells; NF-κB: nuclear factor kappa light chain enhancer of activated B cells; PKC: protein kinase C; PLC: phospholipase; TCR: T cell receptor)

IMMUNOSUPPRESSANTS

Glucocorticoids

Prednisolone and dexamethasone are immunomodulating glucocorticoids. They inhibit transcription of cytokines into macrophages and T cells, used in RA, psoriasis, leprosy, etc.

Drugs Binding to Immunophilins

By preventing T cells from proliferating, cyclosporine A, tacrolimus, and sirolimus function by repressing the gene transcription of cytokines like IL-2. These are used in post-transplantation [graft versus host disease (GVHD)], RA, and amyotrophic lateral sclerosis.

Cytostatics

Azathioprine, cyclophosphamide, mycophenolate mofetil, and leflunomide are the few drugs categorized as cytostatics. These drugs act by inhibiting cell proliferation, and T and B lymphocytes. These are used in active RA, IBD, Churg-Strauss syndrome, autoimmune hepatitis, chronic immune thrombocytopenic purpura (ITP), multiple sclerosis, severe myasthenia gravis, psoriasis, dermatomyositis, pemphigus, and dermatitis.

Monoclonal Antibodies

CD3e: Muromonab (OKT3)—acute allograft rejection

CD20: Rituximab—autoimmune diseases, polychemotherapy—B cell Hodgkins lymphoma, transplantation rejections

CD25: Basiliximab, daclizumab—transplant rejection, multiple sclerosis

CD52: Alemtuzumab—B-CLL (B-cell chronic lymphocytic leukemia)

Immunoglobulin E (IgE): Omalizumab—asthma

IgG1: Palivizumab—respiratory syncytial virus (RSV) prophylaxis

Tumor necrosis *factor alpha (TNF-α)*: Adalimumab, infliximab, golimumab, certolizumab pegol: IBD, RA, ankylosing spondylitis, plaque psoriasis.

IL-4: Pascolizumab—asthma

IL-5: Mepolizumab—asthma

IL-12/23: Ustekinumab—psoriasis, psoriatic arthritis, moderate-to-severe IBD

IL-17A: Secukinumab—plaque psoriasis

Other anti-TNF agents: Abatacept, belatacept, etanercept, etc.—refractory RA

Deactivation or mitigation of immune system substances: Coronavirus disease 2019 (COVID-19), solid transplant rejection, cancers, autoimmune conditions.

Antilymphocytic Antibodies

Polyclonal antibodies and antithymocytes are the common antilymphocytic antibodies used. These drugs act by triggering the effector phase of specific immunity counter lymphocytes—systemic lupus erythematosus (SLE), RA, Sjogren's, primary biliary cirrhosis (PBC), and multiple sclerosis.

Hyposensitization

Allergens are often used for hyposensitization which acts by switch of response from type IgE to IgG (from Th2 to Th1) and depletion in susceptivity to allergens—asthma, rhinoconjunctivitis.

IMMUNOADJUVANTS

These are the agents which are adjoined to a vaccine to expedite the immune response but without any special antigenic activity, i.e., in the truancy of a vaccine, these substances do not manifest any antigen activity.

An example is Freud's adjuvant. These molecules are used to discriminate between Th1 and Th2 cells, cellular and humoral immunity, IgG and IgE, and immunoprotective and immune destructive types of immune actions.

USES OF IMMUNOMODULATORS

In some cases of immunological stimulation, autoimmune processes are modified with immunosuppressive medications. Numerous medications have endured time and have seen widespread use.

Common conditions: These include infections, asthma, IBD, autoimmune disorders like RA, SLE, Sjogren's, psoriasis, psoriatic arthritis, cancer therapy, GVHD, hepatitis, leprosy, etc.

Rare conditions: These include multiple sclerosis, Gullain-Barré syndrome, lupus nephritis, myasthenia gravis, chronic ITP, sclerosing panencephalitis, multiple myeloma, etc.

Corticosteroids, cytotoxic medications such as methotrexate, cyclophosphamide, mycophenolate mofetil, cyclosporin A, and calcineurin inhibitors like tacrolimus, and sirolimus are some of these.

Numerous hematological, renal, neurological, and connective tissue problems have shown these to be helpful.

Myasthenia gravis has been proven to benefit from thymectomy. Ionizing radiation usage is constrained by extreme toxicity. Only pretransplantation procedures are used today.

The antihelminthic medication levamisole enhances the nonspecific immune response. Due to its unexpected effects and potential for agranulocytosis, its use has been restricted.

Thymic peptide extracts with immunostimulatory properties, such as thymosin, thrombomodulin, and thymopentin, may be used to treat RA, small cell lung cancer, fungal and viral infections, and primary immunodeficiency disorders.

The use of OK-432, an extract from a strain of *Streptococcus pyogenes* is used in the management of head and neck, gastrointestinal, and lung cancers.

Mycobacterial heat-shock proteins, for example, exhibit superantigen activity and can stimulate a significant proportion of T cells.

Treatments for leprosy, malignant melanoma, and bladder cancer have benefited from the use of the BCG vaccine.

Infections including hepatitis B, hepatitis C, HHV8 (human herpesvirus 8)—Kaposi's sarcoma, and various hematological cancers, including chronic myeloid leukemia, multiple myeloma, and lymphomas, have all been successfully treated with interferons, the most often used immunostimulatory drugs.

Cell differentiation, cell proliferation, and the expression of cell surface antigens are all significantly influenced by interferons. They increase the activity of NK cells and T-cells that mediate cytotoxicity.

Recent large-scale randomized trials demonstrate that immunomodulators reduce cardiovascular (CV) events among the general population. However, it is uncertain whether these effects apply to RA and if certain treatment strategies in RA reduce CV risk to a greater extent and was found that the addition of either a TNF inhibitor (TNFi) or triple therapy resulted in clinically important improvements in vascular inflammation.

Lenalidomide is an immunomodulator that is recommended for newly diagnosed and relapsed or refractory multiple myeloma. The use of lenalidomide has become widespread as early-line treatment, including as maintenance therapy.

Currently, available disease-modifying therapies (DMTs), all of which have immunomodulatory or immunosuppressive properties, improve the course of relapsing multiple sclerosis.

However, current DMTs fail to benefit the later secondary progressive phase [secondary progressive multiple sclerosis (SPMS)], in which neurodegenerative mechanisms assume overriding clinical importance. Early DMT treatment to control clinical and subclinical inflammatory disease activity has been recommended.

ADVERSE EFFECTS

Due to the rapid withdrawal of corticosteroids after lengthy administration, the adrenal crisis is the most severe, acute adverse consequence of their use. Other side effects mentioned include cataracts, osteopenia with spinal compression, elevated blood pressure, elevated cholesterol levels, intolerance to glucose, diabetes, insomnia, emotional instability, psychiatric disorders, "moon face" (Cushing syndrome), "buffalo hump", acne, and hirsutism.

Azathioprine and 6-mercaptopurine can result in medullar suppression, gastric irritation, pancreatitis, hepatitis, myalgia, and dizziness. Numerous illnesses, including *Pneumocystis carinii* pneumonia, cryptococcal infections, aspergillosis, histoplasmosis, coccidioidomycosis, listeriosis, TB, and cytomegalovirus (CMV), have been reported.

Calcineurin inhibitors like cyclosporine cause hirsutism, gum hyperplasia, hyperuricemia, and hyperlipidemia. Both cyclosporin and tacrolimus cause hypertension, hyperglycemia, nephrotoxicity, neurotoxicity, and hepatotoxicity.

The side effects of methotrexate include flu-like fever, chills, headache, myalgia, bloating, dizziness, lethargy, and diarrhea. It can also have adverse consequences on the liver or lungs.

Tumor necrosis factor antagonists and monoclonal antibodies cause the reactivation of latent infections, like TB.

SUGGESTED READINGS

1. Bascones-Martinez A, Mattila R, Gomez-Font R, Meurman JH. Immunomodulatory drugs: oral and systemic adverse effects. Med Oral Patol Oral Cir Bucal. 2014;19(1):e24-31.
2. Solomon DH, Giles JT, Liao KP, Ridker PM, Rist PM, Glynn RJ, et al; TARGET Trial Consortium. Reducing cardiovascular risk with immunomodulators: a randomized active comparator trial among patients with rheumatoid arthritis. Ann Rheum Dis. 2023;82(3):324-30.
3. San-Miguel J, Dhakal B, Yong K, Spencer A, Anguille S, Mateos MV, et al. CILTA-CEL or standard care in lenalidomide-refractory multiple myeloma. N Engl J Med. 2023;389(4):335-47.
4. Robertson D, Moreo N. Disease-modifying Therapies in Multiple Sclerosis: Overview and Treatment Considerations. Fed Pract. 2016;33(6):28-34.

141

CHAPTER

Recent Advances in Cancer Immunotherapy Management

Vineet Talwar, Arpit Jain

ABSTRACT

Recent strides in cancer immunotherapy have sparked a transformation in cancer treatment approaches, offering renewed optimism to those grappling with this formidable ailment. This manuscript embarks on an exploration of the cutting-edge developments in the management of cancer immunotherapy, delving into a multifaceted array of strategies and breakthroughs that have emerged to leverage the innate potential of the immune system in combating cancer.

This chapter commences by offering a historical perspective, retracing the evolution of cancer immunotherapy from its inception to the contemporary era. Subsequently, it furnishes an all-encompassing survey of diverse cancer immunotherapy modalities, encompassing immune checkpoint inhibitors, chimeric antigen receptor (CAR) T-cell therapy, cancer vaccines, and adoptive T-cell therapy.

In-depth discussions ensue regarding patient selection and the pivotal role of biomarkers in prognosticating treatment responses. Furthermore, the growing significance of personalized medicine within the domain of cancer immunotherapy is examined. The manuscript delves into the captivating realm of combination therapies and the intricacies associated with surmounting resistance to immunotherapy.

Specialized segments are allocated to the deployment of immunotherapy in distinct cancer categories, such as melanoma, lung cancer, and breast cancer, thereby spotlighting the remarkable strides achieved in each domain. Moreover, the document investigates emerging trends, technologies, and ethical considerations inherent in cancer immunotherapy research and clinical implementation.

INTRODUCTION

Recent breakthroughs in cancer immunotherapy have transformed the landscape of cancer treatment, offering new hope to patients battling this formidable disease. This chapter provides an in-depth exploration of the latest advancements in cancer immunotherapy management, covering a diverse array of strategies and innovations aimed at harnessing the power of the immune system to combat cancer. It begins with a historical perspective, tracing the evolution of cancer immunotherapy from its early origins to its current state as a cutting-edge treatment modality. The chapter then offers a comprehensive overview of various types of cancer immunotherapy, including immune checkpoint inhibitors, chimeric antigen receptor (CAR) T-cell therapy, cancer vaccines, and adoptive T-cell therapy, elucidating their mechanisms of action and highlighting notable examples of their successful application.

HISTORICAL PERSPECTIVE

Brief History of Cancer Immunotherapy

This section provides an insightful journey into the origins of cancer immunotherapy, tracing its evolution from the early conceptualizations to the modern era. One key milestone is the pioneering work of William Coley in the late 1800s. Coley's use of bacterial extracts, known as Coley's toxins, to treat cancer patients marked one of the earliest instances of immunotherapy.

Another pivotal moment in the history of cancer immunotherapy occurred in the mid-20th century with the development of the Bacillus Calmette-Guérin (BCG) vaccine for bladder cancer. BCG remains a standard treatment today, illustrating the enduring impact of early immunotherapeutic breakthroughs.

Another noteworthy stride was made with the introduction of monoclonal antibodies, particularly the approval of rituximab for non-Hodgkin lymphoma (NHL) in 1997, signifying a significant step forward in cancer treatment.

Milestones in the Development of Cancer Immunotherapy

One landmark event is the development of the first immune checkpoint inhibitors, such as ipilimumab, which was approved by the Food and Drug Administration (FDA) in 2011 for the treatment of melanoma. This approval marked a turning point in cancer treatment and set the stage for the subsequent development of checkpoint inhibitors like pembrolizumab and nivolumab. The advent of CAR T-cell therapy in the early 21st century is another pivotal milestone. CAR T-cell therapy achieved remarkable success in treating certain hematological malignancies and exemplifies the potential of engineered immune cells in cancer therapy.

TYPES OF CANCER IMMUNOTHERAPY

Immune Checkpoint Inhibitors

Immune checkpoint inhibitors work by blocking inhibitory checkpoints, such as programmed cell death protein 1 (PD-1) and cytotoxic T-lymphocyte-associated protein 4 (CTLA-4). These checkpoints act as "brakes" on the immune response that reactivate the immune response against cancer by blocking specific checkpoint pathways that tumors exploit to evade detection. PD-1 inhibitors, such as pembrolizumab and nivolumab, disrupt the PD-1/programmed death-ligand 1 (PD-L1) interaction on T cells, allowing the immune system to recognize and attack cancer cells while sparing healthy tissues due to their specificity. Similarly, CTLA-4 inhibitors like Ipilimumab prevent CTLA-4 from inhibiting T-cell activation, enhancing the immune response against cancer with precision, as normal cells typically express lower levels of CTLA-4.

Chimeric Antigen Receptor T-cell Therapy

Chimeric antigen receptor T-cell therapy is a cutting-edge approach, involves genetically modifying a patient's T cells to express a synthetic receptor (CAR) that recognizes specific cancer antigens. CARs consist of an antigen recognition domain, typically derived from a monoclonal antibody, linked to intracellular signaling domains that activate T cells upon antigen binding. This therapy harnesses the specificity of CARs to target cancer cells directly. However, challenges in manufacturing consistency, potential toxicities, and cytokine release syndrome must be addressed to maximize its effectiveness, especially in solid tumors.

Chimeric antigen receptor T-cell therapy has yielded remarkable clinical successes, especially in hematological malignancies, such as acute lymphoblastic leukemia (ALL) and NHL. Many patients who had exhausted other treatment options achieved complete remission and long-lasting responses.

Cancer Vaccines

Cancer vaccines encompass various approaches, including peptide-based vaccines, dendritic cell vaccines, and whole-cell vaccines, each designed to harness the immune system against cancer. Peptide-based vaccines use tumor-specific protein fragments to trigger immune responses by presenting them to cytotoxic T cells through antigen-presenting cells. Dendritic cell vaccines involve isolating a patient's dendritic cells, loading them with tumor antigens, and reintroducing them to stimulate a potent immune response. Whole-cell vaccines utilize killed or weakened cancer cells to expose the immune system to a broader array of antigens, enhancing the immune recognition of cancer.

Adoptive T-cell Therapy

Tumor-infiltrating lymphocytes (TILs) are immune cells, primarily T cells that have infiltrated a patient's tumor tissue to mount an immune response against cancer. These TILs are harvested through a surgical biopsy, then expanded and activated in a specialized laboratory in a process called ex vivo expansion. This activation enhances their ability to recognize and target cancer cells. After rigorous quality control, the TILs are reintroduced into the patient, where they can specifically attack cancer cells within the tumor microenvironment.

BIOMARKERS AND PATIENT SELECTION

Biomarkers for Predicting Response to Immunotherapy

Prominent biomarkers like PD-L1 expression, tumor mutational burden (TMB), and microsatellite instability (MSI) are measured through methods such as immunohistochemistry and DNA sequencing, and they hold significance in identifying individuals likely to benefit from immunotherapy. The evolving landscape of predictive biomarkers includes emerging indicators like TILs and genetic signatures, offering insights into the tumor microenvironment and molecular characteristics.

Personalized Medicine Approaches

Personalized medicine in cancer immunotherapy is a tailored approach that considers an individual patient's unique characteristics to optimize treatment outcomes. It relies on biomarkers to select the most appropriate immunotherapies, such as checkpoint inhibitors, for patients. Genetic and molecular profiling identifies specific mutations and alterations that can be targeted precisely, while CAR T-cell therapy customizes treatment to the patient's tumor antigens. This approach revolutionizes cancer treatment by moving away from a one-size-fits-all model and toward a patient-centered, precision medicine approach that aims to improve outcomes and enhance the quality of life for cancer patients.

Challenges in Patient Selection

Patient selection for immunotherapy is a complex process with challenges due to limitations in current biomarkers, including their dynamic nature and the need for standardized testing methods. Additionally, intratumoral heterogeneity can lead to varying biomarker profiles within the same tumor. A multidisciplinary approach involving oncologists, pathologists, and molecular biologists is crucial for informed patient selection decisions. Ethical considerations arise concerning access to personalized treatments and healthcare disparities, as not all patients may have equal access to advanced biomarker testing and therapies.

OVERCOMING RESISTANCE

Mechanisms of Resistance to Immunotherapy

Cancer cells can develop resistance to immunotherapy through a variety of mechanisms. Some of the most common mechanisms include:

- *Loss of antigen presentation*: Cancer cells can lose the ability to present tumor antigens to the immune system. This can happen due to mutations in the genes that encode tumor antigens, or due to changes in the way that cancer cells process and present antigens.
- *Upregulation of alternative immune checkpoints*: Cancer cells can upregulate the expression of immune checkpoints that inhibit the immune response. This can make it more difficult for T cells to kill cancer cells.
- *Development of an immunosuppressive tumor microenvironment*: The tumor microenvironment is made up of tumor cells, immune cells, and other cells. These cells can produce molecules that suppress the immune response, making it more difficult for T cells to kill cancer cells.

Strategies to Overcome Resistance

There are a number of strategies that can be used to overcome resistance to immunotherapy. Some of the most promising strategies include:

- *Combination therapies*: Combining an immune checkpoint inhibitor with a cancer vaccine can help to target cancer cells that have lost the ability to present tumor antigens.
- *Adaptive treatment approaches*: This involves monitoring patients for signs of resistance and adjusting treatment accordingly. This can be done by using biomarkers to track the patient's immune response, or by periodically reevaluating the patient's tumor.
- *Precision medicine*: It involves tailoring treatment to the individual patient. This can be done by identifying genetic mutations or other biomarkers that are associated with resistance to immunotherapy.

Emerging Therapies for Resistant Cancers

Emerging therapies for resistant cancers include bispecific antibodies and engineered immune cells. Bispecific antibodies target both cancer cells and immune cells simultaneously, enhancing the immune response. Engineered immune cells are genetically modified to improve their cancer-killing abilities, either by introducing tumor-specific receptors or modifying their metabolism and signaling pathways. These therapies hold promise in addressing treatment-resistant cancers.

IMMUNOTHERAPY IN SPECIFIC CANCER TYPES

Immunotherapy in Melanoma

Melanoma is one of the most studied and successful applications of immunotherapy. Immune checkpoint inhibitors, such as pembrolizumab and nivolumab, have been shown to significantly improve outcomes for patients with advanced melanoma, including those with metastatic disease. In addition to immune checkpoint inhibitors, other immunotherapies are also being investigated for the treatment of melanoma. These include:

- *CAR T-cell therapy*: This therapy uses a patient's own T cells, which are genetically engineered to express a receptor that binds to a specific protein on the surface of cancer cells. This allows the T cells to recognize and attack cancer cells.
- *Oncolytic viruses*: These are viruses that have been genetically engineered to infect and kill cancer cells.
- *Immunomodulatory drugs*: These drugs work to boost the immune system and help it to fight cancer.

Immunotherapy in Lung Cancer

Lung cancer is the leading cause of cancer death in both men and women worldwide. In 2020, an estimated 2.2 million people died from lung cancer. One significant breakthrough in nonsmall cell lung cancer (NSCLC) treatment has been the development of immune checkpoint inhibitors, such as pembrolizumab and atezolizumab. These drugs target the PD-1 pathway, which plays a crucial role in suppressing the immune response against cancer cells.

Patients with high PD-L1 expression on their tumor cells have shown remarkable responses to immune checkpoint inhibitors. Clinical trials have demonstrated that for some of these patients, immunotherapy with drugs like pembrolizumab can provide durable responses and significantly improved overall survival compared to traditional chemotherapy. As a result, immune checkpoint inhibitors have become a first-line treatment option for select NSCLC patients with high PD-L1 expression, offering hope for better outcomes.

Immunotherapy in Breast Cancer

Triple-negative breast cancer (TNBC) poses significant challenges due to its aggressive nature and limited treatment options. Immunotherapy, particularly immune checkpoint inhibitors targeting PD-L1, has emerged as a promising avenue, especially in PD-L1-positive TNBC cases. Ongoing research explores combinations with targeted therapies like PARP inhibitors and identifies predictive biomarkers, offering hope for improved outcomes in this complex subtype.

Immunotherapy in other Cancer Types

Immunotherapy's application extends to various cancer types. In colorectal cancer, immune checkpoint inhibitors have shown promise in microsatellite instability-high (MSI-H) tumors. In renal cell carcinoma, checkpoint inhibitors have achieved success in advanced disease. Head and neck cancer patients, especially those with recurrent or metastatic disease, have benefited from immunotherapy. These examples illustrate the diverse applications and ongoing research in immunotherapy across various cancer types, each presenting unique challenges and opportunities.

FUTURE DIRECTIONS AND CHALLENGES

Emerging Trends and Technologies

Some of the emerging trends and technologies in cancer immunotherapy include:

- *The development of novel immunotherapeutic agents*: Researchers are developing new immunotherapeutic agents that target different aspects of the immune system. These agents include bispecific antibodies, CAR T-cell therapy, and oncolytic viruses.
- *Advances in genetic editing techniques*: Genetic editing techniques, such as CRISPR-Cas9, are being used to engineer immune cells to improve their ability to fight cancer cells.
- *Innovative drug delivery systems*: Researchers are developing innovative drug delivery systems that can deliver immunotherapeutic agents more effectively to cancer cells. These systems include nanoparticles and gene therapy vectors.

Role of Artificial Intelligence in Immunotherapy

Artificial intelligence (AI) is increasingly integral to cancer immunotherapy, facilitating patient response prediction, drug candidate identification, and treatment plan optimization. AI analyses patient data, including genetic profiles and tumor biopsies, to predict treatment outcomes and personalize care, ultimately improving patient management.

Ethical Considerations in Cancer Immunotherapy Research and Practice

Ethical considerations in cancer immunotherapy encompass the use of experimental therapies, the requirement for informed patient consent, and ensuring equitable access to immunotherapy. Balancing potential risks and benefits of experimental treatments, informed patient participation, and addressing healthcare disparities are central to ethical cancer immunotherapy research and practice.

CONCLUSION

In conclusion, cancer immunotherapy represents a dynamic and rapidly evolving field offering renewed hope to cancer patients. Diverse immunotherapy approaches, including immune checkpoint inhibitors, CAR T-cell therapy, cancer vaccines, and adoptive T-cell therapy, are transforming cancer care. Biomarkers play a crucial role in patient selection, ushering in the era of personalized medicine. Overcoming resistance through combination therapies and emerging treatments holds the promise of better outcomes. Immunotherapy's application in specific cancer types, such as melanoma, lung cancer, and breast cancer, showcases remarkable progress. Future trends, AI integration, and ethical considerations underscore the potential for immunotherapy to continue revolutionizing cancer care, ultimately improving patient outcomes and quality of life.

SUGGESTED READINGS

1. McCarthy EF. The Toxins of William B. Coley and the Treatment of Bone and Soft-Tissue Sarcomas. Iowa Orthop J. 2006;26:154-8.
2. Morales A, Eidinger D, Bruce AW. Intracavitary Bacillus Calmette-Guerin in the treatment of superficial bladder tumors. J Urol. 1976;116(2):180-3.
3. Maude SL, Laetsch TW, Buechner J, Rives S, Boyer M, Bittencourt H, et al. Tisagenlecleucel in Children and Young Adults with B-Cell Lymphoblastic Leukemia. N Engl J Med. 2018;378(5):439-48.
4. June CH, O'Connor RS, Kawalekar OU, Ghassemi S, Milone MC. CAR T cell immunotherapy for human cancer. Science. 2018;359(6382):1361-5.
5. Palucka K, Banchereau J. Cancer immunotherapy via dendritic cells. Nat Rev Cancer. 2012;12(4):265-77.
6. Rosenberg SA, Restifo NP. Adoptive cell transfer as personalized immunotherapy for human cancer. Science. 2015;348(6230):62-8.
7. Riaz N, Havel JJ, Makarov V, Desrichard A, Urba WJ, Sims JS, et al. Tumor and Microenvironment Evolution during Immunotherapy with Nivolumab. Cell. 2017;171(4):934-949.e16.
8. Hodi FS, Chiarion-Sileni V, Gonzalez R, Grob JJ, Rutkowski P, Cowey CL, et al. Nivolumab plus ipilimumab or nivolumab alone versus ipilimumab alone in advanced melanoma (CheckMate 067): 4-year outcomes of a multicentre, randomised, phase 3 trial. Lancet Oncol. 2018;19(11):1480-92.
9. Reck M, Rodríguez-Abreu D, Robinson AG, Hui R, Csőszi T, Fülöp A, et al. Pembrolizumab versus Chemotherapy for PD-L1–Positive Non–Small-Cell Lung Cancer. N Engl J Med. 2016;375(19):1823-33.
10. Emens LA, Molinero L, Loi S, Rugo HS, Schneeweiss A, Diéras V, et al. Atezolizumab and nab-Paclitaxel in Advanced Triple-Negative Breast Cancer: Biomarker Evaluation of the IMpassion130 Study. JNCI J Natl Cancer Inst. 2021;113(8):1005-16.
11. Rabaan AA, AlSaihati H, Bukhamsin R, Bakhrebah MA, Nassar MS, Alsaleh AA, et al. Application of CRISPR/Cas9 Technology in Cancer Treatment: A Future Direction. Curr Oncol. 2023;30(2):1954-76.

142

CHAPTER

IgG4-related Disease: New Thoughts on a Multisystem Disease and Changing the Epidemiology

Bharat Panigrahy, Suryasnata Rath

ABSTRACT

Immunoglobulin G4-related disease (IgG4-RD) is an immune-mediated fibroinflammatory disease. It can affect any organ of the body. The most common organs affected are autoimmune pancreatitis type 1, salivary glands involving parotid and submandibular gland, dacryoadenitis involving the lacrimal gland, orbital pseudomotor, sclerosing cholangitis, and retroperitoneal fibrosis affecting the kidney and aorta.

It usually presents as a mass lesion in organs such as pancreas, biliary tree, orbits, lungs, kidneys, major salivary gland, or lacrimal gland.

Exact cause is not known. Multiple genetic, epigenetic, and environmental factors play a role in the etiopathogenesis of the disease.

There are insufficient data regarding prevalence of IgG4-RD. Most of the data from Japan showing the incidence to be 0.28–1.08/100,000 population. Recently published eleven studies including 1,498 diagnosed patients of IgG4-RD shows that the mean age ranged between 50 and 67 years and male:female ratio mildly favoring the male gender. These studies also showed that more and more cases have been recorded worldwide. Apparently, there are more cases diagnosed in Asia than in Europe or North America.

Diagnosis of IgG4-RD involves clinical, serological, radiological, and histopathological parameters. The typical histopathological features include lymphoplasmocytic tissue infiltration of IgG4 plasma cells and lymphocytes, storiform fibrosis, obliterative phlebitis, and modest tissue eosinophilia. Serum IgG4 > 135 mg is found in most cases.

Glucocorticoid is the first-line treatment. Immunosuppressants such as rituximab and mycophenolate can be tried in high disease activity and relapse cases.

INTRODUCTION

Immunoglobulin G4-related disease (IgG4-RD) is an autoimmune-related fibroinflammatory process. The disease was first diagnosed in 2003 as autoimmune pancreatitis (AIP). Later on the name and definition were recognized in the First International Conference on IgG4-RD in 2011 in Boston. It can affect almost any organ, but pancreas, biliary tree, salivary and lacrimal glands, retroperitoneum, and lymph nodes are usually affected in most cases.

EPIDEMIOLOGY

The exact prevalence of IgG4-RD is not known as it is uncommonly diagnosed. It does not have its own International Classification of Diseases, 10th revision (ICD-10) code. As reported, the incidence in Japan is approximately 0.28–1.08 per 100,000 of population. This disease is predominately found in middle aged and older males. It is also diagnosed in children.

In a recent publication in Annals of Rheumatic Disease, database analysis in USA from 2015 to 2019 found about 524 cases resulting the incidence in 2019 to be 1.39 per 100,000 person years. Mean age being 65 years. The incidence was found to be almost equal to antineutrophilic cytoplasmic antibody (ANCA) associated vasculitis and systemic sclerosis. In comparison to West, Asian origin patients had substantially higher serum concentrations of IgG4.

The major clinical characteristics found in 1,498 diagnosed IgG4-RD patients from eleven studies are summarized in **Table 1**.

In summary, these studies showed that more cases have been diagnosed worldwide. Diagnosis of IgG4-RD is actually found only in tertiary centers. Apparently, more cases diagnosed in Asia than in Europe or North America and this geographical difference has not been clarified.

PATHOGENESIS

The exact pathogenesis of IgG4-RD remains obscure. It is thought to be immune-mediated and like other rheumatic conditions may be an autoimmune disease, although this has yet to be demonstrated.

Both T and B cells play an important role in the pathogenesis. CD4+ T cells producing cytolytic and profibrotic molecules such as granzyme and perforin lead to tissue damage whereas T follicular helper (Tfh) cells are responsible for interleukin-4 (IL-4) production and IgG4 class switch in the germinal centers. This response creates IgG4 secreting plasma blasts and long-lived plasma cells **(Fig. 1)**.

TABLE 1: Clinical characteristics of immunoglobulin G4-related disease (IgG4-RD).

Author	Year	Country	Number of patients	Male:female ratio	Age at onset	Organ involvement	Serum IgG4 >135 mg/dL	
Ebbo	2012	France	25	2.6:1	58	Lymph nodes and pancreas	100%	French registry
Fernández–Codina50	2015	Spain	55	3:1	56	Retroperitoneum, orbital pseudotumor	–	Spanish registry
Lin	2015	China	118	2.3:1	53.1	Lymph nodes, pancreas, and salivary glands	97.5%	Multicenter and prospective
Wallace	2015	USA	125	1.6:1	50.3	Submandibular glands, pancreas, and lymph nodes	51.4%	Single center and retrospective
Quero	2019	Spain	15	4:1	60.7	Submandibular glands, pancreas, lymph nodes, kidney, vascular system, and lungs	–	Single center and retrospective
Campochiaro	2016	Italy	41	1.9:1	62	Pancreas and retroperitoneum	73%	Single center and retrospective
Li	2017	Hong Kong	104	3:1	62	Hepatobiliary, retroperitoneum, lungs, eye, skin, and central nervous system (CNS)	95%	Single center and retrospective
Fong	2018	Singapore	42 (35 definite)	2.9:1	66.3	Pancreas, lymph nodes, bile ducts	77.5%	Single center and retrospective
Inoue	2015	Japan	235	4:1	67	Pancreas, salivary glands, and kidney	88%	Multicenter and retrospective
Wang	2019	China	403	1.69:1	55	Pancreas, liver, gastrointestinal (GI) tract, salivary glands, lung, kidney, retroperitoneum, lymph nodes, prostate, sinus, orbits, skin, and thyroid	–	Prospective
Jamada	2017	Japan	334	1.5:1	63.8	Salivary and lacrimal glands, biliary tree, skin, thyroid lymph nodes, lung, prostate, and retroperitoneum/ periaortic	95%	Multicenter and retrospective

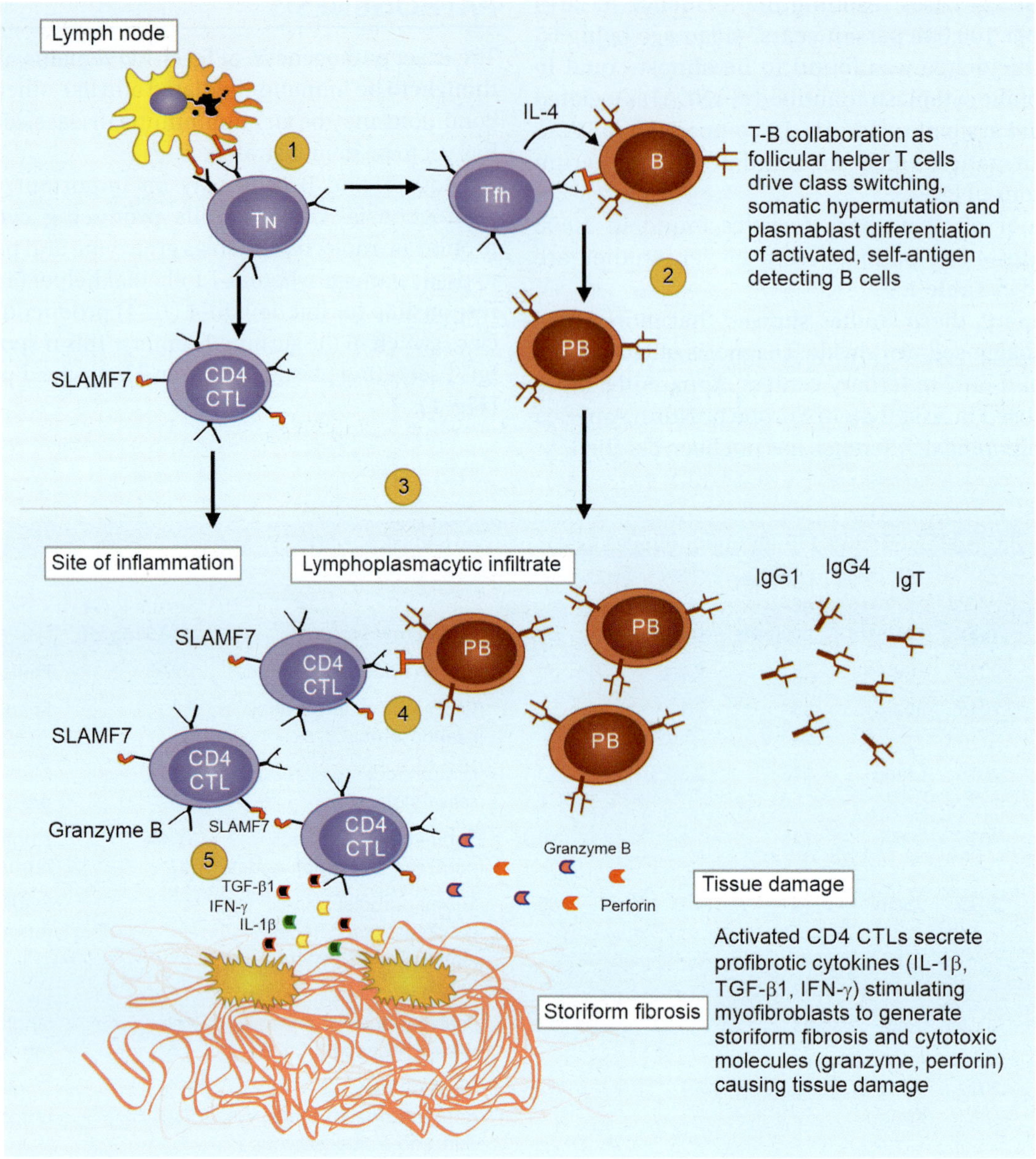

FIG. 1: Pathogenesis of IgG4-RD.

(IFN-γ: interferon-γ; IgG4-RD: immunoglobulin G4-related disease; IL-1β: interleukin-1β; TGF-β1: transforming growth factor-β1)

ENVIRONMENTAL FACTORS

Allergens, infections, and various environmental factors are thought to trigger the immune response. *Helicobacter pylori* has been found to trigger autoantibody activation against the pancreatic ductal epithelium enzyme (CA-II) causing AIP. CA-II antibody is found to be elevated in AIP. Self-antigens such as galectin-3, laminin-511, annexin-A11, and prohibitin have been reported to be involved in IgG4-RD initiation.

GENETIC FACTORS

Most studies have correlated the genetic correlation in AIP. HLA DRB10405 and DQB10401 serotypes have been found to be associated with AIP in Japanese patients whereas HLA-B8 is the only allele significantly associated with IgG4-RD in the Caucasian group.

To summarize in a genetically predisposed individual initial autoantigens include infectious agents and allergic components which activate immune reaction in the target tissue characterized by predominantly T helper 2 (Th2) response. This leads to increased production of IL-2, IL-5, IL-13, and transforming growth factor-β (TGF-β). It also leads to Treg activation and release of IL-10 and elevation of serum immunoglobulin E (IgE). B cell class switching and increased IgG4 production by plasma cells also occurs.

CLINICAL FEATURES

The clinical features vary according to site and severity of the disease. The American College of Rheumatology-European League Against Rheumatism (ACR-EULAR) 2019 describes 11 important sites involved in IgG4-RD. They are major salivary glands, orbits, lacrimal glands, pancreas, bile ducts, retroperitoneum, aorta, kidney, lung, thyroid gland, and pachymeninges.

Immunoglobulin G4-related disease can involve nearly every organ of the body. In 60–90% cases, multiple organs are involved. Patients usually present with subacute mass lesion of the affected organs. The common organs involved are pancreas, lymph nodes, parotid and submandibular salivary glands, lacrimal gland, orbital pseudomotor, kidney, retroperitoneal, biliary tree, and lungs.

Using a cluster analysis four phenotypes has been identified:

- *Phenotype 1*: Pancreato-hepatobiliary disease
- *Phenotype 2*: Retroperitoneal fibrosis and/or aortitis
- *Phenotype 3*: Head- and neck-limited disease
- *Phenotype 4*: Classic Mikulicz syndrome with systemic involvement

DIAGNOSIS

The involved organs share a number of core pathologic features and striking clinical and serologic similarities, including tumor-like swelling of involved organs, a lymphoplasmacytic infiltrate enriched in IgG4-positive plasma cells, and a variable degree of fibrosis that has a characteristic "storiform" pattern.

Diagnosis of IgG4-RD according to the 2019 ACR/EULAR classification criteria requires the integration of clinical, serological, radiological, and histopathological findings. Without biopsy this classification has a specificity of 98.9% but with a substantially reduced sensitivity of 48.6%. However, this classification criteria is not for clinical use.

BOX 1: The 2020 revised comprehensive diagnostic (RCD) criteria for immunoglobulin G4-related disease (IgG4-RD).

Item 1: Clinical and radiological features

One or more organs show diffuse or localized swelling or a mass or nodule characteristic of IgG4-RD. In single organ involvement, lymph node swelling is omitted

Item 2: Serological diagnosis

Serum IgG4 levels >135 mg/dL

Item 3: Pathological diagnosis

Positivity for two of the following three criteria:

1. Dense lymphocyte and plasma cell infiltration with fibrosis
2. Ratio of IgG4-positive plasma cells/IgG-positive cells >40% and the number of IgG4-positive plasma cells >10 per high-power field
3. Typical tissue fibrosis, particularly storiform fibrosis, or obliterative phlebitis

Diagnosis:

- Definite: (1) + (2) + (3)
- Probable: (1) + (3)
- Possible: (1) + (2)

The 2020 revised comprehensive diagnostic (RCD) criteria for IgG4-RD depicted in **Box 1**.

TREATMENT

Asymptomatic, nonprogressive, and limited disease detected incidentally, may be considered for "watchful waiting". However, most of the patients need immediate initiation of treatment.

Prednisone at a dose of 0.6 mg/kg body weight (30–40 mg) is the usual first line of therapy. Usually tapered after 4 weeks gradually with an aim to discontinue entirely within 2–3 months. However, the duration of treatment is controversial due to frequent incidence of relapse. Maintenance dose of 7.5 mg for many months is advocated by many studies. In some Asian studies 5–7.5 mg maintenance therapy is being tried for 2–3 years with minimal relapse rate.

Patients with multiple organ involvement and severe disease may be started with combination therapy of prednisone and mycophenolate mofetil (MMF) or leflunomide. For maintenance MMF, azathioprine can be used.

In relapse cases rituximab is the drug of choice. Rituximab has been also tried in severe disease as a first-line therapy with good result.

SUGGESTED READINGS

1. Kamisawa T, Zen Y, Pillai S, Stone JH. IgG4-related disease. Lancet. 2015;385:1460-71.
2. Della-Torre E, Lanzillotta M, Doglioni C. Immunology of IgG4-related disease. Clin Exp Immunol. 2015;181:191-206.
3. Kamisawa T, Funata N, Hayashi Y, Eishi Y, Koike M, Tsuruta K. A new clinicopathological entity of IgG4-related autoimmune disease. J Gastroenterol. 2003;38:982-4.
4. Umehara H, Okazaki K, Masaki Y. Comprehensive diagnostic criteria for IgG4-related disease (IgG4-RD). Mod Rheumathol. 2011;22(2012):21-30.
5. Fox RI, Fox CM. IgG4 levels and plasmablasts as a marker for IgG4-related disease (IgG4-RD). Ann Rheum Dis. 2015;74:1-3.
6. Hamano H, Kawa S, Horiuchi A, Unno H, Furuya N, Akamatsu T, et al. High serum IgG4 concentrations in patients with sclerosing pancreatitis. N Engl J Med. 2001;44(10):732-8.
7. Carruthers MN, Khosroshahi A, Augustin T, Deshpande V, Stone JH. The diagnostic utility of serum IgG4 concentrations in IgG4-related disease. Ann Rheum Dis. 2015;74(1):14-8.
8. Wallace ZS, Deshpande V, Mattoo H, Mahajan VS, Kulikova M, Pillai S, et al. IgG4-related disease: clinical and laboratory features in one hundred twenty-five patients. Arthritis Rheumatol. 2015;67(9):2466-75.
9. Wallace ZS, Naden RP, Chari S, et al. The 2019 American College of Rheumatology/European League Against Rheumatism Classification Criteria for IgG4-related Disease. Arthritis Rheumatol. 2020;72(1):7-19.
10. Umehara H, Okazaki K, Kawa S, Takahashi H, Goto H, Matsui S, et al. The 2020 revised comprehensive diagnostic (RCD) criteria for IgG4-RD. Mod Rheumatol. 2021;31(3):529-33.

143

CHAPTER

Deficiency of Adenosine Deaminase 2

Paramita Bhattacharya, Iman Kalyan Sarkar

ABSTRACT

Deficiency of adenosine deaminase 2 (DADA2) is a rare autosomal recessive autoinflammatory vasculitis syndrome with diverse manifestations notably early onset ischemic or hemorrhagic stroke, fever, and polyarteritis nodosa (PAN)-like cutaneous manifestations. Adenosine deaminase 2 (ADA2) is predominantly found in myeloid cells and plays a major role in immune regulation by promoting macrophage differentiation, B and T-cell maturation, maintaining vascular integrity and also growth of embryo. DADA2 is caused by loss of function mutation of *ADA2* gene. Diagnosis is based on biochemical assay showing decreased ADA2 activity and genetic testing. As of now, the mainstay of treatment is tumor necrosis factor (TNF) inhibitors in patients with mainly vasculitic and inflammatory manifestations. For severe hematologic manifestations, hematopoietic cell transplantation (HCT) has shown promising results.

INTRODUCTION

Deficiency of adenosine deaminase 2 (DADA2) is a rare, autosomal recessive, and autoinflammatory monogenic vasculitis syndrome. This is caused by loss of function mutation of adenosine deaminase 2 (*ADA2*) gene which was previously known as *CECR1* (cat eye syndrome chromosome region, candidate 1) gene. The disease is characterized by fever, early-onset stroke, variety of cutaneous, and many other systemic manifestations.

Adenosine deaminase 2 was first described in a patient of severe combined immunodeficiency (SCID) due to deficiency of adenosine deaminase 1 (ADA1). ADA enzymes break down adenosine (Ado) and 2'-deoxyadenosine (2'-dAdo) and thus regulates purine metabolism. Deoxyadenosine nucleotides accumulate inside lymphocytes in absence of ADA1 leading to development of SCID. ADA1 and ADA2 are partially homologous. They have different structure and functions. Several studies suggest that ADA2, beside deaminase activity, also has growth factor activities.

EPIDEMIOLOGY

This syndrome was first described in 2014. After that, over 300 cases have been reported. It is estimated that the frequency of deleterious ADA2 mutation variant worldwide is one in 236 persons but disease prevalence is approximately one in 2,22,000 persons.

ADENOSINE DEAMINASE 2 FUNCTION

Adenosine deaminase 2 gene is present on chromosome 22 (22q11.1). It is highly expressed in myeloid cells, lymphocytes, lung, bone marrow, spleen and thymus. ADA2 is a 59-kDa protein that forms homodimers. They are eventually glycosylated, bind to heparin or glycosaminoglycans or cell surface receptors and secreted extracellular space.

The N-terminal of ADA2 is responsible for its growth factor activity. There is high sequence similarities between ADA2 and adenosine deaminase growth factors (ADGFs). ADA2 has role in regulation of proliferation and differentiation of cells and also a possible role in bone marrow differentiation which is yet to be studied for details.

Adenosine deaminase 2 as well as ADA1 have major role in immune cell activation and signaling by binding to proteoglycans and adenosine receptors on immune cells. ADA2 binds to neutrophils, NK cells, B lymphocytes and CD16+ monocytes. ADA2 induces T-cell dependent differentiation of monocytes to macrophages. During inflammatory condition, immune cells of myeloid lineage release ADA2 and it is found in plasma and pleural fluid in high amounts.

GENETICS

Adenosine deaminase 2 is a highly polymorphic gene. It harbors >300 missense and insertion-deletion (indel) mutations. Also there is an overabundance of copy number variants (CNVs) across the gene locus making it highly variable between individuals. Till date, over 60 disease-causing mutations including missense variants in majority, also nonsense variants, splicing mutations and genome deletions have been reported. A subset of carriers of pathogenic ADA2 mutation might exhibit mild disease or late-onset depending on level of ADA2 activity.

Most of the patients suffering from DADA2 are heterozygous for missense mutations. The most common mutations are p.Gly47Arg, p.Gly47Ala etc. All DADA2 patients of Georgian–Jewish descent have been found to have homozygous p.Gly47Arg mutation.

The carrier frequency is about 1:500 in Northern European populations, much lower in African populations, and absent in Asian populations.

PATHOGENESIS

Adenosine deaminase 2 has a major role in development of macrophages from monocytes. In DADA2, there is polarization of monocyte-macrophage toward M1 subset which is known to promote inflammation and tissue damage. There is increased production pro-inflammatory cytokines, disruption of cell junctions and thus significantly increased incidence of intracranial bleeding.

CLINICAL MANIFESTATIONS

Clinical manifestations of DADA2 are so diverse that its early diagnosis remains a challenge most of the time. Mostly it is a disease of childhood but late onset diseases are increasingly being reported. 24% of patients present before the age of 1 year and 77% before the age of 10 years. Mortality is significantly high and life expectancy is <30 years in 8% of those with early onset.

Small and medium vessel vasculitis is the main feature of this disease. Most commonly involved organs are skin and central nervous system (CNS).

Fever, arthralgia, myalgia with increased erythrocyte sedimentation rate (ESR) and C-reactive protein (CRP) were reported in 50% of patients. It may also cause rheumatoid arthritis-like small joint involvement.

Most common feature is cutaneous manifestations which are found in 75% of patients. Livedo reticularis, nodular rash, and macular erythema are described.

Neurological manifestations occur in 50% of patients. Both ischemic and hemorrhagic strokes are reported. Onset of ischemic stroke can be as early as 5 months of age. Typical MRI findings are acute or chronic lacunar infarcts in deep brain or brainstem sparing the subcortical white matter. Other neurological manifestations such as spastic diplegia or paraplegia, ataxia, peripheral neuropathy encephalitis are not so frequent.

Other organs such as kidney, gastrointestinal (GI) tract, and liver are also affected by vasculitis. Arterial hypertension, renal artery aneurysm, renal artery stenosis, glomerular scarring among renal manifestations and inflammatory bowel disease, intestinal necrosis, mesenteric ischemia, stenosis or aneurysm of mesenteric or celiac artery among GI manifestations have been reported. Transaminitis, hepatosplenomegaly, and portal hypertension have also been found in <10% of patients.

Several studies reported occurrence of immunodeficiency with hypogammaglobulinemia and low IgM level some of the patients. There was also decrease in memory B-cells, terminally differentiated B-cells i.e., antibody secreting cells and CD138+ plasma cells. As a result there is recurrent sinopulmonary infections.

Lymphoproliferative disorder including generalized lymphadenopathy and splenomegaly are also an important manifestations of DADA2. Phenotypically similar autoimmune lymphoproliferative syndrome (ALPS) has recently been reported in DADA2 syndrome.

Hematologic manifestations also occur in this disease. Some patients may present with features of cytopenia. Pure red cell aplasia (PRCA) and severe anemia resembling Diamond–Blackfan syndrome have been described. Severe neutropenia is present in close to 10% of patients. Autoimmune hemolytic anemia and thrombocytopenia have also been found in few patients. One patient with DADA2 was found to have MonoMAC syndrome due to associated GATA2 deficiency.

DIAGNOSIS

Diagnosis of DADA2 is suspected in children to young adults with polyarteritis nodosa (PAN) such as vasculitis, livedo with ischemic or hemorrhagic stroke having features of systemic inflammation, cytopenias, and hypogammaglobulinemia. For diagnosis of DADA2, plasma activity of ADA2 should be demonstrated. It is done by high-performance liquid chromatography (HPLC) or enzyme-linked immunosorbent assay (ELISA) assay method. After establishing the deficiency of ADA2, deoxyribonucleic acid (DNA) sequencing should be done. Erythro-9-(2-hydroxy-3-nonyl)adenine (EHNA) is the inhibitor that selectively binds to only ADA1. It is used to differentiate ADA1 from ADA2 activity in biochemical assays.

Differential Diagnosis

- *Stroke or peripheral vasculitis*
  - Sneddon syndrome
  - PAN
  - Behçet's syndrome
  - Antiphospholipid antibodies (APLA)
  - Systemic lupus erythematosus (SLE)
- Pure red cell aplasia
- *Immunodeficiency*
  - Common variable immune deficiency (CVID)
  - GATA2 deficiency

TREATMENT

Patients with Predominant Vasculitis and Systemic Inflammation – TNF Inhibition

Agents: Etanercept, infliximab, golimumab, adalimumab etc.

They significantly decrease inflammatory burden of the disease with decrease in symptoms. They are also associated with a lower risk of stroke.

Glucocorticoids and interleukin-6 (IL-6) inhibitor tocilizumab are also effective in decreasing inflammation but they do not lower the risk of stroke.

Asymptomatic Patients

These patients are detected to have DADA2 by screening of family members. Treatment with tumor necrosis factor (TNF) inhibitors is suggested even without any stroke or other symptoms because of its potential life-threatening events later on.

Symptomatic Carriers

These are the patients with features of DADA2 with single deleterious ADA2 variant and moderate level of ADA2 enzyme activity. No definitive recommendations are present yet. Immunosuppression with glucocorticoids or other agents is suggested.

Patients with Bone Marrow Failure and Immunodeficiency

They are refractory to treatment with TNF inhibitors. Hematopoietic cell transplantation (HCT) and supportive care are recommended. In one study, a cohort of 14 patients who underwent HCT were all alive and well. Their hematologic and inflammatory features also improved significantly and no new vascular events were reported in follow-up of 18 months.

Intravenous immunoglobulin (IVIG), glucocorticoids, granulocyte-colony stimulating factor (G-CSF), and other immunosuppressive agents were not effective in severe hematologic manifestations.

SUGGESTED READINGS

1. Zhou Q, Yang D, Ombrello AK, Zavialov AV, Toro C, ZavialovAV, et al. Early-onset stroke and vasculopathy associated with mutations in ADA2. N Engl J Med. 2014;370(10):911-20.
2. Rama M, Duflos C, Melki I, Bessis D, Bonhomme A, Martin H, et al. A decision tree for the genetic diagnosis of deficiency of adenosine deaminase 2 (DADA2): a French reference centres experience. Eur J Hum Genet. 2018;26(7):960-71.
3. Meyts I, Aksentijevich I. Deficiency of Adenosine Deaminase 2 (DADA2): Updates on the Phenotype, Genetics, Pathogenesis, and Treatment. J Clin Immunol. 2018;38:569-78.